Fundamentals of Nursing

Helen Harkreader, PhD, RN

Professor
Austin Community College
Austin, Texas

W.B. SAUNDERS COMPANY
A Harcourt Health Sciences Company
Philadelphia   London   Toronto   Sydney

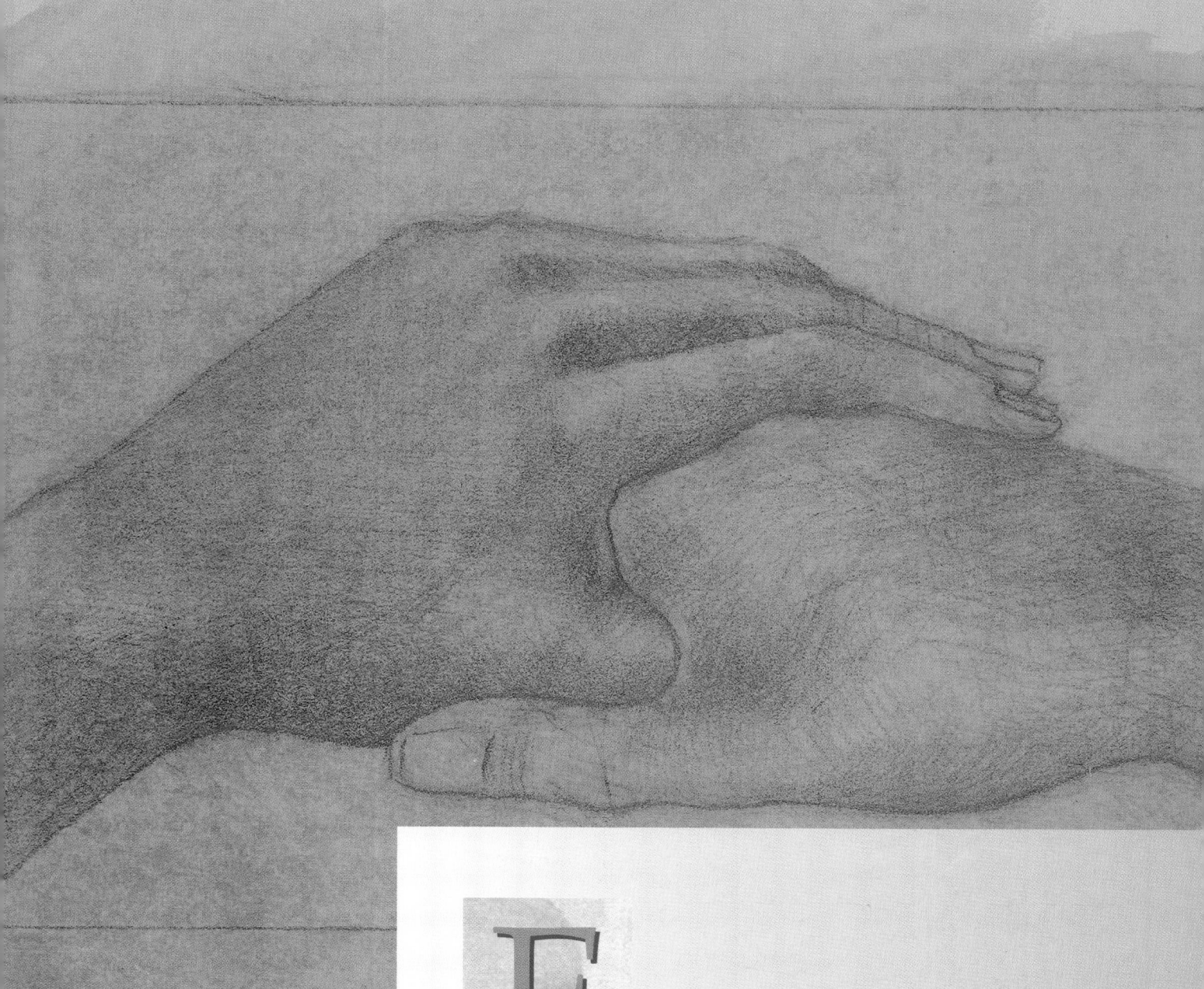

Fundamentals of Nursing

Caring and Clinical Judgment

W.B. SAUNDERS COMPANY
A Harcourt Health Sciences Company

The Curtis Center
Independence Square West
Philadelphia, Pennsylvania 19106

NOTICE

Nursing is an ever-changing field. Standard safety precautions must be followed, but as new research and clinical experience broaden our knowledge, changes in treatment and drug therapy become necessary or appropriate. Readers are advised to check the product information currently provided by the manufacturer of each drug to be administered to verify the recommended dose, the method and duration of administration, and the contraindications. It is the responsibility of the licensed prescriber, relying on experience and knowledge of the patient, to determine dosages and the best treatment for the patient. Neither the publisher nor the editor assumes any responsibility for any injury and/or damage to persons or property.

THE PUBLISHER

Library of Congress Cataloging-in-Publication Data

Fundamentals of nursing: caring and clinical judgment / [edited by] Helen Harkreader.

    p.   cm.

    ISBN 0–7216–8669-9

    1. Nursing—Practice. 2. Nursing. I. Harkreader, Helen Chandler.
    [DNLM: 1. Nursing—United States. 2. Practice Management—United States. 3. United States.   WY 100 F97986 2000]

    RT86.7.F86 2000   610.73—dc21

    DNLM/DLC   99–17270

Vice President, Nursing Editorial Director: Sally Schrefer
Editorial Manager: Thomas Eoyang
Managing Editor: Lee Henderson
Copy Editor: Scott Filderman
Production Managers: Pete Faber, Jeff Gunning
Illustrator: Richard S. LaRocco
Cover Designer: Ellen Zanolle

FUNDAMENTALS OF NURSING: CARING AND CLINICAL JUDGMENT   ISBN 0–7216–8669–9

Printed in the United States of America.

Last digit is the print number: 9   8   7   6   5   4   3   2   1

To my mother, who taught me the value and joy of helping other people.

To my son, who gave my life meaning.

To my husband, who supports me in finding my own path.

To my students, who taught me how to teach.

Helen Harkreader, PhD, RN, has practiced as an acute care adult health nurse in general medicine, intensive care, oncology, gastrointestinal, and surgical nursing units. Having begun her teaching career in 1971, she has taught nursing in both baccalaureate and associate-degree nursing programs. While she has taught at all levels of undergraduate programs in Texas, Arkansas, and Iowa, her primary interest is teaching beginning nursing students. Dr. Harkreader believes that her role as a teacher is to foster the individual growth of nursing students and uses the Myers Briggs Type Indicator as a tool to help students bring their individual strengths to nursing practice. The greatest compliment students can give her is that she has made them think.

Dr. Harkreader has conducted research on the effects of positioning on ventilation-perfusion ratios, caregiver burden as a factor in nursing home placement, and the utilization of vocational nurses.

Dr. Harkreader received her undergraduate degree from Texas Christian University, her master's degree as a Clinical Specialist in Medical-Surgical Nursing from the University of Iowa, and her PhD in adult health nursing from the University of Texas at Austin. She is a member of the American Nurses' Association and is currently serving on the Publications Committee of the North American Nursing diagnosis Association. She serves as Professor of Nursing at Austin Community College in Austin, Texas.

SPECIAL CONSULTANTS

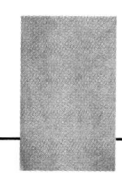

MARY ANN HOGAN, MSN, RN
Clinical Nurse Specialist, Baystate Medical Center,
Springfield, Massachusetts; Adjunct Faculty,
University of Massachusetts Amherst, Amherst,
Massachusetts

ARLENE L. POLASKI, MEd, MSN, RN
Program Director, York Technical College/University
of South Carolina; Lancaster Cooperative Associate
Degree Nursing Program, Rock Hill, South Carolina

MARSHELLE THOBABEN, MS, RN, PHN, APNP, FNP
Professor and Community Health and Psychiatric
Nursing Consultant, Department of Nursing,
Humboldt State University, Arcata, California

V. DOREEN WAGNER, MSN, RN, CNOR
Assistant Professor, Department of Nursing, Georgia
Perimeter College, Clarkston, Georgia

CONTRIBUTORS

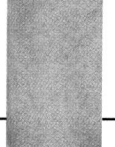

Elizabeth Abrahams, MSN, RN, ONC
Materials Management Clinical Nurse Specialist,
Inova Health System, Falls Church, Virginia
Skin Integrity and Wound Healing

Kay C. Avant, PhD, RN, FAAN
Associate Professor and Chairperson, Family Health
Nursing Division, School of Nursing, The University
of Texas at Austin, Austin, Texas
Making a Nursing Diagnosis

Dee M. Baldwin, PhD, RN
Associate Professor, School of Nursing, Georgia State
University, Atlanta, Georgia
Health Maintenance: Lifestyle Management

Kathleen Barta, EdD, RN
Associate Professor, Eleanor Mann School of
Nursing, University of Arkanas, Fayetteville,
Arkansas
The State of Nursing Science charts

Margaret L. Bell, PhD, RN
Assistant Professor, Department of Chronic Nursing
Care, The University of Texas Health Science Center
at San Antonio School of Nursing, San Antonio,
Texas
The Client With Functional Limitations

Lenore L. Boris, MS, JD, RN
Organizer (Nurse), New York State Public
Employees Federation, Albany, New York;
Lieutenant Colonel, United States Air Force Reserve
Nurse Corps; Nurse Administrator, 439th Medical
Squadron, Westover Air Reserve Base, Massachusetts
The Legal Context of Practice

Laura Bradford, PhD, RNC
Unit Director, Special Care Nursery,
Rush–Presbyterian–St. Luke's Medical Center,
Chicago, Illinois
Health Protection: Risk for Infection

Chyi-Kong Karen Chang, MSN, RN
Teaching Assistant, University of Illinois at Chicago,
Chicago, Illinois; formerly Visiting Assistant
Professor and Assistant Professor, Purdue University,
West Lafayette, Indiana
The Cultural Context of Practice
Evaluating Care

Carolyn Chambers Clark, EdD, ARNP, FAAN, HNC, DBFN
Adjunct Professor, Graduate Program in Nursing,
Schiller International University, Dunedin, Florida;
Faculty Mentor, Doctoral Program in Health
Services, Walden University, Minneapolis, Minnesota
Coping–Stress Tolerance

Jeannette Marie Daly, PhD, RN
Geriatric Nurse Researcher, Department of Family
Medicine, University of Iowa, Iowa City, Iowa
Planning for Intervention
Bowel Elimination

Laura Dulski, MSN, RN
Staff Nurse, New Life Family-Centered Care Unit,
Rush–Presbyterian–St. Luke's Medical Center,
Chicago, Illinois
The Well Child

Carson A. Easley, MS, RN
Instructor of Nursing, Associate Degree Nursing Program, Antelope Valley College, Lancaster, California
The Ethical Context of Practice

Kristen L. Easton, MS, RN, CRRN-A, CS
Assistant Professor of Nursing, Valparaiso University, Valparaiso, Indiana; Community Health Education Director, Porter Memorial Hospital, Valparaiso, Indiana; Doctoral Candidate, Wayne State University, Detroit, Michigan
The Client With Functional Limitations

Shirley Eden-Kilgour, MSN, RN, FNP
Assistant Professor of Nursing, College of Nursing and Health Professions, Arkansas State University, Jonesboro, Arkansas; Retired Professor of Nursing, Loewenberg School of Nursing, University of Memphis, Memphis, Tennessee; Family Nurse Practitioner, Charter Lakeside Behavioral Health Systems, Memphis, Tennessee
Self-Concept

Kathleen A. Ennen, MS, RN
Doctoral Student, University of Illinois at Chicago, Chicago, Illinois; Part-Time Faculty, Parkland College, Champaign, Illinois
The Health Care Delivery System as a Context for Practice

Sally Evankoe, BSN, MS, RN
Instructor, Maternal Child Nursing, College of Nursing, Rush University, Chicago, Illinois
The Well Newborn, Infant, and Toddler

Nancy Evans, BS
Health Science Writer/Editor, San Francisco, California
A Patient's View charts

Joanne H. Frey, PhD, RN
Assistant Professor, University of Massachusetts at Boston, Boston, Massachusetts
Family Coping

Helen Harkreader, PhD, RN
Professor, Austin Community College, Austin, Texas
Assessing the Client: History-Taking
Urinary Elimination
Respiratory Function

Richard Henker, PhD, RN
Assistant Professor, University of Pittsburgh, Pittsburgh, Pennsylvania
Body Temperature

Janet S. Hickman, MS, EdD, RN
Professor and Graduate Program Coordinator, West Chester University, West Chester, Pennsylvania
Critical Thinking and Clinical Judgment

Karen Y. Hill, PhD, RN
Assistant Professor, School of Nursing, Southeastern Louisiana University, Hammond, Louisiana
Documenting Care

Mary Ann Hogan, MSN, RN
Clinical Nurse Specialist, Baystate Medical Center, Springfield, Massachusetts; Adjunct Faculty, University of Massachusetts Amherst, Amherst, Massachusetts
Health Maintenance: Medication Management

Doris Holeman, PhD, RN
Associate Dean and Director, School of Nursing and Allied Health, Tuskegee University, Tuskegee, Alabama
Health Maintenance: Lifestyle Management

Donna D. Ignatavicius, MS, RN, Cm
Clinical Nurse Specialist, Medical-Surgical/Gerontology Nursing, Calvert Memorial Hospital, Prince Frederick, Maryland
Physical Mobility

Susan M. Irvin, MSN, RN
Clinical Coordinator, Ambulatory Surgery Unit, Memphis Veterans Administration Medical Center, Memphis, Tennessee
Self-Concept

Janene Council Jeffery, MSN, RN, CDE
Professor, Austin Community College, Austin, Texas
Loss

Ann Keller, MSN, EdD, RN
Associate Professor and Chair, Department of Nursing, Thomas More College, Crestview Hills, Kentucky
The Well Older Adult

Eileen Klein, MSN, EdD, RN
Assistant Dean, Health Sciences, Austin Community College, Austin, Texas
Cardiovascular Function

Konnie Sue Kyle, MSN, RN, CNRN
Director of Orthopedics, General Surgery, and Neurosurgery, St. Francis Hospital and Medical Center, Topeka, Kansas
Client Teaching

Kathryn A. Lauchner, PhD, RN
Professor, Austin Community College, Austin, Texas
Nursing Research

Delois Laverentz, MN, RN, CCRN
Formerly Assistant Professor, Fort Hays State
University, Hays, Kansas
Sensory/Perceptual Function
Impaired Verbal Communication

Jeanne Lawler-Slack, DnSc, RN
Associate Professor and Practitioner-Teacher, College
of Nursing, Rush University, Chicago, Illinois
The Well Child

Marilyn S. Leasia, MSN, RN, FNP
Nurse Practitioner, Department of Medicine,
Montefiore Medical Center, New York, New York
Assessing the Client: Physical Examination

James Higgy Lerner, RN, LAc
Private Practice, Acupuncture and Oriental
Medicine, Chico, California
Considering the Alternatives charts

Janna Lesser, PhD, RN, CS
Postdoctoral Fellow, UCLA School of Nursing, Los
Angeles, California
Vulnerability

Susan Lewis, PhD, ARNP, CS
Advanced Practice Nurse, Mental Health and
Behavioral Science Service, Department of Veterans
Affairs Medical Center, Louisville, Kentucky
Anxiety

Gwyneth Lymberis, MS, RN, ANP
Assistant Professor, Borough of Manhattan
Community College, The City University of New
York, New York, New York
Sleep and Rest

Nancy J. MacMullen, MSN, PhD, RNC
Associate Professor, Maternal Child Nursing, College
of Nursing, Rush University, Chicago, Illinois
The Well Newborn, Infant, and Toddler

Donna W. Markey, MSN, RN, ACNP-CS
Clinician IV, Surgical Services, University of Virginia
Health System, Charlottesville, Virginia
Delegation Guidelines

Barbara McKinney, MSN, RN
Formerly Clinical Instructor, Ashland Community
College School of Nursing, Ashland, Kentucky
The Nursing Profession as a Context for Practice

Martha Meraviglia, MSN, RN
Doctoral Candidate, School of Nursing, University of
Texas at Austin, Austin, Texas
Spirituality

Beverly M. Miller, MSN, RN
Geriatric Nurse Practitioner, Memphis Veterans
Administration Medical Center, Memphis, Tennessee
Self-Concept

Barbara S. Moffett, PhD, RN
Associate Professor of Nursing, Southeastern
Louisiana University, Hammond, Louisiana
Documenting Care

Frances Donovan Monahan, PhD, RN
Professor and Director, Department of Nursing,
SUNY Rockland, Suffern, New York; Nursing
Faculty, Regents College, Albany, New York
Assessing the Client: Physical Examination

Janet B. Moore, MS, RN, CS
Co-Director, Robin Read Adult Day Health Center,
West Springfield, Massachusetts; Formerly Instructor,
Baystate Medical Center School of Nursing,
Springfield, Massachusetts
Confusion

Virginia Nehring, PhD, RN
Associate Professor, College of Nursing and Health,
Wright State University, Dayton, Ohio
Developing a Framework for Practice
The Well Adult
Spirituality

Beatriz Nieto, MSN, RN, CNS
Assistant Professor, Department of Nursing, The
University of Texas–Pan American, Edinburg, Texas
Health Protection: Risk for Injury

Cecilia A. Prado, MSN, RN
Professor, Austin Community College, Austin, Texas
The Cultural Context of Practice

Laura Roddy Redic, MA, MSN, RNC
Formerly Assistant Professor of Nursing, University
of Arkansas at Pine Bluffs, Pine Bluffs, Arkansas
The Caregiver Role

Betty Kehl Richardson, PhD, RN, CS, AANC
Professor, Austin Community College, Austin, Texas;
Private Practice, Marriage and Family Counseling,
Austin, Texas
Roles and Relationships

Carol F. Roye, EdD, RN, CPNP
Associate Professor, Hunter-Bellevue School of
Nursing, New York, New York
The Well Adolescent

Barbara C. Rynerson, MS, RN, CS
Associate Professor Emerita, The University of North
Carolina School of Nursing, Chapel Hill, North
Carolina
Sexuality and Reproductive Function

Betty Samford, MSN, RN
Doctoral Candidate, School of Nursing, University of
Texas at Austin, Austin, Texas
The Emergency Client

Katherine S. Schulz, RD, MS, LDN
Dietetic Consultant, State of Tennessee, Jackson,
Tennessee
Nutrition

Brenda Leigh Yolles Smith, EdD, RN, CNM, ICCE
Associate Professor, College of Nursing, University
of Tennessee at Memphis, Memphis, Tennessee
Nutrition

Carol E. Smith, PhD, RN
Professor, School of Nursing, University of Kansas,
Kansas City, Kansas
Client Teaching

Nancy Spector, DNFc, RN
Assistant Professor, Loyola University, Chicago, Illinois
Nutritional Deficiency

Karen Stanley, MSN, RN, AOCN
Clinical Nurse Specialist, Pain and Symptom
Management, Kaiser Permanente Fontana Medical
Center, Fontana, California
Pain

Judy Sweeney, MSN, RN
Assistant Professor, School of Nursing, Vanderbilt
University, Nashville, Tennessee
Assessing the Client: Vital Signs
Disuse Syndrome

Rachel A. Taylor, PhD, RN
Formerly Assistant Professor, Department of Health
Care Systems, College of Nursing, University of
Tennessee at Memphis, Memphis, Tennessee
Hygiene

Joyce Z. Thielen, MS, RN, CS
Co-Director, Robin Read Adult Day Health Center,
West Springfield, Massachusetts; Formerly Instructor,
Baystate Medical Center School of Nursing,
Springfield, Massachusetts
Confusion

Marshelle Thobaben, MS, RN, PHN, APNP, FNP
Professor and Community Health and Psychiatric
Nursing Consultant, Department of Nursing,
Humboldt State University, Arcata, California
The Well Adult

Daria Virvan, MSN, RN, CS
Nurse Psychotherapist, Town Center Psychiatric
Associates, Rockville, Maryland
The Nurse-Client Relationship

V. Doreen Wagner, MSN, RN, CNOR
Assistant Professor, Department of Nursing, Georgia
Perimeter College, Clarkston, Georgia
Developing a Framework for Practice
Coping–Stress Tolerance
The Surgical Client

Phyllis Russo Wells, MSN, MEd, MPH, RNC
Women's Health Nurse Practitioner, New Horizons
OB-GYN, PC, Stockbridge, Georgia
The Community as a Client

Bernie White, MSN, RN
Assistant Professor, Creighton School of Nursing,
Creighton University, Omaha, Nebraska
Fluid and Electrolyte Balance

Suzanne S. Yarbrough, PhD, RN
Assistant Professor, School of Nursing, University of
Texas Health Science Center at San Antonio, San
Antonio, Texas
Nursing Management

Charlotte F. Young, PhD, RN
Associate Professor, Department of Nursing, College
of Nursing and Health Professions, Arkansas State
University, Jonesboro, Arkansas
Confusion

Deborah K. Zastocki, BSN, MA, EdM
Nursing Faculty, William Paterson University,
Wayne, New Jersey; Senior Vice President, Clinical
Services and Operations, Chilton Memorial Hospital,
Pompton Plains, New Jersey
The Homebound Client

Sheila Rankin Zerr, BSc, MEd, RN, PHN
Visiting Faculty, School of Nursing, University of
Victoria, Victoria, British Columbia; Visiting Faculty,
School of Nursing, University of British Columbia,
Vancouver, British Columbia
Health Perception

REVIEWERS

Rebecca Lynn Agnew, MSN, RN, CRNPN
Mercy Hospital School of Nursing, Pittsburgh,
Pennsylvania

Stephanie S. Allen, MS, RN
School of Nursing, Baylor University, Dallas, Texas

Ella R. Anaya, MSN, RN, CNS
Kent State University, Kent, Ohio

Susan Appel, MN, RN, CCRN, CS
Carolinas College of Health Sciences, Charlotte, North
Carolina

Alyce S. Ashcraft, MSN, RN, CS, CCRN
Blinn College, Bryan, Texas; Doctoral Candidate,
University of Texas at Austin, Austin, Texas

Margaret Bellak, MN, RN
Indiana University of Pennsylvania, Indiana, Pennsylvania

Nancy Berger, MSN, RNC
Newark Beth Israel Medical Center, Newark, New Jersey

Marcia Bosek, DNSc, RN
Department of Adult Health Nursing, College of Nursing,
Rush University, Chicago, Illinois

Barbara Brillhart, PhD, RN, CRRN, FNP-C
College of Nursing, Arizona State University, Tempe,
Arizona

Barbara A. Brunow, MSN, RN
Providence Hospital School of Nursing, Sandusky, Ohio

JoAnna M. Christiansen, MSN, RN
Formerly East Arkansas Community College, Forrest City,
Arkansas

Julie Doyon, MScN, RN
University of Ottawa, Ontario

Mildred DuBois Fennal, PhD, RN, CCRN
Lander University, Greenwood, South Carolina

Michele A. Gerwick, MSN, RN
Department of Nursing, Indiana University of
Pennsylvania, Indiana, Pennsylvania

Pamala K. Hayes, MSN, RN
John A. Logan College, Carterville, Illinois

Susan S. Johnson, MSN, RN
Guilford Technical Community College, Jamestown, North
Carolina

Carolyn S. Jones, MSN, MEd, RN
Craven Community College, Craven Regional Medical
Authority, New Bern, North Carolina

Roseann Kaminsky, BSN, BSEd, RN
Lorain County Community College, Elyria, Ohio

Kathy Keister, MS, RN
Frances Payne Bolton School of Nursing, Case Western
Reserve University, Cleveland, Ohio; Formerly Assistant
Professor, School of Nursing, Medical College of Ohio,
Toledo, Ohio

Frankie Kellner
Supervisor of Fitness Instructors, British Columbia
Recreation and Parks Association, Delta, British Columbia

Karen P. Kettelman, BAHSA, RN, CNA
Doctors Medical Center, Modesto, California

Joan C. Masters, MA, MBA, RN
Bellarmine College, Louisville, Kentucky

Mary E. Mehok, MSN, RN, CCRN
Mercy Hospital, Pittsburgh, Pennsylvania

Sharon E. Moran, MPH, RN, CS
Hawaii Community College, University of Hawaii, Hilo,
Hawaii

Patricia L. Newland, MS, RN
Broome Community College, Binghamton, New York

Alice B. Pappas, PhD, RN
School of Nursing, Baylor University, Dallas, Texas

Molly R. Parker, BSEd, MHR, RN
Green County Area Vocational Technical School,
Okmulgee, Oklahoma

Bonna Powell, MA, RN, CPNP
Department of Nursing, Marycrest International
University, Davenport, Iowa

Gill Robertson, MS, RD
Registered Dietician, Sun Prairie, Wisconsin

Donna N. Roddy, MSN, RN
Chattanooga State Technical Community College,
Chattanooga, Tennessee

Barbara Ryan, MScN, RN
University of Ottawa, Ottawa, Ontario

Mary E. Sampel, MSN, RN
Formerly School of Nursing, St. Louis University;
Independent Consultant, Missouri Nurses Association, St.
Louis, Missouri

Cindy Seidl, MSN, RN
College of Nursing, University of Nebraska Medical
Center, Lincoln, Nebraska

Carol E. Smith, PhD, RN
School of Nursing, University of Kansas Medical Center,
Kansas City, Kansas

Beth Stevenson, MS, RN, CS
Ohio Department of Health, Columbus, Ohio

Linda M. Stevenson, PhD, RNC
School of Nursing, Baylor University, Dallas, Texas

Catherine Stewart, BN, RN, PHNAA
Boundary Health Unit, South Fraser Health Region, Delta,
British Columbia

Caralee Sueppel, MSN, RN, BLS, CURN
Formerly, University of Iowa Hospitals and Clinics, Iowa
City, Iowa

Marilyn Terrado, PhD, RN, CS
College of Nursing and College of Health Sciences, Rush
University, Chicago, Illinois

Tina Tiburzi, BSN, MBA, RN
Johns Hopkins Hospital, Baltimore, Maryland

Carole J. Petrosky Vozel, PhD, RNC
The Western Pennsylvania Hospital School of Nursing,
Pittsburgh, Pennsylvania

Jane C. Walton, PhD, RNC, CS
College of Nursing, Rush University, Chicago, Illinois

PREFACE

Welcome to the profession of nursing. *Fundamentals of Nursing: Caring and Clinical Judgment* will serve as a guide as you begin the process of developing your practice of nursing. It will give you information about the context of nursing practice, how nurses think, and the people who are recipients of nursing care, as well as the needs and problems that nurses can help people manage. The ideas and techniques in this book should not be taken as the only way to practice nursing but should serve as a beginning to stimulate your creativity to develop a nursing practice that is truly your own.

How the Book Is Structured

Unit 1 is designed to help you understand the context of nursing practice. As with any profession, the *profession* of nursing controls the *practice* of nursing. Chapter 1 describes the profession of nursing and how it developed. Additionally, because nursing is controlled by laws that define and provide constraints to practice, Chapter 2 describes the legal parameters for nursing practice. The profession of nursing is practiced within a code of professional ethics, and Chapter 3 discusses ethics and the basis for the ethical practice of nursing. Nursing also takes place within the context of culture; Chapter 4 therefore introduces you to the concept of culture and teaches you how to provide culturally competent care. Finally, nursing practice takes place within the framework of the prevailing health care delivery system, so Chapter 5 covers health care delivery systems and the role of the nurse as a member of the health care team. In this chapter, the way in which nurses function is shown as interwoven with the roles and functions of other members of the team.

Unit 2 is designed to help you develop a pattern of thinking that will give structure to your practice of nursing. First, in Chapter 6, you will learn about nursing theories that provide a philosophical foundation for practice and that can be used to give structure to

practice. Then, in Chapter 7, you will be introduced to the concepts of critical thinking and clinical judgment, skills that are growing in importance as health care grows in complexity. Chapters 8 through 13 present the nursing process as a method of studying how nurses think. The nursing process is divided into five phases that involve five types of thinking (assessment, diagnosis, planning, intervention, and evaluation); these chapters show the interrelationships among those five types. For example, the process of assessing the client is the process of gathering data and identifying needs to make a diagnosis. Making a diagnosis is related to goal-setting and thinking about what the nurse can do to help the client. Planning involves deciding the who, what, how, when, and where of nursing care, which may require further assessment and consideration of the desired outcomes. Intervening on a client's behalf is not just doing something for the person but doing along with ongoing assessment and evaluation. This unit concludes with a chapter on documentation of the care that you have provided.

Unit 3 discusses some key "tools" used in nursing practice. Although technology is an important part of nursing practice, independent nursing practice primarily uses the tool of a therapeutic relationship with the client (Chapter 15), in which the client makes decisions about health management and learns effective methods of health care. Teaching is a primary nursing intervention, to which Chapter 16 is devoted. Because nursing often occurs in an organized health care setting, nursing management (Chapter 17) is a tool used to ensure efficient and effective nursing practice. Nursing research (Chapter 18) is the final tool that we present to help you continually update your nursing practice.

Unit 4 describes the well client across the life span and examines some of the client's needs to maintain health. Units 5 through 15 present common client problems organized around Marjory Gordon's Functional Health Patterns. These patterns focus your assessment on the client problems that are amenable to nursing care. You can use the Functional Health Patterns to systematically assess your clients, thus ensuring comprehensive assessment for any presenting problem.

Unit 16 will help you integrate the information from Units 5 through 15 to plan care for special client populations. It does this by providing an overview of nursing practice across five areas of practice: caring for clients with functional limitations, caring for surgical clients, caring for clients in emergency situations, caring for populations of clients, and caring for homebound clients. The chapter on clients with functional limitations (Chapter 56) describes concepts associated with rehabilitation nursing, in which clients need assistance in order to take care of themselves and may need prolonged care in the home or an institution. The chapter on the surgical client (Chapter 57) provides general guidelines for the care of a person who is being treated by surgery in an acute care setting. The chapter on the emergency client (Chapter 58) focuses on three diagnoses commonly seen in the emergency setting and helps you establish lifesaving priorities. The chapter on the community as a client (Chapter 59) describes the parameters of nursing care when the "client" is actually a population or community. The chapter on the homebound client (Chapter 60) describes nursing care of clients who are able to maintain function at home only with support and direct care.

Internally, the chapters in Units 4 through 16 of the book are organized in a consistent framework revolving around the application of the nursing process in order to help you establish a systematic pattern of thinking. This framework is described in detail inside the front cover of the book.

Special Features to Facilitate Learning

The amount of information that you will need to assimilate in your fundamentals of nursing course can be daunting. To help you process this information, and to facilitate learning by students with various learning styles, we have developed a series of pedagogical aids that appear throughout the book.

At the start of each chapter in Units 4 through 16, and in selected other chapters, you will find a *chapter-opening case study,* which typically continues with brief vignettes placed throughout the chapter. Included in these vignettes are critical thinking questions, which will help you develop the habit of reflecting critically on client problems and exploring alternative solutions.

In each chapter in Units 4 through 15, a *Nursing Diagnoses* chart introduces you to the nursing diagnoses around which the chapter is organized. For each diagnosis, we provide the official definition approved by the North American Nursing Diagnosis Association (NANDA).

In most chapters in Section 2 of the book, you will find a *Cross-Cultural Care* chart that explores in more detail the implications of culture for the client whose story is introduced in the chapter-opening case study. These charts, which consist of background information, a nurse-client dialogue, and critical thinking questions, introduce you to a wide variety of cultures and subcultures and present true-to-life examples of the impact of culture on health care.

At the ends of chapters in Section 2, a *Nursing Care Planning* chart based on the client in the case study demonstrates how to plan nursing care that addresses the "whole person," including culture. Each of these charts includes culturally sensitive interventions (highlighted in italics) and ends in a series of critical thinking questions.

A key to success in fundamentals of nursing is mastery of clinical nursing skills and procedures. In this book, we highlight the skills and procedures most commonly taught in nursing fundamentals courses in heavily illustrated *Procedures.* Nursing students are typically most comfortable with learning one "right" method of performing a skill or procedure. And most students are more comfortable learning a small number of steps to a procedure rather than an exhaustive list. We have therefore presented each procedure with a small number of key steps, with details under each step for more specific information. Once you have mastered the steps of a procedure, you will need to apply it and adapt it across a variety of situations and practice settings. Under each step, we have therefore included, in *italic* type, rationales, alternative approaches, and decision-making information. This approach will give you a basic structure for practice while introducing you to alternative methods.

As you become a vital member of the health care team, your time will become increasingly valuable. Planning and delegation will become critical to success in your practice. To help you plan your nursing care, we have provided estimates of "Time to Allow" in each *Procedure.* Keep in mind as you are learning these procedures that the estimates for novice nurses are for nurses who have already learned and practiced a skill. Do not expect to perform a skill within the estimated "novice" time frame the first, second, or even third time you perform it! To help you delegate nursing care to nursing assistants and other assistive personnel, each *Procedure* also includes "Delegation Guidelines." These guidelines will tell you what is safe to delegate and under what conditions.

One of the major goals of *Fundamentals of Nursing: Caring and Clinical Judgment* is to convey the human side of health, illness, and health care. As one way to accomplish that goal, we conducted interviews with patients and family caregivers. The resulting charts, which we call *A Patient's View* or *A Caregiver's View,* as appropriate, provide first-person windows into the lives of clients and caregivers. They demonstrate, in the person's own words, how health conditions, medical treatments, and nursing care have affected their lives.

As some of these *Patient's View* and *Caregiver's View* charts attest, modern health care cannot always overcome the effects of illness or the side effects of treatment. Increasingly, people are turning to complementary and alternative therapies. As a nurse, you will need to understand what is known—and what is not known—about these therapies. To introduce you to this topic and to give you the tools to learn more, we have provided a series of *Considering the Alternatives* charts. These charts, which include resource lists, are extended research-based articles written by an expert in the field of complementary and alternative medicine.

Until relatively recently, North American health care professionals have had the luxury of relative insulation from the impact of the cost of care. Physicians and nurses provided the necessary care, and billing departments, insurers, patients, and families worked out the details of payment. Now, however, in the era of managed care and its fallout, nurses must be acutely aware of the cost of health care. As you progress in your nursing education, you will learn much more about these issues. But to introduce you to them at this level, we have provided a series of *Cost of Care* charts, which will begin to give you a sense of the profound impact of cost on health care.

In your practice of nursing you will encounter situations that require immediate action. Throughout the text, we have therefore included *Action Alert!* text highlights, which focus on situations that call for immediate action or immediate physician collaboration.

In fundamentals of nursing you will learn how to formulate nursing diagnoses that accurately identify client health problems and point the way to appropriate intervention. However, students sometimes have difficulty formulating appropriate nursing diagnoses. To help you circumvent that difficulty, we have provided two special features: *Clustering Data to Make a Nursing Diagnosis* charts and *Decision Trees.* The data-clustering charts present a series of client scenarios and corresponding nursing diagnoses. They will teach you how to apply nursing diagnoses to different client scenarios. The *Decision Trees* are unique full-page illustrations that will show you how to work through health care decisions, particularly differential diagnosis involving closely related nursing diagnoses.

To introduce you to the science of nursing research, *Fundamentals of Nursing: Caring and Clinical Judgment* includes not only a separate chapter on nursing research but also a number of special charts entitled *The State of Nursing Science.* These charts will give you an overview of the state of nursing research in various areas of nursing, as well as suggesting research that remains to be conducted in that area.

Nursing, perhaps more than any other health profession, focuses on health—how to achieve it, how to maintain it, and how to restore it after illness. Much of this focus takes the form of client teaching. In this book we have therefore included two types of charts that will sharpen your teaching skills: *Teaching for Wellness* and *Teaching for Self-Care. Teaching for Wellness* charts focus on health promotion and illness prevention. *Teaching for Self-Care* charts focus on restoration of health after illness. Both types of charts model how to convey complex health care information in language that clients and caregivers can easily understand.

A Multimedia Learning Package

For Students

To help you get the most from *Fundamentals of Nursing: Caring and Clinical Judgment,* be sure to use the CD-ROM that is yours at no additional cost. It includes 600 study questions—10 for each chapter—and provides feedback to show you where you need to focus your study before the next test. Also included on the CD-ROM are five interactive tutorials that will guide you through such complex topics as fluid and electrolyte balance and enteral feedings.

You will also want to purchase the *Student Study Guide,* which includes Matching, True or False, Fill-in-the-Blanks, Exercising Your Clinical Judgment, and Test Yourself questions, along with Performance Checklists for all of the major *Procedures* in the textbook.

For Instructors

Instructors adopting classroom quantities of *Fundamentals of Nursing: Caring and Clinical Judgment* will receive an *Instructor's Manual* and instructional CD-ROM.

The *Instructor's Manual* includes four types of innovative exercises:

- Teaching/Learning Activities for the Classroom
- Teaching/Learning Activities for the Learning Laboratory
- Teaching/Learning Activities for the Clinical Setting
- Critical Thinking Exercises

Among the Teaching/Learning Activities for the Learning Laboratory, we have included *Curve Ball* activities—activities that present students with a new twist on a clinical situation and challenge them to think critically. Each chapter also includes the Key Terms, Learning Objectives, and Key Principles from the text, an outline of the chapter, and Resources for Lesson Preparation—a list of Internet addresses to which instructors can turn for up-to-the-minute classroom preparation.

On the instructional CD-ROM, instructors will find a full-featured ExaMaster testing program with 1000 NCLEX-style questions. Also included on the CD-ROM is a LectureView presentation for PowerPoint, which includes 200 images selected from the text, along with 400 word slides to facilitate lecture preparation.

For more information about these resources, instructors may contact their Harcourt Health Sciences sales representative or call Harcourt Faculty Support at 1-800-222-9570.

A New Text for a New Generation of Nurses

Fundamentals of Nursing: Caring and Clinical Judgment is a brand-new text written for a new generation of nurses preparing for practice in the new millennium. As the title suggests, its purpose is twofold: to teach you how to provide nursing care that truly makes clients feel "cared for" in today's fast-paced, high-tech, cost-conscious health care environment and to equip you with the tools you will need to develop a practice based on ongoing learning and sound clinical judgment. I am delighted that you have chosen *Fundamentals of Nursing: Caring and Clinical Judgment* to begin your journey into nursing.

Helen Harkreader, PhD, RN
Austin, Texas

ACKNOWLEDGMENTS

Many people contributed their unique and creative talents to make *Fundamentals of Nursing: Caring and Clinical Judgment* a cohesive blend of the concepts and methods of practice that represent nursing at the dawn of a new millennium. I wish to thank an incredible team of people who contributed to the project. Thomas Eoyang, Editorial Manager, Nursing Books, W.B. Saunders Company, provided an inspiration and support necessary to conceive the project. He listened and asked the right questions. Without his faith in me, the project would not have been possible.

The Saunders developmental team was led by Managing Editor Lee Henderson, who helped me make the ideas a reality. He not only contributed amazing organizational skills but also kept me going when the job seemed impossible. He always knew just when I needed a word of encouragement or some extra help. His sense of humor was invaluable. Developmental Editor Laura Maria Bonazzoli reviewed the content of the chapters and provided organizational and editorial suggestions. Her keen insights into written communication added clarity and cohesion to the ideas. Developmental Editor Catherine Harold refined the writing, ensured consistency with established chapter formats, and prepared the manuscripts for production. Her questions and suggestions late in the development process demonstrated rare insight into the world of nursing. Thanks also to Fran Murphy, who served as photo researcher and coordinated the peer review process, and to Gina Hopf and Adrienne Simon, for ably fielding countless administrative details.

The creative photography of Rick Hastie adds a special dimension to the book that shows professional nurses at work and helps students visualize contemporary nursing practice. Bonnie Hyatt contributed long hours and creativity to setting up the scenes for the photography and ensuring that the clinical procedures were accurately and professionally portrayed.

Rich LaRocco almost singlehandedly created all of the book's digital artwork. Never content to simply recreate images in conventional ways, Rich gave careful thought to each illustration, always searching for new and better ways to illustrate difficult-to-grasp concepts, structures, and processes.

Many expert nurses, representing both nursing education and nursing practice, contributed chapters to the book. Among the contributors, whose individual contributions are acknowledged in the contributor list, are teachers, researchers, nurse practitioners, and clinical specialists, representing expertise from multiple areas of nursing knowledge. Their contributions are to this book what muscle and bone are to the body.

Thanks, too, to the many dedicated nurses who carefully read and critiqued the manuscripts as peer reviewers. Their comments were invaluable and helped us ensure state-of-the-art accuracy in the book.

Particular thanks to my team of Special Consultants: Mary Ann Hogan, Arlene Polaski, Marshelle Thobaben, and Doreen Wagner. These nurses contributed a special blend of expertise to the project, gave unselfishly of their time and energy, and contributed to the overall vision of the book.

Alice Chandler spent long hours at the computer correcting grammar, punctuation, spelling, and format. Her trained eye could always see an extra comma as she glanced through the pages.

I also want to acknowledge the contributions of the production and marketing teams at W.B. Saunders/Harcourt Health Sciences. Copy Editor Scott Filderman edited or oversaw the editing of every line of manuscript, bringing greater clarity and consistency to the text, and helped to pull together the many elements of the book. Production Managers Jeff Gunning and Pete Faber worked closely with the development team, the typesetter, and the printer to transform manuscript into book; we especially appreciated their flexibility and "can-do" attitude, which enabled us to get the book into your hands while the content is fresh. Thanks, too, to Carolyn Naylor, who stepped in for Jeff at a key juncture in the production cycle, and to Illustration Specialist Rita Martello, who coordinated the production of the book's illustrations. Award-winning graphic designers Susan Hess Blaker and Ellen Zanolle worked hand-in-hand, as they do so well, to create and refine the book's interior and cover designs. Their touch brings an uncommon elegance to the printed page. Marketing Manager Tom Wilhelm brought wisdom and expertise to the promotion of the book; we especially appreciate his sharp insights into both the unique strengths of the book and the needs of today's nursing instructor.

Helen Harkreader, PhD, RN

CONTENTS IN BRIEF

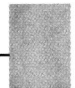

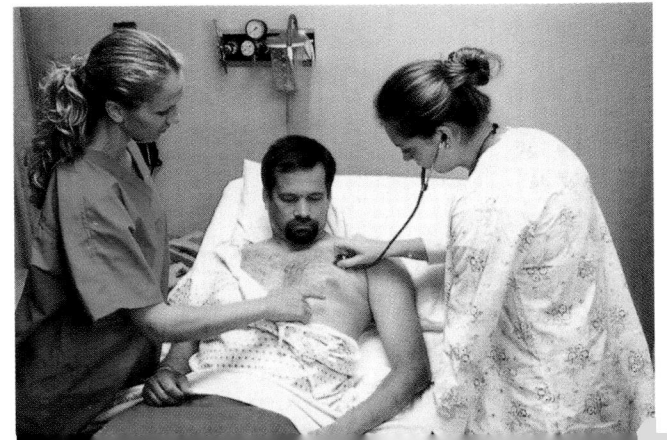

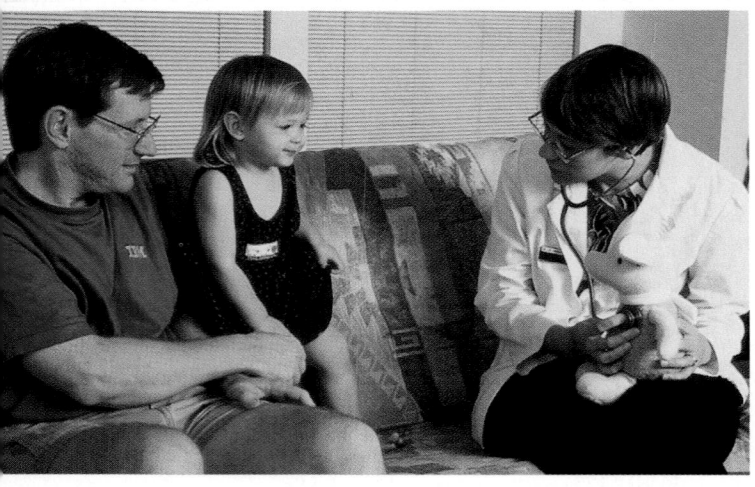

CONTENTS IN DETAIL

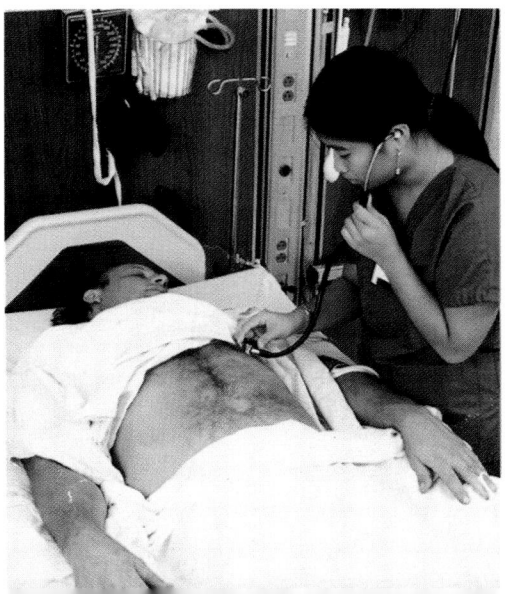

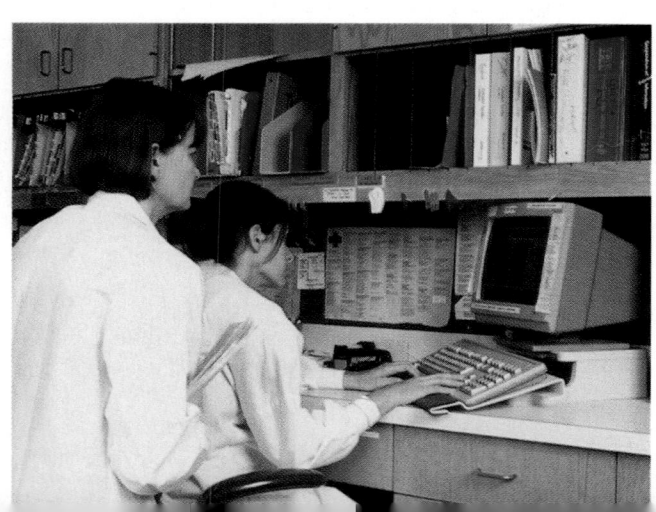

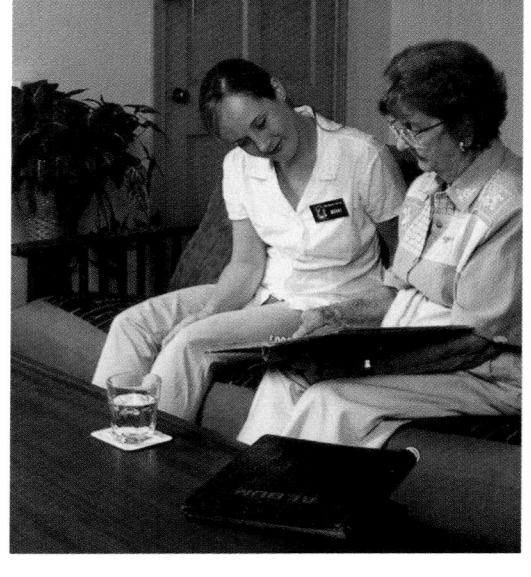

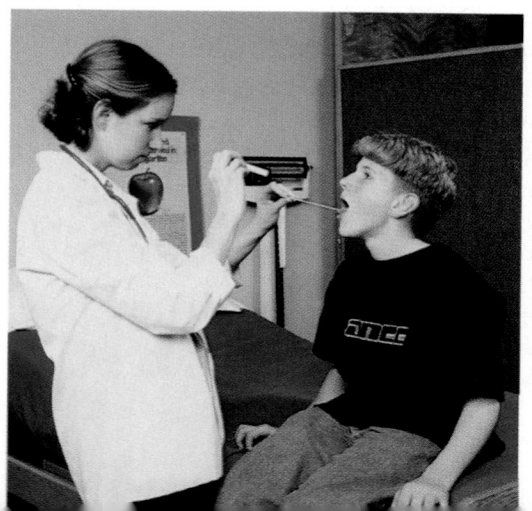

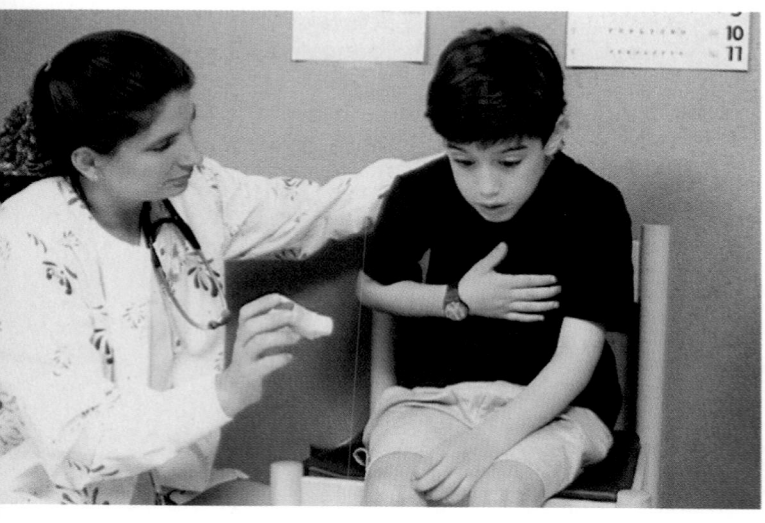

27 Health Protection: Risk for Infection   598

Laura Bradford

28 Health Protection: Risk for Injury   645

Beatriz Nieto

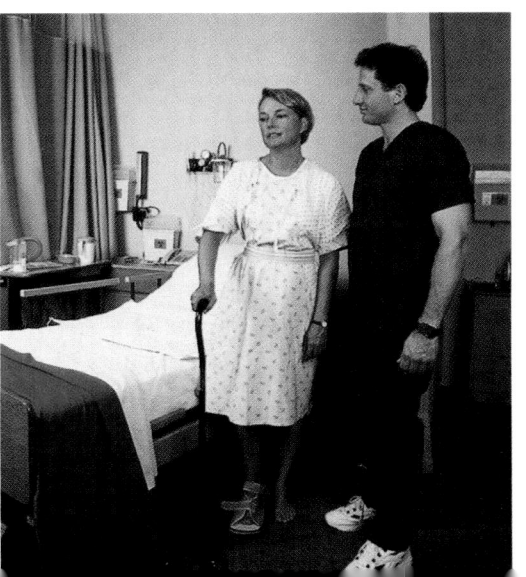

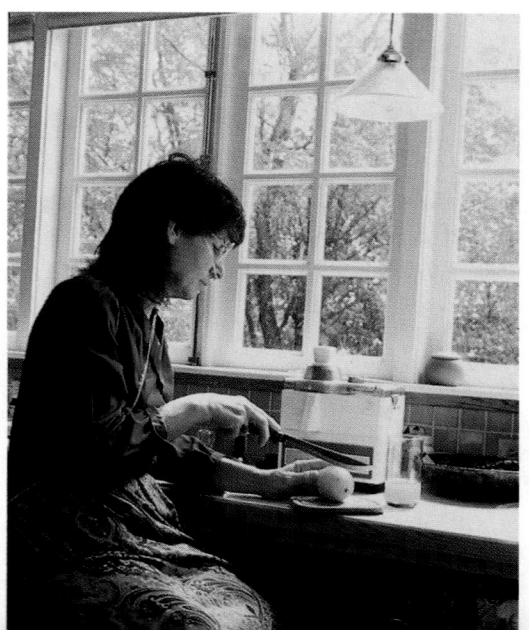

UNIT 8
Activity-Exercise Pattern   923

36 Hygiene   924
Rachel A. Taylor

37 Physical Mobility   970
Donna D. Ignatavicius

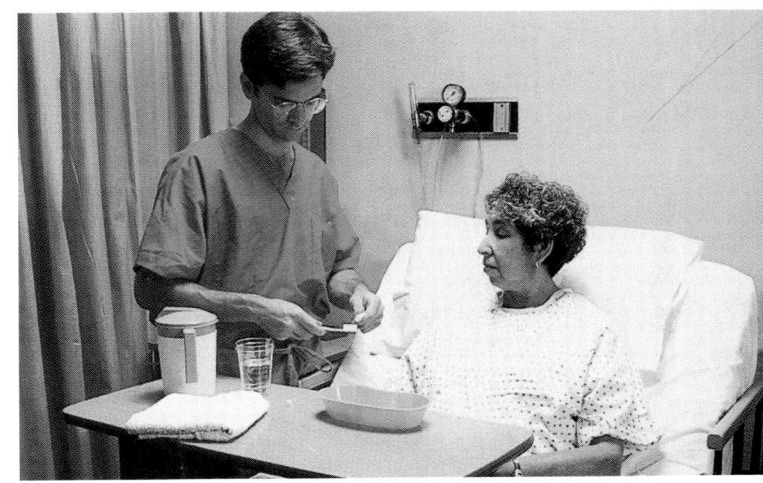

38 Disuse Syndrome   1011

Judy Sweeney

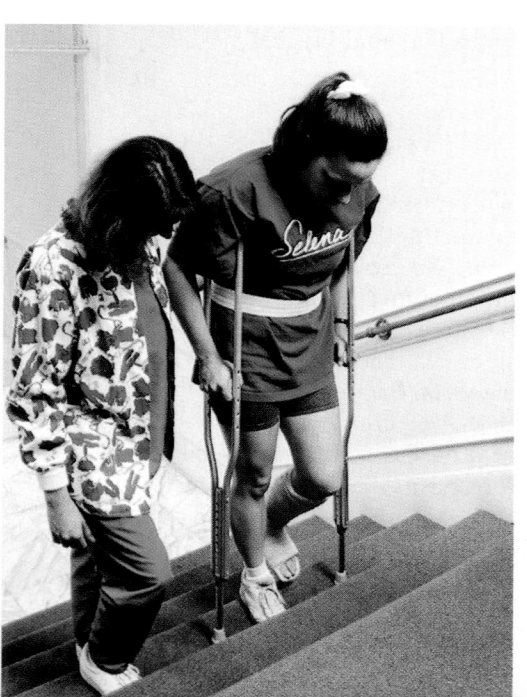

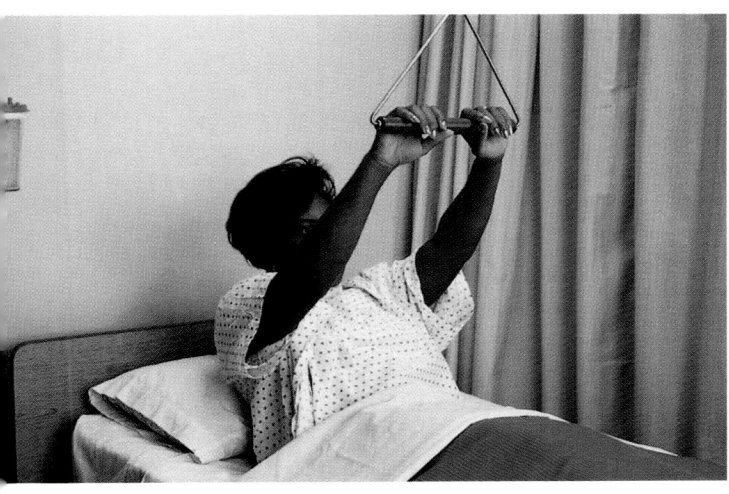

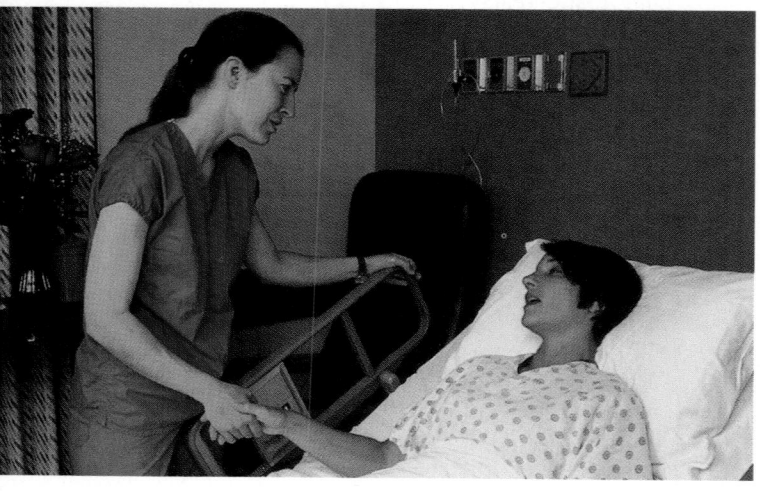

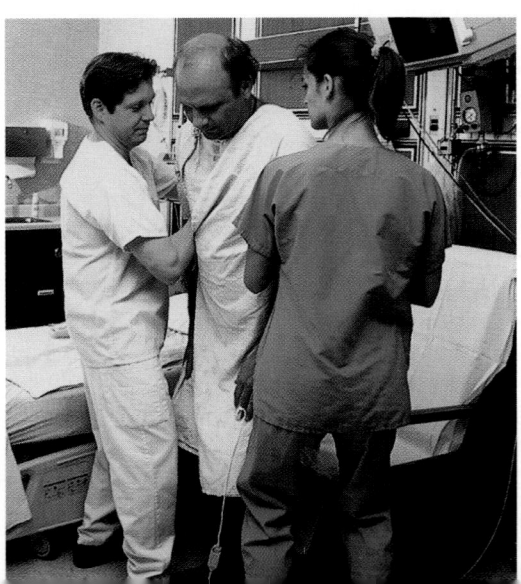

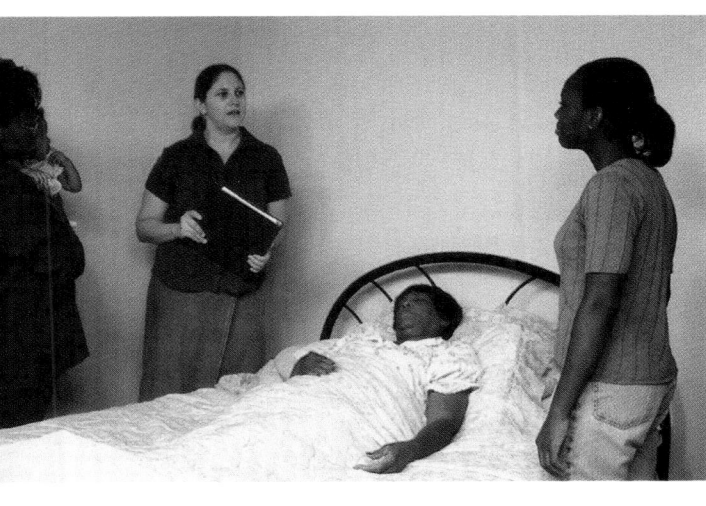

Interdisciplinary Team   1490
Settings of Care   1491
Americans With Disabilities Act   1492
Factors Affecting Functional Limitations   1494
Lifestyle Factors   1494
Environmental Factors   1494
Developmental Factors   1494
Culture/Religious Factors   1494
Psychosocial Factors   1494
Physiological Factors   1495
Assessment   1495
General Assessment of Functional
Limitations   1495
Diagnostic Tests   1497
Diagnosis   1498
Planning   1498
Intervention   1499
Interventions to Prevent Disability   1499
Interventions to Promote Self-Care   1499
Evaluation   1501

57 The Surgical Client   1503
V. Doreen Wagner

Concepts of the Surgical Experience   1504
Settings   1504
Classification of Surgical Procedures   1504
Perioperative Phases   1504
Anesthesia   1507
Informed Consent   1509
Factors Affecting Surgical Outcome   1510
Lifestyle Factors   1510
Cultural and Religious Factors   1511
Developmental Factors   1511
Socioeconomic Factors   1512
Physiological Factors   1512
Psychological Factors   1515
Assessment   1516

General Assessment of the Preoperative
Client   1516
Diagnostic Tests   1517
Focused Assessment for Anxiety   1517
Focused Assessment for Anticipatory
Grieving   1518
Focused Assessment for Risk for Latex
Allergy Response   1518
Focused Assessment for Knowledge
Deficit   1518
Diagnosis   1519
Planning   1519
Expected Outcomes for the Client With
Anxiety   1520
Expected Outcomes for the Client With
Anticipatory Grieving   1520
Expected Outcomes for the Client With Risk
for Latex Allergy Response   1520
Expected Outcomes for the Client With
Knowledge Deficit   1520
Intervention   1520
Interventions to Reduce Anxiety   1520
Interventions to Promote Functional
Grieving   1521
Interventions to Prevent Latex Allergy
Response   1521
Interventions to Increase Client
Knowledge   1522
Evaluation   1527
Intraoperative Phase   1528
Assessment   1528
General Assessment of the Intraoperative
Client   1528
Focused Assessment for Risk for
Infection   1529
Focused Assessment for Risk for Perioperative
Positioning Injury   1530
Focused Assessment for Risk for
Injury   1530
Focused Assessment for Risk for Altered Body
Temperature   1532
Diagnosis   1533
Planning   1533
Expected Outcomes for the Client With Risk
for Infection   1533
Expected Outcomes for the Client With Risk
for Perioperative Positioning Injury   1533
Expected Outcomes for the Client With Risk
for Injury   1533
Expected Outcomes for the Client With Risk
for Altered Body Temperature   1533
Intervention   1533
Interventions to Prevent Infection   1534
Interventions to Prevent Perioperative
Positioning Injury   1534

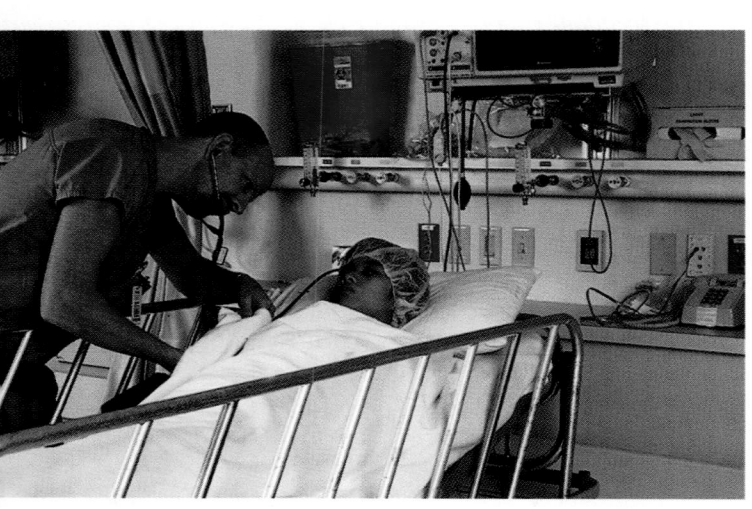

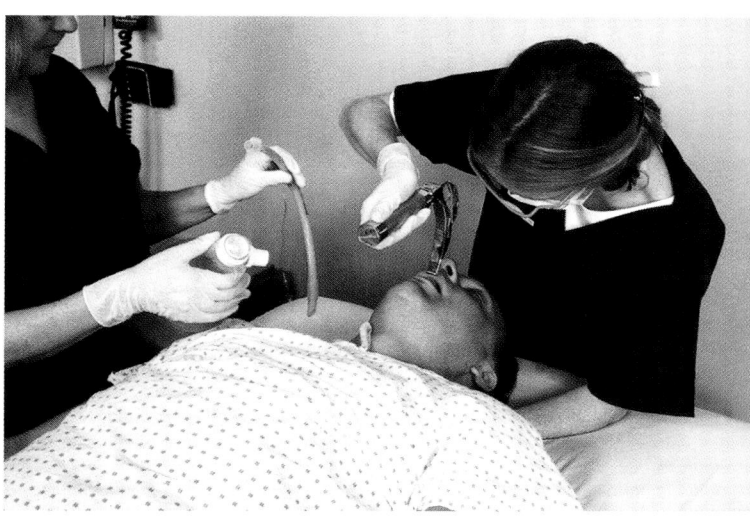

58 The Emergency Client   1551

SPECIAL FEATURES

Considering the Alternatives Charts

The Cost of Care Charts

Cross-Cultural Care Charts

Decision Trees

Nursing Care Planning Charts

A Patient's View/A Caregiver's View Charts

Procedures

The State of Nursing Science Charts

Teaching for Self-Care Charts

Teaching for Wellness Charts

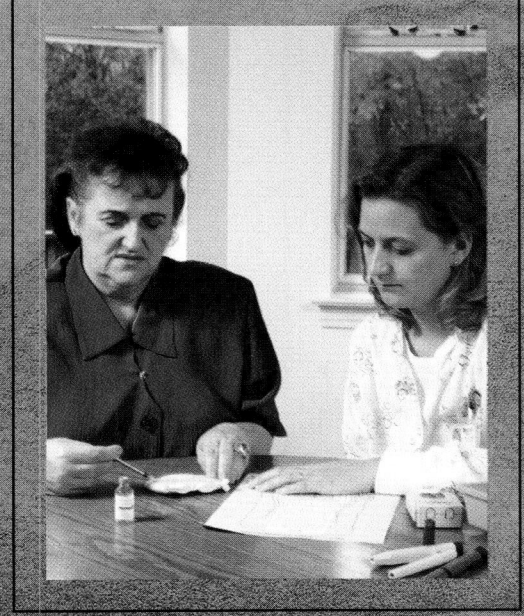

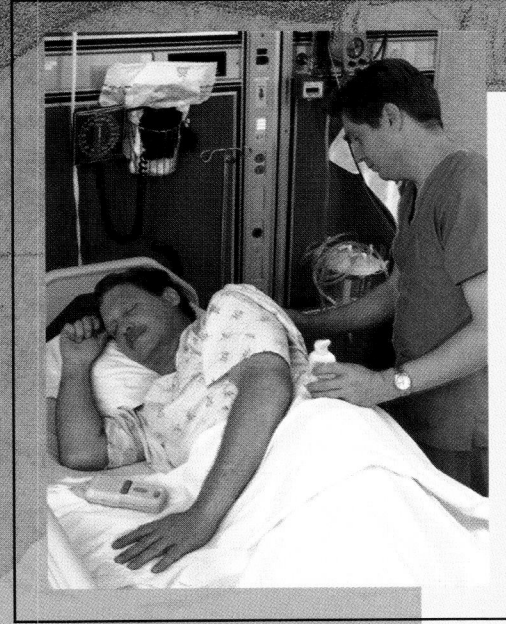

The Context of Nursing Practice

The Social Context of Nursing

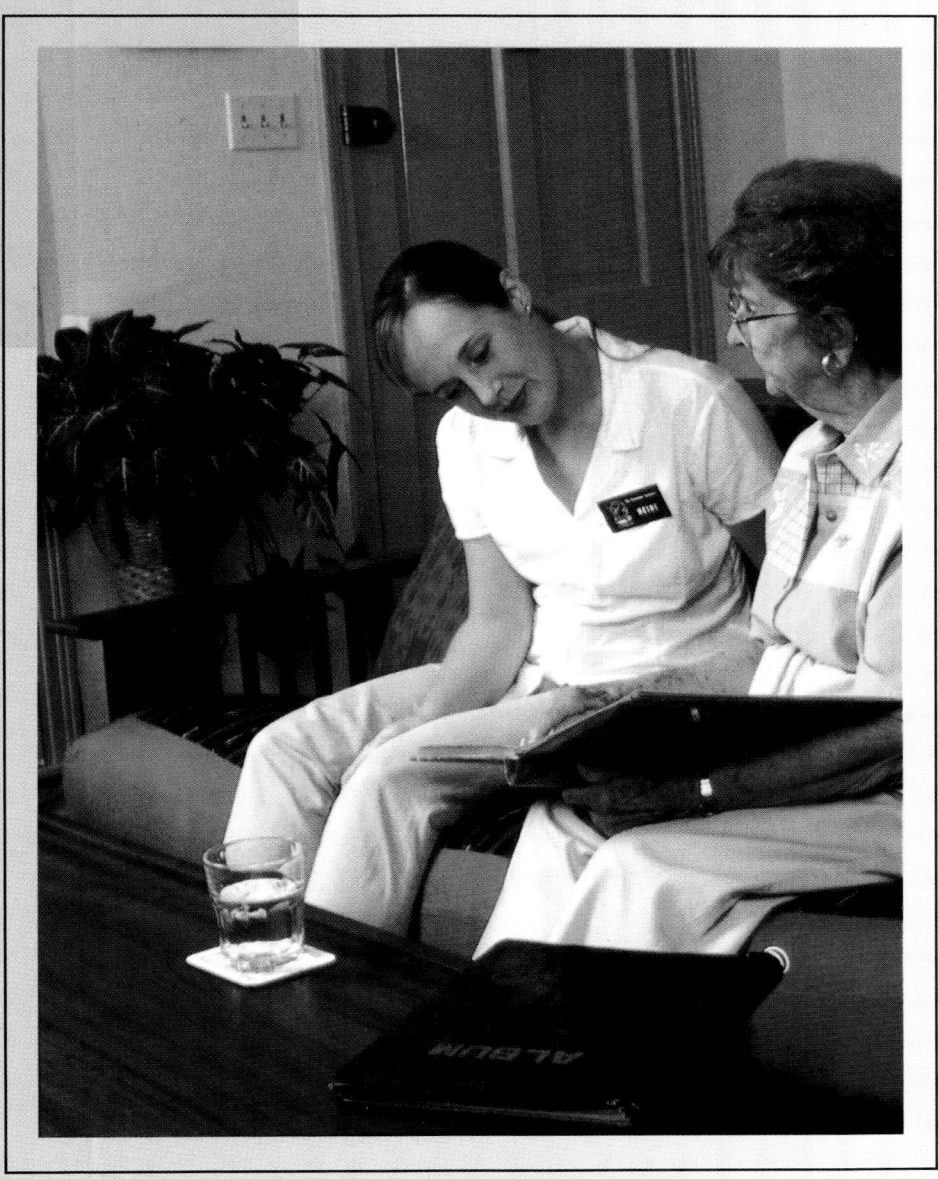

The Nursing Profession as a Context for Practice

Barbara McKinney

Barbara McKinney

Key Terms

client advocate
continuing education
nursing
professionalism

LEARNING OBJECTIVES

After studying this chapter, you should be able to:

1. Describe the evolution of nursing from ancient civilizations to the present, including the influence of religious, scientific, and political developments.

2. Compare the different educational programs in nursing.

3. Identify the effect of professionalism, standards of nursing practice, and nurse practice acts on the profession of nursing.

4. Describe the contribution of at least three professional nursing organizations to the advancement of nursing.

5. Identify nursing roles, components of the health care system, and health care settings.

6. Discuss the social issues and nursing's political agenda.

7. List the predictions for contemporary nursing practice in the 21st century.

Throughout the years, the definition of nursing has changed frequently, yet the common focus of providing humanistic and holistic care has always been preserved. **Nursing** is an accountable discipline guided by science, theory, a code of ethics, and the art of care and comfort to treat human responses to health and illness. *Nursing practice* puts the science and art of nursing into action.

The American Nurses' Association (ANA) represents professional nurses in the United States. The ANA document, *Nursing's Social Policy Statement,* recognizes the contribution of the science of caring in four essential features of contemporary nursing practice as a means of defining nursing:

1. Attention to the full range of human experiences and responses to health and illness without restriction to a problem-focused orientation
2. Integration of objective data with knowledge gained from an understanding of the client or group's subjective experience
3. Application of scientific knowledge to the processes of diagnosis and treatment
4. Provision of a caring relationship that facilitates health and healing (ANA, 1995)

The Canadian Nurses Association (CNA) represents nurses and nursing practice in Canada. The CNA's definition of practice is similar: "Nursing practice can be defined as a dynamic, caring, helping relationship in which the nurse assists the client to achieve and maintain optimal health" (CNA, 1987).

These definitions—nursing and nursing practice—emphasize human response to health and health problems instead of disease processes. Disease is the domain of physicians or the practice of medicine. Nursing and medicine complement one another in the achievement of optimal health for humankind.

EVOLUTION OF THE NURSING PROFESSION

Contemporary nursing practice requires a combination of intellectual achievement, ethical standards, scientific knowledge, technological skills, and personal compassion. Gradually, over centuries, these elements have evolved and blended together. During this evolutionary process nursing practice has been influenced by external factors such as economics, religion, politics, scientific advancements, wars, and changing lifestyles.

This chapter begins with a journey into the evolution of nursing as a profession. Your journey starts with nursing's humble beginnings in ancient civilizations. As Donahue (1985) observes, "From the dawn of civilization, evidence prevails to support the premise that nurturing has been essential to the preservation of life. Survival of the human race, therefore, is inextricably intertwined with the development of nursing."

Nursing in Ancient Civilizations

Anthropologists speculate that in most ancient civilizations, women were responsible for nurturing, nour-

ishing, and providing care to children and ill family members. Nursing in its early history was a community service that preserved and protected the family (Donahue, 1985).

In many cultures, illness was believed to be directly related to religious beliefs and magical myths. A person could also become ill if an evil spirit took control of the body. Medicine men, healers, or shamans exorcised these evil spirits from the sick. They used such methods as incantations, vile odors, massage, charms, and even sacrifices. Women delivered custodial care and seldom assisted the medicine men. This duty typically fell to other males, who generally helped the medicine men (Hamilton, 1996).

Some ancient peoples recognized that illness was at least partly caused by physical factors. The Aztecs, Mayans, and Toltecs, for example, believed health was the result of a balanced body, nature and the supernatural. Illness was treated with massage, blood letting, minerals and herbs, suturing wounds, amputating limbs, extracting teeth, and even trephining, the drilling of holes in the skull (Hamilton, 1996).

Eventually, nursing roles expanded outside the family to the care of tribe members, and the complexity of care increased. According to Dock and Stewart (1925), knowledge provided the initial force for nursing to become an art and science.

Influence of Christianity

Under the influence of Christianity, educated and wealthy women dedicated themselves to caring for the sick and poverty stricken (Donahue, 1985). In fact, the first recorded history of nursing began with passages in the New Testament about women who cared for the sick and injured. The practice of nursing expanded and nurses began to be respected.

In 60 AD, Phoebe, a Roman matron, had the distinction of being named "the first deaconess," a church official ordained to meet the needs of women converts. A secondary function of the deaconess was visiting the sick (Jamieson, Sewall, & Gjertson, 1959). From this role Phoebe became known as the "first visiting nurse." In fact, one of the earliest records of nursing influenced by Christianity was the formation of the Order of the Deaconesses.

Middle Ages

The Middle Ages, the years of 476 AD to 1453, separated ancient from modern times. The first 500 years of this period are often called the *Dark Ages* because of the low level of education of all but the nobles and the clergy and because of the dearth of institutions of higher learning. In addition, the Dark Ages were marked by war, poverty, social injustices, illness, and general misery of the people.

At different times during the Middle Ages, and for a total of 300 years, the bubonic plague killed about one-third to one-half of Europe's population. This widespread disease stimulated hospital construction;

however, these early hospitals had no ventilation, heat, plumbing, or lighting and hardly any sanitation services (Becker & Fender, 1978).

The plague also contributed to the founding of many nursing orders. Gradually, the number of deaconesses diminished as monks and nuns took over the operation of hospitals. The first nursing order, the Augustinian Sisters, was founded. This order provided purely nursing services.

Secular groups also formed to meet and care for the sick and impoverished. The practice of midwifery flourished in the Middle Ages. The Crusades also stimulated expanded nursing and health care. Nurses were also knights and were employed in battle as well as in hospital settings (Doheny, Cook, & Stopper, 1987). Groups of knights, such as the Knights Hospitallier of St. John of Jerusalem, cared for the wounded and ill along the crusade routes (Fig. 1–1). As the number of all-male military nursing orders increased, all-female religious orders were nearly destroyed. A number of religious orders evolved, such as the order of Saint Francis of Assisi, which included Franciscans and Dominicans.

Renaissance and Reformation

The Renaissance started in Italy and expanded to Western Europe. It was a period of renewed interest in

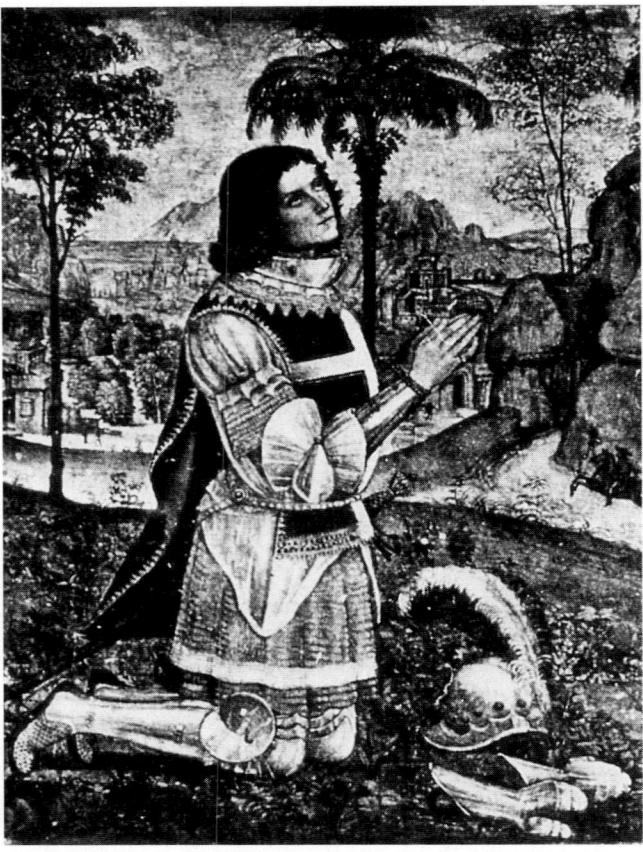

Figure 1–1. A Knight Hospitallier of St. John of Jerusalem. (Courtesy of the National Library of Medicine.)

philosophy, science, and the arts. Learning flourished, and by 1500, a trend toward nursing education had developed. Universities were constructed throughout Europe.

As religious orders became less influential, a need for secular nursing services was recognized (Becker & Fender, 1978). However, even as medicine moved into the university setting, nursing remained behind.

Slowly, monasteries and religious orders declined because of increased Protestantism. Soon male nurses vanished from the nursing profession (Doheny, Cook, & Stopper, 1987). The home became the main locality for nursing care. Only the poor sick were hospitalized. Hospital administrators commonly recruited prostitutes and female criminals to perform nursing functions. The interval between 1600 and 1850 has been described as the *darkest age of nursing*. There was little to no organization, education, or social standing left in nursing.

Colonialism and Revolution

Beginning in the last decade of the 15th century, many European powers sought to expand their territories in the New World. Spain founded colonies around the world, including settlements in Florida, Mexico, Central America, and South America. France established colonies in Nova Scotia, Canada, and Louisiana. England colonized territories in the East, in Africa, Australia, and along the Atlantic coast of North America.

Early colonists experienced some of the same health care problems seen in Europe. Infectious diseases, nutritional disorders, starvation, and complications of pregnancy were common. Folk remedies were the extent of nursing and medical care (Hamilton, 1996).

By the mid-17th century, health care delivery had begun to improve. Medical knowledge began developing in the British colonies. The first colonial hospital was established in what later became New York in 1658 (Selevan, 1984). Typically, the nurses in colonial hospitals were untrained males.

Despite these advances, health care was poor. Physicians were not required to have a license to practice medicine, and medical charlatans were common. Hospital care was available only in the largest colonial cities, and rural colonists relied on visiting physicians and home remedies. The mentally ill went without treatment or were warehoused in hospitals where they were shackled and confined together in filthy, dungeon-like rooms (Hamilton, 1996).

When the 13 American colonies declared their independence from England in 1776, their soldiers were poorly dressed, inadequately armed, hungry, and ill. Soldiers were exposed to impure water, dirty camps, and unsanitary hospitals, and scarlet fever, smallpox, and dysentery devastated their ranks. It has been speculated that more American Revolutionary soldiers died from disease or complications of care than from wounds (Selevan, 1984).

The newly formed United States recognized the need for clean hospitals and trained nurses to supervise soldiers' care while in combat (Chitty, 1993). Nurses played a role in the war by directly caring for soldiers at the battlefront and in hospitals.

Industrialization

The Industrial Revolution began in England and France during the mid-18th century and in Germany and the United States in the 19th century. The Revolution was caused by multiple factors, such as the decline of feudalism, a population explosion following migration from rural to urban areas, scientific advancement, changing work modes, shifting principles of fairness, and adoption of the efficiency idea by agriculture and business (Jamieson, Sewall, & Gjertson, 1959). These factors led to undesirable work conditions and negative attitudes toward the working class and a much lower standard of living. As a result of the Industrial Revolution, families often lived in overcrowded conditions, with poor ventilation, heating, and cooling. In urban areas, water supplies, sanitation, garbage collection, and plumbing were poor. To make matters worse, no adequate method of preserving foods or basic hygiene techniques had been developed yet. Factories paid starvation wages for long hours of dangerous work. Child labor was common. All of the negative factors increased the incidence of illness, injury, and early mortality.

Slowly, consciousness of these barbarous methods began to heighten. At the same time, society's attitude toward health care became more compassionate. Caring for the sick became socially acceptable, even praiseworthy. Hospitals opened to care for the increased illnesses and injuries due to working conditions, and physicians recognized the need for competent hospital nurses. Nursing textbooks on management and techniques were written.

Several groups sought to care for the sick, injured, and poor, such as the Sisters Of Charity, who developed a nurse training program. The Kaiserwerth School of Nursing was established by Pastor Theodor Fliedner in his parish in Kaiserwerth, Germany in 1886. Students from many countries were taught practice, theory, and codes of conduct related to nursing (Doheny, Cook, & Stopper, 1987).

An attempt to organize a school of nursing was made in 1839 by Dr. Joseph Warrington of the Nurse Society of Philadelphia. The classes were taught together with medical students and gave women minimal instruction in obstetrics to enable them to provide maternity nursing services in the home setting (Jenson, Spaulding, & Cody, 1955).

The Influence of War

Advances in military technology in the early 19th century ushered in an age of modern warfare characterized by tremendous escalation in the rates of crippling injuries, loss of limbs, and mortality. This lead to an increased demand for trained military nurses.

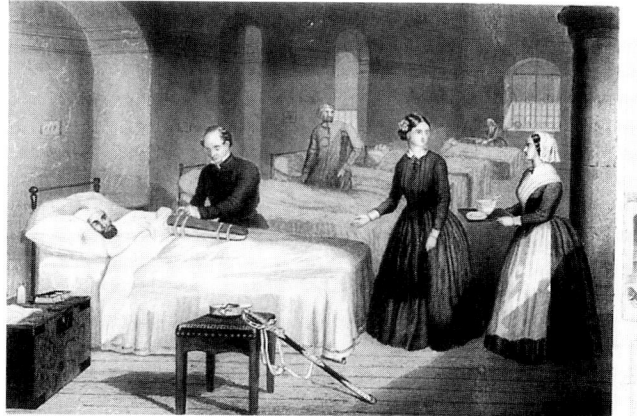

Figure 1–2. Florence Nightingale (1820–1910). (Courtesy of the National Library of Medicine.)

Crimean War

The Crimean War was fought in what is now part of the Ukraine, between 1854 and 1856. Great Britain, France, Turkey, and Sardinia united as allies to defeat Russia. This war is important to any discussion of the history of nursing because of the role played in it by Florence Nightingale. Florence Nightingale is considered the founder of modern nursing (Fig. 1–2).

Florence Nightingale was born in 1820, into an upper-class English family. As a child, she enjoyed wealth, education, and extensive travel. While accompanying her mother to visit the sick, she became aware of the inadequate care of hospitalized patients and expressed the desire to become a nurse. Her parents disapproved and encouraged her to marry, but her desire to become a nurse outweighed her parents' wishes. At age 31, she entered nursing training at Deaconess Institute in Kaiserwerth. In 1853, she completed additional training with the Sisters of Charity in Paris. Shortly thereafter, Nightingale became administrator of a charity hospital for governesses.

In 1854, the Crimean War began. The Secretary of War, a close friend of Nightingale's, recruited her to prepare and lead a group of 38 nurses to British military hospitals in Scutari, Turkey. Their mission was to care for the wounded and to institute reform. Smith (1984) states that once in Turkey, Nightingale found a hospital "so crowded that patients lay on the floor still in bloody uniforms. Bath equipment, sheets, cutlery, and laundry facilities were either nonexistent or nearly so."

With much compassion, Nightingale established sanitary conditions. Hospital units were cleaned and clothing was washed regularly. The clients received nursing care both day and night. Nightingale's reforms reduced the mortality rate of the soldiers from 42.7% to 2.2% in 6 short months (Donahue, 1985; Cohen, 1984; Woodham-Smith, 1951).

Because Nightingale and her nurses made their rounds carrying oil lamps, she became known as "The Lady with the lamp." This remains the symbol of the nursing profession.

After the Crimean War, Nightingale served on several commissions and wrote about health, sanitation, hospitals, and nursing education (Hamilton, 1996). Her most distinguished books are *Notes on Hospitals* (1858) and *Notes on Nursing: What It Is and What It Is Not* (1860).

In 1860, the Nightingale Training School for nurses opened at St. Thomas' Hospital in London. The 1-year course offered classroom and clinical experience, later known as the "Nightingale Plan." This plan became the model for nursing education and was used in the United States and Canada. Three schools of nursing based on her training school model opened in Boston, Connecticut, and New York. The women who graduated from these first schools led nursing into the 20th century.

American Civil War

With the American Civil War (1861–1865), early nursing leaders began to emerge. Table 1–1 summarizes the primary contributions of selected early nursing leaders. These women were willing to take risks when human rights were put in jeopardy or threatened. Women volunteered to care for soldiers on both the Confederate and Union sides of the war. Their contributions included the implementation of sanitary conditions in field hospitals.

It was also during the Civil War that the value of primary prevention became understood in America. A clean surrounding, good nutrition, and nurses in control of the environment were recognized as positive factors for healing. It was clear that training nurses would be beneficial.

After the Civil War, the first schools of nursing based on Nightingale's model began to appear. In Canada, the first training school, St. Catherine's, was founded in Ontario in 1874 (Raab, 1986; Donahue, 1985). A number of Canadians became early nursing leaders in the United States.

One such leader, Isabel Hampton Robb, was a graduate of the Bellevue Hospital Training School in New York (Fig. 1–3). She became the first principal of the Johns Hopkins School of Nursing. In 1894, she wrote a standardized nursing text to be used in America: *Nursing: Its Principles and Practice for Hospital and Private Use* (Donahue, 1985). In 1896, Robb helped found the Nurses Associated Alumnae of the United States and Canada. The Canadian affiliation was removed in 1899. After that, in 1911, it became known as the American Nurses' Association. Robb was instrumental in establishing the National League of Nursing Education that is now known as the National League for Nursing.

Mary Adelaide Nutting, also from Canada, was in the first graduating class at Johns Hopkins School of Nursing. She actively worked for nurses to be educated in the university setting. Nutting was the first nurse to be appointed a university professorship at Columbia University Teachers College and also directed the newly established department of nursing and health (Donahue, 1985).

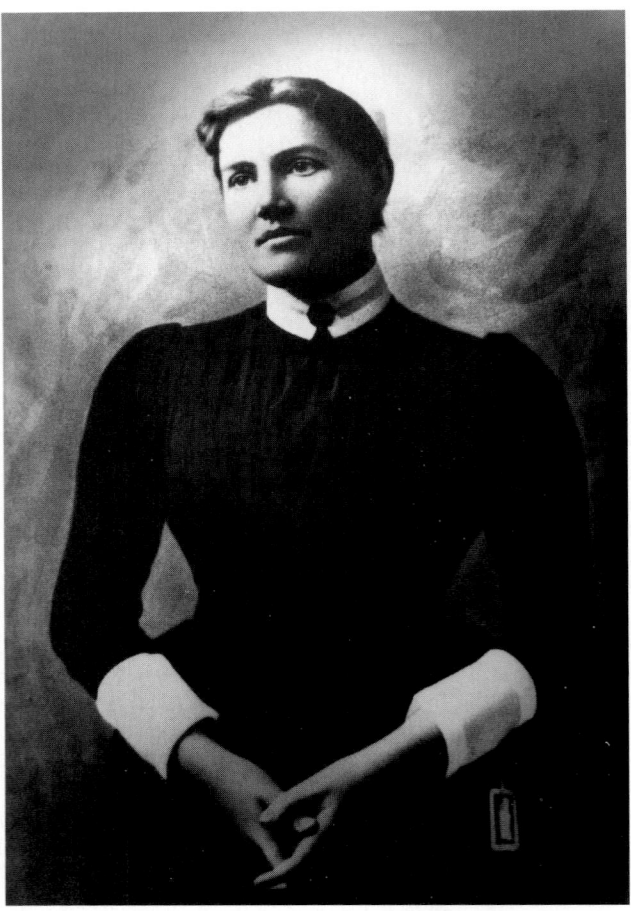

Figure 1–3. Isabel Hampton Robb (1860–1910). (Courtesy of the Alan Mason Chesney Medical Archives of the Johns Hopkins Medical Institutions.)

Mary Mahoney became America's first professional black nurse in 1879. She campaigned for the respect of cultural differences. Today, the ANA bestows the Mary Mahoney Award in recognition of individuals who make significant contributions toward improving relationships among diverse cultural groups.

In 1893, Lillian Wald founded public health nursing when she opened the Henry Street Settlement Service in New York City. Wald, the first community health nurse, recognized the importance of teaching people about health promotion practices and the means to prevent illness. Programs such as tuberculosis control and infant welfare were started. The institutional base later shifted to the government, and public health services were offered through local health departments.

Spanish-American War

The Spanish-American War offered trained nurses an opportunity for employment in military hospitals. The war revealed American deficiencies, namely the lack of emergency nursing reserves. Although the American army casualties were small, their military camps were shattered by epidemic diseases. Typhoid fever and malaria devastated the army camps. Dysentery

TABLE 1–1
Primary Contributions of Selected Early Nursing Leaders

Nursing Leader	Key Date	Contribution
Sojourner Truth	1827	Abolitionist, lecturer, women's rights worker. A black nurse who made enormous contributions during the American Civil War. Worked as a nurse/counselor for the Freedman's Association following the war.
Harriet Ross Tubman	1840	A black nurse who led more than 300 slaves to freedom during the American Civil War. Recognized for her kindness and attention to the sick and suffering.
Florence Nightingale	1854	A war nurse and founder of modern nursing education. A publisher and nurse theorist.
Dorothea Dix	1861	Appointed Superintendent of the Women Nurses of the Army. Devoted herself to the care of the mentally ill and to improvement of jail conditions.
Mary Ann Ball	1861	"Mother Beckerdyke." Known for her nursing skill. Was one of the greatest heroines of the American Civil War. Organized diet kitchens and ambulance services.
Linda Richards	1872	A graduate of New England Hospital for Women and Children. She became the first trained nurse in the United States. Later, developed and established the first nursing school in Japan.
Lavinia Lloyd Dock	1873	A well-known nurse who was actively involved in early 20th-century women's rights issues and the suffragette movement.
Mary Eliza Mahoney	1879	Completed the 16-month training course at the New England Hospital for Women and Children to become America's first black "trained nurse."
Clara Barton	1881	Famous American Civil War nurse who used her work and ideas from the battlefield to develop the American Red Cross.
Mary Agnes Snively	1884	Responsible for the direction of Canadian nursing education. Director of the Toronto General Hospital Canadian Nurses Association.
Isabel Hampton Robb	1886	An outstanding nurse who was first president of the Nurses Associated Alumnae of the United States and Canada. Was first principal of Johns Hopkins School of Nursing, cofounder of the *American Journal of Nursing.*
Betty Moulder and Ada Stewart	1888	First nurses employed as occupational health nurses.
Annie Goodrich	1893	Head of the United States Army School of Nursing in 1918. Was Assistant Professor of Nursing at Teachers College and Dean of Nursing at Yale University. Served as president of the American Nurses Association.
Lillian Wald	1893	Founded the Henry Street Settlement, providing health care for the poor in New York's Lower East Side. Formed the National Organization of Public Health Nursing (the first specialization in nursing) in 1912.
Mary Adelaide Nutting	1894	An early nurse activist at Teachers College. She became known as "the first nursing professor in the world." Influential in raising educational standards for nurses toward undergraduate and graduate nursing degrees.
Namahyoke Curtis	1898	Was the first trained black nurse employed as a contract nurse by the United States War Department during the Spanish-American War.
Clara Maas	1898	A nurse volunteer who participated in the yellow fever research experiment in Havana, Cuba, and lost her life after the Spanish-American War.
Jessie Sleet (Scales)	1900	Became the first black public health nurse.
Martha Franklin	1916	Founded the National Association of Colored Graduate Nurses (NACGN).
Margaret Sanger	1916	Founded the first birth control clinic in America, the forerunner of Planned Parenthood.
Francis Reed Elliott	1918	Became the first black nurse accepted by the American Red Cross Nursing Service.
Frances Payne Bolton	1923	Provided financial support that was instrumental in the development of the nursing school at Case Western Reserve University.
Isabel Maitland Stewart	1925	Conducted research to differentiate between nursing and non-nursing tasks. Successful in influencing upgraded nursing education.
Mary Breckinridge	1925	Founded the Frontier Nursing Service, which provided the first organized midwifery service in the United States.
Lucille Petry	1949	Became the first woman appointed to the position of Assistant Surgeon General of the United States Public Health Service.
Mildred Montag	1952	Conducted research, was instrumental in the development of the first Associate Degree nursing program.

and food poisoning were rampant. The Nurses Associated Alumnae of the United States and Canada offered to help the government to secure skilled nurses. However, the Daughters of the American Revolution had already volunteered their untrained services for nursing care of the troops.

During this time Anita Newcomb McGee, a physician, was appointed in charge of the Army Nursing Service as acting assistant surgeon in the United States Army. Dr. McGee preferred enrolling nurses with a certificate of graduation from a training school for nurses. These nurses were then placed under the direction of the Red Cross, which assisted with their expenses while in service (Jamieson, Sewall, & Gjertson, 1959). Through Congress, the nurses worked on a contract basis receiving $30 per month plus room and meals. Approximately 8,000 volunteer nurses were placed under contract and began what is now the Army Nursing Corps. Dita H. Kinney, head nurse of the United States Army Hospital at Fort Baynard, eventually replaced Dr. McGee.

These nurses and soldiers were continually exposed to typhoid and yellow fever. Clara Louise Maas volunteered to serve in the Spanish-American War as a contract nurse. She became actively involved in yellow fever research experimentation after a mosquito bite and died in 1901. She was the only American and the only woman to die during the experiments.

World War I

In 1917, the United States entered World War I. The number of nurses available could not meet both civilian and military needs. Once again, an untrained volunteer system provided military nursing care. Concerned nursing leaders established the Army School of Nursing in 1918 in order to train volunteers. The school was headed by Annie Goodrich, an assistant professor of nursing at Teachers College.

After the war, the Rockefeller Foundation established a committee to study nursing education. Findings from this study, called the Goldmark Report, revealed the faults associated with hospital nursing programs while identifying lack of funding as nursing's obstacle to higher educational standards (Kalisch & Kalisch, 1986). At this time, the Rockefeller Foundation funded the expansion of nursing programs at Vanderbilt University, Yale University, and the University of Toronto.

During the 1920s, hospitals and nursing schools began to expand. Nursing schools depended on hospitals for support while the hospitals depended on the students to carry nursing's workload. Eventually, this apprenticeship method of educating nurses became increasingly criticized. More and more, male hospital administrators and physicians governed the almost exclusively female student population. This type of paternalism slowed nursing's progress toward professionalism for several decades (Kalisch & Kalisch, 1986).

Many trained nurses became involved in the women's suffrage movement. Women were not considered equals of men, society did not value education for women, and women did not have the right to vote. Lavinia Dock, a well-known early 20th-century nurse, was instrumental in women's issues and the suffrage movement. By the mid-1900s, more women were going to college even though only limited numbers of nursing programs were available in the university setting.

The Great Depression and drought of the 1930s brought financial destruction to a country already exhausted by war. As prosperity diminished, so did the use of private-duty nurses. There was a shortage of funds for visiting nursing services and too many trained nurses on hand. Gradually, hospitals became the primary setting for care for the sick. The decline in home-based nursing care would last until the late 1980s (Chitty, 1993).

World War II

World War II (1939–1945) had an enormous effect on nursing. Qualified nurses were in demand. Training for nurses became associated with classrooms and organized curricula (Fig. 1–4). In 1941, the U.S. Congress passed the Lanham Act to fund nursing education and improve existing educational facilities (Donahue, 1985). Federally subsidized nursing programs were developed to offer women and men a career in nursing while serving their country.

After the war, a small number of nurse officers entered undergraduate and graduate nursing programs. The GI Bill of Rights assisted them in accessing further education. However, many chose to return to traditional homemaking roles. The "baby boom" and economic burst after the war stimulated the construction of hospitals. Within a few years, a shortage of registered nurses created unfavorable working conditions for hospital-based nurses (Chitty, 1993).

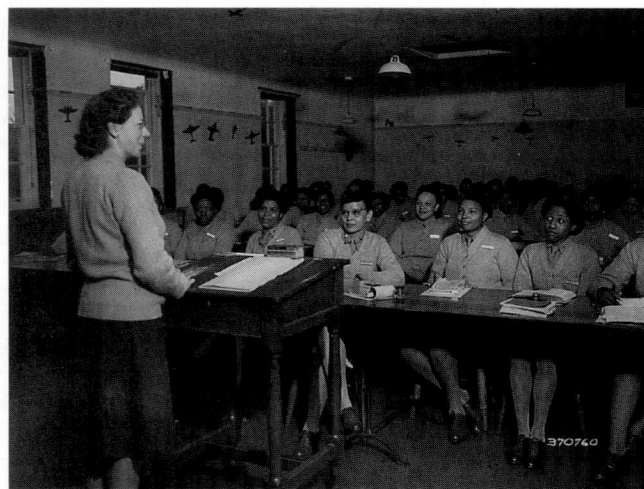

Figure 1–4. During World War II, training for nurses became associated with classrooms and organized curricula. (Courtesy of the National Archives at College Park.)

As dissatisfaction grew, the ANA sanctioned state units to form collective bargaining units. This move created an ethical dilemma for many nurses. Now they would have to decide between their duty to care for clients or their duty to themselves and their families.

In the late 1940s, nursing as a profession was seeking to meet the needs of society and to organize the profession in order to meet those needs. The war years had underlined the requisite for nursing to speak with professional unity. Work began on the professional issues of education and organizational unity.

Korean War

The Korean War was fought between the years 1950 and 1953. The nurses of the U.S. armed forces—Army, Navy, and the new Air Force Nurse Corps—were called on to serve their country. The Army instituted combat emergency teams or units called the Mobile Army Surgical Hospital (MASH). The MASH could be moved at a moment's notice and was usually staffed by 10 physicians, 12 nurses, and 90 corpsmen. It could and did set up anywhere. Within a few hours, 200 to 300 clients could be treated. Hamilton (1996) reports that the success of these units revealed the tremendous contribution of nurses in demanding circumstances. This experience paved the way for development of intensive care units and better emergency or trauma medical treatment.

Fear of a severe nursing shortage was instrumental in an increased recruitment of students to nursing schools to offset the depleted numbers of professional nurses in civilian hospitals. A significant change in nursing education that affected the profession also occurred at this time with the development of associate degree programs in community colleges.

Mildred Montag of Teachers College had developed a new model of nursing education as a result of research she had conducted. She began the piloting of the new model of associate degree nursing programs in 1952, and by 1957 a rapid proliferation of community college nursing programs had begun. The nurse of this new program was to be a nurse technician, operating below the professional nurse but above the practical nurse (Donahue, 1985). Because of major nursing shortages and to meet societal need, however, the associate degreed nurse became the third level of entry into nursing practice.

Vietnam War

From 1957 to 1975, nursing was kept busy with the Vietnam War. The appointment of male nurses to the armed forces nurse corps was made possible by a Congressional bill passed in 1966. As a result of the bill, the number of male nurses increased and some all-male nursing units were even established for short periods of time. Hospitals were fixed facilities during this conflict and helicopters became the means of evacuation and immediate care by medics and flight nurses.

During this time, civilian hospitals expanded rapidly and installed intensive care units and recovery rooms, creating the need for more advanced technical nursing skills. Specialization advanced at a rapid rate as a consequence of the technological changes and new knowledge. This increased specialization introduced constraints in staffing within hospitals. No longer was the nurse able to move freely from one unit to another unless those units had the same kinds of clients and were treated by the same general modes of therapy.

This was a time of professional awakening for nursing. The concept of nursing diagnosis, introduced in the 1950s, contributed to the development of nursing as a science. Masters in nursing programs in clinical specialties and doctoral degrees in nursing were being offered in major universities. Nurse practitioner programs opened, associate degrees in nursing programs proliferated, and financial support from the federal government for nursing education was reaching an all-time high.

Many nurses became employed outside the hospital, and this quickly became the age of nurse entrepreneurship. As nurse-owned businesses grew, the number of certified practitioners working individually and in joint practice with physicians also grew (Hamilton, 1996).

Contemporary Developments

The 1980s involved changes in the medical, technical, and organizational domains of American society that had major effects on who received services, who provided services, and what types of services were available. The introduction of diagnosis-related groups (DRGs) for Medicare by the federal government in 1983 was an effort to contain the rapidly rising cost of health care. DRGs, health maintenance organizations (HMOs), and emergency care centers have all been reflections of the financially driven health care system of the 1980s.

The 1990s were also a decade of profound change in health care delivery and health care settings. This era is characterized by its efforts toward cost containment and heightened efficiency in health care, which eliminated some hospital nursing jobs. However, the increase in jobs for nurses in outpatient and home health agencies has maintained a steady albeit changing nursing work force.

A new trend, *managed care*, emerged while advanced practice nursing specialties grew in an effort to maintain quality health care at the lowest cost. A large number of registered nurses were employed in the role of case manager to review clients' cases and coordinate care in various health settings. Advanced practice nurses, such as the Clinical Nurse Practitioner and Clinical Nurse Specialist, were employed in the traditional and nontraditional health care setting. Third-party payment for these nursing services by insurers was secured as a result of the health care dollar crisis of the 1990s. Home nursing care delivery expanded as a major cost-effective measure during this era.

In 1993, President Clinton focused attention on the need for preventive services in the proposed *Health Security Act of 1993*. Primary prevention was not a new idea for nurses. In an attempt to represent nursing's interest and role, representatives of more than 60 nursing organizations developed their own reform plan called *Nursing's Agenda for Health Care Reform*. The reform focused on primary care, prevention, and community outreach.

PROFESSIONAL NURSING EDUCATION

Since the first schools of nursing opened their doors in the 18th century, nursing education has expanded in response to ongoing changes and advances in health care. Today's nursing roles are more complex and require additional knowledge in the physical, biological, and social sciences, along with nursing practice and theory.

Entry-Level Education

There are currently four types of educational programs that prepare students for entry into practice of professional registered nursing. They are the diploma program, associate degree program, baccalaureate degree program, and graduate degree entry programs.

Diploma Programs

In the United States and Canada, the diploma nursing program is a 3-year program frequently affiliated with a hospital. However, some diploma programs are associated with a college or university and students receive college credit for all non-nursing classes. The programs retain some of the apprenticeship traditions of the past and prepare nurses at a high technical level of practice.

Associate Degree Programs

Associate degree programs in the United States are 2-year programs offered by community colleges as well as colleges and universities. The program's focus is on scientific and practical courses in nursing. Upon graduation, students receive an Associate Degree in Nursing (ADN). Most nurses today graduate from associate degree programs. In Canada, associate degrees are not offered, but similar diploma programs do exist.

Baccalaureate Degree Programs

The basic baccalaureate nursing program is situated within a university or college and requires 4 years of study, including general education courses. In Canada, a Bachelor of Science in Nursing (BScN) or a Bachelor in Nursing (BN) is equal to a Bachelor of Science in Nursing (BSN) in the United States. The focus is on achieving a level of critical inquiry, clinical judgment, decision-making, and clinical knowledge imperative for professional nursing practice.

Many baccalaureate programs admit registered nurses with previously earned diplomas or associate degrees. Some universities offer an independent study program (external degree) without class structure. Most baccalaureate nursing programs accept student transfer credits from accredited universities and colleges. Additionally, transferring students can take challenge examinations for college credit.

Graduate Degree Entry Programs

Master's and doctoral entry-level programs are offered only by a few universities. These programs prepare college graduates who have degrees in disciplines other than nursing as entry-level nurse generalists with advanced knowledge and skill levels. Such programs may offer optional specialization tracks such as nurse practitioners, nurse administrators, and nurse midwives. Regardless of their level of entry into the profession, graduates from all levels of entry take the same registered nurse licensing examination (Fig. 1–5).

Advanced-Practice Education

More nurses are becoming prepared at the master's and doctoral levels in order to continue the expansion of nursing knowledge and expertise as well as provide leadership in the health care policy-making arena in clinical practice and administration. The advanced practice education levels include the master's degree and the doctoral degree.

Master's Degree Programs

A master's in nursing program usually takes about 2 years to complete. Master's degree programs prepare advanced clinical practitioners, nurse educators, or nurse administrators. Special emphasis is given to advanced scientific concepts and clinical practice. Theory and research in nursing form the foundation for the curriculum.

Doctoral Degree Programs

A nurse doctorate requires in-depth inquiry and scientific research into a specific field of learning. Doctoral

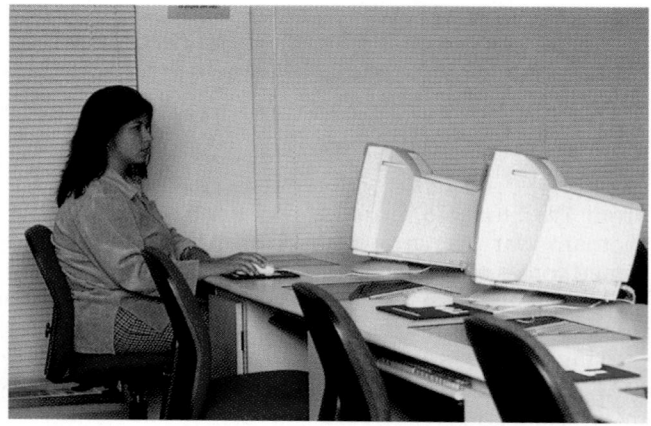

Figure 1–5. A graduate nurse taking the NCLEX-RN exam.

programs produce nurse philosophers, ethicists, theorists, and researchers. Many universities now require that nursing faculty members hold doctorate degrees. Clinical agencies are beginning to ask for doctorally prepared nurses to serve as nurse executives or directors of education and research. Professional organizations are also looking to the doctorate holders to represent them to health policy decision-makers and even consumers.

Continuing Education

Continuing education (CE) is a term used to describe courses that assist professional nurses in developing and maintaining clinical expertise and knowledge that promotes the quality of nursing care. CE is designed to assist nurses in gaining and maintaining knowledge and skills in practice, administration, research, and education.

CE for nurses is offered in forms such as workshops, institutes, short courses, conferences, telecourses, evening courses, and even supplements in professional nursing journals. The use of computers as resources for CE is growing rapidly. CE is mandatory in some states to maintain professional licensure.

Standards of Professional Nursing

Professionalism is behavior that upholds the status, methods, character, and standards of a given profession. But what is a profession? The terms *profession* and *occupation* are often used interchangeably. However, a profession differs from an occupation in two major ways: preparation and commitment (Chitty, 1993). According to Kelly (1981), a profession has the following eight characteristics:

- Services provided are vital to human beings and the welfare of society.
- There exists a special body of knowledge that undergoes continual growth through research.
- The services provided involve intellectual activities and individual responsibility or accountability.
- Practitioners receive education in institutions of higher learning.
- Practitioners have autonomy and control their own policies and activities.
- Practitioners are motivated by the service they provide and consider their work important to their lives (altruism).
- Practitioners' decisions and conduct are guided by a code of ethics.
- High standards of practice are encouraged and supported by an organization.

These characteristics distinguish nursing from occupations. Although nursing has never lacked the quality of altruism, accountability, offering a vital human service, and a code of ethics, nursing is still an emerging profession striving for complete professionalism.

States and provinces regulate the professional practice of nursing through *Nurse Practice Acts*. These acts legally define the scope of nursing practice in a given state. Even though the nurse practice acts differ by locality, they are similar in that they serve to protect the public. They meet the needs of professional nursing as well. The public is guaranteed that minimum standards for entry into the nursing profession are met. The profession is guaranteed that standards of practice with appropriate entry credentialing are met.

Standards of nursing practice are nursing actions that are generally agreed upon by nurses as constituting safe and effective client care. They establish the foundation for the professional practice of registered nurses. The development and implementation of these standards are major functions of nursing's professional organizations. Chapter 13 further discusses standards of Clinical Nursing Practice. Box 1–1 provides the American Nurses Association Standards of Clinical Nursing Practice. Box 1–2 provides the standards for nursing practice of the Registered Nurses Association of British Columbia as an example of standards in Canada.

PROFESSIONAL NURSING PRACTICE

Professional Nursing Organizations

Nursing organizations set standards for nursing practice and education. Nurses display more of a professional commitment if they are actively involved in nursing organizations. Clearly, these organizations empower nurses through educational programs and professional publications. The overall function of a nursing professional organization is to

- Establish, maintain, and improve nursing standards.
- Hold all members accountable for using nursing standards.
- Educate the public to appreciate the nursing standards.
- Protect the public from individuals who have not attained or who willfully do not follow the standards of nursing practice.
- Protect individual members of the profession from one another.

Once the standards of nursing practice are put into effect, they monitor the licensure, accreditation, certification, quality assurance, peer review, and public policy as they relate to the profession of nursing (Phaneuf & Lang, 1985).

According to Merton (1958), "A professional organization is an organization of practitioners who judge one another as professionally competent and who have banded together to perform social functions which they cannot perform in their separate capacities as individuals." The professional organization basically deals with events of concern to the profession.

In North America, there are two similar professional organizations for registered nurses. One is the ANA. Its members are state nurses' associations and

---

AMERICAN NURSES' ASSOCIATION STANDARDS OF CLINICAL NURSING PRACTICE

Standards of Care

STANDARD I. ASSESSMENT

The nurse collects patient health data.

STANDARD II. DIAGNOSIS

The nurse analyzes the assessment data in determining diagnoses.

STANDARD III: OUTCOME IDENTIFICATION

The nurse identifies expected outcomes individualized to the patient.

STANDARD IV. PLANNING

The nurse develops a plan of care that prescribes interventions to attain expected outcomes.

STANDARD V. IMPLEMENTATION

The nurse implements the interventions identified in the plan of care.

STANDARD VI. EVALUATION

The nurse evaluates the patient's progress toward attainment of outcomes.

Standards of Professional Performance

STANDARD I. QUALITY OF CARE

The nurse systematically evaluates the quality and effectiveness of nursing practice.

STANDARD II. PERFORMANCE APPRAISAL

The nurse evaluates one's own nursing practice in relation to professional practice standards and relevant statutes and regulations.

STANDARD III. EDUCATION

The nurse acquires and maintains current knowledge and competency in nursing practice.

STANDARD IV. COLLEGIALITY

The nurse interacts with, and contributes to, the professional development of peers and other health care providers as colleagues.

STANDARD V. ETHICS

The nurse's decisions and actions on behalf of patients are determined in an ethical manner.

STANDARD VI. COLLABORATION

The nurse collaborates with the patient, family, and other health care providers in providing patient care.

STANDARD VII. RESEARCH

The nurse uses research findings in practice.

STANDARD VIII. RESOURCE USE

The nurse considers factors related to safety, effectiveness, and cost in planning and delivering patient care.

American Nurses' Association. (1998). Standards of clinical nursing practice (2nd ed.). Washington, D.C.: Author.

---

individual nurses belonging to the state organization. The ANA sponsors workshops for nurses. It also publishes the *American Journal of Nursing.* The ANA offers specialty certification (Box 1–3).

The Canadian Nurses Association is the national nursing association for Canada. The CNA offers supportive services to all provincial associations. This organization, like the ANA, supports goals such as improved standards of health, high standards of nursing, promotion of professional development and welfare of nurses, nursing education, licensing, and registration of nurses.

The CNA and ANA are part of the International Council of Nurses (ICN). The ICN promotes international associations of nurses and improves nursing practice standards while seeking higher status for nurses. The Council provides nurses with an international power base.

The National League for Nursing (NLN) is a non-professional nursing organization. Nurses on any level, and even non-nurses, can join this organization,

as can nursing agencies. The organization's main function is to promote the improved development of nursing services and education in nursing. In Canada, the Canadian Association of University Schools of Nursing and the Canadian Association of Practical and Nursing Assistants perform similar functions.

The National Student Nurses Association (NSNA) is the pre-professional organization for student nurses in the United States. The Canadian University Student Nurses' Association (CUSNA) is the pre-professional organization for student nurses in Canada. Membership to both organizations requires that students be enrolled in a state-approved nursing education program.

Other organizations include the American Academy of Nurses (AAN), whose purpose is to recognize nurses who have made major contributions to the profession of nursing. The international honor society, Sigma Theta Tau, is a member of the Association of College Honor Societies. Students in the baccalaureate, master's, doctoral, and postdoctoral programs are eligible to be selected as members.

BOX 1–2

STANDARDS FOR NURSING PRACTICE REGISTERED NURSES ASSOCIATION OF BRITISH COLUMBIA

1. Responsibility and Accountability: Maintains standards of nursing practice and professional behavior determined by RNABC and the practice setting.
2. Specialized Body of Knowledge: Bases practice on nursing science and on related content from other sciences and humanities.
3. Competent Application of Knowledge: Determines client status and responses to actual and potential health problems, plans interventions, performs planned interventions, and evaluates client outcomes.
4. Code of Ethics: Adheres to the ethical standards of the nursing profession.
5. Provision of Service to the Public: Provides nursing services and collaborates with other members of the health care team in providing health care services.
6. Self-Regulation: Assumes primary responsibility for maintaining competence and fitness to practice and acquiring evidence-based knowledge and skills for professional nursing.

Registered Nurses Association of British Columbia (1998) Standards for Nursing Practice in British Columbia. Vancouver, B.C.: author pub. no. 128. Reprint with permission from the Canadian Nurses Association. Http://www.rnabc.bc.ca/standard/standind.htm

Specialty nursing organizations in the United States and Canada support specialty practice and often provide certification in their areas (Box 1–4). These organizations focus on specific areas of nursing practice such as oncology nursing. They strive to improve the standard of practice and welfare of nurses in that specialty area.

The National Federation for Specialty Nursing Organizations (NFSNO) represents the largest number of registered nurses practicing in the United States. The organization's goal is to promote excellence in specialty nursing practice. Approximately 39 organizations are members. Each organization is represented by two leaders, plus representatives from the ANA and NLN.

Professional Nursing Roles

In the past, nursing's role consisted of providing care and comfort to clients and performing specific nursing functions. The role of modern nursing has expanded to include a heightened emphasis on illness prevention, health promotion, and concern for the holistic client. Today's nurse functions in approximately eight

inter-related roles: caregiver, advocate, critical thinker, teacher, communicator, manager, researcher, and rehabilitator.

CAREGIVER. The nurse addresses the client's holistic health care needs to promote health and the healing process. In the role of the caregiver, nurses provide treatment for specific disease processes and apply measures to restore the emotional and social well-being of clients.

ADVOCATE. The nurse protects the client by preventing physical and/or chemical injury. In the role of **client advocate,** the nurse assists clients in expressing their rights whenever necessary. The client advocate role requires the nurse to preserve the clients' legal and human rights. Chapters 2 and 3 discuss the legal and ethical contexts of nursing practice.

CRITICAL THINKER. Decision-making and critical thinking skills are used by nurses in conjunction with the nursing process. Prior to the actual provision of care delivery, the nurse plans the best method of care delivery for each client. Look at Chapter 7 for more information on critical thinking and clinical judgment.

TEACHER. The nurse provides clients and family members with information about health, treatment/therapy, and lifestyle changes. As a teacher, the nurse determines if the client understands the information presented and reinforces the learning as necessary. The nurse then evaluates the client's progress. The nurse uses client teaching methods that are compatible with the client's knowledge, education, and literacy levels. For more in-depth information, refer to Chapter 16.

COMMUNICATOR. Open and consistent communication is vital for effective nursing. In order to provide care, rehabilitation, client teaching, comfort, and protection, the nurse must possess excellent communication skills.

MANAGER. Nurses are responsible for the management and coordination of client care. All nurses must have good management skills, whether they supervise others in the provision of nursing care or whether they provide direct care (Fig. 1–6). In Chapter 17 you will learn more about the role of the nurse as manager.

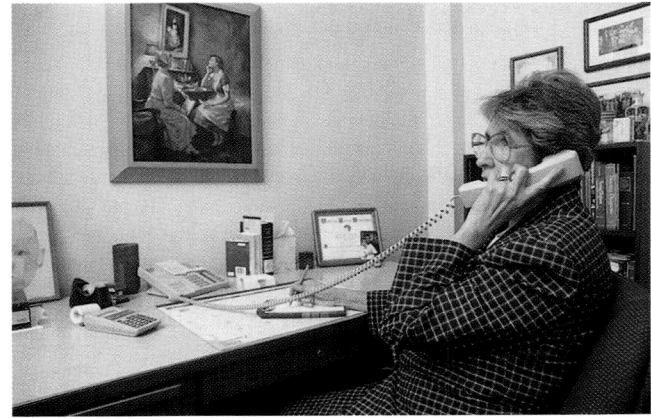

Figure 1–6. Whether a nurse serves as a nurse-manager or as a manager of assistive personnel, management skills are essential.

AMERICAN NURSES' ASSOCIATION CERTIFICATIONS

Generalist Certification

Requirements: RN licensure in United States; effective January 1, 1999, BSN; current clinical practice in specialty; authorized designation RN,C.

General Nursing Practice
Medical-Surgical Nurse (plus continuing education in medical-surgical nursing)
Gerontologic Nurse (plus continuing education in gerontological nursing)
Pediatric Nurse (plus continuing education in pediatric nursing)
Perinatal Nurse (plus continuing education in applicable specialty)
College Health Nurse (plus continuing education in applicable specialty)
School Nurse
Community Health Nurse (plus continuing education in applicable specialty)
Psychiatric–Mental Health Nurse (plus access to clinical consultation, letter of reference, continuing education in applicable specialty)
Nursing Continuing Education/Staff Development (plus BSN)
Home Health Nurse (plus continuing education in applicable specialty)
Cardiac Rehabilitation Nurse (plus advanced Cardiac life support [ACLS] certified, continuing education in cardiac rehabilitation)
Nursing Continuing Education/Staff Development (plus continuing education or academic credit)

Nurse Practitioner Certification

Requirements: RN license in United States; effective 1998, master's degree in nursing; authorized designation RN, CS.

Adult Nurse Practitioner (plus educational preparation as ANP)

Acute Care Nurse Practitioner (plus educational preparation as ACNP)
Family Nurse Practitioner (plus educational preparation as FNP)
School Nurse Practitioner (plus educational preparation as SNP)
Pediatric Nurse Practitioner (plus educational preparation as PNP)
Gerontologic Nurse Practitioner (plus educational preparation as GNP)

Clinical Specialist Certification

Requirements: RN license in United States; effective 1991, master's degree in area of specialty; current clinical practice; authorized designation RNCS.

Clinical Specialist in Gerontologic Nursing
Clinical Specialist in Medical-Surgical Nursing
Clinical Specialist in Community Health Nursing
Clinical Specialist in Adult Psychiatric & Mental Health Nursing (plus consultation/supervision)
Clinical Specialist in Child and Adolescent, Psychiatric & Mental Health Nursing (plus consultation/supervision)
Clinical Specialist in Home Health

Nursing Administration Certification

Requirements: RN license in United States; BS degree; effective 1996, continuing education in nursing administration or master's degree in nursing administration.

Nursing Administration (plus current experience as nurse manager or executive (applicable continuing education or academic credit); authorized designation RN, CNA)
Nursing Administration, Advanced (plus MS degree; effective 1996, continuing education in nursing administration or master's degree in nursing administration; current experience as nurse executive; authorized designation RN, CNAA)

American Nurses' Credentialing Center. (1999). Certification catalog. Washington, D.C.: Author.
Informatics www.nursingworld.org/ancc

RESEARCHER. Nursing research provides the evolving body of knowledge and theory for our profession. Research nurses may be employed in an academic area, community agency, or independent professional agency. The nurse researcher usually conducts studies and investigates problems to improve nursing care. A graduate degree in nursing is usually the minimum educational requirement, although many nurse generalists participate in research. Chapter 18 discusses research as a tool for nursing practice.

REHABILITATOR. Ensuring that a client returns to a maximal state of functioning requires rehabilitative activities administered by nursing along with other disciplines, such as physical therapy. When clients experience alterations in health, the nurse's role is to promote client adaptation and coping.

Nursing and the Health Care Delivery System

In the United States, the health care delivery system is one of the nation's largest industries. The health care delivery system is a complicated social organization, a unique, interdependent system that provides health care for individuals, families, and groups. Health care providers in this system are professionals or para-

BOX 1–4

EXAMPLES OF SPECIALTY ORGANIZATION CERTIFICATIONS*

American Association of Critical Care Nurses (AACN)
  Certified Critical Care Nurse (CCRN)
American Association of Occupational Health Nurses
  (AAOHN)
  Certified Occupational Health Nurse (COHN)
American Association of Nurse Anesthetists (AANA)
  Certified Registered Nurse Anesthetist (CRNA)
American College of Nurse Midwives (ACNM)
  Certified Nurse Midwife (CNM)
American Society of Post-Anesthesia Nurses
  Certified Post-Anesthesia Nurse (CPAN)
Association of Operating Room Nurses (AORN)
  Certified Nurse Operating Room (CNOR)
Association for Practitioners in Infection Control (APIC)
  Certified in Infection Control (CIC)
Association of Rehabilitation Nurses (ARN)
  Certified Rehabilitation Registered Nurse (CRRN)
Emergency Nurses' Association (ENA)
  Certified Emergency Nurse (CEN)
International Association for Enterostomal Therapy
  (AET)
  Certified Enterostomal Therapy Nurse (CETN)

National Association of Pediatric Nurse Associates/
  Practitioners (NAPNAP)
  Certified Pediatric Nurse Practitioner (CPNP)
National Association of School Nurses (NASN)
  Certified School Nurse (CSN)
Oncology Nursing Society (ONS)
  Oncology Certified Nurse (OCN)
The Organization for Obstetric, Gynecologic, & Neona-
  tal Nurses (NAACOG)
  Reproductive Nurse Certified (RNC):
    Ambulatory Women's Health Care
    High-Risk Obstetric Nurse
    Inpatient Obstetric Nurse
    Low-Risk Neonatal Nurse
    Maternal Newborn Nurse
    Neonatal Intensive Care Nurse
    Reproductive Endocrinology/Infertility Nurse
  Neonatal Nurse Practitioner (NP)
  Ob/Gyn Nurse Practitioner (NP)
  Women's Health Care Nurse Practitioner (NP)

*Certificates may be awarded by closely related, but separate and independent, organizations.

professionals with special instruction in health care delivery.

In the recent past, the most common setting for nursing in health care delivery was the acute care hospital. Even today in the United States and Canada, the highest percentage of nurses are employed in hospitals. But today's health care delivery system comprises many other entities such as clinics, practice associations, schools, industries, long-term care facilities, military facilities, independent practitioners' offices, and home health agencies. It is estimated that by 2020, approximately 75% of nurses will be working in the community.

Individuals who receive nursing care are often referred to as consumers, patients, or clients. This is largely determined by the health care setting. A consumer is an individual, group, or community that uses a service. Thus, anyone using health care services or products becomes a health care consumer. A patient is an individual who is waiting to receive or is undergoing care and medical treatment. A client is an individual who employs the services of another qualified to provide the desired service. More information on health care delivery systems is in Chapter 5.

Social Issues Affecting Nursing

Technological advances, demographic changes, and various social movements are current challenges fac-

ing nursing as we enter the 21st century. Ever since World War II, technological advances in equipment, drugs, testing procedures, and treatment modalities have affected health care delivery. Nursing has integrated these technological advances while still focusing on client needs. Nursing has also increasingly assumed the role of helping clients to accept the use of technology in their care.

Demographic changes, such as the population's increasing life span and the growing incidence of chronic long-term illness, have affected health care delivery. In the United States in 1996, the number of people between the ages of 65 and 74 exceeded 18.7 million and the number of elderly persons over the age of 75 exceeded 15.2 million. This increasing elder population, totaling 33.9 million, was mainly a result of effective health promotion and disease prevention techniques. However, although elderly people are living longer, many over 65 have multiple-system medical problems and one or more chronic illnesses. Therefore, geriatric nursing and home health care have become increasingly important nursing specialties.

Since the 1960s, society has scrutinized goods and services of health care. The initial consumer movement in health care sought to address the dehumanization of health care services. More recently, consumer groups have demanded controls on spiraling health care costs. This has prompted diversification in the financing of health care, such as health maintenance organizations and new types of health insurance. Additionally, health care consumers are now more aware of the "client rights," such as the right to information. Nurses also continue to support their clients' rights by acting as a client advocate. Finally, consumers are focusing increasingly on health promotion and illness prevention. Nursing has responded by developing nursing curricula, community programs, specialized health promotion, and preventive teaching for all clients in these two areas.

The women's movement has greatly influenced society. Female clients have assumed more responsibility for their own care. Also, women's health issues are receiving more attention and more research than even a decade ago. The movement has also influenced nursing by inspiring nurses to pursue more autonomy and accountability in their clients' care.

The human rights movement is changing society's attitude toward people who are not representative of the dominant culture or who have special health care needs. Nurses recognize and respond to these clients' special needs by providing holistic care. In addition, advocates lobby for legislation to ensure that all clients receive quality care without sacrificing autonomy, dignity, or other basic human rights.

Nursing's Political Agenda

Politics have always permeated the health care delivery system and the profession of nursing. Today nurses are involved in politics within the work environment, professional nursing organizations, and community as well as at the government level.

In the 1960s, women involved in the feminist movement believed that anyone could utilize personal experience to understand and become involved in the bigger political picture and issues. The personalization of the political process has become a fundamental principle of professional nursing.

Before the 1970s, nurses were not organized. Therefore, they had very little influence on legislation involving health care (Doheny, Cook, & Stopper, 1987). The development of nursing's formalized political action and the establishment of the Nurses Coalition for Action in Politics (N-CAP) in 1974 as a political arm of the ANA changed that. The ANA now has a political action committee, ANA-PAC, which endorses candidates who have exhibited voting records and demonstrated leadership consistent with ANA's political agenda. Endorsement by a group that represents 1.7 million potential voters is important to any candidate; however, nursing's political message is not always heard as one voice. The major nursing associations have formed a special Tri-council to present a united front so that nursing will carry more political weight and have a louder voice.

Until recent years, nurses lacked the political education needed to advance in politics (Mason & Talbott, 1985). Nursing curricula now support nurses' involvement in politics. Professional nursing organizations are also encouraging political involvement. Lobbyists have been employed by many professional nursing organizations to persuade Congress and state legislatures to increase the quality of health care and to address state and federal nursing issues. Nurses are being elected into political offices.

Nursing in the 21st Century

For the nursing graduate, the future holds numerous social, technological, and political changes. The coming changes will shape nursing into a stronger and more efficacious profession. That is, if nursing prepares itself for predicted future trends.

Technology will continue to develop rapidly. Nursing informatics will revolutionize nursing (Fig. 1–7). The front-line clinician will be required to access new information systems and store, retrieve, and interpret client care data. In the future, the Internet will allow nurses to be a part of a global network of people (researchers, families, nurses, and people with disease) all sharing new health information. Nurses will also help consumers to access the information they need and provide them with the knowledge to use it.

Other technological advances, such as genetic engineering, new imaging devices, medical artificial intelligence techniques such as computer-assisted surgery, and new techniques for electrocardiogenic and fetal monitoring, will have a large impact on nursing. Finding a balance between the use of advanced technology and the human needs of our clients is going to continue to cause conflict for nurses. The meshing of "high-touch" with "high-tech" is going to become more of a necessity in the future.

As we enter the 21st century, societies are moving toward globalization. There will be an increased sharing of products, attitudes, and stocks. Third world countries will undergo developmental growth and contribute enormously to the global market (Chitty, 1993). There will be a blending of many cultural lifestyles. Social changes throughout the world will modify the profession of nursing.

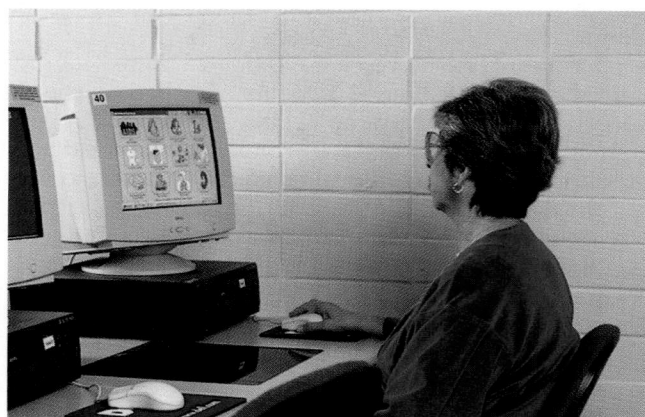

Figure 1–7. In the 21st century, nursing informatics will revolutionize nursing, and computer skills will be essential to nurses at every level of practice.

Clients will make increasingly independent choices about the kind of health care and type of setting they desire. They may choose conventional or alternative healing techniques, such as homeopathy, neuropathy, therapeutic touch, reflexology, Qigong, acupressure, aromatherapy, kinesiology combined with nutritional therapy, physiotherapy, and/or ayurvedic medicine (Sibbald, 1995).

In the future, Western medicine will not have the power it now holds. Physicians will no longer be viewed as "knowing all there is to know" (Fagin, 1992). Sibbald (1995) and other experts on nursing and health care also predict the following:

- Neighborhoods will employ nurses who will work out of 24-hour nurse-managed clinics.
- Nurse practitioners will cross over medical thresholds to provide services usually provided by physicians. This has already happened in Ontario, Canada.
- Nurse therapists and nurse entrepreneurs will provide numerous services for clients and their families.
- Rather than working for one hospital, nurses will be employed by a "service" made up of several institutions.
- Future hospital stays will be exceedingly short and early discharge will become even more important.
- Future nurses will be strong and autonomous practitioners whose practice and care delivery focuses much more on health than illness.

Of course, all of these predictions will greatly influence nursing education and care delivery. Therefore, as a new nurse, you will have the opportunity to cross a threshold into this exciting and rewarding world of nursing. You will become responsible for the future direction of the nursing profession. Your mission, along with that of all future American and Canadian nurses, is to draw strength from your nursing heritage and to unite using your numbers, education, and practice-based research to achieve the very best future together.

KEY PRINCIPLES

- Nursing is an accountable profession guided by science, theory, a code of ethics, and the art of care and comfort to treat human responses to health and illness. Nursing practice puts the science and art of nursing into action.
- The early history of nursing was heavily influenced by religion and by war.
- Florence Nightingale is considered the founder of modern nursing. Because Nightingale made rounds carrying an oil lamp, she became known as "The Lady with the lamp." This became her trademark and remains the symbol of the nursing profession worldwide.
- There are currently four types of educational pro-

grams that prepare students for entry into practice of professional registered nursing. They are the diploma program, associate degree program, baccalaureate degree program, and graduate degree entry programs.
- Graduate nursing programs improve nursing through advancement of theory and science by preparing nurses, clinicians, practitioners, educators, researchers, and administrators.
- Continuing professional education promotes quality and competency in nurses in order for them to provide continued quality of life for the public.
- A registered nurse license is granted after the candidate completes an accredited program of nursing and satisfactorily completes a national licensing examination (NCLEX).
- Nurses function in a variety of roles that are not mutually exclusive but often occur together and clarify the nurse's activities with clients.
- Nursing's professional and nonprofessional organizations and associations fulfill essential functions for the profession as well as for the individual nurse.
- Developments such as alternative methods of health care delivery, the escalating impact of health care costs, and efforts toward health care reform have led to a more politically active and aware nurse.
- By studying nursing history, you are better able to understand the importance of nursing issues such as autonomy, unity within the profession, education, and current practice and can then promote further growth of the profession.

BIBLIOGRAPHY

American Nurses' Association. (1995). *Nursing's social policy statement.* Washington, D.C.: Author.
*American Nurses' Association. (1987). *The scope of nursing practice.* Kansas City, MO: Author.
*Becker, B., & Fender, D. (1978). *Vocational and personal adjustments in practical nursing.* St. Louis: Mosby.
*Bullough, V., & Bullough, B. (1978). *The care of the sick: The emergence of modern nursing.* New York: Prodist.
*Canadian Nurses Association. (1987). *A definition of nursing practice.* Ottawa: Author.
*Carnegie, M.E. (1986). *The path we tread: Blacks in nursing. 1854–1984.* Philadelphia: J.B. Lippincott.
*Chitty, K.K. (1993). *Professional nursing: Concepts and challenges.* Philadelphia: W.B. Saunders.
*Cohen, L.B. (1984). Florence Nightingale. *Scientific American, 250*(128), 137.
Conway-Welch, C. (1996). Who is tomorrow's nurse and where will tomorrow's nurse be educated? *Nursing and Health Care: Perspectives on Community, 17,* 286–290.
*Dock, H.K., & Stewart, I.M. (1925). *A short history of nursing* (3rd ed.). New York: G.P. Putnam & Sons.
*Doheny, M., Cook, C., & Stopper, C. (1987). *The discipline of nursing: An introduction* (2nd ed.). Norwalk, CT: Appleton & Lange.
*Donahue, M.P. (1985). *Nursing: The finest art, an illustrated history.* St. Louis: C.V. Mosby.

*Asterisk indicates a classic or definitive work on this subject.

*Fagin, C. (1992). The myth of superdoc blocks health care reform. *Nursing & Health Care, 13*(10), 542.

Hamilton, P.M. (1996). *Realities of contemporary nursing* (2nd ed.). Menlo Park, CA: Addison-Wesley.

*Jamieson, E.M., Sewall, M.F., & Gjertson, L.S. (1959). *Trends in nursing history.* (5th ed.). Philadelphia: W.B. Saunders.

*Jensen, D., Spaulding, J., & Cody, E. (1955). *History and trends of professional nursing* (4th ed.). St. Louis: C.V. Mosby.

*Kalisch, P., & Kalisch, B.J. (1986). *The advantage of American nursing* (2nd ed.). Boston: Little, Brown.

Kelly, L. (1981). *Dimensions of professional nursing* (4th ed.). New York: Macmillan.

*Levey, S., & Loomba, N.P. (1984). *Health care administration: A managerial perspective.* Philadelphia: J.B. Lippincott.

Mason, D.J., & Talbott, S.W. (1985). *Political action handbook for nurses.* Menlo Park, CA: Addison-Wesley Publishing Inc.

*Merton, R.K. (1958). The function of the professional organization. *American Journal of Nursing, 58,* 50–54.

*Miraldo, P.S. (1991). The nineties: A decade in search of meaning. *Nursing and Health Care,11*(l), 221.

*Molde, S., & Diers, D. (1986). Nurse practitioner research: Selected literature review and research agenda. *Nursing Research, 34*(6), 362.

*Montag, M. (1951). *The education of nursing technicians.* New York: Putnam.

*National League for Nursing. (1990). *Nursing in America: A history of social reform* (videotape). New York: Author.

National League for Nursing Center for Research on Nursing Education and Community Health. (1996). *Nursing Datasource, 1996: Trends in Contemporary Nursing Education* (Vol. I). New York: Author.

*Nightingale, F. (1860). *Notes on nursing: What it is, and what it is not.* London: Harrison. Reprinted in F.L.A. Bishop & S. Goldie (1962). *A bio-bibliography of Florence Nightingale.* London: Dawsons of Pall Mall.

*Phaneuf, M.C. & Lang, M. (1985). *Issues in professional nursing practice: Standards of nursing practice.* Kansas City, MO: Author.

*Roy, C., & Obloy, S.M. (1978). The practitioner movement: Toward a science of nursing. *American Journal of Nursing, 79,* 1698.

Raab, D.M. (1986). *Nursing in Canada: Perseverance in practice.* Health Care.

*Schraeder, B.D. (1988). Entry-level graduate education in nursing: Master of science programs. *Perspectives in Nursing 1987–1989.* New York: Author.

*Selevan, L. C. (1984). Nurses in american history: The revolution. In *Pages from nursing history: A collection of original articles from the pages of Nursing Outlook, the American Journal of Nursing and Nursing Research.* New York: American Journal of Nursing.

Sibbald, B. (1995). 2020 vision of nursing. *The Canadian Nurse, 91*(3), 33–36.

*Smith, F.T. (1984). Florence Nightingale: Early feminist. In *Pages from nursing history: A collection of original articles from the pages of Nursing Outlook, the American Journal of Nursing and Nursing Research.* New York: American Journal of Nursing.

*Woodham-Smith, C. (1951). *Florence Nightingale.* New York: McGraw-Hill.

2

The Legal Context of Practice

Lenore L. Boris

Key Terms

accreditation
advance directive
assault
battery
certification
civil law
common law
confidentiality
contract
credentialing
criminal law
defamation
defendant
false imprisonment
fraud
informed consent

invasion of privacy
law
liability
license
malpractice
negligence
plaintiff
private law
procedural law
professional misconduct
public law
registration
statutory law
substantive law
tort

LEARNING OBJECTIVES

After studying this chapter, you should be able to:

1. Discuss various sources and types of law that directly or indirectly affect nursing practice.
2. Describe four organizations or mechanisms that influence the professional regulation of nursing practice.
3. Discuss a variety of legal regulations that influence nursing practice.
4. Discuss client rights and their influence on nursing practice.
5. Describe two initiatives to improve the quality of nursing care delivered to clients.
6. Summarize actions that can be taken to safeguard one's own nursing practice.

A clear understanding of the responsibilities and obligations imposed by law is essential to the safe, effective practice of professional nursing. As you start your pursuit of a career in nursing, legal directives dictate the educational and entry requirements that you must fulfill before you can practice. Likewise, laws define various roles within nursing, including the licensed practical nurse, the registered professional nurse, the nurse anesthetist, the nurse midwife, and the nurse practitioner. Laws also regulate reimbursement for these services.

Also found within the law are guidelines for the practice of professional nursing and sanctions that can be imposed when nursing practice fails to meet minimum standards. Finally, the basis for lawsuits involving your professional practice are found within the law. Understanding the legal context of your practice of professional nursing is essential to providing safe, efficient, and comprehensive care to your clients. This chapter is a broad overview of the legal and professional guidelines that will influence your practice of nursing.

CONCEPTS OF LAW

Law is a body of rules of action or conduct prescribed by a "controlling authority," in this case the government. In establishing the United States government, the founders created different branches of government and granted them the power to create "rules of action or conduct." These rules or laws govern many of the interactions between individual persons, between people and the government, between people and businesses, between one business and another business, and between one government and another government.

The founding fathers further delineated that certain levels of government should have primary rule over certain types of interactions. The federal government, for example, retains the power to control interstate commerce. This type of law affects the way a large health care organization with sites in several states operates its business. State governments have among their powers the ability to issue licenses to professionals, such as nurses. Understanding the powers granted to the various levels of government enables you to understand and appreciate many of the debates and changes occurring in health care.

There is a specific hierarchy of power within the levels of government, with the federal government having the highest authority. This means that local law cannot contradict or be inconsistent with state law, and state law must be congruent with federal law.

Sources of Law

Four sources of law exist at both the state and the federal level. These sources relate to the branches of government (Fig. 2–1). Laws arising from each of these sources come into being through a distinct process unique to the source. Understanding the source of a

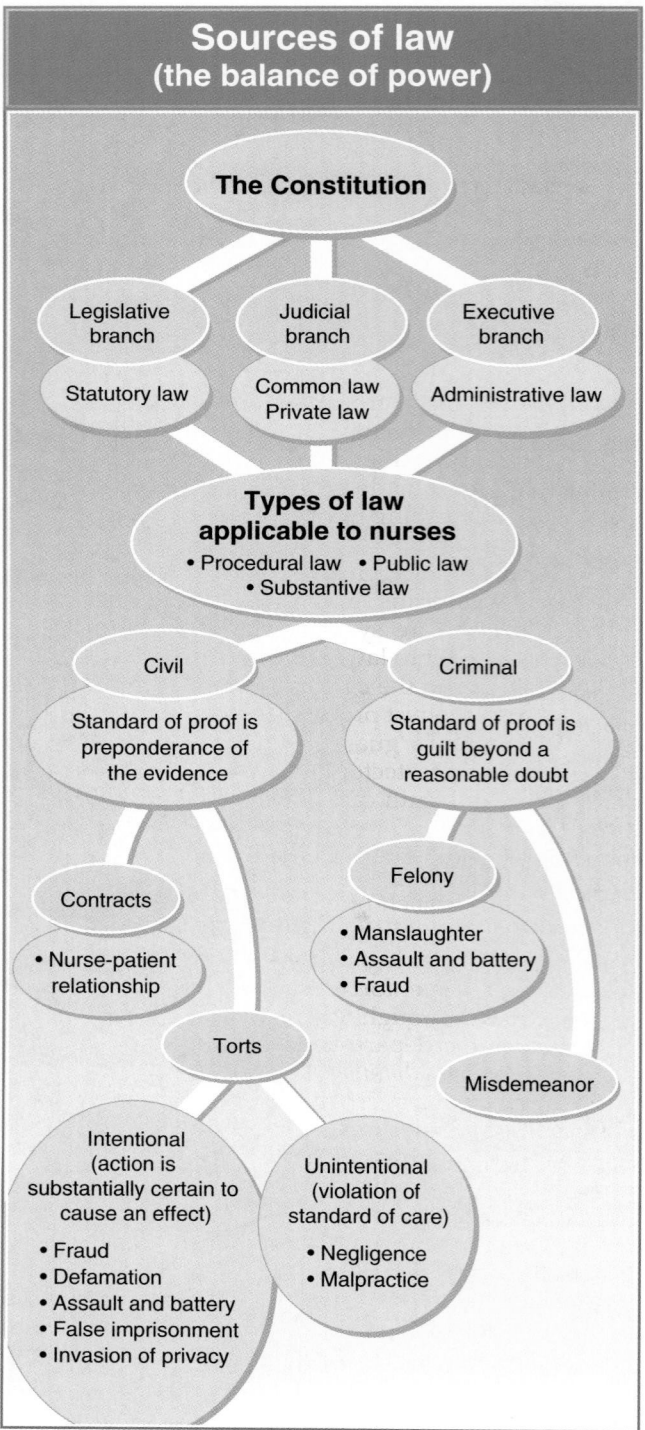

Figure 2–1. Sources of law for nursing practice.

law provides insight into the appropriate process needed to create a new law or to modify or eliminate an existing law.

Constitution

In addition to establishing and outlining the limits of power of different levels of government, the federal and state constitutions grant broad individual rights and responsibilities. Some of the rights particularly pertinent to nursing practice are the rights of privacy, freedom of speech, and due process. The right of privacy is embodied in your obligation to maintain client confidentiality. Freedom of speech relates to a professional registered nurse's right and obligation to share information with clients. Due process gives protection to individuals and guides execution of disciplinary proceedings.

Legislative Branch

The legislative branch of government is an elected body of people who are chosen to represent the interests of their constituents. The legislatures at both the state and the federal level meet and debate proposals to create laws on a wide range of issues. The proposals may have far-reaching implications and represent major shifts in policy.

For example, the perceived need to improve health care for all Americans resulted in proposals to create a national health care system. Although this proposal was not enacted into law, the debate highlighted some of the problems in the current system and, in some instances, more modest proposals were enacted into law. For example, laws guaranteeing hospital stays after childbirth or a mastectomy resulted from the legislative debate on health care.

Executive Branch

The executive branch of government has the dual responsibility of establishing the details of laws enacted by state or federal legislatures (called **statutory law**) and ensuring the enforcement of laws. The executive branch works through various administrative agencies, such as the departments of health, housing, and education, using *administrative law.*

Administrative agencies, whether state or federal, are empowered to establish administrative rules and regulations through specific hearings and rule-making procedures. The resulting rules and regulations conform with enacted law and provide the detail necessary to implement them. For example, statutory laws establish the profession of nursing. State boards of nursing provide the rules and regulations detailing how the profession of nursing will be practiced in each state. These rules and regulations are enforceable as law.

Judicial Branch

The judicial branch of government is responsible for resolving disputes and interpreting all types of laws. The accumulated judicial decisions have created a body of law known as judicial, case, decisional, or common law. **Common law** includes standards and rules applicable to our interactions with one another that are recognized, affirmed, and enforced through judicial decisions.

This court-made law is based on the principle of *stare decisis,* or "let the decision stand." The court's de-cision becomes the rule (law) to follow for subsequent cases involving similar facts. The prior court decision will be applied less rigorously or even not at all if it can be shown that the subsequent case is dissimilar and, therefore, that the law should not apply. With regard to nursing practice, most laws in the areas of negligence and malpractice are judicial.

Types of Law

Laws differ in the topics they address, the procedures used to resolve disputes, and the remedies that are available. For example, a crime such as murder is litigated using criminal procedure. It allows for imprisonment as a possible remedy. A case of defamation is litigated according to the rules of civil procedure. It usually involves a monetary remedy.

The types of law include civil law, criminal law, common law, private law, procedural law, public law, statutory law, and substantive law. These categories are not mutually exclusive, nor is this listing necessarily the only way that various types of laws can be categorized. All types of laws touch on the practice of professional nursing in some way.

Civil Law

Civil law regulates disputes between individuals or individuals and groups. The source of much of civil law is judicial or common law. Civil law involves laws relating to contracts, ownership of property, and other laws. The commonality is that a monetary award is provided for damages or as compensation when injury is caused by another.

TORTS

A **tort** is a civil wrong committed by one person against another person or that person's property. It may be intentional or unintentional. With intentional tort, the injury suffered by the victim was "intended" by the wrongdoer. Intentional torts include fraud, defamation, false imprisonment, assault and battery, and invasion of privacy. Unintentional torts include negligence and professional malpractice.

Intentional Torts

FRAUD. Fraud is the false representation of some fact with the intention that it will be acted upon by another person. It is fraud for a nurse to falsely represent oneself to a client as being certified in a specialty area of nursing. It is fraud to include false statements about past employment on an employment application for the purpose of deceiving the potential employer. It is fraud to include on a resume false information about academic credentials or professional activities as a method to gain employment.

DEFAMATION. Defamation is either a false communication or a careless disregard for the truth that results in damage to someone's reputation. Defamation can take two forms: libel and slander. *Libel* is defamation that occurs through printing, writing, or use of pictures. A nurse who makes false statements about a client or coworkers in the client's record or the local newspaper could be guilty of libel. *Slander* is defamation by the spoken word by either making false statements or making legally unprotected statements damaging to a reputation. An example of slander is telling a client that another nurse is incompetent.

ASSAULT AND BATTERY. Assault is an attempt or threat to touch another person unjustly. **Battery** is the actual willful touching of another person that may or may not cause harm. The terms assault and battery are distinct but are often heard together because an assault precedes a battery. A nurse who threatens a client with an injection or urinary catheterization could be found guilty of an assault. For a nurse to be guilty of battery, the touching must be wrong in some way, such as being done without permission, or done in a way that causes harm or embarrassment. The nurse who proceeds with an injection despite a client's objection could be guilty of battery.

FALSE IMPRISONMENT. False imprisonment involves restraining a person, with or without force, against that person's wishes. Detaining clients against their wishes so they cannot leave a health care facility could be false imprisonment. A different analysis must be applied to clients suffering from diseases that affect judgment, such as Alzheimer's, before determining that a nurse's action constituted false imprisonment.

A less obvious example of false imprisonment is the use of restraints in managing clients. The appropriate use of restraints relates not only to false imprisonment but also to the issue of maintaining client rights and dignity. Concerns about the inappropriate use of restraints have been so great that some states have issued guidelines for their use. These guidelines require a thorough assessment of the client to determine the least restrictive measures to safely accomplish the goal for which restraints are being considered.

If a client or legal representative gives permission for the restraint, there is no liability for false imprisonment. You should carefully document in the client's record the circumstances resulting in permission to restrain and undertake an ongoing assessment of the necessity for continued restraint.

INVASION OF PRIVACY. Invasion of privacy can occur when the client's private affairs are unreasonably intruded upon by the nurse. Soliciting information not required for the client's care and discussing client information with persons not entitled to that information (such as employers or estranged spouses) are two examples of nursing actions that could be interpreted as invasion of privacy. Much information is acquired about a client in the course of providing nursing care. You must exercise prudence in using and sharing this information to protect the client's right to privacy.

Other acts could constitute invasion of privacy and expose you to liability as well. They include unnecessarily exposing a client during transportation between departments in a health facility, failing to ensure the anonymity of clients involved in research projects, or

sharing information about social or rehabilitative services that your client is receiving.

In the course of providing care to clients, photographs are sometimes obtained. You may be eager to share at a professional meeting photographs of an interesting wound or other medical condition. Photographs with clients prominently featured may be used to advertise the opening of a new health care facility. Without permission from the client, photographs featuring clients used for these and other purposes can be deemed an invasion of privacy. Similarly, observing a procedure done to a client is an invasion of privacy if consent has not been obtained.

Unintentional Torts

NEGLIGENCE. Negligence occurs when harm or injury is caused by an act of either omission or commission by a layperson. Negligence can also result from failure to use the kind of care a reasonably prudent person would use in a similar situation. Examples include not locking the brakes on a wheelchair before transferring a client or leaving a baby on an examining table without taking steps to keep him from falling.

Another definition of negligence is failure to do what a person exercising ordinary prudence would have done under similar circumstances. Failing to take the temperature of a client who complains of feeling warm and lethargic is an example of this type of negligence.

MALPRACTICE. Malpractice describes acts of negligence by a professional person as compared to the actions of another professional person in similar circumstances. The difference between negligence and malpractice is significant. Remember that, with negligence, the nurse is judged against what an ordinary, reasonable layperson would do or not do in similar circumstances.

To prove liability for negligence or malpractice, each of four elements must be proven: duty, breach of duty, causation, and damages. *Duty* involves the obligation of the nurse to use due care; that is, to exercise the kind of care a reasonably prudent nurse would use. The kind of care appropriate for a particular client is defined by standards of care. *Breach of duty* is the failure to meet the standard of care. *Causation* is demonstrated when the failure to meet the standard of care results in harm to the client. Finally, for liability to be established, the client must have suffered an actual harm or injury, called *damages*. Table 2–1 provides examples of the elements of liability.

The standard of care is derived from both professional and legal regulation of nursing practice and the employer's expectations for nursing practice. Together these sources outline the kind of care a reasonably prudent nurse would provide for a particular type of client in a particular setting. Compare the following two nurses:

- Nurse A works in a high school. This nurse's practice is guided by, among other things, the nurse practice act, standards developed by the National

TABLE 2–1
Elements of Liability

Element	Example
Duty	The nurse is responsible for accurate assessment and timely reporting of changes in a client's condition.
Breach of Duty	The nurse fails to note that a client's thumb is warm to touch, red, swollen, and painful.
Causation	Failure to note the signs and symptoms of an infection leads to amputation of the thumb.
Damage	Loss of the thumb seriously limits the client's use of his hand.

TABLE 2–2
Areas of Potential Liability for Nurses

	Examples
Failure to Monitor and Assess	• Failure to recognize significant changes in a client's condition. • Failure to report significant changes in a client's condition. • Failure to obtain a complete database. • Failure to monitor a client as indicated by the client's condition.
Failure to Ensure Safety	• Inadequate monitoring of a client. • Improper use of restrictive devices. • Failure to identify a client's risk for injury. • Inappropriate use of equipment.
Medication Errors	• Failure to question medication orders that are unclear. • Failure to adhere to established procedures in medication administration. • Failure to recognize adverse drug reactions. • Lack of familiarity with medication. • Lack of communication in verbal or written medication orders.
Improper Implementation of Skills or Procedures	• Failure to maintain currency in clinical skills. • Failure to adhere to proper techniques. • Failure to follow agency policy. • Performance of unfamiliar skills. • Failure to initiate appropriate actions based on assessment.
Documentation Errors	• Failure to document nursing actions. • Failure to document information relevant to a client's condition. • Failure to document in accordance with agency policies.

Association of School Nurses, Inc., and the school nurse job description. When a high school student sustains a serious injury during football practice, the position requires giving first aid, calling an ambulance, and sending the client to the nearest emergency room.

• Nurse B works in an emergency room. This nurse's practice is also guided by the Nurse Practice Act and the employer's job description. However, the teenager brought from the high school now needs definitive care. Nurse B will provide that care in accordance with standards established by the Emergency Nurses Association.

Liability can ensue for almost any activity involved in the practice of nursing. Further, no practice setting is exempt from potential malpractice litigation. However, there are areas in which allegations of malpractice against nurses occur more frequently. Some of the common areas of concern are outlined in Table 2–2.

When clients believe they have been injured as a result of a nurse's negligence or malpractice, they may start legal proceedings. The **plaintiff,** who is the party bringing a lawsuit, alleges certain facts and outcomes. The **defendant** is the person against whom a lawsuit is filed. The nurse, as defendant, must show that the plaintiff is unable to prove the four elements of negligence or malpractice liability. The procedures for malpractice litigation are complex. Nurses named in a lawsuit are always advised to seek their own legal representation even if their employer is also named as a defendant.

Settlement of the legal action can occur in one of three ways. The parties may negotiate a settlement out of court. A negotiated settlement does not necessarily mean the nurse is guilty of negligence or malpractice. However, the cost of litigation and the potential liability may suggest settlement as the best option. If there is no settlement, the case goes to court. Both plaintiff and defendant attempt to persuade the court to rule in their favor. After hearing all the facts and arguments, a decision regarding liability is made. A third possible method of settling a lawsuit in some states is to present the case to a malpractice arbitration panel.

If you are named in a lawsuit, obtain legal counsel and work closely with your attorney, who probably will want to be present at all discussions of the case, including those with representatives of your health care agency. If the agency requests information, review the request with your attorney before supplying information. Avoid discussion with the plaintiff, the plaintiff's attorney, and witnesses for the plaintiff. Do not attempt to alter or enhance the client's medical record. Rather, try to put in writing everything that you can remember about the case. Your attorney will advise you of your options in each phase of the litigation.

CONTRACTS

A **contract** is an agreement between two or more individuals that creates certain rights and obligations in exchange for goods or services. Contracts can cover many services a nurse offers, either as an employee or as an independent provider of services. Nurse entrepreneurs provide many services, including writing books, providing health teaching, consulting on breast-feeding and infant care, monitoring high-tech venous access devices, and others. A portion of contract law specifically addresses contracts concerning the sale of goods. If the nurse is purchasing goods or products for a business, this latter portion of contract law is relevant.

For a valid contract to exist, several elements must be met. The first element is the requirement for all parties to be capable of entering into a contract. *Capacity* refers to the ability to understand the nature of the contract, its effect, and the obligations incurred by entering into it. Examples of persons who lack the capacity to enter into a contract are minors, persons declared incompetent by the court, or persons with a mental illness determined by a court to render them incompetent.

The second requirement for a contract is *mutual assent.* A clear and direct offer to do something is made and communicated to another person. For example, the nurse can make a written offer to teach a health class or orally offer to provide home care. The person receiving the offer must then voluntarily communicate an acceptance of the offer. The acceptance must be communicated by the same means as that used to make the offer. If the offer was in writing then the acceptance must be in writing; a verbal offering can be accepted verbally.

The next requirement for a valid and enforceable contract is consideration. *Consideration* is a legal term that refers to giving something of value. For example, the nurse can offer a service, such as a workshop on time management for nurses employed in a long-term care facility. The nurse administrator, believing this workshop is a valuable method to enhance the management skills of the nurses, agrees to provide monetary compensation.

A final requirement that must be met is that no defenses exist that could void the agreement. The kinds of defenses that could void a contract are fraud, misrepresentation, illegality, or duress. For example, a nurse could represent herself as an experienced labor-and-delivery nurse and offer to be a woman's personal labor coach for a fee. The contract could be voided if it can be shown the nurse misrepresented that clinical expertise.

Contracts come in many forms; they can be oral or written, implied or express. Whatever the form of a contract, questions can and often do arise concerning whether the parties entered into a legally enforceable contract. The obligations incurred under a contract have value for each party. Hence, if the question arises as to whether there actually was a contract, the answer has serious consequences for both parties.

Additional questions can arise even if there is a valid and enforceable contract in place. *Can the contract be assigned?* Assignment means that one of the parties gives their rights under a contract to another party. For example, instead of receiving payment for services, the nurse could request that the money be donated to a charity. *Can the contract be delegated?* Delegation transfers the duty or obligation under the contract to another person. For example, the nurse may agree to teach a cardiopulmonary resuscitation class but, in the event of illness, can delegate the responsibility to another nurse. Assignment or delegation can be limited by the terms of the contract.

Disagreements can occur in the course of fulfilling the terms of the contract. Attempts are made to use language in a contract so the contract as accurately as possible reflects the intended agreement of the parties. Nevertheless, disputes over interpretation do occur. A number of rules to interpret contract language have developed. For example, the words in a contract will be given their "ordinary meaning." Custom and usage in the particular business and location carry a great deal of weight in determining the contract's meaning.

Finally, legal disputes can occur when one party or the other fails to perform their obligations under the contract. A breach of contract results from a partial or total failure to fulfill one's obligations. When a breach occurs, the nonbreaching party is entitled to damages. Remedies for a breach can include monetary payment or specific performance, which is a court-imposed requirement to perform as originally agreed.

Contract law directly or indirectly influences your practice of nursing. As nurses create new businesses, they are increasingly involved in situations that are governed by contract law. Contract law (and employment law) also governs the relationship between a nurse and an employer. A nurse who breaches contractual obligations faces monetary penalties or loss of employment, but usually is not at risk of losing the license to practice nursing.

Criminal Law

Criminal law defines specific behaviors determined to be inappropriate in the orderly functioning of society. A crime is an act that violates the duties we owe to the community. Generally, our duties are created by statutory law. Examples of criminal acts include larceny, homicide, manslaughter, rape, burglary, kidnapping, and arson.

Punishment for a criminal offense varies with the severity of the crime. Punishment may consist of a fine, probation, imprisonment, or death. A felony is a crime of a serious nature that is likely to be punished by imprisonment or death. A misdemeanor is a crime of a minor nature; it may be punished by a fine, a short prison term, or both.

Some actions that a nurse may take are clearly criminal matters. One example is failure to comply with the mandates of the Controlled Substance Act by engaging in activities such as diverting narcotics for personal use or selling narcotics diverted from clients.

Other nursing actions that are potentially criminal in nature include participating in active euthanasia, bombing an abortion clinic, or disconnecting a life support system. There has even been a recent case of alleged nursing malpractice that was considered so grievous as to warrant criminal charges.

The number of criminal actions that nurses have been involved in are quite small. When they do occur, these cases are monitored closely to determine their impact on the practice of nursing. More frequently, nurses are involved in civil lawsuits.

Common Law

As stated earlier, common law comprises standards and rules applicable to our interactions with one another that are recognized, affirmed, and enforced through judicial decisions. Whether the specific action of a nurse was negligent or constituted malpractice is often determined in court, based on the principles established in prior judicial decisions.

Private Law

Private law controls the relationships between private individuals or private organizations. Examples of private law include torts and contracts.

Procedural Law

Procedural law establishes the manner of proceeding used to enforce a specific legal right or obtain redress. A nurse who is threatened with the potential loss of nursing license for professional misconduct relies on procedural law to ensure a fair hearing. The procedural laws related to civil, criminal, and administrative actions vary in detail and can be quite complex. A nurse facing any kind of legal action will find that procedural laws direct the course of the legal action. However, a nurse who relies on procedural law without the benefit of legal representation is at a disadvantage in any legal action.

Public Law

Public law regulates the relationship of individuals to government agencies and may be administrative, constitutional, or statutory. The defining characteristic is that the law is applicable to a whole group of people. An example of a public law is the requirement that everyone working in a health care setting, including nurses, be tested annually for tuberculosis.

Statutory Law

Statutory law is law enacted by the state or federal legislative branch of government. An example of a federal statutory law relevant to nursing practice is the Americans with Disabilities Act (ADA). To illustrate, a nurse who becomes permanently disabled is protected from employer discrimination because of passage of the ADA. Examples of relevant statutory laws at the state level include nurse practice acts and child or elder abuse reporting laws.

Substantive Law

Substantive law is the part of law that actually stipulates one's rights and duties, in contrast to procedural law, which guides enforcement of one's rights. Substantive law includes the law of contracts, law of real estate, law of torts, law of inheritance, and other types of law. Your obligations as a professional nurse are created by substantive law. To illustrate, your obligation to assess clients and report changes in their status is a matter of substantive law.

Understanding the Law

All levels of government work together to provide the legal framework for the safe practice of professional nursing. However, laws related to the practice of nursing are not permanently fixed. Changes affecting the profession of nursing and its practitioners can and do occur (Fig. 2–2). As a prudent nurse, you must familiarize yourself on an ongoing basis with the legal changes that affect your practice.

As our health care system and medical technology undergo dramatic change, questions arise in the practice of nursing about whether specific situations or tasks are safe and "legal." *Is it legal to staff a 40-bed unit with only one registered nurse (RN) or to have a staffing ratio of one RN per four intensive-care-unit clients? Is it legal for an RN to insert fetal scalp electrodes or to discontinue central lines?* Many people believe that the law provides specific answers to these and hundreds of other questions. But in many instances, the law is subject to interpretation. It is uncomfortable and potentially illegal to practice in the "gray areas" of nursing. Be aware that administrative agencies offer opinions about the intent and interpretation of rules and regulations, and professional nursing organizations often attempt to clarify practice issues. Ultimately, an interpretation may be provided by the courts when a specific ques-

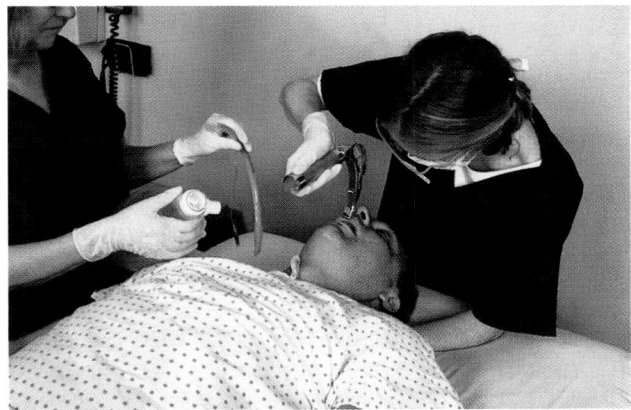

Figure 2–2. As professional practice changes, questions arise about the legal guidelines for practice.

tion is litigated. Understanding your legal obligations and staying abreast of legal changes is the best way to safeguard your professional nursing practice.

Understanding Your Legal and Professional Obligations

Liability is the legal obligation or responsibility to provide care to a client that meets the accepted standards of care. Failure to understand your legal and professional obligations as a nurse could jeopardize your livelihood and your ability to practice as a professional nurse. Illegal practice could result in professional discipline, a civil lawsuit, a criminal lawsuit, or a disciplinary action by your employer. It is important to note that these actions are independent and, therefore, more than one can be brought against you at the same time for the same incident.

Further, a determination of "no wrongdoing" in one action does not mean that you will be cleared of wrongdoing in the other potential actions. Suppose a postpartum client complains to your employer that you did not provide all the care she believed she should have received. The client is angry enough that she decides to report you to the state agency that addresses allegations of professional misconduct. The state agency determines that your practice met the standard of care and declines to take any disciplinary action against you. Meanwhile, your employer, concerned that this is the second time it has received complaints about your nursing care, suspends you from work for 2 days.

All potential legal actions determine the extent to which you meet or fail to meet your legal and professional nursing responsibilities. However, the procedures used to execute each legal action, the possible outcomes, and the law on which the action is based vary. You should be aware that professional discipline, civil or criminal lawsuits, and employer sanctions all represent threats to your license and must be addressed appropriately.

PROFESSIONAL REGULATION OF NURSING PRACTICE

To practice nursing in a safe, efficient, competent manner, you must understand both the legal regulation of nursing practice and the voluntary professional regulation of nursing practice. There are several types and numbers of laws directing nursing practice. Nevertheless, even strict adherence to laws governing nursing practice may be insufficient to guide you in daily efforts to provide quality nursing care. Supplemental guidelines are provided voluntarily by professional nursing organizations, the Centers for Disease Control and Prevention (CDC), employer directives, and educational programs. These guidelines cannot require you to practice outside the limits established by law, but they do provide guidance for your day-to-day efforts to provide competent and legal nursing care.

Professional Nursing Organizations

The American Nurses' Association (ANA) is a professional organization for registered nurses. Registered nurses can also join any of the professional nursing organizations that represent their specialty area. Most of these organizations have established standards of practice that provide more specific guidance to the professional nurse than might be found in the law.

For example, the law may not specify that a nurse working in labor and delivery must take a fetal monitoring course. The standard of practice, however, as outlined by the Association of Women's Health, Obstetric, and Neonatal Nurses recommends a fetal monitoring course for any nurse working in labor and delivery. Although these recommendations do not carry the force of law, they are a standard used to evaluate the quality of care provided by the nurse.

Centers for Disease Control and Prevention

The CDC is a federal health agency of the U.S. Public Health Service. The CDC focuses on epidemiology, prevention, control, and treatment of communicable diseases. It offers guidance to nurses about reporting, treating, and managing communicable diseases—such as sexually transmitted diseases, tuberculosis, and acquired immunodeficiency syndrome (AIDS). Isolation procedures and other infection-control recommendations come from the CDC as well.

Employer Policies and Procedures

Employers should not ask nursing employees to function outside the scope of nursing practice as defined by law. However, employers can and do develop guidelines for the practice of nursing in a specific employment setting. Ideally, these guidelines are within the law and are consistent with established standards of practice.

An employer uses at least two methods to convey its expectations of nurses. First, the employer provides a job description to each new employee. It is important to read and understand what your employer expects of you. Although you may have expertise in starting intravenous (IV) therapy, your new community health employer may not want you to restart an IV line on your home care client. It may seem to you to be a waste of resources to ask the client to leave the home and go elsewhere to have an IV line restarted. Nevertheless, the employer is within its rights to ask you not to perform that task. If you fail to adhere to the job expectation, you may not only lose your job, but you may also be exposed to legal liability.

Employers also use written policies and procedures to convey their expectations about the way you will practice nursing. Occasionally, there is more than one safe and efficient way to perform a specific nursing task. Cost factors, staffing limitations, liability considerations, or other factors may direct an employer to require a specific method for performing a nursing

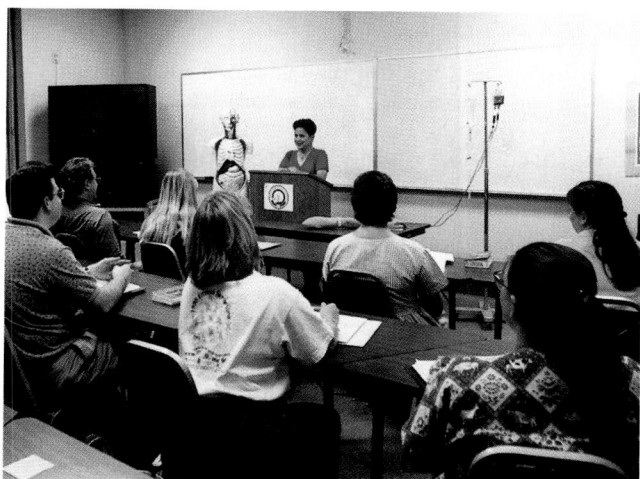

Figure 2–3. Continuing education promotes continued competence in nursing practice.

procedure. To minimize your legal liability, it is absolutely essential to be familiar with your employer's policies and procedures, function within your job description, and practice consistently within established standards.

Educational Programs

Continuing education programs, inservice programs, and professional publications are methods used within the nursing profession to ensure that you practice competently and safely as the nursing profession continues to evolve. Some states mandate continuing education; however, even without this legal requirement, you still have a professional obligation to maintain currency in your nursing practice (Fig. 2–3).

You can obtain the newest information to keep your practice current by attending educational programs, reading professional publications, and maintaining membership in professional nursing organizations. These resources may also provide you with information about legislation that could affect your practice. Evidence of your involvement or lack of involvement in efforts to keep your practice current may affect determinations of your liability in a legal action.

LEGAL REGULATION OF NURSING PRACTICE
Nurse Practice Acts

Among the powers granted to states is the ability to regulate the practice of health care providers, including registered nurses. Regulation of the health care professions serves a dual purpose. First, it protects the public by excluding uneducated or unlicensed persons from practicing in a health care profession. Second, regulation defines the nature and scope of professional practice.

Physicians were the first health care providers to lobby for state regulation of the health care professions

through licensure. The broad definition of medicine contained in legislation had a significant impact on licensure of the other health care professions. The nursing profession and others had to carefully construct practice acts that excluded responsibilities addressed in the previously adopted, well-accepted definition of medical practice. The historic dominance of medicine in defining the health care professions continues to challenge the nursing profession as nurses move into such advanced practice roles as nurse anesthetist, nurse midwife, and nurse practitioner.

Common Features of Nurse Practice Acts

Each state has a nurse practice act, which is the single most important law affecting your nursing practice. However, the definitions and descriptions of nursing contained in those nurse practice acts may differ. The lack of consensus on the definition of nursing has created problems for the nursing profession, particularly when seeking reimbursement for services. If the nursing profession cannot reach consensus on a definition of nursing, how can reimbursement be provided? What services does nursing provide that are unique and therefore should be reimbursable?

Although variations exist in the specifics of each state's nurse practice act, some topics are common. Nurse practice acts usually define terms found within the law, such as "treating" and "diagnosing." A nurse practice act defines the practice of nursing, both registered professional nursing and licensed practical nursing. Historically, some states attempted to list all the tasks registered nurses were legally allowed to perform. Such listings became very restrictive with technical advances in the practice of nursing and the shifting of tasks from the responsibility of physicians to nurses. Subsequent revisions in nursing practice acts allowed flexibility by defining nursing in terms of broad categories of services provided by nurses. These services may include assessing health responses, treating health problems, teaching on health-related topics, and providing supportive care. A nurse practice act also delineates the rules and regulations that govern nursing practice for the licensed practical nurse, nurse practitioner, nurse anesthetist, and nurse midwife.

Often, the relationship of professional nursing to some of the other health care providers is outlined in a nurse practice act. Nurses typically are obligated to implement medical regimens prescribed by physicians and dentists. The care nurses provide to clients independent of a physician's order must be consistent with the treatments ordered by the physician. There is variation from state to state about whether nurses can or must execute the orders of physician assistants, nurse practitioners, respiratory therapists, physical therapists, or other health professionals.

A nurse practice act establishes the requirements for obtaining a license to practice nursing. Completion of a basic educational program is a necessity. A passing score on the NCLEX examination is also required. Sometimes additional requirements, such as good moral character or a minimum age, must be met for licensure in a particular state.

Another common feature of a nurse practice act is the creation of a state board for nursing. The state board is created to assist in matters related to professional licensing and conduct. The specific functions and composition of a state board of nursing vary somewhat from state to state, but a board must comply with the provisions of the nurse practice act that created it. A board does have power to create rules and regulations (administrative law) to execute its responsibilities. It can also modify these rules as the need arises.

Professional Misconduct

Finally, a nurse practice act defines **professional misconduct,** which is a violation of the act that can result in disciplinary action against a nurse. In some states, the actual language for professional misconduct, disciplinary proceedings, curricula, and other topics pertaining to the profession of nursing are not found specifically in the practice act but may be found in education law or health law. These other laws may be referenced in the practice act and always work in concert to create the legal context for professional practice. Unprofessional conduct in the practice of nursing covers a wide array of areas. Some actions viewed as professional misconduct are outlined in Box 2–1. Many states provide a nursing handbook to applicants for nursing licensure that contains the nurse practice act and other relevant law.

BOX 2–1

EXAMPLES OF PROFESSIONAL MISCONDUCT

- Exercising undue influence on the client.
- Moral unfitness.
- Revealing personal information without the client's prior consent.
- Practicing beyond the scope permitted by law.
- Delegating professional responsibilities to a person not qualified to perform them.
- Abandoning or neglecting a client.
- Harassing, abusing, or intimidating a client physically or verbally.
- Failing to maintain a record reflecting evaluation and treatment of a client.
- Failing to exercise appropriate supervision over persons who can only practice under supervision of a licensed professional.
- Guaranteeing satisfaction or cure from the performance of professional services.
- Failing to wear an identification badge.
- Failing to use scientifically accepted infection control techniques.

Disciplinary Actions

Disciplinary actions for professional misconduct are part of administrative procedure. A specific state agency, such as the Board of Nursing, Office of Professional Discipline, or Office of Regulation of the Professions is designated to review and manage allegations of professional misconduct. The state agency investigates the allegation, prosecutes or settles a disciplinary proceeding, and enforces the penalty imposed. The disciplinary proceeding may involve a hearing before an administrative officer if a settlement cannot be reached.

Penalties that a state agency can impose range from relatively mild to quite severe, and they may be temporary or permanent. The state agency can find that allegations are unfounded and take no action. An administrative warning may be issued to resolve a violation involving a minor or technical matter. The most serious penalty is revocation of the nursing license.

Other possible penalties include censure and reprimand, a fine not to exceed a specified dollar amount, a requirement to perform community service, a requirement to complete a specified course of education or training, and an annulment of registration or license. Suspension of license is another penalty that can be imposed. A total suspension can be given for a specified period of time, or until a course of therapy or treatment is completed. A partial suspension is also possible. This means that you could work in nursing, except for the area or task (giving medications, for example) to which the suspension applies. The suspension could last until successful completion of a course of retraining.

Penalties for professional misconduct can have a significant impact on your ability to practice nursing. However, because this type of action is an administrative proceeding and not a lawsuit, nurses sometimes fail to recognize the seriousness of the proceeding, and therefore do not seek legal representation. Any potential disciplinary action must be viewed very seriously. At the first notice that you are under investigation, you should seek legal representation.

Control of the Profession of Nursing

Credentialing refers to the methods by which the nursing profession attempts to ensure and maintain the competency of its practitioners. The nursing profession uses several methods of credentialing, including accreditation, licensure, and certification. These efforts are designed to assure the public that only those persons who have met specified requirements provide nursing care.

Accreditation

Accreditation is a process that monitors an educational program's ability to meet predetermined standards for students' outcomes. The accreditation process examines program length, teaching methods, course objectives, clinical sites, and numerous other factors related to the structure, functioning, and stated outcomes of the educational program. A determination is then made as to whether the educational program meets the minimum standards for basic nursing education. The goals of accreditation include maintaining minimal educational standards and fostering the continuous improvement of nursing educational programs.

Accreditation can be granted by a government agency, such as the state board of nursing, or by a voluntary organization, such as the National League for Nursing (NLN). As a legal requirement, all nursing education programs are accredited by the state. Accreditation by a voluntary organization is often truly voluntary, but may be required by a state for the school to maintain state accreditation.

Although it is not the only organization empowered to accredit nursing education programs, the NLN has been the major program-accrediting body. In recent years, questions have arisen about NLN's ability to adequately monitor nursing education programs. Proposals have been advanced to divest NLN of its role in accrediting programs. Alternative proposals would limit NLN to accreditation of certain educational programs (associate degree programs, for example) and to offer accreditation to baccalaureate programs through another voluntary organization, such as the Commission on Collegiate Nursing Education. Changes in the accrediting body could lead to some dramatic changes in the educational preparation of professional nurses because there would be different accrediting agencies for associate degree programs, diploma programs, and baccalaureate programs.

Licensure

A **license** grants the owner formal permission from a constituted authority to practice a particular profession. The power to grant licenses to professional health care providers is reserved for the state. The state requires the applicant to meet certain criteria to be granted a license, which indicates to the public that this person has met minimal competency standards, thus protecting the public's health and safety. For nurses, licensure requirements vary somewhat from state to state but commonly include educational preparation, passage of the NCLEX examination, good moral character, application, and payment of registration fees.

A major exception to the requirement that you must have a license to practice nursing exists for nursing students. Students enrolled in a recognized, accredited educational program do not need to be licensed to practice nursing, provided such practice is part of the clinical and academic requirements of the educational program and occurs under the supervision and guidance of nursing faculty. Nursing students employed in health care settings in unlicensed roles as aides, client care technicians, and other posi-

tions must be cautioned to avoid applying newly acquired skills belonging solely to the domain of licensed professionals. Legal protection is not available to nursing students practicing nursing outside of their educational programs.

From a historical perspective, someone who wanted to practice nursing in the early 1900s needed only to "register" with the state agency having oversight for nursing. These so-called *permissive* licensure acts allowed the individual to use the initials RN after her name if she registered with the state. Without registration, the person could still practice nursing but could not present herself as an RN. The permissive licensing acts lacked definitions of the scope of nursing practice.

Over time, states have replaced permissive licensing acts with *mandatory* licensing acts. Mandatory licensing acts define the practice of nursing and the requirements for licensure. In practical terms, the difference between permissive and mandatory licensure is moot. All states now have mandatory licensing acts.

States still do require licensed professional nurses to register. **Registration** is a process by which an applicant provides specific information to the state agency administering the nursing registration process. Information may include current address and telephone number, proof of continuing education, testimonies that no legal actions have been taken against the nurse, and other information. After the initial licensing and registration of the professional nurse, registration renewal may be required every 2 to 4 years. In addition to paying a registration fee, you may need to prove the completion of specific coursework (such as an infection-control update) for a particular type of registration.

In some jurisdictions, the terms licensure and registration are synonymous. Technically, however, the terms have different meanings. Licensure is a grant to an individual to practice the profession of nursing. Registration is a method of making sure that the state agency has the most current information about a person to whom they have granted a license. Even in a state that recognizes the distinction between licensure and registration, nurses cannot practice without both a license and a current registration.

With the numerous and dramatic recent changes in the health care delivery system, several current and evolving concerns about nursing licensure have developed. While these issues may seem theoretical and outside the influence of the beginning practitioner, potential changes in nursing licensure may at some point affect your nursing career. You have a professional obligation to be aware of issues involving your nursing license, and thus your livelihood.

An ongoing concern within professional nursing is the concept of institutional licensure for nursing. Currently, the state issues a license to practice nursing to an individual. The boundaries of your professional practice are determined by the state. In effect, you agree to practice nursing according to the rules set forth by the state. As an outcome of this arrangement, you have flexibility to change employers with only minor variations in your professional obligations as a nurse.

In an effort to control the cost, quality, and productivity of the work force, health care institutions have proposed changes in nurse practice acts that, in effect, give them control of nurse licensure. The proposals come in various disguises. Basically, the health care institution would be the gatekeeper, deciding who is qualified to practice nursing within that institution. The institution could review the credentials of the applicant for a nursing position and determine suitability to practice "nursing." Or the institution could provide the education, thus creating a "nurse" tailor-made to the practice setting of the institution. In any event, the individual nurse stands to lose employment mobility, leverage for pay and benefits, and control over individual practice. By decentralizing the practice of nursing, institutional licensure would seriously undermine the collective action of professional nurses to control the defining standards for the professional practice of nursing.

Another ongoing issue in professional nursing is the legal protection of the term "nurse." Licensure of professional registered nurses originally arose to protect the unwary public from uneducated persons seeking employment as nurses. The terms "licensed" or "registered" are used to notify the public that these nurses have met minimal educational and licensing requirements. In some states, however, the term "nurse" is not restricted to persons who have met the educational and licensing requirements of nursing. Thus, someone can advertise and gain employment as a nurse without the appropriate education and credentials. Employers recognize the distinction between a "nurse," a "licensed practical nurse," and a "registered professional nurse." But families seeking a nurse to provide home care to an ailing relative may not be as sophisticated in their understanding of the profession of nursing. They could thus hire someone ill-equipped to provide safe and competent nursing care.

A third licensing issue within the profession of nursing is agreement on the requirements for licensure of persons functioning as nurse practitioners. Nurse practitioners work mainly in primary care settings providing assessment, teaching, and care to a given client population. It can be argued that nurse practitioners are not performing any functions that fall outside the scope of practice of a registered professional nurse and, therefore, do not need a separate license. Yet many nurse practitioners believe that a separate license is needed, particularly if they are prescribing medications. States have approached the licensing of nurse practitioners differently. Educational requirements, licensing, and scope of practice vary among the states. Future efforts may focus on bringing uniformity to these issues.

The dramatic changes in the health care delivery system and the creation of new roles for nurses have created a new licensing concern. Many managed care organizations operate in more than one state. As a case manager or telephone "advice-nurse" for such an organization, you could find yourself working with clients in states other than the one in which you are licensed. If you are considered to be providing professional services to clients in other states, the potential exists that you could be charged with practicing in that state without a license.

Certification

Although not required by law, nurses often seek certification to receive recognition for their expertise in a particular area of nursing. **Certification** is a voluntary process by which a nurse can be granted recognition for meeting certain criteria established by a nongovernment association. A nurse can become certified in many areas of nursing, including geriatrics, pediatrics, emergency nursing, community health nursing, school nursing, maternal-child health, and even such newly identified specialty areas as forensic nursing. Certification is offered through the ANA and many specialty nursing organizations. Requirements vary but typically include specific educational preparation, experience in the specialty area, evidence of continuing education, and successful completion of a certification examination.

In some states, certification can have a second meaning. In New York, for example, certificates are issued to registered professional nurses to reflect their academic preparation as a nurse practitioner. The specific requirements for education and experience to be certified as nurse practitioner are outlined in the law. This legal requirement for certification is entirely different from the certification offered by the professional nursing organizations.

There is a lack of agreement within the nursing profession about the benefits of voluntary or legal certification. Proponents of certification believe it identifies nursing expertise and is analogous to physician board certification. This formalized recognition of nursing expertise could be used to leverage higher salaries. Nurses who have questioned the benefits of certification point out the lack of agreement on what certification means in nursing. Further, certification may be splintering the profession without creating the anticipated economic advantage.

Other Laws Affecting Nursing Practice

Several laws not directly focused on the practice of nursing have a significant impact on the way you must practice nursing. These laws apply not only to nurses but to all health care providers regardless of setting. The Occupational Safety and Health Act, the Controlled Substance Acts, the Health Care Quality Improvement Act, the Americans with Disabilities Act, and Good Samaritan Laws are some of the laws that significantly affect the practice of nursing.

Occupational Safety and Health Act

The Occupational Safety and Health Act of 1970, known as OSHA, established legal standards that define safe and healthful working conditions. The law continues to be periodically updated and expanded. OSHA affects you as a nurse in two ways. First, the law sets standards for the working conditions of nurses as well as other workers. Second, some of the requirements of the law dictate how you manage clients.

OSHA protects you from unsafe or harmful working conditions. For example, OSHA directs the manner in which potentially toxic or flammable chemicals are handled. The use and care of electrical equipment is another area OSHA regulates.

The same OSHA requirements that protect you also protect your clients. For example, OSHA provides standards for the management of contaminated equipment and supplies and the types of isolation techniques used for infectious clients. Promoting health and safety is both your professional obligation and your legal mandate.

Controlled Substance Acts

Several laws have been enacted that address standards for drug development and marketing. These laws affect the process by which new drugs become available to clients. Most significant for you is the Comprehensive Drug Abuse Prevention and Control Act of 1970. This law was enacted to regulate the distribution and use of drugs with the potential for abuse. These drugs include narcotics, depressants, stimulants, and hallucinogens. Your nursing obligations under this law include proper storage and documentation of controlled substances. Failure to meet the requirements of this law are grounds for charges of professional misconduct and potential criminal action against you.

Health Care Quality Improvement Act

One of the difficult issues in attempting to protect the public from unsafe and incompetent health care providers has been tracking information related to adverse licensure actions, malpractice payments, and adverse professional actions. The Health Care Quality Improvement Act of 1986 was created to collect data about unsafe and incompetent practitioners. The law, which does apply to nurses, has limited the ability of health care practitioners who had adverse action taken against them in one state from moving to another state without disclosing their previous performance.

Americans With Disabilities Act

The Americans with Disabilities Act, known as the ADA, passed in 1990, was enacted to protect persons with disabilities from discrimination in such areas as housing, employment, education, and health services. A broad definition of "disability" is included in the Act and includes protection of persons with AIDS or infected with the human immunodeficiency virus (HIV) and persons recovering from drug or alcohol addiction. Many of your clients may be disabled. Consequently, if you work, particularly in an outpatient or community health setting, you may be assisting your clients to assert their rights under this law.

Good Samaritan Laws

Because of your education and experience as a nurse, you may feel a special obligation to provide aid to people in emergency situations. In most states, there is no legal requirement for any person, including a health care provider, to provide assistance at the scene of an emergency. You (just as any other person) could choose to help or to leave the scene. However, a few states have enacted legislation requiring a person trained in health care to stop and aid the injured. It is important for you to know whether your state is one that requires you to provide aid in an emergency. Even without a legal obligation, you may feel an ethical obligation to assist in such circumstances (Fig. 2–4).

Inevitably, the question arises as to your potential exposure for legal liability if you render care at the scene of an accident. To encourage health care providers to assist in emergency situations and to protect providers who do offer care in these circumstances from legal liability, most states have passed "Good Samaritan Laws." Specific laws differ among states, but all Good Samaritan laws offer some protection from the fear of a lawsuit when giving emergency care.

The accident victim may not be able to consent to care, which is a requirement in nonemergency situations. Without such consent, and with the limitations of the situation at hand, you are expected to give the kind of help a reasonably prudent person with your background would give in a similar circumstance. Good Samaritan laws do not provide you with absolute immunity from legal liability. If the care you provide can be shown to be grossly negligent, you could still face liability.

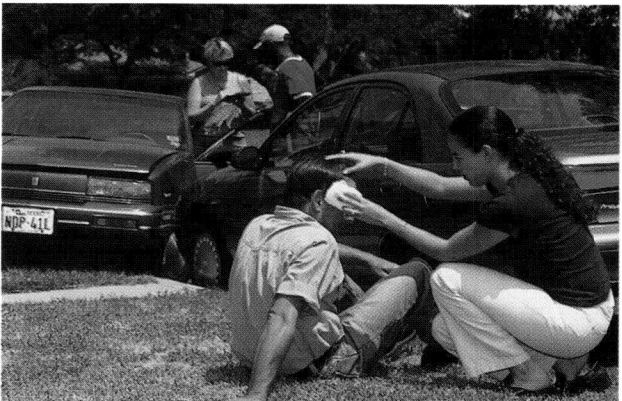

Figure 2–4. Good Samaritan laws offer some protection from legal liability for health care workers who stop to offer assistance at the scene of an accident.

Employment Law

Employment law governs employment practices and encompasses such areas as at-will employment, personal employment contracts, and collective bargaining. It also influences when and how employment may be terminated.

Most nurses work as employees rather than as independent contractors or nurse entrepreneurs. An employee is a person who works for someone else in return for a salary or wages. The agreement to work with the promise of being paid is a contract for hire and can be express or implied, oral or written. The employer has the power to control the details of the work. The employer's expectations as to what work is to be done and in what manner are usually found in the job description and the employer's policies and procedures.

In contrast, an independent contractor agrees to provide a specific service for a fee. The independent contractor has control over the details of providing the service. The employer's control is limited to establishing the end product of the contractor's work. For example, a home care agency can hire a nurse as an independent contractor to monitor any of its clients who have total parenteral nutrition. The independent contractor decides in what order to visit clients, what time of day to see them, and other details of monitoring this particular group of clients. Services must be provided consistent with standards of practice and with the agreement reached with the employer. The contract with the employer may specify details of providing the service; for example, clients must be seen no less than once a day. But the independent contractor can decide that the employer's conditions are not acceptable and refuse to provide services for that particular home care agency.

Nurses who establish a health-related business may find themselves in the position of employer. If they are the sole employee of their business, their activities will be covered by the contracts they develop with their clients. However, if they employ other people in their business, their concerns about employment law will be from the perspective of an employer. The rights and obligations as an employer are covered in a variety of laws, including the Fair Labor Standards Act, Workers' Compensation Laws, the National Labor Relations Act, and other employment-related laws.

Although most nurses still work as employees of hospitals, an increasing number work in community health, ambulatory care, long-term care, and other health care delivery settings. As an employee, you can theoretically have a personal employment contract with an employer, but the number of nurses who do is low. About 10% of registered professional nurses are covered by *collective bargaining agreements,* which are contracts between an employer and a union representing the nurses. Most nurses are at-will employees.

At-Will Employment

The at-will employment doctrine allows both the employer and the employee to terminate the employment relationship at any time and for any reason. Under this doctrine, your employer could terminate you without notice regardless of the length of time you have been employed or the quality of your work, and you would have no legal recourse. Conversely, you could end employment at any time without giving the employer notice. Professional considerations may compel you to give notice of termination, but under the at-will doctrine there is no obligation to do so.

Several exceptions to the at-will doctrine exist. These exceptions are important because they are the basis for a nurse's or an employer's challenge to the discontinuation of the employment relationship. A termination of employment based on discrimination (due to age, gender, or religion, for example) is one exception to the at-will doctrine. Some states have modified the at-will doctrine to permit termination only for "just cause." Another exception is when an implied contract of employment exists. In some cases, courts have decided employer's publications, such as an employee handbook or standard operating policies, have created implied contracts of employment.

The at-will doctrine is not absolute. If you do not have an individual contract and are terminated, you may find one of the numerous exceptions to the doctrine applies to your situation. You could bring a lawsuit challenging your termination as wrongful or retaliatory.

Personal Employment Contracts

Typically, nurse executives, nursing faculty, nurse anesthetists, nurse midwives, and nurse practitioners have individual employment contracts. The contract is between the nurse and the employer. Position responsibilities, terms and conditions of employment, fringe benefits, and other aspects of the employment relationship may be covered in the contract. The contract is a negotiated agreement between the nurse and the employer. The failure of either party to fulfill the duties and obligations of the contract would constitute a breach of contract. The nonbreaching party would be able to seek redress through the courts.

Collective Bargaining

In an employment setting covered by a collective bargaining agreement, the union represents the interests of some or all of the employees of the health care agency. The bargaining unit—that is, the employees represented by the union—may include only registered nurses or it may include other health care professionals (licensed practical nurses, nurse's aides, and other workers in the facility). Excluded from the bargaining unit are persons in management positions within the agency.

The employer and union are obligated to negotiate and reach agreement on the terms and conditions of employment for the bargaining unit members. Terms and conditions of employment cover a broad range of topics that are considered mandatory subjects of bargaining. The terms and conditions include pay and benefits, such as vacations, holidays, health insurance, sick leave, personal leave, and rules pertaining to such issues as lunch breaks, coffee breaks, absenteeism, tardiness, dress codes, overtime work, and safety.

Mandatory subjects of bargaining are not the only conditions of employment that can be negotiated. However, nonmandatory topics can only be negotiated if there is agreement to do so. Examples of nonmandatory subjects include codes of ethics, installation of time clocks, and employee evaluation systems.

The union is the collective voice of members of the bargaining unit and negotiates the collective bargaining agreement. During the life of the agreement, the union provides other services to its members as well. Representation at grievance proceedings and labor-management meetings are major functions of most unions. Unions also track legislation affecting employees, health care issues, and professional practice issues. They lobby legislators to ensure passage of legislation favorable to union membership. Unions also offer such membership benefits as life and disability insurance, discount travel, driver safety training, and discount entertainment tickets.

In exchange for its services, a union collects dues from members. Dues can represent a percentage of an employee's salary or a flat dollar amount. Dues amounts are also sometimes linked to the number of hours an employee works. An employee who opposes the political involvement of the union can pay a fee to the union that excludes that portion of dues earmarked for political activity.

The process of organizing and seeking representation by a union is a lengthy process outlined in labor law. Organizing activity is protected by law, so theoretically nurses seeking to organize for collective bargaining should not face retaliatory action from the employer.

Nurses' opinions vary about the value of collective bargaining. Sometimes nurses cite ethical or moral considerations for opposing union representation of professional nursing. Other nurses believe the clout of a union will ensure that employers hear nursing concerns about client issues and quality nursing care. Nurses are employees and have been granted by law the right to organize collectively for union representation just like other workers. The decision to become organized and be active in a union is an individual choice that should be made after acquiring an understanding of collective bargaining and weighing the benefits and disadvantages of representation (Fig. 2–5).

Employer Actions

As an at-will employee or an employee covered by a collective bargaining agreement, you face three kinds of threats to your livelihood and continued practice of nursing. The first threat involves the employer's right

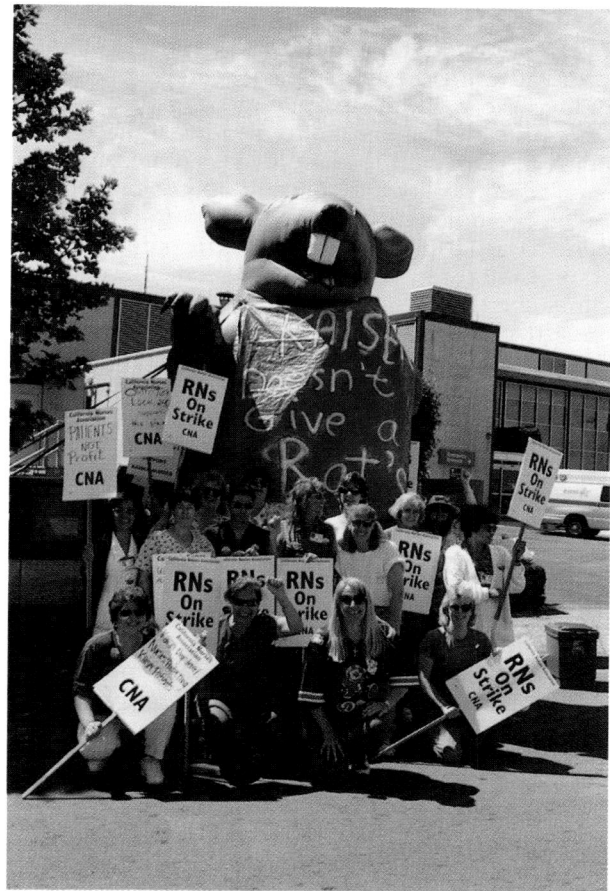

Figure 2–5. The unionization of nurses has both benefits and disadvantages. (Courtesy of David Bacon, Berkeley, CA.)

to terminate your employment. The second involves obligations your employer may have for reporting you to the state agency that handles allegations of professional misconduct. Finally, your employer may be required to provide information damaging to your career during litigation of a lawsuit brought against you.

An employer can terminate your employment for reasons unrelated to your professional practice of nursing. Employment issues common to any employee also affect nurses. Excessive absences or tardiness, failure to notify your employer when you will be absent, poor customer service skills, and poor personal hygiene are the types of issues employers regard as legitimate grounds for termination. Termination for these reasons can occur even if your practice of nursing is flawless.

Employers also terminate nurses for reasons more closely related to the practice of nursing. A nurse who is unable to perform to the employer's expectations as outlined in the job description can face termination. Frequent client complaints, questionable clinical skills, substandard documentation, and failure to master skills needed for that clinical area are examples of grounds for termination. These deficiencies can be justifiable cause for termination of employment, even though they may not result in any client harm.

Usually, an employer does not terminate an employee without first going through a process of notifying and advising the employee of action needed by the employee to continue employment. The process of progressive discipline is addressed in a collective bargaining agreement if the employee is represented by a union. Even without a collective bargaining obligation, most employers have a policy of progressive discipline as a means of avoiding a wrongful discharge lawsuit brought by a disgruntled former employee.

In some instances, nursing practice that is so substandard or results in client harm obligates an employer to report the nurse to the state agency that investigates allegations of professional misconduct. Specific state statutes vary, but allegations of client abuse, substance abuse, illegal activity, or the death of a client under certain conditions are all examples of situations that may obligate an employer to generate a report. This reporting is independent of a termination action the employer may initiate.

Similarly, you may be involved in litigation arising from your employment. The employer is also usually sued. Although the situation that caused a lawsuit occurred in the place of employment, the employer will not necessarily seek to terminate the employment relationship. However, during the course of the lawsuit, the employer may provide evidence damaging to your continuing practice as a nurse.

CLIENT RIGHTS

The health care client has specific rights that affect the relationship between the client and health care provider and between the client and the health care delivery system. These rights protect each client's ability to determine the level and type of care received. Several of these rights interface with your practice of nursing. Informed consent, advance directives, do-not-resuscitate orders, organ transplant, and client confidentiality are among the client's rights that direct, in certain instances, how you must practice nursing.

Informed Consent

Informed consent involves the legal right of a client to receive adequate and accurate information about medical condition and treatment. Such information is necessary for clients to exercise their right to select and consent to particular treatments. The presumption of the law is that all adult clients possess the decision-making capacity to make informed decisions regarding their treatment choices.

If a health care provider believes an adult client is incapable of making informed decisions, an evaluation by a specialist must take place and an opinion rendered before the client is denied the right of informed consent. When the court determines that a client is incapable of making decisions, it may appoint a personal guardian to make decisions on the client's behalf. In some states, statutes have been enacted that identify a rank order listing of whom should be consulted to make decisions. The list may begin with a spouse and continue to adult children, parents, then a brother or sister.

Minor children are viewed under the law as lacking decision-making capacity. Therefore, the parent or legal guardian provides informed consent after receiving all the required information. There are some cases in which minors are able to provide their own consent for treatment, such as for a sexually transmitted disease or when the minor is married or otherwise emancipated.

Courts have established the information to be shared with a client to obtain informed consent (Box 2–2). A physician is responsible for conveying information and obtaining informed consent for medical procedures. If you are involved in obtaining informed consent for a medical procedure, in most states you are only witnessing the signature of the client on the informed consent form. You may be the person who actually ensures that the informed consent form is signed by the client. However, you should only ask the client to sign a consent form if the physician has instructed the client and you have determined that the client reasonably understood the information. You should obtain informed consent for nursing care and procedures.

Advance Directives

An **advance directive** is a written document that provides direction for health care when a person is unable

---

BOX 2–2

INFORMED CONSENT CHECKLIST

The client has received the following information:

☐ Diagnosis.
☐ Name of procedure, test, or medication.
☐ Explanation of procedure, test, or medication.
☐ Reasons for recommending the procedure, test, or medication.
☐ Anticipated benefits.
☐ Major risks of the procedure, test, or medication.
☐ Alternative treatments.
☐ Prognosis if treatment is refused.

The nurse has performed the following duties:

☐ Assessed barriers, such as hearing impediments, transcultural factors, pain, anxiety, and other factors that could influence the client's understanding of the information.
☐ Assessed the influence of education, age, developmental level, and emotional status on the client's ability to understand the information.
☐ Ensured that information was provided in a manner that facilitated understanding.
☐ Determined that the client is voluntarily giving informed consent.

to make personal treatment choices. An advance directive allows clients to express their preferences for health care prior to an event that renders them incapable of indicating their treatment choices. Individual state laws provide for specific kinds of advance directives, including living wills and the durable power of attorney for health care.

A living will provides specific instruction about the care the person does or does not want to receive. Ideally, these preferences are discussed in advance with family and friends who may become involved in decision-making, so the person's wishes are clearly understood by all. A durable power of attorney for health care appoints an agent to make the health care decisions for the client. Again, ideally, the client will have discussed his preferences with the person he appoints as his agent.

Often, a nurse is the first health care provider to become aware that a client has executed an advance directive. Thus, it may be up to you to make sure that a copy of the advance directive becomes part of the client's record. It also may be up to you to inform the physician about the client's advance directive. In any event, you should ensure that both requirements are met.

When working with a client's significant others, it is especially important to ensure that the decision-maker is the person *legally* authorized to make the decisions. Several different family members or significant others may be voicing conflicting opinions about the client's care. Your obligation is to consult with the person legally authorized to make treatment decisions, even when this person is not obviously identifiable.

Organ Transplants

Like other treatments, clients have the right to decline organ transplant as a treatment option. Clients also have the right to determine whether they want to donate their organs and tissues for someone else's benefit at the time of death. The desire to donate organs can be expressed through a written document executed before death. In the absence of an express written directive providing an informed consent for donation, the Uniform Anatomical Gift Act would control the donation of any organ.

The Uniform Anatomical Gift Act is law in all states and provides a list of individuals who can provide informed consent for the donation of the deceased individual's organs. The persons on the list must be contacted in order, usually a spouse first, followed by adult children and parents of the deceased.

Do-Not-Resuscitate Orders

Implicit in the client's right to informed consent is a client's right to refuse treatment. In fact, clients have a right to refuse treatment even if that treatment is needed to sustain life.

Cardiopulmonary resuscitation (CPR) is one type of treatment refused by clients. Most health care agencies have developed policies to guide health care providers when clients choose not to be resuscitated. These policies should include a written order for a do-not-resuscitate (DNR) status, review of the order on a regular basis, and evidence of informed consent by the client or legal representative in requesting a DNR. Additionally, DNR and CPR must be specifically defined, so that the client continues to receive any desired treatment.

Confidentiality

Confidentiality is the client's right to privacy in the health care delivery system. As a nurse, you have an ethical obligation to maintain client confidentiality. You are party to much sensitive and private information about clients and must exercise discretion in sharing that information. Sharing information about a client with people who are not involved in the client's care, such as disclosing information about one client to other clients, is a violation of client confidentiality. Talking about a client in the hallways, cafeteria, grocery store, social club, or anywhere else with people who are not involved in the client's care is also a violation of client confidentiality. Additionally, disclosure of confidential information could expose you to liability for invasion of your client's privacy.

Even if your conversation partner is involved in caring for the client, in public places you must guard against disclosing information within earshot of others. Some nurses mistakenly think that they have not breached client confidentiality if they talk about the client without using a specific name. If sufficient information is conveyed for another person to identify the person under discussion, however, client confidentiality has indeed been violated and charges of invasion of privacy could be forthcoming.

Increasingly, clients are enrolled in health care networks that offer a range of services, including ambulatory care, hospitalization, rehabilitation services, home care services, and other health-related benefits. Ensuring the provision of care falls to case managers, discharge planners, and other care coordinators. Such planning requires access to confidential information. Additionally, third party payers and utilization review departments access confidential information to address payment issues. This information is often transmitted by electronic means to the agencies within the network. The difficulty in maintaining client confidentiality is thus compounded by a greater number of persons accessing sensitive client information and the means by which the information is shared.

Any request for client information you receive should be evaluated very carefully. Address two questions. First, does the person requesting client information have a need to know the information requested? Suppose you work in a home care agency. Client information might be shared with the agency's social worker so the social worker can help the client receive social services. However, the social worker does not necessarily need to know all the details of the client's medical care. Further, the office administrative assistant may recognize your client as a neighbor and ask you probing questions about your client's condition. The state nurse practice act, ethical considerations, and nursing standards of care require you to protect client confidentiality.

The second question to ask yourself is whether the client has authorized the release of information. When clients consent to receive services from a particular health care agency, they usually sign a consent for treatment that includes an authorization for information to be shared with people in the agency involved in the client's treatment. Beyond this, requests for information come from concerned family, friends, or employers. Requests also come from other health care providers, lawyers, insurance companies, and public news sources. Carefully consider whether the client has authorized release of information to these persons. When in doubt, consult with your supervisor.

The confidentiality of some client groups is protected by specific federal or state statutes. Persons receiving treatment for drug and alcohol abuse, mental health care, sexual assault, HIV infection, and AIDS are among the groups whose confidentiality receives additional protection under the law. If you work with clients in these categories, you should familiarize yourself with the particulars of confidentiality requirements.

QUALITY IMPROVEMENT INITIATIVES

Quality improvement initiatives are activities that health care agencies undertake to contain costs, improve quality, and increase competitiveness. Some of the costs an agency seeks to reduce are those related to legal liability arising from adverse occurrences. An adverse occurrence is a term sometimes used to describe errors in practice or the injury or death of a client. Health care agencies have used several methods to manage adverse occurrences. These include incident reports, risk management committees, quality assurance committees, safety programs, and quality improvement programs.

Risk management programs and quality improvement programs are somewhat different in focus, although both can potentially reduce legal liability. Continuous quality improvement, total quality management, and quality initiatives are programs that have proliferated in recent years in health care facilities. These programs focus on improving the quality of client care or the efficient operation of the business by examining the processes used to deliver health care services. For example, a quality improvement initiative might examine how waiting time in an outpatient clinic can be reduced.

In contrast, incident reports and risk management programs identify and analyze risks to be able to take corrective action, reducing legal liability. A risk management program might examine the excessive number of client falls at the entrance to a long-term health care facility. You may become involved in either or both types of programs.

Incident or Adverse Occurrence Reports

An incident or adverse occurrence report is a tool used by health care facilities to document situations that have caused harm or have the potential to cause harm to clients, employees, or visitors. Medication errors, client falls, and needle sticks are common situations documented on an incident report. The report is not part of the client's medical record and should not be referenced in the client's record. These reports are used to identify patterns of risk so that a corrective plan can be developed. The report also serves as a record of the facts surrounding the event should litigation arise at some point in the future.

The nurse who identified the potential or actual harm or who created the situation leading to actual or potential harm completes the incident report. The incident report identifies the people involved in the event (including witnesses), describes the event, and records the date, time, location, actions taken, and other relevant information. A physician may complete the report after examining the client, employee, or visitor if actual or potential injury occurred. Often, suggestions are solicited for how this event can be avoided in the future.

In some instances, incident reports can be used in a court of law. Documentation should be as factual as possible and avoid accusations. Questions of liability are for the court to decide and, therefore, conclusions about who is responsible for the event should be avoided in the incident report.

Risk Management Programs

Risk management programs have several components. An ongoing safety program is essential to ensure the safety of clients, employees, and visitors. Periodic inspections of electrical equipment, monthly fire drills, monitoring of the disposal of hazardous wastes, and other activities are often included in safety programs. Educational programs about potential risks help reduce accidents or injuries. Identification of known risks, such as putting up warning signs for construction or ice on the walkway, are also activities of a risk management program.

A health agency may have a designated risk manager. This person can be an invaluable resource to answer questions regarding potential risks and liabilities.

SAFEGUARDING YOUR PRACTICE

The legal threats to your continuing practice as a professional nurse are very real. Clients deserve and demand that only those persons who are able to provide safe, competent, quality care should practice nursing. Administrative procedures, lawsuits, and disciplinary practices by employers help ensure that unsafe and incompetent nurses are removed from the practice of nursing. Despite the demands and complexity of nursing, you can take steps to safeguard your nursing practice and avoid legal action against you.

Know Your Obligations and Responsibilities

The first step in safeguarding your practice is to thoroughly understand your professional and legal obligations and responsibilities. It is as important to be competent in the professional and legal aspects of your practice as it is to be technically competent. Read your state's nurse practice act. Read your job description and your employer's policies and procedures. Follow legislative bills that may affect your practice. Track court decisions that clarify the specifics of your practice and identify your potential legal exposure. Read the standards of practice that apply to your area of nursing and comply with the guidance provided. These actions are important steps in making sure that your practice conforms to the expectations inherent in your license to practice nursing.

Practice Competently

The competent practice of nursing requires you to expand on the skills and knowledge you acquired as a nursing student as your professional practice develops. You are expected to maintain competency in three domains:

- Technical competency, which involves performing skills accurately, safely, and in a manner consistent with established procedures.
- Cognitive competency, which means that you have acquired the knowledge and information you need to understand the needs of your client and implement appropriate nursing care.
- Interpersonal competency, which requires you to further develop effective communication techniques for working with professional colleagues and maintaining therapeutic relationships with clients.

Keep in mind that clients who believe their nurse is caring and respectful are less likely to sue. The combination of technical, cognitive, and interpersonal competencies applied within the legal limits of nursing practice are an effective safeguard of your nursing practice.

Know Your Strengths and Limitations

The nursing profession is characterized by endless opportunities. The number of work settings, types of clients, specific expectations of a nursing position, conditions of employment, work hours, and any number of other factors combine to create a vast array of nursing opportunities, some of which will match your temperament, skills, knowledge, and interests. The key to finding an appropriate nursing position is an accurate assessment of your professional and personal strengths and weaknesses.

No nurse can function equally effectively in all settings. A nurse accustomed to the collegiality of an institutional setting may find the independence of community health nursing unnerving. An experienced intensive care nurse may feel that work in a physician's office is not challenging enough and may overlook critical elements of practice. A nurse who is mismatched with or overwhelmed by the demands of a particular position or type of client is inviting disciplinary or legal action.

Keep Current

A license to practice nursing signifies that you have met the minimum standards for a beginning practitioner. The expectation is that you will ultimately become a master practitioner of your chosen profession. This can only occur if you acknowledge your role as lifelong learner. Action follows acknowledgment. Attending inservices, pursuing continuing education courses, reading professional publications, and attending professional meetings are evidence of your commitment to continued professional growth.

Projections made about the relevancy of the nursing information you master today suggests that much of what you know will be obsolete in 3 years. Indeed, 20 years ago, standard precautions were unheard of and gloves were worn only to keep your hands clean. At that time, AIDS, Ebola, hepatitis C, and other very serious illnesses had not yet been identified. Nursing is an evolving profession. It is incumbent upon you to keep your practice current. An outdated practice is a practice ripe for a lawsuit.

Document Your Care

Documentation of your activities while practicing nursing will not compensate for failing to render nursing care consistent with established standards of practice. However, timely, accurate, complete, and appropriate documentation of the care you give can provide evidence that you executed your professional responsibilities in accordance with your legal and professional obligations (Box 2–3). Client records are legal documents that may be entered as evidence in a lawsuit. In either a lawsuit or an insurance claim, documentation may be the factor upon which liability determinations are made.

There are many types of documentation formats. In all cases, the content of the documentation requires that you make decisions about the words you use, the relevance of information provided, the completeness of your notations, and the inclusion of certain information. Information conveyed should be an accurate, complete, objective, and relevant assessment of your client and the nursing care you provided. As in other forms of communication, however, excellent documentation takes practice.

The client record is a legal document that should provide a complete and accurate picture of the client's condition and the nursing care provided. Nurses are

---

BOX 2–3

DOCUMENTATION GUIDELINES

The following guidelines are appropriate with any documentation format.

Timing

- Never chart interventions before implementing them.
- Chart as soon after the nursing intervention as possible.
- Chart as frequently as the client's condition warrants.
- Indicate the date and time of entry.
- Indicate the time of pertinent observation or interventions.

Content

- Record facts, such as observations, client behavior, nursing actions, client response, medical visits, status of dressings, amount of drainage, vital signs.
- Use only abbreviations that are accepted by your employing agency.
- Avoid drawing conclusions, such as documenting

that the client is "noncompliant," "angry," or "upset."
- Avoid using words that carry different meanings for different people, such as "good," "bad," or "normal."
- Do not criticize other health care providers.
- Do not make excuses for failing to provide care.
- Do not make derogatory comments about the client.
- Do not reference incident reports or potential lawsuits.

Format

- Never tamper with a medical record.
- Print or write legibly.
- Do not scribble, erase, or use correcting fluid.
- Make sure each page is labeled with the client's name and identification number.
- Do not skip any lines or try to squeeze in an additional line.
- Sign your name and title with each entry.

---

sometimes reluctant to document adverse events that sometimes happen to clients. But falls, medication errors, and other adverse incidents must be documented as completely and accurately as any other information pertinent to the client's care. Document the event in a straightforward manner, including all the steps you took to respond appropriately to the situation.

Purchase Professional Liability Insurance

Despite competent or even expert nursing care, clients are not always satisfied with the outcomes of their health care experiences. Also, the responsibilities and complexities of practice in today's rapidly changing health care environment can create situations that expose you to greater legal risk. While it is virtually impossible to practice flawless nursing, the cost of an error in your practice can be a lawsuit. Increasingly, nurses are being named with the agency and the physician in a lawsuit. Although insurance coverage will not reduce the risk of being sued, at least the financial impact of a lawsuit can be minimized.

In the past, plaintiffs have named in a lawsuit those persons or institutions believed to have the most money. Thus, the hospital and physicians were typically sued, whereas nurses were overlooked because they lacked the so-called "deep pockets." Some people believe that a nurse who has individual liability insurance is more likely to be sued. Yet with the rise in nurses' salaries, the protection against being sued attributed to the "deep pockets" theory is becoming increasingly suspect.

In a variety of employment settings, you may be

told that you are covered by your employer's liability insurance and do not need to purchase individual liability insurance. Your employer's lawyers also may have an excellent record of representing their nurse employees. If you have individual insurance coverage, the approach to management of the lawsuit may differ between your insurance company and your employer. The resulting adversarial relationship between you and your employer could be detrimental to a mutually agreeable resolution of the lawsuit.

Despite these risks, however, there are several sound reasons why you should purchase your own professional liability insurance even if you are covered under an employer's insurance plan. One is to ensure that, if you are named as a defendant in a lawsuit, your best interests will be represented. An employer's first obligation is to reduce or eliminate its own liability. One way of doing that may be to shift responsibility for the incident to you by trying to demonstrate that you practiced incompetently, that you exceeded the limits of your job description, or that you did not follow agency policies and procedures. These would represent attempts to prove that you, and not the agency, should be held liable.

A second reason you should have your own professional liability insurance is to protect you when you are providing care or giving advice outside of work. An employer's insurance will cover only your professional activities while working for the employer. You may want to believe you are a nurse only while at work, but family, friends, and neighbors know otherwise. The first aid you provide at your daughter's soccer game, the health education and screening done during a health fair at the local retirement community, the advice you are asked to give to the neighbor's ailing father you meet at the grocery store, and countless other occasions may expose you to liability. You must protect yourself whether or not you are providing professional services during your employment hours.

KEY PRINCIPLES

- Laws are rules or standards of conduct. Laws are developed by the different branches of government and are statutory, administrative, or judicial, or they arise from constitutions. Governments enact and enforce laws.
- Many different types of law affect the practice of nursing. These include civil, criminal, common, private, procedural, public, statutory, and substantive law.
- Specific laws that secondarily affect the practice of nursing include the Occupational Health and Safety Act, Controlled Substance Act, Americans with Disabilities Act, and Health Care Quality Improvement Act.
- Legal liability may result from intentional torts involving assault and battery, defamation, fraud, false imprisonment, or invasion of privacy.
- Negligence and malpractice are unintentional torts. Liability is determined by proving duty, breach of duty, causation, and damages.
- Voluntary professional standards also regulate nursing practice. Standards of care and practice are developed by professional nursing organizations and organizations that accredit educational programs or institutions.
- Failure to adhere to legal and professional directives regarding the practice of nursing can result in professional discipline, legal liability, or employer disciplinary actions. A nurse may simultaneously be involved in two or more of these actions.
- Employer job descriptions, policies, and procedures direct the practice of nursing in a specific employment setting. These directives should conform to professional and legal practice guidelines.
- Nurse practice acts regulate nursing practice in a specific state and provide mechanisms for disciplinary action against nurses practicing in that state.
- The nursing profession attempts to ensure the competency of its practitioners through individual licensure and certification methods and through educational program accreditation.
- Employment law governs employment practices and encompasses areas such as at-will employment, personal employment contracts, and collective bargaining. It also influences how employment may be terminated.

- Clients have specific rights, including confidentiality, informed consent, use of advance directives, and control over decisions about organ transplant and life-sustaining measures.
- Health care agencies undertake quality improvement initiatives to contain costs, improve quality, and increase competitiveness. They try to reduce potential legal liability through the use of risk management programs and incident or adverse occurrence reporting mechanisms.
- Members of the nursing profession ensure competent and safe professional practice by reading professional publications and attending continuing education programs, professional meetings, and inservice programs.
- Legal safeguards for the nurse begin with competent practice. Additional safeguards include understanding professional responsibilities and obligations, recognizing individual strengths and limitations, keeping knowledge and skills current and accurate, documenting care appropriately, and purchasing individual professional liability insurance.

BIBLIOGRAPHY

Anderson, E.R., & Gold, J. (1996). Medical malpractice insurance: Nurses take on bigger health care role and bigger legal risks. *Journal of Nursing Law, 3,* 27–33.

Ballard, D., & Cohen, J. (1995). Confidentiality of patient records in the computer age. *Journal of Nursing Law, 2,* 49–61.

Bernzweig, E.P. (1996). *The nurse's liability for malpractice: A programmed course* (6th ed.). St. Louis, MO: Mosby–Year Book.

*Black, H.C. (1991). *Black's law dictionary* (6th ed.). St. Paul, MN: West Publishing Company.

Brent, N.J. (1997). *Nurses and the law: A guide to principles and applications.* Philadelphia: W.B. Saunders Co.

Calfee, B.E. (1996). Labor laws: Working to protect you. *Nursing, 26*(2), 34–40.

Dycus, S.J. (1995). Should you be a good Samaritan? *Office Nurse, 8,* 41–42.

Fade, A.E. (1995). Advance directives: An overview of changing right-to-die laws. *Journal of Nursing Law, 2,* 27–38.

Faherty, B. (1995). Advanced practice nursing: What's all the fuss? *Journal of Nursing Law, 2*(3), 9–17.

*Gosfield, A. (Ed.). (1993). *1993 Health law handbook.* Deerfield, IL: Clark Boardman Callaghan.

Infante, M. (1996). The legal risks of managed care. *RN, 59,* 57–59.

Kreplick, J.A. (1996). Unlicensed hospital assistive personnel: Efficiency or liability? Part 1. *Journal of Nursing Law 3,* 7–25.

_____ (1995). Push on to require minimum stays after childbirth. *American Medical News, 38*(29), 16.

Sheehan, J. (1996). Safeguard your license: Avoid these pitfalls. *RN, 59,* 59–62.

Sullivan, G.H. (1996). Risk management: Medical records. *Office Nurse, 9,* 39–41.

University of the State of New York, the State Education Department. (1995). *Nursing handbook.* Albany, NY: Office of the Professions.

Wilkinson, A. (1998). Nursing malpractice. *Nursing, 28*(6), 34–40.

_____

*Asterisk indicates a classic or definitive work on this subject.

The Ethical Context of Practice

Carson A. Easley

Key Terms

autonomy
beneficence
deontology
durable power of attorney for
   health care
ethics
fidelity
justice
living will

morals
nonmaleficence
teleology
values
values clarification
veracity
virtue
virtue theory

LEARNING OBJECTIVES

After reading this chapter, you should be able to:

1. Compare and contrast the concepts of ethics, morals, and values.

2. Compare and contrast three theories of ethics: teleology, deontology, and virtue theory.

3. Identify ethical principles.

4. Discuss the elements of ethical decision-making.

5. Discuss the contents of the American Nurses' Association Code for Nurses.

6. Discuss the concepts of nursing advocacy, accountability, and responsibility.

7. Describe some guides to ethical decision-making, including advance directives, informed consent, and ethics committees and forums.

In nursing, as in life, it is not always easy to determine the best course of action in a given situation. You are dedicated to meeting the needs of your clients, yet institutional policies must be followed, physicians' directives implemented, and professional standards upheld. You also must have a willingness to listen to your own inner wisdom. When two or more of these domains are in conflict, you may face a dilemma of ethics.

Although technical skills are essential for safe and effective nursing care, you must also develop skills in ethical decision-making. You must be able to identify and discuss ethical dilemmas in nursing practice, apply ethical standards to resolve those dilemmas, and provide the rationale for ethical decisions to clients, families, and other health care professionals.

In today's health care arena, ethical issues abound. As technological advances extend life for clients with chronic illnesses, practitioners grapple with the issue of quality of life versus sanctity of life. At the same time, the shrinking health care dollar has led to shorter hospital stays and insurance company restrictions on reimbursement for various tests, equipment, supplies, medications, and procedures. As resources dwindle, the "baby boom" generation is aging. Should care and services be rationed? And if so, how will such decisions be made and by whom?

Organ transplantation, *in vitro* fertilization, genetic engineering, assisted suicide, care of clients with communicable illnesses, umbilical cord blood storage, and allocation of resources are some of the high-profile issues currently being addressed by practitioners. In addition, within your daily practice, you will also confront issues of informed consent, confidentiality (especially with data stored on computer), client advocacy, the competency of caregivers, withholding of food and fluids, and refusal of treatment. Thus, you must be equipped to make decisions about ethical issues in a consistent and objective manner in a rapidly changing and constantly demanding health care delivery system (Federwisch, 1997).

This chapter explores the theories and principles of ethics. It also provides guidelines for ethical decision-making that can be applied systematically to nursing practice.

ETHICS, MORALS, AND VALUES

The words ethics, morals, and values are often used interchangeably to indicate behaviors or ideas that the speaker feels are right, good, just, or proper. Some might say, for example, that it is unethical or immoral to smoke cigarettes in front of children or that anyone who does so lacks values. However, within the domains of philosophy, sociology, and law, these three terms have separate and unique definitions.

Ethical Terms

Ethics

Ethics is the branch of philosophy that attempts to determine what constitutes good, bad, right, and wrong in human behavior (Stewart & Blocker, 1992). The term is derived from the Greek word *ethos*, which means "custom" or "duty." The study of ethics entails the examination of human behavior in terms of what ought to be done in the course of human interactions, and it seeks to provide guidelines or principles as a way to direct human action (Pojman, 1990). Ethical study is a formal analysis of standards for human conduct in a variety of life experiences and conditions.

The following terms are often used in discussions of ethics:

- *Normative ethics*—The development of systems, theories, principles, and rules that provide guidance when deciding whether an action is right or wrong
- *Applied ethics*—The use of ethical systems to make decisions
- *Descriptive ethics*—Ethical behaviors and beliefs
- *Bioethics*—Ethics that are concerned with human conduct in health care (Deloughery, 1995)

Morals

The terms *moral duty* and *moral conduct* are often used to describe ethical behavior. Likewise, the terms *ethics* and *morals* are often used interchangeably when identifying right and wrong. Indeed, in the Greek and Latin origins (*ethos* and *mores)*, both terms mean "customs" or "duties."

However, the terms are used differently by contemporary theorists (Table 3–1). As we have seen, ethics seeks to determine what ought to be done in a given situation. **Morals** are standards of conduct that represent the ideal in human behavior to which society expects its members to adhere (Pojman, 1990).

Moral development is the imprinting of the moral standards put forth by society as the norm for human conduct. Imprinting of moral conduct begins in early childhood. It is seen, for example, when parents teach their children to tell the truth. External forces, such as fear of consequences, may govern adherence to such standards. As we mature, it is expected that moral conduct becomes part of our nature rather than an avenue to avoid unpleasant consequences.

As a nurse, you are expected to be a moral agent. That is, you are expected to perform the duties and functions of nursing within established standards of conduct. You are also expected to possess and use moral standards in making decisions. Therefore, you must first possess the knowledge to recognize a moral conflict. Jameton (1984) identified three components of a moral conflict:

- Moral uncertainty, when a person is unsure what values and principles are applicable or if an ethical problem really exists
- Moral dilemma, when moral principles are in conflict
- Moral distress, when the person understands what ought to be done but no supportive systems are

TABLE 3–1
Terms in Ethics

Term	Definition	Example
Ethics	• Promotes ideal human behavior. • Examines what ought to be done. • Seeks to provide guidelines or principles to direct human action.	• Exploration of ethical principles and moral standards of conduct. • Having a high regard for the uniqueness of the human experience.
Morals	• Standards of conduct that represent "ideal" human behavior. • Standards identified by society as the norm of conduct. • Conduct that is expected regardless of consequences to the individual.	• The expectation that members of society will be honest and tell the truth in all situations, even if they experience negative consequences. • Behaviors that are judged as the "right" thing to do, such as demonstrating respect for clients.
Values	• Ideals, beliefs, and patterns of behavior that are prized and chosen by individuals. • Learned behavior acquired from cultural, family, and community life experiences.	• Personal values, such as belief in strong family connections and the desire to be accepted by others. • Professional values, such as dedication, integrity, and competence.

available to help in reaching a decision or implementing an action

Once you recognize moral conflict, you must then be able to implement moral reasoning. Deloughery (1995) cites research by Rest (1986) that describes moral reasoning in four stages:

• Recognition of a conflict of values or principles
• Selection of an action
• Intention to implement morally correct behavior
• Performance of a selected behavior that resolves the dilemma

Values

Values are ideals, beliefs, and patterns of behavior that are prized and chosen by a person, group, or society. Like morals, values provide a foundation for principled behavior. A discussion of ethics is incomplete without addressing the influence of values on the development of ethical behavior. Values shape decisions in everyday life, from the clothes we wear to the movies we prefer to the food we eat and the cars we buy. Therefore, it is not unusual to expect that our values will be evident in our behaviors.

Types of Values

Values that people hold as important in their private lives are called personal values. They are learned from various experiences in the family and community and are seen as compatible with lifestyle choices. Having strong family connections, having good health, being accepted by others, and being honest are all examples of personal values.

Professional values are qualities that a profession identifies as the acceptable standard of conduct for members of the profession or group. Examples of professional values include integrity, dedication, and fairness. In your position as a health care professional,

you are expected to demonstrate personal and professional values that reflect a respect for human dignity, that honor client rights, that demonstrate care and concern, that support equity, and that honor truth.

Development of Values

Values are learned behaviors that are influenced by culture, ethnicity, education, and life experiences. Values are acquired through structured and unstructured learning, experiences in our homes and communities, and interactions with family, teachers, clergy, and social organizations. As children we are exposed to the values of adults who have influence over our lives. As we mature, we begin to develop our own values, sometimes through trial and error. In childhood a toy may be the most valued object of our young lives. In adolescence, peer opinions begin to be more important than adult and even parent opinions. In adulthood, our behaviors reflect the values we have acquired and use in daily decision-making (Burkhardt & Nathaniel, 1998).

Our values reflect what we hold important and what we believe when we act on them in various situations in daily life. When values are freely chosen, they are demonstrated by our behavior through word and deed. For example, if a physician believes that everyone should have access to quality health care regardless of ability to pay, the medical practice demonstrates that belief by providing quality health services to anyone in need.

You will be exposed to many situations in health care that may produce value conflicts. As noted earlier, moral reasoning requires that you recognize conflicts in values or principles. It is important for you to understand your feelings and be able to identify your values about health, illness, aging, access to care, quality of life, dying, and death. If you understand your values and can express them clearly, you will be better prepared to handle difficult situations and make informed decisions.

Values Clarification

An understanding of personal values forms the basis for ethical decision-making. The process of **values clarification** allows you to identify your personal values and develop self-awareness. This process is essential in nursing because your values provide the platform on which you will make decisions and take action. Raths, Harmon, and Simmons (1979) describe a three-step model for values clarification that includes a seven-step process for identifying values (Table 3–2). Using the model, consider the following situation:

Mary is a 22-year-old college student who is concerned about the weight she has gained during her last semester. Some of her friends have decided to start smoking to control their appetite. Mary is considering this option but finally decides that she values her health and will look for a more health-conscious way to lose weight.

Step 1. *Choosing.* Mary decided to research the issue. After deciding that overall good health is more important to her than a solution that could lead to nicotine addiction and chronic health problems, Mary decides not to smoke. This choice was based on her valuing good health and finding the possible benefit of smoking not substantial enough compared with the overall risk factors.

Step 2. *Prizing.* Mary is proud of her choice. She affirms it by refusing cigarettes when offered. She readily tells her friends of her decision.

Step 3. *Acting.* Mary's makes it clear that she has chosen not to smoke. Her apartment and car have "No smoking" signs. She asks to sit in the nonsmoking sections of restaurants. And when friends ask, "Do you mind if I smoke?," she answers, "Yes."

ETHICAL THEORIES

The Greek philosophers Socrates, Plato, and Aristotle were among the first to examine human behavior in terms of ideal actions, character, and lifestyle. Throughout the centuries, their ideas and writings have formed the basis for ethical debates and discussions and the development of ethical systems. Many philosophers have developed theories that refute, support, or expand on the ethical principles espoused by

TABLE 3–2
Steps in Values Clarification

Choosing	• Choice made freely.
	• Choice made from alternatives.
	• Choice made after considering the consequences of each alternative.
Prizing	• Being proud of choice.
	• Willingly affirming choice.
Acting	• Becomes part of demonstrated behavior.
	• Acted upon frequently.

Modified from Raths, L., Harmon, M., & Simmons, S. (1979). Values and teaching. Columbus, OH: Merrill.

the ancient Greeks. The following is a brief overview of some of these ethical theories and their implications for nursing practice.

Teleology

Teleology is a set of theories that postulate that the outcomes or consequences of an action determine its goodness. The word is derived from the Greek word *telos,* meaning end. These theories are also called consequentialist theories. Inherent within them is the belief that right actions are those that bring good consequences and wrong actions are those that bring bad consequences.

One of the most well known teleological theories is that of utilitarianism. This theory was formulated and advocated by British philosopher John Stuart Mill (1806–1873). Mill believed that actions that resulted in the greatest benefit or happiness for the most people were right and that those that resulted in suffering were wrong. Mill saw right actions as those having the most utility or usefulness for the most people, groups, or societies being affected or influenced by the actions. The right action also produces as little harm as possible to the smallest number of people (Stewart & Blocker, 1992).

One problem with utilitarianism is the subjective definition of right action. There can be no universal, objective standards because what constitutes right and wrong changes continually according to the situation, individual, or society. Additionally, in practice, it is difficult to predict with accuracy that any one action will result in the desired consequences.

Deontology

Deontology is a theory that is not concerned with the consequences of an act but rather with the obligation or duty to perform the act. The word is derived from the Greek word *deon,* which means "duty." Deontological ethics requires that an act be performed because it is morally right to do so. In choosing actions, little regard is given to the desirability of outcomes or the goodness of motives. Behavior is governed by a sense of duty to fellow human beings and respect for one's obligations to others. Human dignity is held in highest regard. Terms often associated with this theory are fidelity, truthfulness, and justice (Stewart & Blocker, 1992).

German philosopher Immanuel Kant (1724–1804) is the best-known deontological theorist. He used the term *categorical imperative* to describe a moral duty that he viewed as a command. To Kant, a categorical imperative requires that you adhere to a moral act regardless of the consequences (Stewart & Blocker, 1992).

In attempting to apply this theory, problems arise when two or more conflicting principles are involved. The person is torn in trying to decide which principle has priority. However, deontology is viewed as the foundation for ethical decision-making in health care because it emphasizes one's duty or obligation to another.

Virtue Theory

Unlike teleology and deontology, which examine actions, **virtue theory** focuses on characteristics that are intrinsic to the person performing the action. **Virtue** may be defined as a practice of conforming life and conduct to moral and ethical principles. Aristotle, who proposed virtue theory, attempted to describe the disposition a person must embody and the *being* that must be evident in their persona for effecting ethical behavior. Virtue-based ethics ask "How should *I* be in order to behave ethically?" (Pojman, 1990). The focus is attainment of excellence.

Deloughery (1995) notes that virtue theory may apply to nursing because attributes such as compassion, caring, empathy, and promise keeping are ascribed to the character of nurses. Thus, nurses are viewed as possessing certain virtues unique to the profession of nursing.

ETHICAL PRINCIPLES

Principles are basic truths or laws that guide conduct and behavior. Ethical principles, also called standards, provide the framework for the practice of professional nursing. Such principles guide actions by providing the basis for rule development within the profession (Yoder Wise, 1995). Following are principles considered essential to the delivery of ethical nursing care.

AUTONOMY

Autonomy refers to a person's right to make individual choices—that is, to self-determine. It is essential that you respect your clients' rights to make their own health care choices. To support autonomy, you provide detailed and realistic information to clients, who then freely choose from the available options. You support clients' decisions even when they are different from your preferences.

BENEFICENCE

Beneficence is the promotion of good. It requires the performance of actions that are of benefit to others. The good of actions must therefore be weighed against any possible harm. For example, failing to turn a bedridden client who complains of pain during such procedures may produce the short-term good of reduced discomfort. But it may also cause the harm of impaired skin integrity and musculoskeletal deformities.

CONFIDENTIALITY

You hear, see, and gather data about clients that is confidential in nature. As described in Chapter 2, confidentiality is the client's right to privacy in the health care delivery system. Confidentiality means maintaining another's privacy by safeguarding information that is entrusted to you. Through the assessment process, you are privy to intimate details about a client's health history. Before you collect data, it is important that clients understand that such information will be documented in the medical record and therefore available to other health care providers. This fact may influence the type and amount of information that a client shares.

It is your responsibility to assure the client that information is held in confidence and used as a means of meeting their health care needs. Because clients have to depend on strangers when they are most vulnerable, you are in a position to protect them from indiscriminate disclosure of health care information that may cause harm. For instance, the disclosure of a client's HIV-positive status could cause the loss of his job and exposure to social isolation and discrimination.

Maintain client confidentiality by not discussing client issues in hallways, elevators, hospital parking lots, or at home with family and friends. Maintaining confidentiality demonstrates the kind of respect that is the cornerstone of the nurse-client relationship (Burkhardt & Nathaniel, 1998).

NONMALEFICENCE

The word *maleficence* means "evil" or "harm." Thus, **nonmaleficence** requires the practitioner to do no harm. Nonmaleficence is the complement of beneficence. It says that your actions should not cause undo harm to clients. Provision of safe and effective nursing care may require you to perform acts that cause fear, discomfort, or pain—inserting a feeding tube, for instance, or giving an injection. The good of these acts (beneficence) is weighed against both the temporary pain and the potential for serious harm if the interventions are withheld. Nonmaleficence also requires that your actions be performed according to acceptable standards of practice because failure to follow such standards could result in client injury.

FIDELITY

Fidelity means honoring agreements and keeping promises. When you say, "I'll give you your pain medication at 9 o'clock" or "I'll be sure to speak with your doctor about your concern," your clients hear them as promises or commitments to their welfare. Keeping such promises is your responsibility. When you cannot honor a promise at the specified time, you must either inform the client and perform the action as soon as possible or have another caregiver complete the task.

JUSTICE

Justice is moral rightness, fairness, or equity. It is therefore concerned with fair and equal treatment of all clients. In applying the principle of justice, you must consider whether it requires that everyone be treated the same or that the same principles and standards be applied to all. For example, equal treatment of two cancer clients may not be possible if one has a strong financial and emotional support system and the other is homeless and mentally ill.

The issue of justice arises in attempts to allocate health care resources and ensure equal access to health care for all. With the aging of the baby boom generation, the need for health care may become greater than available resources. You will have an integral role in promoting equal or fair access to health care. You must therefore be politically astute regarding issues related to resource allocation, and vocal in advocating for equality of access (Fowler & Levine-Ariff, 1987).

VERACITY

Veracity means adhering to the truth. It therefore requires truth-telling consistently and continually. In applying the principle of veracity, you tell the complete truth and not an altered version assumed to be in the client's best interest. Veracity also relates to the principle of autonomy because clients can only make the best decisions for themselves when given complete facts. This issue is most crucial when dealing with terminally ill clients and their right to know their prognosis. Often it is you who must answer clients' questions regarding death and dying.

It is important to remember that respect for others guides the implementation of all ethical principles. When you respect others, you spontaneously ensure freedom of choice, promote good, prevent harm, keep promises, act fairly, and remain truthful (Yoder Wise, 1995).

MAKING AN ETHICAL DECISION

Some decisions in our lives have clearly distinct advantages that provide us with incentives for choices made. For example, choosing to pursue higher education, although not easy, provides a great deal of satisfaction—personally, professionally and, one hopes, financially—upon completion. Many decisions are routine and require little deliberation, such as clothing choices, what to eat for breakfast, and when to retire for the evening. You are often called upon to make decisions that are not as clear-cut and may have choices that conflict (see the Ethics Discussion Scenario, Box 3-1).

When two or more principles are in conflict or when choices are unfavorable, you have an ethical dilemma. That is, no available solution is satisfactory. For example, a geriatric male client is restrained because of his unsteady gait. You are concerned about his risk of injury from falling. The client is oriented and says repeatedly that he does not want to be restrained. In this situation, the principles in conflict are autonomy versus beneficence. You respect the client's right to be autonomous and make his own decisions, yet you are also bound to protect the client from injury and prevent unnecessary harm.

You will face situations like this one daily. You are expected to implement actions that result in good outcomes for the client yet remain in keeping with the client's wishes and desires. Following is a discussion of a six-step ethical decision-making process that will help you identify ethical dilemmas, implement solu-

---

BOX 3–1

ETHICS DISCUSSION SCENARIO

John and Mary both have the chance to obtain the answers to the next exam and secure an "A" in a very difficult course required for completing their degree. John rejects the offer outright. He never considers it as an option because he views it as morally wrong and dishonest.

Mary considers the offer and weighs her options. She has been struggling with work and school and "acing" the next exam would greatly relieve some of the pressure. She knows she is smart enough but has not had enough time to study. She is sorely tempted but finally rejects the offer because she doesn't want to take the chance of getting caught and being expelled from school.

- Is either of these students more moral than the other, because both rejected the offer?
- If so, whom?
- What is the rationale for your choice?
- What values are evident in this scenario?
- Which ethical theory best fits this situation?

---

tions, and evaluate outcomes. It will help you move beyond feelings of uncertainty and helplessness to naming and clarifying the problem and implementing solutions. Review of work by Jameton (1984) provides the basis for following the steps in the ethical decision-making process.

1. *Identify the ethical dilemma.* Is the situation truly an ethical dilemma or is it a legal issue or a problem of faulty communication? Are conflicting principles or values present? Legal and communication issues may be present in any ethical dilemma. However, in the absence of conflicting principles, legal counsel or clarification of communication, rather than ethical analysis, may be appropriate.
2. *Gather pertinent data.* Everyone involved in the case is a source of potentially significant data. Documents such as the health history, nurses' notes, and consent forms are also important to research. Questions to ask include the following:
   - What are the relevant facts at issue in the dilemma?
   - Who are the principal people involved?
   - Are values in conflict with expected outcomes?
   - Is there a clear therapeutic regimen for the client?
   - Do cultural or spiritual factors need to be considered in the decision?
   - Do institutional values and systems support the nursing decisions made?
   - Is there a mechanism for implementing actions?
   - Have policies, procedures, protocols, and economic factors been considered?

3. *Examine the dilemma for the ethical principles involved.* At this point it is important to have a clear understanding of the principles that are key to making an ethical decision in each case. Questions to ask include the following:
   - With whom must the final decision be made, and is that person competent or empowered to make decisions? *(autonomy)*
   - What is the overall good to be accomplished? *(beneficence and nonmaleficence)*
   - Have the principle decision-makers been given all necessary information? *(veracity)*
   - Whose interests are being served? *(justice)*
   - Have there been promises made or are there expectations of behaviors from caregivers? *(fidelity)* Determine which principles are applicable and which are in conflict. Does honoring one over another oppose legal requirements or institutional policies?
4. *Examine all possible solutions.* Explore all possible, reasonable actions in terms of ethical principles. In considering solutions, it is important to evaluate realistically which options you can implement within legal guidelines and agency policy. Activities such as facilitating communication, providing facts, and ensuring that participants are aware of all reasonable options are always within the purview of nursing. Additionally, you must be aware of the likely outcomes of the various possible solutions. Will the consequences of actions taken be those that are intended? Will the intended good be served?
5. *Choose solutions.* After careful deliberation, choose a solution (or solutions) and take action. The chosen solutions must be consistent with ethical principles and be based on ethical analysis.
6. *Evaluate solutions chosen.* Examine solutions chosen for effectiveness. Reflect on whether expected outcomes were reached. Questions to ask include
   - Did solutions chosen resolve the ethical dilemma?
   - What was the effect on those involved?
   - Were additional ethical issues identified?
   - Was the solution chosen the best one in light of the outcomes generated?

Often there is more than one possible solution. The ethical decision-making process assists you in reaching the best solution for a particular situation. The process may also help you to overcome the initial feelings of helplessness that may be experienced when facing an ethical dilemma (see the Case Study, Box 3-2). Keep in mind that a single perfect answer may not result from this process. Instead, you will search for the closest answer to the intended good for the primary parties involved in the dilemma.

ETHICS IN NURSING

You are responsible to society for the provision of safe and effective nursing care. As a profession, nursing has established standards of behaviors that govern the practice. These standards are called codes of ethics.

In the United States, the American Nurses' Association (ANA) Code for Nurses (1985) (see accompanying Box 3-3) is the document governing ethical nursing practice. Although Isabel Hampton Robb wrote a book on ethics for nurses at the turn of the century, it was not until 1950 that the ANA's first Code was adopted. The current edition was adopted in 1985.

The ANA Code for Nurses identifies the goals and values of the profession and sets forth the philosophy of the profession. It includes interpretive statements that explain how each goal is realized in nursing practice. Not surprisingly, the Code focuses on the protection of the client and the identification of standards for a nurse's interactions with clients. Because it identifies the behaviors required for ethical practice, the Code can be used as a guide for evaluating nursing actions. It may also be used as a guide to ethical decision-making. Although the Code is not law, it is the standard by which nursing actions are judged throughout the profession. Sanctions can be imposed against a nurse who is found to be practicing outside the framework of the Code.

Additional codes for professional nursing are the Canadian Nurses Association Code of Ethics for Nursing (see accompanying Box 3-4) and the International Council of Nurses Ethical Concepts Applied to Nursing (see accompanying Box 3-5) As you review, note the similarities. For example, all of the codes address respect for human dignity, rights, confidentiality, competence, and responsibilities of the nurse in the delivery of health care. What other areas are addressed in common? As you can see, all of the codes provide a framework for ethical practice in professional nursing.

Standards of Practice

Part of the mission of the ANA is the establishment of standards of practice for professional nursing in the United States. Standards of practice provide direction for the provision of nursing care, including your role in professional activities. They reflect the nursing profession's autonomy in establishing standards of professional practice. Standards are written statements defining the acceptable level of performance in the profession. Standards also provide a set of expectations that can be consistently applied to evaluate nursing performance. Values of the profession are reflected in practice standards, including the definition of professional nursing (McCloskey & Grace, 1997).

Burkardt and Nathaniel (1998) note that standards may provide a detailed description of specific acts you must perform in care delivery or they may outline the process to be followed. For example, the ANA Standards of Clinical Nursing Practice (1991) delineate that nursing care is provided using the steps of the nursing process. Each step of the nursing process is identified, including descriptive behaviors. The standards can be used as guides to determine if the care provided by

BOX 3–2

CASE STUDY USING THE SIX-STEP ETHICAL DECISION-MAKING PROCESS

Michael R. is a 25-year-old African-American client diagnosed with sickle cell disease who has undergone multiple hospital admissions in the last 2 years. He is admitted to Catherine's med-surg unit for the sixth time in the last 5 months. Catherine has cared for him on his last two admissions. She is again assigned to his care. She is aware that an ongoing issue with Michael is pain management. She is concerned when she reads the pre-scribed pain-management regimen.

His physician prescribed the same regimen during his last two admissions and the client frequently com-plained of inadequate pain relief, asking for more medi-cation before it was time for his next dose. Because of constant pain and inadequate relief, Michael often was angry and frustrated. The nurses have labeled him hos-tile and difficult to work with. They expressed relief that Catherine would provide his care.

Catherine notes that the physician prescribed De-merol, 50 to 100 mg, and Vistaril, 50 mg IM every 4 to 6 hours. She knows that the nurses have a tendency to give the lower medication dose and closer to the 6-hour mark rather than the 4-hour mark. She has read recent research suggesting that morphine is a better medication for pain relief in sickle-cell clients than Demerol.

Catherine also believes that patient-controlled anal-gesia (PCA) would probably be best for Michael. How-ever, he is uninsured and she is afraid that the hospital would not assume the cost of PCA. She is unsure whether the physician would be willing to change the orders or listen to her ideas.

Catherine feels that Michael will have the same issues of pain management arise during this hospital-ization. She is concerned that he is not getting the best possible care for his condition because of the pre-scribed pain management, his financial status, and nursing attitudes. She is unsure of what steps to take or what she should do. What follows is a six-step

ethical decision-making process using this situation as the example.

Step 1: Identify the Ethical Dilemma

What is the situation that raises ethical problems? Is it a matter of ethics, a legal issue, or a question of commu-nication? Are there ethical principles in conflict?

The client is not a private paying client. Some nurses have said that when he rates his pain at 10+ he doesn't appear to be in a great deal of pain. The physician in question is not noted for listening to nurses' opinions about issues that he considers to be medical practice.

Catherine has been feeling dissatisfied with the care that Michael received in the past. She is concerned that she is not protecting his rights or advocating for him. She has voiced her concern to a couple of coworkers, who did not validate her feelings. No formal action has been taken.

Step 2: Gather Pertinent Data

Review all significant data. Identify the relevant facts. Who are the people involved? Is there a conflict of val-ues? Are there cultural influences? What are the eco-nomic and financial implications?

Is the prescribed regimen consistently implemented? Is there a mechanism for implementing action? Are there supportive nursing policies?

Catherine feels that the nursing staff is not showing care and concern. She wonders if the nurses are sensitive to cul-tural variations in expressing pain. She feels that adequate pain management is possible for Michael, but that the current regimen is neither effective nor implemented appropriately. She thinks that Michael should have more involvement in decision-making about his pain management. Nursing poli-cies document standards of nursing practice and nursing care that are helpful guidelines.

Continued

you was in keeping with acceptable practice within the profession.

Accountability and Responsibility

As a nurse, you are responsible and accountable for your actions. That is, you are *responsible* for providing care within established standards of the profession. For example, you are responsible for implementing care using the nursing process. This means you assess client needs, identify nursing diagnoses, identify out-comes, formulate a plan of care, implement actions, and evaluate the effectiveness of nursing care pro-vided (ANA, 1991). As a nursing student, you are re-

sponsible for acquiring the knowledge and skills nec-essary to become a safe practitioner. Included in this knowledge and skill development are the awareness of ethical principles and the process of ethical decision-making. Once you have attained licensure to practice as a registered nurse, you are responsible for maintaining competency in nursing knowledge and skills and demonstrating ethical principles in care de-livery.

Being accountable means that you are answerable for the outcomes of actions taken. You are answerable to clients, institutions, the profession, peers, and soci-ety. In addition you are answerable to yourself in terms of ensuring that your conduct reflects ethical be-

BOX 3–2

CASE STUDY USING THE SIX-STEP ETHICAL DECISION-MAKING PROCESS (continued)

Step 3: Examine the Dilemma for Ethical Principles

What principles are key to making a decision here? What is the overall good to be accomplished (beneficence)? Have the principal decision-makers been given all the necessary information? Whose interests are being served (justice)? What are the expectations from caregivers (fidelity)?

Catherine feels that Michael can expect pain relief. The good of the client should be the primary concern. She also feels that he can expect to be treated with respect and have his dignity maintained.

She remains unsure of the physician's response but thinks he should be approached. She feels that the nursing staff needs more information regarding pain management for clients with sickle-cell disease.

Step 4: Examine All Solutions

What are all the possible and reasonable actions? What options open to Catherine are legal and within agency policy? What are the possible outcomes and consequences of actions taken? Will the intended good be served?

Catherine considers the options open to her:

- *She can voice her concerns to the physician and discuss nursing concerns with the unit staff.*
- *She can consult with the charge nurse and unit director.*
- *She can involve the client in decision-making.*
- *She can consult with the unit's clinical nurse specialist and nursing education department.*
- *She can plan a client care conference.*
- *She can develop a collaborative plan of care using the nursing process.*
- *She can say nothing and not make waves while trying to give Michael the best care possible when she is on duty.*

Step 5: Choose Solutions

After deliberation, choose solutions and act on them. Are solutions chosen consistent with ethical principles?

Catherine chooses to speak with the charge nurse and share her concerns. She shares the research information and asks for a client care conference. She involves the clinical nurse specialist in the conference. The client is involved in the decision-making process and included in the care conference. From the conference, a plan of care is developed that includes recommendation for a referral to a pain-management specialist.

Catherine approaches the physician and discusses her concern. He was aware of the conference but did not choose to participate. He does not change his orders but does make a request for the pain-management specialist to see the client.

Step 6: Evaluate Solutions Chosen

Was the solution effective and the expected outcome achieved? Was the ethical problem resolved or were additional problems identified?

Consultation with the pain-management specialist resulted in a change in the client's pain-management regimen and client education regarding self-care. He was put in a pain-management protocol study and was able to receive a PCA pump.

Catherine observed that Michael experienced effective pain relief. Other nurses said that they found him pleasant and approachable when his pain was managed. Some of the staff voiced that Catherine had gone overboard for one client.

The unit director recommended that nursing forums should be instituted on a quarterly basis to provide information on ethical principles and identify ethical issues. The nurse educator is planning seminars on the topics of pain management and cultural sensitivity.

havior. If you assess that a client has a high risk for injury due to falls and you do not develop and implement a plan of care to protect the client from injury, you are accountable if the client is injured. You are accountable to the client, the family, the nursing service area, and the institution. In this instance, you are also answerable to yourself and the profession because the nursing care provided did not demonstrate implementation of the nursing process or provision of care within ethical principles (nonmaleficence). You are accountable for the outcomes of your nursing judgment and cannot be alleviated from this accountability by physicians' orders or institutional policies (ANA, 1985).

Advocacy

To advocate for someone means to speak for that person when the person is unable to speak for himself or herself. You will often find yourself in the role of advocate for clients when they are incapacitated or diminished by illness. Thus, you may be called upon to assert the client's wishes or desires regarding health care choices. You must be prepared to advocate for clients and families and to provide channels for effective communication of client and family wishes.

You must actively advocate for clients when they are vulnerable and unable to promote their own

BOX 3–3

AMERICAN NURSES' ASSOCIATION CODE FOR NURSES

- The nurse provides services with respect for human dignity and the uniqueness of the client, unrestricted by considerations of social or economic status, personal attributes, or the nature of health problems.
- The nurse safeguards the client's right to privacy by judiciously protecting information of a confidential nature.
- The nurse acts to safeguard the client and the public when health care and safety are affected by the incompetent, unethical, or illegal practice of any person.
- The nurse assumes responsibility and accountability for individual nursing judgments and actions.
- The nurse maintains competence in nursing.
- The nurse exercises informed judgment and uses individual competence and qualifications as criteria in seeking consultation, accepting responsibilities, and delegating nursing activities to others.
- The nurse participates in activities that contribute to the ongoing development of the profession's body of knowledge.
- The nurse participates in the profession's efforts to implement and improve standards of nursing.
- The nurse participates in the profession's efforts to establish and maintain conditions of employment conducive to high-quality nursing care.
- The nurse participates in the profession's effort to protect the public from misinformation and misrepresentation and to maintain the integrity of nursing.
- The nurse collaborates with members of health professions and other citizens in promoting community and national efforts to meet the health needs of the public.

American Nurses' Association. (1985). Code for nurses. American Nurses' Association: Author.

Common Ethical Problems

Nursing care is often provided to clients at risk for ethical dilemmas, such as geriatric clients, terminally ill clients, or clients involved in research studies. Although you will have a certain degree of autonomy in care delivery, it is important to remember that nursing is not practiced in a vacuum. By its very nature, it is provided in collaboration with clients, families, physicians, and other health care practitioners in various practice arenas (Fig. 3–1).

You may find yourself in conflict with clients—for instance, the client with diabetes who refuses to follow the dietary regimen and is frequently readmitted for out-of-control blood glucose levels. You may experience frustration and even anger because of the client's seeming unwillingness to implement self-care measures. If you place a high value on maintaining good health, you may find it difficult to interact with a client who refuses to follow a regimen that manages a chronic illness. Yet, you must also respect the client's right to make his own health care choices. The needs of the client are paramount, and you must put aside feelings of anger and frustration and deliver care that meets the client's needs. Nursing with care and concern is important to the profession and must be demonstrated in spite of personal feelings.

Ethical problems may also stem from your interactions with physicians, such as when physician orders are contradictory to client wishes or when the physician has not informed a terminally ill client of his or her diagnosis and the client constantly questions you. This leaves you feeling caught in the middle and can make you want to avoid the client because of the uncomfortable feelings generated by the client's questions. To whom do you owe loyalty? Is it your responsibility to inform the client of the medical diagnosis? What do you think? In the day-to-day activities of

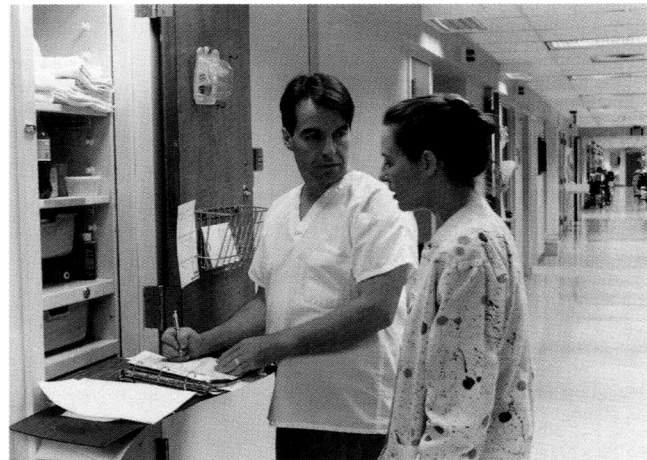

Figure 3–1. Nursing is not practiced in a vacuum but in collaboration with others.

needs. It is important for you to have knowledge of the client's values so you can assist in decision-making that is consistent with the client's lifestyle choices. This may be accomplished by providing necessary information, by helping the client explore options, or by doing both. The overall goal of advocacy is to ensure that the client receives the best possible care and to support the client's right to have health care that is consistent with the client's values and beliefs (Fowler & Levine-Ariff, 1987).

nursing care, ethical problems may also revolve around the following:

- Coworker performance of care or lack of provision of required care
- Unit staffing patterns that negatively influence the provision of safe nursing care
- Insurers that limit the type of care a client may receive or that require discharge when a client would benefit from additional hospital days

As you can see, issues of ethics may be unavoidable in the day-to-day delivery of nursing care. Developing skills to identify when there is conflict of values or ethical principles increases your ability to be effective in care delivery. Also being knowledgeable of the steps in the ethical decision-making process provides you with the tools to ensure that client needs are being served. The next discussion concerns guides that can assist in managing ethical problems.

GUIDES TO ETHICAL DECISIONS IN NURSING

Self-determination has long been valued in Western society, especially regarding health care choices. The American Hospital Association's Patient's Bill of Rights supports this value: *The patient has the right to make decisions about the plan of care prior to and during the course of treatment and to refuse a recommended treatment or plan of care to the extent permitted by law and hospital policy and to be informed of the medical consequences of this action* (AHA, 1992). The ethical principle of autonomy, discussed earlier, is clearly reflected in this passage. Although autonomy calls upon you to respect client health care decisions, this is only possible when the client's choices are made known. As a result of certain injuries or disease states, clients' mental or physical functioning may deteriorate so greatly that they are unable to choose or communicate their desires regarding health care. In these cases, any previously documented information regarding the client's preferences can be invaluable in protecting the client's autonomy.

Advance Directives

Ethical dilemmas arise whenever a client's wishes are not known clearly or understood by those providing care. As described in Chapter 2, an advance directive is a written document that provides direction for health care when a person is unable to make personal treatment choices. However, even an informal discussion between a client and a health care practitioner can be considered a form of advance directive. When you are involved in such discussions, you are responsible for documenting the content of the conversation in the medical record. Formal advance directives, which contain the client's own written instructions for health care, can be more effective than informal discussions. Living wills and durable power of attorney for health care are two such formal advance directives (Hackler,

---

BOX 3–4

CANADIAN NURSES ASSOCIATION CODE OF ETHICS

Values

I HEALTH AND WELL-BEING

Nurses value health and well-being and assist persons to achieve their optimum level of health in situations of normal health, illness, injury, or in the process of dying.

II CHOICE

Nurses respect and promote autonomy of clients and help them to express their health needs and values, and to obtain appropriate information.

III DIGNITY

Nurses value and advocate the dignity and self-respect of human beings.

IV CONFIDENTIALITY

Nurses safeguard the trust of clients that information learned in the context of a professional relationship is shared outside the health care team only with the client's permission or as legally required.

V FAIRNESS

Nurses apply and promote principles of equity and fairness to assist clients in receiving unbiased treatment and a share of health services and resources proportionate to their needs.

VI ACCOUNTABILITY

Nurses act in a manner consistent with their professional responsibilities and standards of practice.

VII PRACTICE ENVIRONMENTS CONDUCIVE TO SAFE, COMPETENT AND ETHICAL CARE

Nurses advocate practice environments that have the organizational and human support systems, and the resource allocation necessary for safe, competent, and ethical nursing care.

Canadian Nurses Association. (1997). Code of ethics for registered nurses. Canadian Nurses Association: Author. Reprint with permission from the Canadian Nurses Association.

BOX 3–5

INTERNATIONAL COUNCIL OF NURSES CODE OF ETHICS FOR NURSES

The fundamental responsibility of the nurse is four-fold: to promote health, to prevent illness, to restore health, and to alleviate suffering.

The need for nursing is universal. Inherent in nursing is respect for life, dignity, and rights of man. It is unrestricted by considerations of nationality, race, creed, color, age, sex, politics, or social status.

Nurses render health services to the individual, the family, and the community and coordinate their services with those of related groups.

Nurses and People

- The nurse's primary responsibility is to those people who require care.
- The nurse, in providing care, respects the beliefs, values, and customs of the individual.
- The nurse holds in confidence personal information and uses judgment in sharing information.

Nurses and Practice

- The nurse carries personal responsibility for nursing practice and for maintaining competence by continual learning.
- The nurse maintains the highest standards of nursing care possible within the reality of a specific situation.
- The nurse uses judgment in relation to individual competence when accepting and delegating responsibilities.

- The nurse, when acting in a professional capacity, should at all times maintain standards of personal conduct that reflect credit on the profession.

Nurses and Society

- The nurse shares with other citizens the responsibility for initiating and supporting action to meet the health and social needs of the public.

Nurses and Coworkers

- The nurse sustains a cooperative relationship with co-workers in nursing and other fields.
- The nurse takes appropriate action to safeguard the individual when care is endangered by a coworker or any other person.

Nurses and the Profession

- The nurse plays the major role in determining and implementing desirable standards of nursing practice and nursing education.
- The nurse is active in developing a core of professional knowledge.
- The nurse, acting through the professional organization, participates in establishing and maintaining equitable social and economic working conditions in nursing.

Moseley, & Vawter, 1989). They are both included in the medical record.

Living Will

A **living will** is a document that provides written instructions about when life-sustaining treatment should be terminated. Additionally, it may indicate when and if a person may be hospitalized and what types of treatment may be implemented. Some living wills may contain general statements requesting that no extraordinary means be used to extend life. The more general the statements, the more open they are to interpretation. California was the first state to recognize living wills with the passage of its Natural Death Act in 1976 (Hackler, Moseley, & Vawter, 1989).

Durable Power of Attorney for Health Care

A **durable power of attorney for health care,** also called a proxy directive, is a document that designates a person to make decisions about the client's medical

treatment in the event that the client becomes unable to do so. The designated person may be a family member, attorney, or friend who is aware of the client's wishes. Like the living will, the durable power of attorney for health care is most effective when the client has written specific instructions (Hackler, Moseley, & Vawter, 1989).

State laws and statutes may vary regarding advance directives. It is important for hospital policies and procedures to be developed and implemented in line with regulatory requirements and for you to become familiar with such policies and procedures.

Informed Consent

As described in Chapter 2, informed consent is a client's legal right to receive adequate and accurate information about his or her medical condition and treatment. Informed consent protects the client's right to autonomy by requiring him to receive information about a treatment or procedure and allowing him to accept or reject it. His consent must be given freely, without coercion. For example, it is essential that clients be given information in language they can understand. Clients must be capable of making health care decisions—that is, they must be mentally competent.

When these criteria have been met, the client's consent is obtained and documented in the medical record in the manner required by hospital policy and procedure. Keep in mind, however, that providing information does not in itself guarantee consent. The health care professional responsible for performing the procedure or prescribing the medical regimen is responsible for obtaining the informed consent (Beauchamp & Childress, 1996).

Institutional Ethics Committees

Institutional ethics committees are multidisciplinary committees of health care professionals within a facility that perform a variety of tasks related to ethical issues within that facility. Nursing is represented on such committees but usually is not in a majority and may only be represented at the administrative level. Ethics committees provide consultation, education, case review, decision-making, and mediation when conflicts arise between health care professionals in the identification and resolution of ethical dilemmas (Fig. 3–2). They are integral to the development of facility policies and procedures regarding ethics and to the implementation of such policies and procedures (Fowler & Levine-Ariff, 1987).

Nursing Ethics Forums

Heitman and Robinson (1997) describe a nursing ethics forum that can provide a mechanism for nurses to identify and address ethical issues that affect delivery of nursing care. These forums are separate from institutional ethics committees and may be hospital-wide or unit-based, involving nursing rounds or case review. Nursing ethics forums focus on assisting you in developing skills in ethical analysis and decision-

making. They may begin informally as discussions of issues that you have identified as ethical dilemmas.

Nursing forums can provide education in ethical theories, principles, and decision-making models. They can help you develop skills in ethical analysis and decision-making by

- Providing education in ethical theories, principles, and decision-making
- Providing a format for nurses to exchange ideas and talk about ethical issues
- Providing a mechanism for early detection of ethical dilemmas
- Creating a format for recommendations to the institutional ethics committee (Heitman & Robinson, 1997)

It is important that you be knowledgeable about concepts of ethical decision-making and able to articulate and apply such concepts in ethical dilemmas. The services of a clinician who has expertise in ethics should be obtained to provide the needed information and instruction.

In many health care settings, you are the primary practitioner with whom clients and families interact. As such, you may be the first to obtain information regarding clients' health care choices. Your nursing skills must include the ability to recognize potential and actual ethical dilemmas. Nursing systems must be able to provide support and direction to you in the deliberation and resolution of identified ethical issues in nursing practice (Heitman & Robinson, 1997).

Providing nursing care within an ethical framework is the cornerstone of professional nursing practice. To practice within such a framework, you must incorporate ethical principles and standards into your nursing behaviors.

KEY PRINCIPLES

- Ethical nursing practice is the cornerstone of professional nursing.
- In the delivery of health care, nurses are often required to make decisions that affect clients; therefore, it is important for nurses to recognize ethical dilemmas and apply ethical standards in resolving those dilemmas.
- Ethics is the branch of philosophy that attempts to determine what constitutes good, bad, right, and wrong in terms of human behavior. The study of ethics helps you determine the correctness of actions in situations that have ethical implications.
- Moral terms are often used to describe ethical behavior. However, morals are standards of behavior to which society expects members to adhere. Moral development requires imprinting of societal expectations about acceptable behavior. Nurses are expected to be moral agents who perform duties within established standards of moral conduct.

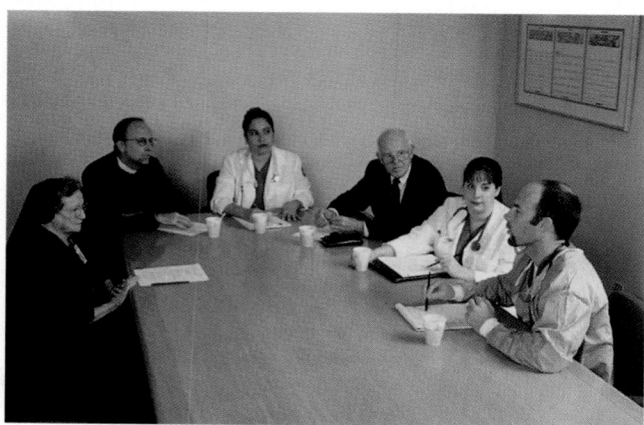

Figure 3–2. An ethics committee at work.

- Values are ideals and beliefs that are chosen and prized by an individual, group, or society. Values form the basis for ethical decision-making. Thus, it is important for nurses to clarify values because they provide the platform from which decisions are made and actions are taken.

- Ethical principles provide the framework for professional nursing and guide nursing actions during care delivery. The principles of autonomy, beneficence, confidentiality, nonmaleficence, fidelity, justice, and veracity are considered essential to nursing.

- In the United States, the American Nurses' Association Code for Nurses governs ethical nursing practice. The Code sets forth the philosophy of the profession and identifies the goals and values of nursing. The Code also provides a guide to ethical nursing practice and can be used to evaluate nursing actions.

- Nurses are responsible for providing care within acceptable standards and are accountable (answerable) for the outcomes of their actions.

- Models for ethical decision-making provide systematic and thoughtful mechanisms to examine issues and determine if ethical dilemmas exist. This systematic analysis helps you in clarifying a problem, identifying possible solutions and actions, and evaluating actions taken.

- Advance directives in the form of the living will and durable power of attorney for health care are methods of identifying client wishes about health care. They support client self-determination (autonomy), which is a key ethical principle. A client's written instructions allow health care providers to be informed about client choices.

- Other guides to ethical decisions in nursing include informed consent, which protects client rights; institutional ethics committees, which help in developing policies, procedures, and other duties related to ethical issues; and nursing ethics forums, which provide a means for nurses to address ethical issues and learn skills needed for ethical decision-making.

BIBLIOGRAPHY

*American Hospital Association. (1992). *Patient's bill of rights.* American Hospital Association: Author.

*American Nurses' Association. (1985). *Code for nurses.* American Nurses' Association: Author.

*American Nurses' Association. (1991). *Standards of clinical nursing practice.* American Nurses' Association: Author.

Beauchamp, T., & Childress, J. (1996). *Principles of biomedical ethics* (4th ed.). London: Oxford University Press.

Burkhardt, M., & Nathaniel, A. (1998). *Ethics and issues in contemporary nursing.* Albany, NY: Delmar Publishers.

Canadian Nurses Association. (1997). *Code of ethics for registered nurses.* Canadian Nurses Association: Author.

Chally, P.S. (1998). Ethics in the trenches: Decision making in practice. *American Journal of Nursing, 90*(6), 17–20.

Deloughery, G. (1995). *Issues and trends in nursing.* St. Louis: Mosby.

DeMarco, R. (1998). Caring to confront in the workplace: An ethical perspective for nurses. *Nursing Outlook, 46,* 27–32.

Federwisch, A. (1997). Making difficult daily choices: Ethics are everywhere. *Nurseweek, 10*(2), 1, 6.

*Fowler, M., & Levine-Ariff, J. (1987). *Ethics at the bedside: A source book for the critical care nurse.* American Association of Critical Care Nurses. Philadelphia: J.B. Lippincott Co.

Gordon, S., & Fagan, C. M.. (1998). Commentary: Preserving the moral high ground. *American Journal of Nursing, 98*(6), 31–32.

Hall, J. (1996). *Nursing ethics and law.* Philadelphia: W.B. Saunders.

*Hackler, C., Moseley, R., & Vawter, D. (Eds.). (1989) *Advance directives in medicine.* New York: Praeger.

Haynor, P. (1998). Meeting the challenge of advance directives. *American Journal of Nursing, 98*(3), 27–32.

Heitman, L., & Robinson, B. (1997). Developing a nursing ethics roundtable. *American Journal of Nursing, 97*(1), 36–38.

Hendin, H. (1999). Suicide, assisted suicide, and medical illness. *Journal of Clinical Psychiatry, 60*(Suppl. 2), 46–50; discussion 51–52, 113–116.

*International Council of Nurses. (1973). *Code for nurses: Ethical concepts applied to nursing.* International Council of Nurses. Geneva, Switzerland: Author.

*Jameton, A. (1984) *Nursing practice: The ethical issues.* Englewood Cliffs, NJ: Prentice-Hall.

McCloskey, J.C., & Grace, H.K. (1997). *Current issues in nursing* (5th ed.) (pp 297–302). St. Louis: Mosby.

Pinch, W. (1996). Is caring a moral trap? *Nursing Outlook, 46,* 130–135.

*Pojman, L. (1990). *Ethics: Discovery of right and wrong.* Belmont, CA: Wadsworth Publishing Co.

*Raths, L., Harmon, M., & Simmons, S. (1979). *Values and teaching.* Columbus, OH: Merrill.

*Rest, J.R. (1986). *Moral development: Advances in research and theory.* New York: Praeger.

Rice, V., Beck, C., & Stevenson, J. (1997). Ethical issues relative to autonomy and personal control in independent and cognitively impaired elders. *Nursing Outlook, 45,* 27–34.

Smith, R., Hiatt, H., & Berwick, D. (1999). Shared ethical principles for everybody in health care. *Nurs Stand, 13*(19), 32–33.

*Stewart, D., & Blocker, G. (1992). *Fundamentals of philosophy* (3rd ed.). New York: Macmillan Publishing Co.

Yoder Wise, P. (1995). *Leading and managing in nursing.* St. Louis: Mosby.

*Asterisk indicates a classic or definitive work on this subject.

CHAPTER 4

The Cultural Context of Practice

Cecilia A. Prado and Chyi-Kong Karen Chang

Key Terms

cultural competence
culture
diversity
ethnic
ethnicity
ethnocentrism

humanistic care
multicultural society
stereotyping
transcultural nursing
universality

LEARNING OBJECTIVES

After studying this chapter, you should be able to:

1. Discuss culture and ethnicity as they relate to the delivery of nursing care.
2. Define humanistic care.
3. Outline the elements and objectives of transcultural nursing.
4. Describe the dangers of stereotyping.
5. List and explain the six concepts included in transcultural assessment.
6. Understand basic aspects of the Irish-American, African-American, Mexican-American, Chinese-American, and Navajo cultures.
7. Anticipate the effects of cultural characteristics on the successful delivery of health care.

CONCEPTS OF CULTURE

Simple observation leads to the conclusion that, although people are all equal, they are not all alike. At least some of the differences among people stem from the behaviors, beliefs, and values learned from their families and other important members of the society around them. Indeed, these cultural and ethnic influences can make people seem very different from one another.

As a nurse, you must be able to transcend the differences among people. You must seek to understand clients of all cultural backgrounds and to provide them with care that enhances their individual health and well-being. To do so, you will need a sound understanding of the effects of culture and ethnicity. And you will need the ability to work comfortably with clients who hold different beliefs and values from your own.

Culture and Ethnicity

Culture can be defined as a patterned behavioral response that develops over time as a consequence of imprinting the mind through social and religious structures and intellectual and artistic manifestations (Giger & Davidhizar, 1995). Culture is shaped by the values, beliefs, norms, and practices held in common by members of the cultural group. It guides a person's thinking, doing, and being and becomes a patterned expression for that person (Giger & Davidhizar, 1995).

Madeleine Leninger, a nurse anthropologist, defines culture as the learned, shared, and transmitted values, beliefs, norms, and lifeways of a particular group that guide thinking, decisions, and actions in a patterned way (Leninger, 1991). Most definitions of culture imply a dynamic, ever-changing process through which a group defines itself through art, music, stories, and lifeways.

For most people, cultural background and ethnic background are intimately related (Spector, 1991). The term **ethnic** refers to groups of people of the same race or national origin within a larger cultural system who are distinctive based on traditions of religion, language, or appearance. A person's **ethnicity** reflects the characteristics a group may share in some combination (Box 4–1).

Multicultural Societies

The United States and Canada are examples of multicultural societies. A **multicultural society** is a society composed of more than one culture or subculture. It includes many groups that participate in and enjoy the larger culture. In such a society, the larger culture provides common interests and values. These shared interests and values help to create a social order that provides benefits to the society at large. In the United States, shared values include a democratic structure, equality among peoples, freedom of speech, and the right to the pursuit of happiness.

The United States contains more than 100 distinct

BOX 4–1

CHARACTERISTICS OF ETHNIC GROUPS

Primary Characteristics

An ethnic group shares one or more of the following:

- Race.
- Color.
- National or geographic origin.
- Religious beliefs.
- Cultural origin.

Secondary Characteristics

Group identity is evident in one or more of the following:

- A sense of identity as a group.
- Distinctive customs, art, music, literature.
- Elements of lifestyles.
- Language, accent, or dialect.
- Style or manner of dress.
- Food preferences, spices, methods of cooking.
- Attitudes derived from group identity.
- Moral values.
- Economic or political beliefs.
- Special political interests as a group.
- Health care practices.

---

ethnic groups and many more that maintain some characteristics of their origins. This is largely because the United States is home to immigrants from every country in the world. Some nations—such as Germany, England, Wales, and Ireland—are well represented. Others—such as Japan, the Philippines, and Greece—have smaller populations in the United States. People from around the world continue to enter the United States, particularly from Vietnam, Laos, Cambodia, Cuba, Haiti, and Mexico, and South and Central American countries (Spector, 1991).

Although the United States was founded and built by peoples from all parts of the world, the social emphasis before the 1960s was on creating a "melting pot" society in which all members would blend together and create a common culture. Various cultures have blended together through marriage, membership in social organizations and, sometimes, adoption. However, a homogenized society runs the risk of losing distinctive contributions from cultural subgroups. In the United States, although cultures have blended to some degree, many cultural groups have remained visible, intact, and a social force within the larger society.

The multicultural societies of the United States and Canada represent all of the cultural and racial groups of the world (Fig. 4–1). But the mix of cultural and ethnic populations is shifting. Experts project that by the

United States

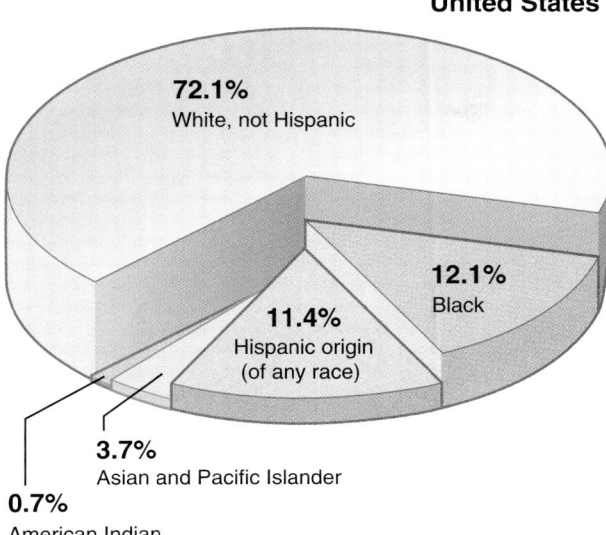

72.1%
White, not Hispanic

12.1%
Black

11.4%
Hispanic origin
(of any race)

3.7%
Asian and Pacific Islander

0.7%
American Indian,
Eskimo, and Aleut

Canada

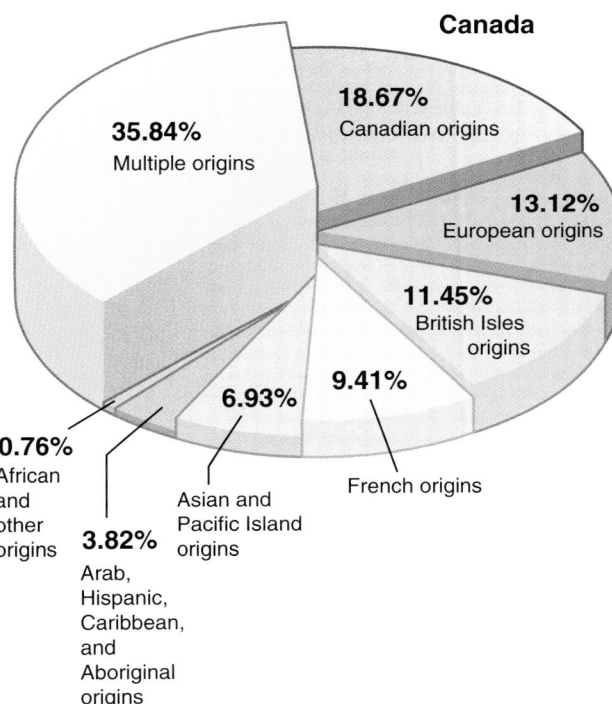

35.84%
Multiple origins

18.67%
Canadian origins

13.12%
European origins

11.45%
British Isles
origins

9.41%
French origins

6.93%
Asian and
Pacific Island
origins

3.82%
Arab,
Hispanic,
Caribbean,
and
Aboriginal
origins

0.76%
African
and
other
origins

Figure 4–1. Racial and ethnic distribution of the populations of the United States and Canada. (Data for the United States from U.S. Bureau of the Census, Population Division, release PPL-91, "United States Population Estimates, by Age, Sex, Race, and Hispanic Origin, 1990 to 1997"; ⟨http://www.census.gov/population/estimates/nation/intfile3-1.txt; data for Canada from Statistics Canada, "Total Population by Ethnic Origin, for Canada, 1996 Census (20% Sample Data)"; ⟨http://www.statcan.ca/english/census96/feb17/eo2can.htm⟩.)

year 2021 the number of Asian-Americans and Hispanic-Americans in the United States will triple, and the number of African-Americans will double (U.S. Dept. of Commerce, Bureau of the Census, 1992).

These projections have important implications for society as a whole—and nursing in particular—now

and into the next millennium. Recognizing the multicultural nature of society may be helpful in improving communication between groups and increasing the likelihood of peoples working together for common concerns and creating ways to solve societal problems. In health care, understanding the cultural context of care for multiple cultural groups will increase your ability to provide individualized care and to reorder health care institutions to meet the needs of diverse groups.

The challenge will be to provide culturally appropriate care to clients with widely diverse backgrounds. To be prepared to meet this challenge, you will need to learn about culture and to understand its relevance to competent care.

Transcultural Nursing

Nursing care is the element of the health care system that seeks to understand each client's unique perspective. Nurses try to understand health problems from the client's point of view. Thus, knowledge of the client's culture becomes a key to optimal client care. **Transcultural nursing** is culturally competent nursing care focused on differences and similarities among cultures, with respect to caring, health, and illness, based on the client's cultural values, beliefs, and practices (Leininger, 1991). To administer culturally appropriate care, you must avoid projecting onto the client your own cultural uniqueness and world view. You must remember that each person is a product of past experiences, beliefs, and values that have been learned and passed down from one generation to the next (Giger & Davidhizer, 1995).

Providing care within the framework of the client's culture can yield a number of benefits:

- Increased understanding of health care behavior that can be used as a basis for practice
- Improved health resulting from internally consistent health practices
- Improved compliance with the health regimen
- Increased satisfaction with services
- Creation of methods or techniques that may be useful cross culturally

Central to the concept of transcultural nursing is the concept of care as the essence of nursing. Care has many meanings, expressions, and forms. To "care for" another person is to take the person under your protection, to attend to the person's needs, or to be responsible for the person. The experience of being "cared about" is to experience empathy, comfort, and presence from another person. Caring has an action component and a component of connectedness between two people. The meaning of care or caring differs across cultures. To give care in the fullest sense of the word requires that you understand the meanings, attributes, characteristics, and practices of care in the context of the client's culture. "All human cultures have some forms, patterns, expressions, and structures of care to know, explain, and predict well-being, health, or illness status." (Leininger, 1991)

Transcultural nursing offers a way to provide humanistic care. **Humanistic care** includes understanding and knowing a client in as natural or human a way as possible while helping or guiding the client to achieve certain goals, make improvements, reduce discomforts, or face disability or death. The goal of a humanistic care is to gain full understanding of human beings and their humanity (Leininger, 1991).

Three elements important to recognize and mold when seeking to provide humanistic care are ethnocentricity, stereotyping, and cultural competence.

Ethnocentricity

Self-esteem means to hold yourself in high regard. Part of the self is produced by the cultural group with which a person identifies and from which the person learned how to behave and what to value. **Ethnocentrism** is the belief that one's own ethnic beliefs, customs, and attitudes are the correct and thus superior ones. Ethnocentricism includes positive regard for that part of yourself that is culturally based. Helping a child to develop self-esteem includes helping the child have pride in the culture that has shaped his life. Children who have pride in their cultural heritage have a good foundation for healthy self-esteem in adulthood (Fig. 4–2).

However, ethnocentrism also has negative effects. In a multicultural society, ethnocentric behaviors produce conflict between cultural groups. One way to overcome the conflict is to identify beliefs and values that are common across all cultures, even those expressed through different behaviors and customs. Social, political, and health care concerns may cross cultures as well.

All cultures have strengths and weaknesses. Strengths of a culture are those elements that enhance the life and well-being of the members of the group. Weaknesses are elements that can have detrimental effects on the group as a whole or on a significant number of people in the group. Most human characteristics can be a strength or a weakness, depending on the circumstances and the behaviors that result from the characteristic.

Stereotyping

The danger in having a little knowledge about culture is in believing that a little knowledge is enough to provide culturally competent care. Instead, it may lead to stereotyping. **Stereotyping** is the assumption that an attribute present in some members of a group is present in all members of a group. Usually, a stereotype is associated with a negative attribute, but not always.

For example, knowing that the Chinese use acupuncture to treat many ailments might lead you to assume that a Chinese-American client would be interested in or even prefer acupuncture as anesthesia for a minor surgical procedure. In reality, both traditional

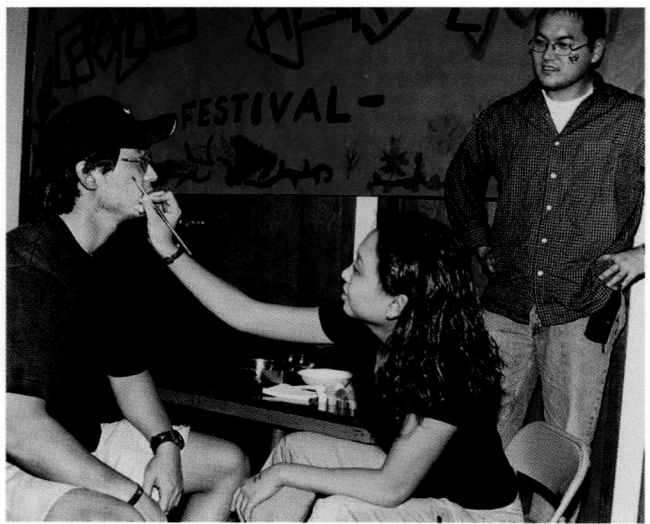

Figure 4–2. Healthy self-esteem in young adulthood is tied to appreciation of one's cultural heritage. These Korean-Americans demonstrate pride in their cultural heritage through participation in a cultural celebration.

and Western medicine is taught in Chinese medical schools, and many Chinese physicians would not use acupuncture.

If you assume that you know something about a person just because that person is Appalachian, Bostonian, Canadian, Mexican-American, male, or a nurse, you are stereotyping. This is a dangerous way of characterizing other people, even when the assumption turns out to be true. In trying to establish rapport, the process of getting to know the person may be as important as the actual knowledge of the person.

Cultural Competence

Cultural competence can be described as having enough knowledge of cultural groups that are different from your own to be able to interact with a member of a group in a manner that makes the person feel respected and understood. However, knowledge alone is not enough. You will need an attitude that values differences before you can see the strengths of a client whose values, beliefs, and behaviors differ from yours.

To be culturally competent, you must be willing to engage actively in seeking understanding of other peoples. Active engagement includes becoming sensitive to differences in styles of communication. You also must be willing to ask about a client's verbal responses and nonverbal behaviors to validate the messages you think you are receiving. And you must clarify your own values as a prerequisite to caring for clients of differing cultures (Table 4–1).

Because it is difficult to acquire enough knowledge of multiple cultures to fully understand the cultural perspective of every client you will encounter as a nurse, it is important to develop positive attitudes that are helpful in working with different peoples. Culturally competent practitioners have five attributes:

TABLE 4–1
Values Clarification: Providing Culturally Competent Care

Value	Related Actions
Make a commitment to providing culturally competent care.	• Make a commitment to providing the best nursing care possible in a manner that respects the values, beliefs, and lifeways of the person for whom you are caring. • Learn about other cultures so you can take a positive approach to their health practices and use group characteristics to improve health. You will see in other cultures what you expect to see; look for strengths. Health teaching is more successful when it builds on strengths. • Examine your own culture—not only the larger common culture but also specific subgroups to which you belong. Review your attitudes and beliefs about health, and objectively assess their origin and logic. • Examine biases, prejudices, and stereotypes that could contribute to ineffective nursing care. Plan ways to avoid the pitfalls that could harm the nurse-client relationship and lead to ineffective care. • Analyze your own communication (including facial expressions and body language) and how it may be interpreted.
Act in concert with the value of culturally competent care.	• Convey respect for the individual and respect for the individual's values, beliefs, and cultural practices. • Recognize that almost any human characteristic can be both a strength and a weakness, depending on the circumstances. • Recognize that cultural symbols and practices can bring comfort. • Support the client's practices, and incorporate them into nursing practice whenever possible.
Honor the value in differences.	• When you encounter different beliefs and values, reserve judgment until you can better understand the source of the beliefs and their meaning in the person's daily life. Do not assume that beliefs and values are wrong simply because they differ from yours. • Recognize differences in the ways clients communicate, and do not assume the meaning of a specific behavior (such as lack of eye contact) without considering the client's cultural background. • Relate your client's differing cultural beliefs to your own. In this way, you convey interest and respect for the client's beliefs.
Validate your perceptions of each client.	• Ask if a cultural practice is acceptable, desirable, or important. • Recognize individual differences. People vary within cultural groups and may make individual choices rather than follow traditional ways. • Learn how each client views health, illness, grieving, and the health care system. • Remember that clients may return to preferred cultural practices during illness; for example, the client who has learned English as a second language may revert to the primary language.

awareness, sensitivity, recognition, respect, and the ability to compromise.

AWARENESS. Awareness includes recognizing the values and beliefs of both your client and yourself. It therefore requires you to clarify your own values, as suggested above, and to actively seek to understand and appreciate the values of others. Thus, becoming aware requires an attitude of discovery, active listening, and the desire to learn.

It is normal to filter observed behaviors through your own values and beliefs. This filtering produces bias or preconceived beliefs about the meaning of behavior or about the beliefs of another person. Bias can be favorable or unfavorable, and it is not necessarily correct.

SENSITIVITY. Sensitivity means recognizing the possibility of different meanings of behavior and look-

ing objectively for cues that suggest the meaning. It also requires you to validate your interpretation with the client.

RECOGNITION. Recognizing the customs and behaviors of clients from different cultures requires knowledge. Obtaining that knowledge requires curiosity. You must have the desire to discover why you are seeing, hearing, or experiencing something about a client.

While you can gain a certain amount of knowledge from books, understanding will be enhanced when you live among and interact with persons of different cultures. Naturally, you will not be able to live among people from all the cultures that you will encounter in nursing practice. However, learning to recognize and value the differences of even one or two other cultures will heighten your observations of all cultures.

RESPECT. Respect may be the most important attitude to convey when working with persons of a different culture. When you respect others, you recognize and acknowledge their worth and uniqueness. You also recognize and honor the rights and privileges of those persons.

Respect dictates that you refrain from interfering with the beliefs and values of another. To develop respect, you must believe that there is value in diversity and then actively look for the value in lifeways that are different from your own.

COMPROMISE. You may need a willingness to compromise when a client's values and beliefs about health care, life, family, responsibility, or medical treatment differ from yours. An attitude of compromise implies that there is more than one right way to do anything.

DIVERSITY AND UNIVERSALITY. Another framework for developing cultural competence is Leininger's theory of diversity and universality. It postulates that "care or caring patterns include assistive, supportive, facilitative, and enabling acts or attitudes that influence the well-being or the health status of individuals, families, groups, and institutions as well as general human conditions" (Leininger, 1991). Caring acts and attitudes can be classified into those that are universal across cultures and those that are diverse. The term **universality** describes a common mode or value of caring or a prevailing pattern of care across cultures. **Diversity** refers to the differences in modes or patterns of care between cultures and includes specific patterns of care within cultural groups.

This model assigns three major modalities to guide culturally sensitive nursing care. *Cultural care preservation/maintenance* includes helping a client to continue cultural practices that have importance to the client. This may include using folk medicine, practicing religious rites, eating traditional cultural foods, or providing interpreters when the client's primary language is not the dominant language.

Cultural care accommodation/negotiation includes changing your behaviors or actions to be more fully understood and accepted by the client. This may include, for example, modifying your manner of addressing the client, extending visiting hours, or ensuring that the client is not interrupted during prayers or meditation.

Cultural care repatterning/restructuring includes helping the client change patterns of living that are not beneficial to healthy life patterns. An example is teaching the client different methods of food preparation, such as steaming or baking instead of frying with saturated fats.

TRANSCULTURAL ASSESSMENT MODEL

The Gigar and Davidhizar (1995) transcultural assessment model considers six cultural phenomena that may vary with application, yet are present in all cultural groups. These phenomena are communication, space, social organization, time, environmental control, and biological variations (Table 4–2).

Communication

Communication difficulties between people of different cultures involve more than speaking a different language. Misunderstanding also arises in the use of idiomatic language that may be peculiar to a dialect, region, or social group. For example, the word "croaked" is slang for "died," and it does not have the same meaning when translated to another language. Nor is it understood by people who have no experience in the social context in which the phrase is commonly understood.

Even nonverbal communication can lead to misunderstandings. Gestures, facial expressions, and body language may carry different, commonly understood meanings in different cultures. Also, clients from different cultures may misinterpret gestures that Western

TABLE 4–2
Elements of Transcultural Assessment

Element	Definition
Communication	A continuous process by which one person may affect another through written or oral language, gestures, facial expressions, body language, space, or other symbols.
Space	The area around a person's body that includes the individual body, surrounding environment, and objects within that environment
Social organization	The aggregate of family and other groups within a society that dictates culturally accepted role behaviors and rules of behavior. Behaviors are prescribed for such significant life events as birth, death, childbearing, and illness.
Time orientation	A person's focus on the past, the present, or the future. Most cultures include all three time orientations, but one orientation is more likely to dominate the cultural perspective.
Environmental control	The perceived ability of an individual or persons from a particular cultural group to plan activities that control nature, such as illness causation and treatment.
Biological variations	Biological differences among racial and ethnic groups may include physical characteristics, such as skin color, and physiological variations, such as lactose intolerance.

From Giger, J., & Davidhizar, R.E. (1995). Transcultural nursing: Assessment and intervention. St. Louis: Mosby.

nurses use to convey empathy and caring. For example, actions such as gentle touch on the hand, maintaining eye contact, or smiling and nodding can feel intrusive, disrespectful, or dismissive to certain clients.

Space

Personal space includes a person's body and the space around the body. The level of discomfort generated when personal space is invaded is highly personal but is also related to culture. Americans, Canadians, and Britons require considerable personal space. Latin Americans, Japanese, and Arabs need a smaller amount of personal space (Watson, 1980). In American society, close personal space is generally reserved for intimate friends or family and is related to the amount of trust one has in another person. Personal space can be used to meet the needs of security, privacy, autonomy, and self-identity.

Three categories of personal space describe our physical distance from others. The intimate zone is within 18 inches of the body. The intimate zone is used when comforting, protecting, or counseling, and it is reserved for people who have a close personal bond. The personal zone is 18 inches to 3 feet from the body and is maintained with friends and some counseling sessions. The social zone is 3 to 6 feet from the body and is used for impersonal business being conducted with people who are working together.

You have probably noticed that you usually begin a nurse-client relationship in the social zone and then move to the personal zone as the relationship is established. Of necessity, you enter the intimate zone when you are providing personal care and therapeutic treatments. Most clients intuitively understand and accept this level of personal space in a health care environ-

ment. However, you cannot assume that all clients will feel this way. Space varies among cultural groups.

Social Organization

Social organization refers to family structure and organization, religious beliefs, and the group's participation in social activities. Among most cultural groups in the United States, the family is the basic unit of organization. However, there is a great deal of variety in the nature and structure of family relationships. For example, many Latin American families have grandparents, aunts, uncles, and cousins in important roles. Similarly, Native Americans have a tribal organization of which the nuclear family is a subunit.

Time

Time can mean many things. It typically refers to measurements, as in the period between one sunrise and the next or the passage of years or decades. Time can also refer to duration, such as how long a person has to complete a task or how long a movie lasts. Time can also refer to specific appointments, such as the time for a meeting or the time to take a medication.

Cultures vary in their awareness of time and how they use this awareness in managing their lives. For some people, time is now. These people are more likely to focus on the task at hand as though there is nothing else to do, giving full attention to the task for as long as it takes to complete. Other people compartmentalize time. These people are more likely to set a specific amount of time for a task and work to get it done in that amount of time.

Additionally, people may be described as past-, present-, or future-oriented (Table 4–3). Culture is only

TABLE 4–3
Selected Consequences of Time Orientation

Orientation	Possible Consequences
Past-oriented	• When traditions conflict with a prescribed treatment regimen, the person may have trouble accepting or maintaining the plan of care. • In contrast, a strong connection with the past may ground the person with others in the same culture and provide a sense of self that encourages positive health practices.
Present-oriented	• A present-oriented person may have little concern for long-term preventive health practices and may respond better to short-term goals. • In contrast, a present-oriented person may be most able to enjoy the here-and-now and may engage fully in exercise, enjoy nutritious food, and appreciate the company of others—all attributes associated with good health.
Future-oriented	• This person has little focus on the difficulties and inconveniences of the present, focusing instead on future goals. • The present is important only if what is happening now will help the person realize long-term goals. • This person may have little trouble following a treatment plan as long as its benefits are clear. • However, the person may have great difficulty dealing with chronic illnesses for which no complete cure is known. • A future-oriented person naturally tends to become more of a present-oriented person with age because, as the future life becomes shorter, the present becomes more important.

one of many factors that influence time orientation. For example, the death of a loved one often focuses a person on the past. Parents who have lost a child may be unable to engage in the present or plan for the future. Poverty focuses a person's attention on the present. Involvement in social, political, or educational activities may focus a person exclusively on the future. Such a person may neglect his or her health in order to achieve the long-term goal. In short, people are found within all cultures who are variously oriented to the past, to the present, and to the future.

Environmental Control

Environmental control refers to both the perception of control over the environment and to methods used to control the environment. Environmental control can be seen in a culture's attitude toward nature and in its commitment to preserving the natural environment. But the environment can also include health care, religion, work, and governmental organizations.

A person's perceived ability to control the environment depends on whether he operates primarily from an internal locus of control or an external locus of control. People with an internal locus of control feel empowered to influence their environment. People with an external locus of control are more likely to believe that events are primarily due to chance, fate, or luck. They may feel helpless to change their environment or circumstances. These people may readily relinquish control to others, allowing you or doctors, for example, to make decisions for them.

Biological Variations

Biologically, humans of all races are the same, with minor variations in skin color, facial features, and body size. These variations provide enough commonality in a given group of people to allow grouping. Genetic variations that produce different health problems in different race are uncommon but do exist. For example, Tay-Sachs disease is more common in people of Jewish ancestry. Thalassemia, a blood disorder, is more common among people of Mediterranean descent. Sickle cell disease is more common among African-Americans.

Most illnesses that are more common in particular groups can be traced to environmental and lifestyle factors. Nevertheless, knowledge of culture is sometimes useful in identifying the lifestyle variables that contribute to disease. It is also useful to direct screening programs at groups that have a high incidence of a particular illness.

UNDERSTANDING SPECIFIC CULTURES

For the most part, a person belongs to a cultural group because he was born into that group. However, culture is partly a matter of choice. An adult may choose to continue to closely identify with the group to which

his parents belonged, or he may adopt the ways of the larger culture around him. This second choice may have benefits but also carries the risk of inducing a feeling of alienation from the part of himself that came from cultural teachings and lifeways. This may require the person to know not only to what group he belongs but also the degree to which he identifies with that group.

The following descriptions provide highly generalized information about certain subgroups of larger cultural groups. Irish-Americans are a subset of white-skinned people of European descent. African-Americans are a subset of black-skinned people. Mexican-Americans are a subset of the rapidly growing Hispanic culture. Chinese-Americans are a subset of the Asian or Oriental culture. Navajos are a subset of the American Indian culture.

Remember that these descriptions may not apply to each person who belongs to each subgroup. Brief descriptions cannot capture the rich cultural heritage and subtle patterns of behavior that are commonly understood in a given culture. Nevertheless, these descriptions may provide a beginning step in your goal of providing culturally competent care.

European-Americans

European-Americans include people whose cultural identity is based on known European ancestors and white people who cannot identify their ethnic origins. This latter group makes up roughly half of the American population (Sowell, 1981). Richard Alba (1990) suggests that European-Americans are in the process of forming a new ethnic group based on the individual's consent to belong rather than on descent. Many of the members of this cultural group have their roots in a combination of European countries, including Germany, England, Italy, Ireland, and others.

European-Americans cannot be understood entirely through considering the whole. Whereas many have integrated into the larger society and are less aware of the influence of their roots, their diverse and multiple origins continue to shape the differences in response to illness and health care seen among the descendants of European-American groups. Additionally, some pockets of European groups have retained a specific cultural identity.

Irish-Americans are an example of a group for whom assimilation has been more the norm than maintaining cultural identity. In 1960, more than half of Irish-American men married outside their cultural group. Today, descendants of the original Irish immigrants identify themselves as Irish-American, as members of other cultural groups, or claim no specific cultural identity. About 16 million people of Irish descent reside in the United States, a figure that represents about 7% of the population (U.S. Dept. of Commerce, Bureau of Census, 1992).

With assimilation into the cultural mainstream of U.S. society, Irish-Americans have gained economic and educational mobility. They are more likely to be professionals or managers and less likely to be laborers, service workers, or factory workers (Blessing, 1980) than were earlier Irish immigrants. Irish-American income is 5% above the national average and their years of schooling are about the same as those of the national average.

Irish immigrants include two distinct groups. The Scotch Irish arrived during the colonial period. They were predominately Protestant and were culturally distinct from the Celtics, who immigrated in the later 19th and early 20th century. When we talk about Irish-Americans today, we are more likely to be describing the Irish Catholics of Celtic origin.

Between 1815 and 1920, 5.5 million Irish immigrated to the United States, largely to escape economic hardship in Ireland. The great potato famine in Ireland in 1845 prompted a massive migration of Catholic Irish, who were largely poor, unskilled laborers; women; children; and elderly. These immigrants did not have the resources to migrate beyond the northeastern cities where they landed. The men took the most menial, difficult, and dangerous jobs, and the women worked as household servants. Westward migration was associated with jobs building canals and railroads. Irish immigrant laborers were often in conflict with other immigrant labor groups, especially the Chinese.

By the early 20th century, second- and third-generation Irish-Americans had moved into white collar jobs. Women were secretaries, nurses, and teachers. Men were skilled laborers, policemen, and firemen. The high percentage of Irish policemen and firemen resulted from political favors granted by officials elected through block voting in the Irish community. Although the Irish had not been well known for an interest in education, higher education became a means of upward mobility for many Irish-Americans. The history of the Irish in America resulted in a belief that assimilation was the route to success in America.

Communication

Although the official language of Ireland is Irish (Gaelic), the British domination of Ireland forced the people to speak English. English is recognized as the second official language and is universally spoken throughout Ireland. About 27% of the population knows both Irish and English (Giger & Davidhizar, 1995). Historically, the Irish had an advantage over other immigrants because of the high percentage who spoke English. Among more recent immigrants, Gaelic may be the spoken language. Learning English is more difficult for the older adult or the adult who is not required to work outside the home.

"Craic" is an Irish expression for good, fun conversation among equals. Irish-Americans are good company because they are often warm, sociable people, with family and friends being an important part of their lives. Wit and humor are a prominent part of

communication that adds to their sociability. The "gift of gab" or "blarney" includes storytelling, laughter, and conversation. Weaving the truth into mythical stories is considered an Irish art form (Sullivan, 1997).

Space

Personal space is associated with the expression of affection. One difficulty noted in Irish-American males is openly expressing love and affection (Giger & Davidhizar, 1995). Some may have more difficulty in expression with close family members than with more distant persons. Others may express feelings easily with a close group but not with persons who are more distant.

When a crisis such as illness occurs, maintaining cultural ties is manifested through heavy dependence on extended family ties. Entrance into the personal space may be reserved for family and others who can honor and understand the cultural perspective (Fallows, 1979).

Social Organization

A repeated theme among Irish-Americans is the significance of family and family structure. Close family bonds exist. Some Irish-Americans tend to delineate roles and behaviors within the family according to gender. Irish-American women may view their role as primary caretaker of the family. When they are ill, their role is greatly compromised. Intermarriage between Irish-American families in the United States is one of the clearest distinctions of social acceptance and social equality in the community. Bachelors and spinsters are infrequent in the Irish-American community.

Irish-Americans have enjoyed a significant rise in the political arena in the United States. This resulted primarily from their strong sense of group solidarity, their fluency with the spoken word, and their personal charm.

Religion and religious views are of paramount importance to some Irish-Americans in maintaining the social integrity of the individual. The lack of recognition of the significance of religious beliefs may serve to augment problems and difficulties encountered with illness (Giger & Davidhizar, 1995).

Time

The Irish are descended from the Celtic tribal culture going back to 3000 B.C. Ancient Celtic tradition is one of individual freedom and personal responsibility. Some Irish-Americans have a high sense of valuing the preservation of their Irish culture and therefore are past-oriented. Indeed, many have a strong allegiance to the past, worship their ancestors, and have a strong family tradition. This is evident in the attitude that nothing happens in the present or will ever happen in the future because it all happened in the far-distant past. Persons in the dominant culture may find it difficult to understand the respect that Irish-Americans have for tradition, and at the same time some Irish-Americans do not appreciate the typical American disregard for tradition (Giger & Davidhizar, 1995).

Environmental Control

Irish-Americans are perceived as having an external locus of control. They tend to cling to a past-oriented value orientation regarding the family and family relationships and tend to consider past values and traditions to be of paramount importance to future growth and development.

Ignoring bodily complaints appears to be a culturally prescribed and supported defense mechanism for some Irish-Americans. The use of the defense mechanisms of ignoring and denying seems to be the typical way of coping with psychological and physiological needs (Giger & Davidhizar, 1995).

Some Irish-Americans may subscribe to folk medicine beliefs that can be perceived as neutral health practices (neither having benefit nor producing harm). Examples are "blessing of the throat" and the wearing of religious medals to prevent illnesses. For some Irish-Americans, the first level of intervention for illness is often home treatment. They may believe that a physician should be seen only in an emergency. Some folk practices may be viewed as beneficial, such as getting plenty of rest and going to bed early, enjoying fresh air and sunshine, and exercising.

Biological Variations

Irish-Americans have been ranked the highest or near the highest in terms of heavy alcohol intake. The use of alcohol is influenced by a variety of factors, including patterns and characteristics of the family and social and economic conditions. Some Irish-Americans drink for reassurance and to escape what is viewed as an intolerable burden.

African-Americans

The term African-American has become popular as a descriptor that suggests pride in a cultural heritage that is a combination of African and American. It can mean the descendants of people who were brought to America as slaves or more recent immigrants from Africa. The earlier term Black American suggested group pride and is still used by some African-Americans to describe their cultural group. The term African-American places the emphasis on cultural heritage, whereas the term Black American emphasizes biological racial identity. African-American will be used in this chapter as a means of emphasizing the cultural characteristics.

African-Americans include immigrants from African countries, the West Indian Islands, the Dominican Republic, Haiti, and Jamaica. The largest importation of slaves to America from the west coast of Africa occurred during the 17th century. The African-American heritage includes courage, persistence, fortitude, and bravery in maintaining human dignity and family solidarity in the bonds of human slavery and its aftermath.

Communication

The African-American dialect is a product of the English learned by slaves from different tribes, different languages thrown together, and the mixing of languages. The syntax and grammar in part reflect the English dialect of southern white Americans. When slavery ended, it was a long time before formal education was available to African-Americans in the United States. Thus, patterns of speech developed that are somewhat unique to African-Americans. The dialect or variation within a language spoken by African-Americans is sufficiently different from standard English in pronunciation, grammar, and syntax as to be classified as "Black English" (Giger & Davidhizar, 1995).

The use of standard English versus Black English varies among African-Americans and may be related to educational level and socioeconomic status. Some speakers move between standard and Black English as though fluent in two languages. The dialect continues to evolve. As with non–English-speaking people, the use of Black English may be one factor that creates educational difficulties among school children.

However, the use of Black English may be a unifying factor for African-Americans in maintaining their cultural identity. It is common for African-Americans to speak standard English when in a professional or social setting with other cultural groups and then revert to Black English in African-American settings. African-Americans who are not comfortable with standard English may become quiet and noncommunicative in mixed social settings.

Most African-Americans use Black English in a systematic way that can be predictably understood by other persons; thus, Black English should not be regarded as substandard or ungrammatical. Some African-Americans use colorful and dynamic speech along with facial gestures, hand and arm movements, expressive stances, handshakes, and hand signals.

When caring for an African-American client, it is important to understand as much of the dialect as possible to gain insight into the culture. You should be cognizant that Black English is an effective means of communication that expresses thoughts in a manner unique to the culture of African-Americans. Thus, it is important for you to avoid labeling and stereotyping the client (Box 4–2).

Space

African-Americans tend to be comfortable with a close personal and social space, at least when interacting with members of their own group. They have a much higher involvement ratio than other cultural groups,

BOX 4–2

STRATEGIES FOR COMMUNICATING WITH CLIENTS FROM DIFFERENT CULTURES

- Take a little extra time to establish a level of comfort between you and the client.
- Ask questions in an unhurried manner. Rephrase a question, and ask it again if the answer seems inconsistent with other information the client has provided.
- Observe for cultural differences in communication, and honor those differences. Use eye contact, touch, and seating arrangements that are comfortable for the client.
- Ask the client about the meaning of health, illness, treatments, and planned care. Investigate how his illness is likely to affect his life, relationships, and self-concept. Find out what he considers to be the cause of his illness. Ask how he prefers to manage illness.
- To establish a therapeutic relationship, listen to the client's perception of his needs, and respect his perspective.
- Listen actively and attentively; try not to anticipate the client's response.

- Talk to the client in an unhurried manner that considers social and cultural amenities.
- Give the client time to answer.
- Use validation techniques to verify that the client understands. Remember that smiles and head nodding may indicate that the client is trying to please you, not necessarily that the client understands you.
- Sexual concerns may be difficult for clients to discuss. Having a nurse of the same sex may facilitate communication.
- Use alternative methods of communication, such as a foreign language phrase book, an interpreter, gestures, or pictures, for clients who do not speak English.
- Learn key phrases in languages that are commonly spoken in your community.

such as German-Americans or Scandinavian-Americans (Giger & Davidhizar, 1995). If you are from a culture where social personal space is larger, you may need to adjust to working in a more intimate personal space when caring for highly involved individuals.

Social Organization

African-Americans tend to be socialized in predominantly African-American environments. Historically, because of prejudice and legalized segregation, African-Americans were isolated from the mainstream of society. Assimilation into mainstream society has been slow because of continued racial prejudice and a desire to build the solidarity of a strong African-American community in predominantly African-American neighborhoods, churches, and schools.

The African-American community has maintained a core of strength through its churches and schools that can be expected to continue as a force in solving the problems of the African-American community. Religion is taken very seriously, and many African-Americans actively participate in church-related activities and believe strongly in the power of prayer.

The family structure of African-Americans in the United States includes the male-headed (patriarchal) family structure and the female-headed (matriarchal) structure. More than half of African-American families have a female head of household. The matriarchal family structure evolved in part because the male historically has had difficulty in gaining employment sufficient to meet the needs of the family. The African-American woman is responsible for maintaining and

protecting the health of family members. Large family networks or community groups, such as churches, provide support during times of crisis and illness.

Grandmothers tend to play an active role in the lives of the African-American family. In fact, children may be raised by grandmothers. Grandmothers may assist with financial support. And they may be actively involved in the care of an ill child. Including a grandmother in the plan of care, therefore, can be of vital importance.

Time

While the perception of time among African-Americans is difficult to characterize, many African-Americans are more present-oriented than past- or future-oriented (Purnell & Paulanka, 1998). Time, especially social time, may be perceived as flexible, but African-Americans can be very time-conscious and take pride in punctuality. Social events often start when everybody arrives and end when everybody leaves, rather than having a set time schedule.

Connections with the past are maintained through the rich heritage of storytelling by elders. They share stories about the family both from the immediate and the distant past. Younger African-Americans may be more future-oriented but are taught to honor the life experiences of the elders.

Environmental Control

The definition of health for many African-Americans stems from African beliefs about life and the nature of being. The Africans believed that life was process rather than a state (Spector, 1991). The nature of a person is viewed in terms of energy force rather than matter. When one possesses health, one is in harmony. Many African-Americans believe in the power of some to heal and help others (McQuay, 1995).

Traditional healers are usually women who use herbs and roots to treat illness. The reliance on healers reflects the deep religious faith of African-Americans. Some belief in voodoo or hoodoo is still present. Health is maintained with proper rest, diet, and a clean environment. Treating illness through prayer and laying on of hands is practiced in some religious groups. Home remedies and folk medicine are used by some African-Americans, and local hospitals are avoided except in extreme emergencies. Fear of hospitals has grown out of lack of access to health care facilities and a continued concern that equal treatment will not be offered.

Lack of access to health care services, low income, and the tendency to self-treat and wait until symptoms become severe tend to increase the morbidity rate among African-Americans (McQuay, 1995). An African-American may perceive receiving health care as degrading or humiliating, and some fear or resent heath care centers. They tend to feel alienated by the system and experience a sense of powerlessness. Some clients may feel they are being "talked down to" by the health care providers and that providers fail to listen to them. Consequently, they choose to "suffer in silence." When a treatment or special diet is prescribed, you must ascertain whether it is consistent with the client's needs, cultural background, income, and religious practices. The treatment plan and rationale must be shared with the client, and it is important that the client understand what is being prescribed.

Biological Variations

The main biological variations for African-Americans are skin color, facial features, and hair texture. Skin color is the most distinctive characteristic among people of different races. It is determined by the amount of melanin or pigment in the skin. Among African-Americans, skin color may vary from a light or "almost white" color to a very dark brown. Melanin provides protection from the effects of the sun. African-Americans and other dark-skinned people have a lower incidence of skin cancer than white-skinned people.

Hypertension is common among African-Americans; they have a higher mortality rate than other groups. Sickle cell disease and lactose intolerance are genetic disorders prevalent in African-Americans; other diseases and disorders common to this culture include cancer, cardiovascular disease, cirrhosis, and diabetes.

African-American children have a tendency to weigh less at birth and be shorter than their white counterparts. These facts may result more from poverty that biological makeup. You must carefully evaluate the growth status of African-American children.

Hispanic-Americans

Members of the Hispanic-American community have their origins in Spain, Cuba, Central and South America, Mexico, Puerto Rico, and other Spanish-speaking countries. This ethnic community is very diverse. It includes people with black skin and people with white skin. Hispanic-Americans are the fastest growing minority group in the United States. The Mexican-American subgroup is one of the most prominent.

Most Mexican-Americans reside in Texas and California. In early U.S. history, Mexican-Americans helped build many southwestern cities. Settlers learned skills such as mining, farming, and ranching. Most Mexican-Americans have remained close to the region of the country that was settled by their ancestors (Giger & Davidhizar, 1995). As new immigrants arrived, they have tended to gather in these areas as well. However, Mexican-Americans have also migrated as farm workers to other areas of the country.

Many Mexican-Americans can trace their ancestry back to Indian groups such as the Incas and Mayas, who developed complex Mexican civilizations before the arrival of the Spanish explorers. Many Mexican-Americans are a blend of both Indian and Spanish European cultures (Giger & Davidhizar, 1995).

Mexican-Americans have been successful at retaining a unique cultural identity within the dominant culture, unlike early European immigrants, who assimilated into the overall U.S. culture. Traditional gender and family roles continue to be part of the heritage that separates Mexican-Americans from other cultural groups. Some Mexican-Americans are well educated, whereas others are migrant workers who move around the country seeking work when crops need to be harvested.

Communication

For many Mexican-Americans, Spanish is the primary language. This language is spoken in many dialects and differs widely among Hispanic groups. Mexican-Americans place a high value on diplomacy and tactfulness (Murillo, 1978) and communicate in a manner that avoids direct confrontation and arguments, which are considered rude and disrespectful. Through the use of elaborate, often indirect communication, the Mexican-American tries to accomplish a communication goal while maintaining politeness and respect. Self-disclosure is avoided with strangers, including health care professionals. In communicating, Mexican-Americans may incorporate the use of senses as well as words, and they are characterized as tactile in their relationships.

Most Mexican-Americans can speak some English, but they may use it selectively. It is not uncommon to use English in the workplace and Spanish at home or with friends. Children of newer immigrants who have not yet mastered English may have a hard time in school. In general, Mexican-American children are more likely to grow up bilingual than European-American children in the same regions. In health care situations, you may observe a client speak to his family in Spanish, to you in English and, when very stressed, to both his family and you in a mix of both English and Spanish.

Space

Mexican-Americans prefer consistent, close relationships and physical touching. They demonstrate a great need for group togetherness. However, there is a strong social value that women not expose their bodies to men or even to other women. A female nurse should always assist a male physician in examining a female client and guard against exposing the client's body parts other than those that are the focus of the examination (Murillo-Rohde, 1977). Men also have strong feelings regarding modesty and may feel threatened if expected to have a complete physical examination (Murillo, 1978).

Social Organization

The strength of the nuclear family (parents and children) is the foundation of the Mexican-American community. For most Mexican-Americans, extended family relationships have special significance, and the family may be the most significant social organization (Murillo, 1978). The Mexican-American family takes pride in family accomplishments and usually does not seek help from outsiders to meet needs or resolve problems. Men assume the dominant role of breadwinner and decision-maker. Even though women often work at jobs outside the home, women also assume the role of homemaker.

Time

Mexican-Americans may be characterized as primarily present-oriented. They may be reluctant to incorporate the distant future into their plans. Thus, you may have difficulties in implementing long-term health care measures. Also, their perceptions of acute and chronic illness may be affected.

Environmental Control

Mexican-Americans are more likely to perceive an external locus of control. They may perceive life as being under the influence of a divine will. There may also be a fatalistic belief that one is at the mercy of the environment and has little control over what happens (Giger & Davidhizar, 1995).

Some Mexican-Americans may view health as purely the result of "good luck" or a reward from God for good behavior. Individuals are expected to maintain their equilibrium in the universe by conducting themselves in the proper way, eating the proper foods, and working the proper amount of time. The prevention of illness is an accepted practice that is accomplished with prayer, the wearing of religious medals or amulets, and keeping relics in the home. Illness may be viewed as an imbalance in the individual's body or as a punishment for wrongdoing.

Some Mexican-Americans believe that an imbalance may exist between hot and cold or wet and dry. These forces are embodied in four body fluids (or humors): blood, which is hot and wet; yellow bile, which is hot and dry; phlegm, which is cold and wet; and black bile, which is cold and dry. When all four humors are balanced, the body is healthy. When an imbalance occurs, an illness is present. If an illness is categorized as hot, it is treated with a cold substance. A cold disease, in turn, must be treated with a hot substance. The classification of what is a hot disease or a cold disease varies from person to person.

Within the Mexican-American folk medicine system, the *curandero* is the folk healer (Fig. 4–3). The *curandero* views illness from a religious and social context rather than the scientific perspective that dominates Western society (Giger & Davidhizar, 1995). The *curandero* is a holistic healer and can be either female or male.

In the folk medicine system, illness may be caused by *susto* (fright), *mal ojo* (evil eye), *envidia* (envy), or *empacho* (gastrointestinal ailment). The most popular form of treatment by folk healers involves herbs, especially when used as teas. Treatments may also include massage, cleanings *(limpias)*, diet, rest, prayers, and supernatural rituals. Rituals include elements of both Catholic and Pentecostal rituals and artifacts: money offerings, confession, candle-lighting, wooden or metal offerings in the shape of anatomic parts *(milagros)*, and laying on of hands. The *herbero* is a folk healer who specializes in the use of herbs and spices for preventive and curative purposes. *Brujos* (male witches) and *brujas* (female witches) are another level of healers. They practice black magic and may not be sought until other forms of healing have been tried.

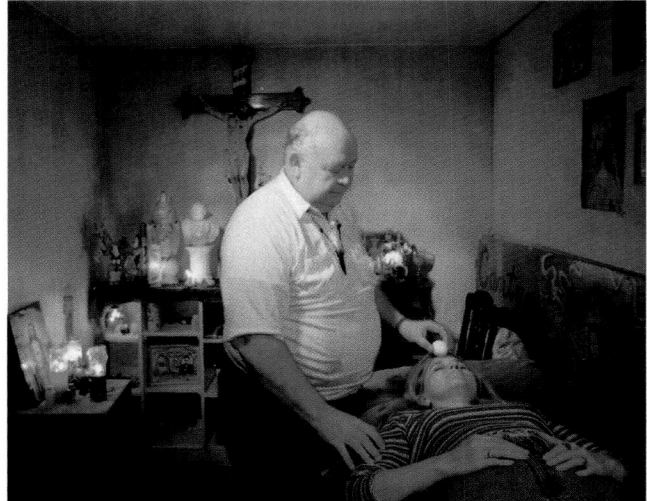

Figure 4–3. Within the Mexican-American folk medicine system, the *curandero* is the folk healer.

Roman Catholicism is the predominant religion practiced by Mexican-Americans. During times of crises, Mexican-Americans may rely on a priest or prayers. Rituals, such as making promises, lighting candles, or visiting shrines, may be practices when a family member is ill.

Biological Variations

The skin color of Mexican-Americans may vary from a natural tan to a dark brown. Those with lighter skin color have more Spanish ancestry; those with darker skin have more Indian ancestry.

The incidence of diabetes among Mexican-Americans is five times the national average, and complications are more frequent. Multiple health problems are of special concern in the Mexican-American population. Hypertension is also found more often among Mexican-Americans. Urban, elderly Mexican-Americans are at risk for many age-related chronic health conditions associated with migrant status, lower levels of education, nutrition, and poverty. Alcoholism is also a crucial health problem among Mexican-Americans (Giger & Davidhizar, 1995). Men are most often affected, because the male role may be correlated with the ability to ingest large amounts of alcohol.

Asian-Americans

Asian-Americans numbered 7.3 million in 1990, and estimates put the population at about 20 million by the year 2020 (Russell, 1996). In 1990, 24% of the Asian-American population was Chinese-American. Chinese-Americans are immigrants and their descendants mainly from Taiwan, Hong Kong, and mainland China.

Chinese-Americans have various degrees of acculturation. Some adhere to Chinese culture, some adopt both cultures, and some adapt entirely to American culture (Chang, 1995). To assess the effect of Chinese culture on the health status and health care behaviors of Chinese-Americans, you should assess communication styles, English proficiency, interpersonal interactions, social support systems, health care practices, the use of Chinese medicines, and biological variations pertinent to Chinese-Americans (Chang, 1995; Grossman, 1996).

Also assess the effect of religious practices on coping with illness. Many religions exist among Chinese-Americans, such as Buddhism, Taoism, Christianity, Islam, and beliefs in myths, fortunes, and worship of ancestors and deified heroes. When they are ill, Chinese-Americans may practice one or more religions to help themselves get well. Respect these practices as long as the client's faith does no harm to health.

The teachings of Confucius form a primary force in Chinese culture. Confucius is a Chinese sage who established rules and codes of ethics for personal and interpersonal behaviors to maintain order and harmony in society. Lao Zi, another Chinese sage, greatly influenced Chinese medicine (Box 4–3). Confucius encouraged people to pursue the virtues of loyalty to family, friends, and the government. He also encouraged filial piety to parents, love, faithfulness, righteousness, and peacefulness. Confucius emphasized harmonious relationships with nature and each other. He suggested accommodating rather than confronting and seeking group consensus rather than advocating individual concerns. A person is expected to demonstrate these virtues, to exert self-control, to be self-reliant, and to behave modestly. Otherwise, one brings shame to one-

---

BOX 4–3

PRINCIPLES OF CHINESE MEDICINE

A Chinese sage named Lao Zi developed a religion called Taoism and influenced the fundamental principles and practices of Chinese medicine (Reid, 1993). Taoism hypothesizes that two opposing and interacting forces—yin and yang—exist in the universe and in the body. Yin is a negative, recessive, female force. Yang is a positive, dominant, male force. In Chinese medicine, a balance between yin and yang yields optimal health. Imbalance between these two forces results in disease (Chang, 1995; Reid, 1993).

The underlying principle of Chinese medicine is to maintain and restore the balance between yin and yang forces in the body. Food, symptoms, diseases, and medicine are classified into yin and yang groups. Yang symptoms or diseases are treated with yin foods and medicines. Yin symptoms or diseases are treated with yang foods and medicines. For example, yang symptoms in-

clude a red complexion, restlessness, thirst, constipation, dark urine, and nervousness. They are treated with foods that have yin qualities, such as oranges, limes, watermelon, and cucumber. Yin symptoms include coldness, loose stools, clear urine, a poor appetite, pallor, and fatigue. They are treated with foods that have yang qualities, such as lamb, beef, chicken, ginger, chili, and peanuts (Chang, 1995; Reid, 1993).

Chinese medicine also believes that an invisible life force or energy, called *qi* (pronounced chee), moves around the universe and within the body. The circulation of *qi* and the quality and quantity of *qi* determine the yin-yang balance. Many forms of exercise, external therapies, and herbal medicines are used to promote the circulation of *qi*, maintain the yin-yang balance, and restore health (Reid, 1993).

self, family members, and society. (Chinese call this "lose face.") Consequently, Chinese-Americans may be group-oriented (Hall, 1976), tending to conform to the group and avoiding conflicts or being different from other people. Chinese-Americans may seem quiet, unassertive, agreeable, and pleasant. They may suppress the exhibition of negative emotions, such as anger, sadness, worry, and depression (Chang, 1995).

Communication

English proficiency and communication styles affect Chinese-Americans' interaction with health care providers and the health care delivery system. Those who are not fluent in English and not familiar with medical terminology or health care services may hesitate to seek medical care until they are very ill. Once Chinese-Americans are in the health care delivery system, they may experience an undue amount of stress. They may not understand their health condition and may be unable to express their concerns or needs. Even when able to express concerns, they may be misunderstood.

To reduce clients' stress, you may help them in the following ways:

- Find a translator who can speak the same dialect as the clients or use family members who are fluent in English to help clients understand their health status and care.
- Use plain and simple English to explain things to the client; avoid jargon or medical terms.
- Provide written materials in addition to verbal information to facilitate clients' and family members' understanding.
- Find resources that are written in Chinese to help clients understand.

During the process of acculturation, some Chinese-Americans may feel shame and develop low self-esteem and feel helpless, powerless, and depressed because of their limitations in English and reduced social support. The Chinese culture emphasizes self-control and self-reliance. Thus, a Chinese-American may feel shame in verbalizing emotional and social problems. The person may only verbalize physical symptoms. You can help by using therapeutic communication skills to identify psychosocial problems underlying physical symptoms (Chang, 1995).

Chinese communication styles tend to be covert and highly contextual (Hall, 1976). Chinese-Americans use implicit, subtle, and indirect communication styles. During communication, they perceive not only explicit information but also implicit clues, such as facial expression, body movements, the use of physical space, gestures, and tone of voice. Because Confucius' teachings emphasize harmonious relationships, respect for elders and authoritative figures, and discourage individual opinions, Chinese-Americans may avoid direct conflicts and may not express their disagreement. If they do, it is considered shameful: they "lose face." Instead, Chinese-Americans may express disagreement in a nonverbal way. They may lose eye contact, change subjects, or appear reluctant (Chang,

1995; Grossman, 1996). When they dislike or disagree with a health care provider, they may switch to another health care provider rather than confront the original one. When communicating with Chinese-Americans, assess their communication style, be sensitive to nonverbal communication clues, and encourage them to verbalize any questions, concerns, or disagreements.

Space

In studies of human spatial relationships, Hall (1976) classified Chinese-Americans as the noncontact group. They tend to maintain a distance between individuals. They have less physical touch and eye contact and speak softly in a controlled tone. Too close a distance, excess touch, too much eye contact, and loud voices may be viewed as impolite or offensive. During nurse-client interactions, if you need to provide care that requires close proximity, frequent touch, or direct eye contact, you should explain yourself to ease the client's feeling of discomfort (Chang, 1995). Also, keep in mind that female Chinese clients prefer to have female nurses and may be uncomfortable with a male nurse. If a female client is assigned a male nurse, she may not verbalize her feelings of discomfort. Instead, she may seem shy, withdrawn, or uneasy.

Social Organization

Chinese-Americans tend to have a hierarchy in the social and family structure. Husbands and elders have authority over wives and children. Elders and people in authoritative positions are highly respected. Chinese culture expects children to take care of their parents when they grow up. If children do not take care of their parents, the parents may feel shame and consider the children disloyal to their family.

Under the influence of democracy and American culture, Chinese-Americans may challenge traditional social structure and values. They may become individual-centered rather than group-centered. They may alter the line of authority in the family. The conflicts between traditional values and American culture may create stress. Some stress may cause physical symptoms and psychological problems. For example, some elder immigrants may lose a sense of respect because they depend on their children for financial, physical, and psychosocial support. As a result of this dependence on their children, the elder immigrants may experience loneliness and emotional isolation. However, they may complain only about problems with sleep or appetite because they may be ashamed to admit emotional problems (Mackinnon, Gien, & Durst, 1996). Some may further develop mental illnesses and commit suicide (Tien-Hyatt, 1987).

When caring for Chinese-Americans, assess their family structure, the line of authority, and social support. You may include family members in the plan of care. You may also involve the person who is authoritative to the client to help the person reach therapeutic goals. To identify psychosocial problems, encourage the client to express thoughts and feelings without feeling shame. For a client with limited social support, help identify available community resources to increase the client's sense of self-reliance and self-esteem (Chang, 1995).

Time

Chinese-Americans perceive time as a dynamic wheel around the past, present, and future (Chang, 1995). They may interpret present events by correlating them with past or future happenings, intuitive understanding, symbolic meanings, and association with fate or myths. For example, to schedule an elective surgery or cesarean section, they may select a lucky day according to a special Chinese calendar. Some may seek divine guidance from a religious temple. Some may wear lucky charms on the neck, wrists, and ankles to ward off evil spirits. Assess whether these practices have any harmful effects on the client's health. If not, seek ways to accommodate them.

Environmental Control

Chinese culture does not emphasize control of the environment but rather maintenance of a harmonious relationship with nature and balance in life. To maintain health, some Chinese-Americans may perform traditional Chinese exercises, such as *tai chi, qi-kung*, or others, to facilitate the flow of *qi* and the yin-yang balance within the body. They believe that fresh air is important for quality *qi*. They usually exercise early in the morning in the park while the air is fresh. They may also prefer to keep windows open to allow the flow of fresh air instead of using air-conditioning (Chang, 1995; Chen, 1996).

When Chinese-Americans are ill, several types of problems may occur. One is that the person may take both Western medicines and Chinese herbal medicines, both of which may have similar effects. Caution the client about overmedication and suggest not taking both types of medicines together.

Some Chinese-Americans may save prescribed medications for later use. They may be afraid of drug side effects or of using too much of the drug. They may not see the need to continue taking medication when they do not feel ill anymore. This practice may be detrimental to health, especially when the medicine is insulin, an antihypertensive drug, a corticosteroid, and so on. Teach clients about medications, and emphasize the importance of taking them as prescribed, without stopping or self-regulating. Encourage the client to work with health care providers for any problems related to medicines.

Some Chinese-Americans may observe the yin-yang quality of foods and eat only foods that can balance the yin-yang quality of their diseases. For example, when post partum (yin quality), some Chinese-Americans may only drink warm milk or hot water (yang quality) and will not drink or eat anything cold (yin quality). Respect this belief, and help the client obtain the preferred foods and drinks.

Some Chinese may use external Chinese medicine, such as acupuncture, moxibustion, skin-scraping, or suction-cupping, to promote the circulation of *qi* and to restore health. Acupuncture uses hair-thin needles inserted into special points. This procedure may leave no marks and has been reported to control pain effectively (Compton's Interactive Encyclopedia, 1996).

Other procedures may produce skin lesions. For example, moxibustion involves placement of a burning moxa (an herb) over vital points. A crater about 1 cm in diameter on the skin may develop. Skin-scraping involves scraping skin firmly at selected points with a blunt spoon or coin until bright red stripes appear. Multiple linear bruises over the neck, the bridge of the nose, along the spine, or over the chest may be observed. Suction-cupping involves the use of an ignited cotton swab inside a glass cup that is quickly placed on a treatment site to create suction. The suction cup is left on the skin 15 to 20 minutes. Circular lesions about 2 inches in diameter may be observed as a result (Boyle & Andrews, 1989; Louie, 1985; Reid, 1993; Spector, 1991). When these lesions are present, do not mistake them as physical abuse. Do provide care as needed to prevent infection.

Biological Variations

Several symptoms or diseases are genetically linked to Chinese-Americans. Mongolian spots (bluish pigmentation, usually at coccyx area) are often observed among Chinese infants. They should not be mistaken as bruises.

More than half of Chinese babies develop neonatal jaundice. The bilirubin level usually peaks at 5 or 6 days (Boyle & Andrews, 1989). Prepare Chinese-American mothers before discharge to be aware of jaundice, and teach them ways to reduce or treat it.

Chinese-Americans typically weigh less than Caucasians. Their drug metabolism may also be different from that of Caucasians. They may develop side effects or toxic effects when they take the dosages usually prescribed for Caucasians. You need to observe if lower dosages are needed to reduce side effects (Chang, 1995; Louie, 1995).

High incidences of lactase deficiency, thalassemia deficiency, and G6PD deficiency have also been reported among the Chinese (Chang, 1995). After drinking milk, some Chinese-Americans may experience abdominal cramps, diarrhea, or flatus. Thus, they may avoid drinking milk. With long-term use, their bodies may develop the enzyme.

Thalassemia deficiency causes rapid red blood cell destruction. Clients require monthly blood transfusions for life. If both parents are thalassemia carriers, infants or mothers may develop complications, such as stillbirth or preeclampsia (Anionwu, 1996).

G6PD deficiency may result in anemia because of rapid red blood cell destruction when some Chinese-Americans take certain drugs (Chang, 1995). Screening for these deficiencies and providing information and genetic counseling are the best preventive care.

Chinese-Americans are at high risks for hepatitis B, tuberculosis, nasopharyngeal cancer, esophagus cancer, stomach cancer, and liver cancer (Chang, 1995; Louie, 1995). The consumption of fermented, moldy, and pickled foods may contribute to the development of esophageal and liver cancers (Chang, 1995). Crowded living arrangements may be one of the contributing factors for tuberculosis. To help Chinese-Americans, you may provide them information about these diseases to reduce their risk and to help them identify these diseases at an early stage.

In summary, when caring for Chinese-Americans, you need to assess the impact of Chinese culture and beliefs on their health status and health care behaviors to help them deal with physical and psychosocial problems, to screen for genetic disorders, and to reduce high-risk diseases.

American Indians

There are about 200 American Indian tribes in the United States, and they are concentrated primarily in western states as the result of forced westward migration. Although many Native Americans live on reservations and in rural areas, just as many live in cities, especially those on the west coast. Oklahoma, Arizona, California, New Mexico, and Alaska have the largest numbers of Native Americans (Spector, 1991). The term Native American implies tribes residing in the continental United States. One of the largest tribes is the Navajo, and elements of their culture are discussed here.

Communication

Many Navajo use English as their primary language, but many are fluent both in the Navajo language and in English. Naturally, those who do not speak English will require the assistance of an interpreter when seeking or receiving health care.

Rather than shaking hands, as is common among many Americans, Navajos tend to extend a hand and lightly touch the hand of the person being greeted. The Navajo culture holds a taboo against touching a dead person or an animal killed by lightning. Consequently, a Navajo client or family member may prefer not to touch articles associated with a dead person or animal.

The Navajo people may appear silent and reserved when first meeting strangers. Warm behavior may be demonstrated once the Navajo individual becomes familiar with you (Giger & Davidhizar, 1995). In the Navajo culture, eye contact is considered a sign of disrespect.

Space

In the Navajo culture, personal space is very important and has no imaginary boundaries. Consequently, Navajo clients may have difficulty adapting to circumstances that place them in unfamiliar spaces. You must familiarize the client with the space provided during hospitalization when personal space is limited.

Social Organization

The Navajo culture is very family-oriented, and the definition of family may have no limits of number or relationship. Navajo people believe that family members are responsible for each other. Therefore, it is not unusual for many relatives to come to the hospital to care for a Navajo client. Decision-making is mutual. The goal of the family is to help its members grow, share resources, and participate in daily activities and significant life events, such as birth, death, marriage, and sickness.

The Navajo culture is neither dead nor static but instead is a living culture, retaining its heritage and advancing with the times. Navajo members may join with other tribes and share their songs and dances as reminders to the Indian people of their old ways and rich heritage. Dancers have always been a very important part of the life of the American Indian (Fig. 4–4). Although dance styles and content have changed, their meaning and importance has not.

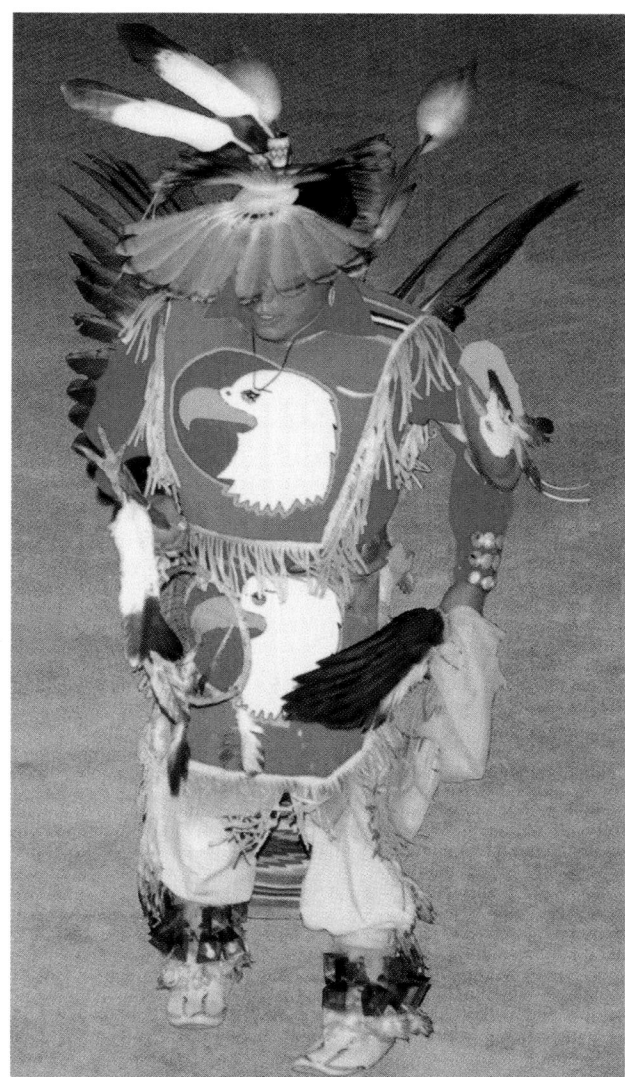

Figure 4–4. Dancers have always been a very important part of the life of the American Indian.

Time

Navajo Indians are viewed as being primarily present-oriented. Time is viewed as a continuum, with no beginning and no end (Primeaux, 1977). Navajo time is casual and relative to present needs that must be accomplished in a present time frame. When a Navajo moves from the reservation to an urban area, a feeling of stress occurs from the cultural conflict concerning time. This conflict is common in health care settings because some Navajos tend to be late for appointments.

Environmental Control

The traditional Navajo belief about health is that it reflects living in total harmony with nature and having the ability to survive under exceedingly difficult circumstances. Illness is viewed as a price being paid for something that happened in the past or for something that will happen in the future. Everything is the result of something else.

Native Americans do not subscribe to the germ theory of medicine. Illness is something that must be. The cause of disease or injury to a person or property, or of continued misfortune of any kind, must be traced back to an action that should not have been performed. Examples of such infractions are breaking a taboo or contacting a ghost or witch. To the Navajo, the treatment of an illness must be concerned with the external causative factors and not with the disease or injury itself (Spector, 1991).

The traditional healer of the Navajo is the medicine man. He is a person wise in the ways of land and nature. He knows the interrelationships of human begins, the Earth, and the universe. He knows the ways of the plants and animals, the moon, and the stars. The medicine man takes his time to determine, first, the cause of the illness, followed by the proper treatment. To determine the cause and treatment of an illness, he performs special ceremonies that may take up to several days. Navajos may rely on traditional tribal medicine, the "white man's medicine," or a combination of both. Conflicts can occur in families when there are different degrees of acceptance for scientific medical treatments.

Navajos may be suspicious of people of European descent. Initial reluctance may dissipate when a health professional respects the client's opinion and demonstrates a sensitivity to the client's point of view. Nurses and caregivers must avoid "interviewing" Navajos to gain information. Often, simply listening helps the person overcome concerns about interacting with health care providers of a different culture.

Biological Variations

Today, Navajos are faced with a number of health problems. Health care skills inherent in the Navajo traditional ways of diagnosing and treating illness have not fully survived the migration and changing ways of life of the Navajo. Because of the loss of these skills and because modern health care centers are not always available, Navajos are frequently in limbo when it comes to obtaining appropriate health care. Additionally, at least a third of Navajos live in abject poverty. With poverty comes poor living conditions, malnutrition, tuberculosis, and high maternal and infant death rates. In 1996, the leading causes of hospitalization for Navajo clients were obstetrical deliveries; accidents, including motor vehicle accidents; respiratory diseases; diseases of the genitourinary system; mental disorders; diseases of the circulatory system; skin diseases; and diseases of the endocrine system (U.S. Dept. of Health and Human Services, Indian Health Service, 1997).

Type II diabetes mellitus is a major health problem for Navajos. It tends to occur early, in the teens or early twenties. As a result, complications also occur early, leading to excessive mortality in the early and middle adult years. According to the U.S. Department of Health and Human Services (1997), the age-adjusted death rate is on the rise (1997). No one knows why diabetes is prevalent among Navajos.

KEY PRINCIPLES

- In a multicultural society, distinct cultural groups retain cultural identity and contribute to the overall society the strengths and lifeways of the group.
- Stereotyping is an unhelpful tendency to assume that an attribute present in some members of a group must be present in all members of the group.
- Culture includes the values, beliefs, norms, and practices shared by a particular group that guide thinking, decisions, and actions in a patterned way.
- Six elements by which to describe cultural diversity are communication, space, social organization, time, environmental control, and biological variation.
- To communicate with persons of other cultures, you should respect each individual's values, beliefs, and cultural practices.
- Communication requires validation that all parties in the communication have been understood.
- There is perhaps as much variation within cultures as between cultures.
- Culturally competent nursing care requires understanding the health care setting from the client's point of view.

REFERENCES

*Alba, R.D. (1990). *Ethnic identity: The transformation of White America.* New Haven, CT: Yale University Press.
Anionwu, E.N. (1996). Sickle cell and thalassaemia: Some priorities for nursing research. *Journal of Advanced Nursing, 23,* 853–856.

*Asterisk indicates a classic or definitive work on this subject.

*Blessing, P. (1980). Irish. In S. Thernstrom (Ed.), *Harvard encyclopedia of American ethnic groups*. Cambridge, MA: Belknap Press.

*Boyle, J.S., & Andrews, M.M. (1989). *Transcultural concepts on nursing care*. Glenview, IL: Scott, Foresman.

Bureau of the Census. (1993). *We, the American Asians*. Washington, D.C.: U.S. Government Printing Office.

Chang, K. (1995). Chinese Americans. In J.N. Giger & R.E. Davidhizar (Eds.) *Transcultural nursing: Assessment and intervention*. St. Louis: Mosby.

*Chen, C.L., & Yang, D.C.V. (1986). The self-image of Chinese-American adolescents: A cross-cultural comparison. *International Journal of Social Psychiatry, 32*(4), 19–26.

Chen, Y.D. (1996). Conformity with nature: A theory of Chinese American elders' health promotion and illness prevention processes. *Advanced Nursing Science, 19*(2), 17–26.

Compton's Interactive Encyclopedia (CD-ROM). (1996). Carlsbad, CA: Compton's New Media, Inc.

*Fallows, M. (1979). *Irish Americans*. Englewood Cliffs, NJ: Prentice-Hall.

Giger, J., & Davidhizar, R. (1995). *Transcultural nursing, assessment and intervention* (2nd ed.). St. Louis: Mosby.

Grossman, D. (1996). Cultural dimensions in home health nursing. *American Journal of Nursing, 96*(7), 33–36.

*Hall, E.T. (1976). *Beyond culture*. New York: Anchor Press/Doubleday.

Leininger, M. (1991). *Culture care diversity and universality: A theory of nursing*. New York: National League for Nursing Press. Pub. No. 15-2402.

*Louie, K.B. (1985). Providing health care to Chinese clients. *Topics in Clinical Nursing, 7*(3), 18–25.

Louie, K.B. (1995). Cultural considerations: Asian-Americans and Pacific Islanders. *Imprint, 42*(5), 41–44, 46.

Mackinnon, M.E., Gien, L., & Durst, D. (1996). Chinese elders speak out. *Clinical Nursing Research, 5*(3), 326–342.

McQuay, J.E. (1995). Cross-cultural customs and beliefs related to health crisis. *Critical Care Nursing Clinics of North America, 7*, 581–594.

*Murillo, N. (1978). The Mexican American family. In C.A. Hernandez, M.J. Haug, & N.N. Wagner (Eds.), *Ethnic nursing care: A multicultural approach* (pp 115–148). St. Louis: Mosby.

*Murillo-Rohde, I. (1977). Care for all colors. *Imprint, 24*(4), 29–32, 50.

*Primeaux, M. (1977). Caring for the American Indian patient. *American Journal of Nursing, 77*, 91–94.

Purnell, L.D., & Paulauka, B.J. (Eds.). (1998). *Transcultural health care: A culturally competent approach*. Philadelphia: F.A. Davis.

Reid, D.P. (1993). *Chinese herbal medicine*. Boston: Shambhala Publications, Inc.

Russell, C. (1996). *The official guide to racial & ethnic diversity*. Ithaca, NY: New Strategist Publications, Inc.

*Sowell, T. (1981). *Ethnic America: A history*. Basic Books.

Spector, R.E. (1991). *Cultural diversity in health and illness*. Norwalk, CT: Appleton & Lange.

Stokes, L.G. (1977). Delivering health services in a Black community. In A.M. Reinhardt & M.B. Quinn (Eds.), *Current practice in family-centered community nursing* (pp 51–65). St. Louis: Mosby.

Sullivan, M. (1997) The Hidden People. http://home.earthlink.net/~maireidsullivan/craig.html

*Takaki, R. (1993). *A different mirror: A history of multicultural America*. Boston: Little, Brown and Co.

*Tien-Hyatt, J.L. (1987). Self-perceptions of aging across cultures: Myth or reality? *International Journal of Aging and Human Development, 24*(2), 129–148.

U.S. Department of Commerce, Bureau of Census. (1992). *Population estimates and projections*. (Publication No. 25-1024). Washington, D.C.: U.S. Government Printing Office.

U.S. Department of Commerce, Bureau of Census. (1992). *Population projections of the United States by age, race, and Hispanic origin: 1990 to 2050* (Publication No. 25-1095). Washington, D.C.: U.S. Government Printing Office.

U.S. Department of Commerce, Bureau of Census. (1993, June 12). News release, *Commerce News*. Washington, D.C.: U.S. Government Printing Office.

U.S. Department of Health and Human Services, Indian Health Service. (1997). *Trends in Indian Health*. www.ihs.gov/PublicInfo/Publications/trends97/trends97.asp.

U.S. Department of Health and Human Services, Public Health Service, National Institutes of Health. (1982). *Diabetes in the 80s*. Report of the National Diabetes Advisory Board. Washington, D.C.; U.S. Government Printing Office.

Walch, J. (1994). *Immigrant America: European ethnicity in the United States*. New York: Garland Publishing, Inc.

*Watson, O.M. (1980). *Proxemics behavior: A cross cultural study*. The Hague, Netherlands: Mouton.

*Asterisk indicates a classic or definitive work on this subject.

The Health Care Delivery System as a Context for Practice

Kathleen A. Ennen

Key Terms

access

ambulatory care center

diagnosis-related group

exclusive provider organization

health maintenance organization

hospice

managed care

Medicaid

Medicare

preferred provider organization

prospective payment system

LEARNING OBJECTIVES

After studying this chapter, you should be able to:

1. Compare and contrast the four types of health care services.

2. Identify health care personnel and describe their training, roles, and responsibilities.

3. Discuss inpatient, outpatient, and community settings for the delivery of health care.

4. Compare and contrast the various types of health care financing, including private insurance, managed care organizations, and government insurance plans.

5. Discuss the effect of demographic and economic factors on the delivery of effective and affordable health care.

6. Identify legal and ethical issues in health care delivery.

7. Discuss various opportunities in health care delivery, including health care reform, technological progress, environmental challenges, and quality improvement.

The American health care delivery system may be viewed in several different ways. Economists may see it as a huge service industry consisting of public and private businesses providing health care services to consumers. Legislators may see it as a drain on public funds and therefore ripe for reform. Social theorists may claim that the system is the property of all citizens, who should be granted universal availability and coverage. Consumers, such as the parents of a child with a serious illness, may view the health care delivery system as a beneficent domain where their child will be nurtured and healed. Each of these descriptions reflects a different perception of the vast, complex system that has evolved for health care delivery in the United States today.

This chapter describes the health care delivery system and current methods of health care financing. It explores some social and economic factors affecting health care, the legal and ethical issues involved in contemporary health care delivery, and some opportunities and advances in health care for the 21st century.

SCOPE OF HEALTH CARE SERVICES

The biomedical model—which presumes the existence of illness or disease—has largely governed health care delivery in the United States. The multiple components of this complex delivery system work together to produce and provide health care services for persons, groups, and communities. There are four major types of health care services: health promotion and illness prevention, diagnosis and treatment, rehabilitation, and supportive care. Each of these will now be discussed.

HEALTH PROMOTION AND ILLNESS PREVENTION. *Health promotion* aims to modify a client's knowledge, attitudes, and skills to adopt behaviors leading to a healthier lifestyle. *Illness prevention* involves the use of immunizations and medications that prevent disease and health screenings that detect disease in its earliest, most treatable stages. Health promotion begins at a client's level of wellness on the continuum of health-illness (Shi & Singh, 1998).

It is difficult to clearly differentiate the concepts of health promotion and illness prevention because health care providers do not use the same models of health and illness. What's more, illness prevention can occur simultaneously with health promotion activities. You approach health promotion and illness prevention with your clients—persons, families, groups, and communities—with jointly developed specific goals of care.

There is ample evidence to suggest that the overall improvement in general health of the past few decades owes less to medical care as such than to positive health behaviors and improved environmental quality. The best national plans for health progress have primarily emphasized illness prevention and health promotion (McBeath, 1991).

DIAGNOSIS AND TREATMENT. Until recently our health care system emphasized diagnosis and treat-ment. Early diagnosis of illnesses has been the focus of physicians' work. Technological advances have allowed physicians to diagnose illnesses far sooner and treat them more effectively than in the past. However, the emphasis on high technology may cause clients to feel the providers' focus is on the machine or procedure at the expense of the person. As a nurse you will be called upon to help your clients understand their diagnosis and treatment and help them participate in their own treatment plans.

REHABILITATION. Many acute illnesses and injuries leave clients with residual physical or mental impairments that affect their ability to function normally. Rehabilitation provides therapies to either restore a client's lost functioning or maintain the remaining levels of physical and mental function and prevent further deterioration (Shi & Singh, 1998).

Rehabilitation activities are applied to a wide range of health problems, such as stroke, joint replacement, burns, or spinal cord injury, which can occur on an acute, chronic, or time-limited basis. Each client's unique goals and needs determine which care providers are needed on the multidisciplinary team. The success of the rehabilitation plan depends on skilled coordination by nurses and active involvement by the client.

SUPPORTIVE CARE. Supportive care is provided to clients still in need of therapy after treatment for acute or chronic illness or are terminally ill. Supportive care includes medical, nursing, psychological, and social services (Andersen, Rice, & Kominski, 1996). This care can be provided in a hospital, a nursing home, a hospice, or in the client's home setting and aims to meet the physical, emotional, and spiritual needs of the client and the family. The objective is to help clients achieve the highest level of functioning permitting the greatest degree of independence and participation in their community.

HEALTH CARE PERSONNEL

In 1994 about 10.6 million people (1 out of every 10 American workers) were employed in health care. Half, 5.3 million, work in hospitals (National Center for Health Statistics [NCHS], 1996). Although physicians remain the most prominent members of the health care system, many other specialties have evolved to participate in today's multidisciplinary team approach to care. Primary members of the health care team include nurses, physicians, and physician assistants. Allied members of the health care team include therapists/technologists and technicians/assistants, pharmacists, alternative practitioners, social workers, and spiritual and religious personnel. Their clinical work is meant to complement the work of physicians and nurses. Many of these allied health workers receive specialized training and education. Currently, allied health workers constitute approximately 60% of the health care workforce in the United States (NCHS, 1996).

REGISTERED NURSES. Nurses are the largest single group of health care professionals in this country. The evolving health care system has created the need for nurses in many specialties. After hospitals, nurses primarily work in long-term care facilities, rehabilitation centers, governmental public and private agencies, schools, ambulatory care centers, and nursing education. The majority of nurses have associate degrees or hospital-based nursing school diplomas. About 600,000 nurses hold baccalaureate degrees, and 160,000 have achieved graduate degrees. There are about 755 Registered Nurses per 100,000 in the U.S. population (NCHS, 1996).

Registered nurses focus on health promotion and disease prevention and are major care providers for sick and injured clients. They may also work as nurse educators, nurse researchers, clinical nurse specialists, and infection control nurses, and they serve as resources for others involved in direct care delivery.

PHYSICIANS. Physicians are the major providers of health services. All states require physicians to be licensed to practice. The number of physicians has steadily increased from 14.1 per 10,000 population in 1950 to 25.2 per 10,000 population in 1994 (Jonas, 1998).

Physicians practice in a variety of settings and arrangements. Some work in hospitals as staff physicians. Others work for federal or state government agencies, public health clinics, community health centers, and prisons. Most physicians are office-based group practitioners.

Increasingly, physicians are specializing. Physicians trained in family medicine, general internal medicine, and general pediatrics are considered primary care providers or generalists. Board certification in a specialty requires additional years of training and a specialty board examination. Common medical specialties include cardiology, dermatology, family medicine, neurology, obstetrics and gynecology, ophthalmology, pediatrics, psychology, radiology, and surgery. Primary care physicians may refer clients to specialists based on evaluation of the client's medical needs.

PHYSICIAN ASSISTANTS. Physician assistants are not meant to be a separate profession such as nursing. The American Academy of Physician Assistants (1996) defines a physician assistant (PA) as "a member of the healthcare team who works in a dependent relationship with a supervising physician to provide comprehensive care." PAs are able to provide care to clients and perform certain medical procedures only under the supervision of a licensed physician. The major services provided by PAs include evaluation, monitoring, diagnostics, therapeutics, and referrals. Physician assistants practice in a variety of settings including physicians' offices, hospitals, ambulatory care centers, nursing homes, government agencies, and community health centers. In 1996 about half of the PA population worked in family practice.

Physician assistants train in one of 80 accredited programs in the United States (AAPA, 1996). Most of these programs grant a baccalaureate degree upon graduation. The National Commission on Certification of Physician Assistants provides PAs with their certification after completion of education and clinical experience requirements.

THERAPISTS, TECHNOLOGISTS, TECHNICIANS, AND ASSISTANTS. Allied health workers can be divided into two broad categories: therapists/technologists and technicians/assistants (NCHS, 1996). Formal requirements for allied health workers range from certificates gained after high school to postgraduate degrees. *Technicians and assistants* are prepared in less than 2 years to perform procedures. They require supervision from therapists or technologists to evaluate the treatment process and its effectiveness. *Therapists and technologists* receive more advanced training. They learn to evaluate clients, diagnose problems, and develop treatment plans. Education for therapists and technologists includes self-development of teaching procedural skills to technicians and assistants (Jonas, 1998).

PHARMACISTS. These professionals have had a traditional role as dispensers of medications prescribed by physicians, dentists, and podiatrists and as advisors on the proper selection and use of medicines. Today, pharmacists also provide education and advice about specific drugs, drug interactions, and generic drug substitution. A pharmacist today takes an active role on behalf of clients by assisting providers in making appropriate drug choices, by effecting distribution of medications to clients, and by assuming direct responsibilities collaboratively with other health care professionals and with clients to achieve the desired therapeutic outcome (American Council on Pharmaceutical Education [ACPE], 1992). All states require licensing of pharmacists, who must be graduates of an accredited pharmacy program, successfully complete a state board examination, and complete a supervised internship (Marcrom, Horton, & Shepherd, 1992).

ALTERNATIVE PRACTITIONERS. This diverse group has become increasingly prominent in recent years. In 1990, 34% of Americans used alternative therapies or complementary medical practices, paying an estimated $10.3 billion out-of-pocket for these treatments (Ernst, 1996). The percentage of clients may have increased to more than 40% today. Client visits amount to 425 million, more than 40 million more visits than to primary care physicians (Gordon, 1996). Viewed by many with skepticism and often labeled as quackery, alternative therapies are still uncommon in typical health care settings, but acceptance is growing, as explained in the accompanying Considering the Alternatives chart. Nontraditional or alternative therapies include homeopathy, herbal formulas, acupuncture, therapeutic touch, and biofeedback. Even meditation imagery, massage, spiritual guidance, and prayer are often included in discussions of nonconventional and alternative therapy options. The use of dietary changes and vitamin supplements to prevent and/or treat health problems is gaining increased acceptance (Neimark, 1997; Gordon, 1996).

CONSIDERING THE ALTERNATIVES
COMPLEMENTARY AND ALTERNATIVE MEDICINE

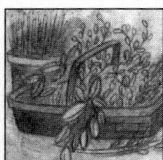

"[The] rapid growth in CAM [complementary and alternative medicine] in many Western countries suggests a degree of public dissatisfaction with what people see as the limitations of orthodox medicine and concern over the side effects of ever more potent drugs. Biotechnical approaches—pharmaceuticals and surgery—often have a limited amount to offer those with chronic, degenerative or stress-related diseases, mental disorders or addiction. In all developed countries there is a widespread recognition of the growing financial, social and personal cost involved, and of the need for a less fragmented, and more participative and humane, approach" (The Foundation for Integrated Medicine, 1997).

Throughout this text you will find "Considering the Alternatives" charts on various subjects pertaining to what are known variously as alternative therapies, complementary therapies, holistic therapies, or unconventional therapies. What are alternative therapies? And why should alternative therapies be of interest to nurses?

Complementary and alternative medicine (CAM) encompasses a broad range of therapies and practices ("Frequently Asked Questions," 1997; Panel on Definition and Description, 1997). Therapies and practices range from medical systems with ancient roots, such as traditional Chinese medicine and acupuncture, to the use of dietary supplements discovered and researched only in recent years, such as glucosamine sulfate for arthritis. CAM includes such familiar techniques as chiropractic, and the less familiar, such as Ayurveda. Many of these practices and techniques are primarily self-care oriented, whereas others rely on practitioners. Many CAM systems include dietary, exercise, and other lifestyle practices that adherents follow, believing such practices to be preventive and health-enhancing.

Although the majority of the practices under the umbrella of CAM are not taught in medical or nursing schools or practiced in hospitals, more and more medical schools are including courses in CAM, and more physicians are including aspects of CAM in their practices (Astin, Marie, Pelletier, Hansen, & Haskell, 1998; Jacobs, Chapman, & Crothers, 1998). A handful of hospitals are beginning to include such practices as acupuncture (Nasir, 1998) and chiropractic within their walls. Insurance companies are also expanding reimbursement for some CAM treatments.

These changes are generated in large part because people are choosing to incorporate complementary and alternative therapies for their own health care in greater and greater numbers and spending increasing amounts of money to do so. Expenditures in the United States on CAM may exceed $15 billion annually, with visits to the wide variety of alternative practitioners rivaling in number those to family and general practitioners, internists, and pediatricians combined. In Australia, more than $1 billion is spent yearly on alternative care, and expenditures on alternative medicines may be twice those for conventional pharmaceuticals (Eisenberg et al., 1998, 1993; MacLennan et al., 1996).

CAM practices have been called *alternative* because they have often been seen as just that—alternatives to the conventional, Western scientific approach to medicine. They have been called *complementary* because many practitioners believe that these practices can complement conventional medicine in many instances, improving health outcomes. The term *holistic* is one used to define a medical or healing system that aspires to take into account all aspects of an individual: body, mind, and spirit. This last is not necessarily outside the realm of conventional medicine and nursing, but many would argue that medicine and nursing may have lost the holistic view and of treatment of patients as people, focusing instead on disease.

As greater numbers of people employ CAM practices, and as research shows what practices are effective, some practitioners believe that we may eventually develop a system of "integrated medicine" that could be truly complementary, allowing the variety of practices that are effective to be used in a given situation for the benefit of clients, without compromising any particular method or philosophy.

It is important for nurses to be aware of alternative therapies and their use by clients for a number of reasons. First, studies performed on the use of alternative medicine have revealed that people often do not inform their caregivers about their use of CAM. This can be dangerous, because certain herbs and vitamins can have interactions with medications (Miller, 1998; O'Hara, Keifer, Farrell, & Kemper, 1998). For example, vitamin E and garlic both possess anticoagulant properties, which could be a problem in a client concurrently taking anticoagulants. So knowing not just what medications but also what vitamins, minerals, and herbs a client takes can be very important. Also, knowledge of the use of alternative therapies by a client can give the nurse a better idea of the client's efforts to manage his or her health and illness. Discussing such use open-mindedly with the client fosters communication and an alliance with the client, with the common goal of the client's well-being. Finally, clients often look to nurses for information about CAM. This open-mindedness, alliance, and information exchanging with clients is, in fact, thera-

(continued)

CONSIDERING THE ALTERNATIVES

COMPLEMENTARY AND ALTERNATIVE MEDICINE (continued)

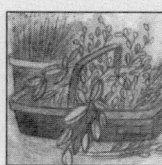

peutic in itself (Galland, 1997). It is our intention, in these Considering the Alternatives charts, to provide background information on complementary and alternative therapies so that you can provide quality information to your clients, who may be "considering the alternatives."

Resources

Publications that can expand and keep your knowledge of CAM current:

Alternative and Complementary Therapies, a bimonthly publication. Mary Ann Liebert, Inc., Publishers, 2 Madison Avenue, Larchmont, NY 10538; 914-834-3100; liebert@pipeline.com.

Alternative Therapies in Health and Medicine, (a peer-reviewed journal). Inno Vision Communications, 101 Columbia, Aliso Viejo, CA 92656; 800-899-1712; alttherapy@aol.com.

HerbalGram, The Journal of the American Botanical Council and the Herb Research Foundation. P.O. Box 201660, Austin, TX 78720; 512-331-8868; www.herbalgram.org.

Scientific Review of Alternative Medicine. Prometheus Books, 59 John Glenn Drive, Amherst, NY 14228-2197; 800-421-0351.

References

Astin, J.A., Marie, A., Pelletier, K., Hansen, E., & Haskell, W.L. (1998). A review of the incorporation of complementary and alternative medicine by mainstream physicians. *Archives of Internal Medicine, 158,* 2303–2310.

Eisenberg, D., et al. (1993). Unconventional medicine in the United States: Prevalence, costs and patterns of use. *New England Journal of Medicine, 328,* 246–252.

Eisenberg, D.M., Davis, R.B., Ettner, S.G., Appel, S., Wilkey, S., Van Rompag, M., & Kessler, R. (1998). Trends in alternative medicine use in the United States, 1990–1997. *Journal of the American Medical Association, 280,* 1569–1575.

The Foundation for Integrated Medicine. (1997). *Integrated healthcare: A way forward for the next five years?*

"Frequently Asked Questions." (1997). NIH Office of Alternative Medicine Clearinghouse, March, 1997.

Galland, L. (1997). *The four pillars of healing* (pp 103–123). New York: Random House.

Jacobs, J., Chapman, E.H., & Crothers, D. (1998). Patient characteristics and practice patterns of physicians using homeopathy. *Archives of Family Medicine, 7,* 531–540.

MacLennan, A.H., Wilson, D.H., & Taylor, A.W. (1996). Prevalence and cost of alternative medicine in Australia. *The Lancet, 347,* 569–573.

Miller, L.G. (1998). Herbal medicinals: Selected clinical considerations focusing on known or potential drug-drug interactions. *Archives of Internal Medicine, 158,* 2200–2211.

Nasir, L. (1998). Acupuncture in a university hospital: Implications for an inpatient consulting service. *Archives of Family Medicine, 7,* 593–596.

O'Hara, M.A., Kiefer, D., Farrell, K., & Kemper, K. (1998). A review of 12 commonly used medicinal herbs. *Archives of Family Medicine, 7,* 523–536.

Panel on Definition and Description, CAM Research Methodology Conference, April 1995. Defining and describing complementary and alternative medicine. *Alternative Therapies in Health and Medicine, 3(2),* 49–57.

SOCIAL WORKERS. Social workers help clients and families cope with problems resulting from long-term illness, injury, and rehabilitation. They also often work in clinical settings as case managers to facilitate appropriate client discharge and follow-up care and to ensure proper use of community services. Social workers may have a bachelor's, master's, or doctoral degree in social work, although a graduate degree is often required for those engaged in clinical practice. Social workers' licensure and scope of practice are regulated in all 50 states. A recent National Association of Social Workers (NASW) survey indicated that approximately 30,000 NASW members are clinical social workers (Sharfstein, Stoline, & Koran, 1995).

SPIRITUAL AND RELIGIOUS PERSONNEL. Pastoral care workers provide spiritual care, which is an integral part of holistic health care. Clients and their families come from diverse religious backgrounds, ranging from Christianity to Taoism, whereas others practice no formal religion at all. The health care team must be comfortable with and receptive to clients' spiritual needs (Sumner, 1998). Many hospitals have a department of full-time pastoral care employees to minister to their clients, families, and staff (Jonas, 1998).

HEALTH CARE SETTINGS

Health care is big business. It is one of the largest industries in the United States, with over $2 billion spent on health care each day. The process of health care delivery occurs within a continuum of health care settings and services.

Inpatient Settings

The term *inpatient* is used to denote care given in the context of an overnight stay in a hospital or other facility. Inpatient treatment is also provided in long-term care facilities such as nursing homes, psychiatric hospitals, and rehabilitation centers.

Hospitals

According to the American Hospital Association (AHA), a hospital is an institution with at least six beds whose primary function is "to deliver patient services, diagnostic and therapeutic, for particular or general medical conditions" (AHA, 1994). A hospital must be licensed, have an organized physician staff, and must provide continuous nursing services under the direction and supervision of registered professional nurses. Federal laws; national codes for building, fire protection, and sanitation; state health department regulations; city ordinances; and the Joint Commission on Accreditation of Healthcare Organizations (JCAHO) govern the construction and operation of hospitals and long-term care facilities (Shi & Singh, 1998).

The modern hospital is the organizational hub of the United States health care system, central to delivery of client care. The hospital represents the community's collective investment in health care resources. Hospitals consume 38% of the nation's health expenditures (Haglund & Dowling, 1993).

The predominant type of hospital today is the general community hospital offering a wide range of medical, surgical, obstetrical, pediatric, and emergency services. Specialty hospitals provide care for a specific disease or population group. Examples of specialty hospitals are children's hospitals, women's and maternity hospitals, and chronic disease hospitals. Public hospitals are owned by agencies of federal, state, or local government. Federally owned hospitals are maintained for special groups of federal beneficiaries: military and governmental personnel, veterans, and Native Americans. State governments generally limit themselves to operating hospitals intended to safeguard public health by isolating mentally ill clients and those with contagious diseases such as tuberculosis. Large urban public hospitals with their outpatient departments are the place of last resort for poor clients located in areas where health resources are in short supply (Haglund & Dowling, 1993).

In the 1980s there was a marked decline in the number of community hospitals and total number of inpatient beds available, largely in response to implementation of the Tax Equity and Fiscal Reimbursement Act (TEFRA) of 1982. Multihospital chains grew during the 1990s in response to the change in reimbursement policies and a need to constrain costs while still providing a variety of health care services within a reasonable geographical area. Shi and Singh (1998) identified three main forces responsible for the continuing downsizing of hospitals: changes in hospital reimbursement, economic constraints faced by community and rural hospitals, and the growth of managed care. **Managed care** is a system that combines the functions of health insurance and the actual delivery of care, where costs and utilization of services are controlled (Shi & Singh, 1998).

Emergency Departments and Trauma Centers

Most hospitals in the United States provide emergency services, and over 93% of community hospitals have emergency departments (EDs) (AHA, 1994). The ED has expanded to provide a range of services for triage care of acutely ill and injured clients. Most major urban communities possess one or more highly developed emergency medical services, including a trauma

center and its system of transportation and uniform communications. Injured clients receive emergency care at the scene and are then moved to a hospital-based ED or trauma center where there are specially trained medical and nursing staffs on duty 24 hours a day. The main purpose of the ED is to provide services around the clock for acutely ill or injured clients as well as walk-in services for less acutely ill clients.

Psychiatric Facilities

Mental illness is the most important group of disorders for which a special subsystem of health care delivery has been organized in the United States (Jonas, 1998). The primary function of a psychiatric inpatient facility is to provide diagnostic and treatment services for clients with psychiatric-related illnesses. Specifically, such an institution must have facilities to provide psychiatric, psychological, and social work services (AHA, 1994). Historically, state governments established facilities for the care of the mentally ill. However, new treatment techniques and issues of cost reimbursement are responsible for the shift from public mental institutions to private psychiatric facilities and the decrease in lengths of stay. Community general hospitals also often provide specialized psychiatric units treating short-term clients with psychiatric diagnoses.

Rehabilitation Centers

Rehabilitation is a long-term service offered to clients who need additional therapy or treatment for recovery from an injury or illness. In 1990 the United States had 128 rehabilitation hospitals or centers and an additional 781 rehabilitation units in the other general and special hospitals with a total of almost 29,000 beds (AHA, 1994). Patients who are discharged from a short-term inpatient stay often continue therapy services for months. They may transfer to a rehabilitation hospital or unit for intense therapy; be transferred to skilled nursing facility to regain strength, then transferred to a rehabilitation center; or sent home and return as outpatient to the hospital or a freestanding rehabilitation center. Rehabilitation hospitals specialize in providing restorative services to rehabilitate chronically ill and disabled clients (Fig. 5–1). Most rehabilitation hospitals also have special arrangements for psychological social work and vocational services.

Long-Term Care Facilities

Long-term care (LTC) describes a range of health and housing services provided to people unable to care for themselves independently (Jonas, 1998). LTC institutions are generically called "nursing homes." Their number has increased significantly since the 1930s, although it is declining today. In 1994 there were about 15,000 nursing homes with about 1.5 million beds. Approximately 75% of nursing homes are under for-profit ownership. More than half of the financial sup-

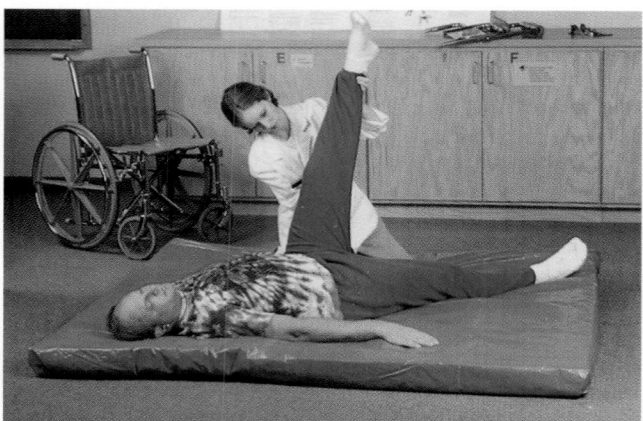

Figure 5–1. Rehabilitation hospitals specialize in providing restorative services to rehabilitate chronically ill and disabled people.

port for nursing homes comes from public funds such as Medicaid. Nursing homes are heavily regulated through licensure and certification requirements (Vladeck, 1996; Richardson, 1995).

In all states, LTC facilities must be licensed to administer medications and provide assistance with activities of daily living. They must also be licensed by the federal government to receive Medicare and Medicaid funding. Institutional LTC is most appropriate for patients whose needs cannot be adequately met in a less acute, community-based setting. It provides a continuum of services depending on the client's level of acuity and dependency. Options today include assisted living facilities, residential care facilities, and retirement centers. Assisted living provides services associated with a resident's activities of daily living. Residential care, also known as sheltered care or board and care, offers some services, such as meals and assistance with taking medicine. Retirement centers provide no nursing or medical services and offer residents the opportunity to maintain their own lifestyle (Shi & Singh, 1998).

A growing component of the LTC continuum is subacute care, which provides services too intensive for the average skilled nursing facility. Subacute care addresses the needs of clients who have recovered from the acute phase of an illness or injury but still require ongoing nursing and medical monitoring and treatment (Walsh, 1995).

LTC units of acute care hospitals may provide subacute care. Nursing homes can open subacute units by raising the staff skill mix. If properly organized, subacute units have the potential for delivering quality postacute services for considerably less cost than the traditional inpatient care in hospitals (Walsh, 1995).

Hospice

Hospice is a cluster of special services that addresses the special needs of dying people and their families. It blends medical, spiritual, legal, financial, and family-

support services. Hospice is a method of care that regards both the client and the family as the unit of care. It is not a location. The venue of care can vary from a specialized facility to a nursing home to the client's own home. Services can be organized out of a hospital, nursing home, free-standing hospice facility, or home health agency (Beresford, 1989).

The idea of providing this comprehensive blend of services to terminally ill clients was first promoted by Dame Cicely Saunders in the 1960s in England. The first hospice in the United States was established in 1974 by Sylvia Lack in New Haven, Connecticut (Beresford, 1989). The hospice movement gathered momentum with the extension of benefit coverage by both Medicare and private insurers because of its lower cost compared with hospitalization. Presently there are approximately 2,000 providers of hospice services (NCHS, 1996).

Outpatient Settings

Outpatient health care services do not require an overnight inpatient stay in a hospital or LTC facility, though these institutions may offer these services. Outpatient services are often called "ambulatory care" and include a wide range of services, from routine tests and treatments to complex procedures and therapies. The managed care environment has made outpatient settings increasingly important in the delivery of health care services.

Physicians' Offices

Private physicians working solo, in partnerships, or in private group practices are the dominant providers of outpatient care. Data from the *Health United States 1995* survey (NCHS, 1996) indicates that 56.8% of all physician contacts occurred in the physician's office. The physician's office is the usual setting for most basic outpatient services, such as physical examinations, diagnostic and screening services, minor illness care, medication administration, counseling and advice, and routine treatment follow-up. Today this office is most likely to be part of a group practice or medical clinic complex.

Ambulatory Care Centers

The **ambulatory care center** provides health services on an outpatient basis to those who visit a hospital or other health care facility and depart after treatment on the same day. This category includes managed care programs and hospital-based ambulatory services, including clinics, walk-in and emergency services, mobile units, and health promotion centers. Freestanding "surgi-centers" and "urgi- or emergi-centers," health department clinics, neighborhood and community health centers, organized home care, community mental health centers, school and workplace health services, and prison health services are additional examples of ambulatory care settings.

Mobile medical services take advanced diagnostic services to clients in rural communities in a convenient and cost-effective manner. For example, mobile eye care and dental care units can be brought to a nursing home site or workplace where they can efficiently serve a large number of clients. Mobile diagnostic services include mammography, magnetic resonance imaging, and cardiac assessment. Other health screening services, such as blood sugar, blood pressure, and cholesterol checks, are provided by trained volunteers. These services are generally provided by nonprofit organizations and are often seen at churches, shopping malls, and fairs, parades, and other public events.

Rural Primary Care Hospitals

Poor economic conditions, isolated rural areas, weather conditions, limited availability of transportation, and long distances affect rural residents' health status and ability to access needed care (Shi & Singh, 1998). It is estimated that more than 20 million rural Americans live in areas deficient in primary health care providers (ANA, 1991; DHHS, 1990). Rural hospitals treat a client mix that is disproportionately poor, elderly, uninsured, and underinsured. These facilities tend to be smaller than urban hospitals and provide fewer services. They also have difficulty recruiting health care providers such as pediatricians, obstetricians, internists, dentists, and nurses. These factors create a climate for financial difficulties and poor health care delivery. Closure of rural hospitals creates further erosion of access to care for rural residents (Summer, 1991).

Emergency and Rescue Systems

Ambulance service and first aid treatment to victims of acute illness, accidents, and disasters by trained emergency medical technicians (EMTs) are the most common mobile medical services. EMTs are trained to provide critical early treatment on site and in transit that is often life-saving. Most urban centers have developed formal emergency medical systems to provide a quick response to emergencies. This system uses hospital-based EDs along with transportation systems and 911 emergency telephone lines to provide immediate access to those needing emergency care. Specialized ambulance services, such as cardiac care units and shock-trauma units, are becoming increasingly prevalent.

Community Settings

Services based in the community are provided through voluntary, public, or proprietary organizations and include adult day care, respite care, congregate meals, transportation, and case management programs. There are a variety of funding sources from Medicare, Medicaid, Title II of the Older Americans Act established in 1965, and other federal, state, and local social services programs. The extent of services provided and the eligibility requirements vary by service, funding source, and locality (Richardson, 1995).

Adult Day Care Centers

Adult day care (ADC) is a daytime program offered in an institutional setting that provides a wide range of health, social, and recreational services to frail (usually elderly) adults who require supervision and care while members of the family or other informal care givers are away at work (Shi & Singh, 1998). The National Institute for Adult Day Care (1984) has defined ADC as "a community-based group program designed to meet the needs of functionally impaired adults through an individual plan of care and program of nursing care, rehabilitative therapies, supervision, and socialization that enables a person to remain in the community." ADC is generally a structured, comprehensive weekday program that provides personal care, midday meals, social services, and transportation in a protective setting. It complements informal care given in the home by family members and helps delay or prevent institutionalization. ADC may also work as respite to help reduce caregiver stress. Many ADC programs provide a mix of medical, maintenance, and social-psychological services. Group socialization and recreational activities are important as well.

Respite Care Services

Respite care is defined as a service that provides temporary relief to informal caregivers such as family members (Shi & Singh, 1998). Respite care is the most frequently suggested intervention to address family caregivers' feelings of stress and burden. ADC, home health care, and temporary stays in nursing homes, hospitals, group homes, or foster care homes are examples of respite care services or programs. In-home respite care provides temporary homemaker, chore, or home health services. The focus of respite care, regardless of how it is provided, is to give the client's informal caregivers time off while meeting the needs for assistance of frail, elderly, or disabled chronically ill clients.

School Health Clinics

The U.S. Bureau of the Census (1995) reports that in 1990 there were over 64.5 million students in over 88,000 primary and secondary schools, colleges, and universities. Almost all educational institutions provide some form of ambulatory health services to students. Services are provided by local health departments or by school boards in conjunction with the local health department.

The work of most school-based health programs is carried out by a registered nurse and confined to basic first aid, case finding, and prevention of certain chronic or epidemic diseases (Fig. 5–2). Very little dis-

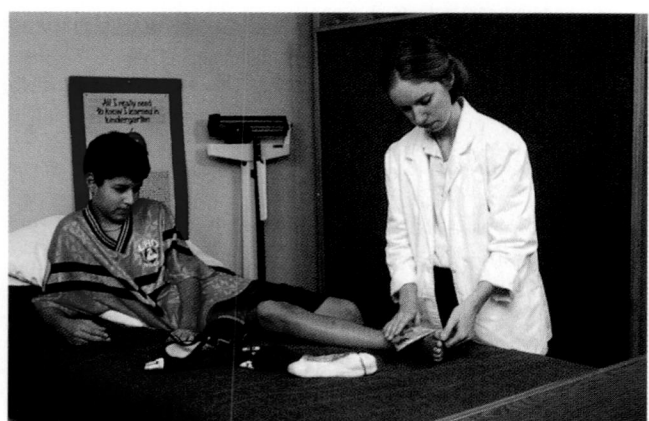

Figure 5–2. The work of most school-based health programs is carried out by a registered nurse and is confined to basic first aid, case finding, and prevention of certain chronic or epidemic diseases.

ease treatment is done in a school health program. Vision and hearing screenings and various immunizations are commonly offered. When indicated, referrals for diagnosis and treatment are made to the student's parents and physician. Colleges and universities provide a broader set of services, including many basic diagnostic and treatment services. In some school settings there are programs to help students deal with mental, physical, and substance abuse problems (Jonas, 1998).

Industrial Health Services

Industrial or occupational health services are provided in most large businesses and factories. The actual number of these "in-plant" health units in the United States is unknown. In smaller firms it may be simply a first-aid box; larger firms may provide systematic health services staffed by industrial nurses and part-time physicians. In a few firms the health services are comprehensive, with complete care for all health disorders, whether or not the disorders are work-related (Jonas, 1998).

Optimal health accomplished through changes in lifestyle works to improve the overall health of America's workforce. Work-site health promotion or wellness programs work to create awareness of health factors, help employees to make lifestyle changes, and develop workplace environments that are conducive to health. There is some evidence that the creation and implementation of industrial health promotion services are cost-effective (Kamen, 1995).

Home Health Care Services

Home health care services, such as nursing, therapy, and health-related homemaker or social services, are brought to clients in their own homes because, generally, these clients are unable to leave their homes safely to get the care they need (Shi & Singh, 1998). Home health care is provided to clients and their families at

their place of residence to promote, maintain, or restore health and minimize effects of disability and illness.

Home health care services are provided mainly to elderly clients. Seventy-five percent of home health care clients are age 65 or over. A profile of the elderly client using home health care services show that 71% were women, 42% were 75 to 84 years of age, 68% were white, 47% were widowed, 93% were living in private residences, and 51% were living with their family members (NCHS, 1996). Without home health care services, the only alternative for many of these clients would be institutionalization in a nursing home.

Neighborhood and Community Health Centers

The Neighborhood Health Center (NHC) movement emerged in the late 1960s as the rallying cry for change in both content and availability of health services for the poor. The NHCs hoped to break the cycle of poverty by also providing jobs and skills and career development opportunities for neighborhood residents. Though the NHC movement did not meet with success, it did provide the basis for the Nixon and Ford administrations' Community Health Center (CHC) Program development (Sardell, 1983).

The CHCs concentrated on the delivery of primary health care services to the community as a whole and to individuals. By the early 1980s there were over 800 CHCs serving over 4.5 million people (Sardell, 1983). In 1996 there were over 600 community and migrant worker comprehensive primary care systems with over 1,600 sites, providing care to nearly 8 million people (Starfield, 1996).

CHCs serve as a primary care safety net for our nation's poor and underserved in both inner-city and rural areas. CHCs have become expert in managing the health care needs of these special populations. Long-standing outreach programs, case management, transportation, translation services, alcohol and drug abuse screening and treatment, mental health services, health education, and social services are provided to roughly 30% of the country's indigent population served by the CHCs nationwide (Shi & Singh, 1998).

Free Clinics

The free clinic, modeled after the 19th-century dispensary, is a general ambulatory care center serving primarily the poor and homeless. A 1991 report found there were 200 free clinics nationwide (Kelleher, 1991). In most of these, trained volunteer staffs give free care to clients. The Hahnemann Homeless Clinics Project in Philadelphia, one of the largest free clinics in the nation, is staffed by nursing and allied health student volunteers from Hahnemann University (Collins, 1995). Another student-run clinic for the homeless is the Arbor Free Clinic in Palo Alto, California, which is entirely managed by medical students from Stanford University (Yap & Thornton, 1995).

HEALTH CARE FINANCING

Over the past few decades a complex blend of private and public mechanisms has arisen to affect how Americans pay for health care. Since the early 1980s, the basic approach for reimbursing hospitals, physicians, and long-term providers of services has been restructured.

After Medicare, private health insurance is the most prevalent source of financing for the United States health care system. Insurance is a mechanism created to help protect against risk. Risk is central to the concept of insurance and refers to the potential substantial financial loss from a low-probability event. A person protected by insurance against a specific risk is called the insured, and the insuring agency that assumes the risk is called the insurer (Shi & Singh, 1998).

Private health insurance plays an important role in influencing the direction and structure of our nation's health care system. The term "health insurance" is often used to mean a wide array of health care financing mechanisms, including the "social insurance" of Medicare and the public assistance of Medicaid, the "self-insurance" plans used by employers, and the managed care programs of health maintenance organizations (HMOs) and preferred provider organizations (PPOs). Clients pay for some of their health care themselves. Persons not covered by either private or government-sponsored health financing programs are called "uninsured."

The American health care system is the most expensive and unique system in the developed world. In 1997 about $4,000 per person was spent on health care as compared with the next most expensive country, Switzerland, which spent $2,500 (Organization for Economic Cooperation and Development [OECD], 1998). However, over the years public outlays for health care financing have increased while private financing has shrunk proportionately. In 1997, the number of people without health insurance increased to 43.4 million, or 16% of the population (U.S. Bureau of the Census, 1997, 1998). There has been a decline in the growth of private health care expenditures since the early 1990s while the government's share of the nation's health care bill in 1997 rose to $507 billion, or 46% of the total, an increase from 40% in 1990. Private resources financed 54% of personal health services, 585 billion dollars in 1997, down from 60% in 1990 (Levit et al., 1998). All of the money to pay for health care services ultimately comes from the American people.

Private Health Insurance

Private health insurance is offered by many types of health plan providers, including commercial insurance companies (such as Travelers), Blue Cross/Blue Shield, self-insurers, and managed care organizations. Group insurance is a policy obtained through an employer, union, or professional organization. Self-insurance is used by a few very large and diversified employers who simply assume the risks by budgeting an amount to cover medical claims incurred by their employees. Individual private health insurance is an important source of coverage for farmers, early retirees, self-employed persons, and employees of businesses that do not offer group health insurance benefits. This category covered about 10.5 million Americans under the age of 65 years in 1994 (General Accounting Office [GAO], 1996).

Managed Care Organizations

Managed care organizations (MCOs) are the single most significant development in America's system of health care delivery in the 20th century. The managed care movement exploded in concert with the persistent rise in health care expenditures. It was not until the 1990s that managed care dominated our nation's health care delivery system.

The fundamental concept behind managed care is the prepayment of services for defined enrolled populations. The approaches to providing health care under MCOs are designed to affect the operation and structure of the health care system and thus to affect use of services by the consumer. These approaches have an impact on quality, access, costs, and other key components of the service delivery system. Many of these approaches have been questioned because of their threat to values such as consumer choice, free access, and avoidance of involvement of insurers in the patient-provider relationship.

The primary care physician assumes the "gatekeeper" role in managed care systems. This provider is responsible for all primary care for the client and determines when referral to specialists is necessary (Fig. 5–3). This provider has the coordinating role for the client's health care needs. The gatekeeper concept manages the patient's use of resources, reduces the self-initiated use of specialty services, and ensures overall coordination, without duplication of care.

HEALTH MAINTENANCE ORGANIZATIONS. HMOs are a type of group health care practice that provides basic and supplemental health maintenance and treatment services to voluntary enrollees who prepay a fixed periodic fee that is set without regard to the amount or kind of services received. HMOs are the most common type of MCO. An HMO has four main characteristics:

- It provides medical care and services to help people maintain their health.
- It requires a fixed fee per month per enrollee for access to a complete range of health care services, which are coordinated and managed.
- All health care is obtained from hospitals, physicians, and other providers participating in the HMO.
- The HMO is responsible for establishing standards for the quality of services provided.

PREFERRED PROVIDER ORGANIZATIONS. PPOs are the most common type of MCO after the HMO. The

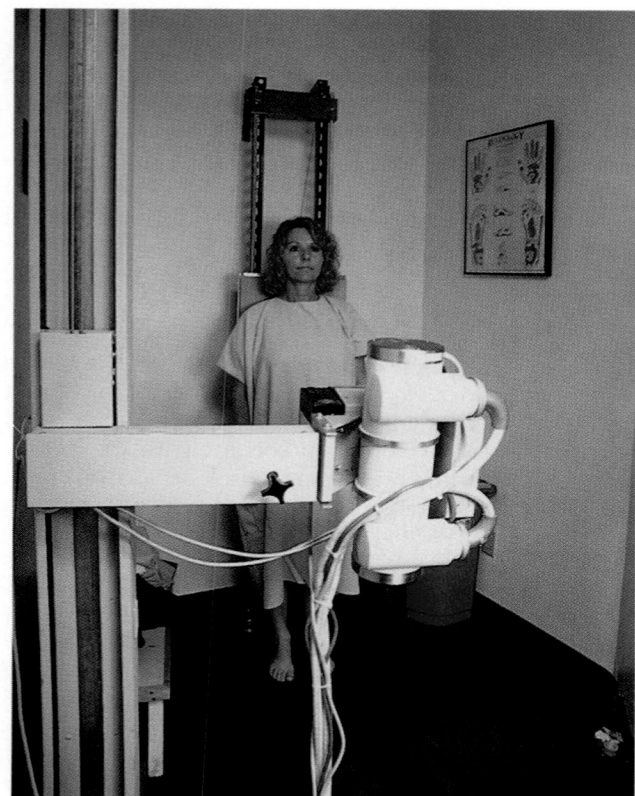

Figure 5–3. Under managed care, the primary care physician serves as a "gatekeeper" for referral for diagnostic procedures and specialty care.

preferred provider organization is an organization of physicians, hospitals, and pharmacists whose members discount their health care services to subscribers (clients). A PPO may be organized by a group of physicians, an outside entrepreneur, an insurance company, or a company with a self-insurance plan. The PPO is the insurance industry's response to the growth of HMOs. PPOs negotiate contracts with companies to lock in the business of treating their employees. The PPO makes contractual arrangements with providers for the delivery of health care services on a discounted fee schedule (Shi & Singh, 1998).

EXCLUSIVE PROVIDER ORGANIZATIONS. Exclusive provider organizations (EPOs) are similar to PPOs in their organization and purpose. However, in an **exclusive provider organization** enrollees are restricted to the EPO's list of providers of health care, called "exclusive providers" Like HMOs, EPOs use a gatekeeping approach to health care service delivery. EPOs have been created by employers whose primary rationale is decreasing costs (Wagner, 1995).

Government Insurance Plans

Public financing of health care services accounts for roughly 46% of the total expenditures on health care in the United States. Governmental spending supports *categorical programs* designed to provide benefits to cer-

tain groups of people. The most well-known examples are Medicare and Medicaid. Like Social Security, Medicare is an *entitlement* program. Because people have contributed toward Medicare through taxes, they are "entitled" to the benefits regardless of the amount of income and assets they may have. In contrast, Medicaid is a welfare program, in which the level of benefits are dependent on a person's income and assets. Medicare and Medicaid purchase government-funded services from the private sector (Shi & Singh, 1998).

MEDICARE. **Medicare** is a federally funded national health insurance program in the United States for people over 65 years of age. Medicare is the first national social insurance program in the United States to finance medical care. Medicare was enacted in 1965 as Title XVIII of the Social Security Act. Additionally, Medicare finances health care services for disabled persons who are also eligible for Social Security benefits and for those who have end-stage renal disease (Koch, 1993).

MEDICAID. Medicaid is the largest health insurer in the United States covering medical services and LTC for 41.3 million people (HCFA, 1996). It was established along with Medicare in 1965 under Title XIX of the Social Security Act. **Medicaid** is a welfare program providing partial health care services for indigent people. It is supported jointly by federal and state governments. The federal government provides matching funds to the states based on the per-capita income in each state. By law the federal matching dollars cannot be less than 50% or greater than 83% of the total state Medicaid program costs. The amount of federal government funding has no preset limits (HCFA, 1996a).

PROSPECTIVE PAYMENT SYSTEMS. A **prospective payment system** (PPS) is a payment system in which what will be paid for, for a specific service, is predetermined. In a retrospective payment system, reimbursement is determined on the basis of costs actually incurred (Shi & Singh, 1998). This system was implemented for short-stay inpatient hospitalizations (Medicare Part A) in the mid-1980s under the Social Security Act of 1983. The predetermined reimbursement amount is set according to **diagnosis-related groups** (DRGs), a system of classification or grouping of patients according to medical diagnosis for purposes of paying hospitalization costs. Payment is based on discharge rather than per diem (per day). Payment is a rate set for "bundled services." It involves approximately 500 DRGs corresponding to the most prevalent diagnoses found in clients using inpatient services (Jonas, 1998). The PPS has enabled Medicare to control the per-case rate of increase for Part A hospital expenditure reimbursement (Davis & Burner, 1995).

OREGON STATE HEALTH PLAN. In 1989, the Oregon state legislature passed a Basic Health Services Act, creating the Oregon Health Services Commission (OHSC) (1991). The OHSC defined basic health care as "a floor beneath which no person shall fall." The OHSC created three levels of health care benefits: "essential," "very important," and "valuable to certain individuals." It also developed a priority list of 709 health services (Hadorn, 1991).

Although Medicaid coverage was expanded to all Oregonians who fell below the poverty level, services are limited to those with the "best cost-to-benefit ratio" (Burton, 1996). This limitation is complex. The Oregon system's priority focuses on prevention and primary care services. It zeroes in on the "change" in quality of life provided by the services of the health care system (Steinbrook & Lo, 1992).

Oregon's health plan was originally seen as extreme, but rationing of health care is no longer seen as radical. Every state is struggling to keep Medicaid costs under control. So far, the Medicaid portion of the Oregon plan has been successful, signing up about 126,000 new members since 1994 (Bodenheimer, 1997; Montague, 1997).

NATIONAL HEALTH INSURANCE PLANS. In the United States, health care is not administered or controlled by a central department or agency of the government. However, many other industrialized countries maintain central control of health care delivery. Three basic types of basic systems are in use.

In the Canadian system, the government finances health care through general taxes, but private providers deliver health care services. Canada's system demonstrates that the use of a national health care budget can be effective in controlling the growth of health care expenditures (Roemer, 1996).

In Great Britain the government National Health Service not only finances the program but manages the infrastructure for the delivery of medical care. Under this system the government operates most of the medical institutions and physicians in this type of system are employees of the government.

In Germany's system of socialized health insurance, employers and employees finance health care through government-mandated contributions. Private providers deliver health care. Private, not-for-profit insurance companies, called "sickness funds," are responsible for collecting the contributions and paying physicians and hospitals (Santerre & Neun, 1996).

Generally, the three national health care systems described have common features: (1) every citizen is entitled to a defined set of health care services, (2) national budgets determine total health care expenditures and allocate resources, and (3) the budget limits determine availability of services and payments to providers. The governments control the proliferation of health care services, especially high technology. Resource allocation determines the extent to which the governments can offer citizens health care services (Shi & Singh, 1998).

ISSUES AND OPPORTUNITIES IN HEALTH CARE DELIVERY

In the last few decades, the United States has experienced great changes in its demographics, family structures, communities, and lifestyles. The conflict between unemployment and poverty with rising health care costs has raised many legal and ethical issues related to the distribution and availability of health care services. The opportunities to influence the future quality and financing of health care services are there (see the accompanying A Patient's View chart).

Demographic Factors Affecting Health Care Delivery

Changes in the composition of a population are important for the planning of health care services. Population change involves three components: births, deaths, and migration. Lower death rates, lower birth rates, and greater longevity occurring together indicate an aging population. The migration of elderly to southern states requires planning of adequate retirement and LTC services in those states (Shi & Singh, 1998).

The United States Constitution mandates that a census be conducted every 10 years. The latest Census Bureau projection (1993) estimates the resident population of the United States at 262.2 million in October 1995. However, despite great efforts, the Census Bureau admits that there is undercounting of some segments of the population, such as Native Americans, as well as people living in public housing and those who are homeless. The resident population will be even larger when undocumented aliens and migrant workers are added (Kelly & Joel, 1996). Population growth calculations estimate only a 0.5% increase by 2040, and if this prediction is accurate the resident population will be about 364 million, an increase of 43% over 1992 (U.S. Bureau of the Census, 1993). These statistics relative to our country's population are a critical ingredient in planning for availability of services to meet the demand for health care.

Increasing Age

The graying of America is considered the most significant population issue facing our country's health care delivery system. In the year 2010, it is predicted that approximately 40 million, or 14% of Americans, will be age 65 years or older, with about 4.3 million age 85 years and older. People in the 85 or older category are the fastest-growing group of the United States population (Kelly & Joel, 1996; Aday, 1993). The number of children under age 18 years in 1990, about 64 million, is similar to that in 1960. The proportion of the United States resident population represented by children has declined from 36% in 1960 to 26% in 1990. By 2010, it is estimated that the proportion of children in the population will be only 23% (U.S. Bureau of the Census, 1993).

The elderly consume more health care services than the younger population. In 1995 Medicare expenditures averaged $5,561 per beneficiary, whereas personal health care expenditures for all Americans were estimated to be $3,219 per capita. A growing elderly

"NO ONE EVER CALLED TO FOLLOW UP WITH ME AFTER THE BIRTH, BUT THE BILLS BEGAN TO ARRIVE ALMOST IMMEDIATELY."

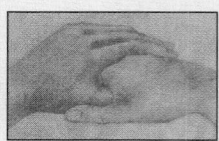 If every pregnancy and childbirth were like my first experience, people would never have big families. As a health science editor, I considered myself well prepared to deal with the health care system, especially during what should be a normal physiological process. Never in my worst nightmares had I imagined what actually happened.

Five months into my pregnancy, I realized I was in the wrong place to get the right kind of care. There was little or no personal interaction or education—I felt like I was just another belly to them, both to the nurses who did the monthly assessments and the physicians who never listened to the baby's heart or anything. If I had a problem or a question, I had to tell it to an answering machine. I have a thyroid disorder that I now know should have been checked each trimester, but wasn't. I had morning sickness 24 hours a day—lost 5 pounds the first trimester, became dehydrated, and passed out one day on the way to work but couldn't reach anyone at the clinic for help. Then I developed a yeast infection, and by that time I was dealing only with medical assistants. I decided it was time to take charge and make a change.

I asked around for recommendations and, based on advice from three different people, went to a practice associated with the university medical center. They made me feel better instantly. There were five physicians, two nurse midwives, four nurse practitioners, and one maternity triage nurse, what I now know was an ideal situation. Whenever I called with a question or a problem, I talked with a person, not a machine. The triage nurse was always available, either immediately or through her beeper. If she couldn't answer my questions, she would consult one of the doctors and get right back to me. She took me on a tour of the hospital, intro-

duced me to everyone in the practice. I think a triage nurse is essential to every medical practice but especially in maternity care.

It's a good thing I changed providers when I did because the complications increased almost immediately. At 27 weeks, after being really sick all week, I became dehydrated and went into preterm labor. I was hospitalized and spent 2 days in labor and delivery, terrified that I would lose the baby. At 31 and 32 weeks, it happened again—2 more days in labor and delivery, complete with monitors, an obstetrics/gynecology (OB) nurse, three OB nurse practitioners, a labor nurse, and a couple of medical residents.

I was working full time, commuting 45 minutes each way every day. When I began having preterm labor every week, my doctor intervened and advised my employer that I needed some flexibility in my work life; otherwise, I was risking a premature birth, a hazardous situation prior to 36 weeks' gestation. Easing my schedule helped a lot; the last month was much easier. In my 40th week, I went into labor on my way to the office.

During the next 38 hours, I saw every doctor in the practice but only two nurses. One of them stayed with me for the entire last day; she was a saint. I was given epidural anesthesia twice—the first one wore off, and the second was given too close to the time when I needed to push, so I felt like I had no legs; I couldn't push. The baby was stuck and they had to use forceps. Then woosh—there she was—beautiful, perfect baby we had hoped for.

In the first hour after delivery, things began to get confusing. I got very brief instruction in breast-feeding and then they had to take the baby away because I was in an older, unsecured section of the hospital. Next morning, two different nurses gave me two different sets of instructions for breast-feeding and strong sug-

(continued)

population will have a serious impact on health care expenditures in the future (HCFA, 1996).

Family Diversity

The last U.S. census showed a trend toward increasing urbanization and persistent rural losses. In 1990, 79% of the population lived in urban areas, up from 63% in 1960. The shrinking average American family, 2.62 people in 1992, is the smallest ever. The number of people residing alone has declined. One-parent families continue to increase and contribute to the small average family size. Only 26% of American households with children under the age of 18 years include a married couple. Women living alone head 11.7% of

all households in the United States and are likely to be part of the 89% of all households receiving at least one noncash benefit such as Medicaid or food stamps (The World Almanac, 1995).

Cultural Diversity

The ethnic composition of the United States is changing. One of every three Americans will be a member of an ethnic minority in 2000 (Furula & Lipson, 1994), and the current minority groups will be the numeric majority by 2050 (Bullough & Bullough, 1994). The immigrants and refugees of the 1990s are primarily Hispanics and Asians and have significantly affected the ethnic population mix in specific

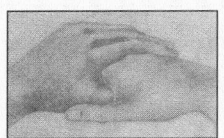

gestions about going home. Although insurance covers a 2-day postpartum stay, they'd really like you to go home the first day.

Finally, the discharge nurse gave me yet another set of instructions about breast-feeding. I thought because she was older and more experienced that she must know what she's talking about. Wrong. Baby and I went home Christmas day, a Thursday, and had no success with breast-feeding because all the various recommendations were so conflicting. I was exhausted, confused, and frustrated. The baby was hungry. My mother was worried and thought the baby looked yellow, so because I knew about jaundice, I called the triage nurse. We took the baby to the pediatrician, who found nothing wrong. I, on the other hand, was a mess. My breasts were engorged and a terrible pain was beginning to build in my abdomen.

By Monday the abdominal pain was excruciating, so I went to the clinic and was examined by my least-favorite physician, who diagnosed the problem as constipation or gas and recommended milk of magnesia. Two days later, on New Year's Eve, my temperature was 102.5°F and I was immobilized by the pain, but I still tried to breast-feed. This time the doctor told me to drink plenty of fluids. Finally, on Friday, I was doubled over in pain, ghostly white, feverish, too weak even to hold my daughter. The doctor said to meet him in Emergency, which I did at 2 PM. After poking and prodding my tender abdomen, he did an ultrasound but was still baffled. Around midnight he concluded that it might be appendicitis and decided to operate.

Surgery solved the mystery: A fibroid tumor on my uterus had caused the preterm labor; fueled by the pregnancy hormones, my uterus began shrinking, causing the tumor to pull at the appendix until it burst.

I was in the hospital for 5 days after the appendectomy. The surgeon thought it was too soon after delivery to remove the tumor; if I hemorrhaged, hysterectomy would be the only option. The nurses on the medical-surgical unit were wonderful, but the surgeons left a lot to be desired. However, each doctor from the OB clinic came in to apologize for not diagnosing my problem sooner, even the "constipation and gas" doctor. During those 5 days, I tried valiantly to maintain my milk supply by using a breast pump (the one they brought in was industrial size!)—a real disaster. Not a single med-surg nurse could remember how to operate the pump.

Later I made two more trips to Emergency because the pain just wouldn't stop. The surgeon said the fibroid would have to come out, but I disagreed. Enough was enough. It took a month just to be able to walk again, and 9 months later I still don't have any feeling in my abdomen.

I did go back to breast-feeding for a time, but it was a struggle. I couldn't sit up and hold my daughter for 40 minutes, so I started to cut back on the amount of time I fed her. Once you do that, you cut back on the amount of fat in the milk, and newborns need that fat. After 4 months, I gave up. With working and traveling, breast-feeding just wasn't practical, but I still have a lot of regrets.

I'm an educated health care consumer. I was in one of the best medical centers in the country—certainly the best in the region—yet my care left a lot to be desired. Not only were my misdiagnosed complications potentially fatal, but the prenatal classes were virtually useless except for the infant CPR classes. No one ever called to follow-up with me after the birth or after the appendectomy, but the bills began to arrive almost immediately. Yet I would recommend that hospital and that ob-gyn group because I believe—sad to say—this may be as good as it gets in today's health care system.

states. If current trends continue, non-Hispanic whites will be a minority in California in 2000. Hispanic-Americans are the youngest population group, with half under the age of 26 years. Most Hispanics reside in Texas, California, and other states in the Southwest. California and Hawaii are the states of choice for most Asian immigrants (U.S. Bureau of the Census, 1993). The melting pot analogy of our country's population (wherein new immigrants assimilate the dominant features of the prevailing culture) is giving way to that of a mosaic, with each ethnic group retaining its culture as a source of identity and support. Some sociologists welcome this phenomenon, whereas others insist that a multicultural society weakens our nation by creating multiple sets of accepted beliefs and values (Kelly & Joel, 1996).

Our health care system is itself a culture and often serves as a barrier to culturally sensitive care. Leininger (1991) states that people of every culture have the right to have their cultural values known, respected, and addressed appropriately in nursing and other health care settings. Culturally sensitive nursing care occurs when you acknowledge the existence of variant value sets and beliefs, develop a sensitivity to each person's fundamental beliefs related to health and illness, and are respectful and understanding of other cultures without judgment.

Lifestyle

Today, thanks to global telecommunications and expanding travel, we live in a world of people who continuously exchange ideas and influence each other's national cultures, languages, and lifestyles. For the consumer, increased options are stimulating and fun. For the major economic powers, a growing world market is an economic bonanza. But even as lifestyles become more similar, there are signs of a backlash against uniformity, a desire to assert the uniqueness of one's culture and language, and a repudiation of foreign influence. The more homogeneous our lifestyles become, the stronger the clinch to our deeper beliefs and values will be (Naisbitt & Aburdene, 1990).

Americans are living longer than ever before. By the year 2010, 14% of the population will be 65 years of age or older. The major causes of death in the United States are chronic diseases such as heart disease, stroke, cancer, and chronic obstructive pulmonary disease (Aday, 1993). At least in part, these illnesses are known as "lifestyle diseases." One in six deaths in this country are attributable to smoking. Dietary practices have a direct role in five of the top-ten causes of death and contribute to three more through alcohol abuse. Lifestyle diseases are the result of human behaviors. The course and outcomes of these diseases can often be altered through positive changes in those human behaviors (Glanz, Lewis, & Rimer, 1990).

The past couple of decades have seen a dramatic increase in public, private, and professional interest in preventing disability and death from these lifestyle-related chronic illnesses. The focus has been on changing peoples' behaviors such as smoking cessation, weight reduction, increased physical exercise, dietary modifications, injury prevention, protected sexual activity, and increased availability and participation in disease-screening and prevention programs. The impetus for change from disease and illness treatment to health promotion and illness prevention is couched in the epidemiological transition from infectious disease to chronic disease as the leading cause of death, our nation's aging population, rapidly escalating costs of illness care, and data linking individual behaviors to increased risks of morbidity and mortality. Five settings today are key arenas for health education and health promotion: schools, communities, work sites, health care settings, and the consumer marketplace (Glanz, Lewis, & Rimer, 1990).

Economic Factors Affecting Health Care Delivery

Economic markets exist for the purpose of allocating scarce resources to pay for the provisions of goods and services. Over most of the 20th century, much political and financial capital has been spent maintaining the primacy of the free market in the American health care delivery system to minimize governmental interference (Ginzberg, 1996). The distribution of and access to health care services for the American people is significantly uneven. For people who live in the right geographic region, have the right health care coverage, and have a disease on which the health care professionals have chosen to focus, the American health care system is the best in the world. Those who live in the wrong place, with no health care coverage, and have diseases or conditions of lesser interest are at greater risk for poor health (Jonas, 1998). In an economy like that of the United States, trends and pressures from within and without affect it daily. Professional nurses are obligated to learn about and understand the disturbing economic trends and pressures affecting our nation and pulling our health care delivery system in many directions.

Employment and Unemployment

American workers' wages have stagnated or declined in recent decades. By some estimates, between 1983 and 1989 more than 60% of the new wealth in this country went to the top 1% of the population while 99% went to the top 20%. The wealth and income in the United States are becoming increasingly concentrated in the hands of just a few people, producing a large gap between those who have and those who do not. The issues of wage stagnation and wealth stratification are not topics that can be adequately addressed here, but they help explain some of the issues and concerns influencing the changes occurring in our health care delivery system (Carville, 1996).

Affluence and Poverty

One in seven Americans lives below the poverty level. One in five children under 18 years and one in four children under 3 years are living in poverty. Two of every five Hispanic children and one of every two black children are poor (The World Almanac, 1995). Many Americans living in poverty are the victims of social and environmental ills such as drug addiction, AIDS, crime, and prostitution. Their children likewise suffer from addiction, low birth weight, and resultant mental and physical problems. Solutions to these ills are often politically motivated, potentially punitive in nature, and wanting for long-term resolution and funding.

Over one-fifth of the elderly population is considered poor or near-poor. Women, blacks, and Hispanics experience poverty at a higher rate and must make do on Social Security benefits. The socioeconomic status of our nation's elderly (older than 65 years) varies dramatically based on their sources of income and assets. LTC institutionalization affects approximately 5% of the elderly population and involves mostly women who are unmarried or widowed.

Vulnerable populations are an increasingly visible reality in our daily experience. The homeless reside under the railroad viaducts. People with AIDS work beside us and live next door. Substance and/or alcohol abuse is a common experience crossing all economic and social levels in our country. Chronically ill and disabled, mentally ill and cognitively impaired, neglected and abused women, children and the elderly make up high-risk categories of vulnerable populations making increasing demands on society as a whole and on the health care system in particular (Aday, 1993).

Increased Costs of Health Care Services

The strengths and weaknesses of our nation's health care delivery system are well documented. Millions of Americans benefit from the care they receive through this system's technological excellence, research, well-educated and diverse group of health care providers, and facilities. This system—for all its wonders—is costly, its quality inconsistent, and its benefits unequally distributed (ANA, 1991).

More than 15% of the gross national product of the United States is consumed by the costs of health care. As a nurse you must understand the economic forces putting pressure on the present system's structure and function. During the 1990s the health care delivery system began a transition from episodic and fragmented care delivered through traditional fee-for-service arrangements to coordinated health care provided by integrated managed care systems. These emerging systems are predicted to be more efficient, focused on preventive and wellness care, and aware of the need to assess quality in outcomes, reduce costs, and adequately meet the needs of the consumer of health care (Buerhaus, 1996).

The expansion of integrated health care delivery systems throughout the country requires clinicians, administrators, educators, researchers, and policy-makers to work together to embrace the needed change and understand the economic forces working in today's market (Buerhaus, 1996). To avoid being shortchanged, nursing must ensure itself a seat at the policy-making table by understanding how economic forces drive change and how the system must continue to evolve to meet the needs of society. By seeing the "big picture," you enhance your position as a member of the health care system of tomorrow and fulfill your responsibility to society as a professional today.

Legal and Ethical Issues in Health Care Delivery

Ethical issues arise in all types of health services organizations. The acute care hospital is the site for the most significant ethical issues. The ever-increasing availability of technology is creating situations that require decision-making under complex and stressful circumstances (Fig. 5–4). Economic constraints and cost-cutting measures exacerbate these ethical problems and raise new ones. Competition pushes health care executives to walk a fine line between what

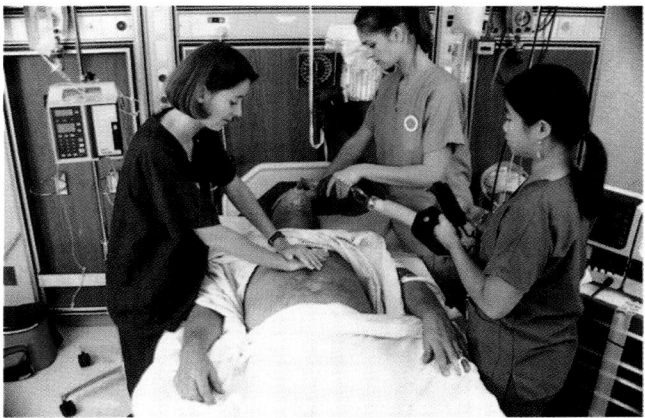

Figure 5–4. Modern technology leads daily to situations that require decision-making under complex and stressful circumstances.

is good for the business and what is ethical. Many ethical issues also have legal ramifications (Darr, 1991).

Access—A Client's Right

Access is a complex construct representing the personal use of health care services and the structures or processes that facilitate or impede that use. It is the link between the health care delivery system and the population the system purports to serve. Understanding access is key to formulating public policy related to the myriad issues of health care services (Andersen & Davidson, 1996). An awareness of the varying degrees and methods of access to health and illness care permits a beginning analysis of who receives what services, the quality of the service, and its outcome for the client (Vladeck, 1996).

Realized access is the actual use of health care providers and services. Equitable and inequitable access are defined according to what determines realized access. For example, to the extent that they are precursors of needs, age, gender, and ethnicity are indicators of equitable access or inequitable access when they determine who obtains access to health care (Andersen & Davidson, 1996).

Effective access is the link between utilization of health care services (realized access) and health outcomes that include enhanced health status and consumer satisfaction. Evaluating the effectiveness of access involves assessment of health care utilization within the context of predisposing, enabling, need, and health behavior variables. Predisposing variables are factors such as age, gender, and social support that could influence a person's health status after treatment. The presence of enabling resources such as health insurance and income can either lead to expeditious medical treatment taking advantage of state-of-the-art technology. Its absence can lead to delays in seeking medical care and result in episodic, fragmented treatment with the potential for negative impact on outcomes and satisfaction with the care received (Andersen & Davidson, 1996).

Legislation

To help formulate public policy that works to enhance access to health services, consumers need to get involved in the political process. For example, the elderly have had a major impact in influencing the political process in our country. As a group they are better educated than ever; organizations such as the Gray Panthers and the American Association of Retired Persons (AARP) have a legislative agenda and their own lobbyists in Washington, D.C., to advance their causes. Their capability to influence legislation and policy relative to specific issues of concern lies in their sheer numbers—their voting power. In contrast, the change in work patterns from a blue-collar manufacturing workforce with dwindling union membership to a white-collar, services-based workforce has affected organized labor's ability to influence politicians and allowed businesses to receive more support for their issues.

To successfully navigate the community-based redesign occurring within the health care delivery system, it is imperative that nurses and other health care providers expand professional relationships and build collegial relationships with community and other professional organizations. Nurses must understand how the government, the workplace, and national and local coalitions simultaneously and independently affect the community as a social unit (Johnson, 1996).

Understanding the political process requires involvement in an issue. Grassroots activism, such as telephone trees, letter writing campaigns, and lobbying of legislators, is spurred by a specific issue of interest and an identified outcome of the activity. No individual or professional organization can effectively go alone to create change. Collaboration with multiple disciplines and health care organizations creates a powerful network through which to effect change through the legislative process.

You have the unique opportunity as patient advocates not only to work in the political arena for accessible and cost-effective health care but also to influence and empower consumers themselves to aid this effort. The ability to create a working relationship among the stakeholders in the health care delivery system will be the key to whether or not nursing can successfully ensure its place at the public policy table (Johnson, 1996).

Ethics of Health Care Financing

The American health care system will continue to face the challenge of balancing three competing goals—containing costs, improving access to health care services, and enhancing the quality of care. The dehumanization of the reformed and re-engineered health care system of the 1990s led to consumer activism in the political areas of patients' rights and patient safety.

Tumultuous change in the health care delivery system requires health care providers, including nurses, to be vigilant to ensure that the level of quality achieved not be left to chance. For their part, consumers must insist that an adequate mechanism for assessing value and effectiveness of care and services be in place to monitor and report to federal, state, and private sector providers. Consumers must be willing to respond to lack of satisfaction in their health care and health services in the same way they would any other product or service, if necessary by lobbying for legislation, legal action, and media campaigns. Today's consumers are better educated, more aggressive, and not limited to thinking that "the doctor knows best" or that illness prevention is the only way to improve their health and overall quality of life.

Opportunities in Health Care Delivery

America's health care system will always be changing, both in financing mechanisms and delivery systems. With an increasing emphasis on health versus illness, the fundamental issue of resource constraints will challenge the system of health service delivery to ensure equitable access, shared costs, and improving quality. Looking to the new millennium, health care professionals must rise to the opportunities presented by health care reform, technological progress, environmental challenges, and quality improvement.

Health Care Reform

The United States health care system is a patchwork of many subsystems loosely connected to provide medical care rather than health care to those who are insured. Although the system is undergoing major changes, most of these are focused on improving delivery of and payment for illness care rather than providing better health care. Reform should look to systems that would integrate services and activities to minimize risks and provide early detection and treatment of emerging diseases. These systems must also place a greater emphasis on wellness and public health for the health care system reform to eventually affect the overall health of the American population (Keck & Scutchfield, 1997).

Technological Progress

The technological advances of recent decades have significantly affected the delivery of health care and its outcomes. Selected developments include computerized clinical laboratory and diagnostic equipment, multiple organ transplants, improved invasive and noninvasive surgical techniques, genetic engineering, and use of lasers. These advances have allowed the health professions to treat certain conditions more quickly, more safely, and more effectively, with less pain and fewer complications.

In spite of their benefits, many fear that "high-tech" equipment and procedures will increase the use of machines and decrease human interaction. It is this fear of depersonalization of health care that is fueling the demand for more humane or "high-touch" care systems, such as hospice care, birthing rooms, and neighborhood clinics. Some high-tech equipment, notably computers, can also be used to increase human contact. For example, electronic mail and Internet services can be used to help people communicate and share information with each other (Kelly & Joel, 1996). The use of computers in health care institutions and agencies is likely to intensify. They have become critical to various functions within a health care organization, such as patient records, billing and accounting, information processing and retrieval, hiring and staffing, and ordering and tracking supplies.

Unquestionably, computers have helped to improve the delivery of health care services in our country. Integrated computerized systems within hospitals and other health care agencies link a patient's care with every department within the facility. Outside the hospital, computer-assisted communication techniques are making speedy transmission of health information and new knowledge a powerful influence in molding public opinion.

Environmental Health Challenges

In addition to the behavioral and biological factors that determine health, a complex array of environmental influences must also be considered. Green and Krueter (1991) find the scope of environmental determinants of health so complex that they divide the environment into three components: physical, social, and psychological. In a health context, the physical environment includes hazards, such as air, noise, and water pollution, with the potential consequences of hearing loss, infectious diseases, gastroenteritis, cancer, emphysema, and bronchitis.

Social and psychological components of environmental health can be combined to address the major issues of behavior modification, perceptual problems, and interpersonal relationships. Crowded living spaces, physical and/or social isolation, rapid and persistent change, and increased social interchange may all contribute to homicide, suicide, decisional stress, and environmental overstimulation, which negatively affects the overall health of the individual and the community. Professional nursing must be involved in policy-making decisions that set standards and controls on responsible agencies and industries directed at control for the potential threats to health and safety in our physical environment.

Quality Improvement

The growth of managed care with its emphasis on cost containment has heightened interest in quality because of the concern that containing costs will diminish and disrupt quality. Defining quality and identifying measurements of quality are hampered by the unequal system attention to cost and access. Differing definitions of quality by clients, providers, and payers translates into different expectations of the health care delivery system and evaluations of its quality. The opportunity is there for health care organizations to minimize these differences in definition and expectation (McGlynn & Brook, 1996).

The basic goal of the health care system in the United States is to provide those services that will optimize the overall health of the resident population. The key to achieving this goal is the commitment to quality—its assurance, monitoring, evaluation, and improvement. The Joint Commission on Accreditation of Healthcare Organizations (JCAHO) has published standards to help health care organizations continuously improve and meet this basic goal.

The future of our health care delivery system and the quality of its services will depend on the ability of health care professionals to work with consumers, policy-makers, and payers. The ethical dilemmas of access, impact of technology, cost versus quality versus amount of service, business orientation of the delivery system, provider turf battles, and availability of alternative health and illness care treatments will challenge everyone to be partners. Professionals, policy-makers, providers, payers, and consumers must act in concert with each other to ensure that basic health care services are delivered by a system that acknowledges the ties between quality and the caring interaction.

KEY PRINCIPLES

- The medical model, or more specifically, the bio-medical model, which presumes the existence of illness or disease, has largely governed health care delivery in the United States.
- *Health promotion* is aimed at modifying a client's knowledge, attitudes, and skills to adopt behaviors leading to healthier lifestyles.
- *Illness prevention* relies on similar strategies described as primary prevention, such as immunizations, health screenings, and medications that prevent disease. The technological advances experienced in the last few decades have enabled medical scientists to improve their accuracy of illness and disease diagnosis and to more effectively treat clients.
- It is thought that the changes in health behaviors and the improvements in environmental quality account for most of the gains in improved health, rather than medical care.
- Registered nurses focus on health promotion and disease prevention and are the major care providers of sick and injured clients and are responsible for planning and delivering direct care to a group of clients.
- Physicians are the major providers of health services playing a central role in the diagnosis and treatment of diseases, illnesses, and injuries.

- The American Academy of Physician Assistants (1996) defines a *physician assistant* as "a member of the health care team who works in a dependent relationship with a supervising physician to provide comprehensive care."
- Allied health workers can be divided into two broad categories: therapists/technologists and technicians/assistants.
- The role of the pharmacist includes instructing clients about medications as well as advising physicians and other health care providers about new and complex pharmaceutical management regimens.
- Social workers help clients and families cope with the problems resulting from long-term illness, injury, and rehabilitation. They also often work in clinical settings as case managers to facilitate appropriate client discharge and follow-up care, working to ensure proper use of community services.
- The term *inpatient* is used in conjunction with an overnight stay in a hospital or other facility. Inpatient treatment is provided in long-term care facilities such as nursing homes, in psychiatric hospitals, and rehabilitation centers.
- Outpatient services do not require an overnight inpatient stay in a hospital or long-term care facility, though these institutions may offer these services.
- Managed care is a system that combines the functions of health insurance and the actual delivery of care, where costs and utilization of services are controlled.
- Changes in the composition of a population are important for the planning of health care services.
- Economic markets exist for allocating scarce resources to pay for the provisions of goods and services.
- The United States health care system will continue to face the challenge of balancing three competing goals—containing costs, improving access to health care services, and enhancing the quality of the delivered health care services.

BIBLIOGRAPHY

*Aday, L.A. (1993). *At risk in America: The health and health care needs of vulnerable populations in the United States.* San Francisco: Jossey-Bass.

*American Academy of Physician Assistants (AAPA). (1996). *PA fact sheet.* Arlington, VA: Author.

*American Council on Pharmaceutical Education. (1992). *The proposed revision of accreditation standards and guidelines.* Chicago: National Association of Boards on Pharmacy.

*American Hospital Association (AHA). (1994). *AHA guide to the health care field 1994 edition.* Chicago: Author.

*American Nurses' Association (ANA). (1991). *Nursing's agenda for health care reform.* Washington, D.C.: Author.

Andersen, R.M., & Davidson, P.L. (1996). Measuring Trends and Access. In R.M. Anderson, T.H. Rice, & G.F. Kominski (Eds.),

Changing the U.S. health care system: Key issues in health service, policy, and management. San Francisco: Jossey-Bass Publishers.

*Beresford, L. (1989). *History of the national hospice organization.* Arlington, VA: The National Hospice Organization.

Bodenheimer, T. (1997). The Oregon health plan—Lessons for the nation. *The New England Journal of Medicine, 337*(9), 651–655.

Buerhaus, P.I. (1996). Creating a new place in a competitive market: The value of nursing care. *Nursing Policy Forum, 2*(2), 13–16, 18–20.

*Bullough, B., & Bullough, V. (1994). *Nursing issues.* New York: Springer.

Burton, L. (1996). The ethical dilemmas of the Oregon health plan. *Nurse Practitioner, 21*(2), 62–72.

Carville, J. (1996). *We're right, they're wrong.* New York: Random House.

Collins, A.C. (1995). The Hahnenmann homeless clinics project: Taking health care to the streets and shelters. *Journal of the American Medical Association, 273*(5), 433.

*Darr, K. (1991). *Ethics in health services management* (2nd ed.). Baltimore: Health Professions Press.

Davis, M.H., & Burner, S.T. (1995). Three decades of Medicare: What the numbers tell us. *Health Affairs, 14*(4), 231–243.

*Department of Health and Human Services (DHHS). (1990). *Health status of the disadvantaged.* DHHS Publication No. (HRSA) HRS-P-DV 90-1. Washington, D.C.: Government Printing Office.

Ernst, E. (1996). The ethics of complementary medicine. *Journal of Medical Ethics, 22*(4), 197–198.

*Furula, B. & Lipson, J. (1994). Cultural diversity in the student body revisited. In J. McCloskey & H. Grace (Eds.), *Current issues in nursing* (4th Ed.) (p 665). St. Louis: Mosby.

General Accounting Office. (1996). *Private health insurance: Millions relying on individual market coverage face cost and coverage trade-offs.* Washington, D.C.: Author.

Ginzberg, E. (1996). The health care market. *Journal of the American Medical Association, 276,* 777.

*Glanz, K., Lewis, F.M., & Rimer, B.K. (1990). *Health behavior and health education: Theory, research, and practice.* San Francisco: Jossey-Bass.

Gordon, J.S. (1996). Alternative medicine and the family practitioner. *American Family Physician, 54*(7), 2205–2212.

*Green, L.W., & Krueter, M.W. (1991). *Health promotion planning: An educational and environmental approach* (2nd Ed.). Mountain View, CA: Mayfield.

*Hadorn, D.C. (1991). The Oregon priority-setting exercise: Quality of life and public policy. *Hastings Center Report, 21*(3), 11–16.

*Haglund, C.L. & Dowling, W.L. (1993). The hospital. In S.J. Williams & P.R. Torreno (Eds.), *Introduction to health services* (4th ed.) (pp 135–176). Albany, NY: Delmar.

Health Care Financing Administration (HCFA). (1996). Medicaid financing and payment. *Health Care Financing Review Statistical Supplement,* 154–165.

Johnson, K.P. (1996). Up close and personal: Making the most of visits to legislators. *Nursing Policy Forum, 2*(2), 7.

Jonas, S. (1998). *An introduction to the U.S. health care system* (4th ed.). New York: Springer.

Kamen, R.L. (1995). *Worksite health promotion economics: Consensus and analysis.* Champaign, IL: Human Kinetics.

Keck, W., & Scutchfield, F.D. (1997). *The future of public health.* Albany, NY: Delmar.

Kelly, L.Y., & Joel, L.A. (1996). *The nursing experience: Trends, challenges, and transitions* (3rd ed.). New York: McGraw-Hill.

Knickman, J.R. & Thorpe, K.E. (1995). Financing for health care. In A.R. Kovner (Ed.), *Jonas' health care delivery in the United States* (5th ed.). New York: Springer.

Koch, A.L., Williams, S.J., & Hylton, H.C. (1993). Marketing prevention to elderly Medicare beneficiaries enrolled in an HMO: The San Diego Medicare Preventive Health Project. *Journal of Health Care Marketing 3*(1), 46–53.

Leininger, M.M. (1991). Culture care diversity and universality: A theory of nursing. Publication No. 15-2402. New York: National League for Nursing Press.

Levit, K., Cowan, C., Braden, D., Stiller, J., Sensenig, A., & Lazenby, H. (1998). National health expenditures in 1997: More slow growth. *Health Affairs, 17*(6), 99–110.

---

*Asterisk indicates a classic or definitive work on this subject.

*Marcrom, R.E., Horton, R.M., & Shepherd, M.D. (1992). Create value-added services to meet patient needs. *American Pharmacy, 532*(7), 48–57.

*McBeath, W.H. (1991). Health for all: A public health vision. *American Journal of Public Health, 81*(12), 1560–1565.

McGlynn, E.A. & Brook, R.H. (1996). Ensuring quality of care. In R.M. Andersen, T.H. Rice, & G.F. Kominski (Eds.), *Changing the U.S. health care system: Key issues in health services, policy, and management* (pp 142–179). San Francisco: Jossey-Bass.

Montague, J. (1997). Why rationing was right for Oregon. *Hospitals & Health Networks, 71*(3), 64–65.

*Naisbitt, J., & Aburdene, P. (1990). *Megatrends 2000: Ten new directions for the 1990's.* New York: Morrow.

National Center for Health Statistics (NCHS). (1996). *Health United States, 1995.* Hyattsville, MD: DHHS Pub. No. (PHS) 96-1236.

*National Institute for Adult Day Care. (1984). *Standards for adult day care.* Washington, D.C.: National Council on the Aging, Inc.

Neimark, J. (1997). On the front lines of alternative medicine. *Psychology Today, 30*(1), 52–57, 67–68.

*Oregon Health Services Commission. (1991). *Prioritization of health services: A report to the Governor and legislature.* Salem, OR: Author.

Organization for Economic Cooperation and Development (OECD). (1998). *OECD health data 1998: A comparative analysis of 29 counties.* Paris: OECD.

Richardson, H. (1995). Long-term care. In A.R. Kovner (Ed.), *Jonas' health care delivery in the United States* (5th ed.) (pp 194–231). New York: Springer.

Roemer, M.I. (1996). Lessons from other countries. In R.M. Andersen, T.H. Rice, & G.F. Kominski (Eds.), *Changing the U.S. health care system: Key issues in health services, policy, and management* (pp 340–351). San Francisco: Jossey-Bass.

Santerre, R.E., & Neun, S.P. (1996). *Health economics: Theories, insights, and industry studies.* Chicago: Irwin.

*Sardell, A. (1983). Neighborhood health centers and community-based care: Federal policy from 1965 to 1982. *Journal of Public Health Policy, 4,* 484–489.

Sharfstein, S.S., Stoline, A.M., & Koran, L. (1995). Mental health services. In A.R. Kovner (Ed.), *Jonas' health care delivery in the United States* (5th ed.) (pp 232–266). New York: Springer.

Shi, L., & Singh, D.A. (1998). *Delivering healthcare in America: A systems approach.* Gaithersburg, MD: Aspen.

Starfield, B. (1996). Public health and primary care: A framework for proposed linkages. *American Journal of Public Health, 86,* 1365–1369.

*Steinbrook, R., & Lo, B. (1992). The Oregon Medicaid demonstration project—Will it provide adequate medical care? *The New England Journal of Medicine, 326,* 340–344.

*Summer, L. (1991). *Limited access: Health care for the rural poor.* Washington, D.C.: Center on Budget and Policy Priorities.

Sumner, C.H. (1998). Recognizing and responding to spiritual distress. *American Journal of Nursing, 98*(1), 26–31.

U.S. Bureau of the Census. (1997, 1998). *Current population reports: Health insurance coverage, 1997 and 1998.* Washington, D.C.: Government Printing Office.

Vladeck, B.C. (1996). The corporatization of American health care and why it is happening. In E.D. Baer, C.M. Fagin, & S. Gordon (Eds.), *Abandonment of the patient: The impact of profit-driven health care on the public* (pp 9–19). New York: Springer.

Wagner, E.R. (1995). Types of managed care organizations. In P.R. Kongstevedt (Ed.), *Essentials of managed health care* (pp 24–34). Gaithersburg, MD: Aspen.

Walsh, G.G. (1995). How subacute care fills the gap. *Nursing, 25*(3), 51.

White, N. & Lubkin, I. (1995). Illness trajectory. In I.M. Lubkin, *Chronic illness: Impact and interventions* (3rd ed.) (pp 51–73). Boston: Jones and Bartlett.

Williams, S.J. (1995). *Essentials of health services.* Albany, NY: Delmar.

Yap, O.W., & Thornton, D.J. (1995). The Arbor Tree clinic at Stanford: A multidisciplinary effort. *Journal of the American Medical Association, 273*(5), 431.

A Framework for Nursing Practice

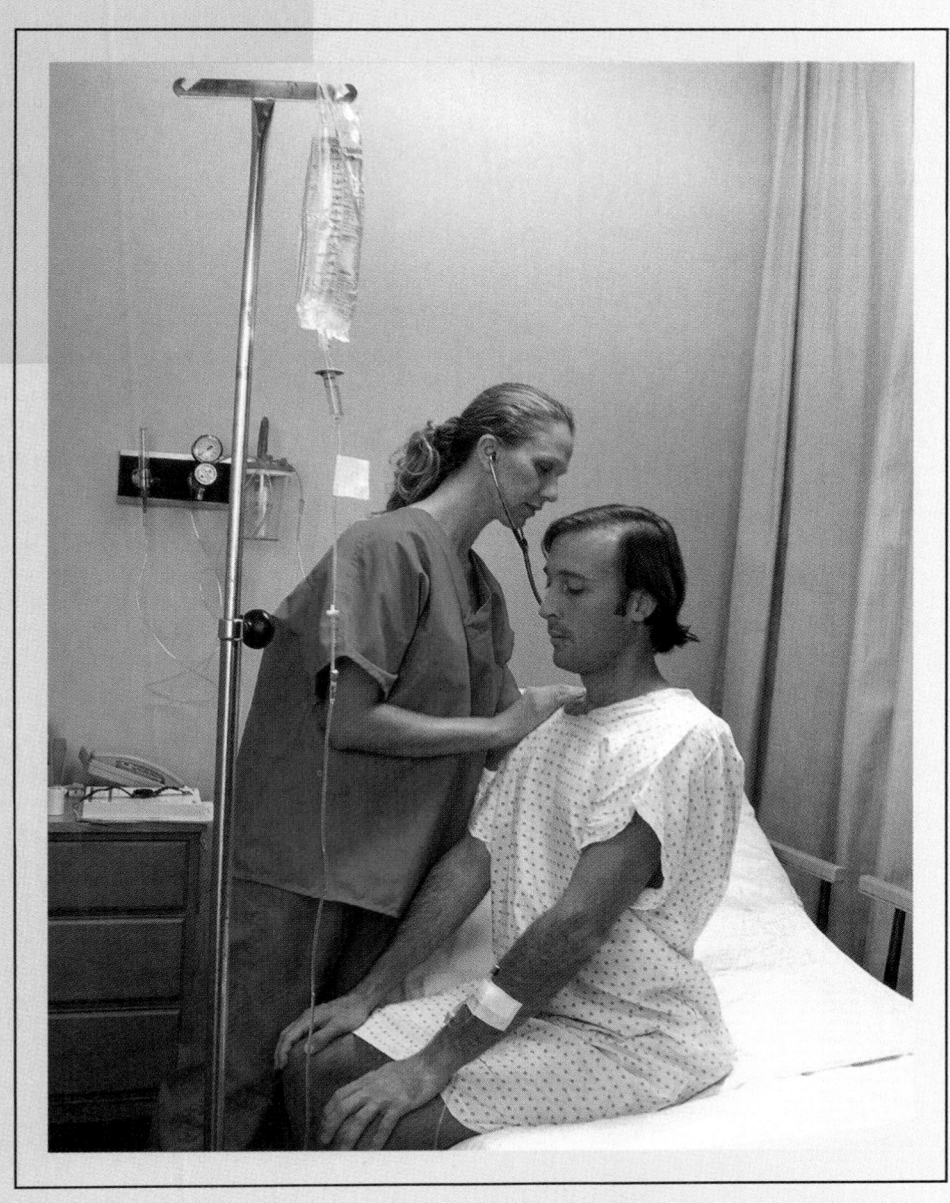

CHAPTER

Developing a Framework for Practice

Virginia Nehring and V. Doreen Wagner

6

Key Terms

conceptual framework
conceptual model
model

paradigm
theory

After studying this chapter, you should be able to:

1. Provide definitions of the terminology used in nursing theory.
2. Describe the four components common to present nursing theories.
3. Discuss the importance of theory in nursing practice.
4. Compare and contrast at least five significant nursing theories.
5. Describe the advantages of multiple theories.
6. Discuss obstacles to implementing nursing theory in practice.
7. Examine the application of three theories to practice.

Early nurse leaders and scholars struggled with the definition, philosophy, and art of nursing. Since World War II, nurse scholars have been diligently establishing a knowledge base for nursing practice in order for nursing to be recognized as a profession and as a science. Nursing as a science has progressed rapidly, and we now have a large body of scientific theory available to guide the practice of professional nursing.

A **theory** is a group of propositions used to describe, explain, or predict a phenomenon. The term *phenomenon* refers to the facts, behaviors, problems, and events that describe a reality. The reality of nursing includes the client, the environment, the health and illness continuum, and nursing actions. Nursing theories therefore interpret and explain the reality of nursing.

Theories of nursing also provide professional autonomy by guiding practice, education, and research activities for nursing as a profession. Theory is useful in demonstrating that nursing is a practice discipline, a profession with a unique body of knowledge, needed and trusted by society to help individuals, families, groups, and communities retain and promote health and intervene when there is illness and disease (Fig. 6–1).

A nursing theory can describe nursing, hypothesize the effects of a nursing intervention, describe the phenomena that nurses treat, or provide a basis for selecting nursing interventions. The theories discussed in this chapter were chosen because they describe a global concept of nursing that gives direction to practice and research. This type of theory usually defines nursing from a philosophical perspective, identifies the concepts of interest to nursing, and hypothesizes a relationship among these concepts. This chapter also shows you how to apply three of the most widely used nursing theories in clinical practice.

FOUNDATION OF NURSING THEORY

There are certain common characteristics related to science development. For example, natural science developed from beliefs about what is present in nature. The science of nursing developed from beliefs about the nature of nursing and the phenomena in nursing practice. Not all nurses share exactly the same philosophy about the nature of nursing practice, but most nurses share common beliefs about the basis for nursing practice. These common beliefs eventually led to theories in nursing. To help you understand nursing theories, the components of a theory are clarified first and then a discussion on how those components are organized follows.

Components of Nursing Theory

Philosophy can be defined as the values and beliefs about the nature of a discipline and the phenomena of concern to the discipline. The philosophy of a discipline determines what is studied and the beginning assumptions about what is true.

Assumptions are beliefs about phenomena that are taken for granted to be true. Nursing theories may assume that quality of life is good, that nursing makes a difference in clients' lives, and that most humans want to maximize their health and well-being. Sometimes for a science to develop, the underlying assumptions need to be questioned and the direction of the discipline challenged.

A *concept* is a complex image of an object, property, or event that is derived from individual experiences. Concepts are a way of naming and describing things that are important in order to understand nursing practice. Concepts typically include two types of definitions: the first definition, called a *conceptual definition,* refers to what the concept is. The second, or *operational definition,* refers to how it is measured or described. For example, stress could be defined conceptually, or in meaningful terms, by saying stress is a feeling of discomfort or distress that results when the person is confronted with overwhelming stimuli. An operational definition of stress might be that stress can be demonstrated in physiological changes such as increased pulse, increased blood pressure, and other "fight or flight" symptoms.

The relationship between the concepts constitutes theory. Concepts, then, can be described as the building blocks of theory. A theory's concepts illustrate that particular theorist's perception of phenomenon and the definition of the concepts make up that reality. This means that to use a theory in the way it is intended, you must know the meaning intended by the concepts.

Because concepts alone do not create a theory, what does? A theory exists when the relationships between concepts that make up the theory are explained in relationship statements. Several terms for relationship statements can be used. *Propositions* are statements that represent the theoretical view of which concepts fit together and how those concepts affects one another. When there are suggestions that a relationship between concepts may exist, that relationship

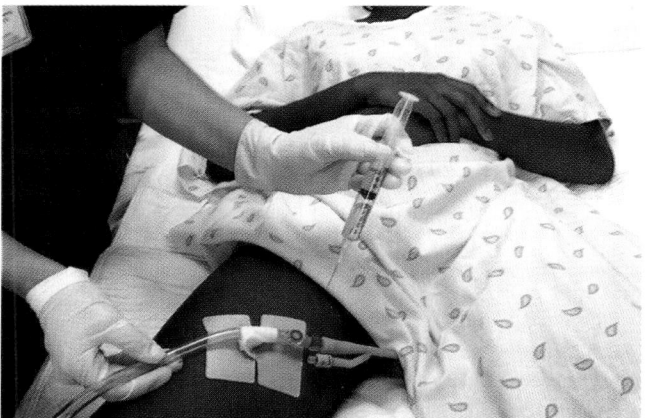

Figure 6–1. Theory is useful in demonstrating that nursing is a practice discipline.

is tested. A *hypothesis* is a relationship statement that can be tested.

A framework is a structure that provides support. A **conceptual framework** is a group of related concepts that support a particular viewpoint or focus. Conceptual frameworks are the structure from which theories are derived.

A **paradigm** is a set of philosophical assumptions from which a scientist studies natural phenomena. A discipline's paradigm includes the knowledge, philosophy, theory, educational experience, practice orientation, research, and literature that is held in common. Nursing's paradigm identifies the common areas of core concern for our discipline.

Use of Theories From Other Disciplines

Historically, nursing was task-oriented and used only basic scientific principles, rules, and traditions for practice. As nursing developed, nursing began to use theories from the behavioral, biological, and physical sciences. Many nursing theories are based on discoveries from other fields, such as knowledge of growth and development from the field of psychology (Fig. 6–2). Nurses have incorporated these theories into their practice.

Early nurse theorists, in the 1950s, dealt with the definition, philosophy, and art of nursing. By the end of the 1960s, the focus of nursing theory was the science of nursing. During the 1980s, theories reflecting humanism and nursing as an art and science were accepted by the profession. Nursing theorists of that time and now found that when non-nursing theory was used with a nursing perspective, the non-nursing theory changes and reflects the uniqueness of our profession. Even with the borrowed concepts or ideas, nursing theory remains about nursing and is our body of knowledge and practice.

Organization of Nursing Theory

The concepts of person, environment, health, and nursing are the most recognized organizing realities of

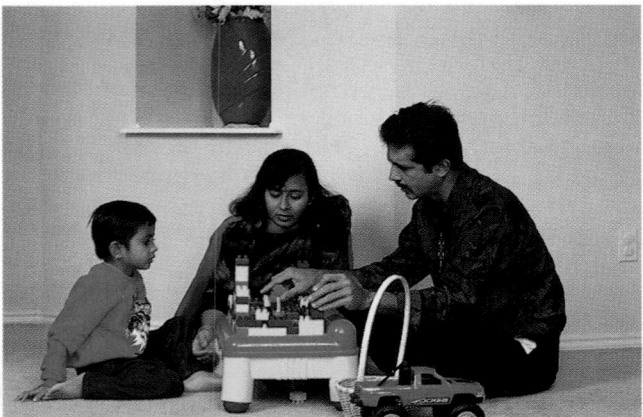

Figure 6–2. Many nursing theories are based on discoveries from other fields, such as knowledge of growth and development from psychology.

nursing theory. These concepts have provided the boundaries and the shared viewpoint and have helped nurses focus their practice over the last half century.

Recently, nurse scientists have added caring to the paradigm for nursing research. Clarification of the caring focus may broaden the boundaries of nursing and reaffirm our long-standing social directive. The major concepts of this new paradigm include self-care, adaptation, mutual goal attainment, culture care, and human becoming. It is these care phenomenon that are beginning to guide research and practice and reaching for further expansion of nursing knowledge. As the dialogue and research continue and a clearer picture emerges, the paradigm of nursing will evolve and change to reflect a more current theoretical practice.

IMPORTANCE OF NURSING THEORIES

Overall, theory is important because it demonstrates that nursing, as a discipline, is a profession with a unique body of knowledge. Nursing theories differentiate the focus of nursing from other professions and are necessary for the continued growth and development of our profession. It enables professional validity and advancement. Present theoretical knowledge and the further development of nursing's knowledge base will also fulfill the expectations of society to help maintain and recover the health of individuals, families, groups, and communities. The importance of theories can also be found in guidance for nursing practice, in the progress of nursing research, and in the development of curricula for nursing education.

Guidance for Practice

The development of nursing knowledge is as important today as it was in 1950. Theories are important to nurses because they help us determine the meaning of clinical experience while providing guidance for our practice. In practice, theory helps you make astute observations, communicate more effectively, work more efficiently, and accomplish the goals of nursing.

Theories guide practice in several ways. First, they prescribe the classes of phenomena that are observed or used in practice. For example, if the theoretical basis for nursing practice didn't include the client's environment, the nurse caring for an elderly woman with a fractured hip would not think it important to know if the home environment was safe and would teach her to use a walker, without thinking of how many stairs she had to climb.

A theory may also determine the relative importance of the phenomena. You may believe that the client's environment is an important determinant of recovery, but how important do you think it is in relationship to her physiological condition? A theory may hypothesize the most appropriate nurse's role. Is nursing primarily doing or is it teaching? Or is it providing an environment conducive to health? Theory can help you define the goals of nursing or even describe the client's role in the relationship.

Precise descriptions of nursing concepts and the organization of concepts help you think clearly and transfer knowledge from one situation to a similar situation. Without organized knowledge and well-defined concepts, you would be forced to memorize unrelated facts for multiple situations. Theoretical thinking strengthens the meaning of nursing and enhances the nurse's role in client care. It provides a framework from which to work with clients. You can choose a specific theory to guide your practice or use ideas from multiple theories.

Theory also gives nurses the structure and the common terminology to communicate nursing goals, actions, and choices, and therefore increases the individual nurse's self-identity and esteem. Much of what nursing does is considered invisible—that is, it goes on inside the nurse's head. By making nursing practice more visible and understandable through theory, nursing becomes more appreciated, valued, and understood by society, other professions, and nurses themselves.

Progress in Research

Nursing theory and research can be viewed as interdependent components of the scientific process. When constructing a theory, the theorist must be knowledgeable about the empirical findings and formalize the available knowledge by validating or verifying knowledge through research activities. A theory is accepted when the consensus of the nursing profession is that the theory provides an adequate description of reality. In the broadest sense, nursing research and theory development are necessary for the continued evolution of nursing as a science.

A conceptual or theoretical framework guides and focuses research. Using a framework for nursing, the known knowledge can be extrapolated, and then the researcher can focus on what is not known. The framework itself may suggest hypotheses that need to be tested or concepts that need to be more clearly defined. Nursing research is the testing of theory based on nursing practice.

Development of Nursing Curricula

To know best what to teach, the first nursing research sought to determine which nursing actions were or were not effective. Nightingale was a superb statistician, keeping detailed statistics on the outcomes of nursing work or interventions. Later research was also used to help determine what should be taught in nursing curricula as well as how best to teach it. Research, theory, and education are interdependent.

Theory is important to nurse educators because it provides a general focus for curriculum design and guides curricular decision-making. Nurse educators may choose one theory on which to base their curricula or may use numerous theories to guide the flow of the nursing program. A theoretical framework can provide the faculty and students with a perspective with which to view client situations, a way to or-ganize client data, and a way to analyze and interpret the information. A theoretical perspective allows faculty to develop a purposeful and proactive curriculum; it gives students an approach from which to learn and begin to practice.

OVERVIEW OF SELECTED NURSING THEORIES

There are many nursing theories, frameworks, and models. This chapter only addresses a few of the major nursing theorists. In the following sections, we will take a brief look at nursing theorists who viewed nursing as philosophy, nursing as interpersonal relationship, nursing as a system, nursing as an energy field, and nursing as care. As you read, you will also get a glimpse into the evolution of nursing theory. For further information about these theories, consult the bibliography for the original works of the theorists.

Nursing as a Philosophy

Florence Nightingale wrote extensively on what she and other nurses were attempting to do during the Crimean War. She gathered statistics on the death rate in the hospital before and after nurses intervened. She was our first researcher, using statistics to show the effect of nursing care. She was also our first theorist, believing the environment crucial to a client's ability to regain health.

Nightingale based the nurse's actions mainly on her recognition of the importance of the environment. She believed environment included all external conditions and influences affecting life including ventilation, food, warmth, odors, noise, and light (Nightingale, 1969). Through being supportive and physically present, the nurses also enhanced a sense of well-being in suffering clients.

To teach new recruits to nursing how to give nursing care, curricula were created to help teach students about nursing using Nightingale's theory, specifically the importance of the environment for client healing. Students were taught how to manipulate the environment and support the client as the client sought health. From the beginning of modern nursing, nurses were involved in the care of clients and seeking health through manipulating the environment.

Virginia Henderson (1955) defined nursing as doing for clients what they would do for themselves if they had the necessary knowledge, will, or strength. Her definition of nursing was adopted by The International Council of Nursing and later by the World Health Organization. Henderson (1955) also identified 14 basic needs of clients that make up the components of nursing care:

Breathing
Eating and drinking
Elimination
Movement
Rest and sleep
Suitable clothing

Body temperature
Clean body and protected integument
Safe environment
Communication
Worship
Work
Play
Learning

Henderson denied having created a theory, but her concept or definition of nursing has been accepted throughout the world.

Faye Abdellah and her colleagues (1960) suggested using a problem-solving approach to deal with the 21 nursing problems she identified in clinical practice. She changed nursing practice when her book *Patient Centered Approaches to Nursing* (1960) was published. This list of nursing problems essentially outlined everything nurses did, from improving nutrition to increasing comfort. Her list served as an organizer for what nurses did. Abdellah's theoretical approach went beyond the medical model of client care as it focused on meeting client needs. It is a very practical theory and was validated by a systematic use of research.

Dorothea Orem (1995) defines nursing as a human service and theorizes that nursing's special concern is in assisting people to achieve self-care. Orem's focus is primarily on the needs of the client and the actions of nursing to meet those needs. Her theory of self-care maintains that nursing care is needed when people are affected by limitations that do not allow them to meet their self-care needs. According to Orem, the need for nursing care stems from a client's self-care deficit.

Orem's conceptual model is widely accepted by nursing because it can be applied to many settings and a broad range of nursing situations. Orem's contribution to theory development is the delineation of nursing function in self-care needs and continued work for empirical support through research. We will be using Orem's model in a client care example later in this chapter.

Nursing as Interpersonal Relationship

Hildegarde Peplau introduced her interpersonal concepts in 1952 and based them on several available theories at that time. She heavily used psychoanalytic theory as well as principles of social learning and concepts of human motivation and personality development to develop her theory of nursing as an interpersonal relationship with clients (Peplau, 1952). Peplau is known as the first to borrow from other scientific fields and relate the data to nursing theory. She was also the first theorist after Nightingale to present a theory for nursing. Peplau's ideas and theory development are the basis for psychiatric nursing.

Peplau saw nursing as a force that is realized as the personality develops through educational, therapeutic, and interpersonal processes. Nurses enter into relationships with clients when clients become aware of health-related needs. In entering into relationships with clients, nurses use the self in a therapeutic way (Fig. 6–3). Peplau believed that in the nurse-client relationship, the nurse assumes many roles: stranger, teacher, resource person, surrogate, leader, and counselor. She also identified four phases of the nurse-client relationship: orientation, identification, exploration, and resolution. Many nurses today use Peplau's theory as a model when working with clients.

Ida Jean Orlando (1961) suggested that all nurses can use interpersonal relationships to meet the needs of the client as defined by that client, not as defined by the nurse. Orlando also introduced the nursing process as a tool for nursing practice. She delineated automatic actions and deliberate actions from the three elements of a nursing situation: client behavior, nurse reaction, and nursing actions. Although many consider the nursing process to be the main framework for practice (Yura & Walsh, 1978a, 1978b), both Peplau and Orlando focused on the nurse-client interaction process. Orlando's theoretical contribution has advanced nursing, from personal and automatic responses to disciplined and professional practice responses.

Nursing as a System

Sister Callista Roy's (1976) adaptation model for nursing was heavily based on Helson's adaptation model. According to Roy, humans are biopsychosocial beings who exist through adaptation within an environment. Her model combines divergent thinking, such as systems, stress, and adaptation, into a convergent view of a client interacting with the environment. Roy's model differentiates nursing from medicine by focusing its activity on client adaptation as opposed to health or illness in themselves. This systems model is a good example of how borrowed knowledge from other disciplines becomes unique when used in nursing.

Roy's theory was originally implemented at Mount Saint Mary's College's School of Nursing in Los Angeles. Based on feedback from students and faculty there, Roy refined her ideas and, consequently as Roy

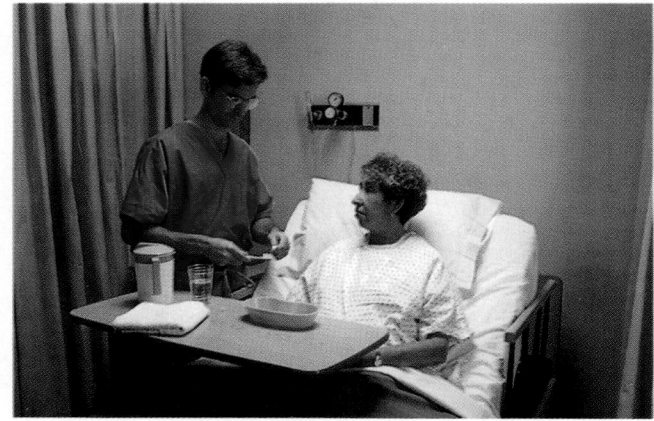

Figure 6–3. In entering into relationships with clients, nurses use the self in a therapeutic way.

published her theory, other schools of nursing as well as clinical agencies began using it and still do today. We will explore the use of Roy's adaptation model in the client care example at the end of this chapter.

In 1970, *Betty Neuman* introduced a comprehensive conceptual model for nursing that is based on a systems point of view to evaluate nursing problems. She views the client as a system functioning harmoniously in relation to environmental influences. The client system is composed of five interacting elements: physiological, psychological, sociocultural, developmental, and spiritual (Neuman, 1995). The focus of this model is the concern with the stability of the client system as it encounters stressors in the environment. The goal of keeping the client system stable is achieved through nursing actions derived from prevention measures.

Neuman's systems model is applicable to many nursing practice settings involving individuals, families, groups, and communities because it promotes the attainment and maintenance of maximum level wellness through purposeful interventions. It is widely accepted by nursing all around the world. Her contribution to theory development in nursing is the recognition of prevention as it relates to stress reduction.

Imogene King's (1971) work can be categorized as a systems model derived from three dynamic interacting systems: personal systems or individuals, interpersonal systems or groups, and social systems or society. King believes the client is a personal system within other systems. Her major concepts are interaction, perception, communication, transaction, role, stress, growth and development, and time and space. The nurse and the client perceive one another and the situation, act and react, interact, and transact. King (1971) defined nursing as a human interaction process between nurse and client, who communicate to set goals, explore actions for reaching the goals, and then agree on which actions to be used. Her theory of goal attainment highlights the importance of the decision-making process and the outcomes of nursing care. King's contribution to nursing is the specification of outcomes for nurse-client interactions.

Nursing as an Energy Field

Myra Levine (1967), in an article published in the journal *Nursing Forum*, distinguished nursing from medical practice by suggesting that all nursing actions were to conserve the client's energy, structural or physiological integrity, personal integrity, and social integrity. Levine's nursing activity analysis resulted in the formulation of *four conservation principles* in helping clients adapt to environment. She saw nurses as manipulating the environment to help clients adapt. She presented the client holistically and as the center of nursing activities. Levine's ideas literally changed nurses' self-perception of what nursing was about and helped nurses organize their thoughts and activities.

Martha Rogers (1970) saw human beings as dynamic energy fields integral or interwoven with environmental fields, both identified and recognized by their pattern, existing in a multidimensional universe. Rogers' theory of unitary human beings has the central focus that humans and their environments are integrated and inter-related energy fields. She clearly emphasized that nursing was not something a person does, but a body of abstract knowledge, a learned profession that is both science and art. Rogers' theory was revolutionary at that time and provided the foundation for a large body of research. Many in our profession regard the theory of nursing as an energy field as having the potential to evolve into a body of knowledge unique to nursing.

Nursing as Care

Madeleine Leininger (1978) was one of the first nursing theorists to stress the importance of *care* in the nurse-client relationship. She believes that caring is the central theme in nursing knowledge and practice. Educated in cultural and social anthropology, Leininger states that caring varies among cultures in its processes and patterns, is largely culturally derived, and is culturally expressed. Leininger's theory of transcultural care focuses on culture-specific and culture-universal nursing practices. She identifies culture as the broadest and most holistic way to view, understand, and be effective with people. She is the founder of *transcultural nursing* and defines this practice as a focused study and analysis of cultures with the goal of developing a scientific and humanistic body of nursing knowledge to better provide culture-specific and culture-universal care. We will discuss Leininger's theory in detail later in this chapter and provide a client care example using this theory.

More recently, *Jean Watson* (1989), in her philosophy and science of caring, wrote that caring must be central to nursing practice to preserve human dignity and humanity. As a moral ideal, nursing practice is based on humanistic or altruistic values in the development of a helping-trust relationship between the nurse and the client. Watson's theory includes 10 *carative factors* that represent both feelings and actions pertaining to the nurse and the client and include things to be felt, experienced, expressed, and promoted by every nurse. Her theory contributes to nursing by sensitizing nurses to humanistic aspects and caring.

Patricia Benner's phenomenological theory describes caring as a common bond between people situated in a meaningful relationship. This situation is essential to nursing. Skill and skilled practice, as defined by Benner (1984), means skilled nursing interventions and clinical judgment skills in actual clinical situations. She sees clinical nursing practice in terms of nurses making a positive difference by being in the situation in a caring way. Benner describes caring in the context of nursing practice and uses examples (she calls them exemplars) to demonstrate five stages of skill acquisition in practice. Novice, advanced beginner, competent, proficient, and expert are the five stages of skill acquisition drawn from Benner's research and found in *From Novice to Expert* as well as numerous publications. Further development of this research led to an interpretive theory of nursing practice that is explained in *The Primacy of Caring: Stress and Coping in Health and Illness.* The primacy of caring is concerned with helping clients cope with the stress of illness.

ADVANTAGES OF MULTIPLE THEORIES

There were alternative viewpoints as nursing evolved as a profession. Some believed that nursing only used borrowed theory—that is, from other disciplines. Other nurses demanded that nursing create its own research methods and knowledge so that nursing concepts would be unique. Today we recognize that no discipline owns knowledge. Therefore, nursing uses knowledge from other fields and shares knowledge with other disciplines.

What the nurse observes, documents, chooses as an intervention, and evaluates depends on the nurse's theoretical perspective guiding nursing practice. Having more than one theoretical perspective increases the nurse's options and choices. The more ways the nurse can analyze the needs of a particular client, the more potential there is for seeing different needs.

Table 6–1 summarizes the work of some of the major nurse theorists.

APPLYING THEORY TO PRACTICE

Perhaps the three most commonly used nursing theories today are those of Leininger, Orem, and Roy. Each is discussed in their application to practice. Whichever theory you choose will influence how you approach nursing care. Obviously, when in a setting that has chosen a particular theory as the basis for practice in that agency, you will also need to use that theory to ensure accurate communication between care providers and to minimize client confusion.

Applying Leininger's Transcultural Care Theory

Leininger recognized from her clinical practice that she was caring for people from many different cultures and ethnic groups. It didn't seem logical that a nurse's actions based on white middle-class cultural beliefs could possibly meet the needs of all the different children and families with which she was involved. Leininger defined culture as the "learned, shared and transmitted values, beliefs, norms and lifeways of a particular group that guides their thinking, decisions, and actions in patterned ways" (Leininger, 1991, 1947). She assumes that the values, beliefs, and practices for culturally appropriate care depend on "the world view, language, religious (or spiritual), kinship (social), political (or legal), educational, economic, technological, ethnohistorical and environmental context" of the culture (1991, 1945). Cultural care is the broadest holistic

nursing theory because it accounts for the totality of life, including social structure, world view, language, and folk and professional systems.

Leininger's influence helped stress the importance of assessing the client's cultural beliefs before planning or implementing nursing care, and this was the basis for creating *transcultural nursing.* Transcultural nursing requires the nurse be able to give care that is deemed culturally acceptable by the client.

Leininger recognized that people from different cultures perceive health, nursing care, environment, and themselves differently. Consequently, to be effective and accepted by the client, nursing care must be given in a way the client can understand so the client can collaborate with the nurse's actions and understand the health goals being sought.

According to Leininger, nurses may choose among three approaches when working with clients from different cultures. First is *cultural care maintenance and preservation,* which is appropriate when the client's cultural beliefs and the nurse's planned interventions are consistent in approach and both can agree on which actions will be taken. *Cultural care accommodation or negotiation* is used when the nurse and the client each work together to negotiate behaviors that will effectively create change to maximize the client's health. Last, *cultural care repatterning or restructuring* includes all those nursing interventions that are respectful but focuses on helping the client change lifestyle behaviors that are culturally appropriate but not, in the client's particular situation, healthy. The accompanying Box 6-1 demonstrates how Leininger's theory might apply to a clinical situation.

Applying Roy's Theory of Adaptation

Roy's theory is one of the most widely used and popular because it is fairly concrete, easy to understand, and immediately applicable in clinical settings. When given a choice, nursing students often choose Roy's theory because Roy's theory "works" in clinical settings.

Roy believes clients are biopsychosocial beings who adapt to the changing environment. The goal of nursing care is helping the client adapt. Therefore, the nurse acts to promote adaptation by manipulating stimuli and the environment. The outcome is adaptation or balance and stability for the client.

Roy defines a person as a biopsychosocial being, an adaptive system in constant interaction with a changing environment. An environment may include three types of stimuli that require the client to adapt. The first kind is *focal stimuli,* which include those immediate stimuli of which the client is clearly aware. Second are *residual stimuli,* or all those ongoing and continuing expectations based on previous successful coping endeavors. Last are *contextual stimuli,* which include everything in the background or environment affecting the situation. A nurse must intervene when a client is not adapting effectively to the demands of the environment.

TABLE 6–1
Overview of Major Nursing Theorists

Theorist	First Theory Publication	Conceptual Focus of Theory
Florence Nightingale *Environmental Theory*	*Notes on Nursing* (1859)	Nursing as *Philosophy.* Environmental manipulation crucial to health and a client's ability to regain health.
Hildegarde Peplau *Psychodynamic Nursing Theory*	*Interpersonal Relations in Nursing* (1952)	Nursing as *Interpersonal Relationship.* First to relate other scientific theory to nursing. During the interpersonal relations between nurse and client, the nurse assumes many roles: stranger, teacher, resource, surrogate, leader, and counselor.
Virginia Henderson *Definition of Nursing*	*The Principles and Practice of Nursing* (1955)	Nursing as *Philosophy.* Known for her definition of nursing. Identified 14 basic needs that are the components of nursing care that help clients gain independence and health.
Faye Abdellah *Twenty-One Nursing Problems*	*Patient Centered Approaches to Nursing* (1960)	Nursing as *Philosophy.* Identified 21 nursing problems that outlined nursing as the care for the whole person. Later revision of theory focused on client need, not nursing tasks.
Ida Jean Orlando *Nursing Process Theory*	*The Dynamic Nurse-Patient Relationship* (1961)	Nursing as *Interpersonal Relationship.* Emphasizes reciprocal relationship between client and nurse using her nursing process theory.
Myra Levine *Four Conservation Principles*	*Introduction to Clinical Nursing* (1969)	Nursing as *Energy Field.* Nurses manipulate the environment and help clients adapt with four conservation principles: Conservation of Energy, Conservation of Structural Integrity, Conservation of Personal Integrity, and Conservation of Social Integrity.
Martha Rogers *Science of Unitary Human Beings Theory*	*An Introduction to the Theoretical Basis of Nursing* (1970)	Nursing as *Energy Field.* Humans and their environments are integrated and inter-related energy fields, and nurses assist clients in the achievement of a maximum level of wellness.
Imogene King *Theory of Goal Attainment*	*Toward a Theory for Nursing: General Concepts of Human Behavior* (1971)	Nursing as a *System.* Decision-making process and outcomes of mutual goal attainment are specified for nurse-client interactions.
Dorothea Orem *Self-Care Theory*	*Nursing: Concepts of Practice* (1971)	Nursing as *Philosophy.* Delineation of the need for nursing care that comes from a client's self-care deficit.
Betty Neuman *Neuman Systems Model*	*A Model for Teaching Total Person Approach to Patient Problems* (1972)	Nursing as a *System.* Client as a system functioning harmoniously in relation to environmental influences. Nursing action based on prevention stabilizes the client.
Sister Callista Roy *Adaptation Model*	*Introduction to Nursing: An Adaptation Model* (1976)	Nursing as a *System.* Clients exist through adaptation to a changing environment, with the nurse as a regulatory mechanism in situations of health and illness.
Madeleine Leininger *Transcultural Care Theory*	*Transcultural Nursing: Concepts, Theories and Practices* (1978)	Nursing as *Care.* Caring is the central theme in nursing knowledge and in culture-specific and culture-universal nursing practice.
Jean Watson *Philosophy and Science of Caring*	*Nursing: Human Science and Human Care* (1979)	Nursing as *Care.* Carative factors come from a humanistic perspective and from scientific knowledge. Nursing is the art and science of a human to human care process.
Patricia Benner *From Novice to Expert*	*From Novice to Expert: Excellence and Power in Clinical Nursing Practice* (1984)	Nursing as *Care.* Phenomenologically describes caring as a common bond between people situated in meaning—a situation that is essential to nursing.

BOX 6–1

APPLYING LEININGER'S TRANSCULTURAL CARE THEORY TO MRS. KELLEY

Maureen Kelly was admitted to your surgical unit after spending 2 immediate postoperative hours in the postanesthesia care unit (PACU). The PACU nurse gives a report after your initial assessment of Mrs. Kelly was completed and you found her stable.

Mrs. Kelly, 56-year-old married homemaker, just underwent a total abdominal hysterectomy with bilateral salpingo-oophorectomy because of fibroids and excessive bleeding resulting in severe anemia. She was experiencing fainting spells before the procedure. One unit of blood was given preoperatively, and she only had 250 mL of estimated blood loss during the surgery. Vital signs have remained stable, and she received morphine for pain twice in the PACU with relief. Abdomen is soft with a bulky, lower abdominal dressing dry and intact. She has an indwelling urinary catheter that has been draining clear yellow urine adequately during and after surgery. Minimal bloody vaginal drainage on the perineal pad during recovery. Her husband and daughter are waiting down the hall in the waiting room. Mrs. Kelly and her husband have fairly strong Irish accents but are easily understood after a little listening. (I do love an Irish accent!) The daughter doesn't have the accent. Other past history includes left leg has limited range of motion and client uses a cane to get about. She was in an auto accident several years ago and apparently had a bad fracture with poor healing. No other chronic conditions. The surgeon wrote orders for postoperative care. The anesthesiologist wrote orders for pain control.

After the report, you go the waiting room and get Mrs. Kelly's family so they can see that she is settled into her room after the surgery.

Since you have been working at the hospital, you have cared for people from all over the world. You recognized the need to be more culturally sensitive and have adopted Leininger's transcultural care theory as a framework for your nursing practice. Having worked

with Irish-Americans before, you recall some of the characteristics the Irish tend to value. A number of these characteristics are listed below:

- Enjoy riddles, limericks, and storytelling and use many words to express a thought with frequent laughter and smiling.
- Less expressive when talking about inner feelings and thoughts.
- Display of emotions and affections in public is avoided and often difficult in private.
- Caring actions are more important than verbal expression of love.
- Use direct eye contact when speaking with others and may interpret not maintaining eye contact as a sign of disrespect or guilt.
- Require distance for personal space.
- Patriarchal family structure is common (women's work in the home and men's work outside the home) with little role sharing.
- Food is an important part of health maintenance—with potential for being high fat.
- Gain meaning in life through home, religion, and the social environment of the pub.
- May ignore illness symptoms and delay seeking medical attention until symptoms interfere with ability to carry out daily activities.
- Wear religious medals to maintain health.
- Behavioral response to pain is stoic, usually ignoring or minimizing it.

In using Leininger's theory, you know that care behaviors, goals, and functions vary transculturally because of the social structure, world view, and cultural values of people from cultures different from your own. So it is important to identify the universal caring behav-

Continued

Roy, in her focus on the process of adaptation, sees two subsystems. The first subsystem is the *regulator,* which is the autonomic nervous system, endocrine system, and perceptual system. The second subsystem is the *cognator* subsystem, which perceives the environment and determines meaning through past learning experiences and current problem-solving, decision-making, and intellectual thought.

Roy identifies four ways the client can adapt. *Physiological needs* constitute the first mode of adaptation. Physiological needs include such processes as activity and rest, nutrition, elimination, oxygenation, and self-preservation. This mode is very concrete and directly related to clinical data. Physiological needs

are typically assessed in the initial nursing history and assessment.

The remaining three modes are a bit more abstract. The second mode is the *self-concept.* The self-concept is the client's beliefs, values, and expectations for the future, the self-image that includes not only those images mirrored by important others such as family and friends but the person's own feelings about the self over time as well. The nurse must interview the client and observe the client's behaviors in order to infer the client's self-concept.

The third mode is *role function.* The role function refers to the social expectations all people have for others, including nurses and clients. Each sees the other

BOX 6–1

APPLYING LEININGER'S TRANSCULTURAL CARE THEORY TO MRS. KELLEY (continued)

iors, beliefs, and values. This is done by recognizing common characteristics and, most importantly, an assessment of the client and family.

To be culturally sensitive, you would begin by using the cultural care maintenance and preservation approach with the Kellys. This means that you and Mrs. Kelly will plan care interventions based on the client's cultural beliefs. Secondly, cultural care accommodation or negotiation will be used to work with the client to negotiate behaviors that will maximize the client's health. You may have to use Leininger's third approach of cultural care repatterning or restructuring to help the client change a lifestyle behavior because it may not be particularly healthy for the client, even though it is a culturally acceptable behavior. Let's follow the care example and see how you will follow these transcultural care approaches.

Mr. Kelly and Sheila, their daughter, are sitting at the foot of the bed in Mrs. Kelly's room when you enter. Mr. Kelly stands and inquires about how his wife is really doing. Mrs. Kelly is moaning and turning her head from side to side. Her hands are on her abdomen. Moving to the client's side, you say "It looks like you are having pain at your surgery site and that is very normal. You just had major surgery and the pain can get very bad if you don't take pain medications routinely at the beginning. Let me look at your dressing and I will also take your vital signs." While you are assessing her, Mrs. Kelly says her pain is bearable and expected. Mr. Kelly says his wife bears pain better than most because she has leg pain all the time since the accident.

You have recognized the client's pain and that her minimizing of the pain may be related to cultural ways. Now you will negotiate with the client and family to help the client receive pain relief. You would explain the reason for the routine administration of the pain medication, that she will not get addicted in the 2

weeks that she will need a strong medicine, and that each day the pain will lessen if it is controlled from the beginning. Mrs. Kelly asks for her St. Christopher medal and her daughter puts it around her mother's neck. You then stress that when Mrs. Kelly has adequate pain relief, she will be able to care for herself instead of others having to tend to all her needs. This was what Mrs. Kelly needed to hear to change her mind about accepting pain medications. You go and get her pain medications.

The next day, you find Mrs. Kelly standing at the sink brushing her teeth. She is pale and perspiring. When you ask if she needs help to the bed, Mrs. Kelly says she can do it herself and lurches to the bed. You end up assisting her into the bed. You have just looked at her laboratory values and saw that she remains severely anemic with an increased triglyceride count and high cholesterol. These physiological factors could delay her recovery and have an impact on her future health. It is important now to talk with Mrs. Kelly about accepting help, changing her diet to a high-iron, lower-fat diet, and possibly taking vitamins with iron.

Mrs. Kelly is being discharged to home on her third postoperative day. She remains weak and reluctantly accepts help with her activities. Her wound is healing with no complications. Mrs. Kelly is quiet and won't say what is bothering her. After speaking with Sheila, her daughter, you realize that Mrs. Kelly is not going to have much assistance during the day because everyone has to work. Her family had taken days off while she was in the hospital and couldn't take more time off from work to help her at home. You contact social services and because of her laboratory results, previous disability, and a possible lack of continuous home assistance the first week after discharge, it is ordered for community health to visit three times with possible reevaluation visits.

person partly in terms of what role that person is currently filling—for example, in the clinical agency, what the client thinks nurses and clients do as well as what the nurse thinks clients and nurses do. These roles are then further defined in terms of both the nurse's and the client's expectations in term of age, gender, race, uniform, and the clinical setting. Nurses often ask clients what the client's goals and expectations are for their meeting with health care professionals.

The last mode is *interdependence*. Interdependence recognizes that such needs as respect, friendship, value, or love needs can only be met through mutual relationships with others. The nurse typically assesses the significant others involved with the client.

Roy suggests a six-stage nursing process (Roy & Andrews, 1991, p. 27): assessment of behavior, assessment of stimuli, nursing diagnosis, goal-setting, interventions, and evaluation.

According to Roy, nursing is needed when the person is ill, the person has the potential for being ill, or a weakened system results in the client's ineffective coping. Roy's model portrays the client as an open system in which stimuli and environmental changes requiring adaptation are the input. You analyze the environment for focal, contextual, and residual stimuli. Using the nursing process, you assess the client's behaviors and influencing factors, concluding with a nursing diagnosis and goal setting. Using those con-

BOX 6–2

APPLYING ROY'S THEORY OF ADAPTATION TO MRS. KELLY

The community health agency is told a new client has just been admitted for home services. The only information given is that the client, Maureen Kelly, has been referred by her physician for follow-up care secondary to hospitalization for a total abdominal hysterectomy with bilateral salpingo-oophorectomy because of fibroids and excessive bleeding resulting in severe anemia.

You make your first home visit using Roy's theory of adaptation as the theoretical basis for practice. From the referral, you know Mrs. Kelly is age 56 and a married housewife whose employed husband has insurance. Making a home visit allows you to also assess the *environment*. The address is a small bungalow in a working-class neighborhood with a good-sized yard. Shrubs and flowers adorn the front yard. No weeds are visible. Flowerpots with blooming plants line the small front porch. After three rings, Mrs. Kelly answers the door. She is dressed in a cotton robe and wearing house slippers, looking both pale and tired. She immediately asks you in and offers you tea, which you decline. Upon being invited to sit down, immediately begin to assess Mrs. Kelly, beginning with Mrs. Kelly's current behavior compared with norms for a woman of her age, physical appearance, probable Irish descent, and apparent working-class economic status. Then a history and physical examination would determine Mrs. Kelly's *physiological mode* functioning. During this examination, sight, sound, touch, smell, and instruments such as a thermometer would be used to assess such factors as Mrs. Kelly's oxygenation, nutrition, elimination patterns, and activity and rest. Verbally you would ask relevant questions related to Mrs. Kelly's self-concept, role function, and interdependence. Questions might include "How would you describe your health?" "What

do you do to keep healthy?" or "How do you spend your leisure time?"

After completing the physical assessment and asking about physiological mode functioning, ask further questions regarding Mrs. Kelly's *role functions* and *interdependence.* Mrs. Kelly responds by discussing her life as a housewife who has never been employed or driven a car. She is responsible for the house and yard including the large garden in back. Her significant other is her husband of 30 years who works in a factory and one married daughter, age 28, who lives nearby. Mrs. Kelly reports she does not get out much since the car accident 5 years ago that gave her a "crippled" leg. She and her husband drive every 2 weeks to pay their utility bills and buy groceries. She talks about the various sales clerks at the stores and utilities, calling them by name, and telling which one is "sweet and nice" and which ones she avoids. The Kellys go to church every Sunday. Her worn Bible sits by a comfortable chair. At the current time she is just trying to keep up with the garden and deal with her postoperative recovery. In comparison with the car accident, she considers the surgery minor. She expresses no regret over the surgery because "I was going through the change anyway." She also shares that her daughter visits each weekend and often brings one of the grandchildren. She loves her daughter and the grandchildren but feels too tired to "have all that noise" around.

Mrs. Kelly's *self-concept* could be assessed through questions related to her perception of her body after the surgery and her feelings or sensations in the surgical area as well as the rest of her body. Feelings related to the surgical site would be reviewed. Women might, for

Continued

clusions and in collaboration with the client, intervene to help the client cope effectively.

The client's open-system throughput includes the regulator and cognator as coping mechanisms, both physiologically and mentally. The four modes, especially the physiological mode, are areas where you may intervene to help the client cope. Finally, the output is either adaptive or ineffective responses by the client as evaluated by the nurse and the client. Health is a state of adaptation that is visible in energy being available to deal with other stimuli. The accompanying Box 6-2 demonstrates how Roy's theory might apply to a clinical situation.

Applying Orem's Theory of Self-Care

Dorothea Orem's theory seems intuitively comfortable and consistent with many nurses' perspectives of nursing. Hence, it is probably among the most widely

used and popular theories of nursing practice, often implemented in hospitals and other clinical settings. Orem's theory focuses on the role of the nurse in helping clients meet their needs. She also carefully distinguishes between the physician's role and the nurse's role, although both physician and nurse see a human being as a rational person with capacities for change. The physician focuses on the client's life processes as they have been disrupted by injury, invading microorganisms, or loss of the will to live. The nurse's special interest is assisting the client with self-care, sustaining the client psychosocially, and meeting individual needs. The nurse includes both the physician's perspective and the client's perspective in planning nursing care.

Orem's theory remains popular because of its usefulness in acute care practice. It uses language and terms with which nurses are familiar and focuses on care of the ill in hospitals. It presumes a list of needs

BOX 6–2

APPLYING ROY'S THEORY OF ADAPTATION TO MRS. KELLY (continued)

example, feel very differently about removal of a uterus than they would removal of a gallbladder. Throughout the initial assessment, carefully note through observation Mrs. Kelly's behaviors and, as appropriate, question her concerning the meaning or purpose of certain behaviors. Mrs. Kelly's perception of the stimuli confronting her would be determined. You would also draw upon your own knowledge concerning the developmental tasks of a 56-year-old woman coping with surgical menopause. Finally, you may want to check environmental considerations, such as drugs the physician may have prescribed to any use of tobacco, alcohol, or other drugs. Recent changes in Mrs. Kelly's life, beyond the surgery, should be determined to be sure all the focal, contextual, and residual stimuli had been assessed. As you draw your conclusions, they should be shared with Mrs. Kelly for validation or correction.

Mrs. Kelly states she is very tired since she returned home and doesn't seem able to get her work done during the day. She feels weak and looks fatigued. She has been just sitting and reading her Bible. She was even too tired to eat breakfast. She states she was too tired to eat lunch the previous day.

Mrs. Kelly emphasizes that caring for the house is her responsibility and it would not be fair to ask her husband for help. You then discuss how Mrs. Kelly might be able to complete her tasks. Discuss when she feels strongest and which tasks have highest priority. A schedule is planned that alternates rest and activity. Point out the extensiveness of the surgery and what might be realistic expectations for Mrs. Kelly after such surgery. Also point out that the surgery was performed to stop the bleeding, which may have led to the anemia

that would also make Mrs. Kelly very tired. Help Mrs. Kelly understand that her role functioning may be temporarily impaired but that she should be able to resume full functioning in a relatively short period of time.

Through discussion with Mrs. Kelly, a short-term goal is set, namely that Mrs. Kelly will be able to do more each day. In addition, you and Mrs. Kelly discuss breakfast and lunch meals that would be easier for her to fix and eat but that would be high in nutrition. Finally, you call the physician to see if there are any contraindications to Mrs. Kelly taking an iron pill with each meal. The physician sees no problem, so Mrs. Kelly calls her husband and asks him to pick up such medication on his way home from the factory. You agree to check back with Mrs. Kelly in about a week to see if her endurance has improved.

Evaluation would be based on whether Mrs. Kelly was able to reachieve her presurgical functioning. Mrs. Kelly's goals might include being able to fulfill the functions involved in her *primary* and *secondary roles*, including being able to cook, care for the house, garden, and be ready for the drive to the grocery store. For rest and relaxation she might use coping methods found in her *tertiary role* as a quilter. If she finds hand quilting relaxing, you might encourage her to continue quilting whenever she was tired from completing tasks related to her primary and secondary roles. As a community health nurse making home visits, you also review appropriate health promotion teaching related to the need for exercise and proper nutrition. The evaluation would conclude successful adaptation if Mrs. Kelly is able to achieve her usual household tasks within 6 weeks of the surgery.

that evolve out of a pathophysiological or medical focus (Meleis, 1997, p. 401). It is less useful in community settings or in health promotion, although Orem (1995) has increasingly made specific how the nurse functions with care of families or in communities. We will use Orem's theory in the community setting to see how it can be used in that practice setting.

Orem writes that she has three theories, the theory of *self-care deficit,* the theory of *nursing systems,* and the theory of *self-care.* The theory of self-care deficit describes clients who can't meet their own care needs because of illness or lack of knowledge. The theory of nursing systems describes and explains nursing actions. Orem defines self-care as "the practice of activities that individuals initiate and perform on their own behalf in maintaining life, health and well-being" (Orem, 1995, p. 104).

Orem's conceptual model has six major concepts: self-care deficit, self-care agency, self-care demand,

nursing agency, nursing system, and self-care, as well as the additional concept of basic conditioning factors, which are the demographic differences among clients.

Orem sees nursing as an art that includes caring for clients, knowledge that can be shared, and being a member of a profession (Orem, 1995). The goal of nursing is to provide care for those unable to care for themselves, to enable the client and family members to become capable of meeting the client's self-care needs to regain health or to maintain health, and to minimize the effects of chronic problems or disability. When the client or family are unable to care for themselves, they have a *self-care deficit* that may requiring nursing care.

Orem sees nurses as having an extensive knowledge base that allows them to understand symptoms and behaviors. Nurses do for others, guide and direct, provide physical or psychological support, provide and maintain an environment that supports further

BOX 6–3

APPLYING OREM'S THEORY OF SELF-CARE TO MRS. KELLY

In applying Orem's theory to the care of Mrs. Kelly, again you would go to Mrs. Kelly's home. Upon being invited in, you would assess Mrs. Kelly with self-care as the focus. Question Mrs. Kelly about significant others who have cared for her in the past or are available at the present time. What are Mrs. Kelly's current goals of self-care? Details related to daily activities and routines are queried while you also assess the home situation. Although the responses would reflect the client's perceptions, you determine the client's physiological functioning as well as the client's perception of herself. As would be done regardless of which theory is being used, a history and physical examination would determine Mrs. Kelly's physiological functioning. Orem (1995) discusses *conditioning factors*, which include age, gender, developmental state, health state, orientation, family lifestyle patterns, typical activities of daily living, resources available, and the immediate environment. As a member of the health care system, you are limited to the resources within the system for which Mrs. Kelly is eligible. However, other self-care agents might be used such as home health aides. Mrs. Kelly might respond in terms of her daily activities during her period of illness as well as during times when she is well in relation to her spouse, children, and household tasks. Mrs. Kelly talks about the care she gives to others as well as care she receives from them.

Based on data analysis, you would make diagnostic conclusions and begin prescribing appropriate interventions. Nursing is done in collaboration or review with the client. Therefore, you establish goals in collaboration with Mrs. Kelly's to meet her self-care deficits. You create a plan for meeting Mrs. Kelly's *health deviation* needs because she is experiencing delayed recovery from her surgery.

Assist Mrs. Kelly with her *universal self-care needs* in any areas where the surgery makes it difficult for her to care for herself. Here, you might engage in a partly compensatory system—for example, if Mrs. Kelly can ambulate only with assistance. However, the nurse would seek to help family members to assist Mrs. Kelly whenever possible because the nurse could not be continuously present in the home.

Finally, examine *developmental self-care* from the perspective of promotion of normalcy—for example, helping Mrs. Kelly understand how hormone replacement therapy may help avoid osteoporosis. Having a community health focus, the home health care nurse would undoubtedly also engage in health promotion teaching—for example, related to the need for rest, sleep, and good nutrition. The evaluation would focus on whether Mrs. Kelly, with the assistance of her family, was able to care for herself.

---

development, and teach others how to maximize health potential. Nursing includes social, psychological, and professional and technological features.

Health itself is a state of being whole, whereas well-being is the person's perception (Orem, 1995 p. 101). A person is distinguished from other living biological entities by the capacity to reflect and seek meaning, symbolize experience, and use symbols to communicate and create. Adults are *self-care agencies*—in other words, responsible for caring for themselves. Each person is responsible for one's own therapeutic *self-care demands*—that is, adults take care of themselves and their dependents to maintain life, health, and well-being. Only when unable to do so do adults become clients.

The purpose of self-care is to fulfill universal, developmental, and health deviation self-care requisites. Nurses must identify the self-care requisites and intervene to meet them. *Universal self-care requisites* are a person's need for such things as air, water, food, activity and rest, and social interaction. *Developmental self-care requisites* are the person's need for continued growth and development or maturation throughout life. *Health deviation self-care requisites* are when the per-

son has symptoms and is aware of a need for assessment and intervention. These include helping the client fulfill the prescription for intervention and care.

Nursing agency is action by nurses, including their determination of what self-care needs the clients have. The *nursing system* is thoughtful and deliberate action to meet the deficit between what clients need and what clients can do for themselves. Orem writes that there are three types of nursing systems, which are dependent on who can or should perform the self-care actions. The first nursing system of *wholly compensatory* care is when the nurse does everything needed for the client. The second nursing system is *partly compensatory* care and is used when the client can meet some needs and the nurse meets the rest. The last nursing system of *supportive educative* care is when the client can perform the care with assistance but needs help with knowing why and how or perhaps assistance with motivation.

Each person, group, and community needs to attain and retain health. Orem's theory implicitly expects each person be self-reliant and responsible for personal care. Families are responsible for care of their family members. When an adult cares for a child, the adult is the dependent care agency and the child is in the developmental stage of dependent care—that is, the child is unable to care for the self without an adult. The accompanying Box 6-3 demonstrates Orem's theory might apply to a clinical situation.

KEY PRINCIPLES

- The basis of any discipline is theoretical. Hypotheses include the philosophy that underlies the discipline, the concepts that are important, and the relationship between and among the concepts.
- Theories help the nurse learn, organize knowledge, apply knowledge, seek new knowledge, and communicate quickly and effectively with other nurses.
- Nursing theory provides a basis for clinical practice.
- Using theory helps the nurse discuss the effectiveness of nursing practice in our current cost-effective health care environment.
- Theory helps determine how best to orient newcomers into the profession of nursing.
- Theory also confirms that nursing, having its own body of knowledge, is indeed a profession.
- More than any other single component, nursing theory helps the nurse to engage in thoughtful, experienced, skillful care of clients, whether that client is an individual, family, or community.
- Using a particular theory helps the nurse ensure that all relevant aspects from the perspective of a client and the environment have been assessed and documented and that all appropriate interventions from that perspective have been planned, implemented, and evaluated in a culturally sensitive approach.

BIBLIOGRAPHY

*Abdellah, F., Beland, I.L., Martin, A., & Matheney, R.V. (1961). *Patient centered approaches to nursing.* New York: Macmillan.

*Ashley, J. (1976). *Hospitals, paternalism, and the role of the nurse.* New York: Teachers College Press.

*Benner, P. (1984). *From novice to expert: Excellence and power in clinical nursing practice.* Menlo Park, CA: Addison-Wesley.

Chinn, P., & Kramer, M. (1995). *Theory and nursing: A systematic approach* (4th ed.). St. Louis: Mosby.

*Dickoff, J., & James, P. (1968). A theory of theories: A position paper. *Nursing Research, 17*(3),197–203.

Fawcett, J. (1995). *Analysis and evaluation of conceptual models of nursing* (3rd ed.). Philadelphia: F.A.Davis.

*Gebbie, K. (Ed.). (1976). *Summary of the second national conference: Classification of nursing diagnosis.* St. Louis: Mosby.

*Gebbie, K.M., & Lavin, M.A. (Eds.). (1975). *Proceedings of the first national conference: Classification of nursing diagnosis.* St. Louis: Mosby.

*Gebbie, K., & Lavin, M.A. (1974). Classifying nursing diagnoses. *American Journal of Nursing, 74*(2), 250–253.

*Hall, L.E. (1963) Center for nursing. *Nursing Outlook, 11,* 805–806.

*Harmer, B., & Henderson, V. (1955). *Textbook of the principles and practice of nursing.* New York: Macmillan.

*Johnson, D. (1959a). A philosophy of nursing. *Nursing Outlook, 7*(4), 198–200.

*Johnson, D. (1959b). The nature of a science of nursing. *Nursing Outlook, 7*(5), 291–294.

Johnson, D.E. (1991). The behavioral system model for nursing. In J.P. Riehl & C. Roy (Eds.), *Conceptual models for nursing practice* (2nd ed.). New York: Appleton-Century-Crofts.

*King, I. (1971). *Toward a theory for nursing: General concepts of human behavior.* New York: John Wiley & Sons.

*Leininger, M.M. (1991). *Cultural care diversity and universality: A theory of nursing.* New York: National League for Nursing.

*Leininger, M.M. (1985). Transcultural care diversity and universality: A theory of nursing. *Nursing and Health Care, 6,* 209–212.

*Leininger, M.M. (1979). *Transcultural nursing.* New York: Masson.

*Leininger, M.M. (1978). *Transcultural nursing: Concepts, theories, and practice.* New York: John Wiley & Sons.

*Levine, M. (1967). The four conservation principles of nursing. *Nursing Forum, 69*(10), 93–98.

Meleis, A.I. (1997). *Theoretical nursing: Development & progress* (3rd ed.) Philadelphia: J.B. Lippincott.

*Neuman, B. (1995). *The Newman systems model.* Norwalk, CT: Appleton & Lange.

*Newman, M. (1986). *Health as expanding consciousness.* St. Louis: Mosby.

Orem, D.E. (1995). *Nursing: Concepts of practice* (5th ed.). St. Louis: Mosby-Year Book.

*Orem, D.E. (1991). *Nursing: Concepts of practice* (4th ed.). St. Louis: Mosby-Year Book.

*Orem, D.E. (1988). The form of nursing science. *Nursing Science Quarterly, 1*(2), 75–79.

*Orem, D.E. (1985). *Nursing: Concepts of practice* (3rd ed.). New York: McGraw-Hill.

*Orem, D.E. (1980). *Nursing: Concepts of practice* (2nd ed.). New York: McGraw-Hill.

*Orem, D.E. (1971). *Nursing: Concepts of practice.* New York: McGraw-Hill.

*Orem, D.E. (1959). *Guide for developing curricula for the education of practical nurses.* Washington, D.C.: U.S. Department of Health, Education & Welfare, Office of Education.

*Orlando, I.J. (1961). *The dynamic nurse-patient relationship.* New York: Putnam.

*Peplau, H. (1952). *Interpersonal relations in nursing.* New York: Putnam.

*Rogers, M.E. (1970). *An introduction to the theoretical basis of nursing.* Philadelphia: F.A. Davis.

*Rogers, M.E. (1964). *Reveille in nursing.* Philadelphia: F.A.Davis.

*Roy, C. (1991). Structure of knowledge: Paradigm, model, and research specification for differentiated practice. In I.E. Goertzen (Ed.), *Differentiating nursing practice: Into the twenty-first century* (pp 31–39). Kansas City, MO: American Academy of Nursing.

*Roy, C. (1984). *Introduction to nursing: An adaptation model* (2nd ed.). Englewood Cliffs, NJ: Prentice-Hall.

*Roy, C. (1976). *Introduction to nursing: An adaptation model.* Englewood Cliffs, NJ: Prentice-Hall.

*Roy, C., & Andrews, H.A. (1991). *The Roy adaptation model: The definitive statement.* Norwalk, CT: Appleton & Lange.

*Yura, H., & Torres, G. (1975). *Today's conceptual frameworks with the baccalaureate nursing programs* (NLN Pub. No. 15-1558, 17–75). New York: National League for Nursing.

*Yura, H., & Walsh, M.B. (1978a). *The nursing process: Assessing, planning, implementing, evaluating.* New York: Appleton-Century-Crofts.

*Yura, H., & Walsh, M.B. (1978b). *Human needs and the nursing process.* New York: Appleton-Century-Crofts.

*Watson, J. (1989). *Nursing: Human science, human care.* New York: National League for Nursing.

*Asterisk indicates a classic or definitive work on this subject.

Critical Thinking and Clinical Judgment

Janet S. Hickman

Key Terms

clinical judgment
critical thinking
decision-making

diagnostic reasoning
nursing process
problem-solving

LEARNING OBJECTIVES

After studying this chapter, you should be able to:

1. Differentiate between critical thinking, problem-solving, decision-making, diagnostic reasoning, and clinical judgment.
2. Describe the elements of the T.H.I.N.K. model of critical thinking.
3. Discuss Benner's stages of skill proficiency in nursing practice.
4. Recognize obstacles to critical thinking.
5. Describe the five interwoven phases of the nursing process.
6. Apply the T.H.I.N.K. model to the nursing process.

As health care becomes more complex, nurses must exercise increasingly complex thinking skills. Indeed, the body of knowledge that nurses need is increasing at such a rate that it is impossible to succeed in nursing simply by applying standardized responses. Even clients who have common needs express those needs in highly individualized ways. Consequently, critical thinking is an important and integral part of nursing practice.

Because critical thinking is an abstract concept rather than something you can observe and measure, defining it can be somewhat difficult. In fact, a number of respected scholars have created somewhat differing definitions of the critical thinking process. However, all definitions of critical thinking include thinking skills that you can learn, practice, and integrate into your nursing care. Using these critical thinking skills will result in sound decisions, safe practice, and creativity in addition to promoting the well-being of your clients.

In this chapter, we will look at some descriptions of critical thinking, the characteristics and attitudes of critical thinking, and how to develop critical thinking skills. We will also explore the relationship of critical thinking to the nursing process, the framework that guides a nurse's thinking.

THE LANGUAGE OF CRITICAL THINKING

Critical thinking is defined as purposeful, self-regulatory judgment that gives reasoned and reflective consideration to evidence, contexts, conceptualizations, methods, and criteria (Facione, 1990).

Critical thinkers examine all elements of a situation and think through alternative strategies to achieve an end. They do not necessarily devise a single solution as the goal of critical thinking but rather a number of scenarios that could occur depending on actions taken or not taken. Rather than one "right" answer, they determine a number of possible outcomes. They use creativity to overcome barriers (Fig. 7–1). Built on the nurse's knowledge, clinical experience, and intuition, critical thinking takes a holistic approach to the client.

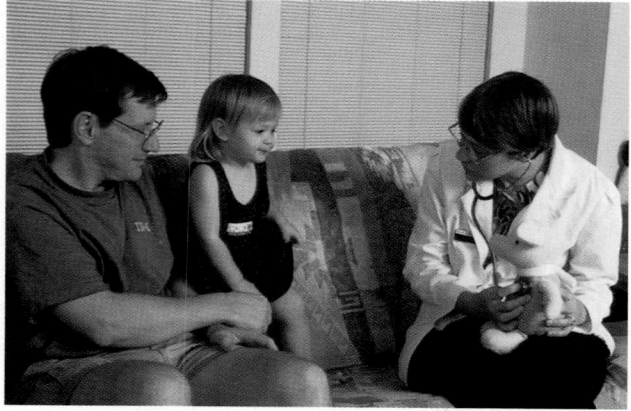

Figure 7–1. A nurse adept at critical thinking uses creativity to overcome barriers to quality nursing care.

Embedded in the broad concept of critical thinking are several more specific thinking skills, including problem-solving, decision-making, diagnostic reasoning, and clinical judgment. Typically, all of these processes take place within the framework of the nursing process.

Problem-solving is defining a problem, selecting information pertinent to its conclusion (recognizing stated and unstated assumptions), formulating alternative solutions, drawing a conclusion, and judging the validity of the conclusion (Watson & Glaser, 1964). Problem-solving is a process used to arrive at an answer or a solution. There is an implied gap of information or action that must be bridged to arrive at the solution. There is also the expectation that the solution be "right" according to a particular standard of measure.

Decision-making involves choosing between two or more options as a means to achieve a desired result. Typically, the decision will be goal-directed, in which case the goal or goals will direct the outcome. For instance, if you were to plan a dinner party, your menu (goal) would direct your decisions in grocery shopping and food preparation. Decision-making in the clinical setting yields approaches for nursing care selected from a variety of possible nursing interventions. You must decide which intervention(s) will be most likely to achieve the desired client outcomes.

Diagnostic reasoning is the process of clustering assessment data into meaningful sets and generating hypotheses about the client's human responses. According to Carnevali and Thomas (1993), diagnostic reasoning can be carried out as a deliberate, conscious activity or it may occur spontaneously with little awareness.

Clinical judgment is a conclusion or an opinion that a problem or situation requires nursing care, determines the cause of the problem, distinguishes between similar problems, or discriminates between two or more courses of action.

The **nursing process** is a critical thinking framework in which you will exercise decision-making, diagnostic reasoning, problem-solving, and clinical judgment. It is composed of five interwoven phases: assessment, diagnosis, planning, intervention, and evaluation. The nursing process provides a framework to guide you to think critically in the clinical setting.

THINKING ABOUT THINKING

To improve your ability to think critically, you need to examine how you think. Thinking about thinking means bringing your mental activities to conscious awareness. It means recognizing thinking patterns that occur in different situations and evaluating the effectiveness of those patterns in achieving desired results. It means understanding yourself and the elements included in your thinking.

Thinking involves multiple mental functions grouped into the following two broad categories:

• Taking in information
• Using information to make decisions

Information is perceived through the five senses and stored in the brain. Storing information requires that the information is processed into meaningful patterns so that it can be retrieved or used in some way. The ways in which you process and understand information form your basic functions of thinking.

People have different preferences for processing information. That is, people seem to create meaning from information more efficiently when they receive that information in the manner that most closely matches their preference. For example, some people process information best when they see it (visual learners), whereas others process information best when they hear it (auditory learners). Think about how you learn best. You may find that you learn better if you have both visual and auditory cues.

Thinking is ever-changing. Before beginning to read this chapter you may have *thought* about the other choices you have for this period of time. You also may have *thought* about whether you would sit at your desk to read or sit in a comfortable chair. You might have *recalled* that a study-skills teacher told you that concentration improves when you study in one consistent place. Making a decision about each of the options requires thinking. Likewise, every action you will take in nursing practice requires thinking. Clearly, that thinking will be enhanced by understanding your thinking process.

Thinking occurs on more than one level of awareness. Sometimes we consciously think by saying to ourselves that a problem must be solved, a decision must be made, or simply that I will pay attention to a symphony. In any event, cognitive activity is occurring in the brain. Appreciating a symphony is a more passive activity than decision-making. However, even when you are making a decision consciously, more passive activity is also going on in your brain to influence the decision.

The T.H.I.N.K. Model

Nursing educators Rubenfeld and Scheffer (1995) have proposed a critical thinking model that incorporates five modes or processes of thinking that occur in combination or simultaneously. Whereas some situations may seem to require only one mode of thinking, the authors emphasize the importance of effectively using all of the thinking modes. Together, the five modes constitute a broad definition of critical thinking. You can use the mnemonic device T.H.I.N.K. to help remember them (Box 7–1).

Total Recall

Total recall involves remembering facts, such as names, dates, normal values, and telephone numbers. Thinking based on total recall is useful when you want to dial a phone number, drive to work, perform a nursing procedure, or obtain complete information during a client interview.

How total your recall is depends on your memory and how you process information into memory. One

---

BOX 7–1

THE T.H.I.N.K. MODEL

T = Total Recall
H = Habits
I = Inquiry
N = New Ideas and Creativity
K = Knowing How You Think

Rubenfeld, M.G., & Scheffer, B.K. (1995). Critical thinking in nursing: An interactive approach. Philadelphia: J.B. Lippincott Co.

---

way to increase recall is to put information into patterns of similar or related items. The pattern of telephone numbers in the United States—a three-digit area code, a three-digit prefix, and a four-digit number—is a pattern that is easier to remember than a string of ten numbers. Similarly, grouping clinical data into patterns can help you remember the data.

Another way to aid total recall is to attach significance to a fact by relating that fact to an experience (Rubenfeld & Scheffer, 1995). For example, most people can remember exactly what they were doing when they first learned of the Oklahoma City bombing. You may remember how to give an injection to a client at your clinical setting because you practiced injection techniques in the learning laboratory. One of the most important aspects of nursing education occurs in the clinical setting where students actualize what they have read in texts and heard in lectures. It is much easier to recall how a client looked and the behaviors she exhibited while in respiratory distress than it is to memorize the signs and symptoms of pulmonary edema. Putting real people's faces in one's memory in the context of the clinical learning setting helps you to learn about clinical practice.

Having total recall of essential facts is crucial to thinking. It allows you to sort information in different ways to solve problems, make decisions, or create scenarios. (Remember, however, that the way you sort or cluster information affects the way you interpret that information.) Ready recall of information also frees your mind to engage in other modes of thinking.

Habits

Habits are accepted ways of doing things that work, save time, or are necessary. Habits are behaviors that have been repeated so many times that they become second nature. When a behavior is habitual, you need not think through the individual steps it involves. Knowing how to drive a car and knowing how to swim are examples of habitual activities. Most of the activities that you learn in the nursing skills laboratory will become professional habits as you gain experience in nursing practice.

Forming habits allows you to do one thing while thinking about another. Much as you can drive a car while having a conversation, you can change a dressing while considering whether the wound has become infected. Naturally, habitual behaviors can be unsafe if unsafe steps become incorporated into the pattern.

Inquiry

Inquiry means examining issues in depth and questioning things that may seem obvious on the surface. It is the primary kind of thinking by which you reach conclusions. Inquiry involves analyzing information to confirm your hunch about a situation. Through feedback and further analysis, you can validate a conclusion. Nurses use this process to verify that the best interpretation is made of the client's clinical situation. Typically, the client will provide the main source of information as well as validation for your perception of reality.

Inquiry also includes the quality of being curious or wondering about the meaning of information. It is a spirit of wanting to know more, to understand, or to be able to explain facts that arise. Having a spirit of inquiry means never being satisfied with an interpretation of facts until you are sure that it is complete and accurate.

New Ideas and Creativity

New ideas and creativity occupy the opposite end of the spectrum from total recall and habit. They emphasize new and different ways of looking at information, and they form the basis for individualized client care. No two clients have identical values, life situations, preferences, and concerns. If you need to teach a person to care for a wound after discharge from the hospital, you need to consider how the client learns, whether the level of anxiety will permit learning to occur at this time, what supplies are available in the home, and the complexity of terminology the client can understand. A creative plan considers all of these variables.

Knowing How You Think

Knowing how you think is called metacognition, which literally means "in the midst of knowing." Knowing how you think means that you recognize when you are using logical reasoning to reach a conclusion. It leads you to ask yourself questions about how you think. Did I get all the facts before making a decision? Am I making assumptions that may not be true? In the example of teaching a client to manage a wound, you recognize that you have made an assumption that all clients want to learn wound care, so you seek validation that the assumption is true. Another question might be, "Do I spend so much time making sure I have all the facts that I am blocked from making a decision?" Box 7–2 lists strategies you can use to gain understanding about how you think.

BOX 7–2

STRATEGIES FOR GAINING UNDERSTANDING ABOUT HOW YOU THINK

- Keep a journal of how you use thinking skills. If you find a principle that works for you, jot it down! If something helps to make a thinking connection for you, jot it down!
- Share your journal with classmates in clinical conference. Compare how different thinking styles work for each of you.
- Discuss with classmates the thinking connections that you find difficult. Share problems and solutions.
- Always consider multiple solutions to any problem.
- Keep at it! Remember that critical thinking is the key to good nursing care and the foundation of accountability.

Critical Thinking as Clinical Judgment

In making a clinical judgment, you form an opinion using critical thinking to identify problems, solve problems, or make decisions. Sound clinical judgments stem from knowledge, clinical experience, and a holistic approach to the client's needs. As you learn to recognize patterns of behavior, the process also begins to include your powers of intuition. Kataoka-Yahiro and Saylor (1994) have proposed a model of critical thinking that helps nurses make the clinical judgments needed for effective nursing care.

The first component of the model is a *specific knowledge base.* Thinking depends on the knowledge base that each individual brings to the thinking process. The nurse's knowledge base includes sciences, liberal arts, and nursing content needed to provide nursing care. Physical sciences help you understand the functions of the body and how humans think and respond to health care situations. The liberal arts provide a basis for understanding human values and cultural variations. Nursing knowledge incorporates these elements, contributes understanding of what it means to be ill, and provides methods of increasing the client's level of wellness.

The second component of the model is *experience.* Each nursing student brings a unique set of individual experiences to the nursing education. Material presented as part of that education will be understood and applied within each student's experience. During nursing education, the student gains additional experiences through the practice of nursing in the clinical setting. Classmates share clinical experiences in formal clinical conferences. Each of these experiences adds to the student's knowledge. As clinical experience increases, so does the ability to think critically in the setting.

The third component of the model is called *competencies* and refers to the cognitive processes used to make clinical judgments. Competencies that you need as a nurse include the following:

- The ability to identify problems caused by illness
- The ability to recognize health needs
- The ability to make decisions about how to improve a client's health
- The ability to recognize when and why nursing care has improved the client's condition

The fourth and fifth components of the model are *attitudes* and *standards* of critical thinking. Attitudes associated with critical thinking include a spirit of inquiry, the desire to understand a situation from more than one perspective, and the valuing or seeking the truth. Paul's (1993) work, discussed shortly, expands on the attitudes and standards of critical thinking.

Characteristics of Critical Thinking

In critical thinking, the most fundamental concern is excellence of thought. The importance of the study of critical thinking is based on two assumptions: first, that the quality of our thinking affects the quality of our lives and, second, that everyone can learn how to continually improve the quality of her thinking. The idea is to systematically form and shape one's thinking to function purposefully to exacting standards. Critical thinking is disciplined, comprehensive, and based on intellectual ideals. As a result of the process of examining critical thinking, well-reasoned thinking develops (Paul, 1993).

Comprehensive critical thinking has the following characteristics:

- It is thinking that is responsive to and guided by such intellectual standards as relevance, accuracy, precision, clarity, depth, and breadth. Without standards to guide it, thinking cannot achieve excellence.
- It is thinking that deliberately supports the development of intellectual traits in the thinker, such as humility, integrity, perseverance, empathy, and self-discipline.
- It is thinking in which the thinker can identify the elements of thought present in the process. For example, the thinker can make logical connections between the elements and the problem at hand. Paul states that the critical thinker will routinely ask probing questions, such as these: What is the purpose of my thinking? What question am I trying to answer? What information am I using? How am I interpreting it? What conclusions am I coming to? What assumptions am I making? If I accept the conclusion, what are the implications and the consequences? Table 7–1 applies these elements to nursing.
- It is thinking that is routinely self-assessing, self-examining, and self-improving. Paul stresses that if students are not assessing their own thinking, they are not thinking critically.

- It is thinking in which there is integrity to the whole system.
- It is thinking that yields a predictable, well-reasoned answer from the comprehensive and demanding process that the thinker pursues.
- It is thinking responsive to the social and moral imperative to argue from alternate and opposing points of view and to seek and identify the weaknesses and limitations of one's own position (Paul, 1993, pp. 20–23).

Attitudes of Critical Thinking

As you develop the habit of thinking critically, you will develop attitudes that continue to foster critical thinking (Paul, 1995, p. 129). These attitudes include independence of thought, fair-mindedness, insight

TABLE 7–1

Paul's Elements of Critical Thinking Applied to Nursing

Element	Application Examples
Assumptions	• The nurse-client relationship is a helping relationship. • Clients have a right to make decisions about their health care.
Information	• Data, facts, and observations about the client. • Knowledge about the pathophysiology and etiology of disease. • Knowledge about human behavior.
Concepts	• Theories, definitions, principles, and laws that give meaning to information and that are used to interpret clinical data and make decisions about effective management of the client's problems.
Purpose of thinking	• To make decisions about data to be collected. • To diagnose problems and make clinical judgments. • To determine client goals or outcomes.
Question of an issue	• Determine the nature of the client's presenting problem. • Identify ethical and legal issues in practice.
Points of view	• The nurse's and client's perception of the clinical situation. • Perspective of health team members.
Interpretation and inference	• Diagnostic reasoning that results in nursing diagnoses, plans, and interventions
Implications and consequences	• Client outcomes and modifications of care

intoegocentricity and sociocentricity, humility and suspension of judgment, courage, integrity, perseverance, confidence in reason, interest in related thoughts and feelings, and curiosity.

Independence of Thought

Critical thinkers need to think for themselves, keeping in mind their own habits and biases. Critical thinkers consider knowledge from a wide variety of disciplines before making judgments about a situation. Nurses should draw on their knowledge base in the sciences and arts when making clinical judgments. These clinical judgments will be validated by the client and can be modified as necessary. Independence of thought in nursing increases with the student's growing knowledge base and clinical experience.

Fair-Mindedness

Critical thinkers are fair-minded, assessing all views of a situation without prejudice. Critical thinkers use the same standards for each situation and remain open to the belief that new evidence could change their minds.

Insight Into Egocentricity and Sociocentricity

Critical thinkers are aware that they have personal biases and actively try to examine their own thinking patterns. They are also aware that other people have personal biases and habits. This is especially true when setting goals with clients. If the nurse operates from only a personal value system without consulting the client, the resulting decision-making will probably fail to address the client's needs precisely. Consequently, the client's behavior is unlikely to change. When you assess which goals the client is interested in achieving, your nursing care is more likely to be successful.

Humility and Suspension of Judgment

Intellectual humility means being aware of the limits of your knowledge. Critical thinkers seek new information and admit when they need to learn. Again, being open to new evidence is part of intellectual humility. In the current health care system, greatly decreased hospital stays have become routine. Based on new evidence, this represents a "new way" of approaching the convalescing client.

Courage

Intellectual courage means having the inner strength to examine one's own views critically. It is the courage to face the idea that your thinking may be wrong. Intellectual courage is especially important when you provide care to persons who hold different values and cultural mores from your own. A person with intellectual courage understands that values and beliefs are not always logical—they are culturally acquired and emotionally bound.

Integrity

Intellectual integrity requires that individuals value good thinking and hold their own thinking to the same standards they use when judging the thinking of others. You must be committed to examining your thinking, becoming aware of flaws in your thinking, and practicing techniques to improve your thinking.

Perseverance

Critical thinkers show intellectual perseverance in finding effective solutions to problems. Perseverance requires a careful and complete gathering of data, sorting of data for patterns, and thinking through alternative solutions and consequences. It is the opposite of going with the first idea. The need for perseverance increases as your knowledge and experience grow.

Confidence in Reason

Critical thinkers believe that careful, thoughtful thinking provides good answers or solutions. Thus, critical thinkers value the development of advanced inductive and deductive reasoning skills and become confident in the thinking process.

Interest in Related Thoughts and Feelings

Critical thinkers are interested in the thoughts that underlie feelings and the feelings that underlie thoughts. From the field of cognitive psychology we learn that thoughts produce feelings. For example, thinking about crime and violence produces fear. On the other hand, feelings often underlie thinking without the person being consciously aware of the values that contribute to the feelings.

Critical thinkers understand that there is an emotional aspect to the thinking process. These emotions need to be explored to determine their origin. Many of the values that a person holds come from growth and developmental stages. Some values are based in reality, and some are not. Critical thinkers explore feelings and consider how they feel about issues. Then they judge which emotions are helpful and which are not.

Curiosity

A critical thinker is a curious person always filled with questions about the world. Never be satisfied that you fully understand why and how people and things work. Additionally, a critical thinker is curious about values and searches for the underlying reasons why people hold certain beliefs.

DEVELOPMENT OF CRITICAL THINKING

Critical thinking is a skill that develops over time and with conscious application of total recall, habits, inquiry, new ideas and creativity, and knowing how you think. As you gain more experience in nursing, your thinking will evolve and advance.

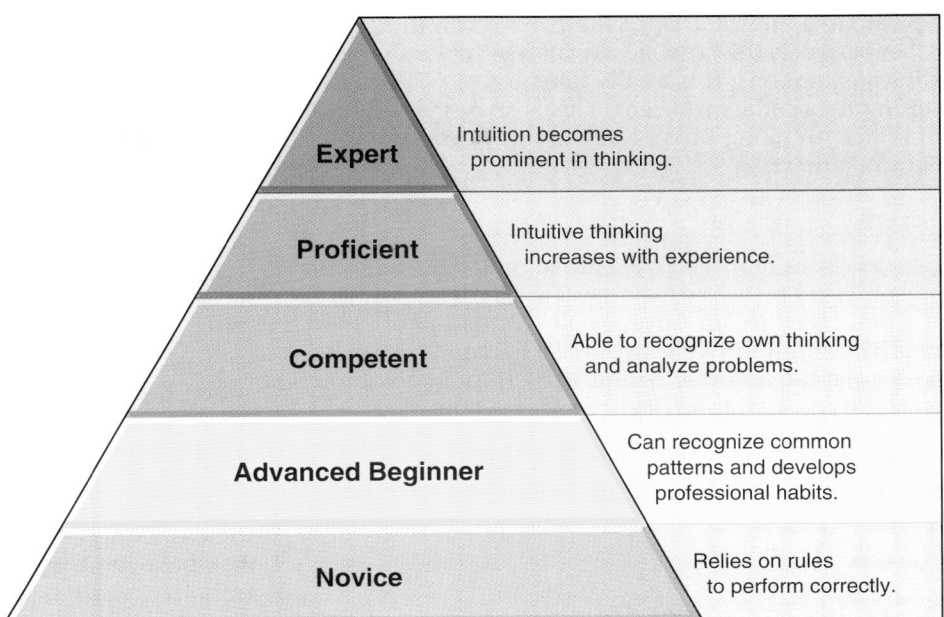

Figure 7–2. Growth in critical thinking from novice to expert. Advancing to expert is not automatic. It requires commitment to continued growth.

Stages of Skill Acquisition

In *From Novice to Expert* (1984), Patricia Benner applies the Dreyfus Model of skill acquisition to nursing practice. The Dreyfus Model suggests that a person passes through five levels of proficiency in acquiring and developing a skill. Applying this model to professional nursing practice, Benner identifies these stages as: novice, advanced beginner, competent, proficient, and expert (Fig. 7–2). Each of these stages requires that the nurse be able to think critically; however, the depth and breadth of the nurse's ability to think critically will evolve with each stage.

Benner's stages of skill acquisition in professional nursing practice reflect changes in three general aspects. The first change is from reliance on abstract principles stored in memory to the use of past concrete experiences to guide actions. The second change is the individual's perception of the situation; it is seen as a whole in which only certain elements are relevant. The third change is from being a detached observer to an involved performer.

Novice

Benner describes the behavior of the *novice* nurse as being rule-governed, limited, and inflexible. Critical thinking operates in the total recall mode. Because the novice has no experience of the situation at hand, rules are used to guide performance. The student nurse follows rules because they are "correct." But, Benner cautions, rules legislate against ultimately successful performance because rules do not specify the most relevant tasks in actual situations.

Advanced Beginner

According to Benner, the *advanced beginner* (or new graduate) has experienced enough real situations to note the recurring meaningful aspects and attributes in a situation. The advanced beginner can formulate guidelines based on experience but may miss their differential importance, thereby treating them equally. Benner states that the advanced beginner benefits from assistance, given by an instructor or a preceptor, in setting priorities. This stage demonstrates the very beginning of the development of professional habits, part of the T.H.I.N.K. process.

Competent

Benner reports that the third stage of proficiency—*competence*—is typified by the nurse who has been in the same or similar position for 2 to 3 years. In this setting, the nurse begins to interpret actions in light of long-range goals or plans about which he or she is consciously aware. The plan dictates which aspects of the current and future situation are most important and which can be ignored. Therefore, the competent nurse can develop a plan based on considerable conscious, abstract, and analytical contemplation of the problem. The competent nurse lacks the speed and flexibility of the proficient nurse but does have a feeling of mastery and the ability to manage the needed nursing care. In this stage, the nurse relies on all modes of the critical thinking process.

Proficient

Benner describes the *proficient* nurse as one who perceives each situation as a whole rather than in its individual aspects. She states that the nurse's perception is the key element in this stage. The perspective is not consciously thought out; instead, it "presents itself" based on experience and recent events. Proficient nurses understand a situation as a whole because they perceive its meaning in terms of long-term goals. They operate in a holistic mode where, based on their clinical experience, they can clearly understand nuances in clinical situations. It typically takes 3 to 5 years in one setting to become proficient. This is an advanced level of critical thinking possibly involving highly complex clinical situations.

Expert

Benner states that the *expert* nurse no longer relies on an analytical principle to connect the understanding of a situation with an appropriate action. The expert nurse has an intuitive grasp of each situation and zeroes in on the accurate region of the problem without wasteful consideration of alternative actions (Fig. 7–3). It takes 5 to 15 years in a setting for a nurse to become expert. Practice at this stage demonstrates the highest level of critical thinking in that the expert nurse knows holistically what to do without consciously thinking through all the data.

Obstacles to Critical Thinking

There are a number of obstacles to developing and exercising your critical thinking skills. By being aware of them, you can ensure that your thinking remains sound.

One of the most common obstacles involves overuse of the habit mode. Nurses tend to develop routines and habits to make sure that work gets done efficiently. However, habits can narrow the focus of your thinking. Unquestioned habits may cause you to miss important cues and could be dangerous to your clients. Every person for whom you provide care is unique. By assuming that habitual behaviors will be correct for all clients, you leave yourself open to mistakes.

Another obstacle to good thinking is anxiety, especially severe anxiety, which can render even the most prepared person unable to perform. Dealing with anxiety requires you to focus on yourself, thus reducing the focus and energy available to your clients.

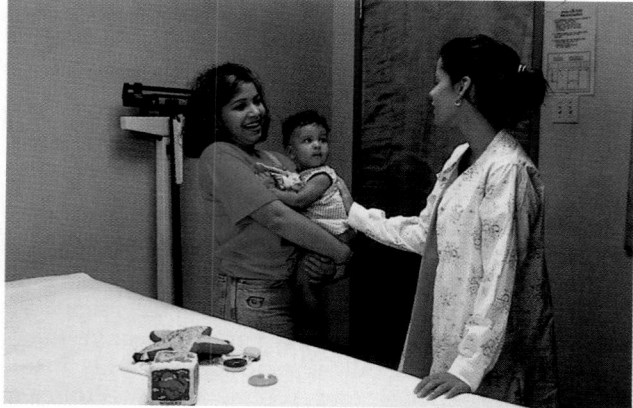

Figure 7–3. An expert nurse uses intuition to ascertain that this mother is happy and the baby is healthy.

Working under deadlines may affect your ability to think critically because you simply may not have enough time to think through all available information before arriving at a solution. You may make decisions prematurely, without all the facts or before the client is ready. Clearly, clinical practice often takes place under time pressures realistic to the setting. One way to overcome this obstacle is to prepare as thoroughly as possible for the clinical experience at hand. Also, you should make good use of your clinical instructor.

Another obstacle to developing critical thinking skills is an overcommitment to ideological, religious, or political principles—to the extent that your mind is closed to other ideas. It is important that you understand your own biases as well as those that your client might have.

Finally, lack of confidence in your thinking can be an obstacle to critical thinking. Nursing students sometimes lack the confidence to stand up for what they believe; it may feel safer to back away from an authority figure (staff nurse, instructor, or physician) than to defend your position. However, if you think clearly, logically, and with consideration for the values of others, then you can always have confidence in your thinking.

CRITICAL THINKING AND THE NURSING PROCESS

In clinical practice, the nursing process provides the structure in which critical thinking, diagnostic reasoning, and clinical judgment take place. It is composed of five interrelated phases: assessment, nursing diagnosis, planning, intervention, and evaluation (Fig. 7–4).

Assessment

The first phase of the process is *assessment*. In this step, you collect data that you then can use to identify client needs that can be managed or treated with nursing care. The focus of your assessment may be narrow or broad and may generate a large amount or a relatively small amount of data, depending on the setting and the client's condition.

A comprehensive assessment is holistic and includes a physical examination, a health history, and a psychosocial-cultural assessment. Client-centered data are usually collected to understand the client's history in the areas of health needs. This health history is organized in a framework that is most pertinent to identify the care needs of the client. Most health care agencies have a form for collecting a health history. Proceeding though scripted questions, you listen for cues that suggest a problem or a need. These cues direct you to explore those areas of concern in more depth. Critical thinking directs this exploration.

The nursing assessment is performed in all nursing specialties and settings. You may encounter clients in the hospital setting where a presenting problem or illness becomes the starting point of the

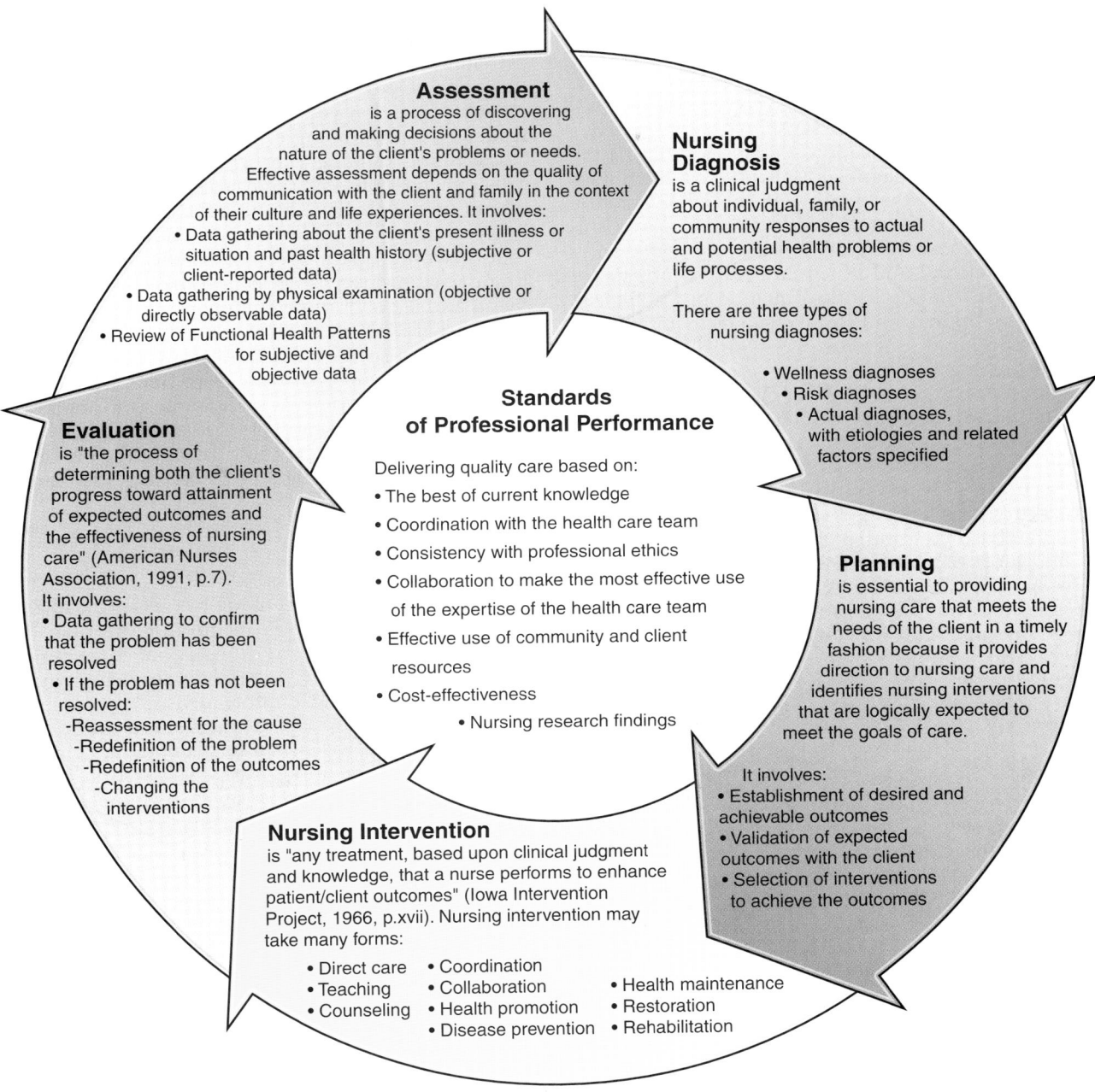

Figure 7–4. The nursing process and standards of professional performance.

assessment. In contrast, in a community setting, you may screen healthy clients for risk factors for a particular disease.

As you collect assessment data, you will engage in critical thinking, mentally grouping data into clusters for specific meaning related to the client's situation. You will listen actively and make observations about the client. As the data pieces form meaningful patterns or information clusters, you will critically analyze them. This is the process of diagnostic reasoning. Diagnostic reasoning is not innate; it is a skill that you

can learn and improve with practice, experience, and an increased knowledge base.

As a result of your assessment, you will arrive at one of the following outcomes:

- You will identify no problem.
- You will identify a potential problem.
- You will identify an actual problem that needs further assessment.

The process of taking a health history is detailed in the next chapter of this tex

Nursing Diagnosis

Once you have clustered the data pieces obtained through assessment, you will assign specific diagnostic labels to those clusters. The North American Nursing Diagnosis Association (NANDA) has adopted a *nursing diagnosis* classification system to promote the standardization of diagnostic labels used by nurses and, consequently, the quality of care delivered by nurses. NANDA defines a nursing diagnosis as a clinical judgment about individual, family, or community responses to actual and potential health problems or life processes. These responses include physiological, cognitive, emotional, and social changes that influence how an individual functions.

Each nursing diagnosis has five components: a label, a definition, a set of defining characteristics (signs and symptoms), a group of related factors, and risk factors. The nursing diagnoses you choose for each client will be based on assessment data for that client; their accuracy depends on the quality and completeness of the data collected. Obviously, the data on which you base your nursing diagnoses should be the best and most reliable available to you.

As specified by NANDA, nursing diagnoses provide the basis for selecting nursing interventions to achieve the outcomes for which you are responsible. Your clinical judgment determines which diagnosis you will attend to first. Chapter 11 focuses on how to identify and write a nursing diagnosis.

Planning

The third phase of the nursing process is *planning*. In this step, you set goals and plan nursing care. Collaboration with the client is essential to successful planning. If a goal that you create on your own holds no importance for the client, the client will have little interest in pursuing the goal and no incentive to become interested (Fig. 7–5). This is why the goals (or outcomes) of the planning process must be client-oriented. The goals you establish should state, in measurable terms, what the client will be doing and how the client will be doing it after nursing care has been delivered. Determining realistic and achievable outcomes means that you can be held accountable for the results of your nursing care.

Planning nursing care involves setting priorities. This can be done by rank-ordering the goals or by identifying goals that should have high, medium, and low priority. High-priority goals would be attended to first or would be the focus of your nursing care. Setting priorities involves critical thinking, clinical judgment, and a good knowledge base.

You will document your plan of care in the client record and also on the nursing care plan so that all nursing personnel can work from the same plan. Because the nursing process is dynamic, information obtained during the planning stage will be added to the assessment data and may, in turn, alter the nursing diagnoses and goals. Chapter 12 describes the planning process in detail.

Intervention

The fourth phase of the nursing process is the *intervention* phase, in which you execute the care plan. *Independent* interventions are those that the nurse is licensed to carry out independently. They include counseling, providing comfort measures, teaching, offering emotional support, managing the environment, and assessing. *Dependent* interventions are those activities carried out under a physician's order. An example is administration of an intravenous infusion. Chapter 12 focuses on nursing interventions.

Evaluation

The final phase of the nursing process is *evaluation*. In this phase, the planned outcomes of nursing care are measured against the actual outcomes. Outcomes can be met, unmet, or partially met and are recorded as such. When outcomes are unmet or partially met, reassessment is necessary to determine why this result occurred. The care plan is then revised accordingly. Clinical pathways and case maps are evaluation tools that can help nurses monitor client progress. These tools show the "average" path that a client with a certain diagnosis would take. These tools provide you with a daily measure of the client's progress on the clinical path. These evaluation tools are examples of building quality assurance measures into nursing care. Chapter 13 describes the evaluation process in detail.

APPLYING T.H.I.N.K. TO THE NURSING PROCESS

You will use each of the five modes of critical thinking outlined in the T.H.I.N.K. model while carrying out the nursing process. Doing so will help you to more

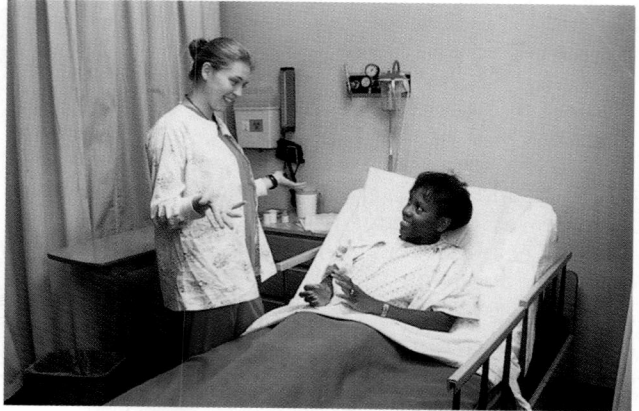

Figure 7–5. Planning for interventions that are acceptable to the client requires the nurse to use creativity to engage the client in the process.

accurately and completely provide for each client's needs.

Using T.H.I.N.K. in Assessment

Total recall is used in assessment when you follow a specific list of questions or guide to collect assessment data. An assessment guide ensures that your assessment covers all essential elements of data collection. *Habits* come into play when you develop consistent patterns of behavior that you use in the assessment process. You use *inquiry* when you explore abnormal findings and form additional questions to obtain more information that may improve your understanding of the problem—and perhaps reveal the cause of the problem. You use *new ideas and creativity* by listening to what is *not* said as well as to what *is* said and by formulating questions that help the client express sensitive feelings or describe embarrassing symptoms. You use *knowing how you think* by asking yourself such questions as: Have I been thorough? Have I identified all the necessary cues? Is there sufficient evidence to support my conclusions?

Using T.H.I.N.K. in Diagnosis

You use *total recall* and *habits* to cluster assessment data into meaningful patterns. *Inquiry* is used as you ask yourself how the data patterns affect the client's health. *New ideas and creativity* are used in the process of diagnostic reasoning to arrive at nursing diagnoses. *Knowing how you think* assists you in the analytical process of diagnosing.

Using T.H.I.N.K. in Planning

You use *total recall* to remember the usual goal for the problems that you have identified. *Habits* help you to develop goals and outcomes that are measurable and achievable. *Inquiry* is used to validate goals with the client, thus making sure that you and the client agree. *New ideas and creativity* may be needed when the client denies that a problem exists or is unwilling to engage in behaviors that improve health. *Knowing how you think* leads to questions about the logic used in connecting the expected outcomes to solving the problems that have been identified.

Using T.H.I.N.K. in Intervention

Total recall is used to remember the steps of a procedure and the principles or elements that are critical to safe and effective intervention. You rely on *habits* to achieve a well-organized, smooth procedure. *Inquiry* helps you to determine if the methods of intervention are the best for the particular client situation. *New ideas and creativity* modify the intervention for client preferences or situational variables. *Knowing how you think* helps you to evaluate the methods of intervention by asking such questions as: Was the client comfortable? Was the intervention successful?

Using T.H.I.N.K. in Evaluation

Total recall and *habits* are used to compare the goals of care with the outcomes of care. *Inquiry* helps you to determine client satisfaction (or dissatisfaction) with the achieved outcomes. *New ideas and creativity* may be necessary to modify the plan of care. *Knowing how you think* helps you to assess an outcome objectively.

KEY PRINCIPLES

- The T.H.I.N.K. model is a mnemonic device that reflects the key elements of critical thinking: total recall, habits, inquiry, new ideas and creativity, and knowing how you think.
- Attitudes that foster critical thinking include independence of thought, fair-mindedness, insight into egocentricity and sociocentricity, humility and suspension of judgment, courage, integrity, perseverance, confidence in reason, an interest in related thoughts and feelings, and curiosity.
- Nurses typically develop skill proficiency in the following order: novice, advanced beginner, competent, proficient, and expert.
- Obstacles to critical thinking include an inadequate knowledge base, an over-reliance on habits, anxiety, too little time to make reasoned decisions, zealous adherence to circumscribed sets of beliefs, and lack of confidence in thinking ability.
- The nursing process is composed of five interrelated phases: assessment, diagnosis, planning, intervention, and evaluation. It provides a framework in which to exercise critical thinking.

BIBLIOGRAPHY

Alfaro-LeFevre, R. (1995). *Critical thinking in nursing: A practical approach.* Philadelphia: W.B. Saunders Co.
Bandman, E.L., & Bandman, B. (1995). *Critical thinking in nursing* (2nd ed.). Norwalk, CT: Appleton & Lange.
*Becker, H.A., & McCabe, N. (1994). Indicators of critical thinking, communication and therapeutic intervention among first-line nursing supervisors. *Nurse Educator, 19*(2), 15–19.
*Belenky, M.F., Clinchy, B.M., Goldberger, N.R., & Tarule, J.M. (1986). *Women's ways of knowing: The development of self, voice, and mind.* New York: Basic Books.
*Benner, P. (1984). *From novice to expert.* Menlo Park, CA: Addison-Wesley Publishing Co.
*Brookfield, S. (1987). *Developing critical thinkers.* San Francisco: Jossey Bass.
Brookfield, S. (1993). On impostership, cultural suicide, and other dangers: How nurses learn critical thinking. *Journal of Continuing Education in Nursing, 24*(5), 197–205.
*Carnevali, D.L., & Thomas, M.D. (1993). *Diagnostic reasoning and treatment decision making in nursing.* Philadelphia: J.B. Lippincott Co.
Chaffee, J. (1997). *Thinking critically* (5th ed.). New York: Houghton Mifflin Co.
Corcoran-Perry, S. & Narayan, S. (1995a). Teaching clinical reason-

*Asterisk indicates a classic or definitive work on this subject.

ing to nurses in clinical education. In J. Higgs & M. Jones (Eds.), *Clinical reasoning in the health professions* (pp 258–286). Oxford: Butterworth Heinemann Ltd.

Corcoran-Perry, S. & Narayan, S. (1995b). Clinical decision making. In M. Snyder & M. Mirr (Eds.), *Advanced practice nursing: A guide to professional development* (pp 69–91). New York: Springer Publishing Company.

*Facione, P.A. (1990). *Executive summary—critical thinking: A statement of expert consensus for purposes of educational assessment and instruction.* Millbrae, CA: The California Academic Press.

*Hammers, J., Abu-Saad, H., & Halfens, R. (1994). Diagnostic process and decision-making in nursing: A literature review. *Journal of Professional Nursing, 10*(3), 154–163.

*Hickman, J.S. (1993). A critical assessment of critical thinking in nursing education. *Holistic Nursing Practice, 7*(3), 36–47.

Higgs, J., & Jones, M. (Eds.). (1995). Clinical reasoning in the health professions. Oxford: Butterworth Heinemann Ltd.

*Jones, S.A., & Brown, L.N. (1993). Alternate views on defining critical thinking through the nursing process. *Holistic Nursing Practice, 7*(3), 71–76.

*Kataoka-Yahiro, M., & Saylor, C. (1994). A critical thinking model for nursing judgment. *Journal of Nursing Education, 33,* 351–355.

Krejci, J.W. (1997). Imagery: Stimulating critical thinking by exploring mental models. *Journal of Nursing Education, 36*(10), 482–484.

Krichbaum, K., Lewis, M., & Duckett, L. (1997). Critical thinking: What is it and how do we teach it? In J.C. McCloskey & H.K. Grace, *Current issues in nursing* (5th ed.). St. Louis: Mosby–Year Book.

North American Nursing Diagnosis Association. (1999). *Nursing diagnoses: Definitions and classification, 1999–2000.* Philadelphia: Author.

*Paul, R.W. (1993). *Critical thinking: What every person needs to know in a rapidly changing world* (3rd ed.). Rohnert Park, CA: Center for Critical Thinking.

*Paul, R.W. (1995). *Critical thinking: How to prepare students for a rapidly changing world.* Santa Rosa, CA: Foundation for Critical Thinking.

Pesut, D.J., Herman, J., & Fowler, L.P. (1997). In J.C. McCloskey & H.K. Grace (Eds.), *Current issues in nursing* (5th ed.). St. Louis: Mosby–Year Book.

Rossignol, M. (1997). Relationship between selected discourse strategies and student critical thinking. *Journal of Nursing Education, 36*(10), 467–475.

*Rubenfeld, M.G., & Scheffer, B.K. (1995). *Critical thinking in nursing: An interactive approach.* Philadelphia: J.B. Lippincott Co.

Vaughn-Wrobel, B.C., O'Sullivan, P., & Smith, L. (1997). Evaluating critical thinking skills of baccalaureate nursing students. *Journal of Nursing Education, 36*(10), 485–488.

Watson, G., & Glaser, E.M. (1964). *Watson-Glaser critical thinking appraisal.* New York: Harcourt, Brace World.

Assessing the Client: History-Taking

Helen Harkreader

Key Terms

active listening

active processing

assessment

biographical data

cardinal signs and symptoms

chief complaint

closed question

cue

data

database

demographic data

functional health patterns

human response patterns

inference

interview

intuition

leading question

minimum data set

nursing history

objective data

open-ended question

orientation phase

signs

subjective data

symptoms

termination

validation

working phase

LEARNING OBJECTIVES

After studying this chapter, you should be able to:

1. Make preliminary decisions to prepare for data collection.

2. Understand assessment as a critical thinking process.

3. Employ interviewing techniques in taking a health history.

4. Develop a systematic framework for organizing data.

5. Document the assessment appropriately.

Assessment is the process of gathering information about a client's health status to identify concerns and needs that can be treated or managed by nursing care (Fig. 8–1). The information gathered may also be known as **data.** It comprises subjective and objective information about the client, such as signs and symptoms of disease. Data collection marks the beginning of the nursing process and continues throughout the process. As data are collected, they are grouped or classified into meaningful clusters that describe the problems to be treated. Thus, assessment involves analyzing data to identify a client's problems and arrive at appropriate nursing diagnoses.

Assessment begins before the actual collection of data; that is, assessment begins with thinking (Fig. 8–2). During this preparatory stage, you will make decisions about the purpose of the assessment, the type of assessment to use, the types of data to be collected, and the sources of data. Consider the difference between assessing a postsurgical client who has requested pain medication and assessing an elderly client who is admitted to a nursing home. Assessment for the client in pain is brief and focused on the experience of pain, whereas assessment for the nursing home client includes the holistic needs associated with daily living.

Assessment is an active mental process requiring

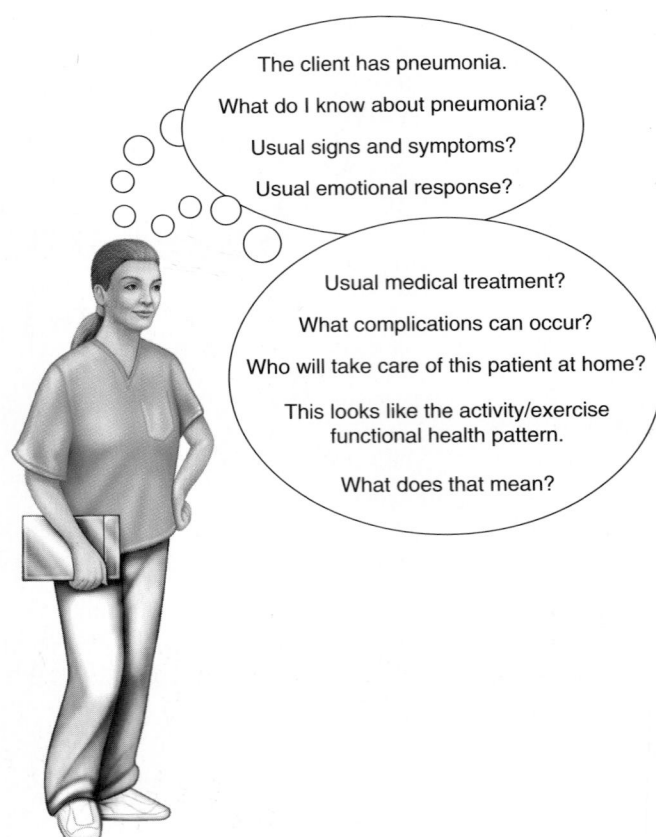

Figure 8–2. Assessment begins with thinking.

critical thinking about the data collected rather than merely obtaining answers to a specific list of questions. To gather information wisely, you need well-developed skills in observing and listening. While doing so, the mental skills of translating, reasoning, intuiting, and validating will make the data meaningful.

Data are more useful when the assessment process is organized in a framework that helps you to identify the nature of data to be collected and classify them into common problem areas. As you collect data in each category prescribed by the framework, you will produce an initial clustering of information about the client. The framework for data collection affects which problems are distinguished or emphasized. For example, if you studied colors by examining red, blue, and yellow, all colors could be put in one of those categories. However, you would not be able to identify or classify the uniqueness of purple, green, and orange, much less the millions of subtle shades in between. In the same fashion, data about a client can be classified by physiological systems, but you might fail to identify social, psychological, and spiritual problems that influence the client's health.

Rarely will you perform assessment as a single isolated step in the nursing process. Rather, as you elicit information about a client, you will begin to consider nursing diagnoses and formulate plans. Also, assess-

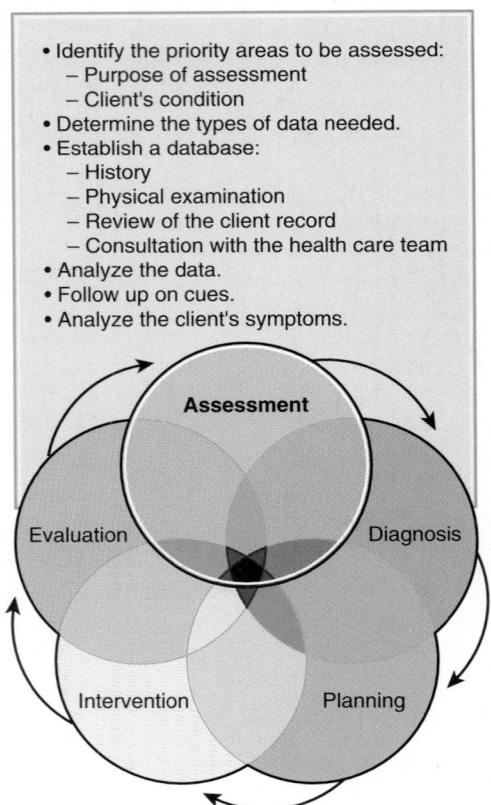

Figure 8–1. Assessment is the process of gathering information about a client's health status to identify concerns and needs that can be treated or managed by nursing care.

ment usually includes giving information to the client. In other words, it is often combined with teaching. In some cases, as when the person has a compromised airway or needs emergency surgery, assessment and implementation may take place almost simultaneously. In all cases, assessment serves to establish priorities for care.

PRELIMINARY DECISION-MAKING

Any time you interact with a client, for virtually any reason, you will assess the person's problems, needs, and concerns. To do so efficiently and correctly, you must make decisions about the type of assessment required, the sources of data to be consulted, how to structure and focus the assessment, and how much information to collect before developing a plan of action.

Purpose of Assessment

An assessment may have a comprehensive focus or a specific, narrow focus. Depending on the purpose, assessment may involve asking two or three specific questions, or it may involve spending an hour in an in-depth conversation with the client. The purpose of the assessment may be to

- Establish a database with which to plan and evaluate comprehensive care.
- Identify actual and potential problems to make nursing diagnoses.
- Focus on a specific problem.
- Determine immediate needs to establish priorities.
- Determine the cause (etiology) of a problem.
- Determine related or contributing factors.
- Identify strengths as a basis for changing behavior.
- Identify the risk for complications.
- Recognize complications.

Types of Assessment

Many professionals classify assessments as initial, focused, emergency, and ongoing. The initial assessment is made at the first contact with the client. A focused assessment is a detailed examination of a specific problem. An emergency assessment identifies or rules out life-threatening problems and those problems that need immediate treatment to prevent complications. Ongoing assessment refers to the data collection that takes place during every contact with the client throughout the client's association with the health care agency.

Initial Assessment

Assessment on initial contact with the client typically is more thorough and comprehensive than subsequent assessments. It begins with the problems that prompted the client to seek nursing services, and it obtains a holistic overview of the client's level of functioning. The nature of the client's problems—and thus

the services to be provided—dictates the course and depth of the assessment. The objective is to rule out as well as to identify problems.

The initial encounter with a client commonly occurs when the client has sought services for a specific problem, desires a general health status evaluation, or seeks wellness care. The client entering the hospital for surgery or for treatment of a medical condition has a specific problem and needs nursing care aimed at managing the treatment for the problem. The client entering a long-term care facility needs a general evaluation of health status to ensure that medical problems are stabilized and to identify the scope of needed nursing care. Wellness services typically take place in community settings, such as schools or clinics, where the nurse may screen for health problems in addition to helping clients manage specific concerns. In any setting, the focus of the nursing assessment is to identify how the nurse can help the client.

The focus of the initial assessment relates directly to the goals of prevention, maintenance, restoration, or rehabilitation. As a screening procedure, assessment is an overview designed to detect risk factors and evidence of certain problems. When prevention is the focus, assessment examines risk and lifestyle factors. A health maintenance assessment examines health and health behaviors. When the goal is restoration, assessment focuses on the need for support of body functions and the detection and prevention of complications. Rehabilitation considers the potential for restoring function and the resources needed to modify the lifestyle. Over the course of an illness, assessment will focus on different goals. For example, for a client recovering from open-heart surgery, restoration of health is the immediate goal. As the client recovers, the goal shifts to rehabilitation.

Not every assessment is comprehensive. In general, the thoroughness of an assessment is directly proportional to the length of expected care. If the client has an acute, short-term problem, such as a need for sutures in an accidentally inflicted minor wound, you will gather only minimal lifestyle information. However, the nurse who cares for clients with serious injuries in a rehabilitation unit will be able to provide better long-term care by knowing the client's health history thoroughly.

Focused Assessment

Once the client's general problems have been identified, you may perform a focused assessment on each problem or problem area. The focused assessment examines the evidence in detail, considers possible etiologies, looks for contributing factors, and considers client characteristics that will help solve the problems. Imagine, for example, that you have identified a diagnosis of *Ineffective individual coping (use of alcohol as primary coping mechanism)* for a client. You then can focus on this diagnosis to gather information about the person's pattern of drinking, defense mechanisms that maintain the behavior, effects on the family, and other information helpful in developing an appropriate plan of care.

Focused assessment also takes place when the client has a complaint or describes a new problem. Common complaints include pain, shortness of breath, difficulty urinating, and visual changes. You must be prepared to assess the severity of the problem, determine a possible cause, evaluate effects on the client's health, and decide on an appropriate course of action.

Emergency Assessment

When the client's situation is life-threatening or time is an important factor in preventing complications, assessment will include only key data directly related to the immediate problem. The initial information you collect will vary, depending on the urgency of the situation. Additional data can be collected after the client's condition is stable. As always, emergency assessment follows the ABCs, which means airway, breathing, and circulation. Naturally, the client needs an open airway to take in oxygen-laden air. The person also must be able to make a respiratory effort. Finally, circulation must be available to transport oxygen to the person's tissues. When you observe an emergency team in action, it may seem that many activities are taking place all at the same time, but the procedure is actually an orderly one based on the ABCs.

Ongoing Assessment

Assessment continues throughout the client's health care experience. Reassessment may occur monthly, weekly, daily, or hourly, depending on the client's condition and the nature of the services being offered. For the critical care client, assessment takes place continually via electronic monitoring equipment. Assessment also takes place continually during and after a client receives anesthesia—until it has worn off and the client has "recovered" from its effects. A client taking a new once-daily medication may need daily assessment until the medication's effects are clear. Weekly assessment may be appropriate for a client on a weight-loss program. Clients in a nursing home may have a formal assessment only once a month.

Nurses routinely make decisions about how often to reassess a client and in what breadth and depth. To make these decisions effectively, you must anticipate the potential for a client's condition to change, the speed at which it could change, and the evidence that would indicate a change. For example, when a client takes a new medication, assessment decisions are based on the expected effects of the medication, how rapidly those effects occur, and potential adverse effects.

Types of Data

As you listen to and interact with a client, you will gather some information that is directly observable and some that is not. Information not directly observ-

able typically comes from the client's description of a problem. Either type of information can provide a **cue,** an indicator of the presence or existence of a problem or condition that represents a client's underlying health status. The data of greatest significance in diagnosing a particular illness, disease, or health problem are called **cardinal signs and symptoms.**

Subjective Data

Information provided by the client that you cannot observe directly is called **subjective data.** When subjective data supplied by the client describe characteristics of disease or dysfunction, those characteristics are known as **symptoms.** Pain, nausea, cramps, dizziness, and ringing in the ears are examples of symptoms because you cannot observe them directly. The client must inform you of their presence.

You may be able to directly observe evidence related to the client's symptom. For example, you may notice grimacing, an increased heart rate, and a doubled-over posture in a client who complains of pain. However, these observations could apply to pain, nausea, or cramps and can only be confirmed by asking the client to name the complaint. You may help the client describe or quantify subjective findings, but you should not make judgments about whether or not the symptom exists. The client is the best—indeed, the only—source of information about subjective findings.

Objective Data

Characteristics about the client that you can observe directly are called **objective data.** When that data indicate characteristics of disease or dysfunction, they are known as **signs.** Objective data can be observed through your senses of sight, hearing, taste, touch, and smell. These data can be measured or quantified, and they can be reliably replicated from one examiner to the next, a concept called *inter-rater reliability.*

For example, you can measure the size of a wound and the amount of drainage it produces. The number of red blood cells in a sample of blood can be counted. Because objective data are clear and factual, they have a high degree of validity. However, objective information is not necessarily superior to subjective information.

Sources of Data

When assessing a client, you will need to make decisions about the most effective use of multiple sources of data, possibly including the client, the client's significant others, your colleagues, and the client's records. You will need to confirm that each data source is appropriate, reliable, and valid for each assessment. Appropriate means that the source is suitable for a particular purpose, person, or occasion. Reliable means that you can trust the information to be accurate and honestly reported. Valid means that the information can be substantiated or confirmed.

Client

Usually, the client is in the best position to provide accurate, reliable, and valid information about subjective data that describe health problems. In fact, some symptoms can be validated and accurately described *only* by the client. Always start by considering the client the primary source of assessment data. However, sometimes a client may be too ill to provide information, may be confused, or may suffer from memory loss or otherwise not be able to provide accurate information.

Significant Others

Especially in these cases, family members may be able to contribute significant information. If the client proves to be an unreliable source of information or simply prefers to have a family member help describe events, you may ask the family for information.

Before discussing the client's problems with family members or significant others, however, you must consider the client's right to confidentiality. Although many times an ill person relies on a family member to help remember details and ask important questions, that client may prefer to maintain some privacy from the family. Making an accurate determination of the client's wishes requires you to respond sensitively to subtle cues that may suggest the client's willingness, even preference, to have a family member remain in the room while you conduct the interview. Remember that you are in a position to ask family members to leave during the interview unless the client expresses the desire to have them stay.

Colleagues

All members of the health care team who have worked with the client can be important sources of data. Each team member will have a unique perspective on the client's problems and therefore may make different observations. For example, the physical therapist may recognize that pain is preventing the client from walking or getting adequate exercise; the dietitian may suggest that pain is interfering with the client's ability to learn important information about a newly prescribed diet.

Nurses who work in the home setting may have fewer opportunities to confer face-to-face with other members of the health care team than nurses who work in institutional settings. Consequently, other forms of communication may become more important in ensuring complete assessment and continuity of care. Usually, the client's record provides the primary method of communication to ensure continuity of care.

Client Records

The client has a right to expect members of the health care team to communicate adequately with each other. Likewise, the client has a right to expect you to be informed about the reason for admission or care. If the client has a medical or nursing record in the agency, you usually will begin by reviewing that record.

For the admission assessment of a hospitalized client, the record will indicate the reason for admission and the physician's admitting orders. In a home health agency, the initial record may show the reason for the referral and a brief history of the current problem. At a follow-up visit in a clinic setting, reviewing the record will help you detect any ongoing problems as well as any new problems. Naturally, clients will feel more confidence in the health care team if you and other members take time to review the record before beginning an assessment. Doing so will also help you avoid collecting data that are already in the record.

Standards of Practice for Assessment

One characteristic of a profession is that it has the means to regulate and control its practice. As the official voice of nurses in the United States, the American Nurses' Association develops and disseminates Standards for Clinical Practice. These standards are broad guidelines that require clinical judgment. They may be used in a court of law when determining what a reasonable and prudent nurse would do in a similar situation. In the area of assessment, these standards require the nurse to do the following:

- Determine priorities from the client's immediate needs
- Gather pertinent data using appropriate assessment techniques
- Collect data from the client and, when appropriate, from significant others and health care providers
- Collect data in a systematic manner that is orderly and thorough
- Continue assessment throughout care
- Document relevant data in a retrievable form

COLLECTING THE DATA

Assessment requires more than obtaining the answers to an established list of questions; it is a process of discovery, of gathering information in a manner that reveals the client's needs. The health assessment forms used by many health care facilities provide plausible and reasonable guides to data collection, but they are only a guide, not a substitute for the critical thinking skills needed for a complete assessment. Whether or not you use a health assessment form, you will gather data using focused forms of listening and processing.

Active Processing

When assessing a client, you will be (1) observing and listening to the client and (2) processing information through translating, reasoning, intuiting, and validating. To accomplish these goals effectively, you will use **active listening.** In other words, you will attend to what the client says and help the client clarify and elaborate and give additional pertinent information.

You will also use **active processing,** which involves a systematic series of mental actions to analyze and interpret the information about the client. When you process information actively, you help yourself form mental impressions by thinking through such questions as "How does this information fit with what I know about a certain disease or health problem?" and "What questions do I need to ask to see how well it fits the pattern?"

Active listening and active processing are closely related concepts that occur simultaneously. Together they require you to use all your senses, to make judgments about the meaning of information, and to validate that meaning. For example, you may see that a client is exhibiting a particular symptom, hear the client describe an alteration in health, and then make a judgment about the meaning of these cues for this client. Finally, you may think about other experiences involving these cues and ask further questions.

As you assess a client, your mind continually shifts back and forth from general or global scanning to focusing on a specific problem. An initial assessment often follows a standardized format that directs your mental activity toward the global scan. Proceeding through specified questions, you listen for cues that suggest a problem, a need, or other cues relevant to the present circumstances. Then you ask questions to follow up on any cues that arise so you can determine whether a problem exists.

After categorizing this specific information in the context of the global assessment, you then continue scanning for problems. Assessment of a specific cue may reveal one of the following three conclusions:

- No problem exists.
- A potential problem exists.
- An actual problem exists and needs further assessment.

Some potential problems may need further assessment; others may need to be noted only for future reference. Box 8–1 illustrates a conversation with a client in which the nurse is actively processing information to guide continued assessment questions.

Observing

Assessment involves using all of your senses to observe the client. You will observe the client's physical condition for cues that need to be followed up with appropriate questions. Observations of difficult breathing, pale skin, or other physical signs help you know how to proceed with the assessment.

Additionally, you will observe the client's behavioral responses. For example, watch for consistency or

---

BOX 8–1

ACTIVE PROCESSING

The line on the simple assessment checklist reads: **Recent weight gain/loss?** Rather than simply placing a check mark on the form to confirm that the client has lost weight recently, the nurse follows up with this conversation.

Nurse: How much weight have you lost?

Client: About 30 pounds in the past 2 months.

Nurse: How do you account for losing so much weight?

(The nurse knows weight loss can be associated with cancer. This question is looking for any other possible cause.)

Client: I don't know. I guess I just haven't had much appetite.

Nurse: Have you had any nausea or vomiting?

(The nurse is still exploring for other possible causes.)

Client: No.

Nurse. Have you had any blood in your stool? Or had black, tarry stools?

(Not finding any explanation for the weight loss, the nurse moves to other warning signs of cancer.)

Client: I haven't seen any blood, but I have sometimes had really dark, sticky bowel movements. Does that mean something?

Nurse: Well, it could be blood. I don't really know what it means. Have you discussed it with your doctor?

(The nurse has begun to explore a plan with the client.)

Client. I know I need to. I guess I don't want to know. My father died of cancer.

(The client has revealed a need for teaching.)

Nurse. Blood can mean several things, only one of which is cancer. How long ago did your father die?

(The nurse is looking for further information before being satisfied with the teaching.)

Client: Oh, it's been 30 years. They didn't know how to treat cancer then. I guess I really should see about it.

Nurse: We can do a screening test for blood in your stool. However, even if it is negative at this time, I want you to make an appointment with your doctor. If there was blood in your stool, it would be best to make sure it is not from cancer. Will you do it?

Client: Yes.

Nurse: Remember that cancer is only one of the possibilities. If it turns out to be cancer, you know that there are many newer treatments than were available when your father died. However, whatever the cause, you need to see the doctor.

The nurse then gives the client a Hemoccult test slide and instructions to collect the specimen.

discrepancy between nonverbal and verbal responses. Interpret eye contact, body language, and facial expressions in the context of what the client says in response to your questions.

Listening

Listening is an active process that involves hearing what the client says and also the meaning behind it. This type of listening requires practice. When you listen actively, you can then formulate questions that help the client describe a problem completely by providing all pertinent information. For example, if the client has difficulty describing the intensity of nausea, you may suggest using a scale from 0 to 10, with 10 being the worst nausea imaginable. It may also be helpful to know if eating makes the nausea better or worse.

Failing to listen attentively to what a client says—and does not say—can keep you from identifying a problem or understanding it completely. Denying the possible seriousness of a problem can cause the client to withhold information. The client may leave out important details, believing that the problem is not important, that certain symptoms are not relevant, or that seeking help was not appropriate.

Naturally, most clients describe their problems from a lay point of view. Consequently, they often include extraneous information. You must decide how long to listen before refocusing the client to more pertinent data. If you interrupt the client too soon or too abruptly, the client may feel misunderstood and will probably feel that you have little interest in helping to identify the problem.

Translating

Assessment also involves translating information into clear, succinct, meaningful statements that will be understood by other health care personnel. The client may express concerns in slang terms or lengthy descriptions. You will then translate and document these descriptions in medical terminology, which has the advantage of abbreviating the description and conveying meanings that are commonly understood by other professionals. However, if you feel that a medical term or interpretation could be misinterpreted, choose instead to document the client's own words.

Grouping data into meaningful patterns is also part of translation. For example, you would group cyanotic skin color, restlessness, and rapid respirations together because they all relate to tissue oxygenation.

Reasoning

Assessment includes actively processing information to make mental connections of the data to diseases, health patterns, or the current situation. Nurses who have a wide knowledge base are more likely to make appropriate mental connections. For example, the nurse who understands pathophysiology can determine whether the client's signs and symptoms are consistent with normal progression of an illness or whether a complication may be developing. Knowing the problems or complications that can occur with an illness, medical treatment, or surgical procedure can help you determine the meaning of the data you collect.

Reasoning also includes recognizing and understanding psychological and social responses to a health problem. These responses must be distinguished from the signs and symptoms of the illness itself.

Reasoning includes making **inferences** from the data, which means that you attach meaning to data or reach a conclusion about data. Inferential reasoning is based on a premise or proposition that supports or helps to support a conclusion. Correct inferential reasoning is based on knowing that the facts are correct, that the premise is correct, and that the known information is sufficient to reach the conclusion. Box 8–2 il-

---

BOX 8–2

UNDERSTANDING INFERENTIAL REASONING

Correct Inferential Reasoning

Fact: Mr. Smith has a bowel movement every 3 days, and the stool is soft and easily passed.
Premise: Constipation is the presence of hard, dry stool that is difficult to pass.
Conclusion: Mr. Smith is not constipated.
Explanation: This correct conclusion can be corroborated by asking whether information included in the premise is sufficient to establish the presence of constipation. Because the premise includes a standard definition of constipation, the conclusion is based on sufficient evidence.

Incorrect Inferential Reasoning

Fact: Mr. Smith has swelling in his ankles and feet.
Premise: Persons with right-sided heart failure have swelling in their ankles and feet.
Conclusion: Mr. Smith has congestive heart failure.
Explanation: Although the premise is correct, the information in both the fact and the premise are insufficient to support the conclusion. Because ankle swelling can result from other problems besides heart failure, more evidence is needed to determine that heart failure has caused Mr. Smith's swollen ankles.

lustrates examples of correct and incorrect inferential reasoning.

You will routinely make inferences about the meaning of information as you collect it. However, reaching a conclusion too rapidly can result in errors. Always validate the data and explore the problem further. Look for evidence that judges the extent of the problem and for logical relationships between the data and the probable causes.

Using Intuition

Intuition is an ability to understand the whole without having systematically examined the parts. It is knowing without always knowing why you know. The knowing comes in a flash of understanding, or a gestalt, without being aware of the thinking that has preceded the understanding. This kind of thinking starts with the whole and then examines the parts to validate that the thinking is correct.

Some people appear to be naturally intuitive thinkers, having developed a preference for intuitive reasoning from early childhood. Poorly developed or untrained intuition skills can lead to faulty reasoning. However, an excessive reliance on intuitive reasoning raises the danger of accepting a conclusion without verifying that the facts support the conclusion. A novice should never rely on intuition alone.

Intuition can be developed through repeated systematic examination of data to arrive at an appropriate conclusion. After multiple experiences with similar situations and similar correct conclusions, you will begin to develop intuitive reasoning as a valid basis for nursing actions.

Well-developed intuitive reasoning distinguishes the expert nurse from the novice (Fig. 8–3). With intuition, the nurse acts correctly, seemingly without thinking, and cannot always explain the basis for the action. Intuition is efficient reasoning that allows the nurse to act quickly to save a life or prevent a complication. It allows the nurse to recognize a client's feel-

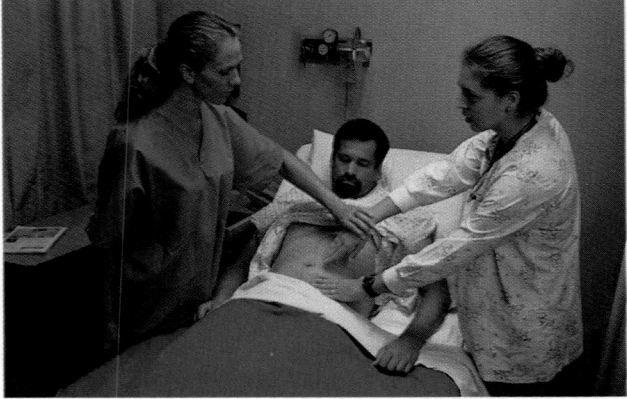

Figure 8–3. Well-developed intuitive reasoning distinguishes the expert nurse from the novice. Here, an expert nurse guides a novice nurse through a systematic physical examination guided by intuitive reasoning.

ings or sense a level of understanding and respond appropriately.

Validating

Validation means substantiating or confirming the accuracy of information using another source or another method. Cross-validation of both objective and subjective data increases the accuracy of the data as a whole. For example, you can validate your interpretation of nonverbal behavior by asking the client about it. When the client reports symptoms (subjective data), you can try to validate them with objective findings. Imagine that a client has reported being constipated; you can look for such objective evidence as lack of a bowel movement, a hard and dry stool, or a distended abdomen.

Sometimes family members or significant others can be used to validate information given by the client. The family can be especially helpful when the client has developed symptoms too gradually to be aware of their onset.

When the client and a family member provide conflicting reports, you must make a clinical judgment about which information to accept. Sometimes you can validate the most accurate account by using other sources, such as the medical record, objective observations, other family members, or the judgments of other team members. For example, suppose a client reports having an occasional alcoholic beverage, whereas a family member reports that the client is a heavy drinker. You check the medical record and find that the client's blood alcohol level on admission indicated heavy drinking. This information does not confirm that the client continually drinks large amounts of alcohol, but it does provide evidence that supports the family member's position.

INTERVIEWING

An **interview** is a planned series of questions designed to elicit information for a particular purpose. Whether you enter a client's room to assess for a complication or a complaint, make a phone call to a home health client, or take an initial history, the interview has a definite purpose. You know in advance exactly what information is needed.

The most formal interview is for the purpose of taking a health history and identifying needs or problems that require nursing intervention. In a setting with a wellness focus, the health history determines specific changes in levels of wellness and patterns of living.

A well-conducted interview helps the client explain his or her own interpretation and understanding of the condition or reason that prompted the visit. The interview usually begins with an open approach that allows the client to talk until you develop an understanding of the client's perspective. Next, you will ask a series of questions while continuing to give the client some control of the interview so you can fully explore the items to be covered. The client should feel like your partner in explaining and defining health problems.

The initial assessment interview begins with information about the client's **chief complaint,** which is the problem that caused the client to seek health services, call the doctor, or request a visit with a nurse; it is the client's description of the problem. The initial assessment typically includes both nursing and medical emphases. The **nursing history** is a narrative of the client's past health and health practices that focuses on information needed to plan nursing care. The medical history focuses on illness and the treatment of disease. The medical and nursing histories have some elements in common. Both types are collected through interviewing the client, using an assessment framework to ensure thoroughness. The physical examination follows the assessment interview.

Phases of the Assessment Interview

A successful interview depends on preparation that anticipates the client's needs and sets the stage for the interview. Additional skills are engaged to ensure that the assessment is comprehensive and the time with the client is productive. Interviewing skills are engaged in each of four phases of the interview process: preparation, orientation, the working phase, and termination.

Preparation

You will need to prepare for each assessment both mentally and physically. Doing so will allow you to assess each client systematically and thoroughly. The extent of your preparation depends on the purpose of the assessment. It may be as brief as asking a colleague to provide one or two pertinent pieces of information before entering a room to assess a client's report of pain. A comprehensive health assessment requires more extensive preparation.

As part of your preparation, you will set the stage for the assessment interview. Ideally, a comprehensive health history should take place in a private setting because some of the conversation may be sensitive or embarrassing to the client.

Naturally, all client information is confidential. Assure the client that the information you solicit will be shared only with the health care team and only for purposes related to providing care. Do not suggest that any information will be kept confidential from the health care team. In some cases, you may need to inform the client of your obligation to share information with legal authorities; as needed, do so before asking for information that may be incriminating.

Additionally, the client should be comfortable and have any immediate needs met before the interview begins. Immediate needs may be as simple as going to the bathroom, or they may require you to treat pain or reposition the client to ease difficult breathing. The client's condition always determines how much information can be collected in one sitting.

Before beginning the interview, assess the client's probable reliability in providing or reporting health information. Obvious problems in reporting result from confusion, disorientation, and poor memory. On the other hand, a high level of stress or anxiety can cause the client to exaggerate symptoms or focus on extraneous information.

Orientation

The **orientation phase** is a brief exchange to establish the interview's purpose, the examination procedures, and the nurse's role in the interview process. The orientation phase in the initial interview is important because it establishes the nurse-client relationship as a legally binding contract. The nurse should be seen as a person who can be trusted with confidential information, trusted to provide competent care, and trusted in some cases with the client's life. The relationship will benefit from establishing an atmosphere that communicates care for the client. Box 8–3 lists key points for the orientation phase.

Therefore, the first step in client assessment is establishing a nurse-client relationship based on mutual trust and understanding. In other words, you must build rapport with the client. Rapport means that there is a sense of understanding and trust between the nurse and client, suggesting that you each have a vested interest in the client's well-being. When rap-

---

BOX 8–3

KEY POINTS FOR THE ORIENTATION PHASE

- Establishing rapport with the client is essential. Rapport implies a sense of understanding and trust between the nurse and the client.
- The initial contact with the client sets the tone for the interview.
- The client who feels acceptance and positive regard is more likely to discuss feelings, thoughts, and values.
- The primary goal in initiating the interview is to establish trust.
- Your tone of voice, body language, choice of words, and dress all give direct messages to the client.
- The psychosocial interview can involve discussing sensitive personal information; privacy is important.
- The interview should have a basic structure and a quality of professionalism.
- Begin by introducing yourself, then describe your credentials, your role in the person's care, and the purpose of the interview.

port is present, the client is more likely to reveal personal information.

Your demeanor can help establish an appropriate rapport and trust; it must portray you as a professional, knowledgeable person who is interested in the client. In a social relationship, flirting, giggling, joking, exchanging personal stories, or talking about sports events are expected forms of interchange. In a professional relationship, however, the conversation focuses on the reason for the relationship: the client. The client should be the most important person in the relationship. A small amount of social interchange can help some clients be more comfortable with you, but you must avoid using a client relationship to meet your own personal or social needs.

Begin the assessment by identifying the client's immediate concerns and addressing them. A mother admitted to the hospital for elective surgery may need to know how to use the telephone to call her children before she will be interested in talking about the upcoming surgery. One client who is admitted for open-heart surgery may be worried about the surgery itself, whereas another may have questions about the postoperative diet and smoking cessation plan. Allow the client's questions and concerns to shape and focus the assessment, but do not limit the interview to these areas.

Working Phase

The **working phase** is the phase of the interview process in which the client and nurse work together to review the client's health history and establish potential and actual problems that will be addressed as part of the care plan. The nurse gains insight about the client's concerns and expectations. The client feels assured these concerns will be addressed.

Termination

Skillfully ending the interview leaves both the nurse and the client feeling satisfied that the purpose has been accomplished, the client has been understood, and there is no unfinished business. The nurse prepares the client for **termination** of the interview by announcing in advance the approximate length of time the interview will take. The client will know how much time the nurse expects to devote to the process. As the interview nears an end, it may be helpful to state that you have just a few more questions. The last phase of the interview allows time for the client to ask questions and address any additional concerns that have not been covered in the interview.

Types of Interviews

You will need to choose the method of conducting an interview based on the type of information you need to collect, the purpose of the interview, and the client's skill in describing problems. Interviews can be primarily directed or nondirected. Most interviews will make use of a combination of approaches.

Directed

In a directed interview, you maintain control over the interview by asking a list of questions that call for specific information from the client. The directed interview is used to elicit specific information and to ensure that the interview covers all relevant areas of assessment. One advantage of the directed interview is its ability to focus the client on information that is pertinent to the immediate concern and avoiding extraneous information. The directed interview is an efficient way to collect data in a short time.

The directed interview makes use of **closed questions,** questions that call for a specific, short response from the client. For example, to assess pain the nurse asks, "Do you have pain? Where is the pain? Describe the pain? How severe is the pain?" The directed interview may also use **leading questions,** questions that suggest a possible appropriate response. An example of a leading question is "You are frightened that the diagnosis will be cancer, aren't you?" Using closed questions can help you collect the most pertinent information in the shortest time.

The directed interview has the disadvantage of not providing the opportunity for clients to freely express their concerns, fears, or feelings. You can obtain the most basic and necessary information, but the client may be left feeling that you are not concerned enough. Clients need to express their feelings and describe their symptoms from their own point of view to feel understood.

Nondirected

The nondirected interview gives more control to the client, thus allowing freer expression of concerns and feelings. Many clients try to "make sense" of their symptoms and may have associated meanings and antecedents to events surrounding the onset of symptoms that may or may not be relevant. The nondirected interview offers the client the opportunity to discuss and seek clarification about these meanings and events.

The nondirected interview uses primarily **open-ended questions** that ask for longer, interpretive responses. Open-ended questions do not call for a specific answer and may be phrased as a request rather than a question, such as "Tell me about the events that brought you to the hospital." or "Describe your symptoms." Open-ended questions are more useful for eliciting information from the client's point of view.

ORGANIZING THE DATA

A **database** is all of the information that has been collected about the client and recorded in the health record as a baseline for the initial plan of care. It typically includes the data from the physician's client history and physical examination, the nurse's assessment, laboratory and diagnostic test results, and input from other members of the health care team. The database is used for comparing the client's response to treatment with the client's baseline condition.

A health care agency establishes a **minimum data set** that specifies information that must be collected from every client entering or being admitted to an institution. There is usually some commonality among clients in a particular setting that directs the decision about what to include in the minimum data set. Many institutions have assessment forms designed to ensure the collection of the minimum data set. Box 8–4 illustrates a typical minimum data set for a hospitalized client.

The Health History

Health care agencies generally use a standardized assessment tool or form on which to record your health history interview. This tool may vary, depending on the goals for care and the type of services offered by the agency. Acute care agencies with short-term stays will need only the information necessary to manage the short-term experience. Some information is gathered for the purpose of helping clients plan their care after discharge. If a client appears to need extensive assistance with discharge planning, additional information may be gathered.

Some agencies use a form organized as a review of body systems, whereas other forms are organized by functional ability or other nursing assessment schemata. In all cases, the goal is to achieve a systematic, comprehensive assessment appropriate to the services of the agency. No matter what organizational framework you use, your assessments will be more efficient when you use a consistent, thorough pattern.

Remember, however, that a structured interview schedule is only a list of questions or cues. Skill in interviewing involves knowing when to move quickly through a list of items and when to ask additional or open-ended questions. You will learn to pick up subtle cues from the client that a problem exists or that the client needs to discuss something further, has questions, or is reluctant to talk about something.

How the assessment is structured will affect the problems that you identify. Assessment forms in health care agencies vary from highly structured to open-ended. In an effort to reduce the time spent documenting, ensure comprehensive assessment, and meet the legal requirements for documentation, assessment forms have been developed that allow you to complete a checklist and possibly write brief notes. Computerized charting systems take the idea one step further, and you may choose from a list to record your findings.

Clearly, assessment can easily become a mechanical process. In such an environment, it is more important than ever for the nurse to have a firmly grounded mental system for assessing the client. Usually, the system begins with an exploration of the client's biographical data, expectations and goals, reason for the visit, and medical and family histories. It then can expand into a holistic approach based on an assessment framework that addresses all aspects of the client's health.

Biographical Data

Biographical data is information that identifies and describes the person, such as name, address, age, gender, religious affiliation, race, occupation, other people residing in the household, and the number of dependent children. This kind of information is also referred to as **demographical data** because it is factual information that can be aggregated to describe populations of clients. Biographical information helps the health provider anticipate problems common to a particular group. For example, difficulty in urinating would have a different probable cause in a 55-year-old male than in a 16-year-old male. Biographical data may also be collected by having the client complete an admission form or by reviewing the client's record.

Expectations and Goals

In describing their symptoms or concerns, clients may provide cues to their feelings about their illness, expectations of the health care encounter, or health care goals. You should listen for information that suggests that the client fears a serious or life-threatening problem. Sometimes you can provide information that calms those fears or helps the client gain a realistic perspective.

The client's goals and expectations are affected by the setting. In home health, the client may be seeking information to decide whether or not to call a physician or determine whether the family has the resources to manage a problem. The family may expect you to give them information or help them manage the problem. The hospitalized client may be expecting a short hospital stay, full recovery, and immediate return to usual activities. Other expectations of the hospitalized client include freedom from pain, to be treated with respect, to be safe, and to receive appropriate treatment for the presenting problem. The nurse needs to know if the client's expectations and goals match those of the health care team.

Social and cultural history provides cues to the person's values and experience with health care (Fig. 8–4). It may also suggest the need to investigate problems that are more likely to occur within a particular group. Care can be planned that is consistent with the client's values.

Reason for the Visit

The health care provider usually begins by finding out the reason for the encounter from the client's point of view. The physician often only writes brief descriptions of the client's problems in the medical record; therefore, you may need a more complete description from the client. Most clients appreciate the opportunity to review the details of the experience that has led them to seek health care.

While listening to the client's account of the reason

BOX 8–4

TYPICAL MINIMUM DATA SET FOR ADMISSION OF A HOSPITALIZED CLIENT

- Admitted from (home, physician's office, emergency medical service, or emergency department)
- Mode of arrival (ambulatory, wheelchair, or stretcher)
- I.D. band on (yes/no)

Present Illness

- Vital signs
- Height and weight
- Time and type of last oral intake
- Chief complaint
- Observations

Allergies

- List drugs, food, other
- Describe reaction
- Allergy band on (yes/no)

Prostheses

- Dentures
- Glasses
- Contact lenses
- Hearing aid
- Walking aid
- Artificial limb
- Artificial eye
- Other

Medication History

- List dose, frequency, date/time of last dose
- Medications brought to hospital
- Disposition
- Valuables (to safe, policy explained, to home [with whom])
- List retained medications

Health History

- Previous illness or hospitalization
- Bleeding tendencies
- Circulatory problems
- Previous transfusion
- Hypertension
- Asthma
- Hay fever
- Arthritis
- Heart problems
- Kidney problems
- Cancer
- Diabetes
- Epilepsy

Functional Status (Activities of Daily Living)

- Primary language spoken
- Diet
- Hygiene (bathing, dressing, grooming)
- Sleeping patterns
- Communication/speaking
- Comprehension
- Seeing/hearing

Mobility (Describe Limitations)

- No limitations
- Unable to sit
- Unable to stand
- Requires walker/cane
- Requires wheel chair
- Requires partial/complete assistance
- Admission instructions given
- Bathroom emergency light
- Visitor policy
- Meals/guest meals
- Smoking
- Room—bed control, phone, call light, TV control, side rails
- Electric appliances O.K. or Maintenance notified of non-U.L. equipment

Social Assessment/Discharge Planning

- Religion
- Are any persons in your home dependent on you?
- Will you need help when you go home?
- Independence in the home setting?
- Obvious family conflicts that may impair health care in the future
- Apparent family support system
- Able to return to previous living situation
- Able to administer all medications
- Indications of possible neglect or abuse
- Do you anticipate any problems after discharge?
- Are you being seen by any health service/agency?
- Do you have any suggestions that will help us with your care here?
- Identified client/family education needs
- Person to notify in emergency
- Respondent (if other than client)

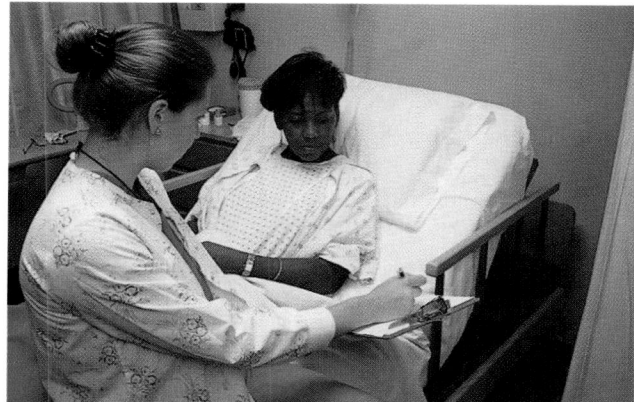

Figure 8–4. The social and cultural history provides important clues to the client's health-related values and to the client's experience with the health care system.

for the visit, you are gathering information about the client's knowledge level and feelings about the problem and areas for teaching. Using active listening techniques, you may discover that the client has misunderstandings about the medical treatment plan. If you cannot remedy these misunderstandings, you will need to share this information with the physician.

HISTORY OF PRESENT ILLNESS

Information about the history of the present illness helps to anticipate problems the client may have and to understand the illness from the client's point of view. Having described the reason for the visit, the client may have given a complete account of the history of the present illness. If not, you can help the client fill in missing information. It is helpful to know when the symptoms began, the severity of the symptoms, and what actions were taken to control the symptoms. The client who enters the hospital may have been managing an illness for a long time through outpatient services, or the symptoms may have had a sudden onset. Helpful questions include: "Have you been seeing a physician for this problem?" "What did the doctor tell you about the problem?" "What medications have you been taking?" "Did the medication help?" "Have you received other treatment?"

ASSESSING THE CHIEF COMPLAINT

You can encourage the client to describe the chief complaint by asking such questions as "How can I help you?", "What brought you to the hospital?" or, "Tell me about your problem." Told in the client's own words, the chief complaint establishes the purpose of the contact, provides direction for the assessment, and establishes the nurse-client relationship.

Then you will gather information to fully describe the client's problem. Ask questions that help the client describe the specific signs and symptoms associated with the problem and provide a history to the present illness. The following seven variables provide a core description of most problems. Although all the variables may not apply to every symptom, using this general pattern of assessment will help you to be thorough.

LOCATION. Symptoms are often associated with a particular body part. Ask the client to be specific about the location of pain, numbness, or other sensation. For example, you might say, "Can you point to the exact location of the pain in your abdomen?" or, "Where does it hurt?" The location of a rash or other lesion may help identify the cause.

QUALITY. You are seeking the client's description of how the symptoms feel. Avoid giving the client words to describe the symptom but, if the client cannot find any words, you can offer choices. People will often describe a symptom by using an analogy, such as "pins pricking my skin," "a knife stabbing me," "something very heavy on my chest," or "something tearing." Clients' choices of analogies are fairly consistent for particular diseases and therefore may provide a definitive cue to the medical diagnosis.

QUANTITY. Measuring quantity is an attempt to determine the intensity or severity of the symptom. Quantity can be elicited as frequency, volume, number, effects on activity, and extent. You might ask, "How severe is your symptom?" or, "How often does it occur?" To get more objective data about pain, it may be useful to have the client rate the pain or other symptom on a scale of 0 to 10, with 10 being the most severe pain imaginable.

CHRONOLOGY. It may be helpful to know how long the client has had the symptom. Was the onset insidious (slow, gradual) or acute (sudden)? Is the symptom constant or does it come in episodes? Does the intensity vary with time? Does the symptom disturb the client's sleep?

SETTING. Where was the client, and what was happening when the symptoms first occurred? The setting may suggest that stress, activity, or environmental pollution is affecting the symptom. For example, the onset of asthma when the person goes to a park may suggest an environmental trigger for the attack.

AGGRAVATING OR ALLEVIATING FACTORS. Ask what the client has found to be helpful in relieving the symptom. What attempts has the client made to relieve the symptom? Is there any activity that makes it worse? Does eating make it worse or better? Does resting help? Was aspirin used to reduce a fever?

ASSOCIATED FACTORS. Look for anything else that might have been missed. Associated factors will vary according to the nature of the problem. You may ask about common associations. For example, for a client with diarrhea and abdominal cramps, ask if that person has recently traveled to a foreign country or eaten a food that might have produced the problem. The client may have an idea about what brought on the problem.

Medical History

A medical history is a review of health problems that required or continue to require treatment by a physician. You are looking for any past medical problems that might influence the present illness by contributing to the problem or altering care for the current problem. A medical history may be elicited through a written checklist of common chronic problems, filled out by either the client or the nurse. Specific questions are asked about each illness in the client's history. By using a checklist, the client is encouraged to be thorough, and the focus of the interview is narrowed to pertinent information.

The medical history also includes a history of allergies to medications, pollutants, foods, and pollens. When the planned treatment includes the administration of medications, it is most important to ask about allergies to medications. If the client reports an allergy, obtain information about the type of reaction and how the reaction has been managed in the past.

Family History

As you ask about the client's medical history, you will also ask about the family history of any illnesses that are genetic or familial. As the name implies, genetic illnesses are passed through genes. Familial illness tend to run in families, but the cause of the increased incidence in a family may be unknown. Familial illness may have a basis in lifestyle, diet, stress, or environmental factors.

Review of Functional Health Patterns

One method of holistic assessment that provides information from a nursing rather than a medical perspective uses **functional health patterns,** a concept that refers to the positive and negative behaviors a person uses to interact with the environment and maintain health. During assessment, you will examine the client's behaviors to determine whether each pattern is functional or dysfunctional. Assessment includes the usual pattern of behavior, complaints, limitations, problems associated with the pattern of behavior, behaviors used to manage the problem, and the client's coping skills. Each pattern is examined for biological, social, psychological, cultural, developmental, and spiritual factors influencing behavior. Box 8–5 lists categories of information to be assessed in each health pattern.

A few key questions in each category may be sufficient to determine that the person does or does not have a problem. If a problem is suggested, then you will ask further questions. However, assessment of functional patterns includes the client's strengths as well as weaknesses, problems, and limitations. Information about methods of health maintenance can be combined with indicators of physical function to develop possible causal relationships between the two. Additional questions are asked not to identify problems, but to elicit the client's usual pattern of function. You need this information to more effectively support the client's usual pattern of functioning while providing care.

BOX 8–5

ASSESSMENT OF FUNCTIONAL PATTERNS

For each functional pattern, assess:

Functional

- Present function.
- Personal habits.
- Culture and lifestyle factors.
- Age-related factors.

Dysfunctional

- History of dysfunction.
- Diagnostic tests.
- Risk factors associated with medical treatment plan.

When a Problem Is Identified in a Functional Pattern

- Relationship to other functional patterns.

Clustering of data by functional health patterns will also help you identify problems responsive to nursing intervention and assign appropriate nursing diagnoses to dysfunctional patterns. Nursing care is more concerned with helping the person manage or function with a health problem than with diagnosing and treating illnesses. Therefore, the focus of functional health patterns is on nursing diagnoses rather than on medical diagnoses.

Marjorie Gordon (1997) introduced a formal framework for assessing functional health patterns in 1982. She identified patterns of human function in 11 categories that address physical, psychological, spiritual, and social needs. Rather than treating the illness, nursing care is aimed at maintaining or improving the client's functional status in each of the 11 areas.

Health Perception–Health Maintenance Pattern

The health perception–health maintenance pattern describes the client's personal view of health and behaviors associated with the quest to be healthy. The client's risk factors for altered health and altered health maintenance should be explored. Health maintenance is inherent in the other 10 patterns of functioning; exploring the health perception–health maintenance pattern gives you the opportunity to focus on health behaviors and risk factors.

Beliefs about health and about the ability to change health directly affect how people manage their health. Important components of this pattern of behavior include the beliefs that a person has about control over health and the actions taken to change the state of health.

Assessment of the client's lifestyle can reveal areas where health can be improved. Knowledge of the client's health-seeking behaviors will provide you with cues to help the client plan care that will improve health. Assessment would include health-related activities in each of the functional patterns.

Assessment of health perceptions may begin by asking the client to describe any current health problems. Information about health perceptions and beliefs may be inherent in the response.

Another way to elicit information about health perceptions is to ask, "Have you had a similar experience in the past?" You may get information about previous illnesses or hospitalizations, including the client's perceptions of these experiences. In eliciting information about the current illness, ask the client to describe it, including the onset and the cause. Ask about previous treatment, whether the client complied with the treatment regimen, and whether the client anticipates having any problems in self-care as a result of the illness. When assessing health perception–health maintenance, you are looking for evidence of a healthy lifestyle.

Asking about the use of alcohol, illegal drugs, over-the-counter drugs, and tobacco products should be a routine part of a health assessment. A nonjudgmental manner is essential to getting truthful information. Accurate information is particularly important if the hospitalized client is expected to have anesthesia or be confined long enough for withdrawal symptoms to occur.

You also need to know whether the client has sufficient information to understand and manage the presenting health problems. Allow time to address the client's concerns, and frequently ask whether the client has any questions. By having the client describe problems and review information received from a physician, you can often detect whether the person has any misunderstandings.

Areas for assessment of the health perception–health maintenance pattern may include the following:

- Client's description of general health
- Health practices
- Use of alcohol, tobacco, and other substances
- Home, school, and occupational safety
- Client's description of the cause of the illness (if present) and actions taken to manage it

Nutritional-Metabolic Pattern

The nutritional-metabolic pattern includes the client's dietary habits in relation to metabolic need. Nutritional patterns are learned from early childhood; they may be modified by lifestyle changes, new knowledge, economics, or health problems. General health is affected by nutritional intake (Fig. 8–5).

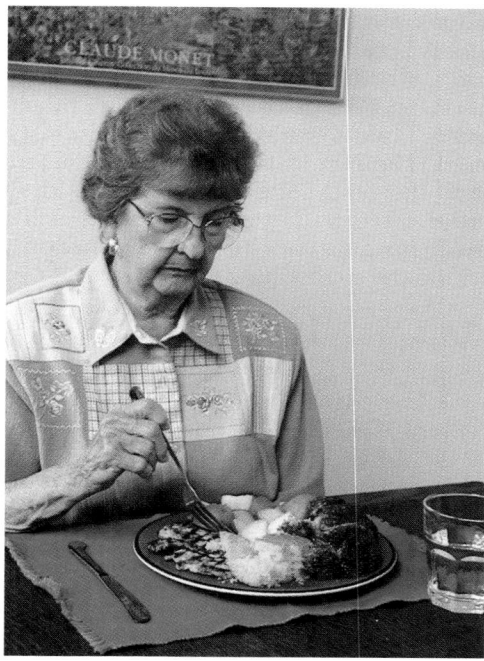

Figure 8–5. General health is affected by nutritional intake. This woman understands the importance of maintaining a well-balanced diet in older adulthood, even though it is difficult on a retiree's fixed income.

You will assess the dietary pattern to ascertain the feasibility of improving the client's general health and in relation to the health problems or potential health problems of obesity, undernourishment, uncontrolled diabetes, or high cholesterol. Metabolism is related to the gastrointestinal system and the endocrine system. Nutrition and metabolism also influence skin by altering the local nutrient supply and wound healing; therefore, the nutritional-metabolic pattern includes examination of the skin and mucous membranes.

Assessment questions for the nutritional-metabolic pattern may include the following:

- Does the client seem well-nourished and well-developed in general appearance?
- Is the client overweight or underweight for the age and height?
- What is the client's usual dietary pattern? Describe typical daily food and fluid intake.
- Does the client adhere to a special diet?
- How does the client's skin look? Are there lesions? Is the skin dry?
- What is the client's body temperature?
- What was the client's recent cholesterol level?
- Does the client have diabetes or a family history of diabetes?
- Does the client have dental problems?

Elimination Pattern

The elimination pattern overlaps with the effects of the nutrition pattern. Nutritional and fluid intake are important determinants of the pattern by which a person eliminates wastes from the body. This pattern includes bowel and bladder habits, the effect of activity on elimination, and the use of laxatives and other aids to elimination. Fluid loss through the skin must also be considered. The elimination pattern is related to the function of the gastrointestinal tract, the kidneys, and the bladder.

Assessment questions for the elimination pattern may include the following:

- What are your usual bowel and bladder habits?
- What is the frequency, consistency, and color of your stool?
- Do you have difficulty with urination?
- Do you experience incontinence?
- How would you describe your use of laxatives or other aids to elimination?
- Do you have a history of bowel or bladder problems?

Activity-Exercise Pattern

The activity-exercise pattern includes the person's ability to be active and the level of activity the person chooses. Energy is expended in exercise, daily routines, leisure, and recreation. The person's ability to engage in activity affects both productivity and the quality of life. The activity-exercise pattern also includes the person's physical capability for self-care, an attribute that also depends on cognitive function, mobility, resources, knowledge, and motivation.

Assessment includes limitations of mobility, type of exercise, duration of exercise, ability to perform activities of daily living, and satisfaction with level of activity. The person's ability to perform activities is related to the musculoskeletal system, the neurological system, the cardiovascular system, and the respiratory system. You may need to assess each of these areas in depth, or you may need only make the observation that the client is or is not capable of adequate self-care.

Assessment questions for the activity-exercise pattern may include the following:

- What are your usual daily activities?
- What is your general level of physical fitness?
- Do you have a history of cardiac or respiratory problems?
- What are your diversional activities?
- Do you need help with home maintenance?
- What is your activity tolerance?
- What is your usual pattern of exercise?
- Do you lead a sedentary lifestyle?
- Are you satisfied with your level of activity?
- Do you smoke? How many packs per day? For how many years?
- Are you able to feed yourself, bathe, go to the toilet, groom yourself, and move about in bed?
- Can you do the shopping and cooking, maintain your home, and achieve general mobility?
- Do you use an assistive device or need help for walking?

Sleep-Rest Pattern

Although the need for sleep and rest varies among individuals, all persons have a need for sleep and rest. Assessment of the sleep-rest pattern includes the usual pattern of sleep and rest, aids to sleep, the person's satisfaction or feeling of being rested, and routines associated with sleep and rest. Problems related to the sleep-rest pattern may form the presenting complaint, or they may be secondary to the chief complaint.

Assessment questions for the sleep-rest pattern may include the following:

- What is your usual pattern of sleep?
- Do you feel rested in the morning?
- Do you use sleep aids?
- Are you able to sleep through the night?
- Do you have trouble falling asleep?

Cognitive-Perceptual Pattern

The cognitive-perceptual pattern includes sensation, perception, and cognition. Sensation is the reception of stimulation through receptors of the nervous system. Sensory functions include vision, hearing, touch, taste, smell, and proprioception (the sense of position). Pain is a sensation and therefore included in this functional pattern. Perception is the ability to receive input from the senses, interpret the information in the brain, and interpret it in a meaningful way. The closely related concept of cognition is the act or process of knowing. Cognitive functions include memory, thoughts, language, and reasoning.

Assessment of the cognitive-perceptual pattern includes neurological assessment and the mental status examination. Additionally, you will assess how a cognitive-perceptual problem alters the client's daily life and how the client compensates for the deficit.

Begin your assessment of the cognitive-perceptual pattern by spending a few minutes getting acquainted and conversing with the client. Listen for cues that the client is hearing and understanding you; is oriented to time, place, and person; and has memory of recent and past events. Evaluate the client's language for unusual speech patterns and reasoning. You may perform this assessment without asking any questions specific to the pattern.

Assessment questions for the cognitive-perceptual pattern may include the following:

- Do you have any difficulty with vision? Do you need glasses for reading or distance vision?
- Do you have any difficulty with hearing? Do you use a hearing aid?
- What is your name? Where do you live? What brought you to the hospital? What day is it?
- How long have you been here?

Self Perception–Self Concept Pattern

The self perception–self concept pattern includes how the person views the self. Self-concept is an attitude, a feeling about self, or an evaluation of self; self-esteem is the affective component of self-concept that describes an attitude, feeling, or evaluation of self-worth. To understand a client's self-concept, you will need information about the person's perception of cognitive, affective, and physical abilities as well as the perception of body image and identity, the general sense of worth, and the general emotional pattern.

When assessing this pattern, you would like to know if the client has mental problems or emotional needs that must be addressed in order to provide the best care. It is particularly important for the home care nurse to recognize depression because this condition has a high potential for interfering with the client's ability to comply with the therapeutic regimen. The hospitalized client is at high risk for anxiety because of the potentially serious nature of problems that require hospitalization. The home care client may have anxiety about managing at home and getting help when it is needed.

You will assess this pattern through active listening rather than by asking specific questions. Listen for negative self talk, lack of confidence, and beliefs about how others regard the client. Also consider body posture, eye contact, voice tone, speech patterns, and general appearance as cues to self-esteem.

Assessment questions for the self perception–self concept pattern may include the following:

- What can you tell me about yourself?
- How will this hospitalization affect your life?
- How would you describe your support systems?
- Who relies on you?
- Where do you go for moral support?
- What do you do to "take care of yourself?"
- How do you feel about being ill? In the hospital?
- Do you have anxiety? How does it affect you?
- Do you have a history of anxiety disorders? Have you used psychotropic drugs? Alcohol? Street drugs?

Role-Relationship Pattern

Roles are the parts played in one's life. Typically, they relate closely to relationships with children, spouse, friends, and coworkers. For example, a person may have the roles of mother, teacher, friend, and colleague. Roles and relationships are the means through which the need for love and belonging is met and self-esteem is developed.

The role-relationship pattern is assessed by examining living arrangements, support systems, and family life. Complaints may include isolation, loneliness, abuse, and marital problems.

Assessment questions for the role-relationship pattern may include the following:

- Who are the members of your household?
- How would you characterize the strength of your marriage?
- Is your family dependent on you? How are they managing during your hospitalization or illness?

- What are the ages of your children? Where do they live?
- Is your family characterized by close family ties?
- When someone is ill, how does your family offer support?
- Do you have trouble sharing your problems and concerns with others?
- Do you have concerns that this illness will affect your ability to perform in your occupation?
- If you are unable to continue in your present occupation, are you in a position to retire?
- Do you have problems with your children that are difficult for you to manage?

Sexuality-Reproductive Pattern

Sexuality is present from birth to the end of a person's life. The expression of sexuality varies among individuals by age, culture, beliefs, health, life circumstances, and social norms. Assessment of the sexuality-reproductive pattern must include the person's satisfaction and perceptions of appropriate sexual and reproductive behavior. Many of the external indicators of sexual patterns may be misleading or lead to stereotypical assumptions that may not be valid.

Generally, the sexuality-reproductive pattern is not assessed specifically unless you have a specific reason to do so. For example, the client may indicate that a potential problem exists or that a potential problem is secondary to the problem for which the client is seeking treatment. Possible indicators include the strength of the client's relationship with a spouse, flirting behavior, an overtly sexy way of dressing, a single parent, children with different fathers, discomfort with persons of the opposite sex, and unmarried adults beyond the usual age for marriage.

Assessment questions for the sexuality-reproduction pattern may include the following:

- How would you characterize your satisfaction with your sexual relationship?
- Would disruption of your sexual relationship with your spouse be a factor in making a decision about having this surgery (taking this medication)?
- What was the date of your last menstrual period?
- At what age did you start menstruation? Are your menstrual periods regular?
- Do you use birth control? What method do you use?
- How many times have you been pregnant? How many live births?

Coping–Stress Tolerance Pattern

Stress is a part of life that results from both positive and negative experiences, from hardships and joys, and from internal and external forces. A person's experience of stress varies with the perception of stress-producing events and the person's skills in managing both the events and the responses to them. During assessment, you would consider the client's evaluation of the current situation and experience with similar situations. How the client managed stressful situations in the past may provide useful information as well.

You may not assess this pattern directly, although hospital nurses commonly ask about previous reactions to hospitalization. In the process of describing the previous experience, the client will often provide cues to how he or she coped with the experience. One client may say, "I don't know how I could have managed without my wife," whereas another may suggest that a warm, friendly relationship with the nurses helped in managing the experience. The home care nurse may get cues from the home environment. A well-ordered, well-planned living environment may suggest that order and planning are a possible coping strategy.

Assessment questions for the coping–stress tolerance pattern may include the following:

- How are you managing (name the current problem or situation)?
- Have you talked to your (significant other) about (the current situation)?
- Have you informed your family and friends of your (current situation)?
- How would you characterize the level of stress in your life over the past year?
- Do you have someone with whom you are comfortable talking about problems or changes in your life?
- Do you use alcohol or other drugs to relieve stress?

Value-Belief Pattern

The value-belief pattern describes the philosophical position that guides a person's choices or decisions in life. The spiritual self is a major component of this pattern. It also reflects what the individual perceives as important to quality of life. Often, values and beliefs are derived from a religious or other formal philosophical base. Family strongly influences the formation of values and beliefs as well. Health care that is consistent with and supportive of the person's value system is most likely to result in positive health outcomes.

Assessment questions for the value-belief pattern may include the following:

- Is your life satisfying? Is your life good?
- What are your plans for the future?
- Do you have a religious affiliation?
- Do you actively practice a religion?
- Is spirituality important in your daily life?
- Will this hospitalization interfere with any religious practices?

Box 8–6 illustrates an example of assessment data for a particular client grouped by functional health patterns.

Documenting the Data

The assessment data that you collect must be documented in the client's medical record to give the entire health care team access to the same information about the client. Thus, the record serves as a means of communication and sharing information for the health care team. The database includes the information contributed by all members of the health care team.

Obviously, it is crucial that data recorded about the client be accurate, complete, and concise. They will be used to make treatment decisions, not just for nursing care, but for medical care, respiratory care, physical therapy, diet therapy, and others. The record should contain all information pertinent to the client's condition. Statements should use the least number of words needed to convey meaning accurately. Often, potential or actual problems identified on an assessment form will need to be described in more detail in your nurse's notes.

Clear documentation differentiates between objective and subjective data. Only factual information should be documented. When the subjective data come from the client, always indicate that the client has stated the information. Carefully consider whether to chart subjective data that stem from your opinions. Almost always, it is better to chart the facts that caused you to develop an opinion rather than the opinion itself. More information on documentation appears in Chapter 14.

KEY PRINCIPLES

- Assessment does not exist in isolation from the other steps of the nursing process; making diagnoses, planning, and establishing outcomes take place simultaneously.
- Critical thinking is a necessary part of assessment to know what questions to ask, what the answers mean, how to follow up, and how to recognize the etiology of the problem.
- The most appropriate format for assessment depends on the purpose and type of the assessment.
- Using multiple sources of data increases the accuracy of the database.
- Prudent health assessment requires that you collect data about sensitive subject matter in a private setting.
- Assessment requires active listening and active mental processing, not merely asking a list of questions.
- During assessment, the client's immediate concerns should occupy your focus of attention.
- Assessment begins with the chief complaint, proceeds to health history, and ends with a physical examination.
- When a symptom is revealed, it should be followed with questions that help the client describe the symptom.
- A systematic method of data collection can help ensure a comprehensive, holistic assessment.
- The collected data are documented in the health record to aid continuity of care and communication with the health care team.

BOX 8–6

DATA ILLUSTRATING FUNCTIONAL HEALTH PATTERNS

A 50-year-old man is admitted to the hospital for abdominal pain. He is being evaluated for a bowel obstruction. Although pain applies specifically to the cognitive/perceptual pattern, it has the potential to affect all other functional patterns as well. Assessing the relationship to other functional patterns might reveal findings such as those listed here.

Pattern	Possible Findings
SELF PERCEPTION–SELF CONCEPT	Client has never been hospitalized and denies that anything could be seriously wrong. "I must have food poisoning. The doctor will probably give me an antibiotic and send me home. One of the guys at work had the same thing." Well-developed muscles emphasized by tight-fitting shirt with rolled-up short sleeves. Attempts to flirt with the nurses.
VALUES-BELIEFS	Lists Christian as religious preference. Wife says she will call the minister if he has to go to surgery, but her husband does not attend church very often.
ROLES-RELATIONSHIPS	States he is angry at his wife because she insisted that he come to the hospital. Is employed as a lineman for the city utility company and is concerned because a recent electrical storm has left a number of power lines down. Has a 30-year-old son who is married and works with his father as a lineman. A 33-year-old daughter is unmarried and lives in another city.
ELIMINATION	Usually has a daily bowel movement after breakfast. Has not had a bowel movement in 5 days. Abdomen hard and distended. Bowel sounds absent. Voids without difficulty. Urine dark and concentrated. Results of abdominal CT scan pending. Father and one uncle died of cancer of colon.
ACTIVITY-EXERCISE	Usually engages in daily weight-lifting but has not exercised since the onset of pain 3 days ago. No history of cardiovascular problems. Has never had cholesterol checked. Vital signs: blood pressure 100/70, pulse 108, respiration 34, temperature 101.2°F. Skin is pale, cool, and clammy. Became dizzy after getting out of bed to go to the bathroom. Hemoglobin and hematocrit levels slightly elevated. Skin turgor sluggish. Eyes sunken. Breath sounds diminished in lung bases.
COGNITIVE-PERCEPTUAL	Complains of severe, diffuse abdominal pain; a 7 on a scale of 1 to 10. Agrees to take pain medication to make his wife happy. Alert and oriented.
NUTRITION-METABOLIC	Has not eaten much for 3 days and nothing for 24 hours. Last meal caused severe nausea followed by vomiting. Appetite is generally good. Often eats in fast-food places for lunch. Coffee, eggs, and toast for breakfast. Wife prepares a balanced meal for supper. No family history of diabetes. Intravenous infusion of D_5W 1/2 NS started in left forearm at 125 mL per hour. Nasogastric tube to low intermittent suction. Serum sodium and potassium levels slightly high.
SEXUALITY-REPRODUCTIVE	Appears to have a close relationship with wife.

BIBLIOGRAPHY

Andrews, M.M., & Boyle, J.S. (Eds). (1995). *Transcultural concepts in nursing care* (2nd ed.). Philadelphia: J.B. Lippincott Co.

Benner, P.A., Tanner, C.A., & Chesla, C.A. (1996). *Expertise in nursing practice: Caring, clinical judgment, and ethics.* New York: Springer Publishing Co.

*Bernstein, L.H. (1992). A public health approach to functional assessment. *Caring, 11*(12), 32–38.

Blewitt, D.K., & Jones, K.R. (1996). Using elements of the nursing minimum data set for determining outcomes. *The Journal of Nursing Service Administration, 26*(6), 48–57.

Coyle, N., Goldstein, M.L., Passik. S., Fishman, B., & Portenoy, R. (1996). Development and validation of a patient needs assessment tool (PNAT) for oncology clinicians. *Cancer Nursing, 19*(2) 81–92.

*Ewing, J.A. (1984). Detecting alcoholism: The CAGE questionnaire. *Journal of the American Medical Association, 252*(14), 1905–1907.

Garrett, M., Schoener, L., & Hood, L. (1996). Teaching strategy to improve verbal communication and critical thinking skills. *Nurse Educator, 21*(4), 37–39.

*Gordon, M. (1997). *Manual of nursing diagnosis 1997–1998.* St. Louis: Mosby–Year Book.

Herrick, C.A., Pearcy, L.G., & Ross, C. (1997). Stigma and ageism: Compounding influences in making an accurate mental health assessment. *Nursing Forum, 32*(3), 21–26.

*Jackson, P.L. (1994). Age-specific well child charting forms. *Nurse Practitioner, 19*(3), 14–18.

Jarvis, C. (2000). *Physical examination and health assessment* (3rd ed.). Philadelphia: W.B. Saunders Co.

Kresevic, D.M., & Mezey, M. (1997). Assessment of function: Critically important to acute care of elders. *Geriatric Nursing, 18*(5), 216–222.

*Maslow, A. (1970). *Motivation and personality* (2nd ed.). New York: Harper & Row.

*Nettis, C., Pavelich, J., Jones, N., Beltz, C., Laboon, P., & Pifer, P. (1993). Family as client: Using Gordon's health pattern typology. *Journal of Community Health Nursing, 10*(1), 53–61.

*Okun, B.F. (1992). *Effective helping: Interviewing and counseling techniques* (4th ed.). Monterey, CA: Brooks/Cole.

Quinn, C. (1997). The nutritional screening initiative: Meeting the nutritional needs of elders. *Orthopaedic Nursing, 16*(5), 13–26.

*Rubinstein, M.F. (1986). *Tools for thinking and problem solving.* Englewood Cliffs, NJ: Prentice-Hall.

Sedlak, C.A., & Ludwick, R. (1996). Dressing up nursing diagnoses: A critical thinking strategy. *Nurse Educator 21*(4) 19–22.

Smith-Battle, L., Drake, M.A., & Diekemper, M. (1997). The responsive use of self in community health nursing practice. *Advances in Nursing Science, 20*(2), 75–89.

* Asterisk indicates a classic or definitive work on this subject.

Assessing the Client: Vital Signs

Judy Sweeney

Key Terms

apical pulse	pulse deficit
auscultatory gap	pulse pressure
basal metabolic rate	systolic blood pressure
bradypnea	tachypnea
diastolic blood pressure	thermogenesis
eupnea	thermolysis
Korotkoff's sounds	vascular resistance

LEARNING OBJECTIVES

After studying this chapter, you should be able to:

1. Safely and accurately measure axillary, oral, rectal, and tympanic temperatures; apical and radial pulses; respirations; and blood pressure.

2. Identify nursing responsibilities related to the assessment of vital signs.

3. Measure vital signs in an organized, accurate manner.

4. Know the normal ranges of each vital sign according to the client's age.

5. Describe the normal physiological features of each vital sign.

6. List factors that influence temperature, pulse, respirations, and blood pressure.

7. Document and report vital sign measurements correctly.

Vital signs are the signs of life; that is, body temperature, pulse, respiration, and blood pressure. Variation in these parameters reflect both physiological and psychological health. Monitoring a person's vital signs is a crucial nursing activity. Your understanding of a client's vital signs will allow you to assess for specific clinical problems and select appropriate nursing interventions. It may also allow you to detect and report the development of life-threatening physical changes.

You may assess clients' vital signs in many settings and locations. You may do so to establish a client's baseline, to detect a change in condition, or to make a nursing diagnosis related to an illness or disease. Some of the many times that you will assess a client's vital signs include the following:

- During any physical examination
- When the client is admitted to a health care facility or hospital unit
- Routinely during the client's stay in a health care facility
- Before and after surgery or an invasive or diagnostic procedure
- Before and after administration of certain medications, especially those known to affect temperature or the cardiovascular or respiratory systems
- When evaluating the effectiveness of a treatment plan
- After specific nursing interventions, such as ambulation
- Any time you suspect the client's condition has changed
- Before discharge from a health care facility

To assess a client's vital signs accurately you should follow methodically and precisely the procedure for assessment. A hurried or careless assessment will offer little data on which to base accurate planning, interventions, and evaluation. Usually, you will assess temperature, then pulse, respirations, and blood pressure. Perform the appropriate procedures to ensure accurate readings and to maintain your safety and that of your client.

INTERPRETING VITAL SIGNS

After measuring a client's vital signs, you will need to make conclusions about the significance of the measurements obtained. You will need to analyze the data and make a nursing diagnosis. This chapter discusses the assessment of each vital sign. However, in practice, the significance of vital signs does not stem from a single value. Rather, the *relationship* of the vital signs to each other and to other assessment findings holds the key to the client's condition. Additionally, the trend of changes in vital signs should guide your conclusions about the client's condition.

First, compare the client's readings with average measurements. Make sure you compare within your client's age group, because normal values may differ for children, adults, and older adults (Table 9–1). For example, 30 respirations per minute are normal for an infant but are abnormally high for an adult.

Next, compare the client's readings with the client's previous readings to consider the trend in the client's vital signs. Have any or all vital signs increased or decreased since the previous measurement? If the previous measurement was recent, is the client's condition changing quickly? If her condition is changing for the worse, how soon will you need to assess her vital signs again to verify the continuing trend? This may be as soon as 5 or 10 minutes. Do you need an emergency plan to prevent serious or fatal consequences?

Next, compare the data you obtained with the client's complete health history and condition. In a client with a history of hypertension, expect a blood pressure that is higher than normal. In a client who just underwent surgery, pain may cause an increased pulse and blood pressure. Perhaps the client is taking a drug that adversely affects her vital signs. Some heart medications, such as digitalis, may slow the heart rate, for example. Others, such as aminophylline, may speed the heart rate. Be sure to review any over-the-counter medications the client may have taken recently. Overall, the goal is to consider whether the client's vital signs coordinate with her history and current clinical

TABLE 9–1
Average Ranges for Vital Signs According to Age Groups

Age Group	Temperature (Oral, in °F)	Pulse per Minute	Respirations per Minute	Blood Pressure (in mm Hg) Systolic	Diastolic
Newborn	N/A	100 to 180 (Mean: 125)	35 to 40	60 to 90	20 to 60
Infant up to age 1	99.4	100 to 160 (Mean: 120)	30 to 60	85 to 105	50 to 65
Toddler ages 1 to 3	99.0 to 99.7	80 to 120 (Mean: 110)	25 to 40	95 to 105	50 to 65
Preschooler ages 3 to 6	98.6	70 to 110 (Mean: 100)	22 to 35	95 to 100	55 to 60
Child ages 6 to 12	98.6	65 to 100 (Mean: 90)	20 to 30	100 to 110	60 to 70
Adolescent ages 12 to 18	97.8 to 98.6	60 to 90 (Mean: 80)	16 to 20	110 to 120	60 to 65
			12 to 16	110 to 130	65 to 80
Adult	98.6 ± 1	60 to 100 (Mean: 75)	12 to 20	110 to 140	60 to 90
Elderly	97.6 ± 1	60 to 100 (Mean: 75)	12 to 20	120 to 140	70 to 90

status. If not, measure her vital signs again to make sure your readings are correct. If changes in the client's vital signs stem from a medication, consult the physician who may change the dose of the medication.

Additionally consider the effects of the environment, level of activity, and mental status on your results. Is the room hot or cold? Does the client appear anxious, angry, or stressed? Has the client been exercising? Is the client a child who is upset and crying?

Action Alert!
For a client who seems nervous, reassess blood pressure and pulse after the client has sat quietly for 10 to 15 minutes.

Your interpretation of vital signs is used to make decisions about the frequency of your assessment. Although a physician's order or facility policy typically specifies the minimum frequency at which vital signs should be measured, you are responsible for assessing vital signs any time a need arises. If a client's vital signs change, you may need to assess them more frequently than the order requires. For example, if the client's temperature rises above 100°F, you should take the temperature again in 60 minutes, even though the physician may have ordered temperature assessment every 4 hours.

Action Alert!
Increase the frequency of vital sign assessment if the client is at risk for a complication or a change in condition. Frequent assessment is indicated for fever, infection, recent surgery, chest pain, or shortness of breath.

COMMUNICATING ABOUT VITAL SIGNS

Whether your client's vital signs are normal or abnormal, you are responsible for communicating your findings to other health care providers. In most cases, you will do so by documenting the vital signs in the client's medical record. Figure 9–1 shows a typical graphic record for recording vital signs.

Action Alert!
Verbally report significantly abnormal vital signs or changes to the physician. Prepare to institute new orders for the client reflecting the change in condition.

You may also be responsible for communicating directly to clients and their families about vital signs and how to measure them. Many clients must track vital signs as part of their ongoing health maintenance. For example, a client who takes an antihypertensive medication may need to routinely measure his blood pressure. Be prepared to provide health teaching about vital signs.

TEMPERATURE

Body temperature reflects the balance between heat produced in the body and heat lost from the body. **Thermogenesis** is the generation of heat from the

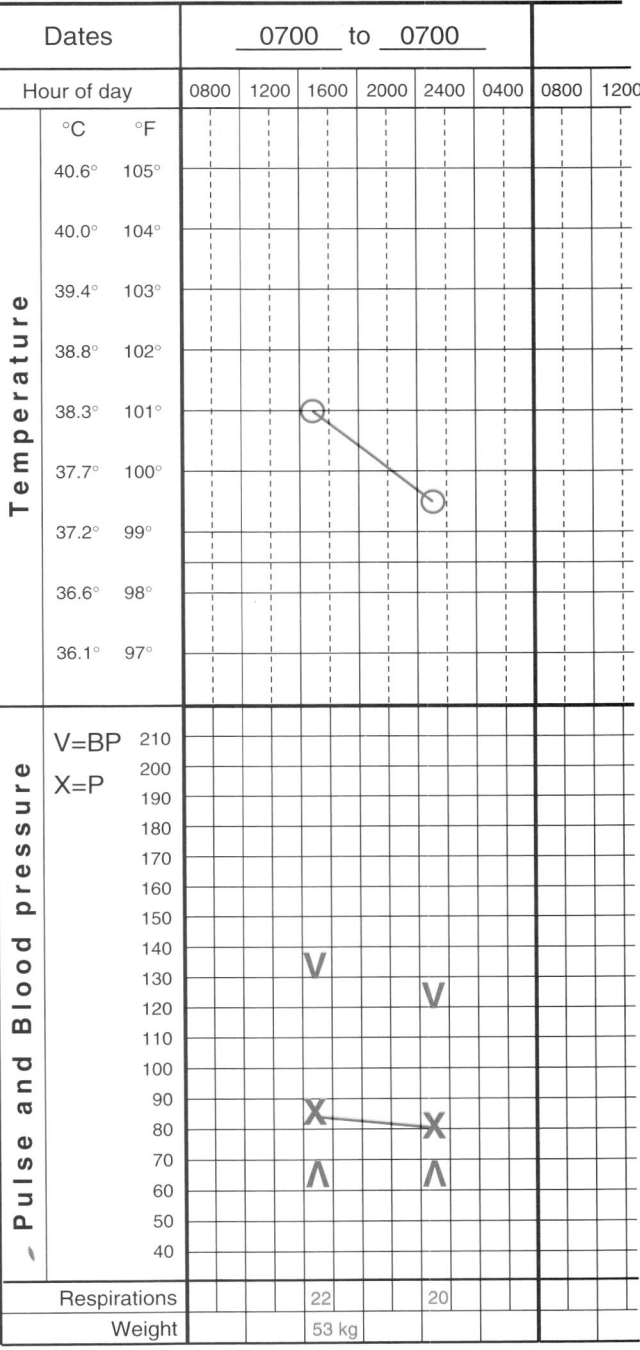

Figure 9–1. An example of how to chart vital signs.

chemical reactions that take place in cellular activity. Heat production is, in part, dependent on the **basal metabolic rate,** or the amount of energy needed to maintain essential basic body functions, expressed as calories per hour per square meter of body surface. It increases with muscular activity, stimulation of the sympathetic nervous system (which produces epinephrine and norepinephrine), and stimulation of the thyroid gland (which produces thyroxine). Heat is dispersed from the body through radiation, conduction, convection, and evaporation, a process called **thermolysis** (see Chapter 33).

Understanding Thermoregulation

Normally, the body balances heat production and heat loss to maintain a temperature between 96.8°F and 99.4°F (36°C to 37.4°C). This process is called thermoregulation. A number of factors can alter a person's temperature. For example, activity alters temperature in a circadian rhythm. For most people, temperature is lowest in the morning because the basal metabolic rate slows during the inactivity of sleep. In the afternoon, the increased activity of the day may raise the temperature by about 1°F. Stress, strong emotions, and exercise can increase cellular activity and thus also raise temperature.

Other factors can alter temperature as well. For example, estrogen causes women to have a slightly higher average temperature than men. Newborns, children, and older adults have a reduced capacity for thermoregulation. A cold environment speeds up heat loss, and a warm environment slows heat loss. Internally, infection and inflammation can raise body temperature through their pyogenic influence on the medulla of the brain.

In response to these many temperature-altering influences, the body can activate a number of psychological (behavioral) and physiological compensatory mechanisms. For example, a behavioral compensatory mechanism is the person's voluntary control over environmental temperature and its effects. If a person is cold, he can adjust the thermostat or put on a sweater.

Physiological compensatory mechanisms are involuntary and intended to help maintain a normal core temperature in the body. The autonomic nervous system helps to keep the core body temperature at 98.6°F (37°C) through receptors in the skin, abdomen, and spinal cord. These receptors sense internal and external temperature changes and send this information through the nervous system to the hypothalamic region of the brain. The data are integrated, and the appropriate effector mechanisms (such as blood vessels, sweat glands, and skeletal muscles) are activated.

The cardiovascular system plays an important role in maintaining body temperature through its vast network of blood vessels. An increase in body temperature causes blood vessels near the skin surface to dilate, a process called vasodilation. By bringing an increased volume of warmed blood to the skin surface, vasodilation enhances heat loss. In contrast, a decrease in body temperature causes vasoconstriction that keeps warmed blood closer to the center of the body, thus maintaining its core temperature. By insulating the body, fat helps to control heat loss as well.

Keep in mind that the body's cells function within a relatively narrow range of normal temperatures (Fig. 9–2). Often, the cells can tolerate extreme temperature for a short time and may even benefit from it. For example, the increased heat of a fever is thought to benefit the immune system and increase its activity. How-

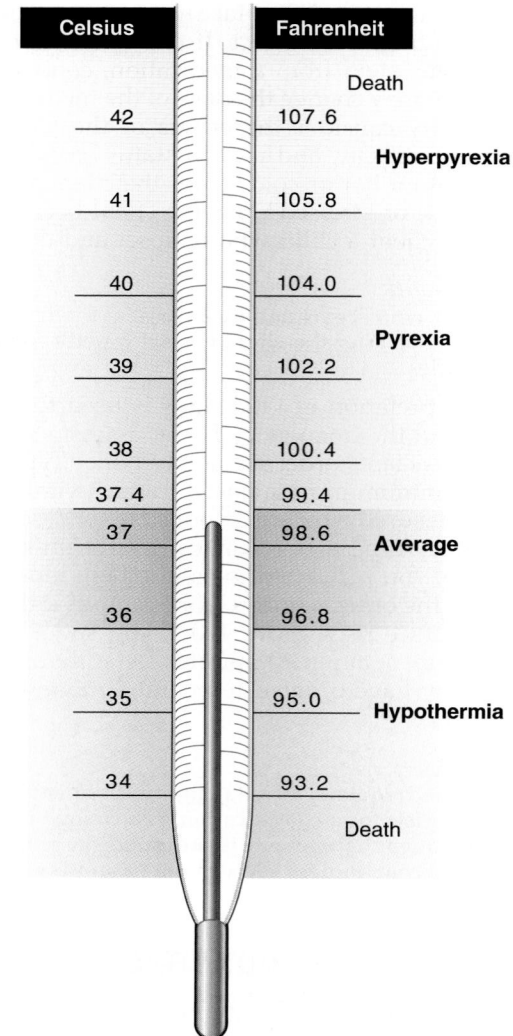

Figure 9–2. Range of normal body temperature and alterations in body temperature on the Celsius and Fahrenheit scales.

ever, prolonged temperature elevation (hyperthermia) or reduction (hypothermia) can lead to tissue damage and death. High temperatures damage cells by inactivating proteins and enzymes. Low temperatures damage cells when ice crystals form and puncture the cell membranes.

Naturally, if a client cannot alter his temperature, is unconscious, or is unaware of the environment, you may need to intervene and help the client with temperature regulation. Even for a client who can regulate temperature normally, your assessment of temperature offers vital information about his condition.

Measuring Temperature

As you know, temperature can be measured using either the Fahrenheit or the Celsius (also called Centigrade) scale (see Fig. 9–2). Any reading can be converted from one scale to another by completing a simple calculation (Box 9–1). Depending on your cli-

BOX 9–1

CONVERSION FORMULAS FOR FAHRENHEIT AND CELSIUS TEMPERATURES

Converting from Fahrenheit to Celsius:

- Subtract 32 from the Fahrenheit reading
- Multiply the resulting number by 5/9

For example, the following formula shows the conversion of 98.6°F to Celsius:

$$98.6 - 32 = 66.6 \times 5/9 = 37°C$$

Converting from Celsius to Fahrenheit:

- Multiply the Celsius reading by 9/5 (1.8)
- Add 32 to the resulting number

For example, the following formula shows the conversion of 37°C to Fahrenheit:

$$37 \times 9/5 = 66.6 + 32 = 98.6°F$$

ent's needs, you may use a standard glass thermometer, an electronic thermometer, a tympanic thermometer, chemical dots, or an intravenous catheter to measure temperature.

Glass Thermometer

This device is a hollow glass cylinder. At its base is a bulb filled with mercury. When the mercury is heated, it expands, forcing a column of mercury to rise in the hollow tube. The height to which it rises on a calibrated column reveals the client's temperature.

Figure 9–3A shows oral and rectal thermometers. The rectal thermometer is the same as the oral thermometer except that it is color coded red to alert you not to take oral temperatures with a thermometer that has been used to take rectal temperatures. The tip is blunt to avoid trauma to delicate membranes.

Glass thermometers are inexpensive, easy to use, easily disinfected, and can be used multiple times for the same client. The main disadvantage is that the glass can break and release mercury, a poisonous substance. Also, this type of thermometer cannot be shared between clients. It can also be difficult to read the small calibrations. The readings are recorded to the nearest 0.2°F.

Electronic Thermometer

This device has a heat-sensitive probe attached by a thin wire to a battery-powered control unit (Fig. 9–3B). It offers a convenient, safe, accurate, and fast method for measuring temperature. The reading is quickly displayed on the unit and is easy to read. Typically, the unit beeps when the measurement is complete. Readings can be measured to the nearest 0.1°F.

An electronic thermometer can be used for oral, axillary, or rectal temperature measurements and with multiple clients. The use of disposable probe covers (also called sheaths) avoids the transmission of microorganisms between clients. For visually impaired clients, electronic thermometers are available that give auditory temperature readings. The disadvantage of electronic thermometers is their cost and required maintenance.

Tympanic Thermometer

Another safe and accurate device for temperature measurement is the tympanic probe. A heat-sensitive probe is placed into the ear canal to measure the temperature of blood in the tympanic membrane (Fig. 9–3C). Readily visible measurements are displayed on the unit and reflect temperature to the nearest 0.1°F. The unit can be used for multiple clients. Disposable probe covers avoid the transmission of microorganisms between clients.

The disadvantage of tympanic thermometers is that they are fragile and can be costly. To retain its accuracy and reliability, the thermometer must be maintained according to the manufacturer's guidelines.

Temperature Strip and Chemical Dot

A temperature strip or chemical dot is typically used for a client in an isolation unit or for home measurement of temperature (Fig. 9–3D). As the client's temperature rises or falls, the strip or dot changes color.

These devices are inexpensive and usually disposable. The disadvantage is that they provide less accurate readings, and they may vary widely. In addition, sweating can alter the contact between the device and the client's skin, a change that also may alter the temperature reading.

Intravenous Catheter

A central intravenous catheter can be used to measure core temperature: the temperature of blood flowing through the heart. It uses a thermistor attached to the central line. It is the most accurate and reliable method for measuring core temperature, but it is used only for clients in intensive care units because of the potential complications of infection and air emboli.

Routes for Measuring Temperature

Usually, you will obtain a client's temperature reading by the oral, rectal, axillary, or tympanic route (Procedure 9–1). Placement of the thermometer (glass or electronic) under the tongue is the most common, convenient, and accepted method for temperature measurement in adults. The client must be able to follow directions and breathe through her nose. Nasal oxygen cannulae and nasogastric tubes do not seem to affect the reading adversely.

If the client has just eaten, ingested fluids, or smoked a cigarette, wait 15 to 30 minutes before ob-

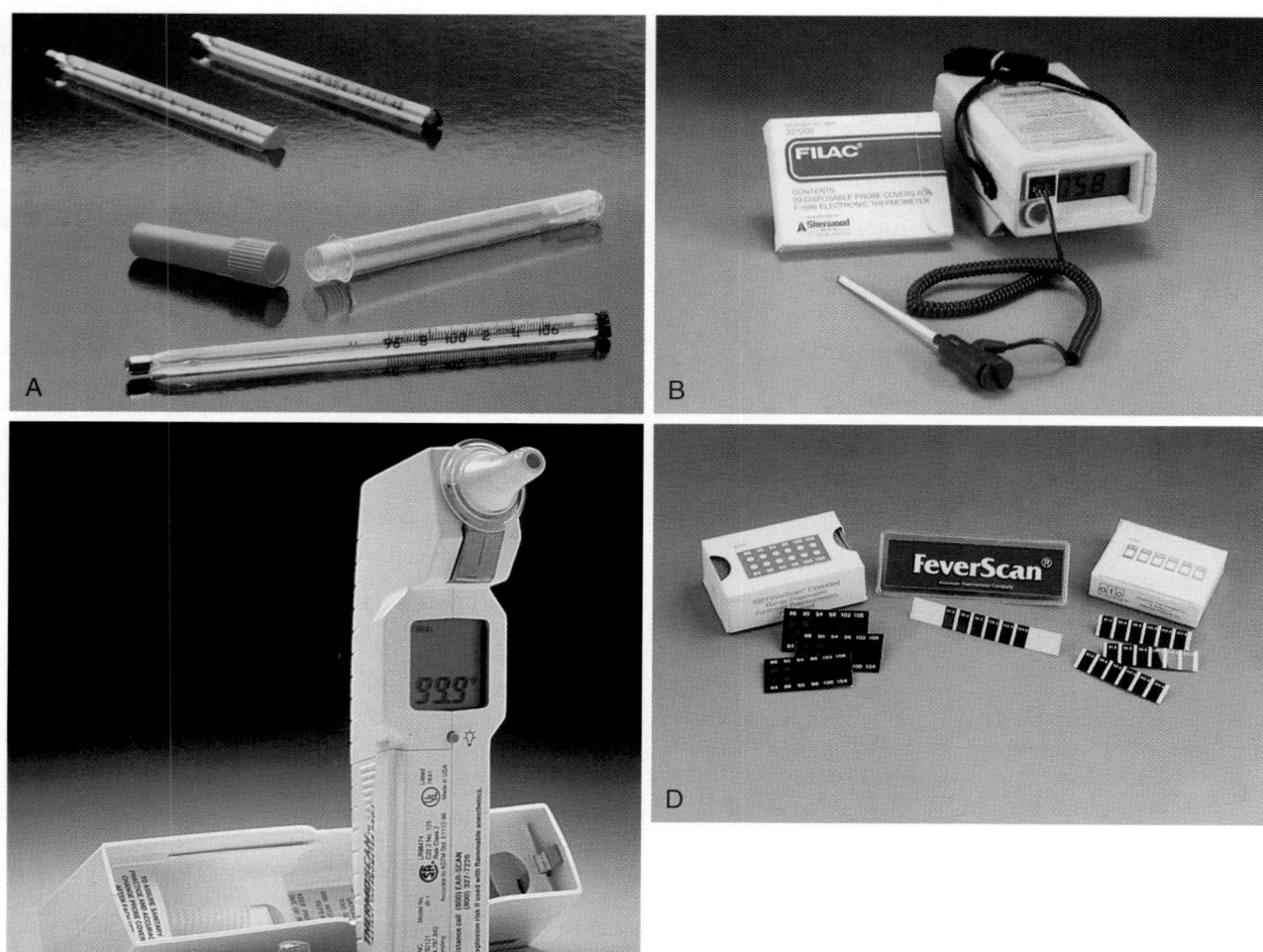

Figure 9–3. Types of thermometers. A, Glass thermometers; B, electronic thermometer; C, tympanic thermometer; D, disposable temperature strips. (A, Courtesy of American Diagnostic Corporation, Smithtown, NY; B through D, Courtesy of Medline Industries, Mundelein, IL.)

taining the temperature reading. Avoid using this method for any client who could be injured by the thermometer, who cannot close her mouth to breathe, or who cannot follow simple instructions.

The rectal route is used for infants and for small children who cannot hold a thermometer safely in their mouths. It is also used for adults who are unconscious or confused, have respiratory difficulty, or have had recent oral surgery. The rectal route is contraindicated for clients who have had rectal or perineal surgery or injury and clients who have severe hemorrhoids. It is also not used with cardiac clients because the thermometer can stimulate the vagus nerve, slowing the heart rate.

The axillary route can be used for all clients, including newborns. However, it offers less accurate readings because it measures only surface body heat. It is contraindicated if the client is uncooperative or combative.

The use of the ear canal and tympanic membrane is fast, safe, easy, and noninvasive. A tympanic ther-

mometer can be used for children and adults. It is considered very reliable and accurate. However, it is contraindicated for clients who have had a recent ear infection or ear surgery.

After obtaining a client's temperature by any route, document your reading in the client's medical record. Temperature is usually charted on a graph. Each temperature is connected to the previous one with a line to show trends over time (see Fig. 9–1). Rectal and axillary temperatures are charted with the designations R and Ax, respectively. Chart other information about the client's temperature on your nurse's notes or a progress report.

PULSE

Each time the heart muscle contracts (systole), a bolus of blood is forced into the arterial system. That movement creates a pulse wave that starts at the heart and travels throughout the arterial system. By placing your fingers over an artery, particularly at a location where

PROCEDURE 9–1

Assessing Temperature

TIME TO
ALLOW
▼
Novice:
2 min.
Expert:
2 min.

A person's temperature reflects the balance between heat produced in the body and heat lost from the body. Because a number of disorders and medications can upset this balance, measuring a person's temperature can give you important information about his health.

Delegation Guidelines

The measurement and recording of body temperature is a simple, low-risk procedure that you may delegate to a nursing assistant. Be sure to indicate the route by which the temperature is to be taken. You remain responsible for your knowledge of the temperature measurement and your assessment of changes in the client's temperature.

Equipment Needed

- Thermometer (oral, rectal, electronic, tympanic)
- Water-soluble lubricant
- Disposable probe covers
- Clean gloves and tissues
- Watch with sweep second hand

---

1 Select an appropriate route, and obtain a corresponding thermometer.

You may use the oral, rectal, axillary, or tympanic route. Choose the route that is safest and most convenient for the client. For consistency of results, use the same route for succeeding temperature measurements.

2 Prepare the thermometer.

Glass Thermometer

a. Ensure that the thermometer is clean and free of defects. Follow agency policy for storage and cleaning. A common practice is to provide each client with an individual thermometer. The thermometer is cleansed with an alcohol wipe between uses, wiping from the bulb to the stem using a rotating motion. Any disinfection should be thoroughly rinsed away in cool water before use.

Hot water will expand the mercury and can break the glass. Consider covering the thermometer with a disposable sheath to protect both you and the client. The thermometer is covered with a clean sheath for each use. A well-designed sheath inverts on itself as it is removed, thus preventing you from contact with oral mucus. The sheath helps contain the glass and mercury if the thermometer breaks.

b. Ensure that the mercury is confined to the bulb (registers ≤96°F/35.6°C). Hold the thermometer firmly by the tip. Using a flicking wrist motion, shake the thermometer. This action forces the mercury into the bulb. Check the reading on the thermometer to ensure that it is below body temperature.

Hold the thermometer with the numbers positioned to be read from left to right. Slightly rotate the thermom-

eter toward yourself until the column of mercury is visible. Most thermometes have a white or yellow background to increase visibility of the mercury. You should be viewing the background against the mercury.

Electronic/Tympanic Thermometer

a. If using an electronic thermometer (see Fig. 9–3B), turn on the device by removing the probe. If using a tympanic thermometer, turn on the unit (see Fig. 9–3C).

b. Place a disposable sheath or cover over the probe.

A probe cover prevents transmission of microorganisms between clients.

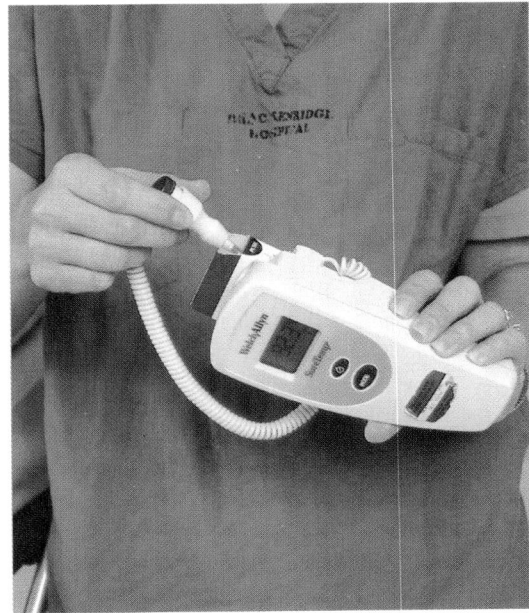

Placing a disposable sheath, or cover, on the probe.

Continued

PROCEDURE 9–1 *(continued)*

Assessing Temperature

3 Measuring temperature.

Oral route: place the glass thermometer under the client's tongue sublingual pocket next to the frenulum for 2 to 4 minutes or according to your facility's policy. Leave the electronic probe in place until the unit beeps.

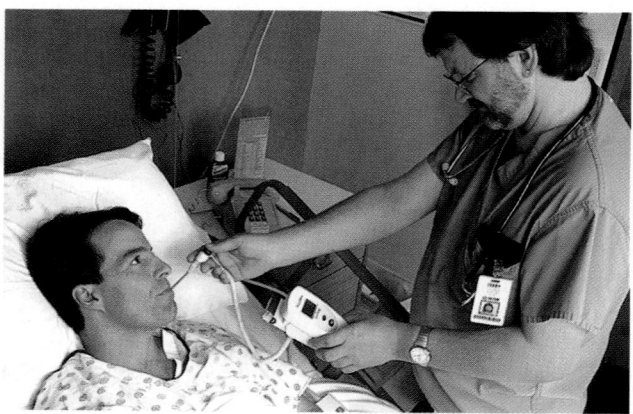

Holding the probe in place for oral temperature assessment.

Have the client close his mouth and hold the thermometer in place with his lips. Make sure the bulb remains in direct contact with the sublingual tissue. Warn the client not to bite on the thermometer, especially a glass one, because the glass could break and allow mercury to enter the client's mouth.

Rectal route: lubricate the thermometer, and position the client in the sidelying position.

a. Put on clean gloves.

   Rectal temperature has a higher risk of contact with fluid from mucous membranes.

b. Lubricate the bulb of the thermometer with water-soluble jelly.

   Lubrication prevents rectal trauma.

c. Place the client in left Sims' position, and drape him for privacy.

   Left Sims' position allows easy access to the client's anus. Appropriate draping helps to minimize the client's discomfort.

d. Gently insert the thermometer about 1.5 inches into the rectum.

   Angle the thermometer toward the client's umbilicus during insertion.

e. Hold the thermometer in place for 2 to 4 minutes or according to your facility's policy.

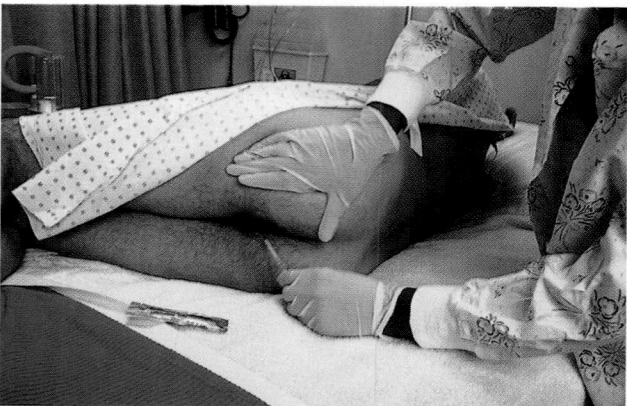

Holding the probe in place for rectal temperature assessment.

Axillary route: place the thermometer in the center of the client's axilla, and leave it in place for 8 to 10 minutes or according to your facility's policy.

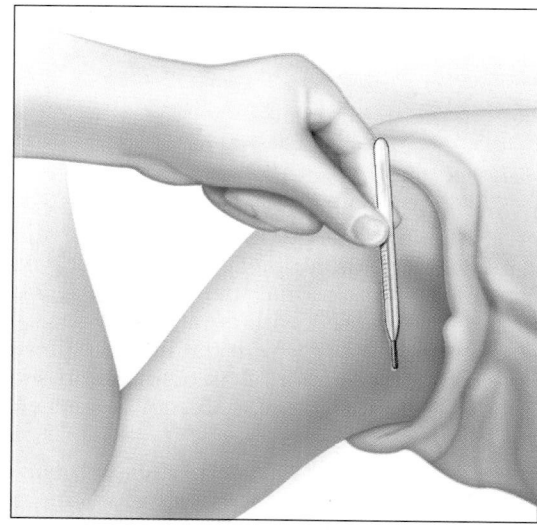

Placing the probe for axillary temperature assessment.

To secure the thermometer and make sure the bulb of the thermometer remains in contact with the axillary skin, have the client cross his arm across his chest.

Tympanic route: pull the client's auricle back, and then gently obtain the temperature measurement.

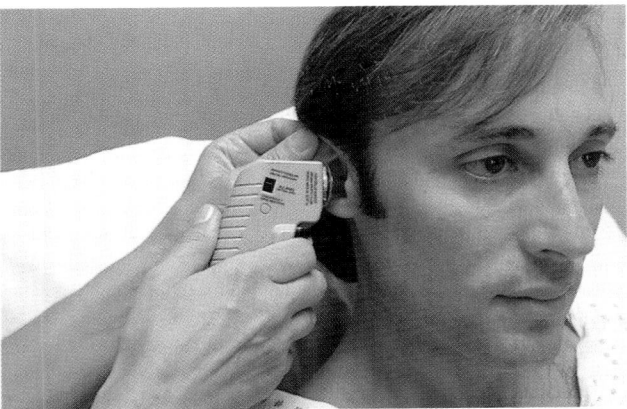

Inserting the tympanic probe into the ear canal.

For a child, pull the auricle down and back. For an adult, pull the auricle up and back. Doing so will straighten the ear canal and help to direct the probe toward the tympanic membrane.

a. Place the probe into the ear canal, pointing the tip of the probe toward the client's nose.

   The probe must be directed on the tympanic membrane. Errors in measurement occur when it is directed toward the wall of the ear canal.

b. Holding the probe steady, quickly press the activation button.

c. A buzzer will sound when the temperature has been measured.

   A tympanic reading usually takes only 2 or 3 seconds.

4 Read the temperature measurement.

a. After an appropriate time or after the electronic thermometer beeps, remove the thermometer from the client's mouth, axilla, ear canal, or anus.

b. After removing a glass rectal thermometer, wipe it with a tissue, using a rotating motion from stem to bulb. Discard the tissue, or remove the disposable sheath.

   This pattern moves from clean to contaminated areas of the thermometer and prevents transmission of microorganisms.

c. Read the temperature measurement indicated on the thermometer. If using an electronic thermometer, obtain the measurement, and then discard the probe cover directly into the trash by pressing the release button.

   This prevents transmission of microorganisms.

5 Document the client's temperature in his medical record as soon as you obtain the reading.

Note whether the reading was oral, rectal, or axillary by writing oral, R, or Ax next to the measurement.

6 Report an abnormal temperature to a charge nurse or physician.

A normal oral temperature is 98.6°F (37°C), a normal rectal temperature is 99.6°F (37.5°C), and a normal axillary temperature is 97.6°F (36.5°C).

TABLE 9–2
Pulse Patterns

Pattern	Description
Pulsus paradoxus	A regular rhythm of an increase, then decrease, in the pulse *amplitude* associated with respirations (may also be heard on the blood pressure measurement). May be a sign of a serious cardiac or respiratory condition.
Pulsus alternans	A regular rhythm with a pattern of a strong normal pulse followed by a weak pulse. (Every other beat is strong). One of a group of signs that indicate a failing heart.
Pulse bigeminy	Cardiac arrhythmia results in an irregular rhythm with a pattern of a strong normal pulse (beat originating in the sinus node) followed quickly by an early, weak pulse (beat originating elsewhere in the heart). May progress to ventricular fibrillation and death.
Sinus rhythm	The electrical impulse is generated in the normal pacemaker (sinus node). Usually a regular rhythm with a rate between 60 and 100 beats per minute for an adult.
Tachycardia	Regular rhythm with a rate higher than 90 to 100 beats per minute for an adult. Decreases cardiac output by decreasing ventricular filling time. If prolonged, may lead to shock.
Bradycardia	Regular rhythm with a rate less than 50 to 60 beats per minute for an adult. Rate is insufficient to meet the demands for oxygen. May lead to cardiac standstill.
Sinus arrhythmia	Slightly irregular rhythm that speeds up and slows down with respirations. Originates in the sinus node. Does not usually affect cardiac output or vital signs.

it crosses a bone, you can feel the pulse waves created by myocardial contractions. Thus, the pulse is a rhythmic fluctuation of fluid pressure against the arterial wall created by the pumping action of the heart muscle. Between contractions, the heart muscle rests (diastole), and the pulse wave disappears.

Understanding Pulse Characteristics

The characteristics of the pulse are rate, rhythm, and strength. Examining these characteristics gives you information about the function of the heart, the volume of blood in the vascular system, and the patency and resiliency of blood vessels. A number of abnormal pulse patterns may develop, based on changes in the client's heart rate, rhythm, and strength (Table 9–2).

Rate

Because pulse waves stem directly from the heart's contractions, a client's pulse offers direct information about the action of his heart. A normal rate is generally considered to be 60 to 90 beats per minute, although the range of normal may extend from 50 to 100. The heart rate is controlled primarily by the autonomic nervous system. The sympathetic nervous system increases the heart rate, and the parasympathetic system decreases the heart rate. Both of these changes stem largely from the body's response to the cells' need for oxygen.

TABLE 9–3
Factors That Influence Pulse

Factor	Influence
Age	Infants and children have a slightly higher heart rate than adolescents and adults. As the client ages, the pulse rate gradually decreases.
Emotions and stress	Anxiety, fear, anger, and pain stimulate the sympathetic nervous system and cause the pulse rate to increase. Relaxation stimulates the parasympathetic nervous system and decreases the rate.
Exercise	Exercise increases the oxygen demand, and the rate increases. A conditioned athlete can have a slow but effective resting heart rate.
Rest and sleep	During rest and sleep, oxygen needs decline, and the rate decreases.
Temperature	Hyperthermia and fever increase the heart rate. Hypothermia decreases the heart rate.
Dehydration, shock, and hemorrhage	Decreases in blood volume or cardiac output result in an increased pulse rate because of sympathetic stimulation.
Hypoxia and hypoxemia	When oxygen levels in the blood decrease, the heart rate increases in an attempt to compensate.
Vomiting	Vomiting stimulates the vagus nerve and causes the pulse rate to drop.
Head injury and increased intracranial pressure	Head injuries cause the pulse to decrease.
Electrolyte balance	Changes in potassium and calcium affect the pulse rate and rhythm.
Medications	Certain medications cause the heart rate to increase, such as adrenalin and atropine, and others decrease the pulse, such as digitalis.

Any psychological stressor (producing anxiety, fear, or anger) or physiological stressor (such as exercise or a loss of blood) causes the body's compensatory mechanisms to launch a "fight-or-flight" response. Information is relayed to the cardiac center in the medulla, and the sympathetic nervous system is stimulated. These changes are reflected by changes in the client's pulse.

Other factors can influence the pulse rate as well (Table 9–3). For example, infants and children have a higher basal metabolic rate and, thus, a slightly higher pulse rate than adults. Some medications (such as digitalis) slow the heart rate, and others (such as amphetamines) increase the rate. Low blood pressure, dehydration, fever, and pain can each stimulate the sympathetic nervous system. In contrast, rest and relaxation can stimulate the parasympathetic nervous system.

Rhythm

Normally, the heart beat is initiated in the sinus node in the atrium and produces a regular rhythm. However, chemical disturbances, such as inadequate oxygen in the heart muscle and electrolyte imbalance, may cause the heart to beat irregularly. Some children have a normal disrhythmia in which the heart rate increases with inhalation and decreases with exhalation. Even so, all irregular pulse rhythms should be reported to a physician.

Strength

The quality of the pulse reflects the strength of the cardiac contraction and the volume of blood available in the vascular system. A normal contraction of the heart muscle combined with an adequate blood volume will create a strong pulse wave. A weak heart contraction combined with a low blood volume will create a small, weak, thready pulse wave. An increased heart contraction combined with a large blood volume will create a large, bounding pulse wave.

A number of conditions can alter the strength of a client's pulse. For example, heart failure can cause the strength of the heart's contraction to vary on alternating beats while the rhythm remains regular, a condition called pulsus alternans.

You also may detect an abnormality (in adults) in which the strength of the client's pulse wave increases during inhalation and decreases back to normal during exhalation, a condition called pulsus paradoxus. This can also be heard when measuring blood pressure. Finally, the nervous system can alter the strength of the client's pulse. Stimulation of the sympathetic nervous system increases the force of myocardial contraction, increasing the amount of blood ejected from the heart with each beat (stroke volume) and creating a large pulse. Stimulation of the parasympathetic nervous system decreases the force of contraction, thus decreasing stroke volume and creating a small pulse.

Measuring Pulse

It is essential that you maintain a high degree of accuracy when assessing a client's pulse. Crucial clinical decisions, such as the administration of oxygen and medications, are based on pulse values. To facilitate accurate pulse measurement, you should compress the client's artery with the pads of your two middle fingers. Press firmly without occluding the artery. If you use your thumb or index finger, you will sometimes feel your own pulse rather than the client's (Procedure 9–2).

Peripheral Pulses

Peripheral pulse sites are located where arteries lie over bony surfaces. Eight sites are available to assess peripheral pulses: the carotid artery in the neck; the brachial, radial, and ulnar arteries in the arms; and the femoral, popliteal, dorsalis pedis, and posterior tibial arteries in the legs (Fig. 9–4).

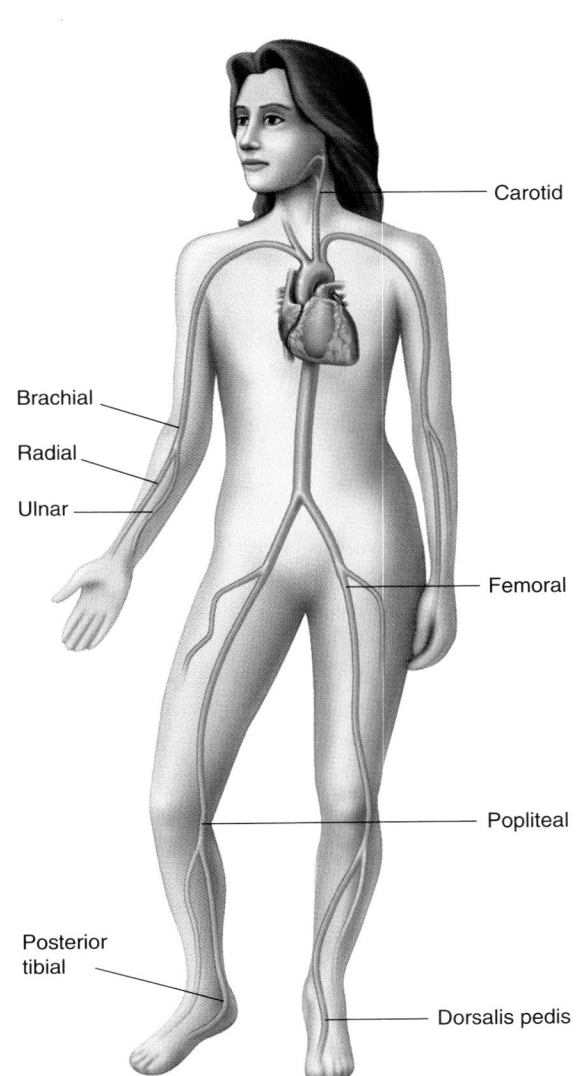

Figure 9–4. The eight sites commonly used to assess peripheral pulses.

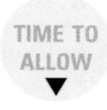

Assessing Radial and Apical Pulses

TIME TO
ALLOW
▼
Novice:
1 min.
Expert:
1 min.

A person's pulse reflects the function of his heart and the condition of his arterial system. Usually, you will measure a client's radial pulse in his wrist. In some cases, however, you will need to measure his apical pulse instead of or in addition to his radial pulse.

Delegation Guidelines

The measurement and recording of the radial and apical pulse rate is a simple procedure that you may delegate to a nursing assistant who has received training in this technique. Training should include specific instructions on findings that necessitate your immediate notification. You *remain responsible for knowledge of the pulse measurement and your assessment of a client with any reported irregularities.*

Equipment Needed

- Stethoscope
- Watch with sweep second hand

---

1 Prepare the client for pulse measurement.
a. Place the client in a comfortable position.
b. Have the client relax.

If the client is not relaxed, wait 10 or 15 minutes before obtaining the pulse reading. This will enhance the accuracy of your reading by preventing false elevations caused by stress or anxiety.

Radial Pulse Measurement

2 Place the client's arm across his abdomen.

3 Locate the client's radial pulse.
a. Place the pads of your middle fingers on the inside of the client's wrist.

Do not use your thumb or first finger to palpate the pulse because they each have a pulse of their own.

b. Compress the radial artery firmly against the underlying bone.

c. Occlude the pulse, and then gradually release pressure until the pulse becomes palpable.

Occluding and then restoring the pulse verifies its presence.

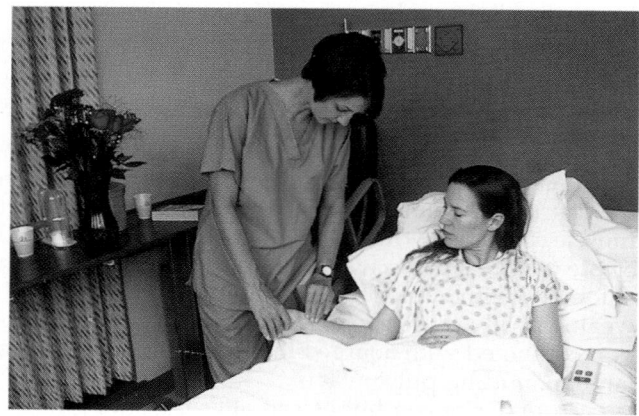

Locating the radial pulse.

The most common site for assessing the pulse is the radial artery. Other frequently used sites are the carotid, femoral, and cardiac apex. The radial artery, on the inner surface of the wrist on the thumb side, is accessible and easily palpated.

Other pulses have specific uses. The brachial artery, located in the antecubital fossa of the inner aspect of the elbow, is used for blood pressure assessment. The popliteal artery, located behind the knee, can also be used for blood pressure assessment. In an emergency or during cardiopulmonary resuscitation

(CPR), you may assess the client's heart rate, using the carotid pulse in an adult or the brachial pulse in an infant. The dorsalis pedis and posterior tibial arteries are used to assess the status of the peripheral vascular system.

No matter how you measure a client's pulse, always document your findings immediately in the client's medical record (see Fig. 9–1). If you obtained an apical pulse, note it with an A. Place other information about the client's pulse in your nurse's notes or a progress report.

4 Assess the quality of the client's radial pulse.
a. Palpate to determine the rhythm and strength (amplitude) of the client's pulse.
b. If the radial pulse is irregular or weak, you will need to assess the client's apical pulse.

5 Count the client's pulse.
If the radial pulse is regular and of normal strength, count the number of beats for 30 seconds, and then double the result to obtain the client's pulse per minute. If it is irregular, count for a full minute.

Apical Pulse Measurement

6 To assess apical pulse, place the client in the supine position, turned slightly onto the left side. Alternatively, have the client sit up and lean forward slightly.
A left-lying position or forward-leaning position enhances transmission of heart sounds through the chest wall.

7 Locate the apical pulse.
a. Keep the client covered appropriately, exposing the chest only as needed.
b. Locate the apical pulse at the fifth intercostal space to the left of the midclavicular line on the client's anterior thorax.
c. If necessary, lift a female client's breast to find her apical pulse.
Finding the correct anatomic location of the apex increases the accuracy of apical pulse measurement.
d. Place the diaphragm of your stethoscope firmly against the client's chest. Avoid rubbing against clothing or linen.
The diaphragm is used for high-pitched sounds, such as heart tones. Firm skin contact enhances sound transmission. Clothing may cause interfering noises.

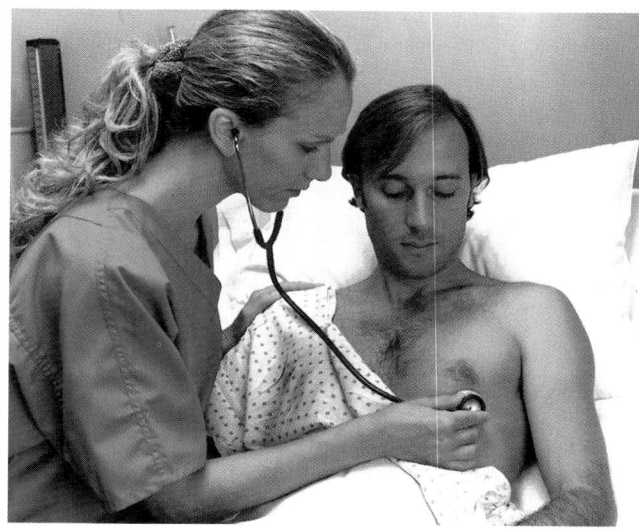
Locating the apical pulse.

8 Assess the rhythm of the client's apical pulse.
The apical pulse is the most likely to reveal irregularities of heart rhythm.

9 Count the apical pulse for 1 full minute.
This will increase the accuracy of your reading.

10 Document the client's pulse in his medical record as soon as you obtain the reading. Note any abnormality of rhythm or strength.
A normal pulse is 60 to 100 beats per minute and regular.

11 Report an abnormal pulse to a charge nurse or physician.

Apical Pulse

The **apical pulse** is the heart rate counted at the apex of the heart on the anterior chest. If a client has weak or ineffective heart contractions, cardiac disease, an irregular heart rhythm, or a history of taking cardiac medications that affect the heart's action, you may not be able to palpate all beats at the radial pulse location. For these clients, apical pulse measurement provides a more accurate means of assessment. The apical pulse is preferred for infants and children because it can be difficult to palpate their peripheral pulses. Of course,

you may choose to perform an apical pulse measurement instead of a radial pulse measurement on any client for whom you think it would be helpful.

To take an apical pulse you will need a stethoscope. A stethoscope consists of ear pieces connected to two stiff tubes that join with a single flexible tube that ends in a sound-transmitting device that has a diaphragm on one side and a bell on the other (Fig. 9–5). Place the ear pieces into your ear canals with the ends pointing slightly toward your nose, not the back of your head. Use the bell to assess low-frequency sounds and the

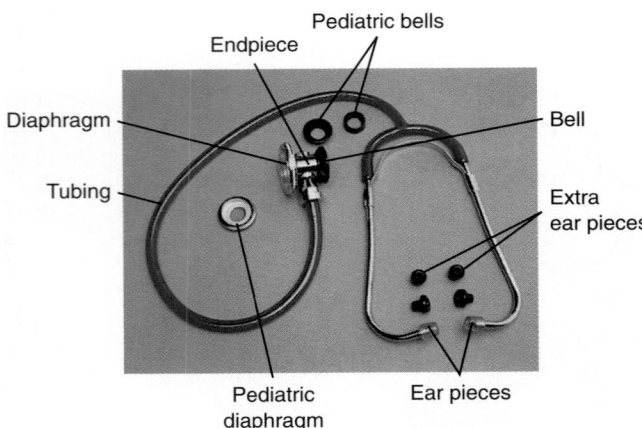

Figure 9–5. Components of a stethoscope.

diaphragm to assess high-frequency sounds. Remember that a stethoscope does not magnify heart sounds. It simply focuses them into the end piece and eliminates outside sounds. To decrease the transmission of microorganisms, wipe the ear pieces, diaphragm, and bell with alcohol between clients.

When you listen to the client's anterior chest, you will hear two sounds produced by a normal heart. The first heart sound, called S_1, results when the mitral and tricuspid valves close during systole. This creates the "lub" of the "lub-dub" heart sound. It can be heard best at the apex of the heart, fifth intercostal space, just left of the midclavicular line. The second heart sound, called S_2, results when the aortic and pulmonic valves close during diastole. This creates the "dub" of the "lub-dub" heart sound. It can be heard best at the base of the heart, second intercostal space, right or left of the sternal border. When assessing a client's apical pulse rate, count S_1 and S_2 together ("lub-dub") as one beat.

Apical-Radial Pulse

To gain further information about the effectiveness of the heart as a pump in the event of dysrhythmias and cardiac disease, take an apical-radial pulse to assess for a pulse deficit: a discrepancy between the apical pulse rate and the radial pulse rate. You will be able to detect the weak contraction by simultaneously listening to the heart and feeling the pulse. When the apical pulse rate exceeds the radial pulse rate, this difference is described as a **pulse deficit.** To assess apical-radial pulse, you and a colleague will work together. One of you auscultates the apical rate while the other palpates the radial pulse. Both of you start counting at the same time, count for a full minute, and compare your findings. The difference is documented as a pulse deficit.

Pulse Quality

A weak pulse is caused by any condition that slows or restricts the blood flow, such as decreased blood volume, weak heart contractions, or partial obstruction of arteries (Table 9–4). For example, vasoconstriction can cause the artery to become so narrowed that the pulse wave is difficult to feel. Likewise, in shock, the blood volume may be reduced to the point where you can no longer feel the pulse wave. In contrast, in vasodilation and overhydration, the extra blood volume can make the pulses very pronounced.

Additionally, to produce a palpable pulse, the wall of an artery must have enough elasticity to respond to the pulse wave. The more elastic the walls of the artery, the more easily the wave can distend the artery and create a pulse wave. The harder and stiffer the wall of the artery, the less the pulse wave can distend it. The result will be a weak pulse that is difficult to palpate.

When you have trouble palpating a pulse wave, you may need to use a Doppler ultrasound stethoscope to assess the weakened pulse (Fig. 9–6). By enhancing pulse sounds, it can also enhance the accuracy of your assessment. The Doppler stethoscope can help you detect a pulse when you cannot palpate one. It may be especially helpful for a client who has a total occlusion of an artery. To use the device, place the transducer over the artery while listening through the earpieces. A sensor picks up the arterial pulse wave and magnifies the sound, giving it a "whooshing" sound.

RESPIRATION

To survive, the cells of the body must receive enough oxygen to meet their metabolic needs. They must also release carbon dioxide, the major byproduct of metabolism. As you know, breathing—also known as respiration—accomplishes these purposes.

TABLE 9–4
Factors That Influence the Palpation of Pulses

Factor	Influence
Heart failure and myocardial infarction	Injury to the heart muscle impairs contractility and decreases the stroke volume. Ineffective contractions may be unable to transmit a palpable fluid wave to the peripheral pulse sites. Pulses may be difficult to palpate, and the client may have an apical-radial pulse deficit.
Artery patency	A clot in an artery causes the pulse to be absent distal to the occlusion.
Arteriosclerosis	Hardening and stiffening of the artery makes palpation more difficult.
Low blood volume	The client will have a weak, thready pulse that may be difficult to palpate.
High blood volume	The client will have an overly strong, bounding pulse.

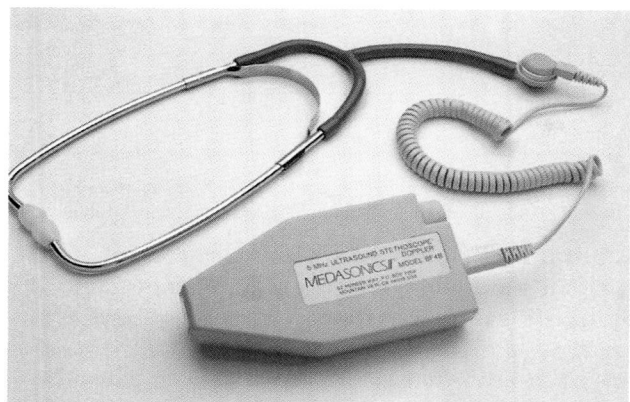

Figure 9–6. A Doppler ultrasound stethoscope. (Courtesy of Medasonics, Inc., Newark, CA.)

Understanding Respiration

A person's respiratory rate and depth vary with the cellular demand for oxygen and with levels of carbon dioxide and hydrogen ions (pH) in the blood (see Chapter 39). Receptors throughout the body feed information to the brain about the level of oxygen available to cells. The brain, in turn, regulates the person's respiratory rate. For example, peripheral chemoreceptors located in the aorta and carotid arteries are especially sensitive to low blood levels of oxygen (hypoxemia). Central chemoreceptors in the medulla are especially sensitive to high levels of carbon dioxide (hypercapnia) and changes in pH. When these receptors sense a change in oxygen, carbon dioxide, and hydrogen ions, they communicate via the autonomic nervous system to the respiratory center in the medulla for integration. As a result, the rate, depth, rhythm, or effort of respiration may change. During rest and sleep, cells need less oxygen, and respirations become shallow, quiet, and slow.

Measuring Respirations

The act of breathing is primarily involuntary. In fact, people usually are not aware that they are breathing. When you measure respirations, you are assessing this natural, involuntary function. However, breathing can come under voluntary control as well. When a person concentrates on her breathing, the rate may change. Consequently, when you assess a client's respirations, you should do so when the client is not aware of your actions. This ensures that you will be assessing the client's natural respirations. To keep the client unaware of your assessment, try counting respirations just after you take the client's pulse, while still holding her wrist (Procedure 9–3). Count one cycle of inspiration and expiration as one breath. Make sure to assess the client's complete breathing pattern, including rate, rhythm, depth, and effort.

The normal respiratory rate for an adult is between 12 and 20 breaths per minute, a status known as **eupnea.** A rate of more than 20 breaths per minute is called **tachypnea,** and a rate less than 12 breaths per minute is called **bradypnea.** Children normally have slightly higher respiratory rates than adults.

Normally, breathing occurs at a regular rhythm. Irregular breathing in an adult can result from head injury, increased intracranial pressure, or cardiovascular complications (Table 9–5). Report irregular breathing to the nurse in charge or a physician immediately. Infants and children normally have a slightly irregular pattern of breathing.

The depth of ventilation, called tidal volume, indicates the volume of air exchanged with each breath. Normally, it is about 500 cc. Because you will not be able to measure this volume while taking vital signs, you will need to estimate whether the client is exchanging an adequate volume of air with each breath. With normal depth, you will see a moderate amount of chest movement. With deep breathing, the chest expands fully. With shallow breathing, you may see little chest movement at all. Fast, deep breathing is known as hyperventilation or hyperpnea (see Chapter 39). Slow, shallow breathing is known as hypoventilation (see Chapter 39). Normal respiration includes periodic deep breaths known as sighing. Sighing is a protective mechanism that periodically expands unused alveoli and prevents their collapse.

Normal ventilation is effortless and quiet. It results from movements of the intercostal muscles and diaphragm. Accessory muscles are not used. Exercise, shortness of breath (dyspnea), or respiratory diseases can lead to an exaggerated respiratory effort to breathe. Infants and children often flare their nostrils if they are having difficulty breathing.

On occasion, you may use a stethoscope to count a client's respirations, especially if they are shallow and slow. You also may use palpation to assess slow, shallow respirations. Place your hand on the client's lower chest or abdomen and feel for a slight rise and fall with each breath. No matter which assessment method you use, document the client's respirations immediately after obtaining the reading (see Fig. 9–1). Other information about the client's respiration can be documented in your nurse's notes or a progress report. For example, you would document other indicators of respiratory status, such as arterial blood gas measurements, a blue tinge to the client's skin or mucous membranes, and restlessness.

BLOOD PRESSURE

As it flows through the body, blood exerts pressure against the inner walls of blood vessels, especially on the arterial side of the circulation. The intensity of this pressure offers you important information about the person's cardiovascular and circulatory status.

During myocardial contraction (systole), when blood is ejected from the heart and into the arteries of the body, blood pressure reaches its height. During diastole, when the heart rests, blood pressure falls to its baseline level. This is why blood pressure measurements have two values, known as **systolic blood pres-**

Assessing Respirations

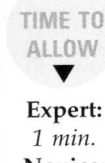

TIME TO ALLOW
▼
Expert:
1 min.
Novice:
1 min.

Respiration is a largely involuntary process, but it may come under voluntary control at times. By assessing respirations without the client's knowledge, you can gain important information about the client's respiratory and cardiovascular systems.

Delegation Guidelines

The measurement and recording of the client's respiratory rate is a simple procedure that you may delegate to a nursing assistant who has received training in this technique. Training should include specific instructions on findings that necessitate your immediate notification. You must complete the full respiratory assessment if one is indicated.

Equipment Needed

• Watch with a sweep second hand

---

1 Make sure the client is relaxed and quiet.

If necessary, wait 10 or 15 minutes before counting respirations. Anxiety, discomfort, and exercise increase the rate and depth of respirations and may result in a false reading.

2 Make sure that the client's anterior thorax is easily visible and that the lungs can complete the full excursion of respiratory movement without hindrance.

The client may be sitting or lying down, whichever makes it easier for you to observe the chest moving.

3 Make sure the client does not know you are counting his respirations.

If aware, the client may alter his respirations or concentrate on them, which can alter their natural number. Many nurses simply continue holding a client's wrist after taking a pulse measurement. The client thinks the pulse measurement is still continuing while the nurse has begun counting respirations.

4 Watch the rise and fall of the client's chest. Count each cycle of inhalation and exhalation as one breath.

If necessary, you may place your hand on the client's lower thorax or abdomen and palpate the movement.

5 Count the client's respirations.

For an adult with a regular rhythm, count for 30 seconds, and multiply your result by 2. For an infant, a child, or an adult with an irregular rhythm, count for a full minute to obtain the most accurate reading. Infants and children normally have a slightly irregular rhythm.

6 Perform the post-skill activities outlined in Procedure 9–1.

7 Document the client's respirations in his medical record as soon as you obtain the reading.

Normal respirations are 12 to 20 per minute, regular, of moderate depth, and effortless.

8 Report abnormal respirations to a charge nurse or physician.

---

sure and **diastolic blood pressure.** The difference between systolic and diastolic blood pressures is known as the **pulse pressure.** For an adult, systolic pressure normally varies from 100 to 140 mm Hg. Diastolic pressure normally varies from 60 to 90 mm Hg. Pulse pressure is normally about 30 to 50 mm Hg. By correlating a client's blood pressure readings with his history and other signs and symptoms, you can make important conclusions about changes in his health.

Understanding Blood Pressure

Several factors combine to form the reading that you recognize as a person's blood pressure (Fig. 9–7). One of the most important is the volume of blood in the person's vascular system. Less blood yields a lower blood pressure; more blood yields a higher blood pressure. A second factor is the action of the heart. An increased cardiac output raises blood pressure, and a decreased cardiac output lowers it. A third factor is the resistance of the blood vessels to distension, known as **vascular resistance.** When vascular resistance increases, blood pressure rises, and vice versa.

Compensatory mechanisms involving the brain, kidneys, and adrenal glands combine with these factors to help keep blood pressure in the normal range. For example, when nervous system receptors (baroreceptors) in the great vessels sense a drop in blood pressure, they relay that information to the pressure center in the medulla. The sympathetic nervous system is

TABLE 9–5
Breathing Patterns

Pattern		Description
Eupnea		Between 12 and 20 breaths per minute in regular rhythm and of moderate depth for an adult.
Bradypnea		Regular rhythm of less than 12 breaths per minute for an adult.
Tachypnea		Regular rhythm of more than 20 breaths per minute for an adult.
Apnea		Absence of respirations that leads to respiratory arrest and death.
Hypoventilation		Rate and depth are decreased, reducing the volume of air available for gas exchange and possibly leading to retention of carbon dioxide and respiratory acidosis.
Hyperventilation Hyperpnea		Rate and depth are increased, increasing the volume of air available for gas exchange and possibly leading to respiratory alkalosis from the blowing off of excess carbon dioxide. It is usually associated with exercise or anxiety.
Cheynes-Stokes		Alternating periods of apnea, hypoventilation, and hyperventilation usually associated with head injury or heart failure.
Kussmaul		Rate and depth are increased. Usually associated with diabetic ketoacidosis as a compensatory mechanism to eliminate excess carbon dioxide.

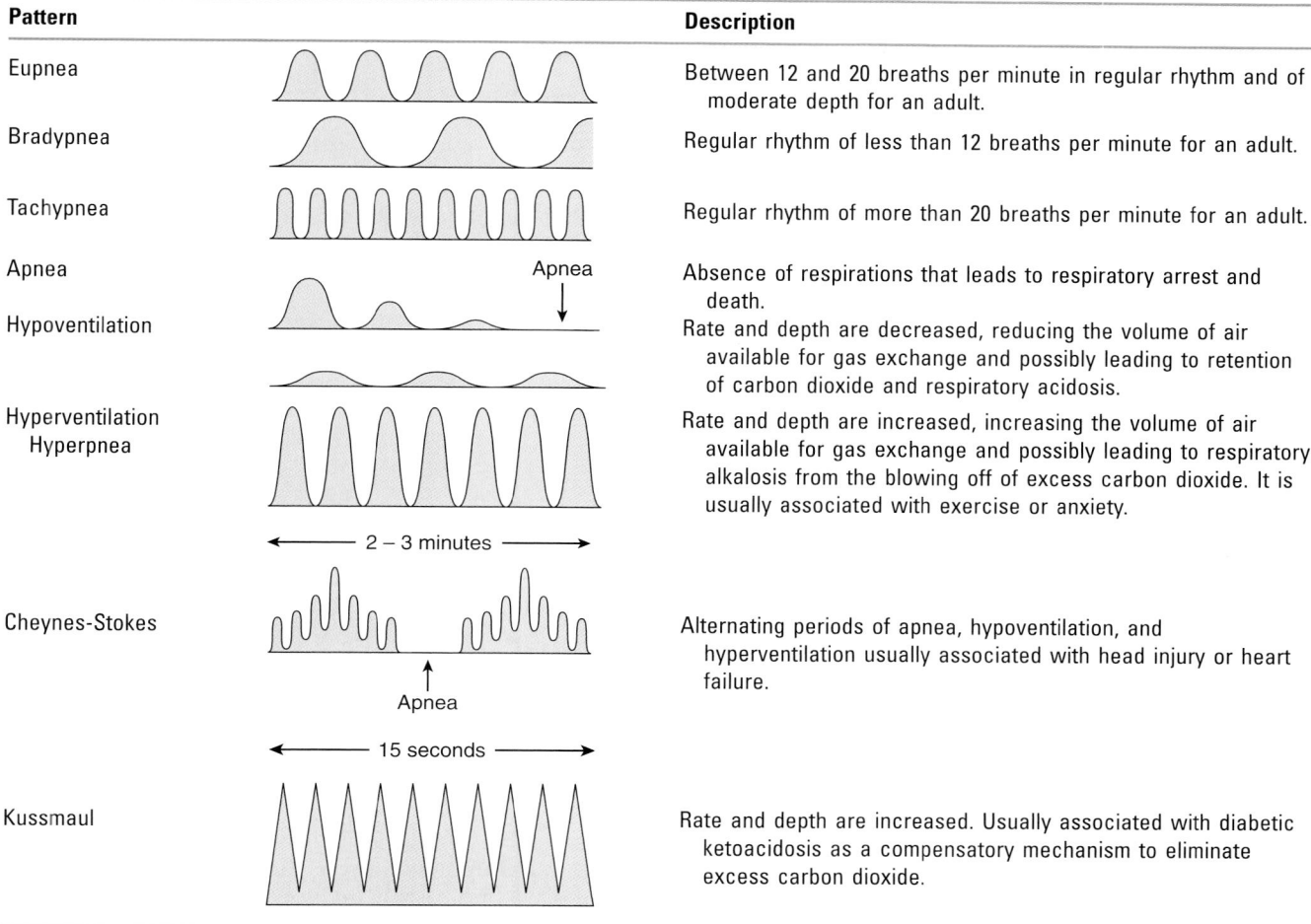

then activated. In response, blood vessels constrict, and blood volume rises in response to sodium retention by the kidney and catecholamine (epinephrine and norepinephrine) production by the adrenal glands. When the parasympathetic nervous system is activated, a series of events occurs to cause the blood pressure to decrease.

Other factors that help to regulate blood pressure to some degree include the viscosity of blood; the velocity of blood flow; levels of oxygen and carbon dioxide in the blood; the client's age, emotions, pain, and exercise; time of day; and medication use (Table 9–6). Finally, hemorrhage, shock, dehydration, and blood loss reduce blood pressure by lowering the circulating blood volume. Renal failure and other causes of fluid overload can raise blood pressure. Head injuries can raise blood pressure as well, by interfering with regulatory mechanisms in the medulla.

Measuring Blood Pressure

To measure a person's blood pressure, you will use a sphygmomanometer and stethoscope to listen to a se-

ries of sounds, usually in the client's brachial artery. A sphygmomanometer includes a pressure manometer (Fig. 9–8), an inflatable cuff, and a pressure bulb. The manometer can function either with air (aneroid) or mercury. Both measure blood pressure in millimeters of mercury (mm Hg). Before taking a person's blood pressure reading, you should calibrate the manometer to zero to avoid a false high reading.

You will also need to choose a blood pressure cuff of appropriate size for your client (Procedure 9–4). Cuffs come in newborn, infant, child, and adult sizes for both arm and leg measurements. The inflatable bladder inside the cuff should be long enough to almost encircle the limb. The cuff's width should be about two-thirds the length of the upper arm or thigh. A too-narrow cuff will produce a false high reading. A too-large cuff will produce a false low reading. Place the cuff directly over the client's brachial artery to ensure complete and equal compression.

To hear the sounds on which you will base your blood pressure measurement, you will need to know how to use a stethoscope correctly. Some of the sounds are very faint, and the possibility of error is

Factors That Increase Blood Pressure

- Increased peripheral vascular resistance
  - Vasoconstriction
  - Increased blood viscosity

- Increased blood flow
  - Increased cardiac output
  - Increased blood volume

Factors That Decrease Blood Pressure

- Decreased peripheral vascular resistance
  - Vasodilation

- Decreased blood flow
  - Decreased cardiac output
  - Decreased blood volume

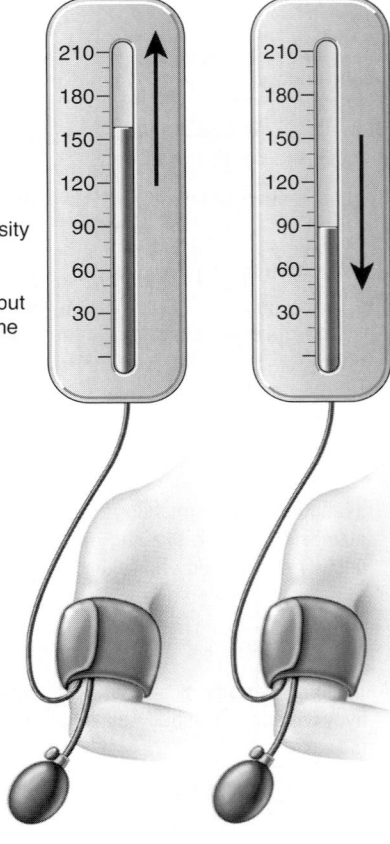

Figure 9–7. Physiological factors affecting blood pressure.

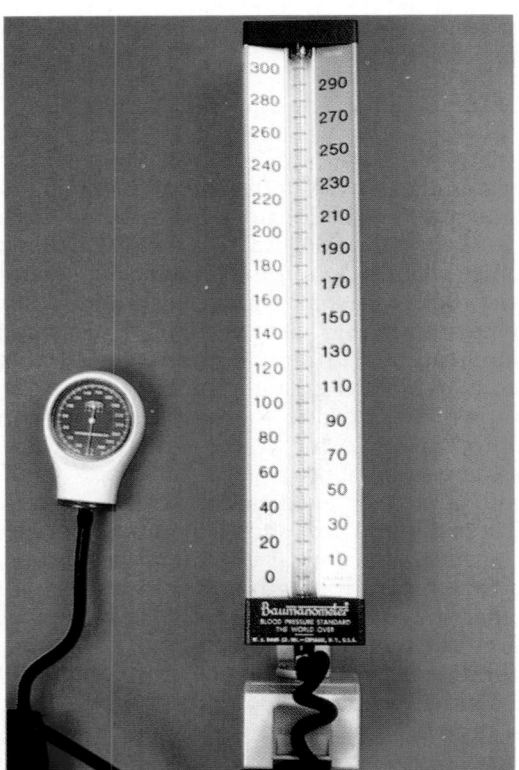

Figure 9–8. Manometers: aneroid (left) and mercury (right). (From Polaski, A.L., & Warner, J.P. [1994]. *Saunders fundamentals for nursing assistants: Slide package.* Philadelphia: W.B. Saunders Co.)

considerable (Table 9–7). To ensure the accuracy of your measurement, insert the stethoscope earpieces so the tips point toward your nose, not the back of your head. Turn the television or radio down or off and, if necessary, ask people in the room to be quiet. You will need to practice and refine your technique for measuring blood pressure to make sure you can do it accurately.

The five distinct sounds you will listen for when measuring blood pressure are called **Korotkoff's sounds** or Korotkoff's phases. When blood is flowing freely through an artery or the artery is totally obstructed, no sound can be detected even with a stethoscope. However, if you partially constrict the artery, turbulent blood flow vibrates the walls of the artery and produces sound. Thus, the blood pressure cuff is used to temporarily obstruct the artery. As you slowly release pressure from the cuff, the obstruction is gradually reduced, and the sounds change. When the blood flows freely again, the sound disappears.

The first sound you will hear as turbulent blood begins flowing through the partially compressed artery is Korotkoff I, a clear tapping sound (Fig. 9–9). As you continue to release pressure, the other sounds follow. Korotkoff II is a murmur or swishing sound. Korotkoff III is a clear, intense tapping. Korotkoff IV is a distinct change to a muffled sound and indicates the first diastolic blood pressure. Korotkoff V is the disappearance sound caused by freely flowing blood; it indicates the second diastolic blood pressure.

TABLE 9–6
Factors That Influence Blood Pressure

Factor	Influence
Age	Newborns and infants have the lowest blood pressure. Blood pressure increases as age increases. It is highest in the elderly because of a decrease in the elasticity of vessels, which causes an increase in resistance to blood flow. However, even in the elderly a blood pressure above 140/90 should not be considered normal.
Stress and emotions	Anxiety, pain, tension, worry, and stress raise blood pressure by stimulating the sympathetic nervous system, which causes vasoconstriction and a resulting increased heart rate.
Medication	Medications that lower blood pressure include narcotics, tranquilizers, hypnotics, diuretics, antihypertensives, and certain cardiac medications (particularly vasodilators). Medications that raise blood pressure include antihistamines, estrogen, and corticosteroids (glucocorticoids and mineralocorticoids).
Diurnal variation	Blood pressure is typically lowest in the early morning, with decreased activity, and highest in the afternoon or evening, with increased activity.
Gender	After puberty, males tend to have higher blood pressure than females. After menopause, women tend to have higher blood pressure than men of the same age.
Environment	A hot environment can lower blood pressure by causing vasodilation. A cold environment can raise it by causing vasoconstriction.
Exercise	Blood pressure increases with activity and exercise because the sympathetic nervous system responds to the body's increased need for oxygen.
Body position	Blood pressure is lowest in the recumbent position. It is slightly higher in the standing position because of sympathetic nervous system stimulation.
Right versus left arm	About one-fourth of the population has a difference of 10 (±5) mm Hg between the right and left arm.
Arm versus leg	There is a difference of 10 to 40 mm Hg in systolic blood pressure between measurements taken using the arm and measurements taken using the leg.
Vasodilation	Parasympathetic nervous system stimulation causes blood vessels to increase their lumen diameter, thus lowering blood pressure. This may happen in response to warm temperatures, fever, and relaxation, for example.
Vasoconstriction	Sympathetic nervous system stimulation causes blood vessels to decrease their lumen diameter, thus raising blood pressure. This may happen in response to cold temperatures, for example.
Head injury	Injuries to the head and increased intracranial pressure result in increased blood pressure.
Reduced blood volume	Blood pressure decreases if the circulatory system contains an inadequate volume of blood, as from low cardiac output, hemorrhage, or shock.
Increased blood volume	Too much fluid in the cardiovascular system increases blood pressure.

To assess a client's cardiovascular function fully, you may need to check for orthostatic hypotension, in which blood pressure drops by 20 mm Hg or more with position changes (see Chapter 38). You will do so by measuring his blood pressure in lying, sitting, and standing positions. Wait about 2 minutes between position changes before you take the next reading to allow the client's compensatory mechanisms to stabilize his blood pressure. Orthostatic hypotension may result from a reduced blood volume or certain medications.

A*ction* A*lert!*
Ensure safety of the client with orthostatic hypotension when getting out of bed.

If the client has hypertension, you may not hear Korotkoff II. This absence is called an **auscultatory gap.** You will hear a faint first Korotkoff sound, then silence until the third Korotkoff sound comes in loud and crisp. The cause of this gap is unknown. However, recognizing it is crucial. If you fail to recognize it, you could mistake the third Korotkoff sound (instead of the first) as the client's systolic pressure. Doing so produces a false low systolic reading.

If the normal tapping sounds disappear on inspiration and return on expiration, the client has pulsus paradoxus. Slowly decrease the cuff pressure and listen for the paradoxical pulse to cease. If it is present for more than 10 mm Hg, it may be a sign of serious cardiovascular problems.

If you cannot use the client's arm to measure blood pressure, you may need to use the popliteal artery behind the knee. Use an appropriate thigh-sized cuff. Systolic pressures in the leg can differ by 10 to 40 mm Hg from pressures in the arm. When documenting your findings, make sure to note that your reading is from the client's leg.

Finally, if you have trouble hearing the Korotkoff sounds, you may need to use Doppler ultrasound to measure the client's blood pressure. This problem may result from severe hypotension, shock, or circulatory instability. The Doppler transducer picks up and amplifies blood pressure sounds so you can hear them. However, you will be able to determine only a systolic pressure measurement with this device. If you need to

PROCEDURE 9–4

Assessing Blood Pressure

TIME TO
ALLOW
▼
Novice:
2 min.
Expert:
2 min.

Blood pressure is the pressure exerted by blood against the inner walls of the arteries. Measuring a client's blood pressure will give you information about the health of the cardiovascular, circulatory, and renal systems.

Delegation Guidelines

The measurement and recording of the client's blood pressure is a simple, low-risk procedure that you may delegate to a nursing assistant who has received training in this technique. Training should include specific instructions on findings that necessitate your immediate notification. You *remain responsible for assessing any variance or irregularities in the client's blood pressure.*

Equipment Needed

* Sphygmomanometer with cuff of correct size
* Stethoscope

---

1 Select a cuff of correct size for the client and the limb you intend to use.
a. Select a bladder that fits almost completely around the client's arm.
b. Select a cuff width that is about two-thirds the length of the client's upper arm.

A cuff that is too wide will result in a false low reading. A cuff that is too narrow will result in a false high reading.

2 Choose the arm on which you will take the blood pressure reading.

Avoid taking a blood pressure measurement on an arm that is used for hemodialysis or has a shunt, burn, cast, intravenous line, or traumatic injury. Also avoid using an arm contiguous with the site of breast or axillary surgery. If you cannot use one of the client's arms to take a blood pressure reading, use a leg, and measure blood pressure at the popliteal artery.

3 Position the client's arm so it is level with the heart, palm up, in a relaxed and comfortable fashion. If the client is supine, you may place his arm on the bed. If the client is sitting or standing, position the arm on an overbed table, or hold it with your elbow.

Positioning the arm below heart level will result in a false high reading. Positioning it above heart level will result in a false low reading. Positioning it with palm up exposes the brachial artery.

4 If the client is changing from a lying to a sitting position, wait at least 2 minutes before taking the blood pressure measurement.

This time allows the body's compensatory mechanisms to stabilize the blood pressure.

5 Affix the cuff onto the client's arm.
a. Do not place the cuff over the client's clothing.
b. Place the bottom edge of the cuff 1 inch above the client's antecubital fossa.

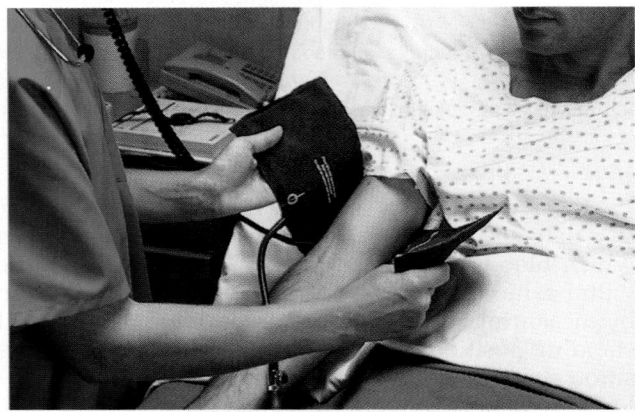

Placing the cuff 1 inch above the antecubital fossa.

c. Place the center of the cuff directly over the brachial artery.
d. Wrap the cuff snugly around the client's arm while allowing space to place the stethoscope over the brachial artery.

This ensures uniform and complete compression of the brachial artery. A cuff that is too loose will result in a false high reading.

6 Position the sphygmomanometer at eye level. The mercury in a manometer or the needle of an aneroid gauge should be at zero.

Positioning the manometer above eye level results in a false high reading. Positioning it below eye level results in a false low reading.

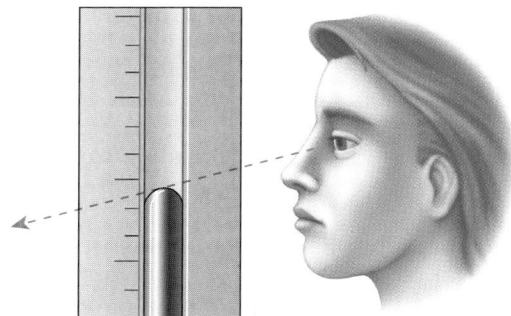

Falsely low reading

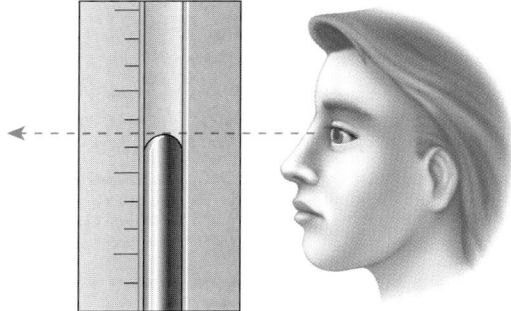

Accurate reading

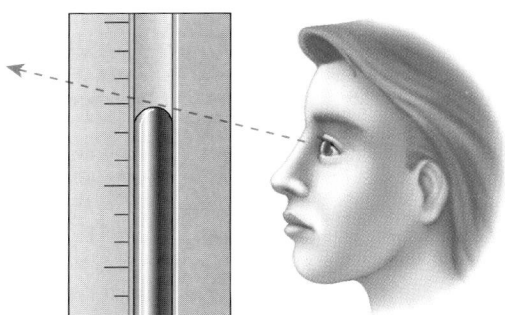

Falsely high reading

Effect of viewing the meniscus at different levels. Viewing at eye level gives the most accurate reading.

7 Obtain the palpatory systolic blood pressure.
a. Palpate the brachial or radial pulse.
b. Inflate the cuff until the pulse disappears.
c. Release the pressure slowly until the pulse returns, and note this reading.
d. Quickly release the cuff.

Palpatory blood pressure should be performed on all clients when taking a blood pressure reading for the first time. It ensures that the cuff will be sufficiently inflated to give you an accurate systolic reading by auscultation. It also provides information about an auscultatory gap. Failure to identify such a gap will result in a false low systolic reading.

8 Obtain the blood pressure reading.
a. Wait 30 to 60 seconds after obtaining the palpatory systolic blood pressure.

If you attempt to obtain the blood pressure reading too soon after obtaining the palpatory systolic blood pressure, you will receive a false high reading.

b. Place the bell of your stethoscope lightly over the brachial artery.

The bell of the stethoscope is used for low-pitched sounds, such as blood pressure tones.

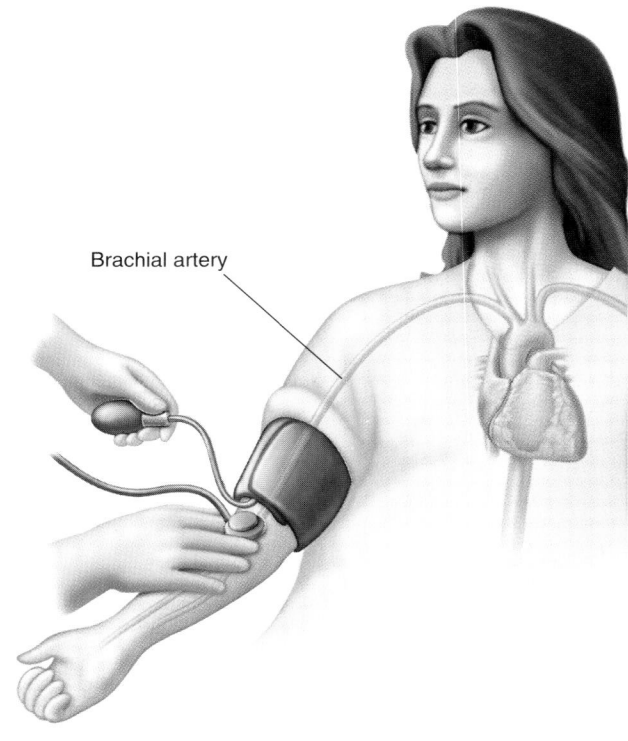

Brachial artery

Positioning the stethoscope over the brachial artery.

Continued

PROCEDURE 9–4 *(continued)*

Assessing Blood Pressure

c. Tighten the screw clamp, and quickly inflate the cuff to 30 mm Hg above the palpatory systolic blood pressure reading.

The auscultatory systolic blood pressure should be slightly higher than the palpatory reading. Slow inflation can result in an inaccurate reading.

d. Deflate the cuff slowly and steadily at 2 to 3 mm Hg per second until you hear a soft, tapping sound. This is the first Korotkoff sound and indicates the client's systolic blood pressure.

Deflating the cuff too rapidly results in a false low systolic reading. Deflating the cuff too slowly results in a false high diastolic reading.

e. Continue deflating the cuff slowly. Listen for a murmur or swishing sound (Korotkoff II), a clear tapping (Korotkoff III), and a muffling of sound (Korotkoff IV).

Muffling of sound correlates with the beginning of diastole and is the best indicator of diastolic blood pressure in children.

f. Continue deflating the cuff slowly, listening for the sounds to stop.

Cessation of sounds correlates with the end of diastole (Korotkoff V) and is the best indicator of diastolic blood pressure in adults. In children and athletes, the sounds of phase V may continue all the way to zero.

9 Deflate the cuff quickly and completely. If you must take another blood pressure reading, wait 1 to 2 minutes before doing so. Continued pressure on the blood vessels will decrease circulation to the hand, causing the client discomfort. Waiting a minute or two allows normal circulation to return to the hand.

10 Document the client's blood pressure in his medical record as soon as you obtain the reading. If you identify an auscultatory gap, document the mm Hg that corresponds to the length of the silence.

Normal systolic blood pressure is 100 to 140 mm Hg. Normal diastolic blood pressure is 60 to 90 mm Hg. Some facilities require that you document three sounds: systolic blood pressure, muffling, and diastolic blood pressure.

11 Report an abnormal blood pressure to a charge nurse or physician.

Phase I - Clear tapping		**128 mm Hg** **Systolic**
Phase II - Murmur or swishing sound		110 mm Hg
Phase III - Clear, intense tapping		100 mm Hg
Phase IV - Distinct sound changes to a muffled sound		**88 mm Hg** **First diastolic**
Phase V - Silence		**80 mm Hg** **Second diastolic**

Blood pressure = 128/88/80

Figure 9–9. The Korotkoff sounds (also called phases).

TABLE 9–7

Blood Pressure Measurement: Sources of Error and the Effect on Results

Source of Error	Effect on Blood Pressure Reading
Cuff size too wide	False low
Cuff size too narrow	False high
Cuff wrapped too loose	False high
Arm below heart level	False high
Arm above heart level	False low
Manometer below eye level	False low
Manometer above eye level	False high
Cuff deflated too rapidly	False low systolic
Cuff deflated too slowly	False high diastolic
Failure to wait 30 to 60 seconds between successive blood pressure readings	False high
Failure to identify an auscultatory gap with a palpatory systolic blood pressure measurement	False low systolic
Defective equipment, poorly calibrated manometers, hearing impairment, or improper use of stethoscope	Inaccurate readings

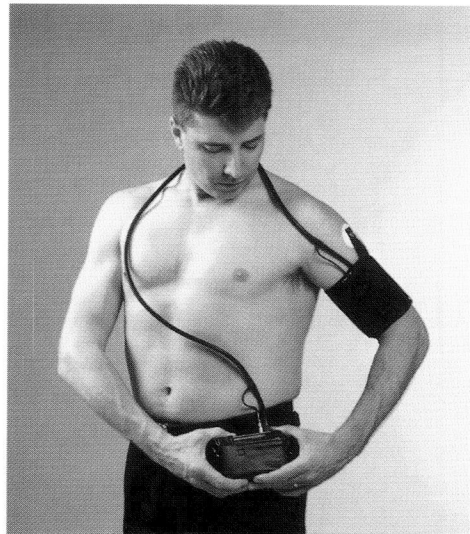

Figure 9–10. An automated blood pressure monitor. (Photo courtesy of Welch Allyn, Inc.)

take frequent blood pressure readings, you may want to use an automated blood pressure machine to obtain quick, accurate measurements (Fig. 9–10).

In all cases, document your client's blood pressure as soon as you obtain the reading. Make sure you follow your health care facility's policy when documenting pressures. Most continue to use the two-part measurement that lists systolic and diastolic levels. However, a growing number of facilities require a three-part documentation. If yours does, you will need to chart systolic, muffling, and diastolic readings. Along with the numerical readings, you should also document the location from which you took the reading and the client's position.

KEY PRINCIPLES

- Assessment of vital signs provides you with crucial information about a client's psychological and physical state of health.
- The body's temperature is a balance between heat production and heat loss.
- Body temperature is affected by the client's health, age, stress, and time of day.
- Common types of thermometers are glass, electronic, and tympanic.
- Routes for temperature measurement are oral, axillary, rectal, and tympanic.
- The pulse is a wave of blood in the arteries created by the pumping action of the heart.
- Assessment of the radial and apical pulse includes the rate, rhythm, and strength.
- The rate and depth of respirations change according to the body's need for oxygen, the release of carbon dioxide, and the person's emotions.

- Blood pressure is largely a reflection of blood volume, cardiac output, and vascular resistance.
- Blood pressure measures the highest pressure (systolic) and the lowest resting pressure (diastolic) of the fluid in the vessels.
- Accurate documentation is essential for communication of vital sign data to other health care providers.

BIBLIOGRAPHY

Bayne, C.G. (1997). Technology assessment: Vital signs: Are we monitoring the right parameters? *Nursing Management, 28*(5), 74–76.

Beaudry, M., VandenBosch, T., & Anderson, J. (1996). Research utilization: Once-a-day temperature for afebrile patients. *Clinical Nurse Specialist, 10*(1), 21–24.

Braun, S.K., Preston, P., & Smith, R.N. (1998). Getting a better read on thermometry. *RN, 61*(3), 57–60.

Dunbar, S.B., & Farr, L. (1996). Temporal patterns of heart rate and blood pressure in elders. *Nursing Research, 45*(1), 43–48.

Erickson, R.S., Meyer, L.T., & Woo, T.M. (1996). Accuracy of chemical dot thermometers in critically ill adults and young children. *Image Journal of Nursing Scholarship, 28*(1), 23–28.

Flo, G., & Brown, M. (1995). Comparing three methods of temperature taking. *Nursing Research, 44*(2), 120–122.

Henker, R., & Coyne, C. (1995). Comparison of peripheral temperature measurements with core temperature. *AACN Clinical Issues, 6*(1), 21–30.

Irvin, S.M. (1999). Comparison of the oral thermometer versus the tympanic thermometer. *American Journal of Nursing, 13*(2), 85.

Lanham D.M. (1999). Accuracy of tympanic temperature readings in children under 6 years of age. *Pediatric Nursing, 25*(1), 39–42.

McConnell, E.A. (1995). Monitoring peripheral pulses with a Doppler ultrasound device. *Nursing, 25*(3), 18.

McConnell E.A. (1998). Automated vital sign monitoring devices. *Nursing Management, 29*(2), 49–51.

Murphy, L., & Linn, L. (1996). Managing vital signs monitoring problems. *Nursing, 26*(11), 32gg–32jj.

Roper, M. (1996). Back to basics: Assessing orthostatic vital signs. *American Journal of Nursing, 96*(8), 43–46.

Schmitz, T., Blair, N., Falk, M., & Levine, C. (1995). A comparison of five methods of temperature measurement in febrile intensive care patients. *American Journal of Critical Care, 4*(4), 286–292.

Schumacher, S.B. (1995). Monitoring vital signs to identify postoperative complication. *MEDSURG Nursing, 4*(2), 142–145.

Sneed, N.V., & Hollenbach, A.D. (1995). Measurement error in counting heart rate. *Critical Care Nurse,* February 1995, 36–40.

*Solomon, J. (1994). Consult stat: This nurse's ears aren't deceiving her. *RN, 57*(11), 67–71.

Solomon, J. (1995). Consult stat: Variations of blood pressure technique. *RN, 57*(7), 63–64.

Thomas, D.O. (1996). Assessing children: It's different. *RN, 59*(4), 38–45, 53.

Thomas, S.A., & DeKeyser, F. (1996). Blood pressure. *Annual Review of Nursing Research, 14*, 3–22.

Winslow, E.H. (1995). Research for practice: Are 60-second pulse counts necessary? *American Journal of Nursing, 95*(1), 53.

Winslow, E.H., Jacobson, A.F., & Beazlie, M.A. (1997). Research for practice: Tympanic thermometers: Accuracy is questionable. *American Journal of Nursing, 97*(5), 71.

Zaiser, D.K. (1996). Skills primer: Patient assessment pitfalls. *Emergency, 28*(10), 26–31.

*Asterisk indicates a classic or definitive work on this subject.

CHAPTER 10

Assessing the Client: Physical Examination

Marilyn S. Leasia and Frances Donovan Monahan

Key Terms

auscultation
inspection
lesion
ophthalmoscope
otoscope

palpation
percussion
point of maximum impulse
precordium
turgor

LEARNING OBJECTIVES

After studying this chapter, you should be able to:

1. Define and describe each of the four techniques used in physical examination: inspection, palpation, percussion, and auscultation.
2. Identify and understand the primary instruments used in physical assessment.
3. Acquire courteous nonthreatening techniques to ensure client comfort and prepare the client for each regionally focused area of a complete physical examination.
4. Perform a complete physical examination on a client using a head-to-toe approach.
5. Recognize normal physical findings.
6. Recognize when physical findings deviate from normal.

The physical examination is a systematic means of collecting objective assessment data. Objective data may be used to verify findings from the history or to determine the meaning of the findings. Although the history and the physical examination are usually conducted as separate procedures, the information is synthesized to identify and explain the client's problems, which may have psychological, social, or spiritual components.

As you collected the nursing history, you identified problems and possible problems in the client. In doing a physical examination, you are now looking for objective evidence commonly associated with these problems. Your findings may confirm the problems you suspected or at least add evidence to substantiate your hypotheses.

Physical assessments can be either *comprehensive* or *focused*. Ideally, every physical assessment should be comprehensive; that is, it should evaluate every body system and every area of function. However, a comprehensive physical assessment is often limited to the first time that a client sees a specific health care provider or enters a health care agency. Subsequently, assessment is focused on the reason for the visit and the client's current needs. When a client presents in acute distress with need of immediate intervention for a specific problem, assessment is focused on the most important data for the immediate problem.

How quickly you narrow the focus may depend on the client's needs and your knowledge level. A focused assessment assumes you have the knowledge to rule out the need for examination of particular body parts or function.

Regardless of type, all physical assessment is aimed at detecting problems related to altered function, establishing baseline data against which subsequent data can be compared to judge whether the client's condition is improving or worsening, and identifying factors that place the client at risk for additional health problems. To learn to perform physical assessment, you must first learn to recognize normal findings. As you continue to study each normal health pattern, you will add knowledge of some common abnormal findings.

PREPARATION FOR PHYSICAL EXAMINATION
Techniques of Physical Examination

The four basic techniques used in physical examination are inspection, palpation, percussion, and auscultation, and they are performed in order. Inspection is always done first. Palpation follows, except during examination of the abdomen when it is done last so that it does not alter bowel sounds and change the findings on percussion and auscultation.

Inspection

Inspection is the systematic visual examination of the client. It involves observation of color, shape, size, symmetry, position, and movement. For inspection to yield accurate findings, the area to be inspected must be fully exposed and the environmental light must be good. Use natural light because it does not distort color. Use tangential lighting (lighting that shines from one side and casts shadows) to increase your ability to detect variations in body surface such as changes in abdominal contour (Fig. 10–1).

Palpation

Palpation is examination of the body through the use of touch or feeling with the hand. It is used to obtain information regarding temperature, moisture, texture, consistency, size, shape, position, and movement. Use palpation to assess pulses as well as to check for tenderness, guarding, abdominal distention (enlarged or swollen abdomen), masses, and edema.

When checking temperature, use the back of your hand, as it is usually more sensitive than the palm. When assessing factors such as texture, shape, size, muscle tone, movement, or tenderness, use the pads of your fingers.

Palpation may be either light or deep. Use light palpation to examine lesions or masses on the surface of the skin or lying immediately under the skin. A light touch helps you avoid changing the shape of the lesion or mass. For light palpation, place your hand, fingers together, parallel to the area to be palpated. Press your finger pads into the area to a depth of 1 to 2 cm (½ to ¾ inch). Repeat this action in ever widening circles until you have palpated the entire area to be examined. Use light palpation to check muscle tone and to check for tenderness. It is always done prior to deep palpation.

Use deep palpation to identify abdominal organs and abdominal masses. With deep palpation, hold your hand at a 60-degree angle, fingers together, and

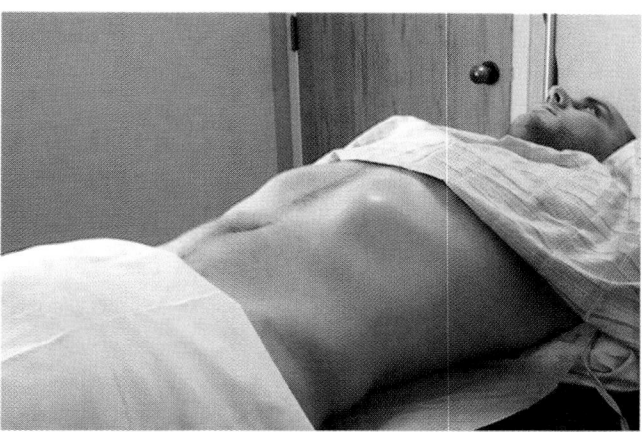

Figure 10–1. Tangential lighting (lighting that shines from one side and casts shadows) increases your ability to detect variations in body surface, such as changes in abdominal contour.

use your finger pads and fingertip to press inward to a depth of 4 cm (2 inches). For two-handed deep palpation, place one hand on top of the other and palpate as just described. Two-handed palpation may help you keep the lower hand relaxed and thus more sensitive to underlying structures.

Before performing palpation, wash and warm your hands. Make sure your fingernails are short to avoid scratching the client's skin. During palpation, tell the client to take slow deep breaths through his mouth to decrease muscle tension, which can interfere with palpation. Palpate any tender areas last, and stop palpating if the client has pain at any point during the examination.

Percussion

Percussion is the use of short, sharp strikes to the body surface to produce palpable vibrations and characteristic sounds. Percussion is used to determine the size and shape of a body organ or to elicit pain and tenderness. Additionally, it can be used to detect whether tissue is fluid-filled, air-filled, or solid. Generally, as the amount of air present in the area being percussed increases, the sounds produced become louder, longer, and deeper. Softer, higher, shorter sounds are produced from more solid areas.

The five types of percussion sounds are *resonance* (hollow sound), *hyper-resonance* (booming sound), *tympany* (musical or drum sound), *dullness* (thud), and *flatness* (extremely dull sound). Resonance is heard over the normal lung; hyper-resonance is heard over an emphysematous lung; tympany is the sound produced by air-filled bowel; dullness is heard over dense structures such as the liver and heart; and flatness is heard over very dense structures such as skeletal muscle and bone.

You will perform percussion to determine the size, shape, density, and location of underlying structures. It is also used to elicit tenderness and to detect the presence of air or fluid in a body cavity. The two types of percussion are direct and indirect.

Direct percussion uses a sharp, rapid movement of the wrist in which you use the pad of your middle finger to strike the area of the client's body to be percussed (Fig. 10–2A). This striking finger is called the plexor. Direct percussion is used primarily to assess the sinuses in adult clients, for example.

Indirect percussion involves two hands. In this type of percussion, you place a finger of your nondominant hand in contact with the client's body, then use your plexor to strike your own finger on the client's body (Fig. 10–2B). The finger in contact with the client's body is called the pleximeter and it is struck by the plexor (the middle finger of your dominant hand) just behind the nail bed at the distal interphalangeal joint, which is hyperextended.

Strike the pleximeter with the plexor at a right angle, then withdraw it immediately to avoid dampening the resulting vibrations. When performing indirect percussion, strike each area twice and then move to a new area. Keep your other fingers and the palm of your hand off the body part being percussed, as this will dampen the vibrations. Generally the thicker the body wall is in the area being percussed, the greater the force of strike needed to produce a clear tone.

Percussion that uses either the ulnar surface of the hand or the fist to strike the surface to be percussed is called blunt percussion. If the area to be percussed is struck directly, it is direct blunt percussion. It is indirect blunt percussion when the palm of the nondominant hand is placed flat on the area to be percussed and the back of the hand is struck.

Again, make sure your hands are washed and warmed, and that your fingernails are short.

Auscultation

Auscultation is the process of listening to sounds generated within the body. Examples of such sounds are those produced by the passage of air in and out of the lungs (breath sounds), those produced by the flow of blood through the heart and blood vessels (heart and vascular sounds), and those produced by the move-

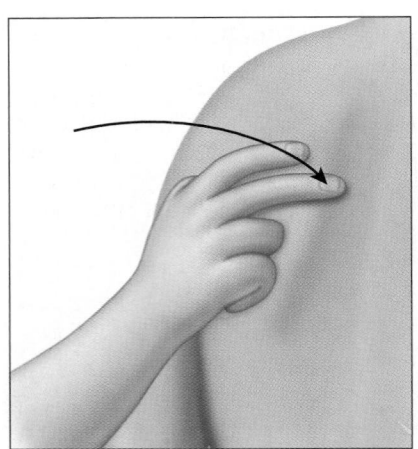
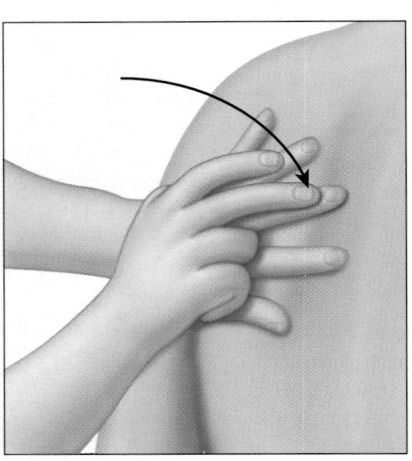

A   **B**

Figure 10–2. Technique for direct percussion (A) and indirect percussion (B).

ment of fluid and gases through the intestinal tract (bowel sounds). Each auscultated sound is described in terms of loudness, pitch, quality, frequency, and duration. Auscultated sounds can be abnormal based on where they are located or on changes in one or more of these characteristics.

Auscultation is most often done using a stethoscope, which we will discuss in the next section. However, you may also listen without a stethoscope to detect breath sounds, clicking or popping sounds from joint movements, and other sounds of body functions.

Equipment for Physical Examination

To perform a physical examination, you will rely heavily on the use of your five senses, particularly your ability to observe. Much of the examination is a mental activity rather than something you actually do. However, some equipment is used for specific aspects of the basic physical examination and additional equipment may be used for specialized parts of the examination (Fig. 10–3).

For most purposes, you will need a stethoscope,

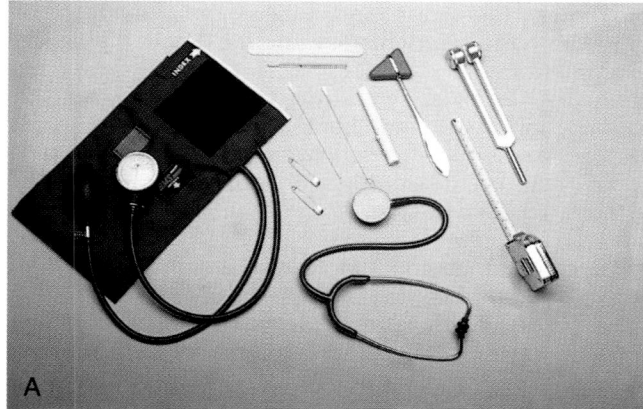

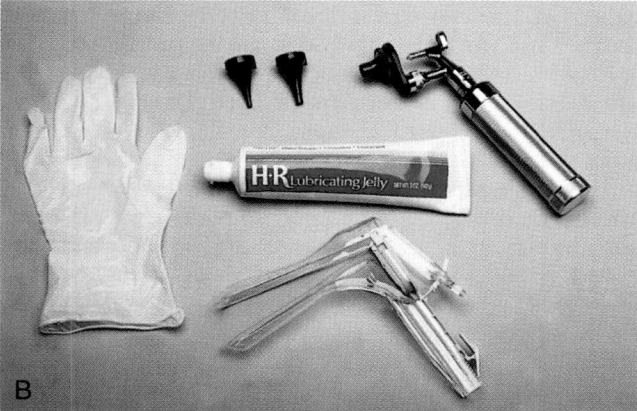

Figure 10–3. A, Equipment used for a basic physical examination: Sphygmomanometer, stethoscope, tongue blade, thermometer, safety pins, cotton-tipped applicators, penlight, percussion hammer, tape measure, and tuning fork. B, Equipment used for specialized aspects of the physical examination: clean gloves and water-soluble lubricant, otoscope, and vaginal speculum.

sphygmomanometer, and thermometer to take vital signs. A tongue blade and penlight are useful to examine the oral cavity and throat. The tuning fork, cotton-tipped swabs, and safety pins are only needed for the neurological examination.

For safety and accuracy, conduct the examination in a manner that is both time-efficient and conducive to client comfort and satisfaction. It is essential that all equipment be clean or sterile, accessible, in working order, and warmed if it will touch the client. Most nurses carry a stethoscope and a penlight as the most commonly used equipment.

You will need to become proficient in using a stethoscope to detect the sounds created within body cavities and blood vessels. The ear pieces should fit snugly to occlude noises other than those transmitted through the tubing, but should not be uncomfortably tight. An ear piece that is too small may slip into the auditory canal and totally occlude sound. An ear piece that is too large may not occlude outside noises well.

Many stethoscopes have both a bell and a diaphragm. The bell is used to improve detection of relatively soft, lower pitched sounds such as extra heart sounds or murmurs. The diaphragm improves detection of relatively higher pitched sounds such as breath sounds, bowel sounds, and normal heart sounds. Thus, the diaphragm is used more often than the bell.

The thickness and length of the tubing can affect the quality of sound transmission. The tubing should be thick with an internal diameter of ⅛ inch. Twelve to 14 inches is considered to be the ideal length. You will need to purchase a reasonably good quality stethoscope with interchangeable ear pieces to be successful in detecting subtle sounds.

To use a stethoscope you will need to control for extraneous sounds. The room should be quiet. This may include turning off suction devices that are being used on the client. Ascertain the safety of turning off the suction. Additionally, the room should be warm. Shivering may distort the sound. Listening through clothes can create extraneous sound and dampen the sounds. Hair on the chest can mimic abnormal lung sounds.

Practice listening to sounds that are familiar until you can hear very quiet, soft sounds. Place the stethoscope firmly, but not pressing, on the client's skin and keep the tubing still. As you practice using your stethoscope you will become more proficient at hearing sounds. As you listen to normal body sounds imagine the normal function that is occurring and associate the sound with the function. You should mentally "see" what is happening in the body.

CONDUCTING THE PHYSICAL EXAMINATION

It is critical that the physical examination be conducted in a manner that will promote collection of complete, accurate assessment data. This means that you should follow a regular pattern of examination, position the client for the most accurate collection of data, and describe your findings in a manner that can be understood by other health care providers.

There is no one correct pattern for physical examination; the importance of the pattern is to ensure a comprehensive assessment through systematic data collection. The pattern may be modified as appropriate to the physical condition of the client and the information that is needed. A head to toe, body systems, or other approach may be used. What is important is that the approach chosen becomes second nature to you, thus helping to ensure that no aspect of assessment is overlooked and that data are organized in a meaningful fashion. Proceeding from head to toe helps you proceed from clean to dirty. Thus you are not examining the mouth with a hand that has touched a foot.

Both the environment and the client must be prepared. The environment needs to be well lighted and at a comfortable temperature. It must also provide privacy, be free of interruptions, and be quiet enough to allow auscultation as well as easy communication of questions, answers, and instructions between you and the client.

To prepare the client, introduce yourself and describe what the examination will involve. Ask the client about any cultural practices that need to be followed during the examination, and plan accordingly. Reassure the client about the confidentiality of the examination and your desire to keep him as comfortable as possible. Ask the client to immediately report any fatigue or discomfort.

Before starting the examination, provide the client with the opportunity to use the bathroom and to assume a comfortable position. Throughout the examination, drape the client for privacy and position him correctly for the part of the body being examined (Table 10–1).

For the ambulatory client, the physical examination usually starts in the sitting position. For the hospitalized client, the examination is often started with the client lying in bed. You need to plan the examination to avoid having the client change positions any more than necessary while still allowing you to obtain all needed data.

To accurately describe the findings of a physical examination, you need to use terms that have a common meaning to other health care providers. To help you describe the location of the area you are examining, the body is divided by three planes. These planes divide the body into anterior-posterior, inferior-superior, and medial-lateral aspects (Fig. 10–4).

The frontal plane divides the body into anterior and posterior surfaces. The anterior surface is called the ventral surface and the posterior surface is the dorsal surface.

The transverse plane divides the body into inferior and superior aspects. Inferior and superior are used in relation to a point of reference. For example, the knee is inferior to the thigh and superior to the foot. Distal

and proximal are also used in relation to a reference point. Distal means away from, usually with reference to a point of origin. In other words, the hand is distal to the elbow. Proximal means nearer to a point of origin. The elbow is proximal to the hand. The reference point is usually the heart or the thorax.

The sagittal plane divides the body into right and left halves. The sagittal plane is described as the midline. While medial refers to the center of the body and lateral to the sides, the terms medial and lateral are also used in relation to a point of reference. For example, you might describe a lesion as on the lateral aspect of the right thigh two inches distal to the patella.

General Survey

The general survey is the first step in physical assessment. It provides information on the overall state of the client. It begins on first meeting the client and continues through the health history interview and includes the measurement of height, weight, and vital signs. The general survey provides a basic impression of the client derived from overall physical appearance relative to age, body development, height, weight, movement, behavior, and vital signs, which helps guide both the health history and the detailed physical examination.

Inspection of body posture may reveal significant information about the client's emotion and physical status. Assess it as the client enters the examination room or sits on the examination table, on the bed, or in a chair. Observe posture frontally, laterally, and posteriorly.

Record the client's height and weight as parameters of general health status (Fig. 10–5). Measure the height and weight rather than relying on the client's report. However, if it is not possible to weigh and measure the client, record the client's report and note that it is approximate. Medication doses may be calculated based on the recorded height and weight.

A standardized balanced scale is preferable to a spring-loaded scale. This scale can easily be checked for balance at the zero mark each time a client is weighed. More accurate and consistent weights are obtained. Ideally a person is weighed at the same time of the day, with the same clothes, on the same scale, and immediately before eating. To measure a client, be sure the client is standing erect and looking straight ahead. No shoes should be worn for the most accurate measurement.

Scales are available to suspend a bedridden client in a sling, to lay an infant on a platform, to roll a wheelchair on a platform, or even as part of high-tech hospital beds. If sheets, clothes, wheelchairs, or items are weighed with the client, weigh the item separately and subtract the amount for the person's total weight.

Height and weight are important measures in children to determine that growth and development are proceeding at a normal rate. In both children and adults, compare the height and weight to determine

TABLE 10–1
Client Positions for Physical Examination

Position	Description and Use
Dorsal recumbent	Can be used to examine head and neck, anterior thorax, breasts, abdomen, arms, and legs. Turn the client to examine the back and posterior thorax. With client's knees flexed, can be used to relieve strain on the lower back during the examination. (Perineal and vaginal examination can be done in this position.)
Sitting	Client sits on the end of an examination table or the side of a bed. Better position of anterior and posterior chest than dorsal recumbent position. Client will need to lie down for abdominal examination.
Lithotomy	The feet and legs are put in stirrups. Used for vaginal and rectal examination in a female.
Genupectoral (knee-chest)	Used for a rectal examination.
Prone	Can be used to examine the posterior thorax in this position. Most common use is for range of motion in hip.
Sims'	Can be used to examine the posterior thorax. Used as an alternative position for vaginal and rectal examination when lithotomy position is contraindicated.

whether the person is overweight or underweight. This is one indicator of general health and nutrition.

Signs of Acute Distress

The general survey begins with observing the client for obvious signs of distress. These include cyanosis, labored breathing, bleeding, diaphoresis, writhing, moaning, or guarding of a body part. If any of these signs is present, determine whether immediate intervention is needed. If no sign of distress requiring im-

mediate intervention is present, the general survey continues.

Age and Developmental and Nutritional Status

Assess the client in terms of apparent age versus reported age. This assessment is based on signs of aging such as skin changes, gait, posture, muscle strength, and mental alertness. It answers the question, "Does the client look older or younger than actual chronological age?" Obtain height and weight measurements

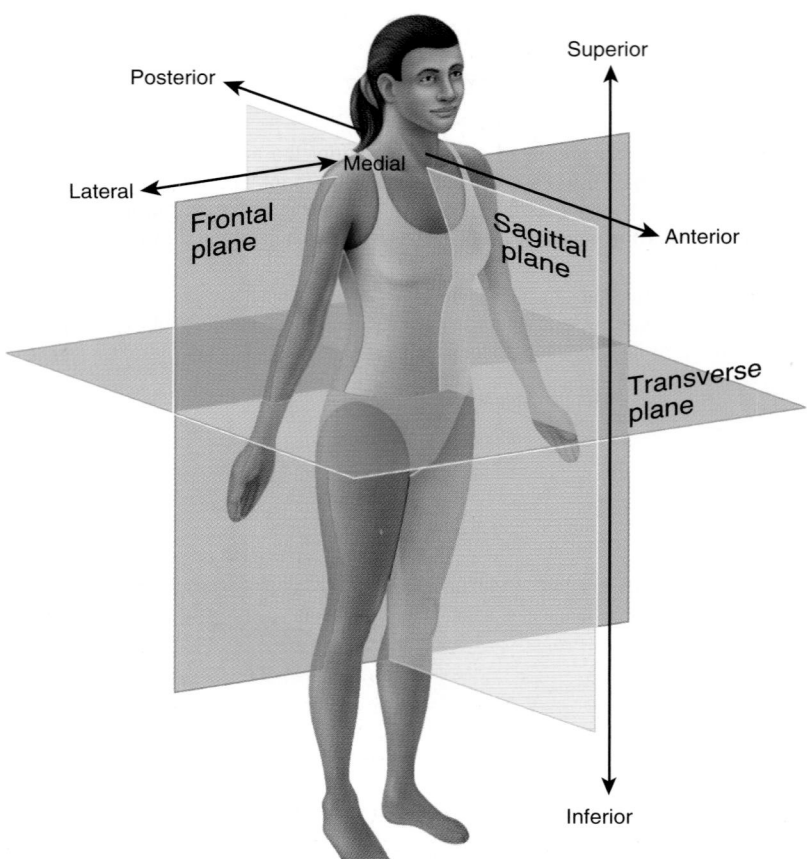

Figure 10–4. The body is divided by three planes. The frontal plane separates the body into anterior and posterior aspects. The transverse plane separates the body into inferior and superior aspects. The sagittal plane runs through the midline and separates the body into left and right halves and lateral and medial aspects.

and note general body shape, muscular development, and fat distribution. Draw an impression regarding the client's apparent nutritional status. Does he seem to be well-nourished, malnourished, obese, thin, emaciated (see Chapter 29)?

Related assessments that are part of the general survey are concerned with sexual development. Note the client's secondary sexual characteristics, such as facial hair, breast size, and voice quality. Are they appropriate for the client's age and gender?

Observe for normal body proportion, the size and symmetry of facial features, facial mobility, length of limbs, and symmetry of body parts. Also observe the symmetry, smoothness, and coordination of movement, as well as the absence of involuntary movement of the head and limbs; posture both sitting and standing; balance on standing and walking; speed, smoothness, and style of gait; and use of assistive devices or prosthetic limbs.

Skin color and condition as well as personal hygiene and dress and the presence of body and breath odors are all components of the general survey. On encountering a person with a body odor, you must consider cultural variation. Typical American values dictate freedom from body odor as the norm. In many other cultures, however, the presence of normal body odor is the norm. For persons of all cultural groups, however, a fecal, urinary, or other than normal body odor is an abnormal finding. Similarly, breath

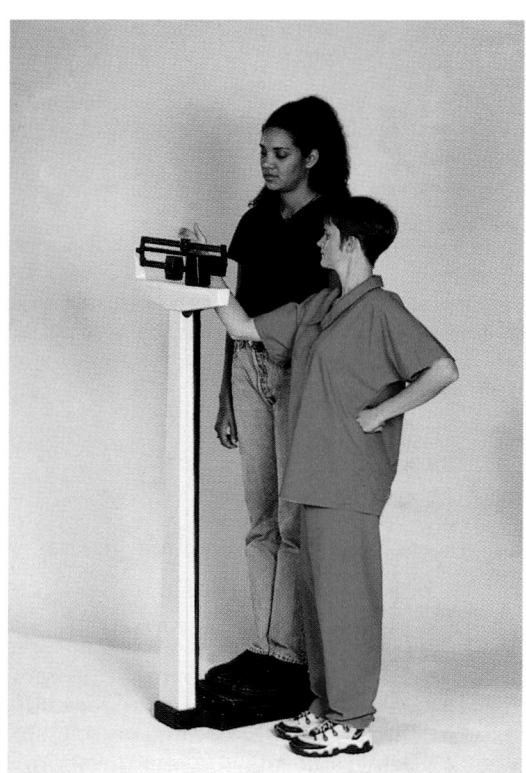

Figure 10–5. In both children and adults, as one indicator of general health status and nutrition, compare height and weight to determine whether the person is overweight or underweight.

odors, such as a sweet smell, or the smell of alcohol, acetone, or ammonia are abnormal findings. Be alert to the excessive use of colognes or perfumes and determine whether they are used to disguise an abnormal odor.

Orientation, Mood, Manner, Affect, and Speech

Assess the client's level of consciousness (Box 10–1). For example, is the client oriented, alert, aware, and able to respond to questions and instructions quickly and appropriately? This information is evident through observation and responses to routine questions in the health history.

Observation of the client's mood, manner, affect, and speech is also a part of the general survey. Mild anxiety with a cooperative, attentive attitude, and with mood and affect appropriate to the situation are normal findings. Abnormal findings include marked nervousness, restlessness, agitation, combative or uncooperative behavior, bizarre mannerisms, apathetic, depressed, or euphoric attitude, and stooped posture. In observing the client's speech, note the speech pattern, pace of speech, use of words, thought pattern, and sentence structure. Also note the tone, clarity, and strength of the voice and whether the client has any speech defects.

Abnormal findings include excessively slow or fast speech; halting, slurred, garbled, or very deliberate speech; an excessively soft or loud voice; or a voice that is weak, hoarse, high-pitched, or monotone. Aphasia, dysphasia, use of inappropriate vocabulary, stuttering, and lisping are also abnormal findings.

Mental Status

The mental status examination provides a detailed description of the client's cognitive functioning at a given time. You can ascertain whether the client understands what is happening and how well the client can cooperate with the treatment plan. The depth of the mental status examination depends on the reason the client is being seen, the relevant medical problems, and the expected goals for treatment. If mental status is part of the chief complaint or related to the chief complaint, then a thorough mental status examination should be conducted. For example, in the confused client the following should be considered in evaluating the client:

The client's general *appearance* may provide a clue to the client's level of functioning. Poor hygiene and grooming can suggest depression, schizophrenia, organic brain disease, or lack of sufficient cognitive functioning to care for the self. Bizarre dressing and make-up may be seen in manic-depressive illness.

Assess whether or not the *behavior* is appropriate for the client's reference group, age, and social situation. Unusual, bizarre, or inappropriate behavior may indicate a mental disturbance.

Assess whether or not the client is able and willing to *cooperate with the interviewer.*

Affect refers to the external expression of emotion attached to ideas or mental representation of ideas. Affect is normally an expression of the internal mood of the person. Assess whether the affect is appropriate for the topic of conversation or situation. Inappropriate affect is inconsistent with content of the client's speech or ideas, such as laughing at a sad story. A flat affect is a lack of emotional expression and is associated with depression.

Assess the *speech* for clarity, choice of words, rate of speech, and any unusual speech patterns. Speech may be slowed in depression or rapid in manic-depressive illness. The person with organic brain damage may have difficulty speaking.

Orientation is the most basic assessment. Ask direct question to determine whether the client knows who he is, where he is, and whether he has some orientation to time (Box 10–2). Orientation to time should take into consideration the normal tendency to lose track of time without the usual cues to the time of day. Most people will normally have some frame of refer-

---

BOX 10–1

DESCRIBING A CLIENT'S LEVEL OF CONSCIOUSNESS

Awake and Alert: The client is aware of the surroundings and can respond appropriately to internal and external stimuli. Awake means not asleep and should not be confused with alert.

Lethargic or Somnolent: Easily drifts off to sleep or is not fully alert even though awake. This person may appear to be asleep but can be aroused with difficulty.

Obtunded: More difficult to arouse than lethargic. Technically refers to someone who is heavily dosed with narcotics and may not only be difficult to arouse but also may not be breathing adequately.

Stupor, Semi-Coma, Comatose: A state of almost complete unconsciousness. May respond to strong stimuli such as loud noise, shaking, or pain. These terms may represent a continuum, with stupor being the most arousable; however, they are hard to distinguish. For this reason, record precisely the observations you make, such as spontaneous movement, opening eyes, attempts to speak, or level of pain that elicits a response.

Coma: A state of unconsciousness from which the client cannot be aroused even by painful stimulus. Painful stimulus is applied by rubbing deeply on the chest. If there is no response, the coma is deep.

Orientation: If the mental status is not certain, ask the person to identify time, place, and person. Ask the client to state his name, where he is, and what day it is.

BOX 10–2

BRIEF MENTAL STATUS EXAMINATION

Ask the client to respond to the following instructions and questions:

- State your full name.
- Where are we? Hospital? City? State?
- What is the date today? Month? Year?
- What day of the week is it?
- I am going to name three objects and I want you to repeat them back to me when I ask you.
- Where do you live? Address? City? State?
- How old are you?
- Name the three objects I listed for you.
- Count backward from 100.

---

ence like it is after lunch or night time. However, not knowing the day of the week may be a function of a lifestyle in which keeping up with the day of the week is not important.

Cognitive functioning refers to the client's patterns of thinking. Assess for logic, relevance, organization, and coherence of the pattern of thinking.

Ask the client if he has any problems with *memory* or concentration or if he has noticed any changes in memory. Assess the recent and remote memory. Recent memory is assessed by asking the client if he remembers events, such as what was eaten for the evening meal or what occurred on a recent news program. Remote memory is generally considered to be memory of events from 6 months or more in the past. The client's birth date, names of children, and names of past presidents may serve as reference points.

Intellectual functioning includes abstract thinking, concentration, content and process of thinking, perceptions, social judgment, and insight.

- *Abstract thinking* is frequently assessed by giving the person a proverb and asking what it means. The client who can do abstract thinking will give the nonliteral meaning.
- *Concentration* is tested by asking the person to remember a series of numbers or unconnected words and asking him to repeat them later in the examination.
- *Thought* is examined for content and process. Abnormality in content includes looking for delusions. Abnormalities of process means that associations between thoughts are vague, or thoughts are loosely connected, poorly organized, or illogical.
- *Perception* is the ability to see the environment as it is; assessment includes asking about illusions and hallucinations. Illusion is misinterpreting external sensory stimuli. Hallucinations are false perceptions of any of the five senses: vision, hearing, taste, touch, or smell.

- *Social judgment* is whether or not the client can compare and evaluate alternatives, make and carry out reasonable decisions, and behave in an appropriate manner for a given social situation.
- *Insight* refers to the client's ability to evaluate and understand the events and behavior that resulted in the present situation.

Vital Signs

The final component of the general survey is vital signs: temperature, pulse, respiratory rate, and blood pressure. Vital signs are an important determinant of the person's overall health.

Assessment of the Skin, Hair, and Nails

Assessment of the skin requires that you be able to recognize a vast array of normal variations in skin color, tone, distribution of pigmentation, effects of the sun, hair growth, and distribution of hair. Physical assessment of the skin, hair, and nails involves the following activities:

- Inspecting the skin for color, cleanliness, hair distribution, and presence of lesions
- Palpating the skin to determine moisture, temperature, texture, mobility, and turgor
- Inspecting the hair for quantity, distribution, color, and cleanliness
- Checking the texture of the hair
- Inspecting the scalp for cleanliness, parasites, and lesions
- Inspecting the fingernails and toenails for color, shape, contour, smoothness, uniformity of thickness, and presence of lesions

Skin

APPEARANCE

To inspect and palpate the skin, expose and cleanse areas as needed. Use good, preferably natural, light to avoid distortion of color. Make the room temperature comfortable to prevent color or other changes due to excessive heat or cold. In assessing skin color, note general color as well as local or patchy variations.

Normally skin is intact, free of lesions, and pink toned in light-skinned persons and light to dark brown or olive in dark-skinned persons with an underlying healthy glow. Light-toned lips, palms, nail beds, and soles are common among dark-skinned persons, as are areas of blue-black discoloration over the sacrum and pigmented spots on the nail beds and in the sclera.

Abnormalities of skin color include pallor, cyanosis, flushing, and yellowing. Pallor, which appears as a loss of red tones in dark skin, is best seen in the nail beds, lips, oral mucous membranes, and palpebral conjunctivae. Cyanosis or blueness in light skin is seen as ash gray in dark skin. Central cyanosis is best seen in lips, buccal mucosa, and the tongue. Peripheral cyanosis is best observed in the nail beds and in the skin of the arms and legs. Jaundice (yellow skin from liver disease) is seen in the bulbar conjunctiva, lips, and hard palate as well as the skin.

LESIONS

Many different types of lesions occur in the skin. A **lesion** is a wound, injury, or pathological change in the body. A thorough description of a lesion is useful in determining whether the lesion is primary or secondary and whether it is benign or malignant. A primary lesion arises from the original source, condition, or set of symptoms in a disease process. A secondary lesion arises as a result of complications from the primary condition. The characteristics of a lesion may help determine the nature of an injury or of the disease process. Observe the lesion for size, shape, and color. Then palpate to determine whether it is hard, soft, freely mobile with the skin, or attached to underlying structures. Also palpate for temperature. The various types of lesions are illustrated in Figure 10–6.

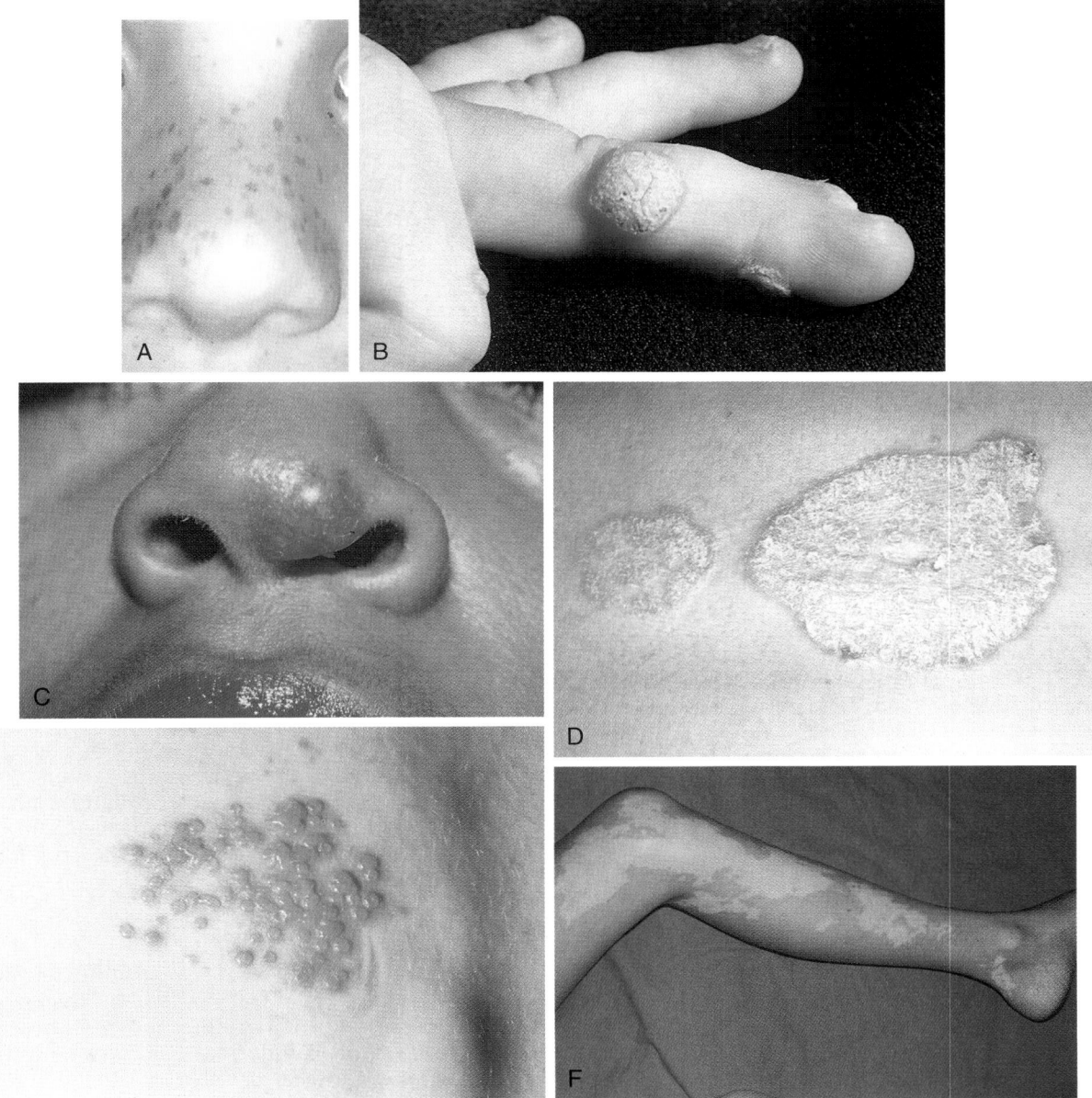

Figure 10–6. Examples of skin lesions. A, macules (freckles); B, papule (common wart); C, nodule (sarcoidosis); D, plaque (psoriasis); E, vesicles and bullae (herpes simplex); F, patches (vitiligo). (A from Hurwitz, S. [1993]. Clinical pediatric dermatology: A textbook of skin disorders of childhood and adolescence [2nd ed.]. Philadelphia: W.B. Saunders; B, D, and E from Lookingbill, D.P., & Marks, J.G., Jr. [1993]. Principles of dermatology [2nd ed.]. Philadelphia: W.B. Saunders; C and F from Callen, J.P., Greer, K.E., Hood, A.F., Paller, A.S., & Swinyer, L.J. [1993]. Color atlas of dermatology. Philadelphia: W.B. Saunders.)

Illustration continued on following page

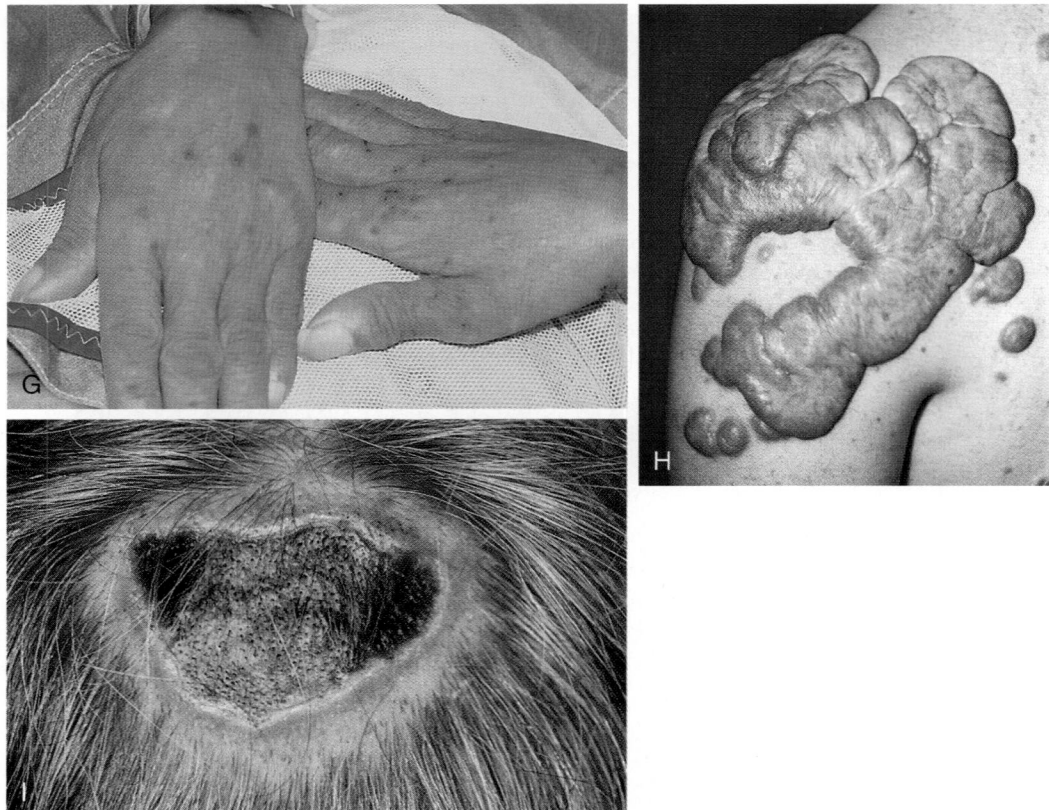

Figure 10–6 *Continued.* G, petechiae; H, keloid; I, necrosis (pressure necrosis after coronary artery bypass). (I from Callen, J.P., Greer, K.E., Hood, A.F., Paller, A.S., & Swinyer, L.J. [1993]. Color atlas of dermatology. Philadelphia: W.B. Saunders; G Courtesy of Dr. Beverly A. Johnson, Washington, D.C.; H from Ignatavicius, D.D., Workman, M.L., & Mishler, M.A. [1999]. Medical-surgical nursing across the health care continuum [3rd ed.]. Philadelphia: W.B. Saunders.)

MOISTURE, TEXTURE, AND TEMPERATURE

Assess the moistness and texture of the skin using the pads of your fingers. Normally, the skin is dry, soft, smooth, and even. Excessively dry, damp, sweaty, oily, or rough, thick, uneven skin is an abnormal finding. Check skin temperature with the back of your hand. It is normally warm or cool, not hot or cold. General skin temperature as well as temperature of any reddened areas should be checked bilaterally.

TURGOR AND MOBILITY

Skin **turgor** is a reflection of the skin's elasticity, measured as the time it takes for the skin to return to normal after being pinched lightly between the thumb and forefinger. To check skin turgor and mobility, pinch and lift a fold of skin on the hand or forearm, over the sternum, or over the clavicle. Observe the ease of moving the skin and the speed with which it returns to its original position (Fig. 10–7). If mobility is normal, the skin moves easily. If turgor is normal, the pinched up skin fold immediately returns to normal position. Turgor is abnormal if the skinfold remains tented up (elevated) for more than 3 seconds. If you have doubts about the results obtained on the hand or forearm in an elderly client with loose skin, use the skin over the sternum.

Hair and Scalp

To assess the hair and scalp, ask the client to remove any wig, hairpiece, or other head covering being worn. Observe the quantity, distribution, and color of the hair, then palpate the hair to determine its texture. Abnormal findings include patchy or sudden hair loss, and brittle hair. Next, part the hair in several areas and inspect the scalp. It should be smooth, clean, and intact. Look for discolorations, lumps, scaliness, or open areas. Inspect the base of the hair shaft for nits, which are tiny, white, opaque eggs of head lice found attached to the hair shafts. Palpate the skull for lumps or tender areas.

Nails

Inspect the fingernails and toenails to determine their color, shape, contour, smoothness, thickness, and cleanliness. Abnormal findings are described by comparing the nail to a normal nail. Normally they are clean, curved, and hard, with a pink to light brown nail bed. The angle between the nail and its base is 160 degrees. Abnormal findings include soft or brittle nails, inflammation, and pale or cyanotic nail beds. Cleanliness and grooming of nails are a cue to hygienic practices. Examples of abnormal changes in nails include

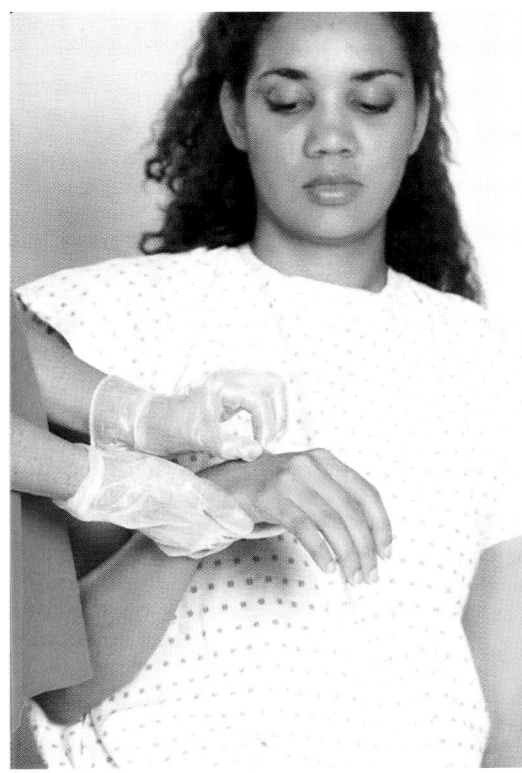

Figure 10–7. Checking skin turgor and mobility.

spoon-shaped nails, Beau's lines, splinter hemorrhages, paronychia, and clubbed nails (Fig. 10–8).

Assessment of the Head and Neck

Physical assessment of the head and face involves the following activities:

- Observing the size, symmetry, position, and movement of the head as a whole and of the facial features
- Palpating the skull
- Checking for tenderness of the temporal artery
- Checking the function of the temporomandibular joint
- Checking the function of cranial nerve VII (facial)
- Checking the function of cranial nerve V (trigeminal).

Head and Face

Assessment of the head and face begins with observation of size, position, and symmetry. The head should be normal in size, not abnormally small (microcephalic) or large for the person's age. In the elderly, the nose and brows are often prominent and the lower face may appear small, with the mouth shrunken if the person is edentulous (without teeth).

The head should be in a normal upright position, not tilted backward, forward, or to the left or right side. It should also be symmetrical in shape, that is, the

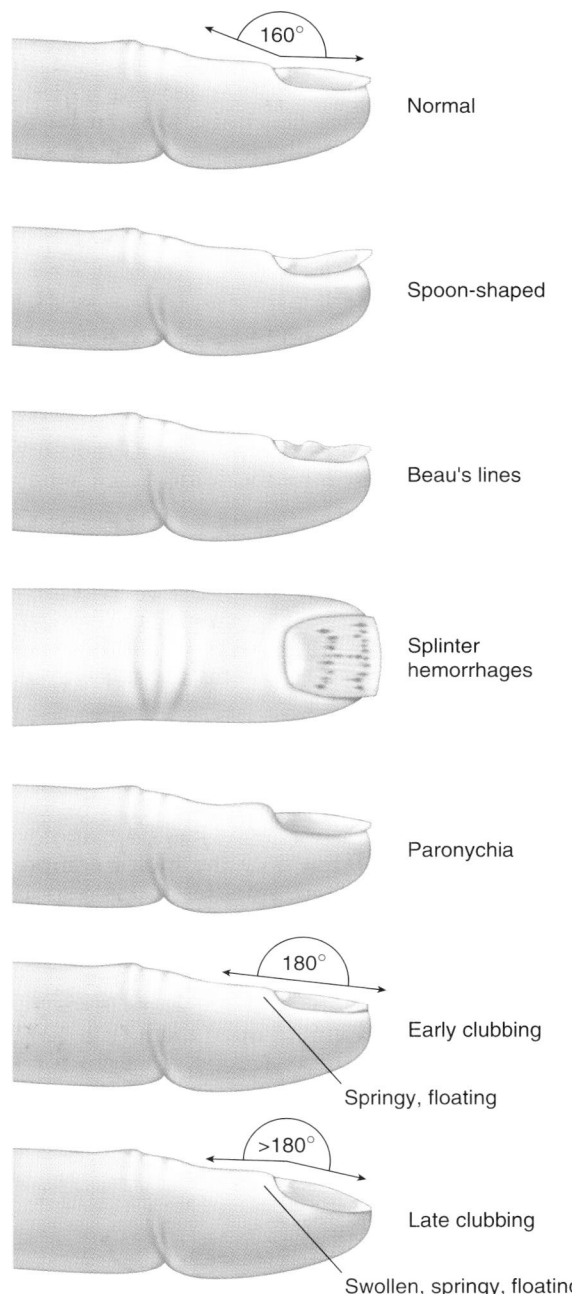

Figure 10–8. Comparing normal and abnormal nails. Examples of abnormal changes in nails include spoon-shaped nails, Beau's lines, splinter hemorrhages, paronychia, and clubbing.

same on the right and the left side. The eyebrows, palpebral fissures, and nasolabial folds should be equal in size, shape, and position. The sides of the mouth should be similar in appearance and free of any abnormal one-sided droop or sag. Facial movements and expressions should be free, variable, and symmetrical. Distorted, absent, or asymmetrical movement or expression is abnormal. Involuntary movement is also abnormal, although in the elderly mild rhythmic tremors are common.

Temporal Artery

The temporal artery is not routinely assessed. To do so, palpate the temporal artery, located superior to the temporalis muscle. The pulsation can be felt in front of the ear. Normally it is nontender, smooth, and pliable. Tenderness or hardness is abnormal. The temporal arteries are often prominent and tortuous in the elderly.

Temporomandibular Joint

Examine the temporomandibular joint to determine its range of motion and to check for any swelling or tenderness. To do this, place the tips of your index fingers on each side of the client's face just in front of the tragus of the ear. Ask the client to open his mouth while your fingertips slide into the joint space when the mouth opens.

Normally the mouth will open 3 to 6 cm and the lower jaw can move laterally 1 to 2 cm. Snapping or popping sounds when the mouth is opened are common and not pathological. Restricted motion, deviation of the lower jaw to one side when the mouth is opened, pain, or crepitus (crackling or rubbing sound) are abnormal findings.

Cranial Nerve VII

Cranial nerve VII (facial nerve) is routinely tested. It is a mixed nerve, which means it has both motor and sensory components, but only the motor component, which innervates the facial muscles and is responsible for closing the eye and for labial speech, is routinely tested. To test motor function of cranial nerve VII, ask the client to smile, frown, raise his eyebrows, show his upper and lower teeth, and keep his eyes tightly closed while you attempt to open them (Fig. 10–9). As the client performs these actions, observe for symmetrical strength and movement. Ask the client to puff out his checks. Then use your finger pads to press the

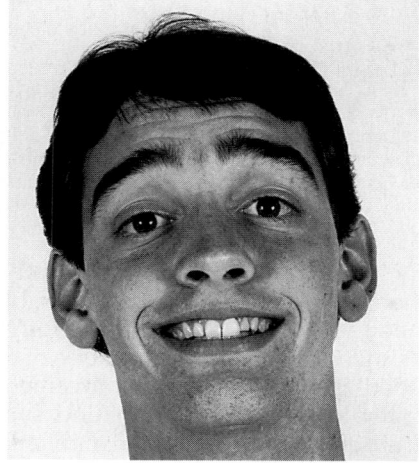

Figure 10–9. Assessing cranial nerve VII function. (From Jarvis, C. [2000]. Health assessment and physical examination [3rd ed.]. Philadelphia: W.B. Saunders.)

puffed cheeks in. Air should escape equally from both cheeks with this maneuver.

Cranial Nerve V

Cranial nerve V (trigeminal nerve) is also a mixed nerve. Its motor component innervates the muscles of mastication while its sensory component is responsible for sensation in the face, scalp, cornea, and the mucous membranes of the mouth and nose. Its motor function is tested by asking the client to clench his or her teeth together while you push down on the chin to try to separate the jaws. Normally the jaw cannot be separated and muscle strength is equal on both sides of the jaw.

Sensory function of cranial nerve V is tested in two ways. First, ask the client to close his eyes and then touch his chin, cheeks, and forehead with a sterile pin or cotton ball. Ask the client to describe what is felt and where it is felt. The client should be able to distinguish sensations of light touch, dullness, and sharpness and identify their location as on the forehead, cheeks, or chin. Absent, decreased, or unequal sensation is abnormal.

The second test of sensory function involves touching a wisp of cotton to the cornea and observing for the normal blink in response to the touch. For this test, contact lenses must be removed, and the client looks straight ahead while the cotton wisp is brought in from the side to prevent the natural blinking response. This test is often omitted during a normal screening examination.

Eye

People under age 40 should have their eyes tested every 3 to 5 years. After age 40 the eyes should be examined every 2 years. More frequent examinations are needed if the person has hypertension, diabetes, glaucoma, other eye disease or bleeding disorders. Physical assessment of the eye involves the following activities:

- Testing visual acuity for distance vision and near vision
- Inspecting the outer eye structures, including lids, lashes, sclera, conjunctiva, cornea, iris, and pupil
- Testing pupillary response to light
- Testing pupillary response to light and accommodation
- Checking extraocular muscular function
- Checking visual fields
- Examining the ocular fundus

DISTANCE VISION

Visual acuity is the clearness of the visual image or the degree of detail the eye can discern in an image, which allows the eye to discriminate between forms. The Snellen chart is used to screen for acuity of distance vision. This chart consists of lines of print that become progressively smaller as one reads from the top to the bottom of the chart. There are three versions of the

Snellen chart: one for the preschool child, which has commonly recognized symbols instead of letters; the Snellen E chart, which can be used for the preschool child or others who cannot read; and the standard Snellen chart, which consists of random letters.

The client is positioned 20 feet in front of the chart and is directed to cover one eye with a cover card and read the smallest line of print possible with the other. Acuity is recorded as 20 (distance from the chart) over the number printed by the side of the smallest line of print the client can read with at least 50% accuracy. This is followed by a minus sign and the number of letters of this line that the client read incorrectly.

An example is 20/80-1, which means that the client was able to read with one error at 20 feet a line of print which a person with normal vision could read at 80 feet. This procedure is repeated for the other eye. If corrective lenses, glasses, or contacts are worn, distance vision is tested both with and without them and CC (with correction) or SC (without correction) is recorded after the acuity ratio. Normal acuity is 20/20. Legal blindness is defined as 20/200 with correction in either eye. If the client cannot see any print on the Snellen chart, finger counting ability, hand motion, and light perception are tested.

NEAR VISION

Acuity of near vision is tested in adults over age 40 and in those who present with a complaint of difficulty reading. This is done by asking the client to read lines of print of different sizes on a Jaeger chart, which the client holds 14 inches in front of his or her face. A Jaeger card is similar to a Snellen chart, but the print size is scaled to equal the print size at 20 feet when read at 14 inches. Results are recorded as the smallest line the client can read, that is, as J1 (smallest letters) through J12 (largest letters). Normal near vision acuity is reading J1 with each eye without moving the card or hesitating in reading. Near vision acuity can also be checked by having the client hold and read any printed materials at a comfortable distance from the face. If this type of test is used, the type of material and the distance it is held from the face is recorded.

OUTER EYE STRUCTURES

To examine the structures of the eye, begin with the outer structures and work your way inward. Inspection of the outer eye structures begins with noting the position of the eyelids in relationship to the globe. Normally, no sclera (white) is visible between the upper lid and the iris. The lids are also observed for the presence of abnormalities such as ptosis (drooping of the upper lid), incomplete closure, redness, swelling, and presence of discharge or other lesions. The eyelashes are observed for even distribution and outward curve. Uneven distribution, inward growth touching the globe, crusting, or other lesions are abnormal findings.

The globe, conjunctiva, sclera, iris, and pupil are also inspected. The right and left globes should be aligned and neither sunken nor protruding. The sclera

and conjunctiva are inspected by separating the lids between the index finger and the thumb and asking the client to look up, down, and to each side. The palpebral (eyelid) conjunctiva is inspected by everting the lower lid with your thumb while asking the client to look up. The sclera should be smooth, moist, and glossy and the conjunctiva clear, pale pink, and glistening, often with small blood vessels visible. The irises should be similar in shape, color, clarity, and markings. The pupils should be 3 to 5 mm in diameter, round, and equal in size in both eyes. Excessively dilated or constricted pupils as well as irregular or unequal pupils are abnormal. The clarity of the cornea is checked by shining a light from the side onto each eye and observing for cloudiness or opacities.

PUPILLARY RESPONSE TO LIGHT AND ACCOMMODATION

Pupillary response to light is tested by bringing a bright light in from the side to directly in front of each pupil while the client is looking straight ahead into the distance. The pupil into which the light is shone should constrict. This is called the direct response. Simultaneously, the other pupil should also constrict. This is called the consensual response. Speed and degree of constriction should be equal in both pupils and should be followed by equal dilation. Absence of constriction or an asymmetrical response is abnormal. Degree of constriction is recorded as millimeters before and after exposure to the light and speed is described as brisk or sluggish.

Accommodation is adjustment of the eye for seeing objects at various distances. To test accommodation, hold a finger or an object such as a pen 10 to 15 cm (4–5 inches) in front of the client's nose. Then tell the client to look ahead into the distance and then to quickly look at the finger or other object. If accommodation is normal, both eyes converge (move medially) and the pupils constrict. Normal pupillary findings are recorded as PERRLA, which means "pupils equal, round, and reactive to light and accommodation."

EXTRAOCULAR MUSCLE FUNCTION

Extraocular muscle function is tested by checking for parallel gaze, coordinated eye movement, and convergence. Checking for parallel gaze, also referred to as checking the corneal light reflex, is done by shining a light straight into the client's eyes from a distance of 31 cm (12 inches) while the client looks straight ahead. Normally the light is reflected on or just medial to the pupil in both eyes. Reflection of the light in a different location in each eye is abnormal.

Coordinated eye movement is checked by holding a finger 31 cm (12 in) in front of the client and moving it from the center to one of the eight locations, holding a moment, and then returning it to center (Fig. 10–10). This action is repeated for each of the eight locations while the eyes are observed for normal parallel movement. As the gaze moves up and down, the upper lid is observed and should be seen to overlap the iris at all times. Both eyes should remain parallel as the finger is tracked through the eight locations. Weakness of ex-

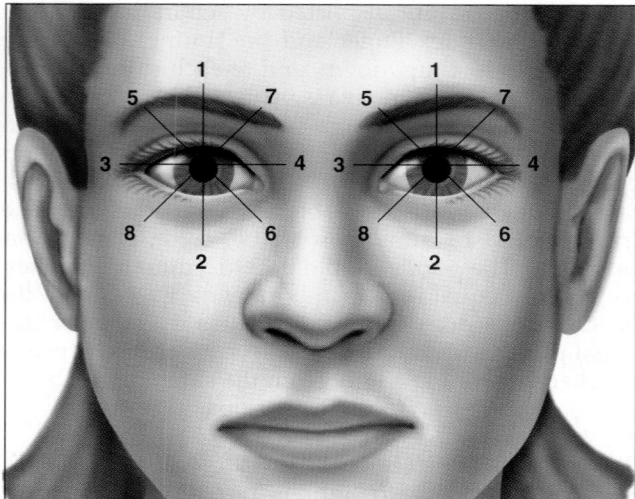

Figure 10–10. The eight cardinal directions of gaze, which are used in checking for coordinated eye movement.

traocular muscles or cranial nerve dysfunction will result in nonparallel tracking. Additionally, you should look for nystagmus, which is involuntary, rapid, rhythmic movement of the eyeball.

Convergence is then tested by asking the client to watch your finger as you move it from out in front of the client's eyes in toward the bridge of his nose. The iris of both eyes should converge or move toward midline as the finger moves toward the nose.

VISUAL FIELDS

The visual field is the entire area seen by the eye in a fixed position. Visual fields are checked by means of a confrontation test. Position yourself in front of the client so that your faces are at the same level. Then direct the client to cover his right eye while looking with his left eye into your right eye. Then cover your left eye and bring a raised finger, pen, or other object held at arm's length between yourself and the client from several points in the right periphery into the visual field. Tell the client to say "Now" when the object comes into view. This should be at the same time the object enters your field of vision. Thus, you can use your visual field to test your client's. This gross check of visual fields is repeated for the other eye. Normal findings are recorded as "Visual fields full to confrontation." Normal results are about 50 degrees upward, 90 degrees temporal, 70 degrees down, and 60 degrees nasal.

OCULAR FUNDUS

You can examine the inner eye by directing a light through the window of the pupil to view the lens, anterior chamber, vitreous, and the ocular fundus. The examination of the inner eye (funduscopic examination) is not routinely performed by registered nurses. However, it may be performed by advanced practice nurses and other nurses who have received special training.

The ocular fundus is the back portion of the interior of the eyeball visible through the pupil by examination with an ophthalmoscope. The **ophthalmoscope** is an instrument used to visualize the retina including the optic disk, macula, and retinal blood vessels through the pupil. The examination is done in a darkened room and begins with you about 15 inches away from the client and slightly to the side of the client's line of vision. As the light beam from the ophthalmoscope is shone on the pupil of the eye to be examined, an orange-red glow called the red reflex appears in the pupil. This glow should be uninterrupted and fill the pupil. Dark shadows or black dots interrupting the glow are abnormal.

The client must be able to cooperate and hold the eyes still by looking at a distant object identified by you and that holds the gaze about 20 degrees upward and to the side. Hold the ophthalmoscope in your right hand and use your right eye to examine the client's right eye (Fig. 10–11). The ophthalmoscope is used as an appendage to your own eye. To prevent losing the fundus during the examination, stabilize the ophthalmoscope on your eyebrow or nose and move the head and instrument as one unit. Rest the index finger on the lens wheel to easily focus during the examination and your thumb on your lower jaw. The light should be adjusted to maximum if tolerated by the client.

The ophthalmoscope contains a set of lenses to control the units of measurement (dioptrics), thus focusing for vision from near to far. The black numbers are positive dioptrics for focusing on objects nearer in space and the red numbers are negative dioptrics for focusing on objects further away.

Start with the lens set at zero and adjust upward for better focus on details found in the examination. Begin about 10 inches from the client at an angle of 15 degrees lateral to the person's line of vision. When you have found the red glow (the reflection of the light off the inner retina), move closer to the client until your heads are almost touching. If you lose the red glow, move back, relocate the glow, and move forward again.

As you advance, adjust the lens to plus 6 and note any opacities in the lens. These appear as black areas

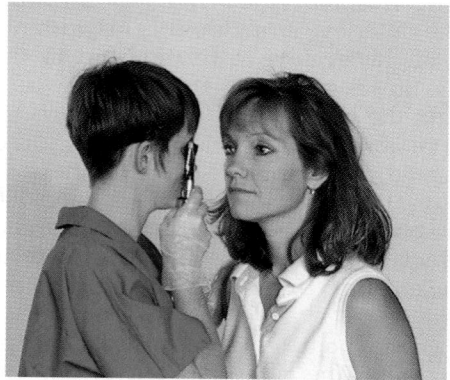

Figure 10–11. Ophthalmoscopic examination.

or dark shadows interrupting the red reflex. Continue to move forward until your forehead almost touches the forehead of the person you are examining. Adjust the lens setting (diopter) to bring the fundus into focus. When both you and the client have normal vision, this should be at 0. Adjust to red dioptrics for nearsighted eyes and to black for farsighted eyes.

Begin the examination of the optic fundus by finding the optic disk (Fig. 10–12). The optic disk is an area on the nasal side of each retina. The blood vessels of the retina converge at the optic disk. If you do not see the optic disk, track a blood vessel as it grows larger and it will lead you to the optic disk. Outside the optic disk, the retina is light red to dark brown-red with the shade varying in accord with skin color.

Assess the structures in the ocular fundus: optic disc, retinal vessels, general background, and macula. The optic disk is normally yellow-orange to creamy-pink in color with distinct margins except at the nasal edge. Pallor, hyperemia, irregular shape, or blurred margins are abnormal findings. Retinal vessels visualized should consist of one artery and vein passing to each quadrant of the retina with a progressive decrease in the diameter of both veins and arteries as they extend toward the periphery. Arteries are brighter red than veins. Abnormal findings would include the absence of major arteries, constricted arteries, dilated veins, and extreme tortuousness. The general background should be free of lesions such as hemorrhage or exudate. The macula lutea is an irregular yellowish depression on the retina, lateral to and slightly below the optic disk. It receives and analyzes light only from the center of the visual field. At the macula, which is about 1 DD (one disk diameter, i.e.,

the size of the diameter of the optic disk), the color may be darker than the rest of the retina, but all areas should be free of clumped pigment, which occurs with aging, trauma, or retinal detachment. Hemorrhage or exudate may represent macular degeneration. For further detail on examination of the ocular fundus, a specialty text on physical assessment should be consulted.

Ear

Physical assessment of the ear involves the following activities:

- Inspecting and palpating the external ear
- Inspecting the external auditory meatus
- Using an otoscope to examine the external auditory canal and the tympanic membrane (eardrum)
- Testing the acuity of hearing (cranial nerve VIII)

EXTERNAL EAR

Inspection of the external ears involves noting their placement on the sides of the head, their alignment with each other, and their size, shape, symmetry, and skin color. The top of the pinna (the projecting part of the ear; also called the auricle) is normally level with the outer corner of the eye and the whole ear angled at less than 10 degrees toward the occiput. The skin of the external ear should be the same color as the face and should be intact, smooth, and free of drainage or lesions. In the elderly, ear lobes may be pendulous and coarse and stiff hairs may be present on the external ear.

Next, the external ear is palpated to identify nodules or other irregularities. The pinna is moved up and down, the tragus (the cartilaginous projection anterior to the ear canal) is pressed, and the area behind the ear is pressed with normal findings being no pain or tenderness on manipulation. The external auditory meatus is inspected for redness, swelling, discharge, and foreign body, which, if present, constitute abnormal findings. The size of the opening is noted and should be unobstructed.

EXTERNAL AUDITORY CANAL

The external auditory canal is examined using an otoscope fitted with the largest speculum that can be inserted comfortably into the auditory canal. An **otoscope** is a hand-held instrument used to examine the external ear, the eardrum, and, through the eardrum, the ossicles of the middle ear. It consists of a light, a magnifying lens, a speculum, and sometimes a device for insufflation.

With the client in a sitting position, move to the side and slightly to the back of the ear to be examined. Ask the client to tip his head toward the shoulder on the opposite side (Fig. 10–13). Grasp the top of the pinna and pull it up and slightly away from the head with your nondominant hand. This pull straightens the ear canal in the adult and is maintained throughout the examination. In the infant, the pinna is pulled downward since the canal is directed downward.

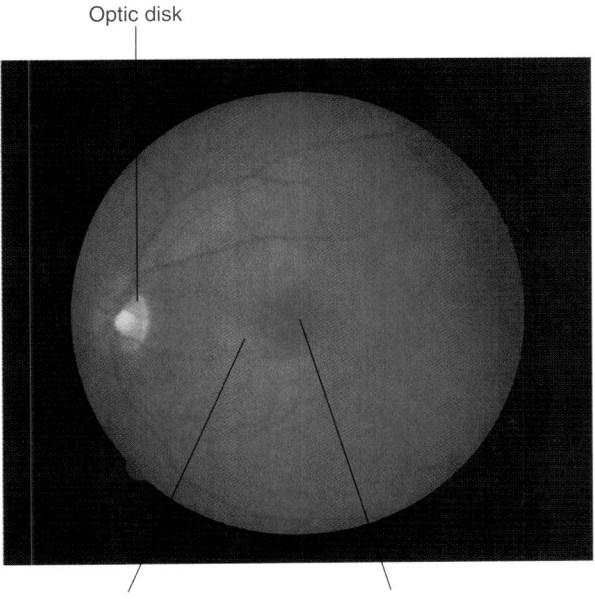

Optic disk

Macula lutea   Fovea centralis

Figure 10–12. Normal ocular fundus, as seen on ophthalmoscopic examination. Note the location of the optic disk. (Courtesy of Dr. Harry Kaplan and Dr. Lawrence P. Roach, Philadelphia, PA.)

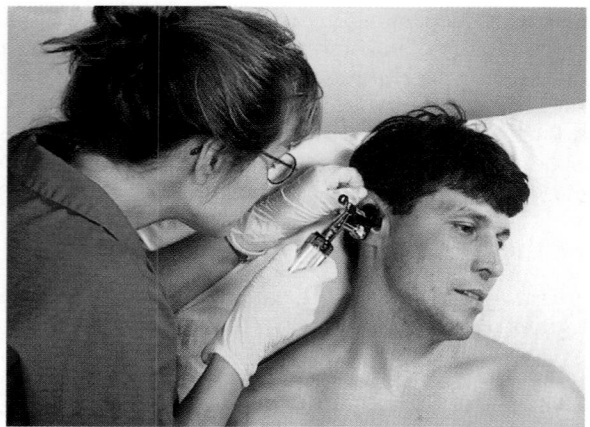

Figure 10–13. Otoscopic examination.

The otoscope is commonly held in an upside down position in the dominant hand and the hand is kept firmly braced against the side of the client's head so that if the head moves so does the otoscope, thus preventing accidental trauma to the auditory canal. The speculum is slowly inserted at a slightly downward and forward angle approximately ½ inch into the auditory canal. Because of its sensitivity to pain, avoid touching the medial wall of the canal. Watch the insertion and then put your eye to the otoscope.

Once the speculum is inserted, the canal can be observed. If you cannot see anything but the wall of the ear canal, angle the otoscope slightly toward the client's nose. You may need to rotate the otoscope to see all of the eardrum.

Normally, the walls are pink and uniform, with small to moderate amounts of cerumen present. Cerumen or ear wax is moist and honey-colored to dark brown or black in most white or black individuals and dry, gray, and flaky in most Asians and Native Americans. Large amounts of ear wax, swelling, redness, discharge, foreign bodies, or other lesions are abnormal, as are marked pain on insertion of the speculum and foul odor. Sometimes you will have to remove ear wax for good visualization. Ear irrigations are discussed in Chapter 43.

TYMPANIC MEMBRANE

Following inspection of the external auditory canal, the tympanic membrane (eardrum) is also inspected with the otoscope and the positions of the handle of the malleus, the umbo, the short process, and the cone of light are noted. The tympanic membrane separates the external and middle ear and is tilted obliquely to the ear canal. Normally the tympanic membrane is intact, pearly gray, shiny, translucent, and conical, although in the elderly it may be whiter, duller, and thicker than in the younger adult.

Assess for landmarks. The cone of light at 5 o'clock in the right ear and 7 o'clock in the left ear is a reflection of the otoscope light. The malleus is the primary landmark. The short process of the malleus stands out as a knob. The manubrium or the handle of the malleus extends downward from the short process to the

umbo (Fig. 10–14). Mobility of the eardrum is assessed by having the client hold the nose and swallow; the membrane should be seen to flutter. Abnormal findings include perforations, scarring, dullness, blue, red, or amber coloring, retraction with accentuated landmarks, bulging with partially occluded landmarks, or a fluid level in the middle ear.

HEARING ACUITY

Hearing is mediated by the acoustic nerve, which is cranial nerve VIII. Testing of hearing acuity involves checking gross acuity, checking ability to lateralize sound, and comparing air and bone conduction of sound.

Gross hearing is evaluated during the course of normal conversation. The voice test is a more specific measure of gross hearing acuity. For this test, occlude one of the client's ears by pressing on the tragus with your index finger to occlude the auditory canal. Stand one to two feet from the client's ear. With the client's eyes closed or your mouth covered to prevent lip reading, exhale and whisper words of two equally accented syllables toward the ear being tested. The same procedure is used for the other ear. Normally the client can repeat the whispered words accurately. Repeat with spoken words. Whispered words are higher tones than spoken words and are the more common lost tones.

Lateralization of sound is evaluated by means of the Weber test. For this test, set a 512 or 1024 Hz tuning fork lightly vibrating by tapping the tines against your hand. The base of the tuning fork is then placed in the middle of the top of the client's head or in the middle of the forehead. Ask whether the client hears

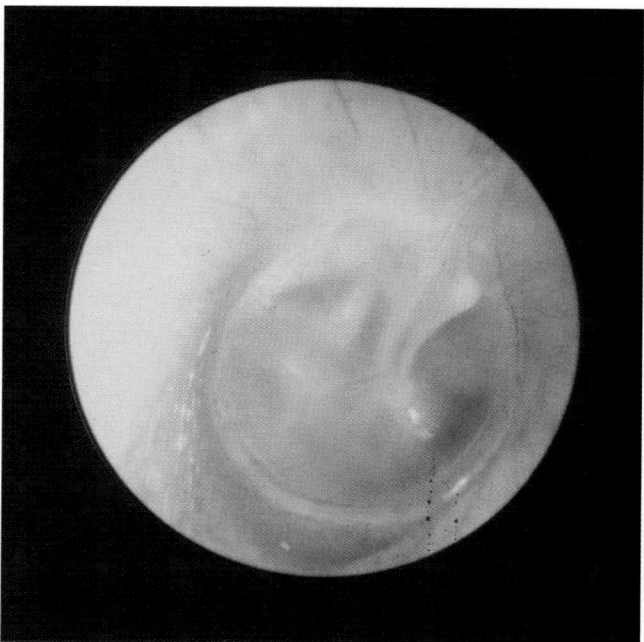

Figure 10–14. Normal tympanic membrane as seen on otoscopic examination. (From Swartz, M.H. [1994]. Textbook of physical diagnosis: History and examination [2nd ed.]. Philadelphia: W.B. Saunders.)

the tone only in the right ear, only in the left ear, equally in both, or more in one ear than in the other (specify). Normally the tone is heard equally in both ears. If a conductive hearing loss exists, the tone is lateralized to the affected ear because the normal ear is more likely to be distracted by room noises. In the case of sensorineural hearing loss, the sound is lateralized to the unaffected ear.

Air and bone conduction are compared by means of the Rinne test. In this test, a lightly vibrating tuning fork is placed on the client's mastoid process and the client is asked to indicate when the tone is no longer heard. When the client indicates the tone is no longer heard, quickly move the tuning fork so that the tines are in front of the auditory meatus. Then ask the client if a tone is heard; if so, have him indicate when it ends. Then repeat the procedure for the other ear.

Normally air conduction is twice as long as bone conduction, so the client is able to hear the tone when the tines are placed in front of the auditory meatus for as long as the tone was heard when the tuning fork was on the mastoid process. In sensorineural hearing loss, air conduction is longer than bone conduction but not twice as long. It is equal to or shorter than bone conduction in conductive hearing loss.

Nose and Sinuses

Physical assessment of the nose and sinuses involves the following activities:

- Checking patency of the nares
- Inspecting the outside and the inside of the nose
- Palpating the sinuses for tenderness
- Testing the function of cranial nerve I

NOSE

Observe the external aspect of the nose for abnormalities such as asymmetry, lesions, or signs of inflammation. Check the patency of the nares by asking the client to close his mouth and then occluding each naris in turn while feeling for exhaled air from the nonoccluded naris. Next, inspect the inside of the nose using an otoscope fitted with a short, wide nasal speculum and magnifying lens. With the client's head tilted back and the handle of the otoscope held to the side, insert the speculum 1 cm into each naris without touching the nasal septum. Direct it back and somewhat upward to allow both the upper and lower nose to be seen.

Normally the mucosal lining of the nose is intact, smooth, and deep pink; the nasal septum is straight, and the turbinates are smooth and colored like the rest of the mucosa. The nasal mucosa is redder than the oral mucosa. The septum is somewhat deviated in most adults. The lateral wall of the nose consists of inferior, middle, and superior turbinates. The inferior turbinate is the largest and lies like a finger along the lower lateral wall of the nose.

Pale, bright red, or gray mucosa is abnormal. Bogginess, exudate, swelling, bleeding, ulcers or fissures, presence of polyps, or a perforation or deviation of the septum are other abnormal findings.

SINUSES

The paranasal sinuses are pockets within the cranium that lighten the weight of the skull. They are lined with a ciliated mucous membrane and communicate with the nasal cavity. The frontal and maxillary sinuses are within the frontal and maxillary bones (Fig. 10–15). The sphenoid sinuses are deep within the

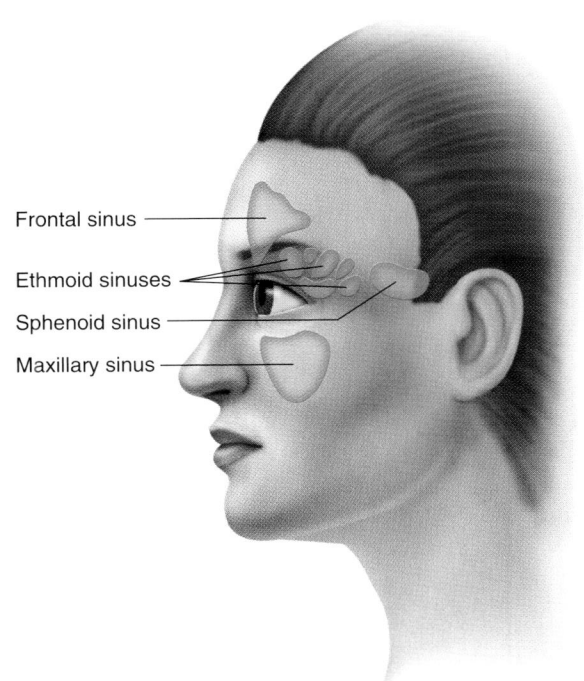
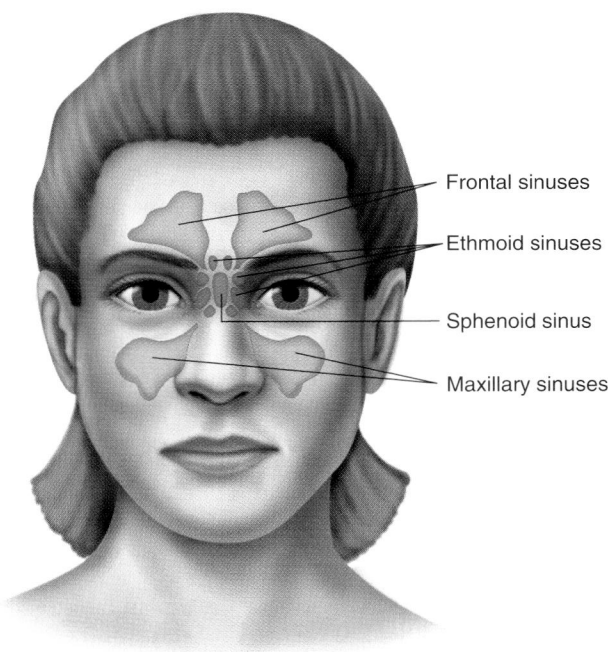

Frontal sinus

Ethmoid sinuses

Sphenoid sinus

Maxillary sinus

Frontal sinuses

Ethmoid sinuses

Sphenoid sinus

Maxillary sinuses

Side view

Front view

Figure 10–15. The paranasal sinuses.

skull in the sphenoid bone, and the ethmoid sinuses are between the orbits of the eyes.

Examination of the sinuses is performed by indirect methods of inspection and palpation of the overlying soft tissues (frontal and maxillary sinuses) and by noting secretions that may drain from the nose. Use the pads of your thumbs to palpate the frontal and maxillary sinuses. Palpate the frontal sinuses by pressing up from under the medial aspect of the brow ridges. Palpate the maxillary sinuses by pressing up and in under the zygomatic arch. Normally the sinuses are nontender on palpation.

CRANIAL NERVE I

To test cranial nerve I, the olfactory nerve, the client closes his eyes while you occlude one naris and hold a substance with a familiar odor under the other. Ask the client if he smells anything and, if so, to identify it. The procedure is then repeated for the other naris. Normally familiar odors such as coffee or vanilla can be distinguished. The sense of smell is often decreased in the elderly.

Mouth and Throat

Physical assessment of the mouth and throat involves the following activities:

- Inspecting the lips, gums, teeth, buccal mucosa, roof and floor of the mouth, top, bottom, and sides of the tongue, throat, tonsils, and uvula
- Checking motor function of the palate, pharynx, and larynx (cranial nerve X)
- Testing the client's ability to move the tongue (cranial nerve XII)

LIPS

Observe the color and moistness of the client's lips. Also inspect them for cracking, ulcers, and lumps. Normally the lips are smooth, pink, moist, intact, and free of lesions. A blue tinge to the pink coloration due to the presence of melanin pigment is a normal finding in some dark-skinned people. Abnormal findings include dryness, cracks, fissures, pallor, cyanosis, drooping, and involuntary movements. Inspect the oral mucosa of the lower lip for color and lesions by everting the lip (Fig. 10–16*A*).

MOUTH AND THROAT

Ask the client to remove any dentures and open his mouth. Inspect the buccal mucosa, gums, teeth, roof of the mouth, top, bottom, and sides of the tongue, and floor of the mouth. To allow good visibility of the buccal cavity, good light and a tongue blade are essential (Fig. 10–16*B*). This action exposes the buccal mucosa, which can then be inspected for color, intactness, or presence of lesions.

Like the lips, the buccal mucosa is normally intact, smooth, moist, and pink with areas of dark pigmentation in black-skinned clients. The tongue should be shiny, pink, and moist with even distribution of papillae arranged in an inverted V.

Inspect the teeth for dental caries (cavities) and periodontal disease (pyorrhea). The enamel should be smooth, white, and shiny. Brown or black discoloration of the enamel may indicate staining or the presence of caries. Periodontal disease is characterized by red, swollen gums (gingivitis), bleeding, receding gum lines, and the formation of pockets between the teeth and gums. In advanced periodontal disease, the teeth may be loose and pus may be present.

You should also assess for other inflammatory conditions of the mouth. Glossitis is inflammation of the tongue. Stomatitis is inflammation of the oral mucosa. Fungal infection or oral candidiasis is a common cause of stomatitis. Parotitis is inflammation of the parotid gland (the largest of the salivary glands) and results in obvious swelling of the lower cheek. The most well known infection of the parotid gland is mumps.

To assess the oropharynx, have the client tilt his head back and open his mouth. Use the tongue blade to depress the tongue about halfway back and shine a penlight on the throat (Fig. 10–16*C*). Depress one side at a time to avoid eliciting the gag reflex. In the oropharynx, or throat, the uvula should be midline. The lingual tonsils lie on either side of the dorsal surface of the tongue. These tonsils normally do not protrude beyond the tonsillar pillar and are of the same color as the rest of the oropharynx. The tonsils may have crypts with exfoliated epithelium, giving a white appearance. Examine the throat for redness, swelling, and the presence of lesions, plaque, or exudate. The tonsils are graded from 1 to 4. Grade 1 is normal. In grade 2, the tonsils are between the pillars and the uvula. In grade 3, the tonsils touch the uvula. In grade 4, one or both tonsils extend to the midline of the oropharynx.

Neck

The neck contains a number of important structures. The major blood vessels supplying the head are the carotid artery and jugular vein. The neck is also highly lymphatic, receiving lymph drainage from the head. The esophagus and trachea course through the neck supported by the cervical spine. Strong muscles support the head and assist with multidirectional range of motion. Figure 10–17 shows the structures of the neck. Physical assessment of the neck involves the following activities:

- Observing the shape, symmetry, position, and motion of the neck
- Inspecting the carotid artery and jugular vein
- Inspecting and palpating the trachea
- Inspecting and palpating the thyroid gland
- Palpating cervical lymph nodes

APPEARANCE AND MOTION

With the client in an upright position, begin your assessment of the neck by observing for symmetry and proportion to the head and shoulders. To assess for normal movement, direct the client to put his head back to check extension, put the chin on the chest to

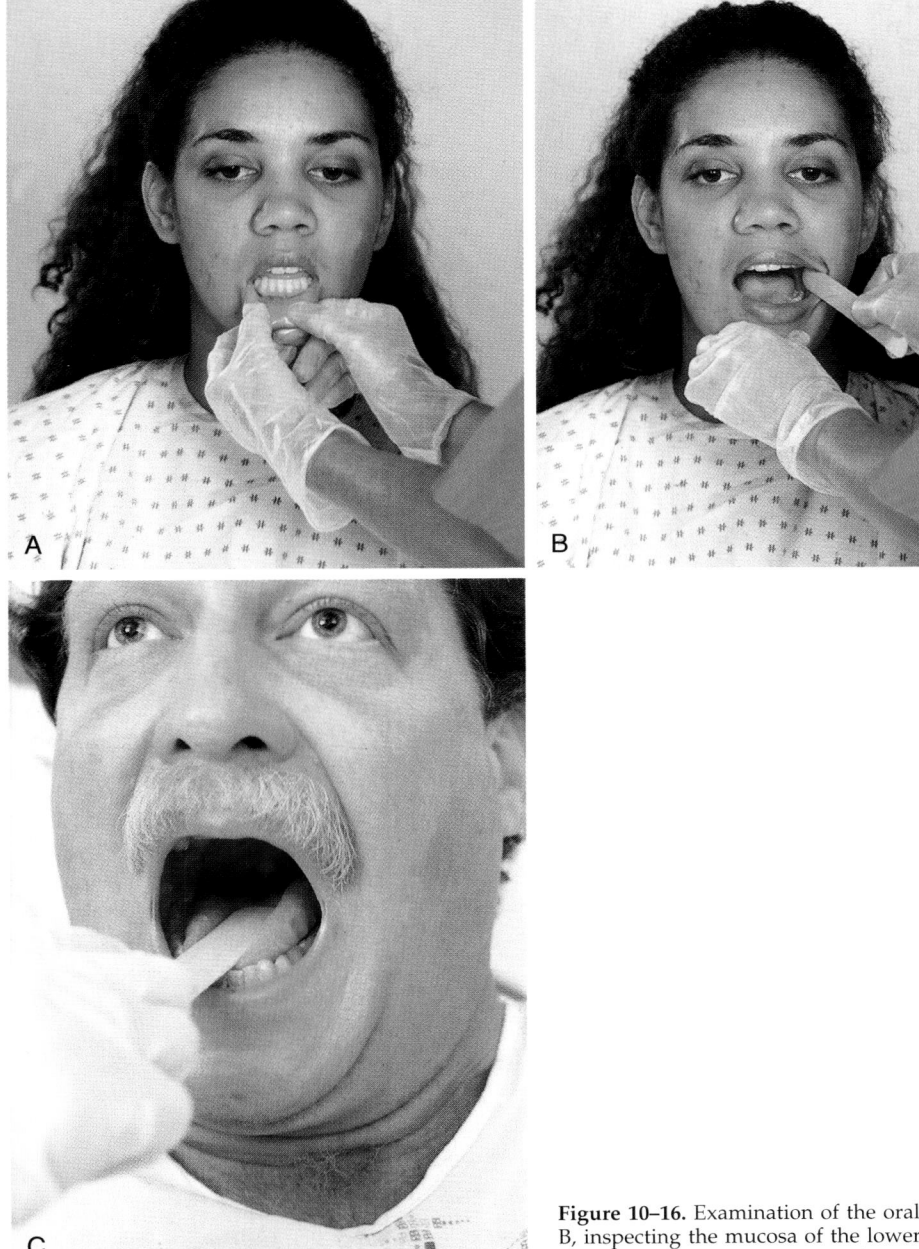

Figure 10–16. Examination of the oral cavity. A and B, inspecting the mucosa of the lower lip (A) and buccal cavity (B). C, assessing the oropharynx.

check flexion, touch the chin to each shoulder to check rotation, and bend the right ear to the right shoulder and the left ear to the left shoulder without raising the shoulder to test lateral abduction.

Normally the neck flexes 45 degrees, extends 55 degrees, laterally flexes 40 degrees, and rotates 70 degrees (and is free of uncoordinated, uncontrolled movements). This check of range of motion must be performed slowly in geriatric clients since they may become dizzy with the lateral movements.

Assess for muscle strength by having the client turn his head to one side against the resistance of your hand. Ask the client to shrug his shoulders against the resistance of your hands. The strength should be equal on both sides.

Abnormal findings include unusual shortness of the neck, lack of symmetry, fullness, edema, masses, and scars. In geriatric clients, the neck may appear shortened. This is a normal finding that occurs as a result of muscle atrophy, compression of vertebrae, and loss of fat.

JUGULAR VEIN AND CAROTID ARTERY
Observe the side of the neck over the jugular vein and the carotid artery. Normally the jugular vein is not distended and only a mild pulsation of the carotid artery

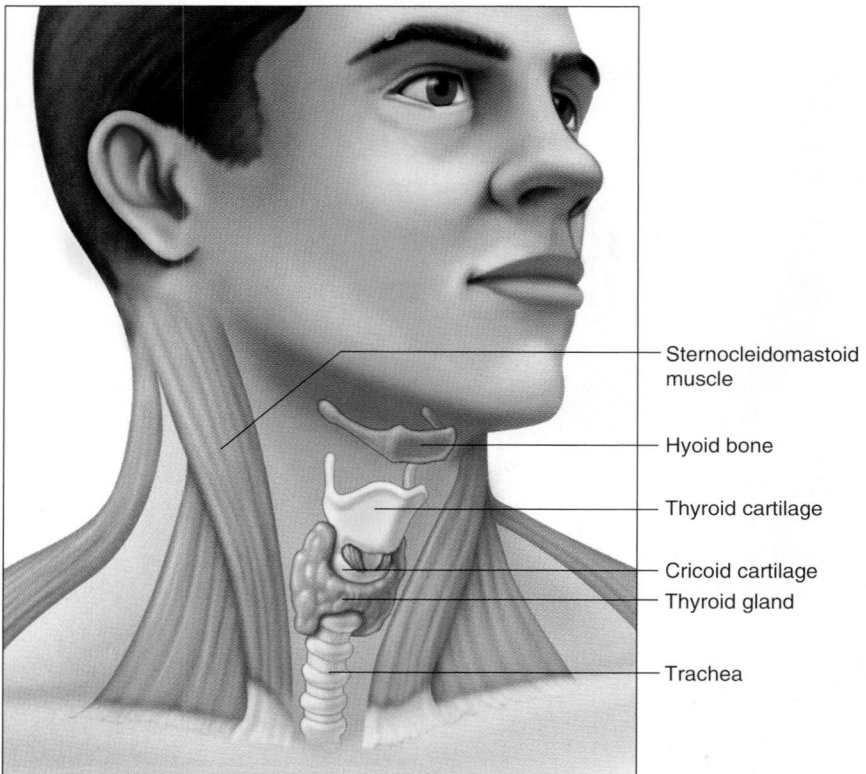

Figure 10–17. Major structures of the neck.

can be seen. A distended jugular vein or marked pulsations of the carotid are abnormal.

TRACHEA

Observe the middle front of the neck and then palpate for any sign of tracheal deviation from the midline. To palpate for tracheal deviation, place your index finger along one side of the trachea and note the distance between the side of the trachea and the sternocleidomastoid muscle. Repeat this action on the other side and compare the two distances. Normally the distances should be equal and the trachea nontender with distinct rings palpable. Soreness or swelling indicated by nonpalpable rings is abnormal.

THYROID

The thyroid gland has two lobes lying on either side of the trachea. The thin isthmus that connects the lobes lies over the trachea just below the cricoid cartilage.

To assess the thyroid gland, ask the client to lift his chin so you can observe his neck for a visible thyroid. You may also ask the client to take a sip of water, lift his chin, and then swallow while you watch the movement of the thyroid in his neck. Normally the thyroid is not visible on inspection.

Next, palpate the size, shape, and consistency of the thyroid. This is done by standing behind the client and asking him to tilt his head back slightly. Place the fingers of both hands on the sides of the client's neck with the index fingers just below the cricoid cartilage (Fig. 10–18). Then ask the client to swallow while you feel for the thyroid isthmus to rise. Then move your

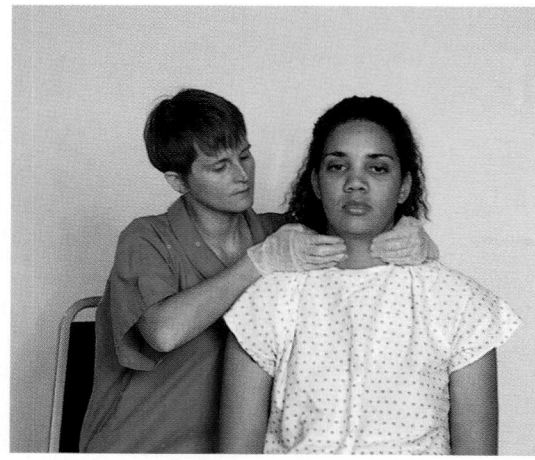

Figure 10–18. Palpating the thyroid gland.

fingers downward and laterally to identify any palpable parts of the lateral lobes.

The normal thyroid feels smooth and rubbery. If palpable, the lobes should be symmetrical and painless.

CERVICAL LYMPH NODES

Lymph nodes in the neck collect lymph from the head and neck (Fig. 10–19). There are 10 major groups of superficial cervical lymph nodes:

- Preauricular (in front of the ear)
- Parotid

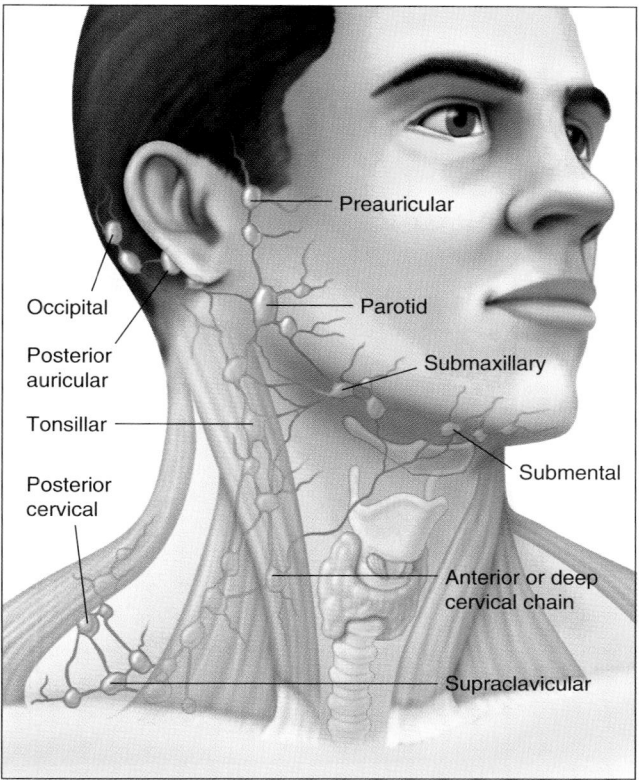

Figure 10–19. The cervical lymph nodes.

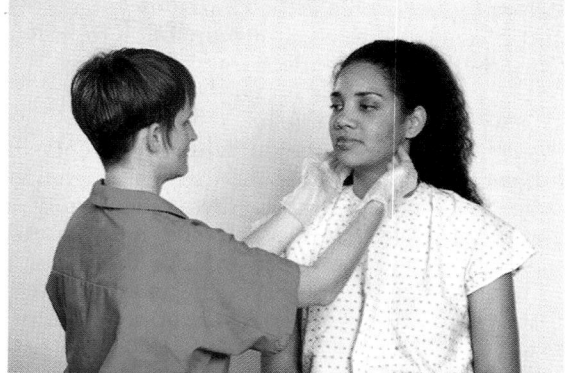

Figure 10–20. Palpating the cervical lymph nodes.

- Submaxillary
- Submental (midline, beneath the tip of the mandible)
- Anterior or deep cervical chain
- Supraclavicular (between the sternocleidomastoid muscle and the trapezius muscle at the base of the neck)
- Occipital (at the base of the skull)
- Posterior auricular (behind the ear, over the mastoid process)
- Tonsillar
- Posterior cervical (between the sternocleidomastoid muscle and the trapezius muscle in the middle of the neck)

Cervical lymph nodes are assessed by palpating both sides of the neck simultaneously using the pads of your index and middle fingers. Bend the client's head slightly forward or to the side to relax the soft tissues and muscles around the area being examined.

To examine the submental and submandibular nodes, place your fingertips under the mandible and move the skin over the nodes. To assess the supraclavicular nodes, have the client flex her neck forward. Exert light to moderate pressure and move the skin over the underlying tissues beginning in front of the ear and progressing systematically over the areas of the neck where the groups of cervical lymph nodes are located. There is no one right order for palpation of cervical nodes (Fig. 10–20). It is simply important that an order be selected and used consistently so that no area is accidentally missed.

Normally, cervical lymph nodes are either not palpable or are smooth, firm, less than 1 cm in diameter with definite margins, mobile, and nontender. In geriatric clients, submandibular salivary glands commonly prolapse and may be felt as soft masses in the upper neck, below the jaw.

Enlargement of the lymph nodes is called lymphadenopathy. Describe the location, size, presence of tenderness, consistency, inflammation, and whether they are freely moveable. It can result from infections or neoplasms of the oral pharynx or nasopharynx, systemic diseases, or infections such as mononucleosis or measles. Infection of the mouth or oropharynx is the most common cause.

Assessment of the Breasts and Axillae

Breasts

The breasts of both men and women are composed of glandular, fibrous, and adipose tissue. Women of course have more adipose and glandular tissue and the glandular tissue is mature. However, the breasts in both sexes should be inspected and palpated for malignancy. Breast cancer is rare in men, but one of nine women will acquire breast cancer at some point in her life. Therefore, women should be taught breast self-examination (see Chapter 51).

The glandular tissue in the female breast is concentrated in the upper outer quadrant, where a tail of breast tissue projects into the axilla and is known as the tail of Spence. The breast is drained by four groups of axillary lymph nodes: central axillary nodes high in the midaxilla; pectoral, along the outer edge of the pectoral muscle at the anterior axillary line; subscapular, along the posterior axillary line at the lateral edge of the scapula; and lateral, inside the upper arm along the upper humerus.

Physical assessment of the breasts involves the following activities:

- Observing the size, contour, symmetry, skin color and appearance, and vascularity of the breasts
- Observing the areolae for shape, color, and hair
- Observing the size, shape, symmetry, and direction of point of the nipples

- Palpating each breast for consistency, tenderness, and presence of masses or palpable lymph nodes
- Checking for nipple discharge

SIZE, SHAPE, AND APPEARANCE

To inspect the breasts, begin with the client sitting with her arms at her sides and then ask the client to raise her arms over her head, lower them, and press her hands against her hips. If she has pendulous breasts, ask her to lean forward. As the client performs these actions, observe the size, symmetry, contour, vascular pattern, and skin appearance of the breasts.

Normal breasts are symmetrical, although one may be larger than the other. They are conical to pendulous in shape, even in contour, and similar to normal skin on the trunk with a faint, symmetrical vascular pattern evident.

Asymmetrical breasts; breasts markedly different in size; areas of retraction, dimpling, or flattening; erythematous or peau d'orange (orange peel appearance) skin; and asymmetrical vascular dilation are all abnormal findings.

PALPATION

Palpate the breasts first with the client sitting with her hands at her sides and then lying on her back with the arm on the side being examined raised and positioned with the hand behind her head and a pillow under her shoulder. This position allows the breast tissue to flatten evenly over the chest wall (Fig. 10–21). Palpation must be done in a specific pattern, such as a spiral working out from the areola, horizontal or vertical lines up and down the breast, or as spokes of a wheel from the areola to the periphery, to ensure that all four quadrants and the axillary tail of Spence are assessed (Fig. 10–22). In palpating the breasts, move the pads of your fingers in a firm circular motion to slide the skin over the breast tissue. In judging the findings, one breast must be compared with the other.

Normally, breast tissue feels uniformly loose or dense, smooth, and either firm or soft. The finding of

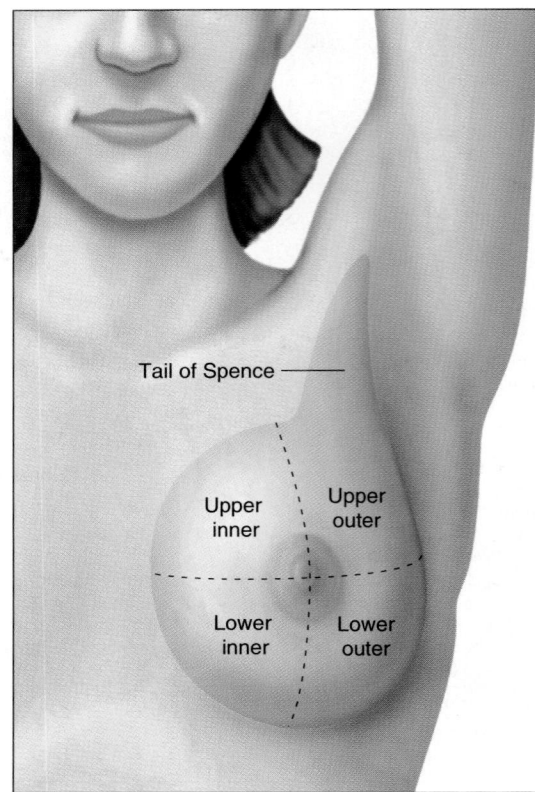

Figure 10–22. The four breast quadrants and the axillary tail of Spence.

areas of thickening, palpable masses, or tenderness or pain on palpation except in the premenstrual female is abnormal. Following palpation, the nipple of each breast is gently compressed between the thumb and forefinger to check for nipple discharge. With the exception of lactating women, the appearance of discharge with or without nipple compression is abnormal, as is retraction, deviation, or recent inversion of a nipple.

Axillae

Physical assessment of the axillae involves the following activities:

- Inspecting the condition of the axillae
- Palpating the axillae for masses and tenderness

INSPECTION

Inspect each axilla for cleanliness, hair distribution, and skin condition. Axillary hair is a secondary sex characteristic, and thus is absent prior to puberty. In the elderly, axillary hair is normally sparse and gray. In persons of all ages, the skin of the axilla should be free of redness, crusts, rashes, or other lesions.

PALPATION

Palpate the axillae after inspecting them. Have the client sit with her arms hanging at her sides. Support the client's arm on the side to be examined with one hand

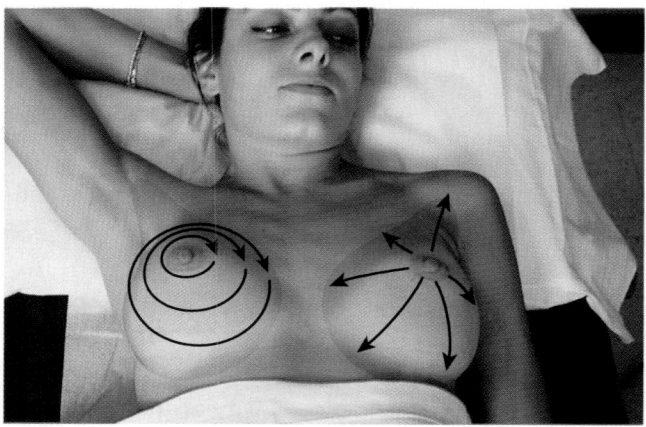

Figure 10–21. Client position and assessment patterns for breast palpation.

and use the fingertips of the other hand to palpate the axilla. With your fingers together, slightly cupped, and as high up in the axilla as possible, press inward toward the chest wall and move your fingers downward. Repeat this action down the anterior border of the axilla, along the inner aspect of the upper arm and, standing behind the client, down the posterior border of the axilla. Usually no lymph nodes are felt; however, one or more soft, nontender central nodes are an occasional insignificant finding.

Assessment of the Thorax

Assessment of the thorax includes the chest wall, the lungs, the heart, and the great vessels. Begin with either the anterior or posterior chest using the techniques of inspection, palpation, percussion, and auscultation, then proceed to the opposite chest wall. In the hospitalized client, it is common to begin with the anterior chest for convenience when the client is lying in bed.

Examining the organs within the chest cavity is an indirect examination based on knowledge of the location of the underlying structures. You must become familiar with the landmarks on the chest wall to associate findings with the underlying structures. Using imaginary reference lines, you will be able to describe the location of your findings in a manner that will have the same meaning to anyone reading your description. Useful landmarks include the ribs, the sternal notch, the angle of Louis, the thyroid process, the vertebra prominens, and the scapula.

As you begin learning to identify key locations on the chest wall, it is useful to count the ribs. Once you are comfortable with the locations, you will no longer need to count. The first rib is hidden beneath the clavicle; therefore, the first space is the first intercostal space, and the first rib to be felt is the second rib. The angle of Louis separates the manubrium from the body of the sternum. The second intercostal space is at the same level as the angle of Louis. Additionally, the trachea bifurcates at the angle of Louis. Posteriorly, all 12 ribs articulate with the thoracic spine.

The right lung has three lobes and the left lung has two lobes. Figure 10–23A helps you locate the lobes of the lungs using landmarks on the anterior surface of the chest wall. On the right, the horizontal fissure that divides the upper lobe from the middle lobe follows the fourth rib. The fissure between the middle and lower lobe starts at the midclavicular line under the sixth rib and angles diagonally to the midaxillary line in the axilla. On the left, the heart occupies the space that would otherwise be the middle lobe. Only a small portion of the lower lobes are accessible anteriorly on both the right and left side.

Posteriorly, you primarily have access to the lower lobes. With the client's arms raised over the head, the division between the upper and lower lobes starts at the third thoracic vertebra and runs obliquely following the edges of the scapulae (Fig. 10–23B).

On the lateral left side, the upper and lower lobes are divided obliquely from the midclavicular line at the sixth rib to the axilla at the level of the third thoracic vertebra (Fig. 10–23C). The same line on the right side divides the upper and middle lobes from the lower lobe. The upper and middle lobes are divided by a horizontal line from the fourth rib to the fifth rib at the midclavicular line (Fig. 10–23D). The best access to the right middle lobe is on the right side.

Chest Wall and Lungs

Physical assessment of the chest wall and lungs should include the following:

- Inspection and palpation of the chest for shape, contour, and symmetry
- Inspection of the pattern of breathing
- Palpation of tactile fremitus
- Palpation of respiratory excursion
- Percussion of the posterior and anterior thorax
- Auscultation of the posterior and anterior thorax

INSPECTION AND PALPATION
Assessment of the thorax and lungs requires evaluating the anterior, posterior, and lateral areas of the thorax, using the techniques of inspection, palpation, percussion, and auscultation.

Anterior Landmarks
The anterior chest is divided into vertical imaginary lines, which serve as anatomic landmarks (Fig. 10–24):

- the midsternal line, drawn vertically through the center of the sternum;
- the left and right midclavicular lines, drawn vertically through the midpoint of the left and right clavicles and running parallel to the midsternal line; and
- the left and right anterior axillary lines, drawn vertically through the anterior axillary folds and running parallel to the midsternal line (see Fig. 10–26).

Additional anterior anatomic landmarks include the manubriosternal junction (often called the angle of Louis), the suprasternal notch, the costal angle, the clavicles, and the ribs. Anteriorly, the ribs articulate with the manubrium and sternum. Posteriorly, they articulate with the vertebral processes. The first seven ribs articulate with the manubrium and body of the sternum and the last five ribs are fused into a bony and cartilaginous costal angle anteriorly. They are supported and connected by the intercostal muscles and attached to each other by costal cartilage. The exceptions are the 11th and 12th ribs, which remain unattached (or floating) anteriorly. The palpable spaces between the ribs are called intercostal spaces (ICSs) and are numbered in ascending order beginning at the base of the neck and moving downward (i.e., the first left or right ICS, second left or right ICS, etc.). They are used as anatomic landmarks.

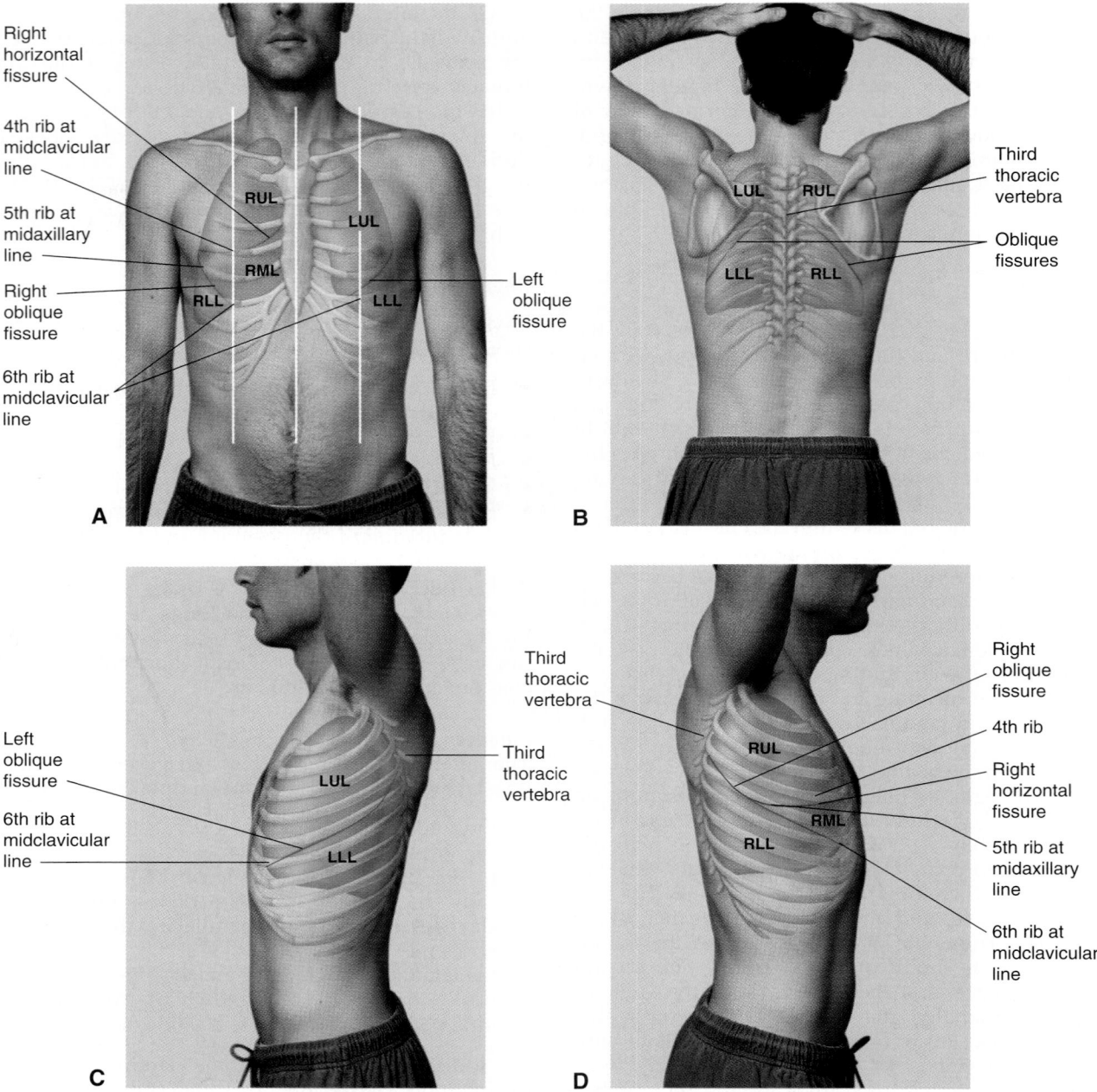

Figure 10–23. Chest landmarks: A, anterior chest landmarks and underlying lungs; B, posterior chest landmarks and underlying lungs; C, left lateral chest landmarks and underlying lungs; D, right lateral chest landmarks and underlying lungs.

Posterior Landmarks

The posterior chest is divided similarly into three vertical and parallel imaginary lines that serve as landmarks (Fig. 10–25):

- the vertebral or midspinal line, running through the center of the spinous processes; and
- the left and right midscapular lines, which run vertically through the midpoint of the inferior angle of the scapulae and parallel to the vertebral line.

Additional posterior landmarks include the scapulae, the spinous processes, and the intercostal spaces of the ribs. All 12 of the ribs articulate posteriorly with the thoracic vertebrae.

Lateral Landmarks

The lateral chest is divided similarly into three imaginary lines (Fig. 10–26). The midaxillary line is drawn vertically through the midpoint of the left and right axillae. The anterior axillary line is drawn vertically through the anterior axillary folds and parallel to the midaxillary line. Finally, the posterior axillary line is drawn through the posterior axillary folds parallel to the midaxillary line.

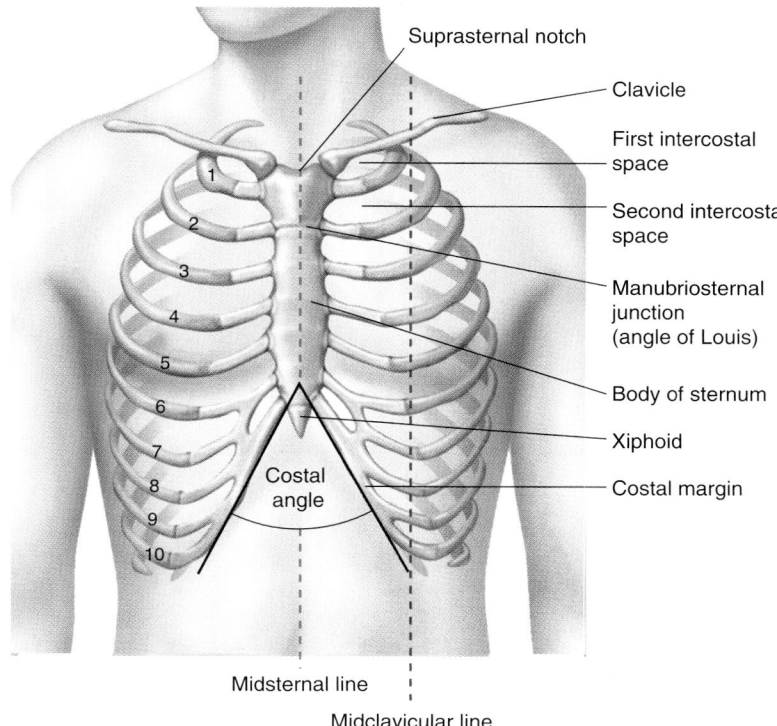

Figure 10–24. Anterior chest landmarks.

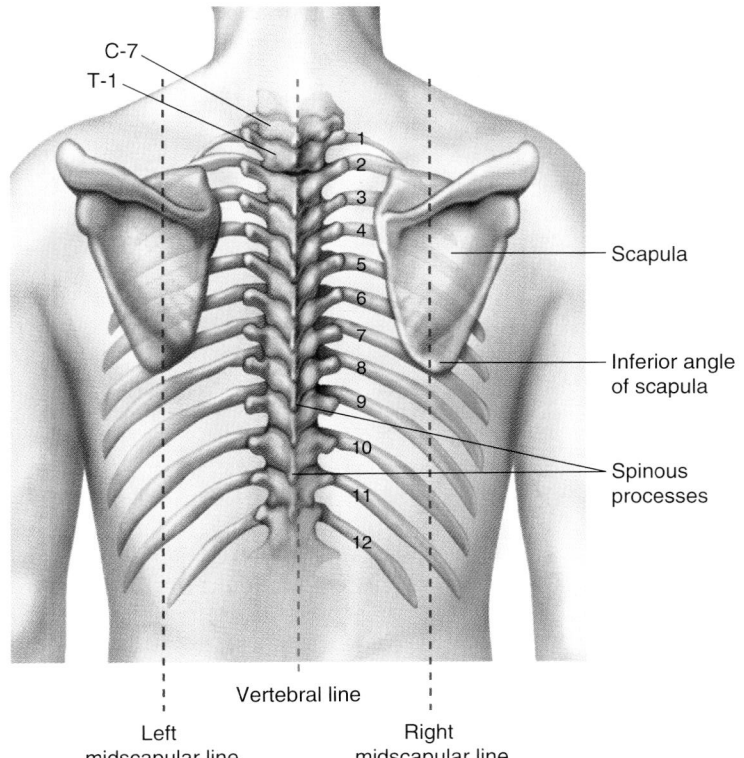

Figure 10–25. Posterior chest landmarks.

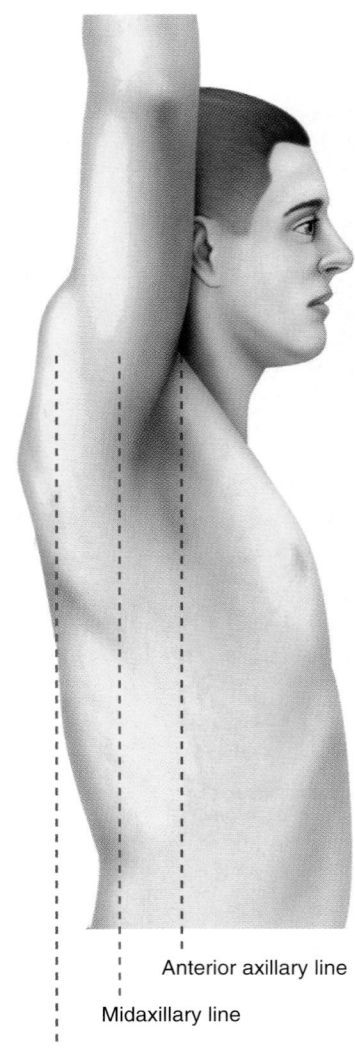

Anterior axillary line

Midaxillary line

Posterior axillary line

Figure 10–26. Lateral chest landmarks.

Shape, Contour, and Symmetry

Begin your assessment of the chest and lungs with the client undressed from the waist up and sitting up on the examining table. Observe the posterior thorax from a midline position behind the client. Observe the anterior thorax with the client lying supine. Note whether the chest is of normal size and contour (Fig. 10–27A and B). Does the chest appear asymmetrical? Normally, the anteroposterior to lateral ratio should be 1:2 or 5:7.

Note whether there are congenital anomalies, past traumatic injuries, disfigurements, or surgical alterations. Inspect and palpate the thorax, clavicles, scapulas, ribs, and spine for contour and abnormalities. Note any congenital abnormalities, traumatic injuries, post-surgical alterations, masses, lesions, tenderness, or abnormal slopes or contours. Ask the client to bend over at the waist to further inspect the curvature of the spine.

Figure 10–27C through F illustrates normal variations and abnormalities of chest configuration. Pigeon chest (Fig. 10–27C) and funnel chest (Fig. 10–27D) are considered normal congenital variations and are not corrected unless the deformity interferes with cardiopulmonary function or the client desires correction for cosmetic reasons. Barrel chest (Fig. 10–27E) is associated with chronic obstructive pulmonary disease. Kyphosis (Fig. 10–27F) and scoliosis (shown in Fig. 37–5) can be severe enough to interfere with breathing.

Pattern of Breathing

Inspect the client's breathing pattern. Attempt to observe the client without making him aware that you are observing his respirations. A commonly used technique is to pretend you are taking the client's pulse while you are actually observing his respiratory pattern. Note any abnormalities of breathing rate or rhythm. A rate of 12 to 20 breaths per minute is considered normal for an adult. A regular breathing rate for an adult will be evidenced by approximately equal lengths of expiration and inspiration.

Any variations in rate and rhythm, such as tachypnea (rapid breathing), bradypnea (slow breathing), hyperpnea (sighing), hyperventilation (rapid deep breathing), apnea (periods of cessation of breathing), Cheyne-Stokes respirations (irregular breathing with long pauses), Kussmaul's respirations (rapid, deep breathing seen in diabetic ketoacidosis), wheezing (squeaking or whistling), respiratory lag or pauses, prolonged expiration, bulging of the intercostal spaces, or use of accessory muscles to breathe should be clearly noted.

Tactile Fremitus

Palpate for tactile fremitus (also called vocal fremitus). **Tactile fremitus** is a vibration, as in the chest wall, over an area of secretions, felt on the thorax while the client is speaking. Ask the client to repeatedly say "99" as you place the ball of your hand (posterior palm near the proximal finger joints) on each of the target areas as diagrammed. Figure 10–28 shows the systematic pattern for palpating for tactile fremitus; this pattern will later be repeated for percussion and auscultation.

Compare the transmission of the client's voice through the chest wall in opposite symmetrical areas of the chest. The vibratory transmission of the voice should be equivalent in symmetrical areas. Sensations will be decreased in clients with a soft voice, laryngeal disease or obstruction, bronchial obstruction, chronic obstructive pulmonary disease (COPD), effusions (fluid), fibrosis (thickening), pneumothorax (air), or infiltrating tumor. Vibratory sensations will be increased with conditions that would increase the transmission of sound, such as a consolidated lung (lobar pneumonia).

Respiratory Excursion

Palpate for **respiratory excursion,** which is the ability of the lungs to expand as evidenced by the degree to which the chest wall expands. To do this, stand behind the client with your thumbs placed on the spinous processes at the level of the tenth ribs. Spread your fingers apart over the lateral thorax with your thumbs pointing toward each other and your fingers pointing away from each other (Fig. 10–29). Press your palms inward toward the spine, moving your thumbs closer together with only a small skin-fold between them. Now ask the client to exhale and then take a deep breath and hold it. Observe the movement of your thumbs and note the expanded distance between them. Normal respiratory excursion will separate the thumbs by 1¼ to 2 inches. Limited respiratory excursion may occur with chronic fibrotic disease of the lungs, COPD, emphy-sema, pulmonary tumors, abdominal mass, or superficial pain.

PERCUSSION

Percuss the posterior and anterior thorax to reveal the nature of underlying tissue. To obtain a percussion "note," press the middle finger of your left hand firmly on the surface. Cock the middle finger of your right hand and strike the middle finger of your left hand between the distal joint and your fingernail. Work your way down the posterior and then the anterior thorax, striking at least twice in each of the percussion target areas in intercostal spaces. Listen for dullness, resonance, or tympany (Fig. 10–30). Dullness will be heard over solid or fluid-filled tissue (such as

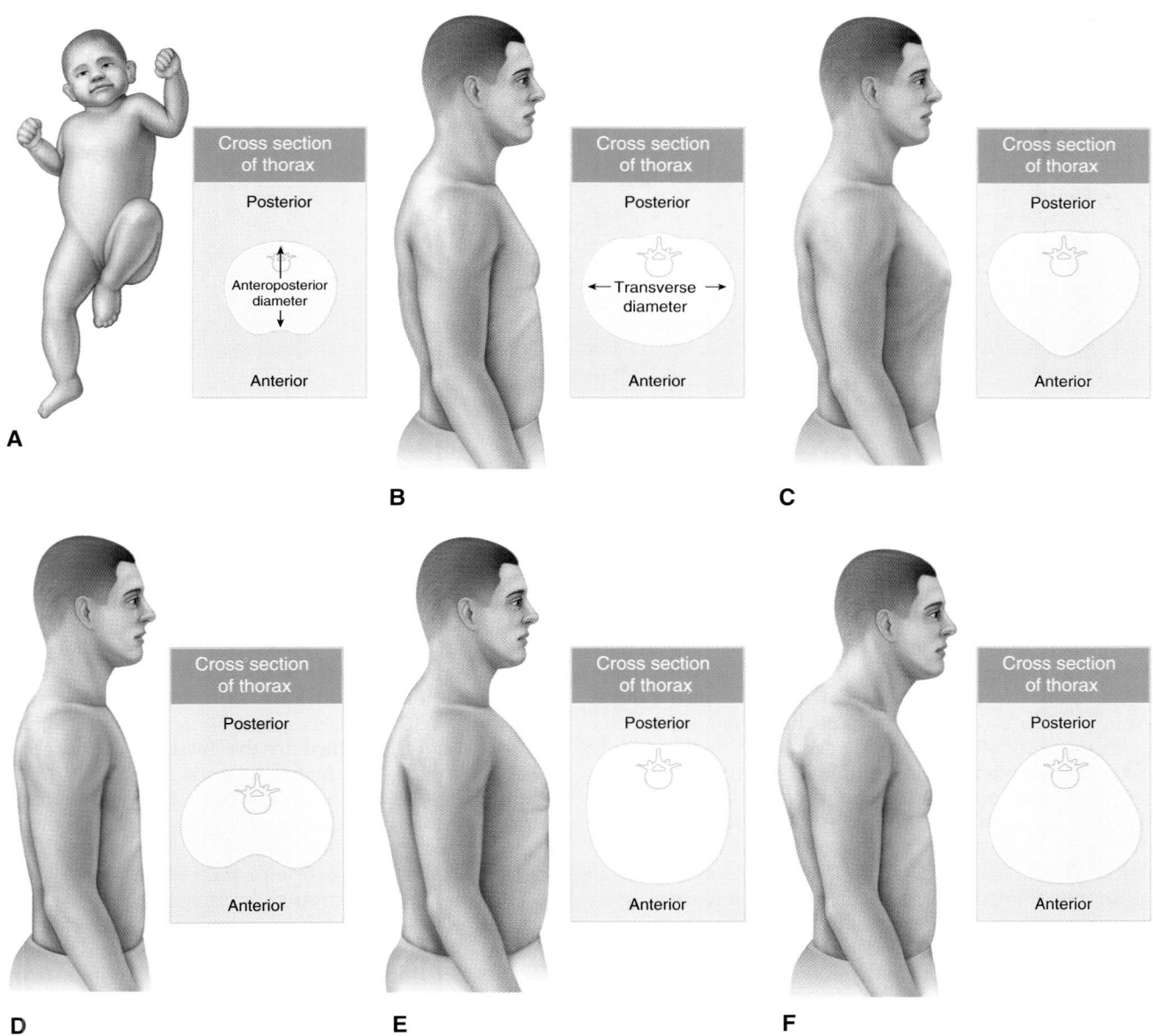

Figure 10–27. A and B, normal configuration of the thorax in an infant (A) and an adult (B). C through F, normal variations and abnormalities of chest configuration. C, pigeon chest; D, funnel chest; E, barrel chest; F, kyphosis.

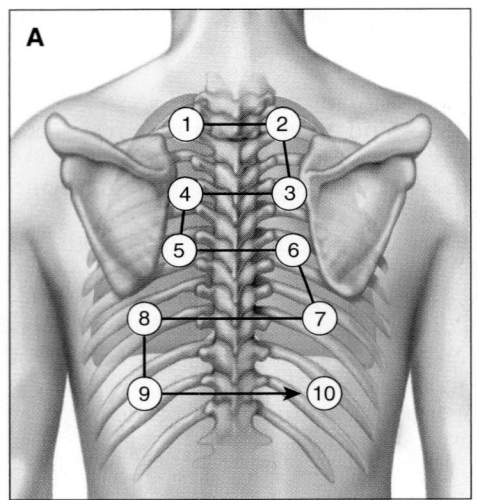

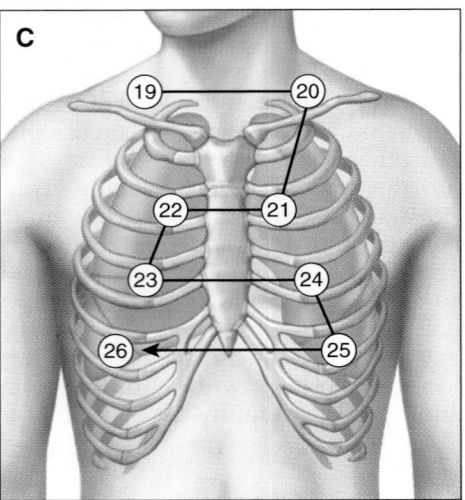

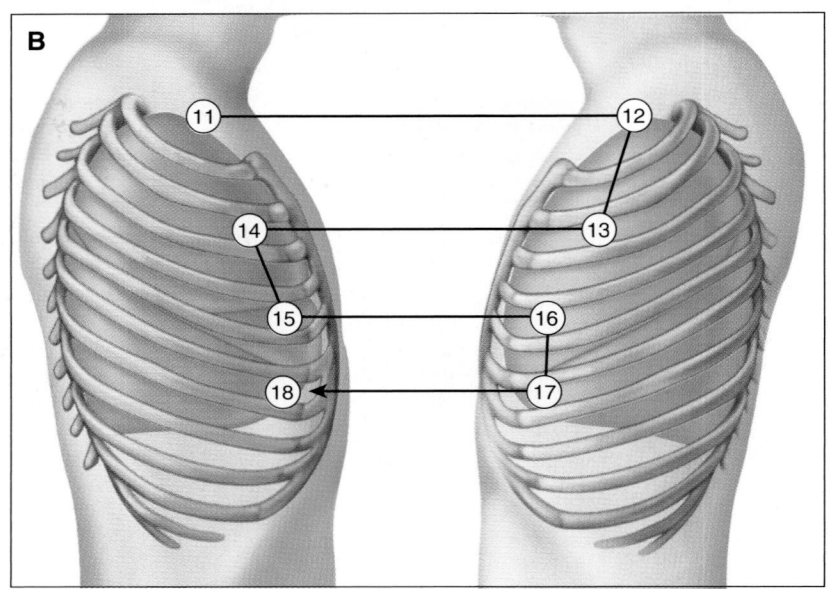

Figure 10–28. Systematic pattern for palpation of tactile fremitus, percussion, and auscultation on the chest. A, posterior; B, lateral; C, anterior.

large underlying organs such as the liver or heart). Resonance will be heard over air-filled tissue (such as most of the lung spaces). Tympany will be heard over tissue that is hyperinflated with air or where a large amount of air is common, such as the gastric air bubble.

Percuss for diaphragmatic excursion or the ability of the lungs to expand as evidenced by the movement of the diaphragm. Ask the client to exhale and hold it. Percuss downward from a point of resonance toward the diaphragm. Mark the point where dullness is initially heard. Ask the client to then inhale and hold it. Again percuss downward from a point of resonance to the area where diaphragmatic dullness is initially heard. Mark this point and measure the distance between both points. Normally the diaphragm will descend 3 to 6 cm. Excursion is decreased in COPD.

AUSCULTATION

Auscultate the posterior and then the anterior thorax in the fashion diagrammed. Sit the client up for both posterior and anterior chest auscultation, since abnormal findings may be masked in a supine client. Undress the client from the waist up. With the diaphragm of the stethoscope on bare skin, listen to the client breathing. Move across and down the posterior and then the anterior chest in the fashion diagrammed. Discern whether artifactual sounds are occurring and eliminate them before proceeding. Artifactual sounds are those made inadvertently from clothing, muscle contractions, paper, scratching, or from your fingers resting on the stethoscope or the client's chest.

Identify and distinguish bronchial, bronchovesicular, and vesicular breath sounds (Fig. 10–31) from artifactual and abnormal breath sounds. Bronchial breath sounds are normal sounds heard with a stethoscope over the main airways, including trachea and sternum. Expiration and inspiration produce noise of equal duration, sounding like blowing through a hollow tube. Bronchovesicular breath sounds are normal breath sounds that occur between sounds of the bronchial tubes and those of the alveoli, or a combination of the two sounds. Vesicular breath sounds are a normal sound of rustling or swishing heard with a stethoscope over the lung periphery, characteristically higher pitched during inspiration and falling rapidly during expiration.

Adventitious is derived from a Latin word meaning from an outside source. Thus, adventitious breath sounds are produced by a source other than normal lungs. There are basically three types of adventitious breath sounds: discontinuous, or coarse and fine crackles that indicate the presence of fluid in the lung spaces; continuous, including high- and low-pitched wheezes, which indicate narrowing or partial obstruction of the airways from inflammation, mucus, edema, foreign body, or mass; and rubs, grating sounds heard both on inspiration and expiration that are caused by the rubbing together of inflamed pleural surfaces. Note any adventitious sounds, their timing (inspiratory or expiratory), location, and whether they clear with coughing, deep breathing, or position changes. Adventitious sounds are discussed in Chapter 39.

Heart

Examination of the heart should include the following steps:

- Inspect and palpate the anterior chest including all six anatomic landmarks.
- Palpate the apical impulse or point of maximum impulse.
- Palpate the carotid pulse.
- Percuss the cardiac border to assess the size of the heart.
- Auscultate the heart for rate and rhythm.
- Compare the apical and radial pulse if the rhythm of the heart is found to be irregular.
- Compare the apical and radial pulse if the rhythm of the heart is found to be irregular.
- Auscultate the heart in each of the six anatomic landmarks.
- Identify and auscultate S_1 and S_2.
- Identify and auscultate systole and diastole.
- Auscultate for extra heart sounds.
- Auscultate and evaluate any heart murmurs.

ANATOMIC LANDMARKS

The location of the heart in the anterior chest begins with identifying anatomic landmarks. The **precordium** is the area on the anterior chest overlying the heart and great vessels. The heart extends from the right border of the sternum to the left midclavicular line and from the second intercostal space to the fifth intercostal space. It is inverted in the chest with the base at the top and the apex pointing down and to the left. It is rotated with the right side anterior and the left side posterior.

The sounds produced by the heart are associated with the heart valves. The areas to listen to for the sounds are not directly over the valves, but are over the area where the sound produced by the valve is transmitted (Fig. 10–32). Sound is transmitted in the

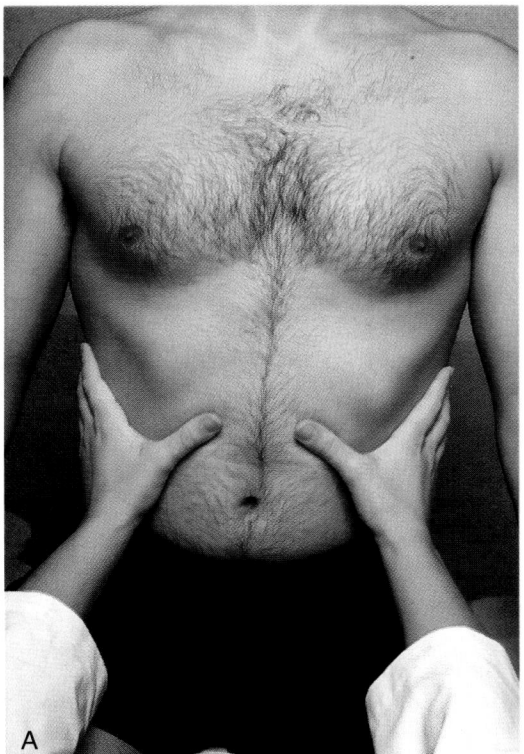
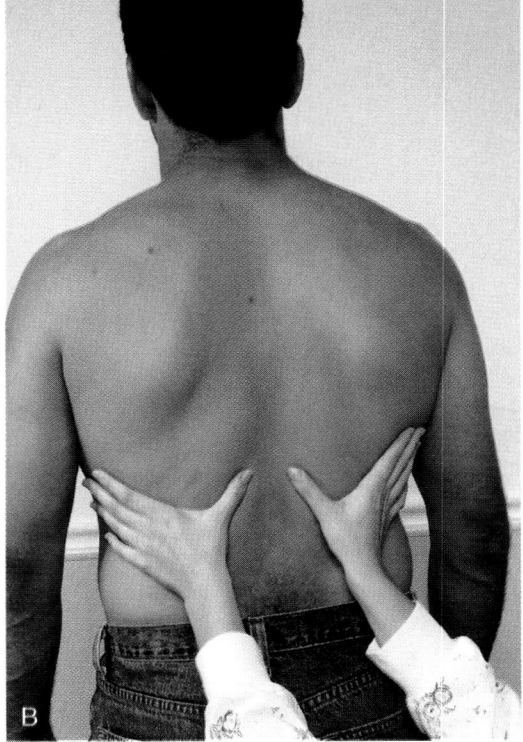

Figure 10–29. Position of the hands for assessing respiratory excursion on the anterior thorax (A) and posterior thorax (B).

direction of blood flow. The area associated with the pulmonic valve is the second intercostal space to the left of the sternum. The area associated with the aortic valve is the second intercostal space to the right of the sternum. The area associated with the triscupid valve is the fifth intercostal space at the sternal border. The area associated with the mitral valve is the fifth intercostal space at the midclavicular line. As an additional area where some murmurs may be best heard, Erb's point is located in the third intercostal space on the left sternal border.

EVENTS OF THE CARDIAC CYCLE

The heart is evaluated in relationship to the events of the cardiac cycle. The cardiac cycle is the time from the beginning of the contraction of the ventricles to the beginning of the next contraction. Systole is the contraction phase and diastole is the relaxation phase. When the ventricles contract, pressure immediately increases in the ventricles, causing the mitral and triscupid valves to close and the aortic and pulmonic valves to open. When the ventricles relax, the pressure drops to below that of the aorta and pulmonary vein, causing the aortic and pulmonic valve to close. The greater pressure in the atria opens the mitral and tricuspid valves.

Two heart sounds are produced by the events of the cardiac cycle. The first heart sound, S_1, is the heart sound produced by the vibration of the chest wall set in motion by the closure of the mitral and tricuspid valves. S_2 is the second heart sound, produced by the vibration of the chest wall set in motion by the closure of the aortic and pulmonic valves. Thus, S_1 is associated with systole and S_2 is associated with diastole. The heart sounds are often described as a lubb-dupp sound with the lubb being S_1 and the dupp being S_2.

INSPECTION AND PALPATION

Begin the assessment of the heart with inspection and palpation of the anterior thorax. Have the client un-

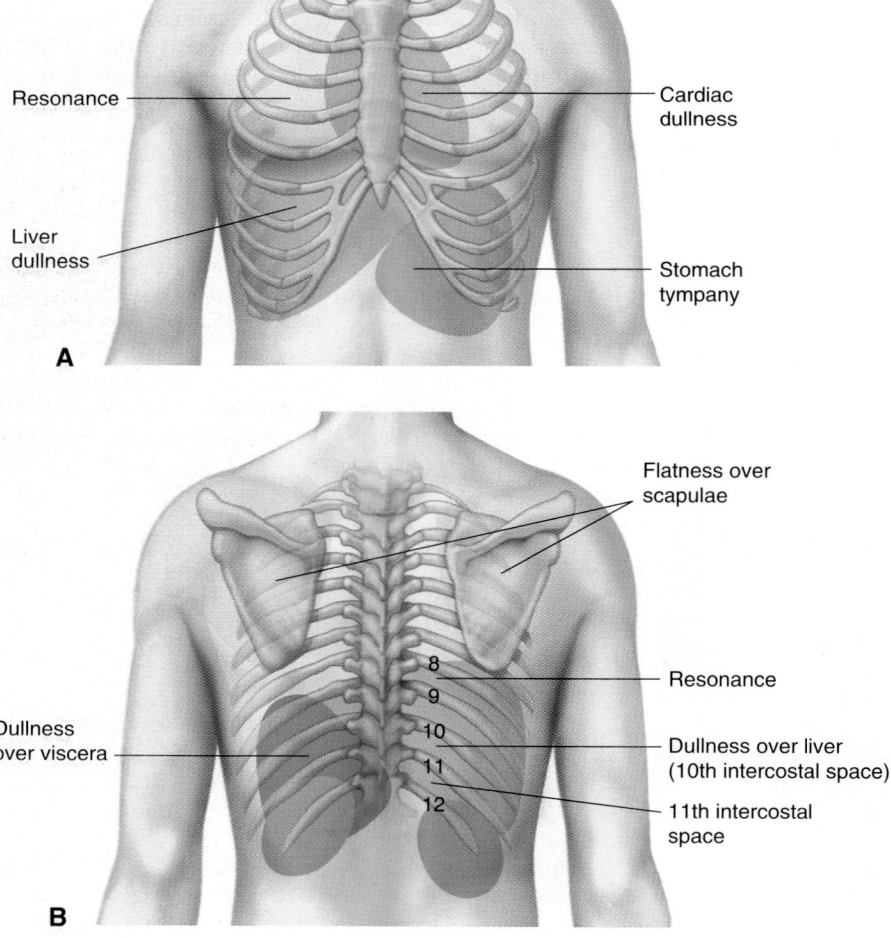

Figure 10–30. Normal percussion notes over the anterior (A) and posterior (B) chest and upper abdomen.

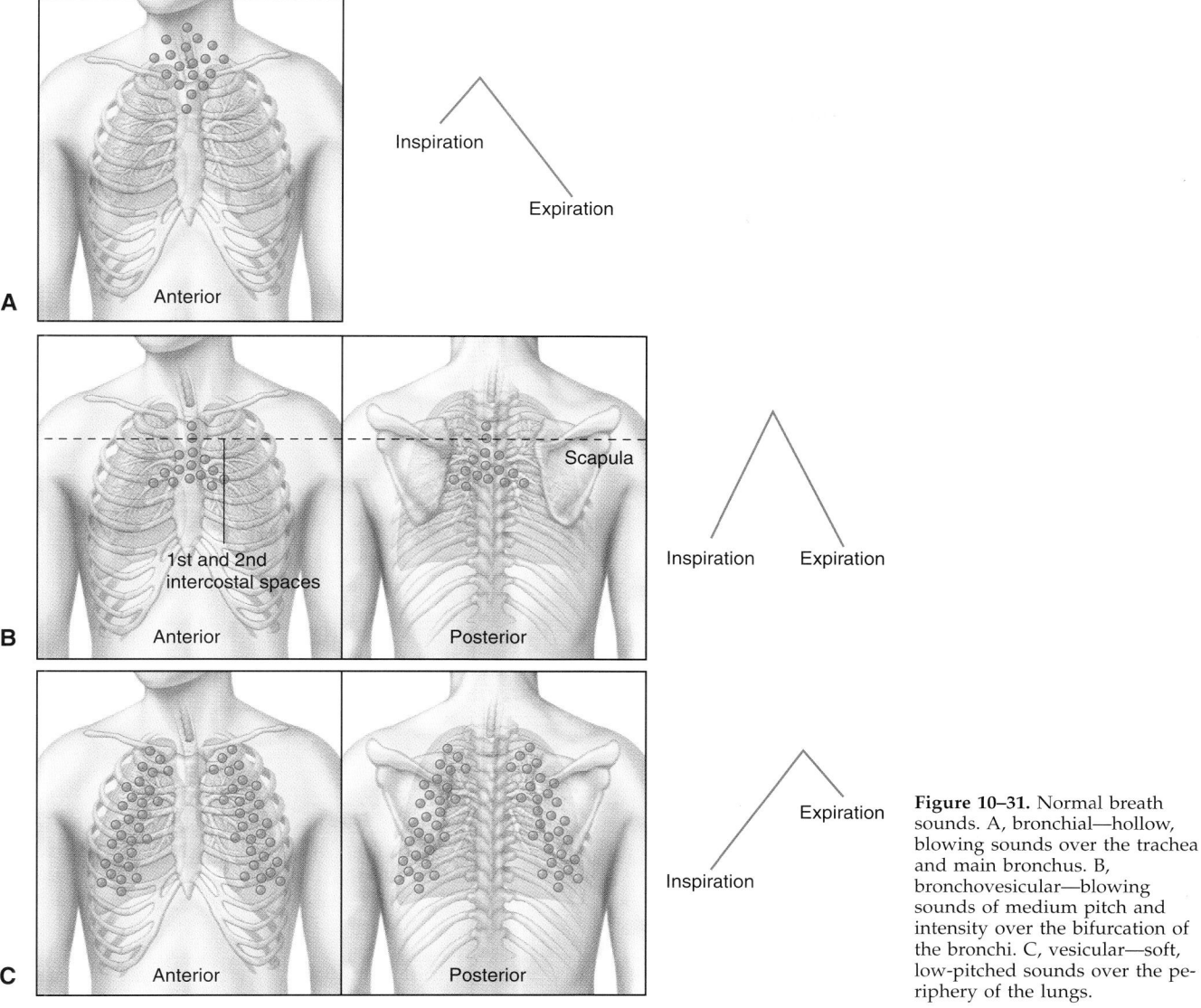

Figure 10–31. Normal breath sounds. A, bronchial—hollow, blowing sounds over the trachea and main bronchus. B, bronchovesicular—blowing sounds of medium pitch and intensity over the bifurcation of the bronchi. C, vesicular—soft, low-pitched sounds over the periphery of the lungs.

dress to the waist and examine the client first sitting up, then lying down under adequate lighting. Be sure to inspect the client from the side and at an angle to take full advantage of lighting.

Inspect and palpate the aortic area, the pulmonic area, Erb's point, the tricuspid area, the apical area, and the epigastric area just below the tip of the sternum. Palpate the anatomic landmarks of the precordium. Palpate the chest and anatomic landmarks using the ball of the hand and posterior side of the proximal finger joints placed lightly on the chest surface in each area. Time the occurrence of any perceived pulsations, heaves, or thrills during systole and diastole by simultaneously auscultating the heart or palpating the carotid artery.

Heaves are forceful pulsations that bound up against your hand. Thrills are vibrations. Normally no lesions, masses, or abnormalities should be noted. There may be a light tapping sensation in the apical landmark (fourth or fifth intercostal space at the mid-

clavicular line); however, any heaves, thrills anywhere in the precordium, or any pulsations palpable in any location other than the apical landmark should be considered abnormal.

Apical Pulse

As defined in Chapter 9, the *apical pulse* is the heart rate counted at the apex (the point of maximum impulse) of the heart on the anterior chest. The **point of maximum impulse** (PMI) is the point where the heart comes the closest to the chest wall at the apex of the heart. Palpate and evaluate the apical impulse by placing your hand over the fifth intercostal space at the midclavicular line. Usually you will feel a light tapping sensation occurring in the apical area at the left fifth intercostal space at the midclavicular line. Normally the tapping sensation is limited to 1 to 2 cm in diameter and confined to one intercostal space. Displacement of the apical impulse or an impulse felt in an area that is larger than 2 cm in diameter may be

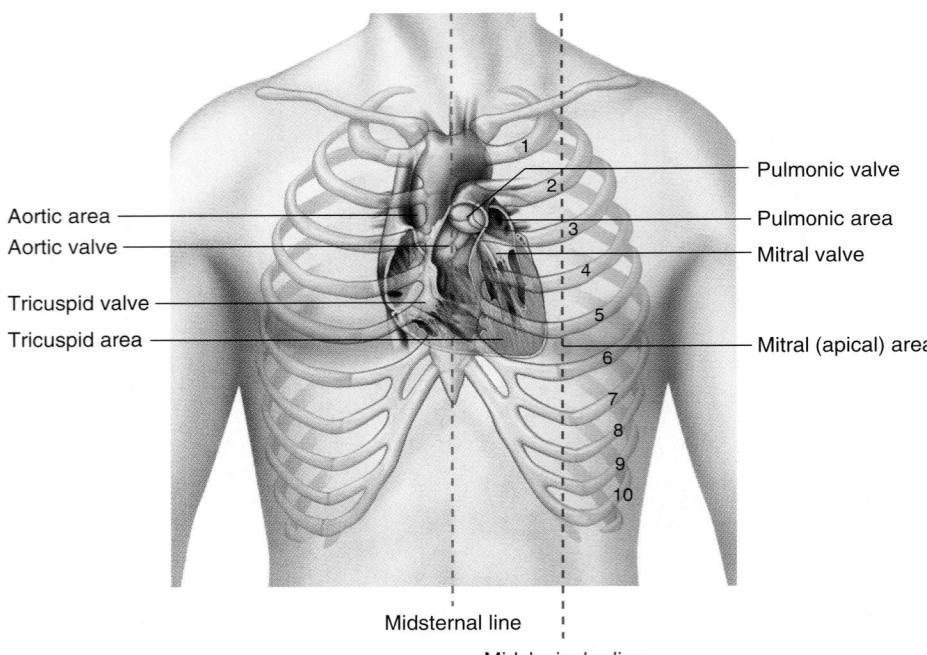

Aortic area

Aortic valve

Tricuspid valve

Tricuspid area

Pulmonic valve

Pulmonic area

Mitral valve

Mitral (apical) area

Midsternal line

Midclavicular line

Figure 10–32. Anatomic sites for assessment of the precordium.

secondary to abnormal curvatures of the spine, cardiomegaly, emphysema, obesity, increased musculature, or enlarged breasts. The PMI may also be faint or barely perceptible secondary to pericardial effusions, pulmonary effusions, tumors, or any condition that may increase tissue mass or fluid between the heart and the chest wall.

Carotid Pulse

Palpate and evaluate the carotid pulse. The carotid artery is located in the groove between the trachea and the sternomastoid muscle and can usually be easily felt anywhere along this groove. To locate the most prominent pulse, ask the client to turn his head away from the side chosen for palpation. Observe the neck for pulsations. Place the tips of two fingers held together (usually the index and second finger) lightly over the pulsations. Figure 10–33 shows the major arteries and veins of the right side of the neck. Auscultate the heart simultaneously and determine whether the carotid pulse is regular and synchronous with S_1.

PERCUSSION

Rarely is the technique of percussion employed to determine cardiac size in current practice because chest x-rays now provide a much more reliable assessment of cardiac size and contour. However, in areas where chest x-rays are not readily available, this may be a useful technique to know.

Using the percussion technique described previously, percuss out the borders of cardiac dullness and assess the size of the heart. The heart tissue will be dull to percussion amid surrounding resonant lung tissue. The left border of cardiac dullness is usually at the fifth intercostal space at the midclavicular line and

second intercostal space at the sternum. The right border of cardiac dullness is usually at the sternum.

A number of conditions, such as cardiomegaly (enlarged heart), left ventricular hypertrophy (enlarged left ventricle), pericardial effusions (fluid surrounding the heart), or a cardiac mass, may account for increased heart size. A small number of clients may have congenital anomalies such as dextrocardia (abnormally rotated or positioned heart) or situs inversus (organs located on the opposite sides), which will result in markedly abnormal findings.

AUSCULTATION

Auscultate the heart for rate and rhythm. Using the diaphragm of the stethoscope, auscultate the apical area of the heart for the rate and rhythm, counting the first heart sound (S_1, lubb) and the second heart sound (S_2, dupp) in combination as one beat, lubb-dupp.

Assess the apical heart rate by counting the number of beats there are in 1 full minute. Assess the cardiac rhythm. Listen to several full cycles, paying particular attention to the length of the systolic pauses between S_1 and S_2. The length of both the systolic and the diastolic pause should be consistent in all cycles. Any variation in length of systolic or diastolic pauses, abnormally long pauses, or sudden increase in heart rate over 100 cycles constitutes an irregular rhythm.

The average heart rate for adults is between 60 and 100 beats per minute (bpm). The average heart rate for children varies depending on age. Sinus bradycardia, or heart rate less than 60 bpm may be normal in well-conditioned athletes but is abnormal when associated with hypothermia, hypothyroidism, and drug overdoses (narcotics and digoxin). Sinus tachycardia or a heart rate greater than 100 bpm may be normal with increased exercise; however, it is abnormal in association with increased caffeine intake, stimulant overdoses, fever, pain, hyperthyroidism, anxiety, shock, and heart disease. A sinus dysrhythmia, in which the pulse rate changes with respirations, increasing at the peak of inspiration and decreasing with expiration, often occurs in children and young adults as a normal variant. Ventricular premature contractions result in irregular heart rhythms perceived as beats that occur out of sequence and may occur singularly or in couplets. They may occur frequently or infrequently and are caused by abnormal electrical conduction through the ventricular tissue and may indicate or be a precursor to a serious arrhythmia.

If the rhythm of the heartbeat is found to be irregular, compare the apical and radial pulses. Compare the rate (or beats per full minute) between the apical and radial pulses. Usually the apical and radial pulses will be equivalent in rhythm. If a pulse deficit occurs, it is always the radial pulse that has the lower rate.

Auscultate the heart in each of the six anatomic landmarks using first the diaphragm of the stethoscope and then the bell. Apply firm pressure when using the diaphragm and light pressure when using the bell. At each site, listen for the rate and rhythm, S_1, S_2, systole and diastole, extra heart sounds, and murmurs. Since the sounds produced by the closing of heart valves may often be heard throughout the precordium, it is now advised to edge the stethoscope across the base of the heart and down the chest to the apex in a Z-like pattern, which will include the anatomic landmarks while at the same time cover more surface area of the heart.

Heart Sounds

Identify and carefully auscultate S_1 and S_2. The first heart sound (S_1, or lubb) occurs at the same time as the carotid pulse. It is heard best at the apex of the heart and is louder than the second heart sound (S_2, or dupp) at the apical and tricuspid area and at Erb's point. It is softer than S_2 at the pulmonic and aortic areas. The second heart sound (S_2, or dupp) is heard best in the aortic area. It is louder than S_1 in the aortic and pulmonic areas and at Erb's point.

As you listen to the heart sounds, listen to S_1 and S_2 carefully and separately. Identify and auscultate systole and diastole. Systole is the shorter pause between S_1 and S_2. Diastole is the longer pause between S_2 and S_1. Usually systole and diastole are silent. Figure 10–34 will help you compare the heart sounds to the events of the cardiac cycle and the electrocardiogram.

Once you have identified S_1 and S_2, note whether the heart sounds are normal, accentuated (loud), or split. A split sound means you can distinguish more than one sound in S_1 or S_2. A physiological split of S_2 can occur with respiration. The change in intrapulmonary pressure causes blood to sequester in the lungs with inspiration, resulting in late closure of the pulmonic valve. Hence, closure of the aortic and pulmonic valves are heard separately. A physiological split of S_2 is easily identified because it varies with respiration.

Extra Heart Sounds

Auscultate for extra heart sounds. Note whether there are split sounds, third (S_3) or fourth (S_4) heart sounds, or audible clicks. S_3 is a third heart sound thought to

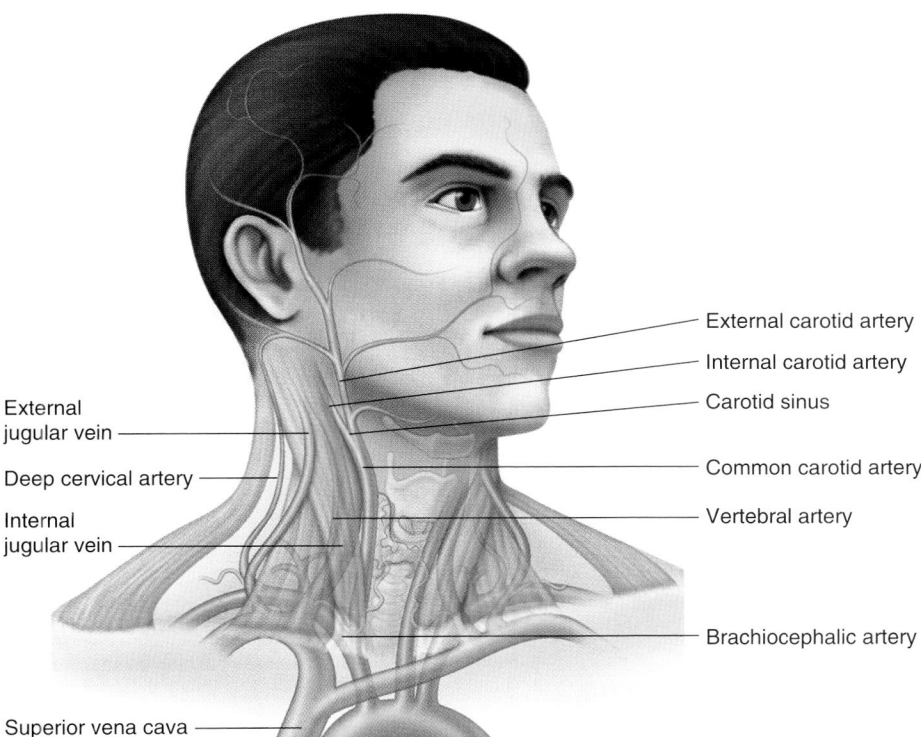

External jugular vein

Deep cervical artery

Internal jugular vein

Superior vena cava

External carotid artery

Internal carotid artery

Carotid sinus

Common carotid artery

Vertebral artery

Brachiocephalic artery

Figure 10–33. Arteries and veins of the right side of the neck.

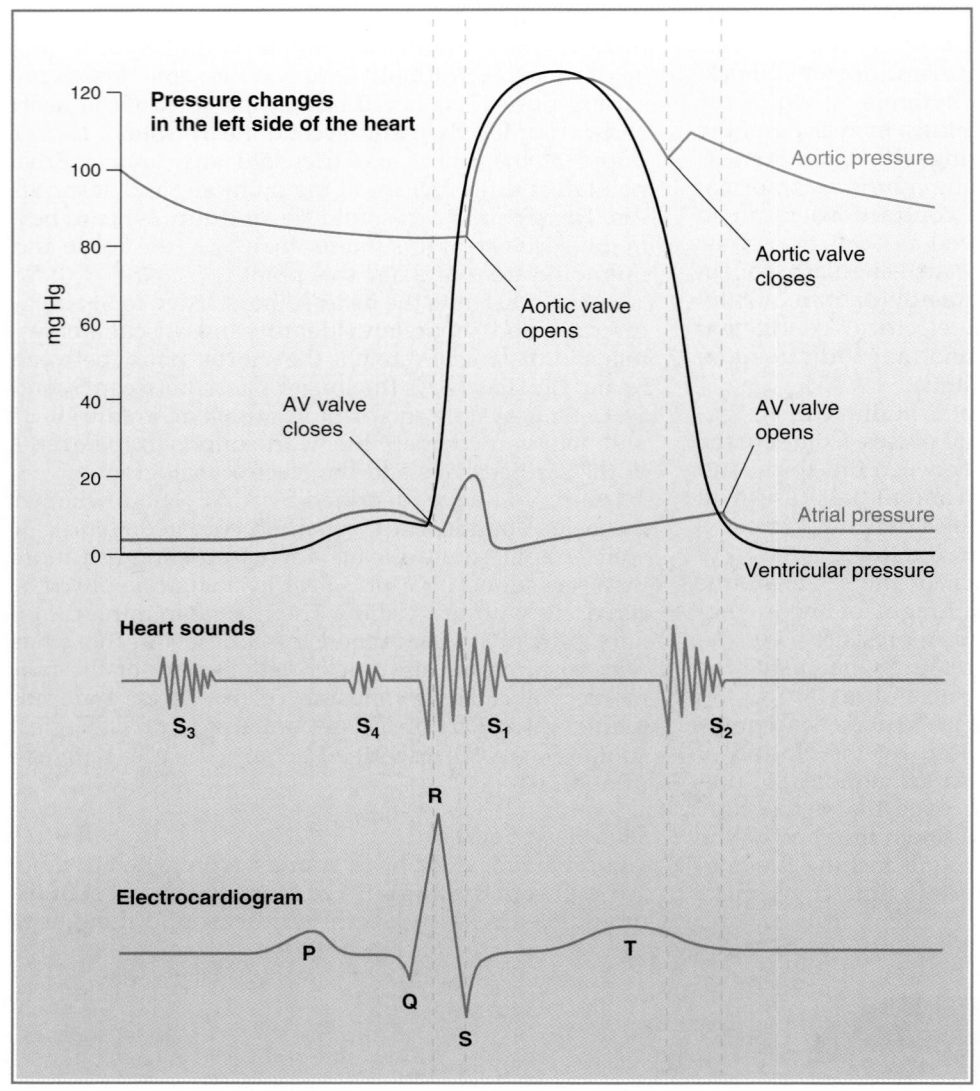

Figure 10–34. Relationship of heart sounds to the events of the cardiac cycle and the electrocardiogram.

be caused by vibrations of the ventricle walls when they are suddenly distended by blood from the atria and is heard most clearly at the apex of the heart. Third heart sounds may be heard just after S_2. S_4 is a fourth heart sound that may be heard at the apex of the heart during expiration and is caused by vibrations of the atria after contraction. The fourth heart sound may be heard just before S_1.

S_3 and S_4 are called gallop rhythms because the sound produced resembles the galloping of a horse. S_3 is a ventricular gallop. An atrial gallop is an abnormal cardiac rhythm in which a low-pitched, extra heart sound (S_4) is heard late in diastole, just before the S_1.

An S_3 can be heard when the atrioventricular valves open and blood rushes into the ventricles. It occurs when the ventricles are resistant to filling during the early rapid filling phase of diastole. S_3 is best heard at the apex in the lateral position or lower left sternal border. S_3 is normal in children and in young adults but after age 40 is usually taken as a sign of heart failure. The sound of an S_3 can be simulated by rapidly repeating LUBB-dupp-pa.

S_4 is also a sound produced by ventricular filling, but it results from contraction of the atria late in diastole. It is heard immediately before S_1 when the atria contract to finish filling the ventricles immediately before contraction. A physiological S_4 may occur in adults over the age of 40, particularly after exercise, but it usually indicates a pathological condition such as hypertension, fluid overload, or heart failure. An S_4 can be simulated by rapidly repeating deeLUBB-dupp.

Murmurs

Auscultate for heart murmurs. Murmurs occur when there is turbulent blood flow in the heart or great vessels. When auscultated, they are heard as a soft swooshing or blowing sound rather than the clear lubb-dupp of the first and second heart sound. Three conditions can cause murmurs: increased velocity of the blood, decreased viscosity of the blood, and structural defects in the valves or unusual openings in the heart chambers.

Evaluate all murmurs for intensity, pattern quality, location, radiation, and posture. The intensity (loud or soft) of a murmur may be high, medium, or low, depending on the pressure and rate of blood flow. To more accurately describe their intensity, murmurs can be graded on a scale of 1 to 6 according to the following criteria:

Grade 1: Barely audible

Grade 2: Audible but faint

Grade 3: Moderately loud

Grade 4: Loud and associated with a thrill

Grade 5: Loud and heard with the edge of the stethoscope lifted off the chest wall

Grade 6: Loudest and heard easily without a stethoscope or with a stethoscope held just above the chest wall

Murmurs may also vary in their pattern intensity (Fig. 10–35). They may grow louder in intensity (cre-

scendo), taper off in intensity (decrescendo), or increase in intensity to an apex and then taper off all within one systolic or diastolic pause (crescendo-decrescendo or diamond-shaped). The murmur may be pansystolic or holosystolic (or pandiastolic or holodiastolic). In other words, it occurs throughout the entire length of the systolic (or diastolic) pause, or it occurs in the early, middle, or late part of systole or diastole. Whatever pattern the murmur exhibits, it should be carefully and accurately described to help differentiate the possible underlying causes. This chapter introduces some patterns of intensity. However, it is beyond the scope of this chapter to provide more detailed explanations of the characteristic murmurs associated with each cardiac abnormality.

Location refers to the location within the cardiac cycle. A murmur heard during the lubb, or systolic phase, is a systolic murmur; one heard during the dupp, or diastolic phase, is a diastolic murmur.

A murmur can radiate downstream of the blood flow and be heard on a different area of the precordium.

The degree to which a murmur can be heard can vary with posture. Therefore, a thorough examination of the heart includes listening with the client in the supine, forward sitting, and side-lying positions (Fig. 10–36).

Assessment of the Peripheral Vascular System

Include the following in the assessment of the peripheral vascular system:

- Assessment of the client's blood pressure
- Inspection and palpation of the carotid arteries
- Assessment of the jugular venous pulsations
- Assessment of the peripheral venous circulation
- Assessment of the peripheral arterial circulation

Ask the client to undress to his underwear and examination gown. He will need to sit, stand, or lie down as necessary throughout the examination of the peripheral vascular system.

Blood Pressure

Using your stethoscope and sphygmomanometer, assess the client's blood pressure while the client is relaxed and sitting and again just after standing. Blood pressure will normally vary among individuals. In general, systolic pressure in the adult varies from 95 to 140 mm Hg, and diastolic pressure varies from 60 to 90 mm Hg. Compare the blood pressures in each arm. A difference of 15 mm Hg or less systolic and 5 mm Hg or less diastolic while the client is standing and a difference of 5 to 10 mm Hg or less while the client is sitting are considered normal. Assess whether there are orthostatic changes in blood pressure (represented by a change of greater than 10 mm Hg in diastolic pressures taken from the same arm while the client is sit-

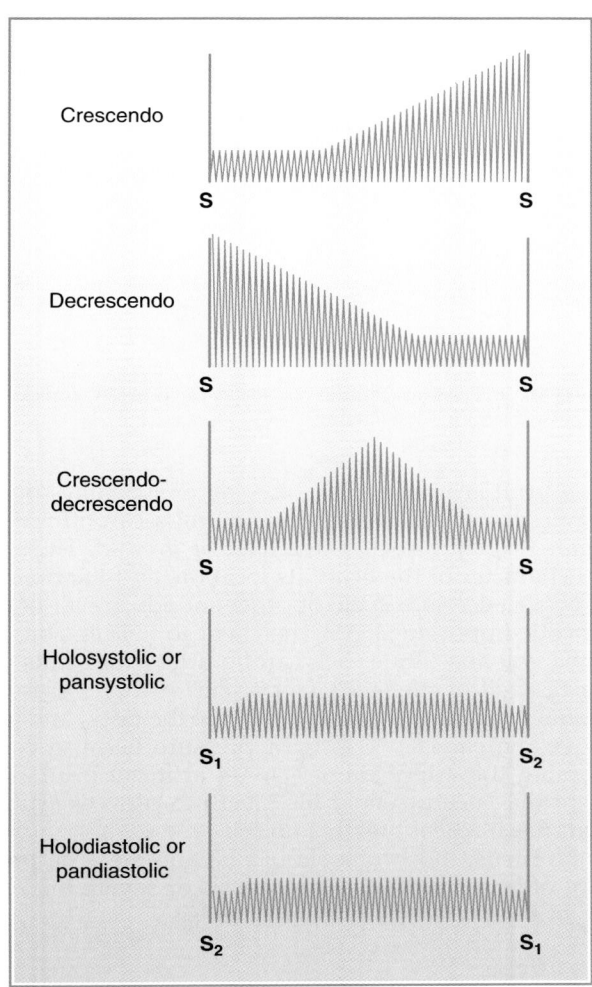

Figure 10–35. Characteristics of heart murmurs.

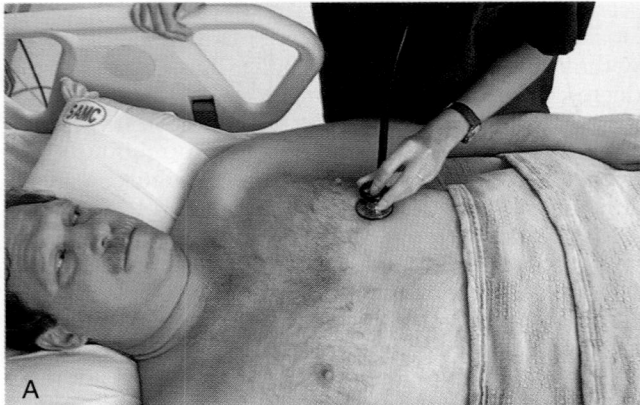

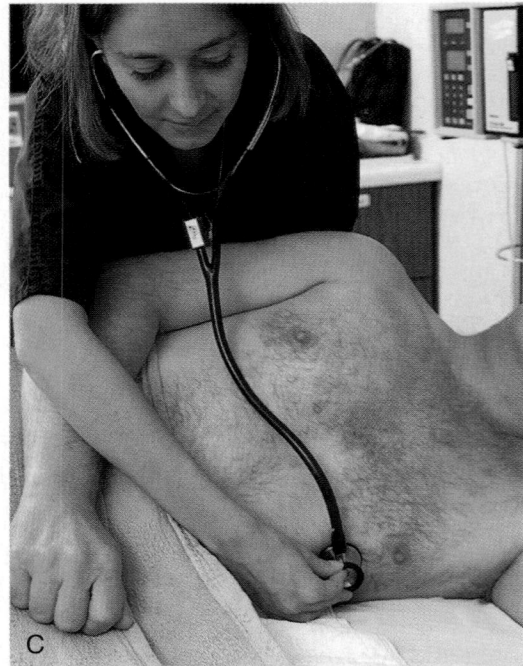

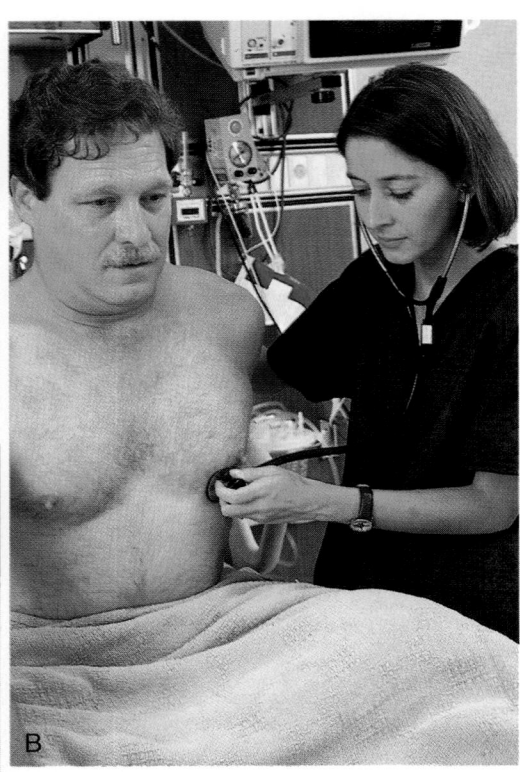

Figure 10–36. Positions for auscultation of the heart. A, supine; B, forward-sitting; C, side-lying.

ting and standing). Refer to Chapter 9 for a more thorough discussion of blood pressure and vital signs.

Carotid Arteries

Inspect and palpate the carotid arteries. With the client sitting, inspect and palpate the pulsations of the carotid arteries. Use the index and middle fingers together to gently palpate the carotid arteries on either side of the neck near the medial edge of the sternocleidomastoid muscle.

Examine one artery at a time. It may help to turn the client's head slightly away from you for inspection and then back toward you for palpation. Compare and note the rate, rhythm, and strength of pulsations of both carotid arteries. A normal rate will vary between 60 and 90 bpm bilaterally. The carotid pulsations should feel strong, elastic, and regular. Note whether the rate is synchronous with the client's heartbeat and whether the rate changes with inspiration or expiration.

A bruit is an abnormal blowing or swishing sound or murmur heard while auscultating a carotid artery, organ, or gland, such as the liver or thyroid. The special character of the bruit, its location, and the time of its occurrence in a cycle of other sounds are all of diagnostic importance. Ask the client to hold his breath while you auscultate each carotid artery for bruits using the bell of the stethoscope (Fig. 10–37). Assess at the angle of the jaw, middle third of the neck, and just above the clavicle. Use light pressure because compressing the artery can create an artificial bruit. The client may need to hold his breath to prevent artifact from the tracheal breath sounds.

Normally, no bruits should be audible. The presence of bruits indicates thrombosis or severe thickening of the lumen from atherosclerosis.

Neck Veins

Assess the jugular venous pulsations. Inspect the jugular veins with the client sitting up at a 90-degree angle

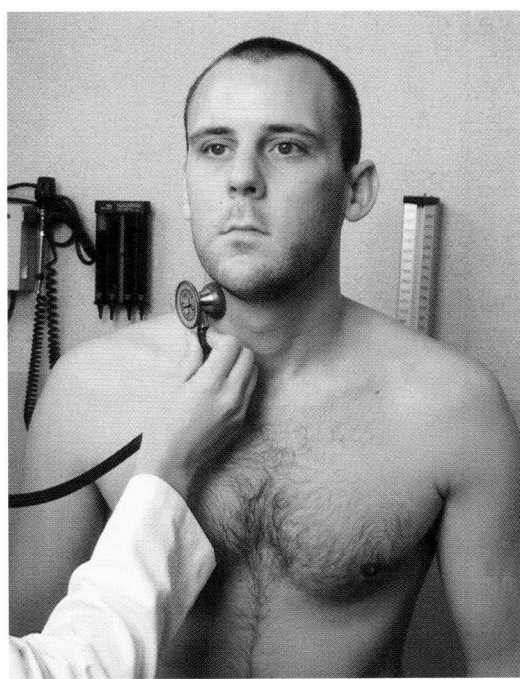

Figure 10–37. Assessing for a carotid bruit.

and again with the client lying down with the head raised slightly at a 30-degree to 45-degree angle. Assess the level for jugular vein distention on both sides using the two-ruler method. Note any pressures that measure greater than 3 cm, or 1¼ inches. Normal jugular venous pressure is usually less than 2.5 cm, or 1 inch. Chapter 40 further discusses jugular vein distention.

Peripheral Veins

Assess the peripheral venous circulation. Inspect and palpate for signs of peripheral venous insufficiency (changes in the skin, changes in temperature, presence of edema, varicosities, phlebitis, and thrombosis). Assess the skin, nail beds, and extremities for signs of venous insufficiency. Note whether there is pallor, cyanosis, stasis, dermatitis, ulcers, necrosis, edema, or cellulitis. Note whether there is clubbing of the client's fingers or toes, and whether temperature changes are unilateral of bilateral.

Note whether there is any edema of the lower extremities. Assess whether it is pitting or non-pitting. Note the extent of involvement. The edema of peripheral vascular disease is usually ascending. It may begin in the ankles and ascend up the legs, depending on the severity of the vascular compromise. Chapter 40 discusses edema in greater detail.

Inspect and palpate the lower extremities for varicosities. Varicose veins are swollen, distended, and knotted veins resulting from incompetent valves that allow the blood to back-flow, thus distending and stretching the veins. They appear as swollen, thick, tortuous veins easily seen and palpated along the surface of the lower extremities. Inspect and palpate the

superficial veins for signs of phlebitis or inflammation. Look for reddened, thickened, or tender veins. If varicosities are present, palpate the vessel with one hand while pressing down on the vessel with your second hand at a point just above the first hand. Palpate for the impulse of blood flow. Normally there should be none. If any varicosities occur in the lower legs, assess for phlebitis.

To check for the presence of phlebitis (inflammation of a vein), *gently* squeeze the calf muscle against the tibia and note the presence of any tenderness. Additionally, you can perform a special maneuver to detect a deep vein thrombosis (DVT). With the client's knee slightly flexed, dorsiflex the foot. In the presence of a deep vein thrombosis, there will be characteristic sharp calf pain, which is described as a positive Homans sign (Fig. 10–38). A positive Homans sign suggests DVT but is not definitive.

Peripheral Arteries

Assess the peripheral arterial circulation. Inspect and palpate for signs of peripheral arterial insufficiency. Inspect the skin and nails. Note the presence of thin shiny skin, scaly skin, decreased hair growth, or thickened nails. Note whether the extremities are cool to the touch. Note whether the client demonstrates any sensory deficits. Test the client's ability to perceive soft, dull, sharp, and vibratory sensations with his eyes closed.

Check each of the peripheral pulses (radial, ulnar, brachial, femoral, popliteal, dorsalis pedis, and posterior tibial pulses). Since each person's anatomy varies slightly, pulses are located primarily by touch. Exert light pressure with your index and middle fingertips held together and palpate the arterial pulses. You may need to use deep palpation to locate the temporal artery. Compare all contralateral or paired pulses for rhythm, strength, and equality. If the pulse is difficult to find or not readily palpable, you may need to use a Doppler or ultrasound stethoscope to amplify the sound of the arterial pulsations.

Palpate the radial pulse along the radial groove on the palmar and radial side of the wrist. Palpate the ul-

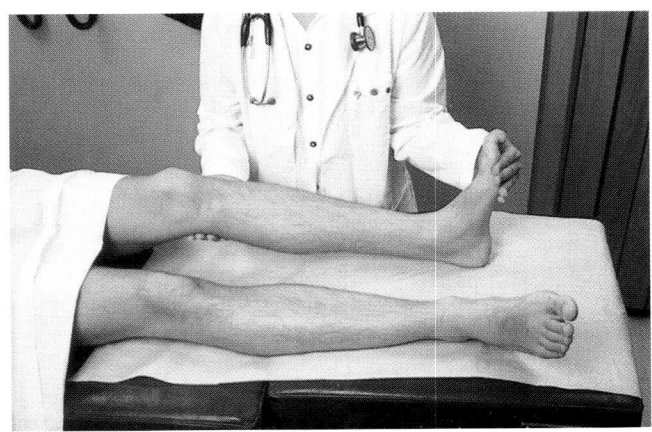

Figure 10–38. Assessing for Homans' sign.

nar pulse on the palmar and medial side of the wrist. Palpate the brachial pulse at the antecubital fossa between the biceps and triceps muscles. Palpate the femoral pulse with the client supine just below the inguinal ligament and halfway between the symphysis pubis and the anterior superior iliac spine. Palpate the popliteal pulse located behind the knee with the client supine or prone. Ask the client to relax the leg muscles and slightly flex the knee. Palpate the dorsalis pedis pulse with the client supine. It can be found on the anterior or upper aspect of the foot, halfway between the base of the ankle and the second metatarsophalangeal joint. Palpate the posterior tibial pulse just below and behind the medial malleolus with the foot relaxed and slightly extended.

Assessment of the Abdomen

The abdomen is a large oval cavity extending from the diaphragm to the floor of the pelvis. It is lined with the parietal peritoneal membrane covering the wall of the abdomen and is continuous with the visceral peritoneal membrane that covers the organs of the abdomen. To assess the abdomen, you must know the precise location of the visceral organs underlying the skin and abdominal muscles.

The abdomen can be divided into four or nine quadrants. Commonly the abdomen is divided into four quadrants by vertical and horizontal lines at the umbilicus (Fig. 10–39). However, the older nine-quadrant method may be useful to describe findings in a more precise manner. For more information on the nine-quadrant method, consult a physical assessment text.

The liver and gallbladder are in the upper right quadrant and are protected by the lower ribs. Only the lower border is normally palpable. The spleen is protected by the lower ribs on the left. The organs of the abdominal cavity are not normally palpable. The lower left colon may be palpable if filled with feces and the bladder if filled with urine. The uterus and ovaries are palpable with a bimanual vaginal examination.

The following should be included in assessment of the abdomen:

- Inspection of the abdomen
- Auscultation for bowel sounds and bruits
- Percussion of the abdomen
- Percussion of the size and span of the liver
- Percussion of the gastric air bubble
- Percussion of the kidneys
- Percussion of the spleen
- Palpation of the abdomen in all four quadrants using light and deep palpation techniques
- Palpation of the umbilicus
- Palpation of the liver
- Palpation of the gallbladder
- Palpation of the spleen
- Palpation of the aorta
- Palpation for ascites in the distended abdomen
- Ballottement of a suspected mass

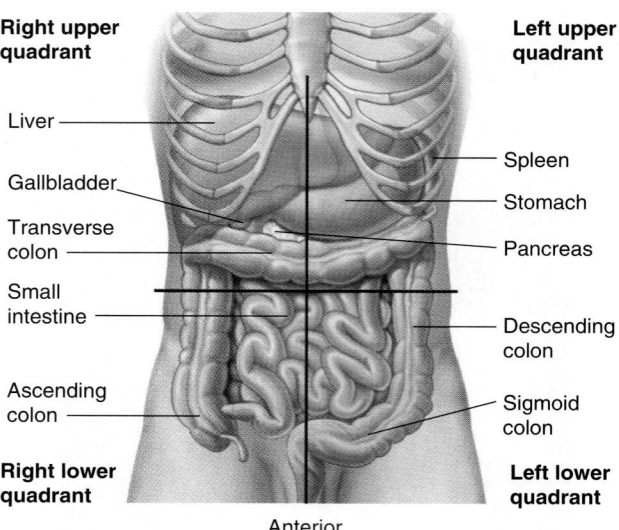

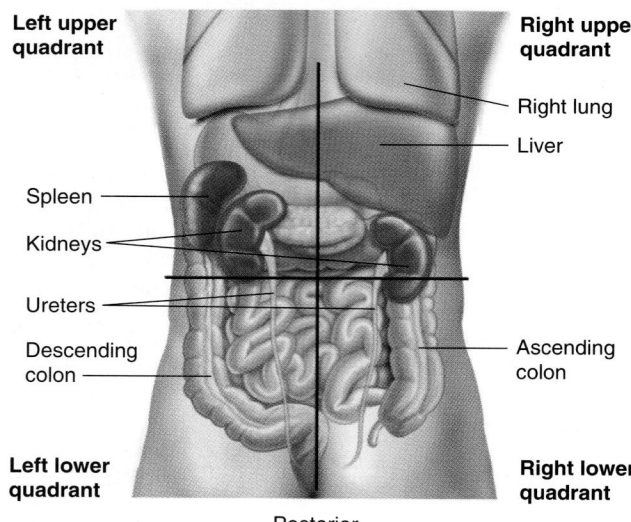

Figure 10–39. The four abdominal quadrants and the underlying organs.

Inspection

To prepare the client for an examination of the abdomen, ask him to undress to the waist and don an examination gown. Cover the legs and genitalia with a sheet and have the client lie supine with knees slightly flexed and arms at the side or folded across the chest. You may need to provide pillows for the head and knees to make the client more comfortable. Ask the client to locate any tender areas before proceeding and examine these areas last. Examine the client with warm hands and a warm stethoscope. Try to distract the client with conversation throughout the examination, while watching his facial expressions for any grimaces or confirmations of pain.

Observe the client's posture. Note whether the client is guarding or splinting the abdomen, lying perfectly still, constantly changing positions, frequently leaning forward, or favoring one side or position.

Inspect the skin. Note the color of the skin, turgor, and presence of erythema, ecchymosis, lesions, masses, striae (stretch marks), old scars, or venous abnormalities (refer to the section on skin and nails). Note whether the client has markedly diminished or excessive adipose tissue. Jaundice or a yellow hue to the skin and sclera may indicate an underlying liver or gallbladder disease. A bluish tinge to the abdomen (Cullen's sign) may indicate internal bleeding. Bruising of the flank (Grey Turner sign) may indicate pancreatitis or internal bleeding.

Assess for abdominal distention. Inspect the abdomen from all angles while the client is lying supine and again while the client holds a deep breath. Abnormal distention of the abdomen occurs with the accumulation of fluid, feces, or gas or the presence of a tumor (as with ascites, bowel obstruction, and cancer). Mild distention of the abdomen below the umbilicus may be normal and secondary to a full bladder or stool in the colon. A glistening taut abdomen might indicate the presence of ascites. Ascites is the abnormal accumulation of serous (edematous) fluid within the peritoneal cavity. Note the symmetry, the contour (flat, convex, or concave), the presence of surface movements (breathing, peristalsis, aortic pulsations), bulging, or masses (hernias, cysts, tumors), obesity, and distention (obstruction, ascites). It is normal to see the pulsation of the aorta and waves of peristalsis in thin persons.

Asymmetry above the umbilicus may indicate gastric dilation, pancreatic cyst, or malignancy. Asymmetry below the umbilicus may indicate pregnancy, fibroid uterus, ovarian cancer, bowel or bladder obstruction, hernias, tumors, or cysts.

Auscultation

Auscultate the abdomen for bowel sounds with the diaphragm of the stethoscope. It is important to auscultate the abdomen prior to palpation and percussion so as not to disturb abdominal contents and the peristaltic waves.

Using the diaphragm of the stethoscope, auscultate the abdomen in all four quadrants. Begin in the left lower quadrant (LLQ) and listen for several minutes. Bowel sounds are gurgling, high-pitched sounds occurring as gas passes through the intestine. Occurring irregularly, there may be anywhere from 5 to 20 a minute. After eating, the bowel is active and produces more frequent sounds. The loud, audible sound of the stomach "growling" is termed borborygmus and is the same type of sound heard with a stethoscope. If bowel sounds are present, note their character and frequency and whether they are normal, hyperactive, or hypoactive. Hypoactive sounds are quiet and infrequent. Hyperactive sounds are loud and frequent. Normal is somewhere in between. The complete absence of bowel sounds indicates a nonfunctional intestine. Listen for 5 minutes before deciding that bowel sounds are absent.

If they are absent after 1 to 1½ minutes in one quadrant, make note of this and proceed to the other

three quadrants. Bowel sounds normally do not occur in all four quadrants but should occur in at least one. However, hyperactive bowel sounds, or borborygmi, may occur in response to inflammation of the bowel, laxative abuse or overuse, and certain spicy foods. Hypoactive bowel sounds or the complete cessation of bowel sounds may occur in response to conditions that decrease the gastric motility, such as pancreatitis, paralytic ileus, or an obstruction.

Auscultate for abdominal bruits. Using the bell of the stethoscope, auscultate for abdominal bruits in the target areas diagrammed. Listen carefully for bruits, hums, and friction rubs in the epigastric area and all four quadrants over the aortic, renal, iliac, and femoral arteries and the thoracic aorta. Normally no bruits will be heard. If bruits, venous hums, or friction rubs are present, they may indicate an underlying stricture, thrombosis, or aneurysm. If bruits are present, notify the physician and do not further palpate the abdomen, as this may damage an existing aneurysm.

Percussion

Percuss the abdomen using the percussion techniques previously described. Percuss all four quadrants of the abdomen to determine the nature of underlying tissue. Hollow organs such as the gastric air bubble in the left upper quadrant (LUQ) will produce tympanic sounds, and solid or fluid-filled tissue, such as the liver, kidneys, spleen, pancreas, and distended bladder, will produce a dull sound.

Percuss the size and span of the liver. Begin at a point just below the umbilicus on the right midclavicular line and percuss upward to the lower liver edge. Mark the area where the dullness of the upper liver edge begins. Next, percuss downward from an area of resonant lung to the upper liver edge. Mark the area where the dullness of the upper liver edge begins. Measure between the two marks with a ruler or tape measure. Record this measure as the liver span. The liver is normally dull to percussion. The normal liver span should be from 6 to 12 cm, or 2½ to 5 inches, in width. An enlarged liver (>12-cm span) may indicate cirrhosis, hepatitis, hepatoma, cyst, abscess, or other extrinsic mass or malignancy that impinges on the liver.

Percuss over the LUQ, the left anterior rib cage, and the left epigastric area for the gastric air bubble. It will produce tympany in a small area of the LUQ.

Percuss the kidneys. Ask the client to sit or stand and percuss the posterior costovertebral angle at the scapular line. The kidneys should be dull and painless to percussion. Tenderness of the costovertebral angle may indicate acute pyelonephritis or glomerulonephritis.

Percuss the spleen in the area of the left tenth rib just posterior to the midaxillary line. Identify the small oval area of splenic dullness. You may also assess for splenic enlargement by percussing the normally tympanic area in the lowest left interspace on the left anterior axillary line. If this area grows dull when the client takes a deep breath, the spleen may be enlarged.

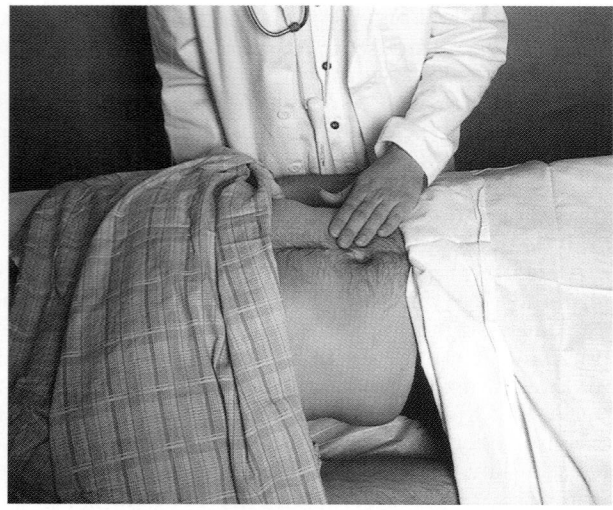

Figure 10–40. Light palpation of the abdomen.

Palpation

Palpate the abdomen in all four quadrants using the technique of light palpation (Fig. 10–40). Use the fingerpads or palmar surface of three or four fingers held together. Move methodically through each quadrant, depressing the abdomen not more than ½ to 1 inch, while using dipping or circular motions. Identify and note the size and location of any abnormalities and areas of increased resistance or tenderness. While distracting the client, return to and further evaluate areas of increased resistance and tenderness to determine whether the resistance is voluntary or involuntary. With the client relaxed, palpate for any abnormal rigidity of the rectus muscles.

Palpate the abdomen in all four quadrants using the technique of deep palpation (Fig. 10–41). Using the palmar surface or fingerpads of three or four fingers held together, deeply palpate the abdomen, depressing underlying tissue 1 to 3 inches as you move me-

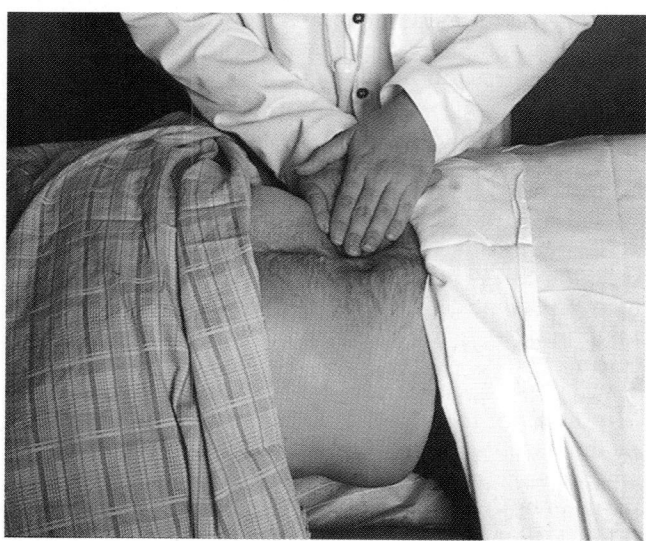

Figure 10–41. Deep palpation of the abdomen.

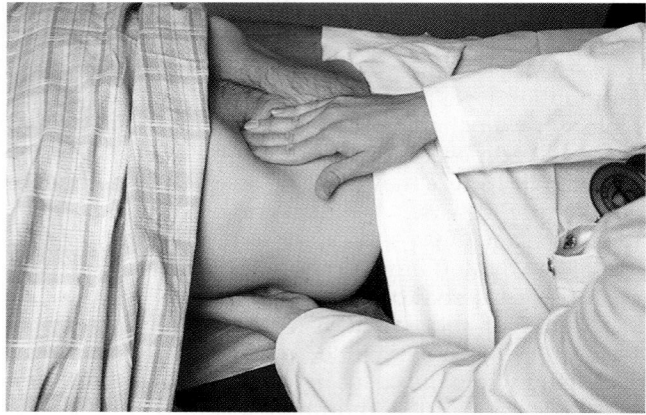

Figure 10–42. Palpating the liver.

thodically through each quadrant. Move your fingers back and forth over underlying tissue to delineate organs and detect less obvious masses. Deeply palpate for rebound tenderness, which will occur after the sudden release of deep pressure on the abdomen if an acute inflammatory process is present. Proceed cautiously and avoid deeply palpating any areas of known severe tenderness, pulsating masses, or recent surgical incisions.

Palpate the umbilicus for tenderness, masses, bulges, hernias, lesions, and discharge.

Palpate the liver. Place your left hand under the client's right posterior thorax parallel to and at the level of the 11th and 12th ribs. Place your right hand on the client's right upper quadrant (RUQ) over the midclavicular line with fingers pointing toward the head and positioned below the lower edge of liver dullness. Ask the client to take a deep breath while you press inward and upward with the fingers of your right hand. With inspiration, the liver descends lower in the abdomen. Attempt to feel the edge of the liver as it descends (Fig. 10–42). The liver edge may normally descend up to 1 inch on deep inspiration, but often it is not palpable, which is also normal. When palpable, the liver edge should feel smooth, firm, and nontender and have a regular contour. A liver palpated more than 1 or 2 cm (fingerbreadths) is abnormal. Abnormalities may indicate the presence of cirrhosis, hepatitis, hepatoma, cyst, abscess, malignancy, or other extrinsic mass compromising the integrity of the liver.

Palpation of the gallbladder is usually not performed on routine physical examinations. This technique is usually left to highly experienced practitioners and is performed in the following manner. Ask the client to take a deep breath and palpate deep below the liver margin for enlargement of the gallbladder. Since the gallbladder is usually not palpable, a palpable gallbladder is more than likely enlarged. An enlarged, palpable, tender gallbladder may indicate cholelithiasis (gallstones), cholecystitis (infection), malignancy, abscess, or obstruction by an extrinsic mass or malignancy. A positive Murphy sign (abrupt cessation of inspiration during deep palpation of the gallbladder) is further indicative of an acute process.

Palpate the spleen. Place your left hand under the client's left costovertebral angle and your right hand on the abdomen below the left costal margin. Ask the client to take a deep breath while you press the fingertips of your right hand inward. Palpate the edge of the spleen as it descends with inspiration. The spleen is often not palpable; if it is palpable, it may be enlarged.

Palpate the aorta. Use your thumb and forefinger to palpate the aorta by pressing deeply just to the left of the vertical midline of the abdomen. Unless the client is morbidly obese, the aorta will be palpable with strong and regular pulsations. Faint or irregular pulsations may indicate cardiovascular disease. A distinct pulsating mass indicates an aneurysm and should not be further palpated, to avoid possible inadvertent rupture.

Palpate the bladder. Palpate the area above the pubic symphysis if the client's history indicates possible urinary retention. You may be able to feel the top of a full bladder because it rises above the symphysis pubis. Sometimes it will deviate to one side or the other. The alert client will be able to describe the sensation of the urge to urinate when you press on a full bladder.

If the abdomen appears distended, palpate for ascites. Ask the client to lie supine. Have a colleague assist you by pressing his hand and forearm firmly along the vertical midline of the abdomen. Place your hands on either side of the client's abdomen. Strike one side of the client's abdomen forcefully with your fingertips and, with the other hand, feel for the rebounding impulse of a fluid wave. Another technique for determining the presence of ascites is to percuss "shifting dullness" in the abdomen. With the client lying supine, percuss from the midline of the abdomen to the flank. Mark the level of dullness. Ask the client to lie on his side and percuss again over the same area, this time from the flank to the vertical midline of the abdomen (Fig. 10–43). Note any change in the level of dullness. If ascites is present, the level of dullness will be slightly higher with the client lying on his side. The presence of ascites may result from a number of medical problems, primarily liver disease, congestive heart failure, or ovarian cancer.

Perform ballottement for any suspected masses. It may be difficult to palpate a suspected mass in a person with marked ascites. In this situation, ballottement may prove helpful in determining the presence of a mass. To perform ballottement for a suspected mass, thrust the fingers of the right hand quickly and firmly into the area of the suspected mass. If the mass is freely mobile, it will initially retreat into the abdomen, and then immediately rebound back against your fingers.

Assessment of the Musculoskeletal System

Include the following in your assessment of the musculoskeletal system:

- Assessment of the client's posture, stance, and gait
- Inspection for gross abnormalities

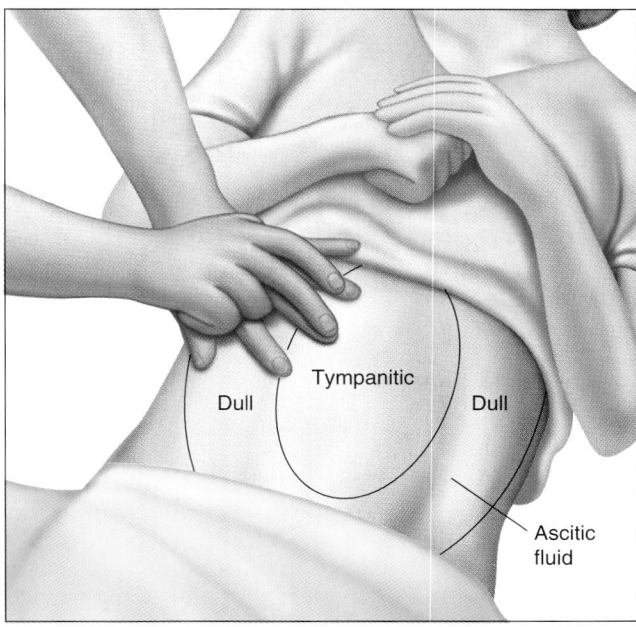

Figure 10–43. Assessing for ascites.

- Inspection of the skin and surrounding tissues of all the bones, joints, and muscle groups
- Inspection of the temporomandibular joint (TMJ) and jaw and assessment of its range of motion
- Inspection of the neck and spine and assessment of their range of motion
- Inspection of the upper extremities and assessment of their range of motion
- Inspection of the lower extremities and assessment of their range of motion

Posture, Stance, and Gait

Assess the client's posture, stance, and gait by observing the client inconspicuously as he enters the examining room. The client should be able to stand erect with his head up, face forward, arms hanging straight at the sides, shoulders and hips parallel, and legs straight with both knees and feet side by side and a few inches apart.

The client's contralateral (matching) extremities should appear grossly symmetrical, equal in size, shape, and length. Note whether the client appears unable to stand erect or exhibits a hunched, bent, or stooped posture. Note any apparent abnormal curvature of the spine as in kyphosis (accentuated lordosis), or scoliosis (a lateral bending of the spine). Also note any contractures or deformities of the extremities. Note whether the client is able to stand on both feet comfortably without assistance or support and without any swaying or loss of balance. Note whether the client is able to stand on one foot at a time without difficulty. Note any evidence of uneven distribution of weight, swaying, stumbling, or loss of balance, favoring one foot, standing on the heels, toes, or edges of the feet, uneven depth of footprints, or toes pointing either laterally or medially rather than straight ahead.

Assess the client's gait by asking the client to walk across the room. The client should be able to walk with equal and symmetrical strides with respect to timing, weight bearing, and distance. The client's steps should consist of a rhythmic planting of first the heel and then the toe of the foot with the toes pointing forward. While walking, the client may sway slightly as he shifts weight from foot to foot but should not demonstrate an unsteady gait, loss of balance, shuffling, limping, propulsive walking, veering off in one direction, foot drop, foot lag, or any irregularity in the timing of the stride.

Gross Abnormalities

Inspect for any gross or obvious abnormalities that are easily noticed on an initial head-to-toe inspection (such as amputation, congenital deformities, contractures, paralysis, and so on). Inspect and palpate the skin and surrounding tissues of all the bones, joints, and muscle groups (refer to the section on assessment of the skin and nails). Inspect for color, temperature, swelling, edema, skinfolds, and lesions. Note any abnormalities.

Muscle Tone and Strength

Assess all muscle groups for contralateral symmetry, tone, and strength. Contralateral muscle groups, or those muscles identically paired, as in the left and right biceps, should be symmetrical in size, shape, contour, position, and alignment of like joints. Note any variances.

Assess all muscle groups for muscle tone. You can assess muscle tone and strength at the same time as range of motion by noting the degree of resistance felt on passive range of motion (Fig. 10–44). Normally, a slight resistance is felt.

Assess muscle strength by asking the client to pull away from or push against an opposing force that you impose. Repeat these same maneuvers with the contralateral joint and assess bilateral muscle strength. Normally, a particular muscle group will have normal tone if slight resistance is demonstrated against passive range of motion. A hypertonic muscle exhibits increased resistance to passive range of motion. A hypotonic muscle presents as a boggy, flat, flabby, or flaccid muscle that offers little or no resistance against passive range of motion.

Assess the strength of all muscle groups. Each muscle group should be relatively equal when compared to the muscle group on the contralateral side. The dominant hand or arm may normally be slightly stronger. Measure, when possible with a tape measure, the size (diameter) of any muscle or muscle group that demonstrates weakness. A smaller size of a particular muscle or muscle group may indicate atrophy. Con-

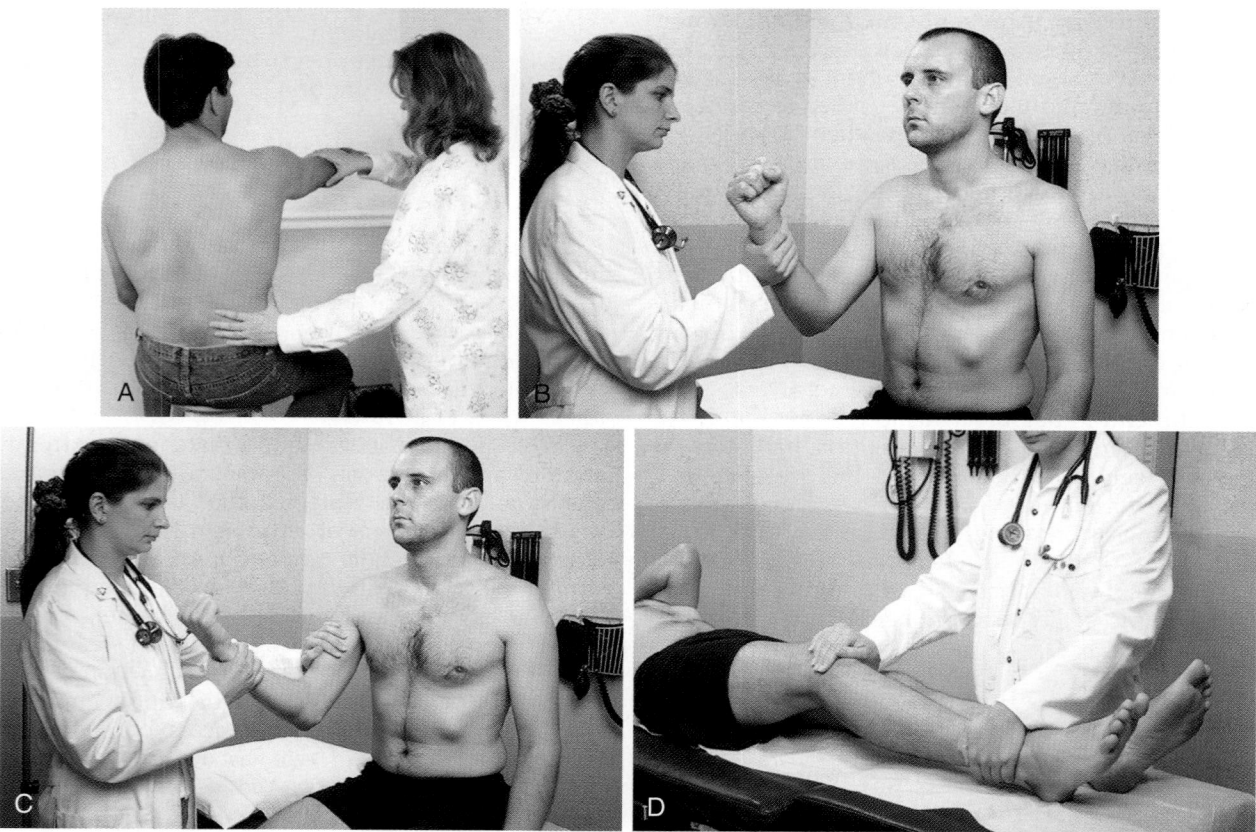

Figure 10–44. Assessing for muscle tone and strength. A, ask the client to flex his shoulder muscle against your hand as you apply resistance. B, ask the client to extend his elbow as you apply resistance. C, ask the client to flex his elbow as you apply resistance. D, ask the client to raise his knee as you apply resistance.

versely, an unusually large muscle may indicate hypertrophy.

Contralateral Bones and Joints

Assess the contralateral bones and joints for symmetry with respect to size, shape, position, alignment, stability, and range of motion. Asymmetry may be the result of congenital anomalies, arthritis, bony tumors, fractures, dislocations, adhesions, or surgery. Malalignment may be secondary to fracture dislocation, congenital anomalies, or surgical procedures. The joints should be able to be moved passively in all directions and degrees expected for the specific groups. There should be no abnormal movements or sounds produced by movement or manipulation of the joints. Any pain or stiffness elicited upon movement of a joint that has no associated fracture or dislocation usually indicates arthritis or tendon or ligament damage.

Assess the stability of each joint. To do this, grasp and stabilize the joint on the proximal side with one hand while attempting to move the joint with the other hand from the distal end. Note any abnormal movements, unusual sounds, crepitus, or abnormal range of motion or tenderness associated with these movements.

Finally, assess each joint for full passive range of motion (ROM). Note the angle at which the joint is freely able to bend in each position. (Use a goniometer for more accurate measurements if desired.) When doing a musculoskeletal assessment, it is often easiest to begin with the temporomandibular joint and jaw and then progress from head to toe. For example: assess the neck, then the spine, then the upper extremities, and then the lower extremities.

Jaw and Temporomandibular Joint

Inspect and palpate the jaw and temporomandibular joint (TMJ). Place two or three fingertips of each hand over the TMJs simultaneously. Ask the client to open and close his mouth widely two or three times while your fingertips are in place. Palpate for any unusual clicking sounds, sliding, or "catching" of the joint. With the client's mouth open as wide as possible, ask the client to vertically insert three fingers held side by side between the upper and lower teeth. Ask the client to slide the lower jaw forward and from side to side. The lower teeth should be able to be moved beyond and overlap the upper teeth in each instance. Note any malalignment of the upper jaw and lower jaw, inability to move the lower jaw sideways or forward (lockjaw), inability to open or close the jaw, or pain on mastication or movement of the jaw.

Neck, Cervical Spine, Thoracic Spine, and Lumbar Spine

Inspect and palpate the neck, cervical spine, thoracic spine, and lumbar spine, first with the client standing erect and then with the client bending over at the waist. Inspect from directly behind the client and again from the side view. Normally the cervical spine is concave, the thoracic spine convex, and the lumbar spine concave. Note any abnormal curvatures, palpable masses, compression fractures, or lesions or any pain along the spine. An abnormal curvature of the spine may be a result of kyphosis (an accentuated posterior curvature of the thoracic spine), sway back or lordosis (an accentuated lumbar curvature), scoliosis (a lateral curvature of the spine), ankylosing spondylitis (evidenced by persistence of the lumbar concavity and failure of the spinous processes to separate when the client bends over at the waist), or spondylolisthesis (a forward slipping and fusing of the vertebrae).

Assess the range of motion of the neck and spine. Assess flexion by asking the client to touch his chin to his chest. Assess hyperextension by asking the client to bend his head backward with his chin pointing up toward the ceiling. Assess rotation by asking the client to turn his head as far as possible to the left and then to the right with the ears facing the front and back. Assess lateral bending by asking the client to bend the head laterally, attempting to touch the ear to the shoulder. The normal range of motion for flexion is 70 to 90 degrees, for hyperextension 55 degrees, for rotation 70 degrees, and for lateral bending 35 degrees.

Assess the range of motion of the spine. To assess flexion, ask the client to bend forward at the waist; to assess extension, ask the client to bend backward at the waist. To assess rotation, ask the client to stand with his feet planted and toes pointed forward and attempt to rotate the torso so that the shoulders attempt to face forward and backward. To assess lateral bending, ask the client to bend laterally at the waist with shoulders pointing toward the floor or feet. Normal range of motion for flexion is 75 degrees, for extension 30 degrees, for rotation 30 degrees, and for lateral bending 35 degrees.

Upper and Lower Extremities

Following the assessment of the neck and spine, assess the upper and then the lower extremities. Work your way down from top to bottom, assessing first the right side and then the left side. For example, assess the right and then the left shoulder, then move to the elbows, then the wrists, then the fingers, then the hips, then the knees, then the ankles, and then the toes. After inspection and palpation of each joint and muscle group, assess each for range of motion and muscle strength.

Shoulders

Assess the shoulders for range of motion and muscle strength. Assess flexion by asking the client to lift the arm forward and above the head with the arm straight and horizontal to the floor, then move the arm backward to the spine. Assess extension by moving the arm backward with the arm straight. Assess horizontal extension by asking the client to abduct the arm horizontal to the floor and then bring the arm across the chest.

To assess abduction, lift the arm straight up above the head. To assess adduction, adduct the arm toward the midline of the trunk. Note any pain, which may be secondary to arthritis, inflammation, infection, bursitis, tendinitis, bony spurs, calcific deposits, masses, fractures, and dislocations. A frozen shoulder, evidenced by the inability of the client to abduct the arm without characteristic "shrugging" suggests a rupture of the supraspinatus tendon or rotator cuff injury. Normal range of motion for the shoulders can be expected to be 180 degrees for flexion, 130 degrees for horizontal flexion, 60 degrees for extension, 45 degrees for horizontal extension, 180 degrees for abduction, and 45 degrees for adduction.

Elbows

Assess the range of motion for the elbows. Assess flexion by asking the client to bend the lower arm up toward the biceps. Assess extension by asking the client to open his arm to a fully extended resting position. Assess hyperextension by asking the client to extend his arm beyond the normal resting position. Assess supination by asking the client to turn the lower arm so that the front faces upward. Assess pronation by asking the client to turn the lower arm so that the front faces downward. Normal range of motion for the elbows is expected to be 150 degrees for flexion, 150 degrees for extension, 0 to 10 degrees for hyperextension, 90 degrees for supination, and 90 degrees for pronation.

Wrists

Assess the range of motion for the wrists. Assess flexion by asking the client to flex the wrist toward the lower arm. Assess extension by asking the client to extend the wrist backward. Assess radial deviation by asking the client to deviate the wrist toward the radius. Assess ulnar deviation by asking the client to deviate the wrist toward the ulna. Normal range of motion for the wrists is expected to be 80 to 90 degrees for flexion, 70 degrees for extension, 20 degrees for radial deviation, and 30 to 50 degrees for ulnar deviation.

Fingers

Assess the range of motion for the fingers. Assess flexion by asking the client to close his fingers into a fist. Assess extension by asking the client to fully open his fingers. Assess abduction by asking the client to spread his fingers apart. Assess adduction by asking the client to cross the fingers together so that they touch and overlap. Assess opposition by asking the client to touch each finger with the thumb of the same hand. Normal range of motion for the fingers is expected to be 80 to 100 degrees for flexion, 0 to 45 degrees for extension, and 20 degrees for abduction. Normal adduction is demonstrated if the client is able to cross his fingers. Normal opposition is demonstrated if the client is able to touch each finger to the thumb of the same hand.

Hips

Assess the range of motion of the hips. Assess flexion with both a straight knee and a bent knee. Ask the client to first raise his leg straight up without bending the knee and then to raise it again with the knee bent. Assess extension by asking the client to lie prone and then extend the leg backward. Assess abduction by asking the client to abduct a partially flexed leg outward. Assess adduction by asking the client to adduct a partially flexed leg inward. Assess internal rotation by asking the client to flex the knee and swing the foot toward the midline. Assess external rotation by asking the client to flex the knee and swing the foot away from the midline. Normal range of motion for the hips is expected to be 90 degrees for straight knee flexion, 110 to 120 degrees for bent knee flexion, 30 degrees for extension, 45 to 50 degrees for abduction, 20 to 30 degrees for adduction, 35 to 40 degrees for internal rotation, and 45 degrees for external rotation.

Knees

Assess the range of motion of the knees. Assess flexion by asking the client to fully bend the knee so that the posterior calf and posterior thigh are nearly touching. Assess hyperextension by asking the client to extend the knee beyond the normal point of extension. Assess internal rotation by asking the client to rotate the knee and lower leg toward the midline. Assess external rotation by asking the client to rotate the knee and lower leg away from the midline. Normal range of motion is expected to be 130 degrees for flexion, 15 degrees for hyperextension, and 10 degrees for internal rotation.

Ankles

Assess the range of motion of the ankles. Assess dorsiflexion by asking the client to bend the ankle of the foot so that the toes point toward the head. Assess plantar flexion by asking the client to bend the foot downward with the toes pointing downward. Assess eversion by asking the client to turn the foot away from the midline. Assess inversion by asking the client to turn the foot toward the midline. Normal range of motion is expected to be 20 degrees for dorsiflexion, 45 degrees for plantar flexion, 20 degrees for eversion, and 30 degrees for inversion.

Toes

Assess the range of motion of the toes. Assess flexion by asking the client to curl his toes under his foot. Assess extension by asking the client to lift the toes to point upward. Assess abduction by asking the client to spread the toes apart. Normal range of motion is expected to be 35 to 60 degrees for flexion, 0 to 90 degrees for extension (depending on the specific joint), variable capability for abduction, and inability to adduct the toes.

Reflexes

A muscular reflex is an involuntary response to a stimulus in which the sensory nerve carries the message to the spinal cord and directly back to cause a contraction in a muscle. All muscles will contract reflexively when stimulated. However, only a few reflexes are tested clinically as indicators of motor function (Fig. 10–45).

Reflexes are classified as superficial and deep tendon reflexes. Superficial reflexes are elicited by stroking or stimulating the skin. Deep tendon reflexes are elicited by stretching a tendon by tapping with a percussion hammer. Testing reflexes requires sensitivity to slight contractions of muscles. Reflexes are classified as 0, no response; 1+, slightly diminished; 2+, normal; 3+, brisker than normal; and 4+, hyperactive. This scale is subjective and the rating may vary between examiners and with experience.

The biceps, triceps, and brachioradialis reflexes provide information about the function of the nerves of the cervical spine (C-5, C-6, C-7, C-8). All three are deep tendon reflexes. To test the biceps reflex, have the client partially flex the elbow and rest the arm on his own thigh or on your forearm. Place your thumb in the antecubital space over the biceps tendon. Tap your thumb with the percussion hammer. A positive response is slight movement of the forearm with contraction of the biceps muscle.

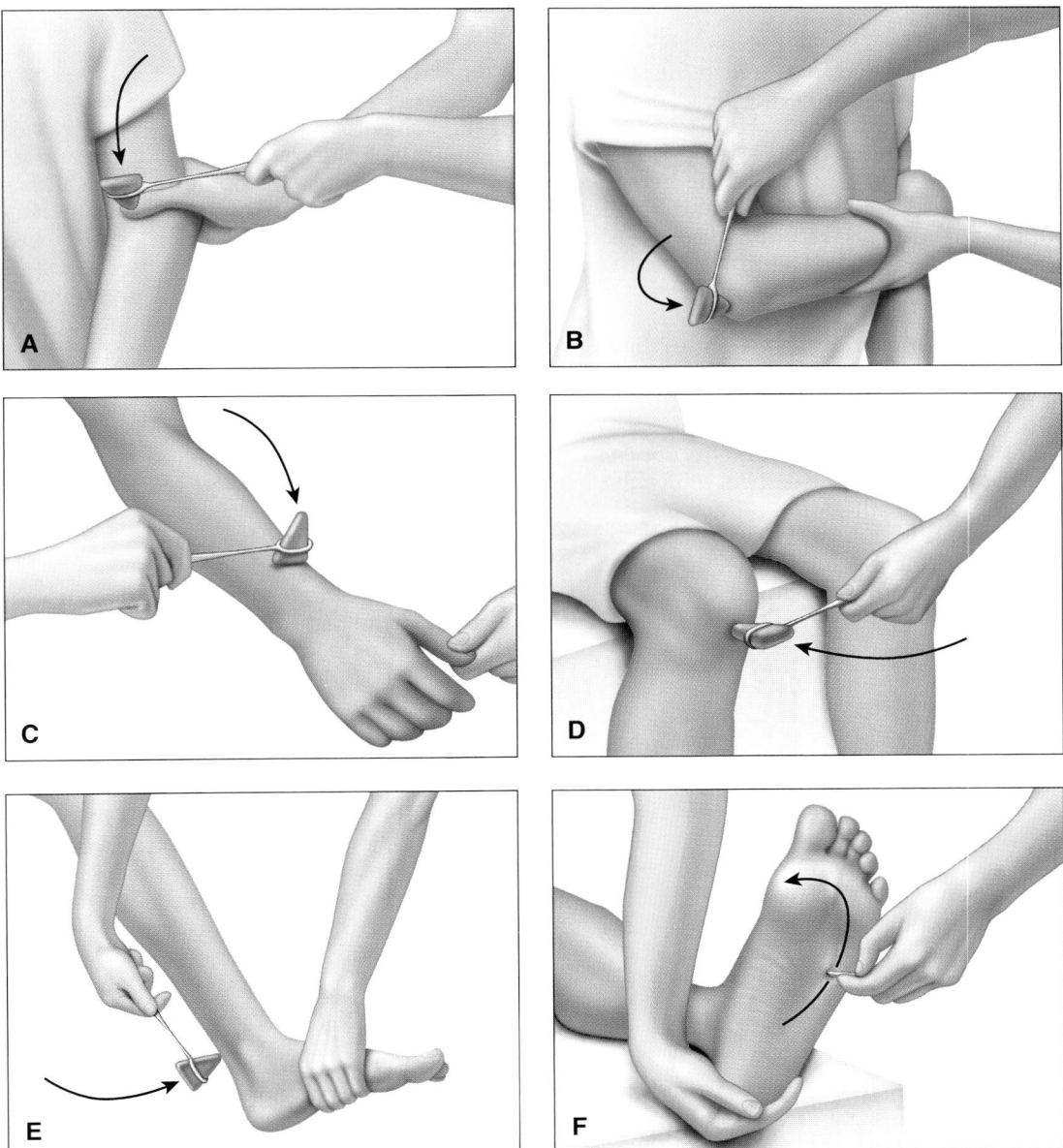

Figure 10–45. Assessing reflexes: A, biceps reflex; B, triceps reflex; C, brachioradialis reflex; D, patellar reflex; E, Achilles reflex; F, plantar (Babinski's) reflex.

To test the triceps reflex, flex the client's arm at the elbow and hold it suspended at a right angle to the shoulder. The arm should be relaxed with the forearm hanging freely. Directly tap the triceps tendon just above the elbow. The forearm should extend slightly. Alternatively, you may have the client hold the forearm across the chest, flexed 90 degrees at the elbow.

To test the brachioradialis reflex, have the client rest the forearm on his thigh. Grasp the thumb to suspend the forearm in a relaxed position. Tap the forearm directly on the lateral aspect of the radial bone 2 to 3 cm above the joint. The forearm should flex slightly, turning toward the supinated position.

In the lower extremity, the knee jerk, Achilles, and plantar reflexes are tested. The knee jerk or patellar reflex tests function of L1, L2, and L3 nerves. The Achilles reflex tests function of S1 and S2 nerves. These are deep tendon reflexes. To test the patellar reflex, have the client sit on a table or bed from which the foot and lower leg can hang freely. Strike the tendon directly below the patella (knee cap). The lower leg should extend.

To test the Achilles reflex, position the person supine with the hip externally rotated and the knee flexed. Hold the foot in a relaxed dorsiflexed position and strike the Achilles tendon with the percussion hammer. You should feel the foot plantar flex against your hand.

The plantar, or Babinski, reflex is a superficial reflex that is present in the first 8 to 10 months of life, then disappears and should be absent in adults. This reflex should be tested with the patient in a relaxed supine position. With a blunt instrument, apply firm pressure and draw a line from the heel along the lateral aspect of the sole of the foot and across the foot pad under the toes. With a positive response, the toes spread outward and the big toe moves upward. This finding indicates upper motor neuron disease of the pyramidal tract.

Assessment of the Anus, Rectum, and Prostate

The following should be included in the assessment of the anus, rectum, and prostate:

- Inspection and palpation of perianal tissue and perineum
- Inspection for the appearance of protrusions of masses with straining
- Digital examination to palpate the anus, rectum, and prostate
- Assessment of the tone and musculature of the anal sphincter
- Palpation of the muscular anal ring and rectum
- Palpation for high masses
- Palpation of the prostate in men
- Palpation of the uterus and cervix in women
- Examination of the fecal material

Perianal Tissue and Perineum

Inspect and palpate the perianal tissue and perineum. Position the client (male or female) on his or her side in the Sims position with knees slightly flexed. Gently retract the buttocks with your gloved hand, and inspect the anal and perianal tissue. Note color, texture, lesions, masses, prolapse, hemorrhoids, erythema, ecchymosis, skin breakdown, decubitus ulcers, fistulas, sinus tracts, abscesses, masses, lesions, and any evidence of poor hygiene. Perianal tissue may appear slightly darker in pigmentation, and anal tissue is slightly reddened normally.

Ask the client to bear down as though attempting a bowel movement and inspect for the appearance of protrusions, masses, hemorrhoids, prolapse, or polyps.

Digital Rectal Examination

Perform a digital examination to palpate the anus, rectum, and prostate. Press gently against the anal sphincter with your gloved and lubricated index finger pad. Ask the client to bear down and gently press your fingertip into the opening of the anus. Assess the tone and musculature of the anal sphincter. (Normally the anal sphincter will tighten firmly around the inserted finger and the client may express the urge to defecate.) Palpate the entire surface of the anal sphincter. Ask the client to tighten the buttocks around your finger to allow assessment of tone and strength of the sphincter.

Palpate the musculoanal ring and rectum. Palpate the entire surface of the musculoanal ring by turning the finger in a circular motion around its own axis. Then, move further inward to the rectum and repeat. Note any palpable lesions, masses, lacerations, or abnormalities or a palpable rectal shelf (often secondary to peritoneal metastatic disease).

Palpate for high masses. With your gloved finger as far into the rectum as possible, ask the client to bear down and palpate for any descending masses. Note the presence of any high mass descending against the inserted fingertip when the client bears down.

Palpate the prostate in men (only after the onset of puberty). Turn your finger to palpate the anterior rectal wall. Gently palpate the prostate (Fig. 10–46). Try to identify the two lateral lobes and the median sulcus. Normally the prostate will feel rubbery and smooth to palpation and less than 1 cm of the prostate tissue will be palpable protruding into the rectal wall. Note any enlargement, irregularity in shape, palpable mass, tenderness, or softening (bogginess).

Palpate the uterus and cervix in women. Turn your finger to palpate the anterior rectal wall. Gently palpate the uterus and cervix. Normally, they will feel rubbery and smooth. Note any enlargement, irregularity in shape, palpable mass, tenderness, or softening (bogginess).

Withdraw your gloved finger and examine the fecal material on the glove for color (brown, gray, yellow, black) and consistency (watery, loose, greasy,

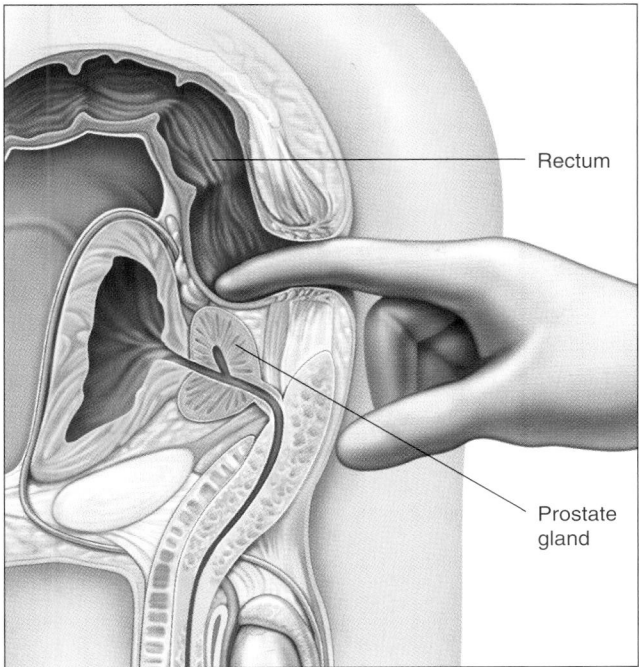

Figure 10–46. Palpating the prostate gland through the anterior wall of the rectum.

formed, hard, impacted). Using a Hemoccult card, test the fecal material for occult blood. Normally, the stool should appear brown, feel formed, and contain no evidence of frank or occult blood.

Assessment of the Female Genitalia

The following should be included in the assessment of the female genitalia:

- Inspection and palpation of the vulva for lesions, masses, and abnormalities
- Inspection of the pubic hair for infestations, density of growth, and sexual maturity
- Inspection and palpation of the labia majora for lesions, masses, inflammation, swelling, and abnormalities
- Inspection of the labia minora
- Inspection of the clitoris
- Inspection of the urethral meatus and Skene's glands
- Inspection of the hymen and vaginal introitus
- Inspection of Bartholin's glands
- Inspection of the cervix
- Inspection of the vaginal wall
- Palpation of the cervix
- Palpation of the ovaries and adnexa
- Palpation of the uterus

External Genitalia

Prepare the client for the examination. Ask the client to urinate and empty her bladder. Have her undress from the waist down and assume a semirecumbent position on the examining table with her knees and thighs draped and her feet in the stirrups. Ask the client to rest her hands on her waist and to relax her knees and let them fall to the side as far as possible.

Wear gloves to inspect and palpate the vulva for lesions, masses, and abnormalities. Touch the client's thigh initially to avoid startling her, then proceed with the examination, parting the pubic hair as necessary to facilitate thorough examination. Palpate any noticeable masses, lesions, swelling, or abnormalities. Normally, the skin is smooth, warm, and pink in light-skinned people and olive to brown in dark-skinned people, and it may be lighter in color than the rest of the body because of lack of exposure to sun. Note any hematomas, ecchymosis, irregular pigment, macules, papules, wheals, vesicles, ulcers, or other rashes.

Inspect the pubic hair for infestations, density of growth, and sexual maturity. Part the pubic hair to look for infestations of pubic lice often found at the base or root of the pubic hair. Also inspect for nits (tiny teardrop-shaped white or gray eggs) adhering to the hair stalks. Assess the sexual maturity of the client.

Inspect and palpate the labia majora and labia minora for lesions, masses, inflammation, swelling, and abnormalities. It may be necessary to grasp the labia majora between two fingers to accomplish a thorough examination. Part the labia majora with your gloved fingers to inspect the labia minora. Note and thoroughly palpate any observed lesions or abnormalities.

Inspect the clitoris for position, size, lesions, masses, and abnormalities. The clitoris can be found between the anterior junction of the labia majora and the labia minora. Normally, the clitoris will appear to be a small pink nodular form that does not exceed 0.5 cm in width and 2 cm in length. (In some cultural groups the clitoris may have been ceremonially excised.)

Separate the labia minora and locate the urethral meatus, a small orifice, just below the anterior junction of the labia minora. Inspect for lesions, prolapse, polyps, fistulas, edema or tenderness, masses, or discharge. If there is inflammation or urethritis is suspected, milk the urethra gently by inserting a gloved finger into the vagina and stroking its posterior side in a downward motion toward you. Culture any discharge for gonorrhea, chlamydia, and bacteria. Perform a potassium hydroxide and wet prep to discern the presence of yeast or *Trichomonas,* respectively.

Inspect the hymen and vaginal introitus. The hymen may be intact in children and virgins; however, usually only remnants of the hymen remain in sexually active women. If the hymen is edematous, torn, or absent in small children, sexual abuse must be considered as a possible cause.

With the labia separated by your gloved finger, inspect the vaginal introitus or vaginal opening. Ask the client to bear down to allow the support of the vaginal outlet to be evaluated. Observe and note any abnormal swelling or bulging. The introitus is usually open and unobstructed, but in older, multiparous women it is not uncommon to observe a cystocele (a bulging mass arising from the anterior wall of the vagina) or a rectocele (a bulging mass arising from the posterior vaginal floor). Both a cystocele and rectocele are caused by inadequate support of the vaginal outlet. A large, smooth, pink, protruding mass may actually be a uterine prolapse with the cervix visible in the vaginal canal. Uterine prolapse can be staged as first degree, second degree, or third degree depending on the severity of drop in the vaginal vault. In first degree prolapse, the cervix is palpated slightly lower than usual in the vaginal vault; in second degree prolapse the cervix can be palpated halfway down the vaginal vault; and in third degree prolapse the cervix is at the introitus or sometimes even visibly protruding from the vaginal opening.

Inspect the Bartholin glands located bilaterally at the base of the vaginal opening. The Bartholin glands are normally not visible other than a small pinpoint duct opening inside the labia. Palpate the glands between your gloved index finger and thumb by placing one finger inside the vaginal opening and one on the outside of the labia majora. Normally the Bartholin glands will be nontender and not palpable. Note any pain, swelling, masses, or discharge. A large nontender unilateral mass may be a Bartholin cyst. A large tender fluctuant unilateral or bilateral mass may be a Bartholin abscess. The abscess may have tracked, spontaneously ruptured, or remained exquisitely tender and fluctuant. Gently compress the glands between two gloved fingers and culture any discharge exuding from the duct openings for gonorrhea, chlamydia, and bacteria.

Internal Genitalia

After you have completed your examination of the external genitalia, prepare to perform the speculum examination of the internal genitalia. Figure 10–47 illustrates a vaginal speculum used to hold the vagina open to visualize the cervix. Lubricate your gloved fingers and speculum with water. Water is used as the lubricant to prevent contamination when a smear for cytology is part of the examination. Insert one or two fingers into the vaginal opening and press downward on the posterior aspect to further open the introitus and facilitate the insertion of the speculum. With the speculum closed and held so that the blade width is in a vertical position, insert the speculum. Gently push in a downward and sloping fashion, while at the same time rotating the blade so that the width is now in a horizontal position. Follow the vaginal canal to the cervix. Open the speculum and manipulate the cervix into position and secure by clamping. Observe the cervix, obtain specimens for cytology, and culture any discharge.

The cervical os appears as a small rounded opening within a central depression on the cervix in nulliparous women. It takes on a more "fish-mouthed" appearance in multiparous women. There are usually no lesions, masses, erythema, or cervical motion tenderness. Usually the cervix will appear as a smooth,

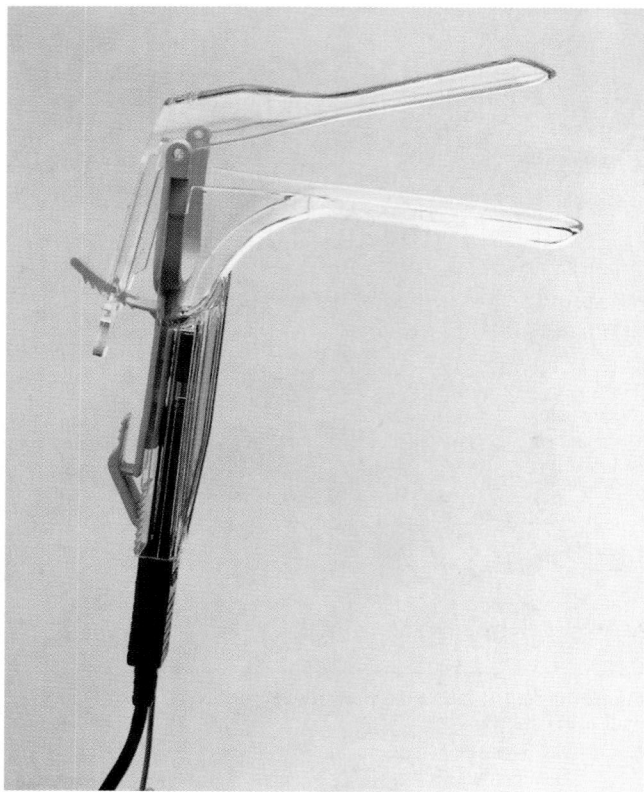

Figure 10–47. A vaginal speculum. (Courtesy of Welch Allyn, Inc.)

rounded, pink, moist, sometimes glistening, and firm mass. Although the cervix usually remains about 1 inch in diameter in size, it enlarges, softens, and becomes bluish-tinged normally in pregnancy and may appear pale during menopause.

The Papanicolaou smear, or Pap smear, is a cytology test to screen for cervical cancer. To obtain a specimen for a Pap smear you will use a cytobrush and an Ayre speculum to collect specimens from three sites. Each specimen is placed on a separate glass slide, sprayed with fixative within 2 seconds, and labeled with the source. A Pap smear should not be done during the menstrual period or if the client has infectious discharge. Ideally the woman should not have intercourse, douche, or put anything in the vagina 24 hours prior to the test.

Unclamp the speculum and hold it open as you withdraw it slowly from the vaginal canal. As you withdraw the speculum, inspect the walls of the vaginal canal. Use a gooseneck lamp or penlight to better illuminate the canal.

Normally you will see rugate homogeneous tissue with thin, clear or cloudy, odorless secretions, which will likely be more profuse in pregnant women. Note any abnormal findings of masses, lesions, vesicles, papules, warts, or thick, foul-smelling discharge. Palpate the vaginal wall by inserting the lubricated and gloved middle and index finger of the right hand into the vagina (Fig. 10-48). Palpate the anterior, posterior, and lateral walls of the vaginal canal.

Palpate the cervix with the tips of your fingers. Note the position, shape, consistency, and mobility of the cervix. Gently move the cervix from side to side and test for cervical motion tenderness, which can be a telltale sign of a pelvic inflammatory disease or other acute pelvic process. Attempt to admit one fingertip into the cervical os to determine its patency. Usually the cervical os remains closed and will offer tight resistance. If the os admits one fingertip, or offers no resistance, it is considered open and may indicate a threatened or inevitable abortion or incompetent cervix.

Palpate the ovaries and adnexa. Place your left hand on the client's abdomen about halfway between the umbilicus and the symphysis pubis. Push inward and downward toward the symphysis pubis while at the same time pushing upward on the vaginal mucosa lateral to the cervix with the fingers of your right hand. Try to palpate the small almond-shaped ovary on either side. Palpate for the adnexa. Normally it will not be palpable unless there is an adnexal thickening or mass.

Palpate the uterus with your hands positioned as described above. Push downward toward the symphysis pubis with your left hand while pushing upward on the cervix with the fingers of your right hand. Attempt to grasp the uterus between the fingers of your two hands. Note the position, size, shape, consistency, and mobility of the uterus. Note also whether the uterus is tender. The fundus will not be palpable above the symphysis pubis (pubic bone). If it is enlarged, soft, or tender, it may indicate pregnancy, fibroids, hydatidiform mole, or the presence of a mass.

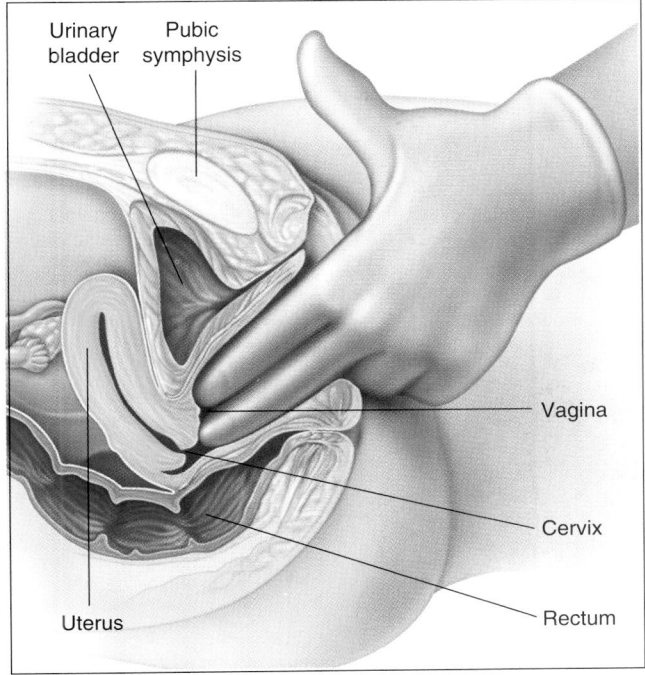

Figure 10–48. Palpating the uterus and cervix.

Assessment of the Male Genitalia

The following should be included in assessment of male genitalia:

- Assessment of sexual maturity
- Assessment of the prepuce or foreskin
- Assessment of the glans penis
- Assessment of the urethral meatus
- Assessment of the penile shaft
- Assessment of the scrotum and testes
- Assessment of the presence of hernias

Sexual Maturity

Assess the external genitalia for sexual maturity. Note the distribution and quantity of pubic hair. Pubic hair will be absent in infants and children and will be thick, extending onto the thighs, in adults. The density of growth and distribution of hair should be consistent with that expected for the client's age group. An abnormal quantity or distribution may indicate hormonal imbalances, chronic disease, dermatitis, or a response to medications. Hair loss may be symmetrical and nonscarring, or asymmetrical and scarring.

Penis

Note the shape and size of the penis. The penis will attain adult size and shape after puberty. Note the size, color, and texture of the scrotum. The scrotum darkens and develops rugae after puberty. Assess the sexual maturity (see Chapter 51).

Part the pubic hair as necessary to facilitate thorough examination of the skin. Inspect and palpate the skin for color, temperature, lesions, masses, excoriations, lacerations, abnormalities, infestations, or lack of hygiene. Gently move and manipulate the penis and scrotum to allow visualization of their posterior sides. Palpate thoroughly and note the type and location of any lesions, macules, papules, ulcers, vesicles, rashes, lacerations, excoriations, or masses. Hot red skin may indicate cellulitis, infection, or inflammation. The presence of lesions may indicate dermatitis or sexually transmitted disease (STD).

Inspect and palpate the prepuce and foreskin in uncircumcised males. Note any lesions, swelling, edema, lacerations, erythema, or ecchymosis. Gently retract the foreskin. Inspect the interior. Smegma, a whitish, pasty exudate may normally be present. Pay particular attention to the junction between the prepuce and the glans, as this is often a common site for lesions related to sexually transmitted diseases. Any difficulty in retracting or inability to retract the foreskin (phimosis), or difficulty in replacing or inability to replace a retracted foreskin (paraphimosis) is abnormal and should be noted and further evaluated.

Inspect and palpate the full surface of the glans. The glans will normally appear moist and pink in uncircumcised males. Note the presence and exact location of any lesions, masses, swelling, edema, abnormalities, erythema, ecchymosis, or balanitis (inflammation of the glans with marked erythema and edema).

Note the location of the urinary meatus. It will normally appear as a pink slit-like opening located in the center of the glans. Check for hypospadias, congenital displacement of the urethral meatus (usually found on the posterior side of the glans or penile shaft). Note the location and type of any lesions or abnormalities. Inspect for urethral prolapse, a perceivable small rosette of prolapsed membranes protruding from the meatus. Inspect also for fissures and fistulas. Open the meatus slightly by gently compressing the glans between your thumb and finger (or allow the client to do this). Inspect the color of the lining of the meatus and culture and describe any obvious discharge (e.g., yellow, white, clear, blood-tinged), which likely indicates the presence of a urethritis. Discharge should be cultured for gonorrhea, chlamydia, and bacteria, and a potassium hydroxide and wet prep should be performed at this time to assess for the presence of yeast and *Trichomonas,* respectively. If the client has complained of discharge and none is seen, you may need to gently "milk" the shaft of the penis to produce a bead of discharge for culture.

Inspect and palpate the shaft of the penis. Gently manipulate and lift the penis to allow inspection and palpation of the entire surface area. Note the exact location and type of lesions, masses, or abnormalities. Palpate for induration and tenderness along the ventral surface of the penis. In infants and children, this may be omitted. Tenderness or induration along the ventral surface may indicate urethral stricture and periurethral inflammation, or carcinoma.

Scrotum and Testes

Inspect and palpate the scrotum and testes. Gently palpate the testicles by grasping them between your thumb and forefinger. Palpate the epididymis, spermatic cord, and vas deferens. Note any lesions, masses, tenderness, or enlargement. Transilluminate the scrotum and testicle if a mass is suspected or an enlargement is observed. A fluid-filled mass will illuminate well, while a mass filled with blood, pus, or solid tissue will not.

Normally, the scrotum consists of coarse loose rugate skin of slightly darker pigmentation than the rest of the body. The left testicle is normally lower than the right. When compressed gently between the examiner's two fingers, the testes will be sensitive but not painful and should not feel much greater than 1 inch in diameter. Check for undescended testicles (cryptorchidism) and poorly developed scrotum on one or both sides. Note any nontender swelling or masses such as hydrocele or spermatocele (fluid-filled cysts of the tunica vaginalis and epididymis, respectively). Both hydroceles and spermatoceles will transilluminate when a penlight is held up against the scrotal sac.

Palpate for testicular cancer, a hard palpable nontender nodule usually favoring the anterior side of the testes. Note any tender swelling or mass. This may be caused by scrotal edema (from congestive heart failure, chronic renal failure, or nephrotic syndrome), epididymitis (an acute bacterial infection of the epididymis), or testicular torsion (a painful swelling caused by torsion or twisting of the spermatic cord).

Palpate the vas deferens and spermatic cord. Note any thickening, which may occur with chronic infections and tuberculosis. Note the presence of a varicocele, a string of bead-like nodules or varicosities (which feel characteristically like a "bag of worms"), palpated usually on the left side.

Inguinal Canal

Inspect and palpate for hernias. Figure 10–49 illustrates the structures of the inguinal area. Ask the client to stand and bear down as though having a bowel movement. Inspect the inguinal areas and scrotum for any bulging or masses. With one finger, press inward on the loose skin at a low point on the scrotum. Follow the spermatic cord upward by invaginating loose scrotal skin until you can palpate the external inguinal ring. If possible, follow the inguinal canal to the internal inguinal ring.

Ask the client to bear down and again feel for any bulging or masses. If a hernia is palpable, apply gentle pressure and note whether it is reducible. Never force your finger into the inguinal canal. If you meet with resistance or the client complains of pain, discontinue the examination.

Identify any existing hernias. A direct inguinal hernia is palpated above the inguinal ring, bulges anteri-

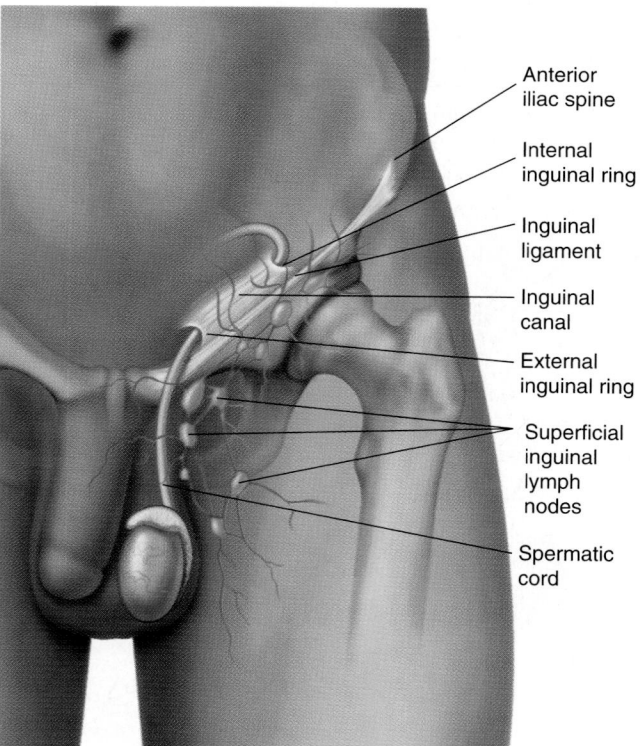

Figure 10–49. Structures of the inguinal area.

orly, does not travel down the inguinal canal, and may, but rarely does, invade the scrotum. An indirect inguinal hernia is palpated above the inguinal ligament close to the internal inguinal ring; it travels down the inguinal canal and often invades the scrotum. A femoral hernia is palpated below the inguinal ligament and appears more lateral than inguinal hernias and is often difficult to distinguish from enlarged inguinal lymph nodes. All hernias may become painful if strangulation occurs either by torsion of the bowel or by compression by surrounding tissues.

KEY PRINCIPLES

- The physical examination is a systematic means of collecting objective assessment data.
- The four basic techniques used in physical examination are inspection, palpation, percussion, and auscultation and are performed in that order.
- To perform a physical examination you will rely heavily on the use of your five senses, particularly your ability to observe.
- Physical examination should be conducted following a regular pattern of examination and with the client positioned for the most accurate collection of data.
- The general survey provides information on the overall state of the client.
- The mental status examination provides a detailed description of the client's cognitive functioning at a given time.
- Good, preferably natural, light should be used to avoid distortion of color when inspecting the skin.
- A thorough description of a lesion is useful in determining if the lesion is a primary or secondary lesion and whether it is benign or malignant.
- Specific tests for hearing are only performed if gross hearing testing suggests a problem.
- Assessing the heart provides cues to the structure and function of the heart that are useful in anticipating changes in cardiac output.
- Assessment of the peripheral vascular system focuses on the blood pressure and the pulses (and other signs of peripheral circulation) in relationship to the cardiac function.
- Assessing the function of the veins is part of assessing venous return to the heart.
- Abdominal assessment determines function of the bowel and detects abnormalities of other organs and structures in the abdomen.
- Assessment of the musculoskeletal system detects abnormalities of the structure and function of bones, muscles, and joints.

BIBLIOGRAPHY

Balakas, K., & Schappe, A. (1995). Procedures in home care. Well baby assessment. *Home Healthcare Nurse, 13*(5), 82–84.
Bates, B. (1997). *A guide to physical examination and history taking* (6th Ed.). Philadelphia: J. B. Lippincott.
Csokasy, J. (1999). Assessment of acute confusion: use of the NEECHAM confusion scale. *Applied Nursing Research, 12*(1), 51–55.
Dienger, M. J., & Llewellyn, J. (1995). Increasing compliance with breast self-examination. *MEDSURG Nursing, 4*(5), 359–366.
Fowlie, P., & Forsyth, S. Examination of the newborn infant. *Modern Midwife, 5*(1), 15–18.
Kelsher, K. C. (1995). Primary care for women: environmental assessment of the home, community, and workplace. *Journal of Nurse Midwifery, 40*(2), 59–64, 88–96.
Ludwig, L. M. (1998). Cardiovascular assessment for home healthcare nurses. Part II: Assessing blood pressure and cardiac function. *Home Healthcare Nurse, 16*(8), 547–554.
Mahon, S. M. (1998). Cancer risk assessment: conceptual considerations for clinical practice. *Oncology Nursing Forum, 25*(9), 1535–1547.
Misulis, K. E. (1996). *Neurologic localization and diagnosis.* Boston: Butterworth-Heinemann.
Nicoteri, J. A. (1999). Rising above "soar" throats. Take a common-sense approach to assessing young adults with sore throats. *American Journal of Nursing, 99*(3), 18–20.
O'Hanlon-Nichols, T. (1998). Basic assessment series. A review of the adult musculoskeletal system. *American Journal of Nursing, 98*(6), 48–52.
O'Hanlon-Nichols, T. (1998). Basic assessment series. The adult pulmonary system. *American Journal of Nursing, 98*(2), 39–45.
Poncar, P. J. (1995). Who has time for a "head-to-toe" assessment? *Nursing, 25*(3), 59.
Pressman, E. K., Zeidman, S. M., & Summers, L. (1995). Primary care for women: Comprehensive assessment of the neurologic system. *Journal of Nurse Midwifery, 40*(2), 59–64, 163–171.
Rice, K. L. (1998). Sounding out blood flow with a Doppler device. *Nursing98, 28*(9), 56–57.
Scott, A., & Hamilton, K. (1998). Nutritional screening: an audit. *Nursing Standards, 12*(48), 46–47.
Seidel, H. M., Ball, J. W., Dains, J. E., & Benedict, G. W. (1999). *Mosby's guide to physical examination* (4th Ed.). St. Louis: Mosby.
Silverman, M. E., & Hurst, J. W. (1995). *Clinical skills for adult primary care.* Philadelphia: Lippincott-Raven.
Springhouse Corporation. (1996). *Assessing patients.* Springhouse, PA: Author.
Stevenson, C. (1998). Abdominal assessment clarifications. *Home Healthcare Nurse, 16*(6), 363.
Vessey, J. A. (1995). Primary care approaches: developmental approaches in examining young children. *Pediatric Nursing, 21*(1), 53–56.
Weilitz, P. B., & Lueckenotte, A. (1995). Respiratory assessment of older adults: Part II. *Perspectives in Respiratory Nursing, 6*(2), 1, 3–4.

Making a Nursing Diagnosis

Kay C. Avant

Key Terms

clinical judgment
collaborative problem
cue
defining characteristic
diagnostic label
diagnostic reasoning
differential diagnosis

nursing diagnosis
qualifier
related factors
risk factors
"risk for" nursing diagnosis
taxonomy
"wellness" nursing diagnosis

LEARNING OBJECTIVES

After studying this chapter, you should be able to:

1. Discuss the classification of nursing diagnoses.
2. Describe the five components of a NANDA nursing diagnosis.
3. Compare and contrast four types of nursing diagnoses.
4. Describe the process of diagnostic reasoning.
5. Discuss several sources of diagnostic error and how to avoid them.

As part of professional nursing practice, you must be able to recognize a variety of client problems and identify those that are amenable to treatment with nursing care. This is done by using the nursing process as a problem-solving or clinical decision-making model. Although you may think of nursing diagnosis as the second phase of the nursing process, it is actually the end result of assessment. As you gather assessment data about a client through the nursing history and physical examination, you recognize interrelationships among pieces of data and group them into clusters to form nursing diagnoses. A nursing diagnosis implies that you have made decisions about the nature of a client's problems and have given those problems names.

Making a nursing diagnosis may be as simple as giving a name to an obvious problem or client need. At other times it may require complex thinking skills to correctly identify the problem, its cause, and factors that contribute to the problem. One of the most important skills that you must possess as a nurse is the ability to think through problems and make sound clinical judgments about the needs of clients under your care.

In a constantly changing health care environment driven by economic constraints, providing quality care requires that you have strong skills in critical thinking (see Chapter 7). Making nursing diagnoses helps you think critically in nursing practice. Nurses who cannot think critically about all aspects of nursing may not be safe practitioners.

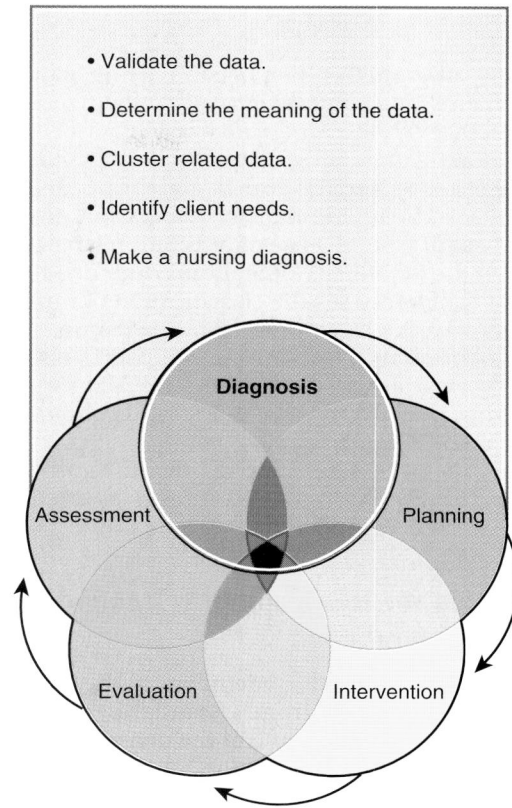

- Validate the data.
- Determine the meaning of the data.
- Cluster related data.
- Identify client needs.
- Make a nursing diagnosis.

Figure 11–1. Nursing diagnosis is the second step of the nursing process.

CONCEPTS OF STANDARDIZED NURSING DIAGNOSIS LANGUAGE

Nurses use a specific process of clinical decision-making called the nursing process. Chapters 8, 9, and 10 focused on aspects of the assessment process. This chapter explains how to make sense of assessment data by using the second phase of the nursing process: nursing diagnosis (Fig. 11–1). The North American Nursing Diagnosis Association (NANDA) defines a **nursing diagnosis** as a clinical judgment about individual, family, or community responses to actual or potential health problems or life processes. A nursing diagnosis provides you with a basis for selecting nursing interventions to achieve outcomes for which you are accountable (NANDA, 1999, p 149). To make a nursing diagnosis, critical thinking is the primary skill needed.

One of the basic concepts to understand about nursing diagnoses is that they are human responses. This means that you are concerned with the way clients respond to life and health conditions. Nursing diagnoses refer not to the problems nurses encounter while working with clients but rather to the problems clients have.

Another basic concept of nursing diagnoses is that they identify problems for which you are accountable and are capable of diagnosing and treating *independently*. A **collaborative problem** is a clinical problem

that cannot be solved by you alone (or by the nursing staff) but that instead requires medications or treatments that you are unable to do or not licensed to order. All states, the American Nurses' Association, and many specialty nursing organizations have standards of practice that help nurses identify the scope of practice and the appropriate nursing actions for independent practice.

Nursing diagnoses are a *part* of the nursing process. The phases of the nursing process are interlinked and function as a whole to help you make sound clinical judgments. Making a nursing diagnosis establishes a link between assessment and planning interventions. Without accurate diagnoses, you will be unable to determine appropriate interventions.

Evolution

If nursing diagnosis is a technique for describing areas of human concern that nurses are qualified to help clients to manage, then nurses have been making diagnoses since nursing practice began. Until the 1950s, however, nurses were reluctant to use the term *diagnosis* because it could create confusion between medical practice and nursing practice. Virginia Henderson and Fay Abdellah are credited with advancing nursing as a profession by providing the beginnings of a language that encouraged nurses to identify *client-centered prob-*

lems instead of nursing tasks as the focus of nursing practice.

Many other nurses then began writing about nursing problems, and some began calling them nursing diagnoses. By 1971, the American Nurses' Association included making a nursing diagnosis in its standards for nursing practice, and the term began to appear in nurse practice acts. Believing that the profession of nursing would benefit from the use of a common language, the faculty at the University of St. Louis organized the first national conference for the classification of nursing diagnosis in 1973. Developing from this conference, the North American Nursing Diagnosis Association (NANDA) was established in 1983. NANDA's purpose at that time was to develop, refine, and promote a taxonomy of nursing diagnostic language that could be used by all professional nurses (Kim, McFarland, & McLane, 1984). This group continues to meet every other year to accomplish its ongoing work.

Rationales for Developing a Standardized Nursing Language

Nurses, clients, and other members of the health care team all reap benefits from a standardized language for nursing diagnoses. Some of the benefits of a shared diagnostic language include the following:

- It provides a common language for nurses to communicate with each other and the health care team.
- It ensures that nursing care is documented in a manner that is recognizable and retrievable for quality improvement studies.
- It facilitates nursing research by enabling retrieval of nursing data from a computerized medical record to document the effectiveness of nursing care.
- It places the emphasis on nursing care to solve the client's problem rather than on completing tasks.
- It increases the likelihood of using creative approaches to nursing rather than repetition of the usual interventions, especially when those interventions are not working.
- It paves the way for third-party reimbursement for nursing care that can be proved to be beneficial and cost-effective.
- It provides a method for identifying the focus or goal of nursing activity.
- It defines the nursing body of knowledge.
- It contributes to the autonomy and self-regulatory capacity of nursing.

The advent of computerized medical record systems has further increased recognition of the benefits of a standardized nursing language. Because nursing is the primary service offered by home health agencies, their medical record systems clearly need to identify and document client problems treated by nurses. On the other hand, hospitals typically emphasize a medical model or multidisciplinary approach to medical records. Nursing care is subsumed into the care of other practitioners, particularly physicians, and as a result is virtually invisible. (Recently, some hospital record-keeping systems have begun to use the NANDA system as a means of reflecting nursing practice.)

When the system of naming problems does not reflect any nursing options, the nurse is challenged to enter data into the system that shows the benefit of nursing care to the client. If these benefits cannot be named or identified, then they certainly cannot be controlled, financed, researched, or put into public policy (Clark & Lang, 1992).

Taxonomies

A **taxonomy** is a system of identification, naming, and classification of phenomena. In nursing, the phenomena are human responses, physiological and behavioral, for which nursing care can be beneficial. A taxonomy is useful to nursing scientists in distinguishing various client problems and improving methods of nursing practice. There are three major taxonomies for nursing diagnoses and a taxonomy of psychiatric nursing diagnoses. Taxonomies also exist for nursing interventions and nursing outcomes.

NANDA System

NANDA is the organization officially sanctioned by the American Nurses' Association as the body responsible for developing a system of classification of nursing diagnoses. Thus, this system is widely accepted and used.

REVIEW PROCESS

NANDA actively solicits new nursing diagnoses for review and incorporation into the nursing diagnosis database. After submission, proposed new diagnoses or proposed revisions of current diagnoses undergo a systematic review to determine if they are consistent with the criteria for a nursing diagnosis. Each diagnosis is then reviewed and staged into one of four levels by the Diagnostic Review Committee (DRC) based on the amount of supporting evidence available for the level of development and validation:

- Level 1 incorporates a nursing diagnosis from the time it is recommended with a label until it is placed on the taxonomy list for study.
- Level 2 incorporates nursing diagnoses that have been accepted for clinical development and are undergoing clinical study.
- Level 3 incorporates nursing diagnoses that have undergone clinical development and testing.
- Level 4 incorporates nursing diagnoses that have been refined or revised.

Once a nursing diagnosis is staged by the DRC, the taxonomy committee classifies the diagnosis in the taxonomy. The diagnosis list is revised every 2 years.

STRENGTHS AND LIMITATIONS OF THE NANDA SYSTEM

Like any other organization, NANDA and its classification system are constantly evolving. Since its inception in 1983, NANDA has responded to the expanding role of nursing in health care. As the climate of health care continues to change, more progress with nursing diagnoses, especially in the areas of wellness and community diagnosis, is needed.

Currently, the strengths of NANDA include the following:

- Membership in the organization is open to all nurses.
- It has a process for revising, refining, and introducing new nursing diagnoses.
- It is not specific to one nursing specialty.
- It has been widely accepted, especially in nursing education.
- It includes international members.
- It broadens the scope of nursing practice beyond what is currently reimbursable.
- It is endorsed by the American Nurses' Association as the "official" nomenclature.

Currently, the limitations of NANDA include the following:

- It does not comprehensively include wellness diagnoses.
- It does not comprehensively include community health diagnoses.
- It does not comprehensively include psychiatric diagnoses.
- Its language is not readily recognized and understood by other members of the health care team.
- Different levels of abstraction can make the system confusing. (Some diagnoses are very general and could include a range of problems, whereas others are very specific.)
- The language is verbose and contains jargon.
- It requires writing a "related to" statement in many cases to achieve the specificity needed to plan nursing care.

Omaha System

The Omaha System is a classification system developed by the staff of the Visiting Nurse Association (VNA) of Omaha, Nebraska, as a documentation and data management system that conveys the autonomy of community health nursing practice. The project to develop the system represents 15 years of research, much of which was federally funded. The system includes a problem classification scheme that is a taxonomy of nursing diagnoses valuable to community health nurses. Thus, the domains within the scheme reflect the home and community practice setting. For example, diagnoses within the environmental domain address material resources, physical surroundings, and the client's community. This system has the ad-

vantage of having been developed from what visiting or home health nurses actually do within the framework of reimbursable nursing practice (Martin & Scheet, 1992).

Saba System

The Saba Nursing Diagnoses for Home Health Care: Classification and Coding Scheme was developed through a federally funded project that reviewed 8,961 clients of home care agencies. The system consists of nursing diagnoses and interventions that serve as a framework for home health nursing practice. Like the Omaha System, the Saba System is closely linked to services provided under Medicare and also has the advantage of communicating what home health nurses actually do. Many of the Saba nursing diagnoses are identical to those of NANDA.

Psychiatric Nursing Diagnoses

A task force was formed in 1984 under the American Nurses' Association to develop psychiatric nursing diagnoses. In 1994, this group turned its work over to NANDA for further refinement and development. Because psychiatric nurses find the *Diagnostic and Statistical Manual of Mental Disorders* useful, the psychiatric group has proposed that some of the diagnoses from this manual be recognized as nursing diagnoses. That group of nursing diagnostic labels is listed in the 1999–2000 NANDA manual as undergoing development (NANDA, 1999).

COMPONENTS OF A NURSING DIAGNOSIS

A nursing diagnosis has five components: a label, a definition, a set of defining characteristics, a group of related factors, and risk factors (Box 11–1). Note that not all of these components are documented in the client's plan of care.

Label

The **diagnostic label** is the name of the nursing diagnosis. It is a concise term or phrase that represents a pattern of related cues that are signs and symptoms. It may include a **qualifier,** which is a word such as *impaired, altered, decreased, ineffective, acute,* or *chronic,* that gives the nursing diagnosis greater specificity (NANDA, 1999).

Definition

The *definition* of the diagnosis provides a full, precise description of the pattern of signs and symptoms, delineates the meaning of the label, and helps to differentiate it from similar or related diagnoses (NANDA, 1999). The definition is not documented in the client's plan of care.

BOX 11–1

COMPONENTS OF A SAMPLE NANDA NURSING DIAGNOSIS

Taxonomy Heading

1.3.2.1.3

Diagnostic Statement

Urge incontinence (1986)

Definition

The state in which an individual experiences involuntary passage of urine occurring soon after a strong sense of urgency to void.

Defining Characteristics

Urinary urgency; frequency (voiding more often than every 2 hours); bladder contracture/spasm.

Nocturia (more than two times per night); voiding in small amounts (less than 100 mL) or in large amounts (more than 550 mL); inability to reach toilet in time.

Related Factors

Alcohol; caffeine; decreased bladder capacity (e.g., history of pelvic inflammatory disease, abdominal surgeries, indwelling urinary catheter); increased fluids; increased urine concentration; irritation of bladder stretch receptors causing spasm (e.g., bladder infection); overdistention of bladder.

From North American Nursing Diagnosis Association. (1999). Nursing diagnoses: Definitions and classification 1999–2000. Philadelphia: Author.

BOX 11–2

QUESTIONS TO CONSIDER WHEN IDENTIFYING RELATED FACTORS

- Do the related factors allow me to understand the etiology, or cause, of this client's human response?
- Is the cause of the problem clear?
- Will removing or ameliorating the cause solve the problem?
- Do the related factors help me decide which interventions are most appropriate?
- Can any of the related factors be changed by nursing care?
- If so, which factors can be changed by nursing care?
- Does the information make a difference in the interventions that will be performed for this client?
- Will changing the related factors solve the problem, manage the problem, or help the client tolerate the problem until a definitive solution can be found?

Defining Characteristics

Defining characteristics are descriptors of a client's behavior that determine whether a nursing diagnosis is present and whether a particular diagnosis is appropriate or accurate. Defining characteristics are either directly or indirectly observable clinical cues (NANDA, 1999). **Cues** are the indicators of the presence or existence of a problem or condition that represents a client's underlying health status. Signs and symptoms of a problem provide the clinical cues that a problem is present. Signs are directly observed, and symptoms are reported by the client.

Related Factors

Related factors are "those factors that appear to show some type of patterned relationship with the nursing diagnosis" (NANDA, 1999, p 150). They help define

how the problem should be managed. Such factors may also be described as being antecedent to (prior to), associated with, contributing to, or abetting the nursing diagnosis (NANDA, 1999). Related factors may also be called etiologies; however, etiologies are strictly causative factors. The etiologies of nursing diagnoses are often medical diagnoses. Using *related factors* suggests a broad approach to nursing management in treating responses to medical diagnoses. Writing the "related to" part of the nursing diagnostic statement may be difficult at first (Box 11–2).

Risk Factors

Risk factors are internal or external environmental factors that increase the vulnerability of a person, family, or community to an unhealthful event (NANDA, 1999). A significant part of nursing practice is preventive, so nursing language must be able to express client problems that require prevention.

TYPES OF NURSING DIAGNOSES

There are several types of nursing diagnoses. They can be described as actual, risk for, or wellness diagnoses to represent the different spheres of nursing care. Because nursing care focuses on prevention, restoration of health, and maintaining wellness, nursing diagnoses take these forms. Nurses also help to manage problems where collaboration with the physician is necessary.

Actual Nursing Diagnoses

Actual nursing diagnoses describe "human responses to health conditions/life processes that exist in an individual, family or community." (NANDA, 1999, p 149). Actual nursing diagnoses describe a current client problem. When a client has an actual diagnosis, you can identify the signs and symptoms (defining characteristics) that indicate the presence of the diagnosis.

"Risk for" Nursing Diagnoses

A **"risk for" nursing diagnosis** describes human responses that *may* develop in a vulnerable person, family, or community. "Risk for" diagnoses are supported by risk factors that contribute to increased vulnerability (NANDA, 1999). "Risk for" nursing diagnoses are used when the client does not have a sufficient number of defining characteristics present to justify making the actual nursing diagnosis. Thus, "risk for" diagnoses are used to help you plan nursing care aimed at *preventing* the problem.

For instance, an elderly woman in a nursing home might have a risk for impaired skin integrity. The client does not actually have any broken skin or abraded areas visible. Nonetheless, she is very thin, eats poorly, is confined to bed, is not using pressure-relieving devices, and sometimes wets the bed at night. All of these factors predispose her to skin breakdown. The nursing diagnosis *Risk for impaired skin integrity* alerts the nursing home staff that preventive measures should be taken to reduce the risk of skin breakdown.

Although the current NANDA taxonomy lists 30 risk-for nursing diagnoses, the words "risk for" may be added to almost any nursing diagnosis for a client who does not actually have the problem but for whom the risk is present. Many nurses believe that making diagnoses that define the client's risk enhances their ability to communicate this important information to clients and to institute a plan of preventive care. Others argue that nursing diagnoses should be made only when actual problems exist.

Wellness Nursing Diagnoses

A **wellness nursing diagnosis** "describes human responses to levels of wellness in an individual, family, or community that have the potential for growth and/or the potential for enhancement to a higher state" of well-being (NANDA, 1999, p 149). For example, the nursing diagnosis *Family coping: potential for growth* might be used with a family whose 7-year-old son is recovering from a serious automobile accident. The child is going home in a body cast, and the parents are interested and involved in the child's care and are fostering the child's intellectual and developmental needs by devising activities that the child can do even while immobilized. They have been bringing his homework to him daily in the hospital so that he will not fall behind his peers in school. They have con-tacted an organization that provides car seats and wheelchairs for disabled children, and they plan to maintain the child's involvement in school and community activities. The parents see taking the child home as a challenge to their ingenuity and creativity. This diagnosis, then, reflects the family's ability to cope with and grow from the stressful experience.

Collaborative Problems

In some client situations, the problems to be resolved require the interventions of more than one member of the health care team. In such cases, health team members share the responsibilities associated with solving those problems. There is overlap between medical and nursing diagnoses and problems identified by such others as physical therapists, nutritionists, and social workers. Carpenito (1997) calls these *collaborative problems*. They are collaborative because they require interventions from several members of the team to solve the problem (Fig. 11–2).

Collaborative problems require a different level of autonomy on your part. That is, you work interdependently with all health team members needed to solve the problem. This is in contrast to your independent functioning, when you work alone or with other nursing colleagues to solve the problem, and your depen-

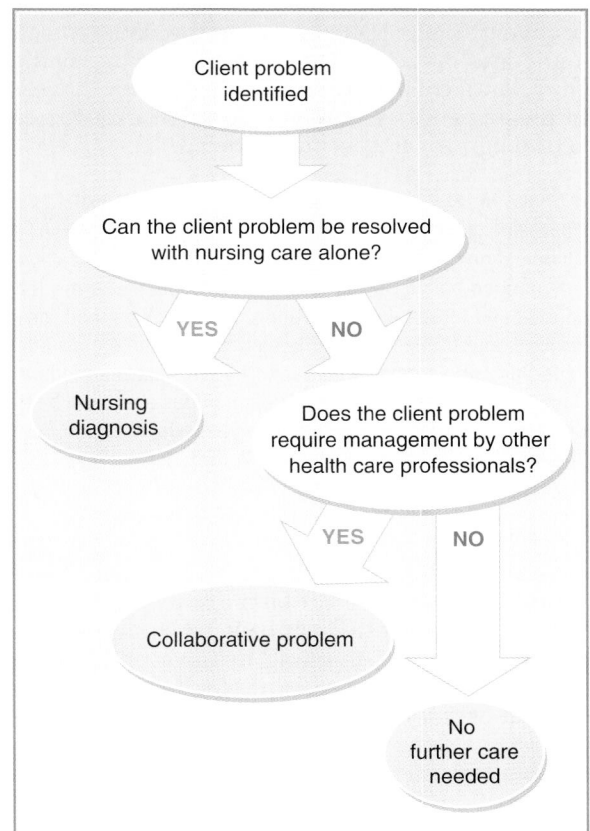

Figure 11–2. Differentiating between nursing diagnoses and collaborative problems.

TABLE 11–1

Example of the Relationship Among Medical, Collaborative, and Nursing Problems and the Dependent, Interdependent, and Independent Functions of the Health Care Team Members

Medical Problem/Dependent Function	Collaborative Problem/Interdependent Function	Nursing Problem/Independent Function
Pain: Physician orders pain medication. Nurse administers medication safely.	*Pain:* Physician orders pain medication. Nurse teaches client how to use medication at home.	*Pain:* Nurses teaches relaxation techniques and positioning methods to reduce the need for pain medication.
Impaired physical mobility: Physician orders physical therapy. Physical therapist carries out orders.	*Impaired physical mobility:* Physical therapist determines types of therapy needed and initiates a treatment plan. Nurse helps client understand how to do exercises at home.	*Impaired physical mobility:* Nurse helps client decide how client will manage daily activities at home and in school while the cast is on.
	Knowledge deficit: Physical therapist teaches client how to ambulate on crutches. Nurse encourages client to practice crutch walking in the corridor before going home.	*Knowledge deficit:* Nurse assesses client's knowledge about bone healing and provides information about the relationship between diet and bone growth.

dent functioning, when you follow someone else's orders (usually those of a physician). In the dependent function, you do not write the order, but you are responsible for carrying it out in a safe and competent manner.

A case example may illustrate how medical, nursing, and collaborative problems require the use of dependent, independent, and interdependent functions, respectively. Table 11–1 organizes the data from this example into diagnoses. Please note that the medical, nursing, and collaborative diagnoses may have exactly the same labels, but the focus of care for each type of diagnosis is specific to the specialty.

John Chase breaks his leg in football practice. A physician sets the bone, puts a cast on the leg, and orders physical therapy and pain medication. The physical therapist must decide the physical therapy needed based on the type of cast applied and the length of the cast and must then teach John the proper method for getting around on crutches or in a wheelchair. The nurse must administer the pain medication, teach John how to use the medication at home, assess his knowledge of broken bones and bone healing, enhance this knowledge as needed, and help John decide how he will manage his daily activities while in the cast.

DIAGNOSTIC REASONING PROCESS

The reasoning process that nurses use when identifying nursing diagnoses is different from everyday, ordinary mental activities. Diagnostic reasoning skills require logical, flexible thinking to solve problems and plan nursing care that accounts for individual client needs and uses the individual strengths of both client and nurse to the fullest extent possible (Alfaro-LeFevre, 1995).

Diagnostic reasoning in nursing is somewhat different from diagnostic reasoning in medicine. Although the steps are similar for both medicine and nursing, the contexts and the factors under consider-

ation are different. The task of medical diagnosis is one of assessing, identifying, and labeling disease states. The physician generates hypotheses based on signs and symptoms that are part of a well-defined and widely shared vocabulary. The steps in medical diagnostic reasoning are to do the following:

- Assess the signs and symptoms present
- Generate hypotheses about what the disease state might be
- Sort through and evaluate potential disease labels
- Select the best disease label that describes the client's set of signs and symptoms
- Select the best treatment for the disease based on the underlying cause(s) of the disease (Feinstein, 1967)

Even though advanced practice nurses (such as nurse practitioners) can diagnose some diseases, and even registered nurses can often identify specific disease states in some clients, the nurse's function is not to diagnose disease. The process of diagnostic reasoning in nursing requires the same clear, logical steps in thinking that is required for medical diagnosis. The difference, however, is that nurses diagnose the *human responses* to actual and potential health problems that *result from* or have *an impact on* disease, lifestyle, and life situations. Human responses include physiologic, cognitive, emotional, and social changes that have to do with the meaning of health and illness to the person as well as how the person is able to function.

Because you must take into account the psychosocial and life circumstances of the client (in addition to the medical diagnosis) when making any nursing diagnoses, nursing diagnosis often requires both complex and creative critical thinking. In contrast to medicine, making a nursing diagnosis does not necessarily limit the possibilities for treatment to a narrow choice of known protocols. The choices for nursing interventions are more numerous because a narrow choice of well-documented treatments is not always available. Diagnostic reasoning in nursing takes into account both the assets and deficits of each client, and it occurs in cycles that are repeated until the problem is resolved.

Critical Thinking, Diagnostic Reasoning, and Clinical Judgment

Critical thinking is defined by van Hooft, Gillam, and Byrnes (1995) as reasonable and reflective thinking that is "rational and practical as well as theoretical, committed, self aware, sympathetic to the commitments of others, conducive to dialogue" and focused on deciding what to do. This definition is helpful because it links the idea of rationality, reasonableness, and reflection to the practical decision-making necessary in a discipline like nursing. In addition, it makes clear that critical thinking in nursing must be done within the context of the nurse-client interaction and the interdisciplinary health care system.

The critical thinking that you engage in each day to make sound clinical judgments is more advanced than the critical thinking needed to answer a difficult question on a test. The level of critical thinking needed to make clinical judgments about a client's life and health requires that you have a higher level of ability than nonprofessionals do. This higher level of critical thinking is what is entailed in diagnostic reasoning and clinical judgment. They use steps similar to those used for diagnostic reasoning in medicine. You will do the following:

- Collect and review client assessment data
- Generate clusters of cues and form hypotheses about the client's human responses
- Sort through and evaluate potential nursing diagnostic labels that reflect the cue clusters generated
- Select the best labels to describe the client's human responses
- Determine the causes or related factors for each diagnosis chosen
- Plan interventions based on the diagnosis and related factors (Carnevali, Mitchell, Woods, & Tanner, 1984)

The hardest parts of the process for the beginner are clustering client assessment data into meaningful sets and generating hypotheses about the client's human responses. Clustering cues is harder when you have little clinical experience and are using knowledge primarily gained from a textbook. Using the health patterns in this textbook or the NANDA book, which give examples of diagnoses with the appropriate cue clusters or defining characteristics, will help you to learn patterns of cues that commonly occur together.

Nursing diagnoses, then, are the labels you apply to the cue clusters generated. Thus, the client's assessment data and defining characteristics of the diagnostic label chosen should be directly comparable. There should be a good match, or "fit," between the actual client data and the defining characteristics of the diagnosis. The diagnoses are then linked to the factors that caused or are related to the diagnoses. Nursing interventions are planned based on those causal or related factors.

Novice nurses tend to reason from only one cue or symptom rather than a cluster of cues. However, once you can recognize common patterns of cue clusters, your diagnostic reasoning ability will improve rapidly.

A **clinical judgment** is a conclusion or an opinion that a problem or situation requires nursing care and that determines the cause of the problem, distinguishes between similar problems, or discriminates between two or more courses of action. Clinical judgments involve making decisions about what to observe, prioritizing problems, and deciding what to do in a clinical situation (Tanner, 1993). Clinical judgment is a broader concept than either critical thinking or diagnostic reasoning, and it encompasses both.

As a novice, you cannot expect to have the same clinical judgment abilities as an experienced nurse; however, even a novice is capable of quite sophisticated judgments given practice, time, and good supervision. The more experience you have with a particular client population, the more sensitive, specific, and expert your clinical judgments will be about the clients under your care.

Steps in the Diagnostic Process

The process of arriving at a nursing diagnosis involves several interrelated steps; no step exists in isolation from the whole. The process is also ongoing: each step is repeated until you are satisfied that the plan of care is the best one possible based on the data available.

In the initial contact with the client, often on admission to a facility or service, the emphasis is on gathering assessment data and generating tentative diagnoses. Making the first set of nursing diagnoses for a client takes more time and effort than updating and changing the care plan. Schedule extra time to generate the initial care plan, because the data are new. A carefully constructed initial care plan will save you time in the long run. It is easier to update and revise a good care plan than to create the care plan on an ad hoc basis.

In the following paragraphs, we discuss the steps in the diagnostic reasoning process. Box 11–3 illustrates an example of how to use the diagnostic reasoning process.

Reviewing the Assessment Data

The first step in making a nursing diagnosis is to review all the assessment data available about the client. This includes the medical history and physical examination data, laboratory analyses, and data obtained from the nursing history and assessment. The amount of data may seem overwhelming at first, but as you review the data, you will be able to make distinctions between relevant and irrelevant data by asking two

BOX 11–3

MAKING A NURSING DIAGNOSIS: A CASE EXAMPLE

Mrs. Brown is a 45-year-old woman who was admitted to the hospital last night from the emergency department with a medical diagnosis of "moderately severe vaginal bleeding secondary to fibroadenoma." She was sent directly to the operating room, where she underwent an abdominal hysterectomy. She was transferred to the surgical nursing unit from the post-anesthesia care unit (PACU). She had an IV of D$_5$ lactated Ringer's solution running in her left arm, a surgical dressing on her abdomen that was clean and dry, and an indwelling catheter in her bladder. She responded to verbal commands but was still very sedated when she arrived on the nursing unit. Her color was pale. Her vital signs were: blood pressure 126/78, pulse 88, temperature 97.8°F.

Step 1: Review the Assessment

When the nurse, Janine Cole, comes on duty 2 hours later, she reviews Mrs. Brown's chart. She finds that Mrs. Brown began bleeding suddenly and heavily the night before and was driven to the hospital by her husband. Her estimated blood loss before surgery was 500 mL. Blood loss during surgery was estimated at less than 500 mL. She received one unit of whole blood during surgery. Her hemoglobin value in the PACU was reported as 9.0. Her hematocrit level was 40%.

When Janine enters Mrs. Brown's room, she finds Mrs. Brown awake but drowsy. Her husband is in the room with her. He looks very tired and worried. Janine introduces herself to Mr. and Mrs. Brown and then checks Mrs. Brown's vital signs, abdominal dressing, IV, and catheter drainage. The client's vital signs are: blood pressure 110/76, pulse 78, and temperature 98.6°F. Her color is pink. Her capillary refill rate is less than 3 seconds. The dressing has a slight pink area near the center but is dry. Her urine output was 50 mL in the last hour.

Mrs. Brown is restless and complains of discomfort. She is reluctant to move or to have Janine touch her or the bed because she says it hurts when the bed is jostled. Aside from her discomfort, she seems to be primarily worried about her husband. She keeps asking him if he is all right and encouraging him to go home and rest. She tells Janine that he has been up all night and has had no sleep.

Step 2: Cluster the Data

Janine clusters data under the appropriate functional health patterns. She does not have data on some of the health patterns, so she uses only the ones that are appropriate at this time.

Health Perception-Health Management: Postoperative state.

Nutritional-Metabolic: NPO last night and until 9 AM this morning, IV 5% R/L at 20 gtt/min, now taking small sips of clear liquids. Temperature is 98.6°F, abdominal wound present, dressing slightly pink in one spot but dry.

Elimination: Indwelling catheter drainage is 50 mL in the last hour, intake from IV was 1200 mL, no evidence of bowel sounds on auscultation as yet.

Activity-Exercise: Has been immobile in OR, still recumbent and inactive due to IV catheter, sedation. Pulse is 78, blood pressure is 110/76.

Cognitive-Perceptual: Drowsy but alert to surroundings. Restless, complains of discomfort, reluctant to move or have bed touched.

Self-Perception–Self-Concept: No data on how she feels about hysterectomy and impact this will have on her sense of self as woman.

Role-Relationship: Husband is present and concerned. She is more concerned about him than her own discomfort.

Step 3: Select Possible Nursing Diagnoses

Janine considers the data clusters and makes the following list of possible nursing diagnoses: *Impaired skin integrity, Risk for infection, Pain, Altered urinary elimination, Impaired physical mobility, Bathing/hygiene self-care deficit,* and *Anxiety.* Some of these diagnoses may be ruled out when Janine compares the actual data about Mrs. Brown with the defining characteristics of the diagnoses initially selected (see Table 11–4).

Step 4: Differentiate Among Possible Diagnoses

Janine then compares the defining characteristics of the possible diagnoses with the actual data she has about Mrs. Brown.

Continued

questions: What is the significance of these data for nursing care? What problems could the client have based on this information?

As you review the assessment data, you are looking for subjective and objective cues. Some examples of cues may be a cough, a pattern of bruises, or a client's report of stress caused by an impending divorce.

Clustering the Data

A single cue often alerts you to a problem. However, it is almost never enough to make a definitive diagnosis and is certainly not enough to associate the diagnosis with a related factor. Thus, the next step in generating nursing diagnoses is to mentally organize the data into

BOX 11–3

MAKING A NURSING DIAGNOSIS: A CASE EXAMPLE (continued)

Step 5: Identify Appropriate Diagnoses

Janine compiles the final list of nursing diagnoses and arranges them by priority:

1. *Pain.*
2. *Risk for infection.*
3. *Impaired physical mobility.*
4. *Impaired skin integrity.*
5. *Bathing/hygiene self-care deficit.*

Anxiety and *Altered urinary elimination* were removed from list as not valid.

Other nurses may have prioritized this list somewhat differently; however, it is clear that the highest priority is to help Mrs. Brown get comfortable and become free of pain. When she is no longer uncomfortable, it will be easier to help her groom herself and get out of bed.

Step 6: Determine Related Factors

Janine now links the nursing diagnoses with their "related to" factors or etiologies and comes up with the following final list of diagnoses:

- *Pain related to recent abdominal surgery.*
- *Impaired skin integrity related to operative incision into the abdomen.*
- *Impaired physical mobility related to pain from abdominal incision, IV in arm, indwelling catheter in bladder.*
- *Risk for infection related to impaired skin integrity, history of blood loss, and presence of indwelling catheter.*
- *Bathing/hygiene self-care deficit related to presence of IV in one arm, indwelling catheter in bladder, pain, and sedation due to recent operative procedure.*

Step 7: Discuss the Diagnoses With the Client

Janine returns to Mrs. Brown's room to administer her pain medication and to verify the other nursing diagnoses she has made. Although the diagnoses of *Impaired skin integrity, Risk for infection,* and *Bathing/hygiene self-care deficit* are based on objective evidence and might not require validation from the client, Janine discusses

them with Mrs. Brown to be sure their priorities are congruent. Mrs. Brown agrees with the diagnoses of *Impaired skin integrity, Risk for infection, Bathing/hygiene self-care deficit,* and *Impaired physical mobility.* She is eager to get her IV and catheter removed so she can get out of bed. Mrs. Brown says that she is not anxious about anything, just worried that her husband has been up all night and has not had any sleep. Once Mrs. Brown has validated the nursing diagnoses, Janine enters them into the nursing care plan.

Step 8: Plan the Nursing Care

Janine plans her nursing care for Mrs. Brown based on the etiologies of the nursing diagnoses. Because the highest priority was Mrs. Brown's pain, which resulted from the recent abdominal surgery, Janine gave the pain medication ordered. The diagnoses *Impaired skin integrity* and *Risk for infection* share "related to" factors: the abdominal wound and the catheter. In addition to maintaining strict asepsis with dressing changes and catheter care, Janine plans to urge Mrs. Brown to deep-breathe frequently to reduce the risk of postoperative pneumonia. A third intervention she plans will be to ambulate Mrs. Brown as soon as possible to increase bowel peristalsis and reduce the risk of paralytic ileus.

Janine also plans to assist Mrs. Brown with her bath today to alleviate the *Bathing/hygiene self-care deficit* diagnosis; the presence of an IV in one arm, a painful abdominal wound, and a catheter significantly reduce Mrs. Brown's ability to manage her own hygiene. Finally, Janine will help Mrs. Brown get out of bed and move around several times during the day to help her increase her physical mobility.

Janine will continue to monitor Mrs. Brown's progress and will alter, delete, or add to the list of nursing diagnoses as needed throughout Mrs. Brown's hospital stay. Reviewing the nursing process steps frequently (at least once a shift or more often if needed) during a client's stay is crucial to maintaining an accurate picture of the client's needs and giving the best possible care based on those needs.

---

clusters of cues that seem to fit logically together and lead to insights or inferences about the client's condition. For example, a cough could be a cue to a number of nursing diagnoses. If the client also has wheezing, dyspnea, cyanosis, and a history of asthma, an experienced nurse would consider the nursing diagnosis *Impaired gas exchange related to airway obstruction secondary to asthma.*

Remember that not all cues are needed or useful.

Do not try to force all of the cues into meaningful clusters. On the other hand, some important cues may not be available. Thus, you may have to reassess the client to obtain the missing information at a later time.

Before moving on to the next step, review the clusters you have generated. Do they make sense conceptually and logically? Do they provide insights into the client's condition? Do the clusters indicate potential nursing diagnoses?

Selecting Possible Nursing Diagnoses

After answering these questions, review each potential problem represented in a data cluster. Think critically about which nursing diagnoses might be relevant to the situation. Remember that diagnoses cannot be selected in isolation from the goals of care. When you understand the client's reason for seeking service, goals for health, preferences in managing care, and lifestyle, you will be more likely to choose a diagnosis that is appropriate for the individual client in each particular situation.

The possible diagnoses you choose should be realistically manageable within the care setting. The hospital nurse probably does not often use the diagnosis of *Impaired home maintenance management*, and the school nurse may have little use for *Decreased cardiac output.*

If no diagnosis seems to fit a particular data cluster, you may need to create a new diagnostic label that captures the meaning of the cluster. However, make sure to carefully review the currently available diagnoses before creating a new diagnosis. If a new label is necessary and it seems to work well for a particular population over time, consider submitting it to NANDA for review and development.

Differentiating Among Possible Diagnoses

Once you have identified possible nursing diagnoses for your client, you will need to differentiate among them and narrow the possibilities until you identify the most appropriate diagnosis for each problem. Finding the most useful nursing diagnosis involves ruling out several possible diagnoses. **Differential diagnosis** is the term used to describe the process of deciding among several possible diagnoses to most accurately describe the client's problem. This process involves pattern matching of the client's assessment data with the defining characteristics of possible diagnoses to determine which one has the best fit. The process is described in detail later in the chapter.

The following questions and steps will be useful in differentiating between diagnoses:

- Does the cluster of cues match one of the diagnoses better than the others? If so, this is probably the correct diagnosis.
- If the cluster of cues does not match perfectly any of the diagnoses under consideration, where does the problem lie? Perhaps there are not enough data available to choose appropriately.
- If not enough data are available, determine which data you need to make a decision. Then collect the data.
- Review the defining characteristics and data again to find the best match. Perhaps there is now a high probability of two or more different diagnoses being correct. If additional new data cannot be found to help solve the problem, you must take one of two approaches. First, you can keep both diagnoses in the care plan until the situation becomes

clearer. Second, you can consult with the client about which diagnosis is correct.

Identifying Appropriate Diagnoses

After selecting possible diagnoses and undertaking the process of differentiating between them, you will reach the point of identifying the nursing diagnosis or diagnoses most appropriate for your client. It is at this point that you will need to exercise clinical judgment; not all of the nursing diagnoses may be amenable to immediate intervention at this time. Not all possible diagnoses may be relevant to the current situation. Consequently, they need not be included in the care plan. Finally, some diagnoses will be of lower priority than others. Exercise your judgment when prioritizing diagnoses, setting goals for care, and planning nursing interventions to meet those goals.

Determining Related Factors

Next, determine what the "related to," or etiologic (causal), factors are for the diagnoses you have selected. The "related to" or etiologic statement is very important because it gives direction to nursing care, guiding your choice of nursing interventions to alleviate the client's health concern.

When selecting a related factor, it might be helpful to ask yourself, "Does this information help me decide which interventions are most appropriate?" For example, selecting the diagnosis *Risk for infection related to postoperative care* is neither desirable nor useful. It focuses on nursing actions, not the client's problem. A better choice would be *Risk for infection related to shallow breathing, use of indwelling catheter, and surgical incision.* Selecting the more specific and client-focused factors makes determining interventions more efficient.

A second question to ask yourself is, "Does this information make a difference in the interventions that will be performed for this client?" For example, with a client who has had a total joint replacement and must learn to walk again, you would select the diagnosis *Impaired physical mobility related to pain.* This diagnosis reflects your knowledge that pain management will be a major factor in helping the client begin to walk. It therefore focuses nursing care on pain management. The diagnosis *Impaired physical mobility related to a total hip replacement* fails to reflect your knowledge that the hip is stable and that the client *can* walk but does not want to because of the pain.

In some cases, nursing interventions are methods of implementing medical therapy for a specific medical diagnosis. For example, given the diagnosis *Altered thought processes related to stage three Alzheimer's disease,* you must recognize that neither you nor the physician can change the client's advanced Alzheimer's disease. This diagnosis tells you that the change in thinking is irreversible, so the plan of care focuses on helping the client manage within the limitations imposed by the illness. Now consider the same label with a different etiology: *Altered thought processes related to lithium tox-*

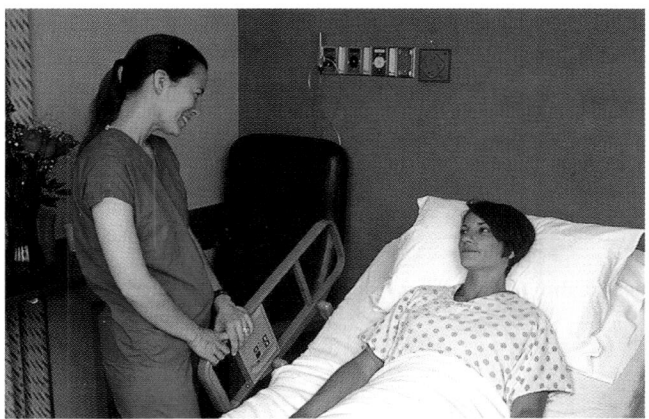

Figure 11–3. Discussing nursing diagnoses with the client and family ensures that your goals and those of the client and family match.

icity. This diagnosis reveals that the client has a reversible problem. The nursing interventions, therefore, focus on the client following the physician's treatment plan for hydration, helping the client cope, reducing the client's anxiety, and maintaining the client's safety.

Discussing Nursing Diagnoses With the Client

Finally, discuss your nursing diagnoses with the client and family (Fig. 11–3). Does the client agree with your inferences? If so, set nursing care goals with input from the client. This is a sound method for validating your nursing diagnoses and ensures that your goals and those of the client match. Table 11–2 summarizes the diagnostic reasoning process.

Writing the Nursing Diagnostic Statement

Writing a useful nursing diagnosis means identifying the client's problem clearly so that all nurses who use the nursing care plan have the same understanding of the client's problems. How the problem is stated focuses nursing care and provides a basis for evaluating the effectiveness of the chosen care. As noted earlier, the related factor is especially important in providing needed clarity. The following paragraphs provide some useful tips for writing diagnostic statements that are meaningful and useful.

Identifying the Client's Needs

The diagnosis should identify client needs or problems rather than nursing problems. One of the advantages of using NANDA diagnoses is that they focus on client problems and human responses. You may be tempted to write the "related to" statement in terms of services or procedures; however, stating the need for services as a nursing diagnosis will not help you make decisions about how to provide those services.

You may also be tempted to write the "related to" statement in terms of the technology being used. Again, the management of technology is your prob-

lem, not the client's problem. Asking yourself why the technology is being used may help you identify the client's problem.

Avoiding Legally Inadvisable Statements

State all of your nursing diagnosis in a manner that meets the legal guidelines for entries into the health record. Your related factors should not place a value judgment on the client's behavior or make a judgment that could be construed as libel in a court of law. Also avoid statements suggesting that nursing care has been or is potentially negligent. Table 11–3 gives examples of legally inadvisable nursing diagnostic statements.

SOURCES OF DIAGNOSTIC ERROR

Naturally, it is possible to make errors during the process of making a nursing diagnosis. Errors can occur during data collection, clustering, or interpretation. It is also possible to overdiagnose or underdiagnose the client's nursing problems.

Errors in Data Collecting

You may be tempted to begin with a medical diagnosis and anticipate a client's problems based on that diagnosis. Although this may be a good way to begin identifying possible nursing diagnoses, additional assessment is always needed. Relying on the medical diagnosis may lead to premature termination of data collection and analysis, thus reducing the likelihood of a comprehensive assessment. As a result, client problems unrelated to or unexpected from the medical diagnosis may be missed.

A second error in data collection occurs if you fail to collect adequate data from which to make inferences. This leads to two potential problems. The first problem is making an inferential leap to the wrong diagnosis based on insufficient data. Table 11–4 gives some examples of this type of error. The second problem is that you may fail to make a needed diagnosis because you lack the necessary clinical cues (see the following paragraph). Except in an emergency situation, always take the time to do an adequate assessment.

Errors in Cue Clustering

Errors in cue clustering often result from inadequate data, poor critical thinking, or lack of familiarity with either the clinical population or the nursing diagnosis language. If cues from assessment data are incorrectly clustered, you may name the cluster incorrectly and choose the wrong nursing diagnosis. Choosing the wrong diagnosis results in ineffective interventions. This does not serve the client well because the problem does not get resolved. It does not serve you well either, because your time and energy are wasted on ineffective nursing care.

TABLE 11–2
Applying the Diagnostic Reasoning Process*

Actual Client Data	Possible Nursing Diagnosis	Defining Characteristics	Nursing Decision
Client has broken skin and traumatized tissue due to abdominal surgery. Indwelling catheter is inserted in bladder.	*Impaired skin integrity*	*Present:* Disruption of skin surface; invasion of body structures. *Not present:* Destruction of skin layers.	This is a valid diagnosis. Two out of three of the defining characteristics are present.
Client has broken skin and traumatized tissue due to abdominal surgery. Indwelling catheter is inserted in bladder. Altered bowel peristalsis due to general anesthesia and abdominal surgery; hemoglobin is decreased, surgery is an invasive procedure, and no antibiotics ordered at present.	*Risk for infection*	*Present:* Inadequate primary defenses (broken skin, traumatized tissue), inadequate secondary defenses (decreased hemoglobin, altered peristalsis), tissue destruction and increased environmental exposure (invasive procedure). *Not present:* Inadequate primary defenses (decrease in ciliary action, stasis of body fluids, change in pH secretions); inadequate secondary defenses (leukopenia, suppressed inflammatory response) and immunosuppression; chronic disease; malnutrition; pharmaceutical agents; trauma; rupture of amniotic membranes; insufficient knowledge to avoid exposure to pathogens.	This is a valid diagnosis for most postoperative clients for at least the first few days, especially for those who are not receiving antibiotics. The client is at risk for wound infection, respiratory infection (since abdominal surgery may decrease ability to breathe deeply), paralytic ileus (intestinal paralysis caused by handling of the bowel during surgery), and urinary tract infection owing to a catheter.
Verbalized discomfort, expressed concern about movement causing pain, reluctance to let anyone touch the bed, and restless behavior.	*Pain*	*Present:* Verbal or coded reports; protective behavior. Expressive behavior, such as restlessness. *Not present:* Observed evidence; antalgic position and gestures; guarding behavior; facial mask; sleep disturbance. Self-focus; narrowed focus; distraction behavior, autonomic alteration in muscle tone; autonomic responses; changes in appetite and eating.	This is a valid nursing diagnosis. There are several defining characteristics present.
A hysterectomy results in edema in the pelvic region, which may result in difficulty in passing urine. Preventive measure (an indwelling catheter) is in place.	*Urinary retention*	*Present:* None *Not present:* Retention; inability to pass urine.	The diagnosis is not valid. Write the diagnosis as *Risk for urinary retention* and institute when indwelling catheter is discontinued.
Client is reluctant to move, intravenous catheter in arm, indwelling urinary catheter in bladder, abdominal incision, pain.	*Impaired physical mobility*	*Present:* Inability to purposefully move within the physical environment, including bed mobility, transfer, and ambulation; reluctance to move; imposed restriction of movement. *Not present:* Limited range of motion; decreased muscle strength, control, or mass.	This is a valid diagnosis. The client will likely need help to get out of bed and to ambulate the first time or two. However, this diagnosis will likely be valid only for a short time because the client will be encouraged to be out of bed as soon as possible.

TABLE 11–2
Applying the Diagnostic Reasoning Process* *Continued*

Actual Client Data	Possible Nursing Diagnosis	Defining Characteristics	Nursing Decision
Intravenous catheter in left arm; indwelling catheter in bladder; surgical incision making movement difficult; pain.	*Bathing/hygiene self-care deficit*	*Present:* Inability to wash body or body parts; inability to obtain water or get to water source; inability to regulate water temperature or flow	This is a valid diagnosis. It will be used short-term until the client can bathe.
Client is restless and expresses concern about spouse and pain.	*Anxiety*	*Present:* Apprehension (about spouse); distress (about pain and about spouse's welfare); worried; restless. *Not present:* Increased tension; painful or persistent helplessness; fearful; regretful; overexcited; rattled; jittery; feelings of inadequacy; shakiness; fear of unspecific consequences; expressed concerns due to change in life events; sympathetic stimulation; insomnia; glancing about; poor eye contact; trembling; facial tension.	This is probably not a valid diagnosis. The client's concern is more likely worry than anxiety because there are few defining characteristics of anxiety. To verify, you could ask the client if client feels anxious about anything. If client voices concern that spouse has been up all night and needs to rest, you would confirm the diagnosis as inappropriate.

*This table shows a comparison between actual client data, possible diagnoses, defining characteristics of possible diagnoses, and nursing decisions about the validity of choosing the diagnoses.

TABLE 11–3
Examples of Legally Inadvisable Nursing Diagnostic Statements

Inadvisable Diagnosis	Problem	Appropriate Diagnosis
Ineffective airway clearance related to infrequent suctioning	Suggests negligence	*Ineffective airway clearance* related to shallow breathing
Risk for infection related to improper aseptic technique	Implies lapse in standards of care	*Risk for infection* related to operative incision in abdomen
Ineffective infant feeding pattern related to poor mothering	Judgmental and derogatory	*Ineffective infant feeding pattern* related to poor suck/swallow rhythm
Bathing/hygiene self-care deficit related to poverty	Judgmental	*Bathing/hygiene self-care deficit* related to lack of running water in home
Ineffective breastfeeding related to maternal self-absorption	Implies mother is neglectful	*Ineffective breastfeeding* related to maternal uncertainty and anxiety

Another error in cue clustering made frequently by novices is making a nursing diagnosis on the basis of a single cue. Only rarely are accurate diagnoses based on a single cue. There is almost always more data needed before inferences can be drawn. Validate or confirm your diagnoses with the client as one means of avoiding cue clustering errors.

Errors in Interpretation

A frequent source of error is interpreting cues inappropriately. In some cases, assessment data may be ambiguous and difficult to interpret, or the data may lead you to infer two or more equally possible diagnoses. The best solution is to verify the possible diagnoses with the client or the client's family.

Failure to identify and include client health strengths in your analysis of cues is another source of inappropriate interpretation. Clients have strengths and resources that nurses do not always know about. These strengths can have a significant impact on their health status and their ability to cope with health problems and life processes. Failure to assess for strengths as well as problems often leads to misinterpretation.

TABLE 11–4
Selected Sources of Diagnostic Error

Cues Used To Form Diagnosis	Incorrect Diagnosis	Diagnostic Error	Cues Ignored in Forming Diagnosis	Correct Diagnosis
Heart rate 50 beats per minute	*Decreased cardiac output*	Inferential leap; failure to consider all significant cues	Skin warm and dry, blood pressure 125/80, color pink, usual heart rate 52.	None needed; cue reflects normal function
Client asks to be left alone	*Social isolation*	Inappropriate interpretation of cues	Client did not sleep last night and needs a nap.	*Fatigue*
Urine output 30 mL per hour	*Fluid volume deficit*	Insufficient cues	Client has a history of renal failure and is developing edema	*Fluid volume excess*
Client appears uncomfortable and is restless after surgery for a fractured hip.	*Pain*	Inaccurate cue grouping	Further assessment reveals that the bladder is full and the client needs a bedpan.	*Self-care deficit (toileting)*
The client has not had a bowel movement in 3 days.	*Constipation*	Use of a single cue as the basis of the diagnosis	The client normally has a bowel movement every 3 days.	None needed; cue reflects normal function.
Client has not monitored blood glucose levels for last 10 days and expresses frustration and anger with managing diet and insulin.	*Ineffective management of therapeutic regimen*	Inconsistent or ambivalent cues	Client has been well controlled and able to manage in the past. Client separated from spouse last week.	*Ineffective individual coping*
Client is immobilized from a fractured leg and has a long leg cast in place	*Impaired home maintenance management*	Inferential leap from insufficient data	Family has housekeeper, but all bedrooms are located upstairs.	*Impaired physical mobility*

Underdiagnosing and Overdiagnosing

Underdiagnosing can occur because of problems in the client assessment. To ensure comprehensive care, you need a systematic method of assessing and documenting the client's health status to avoid missing problems. If the documentation method lacks a sufficient number of categories, important areas may be subsumed in a larger category and be overlooked. Broad categories should have subcategories. For example, if one category is physiological, the body systems can be used as subcategories to make sure the physical assessment is complete.

If you have an insufficient knowledge base, you may miss the significance of important cues. The more you know about the client's medical problem and responses to that problem, the more specific and sensitive your nursing diagnoses will be.

Overdiagnosing occurs when you anticipate possible problems and fail to validate their actual existence. This approach suggests inadequate assessment. A second kind of overdiagnosing occurs when you simultaneously attempt to diagnose every problem the client has now, may have soon, and could have at any time in the future. This results in a very long list of diagnoses, many of which are irrelevant to the client's immediate problem. Determine which problems have the highest priorities, and remove the others until the most immediate concerns are dealt with. Always try to validate nursing diagnoses and goals with the client.

KEY PRINCIPLES

- As a nurse, you must be able to think through problems and make sound clinical judgments about the clients under your care.
- A nursing diagnosis is a clinical judgment about individual, family, or community responses to actual or potential health problems or life processes. It provides the basis for selecting nursing interventions to achieve outcomes for which you are accountable.
- Nursing diagnoses are human responses, the way clients respond to the life- and health-related conditions. Nursing diagnoses are not problems that *nurses* have but that *clients* have.
- Nursing diagnoses are *part* of the nursing process. Making a nursing diagnosis is the link between assessment and planning interventions. Without ac-

curate diagnosis of the client's problems, you cannot determine appropriate interventions.

- Nursing diagnoses identify problems for which you are accountable.
- There are five components of a nursing diagnosis: a label, a definition, a set of defining characteristics, a group of related factors, and risk factors.
- Diagnostic reasoning consists of collecting and reviewing client assessment data; generating clusters of cues and forming hypotheses about what the client's human responses might be; evaluating potential nursing diagnosis labels that reflect the cue clusters generated; selecting the best labels to describe the client's human responses; determining the related factors for each diagnosis; and planning interventions based on each diagnosis and its related factors.
- Common errors in nursing diagnosis occur when data are incorrectly collected, clustered, or interpreted. Other common errors include underdiagnosing or overdiagnosing the client's condition.

BIBLIOGRAPHY

*Alfaro-LeFevre, R. (1994). *Applying the nursing process: A step-by-step guide* (3rd ed.). Philadelphia: J.B. Lippincott Co.

Alfaro-LeFevre, R. (1995). *Critical thinking in nursing: A practical approach.* Philadelphia: W.B. Saunders.

Aquilino, M.L. (1997). Cognitive development, clinical knowledge, and clinical experience related to diagnostic ability. *Nursing Diagnosis: The Journal of Nursing Language and Classification, 8*(3), 110–119.

*Avant, K. (1990). The art and science in nursing diagnosis development. *Nursing Diagnosis: The Journal of Nursing Language and Classification, 1*(2), 51–55.

*Carnevali, D.L., Mitchell, P.H., Woods, N.F., & Tanner, C.A. (1984). *Diagnostic reasoning in nursing.* Philadelphia: J.B. Lippincott Co.

Carpenito, L.J. (1997). *Nursing diagnosis: Application to clinical practice.* Philadelphia: Lippincott-Raven.

Clark, J., & Lang, N. (1992). Nursing's next advance: An internal classification for nursing practice. *International Nursing Review, 39*(4), 109–112.

Coenen, A., Ryan, P., Sutton, J., Devine, E.C., Werley, H.H., & Kelber, S. (1995). Use of the nursing minimum data set to describe nursing interventions for select nursing diagnoses and related factors in an acute care setting. *Nursing Diagnosis: The Journal of Nursing Language and Classification, 6*(3), 108–114.

Cox, H.C., Hinz, M.D., Lubno, M.A., Newfield, S.A., Ridenour, N.A., & Sridaromont, K.L. (1997). *Clinical applications of nursing diagnosis: Adult, child, women's, psychiatric, gerontic, and home health considerations.* Baltimore: Williams & Wilkins.

*Feinstein, A.R. (1967). *Clinical judgment.* New York: Robert Krieger Publishing Co.

Fowler, S.B. (1997). Impaired verbal communication during short-term oral intubation. *Nursing Diagnosis: The Journal of Nursing Language and Classification, 8*(3), 93–98.

Gordon, M. (1997). *Manual of nursing diagnosis 1997–1998.* St. Louis: Mosby.

*Gordon, M. (1984). *Nursing diagnosis: Process and application.* New York: McGraw-Hill.

*Hamers, J.P., Huijer Abu-Saad, H., & Halfens, R.J. (1994). Diagnostic process and decision making in nursing: A literature review. *Journal of Professional Nursing, 10*(3), 154–163.

*Kim, M.J., McFarland, G.K., & McLane, A.M. (1984). *Classifications of nursing diagnoses: Proceedings of the second national conference.* Philadelphia: North American Nursing Diagnosis Association.

*Martin, K.S., & Scheet, N.J. (1992). *The Omaha system: Applications for community health nursing.* Philadelphia: W.B. Saunders.

Meltzer, M., & Palau, S.M. (1996). *Acquiring critical thinking skills.* Philadelphia: W.B. Saunders.

North American Nursing Diagnosis Association. (1999). *Nursing diagnoses: Definitions and classification 1999–2000.* Philadelphia: Author.

*O'Neill, E.S. (1994). The influence of experience on community health nurses' use of the similarity heuristic in diagnostic reasoning. *Scholarly Inquiry for Nursing Practice, 8*(3), 261–273.

Pehler, S.R. (1997). Children's spiritual response: Validation of the nursing diagnosis spiritual distress. *Nursing Diagnosis: The Journal of Nursing Language and Classification, 8*(2), 55–66.

*Radwin, L.E. (1990). Research on diagnostic reasoning in nursing. *Nursing Diagnosis: The Journal of Nursing Language and Classification, 1*(2), 70–77.

Rantz, M., & LeMone, P. (Eds). (1995). *Classification of nursing diagnoses: Proceedings of the eleventh conference.* Glendale, CA: CINAHL Information Systems.

Simon, J.M., & Baumann, M.A. (1995). Differential diagnostic validation: Acute and chronic pain. *Nursing Diagnosis: The Journal of Nursing Language and Classification, 6*(2), 73–79.

Tanner, C.A. (1993). Rethinking clinical judgment. NLN Publications, Apr. (14–2511): 15–41.

van Hooft, S., Gillam, L., & Byrnes, M. (1995). *Facts and values: An introduction to critical thinking for nurses.* Sydney, Australia: Maclennan & Petty.

Woodtli, A. (1995). Stress incontinence: Clinical identification and validation of defining characteristics. *Nursing Diagnosis: The Journal of Nursing Language and Classification, 6*(3), 115–121.

*Asterisk indicates a classic or definitive work on this subject.

Planning for Intervention

Jeannette Marie Daly

Key Terms

care plan conference
clinical pathway
collaboration
computerized care plan
consultation
direct care intervention
discharge planning
indirect care intervention

individualized care plan
nurse-initiated intervention
nursing care plan
nursing intervention
physician-initiated
 intervention
standardized care plan

LEARNING OBJECTIVES

After studying this chapter, you should be able to:

1. Describe types of planning for individual clients and client groups.
2. Identify priorities for planning client care.
3. Describe the process of establishing client expected outcomes.
4. Discuss the essential skills needed to implement client care.
5. Describe types and components of interventions to individualize care for each client.
6. Describe the development of a nursing care plan.

Planning is the phase of the nursing process during which you will identify the goals of nursing care and the actions to attain those goals (Fig. 12–1). The American Nurses' Association (ANA) supports planning as a means to use theoretical and research-based understandings to prescribe interventions to attain expected outcomes (ANA, 1995).

The result of the planning process is a guide for health care that identifies client problems in need of nursing care (specified by nursing diagnoses), predicts outcomes that are sensitive to nursing care, and lists interventions that will result in the expected outcomes or a **nursing care plan.** A **nursing intervention** is "any treatment, based upon clinical judgment and knowledge, that a nurse performs to enhance [client] outcomes" (Iowa Intervention Project, 1996, p. xvii). The nursing care plan is recorded in the client's health record and serves as a tool to communicate the plan of care to all members of the health care team.

Planning is essential for determining and providing optimal nursing care. As health care resources become more limited, planning becomes even more important. Systematic planning allows you to make the best use of the resources available while avoiding use of ineffective—and therefore wasted—resources.

Although planning is labeled specifically as the third phase of the nursing process, it does not take place in isolation. Indeed, planning is interwoven with all phases of the nursing process. You will begin planning and continue doing so throughout the process of gathering assessment data and identifying client problems.

TYPES OF PLANNING

Planning applies both to individual clients and to groups or client populations that are served by a health care agency. For an individual client, planning involves identifying the person's health problems and developing a plan of care to address them. For a group, planning involves identifying characteristics common to the population and making decisions about the services to be offered, the environment in which care will take place, and the staffing needed to accomplish that care.

Planning for Individuals

Nurses plan care both independently and together with other members of the health care team. For each client, you will begin planning for nursing care at or even before your initial contact. You will continue planning throughout the client's stay in the hospital or other health care facility, and you may plan for home or community care after the client's discharge.

As the client's condition changes, plans must be reviewed and modified, sometimes together with other members of the health care team. Planning for discharge begins during the initial contact with the client by establishing the expected outcomes and anticipating follow-up care that may be needed.

Initial Planning

Your first contact with a client allows you to begin assessing the client and his problems. You will complete a thorough history and perform a physical examination to gather data needed to identify problems. While doing so, you will begin to form impressions about the client's most acute or important problem. Naturally, you should also ask the client what he considers to be his most urgent or important problem. If his perception differs from yours, the two of you will need to work together to identify his real and perceived needs.

Next, you will develop an overall plan of care for the client that spans his length of stay or duration of services. The nursing plan includes steps needed to support the client during medical care and to help the client become independent in self-care.

Although the plan addresses mainly the reason for admission, it also should include strategies to manage other problems that could influence the resolution of the client's primary problem. Consequently, plans also should include other members of the health care team and referrals to other settings for additional services.

As an example, consider an elderly client admitted to the hospital with fractured ribs and difficulty breathing after falling at home. When assessing the client, the nurse immediately notices rapid respirations and shortness of breath. The client complains of severe pain. In this case, the nursing plan would include oxy-

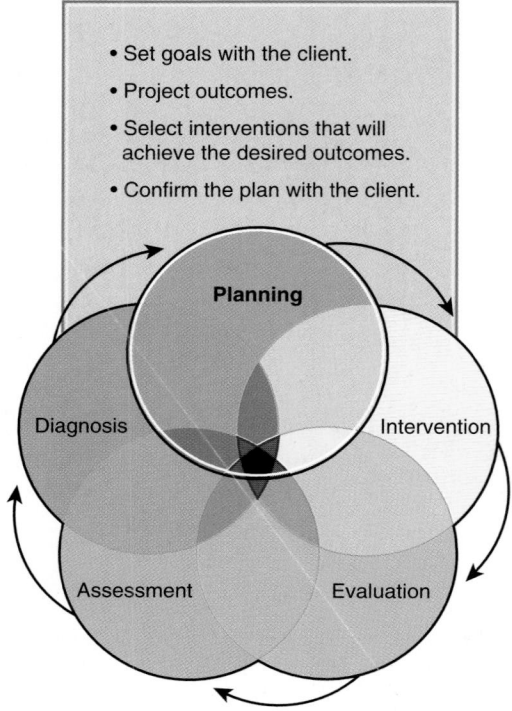

Figure 12–1. During the planning phase of the nursing process, you will set goals with the client, project expected outcomes, select interventions to achieve the desired outcomes, and confirm the plan with the client.

gen therapy and pain medication. The nurse calls a respiratory therapist to begin oxygen therapy while giving the client her prescribed pain medication. At the same time, the nurse begins to formulate a plan to investigate reasons for the fall and to prevent future falls.

All initial plans should be documented in the client's record to ensure coordination of care among members of the health care team. However, remember that planning occurs whether or not the plan is recorded in the client's record. In the example given above, the nurse would record the interventions applied and results attained rather than the plan to treat pain and administer oxygen. However, the plan to assess why the client fell and ways to prevent future falls would be recorded.

Ongoing Planning

During a client's stay in a health care facility, planning is ongoing because the client's health condition may change. These changes must be monitored, and interventions must be altered and implemented as appropriate.

In an acute care setting, a client's condition may change rapidly, thus altering your initial plan. For example, you may plan to check a client's vital signs twice daily, only to find that the client has become weak and dizzy in the interim. If you determine that his vital signs must be checked more often than originally planned, you will need to revise the written plan in the client's record so other members of the health care team are aware of the change.

In a long-term care setting, where changes are often gradual and sometime subtle, ongoing planning may be more formal. If a client's functional abilities decline in two areas, a change-of-status assessment and a revised care plan must be initiated. For example, if your client's mental function declines and his ambulation changes from steady to unsteady, you would need to create a new plan of care. Prompt revisions to the client's plan of care not only ensure the correct care but also help maintain the proper source of funding for the client's care (Department of Health and Human Services, 1991).

Discharge Planning

At the moment a client enters the health care system, you will begin planning for his discharge. **Discharge planning** means "preparation for moving a client from one level of care to another within or outside the current health care agency" (Iowa Intervention Project, 1996, p. 207). Although discharge planning is an independent nursing activity, the prudent nurse seeks input from many members of the health care team. Activities for discharge planning appear in Box 12–1.

Discharge planning addresses client needs that will continue after the present services end. Such planning may include arranging for home care to help the client recover fully after hospital discharge. It may include

---

BOX 12–1

DISCHARGE PLANNING INTERVENTION

Discharge Planning

DEFINITION

Preparation for moving a client from one level of care to another within or outside the current health care agency.

ACTIVITIES

- Help the client, family, and significant others to prepare for discharge.
- Collaborate with the physician, client, family, significant others, and other health team members in planning for continuity of health care.
- Coordinate efforts of different health care providers to ensure a timely discharge.
- Identify client's and primary caregiver's understanding of knowledge or skills required after discharge.
- Identify client teaching needed for post-discharge care.
- Monitor readiness for discharge.
- Communicate the client's discharge plans, as appropriate.
- Document the client's discharge plans, as appropriate.
- Document the client's discharge plans in the chart.
- Formulate a maintenance plan for post-discharge follow-up.
- Assist the client, family, and significant others in planning for the supportive environment necessary to provide the client's post-hospital care.
- Develop a plan that considers the client's health, social, and financial needs.
- Arrange for post-discharge evaluation, as appropriate.
- Encourage self-care, as appropriate.
- Arrange discharge to next level of care.
- Arrange for caregiver support, as appropriate.
- Discuss financial resources if the client needs health care after discharge.
- Coordinate referrals relevant to linkages among health care providers.

Iowa Intervention Project. (1996). Nursing interventions classification (NIC). St. Louis: Mosby-Year Book.

---

rehabilitation services for a client recovering from a stroke, being fitted for an artificial leg, or learning to walk on an implanted hip joint.

In addition to specifying which services a client will need, discharge planning also addresses the setting in which those services should be delivered. Typical settings include inpatient facilities, outpatient facilities, and the client's home. The client's support system, home environment, and transportation options are all important considerations in planning for safe ongoing care after discharge.

Collaborative Planning

Collaboration is the act of two or more health care professionals performing work cooperatively to achieve a common goal. It implies a partnership of professionals who each recognize and acknowledge the expertise of other members of the health care team. Authority in a collaborative situation is derived from professional knowledge, sphere of activity, and responsibility rather than from a hierarchical relationship.

Collaborative planning occurs in every clinical setting and may involve other nurses, physicians, dietitians, respiratory therapists, social workers, and other team members. Collaborative planning ensures continuity and coordination of care.

Consultation

Consultation is the act of two or more health care professionals deliberating for the purpose of making decisions. When the nurse lacks the knowledge or expertise to solve a problem or determines that a plan of care is not effective, it is appropriate to consult with a person who has more experience in the problem area. Nurses working in institutional settings have multiple nursing resources available for consultation. Head nurses, charge nurses, supervisors, and clinical nurse specialists all provide consultation in the planning process. Consultation may occur during all phases of the nursing process, but it is very important in the planning process.

Consulting with specialists and experts provides optimal care for each client by helping to solve difficult problems. Each consultant brings a different viewpoint and area of expertise to the development of the care plan. For example, an enterostomal therapist could provide information on special paste to facilitate adhesion of a stomal wafer to the skin for bag attachment. A physical therapist could discuss the benefits of using a transfer board instead of a lift for moving a client from bed to chair.

Successful consultation has five major elements. First, the nurse identifies an appropriate person with expertise in the problem area. Second, the nurse provides the consultant with factual information about the client and the nature of the problem. Third, the nurse allows the consultant to make an independent judgment about the nature of the problem and possible solution. Fourth, after the consultant has made a judgment, the nurse and consultant discuss the differences in their findings. Fifth, the nurse and consultant decide who should implement the care recommended.

Care Plan Conferences

A **care plan conference** is the action of a group conferring or consulting together to plan care for the client

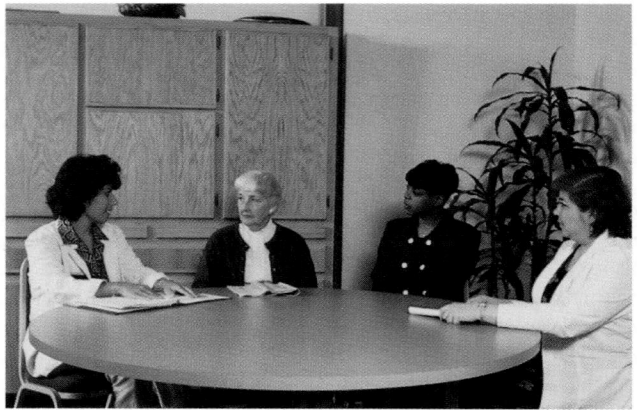

Figure 12–2. A care plan conference allows members of the health care team to discuss and revise the client's care plan as needed. Commonly, the client or a family member is invited to attend.

(Fig. 12–2). Various members of the health care team may organize a care plan conference to review the client's problem list and to plan further strategies to achieve the outcomes established for the client. Typically, the client, family members or significant others, and any team members involved in the client's recovery are invited to the care plan conference.

The frequency and attendees of care plan conferences vary with the setting and the client's situation. A conference may include a nurse, a physician, and a family member who meet in the hall to discuss the client's care. Or a conference may be a formal meeting in which all persons involved in the client's care agree to meet at a specific place and time.

In long-term care, formal care plan conferences are held when the client is admitted to the facility, at 3-month intervals, and when the client's condition changes. Health care professionals who usually attend these meetings include the nurse, activity director, social worker, dietitian, and other therapists, such as a physical therapist or speech therapist. The client has the right to be included in the conference or may be represented by a family member. The physician may also be involved.

In the hospital setting, formal conferences are less common but may occur in special situations. For example, in some hospitals, interdisciplinary teams work together to plan for the treatment of child abuse and neglect. The composition of these teams varies but may include nurses, social workers, psychiatrists, abuse counselors, physicians, and teachers.

Teamwork is needed to facilitate these conferences. The group leader can facilitate the interdisciplinary team meeting by keeping the group focused on important issues and concluding the meeting in a reasonable time. Consultation with team members during the meeting ensures that outcomes are consistent with the plans of the entire team.

Planning for Groups

Although planning for individual clients provides a strong foundation for meeting individual needs, planning for groups of clients improves the overall ability of staff to provide efficient, well-organized care. Planning to meet the needs of a group includes the types of services needed by the population, staffing needed to provide care, and the environment required.

Client Populations

Broad categories of service, such as post-surgical care, rehabilitation, or long-term care, serve clients with some characteristics in common. Planning can reflect the needs of the clients as a group. Planning includes developing a pattern of care to meet the needs of special client populations.

Nurses work collaboratively with other members of the health care team to plan care for groups of clients. For example, because surgical clients have a common set of problems, nurses can establish routines for the unit to meet clients' common needs quickly and in a standardized manner. They also can implement a general care plan that applies to most clients in the unit. Then, as the nurse develops a care plan for each individual client, only information unique to that client must be documented.

Clients who need long-term care, whether in the home or in an institutional setting, have different needs than clients in the acute care setting. Long-term care must fit individual lifestyles, accommodate personal preferences, and maximize each person's self-care ability. Nursing home care involves creating a home-like environment and planning for diversional activities, maintaining competencies, and enhancing the quality of life.

In all cases, planning services to meet the common needs of groups of clients can increase the efficiency and quality of care. It also allows nurses to individualize care, as needed, with relative ease.

Staffing

Planning includes the process of determining the most appropriate person or persons to provide that care. The level of care required determines the type and number of personnel needed. Level of care is defined by answers to the following questions:

- How complex is the care needed?
- Does the care involve procedures with a high risk for complications?
- How time-intensive is the care needed?
- Is the client's condition likely to change rapidly?
- Does the client have other medical problems that require monitoring for drug interactions?
- Is the client able to provide any self-care?

Then the level of care is tied to the staff needed to provide the care with consideration of the following:

- The knowledge, training, and experience of personnel available
- The level of supervision required to ensure safe, effective care
- The job description and legal limitations of the scope of practice of available personnel.

Environmental Planning

In institutional settings, planning begins well before clients undergo assessment and care. Indeed, it begins with the initial design of the facility, which should be fully focused on accommodating the needs of clients served.

A unit or wing of the facility may be reserved for persons who have had heart surgery or orthopedic surgery or who are in renal failure. Special features in this unit will be designed to meet common care needs of the intended population. For example, unit planning may include an exercise room in the heart unit or a dialysis area in a renal unit.

Some factors to be considered include lighting, emergency response systems, safety features, and client comfort. Examples of design goals that reflect planning for client needs include, but are not limited to, the following:

- Elevators used for transferring clients must be large enough to hold a bed and accompanying personnel.
- The surgical recovery area should be on the same floor as the surgical suite to avoid the need to transport an unstable client in an elevator.
- A family waiting room should be located adjacent to the surgical recovery area.
- Handrails should line the hallways, and grab bars should be installed in bathrooms, along with emergency call lights.
- The nurse's station should occupy a central location.
- A secure environment should be available for clients with cognitive impairments.

Naturally, when decisions are made about designing or remodeling a nursing unit, nurses are part of the team. They contribute knowledge of work patterns and client needs to help finalize a practical, efficient environmental design.

Even in the home setting, the nurse can help the client and family members identify and accomplish appropriate modifications for safety and convenience. Planning in the home may mean modifying the care to fit the environment.

THE PLANNING PROCESS

Planning for individual client care includes establishing priorities, making decisions about the desired results of care, and selecting the interventions most likely to achieve those results. The client's care must be organized based on the priority of activities essential for life and recovery. It also must consider the client's perceptions and self-care abilities.

Establishing Priorities

You must make decisions about which diagnoses need immediate attention, which can be safely postponed, and which should be treated in another setting. During the planning process, you will need to establish priorities.

Establishing priorities means that you rank the nursing diagnoses in order of importance. The meaning of importance varies with the setting, the client's condition, and the client's needs. Importance can mean the diagnosis that should be treated first or the diagnosis that should receive the most time and energy.

Threats to Physiological Integrity

When a client has a threat to physiological integrity, her physical needs demand highest priority. Basic human needs include air, water, and food. Among these basic needs, the first priority is any threat to the vital functions of breathing, heartbeat, and blood pressure. Obviously, a person having difficulty breathing will not want a nurse to discuss his sense of self-worth. The immediate need is to relieve the difficult breathing.

Imagine a client with lung cancer who is struggling to breathe, nauseated from chemotherapy, too weak to rise from bed unassisted, and aware that she will die in a short time. The following is a prioritized list of diagnoses for this client:

- Ineffective breathing pattern related to obstructed airway
- Altered nutrition: less than body requirements, related to nausea and vomiting
- Impaired physical mobility related to generalized weakness
- Hopelessness related to coping with the diagnosis of a terminal illness
- Bathing/hygiene self-care deficit related to generalized weakness

All of the problems listed are important, but breathing is basic to life. If the breathing pattern is life-threatening, this diagnosis will have the highest priority. Getting enough to eat is secondary in importance at that moment. When vital functions are stable, attention can be turned to the other physiological systems. Mobility is important for the client to move about safely in the environment.

Action **A**lert!
Basic survival needs take first priority when your client has a threat to physiological integrity.

When planning a client's care, be prepared to shift priorities as her condition and needs change. Indeed, only rarely are priorities clear and stable. You must consider the strong interrelationship among nursing diagnoses when establishing priorities. In the diagnoses just listed for lung cancer, hopelessness is placed low on the list of priorities. However, hopelessness may need to be treated before the client is interested in food. Recognizing that one diagnosis has priority does not mean the remaining diagnoses are ignored or delayed.

Commonly, you may find yourself accomplishing several interventions at once. For example, while suctioning a client, you can monitor an intravenous feeding and give hope and comfort through your touch and tone of voice.

The Health Care Setting

Priorities also tend to vary with the health care setting involved. In an intensive care unit, for example, the nursing diagnosis *ineffective breathing pattern* may be the top priority of nurses working to sustain the client's life. After discharge, the client may have the same diagnosis. However, the diagnosis *knowledge deficit related to inexperience with managing a medical condition* may become the higher priority because the client's breathing pattern has stabilized and the focus of home care shifts to health education.

For the hospital nurse, priorities are more likely to involve physiological diagnoses, and care typically addresses physical needs. As physical needs are stabilized, other problems can be managed. The priority of care can change daily or even hourly as the person's condition improves or worsens.

In a long-term care setting, where the client's physical needs are stable, quality-of-life issues may take on greater importance than physical care. A care plan in a long-term care setting could have the following nursing diagnoses:

- Altered thought processes
- Bathing/hygiene self-care deficit
- Dressing/grooming self-care deficit
- Impaired physical mobility

Responding to each of these diagnoses requires increasing the client's independence. It becomes your priority for care. Being perfectly groomed may not be as important as the client being able to manage self-care. Thus, a plan that seeks to improve the altered thought processes and impaired mobility would help to accomplish the main priority—independence.

Client's Perception of Need

Another consideration in planning priorities for nursing diagnoses is the client's perception of the situation. If a client has just come to a nursing unit following an emergency appendectomy and complains of pain, you would place a high priority on his physical safety and would respond to his concern by establishing pain as a priority diagnosis. Alternatively, if the long-term care client prefers not to participate in social activities, he would not choose *social isolation* as a diagnosis to receive high priority.

Clearly, considering a client's input helps you to provide care that is individualized and satisfying to the client. However, the planning process also allows you to help clients recognize problems and accept help.

Client's Self-Care Ability

For the client able to provide self-care, some diagnoses will have a lower priority in your plan. For instance, *bathing/hygiene self-care deficit* may have a high priority for a post-surgical client but not for a client who can care for himself independently. (If surgery involved his arms or shoulders, he may not have his usual self-care abilities, which would raise the diagnosis to higher priority.)

Determining which nursing diagnoses take precedence over others is a decision-making process that may change repeatedly depending on the client's condition. Learning to set priorities accurately, however, will reap many benefits as you plan your client's care.

Establishing Outcomes

As part of the planning process, you will establish the desirable end result of nursing care—the expected outcome—for each nursing diagnosis. By devising an expected outcome, you express a reasonable expectation that nursing care can produce the intended result. In other words, you can be held accountable for the results of the care you planned. Always apply the following criteria when deciding whether your outcomes qualify as appropriate and expected results of nursing care.

The expected results should be *realistic* or *achievable*. Realistic expectations are based on a review of the entire database and the nursing diagnoses relevant to each client to determine if the outcome can be expected for this client. Carefully evaluate the person's disabilities, resources, and unique life circumstances. Logical reasoning should verify that nursing care can achieve the result predicted.

Ideally, your expected outcomes will describe results of nursing care that are *measurable* and can be directly observed. Another member of the health care team should be able to read the outcome and have the same image of the expected results as you did when you developed it.

Use two components to describe what you want to accomplish in measurable terms: an action and a qualifier that describes the health state to be achieved. Choose verbs to describe cognitive, affective, and psychomotor actions (Box 12–2).

For example, if the nursing diagnosis is *knowledge deficit related to lack of experience in giving insulin,* you would expect your nursing care to result in the client knowing how to self-administer insulin. However, if you use the verb *to know* when phrasing your outcome, you have no way to measure the client's behavior. Instead, use a measurable action verb. In cognitive terms, your outcome could say, "the client will state the steps needed to self-administer insulin." In terms of psychomotor performance, your outcome could say, "the client will correctly administer insulin to himself."

The expected results should be *acceptable* to the client. Always remember that planning is done not only for the client but also with the client (Fig. 12–3). Establishing expected results in collaboration with the client can favorably affect treatment results and client satis-

---

BOX 12-2

VERB SUGGESTIONS FOR GOAL STATEMENTS

Cognitive Domain

Knowledge: defines, describes, identifies, labels, lists, matches, names, outlines
Comprehension: converts, defends, distinguishes, estimates, explains, gives examples
Application: changes, computes, demonstrates, discovers, manipulates, predicts, shows
Analysis: diagrams, discriminates, identifies, illustrates, infers, outlines, relates
Synthesis: categorizes, combines, compiles, organizes, plans, rearranges, revises, tells
Evaluation: appraises, compares, concludes, criticizes, explains, interprets, relates

Affective Domain

Receiving: asks, chooses, describes, follows, gives, holds, locates, names, selects
Responding: answers, assists, greets, helps, performs, presents, reads, recites
Valuing: completes, describes, differentiates, explains, joins, justifies, proposes, reads

Organization: adheres, alters, arranges, combines, defends, integrates, modifies, orders
Characterization by a Value: acts, discriminates, displays, influences, proposes, uses

Psychomotor Domain

Perception: chooses, detects, distinguishes, isolates, relates, selects, separates
Set: begins, displays, explains, moves, proceeds, reacts, responds, shows, starts
Guided Response: assembles, builds, calibrates, constructs, dismantles, heats, measures
Mechanism: assembles, builds, calibrates, constructs, dismantles, heats, measures
Complex Overt Response: assembles, builds, calibrates, constructs, dismantles, heats
Adaptation: adapts, alters, changes, rearranges, reorganizes, revises, varies
Origination: arranges, combines, composes, constructs, creates, designs, originates

Gronlund, N. E. (2000). How to write and use instructional objectives (6th ed.). Upper Saddle River, NJ: Prentice Hall.

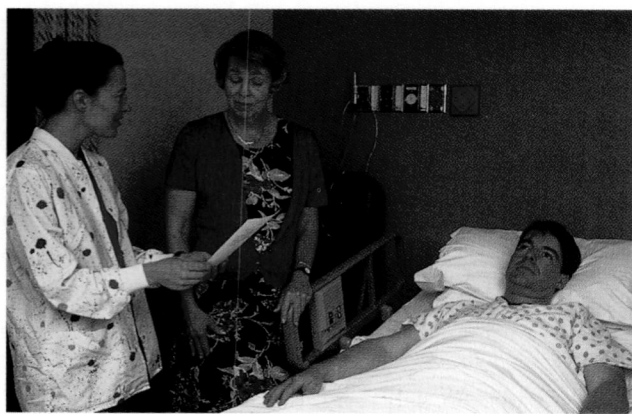

Figure 12–3. Planning is done not only *for* the client and family but *with* the client and family. Mutual goal-setting ensures that the nurse, client, and family are working together.

faction. Although you can help a client by setting realistic expectations, the client must participate actively in planning to be a full partner in care.

To elicit a client's enthusiastic participation in the program of care, listen to his concerns, talk frankly, negotiate, and sometimes compromise. Many people welcome the opportunity to be more actively involved in decision-making. Including the client's family and friends in setting goals and outcomes may be helpful as well. Significant others are often responsible for carrying out the nursing plan following discharge. They may be more willing to continue the therapeutic regimen at home if they understand its rationale and have had input into the decision-making process.

Finally, your planning should include decisions about the *time frame* during which the intended results will be achieved. Terms commonly used to emphasize a time frame include short-term goals and long-term goals. A short-term goal can be met in an hour, a day, or a week. A long-term goal may take a few weeks or months. Especially in a rehabilitative or long-term care setting, a long-term goal may be ongoing.

It is essential that you be able to determine realistic time frames for attaining expected outcomes. Specifying the date for achieving an expected outcome reflects your best judgment about the time needed. This judgment is based on knowledge about the problem, the person's condition, the support systems available, and the necessary nursing interventions.

For example, consider the expected outcome that the client will no longer have hard, dry stools. If the client takes a cathartic medication, the time frame for evaluation of the expected outcome could be 3 days. If the client prefers to resolve the problem by changing her diet and increasing activity instead of taking a medication, the time frame may extend.

In a general sense, setting appropriate time frames can provide benefits beyond those inherent in achieving an expected outcome. For example, setting a time frame can accomplish the following:

- Motivate people to strive toward resolution of the problem

- Provide the client (and nurse) with a sense of accomplishment
- "Pace" nursing care and encourage focus on continued progress
- Prompt the nurse to evaluate the achievement of the outcome.

If an expected outcome is unmet, it means that the time frame must be reconsidered, the expected outcome must be modified, or new interventions must be devised. Of course, expected outcomes must be revised as the client's health status changes.

Defining Outcomes

The term *outcome* has come into popular use from the idea that nurses should be able to demonstrate the results of care in specific, measurable terms. The best of nursing care may not be worthwhile if it fails to result in measurable changes in the client's behavior or condition.

Goal is another word used to describe something that you expect to happen or desire as a result of nursing care. Commonly, however, goals are broad, general statements about the desired results of nursing care; expected outcomes offer specific criteria for measuring results.

For example, if the nursing diagnosis is *activity intolerance related to ineffective breathing secondary to emphysema*, the goal would be to increase the client's activity tolerance. To meet that broad goal, you would devise a set of expected outcomes that allow you to measure the improvement in activity tolerance. Specific outcomes might include the following:

- Client takes bronchodilator on a regular schedule.
- Client correctly uses inhaler before attempting exercise.
- Client can walk one block without shortness of breath.

The overall goal comes from the client's description of the problem and could be something like, "I want to be able to walk to the park to visit with my friends." The expected outcomes in this case illustrate specific ways to accomplish—and measure the accomplishment of—that goal.

Regional and institutional differences in the use of terminology and documentation systems may determine your use of goals, outcomes, and other terms. The important idea that remains, however, is that concrete descriptions of client behaviors are used to demonstrate when the plan of care has been successful. The outcomes or goals that you devise should be linked to your nursing diagnoses and direct interventions to demonstrate the desired changes.

Types of Outcomes

The measurement of health care outcomes has developed over time. Earlier in the 20th century, common outcome measures included morbidity, mortality, length of client stay, and infection rate. However, as the health care industry has become more sophisticated and the consumer more knowledgeable, these measures of success have been deemed inadequate to capture the complexity of health care and measure the specific outcomes produced.

Now, client satisfaction forms an important outcome measure as well. Global multidisciplinary measures describe the client's satisfaction with care, the hospital stay, activities of daily living, and cognitive function. Other outcome measures may include structural or process characteristics that judge the effectiveness and efficiency of a health care setting. Such outcomes in this situation may be cost, profit, unscheduled readmissions, unscheduled repeat surgeries, and unnecessary procedures. Global measures are adequate for assessing the effectiveness of a health care system but are not specific for measuring the results of nursing care or specific outcomes for individual clients.

Outcomes that are discipline-specific can be influenced and changed by the discipline involved. A nursing-sensitive client outcome is "a measurable client or family caregiver state, behavior, or perception that is conceptualized as a variable and is largely influenced by and sensitive to nursing interventions" (Iowa Outcomes Project, 1997, p. 22). In your nursing care plans, you would choose only outcomes that are sensitive to nursing interventions when describing the client's state.

Nursing Outcomes Classification System

Increasingly, nurses and facilities are recognizing the benefits of using a standardized outcome classification system. The research-based Nursing Outcomes Classification (NOC) system from the Iowa Outcomes Project is the best known and most highly developed system available.

NOC outcomes are one-word or two-word generalizations that describe the results of nursing care, followed by measurement criteria for each one. The NOC project describes outcomes as "client states, behaviors, or perceptions that follow and are expected to be influenced by an intervention" (Iowa Outcome Project, 1997). Outcomes are at a higher level of abstraction than the measurement criteria to help you link the outcome to the client's problem or nursing diagnosis. For each outcome, you can select indicator behaviors for an individual client.

The NOC system offers a beginning list of expected outcomes that allow you to evaluate whether a nursing diagnosis has been resolved. Examples of outcomes include bowel elimination, cognitive orientation, compliance behavior, coping, fear control, grief resolution, respiratory status, gas exchange, and vital sign status. Table 12–1 illustrates an NOC outcome for vital sign status.

The classification of nursing-sensitive client outcomes is a four-tiered structure with domains, classes, outcomes and indicators. Each domain and class has a definition that helps to place and locate specific outcomes (Table 12–2). The fourth level includes indicators written in concrete, measurable terms.

NOC outcomes have several advantages. They are understandable to all health care professionals. They are measured on a scale to allow measuring negative or positive changes or a lack of change resulting from nursing interventions (Iowa Outcomes Project, 1997, p. 23).

The indicators define the client outcome and list aspects of a client state that are needed to measure the outcome. All of the indicators are not required to assess the outcome state in every circumstance, depending on the nursing diagnosis, the interventions, and the care setting. Therefore, indicators can be modified, deleted, or added in a given clinical situation.

TABLE 12–1
Example of Nursing-Sensitive Client Outcomes

Vital Signs Status

Definition

Temperature, pulse, respiration, and blood pressure within expected range for the individual.

Scale:	Extreme Deviation From Expected Range	Substantial Deviation From Expected Range	Moderate Deviation From Expected Range	Mild Deviation From Expected Range	No Deviation From Expected Range
Indicators:					
Temperature	1	2	3	4	5
Apical pulse rate	1	2	3	4	5
Radial pulse rate	1	2	3	4	5
Respiration rate	1	2	3	4	5
Systolic blood pressure	1	2	3	4	5
Diastolic blood pressure	1	2	3	4	5
Other (specify)	1	2	3	4	5

Johnson, M., & Maas, M. (1997). Nursing outcomes classification (NOC). St. Louis: Mosby.

TABLE 12–2
Taxonomy of Nursing Outcomes Classification

	Domain 1	Domain 2	Domain 3	Domain 4	Domain 5	Domain 6
Level 1 Domains	**Function Health** Outcomes that describe capacity for and performance of basic tasks of life.	**Physiologic Health** Outcomes that describe organic functioning.	**Psychosocial Health** Outcomes that describe psychological and social functioning.	**Health Knowledge and Behavior** Outcomes that describe attitudes, comprehension, and actions with respect to health and illness.	**Perceived Health** Outcomes that describe impressions of an individual's health.	**Family Health** Outcomes that describe health status, behavior, and functioning of the family as a whole or of an individual as a family member.
Level 2 Classes	**Energy Maintenance** Outcomes that describe an individual's energy rejuvenation, conservation, and expenditure.	**Cardiopulmonary** Outcomes that describe an individual's cardiac, pulmonary, circulatory, or tissue perfusion status. **Elimination** Outcomes that describe an individual's waste excretion and elimination patterns and status.	**Psychological Well-Being** Outcomes that describe an individual's emotional health.	**Health Behavior** Outcomes that describe an individual's actions to promote, maintain, or restore health.	**Health and Life Quality** Outcomes that describe an individual's health status and expressed satisfaction with health and related life circumstances.	**Family Caregiver Status** Outcomes that describe the health and performance of a family member caring for a dependent child or adult.
	Growth and Development Outcomes that describe an individual's physical, emotional, and social maturation.	**Fluid and Electrolytes** Outcomes that describe an individual's fluid and electrolyte status.	**Psychosocial Adaptation** Outcomes that describe an individual's psychological and/or social adaptation to altered health or life circumstances.	**Health Beliefs** Outcomes that describe an individual's ideas and perceptions that influence health behavior.	**Symptom Status** Outcomes that describe an individual's ability to constrain objective and subjective states triggered by disease or illness.	**Maltreatment Resolution** Outcomes that describe an individual's physical, social, and emotional recovery from any type of neglect or abuse.

Mobility
Outcomes that describe an individual's physical mobility and the sequelae of restricted movement.

Self-Care
Outcomes that describe an individual's ability to accomplish basic and instrumental activities of daily living.

Immune Response
Outcomes that describe an individual's physiological reaction to substances that are foreign or interpreted by the body as foreign.

Metabolic Regulation
Outcomes that describe an individual's ability to regulate body metabolism.

Neurocognitive
Outcomes that describe an individual's neurological and cognitive status

Nutrition
Outcomes that describe an individual's nutritional status.

Tissue Integrity
Outcomes that describe the condition and function of an individual's body tissues.

Self-Control
Outcomes that describe an individual's ability to restrain behavior that may be emotionally or physically harmful to self or others.

Social Interaction
Outcomes that describe an individual's relationships with others.

Health Knowledge
Outcomes that describe an individual's understanding and skill in applying information to promote, maintain, and restore health.

Risk Control and Safety
Outcomes that describe an individual's safety status and/or actions to avoid, limit, or control identifiable health threats.

Iowa Outcomes Project. (1997). Taxonomy of nursing outcomes classification (NOC). Iowa City, IA: Author.

INTERVENTION

Intervention is the action phase of the nursing process, in which you provide the services to reach the goals of supporting and protecting your client (Fig. 12–4). Having recognized an actual or potential health problem, you intervene to change the client's level of physical, psychosocial, or spiritual functioning in the context of the family. An intervention may help the client make lifestyle changes, support physical function, support homeostasis, support psychosocial well-being, support the family unit, and make effective use of the health care delivery system to solve problems (Iowa Intervention Project, 1996). Effective intervention in each of the domains requires the use of nine skills.

Identifying nursing interventions involves selecting actions that enable the client to achieve outcomes and to resolve the related factors in nursing diagnoses. These actions are also called nursing orders, nursing activities, and nursing approaches. To be clearly communicated to the nursing team, the intervention should contain elements that clearly explain the action to be performed.

Skills of Intervention

The skills you will need to intervene are used in all of the domains of intervention. These skills involve being able to function in the areas of cognitive (thinking) processes, technical (psychomotor) activities, and interpersonal relationships.

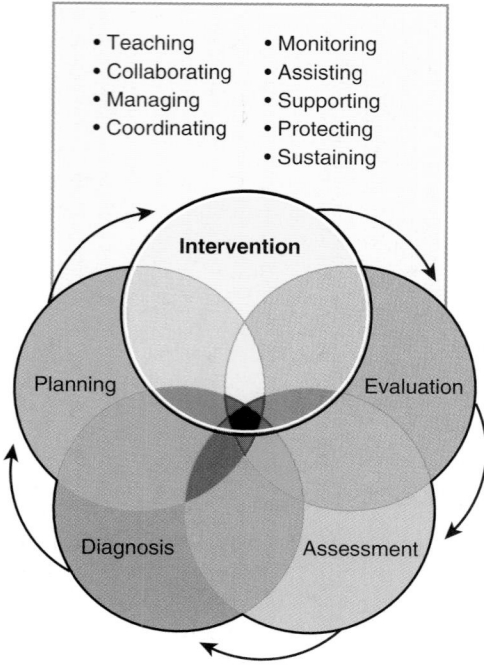

- Teaching
- Collaborating
- Managing
- Coordinating
- Monitoring
- Assisting
- Supporting
- Protecting
- Sustaining

Intervention

Planning

Evaluation

Diagnosis

Assessment

Figure 12–4. Intervention is the action phase of the nursing process. During the intervention phase, you provide the services identified during the planning process to support and protect your client. Intervention involves teaching, collaborating, managing, coordinating, monitoring, assisting, supporting, protecting, and sustaining.

Teaching

Highly developed teaching skills are one of a nurse's most important assets. Today's client expects to receive complete information and participate in the decision-making process. Accomplishing this goal helps everyone. For example, safety improves when the client has knowledge of the benefits and risks of care. Likewise, complications are fewer when the client knows how to manage a disorder or monitor a recovery period at home.

Collaborating

Sometimes you will intervene for your clients by collaborating with colleagues. Collaboration is the professional method of asking for and receiving assistance to ensure the best possible care for your client.

Managing

You can intervene for a client by managing care provided by others, and parts of your nursing care plan can be delegated to other health care workers. For example, a nursing assistant may intervene by bathing the client. Although the intervention is delegated, you are still accountable for the activity. You need to know that the intervention was completed; the nursing assistant needs to report any irregularities that arose during the intervention.

Coordinating

When multiple health team members are involved in the client's care, intervention involves coordination of the client's care. Commonly, a nurse takes charge of that coordination. Nurses have broad general knowledge of the roles and functions of the health care team and are in the best position to coordinate the various services that might be needed by the client.

Monitoring

Surveillance or monitoring is a primary nursing intervention, particularly in acute care settings. Monitoring the client's status and reporting changes to the physician is a major component of nursing. It ensures that the physician receives the information necessary to accomplish the client's health goals and to prevent complications. The purposes of monitoring are to detect complications, to evaluate the effectiveness of the interventions, and to ensure the interventions are carried out correctly.

Assisting

Interventions may involve assisting a client who is partially or fully unable to care for himself. The client may be disabled and need assistance to perform the basic activities of daily living, or he may lack the manual dexterity to perform medical treatments. You would provide assistance when the client needs help to take medications, seek health related services, or plan for the management of a health problem.

Supporting

Interventions may be primarily supportive when the client is able and has the knowledge but lacks willpower, resilience, or the motivation to care for himself. Supportive care makes the client feel able to face adverse circumstances, find inner strength, and believe in self-efficacy. To give supportive care you do not necessarily change your client's methods of self-care; rather, you strengthen the client to get his/her needs met.

Care is also classified as supportive when a client's physiological processes are marginally functional, and she needs care to maintain life functions. Physiological support involves implementing the physician's plan. You may give intravenous fluid or blood to maintain blood pressure or medications to strengthen the heart or control arrhythmias.

Protecting

Nurses play a major role in protecting clients from harm. The hospital (or other health care institution) environment should be the safest environment whether the person is critically ill, having surgery, learning to walk after a stroke, learning to cope with blindness, or needs protected living in old age. However, medical treatment always involves some degree of risk, which means that clients need constant surveillance and intervention to prevent harm. Among the many examples, you may act to prevent the complications of bed rest, adverse effects of medications, and injuries.

Sustaining

Nursing interventions sustain life and physical function when the client's condition is critical. The most obvious example is the implementation of cardiopulmonary resuscitation when the heartbeat or respiration has stopped. Critical care, recovery room, and emergency room nurses are involved in life-sustaining procedures.

Types of Interventions

Nursing interventions can be direct or indirect and may originate with a nurse, a physician, or another type of health care provider.

Direct Care Nursing Interventions

A **direct care intervention** "is a treatment performed through interaction with the client(s)" (Iowa Intervention Project, 1996, p. xvii). Direct care interventions include both physiological and psychosocial nursing actions designed to improve the client's health or modify the environment in a way that is conducive to health or that prevents disease.

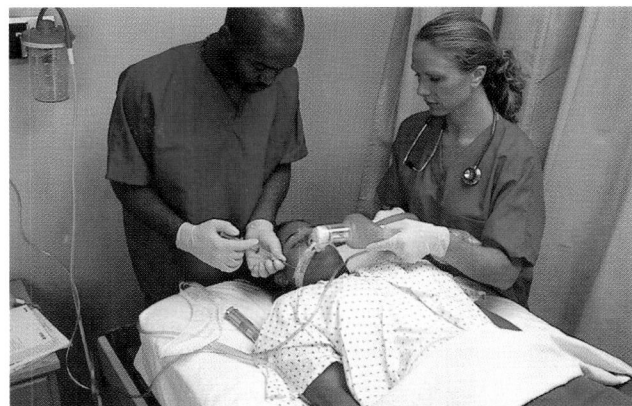

Figure 12–5. In today's health care environment, nurses must be prepared to accomplish highly technical direct care interventions. Remember, however, that a highly technical setting makes sensitive psychosocial interventions more important than ever.

Examples of physiological direct care nursing interventions include bowel training, cast care, cardiac precautions, constipation/impaction management, ambulation, eye care, and self-care assistance (toileting, for example). Examples of psychosocial direct care nursing interventions include counseling, emotional support, hope instillation, humor, and presence. Figure 12–5 shows a nurse performing a direct care intervention.

Indirect Care Nursing Interventions

Nursing includes many activities intended to maintain a safe environment and to coordinate the client's care. Even though these activities are not at the client's bedside and may not even be specific to an individual, they are necessary for client welfare. An **indirect care intervention** "is a treatment performed away from the [client] but on behalf of a [client] or group of [clients]. Indirect care interventions include nursing actions aimed at management of the [client] care environment and interdisciplinary collaboration" (Iowa Intervention Project, 1996, p. xvii). Examples of indirect care nursing interventions include delegation, emergency cart checking, shift report, and telephone consultation. Box 12–3 shows an example of an indirect care intervention needed for continuity of care in an acute care facility.

Nurse-Initiated and Physician-Initiated Nursing Interventions

Nurses provide two types of care for their clients. Independent care is within the scope of nursing practice and does not require a physician's order. Dependent care is within the scope of nursing practice but is carried out only as part of a physician's treatment plan. Both types of actions are correctly described as nursing care because these actions require a nurse's expertise to ensure the client's safety.

A **nurse-initiated intervention** is within the scope of nursing practice and is prescribed by the nurse in-

BOX 12–3

EXAMPLE OF AN INDIRECT CARE NURSING INTERVENTION

Shift Report

DEFINITION

Exchanging essential client care information with other nursing staff at change of shift.

ACTIVITIES

* Review pertinent demographic data, including name, age, and room number.
* Identify chief complaint and reason for admission, as appropriate.
* Summarize significant health history, as necessary.
* Identify key medical and nursing diagnoses, as appropriate.
* Identify resolved medical and nursing diagnoses, as appropriate.
* Present information succinctly, focusing on recent and significant data needed by nursing staff assuming responsibility for care.
* Describe treatment regimen, including diet, fluid therapy, medications, and exercise.
* Identify laboratory and diagnostic tests to be completed during the next 24 hours.
* Describe health status data, including vital signs and signs and symptoms present during the shift.
* Describe nursing interventions being implemented.
* Describe client and family responses to nursing interventions.
* Summarize progress toward goals.
* Summarize discharge plans, as appropriate.

Iowa Intervention Project. (1996). Nursing interventions classification (NIC). St. Louis: Mosby-Year Book.

BOX 12–4

EXAMPLE OF A NURSE-INITIATED NURSING INTERVENTION

Dressing

DEFINITION

Choosing, putting on, and removing clothes for a person who cannot do so independently.

ACTIVITIES

* Identify areas where client needs assistance in dressing.
* Monitor client's ability to dress independently.
* Dress client after personal hygiene completed.
* Encourage participation in selection of clothing.
* Dress affected extremity first, as appropriate.
* Dress in nonrestrictive clothing, as appropriate.
* Dress in personal clothing, as appropriate.
* Change client's clothing at bedtime.
* Select shoes or slippers conducive to ambulation.
* Offer to launder clothing, as necessary.
* Continue giving assistance until the client can assume full responsibility for dressing.

Iowa Intervention Project. (1996). Nursing interventions classification (NIC). St. Louis: Mosby-Year Book.

dependent of the physician. It is "an intervention initiated by the nurse in response to a nursing diagnosis; an autonomous action based on scientific rationale that is executed to benefit the client in a predicted way related to the nursing diagnosis and projected outcome" (Iowa Intervention Project, 1996, p. xvii). Helping the client to dress is an example of a nurse-initiated intervention (Box 12–4).

A **physician-initiated intervention** is within the scope of nursing practice but requires a physician's order for the nurse to implement. A "physician-initiated treatment is an intervention initiated by a physician in response to a medical diagnosis but carried out by a nurse in response to a 'doctor's order.' Nurses may also carry out treatments initiated by other providers,

such as pharmacists, respiratory therapists, or physician assistants" (Iowa Intervention Project, 1996, p. xvii). An example of a physician-initiated intervention is management of the client's diet when the client is recovering from an illness that has caused a medical need for dietary limitations (Box 12–5).

Nursing Intervention Classification System

The words that describe nursing interventions are as much a part of the language of nursing as are nursing diagnoses. For nurses to communicate with each other and to describe nursing to the health care team, the language of nursing needs to have a common meaning among nurses.

A standardized language is useful to assist nurses in documenting care. Rather than writing a sentence or two to describe care, the nurse can use a few words to describe an array of activities on the client's behalf.

A standardized language provides a common language for communication. The communication could be for care-plan development, research, staff education, or curriculum development. The nursing intervention classification (NIC) system, developed at the University of Iowa, is a standardized language appropriate for computerized client information systems to describe the component of client care that is nursing practice.

BOX 12–5

EXAMPLE OF A PHYSICIAN-INITIATED NURSING INTERVENTION

Diet Staging

DEFINITION

Instituting required diet restrictions with subsequent progression of diet as tolerated.

ACTIVITIES

- Determine presence of bowel sounds.
- Institute NPO status, as needed.
- Clamp nasogastric tube and monitor tolerance, as appropriate.
- Monitor for alertness and presence of gag reflex, as appropriate.
- Monitor tolerance to ingestion of ice chips and water.
- Determine if client is passing flatus.
- Collaborate with other health care team members to progress diet as rapidly as possible without complications.
- For adults and children, progress the diet from clear liquid to full liquid to soft diet to regular or special diet, as tolerated.
- For babies, progress the diet from glucose water or oral electrolyte solution to half-strength formula and then to full-strength formula.
- Monitor tolerance to diet progression.
- Offer six small feedings rather than three meals, as appropriate.
- Post the diet restrictions at bedside, on chart, and in care plan.

Iowa Intervention Project. (1996). Nursing interventions classification (NIC). St. Louis: Mosby-Year Book.

Most of the NIC interventions are appropriate for use in any health care setting or specialty area. Common core interventions across specialties are active listening, emotional support, infection control, vital signs monitoring, infection protection, and medication management (Bulechek, McCloskey, Denehy, & Titler, 1994).

By classifying nursing interventions into broad categories, the NIC taxonomy describes the scope of nursing practice. The classification of nursing interventions includes domains, classes, interventions, and nursing activities. The domains include classes or groups of related nursing interventions. Each domain and class has a definition to help you select specific, appropriate nursing interventions for a nursing diagnosis (Table 12–3).

Although the NIC taxonomy is useful for describing the nursing management of a client, it does not

prescribe interventions for particular nursing diagnoses. The nurse makes a judgment about which interventions will most effectively manage a diagnosis. Sometimes several interventions may be required to plan care for a nursing diagnosis.

Elements of an Intervention

Planning involves making decisions about the *who, what, where, when, why,* and *how* of client care. *Who* refers to the person providing care. The best person to provide care may be a physical therapist, a nurse, a nursing assistant, a family member, the client, and so on. *What* refers to the care that will most effectively meet the client's needs. *Where* could be the client's home, a clinic, or a hospital. *When* refers to the time that the care is delivered or to the sequence of events required. The time may be before the client is admitted to a hospital, during a hospital stay, after discharge, during a clinic or office visit, or at a particular time of day. *Why* provides the rationale for care and includes evidence that the care is important, will work, or will meet individual client needs. *How* defines the methods of intervention required and may specify measures needed to individualize a client's care.

THE NURSING CARE PLAN

The nursing care plan consists of three components: client problems (nursing diagnoses), expected outcomes, and interventions. The list of client problems may be a common list with input from the entire health care team, or it may list only problems identified by nurses. The use of a common list facilitates a multidisciplinary team approach. The advantage of a separate list is that it clearly identifies the contribution of nursing to client care.

The problem list may identify nursing diagnoses using the North American Nursing Diagnosis Association (NANDA) taxonomy, or it may adopt another system for naming problems treated by nurses. NANDA diagnoses are more likely to appear when nursing writes a separate list; however, some agencies use NANDA language even in a common problem list.

Outcomes statements may be developed by the nurse who writes the care plan, or the nurse might use NOC language to identify outcomes on the care plan. The language for interventions can be taken from the NIC system, the Omaha system, or the Home Healthcare Classification system (Iowa Intervention Project, 1996; Martin & Scheet, 1992; and Saba et al., 1991). Interventions should be written specifically enough that care can be administered consistently by all nurses assigned to the client's care over a period of time.

Guidelines for Developing Care Plans

The plan of care establishes priorities and guides the efforts of the client, the nurses, and other members of the health care team. As these decisions are made, the care plan is written to provide documentation for all

TABLE 12–3

Nursing Intervention Classification Taxonomy of Nursing Interventions

Level 1 Domains	Domain 1	Domain 2	Domain 3	Domain 4	Domain 5	Domain 6
	1. Physiological: Basic Care that supports physical functioning.	**2. Physiological Complex** Care that supports homeostatic regulation.	**3. Behavioral** Care that supports psychosocial functioning and facilitates life-style changes.	**4. Safety** Care that supports protection against harm.	**5. Family** Care that supports the family unit.	**6. Health System** Care that supports effective use of the health care delivery system.
	A. Activity and Exercise Management: Interventions to organize or assist with physical activity and energy conservation and expenditure.	G. Electrolyte and Acid-Base Management: Interventions to regulate electrolyte/acid-base balance and prevent complications	O. Behavior Therapy: Interventions to reinforce or promote desirable behaviors or alter undesirable behaviors.	U. Crisis Management: Interventions to provide immediate short-term help in both psychological and physiological crises	W. Childbearing Care: Interventions to assist in understanding and coping with the psychological and physiological changes during the childbearing period.	Y. Health System Mediation: Interventions to facilitate the interface between client/family and the health care system
	B. Elimination Management: Interventions to establish and maintain regular bowel and urinary elimination patterns and manage complications due to altered patterns.	H. Drug Management: Interventions to facilitate desired effects of pharmacological agents.	P. Cognitive Therapy: Interventions to reinforce or promote desirable cognitive functioning or alter undesirable cognitive functioning.	V. Risk Management: Interventions to initiate risk-reduction activities and continue monitoring risks over time.	X. Life-Span Care: Interventions to facilitate family unit functioning and promote the health and welfare of family members throughout the life span	a. Health System Management: Interventions to provide and enhance support services for the delivery of care.
	C. Immobility Management: Interventions to manage restricted body movement and the sequelae.	I. Neurologic Management: Interventions to optimize neurological functions.	Q. Communication Enhancement: Interventions to facilitate delivering and receiving verbal and nonverbal messages.			b. Information Management: Interventions to facilitate communication among health care providers.

D. Nutrition Support: Interventions to modify or maintain nutritional status.

E. Physical Comfort Promotion: Interventions to promote comfort using physical techniques.

F. Self-Care Facilitation: Interventions to provide or assist with routine activities of daily living.

J. Perioperative Care: Interventions to provide care before, during, and immediately after surgery.

K. Respiratory Management: Interventions to promote airway patency and gas exchange.

L. Skin/Wound Management: Interventions to maintain or restore tissue integrity.

M. Thermoregulation: Interventions to maintain body temperature within a normal range

N. Tissue Perfusion Management: Interventions to optimize circulation of blood and fluids to the tissue.

R. Coping Assistance: Interventions to assist another to build on own strengths, to adapt to a change in function, or to achieve a higher level of function.

S. Client Education: Interventions to facilitate learning.

T. Psychological Comfort Promotion: Interventions to promote comfort using psychological techniques.

Iowa Intervention Project. (1996). Nursing interventions classification (NIC). St. Louis: Mosby-Year Book.

health care personnel who will be caring for the client.

The traditional nursing care plan is formatted in three columns, with additional columns for the date and signature of the person who developed the plan and for the dates when outcomes are achieved. When the problem is resolved, it is documented on the nursing care plan. Evaluation data are charted in nursing progress notes or, in student care plans, they may be written in a fourth column.

Purposes of a Written Care Plan

The written care plan has evolved as a tool for providing current information for client care. The purpose of a nursing care plan is to communicate the planned care to the health care team, thus ensuring continuity of care. A written plan should be concise to communicate information efficiently. On the other hand, it should provide enough information that everyone providing the care will provide the same care. The purposes of a care plan can also include the following:

- Identify all problems being treated
- Provide a detailed guide for nursing care
- Individualize the care provided
- Set priorities
- Coordinate care among all health care workers

- Guide evaluation of care
- Provide for individual and family participation in planning
- Document current nursing practice

Types of Care Plans

There are different types of care plans in practice today, with their own sets of advantages and disadvantages. These types of care plans have varying degrees of individualization and standardization.

Individualized Care Plans

An individualized care plan is one written specifically for each client who enters a health care facility. This type of care plan is developed from the admission history, physical and functional assessment, and problems anticipated based on the physician's treatment plan.

Individualized care plans allow you to identify the unique problems of each client, to decide on the outcomes to be achieved, and to identify which nursing interventions will be appropriate to achieve those outcomes. These plans contain only the applicable nursing diagnoses, outcomes, and interventions. The dis-

---

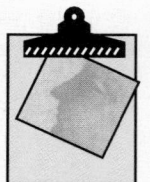

NURSING CARE PLANNING
SAMPLE INDIVIDUALIZED NURSING CARE PLAN

Nursing Diagnosis	Expected Outcomes	Interventions	Evaluation (After 24 Hours of Care)
Constipation related to decreased oral intake, decreased activity, use of constipating medications.	Has daily bowel movement with stool soft and formed. Reports no difficulty passing stool.	Activities: Monitor bowel movements including frequency, consistency, shape, volume, and color, as appropriate.	Client reported that he had a hard-formed stool this morning after breakfast and wanted to increase prunes in diet. Will continue plan.
		Identify factors (e.g., medications, bed rest, diet) that may cause or contribute to constipation.	Has been on bed rest for 3 days. Increased activity by walking in hall three times in last 24 hours. Client participated in developing plan.
		Encourage increased fluid intake.	Fluid intake 1500 mL last 24 hours.
		Instruct client/family on appropriate use of laxatives.	Not interested in trying laxatives. Requested and ate prunes.

advantage of individualized care plans is the time required to write them.

Standardized Care Plans

Standardized care plans typically are written by a group of nurses who use their collective expertise to produce a plan to direct nursing care for clients with specific medical diagnoses (such as myocardial infarction) or nursing diagnoses (such as pain or anxiety). They also are developed for clients undergoing special procedures (such as cardiac catheterization).

These care plans are duplicated and made available to the appropriate units in the health care facility. The format is designed with extra space so you can individualize the plan by filling in specific client characteristics, related factors associated with the nursing diagnosis, deadlines for the outcomes, and additional details in the interventions. For example, you can individualize interventions by adding frequencies, amounts, times, and client preferences.

Standardized care plans have the advantage of saving you time by reducing the amount of writing required. They also are particularly helpful to nurses working in unfamiliar areas. The main disadvantage of standardized care plans is the lack of individualization. Not all of the nursing diagnoses, outcomes, and interventions listed on the standardized care plan will pertain to every client. Using a standardized care plan requires you to critically analyze its applicability to an individual.

Computerized Care Plans

A **computerized care plan** is a standardized care plan or a care plan created by a computer program. Many software vendors have developed computerized care plans. They are usually written by expert clinicians.

A computerized care plan has nursing diagnoses, client outcomes, and nursing interventions, and it also allows for the relevant dates to be inserted. You choose the appropriate nursing diagnoses, outcomes, and interventions for the individual client.

Advantages of computerized care plans include their legibility and the ease with which they can be changed or updated. They also allow nurse researchers to collect data about groups of clients. The disadvantage of computerized care plans is the same as for standardized care plans—namely, their lack of individualization. However, computerized care plans can be simpler to individualize than standardized forms.

The Institute of Medicine's report (1991) on computer-based client records identified that the prerequisite for computerized client records is standardized health care vocabularies. The NANDA system, NIC system, NOC system, Omaha system, and Home Healthcare Classification system are the most widely recognized standardized languages for nursing (NANDA, 1996; Iowa Intervention Project, 1996; Iowa Outcomes Project, 1997; Martin & Scheet, 1992; and Saba et al., 1991).

The basic goal of the medical informatics community is the development of information systems that will facilitate useful retrieval of biomedical information. Ideally, nursing would have a unified, single language system that could be used throughout the country. All nurses could communicate the function of nursing in a unique language. Nursing information could be retrieved from large, distributed information spaces, and nursing would be able to articulate with classifications from other disciplines.

Case Management Plans

Case management is a model of nursing practice that gives one person the responsibility for overseeing the client's care over the course of an illness. The case manager ensures that the client's care is well coordinated, with no gaps or overlaps in service.

Case management may describe many different things in different health care settings. It may be a group of activities nurses perform in one setting, a client care delivery system, a professional practice model, or a separate service set up by independent practitioners or insurance companies. Case management is used across the health care continuum from home health to long-term care to hospitals.

Indeed, case management models exist on a continuum from working with an individual client to managing a system of service delivery. At the client end, a hospital case manager may be responsible for client care from preadmission to post-discharge. In another model, the case manager may focus on services provided to groups of clients and planning for a system that controls costs and reduces the length of hospital stay. At the extreme business end of the spectrum is outcome management. An outcome manager's function is similar to that of a case manager but is more focused on researching and analyzing cost-effective ways to produce desired outcomes among large groups of clients.

Nursing case management was introduced in the acute care setting in 1985 to respond to the prepaid health movement, which seeks to ensure quality care in a health care system focused on cost control. In most settings, case management is still performed by nurses. The ANA defines case management as "a system with many elements: health assessment, planning, procurement, delivery and coordination of services, and monitoring to assure that the multiple service needs of the client are met" (ANA, 1988).

Nurses who are case managers use the nursing process and nursing terminology to develop plans of care for clients. These plans of care include the activities of other professionals and provide care for the client in multiple settings over a period of time (Goodwin, 1994). For example, a client with chronic obstructive pulmonary disease may have home health services and be admitted for an acute exacerbation of the disease. He may then be discharged to long-term care before being able to go home. The nurse case manager would plan this entire span of services.

Text continued on page 261

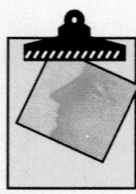

NURSING CARE PLANNING
SAMPLE NURSING CARE PLAN USING STANDARDIZED LANGUAGE

Mrs. Worden tripped over her space heater at home and fell. She burned her left anterior thigh on the space heater and fractured her right hip. Her frail elderly husband called the emergency number (911), and an ambulance responded. Mrs. Worden was admitted to the local hospital, where she underwent an open reduction and internal fixation to repair the fractured right hip. Treatment was also started for the second-degree burn on her left hip. After 4 days on the inpatient surgical unit, she was ready for discharge but not independent enough in mobility or activities of daily living to return home. She was discharged to a skilled unit in a local nursing home.

Admission data included the following:

- White female, age 84. Height 5 ft. 3 in. Weight 128 pounds.
- BP 148/72, T 97.6, RP 68 and regular, R 18.
- Wound anterior thigh measured 4 cm × 3 cm with a depth of 0.5 cm.
- Incision right hip measured 9 cm in length with 13 sutures intact. Skin was pink with no signs of infection. Skin edges approximated.
- Range of motion all extremities within normal limits except right hip abduction was only 20 degrees and right knee flexion was only 45 degrees. Pain noted on movement of right leg during range of motion.
- Ambulated 4 yards with pain and fatigue.
- Is continent of bladder and bowel.
- Oral intake has been a regular diet with intake of 75 to 100% at each meal.
- Last known bowel movement was 2 days prior with a usual routine of daily defecation.
- Oriented to time, person, and place.
- Very upset that she could not go home for physical and occupational therapy rather than going to the nursing home.

The following is an individualized care plan for Mrs. Worden using the NANDA, NIC, and NOC standardized languages. Notice that less documentation is needed because the standardized language has a common meaning for all users of the plan.

Nursing Diagnoses (Prioritized)

Nursing Diagnosis: Pain related to injuring agent (burn on left hip) as manifested by verbal report of pain rated at 3 on scale of 0 to 10 during dressing changes.
Outcome: Pain level.
Nursing Interventions: Analgesic administration, Pain management.

Nursing Diagnosis: Constipation related to decreased mobility as manifested by hard formed stool, straining at stool, and report of no defecation in last 2 days.
Outcome: Bowel elimination.
Nursing Interventions: Constipation/impaction management, Exercise therapy: ambulation.

Nursing Diagnosis: Impaired physical mobility, level 3, related to decreased strength and endurance and pain on movement as manifested by inability to ambulate independently.
Outcome: Ambulation: walking.
Nursing Interventions: Exercise therapy: ambulation, Exercise therapy: Joint mobility.

Nursing Diagnosis: Impaired skin integrity related to mechanical factor of falling on electric heater as manifested by wound anterior thigh measuring 4 cm × 3 cm with depth of 0.5 cm.
Outcome: Wound healing: primary intention.
Nursing Interventions: Wound care.

Nursing Diagnosis: Impaired skin integrity related to surgical procedure right hip as manifested by incision right hip measuring 9 cm.
Outcome: Wound healing: primary intention.
Nursing Interventions: Incision site care.

VALLEY BAPTIST MEDICAL CENTER
Harlingen, Texas

ADMISSION ORDERS - PNEUMONIA

1. ☐ Admit to medical floor.　　　☐ Other _____

2. ☐ Admit to the service of Dr. _____

3. Diagnosis _____

_____

4. ☐ Initiate Pneumonia Restorative Care Path.

5. LAB:　☐ ER Profile (CBC w/diff, Chem 14)
　　　　　☐ Blood cultures X 2, 15 minutes apart - separate sticks
　　　　　☐ Aminophylline Level, if patient taking.
　　　　　☐ Sputum C&S / Induction p.r.n. by RT.
　　　　　☐ UA
　　　　　☐ If SpO_2 <92%, collect ABG
　　　　　☐ _____

6. ☐ Chest X-ray

7. ☐ O_2 at _____ LPM via _____　　　☐ Follow O_2 Protocol

8. ☐ Respiratory Treatment: _____

　　☐ Bronchodilator Protocol　　　☐ Suction p.r.n.

9. ☐ Diet: _____

10. ☐ IV: _____

11. ☐ Antibiotic Therapy: _____

_____

　　☐ Initial Dose NOW

12. ☐ Acetaminophen gr X, 1 suppository or 650 mg P.O. for Temp >100.6F° q 4 hrs p.r.n.

13. ☐ Old charts to the floor.

14. ☐ Vital signs q 4 hours until stable, then routine.

15. Activity: ☐ Ambulate at least BID　☐ Bathroom with assistance　☐ Bed rest

16. ☐ Social Service to evaluate.

17. _____

_____

Date _____ Time _____　　_____ M.D.
　　　　　　　　　　　　　　　　　　　　　　　　　　Physician Signature

VBMC 1965-129-0396

A

Figure 12–6. An example of a clinical pathway for a client with pneumonia. A, admission orders. (Courtesy of Valley Baptist Medical Center, Harlingen, TX.)

Illustration continued on following page

VALLEY BAPTIST MEDICAL CENTER
Harlingen, Texas

RESTORATIVE CARE PATH
PNEUMONIA > 17 Years of Age

KEY: Initials=Completed; N/A = Not Applicable; 0 - Variance

Page 1 of 2   VBMC 1620-005-0196

DRG: 79 and 89   Special Considerations:

	Day 1 / Date: RN Review	Day 2 / Date: RN Review	Day 3 / Date: RN Review	Signature/Status	Initial	Day 4 / Date: RN Review	Day 5 / Date: RN Review	Signature/Status	Initial	EXPECTED OUTCOMES
Consults	Call Internal Medicine or primary MD to admit	If not improved 48 hrs after admission, consider pulmonary consult	------> All consults notified			------>	------>			All consults notified
Tests	ER Profile; Blood Culture X 2 (separate sticks) 15 min. apart; Aminophylline Level (if taking); UA; Sputum C&S / Induction p.r.n. by RT; CXR; If O$_2$Sat <92, collect ABG	Call MD for abnormal labs; ABGs p.r.n.; Swab for MRSA for nursing home patients or transfers; If sputum not collected, in 4 hrs, notify MD	Call MD for abnormal labs; In 48 hrs, if no clinical improvement, consider CBC, CXR, alternate means of sputum collection			------>	------>			All labs WNL or stable for patient.
Assessment & Evaluation	Initiate Database; Vital signs q 1 hr or as indicated; F/C if unable to void; I&O; Assess for TB risk factors	Vital signs q 4 hrs; Check voiding	------>			If pt afebrile X 24 hrs, consider disch; ------>	------>			Pt afebrile, consider disch; Voiding adequate; I&O WNL
Activity / Safety	Bed rest with BRP	------> Activity as tolerated	------>			------>	------>			Return to previous activity level
Treatments	O$_2$ _____ L/min (NC / Mask / Trach); Resp. Tx.; O$_2$ Sat Monitor; Suction p.r.n.	O$_2$ protocol	------>			------>	------>			Respiratory status stable
Diet	Assess nutritional status; Dietitian? ☐ Yes ☐ No	Diet _____	Diet _____			Diet _____	Diet _____			Patient tolerates prescribed diet

Case Manager

B(1)

Figure 12–6 *Continued.* B, restorative care path. (Courtesy of Valley Baptist Medical Center, Harlingen, TX.)

VALLEY BAPTIST MEDICAL CENTER
Harlingen, Texas
RESTORATIVE CARE PATH
PNEUMONIA > 17 Years of Age

VBMC 1620-005-0196

Page 2 of 2

	Date: ☐ ER ☐ PATT ☐ Direct Adm Day 1: RN Review	Date: Day 2: RN Review	Date: Day 3: RN Review	Date: Day 4: RN Review	Date: Day 5: RN Review	EXPECTED OUTCOMES
Meds / IV Fluids	___ Start IV ___ Start Antibiotic Protocol ___ @ ___ hr ___ Continue IV antibiotics ___ List Home meds ___ ER Fever Protocol ___ Adjust antibiotics per culture results.	___ Reevaluate antibiotic therapy if no clinical improvement ---->	___ Consider Saline lock ___ Consider P.O. antibiotics ---->	----> ---->	----> ---->	D.C. with P.O. antibiotics
Pain Management	___ Medicate as ordered; document effect.	---->	---->	---->	---->	Prescription for pain meds as needed.
Patient/Family Education	___ Explain procedures, meds & equipment. ___ Provide educational materials ___ Reinforce teaching ___ Provide opportunity for questions. ___ Return demo & document progress ___ Provide patient pathway	----> ---->	----> ---->	----> ---->	----> ---->	Pt/family verbalize understanding of D/C instructions, follow-up appointment/classes.
Psychosocial	___ Allow verbalization of feelings ___ Consider referral to Pastoral Services.	----> ---->	----> ---->	----> ---->	No anxiety ---->	No anxiety noted
Discharge Planning / Continuum of Care	___ Obtain old chart & send to floor with patient. ___ Social Service Consult ___ Discharge Planning Assessment ___ Discharge home ___ Admit (consider STO)	---->	---->	___ Consider discharge	---->	Discharge: ☐ Home ☐ NHP ☐ Home Health ☐ Transfer ☐ Rehab ☐ Other ☐ Records faxed ☐ Report called ☐ D.C. instructions given.
Signatures 7 - 3						
Signatures 3 - 11						
Signatures 11 - 7						

B(2)

Figure 12–6 *Continued.* See legend on opposite page

Illustration continued on following page

	EMERGENCY ROOM	DAY 1	DAY 2	DAY 3	DAY 4	DAY 5
Activity		• You will be on bed rest. • Your nurse will raise the head of your bed to help you breathe easier.	• Activity will be encouraged, however, **PLEASE ASK** for assistance to prevent a fall or injury.	• Your activity level will be increased daily. • If you need assistance, please use the call bell.	• Your activity level will be increased daily. • If you need assistance, please use the call bell.	• Your activity level will be increased daily. • Use the call bell if needed.	• Your activity level will be increased daily.
Treatments		• Nurses or Respiratory Therapist (RT) may start oxygen. • RT will check the oxygen level by either a blood test or monitor. • You will be expected to try to produce some sputum for lab testing. • If you are unable to produce sputum, RT may be asked to help you.	• Your nurse will be checking blood pressure, heart rate, temperature and respirations. • Your nurse may measure your fluid intake and urine output. • RT will continue to check your oxygen level.	• Nurses will continue to check blood pressure, heart rate, temperature and respirations. • RT will continue to check your oxygen level.	• Nurses will continue to check blood pressure, heart rate, temperature and respirations. • Oxygen checks continued. You will be slowly taken off oxygen. • Continued monitoring of intake & output.	• Nurses will continue checking blood pressure, heart rate, temperature and respirations. • You will be slowly taken off oxygen.	• Nurses will continue to check blood pressure, heart rate, temperature and respirations.
Tests		• Your doctor may order urinalysis, blood tests, chest x-rays and respiratory treatments. • Your family doctor may be called to admit you. If you do not have a doctor, one will be provided for you.	• If you were unable to cough up any sputum, you will be asked to try again. • If you were unable to urinate, a tube called a foley catheter may be inserted into your bladder.	• You may have more blood tests, another chest x-ray, and possible re-collection of sputum.			
Medications		• Your nurse will start an IV in a vein to administer antibiotics. • The doctor may order medication for pain or fever. • If you have a list of your home medications, please give it to your nurse.	• Your nurse will continue to monitor your IV on a regular basis. • You may be started on some of your own home medications given by the nurses.	• The nurse will continue monitoring your IV or you may begin taking antibiotics by mouth.			
Teaching		• Your doctor or nurse will explain procedures, medications and equipment. • You will be given an opportunity to ask questions. • Instructions will be reviewed with you and your family.					
Diet			• A dietitian may be asked to visit with you about your eating habits.			
Discharge Planning		• You should expect to stay in the Emergency Room for a limited period of time, then be taken to a room in the hospital.	• A social worker and/or case manager will meet with you to discuss any discharge needs.	• Social services will continue to provide referrals and/or arrangements as needed.	• Social Services continues referrals/arrangements. • If your condition has improved sufficiently, you may be discharged.	• Discharge plans/referrals completed. • If improved sufficiently, you may be discharged.	• Referrals and all arrangements completed. • Discharged to home.

C

Figure 12–6 *Continued.* C, patient pathway. (Courtesy of Valley Baptist Medical Center, Harlingen, TX.)

Clinical Pathways

A **clinical pathway** is a standardized multidisciplinary care plan that projects the expected course of the client's treatment and progress over the hospital stay. It is a method for describing the plan of care by predicting the course of the client's hospital stay and prescribing the care and outcomes on a day-by-day basis. Clinical pathways are guidelines for health professionals in hospitals, home care, and long-term care.

You may hear clinical pathways called care maps, clinical paths, critical paths, critical pathways, collaborative care plans, and multidisciplinary care plans. All have the commonality of containing all the critical elements of the client's care. No matter which name is applied to it, a clinical pathway is a "written plan that functions as a map and timetable for efficient and precise delivery of health care" (Vantassel, 1990, p. 5). This type of plan is seen by many as a way to maintain quality care and coordinate services while controlling costs.

Most clinical pathways are written on a grid that lists the client's problems, outcomes, and interventions by multidisciplinary staff along a specified time line. Figure 12–6 shows an example of a clinical pathway. Usually, the facility's pathway is developed by a group of multidisciplinary clinicians who care for clients with specific illnesses. In fact, the pathway's primary value lies in its multidisciplinary approach. Ideally, the clinical pathway should include each discipline's standardized language.

Clinical pathways are available for procedures, conditions, illnesses, and diagnosis-related groups. Time lines can range from a few hours or days to a period covering weeks or months, depending on the condition or procedure for which the pathway was developed. For example, a clinical pathway for a client having a sigmoidoscopy would cover just a few hours. A clinical pathway for a client having a total hip replacement may include a 3- to 4-day acute care phase after surgery, followed by another 4 days of skilled nursing care before discharge.

KEY PRINCIPLES

- The planning phase of the nursing process is used to set priorities, develop outcomes, designate deadlines, and identify nursing interventions.
- Planning for individuals is initiated with entry to the health care system, continues throughout the length of service, and ensures ongoing care through discharge planning.
- Planning for individuals is a team effort through collaboration, consultation, and care plan conferences.
- Planning for groups of clients with a common set of needs involves designing services for the population being served, determining the level of staffing, and designing the environment of care.
- The planning process involves setting priorities based on the client's physical needs, the services expected in the setting, the client's perception of need, and the client's ability to provide self-care.
- Predicting the outcomes of nursing care implies that nursing can be held responsible for nursing-sensitive outcomes, not just for the provision of nursing care.
- The Nursing Outcome Classification system is a standardized method of stating nursing-sensitive outcomes.
- The skills required for successful intervention are cognitive, technical, interpersonal, and ethical/legal.
- Implementation always includes reassessment and the continuation of the planning phase.
- Intervention is not complete until the care is documented.
- Nurse-initiated and physician-initiated interventions treat the related factors to resolve the signs and symptoms that define the nursing diagnosis.
- The Nursing Intervention Classification system is a standardized method of identifying nursing interventions.
- A nursing care plan is a guide to client care that coordinates the actions of the nursing team and improves continuity of care over the course of an illness.
- A nursing care plan includes nursing diagnoses, expected outcomes, and interventions.
- The type of nursing care plan is less important than the goal of providing comprehensive care designed to meet the needs of the individual client.

BIBLIOGRAPHY

Adams, C.E., & Wilson, M. (1995). Enhanced quality through outcome-focused standardized care plans. *Journal of Nursing Administration, 25*(9), 27–34.
*American Nurses' Association. (1988). *Nursing Case Management.* Publication No. NS-32. Kansas City, MO.
American Nurses' Association. (1995). *Nursing's Social Policy Statement.* Washington, D.C.: American Nurses Publishing.
Becker H., Payne, D., Adams, M.L., & Grobe, S. (1996). Evaluating outcomes of services. *Nurse Practice, 21*(11), 153–155.
Beyea, S.C., & Nicoll, L.H. (1998). Developing clinical practice guidelines as an approach to evidence-based practice. *AORN Journal, 67*(5), 1037–1038.
Bulechek, G.M., McCloskey, J.C., Denehy, J.A., & Titler, M. (1994). Report on the NIC project: Nursing interventions used in practice. *American Journal of Nursing, 94*(10), 59–66.
Carroll, D., & Seers, K. (1998). Relaxation for the relief of chronic pain: A systematic review. *Journal of Advanced Nursing, 27*(3), 476–487.
Castle, N.G., & Mor, V. (1998). Physical restraints in nursing homes: A review of the literature since the Nursing Home Reform Act of 1987. *Medicare Residents Review, 55*(2), 139–170.
Cimino, J.J., & Clayton, P.D. (1994). Coping with changing controlled vocabularies. *Proceedings Eighteenth Annual Symposium on Computer Applications in Medical Care.* Philadelphia: Hanley & Belfus, Inc.

*Asterisk indicates a classic or definitive work on this subject.

*Daly, J.M. (1993). *NIC Interventions Linked to NANDA Diagnoses,* Iowa City, IA: Iowa Intervention Project.

Daly, J.M., Maas, M., & Buckwalter, K. (1995). What nursing diagnoses do nurses use in long term care? *The Director, 3*(3), 115, 118–120, 123.

Daly, J.M., Maas, M.L., & Johnson, M. (1997). Nursing Outcomes Classification: An essential element in data sets for nursing and health care effectiveness. *Computer Nursing, 15*(2), S82–S86.

Daly, J.M., Maas, M., McCloskey, J.C., & Bulechek, G. (1996). A care planning tool that proves what we do. *RN, 59*(6), 26–29.

Denehy, J. (1998). Integrating Nursing Outcomes Classification in nursing education. *Journal Nursing Care Quality, 12*(5), 73–84.

*Department of Health and Human Services. (1991). Medicare and Medicaid: Requirements for long term care facilities and nurse aide training and competency evaluation programs, final rules. *Federal Register, September 26,* 48826–48922.

Gibbs, B., Lonowski, L., Meyer, P.J., & Newlin, P.J. (1995). The role of the clinical nurse specialist and the nurse manager in case management. *Journal of Nursing Administration, 25*(5), 28–34.

Goodwin, D.R. (1994). Nursing case management activities. *Journal of Nursing Administration, 24*(2), 29–34.

Grobe, S.J. (1995). Informatics: The infrastructure for quality assessment and quality improvement. *Journal of the American Medical Informatics Association, 2*(4), 267–268.

Grobe, S.J. (1996). The nursing intervention lexicon and taxonomy: Implications for representing nursing care data in automated patient records. *Holistic Nursing Practice, 11*(1), 48–63.

*Hildman, T.B., & Ferguson, G.H. (1992). Registered nurses' attitudes toward the nursing process and written/printed nursing care plans. *Journal of Nursing Administration, 22*(5), 5.

*Institute of Medicine. (1991). *The computer-based patient record: An essential technology for health care.* Washington, D.C.: National Academy Press.

Iowa Intervention Project. (1996). *Nursing interventions classification (NIC).* St. Louis: Mosby-Year Book.

Iowa Outcomes Project. (1997). *Nursing Outcomes Classification (NOC).* St. Louis: Mosby-Year Book.

*Johnson, P.A., Stone, M.A., Larson, A.M., & Hromek, C.A. (1992). Applying nursing diagnosis and nursing process to activities of daily living and mobility. *Geriatric Nursing 13*(1), 25–27.

Johnson, S.J., Brady-Schluttner, K., Ellenbecker, S., Johnson, M., Lassegard, E., Maas, M., Stone, J.L., & Westra, B.L. (1996). Evaluating physical functional outcomes: One category of the NOC system. *Medsurg Nursing, 5*(3), 157–162.

Maas, M.L. (1997). Advancing nurse's accountability for outcomes. *Outcomes Management Nursing Practice, 1*(1), 3–4.

Maas, M.L., Specht, J.P., Weiler, K., Buckwalter, K.C., & Turner, B. (1998). Special care units for people with Alzheimer's disease: Only for the privileged few? *Journal of Gerontology Nursing, 24*(3),28–37.

Martin, K.S., & Norris, J. (1996). The Omaha System: A model for describing practice. *Holistic Nursing Practice, 11*(1), 75–83.

*Martin, K.S., & Scheet, N.J. (1992). *The Omaha System: Applications for Community Health Nursing.* Philadelphia: W.B. Saunders Co.

McCloskey, J.C. (1995). Nurse executive: The discipline hearts of a multidisciplinary team. *The Journal of Professional Nursing, 11*(4), 202.

McCloskey, J.C. (1996). Standardizing nursing language for computerization. In M.E.C. Mills, C.A. Romano, & B.R. Heller (Eds.), *Information management in nursing and health care* (pp 16–27). Springhouse, PA: Springhouse Corporation.

McCloskey, J.C., Bulechek, G.M., Moorhead, S., & Daly, J. (1996). Nurses' use and delegation of indirect care interventions. *Nursing Economic$, 14*(1), 22–33.

Micek, W.T., Berry, L., Gilski, D., Kallenbach, A., Link, D., & Scharer, K. (1996). Patient outcomes: The link between nursing diagnoses and interventions. *Journal of Nursing Administration, 26*(11), 29–35.

Moorhead, S., Clarke, M., Willits, M., & Tomsha, K.A. (1998). Nursing Outcomes Classification implementation projects across the care continuum. *Journal of Nursing Care Quality 12*(5), 52–63.

North American Nursing Diagnosis Association. (1999). *Nursing Diagnoses: Definitions and Classification 1999–2000.* Philadelphia: Author.

Prophet, C.M., & Delaney, C.W. (1998). Nursing Outcomes Classification: Implications for nursing information systems and the computer-based patient record. *Journal of Nursing Care Quality, 12*(5), 21–29.

Reed L., Blegen, M.A., & Goode, C.S. (1998). Adverse patient occurrences as a measure of nursing care quality. *Journal of Nursing Administration, 28*(5), 62–69.

Robbins, B.T. (1997). Application of nursing interventions classification (NIC) in a cardiovascular critical care unit. *Journal of Continuing Education Nursing, 28*(2), 78–82.

*Saba, V.K., O'Hare, P.A., Zuckerman, A.E., Boondas, J., Levine, E., & Oatway, D.M. (1991). A nursing intervention taxonomy for home health care. *Nursing and Health Care, 12*(6), 296–299.

Swearengen, J. (1997). Using quality indicators to improve quality of care. *Provider, 23*(2), 47, 49.

Timms, J.A., & Behrenbeck, J.G. (1998). Implementing the Nursing Outcomes Classification in a clinical information system in a tertiary care setting. *Journal of Nursing Care Quality. 12*(5), 64–72.

Vantassel, M. (1990). Effective applications of critical pathways. *Michigan Nurse, 3*(5), 5–6.

Evaluating Care

Chyi-Kong Karen Chang

Key Terms

case management
concurrent audit
continuous quality
    improvement
evaluation
peer review
performance appraisal
policy
procedure

protocol
quality assurance
retrospective audit
standards of care
standards of client care
standards of practice
standards of professional
    performance
variance

LEARNING OBJECTIVES

After studying this chapter, you should be able to:

1. Describe the purposes and process of establishing expected outcomes.

2. Evaluate yourself regarding factors affecting outcome attainment.

3. Discuss the process of evaluating care you provided.

4. Evaluate yourself regarding the compliance of standards established by the American Nurses' Association.

5. Describe the evaluating process of the Joint Commission on Accreditation of Healthcare Organizations regarding an organization's quality of care.

6. Discuss the purposes and types of internal standards established by health care organizations.

7. Discuss the methods that an organization uses to evaluate compliance with internal standards.

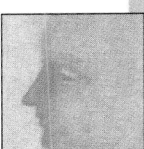

Mr. Scott Stanley, a 47-year-old male, had a left total knee replacement. To control pain, his doctor prescribed intravenous (IV) patient-controlled analgesia (PCA) morphine sulfate (MS) 1 mg every 10 minutes.

The nursing diagnosis is pain related to edema and muscle spasm secondary to surgery. The expected outcome is that the client will verbalize that pain has been reduced or controlled during the hospital stay. The next morning you are assigned to care for Mr. Stanley during his first postoperative day. How will you evaluate whether his pain has been controlled or reduced?

- Determine the client's progress toward the attainment of expected outcomes.
  - Reassess the client.
  - Compare your findings to the expected outcomes.
  - Determine the client's status.

- Determine the effectiveness of nursing care.
  - Assessment:
    Was assessment accurate and thorough?
  - Diagnosis:
    Was the diagnosis derived from the data, and did it accurately identify the problem?
  - Planning:
    Were the expected outcomes measurable, realistic, and appropriate?
  - Intervention:
    Were the interventions appropriate and appropriately implemented?

- Continue the plan or revise the diagnosis, expected outcomes, or interventions.

Figure 13–1. The process of evaluation.

Evaluation is a systematic and ongoing process of examining whether expected outcomes have been achieved and whether nursing care has been effective (Fig. 13–1). However, evaluation must also examine the quality of nursing care delivery and link positive client outcomes to quality care.

To evaluate the client's progress toward attaining expected outcomes, you will first need to review the expected outcomes for each diagnosis. Recall from Chapter 12 that expected outcomes are defined as a specific client status to be achieved at a specified time after interventions (ANA, 1995). The purposes of expected outcomes are to direct nursing interventions, to maintain continuity of nursing care, and to measure the effectiveness of nursing interventions (ANA, 1998). Keep in mind that accurate, meaningful evaluation relies on expected outcomes that are measurable, realistic, and attainable in relation to a client's capabilities and available resources.

Standards are established to evaluate the quality of care and to guide nursing practice. Nurses must agree on the standards and consistently practice according to the standards if nursing care is to be identified as the cause of positive outcomes. This chapter introduces evaluation by outcomes and by standards of practice.

EVALUATING CLIENT OUTCOMES

The process of evaluating nursing care reconsiders each phase of the nursing process. Was assessment accurate and thorough? Was the nursing diagnosis derived correctly from the data, and did it accurately identify the problem? Were the expected outcomes measurable, realistic, and appropriate? Were the interventions appropriate and appropriately implemented? During the evaluation phase, ask yourself the following key questions:

- What are the client's responses to interventions in relation to expected outcomes? Are the responses desirable or undesirable?
- Are the interventions effective in meeting expected outcomes? If not, why are the interventions ineffective? Is it necessary to revise outcomes or interventions?
- Is the nursing diagnosis still active? Is it necessary to revise or to add new nursing diagnoses?

Examining the Client's Responses to Interventions

Interventions include both medical and nursing interventions. After intervening, you should evaluate both the client's physical and psychosocial responses and document responses that are desirable or undesirable. Desirable responses indicate that the purposes of interventions are achieved and the client is progressing toward expected outcomes. Undesirable responses indicate poor progress toward expected outcomes or the occurrence of complications or side effects.

To assess physical and psychosocial responses to medications or treatments, you evaluate whether the purposes of medications or treatments have been achieved, the occurrence of complications or side effects, and the client's understanding of medications or treatments. Through the process of continuous evaluation, you may identify problems that need additional care. For example, some clients stop taking antibiotics or antihypertensives when their symptoms have subsided. When you evaluate the client's psychosocial responses to medications, you identify the problem of lack of understanding of medications.

Evaluating responses to diagnostic tests or procedures is another important aspect of nursing care. Throughout tests or procedures, the client may have many questions or concerns and may develop complications. Care can then be provided to ease the client's anxiety, increase the client's understanding, or detect complications or side effects at an early stage.

After providing nursing interventions, you should evaluate responses of the client and family members. After the client or family members have received health teaching, evaluate their understanding of the teaching. They may not understand the information completely or may have some misunderstanding. Some families may need further information. Others may need reinforcement to perform appropriate health behaviors.

Evaluating the client and family member's perceptions of care provided is also important. You may perceive that good nursing care has been provided, but the client or family members may think otherwise. The client's perceptions of nursing care influence his satisfaction with nursing care. Client satisfaction with nursing care is considered a quality indicator (ANA, 1995). Therefore, feedback from the client or family members needs to be sought to understand their perceptions of the care received and to help improve client satisfaction with nursing care. If a client or family member is dissatisfied with his care, you will need to identify the causes of his dissatisfaction and seek ways to reduce it.

Appraising the Success of Interventions

After evaluating the client's responses to interventions, you must judge the success of the interventions in achieving expected outcomes. Continue effective interventions and examine the reasons why others may be ineffective. Interventions may be inappropriate or insufficient to meet the goals and thus need to be discontinued or revised.

Outcomes may be completely met, partially met, or not met. When the client responds as expected, outcomes are completely met. When client's responses indicate some progress toward the goals, outcomes are partially met. When client's responses do not show any progress toward attaining goals, none of the outcomes are met. If the expected outcomes were not appropriately customized to the client's health status, for example, they may need to be revised.

Continuing, Revising, or Resolving the Care Plan

After evaluating the success of interventions, you will need to decide whether the nursing care plan should be continued or revised (Fig. 13–2). If the client attained the expected outcomes, the nursing diagnosis can be resolved. If the expected outcomes were only partially attained, you may need to revise interventions, add new ones, or discontinue others (Table 13–1). However, there may be justification for continuing interventions when the problem is not resolved.

When your evaluation identifies new problems, you will need to revise the client's existing care plan to address those problems. For example, acute pain is a common problem after surgery, and narcotics usually control surgical pain. However, clients commonly develop constipation. You will need to develop plans to manage constipation.

Recall Mr. Stanley from the beginning of the chapter. Mr. Stanley states that he did not sleep last night because of the pain in his left knee. On a scale of 0 to 10, he describes the pain intensity as "8 most of the time." He cannot find a comfortable position. The ice pack does not relieve the pain. At 8:00 AM, you note that Mr. Stanley activated the MS-PCA 19 times since 6:00 AM and has received 12 doses (i.e., he has been using PCA every 10 minutes). During the night Mr. Stanley had a problem urinating and was catheterized at 1:00 AM. He cannot void in bed. You observe that his lower abdomen is distended. You conclude that lack of sleep and having difficulty voiding are aggravating factors for his pain.

You plan to help Mr. Stanley void so that his pain may be controlled. The physician's orders include naloxone (Narcan) IV 1 mg q 10 minutes × 5 to relieve respiratory depression or urinary distention and that Mr. Stanley may stand up to void. You give 1 mg Narcan to counteract the side effect of the anesthetics and help him to stand up to void. Mr. Stanley voids 1,000 mL of clear yellow urine. He feels better but states that the pain is a 6 on a scale of 0 to 10. You conclude that the outcome is partially met.

You call the physician and receive an order to increase MS-PCA to 1 mg q 9 minutes. Later, Mr. Stanley is able to void in bed with a urinal. He states that he is more comfortable now and that his pain is much reduced. One hour later, Mr. Stanley is listening to music and falls asleep. The outcome is fully met. You conclude that the pain may recur; therefore, the current care plan should be continued.

FACTORS AFFECTING OUTCOME ATTAINMENT

Many factors affect the attainment of client outcomes. Evaluate yourself frequently to see if you are enhancing or impeding outcome attainment.

Facilitators

Stated clearly, realistic outcomes facilitate evaluations. A clear understanding of the client's illness and treatments will help you to select reasonable expected outcomes. After thoroughly identifying the client's problems and gathering adequate supporting data, you will be able to establish individualized and realistic outcomes.

Thinking of evaluation as a continuous process facilitates evaluation (Fig. 13–3). It requires frequent monitoring to gauge the client's progress in attaining an expected outcome. Observe for signs that progress is being made or that the client's condition is conducive to progress.

Maintaining continuity of care facilitates outcome attainment. Because all of a client's health problems may not be resolved with one episode of care, document all pertinent information about the client's problems, care plans, and progress toward expected outcomes. That way, the client's care plan can be continued, and his progress toward attaining his expected outcomes can be continuously assessed.

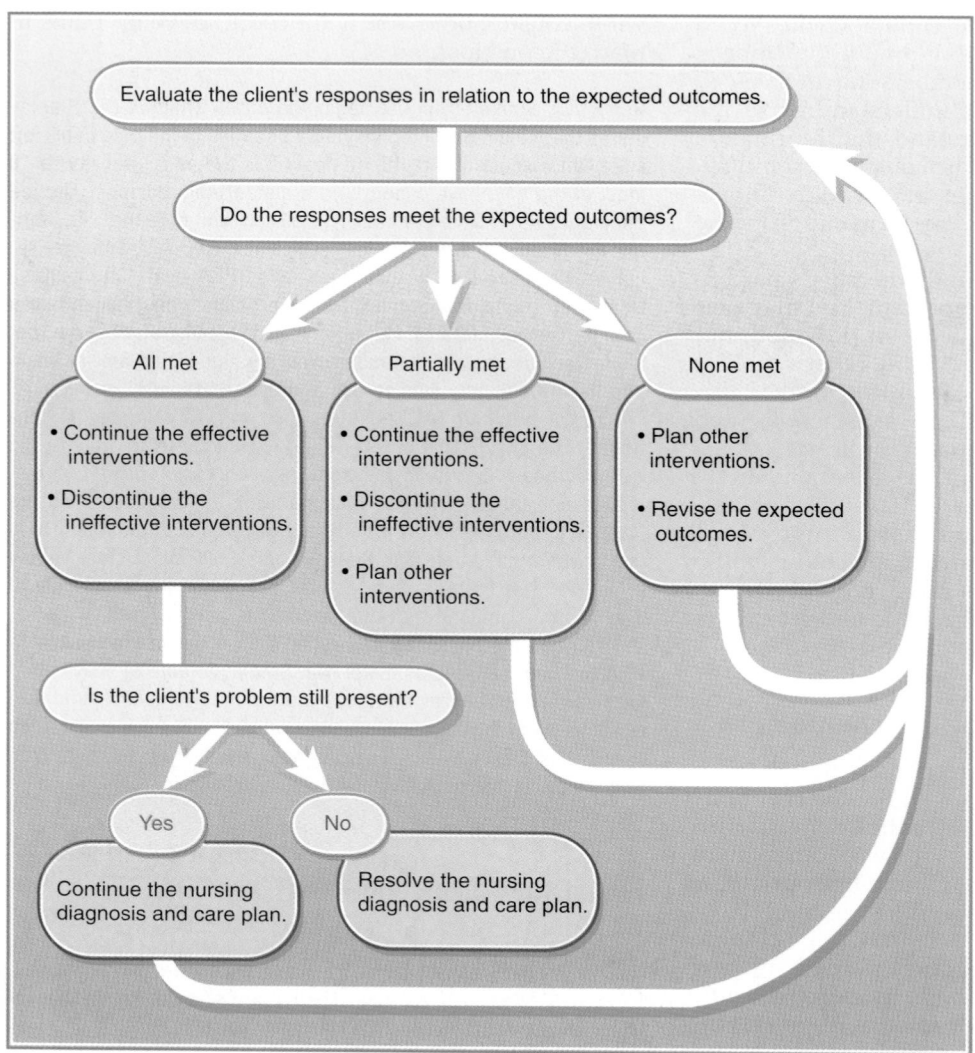

Figure 13–2. The process of evaluating a care plan.

Collaborating with other health care professionals is also crucial for facilitating outcome attainment. You should not only work closely with physicians but also recognize the client's needs for other health professionals. Using an interdisciplinary approach to meet the client's needs will expedite his recovery.

Client participation facilitates attaining outcomes. When the client understands what you seek to accomplish through the interventions applied, he will be more motivated to reach the goals. Box 13–1 summarizes factors facilitating outcome attainment.

Barriers

Barriers that impede the attainment of expected outcomes need to be evaluated as well. Barriers involve you and your colleagues more than the client and his condition. For example, a lack of critical thinking can leave you unaware of the client's problems and uncertain about why he may not be attaining his goals. Avoid focusing on routine tasks, such as taking vital signs or giving medications and treatments. Instead,

think critically as you work through the nursing process to identify and solve the client's problems. Ask yourself wide-ranging questions as you evaluate the success of the nursing process in your client's care (Box 13–2).

Lack of knowledge about client care, diseases, and treatments is another barrier affecting outcome attainment. To think critically, you will need to equip yourself continuously with knowledge relevant to client care. You can use many methods to keep your knowledge current and comprehensive.

Fragmented nursing care is another factor that hinders outcome attainment. In today's fast-paced clinical settings, interventions may not be consistently implemented, documented, and reassessed from shift to shift. Consequently, client problems may take longer than necessary to be resolved (Fig. 13–4).

To avoid fragmented care, you need to improve the team's working relationship and to maintain continuity of care. Strive to develop a system to facilitate verbal and written communication among the staff regarding each client's care. Some health care institu-

TABLE 13–1
An Example of Revising Interventions for an Unmet Expected Outcome

Client Data: A 72-year-old male with deep vein thrombosis in the left leg and a history of a brain tumor; hospitalized for 3 days.

Nursing Diagnosis	Expected Outcomes	Interventions	Evaluation and Charting
Altered nutrition: less than body requirements related to poor appetite and decreased oral intake	Client will increase oral intake by eating 75% of each meal. Client will identify causes of poor appetite.	Assess the causes of poor appetite. Assess daily intake and output status. Assess client's favorite foods and drinks and assist client to obtain them. Explain the importance of proper nutrition and fluid intake in avoiding further blood clots and facilitating recovery.	8:00 AM. Refuses to eat breakfast. Has no appetite. Oral intake has been less than 25% with each meal since admission. Last 24-hr intake is 900 mL and output is 1,200 mL. Has had no appetite for about 1 month since radiation therapy. Likes to eat sherbert and chocolate milk. Offered orange sherbert and chocolate milk. Drinks 50 mL of milk and half cup of sherbert. Explained to client the importance of nutrition and hydration. States that he does not have appetite but will try to drink more fluid. Discussed with client whether he can meet a goal to eat at least 25% of each meal and to drink a cup of his favorite fluid every 2 hours when he is awake. States that he will try. 10:00 AM. Does not want to drink chocolate milk anymore. Offered cranberry juice. Drinks 20 mL. 12:00 PM. Ate 10% of lunch. States feeling tired. Continues to have poor nutritional intake. Needs further interventions.
Nursing diagnosis added: *Altered oral mucous membrane* related to dryness	Expected outcome may be revised as: Client will increase oral intake by eating 25% of each meal.	Interventions may be revised to add the following interventions: Assess oral conditions, such as dryness and ulcers, and the side effect of medications. Provide oral care before and after each meal. Discuss with the physician the possibility of parenteral nutrition or a consult with a dietitian.	

tions use clinical care guidelines and computerized client records to facilitate continuity of care.

Lack of communication among professionals in differing disciplines can also deter outcome attainment. When health professionals fail to communicate or to make adequate referrals, the client's problem may not resolve appropriately.

Lack of involvement by the client himself is another barrier to outcome attainment (Box 13–3). Usually, that lack of involvement stems from a lack of adequate information. Most clients want to be informed about their condition, their treatment, and what they can do to improve their health or prevent problems. Most clients also want to be involved in making decisions about their care. To help a client reach his expected outcomes, explain the plan of care and encourage the client to participate in it. Encourage him to ask any questions he has and to clarify anything he finds confusing.

EVALUATING THE QUALITY OF NURSING CARE

Evaluation applies to more than the nursing process. It also applies to health care organizations and to the nurses who work there. Each health care organization is responsible for protecting the public from unsafe, incompetent, and illegal nursing practice. The organization first develops standards to describe the mini-

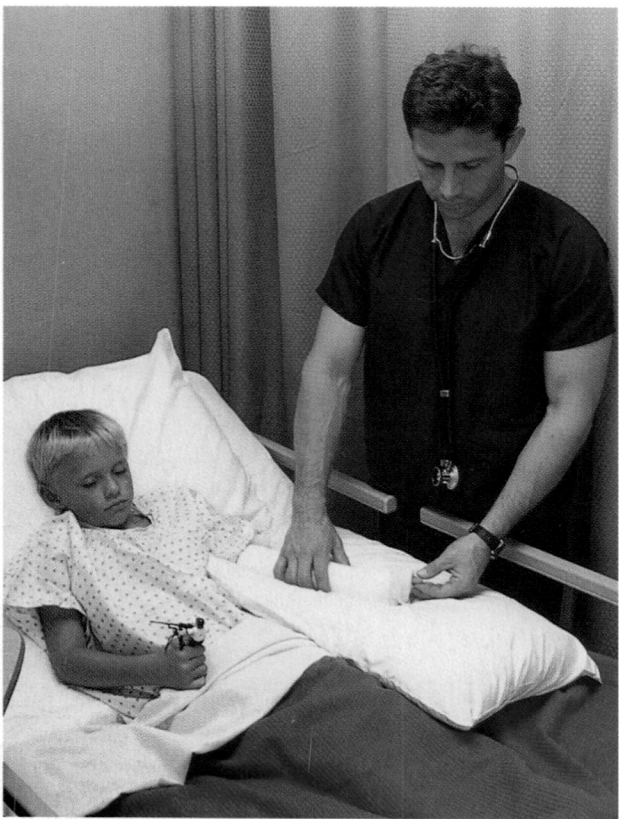

Figure 13–3. Evaluation is a continuous process. This nurse evaluates the circulation in a child's casted arm in an ongoing, regular manner.

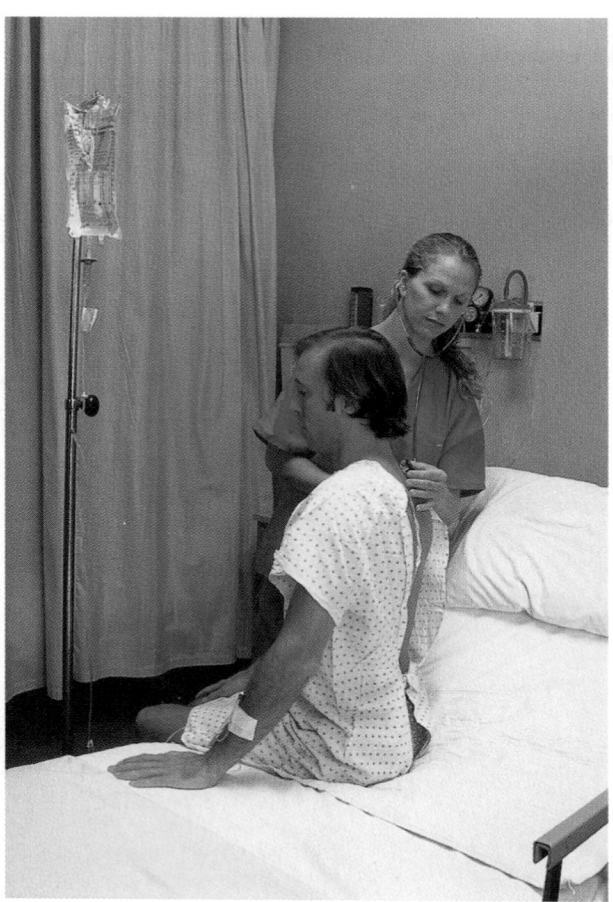

Figure 13–4. Avoidance of fragmented nursing care is critical to the achievement of expected outcomes. This nurse continuously reassesses and documents her client's respiratory status.-

mum levels of quality required. The standards are then used to evaluate individual nurses' performance in delivering quality nursing care.

The internal nursing standards created by health care organizations are influenced by external stan-

---

BOX 13–1

FACTORS FACILITATING OUTCOME ATTAINMENT

- Understand clearly the expected outcomes for each problem.
- Understand the client's disease and treatments.
- Assess the client accurately and thoroughly.
- Identify all pertinent problems.
- Formulate realistic and individualized outcomes.
- Revise outcomes and interventions when necessary.
- Maintain the continuity of care.
- Work as a team with other health care professionals.
- Encourage the client's participation in setting goals.

---

dards already established by each state's nurse practice act, by the nursing profession, and by federal, state, and private regulatory agencies (ANA, 1994). The standards established by the American Nurses' Association (ANA) are the most influential in the profession. Many specialty nursing professional organizations, such as those of pediatric clinical nursing, gerontological nursing, acute care nursing, oncology nursing, and others, derive their standards from those created by the ANA. Professional standards are not legally binding; however, the nurse practice act and regulations adopted by each state do have the power to be legally binding.

The health care organization's standards also reflect federal, state, and private regulatory requirements. The organization must comply with these agencies to continue operating. For example, standards set by the Health Care Financing Administration, the state board of nursing, the state department of health, and the Joint Commission on Accreditation of Healthcare Organizations (JCAHO) influence the development of the organization's standards. ANA and JCAHO standards are the most influential. However, you will be responsible for meeting both internal and external standards in any health care organization you serve.

EVALUATING THE SUCCESS OF THE NURSING PROCESS

Assessment

- What is the pathophysiology of my client's medical diagnoses? What is the relationship between the client's diagnoses and treatments?
- What are my client's physical and psychosocial responses to present illness, diagnoses, and treatments?
- What diagnostic tests has the client had? What are the relationships between abnormal results, the client's responses, and treatments?
- What are my client's treatments (i.e., diet, routine and PRN medications, activity, and so on)? Why are these prescribed? What are the client's responses to these treatments?

Diagnosis

- What actual and potential problems can I identify from assessment data?
- What is the priority of these problems?
- How do I describe these problems with nursing diagnoses approved by the North American Nursing Diagnosis Association?
- Do I have sufficient evidence (contributing factors, signs, symptoms) to confirm the diagnoses?
- Do I need to seek further data from current or past medical records, other health team members, family members, or other references to confirm or to rule out the nursing diagnoses?

Planning

- Are these outcomes client-focused? Is my client aware of the expected outcomes? Is my client ready to par-

ticipate in setting specific goals (outcome criteria)?
- Are these outcomes measurable and achievable in the short term or long term?
- Are these outcomes aimed to restore, maintain, or promote my client's health?

Intervention

- What interventions can be implemented to achieve expected outcomes?
- Do these interventions conform to professional standards and organizational standards and protocols?
- How should I implement these interventions safely and effectively?
- What can I do to maintain the continuity of care?

Evaluation

- What are the client's responses to interventions in relation to the expected outcomes?
- Are outcomes all met, partially met, or not met? Is it necessary to revise some outcomes to make them attainable?
- Are these interventions effective to achieve the expected outcomes? Are there problems with interventions? Are there better ways to implement these interventions?
- Are there alternative approaches to reach the goals?
- Should I continue, revise, or discontinue these interventions?
- Should I continue or resolve the nursing diagnoses?
- Has evaluation identified any new problems that require a nursing response?

BARRIERS TO THE ATTAINMENT OF EXPECTED OUTCOMES

- Lack of critical thinking to understand the client's problems, expected outcomes, and interventions.
- Inadequate knowledge about the client's responses to interventions.
- Fragmented nursing care.
- Lack of collaborative work with other health care professionals.
- Lack of client's involvement.

ANA Standards

The ANA published the first standards of practice for the nursing profession in 1973. They defined the nursing professional's accountability to the public and described the nursing professional's responsibilities. To clarify the nature and scope of nursing practice, the ANA revised and elaborated on the original standards in 1991 and 1998. The revision addressed two dimensions: standards of care and standards of professional performance. The Canadian Nurses Association published standards for nursing practice in 1987. This organization recently decided not to update its standards. Standards for Canadian nurses will come from provincial nursing organizations.

Standards of Care

The ANA defines **standards of care** as "authoritative statements that describe a competent level of clinical

BOX 13–4

STANDARDS OF CARE

Standard I. Assessment

THE NURSE COLLECTS PATIENT HEALTH DATA

Measurement Criteria

1. Data collection involves the patient, family, and other health care providers, as appropriate.
2. The priority of data collection activities is determined by the patient's immediate condition or needs.
3. Pertinent data are collected using appropriate assessment techniques and instruments.
4. Relevant data are documented in a retrievable form.
5. The data collection process is systematic and ongoing.

Standard II. Nursing Diagnosis

THE NURSE ANALYZES THE ASSESSMENT DATA IN DETERMINING DIAGNOSES

Measurement Criteria

1. Diagnoses are derived from the assessment data.
2. Diagnoses are validated with the patient, family, and other health care providers, when possible and appropriate.
3. Diagnoses are documented in a manner that facilitates the determination of expected outcomes and plan of care.

Standard III. Outcome Identification

THE NURSE IDENTIFIES EXPECTED OUTCOMES INDIVIDUALIZED TO THE PATIENT

Measurement Criteria

1. Outcomes are derived from the diagnoses.
2. Outcomes are mutually formulated with the patient, family, and other health care providers, when possible and appropriate.
3. Outcomes are culturally appropriate and realistic in relation to the patient's present and potential capabilities.
4. Outcomes are attainable in relation to resources available to the patient.
5. Outcomes include a time estimate for attainment.
6. Outcomes provide direction for continuity of care.
7. Outcomes are documented as measurable goals.

Standard IV. Planning

THE NURSE DEVELOPS A PLAN OF CARE THAT PRESCRIBES INTERVENTIONS TO ATTAIN EXPECTED OUTCOMES

Measurement Criteria

1. The plan is individualized to the patient (e.g., age-appropriate, culturally sensitive) and the patient's condition or needs.
2. The plan is developed with the patient, family, and other health care providers, as appropriate.
3. The plan reflects current nursing practice.
4. The plan provides for continuity of care.
5. Priorities for care are established.
6. The plan is documented.

Standard V. Implementation

THE NURSE IMPLEMENTS THE INTERVENTIONS IDENTIFIED IN THE PLAN OF CARE

Measurement Criteria

1. Interventions are consistent with the established plan of care.
2. Interventions are implemented in a safe, timely, and appropriate manner.
3. Interventions are documented.

Standard VI. Evaluation

THE NURSE EVALUATES THE PATIENT'S PROGRESS TOWARD ATTAINMENT OF OUTCOMES

Measurement Criteria

1. Evaluation is systematic, ongoing, and criterion-based.
2. The patient, family, and other health care providers are involved in the evaluation process, as appropriate.
3. Ongoing assessment data are used to revise diagnoses, outcomes, and the plan of care, as needed.
4. Revisions in diagnoses, outcomes, and the plan of care are documented.
5. The effectiveness of interventions is evaluated in relation to outcomes.
6. The patient's responses to interventions are documented.

Reprinted with permission from American Nurses' Association. Standards of clinical nursing practice (2nd ed.). Copyright 1998 American Nurses' Publishing, American Nurses' Foundation/American Nurses' Association, Washington, D.C.

nursing practice demonstrated through assessment, diagnosis, outcome identification, planning, implementation, and evaluation" (ANA, 1998, p. 2). These standards emphasize the nurse's practice in caring for the client regardless of the nurse's educational background. In other words, every nurse is expected to demonstrate competent practice in these standards.

The ANA outlines six standards of care: assessment, diagnosis, outcome identification, planning care, implementation, and evaluation (Box 13–4). The

BOX 13–5

A COURT CASE THAT USED STANDARDS OF CARE TO EVALUATE THE QUALITY OF NURSING CARE

A 64-year-old male client who underwent five-vessel coronary artery bypass surgery in a Louisiana hospital developed respiratory complications after surgery. He was transferred to a medical/surgical unit 12 days after surgery. At 4 PM, the nurse noticed that the client had crackles in his lungs and rapid respirations. At 5:30 PM, the client was restless and vomited. The nurse contacted the physician and gave the client a suppository to control nausea and vomiting. The assessment did not include vital signs.

Between 5:30 PM and 6:45 PM, the client's wife stated that she used the call light 10 to 12 times and was told that the nurse was taking a dinner break. When the nurse returned at 6:45 PM, she noted that the client's eyes were rolled back, and she paged a respiratory arrest code. The client died 2 days later. The client's wife and daughter sued the hospital for nursing negligence.

An expert in general nursing found two deficiencies in nursing standards of care in the documentation. First, there was no documentation assessment between 5:30 PM and 6:45 PM. Second, the nursing care plans did not address *Risk for aspiration,* nor did the notes address the problem that the client vomited at 5:30 PM. The court concluded that sufficient evidence indicated that the nursing staff had breached the standards of care and awarded the client's wife $150,000 and her daughter $50,000 for damages.

From Miller, E., Flynn, J.M., & Umadac, J. (1996). Not documented, not done: A silent chart undermines a nurse's credibility. Nursing96, 26(10), 70. With permission from Nursing96, Springhouse Corporation.

organization also lists criteria to measure the nurse's practice in each standard. Competent practice of these standards reflects competent use of the nursing process. The criteria to measure competent practice of the standards are called indicators (ANA, 1998).

Standards of care (internal and external) are used in court cases to evaluate the quality of care delivered and the competence of the nurses delivering it (Guido, 1997). When the evidence indicates that nurses failed to meet these standards, the duty of care has been breached. The nurse or nurses involved are then guilty of malpractice (Guido, 1997). Box 13–5 describes a court case that used standards of care to evaluate the quality of nursing care delivered (Miller, Flynn, & Umadac, 1996). As this case illustrates, nurses are responsible for performing—and documenting—com-

petent care that meets all internal and external standards.

Standards of Professional Performance

Standards of professional performance are defined as "authoritative statements that describe a competent level of behavior in the professional role, including activities related to quality of care, performance appraisal, education, collegiality, ethics, collaboration, research, and resource utilization" (ANA, 1998). Box 13–6 lists behaviors that demonstrate the standards of professional performance (ANA, 1998).

To comply with Standard I, you should evaluate yourself regarding client care and the quality of care provided in the organization. You also can participate in activities that evaluate and improve the quality and effectiveness of nursing care in the organization. Typically, these activities include identifying indicators of quality and effectiveness and collecting data related to those indicators. When the data reveal problems with nursing care, you will need to identify ways to improve its quality and effectiveness. The results of such data analysis can also be used to refine policies

BOX 13–6

THE STANDARDS OF PROFESSIONAL PERFORMANCE

Standard I: The nurse systematically evaluates the quality and effectiveness of nursing practice.

Standard II: The nurse evaluates one's own nursing practice in relation to professional practice standards and relevant statutes and regulations.

Standard III: The nurse acquires and maintains current knowledge and competency in nursing practice.

Standard IV: The nurse interacts with and contributes to the professional development of peers and other health care providers as colleagues.

Standard V: The nurse's decisions and actions on behalf of patients are determined in an ethical manner.

Standard VI: The nurse collaborates with the patient, family, and other health care providers in providing patient care.

Standard VII: The nurse uses research findings in practice.

Standard VIII: The nurse considers factors related to safety, effectiveness, and cost in planning and delivering patient care.

Reprinted with permission from American Nurses' Association. Standards of clinical nursing practice (2nd ed.). Copyright 1998 American Nurses' Publishing, American Nurses' Foundation/American Nurses' Association, Washington, D.C.

and procedures intended to reinforce safe, high-quality nursing care.

To demonstrate compliance with Standard II, critically evaluate your nursing practice in relation to standards of care and standards of professional performance. Self-evaluation can help you identify the strengths of your own practice and areas in which you can improve.

To show compliance with Standard III, pursue continuing education opportunities, and study professional journals to update your knowledge and skills. Some states require continuing education for license renewal; others do not. However, learning is a lifelong process. As a competent professional nurse, you should continue to seek learning opportunities—whether your state requires it or not—because of your own desire to improve your clinical competency and expertise.

According to Standard IV, you should strive to share your knowledge and skills with colleagues and nursing students (ANA, 1998). You can formally or informally share with colleagues the information you gain from workshops, published articles, or books. You can also help each other by offering or receiving constructive comments to improve professional development.

To evaluate your compliance with Standard V, you need to be familiar with the Code for Nurses (ANA, 1985). You also need to evaluate your ethical behavior, such as respecting the client and the client's rights, being sensitive to the client's needs and preferences, protecting the client, maintaining the client's confidentiality, and being the client's advocate (ANA, 1998). When ethical dilemmas occur, you will need to refer to the institution's policy or consult with ethics experts in the institution to seek the most appropriate decision for the client.

To comply with Standard VI, you will need to work with the client, family members, and other health care professionals to meet each client's needs. When the client's needs require interventions from other health care providers, contact those professionals. For example, if a pain medication fails to relieve a client's pain, discuss this finding with the physician, and seek other medications or methods to control the client's pain.

To comply with Standard VII, apply research findings that improve nursing practices, and participate in research activities that contribute to the development of nursing knowledge (ANA, 1998). Work to stay current with research related to your practice area (Fig. 13–5). When reading nursing research reports, use your own knowledge and experience to discern whether you think the findings are valid and reliable, and evaluate whether these findings can be generalized to other clinical settings.

To demonstrate competent behaviors in compliance with Standard VIII, evaluate your practice in relation to safety, effectiveness, and cost. You can contribute to the control of health care costs by reducing the use of unnecessary equipment and supplies. Evaluate the impact of reduced health care costs on

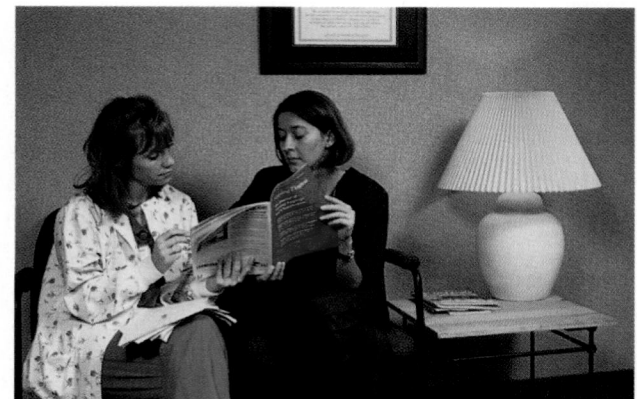

Figure 13–5. To comply with Standard VII, these nurses are keeping themselves up to date on research related to their practice area.

client health. Never choose a cost-saving strategy that will have negative effects on the client's welfare. When these strategies jeopardize a client's health or safety, evaluate and document that fact, and seek other solutions constructively within the institution. If the problem cannot be solved within the institution, seek external authorities to solve the problem (ANA, 1994).

JCAHO Standards

Health care organizations are concerned about being accredited by JCAHO. Being accredited is not only prestigious but also a necessity for the organization to continue to operate. Although JCAHO is a voluntary accreditation organization, federal and state regulatory agencies and insurance carriers require that health care organizations be accredited by JCAHO to be certified, to be licensed, or to receive reimbursement.

JCAHO evaluates each health care organization every 3 years. The extent of an organization's compliance with JCAHO standards determines the organization's accreditation status. In the past, when the organization received accreditation, it indicated that the organization had the capabilities to provide quality care. However, the public demands the evaluation of actual performance or outcome information instead of potential capabilities. Thus, JCAHO continuously improves and revises its standards so that an organization's accreditation reflects its actual performance of quality care (JCAHO, 1994a).

During the accreditation process (O'Leary, 1996), JCAHO examines the organization's performance in *doing the right thing* and *doing the right thing well*. The characteristics of doing the right thing are efficacy and appropriateness. The characteristics of doing the right thing well are availability, effectiveness, timeliness, safety, efficiency, continuity, respect, and caring. JCAHO believes that the organization demonstrating these characteristics is more likely to provide high-quality care with optimal client outcomes and efficient resource use.

Internal Standards

An organization assures quality of care by developing specific standards and evaluating compliance with these standards. Each organization integrates the ANA standards and regulatory agencies' standards, especially JCAHO's standards, to formulate its internal standards. The relationships among external standards, internal standards, and evaluating compliance with standards are summarized in Figure 13–6.

The organization's internal standards are further clarified to guide or to standardize staff performance through standards of practice, standards of client care, policies and procedures, protocols, case management, and clinical pathways.

Standards of Practice and Standards of Client Care

The nursing department usually develops its standards of practice and standards of client care from ANA standards to provide general guidelines for nursing practice. **Standards of client care** are the essential elements of *nursing care* prescribed for specific client populations. **Standards of practice** describe what the nursing staff should assess, plan, implement, and evaluate during daily and ongoing care for specific client populations. The content of these standards overlaps.

Policies and Procedures

Organizations develop policies and procedures based on standards of practice and standards of client care. A **policy** is a set of rules and regulations that govern nursing practice and nursing care. Policies may pertain to clients, such as the client's bill of rights, or to the nursing staff, such as the staff's employment, deployment, and assignment; staffing patterns; staff mix (the number of registered nurses, licensed professional nurses, and nursing assistants); attendance; sick leave; chemical dependency; incident reports; and floating to other units.

A **procedure** is a detailed description of a specific method of performing nursing care. Procedural guidelines, such as medication administration, insertion of nasogastric tubes or urinary catheters, and isolation, are published in a procedure manual. The procedure manual describes who is responsible for performing

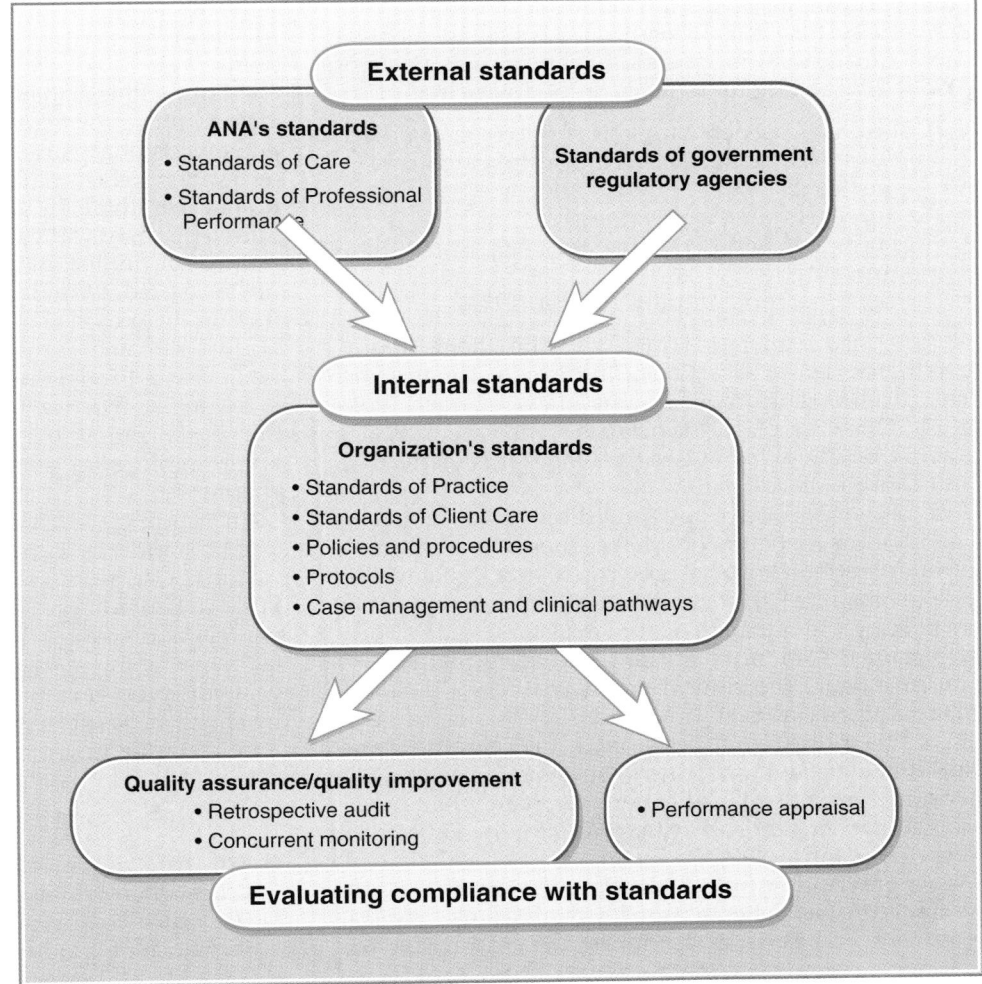

Figure 13–6. Relationships between external standards and internal standards and evaluating compliance with standards.

the procedures, what equipment or supplies are necessary, and what information should be assessed and documented.

Protocols

A **protocol** contains detailed guidelines for nursing care for clients with specific conditions. For example, protocols may be developed for alcohol withdrawal, cardiac catheterization, fall risk, skin risk, restraints, surgical client management, and chest pain. Protocols are also developed to allow nurses to perform procedures beyond the legal scope of nursing practice. For example, the critical care unit may develop a protocol that allows the nurse to treat life-threatening arrhythmias before the physician arrives. This protocol defines life-threatening arrhythmia, the dosage and frequency of medications or treatments to be used, the staff responsible for administering the medication or treatment, and the assessment and documentation to be done.

Case Management and Clinical Pathways

Recently, case management and clinical pathways have been developed to reduce costs while ensuring quality of care. **Case management** is defined as a care delivery system that focuses on the management of client care across an episode of illness. The goals of case management are to achieve the following:

- Coordinate needed care and services across disciplines to reduce fragmented or duplicated care
- Achieve satisfactory clinical outcomes
- Reduce cost per case
- Reduce the length of hospital stay and use resources effectively
- Reduce readmission rates (Bower, 1994).

The case manager works with the client, family, health care team, and payers to develop client goals. The case manager then designs plans to reach those goals. Once the plan is formulated, the case manager carries out the plan, revises the plan if it is ineffective, and coordinates all care.

Clinical pathways are interdisciplinary plans of care that prescribe the optimal sequencing and timing of interventions for a category of clients (Ignatavicius & Hausman, 1995). A clinical pathway is a process of evaluating the outcome of care measured against predetermined standards and implementing methods of improvement. The clinical pathway offers a detailed, standardized care plan from admission to discharge. It links diagnoses, outcomes, and interventions and specifies expected outcomes to be achieved in a predetermined period. All health care personnel that are involved in client care are expected to follow the recommended paths.

Any deviation from a clinical pathway is called a **variance.** When clients are deviated from a clinical pathway, you need to document the reasons for the variance. Aggregated data on variances are used to identify the common causes of variances. This information will then be used to seek ways to reduce variances. The causes of variances are usually related to clients, health care providers, or health care delivery systems. These may include complications, unresponsiveness to treatment, a physician's delay, a nurse's delay, or scheduling problems.

Case management and clinical pathways are used for different types of client populations. In general, case management is used to manage clients who:

- Require complex care and costly services
- Have a frequent need for inpatient or outpatient health care services
- Lack social support or financial resources
- Vary significantly from clinical pathways

On the other hand, clinical pathways are used for high-volume clients who are expected to achieve predetermined outcomes in a specified time.

Positive findings have been reported from the implementation of clinical pathways. These include reduced delays in client care, more standardization in client care or treatment, better collaboration among health care personnel, fewer complications, and reduced lengths of stay and client charges. Thus, many organizations now use clinical pathways, either commercially available standardized plans or pathways developed in-house for certain diagnoses and treatments.

Many clinical pathways have been developed, such as those for abdominal hysterectomy, cholecystectomy, coronary artery bypass graft, cerebral vascular accident, chest pain, myocardial infarction, pneumonia, and total hip replacement. However, clinical pathways may differ among organizations. Some pathways only list specific interventions to be carried out at a predetermined day or time. Some describe nursing diagnoses and collaborative problems, client/family outcomes, and interventions to be implemented at a predetermined time or day. You need to be aware of the type of clinical pathways in use in your organization to help guide your nursing practice. An example of a clinical pathway is presented in Chapter 12.

In summary, each organization develops its own specific standards to guide and to standardize nursing practice. You need to be familiar with all these standards to provide care as defined by the institution. If you feel that an organization's standards conflict with national nursing standards, you will need to communicate the problem and the potential adverse effects on the client. If possible, propose a solution to revise the current standard.

Evaluating Compliance

Health care organizations use two common approaches when evaluating compliance with standards: (a) performance appraisal to evaluate an individual's performance of quality care and (b) quality assurance and quality improvement activities to evaluate the quality of care delivered by a group of nurses in a specific setting.

Performance Appraisal

A **performance appraisal** is a systematic and standardized evaluation of an employee's work contribution, quality of work, and potential for advancement, made by the employee's supervisor (Albrecht, 1972). Performance appraisals focus on each staff member's consistent compliance with standards. They may be used formally or informally to identify performance strengths and areas for improvement. Often, the results of a performance appraisal are used to determine promotion, selection, termination, or pay raise. When appraisals indicate that a nurse consistently fails to comply with standards, this nurse becomes a problem employee and requires disciplinary action and frequent evaluation.

The process of performance appraisal varies with each organization. The organization defines a job description for its staff based on its institutional standards. Performance appraisal is then conducted regularly according to the job description (Huber, 1996). The process of performance appraisal must be described in the policy and procedure manual (JCAHO, 1994b).

Each organization determines how each staff member should be evaluated. In general, nurses are expected to perform self-evaluation according to the institution's performance appraisal form. The nursing supervisor uses the same form to evaluate nurses' performance. Some organizations may also require each nurse to perform peer reviews. A **peer review** is the evaluation of the performance of one staff member by another staff member to judge the quality of care provided.

Each organization uses its own form of performance appraisal. It may include anecdotes, open-ended essays, checklists, and rating scales (Huber, 1996). In anecdotal notes, the evaluator documents details of events, behaviors, or attitudes that reflect a nurse's performance. These notes are often used to complement other forms of performance appraisal. Open-ended essays ask the evaluator to describe the nurse's performance in response to standard questions. The checklist requires the evaluator to indicate the presence or absence of a nurse's performance. The rating scale includes various types of measuring criteria, such as "excellent, good, average, below average, and poor." The evaluator rates each nurse's performance according to the categories supplied.

Quality Assurance and Continuous Quality Improvement

Quality assurance (QA) is a process of evaluating the outcome of care measured against predetermined standards and implementing methods to achieve these standards (Coyne & Killien, 1987). Three main steps are involved. First, each nursing unit selects aspects of care to represent the standards, criteria for achievement of the standards, and methods of monitoring. Second, the nursing department analyzes the data to determine potential causes of poor compliance. Third, the unit seeks ways to improve compliance with the standards.

Retrospective audits and concurrent audits are used to conduct QA activities. The **retrospective audit** is an evaluation method to inspect the medical record for documentation of compliance with the standards. This method requires less time than a concurrent audit and thus is used most often by the health care organization. The **concurrent audit** is an evaluation method to inspect the nursing staff's compliance with predetermined standards and criteria while the nurses are providing care. The auditor compares the performance against other nurses' performance and over time.

Generally, each organization designates responsibilities for conducting an audit to the QA staff, the head nurse, the charge nurse, or the nurse educator. However, a peer review approach in which every member of the nursing staff is involved in auditing for quality of care is a growing trend (Fig. 13–7).

The following example (Atkins, Nadzam, & Ceccio, 1991) illustrates the process of QA activities. A unit selects client safety regarding intravenous (IV) therapy as the important aspect of care. Indicators of compliance are following the policy for IV therapy and evidence of IV complications. The criteria to be monitored are the following:

- Tubing changed every 72 hours
- Sites rotated every 72 hours
- Bags or bottles changed every 72 hours
- Dressings changed every 72 hours

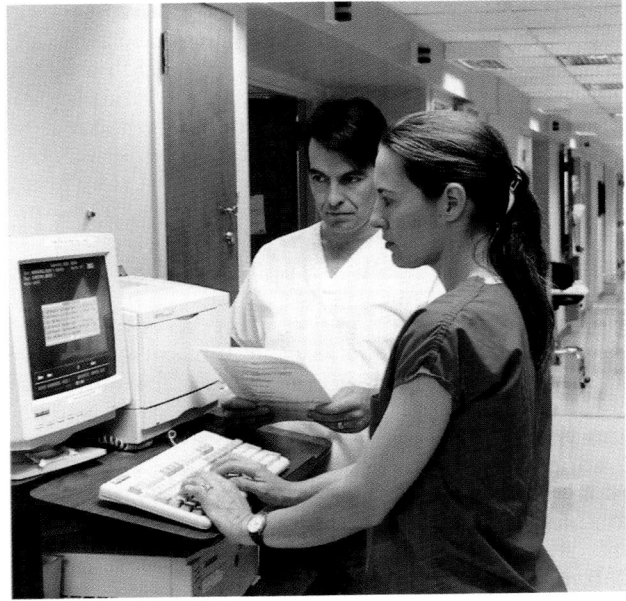

Figure 13–7. Recently, nursing staff members have become involved in auditing the performance of other staff members through the review of client records.

- Daily inspections for complications
- No complications related to IV therapy

Using the retrospective audit method, every member of the nursing staff randomly selects three charts per month to determine if the documentation complies with the criteria. This unit predetermines that 90% of the selected charts must comply with the standard. Thus, when less than 90% of the charts comply with the standard, this unit will analyze the causes of substandard performance. The staff members who did not perform according to the criteria will be identified and advised by the head nurse or charge nurse. Reasons for not performing according to the standards and ways to improve compliance will be identified.

The concurrent audit method is often used for members of a nursing staff during their orientation period. When the new nurses are performing IV therapy, they are expected to find the nurse educator or a mentor nurse to observe their performance and to ensure that their performance complies with the standard of IV therapy.

Because QA activities require tedious, comprehensive evaluation of documentation to show compliance with standards, they may have a delayed impact on quality of care. Thus, QA activities have been gradually replaced with continuous quality improvement activities. **Continuous quality improvement** (CQI) is a systematic approach to control and to improve quality from both professionals' and clients' perspectives. It is also called *total quality improvement* or *total quality management*. It incorporates professionals' and clients' perspectives of quality to set desirable outcomes. It uses statistical methods to measure processes of care and outcomes. And it involves relevant health care personnel to continuously improve processes of care to achieve predetermined outcomes. CQI is based on two main assumptions: (a) quality can always be improved, and (b) the health care delivery system often prevents health care providers from providing quality care. Thus, CQI works on the system to improve the quality of care. When predetermined outcomes are not achieved, all relevant health care personnel work together to identify the problems with the system and to seek ways to improve the system until desirable outcomes are achieved.

The following example illustrates the process of CQI in an acute care setting. A satisfaction survey of clients discharged from an orthopedic unit indicated that clients were dissatisfied with nurses' responses to call lights (Van Handel & Krug, 1994). The staff in this unit decided to improve the outcome: client satisfaction with nurses' responses to call lights. First, they conducted a study. The first step of this study determined the nature of clients' call lights and the most common times when clients used call lights. Call light tally sheets were developed to collect data. All nursing staff in this unit participated in the study. Results indicated that clients' use of call lights related primarily to the immediate physical environment and that clients used call lights most often at the change of shifts and around suppertime. The staff then held several meetings and developed three strategies to solve the problem. First, staff members were reminded to anticipate and meet each client's needs before leaving the room. Second, two new unit assistants were hired to help answer call lights at the most common time. Third, staff members were encouraged to take flexible breaks and meal times to help keep more people available to answer call lights. After the implementation of these strategies, this unit's client satisfaction with call lights was remarkably improved. The unit continued to seek improvement in client satisfaction, developed guidelines for staff to deal with client complaints, and conducted a client focus group to seek clients' input for better client care.

KEY PRINCIPLES

- Evaluation is a systematic and ongoing component of the nursing process to determine if the client's progress toward expected outcomes is achieved, if interventions provided are effective in meeting expected outcomes, and if nursing care is provided according to standards of practice.
- Expected outcomes should be established before evaluation. Outcomes should be measurable and individualized and have an estimated time frame.
- After interventions are implemented, the client's physical and psychosocial responses to the interventions are evaluated. Desirable and undesirable responses are noted, and interventions for undesirable responses are made.
- The success of interventions should be appraised and a determination made to continue, revise, or resolve care plans.
- Nurses should evaluate themselves frequently regarding facilitators and barriers of outcome attainment.
- The internal standards of each health care organization are influenced by external standards, such as ANA standards and standards of federal, state, and private regulatory agencies.
- ANA standards consist of standards of care and standards of professional performance. Standards of care describe competent practice of nursing process. Standards of professional performance depict competent professional behaviors.
- The JCAHO surveys health care organizations to assess certain dimensions of the organization's performance. The demonstration of these characteristics indicates that the organization is likely to provide high-quality care.
- An organization develops internal standards to guide and standardize nursing practice, such as standards of practice, standards of client care, policies, procedures, protocols, case management, and clinical pathways.
- An organization evaluates compliance with standards through two approaches: performance ap-

praisal to evaluate each nurse's compliance with standards, and QA or CQI to evaluate the quality of nursing care provided by a group of nurses.

BIBLIOGRAPHY

*Albrecht, S. (1972). Reappraisal of conventional performance appraisal. *Journal of Nursing Administration, 2*(2), 29–35.

*American Nurses' Association. (1985). *Code for nurses with interpretive statements.* Kansas City, MO: Author.

*American Nurses' Association. (1994). *Guidelines on reporting incompetent, unethical, or illegal practices.* Washington, D.C.: Author.

*American Nurses' Association. (1995). *Implementation of nursing practice standards and guidelines.* Washington, D.C.: Author.

American Nurses' Association. (1998). *Standards of clinical nursing practice,* 2nd ed. Kansas City, MO: Author.

Atkins, P.M., Nadzam, D.M., & Ceccio, C.M. (1991). the pyramid for nursing quality assurance. In P. Schroeder (Ed.), *The encyclopedia of nursing care quality, volume 7.* (pp 81–99). Gaithersburg, MD: Aspen Publishers.

Bower, K.A. (1994). Case management and clinical paths: definitions and relationships. In P.L. Spath (Ed.), *Clinical paths—tools for outcomes management.* (pp 25–32). Chicago, IL: American Hospital Publishing.

The Canadian Nurses Association. (1987). *A definition of nursing practice: Standards for nursing practice.* Ottawa, Ontario: Author.

*Coyne, C., & Killien, M. (1987). A system for unit-based monitors of quality of nursing care. *Journal of Nursing Administration, 17*(1), 26–32.

Forsyth, T.J., Maney, L.A., Ramirez, A., Raviotta, G., Burts, J.L., & Litzenberger, D. (1998). Nursing case management in the NICU: Enhanced coordination for discharge planning. *Neonatal Network, 17*(7), 23–24.

Gardner, K., Allhusen, J., Kamm, J., & Tobin, J. (1997). Determining the cost of care through clinical pathways. *Nurse Economist, 15*(4), 213–217.

Guido, G.W. (1997). *Legal issues in nursing.* Stanford, CT: Appleton & Lange.

Haag-Heitman, B., & Kramer, A. (1998). Creating a clinical practice development model. *American Journal of Nursing, 98*(8), 39–43.

Homes, L.M., & Hollabaugh, S. K. (1997). Using the continuous quality improvement process to improve the care of patients after angioplasty. *Critical Care Nurse, 17*(6), 56–65.

Huber, D. (1996). Performance appraisal. In *Leadership and nursing care management* (pp 529–546). Philadelphia: W.B. Saunders Co.

Ignatavicius, D., & Hausman, K. (1995). *Clinical pathways for collaborative practice.* Philadelphia: W.B. Saunders Co.

*Joint Commission on Accreditation of Healthcare Organizations (1994a). *Framework for improving performance: A guide for nurses.* Oakbrook Terrace, IL: Author.

*Joint Commission on Accreditation of Healthcare Organizations (1994b). *Accreditation manual for hospitals: Volume I standards.* Oakbrook Terrace, IL: Author.

Kobs, A.E. (1998). Getting started on benchmarking. *Outcomes Management in Nursing Practice, 2*(1), 45–48.

Miller, E., Flynn, J.M., & Umadac, J. (1996). Not documented, not done: A silent chart undermines a nurse's credibility. *Nursing96, 26*(10), 70.

O'Leary, D.S. (1996). President's Column: CQI—a step beyond QA. *Joint Commission Perspectives, 10,* 2–3.

Parsley, K. (1998). In search of pathways. *Nursing Times, 94*(32), 40–41.

Rosenberg, M.L. (1998). Developing behavioral health clinical guidelines for depression: Emerging standards for guiding care. *Nursing Case Management, 3*(5), 204–207.

*Van Handel, K., & Krug, B. (1994). Prevalence and nature of call light requests on an orthopaedic unit. *Orthopaedic Nursing, 13*(1), 13–20.

*Asterisk indicates a classic or definitive work on this subject.

14

Documenting Care

Barbara S. Moffett and Karen Y. Hill

Key Terms

admit note
APIE charting
charting by exception
discharge note
documentation
flow sheet
focus charting
interval or progress note

narrative charting
PIE charting
problem-oriented medical
   records
SOAP charting
source-oriented medical
   records
transfer note

LEARNING OBJECTIVES

After studying this chapter, you should be able to:

1. **Explain the purpose of documentation.**
2. **State the purpose of using appropriate medical terminology and standard abbreviations when documenting care.**
3. **Discuss the importance of recording information legibly, concisely, completely, and sequentially.**
4. **Identify significant data that should be documented in clients' records.**
5. **Explain the value of recording complete data entries using clear and objective terms.**
6. **Relate the need for variation in documenting for special populations and facilities.**
7. **Differentiate among various charting formats.**
8. **Describe the usefulness of various types of flow sheets.**

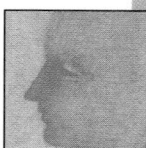

Geraldine Peters, age 68, lives alone and was working in her garden when she fell and fractured her left hip. She was taken to the emergency department of a hospital nearby, where she was admitted. She was scheduled for an open reduction and internal fixation of her left hip the following morning. There are a number of considerations you need to make in documenting Ms. Peters' care and her responses to that care. This chapter addresses the purposes, principles, and methods of documenting client care.

Documentation (or charting) of client care refers to the recording of information relevant to data collection, planning, implementation, and client response to care given. Record-keeping systems vary among health care agencies. Documentation systems have evolved in an effort to adjust to changes in health care delivery, reflect changes in nursing practice, and incorporate regulatory agency requirements (Iyer & Camp, 1995).

PURPOSES OF DOCUMENTATION

Accurate documentation of information is essential in order to communicate information to all members of the health team, to ensure legal accountability, and to demonstrate effective use of the nursing process and appropriate standards of care.

Communication

Documentation of a client's care is useful in providing a means of communication among health team members. Clients in health care settings may be cared for by more than one nurse and seen by several other health care providers. It is essential that all personnel provide written documentation of actions and observations to ensure coordination of activities and continuity of care. Proper documentation informs appropriate personnel about a client's condition and response to illness, interventions implemented, and the results of care and treatment given. The American Nurses' Association (ANA) Standards of Clinical Nursing Practice (1998) require the use of the nursing process in providing care to clients. Communication of the use of this process is primarily through documentation in the client's medical record.

Quality Assurance

Quality assurance focuses on providing care according to established standards. Standards of care are guidelines that represent generally accepted practice and are derived from a variety of sources including the ANA, state statutes, accrediting agencies, and agency policy or procedure manuals. ANA Standards of Care relevant to documentation are summarized in Box 14–1.

Evaluation of care is critical in providing quality assurance in client care and is necessary in order to ensure that standards of care are met. In addition, many health care accrediting agencies require regular quality assurance audits of client care. Documentation serves as the basis for collecting quality assurance data. Client outcomes serve as the measure of quality and are monitored through complete and accurate documentation. The record provides evidence that professional and agency standards have been incorporated into the client's care. The record should reflect initial and ongoing assessment, the problems identified through assessment, expected outcomes of care, interventions, and evaluation of progress toward expected outcomes.

BOX 14–1

ANA STANDARDS OF CARE RELEVANT TO DOCUMENTATION

Standard I. Assessment

Relevant measurement criterion: Relevant data are documented in a retrievable form.

Standard II. Diagnoses

Relevant measurement criterion: Diagnoses are documented in a manner that facilitates the determination of expected outcomes and plan of care.

Standard III. Outcome Identification

Relevant measurement criterion: Outcomes are documented as measurable goals.

Standard IV. Planning

Relevant measurement criterion: The plan is documented.

Standard V. Implementation

Relevant measurement criterion: Interventions are documented.

Standard VI. Evaluation

Relevant measurement criterion: Revisions in diagnoses, outcomes, and the plan of care are documented. The patient's responses to interventions are documented.

From American Nurses' Association. (1998). Standards of clinical nursing practice (2nd ed.). Washington, D.C.: Author.

Legal Accountability

Documentation of care is necessary as a source of legal accountability for you. Accountability for client care requires that standards of care be met. Documentation should, therefore, verify the need for interventions, verify the type of care given, and allow examination of progress toward expected outcomes.

Common liability issues for nurses include protection from avoidable injury, monitoring and reporting changes in condition, and performing interventions correctly. The record should document assessment of clients at risk, safety measures implemented, and the use of any restraints. If errors or injuries occur, the record should include careful documentation of the occurrence as well as what was done in response to the situation.

Action Alert!
Remember that the chart is a legal record and protects the client, the nurse, and the health care agency.

Reimbursement

Reimbursement for client care by Medicare, Medicaid, health maintenance organizations (HMOs), or insurance companies is often determined by review of clients' records. As cost-containment efforts intensify, documentation of nursing care is used to determine and justify the need for services. Utilization review committees often monitor lengths of stay and services.

Action Alert!
If there is inadequate documentation of the client's condition, nursing activities, or treatments and procedures, appropriate reimbursement for services may be denied.

Cost awareness has increased the emphasis on what care is necessary and how care is to be implemented. Clear, concise, and accurate documentation is essential for capturing scarce resources for client care. Complete data related to admission, supplies used, monitoring activities, follow-up, education, and discharge planning are necessary for appropriate reimbursement.

Research

Nursing research in recent years has resulted in new approaches to client care as well as increasing professional knowledge. This research depends on complete and accurate documentation of client data (Eggland & Heinemann, 1994). Research has led to development of standardized formats for collecting and recording data and allows researchers to trend data to better predict health care needs of the community. In addition, research questions are often generated through review of aggregate data obtained from medical records.

FUNDAMENTALS OF CHARTING

No matter what format is used for documentation, the principles of documentation, such as legibility, brevity, sequence, corrections, omissions, signing, and confidentiality, remain the same. The client's chart is a legal record and therefore must conform to certain legal standards. Because ink indicates permanency, all entries in the record should be entered in black ink, unless the agency has a different policy. Black ink allows the chart to be easily copied and the record to be microfilmed with adequate readability.

Terminology

Entries include medical terminology and abbreviations in order to facilitate communication. Standard abbreviations are terms consistently used in the medical profession in an abridged format. Consistency in their use saves time and space. Health care facilities compile their own acceptable abbreviation lists that are used as much as possible in charting. It is your responsibility to become acquainted with accepted abbreviations in a particular agency. When in doubt, ask your nursing instructor and/or use the full term that will be understood regardless of where it is read.

Action Alert!
What may be an acceptable medical abbreviation in one geographical area or specialty area may be unheard or used differently in another area. For example, "PAT" is a fairly common abbreviation for paroxysmal atrial tachycardia, but this term may also be used on obstetrical units to abbreviate "pregnancy at term."

Symbols and medical terms comprising root words, prefixes, and suffixes are used to condense charting entries. When you break down words into root words and understand prefixes as well as suffixes added to root words, it helps you to decipher what unfamiliar words mean. Knowledge of these word parts assists in building an extensive vocabulary and should be committed to memory (Table 14–1).

Principles

Legibility

Legibility is essential when documenting in the health care record. Entries may be made in script or print—whichever is more legible. Proper use of terms and correct spelling are extremely important. Poor handwriting and spelling reflect negatively on you and could be translated by a jury as inadequate nursing care.

Action Alert!
Consider the consequences of trying to interpret charting that is not readable. Recalling information from illegible entries may be difficult or even impossible if the record is requested in a court of law several years after the entries were made.

Brevity

Charting entries should be as brief as possible. Sentences are stripped to essential components, eliminating all words that can be stripped without changing the intended meaning of the entry. This includes articles such as "a" and "the" as well as the subject of the sentence.

```
7/16/00   0700    Dentures removed/cleaned
                  with Polident. Oral
                  mucous membranes smooth,
                  s̄ lesions. Assisted c̄
                  bed bath, linens
                  changed.
                          —C. Lott, RN
```

TABLE 14–1
Symbols, Root Words, Prefixes, and Suffixes Used in Documentation

Term	Meaning	Term	Meaning
Symbols			
>	greater than	+	positive
<	less than	−	negative
↑	increase	M	murmur
↓	decrease	2°	secondary to
△	change	✔	check on
~	approximately		
Root Words			
adeno	gland	-oma	tumor
angio	vessel	ophtha	eye
arterio	artery	ortho	straight
artho	joint	osteo	bone
cardio	heart	oto	ear
cerebro	brain	-oxia	oxygen
cyst	bladder	patho	disease
cyto	cell	phlebo	vein
derma	skin	pnea, pneum	breathing, lungs
hemo	blood	pyelo	renal pelvis
hepato	liver	pyo	pus
hystero	uterus	pyro	heat
lith	stone: calculus	reno	kidney
meningo	meninges	thrombo	blood clot
myelo	bone marrow, spinal cord	thora	chest
myo	muscle	uro	urine
nephro	kidney	vaso	vessel
neuro	nerves	veno	vein
Prefixes			
a- or an-	without	hypo-	decreased
anti-	against	leuko-	white
bi-	twice, two	noct-	night
bio-	life	olig-	deficiency
brady-	slow	para-	beside
chole-	bile; gall	peri-	around
di-	double	poly-	many, multiple
dys-	difficult, painful	retro-	backward
ecto-	outside	supra-	above
endo-	within	tachy-	fast
hemi-	half	trans-	across
hyper-	above; excessive	uni-	one
Suffixes			
-cele	swelling, protrusion	-ostomy	artificial opening
-ectomy	removal	-otomy	incision of; cutting into
-emesis	vomiting	-penia	deficiency; lack of
-emia	blood	-plasty	repair of
-graph, -gram	tracing	-rhea	discharge
-itis	inflammation	-uria	urine

Note that neither the client's name nor the word "client" nor "patient" was charted because *all* entries are about the client. If necessary, the name of the person notified when the client is admitted, results of laboratory work, or any important detail that is to be reported by orders of the physician may be used in the charting. Using an actual name should be followed by the title or position of the person. This is not absolutely necessary but does eliminate confusion if the physician did not receive the information requested. An example would be the following:

```
7/16/00   0900   Report of STAT CBC
                 called to Jane Doe, RN
                 at Dr. Smith's office.
                            —C. Lott, RN
```

Completeness

Although brevity is essential, you should document all information necessary to explain the events of a shift. Anyone reading the documentation should have a clear picture of what took place or is being described. If necessary, direct quotes can be used to describe what a client said. The need for complete entries is critical when a record is used in a court of law. Recall of care provided several years after the event is difficult, if not impossible.

Action Alert!
From a legal perspective, entries not made in a client's record imply actions not taken or treatments not given. It is usually helpful to remember the saying "If you didn't chart it, you didn't do it."

Sequence and Timeliness

Recording of information on the client's record should be sequential. Noting the time and date are important for evaluating client care and legally. Every charting format has a single place for the date to be recorded, thus eliminating the need for documenting the date with every entry. The year should be included with the month and day because the chart is a legal document. However, the time must be included with each entry and should include AM or PM unless military time is used. It is best to note the exact time for each event.

The exact time events occur during the shift becomes critically important when pain medication is given, any follow-up care is necessary, a client's condition changes, or vital procedures are being planned such as organ transplants. The amount of time between events becomes crucial when certain medications are given or the chart is reviewed for auditing purposes.

Charting statements should be logically organized according to time (0800, 0830, 0900, etc.) and content. Just as you must use an organized sequence in order not to omit any information when assessing a client, documentation of data collection should also be logical in sequence. The statement is also more easily read when written in a logical pattern.

Entries should be logical according to whichever format of charting is being used (e.g., head-to-toe approach, body systems). If an entry is accidentally omitted, making the entry out of sequence, an addendum should be made.

Corrections

Two types of corrections usually made to a record are correcting a written entry and adding an entry later. First, individual agency policy may vary in the correct format to use in correcting an entry. Common policies include drawing a single line only or drawing a single line and writing the word "void" or "error" in the space above the incorrect entry, followed by the initials of the writer. The word "error" may still be used by an agency but is not recommended because it implies a wrong (Iyer & Camp, 1995). A single line instead of multiple lines is required in order to keep the incorrect entry legible.

Action Alert!
The use of erasures, "whiting out," or blackening the entry are not permitted because of the implication of "covering up" an error or mistake.

Second, in the event an entry needs to be made on the client's record for 0830, but another nurse has already made a notation for 0915, an addendum must be made. It would be incorrect to avoid entering the note on the chart. This information can and should be noted as an addendum. Consider the following example:

```
7/16/00   0910   Abdominal dressing
                 changed per Dr. Jones.
                 Suture line intact with
                 small amt.
                 serosanguineous drainage
                 noted at proximal edge.
                            —C. Lott, RN

          0930   Addendum 0830. Assisted
                 to chair per P.T. c̄
                 assistance X2 and use of
                 walker. C/O weakness and
                 instructed not to weight
                 bear on Ⓛ leg.
                            —C. Lott, RN
```

Note that in the previous example, the time of each entry remains sequential (0900, then 0930) although the appropriate time of the entry (0830) being documented late is made after the word *addendum*. This time (0830) is when the nursing action actually occurred. An addendum should be avoided as much as possible. However, it may be necessary to make an important late entry that makes the charting out of sequence. Charting in a timely manner throughout the shift instead of once or twice toward the end of the shift usually prevents entries from being out of sequence.

If information that is omitted is recalled a day or several days later, it should be noted in the current notes with the current date and time, followed by "addendum to nurse's notes of [month, day, and year]," followed by the entry. Agency policy will specify whether the term "late entry" rather than "addendum" should be used.

In rereading an entry, you often discover that certain words needed to clarify an entry have been accidentally omitted. An omitted word or phrase must not be squeezed between words in small letters or inserted above or below a written line. An addendum would need to be made to clarify the entry with the necessary description.

Omissions

Blank spaces are not to be left on the chart. As much as possible, you should write to the end of a line instead of leaving a blank space. Avoid writing outside of the lines (in the margin) of the charting form. A horizontal line is drawn through any empty space to the right margin in order to prevent later entries from being made in front of a signature.

Consider the following correct example:

```
7/16/00    0910    Penrose drain intact,
                   depressed, & draining
                   400 mL fluid. Reports no
                   discomfort. Foley
                   draining clear, yellow
                   urine with 300 mL output
                                   —C. Lott, RN
```

If a part of a page is blank at the end of the 24-hour time period, an "X" should be drawn through the remainder of the page. Notes should flow from shift to shift and a new set of notes started after 24 hours.

If it is necessary to recopy a page of the chart, the person copying the page should date and time the entry and write "Copied by . . ." followed by his or her signature. Copying a chart usually requires written consent by the client or responsible party.

Signing

The correct way to sign a notation in the client's record is using the first initial and full last name, followed by the abbreviation of the health care worker's position title (RN, LPN, SN). Some agencies require the full first and last names followed by an abbreviation of the individual's current position. You usually sign to the far right of the entry once it is complete.

Traditionally, SN has been the accepted abbreviation for student nurse. Even if the student has another title such as LPN (Licensed Practical Nurse), he or she is to use the abbreviation for student nurse when functioning in that capacity. The student nurse may also be required to write the initials of the school affiliation along with the title SN. A written signature must follow every entry into a client's record.

The correct format would be as follows:

```
7/16/00    1530    Awake & oriented to
                   time, place, & person.
                   Skin warm and dry.
                                   —C. Lott, RN

           1600    CBC drawn per lab.
                                   —C. Lott, RN

           1645    To radiology via
                   wheelchair for CXR.
                                   —C. Lott, RN
```

Confidentiality

All client records are confidential files that require permission and often a signature from the client in order to be copied. Information within the chart is often of a personal matter as well as legal evidence of the care provided and should be available to the health team members only. Client records are not accessible to insurance companies, significant others, research teams, or third parties without the written permission of the client. Clients themselves must sign and submit a request for their information from a medical file.

Action Alert!
It is the responsibility of the nurse and other health team members to maintain the confidentiality concerning medical records within any medical facility.

Do's and Don't's of Charting

Proper charting should follow the principles of effective documentation and use correct terminology as well as abbreviations. Charting quickly may lead to incomplete entries or rather odd-sounding statements that do not imply the meaning intended. Thinking through the entry before writing it and rereading the entry may eliminate notations that may sound strange or even funny and avoid embarrassment. Documentation that is clear, accurate, and legally sound requires following certain do's and don't's of charting (Box 14–2).

CONTENT OF CHARTING

Although agencies vary in specific requirements about what needs to be charted, you should develop a systematic approach to documentation of client care. The system may involve head-to-toe, body systems, problem-oriented, human needs, functional health patterns, or any other organized approach for deriving significant data to be documented. Regardless of the choice of organizational method, there are guidelines that should be followed. All significant client care should be documented either in narrative (progress) notes or on **flow sheets** (forms used to document data

---

BOX 14–2

DO'S AND DON'T'S OF CHARTING

DO check the name on the chart before making an entry.

DO chart brief, concise, and complete entries. Eliminate all unnecessary words.

DO sign each entry or follow agency policy for initialing entries.

DO use objective, measurable terms.

DO use black ink.

DO write neatly and legibly.

DO use standard abbreviations whenever necessary and only those acceptable to the agency.

Do use quotes to relate what the client actually said whenever necessary.

DO write entries logically and sequentially.

DO make addendums as needed.

DO make entries about nursing care as close to the time of delivery as possible.

DO report failure of client to follow treatment regimens and to take medications or receive treatments, and the rationale given by the client.

DON'T sign anyone else's entry or document for someone else.

DON'T skip lines.

DON'T use the word "client" or "patient" throughout the document.

DON'T write opinions or biased statements.

DON'T make entries suggesting an error or unsafe practice.

DON'T repeat narratively if flow sheets and other forms are used for the same information.

---

that can be more easily followed in graphic or tabular form).

Upon admission to a facility, most health care agencies require a health history to be completed followed by a current needs assessment. These may be combined or on separate forms. The format and degree of detail will vary according to the health care agency. The registered nurse on the unit usually completes the initial health history form, which then becomes a permanent part of the chart. The current needs assessment may be completed by the same person taking the health history or the person assuming responsibility for care of the client. Structured forms usually provide a checklist format with which you can easily check or circle observations. Unstructured forms usually list areas to be assessed, with you writing narrative observations. The initial assessment leads to identification of the client's problems. If no specific form is used by the agency for this purpose, it is written in the narrative notes. Following these ad-

mission forms, documentation of the client's arrival and subsequent care needs to be made.

Types of Entries

Various types of entries compose the documentation made by you: admit notes for a newly admitted client, change-of-shift notes, assessment findings, interval or progress notes, transfer and discharge notes, client teaching notes, and descriptions of observations.

Admit Notes

Upon assuming responsibility for a new client who just entered the facility, you usually record an admit note. An **admit note** is the opening nurse's note acknowledging the arrival of a new client. Following the admit note, a narrative entry noting the complete assessment is made and followed by notes regarding the client's current status at intervals with notations of any changes in condition. If the admission history or assessment form provides a place for this information, an additional narrative note is not necessary.

The admit note usually includes the following: age, gender, how the client arrived, where the client came from, medical diagnosis, chief complaint, general appearance, treatments in progress, allergies, vital signs (if required by the agency or if abnormal), notification of physician, and STAT laboratory work or orders that have been completed (Fig. 14–1).

Change-of-Shift Notes

At the change of shift, you do not need to document an opening admit note for a client who has been in the facility for a period of time. Instead, you usually begin the documentation with the client assessment made on rounds. Any format is acceptable but should include a thorough assessment of the client's current status followed by interval notes regarding any change in the client's status. It may be a requirement of the facility to note that a report was received or given and by whom.

```
7/16/00   0830   Shift report received
                 from S. Smith, RN. Awake
                 & alert on rounds . . .
                 [continue note with
                 current assessment data]
```

Assessment Notes

After an opening admit note or beginning shift note, a complete assessment of the current status of the client should follow. Documentation of the complete assessment may be entered using different formats: narrative, flow chart, or both. Various methods for charting any entry narratively are acceptable: head-to-toe as-

7/14/00 | 1400 | 68-year-old female admitted to room 268A via stretcher from ER with dx. Fx. Ⓛ hip. P 92, BP 142/89, R 21, T 98.8 C/O pain to Ⓛ hip from mid-thigh to greater trochanter area, marked bruising noted in same area s̄ edema at present. Stated fell while gardening and unable to "get up again," lives alone, neighbor called 911. IV of D5W infusing at TKO rate to Ⓡ upper arm s̄ signs of infiltration or inflammation c̄ 950 cc TBA. Nursing history and assessment noted, NKA, Dr. Parker notified of admit, new orders noted. ————————— C. Lott, RN

Figure 14–1. Example of an admit note.

sessment, body systems, functional health patterns, or nursing diagnosis (Fig. 14–2).

Interval or Progress Notes

After the complete assessment is made, interval notes should be entered. Agencies may use either the term *interval notes* or *progress notes*. **Interval notes** or **progress notes** are nursing notes entered at various times during a shift that reflect any aspect of change in client condition or anything affecting the client such as tests, STAT or PRN medications, and procedures. Content to include in an interval note is determined by you and the condition of the client but may include the following: treatments, medications, new orders, ambulation, periods of rest, presence of visitors, and client symptoms.

When you make rounds on clients, the status of their condition is noted. Documentation at intervals usually means every 2 to 4 hours. This will vary depending on the documentation format used by the agency and perhaps the unit within the agency. In more critical situations, or whenever a client's condition changes, entries may be required more often than every 2 hours. Charting more frequently is a nursing judgment as long as the agency guidelines are followed for the minimal amount of documentation needed.

If the interval is too long between notations or there is lack of sufficient explanation leading up to a serious change in status, the documentation is not acceptable. The status of the client may remain unchanged on rounds and can be noted as such by you.

Transfer and Discharge Notes

When a client is transferred to another facility or to another unit, whether temporarily or permanently, you should write a transfer note. A **transfer note** is a nursing note that reflects the movement of a client from one location to another either within the agency or to another agency. Policies should exist on every unit for specific content to include in a transfer note. Generally, the notation includes reason for transfer, method of transportation, person receiving report, notification of physicians or family members, and the general condition of the client, including vital signs and treatments in progress (Fig. 14–3).

A similar notation should be made when a client is sent for a test within the same facility, but less information is usually required. Information to be included depends on the client's condition and may include place (e.g., laboratory, x-ray), method of transfer (e.g., wheelchair, stretcher), persons accompanying the client, attachments, level of consciousness, and vital signs.

When the client returns to a unit, a note should be made that includes appropriate assessment of the condition, time of arrival, method of transfer, and attach-

7/14/00	1430	Awake, alert, oriented x3. PERRLA. Stated feels "tired and exhausted from experience." Resp. even, non-labored. Lungs clear in all lobes. Heart sounds normal S1 and S2, regular rhythm. Radial pulses equal, regular, and palpable + 2/3. IV to (R) upper arm of D5W infusing at TKO rate c̄ 900 cc TBA. Capillary refill <3 sec. bilaterally. Abdomen soft c̄ active bowel sounds in all 4 quadrants. Denies difficulty c̄ bowel or bladder. (L) hip bruised, non-edematous, painful to touch. Trochanter roll in place to keep leg aligned. Peripheral pulses palpable, + 2/3, equal. No edema to extremities. Feet warm and dry c̄ capillary refill <3 sec. SR up x2, neighbor at bedside. ——— *C. Lott, RN*

Figure 14–2. Example of an assessment note.

ments. Depending on the reason for the absence from the unit, specific assessment findings may need to be included in this entry, such as vital signs, level of consciousness, and ability to swallow.

When a client is discharged from the hospital, a discharge note should be made to close the chart. A **discharge note** is a nursing note that reflects the circumstances around the release of a client from a facility. This entry should not be made until all other necessary entries have been completed. The specific information needed for a discharge note may vary according to the type of facility. Some agencies may require a summary of the client's stay showing her improvement or reason for discharge, client teaching, and a note addressing the client's understanding of the self-care needed. Similar to the transfer note, a discharge summary should generally include preparations for the discharge, the time of departure, method of transportation, family members present, condition of the client, vital signs, and any necessary paperwork given to the client, which may include prescriptions (Fig. 14–4).

Client Teaching Notes

Instructions given to a client and perhaps even a family member need careful documentation. Client teaching may include medications, wound care, diabetic care, activity restrictions/progression, or diet. The method of teaching may include videos, discussion, reading, demonstration, and return demonstration. The content that is taught as well as the method of teaching needs to be documented. In addition, the time frame, person responsible for teaching, and the results of the teaching need to be charted. If more than just the client is involved, noting who attended the teaching session is important. If pamphlets or booklets are given to the client for further reading, these should be noted. How the client responds to the teaching should be documented. Whether the client and/or family can return-demonstrate a skill such as wound care or explain the content in their own words is essential to evaluate the teaching. All teaching that occurs should be noted, including reinforcement of information already taught. Special forms may be used in an agency by staff assigned to this responsibility.

| 7/18/00 | 0900 | Transfer arrangements to skilled facility for services of Dr. Warren complete. Hospital chart copied, to be sent with client. ——————— ——————————— C. Lott, RN |
| | 1110 | Transferred to skilled facility by stretcher per AST Ambulance Service. Neighbor present, copy of hospital chart given to ambulance attendant, J. Wild. No treatments in progress. No acute distress, skin warm and dry. Color flesh-toned. Ⓛ hip incision clean and dry s̄ irritation or redness. Denies pain at present. Peripheral pulses palpable, + 2/4, and equal. T 98.9, P 76 , R 18, BP 132/78. ——— ——————————— C. Lott, RN |

Figure 14–3. Example of a transfer note.

| 7/30/00 | 1530 | Dr. Warren visited c̄ orders to d/c current meds. Neighbor notified and on the way. Home health nurse S. Beil, RN, notified of discharge and arrangements for first visit made. PT visited concerning walker and reinforced proper use. ——— K. Smith, RN |
| | 1615 | Neighbor present. HL in Ⓡ upper arm discontinued. Site s̄ redness or warmth. T 98⁶, P 68, R 22, BP 110/72. No complaints. Skin warm and dry. Ⓛ hip incision healing, intact s̄ inflammation or irritation. Pedal pulses + 2/3, equal, feet warm and dry. Discharge instructions given c̄ prescription for meds. Neighbor stated she would pick up her prescriptions on the way home. Discharged per wc s̄ distress. ——— K. Smith, RN |

Figure 14–4. Example of a discharge note.

Even when client educators teach the client and/or family, you should note their presence in the narrative.

Descriptions of Observations

Nurses' notes should be recorded objectively. You state observations rather than opinion. For example, if you believe that a client is less alert today than yesterday, you should describe the client's response today rather than stating "not as alert today."

Although subjective data presented by the client are included in the nurse's notes, they should be clearly labeled as such. This could be denoted by preceding the subjective data by "states," indicating that the client is relating this information or by using quotation marks around the client's exact words.

Vague documentation should be avoided at all times. Words such as "seems to be" or "apparently" should not be used. It is more descriptive to document the behavior that led to that conclusion. Similarly, adjectives such as *good, some, a little, bad,* and *better* should be avoided because these terms are relative and may have different meanings for people using them.

Although the term *normal* may be used to describe some physical assessment, it is usually not the best choice for most entries. Of course, unflattering adjectives that characterize the client's behavior (e.g., obnoxious, ignorant) should never be used.

Action Alert!

Nurse's notes should be written so that anyone reading them would have an accurate, objective picture of the client or the facts pertaining to a client situation.

SYMPTOMS AND COMPLAINTS

Any symptom or complaint should be documented in detail. These may include subjective or objective data and should be specific in terms of location, duration, intensity, amount, size, and frequency (as indicated).

DRESSINGS, TUBES, OR ATTACHED DEVICES

Observations of tubes should be documented in the initial entry of each shift and at least every 2 hours thereafter. Documentation should be more frequent when the condition is warranted. Notations about dressings should include the location of the dressing, secure attachment of dressing to client, and amount as well as a description of any drainage observed. If a dressing is removed, the condition of the skin under the dressing should be described (e.g., edges are approximated; any redness, edema, drainage, sutures, or staples) (Fig. 14–5).

Tubes providing intravenous, nasogastric, or gastrostomy feeding should be observed for what is being administered and the rate of flow. In addition, the infusion site should be noted for any tenderness, redness, edema, or warmth. An IV site is usually assessed at least every 2 hours. Notation of the IV access may be included on the flow sheet. The type and condition of any feeding or gastrostomy tube (e.g., Levin, Keo-feed,

Peg) should also be recorded, along with documentation of patency and proper placement. Use of a pump with any tubing should be noted for reimbursement purposes (see Fig. 14–5). If an agency policy requires the use of a pump with certain age groups or clients with specific conditions, this can be noted as "use of a pump according to policy."

Notations concerning any drainage tubes should include location and patency of the tube, attachment to any drainage or suction system, and a description of any drainage. Description of drainage should include color, character, and amount. Specific amounts are recorded on the intake and output (I&O) flow sheet at specified intervals (see Fig. 14–5).

MEDICATIONS AND TREATMENTS

Most agencies maintain a medication administration record for the purpose of documenting all medications and treatments. When a medication/treatment is given STAT or "as needed" (PRN) based on your judgment, a statement should also be charted in the progress notes as to the events that led to this decision. For example, if a client is given a medication that has been ordered PRN for pain, you should document the need for the medication along with an adequate description of the pain (e.g., location, type, intensity). A follow-up note should also be recorded at an appropriate interval in order to evaluate the effectiveness of the medication or treatment. When documenting the effects of a medication or treatment, care should be taken to record the information objectively (see Fig. 14–5).

There are times when a medication or treatment may not be given as ordered. This may be due to your judgment that it would be harmful for the client at that time, or perhaps the client refuses the treatment. In any case, withholding of the treatment should be documented along with the explanation for the action. It is also appropriate to notify the physician if any routine medication is withheld and this, too, should be documented. An example for Mrs. Geraldine Peters might be as follows:

```
7/16/00   0900   C/O sharp, constant pain
                 in Ⓛ hip, requesting
                 pain medication. BP
                 98/50, P 62, RB 10.
                 Oriented X3. Responds to
                 verbal stimuli but
                 easily returns to sleep.
                 Need to wait for pain
                 medicine explained due
                 to low BP & resp. and
                 length of time since
                 last injection 3 hours
                 (order is for q4 hrs).
                 Will reassess in 15
                 minutes.
                        —C. Lott, RN
```

Dressing	7/15/00	2030	Dressing on ⓛ hip c̄ red dime-sized area of drainage. Dressing changed. Staples present, incision c̄ dime-shaped area of redness noted at lateral end. ———————— ————————— S. Richards, RN
Tubes	7/15/00	2030	IV D5W in ® antecubital space infusing at 50 cc/hr c̄ 300 cc TBA. Site free of redness or edema. Hemovac to ⓛ hip intact, depressed c̄ 50 cc red drainage. — ————————— S. Richards, RN
Attached Devices	7/15/00	2030	Foley catheter to GU bag patent and draining 300 cc clear, amber urine. ——— ————————— S. Richards, RN
Medication and Treatment	7/15/00	2030	Holding ⓛ leg and C/O throbbing pain at incision area. Tylox tabs ii given PO. SR up x4, instructed not to get OOB s̄ assistance, call bell in reach. ——— ————————— S. Richards, RN
		2245	States "feels much better." No nonverbal expression of discomfort noted. ——— ————————— S. Richards, RN
Valuables	7/14/00	1430	Jewelry and keys placed in folder #2396, sent to admit office c̄ J. Zimmerman, clerk. ——— S. Richards, RN

Figure 14–5. Descriptions of observations.

In the event of a medication error, documentation of the error, the follow-up, assessment of the client, and notification of the physician must be completed. Most facilities require that an incident report be filed describing carefully and objectively the error or incident, the action taken, assessment findings, and follow-up information. All medications, whether ordered or in error, are usually noted on the Medication Administration Record (MAR). Documenting in the narrative that an error was made and that an incident report was completed is not necessary and never recommended.

OBSERVATIONS OF PSYCHOSOCIAL STATUS

In addition to physical needs, you should document significant data related to psychosocial status. You assess the client's sensorium in relation to level of consciousness and orientation to time, place, and person. Any confusion or change in consciousness is significant and should be documented specifically.

The safety and security needs of clients seeking health care are frequently threatened, resulting in anxiety. Any evidence of fear or anxiety should be documented on the client's record. If a client decides to leave the facility against the advice of her physician (unless ordered by law to be admitted), you note the same information as a discharge but chart "left AMA" (which stands for "against medical advice"). If the client states a reason for leaving, this should be included in the narrative. The physician should be notified of any AMA situation and an entry made in the chart as to this notification.

ACTIVITIES OF DAILY LIVING

Activities of daily living (ADLs) are documented primarily on flow sheets and may be recorded by anyone administering care. If a flow sheet is not available, ADLs should be noted in the narrative charting, which is described later in this chapter. You should, however, check that AM and PM care are administered and charted. Information recorded related to AM care includes type of bath, oral hygiene, change of linen, and the type of assistance needed. The type of assistance and the number of health care workers needed to move a client from place to place should also be included. Information recorded related to PM care includes oral hygiene and toiletry essentials.

Examples of ways to note transfer needs include independent, minimal supervision and/or assistance; continuous supervision and/or assistance of one person; continuous assistance of two persons; or total care. ADLs can also be charted (using similar terminology) as to the client's degree of independence.

VALUABLES

Describe any valuables such as jewelry in general terms. Instead of "solid gold, one-carat diamond ring," a better description might be "yellow ring with clear stone." When a client enters a facility with jewelry or valuables that need to be secured during his or her stay, an entry should be made that these items were sent to the appropriate department. The detailed description of specific items should be included with the belongings rather than charted (see Fig. 14–5). The actual description of the jewelry, as well as the items and amount of money in the wallet, is usually described on the outside of the folder in which they are placed. Agencies may require the signature of two health care professionals on any documentation of valuables with a copy placed in the client's chart. If valuables are sent home with a family member, it is important to document the name of the person who took the valuables and the relationship to the client.

SPIRITUAL CARE

Spiritual care is often neglected in documentation but is an important entry for many clients. Entries may need to be included that describe signs and symptoms of spiritual distress, symbols or articles of spiritual meaning, rituals practiced, source of hope, and expressions of grief.

SAFETY CONCERNS

A significant area needing detailed and complete documentation is that of safety issues for the client, particularly the elderly or immobile client. Although flow sheets now include many of these safety concerns, narrative charting may still be needed. Regardless of where the information is written, documenting safety measures taken for each client while in a facility is essential. Examples of important safety concerns include side rails, ambulation, past medication or surgery, ability to use call lights, knowledge of emergency call lights, use of restraints, offering toiletry if immobile, falls, and transporting clients. Client teaching about safety should be adequately documented.

Many facilities have special guidelines for including safety concerns, and these may be mandatory notations for every client. However, you have the right and responsibility to note safety issues in a factual manner as often as needed (Table 14–2). The policies for documenting safety issues should be clear to all employees.

An *incident form* is usually required for documentation in the event of a client fall or accident. In addition to this form (which usually stays with the agency and not on the chart), a narrative entry should be made that lists factual information about the incident. A notation that an incident form was filled out is not

TABLE 14–2
Necessary Charting Entries for Safety Concerns

Medication administration	SR placed up if sedating, instructions given not to get OOB without assistance.
Transporting client	SR placed up, attendant with client at all times.
Admit	Instructions given on using call light and the difference in regular and emergency light.
Restraints	Notation every 2 hours; offered water, meal, bathroom privileges; ROM checked.
Ambulation	Assistance required, use of house shoes, use of assistive devices such as walker, cane.
Change in LOC or sensorium from a recent major event such as surgery	Instructions given not to get up the first time without health care assistance. VS taken if dizziness experienced or change in LOC. SR up if disoriented, notification of doctor if status changes, presence of sitter or family member.
Falls	Actual facts as reported by client, family, and health care worker should be included. Actual assessment findings upon first discovering the accident, including the position client was in when found, notification of physician, family, or house supervisor. Also specific accounts leading up to the event. Report what was done, such as x-rays and notification of physician. Note the history of falls during last hospitalization or at home when admitting a client.

documented because incident forms are for agency use only. You should present the facts related to the event and accurate assessment findings after the incident. It is often necessary and suggested that actual quotes from the client be used. Entries should be as objective as possible, particularly if the accounts of the incident are inaccurate or different between the health care workers and the client.

Significant Notations for Special Populations

Documentation entries may need to be made for special groups such as the elderly, children, and culturally diverse clients. Issues specific to a client such as language barriers or dietary customs of a specific culture may need to be noted. Life span considerations in the elderly as well as children are often a part of the charting that may not be as necessary for other clients.

Elderly Clients

Special attention should be taken to include accurate and complete descriptions of the skin, ADLs, mobility, mental status, and the affective behavior of elderly clients. Notes should include how prepared an elderly

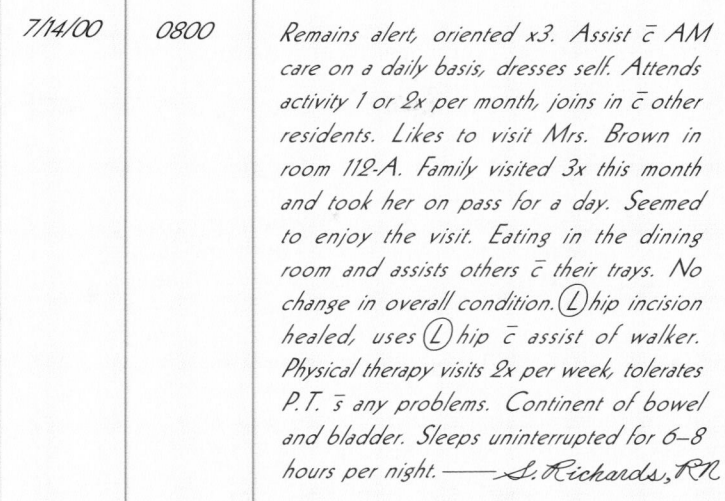

| 7/14/00 | 0800 | *Remains alert, oriented x3. Assist c̄ AM care on a daily basis, dresses self. Attends activity 1 or 2x per month, joins in c̄ other residents. Likes to visit Mrs. Brown in room 112-A. Family visited 3x this month and took her on pass for a day. Seemed to enjoy the visit. Eating in the dining room and assists others c̄ their trays. No change in overall condition. (L) hip incision healed, uses (L) hip c̄ assist of walker. Physical therapy visits 2x per week, tolerates P.T. s̄ any problems. Continent of bowel and bladder. Sleeps uninterrupted for 6–8 hours per night.——S. Richards, RN* |

Figure 14–6. Example of an entry in a long-term care facility.

client is to go home, discharge planning beginning from the day of admittance, and any emotional needs. Progress in the ability to carry out ADLs is essential throughout a client's stay to show adequate ability to perform self-care upon discharge.

Pediatric Clients

Special attention should be paid to including observations about the relationship between the parents and child, dependence of the child on the parent, developmental level of the child for age, ability of child to play, language used by child and parents, and any excessive emotional needs for pediatric clients. Examples might include the following: mother rocking child and reading a book; speaks in complete, simple sentences; or child noted to be able to stack blocks, play hide and seek, and entertain self with colors. Accurate and descriptive documentation of the physical assessment of children in emergency departments is crucial, especially if abuse is suspected.

Clients From Nondominant Cultures

Suggested areas for documentation with culturally diverse clients include fluency of English, ability to read and write, native language, beliefs about cause of illness, special concerns related to religious beliefs, dietary differences (foods excluded or preferred), and the need for individualized, uninterrupted time for meditation.

Extended and Long-Term Care

The use of a classification system to show acuity and specifications of the amount or type of equipment/supplies is often included in the documentation for extended-care and long-term care facilities. Extended-care facilities may have additional special forms that are used to document group sessions with family members, planning a home visit in preparation for discharge, or visits with social workers to discuss dis-

charge options. Long-term care facilities may require weekly or monthly charting in a summary manner as opposed to daily. You generally make a narrative entry about such items as the client's abilities, progress, or degenerative changes (Fig. 14–6). Interval or progress notes as described earlier are also made throughout the shift to note the client's condition. Box 14–3 is a list of guidelines for documentation in these types of facilities.

BOX 14–3

GUIDELINES FOR EXTENDED AND LONG-TERM CARE

- Know requirements of the regulating body of the agency: quarterly reviews, when to document.
- Note phone calls, relative visits, interaction with other clients.
- Verify how nurses spend their time with the client on a visit and issues concerning reimbursement.
- Be specific in indicating progress or lack thereof: ambulated 10 feet on 7/21/99, progressed to 15 feet on 7/22/99.
- Record supplies used.
- Note activities performed by nurses for other departments on the weekends including CPM machines, physical therapy, ECGs, etc.
- Describe a clear picture that includes fine details: Could not open milk carton or use utensils; after meat cut and packages opened, client fed self without problems.
- Include entries that reflect progress or lack of progress of client goals and objectives as reflected on the plan of care.
- Include the client's response to drug therapies.

Home Health Guidelines

Documentation in a home health care situation is often different from documenting in an acute care facility because of the need to justify the visit by a professional nurse. Home health nurses usually document an initial assessment with a complete database. Visits thereafter are usually progress notes for each visit and include direct care, teaching or instructions given, performance of skills, and evaluation of homebound status. Home health nurses use progress notes written in narrative format that should be consistent with other disciplines charting on the same client. With each visit, the need for the help of a professional health care worker should be mentioned. Reimbursement for the visit is directly related to the accuracy and wording of the documentation showing a need for professional assistance. General guidelines are offered for beginning nurses in a home health setting (Table 14–3).

Additional suggestions for effective charting in a home health situation include the following:

- Leave out extraneous information that could affect reimbursement.
- Record all equipment and supplies used at the visit.
- Avoid vague statements like "doing better" or "no acute distress."
- Monitor new procedures to see if all personnel are doing the same thing.
- Note safety concerns such as "throw rugs removed from path to BR."

TABLE 14–3
Guidelines for Beginning Nurses in a Home Health Setting

Direct skilled care: Diverse and involved care that can be provided only by trained professionals	Catheter changes, catheter care Wound care Treatments: venipuncture, suctioning Injections/administering medications Ostomy care Aseptic technique Heat treatments Tube feedings
Client teaching: A part of any skill done	Inclusion of client and family Response to information Ability to perform activity independently Verbalizes understanding of the instruction Booklets or educational material left for client or family
Homebound status: Inability to leave home to obtain similar health care services at a clinic, doctors office, or outpatient clinic	Reason for status on admit and weekly thereafter Support of other disciplines Evaluation

- Key terms in home health include *assessment, instructions,* and *skilled care.*
- Know which medical equipment can be provided and document why.
- Home health nurses must be especially confident in knowing definitions and in medication administration. All charting should be made with the assumption that the documents will probably be audited.

Following is an example of home health charting:

```
7/16/00   0900   Wound area remains open,
                 wound edges irregular;
                 sacral wound area
                 intact, stage 2 has
                 decreased in size: 2 cm
                 L and 2 cm W since
                 1/15/00. No change in
                 size of (L) heel pressure
                 ulcer. Family turning
                 client q 2 hours and
                 keeping heels clear of
                 mattress as directed.
                 Caregivers still unable
                 to perform wound care.
                         —K. Hobson, RN
```

Problem areas frequently identified in charting for home health care clients include

- Lack of a clear picture of what is going on with the client.
- Discrepancies between what went on with the client and what appeared in the chart.
- Difficulty in determining the client's status, functional limitations, current level of activity, or homebound status.
- Why the nurse is seeing and needs to continue seeing the client.
- Failure to document for Medicare reimbursement.

Special Entries

Finally, several situations require special notations in which you should make complete and accurate explanations. First, notification of physicians should include the time, how they were notified (e.g., direct call, beeper), and why. When the physician responds and what action was taken should be noted as a follow-up to the phone call. Failure on the part of the physician to respond should be noted as well. Second, any follow-up entry should emphasize why actions were taken, what was done, and the client's response.

Third, charting results of specific laboratory tests or nursing actions when administering certain classifications of medications is generally expected (Table 14–4). For example, adjusting a heparin drip according to

TABLE 14–4
Examples of Charting Entries for Medications

Irritating medications such as hydroxyzine (Vistaril) or iron	Must chart IM "z-track"
Antiarrhythmics	Change in the cardiac rhythm
Pain medication	Safety measure after administered, vital signs, relief obtained
Antianginals/ antihypertensives	Vital signs
Insulin administration	Glucose value before administration, condition of client during peak times
Diuretics	Recent electrolyte values, signs or symptoms of electrolyte loss
Heparin or anticoagulants	Coagulation laboratory tests: PT, PTT
Allergies	What specific response the client has

a sliding scale order would include noting the partial thromboplastin time (PTT) value and the adjusted rate of the heparin. Documentation of a blood pressure or pulse is required for many classes of cardiac medications such as digoxin (Lanoxin) or antihypertensives.

MEDICAL RECORD AND DOCUMENTATION FORMATS

Types of Medical Records

Medical records have traditionally been organized in one of two ways: source-oriented or problem-oriented. The emergence of case management has introduced critical pathways as another method of organizing client care information.

Problem-Oriented Records

Problem-oriented medical records are a form of documentation originally designed to organize information according to identified client problems, with all members of the health team documenting information sequentially. Problem-oriented records consist of four components: the database, the problem list, initial plans for each problem, and progress notes. All members of the health care team make entries on the same record using the same problem list. Problems are added to the list using the language appropriate for the health care provider making the entry. For example, physicians could add medical diagnoses, whereas nurses could use the form of nursing diagnoses. The primary advantages of this system are the inclusion of a common problem list and that progress related to each problem can be monitored more easily.

Source-Oriented Records

Source-oriented medical records are a type of medical record with separate divisions according to health discipline (e.g., medicine, nursing, laboratory, respiratory care). These records include information about care given, the client's response to care, and other events documented chronologically and sequentially in a specific location in the record designated for the particular health team member making the entry.

Clinical Pathways

Clinical pathways, also called critical pathways, may be recorded using an interdisciplinary approach or organized by health care discipline. Outcomes and interventions are derived collaboratively and reviewed and updated regularly. Any exceptions (variations) are documented along with suspected causes for the variance and actions taken in response.

Charting Formats

Regardless of the organization of the medical record itself, health care agencies may choose from a variety of formats for documentation. The format chosen depends on the type of agency, the primary purposes of documentation, and the types of health care workers involved. Regardless of the format, the principles, the mechanics, and generally even the content remain the same. How the content is recorded, however, depends on the format chosen. This discussion addresses several formats currently used as well as the use of flow sheets for documenting relevant data.

Formats for documentation may be narrative, problem-focused or process-focused, or a combination of these. Source-oriented records that separate parts of the chart by disciplines might still use a problem-oriented approach to documentation of nursing care. Most formats also incorporate flow sheets to some extent.

Narrative Charting

Narrative charting is a method of charting that provides information in the form of statements that describe events surrounding client care. It is relatively unstructured, providing you with flexibility in determining how information is recorded. It allows anyone reading the record to easily follow a sequence of events. Medical as well as nursing interventions may be included and may relate to more than one identified problem at the same time. It also allows inclusion of significant events related to the client that might not be directly related to an identified client problem.

There are, however, some disadvantages to the use of narrative notes. This method is time-consuming and makes retrieval of information and tracking of progress and outcomes more difficult. In addition, the lack of specific prompting of notations in terms of times or identified problems often leads to entries that fail to sufficiently address client problems. Entries may also include unnecessary or meaningless notations simply because you feel compelled to write "something" at periodic time intervals. You should

| 7/17/00 | 0220 | Awake, alert, and oriented x3. Skin warm and dry. IV D5W infusing in Ⓡ lower arm @ 100 cc/hr c̄ 450 cc TBA. Site s̄ redness or edema. Reports pain in Ⓛ hip. States pain is 8 on a scale of 1–10. Tylox tabs ii given PO. ——————— S. Richards, RN |
| | 0245 | Sleeping. Siderails ↑ x4. ——————— S. Richards, RN |

Figure 14–7. Example of narrative charting.

avoid duplication of content already included on the record in order to reduce discrepancies in data.

Narrative documentation can easily be combined with flow sheets, however, to retain the advantage of complete descriptions when desirable with the brevity of the flow sheet when descriptive data is not needed (Iyer & Camp, 1995). An example of notations using the narrative approach is found in Figure 14–7.

Charting by Exception

Charting by exception provides documentation in progress notes only if data are significant or abnormal. This format reduces lengthy and repetitive charting and allows client progress to be followed more easily. This system provides comprehensive flow sheets for documentation of both medical and nursing orders. Provided assessment is within normal limits or unchanged from the previous assessment, no narrative progress notes are necessary. Charting by exception is predicated on establishment of norms for assessment, with forms varying by agency. For example, the 24-hour assessment example included in Figure 14–8 and the entry made in Figure 14–9 are examples of charting by exception.

The flow sheet provides a column for each hour in a 24-hour period. You simply place a check mark (✔) or initials in each block to indicate findings at a given time. If assessment findings are normal, no other documentation is needed. Specific notations can be included in the block that indicate specific observations. In Figure 14–8, the notation of 100% is included under diet to indicate the proportion of food consumed. An arrow (↓) is placed in the block indicating bed position. If the nurse initials findings considered abnormal, a detailed description is required in the progress notes.

Although charting by exception is time-efficient and reduces duplicative entries, it is more difficult to identify omissions in care, and details are often limited. It is also more difficult to follow the nursing process using this format (Tammelleo, 1994).

APIE and PIE Charting

APIE charting and **PIE charting** are methods of charting that evolved from the problem-oriented type of medical record and that are designed to allow docu-

mentation using the nursing process. The acronym APIE stands for

A = assessment
P = problem identification
I = interventions
E = evaluation

The acronym PIE stands for

P = problem identification
I = interventions
E = evaluation

The process begins with an admission assessment that is usually completed on a separate form and initiation of a problem list (may be in the form of nursing diagnosis or problem statement) based on the initial assessment. An example of a problem list for Ms. Peters is found in Figure 14–10, followed by examples of data entries using the APIE format (Fig. 14–11).

Some agencies include data to support the problem identified by adding "as evidenced by (AEB)" to the diagnosis. For example, *Pain related to surgical incision AEB. guarding of incision and verbal complaints of pain.* Some problem lists may also include goals or expected outcomes for each problem.

Documentation of client care is focused on interventions and evaluation related to problems listed. Each entry in the progress notes is preceded by the date, time, and problem number, along with the indication as to whether the entry relates to implementation or evaluation (see Fig. 14–11).

Each problem should be evaluated at least once per shift (and some agencies may require more frequent entries). Only information related to implementation or evaluation of problems on the problem list are included in the progress notes. Once the initial or admission assessment is complete, routine assessment is recorded each shift on a flow sheet. An "assessment" entry is not required in the progress notes unless there is a change in the client's status. For example, if the client in the situation just introduced complains of constipation, it would be noted as in Figure 14–11. Problem No. 4 would also be added to the problem list. As problems are resolved, the date is indicated on the problem list.

Advantages of the APIE format include easy reference to specific problems and use of the nursing pro-

DATE: 7/15/00 DIAGNOSIS ORIF (L) hip

ALLERGIES NKDA

SIGNATURES:

	7a - 7p	Initials		7p - 7a	Initials
NURSE	C Lott, RN	(CL)			( )
NURSE		( )			( )
TECH/ASST		( )			( )
OTHER		( )			( )

NURSING 24 HOUR ASSESSMENT

SYSTEM		7A	8	9	10	11	12P	1	2	3	4	5	6	7	8	9	10	11	12A	1	2	3	4	5	6
NEUROLOGICAL		7A	8	9	10	11	12P	1	2	3	4	5	6	7	8	9	10	11	12A	1	2	3	4	5	6
NORMAL	ALERT-APPROP. FOR AGE										CL														
	ORIENTED X3										CL														
	MAEW										CL														
ABNORMAL	LETHARGIC																								
	DISORIENTED																								
	UNRESPONSIVE																								
	PAIN SCALE (Rate 1-10)										8	4													

Discharge Outcome: Patient will demonstrate optimal contact with reality; maintains usual reality orientation; regains/maintains usual level of consciousness free of adverse neurologic symptoms/complications.

CARDIOVASCULAR		7A	8	9	10	11	12P	1	2	3	4	5	6	7	8	9	10	11	12A	1	2	3	4	5	6
NORMAL	HEART RATE (WNL For Age)										CL														
	CAPILLARY REFILL (2-3 SEC)										CL														
	RAD. PULSES EQUAL & STRONG R, L, Bil.										CL														
	PED. PULSES EQUAL & STRONG R, L, Bil.										CL														
ABNORMAL	IRREGULAR RATE																								
	WEAK PULSES																								
	ABSENT PULSES																								
	EDEMA																								
	ECG RATE																								
	ECG RHYTHM																								

Discharge Outcome: Patient displays vital signs within patient's normal range. • Patient demonstrates adequate perfusion as individually appropriate.

PULMONARY		7A	8	9	10	11	12P	1	2	3	4	5	6	7	8	9	10	11	12A	1	2	3	4	5	6
NORMAL	B.S. CLEAR: R, L, Bil.										CL														
	B.S. EQUAL BILATERALLY										CL														
	RATE REGULAR (WNL for Age)										CL														
	Pulse Ox O₂ Sat.																								
	Probe Placement Site																								
	O₂ Device																								
	FiO₂ or l/m																								

**Call MD if O₂ Sat. is 92% or less, unless otherwise ordered by physician. If patient's O₂ Sat. is <93% - - assess patient which would include B.S., respiratory effort, vital signs, and the need for respiratory treatment.

ABNORMAL	COUGH																								
	SHALLOW RESP.																								
	LABORED RESP.																								
	IRREGULAR RESP.																								
	SPUTUM-DESCRIBE:																								
	ADVENTITIOUS BREATH SOUNDS																								
	DECREASED BREATH SOUNDS																								

Discharge Outcome: Patient will maintain effective breathing pattern with respiratory rate within normal range for patient.

GASTROINTESTINAL		7A	8	9	10	11	12P	1	2	3	4	5	6	7	8	9	10	11	12A	1	2	3	4	5	6
NORMAL	ABDOMEN SOFT										CL														
	BOWEL SOUNDS ALL QUADRANTS										CL														
	FLATUS																								
ABNORMAL	FIRM																								
	TENDERNESS																								
	DISTENDED																								
	BOWEL SOUNDS ABNORMAL																								
	STOOL ABNORMAL																								
	NAUSEA &/OR VOMITING																								

Discharge Outcome: Patient will establish/maintain normal patterns of bowel functioning for patient.

#035

1808.4 • 9/08/97

Figure 14–8. Nursing 24-hour assessment. (Courtesy of North Oaks Health System, Hammond, LA.)

Illustration continued on following page

DATE: 7/15/00

SIGNATURES:
	7a - 7p	Initials	7p - 7a	Initials
NURSE	CLott, M	(CL)		( )
NURSE		( )		( )
TECH/ASST		( )		( )
OTHER		( )		( )

NURSING 24 HOUR ASSESSMENT

NORMAL	GENITOURINARY	7A	8	9	10	11	12P	1	2	3	4	5	6	7	8	9	10	11	12A	1	2	3	4	5	6
	INDWELLING FOLEY																								
	URINE CLEAR										CL														

ABNORMAL	GENITOURINARY	7A	8	9	10	11	12P	1	2	3	4	5	6	7	8	9	10	11	12A	1	2	3	4	5	6
	INCONTINENT																								
	CLOUDY URINE																								
	BLOODY URINE																								

Discharge Outcome: Patient will maintain/regain effective pattern of elimination.

	SKIN	7A	8	9	10	11	12P	1	2	3	4	5	6	7	8	9	10	11	12A	1	2	3	4	5	6
NORMAL	WARM, DRY										CL														
	INTACT																								
	GOOD TURGOR										CL														
	MUCUS MEMBRANES MOIST																								
	COOL																								
ABNORMAL	FLUSHED, HOT																								
	GRAY, CYANOTIC																								
	DIAPHORETIC																								
	RASH/LESION																								
	ABRASION, BRUISES																								
	COLD																								
	CLAMMY																								

Braden Scale: Circle Appropriate Score
1. **If Braden score is 17-23,** pressure ulcer prevention precautions will be implemented.
2. **If Braden score is 12-16,** moderate pressure ulcer prevention precautions will be implemented.
3. **If Braden score is 0-11,** strict pressure ulcer prevention precautions will be implemented.
Previous Score:_____ Today's Score:_____

SKIN INJURY/WOUND ☐ YES ☐ NO
IF YES, REQUIRES SKIN INJURY/WOUND ASSESSMENT FLOWSHEET AND NARRATIVE DOCUMENTATION.

CLINICAL CONDITION PARAMETERS

SENSORY PERCEPTION: RESPONSE TO PRESSURE-RELATED DISCOMFORT
Completely Limited (unresponsive, quad, coma)	1
Very Limited (Responds only to painful stimuli, paraplegic, semicoma)	2
Slightly Limited (Responds with some sensory impairment CVA)	3
No Impairment (No limiting sensory deficit)	(4)

MOISTURE DEGREE TO WHICH SKIN IS EXPOSED TO MOISTURE
Constantly Moist (Always incontinent, 2 or more linen changes every 8 hours)	1
Moist (Often Incontinent, linen change every 8 hours)	2
Occasionally Moist (Seldom incontinent, linen changes 2 every 24 hours)	3
Rarely Moist (Skin is dry, routine linen change)	(4)

ACTIVITY: DEGREE OF PHYSICAL ACTIVITY
Bedrest (Confined to bed)	(1)
Chairfast (Minimum weight bearing, ambulatory w/assist)	2
Walks Occasionally (Ambulatory short distance, sits mostly)	3
Walks Frequently (Ambulatory outside room, BID)	4

MOBILITY: ABILITY TO CONTROL, CHANGE BODY POSITION
Completely Immobile (Cannot move self)	1
Very Limited (Makes insignificant movements)	2
Slightly Limited (Makes slight changes independently)	(3)
No Limitation (Makes major, independent changes)	4

NUTRITION: USUAL FOOD INTAKE PATTERN
Very Poor (NPO, IV > 5 days, < 1/3 meals)	1
Probably Inadequate (Needs assistance, < 1/2 meals)	2
Adequate (TPN, enteral needs met, > 1/2 meals)	3
Excellent (No supplement, eats most meals)	(4)

FRICTION AND SHEAR: ABILITY TO MAINTAIN BODY POSITION
Problem (Requires complete assist., slides down in bed/chair)	1
Potential Problem (Requires maximum assist., sometimes slides down in bed/chair)	2
No Apparent Problem (Moves independently, maintains good position in bed/chair)	(3)

Discharge Outcome: Patient will display timely wound healing; maintain intact skin or regain skin integrity; maintain circulation to skin; or the patient will be free from skin impairments or decubitus ulcers.

	NUTRITION	7A	8	9	10	11	12P	1	2	3	4	5	6	7	8	9	10	11	12A	1	2	3	4	5	6
	DIET (% EATEN)											100%													
	SNACKS (% EATEN)																								
	DIET/SNACKS OFFERED																								
	FLUIDS REFUSED																								
	NOURISHMENT REFUSED																								

Discharge Outcome: Patient will demonstrate stable weight/or progressive weight gain with normalization of lab values and free of signs of malnutrition. Obesity assessed.

Figure 14–8 Continued

NORTH☘OAKS

DATE: 7/15/00

SIGNATURES:	7a - 7p	Initials	7p - 7a	Initials
NURSE	C Lott, RN	(CL)	_____	( )
NURSE	_____	( )	_____	( )
TECH/ASST	_____	( )	_____	( )
OTHER	_____	( )	_____	( )

NURSING 24 HOUR ASSESSMENT

	PSYCHOSOCIAL	7A	8	9	10	11	12P	1	2	3	4	5	6	7	8	9	10	11	12A	1	2	3	4	5	6
NORMAL	COOPERATIVE										CL														
	APP. EMOTIONAL RESPONSE																								
	APP. SOCIAL INTERACTION																								
	AWAKE										CL														
	ASLEEP																								
	DROWSY/RESTING																								
ABNORMAL	RESTLESS/ANXIOUS																								
	WITHDRAWN/DEPRESSED																								
	UNCOOPERATIVE																								
	HOSTILE/COMBATIVE																								
	NONCOMPLIANT																								
	CRYING																								
	HALLUCINATIONS																								
	CONFUSION																								
	CURSING																								
	THREATENING																								

Discharge Outcome: Patient will maintain/regain bio-psychosocial homeostasis.

HYGIENE	7A	8	9	10	11	12P	1	2	3	4	5	6	7	8	9	10	11	12A	1	2	3	4	5	6
COMPLETE BATH																								
ASSISTED BATH										CL														
SELF																								
SHOWER/TUB/SITZ BATH																								
PERI-CARE/CATHETER CARE																								
ORAL-CARE																								
LINENS CHANGED										CL														

Discharge Outcome: Patient will resume/perform self-care activities within level of own ability or if unable, patient will receive help to maintain personal hygiene.

SAFETY	7A	8	9	10	11	12P	1	2	3	4	5	6	7	8	9	10	11	12A	1	2	3	4	5	6
PATIENT SAFETY CHECK q2H										CL														
ID BAND CHECKED q SHIFT										CL														
SIDE RAILS UP X 2										CL														
FAMILY (F), SITTER (S), OTHER (O)																								
BED POSITION ↑↓										↓														
BED WHEELS LOCKED										CL														
SEIZURE PRECAUTIONS																								

Discharge Outcome: Patient will remain free of injury during hospital stay.

ACTIVITY	7A	8	9	10	11	12P	1	2	3	4	5	6	7	8	9	10	11	12A	1	2	3	4	5	6
TURN: R, L, B, A																								
UP IN CHAIR																								
AMBULATED																								

Discharge Outcome: Patient will be able to perform schedule of activities appropriately for condition and mental readiness.

IVs, TX, & DRESSINGS	7A	8	9	10	11	12P	1	2	3	4	5	6	7	8	9	10	11	12A	1	2	3	4	5	6
IV SITE CHECKED: (WNL)										CL														
INFUSION PUMP																								
IV SITE ROTATED																								
Dressing ® hip										CL														

Discharge Outcome: IV/wound sites will be free of S/S of complications/infections; patient will receive parenteral therapy safely and comfortably; patient will regain fluid and electrolyte balance; patient will be free from preventable complications of IV Therapy.

MD VISIT		TIME		TIME		TIME		TIME		TIME

Figure 14–8 *Continued*

| 7/15/00 | 1600 | C/O pain in ⓛ hip. States 8 on a scale of 1–10. Instructed to use PCA as needed. Dressing to ⓛ hip c̄ mod. amt. serous drainage (6-cm diameter). Dressing reinforced. IV D5W @ 100 cc/hr c̄ 450 cc TBA. ————————— S. Richards, RN. |
| | 1630 | States mild discomfort. Pain rated 4 on a scale of 1–10. Reinforcement to dsg. clean and dry. ————————— S. Richards, RN. |

Figure 14–9. Example of charting by exception.

cess. One disadvantage nurses cite is that all entries must relate to a specific problem on the problem list, making it difficult to document events unrelated to an identified problem. The format also omits documentation of the planning portion of the nursing process that identifies expected outcomes. Some agencies use the acronym PIEP, which adds a *Plan* element that addresses the concern about follow-up. The system also requires charting about problems periodically, even if unchanged. Therefore, this format may not be the most efficient for some settings, particularly long-term care. If several problems are included on the problem list, documentation may be lengthy (Iyer & Camp, 1995).

Focus Charting

Focus charting is a method of charting that addresses client problems or needs and includes a column that summarizes the focus of the entry. It may not necessarily require the use of a nursing diagnosis (some agencies use nursing diagnosis for the "focus"; others do not). This focus can include a nursing diagnosis, activities or concerns of the client, or other incidents. The format requires using DAR or DAE, acronyms for

D = data
A = action
R = response

or

D = data
A = action
E = evaluation

Data include any subjective or objective observations, whereas action indicates any interventions resulting from the observations. Response or evaluation entries document the effect of the intervention on the client and may be recorded immediately or at a later time if appropriate. For example, if medication is given for pain, the response will not likely be assessed until sufficient time has been allowed for the medication to be effective. This format also employs flow sheets for documentation of routine observations and interventions. Figure 14–12 is an example of focus charting.

Advantages of focus charting include flexibility, easy data retrieval, and close alignment with the nursing process. One disadvantage is the possibility of inconsistency in labeling of problems.

SOAP Charting

SOAP charting is a method of charting used to record progress notes with problem-oriented medical records; it includes subjective data, objective data, assessment, and plan. The progress notes include narrative notes as well as flow sheets that are used by all members of the health team. The narrative notes are specifically related to the problem list and are numbered and titled

Date/Initials	Problem #	Nursing Diagnosis	Date Resolved/Initials
7/15/00 BSM	#1	Pain related to surgical incision. ———————	
7/15/00 BSM	#2	Risk for infection related to surgical incision. ———	
7/15/00 CRT	#3	Impaired home maintenance management related to impaired mobility. —————————	

Figure 14–10. Example of an APIE problem list.

Date	Time	Problem #	Remarks
7/16/00	1600	#1	I = Tylox i given PO for C/O incisional pain. ———S. Richards, RN
	1630	#1	E = Sitting in chair at bedside. States pain relieved. ———S. Richards, RN
		Assessment	States she feels constipated. Last BM 7/12. Abdomen firm. ———
		P#4	Constipation related to decreased activity and change in diet. ———
		I#4	Dr. Alvarez notified. Stool softener adm. as ordered. Encouraged to ↑ fluid intake. ———S. Richards, RN

OR

Date	Time	Problem #	Remarks
7/16/00	1600	IP#1	Tylox i given PO for C/O incisional pain. ———S. Richards, RN
	1630	EP#1	Sitting in chair at bedside. States pain relieved. ———S. Richards, RN
		Assessment	States she feels constipated. Last BM 7/12. Abdomen firm. ———
		P#4	Constipation related to decreased activity and change in diet. ———
		IP#4	Dr. Alvarez notified. Stool softener adm. as ordered. Encouraged to ↑ fluid intake. ———S. Richards, RN

Figure 14–11. Example of APIE data entries.

Date	Time	Focus	Notes
7/16/00	1600	Pain	D = C/O pain at incision site (L) hip. Requests pain medication. ——— ———S. Richards, RN A = Tylox ii given PO. ——— ———S. Richards, RN
	1600	Dressing	D = Abd. dressing c̄ mod. amt. serous drainage.———S. Richards, RN A = Dsg. reinforced. ——— ———S. Richards, RN
	1630	Pain	R = States pain relieved.——— ———S. Richards, RN
		Dressing	R = Dsg. dry and intact. ——— ———S. Richards, RN

Figure 14–12. Example of focus charting.

accordingly. For example, any reference made to a client's surgical incision would be preceded by the number of the problem (from the problem list) and/or the name of the problem (e.g., #1 Open Reduction and Internal Fixation . . .).

In this particular format, progress notes are written in a specific format that contains four parts, easily remembered by the acronym SOAP, which, as was noted earlier, stands for

S = subjective data
O = objective data
A = assessment
P = plan

Subjective data describe the client's problem as the client sees it. The data are not observable or measurable and, therefore, must be related to the health care provider by the client. Objective data are those items of information that are measurable and observable by another person. Laboratory findings are also examples of objective data. The assessment component in the SOAP note summarizes conclusions based on the data presented, whereas the plan outlines actions that will address the identified problem. For example, the plan may include further diagnostic tests, therapeutic medical or nursing interventions, or client education. Often the plan is simply to continue the previously outlined plan.

There are times when not all SOAP elements may be present or appropriate. For example, if there are no objective data to support a problem, "none" is written by the "O" in the SOAP note. One example of a progress note in the SOAP format is found in Figure 14–13. Advantages of the SOAP format include a uniform problem list used by all personnel and easy reference to data related to specific problems. Disadvantages include lack of flexibility (similar to the APIE method), with all documentation directed toward a specific problem.

Flow Sheets

Regardless of the format, flow sheets are often used to document data that can be more easily followed in graphic or tabular form. They are used in many agencies to facilitate documentation of routine assessment data and nursing interventions in checklist format. Trends related to ADLs, body systems review, and other nursing observations and activities can be easily

followed using flow sheets. Checklists and flow sheets provide a method for summarizing client progress in an abbreviated manner that saves time and often improves the quality of documentation (Charting tips, 1988). Not only are flow sheets often more legible but they facilitate consistent documentation of assessment and interventions.

The format of the flow sheet may be relatively unstructured, with you adding categories as needed, or it may be very structured, requiring checks in appropriate columns. Structured formats provide reminders for you of certain data that should be included at regular intervals and reinforce standards of care. All flow sheets require date and signature of you making the observation. Some observations will still require further description in narrative progress notes.

Graphic Records

Graphic records are used to record vital signs in most agencies. Although graphs may vary among agencies, Figure 14–14 is one example. Some graphic forms will also provide a graph for documentation of pulse and respiration, but most simply provide a space to write the number value for pulse, respiration, and blood pressure. Some agencies may use tabular forms for recording all vital signs or may use such forms when vital signs are to be recorded at more frequent intervals than the graph allows.

Other Types of Flow Sheets

Other common flow sheets used for recording data include the following:

- I&O (see Fig. 14–14)
- Wound assessment (Fig. 14–15)
- Medication administration records
- Intensive vital signs
- Neurological checks

Documentation by Computer

The use of computer systems for documentation in health care agencies varies in scope depending on the agency. Most health care agencies have incorporated information systems for management of admissions, billing, and communication of orders for diet, pharmacy, and diagnostic tests. Use of these systems allows departments within an institution to interact as

Date/Time	Problem	Progress Note
7/16/00 1600	#1 Pain related to surgical incision	S = States discomfort in Ⓛ hip. ——— O = Grimaces c̄ movement to Ⓛ side. Requests pain medication q3h. ——— A = No change. ——— P = Continue pain meds prn. ——— ——— S. Richards, RN

Figure 14–13. Example of a progress note in SOAP charting.

NORTH🍂AKS
12-HOUR GRAPHIC AND I&O RECORD

		7A-7P			7P-7A			7A-7P			7P-7A			7A-7P			7P-7A			7A-7P			7P-7A			7A-7P			7P-7A		
Date																																		
Hour		8	12	4	8	12	4	8	12	4	8	12	4	8	12	4	8	12	4	8	12	4	8	12	4	8	12	4	8	12	4		

Temperature (105, 104, 103, 102, 101, 100, 99, 98, 97)

Pulse										
Respiration										
Blood Pressure										
Weight										
Bowel Mov't										

	7a–7p	7p–7a	7a–7p	7p–7a	7a–7p	7p–7a	7a–7p	7p–7a	7a–7p	7p–7a
Intake Parenteral										
Oral										
Blood/Plasma										
Piggy Back										
Tube Feeding										
G.U. Irrigant										
12 Hr. Total										
24 Hr. Total										
Output Catheter										
Emesis										
Suction										
Voiding										
Drain										
12 Hr. Total										
24 Hr. Total										
Meals	B___% L___% D___%		B___% L___% D___%		B___% L___% D___%		B___% L___% D___%		B___% L___% D___%	

Instock #001   3132.2 · 11/9/98

Figure 14–14. Example of a graphic record. (Courtesy of North Oaks Health System, Hammond, LA.)

NORTH OAKS

Attachment D: Skin Injury/Wound Assessment Flowsheet

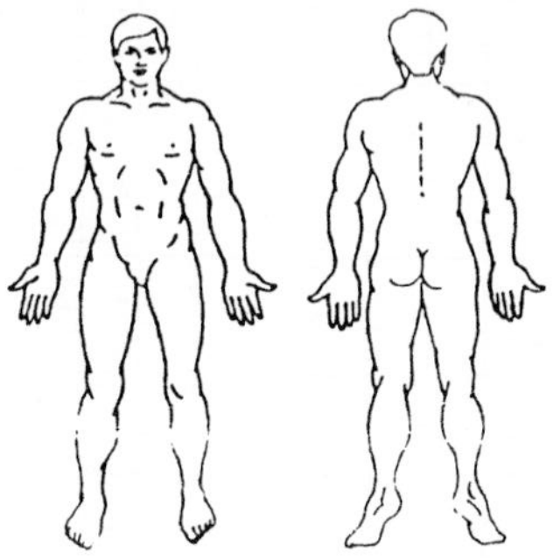

STAGE 1: Nonblanchable erythema of intact skin.

STAGE 2: Partial thickness skin loss involving epidermis and/or dermis.

STAGE 3: Full thickness skin loss involving damage or necrosis of subcutaneous tissue that may extend down to, but not through, underlying fascia.

STAGE 4: Full thickness skin loss with extensive destruction tissue necrosis or damage to muscle, bone or supporting structures.

*: Unable to stage due to eschar covering wound.

R   L   R

Number each injury/wound on the diagram. Complete a full row of information for each injury/wound.

Injury/Wound Types	Drainage	Odor	Color
Stasis Ulcer Pressure Ulcer Arterial Ulcer Surgical Wound Laceration	Bruises Skin Tear Rash Hematoma Other: Specify.	Serous Purulent None Other: Specify.	Mild Foul None Other: Specify.	Pink Red Black Eschar Other: Specify.

Date	Site#	Injury/Wound Type (Specify)	Stage	Length Width cm	Depth cm	Tunneling Yes/No	Color	Drainage Amt/Type	Odor	Culture Date	Treatments & Comments	Signature & Title

JOB#2841.4+(2/18/98)

Figure 14–15. Example of a skin injury/wound assessment flow sheet. (Courtesy of North Oaks Health System, Hammond, LA.)

well as provide a database for research and quality assurance. In addition, agency-wide computer information systems are more efficient in that information entered in the system can be automatically transferred to other areas (Thede, 1998).

Many agencies have incorporated software for documentation of client care. Systems may include options for generating individualized care plans, automated Kardex, and acuity levels, as well as providing a mechanism for recording ongoing assessment data. Although some systems provide for computer input only at the nurses' desk, bedside systems—including hand-held systems (Fig. 14–16)—are becoming more common. Bedside charting systems, also referred to as point-of-care systems, often include prompts for you to input data that provide more accurate and complete records. In addition, charting at the bedside saves time for you and allows current information to be immediately available to all who need access to client information. Some systems automatically retrieve and record information from electronic devices (vital signs) and place the information in more than one place on the record simultaneously, avoiding duplication of effort. Legibility of information is an added benefit from computer documentation systems (Eggland & Heinemann, 1994).

Although charting by computer provides an efficient method of documentation, there is increased concern for security of information in order to protect client rights. Documentation on the client's computerized record requires the individual charting to have a log-in and password for entering the computer record system. It is imperative that this password not be shared with anyone because anything entered will be credited to the person to whom the password or signature is assigned. In addition, you should log off the computer before leaving the terminal in order to ensure that information about a client is not displayed on the monitor for others to view.

Computer-generated printouts should also be protected so that information about clients is not indiscriminately duplicated or distributed. Most agencies using computer charting incorporate a system for logging and tracking computer printouts. Charting procedures for computer records systems vary by agency.

KEY PRINCIPLES

- The purposes of charting are communication, quality assurance, legal accountability, reimbursement, and research.
- All documentation entries should follow standard medical terminology and abbreviations.
- Common principles of good documentation include legibility, brevity, sequence, making corrections appropriately, omitting blank spaces, and signing properly.
- All medical records are confidential.
- Content can be documented using several types of entries: admit note, change-of-shift note, assessment findings, and interval notes.
- Special notations should be made when a client is transferred or discharged or when client teaching is received.
- All objective and subjective observations should be documented completely, accurately, and specifically.
- Significant data concerning psychosocial status, ADLs, valuables, spiritual care, and safety concerns should be documented in narrative form as needed.
- Entries about special groups such as the elderly, children, and culturally diverse clients need to be specific notations particular to that population.
- Documentation for extended-care, long-term, and home health agencies should include life span issues, support for reimbursement, and key terms specific to the various types of agencies.
- Entries can be made using various formats for documentation.
- Flow sheets are used to summarize data in an abbreviated form and allow a quick reference for specific data.
- Computerized records allow for systematic data entry and retrieval and facilitate consistency for purposes of quality assurance and research.

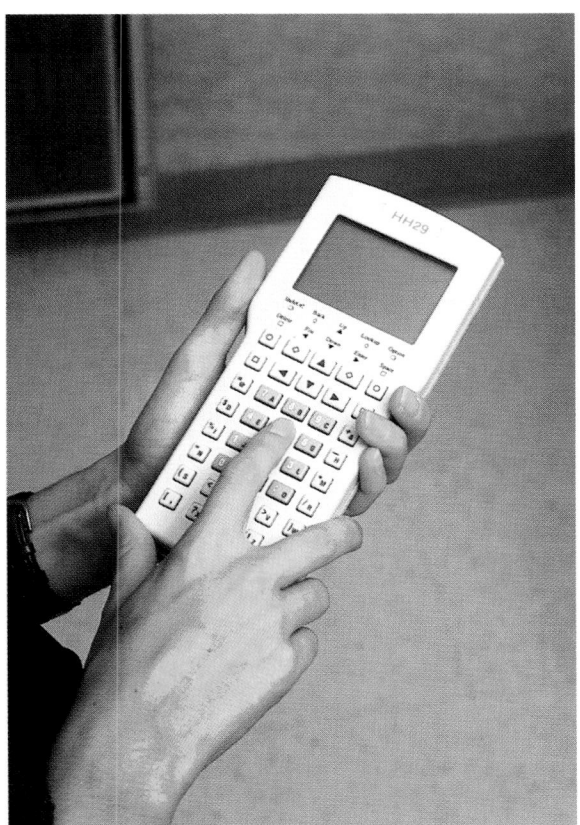

Figure 14–16. A hand-held computer documentation system.

BIBLIOGRAPHY

*American Nurses' Association. (1999). *Standards of clinical nursing practice* (2nd ed.). Washington, D.C.: Author.

Buchauer, A., Pohl, U., Kurzel, N., & Haux, R. (May, 1999). Mobilizing a health professional's workstation—results of an evaluation study. *International Journal of Medical Informatics, 54*(2), 105–114.

Charting tips: Using flow sheets correctly. (June, 1998). *Nursing 98,* 76.

Cox, H.C., Hinz, M.D., Lubno, M.A., Newfield, S.A., Ridenour, N.A., Slater, M.M., & Sridaroment, K.L. (1997). *Clinical applications of nursing diagnosis.* Philadelphia: F.A. Davis.

———————————

*Asterisk indicates a classic or definitive work on this subject.

*Eggland, E.T., & Heinemann, D.S. (1994). *Nursing documentation: Charting, recording and reporting.* Philadelphia: J.B. Lippincott Company.

Griffiths, J., & Hutchings, W. (1999). The wider implications of an audit of care plan documentation. *Journal of Clinical Nursing 8*(1), 57–65.

Iyer, P.W., & Camp, N.H. (1995). *Nursing documentation* (2nd ed.). St. Louis: Mosby.

Stahl, D. (1995). Maximizing reimbursement for subacute care. *Nursing Management, 26*(4), 16–19.

*Tammelleo, A.D. (1994). Charting by exception: There are perils. *RN, 57*(10), 71–72.

Thede, L.Q. (1998). *Computers in nursing.* Philadelphia: Lippincott Williams & Wilkins.

Van Tassel, M., & DeSantis, S. (1995). Tackling hospital costs and delays. *Nursing Management, 26*(3), 24–28.

Weintraub, M.I. (1999). Documentation and informed consent. *Neurologic Clinics, 17*(2), 371–381.

The Tools of Practice

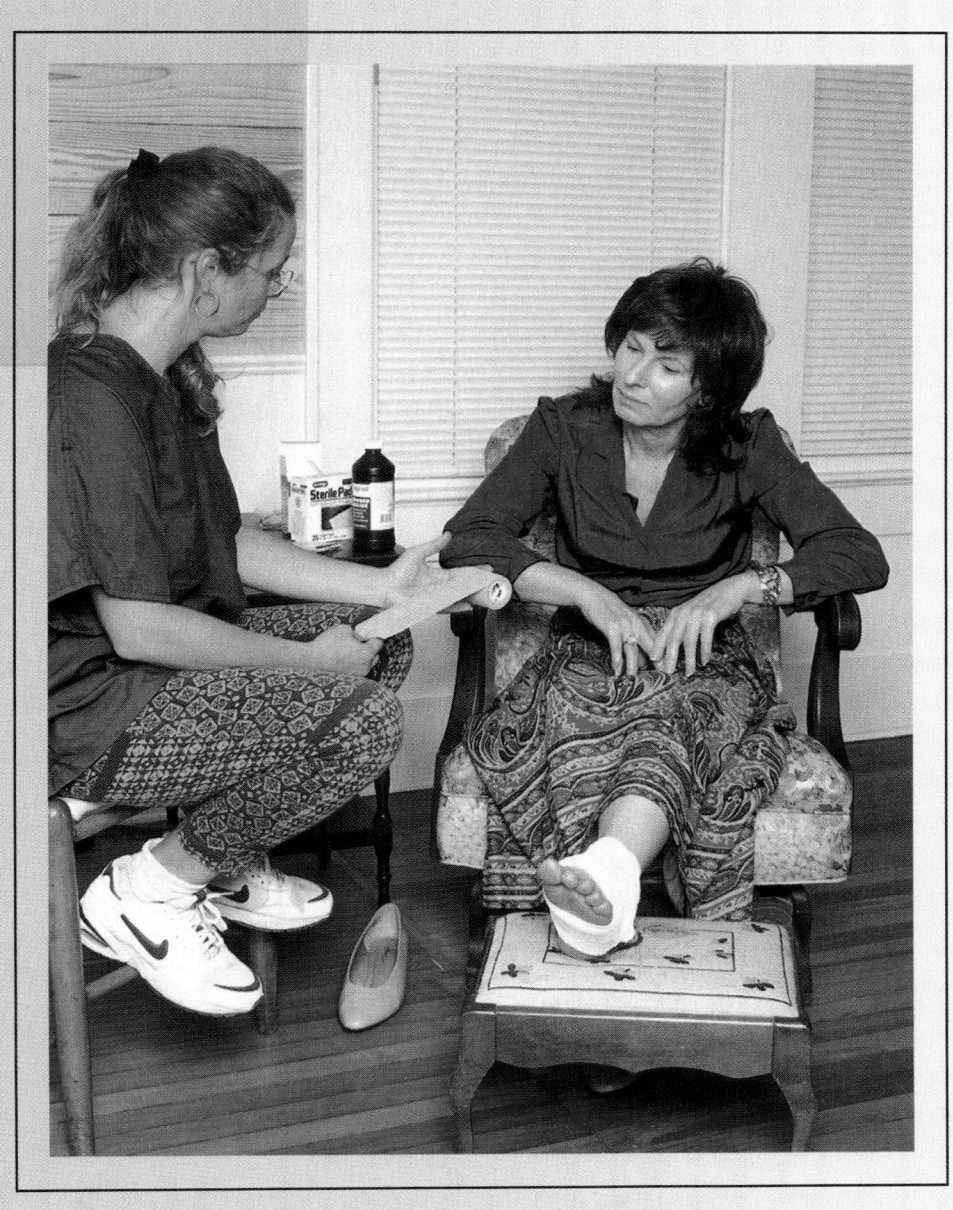

The Nurse-Client Relationship

Daria Virvan

Key Terms

acting-out behaviors
attending behaviors
body language
context
decoder (receiver)
empathy
encoder (sender)
feedback
language
message

nonverbal communication
paralanguage
personal space
positive listening
sensory channel
therapeutic rapport
therapeutic relationship
unconditional positive regard
verbal communication

LEARNING OBJECTIVES

After studying this chapter, you should be able to:

1. Identify the tasks associated with each of the three phases of the therapeutic relationship.

2. List and describe the six elements of the communication process.

3. Identify how Peplau, Travelbee, Satir, and Watzlawick contributed to an understanding of the nurse and the client and communication.

4. Compare and contrast the two main forms of verbal communication.

5. Identify the elements of body language and paralanguage.

6. Describe the nursing attitudes and action-oriented characteristics that facilitate effective therapeutic techniques.

7. Identify some techniques that impair therapeutic communication.

8. List and give examples of seven techniques that enhance therapeutic communication.

9. Identify a variety of characteristics of effective communication techniques.

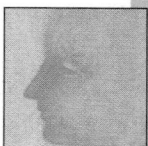

Jane Smith, RN, was dispensing bedtime medications in a busy medical-surgical unit. As Mr. Lewis took his pills quietly he commented, "I feel pretty scared about my operation tomorrow." Ms. Smith looked at him condescendingly. "That surgery is a piece of cake," she said. "You have nothing to be afraid of." Mr. Lewis didn't respond, but when Ms. Smith came to work the next day she learned that her client had had a sleepless night. "We all tried to talk to him about what was bothering him," reported the day nurse, "but he said nobody at this hospital cared enough to talk to him." What went wrong?

Had Ms. Smith been more aware of therapeutic communication techniques, she might have avoided upsetting her client. What could she have done better? What did she do that she should not have done? How might she have responded in a more sensitive and empathetic manner? The answers to these questions lie in an understanding of therapeutic communication.

This chapter will orient you to beginning theories, principles, and techniques of therapeutic communication related to the nurse-client interaction. Because you will be expected to use therapeutic communication techniques throughout your professional life, it is vital that you begin to learn these techniques early in your student experience. As with most skills you learn in nursing, you will continue to develop competence and gain mastery of these techniques as you practice them in the clinical setting over time. Also, the more you practice, the more confident you will be, and the better the outcomes will be.

THE THERAPEUTIC RELATIONSHIP

A **therapeutic relationship** is a helping relationship. Nurses are helpers, and clients are those seeking help. A therapeutic relationship is personal, client-focused, and aimed at realizing mutually determined goals.

In a therapeutic relationship, people who are seeking help bring their own life experiences, intelligence, achievements, values, beliefs, and motivations for change to the relationship. You bring experience, understanding, and skills. You and your client can be viewed as unique systems that intersect on a common ground: the therapeutic nurse-client relationship.

Although it is true that people often help each other in social relationships, this kind of help differs from that occurring in therapeutic relationships. Social relationships may involve an infinite range of nonspecific helping activities, such as walking the neighbor's dog or helping a person who is using a walker to cross the street safely. Social helping may give the helper more satisfaction from the interaction than the person being helped. And social helping is often only a small part of the total relationship. In contrast, the help provided in the therapeutic relationship is the main reason for the relationship; it is focused on the client and has a specific purpose.

*A*ction *A*lert!
To establish a therapeutic relationship, remain focused on eliciting the client's feelings, thoughts, and values, and center on achieving the client's goals.

Another difference between social and therapeutic relationships is that the social relationship is more reciprocal, with both persons sharing personal beliefs, feelings, and opinions with each other. This is not true of the therapeutic relationship. You may share feelings with the client, but only when such sharing is appropriate for the benefit of the client.

Phases of the Therapeutic Relationship

Therapeutic relationships develop and evolve over time. This time may be brief, or it may extend over weeks, months, or even years. Regardless of the length of time, there are three distinct phases to the relationship: the orientation phase, the working phase, and the termination phase. Because relationships are fluid, the phases flow into each other; nevertheless, each phase may be recognized by the tasks associated with it.

Orientation Phase

In the orientation phase of the therapeutic relationship, you and the client make a verbal agreement to work together to solve one or more of the client's problems. This agreement initiates a working relationship and forms the basis for the work you will do together.

As you enter into a relationship with a client, it is helpful to be aware of the personal feelings that can arise at these times. Both of you may be anxious and uncomfortable during this phase. You may feel inadequate, and the client may feel unsure about you and may need to know that you are willing and able to help.

A primary goal of the orientation phase is the establishment of trust (Fig. 15–1). Trust is enhanced when you connect with the client in a respectful and nonintrusive manner that conveys personal consideration and concern.

Honesty and enthusiasm help establish trust. You can convey these two traits in such responses as "I don't know the answer right now, but I will find out and let you know in an hour," or "I cannot promise I can help solve your problem, but I can listen and I do care."

*A*ction *A*lert!
Do not pretend to know an answer to a client's question. This deception will erode the client's trust. Your candor is necessary to promote client confidence.

Trust is also promoted when you establish confidentiality as a ground rule for the relationship. How-

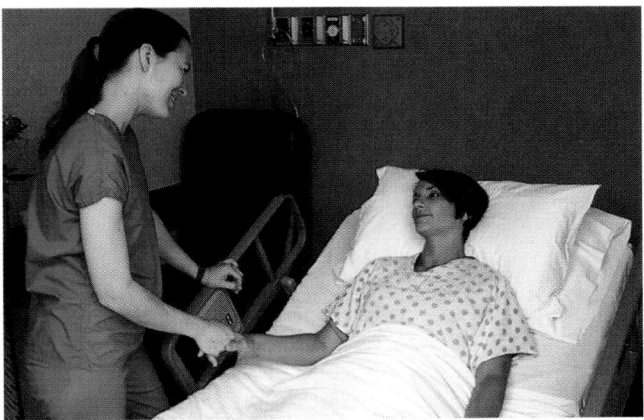

Figure 15–1. Establishing trust with the client is a key goal of the orientation phase of a therapeutic relationship. You can do this by conveying respect, personal consideration, and concern for the client's needs.

ever, confidentiality must be handled carefully. Sometimes, in a desire to have the client trust you, you become tempted to promise complete confidentiality, and then you are placed in an ethical dilemma when the client confides something that must be revealed to others for the client's protection or for the protection of others. For example, what would you do if you had pledged unconditional confidentiality to a client, only to have him confide that he has active tuberculosis and works with AIDS patients? If you do not report this information, you risk the possibility of an infectious disease catastrophe. If you do reveal it, you have broken your word and violated the client's trust.

Confidentiality is an ethical obligation to share health care information about a person only with other persons who have a professional need to know the person's health status. It is unrealistic to promise a client that you will never tell anyone about anything that occurs between you. However, you may safely promise that you will respect your client's privacy and will share information only when there is a medical need to do so. It is important to tell your clients that you cannot maintain confidentiality if doing so would endanger the health and well-being of themselves or others. Such a caveat should make clients feel that you will protect them and will not allow them to hurt themselves or others. If clients feel safe, they will feel a sense of trust, and the relationship will be reinforced.

Besides establishing trust, you should establish the ground rules for the relationship. If you will be meeting with a client frequently, be sure to specify clearly where, when, and for how long each meeting will be. For example, a primary nurse might say, "I will be teaching you how to care for your Hickman catheter. We will meet here for an hour tomorrow at 10:00 AM so I can assess your current knowledge. After tomorrow, we will work together 30 minutes a day for 5 days until you can comfortably and safely take care of your catheter."

As you establish meeting times and places, honesty and achievability are paramount. Do not promise what you may not be able to do. It is better if the client can rely on meeting with you 15 minutes each day than for you to promise 30-minute sessions that you may not have the time for.

At any time in the relationship, you may begin to feel a bond with your client. **Therapeutic rapport** is a special bond that exists between a nurse and a client who have established a sense of trust and a mutual understanding of what will occur in their relationship.

Working Phase

Once rapport has been established and the relationship has been structured, the working phase (middle phase) of the therapeutic relationship begins. In this phase the nurse performs additional client assessment and analyzes the resulting data. The client's covert feelings, values, beliefs, and attitudes are sought out and examined.

Often during this phase, initial nursing diagnoses are corrected, or additional nursing diagnoses are for-

mulated. However, the working phase is mainly a time for completing nursing interventions that address expected nursing outcomes. You respond to clients mainly by presenting information and by helping them validate and clarify their understandings. Rather than directing clients, you attempt to help them become self-directed. It is a time when clients can formulate and test solutions to their problems. Evaluation also occurs in this phase of the relationship and, when necessary, the care plan is revised.

Termination Phase

The termination phase of the therapeutic relationship occurs near the end of the relationship, when the work of the client and nurse is coming to a close. The termination itself should not be abrupt or unexpected and should be acknowledged from the beginning of the relationship by both you and the client.

Recall the example given in the orientation phase. The primary nurse clearly stated she would work with the client on catheter care for a certain time each day for a specified number of days. She did not say she wanted to meet with the client "every weekday." No one should have interpreted her offer to meet with the client as extending beyond the hospital stay. She was saying, in effect, "I will be meeting with you only until you are discharged." Clear communication helps to clarify expectations from the start of the relationship.

Even when the termination is thoughtfully planned, it may still be difficult to end a meaningful interaction. You and the client are aware that this phase precedes a permanent separation, and you both may feel anxiety, sadness, and a sense of loss.

How the client reacts to the termination depends on the meaning assigned to it, the length of the relationship, and whether or how outcomes were achieved. Some clients may display denial and regret and may engage in acting-out behaviors. **Acting-out behaviors** are inappropriate or unexpected client behaviors that communicate about the client's true or subconscious feelings and concerns. A client who is acting out during termination may refuse to talk when meeting with you, fail to keep appointments, and become more forgetful. At such times, you may help the client to recognize feelings about parting while emphasizing positive changes that have occurred during the relationship. It may be helpful to offer support and express optimism for the future. At the same time, it is important to be clear about ending the relationship without offering false hope for continuation. Although this process can be uncomfortable for you, it provides the client with clear boundaries and expectations.

Elements of the Therapeutic Relationship

Three elements are present in all phases of the therapeutic relationship: you, the client, and communication between the client and you. You are a helper trained in skills that facilitate client growth; the client is seeking help with personal growth; and communication is the meaningful interaction between two people that leads to such growth.

The Communication Process

A widely accepted model for the communication process consists of the following six elements (Fig. 15–2):

- **Encoder (sender):** This person initiates a transaction to exchange information, convey thoughts and feelings, or engage another person.
- **Message:** This is the content a sender wishes to transmit to another person (the receiver) in the process of communication. The message must be encoded in a language of symbols or cues that are understandable to both sender and receiver.
- **Sensory channel:** This is the means by which a message is sent. The three primary channels are visual, auditory, and kinesthetic. Using these three channels, a wink, a tone of voice, and a hand gesture can all effectively convey a message without benefit of words.
- **Decoder (receiver):** This is the person to whom a message is aimed. This person must be able to decode the message sent to understand it clearly. If the message that the sender transmits is what the receiver understands, then clear and effective communication has occurred.
- **Context:** This is the condition under which a communication occurs.
- **Feedback:** This is the process by which effectiveness of communication is determined.

The feedback process is so important to communication that it deserves additional attention. There are four types of feedback: internal, external, positive, and negative.

Internal feedback is a mechanism of self-perception. When you communicate, you automatically assess what you have said or done. For example, if you make a verbal blunder, you react self-consciously after realizing your mistake. If, however, you feel you have communicated clearly what you meant, you are pleased and satisfied with the effort.

External feedback is received from another or others, in the form of visual, auditory, or kinesthetic information. The response to the message sent gives information about how effectively you transmitted the message.

Positive feedback affirms your efforts to communicate by rewarding and reinforcing successful communication. If your messages are met with a smile or exclamation of relief, you feel good and continue to use those communication behaviors.

Negative feedback is a response that tells you your original message was poorly transmitted or received and needs to be modified. However, there is more to negative feedback than just a message telling you the original message was garbled. Negative feedback may also be judgmental and indicate that the receiver disagreed with your message.

It is important to note that both sender and receiver can seek feedback and clarify and qualify the message as needed. For example, consider the following interaction between Mrs. Herbert and Rick Jones, RN, after Mr. Jones completes Mrs. Herbert's diabetic teaching:

> Mrs. Herbert: "I think I understood the procedure better yesterday."
> Rick Jones, RN *(insulted by an unfavorable comparison to another nurse and seeking clarification)*: "Are you thinking that I have confused you with today's teaching?"
> Mrs. Herbert *(realizing that Mr. Jones misunderstood)*: "I wasn't saying it was your fault. I was just more with it yesterday."

Had Mr. Jones not clarified what Mrs. Herbert meant, he might have left the interaction with negative feelings about Mrs. Herbert and about his own ability to do diabetic teaching.

With this example, you can see how disruptive it could be to an interaction, and even to a relationship, if an unclear message is not clarified by seeking and receiving feedback or correction. It is unfortunate in this situation that the client had to be the one to seek feedback and to clarify, because this should be done by the nurse.

*A*ction *A*lert!
Ensure that communication with clients is both clear and therapeutic.

Theories Concerning the Nurse-Client Relationship

Several theorists have provided us with a better understanding of the nurse, the client, and communication and of the interaction among these elements in a therapeutic relationship. Here are selected examples.

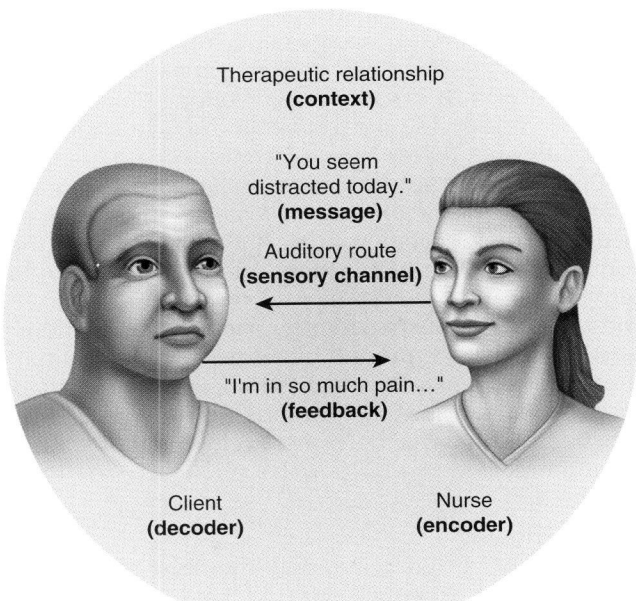

Figure 15–2. This diagram shows the six elements of communication within the therapeutic relationship: the encoder (sender), the message, the sensory channel, the decoder (receiver), feedback, and context.

PEPLAU'S THEORY

Hildegard Peplau, a psychiatric nurse and one of the first nurse theorists, identified six roles that are assumed by the nurse in relation to the client in a therapeutic relationship (Peplau, 1952):

- *The stranger:* This role is shared by both the nurse and the client entering the therapeutic relationship. The nurse offers the client respect, interest, and acceptance in a nonpersonal manner. The client is assumed to be emotionally intact unless conflicting evidence arises.
- *The resource:* The nurse assumes the role of a resource person, helping the consumer-client to negotiate the health care system by providing care and offering answers to specific questions.
- *The teacher:* The nurse assumes the role of teacher to help educate the client and help the client understand and use experiences within the health care system.
- *The leader:* The nurse assumes the leadership role to help the client-follower to contribute to and participate in a democratic nursing process.
- *The surrogate:* The nurse assumes the surrogate parent role to help the client resolve interpersonal problems that need to be safely worked out in the presence of an understanding other and to give the client a corrective interpersonal experience.
- *The counselor:* The nurse assumes the counselor role to help integrate reality and the client's emotional responses to illness into the total life experience.

Peplau believed that nurses who related with clients in a healthy way could provide corrective interpersonal experiences for them; that if clients had positive relationships with nurses they could then have healthier relationships with others. She encouraged nurses to promote trust in their relationships by relating to their clients in an authentic manner. For Peplau, relating in an authentic manner meant sharing feelings and thoughts appropriately. For example, note how Mrs. Lyons, a renal nurse, shares her feelings with Mr. Little when he learns his second kidney transplant is failing. He is red-eyed and clenching his fists but is unable to verbalize his feelings.

Mrs. Lyons *(making eye contact with Mr. Little):* "This is a hard piece of news for you."
Mr. Little *(silent, but starts to cry)*
Mrs. Lyons: "I feel sad too, Mr. Little. Having two transplants fail is very hard."

Peplau noted that closeness in a therapeutic relationship builds trust, increases the client's self-esteem, and leads to new personal growth for the client.

TRAVELBEE'S THEORY

Joyce Travelbee, another noted nurse theorist, pointed out that the nurse is a human being who is vulnerable to stereotypes, labels, and generalizations (Travelbee, 1966). Travelbee noted that it is not possible for a ster-

eotype (of a nurse) to relate to another stereotype (of a client) in a human way. In this example, Miss Lane is a nurse working with paralyzed adults. In Miss Lane's stereotyped view, paralyzed clients have enough problems and should not be overly challenged. She also believes she is overworked and underpaid and that her clients should be grateful for the care she gives. Miss Lane is assigned to work with Lisa Simmons, a 28-year-old woman recovering from a devastating car crash. Lisa is alert, bright, and highly motivated.

Miss Lane: "Good morning, Lisa. Let me cut up your breakfast for you."
Lisa: "My arms are fine, it's my legs that don't work."
Miss Lane *(to herself):* You poor thing, you need all the help you can get. You're lucky I'm your nurse today. *(to Lisa)* "No sweetie, let's do it my way, I don't have all day for this."

Not only has Miss Lane not related to Lisa as another human being who is deserving of respect and consideration, but she has also given Lisa a reason to view other nurses as callous, rude, and insensitive.

Travelbee noted that one nursing goal is to change the distorted beliefs others have about nurses and nursing. According to Travelbee, the client is the help-seeker whose overt and covert needs are the focus of the therapeutic relationship. She proposed that understanding the individual client's experience is paramount and that people cannot be known if their uniqueness is not appreciated. Your task, then, is to see the individual "with fresh eyes" and without labeling or stereotyping.

An important component of Travelbee's theory concerns the process of *human reduction*. This term, a synonym for dehumanization, refers to viewing the client as other than a human being. Viewing the client as an illness ("the heart attack in Room 210"), a task ("the bed-bath-and-dressing-change on Team B"), or a stereotype ("all amputees") are three examples of human reduction. It is only in overcoming assigned labels that you and the client can relate on a human level and establish a therapeutic relationship.

Like Peplau, Travelbee conceptualized the communication process as a means of fostering the development of human relationships. She believed that the human-to-human relationship allows the nurse to help clients and their families cope with illness and to find meaning in the experience. She believed communication to be reciprocal, dynamic, and influential. Travelbee recognized that each interaction has differences and similarities that prohibit forming rigid rules of action but that does permit development of skill as a communicator.

SATIR'S THEORY

Virginia Satir, a dynamic family therapist and expert communicator, described effective communication as a transaction in which the sender of the message makes a clear request or statement, which the receiver accurately receives (Satir, 1971). If communication is effective, what the sender intends and what the receiver receives match. Satir described four types of ineffective communicators:

- *The placator:* This person feels vulnerable to rejection and avoids it by always seeking to please others.
- *The blamer:* This person feels like a failure but hides it by being unreasonable and controlling to others.
- The *super-reasonable:* This person intellectualizes events so feelings are not experienced. This refusal to feel conceals inner feelings of vulnerability.
- *The irrelevant posture:* This person focuses the communication away from feelings and current reality. By pretending a stressor does not exist, the person can ignore feelings of alienation.

For an example of these four dysfunctional patterns, consider Mrs. Elliot. Mrs. Elliot is a hospital volunteer guiding her cart of books and magazines in a busy hallway, and a child darts in front of her and narrowly avoids being injured. The child's mother turns angrily to Mrs. Elliot. Mrs. Elliot might reply in any one of the following ways, according to the four different dysfunctional patterns:

- *Placating:* "I'm sorry! Let's check your poor darling and make sure he's not hurt."
- *Blaming:* "Why don't you watch your kid? He could hurt somebody."
- *Super-reasonableness:* "My goodness, children can be a challenge to watch."
- *Irrelevant:* "I've got lots of children's books here on this cart."

Each of these dysfunctional patterns of reaction results in impaired communication by relaying inaccurate information about Mrs. Elliot's true feelings of concern and anxiety. With such persons, it is necessary for you to help the clients understand and communicate their true feelings before progress can be made.

WATZLAWICK'S THEORY

Paul Watzlawick, a noted communication theorist, wrote extensively about the pragmatics of communication. He believed communication to be inevitable. He noted the following:

- All behavior has message, value, or meaning.
- You are always behaving. You cannot fail to behave.
- Inasmuch as you cannot stop behaving, you cannot stop communicating.
- Therefore, communication is inevitable.

TYPES OF COMMUNICATION

There are generally two types of communication: verbal and nonverbal. Each type has several components.

Verbal Communication

Verbal communication involves the use of words to convey messages. This type of communication is achieved by speaking or writing in a code that is mutually understood by sender and receiver. The tool of verbal communication is language. **Language** is a set of words that have meanings that are comprehensible within a group. Because a word has a definition, however, does not guarantee that its meaning will be interpreted in the same way by all group members. For example, in the English language, the word *hot* could mean something is very warm, stolen, or sexually attractive. It is important, therefore, to validate meaning between you and the client.

TALKING. Talking is the act of verbalizing symbols to convey thoughts, feelings, or ideas. It is a skill so taken for granted that it is almost impossible to communicate without it. This sense of helplessness can be overwhelming for clients who are intubated, who do not speak the dominant language, or who are rendered speechless by surgery or a neurological disorder.

WRITING. Written communication transfers a thought or spoken symbol into printed form. Being able to communicate accurately and clearly in writing is critical for you (e.g., in documenting nursing care). It can be especially useful in communicating with clients who are unable to hear or speak clearly, if at all. If you communicate with clients by writing, you should communicate as clearly as if you were speaking to the person. For example, it is important that you use clear language, use an appropriate vocabulary, and speak at the client's level of understanding. Correct spelling is vital to clear written communication.

When communicating with clients in writing, you should ensure that your printing is large enough and dark enough to be legible, that the room lighting is conducive to reading, and that the client is wearing reading glasses, if needed.

Nonverbal Communication

Nonverbal communication is a set of behaviors that conveys messages either without words or by supplementing verbal communication. Nonverbal communication consists of body language, paralanguage, and any other means by which one communicates with others without the use of words. As a health care professional, you are mainly concerned with body language and paralanguage.

Body language refers to nonverbal communication behaviors that are accomplished by the movement of our bodies or body parts, by the presentation of ourselves to the world, and by the use of our personal space (see later). Common body language behaviors include personal appearance; conscious and unconscious changes in facial expressions; body posture and gestures; the distance maintained from others; and how others are touched by us (Fig. 15–3). **Paralanguage** refers to nonverbal components of spoken language. These components give speech its rhythm and humanness and include stress, accent, pitch, pause, intonation, rate, volume, and quality.

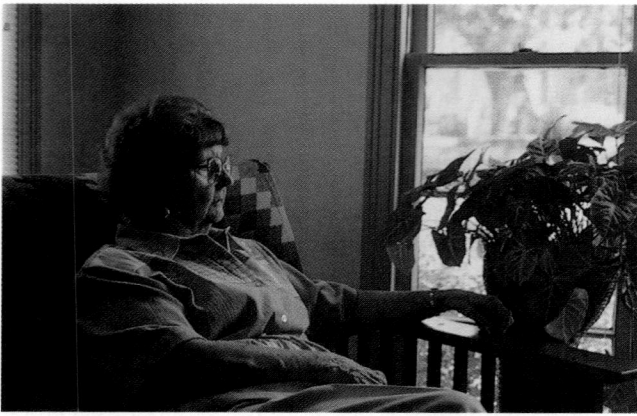

Figure 15–3. Body language is one important form of nonverbal communication. What might this woman's body language be saying?

Action Alert!
Carefully observe a client's nonverbal behavior. Because it is unconscious and therefore more difficult to control than verbal communication, it often provides a more reliable indication of the person's true message.

Body Language

Clients typically communicate a great deal with body language; therefore, messages sent by this means can be important in the overall assessment of the client. A few examples of the general areas you may assess follow.

PERSONAL APPEARANCE

A rapid assessment of the client's general appearance gives an initial impression of factors as varied as social standing, self-esteem, and emotional status. Because most persons are aware of being judged by their general appearance, they usually take steps to alter their appearance to create a more favorable impression, even in a health care setting. Rare is the mother who has not warned her child to wear clean underwear so that in the event of an accident, the emergency room doctor will not think badly of the child.

You can obtain useful information about a client's condition by observing whether the client has attended to good grooming. For example, the client who has neglected personal appearance may lack the means to do so (no bathing facilities), awareness of its importance (as in mental illness), the ability (due to physical handicap), the desire (from a lack of appropriate socialization), the energy (due to severe depression, physical weakness or handicap, or disease), or the time (before a sudden trip to the emergency room or delivery room).

Of course, you must be careful not to judge the client based on external appearances. For example, you might decide that a woman arriving in the emergency department who is totally filthy is too depressed to take care of her own hygiene. She may have just suffered a stroke after spending 9 hours digging up and rearranging her garden, in the hot sun, while wearing her oldest clothes. To avoid hasty judgments, it is always useful to validate impressions with additional data.

FACIAL EXPRESSIONS

Assessing a client's eyes and facial movements can also yield valuable information. When you assess these areas, note whether the movements are voluntary or involuntary (winks or smiles versus tics or twitches). Note whether the client can focus and maintain eye contact. Observe the eyes for redness, clarity, and tearing and the face for the raising and lowering of eyebrows or the presence of a smirk, smile, or frown.

A client can communicate pain, fear, anger, sadness, happiness, contentment, or excitement with the eyes and with facial muscular activity. Do not be too quick to assign meaning to facial expressions alone, however, because reading body language is not an exact science. For example, if you note a client's eyes are red-rimmed and teary and that he has difficulty making eye contact with you, further investigation is warranted. It may be that the client is embarrassed that he has been crying, or he may be a bashful person who is suffering from a seasonal allergy. Other possibilities exist to explain these few observations. Use your observations of facial expressions as cues to let you know where further assessment might be needed.

BODY POSTURE

As is true of facial movement, body posture and stance can also provide cues to a person's physical and emotional state. To assess body posture, note whether the person is standing straight, is slumped, or is hunched over. An erect posture usually signifies a feeling of fitness and confidence. Slumping often occurs in persons who are physically exhausted, weak, emotionally depressed; hunching can signal a desire to be left alone. A client who is hunching with forearms crossed over the abdomen may be guarding a painful abdomen. A more severely hunched posture, with head down, forearms brought up across the chest, and knees brought up to guard the abdomen (a fetal position), may indicate extreme fear or depression.

GESTURES

Observe the types of gestures used by your clients. Some clients talk with their hands by gesturing while they speak. Emphatic gestures often convey messages of urgency. The urgency may be accompanied by distress, great happiness, or excitement. Urgent hand gestures may represent the conversion of pent-up emotional energy into physical energy that can be released. Thus, urgent hand gestures can be a sign that the client has strong needs to be heard (and perhaps assisted). They may also be a means of client coping when the person is unable to adequately convey urgent messages verbally. It is also important to understand what gestures mean within different cultures to avoid misunderstanding when communicating with clients from diverse backgrounds.

PERSONAL DISTANCE

Everyone has a **personal space,** a private zone or "bubble" around our body that we believe is an extension of ourself and that belongs to us. We carry this personal space around with us at all times. A select number of other people are allowed to enter this space at certain times, and we tend to be uncomfortable if others enter this space at all. Therefore, we behave in ways to prevent this from happening. At certain times and in certain situations, we expand our personal space, and to maintain comfort most people must stay even farther away from us than usual.

The size of this space appears to be culturally determined at least in part, and it can vary considerably from culture to culture. People within each culture respect others' personal spaces and use culturally determined body language signals to help maintain appropriate distances from each other. In Western culture, most people maintain similar distances from each other according to their relationships and to the activities involved. As an example, two men who are strangers on opposing teams might grapple together on a football field when they would never think of allowing their bodies to come into contact in the shower after the game.

TOUCHING

Nurse-client touching is an issue that requires great sensitivity. Because nursing is a hands-on profession, it is daily practice to touch clients often and intimately. However, be constantly aware that touch conveys many meanings to clients. It may indicate agreement, caring, loving, or even sexual desire.

Many clients are hungry for a handclasp or other form of human touch and will demonstrate this by reaching out to you (Fig. 15–4). Most clients desire or

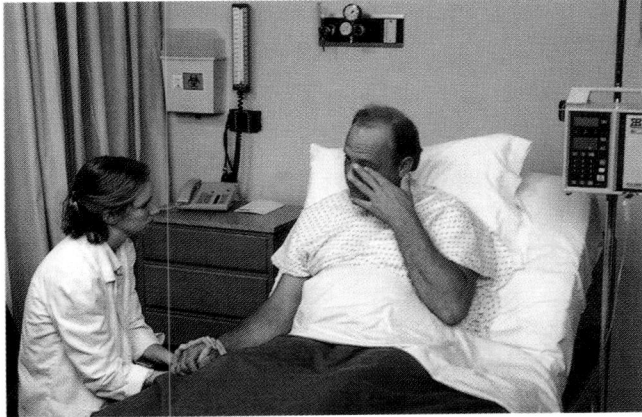

Figure 15–4. Many clients are hungry for a handclasp or other form of human touch. By touching the client when appropriate, you can convey warmth and empathy. However, if the client feels touch is inappropriate, draw back and respect the person's feelings. Otherwise, you risk undermining your attempt to communicate.

feel neutral about a casual touch such as a pat on the arm during the course of normal conversation. However, clients who have been physically or sexually abused tend to see uninvited touch as a boundary violation.

If a client has not indicated a specific desire to touch or be touched, assess the client's feelings about touch before using it. A rule of thumb is to ask permission before touching. It is easy to ask, "May I touch your arm?" Asking can help avoid possible problems. In certain settings it is appropriate to say, "I'd like to give you a hug. May I?"

Touch may be accepted more or less readily in different situations. For example, a hug may be greeted with relief by a family member in a hospice when support is needed most, but it would probably be perceived as a violation of personal space in an initial meeting with a client in a clinic. Touching can soothe or disturb people to their very depths. Therefore, it must be used judiciously, based on assessment of the client's needs and wishes.

Paralanguage

Clients may communicate a great deal with verbal messages as they attempt to relate the content of their thoughts. Even better communication can occur when appropriate use is made of nonverbal components of speech, or paralanguage. An understanding of paralanguage can help you grasp the content of the client's message, and it can sometimes help you tune in to the emotional component of the message—the client's mood.

STRESS. *Stress* refers to the part of a word, phrase, or sentence that is highlighted by changing pitch or elongating the syllable. Words that are stressed are generally the more important words. For example:

"Nice to meet you." (with no particular stress)
"*Nice* to meet you."
"Nice to *meet* you."
"Nice to meet *you.*"

All these statements have slightly different meanings because of the way stress is used.

ACCENT. *Accent* refers to the different pronunciation of syllables used by non-native speakers of a language. Accent alone can cause a loss of clarity that can result in a breakdown in communication. Do not pretend that you understand what someone has said when you do not. Seek to clarify what has been said by asking the person to repeat what was said, use different words, or write out the troublesome phrase.

PITCH. *Pitch* refers to whether the voice is high or low. Pitch results from the speed of vocal cord vibrations. Pitch is gender-related in that most men's voices are pitched lower than most women's voices. It is also age-related in that children's voices are usually pitched higher than adults' voices. In any individual, changes in pitch can alter the meaning of the content of a message. For example, pitch rises at the end of a question (interrogative sentence) and stays the same or lowers in making a statement (declarative sentence). Thus, "You have tuberculosis?" and "You have tuberculosis." are very different in meaning.

PAUSE. *Pauses* punctuate speech with periods of silence or non–word sounds, such as "Let me see . . ." or "Hmm, I believe you are right." Often a pause indicates that the person is still considering something, is considering whether to share something, or is searching for the words to use to encode properly what is to be told. At other times, pauses are used for effect as part of varying intonation. In any event, the pause should be respected and the person given adequate time to complete the communication interrupted by a pause.

INTONATION. *Intonation* is the variety of stress and pause patterns within a phrase or sentence. For example, people often use one intonation when giving a formal speech and other intonations when communicating with a superior at work or with a close friend.

RATE. The *rate* of speech refers to how many syllables are spoken per unit of time. Rate also takes into account the number of pauses made. Increased rate of speech may indicate nervousness or agitation. It is sometimes possible to control anxiety by focusing on a rapid speech rate and slowing it.

VOLUME. *Volume* comprises the loudness and intensity associated with the speaking voice. Intensity is a measure of forcefulness and can convey a message about the speaker's emotions. Generally, a loud voice indicates anger or frustration, and the speaker uses it as if loudness could somehow increase the power of the words to control the listener or others. Changes in volume (either up or down) may also occur in anxiety.

QUALITY. Voice *quality* is a measure of clarity, hoarseness, or nasality in the speaker's voice. Physical and emotional conditions can cause a change in voice quality. For example, the voice often becomes husky with deeply felt emotions, harsher with anger, and more nasal with a cold.

FACILITATING EFFECTIVE THERAPEUTIC COMMUNICATION

Nursing Attitudes That Promote Communication

Therapeutic communication is enhanced when you adopt helpful attitudes to indicate interest in and regard for the client. Before entering into the nurse-client relationship, it is useful to know about these communication-enhancing strategies. These nursing attitudes are sometimes referred to as *responsive attitudes.*

AWARENESS. Awareness of clients is necessary before human relationships with them are possible. In showing awareness, you acknowledge the presence of your client. It is best demonstrated by displaying attending behaviors. **Attending behaviors** show that you are paying attention and listening to what the client is saying. You demonstrate attending behaviors, for example, by facing the client, leaning toward the client, using appropriate eye contact, keeping your

eyes open with eyebrows raised, and maintaining an *open body posture,* a body position in which the arms and legs are uncrossed.

ACCEPTANCE, RESPECT, AND UNCONDITIONAL POSITIVE REGARD. Acceptance is an openness to the unique qualities and attributes of individual clients. Acceptance does not mean condoning inappropriate client behaviors. It means that clients are accepted for who they are, even if their behavior is undesirable. Respect is more than an attitude of acceptance. It also includes valuing, highly regarding, or esteeming clients for who they are.

Unconditional positive regard, a term coined by the psychologist Carl Rogers, describes respect for the client that is not dependent on the client's behavior. You learn to value and care for clients simply because their humanity warrants your care.

You avoid being critical, derogatory, or judgmental. You understand that the client's imperfections are part of the total picture; the imperfections may be undesirable behaviors, but they are coping mechanisms the client needs at the time. Many clients struggle with the dehumanizing aspects of illness and dependency. You empower clients by showing respect and by appreciating their humanness without ridiculing or demeaning them.

Another reason why you should not judge the client is simply that the client should not view you as a judge. In such a relationship, the client seeks to please you, which diverts attention from the objective of focusing on the client's growth.

EMPATHY. **Empathy** is the accurate perception of the client's feelings. It is the ability to "be in the other person's shoes" without taking on the client's feelings or thoughts. Empathy is not sympathy, wherein you feel pity or compassion for the client. Rather, it is a sense of understanding or "being with" the client. Evans, Witt, Alligood, and O'Neil (1998) identify two types of empathy, *basic* and *trained.* Basic empathy is a raw "feeling for" sense of where and how the client is emotionally. Not everyone is born with equal amounts of basic empathy, but it is possible to learn trained empathy. This is based on learning a role and a way to respond to clients in the nurse-client relationship. You can learn to assess and respond to client feelings empathetically even if you are not a "natural" at it. In your career, you will experience both empathy with and sympathy for clients, but empathy will help you build important bridges.

RELATEDNESS. Relatedness is the recognition of similarities between you and the client and the forging of emotional connections based on those similarities. Relating to clients helps to establish human-to-human ties that make communication possible. Common experiences make you and the client more readily known to each other.

CARING. Caring is taking an emotional risk to feel a personal interest in the client's welfare. By investing yourself in the client, you consciously decide to take emotional risks and give of your skills, compassion, and experience. Such concern can be draining, and you must continually assess personal psychic energy and emotional resources to prevent exhaustion.

OBJECTIVITY. Objectivity is an unbiased, reality-based stance that allows you to assess the facts of a client's situation without being emotionally pulled into the client's difficulties. You can be objective and still have warm feelings for the client and attend to the client's thoughts and feelings. Thinking about the client objectively allows you to understand client experiences and to identify areas of difficulty in order to guide the client toward developing appropriate problem-solving skills.

PROTECTIVENESS. Protectiveness leads you to shield the fragile and vulnerable client during the person's recovery from illness. There is a fine line between protectiveness and fostering dependence. Protectiveness is a caring attitude that should be used judiciously while you continue to evaluate the client's capacity to defend the self.

GENUINENESS. Genuineness is your ability to be honest, open, and sincere in self-presentation. The phrase "what you see is what you get" describes the demeanor of a genuine person. It is important not to confuse being genuine with being totally self-disclosing or casually spontaneous, as one would be with friends or family. For example, you may share a family's joy on the birth of a baby and demonstrate it with warm congratulations for the parents and admiration for the baby.

OPENNESS. Being open with a client reflects your ability and willingness to be real, genuine, and emotionally accessible. Openness does not mean that boundaries are violated. It means that you choose what to share with the client and share it in an authentic manner. When you are open with a client, the client tends to lower defenses and to relate more honestly to you.

PROFESSIONAL CLOSENESS OR DISTANCE. There is a delicate balance between maintaining objectivity and the firm boundaries associated with professional distance and the warmth, openness, and availability associated with professional closeness. You should be accessible to the client, but the therapeutic relationship is not a friendship. Friendships are social rather than therapeutic relationships. This does not mean, however, that you must be impersonal or treat clients with indifference.

Professional closeness and stance vary throughout the relationship as you and the client come together as strangers, work on mutual goals, and proceed to termination. New nurses may feel uncomfortable with attempts at maintaining professional closeness and stance. A good rule to follow is to become invested without being engulfed. This means caring about clients and allowing yourself to know their concerns, but it does not mean taking their thoughts, feelings, or attitudes as your own.

SENSE OF HUMOR. Many have questioned the appropriateness of using any form of humor in a therapeutic relationship. Certain types of "humor" must be avoided, such as morbid humor, humor based on sarcasm, or humor that degrades anyone. These are inappropriate and unprofessional. However, you must be able to laugh at yourself and at the humorous situations that can arise. Being a role model of this openness and demonstrating the appropriate use of humor can be therapeutic for clients just as it is for yourself.

Appreciation of the humorous side of life can be a desirable attitude for you. However, the ability to use humor therapeutically is a talent that not all nurses possess. When you are comfortable with the sensitive use of humor, you can sometimes use it to put clients at ease, defuse emotionally loaded situations, or simply inject a light note into an otherwise difficult day. You must assess each client's readiness for humor. If the client is likely to perceive any levity as a put-down, it is much better to maintain a more serious demeanor. Although clients can appreciate wit as much as anyone, they must first feel that you are trustworthy, dependable, and on their side.

Action-Oriented Characteristics

We have reviewed 11 responsive attitudes that promote therapeutic communication. In addition, you must possess three action-oriented characteristics in order to achieve successful therapeutic communication. These characteristics—concreteness, immediacy, and confrontation—must be used with the responsive attitudes if they are to be effective without alienating the client.

CONCRETENESS. Concreteness refers to communicating concerns in specific and personal language rather than in generalities. You can help the client to be concrete by role-modeling concreteness and by asking the client to remain in the "here-and-now" during discussions. You can do this by discouraging vague or general references to events and seeking information as explicitly as possible. For example, rather than saying to a client, "Tell me about yourself," you might say, "Tell me how that (event) affects you personally at this time." Concreteness helps keep communication clear and helps the client cope with experiences in measurable terms.

IMMEDIACY. Immediacy requires direct attention to the specific dynamics existing within the relationship between you and your client. If you have difficulty working with a client or if there has been tension in the relationship, it is easier to ignore the conflict and avoid the client. However, this is mutually counterproductive. To practice immediacy, try to elicit information about what is interfering with your interactions. For instance, if you have gently confronted a diabetic client about consistently high blood sugars and then find the client is avoiding you, you might say, "I've noticed we haven't spoken in the last 2 months. I wonder what's going on between us that makes it difficult for us to talk." You are not focusing on the client or yourself but on what is occurring between the two of you.

CONFRONTATION. Confrontation is a process in which you sensitively point out inconsistencies in a client's behavior. This type of confrontation is not angry, attacking, or demeaning. It should not be used before trust is established. In a therapeutic relationship, you can use confrontation to enlighten the client about conflicting verbal and nonverbal behaviors. For example, you might say, "I see you have tears in your eyes and your shoulders are shaking, but you told me you were calm. Now I am wondering what it is that you really feel."

Respecting Differences

You must develop effective communication skills to enhance your work with clients of different groups, of different cultures, and at different stages of health.

DEVELOPMENTAL DIFFERENCES. As has been mentioned, communication techniques must be appropriate for the client's stage of development, or communication can be diminished. Examples of how to apply therapeutic techniques to children, adolescents, and adults of all ages have been provided in the tables appearing later in this chapter.

CULTURAL DIFFERENCES. Clients from different cultures may or may not speak a different language but will most often have differing customs, values, mores, and social structures, all of which can affect communication. Obviously, the more you understand about the culture of your client, the better you will be able to communicate. It is helpful to learn crucial words and sentences in the client's language or to have a translator write out cards with commonly used bilingual sentences. However, understanding the non-native client requires more than just learning a few new phrases. You must be aware of any personal biases to avoid stereotyping and labeling these clients. Respect for the client's experience and acceptance of the differences that exist between you can help establish a safe, therapeutic environment in which maximum communication can occur.

GENDER DIFFERENCES. Men and women communicate differently, and understanding these differences enhances therapeutic relationships. Deborah Tannen, a popular author and communication expert, pointed out that men and women have different styles of intimacy and independence. According to Tannen, men seek dominance in a hierarchical structure to be independent; women avoid being dependent and subordinate but do not need to dominate. Intimacy to women means a free sharing of thoughts, hopes, and feelings. Men avoid such sharing to preserve personal freedom (Tannen, 1990).

Tannen's theories can help you to negotiate hierarchy and power issues delicately when talking with persons of both genders. For example, Tannen referred to *rapport talk* and *report talk*. Rapport talk, more comfortable to women, is a way of connecting with others and negotiating relationships. Examples of rapport talk are the techniques of offering self, suggesting collaboration, exploring, and focusing. Report talk, the demonstration of knowledge and skill, is the preferred conversational style of men. Examples of report talk

are presenting reality, encouraging formulation of a plan, and summarizing. In short, women speak to connect; men speak to preserve status and independence (Tannen, 1990). You must recognize the validity of both styles. A respectful awareness that gender affects style as well as a willingness to "read between the lines" promotes more effective communication with both sexes.

TECHNIQUES THAT IMPAIR THERAPEUTIC COMMUNICATION

Before you begin to learn about therapeutic communication techniques, it is imperative that you understand what not to do. This is because there is no single set of words or phrases that will always be helpful to all people, in all situations, at all times. You can be given only generally accepted guidelines and examples, and you must practice your therapeutic techniques within these guidelines, using your own words. It is difficult to know which of your own words might be hurtful, or merely less than helpful, unless you have a good grasp of what should not be done.

Nontherapeutic communication techniques impair the flow of communication in what would otherwise be a progressive movement toward client growth. Some nontherapeutic techniques thwart communication by undermining you, for example, by calling into question your honesty or by diminishing the client's trust in you. Other nontherapeutic techniques thwart communication by undermining the client. Nontherapeutic techniques that undermine the client are those that are demeaning, those that reinforce or strengthen irrational ideas or beliefs, those that tend to raise client anxiety levels, and those that tend to make the client dependent on you. Still other nontherapeutic techniques block the flow of ideas between the client and you. Some nontherapeutic techniques block communication in more than one way. Table 15–1 describes many nontherapeutic communication techniques along with selected examples that might be used with pediatric, adolescent, and adult clients.

TECHNIQUES THAT ENHANCE THERAPEUTIC COMMUNICATION

To maximize therapeutic communication you need to use techniques that encourage clients to open up and speak more freely. A number of such techniques of therapeutic communication are generally considered helpful for you to use and are listed in Table 15–2. Like any other tools, if they are used inappropriately, they can impede communication instead of enhancing it. It is helpful to know what to do and what not to do when using them. Here are some guidelines:

- Individualize each technique to your client's level of understanding. For example, you might tell a 40-year-old man, "I will demonstrate the correct technique for injecting your insulin," but to a 6-year-

TABLE 15–1
Nontherapeutic Communication Techniques

Technique	Description/Definition	Example
Belittling feelings expressed	The nurse minimizes the degree of the client's distress or discomfort, thereby implying that the client's feelings are insignificant.	*Nurse with child:* Child: "I hate shots." Nurse: "You are not the only one." *Nurse with adolescent:* Adolescent: "There is no reason to go on." Nurse: "Aren't you being a little dramatic?" *Nurse with adult:* Adult: "My life means nothing." Nurse: "If you take a walk, you will feel better."
Reassuring	The nurse implies that the anxious client has no cause for worry or concern.	*Nurse with child:* "No need to fuss over such a small needle." *Nurse with adolescent:* "One day you will look back at this and laugh." *Nurse with adult:* "Your chest pain isn't a heart attack."
Parroting	The nurse mechanically repeats the client's words without evaluating what has been said and without helping the client to think things through. It indicates a lack of interest, respect, and relatedness on the nurse's part.	*Nurse with child:* Child: "My mommy left." Nurse: "Your mommy left." *Nurse with adolescent:* Adolescent: "I am not going for dialysis." Nurse: "You are not going for dialysis." *Nurse with adult:* Adult: "I do not see any options for treatment." Nurse: "You do not see any options for treatment."
Disapproving	The nurse makes a negative value judgment about the client's behavior or thinking.	*Nurse with child:* "Shame on you!" *Nurse with adolescent:* "I cannot believe you did that." *Nurse with adult:* "Why don't you stop all this foolishness?"
Disagreeing	The nurse opposes the client's thinking. The nurse's disagreement implies the client is wrong and must defend the position	*Nurse with child:* "I think you are wrong about this." *Nurse with adolescent:* "You can say what you like, but it does not make it right." *Nurse with adult:* "I definitely disagree with you."
Rationalizing feelings expressed	The nurse provides a seemingly rational (but untrue) excuse for the client's expression of emotions in order to avoid an emotional reaction to the client's feelings or to avoid having to respond appropriately to the client. This rationalizaiton of feelings robs affective material shared by the client of its power.	*Nurse with child:* Child: "I'm mad." Nurse: "Maybe you are just tired." *Nurse with adolescent:* "Jack, crying because you hurt will only make it worse." *Nurse with adult:* Adult: "Now I am just a heart patient." Nurse: "Wouldn't you be worse off if you had AIDS?"
Interpreting	The nurse attempts to tell the client the meaning of the client's experience by seeking to make conscious that which is unconscious.	*Nurse with child:* "What you really mean is . . . ." *Nurse with adolescent:* "Your true feelings are . . . ." Nurse with adult: "On a deeper level, you believe. . . ."
Advising	The nurse literally tells the client what to do. This implies that the nurse knows best and the client is incapable of independent problem solving.	*Nurse with child:* "Tell the doctor how much better you feel today." *Nurse with adolescent:* "Stop eating sweets and you will lose weight." *Nurse with adult:* "I would choose option A."

Table continued on following page

TABLE 15–1
Nontherapeutic Communication Techniques *Continued*

Technique	Description/Definition	Example
Blaming	The nurse inappropriately expresses feelings of anger or impatience with the client as a means of faulting the client because the nurse-client relationship is not progressing well. This is a therapeutic dead-end that negates the nurse's role as a client advocate, destroys trust, and takes away client motivation to work with the nurse to identify and explore sensitive topics.	*Nurse with child:* "Well, you can't expect a sticker when you cry every time I come near you." *Nurse with adolescent:* "Get your act together, and things will go better for you." *Nurse with adult:* "Nobody told you to pull your back out, did they?"
Moralizing	The nurse judges the client according to personal moral values. Because the client must feel free to discuss issues within the therapeutic relationship, this moralizing oversteps appropriate limits and places the relationship in jeopardy.	*Nurse with child:* "Eating too many sweets is very bad for you." *Nurse with adolescent:* "Your crazy behavior is bound to get you in trouble." *Nurse with adult:* "Birth control pills will just promote irresponsible sexual behavior."
Patronizing	The nurse treats the client in a condescending manner, thereby demeaning the client. This makes acceptance, respect, and mutual decision-making impossible.	*Nurse with child:* "Just go play somewhere now." *Nurse with adolescent:* "Of course your ideas are important to me sweetie." *Nurse with adult:* "Let's put on our slippers before we fall."
Making stereotypical comments	The nurse makes empty conversation using trite phrases and cliches, thereby encouraging the client to do the same rather than honestly exploring issues.	*Nurse with child:* "You will thank me later." *Nurse with adolescent:* "Pretty is as pretty does." *Nurse with adult:* "Let a smile be your umbrella."
Introducing an unrelated topic	The nurse changes the subject when the client brings up material the nurse prefers not to discuss.	*Nurse with child:* Child: "What is sex?" Nurse: "Finish your lunch before it gets cold." *Nurse with adolescent:* Adolescent: "What is my diagnosis?" Nurse: "Did you see the game last night?" *Nurse with adult:* Adult: "The doctor says that I am dying." Nurse: "Time for a bath."
Using jargon	The nurse excludes the client and makes the interaction incomprehensible by using nursing jargon (the specialized language used by a group).	*Nurse with child:* "Do not regurgitate your nutritional supplement." *Nurse with adolescent:* "Your increased sexual preoccupation indicates progression towards full maturation." *Nurse with adult:* "Coronary abnormalities are indicated on the angiogram."
Giving literal responses	The nurse responds to the client's figurative statement as though it were factual. The nurse misses a chance to explore material with the client.	*Nurse with child:* Child: "My insides are exploding." Nurse: "That sounds messy." *Nurse with adolescent:* Adolescent: "I am losing my mind." Nurse: "Find it." *Nurse with Adult:* Adult: "My world is ending" Nurse: "The world is not ending."

TABLE 15–1

Nontherapeutic Communication Techniques *Continued*

Technique	Description/Definition	Example
Requesting an explanation	The nurse asks "why" of the client, thereby asking for a reason for feelings and behaviors when the client may not know the reason.	*Nurse with child:* "Why don't you stop crying?" *Nurse with adolescent:* "Why are you upset?" *Nurse with adult:* "Why can't you fall asleep?"
Probing	The nurse digs for information or persistently questions the client even after the client indicates unwillingness to discuss the issues.	*Nurse with child:* Nurse: "Tell me about the test." Child: "I do not want to." Nurse: "Tell me anyway." *Nurse with adolescent:* "Tell me more about that terrible event." *Nurse with adult:* "I cannot help you if you do not give me all the information about your drug habit."
Challenging	The nurse insists the client provide a rational basis for irrational thinking. The client then becomes defensive, and issues are closed to exploration.	*Nurse with child:* "If the doctor is bad, then why is he nice to me?" *Nurse with adolescent:* "What makes you think 85 pounds is too fat?" *Nurse with adult:* "If you are not diabetic, then why is your blood sugar so high?"
Testing	The nurse tests the client's capacity for insight by first assuming that the client has no insight and then expecting the client to agree.	*Nurse with child:* "What color is this blue glass?" *Nurse with adolescent:* "Have you figured this out yet?" *Nurse with adult:* "You think you still believe . . . ?"

old girl you would say, "I will show you how to give your doll a shot."

- Vary the communication technique. Avoid using a single technique repeatedly. For example, saying "Tell me more" shows interest in what the client is saying and is therapeutic. But if you say "Tell me more" after everything the client says, it demonstrates that you are not giving a thoughtful response to each of the client's answers. Too many "Tell me more's" (or any similar phrase) can be counterproductive.
- Use paralanguage appropriately to convey your intended meaning. For example, you may say something generally considered to be therapeutic, such as "I see," and say it sarcastically, icily, or in some other tone that is nontherapeutic. Another nurse may say something generally considered to be nontherapeutic but say it so warmly and with such caring that it is actually therapeutic for the client. Two nurses may say the exact same words and one will be seen as helpful and the other as condescending. In such cases, paralanguage may make the difference.
- If you are using therapeutic techniques correctly, your client will be doing most of the talking as you listen and guide the interaction. If you find you are doing most of the talking, something is wrong, and you need to pause and reflect about how to get back on track.
- You will probably make mistakes in talking with clients, and you will say some things that are not the best possible responses. In fact, there may be times that you will be angry with yourself because you said something so nontherapeutic. However, if you have a genuinely therapeutic relationship with the client, the relationship will survive an error or two.
- As you enter the clinical area to talk with a client for the first time, relax and realize that most clients want very much to talk to you.
- Any specific techniques of communication might be used at any time, according to the client and the situation, but some techniques tend to be more helpful at the beginning of an interaction, and some tend to be more helpful in the middle or at the end of an interaction.

Beginning the Interaction

OFFERING SELF. Offering self is a technique in which you offer to stay with the client and either talk or just sit quietly. In offering self, you need to clearly

TABLE 15–2

Therapeutic Communication Techniques

Technique	Description/Definition	Example
Offering self	The nurse offers to stay with the client and either talk or just sit quietly.	*Nurse with child:* "Let's sit in the playroom together and play for 10 minutes." *Nurse with adolescent:* "Let's have a soda together." *Nurse with adult:* "I'll be back in 15 minutes to sit with you."
Providing broad openings	The nurse invites the client to select a topic.	*Nurse with child:* "What will we talk about today?" *Nurse with adolescent:* "Tell me what I can teach you about your dialysis." *Nurse with adult:* "What shall we cover next?"
Providing silence	The nurse allows the verbal conversation to stop to provide a time for quiet contemplation of what has been discussed, for formulation of thoughts about how to proceed, or to reduce tension.	(Silence)
Focusing	The nurse selects one topic for exploration from among several possible topics presented by the client.	*Nurse with child:* "Tell me your favorite food for breakfast before you tell me about lunch." *Nurse with adolescent:* "You mentioned several things you like about school. What do you like best?" *Nurse with adult:* "You mention several advantages to your hip surgery. What is the single greatest improvement you have noticed?"
Asking for clarification	The nurse lets the client know that what was said was unclear. If necessary, the nurse asks for clarification or suggests ways to make the message clearer.	*Nurse with child:* "I did not understand what you said. Would you say it again for me?" *Nurse with adolescent:* "Maybe you would explain more about what you mean so I can be more helpful." *Nurse with adult:* "Let me tell you what I heard you say to me."
Reflecting	The client asks a question, and the nurse turns the question around and reflects it back to the client, or the client makes a statement, and the nurse selects one or more words to reflect back to the client for consideration. This technique strengthens the client's confidence.	*Nurse with child:* Child: "Should I wear blue or green?" Nurse: "Which would you like to wear?" *Nurse with adolescent:* Adolescent: "My mom won't let me pierce my tongue." Nurse: "What would it be like to have a pierced tongue?" *Nurse with adult:* Adult: "What should I tell the doctor?" Nurse: "What would you like to tell the doctor?"
Placing events in time or sequence	The nurse asks the client to explain more about when an event occurred (placing the event in time) or to explain the sequence of events (placing events in sequence) to clarify for the nurse.	*Nurse with child:* "Did you get sick before or after you ate?" *Nurse with adolescent:* "Tell me the steps you followed in changing your dressing." *Nurse with adult:* "Did your blood sugar go up after breakfast today or yesterday?"
Restating	The nurse paraphrases what the client has said. This paraphrased message may be fed back to the client in the form of a statement or a question to provide the client the opportunity to agree or disagree and clarify further.	*Nurse with child:* Child: "I want my blankie." Nurse: "You would like your blankie." *Nurse with adolescent:* Adolescent: "I just puked." Nurse: "You were sick to your stomach." *Nurse with adult:* Adult: "It's no use." Nurse: "You are pretty discouraged."
Seeking consensual validation	The nurse attempts to verify with the client that a certain term means the same thing to both parties.	*Nurse with child:* "You want Baby Lisa? Is she your doll?" *Nurse with adolescent:* "When you say you were high, did you mean you had just taken some drugs?" *Nurse with adult:* "Tell me if I understand your meaning correctly."

TABLE 15–2
Therapeutic Communication Techniques *Continued*

Technique	Description/Definition	Example
Encouraging descriptions of perceptions	The nurse asks the client to describe perceptions and associated emotions. This is particularly useful in understanding a client's experiences during hallucinations.	*Nurse with child:* "Tell me what you saw when I turned off the light." *Nurse with adolescent:* "How do think the other kids feel about you?" *Nurse with adult:* "Describe what it is like when your hear the messages from God."
Voicing doubt	The nurse questions how something the client has misperceived could possibly be true. This is done by questioning the truthfulness of what was perceived without questioning the truthfulness of the client.	*Nurse with child:* "When I sit in the dark with you, I don't see a monster." *Nurse with adolescent:* "I have never heard other kids say anything unkind about you." *Nurse with adult:* "I haven't really known of anyone getting direct messages from God."
Presenting reality	When a client has had an unrealistic perception of reality, the nurse accepts the fact that the client has misperceived something but indicates that the nurse did not have a similar perception. When something in the environment is stimulating the misperception, the nurse attempts to point this out.	*Nurse with child:* "I think that shadow on the wall might look like a monster to you." *Nurse with adolescent:* "The other kids tell me they worry that you don't seem to like them." *Nurse with adult:* "I have heard that God usually speaks to our hearts instead of our ears."
Summarizing	The nurse briefly states, in an orderly manner, what has been discussed. The purpose is to help ensure that client and nurse are in agreement about what went on, what decisions were made to help ensure that nothing was omitted, and to bring the relationship to a close.	*Nurse with child:* "Tomorrow we will do your bath before breakfast and cartoons." *Nurse with adolescent:* "Let me review the steps for coughing and deep-breathing exercises." *Nurse with adult:* "You have told me all the appropriate things to do to take care of that wound. I think you are ready to do it by yourself from now on."

establish parameters for the amount of time offered. For example, "I have 30 minutes available to talk with you at 10 o'clock today" or "I will stay with you while you wait for your family." Additional examples are found in Table 15–2.

In some cases, it is therapeutic to give the client a choice about your offer. Say, for example, "Would you like to meet with me for 20 minutes at one o'clock today?" However, some clients, such as those who are depressed, very much need to have you with them but will tend to reject your offer. Others should not be asked to make decisions about anything, because it raises their anxiety level. As you learn more and more about you clients and their individual needs, you will learn who can be asked and who should just be told that you are there for them. Until you do know, or if you are ever in doubt, it is always safe to offer self without allowing a choice.

Offering self can be very helpful when you are talking with someone who seems unable to express their thoughts or who does not want to talk at the mo-

ment. You can say something like, "It is okay if you don't feel like talking right now. I'll just stay here with you for 20 minutes." If you make this time commitment, be sure that you honor it for as long as you said you would. This helps establish that you are someone who can be trusted.

PROVIDING BROAD OPENINGS. Early in a meeting with a client, it may be useful to provide a broad opening. In this case, you invite the client to select a topic for discussion. Here, too, it is therapeutic to set some parameters concerning what you are willing to discuss. For example, in most instances, it would not be helpful for the client to discuss personal information about you or for you to engage in social-level small talk with the client. Therefore, it is not always appropriate to say, "We can talk about anything you like." It is better to say, for example, "We can discuss the issues that are bothering you." The latter is a very broad, client-focused opening.

MAKING OBSERVATIONS. In making observations, you acknowledge that something or someone exists or has changed in some way. You make an observation without appearing to judge either positively or negatively. For example, you comment that your client required only two doses of pain medication today when four were needed 2 days ago. When the observation pertains to the client, this technique may be termed *giving recognition*. However, the term *recognition* is less desirable because it may be misconstrued by the client as receiving approval or praise from you. The acknowledgment you give when making an observation should open communication about the subject at hand but not provide the client with any specific positive reinforcement.

SUGGESTING COLLABORATION. Suggesting collaboration is a technique in which you offer to work together with the client. This technique is useful in beginning a relationship with a client because it establishes that you and the client will work together as a team. Initially, the work may involve discussing some of the issues of concern to the client. Later, as problems are identified and nursing diagnoses are made, the work may shift to establishing and meeting client outcomes. At all times, the work focuses on the client.

Action Alert!
Begin any therapeutic interaction with clarity, and focus on the client.

Continuing the Interaction

PROVIDING SILENCE. Providing silence in a therapeutic manner allows the verbal conversation to stop and provides a time for quiet contemplation of what has been discussed or for formulating thoughts about how to proceed. The silence can also provide an opportunity for reducing tension when the interaction has been concerned with powerful issues and when emotions have been particularly deep.

Many people (nurses as well as clients) are uncomfortable with silence and will talk continuously about nothing in particular just to avoid it. This is obviously not a therapeutic approach for you to take. If you find that you are uncomfortable with silence, think about what has been going on during the silence, and use it constructively to think about what you will say next. You will find that, with practice, you can become more and more comfortable with silence.

ACCEPTING MESSAGES. Accepting messages is a way of providing feedback to acknowledge to the client that you have heard and understood what the client said. The acknowledgment is done in a manner that is neutral in tone, without agreeing, disagreeing, or providing any judgments about the message. The accepting may be done verbally or nonverbally. Your method of accepting messages should be brief and should allow the client to continue on with a train of thought without any real interruption.

PROVIDING GENERAL LEADS. In ordinary social communications, people take turns communicating. After your clients have spoken for awhile, they may hesitate because they are uncertain about whether it is appropriate to continue or whether they should try to draw you into the conversation. It is your task to keep clients focused on their own issues and to ensure that they continue to feel comfortable discussing them. To do this, you may use the technique of providing general leads. General leads are brief interjections ("Yes, I see," or "And then what happened?") that let clients know that they are on the right track and should continue. The leads provided should not cause real interruptions in the train of thought as they urge clients forward.

EXPLORING. As clients are talking, they may mention something that you believe is significant enough to warrant further attention. If they have introduced the subject and have not indicated that further discussion is undesirable, it is appropriate to attempt to delve into the matter in greater detail. To do this, you use the technique of *exploring*. To explore, you ask the client to describe something in more detail or to discuss it more fully. However, be careful not to use the nontherapeutic technique of *probing*. If your client gives an indication that further discussion is off-limits, honor this, and use another technique, such as providing a general lead to get the client to continue with what he was saying. For example, if your client says, "I won't discuss what that doctor told me," it is counterproductive and disrespectful to ask further questions about that subject.

FOCUSING. When clients are talking with you, they may start bringing up many different topics or concerns at once. These may all be worth exploring further, but you cannot explore them simultaneously. When this happens, it is best to select one subject to explore further while keeping others in mind for future discussion. Selecting one subject for exploration from among several is termed *focusing*.

For example, an adult client may say, "Things really fell apart after my second heart attack. I knew if I didn't control my diabetes that I would wind up near dead. You know, diabetics can lose their kidneys if they are not careful. I have two uncles who went bad from too much sugar. I think I'm a goner." How do you decide which point to explore? You may choose to focus on how the client feels about being diabetic, about the obvious concerns raised about its possible effects, about issues related to having had two heart attacks, or about the client's feelings with regard to mortality.

If you focus on one point, you can always return to other issues later on. You might prepare the client for this by making an observation, focusing, and then requesting further exploration in the future. For example, you might say, "You have given me a great deal to think about, and much of it seems worth talking about (making an observation). For now, I would like to know more about your most recent heart attack (focusing), and later on, perhaps we can discuss your other concerns (requesting further exploration in the future)."

Action Alert!
Use the above techniques to give the client permission to discuss his concerns. Keep the interaction client-centered, and clarify without speaking for the client.

ACTIVE LISTENING. Listening is the process in which spoken and other auditory information is received. Listening is an integral part of therapeutic communication. **Positive listening** is simply understanding the auditory messages sent by a sender. Being lonely, frightened, or doubtful can be an uncomfortable experience unless someone is there to receive these messages. Active listening plays a role in helping the client communicate thoughts, feelings, and beliefs. You take an active part in listening by eliciting details from the client and by inviting the client to think more about what is being said. It is more than positive listening.

Active listening is a means of "being with" the client and indicating acceptance and agreement, using verbal and nonverbal cues. It is an art and the key to therapeutic interaction. To use active listening, you must understand and use all of the other therapeutic techniques of communication. Compare the following examples:

Passive listening:
  Client: "I just learned I have cancer."
  Nurse: "I see."
  Client: "I'm afraid I will die."
  Nurse: "Hmm."
Active listening:
  Client: "I just learned I have cancer."
  Nurse *(With concern in voice and turning to face client):* "I wonder how you're feeling about this."
  Client: "I'm afraid I will die."
  Nurse: "Dying feels like a real possibility to you."
  Client: "My mother died of cancer when I was eight, and I have an eight-year-old."
  Nurse: "This really hits close to you."

Note how active listening brought out information not available to the passive listener. This is truly the basis for therapeutic interaction.

Action Alert!
Actively listening to what the client says and responding to it in a considered way demonstrates your care and concern for the client and his message.

KEEPING COMMUNICATION CLEAR
ASKING FOR CLARIFICATION. Sometime clients say things that are unclear, have more than one specific meaning, or are simply vague. These garbled messages can impede communication. When this occurs, you can use several techniques to help clarify the message for both you and the client. The most straightforward technique is asking for clarification. Simply let the client know that you are not certain about what was said and, if necessary, request that the client clarify anything that is obscure. If the client does not understand what was unclear, you may have to tell the client how it could be clarified for you. For example, if you are unsure about whether the client said "I saw the patient's mail" versus "I saw the male patient," you may have to ask the client to repeat the statement, spell the word ("male" or "mail"), or rephrase the concept.

RESTATING. Another way to clarify is to use the therapeutic technique of *restating,* or paraphrasing, what the client has said. To do this, you alter the client's words so that the meaning is the same as how you understand the client's meaning. You may feed this back to the client in the form of a statement or a question and provide the client the opportunity to agree or disagree that this was the intended message and, if necessary, to clarify further.

SEEKING CONSENSUAL VALIDATION. Sometimes, when a certain term used by a client has been unclear, you can use the technique of seeking consensual validation to help ensure that both you and the client agree on the meaning of the term. For example, at the end of a lesson about insulin injection, a client might say, "I'm through." You may interpret this in one of three ways: the client has learned the information well enough to self-inject insulin, the client is feeling tired after intense teaching, or the client is feeling discouraged and needs extra support. Focus on one of these three, and seek to verify whether or not that is what the client meant. You might ask, "When you say you are through, I understand that you are tired. Is that correct?" This gives the client the opportunity to agree or disagree and clarify further.

PLACING EVENTS IN TIME OR SEQUENCE. Often in describing an event or a series of events, clients fail to relate the story in strict chronological order. This can make the client's message about the occurrence difficult to follow. When this happens, you can ask the client to explain more about when the event occurred (placing the event in time) or to explain the sequence of a series of events (placing events in sequence).

HELPING THE CLIENT INCREASE SELF-AWARENESS
VERBALIZING THE IMPLIED. With the technique of *verbalizing the implied,* you understand the words the client has said but believe the words have an underlying meaning that was hinted at but not voiced specifically. You may need to verbalize this underlying message. The client may then verify that the message you received was indeed true. This frees the client to discuss with you some underlying feelings that had not been voiced before. Conversely, it is possible that the client did not mean to imply anything more than the actual words expressed. In this case, verbalizing the implied allows the client to verify that you have an inaccurate perception of the message.

ENCOURAGING ASSESSMENT OF EMOTIONS. It is important for people to be in touch with their own feelings. Too often, to cope with overwhelming feelings, clients wall themselves off from all emotions. This can be very unhealthy. To help clients get back in touch with their feelings, use the technique of encouraging assessment of emotions. To do this, ask clients to focus on their feelings, and ask them how they feel.

TRANSLATING INTO FEELINGS. Sometimes clients find it difficult or impossible to express their feelings verbally by using appropriate terms for common emotions. You can help the client by translating their messages into verbal expressions of feelings. However, you should always be open to correction if the client finds the translation inaccurate.

REFLECTING. In this technique, you reflect questions and statements back to the client to help the client to think about them and come to a conclusion. This helps the client gain confidence in making assessments and decisions and encourages the client's self-reliance.

There are two forms of reflection. One form is used when the client asks a question and the question is turned around and reflected back to the client. For example, the client might ask, "How am I doing with my physical therapy?" and you might reflect back with, "How do you think you're doing?" This demonstrates that you value the client's opinion.

The second form reflects back to the client some of their own words. This should not be confused with *parroting*, in which all of the client's words are directed back without thought on your part. With reflection, however, you think about the message and select the word or words that are important for the client to think about. This requires active involvement by both you and the client. For example, the client might say, "I'm scared about my surgery tomorrow." With reflection, you might ask, "Scared?" and suggest that the client consider and further discuss the feeling of being scared.

ENCOURAGING COMPARISON. To help clients integrate new experiences into what they know of life and to help them learn, you can encourage comparison. To do this, you may ask the client to compare or contrast a certain life experience with another.

HELPING THE CLIENT MAINTAIN CONTACT WITH REALITY

ENCOURAGING DESCRIPTIONS OF PERCEPTIONS. Sometimes clients will perceive things that others do not. It can be helpful for the client to describe such perceptions and the emotions attached to them. This technique of encouraging descriptions of perceptions is suitable when working with clients who have hallucinations of various types. It is not recommended that you attempt to communicate with a client who is actively hallucinating. If you know this is happening, wait until the hallucination has ended before attempting to elicit the client's perceptions and emotions.

VOICING DOUBTS. Sometimes clients have a wrong perception of reality. You know that it is nontherapeutic to disagree with clients because it risks strengthening their resolve to convince you that they are correct. Instead of *disagreeing* with a client who reports seeing something that is not there and asks whether you also see it, you can use the therapeutic technique of *voicing doubt.* To do this, you do not agree or disagree. You accept the fact that the client has perceived something that you have not, and you let the client know that you have difficulty understanding how the client's percep-

tion could be real. You do not doubt the client, but you do doubt the reality of the client's perception. You also make the client understand that while you question the validity of the client's perception, you still accept the client as a person of worth. It is always the reality of the perception that is questioned and never the person's truthfulness about the perception. Say, for example, "I just can't believe such a thing could be," not "I just can't believe you."

PRESENTING REALITY. In situations where you are with clients when a misperception of reality occurs, you can be the person who can help these clients identify what is real and what is not. This technique, called *presenting reality,* can be very reassuring to some people. Similar to the technique of voicing doubt, you accept the fact that the client has perceived something that you have not perceived, but you let the client know that you did not have a similar perception. You might say, for example, "It must be very frightening for you to hear sirens wailing, but I don't hear anything."

Concluding the Interaction

ENCOURAGING FORMULATION OF A PLAN OF ACTION. Once you enter the working phase of the relationship, and once you and the client have identified problems, diagnoses, and desired outcomes, you need to encourage formulation of a plan of action. This technique calls for encouraging the client to formulate the plan. It is more therapeutic and more likely to be successfully carried out if the plan comes from the client rather than from you.

To encourage formulation of a plan of action, you ask the client to consider what might be the best thing to do in a future situation. This future situation might be one that the client has never experienced, or it might be one that the client has experienced but was not able to handle successfully. This allows the client to think things out in advance and to be prepared.

This technique may also be used near the end of a relationship in which the client has had an opportunity to try out a plan and has not been successful. After evaluating with the client what went wrong, you might suggest formulation of a new plan of action. This helps the client to see that new approaches can always be tried.

SUMMARIZING. One therapeutic technique that might be done at intervals is summarizing. In this technique you summarize by briefly stating, in an orderly manner, what you and the client have discussed to that point in the interaction. One usually thinks of this as a final activity, but if a client presents a great deal of data to you, it is often helpful to stop and summarize briefly at opportune times. This helps ensure that you and the client agree about what went on and what decisions were made. It also helps to ensure that you covered all of the information you both wanted to discuss. Of course, summarizing can help bring closure in the termination phase of a therapeutic relationship.

KEY PRINCIPLES

- The three phases of the therapeutic relationship are the orientation phase, the working phase, and the termination phase. Each phase has certain tasks associated with it.
- The six elements of communication are: encoder, message, sensory channel, decoder, feedback, and context.
- Body language is a form of nonverbal communication that consists of human communication by alterations in personal appearance, changes in facial expressions, changes in body posture, use of gestures, maintenance of personal distances, and use of touching; paralanguage is a form of nonverbal communication that consists of the elements of stress, accent, pitch, pause, intonation, rate, volume, and quality.
- Nursing attitudes that facilitate effective therapeutic communication include awareness, acceptance, respect, unconditional positive regard, empathy, relatedness, caring, objectivity, protectiveness, genuineness, openness, appropriate professional closeness or distance, and a sense of humor. Action-oriented characteristics that facilitate effective communication include concreteness, immediacy, and confrontation.
- It is vital to recognize nontherapeutic communication techniques in order to avoid using them as you begin to learn and practice therapeutic communication techniques.
- Inappropriate use of therapeutic communication techniques can turn them from therapeutic techniques into nontherapeutic techniques; therefore, it is important to adhere to the guidelines for their correct use.
- Although any specific therapeutic technique might be used at any time, some techniques tend to be more helpful at the beginning, middle, or at the end of an interaction.

BIBLIOGRAPHY

Abdullah, S.N. (1995). Towards an individualized client's care: Implication for education. The transcultural approach. *Journal of Advanced Nursing, 22,* 715–720.

Arnold, E., & Boggs, K. (1995). *Interpersonal relationships: Professional communication skills for nurses* (2nd ed.). Philadelphia. W.B. Saunders.

Doak, L., Doak, C., & Root, J. (1996). *Teaching patients with low literacy skills.* Philadelphia: J.B. Lippincott.

Dzurec, L.C., & Coleman, P. (1995). What happens after you say hello? A hermeneutic analysis of the process of conducting clinical interviews. *Image: Journal of Nursing Scholarship, 27*(3), 245.

Evans, G.W., Witt, D.L., Alligood, M.R., & O'Neil, M. (1998). Empathy: A study of two types. *Issues in Mental Health Nursing, 19*(5), 453–61.

Gobis, L.J. (1997). Reducing the risks of phone triage. *RN, 60*(4), 61–63.

Juliana, C.A., Orehowsky, S., Smith-Rogojo, P., Sikora, S.M., Smith, P.A., Stein, D.K., Wagner, D.O., & Wolf, Z.R. (1997). Interventions used by staff nurses to manage "difficult" patients. *Holistic Nursing Practice, 11*(4), 1–26.

Katz, J.R. (1997). Back to basics: Providing effective patient teaching. *AJN, 97*(5), 33–36.

Kelly, D. (1995). Three tips for closer caring. *Nursing95, 25*(5), 72.

Morse, J.M., & Intrieri, R.C. (1997). Talk to me: Patient communication in a long-term care facility. *Journal of Psychosocial Nursing, 35*(5), 34–39.

*Peplau, H. (1952). *Interpersonal Relations in Nursing.* New York: McGraw-Hill.

*Satir, V. (1971). *Peoplemaking.* Palo Alto, CA: Science and Behavior Books.

Sears, M. (1996). Relationships: Using therapeutic communication to connect with others. *Home Healthcare Nurse, 14*(8), 614–617.

Sully, P. (1996). The impact of power in therapeutic relationships. *Nursing Times, 92*(41), 40–41.

*Tannen, D. (1990). *You just don't understand: Women and men in conversation.* New York: Ballantine Books.

*Travelbee, J. (1966). *Interpersonal Aspects of Nursing.* Philadelphia: F.A. Davis.

Watzlawick, P., Jackson, D.D., & Bandas, J.B. (1967). Pragmatics of human communication: A study of interactional patterns, pathologies, and paradoxes. New York: Norton.

Wichowski, H.C., & Kubsch, S. (1995). Improving your patient's compliance. *Nursing95,* 66–68.

*Asterisk indicates a classic or definitive work on this subject.

CHAPTER 16

Client Teaching

Carol E. Smith and Konnie Sue Kyle

Key Terms

affective learning domain
cognitive learning domain
learning
learning contract
learning objectives

perceptual learning domain
psychomotor learning domain
teaching
teaching plan

LEARNING OBJECTIVES

After studying this chapter, you should be able to:

1. Discuss the rationale for client teaching, including its benefits and purpose.
2. Describe the teaching and learning process, including domains of learning and principles of effective teaching.
3. Summarize the client characteristics to consider when assessing teaching needs.
4. Compare and contrast factors that facilitate learning and those that are barriers to learning.
5. Discuss the nursing diagnosis *Knowledge deficit* and compare it to a related diagnosis.
6. Develop a teaching plan for a client.
7. Discuss strategies for implementing client teaching effectively.
8. Write sample documentation for teaching and learning processes.
9. Discuss methods for evaluating, teaching, and learning.

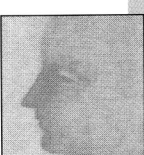

Charlotte Avery is an 82-year-old Jamaican-American woman who lives in Boca Raton, Florida. Mrs. Avery is a retired restaurant manager. She lives alone in the home she shared with her third husband, Charles, who passed away 2 years ago. Mrs. Avery was recently diagnosed with insulin-dependent diabetes mellitus. She needs information about her condition and self-care. The nurse makes the diagnosis of *Knowledge deficit*.

TEACHING AND LEARNING NURSING DIAGNOSES

Knowledge deficit (specify): Absence or deficiency of cognitive information related to specific topic.

From North American Nursing Diagnosis Association. (1999). NANDA nursing diagnoses: Definitions and classification 1999–2000. Philadelphia: Author.

CONCEPTS OF CLIENT TEACHING

Public access to health care information has never been greater. Bookstore shelves are crowded with self-help books and medical reference texts. The latest medical research findings are published in newspapers and magazines and even reported on the evening news. Pharmaceutical companies advertise prescription drugs in television commercials, encouraging consumers to ask their family health care providers for more information. Via the Internet, consumers can retrieve information from around the world on any topic within minutes.

At the same time, the public need for health care teaching has also continued to rise. Hospitals that discharge clients earlier than ever must make sure that those clients can care for themselves at home. Such factors as illiteracy, an aging population, and an emphasis on preventive health care challenge nurses to meet clients' growing learning needs while recognizing that health care information is the basic right of every client.

Client Rights and Nursing Standards

Indeed, the American Hospital Association (AHA) has sought to formalize that right, along with other health care providers who support the public in its demand for information. In 1975, the AHA published the Patient's Bill of Rights. More than half of these rights pertained to the client's right to information (AHA, 1975). For example, the bill asserted the client's right to receive information from his physician necessary for informed consent before the start of a procedure.

Although this bill of rights is a position statement of the AHA and is not legally binding, it has dramatically expanded the nurse's role in providing health care information. Since 1975, nurses have become directly involved not only in client teaching but also in deciding what information clients and families receive and how it is presented.

The role of the nurse in client education is a legal mandate. The nurse practice act in each state indicates that teaching is the primary role for the registered nurse (Smith, 1987, 1989). The Joint Commission on Accreditation for Healthcare Organizations (JCAHO), which accredits hospitals, includes a statement that clients and their significant others must receive education specific to their health care needs throughout their stay (Cornette, 1994).

Benefits of Client Teaching

The benefits of teaching are well documented. Benefits of health teaching and learning include positive client outcomes and decreased readmissions to the hospital. Client teaching also helps to control costs and maintain quality care.

Cost Control

Client teaching has become an important factor in controlling costs within health care systems. Education helps control costs by means of the following:

- Preventing illnesses that may require expensive care
- Enabling the client to manage a prescribed treatment regimen after discharge from an acute care facility
- Preparing the client to anticipate and recognize complications, to seek help early, and to prevent hospital readmission
- Increasing the care that can be given at home, including high-technology care and diagnostic testing
- Increasing compliance with the treatment regimen, thus reducing the need for more costly medical procedures

Quality Control

Client teaching has also become a critical component of maintaining quality of care. Education helps maintain quality by means of the following:

- Encouraging the client and family to be active partners in the delivery of health care, thus improving the outcome
- Increasing client satisfaction by helping the client understand what can reasonably be expected from the health care system
- Increasing the client's sense of control, which is derived from knowledge
- Ensuring that clients have the knowledge they need to provide self-care
- Increasing communication between the client and provider
- Increasing client satisfaction through a mutually respectful relationship

THE TEACHING AND LEARNING PROCESS

Teaching and learning are mutually dependent aspects of a dynamic, interactive process. **Teaching** is a set of planned activities performed to influence knowledge, behavior, or skill. To teach effectively, you must understand the subject to be taught, accurately assess the client's learning needs, control the learning environment, and use methods appropriate for the client's needs.

Learning is the acquisition of knowledge, behavior, or skill through experience, practice, study, or instruction. It is an all-encompassing experience that involves acquiring new knowledge, information, and skills, and thus changing one's behavior. Learning may cause people to change their attitudes, perceptions, habits, and methods of problem-solving.

Coherence With the Nursing Process

The teaching and learning process is coherent with the nursing process (Table 16–1). In the assessment phase, you gather subjective and objective data related to the client's knowledge base and learning needs. In the diagnosis phase, you identify specific learning needs. You then develop a plan, take appropriate actions to implement the plan, and evaluate the teaching and learning process.

Domains of Learning

Learning theorists have identified four domains of learning. By integrating all four of these domains into your teaching plans, you will improve the quality of your teaching. Each domain represents a broad classification of human behavior. The domains are the following:

- Perceptual domain: the ability to discern, distinguish, or differentiate information
- Cognitive domain: the ability to make sense of and use information
- Affective domain: the feelings and values associated with information
- Psychomotor domain: manipulative and motor skills

Within each domain, behaviors can be classified from simple to complicated stages of learning. We will now explore each of the domains in more detail.

Perceptual Domain

Bloom (1956) developed a three-domain classification system to help educators teach more effectively. He thoroughly describes the cognitive, affective, and psychomotor domains. More recently, theorists have recognized a perceptual domain as separate from the cognitive domain. The **perceptual learning domain** involves the ability to perceive (see, hear, understand, and respond) written words, spoken words, pictures, or symbols. The perceptual learning domain is essential for acquiring information.

Nurses teach in the perceptual domain when they determine whether clients can see, hear, and perceive the meaning of the information given and can connect the meaning to their own situation (Fig. 16–1). You

TABLE 16–1

Comparison of the Nursing Process and the Teaching Process

Step	Nursing Process	Teaching Process
1	• Collect and analyze data. • Assess client needs.	• Collect and analyze data about client's knowledge. • Identify learning needs.
2	• Label needs with nursing diagnoses.	• Make an educational diagnosis, such as *Knowledge deficit, Altered health maintenance,* or *Health-seeking behaviors.*
3	• Identify desired outcomes. • Plan nursing interventions.	• Prepare a teaching plan by writing objectives, content, time frame, teaching format, and how to teach content, such as by using audio-visual equipment.
4	• Implement nursing care.	• Implement the teaching plan and delivery of content.
5	• Evaluate clients' outcomes. • Reassess as needed.	• Evaluate client learning based on objectives. • Reassess as needed.

cannot always make an assumption that a client can look at a picture or a printed page and comprehend the meaning of the symbols or words that appear there.

The classification system for the perceptual domain was developed by an educational theorist named Moore (1970). Following are the aspects of perceptual learning described in terms of behavior that you can observe:

- **Sensing information.** The client who can sense information will demonstrate that ability by using the senses of seeing, hearing, and fine motor ability or touch.
- **Sensing changes.** The client also uses those senses to determine that changes have occurred.

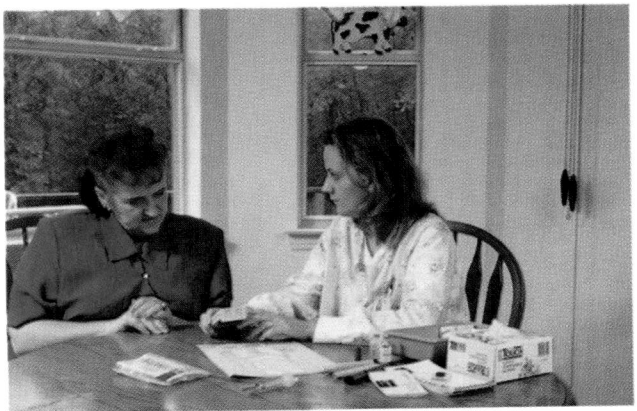

Figure 16–1. In the *perceptual* domain, the client sees the glucometer reading and recognizes that it is abnormal for her.

- **Responding.** The client responds to visual and auditory stimuli, such as pictures, words, and faces. These responses demonstrate her ability to recognize symbols and figures.
- **Associating meaning.** The client associates perceived symbols with having personal significance.
- **Making decisions.** The client makes decisions based on accurate observations. This last level of the perceptual domain may be assessed concurrently with the other domains.

Cognitive Domain

The **cognitive learning domain** includes acquiring knowledge, comprehending, and using critical thinking skills (Fig. 16–2). Learning takes place at several levels in the cognitive domain:

- **Acquisition.** To acquire knowledge, the client obtains information, commonly by memorizing terms, facts, principles, and procedures.
- **Comprehension.** Comprehension implies understanding of new information. When people comprehend new information, they can repeat the content back in their own words, relate the information to something already known, or attach meaning to the information.
- **Application.** Application of knowledge is the intellectual ability to use acquired information in similar but differing situations.
- **Analysis.** Analysis, the fourth level of cognitive learning, is the ability to separate information into components of the whole.
- **Synthesis.** Synthesis is reassembling parts to identify a new whole. The client uses the information that you provide and communicates a creative and unique use of the information.
- **Evaluation.** Evaluation involves making judgments about the effects of the treatment.

Synthesis and evaluation represent the highest levels of cognitive ability. Although nurses routinely synthesize and evaluate information at these levels, cli-

ents—especially sick clients—are not always able to reach this level of learning (Dollahite, Thompson, & McNew, 1996). A client may only be able to comprehend the steps of a carefully prescribed routine; she may not be able to analyze or modify that routine. When teaching such a client, limit yourself to essential information, such as the cause of an illness, lifestyle changes needed to prevent complications, basic symptom management, and specific skills as needed, such as how to irrigate a colostomy. Usually, the client can function when given this amount of information; indepth explanations can be added as the client asks questions.

Affective Domain

The **affective learning domain** includes the ethics, principles, and reasoning that determine and guide moral or "right" behavior. The affective domain includes values, beliefs, feelings, and attitudes (Fig. 16–3). Thus, teaching in the affective domain can address a client's health-seeking behaviors and choices at a deep and powerful level.

Emotions are also addressed in the affective domain. Feelings that arise in response to health care situations need to be recognized and managed. Anger, frustration, relief, and joy are often experienced as part of obtaining health care, being diagnosed with illness, or even receiving a clean bill of health. Helping a client understand and manage feelings is essential to integrating new learning into activities of daily living.

Within the affective domain, there are five levels of learning. These levels are described in terms of behavior that you can assess:

- **Receiving.** Affective learning begins with the process of receiving. The person names the feeling or emotion and recognizes that the emotion may be interfering with action.
- **Responding.** Responding occurs when the client can freely discuss feelings.
- **Valuing.** Valuing occurs when a person freely chooses a particular action from among several alternatives.

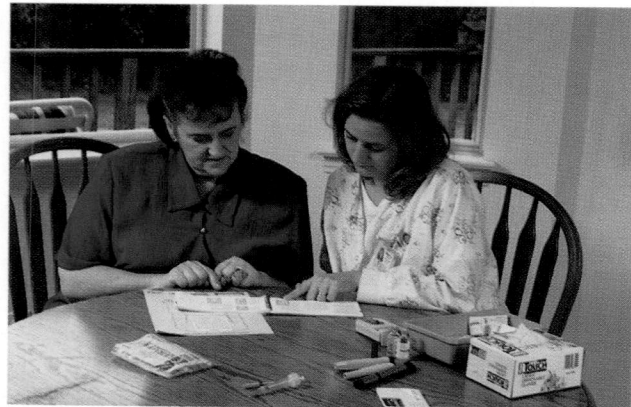

Figure 16–2. In the *cognitive* domain, the client is able to discuss the signs and symptoms of low blood sugar.-

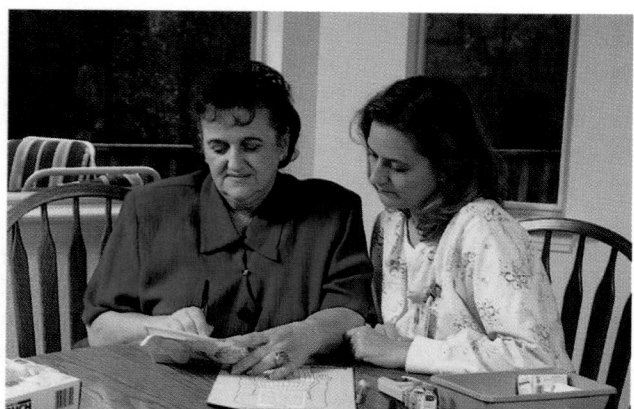

Figure 16–3. In the *affective* domain, the client commits to performing daily self-injections.

- **Organizing.** Organizing integrates a value into everyday life.
- **Characterizing.** Characterizing refers to the client's ability to internalize values into a philosophy of life, making it possible to behave consistently in accordance with those values.

You can promote a client's health and well-being by facilitating high-level learning in the affective domain. To do so, you must accomplish the following three personal goals:

- Understand your own value system, and provide information to clients in a manner that minimizes your own biases.
- Respect the validity and uniqueness of each person's value system, even when it differs from yours.
- Provide accurate and complete information about health and illness, thereby setting the stage for affective learning.

Learning in the affective domain can be difficult to evaluate and typically must be an ongoing process. Some clients may take years to internalize feelings and values fully enough to change their behavior.

Psychomotor Domain

The **psychomotor learning domain** includes physical and motor skills, such as giving injections (Fig. 16–4). These skills may require varying levels of dexterity, coordination, and the ability to manipulate equipment and objects. Teaching can be individualized to meet client needs by understanding the six levels of learning within the psychomotor domain:

- **Set.** Set is the level in which the client shows a readiness to take on a particular skill or task.
- **Guided response.** At this level, the client tries to imitate the behavior portrayed by the nurse.
- **Mechanism.** At this level, the client has successfully achieved a task or skill. This skill will then become a habit and a change from previous behavior.

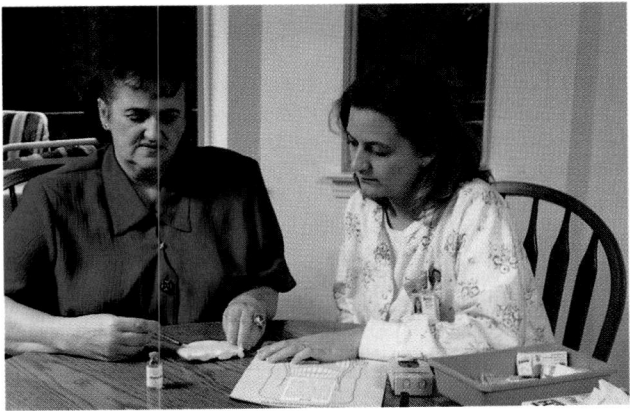

Figure 16–4. In the *psychomotor* domain, the client manipulates the equipment to perform self-injection.

- **Complex overt response.** Here, the client can perform the task or skill independently, without having to give attention to the task.
- **Adaptation.** At this level, the client has mastered the skill so proficiently that she can adapt the task to varying physical conditions or situations.
- **Origination.** This level of the psychomotor domain challenges the client to create new ways or acts of manipulating the skills or abilities.

Proficiency at each level of the psychomotor domain is necessary to master many manual skills. Once mastered, the psychomotor skill then becomes a means to the end.

A clear understanding of the interdependence of perceptual, cognitive, affective, and psychomotor domains of learning will enable you to assess each client's learning needs with confidence. When those needs are accurately identified, learning objectives can be mutually negotiated and teaching in all domains implemented.

FACTORS AFFECTING CLIENT TEACHING

Many factors can influence the effectiveness of your teaching, including you, your client, the family or significant others, and the situation. Additionally, time to teach is a factor. You will have limited interaction with clients. Therefore, you must maximize your teaching effectiveness to compensate for the short teaching time available.

Client Characteristics

Many characteristics can influence a client's approach to learning, such as age, race, gender, medical diagnosis, and clinical progress. Likewise, religious beliefs and cultural background may alter the client's learning needs and therefore affect the methods by which you present materials in particular content areas. Other important assessment factors include literacy, education, developmental level, and learning style.

Literacy Level

You may encounter clients who cannot read or who cannot read English. Clients who can read will have varying abilities, from very basic to very advanced. Most clients will be embarrassed to admit their inability to read educational materials. Consequently, you must determine each client's ability to read and comprehend educational materials. Be prepared to provide privacy and the educational methods that complement each client's learning ability.

Level of Education

Before you start teaching a client, assess her general health knowledge, her perception of her current illness, and the type of teaching that will be most helpful and easily understood. To make this assessment, you most likely will want to consider the client's level of formal education. However, you cannot assume that a well-educated person is a well-informed person when it comes to health education.

In addition to assessing a client's educational level, determine the following:

- What he has been told by a physician or has learned from media sources
- What he knows about his illness
- What is his previous experience with illness, the health care system, or hospitalization

Although unrelated to formal education, these areas influence a client's learning process. It is in this "educational realm" that you as the nurse may determine the client's readiness to learn, goals for learning, and learning needs.

Developmental Level

Learning can also be influenced by whether the client is a child, adolescent, adult, or elderly adult.

CHILDREN

For children, the teaching and learning process can be fundamentally different than that used by adults. You must adjust the complexity and volume of information taught to each child's age and cognitive level. You also must carefully choose terms and examples to keep them appropriate for the child's age level.

For example, young children may learn best by playing games, drawing, or watching video-modeling of behavior. The use of dolls, stuffed animals, or other toys may be helpful. Many children are receptive to instruction that involves role-playing. This type of interaction may be therapeutic as well as educational. Children and their parents may require specialized teaching approaches (Box 16–1). Note that parents may need affective domain assessment for their emotional reactions to their children's problems.

ADOLESCENTS

The first approach to effective teaching with adolescents is to develop a trusting relationship. Privacy is essential when discussing personal matters, such as self-esteem. How a teen "looks" to his peers is of utmost importance because peers play a vital role in the life of teenagers.

Adolescents expect honesty, openness, and the truth about their illnesses. Thus, you will want to allow adolescents to have as much control as possible in the health care arena. This includes letting them choose what they want to wear and eat, within reason. If possible, let them visit with friends.

ADULTS

Knowles (1980) identified four assumptions that characterize adult learning. These four assumptions will help you in planning to teach adults. Remember, how-

---

BOX 16-1

TIPS FOR TEACHING CHILDREN

- Trust is essential to a therapeutic relationship with a child.
- In general, the younger the child, the shorter the attention span.
- Children are exposed to various levels of information about health care. Be sure to assess the child's knowledge.
- Children form misconceptions easily. A child's imagination may create greater fear than the truth, told directly and simply.
- Parents can often provide cues to the child's emotional response and capacity for understanding information. However, some parents may underestimate or overestimate their child's capacity.
- Children may regress developmentally in a situation of illness.
- Children may better manage uncomfortable information through role-playing with dolls and models.

---

ever, that adults are highly variable; not all of the following descriptions may apply.

LEARNING IS SELF-DIRECTED. As people mature, their learning becomes increasingly self-directed, largely because changes in self-concept take the learner from a state of dependency to a state of increasing independence. In general, adults identify their learning needs and then take action to acquire the knowledge they know they need.

LEARNING IS BUILT ON PREVIOUS KNOWLEDGE. The adult learner brings a lifetime of accumulated learning to each new learning experience. Indeed, as adults, we define or characterize ourselves largely by our experiences. The older we become, the more ingrained our previous experiences become. Therefore, to facilitate adult learning, you should make use of previous learning and experiences as resources to enhance present learning.

LEARNING IS PRACTICAL. Learning is more likely to happen when an adult is ready to learn. That readiness results in part from an adult's realization that she needs certain knowledge to perform effectively in a chosen role. Health education receives attention when the adult needs the information and knows she needs it. Learning has then become meaningful. Therefore, health education is more effective when the person has signs and symptoms of an illness and needs to know about the illness.

LEARNING IS PURPOSEFUL. Closely related to readiness to learn is the fourth assumption, that learning is purposeful. Adult learning is based on real-life problems and obtaining immediate results. This problem-centered learning differs from the type of learning accomplished in school, which is subject-oriented and has a delayed application. For adults, learning must have a purpose.

These characteristics of adult learners should be integrated sensibly into the learning process. By applying these assumptions when integrating with adult learners, you can create a supportive learning environment.

ELDERLY ADULTS

Although intelligence may actually increase as a person ages, the capacity to learn is affected by changes in function. These changes may not appreciably affect performance until a person's eighties or nineties. However, the incidence of chronic and debilitating diseases will alter intellectual abilities for an individual.

Reaction time, or the amount of time required for a response to a stimulus, will slow with age. The person will need more time to process information and perform psychomotor skills. It may take longer to make decisions, especially if the decision requires consideration of multiple aspects of a problem. Instructions need to be free of unnecessary detail and explanations. The person can become confused by paying too much attention to irrelevant detail.

Although memory may not be severely impaired, an older person often experiences slowness in acquiring, storing, and recalling new information. To compensate, the person uses selective attention to screen out extraneous information, thus sometimes missing information that is actually important. By slowing the pace of receiving new information, older persons can often compensate for a decline in learning new information.

The capacity to learn is affected by stress and fatigue. The older person often fatigues more easily, and thus has more difficulty paying attention to new information than he did earlier in life. Additionally, stress is associated with multiple stimuli or trying to think about a number of things at the same time. When the activities of daily living are requiring more thinking time and energy, the older adult may be less able to screen out thoughts and concentrate on learning new information.

Remember that changes with aging are highly variable. Older adults have written a first novel, taken up painting, and otherwise developed new skills.

Learning Styles

Every client has an individual learning style, a way that she prefers to learn or learns best (Brown, Wright, & Christensen, 1987). You can enhance the effectiveness of your teaching by discovering this style for each client early in the course of teaching. Unfortunately, many nurse educators use a teaching strategy that is most comfortable for them, rather than individualizing their strategy to accommodate the client's style of learning.

Some clients will prefer to hear you talk about a topic. Others will prefer to read a pamphlet or hand-out, then ask questions after their independent study is complete. To increase your effectiveness, ask your clients how they most enjoy learning new information, then adapt your teaching strategy to their preference.

Nurse educators agree that education is a process. Meaningful interactions will provide creative ways for mutual understanding, problem-solving, and decision-making. Adapting yourself into the nurse educator role means that you find the learning style that is best for your client and that you adapt the teaching material to accomplish a behavior change (Colucciello, 1993).

Factors That Facilitate Learning

To teach effectively, you must understand and use factors that facilitate learning. They can guide your decisions about teaching children, adults, families, groups, and communities. They include readiness and motivation.

Readiness

The client must be both physically and emotionally ready to learn. The client must desire to know, be physically and mentally alert, be able to concentrate and focus on the information, and have a frame of reference for the information.

Motivation

Clients learn more if they have a genuine desire or motivation to learn. Motivation is greatest in clients who recognize their learning needs and perceive the available teaching as meaningful.

Motivation can be difficult to measure and, usually, you must rely on indirect signs. Strategies to assess motivation include asking questions or engaging the client in a conversation about the topic. An unmotivated client will become distracted, change the subject, or otherwise show signs of not paying attention. Some clients will suggest that you give the information to their spouse or significant other.

People differ in the amount and type of information they can tolerate concerning their illness or behavior. Some people become anxious if they feel uninformed about their illness, including its cause, prevention, and treatment. Others become anxious if you try to talk about their disorder. When anxious clients resist instruction, wait until they begin asking questions or show other signs of readiness. At this point, their anxiety may have lessened, and they may be more receptive to new information.

Clients' motivation to learn increases in an atmosphere of acceptance. Clients need to feel that you are genuinely interested in helping them learn. They also need time to assimilate ideas and develop new skills. They have the right to make mistakes and even to fail at a task without "losing face." You can increase their motivation by acting as a facilitator, not as a judge.

Factors That Inhibit Learning

Barriers to learning may include physiological, psychological, cultural, environmental, socioeconomic, and teaching factors.

Physiological Factors

Clients who are critically ill, in severe pain, restless, oxygen-deprived, fatigued, weak, deaf, or vision-impaired face physical obstacles to learning. These obstacles interfere with readiness to learn because they reduce the person's ability to concentrate, and they deplete energy. All but the most simple information must be postponed until the client is able to attend to learning. Any information provided during a serious illness should be repeated as the client recovers.

Physiological barriers include perceptual problems. Always assess hearing and visual acuity. If the client has a sensory deficit, the nurse considers this factor when selecting visual aids or teaching strategies.

Psychological Factors

Psychological barriers are related to motivation. Attitude changes throughout the course of a serious illness and also when a person moves from being well to being ill. It is helpful to understand what the client's personality and self-image were like before the onset of the present illness. Clients sometimes experience a personality change as a result of a real or perceived threat to their self-esteem or present lifestyle.

Teaching content may be altered by the medical or nursing prognosis. A client who is terminally ill may have different learning needs and capabilities than those of a client not facing death. Unfortunately, because the learning needs of the dying client are different, often they are ignored altogether.

Psychological stresses also interfere with concentration. People who feel anxious, fearful, and angry about their illness may have difficulty learning. Those who have trouble adjusting to a new diagnosis may experience denial, which postpones their readiness to learn.

Cultural Factors

Teaching and learning can be complicated when clients speak languages that are different or have cultural or ethnic backgrounds and values that differ from yours. In all cases, you and your clients will benefit from your awareness of cultural differences and your willingness to obtain assistance with teaching when needed.

Some ethnic groups follow unique beliefs and practices, many of which involve diet, nutrition, health, and illness. Certain foods may be forbidden; certain health rituals may be required. At all times, consider cultural and religious values when assessing overall teaching and learning needs. However,

avoid stereotyping clients by their ethnic or cultural background (Chachkles & Christ, 1996).

Also recognize that the values you hold may—and probably do—vary from those of your clients. For example, you may value self-care and independence; the client may not. You may have trouble identifying with a client who says, "Just tell my wife. She gives me all my pills." Yet you must regard each client as a unique individual with valid wishes about teaching and learning.

Environmental Factors

Learning is facilitated in a pleasant, quiet environment, free from distractions. The teaching area should be well lit, comfortably warm, and (if possible) away from the hub of activity.

Lack of privacy, noise, and interruptions can seriously disrupt teaching sessions. When the room is too hot or cold, the client may be too uncomfortable to concentrate. In group teaching sessions, some clients may be distracted by the movements and noises of others in the room.

Distractions from the teaching process may arise in a variety of settings. Imagine the distractions possible in a homeless shelter or in a client's cluttered home with barking dogs, small children, and a loud television. Even a hospital room does not always offer the privacy and quiet needed for teaching because visitors, physicians, and other nurses enter the room to complete their roles. Reducing stimuli to gain your clients' full attention may challenge you to be creative for your teaching and learning sessions.

Socioeconomic Factors

When teaching a client about his illness and the care he requires, it helps to consider his home situation, living arrangements, and usual activities. Evaluate his relationships with significant others to determine the strength of his personal support system. Assess the type of work he does as well as his level of stress. Knowing the person's financial situation enables you to plan cost-effective health and maintenance care when possible. Keep in mind, however, that some clients are very private about their financial matters. Be prepared to explain your need to know about the client's financial condition.

Teaching Factors

Teaching factors that inhibit learning include lack of knowledge and preparation, lack of planning, overuse of technical words, delivery of poorly prepared and fragmented presentations, unwillingness to draw the learner into discussion, hurried or poorly planned demonstrations, and a condescending attitude toward the learner.

ASSESSMENT

For a client with learning needs, you will follow the phases of the nursing process just as you would for a

A PATIENT'S VIEW
"THE CLINIC NURSES HAVE TAUGHT ME SO MUCH ABOUT HOW TO MANAGE DIABETES"

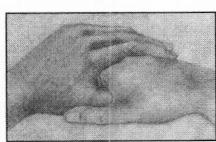 When I was 48, I began to feel like my body was shutting down. I was tired all the time, I had no energy, and I was losing weight. But my doctor didn't seem concerned, so I just chalked it up to stress. And there was plenty of that. My dad was dying of a brain tumor, my mother had been diagnosed with Alzheimer's and, as the oldest daughter, I was the primary caregiver.

After Dad died in 1991, I took my mother to Vermont to visit my brother and his family. We had always taken walks and hikes together, and she still enjoyed that, even though she would lose her way home without me. One afternoon as we were walking through the woods, I slipped and grabbed onto a nearby tree branch to keep from falling. Unfortunately, a thorn on the branch pierced my hand. It wasn't terribly painful, so I just put some ointment and a bandage on it and thought nothing more about it. The next morning, my arm was twice its normal size! A local doctor gave me a shot of antibiotics and a prescription and told me to check in with my regular doctor as soon as I got home, which I did. He couldn't explain why I had experienced such an extreme reaction but thought that maybe I had multiple sclerosis. A few months after that, however, he came up with the real diagnosis: diabetes. I later learned that the incident with my arm was a classic sign of diabetes, and my doctor missed it.

As soon as my doctor figured out what the problem was, he put me on 130 units of insulin a day. Almost immediately, I began to gain weight, even though I was walking three to five miles a day; eventually, I gained a hundred pounds. My vision began to deteriorate, because the blood vessels in my eyes were hemorrhaging. So the doctor sent me to a specialist who did laser treatments to stop the hemorrhaging. It was $1,500 a treatment. My vision loss made it impossible for me to work, so it wasn't long before I ran out of money and was forced to go to a public clinic for all my medical care. Ironically, that turned out to be the best thing that could have happened to me.

The clinic I go to is run by nurses, and it is wonderful. I can't say enough good things about the way they treat you. Everyone there is friendly. They always call you by name. They take time to listen. You never feel rushed.

They pay attention to what's happening in your day-to-day life. They make sure that you're scheduled for routine screenings, such as Pap smears, mammograms, and so on. They recognize that people's circumstances change, and they don't punish you because you don't have money. What's more, I get better care now than when I did have money!

The doctors who work at my clinic are all volunteers, and they are excellent. My endocrinologist is a woman, and she keeps up on all the latest research. My former doctor was not good at controlling my diabetes; over a period of time, my clinic doctor has gotten me totally off insulin and onto oral medications. My diet was pretty good, but she fine-tuned it. She also suggested that I find an additional caregiver for my mother. Those changes have made a huge difference in my life, in my weight, and in my blood sugar.

The clinic nurses have taught me so much about how to manage diabetes: to watch my feet for sores that don't heal, to take my vitamins (A, B, C, E, and a combination supplement of calcium, magnesium, and zinc). And every 3 months I have tests for long-term blood sugar control and liver function because of the oral medications I'm taking. So far, my diabetes is under really good control.

Another thing about this clinic: When you know something is wrong but you can't put your finger on it, they go after it. I'm probably one of the few adults over age 50 with tonsils. When I had tonsillitis as a child, the doctor used radiation treatments to shrink them instead of surgically removing them. The treatment backfired, and the tonsils grew to four times their normal size. That meant that tonsillitis almost closed my throat. My new clinic doctor noticed that and suggested a tonsillectomy, but they could remove only one, because the carotid artery was tangled in the other one. But even removing one was a big improvement.

Living with diabetes has changed my life forever. I have cataracts and am losing my near vision. Even with bifocals, I can barely see the pupils in my eyes when I'm three inches from the mirror. I can still read if the light is bright enough and the print is black enough. Any color other than black just fades away. I'm hopeful that when the cataracts are removed in a year or two, I'll be able to see enough to work again. I'm 56 years old.

client with physiological needs. Several nursing diagnoses can be applied to clients with learning needs, but *Knowledge deficit* is the most common. In certain client situations, a related diagnosis—such as *Noncompliance* or *Self-care deficit*—may be more appropriate. *Knowledge deficit* is defined as "the absence or deficiency of cognitive information related to [a] specific topic" (NANDA, 1998).

Focused Assessment for Knowledge Deficit

Any client can have a need for health-related knowledge; however, several factors may increase the risk of a *Knowledge deficit*. Clients at greatest risk include those with chronic illnesses that require complex treatment regimens, those needing special procedures, and those for whom preventive measures are important, such as pregnant clients, elderly clients with respiratory disease, and clients with impaired immunity.

Generally, the uneducated client is thought to be at greater risk, but highly educated clients often do not have experience with or understanding of medical or health problems. Family members, including children, also need information, as does anyone who acts as the client's caregiver.

Defining Characteristics

Verbalization that a client has no knowledge, incomplete knowledge, or incorrect knowledge is a defining characteristic for the nursing diagnosis *Knowledge deficit*. The client may tell you directly that he needs knowledge, or he may ask questions that indicate the specific knowledge sought. Look for objective clues that the client does not have appropriate knowledge or does not understand. The evidence may be direct, as in the client who fails to follow instructions accurately or who performs poorly on tests or return demonstrations.

Related Factors

Related factors may give direction to your choice of interventions. These factors may require you to modify your teaching to minimize the effect of a factor or remove it before implementing the teaching plan. Related factors for *Knowledge deficit* are the following:

- Cognitive limitation
- Information misinterpretation
- Lack of interest in learning
- Lack of motivation
- Lack of recall
- Limited exposure to information (specify)
- Limited practice of skill
- Unfamiliarity with information resources
- Unreadiness to learn

Focused Assessment for Related Nursing Diagnoses

Altered health maintenance is closely related to *Knowledge deficit*. Assess the client's ability to identify an adaptive behavior, manage a health-related behavior, or seek assistance (NANDA, 1998). Client teaching is a pertinent intervention when you identify the related factor as a lack of material resources, a lack of or significant alternation in communication, and a lack of effective individual coping. All affect the nurse educator in the teaching and learning process.

Assess the client for *Health-seeking behavior*. Does the client need assistance to actively seek ways to alter personal health habits and/or the environment to move toward a higher level of health (NANDA, 1998)? Assess the client's knowledge of ways to achieve his health goals or change unhealthy behaviors.

Assess for *Ineffective individual coping*. Identify adaptive behaviors and abilities of the client to meet life's demands and roles (NANDA, 1998). Teaching may be needed to develop good nutrition habits, to manage stress, and to develop coping strategies.

DIAGNOSIS

Although teaching is an appropriate intervention for almost all nursing diagnoses, *Knowledge deficit* is the nursing diagnosis identified most often for clients with learning needs. You must consider the goal of client teaching before selecting the diagnosis. If the goal of teaching is to maintain health, the diagnosis should be *Altered health maintenance*. If the goal of teaching is to ensure compliance with the treatment regimen, the diagnosis should be *Ineffective management of therapeutic regimen*. If the goal of teaching is to convince the client of the value of continuing with treatment, the diagnosis is *Noncompliance*.

The diagnosis can be *Knowledge deficit* when the need is to remove barriers to learning; for example, limited vision that interferes with reading labels or situational depression that interferes with the client's desire to learn about illness. When the goal of care is to help the client learn, it is appropriate to identify the diagnosis as *Knowledge deficit*.

In other cases, the need for knowledge is only part of a multifaceted problem. Ineffective denial is a good example. Denial of an illness may keep the client from engaging in health-seeking behaviors. Lack of knowledge may be only one facet of the problem. In fact, the client in denial may dismiss knowledge already gained or may fail to perceive the relevance of knowledge.

PLANNING

After selecting the appropriate nursing diagnosis, you must then decide what to teach the client, when to teach it, and how to teach it. Together with the client, develop a specific teaching plan that (1) builds on the client's present knowledge base, (2) provides new information, and (3) increases the client's level of understanding about his health status.

What to Teach

Select the teaching topics appropriate to the client's learning needs. Develop a teaching plan based on specific, measurable, learning objectives.

Topics

The hospitalized client and her family may need information about the following topics:

- Basic anatomy and physiology
- The causes of her symptoms
- Characteristics of her illness that could alter her lifestyle
- Her prognosis
- The hospital environment, including bedside equipment and how it works; the locations of bath-

rooms, cafeteria, and chapel; and hospital policies and routines

- The staff, including the names of her nurses, the nursing supervisor, the clinical director or manager, the dietitian, the team leader, the chaplain, and others as needed
- Diagnostic tests that she will need, steps needed to prepare for those tests, and the meaning of their results
- The expected duration of her hospitalization and ongoing care
- Her prescribed medications, including administration guidelines and adverse effects that may develop
- The goals of her treatment program
- Steps to avoid or overcome complications
- The cost of her care
- Home care, community resources, and needed follow-up

Continually assess your clients' learning needs and identify other areas of interest unique to each client. Asking clients for input into the teaching plan helps to ensure that their content is interesting and relevant to their needs.

Teaching Plan

A **teaching plan** is an organized, individualized, written presentation of what the client must learn and how the instructions and information needed will be provided. It should be outcome-oriented, with individualized goals set by the nurse and the client. Like a nursing care plan, it follows the steps of the nursing process. A standardized teaching plan may be designed for groups of clients, such as clients newly diagnosed with diabetes or clients who have had coronary bypass surgery; however, each plan should be individualized for the specific client. See the sample teaching plan for Mrs. Avery, who is beginning insulin therapy for her diabetes (Chart 16–2).

In general, clients will be more successful in remembering and assimilating information if you begin with the simple and proceed to the complex. In a well-developed teaching plan, each concept presented is based on a broader and more fundamental concept. Clearly, a person cannot understand abnormalities of function without first understanding normal function. Likewise, a client will not comprehend the treatment and prevention of a disease without first learning about its cause. Thus, when teaching someone about illness and therapy, you should begin with a broad discussion of the normal anatomy and physiology of the diseased organ or system. Then proceed to describe factors that cause the disease, and end the discussion with a presentation of how the client can take part in her treatment and rehabilitation program.

Learning Objectives

Learning objectives are essential to an effective teaching plan and are written like client goals in a nursing care plan. A **learning objective** is a statement that describes the intended results of learning rather than the process of instruction. It documents in a clear, realistic, and measurable manner the performance that proves a client's competency in a certain area. It must be client-centered and stated in behavioral terms to allow measurement and evaluation of the client's progress. A well-written learning objective includes the following elements:

- The expected performance
- Conditions in which the behavior will be performed
- Criteria by which the performance will be evaluated

Consider the following learning objectives:

- *Objective 1:* Mrs. Avery will understand about diabetes mellitus before discharge from the health care facility.
- *Objective 2:* By the end of the second teaching session, Mrs. Avery will be able to state the signs and symptoms of hyperglycemia (high blood glucose) with 100% accuracy.

The first objective is vague and ambiguous and therefore difficult to evaluate. The second objective is specific and measurable, with a clearer statement of the desired outcome. It incorporates the characteristics of a well-written objective. It lists all the necessary characteristics, including these:

- *Performance:* State the signs and symptoms of hyperglycemia
- *Condition(s):* By the end of the second teaching session
- *Criterion:* 100% accuracy

A clear objective that includes measurable terminology will allow you to evaluate whether the desired learning has occurred. Additionally, Mrs. Avery will know the goals of your teaching sessions, and she will be able to focus her efforts on meeting those goals. Because the management of diabetes mellitus requires a number of procedures, you will need several learning objectives to help Mrs. Avery learn to assume the responsibility for self-care. Examples of such objectives might include the following:

- By the end of the first teaching session, Mrs. Avery will correctly explain the pathophysiology of diabetes in terms appropriate to her level in the cognitive domain.
- Each morning before breakfast, Mrs. Avery will correctly test her blood glucose level, using the fingerstick method, sterile technique, the proper equipment, accurate interpretation of the results, and correct documentation of the findings.
- On the day before discharge, Mrs. Avery will use a list provided to her to choose appropriate foods to plan a sample breakfast, lunch, and dinner menu with 100% accuracy.

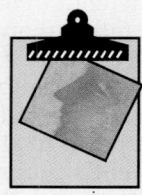

NURSING CARE PLANNING
TEACHING PLAN FOR A DIABETIC CLIENT BEGINNING INSULIN THERAPY

Admission Data

Charlotte Avery is an 82-year-old Jamaican-American woman who lives in Boca Raton, Florida. After Mrs. Avery's parents died, she became the proprietor of her family's restaurant business. Mrs. Avery retired 7 years ago. Her son now runs the restaurant, and she cares for two great-grandchildren. When Mrs. Avery fainted in her home 3 days ago, her 9-year-old great-grandchild called 911. It was later found that Mrs. Avery's diabetes was out of control. Her physician told her that she would no longer be able to control her diabetes with diet and oral medications alone. She must now learn to monitor her blood sugar and self-administer insulin. The nurse developed the following teaching plan for Mrs. Avery.

TEACHING PLAN

Nursing Diagnosis Affective Domain	Expected Outcomes	Interventions	Evaluation
Knowledge deficit (affective) related to readiness to learn to self-administer insulin and manage a diabetic diet	Mrs. Avery will discuss her feelings about taking insulin.	Provide a quiet environment that supports the discussion of feelings. *Show confidence in ability for self-care.	States she has handled the birth of five children and the death of three husbands and has recovered from the loss of her first restaurant by fire. This seems like a minor problem.
	Mrs. Avery will accept the need for insulin and dietary change.	Assess the client's desire to learn to self-administer injections.	States that she cares for two great-grandchildren and must stay healthy.
	Mrs. Avery will articulate and demonstrate confidence in her ability to self-administer subcutaneous injections.	Provide constructive and positive feedback in the learning process.	States: "She knows she can learn, but it is very confusing."
	Mrs. Avery will make a commitment to keep daily records of insulin injections, glucose monitoring, and insulin reactions.	Provide a record book for recording.	Records sample data accurately in her record book.
Cognitive Domain			
Knowledge deficit (cognitive) related to new experience of managing diabetes with insulin	Mrs. Avery will complete a multiple-choice test of knowledge of diabetes.	Provide the multiple-choice test, and explain the instructions.	Test results reveal general knowledge of diabetes; lacks understanding of need for a balanced diet and meals at regular intervals; past control had been achieved by avoiding sugar.
		Assist with understanding the questions, but avoid giving the answers.	Unable to take test independently; discussion of questions revealed areas of knowledge deficit.

Continued

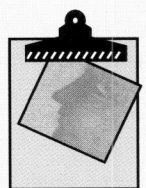

NURSING CARE PLANNING
TEACHING PLAN FOR A DIABETIC CLIENT BEGINNING INSULIN THERAPY *(continued)*

TEACHING PLAN *(continued)*

Cognitive Domain	Expected Outcomes	Interventions	Evaluation
	Mrs. Avery will list the differences between regular insulin and long-acting insulin.	Describe the difference between regular insulin and long-acting insulin. Simultaneously provide the information in written form.	Listened intently to information about regular and long-acting insulin and said, "NPH will last all day. Regular is only good for one meal."
Psychomotor Domain			
Knowledge deficit (psychomotor) related to lack of experience with administration of insulin and glucose monitoring.	Mrs. Avery will inject insulin using correct technique.	Demonstrate insulin injection technique. Immediate return demonstration; coach through return demonstration; repeat return demonstration independently.	Able to draw up regular insulin but inaccurate in adding long-acting insulin to the syringe; asked nurse to draw up insulin; correctly injected insulin. States "I will do it next time."
	Mrs. Avery will demonstrate blood glucose testing with a glucometer.	Demonstrate fingerstick, applying blood to test strip, and reading results; immediate return demonstration.	States "That looks easy enough. Let me try it." Requires some coaching for return demonstration.

*Italicized interventions indicate culturally specific care.

Critical Thinking Questions

1. The following is documented during a follow-up visit to the clinic: *Verbalized that she had an episode of low blood sugar last weekend. Action taken was to check her blood sugar (which was 42), drink a glass of orange juice, eat two peanut butter crackers, and rest. Repeated her blood sugar 30 minutes later; reading was 96. Stated she felt better and continued her housework.* From this documentation, how would you evaluate the effectiveness of the teaching plan for Mrs. Avery?

2. Considering the change that can occur in learning with aging, how many teaching sessions would you need before Mrs. Avery self-injects her insulin? Can Mrs. Avery be expected to administer her insulin independently? How would you explain the pathological changes associated with diabetic complications?

When to Teach

Keep in mind that teaching can take place at any time. It can be scheduled or unscheduled. For example, instruction can be given at specific times that are formally designated and spaced throughout the day or informally when a person asks questions or encounters new experiences. In general, however, try to avoid noisy, hectic times when clients are distracted (such as during meals or after administration of pain medication). You must decide when learning will be optimum. Research studies indicate that teaching at the time when family members or significant others are available is an advantage (Grieco, 1996; Mayo, 1993).

How to Teach

Many avenues are available for making the best use of your teaching time. Depending on the client's needs and the resources available, you can use one-to-one instruction, group lectures, printed materials, programmed instruction, computerized teaching, other teaching aids, and other expert teachers. Sometimes your clients will benefit from more than one mode of instruction.

One-to-One Instruction

Formal or informal, one-to-one instruction allows you to pace and customize your teaching to the client's learning rate.

Group Instruction

This method requires a meeting place, handout materials, a meeting agenda and lesson plan, and seating that facilitates group interaction (chairs placed in a circle, for example). You must deliver a prepared lecture on the chosen topic, lead a discussion, review major points covered in the discussion, and arrange for the next meeting.

The three major advantages of group meeting are the economy of teaching time, the possibility of delivering a large amount of factual information, and the opportunity for clients with similar problems to share experiences, viewpoints, and opinions with each other. Two disadvantages are the lack of ability to pace your teaching to individual learning rates and the possibility that some clients will be too intimidated to ask questions in front of the group.

Printed Materials

Printed materials—such as pamphlets and brochures—allow the client to read and study at his own pace. They are affordable, are portable, and can be used to teach or reinforce a learning experience. Also, clients can share the materials with family and significant others so that all have similar information.

Programmed Instruction

Highly effective with bright, self-directed people, programmed instruction involves a prepared program of study that lists learning objectives and provides activities to meet those objectives. It may include a pre-test and post-test for self-evaluation.

Using this method, learners can study at their own pace, proceeding to more difficult concepts once they understand basic ones. Consider providing a discussion period or question-answer session to clarify or amplify the content as needed.

Computerized Instruction

This method is similar to programmed instruction, except that the learner uses a computer program. It allows self-study and self-pacing, and it may also provide an interactive component that printed materials cannot. Computerized learning packages are finding increased use at all educational levels. They are likely to enjoy broader usage as client education software becomes more common.

Research has shown that on-line computer systems placed in public areas can provide important health care information on such subjects as preventing cancer, controlling hypertension, and understanding medication safety. The lack of supervision at the terminal and the novelty of the system did not keep clients from using the system (Peterson & Rippey, 1992).

Computer programs, such as The Comprehensive Health Enhancement Support System (commonly called CHESS), were developed in response to a needs assessment. CHESS supplies education via modem on personal computers to teach about breast cancer, HIV/AIDS, Alzheimer's disease, and heart disease. Experts consider the program successful because it presents high-quality, well-organized health information at a literacy level that meets all clients' needs (Boberg et al., 1997).

Teaching Aids

Teaching can be enhanced by the proper use of aids, such as drawings, models of organs, charts, graphs, audiotapes, a bulletin board, a blackboard, posters, pictures, an overhead projector, slide shows, films, videotapes, closed-circuit television, flash cards, programmed instruction, and games (Bernier, 1996; Johnson, Rice, Fuller, & Endress, 1978).

Resource People

The use of a specialized resource person can be extremely helpful to a client's learning process. For example, when teaching about a special diet, you could have a dietitian attend your session and share information as needed. Physicians, physical therapists, and occupational therapists all make significant contributions to teaching and learning.

Other clients can help as well, especially those who have successfully managed a similar condition. These experienced people can help your client know that it is possible to change behaviors and manage difficult disorders. For example, someone who has successfully managed lifestyle changes after having cardiac bypass surgery might be called to talk with a client preparing for the surgery.

INTERVENTION

To implement your teaching, you will need to use effective strategies and appropriate learning activities. Teaching is documented in the health record.

Strategies for Effective Teaching Intervention

As the teacher, your behaviors have a profound influence on your client's ability to learn. By employing the following strategies for effective teaching intervention, you can maximize the learning process.

Selecting Appropriate Teaching Methods

Selection of a teaching method depends on the subject matter and on the client's background, personality, and needs. Teaching may involve formal lectures and demonstrations. However, informal individual or group discussions are more appropriate for most clients in a health care setting.

Audiovisual aids and printed information can enhance the discussion and facilitate learning. Audiotapes, videocassettes, and in-house television channels are available for client teaching (Chang & Hirsh, 1994;

Mahler & Kulik, 1995). Computer programs also are becoming available for client education.

When using adjunct methods, it is wise to be available afterward to answer questions and evaluate what clients have learned. Before using print or video teaching aids, verify their content and assess their comprehension level. Typically, a reading level between grade 4 and grade 6 is best. For each client, do your best to provide accurate, current, and relevant information at the level and in the style most likely to fulfill the person's unique learning needs.

Rewarding Positive Behaviors

Rewards for correct behaviors reinforce learning. Behaviors that are rewarded are more likely to be repeated. For ill clients, rewards tend to involve the following:

- Reduced pain or other symptoms
- Return of a normal or near-normal lifestyle
- Avoidance of complications
- Positive regard from a nurse or physician

Immediate rewards provide better reinforcement than delayed rewards. Therefore, you should compliment a client immediately after she asks a thoughtful question, demonstrates something she learned about her illness, or performs a procedure satisfactorily.

Encouraging Active Participation

People learn more effectively when they participate in their health education program. Active participation generates interest; lack of participation generates boredom.

There are a number of ways to encourage participation. For instance, when presenting written material, make sure the client understands it. Clients who are merely handed a list of instructions may or may not follow them. Most instructions require discussion about why they are important. After demonstrating a procedure, ask the client to work through each step with you rather than wait for a return demonstration.

Repeating Key Facts and Concepts

Repetition of key facts and concepts reinforces learning. Likewise, practice reinforces new skills. Reviewing materials presented earlier prepares the client for receiving new materials. Encourage your clients to repeat, practice, and review.

Encouraging Immediate Practice

Clients retain new information and skills longer when they put them into practice right away. In contrast, when clients cannot use their knowledge right way, they tend to forget what they have learned. For example, in many obstetric units, it is common practice for new mothers to begin caring for their infants almost immediately. Under supervision, mothers learn how to bathe, feed, and diaper. New mothers are encouraged to practice skills right away, under supervision, instead of being sent home to flounder alone.

Helping the Client Surmount Learning Plateaus

Clients occasionally reach learning plateaus, where it may appear that they have lost interest. The person may even seem discouraged. Remember, however, that learning plateaus are normal. To surmount them, use visual aids, movies, or other stimulating methods of presentation to give the client a break from structured learning until the previous level of enthusiasm returns.

Negotiating

By actively involving clients in the decision-making process, nurses stimulate their motivation to learn. Clients are more apt to be enthusiastic about learning information that they have identified as important to them. Combining client interests with content necessary to reach health care goals makes the teaching and learning process mutually gratifying.

Some clients may resist learning. Perhaps they are still in denial about the disease process or feel angry at the adjustments they must make in their lifestyle. Or they may resist for other reasons: they "don't have time," they are presently asymptomatic, or they lack family support, for example. For these individuals, contracting may be an effective way to elicit their participation. In a **learning contract,** much like any business contract, each party (nurse and client) agrees to contribute certain things to the agreement. The nurse provides information, and the client agrees to use that information.

Mager (1975) states that instruction is effective to the degree that it succeeds in changing behavior in the desired direction. If teaching (instruction) does not lead to learning or changes in behavior, then it has no effect, no power (Redman, 1993). The contract helps the client commit to goals to achieve the desired outcomes in the learning situation. The nurse prioritizes the most essential aspects of care within the contract. As times goes by, the contract helps the client experience the satisfaction or reward of accomplishment in learning, and the contract can be changed to include other learning needs.

Learning Activities

Clearly, teaching and learning can take place in many manifestations. Three of the most important activities for any form of learning are discussion, demonstration, and role-playing.

Discussion

Discussion encourages clients to participate actively in the health education program. You can draw a client into a discussion by asking for her response to something you just taught. For example, you might ask a client to share ways in which the content applies to her life or examples of personal experiences or opinions that relate to it. In a class for clients receiving radiation treatment, for example, you might ask how they coped with their hair loss.

Demonstration

Demonstrations provide the best method for teaching motor skills, such as how to give a self-injection or how to transfer safely from a bed to a wheelchair. To prepare for a demonstration, complete the following steps:

- Make notes, and organize your thoughts so you can narrate your demonstration clearly.
- Obtain the needed equipment, and make sure it works.
- Outline the procedure on a handout so your client can follow along with you.
- Practice the demonstration until you can do it skillfully.

When giving the demonstration, make sure the client can see it clearly. Proceed slowly, allowing questions as you go. Afterward, immediately reinforce learning by having the client return the demonstration to the best of her ability.

Role-Playing

Role-playing is a creative learning activity in which a person can act as different people (physician, nurse, spouse, employer) in a variety of real-life situations to help learn new behaviors or solve problems. Initially, some people may feel shy or embarrassed about role-playing. As they become comfortable, however, they discover that it can be a very effective strategy for gaining new insights in a "safe" environment. Role-playing can be effective in teaching, parenting, and other interpersonal skills.

Documentation of Teaching

Documentation records the progress when teaching is done in multiple sessions. Additionally, the documentation records the cost-effectiveness of your teaching for quality evaluation, confirms the outcomes of the teaching and learning process, and provides legal material that could be considered in a court of law. As in other areas of nursing, accurate and complete documentation of your teaching is crucial.

EVALUATION

Evaluating how well the nurse and the client have met teaching and learning goals is an important part of the teaching and learning process (Boswell et al., 1996). Remember that it is important to develop learning objectives in terms of behaviors and measurable outcomes *before* beginning the teaching and learning process. Then, after the program, you can evaluate the success of the teaching and how well the client has

made positive life changes. Ideally, evaluation should determine that *learning has occurred* and that you were effective as a teacher. If discrepancies exist between the desired and actual outcomes, systematic problem-solving can help to rectify them and strengthen the teaching and learning process yet more.

Evaluation of Teaching

Evaluation of the teaching process measures whether the short-term learning goals have been met and whether the knowledge results in long-term behavioral changes. Evaluation also examines the effects of the change in behavior on health status and whether resources used to produce the change in health status are the most cost-effective method of treatment.

Short-Term Goals

Ask yourself a variety of questions to determine whether short-term learning has occurred and is being acted on. These may include the following:

- Has the client been given the necessary information for a safe discharge?
- Has the client accomplished the learning objectives?
- Can the client demonstrate proficiency in the skills needed to maintain self-care?
- Is there a measurable difference in the client's attitude about his highest level of health?
- Can the client cope with limitations imposed by the illness? Does the client show a willingness to make necessary lifestyle changes?
- Do the client's significant others understand the client's problems and demonstrate readiness to provide appropriate support?

Long-Term Goals

If you focus only on the evaluation of short-term learning (what a client learns before discharge), you will neglect the importance of long-term changes in behavior.

Nurses can help to determine the long-term effectiveness of teaching strategies (Agars & McMurray, 1993). However, the client, the facility staff, the outpatient nurse, and the physician all share responsibility for reinforcing long-term learning and evaluating its success over time.

Long-term evaluation may involve follow-up questionnaires or telephone calls at selected intervals after discharge. This method allows clients to demonstrate the success of learning in a real-life situation. Many times, when clients are in a health care facility and away from the demands of everyday living, they assume that a behavioral change will be easy to implement. However, the "ideal" is seldom encountered at home or in the workplace. Additional learning, problem-solving, and creativity may be necessary to integrate the desired change at home. On the other hand, in the relaxed and familiar home environment, the person may discover a "readiness to learn" that was not present during the stress of the institutional environment.

The fact is that short-term outcomes may differ from the long-term reality. Clients may "know" what is needed at the time of discharge, but they may forget or neglect that need over time, especially if they lack support or reinforcement. Long-term follow-up can be used to renew information learned in the hospital. By reinforcing what is learned in institutional teaching programs, the primary care nurse in the community provides continuity and promotes retention of learning.

Feedback received from clients after they have been discharged also provides tremendous benefits to the nurses responsible for the original teaching. In short, feedback allows nurses to evaluate the effectiveness of hospital teaching by identifying relevant content and effective teaching strategies.

Evaluation of Learning

Helpful methods to evaluate a client's learning include discussion, oral tests, written tests, and return demonstration. Testing should be fun, easy, and non-threatening. It should give the client positive reinforcement that learning has occurred rather than focus on what needs to be learned. In client education, testing is more a teaching tool than it is an evaluation process.

Discussion

In the evaluation process, the discussion method is used to review what has been learned. Review three or four main points. Ask questions of the client to evaluate whether learning has occurred. Observe the client's comfort level with the information and evaluate the client's ability to apply the information to his own health care concern and, as a result, change his behavior.

Oral Tests

Oral testing requires preparation on your part and can be quite time-consuming because it is accomplished one-to-one with the client. Large-group oral testing may be ineffective because not all clients will be able to answer. If a client has trouble articulating answers, outcomes are then difficult to evaluate.

Oral testing can be beneficial when a reading level cannot be matched to a written test or the client has visual deficits. The desired outcome is for the client to verbalize the key points and to apply the knowledge.

Written Tests

Written tests are prepared for individuals or groups and require that clients be able to read. Written tests can be in the form of multiple choice, true-or-false, matching, or essay questions. They require a space that is quiet, comfortable, and conducive to thinking

because they ask the client to recall teaching. The goal of written testing is to reflect what the client has learned and give the client a sense of satisfaction.

Return Demonstration

Return demonstration is an excellent means of evaluating a skill or task. You demonstrate the skill or task and then ask the client to return or "mirror" the skill. Written steps or instructions are valuable along with the demonstration to enhance recall once the demonstration is finished. The desired outcome is for the client to perform all the steps independently without error.

KEY PRINCIPLES

- Nursing standards for practice include client education. They assume that clients have a right to information and that nurses have a legal mandate to provide client education.
- In addition to the client's right to information, client education benefits health care through cost control and quality control.
- The purposes of client education are to promote health, prevent illness, restore health, and help clients cope with illness.
- Learning theorists have identified four domains of learning: perceptual, cognitive, affective, and psychomotor.
- Client characteristics affecting teaching are literacy, level of education, developmental level, and learning style.
- Readiness to learn and motivation facilitate learning.
- The client must be physically and psychologically able to learn.
- Cultural and environmental factors can inhibit learning.
- The ability of the nurse as an educator affects learning.
- *Knowledge deficit* is diagnosed when the client lacks knowledge of health management practices that are necessary to achieve or maintain health.
- Other nursing diagnoses commonly used for client education are *Altered health maintenance, Health-seeking behaviors,* and *Ineffective individual coping.*
- Planning to teach includes selecting topics, developing a teaching plan, and writing learning objectives.
- Although most client teaching is one-to-one instruction, there are multiple teaching methods available to maximize efficiency and effectiveness.
- Strategies for effective implementation include selecting appropriate teaching methods, rewarding positive behaviors, encouraging active participation, repeating key factors and concepts, encouraging immediate feedback, helping the client surmount learning plateaus, and negotiating.

- Evaluation of learning requires evaluating both the short-term goal of acquiring knowledge and the long-term goal of changing behavior.
- The method of evaluation should reinforce learning.

BIBLIOGRAPHY

*Agars, J., & McMurray, A. (1993). An evaluation of comparative strategies for teaching breast self-examination. *Journal of Advanced Nursing, 18*(10), 1595–1603.

American Hospital Association. (1975). *A Patient's Bill of Rights.* Chicago: Author.

Beggs, V.L., Willis, S.B., Maislen, E.L., Stokes, T.M., White, D., Sanford, M., Becker, A., Barber, S., Pawlow, P.C., & Downs, C. (1998). Patient education for discharge after coronary bypass surgery in the l990s: Are patients adequately prepared? *Journal of Cardiovascular Nursing, 12*(4), 72–86.

Bernier, M.J. (1996). Establishing the psychometric properties of a scale for evaluating quality in printed educational material. *Patient Education and Counseling, 29*(3), 283–299.

*Bloom, B.S. (1956). *Taxonomy of educational objectives. Book 1: Cognitive domain.* New York: Longman.

Boberg, E.W., Gustafson, D.H., Hawkins, R.P., Bricker, E., Pingree, S., McTavish, F., Wise, M., Owens, B., & Botta, R. (1997). CHESS: The Comprehensive Health Enhancement Support System. In P.F. Brennan, S.J. Schneider, and E. Tornquist (Eds.), *Information networks for community health* (pp 171–188). New York: Springer-Verlag.

Boswell, E.J., Pichert, J.W., Lorenz, R.A., Schlundt, D.G. Penha, M.I., Alexander, S., Davis, D.E., Evangelist, J.L., Haushalter, A.R., Lindsay, L.C., Palm, M., & Sauve, D. (1996). Evaluation of a patient teaching skills course disseminated through staff developers. *Patient Education and Counseling, 27*(3), 247–256.

*Brown, C., Wright, R., & Christensen, D. (1987). Association between type of medication instruction and patients' knowledge, side effects and compliance. *Hospital and Community Psychiatry, 38*(1), 55–60.

Chachkles, E., & Christ, G. (1996). Cross cultural issues in patient education. *Patient Education and Counseling, 27*(1), 13–21.

*Chang, B.L., & Hirsh, M. (1994). Video intervention: Producing videotapes for use in nursing practice and education. *Journal of Continuing Education in Nursing, 25*(6), 263–267.

Clayton, M. (1998). Encouraging children to use cycle helmets. *Paediatric Nursing, 10*(3), 14–16.

---

* Asterisk indicates a classic or definitive work on this subject.

*Colucciello, M.L. (1993). Learning styles and instructional processes for home healthcare providers. *Home Healthcare Nurse, 11*(2), 43–50.

Conrad, S.A., & Rensink, Y. (1997). Using intranet technology in the ICU. *Nursing Management, 28*(7), 34–36.

*Cornette, S. (1994). Organizational strategies for compliance with JCAHO standards. *Patient Education Update, Fall,* 8.

Dollahite, J., Thompson, C., & McNew, R. (1996). Readability of printed sources of diet and health information. *Patient Education and Counseling, 27*(2), 123–134.

Ellison, G.C., & Rayman, K.M. (1998). Exemplars' experience of self-managing type 3 diabetes. *Diabetes Education, 14*(2), 325–330.

Grieco, A.J. (1996). Editorial: The importance of the family in patient education and care. *Patient Education and Counseling, 27*(1), 1–3.

*Johnson, J., Rice, V., Fuller, S., & Endress, M. (1978). Sensory information: Instruction in a coping strategy and recovery from surgery. *Research in Nursing and Health, 1*(1), 4–17.

*Knowles, M. (1980). *The adult learner: A neglected species* (2nd ed.). Houston: Gulf Publishing.

Lightfoot, J., & Bines, W. (1998). Keeping children healthy: Role of the school nurse. *Nursing Times, 94*(21), 65–68.

*Mager, R.F. (1975). *Preparing instructional objectives* (2nd ed.). Belmont, CA: Fearon-Pitman Publishers.

Mahler, H.I.M., & Kulik, J.A. (1995). The development and validation of three videos designed to psychologically prepare patients for coronary bypass surgery. *Patient Education and Counseling, 25*(1), 59–66.

*Mayo, A.M. (1993). Teaching family–significant other nursing. *Journal of Continuing Education in Nursing, 24*(1), 27–31.

*Moore, M.R. (1970). The perceptual-motor domain and a proposed taxonomy of perception. *Audio Visual Community Review, 18*(5), 379–413.

North American Nursing Diagnosis Association. (1999). *NANDA Nursing diagnoses: Definitions and classification 1999–2000.* Philadelphia: Author.

*Peterson, M.G.E., & Rippey, R.M. (1992). A computerized cancer information system. *Patient Education and Counseling, 19*(1), 81–87.

Posel, N. (1998). Preoperative teaching in the preadmission clinic. *Journal of Nursing Staff, 14*(1), 52–56.

*Redman, B.K. (1993). Patient education at 25 years: Where we have been and where we are going. *Journal of Advanced Nursing, 18*(5), 725–730.

Richards, B., Colman, A.W., & Hollingsworth, R.A. (1998). The current role of the Internet in patient education. *Internet Journal Medical Information, 50*(1–3), 279–285.

Ryan, J.M., & Southern, J. (1998). A & E nursing and the Internet. *Accident Emergency Nursing, 6*(2), 106–109.

*Smith, C.E. (1987). Patient teaching: It's the law. *Nursing, 17*(7), 67–68.

*Smith, C.E. (1989). Overview of patient education: Opportunities and challenges for the twenty-first century. *Nursing Clinics of North America, 24*(4), 583–587.

Nursing Management

Suzanne S. Yarbrough

Key Terms

accountability

authority

delegation

leadership

management

nurse manager

responsibility

risk management

LEARNING OBJECTIVES

After studying this chapter, you should be able to:

1. Discuss theories and types of management.

2. Describe the characteristics of managers.

3. Explain the role of the nurse manager in ensuring quality client care, managing budgets, and managing people.

4. Describe the change process and strategies for managing resistance to change.

5. Explain the nurse manager's role in managing risk.

6. Compare and contrast the roles of nurse managers and nursing leaders as participants in multidisciplinary health care teams.

A **nurse manager** is a nurse responsible for managing the operation and expenses of a health care organization that employs nurses as the means to produce health. Nurse managers plan, organize, staff, direct, coordinate, and control the way in which nursing resources are allocated to achieve a health care institution's mission. They use strategies and techniques to inspire or elicit work from others. These strategies must fit with the institution's policies and the factors that motivate employees to work. Nurse managers want to inspire work, and they want to encourage those who work for them to remain with the institution. Nurse managers are responsible (held answerable) for the delivery of client care.

Beliefs about power and motivation to work and about how to retain employees stem from the study of management theories. **Management** is defined as the implementation of strategies that promote effective and efficient use of resources (staff, technology, supplies, and time) to achieve organizational goals. Management theories define basic concepts about human motivation to work, associated management strategies, and organizational structures that result in increased productivity and employee satisfaction (Grohar-Murray & DiCroce, 1997; Spitzer-Lehman, 1994).

THEORIES OF MANAGEMENT

According to Grohar-Murray and DiCroce (1997), there were two original management theories. Theory X proposed that workers were negatively motivated. Thus, they needed strong managerial direction and control. That theory led to tightly constructed bureaucratic organizational structures with hierarchical management levels. Theory Y proposed that workers were positively motivated and self-directed. Thus, tightly controlled organizational structures were less necessary to motivate them. However, bureaucratic management schemes were necessary to provide direction.

Later theorists explored motivation more deeply. Ouchi (1981) proposed theory Z after comparing Japanese management methods—and the higher productivity they yielded—with American management methods based on theories X and Y. Theory Z was intended to enhance American productivity by incorporating some Japanese methods and ideals. It moved beyond theory Y by allowing motivated workers to participate in decision-making processes that affected production. It proposed that productivity and quality are enhanced when workers feel trusted by management and are asked to participate in organizational planning. This theory reflected less need for managerial control and direction.

The objective of management, according to theory Z, is to provide well-defined objectives and allow workers great latitude in how they accomplish those objectives. Managers remain open to input from workers and accept them as an integral part of decision-making. Communication is a two-way process between management and employees. Managers can accept criticism and make changes for the good of the organization based on worker input.

Rather than having to motivate employees, managers recognize the inherent motivation of those who work for the organization. They recognize that employees who feel trusted will behave more responsibly (Fig. 17–1). Managers make difficult decisions, employing ethical reasoning as a means to fulfill obligations to the public they serve. They inspire or facilitate work based on the assumption that workers share their views about the organization's obligations to its consumers (Ouchi, 1981).

Common assumptions about employee motivation typically indicate a tendency toward theory Y or theory Z. One belief is that employees who are trusted to be responsible for personal job performance will be more productive than those who are coerced and tightly controlled. A second belief is that the structure of the organization should not impede employee performance by being rigid. Therefore, as management theories have evolved, so have organizational structures and management styles or strategies. This is true for nursing management as well.

Based on theory Z, organizational structures in health care have become more flattened. Fewer management layers move decision-making closer to the front-line workers. As a result, lines of communication and control over work have become less centralized. Rather than one manager assuming control from the center of the organization, many managers or teams take charge of their work units. Decision-making within these structures is shared. Nurse managers have become consensus builders who facilitate client care rather than act as control agents. All staff share in problem-solving, planning, organizing, evaluating outcomes, and attaining goals.

TYPES OF MANAGERS

Managers influence the ways in which groups of people work together to create an organization's product. The manager oversees the work unit or team, in-

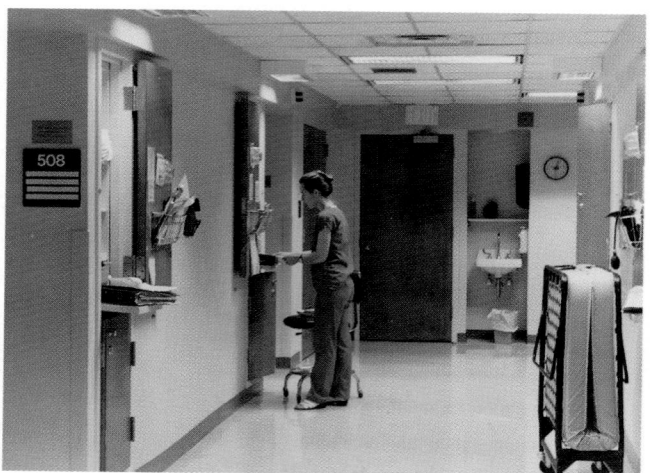

Figure 17–1. Employees who feel trusted will behave more responsibly. This nurse is working independently to help accomplish the organization's mission.

TABLE 17-1
Characteristics of Nurse Managers at Different Levels

Level of Management	Title	Educational Preparation	Tasks
Front-Line Manager	• Team leader • Case manager • Charge nurse	• RN • 1 to 2 years of nursing experience	• Manage client care • Supervise team members • Know status of all clients • Know all team members' roles
Middle Manager	• Unit manager • Supervisor	• RN • BSN or MSN preferred • 1 to 5 years of nursing experience	• Supervise nurses and ancillary staff • 24-hour accountability • Manage resources • Motivate others • Act as change agent • Manage quality • Manage risk
Nurse Executive	• Director of nursing • Vice president for nursing • Nursing CEO	• RN • MSN or PhD in allied health preferred • Management experience	• Operationalize nursing • Provide resources • Facilitate quality care • Facilitate efficiency

cluding the financial aspects of its operation, and implements strategies to meet the goals of the organization. In health care, management involves implementing strategies to promote effective uses of nurses and other staff in environments ranging from tertiary care hospitals to clients' homes. In all cases, the goal is to promote health.

Nurses can assume varying roles in management, ranging from front-line nurse manager to nurse executive. Table 17–1 lists characteristics of three levels of nurse managers.

Nurse Executives

A top-level nurse manager is called a nurse executive. This person may be called the director of nursing services or the vice-president for client care services. Nurse executives supervise multiple departments in which professionals of various disciplines provide care for all those served by the organization. Usually, a person must have an advanced degree in nursing and several years of clinical and middle-management experience before receiving an executive position.

The nurse executive works closely with the organization's administrative team and may have equal ranking with other executives who manage broad organizational functions, such as the chief financial officer, who oversees the budget, and the chief operations officer, who oversees the physical plant. The nurse executive ensures that all client care provided by nurses is carried out in keeping with the objectives of the entire health care organization.

Middle Managers

Middle-level nurse managers oversee care delivered by a smaller groups of nurses and ancillary staff in a specified segment of the organization. Middle managers typically report to the nurse executive. In a hospi-

tal, a middle manager may oversee the day-to-day operation of several client-care units. In a home health agency, a middle manager might oversee the operation of a specific office or area. In all cases, their responsibilities include managing the staff (nursing and ancillary personnel who provide client services) and the budget.

Middle-level nurse managers can hire and fire staff. They prepare work schedules. And they act to maintain the quality of client services. They do so in part by writing and implementing policies that guide client care and unit operations. The nurse manager must balance the priorities of nurses (caring for people who are responding to actual or potential health threats) with the priorities of the organization (financial health) and the public mandate to control health care costs.

Most middle managers have at least a bachelor of science degree; some have an advanced degree in nursing. Usually, a middle-level manager has had some experience in nursing and has shown leadership qualities in addition to clinical competence.

Front-Line Managers

A front-line manager typically works as a charge nurse, team leader, or client care coordinator—a role that is closely identified with the actual delivery of client care (Fig. 17–2). This person's duties are established by the middle-level nurse manager.

In a hospital or unit-based setting, the front-line manager coordinates the activities of all staff who provide client care (RNs, LPNs, and nursing assistants). The front-line manager makes client-care assignments, knows about all of the clients receiving care, and makes sure that appropriate services are provided. This manager may interact with physicians and other health care providers and may consult with the nurses who provide the client's care.

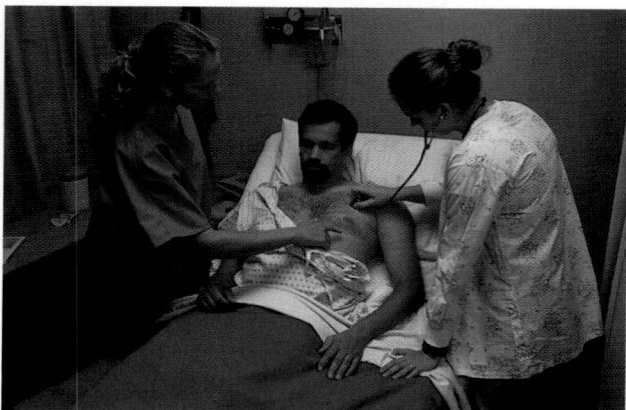

Figure 17–2. Front-line managers are identified with the actual delivery of care. Here, a front-line manager works side-by-side with a staff nurse in direct client care.-

CHARACTERISTICS OF MANAGERS

Regardless of their specific position in an organization, nurse managers are excellent clinicians able to direct the work of others. By applying nursing process strategies and management theories, nurse managers assess and analyze problems related to the delivery of client care. By doing so, they can plan, organize, and lead others in implementing interventions that benefit clients and achieve institutional goals (Katz & Green, 1997). Nurse managers understand how the organizational structure is designed to benefit clients.

Nurse managers also understand the contributions made by bedside nurses and support staff to the overall success or failure of the organization. They use their knowledge of professional, legal, and ethical models to direct the activities of nurses and support staff. They use their expertise to maintain safe, efficient, and cost-effective clinical services (Spitzer-Lehman, 1994). They also can recognize problems within work groups and can implement strategies to solve those problems before they disrupt the flow of client care.

In whatever positions they hold, successful nurse managers possess a number of characteristics important to fulfilling their duties. These characteristics include responsibility, accountability, leadership, and a commitment to quality care.

Responsibility and Accountability

Responsibility is the obligation to act or direct to accomplish a goal. Nurse managers are held accountable for their own actions, the actions of those they oversee, and the appropriate delivery of client care that achieves outcomes. Having **accountability** means being held answerable for personal actions or the actions of others. A nurse manager's level of responsibility is defined by the organizational structure and the level of assigned authority. **Authority** is the ability or legitimate power to make decisions, implement strategies, and elicit work from others. Nurse managers have the

authority to direct the work of others as a way to balance their accountability and responsibility for client care.

Nurse managers, particularly those at the executive and middle management levels, are fiscally responsible and accountable. They have authority to direct the allocation of resources (equipment, supplies, technology, time, and staff). They use rules of fiscal management to plan, implement, and evaluate budgets and delivery systems. For example, a unit manager who wants to hire a new nurse would be expected to justify the expense by providing data about the amount of care required by clients in the unit, the number of nurses available to provide that care, and the effect of current staffing patterns on client outcomes.

Nurse managers plan for the future while participating in current design, implementation, and evaluation systems for the delivery of care. The bottom line issue is productivity. Nurse managers are responsible for making sure that everyone is working at their maximum capacity. Nurse managers are accountable for ensuring that clients receive care in a manner that produces the best possible outcome, the highest degree of satisfaction, and the lowest cost (Spitzer-Lehman, 1994).

Leadership

Although managers incorporate ideals and strategies to help move work in the direction of an organization's objectives, leaders go further. They incorporate interpersonal interactions and strategies that inspire others to work toward those goals. Management involves implementing strategies to accomplish organizational goals; **leadership** involves showing others the way, directing others in a course of action, going before others, or going with and inspiring others. Successful nurse managers employ these leadership skills and characteristics to increase their effectiveness as managers.

Various theories exist to explain leadership. The consensus is that leaders incorporate communication skills, understanding of the group process, and a strong vision for health care as the means to effect group movement in a specific direction (Grohar-Murray & DiCroce, 1997). Leaders use open, honest, clear, and concise communication. They listen actively to learn about the wishes of a group. They use group process to build consensus and stimulate enthusiasm for projects. Nurse leaders understand the importance of their work and incorporate the values of the profession in all aspects of their professional life.

Because the position of a nurse manager involves inspiring others to work, all nurse managers should be leaders. However, leaders do not always hold management positions. Leaders can do the work of inspiring others from any position (Grohar-Murray & DiCroce, 1997). Indeed, nurses have many opportunities to be leaders in health care.

For example, a bedside nurse with no role in managing the organization may be a leader in a nursing organization, such as the American Nurses' Association. These leaders work to influence political activities that affect health care policies at the local, state, or national level. Or a nurse may be a leader among a group of peers, influencing the way the group goes about the daily activities of providing for clients. Leaders work to create change that benefits clients throughout the health care industry. Leadership qualities are an essential component of the effective nurse manager's storehouse of strategies for promoting health care.

Commitment to Quality Care

Nurse managers are vital to the process of maintaining quality in health care. As nurses, they can use their knowledge of health and the human health experience to implement structures (such as policies and staffing patterns) and processes (steps in identified tasks) that improve health outcomes. As managers, they can evaluate client outcomes using statistical and research methods to identify strategies that promote quality in health care.

Naturally, nurse managers must be excellent clinicians. From that base, they can influence the development of the organization's goals while contributing to the attainment of those goals. They manage the cost-effective delivery of care by creating budgets, allocating nursing resources, and overseeing the delivery of care. They contribute to improvements in the quality of client care both personally and in the supervision they give.

As managers, nurses must think critically. They employ ethical decision-making models as the means to maintain legal and professional standards. They implement management strategies that incorporate nursing, management, leadership, economic, and quality improvement theories that promote effective and efficient health care delivery.

ROLES OF MANAGERS

Nurse managers—whether front-line managers, middle managers, or executives—have a position within the organizational hierarchy of a health care institution. An organization is defined as a social system deliberately established to carry out some defining purpose (Grohar-Murray & DiCroce, 1997, p. 125). In health care, examples of organizations include hospitals, long-term care facilities, home care agencies, and community agencies. Health care organizations are social systems designed to provide services for clients.

A hierarchy is a way of looking at relationships in terms of who directs or has authority over whom. An organizational hierarchy shows how members of an organization relate to one another. Most organizations create a diagram called an organizational chart that depicts the hierarchical arrangement of its managers. Figure 17–3 is an example of an organizational chart.

An organizational chart is used to delineate levels of authority and responsibility by showing relation-

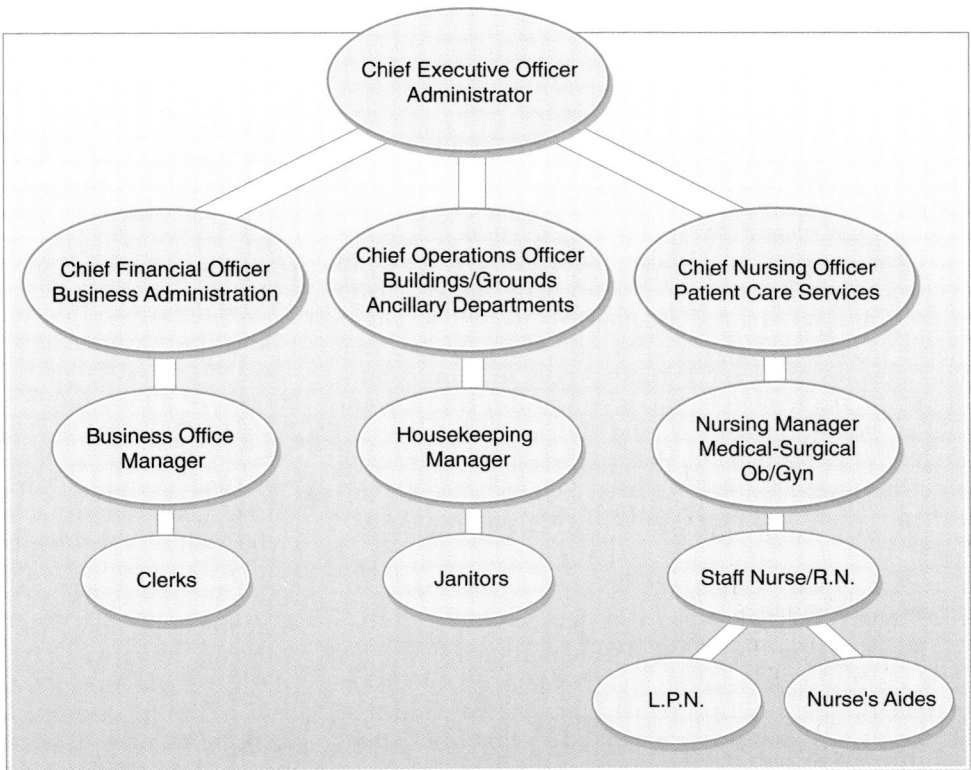

Figure 17–3. A sample organizational chart.

ships among levels of management. Most health care organizations are headed by an administrator. The nurse executive would answer to and receive direction from the administrator. Depending on the size of the organization, the nurse executive may direct the activities of nurse managers who, in turn, oversee the work of groups of nurses and ancillary staff who provide client care. At each level, the manager receives direction from the person directly overhead on the organizational chart.

The way in which a health care institution outlines and defines its organizational hierarchy dictates the leadership styles and management techniques that nurse managers will use to achieve the institution's mission. For example, a small long-term care facility with three client care units might have a director of nursing who assumes authority, accountability, and responsibility for all nursing activities. The director of nursing might delegate certain management tasks to another RN who functions as supervisor for all client care activities in the facility during each shift. The supervisor prepares assignments for each of the units and oversees all client care activities for that shift. Nurses who provide direct client care would address questions about that care to the supervisor. However, in this small institution, they would address questions about scheduling or overall facility operation to the director of nursing. This is an example of a flat organizational hierarchy.

The roles filled by a nurse manager result largely from the responsibilities incurred at various levels of the organization's hierarchy. In general, however, those roles involve managing quality, budgets, people, change, and risk.

Managing Quality

Quality assurance is a process of evaluating the outcome of care measured against predetermined standards and implementing methods of improvement. A quality assurance program is based on a clear definition of quality and the reliable and valid outcomes used to measure it. Although the current trend in health care is toward cost containment, the goal is to do so without reducing the quality of client services.

Managing quality means accentuating positive outcomes as well as avoiding negative outcomes. Quality management begins when health care organizations define themselves and the product that they intend to deliver. They define themselves by their mission (the product), their values (their view of the importance of the product), and their goals and objectives.

Mission Statement

The overall definition of the business of health care for each institution is written in the form of a mission statement. The service provided and the value of that service to health care are specified in this brief statement (Box 17–1).

BOX 17–1

SAMPLE MISSION STATEMENT FOR A HOME HEALTH AGENCY

- To be dedicated to the provision of excellent home health care for older adults of the community.
- To serve as one of the community's best resources for elder assistance.
- To help elderly adults in the community maintain desired level of independence.
- To provide nursing and allied health services that will facilitate maximal independence for elderly adults in the community.
- To provide care in a fiscally responsible manner, maintaining profit for the agency.

The mission statement is a means for communicating the institution's overall philosophical stance along with the aspects of health care that are most valued by the institution. For example, the mission of a home health agency may be to help maintain the independence and functional ability of elderly residents of a specified town. That statement reflects a philosophical perspective that values elderly clients and their abilities to maintain self-determination.

The mission statement is used to identify institutional goals. Goals are statements that specify the desired results of service, practice, and management within the institution. Goals are translated into specific objectives to guide the day-to-day operation of the work units.

Ordinarily, the mission statement and goals for the organization are written, and all staff are aware of them. Often, mission statements are posted in areas frequented by staff and visitors so that everyone is reminded of them frequently.

Goals and Objectives

Goals define and describe the means used to ensure that values expressed in the mission statement are upheld in the delivery of services. In other words, the home health agency's goals would specify ways to help the elderly. For example, one goal might be to develop a day care program for those unable to manage total independence. Another goal might be to have a nurse gerontologist available to consult with nurses who visit elderly clients.

Health care institutions base their goals for providing service on the values reflected in their mission statement. A home care agency's goal is to provide nursing, therapy, and social services that help the elderly remain functionally independent. At the other end of the spectrum, a tertiary care hospital's mission may be to provide state-of-the-art technology to improve the survival of certain client populations. The hospital's goals would therefore be to obtain or develop the technology needed to maintain that client population. Another goal would be to associate with a university where nurses and physicians are educated about that client population and where research is conducted to benefit that client population.

Goals are global statements about how the institution will strive to achieve its mission. In contrast, objectives specify the means for achieving each goal. They define numbers and types of nurses, for example, and the ancillary staff needed to accomplish a goal. Objectives are also used to define nursing roles in providing individualized client care.

For example, if the mission reflects a philosophy that values individualized client care, a goal would be to facilitate nurse-client relationships that promote individual knowledge of clients. The objective would be to specify and implement a method of delivering nursing care that is expected to increase individualized care. The staff could evaluate a team or primary care model for specifying the relationship that a nurse and client have and the way that ancillary staff assist the nurse in client care.

In the primary nursing care model, one nurse assumes responsibility for a client throughout that client's health care experience by assessing the client's needs and overseeing all aspects of the nursing care plan. Anyone providing care for that client collaborates with the client's primary care nurse. On the other hand, team nursing care models divide tasks or client care needs according to team members' skills and competencies. No individual staff nurse accepts full responsibility for that client's care plan. Because the primary care model tends to promote individualized care, the objective for this facility would be to use a primary care nursing model to deliver individualized client care.

Policies and Procedures

Objectives are implemented through written documents called policies and procedures. Policies and procedures are rules and outlined processes that define the steps taken to meet objectives, to achieve goals, and therefore, to accomplish the institutional mission (Fig. 17–4). Policies specify roles and operations within the organization. Procedures outline the steps in specific tasks. Each is based on accepted standards of care.

For example, the objective to provide primary nursing care would be implemented through policies that specify the number of clients a primary nurse will be responsible for and the licensure or educational requirements for primary care nurses. Related procedures might list steps required in a nursing care plan and care to be provided by non–primary nurses.

Because nurse managers are responsible and accountable for achieving goals and objectives, they must have the authority to implement policies and procedures that help their work units accomplish the mission. Policies and procedures are written for virtu-

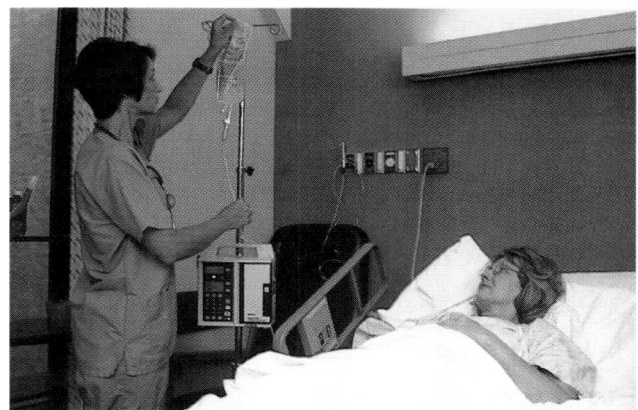

Figure 17–4. This nurse manager is evaluating a client's intravenous therapy to validate the effectiveness of her institution's policy for intravenous therapy.

ally every element of client care, even hand-washing. Nurse managers make sure that policies and procedures are carried out. To do so, they must ensure that appropriate resources are available to staff, such as soap and sinks for washing hands.

Policies and procedures are based on legal and professional standards regarding safe and effective client care. Nurse managers must know the legal, ethical, and professional implications of their actions and the actions of those they manage. They must effectively communicate that knowledge to others in the institution to ensure that policies and procedures adhere to those standards while contributing to attainment of institutional goals.

Nurse managers evaluate how well policies and procedures facilitate the attainment of goals by measuring outcomes. For example, a home health agency that specializes in providing infusion therapy in clients' homes might document the percentage of clients who developed phlebitis or systemic infections following infusions. The nurse manager would report the results for a specified period to show that the goal (no adverse effects) had or had not been met. Administrative staff and agencies that pay for health care could then use that data to evaluate the effectiveness of related policies and procedures.

For example, the agency's policies might specify that only RNs with special training in venipuncture can start the infusion but that LPNs trained in infusion therapy could maintain the infusion after the venipuncture. The agency probably would also have a procedure that specifies the steps for a venipuncture and for maintaining the venous access once established. Based on outcomes, the management team may change policies and procedures. Likewise, the third-party paying organizations can use outcomes to determine future use of the agency's services.

Nurse managers have a very important role in implementing standards and procedures as well as monitoring and measuring success in carrying out the institutional mission. Nurses must justify their importance in the provision of health care by demonstrating that nursing care is appropriate, safe, effective, and efficient. Nurse managers use tools for gathering that data, such as statistical and research methods, with the ultimate goal of identifying opportunities for improving structures (policies), processes (procedures), or outcomes. In other words, nurse managers use quality indicators to identify problems in the delivery of nursing services, to implement strategies to correct problems, and to evaluate the effectiveness of those strategies.

Managing Budgets

In 1966, the federal government introduced health insurance programs for the elderly and the poor: Medicare and Medicaid. Until that time, health care had been financed by private individuals or private insurance programs that held the cost of care at a level that was affordable for most people. Medicare and Medicaid greatly improved access to health care for certain population groups. These programs also ensured that health care providers would be paid for the services they provided.

However, according to Feldstein (1993), these changes in access to care and reimbursement caused health care costs to rise at a rate greater than that of inflation. Neither the government, which finances about 40% of health care, nor private insurance companies have been able to keep pace with the rising cost of health care. New laws, government activities, and types of health insurance have attempted to regain control of health care costs.

Cost Containment

Cost containment remains a major goal in health care today and affects all health care practitioners (Feldstein, 1993). The challenge for nurses, especially nurse managers, is to balance the value of nursing and the quality of care with the cost of providing care, while continuing to fulfill their obligation to be client advocates.

Nurse managers strive to ensure the highest quality care at the lowest possible cost. As health care costs have risen, government agencies, and now insurance companies, have become more careful about seeking justification for expenditures.

Agencies that pay for health care (such as insurance companies) also expect health care providers, and nurses in particular, to carefully document and justify the necessity of all services provided to a client. Nurse managers must understand all factors that influence a unit's operation to be able to mount effective arguments for or against changes that influence the unit's function. Nurse managers also must use budgeting and accounting principles to justify staffing patterns. They must project the number and types of staff needed to produce quality health care. They also must project and justify the supplies and equipment needed. In short, they must provide a reasoned argument to convince those in control of the purse strings

that the best quality nursing care is being delivered in the most efficient way possible.

Forecasting

Nurse managers apply methods of accounting and budgeting to accomplish the task of financial management. Box 17–2 lists and defines common financial management terms used in this process. The nurse manager consults the mission statement of the institution, quality goals, and productivity standards as the basis for establishing budgets. For example, consider an agency that provides adult day care and has the goal of realizing a 5% profit on that care. The nurse manager's job would be to implement strategies that facilitate care while keeping the cost of operations at least 5% less than the revenue recovered for services.

Productivity is the measure of efficiency that drives all budgeting strategies. It is measured by subtracting the cost of providing care (salaries, maintenance, cost of supplies and equipment, and so on) from the amount of money received in payment for services. The overall process for measuring productiv-

---

BOX 17–2

FINANCIAL MANAGEMENT TERMS

- **Budget**—A financial plan used to estimate the cost of services, expected revenues, and potential profits for a prescribed time.
- **Revenues**—Monies received during a specified time.
- **Expenses**—Monies spent in the provision of services, such as the cost of salaries and benefits for staff, the cost of maintaining the work environment (heat and electric), and the cost of equipment and supplies.
- **Break-even point**—The point at which revenues equal expenses.
- **Profit margin**—The percentage by which revenues exceed expenses.
- **For-profit health care organization**—An institution that seeks to make a profit during specified periods.
- **Fiscal year**—The 12-month time during which a specific budget is in effect.
- **Variance**—The difference between a forecasted budget (revenue over cost) and actual balance.

Information from Huber, D. (1996). Leadership and nursing care management. Philadelphia: W.B. Saunders Co.; Marquis, B.L., & Huston, C.J. (1996). Leadership roles and management functions in nursing: Theory and application. (2nd ed.). Philadelphia: Lippincott-Raven; Grohar-Murray, M.E., & DiCroce, H.R. (1997). Leadership and management in nursing. Stamford, CT: Appleton & Lange.

ity is accomplished through accounting. Budgeting and accounting strategies are used to forecast the amount of income that will be produced by a work unit minus the cost of maintaining that work unit. Administrative fiscal managers allocate resources (staff, supplies, and equipment) based on these projections.

Nurse managers may be responsible for part or all of the budgeting and accounting process. They must forecast nursing expenses that will be incurred while providing quality client care. And they must forecast the approximate numbers and types of clients to estimate revenues. If the cost of care turns out to exceed revenues, nurse managers then must explain the reason for the variation from budgeted projections.

Nurse managers understand budgeting and accounting principles and accept responsibility and accountability for managing profits and losses for their work units. As leaders in health care, nurse managers provide reasoned explanations of balance sheets, and they help build institutional policy to optimize the quality and efficiency of nursing care.

Managing People

Nurse managers are more than excellent clinicians and astute fiscal managers. They also must manage people. This objective requires multiple tasks, including planning, organizing, staffing, directing, coordinating, and controlling nursing processes to produce cost-effective, quality health care. Nurse managers assume responsibility for nursing productivity on a continual basis as opposed to limiting that responsibility to only the time when the manager is physically present.

Nurse managers are responsible for evaluating performance and possibly for hiring and firing as well. They not only evaluate but also coach or counsel health care providers. They assume responsibility for staff development and education and the implementation of standards of care. They collaborate with other departments and disciplines in the interest of client care management. And nurse managers represent the health care institution and nursing as leaders. All of these tasks require that nurse managers be capable leaders who can communicate, organize, and delegate (Grohar-Murray & DiCroce, 1997).

Leadership Style

Accomplishing multiple complex functions in participatory management environments requires a leadership style that empowers others and encourages their participation. Effective nurse managers tend to be consensus builders. That is, they encourage discussion or debate that promotes productivity. They solicit input from all levels of staff in the decision-making process. They seek data from multiple sources before implementing strategies to promote productivity. Consensus-building managers are good negotiators and function as change agents.

Pugh and Woodward-Smith (1997) made a distinction among assertive, aggressive, passive, and passive-aggressive leadership styles. Table 17–2 lists characteristics of each style.

Assertive nurse managers recognize each person's right to be treated as an autonomous participant in the process of client care, leading to the achievement of outcomes. They strive to achieve a balance between involvement with the process of health care and realization of the desired outcome. Therefore, they try to have team members work together to implement processes that contribute to the greater good of attaining organizational goals. Assertive nurse managers are consensus-building managers. They understand their role and the role of other health care employees. They can discuss issues openly, accepting other viewpoints. They fit the management profiles suggested by Ouchi (1981) in theory Z. These managers accept that all employees wish to produce a quality product, and they work with the team to create that product.

In contrast, aggressive nurse managers are interested only in achieving organizational goals (Pugh & Woodward-Smith, 1997). Individual rights of employees are negated in the interest of achieving the goal. Aggressive managers do not trust those working for them. They attempt to control behavior in an authoritarian manner rather than facilitating work.

Passive nurse managers are less interested in processes or products than they are in maintaining employee satisfaction and harmony in the workforce (Pugh & Woodward-Smith, 1997). These managers are unable to build consensus or cohesiveness because of their need to please each individual or avoid conflict. Ironically, disharmony commonly results from this lack of leadership because each individual strives to have the ruling view or the manager's favor. Productivity is sacrificed in the interest of friendships.

Passive-aggressive managers vacillate between being authoritarian and outcome-oriented and maintaining peace and harmony (Pugh & Woodward-Smith, 1997). They—and the employees they supervise—have no clear view of the mission or the means of achieving it. There is chaos as each employee strives either to gain the manager's favor or to avoid authoritarian judgment.

Communication

Communication is the key to an assertive, democratic leadership style. Communication facilitates all other management activities. It is a process of giving and receiving messages for the purpose of transmitting or exchanging information. An assertive nurse manager can communicate goals, delegate responsibilities and authority, coach, and inspire others through words and actions. An assertive manager also can obtain information by being an active listener and an acute observer. Table 17–3 provides examples of assertive communication.

Pugh and Woodward-Smith (1997) described the attributes of an assertive communicator. That person uses messages that indicate personal ownership of beliefs, values, and needs. For example, the person says,

TABLE 17–2
Leadership/Management Types and Strategies

Assertive	Aggressive	Passive	Passive-Aggressive
• Democratic	• Autocratic	• Laissez faire	• Vacillates between autocratic and laissez faire
• Balances goals and process	• Focused on goals	• Focused on process	• Vacillates between goal and process
• Empowers others	• Authoritarian	• Maintains harmony	
• Facilitates participation	• Demands or coerces	• Manipulates	• Vacillates between authority and harmony
• Encourages discussion	• Tells	• Implies	
• Encourages staff input	• Makes rules	• Adopts most popular view	• Vacillates between demanding and manipulating
• Uses data to solve problems	• Accuses	• Defensive	• Vacillates between telling and implying
• Delegates	• Forces	• Does jobs rather than asks	
• Listens	• Talks	• Listens but does not hear	• Vacillates between ruling and following
• Observes	• Monitors and watches	• Attends to popular view	
• Communicates beliefs	• Imposes rules	• Follows	• Vacillates between accusing and defending
• Communicates expectations	• Demands results	• Begs for compliance	• Either demands or does job rather than ask
• Gives factual messages	• Selects information	• Uses emotion-based messages	
• Has positive attitude	• Has negative attitude	• Has negative attitude	• Either talks or listens without hearing
• Trusts	• Distrusts	• Distrusts	• Either monitors or attends to popular view
• Builds consensus	• Dictates	• Wants to be popular	• Vacillates between imposing rules and following
			• Vacillates between demanding and begging
			• Vacillates between selecting and emoting
			• Has negative attitude
			• Distrusts
			• Either dictates or wants to be popular

TABLE 17–3
Assertive Communication Techniques

Effective Messages	Less Effective Messages
"I observed that you were able to manage your clients' care today but that you have to stay past work hours to complete your nurse's notes most days. I believe that work assignments should be set up in a way that lets us complete all of our duties within the scheduled work time. Is there something that we can do to help you accomplish that goal?"	"You never get your nurse's notes written during your shift. You need to get organized so you can get done on time. I won't pay you overtime for notes any more."
	OR
	"I'll have Mary Jane change your assignment since you always have to stay overtime to finish your nurse's notes."
"Our client census is at a peak right now, with some acutely ill clients. We are going to need one more nurse than usual for the next three shifts. These are the options available to us. . . ."	"I need three nurses to work overtime, with the way the census is running. This is the new staffing schedule."
	OR
	"Can anybody work an extra shift to cover the increased census? My husband told me that he won't tolerate my covering all of the extra shifts for the unit any more."
"The team worked well together on this project. Through your efforts, we accomplished the changes in client outcomes that we needed."	"Lucky for you guys we met our goals somehow."

"I want" or "I need" rather than "you must" or "you didn't." An assertive manager also communicates beliefs and expectations about values and goals. This promotes group participation rather than imposing values and coercing work. Assertive nurse managers do not accuse. They state an observation and discuss alternatives. They listen to complaints and concerns. They discuss alternative solutions rather than becoming defensive.

Clear communication is facilitated by structuring messages to make them more understandable. One way is to avoid jargon, especially when communicating with people from other disciplines. Using jargon or abbreviations can lead to misinterpretation or confusion. Another way is to keep messages factual, using appropriate details rather than global metaphors to present information. Also, assertive managers avoid the use of emotions when communicating about work (Spitzer-Lehmann, 1994).

In summary, assertive nurse managers actively seek employee input about policies and procedures rather than imposing rules without regard for their applicability (Pugh & Woodward-Smith, 1997). They maintain a positive attitude toward work and a satisfying work environment. Responsibilities are shared rather than imposed. They trust that others are capable of and motivated to produce a quality product. And they can risk their sense of control, or authority, in the interest of promoting a cohesive work unit (Grohar-Murray & DiCroce, 1997).

Organization and Delegation

Assertive nurse managers employ other management skills to implement processes that lead to quality outcomes. They do so because nurse managers must manage multiple tasks to accomplish their mission. Thus, they must use time effectively and maximize productivity. Time management requires organization and judicious delegation of tasks. Box 17–3 lists key time management tips.

Organization requires the nurse manager to identify tasks, obligations, and activities that must be accomplished in a given period. Then the manager must estimate the time required by each task and rank the tasks, obligations, and activities in priority order. In general, the order should follow the institution's goals and objectives. Activities essential to achieving a goal must take place sooner than activities less essential to achieving the goal. Once the manager has identified times and priorities, the next step is to establish a plan for accomplishing the tasks and activities.

Some tasks need not be done specifically by the nurse manager and can be delegated. **Delegation** involves assigning responsibility for certain tasks to other people, thereby allowing the manager to concentrate on organizational goals and productivity—tasks that can be accomplished only by a nurse manager (Spitzer-Lehman, 1994). Box 17–4 lists strategies for effective delegation.

When a nurse manager delegates a task to another

BOX 17–3

TIME MANAGEMENT TIPS

- Identify tasks, obligations, and activities.
- Write them down.
- Identify which must be completed in specified time frames.
- Prioritize according to importance.
- Work on the most important first.
- Cross tasks off as they have been accomplished (a very satisfying activity).
- Delegate tasks that do not require your expertise. Remember to give specific directions and to follow up on progress regularly.
- Do not accept assignments that you are not capable of completing.
- Avoid the need to be perfect.

---

member of the health care team, the manager must communicate all aspects of that task to the person charged with accomplishing it. A clear understanding of the manager's expectations will help the person accomplish the task independently and successfully. The person to whom the task is delegated should have the freedom to decide on a course of action for accomplishing the task. Therefore, that person should have ability, knowledge, and motivation to accomplish the delegated task.

The manager must know each employee's capabilities and the practice constraints dictated by licensure and education level. No nurse should delegate responsibility to ancillary personnel who lack the ability, education, or licensure to make appropriate nursing decisions. If the task requires nursing judgment, the task either should not be delegated or the individual to whom the task was assigned should be instructed to report specific information back to the delegating nurse.

For example, a manager may ask a personal care assistant—a nurse's aide—to take morning vital signs for all clients. However, although the assistant may be able to take and record blood pressures, this person does not have the ability to make judgments about the values obtained. Therefore, the delegating nurse must devise a specific mechanism for the assistant to report all morning vital signs to an identified nurse before delegating the task. The ultimate responsibility for a task lies with the person who delegated it.

In a general sense, work does flow more easily when shared with others. Consequently, nurse managers who use their knowledge of others, the work to be accomplished, and tasks appropriate for delegation will work more effectively and efficiently. In addition, they can accept responsibility and accountability for the work of others because tasks will have been delegated appropriately.

BOX 17-4

DELEGATION

Delegation—a management tool that allows managers to distribute work (responsibility, accountability, and authority for the means of accomplishing goals) by assigning tasks to others in accordance with their abilities, knowledge, and credentials.

Steps in Effective Delegation

- Identify the task.
- Analyze the skill and knowledge needed to accomplish the task.
- Identify the person who has the skills, knowledge, and time to accomplish the task.
- Assign the task. Provide clear and concise details about the task, including the time frame and expected outcome, the purpose of the task, and any limitations in responsibility or authority for accomplishing the task.
- Validate the person's understanding.
- Let the person complete the task with occasional follow-up and feedback.

DO NOT delegate a task if you feel uncomfortable about someone else having control over how it will be completed.

Information from Huber, D. (1996). Leadership and nursing care management. Philadelphia: W.B. Saunders Co.; Marquis, B.L., & Huston, C.J. (1996). Leadership roles and management functions in nursing: Theory and application. (2nd ed.). Philadelphia: Lippincott-Raven; Grohar-Murray, M.E., & DiCroce, H.R. (1997). Leadership and management in nursing. Stamford, CT: Appleton & Lange.

Managing Change

The one constant in health care delivery is change. Quality management programs are based on the ideal of continuously improving processes to continuously improve outcomes. To achieve that ideal, policies and procedures must be continuously evaluated and revised so institutions will function more effectively and efficiently. Deficiencies identified in quality indicators are viewed as opportunities for improvement and the impetus for change.

Nurse managers, acting as change agents, are obligated to influence the direction of change and maintain professional nursing standards. Change occurs more readily when it is planned and managed. Changes that are allowed to happen without planning result in chaos. Consequently, effective nurse managers use steps similar to the nursing process to plan and accomplish changes in policies and procedures for their work units. Box 17–5 lists steps in the change process.

BOX 17-5

STEPS FOR MANAGING CHANGE

Planned Change

- Identify the need for change (assess).
- Identify the potential causes of a problem or opportunity for improvement (analyze structures and processes).
- Identify potential actions (plan).
- Implement actions (implement).
- Evaluate outcomes (evaluate).
- Incorporate new behaviors into new structures or processes (evaluate).

The Change Process

The manager identifies the need for change through assessment. Quality indicators, usually client outcome data, are assessed to detect trends that suggest a need for improvement. For example, an agency providing telephone home care visits to clients with congestive heart failure may decide that their clients have a decreased ability to function because of dyspnea. Therefore, the agency may decide to measure client dyspnea when they admit clients for nursing care, at specific intervals during nursing care, and the time of discharge from telephone home care. The agency would expect to see a trend indicating that nursing interventions caused an overall decrease in client dyspnea. When that fails to happen, the nurse manger would assess, analyze, and diagnose possible reasons for that variance from the expectation.

Assessment would include looking at the numbers and types of clients admitted with dyspnea, nursing interventions (procedures) implemented to alleviate dyspnea, and the types of nurses who cared for the clients (RN versus LPN, for example). Next, the nurse manager would analyze the assessment data in order to identify possible causes of the problem and the variance from expectation. For example, the manager might find that clients talked to a different nurse each time they were called, with the result that care plans were not being followed as written. Further analysis might indicate which policies or procedures caused the variance, such as staffing patterns for the time in question. The problem is identified in the same way that a nursing diagnosis is identified.

Once problems have been identified, actions can be taken to resolve them. That may mean planning new policies. In the dyspnea example, the nurse manager might change the schedule so the same nurse always calls on specific clients. Or the manager may examine research on interventions appropriate for dyspnea and, as needed, alter those provided to clients of the agency.

In most cases, the nurse manager would act as a

member of a process-improvement team. Staff nurses also participate in these teams in the interest of promoting democratic change. The planning phase of the process includes formulating how the policy or procedure should be rewritten, in keeping with professional standards, and how the rewritten version should be implemented. If the team decides that one more nurse is needed to cover a certain number of calls, the process must also involve budget analysis to justify the expense of hiring another nurse, plans for advertising and hiring a new nurse, instituting policies and procedures for orienting the new nurse once hired, and staffing patterns for the entire team once the new nurse is oriented.

Once the plans are made, the next step is to implement them. In this example, the new nurse would be hired. The change process does not end with implementation of the new policy or procedure, however. The next step entails evaluating the effectiveness of the planned change. And in the final step, further evaluation reveals either the need for more planning if the new process fails to improve the outcome or the means to incorporate successful new behaviors into practice. Theoretically, when employees see the value of a planned change, they are more likely to accept the change and incorporate the new behaviors it represents.

This process closely resembles the nursing process. Data are gathered and analyzed as the means for identifying a problem (nursing diagnosis). Nursing interventions are implemented, using a plan to alter factors that caused the problem. Interventions and change tactics begin with realistic, measurable objectives or goals planned to occur within a specified period. Once interventions have been implemented, their effectiveness is evaluated, and the plan is either accepted as effective and incorporated into practice or reassessed and revised because it did not have the desired effect.

Controlling Anxiety

Nurse managers understand that change, even when planned carefully, causes anxiety, Indeed, the natural response of employees—virtually all humans, in fact—is to resist change. As the change agent, the nurse manager can initiate changes successfully by soliciting input from staff affected by the change, implementing the plan in stages, and demonstrating the effectiveness of the change through evaluation, thereby decreasing anxiety related to the change.

Several theories have been proposed to address resistance to change and ways to overcome that resistance. Change is brought about effectively in systems or organizations when the need for a change is recognized and accepted by those affected by the change: the employees. The first steps of the change process (assessment and analysis) help the manager raise the employees' awareness of a need for change. This initial step starts the process of overcoming resistance.

Once employees have begun to recognize and accept the need for change, the nurse manager seeks in-put from them about how to implement the change. By facilitating employee involvement in the process, the nurse manager allows resistance to be addressed directly. People involved in the change process are more likely to become invested in the new process and accept the change when their concerns are heard and addressed as part of the planned change. Instituting changes in a stepwise manner also makes the process less threatening and therefore more acceptable. Finally, changes are most likely to be accepted and incorporated into new behaviors when evaluation shows the new plan to be effective.

The nurse manager is responsible for implementing the change, but the change itself requires the cooperation of everyone involved; it also requires the understanding that change is continuous. To help accomplish changes peacefully, the nurse manager needs leadership skills, communication skills, and education to influence acceptance of the change. Trusting relationships that result from a democratic, assertive leadership style and a consensus-building outlook form the basis for effective change (Spitzer-Lehman, 1994).

Managing Risk

Risk management is the process of identifying, evaluating, and reducing or financing the cost of predictable losses. These losses include losses from litigation (lawsuits). Although risk management can be performed at the individual level to prevent personal lawsuits, the nurse manager implements risk management strategies at the institutional level.

The nurse manager must be keenly aware of competing professional, legal, and ethical claims. Nurse managers must evaluate all new programs, policies, and procedures in terms of their potential for doing good or causing harm or both.

Malpractice and Negligence

The major legal issues faced by bedside nurses involve avoiding malpractice or negligence claims. Nurse managers are responsible for overseeing the legal practices of the health care providers they manage. They also must consider the legal implications of client care decisions and management practices when delegating care to other providers. Box 17–6 lists steps taken by nurse managers to minimize legal risk. The best protection comes from following professional standards of safe care when instituting policies and procedures used to guide nursing practice. Managing the legal risks in client care is closely tied to quality management activities.

Both technical and interpersonal aspects of quality health care have been at issue when clients have sued institutions or individual health care practitioners (Spitzer-Lehman, 1994). Therefore, the nurse manager is responsible for creating an environment in which clients perceive both technical competence and an ethic of caring. Nurse managers have to assume a pro-

---

BOX 17–6

RISK MANAGEMENT/QUALITY ASSURANCE STRATEGIES

- Determine quality indicators essential to client care in this institution.
- Determine methods for measuring those indicators.
- Implement measurement strategies (measuring indicators and mapping trends).
- Assess and analyze variations from expected norms.
- Plan and implement strategies for improving performance.
- Gather data related to occurrences (indicators of potential problems, such as medication errors or employee injuries), and follow procedures to assess, analyze, plan, and implement strategies to alter the causes of the unusual occurrences.

active stance in monitoring, evaluating, and correcting the services rendered by other health care providers. Nurse managers must ensure that providers have the tools (education, supplies, policies, and procedures) that enable them to provide the best possible care, technically and emotionally.

Discrimination and Safety

In their agency advocacy role, nurse managers also must act to avoid litigation brought by employees. Indeed, they are obligated to abide by federal, state, and local laws governing health care. The Equal Employment Opportunity Act, Americans with Disabilities Act, and Family Leave Act all provide guidelines that help to ensure fair and impartial treatment to all employees.

Most institutions have human resource departments that help nurse managers resolve issues related to gender, race, age, or disability discrimination. Nurse managers who are proactive about maintaining quality health care—who use assertive communication styles to manage employees—will be more effective in avoiding legal problems related to infringement of an employee's rights.

Nurse managers must know and abide by Occupational Safety and Health Act (OSHA) regulations regarding maintenance of a safe work environment. That includes implementing policies about infection control, the use of chemical and biological agents, and the use of special equipment.

Licensure and Certification

It is often easy to think of potential good and harm only in terms of the effect on clients. However, nurse managers must promote good and avoid harm for the

institution as well when implementing policies and procedures. Loss of revenue is only one type of harm that could befall the institution. Other issues can reduce the longevity of any health care agency as well. For example, governmental rules and regulations must be followed to maintain licensure or certification.

Nurse managers are obligated to know and abide by regulations imposed by those who pay for health care, such as the Health Care Financing Agency (HCFA) of the federal government. HCFA regulates Medicare and Medicaid as well as payment for services provided under those programs. Each insurance program, health maintenance organization, preferred provider service, and so on, also imposes rules regarding allowed services and the means by which they are provided.

Agencies such as the Joint Commission for Accreditation of Health Care Organizations (JCAHO) also impose stringent guidelines regarding the provision of client care services. Nurse managers must know all of these regulations and the influence they have on practice in each environment. Any health care agency found to be out of compliance with these regulations could lose the license or certification that is required to do business.

Therefore, nurse managers utilize leadership strategies to help other health care providers understand the rules and regulations and incorporate strategies to promote compliance. In an overall sense, they must use their knowledge of professional standards, legal implications of nursing practice and management, and ethical models to balance their obligation to act as client advocates with their obligation to promote the health care agency.

MANAGERS IN COLLABORATIVE HEALTH CARE TEAMS

Regardless of the type of health care facility involved, nurses are expected to participate in collaborative (multidisciplinary or interdisciplinary) health care teams as managers and as leaders. Client care is no longer the domain of one or two health care disciplines. Today, more people are living with chronic health conditions than ever before. And they require more assistance than that provided by physicians and nurses.

For example, someone surviving a stroke may go to a rehabilitation facility where he receives care from nurses, physical therapists, occupational therapists, speech therapists, social workers, pastoral care practitioners, discharge planners, case managers, and even dietitians. Ancillary staff might include personal care providers, home health aides, and laboratory and radiology technicians. Each provider has a plan of care for the client. To achieve the desired overall outcome, all of the care plans must be implemented in a coordinated fashion.

Collaborative health care teams have evolved as the means to ensure coordination of services and suc-

BOX 17–7

MULTIDISCIPLINARY HEALTH CARE TEAMS

Goal—To facilitate client's achievement of therapeutic goals, to improve client services, and to avoid overlap of client care services.

Membership—Those participating in the care of a single client or a group of clients being served by an institution or by a unit within an institution.

Purpose—Planning client care. Each discipline shares data of their care plan: client's progress toward therapeutic goals, response to individualized interventions. The entire team evaluates progress and plans future interventions.

Roles—Team members have a clear knowledge of their professional roles and the standards that guide their practice, which they share with the other team members in planning client care.

Nursing role—Nurses share nursing processes, nursing theories, and nursing research that influence their choice of interventions. They offer input regarding the standards and regulations that affect their practice in each unique client care setting.

Essential Components for a Successful Team Effort

- Shared goals.
- Shared commitment to client care.
- Shared accountability for client outcomes.
- Open communication about interventions (care plans).

Common Members of a Multidisciplinary Team

- Nurse.
- Physical therapist.
- Occupational therapist.
- Speech therapist.
- Social worker.
- Pastoral care provider.
- Dietitian.
- Physician.
- Client.
- Client's family.

cessful outcomes for clients. Box 17–7 lists the essentials of a multidisciplinary health care team. Each discipline is responsible and accountable for the outcomes of its specific interventions. No one discipline has the power or right to negatively influence work being done with a client by another. Therefore, it is extremely important that all providers work together to avoid overlapping services. They need a shared goal to produce the best client outcome efficiently and effectively.

In keeping with management theories, such as theory Y and theory Z, health care organizations have adopted collaborative team models that promote and protect professional autonomy for each discipline (Aroian, Meservey, & Crockett, 1996). In these models, all disciplines meet and confer about client care. Each member has an equal part but a different role in the client's care. No member of a team is more important than another, although, depending on the client's problem, one team member may be more involved at a given time. In the stroke example, the physical therapist may play a larger role in helping a client who has lost the function of a limb. The speech therapist might be more involved with a client who has impaired swallowing.

Members of collaborative health care teams share their expertise with other group members to plan, implement, and evaluate care strategies. Clients are involved as equal participants in the process. Nurses share their care plans and their observations about client's holistic human response to all interventions. As

experts in alleviating factors that affect the human response to health threats, nurses provide data about human responses and the means to ease the factors that cause those responses. In the stroke example, nurses on the team would observe the client's overall response to therapies. The client's primary nurse might make recommendations to therapists about personal factors that affect the client's motivation to participate in therapies.

Nurse managers, who might function as facilitators for collaborative health care teams, can maximize the benefits of teamwork through activities based on group-process theories. Clear communication of objectives is the cornerstone for enhancing the group process. Each member must understand his or her special role in the process and be able to communicate it to the other team members. Each member should share a commitment to quality care, and each should accept the views and roles of other team members. Groups that work together, showing respect and appreciation for the ideas of all members, can be extremely effective in achieving goals.

Nurses have the opportunity to function as health care leaders in collaborative teams. Nurse managers, in the facilitator role, can provide education and guidance. They can model the behaviors that enhance communication and group cohesiveness. And they can evaluate the performance of nurses on these teams and coach them in improving communication and group participation. Nurse managers may also provide expert views on reimbursement, legal issues, professional standards, and organizational issues that affect team activities. Nurse managers make use of all of the elements of management—quality, budgets, people, change, and risk—as tools to facilitate nurse participation and leadership in collaborative teams and all areas of practice.

KEY PRINCIPLES

- Nurse managers derive their style of management from the health care institution's policies about employee motivation. Many administrators now believe that employees work best when they share in the institution's goals. Assertive management styles are considered to be more effective in motivating others.
- Successful nurse managers have the characteristics of responsibility, accountability, leadership, and commitment to quality.
- Nurse managers have an important role in the delivery of client care regardless of the health care setting. Their roles and responsibilities are defined according to the mission, goals, and objectives of the health care institution.
- The nurse manager, in keeping with institutional goals and objectives, ensures quality client care by implementing policies and procedures that create specified health care outcomes. Nurse managers have a role in initiating policies and procedures and in measuring outcomes.
- Nurse managers are also responsible for maintaining efficient delivery of health care. They must understand and apply budgeting principles to justify expenses that influence profitability.
- Accomplishing multiple complex functions in a participatory management environment requires a leadership style that empowers others and encourages their participation.
- Communication is the key to an assertive, democratic leadership style.
- Change theories direct nurse managers through processes in which they recognize the need for change, plan for change, implement strategies for change, and motivate employees to embrace change.
- Nurse managers know and use ethical and legal models as they implement nursing care within the limitations of professional practice standards.
- In collaborative health care teams, client care is never exclusively the domain of any single health care discipline.

BIBLIOGRAPHY

Aroian, J., Meservey, P.M., & Crockett, J.G. (1996). Developing nurse leaders for today and tomorrow. *Journal of Nursing Administration, 26*(9), 18–26.
Blancett, S.S., & Flarey, D.L. (1995). *Reengineering nursing and health care: The handbook for organizational transformation.* Gaithersburg, MD: Aspen Publishers.
*Brimelow, S. (1998). Research strategy. *Nursing Management, 4*(10), 21.
Canavan, K. (1997). Proving nursing's value. *American Journal of Nursing, 97*(7), 57–58.
Donabedian, A. (1995). In N.O. Graham (Ed.), *Quality in health care: Theory, application, and evolution.* Gaithersburg, MD: Aspen Publishers.
Dunham-Taylor, J. (1995). Identifying the best in nurse executive leadership. *Journal of Nursing Administration, 25*(7/8), 24–31.
*Feldstein, P.J. (1993). *Health care economics* (4th. ed.). Irvine, CA: Delmar Publishers.
Flarey, D.L. (1995). *Redesigning nursing care: Transforming our future.* Philadelphia: Lippincott-Raven.
Fowler, J. (1996). The organization of clinical supervision within the nursing profession: A review of the literature. *Journal of Advanced Nursing, 23*(3), 471–478.
*Frommer, A.G. (1996). Benchmarking, monitoring and moving through the continuum of the clinical pathway system. *Best Practice Benchmarking Healthcare, 1*(3), 157–160.
Grohar-Murray, M.E., & DiCroce, H.R. (1997). *Leadership and management in nursing.* Stamford, CT: Appleton & Lange.
*Hankins, R., Brady T., & Saucier B. (1998). Finance and accounting for nurses. Part 4. *Nursing Management, 5*(1), 22–25.
Huber, D. (1996). *Leadership and nursing care management.* Philadelphia: W.B. Saunders Co.
Katz, J.M., & Green, E. (1997). *Managing quality: A guide to system-wide performance management in health care* (2nd ed.). St. Louis: Mosby.
*Malby, B., & Manning, S. (1998). Promoting change through peer review. *Nursing Management, 5*(2), 24–25.
Marquis, B.L., & Huston, C.J. (1996). *Leadership roles and management functions in nursing: Theory and application* (2nd ed.). Philadelphia: Lippincott-Raven.
McMican, A. (1998). The quality measurement matrix: An elegant planning and educational tool. *Journal of Nursing Care Quality, 12*(4), 1–3.
Neubauer, J. (1995). The learning network: Leadership development for the next millennium. *Journal of Nursing Administration, 25*(2), 23–32.
*Ouchi, W.G. (1981). *Theory Z: How American business can meet the Japanese challenge.* Menlo Park, CA: Addison-Wesley Publishing Co.
Porter, N. (1998). Providing effective clinical supervision. *Nursing Management, 5*(2), 22–23.
Pugh, J.B., & Woodward-Smith, M. (1997). *Nurse manager: A practical guide to better employee relations* (2nd ed.). Philadelphia: W.B. Saunders Co.
*Rinomhota, A.S. (1998). Staff attitudes to clinical placements. *Nursing Management, 5*(2), 12–13.
*Spitzer-Lehman, R. (1994). *Nursing management desk reference: Concepts, skills, and strategies.* Philadelphia: W.B. Saunders Co.
Westrope, R.A., Vaughn, L., Bott, M., & Taunton, R.L. (1995). Shared governance: From vision to reality. *Journal of Nursing Administration, 25*(12), 45–54.

* Asterisk indicates a classic or definitive work on this subject.

Nursing Research

Kathryn A. Lauchner

Key Terms

abstract
data
data collection
dependent variable
experimental research
hypothesis
independent variable
informed consent
institutional review board
instruments

nonexperimental research
operational definition
qualitative research
quantitative research
quasiexperimental research
research design
research problem
sampling
theoretical framework

LEARNING OBJECTIVES

After studying this chapter, you should be able to:

1. Describe the importance of nursing research.
2. Identify the influence of ethical dilemmas in nursing research and the mechanisms for the protection of human subjects.
3. Describe the personnel involved in research studies, types of studies, and the parts of a typical research study.
4. Discuss the steps of the research process.
5. Identify ways of implementing nursing research findings in your nursing practice.

Imagine that you are in the library, and you take a break from studying your fundamentals text. In the study carrel you find a nursing research journal and, as you flip through the journal, you come upon the following text:

"The purpose of this study was to determine the accuracy and reliability of three types of thermometers: IVAC (IVAC Corp., San Diego, CA), TempraDOT (PyMaH Corp., Somerville, NJ), and an off-the-shelf mercury thermometer used to take oral temperatures. Roy's Adaptation Model provided the theoretical basis for the study. The convenience sample consisted of 35 adults who volunteered for the study. Information was collected by two registered nurses following the manufacturers' recommendations required for an accurate reading. Results indicated no differences in the validity and reliability of the three types of thermometers."

Just then, your instructor stops by your carrel and says, "I see you're reading the study about thermometers." She asks you the following questions:

- Do you think a sample of 35 adults is large enough that you could use this research with adult clients?
- If you were working in pediatrics, could you use this study to guide your practice with children?
- Do other factors besides the recommendations made by the manufacturer affect the accuracy of temperature measurement?
- How do you know which of the temperature readings is the correct one if the readings varied from one thermometer to another?
- If you were going to take rectal or axillary temperatures, would an IVAC and a mercury thermometer be equally accurate?

How would you answer?

Welcome to the world of nursing research. It shapes your daily practice in ways you never imagined. Indeed, it forms the basis for most of the nursing knowledge you will use in your nursing career and for many of the facts and concepts presented in your nursing courses.

Research has the potential to improve nursing practice. However, before you can begin to incorporate research successfully into your practice, you must be able to evaluate research. Questions such as those asked above and many others need to be answered before you can accept any research study as a valid basis to change your practice. The purpose of this chapter is to help you ask the right questions and evaluate the answers before you use nursing research in your practice.

IMPORTANCE OF NURSING RESEARCH

Nursing research is the method used to develop or search for knowledge about issues important to nurses and nursing practice today and into the future. More than ever before, nurses are being asked to determine and document their role in the delivery of health care. To define that role, nurses need a distinct body of

knowledge that separates nursing from other health professions. Nurses must be able to articulate what they do and how their actions improve the health of their clients.

Additionally, research can provide a guide when making the many decisions inherent in nursing practice. Research can help you answer such important questions as: What should I assess? Which clients can reach certain goals? Which interventions produce the best client outcomes? When should evaluation take place? Nursing research also has the potential to identify the importance of the caring component of health care delivery in achieving the outcome of a healthier society.

Historical Perspective

The first acknowledged nurse researcher was Florence Nightingale, who systematically demonstrated the importance of nursing in reducing the morbidity of wounded soldiers in the Crimean war (Rogers, 1989). When she arrived at the British military hospital at Scutari in November 1854, Nightingale found a hospital that was designed for 1,700 clients but filled with nearly 4,000 people (Fig. 18–1).

The hospital had no furniture, eating utensils, or blankets, but it did have lice, maggots, rats, and other vermin. Men lay naked on the floor in their own excrement, and filth covered the walls. It was later determined that 75% of all the casualties suffered by the British army resulted from diseases contracted in the hospital, such as dysentery, typhoid, and cholera (Kalisch & Kalisch, 1978).

Nightingale implemented reforms and collected information on the factors that influenced soldier morbidity and mortality. She considered the effects of cleanliness, ventilation, nutrition, temperature, and humidity. When she arrived, the mortality rate at the hospital was 60 percent. When she left, the mortality rate was just over 1 percent. Her interventions reduced the total mortality rate from 42 percent in February 1885 to 2 percent in June of the same year (Hebert, 1981).

Nightingale presented her findings in tables, charts, and graphs that were quite sophisticated by 1850s standards (Rogers, 1989). To influence Parliament and the British army, she wrote a study entitled *Notes on Matters Affecting the Health, Efficiency and Hospital Administration of the British Army*, which was later published as *Notes on Hospitals* (1859). As a result of Nightingale's research, the views of the British army changed.

From the time of Nightingale until the 1950s, few nurses conducted nursing research. That was largely because the nursing education did not include information about research and research techniques. In the 1920s, *The American Journal of Nursing* began publishing case studies, which were the earliest form of published nursing research. Case studies involved the analysis of one or more clients to increase nursing knowledge of clients with similar conditions.

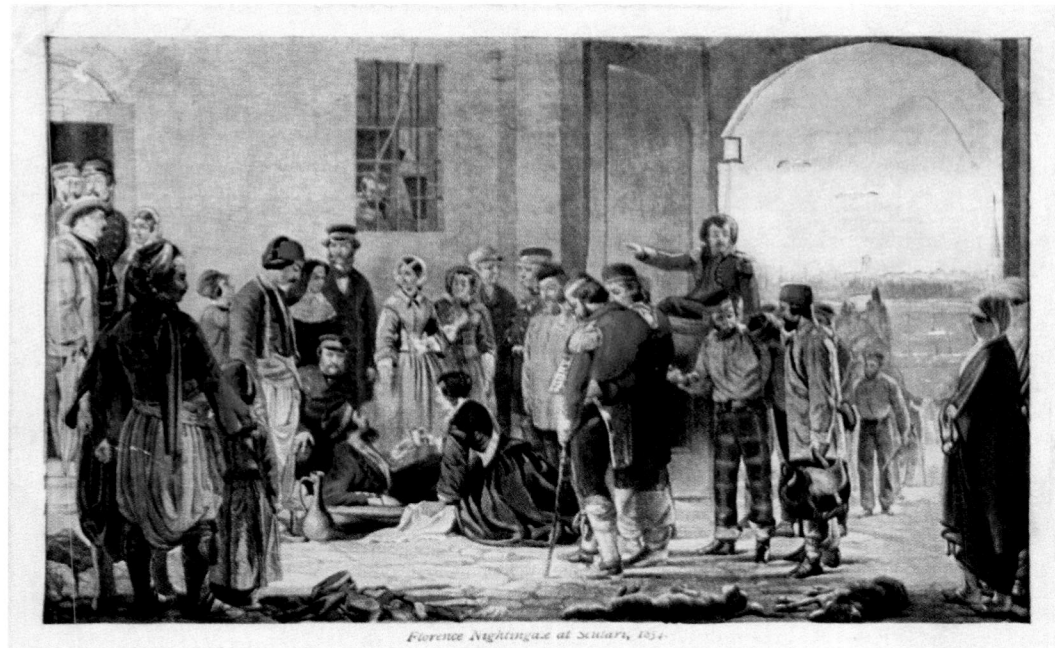

Figure 18–1. Florence Nightingale at Scutari Hospital. (Reprinted by permission of Zwerdling Nursing Archives.)

In 1923, the Goldmark Report advanced nursing as a scientific discipline by recommending that more schools of nursing be established in university settings. The baccalaureate degree in nursing provided for the development of graduate nursing education. The first Master of Nursing degree was offered by Yale University in 1929. Teachers College at Columbia offered the first doctoral program for nurses in 1924, with a degree in education to prepare doctoral nurse educators. The Association of Collegiate Schools of Nursing was organized in 1932 and encouraged nurses to conduct research to improve education and practice. In 1952, this organization sponsored the publication of the first research journal, entitled *Nursing Research.*

During the 1950s, nursing research focused on nursing education, primarily because nurses with the knowledge to conduct nursing research were nurse educators. With the beginning of clinical specialty groups, such as medical-surgical, psychiatric, pediatric, and obstetric, nursing research began addressing specific client care issues. The combination of all of these factors promoted nursing research.

In 1965, the American Nurses' Association (ANA) sponsored the first in a series of research conferences. These conferences stimulated an increasing number of clinical studies to focus on the quality of client care and nursing interventions. These conferences continue today, along with many others at which nursing research is presented.

The 1970s were marked by a growth in nursing research. The number of nurses with master's degrees in practitioner and clinical nurse specialist programs increased rapidly, along with the number working at the doctoral level. These nurses had the knowledge to conduct research and to use research in nursing practice.

In 1972, the ANA Commission on Nursing Research established the Council of Nurse Researchers to advance research activities, provide an exchange of ideas, and recognize excellence in research. The commission also prepared position papers on subjects' rights in research and guidelines concerning research and human subjects.

The conduct of clinical nursing research was the primary focus of the 1980s. In 1980, the American Nurses' Association Commission on Nursing Research identified priorities that helped focus research on clinical nursing practice. In 1985, the same group, known as the ANA Cabinet on Nursing Research, expanded the priorities for nursing research. Currently, the ANA Council on Nursing Research has established the priorities presented in Box 18–1.

The number of clinical journals publishing nursing research and the body of nursing knowledge generated through research have increased rapidly. In 1985, the National Center for Nursing Research (NCNR) was created under the National Institutes of Health. The purpose of the NCNR was "the conduct, support, and dissemination of information regarding basic clinical nursing research, training, and other programs in patient care research" (Bauknecht, 1985, p. 2).

During the early 1990s, the NCNR brought together prominent nurse scientists for two Conferences on Research Priorities (CORP). CORP priorities are listed in Box 18–2. In 1993, the NCNR became the National Institute of Nursing Research (NINR). The change in title increased the recognition of nursing as a research-based health profession.

BOX 18–1

ANA NURSING RESEARCH PRIORITIES

Generation of knowledge enabling nurses to do the following:

- Develop and test nursing and multidisciplinary models for care delivery that are clinically effective, cost-effective, and accessible.
- Develop culturally sensitive instruments to measure client/family variables and outcomes sensitive to nursing interventions across all settings of care delivery.
- Evaluate approaches to nursing education for general as well as specialty practice.
- Identify and test strategies that foster healthy behaviors and self-care among all age, social, and cultural groups.
- Identify and test interventions to minimize or prevent environmentally induced health problems.
- Evaluate the effects of health technologies in acute and chronic illness.
- Develop and test primary nursing strategies for health promotion and disease prevention in children and adolescents, especially related to infectious and sexually transmitted diseases, trauma, and lifestyle-related disease risks.

- Test models of nursing management for major health problems in vulnerable populations; particularly, frail older adults, women and children living with violence, inner city urban and rural groups, and under-represented (by reason of race, culture, socioeconomic status, geographic location, and mental or physical status) societal groups.
- Develop databases of health care use and critical health status indicators in vulnerable populations.
- Investigate health care decision-making of providers and clients, and test collaborative decision-making models for their effect on improved client/family outcomes.
- Analyze home health care services and data on elders at home and in long-term care facilities.
- Evaluate outcomes of care delivered to elders at home and in long-term care facilities.
- Test models of care that are affordable without compromising adequate quality.
- Identify quality indicators that reflect appropriate nursing skill and staff mix.

Reprinted with permission from American Nurses' Association Council on Nursing Research. (1997). Directions for nursing research: Toward the twenty-first century. Copyright 1997 by American Nurses Publishing, American Nurses Foundation/American Nurses' Association, 600 Maryland Ave., SW, Suite 100W, Washington, D.C. 20024-2571. To order, call 800/637-0323.

BOX 18–2

RESEARCH PRIORITIES FROM THE NATIONAL CENTER FOR NURSING RESEARCH FROM 1995 THROUGH 1999

- Developing and testing community-based nursing models.
- Assessing the effectiveness of nursing interventions in HIV and AIDS.
- Developing and testing approaches to remediating cognitive impairment.
- Testing interventions for coping with chronic illness.
- Identifying biobehavioral factors and testing interventions to promote immunocompetence.

From National Center for Nursing Research. (1993). Research priorities from the National Center for Nursing Research. Bethesda, MD: Author.

Today, nursing research is focusing on health promotion and illness prevention as well as traditional health restoration. The number of clinical nursing studies continues to increase. Nurses are developing an increasingly strong scientific base of knowledge for nursing practice.

Contributions to Society

Nursing research has improved the quality of life for many people. Through nursing research, new knowledge has been developed to improve nursing care for clients of all ages and cultures. Neonatal research has provided nurses with new methods for stimulating respiration in low-birth-weight infants. It has yielded new knowledge about the effects of parental touch and environmental lighting for preterm infants. Children and adolescents have benefited from studies about the psychosocial stress of being hospitalized or isolated because of a chronic illness. Adults have benefited from studies about spousal and elder abuse and about adaptation to pain.

Nursing research has addressed the topics of concern to our clients. A body of nursing research knowledge exists to improve the physical and psychosocial well-being of clients with many types of illnesses or conditions. Many client teaching pamphlets and videos are based on the findings from nursing research studies.

Advancement of Nursing Profession

In addition to contributing to society, nursing research also advances the profession of nursing by expanding the body of nursing knowledge. Nurse researchers develop and share knowledge with other nurses seeking answers to the same questions. Extension of the knowledge base is essential for the continued growth of the profession and for the improvement of nursing care. Through nursing research, nurses learn new ways to solve old problems and address current professional issues. Without nursing research, nurses would not have valid and reliable information to serve as the basis for nursing decisions.

Nursing research contributes to the profession by expanding the scientific basis for nursing. Through research, nurses have discovered personal characteristics related to compliance with therapeutic regimens, identified groups at risk for specific health problems, designed effective nursing interventions for particular types of clients, and demonstrated how cultural beliefs influence health care. Solutions to clinical problems are commonly found in nursing research.

Finally, nursing research contributes to the profession by developing theories of nursing practice. Although the accumulation of facts is important, the organization of facts into theories increases our understanding of these facts. Nursing theory is the way the nurse theorist views the world of nursing and its influence on client care.

ETHICS OF NURSING RESEARCH

Ethical standards are especially important in nursing research because studies of human health patterns involve the use of human subjects whose rights must be protected. Many of these subjects are especially vulnerable. For example, if psychiatric clients are the subject of a study on medication compliance, the researcher is ethically obliged to question the ability of these clients to fully consent to the study. Infants, children, clients in pain, terminally ill clients, and very old clients are other especially vulnerable populations. The Tuskegee syphilis study illustrates the importance of maintaining ethical standards in research.

The Tuskegee study was conducted between 1938 and 1972 and was supported by the U.S. Public Health Service. It involved 400 poor African-American men from Tuskegee, Alabama, who had contracted syphilis. Their medical treatment was withheld so researchers could study the course of the disease. The subjects were examined periodically but did not receive treatment, even after penicillin was found to be effective. Many of the subjects who consented to participate in the study were not informed about the purpose and procedures of the study. Some were unaware that they were subjects at all (Vessey & Gennaro, 1994). No effort was made to stop the study, even though findings from the study were published every 4 to 6 years. As late as 1969, the Centers for Disease Control decided that the study should continue.

Too often, researchers' desires for knowledge or advancement have led to injury, increased illness, and even death among research subjects. Consequently, researchers now must adhere to strict guidelines intended to protect those who take part in studies.

Codes of Ethics

To protect research subjects from ethical violations, many disciplines have established their own codes of ethics. A code of ethics serves to guide researchers in protecting the rights of human subjects. In 1975, the ANA published *Human Rights Guidelines for Nurses in Clinical and Other Research* (Box 18–3). Likewise, the American Sociological Association (1984) and the American Psychological Association (1982) published codes of ethics for sociological and psychological research. Although the principles of ethical human research are common across disciplines, these three documents each address the particular concerns of their disciplines.

In addition, the National Commission for the Protection of Human Subjects of Biomedical and Behavioral Research (1978) issued a code of ethics that formed the basis of regulations for research sponsored by the federal government. Known as the *Belmont Report,* this document has served as the model for codes of ethics for many disciplines.

Risk/Benefit Ratio

Conducting ethical research involving human subjects requires analyzing the risk/benefit ratio. This ratio measures whether the risks to research subjects outweigh the possible benefits to society and the nursing profession. The risk to subjects should never exceed the value to society. For nurse researchers, this principle can be interpreted to mean that the topic of the research should be significant and have the potential to improve client care. If the research topic does not have the potential to improve client care, the research should not be conducted.

All research involves risks to the subjects. In most cases the risks are minimal, but researchers should always try to reduce even minimal risks. The most common types of risks to subjects include the following:

- Psychological factors, such as fatigue, anxiety caused by self-disclosure, anger at the type of questions being asked, or the loss of privacy.
- Physical factors, such as physical harm, discomfort, or adverse effects.
- Sociological factors, including the loss of time and financial costs for extra laboratory tests or transportation.

BOX 18–3

ANA HUMAN RIGHTS GUIDELINES FOR NURSES IN CLINICAL AND OTHER RESEARCH

Guideline 1: Employment in Settings Where Research Is Conducted

Conditions of employment in settings where research is conducted need to be spelled out in detail for all potential workers . . . Anyone employed in work that carries the potential of risk to others needs to be advised as to the types of risks involved, the ways of recognizing when risk is present, and the proper actions to take to counteract harmful effects and unnecessary harm.

Guideline 2: Nurses' Responsibilities for Vigilant Protection of Human Subjects' Rights

In all instances, the prospective subject must be given all relevant information prior to participation in activities that go beyond established and accepted procedures necessary to meet the subject's personal needs . . . . Nurses must be increasingly vigilant in their concern for subjects and clients who by reason of their situation and/or illness are not able to protect themselves effectively for externally imposed threat or injury. They must be sensitive to the tendency toward exploitation of "captive" populations such as students, clients, and inmates in institutions and prisons. All proposals to be used need to be discussed with the prospective subject and with any worker who is expected to participate as a subject or data collector or both. Special mechanisms must be developed to safeguard the confidentiality of information and protect human dignity.

Guideline 3: Scope of Application

The persons to whom these human rights guidelines apply include all individuals involved in research activities and include the following groups: clients, donors of organs and tissue, informants, normal volunteers including students, and vulnerable populations that are "captive" audiences, such as the mentally disordered, mentally retarded, and prisoners.

Guideline 4: Nurses' Responsibility to Support the Accrual of Knowledge

Just as nurses have an obligation to protect the human rights of clients, so do they also have an obligation to support the accrual of knowledge that broadens the scientific underpinning of nursing practice and the delivery of nursing services.

Guideline 5: Informed Consent

To safeguard the basic rights of self-determination, nurses must obtain consent from the prospective subject or the subject's legal representative to participate in research of unusual clinical activities. The subject needs to receive:

- A description of any benefit to the subject or the development of new knowledge that might be expected
- An offer to discuss or answer any questions about the study
- A clear statement so that the subject is free to discontinue participation at any time the subject wishes
- Full freedom from direct or indirect coercion and deception

Guideline 6: Representation on Human Subjects Committee

There is increasing public support for systematic accountability to ensure that individual rights are not denied to human subjects who participate in research studies. In most instances, the protective mechanism takes place through a committee judged competent to review studies and other investigative activities that involve human subjects. The profession of nursing has an obligation to publicly support the inclusion of nurses as regular members of institutional review committees of this kind.

Adapted and summarized from American Nurses' Association. (1975). Human rights guidelines for nurses in clinical and other research. Copyright 1975 by American Nurses Publishing, American Nurses Foundation/American Nurses' Association, 600 Maryland Ave., SW, Suite 100W, Washington, D.C. 20024-2571. To order, call 800/637-0323, publication code D-46 5M 7/75.

In addition to the benefits to society and the nursing profession, the subjects themselves may benefit from participation in the study. These benefits may include increased knowledge about themselves, knowledge that they may be helping others, enhanced self-esteem, access to an intervention that may be available only through research, comfort in being able to discuss their concerns with a nonjudgmental researcher, and direct monetary or material gains. Some researchers give study participants a small honorarium or other token rewards for their time.

Review Boards

Most hospitals, universities, and other institutions where research is frequently conducted have formed review boards to protect the rights of subjects. These review boards are formal committees with protocols for reviewing research proposals and plans. Review boards are sometimes called *human subjects committees*.

Research supported by federal funds is subject to strict guidelines concerning the use of human or animal subjects. An **institutional review board** (IRB) is a committee whose duties include making sure that proposed research meets the federal requirements for ethical research. The committee is mandated by the federal government if the institution is receiving federal funds for research.

Before beginning the research, the researcher must submit a proposal about the research to the IRB. In addition to verifying the ethical treatment of humans, the IRB will monitor research progress to ensure adherence to the approved procedures. Federal requirements stipulate that an IRB must consist of five or more members, one of whom is not affiliated with the institution personally or through family, and one of whom is not a researcher. The IRB members cannot be all male or all female, and the members may not all belong to the same profession (Code of Federal Regulations, 1983).

Because not all research receives federal support or is conducted in institutions with review boards, some studies may not undergo formal review. Regardless of the lack of a formal review process, all researchers have the responsibility to ensure that their research plans adhere to ethical guidelines. Many solicit an external review even when not required to do so.

When publishing research, most authors acknowledge that the study was reviewed by an IRB or human subjects committee. When the author identifies a formal review by a committee, you can assume that the study was reviewed for ethical considerations.

Informed Consent

Informed consent means that the subjects have been given sufficient information about the research to enable them to consent voluntarily to participate or decline to participate. Subjects must have the ability to comprehend the information they are given about the study. They also have the right to know the following (Polit & Hungler, 1995):

- The purpose of the study
- The type of information to be collected
- The use of that information in a scientific study
- The amount of time or money that will be required of the subject
- The procedure for collecting information
- The way in which subjects are selected
- The potential physical or emotional harm or discomforts that may be associated with the study
- The potential alternative treatments available, if relevant
- The potential benefits to the subject, including monetary or other token rewards
- The potential benefits to others
- The names of the researchers, institutional affiliations, whom to contact, and the method of contact for additional information or complaints
- A description of the voluntary participation in the study and the right to withdraw at any time without reason or penalty
- A description of how confidentiality will be maintained throughout the study

Most researchers will provide subjects with a written consent form, which the researcher will ask the subject to sign before joining the study. This document is kept by the researcher, and a copy is retained by the subject. A sample research consent form is shown in Figure 18–2.

The above procedure protects the rights of most subjects, but sometimes researchers are interested in studying special vulnerable groups of subjects who may be incapable of giving fully informed consent. Vulnerable groups typically include infants; children; mentally, emotionally, or physically disabled individuals; pregnant women; the terminally ill; and institutionalized or hospitalized clients. With these vulnerable subjects, the researcher may be required to undertake additional procedures and be especially sensitive about protecting subjects' rights. The researcher should make sure that risks are minimal and possible benefits are pronounced.

Ethical Dilemmas in Nursing Research

Nurse researchers rarely decide purposely to violate the ethical principles of research. However, enthusiasm for conducting research may pose ethical dilemmas for the nurse researcher who comes to believe that the knowledge gained from research is more important and beneficial than the rights of subjects or ethical principles. Following are some examples of research questions and associated ethical dilemmas.

Research question: Do maternity clients discharged 24 hours after childbirth experience fewer complications when visited by a home health nurse? *Ethical dilemma:* If some clients will be visited by a home health nurse, then other clients will not be visited. If one group is receiving treatment, and the other group is not receiving treatment, are there potentially hazardous consequences to the group not receiving treatment? If the answer to this question is yes, the researcher is endangering the group not receiving treatment. How can this problem be resolved?

Research question: How do clients cope with the new diagnosis of an impending terminal illness? *Ethical dilemma:* Clients diagnosed with a terminal illness are very vulnerable. To answer this question, the researcher may need to ask intrusive questions. By asking these questions, the researcher may cause psychological trauma and increase the client's anxiety level. However, the results of this study may give nurses valuable insight into the coping mechanisms used by newly diagnosed terminally ill patients. Is this study fair to the subjects?

As these examples illustrate, nurse researchers frequently encounter ethical dilemmas. Ethical codes and IRBs help to guide researchers in resolving these dilemmas and protecting the rights of subjects.

THE RESEARCH STUDY

The research project itself is usually called a study or an investigation. The tools that the researcher uses to conduct a study are called **instruments.** Instruments can be thermometers, laboratory tests, a list of ques-

---

CONSENT TO PARTICIPATE IN A RESEARCH STUDY

In signing this consent form, I understand that I will be part of a research study that will focus on the effects of exercise on weight loss. I understand that I am agreeing to participate in the study for a total of six weeks, during which I will be asked to consume only prepackaged meals and snacks totaling 2000 calories per day. The foods and snacks will be provided for me free of charge, and I will be able to select the foods from a list that will be provided. I understand that I will keep a record of all foods and fluids consumed by me and will present this record weekly. I also understand that I will need to be present at the Tomlinson Health Sciences Center each Monday morning during the length of the study between 6:00 a.m. and 6:30 a.m., where I will be weighed without clothes, after emptying my bladder, and before I have consumed any food or liquids. I understand that I may or may not be asked to walk continuously for 30 minutes on Mondays, Wednesdays, and Fridays.

I have been informed that participation in the study is entirely voluntary, and that even after the study begins I can terminate my participation at any time. I have been told that my weight and records will not be given to anyone else and that no reports of this study will ever identify me in any way.

This study will help to develop a better understanding of the relationship between weight loss and exercise. I understand that the results of this research will be given to me if I ask for them and that Dr. Kathy Lauchner is the person to contact if I have any questions about the study or about my rights as a study participant. Dr. Lauchner can be reached by collect call at 1-800-555-1212.

Date: _____ Participant's Signature _____

Researcher's Signature _____

Figure 18–2. A sample research consent form.

---

tions, or a checklist. The term **data** is used to designate the information the researcher is interested in collecting. Data may take the form of words, or they may have numeric value.

The people being studied are called subjects, study participants, or informants. Subjects are enlisted from *populations*, the groups of individuals that the researcher is studying. For example, if a researcher wants to understand the reasons abused wives stay in relationship with their abusers, a sample of abused wives will be asked to participate in the study. If the sample truly represents the population of abused wives, the researcher can derive conclusions about the whole population from the sample.

Personnel

The person who undertakes a research project is usually called a researcher but is sometimes called an *investigator*. When a team of people undertakes a research project, the person directing the study is called the *principal investigator* or *project director*.

Types of Studies

The type of research depends on the questions asked by the researcher and the topic under study. Some research questions may be asked in different ways, which influences the type of research. Not all types of

TABLE 18–1
Types of Research

Types of Design	Characteristics
Correlational	Examines the relationship between two or more variables to see if, when one variable changes, the other variable also changes without any active intervention.
Descriptive	Accurately identifies and describes the characteristics of individuals, situations, or groups.
Case study	Involves the detailed investigation of an individual, group, or institution to understand which variables are important to the subjects' history, care, or development.
Historical	Examines events that have occurred in the past through systematic collection of data and critical evaluation.
Needs assessment	Involves the collection of data to estimate the needs of a community or an organization so that decisions can be made.
Survey	Collection of data from a sample of subjects who resemble the population in terms of variables being studied; studies to examine opinions, attributes, behavior, or characteristics of a population.

research lend themselves to all questions. The major types of research used by nurse researchers appear in Table 18–1.

Research studies range from experimental to non-experimental. **Experimental research** is a study in which the researcher manipulates a treatment or intervention, randomly assigns subjects to either a control or experimental group, and has control over the research situation. Because nurse researchers study human subjects, often in health care situations, a true experimental design is difficult. Consequently, nursing research is most commonly quasiexperimental or non-experimental research. **Quasiexperimental research** is a type of study in which the researcher manipulates a treatment or intervention but is unable to randomize subjects into groups or lacks a control group. **Nonexperimental research** is a type of study in which the researcher collects data without the introduction of a treatment or intervention.

Parts of the Study

A research report begins with an **abstract,** which is a short summary that contains brief information about the purpose of the study, the number of subjects, the methodology used to select subjects, the type of study conducted, and the major results obtained from the study. The abstract is used by the reader to decide whether the study contains information of interest. Some nursing journals print only the abstract of a

study along with a reference that readers use to locate the full study report. An example of an abstract appears in Figure 18–3.

If the entire study is included in the journal, you will typically find the following parts:

- *Introduction:* Usually, this section describes the research problem, presents the purpose of the study, gives a literature review, outlines the theoretical background, and explains the research questions.
- *Methods:* This section describes how the researchers sought to answer the research questions. This section also includes the sample size, how the sample was selected, how the data were collected, and the instruments used to collect data.
- *Data analysis:* Here you will see how the data were analyzed and which statistical tests were used to analyze the data. This section frequently includes tables, charts, or graphs.
- *Results:* This section describes the results obtained by the study, usually by addressing each research question individually.
- *Discussion:* This section includes the researchers' interpretation of the results, any conclusions drawn from the study, the relationship of the study findings to the theoretical background, and suggestions for future research.
- *References:* Here you will find all the references used in the study.

Many of the research reports found in current nursing literature will be primary sources. A *primary source* is the original research report written by the researchers. A *secondary source* is any other published material that reports on the study. When a research report or textbook cites a study, it become a secondary source. A secondary source is an adaptation of the primary source and may contain another person's interpretation of the research.

STEPS IN THE RESEARCH PROCESS

The research process follows a series of unique and essential steps. Although these steps may vary with the type of research conducted, a typical research study will follow this order:

- State the research problem.
- Review the literature.
- Develop a theoretical construct.
- Identify variables.
- Clarify operational definitions.
- Formulate research questions.
- Select a research strategy.
- Collect data.
- Analyze data.
- Interpret findings.

These steps help the researcher address a problem in an orderly way. They also help consumers of research to understand and evaluate the study. Most research articles will be organized and written according to these steps. The steps are common to all research, not only nursing research.

Effects of Exercise on Weight Loss

ABSTRACT: The purpose of this 6-week study was to determine the effects of 30 minutes of walking, three times a week, on weight loss. A random sample of 100 adult males and females, enrolled in a structured weight loss program, participated in the study. All of the subjects continued their normal activity levels, while one-half of the subjects agreed to increase their exercise level by walking three times a week. The Roy adaptation model served as the theoretical framework. Results indicated that those subjects who walked three times a week had a significantly greater weight loss than those subjects who maintained their normal activity.

Americans are increasingly striving to lose weight. The majority of the population is overweight, and Americans spend approximately $30 million each year on weight loss medications and dietary aids (Sampson, 1997). Obesity is a major health problem in the United States and one that influences the physical and mental health of the population. The purpose of this study was to determine the effects of 30 minutes of walking, three times a week, on subjects enrolled in a weight-loss program consisting of a 2000-kcal/day diet. The hypothesis was that people who walked 30 minutes three times a week would lose more weight than people who did not.

Several researchers have studied the effects of exercise on weight loss. Johnson (1995) studied 400 adults over the age of 65 who attended a 30-minute exercise class a minimum of once a week for a 6-month period. The results of that study indicated that subjects who attended the exercise class a minimum of three times a week lost weight, while those who attended less than three times a week did not lose weight. Likewise, Smith (1997) found that children who played baseball three times a week also lost weight, while children who played baseball less than three times a week did not lose weight.

The theoretical framework for the current study is the Roy adaptation model. According to Roy (Roy & Andrews, 1996), focal, contextual, and residual stimuli influence adaptation in the physiological, self-concept, role function, and interdependence modes. This study examined the need for nutrition and activity and rest in the physiological mode. The researchers viewed weight loss as an adaptation in the physiological mode, diet as a focal stimulus, and exercise as a contextual stimulus.

Methods

During the 6 weeks of the study, all 100 participants consumed prepackaged meals and snacks totaling 2000 kcal/day. On a flowsheet designed for this study, each subject was required to record all food and fluid intake immediately upon consumption. In addition, the subjects assigned to an exercise group were required to walk for 30 minutes on Mondays, Wednesdays, and Fridays for the 6 weeks of the study. Each participant in the exercise group was given a stopwatch to time the length of the walking. All participants were weighed using the same scale each Monday morning between 6:00 a.m. and 6:30 a.m. without clothes, after emptying their bladders and before consuming any foods or fluids.

Approval of the institutional review board was obtained for this study. All research data were collected by the researcher, who explained the study to each participant and procured informed consent.

Subjects for the study were solicited from an advertisement in a local newspaper. Of the 400 adults who responded to the advertisement, 150 met the criteria established by the researcher. These criteria included willingness to follow the study protocol, absence of physical or mental illnesses, and ability to pass a physical examination conducted by the researcher. Of the 150 respondents who met the criteria, 100 were randomly selected for inclusion in the study and randomly assigned to either the exercise or nonexercise groups. All of the subjects completed the study.

Subjects ranged in age from 22 to 64 and included 56 females and 44 males. The majority of the subjects, 82%, were employed outside the home, and education levels ranged from completion of the sophomore year of high school to a master's degree.

Instrumentation used to gather data included a Brice-Jones scale and Olympic stopwatches. The scale was calibrated by a technician from the state Bureau of Weights and Measurements each Monday morning prior to collecting the weight data . Between each subject the scale was reset at the 0 level. During the time of the study, the scale was not moved. New stopwatches were used for the study. Prior to the beginning and at the end of the study, each stopwatch was tested by a computer timing devise to ensure accuracy.

Data Analysis

The data were analyzed using a t-test. The mean weight loss for the nonexercise group was 6 lb, while the mean weight loss for the exercise group was 9 lb. These results were significant ($p < .05$).

Results

The results of this study indicate that exercising three times a week for 30 minutes contributed to weight loss. The weight loss for the exercise group was

Figure 18–3. Example of a brief research article.

approximately one-third greater than for the nonexercise group. The flowsheets for both groups indicated that study participants adhered to the study protocol and consumed only the prepackaged meals. The amount of fluids consumed by the subjects varied from 1400 mL to 3200 mL, with the mean consumption being 2200 mL. One subject in the exercise group was unable to exercise on the specified day, but did exercise the following day.

Discussion of the Results
The findings from this study suggest that exercise does influence weight loss. These finding support the previous studies conducted by Johnson (1995) and Smith (1997). Exercise seems to increase weight loss in adults, as well as in children and older adults. These three studies may represent a beginning body of knowledge about the effects of exercise on weight loss.

The amount of fluids consumed by the subjects varied greatly, and may have influenced weight loss. The effect of fluid consumption on weight loss is an area for further study. In addition, the ability of the subjects to adhere to the diet deserves further consideration. The researcher acknowledges that in most studies, the subjects do not report such strict adherence to the diet. The adherence in this study may be due to the limited time frame of the study or to the prepackaged meals. This too is an area for further research.

This study supports the Roy model. The exercising subjects lost weight, and the researcher viewed this weight loss as a physiological adaptation to the focal stimulus of diet and the contextual stimulus of exercise.

References
Johnson, K. N. (1995). Exercise and weight loss in children. *Journal of Pediatric Conditions*, *65*(5), 332–336.
Roy, C., & Andrews, H. A. (1996). *The Roy adaptation model* (2nd Ed.). Norwalk, CT: Appleton & Lange.
Sampson, T. R. (1997). *American weight loss statistics.* Bluffs, MT: Sanderson.
Smith, P. T. (1997). Weight loss in older adults. *Journal of Gerontological Physiology*, *6*(4), 11–28.

Figure 18–3 *Continued.* See legend on opposite page.

State the Problem

A **research problem** is an observation, situation, occurrence, or even a hunch that an investigator chooses to research. Initially, it may simply be an area of interest that the researcher then further defines. Most problems begin with something the researcher has observed in practice. For example, if in clinical practice a nurse observes that some diabetic patients are better able to control their blood glucose levels than others, the researcher might question the reason for this difference.

In addition to the significance of the study, researchers must consider whether it is possible to design a study to research the problem. Not all problems are amenable to research methods. For example, issues that are of a moral or ethical nature are not researchable.

Another consideration that researchers must address is the feasibility of conducting the research. All researchers face limitations, such as time, availability of subjects and resources (such as equipment), the cooperation of institutions, financial support, and the facilities needed to conduct the research. Many researchers change or limit their research problems based on the availability of resources.

The research problem or purpose of the research should be stated early in the research report. In the problem or purpose statement, the researcher should clearly identify the variables under study, the suspected relationship of these variables, and the population of interest. For example, a purpose statement might be: *The purpose of this study is to compare the effects of grief on the physiological health of women who experienced the death of a spouse within the preceding 12 months and the effects of grief on the physiological health of women who experienced the death of a child within the preceding 12 months.*

The researcher's use of verbs in the purpose statement often identifies the state of the knowledge about the subject or the manner in which the researcher sought to solve the problem. The verbs *explore* or *describe* usually indicate a topic about which little is known, whereas *test* or *compare* suggests a more thoroughly developed knowledge base. Verbs such as *show, prove,* or *demonstrate* indicate possible researcher bias and should not be used.

Review the Literature

The researcher begins to study the problem by reviewing what has already been studied about it. A literature review is essential to all types of research and serves as the foundation for the research study. The researcher conducts the review by thoroughly examining all available literature related to the research problem. The purposes of the literature review are to help the researcher identify or refine the research problem, strengthen the rationale for the research, develop a conceptual framework, and provide a useful approach for the study.

The researcher may conduct the literature review using manual or computer search methods. They are the same methods you would use to look for information about any nursing topic of interest.

Manual Searches

Manual search may be time-consuming, but it is an inexpensive method for locating and reviewing nursing research literature. This type of search requires familiarity with the library and various index tools, such as card catalogs, medical and nursing indexes, abstracts, and bibliographies. In many libraries, card catalogs are available on computer.

Indexes are organized according to subject and author; they are the researcher's main source for locating articles published in journals. Researchers and nurses frequently read abstracts to determine the potential usefulness of an article. To fully evaluate the research, however, the entire article must be examined. Bibliographies contain lists of publications on a specific topic. Sources of bibliographies include indexes, articles, books, dissertations, and theses. A list of indexes, abstracts, and bibliographies frequently used by nurses appears in Table 18–2.

Computer Searches

Computer searches are used to reach bibliographic information stored in databases. Many computer databases offer the same information found in indexes and abstracts, but the information accessed through a computer may be more current. A computer search may be completed at any computer that has access to the database. Library computers usually have access to databases, or the librarian can help to access the desired database.

To locate information, the topic must be narrowed and key words determined. Key words are used to search the database. After searching the database, the researcher can obtain an on-line printout immediately or an off-line printout in 3 to 5 days. The cost of the search depends on the database being searched and the time spent doing the search. Table 18–3 identifies databases of interest to nurses.

Develop a Theoretical Framework

A **theoretical framework** is a logical but abstract structure that suggests the relationship among the variables in a research study. It allows for the organization and explanation of all of the information included in the study. Working within a framework enables the researcher to tie the research to the body of nursing knowledge. Thus, the study findings can be generalized to similar populations. All frameworks are based on key concepts and the relationships among those concepts.

For example, a researcher who wants to examine the effect of poor health on life satisfaction must recognize that both poor health and life satisfaction are abstract concepts. Such concepts are frequently organized into theories. In this example, the researcher might want to use the Roy Adaptation Model (Roy & Andrews, 1996) as the theoretical basis for the study. In this model, poor health would be viewed as a focal

TABLE 18–2
Manual Literature Search Resources: Indexes

Source	Types of Listings
Indexes	
Cumulative Index to Nursing and Allied Health Literature	More than 300 nursing and allied health journals
International Nursing Index	Nursing literature from around the world
Nursing Studies Index	Nursing literature from 1900 to 1959
Index Medicus	More than 2,600 biomedical journals
Hospital Literature Index	References on health care and administration
Education Index	More than 300 education journals
Social Science Citation Index	More than 1,500 social science journals
Science Citation Index	More than 100 science journals
Abstracts	
Nursing Research Abstracts	Abstracts of nursing-related studies from 1960 to 1978
Nursing Abstracts	Abstracts of nursing research studies published since 1979
Excerpta Medica	Abstracts from basic biological sciences
Current Index to Journals in Education	Abstracts of education literature
Psychological Abstracts	Abstracts from more than 900 periodicals and 1,500 books on psychology and related disciplines
Sociological Abstracts	Abstracts from more than 1,200 journals on sociology and related disciplines
Dissertation Abstracts International	Abstracts from doctoral dissertations published throughout the world
Bibliographies	
Bibliography on Nursing Research 1950 to 1974	Includes more than 1,000 sources organized according to 22 broad classifications
A Bibliography of Nursing Literature 1859–1960 and A Bibliography of Nursing Literature 1961–1970	Contains more than 1,000 publications useful for historical research
Specialized Bibliography Series	Contains a broad range of topics and is available through the National Library of Medicine

TABLE 18–3
Computer Search Database Resources

Database	Types of Listings
CINAHL	Corresponds with the information in *Cumulative Index to Nursing and Allied Health Literature* from 1983 to present.
MEDLARS/MEDLINE	Corresponds with the information in *Index Medicus, International Nursing Index,* and *Index to Dental Literature* from 1966 to present.
EMBASE	Corresponds with the information in *Excerpta Medica* from 1974 to present.
HEALTH	Corresponds with the information in *Hospital Literature Index* from 1975 to present.
ERIC	Corresponds with the information in *Resources in Education* and *Current Index to Journal in Education* from 1966 to present.
SOCIAL SCISEARCH	Corresponds with the information in *Science Citation Index* from 1965 to present.
PsycINFO	Corresponds with the information in *Psychological Abstracts* from 1967 to present.
Sociological Abstracts	Corresponds with the information in *Sociological Abstracts* from 1963 to present.
Dissertation Abstracts Online	Corresponds with the information in *Dissertation Abstracts International* from 1961 to the present
BIOETHICSLINE	Includes citations from 1973 to present concerning ethical questions in health care; housed at the National Library of Medicine and the Kennedy Institute of Ethics.
CANCERLIT	Includes all cancer-related literature from 1963 to present.

stimulus to trigger some kind of adaptation and lead to either life satisfaction or a lack of satisfaction. Without the model, it might be tempting to look only at the negative effects of poor health. Using a theory helps researchers clarify relationships and explain relationships. In addition, using a theory helps contribute to the testing of that theory, which increases nursing knowledge.

Identify Variables

The concepts under investigation in research studies are called variables because they are expected to change or differ from one person to another or from one time to another. The researcher is often trying to study how variation in one concept produces change in another concept. Almost anything in people and their environments may vary and, thus, be considered a variable. If all humans were 5 feet tall and weighed 100 pounds, then height and weight would not be variables. Disease conditions are variables because not all people have the disease; those that do may have varying degrees of severity. Other examples of variables include temperature, weight, knowledge, nursing interventions received, self-concept, health, and grief.

Researchers talk about independent and dependent variables rather than about cause and effect because, even though a relationship may exist between two variables, that does not prove cause and effect. An **independent variable** may change during the study, but the change is expected to remain constant or to cause change in another variable. A **dependent variable** is expected to change with the treatment; thus, to have been caused by an independent variable. Following are three easy ways to distinguish between dependent and independent variables:

- The independent variable is the cause, and the dependent variable is the effect.
- The independent variable is what the researcher will manipulate, and the dependent variable is the outcome of that manipulation.
- Changes in the dependent variable depend on changes in the independent variable.

Now apply these criteria to a research problem: Do clients who receive home nursing care after discharge experience fewer complications? *Home health nursing* is the independent variable, because it may be the cause of fewer complications, and it is what the researcher will manipulate. *Complications* is the dependent variable because it is the effect. It depends on changes in the independent variable. For more practice in determining independent and dependent variables, see Table 18–4.

Clarify Operational Definitions

Research requires precision in how the concepts are being measured. An **operational definition** is the meaning of the concept precisely as it is being used in the study, defined in a manner that specifies how the concepts will be measured. For example, if the researcher has identified height as a variable for a study, the operational definition may be the distance from the bottom of the feet to the top of the head as measured in inches. This definition specifies that information will be collected in inches, not centimeters. Also, this definition specifies to other researchers and readers exactly how this term is used in this study, allowing for the replication of the study in the future.

Operational definitions are even more important when researchers are studying variables that are not as easily defined as height. Variables such as self-concept, pain, grief, stress, and adaptation are very difficult to operationalize. For example, in a thesis, psychosocial adaptation was defined as: "overall ad-

TABLE 18–4

Examples of Independent and Dependent Variables

Research Question	Independent Variable	Dependent Variable
Does involvement in health-promotion activities increase the level of adaptation?	Involvement in health-promotion activities	Adaptation
How does the client's culture affect the request for pain medication?	Client's culture	Request for pain medication
Do clients who receive pain medication frequently after surgery experience fewer postoperative complications?	Receiving pain medications	Experience fewer complications
Does cigarette smoking cause lung cancer?	Cigarette smoking	Lung cancer
Do mothers experiencing the birth of their second child feel less anxiety than mothers experiencing the birth of their first child?	Birth of the first or second child	Anxiety

justment to health care orientation, vocational environment, domestic environment, sexual relationships, extended family relationships, social environment, and psychological distress" (Huckstein, 1995). These concepts were measured by a Psychosocial Adjustment to Illness Scale that gave specific meaning to each of the concepts. In this example, the researcher clarified what was meant by psychosocial adaptation, and how the term was to be measured. Another researcher could repeat this study using precisely the same method of measurement.

Formulate a Hypothesis

A **hypothesis** is a tentative prediction of the relationship between two or more variables being studied. It includes independent and dependent variables. In a previous example, the research problem was to compare the effects of grief on the physiological health of women who had experienced the death of a spouse versus a child during the preceding 12 months. The hypothesis for this problem could be: Women who have experienced the death of a child in the past 12 months will report less grief and better physiological health than women who have experienced the death of a spouse in the past 12 months. If the hypothesis fails to propose a relationship between two or more variables, it cannot be tested.

A hypothesis should be based on previous research or should be deduced from a theory. The researcher should present a sound, justifiable, logical rationale for the study hypothesis.

Select a Research Design

A **research design** is a researcher's strategy for testing a hypothesis. The hypothesis should guide the design, but the researcher must decide what design would be best for the study. Research designs are categorized as either quantitative or qualitative. **Quantitative research** is a type of study that uses variables analyzed as numbers, and **qualitative research** is a type of study that uses ideas that are analyzed as words. Quantitative designs usually are best suited to studies that focus on determining cause-and-effect relation-

ships, whereas qualitative designs are best suited to studies that focus on discovery or exploration.

Collect Data

Data collection is the process by which the researcher acquires subjects and collects the information needed to answer the research question. It is the actual measurement of the study variables. Researchers use various instruments—such as questionnaires, interviews, scales, observations, and physiological measurements—to collect data.

Any instrument used in research should be reliable and valid. *Reliability* is the degree of consistency and accuracy with which an instrument measures a variable. For example, if an instrument is used to measure temperature, that instrument (in this case a thermometer) should measure the temperature accurately each time it is used. With physiological measures, instruments are usually straightforward. Concepts, such as health or stress, can be difficult to measure. *Validity* is the ability of an instrument to measure what it is designed to measure. For example, a valid measure of self-concept must measure a person's perception of the self, not another person's assessment of the study subject's belief's about self. One method of addressing validity is to ask experts to evaluate these instruments. To evaluate an instrument's validity, the reader of the research must decide if the experts are in fact experts, if the number of experts was sufficient, and if the author revised the instrument based on input by the experts.

Sampling is the process of selecting the subjects from the population being studied. It is an economical and efficient means of collecting data when use of an entire population is not feasible. Sampling techniques and the criteria used to define the population affect whether the findings can be *generalized* as being true of the whole population. The sample should reflect the same variations as those of the population. Generally, the largest sample size possible is the best.

There are two basic sampling techniques used in nursing research: random or probability sampling, and nonrandom or nonprobability sampling. *Random sampling* is the only method of obtaining a representative sample. In a randomly selected sample, each member of the population has an equal chance of appearing in the sample. It reduces the possibility of researcher bias. *Nonrandom sampling* involves the selection of subjects using nonrandom techniques. It is less rigorous and results in a less representative sample. The major disadvantage of nonrandom samples is that they limit the researcher's ability to generalize from the study results.

Analyze Data

The primary purpose of data analysis is to impose order on the quantity of data so that conclusions can be made and communicated. The researcher's choice of research design determines how the data should be analyzed. Quantitative research should be analyzed by numbers and statistics. Quantitative data analysis uses statistical computation to summarize the collected data, compare and contrast the data, test theoretical relationships, generalize about the population based on sample findings, and evaluate possible cause-and-effect relationships. Most researchers use computers to help with statistical analysis.

Qualitative research should be analyzed through words and logic. It depends on intuitive and analytical reasoning to guide the organization, clustering, and reduction of data. *Reduction* is the organization of volumes of narrative data into concepts that allow the researcher to deduce meanings. After the data are reduced, they may be displayed using tables, graphs, and matrices. From the data display, the researcher then draws conclusions and attaches meaning to the findings.

Interpret Findings

To interpret research findings, the researcher examines, organizes, and attaches meaning to the results obtained from the data analysis. Study findings should be drawn from the data analysis and related back to the theoretical framework.

The researcher forms conclusions from the current study coupled with information learned from previous research studies. When forming conclusions, the researcher must clearly state that the research supports or does not support a position; the researcher must not state that the research *proves* a position. Also, conclusions should result from a logical deduction of the data and not extended to include variables not addressed in the study. When formulating conclusions, the researcher should provide practical suggestions for implementing the findings in nursing. The areas of nursing where the findings can be implemented should be identified as well as implications for nursing education and further nursing research.

RESEARCH IN NURSING PRACTICE

The goal of nursing research is to improve nursing practice. Consequently, nurses must incorporate the findings from nursing research into their practices. Nursing practice identifies areas for research, and nursing research helps solve clinical practice problems. This reciprocal relationship improves practice and provides for new professional knowledge.

Research Functions According to Level of Practice

All nurses, including nursing students, share the responsibility for improving practice. All can contribute to nursing research. Students and practicing nurses are commonly unsure of their role in nursing research. In an attempt to clarify this confusion, the ANA has identified the investigative functions of nurses at various educational levels (Table 18–5).

Nurses at all educational levels can contribute to nursing research by collecting data for an ongoing research study. It is important for all nurses to understand the factors that can affect research results and to make sure that the data collected will be as accurate as possible.

When assisting with research data collection, it is critical that you follow the research protocol. Slight differences in protocol may make significant changes in study results. If, for example, the research protocol states that blood must be drawn 30 minutes after the administration of a medication, and you draw the blood 60 minutes afterward, the study results may be invalid. If the study protocol cannot be followed, contact the principal investigator to determine what to do with the data. Never just assume that 30 minutes make no difference. The value of research depends on accurate, precise data collection.

Identifying Nursing Research Problems

Nursing research problems begin as questions that need to be answered or problems that need to be solved. The nurse's everyday experience provides a rich supply of problems for investigation. Student nurses and practicing nurses encounter occurrences or situations that are puzzling or problematic. As a student, you have probably asked such questions as, "Why is this procedure done this way?" "Is there a better way?" "Why did this happen?" "What would happen if . . . ?" These questions are frequently the beginning of research problems.

Research problems may also come from nursing literature. Most research articles include recommendations for further research, in which the author discusses areas of related research that, if conducted, would build on current knowledge. Also, inconsistencies in the findings of reported research often provide ideas for further study. Similar studies may yield conflicting results, possibly because of the different samples or different situations. Nursing knowledge benefits from the replication of studies with different samples and in different situations to establish the validity and generalization of previous findings.

TABLE 18–5
Investigative Functions of a Nurse at Various Educational Levels

Associate Degree in Nursing	• Demonstrates awareness of the value of research in nursing. • Assists in identifying problem areas in nursing practice. • Assists in collecting data within an established, structured format.
Baccalaureate Degree in Nursing	• Reads, interprets, and evaluates research for applicability to nursing practice. • Identifies nursing problems that need to be investigated and participates in the implementation of scientific studies. • Uses nursing practice as a means of gathering data to refine and extend practice. • Applies established findings of nursing and other health-related research to nursing practice.
Master's Degree in Nursing	• Analyzes and reformulates nursing practice problems so that scientific methods can be used to find solutions. • Enhances the quality and clinical relevance of nursing research by providing expertise in clinical problems and by providing knowledge about the way in which these clinical services are delivered. • Facilitates investigations of problems in clinical settings by contributing to a climate that supports investigative activities, collaborating with others in investigations, and enhancing nursing access to clients and data. • Conducts investigations to monitor the quality of nursing practice in a clinical setting. • Helps others apply scientific knowledge in nursing practice.
Doctoral Degree in Nursing or a Related Discipline	• Provides leadership for the integration of scientific knowledge with other sources of knowledge for the advancement of practice. • Conducts investigations to evaluate the contribution of nursing activities to the well-being of clients. • Develops methods to monitor the quality of nursing practice in a clinical setting and to evaluate contributions of nursing activities to the well-being of clients.
Graduate of a Research-Oriented Doctoral Program	• Develops theoretical explanations of phenomena relevant to nursing by empiric research and analytic processes. • Uses analytic and empiric methods to discover ways to modify or extend existing scientific knowledge so that it is relevant to nursing. • Develops methods for scientific inquiry of phenomena relevant to nursing.

Adapted from American Nurses' Association Commission on Nursing Research. (1981). Guidelines for the investigative functions of nurses. Copyright 1981 by American Nurses Publishing, American Nurses Foundation/American Nurses' Association, 600 Maryland Ave., SW, Suite 100W, Washington, D.C. 20024–2571. To order, call 800/637-0323.

A third source of research problems comes from nursing theory. To be useful in practice, theories must be tested through research. When theory is used as a basis for research, deductions from the theory must be developed. The researcher would ask such questions as, "If I use this theory, what behavior would I expect in this situation under this condition?" "Can I predict what would happen using this theory?" "What study findings would provide support or nonsupport for this theory?"

Another source for identifying nursing research problems is external. Some organizations or government agencies sponsor funded research and may identify topics for research based on current social concerns or problems. For example, in the last few years many government agencies have requested a variety of AIDS-related research projects. Research ideas may represent a response to priorities established by the nursing profession. The NINR funds research based on the priorities listed in Box 18–2. In addition, many nursing specialty practice groups fund research related to the specialty area.

Evaluating Research Findings

Research in a practice profession, such as nursing, provides information needed to improve practice. For research to improve practice, researchers need to study problems that have been identified by practicing nurses. The practicing nurse needs to have the skill to evaluate research findings and develop interventions that make appropriate use of the information. Nursing research has relevance for all nurses, not just the minority of nurses who are nurse researchers. The following sections offer an introduction to the evaluation of nursing research.

Tentative Nature of Research Findings

The results of research never prove that a hypothesis or theory is true. Rather, all research results are tentative. A hypothesis tests only one small part of a theory, and researchers cannot even state that the small part of the theory tested by the hypothesis is true. The hypothesis may be faulty, the sample may be too small, the sample may not be representative of the population, or there may be another serious flaw in the study.

For example, suppose that an undiscovered enzyme controls blood cholesterol levels, but researchers report that blood cholesterol levels have been proven to result from diet, exercise, metabolism, and family history. What the researcher considered proof would be false. The results of the study were not proof. They merely indicated that a relationship existed for this sample. Instead of indications of proof, watch for phrases such as *the data support* or *the data indicate* as you read studies. Research results are always tentative and are based on the sample and study involved.

Research Bias

Bias is a factor that can change or distort the results of a study. In a good research study, you can feel confident that a change in the dependent variable is because of the independent variable. However, when a researcher does not attempt to control for bias, this relationship may not be true. Bias may result from the researcher's conscious or unconscious desire to demonstrate a relationship between variables (Kelber & Pearson, 1996). Bias is commonly introduced when studies are designed to elicit specific results.

Another source of bias is the difference among subjects in groups that are being compared. When groups are formed on a nonrandom basis, the risk of bias is always present. For example, in a study in which blood cholesterol level is the dependent variable and diet and exercise are the independent variables, a major concern is that individuals with high cholesterol may differ from those with low cholesterol in ways not connected with the independent variables. Other differences, like metabolism and family history, may cause high or low cholesterol. Unless these other differences, called extraneous variables, are controlled, the resulting biases make it difficult for the researcher to conclude that lower cholesterol levels are related to diet and exercise.

When study data are collected by observation, the researcher's beliefs may unconsciously bias objective collection. To prevent bias from occurring, a *double-blind* technique is often used. The double-blind technique removes observer bias because both the subject and the person collecting the data are "blind" to the research objective. If this technique cannot be used, many researchers will use two or more independent observers to reduce or eliminate observer bias.

Threats to Validity

If a study has validity, it actually measures what it was designed to measure. When evaluating research, you should examine factors within the design and factors external to the study that could affect the results. These two types are called internal and external validity.

Internal validity depends on the extent to which a change in the dependent variable can be attributed to the independent variable. True experiments possess a high degree of internal validity because of the use of control groups and randomization. This enables the researcher to control for extraneous variables, thereby ruling out most alternative explanations for the study results.

Other research designs always have alternative explanations for the study results because extraneous variables in addition to the independent variable could cause a change in the dependent variable. These alternative explanations are called threats to internal validity and have been grouped into several classifications:

- History: Have any extraneous variables occurred during the time of the study? Were there any changes in the environment that could have influenced the study findings?
- Maturation: Has the passage of time since the beginning of the study affected the results? Are there any internal changes in subjects—such as aging, growth and development, or wound-healing—that would affect the study results?
- Mortality: Did the loss of subjects from different groups during the study affect the results? Was the loss of subjects from each group approximately equal?
- Selection: If the subjects were not randomly assigned to groups, were there pre-existing differences between groups?
- Testing: Were the pre-tests and post-tests identical? Could the subjects remember the material from the pre-test to the post-test?
- Instrumentation: If the pre-test and the post-test were not identical, where they equal? If different observers were collecting data, how were these people trained to ensure that each used the same technique and scored the data in the same manner?

External validity refers to the extent to which findings can be generalized to other populations, samples, or situations. Researchers almost never conduct studies to use the findings with only one group of subjects. Researchers hope that study findings can be used by other nurses in similar situations. There are several threats to external validity, two of which will be discussed here.

- Sample inadequacy: Does the sample represent the population? Is the sample large enough for the researcher to draw conclusions?
- Hawthorne effect: Did the study cause the subjects to act differently than they would have usually acted?

Faulty Statistics

Statistical analysis allows the researcher to make quantitative data meaningful. It allows the researcher to summarize, organize, compare, evaluate, and communicate numerical data. Without statistics, data would be a mass of numbers with little or no meaning.

Statistics are classified as either descriptive or inferential. Descriptive statistics are used to describe data. Examples of descriptive statistics include averages and percentages. When researchers use statistics to make inferences or draw conclusions about a population, inferential statistics are used. The difference between the two is that descriptive statistics are concerned only with characteristics of the data obtained by the researcher, whereas inferential statistics are concerned with generalizations to a population larger than that of the data.

Scientists have developed a classification system for different types of data resulting from instruments. This classification system is important because the statistical tests performed on data depend on the measurement level. A faulty statistic can result when the researcher uses the wrong measurement level.

In addition, when researchers use inferential statistics to generalize findings to a population, the statistical tests used have assumptions that should be met in order to use the test. If these assumptions are violated, then the results of the test may be questionable. If the researcher uses an inappropriate measurement level or violates major statistical assumptions, then the study results may be invalid.

Implementing Research Findings

The responsibility for implementing research findings is shared by all nurses (Fig. 18–4). In fact, nurses' behaviors and attitudes are critical to the success of any efforts to base nursing practice on research findings (Thompson, 1996). Individual nurses can contribute to implementing research findings by the following:

- Reading and evaluating nursing research articles
- Attending professional research conferences
- Supporting nursing research projects
- Participating in institutional research projects
- Sharing research findings with other nurses

Expanding Professional Knowledge Base

Nursing students and staff nurses who read research reports and look for opportunities to apply sound re-

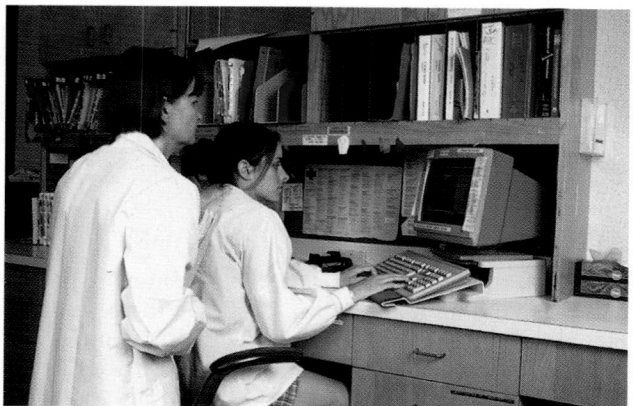

Figure 18–4. All nurses share the responsibility for implementing the findings of nursing research.

search findings make an important contribution to the expansion of nursing knowledge in addition to improving their own clinical practice (Beyea & Nicoll, 1997). Nurse researchers are usually not interested in pursuing knowledge for its own sake but want their findings to improve practice.

When research findings are incorporated into individual clinical practice, nursing knowledge expands. Nurses identify when particular findings seem to work or not to work. From this evaluation, new hypotheses are formed, ideas are generated, and the nursing profession is revitalized. Some of the new hypotheses and ideas may never be tested in a controlled research study but, as nurses communicate new and different methods, nursing practice is improved, and the knowledge base of nursing is expanded.

Every nurse has an important role to play in making use of nursing research. Research originates from questions being asked by practicing nurses. Every nurse has not only the right but also the responsibility to ask for evidence that practices and procedures are effective. Clinical decisions must be based on sound rationales. Practices and procedures must be challenged and changed based on current knowledge rather than simply accepted because "it's always been that way."

Making Clinical Decisions

There is tremendous potential for using nursing research to make clinical decisions. The nursing process requires nurses to make many decisions. What will be assessed? What are the priority nursing diagnoses? What plan of care will produce the best outcomes? What interventions are necessary? How will the results be evaluated? When will the results be evaluated? Nursing research plays an important role at each phase of the nursing process by helping nurses make informed decisions when carrying out the nursing process.

Research-based nursing decisions begin when clinical problems are identified. If the problem has minimal significance to nurses, or if making a change or introducing a new intervention will not benefit clients or nurses, there is little point in implementing the change. However, when an important problem has been identified, you can proceed by identifying and critiquing the current research literature for information that will help you make decisions. To decide if the information is useful in solving your problem, ask questions about the transferability, feasibility, and cost/benefit ratio (Cullum & Sheldon, 1996).

Transferability simply refers to whether it makes good sense to attempt an innovation in your practice situation. Feasibility refers to the practical concerns about the availability of resources to implement the innovation. If the resources are not available, can they be obtained? The cost/benefit ratio encompasses the likely costs and benefits to various groups, including nurses, clients, and the institution as a whole. Clearly, the client is of utmost importance. The benefits to the client should be high, with minimal risk.

After determining the transferability, feasibility, and cost/benefit ratio, assess the potential for implementation for the innovation, and plan to include the innovation in your practice. Implement and evaluate the innovation. Then, make a rational decision about adopting the innovation based on your evaluation. Remember that implementing change is sometimes difficult and frequently takes longer than is originally thought.

Improving Quality of Care

As a student, the best way for you to use nursing research to improve the quality of your practice is to identify an area of nursing where you have unanswered questions. Go to your library, and conduct a literature search using both manual and computer techniques. Your reference librarian can help you locate the various indexes and provide information and assistance with computer searches. Once you have located several research articles of interest, consult the listing of periodicals for your library, and select one or two journal articles. If your library does not have research journals, the reference librarian may be able to help you obtain them through an interlibrary loan. After you have obtained the articles, it is helpful to photocopy them so that you can make notations in the margins. As you read the articles, try to identify the positive and negative aspects of the articles and any flaws in the research. Pay particular attention to the implications for clinical practice. Then identify how you can use the research to improve the quality of care you provide to your clients. Incorporating nursing research into your clinical practice provides constant renewal of your nursing knowledge and that of the profession at large.

KEY PRINCIPLES

- Nursing research is important because it serves the public through improved health care, and it establishes a scientific basis for nursing practice.
- Ethical research protects study participants by rigidly following protocols that maintain the rights of subjects.
- Because of the nature of the issues studied, nursing research is often descriptive rather than experimental.
- The steps of the research process follow a standard format that reflects the scientific method and produces rigorous, disciplined study that can be replicated.
- Every nurse has a role to play in advancing the profession of nursing through research, whether it be as a principal investigator or by creating effective interventions based on the findings of researchers.

- Research problems ideally come from problems encountered in a clinical practice setting, the resolution of which would improve the outcomes of client care.
- A single research study can offer evidence that supports a position, fact, or belief about nursing care but cannot be used to prove the truth of a hypothesis.
- Research contributes to practice by generating ideas about the nature of human responses, naming and describing the human responses treated by nurses, validating methods of intervention, and demonstrating nursing sensitive outcomes.

BIBLIOGRAPHY

*American Nurses' Association. (1975). *Human rights guidelines for nurses in clinical and other research.* Kansas City, MO: Author.

*American Nurses' Association Commission on Nursing Research. (1981). *Guidelines for the investigative functions of nurses.* Kansas City, MO: American Nurses' Association.

*American Nurses' Association Council on Nursing Research. (1997). *Directions for nursing research: Toward the twenty-first century.* Washington, D.C.: American Nurses' Association.

*American Psychological Association. (1982). *Ethical principles in the conduct of research with human subjects.* Washington, D.C.: Author.

*American Sociological Association. (1984). *Code of ethics.* Washington, D.C.: Author.

*Bauknecht, K.L. (1985). Capitol commentary: NIH bill passes, includes nursing research center. *American Nurse, 17*(2), 2.

Beyea, S.C., & Nicoll, L.H. (1997). Research corner: Research utilization begins with learning to read research reports. *AORN Journal 65*(2), 402–403.

*Code of Federal Regulations. (1983). *Protection of human subjects: 45 C.F.R. 46* (revised as of March 8, 1983). Washington, D.C.: Department of Health and Human Services.

Cullum, N., & Sheldon, T. (1996). Clinically challenged: Gap between nursing research and practice. *Nursing Management, 3*(4), 14–16.

*Goldmark, J. (1923). *Nursing and nursing education in the United States.* New York: Macmillan.

Goode, C.J., & Tiller, M.G. (1996). Moving research-based practice throughout the health care system. *Medsurg Nursing, 5*(5), 380–383.

*Hebert, R.G. (1981). Introduction. In R.G. Hebert (Ed.), *Florence Nightingale: Saint, reformer, or rebel?* Malabar, FL: Robert Krieger Publishing Co.

Huckstein, M.E. (1995). *The relationship between hardiness and adaptation to lifestyle changes in multiple trauma patients.* Master's thesis. Miami, FL: Florida International University.

*Kalisch, P., & Kalisch, B. (1978). *The advance of American nursing.* Boston: Little, Brown & Co.

Kelber, S.T., & Pearson, B.D. (1996). Translating research into practice: Ways bias may occur in research. *Journal of Urological Nursing, 15*(1), 1216–1221.

*National Center for Nursing Research. (1993). *Research priorities from the National Center for Nursing Research.* Bethesda, MD: Author.

*National Commission for the Protection of Human Subjects of Biomedical and Behavioral Research. (1978). *Belmont report: Ethical principles and guidelines for research involving human subjects.* Washington, D.C.: U.S. Government Printing Office.

*Nightingale, F. (1859). *Notes on Hospitals.* London: Longman.

*Asterisk indicates a classic or definitive work on this subject.

Polit, D.F., & Hungler, B.P. (1995). *Nursing research: Principles and methods* (5th ed.). Philadelphia: J.B. Lippincott Co..

*Rogers, B. (1989). Florence Nightingale and research. *AAOHN Journal, 37*(6), 238–239.

*Rothman, D.J. (1982). Were Tuskegee and Willowbrook studies in nature? *Hastings Center, 12*(2), 5–7.

Roy, C., & Andrews, H. (1996). *The Roy adaptation model* (2nd ed.). Norwalk, CT: Appleton & Lange.

Thompson, D.R. (1996). Getting research into practice. *Intensive and Critical Care Nursing, 12*(4), 191–192.

*Vessey, J., & Gennaro, S. (1994). The ghost of Tuskegee: The Tuskegee study of untreated syphilis in the Negro male. *Nursing Research, 43*(2), 67.

*Asterisk indicates a classic or definitive work on this subject.

The Well Client Across the Life Span

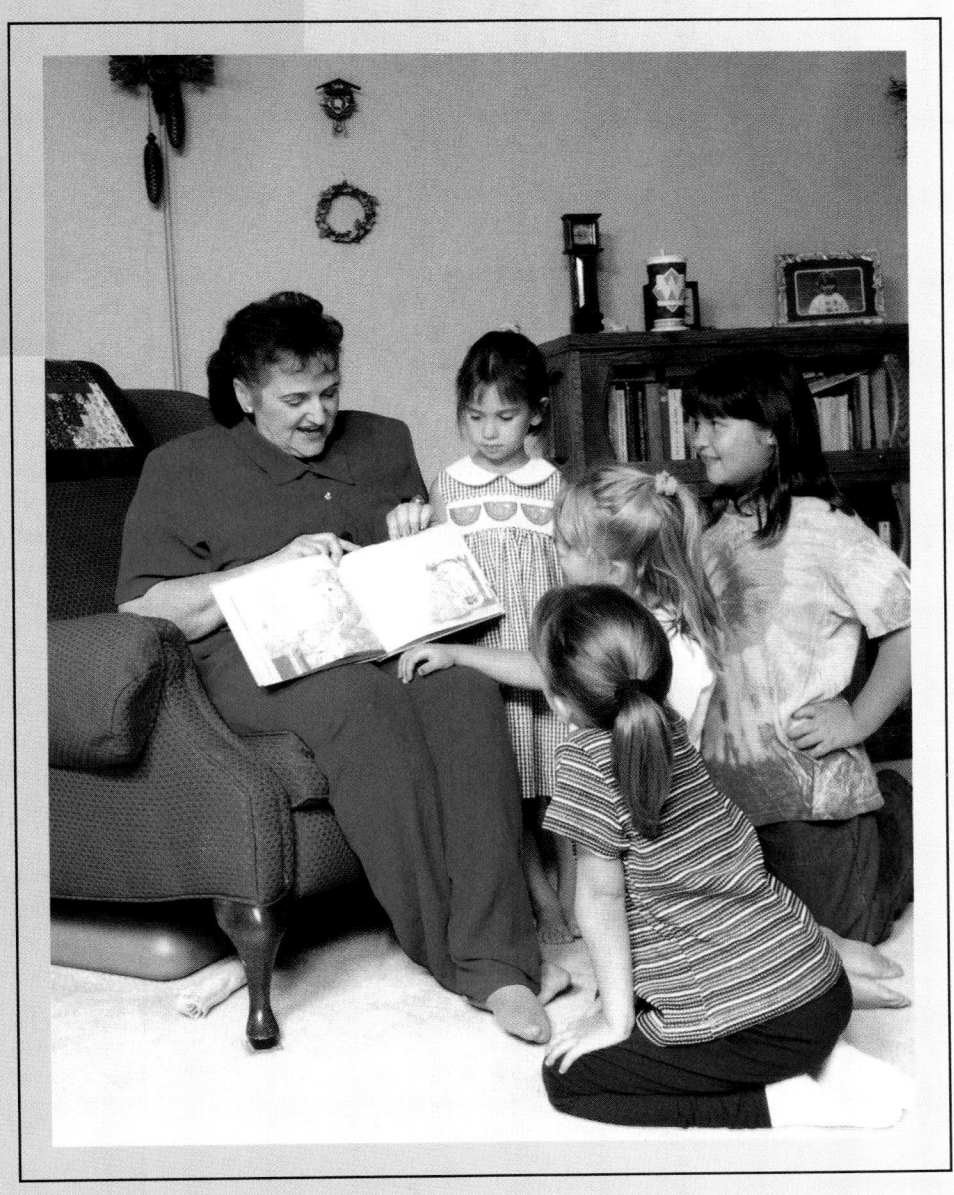

The Well Newborn, Infant, and Toddler

Nancy J. MacMullen and Sally Evankoe

Key Terms

accommodation
adaptation
assimilation
attachment
bonding
cephalocaudal
cognitive development
critical periods
development
developmental milestones
developmental task

differentiated development
growth
infant
newborn
object permanence
proximodistal
psychosocial development
sensory stimulation
teratogen
toddler

LEARNING OBJECTIVES

After studying this chapter, you should be able to:

1. Compare and contrast three significant theories of growth and development.
2. Identify developmental milestones in the newborn, infant, and toddler.
3. Describe environmental, socioeconomic, nutritional, and physiological factors affecting growth and development.
4. Describe the assessment of growth and development in the newborn, infant, and toddler.
5. Discuss assessment strategies to detect altered growth and development.
6. Select an appropriate nursing diagnosis for a newborn, infant, or toddler with problems in growth and development.
7. Plan interventions to promote maintenance of a newborn's, infant's, or toddler's health.
8. Evaluate outcomes for a newborn, infant or toddler with altered health maintenance.

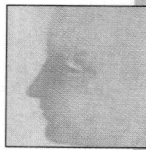

Yung Hi is a 33-month-old Korean girl who has been in the United States for only 6 months. She and her mother, maternal grandmother, and brother joined her father, who has been employed as a physics professor at the local state university for more than a year. Dr. Hi speaks fluent English, but the rest of the family understands more English than they can speak.

Yung fell while playing in the parking lot of their apartment complex. Her older brother tripped and fell on her outstretched leg as it extended over the curb. Yung's mother witnessed the accident. When Dr. Hi attempted to move her and was unable, he called for an ambulance.

Yung is admitted to the hospital with a diagnosis of a displaced fracture of the right femur. She will be in Buck's traction for 8 weeks after closed reduction of the fracture and placement of Steinmann's pins. Because Yung Hi will be immobilized for 8 weeks, there is concern that her normal developmental activities will be interrupted. Therefore, the nurse considers the nursing diagnoses Risk for altered growth and development and Altered health maintenance.

(continued)

Besides being skilled in orthopedic nursing, to care for Yung Hi you must understand the concepts of growth and development. Knowing the hallmarks of human maturational periods will enable you to provide comprehensive care. Assessment of growth and development will help you consider a child's physiological, developmental, and psychosocial needs; to identify risk factors; and to prevent complications. Most important, armed with an understanding of growth and development, you can provide holistic care to promote the client's health.

WELL NEWBORN, INFANT, AND TODDLER NURSING DIAGNOSES

Altered Growth and Development: The state in which an individual demonstrates deviations in norms from his/her age group.

Altered Health Maintenance: Inability to identify, manage, and/or seek out help to maintain health.

From North American Nursing Diagnosis Association (1999). NANDA nursing diagnoses: Definitions and classification 1999–2000. Philadelphia: Author.

CONCEPTS OF GROWTH AND DEVELOPMENT

The words growth and development have separate and distinct definitions even though they are often used simultaneously. Human growth and development is a dynamic process and continues through the life span. **Growth** is the physiological development of a living being and is the quantitative (measurable) change seen in the body. It refers to an increase in specific parameters, such as height and weight. Variations in growth occur with each person. It is often sporadic, with rapid growth spurts occurring at several points, such as the prenatal, neonatal, infant, and adolescent stages.

Development is a progression of behavioral changes that involve the acquisition of appropriate cognitive, linguistic, and psychosocial skills. Development is a qualitative change in and refers to increasing competence in behavioral functioning. During each developmental stage, certain goals must be achieved. Attainment of these hallmarks of development indicates whether a child is progressing normally. The following principles are important for you to know about the basic processes of growth and development:

- Human growth and development follows predictable, continuous, and expected sequential patterns that are influenced by genes, environment, and positive or negative factors that are present or absent in a person's life.
- Each stage of development depends on adequate completion of the previous stage and is itself the foundation for the development of new skills.
- Neuromuscular growth and development starts at the head and moves toward the feet, a pattern called **cephalocaudal.** For example, infants first achieve head control and then shoulder and trunk control before learning to sit or walk.

- Skill development starts at the midline of the body and moves outward, a pattern called **proximodistal.** Infants begin to move their arms and then to use their hands together before using each arm separately or beginning to use the fingers to manipulate objects.
- Periods of time when a person has an increased vulnerability to physical, chemical, psychological, or environmental influences are called **critical periods.** Growth or development may stop temporarily or regress during stressful life events.
- Development becomes increasingly differentiated over time, starting with a generalized response and progressing to a skilled specific response. This is called **differentiated development.** For example, a newborn's initial response to a playful stimulus involves the total body, whereas a 3-year-old can respond more specifically with laughter.

Theories of Growth and Development

Stages of physical growth usually correspond to certain developmental changes. A variety of theories propose to explain how a person develops. Three of the major developmental theories are included in this chapter. They are the psychosocial, the cognitive, and the developmental task theories.

Psychosocial Theory

Psychosocial development involves subjective feelings and interpersonal relationships. Erik Erikson described a series of psychosocial stages to outline the emotional and social development of the personality. Each stage defines a task that must be achieved. The resolution of the task may be successful, partial, or unsuccessful. Successful completion or mastery of each of these stages is built on the satisfactory completion of the previous stage. Erikson believed that the greater the task achievement, the healthier the personality of the individual; failure to achieve a task influences the person's ability to achieve the next task (Erikson, 1968). Erikson's theory is useful to nurses, because it describes expected emotional behaviors from birth through later adulthood.

Erikson describes eight major psychosocial crises experienced by people as they progress in their development. The stages reflect both positive and negative aspects of the critical periods every person goes through. Resolution of the conflicts at each stage enables the person to function effectively in society. Newborns to children 3 years of age experience the first two stages, trust versus mistrust and autonomy versus shame and doubt.

The stage of trust versus mistrust occurs from birth to age 1. The most important person for the infant at this stage is the mother or primary caretaker, and the quality of this relationship is extremely important. While building this relationship, an infant receives information through all the senses. **Sensory stimulation** is the activation and exhilaration of the senses. An appropriate amount of sensory stimulation enables the infant to develop trust. If the infant's needs are not met, either through overstimulation or neglect, then some degree of mistrust develops.

The second stage of autonomy versus shame and doubt applies to children from ages 2 to 3. This stage is influenced by the toddler's maturing muscle system, which gives the child a sense of control over his or her body. This mastery enables the toddler to experience a sense of power and, thus, autonomy.

Cognitive Theory

Cognition is characterized by the intellectual process of knowing, which includes perception, judgment, use of language, and memory. **Cognitive development** represents a progression of mental abilities from illogical thinking to logical thinking, from simple to complex problem-solving, and from understanding concrete ideas to understanding abstract ideas.

The theorist best known for exploring cognitive development is Jean Piaget. He described cognitive development as involving the increasing ability to think and reason in a logical manner. Piaget believed that intellectual development is an adaptive process that occurs as a regulatory function of both physiological and intellectual growth.

According to Piaget, a person uses three abilities during cognitive development: assimilation, accommodation, and adaptation. **Assimilation** is the process of learning from new experiences. People acquire knowledge and skills as well as insight into the world around them. **Accommodation** is a process of change or modifying old ways of thinking to fit new situations. This adjustment is possible because new knowledge has been assimilated. **Adaptation,** or coping behavior, is the change that occurs as a result of assimilation and accommodation.

BOX 19–1

HAVIGHURST'S DEVELOPMENTAL TASKS OF INFANCY AND EARLY CHILDHOOD

Learning to take solid foods
Learning to walk
Learning to talk
Learning to control elimination of body wastes
Learning gender differences and sexual modesty
Achieving psychological stability
Forming concepts of social and physical reality
Learning to relate emotionally to others
Learning to distinguish right from wrong and developing a conscience

---

Developmental Task Theory

Robert Havighurst believed that living and growing are based on learning and that people must continuously learn to adjust to the changing society around them. He described these learned behaviors as developmental tasks. A **developmental task** is an important activity that arises at a certain period in life (Box 19–1). Successful achievement of these tasks leads to happiness and success in later tasks, whereas failure leads to unhappiness, societal disapproval, and difficulty with later tasks (Havighurst, 1972).

People progress from birth to death by working their way from one stage of development to the next by solving problems encountered at each stage. Tasks arise mainly from the biological nature of the human, but they can be derived from cultural patterns as well. Thus, lists of developmental tasks will not be the same for all cultures. Infancy and early childhood represent the first two of six life stages, each associated with essential developmental tasks.

Developmental Milestones

Growth and development are evaluated by comparing an individual's characteristics with the range of growth and developmental characteristics expected for a person in the same age group. **Developmental milestones** are the predictable patterns of normal development according to age. This section discusses these growth and development characteristics for newborns, infants, and toddlers (Table 19–1).

Newborns

A **newborn** is a child born within the previous 28 days. Growth and development of the newborn is usually followed intensely and enthusiastically by the child's parents. They may have many questions about the "normalcy" of their baby's behavior. Even so, they are often able to provide you with significant cues to the progression of the child's development.

TABLE 19–1

Developmental Milestones for Newborns, Infants, and Toddlers

Age	Developmental Milestone
0 to birth	• Differentiates between light and dark. • Turns toward direction of sound. • Responds to touch.
1 to 3 months	• Supports upper body with arms when prone. • Raises head and chest. • Brings hand to mouth. • Opens and shuts hands. • Begins hand-eye coordination. • Begins babbling and cooing.
4 to 7 months	• Rolls from stomach to back. • Sits with support and then sits independently. • Finds hidden object. • Babbles, laughs, and squeals. • Performs social play (such as peek-a-boo).
8 to 12 months	• Rocks. • Moves from sitting or crawling to a prone position. • Makes initial walking effort. • Uses pincer grasp. • Mimics gestures. • Shakes, throws, and drops objects. • Drinks from cup. • Responds to verbal cues.
1 to 2 years	• Walks alone. • Climbs. • Scribbles. • Sorts objects. • Shows return of separation anxiety. • Imitates others.
2 to 3 years	• Runs. • Peddles tricycle. • Screws and unscrews jar lids or objects. • Holds writing instrument. • Begins to make circular and horizontal strokes.

GROWTH PARAMETERS

At birth, the average weight for a European-American female is 7.5 pounds (3.4 kg) and, for a male, 7.7 pounds (3.5 kg). Normal weights may range, however, from 5.5 pounds (2.5 kg) to 8.5 pounds (4 kg). Newborns of Asian and Native American descent are somewhat smaller. Because most (70 to 75%) of a newborn's weight is from water, the typical newborn loses 5 to 10% of her weight in the first few days after birth. This weight loss is normal, and newborns usually regain that weight in about 1 week (Pomerance, 1995).

A newborn's length is measured from head to heel (Fig. 19–1A). Average normal lengths range from 19 to 21 inches (48 to 53 cm). Female babies are, on average, smaller than male babies. For the most accurate mea-surement of length, newborns should be placed flat on their backs with at least one leg extended.

At birth, a newborn's head is about one-third the size of an adult's head. Measurement of head circumference is of particular importance in babies to determine the growth rate of the skull and the brain (Fig. 19–1B). The usual newborn head circumference ranges from 12.5 to 14.5 inches (32 to 37 cm). The head circumference should be about 1 inch (2.5 cm) less than the chest circumference. A newborn who deviates from this normal range may have central nervous system anomalies (Pomerance, 1995).

SENSORY DEVELOPMENT

A newborn can smell at birth, as soon as the nose is cleared of mucus and other fluids. Newborns can recognize the smell of their mother's milk and respond to this smell by turning toward the mother.

Familiar sounds are recognizable, and the newborn often turns toward the sound. Neonates with intact hearing will react with a startle to a loud noise, referred to as the *Moro reflex*. Usually they can distinguish between their mother's voice and another woman's voice within a few days.

Newborns can follow large moving objects and blink in response to bright lights. A newborn's pupils respond very slowly, however, and the eyes cannot focus on close objects. Because color vision is not fully developed, newborns prefer to focus on black and white objects, especially geometric shapes and checkerboards.

A neonate's sense of touch is well developed at birth. The baby's positive response to the warmth and security of swaddling, holding, and touching demonstrates the importance of touch for healthy development. The neonate is also sensitive to temperature extremes and pain. Babies cannot isolate the discomfort and react with a generalized response.

MOTOR DEVELOPMENT

The development of the newborn's ability to move and to control the body is called *motor development*. Initially, the newborn has uncoordinated body movement. A neonate's normal motor activity includes involuntary reflexes and turning the head from side to side when in a prone or supine position. As the baby obtains more muscle control, body movements become smoother and more purposeful.

REFLEXES

Reflexes in the newborn are involuntary responses. The presence of these specific reflexes indicates normal nervous system development in the newborn. The natural progression of neural development is cephalocaudal, proximodistal, and general to specific. Also present at birth are the abilities to yawn, stretch, sneeze, burp, and hiccup.

PSYCHOSOCIAL DEVELOPMENT

Psychosocial development in the neonate is initiated with the process of attachment. **Attachment** is the de-

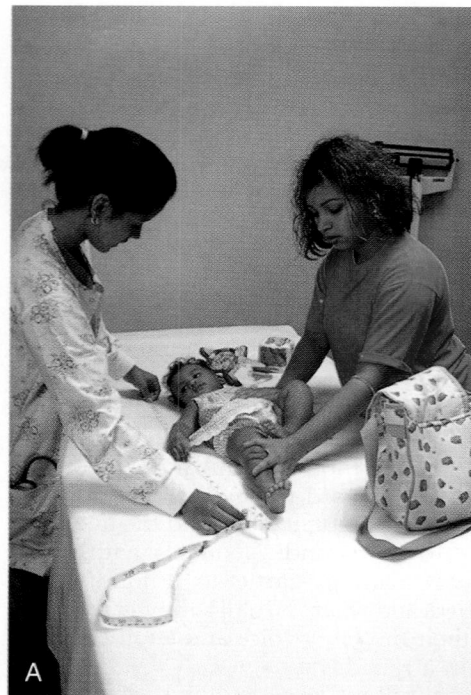
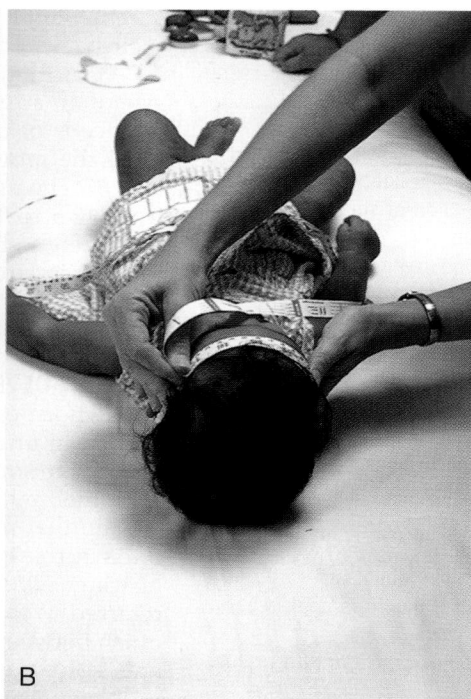

Figure 19–1. Measuring growth. A, Body length; B, head circumference.

velopment of strong ties of affection of an infant with a significant other (mother, father, sibling, caretaker). This is a psychological rather than a biological process. Bowlby (1969) studied the process in which the infant or child forms an attachment by seeking proximity with a specific figure.

Recognizing that attachment occurs both from infant to parent and from parent to infant, researchers developed the concept of mutual bonding through observation of premature infants. **Bonding** is a process of forming an attachment between parent and newborn. While bonding was initially studied as occurring during the first hours after birth, bonding continues to develop during the first year and possibly beyond.

The emotional bond between mother and newborn is developed and sustained through cyclical cues and communication from one to the other (Fig. 19–2). Even at this early stage, newborns attempt to communicate and are consoled by gentle human touch. Crying is the primary means by which newborns make their needs and wants known. Parents are often able to distinguish between different types of cries, such as those of hunger and discomfort.

COGNITIVE DEVELOPMENT
Cognitive development in the neonate is primarily reflexive. However, the newborn reacts socially to caregivers by paying attention to the face or voice and by cuddling when held. The baby is able to interact with the environment by responding to various stimuli, such as touch and sound. The neonate displays displeasure by crying and shows satisfaction by quieting and making soft vocalizations. According

to Piaget, neonates are active participants in learning through their senses. Additionally as motor function progresses from reflexes to purposeful activities, the child rapidly increases interactions with the environment.

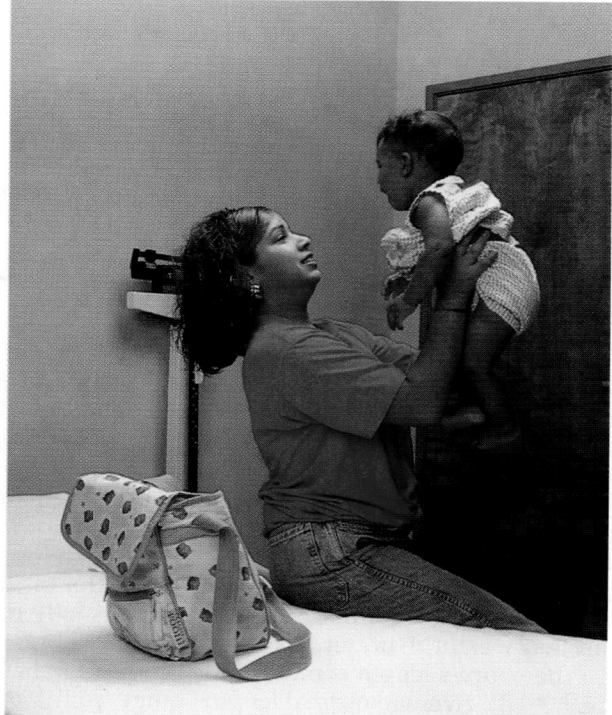

Figure 19–2. The emotional bond between mother and infant is developed and sustained through cyclical cues and communication from one to the other.

Infants

An **infant** is a child from the age of 1 month to the end of 12 months. Infancy is a time of continuous and rapid growth and development. Most parents of infants carefully monitor their baby's height and weight throughout the first year and celebrate the achievements of numerous developmental milestones.

GROWTH PARAMETERS

Height and weight are predictable along a growth curve. An infant usually gains 5 to 7 ounces weekly for about the first 4 to 6 months. By 4 to 7 months the birth weight doubles (Wong & Perry, 1998). By 1 year of age, the normal infant weighs about three times its birth weight. The average male baby weighs 22 pounds (10 kg), and the average female baby weighs 21 pounds (9.5 kg) by the first birthday (Pomerance, 1995).

The rate of increase in height is largely influenced by the baby's size at birth and by nutrition. By the end of the infant's first year, recumbent length has increased 50% since birth, and the average range is 28 to 32 inches. Head growth begins to slow down between 8 and 12 months of age. By 10 months, head and chest circumferences are about the same. Head circumference is usually 18 inches (47 cm) by the end of infancy (Pomerance, 1995). Because the rate of growth for each child differs, these measurements should be compared with the percentile curves on a growth chart.

SENSORY DEVELOPMENT

The senses of smell and taste continue to develop throughout the first year. Many new smells and tastes are introduced with the taking of solid foods at 4 to 6 months of age. With each new food experience, the infant begins to show discrimination toward favorite tastes and smells.

Eyes begin to focus and fixate at 4 months. The infant can recognize familiar objects and follow moving ones. Most 9-month-old babies can recognize facial characteristics and often smile in response to a familiar face. By the end of the first year, depth perception has developed, and the infant will be able to recognize a change in level, such as the start and finish of a step or the edge of a bed.

At about 5 months, the infant will pause while feeding to listen to the mother's voice. A 9-month-old baby will locate the source of sounds and be able to recognize familiar sounds or voices. By 1 year of age, the infant listens to sounds, begins to distinguish words, and can respond to simple commands.

Touch remains important. Infants continue to demonstrate positive responses to the security of being held and cuddled. Babies are also positively stimulated by touching different textured fabrics and object shapes. Exploration through touch and placing items in the mouth to further explore them begins at 3 months of age and may last through toddlerhood.

MOTOR DEVELOPMENT

From 1 to 3 months of age, the infant attains additional physical skills and becomes more neurologically so-

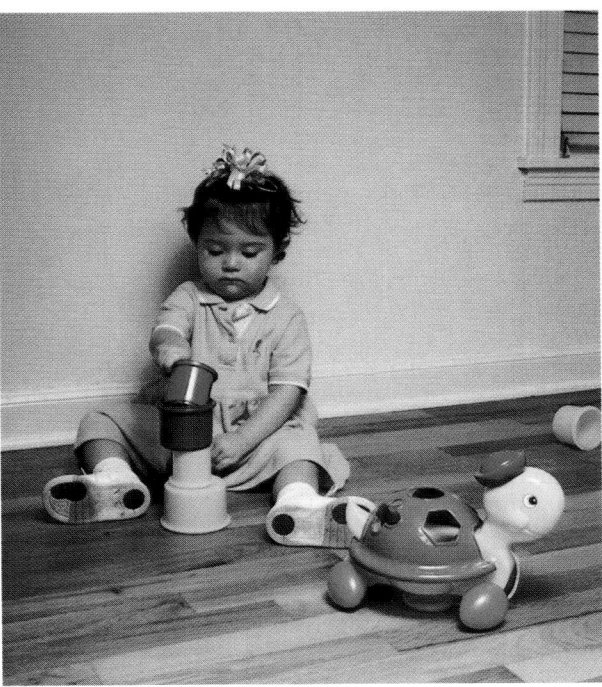

Figure 19–3. With development of the pincer grasp, the infant takes great pleasure in stacking objects and putting objects into containers and removing them.

phisticated. In the prone position, the infant can raise her head and chest and support her upper body with her arms. By 4 to 7 months, the infant can roll from her stomach to her back and vice versa. By 5 months, an infant can sit with support. By the end of 7 months, most infants can sit without support.

From 8 to 12 months of age, infants make great developmental strides. They can get up on their hands and knees and rock back and forth on both knees. Crawling begins by the 10th month. Infants of this age can move from a sitting to a crawling to a prone position. The infant makes her first efforts toward walking, such as pulling to stand, standing briefly with support, cruising along furniture, and walking two to three steps unassisted. The pincer grasp is developed, and the infant takes great pleasure in stacking objects, putting objects into containers, and removing them (Fig. 19–3). Parents can encourage the development of this skill by offering items that promote grasping, such as cereal bits.

REFLEXES

As the infant develops neurologically, the primitive or neonatal reflexes begin to disappear. Later infant reflexes develop at 3 months of age, beginning with the Landau reflex (lifts both head and legs when suspended prone with support under abdomen).

PSYCHOSOCIAL DEVELOPMENT

Psychologically, the infant begins to communicate through body language. There are attempts to imitate some facial expressions and movements, such as a social smile, by the end of the second month. The

4-month-old infant enjoys interacting with people and will vocalize displeasure when left alone. Infants mimic gestures, babble with inflection, say "mama" and "dada," and try to imitate other words by about 6 months of age. The infant responds to simple verbal cues and uses simple gestures, such as shaking the head "no" and waving "bye-bye." Smiling, laughing, waving, and reaching out to others are examples of purposeful interactive social behavior.

Self-esteem develops through trust and increasing control of the body. Trust develops when the parent or caregiver can be counted on to provide essential needs. However, by 6 to 9 months the infant begins to have a greater awareness of self as separate from mother or father. *Separation anxiety* emerges as crying when the infant is separated from parents or approached by strangers. Thus, self-esteem requires the development of a sense of control.

COGNITIVE DEVELOPMENT

Infants learn about their world through their activities. They anticipate feeding times and going "bye-bye." They become excited when they see their parents. They have an increasing ability to concentrate and to recognize and respond to a familiar environment or a friend of the family.

Rudimentary language skills are developing. Babies begin to coo and make sounds soon after birth, and by 12 months they can convey their wishes through several key words. Use of syllable repetition (ma-ma, da-da), early phonetic expression (babbling), and imitation of intonations and sounds are characteristic of the language development of infants.

Piaget's first stage of cognitive development, the sensorimotor stage, has six substages. The first substage is reflexive. The second substage is the primary circular stage and spans the 1-month to 4-month range. During this time, the infant discovers enjoyment of random behaviors, such as sucking a thumb, and repeats them. Piaget's third substage, the secondary circular stage, is demonstrated by the 4- to 8-month-old when she relates her own behavior to change in the environment, such as shaking a rattle to hear the sound.

By 8 to 12 months, an infant can coordinate more than one thought pattern at a time to reach a goal, such as repeatedly throwing an object on the floor. This substage is termed coordination of secondary schemes. Infants in this substage are also beginning to develop a sense of object permanence. **Object permanence** is the awareness that unseen objects do not disappear and is evidenced by the infant searching for an object that has been moved out of sight.

Toddlers

A **toddler** is a child ages 1 to 3 years. The term toddler refers to the pattern of locomotion of children in this age group. Toddlers walk with their feet several inches apart and their arms held out to maintain balance. The ability to walk is an important developmental milestone for toddlers. Toddlers move toward the increas-ing independence of childhood, leaving the dependency of infancy behind.

GROWTH PARAMETERS

The most noticeable physical change during the toddler years occurs as head growth slows down and the relatively short legs and trunk of an infant begin to lengthen. Baby fat begins to decrease. The abdomen continues to be prominent, as it was in infancy, but appetite changes. Physiological growth and development continues steadily, but the pace of the gains is considerably slower than during infancy. Weight gain is about four pounds (2 kg) yearly, with height increases averaging 2.2 inches (6 cm) yearly. By age 2, the female toddler will be about 34 inches (86.4 cm) tall and weigh 27 pounds (12.2 kg). Males will average 34 inches (86.4 cm) and almost 28 pounds (12.9 kg) by age 2 (Pomerance, 1995).

SENSORY DEVELOPMENT

All of the senses continue to develop and become more associated with each other during the toddler stage. Toddlers use all of their senses to explore their environment. Walking enhances their ability to explore without relying on others. Vision is fairly well established by ages 1 and 2. Visual acuity is about 20/40. The ability to focus on near and far objects is fairly well developed by 18 months and continues to develop with age. Hearing is at adult levels by age 3.

The toddler's taste buds are sensitive to the natural flavors of food, and taste preferences begin to emerge. She is less likely to try a new food if the food has an unfamiliar appearance, smell, texture, or taste. Touch is also a very important sense to the toddler. A distressed toddler often uses tactile sensations as a self-comforting technique, such as stroking the satin ribbon on a favorite stuffed animal.

MOTOR DEVELOPMENT

Fine muscle coordination (fine motor) and large muscle activity (gross motor) improve during toddler-hood. At 18 months of age, a toddler can pick up beads and put them in a cup. She can also hold a spoon and a cup and walk up stairs with assistance. By age 3, fine motor skills have continued to improve and include turning a book one page at a time, screwing and unscrewing objects, turning handles, and making vertical, circular, and horizontal strokes with a writing instrument. Gross motor skills of the 3-year-old include climbing, walking up and down stairs unassisted, running easily, bending over without falling, peddling a tricycle, and kicking a ball.

Remember that Yung Hi is in the toddler stage of her growth and development. She had been running and playing with her brother when the accident occurred. What type of activities will Yung be able to accomplish while in traction? How can you help her maintain the developmental milestones she has already achieved?

REFLEXES

Neural growth continues during the toddler years, with additional myelinization and cortical brain development. Neurological growth and musculoskeletal development allow the toddler to perform more complex physical tasks. The primitive reflexes of infancy must disappear before voluntary behaviors appear. For example, children do not walk until the involuntary stepping reflex disappears. By age 3, deep tendon reflexes (biceps, triceps, patellar, and Achilles) are well developed.

PSYCHOSOCIAL DEVELOPMENT

Havighurst's developmental task during toddlerhood shows the child learning to control the elimination of urine and feces (toilet training), learning gender differences, forming concepts, learning language, and distinguishing right from wrong. According to Erikson, toddlers enter the stage of autonomy versus shame and doubt. Independence increases and is demonstrated by the toddler's self-feeding, walking, talking, and toileting. Children who do not feel autonomous may be reluctant to explore and be fearful of activities and people. A major developmental gain for this age is the achievement of a sense of independence and autonomy.

The struggle between choosing independence over dependence is a frustrating decision for the toddler. Toddlers tolerate their parents being out of sight in a comfortable setting and revel in their independence, but the return of separation anxiety can be a significant problem if the settings or people are unfamiliar. The fear of abandonment is great during early toddler years. Separation anxiety can be very traumatic for both parents and children and is frequent during these years.

Toddlers also begin to develop their sense of autonomy by asserting themselves with frequent use of the word "no." It may be used to refuse a request, to demonstrate lack of understanding, or to practice a word that the child notices has a dramatic effect on others. They can become very negative, practicing the power of "no" every day for months.

Temper tantrums usually make their appearance at about age 2. Tantrums stem from the child's striving for power and control and the sudden loss of both. There are so many activities toddlers want and struggle to do but are not developmentally ready to perform.

Toddlers enjoy playing near others, but frequently do not share objects or engage in close interactive activities with other children. In *parallel play,* toddlers play beside but not with their friends. The types of play that appeal to toddlers are those that allow them to use large muscles, those that include repetitive and rhythmic motions, and those involving language. Play is a natural way to enhance the toddler's physical and psychosocial development.

Self-concept and body image are also part of psychosocial development. Toddlers develop their sense of self-esteem not only through others' responses to them but also through pleasure in their accomplishments. Mastering toilet training, gaining motor skills, and making choices all enhance a toddler's self-confidence. Sexuality is another aspect of toddler development. Toddlers begin to develop some gender-based expectations, can describe themselves as a girl or a boy, and can accurately apply gender labels to those around them.

COGNITIVE DEVELOPMENT

According to Piaget, the toddler completes the sensorimotor phase and starts the preoperational stage. By completing the sensorimotor phase, the toddler moves from solving problems by trial and error to using mental processing. For example, a toddler will not handle a toy immediately to see how it works but will look at it carefully to think about how it works. The toddler is becoming more differentiated from the environment. She will search for a hidden object where she last saw it, showing her increasingly thorough understanding of object permanence.

By the end of the second year, the toddler enters the first part of the preoperational stage with *preconceptual thinking.* This stage is characterized by the beginning use of symbols, mental imagery, and increased language skills. A toddler continues to be very concrete and egocentric in thinking, and her logic is the source of many miscommunications between parent and child.

During this time, language skills increase tremendously. The toddler engages in collective monologues by herself or with a group of children. The understanding of language increases. Toddlers can follow a two- or three-word command and can understand many sentences. The understanding of physical relationships begins with concepts, such as "on," "in," and "under." A 3-year-old can say her name, age, and gender and use four- to five-word sentences. Strangers are beginning to understand what the toddler is trying to say. The child at this age can recognize all common objects and pictures.

Yung cries occasionally and remains nonverbal with the nurses. She speaks Korean with her parents and clings to her mother. Yung's father has been attempting to explain the traction and hospital room to his wife and child. This may be a good time to have the father translate and assess for developmental data that will help you determine how to make Yung's long stay less traumatic.

FACTORS AFFECTING GROWTH AND DEVELOPMENT

Many factors, such as environment, socioeconomic status, nutrition, and physiological status, influence a newborn's growth and development. The interaction of these factors greatly affects how a person responds to everyday situations. These factors also influence the choices a person makes regarding health care behaviors.

Environmental Factors

Family dynamics, community structure, cultural and religious beliefs, and educational opportunities are all part of the environment in which the infant and child interact.

Family Dynamics

The family has long been seen as an essential environment for healthy growth and development. Family has a crucial influence on the formation of a child's identity and feelings of self-esteem (Friedman, 1998). A child's ability to feel secure about self and relate to others depends on how well her identity is established and how supportive the family members are of the child.

Community Structure

Community structure can help or hinder the child's growth and development. The community should be a safe place for the child to play, worship, and go to school. The family's community network includes all those persons, activities, and institutions that have the potential to support, harm, or drain energy from the family and therefore affect the child.

Culture and Religion

Culture influences everything people do, produce, know, and believe in as they grow and develop as members of social groups. Characteristics of culture are not instinctual; they are passed from one generation to another through a complicated process of social interaction. Through this socialization, children learn the intellectual, physical, and social skills needed to function in their society (Erikson, 1963). As children become familiar with the patterns of behavior associated with their culture, they also develop distinctive personalities, thoughts, and feelings, as suggested in the accompanying Cross-Cultural Care chart.

Religious development refers to the acceptance of specific beliefs, values, rules of conduct, and rituals. Religious values may also be part of the cultural values of groups that have one dominant religion. These beliefs can influence lifestyle, attitudes, and feelings about health and wellness activities in the family. Toddlers may be aware of some religious practices and learn to recognize and name the symbols of the family's religion, develop a concrete idea of their family's reverence for a Supreme Being, and distinguish good behavior from bad behavior.

Educational Opportunities

Growth and development are affected by the type and amount of stimuli offered to an infant and toddler. The child's developmental level and cognitive abilities will determine the concepts the child can learn. Short attention spans warrant presenting information in small bits, with frequent reinforcement and opportunities for doing rather than just listening. For the infant, a variety of sensory stimuli, such as colorful mobiles, musical toys, soft stuffed toys, and frequent parent-child play, encourages learning by interacting with the environment. For the toddler, the family promotes language development, teaches toileting skills, and encourages development of cognitive and intellectual skills by providing a variety of age-appropriate experiences and stimuli.

Socioeconomic Factors

Socioeconomic factors, such as income, educational level, and single parenthood, influence the growth and development of children. A child who grows up in an economically deprived home may have impairments in physical, psychosocial, and cognitive development. Low-income parents also may not have the resources to obtain appropriate health care for their child. Failure to obtain immunizations and treatments leaves the child open to increased illnesses and complications.

Poorly educated parents may be less likely to know about or take preventive measures to promote wellness and avoid injuries, accidents, or disease. Lack of parental knowledge about a child's developmental needs and the importance of age-appropriate stimulation to promote growth and development may cause developmental delays. Inadequate educational resources can influence parenting skills, finances, and basic knowledge of a child's developmental needs.

A single-parent family consists of one parent, either father or mother, and one or more children. Problems associated with single-parent families include finances, child care, and loneliness. Families with infants and toddlers have a major task of providing a safe, secure, and loving environment, as well as providing varied stimulation for normal growth and development. A single parent may have difficulty meeting all these needs because of a greater emphasis on work to acquire the physical necessities of life.

Nutritional Factors

Nutritional concerns for the child begin during pregnancy and continue after birth, when the parents decide what method of feeding to choose. Human milk is the most desirable for the first 12 months of life. Breast milk has several benefits over commercially prepared formulas:

- It offers immunologic benefits.
- It is more easily digested because of smaller curds than those in formula.
- It enhances absorption of fat and calcium.

In addition, breast milk is economical and readily available to the baby. If the parents choose not to breast-feed, commercially prepared iron-fortified formulas are available. Special formulas are also available for infants with malabsorption problems, hypersensitivity to protein, or lactose intolerance.

Solid foods are introduced gradually, beginning at about 4 months. Rice cereal is most often tried first, because it has the fewest allergic responses. It is usually mixed with formula or expressed breast milk. Iron-fortified cereals are usually recommended by 6 months. After that, strained, puréed infant foods are gradually added, one at a time, usually one every 5 days. As each new food is added to the infant's diet, the parent should observe for signs of intolerance or allergy.

The toddlers' growth rate slows, decreasing slightly the need for calories, fluids, and protein. Most tod-

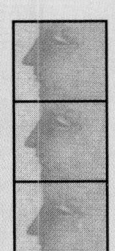

CROSS-CULTURAL CARE
CARING FOR A KOREAN TODDLER

Yung Hi, the young client presented in this chapter, and her family are Korean and new to the United States. Koreans, like many Asian peoples, are of Mongolian-Tungus descent. Although each person is unique, Korean people are generally characterized as being generous, kind, and resourceful. The following behaviors also have been identified as culturally characteristic and valued by Korean people:

- Putting the family's welfare ahead of the individual
- Viewing infants and young children as passive and dependent
- Having a strong sense of self-respect and self-control
- Maintaining a stoic demeanor and offering few complaints
- Being polite by giving a person the response she is expecting
- Avoiding physical contact
- Upholding men as authority figures, with women expected to be obedient
- Believing that education is important
- Viewing health as a balance between positive and negative energy forces (yin and yang)

Yung's nurse, Wanda, works with and cares for the parents, too. See if you can recognize cultural sensitivity to the Hi family's cultural values:

Wanda: [Stops at the foot of the bed, staying a distance away from parents] Good afternoon, Yung. I see you are drawing a picture. I really like the colors you picked! *[Yung smiles shyly with head held down; stops drawing]* Hello, Dr. Hi and Mrs. Hi. I'm glad you are both here. I would like to discuss something with you.

Dr. Hi: How are you? What would you like to tell us? *[Stands and moves behind his chair, then turns to wife and translates]*

Wanda: Dr. Rowen has prescribed play therapy for Yung. It will help her stay as mentally and physically healthy as possible for her age while she is in the hospital. A therapist should be in this afternoon to begin

with Yung. Will you be here for the next hour? Jill, the therapist, is coming at 4:30.

Dr. Hi: [Finishes translating to his wife] The doctor ordered this for our daughter. We will be here.

Wanda: I'm very glad you can stay. Mrs. Hi, I've seen you play a finger game with Yung that has a very sweet song with it. That type of activity is what the therapist will be doing, playing and helping Yung use her new talking skills and finger movements. We want her to be as active in mind and body as she possibly can during the time she's in traction. Does Yung have a favorite game or song that we could share with the therapist when she comes? *[Touches Yung's feet and assesses pedal pulses]*

Dr. Hi: Are her feet okay? Why do you touch them?

Wanda: I'm sorry, I should have told you first what I was going to do. I'm making sure her leg is healing and the circulation is the same in the hurt leg as in the good leg.

Dr. Hi: Okay . . . *[Dr. Hi speaks a few words to his wife and then translates her response]* To answer what you asked, Yung likes to sing and pretend to be a mother to her stuffed animal rabbit. My wife will work with Yung to learn the new playthings the therapist will introduce.

Critical Thinking Questions

- Did Dr. Hi and his wife demonstrate any behavior that may be considered characteristic of Koreans?
- What did Wanda do that was culturally sensitive or insensitive while discussing the client's care with the parents?
- Do you think Wanda has a more significant cultural barrier to overcome because of Mrs. Hi's and Yung's inability to speak English?

Reference

Leininger, M. (1991). *Culture care diversity and universality: A theory of nursing.* New York: National League for Nursing Press.

dlers are eating the same food prepared for the family and using a cup.

Physiological Factors

Most children grow and develop without problems. However, a variety of physiological factors may influence a child's growth and development. One of the most difficult—and most costly—stems from preterm birth, as discussed in The Cost of Care chart. With a term birth, some problems may be apparent immediately, whereas others will become evident

during the first months or years of a child's life. These latter problems may be caused by a defect in the child's genes or acquired during gestation, birth, or shortly after birth because of infection, failure to thrive, or abuse.

Birth Defects and Genetic Disorders

Birth defects, also called congenital anomalies, are abnormalities present at birth. The term typically refers to structural problems inherited genetically or caused during gestation, or the birth process.

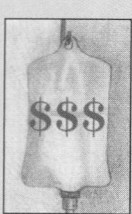

THE COST OF CARE
PRETERM INFANTS

Of the billions of dollars spent each year on health care in the United States, about one-third goes to caring for preterm infants during their first year of life. Nurses are studying nursing costs for preterm infants receiving conventional care compared with those receiving developmental care.

Developmental care focuses on light and noise management, coordination of interventions to minimize sleep interruptions, and positioning and bundling of the infant to promote self-regulation. When compared with 60 preterm infants who received conventional care, the 60 who received developmental care from nurses and developmental care specialists showed improved physiological stability and fewer days in the neonatal intensive care unit.

Also, the group that received developmental care moved from the intensive care unit to a transitional unit earlier than the group that received conventional care. The former group's nursing intensity needs were also lower than those of the latter group. The study's authors concluded that receiving developmental care rather than conventional care led to an average cost savings of $4,340 per infant during the first 35 days of life or less.

Current and future health care trends create many challenges for nurses. Developmental care for all age groups is an approach that nurses may find raises quality while lowering cost. In the 21st century, nurses are in a position to emerge as leaders in providing cost-effective, needs-based, health care services aimed at improving the health of communities.

Reference

Petryshen, P., Stevens, B., Hawkins, J., & Stewart, M. (1997). Comparing nursing costs for preterm infants receiving conventional versus developmental care. *Nursing Economics, 15*(3), 138–145, 150.

The *cerebral palsies* are an example of a birth defect. They are a group of disorders of posture and movement caused by a nonprogressive lesion of the brain (Liptak, Miller, and Couch, 1997, p 432). The conditions range from involving a single limb to producing total disability and are classified from an event during pregnancy, at birth, or shortly after birth. Postnatal factors (after 28 days) are thought to cause 10% of cases. These factors include infections, asphyxia, and accidental injuries. Cerebral palsy occurs in about 2 to 2.5 cases per 1,000 live births. The child may or may not be mentally retarded in addition to having physical problems (Liptak Miller, and Couch, 1997).

The two most common musculoskeletal birth defects are *clubfoot* and *congenital hip dysplasia.* Clubfoot is a deformity not only of the foot but also of the entire lower leg. Mild forms of clubfoot result from improper positioning in the uterus (Thompson, 1995).

Congenital hip dysplasia is dislocation of the hips. The head of the femur is partially or completely displaced from the acetabulum (hip socket). A special harness is used to keep the hips abducted and allow the head of the femur to remain in the socket. Over time, this constant pressure enlarges and deepens the acetabulum, thus correcting the dislocation (Thompson, 1995).

A **teratogen** is an agent or influence that causes physical defects in the developing fetus. A variety of drugs, diseases, and irradiation are teratogens. Congenital infections, such as syphilis and rubella, are teratogenic. The neonate born to a mother who smokes cigarettes, drinks alcohol, or uses drugs is of special concern. These teratogens may cause developmental deficits as well as complications during birth. Nicotine doubles the risk of low birth weight and may be a factor in the development of cleft palate. Fetal alcohol syndrome in the neonate is believed to be a leading cause of birth defects, including growth retardation, developmental delay, and impaired intellectual ability. Genetic disorders occur in about 5% of live births (Thompson, 1995).

Chromosomal abnormalities are defects in the structures called chromosomes, which carry genetic material. Entire chromosomes or large segments may be missing, duplicated, or otherwise altered. *Down's syndrome* is one of the most common chromosomal abnormalities. These children have mental retardation, a protruding tongue, a flat nasal bridge, small ears, short digits, and other deformities.

Phenylketonuria is a genetic disorder of amino acid metabolism in which phenylalanine cannot be converted to tyrosine because of a deficiency of the enzyme phenylalanine hydroxylase. If undetected, phenylketonuria results in severe, irreversible mental retardation. A simple blood test required by all states is performed to detect this disorder. Treatment is through dietary management (a low-phenylalanine, tyrosine-enriched diet) and frequent monitoring of serum phenylalanine concentration (Thompson, 1995).

Infection and Communicable Disease

Common sites of infections in infants include the ears, upper respiratory tract, and gastrointestinal tract. More than 75% of children have at least one episode of *otitis media,* an infection and inflammation of the middle ear. With antibiotic treatment, most of these cases resolve, but others progress to chronic hearing loss that requires intervention (Weiss, Chute, and Parisier, 1997).

A*ction* A*lert!*
When a child fails to startle at loud noises, does not always respond when called, or has delayed or difficult understanding of speech, there is a probability of a hearing deficit in one or both ears.

Infants who are not immunized or who are incompletely immunized are at risk for the acute illnesses and long-term complications of childhood communicable diseases. During the toddler period, immunizations continue to be an important aspect of health protection and maintenance.

Acquired immunodeficiency syndrome (AIDS) is a communicable disease caused by the human immunodeficiency virus, type 1 (HIV-1). Up to 2,000 HIV-infected infants are born in the United States each year. Perinatal transmission, from infected mothers to their infants via the placenta, is the primary mode of transmission, although not all babies born of infected mothers have the disease. From 7 to 40% of infants born to HIV-positive mothers become infected. Half of these infected infants, if untreated, develop AIDS in the first months of life and die soon thereafter. The other half remain relatively well during infancy but gradually become chronically ill during childhood (Maldonado, 1997).

Failure to Thrive

Failure to thrive is a severe slowing of growth and development resulting from conditions that interfere with normal metabolism, appetite, and activity (Thompson, 1995). Failure to thrive is thought to be caused by maladaptive parent-child interaction, such as when the child receives inadequate nutrition because of the parents' lack of knowledge or concern. It also relates to the parents' inability or unwillingness to provide for the child's emotional needs. Identification of an infant who fails to thrive is based on careful observation and documentation of inconsistent growth patterns and the ruling out of underlying physical causes.

Child Abuse

Abuse of children includes physical abuse, physical neglect, sexual abuse, and emotional maltreatment. Most child abuse begins in infancy. All categories of child abuse endanger the child's physical and emotional health and development. Each state has its own laws related to the various categories of child abuse. Nurses in all states must report known or suspected child abuse (Greipp, 1997).

Physical abuse typically occurs when a parent or caregiver becomes frustrated or angry. In these instances, the injury commonly results from shaking, striking, or throwing the child. Physical injury can also represent intentional, deliberate assault, such as burning, biting, cutting, twisting limbs, or torturing.

Physical neglect refers to maltreatment that can harm or threaten harm to a child's health or welfare. Neglect includes such dangers as intentional failure to provide adequate nutrition, clothing, shelter, or medical care. A key factor in neglect is the extreme or persistent presence of these conditions in the child's home (Dubowitz and Finkel, 1997).

Sexual abuse is defined as acts of sexual assault, sexual exploitation of minors, or both. Sexual assault includes rape, incest, sodomy, oral copulation, and penetration of the genital or anal opening by a foreign object. Sexual exploitation includes activities such as pornography that depicts children.

There are two forms of emotional maltreatment: emotional abuse and emotional deprivation. Emotional abuse is characterized by excessive and distorted parental attitudes and actions that lead to emotional and behavioral problems. Parents can emotionally abuse their children by subjecting them to unpredictable responses, double messages, and verbal insults such as belittling, terrorizing, or blaming. Emotional deprivation occurs when parents ignore or reject their child for any number of reasons, including drug use, personal problems, psychiatric disturbances, or other preoccupying situations (Thompson, 1995).

Abuse occurs in all levels of society. Certain factors have been associated with increased potential for abusive behavior:

- Parents under stress from unemployment, marital problems, or substance abuse
- Lack of knowledge about parenting and childhood development
- Children who cry frequently, who wet the bed, or who have physical, emotional, or cognitive disabilities

Action **A**lert!
A child who has repeated or unreported injuries may be a victim of child abuse.

ASSESSMENT

Assessment of the physical, cognitive, and psychosocial capabilities of the neonate, infant, and toddler is routinely completed at well-baby visits to the physician or advanced practice nurse. The purpose of the well-baby examination is health promotion and disease prevention.

General Assessment of Growth and Development

Infants are usually assessed at least six times during the first year. Usually, this assessment takes place at 2 weeks, 2 months, 4 months, 6 months, 9 months, and 12 months. Toddlers are seen at 15 months, 18 months, 24 months, and 36 months. Components of the well-baby examination include the health history and the physical examination.

Health History

Perform a health history in a setting conducive to interaction with the child and the parents, such as a brightly lit room with comfortable chairs and toys. A short introduction and explanation of what will occur during the visit make the parents and child feel at ease. When appropriate, include the child in the inter-

BOX 19–2

EXAMPLE OF HEALTH HISTORY QUESTIONS

- *Reason for contact:* Why did the child come to the health care provider? Was it for a health maintenance visit or complaint of illness?
- *Present illness, chief concern:* What are the signs and associated symptoms? What makes them better or worse? Which over-the-counter drugs were taken? How long did the symptoms persist? What was done for the problem?
- *Family history:* What is the health status of siblings, parents, and grandparents? Are there significant illnesses or genetic problems in the family? Any heart, kidney, or congenital diseases? Does anyone in the family have seizures, mental retardation, or mental illness? Is there a family history of tuberculosis, diabetes, or sexually transmitted disease? Do allergies run in the family? If they do, inquire further about specific symptoms.
- *Prenatal and childbirth history:* Were there any medical, surgical, or pregnancy problems? Has the mother had any miscarriages or stillbirths? Ask the mother about the pregnancy with this child. Did she use cigarettes, alcohol, or drugs while pregnant? If so, how much?

Was this pregnancy planned? What was the labor like? How long was it? Were there any complications? What type of analgesia or anesthesia was used?
- *Neonatal history:* Were there any unusual circumstances during the newborn period? When did the baby sleep through the night? Was the baby unusually fussy? At what time of the day was the baby most fretful?
- *Social history:* What is the home situation like? Who are the significant others in the child's life? In what activities is the child engaged? Does the child attend day care? How does the child like it?
- *Nutritional history:* What type of infant feeding is or was being done? What is a typical menu for 24 hours? What foods does the child like or dislike? Are there any food allergies?
- *Developmental history:* Were typical developmental milestones achieved? When did they occur? Were there any significant developmental delays?
- *Immunization history:* What immunizations were given? Do they need to be updated? Were there any untoward reactions?

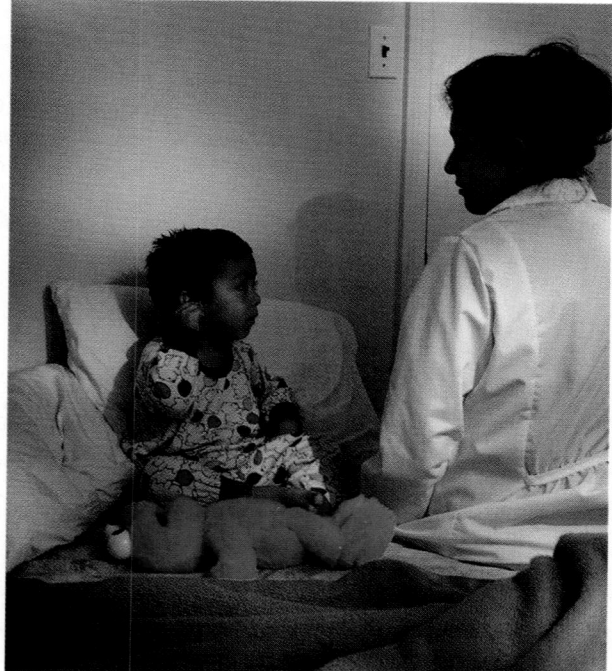

Figure 19–4. During the history and physical examination, an older toddler can sometimes provide helpful information. This toddler tells the home care nurse "where it hurts."

view. Older toddlers can sometimes give helpful information during the history and physical examination, such as pointing to "where it hurts" (Fig. 19–4).

A comprehensive health history includes many components (Box 19–2). Typically, the health care provider obtains a complete history during the initial health care visit and updates it on subsequent visits. For an ill child, the history focuses on the current complaint. Close the health history with a review of systems.

Physical Examination

Before beginning the physical examination, make sure the child is warm and comfortable. Make adjustments for the child's age. For example, when examining an infant, instead of proceeding from head to toe, you may need to begin with the heart rate to avoid difficulty counting if the baby should start to cry. Assess the child's general appearance. Determine the child's body build, size, alertness, and activity level. Obtain vital signs, height, and weight. Proceed to examine each body system thoroughly and accurately, using inspection, palpation, percussion, and auscultation.

GROWTH

Instruments used to assess growth include a tape measure, a height marker, and a scale. Use a tape measure to obtain height (or length) and head circumference. At age 3, measure the child's standing height.

Weigh an infant or small child without clothing on a hygienic paper liner, because diaper weights can vary by 10% or more. By age 3, the child, dressed only in underpants, should be weighed on a standing scale. Scales used for weighing children may be self-adjusting, or they may need to be balanced before each use.

Measure an infant's head circumference until she reaches age 1. Place the measuring tape around the largest circumference of the head, just above the eyebrows and the posterior prominence of the occiput. The tape should remain horizontal from front to back.

Compare the child's height and weight with growth charts to detect risks from slow or accelerated growth. Initial measurements are done immediately after birth and compared with a graph of the relationship between gestational age in weeks and birth weight to determine if the newborn is average, small, or large for gestational age. During frequent health visits from newborn through toddler stage, the relationships between height and weight continue to be measured and recorded on charts to diagnose any disorders related to physical, emotional, environmental, or social deficiencies.

DEVELOPMENT

The simplest and most efficient method of assessing developmental milestones is to obtain a developmental history. Ask parents to recall when developmental events occurred in their child's life.

Various methods and instruments are available to ascertain developmental milestones in children. Monitor development using valid, reliable tests that have a developmental focus, such as developmental screening tests.

Developmental Screening Tests

Screening is a method of employing a test to identify children who appear healthy but who may have an increased risk of significant problems. Good screening tests are easy to use, accurate, and predictive. Screening tests are not diagnostic in themselves but point the way to further testing to determine a diagnosis. A number of screening tests can be used on children, beginning with the first few days of life and continuing into adolescence. Three such tests are described as follows.

Neonatal Perception Inventories

These tests measure maternal perceptions of the newborn. They may be used as a screening instrument for infants at high risk for psychosocial disorders in the mother-infant relationship. The mother rates the "average baby" on factors such as feeding, crying, and sleeping. Then she rates her own infant. When a mother compares her infant unfavorably with the average baby, the infant is considered to have a high risk for impairment in the mother-infant relationship. This leads to a potential disruption of attachment in later months (Overby, 1996).

Denver Developmental Screening Test

This test detects developmental delays by evaluating four skill areas: gross motor skills, fine motor–adaptive skills, language skills, and personal-social skills. It indicates normal age ranges for developmental tasks and, depending on the child's performance, can identify potential problems and the need for a more in-depth examination (Bradshaw, 1982).

Brazelton Neonatal Behavioral Assessment Scale

This test was developed to assess the social and interactive behavior of newborn infants. The instrument is composed of reflex items, behavioral response items, ratings of infant states during the examination, infant interactive attractiveness, the need for stimulation, intervening variables during the examination, and a description of self-quieting activities. The text can be used as a teaching tool to point out to parents the unique characteristics and responses of their newborn, thereby enhancing parental interaction (Walker, 1982).

Focused Assessment for Altered Growth and Development

Assessment of growth and development is a routine part of a well-child assessment in the first 3 years after birth. Children who experience alterations in growth or development are at risk. Focused assessment for altered growth and development occurs when you identify risk factors and diagnostic cues.

Children who have chronic illnesses, unstable family lives, teenage mothers, or multiple caregivers are at risk for altered growth and development. If you practice in a hospital, you will know that a child who is withdrawn or whose behavior is inappropriate for her age may be reacting to the hospital or may have a larger developmental problem. During the child's health maintenance visit in the clinic, you can pick up cues by listening to the parent's description of the child and by observing the child's behavior.

Defining Characteristics

The defining characteristics related to the nursing diagnosis *Altered growth and development* are observed behaviors that indicate that the individual is experiencing an alteration in growth and development. They include the following:

- Delay or difficulty in performing skills (motor, social, or expressive) typical of the child's age group
- Altered physical growth (weight or height)
- Inability to perform self-care or self-control activities appropriate for the child's age

Related Factors

Related factors for *Altered growth and development* can be divided into two categories: those of the parent and the child. You decide whether the problem of *Altered growth and development* can best be solved by working directly with the child or with the parent. Parenting style and parenting skills are basic related factors for *Altered growth and development*. Physiological considerations should be considered if a disability or chronic disease is present. The care plan would then include modifications that take the disability into account. Below are characteristics of the child and of the parent that may be related factors associated with a child's altered growth and development. Characteristics of a child include the following:

- Environmental and stimulation deficiencies
- Prescribed dependence
- Separation from significant others
- Effects of physical disability
- Prematurity

Characteristics of a parent or caregiver include the following:

- Disadvantaged social environment
- Poor support system
- Inadequate caretaking
- Indifference
- Inconsistent responsiveness
- Multiple caregivers

Upon assessment of Yung Hi, you see many of the related factors characteristic of a child with *Altered growth and development*. Yung is a toddler in a private room and is on complete bedrest, with 8 weeks of traction to endure. She must depend totally on others. She is separated from her home and usual routine. Yung's physical disability limits her level of activity, and she cannot speak English. Her mother spends most of the day with her; however, when her father comes to visit in the evenings, he takes Yung's mother home with him. Have you determined any other related factors?

Focused Assessment for Altered Health Maintenance

The nursing diagnosis *Altered health maintenance* refers to an inability to identify, manage, and/or seek out help to maintain health. It is a state in which a person experiences, or is at risk of experiencing, a disruption in wellness from an unhealthy lifestyle. An alteration in health maintenance is almost never under the control of infants or toddlers; therefore, you will need to assess the parent or family.

Defining Characteristics

Defining characteristics for *Altered health maintenance* appropriate to the adult caring for an infant or toddler include demonstration of an unhealthy lifestyle, lack of interest in health maintenance, and reported or observed inability to take responsibility for meeting basic health needs in any or all functional pattern areas. Other parental characteristics may include an inability to follow instructions, impaired cognitive functioning, and a lack of adaptive behaviors to internal or external environmental changes.

The well child may have risk factors for altered health maintenance caused by family health practices. Parents who lack education, have a history of substance use or abuse, are single parents, lack support systems, have financial distress, or have a chronic illness may present problems for the child's health and wellness. You can pick up further cues when discussing child immunization schedules with the parent, such as the parent's inability to concentrate or follow instructions or a lack of interest in making the next scheduled well-baby visit that includes immunizations.

Related Factors

Related factors for *Altered health maintenance* involve the child's parents and may include the following:

- Lack of ability to make deliberate and thoughtful judgments
- Ineffective individual or family coping
- Disabling spiritual distress
- Lack of material resources

DIAGNOSIS

Once the components of the well-baby or child assessment are completed, you will determine a nursing diagnosis, as demonstrated in the accompanying Data Clustering chart. The choice of a nursing diagnosis involving a child's growth and development in the first 3 years after birth depends on the identification of any problems and the etiologic factors of the diagnosis. When the history and physical examination reveal abnormal growth or development parameters resulting from environmental deprivation, physical disability, or an acute problem, *Altered growth and development* is an appropriate choice for a nursing diagnosis.

Because parenting style and parenting skills are related factors for altered growth and development, you will need to distinguish the diagnoses *Altered parenting* and *Ineffective family coping* from *Altered growth and development*. If the problem involves family functioning, such as an alcoholic or abusive family, you may choose *Ineffective family coping*. The approach to treatment then becomes family-centered. If you are working primarily with the parent and indirectly with the children, the diagnosis is more likely to be *Altered parenting*. The defining characteristics of *Altered parenting* suggest that the diagnosis refers to more serious behaviors that define a parent's inability to relate positively to the child.

The nursing diagnosis *Altered health maintenance* is directly related to growth and development, but it has a different focus. Positive health practices help to ensure that growth and development proceed normally. This diagnosis is typically used for a well child who has no obvious problems. However, family health practices may place the child at risk for growing up unhealthy or for contracting specific illnesses or health problems of childhood, such as measles or dental caries.

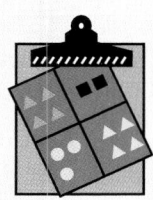

CLUSTERING DATA TO MAKE A NURSING DIAGNOSIS
GROWTH AND DEVELOPMENT PROBLEMS

Data Cluster	Diagnosis
30-month-old male admitted to hospital for malnutrition. Height and weight below 15th percentile on growth charts. Child is lethargic and nonverbal. Mother reports withholding food when he cries.	*Altered growth and development* related to parental indifference and lack of caregiving
Unemployed teenage mother of 2-year-old unable to present immunization health record. Mother expresses lack of knowledge about "kids needing shots." Toddler diagnosed with mumps.	*Altered health maintenance* related to lack of knowledge and financial resources
10-month-old infant admitted to hospital after falling from second-story window. She had multiple fractures and a closed-head injury.	*Diversional activity deficit* related to long-term hospitalization and recuperation
Parents make and meet each scheduled immunization appointment for their infant. Child's immunizations are complete.	*Health-seeking behaviors* related to desire to obtain higher level of wellness through prevention

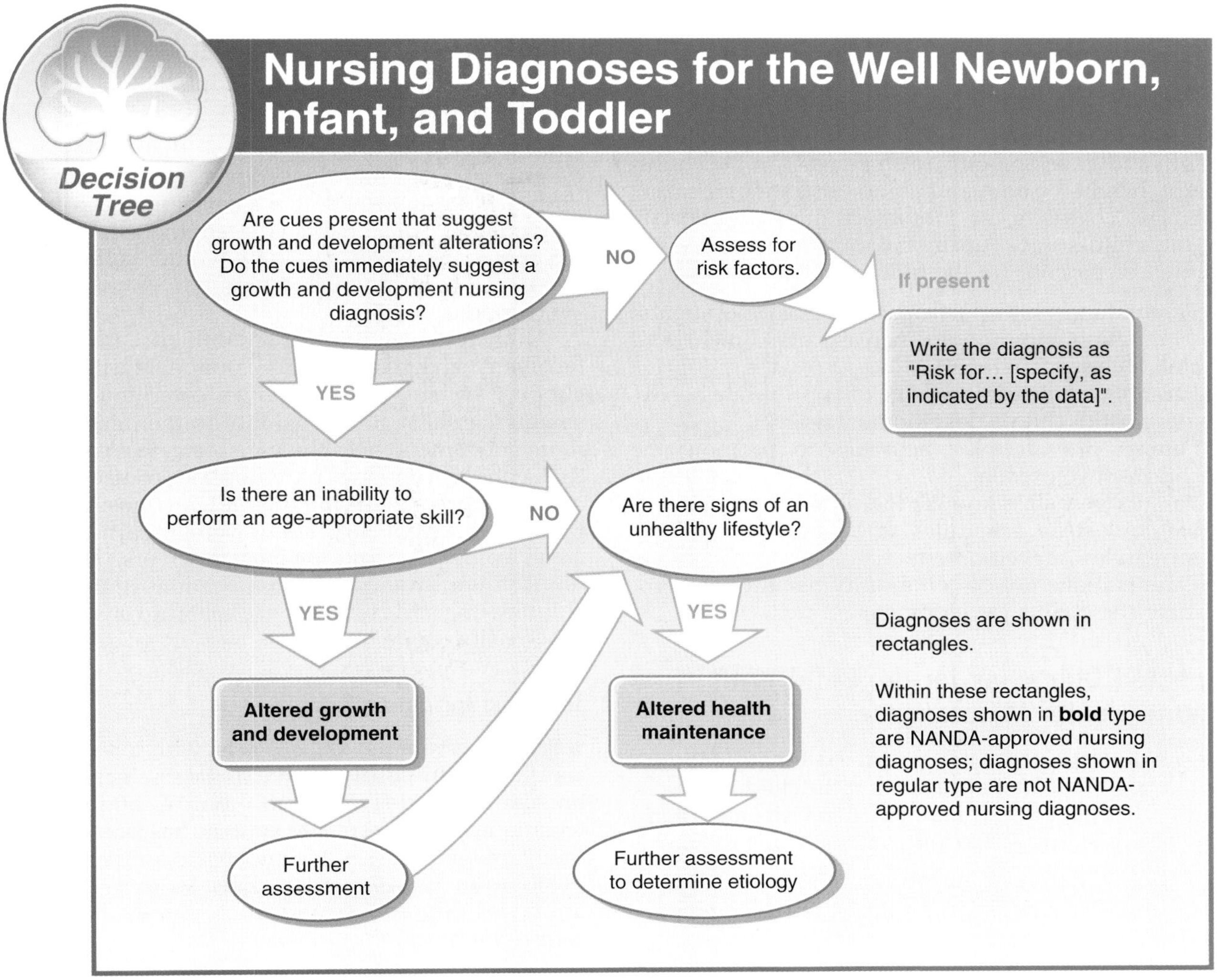

Nursing Diagnoses for the Well Newborn, Infant, and Toddler

Decision Tree

Are cues present that suggest growth and development alterations? Do the cues immediately suggest a growth and development nursing diagnosis?

NO → Assess for risk factors.

If present

Write the diagnosis as "Risk for... [specify, as indicated by the data]".

YES

Is there an inability to perform an age-appropriate skill?

NO → Are there signs of an unhealthy lifestyle?

YES

Altered growth and development

YES

Altered health maintenance

Further assessment

Further assessment to determine etiology

Diagnoses are shown in rectangles.

Within these rectangles, diagnoses shown in **bold** type are NANDA-approved nursing diagnoses; diagnoses shown in regular type are not NANDA-approved nursing diagnoses.

Diversional activity deficit may be the nursing diagnosis for a child experiencing a restriction in or decreased stimulation from recreational or play activities. Diversional activity deficit influences developmental growth and is associated with any prolonged hospitalization, as with Yung Hi, whose fractured femur required 8 weeks of traction. It is also an appropriate diagnosis for a home-bound child with a chronic or disabling condition. Defining characteristics include isolation with limited ability to leave the room; lack of age-appropriate toys at the bedside; physical limitations affecting participation in usual activities; and irritability, moodiness, and inactivity.

You may find that *Diversional activity deficit* is also a related factor for other nursing diagnoses.

PLANNING

One of the most important elements in providing care for children is planning. When your client is age 3 years or younger, you naturally will need to assess the parents, their perceptions of health, and their cultural belief systems. Planning a comprehensive, consistent care plan for the newborn, infant, or toddler with altered growth and development or altered health maintenance is discussed below.

Expected Outcomes for the Child With Altered Growth and Development

The expected outcome criteria for a child with altered growth and development are an increase in the child's weight, height, or both and a demonstration of social, language, cognitive, or motor activities appropriate for the child's age. Additional outcome criteria for children or parents are the following:

- Parents and child participate in a developmental stimulation program to increase attachment and skill levels.
- Parents verbalize knowledge of appropriate behaviors for the child's developmental level.
- Parents provide play activities to promote the child's development.
- Parents verbalize knowledge of appropriate feeding and sleep schedules to promote the child's growth and development.
- Parents make use of community resources to promote the child's development.

Expected Outcomes for the Child With Altered Health Maintenance

The overall expected outcome criteria for a client with altered health maintenance are that the child is present for all scheduled health maintenance visits and maintains health status. Other outcomes for this diagnosis are the following:

- Parents describe appropriate health maintenance program.

- Parents demonstrate behaviors needed to manage the child's health alteration.
- Parents identify health resources available, such as pediatric nurse practitioner, nutritionist, and dentist.
- Child receives all scheduled immunizations.
- Parents use appropriate safety measures, such as car seats and age-appropriate toys.

INTERVENTION

Implementation of your care plan to promote healthy growth and development as well as health maintenance will involve working closely with the child's parents. Education of parents is the primary choice of intervention for both diagnoses.

Interventions to Promote Growth and Development

Nurses play an important role in promoting healthy growth and development through informing and teaching parents of newborns, infants, and toddlers. Appropriate parenting skills in relation to attachment, play, nutrition, toilet training, rest and sleep, caring for a sick child, and referrals are the interventions discussed below.

Promoting Attachment

Attachment is an ongoing process that begins during pregnancy and intensifies during the months after birth. Once established, it is a constant and consistent relationship. Attachment is strengthened by intense communication between parent and child through eye-to-eye contact, touch, voice, odor, and reciprocal, synchronous activity.

Numerous conditions may influence or hinder attachment, such as a parent's emotional health, level of support system, competency in communication and caregiving skills, and proximity to the infant. To promote attachment, help the parent create environments that enhance positive parent-infant contact. Provide quiet and privacy during their interactions. Instill confidence by supporting parents as they learn how to become competent and loving caregivers. Familiarize yourself with any cultural implications in the parent's childbearing and child-rearing beliefs to ensure culturally sensitive care.

Teaching Parenting Skills

Teaching parenting skills starts with preparing the couple for childbirth. Prenatal classes include topics on labor and delivery, pain control, and breathing techniques. Newborn care content has been added to many prenatal classes to compensate for the shortened postpartum stay of mothers. Even so, these days there are fewer opportunities to teach parents basic baby-care techniques.

Another opportunity for parent education occurs during each well-child visit. Take time to answer parents' questions about child care and child-rearing issues, such as discipline, sleep disturbances, and nutritional needs. Act as a role model by demonstrating skills in relating to the child. Suggest classes, support groups, literature, and other resources.

CREATIVE PLAY

Each infant and toddler is a unique individual. Encourage parents to respect and enjoy their baby's individuality. This will help parents to establish the best possible foundation for their child's development, high self-esteem, and healthful relationships with others. Discuss with parents appropriate toys available to stimulate the infant's and toddler's nervous system to achieve developmental milestones (Table 19–2).

Newborns enjoy mobiles with highly contrasting patterns hanging above the crib or a mirror attached securely to the inside of the crib. The newborn also loves to hear soft music from a music box, compact disk, tape, or a parent singing a lullaby. Toys that are brightly colored, soft, and make gentle sounds are soothing to newborns.

The 1- to 3-month-old is partial to brightly colored mobiles and pictures. Infants like a variety of music and enjoy having someone sing to them. By 3 months, infants begin to reach for and grasp objects such as rattles.

Tell parents that textured toys that make sounds and have finger holds are appropriate for a 4- to 8-month-old. Infants enjoy looking through rattles that show pieces making noise. Baby books with vinyl, cloth, or board pages are of interest to this age group. Musical toys, such as bells and maracas, create amuse-

ment for the infant. Warn parents to be careful that none of the parts, such as beads or buttons, can come loose.

Explain to parents that their 8- to 12-month-old is able to stack objects in different sizes, shapes, and colors, so soft blocks and similar toys are helpful. Infants of this age are also fascinated by toys that float, squirt, or hold water in the bathtub. "Busy boxes" that open, squeak, or move keep infants' hands busy. Infants at this age are also interested in plastic cups, pails, paper tubes, empty boxes, magazines, and bottles of different sizes.

Tell parents of the 1- to 2-year-old to expect their toddler to begin to engage in make-believe. Toys that foster make-believe are kitchen sets, tool sets, brooms, dress-up clothes, dolls, cars, and trains. By age 2, toddlers enjoy spending time playing outdoors on swings or slides, in a sandbox, or riding a tricycle. By age 3, toddlers are learning to put things together and take them apart. Toys that encourage this skill include simple shape-sorters, pegboards, connecting links, or nesting toys. Toddlers also can put together simple jigsaw puzzles.

A 2- to 3-year-old becomes more creative in "pretend play" and imitation of adult behaviors (Fig. 19–5). Additionally, this child begins to notice and play

TABLE 19–2
Age-Appropriate Toys

Age	Appropriate Toys
0 to 3 months	• Mobiles. • Soft toys.
4 to 7 months	• Toys with sounds and fingerholds. • Rattles. • Vinyl books.
8 to 12 months	• Toys that float, squirt, or hold water. • Busy boxes. • Different-sized containers or cups. • Books.
1 to 2 years	• Kitchen and tool sets with large parts. • Dress-up clothes. • Trucks, cars, and dolls. • Books. • Sandbox.
2 to 3 years	• Pegboards with large pegs. • Shape sorters. • Nontoxic paints, crayons. • Simple jigsaw puzzles. • Tricycle.

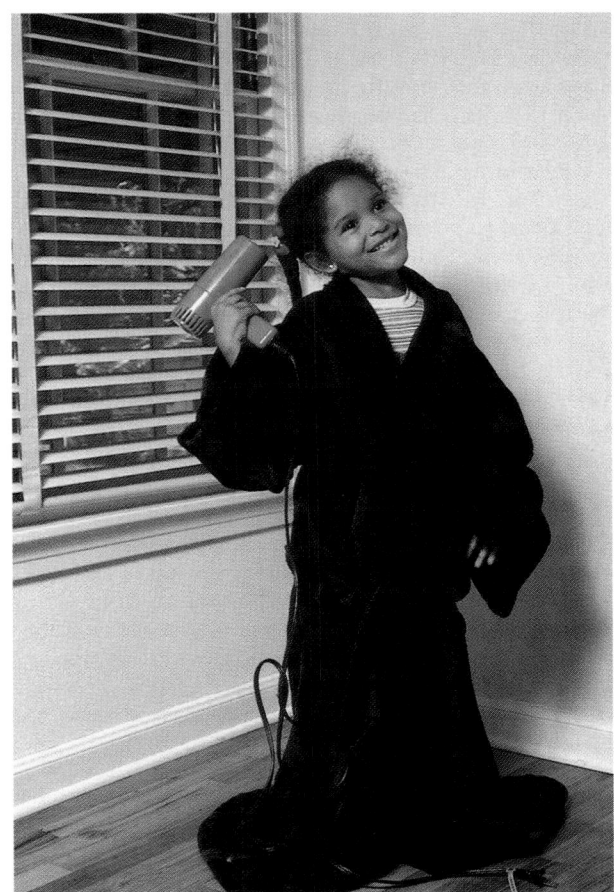

Figure 19–5. A 2- to 3-year-old becomes both more creative and more imitative of adult behavior in her make-believe play.

alongside other children. This parallel play remains egocentric, but some interaction begins with such games as hide-and-seek or tag. Parents can enable this important change in interaction by taking their toddlers to day care, parks, and civic events for children.

To increase their child's self-esteem and confidence, parents should be encouraged to form play groups or have their child attend day care. Toddlers can learn new things and interact with other children their age. Encourage parents to let their child move at her own pace when joining group activities. The more confident and secure children feel, the more independent and well-behaved they are likely to be.

FEEDING AND ELIMINATION

Inform parents that human milk or formula is all that is necessary for the first 4 to 6 months. Single-grain rice cereal is usually the first food introduced because of its high iron content, easy digestibility, and low rate of allergic reactions. Tell parents that citrus fruits, meat, and eggs should be introduced only after the infant reaches 6 months because of the possibility of allergic reactions.

At 6 months, teething foods may be offered. Finger foods are introduced beginning at 8 to 9 months. Instruct parents to encourage the child to feed herself, even though it can be a messy experience. Inform parents that this is all a part of the learning process. By the end of the first year, the child can tolerate table foods.

Inform parents that, when their child reaches 12 to 18 months, the growth rate begins to slow, decreasing the child's need for fluids and calories. Because of this decrease in nutritional needs, most children exhibit a decrease in appetite.

As the child becomes a toddler, she will begin to feel a need to be in control of her abilities. By about 18 months, most toddlers become more picky and fussy in their eating. They are influenced by more than simply how food tastes. Food on the plate must be separated; the child may wish to eat from the same cup, dish, or bowl at each meal; and mixed foods such as casseroles are not usually favored. Tell parents that some days their toddler will eat large amounts of food and other days almost nothing. Many times a noted increase in appetite corresponds with a growth spurt.

Inform parents that good eating habits are established in the first 3 years after birth. By giving their child nutritious meals and snacks, they will be helping to set the stage for future food consumption. Choose nutritious finger foods, such as crackers, cereal bits, or teething biscuits, rather than cookies. Encourage parents to avoid using food as a reward. Tell them that it is not necessary for infants to finish every drop in their bottle or for their toddler to clean the plate.

Instruct parents that an infant should have six to eight wet diapers a day, sometimes more. Whether their infant is breast- or bottle-fed will determine how many bowel movements a day. Breast-fed babies have more frequent stools. Tell parents that they will begin to notice a regular pattern in bowel and bladder elimination at around 8 months.

Inform parents that, as their infant becomes a toddler, they can begin to assess for toilet-training readiness. Not only does their toddler have to show signs of physical, mental, and psychological readiness, but the parents must also be ready. The toddler shows physical signs of readiness by having regular bowel movements, being able to remove her own clothes, and staying dry for at least 2 hours or waking up dry from a nap. Mental readiness consists of being able to recognize the urge to urinate or defecate and to communicate, either verbally or nonverbally, the need to use the toilet. Psychologically, the toddler will show curiosity about siblings' or adults' toilet habits. The toddler tends to become impatient with a soiled or wet diaper and wants to be changed immediately.

Besides recognizing the child's readiness for toilet training, the parents need to be willing to invest the time needed for toilet training. Parents should make this process as positive, natural, and nonthreatening as possible. Instruct parents that their toddler should be ready to begin between ages 18 and 24 months. Bowel training is usually accomplished before bladder training because it is more predictable and has a regular pattern.

Yung's father tells you that he is sad to see lost all the toilet training Yung accomplished these past 4 months. Because Yung is unable to get out of bed, she is using diapers again. What could you do to promote more independence and self-confidence related to toilet training with Yung while she is in traction?

REST AND SLEEP

Inform parents that, at first, newborns sleep about 16 hours a day in 3- to 4-hour stretches between feedings. As they get older and their stomachs grow, they go longer periods between feedings. By 2 months, they are more alert and social and will be awake more during the day. Because of the increased stomach capacity, they may skip a night feeding. By 3 months, parents will be happy to know that their child may be sleeping through the night.

At 4 months, parents should expect their infant to need only two naps a day, each lasting 1 to 3 hours. A consistent bedtime routine will help their infant to wind down at the end of the day. Such a routine may consist of a warm bath, rocking, stories, or soft music.

As the infant approaches 8 months, separation anxiety begins to increase. The child may resist going to bed and may wake up more often, looking for a parent. This is the time to introduce a transitional object (such as a blanket or teddy bear) to comfort the child when parents are not present. Stress the importance of following a consistent pattern or bedtime ritual.

As the child becomes a toddler, delaying tactics may be used. Tell parents to stick to the bedtime routine. During this age, dreams begin. Cutting teeth, a change in routine, or illness can also make an infant or toddler awaken more frequently in the night. Encourage parents to give attention to the child's distress, but let the child know she is to keep to her bedtime routine.

Yung is alone at night. After the night nurse told the parents about Yung's distress at night, Yung's mother brought in her favorite stuffed animal, a white rabbit with purple overalls and red bow tie. Yung had been whimpering and rocking back and forth in the bed. The night after her mother brought in the favorite bunny, Yung clutched the rabbit to her chest, rubbed the satin bow tie, and hummed herself to sleep. She kept the stuffed rabbit with her at all times after that night.

At 2 to 3 years, the child may take a single 1- to 2-hour nap around lunchtime. Some children may give up naps entirely. Again, inform parents that their child may begin to resist going to sleep. Part of this is from separation anxiety and part from the negativity stage of development. Giving the child choices at bedtime helps. A night light may become necessary. Nightmares may also awaken toddlers. Parents should hold and comfort their child until they are calm enough to fall back to sleep.

CARE OF THE SICK CHILD

Teach parents caring for an ill child at home that age-appropriate activities can help the child feel more secure and comfortable during recovery. When a sick child is hospitalized, you act in partnership with parents to provide interventions that will meet the child's psychosocial and developmental needs (Fig. 19–6). Hospitalization brings more far-reaching concerns: pain, separation, fear, and the potential loss of autonomy.

Eliminating pain totally for the infant or child may be impossible. However, there are some interventions that may prove helpful in alleviating pain temporarily. Visual pain-scale instruments to measure pain are available for pediatric patients and may be needed if the child is unable to verbalize. Once assessment is completed, administer pain medication as ordered. Complementary techniques for pain management, such as guided imagery, distraction, reading, and creative use of touch (such as massage or position changes), are helpful in potentiating pharmacological relief.

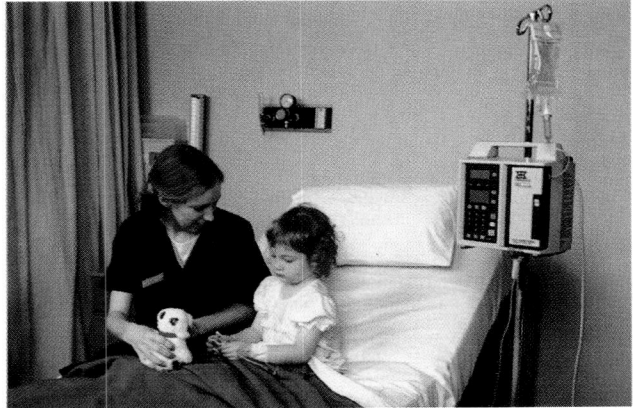

Figure 19–6. When a child is hospitalized, you will partner with parents by engaging the child in play that will promote continued growth and development and provide comfort.

Yung's father asked a friend to perform acupuncture on Yung to help with the pain she was experiencing because of the fracture. Yung was quiet during the acupuncture and slept for 3 hours after the treatment. How do you feel about alternative or complementary forms of health care? Was acupuncture important to the Hi family?

Encourage parents to participate in their hospitalized child's care. Separation from parents is a very difficult issue for infants and toddlers. Relieve parents' anxiety about the unfamiliar setting and procedures so they can better relieve their child's anxiety. Encourage parents who cannot actively provide care to visit with their child as often as possible, but do not dictate parental behavior. Ask the parents about the child's usual daily routine and strive to maintain it during the hospitalization. Doing so will help make the child feel more secure.

Communicating with infants and toddlers is a nursing challenge, but it is necessary to provide even minimal nursing care. Ask parents what indecipherable words mean. Knowing the child's words for elimination, pain, hunger, mother, father, and so on, will increase your understanding of the child's statements and requests.

Knowing a child's food preferences will help to promote good nutrition while the child is hospitalized. Make note of any specific dislikes, allergies, or food intolerances. If possible, encourage parents to bring the child's favorite food to the hospital. Consider the child's developmental level before attempting to feed the child. Ask the parents whether the child uses a bottle, cup, spoon, or fork. Also ask about the child's favorite finger foods at home, and arrange for them to be given to the child in the hospital.

The hospitalized child needs to progress developmentally even while experiencing an illness. Consider the child's developmental stage when performing nursing interventions, particularly those that require the child's cooperation.

Providing Client Referrals

An important aspect of your role as patient advocate is providing client referrals. You are the primary source of information for parents. Direct them to appropriate programs, and provide necessary information about the care of their children. This may include formal educational classes, support groups, counseling services, printed materials, videos, and computer programs on the desired topic.

Interventions to Promote Health Maintenance

Interventions related to health maintenance include assisting parents with scheduling health maintenance visits so their children can receive preventive health. You also will teach parents about immunizations, child safety, and dental care. Again, education of the parents is the primary intervention.

Immunizations

One of your most important tasks is to inform parents of the reasons for routine immunizations. Children are susceptible to disease because they have an immature immune system. Immunization protects the child from being infected and prevents the infection of others at day care centers.

When administered properly, immunizations provide the most cost-effective contribution to the health of children worldwide. They are recommended in an established schedule for healthy infants and children (Fig. 19–7). Instruct parents on the importance of completing all scheduled immunizations. Give them an immunization schedule. Inform parents of the common side effects of each vaccine. Although most side effects are mild, the parents need to know what to expect. Mild discomfort is normal, with slight fever, rash, or soreness at the site of injection. Serious reactions to vaccines are rare. If the child is immunodeficient from AIDS, an organ transplant, or immunosuppressive therapy, the parents should consult their physician about vaccines for their child.

Parents should retain a vaccination record and have it updated each time the child receives a scheduled vaccination. A vaccination and health record will help the parents when they move to a new area or have a change of health care provider or when their child attends day care, preschool, or elementary school. Work closely with parents to establish and maintain a schedule for immunizations.

Child Safety

Accidents are a leading cause of death of infants and toddlers. Many accidents result from a child's natural curiosity and exploration of the environment. Some common accidents are aspiration, choking, falls, burns, car accidents, and drowning. A vital part of assessing for potential accidents is to ask parents about safety hazards in the child's environment. For example, do the parents ever leave their baby or toddler unattended in the bath?

To give yourself a baseline for educational interventions, determine the parents' knowledge about safety and accident prevention. Many parents are unaware of the potential dangers that can be found in a home. The potential for serious injury is ever-present. If parents are made aware of these dangers, they may be able to prevent devastating consequences.

Vaccines[1] are listed under routinely recommended ages. Bars indicate range of recommended ages for immunization. Any dose not given at the recommended age should be given as a "catch-up" immunization at any subsequent visit when indicated and feasible. Ovals indicate vaccines to be given if previously recommended doses were missed or given earlier than the recommended minimum age.

Age ▶ Vaccine ▼	Birth	1 mo	2 mos	4 mos	6 mos	12 mos	15 mos	18 mos	4-6 yrs	11-12 yrs	14-16 yrs
Hepatitis B[2]	Hep B	Hep B		Hep B		Hep B				Hep B	
Diphtheria, Tetanus, Pertussis[3]			DTaP	DTaP	DTaP		DTaP[3]		DTaP	Td	
H. influenzae type b[4]			Hib	Hib	Hib	Hib					
Polio[5]			IPV	IPV		Polio[5]			Polio		
Rotavirus[6]			Rv[6]	Rv[6]	Rv[6]						
Measles, Mumps, Rubella[7]						MMR			MMR[7]	MMR[7]	
Varicella[8]						Var				Var[8]	

Approved by the Advisory Committee on Immunization Practices (ACIP), the American Academy of Pediatrics (AAP), and the American Academy of Family Physicians (AAFP).

Figure 19–7. Recommended childhood immunization schedule, United States, January–December 1999. (Recreated from Centers for Disease Control and Prevention Recommended Childhood Immunization Schedule, United States, January–December 1999. Available at http://www.cdc.gov/nip/pdf/child_imm_sched_99.pdf. Accessed February 2, 1999.)

Exploration plays an integral part in the infant's and toddler's psychological development. As soon as locomotion is established, the parents should use gates as a means to control the infant's access to various areas. Instruct parents about safety latches that can be applied to drawers and cupboards that contain dangerous materials. Give parents the telephone number of the local poison control center and emergency department, and tell them to post the number near the telephone. Also, tell parents to keep syrup of ipecac in the medicine cabinet, and give them guidelines for its use.

Playthings, although valuable in enhancing a child's development, may also cause injuries, accidents, or death. Teach parents to screen toys for age-appropriateness. Children younger than age 3 should not have toys with small, removable parts on which they could choke. Instruct parents to check toys routinely for loose parts or sharp edges. All paints, crayons, molding clays, and other craft items should be nontoxic.

Accidents can occur when food is ingested too quickly or is too large to be swallowed safely. Therefore, food should also be age-appropriate. As the infant progresses from liquids to solids, parents may mash, grind, or cook food until it is soft enough to swallow without chewing. When prepared appropriately, toddlers can eat many of the same foods their parents eat.

Accidental drowning is one of the leading causes of injury and death of children ages 1 to 3. Warn parents that an infant or toddler can drown in only a few inches of water. Bathtubs, toilets, water buckets, and swimming pools are the usual sites of drowning (Castiglia, 1995).

Burns are another source of injury common to infants or toddlers. Instruct parents that they should never hold an infant or toddler when smoking, holding hot liquids, or cooking. Hot liquids or food should never be left near the edge of tables or counters. Tell parents to test bath water before putting a child into it. Also tell them to set their hot water heater at 120°F or lower.

Just as safety is important in the home, it is also important when traveling. A federally approved, properly installed car seat must be used at all times. The infant should sit facing backward in the car until he or she can sit independently. No infant or child should sit in the front seat of a car with a passenger-side air bag. A car seat should be used throughout the toddler stage of development.

Dental Care

Dental health is important even for infants and young children. By age 3, some children already show alarming tooth decay. Neglected dental problems can lead to infection and subsequent tooth loss. Teach parents that healthy "baby teeth" influence the formation of healthy gums and permanent teeth. Ask the parents if the child has any history of dental problems or mouth pain. Ask if the infant or child is given fruit juice when put to bed. To prevent cavities, instruct parents to never let their child fall asleep with a bottle. This habit promotes decay because fluid pools around the teeth.

Inform parents that dental hygiene is essential from the time of their child's first feeding. Even before the first teeth erupt, the child's mouth should be cleaned with a damp gauze or cloth after each feeding. On average, the first tooth erupts at 6 months. Some children show mild signs of drooling and increased finger sucking when teething. Other children become irritable and may refuse to eat. At the eruption of the first tooth, parents should begin to brush the tooth with a soft toothbrush and continue to assist their child with brushing through age 3.

Early screening for signs of caries or cavity development, starting during the first year after birth, could identify infants and toddlers who are at risk of developing early childhood caries. High-risk children include those with early signs of tooth decay, poor oral hygiene, limited exposure to fluorides, and frequent exposure to sugary snacks and drinks (Ismail, 1998).

EVALUATION

To objectively evaluate the degree of success in achieving a goal or outcome, you would assess the infant or toddler for the presence or absence of the desired behavior or response and determine the level of agreement between the outcome criteria and the child's actual response. Knowledge of the principles of growth and development and health maintenance will ensure your progress in meeting the goal of providing comprehensive care to newborns, infants, and toddlers.

The discharge note for Yung Hi might look like this:

Child is smiling and says "thank you" in English and "go home" in Korean. Back to demonstrating how to stack only the red blocks "high" (in English) to her stuffed bunny while standing at the bedside in a single hip spica cast. To discharge home with parents in attendance. Pediatric home health nurse to see every day for 1 week, then every week till cast removed. To visit physical therapist and orthopedic physician in 1 week. No medication orders given. Written cast-care instructions reviewed with parents (father translated to mother and client). Lungs clear to auscultation, vital signs stable and within normal limits. Spica cast intact with equal pedal pulses palpated and right shoulder/arm with full range of motion. Free from cast rub. Nutritional and developmental status intact.

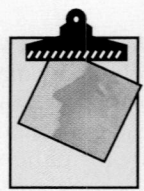

NURSING CARE PLANNING
A CLIENT AT RISK FOR ALTERED GROWTH AND DEVELOPMENT

Admission Data

Yung Hi is admitted from the postanesthesia care unit to the orthopedic unit. The unit nurse receives the following report:

33-month-old Asian female child admitted to ER with displaced fracture of the right femur. No known allergies or medical conditions. Toddler had been playing in playground of apartment complex when she fell, and her older brother tripped and fell on her outstretched leg. No reported loss of consciousness. Mother witnessed the fall and (through translation) said that the child did not hit her head. The father attempted to move child and, when unable, called for an ambulance. Right thigh demonstrated deformity with apparent misalignment of femur and no break in skin integrity. Closed reduction and placement of Steinmann's pins to right tibia for Buck's traction of right femur under general anesthesia in OR. Stable during procedure and while in recovery. Vitals: BP 92/48, pulse 146, respirations 38. Popliteal, posttibial, and pedal pulses present bilaterally with right pulses +2 and left +3. No other significant physical findings. Call in to physical therapy to place traction in room.

Physician's Orders

Admitting diagnosis: displaced fracture of right femur.
Surgical procedure: closed reduction right femur with Steinmann's pin placement right tibia.
Bedrest with balanced suspension traction to Steinmann's pins, 5 lb to each weight.
Do not elevate head of bed until further notice.
Neurovascular checks to right leg every 30 minutes × 4; every 1 hour × 4, then every 4 hours.
Diet as tolerated.
Children's Tylenol with codeine 5 mL PO q3–4h prn pain.
Colace elixir 30 mg PO every day.

Nursing Assessment

Drowsy and nonverbal. Mother at bedside. Mother reports no pain expressed. Vital signs stable. Traction in place to right leg with 5 lb to each weight. No redness, drainage, or swelling around pin sites at right tibia. Able to wiggle toes. Leg and foot pink and warm to touch, capillary refill approximately 2 seconds. Pedal and posttibial pulses strong (+2) bilaterally. Edema +1 noted to right leg and foot with large ecchymosis noted medial right thigh. Lung sounds clear bilaterally A & P. Positive bowel sounds, voiding adequate amounts clear yellow urine in diaper. No skin breakdown noted over bony prominences at sacrum, heels, and scapulae.

NURSING CARE PLAN

Nursing Diagnosis	Expected Outcomes	Interventions	Evaluation (After 24 Hours of Care)
Risk for altered growth and development related to diversional activity deficit and immobility secondary to traction	Continue to demonstrate physical, psychosocial, and cognitive skills of previous stage of growth and development.	*Ask family members to bring child's favorite toys, family pictures, and other objects from home to place at bedside.*	Parents brought in favorite stuffed bunny and blanket, pictures of each family member, and favorite book.
	Maintain range of motion and strength.	Consult physical therapist (PT) for strength and range-of-motion exercises.	PT consulted. Will work with client t.i.d. *Asked parents to be present to learn exercises and to help translate to client.*
	Participate in age-appropriate play.	Consult play therapist and *have therapist come when both parents present.*	Play therapist met with parents and child. Favorite toys, music, and activities discussed.
	Demonstrate increased understanding of treatments.	Provide child with opportunities for therapeutic play.	Played nurse and doctor with favorite stuffed rabbit as the client in traction.

Continued

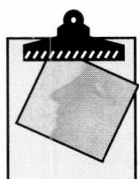

NURSING CARE PLANNING
A CLIENT AT RISK FOR ALTERED GROWTH AND DEVELOPMENT *(continued)*

NURSING CARE PLAN *(continued)*

Nursing Diagnosis	Expected Outcomes	Interventions	Evaluation (After 24 Hours of Care)
	Select and play with age-appropriate toys.	Place developmentally appropriate toys conducive to immobility at the bedside.	Crayons, paints, pegboard, books, and stuffed animals at bedside.
	Express enjoyment in selected play activities.	Schedule times to engage child in developmental play during day and early evening shift.	Met with client and played at 10 AM, 1 PM, and 7 PM. Parents, PT, and play therapist also with client and conducted play and physical activity.
	Achieve developmental tasks appropriate to age.	Monitor developmental status and progress at regular intervals.	Age-appropriate play, talks with mother and father, sings. Says "thank you" in English and nods head at same time.

Italicized interventions indicate culturally specific care.

Critical Thinking Questions	**1.**	Which developmental theory would you apply to Yung to assist you in caring for her? Why would you choose one theory over the other?
	2.	Yung wanted to keep her stuffed rabbit in traction after the therapeutic play session was over. Why do you think Yung wanted to do this?

The above example shows documentation of a happy child demonstrating age-appropriate behaviors for an "almost" 3-year-old, such as verbalizing new words learned, stacking blocks, interacting with her stuffed rabbit, and recognizing going home. Follow-up care and referral information for meeting new recovery goals at home were provided to the parents. You can use this data to document that the expected outcomes for *Risk for altered growth and development* were met by discharge.

If the overall outcome was not met, reassessment and changes in the plan of care would be warranted. It may be that another nursing diagnosis would be a better choice. Refer to the Nursing Care Planning chart for Yung Hi to see an example of nursing process in action.

KEY PRINCIPLES

- Although the terms *growth* and *development* are often used synonymously, they have separate and distinct definitions. Growth refers to a physiological process, whereas development involves the maturation of body organs and the acquisition of appropriate cognitive, linguistic, and psychosocial skills.
- Developmental theories attempt to explain how the human organism matures and acquires appropriate cognitive, linguistic, and psychosocial skills.
- The environment, whether family, community, or culture, is a crucial factor in supporting healthy development.
- Socioeconomic factors influence growth and development. Families who have limited incomes may fail to obtain health care, resulting in a loss of services that could promote growth and development.
- Many physiological factors affect growth and development. These include congenital anomalies, communicable diseases, failure to thrive, and child abuse. Physiological data for measuring growth include those of weight, height, and head circumference. Psychological testing for development may include cognitive and developmental tests.
- The choice of a nursing diagnosis to guide the management of problems involving growth and development or altered health maintenance during

the first 3 years after a child's birth depends on the objective and subjective data gathered.

- Planning nursing care for a newborn, infant, or toddler depends on the nursing diagnosis chosen and realistic and measurable goals or outcomes.
- Interventions to promote growth and development are related to promoting attachment, teaching parenting skills, and providing referrals.
- Interventions to promote health maintenance are immunizations, child safety, and dental care.
- Evaluation of nursing care provided to clients with altered growth and development or altered health maintenance involves comparing desired goals to the actual outcome of nursing care.

BIBLIOGRAPHY

*Bowlby, J. (1969). *Attachment and loss.* New York: Basic Books.

*Bradshaw, M.M. (1982). Denver Developmental Screening. In S.S. Humeneck (Ed.), *Analysis of current assessment strategies in the health care of young children and childbearing families.* Norwalk, CT: Appleton-Century-Crofts.

Castaglia, P. (1995). Drowning. *Journal of Pediatrics, 9*(4), 185–186.

Dubowitz, H., & Finkel, M. (1997). Child abuse and neglect. In R.A. Hoekelman, S.B. Friedman, N.M. Nelson, H.M. Seidel, & M.L. Weitzman (Eds.), *Pediatric primary care* (3rd ed.) (pp 621–626). St. Louis: Mosby.

*Erikson, E.H. (1963). *Childhood and society* (2nd ed.). New York: W.W. Norton.

Friedman, J. (1998). *Family nursing: Research, theory and practice.* Norwalk, CT: Appleton & Lange.

Greipp, M.E. (1997). Ethical decision making and mandatory reporting in cases of suspected child abuse. *Journal of Pediatric Health Care, 11*(6), 258–265.

*Havighurst, R.J. (1972). *Developmental tasks and education.* New York: David McKey.

Hickey, J., & Goldberg, F. (1996). *Ultrasound review of obstetrics and gynecology.* Philadelphia: Lippincott-Raven.

Hoekelman, R.A. (1995). The physical examination of infants and children. In B. Bates, *A guide to physical examination and history taking* (6th ed.) (pp 555–625). Philadelphia: JB Lippincott.

Ismail, A.I. (1998). Prevention of early childhood caries. *Community Dentistry and Oral Epidemiology, 26*(1), 49–61.

Jorde, L.B., Carey, J.C., & White, R.L. (1995). *Medical genetics.* St. Louis: Mosby.

Kenny, T.J., & Nitz, K. (1997). Mental retardation. In R.A. Hoekelman, S.B. Friedman, N.M. Nelson, H.M. Seidel, & M.L. Weitzman (Eds.), *Primary pediatric care* (3rd ed.) (pp. 409–412). St. Louis: Mosby.

*Klaus, M.H., & Kennell, J.H. (1982). *Parent-infant bonding* (2nd ed.). St. Louis: C.V. Mosby.

Landrigan, J., & Carlson, J.E. (1995). Environmental policy and children's health: The future of children. *Critical Issues for Children and Youth, 2*(5), 34–52.

Leininger, M. (1991). *Culture care diversity and universality: A theory of nursing.* New York: National League for Nursing Press.

Liptak, G.S., Miller, G., & Couch, S. (1997). Cerebral palsy. In R.A. Hoekelman, N.M. Nelson, H.M. Seidel, & M.L. Weitzman (Eds.), *Primary pediatric care* (3rd ed.) (pp 432–438). St. Louis: Mosby.

Maldonado, Y. (1997). Epidemiology of HIV infection in children and adolescents. In S.S. Long, L.K. Pickering, & C.G. Prober (Eds.), *Principles and practice of pediatric infectious diseases* (pp 738–749). New York: Churchill Livingstone.

Manning, F. (1995). *Fetal medicine: Principles and practice* (pp 307–341). Norwalk, CT: Appleton & Lange.

McFarland, G.K., and McFarlane, E.A. (1997). *Nursing diagnosis and intervention: Planning for patient care* (3rd ed.). St. Louis: Mosby.

McManaway, J.W. (1997). Visual problems. In R.A. Hoekelman, N.M. Nelson, H.M. Seidel, & M.L. Weitzman (Eds.), *Primary pediatric care* (3rd ed.) (pp 1148–1151). St. Louis: Mosby.

*Mercer, R. (1982). Parent infant interaction. In L. Sonstegard (Ed.), *Women's health and childrearing,* vol. 2. New York: Grune & Stratton.

North American Nursing Diagnosis Association. (1999). *NANDA nursing diagnoses: Definitions and classification 1999–2000.* Philadelphia: Author.

Overby, K. (1996). Screening. In A.M. Rudolph, J.I.E. Hoffman, & C. Rudolph (Eds.), *Rudolph's pediatrics* (pp 3–36). Norwalk, CT: Appleton & Lange.

Petryshen, P., Stevens, B., Hawkins, J., & Stewart, M. (1997). Comparing nursing costs for preterm infants receiving conventional versus developmental care. *Nursing Economics, 15*(3), 138–145, 150.

Pomerance, H.H. (1995). Growth and its assessment. *Advances in Pediatrics, 42,* 545–573.

*Singer, D., & Revenson, T. (1978). *A Piaget primer: How a child thinks.* New York: The New American Library.

Steward, D.K. (1997). Nonorganic failure to thrive: A theoretical approach. *Journal of Pediatric Nursing, 12*(6), 342–347.

Thompson, M.L. (1995). *Concepts in pediatric nursing.* Springhouse, PA: Springhouse Corp.

*Walker, L.O. (1982). Brazleton neonatal behavioral assessment scale and neonatal perception inventories. In S.S. Humenick (Ed.), *Analysis of current assessment strategies in the health care of young children and childbearing families* (pp 149–161). Norwalk, CT: Appleton-Century-Crofts.

Weiss, M.H., Chute, P.M., & Parisier, S.C. (1997). Hearing loss. In R.A. Hoekelman, S.B. Friedman, N.M. Nelson, H.M. Seidel, & M.L. Weitzman (Eds). *Pediatric primary care* (3rd ed.) (pp 991–993). St. Louis: Mosby.

Wong, O.L., & Perry, S.E. (1998). *Maternal-child nursing care.* St. Louis: Mosby.

*Asterisk indicates a classic or definitive work on this subject.

The Well Child

Jeanne Lawler-Slack and Laura Dulski

Key Terms

attention-deficit/hyperactivity disorder
concrete operations
conservation
decentering accommodation
latchkey children

learning disability
preschooler
school-aged child
sibling rivalry
symbolic play

LEARNING OBJECTIVES

After studying this chapter, you should be able to:

1. **Describe the normal growth and development of the preschool and school-aged child.**

2. **Identify factors affecting growth and development of the preschool and school-aged child.**

3. **Discuss assessment of growth, development, and health maintenance for the preschool and school-aged child.**

4. **Plan nursing care that demonstrates knowledge of normal growth and development of the preschool and school-aged child.**

5. **Identify areas in which the parents of preschool and school-aged children can benefit from the nurse's anticipatory guidance.**

6. **Describe evaluation of expected outcomes for the preschool and school-aged child experiencing *Altered growth and development* or *Altered health maintenance*.**

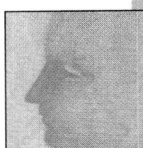

During a family vacation, 4-year-old Timmy Smith was injured in a water-skiing accident and brought to the emergency room (ER) of the local hospital. His parents told the ER nurse they were teaching him to water ski when he fell in the water and sprained his ankle and wrist. Timmy was not seriously injured, but the ER nurse was concerned that his parents were being unrealistic about young Timmy's athletic abilities. Timmy admitted to the nurse that he was afraid that his parents were angry with him for failing to learn to water ski. Although he had just completed a swimming course, he was still afraid of drowning. Timmy's parents told the nurse they thought they remembered being able to water ski at his age and were surprised that he was having so much difficulty. They told her "he just needed more practice."

Because the nurse is concerned that Timmy's parents were expecting him to engage in sports activities that were beyond his ability, thereby adversely affecting his growth and development, she assesses for *Altered growth and development or Risk for altered parenting.* The Nursing Diagnoses chart defines these two NANDA nursing diagnoses.

CONCEPTS OF CHILDHOOD DEVELOPMENT

This chapter focuses on the principles of child growth and development. Knowledge of normal growth and development of well children will help you to promote their health, establish healthful behavior patterns, and detect abnormalities. This knowledge will also help you individualize your care of children and their families. During the preschool and school years, children continue their physical, motor, cognitive, linguistic, and psychosocial growth.

Development of Preschoolers

Physical Development

A **preschooler** is a child between the ages of 3 and 5 years. During this period, a significant change in body contour occurs. The prominent lordosis and protuberant abdomen characteristic of the toddler change to slimmer, taller, and more child-like proportions. The child's future body type becomes more apparent. Body types may be *ectomorphic* (lanky body build), *mesomorphic* (medium muscular body), or *endomorphic* (large build). Weight, height, and growth differentials depend on genetic factors (e.g., tall parents generally have tall children), cultural and ethnic characteristics, dietary habits, and the general health of the child. In the United States, African-American children tend to be taller than European-American children, who, in turn, are taller than Asian-American children (Rice, 1996).

WEIGHT AND HEIGHT

The average preschool child gains weight slowly, only 2 kg (4.5 lb) a year. It is not unusual for parents to perceive that the child is losing weight during this developmental period, whereas they are actually seeing age-appropriate changes in body contours. Preschoolers also grow slowly, gaining only 2 inches (51 mm) to 3.5 inches (89 mm) in an average year.

PHYSIOLOGICAL CHANGES

Preschool-aged children undergo many physiological changes. Increased growth of lymphatic tissue increases the levels of antibodies in the child, so illnesses become more localized as in a runny nose with diminished systemic reaction such as fever. Heart murmurs may be heard on auscultation; this is because the heart changes its size in relation to the thorax, and murmurs at this stage are not normally a cause for concern. The heart rate decreases to about 85 beats/minute while blood pressure stabilizes at about 100/60 mm Hg. The bladder is still quite small, so voiding occurs about 8 to 10 times daily; this explains why preschool children forget to use the toilet when they become absorbed in an activity and instead wet their clothes.

DENTITION

Preschoolers generally have all 20 of their deciduous teeth by age 3 years. Rarely do new teeth erupt during this period. At age 3, children should begin annual dental check-ups. The teeth should be brushed at least twice daily and the family should help the child learn to floss daily.

Motor Development

Preschoolers experience tremendous improvement in large and fine muscle coordination. They can run well, walk up and down stairs, and learn to hop. By age 5 years, they can usually skip and throw and catch balls (Table 20–1). Improving fine-motor skills and hand-eye coordination enables them to copy circles, squares, and triangles and to print letters and numbers. Their motor development depends primarily on overall physical maturation and is influenced by their opportunities for exercise and practice of activities such as skipping and hopping.

Cognitive Development

Cognition is the act or process of knowing. Jean Piaget (1896–1980), a Swiss developmental psychologist, constructed the Piagetian approach to cognitive development in children (Piaget & Inhelder, 1969; Piaget, 1950). He believed that cognitive development is the combined result of maturation of the brain and nervous system and of adaptation to our environment. Piaget outlined four stages of cognitive development. To progress from one stage to the next, children reorganize their thinking processes to bring them closer to reality. This chapter focuses on the *"Preoperational Stage"* (2 to 7 years), discussed here, and the *"Concrete Operational Stage"* (7 to 11 years), discussed further in the section on school-aged children.

TABLE 20–1
Motor Skills of the Child 4 to 11 Years Old

Age	Motor Skill
4 years	Walks on tiptoes
	Alternates feet when descending stairs
	Hops or jumps forward
	Holds a pencil with control
	Can cut and paste
5 years	Skips
	Throws overhand with some accuracy
	Can catch a bounced ball
	Handles scissors with skill
	Rides a tricycle
6 years	Ties own shoes
	Runs, jumps, climbs
	Skips
	Rides a bike with training wheels
	Learns to swim
7 to 8 years	Can use inline skates
	Rides a bicycle
	Swimming improves
	Continues to refine small muscle control—is more graceful
	Can throw and hit a baseball
9 to 11 years	Can participate in most sports
	Has good hand/eye coordination
	Refines gross and fine motor skills
	Can do craft projects
	Can catch a ball in one hand

The preoperational stage is divided into the preoperational phase, ages 2 to 4, and the phase of intuitive thought, ages 4 to 7. During the preoperational phase, children shift from totally egocentric thought to social awareness and the ability to consider others' viewpoints. They acquire language and learn that they can use thought to deal with the world symbolically. They use words to describe actions and mentally and symbolically accomplish actions through the use of words. They develop the ability to imagine an action instead of performing the act. For example, they can imagine pulling a toy even if they do not actually have the toy to pull. At about age 4, preschoolers first begin to think about the future and start to plan what they will be doing later in the day or in a few days, instead of concentrating on the here and now. This reflects their increasing ability to think. Around age 5 they show increasing ability to use language to describe their emotions. An important requirement for preschoolers' mental development is that they be reared in an intellectually stimulating environment.

Action Alert!
Counsel parents to give their children age-appropriate materials and to encourage them to explore their environment. Maximum mental growth takes place when they are stimulated mentally, year after year.

Language Development

By age 5, preschoolers have a vocabulary of more than 2,000 words. They can use all parts of speech correctly. They tend to use more verbs than nouns. Their sentences average four to five words in length. They can define familiar objects, identify colors, and express their feelings. They understand the concepts of "under," "over," "up," and "down" and of opposites, such as "open" versus "closed." The pattern of asking questions is at its peak and they will repeat a question until they receive an answer.

Psychosocial Development

The psychosocial development of preschoolers is marked by an increasing sense of personal identity and willingness to work with others. Ideally, they have mastered the tasks of "sense of initiative."

PEER RELATIONSHIPS
The development of peer relationships is one of the most important aspects of a child's social development. Four-year-olds continue to play in groups but may become involved in more arguments as they begin testing their roles in the group. The increasing conflict may cause parents to worry that their child is regressing, but it is really a forward movement. Five-year-olds begin selecting their "best" friends. They depend less on parents and more on peers for social interaction. They tend to offer approval, make demands on one another, and demonstrate the ability to show empathy when others are distressed (Rice, 1996).

GENDER-ROLE DEVELOPMENT
At ages 4 to 5, preschoolers develop gender-role identification and begin to assume the roles of persons of their own sex. Kohlberg (1966) states that the child's self-categorization as a boy or girl is the basic organizer of the gender role attitudes that develop. Children act consistently in accordance with gender expectations communicated to them by family members and society. Boys and girls are socialized differently from birth. In the United States, boys are often expected to be more active and aggressive, whereas girls are expected to be polite and less aggressive. Such gender expectations have continued throughout the 1990s (Fagot & Hagan, 1995).

PLAY
Play provides for physical, social, and mental development of preschoolers. Five-year olds continue to enjoy the rough-and-tumble play that they participated in at age 4, but they become more interested in group games, such as board games or sports such as soccer. This helps them learn to take turns and to be able to accept losing or winning and to cooperate with other children in a group. Active play is important for their physical growth, refinement of motor skills, and releasing pent-up energy; the use of tricycles, wagons, sports equipment, and water play can help develop

muscles and coordination. Play time also helps them to learn to control their impulses and feelings and to express them in socially acceptable ways. Imaginative play is a healthy outlet for ill children because it allows them to think of creative solutions to their illness experiences and to develop problem-solving skills.

Action Alert!
Inform parents that play time is especially significant for the child who is ill. Through play, children can express and work out fears, anger, and misunderstanding about their illness.

Symbolic play is pretend or imaginative play that enables preschool children to recreate experiences and to try out roles (Fig. 20–1). They create imaginary companions that they talk to, they play with, and become a regular part of their daily routines. Reassure parents that it is normal for their preschoolers to create imaginary playmates and that it helps the child differentiate between fantasy and reality.

FEARS
Common fears that develop at this time include fear of the dark, separation from parents, or in some cases fear of bodily harm.

FEAR OF THE DARK. The vivid imagination of the preschool-aged child can turn a stuffed toy by day into a threatening monster in the dark. Parents must be prepared for this fear and understand that it is a normal phase of growth. They may need to reassure their child who is reluctant to go to sleep unless a light is on or who wakes up screaming from a nightmare.

FEAR OF SEPARATION OR ABANDONMENT. Fear of separation continues to be a concern for preschoolers because they do not have a sense of time and are not comforted by mother's reassurances that she will return to preschool in 2 hours.

FEAR OF MUTILATION. Some preschoolers have a fear of bodily harm that may make it difficult for them to cooperate with medical personnel and treatments, such as needlesticks or an otoscopic examination. They cry out not only from the pain but also from the sight of injury.

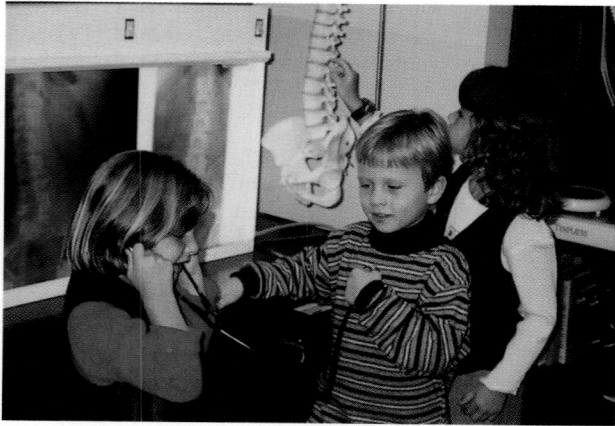

Figure 20–1. Symbolic play enables preschool children to recreate experiences and try out various adult roles.

Action Alert!
Encourage parents to thoroughly prepare their children for any separation experiences, such as being admitted to the hospital.

Moral Development

Piaget (1997) describes the development of moral judgment as a gradual cognitive process enhanced by the increasing social relationships of children. Early in their moral development, children are constrained by the "rules of the game." As children develop, they learn that rules are not absolute but can be altered by social consensus and that adult rules are no longer sacred (Helwig, Tisak, & Turiel, 1990). At the age of 4 to 5 years, children begin to understand that society considers certain behaviors right and certain other behaviors wrong, and they begin to label their own behaviors and those of others as right or wrong.

Preschoolers begin to have an elemental concept of God if they have been provided some exposure to religion. This belief in an outside force aids the development of conscience (Kohlberg, 1981). They tend to do good out of self-interest rather than because of spiritual motivation. They enjoy the security of religious rituals, such as grace said before meals. Praying to God and observing religious traditions can help children through stressful periods such as hospitalization.

Development of School-Aged Children

Physical Development

A **school-aged child** is a child in the developmental stage between 6 and 11 years old. Although some girls begin puberty during the end of this period, most researchers consider these girls developmentally preadolescent despite their physical changes.

During the school years, children's rate of physical growth is steady but is slower than at any time since birth and their motor, cognitive, and psychosocial development progresses rapidly.

WEIGHT AND HEIGHT
On average, school-aged children grow 1 to 2 inches (25 to 51 mm) and gain 3 to 5 pounds (1.36 to 2.27 kg) per year. Boys are slightly taller and heavier than girls during the early school years, but by age 9, girls experience an acceleration in skeletal growth and begin to be taller and heavier than boys. Boys experience an acceleration in growth around 12 years of age (Beck, 1998).

PHYSIOLOGICAL CHANGES
Cardiovascular function is usually stable in school-aged children. Growth of the brain is complete around age 10, and this results in the refinement of fine motor coordination. Maturation of the respiratory system leads to increased oxygen–carbon dioxide exchange, increasing exertion ability and stamina. The frontal sinuses are developed, and sinus-caused headaches become a possibility.

DENTITION

During the school-aged years, all primary teeth are lost and the majority of permanent teeth have erupted. The timing is somewhat variable, depending on both heredity and nutrition (Fig. 20–2). Children need to brush and floss daily to maintain healthy teeth and gums. A dentist needs to be consulted about jaw malformations or misaligned teeth.

> A*ction* A*lert!*
> Remind parents that children should have a dental examination and teeth cleaning annually.

SEXUAL MATURATION

About 10 years of age, the hypothalamus transmits an enzyme to the anterior pituitary gland to begin production of gonadotropic hormones, which activate changes in testes and ovaries (Cunningham, 1996). Timing of sexual maturity varies widely between 10 and 14 years of age. Puberty is occurring increasingly earlier, and it would not be unusual to find school-aged girls already menstruating at age 11 or earlier (see Chapter 21).

> A*ction* A*lert!*
> Encourage parents to discuss sexual responsibility with the child. Children at this age should also be reminded that their body is their own to be used only in the way they choose.

Motor Development

As musculature increases in size, coordination continues to improve. Most 6- to 11-year-olds can learn to in-line skate; play baseball, soccer, or tennis; and do gymnastics. Fine-motor skills continue to develop as well. School-aged children can sew, learn to use garden tools, handle a hammer and a saw, draw in proportion, and master penmanship in writing. Reaction time depends on brain maturation, which is why so many children aged 5 to 7 have trouble catching a ball. Any sport that requires quick reactions, distance judgment, and hand-eye coordination may be difficult for younger school-aged children.

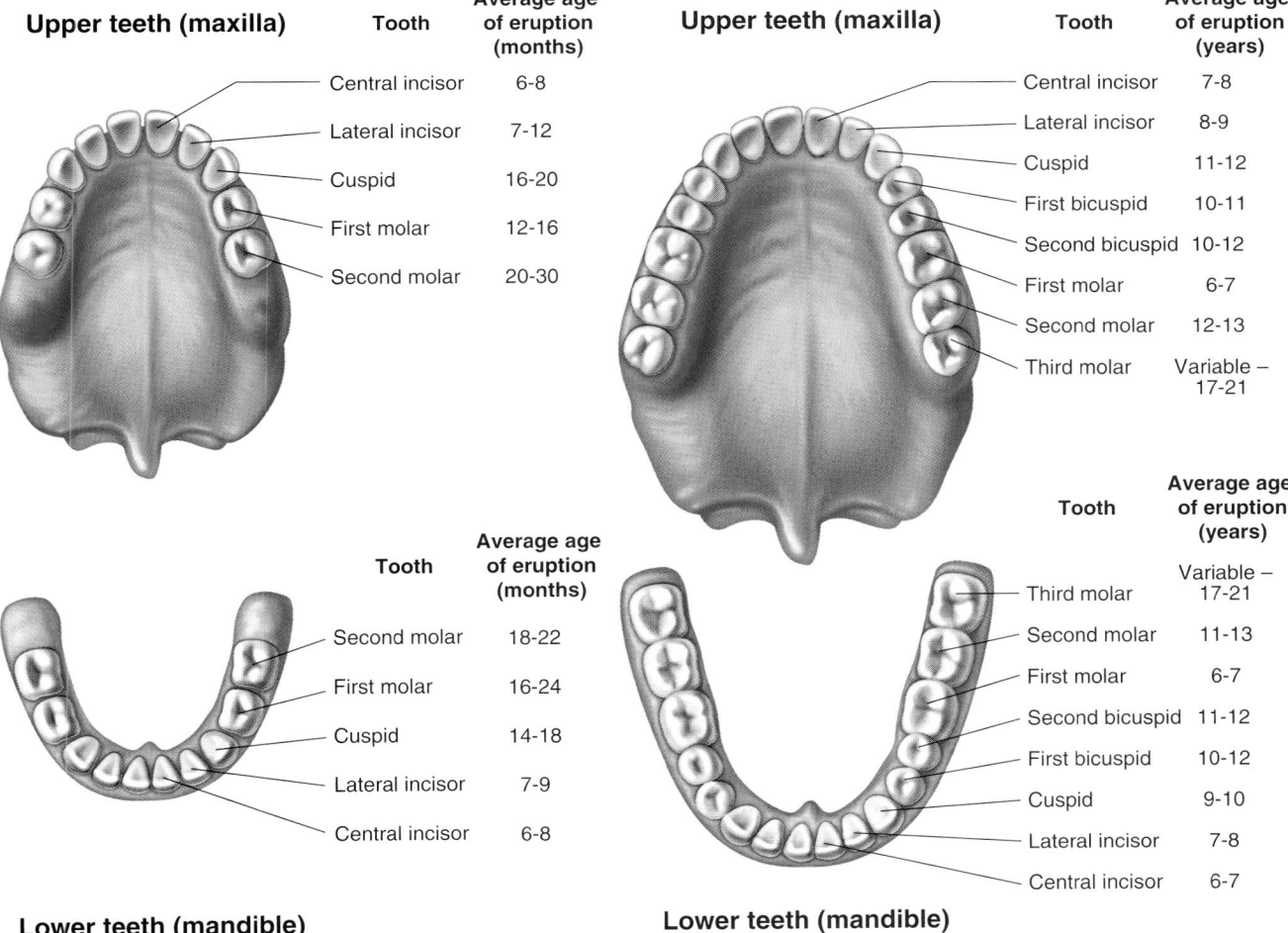

A

B

Figure 20–2. Sequence of eruption of primary (A) and secondary (B) teeth.

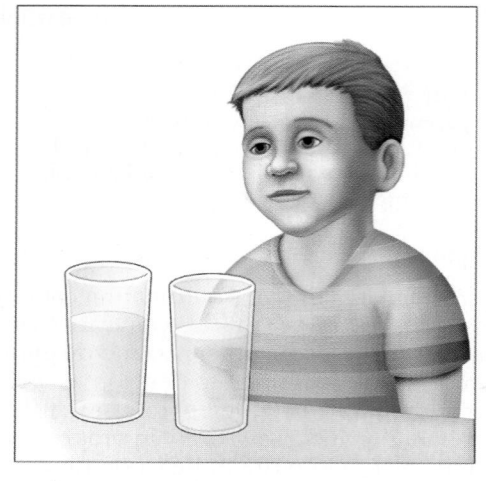
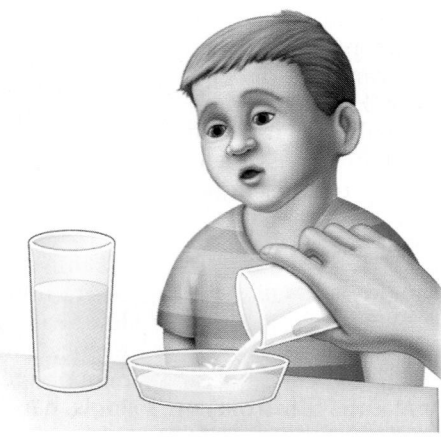

A   **B**

Figure 20–3. The preschool child does not yet understand the principle of conservation. A, The preschooler is able to understand that two glasses of the same size contain equal amounts of liquid. B, However, when the content of one of the glasses is poured into a dish of equal volume, the child becomes perplexed because he does not understand that changing the shape of a substance does not change its volume.

Cognitive Development

According to Piaget (1980), school-aged children are in the *concrete operational* stage of development. **Concrete operations** is the stage of cognitive development at which children begin to project the self into other people's situations and realize that their own way of thinking isn't the only way. **Decentering accommodation** is a child's ability to adapt thought processes to perceive more than one reason for a person's actions.

At this time childrens' thoughts become increasingly logical and coherent and they are able to classify, sort, and organize facts. However, they still lack the capacity to generalize or deal in abstract ideas. School-aged children are able to increase their understanding of many concepts associated with objects. *Class inclusion* is a child's ability to understand that objects can belong to more than one group. The ability to group things into categories enables the child to expand knowledge through category-based indicators, which enables them to solve problems. **Conservation** is a child's ability to understand that changing the shape of a substance does not change its volume. Preschool-aged children lack this perception (Fig. 20–3). Understanding this concept helps limit sibling arguments over who has more milk when two different-shaped glasses of equal volume are presented.

> *A*ction *A*lert!
> Teach parents to understand that their school-aged child may demonstrate a varying ability to handle problems and can most effectively handle one major problem at a time.

Language Development

At age 6, the child's vocabulary is quite large—about 10,000 words—and reaches about 40,000 by adolescence. School-aged children enlarge their vocabularies by analyzing the structure of complex words and thinking about them and using them more precisely. They appreciate the multiple meanings of words. Their conversational strategies become more refined. Children have generally mastered most of the grammar of their language when they enter school, and the use of complex grammatical constructions improves (Beck, 1998).

Psychosocial Development

According to Erikson's stages of development, discussed in Chapter 19, the developmental task of the school years is the establishment of a *sense of industry*, in which the child is motivated to expend effort in a purposeful activity. During this stage, a child masters social and cognitive skills. However, there is a risk that the child will not gain competency at a chosen task and develop a sense of inferiority rather than of industry. Successful completion of this stage of development enables children to recognize their abilities as well as their liabilities and to develop a sense of competence. Competition is also important; by comparing themselves to their peers, children can understand their own personal strengths and weaknesses.

PEER RELATIONSHIPS

Learning to understand and get along with children who are different from themselves are important developmental tasks. Parents of school-aged children are usually very interested in the kinds of friends that their children want to visit with or invite home. This concern is appropriate because peer group influence over children grows stronger throughout the school years. Their acceptance by their peers is very important and influences their adjustment during adolescence. Box 20-1 lists behavior characteristics that promote peer acceptance. When school children have negative reputations and poor relationships with peers, they experience lower self-esteem and loneliness and find the experience of school very stressful (Rice, 1996).

GENDER-ROLE DEVELOPMENT

Gender stereotypes are learned through parents, teachers, peers, and the media. Although the standards of "maleness" and "femaleness" are undergoing gradual change, with some mixing of male and female

BOX 20–1

BEHAVIORAL CHARACTERISTICS THAT PROMOTE PEER ACCEPTANCE

- Outgoing, socially interactive.
- Physically attractive (girls); athletic ability (boys).
- Has a high level of energy.
- Early participation in social events.
- Has a good sense of humor and is good natured.
- Accepts others even when they are not like one-self.
- Performs well in school.
- Has the ability to communicate effectively.

traits and roles, traditional behaviors continue to predominate. Children's understanding of gender roles broadens, and their gender role identities change as they think more about people as personalities. Their ability to classify flexibly enables them to have a more open-minded view of what boys and girls can do than they did at a younger age (Beck, 1998).

PLAY

During the school years, group activities dominate play time. Through group dynamics, school-aged children learn to work cooperatively toward a common goal. Success in physical and cognitive play is important. At this age they discover reading as an enjoyable activity that opens doors to other worlds. They develop an interest in collecting items, such as Beanie Babies or sports cards, and value the quantity of the collection. As they approach adolescence, they become more interested in listening to music and developing the ability to perform popular dances. They spend more and more time with friends in activities outside of the home.

FEARS

As children explore the world around them, having new experiences and confronting new challenges, fears and anxieties are an unavoidable part of growing up. Children between the ages of 6 and 11 have many fears and concerns, such as fear of darkness, animals, high places, or thunderstorms. The death of a close friend or family member may cause them much anxiety about the health of those around them. Other children who see news reports on TV and in the newspapers may feel threatened by burglars, kidnappers, or violence in the classroom. They strongly identify with others their age. Stories about child abuse or school-yard shootings can confuse and frighten them. Children want to be reassured that these terrible things will not happen to them. It is important to let children talk about a frightening situation and to share what is on their minds. The child's questions can guide the depth and details of your answers.

Action Alert!
When children are concerned about what they see on TV or read in the newspaper, encourage parents to reassure their children and provide them the perspective they need to understand what they are viewing.

Most fears wax and wane during childhood, but sometimes the fears can become so extreme, persistent, and focused that they develop into phobias. Phobias are strong and irrational fears that can significantly influence and interfere with a child's daily activities. For example, a child with a phobia about dogs might be so frightened as to refuse to go outdoors because a dog might be nearby. If talking with the child and providing reassurance is not successful, help from a therapist who specializes in treating phobias may be necessary.

To handle terrifying and confusing situations, children take their emotional cues from the adults around them. When parents admit to some of their fears and concerns and show how they are responding to their emotions in positive ways, they are teaching their children that their own fears can be overcome.

Moral Development

As children progress in cognitive development, they also move through stages in the development of conscience and moral standards. At age 6 or 7, children know the rules and behaviors that are expected of them but they do not understand the reasons behind them. Rewards and punishments guide their judgments. They believe a "bad act" is one that causes harm or breaks a rule. Consequently, they may interpret an accident or other misfortune as a punishment for a "bad act" committed earlier. Older school-aged children are able to understand what prompts an action and therefore do not judge an action only on its consequences. Rules become less absolute, and actions are based on the needs and wants of others. School-aged children consider their motivations when making judgments about how their behaviors affect themselves and others. They are able to understand the concept of treating others as they would like to be treated.

FACTORS AFFECTING CHILDHOOD GROWTH AND DEVELOPMENT

Environmental Factors

FAMILY DYNAMICS. Family dynamics is the pattern of interpersonal relationships within a family. This pattern is affected by the structure, size, and composition of the family.

FAMILY STRUCTURE. Family structure affects the child's growth and development. Each individual has a position in the family structure and plays a defined role in interactions within the family group. Structure includes traditions and values that set standards for interaction within and outside the group. When family ties are strong, social control is effective and members conform to their roles. Conflicts arise when people do not fulfill their roles in ways that meet the expectations of other family members.

Family size and composition also influence child development. No two children grow up in exactly the same environment. Birth position of children has been shown to affect the child's personality. Parents treat children differently, and sibling interactions vary depending on the child's position within the family.

Parenting practices vary with family size. In smaller families, more emphasis is placed on individual development of the children and they are often pressured to measure up to family expectations. They often experience more democratic participation in family decisions. In large families, there is greater emphasis on organization and a more authoritarian approach to control and there is less one-to-one contact between the parent and any individual child. There is usually a dominant parent or older child. Siblings rely on each other to meet their needs. They are usually made more aware of what constitutes misbehavior and disapproval by another sibling, and this is often more meaningful than parental disapproval. Children in large families develop the ability to adjust to a variety of changes and unexpected happenings. Cooperation is essential because a large number of individuals share a limited amount of space.

Age differences between siblings affect the childhood environment. The arrival of a baby brother or sister has the greatest impact on the older child, and a 2- to 4-year difference in age appears to be most threatening. In general, the narrower the spacing between siblings, the more the children influence one another; when they are close in age and of the same gender, they often have access to common life events.

DISCIPLINE. The term *discipline* means to adhere to a set of rules for conduct and it describes actions taken to enforce the rules after noncompliance. *Limit-setting* means establishing guidelines for behavior. Children want and need limits. These limits must be clear and enforced consistently for children to adhere to the rules. They test limits that are set to learn the extent to which they can manipulate their environment, and they are reassured when they know that others will be there to protect them from potential harm. Parents who maintain firm control and use consistent limit-setting tempered by reasonableness are generally most successful.

SIBLING RIVALRY. Sibling rivalry refers to the competition of brothers and sisters for the attention, approval, and affection of the parents. It is common in families but varies in degree of severity. Because each child occupies a special place within the family and each child has a different personality and temperament, it is impossible for parents to treat their children exactly the same. Differences in parental response can cause one child to envy or fear the other, who is perceived to be receiving more physical or emotional care and benefits from parents than the other. Box 20-2 provides some strategies to teach parents for dealing with sibling rivalry.

BOX 20–2

STRATEGIES FOR SIBLING RIVALRY

Parents should

- Be fair.
- Not compare children.
- Encourage children to work out differences.
- Set guidelines on how conflicts can be resolved.
- If discipline (reprimand) is necessary—do it in private with the child.
- Have regular family meetings with all members present to express thoughts and to give positive recognition.

SCHOOL SYSTEM. Many factors influence a child's school experience, including hereditary and physical factors, achievement motivation, family background, and sociocultural factors. Because more mothers work outside the home, parents are placing their children in some kind of child care arrangement, and the number of children in early childhood education programs has grown tremendously. Additionally, many parents have come to recognize the benefits of preschool education, which can provide enriched intellectual and social experiences.

An important characteristic of successful schools is that they emphasize academic excellence. They have high expectations of the students and devote a high proportion of classroom time to active teaching. Ideally, they pay attention to the needs of individual students and can adjust teaching accordingly. Teachers are expected to respect their students and to help them to have pride in themselves.

COMMUNITY. Children and their families reside in a community in which residents share and are influenced by a common environment. The community can encourage a positive outcome for children or it can stunt it. Children living in high-risk neighborhoods have more social and behavioral problems than those in low-risk neighborhoods. For example, a school-aged child who lives in a high-crime area is more likely to experience violence or become involved with substance abuse. Lack of community resources can affect a child's health in other ways—for example, a 5-year-old child may experience measles because there were no affordable immunization services in the community.

SOCIOECONOMIC FACTORS. One of the most adverse influences on health is low socioeconomic status. Low *socioeconomic status* (SES) persons suffer from more health problems at any one time than people in any other group. Low-SES families often have poor medical care, higher mortality rates, and higher rates of psychological and mental illnesses. Low income generally means inadequate, crowded housing in poor neighborhoods, where crime and social and family problems abound. Low-SES families strive for security with basic necessities of life. Such families are most often headed by a single parent.

As a result of unfavorable life circumstances, low-SES parents have more stresses, which impairs parental functions. One study of 585 children from the lowest socioeconomic class found that low SES was significantly correlated with eight factors in the child's socialization and social context, including harsh discipline, lack of maternal warmth, exposure to aggressive adult models, maternal aggressive values, family life stressors, mother's lack of social support, peer group instability, and lack of cognitive stimulation (Dodge, Pettit, & Bates, 1995).

Physiological Factors

RESPIRATORY AILMENTS. It is not unusual for children to experience cold symptoms, but if the small airways become inflamed, expiratory obstruction, wheezing, and pneumonia can develop. The incidence of childhood asthma is on the rise.

EAR INFECTIONS. Otitis media (inflammation of the middle ear) is one of the most common ear problems in children and is one of the frequently identified reasons parents seek medical care for their children. By age 3, most children have had one or more episodes of otitis media. Prompt evaluation and treatment can prevent hearing loss from this disorder.

HEAD LICE. Children are susceptible to pediculosis capitis, which is caused by the head louse. The most common symptom is intense itching on the back of the head or neck. Infestation results from direct contact with infested persons or their personal belongings, particularly clothing and headgear. If a louse infestation is suspected, every member of the family should be checked and treated with a pediculicide, if necessary, and clothing and bedding should be carefully washed.

Action Alert!
Instruct parents how to safely and properly treat their childrens' lice-infested hair and how to launder their infested clothing and bedding.

ANIMAL AND INSECT BITES. Dog bites are the most common animal bite wounds, followed by cat bites. Dog bites are most common in children aged 5 to 14 years. A child bitten by a dog or cat usually presents with limited cellulitis, and 15 to 20% of these wounds become infected (Dershewitz, 1998; Fineberg, 1998). Because of the sharp teeth of cats, puncture wounds are common and, if untreated, may lead to osteomyelitis and septic arthritis. The risk of rabies and tetanus should be also considered with animal bites. Children will require a tetanus immunization if they have not had a booster within 5 years. In the United States, rabies is predominantly a disease of wild animals such as raccoons, skunks, and bats. Check with the local state health department to obtain the latest information concerning the presence of rabies in a given animal population.

Insect bites are fairly common, especially during the summer. Lesions are commonly found on exposed areas of the body. Some insects, such as mosquitoes, carry the encephalitis virus in various areas of the country.

Action Alert!
Teach parents to have their children wear long sleeves and pants, especially if they are outside at sundown when biting insects are most active. Also advise them to apply a children's strength insect repellent to exposed skin if mosquitoes are suspected of carrying the encephalitis virus.

ENURESIS. Children usually achieve urinary continence by age 5 to 6. *Enuresis* is recurrent involuntary urination that occurs during sleep. Children are considered to have enuresis when they experience persistent involuntary voiding of urine into the bed or clothes beyond the age of expected control. Primarily an alteration of neuromuscular bladder functioning, enuresis is the most common voiding abnormality in children and is best viewed as a symptom rather than a disorder. If left untreated, most enuretic children eventually develop complete control (Houts, 1995). There are three subtypes of enuresis: nocturnal only (night-time), diurnal only (daytime), or both. Nocturnal enuresis is common and declines in frequency as children grow older. Approximately 3% of children at 12 years of age still experience nocturnal bedwetting. Medical problems such as diabetes and kidney or bladder problems should be ruled out as possible causes of nocturnal enuresis (Rushton, 1995).

Behavioral techniques are used extensively in the treatment of enuresis. Treatment is individualized to the child's wetting pattern, social environment, and family resources and attitudes. Parents must learn how to respond nonjudgmentally to their child's wetting accidents and noncompliance with treatment. For the child who wets intermittently during the day, a 1- to 3-hour voiding schedule is useful. An inexpensive digital watch can be set to chime at scheduled voiding times. A reward system is useful for reinforcing correct behavior.

For nocturnal enuresis, behavioral treatment involves the use of a urine alarm to teach the child to respond to a full bladder by awakening the child when there is contact with the first few drops of urine. This method is appropriate for children 6 to 7 years of age and older. The process usually takes 2 to 4 weeks and is successful with over 80% of children.

Lifestyle Factors

NUTRITION. Poor nutrition may cause a child to tire easily, have a poor appetite, experience slower growth, or become ill because of an inability to resist pathogens and infections. As children grow older, poor eating habits can contribute to the development of obesity. Obese children do not necessarily eat more food, but they prefer calorific foods high in fats, starches, and sugars such as junk foods (e.g., potato chips, sweets, and soft drinks). Teach parents the importance of providing children with nutritious foods and of not bringing junk foods in the house. Instead, snacks should consist of fruits and low-fat foods. Parents should also encourage children to drink more water and fewer soft drinks.

Eating problems may develop when parents excessively encourage children to eat, fail to provide nutritious meals, or are overindulgent and give children whatever they want to eat. Parents must recognize that children's appetites vary—sometimes they eat a lot, sometimes a little. Children should not be bribed with rewards for eating. The less fuss that is made about eating the better. If a child has poor appetite, encouraging physical activity can stimulate the appetite.

ACTIVITY AND EXERCISE. Parents should encourage their children to exercise and become involved in enjoyable and vigorous activities that promote their physical development, preferably with other children at the same developmental level. Activities should help children develop motor skills that will enable them to reach their full physical potential. They should provide them with basic skills and habits that will make fitness an enjoyable, lifelong activity.

Parents of preschool-aged children need to make a systematic effort to teach them physical and athletic skills. They should be highly active and be given plenty of opportunity for running about and exercising growing muscles. School-aged children need daily exercise but not necessarily organized sports; bike riding and playing at a playground can provide exercise.

From about age 5 to 8, children become more interested in organized group play and team sports, like community leagues for soccer and T-ball (Fig. 20–4). Their physical and cognitive development are not ready for serious competition, but participation in organized activities builds socialization and self-esteem.

SLEEP AND REST. The number of hours per day spent sleeping varies with individual children and with different age groups. The preschool-aged child sleeps approximately 11 hours, gradually decreasing during the school-aged years to 9 or 10 hours. Sleep disorders develop in children due to a variety of altered biologic and emotional states. Lack of sleep may lead to fatigue, irritability, and emotional and physical problems. Sleep problems affect 25 to 40% of infants and children (Blum, Ditmar, & Charney, 1997). Parents' sleeping patterns may also be disrupted due to their child's problem.

SUBSTANCE ABUSE. When children begin to experiment with drugs, they often mistakenly think they can control their use. They believe that the use of cigarettes is better than alcohol or marijuana, which is illegal. Children at risk for drug use are those who have poor self-concept or a strong need for acceptance and approval of their peers. Children who have school or family stresses may find relief in the use of controlled substances.

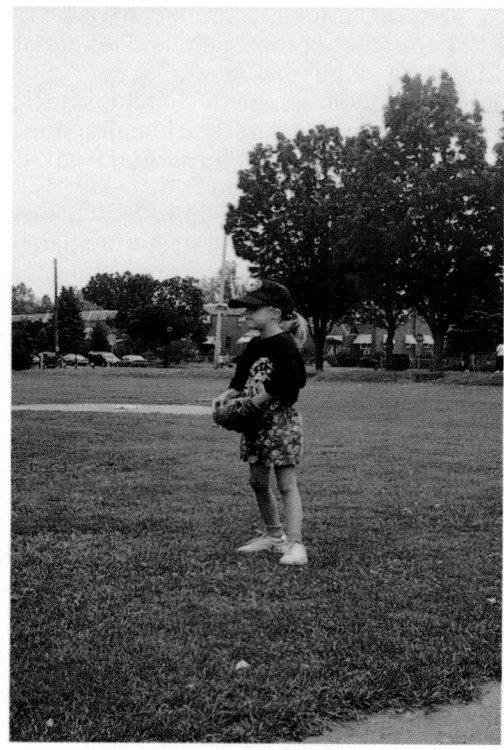

Figure 20–4. From about ages 5 to 8, children become more interested in organized group play and team sports. Sports help the school-age child develop physical skills, a healthy sense of competition, an understanding of the importance of following rules, and the importance of teamwork.

*A*ction *A*lert!
Encourage parents to discuss the risks of tobacco, alcohol, and other drugs with their children.

Common Behavioral Concerns

ATTENTION-DEFICIT/HYPERACTIVITY DISORDER. Attention-deficit/hyperactivity disorder (ADHD) is a neuropsychological disorder associated with disturbances in attention, impulsivity, and hyperactivity. ADHD is estimated to affect 6 to 9% of children and adolescents, and is more prevalent in boys. Preschoolers are frequently referred to therapists for hyperactivity, impulsivity, and aggressiveness. School-aged children often have marked inattention, easy distractibility, impatience, low frustration tolerance, and frequent shifting of activities; they talk excessively and intrude into others' conversations and personal space. Children with ADHD are at risk for developing emotional and behavioral problems, such as conduct or antisocial behaviors, substance abuse, depression, and anxiety disorders (Jellinek, 1998; Voeller, 1996).

ADHD appears to serve as an umbrella diagnosis for a variety of behavioral-attention problems with a variety of causes. They include psychologic adversity, perinatal insults, and other yet unknown biologic causes. Data from family, genetic, twin, and adoption studies suggest a genetic origin in 20 to 50% of cases (Murphy & Hagerman, 1996). Both drug and behavior-modification treatment methods have been used with success, which may support the theory of varying causes. Parents need to be supported and taught behavioral management strategies. Medications most often employed for ADHD include the psychostimulants, antidepressants, and antihypertensives (Spencer, Biederman, & Wilens 1996).

LEARNING DISABILITY. According to the Learning Disabilities Association of America (1999), a **learning disability** is a lifelong disorder that affects the manner in which people of normal or above-average intelligence select, retain, and express information. It has been estimated that approximately 5% of public school children have a learning disability (Shaywitz, Fletcher, & Shaywitz, 1995). They may result from abnormalities in the structure or function of the brain that are congenital or acquired, such as head trauma and intracranial infections.

Parents usually report that their child is unable to learn basic school material at the expected age and grade level. The deficiency usually occurs in specific areas such as reading, although related skills such as writing and mathematical concepts may also be affected. An evaluation may reveal that their overall ability as measured by IQ tests is not abnormal but standardized academic achievement tests demonstrate areas of weakness. The evaluation should exclude other causative factors such as hearing or visual defects, psychological factors, and inadequate teaching.

ASSESSMENT

General Assessment of Children

Optimum childhood growth and development and prevention of accidents and illness are the objectives of pediatric health supervision.

Health History

The health history aims to review the child's past physical and psychosocial history and to determine whether the parents or the child has any complaints or concerns. It includes a complete nutritional assessment, exercise habits, sleep patterns, and growth and development milestones. Progress in school and the child's social interactions with family and peers should also be evaluated.

The depth and extent of a nursing health history vary with its intended purpose. The format used for history taking is usually a combination of direct and indirect techniques to elicit information about each of the functional health patterns. The school-aged child should be able to cooperate fully with you, whereas the younger child may be more challenging.

Physical Examination

The American Academy of Pediatrics recommends that preschoolers and school-aged children have a routine well-child examination at least every 2 years, with at least four examinations being conducted between the ages of 4 and 11 years. The well-child visits provide an excellent opportunity for you to become acquainted with the child and family, to develop a database on the child, and to teach the child and parents about preventive health care.

The well-child examination involves several evaluations. The immunization history is reviewed to be sure the child is current. Measurements of the child's height, weight, and blood pressure are obtained, and vision and hearing are screened. A complete physical examination is performed.

Diagnostic Tests

Additional diagnostic tests may be performed, but there is some variability in the tests performed at each visit. The following are examples of such tests.

CHOLESTEROL SCREENING. Parents are increasingly becoming aware that risk factors for cardiovascular disease, particularly coronary artery disease related to dietary cholesterol intake, may be present in their children. However, there is no consensus regarding the efficacy of universal cholesterol screening in children.

A*ction* A*lert!*
Advise parents of young children to provide diets low in cholesterol and saturated fat and recommend an active lifestyle for children and the avoidance of smoking, including second-hand smoke.

BLOOD TESTING FOR LEAD POISONING. According to the Centers for Disease Control and Prevention, or CDC (1998), 890,000 American children aged 1 to 5 have elevated blood lead levels, and more than one-fifth of African-American children living in housing built before 1946 have elevated blood lead levels. The major sources of lead exposure are deteriorated lead-based paint in older housing and dust and soil that are contaminated with lead from old paint and from past emissions of leaded gasoline. Lead poisoning can cause learning disabilities, behavioral problems, and at very high levels, seizures, coma, and even death. The CDC recommends that at-risk children undergo a blood lead test (CDC, 1998).

TUBERCULOSIS SCREENING. In the United States, tuberculosis (TB) occurs in less than 1% of children. However, all children should have a careful history to ascertain their risk and should be screened three times during childhood for TB: at 12 to 15 months of age, before entering kindergarten, and at 14 to 16 years of age. The multipuncture Mono-Vac is adequate for routine screening rather than the purified protein derivative (PPD) test. Children found to be at risk should be identified and screened yearly.

INTELLIGENCE TESTING. The most common test of intelligence in the United States is the Stanford-Binet Intelligence Scale. It is used with persons from age 2 through adulthood. This test yields scores in verbal reasoning, quantitative reasoning, abstract visual reasoning, and short-term memory. It also provides a composite score that can be interpreted as an "Intelligence Quotient" (IQ) that reflects overall intelligence.

Intelligence testing of children usually begins during preschool years. Children's maturation and educational experiences have to be considered when interpreting the result. There is a high correlation between the measures of intellectual performance in the preschool years and academic progress in later years (Rice, 1996) (Fig. 20–5). However, test results do not predict children's ability to get along with other people, adaptability to different situations, or emotional stability.

Focused Assessment for Altered Growth and Development

Children are at risk for problems of growth and development from both internal and external factors. Physical development requires health, nutrition, and exercise. Psychosocial development requires opportunities to complete developmental tasks with a warm, caring adult to guide the way. The particular risks that are common for children are illness, lead poisoning, substance abuse, TB, safety, home life, and school.

Defining Characteristics

When working with young children you need a quick, reliable method for checking a child's developmental progress to decide if more in-depth assessment is necessary to determine a need for special services. The most widely used developmental screening tests are reviewed in Chapter 19. The lack of a single overall description of physical growth during this period makes comparison of individual characteristics to an established norm more difficult. Growth patterns established in the earlier years can be a better guide to assessment than a child's current measurements. During the school years, individual differences due to genetics and environment become more apparent.

Related Factors

If the parents lack the skills to provide a healthy growth-producing lifestyle or are just indifferent to the

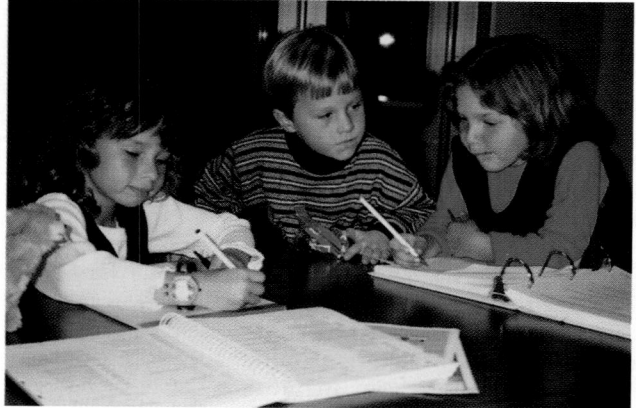

Figure 20–5. There is a high correlation between the measures of intellectual performance in the preschool years and academic progress in later years

child's needs, development may be hampered. Consistency is important in parenting. Parents who respond sporadically to the child's needs or vacillate between positive and negative responses will not provide the child with a consistent pattern of caring against which to gauge behavioral choices.

Children need to be able to rely on their caretakers. Foster children and other children who experience multiple caretakers have difficulty meeting the developmental tasks for their particular age group. Separation from significant caregivers will likewise result in delayed development of skills or regression to a previous stage of development. Regression to an earlier stage or behavior often occurs in the hospitalized child.

Focused Assessment for Altered Parenting

A health maintenance visit for the school-aged child includes an assessment of the parent's ability to provide a constructive environment that nurtures the growth and development of the child. You should be aware that inappropriate parenting behaviors may be a reaction to an unfamiliar setting or part of a larger parenting role problem. During the health maintenance visit, you pick up cues from observing the interaction between the child and parent and from listening to child and parents' descriptions of developmental issues and concerns.

Defining Characteristics

The defining characteristics of *Altered parenting* are observed delays in growth and development, observed inappropriate parenting behaviors, or concern with parenting skills expressed by the parent. Evidence of child abuse is a clear defining characteristic of *Altered parenting*.

Related Factors

The difficulty in parenting can be related to a lack of knowledge or lack of exposure to positive parenting practices. The parents may be single, young, and immature. They may have problems that interfere with parenting, such as emotional disturbances, addictions, illness, or disability. They may have a child of undesired sex, undesired characteristics (hyperactive or rebellious), or who is physically handicapped or seriously or even terminally ill. Situational or personal factors may contribute to parental role conflicts, including a parent separated from the nuclear family, lack of an extended family, unemployment or economic problems, or recent separation or divorce.

DIAGNOSIS

Once the components of the well-child assessment are completed, you will use the health history, vital signs, physical examination, and results of diagnostic tests, if needed, to develop a database to differentiate among the three nursing diagnoses. The nursing diagnosis *Al-*

tered growth and development is appropriate for the child who is not achieving normal physical growth or is not achieving the developmental tasks of the particular age group. You must be knowledgeable about age-appropriate developmental expectations to diagnose such problems.

The nursing diagnosis *Altered parenting* is used when the family environment does not provide the basic needs for a child's physical growth and development. The child may not be provided with stimulation that enables the child to grow cognitively, emotionally, or socially or who may not be provided with a consistent, stable, nurturing environment.

PLANNING

Once the nursing diagnoses have been identified, a plan of care is developed and outcomes are established for each diagnosis. Each plan of care is individualized depending on the child's needs. You will need to work collaboratively with the parents and the child, depending on the developmental level of the child, to foster the child's growth and development.

Expected outcomes for well children might include the following:

- The parents understand normal growth and development in their preschool-aged child and the signs and symptoms of common illnesses.
- Children's participation in daily physical activities is appropriate for their age.
- The child experiences no injuries (other than normal cuts and bruises) from play activities or other activities of daily living.
- Parents will bring their child to a dentist at least once a year, and the child brushes and flosses teeth (under adult supervision) at least once daily.
- Parents will bring their child for recommended screening tests at appropriate times.
- An older school-aged child understands his growth and development patterns.
- Children progress to at least their average performance levels in schoolwork and activities.

INTERVENTION

Through the use of a thorough assessment process, you identify problems that affect children's growth and development. Your interventions will be based on establishing a trusting relationship with your clients and their families and incorporating their cultural beliefs in your interventions. The main interventions for *Altered growth and development* and *Altered parenting* are health education and counseling.

Interventions to Promote Health

Education and anticipatory guidance are the best preventive measures for parents of preschool and school-aged children. Families need to understand normal growth and development and nurturing child care practices. They may have many concerns about smok-ing; child safety inside and outside the home; school adjustment; violence; use of TV, video games, and other media; latchkey children; and a number of other issues presented in this chapter. Parents who receive early guidance with their children build competence in their parenting skills. Teaching parents when it is necessary to contact health care providers promotes decision-making about self-care. Box 20-3 lists selected reasons for parents to contact a health care provider.

TEACHING ABOUT PROPER NUTRITION. Parents need to teach their child to eat properly by modeling the principles of healthy nutrition. They can provide healthy meals and snacks and low-fat foods rather than focusing on the "forbidden" junk foods. Teach parents the importance of teaching children to eat nutritious foods by using the food guide pyramid: milk and dairy products, lean meat, fish, poultry, fruits and vegetables, and breads and cereals.

ENCOURAGING ACTIVITY AND EXERCISE. Parents should encourage their children in lifetime fitness activities such as walking, running, bicycling, skating, swimming, golf, or tennis. They should encourage children to participate in physical activities and sports in school or local community sport programs. Not only will this promote physical activity but it will promote psychosocial development through interaction with other age-appropriate children.

A*ction* A*lert!*
Encourage parents whose children are obese to participate in physical activities. Obese children tend to be less active, which reduces food metabolism and increases fat accumulation.

PROMOTING SLEEP AND REST. Parents are responsible for seeing that their children get enough sleep to function effectively during the day. They must promote regular sleeping habits in their children. You can recommend that they establish relaxed bedtime routines that occur at the same time each night. Children

---

BOX 20–3

REASONS FOR PARENTS TO CONTACT A HEALTH CARE PROVIDER

- Routine well-child examinations and immunizations.
- Drastic changes in their child's behavior.
- Severe pain.
- Severe or worrisome injury.
- Prolonged high fever (over 102°F [48.8°C]).
- Persistent cough.
- Foul-smelling drainage from the nose, eyes, ears, or anywhere else.
- Persistent vomiting.
- Unexplained persistent rash.
- Prolonged diarrhea.
- Blood in urine or stool.

are often upset by variations in routines. Violent and frightening bedtime stories and television programs may precipitate nightmares in children and should be avoided. Activities that are excessively stimulating or disturbances in parent-child relationships may make it difficult for children to sleep.

DISCOURAGING SMOKING. The hazards of smoking at any age are undisputed. Antismoking efforts must begin before adolescence. It is important to talk with school-aged children about the adverse health effects of smoking and how children can resist peer pressures. Instead of just going along with the crowd, the child needs the skills and confidence to make correct decisions.

PROMOTING APPROPRIATE USE OF TELEVISION, COMPUTERS, AND VIDEO GAMES. Children's early years are a critical time for the socializing effects of television, computer games, movie and video game viewing habits. Children learn about what to watch and how much to watch from parents and siblings. Encourage parents to set reasonable limits on the amount of time their children watch TV, use a computer, or play video games. Encourage them to watch programs with their children. For example, many computer programs are cartoon-like and computer games may consist of mindless button-pushing. Quality educational software for computers generally provides one or more educational activities. Such products help children practice basic skills in math, reading, and other subjects; facilitate writing and publishing skills; stimulate creativity; challenge higher-order thinking skills such as deductive reasoning and problem-solving; encourage an understanding of complex inter-relationships within systems; and offer ways to explore the online world (Fig. 20–6).

Parents need to discuss with their children the potential dangers of using the Internet. Advise parents to warn their children that E-mail is not as private as it seems. Have them discourage their children from sharing their password to an E-mail address, even with close friends. Most services make it easy to change a password. All users, including adults, should change passwords frequently to reduce the chances of their being stolen. Have parents tell the children not to share family secrets in their E-mail messages. Parents can find out more about Internet safety issues from the Online Safety Project at *www.safekids.com* and *www.safeteens.com* (Burzynski, 1998).

Action **A**lert!
Advise parents that when their children spend hours in front of a TV, computer, or video game, they are missing the opportunity to develop their physical and social skills by playing with siblings or friends instead of being sedentary and solitary.

Interventions to Promote Effective Parenting

HELPING PARENTS DISCIPLINE THEIR CHILD. The purpose of discipline is to instruct children in proper conduct or action rather than to punish children. The ultimate goal of disciplinary action is to teach children to develop a sense of inner control so that they can follow generally accepted standards of behavior and live in accord with the rules and regulations established by the group (Blum, 1995). When discussing ways to enhance the parents' ability to help the child develop inner control, keep in mind several principles. Children respond more readily to parents within the context of a loving, trusting relationship of mutual self-esteem. Learning is enhanced if responses involve rewards and punishments. Discipline is more effective if it is applied consistently rather than erratically, and it is most effective when it is applied soon after the offense occurs. Severe punishment that is cruel and abusive is counterproductive, resulting in similar harsh behavior on the part of the child.

HELPING PARENTS PREPARE THEIR CHILD FOR SCHOOL. During the preschool years, it is important that a child have opportunities for peer interaction. A preschool child who has learned to be comfortable in groups is better able to learn in kindergarten. Explain to parents that interacting with older siblings is not the same as interacting in a group experience with peers.

At the end of the preschool period, children will begin a formal school experience. It is wise for parents to begin preparing the child for changes in daily routine well in advance of the beginning of school. The child may need to wake up earlier and go to bed earlier and may be taking a bus to school or be required to select a lunch from a buffet-style meal. It is helpful for parents to rehearse with their child some of the routines required for school; this will help limit the number of distractions early in the school year.

Parents should also be familiar with the developmental expectations of the school. Are the children expected to tie their own shoes or print their name on their papers? Encourage parents to meet with school administrators and teachers before the school year begins to discuss expectations. The most important task of parenting at this time is to instill in the child the concept that learning is fun and that new experiences are exciting. Parents who are fearful for their child's

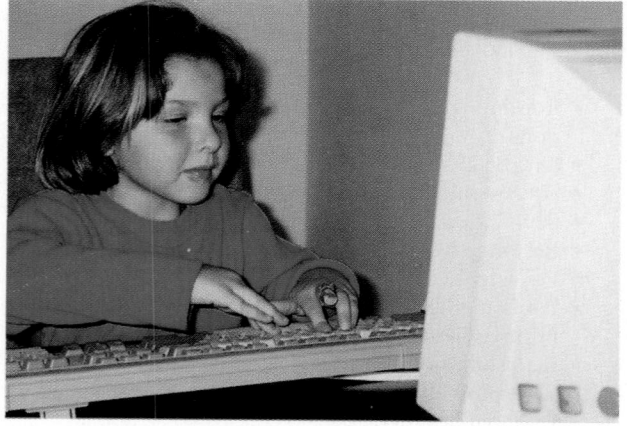

Figure 20–6. This preschooler already knows how to use a computer and educational software.

safety or anxious about their child's performance will communicate this message to their child. Remind parents that the best way to reduce their anxiety is to stay involved in their child's learning.

The most important task for children in early school years is learning to read. Parents can serve as role models by reading books, magazines, and newspapers instead of watching television. Encourage parents to read aloud to their children at bedtime, to play word games with them, and to have them read simple directions to them. Refer parents to reading programs and events sponsored by their local library.

The early school years can be stressful for a child. Encourage parents to spend time with their child to learn how the child perceives the school experience. If signs of stress such as nail biting or thumb sucking appear, the parent should try to identify the underlying stress and assist the child in identifying coping strategies.

Some children may experience school phobia, the fear of attending school. Because fear is one of the most powerful negative human emotions, children may use physical symptoms such as vomiting, headache, or abdominal pain as an excuse to stay home from school. Explain to parents that they must determine the reason for their child's resistance to school before they can help the child to overcome the fear. Refer the child and family to a counselor if the phobia persists.

Interventions to Prevent Injury

No child can be considered free from risk of injury. Your awareness of some injury patterns may be helpful in counseling parents. The type of injuries to which a child is most vulnerable varies with personal circumstance, age, the child's size, and developmental ability. Parents of preschool-aged children must realize that although their children's skills are becoming sophisticated, their judgment is not. Preschoolers cannot be relied on to recognize danger. In contrast, school-aged children are less likely to experience unintentional injuries because they have developed more refined muscular coordination and have the cognitive abilities to avoid injuring themselves. It is often difficult for parents to maintain a balance between the level of supervision and restriction and their children's need for independence.

Action Alert!
Teaching parents about child safety should be part of every well-child visit. Most accidents occur because parents over- or under-estimate their child's abilities.

Promoting Home Safety

The following are safety tips you should share with parents during well-child visits to prevent future injury.

FIRE SAFETY. Fires destroy 400,000 homes each year, and these disasters occur most commonly during the winter months. Fire spreads quickly; you have only 2 minutes to escape after you hear a smoke alarm and 3 to 5 minutes before it may be impossible to escape from the interior of a home (Laliberte, 1998). Fires present a special danger to young children, who cannot be depended on to react quickly in an emergency. When a fire occurs, children who have not been trained for a fire emergency may mistakenly try to hide in a "safe place." Every year more than 800 children age 14 and under die in home fires; the victims are often found under beds or in closets where they fled to escape the smoke and flames. Another 47,000 children are injured (Laliberte, 1998).

Teach parents that the best protection against fire-related injuries is to equip homes with smoke detectors. Smoke detectors should be placed in all hallways adjacent to bedrooms as well as near the kitchen area and the garage. Children should be instructed to leave the house at once in the presence of smoke or fire, even if the fire is small. Calls to 911 can be made from another home. Ask the family if fire drills are held regularly so that children can plan and rehearse all possible escape routes. Children should be taught to "stop, drop, and roll" if their clothing should catch fire. House fires are not the only threat. Many children are burned when they accidentally upset a cooking pot, touch a hot grill, or play with fireworks. Portable heaters are another source of danger.

Action Alert!
Teach children to avoid playing with matches, to know fire escape routes, and to practice fire escape drills at home. Teach them to avoid hot stoves and to avoid playing with flammable substances.

FIREARM SAFETY. In the United States, unintentional shootings kill about 500 children and severely injure many more children each year (Johnson & Oski, 1997). Rates for unintentional firearm deaths are 10 time higher in low-income areas. Children cannot be trusted to handle a gun safely, even though they have the mechanical skill and strength to fire one. You need to ask parents about whether they own guns. If so, instruct them that guns should be locked away unloaded and separate from the ammunition.

SAFETY OF LATCHKEY CHILDREN. The term **latchkey children** describes children in elementary school who spend some part of their time before or after school without adult supervision. The name arose from children who carried keys to let themselves into their homes before the parents returned from work. The lack of affordable day care contributes to this phenomenon today, and about 2 to 5 million children between the ages of 6 and 13 are latchkey children (Wong, 1999). Many of these children report that they are afraid and lonely while at home alone. A major concern is that unsupervised children are at risk for accidents and injuries and impaired school performance, and these children are more likely to use alcohol or other illegal drugs.

Educate parents about both the positive and negative aspects of leaving their children home alone. Parents need to be sure that their child is not extremely fearful, impulsive, or unable to solve problems that may arise. If the older school-aged child is mature, feels safe in the community, and knows how to act responsibly, the opportunity for a short period of independence every day can be a positive experience. Review with parents the safety guidelines for latchkey children summarized in Box 20-4.

Inform parents of community resources available to latchkey children. For example, many communities have organized after-school programs or telephone programs staffed by volunteer adults who are available to answer telephone calls from latchkey children or to periodically call the children at home.

Promoting Safety at Play

BICYCLE SAFETY. Bicycling injuries begin to take their toll during the early school-aged years. Children of this age are still not capable of making accurate judgments about speed and distance. In order to fit in with their peer group, these children may neglect to wear helmets. Bicycle injuries account for approximately 600,000 ER visits and more than 1,200 deaths annually. Approximately 70% of the bicyclists treated in ERs are under age 15 (Wong, 1999). Deaths usually result from head injuries and almost always are the result of collisions between bicycles and motor vehicles.

The best way to avoid bicycle accidents is knowing how to ride a bike safely. Instruct parents to require

---

BOX 20-4

GUIDELINES FOR PARENTS OF LATCHKEY CHILDREN

- Keep a list of emergency telephone numbers by the telephone.
- In case of a power failure, prepare a safety kit. Be sure a flashlight and extra batteries are included. (You do not want a child lighting candles during a power failure.)
- Keep firearms locked and inaccessible to children. Teach firearm safety.
- Plan after-school snacks that do not require cooking.
- Designate a neighbor or a relative who is home at that time for the child to call or go to if necessary.
- Leave a written list of the rules for after-school time. Be clear about play activities and homework time.
- Practice how to report a fire and telephone police.
- Rehearse activities that may be required of the child while home alone (e.g., a light bulb is burned out, or the circuit breaker needs resetting).
- Plan after-school activities at least two afternoons a week to increase socialization.

---

helmet use and to teach their children that bicycle riding is an important responsibility. Children should demonstrate safe riding skills and understand traffic safety laws before being allowed to ride a bicycle on the street. Inform parents of community guidelines for bicycle safety. Pamphlets and videos can help parents teach bicycle safety to their children.

Action **A**lert!
Remind parents that they must select the proper equipment and see that their child learns and obeys traffic laws when riding a bicycle.

SKATEBOARD AND IN-LINE SKATE SAFETY. The use of skateboards and in-line skates by school-aged children puts them at risk for injuries to the arms, legs, head, and neck. If a child uses a skateboard or in-line skates, a helmet is mandatory because this activity takes place on hard surfaces such as concrete and there is great risk of head injury. Homemade ramps on hard surfaces can be very hazardous. Wrists, knees, and elbows also need protective gear. Children under age 5 should not use skateboards or in-line skates because they are not developmentally prepared to protect themselves from injury.

Action **A**lert!
Advise parents to enforce safety guidelines such as prohibiting their children to use their in-line skates or skateboards on streets and highways.

WATER SAFETY. Drownings are a leading cause of death among preschool and school-aged children. Warn parents that most drownings occur when children swim without adequate adult supervision. In most cases, the parents have overestimated the child's swimming ability and knowledge of water survival skills. Advise parents that their children should learn how to swim from an experienced and qualified swimming instructor. When children ride in a boat, they should always wear a personal flotation device. Remind parents that children learn by example, so it is important that adults also follow safety guidelines.

EVALUATION

Evaluation is a systematic, ongoing process in which you evaluate your client's progress toward attainment of goals. At this time you and the child's parents review the problems identified at the last visit and discuss whether and how they were resolved. It is not unusual for some problems to be resolved, only to be replaced by new and different concerns. If the expected outcomes are not achieved within the defined time, reassessment may find reasonable explanations for the lack of progress. New assessment data are used to revise nursing diagnoses, outcomes, and the plan of care. The effectiveness of your nursing interventions is evaluated with respect to your client's and the parents' responses and their attainment of goals.

Finally, as part of the well child's annual evaluation, you should assess how the parents are adjusting to their changing role as their child grows and develops. It is important that the parents' expectations be realistic and that they promote their children's growth and development.

KEY PRINCIPLES

- Children progress through similar stages of growth and development, but the rate of progression and the behaviors observed vary with the person.
- Understanding children's growth and development enables the nurse to individualize approaches to the child's health care needs based on developmental variations in each stage.
- Social development of the preschooler includes further individualization—separation, more sophisticated language, greater independence, and more imaginative forms of play.
- Preschoolers have a number of universal fears: fear of the dark, mutilation, and abandonment.
- Preschoolers operate at a cognitive level that prevents them from understanding the principle of conservation.
- Preschoolers are self-centered, and this makes it difficult for them to share and accept other people's viewpoints.
- During the school-aged years, development slows but there is a steady gain in height and weight with maturation of body systems. The primary teeth are lost and replaced by permanent teeth.
- School-aged children develop a sense of industry or accomplishment.
- School-aged children have a limited capacity for abstract thought but can solve more complex problems, make judgments based on reasoning, and accept a viewpoint different from their own.
- The school-aged child develops a conscience and understands what is morally right and wrong.
- Cooperative team play, acquisition of skills, and adhering to the rules are the major focus of play for the school-aged child.
- The nursing diagnosis *Altered growth and development* is appropriate for the child who is not achieving normal physical growth or is not accomplishing the developmental tasks of the particular age group.
- The nursing diagnosis *Altered parenting* is used when the family environment does not provide the basic needs for a child's physical growth and development.
- Growing and learning between the ages of 4 and 11 require a certain amount of risk, but the risk is manageable if the child is taught about safety.
- Evaluation of the well child is a systematic, ongoing process in which the nurse evaluates the child's progress toward attainment of goals. The nurse

and the child's parents review the problems identified at the last visit, discuss their resolution, and make adjustments as needed.

BIBLIOGRAPHY

*Allshouse, M., Rouse, T., & Eichelberger, M. (1993). Childhood injury: A current perspective. *Pediatric Emergency Care, 9*(3): 159–164.

American Academy of Pediatrics. (1998). *AAP recommends targeted lead screening, universal screening in high-risk areas.* http://www.aap.org/advocacy/archives/junpol.htm. (4/8/99).

Beck, L.E. (1998). *Development throughout the lifespan.* Needham Heights, MA: Allyn & Bacon.

Blum, N.J. (1995). Disciplining young children: The role of verbal instructions and reasoning, *Pediatrics, 96*(2), 336–341.

Blum, N.J., Ditmar, M.F., & Charney, E.B. (1997). Behavior and development. In R.A. Polin & M.F. Ditmar (Eds.), *Pediatric secrets* (2nd ed.). St. Louis: Mosby.

Burzynski, J. (1998). World of computers and the internet: Guidelines are necessary. *Chicago Parent, 15*(11), 39–42.

Centers for Disease Control and Prevention (CDC). (1998). CDC's lead poisoning prevention program. *http://www.cdc.gov/nceh/pubcatns/97fsheet/leadfcts/leadfcts.htm.* (4/10/99).

Cherow, E., Dickman, D.M., & Epstein, S. (1999). Organization resources for families of children with deafness or hearing loss. *Pediatric Clinics of North America, 46*(1), 153–162.

Cunningham, F.G. (1996). *Williams obstetrics* (20th ed.). Norwalk, CT: Appleton & Lange.

Dershewitz, R.A. (Ed.). (1998). *Ambulatory pediatric care* (3rd ed.). Philadelphia: J.B. Lippincott.

Desselle, D.D., & Pearlmutter, L. (1997). Navigating two cultures: Self esteem and parents' communication patterns. *Social Work Education, 19*(1), 23–30.

Dodge, K.A., Pettit, G.S., & Bates, J.E. (1995). Socialization mediators or the relation between socioeconomic status and child conduct problems. *Child Development, 65,* 649–665.

Fagot, B.I., & Hagan, R. (1995). Observations of parent reactions to sex-stereotype behaviors: Age and sex effects. *Child Development, 62*(3) 617–628.

Fineberg, R. (1998). Animal exposures. In R. Finberg (Ed.), *Saunders manual of pediatric practice.* Philadelphia: W.B. Saunders.

*Helwig, C.C., Tisak, M.S., & Turiel, E. (1990). Children's social reasoning in context: Reply to Gabbennesch. *Child Development, 61,* 2068–2078.

Houts, A.C. (1995). Nocturnal enuresis as a biobehavorial problem. *Behavioral Therapy, 30,* 133–151.

Jellinek, M. (1998). Attention-deficit hyperactivity disorder. In R.A. Dershewitz (Ed.), *Ambulatory pediatric Care* (3rd ed.). Philadelphia: J.B. Lippincott.

Johnson, K.B., & Oski, F.A. (1997). In K.B. Johnson & F.A. Oski (Eds.), *Oski's essential pediatrics.* Philadelphia: Lippincott-Raven.

Keefer, C.H. (1998). The well child. In R.A. Dershewitz (Ed.), *Ambulatory pediatric care* (3rd ed.). Philadelphia: J.B. Lippincott.

*Kohlberg, L. (1966). A cognitive developmental analysis of children's sex role concepts and attitudes. In A. Macroby (Ed.), *The development of sex differences.* Palo Alto, CA: Stanford University.

*Kohlberg, L. (1981). *Philosophy of moral development: Moral stages and the idea of justice.* New York: Harper & Row.

Laliberte, R. (1998). Fire: How safe is your family? *Parents Report,* December, 57–62.

Learning Disabilities Association of America (LDAA). (1999). *When learning is a problem.* http://www.ldanatl.org/pamphlets/learning.html. (4/10/99).

Locker, D., Liddell, A., Dempster, L., & Shapiro, D. (1999). Age of onset of dental anxiety. *Journal of Dental Research, 78*(3), 790–796.

*Asterisk indicates a classic or definitive work on this subject.

Marcus, S.M. (1998). Lead poisoning. In R.A. Dershewitz (Ed.), *Ambulatory pediatric care* (3rd ed.). Philadelphia: J.B. Lippincott.

Murphy, M.A., & Hagerman, R.J. (1996). Attention deficit hyperactivity disorder in children: Diagnosis, treatment and follow-up. *Journal of Pediatric Health Care, 10*(1), 2–11.

North American Nursing Diagnosis Association. (1999). *NANDA nursing diagnoses: Definitions and classifications, 1999–2000.* Philadelphia: Author.

Piaget, J. (1997). *The moral judgement of the child.* Glencoe, IL: Free Press.

*Piaget, J. (1950). *The psychology of intelligence.* London: Routledge and Kegan Paul.

*Piaget, J., & Infelder, B. (1969). *The psychology of the child.* New York: Basic Books.

*Piaget, J. (1980). Intellectual evolution from adolescence to adulthood. In R.E. Muuss (Ed.), *Adolescent behavior and society: A body of readings* (3rd ed.). New York: Random House.

Rice, F.P. (1996). *Child and adolescent development.* Englewood Cliffs, NJ: Prentice Hall.

Rushton, G.H. (1995). Wetting and functional voiding. *Urologic Clinics of North America, 22,* 75.

Shaywitz, B.A., Fletcher, J.M., & Shaywitz, S.E. (1995). Defining and classifying learning disabilities and attention-deficit/hyperactivity disorder. *Journal of Child Neurology, 10*(Suppl. 1), S50–S57.

Spencer T.J., Biederman J., & Wilens T.E. (1996). Pharmacotherapy of ADHD across the life cycle: A literature review. *Journal of the American Academy Child and Adolescent Psychiatry, 35,* 409.

TV-Free America. (1999). *Television statistics.* Available from: *http://www.tvfa.org/stats.html.* (4/10/99).

Voeller, K. (1996). The neurological basis of attention deficit hyperactivity disorder. *Internal Pediatrics, 15*(2), 171–176.

Wong, D.L. (1999). *Whaley & Wong's nursing care of children* (6th ed.). St. Louis: Mosby.

The Well Adolescent

Carol F. Roye

Key Terms

adolescence
anorexia nervosa
bulimia nervosa
constitutional delay of puberty
egocentrism
familial short stature
formal operations

gynecomastia
menarche
nocturnal emission
obesity
puberty
scoliosis

LEARNING OBJECTIVES

After studying this chapter, you should be able to:

1. **Describe the normal growth and development of an adolescent.**
2. **Discuss factors that affect adolescent growth and development, including environmental, socioeconomic, lifestyle, psychosocial, and physiological factors.**
3. **Describe the general assessment of adolescents for normal function and risk factors.**
4. **Compare and contrast nursing diagnoses that may be especially appropriate for use with adolescents.**
5. **Plan nursing interventions to maintain wellness and reduce risk factors for adolescents.**
6. **Discuss interventions to improve adolescents' access to health care.**
7. **Evaluate nursing care using outcome criteria.**

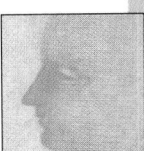

Malik Mirad is an 18-year-old high school senior whose father came to the United States from Saudi Arabia to study engineering, married a U.S. citizen, and stayed in the United States. Malik is 6'2" and is described by many as handsome. He is studying to be a biology major and has an overall A− average. He plays soccer and is vice president of the student body. He comes to the school nurse's office for his sports physical examination.

During his interview, Malik reports feeling a little stressed about graduating, drinking with his friends on weekends, and engaging in unprotected sexual intercourse with multiple girls. He says, "I don't believe I can get AIDS or other diseases from my girlfriends because they have all been virgins." The school nurse chooses the nursing diagnosis *Altered health maintenance* to address the issues that Malik is facing in adolescent development and considers a variety of related diagnoses, including *Ineffective individual coping* and *Risk for infection*. Malik made a follow-up appointment with the school nurse (see Well Adolescent Nursing Diagnoses).

WELL ADOLESCENT NURSING DIAGNOSES

Altered Growth and Development: The state in which an individual demonstrates deviations in norms from his or her age group.

Altered Health Maintenance: Inability to identify, manage, and/or seek out help to maintain health.

Body Image Disturbance: Confusion in the mental picture of one's physical self.

Ineffective Individual Coping: Inability to form a valid appraisal of the stressors, inadequate choices of practiced responses, and/or inability to use available resources.

Risk for Infection: The state in which an individual is at increased risk for being invaded by pathogenic organisms.

Self-Esteem Disturbance: Negative self-evaluation/feelings about self or self-capabilities, which may be directly or indirectly expressed.

From North American Nursing Diagnosis Association. (1999). NANDA nursing diagnoses: Definitions and classification 1999–2000. Philadelphia: Author.

CONCEPTS OF ADOLESCENT DEVELOPMENT

Adolescence is the period of transition between childhood and adulthood. It is a period of rapid growth and dramatic change, both physically and psychologically. For the purpose of discussion, this chapter defines adolescence as being between ages 12 and 21. Keep in mind, however, that children grow and develop at different rates, and any definition of adolescence should be flexible on both ends.

Developmental Milestones

The three stages of adolescence are the following:

- Early adolescence, from about ages 12 to 14, when the adolescent has not entirely left the world of childhood
- Middle adolescence, from about ages 15 to 17, when the adolescent undergoes a time of consolidation
- Late adolescence, from about ages 18 to 21, when the adolescent reaches the threshold of adulthood and begins to establish himself as an independent person

Physical Development

The hallmark of adolescence is a physical process known as **puberty**—the sequence of physiological events that cause the reproductive organs to mature, making conception and childbirth possible. In girls, menarche is the hallmark event of this change. **Menarche** is the time of the first menstrual period; it occurs at an average age of 12 years and 4 months, although it may range from ages 9 to 17. In boys, the first nocturnal emission marks the transition to puberty. A **nocturnal emission** is a discharge of semen during sleep;

it occurs at an average age of 13 years and 4 months, but it may range from ages 11 to 15.

During adolescence, secondary sexual characteristics appear. These are changes in bodily features induced by sex hormones, such as pubic hair, axillary hair, and fully developed breasts and penis. Secondary sexual characteristics develop in the same sequence in all adolescents, although the timing differs from person to person. The sexual maturity scale developed by Tanner identifies five stages of pubertal development that focus on breasts in girls and scrotal and penile development in boys (Fig. 21–1). Pubic hair can be assessed in both genders but offers less important information in the overall physical assessment.

Adolescents experience a rapid growth in height called the pubertal growth spurt. It begins before menarche or the first nocturnal emission and accounts for 15 to 25% of the final adult height. Body fat is also affected. In girls, the amount of adipose tissue increases, reducing the proportion of lean body mass. In boys, the lean body mass increases during this time.

Girls begin their growth spurt at an earlier age than boys but commonly reach a shorter adult height because of a lower velocity of growth and a shorter period of growth. The cardiorespiratory system grows at a disproportionate rate to the rest of the body, making aerobic activity at this age an important part of physical fitness.

Motor Development

During early puberty, many adolescents experience some awkwardness because the feet, legs, and arms begin the growth spurt before the height catches up. This tendency is what gives many young teens a spindly appearance. The musculoskeletal system is also most vulnerable to injury during the period of peak height velocity, which occurs during Tanner stage III.

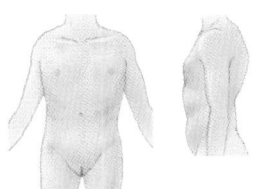

Stage I
Breasts: Preadolescent; elevation of the papilla only
Pubic hair: None

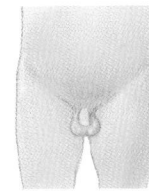

Stage I
Penis: Childhood size and proportion
Testes and scrotum: Childhood size and proportion
Pubic hair: None

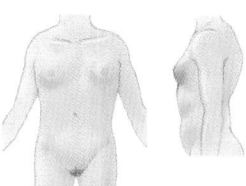

Stage II
Breasts: Breast budding (thelarche); small mound formed by elevation of the breast and papilla, with enlargement of the areolar diameter
Pubic hair: Sparse growth of long, downy pubic hair over mons veneris or labia majora; may occur with breast budding or several weeks or months later (pubarche)

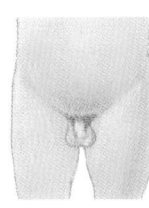

Stage II
Penis: Slight or no enlargement
Testes and scrotum: Enlargement; scrotal skin reddens, changes in texture
Pubic hair: Sparse growth of long, downy pubic hair mainly at the base of the penis

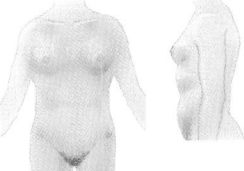
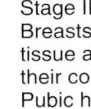

Stage III
Breasts: Further enlargement of breast tissue and areola with no separation of their contours
Pubic hair: Increased amount of hair and changes in the character of the hair (darker, coarser, and more curly), spread sparsely over junction of pubes

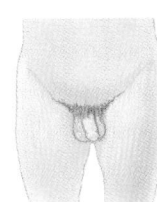

Stage III
Penis: Enlargement, particularly in length
Testes and scrotum: Further enlargement
Pubic hair: Darker, coarser, curlier hair spread sparsely over the pubic symphysis

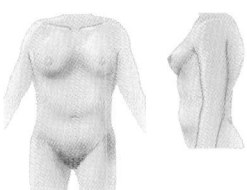

Stage IV
Breasts: Double contour form: projection of areola and papilla form a secondary mound on top of breast tissue
Pubic hair: Adult appearance but less area covered; no spread to medial aspects of thighs

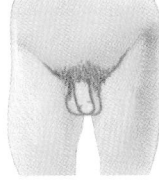

Stage IV
Penis: Further enlargement in length and breadth, with development of the glans
Testes and scrotum: Further enlargement
Pubic hair: Coarse and curly hair; greater area covered than in Stage III, but still less than in an adult, with no spread to thighs

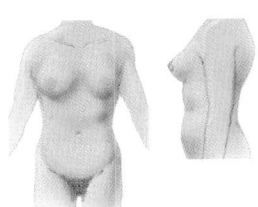

Stage V
Breasts: Larger, more mature breast with single contour form
Pubic hair: Adult distribution and quantity, with spread to medial aspect of thighs

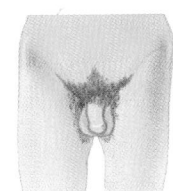

Stage V
Penis: Adult in size and shape
Testes and scrotum: Adult in size and shape
Pubic hair: Adult distribution and quantity, with spread to thighs but not to abdomen

A   B

Figure 21–1. Tanner stages of physical development: A, female; B, male. (Bowden, V.R., Dickey, S.B., & Greenberg, C.S. [1998]. Children and their families: The continuum of care. Philadelphia: W.B. Saunders.)

Action Alert!
Adolescents in early puberty should avoid collision sports and intense, prolonged physical training.

Cognitive Development

During early adolescence, most youngsters acquire the stage of thinking that Piaget and Inhelder (1958) call **formal operations.** It is the ability to reason abstractly. For example, the adolescent can engage in "if-then" deliberations, recognizing that if one event has occurred, another will likely follow. For example,

if Mom's car will not start in the morning and she says that the battery is probably dead, then the adolescent will realize that other accessories in the car—such as the radio and lights—also will not function.

Similarly, adolescents develop the ability to reason and question constructs that they previously took for granted, such as the belief that parents are always correct. They begin to question others. They also develop the ability to see another person's perspective. In addition, they begin to think about thinking and to think about their own thoughts.

Another hallmark of adolescent cognitive development is **egocentrism,** which refers to the tendency to spend so much time thinking about and focusing on your own thoughts and changes in your own body that you come to believe that others are focused on them as well. As a result, young adolescents construct what Elkind (1992) has termed the "imaginary audience." This is a belief that everyone in your proximity is deeply interested in your every thought and action. This leads adolescents to believe that they must be very special because everyone else is so fascinated by them. Several types of "typical" adolescent beliefs result from this type of thinking, such as "No one has ever experienced what I'm feeling" and "Other people will die, but not me." The belief in the uniqueness of oneself is referred to as the personal fable. Although most people never completely lose their personal fables, they decline in influence as they progress through adolescence and share experiences with others. Egocentrism similarly decreases from early through late adolescence.

Psychosocial Development

Erik Erikson, the foremost theorist on psychosocial development, describes the chief developmental task of adolescence as the development of identity versus identity diffusion. To achieve a sense of identity, the adolescent must be able to integrate past, present, and future selves. During this period, the adolescent gradually becomes less reliant on family and more reliant on herself and others. A sense of group identity becomes strong and may lead to specific behaviors, styles of hair and dress, and activities (Fig. 21–2). However, the family still influences an adolescent's basic values and provides important emotional support, regardless of whether the adolescent consciously recognizes this influence. Gender identity also becomes consolidated during adolescence, and young people may begin to have heterosexual relationships, homosexual relationships, or both.

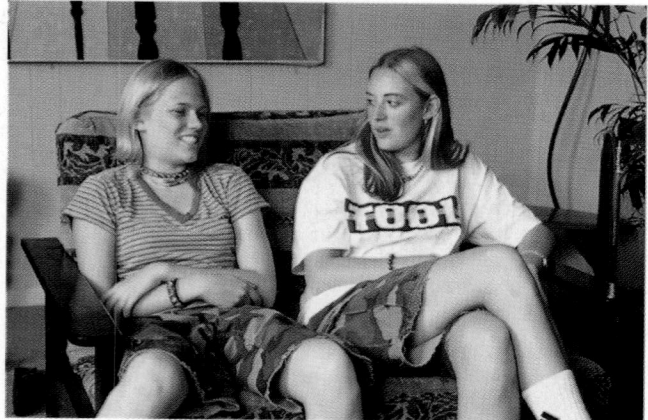

Figure 21–2. Peers have a strong influence on an adolescents' clothes, hairstyle, and manner of speech.

FACTORS AFFECTING ADOLESCENT GROWTH AND DEVELOPMENT
Environmental Factors

FAMILY. Parents who are nurturing, supportive, and consistent in enforcing rules will help to foster adolescent development. These parents show respect for individuality by reasoning with the adolescent, allowing self-expression, considering the adolescent's point of view, and negotiating with the adolescent.

Parents are neglectful when they fail to take an active role or interest in the adolescent's life, are unresponsive, or have few or no expectations of the adolescent. When parents physically, sexually, or emotionally abuse an adolescent, they place the teen at high risk for altered growth and development because they destroy trust and leave the teen with feelings of low self-esteem and helplessness.

Action **A**lert!
Adolescents who are abused or neglected are at high risk for *Altered growth and development.*

COMMUNITY. Community attributes also affect adolescent development. To develop a sense of future goals, teens must have role models in the community. They should see neighborhood adults going to work and having satisfying jobs. Especially in impoverished areas, teens may not have such role models, and their own sense of future goals can be severely limited. Some teens may then turn to illegal job markets, especially the drug trade (Brookins, Petersen, & Brooks, 1997).

SOCIOECONOMIC CONDITIONS. Studies indicate that people with lower income or education have a higher prevalence of health-risk behaviors, such as smoking, being overweight, and leading a sedentary lifestyle. Adolescents who live in poverty typically have limited access to heath care, poor nutrition, and substandard housing. This puts them at high risk for altered growth and development (Centers for Disease Control and Prevention [CDC], 1998b; Papalia & Olds, 1998).

Physiological Factors

Physiological factors and acute or chronic illness may affect the adolescent's growth and development as well.

Delayed Puberty

CONSTITUTIONAL DELAY OF PUBERTY. As mentioned earlier, the average age of the onset of puberty is 12 in girls and 13 in boys. A delay of more than 2 or 3 years from this norm may cause adolescents tremendous anxiety. **Constitutional delay of puberty** is defined as an absence of early signs of puberty, such as Tanner stage II breasts by age 13 for girls or Tanner stage II genitalia by age 14 for boys. This constitutional delay causes more than 9 in 10 cases of delayed puberty. The adolescent has no underlying pathology but is simply a "late bloomer."

Boys are affected by a constitutional delay of puberty more often than girls, and the condition is more likely to arise in a family in which the pubertal development of the same-sex parent was delayed. In other words, the adolescent's parent reports being small as a teenager and going through puberty later than his or her peers.

Youngsters with a constitutional delay of puberty also have a delayed bone age. Because they are small for their age, their physical presentation is that of a younger child. Not surprisingly, they have more growth left than a child of the same age who does not have delayed puberty.

Although benign and self-limiting, constitutional delay of puberty can cause psychological problems, such as body image disturbance, self-esteem disturbance, negative emotional reactions, long-term dependency on parents, and failure to acquire appropriate social skills. It is important to reassure adolescents and their parents that this condition is self-limiting and that the adolescent is normal.

Action Alert!
Reassure adolescents with constitutional delay of puberty that they are normal.

PATHOLOGICAL DELAY OF PUBERTY. Many disorders can delay puberty, but all are rare. For example, chronic renal or cardiac disease, regional enteritis, or sickle cell disease can delay puberty and restrict growth. Malnutrition and certain chromosomal abnormalities—such as Turner's syndrome and Klinefelter's syndrome—also delay puberty.

Short Stature

Most cases of short stature result from heredity and not an underlying disease. **Familial short stature** is a term used to describe a height below the 3rd percentile on the growth chart. Most adolescents with familial short stature have a family history of short stature, a growth curve that parallels the 3rd percentile, a history of birth weight and length at the 3rd percentile, and a bone age that is appropriate for their chronological age. Their physical examination is normal.

The same conditions that can cause a pathological delay of puberty are responsible for pathological short stature. They include renal disease, regional enteritis, chromosomal abnormalities, and hypothyroidism. Growth hormone deficiency is one of several causes of dwarfism, which is characterized by short stature.

Gynecomastia

A common complaint of adolescent boys is **gynecomastia,** which is a benign increase in breast tissue associated with puberty. It results from an imbalance in circulating estrogens and androgens. Occasionally, it is caused by other entities or drugs, such as the following:

- Anabolic steroids
- Antineoplastic agents
- Drugs of abuse, such as marijuana and amphetamines
- Renal failure and dialysis
- Klinefelter's syndrome

Gynecomastia can be unilateral or bilateral, and the breasts are frequently tender when touched, even by clothing. Most cases resolve spontaneously within 12 to 18 months. Occasionally the breasts become very large, a condition known as macromastia. When this occurs, drug treatment or surgery is indicated.

The main sequelae associated with gynecomastia are psychological. Adolescent boys become self-conscious about their breasts, particularly if they are large. They may not want to remove their shirts during gym and may be teased by peers. Counseling may be helpful.

Action Alert!
Assure boys with gynecomastia that the condition is a normal and relatively common part of puberty and that it usually goes away by itself within about 12 to 18 months.

Acute Illness

Fortunately, most acute illnesses during adolescence are short-lived and easily treated. However, mononucleosis deserves special mention because it is most prevalent during the adolescent and young adult years. The vast majority of cases of mononucleosis are caused by Epstein-Barr virus. Transmission typically occurs through saliva during direct, prolonged contact with oropharyngeal secretions.

A teen infected with Epstein-Barr virus usually presents with fever, fatigue, a sore throat, and enlarged lymph nodes. Some clients also have an enlarged spleen. Care is generally symptomatic and includes rest and analgesics. The disorder usually runs its course in 2 to 4 weeks. Adolescents who have had an enlarged spleen should not return to sports until the spleen is completely normal (Neinstein, 1996).

Chronic Illness

The number of adolescents living with chronic illness has increased, not because the incidence of disease has changed but because more children with chronic conditions are surviving. Experts believe that one in four or five adolescents today are affected by chronic illness. The most common are asthma, diabetes mellitus, congenital heart disease, sickle cell disease, chronic renal disease, epilepsy, and hemophilia. Advances in treatment have transformed many diseases that once were almost always fatal (such as leukemia and other childhood cancers) into chronic, treatable conditions.

Studies have shown that, in general, adolescents with chronic illnesses are as well-adjusted as their healthy peers. However, chronically ill, disabled adolescents do have a higher-than-average risk of psychological disorders. They are more likely to have trouble with tasks related to achieving independence, such as planning for the future, dating, and remaining in school. They also have more difficulty achieving satisfying relationships with family. Depending on the nature of the illness, they may have trouble forming a healthy self-image and developing healthy peer relationships and sexuality.

Certain factors increase the risk of psychological problems in the chronically ill adolescent, whereas other factors appear to be protective. Parental or family problems increase the adolescent's vulnerability. In contrast, factors that reduce vulnerability include academic success, self-confidence, a supportive relationship with at least one parent, and family closeness.

Lifestyle Factors

The primary causes of adolescent morbidity and mortality are preventable health-risk behaviors (Fig. 21–3). According to the CDC (1998a), the three top causes of death for adolescents are unintentional injuries (especially motor vehicle accidents), homicide, and suicide.

In addition, adolescents sustain many injuries that receive treatment in outpatient settings, at school, or at home. These injuries include drowning (the second leading cause of nonintentional injury and death); bicycle, motorcycle, and skateboard accidents; and sports-related injuries. Football causes the highest number of injuries in boys, followed by wrestling. Softball and gymnastics cause the most injuries in girls (Neinstein, 1996).

The CDC (1998a) monitors the health-risk behaviors of high school students with the Youth Risk Behavior Surveillance System. As part of its 1998 analysis, the CDC conducted a national school-based youth risk survey. The results indicate that many high school students engage in behaviors that increase their likelihood of death or injury. The survey found that

- 50.8% had drunk alcohol.
- 48.4% had had sexual intercourse, of which 43.2% had not used a condom during the last encounter.
- 36.6% had ridden in a motor vehicle with a driver who had been drinking alcohol.
- 19.3% had rarely or ever worn a seat belt.
- 18.3% had carried a weapon during the 30 days preceding the survey.
- 7% had attempted suicide during the 12 months preceding the survey.

Recall Malik, the adolescent in our case study. What behaviors of Malik's presented health risks?

OBESITY. Obesity is defined as body weight or body fat percentage that exceeds a chosen reference point. There is no standard definition of obesity,

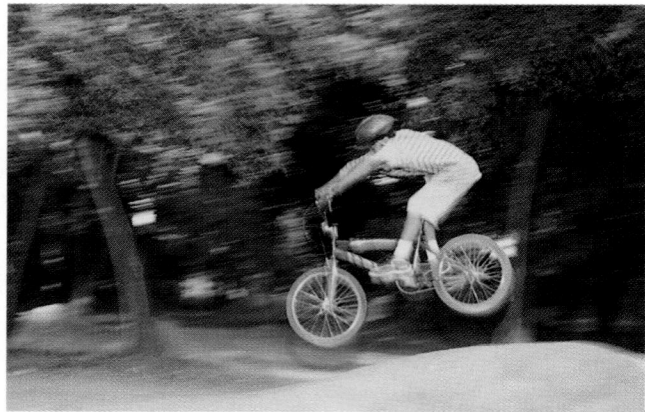

Figure 21–3. Adolescents have a high rate of accidents because of their participation in sports and other health-risk behaviors.

although many researchers define it as a body weight more than 20% above the ideal body weight (MacKenzie & Neinstein, 1996; Neinstein, 1996). Among adolescents aged 12 to 17, about 12% are overweight, a figure that represents a 6% increase over the previous decade (National Center for Health Statistics [NCHS], 1998). These teens tend to eat very quickly and for emotional comfort. Usually, they eat while engaged in other activities such as watching television, overindulge in fast foods, and skip breakfast and lunch only to consume many calories at night (Klish, 1998).

Therapy for these adolescents is a formidable task. Counseling should include nutritional teaching as well as promoting exercise. Because adolescents are usually not the ones who buy and prepare food, it is helpful to involve the parents in treatment as well.

SUBSTANCE ABUSE. Substance abuse is a primary risk factor for altered growth and development because it interferes with biological, psychological, and sociocultural integrity. It is a cofactor in the most common causes of deaths and injuries in this age group, including motor vehicle and other accidents, homicide, suicide, and the diseases that can result from unprotected sexual intercourse. Not all teenagers who use alcohol or other drugs become abusers or dependent. Experts estimate a 3.5% rate of alcohol abuse and a 2% rate of drug abuse among teens ages 14 to 16. For ages 17 to 20, the estimated rate rises to 15% for alcohol and 4% for other drugs. The goal of treatment is to diagnose the problem early, to stop the alcohol or drug use, and to determine if other environmental or psychiatric problems are related to the substance use. Treatment usually includes self-help groups or outpatient counseling for the teen and family (Weinberg, Rahdert, Colliver, & Glantz, 1998).

The American Academy of Child and Adolescent Psychiatry has reported that parents are often unaware that their adolescent children are using alcohol and other drugs. They were more aware of the problem when adolescents used substances frequently, were younger, were having social problems, or used more than one substance. Parents were more likely to be aware of alcohol-related problems, such as drunk driving, and of marijuana and hallucinogen use, compared with cocaine or opioid use. Characteristics that have been linked to an increased risk for substance abuse include difficulties with judgment and foresight, aggression, disruptive behavior, and psychiatric disorders, such as a conduct disorder or depression. Signs of substance abuse included loss of inhibitions, lethargy, hyperactivity, agitation, sleepiness, and over-alertness (Weinberg, Rahdert, Colliver, & Glantz, 1998).

TOBACCO USE. Cigarette smoking is another serious health problem among adolescents that has profound implications for their adult health. The prevalence of smoking remains high among all groups of adolescents. The 1998 youth risk survey reported that 28% of male students and 20.9% of female students had smoked before age 13. Because nicotine is a highly addictive substance, most young people who begin smoking during adolescence will become regular smokers (CDC, 1998a).

VIOLENCE. Homicide is the second leading cause of death among 15- to 24-year-olds and the leading cause of death for African-American and Hispanic teenagers. Risk factors for homicide include the use of alcohol or drugs, exposure to media violence, a personal history of child abuse, witnessing violence (particularly in the home), and poverty. A sense of helplessness pervades many young people who grow up in poverty (Neinstein, 1996).

SEXUAL BEHAVIOR. Another prominent cause of morbidity and mortality in adolescents is their sexual behavior. More than 7% of teens reported having intercourse before age 13. Estimates vary, but most studies agree that at least half of adolescents in the United States engage in intercourse during their high school years, and 43.2% had not used a condom at last sexual intercourse. Sixteen percent reported having intercourse with four or more partners.

Rates of sexual activity differ by race, gender, and socioeconomic status. Male adolescents are more likely to engage in intercourse than females. Overall, African-American teens (72%) were more likely to have had intercourse than Hispanic or white students (52% and 44%, respectively). Teenagers who engage in early sexual activity may have unwanted pregnancies and become infected with sexually transmitted diseases (STDs), including the human immunodeficiency virus (HIV) (CDC, 1998a).

Adolescents are in the age group at greatest risk for acquiring STDs. Girls have an increased risk compared with adult women because the uterine cervix has immature cellular properties that increase its susceptibility to infection. Adolescents are more likely to have multiple sexual partners and to engage in unprotected intercourse than their adult counterparts, both of which are risk factors for STDs. Chlamydia is the most common STD among teenagers. Young women make up the largest category of new AIDS cases, which is attributed to the number of girls and women infected as teenagers. Hispanic and African-American women are at greatest risk (Wortley & Fleming, 1997).

Recall that Malik admitted to having multiple girlfriends with whom he had unprotected intercourse. For what conditions might he be putting himself at risk?

Each year, more than a million American teenagers (more than 1 in 10 of all 15- to 19-year-olds) become pregnant. According to the CDC (1998a), African-American teenagers (15%) were more likely to have been pregnant or to have gotten someone pregnant than Hispanic (7%) or white teenagers (6%).

Preventing teenage pregnancy requires much more than a "just say no" approach. Parents do not have to condone their adolescents' behaviors, but neither can they simply ignore the possibility that their teenagers may be involved in sexual activity. Encourage parents to talk with their teens about sexual activity in a nonjudgmental and informative manner, including discussions of both abstinence and methods of birth control. Suggest that parents encourage their teenagers to come to them first if pregnancy occurs. Parents need to convey the message that they will "be there" for their teens no matter what the crisis (Brody, 1996).

Action **A**lert!
Encourage parents to talk with their teenagers about sex in a nonjudgmental and informative manner.

Psychological Factors

SUICIDE. It is difficult to estimate how many adolescents commit suicide because of the number that go unreported—a single-car accident that actually was a suicide, for example. Adolescent girls make more suicide attempts than boys. The usual pattern is to take an overdose of available medication, often an over-the-counter medication such as acetaminophen. Males are more likely to complete the suicide because they tend to use more lethal methods, such as shooting, poisoning, or hanging. Risk factors include a family history of suicide (with an increased risk around the anniversary of the death), alcohol or other drug use, chronic physical illness, psychiatric disorders (such as an anxiety disorder or depression), and the loss of a significant person or relationship. A history of a previous suicide attempt is another important risk factor (CDC, 1998a; Shaffer, 1996).

ANOREXIA NERVOSA. Anorexia nervosa is a complex disorder characterized by self-induced weight loss driven by a morbid fear of becoming fat. Of the adolescents suffering from this affliction, 90% are female. These teenagers are preoccupied with food and weight and have a distorted body image. They believe that their morbidly thin bodies are too heavy. They have a revulsion for food that yields a weight loss of 25% or more of the normal body weight with no other apparent illness or psychiatric disorder. They may exercise compulsively to work off any food eaten.

Anorexia is the third most common chronic condition among adolescent girls (after obesity and asthma). The syndrome can begin in children as young as age 9. It can have serious or even life-threatening complications, such as cardiovascular problems (bradycardia, arrhythmia, cardiac muscle damage, mitral valve prolapse, and sudden death, probably secondary to arrhythmias) and kidney damage. Virtually all girls with anorexia become amenorrheic early in the course of the illness. The resulting low levels of estrogen can lead to osteoporosis later in life (Fisher et al., 1995; Schreiber et al., 1996).

BULIMIA NERVOSA. Bulimia nervosa is a disorder characterized by binge eating coupled with purging via emetics, laxatives, or self-induced vomiting. It may be a subtype of anorexia, and it has a similar etiological pattern. It has a slightly older age of onset, with college-aged women more likely to present with this disorder than girls of high school age or younger.

Although they can experience mild weight loss or gain, girls with bulimia often have a stable weight. They may suffer from gastric or esophageal rupture, parotid gland enlargement, hypokalemia, erosion of dental enamel from induced vomiting, scars on the knuckles of one hand, and amenorrhea or irregular menses. Death has been reported from abuse of ipecac taken to induce vomiting (MacKenzie & Neinstein, 1996).

ASSESSMENT

General Assessment of Adolescents

Health History

Most health problems encountered by well adolescents are caused by health-risk behaviors. If possible, interview an adolescent client without the parents present, and reassure the client that your conversation will be confidential (unless the teen is suicidal or homicidal). Most adolescents would prefer not to divulge certain information in front of their parents, such as grades, drug use, sexual behavior, and suicidal thoughts. You may want to interview the parents separately to determine their concerns.

Do not be afraid to ask adolescents about illegal, unsafe, or otherwise undesirable behavior. Research has shown that they will not interpret the question as tacit approval to engage in that behavior. For example, asking an adolescent whether he has ever had a sexual relationship will not encourage him to begin a sexual relationship.

Adolescents are more likely to be honest when respected and questioned honestly. They are very sensitive not only to what you actually say to them, but to what they think your perceptions are of them. It is important for you to remain nonjudgmental. Teens who believe they are being criticized are unlikely to return for care.

When you assess an adolescent, ask the least personal questions first to allow her to become comfortable talking with you. For example, ask about home, education, and other activities first, before you ask about drug use, sexuality, and suicide risk (see Box 21-1 concerning Sample Health History Questions for an Adolescent). Ask the teen's perceptions of her

weight, her ideal weight, and what measures, if any, she has taken to alter her weight. Finally, question the teen's risk for injury. Also assess the adolescent's developmental level. Is he operating at an earlier cognitive level than you would expect? Is she more physically mature than the average teenager her age?

Physical Examination

Make sure to assess the adolescent's physical, cognitive, and psychological functioning, beginning with a general assessment of appearance. Monitor the teen's vital signs, vision, and hearing, and obtain the results of any other diagnostic screening tests. Obtain height and weight, and assess for anorexia or bulimia if the client has a weight loss of more than 10% of previous weight or her body weight is in the 5th percentile.

Pay particular attention to the adolescent growth spurt, which peaks in girls at about age 12 and in boys at about age 14. During this period, adolescents experience many physical changes. Boys gain an average of 8 inches in height and more than 40 pounds in weight, whereas girls gain somewhat less height and weight. Boys' voices begin to deepen, and facial hair appears on the upper lip and then on the cheeks and lower lip. Pubic hair begins to develop, and the penis, testes, and scrotum enlarge. Some boys experience gynecomastia. Girls' breasts and pubic hair begin to develop. Menarche usually takes place during Tanner stage III or IV.

Depending on the reason for your examination, you should pay particular attention to certain areas. For example, if you were administering a sports physical, you would assess the teen's heart, lungs, and abdomen for any abnormalities, and you would test all of the joints for range of motion, flexibility, strength, and reflexes. The type of diagnostic tests performed or ordered is discussed under the next heading.

Scoliosis is a structural lateral curvature of the spine. More than 60% of cases occur in girls. It often first appears during late childhood or adolescence, so all adolescents should be appropriately screened. Many states mandate scoliosis screening in the schools.

Diagnostic Tests

All teens should have a hearing, vision, and blood pressure screening annually and be encouraged to have dental checkups and perform good dental care. They should be up to date with immunizations, including tetanus and diphtheria (every 10 years), hepatitis B, measles, mumps, rubella (the second inoculation), and varicella (if there is no history of chicken pox). They should also be screened for tuberculosis.

Iron-deficiency anemia is a relatively common problem in adolescents, especially girls. This is usually due to menstrual blood loss and lack of iron in the diet. All teens should have a hemoglobin or hematocrit level yearly to check for this condition. Adolescents whose parents have a serum cholesterol level greater than 240 mg/dL and adolescents who are over 19 years of age should be screened for total blood cho-

BOX 21–1

SAMPLE HEALTH HISTORY QUESTIONS FOR AN ADOLESCENT

Home

- Where do you live and who lives there with you?
- Do you get along?
- Do you have privacy in your home?

Education

- What grade are you in?
- What are you good at in school? What is hard for you?
- What kinds of grades do you get?

Activities

- What do you do after school?
- What do you do with your friends?

Alcohol

- Do you know anyone who has tried drugs, alcohol, or cigarettes?
- Have you ever tried drugs or alcohol?
- Do you drink alcohol? What do you usually drink, and how often? Alone or with friends?

Sexual Behavior

- Many young people become interested in sexual relationships at your age. Do you currently have, or have you ever had, a boyfriend or girlfriend? (Include both options for all clients.)
- Have you ever been worried that you had a sexually transmitted disease or that you were (or were responsible for someone becoming) pregnant?

- Have you used anything to prevent disease or pregnancy?
- What did you use?

Suicidality

- Everybody feels sad or depressed sometimes. Do you think that you feel that way more often than other young people your age?
- Have you ever felt that life was not worth living?
- Have you ever wanted to kill yourself? If yes, have you made a plan to kill yourself?

Weight

- Do you feel that your weight is just right, too low, or too high?
- Have you ever tried to do anything to change your weight?
- Do you think about food a lot?

Injuries

- Do you know students in your school who have guns or other weapons?
- Do you have a gun? Are there guns in your home?
- Have you ever been the victim of violence or seen someone being assaulted?
- Do you or any of your friends drive a car? Do they ever drive after drinking?
- Have you ever gotten in a car with a driver who has been drinking?
- Do you ever drive after having had something to drink?

---

lesterol level at least once (American Medical Association [AMA], 1995).

Testicular cancer is a disease of adolescents and young men. It is readily treatable when detected early. Adolescent males should be screened for this disorder and taught how to examine their testicles so they can perform a self-examination regularly.

Although breast cancer is exceedingly rare in adolescents, all girls who have reached Tanner stage II of breast development should have a breast examination as part of their regular physical. This also enables you to monitor breast development during puberty. All adolescent females should be taught to perform a breast self-examination and to make it a routine part of their health behaviors.

All adolescents should be asked annually about involvement in sexual behaviors that may result in unwanted pregnancy and STDs, including HIV infection. To screen for STDs, female adolescents should have a cervical culture and males should have urine leuko-

cyte esterase analysis to screen for gonorrhea. The frequency of screening for STDs depends on the sexual practices of the adolescent involved. All sexually active females or any female 18 years or older should be screened annually for cervical cancer with a Papanicolaou (Pap) test. Adolescents at risk for HIV infection should be offered confidential HIV screening (AMA, 1995).

Focused Assessment for Altered Growth and Development

Defining Characteristics

Defining characteristics for the diagnosis *Altered growth and development* include the following:

- Altered physical growth
- Delay or difficulty in performing skills (motor, social, expressive) typical of age group

- Inability to perform self-care or self-control activities appropriate for age
- Flat affect, listlessness, or decreased responses

Related Factors

Factors related to the diagnosis *Altered growth and development* include the following:

- Prescribed dependence
- Indifference
- Separation from significant others, inadequate caretaking, or multiple caretakers
- Environmental and stimulation deficiencies
- Effects of physical disability
- Inconsistent responsiveness

Focused Assessment for Altered Health Maintenance

Adolescents have an increased risk for the diagnosis *Altered health maintenance* because of their high-risk health behaviors, such as substance abuse, poor nutrition, or reckless driving. They often have feelings of invulnerability coupled with peer pressure to engage in high-risk behaviors, putting themselves at risk for physical illness, psychosocial problems, or death.

Defining Characteristics

Defining characteristics for the diagnosis of *Altered health maintenance* include the following:

- History of lack of health-seeking behavior
- Reported or observed lack of equipment, financial, and/or other resources
- Reported or observed impairment of personal support systems
- Expressed interest in improving health behaviors
- Demonstrated lack of knowledge regarding basic health practices
- Demonstrated lack of adaptive behaviors to internal/external environmental changes
- Reported or observed inability to take responsibility for meeting basic health practices in any or all functional pattern areas

Related Factors

Factors related to the diagnosis *Altered health maintenance* include the following:

- Ineffective family coping
- Perceptual/cognitive impairment (complete/partial lack of gross and/or fine motor skills)
- Lack of, or significant alteration in, communication skills (written, verbal and/or gestural)
- Unachieved developmental tasks
- Lack of material resources
- Dysfunctional grieving
- Disabling spiritual distress
- Lack of ability to make deliberate and thoughtful judgments
- Ineffective individual coping

Focused Assessment for Related Nursing Diagnoses

The diagnosis *Ineffective individual coping* is appropriate for adolescents who seem to have trouble solving problems, meeting role expectations, or meeting their own basic needs. Peer pressure, the ready availability of drugs and alcohol, and the portrayal of sexual relations in the media all send conflicting messages. The stress of making good grades, making the team, or getting into a good college may further challenge adolescents.

Self-esteem is still developing in the adolescent and depends on the successful completion of Erikson's final task of the adolescent period, the development of identity. Any of the risky behaviors that are common in adolescence may have roots in poorly developed self-esteem. Additionally, the negative consequences of these high-risk behaviors will further damage or retard the development of self-esteem. Therefore, the nursing diagnosis *Self-esteem disturbance* may apply to the adolescent client.

Adolescents are also at risk for the diagnosis *Body image disturbance,* which is a feeling that the body is the wrong size, the wrong shape, at the wrong time. Images of "perfect" adolescent bodies flood magazines and television shows, and many adolescents may come to feel that they cannot "measure up." They are too fat or too thin, their hair is too straight or too curly, girls' breasts are too large or too small, boys are too short or too scrawny.

The increased prevalence of sexual intercourse at young ages, coupled with other risk behaviors for STDs discussed earlier, may make the diagnosis *Risk for infection* appropriate.

The diagnosis *Altered sexuality patterns* would be applicable for an adolescent experimenting with sexual relationships; however, this label seems to defy the nonjudgmental attitude needed to work successfully with this population.

DIAGNOSIS

The Data Clustering Chart provides suggestions for choosing the appropriate diagnoses for adolescents.

PLANNING

Plan primary prevention strategies with adolescents, with the goal of discouraging them from participating in high-risk behaviors. When planning care for well adolescents, focus your teaching on specific high-risk behaviors while incorporating teaching about all risk behaviors in an effort to prevent them. Because adolescence is normally a time of risk-taking, chronically ill teens may have the additional problem of engaging in risk-taking behavior by failing to comply with their treatment regimen.

It is essential to include the adolescent as an active partner in developing appropriate responses to the

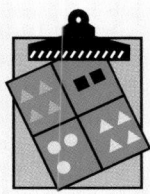

CLUSTERING DATA TO MAKE A NURSING DIAGNOSIS
ADOLESCENT PROBLEMS

Data Cluster	Nursing Diagnosis
Joan is 14, well developed, popular, and has been going steady with a 16-year-old who drives his own car. At an appointment with the school nurse, Joan says that her period is late and that she has not used contraceptives.	*Altered health maintenance* related to having unprotected sex
Jose is a 16-year-old who has had above-average grades until this year. When his friends made the football team, he started hanging out with a different group. He has been arrested for reckless driving and possession of marijuana. His physician referred him to a psychiatric nurse practitioner for counseling.	*Ineffective individual coping* related to establishing peer relationships through reckless behavior
Marie is 17. She has made straight A's throughout school and is on the school choir, the newspaper staff, and the drill team. Marie is thin and appears underdeveloped for her age. The nurse records her height at 5'8" and weight at 98 lbs in an exam gown. Marie says that she thinks a lot about how fat she is.	*Body image disturbance* related to a distorted belief about her weight
William has been cutting classes and not doing his homework. His affect is flat; he says he wakes up at 4 in the morning and is tired all the time. His mother is afraid he is using drugs and brings him to a nurse practitioner for a physical exam. William denies using drugs but admits to planning his death, probably by taking his father's medication.	*Risk for violence* related to suicidal ideation

risk situation. The teen should be able to identify positive responses, such as, "Thanks for asking me to go to the beer party, but I have other plans." He might want to find new activities—such as trying out for a team or auditioning for the school play—to find a set of friends and a situation in which drinking is not the goal. Some schools have peer education or peer support programs in which teens are trained to teach or support classmates who are having difficulties with risk behaviors. The peer educators are under the supervision of the faculty (Siegel, Aten, Roghmann, & Enaharo, 1998).

Reflect back on Malik from our case study. Why did the nurse choose the diagnosis *Ineffective individual coping* for Malik?

INTERVENTION

Interventions to Prevent Illness

Primary prevention is clearly a key issue in adolescent health because most of the morbidities of adolescents are behavioral and therefore preventable. Client teaching is important, but research has repeatedly shown that knowledge alone does not result in behavior change. You must also be skilled in the techniques of primary prevention (see Box 21-2 concerning Primary Prevention for Adolescents).

The Health Belief Model (Janz & Becker, 1984) offers insight into what motivates clients to change their high-risk behaviors. According to this model, four factors must be present for clients to change their behavior. They must perceive the seriousness of their high-risk behavior, perceive their susceptibility, perceive that the barriers to changing their behavior are not overwhelming, and perceive that there are benefits from changing their behavior.

How would you would attempt to help Malik understand the dangers inherent in his drinking, including the dangers of physical intoxication and impaired judgment?

Using this theory, adolescents must first acknowledge that their present behavior truly threatens their health. Otherwise, they will feel they have no reason to change. Second, adolescents must believe that they are susceptible to the poor health outcome. This belief can be difficult to instill in teens, who often feel invulnerable. Third, if there are barriers to changing the behavior that seem overwhelming to teens, they most likely will not adopt the safer behavior. For example, if a young woman thinks that her boyfriend will leave her if she asks him to use a condom, she may feel that it is not worth it to ask him. And finally, the benefits of the behavior change must appear to be worthwhile, or teens will feel there is no point in adopting the behavior.

Action Alert!
Consider the factors that motivate adolescents to change their high-risk behaviors as you develop your health education strategies.

Interventions to Overcome Health Care Barriers

A barrier to implementing care for adolescents is their perceived lack of access to health care providers. Some adolescents do not seek health care because they feel uncomfortable in both their pediatrician's office, where they were treated as a child, and clinics that primarily serve adults. They may also be uncomfortable divulging personal information about a potentially embarrassing topic such as a suspected pregnancy to either their parents or health care providers. Some adolescents are unaware of where to obtain care. Others may not live where clinics are conveniently located. Still others have parents who may not be aware of the health needs or concerns of their adolescents.

What barriers might you need to overcome to ensure Malik's adherence to the plan of care?

Interventions Through School-Based Clinics

Studies have shown that school-based clinics are an effective means of providing care to adolescents. They are often an integral part of the school where adolescents seek care and the most common place where

---

BOX 21–2

PRIMARY PREVENTION FOR ADOLESCENTS

- Yearly health checkup to include complete blood count, blood pressure, height, weight, Tanner stage.
- Immunizations to include tetanus and diphtheria every 10 years, hepatitis B series, measles, mumps, rubella, hepatitis A for high-risk persons (including those traveling to endemic areas), and tuberculosis.
- Health education about the risks of weapons, dangers of alcohol and drug use, drunk driving.

---

teachers and administrators refer students who are having health problems. Many clinics are multidisciplinary, with on-site social workers and health educators. In most clinics, primary care health services are provided by nurse practitioners who consult with physicians. They provide reproductive health services aimed at reducing rates of teen pregnancy and STDs, and they often provide primary care health services, care for chronic and episodic illnesses (such as asthma and ear infections), health education, and mental health services. Most school districts mandate health education programs. In addition to one-to-one care, the group approach used in schools is a very effective one for teens because they are peer oriented.

Interventions for the Ill Adolescent

Hospitalized Adolescents

An important goal of care for hospitalized adolescents is to avoid disruption of their psychosocial development. The principles of communication with well adolescents should be maintained during their hospitalization. Withhold judgments about teens' behaviors and treat them with respect. Consult them on treatment decisions instead of dealing only with their parents, because they are in the process of gaining independence from their families. They will be more likely to comply with the treatment regimen when they take part in the decision-making process.

Certain structural adjustments on the hospital unit can help. Teens prefer being with other teens. They often feel uncomfortable sharing a room with a much younger child or an older person. Even a few rooms at one end of the hall, for teens only, can be helpful. Leisure activities geared to their age level are facilitated by this room arrangement. In this way, they can continue to engage in peer activities. Privacy is a very important concern for teens. They should be in a bed with full curtains. In addition, most adolescents have very hearty appetites and should have frequent access to snacks. They should know that (if possible) they can wear their own clothes and have their friends visit.

Adolescents With Chronic Illness

Although an important goal is to help chronically ill adolescents establish independence, you also need to consider the importance of parents in the care of adolescents and their concerns about their adolescents. Many parents of chronically ill children are overly protective and very anxious. You can help them understand normal adolescent developmental needs so that parents can avoid impeding the teen's growth.

Because chronically ill adolescents often have delayed puberty, they may have difficulty establishing self-identity and peer relationships with members of the same and the opposite sex. They may need counseling in coping with these issues.

Action Alert!
Encourage chronically ill adolescents to discuss any concerns about their development.

Adolescence is often an especially perilous period for the chronically ill adolescent. Because adolescence is normally a time of risk-taking, adolescents with a chronic illness may engage in risk-taking by failing to comply with their treatment regimen. For example, a teen with diabetes mellitus may eat foods that are too high in sugar, fail to monitor blood glucose levels, or fail to take insulin as directed. Asthmatics may take up smoking or fail to use an inhaler before sports activities.

You can take several steps to minimize these unhealthy behaviors. The most important steps in achieving compliance is to involve the adolescents in making decisions about care and in providing self-care. To help an adolescent reduce high-risk behaviors, apply the Health Belief Model. Adolescents must understand the nature of their illness, the seriousness of noncompliance, and their susceptibility to adverse outcomes. You, therefore, must understand adolescents' perceptions of barriers to care so that you can help the client address these. For example, you can obtain from the American Dietetic Association lists of approved items served at the major fast-food chains; this step allows the diabetic teen to go out with friends but make appropriate food choices. Or you can encourage an asthmatic soccer player to use her inhaler in the restroom, before going out on the field. Finally, help adolescents to understand the benefits they will reap from complying with their treatment regimen.

A*ction* A*lert!*
The most important way to foster compliance is to have adolescents involved in making decisions about care and in providing self-care.

EVALUATION

Evaluation is a systematic, ongoing process in which you evaluate the adolescent's progress toward the attainment of goals. With many of the behavioral problems of adolescence, you will not have an objective, accurate measure of the outcome. For example, to evaluate a change in drinking habits, you will need to rely on the client's report. However, if he does not feel completely comfortable with you, you may receive an inaccurate report. One objective way to look for a change in a teen's weekend drinking would be to check his attendance record on Mondays. Likewise, an objective way to evaluate an increase in condom use would be to check for a change in the frequency of the client's STDs.

During a follow-up visit with Malik, how would you assess whether he is following through with your mutually established plan?

KEY PRINCIPLES

- Adolescence is a period of transition between childhood and adulthood. It is a period of rapid and dramatic change, both physically and psychologically.

- The hallmark of adolescence is puberty, which is the sequence of physiological events that cause the reproductive organs to mature, making conception and childbirth possible.
- The chief developmental task of adolescence is the development of identity versus identity diffusion.
- Substance abuse and cigarette smoking are serious health problems among adolescents and have profound implications for their adult health.
- The top causes of death for adolescents are motor vehicle accidents and other unintentional injuries, homicide, and suicide.
- Sexual behaviors, including initiation of intercourse at an early age, STDs, and teen pregnancy are all problems affecting the health of adolescents in the United States.
- Several principles should guide your assessment of the adolescent: assuring confidentiality, ordering the questions from least personal to most personal, not being afraid to ask, and being respectful and nonjudgmental.
- *Altered growth and development* and *Altered health maintenance* are key nursing diagnoses during adolescence.
- When planning care for adolescents, focus your teaching on the teen's specific risk behaviors and nursing diagnoses while incorporating teaching about all risk behaviors to help prevent them before they begin.
- Primary prevention is a key issue to adolescent health.
- Look for objective measures of outcome attainment in adolescents.

BIBLIOGRAPHY

American Medical Association. (1995). *Guidelines for adolescent preventive services (GAPS): Recommendations for physicians and other health professionals.* Available from http://www.ama-assn.org/adolhlth/recommend/monogrfl.htm 1/31/99.
Brody, S. (1996). The evolution of character. *Journal of the American Psychoanalytical Association, 44*(3), 1003–1006.
Brookins, G.K., Petersen, A.C., & Brooks, L.M. (1997). Youth and families in the inner city: Influencing positive outcomes. In H.J. Walberg, O. Reyes, & R.P. Weissberg (Eds.), *Children and youth interdisciplinary perspectives* (pp 45–66). Thousand Oaks, CA: Sage Publications.
Burstein, G.R., Gaydos, C.A., Diener-West, M., Howell, M.R., Zenilman, J.M., & Quinn, T.C. (1998). Incident chlamydia trachomatis infections among inner-city adolescent females. *Journal of the American Medical Association, 280*, 521–526.
Centers for Disease Control and Prevention. (1998a). CDC surveillance summaries: Youth risk surveillance, United States, 1997. *Morbidity and Mortality Weekly Review, 47*(SS-3). Available from http://www.cdc.gov/epo/mmwr/preview/ss4703.html 1/31/99.
Centers for Disease Control and Prevention. (1998b). *Socioeconomic status and health chartbook in health, United States, 1998.* Available from http://www.cdc.gov/nchswww/products/pubs/pubd/hus/2010/98chtbk.htm 2/1/99.
Cohen, E., Mackenzie, R.G., & Yates, G.L. (1991). A psychosocial risk assessment instrument: Implications for designing effective intervention programs for runaway youths. *Journal of Adolescent Health, 12*(7), 539–544.

Cohen, E. & Neinstein, L.S. (1996). Homosexuality. In L.S. Neinstein (Ed.), *Adolescent health care: A practical guide* (pp 641–655). Baltimore: Williams & Wilkins.

Division of adolescent and school health, National Center for Chronic Disease Prevention and Health Promotion, CDC. *Morbidity and Mortality Weekly Review, 41*(46) http://www.cdc.gov/epo/mmwr 866–868.

Division of HIV/AIDS Prevention, National Center for HIV, STD, and TB Prevention, Centers for Disease Control and Prevention. (1996). *HIV/AIDS surveillance report.* Rockville, MD: CDC.

*Elkind, D. (1992). Cognitive development. In S.B. Friedman, M. Fisher, & S.K. Schoenberg (Eds.), *Comprehensive adolescent health care* (pp 24–26). St. Louis: Quality Medical Publishing.

Fisher, M., Golden, N.H., Katzman, D.K., Kreipe, R.E., Rees, J., Schebendach, J., Sigman, G., Ammerman, S., & Hoberman, H.J. (1995). Eating disorders in adolescents: A background paper. *Journal of Adolescent Health, 16,* 420–437.

*Janz, N.K., & Becker, M.H. (1984). The health belief model: A decade later. *Health Education Quarterly, 11,* 1–47.

Klish, W.J. (1998). Childhood obesity. *Pediatrics In Review, 19,* 312–315.

Kulin, H.E. & Muller, J. (1996). The biological aspects of puberty. *Pediatrics in Review, 17*(3), 75–86.

MacKenzie, R., & Neinstein, L.S. (1996). Anorexia nervosa and bulimia. In L.S. Neinstein (Ed.), *Adolescent health care: A practical guide* (pp 564–583). Baltimore: Williams & Wilkins.

National Center for Health Statistics. (1998). *Student use of most drugs reaches highest level in nine years—more report getting "very high, bombed or stoned".* PRIDE, Inc. Press Release, September 25, 1996. Available at http://www.cdc.gov/nchswww/default.htm.

Neinstein, L.S. (1996). Vital statistics and injuries. In L.S. Neinstein (Ed.), *Adolescent health care: A practical guide* (pp 110–138). Baltimore: Williams & Wilkins.

Neinstein, L.S., & Anderson, M.M. (1996). Adolescent sexuality. In L.S. Neinstein (Ed.). *Adolescent health care: A practical guide* (pp. 627–639). Baltimore: Williams & Wilkins.

Neinstein, L.S., Juliani, M.A., & Shapiro, J. (1996). Suicide. In L.S. Neinstein (Ed.), *Adolescent health care: A practical guide* (pp 1116–1123). Baltimore: Williams & Wilkins.

Neinstein, L.S. & Kaufman, F.R. (1996). Abnormal growth and development. In L.S. Neinstein (Ed.), *Adolescent health care: A practical guide* (pp 165–193). Baltimore: Williams & Wilkins.

Neinstein, L.S. & Kaufman, F.R. (1996). Normal physical growth and development. In L.S. Neinstein (Ed.), *Adolescent health care: A practical guide* (pp 3–39). Baltimore: Williams & Wilkins.

Neinstein, L.S. & Pinsky, D. (1996). Alcohol. In L.S. Neinstein (Ed.), *Adolescent health care: A practical guide* (pp 1009–1017). Baltimore: Williams & Wilkins.

Neinstein, L.S., Rabinovitz, S.J., & Schneir, A. (1996). Teenage pregnancy. In L.S. Neinstein (Ed.), *Adolescent health care: A practical guide* (pp 656–676). Baltimore: Williams & Wilkins.

Neinstein, L.S. & Zeltzer, L.K. (1996). Chronic illness in the adolescent. In L.S. Neinstein (Ed.), *Adolescent health care: A practical guide* (pp 1173–1195). Baltimore: Williams & Wilkins.

North American Nursing Diagnosis Association. (1999). *NANDA nursing diagnoses: Definitions and classification 1999–2000.* Philadelphia: Author.

*Piaget, J., & Inhelder, B. (1958). *The growth of logical thinking from childhood to adolescence.* New York: Basic Books.

Papalia, D.E., & Olds, S.W. (1998). *Human development* (7th ed.). Boston: McGraw-Hill.

Resnick, M.D., Bearman, P.S., Blum, R.W., Bauman, K.E., Harris, K.M., Jones, J., Tabor, J., Beuhring, T., Sieving, R.E., Shew, M., Ireland, M., Bearinger, L.H., & Udry, J.R. (1997). Protecting adolescents from harm. *Journal of the American Medical Association, 278,* 823–832.

Roye, C. (1995). How to care for your adolescent patient. *American Journal of Nursing, 95,* 18–23.

Santelli, J., Morreale, M., Wigton, A., & Grason, H. (1996). School health centers and primary care for adolescents: A review of the literature. *Journal of Adolescent Health, 18*(5), 357–366.

Schreiber, G.B., Robins, M., Striegel-Moore, R., Obarzanek, E., Morrison, J.A., & Wright, D.J. (1996). Weight modification efforts reported by Black and White preadolescent girls: National Heart, Lung, and Blood Institute Growth and Health Study. *Pediatrics, 98,* 63–70.

Shaffer, D. (Nov. 9, 1996). *Teen Suicide.* (Presented at Child Psychiatric Disorders: Recognition and Treatment.) Columbia Presbyterian Medical Center, New York.

Siegel, D.M., Aten, M.J., Roghmann, K.J., & Enaharo M. (1998). Early effects of a school-based human immunodeficiency virus infection and sexual risk prevention intervention. *Archives of Pediatric and Adolescent Medicine, 152,* 961–970.

Spitz, A.M., Velebil, P., Koonin, L.M., Strauss, L.T., Goodman, K.A., Wingo, P., Wilson, J.B., Morris, L., & Marks, J.S. (1996). Pregnancy, abortion, and birth rates among U.S. adolescents—1980, 1985, and 1990. *JAMA, 275*(13), 989–994.

U.S. Department of Health and Human Services (HHS). (1999). *YouthInfo Directory.* Available from: http://www.youth.os.dhhs-.gov/youthinf.htm 1/31/99.

Warf, C. (1996). Youth violence. In L.S. Neinstein (Ed.), *Adolescent health care: A practical guide* (pp 1107–1115). Baltimore: Williams & Wilkins.

Weinberg, N.A., Rahdert, E., Colliver, J.D., & Glantz, M.D. (1998). Adolescent substance abuse: A review of the past 10 years. *Journal of the American Academy of Adolescent Psychiatry, 37*(3), 252–261.

*Winer, G.A. (1986). Cognitive and psychosocial development during adolescence. In C.S. Shuster & S.S. Ashburn (Eds.), *The process of human development* (pp 527–546). Boston: Little, Brown.

Wortley, P.M., & Fleming, P.L. (1997). AIDS in women in the United States: Recent trends. *JAMA, 278*(11), 911–916.

Yusuf, H., Averhoff, F., Smith, N., & Brink, E. (1998). Adolescent immunization: Rationale, recommendations, and implementation strategies. *Pediatric Annals, 27,* 436–444.

*Asterisk indicates a classic or definitive work on this subject.

The Well Adult

Marshelle Thobaben and Virginia Nehring

Key Terms

fetal alcohol syndrome
menopause
middle adulthood

midlife crisis
sandwich generation
young adulthood

LEARNING OBJECTIVES

After studying this chapter, you should be able to:

1. **Discuss the developmental tasks a young adult must complete.**
2. **Describe the developmental tasks of the middle years.**
3. **Identify a variety of factors affecting adult development.**
4. **Describe the assessment of a well adult for normal function and risk factors.**
5. **Differentiate among the variety of nursing diagnoses appropriate for middle adults seeking knowledge or health care related to growth and development.**
6. **Plan nursing interventions to maintain wellness and reduce risk factors as appropriate to the adult's developmental level.**
7. **Evaluate nursing care using outcome criteria.**

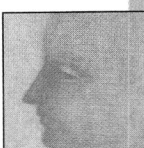

Mr. Edward Biaggio, a 42-year-old obese Italian-American man, is married with two children who are in high school and living at home. He recently began working as a chief accountant at a large insurance company. The occupational health nurse began to monitor his blood pressure after he came in for a routine yearly health screening and was diagnosed with borderline hypertension. His blood pressure reading is 148/96. He is 5'10" tall and weighs 227 pounds.

He has not had a physical examination since college. He smokes two packs of cigarettes a day and reports, "I don't eat many fruits and vegetables. I just never liked them." His diet is high in fat, and he has not exercised for "years." Mr. Biaggio says that he's surprised he has high blood pressure because he is not feeling bad. He knows he should lose a little weight, quit smoking, and get some exercise.

Possible nursing diagnoses for Mr. Biaggio's situation are defined in the accompanying nursing diagnosis chart.

WELL ADULT
NURSING DIAGNOSES

Altered Growth and Development: The state in which an individual demonstrates deviations in norms from his/her age group.

Altered Health Maintenance: Inability to identify, manage, and/or seek out help to maintain health.

Altered Nutrition: More Than Body Requirements: The state in which an individual is experiencing an intake of nutrients that exceeds metabolic needs.

Altered Parenting: Inability of the primary caregiver to create an environment that promotes the optimum growth and development of the child.

Caregiver Role Strain: A caregiver's felt or exhibited difficulty in performing the family caregiver role.

Ineffective Management of Therapeutic Regimen: Individuals: A pattern of regulating and integrating into daily living a program for treatment of illness and the sequelae of illness that is unsatisfactory for meeting specific health goals.

Knowledge Deficit (Specify): Absence or deficiency of cognitive information related to a specific topic.

From North American Nursing Diagnosis Association (1999). NANDA nursing diagnoses: Definitions and classification 1999–2000. Philadelphia: Author.

CONCEPTS OF ADULT DEVELOPMENT

Each adult's growth and development are unique and complex because they are influenced by genetics, socioeconomic status, ethnic group, religious faith, and social expectations. Growth refers to the quantitative change a person undergoes, and development refers to the progressive increase in skill and capacity to function. Always, a person's growth and development represent the interaction of genetic makeup and environment.

Tasks of Young Adulthood

Young adulthood refers to the period from ages 20 to 35. In 1998 the U.S. Census Bureau (USCB) reported that more than 56 million Americans, almost 21% of the population, were between ages 20 and 34. By 2005, this age group will most likely decline to less than 20% of the population (USCB, 1998c).

This development stage ranges from the end of adolescence to the beginning of middle adulthood. Young adults face a variety of developmental tasks that center around the assumption of adult roles and responsibilities (Fig. 22–1). During this period, most people are in search of self. They need to establish autonomy from parents or parent surrogates, develop philosophies of life and personal lifestyles, choose and prepare for employment, marry or establish other types of significant relationships, develop parenting behaviors, and become participatory citizens.

There is considerable variability in how and when different people accomplish these tasks. Young adults are expected to perform many roles, including parent,

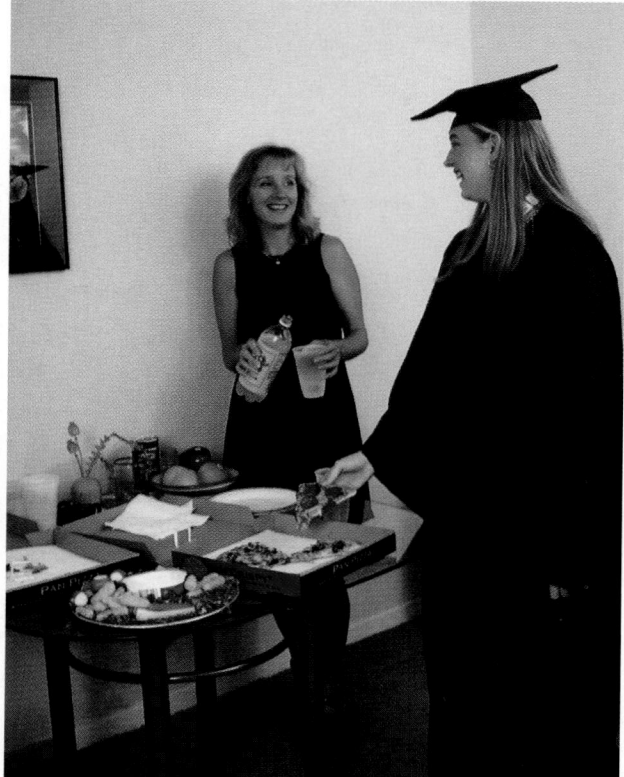

Figure 22–1. For many young adults, graduation from college is an important milestone that marks the end of adolescence and the beginning of adult roles and responsibilities.

TABLE 22–1
Erikson's Stages of Development for the Young Adult and Middle Adult Years

Stage	Age	Description
VI	Young adult years	• Intimacy versus self-absorption, later called intimacy versus isolation. • Significant relationships are partners in friendship, sex, and competition and cooperation and ability to engage in a trusting fellowship. • The young adult seeks a permanent life partner with whom to give and receive love and support. • The primary issue is love.
VII	Middle adult years	• Generativity versus stagnation, which is a creative giving of the self to the world in a participatory way. Generativity is helping and guiding the next generation. • Unless such concern develops, the person focuses on self, stagnates, and commonly regresses. • Middle adults share tasks and divide necessary labor. • The primary issue is care.

Erikson, E.H. (1963). Childhood and society (2nd ed.). New York: W.W. Norton; and Erikson, E.H. (1982). The life cycle completed. New York: W.W. Norton.

grandparent, spouse or companion, son or daughter, citizen, civic leader, friend, and employee or employer.

Tasks of Middle Adulthood

Middle adulthood is the period from ages 35 to 64. In 1998 the USCB reported that more than 101 million people, more than 37% of the population, were between ages 35 and 64. By 2005, this age group will most likely increase to nearly 40% of the population (USCB, 1998c).

During this period, generativity expands. It began early in adulthood, particularly with childbearing, child rearing, and establishing a career. Mature adults are concerned with establishing and guiding the next generation in their roles as parents, teachers, mentors, civic leaders, and guardians of the culture. If this is not accomplished, they may feel a sense of personal impoverishment.

Theories of Adult Development

Traditionally, biologists have divided the life span into the following three phases:

• Progressive growth from birth to age 25
• Stability almost to age 45
• A decline of physical capabilities after age 45

Other biologists have suggested the acquisition, possession, and loss of reproductive ability as the three stages of life.

In his theory of psychosocial development, Erik Erikson (1963) identified eight stages of development from birth through death, two of which apply to young and middle-aged adults (Table 22–1). He believed that psychosocial development was a continuous process and that delays or crises in one stage could delay or diminish the achievement of other stages.

Erikson's adult stages focus on intimacy versus isolation (young adult) and generativity versus stagnation (middle adult). During the stage of intimacy versus isolation, young adults are in an intense search

for self and focus on developing their capacity for reciprocal love and close personal relationships based on commitment to others. They experience conflicting values as they try to sort out what life means to them. They must resolve the conflict of balancing independence and intimacy as they form significant relationships with partners, with the aim of providing a nurturing environment for children. These tasks are relevant in a variety of lifestyles, including heterosexual marriage, homosexual and heterosexual cohabitation, and voluntary childlessness.

Erikson's seventh stage of psychosocial development, generativity versus stagnation, is reached during middle adulthood. The person tends to assess generativity by focusing on creativity, productivity, procreation, and the development of a capacity to care for others (Fig. 22–2). The individual must balance the feeling that life is personally satisfying and socially meaningful with the feeling that life is without meaning. If stagnation occurs, the person may become egocentric and self-absorbed.

Levinson (1978, 1986) conceived of development as a sequence of qualitatively distinct eras or seasons, each of which has its own time and brings certain psychological challenges to the forefront of a person's life (Table 22–2). He identified three eras in adult life: early adult, middle adult, and late adult.

Review the opening case study and consider Mr. Biaggio's stage of development. What questions might you ask to determine if his struggle with the developmental tasks of his stage of life are affecting his health?

FACTORS AFFECTING ADULT DEVELOPMENT

Life expectancy for Americans has risen to 76 years, primarily because of advances in public health, such as improved housing, sanitation, and immunizations. Today, risk factors that contribute to premature adult morbidity and mortality include high-risk lifestyle practices and other physiological, psychosocial, socioeconomic, and environmental factors.

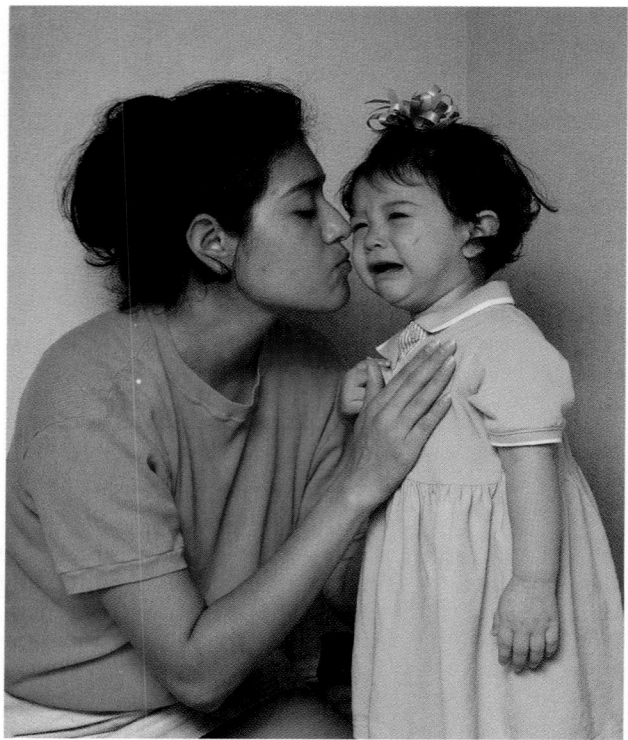

Figure 22–2. The stage of generativity involves the development of a capacity to care for others.

Action Alert!
If people avoid the behaviors that increase their risk for chronic diseases, they can expect to have healthier and longer lives.

High-Risk Lifestyle Practices

Unhealthy Diet

The U.S. Public Health Service (PHS) estimates that one in three people ages 20 and older are overweight (PHS, 1995). Minority populations, especially women, are affected disproportionately; nearly half of African-American, Mexican-American, and Native American adults are overweight. Diet-related health conditions cost an estimated $250 billion annually in medical costs and lost productivity in the United States.

Four of the ten leading causes of death in the United States are linked to diet: heart disease, stroke, diabetes, and certain cancers, especially colorectal, endometrial, and ovarian cancer. The risks of developing hypertension or diabetes nearly triple for adults who are 20% or more overweight. Being overweight also increases the risk of gout, gallbladder disease, hip fractures, and osteoarthritis. Together, these diseases account for nearly two-thirds of the two million annual deaths in this country.

Being too thin can raise the risk of health problems as well. Anorexia nervosa, loss of appetite, and similar disorders are linked to menstrual irregularities and osteoporosis in women and to a greater risk of early death in both women and men.

Our client, Mr. Biaggio, needs help with his diet. What do you know about the dietary patterns in the Italian culture? How could you find out more about Mr. Biaggio's pattern of eating? How can you motivate him to change?

Action Alert!
Teach clients to choose a diet with plenty of grain products, vegetables, and fruits. The diet should be low in saturated fat and cholesterol, moderate in sugars, and moderate in sodium.

Cigarette Smoking

The Centers for Disease Control and Prevention (CDC) report that at least one in every five deaths in the United States is related to cigarette smoking and that an average of 430,700 people die from smoking-related illnesses each year (CDC, 1997). About half of all lifelong smokers will die from smoking. Since the first surgeon general's report on smoking and health in 1964, about 10 million Americans have died from smoking-related causes, such as lung cancer, other smoking-related cancers, heart disease, emphysema, and other respiratory diseases. The direct medical costs associated with smoking are estimated at $50 billion annually, or 7% of total U.S. health care costs (CDC, 1997).

Among adults of ethnic minority groups, tobacco use varies (CDC, 1998c). Cigarette smoking is a major cause of death among African-Americans, American Indians, Alaska Natives, Asian-Americans, Pacific Islanders, and Hispanics. American Indians and Alaska Natives have the highest prevalence of tobacco use, followed closely by African-American and Southeast Asian men. Asian-American and Hispanic women have the lowest prevalence.

Action Alert!
Cigarette smoking is the single most preventable cause of premature death in the United States.

Substance Abuse

Adults who abuse alcohol increase their risk for hypertension, stroke, heart disease, certain cancers, accidents, violence, suicides, birth defects, and overall mortality. Alcohol abuse may cause cirrhosis of the liver, inflammation of the pancreas, damage to the brain and heart, and malnutrition. It may alter the effectiveness of medicines or increase the risk of toxic reactions. Some medications may increase blood alcohol levels or increase the adverse effect of alcohol on the brain.

Of every 1,000 live births, one to three infants has **fetal alcohol syndrome,** a distinct cluster of physical and mental impairments caused by prenatal exposure to alcohol (SAMHSA, 1998).

Action Alert!
Teach women who are pregnant or trying to conceive to avoid alcohol and illicit drugs. Heavy drinking during pregnancy has been linked to major birth defects and fetal alcohol syndrome.

TABLE 22–2
Levinson's Development Phases

Approximate Age	Tasks
20 to 24	• Leaving the family. • Making the transition between adolescence and the adult world. • Those who go to college or military service have an intermediate experience.
25 to 29	• Getting into the adult world. • Building an initial life structure, deciding on an occupation, and working on intimacy versus isolation. • A time of exploration and initial choice.
30 to 35	• Age 30 transition. • Person either confirms earlier choices or may choose to modify or change the initial structure. • Person has vision of the future. • Person realizes extent to which he is dependent on and shaped by others, a de-illusioning process. • A mentor can be very helpful at this stage.
35 to 39	• Settling down. • Person may build a second, and more stable, early adult life structure. • Becomes "one's own person." • Person moves from being mentored to being able to mentor.
38 to 42	• Midlife transition. • Person realizes that earlier choices cannot fulfill all of the self and that parts of the self were repressed or dormant. At some point, life must be restructured to express more of the self. • The adult reappraises, modifies, and rediscovers important neglected parts of the self and makes choices that provide for a new life structure. There may be a sense of compromise of the dream as person searches for what he really wants. • There is a sense of bodily decline and a need to confront one's mortality. The person recognizes that he is no longer young.
44 to 46	• Restabilization. • The fullest and most creative period of life. • Time represents both the possibility for further development and a threat to the self. • Person is building and living with a first provisional life structure for middle adulthood.
47 to 59	• Stable period of fulfillment.
60 to 65	• Preparing for retirement and death.

Information from Levinson, D.J. (1978). The seasons of a man's life. New York: Alfred A. Knopf; and Levinson, D.J. (1996). The seasons of a woman's life. New York: Alfred A. Knopf.

Illicit drug use and its consequences threaten Americans of every socioeconomic background, geographic region, educational level, and ethnic or racial identity. Among Americans age 12 and older, 34.8% have used an illegal drug in their lifetime; of these, more than 90% used either marijuana or hashish, and about 30% tried cocaine. Researchers estimate the number of chronic drug users at 3.6 million for cocaine and 810,000 for heroin (SAMHSA, 1998).

Drug-related deaths have increased 42% since 1990, to more than 14,000 in 1995. Accidents, crime, domestic violence, illness, lost opportunity, and reduced productivity are the direct consequences of substance abuse. Drug abuse and trafficking hurt families, businesses, and neighborhoods; impedes education; and burdens the criminal justice, health, and social service systems.

Chronic drug users are particularly susceptible to infectious diseases and are considered high-risk transmitters. They and their sexual partners have higher risks of contracting hepatitis, tuberculosis, gonorrhea, syphilis, and other sexually transmitted diseases. High-risk sexual behavior associated with crack co-

caine and the injection of illegal drugs enhances the transmission and acquisition of human immunodeficiency virus (HIV). About 40% of new HIV cases are directly or indirectly linked to injecting drugs (SAMHSA, 1998).

Substance abuse is a common problem among families reported for child maltreatment. Researchers have found that 25 to 50% of men who commit domestic violence also have substance abuse problems. Also, women with substance abuse problems are more likely to become victims of domestic violence. To make matters worse, Americans who lack access to comprehensive health care and have smaller incomes may be less able to afford treatment to overcome drug dependence.

Psychological Factors

Stress

Stress is the most common cause of illness in our society, probably underlying as much as 70% of all visits to primary care providers (Posen, 1995). It is a major risk factor for the development of physical and psychological problems. Stress encompasses the negative cognitive and emotional states that result when clients feel that the demands placed on them exceed their ability to cope (Posen, 1995).

Stress can be caused by external and internal influences. External stressors may stem from the following:

- The physical environment, such as loud noises, bright lights, excessive heat, and confined spaces
- The social environment, such as aggressiveness on the part of someone else
- The work environment, such as deadlines or "red tape"
- Major life events, such as the death of a relative, a lost job, a promotion, or a new baby
- Daily hassles, such as heavy traffic, misplaced keys, or a flat tire

Internal stressors commonly stem from lifestyle choices, such as drinking caffeinated beverages, getting too little sleep, or overloading the daily schedule. Stress may also stem from negative self-talk, such as pessimistic thinking and self-criticism, or from stressful personality traits, such as being a workaholic (Posen, 1995).

Think about Mr. Biaggio again. He has just taken a new job in an important position. Can you list possible stressors in his life?

Action **A**lert!
You can help clients reduce the negative effects of stress by teaching them to reduce their perceived pressures, increase their coping resources, or both.

Depression

About 5 to 12% of men and 10 to 20% of women in the United States will experience a major depressive episode at some time in their lives. About half of these people will become depressed more than once, and up to 10% of them (1 to 1.5% of Americans) will experience manic-depressive illness or bipolar disorder. Depression is a potential killer; as many as 15% of those who develop it commit suicide each year. In 1996, the CDC listed suicide as the ninth leading cause of death in the United States. Most researchers, however, believe this number is too small (Nemeroff, 1998).

Growing findings indicate that severe depression also heightens the risk of dying after a heart attack or stroke and reduces the quality of life for clients who have cancer and might reduce their survival time. Clients who are depressed experience a great deal of functional impairment, resulting in lost work time, decreased job performance, and decreased family and social functioning. Encourage clients to seek treatment for depression; effective treatment is available (Nemeroff, 1998).

Action **A**lert!
Remember to screen clients for depression when they have a history of depression, chronic illness, a recent loss, a sleep disorder, chronic pain, or multiple unexplained somatic complaints.

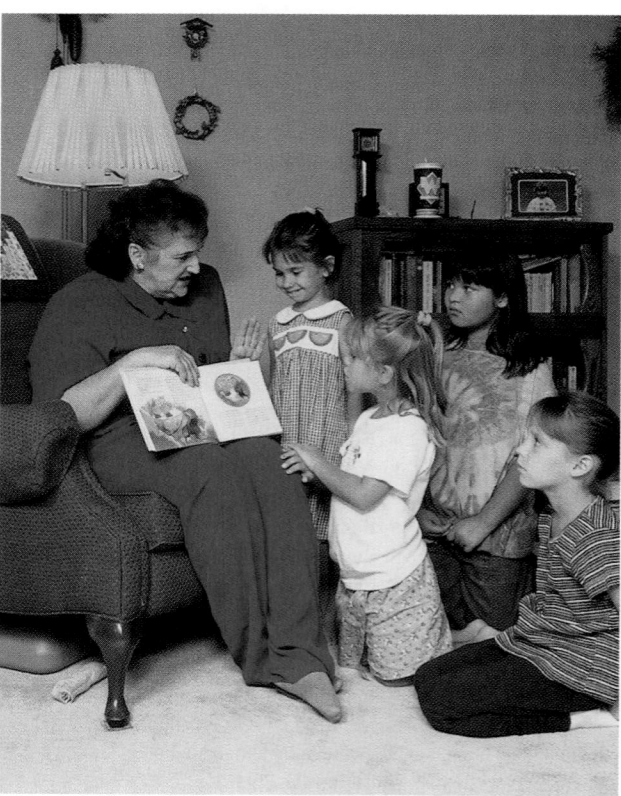

Figure 22–3. Although some older adults may feel that they have become a burden or inconvenience to their families, they can still play an important role in the family by building into the lives of future generations.

Midlife Crisis or Transition

Some adults experience a midlife crisis, also called a midlife transition. **Midlife crisis** is a stressful life period during middle adulthood, precipitated by the review and reevaluation of one's past, including goals, priorities, and life accomplishments, during which the person experiences inner turmoil, self-doubt, and major restructuring of personality. Typically, a midlife crisis occurs in the early to middle forties but may not occur until the fifties.

As a group, middle-aged adults are commonly called the **sandwich generation.** They are caught between the needs of adjacent generations, caring for ill or frail parents while handling the competing demands of children and employment. Their responsibilities may range from financially supporting a retired parent to taking physical care of a frail, demented, dependent parent while caring for their own children.

All generations feel the effects of this sandwiching. For example, some elderly parents may feel that they have become a burden or inconvenience to their families but try to help their families any way then can (Fig. 22–3). The children may feel neglected by their parents and resentful or jealous of their grandparents.

The middle-aged adult is caught in the middle, trying to please everyone, but feels unsupported and unappreciated.

Depending on the family's financial situation and the type of health insurance the elderly family member has, home health services can ease some of the middle-aged adult's caregiving tasks. Individual counseling and participation in support groups can help to relieve some of the family's stress and provide encouragement in difficult times.

Socioeconomic Factors

Poverty

More than 35 million people in the United States (about 13% of the population) live below the poverty line. In 1997 this line was set at $16,400 for a family of four and $12,802 for a family of three in annual income (USCB, 1998b). Almost 7% of families (nearly 4 million) with children younger than age 18 lived in homes maintained by the grandparents. Of these, 27% of the children lived in poverty and received public assistance (Casper & Bryson, 1998).

Poverty is associated with limited access to heath care, poor nutrition, substandard housing, and inadequate prenatal care. If clients have no health insurance, they tend to receive substandard medical care, putting them at risk for medical problems. Clients who are better educated and more affluent can afford a healthier diet, better preventive health care, and more prompt medical treatment. However, these advantages do not mean that their lifestyle practices will prevent chronic diseases and premature morbidity and mortality (Papalia & Olds, 1998).

Health Insurance

Adult clients may have health insurance coverage through their employer, by private pay, or by federal or state health plans. Employment is the leading source of health insurance coverage. Among the general population age 18 to 64, workers (full-time and part-time) were more likely to be insured than nonworkers. Among the working poor, however, there was less probability of being insured than among nonworkers. The primary reason is that employers failed to provide health insurance, or that the financial burden on employees to buy their company's plan was prohibitive. Almost half of poor full-time workers were uninsured in 1997. Overall, more than 43 million Americans (16.1% of the population) were without health insurance coverage during 1997 (Kuttner, 1999; USCB, 1998b).

Despite the Medicaid program, nearly a third of all poor people (more than 11 million) had no health insurance in 1997. The highest uninsured rate was among people of Hispanic origin. More than a third of Hispanics were uninsured, compared with about 12% for non-Hispanic people.

Environmental Factors

Employment

The U.S. Department of Labor's Bureau of Labor Statistics (1998) reported that 82% of U.S. families had at least one worker in 1997. The rate of working mothers was 72%, and the rate for unmarried mothers (single, widowed, divorced, or separated) was 75%. Among mothers with children younger than age 1, 58% were working or looking for work. The U.S. Department of Labor's Bureau of Labor Statistics (1999) reported that the unemployment rate was 4.3% as of December 1998, the lowest in more than three decades.

Work-Related Injuries and Deaths

According to the ODPHP (1995), work-related injury deaths are 5 per 100,000 workers. Nonfatal work-related injuries occur at a rate of 7.9 per 100 workers. The leading work-related diseases and injuries are occupational lung disease, musculoskeletal injuries, traumatic injury or death, cardiovascular disease, disorders of reproduction, neurotoxic disorders, loss of hearing, dermatological conditions, and psychological disorders (Clemen-Stone, McGuire, & Eigsti, 1998).

In the 1995 revision to the *Healthy People 2000: National Health Promotion and Disease Prevention Objectives* (U.S. Department of Health and Human Services, Public Health Service), a new objective to reduce the rate of homicides occurring in the workplace was added. Homicide is the third leading cause of fatal injury for male workers, and it is the leading cause of injury and death for women in the workplace (ODPHP, 1995).

Nearly half of all worker-compensation costs reported to the Bureau of Labor Statistics each year represents ergonomic-related disorders. The Occupational Safety and Health Administration reports more than 300,000 new cases of cumulative-trauma disorders each year, including injuries to the back, hand, wrist, forearm, and neck. The repeated trauma results largely from poorly designed work environments, poorly designed tools, and individual health problems (Van Fleet & Bates, 1995).

Cultural/Religious Factors

Chronic disease has an increased impact on racial and ethnic minority groups. For example, the prevalence of diabetes among African-Americans, Hispanics, American Indians, and Alaska Natives is significantly higher than for white Americans. In one recent study, the cancer survival rate among African-Americans was about 44% compared with 59% for white Americans. This difference can be attributed largely to late diagnosis in minority groups (CDC, 1998b).

No single factor negatively affects the growth and development of people in racial and ethnic minority groups. Growth and development result from a complex interaction of factors, such as socioeconomic status, cultural characteristics, acculturation, stress, biological elements, targeted advertising, and varying capacities of communities to promote healthy lifestyle practices (CDC, 1998b).

Clients' cultural and religious beliefs influence their health care beliefs, values, customs, and practices. You need to be aware of each client's cultural belief patterns so you can recognize and understand them. Unless you incorporate these belief patterns into your care plans, you may create a conflict between your nursing interventions and your clients' cultural backgrounds.

Physiological Factors

Heart Disease

High blood cholesterol is an important modifiable risk factor for coronary artery disease, which is the leading cause of death for men and women in the United States. Risk factors include a family history of very high cholesterol levels, premature coronary artery disease in a first-degree relative (before age 50 in men or age 60 in women), diabetes, smoking, or hypertension. Annually, about 1.5 million Americans have a new or recurrent myocardial infarction; about a third of these people die (ODPHP, 1998).

Hypertension

About 50 million Americans need monitoring or medication because they have elevated blood pressure. They are at increased risk for coronary artery disease, peripheral vascular disease, stroke, renal disease, or retinopathy. Treatment of hypertension is very effective, although it must commonly be tailored to meet individual needs and responses. Antihypertensive therapy has contributed to a 59% reduction in the age-adjusted stroke mortality rate and a 50% reduction in the mortality rate from that of coronary artery disease since 1972 (ODPHP, 1998).

*A*ction *A*lert!
Advise clients (men aged 35 to 65 and women aged 45 to 65) to have a periodic cholesterol screening and normotensive adults to have blood pressure checked at least every 2 years (Report of the U.S. Preventive Services Task Force, 1996).

Mr. Biaggio is advised to lower his blood pressure with diet and exercise. How often would you suggest that Mr. Biaggio have his blood pressure checked?

Leading Causes of Death in Adults

Chronic diseases account for 70% of all deaths in the United States, more than 60% of total medical care expenditures, and decreased quality of life for millions of Americans (CDC, 1998b). The leading causes of death in young adults are acquired immunodeficiency syndrome (AIDS), accidents, cancer, heart disease, suicide, and homicide (Papalia & Olds, 1998). The leading causes of death in middle-aged adults are heart disease, lung cancer, cerebrovascular disease, breast can-

cer, colorectal cancer, and obstructive lung disease (Mandle, 1998).

*A*ction *A*lert!
Teach clients that living healthfully and avoiding behaviors that increase the risk of chronic disease will result in longer, healthier lives.

ASSESSMENT

General Assessment of Young and Middle Adults

Well adults need nursing assessments just as ill adults do. By assessing a well adult, you can help to prevent or manage chronic diseases and acute illnesses (Fig. 22–4). You may assess a well adult in many settings and for many reasons. Well adults may obtain health care at a physician's office, community health clinic, nursing center, college health center, or occupational health center, to name a few.

Some clients need a preemployment examination before starting a new job. Some need annual screenings to detect any changes in their health. Both men and women need physical examinations to participate

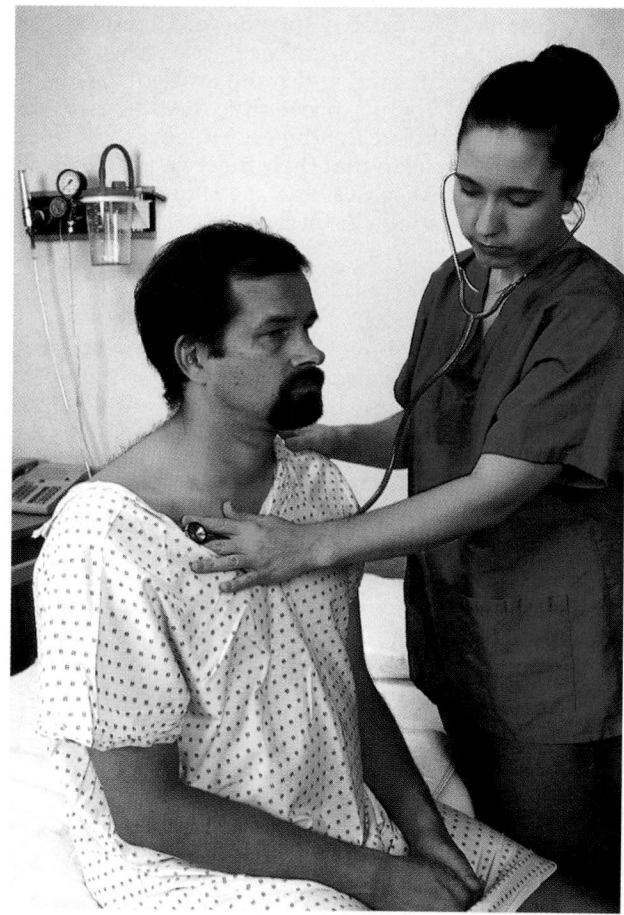

Figure 22–4. You will assess a well adult to help prevent or manage chronic conditions and prevent acute illness.

in college sports. Women who wish to use contraception usually need annual physical examinations, and those who are pregnant are encouraged to seek prenatal and postnatal care.

As adults age, they often seek care to learn how to maintain their health or adjust to the physical changes they are experiencing. When clients have an illness, they are assessed to determine any problems they might have or if the recommended interventions are effective in restoring or maintaining health.

Health History

Any nursing assessment normally begins with a health history. The history includes the client's biographical data, past health history, chief complaint, and present health status. Depending on the reason the client is seeking care, the assessment may include a family history and dynamics. The completeness of the health history is determined by the client's health status, his ability to answer your questions, and his trust in the relationship he has with you. To obtain a thorough and accurate health history, you need to develop a trusting relationship with the client.

Start by asking the client to describe his health. In his opinion, is it poor, good, or excellent? Ask how much control he believes he has over his own health. Inquire about any illnesses within the past year that have prevented the client from pursuing his normal activities. Ask what he does to keep himself healthy. Specifically mention breast or testicular self-examinations. Ask whether he uses alcohol or other drugs, and how much. Ask whether he smokes, how much, and for how long.

Especially as an adult ages, body function becomes a subject of concern as various body parts fail to perform as they did in youth. Often, the middle-aged adult becomes interested both in maximizing health and physical functioning and in seeking information about other health-seeking behaviors. Ask whether the client feels the need to improve his health or physical function.

You can use Gordon's functional health patterns as a framework to obtain the client's specific health history (see Chapter 8).

Physical Examination

The type of physical examination you perform for a well adult depends largely on the reason for the examination. For example, when you give a person a sports physical, you will screen for previous and current injuries, sexually transmitted diseases, and alcohol and other substance abuse. You would assess all joints for range of motion, flexibility, strength, and reflexes. You would listen to the person's heart and lungs and examine his eyes, ears, and abdomen for any abnormalities.

An annual physical examination for a woman of childbearing age would include questions about possible domestic violence and increased risks for sexu-

ally transmitted diseases. You would take her vital signs, including an accurate height for osteoporosis prevention. You would assess her heart, lungs, thyroid gland, breasts, abdomen, and genital and rectal areas for any abnormalities. She would need a Papanicolaou test (also called Pap test) if it has been 3 years since her last test—fewer, if she has an increased risk of cervical cancer (Report of the U.S. Preventive Services Task Force, 1996).

In all well adult examinations, you should also assess the client's general health and cognitive and emotional functioning. Begin by assessing the client's appearance. Observe his behaviors and apparent mental status. Consider whether his vision and hearing seem to be within normal limits. Obtain his vital signs, height, weight, and the result of any diagnostic screening tests, such as a mammogram or cholesterol screening.

By their mid-twenties, most adults are fully developed and at peak functioning. From then, the person will experience a gradual decline in touch sensitivity and respiratory, cardiovascular, and immune system functions. Athletic ability peaks in the twenties and then begins to decline.

During the thirties and forties, vision and hearing begin to change. The accommodative ability of the ocular lens declines; by the fifties and sixties, it no longer exists. Color discrimination declines as well, and most people have an increased sensitivity to glare during their forties and fifties (Berk, 1998). Hearing begins to decline in the thirties and forties, initially involving mostly high frequencies. By the fifties and sixties, hearing loss may include all frequencies, although still most pronounced at high frequencies.

Skin changes, especially lines and sagging, become more pronounced in the forties and fifties. Age spots begin in the fifties and sixties. Hair begins to gray and thin in the early forties, a process that continues throughout adulthood. An adult's height begins to decline in the thirties and forties; because of the compression of disks in the spinal column, height may drop an inch during the fifties and sixties (Berk, 1998).

Sexual activity increases during the twenties and thirties and begins to decline in the thirties and forties. Men experience a decrease in the quality of semen and sperm after age 40. The inability to obtain an erection can occur at any age, but it becomes more common in midlife.

Fertility problems for women increase sharply in their forties. As basal metabolism declines in the forties and fifties, weight increases, and muscle and bone mass decline. This process accelerates in women after menopause. **Menopause** is the stage in the female climacteric, during which hormone production is reduced, the ovaries stop producing eggs, and menstruation ceases. The woman's reproductive ability has now ended. Menopause usually occurs between ages 50 and 55, although it ranges from ages 40 to 59. After menopause, the rate of osteoporosis increases.

Diagnostic Tests

A key to wellness for the adult is appropriate screening, especially for clients in high-risk groups. You may be directly involved in screening or in teaching clients about the importance of screening tests (Table 22–3).

Coronary artery disease is the leading cause of death in the United States. Consequently, clients should be screened regularly for elevated cholesterol level, a major modifiable risk factor for heart disease. If the total cholesterol level is increased, then the client should be tested for other lipid abnormalities as well.

Hypertension is a risk factor for coronary artery disease, congestive heart failure, stroke, ruptured aortic aneurysm, retinopathy, and renal disease. All adults should be screened for hypertension at least every 2 years. If the diastolic reading is 85 and the systolic reading is 140 or below, screening every 2 years is sufficient. Hypertension is never diagnosed based on a single reading.

Mr. Biaggio, from our case study, was being monitored by the occupational health nurse after he was diagnosed with borderline hypertension. He is self-monitoring his blood pressure and has obtained readings of 140/90, 160/88, and 150/92 in a single day. He says, "See, it isn't too bad for a man my age." How would you respond?

TABLE 22–3

Health Screening Guidelines for Well Adults

Test	Young Adulthood (Ages 20 to 35)	Middle Adulthood (Ages 35 to 64)	Comments
Body measurement	Measure height and weight periodically	Measure height and weight periodically	Obesity is a major public health problem.
Blood pressure	At least every 2 years for normotensive adults or annually for borderline hypertension. Others should seek the advice of a physician.	At least every 2 years for normotensive adults or annually for borderline hypertension. Others should seek the advice of a physician.	About 50 million Americans have hypertension that warrants monitoring or drug therapy.
Breast examination	Every 3 years. More frequent for high-risk groups.	Mammography and clinical breast examination every 1 to 2 years (age 50 to 69). Breast self-examination alone is useful but not reliable.	Breast cancer is the most common type of cancer in women and the second leading cause of death.
Cholesterol level	Should seek the advice of a physician. High-risk groups may need screening.	Periodic screening for men ages 35 to 65 and women ages 45 to 65. High-risk groups should seek the advice of a physician.	High blood cholesterol is a modifiable risk factor for heart disease.
Papanicolaou test	All women who are age 18 or older or sexually active and who have a cervix should have a Pap test every 3 years.	All women who are age 18 or older or sexually active and who have a cervix should have a Pap test every 3 years.	The major risk factor for cervical cancer is sexually transmitted infection with human papillomavirus.
Prostate-specific antigen test		Annual test together with rectal examination beginning at age 50; earlier for men at high risk	Prostate cancer is the second leading cause of cancer death in men.
Sigmoidoscopy		Every 3 to 5 years beginning at age 50 (age 40 for those with a family history of colorectal cancer, along with fecal occult blood tests, sigmoidoscopy, colonoscopy, or barium enema)	Colorectal cancer is the third leading cause of cancer death in the United States, most often among people older than age 40.
Tuberculosis	Skin testing for all persons at high risk.	Skin testing for all persons at high risk.	Control depends on screening high-risk populations and providing preventive therapy.
Vision	Comprehensive eye and vision examination every 2 to 3 years; more often if increased risk factors present.	Comprehensive eye and vision examination every 2 years; more often if increased risk factors present.	Vision loss is common in adults, especially with advancing age.

Based on recommendations from U.S. Department of Health and Human Services, Public Health Service, Office of Disease Prevention and Health Promotion. (1998). Clinician's handbook of preventive services (2nd ed.). Available from: http://text.nlm.nih.gov/ftrs/tocview 1/18/98; Report of the U.S. Preventive Services Task Force. (1996). Guide to clinical preventive services (2nd ed.). Baltimore: Williams & Wilkins.
Note: Recommendations of other groups will differ.

The annual incidence of breast cancer increases with age. Screening for breast cancer is recommended every 1 to 2 years for women ages 50 to 59. Screening includes a breast examination by a health practitioner and a mammogram (Report of the U.S. Preventive Services Task Force, 1996). Screening in younger women is recommended when there is a family history of breast cancer, especially premenopausal breast cancer. Older women may be selected for screening based on risk factors, health, and expected longevity. All women should be encouraged to do a breast self-examination every month.

All people older than age 50 should be screened for colorectal cancer every 3 to 5 years beginning at age 50 (40 if they have a family history of colorectal cancer). The most common screening methods are the fecal occult blood test and sigmoidoscopy. When the finding is positive, a colonoscopy may be performed. Other screening methods include a digital rectal examination and barium enema. For people who have first-degree relatives with colorectal cancer, more thorough screening may be recommended.

Screening for cervical cancer is recommended for all women with a cervix who are sexually active or have reached age 18, whichever comes first. A Papanicolaou test performed every 3 years is as effective as having the test annually. Risk factors of multiple sex partners, an early onset of sexual intercourse, low socioeconomic status, and HIV infection suggest the need for more frequent screening.

All men should have an annual prostate-specific antigen test and an annual rectal examination beginning at age 50, or earlier with men at high risk.

Rubella contracted during the first 16 weeks of pregnancy causes serious complications, including miscarriage, abortion, stillbirth, and congenital rubella syndrome. All women of childbearing age should have either a documented history of rubella or a rubella titer. Offering nonpregnant women the rubella vaccine is an acceptable alternative.

All adults should be screened for problem drinking of alcohol. Heavy drinking is defined as more than five drinks per day, five times per week (Report of the U.S. Preventive Services Task Force, 1996). Medical problems due to alcoholism include hepatitis, cirrhosis of the liver, cardiomyopathy, and withdrawal syndrome. Heavy drinking and alcoholism (dependency) have dire social consequences as well, including suicide, divorce, depression, domestic violence, unemployment, and poverty.

All clients should be screened for tobacco use, and those who use tobacco products should be advised to quit and encouraged to develop a plan to quit. Many methods are used to help tobacco users quit the habit, but success is directly related to the person's determination to quit rather than to the method itself. Most people try more than once before actually quitting.

All clients should be assessed for their immunization status. All clients need a diphtheria-tetanus vaccination every 10 years.

Vision loss is common in adults, and the prevalence increases with advancing age. Young, normal-risk adults should have a comprehensive eye and vision examination every 2 to 3 years. Middle-aged, normal-risk adults should have such an examination every 2 years.

High-risk clients should be screened for tuberculosis. These include people who have close contact with someone known or suspected to have tuberculosis, people infected with HIV, people who inject illicit drugs, people who live or work in high-risk group settings (such as a nursing home or child care center), and people who are medically underserved. Controlling tuberculosis depends on thorough screening of high-risk populations and providing preventive therapy.

Focused Assessment for Altered Growth and Development

Asking questions about the client's family will help you determine the developmental stage of the family and the client. Clients may have psychosocial problems accepting adult roles and responsibilities. The client may lack knowledge about his current developmental stage or have decisional conflicts related to the transitions associated with the stage.

Adulthood is a time of almost constant role transitions, from becoming independent from parents, forming a significant love relationship, becoming a parent, and launching a child into the world, to becoming a grandparent and caring for elderly parents. Adults must also learn to accept their role in the work world and as citizens.

Adulthood is a time of continued physical development as well. Throughout, there is a gradual decline in the adult's touch, sensitivity, respiratory, cardiovascular, and immune system functions. Adults who have been involved in high-risk behaviors, such as smoking, poor dietary habits, and drug abuse, may have difficulty with their physical development and may develop chronic diseases.

When a client's physical or psychosocial development is altered, you should consider the nursing diagnosis *Altered growth and development*. Risk factors for this diagnosis include the following:

- Failure to achieve previous developmental stages
- Choosing a lifestyle different from cultural or societal norms
- Transition crises, such as childbirth, parenting, or midlife crisis
- High-risk lifestyle behaviors, such as smoking or substance abuse
- Chronic illness or disability
- Violence
- Unwanted pregnancy
- Exposure to environmental and occupational risk factors
- Expression of dissatisfaction with life, health, or achievement of goals

Defining Characteristics

Defining characteristics for *Altered growth and development* include the following:

- Altered physical growth
- Delay or difficulty in performing the skills (motor, social, expressive) typical of one's age group
- Inability to perform self-care or self-control activities appropriate for one's age
- A flat affect
- Listlessness or decreased responses

Related Factors

Factors related to the onset of *Altered growth and development* include the following:

- Prescribed dependence or physical disability
- Indifference or inconsistent responsiveness
- Separation from significant others
- Deficiencies of environment or stimulation
- Inadequate caretaking or multiple caretakers

Focused Assessment for Altered Health Maintenance

A focused assessment for a client with *Altered health maintenance* includes looking at the client's ability to identify, manage, and or seek out help to maintain his health (NANDA, 1999). Ask questions that will provide cues to the client's ability and motivation to take responsibility for his own health. For example: Have you engaged in a healthy lifestyle in the past? For what reasons did you seek health care in the past? Did you adopt the recommended interventions? Why or why not? Do you receive support from your family or significant other? How do family members or friends make it easy (or difficult) to maintain good health practices?

Review common causes of adult illness and injury, and discuss ways to reduce their risks. Determine the client's level of interest in improving his health and reducing his risks. This will also help you assess the client's level of knowledge. Assess whether the client faces barriers to taking effective health actions, such as finances or health care resources.

Keep in mind the common causes of illness and death for adults. They include the following:

- Accidents, AIDS, homicide, and suicide
- Substance abuse that interferes with productivity and relationships and raises the risk of injury, especially domestic violence, and death
- Unsafe sexual practices, which raise the risk of unwanted pregnancies and sexually transmitted diseases, including HIV infection
- Family, lifestyle, or occupational risk factors for cancer or heart disease (such as obesity, a sedentary lifestyle, tobacco use, alcohol abuse, and poor nutrition)

Defining Characteristics

Defining characteristics for *Altered health maintenance* include the following:

- History of a lack of health-seeking behaviors
- Reported or observed lack of equipment, finances, or other resources
- Reported or observed impairment of personal support systems
- Expressed interest in improving health behaviors
- Demonstrated lack of knowledge regarding basic health practices
- Demonstrated lack of adaptive behaviors to internal or external environmental changes
- Reported or observed inability to take responsibility for meeting basic health practices in any or all functional pattern areas

Related Factors

Factors related to the onset of *Altered health maintenance* include the following:

- Ineffective individual or family coping
- Perceptual or cognitive impairment
- Impaired gross or fine motor skills
- Lack of or significant alteration in communication skills
- Unachieved developmental tasks
- Lack of material resources
- Dysfunctional grieving or disabling spiritual distress
- Lack of ability to make deliberate and thoughtful judgments

Focused Assessment for Related Nursing Diagnoses

To effectively address a client's altered growth and development, you may need to assign other, specific nursing diagnoses. When the client needs to make dietary modifications to improve health, for example, the diagnosis *Altered nutrition: more than (less than) body requirements* is used. When the person needs knowledge to change his lifestyle, the diagnosis *Knowledge deficit* is used. When the person is a parent who needs help with parenting skills, the diagnosis is *Altered parenting*. When the person is overwhelmed with the stress of caring for a dependent person, the diagnosis is *Caregiver role strain*. When the person is not managing an acute or chronic illness effectively, the diagnosis is *Ineffective management of therapeutic regimen*.

DIAGNOSIS

Keep in mind that the diagnosis *Altered growth and development* is a broad category applicable to a client with multiple issues. Often, however, a single issue is the focus of nursing care. In this case, you will want to use a more specific nursing diagnosis, such as those

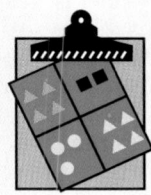

CLUSTERING DATA TO MAKE A NURSING DIAGNOSIS
HIGH-RISK LIFESTYLE CHOICES

Data Cluster	Diagnosis
A 52-year-old male client smokes two packs of cigarettes daily. He has not exercised regularly since he was in college, and he cannot remember when he last had a physical examination.	*Altered health maintenance* related to lifestyle/habits.
A 64-year-old female client has had three consecutive blood pressure readings above 140/90. She says she feels fine and finds it hard to believe that anything is wrong.	*Knowledge deficit* regarding causes of hypertension related to perception of health.
A 36-year-old male client, 5'10" in height, weighs 237 pounds. He reports eating fast food every day for breakfast and lunch. He says that he eats fresh vegetables and fruits about three times a week.	*Altered nutrition:* more than body requirements related to lifestyle management.

described above. Group the client's diagnostic cues to help determine the best nursing diagnosis, as described in the accompanying data clustering chart.

PLANNING

Each plan of care must be individualized to a client's needs, age, and culture. Address the client's concerns first. Then, together with the client, develop a care plan that includes achievable short- and long-term goals designed for success. Explore options with the client to help him achieve his goals by changing behaviors (reducing weight, stopping tobacco use, increasing exercise, preventing unwanted pregnancy, and so on). With your assistance, the client should prioritize his goals and specify time frames for achieving them.

Mr. Biaggio decided that his primary goal was to start an exercise program. He thought he would feel better about himself by taking brisk walks 3 days per week after dinner. He felt he would then be able to try to stop smoking because he would have more confidence in his ability to quit. How would you respond to Mr. Biaggio? Is his plan reasonable or unrealistic?

INTERVENTION

Client interventions are based on developing trusting relationships. Your client relationships must be based on honesty, acceptance, respect, empathy, and cultural sensitivity. First, assess your own cultural beliefs, and become aware of regional, ethnic, and religious beliefs as well as of practices of groups in the area where you work. This aids you in the development of culturally specific interventions.

Interventions to Change Lifestyle

Changing a client's high-risk behaviors involves more than giving information. Knowledge is necessary but not sufficient to change health behaviors. Thus, one set of interventions will not be effective for all clients. Instead, you will need to adapt your teaching and recommendations to each client's perceptions of his health and his ability to change. The best way to improve a client's health status and health behavior is by enhancing his self-efficacy (ODPHP, 1998).

The main interventions for *Altered growth and development* and *Altered health maintenance* are health education and counseling for prevention of health risks. The two major objectives for these interventions are to change clients' health behaviors and improve their health status. Several strategies can help you do this.

Education

When teaching a client about interventions to change lifestyle choices, give specific, informational instructions to help maximize compliance. For example, explain the purposes and expected effects of interventions you recommend to the client, and tell him when to expect these effects. This is especially important if the benefits of an intervention will not be immediate. Otherwise, the client may become discouraged and abandon the intervention. Many interventions have benefits that are not apparent for several months, such as those of a regular exercise program.

If there is a possibility that a client will experience side effects from an intervention, such as those of medication for depression, tell the client what to expect and under what circumstances he should stop the intervention and consult a health care provider (ODPHP, 1998).

Also, suggest small changes rather than large ones. Ask the client to do only slightly more than he is already doing. By achieving a small goal, the client has initiated positive change. This change will encourage him to continue.

Successful persuasion involves not only increasing a client's belief in his capacities but also structuring interventions so that they are likely to be successful. Sometimes, rather than eliminating established behaviors, it is better to add new behaviors. For example, it might be better to suggest that an overweight client add exercise to his day rather than suggesting that he eat less. Also, link new behaviors with old ones. For example, you might suggest that a client take his medication in the morning while brushing his teeth (ODPHP, 1998).

Finally, use a combination of strategies to help educate the client, such as oral and written instructions, audiovisual aids, individual and group counseling, and community resources. Multiple techniques are more likely to foster the client's success than single strategies. Refer clients to community agencies, voluntary health organizations (such as the American Heart Association), instructional references (such as books, videotapes, or the Internet), or to support groups for clients with similar problems (ODPHP, 1998).

If Mr. Biaggio succeeds in taking brisk walks three times a week for a month but makes no other changes, he is not likely to have lost much weight. However, he may have achieved other benefits. Can you think of any?

Counseling

Research suggests that clients have only a few important beliefs about any one subject. To persuade clients to change their behavior, it is first necessary to identify their beliefs relevant to the high-risk behavior and to provide information based on this foundation. An example is asking a client, "What gets in the way of you eating a low-fat diet?" Once the clients' concerns and an understanding of their issues are apparent, you can appropriately focus your teaching (ODPHP, 1998).

Behavior change will be enhanced by fully explaining the regimen and its rationale, demonstrating it clearly, and writing down the instructions. Once the client fully understands the intervention, ask him for a specific commitment. Ask him to describe specifically what he plans to achieve. Doing this encourages him to begin thinking about how to integrate a new behavior into his daily schedule.

Also ask the client if he is willing carry out the commitment. Clients with a high degree of certainty are more likely to follow through. If your client expresses uncertainty, you can explore the problems that might be encountered in carrying out the regimen (ODPHP, 1998).

Use the power of your profession. Research studies have indicated that your individual attention and feedback to the client are more useful than news media or other communication media in changing the client's knowledge and behavior. Most clients respect nurses and believe that what you say is important. However, some clients lack confidence in their ability to make lifestyle changes. Be empathic and supportive while providing firm, definite recommendations for changing high-risk behaviors. For example, you can say, "I want you to quit smoking." The message is simple and specific. You also need to monitor the client's progress through follow-up contact, either by appointment or telephone call, within a few weeks to evaluate progress, reinforce successes, and identify and respond to problems (ODPHP, 1998).

Recognizing Barriers

Many barriers exist to making a change in unhealthy lifestyle behaviors. The client may feel unwilling to take responsibility for accomplishing day-to-day preventive behaviors for many reasons. Such unwillingness may result from lack of motivation, lack of readiness, inadequate health care teaching, lack of support, and lack of financial resources.

In clinics and other health care settings, barriers to implementing a preventive health program include an emphasis on curing illness and injury rather than prevention. You or your agency may not have an adequate system for tracking, monitoring, and following up on a client's progress. Your clients may lack health insurance, or their insurance may not pay for preventive services (ODPHP, 1998).

Other barriers include you or other health care providers lacking training in preventive health services or being confused over conflicting recommendations for adult health screening tests. You or other health care providers may not have confidence that prevention interventions work. Or you may lack time in the face of competing demands to do follow-up care with essentially well adults (ODPHP, 1998).

EVALUATION

Evaluation is a systematic, ongoing process in evaluating the client's progress toward the attainment of goals, as suggested in the accompanying nursing care plan. Clients and their families, when appropriate, are involved in the process. The ongoing assessment data you gather are used to revise nursing diagnoses, outcomes, and the plan of care. Evaluate the effectiveness of your interventions by considering your client's responses to them as well as the attainment of goals.

KEY PRINCIPLES

- Biologically, development is seen as growth, stability, and decline.
- Adult development is influenced by the social expectations for adults in the social climate present during the developmental years.

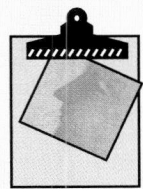

NURSING CARE PLANNING
A MIDDLE-AGED ADULT WITH BORDERLINE HYPERTENSION

Assessment Data

After performing an assessment at the client's worksite, the occupational nurse records the following report:

Mr. Biaggio is a 42-year-old obese Italian-American man, is married with two children who are in high school and living at home. He works as an accountant at a large insurance company, smokes two packs of cigarettes/day, eats a diet high in fat, and has not exercised for "years." "I don't many eat fruits and vegetables. I just never liked them." Mr. Biaggio states he does not understand why he has high blood pressure and that he is not feeling bad. He knows he should lose a little weight and get some exercise. He knows that smoking is not good for him, but he has been unable to quit in the past. BP is 140/90. Height is 5' 10", and weight is 220 lbs.

Nursing Orders	Health teaching about hypertension, low-salt diet, and weight reduction Recommendations for smoking cessation and exercise	Follow-up appointment in 1 month Refer to private physician for follow-up care

NURSING CARE PLAN

Nursing Diagnosis	Expected Outcomes	Interventions	Evaluation (After 1 Month)
Altered health maintenance	Client will have appropriate screenings and immunizations done within the next 6 months	Review appropriate screening tests and immunizations for client's age group	Client has scheduled an appointment for a physical examination with his private physician
	Client will eliminate high-risk behaviors within 1 year	Counsel client on recognizing high-risk behaviors and understanding their connection to chronic illness. *Review his eating habits, including who cooks and how the food is prepared.*	Client can describe connection between smoking, high-fat diet, lack of exercise, and hypertension, hear disease, cancers, and other chronic diseases

Italicized interventions indicate culturally specific care.

Critical Thinking Questions	1. How might the family affect Mr. Biaggio's compliance with the treatment regime? 2. What other resources might be useful for him? 3. What approach would you use to help Mr. Biaggio stop smoking? 4. How is smoking related to Mr. Biaggio's hypertension?

- Accepting adult status means giving up the desire to keep options open and postpone important choices.
- Young adults take multiple paths to achieving the developmental tasks of choosing a mate, developing a career, starting a family, and defining a marriage.
- The developmental tasks of the middle years depend in part on choices made during the young adult years. They may include raising children, being a grandparent, managing physical changes, or caring for older parents.

- Assessment of the well adult is a process of holistic assessment of all functional health patterns.
- Problems of adult development are diagnosed as *Altered growth and development* or a more specific diagnosis to address individual problems.
- Planning for the well adult is centered around the goals of maintaining health and preventing illness.
- Teaching the well adult requires understanding of the client's culture, motivation to change behaviors, knowledge of the developmental stage, and motivation to learn.

- Health screening is a key to prevention of illness.
- The main interventions for *Altered growth and development* and *Altered health maintenance* are health education and counseling for prevention of health risks.
- Barriers to adult preventive health care may be related to the client's reluctance to change and also to the agency's emphasis on treatment of illness.
- Evaluation is a systematic, ongoing process.

BIBLIOGRAPHY

American Nurses' Association. (1998). *Position statements: Discrimination and racism in health care.* Available from:http://nursing-world.org/readroom/position/ethics/etdisrac.htm 1/16/99.

Berk, L.E. (1998). *Development through the lifespan.* Boston: Allyn and Bacon.

Casper L.M., & Bryson, K.R. (1998). Co-resident grandparents and their grandchildren: Grandparent-maintained families. *Population division working paper no. 26.* Available from: http://blue.census.gov/search97cgi/s 1/16/99.

Clemen-Stone, S., McGuire, S.L., & Eigsti, D.G. (1998). Occupational health nursing. In *Comprehensive community health nursing* (5th ed.). St. Louis: Mosby, Inc.

Edelman, C.L., & Mandle, C.L. (1998). *Health promotion throughout the lifespan* (4th ed.). St. Louis: Mosby.

*Erikson, E. (1959). Growth and crises of the healthy personality. *Psychological Issues, 1,* 50–100.

*Erikson, E.H. (1963). *Childhood and society* (2nd ed.). New York: W.W. Norton Co.

*Erikson, E.H. (1982). *The life cycle completed.* New York: W.W. Norton Co.

Kelley, F.H. (1997). *11 ways to keep your New Year's resolution to quit smoking.* Available from: http://www.quitsmoking.com 1/23/99.

Knox, C., & Thobaben, M. (1997). Partnerships between home care providers and client families. *Home Care Provider, 2(2),*57–59.

Kuttner, Robert. (January 21, 1999). The American health care system: Employer-sponsored health coverage. *New England Journal of Medicine, 340,* 3. Available from: http://www.nejm.org/content/1999/0340/0003/0248.asp 1/23/99.

*Levinson, D.J. (1978). *The seasons of a man's life.* New York: Alfred A. Knopf.

*Levinson, D.J. (1986). A conception of adult development. *American Psychologist, 41,* 3–13.

Levinson, D.J. (1996). *The seasons of a woman's life.* New York: Alfred A. Knopf.

*Levinson, D., Darrow, C., Klein, E., Levinson, M., & McKee, B. (1986). Periods in the adult development of men: Ages 18–45. *The Counseling Psychologist, 6(12),* 21–25.

Lipson, J.G., Dibble, S.L., & Minarik, P.A. (1996). *Culture and health care: A pocket guide.* San Francisco, CA: UCSF Nursing Press.

Mandle, C.L. (1998). Middle-age adult. In C.L. Edelman & C.L. Mandle (Eds.), *Health promotion throughout the lifespan* (4th ed.). St. Louis: Mosby.

Nemeroff, C.B. (June 1998). The neurobiology of depression. *Scientific American.* Available from: http://www.sciam.com/1998/0698issue/0698nemeroff.html 1/24/99.

North American Nursing Diagnosis Association. (1999). *NANDA nursing diagnoses: Definitions and classification 1999–2000.* Philadelphia: Author.

Papalia, D.E., & Olds, S.W. (1998). *Human development* (7th ed.). Boston: McGraw-Hill.

Posen, D.B. (1995). Stress management for patient and physician. *The Canadian Journal of Continuing Medical Education.* Available from: http://www.mentalhealth.com/mag1/p51-str.html 1/24/99.

Report of the U.S. Preventive Services Task Force (1996). Guide to Clinical Preventive Services. (2nd ed.). Baltimore: Williams & Wilkins.

U.S. Department of Commerce, U.S. Census Bureau (USCB). (1998a). *Health insurance coverage: 1997.* Available from: http://blue.census.gov/search97/cgi/s97 1/17/97.

U.S. Department of Commerce, U.S. Census Bureau (USCB). (1998b). *News: Poverty rate down, household income up: Both return to 1989 pre-recession levels, Census Bureau Reports.* Available from: http://www.census.gov/Press-Release/cb98-175.htm 1/16/99.

U.S. Department of Commerce, U.S. Census Bureau (USCB). (1998c). *Resident population of the United States: Estimates, by age and sex.* Available from: http://www.census.gov/population/estimates/nation/intfile2-1txt 1/9/99.

U.S. Department of Health and Human Services, Health Care Financing Administration (HCFA). (1998). *Medicaid.* Available from: http://www.hcfa.gov/medicaid/medicaid.htm 1/20/99.

U.S. Department of Health and Human Services, Public Health Services (PHS). (1995). *Keys to healthy weight: Balance food energy and physical activity.* Available from: http://odphp.osophs.dhhs.gov/pubs.prevrpt.95sum1.htm 1/9/1999.

U.S. Department of Health and Human Services, Public Health Services, Centers for Disease Control and Prevention (CDC). (May 23, 1997). *Facts about cigarette mortality.* Available from: http://www.cdc.gov/od/oc/media/fact/cigmortl.htm 1/24/99.

U.S. Department of Health and Human Services, Public Health Services, Centers for Disease Control and Prevention (CDC). (CDC, 1998a). *Physical activity and good nutrition: Essential elements for good health.* Available from: http://www.cdc.gov/nccdphp/dnpa/dnpaaag.htm 1/11/99.

U.S. Department of Health and Human Services, Public Health Services, Centers for Disease Control and Prevention, National Center for Chronic Disease Prevention and Health Promotion (CDC, 1998b). *Chronic diseases and their risk factors: The leading causes of death: A report with state-by-state information.* Available from: http://www.cdc.gov/nccdphp/statbook/statbook.htm 1/24/99.

U.S. Department of Health and Human Services, Public Health Services, Centers for Disease Control and Prevention, National Center for Chronic Disease Prevention and Health Promotion, Office on Smoking and Health (CDC, 1998c). *A report of the surgeon general: Tobacco use among U.S. racial/ethnic minority groups.* Available from: http://www.cdc.gov/nccdphp/osh/sgr-minaag.htm 1/24/99.

U.S. Department of Health and Human Services, Public Health Services, Office of Disease Prevention and Health Promotion (ODPHP). (1998). *Clinician's handbook of preventive services* (2nd ed.). Available from: http://text.nlm.nih.gov/ftrs/tocview 1/18/98.

U.S. Department of Health and Human Services, Public Health Services, Office of Disease Prevention and Health Promotion (ODPHP). (1995). Priority Area 7: Violent and Abusive Behavior. Available from: http://odphp.osophs.dhhs.gov/pubs/hp2000/prior.htm 6/17/99.

U.S. Department of Health and Human Services, Substance Abuse & Maternal Health Services Administration, The National Clearinghouse for Alcohol and Drug Information. (SAMHSA). (1998). *The national drug control strategy, 1998.* Available from: http://www.health.org/ndc98/contents.html. 1/12/99.

U.S. Department of Labor Bureau of Labor Statistics (USDLB). (May 1998). *Employment characteristics of families summary.* Available from: http://stats.bls.gov/news.release/famee.nws.htm 1/17/99.

U.S. Department of Labor Bureau of Labor Statistics (USDLB). (January 1999). *The employment situation: December 1998.* Available from: http://stats.bls.gov/news.release/empsit.nws.htm 1/17/99.

Van Fleet, E. & Bates, R. (1995). *Ergonomic and cumulative trauma disorders. National safety council facts and resources.* Available from: http://www.nsc.org/mem/educ/ergon.htm 1/17/99.

Wichowski, H.C., & Kubsch, S.M. (1997). The relationship of self-perception of illness and compliance with health care regimens. *Journal of Advanced Nursing, 25,* 548–553.

*Asterisk indicates a classic or definite work on this subject.

The Well Older Adult

Ann Keller

Key Terms

ageism
older adult

polypharmacy
retirement

LEARNING OBJECTIVES

After studying this chapter, you should be able to:

1. Describe the older adult by stages of life and demographics.
2. Discuss factors affecting health in older adults.
3. Describe modifications of the health history and physical examination for the older adult.
4. Discuss nursing diagnoses relevant to health maintenance for the older adult.
5. Plan for goal-directed interventions for health maintenance of the older adult.
6. Evaluate the outcomes that describe progress toward the goals of health maintenance.

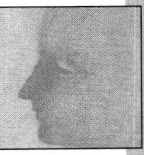

Betty Ellerton, an 81-year-old African-American widow of 6 months, lives alone in her house. At the time of her husband's death, she canceled her ophthalmologist appointment to change her eyeglass prescription. Several months later, while still wearing the old glasses, she tripped and fell to her knees, sustaining a hairline fracture of the left tibial head. After being hospitalized for 2 days, she spent 3 weeks in a rehabilitation facility learning how to walk with a walker, non–weight-bearing on her left leg, and how to remove and apply her air cast.

She is discharged from the rehabilitation facility after demonstrating competency in her leg-strengthening exercises, which she has been instructed to do four times a day. She is able to move from her wheelchair to the toilet, chair, and bed. She has also realized her therapy goal of three-point ambulation with the walker for 150 feet, without fatigue. Her house has many steps at the entrances and therefore is inappropriate for her 3-month rehabilitation. Because of financial constraints, Betty opts to live with her daughter in an easily accessed, single-story dwelling 3 hours from her home.

While her daughter is at work, Betty falls while ambulating with her walker. After returning from the physician's visit to check her leg, she goes to bed and refuses to get up, doing so only to go to the bathroom. Betty refuses to continue her leg exercises and ambulation. One of the diagnoses listed by the home health nurse is *Altered health maintenance* as defined in the accompanying Nursing Diagnosis chart.

**WELL OLDER ADULT
NURSING DIAGNOSES**

Altered Health Maintenance: Inability to identify, manage, and/or seek out help to maintain health.

From North American Nursing Diagnosis Association. (1999). NANDA nursing diagnoses: Definitions and classification 1999–2000. Philadelphia: Author.

CONCEPTS OF OLDER ADULTHOOD

Many people use the term *elderly* when describing an older person, especially when that person is frail, chronically ill, and in need of assistance from others. In this book, we prefer the term **older adult,** used to describe any person age 65 or older. Indeed, no matter what term is used to describe an older person, whether elder, senior citizen, Gray Panther, or just plain old, the stereotypical conception of older adults as frail and needy must change—and is changing—as life expectancy increases.

Many people now live healthy, productive lives well into their 80s. The typical older adult is actively engaged in life, learning new things, and developing a level of understanding that is not possible for a person with less life experience. Freed from the uncertainties of youth and the burdens of middle age, many people find that old age is a time of joy and peace that comes with reflection, shared community, and increased spirituality.

When aging is viewed in the context of normal human development and not in the framework of abnormal decline, older adults can be seen as experts in the field of living. Successful aging can then be appreciated as a process of creating a positive relationship with the Self as we physiologically and psychosocially experience growth, change, and loss.

At the same time, the biological effects of age do cause people to redefine health and health maintenance goals with each decade. Although most people do not fear old age itself, most do fear the infirmity that can accompany old age. A major concern in old age is being unable to care for oneself. Health takes on a new meaning that is associated with one's ability to function and be actively involved in living. In fact, although approximately 85% of older adults have some chronic health problem, most do not define themselves as ill. In a Canadian study, 76% of respondents ages 60 to 69 and 74% of those over age 70 reported that their health was good to excellent in comparison with others of their age group (Epp, 1986). Nursing care of the older adult is aimed at helping clients maintain or improve this perceived level of wellness, and at forestalling the effects of chronic illness for as long as possible.

Stages of Older Adulthood

As discussed in the previous chapter, physical changes associated with aging begin as early as the 40s. In their 40s, 50s, and 60s, many people begin to wear prescription glasses, and some begin to notice hearing loss. These adults begin to recognize the need to exercise regularly to maintain physical agility. In their 50s, people notice the onset of chronic illness, either personally or in their friends and relatives, and they recognize the need for preventive care and a healthy lifestyle. In their 60s, healthy adults look forward to **retirement**—the permanent withdrawal from one's job—by making plans to travel, garden, learn new skills, and so on. Although grandparenting can be part of a person's life from the late 30s, an active relationship with grandchildren or great grandchildren is common into the 60s and beyond.

For the person who can maintain her health, the 70s continue to provide opportunities for an active, fulfilling lifestyle, despite the increased likelihood of health problems. Chronic illness becomes more probable, the person may be acutely aware of health problems among friends and relatives, and attending the funerals of acquaintance and friends becomes a more common event. If the person has not yet had cataract surgery or a need for hearing aids, this decade carries a high likelihood that these aids will be needed. However, because cataract surgery has become relatively simple and hearing aids more effective, the person's lifestyle is not necessarily hampered. People in their 70s continue to learn new skills, run for political office, and make significant contributions through volunteer work. Many are still active in such sports as golf, swimming, and horseback riding.

The 80s are more likely to be a time of slowing down, although the change is gradual and not necessarily significant for all people. Major surgery is common at this time, with such procedures as total hip and knee replacement, coronary artery bypass, and endarterectomy being used to help extend the person's period of active living. A change in motor coordination is noticeable, and the incidence of Alzheimer's disease increases. For many, the 80s are associated with giving up driving a car, a major loss of freedom and independent living. Some people in their 80s move to retirement homes and make a gradual transition to assisted living.

Even the healthiest older people recognize a significant decline in physical function during their 90s, and they spend at least some time anticipating death. Activities are usually more limited than in the 80s, and the person is less likely to be able to contribute to the family's general welfare, at least in terms of physical labor. Maintaining mobility and activity becomes more difficult. Major surgery is performed successfully on people in their 90s, but a decision to manage a health problem conservatively is more likely. Maintaining independent healthy living in the 90s requires the use of alternative strategies for managing the tasks of daily living, such as housekeeping, grocery shopping, cooking, and seeking medical care. An income that was adequate when the person retired at age 65 may be inadequate to manage independent living and the increased costs of health care some 30 years later. Typically, a person in her 90s has become the oldest living relative in a family unit. Her quality of life is maintained through simple pleasures: the company of significant others, sharing life stories, dining with others, and maintaining an interest in the affairs of the world.

Demographics

In 1996, according to the U.S. Bureau of the Census, about 13% of the population of the United States was age 65 or older (Fig. 23–1). This represents about 33.5 million people. More significantly, the population of older Americans is increasing. Studies estimate that, by the year 2030, 20% of the population will be age 65 or older (Fig. 23–2). The fastest growing segment of the population in the United States will continue

to be those over age 85 (U.S. Bureau of the Census, 1996).

At present, women constitute the majority of the 65-and-older group. This is projected to continue through 2025, by which time the ratio of men to women will be 83 : 100 (U.S. Bureau of the Census, 1996). Many older adult health issues are therefore the health issues of women. Statistics indicate that many older women who suffer from chronic diseases and disability live in poverty (Sitzes, 1995). Indeed, seven of 10 poor people age 65 and older are women whose income dropped as they aged. Moreover, nearly one of four women age 85 and older have incomes below the poverty level. This is thought to be due, in large part, to the lower economic status of these women throughout their lives. Obviously, this has a compromising effect on their ability to obtain—and pay for—adequate health care.

However, as discussed earlier, older adults in general maintain a high level of functional health that allows independent living. Although about 35% will, at one time or another, use a long-term-care facility, only 5% are institutionalized at any one time. This means that 95% of this age group is living in the community. Of these, 31.5% live alone, 54.7% live with their spouse, 14.6% live with someone else, and 0.1% live in group quarters other than institutions (U.S. Bureau of the Census, 1996).

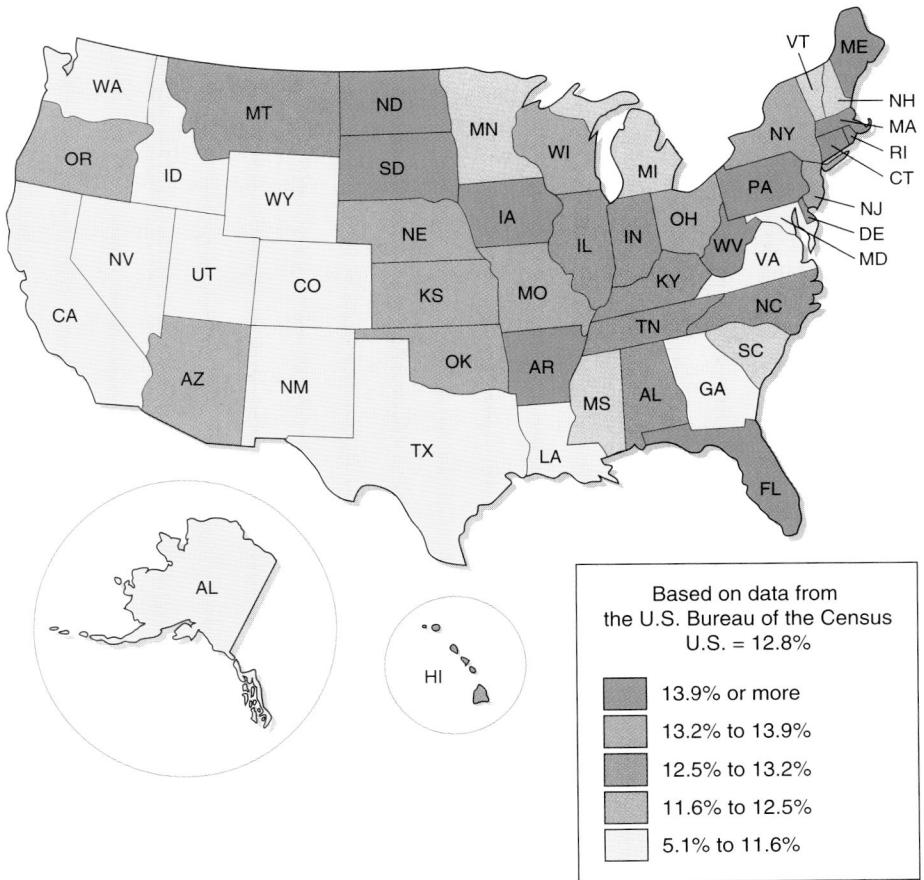

Figure 23–1. Percentage of Americans age 65 and over by state in 1996. Nationally, 12.8% of Americans are 65 or over. (Redrawn from Administration on Aging. Statistical information on older persons. Available at http://www.aoa.dhhs.gov/aoa/stats/96pop/96percentmap.html.)

Based on data from the U.S. Bureau of the Census
U.S. = 12.8%

13.9% or more
13.2% to 13.9%
12.5% to 13.2%
11.6% to 12.5%
5.1% to 11.6%

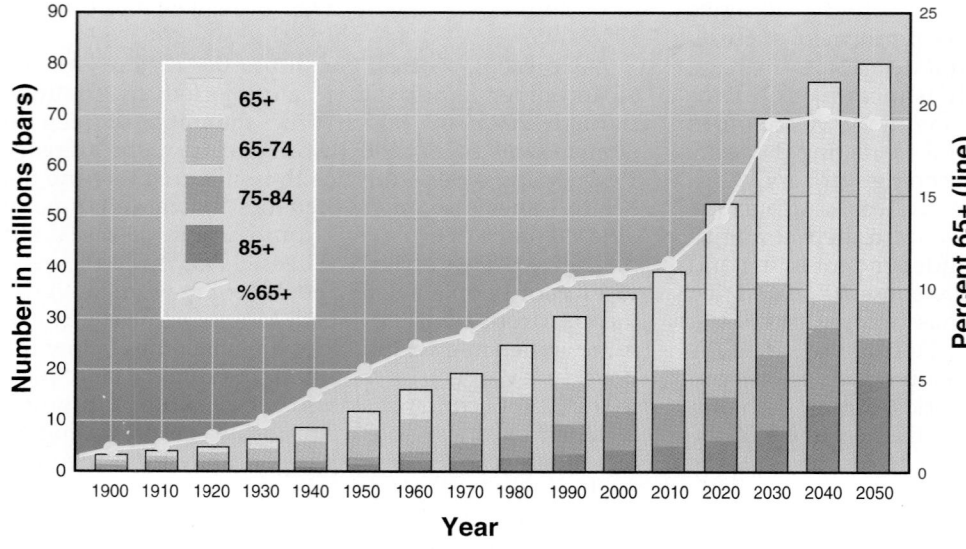

Figure 23–2. Growth of the U.S. population age 65 and over by age group from the year 1900 to 2050. (Source: U.S. Bureau of the Census: "Sixty-Five Plus in America," P23-178RV; "Population Projections of the United States, by Age, Sex, Race, and Hispanic Origin: 1993 to 2050," P25-1104, Census data [1900–1990] are as of April 1, projections [2000–2050] are as of July 1. Redrawn from Administration on Aging. Statistical information on older persons. Available at http://www.aoa.dhhs.gov/aoa/stats/growthcart97.gif.)

FACTORS AFFECTING OLDER ADULTS

Several important factors affect the life and health of older adults. They include lifestyle, environmental factors, culture and religion, socioeconomic factors, physiological factors, and psychosocial factors.

Lifestyle Factors

Nutrition and Fluids

Nutritional status has a large impact on the older adult's overall health. In 1993, the Urban Institute did a national survey that suggested that almost 5 million older Americans suffer food insecurity, in which the household does not always have adequate food. More than 1.5 million older Americans had some food deprivation within 6 months of the survey.

Do not assume that, if a household is above the poverty line, the family members always have adequate food. About 4 million older adults take actions such as eating less, borrowing from relatives, or going to senior meals programs because they are without food or expect to be very soon.

Several factors can contribute to poor nutritional status in the older adult. They include poor oral health; use of multiple medicines, which can alter the absorption of vitamins and minerals; and reduced mobility, which makes obtaining and preparing meals challenging, especially for the older adult who lives alone.

Activity and Exercise

Physical activity is an important factor in the older adult's ability to maintain health and independence. Regular exercise promotes appetite, mental health, and balance. It also helps to decrease stress (Mezinskis, 1996; Yen, 1996).

The person's current level of mobility can provide direction in determining an appropriate exercise pro-

---

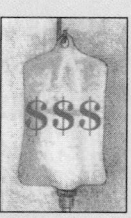

THE COST OF CARE

FINANCING HEALTH CARE FOR OLDER ADULTS

For older persons, the average cost of long-term care exceeds $30,000 a year. In 1991, $59.9 billion was spent on nursing home care, with nursing home residents and their families paying $25.8 billion. Medicaid spent $28.4 billion, and Medicare spent $2.7 billion. Private insurance paid $600 million.

When surveyed, older people prefer home and community care to long-term care in a nursing facility. However, most public and private insurance funds are spent on institutional care for the elderly. The Urban Institute estimated that, in 1993, $75 billion was spent on nursing home care and $33 billion was spent on home-based care, for a total of $108 billion spent on long-term care in both settings. The United States government spends nearly $10 in nursing homes for every $1 spent for home and community care.

Discussion

Nurses need to be involved in policy-making for long-term-care funding. Nurses would be able to contribute knowledge of the needs of the elderly to the planning process.

Reference

White House Conference on Aging, 1995. (May, 1995). *Background materials.* Washington D.C.: White House Conference on Aging Policy and Advisory Committee.

gram for an older adult. A careful assessment to match an older adult with the proper program is essential to get the most from it (Coleman, Buchner, Cress, Chan, & deLateur, 1996). Even chair-bound older adults can do range-of-motion exercises. More mobile adults can benefit from more advanced exercise programs that have been adapted to their needs.

Alcohol Abuse

The use of alcohol by older adults varies widely from person to person. However, although statistical results are mixed, studies suggest that about 3 million older adults are affected by alcoholism (Ruppert, 1996).

Usually, it is difficult to detect alcohol abuse. This is especially true of older adults, who require less alcohol to achieve higher blood alcohol concentrations than when they were younger. This change results from a loss of protective mucus in the stomach and a decrease in total body water (Ruppert, 1996). Also, alcohol typically is metabolized more slowly in an older adult, resulting in a longer exposure time and a higher rate of tissue damage (Hoffman, 1995).

Action Alert!
Teach the client to avoid drinking alcohol when taking any medications. Alcohol can interact with medications and alter the way they are metabolized.

Signs and symptoms of alcohol misuse may be similar to or mistaken for other clinical concerns (Ruppert, 1996). Often, however, alcoholism simply goes undetected by health care providers, either because they fail to look for this problem among older adults or because older adults who drink heavily tend to be socially isolated.

Sleep and Rest

Just as activity is important to the older adult, so too is rest. Older adults need 5 to 7 hours of sleep daily. As age increases, so can the need for rest periods throughout the day.

Age-related changes that can affect a person's ability to sleep at night include nocturia, muscle cramps, and anxiety (Eliopoulis, 1997). The length of Stage 4, the deep restful sleep, may decrease with age as well (Johnson, 1996). To help increase sleeping time, the older person may benefit from avoiding physical exertion near bedtime, effective toileting, avoiding stimulants (such as caffeine) after supper, and obtaining needed pain relief before trying to fall asleep.

Environmental Factors

The environment has a great effect on us, young or old. As adults age, they may spend more time at home because of retirement or altered health and mobility. Age-related changes and the increased amount of time spent at home make it increasingly important to ensure the safety of an older adult's environment. Usually, you can do so by enhancing basic safety practices already in place for other age groups. Your goal is to

mitigate the effects of age-related changes while maintaining as much independence as possible for the older person.

Home Safety

An older adult's environment probably will need more attention to safety than may have been necessary at other times in her life. Often, the older person's safety can be enhanced simply by encouraging the use of health aids already in place. For example, regular battery replacement in smoke and carbon monoxide detectors will increase warning systems to support safety. Encourage the person to wear a hearing aid and glasses, if she needs them, to increase her sensory awareness.

Housing Safety

Housing is directly related to the older adult's income. The more affluent the person, the higher the adequacy of the housing. Likewise, the lower the income, the more inadequate the housing may be. Plus, if the neighborhood around the home declines as the house and the older adult age, the person's safety may suffer. Without any hope of an increase in income, however, the person may be forced to remain in that area. The person may be forced to stay indoors more if she fears moving about in the neighborhood.

Some older adults have begun to share housing to address the problems of aging on fixed or decreasing incomes. This can be accomplished by home sharing, renting portions of the home to other older adults who have similar needs and interests. Some older adults sell their houses and move in with family members.

Driving Safety

Driving safety is a major independence issue. Because many older adults need to provide their own transportation to maintain their interests and their lifestyle, driving skills need to be safe. The national crash involvement average for drivers age 65 and older is 36 per 1,000 driving years (Foley, Wallace, & Eberhard, 1995). This rate is higher than in some other age groups, but not the highest. However, motor vehicle accidents increase with visual changes and increased arthritis, as manifested by back pain and the use of anti-inflammatory drugs (Foley, Wallace, & Eberhard, 1995). Increasing pharmaceutical use may alter the older driver's safety level as well, especially if she also uses alcohol.

Action Alert!
Assess the client for prescription drug history, alcohol intake, and driving behaviors. People of all ages should never mix drinking and driving.

Cultural/Religious Factors

Culture and ethnic origin are more likely to be important influences in older adults, especially when the person is a first-generation American. Aging people have lived as the people they are for a long time. The beliefs and norms of the groups to which each client belongs have shaped ideas about health, diet, education, illness, pain, silence, symptom reporting, family support, death, health care providers, and the elderly and aging. Within the context of the assessment, you can determine the strength of the client's affiliation to an ethnic group, health practices, and beliefs about health care (Evans & Cunningham, 1996).

An example of this would be setting up living arrangements in a care plan for Betty Ellerton, the African-American client introduced at the start of the chapter. After you investigate and understand Mrs. Ellerton's and her daughter's sense of family and family caring, you can use that basic information as a starting point in building a care plan that reflects their thoughts and beliefs about these issues.

Socioeconomic Factors

Historically, each new generation of older American adults has had more financial resources than the previous cohort. Therefore, the present generation is the most financially secure group of older adults in our nation's history. The reasons for this include the economic boom that followed World War II, maturation of Social Security and private pensions, health benefits provided by Medicare (starting in 1965), and an increase in housing values in the late 1970s. More than three-fifths of people ages 65 and older depend on Social Security to provide half or more of their income (White House Conference on Aging, 1995).

However, in these times of increased economic security for some older adults, about 12% of the noninstitutionalized population ages 55 and older lives below the poverty level. Increased age (above 55), being

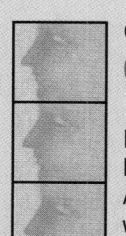

CROSS-CULTURAL CARE
CARING FOR AN OLDER AFRICAN-AMERICAN WOMAN

Betty Ellerton, the client whose story we have been following through the chapter, is an older African-American woman. Her choice to live with her daughter comes from her belief in relying on family members who are concerned and involved in her life. Mrs. Ellerton expects her daughter to be available and supportive of her needs at this difficult time. Her expectation that her daughter's home would be available to her as long as it is needed is not considered inappropriate by either of them. Indeed, the daughter is honoring Mrs. Ellerton by opening her home to her mother as she cares for her.

Mrs. Ellerton's depression and feelings of defeat with the fall during her rehabilitation could be based in feeling out of control and needing continued help to do her self-care. She might feel unhappy with the prospect of more interaction with health care providers when she felt that she had been becoming independent from them.

Although every client is unique, many older African-Americans have a tendency to hold the following values:

- Religion, including prayers and music for spiritual strength.
- Technology.
- A concerned and supportive family, possibly including an extended family network.
- Reliance on family members for daily survival.
- Folk healing and use of home remedies.
- Endurance of the inevitable pain and suffering experienced in life.
- Assistance with self-care.
- Caution, sometimes suspicion, when interacting with unknown health care providers.

Let's see how Mary, Mrs. Ellerton's nurse, demonstrated sensitivity to her client's cultural values:

Mary: How do you feel about staying at your daughter's home?

Mrs. Ellerton: We'll manage. She'll be able to take care of me.

Mary: When do you plan to do your leg exercises?

Mrs. Ellerton: I might do them before I eat; I don't know, I'm pretty tired.

Mary: Do you feel strong enough to walk with the walker?

Mrs. Ellerton: I won't walk too much. I'm used to watching a lot of television. I don't have many visitors.

Mary: Let's talk about living alone.

Critical Thinking Questions

- Mrs. Ellerton's daughter is concerned about her mother's motivation for self-care, but does not want her to fall again. How can you help?
- How could you use Mrs. Ellerton's cultural values to strengthen her motivation for self-care?
- If Mrs. Ellerton's reliance on her daughter is a cultural value, should you encourage self-care?

References

Leininger, M. (1991). *Culture care diversity and universality: A theory of nursing.* New York: National League for Nursing Press.
Campinha-Bacote, J. (1998). In Purnell, L.D., & Paulanka, B.J. (Eds.). *Transcultural Health Care.* Philadelphia: F.A. Davis Co.

female, and being either African-American or Hispanic all raise the risk of poverty and the severity of the poverty experienced. Three of four adults ages 65 and older living below the poverty level are women. Among African-American women ages 85 and older who live alone, 40% live in poverty (White House Conference on Aging, 1995).

Health care for older adults is becoming increasingly expensive and complex. The levels of health care deductibles are increasing, making it more difficult for even employed older adults to pay them. For those not working, paying the deductibles takes a larger percentage of their income. For both groups, the rising cost and use of medications is unpredictable.

Those older adults, now in poverty, will have a more difficult time meeting their basic survival needs, as well as their health care needs. Increasingly, working older adults are discovering that more of their after-tax dollars are spent on health care.

Physiological Factors

Older adults must adapt to a number of physiological changes associated with aging (Fig. 23–3). These changes include chronic illnesses, sensory deficits, cognitive and intellectual changes, and changes in mobility.

Chronic Illness

Chronic illnesses, such as arthritis, hypertension, heart disease, and diabetes, can be major concerns for older

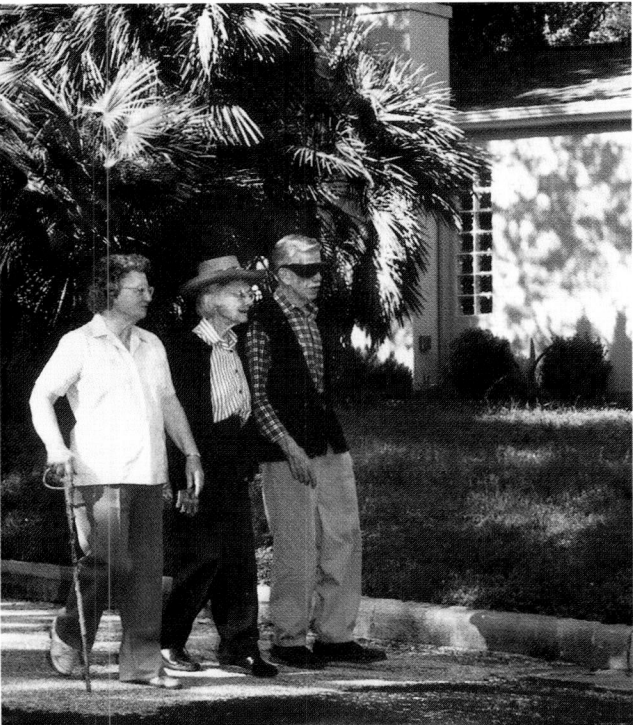

Figure 23–3. These older adults demonstrate some common adaptations to the physiological changes of older adulthood.

adults. Beckerman and Northrop (1996) found that the older adult's level of hope, life satisfaction, and self-concept influenced the adjustment to such a disease process. Most older adults have at least one chronic disease. Even so, 51% of all older adults are not limited in their self-care by the disease process (U.S. Bureau of the Census, 1995). It seems that the elderly are effectively managing many of these disease processes. The goals for older adults who have chronic illness are to maintain self-care, prevent complications, delay decline, and achieve the highest possible quality of life.

Sensory Deficits

Visual changes with aging include a decrease in visual acuity and accommodation, the ability to focus at various distances. This loss of accommodation is called presbyopia, and it results from a loss of flexibility in the lens. Commonly, it begins to appear in a person's 40s, when reading glasses become necessary. A variety of techniques can help you interact most effectively with an older adult who has a visual or other sensory deficit (Box 23–1).

Other visual changes may occur as well. For example, the older person's pupils may become less responsive to light, reducing her ability to see well in dimly lit areas or at night. The person may need more light for reading and fine work. Difficulty in seeing at night can change or decrease the older adult's level of independence. If night driving becomes too challenging, for example, the person may need to make plans, or alter them, to avoid driving at night.

Cataracts, or clouding of the lens, are a common age-related change. They can cause blurring and decreased light and color perception. Correction of this condition, the surgical removal of the clouded lens, commonly can be performed as same-day surgery. Afterward, the person may receive a lens implant or wear corrective lenses.

Glaucoma, also common in the older adult, is a degenerative disease of increasing intraocular pressure that arises when aqueous humor is unable to drain properly from the anterior chamber of the eye. Glaucoma can lead to optic nerve damage if untreated. Yearly checks of intraocular pressure should be encouraged for all people age 40 and older, but especially for African-Americans, who have a high risk for this condition. Medication commonly controls the disease process, but careful monitoring is essential for the rest of the person's life (Thames, 1996).

> **A**ction **A**lert!
> If your client needs extra light to read comfortably, teach her to position a 300-watt bulb so that it shines forward from behind her shoulder.

Loss of hearing is not a normal part of aging. However, it is not uncommon to gradually lose the ability to hear high-frequency sounds. Because of the gradual nature of this change, many older adults adapt to it without much difficulty. However, reduced hearing in older adults also can result from secretion of a drier

BOX 23–1

TIPS FOR INTERACTING EFFECTIVELY WITH OLDER ADULTS WHO HAVE SENSORY DEFICITS

The Visually Impaired Older Adult

- Identify yourself each time you enter the client's space.
- Tell the client when you are leaving.
- Maximize available lighting.
- Use color-contrasted toiletries and kitchen utensils as visual cues.
- Do not move objects in the client's space without permission.
- Verbally cue the client before you hand her an object.
- Describe objects, such as food on plate, as if they were on a clock face, to enhance communication.
- Make sure the client's glasses are clean.

The Hearing-Impaired Older Adult

- When talking with the client, face her at her level. Make sure the area is well lit, and keep your hands away from your face.
- Eliminate as much competing noise as possible.
- Speak at a moderate speed, articulate clearly, and use short sentences.
- Pause between sentences.
- Make sure that only one person speaks at a time.
- Use creative facial and hand gestures.
- Assess the use and function of hearing aids.
- Do not shout.

Adapted from Ebersole, P., & Hess, P. (1998). Toward healthy aging. (5th ed.). St. Louis: Mosby; and Miller, C. (1995). Nursing care of older adults. Philadelphia: Lippincott-Raven.

type of cerumen than what was produced when they were younger. These secretions can be more difficult to remove and, if they accumulate, can cause difficulty in hearing (Thames, 1996).

Action Alert!
When an older adult fails to answer your questions appropriately, suspect hearing loss. When talking with the person, face her and use short, direct phrases while you assess her hearing acuity.

Cognitive and Intellectual Development

Patterns of adult intellectual development have been studied seeking to understand peak intelligence times, effect of life experiences on learning, who is at risk for cognitive impairment, and the effect of intervention strategies on cognition. Measuring cognition, memory, and learning in older adults has evolved throughout the 20th century. Cognitive performance remains diffi-cult to predict because of the many factors that must be considered (see Chapter 45 for more information).

When tests are judiciously chosen and test-taking conditions are conducive to the older adult, the result typically finds that intelligence does not decrease with age. Two of the more reliable and validated tools for assessing cognitive function in the older adult are the Mini-Mental State Examination developed by Folstein, Folstein, and McHugh (1975), and the Short Portable Mental Status Questionnaire developed by Pfeiffer (1975).

What has been documented is that healthy older adults do not demonstrate a decline in such intellectual abilities as wisdom, judgment, and common sense. They may have a slight, gradual decline in short-term memory, calculation ability, word fluency, and abstraction beginning at about age 60. Older adults can learn new skills, but it may be at a slower pace. Sensory deficits and lack of relevance to their daily life must be factored into the teaching plan when working with the older adult client (Miller, 1995a).

Mobility Concerns

Normal aging does not necessarily limit mobility. The extent to which age-related changes affect movement is often determined by movement patterns established before entering old age. Thus, remaining active throughout one's life is a way to maintain healthy movement in old age (Fig. 23–4).

As a person ages, gait changes can result from changes in muscles and joints. Muscle strength, flexibility, stability, and cognition are some of the factors that contribute to mobility. When illness affects any of these factors, mobility may decline and the risk of falls may rise. Falls cause about one-third of serious illnesses in people over age 75 (Baldwin, Craven, & Dimond, 1996). They are the primary cause of femoral neck fractures (Nyberg, Gustafson, Berggren, Brannstrom, & Bucht, 1996).

Among clients who fracture a hip as a result of a fall, only about half of those walking independently before the fracture can do so after the surgical repair. Many can walk only with assistance (Tideiksaar, 1996). Therefore, prevention of falls has a great influence on keeping older persons healthy.

Psychosocial Factors
Self-Concept and Self-Image

Self-concept in the older adult is dependent on self-concept throughout life. However, it is also affected by the society's image of aging. **Ageism** is a stereotype, prejudice, or discrimination against people, especially older adults, based on their age. Like sexism and racism, ageism is based on a very narrow definition of how a certain age group is or lives. That definition is then used to view all members of this group as having the same characteristics, behaviors, or both.

Ageism is deeply embedded in Western culture. In a society that values youth and beauty to an obsessive

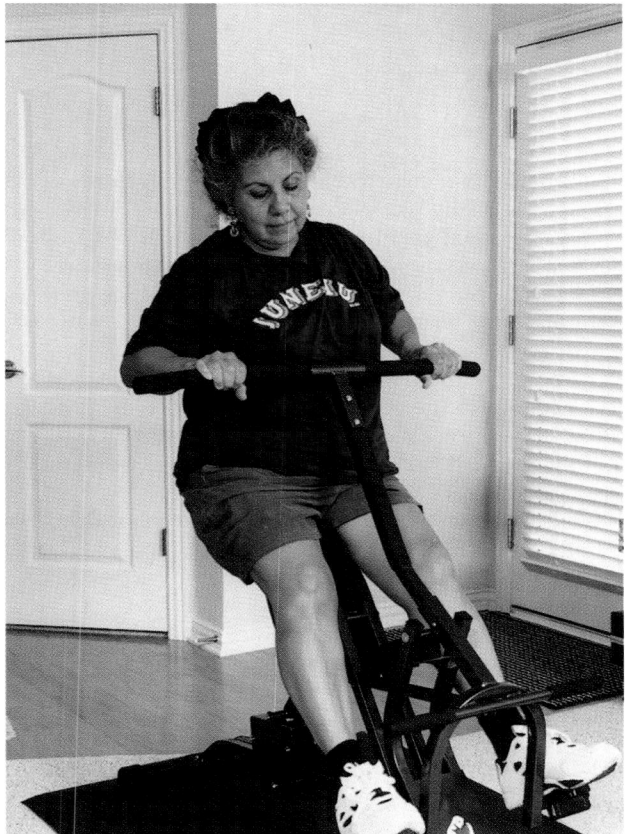

Figure 23–4. Remaining active throughout life is a way to maintain healthy movement in old age.

degree, being old can be seen as a negative. Older adults, as they have aged, have been participants in their culture. As with other victims of prejudice, the effects of discriminatory thinking about being old can damage one's self-esteem. It is not uncommon to have ageist thinking present in older adults who are successfully adjusting to developmental changes but who see themselves as disconnected from their age cohort.

*A*ction *A*lert!
Constant ageist statements about oneself or one's age cohort is a sign of low self-esteem. Encourage self-expression about individual strengths and weaknesses.

Roles and Relationships

Work is a large part of how people define themselves and construct their self-esteem. An older adult's evaluation of the work she does and the work she did as an employee will greatly affect her feeling of connection to the world. However, retirement has changed in ways that give new meaning to life after work. Now it is not unusual to spend more than 20 years as a retiree. How many years a woman or man spent on the job, how the person left the job (willingly, by force, or because of health concerns), and the person's financial and marital status affect adjustment to retirement.

The role of grandparent has taken on renewed significance because of the many changes occurring in the role of parent and the gaps in families created by later marriages and child-rearing (Longino & Earle, 1996). Older adults today can be increasingly involved with children and grandchildren because of the increase in divorce, remarriage, and health care needs (Pruchno & Johnson, 1996; Longino & Earle, 1996). In addition, grandparents often provide support, advice, and a view of the world held only by their particular age cohort.

For the older adult, the role of the spouse changes from earlier configurations. Although long marriage may result in a strong relationship, age-related health changes can bring new challenges for a couple. The death of a spouse is a common consequence of a long life, and one of the most stressful passages for the older adult.

Personal Loss

The death of a spouse is a profound loss. Living alone as a result of the death affects more women than men, both because women have a longer life span and because most men remarry. Men adjust to the loss of a spouse differently than women. Most men remarry and usually marry women younger than their age cohort. The wife may have been in charge of monitoring his care. With her death, the husband also may lose his social agent and might be prone to isolation. For a woman the loss of a spouse may mean learning to manage finances and home repairs. It also means the loss of a companion and caretaker.

*A*ction *A*lert!
Assess a bereaved widow or widower who feels unable to live without the deceased spouse for dysfunctional grieving.

Depression

Depression, although not a normal part of aging, is the most common problem in older adults. Estimates claim that 10 to 65% of people over age 60 have depressive symptoms at some time during their old age. The incidence is higher among nursing home residents than among older adults who live in the community (Reynolds, 1996; Devons, 1996).

Because depression commonly occurs simultaneously with other diseases, it can be misdiagnosed or overlooked. Research shows that medical illness is the most common factor in late-life depression. As well, depressive disorders may cause or contribute to medical illnesses (Lyess et al., 1996). Another possible source of depression is drug therapy. The type of drug an older adult may be taking, or a number of drugs taken for treating multiple problems, can contribute to depression. Several drugs taken for high blood pressure, heart disease, and insomnia are known to cause depression in some people. When assessing for depression and its causes, make sure you take a thorough drug history (Miller, 1995b).

Teaching for WELLNESS

HELPING AN OLDER ADULT MAINTAIN HEALTH

Purpose: To maintain a healthy lifestyle.

Rationale: A healthy lifestyle enhances the quality of life. Teaching should support health promotion and disease prevention.

Expected Outcome: The client will maintain her present level of functioning.

Client Instructions

Your client can do many things to maintain her health well into old age. You can help her by offering these suggestions:

- Maintain your social relationships. Use the telephone to call your family and friends. Attend family functions, church activities, and senior citizen events in your community.
- Exercise every day. Walking is one of the best exercises. Wear sturdy shoes and work up to walking three to four times a week for 20 minutes each time.
- Relax. Take deep breaths and practice relaxation exercises. Visualize a peaceful outdoor scene or a happy family event. Decrease stressors in your life and share problems with a trusted person, such as your clergy.
- Eat sensibly. Eat from the five food groups. It may be easier—and better—to eat six small meals and one or

two snacks than three meals each day. Drink plenty of fluids, especially water.
- Stop smoking. Do not be afraid to seek help, such as a smoking cessation class or a nicotine replacement plan, to help reduce the need for smoking. See your physician for help.
- Sleep well at night. To do so, try not to nap in the late afternoon or evening. Do not eat right before bed. Limit fluids in the evening hours to reduce the need to urinate during the night. If you wake up at night and do not fall back to sleep right away, get up and read or watch television until you become sleepy.
- Avoid constipation. Eat fruits and vegetables, drink fluids, and maintain a walking program, if possible. A stool softener, if suggested by your physician, can help with gentle elimination of stool.
- Maintain a comfortable environment. Use your heating and cooling system for adequate warmth in winter and a cool environment in very hot, humid weather.
- Practice health maintenance. Take medication as ordered. Schedule and keep appointments with your physician. Comply with suggested standards for screening tests, flu shots, and so on. Be alert to changes in your body, and seek help from your healthcare provider as soon as possible.

Coping Strategies

Older adults have lived a long life, taking care of themselves successfully. They have handled many crises, overcome many adversities, and made countless decisions. In place in their lives are a series of coping strategies that they have developed to meet each challenge. As you work with older adults, you must assess these strategies and try to support each older adult as she applies them. Embedded in the client's choice of strategies will be her values and culture-specific needs.

Only if a client cannot successfully handle a situation alone will you step in to help her strengthen her weaknesses so she can overcome her restrictions and draw on a lifetime of experience to meet the current challenge. Allowing the client as much participation as possible ensures the success of this strategy.

ASSESSMENT
General Assessment of Older Adults

Before undertaking an assessment of an older adult, it is important to establish a trusting relationship (Fig. 23–5). Prepare the environment to promote the client's comfort. Make sure the client has all the equipment

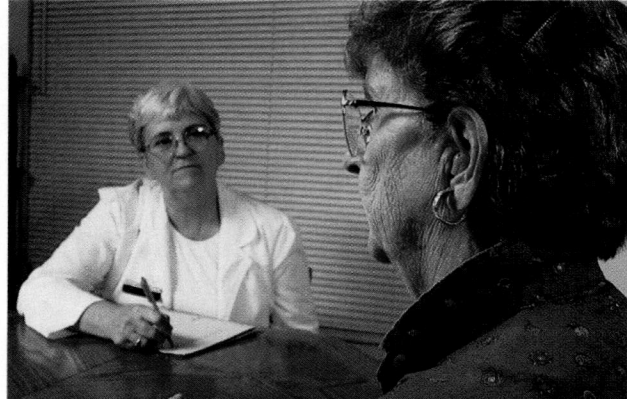

Figure 23–5. Establishing a trusting relationship with the client is an important component of assessing the older adult. This nurse takes the time to develop a relationship with her client before beginning the assessment.

she needs to function at her highest level during the assessment, such as eyeglasses, hearing devices, and mobility supports. The room should be private, well lit, quiet, and warm.

Also, organize your assessment to eliminate repetition and to conserve the client's energy. A printed assessment form will help you be organized. Being efficient helps build trust between you and your client.

As you begin to interact with the older adult, it is important to be client-centered. Giving her choices during the assessment and asking for her input about the pace, rhythm, and order of the questions will help her to feel that she has control of this activity. Observing how she answers your questions will give you additional information. Asking the client about her comfort helps her maintain power over her body and her personal story.

The purpose of the assessment is to identify strengths and limitations so you can plan nursing interventions to optimize function and independence. Consequently, you should focus your assessment on function, not on the changes of aging. Structure your questions to elicit functional data. And make sure your older client understands the purpose of the assessment; her understanding is vital to the success of your assessment. At the end of your assessment, allow time for her to ask questions and clarify any confusing aspects of your conversation

Health History

Health maintenance assessment includes a review of behaviors the client uses to adapt to physical and environmental changes. The older adult has fixed values and beliefs that may make it difficult to learn new skills and cope with a changing world. For example, the use of an electronic gadget for triggering an emergency call response may represent a new way of coping. New knowledge about beneficial health practices may require a lifestyle adjustment.

Take a history of the person's lifetime health-seeking behaviors. Older persons with a history of a healthy lifestyle may have less difficulty adjusting to changes in the methods used to maintain health. The person who values good health will often express interest in learning health maintenance activities.

Assess for the physical and social resources needed to maintain health. The client may need a wheelchair, walker, or cane to maintain mobility. A home environment may require modifications to make it easy and safe for the person to move around. The presence and use of support systems is directly related to the success of health maintenance activities. For the well older adult, belonging to a group of senior citizens who are experiencing similar problems in maintaining health can be a major source of support.

Assess for past health history that is important to understanding the current health status. With the older adult you should structure questions to gather information in a focused manner and help the person concentrate on events that might influence the client's current health. You can create a balance between allowing the client to talk and gathering relevant data.

Functional assessment identifies the older adult's strengths and weakness in the activities of daily living (ADL). These include the activities involved with eating, grooming, dressing, toileting, mobility, social interaction, and problem-solving.

Assessment of the person's medication history should begin with a review of her medications, in their containers, to confirm the drug name, dosage, time taken, purpose, and side effects. Encourage the client to talk with you about her prescriptions and any over-the-counter (OTC) medications she takes. Doing so will help you determine her level of understanding and beliefs about the drugs she takes. This will help you identify potential, as well as actual, problems.

Physical Examination

The physical examination is essentially the same as for a younger person. However, as you perform the examination you should be aware of age-related changes.

HEAD AND NECK

As you perform the examination you may see age-related changes, such as retraction of the gingivae, shrinkage of the roots of teeth, and atrophy of taste buds. These changes can lead to degeneration of tissues around the teeth, leading to loss of teeth and loss of taste discrimination. Determine the client's ability to swallow without choking.

COGNITIVE FUNCTION

Measuring cognitive function in the older adult should be done carefully because of some potential problems caused by physical needs. For example, if the older adult tires easily, it may be advantageous to perform the testing in several sittings at different times.

Gerontologists have been concerned about the testing of older adults because of some important differences between testing younger and older adults. Older adults need a quiet, well-lit, and temperate environment, with no distractions. The testing environment should also be emotionally nonthreatening to reduce the client's anxiety. Before testing, it may be beneficial to both you and the older adult to have some relaxed time together to get to know one another. Under these conditions, the test taker can be motivated to work to maximum capacity (Foreman, Fletcher, Mion, & Simon, 1996). (See Chapter 45 for more information.)

Action **A**lert!
Observe for confusion. In an older adult, it can signify the presence of an infection even before body temperature changes.

CARDIOVASCULAR FUNCTION

Age-related changes that occur in the cardiovascular system include thickening and stiffening of the heart valves. More time is needed for the maximum heart rate to return to its resting rate. Cardiac output may be reduced during stress. The blood vessels become more rigid, which can increase the systolic blood pressure (Pena, 1996).

RESPIRATORY FUNCTION

Age-related changes in the older adult include increased airway resistance, a decreased exchange of oxygen and carbon dioxide (caused by diminished pulmonary circulation), and decreased strength in the respiratory accessory muscles, which causes rigidity in breathing. These changes can lead to other changes:

- A decrease in vital capacity, which is the maximum amount of air that can be expired after maximal inspiration.
- A decrease in residual volume, which is the volume of gas left after maximal expiration.
- A decrease in functional capacity, which is the amount of air left in the lungs after normal expiration.

MUSCULOSKELETAL FUNCTION

Age-related changes in bones include a loss of bone mass and density, increased bone reabsorption, and decreased calcium absorption. As they age, muscles become smaller and have decreased numbers of muscle fibers, which presents as less muscle mass. Cell membrane deterioration results in a loss of fluid and potassium from cells. Slower movements are the result of prolonged contraction and relaxation time. Whether these changes are age-related or result instead or in part from inactivity is still under investigation (Hermansen & Luggen, 1996).

GASTROINTESTINAL FUNCTION

Age-related gastrointestinal changes may include inflammation of the gastric membrane from drug treatments. This can lead to ulcers or gastritis. Diverticulitis can result from obesity or from straining at bowel movements, a problem typically caused by the intake of too many refined, low-fiber foods. An age-related contributing factor can be a decrease in the colon's muscular strength.

BOWEL FUNCTION

Assessment of the abdomen may reveal loss of abdominal muscle tone, and decreased muscle tone in the colon may result in hypoactive bowel sounds. Loss of muscle tone increases the risk for constipation. Weakness of the internal anal sphincter may be a factor in controlling intestinal elimination. Assess for an abdominal mass in the left lower quadrant suggesting constipation. The elderly are also more prone to diverticulitis.

URINARY FUNCTION

Keep in mind that urinary incontinence (involuntary urination) is not a normal age-related change in the older adult. There are several types of urinary incontinence. They can be identified through a good health assessment and history, including a drug history. When taking the health history, check the client's daily pattern of urinating, including amount, times, frequency, and whether incontinence occurs. If it does occur, assess precipitating factors, time of day, and presence of blood in urine (Penn, Lekan-Rutlege, Joers, Stolley, & Amhof, 1996). If the older adult takes a medication with diuretic effects that could contribute to her risk of incontinence, consult with the physician who prescribed the medication (Miller, 1995b).

SEXUAL FUNCTION

Include an assessment of the older adult's sexual activity and function. Sexuality and interest in sexual intercourse do not necessarily decrease as a person ages. Important to a wellness lifestyle is having a relationship that meets the adult's sexual needs. Sexual activity and mental health are the most important predictors of sexual satisfaction (Matthias, Lubben, Atchinson, & Schweitzer, 1997).

The physical ability to maintain sexual function does not necessarily change with aging. Nursing research has found that older adults are as interested in sexual activity as they were throughout their life, and that patterns remain fairly constant into old age (Bernhard, 1995).

Focused Assessment for Altered Health Maintenance

Defining Characteristics

Assess the older adult for current knowledge of health care. The older adult tends to continue to use the knowledge of health practices acquired early in life. The onset of chronic disease and changing scientific knowledge of health suggest that the older adult could benefit from changing health practices.

Assess for health-seeking behaviors. To what extent does the older adult believe that maintaining and improving health is possible despite advancing age?

Assess the client's ability to adapt to a changing environment. Does the client have the ability to learn to use a computer to seek health information? Can the person learn to take new routes to participate in an exercise class? What compensatory mechanisms has the person tried? For example, many older adults will arrange to take a route at a time of day that avoids heavy traffic. Others may practice driving to the location of a special event at a time when there is no pressure to arrive at a certain time.

Assess for the resources to manage health. Does the client need financial assistance to obtain medication? Does the client have interpersonal relationships and activities with others in which there are stress-buffering benefits and sharing of health information?

The home health nurse visiting Mrs. Ellerton saw a change in her behavior. She had been walking and now refused. She had been interacting with her daughter throughout the home and now was confining herself to her bedroom. These are characteristics that define the nursing diagnosis of *Altered health maintenance*. The nurse must assess Mrs. Ellerton's level of dependence, ascertain recent changes, and determine what adaptive behavior she has or can develop to readjust. Mrs. Ellerton's relationship with her daughter is strong and can be used to help the client with her feelings of frustration and depression, to reset goals for ambulation, and to get her glasses fixed.

Related Factors

Altered health maintenance may be related to ineffective coping strategies. What worked, perhaps marginally, when the person was young is no longer viable or productive. Behaviors in an older person are often the same or exaggerated versions of the behavioral patterns of their younger life. Borderline depression becomes clinical depression.

The selection of interventions will depend on the person's cognitive and perceptual ability as well as her level of gross and fine motor skills needed to engage in health maintenance behaviors. If the person is forgetful, she may need strategies to remind her about medications, meals, or exercise. If she has periods of confusion, totally independent living may not be possible. Safe use of a stove and other appliances should be considered. The person's communication skills (written, verbal, or gestural) are important in selecting health maintenance strategies. The lack of ability to make deliberate and thoughtful judgments is a determining factor for totally independent living.

Examples of related factors for *Altered health maintenance* may include a lack of knowledge about the importance of bathroom lighting and plumbing maintenance or an inability to afford new glasses.

DIAGNOSIS

There may be justification for more specific nursing diagnoses that will need to be managed to be able to effectively resolve *Altered health maintenance*. Examples include *Ineffective individual coping, Ineffective family coping, Dysfunctional grieving*, and *Spiritual distress*.

PLANNING

When working with an older client, planning forms an integral part of constructing an effective nursing care plan with appropriate nursing diagnoses. For the older client at risk for *Altered health maintenance*, the goal is for her to demonstrate the knowledge she needs to improve her health behaviors.

INTERVENTION

Interventions to Prevent Illness

Noe and Barry (1996) identify three goals of prevention through screening, immunizations, and health education:

- Improving quality of life
- Maintaining function
- Delaying or preventing age-related conditions

A preventive regimen for the older adult should be individualized based on her physiological status. Although controversy exists around some screening techniques, a careful and constant monitoring of the older adult's health status is important.

Promoting Cancer Screening Tests

Breast cancer in women over age 65 represents 45% of new cancers diagnosed. Annual breast examinations should be performed, and women should have a mammogram every 1 or 2 years up to age 75 (Noe & Barry, 1996). The reduction of morbidity and mortality from breast cancer is still best accomplished by early detection and treatment. Because it is the women themselves who find 90% of all breast cancers, it is imperative that older adult women have the skill for early detection.

Educating women about self-care is vital in their accessing the health care system in a timely manner to get early treatment. As you teach breast self-examination, remain sensitive to the older woman's sensory needs and her sense of privacy about her body. Include in your client education how often to get a mammogram and how cancer can be detected (Sitzes, 1995). Most older women have not received information about cancer in much detail throughout their lives because, until about 1970, medical care was used only when the person was ill.

Papanicolaou (Pap) tests should be performed every 1 to 3 years until age 65. If three or more consecutive tests are normal, they may be done less often (Noe & Barry, 1996). After age 65, Pap tests should be done yearly. Older women who reached their childbearing years between 1930 and 1950 may not have been accustomed to yearly Pap tests. You must urge each older woman to get Pap tests. Talk with her and allow her to express her concerns about privacy during a pelvic examination.

The diagnosis of prostate cancer, the most common cancer in men, is currently being re-evaluated. Typical screening tests include a digital rectal examination and a prostate-specific antigen blood test. However, recently studies have shown that age and ethnic origin may affect the success of these strategies, and the older male client should consult with his physician to obtain the highest degree of accuracy in predicting prostate cancer from these tests.

You should teach older men that it is very important to monitor their prostate health. Encourage them to discuss with their doctor and, in collaboration, consider what strategies about prostate health should be a part of an annual individualized health screening for men over age 50 (Urich, 1997).

Skin and oral cancer screening should take place yearly for those who are at high risk or who identify a suspicious lesion themselves. High-risk clients are those with a family history, or those who have smoked or had high alcohol intake for a number of years. When you teach preventive measures to older adults, teach them to inspect their skin for suspicious lesions and to report any change to their physician or primary nurse practitioner.

Encouraging Immunization

Immunizations can be used to protect older adults from disease or to minimize the effect of disease. Appropriate immunizations and the schedule for each older adult to maximize their level of wellness is an individualized plan, based on their strengths and needs. An over-riding concern in health screening of

TABLE 23–1
Preventive Health Measures for Older Adults

Recommended Interval	Client Gender	Preventive Measure
Once	Both	Pneumococcal pneumonia vaccination
		Tetanus booster (every 10 years)
		Hepatitis B series vaccination
Every 3 to 5 years	Both	Sigmoidoscopy after age 50
Every 2 years or less	Both	Hearing ability
		Visual ability
Yearly	Both	Physical examination
		Stool test for occult blood
		Dental examination and cleaning
		Influenza vaccination
		Cholesterol level
		Two-step tuberculin testing
	Female	Pelvic and breast examination
		Mammogram
		Digital rectal examination
		Papanicolaou test
	Male	Prostate screening in consultation with physician
		Testicular examination
Monthly	Female	Breast self-examination
	Male	Testicular self-examination

Information from Ebersole, P., & Hess, P. (1998). Toward healthy aging (5th ed.). St. Louis: Mosby; Eliopoulos, C. (1997). Gerontological nursing (4th ed.). Philadelphia: Lippincott; Murray, R., & Zentner, J. (1997). Health assessment & promotion strategies. Stamford, CT: Appleton & Lange.

the older adult is regular contact with a primary health care provider. The best health maintenance plan is developed collaboratively between the older adult and the health care provider, nurse practitioner, or physician. Table 23–1 outlines preventive measures for older adults.

Teaching About Nutritional Needs

Periodic nutritional assessments ascertain whether the older adult is able to obtain and prepare food and whether she consumes adequate protein, calories, minerals, and vitamins. Additionally, sufficient fluid intake is especially important for the older adult (White House Conference on Aging, 1995). Also assess for special problems like milk intolerance.

CALORIC NEEDS
Calories are the energy-producing units of food. A person's caloric needs are affected by gender, physical activity, and position on the wellness-illness spectrum. Caloric needs typically decline as a person ages, commonly because of a decrease in physical activity. An important factor to consider, however, is that older adults should decrease their empty calorie intake and use their calories to consume foods with a higher nu-

tritional content than when they were younger and possibly more active.

EATING HABITS
How and what an older adult eats is decided by a variety of factors. Decrease in taste and smell can reduce appetite. Additionally, decreased income, difficulty getting to the market, and decreased mobility can affect an older adult's eating habits.

Cultural influence on diet for the older adult usually does not change with aging. An older adult who has followed dietary laws throughout her life will continue to choose foods according to that diet.

Nutrition can be negatively affected by the physiological effects of medications. Work with the older adult to reduce side effects of the medications that might affect the appetite.

Nursing interventions that can help homebound older adults obtain necessary food include connecting them with community services that can provide transportation to shopping areas, or with agencies that deliver prepared meals, such as Meals on Wheels. When your nutritional assessment finds inadequate nutritional intake, you should work with the health care team to encourage and educate the client about the use of calorie supplements, vitamin supplements, and mineral supplements.

FLUID NEEDS
Teach clients about the need for adequate fluid intake. An elderly client may drink less to decrease the number of trips to the bathroom. Perhaps the client never developed the habit of drinking plenty of fluids. Explain that six to eight glasses of fluid (8 ounces in each glass) help bathe the cells in fluids, break down food in the body, and flush the kidneys.

Establishing Home Safety

Collaboratively, you, the client, and the client's family can increase home safety, often without much cost. Teaching older adults to use their spaces wisely is often all it takes for them to focus on current needs and age-related changes. Controlling clutter, using available lights, and repositioning electrical cords may be a change from how they are used to thinking about moving through their space but can be the start of placing a higher value on safety. The client might need teaching about the use of nonslip shoes and slippers, as well as the importance of protecting the feet by wearing shoes.

As Betty Ellerton's wellness level increases and she thinks about returning to her own home to continue to live alone, the home health nurse at her daughter's house can design a nursing care plan together with Betty and her daughter. The home health nurse in Betty's home town will benefit from the plan as well and can use it to ensure continuity of care for the client. The new home health nurse could do a home safety assessment with Betty and her daughter in Betty's home, so that everyone involved has increased sensitivity to Betty's needs.

Helping the Client Manage Medications

It is possible that up to one third of hospital admissions are caused by adverse drug reactions and interactions (DeMaagd, 1995). The explanation for this may lie in **polypharmacy,** the use of more drugs than is clinically indicated (Carlson, 1996), or in age-related changes that cause unexpected reactions.

Many of the nursing interventions for the older adult involve education about medications. At home, older adults need to be assessed by the visiting nurse regarding their understanding about their drug regimen. After performing an assessment, you must educate the older adult about any misconceptions she might have about prescribed medications. Teach her about the interactions of prescribed drugs and the effects of taking over-the-counter drugs with those prescribed. You also will need to teach the client how to avoid medication errors and interactions, as outlined in the Teaching for Wellness chart.

Teach the client to drink plenty of fluids when taking medications. To enhance compliance, it would help the client to know that with aging there is decreased absorption, and it takes longer for drugs to take effect. In addition, kidney function decreases, so drugs take longer to leave the body. Also, because albumin (protein) levels are decreased, there is less protein for drugs to bind to, so there may be more of the drug floating in the blood, thus leading to drug toxicity.

Instruct older adults to carry a complete list of all their medications (prescriptions and over-the-counter) being taken, so that all health care providers stay informed about the medication regimen. Work with the client to monitor and attempt to maintain the least amount of medication possible for the greatest effect. This takes effective communication between you, the client, the client's family, and the client's physician.

If you care for an older client in a short-term or long-term facility, you will work together with pharmacists and physicians to identify interactions, adverse reactions, and duplication of drug effects.

Interventions to Promote Health Maintenance

Helping the Client Maintain Mobility

When an older adult seeks health care, it is vitally important that, from the first interaction, you collaborate with the client to make sure she receives the support she needs to maintain her mobility. If she needs assistive equipment at home, you can work with the client and family to make it available in the health care facility. The client's wheelchair, walker, or cane should be brought with the client, so she feels comfortable as she adjusts to a new environment, whether it be just for tests or for a longer stay.

Adjusting to new surroundings and new equipment simultaneously increases the risk for falls, a problem you should consider often with this age co-hort. Make sure the client wears supportive, nonskid shoes or sneakers. A risk assessment for falls should be done upon admission for any older adult in a care facility.

Scheduling Health Maintenance Visits

Plan with the older clients for regular visits with a primary health care provider for screening and evaluation, including vision checks, physicals, immunizations, and foot care. Teaching the older client to arrange annual checkups and immunizations at the same time yearly helps the client remember her immunizations. Consistent scheduling will help the client with arrangements that must be made in advance to keep the appointment. If community support services must be included, they can be arranged in advance.

Providing Group Teaching

Nurses in primary settings can help older adults maintain a high level of health and wellness by teaching them about vaccines available against common diseases. Influenza kills 16,000 to 18,000 persons over age 65 each year (Noe & Barry, 1996). Hughes and Tartasky (1996) state that 80 to 90% of all influenza-associated deaths occur in the 65-and-older age group.

A vaccine for influenza has been available since 1940, yet influenza immunization rates have remained very low. A goal for *Healthy People 2000* is to reduce influenza-related deaths. If older adults used the annual vaccine, many could avoid this potentially dangerous disease. You can help older adults by reminding them to make and keep appointments for this vaccination. It is not uncommon for senior citizen groups, Kiwanis clubs, councils on aging, and even local grocery stores to support the offering of flu shots as a community project. This can make access to the vaccination easy and inexpensive.

People age 65 and over are also in the highest risk group for pneumococcal pneumonia. Obtaining a vaccination against it is a safe and cost-effective way to decrease the risk of getting this disease, which kills about 40,000 people yearly. Older adults who have not had this vaccine in the past 6 years should be revaccinated.

The tuberculosis (TB) seen most often among older people is reactivation TB. It results either from becoming reinfected by a person with active TB or from reinoculation by an infection the older adult had previously (Goodwin, 1996). When you teach older adults about this, make sure they understand the importance of an annual two-step skin test.

Nurses in nonprimary settings also have the opportunity to assist older adults in health-promoting activities. Many older adults may benefit from alternative and complementary therapies, including some forms of nutritional supplementation, as discussed in the Considering the Alternatives chart. Group settings may be especially beneficial for stimulating discussion of health promotion and sharing of experiences by older adults. You can bring information to the group on health promotion that may not have been part of the life experience of the group. The group contributes a sense of commonality about the problems faced by older adults, provides a philosophical perspective, and contributes successful ways of coping through sharing similar experiences. It is important to let the group set the agenda and plan the sessions. Some of the topics that are likely to be selected by the group follow.

Because stress is associated with increased disease, stress management is an important component of health promotion activities. Daily hassles are more associated with health problems than are stressful life events because daily hassles maintain a high level of stress over a long period of time. Daily hassles for older adults include concerns for safety and maintaining relationships with others. Unwanted intrusions in the form of door-to-door solicitation, computerized telephone advertising, and other telemarketing techniques are disturbing because of the invasion of privacy at home. For the older adult who lives alone, fears arise that the intruder will take advantage of her or is seeking to learn information that will be helpful in a robbery.

Estate planning can be a source of stress as well. The older person has spent a lifetime accumulating possessions and probably feels that it is important to leave something of value to significant others. It is important both to be remembered and not to have the usually small amount of money or property go to pay for lawyers and court costs. Planning and making advanced arrangements for burial is also an important topic.

The threat of an illness that results in hospitalization is a source of stress. Hospitalization is disruptive, frightening, and has the potential to significantly reduce any savings the person may have accumulated. Even though Medicare and supplemental health insurance pay a significant portion of medical expenses, hospitalization can be expensive. Perhaps the greatest source of stress associated with hospitalization is the vulnerability to death or loss of independence. Hospitalization for a fractured hip is particularly frightening because most older people know someone who sustained a fracture and had to enter a nursing home.

A simple problem-solving model can be helpful when discussing the hassles and stressors of life for older adults. The group can together define the problems and discuss possible solutions. Health promotion includes a discussion of food, because the need to change the diet often accompanies chronic health problems. Women enjoy sharing recipes and discussing how to modify old favorites to reduce fat, sodium, and cholesterol. Older men often become more interested in food, nutrition, and cooking and may seek information on diet and meal-planning as well as recipes and food preparation.

The use of exercise to manage stress and maintain activity is a popular topic of discussion. Older people will quickly realize the benefit of a program of activity and exercise because the change in energy level can be quick and dramatic when the person starts exercising.

When she returns home, or even at her daughter's house, Mrs. Ellerton might enjoy and probably would benefit from talking with other older adults experiencing the same issues of temporary or dramatic changes in mobility status. Betty is a private person who values her family, but being able to complain away from the worried ears of her daughter about all of the transitions she has had to endure might lift her spirits.

For the older person who lives alone or even with another person, loneliness can be a problem. Supportive relationships and friendships are critical to well-being. Developing support systems can be a beneficial effect of health promotion groups. Older people can develop the wisdom to form friendships and peer support without the burden of concern about social or economic class. The group itself may result in mutual support and friendship that extends beyond the class.

Action Alert!
Talking only of failures in life is a sign of possible despair. Institute meditation focused on a peak life experience.

EVALUATION

Evaluation involves ongoing reassessment of the older adult to establish that expected health outcome criteria are being met.

The nursing notes on Mrs. Ellerton's altered health maintenance include the following: Using walker, walks 45 feet to living room, five times a day, four for doing leg exercises, and once for watching evening news with daughter. Client wrote a letter requesting that her medical records be transferred to local ophthalmologist. Made appointment for eye examination.

In the above example, the nurse documented that Mrs. Ellerton has reached the previously set goals: she is walking and doing her exercises. She has begun to work on getting her eye health evaluated, another desired outcome.

If a client's expected outcomes are not achieved within the defined time frame, reassessment is needed to examine the impediments to her progress. For example, when Mrs. Ellerton fell in her daughter's home and went to bed, refusing to continue in a progressive manner, the home health nurse might assess the situation and set alternative expected outcomes within the context of Mrs. Ellerton's evolving, dynamic needs. The nurse might readjust the number of times the client is expected to leave her room. The nurse, the client's daughter, and the client might renegotiate the amount of assistance given during ambulation, until Mrs. Ellerton regains confidence. Re-evaluation of gait strength and feelings about ambulation could be set for a week hence.

Keeping the nursing care plan dynamic is essential for assisting older adult clients to their highest level of function. Interventions are implemented to help cli-

COMPLEMENTARY AND ALTERNATIVE MEDICINE: HEALTH CARE AND THE OLDER ADULT

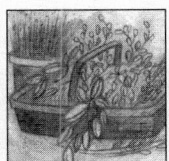

In the United States, the fastest growing population group consists of those over age 85. By the year 2030, there may be more than 70 million Americans over age 65 (Luskin et al., 1998). Other countries in the world, such as Japan and China, also have growing populations of older adults.

Many factors contribute to increased longevity. In this feature, we examine a number of factors that can contribute to improved quality of life for older adults—itself a factor in increasing the *quantity* of life. And, in truth, many of the things that enhance the quality of life for older adults are also healthy for younger people.

A basic contributor to health at any age is physical activity. Although this seems very basic, in the past few years research has been showing a number of important and specific effects of exercise. Physical activity has been shown to reduce the risk of breast cancer in women (Thune, Brenn, Lund, & Gaard, 1997). Although the reduction was greatest in younger, premenopausal women, Thune and colleagues noted that women who exercised regularly were leaner, and that the protective effects of exercise against breast cancer would extend to lean postmenopausal women as well. The regular exercisers also had improved serum lipid profiles that could be beneficial in other ways, such as reduced heart disease.

The benefits of exercise in the prevention of heart disease are well known. Exercise is now accepted as a part of cardiac rehabilitation after myocardial infarction, as well as a measure to prevent heart disease in the first place. A review of the literature on exercise and its relation to depression found that exercise tends to provide a mild antidepressant effect for people of all ages. While cautioning that further research is necessary, the authors cited conclusive evidence that exercise was a better treatment for depression than no treatment at all (Moore & Blumenthal, 1998).

A specific exercise that has been studied in relation to older adults is the Chinese dance-like soft martial art form known as *taijiquan (tai chi chuan). Taijiquan* consists of a series of movements performed slowly, while breathing naturally, often learned and practiced in a group. Numerous studies have found that *taiji* and a related form known as *tai chi chih* offer such benefits as improving balance, reducing the fear of falling, delaying the onset of falls, lowering blood pressure, improving mood, and improving cardiorespiratory function. One study found a 47.5% reduction in the risk of multiple falls in a group with a mean age of 76 who practiced *taijiquan* (Wolf et al., 1996; Schaller, 1996; Lai, Lan, Wong, & Teng, 1995).

These and numerous other studies may explain why each day in China millions of people of all ages practice *taiji*, and also may offer support for the claims of im-

proved flexibility in those practicing *taijiquan*. Also, *taijiquan* has been shown to be equivalent in effect to moderate aerobic exercise, but it is a low-impact form of exercise that reduces the risk of falls and joint injury.

A number of mind-body therapies, such as those discussed in the Considering the Alternatives chart in Chapter 52, have been shown to benefit older adults. Social support networks and spirituality also have been found to offer positive health effects. Taken together, these factors can contribute to what has been called "successful aging" (Luskin et al., 1998).

Diet, another basic ingredient of good health (see the Considering the Alternatives chart in Chapter 29) is certainly important for healthy aging. A majority of older Americans are said to be hypertensive. When older people lower their salt intake moderately and lose about 10 pounds, they may greatly reduce their risk of hypertension, heart attacks, and strokes. In many cases, they may reduce or eliminate the need for antihypertensive medication (Whelton et al., 1998).

Various studies have found particular nutritional deficiencies in the older population, not always clearly revealed by serum vitamin levels (Naurth et al., 1995). For example, researchers have found that administering vitamins B_6 and B_{12} and folic acid to older adults can improve cognitive function, and that what is at times diagnosed as senile dementia may in fact be vitamin deficiency (Bland, 1998). Intake of a nutrient such as vitamin C, or lack of adequate intake, can be related to problems such as diabetes, heart disease, and the formation of cataracts (Cheraskin, 1998). Folic acid has been shown to reduce plasma homocysteine levels, which are related to cardiovascular disease (Malinow et al., 1998). Vitamin E supplementation apparently reduced heart disease, the risk of prostate cancer, and deaths from prostate cancer in one recent study (Gey, Puska, Jordan, & Moser, 1991).

An editorial in the *New England Journal of Medicine*, focusing on folic acid, addressed the issue of whether adults should be encouraged to take a daily multivitamin, pointing out that those who do so seem to experience better health (Oakley, 1998). It is possible that nutritional interventions such as these could save enormous amounts of money by reducing disease and disability. It is thus important that we pay careful attention to the diets of our older clients.

In addition to proper diet and possible nutritional supplementation, some research supports the use of other substances by the elderly. One of these substances is the herb gingko biloba, which has been shown to improve cerebral blood flow. It thus shows promise in the treatment of memory loss, tinnitus, depression, dizziness, and other problems related to impaired cerebral blood flow. It has also shown promise in treating intermittent claudication, which causes leg cramps. Preliminary reports show promise in the treatment of Alz-

(continued)

COMPLEMENTARY AND ALTERNATIVE MEDICINE: HEALTH CARE AND THE OLDER ADULT (continued)

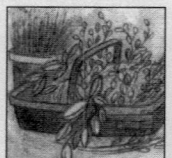

heimer's disease and multi-infarct dementia (Kanowski et al., 1997).

Garlic has been used and studied for years for its cholesterol-lowering and triglyceride-lowering effects, as well as for possible effects in preventing cancer (Brown & Yarnell, 1996). Coenzyme Q10, also known as ubiquinone, is synthesized in human cells. Deficiencies of it apparently occur in a number of human diseases, and supplementation may be helpful in reducing the symptoms of heart disease, such as angina (Murray, 1994b).

One important fact to keep in mind with older clients—and others—is that gingko biloba, garlic, vitamin E, and coenzyme Q10 all have anticoagulant properties, properties that likely account for part of their therapeutic effect. However, in conjunction with pharmaceutical anticoagulants, this effect can lead to changes in International Normalized Ratio levels and bleeding. This danger underscores the importance of being aware of, and knowledgeable about, the herbs and supplements that our clients may be taking. Of note in relation to this is that many Chinese medicinal herbs used in treating the elderly are considered "blood movers" and have circulatory effects (Miller, 1998). And blood flow, which is also enhanced by exercise, is recognized as essential for health, especially in the elderly.

Another supplement of particular interest for the elderly is glucosamine sulfate. It has been shown to be effective in treating arthritis, with minimal toxicity and a greater degree of safety than nonsteroidal anti-inflammatory drugs such as ibuprofen and naproxen. It seems to provide material that can be taken up and incorporated into the joint surfaces, thus reducing inflammation and pain (Murray, 1994a).

It is important that, as nurses, we not succumb to the "pathologizing" of age, that is, simply writing off complaints and symptoms to "getting old" alone. Too often, treatable symptoms are dismissed by clients, the public, and even health professionals in this way. Old age and decline are inevitable, as is death. However, complementary and alternative medicine offers many useful practices and interventions that encourage activity of the body and mind for older adults. Together with informed self-care and informed professional care, aging can be truly successful. The opportunities for "successful aging" have never been greater.

Resources

Publications that can expand and keep your knowledge of complementary and alternative medicine current:

Friedan, B. (1993). *The fountain of age.* New York: Simon and Schuster.

Lock, M. (1993). *Encounters with aging.* Berkeley, CA: University of California Press.

References

Bland, J. (1998). The use of complementary medicine for healthy aging. *Alternative Therapies in Health and Medicine, 4*(4), 42–48.

Brown, D.J., Yarnell, E. (1996). *Phytotherapy research compendium.* Seattle: Natural Product Research Consultants.

Cheraskin, E. (1998). Vitamin C . . . who needs it? *Natural Medicine Journal, 1*(5), 18.

Gey, K.F., Puska, P., Jordan, P., & Moser, U.K. (1991). Inverse correlation between plasma vitamin E and mortality from ischemic heart disease in cross-cultural epidemiology. *American Journal of Clinical Nutrition, 53,* 326S–334S.

Kanowski, S., Herrmann, W.M., Stephan, K., Wierich, W., & Horr, R. (1997). Proof of efficacy of the *Ginkgo biloba* special extract EGb 761 in outpatients suffering from mild to moderate primary dementia of the Alzheimer type or multi-infarct dementia. *Phytomedicine, 4*(1), 3–13.

Kleijnen, J., & Knipschild, P. (1992). Gingko biloba. *The Lancet, 347,* 292–294.

Lai, J.S., Lan, C., Wong, M.K., & Teng, S.H. (1995). Two-year trends in cardiorespiratory function among older Tai Chi Chuan practitioners and sedentary subjects. *Journal of the American Geriatrics Society, 43*(11), 1222–1227.

Luskin, F.M., Newell, K.A., Griffith, M., Holmes, M., Telles, S., Marvasti, F.F., Pelletier, K.R., & Haskell, W.L. (1998). A review of mind-body therapies in the treatment of cardiovascular disease. Part 1: Implications for the elderly. *Alternative Therapies in Health and Medicine, 4*(3), 46–61.

Malinow, M.R., Duell, P.B., Hess, D.L., Anderson, P.H., Kruger, W.D., Phillipson, B.E., Gluckman, R.A., Block, P.C., & Upson, B.M. (1998). Reduction of plasma homocysteine levels by breakfast cereal fortified with folic acid in patients with coronary heart disease. *New England Journal of Medicine, 338,* 1009–1015.

Miller, L.G. Herbal medicinals: Selected clinical considerations focusing on known or potential interactions. *Archives of Internal Medicine, 158,* 2200–2211.

Moore, K.A., & Blumenthal, J.A. (1998). Exercise training as an alternative treatment for depression among older adults. *Alternative Therapies in Health and Medicine, 4*(1), 48–56.

Murray, M. (1994a). Glucosamine sulfate: Effective osteoarthritis treatment. *The American Journal of Natural Medicine, 1*(1), 10–14.

Murray, M. (1994b). *Natural alternatives to over-the-counter and prescription drugs.* New York: William Morrow.

Naurth, H.J., Joosten, E., Riezler, R., Stabler, S.P., Allen, R.H., & Lindenbaum, J. (1995). Effects of vitamin B_{12}, folate, and vitamin B_6 supplements in elderly people with normal serum vitamin concentrations. *The Lancet, 346,* 85–89.

Oakley, G.P. (1998). Eat right and take a multivitamin. *New England Journal of Medicine, 338,* 1060–1061.

Schaller, K.J. (1996). Tai chi chih: An exercise option for older adults. *Journal of Gerontological Nursing, 22*(10), 12–17.

Thune, I., Brenn, T., Lund, E., & Gaard, M. (1997). Physical activity and the risk of breast cancer. *New England Journal of Medicine, 336,* 1269–1275.

Whelton, P.K., Appal, L.J., Espeland, M.A., et al. (1988). Sodium restriction and weight loss in the treatment of hypertension in older persons. *JAMA, 279,* 839–846.

Wolf, S.L., Barnhart, H.X., Kutner, N.G., McNeely, E., Coogler, C., & Xu, T. (1996). Reducing frailty and falls in older persons: An investigation of Tai Chi and computerized balance training. *Journal of the American Geriatrics Society, 44*(5), 489–497.

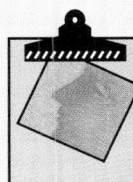

NURSING CARE PLANNING
AN OLDER ADULT WITH ALTERED MOBILITY AND ALTERED PSYCHOSOCIAL WELL-BEING

Assessment Data

The home health nurse visits Mrs. Ellerton in her daughter's home to follow up on her ambulation progress. Her report is as follows.

Mrs. Ellerton is an 81-year-old African-American woman, recently widowed, with altered mobility and psychosocial well-being.

Physician's Orders
Diagnosis: fracture of tibial head
Ambulation as tolerated
Continue rehabilitation leg strengthening exercises q.i.d.
Diet as tolerated

Nursing Assessment
Mrs. Ellerton reports no desire to walk around her daughter's home because there is no reason to do so. She says she is more comfortable just staying in bed, watching TV. She states she is able to ambulate as much as necessary. She does not walk into the living room because the better TV is in her bedroom. She lies close to the screen because she states her glasses are not strong enough. The bathroom is closer to the bedroom than the living room. She has stopped doing her leg exercises. Mobility is to be non–weight-bearing on left leg, using walker. Away from home and friends, in bed, refusing to do exercises, exhibiting signs of despair. Cancelled eye appointment, glasses inadequate, fell in home, withdrawn from daughter, changed rehabilitation behavior pattern, staying in bed.

NURSING CARE PLAN

Nursing Diagnosis	Expected Outcomes	Interventions	Evaluation (After 2 Weeks of Care)
Altered health maintenance related to lack of motivation for self-care.	The client will resume leg exercises four times a day.	Reinforce importance of exercise to health lifestyle, returning home. Obtain a volunteer from her church to come once a day and assist with exercises. Arrange for Meals on Wheels to bring lunch.	Mrs. Ellerton agrees that exercise is important for health. A college student from her daughter's church agrees to visit at 8 AM three days a week. Meals on Wheels will bring lunch 3 days a week.
	Walks to living room four times a day.	Contract with the daughter to insist that the evening meal be eaten in the kitchen. Place good TV in living room so client can watch with daughter.	Mrs. Ellerton reluctantly comes to the kitchen for meals but still refuses to exercise with her daughter. Watches TV in the living room on the days she is expecting Meals on Wheels.
	Prescription obtained for corrective lenses.	Get eye examination and glasses adjusted while at daughter's house.	Records sent from home physician to new physician locally.
	Increase motivation for self-care.	Contract with the daughter to plan for a social occasion, possibly with grandchildren.	Mrs. Ellerton is making plans to have Thanksgiving at her grandson's house.

Critical Thinking Questions

1. How might the client's depression affect compliance with the treatment regimen?
2. Given her present state of depression and despair, how might Mrs. Ellerton feel if she could not return to her own home?
3. What other assistance would the daughter need to more efficiently manage Mrs. Ellerton's care at home?

ents attain expected outcomes within a specific time frame. Ongoing evaluation of this process supports progress and identifies new problems to be solved.

KEY PRINCIPLES

- About 13% of the population in the United States is age 65 or older.
- Women usually live longer than men in all ethnic and racial groups.
- Ageism is a way of thinking, common to both young and old people in Western culture, that abounds with inaccurate, harmful stereotypes and prejudices.
- As with many adaptations to getting old, older adults may re-examine their relationships with friends and family members, with social organizations, and with living spaces.
- An older adult's self-esteem is rooted in many complex relationships, including cultural, religious, racial, and ethnic identities, uniquely constructed by each individual.
- An important concern in aging may include adapting the personal environment to age-related changes to support safety and independence.
- Health services for older adults, in the community or within facilities, need to be matched holistically to each individual's unique needs.
- Multidimensional assessment, focused on functional abilities, captures age-related changes within the context of adaptation.
- Cognitive function should be assessed carefully, in an environment that supports maximum function, using tools that are specifically designed for accuracy with older adults.
- Health-seeking behaviors present in older adults should be evaluated for accuracy and supported when appropriate. Health education is an integral part of nursing intervention with older adults.
- Medication history is a part of health assessment, to check communication in the health care team and examine the older adult's understanding of drug therapies.

BIBLIOGRAPHY

Baldwin, R., Craven, R., & Dimond, M. (1996). Falls: Are rural elders at greater risk? *Journal of Gerontological Nursing, 22*(8), 14–20.

Beckerman, A., & Northrop, C. (1996). Hope, chronic illness and the elderly. *Journal of Gerontological Nursing, 22*(5), 19–25.

Bernhard, L. (1995). Sexuality in women's lives. In C.I. Fogel & N.F. Woods (Eds.), *Women's health care* (pp 475–491). Thousand Oaks: Sage Publications.

Campbell, J., & Huff, M. (1995). Sexuality in the older woman. *Gerontology & Geriatrics Education 16*, 71–81.

Campina-Bacote, J. (1998). African-Americans. In L.D. Purnell & B.J. Paulanka (Eds.), *Transcultural Health Care*. Philadelphia: F.A. Davis.

Carlson, J.E. (1996). Perils of polypharmacy: 10 steps to prudent prescribing. *Geriatrics, 51*(7), 26–35.

Coleman, E., Buchner, D., Cress, M.E., Chan, B., deLateur, B. (1996). The relationship of joint symptoms with exercise performance in older adults. *Journal of the American Geriatric Society, 44*, 14–21.

DeMaagd, G. (1995). High-risk drugs in the elderly population. *Geriatric Nursing 16*, 199–207.

Devons, C. (1996). Suicide in the elderly: How to identify and treat patients at risk. *Geriatrics 51* (3), 67–72

Ebersole, P., & Hess, P. (1998). *Toward healthy aging*. St. Louis: Mosby.

Eliopoulos, C. (1997). *Gerontological nursing* (4th ed). Philadelphia: Lippincott.

*Epp, T. (1986) *Achieving health for all: A framework for health promotion*. Ottawa Ministry of Supply and Services.

Evans, C.A., & Cunningham, B.A. (1996). Caring for the ethnic elder. *Geriatric Nursing, 17*(3), 105–110.

Foley, D., Wallace, R., & Eberhard, J. (1995). Risk factors for motor vehicle crashes among older drivers in a rural community. *Journal of the American Geriatrics Society, 43*, 776–781.

*Folstein, M.E., Folstein, S.E., & McHugh, P.R. (1975). Mini-mental state: A practical method for grading the cognitive state of patients for the clinician. *Journal of Psychiatric Research, 12*, 189–198.

Foreman, M., Fletcher, K., Mion, L., & Simon, L. (1996). Assessing cognitive function. *Geriatric Nursing, 17*(5), 228–233.

Goodwin, J. (1996). Respiratory issues of older adults. In A.S. Luggen (Ed.), *Core Curriculum for Gerontologic Nursing*. St. Louis: Mosby.

Gratton, B., & Haber, C. (1996). Authority, burden, companion. *Generations, Spring*, 7–11.

Hermansen, S., & Luggen, A.S. (1996). In A.S. Luggen (Ed.). *Core Curriculum for Gerontologic nursing* (pp. 449–461). St. Louis: Mosby.

Hoffman, A. (1995). In M. Stanley & Beare, P.G. (Eds.), *Gerontological Nursing* (pp 439–453). Philadelphia: F.A. Davis Co.

Hughes, D., & Tartasky, D. (1996). Implementation of a flu immunization program for homebound elders: A graduate student practicum. *Geriatric Nursing, 17*(5), 215–221.

Johnson, B. (1996). Older adults and sexuality: A multidimensional perspective. *Journal of Gerontological Nursing, 22*(2), 6–15.

*Leininger, M. (1991). *Culture care diversity and universality: A theory of nursing*. New York: National League for Nursing Press.

Longino, C., & Earle, J. (1996). Who are the grandparents at century's end? *Generations, 20*(1), 13–16.

Lyess, J., Bruce, M., Koenig, H., Parmelee, P., Schulz, R., Lawton, P., & Reynolds, C. (1996). Depression and medical illness in late life: Report of a Symposium. *Journal of the American Geriatric Society, 44*, 198–203.

Matthias, R., Lubben, J., Atchison, K., & Schweitzer, S. (1997). Sexual activity and satisfaction among very old adults: Results from a community-dwelling Medicare population survey. *The Gerontologist, 37*(1), 6–14.

Mezinskis, P. (1996). Promotion of self-care and independent functioning. In A.S. Luggen (Ed), *Core Curriculum for Gerontologic Nursing*. St. Louis: Mosby.

Miller, C. (1995a). *Nursing Care of Older Adults*. Philadelphia: J.B. Lippincott Co.

Miller, C. (1995b). Medications can cause or treat urinary incontinence. *Geriatric Nursing, 16*(5), 253–255.

Miller, C. (1996). Multiple choices in over-the-counter drugs. *Geriatric Nursing 17*(5), 251–253.

Murray, R.B., & Zentner, J.P.(1997). *Health assessment & promotion strategies: Through the life span.* (6th ed). Stamford: Appleton & Lange.

Noe, C., & Barry, P. (1996). Healthy aging: Guidelines for cancer screening immunizations. *Geriatrics, 51*(1), 75–83.

North American Nursing Diagnosis Association. (1999). *NANDA nursing diagnoses: Definitions and classification 1999–2000*. Philadelphia: Author.

Nyberg, L., Gustafson, Y., Berggren, D., Brannstrom, B., & Bucht, G. (1996). Falls leading to femoral neck fractures in lucid older people. *Journal of the American Geriatric Society, 44*, 156–160.

Pena, C. (1996). Cardiovascular disease in the older adult. In Luggen, A.S. (Ed.). *Core Curriculum for Gerontological Nursing* (pp 406–419). St. Louis: Mosby.

*Asterisk indicates a classic or definitive work on this subject.

Penn, C., Lekan-Rutlege, D., Joers, A., Stolley, J., & Amhof, M. (1996). Assessment of urinary incontinence. *Journal of Gerontological Nursing, 22*(1), 8–19.

*Pfeiffer, E. (1975). A short portable mental status questionnaire for the assessment of organic brain deficits in elderly patients. *Journal of the American Geriatric Society, 23*, 433–441.

Pruchno, R., & Johnson, K. (1996). Research on grandparenting: Review of current studies and future needs. *Generations, 20*(1), 65–69.

Reynolds, C. (1996). Depression: Making the diagnosis and using SSRIs in the older patient. *Geriatrics, 51*(10), 28–34.

Ruppert, S.D. (1996). Alcohol abuse in older persons: Implications for critical care. *Critical Care Nursing Quarterly, 19*(2), 62–70.

Sitzes, C. (1995). A community-based breast cancer education and screening program for elderly. *Geriatric Nursing, 16*(4), 151–154.

Thames, D. (1996). Sensorimotor stimulation. In Luggen, A.S. (Ed.) *Core Curriculum for Gerontological Nursing* (pp 308–313). St. Louis: Mosby.

Thompson, J., & Wilson, S. (1996). *Health Assessment for Nursing Practice.* St. Louis: Mosby.

Tideiksaar, R. (1996). Preventing falls: How to identify risk factors, reduce complications. *Geriatrics, 51*, 43–53.

Urich, V. (1997). Should prostate-specific antigen be routinely measured in elderly men? *Clincial Geriatrics, 5*(6), 50–57.

White House Conference on Aging, 1995. (May, 1995). *Background materials.* Washington D.C.: White House Conference on Aging Policy and Advisory Committee.

U.S. Bureau of the Census, Statistical Abstract of the U.S.: 1996 (116th ed.). Washington, D.C.

Yen, P. (1996). The marriage of nutrition and activity. *Geriatric Nursing, 17*(3), 143–144.

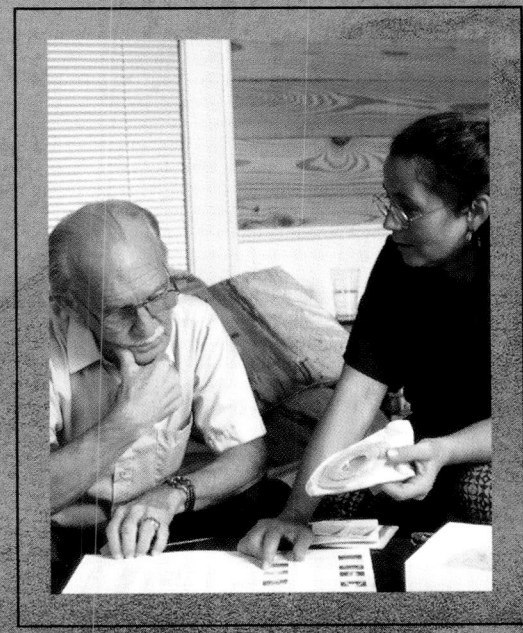

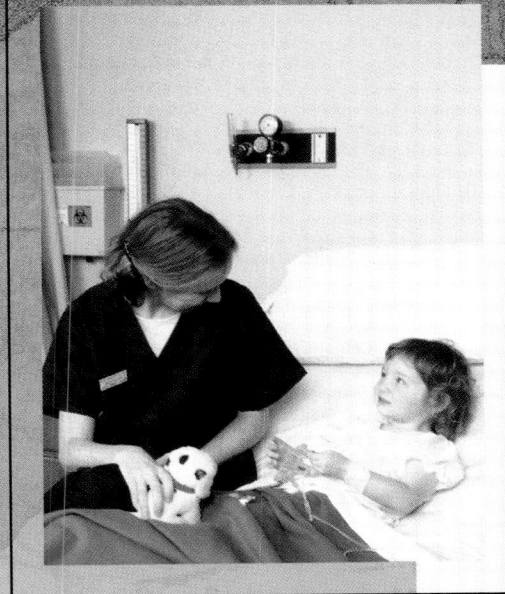

Nursing Care for Functional Health

Health Perception–Health Management Pattern

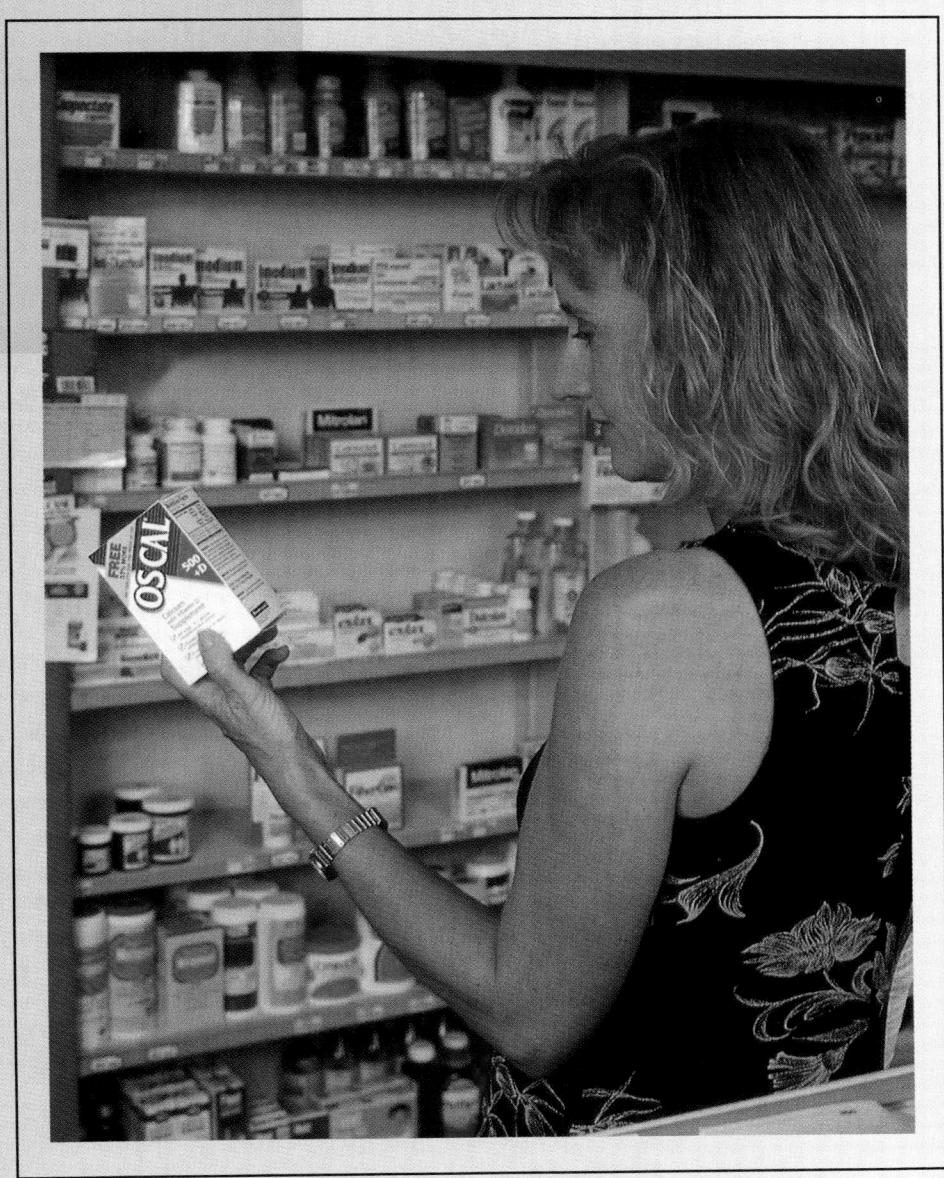

Health Perception

Sheila Rankin Zerr

Key Terms

disease
etiology
health goals
health-illness continuum
health perception
health promotion
health within illness
illness
longevity statistics

population health
preventive health care
primary health care
primary prevention
secondary prevention
tertiary prevention
well-being
wellness

LEARNING OBJECTIVES

After studying this chapter, you should be able to:

1. Describe the perception of health for individuals, families, and communities.
2. List factors that affect health.
3. Understand the focus of assessment of health in the individual, family, and community.
4. Identify health goals and expected outcomes when planning for individuals, families, and communities.
5. Discuss the use of the nursing diagnosis *Health-seeking behaviors.*
6. Identify methodologies of intervention for improving the health of individuals, families, and communities.
7. Evaluate health outcomes in individuals, families, and communities.

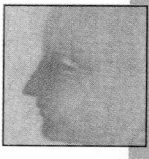

An advertisement appearing in a local newspaper invites citizens to a public forum organized by the local health council and regional health board. The purpose of the forum is to identify local and community health goals. The community, called Delta, is a local division of a Canadian province, but it could be anywhere in the United States. The community has a population of 46,000 and consists of a mix of farming and light industry. Many residents work in a nearby city.

At the public forum, 30 interested citizens gather. They include health professionals, municipal politicians, and lay citizens. The chairperson of the health council outlines the evening's agenda. First, participants will review individual and family health perceptions and how they relate to community health goals. Next, participants will be introduced to government health initiatives that are currently under development. These documents will serve as a resource and basis for discussion.

The group is beginning a process that will include assessing the perception of health in the community and identifying community needs; identifying local health goals and priorities; identifying expected outcomes of community health actions; determining the methodology (programs and services) to achieve identified outcomes; and evaluating the results.

The nurses involved in this group contribute their perception of health to the planning process. If they identified a nursing diagnosis for the community with which they were working, it might be *Health-seeking behaviors.*

CONCEPTS OF HEALTH

Health is important to individuals, families, and communities. It is important to individuals to feel good, to be able to perform needed work, and to enjoy life. It is important to families to meet the needs of their members by providing love, belonging, food, shelter, and safety and by helping family members achieve their highest potential. Health is important to the community, both from the standpoint of quality of life and the economic well-being of its citizens. Additionally, health has been described as the bedrock on which social progress is built. Healthy people can do things that make life worthwhile, and as the level of health increases, so does the potential for happiness. **Health perception** is the knowledge and experience of one's state of wellness and well-being.

Nurses are involved in health care planning and decision-making for individuals, families, and communities. To fulfill the nursing role at any of these three levels, you will need to understand the meaning of health to the individual, the family, and the community. As you begin to study this chapter on the perception of health, consider your own perception of health. Ask yourself important questions about health, such as these: "What does it mean when I say I am healthy? Could I be healthier? How could I make that happen? Is it worth the effort? What would I need to sacrifice to become healthier? Are there factors in my environment that would hinder me from becoming a healthier person?"

Also think about your family and community. What factors would you use to describe a healthy family? A healthy community? What would need to change in your community to increase the health of the people with whom you live and work? To answer these questions, you need to consider the influences of living and working conditions, natural environment, health services, biological influences, and individual capacities and skills (Fig. 24–1).

As a world culture, our ideas about health and illness have changed over the past century. At the beginning of the century, society thought in terms of a dichotomy of healthy or ill. Health care was focused on conquering the most prevalent diseases. Around the middle of the 20th century, the death rate from acute disease declined below that of chronic illness. Thus, it became more important to identify the risk factors and change lifestyle factors to prevent chronic illness. In the 1980s, the emphasis in health care shifted to chang-

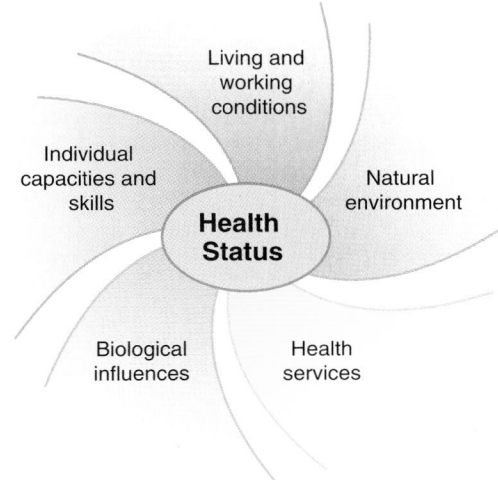

Figure 24–1. Influences on health. (Redrawn from Province of British Columbia. [1995]. Health goals for British Columbia: Identifying priorities for a healthy population—a draft for discussion. Office of the Provincial Health Officer. Victoria, BC: Author.)

ing behaviors and health habits as a way to prevent illness and prolong life. Today, the importance of a comprehensive program of health promotion is recognized as a means to manage all the factors that determine whether or not we are healthy and live in a healthy community. **Health promotion** is the advancement of health through the encouragement of activities that enhance the wellness of individuals, families, and communities.

Health as a National and an International Goal

As citizens of the world, we can no longer view health only from an individual or local community perspective. A global economy and growing international mobility suggest that the health concerns of one country must be adopted by other countries as well. The industrialized nations of the world look to each other for ideas about how to improve the health of their citizens and those in less developed countries. They also must monitor the threat of pathogen transmission across international boundaries.

The World Health Organization (WHO) has defined health as a state of complete physical, mental, and social well-being, and not merely the absence of illness. This holistic definition recognizes that being healthy involves more than simply physiological functioning. The need for comprehensive health goals to address these determinants of health has been well recognized. **Health goals** outline broadly what needs to be done to achieve health for individuals, families, and communities.

WHO also declared that health is a fundamental human right and established a social goal to attain the highest possible level of health by all people by the year 2000 (WHO, 1978). This goal was subsequently adopted by many nations, including the United States and Canada (Box 24–1). WHO further promoted primary health care as the key to attaining the target of health for all by the year 2000.

In 1990, the U.S. Public Health Service released target health objectives for the United States in a document entitled *Healthy People 2000: National Health Promotion and Disease Prevention Objectives.* This document outlined 21 priority areas and established scores of specific health objectives for the country (Table 24–1).

A consortium of more than 300 organizations worked with local, state, and federal government agencies to develop national goals for a preventive health agenda.

An interim progress report released in 1995 listed specific steps by which premature deaths could be reduced (Box 24–2). Full evaluation of the *Healthy People* objectives is currently in progress, with new targets now being established for the year 2010 in a set of objectives called *Healthy People 2010.*

The first year of *Healthy People 2010* was a time of listening, and it began a broad consultation process for a decade-long agenda. The overarching goal of *Healthy People 2010* is "increasing the quality and years of healthy life," but it will also strengthen the goal of "reducing health disparities" to "elimination of health disparities."

Canada formally adopted WHO health goals with the 1986 document *Achieving Health for All: A Framework for Health Promotion* (Epp, 1986). Some provinces, including Ontario, Quebec, and British Columbia, have initiated the process of establishing health goals.

Definitions of Health

Whether a client is an individual, family, or community, your understanding of different perspectives of health will help you to manage health and health care from the client's perspective. The client's goals for health are derived from the definitions of health.

BOX 24–1

HEALTH GOALS OF THE UNITED STATES AND CANADA

In the United States, health care planning is commonly based on the goals of *Healthy People 2010.* Canada's national health care system, and the Canada Health Act on which it was built, reflects five established principles. Although the health care systems of the United States and Canada differ, the principles of community planning are the same in both countries. In the United States, community planning initiatives are more likely to exist at the local and state level rather than at the national level.

United States' Goals (2010)

OVERARCHING GOALS

- To increase the span of healthy life.
- To eliminate health disparities among different populations.

ENABLING GOALS

- To promote healthy behaviors.
- To protect health.
- To ensure access to quality health care.
- To strengthen community prevention.

Canada's Principles

- *Universality.* Essential health services must be available to all persons normally resident in Canada with-

out regard to age, risk category, present health status, or ability to pay.
- *Comprehensiveness.* Essential health services must be provided and include the following range of services: health promotion, disease/accident prevention, curative care, rehabilitative care, and supportive care.
- *Accessibility.* Essential health services must be available to all those eligible to receive them, with no unreasonable geographic barriers and no financial barriers.
- *Portability.* Essential health services should be available to those eligible when they are away from home, at least to the level the services would be available at home.
- *Public administration.* Essential health services should be planned, funded, and supervised on a nonprofit basis by public authorities.

References

Maiese, D.R., & Fox, C.E. (1998). *Laying the foundation for healthy people 2010—The first year of consultation. Public Health Reports, (113)*92–95. Can be accessed at http://web.health.gov/healthypeople/2010article.htm.

Canada Health Act Overview. (1992). In *Health and Welfare Canada. Canada Health Act Annual Report 1991–1992.* Ottawa: Ministry of Supply and Services Cat HI-4/1992.

TABLE 24–1
PRIORITY AREAS ESTABLISHED BY *HEALTHY PEOPLE 2000*

Health Promotion	*Physical Activity*	• More people exercising regularly. • Fewer people never exercising.
	Nutrition	• Fewer people overweight. • Lower-fat diets.
	Tobacco	• Fewer people smoking cigarettes. • Fewer youth beginning to smoke.
	Alcohol and Other Drugs	• Lower rate of alcohol-related automobile deaths. • Less alcohol use among youth ages 12 to 17. • Less marijuana use among youth ages 12 to 17.
	Family Planning	• Lower teen pregnancy rate. • Fewer unintended pregnancies.
	Mental Health and Mental Disorders	• Lower suicide rate. • Fewer people reporting stress-related problems.
	Violent and Abusive Behavior	• Lower homicide rate. • Lower assault injury rate.
	Educational and Community-Based Programs	• More schools with comprehensive school health education. • More workplaces with health promotion programs.
Health Protection	*Unintentional Injuries*	• Lower rate of unintentional injury deaths. • More people using automobile safety restraints.
	Occupational Safety and Health	• Lower work-related death rate. • Lower work-related injury rate.
	Environmental Health	• No children with blood lead levels of 25 µg/dL or above. • More people with clean air in their community. • More people in radon-tested houses.
	Food and Drug Safety	• Fewer *Salmonella* outbreaks.
	Oral Health	• Fewer children with dental caries. • Fewer older people without teeth.
Preventive Services	*Maternal and Infant Health*	• Fewer newborns with low birth weight. • More mothers with first-trimester care.
	Heart Disease and Stroke	• Lower death rate from coronary artery disease. • Lower death rate from cerebrovascular accident. • Better control of high blood pressure. • Lower cholesterol levels.
	Cancer	• Lower rate of cancer deaths. • Increased screening for breast cancer for women over age 50. • Increased screening for cervical cancer for women over age 18. • Increased testing for fecal occult blood for people over age 50.
	Diabetes and Chronic Disabling Conditions	• Fewer people disabled by chronic conditions. • Lower rate of diabetes-related deaths.
	Infection With Human Immunodeficiency Virus (HIV)	• Slower increase in HIV infection rate.
	Sexually Transmitted Diseases	• Lower gonorrhea infection rate. • Lower syphilis infection rate.
	Immunization and Infectious Diseases	• No measles. • Lower pneumonia and influenza death rates. • Higher immunization levels for children ages 19 months to 35 months.
	Clinical Preventive Services	• No financial barriers to recommended preventive services.

From United States Public Health Service. (1990). Healthy people 2000: National health promotion and disease prevention objectives. Washington, D.C.: Government Printing Office.

STEPS TO ALTER THE UNDERLYING CAUSES OF PREMATURE DEATH

Of the 2.1 million deaths in the United States in 1992, about one-third resulted from heart disease and one-fourth from cancers. In theory, many lives could be saved by altering the underlying causes of these and other leading causes of death. Here are some examples.

- Elimination of tobacco use, either by preventing its initial use or by stopping its current use, could prevent more than 400,000 deaths annually from cancer, heart and lung diseases, and cerebrovascular accident (stroke).
- Improved diet and exercise patterns could prevent 300,000 deaths annually by reducing the effects of heart disease, stroke, diabetes, and cancer.
- Prevention of underage drinking and excess alcohol consumption could prevent nearly 100,000 deaths, especially those involving motor vehicle crashes, falls, drownings, and other alcohol-related injuries.
- Improved safety measures and worker training could prevent numerous deaths from injuries at work sites, at home, in recreational settings, in communities, and on roadways.
- Immunizations could prevent 63,000 of 90,000 deaths caused by infectious diseases affecting children and adults.
- Reduction of the use of firearms—in murders, suicides, and accidental discharges—could prevent 35,000 deaths annually.
- Safe sexual intercourse could prevent 30,000 deaths annually from unintended pregnancies, acquired immunodeficiency disease, and other sexually transmitted diseases.

From United States Department of Health, Education and Welfare. (1995). Healthy people 2000: 1995 report and progress. Washington, D.C.: Author.

Health as the Absence of Disease

Health and illness can be viewed as a dichotomy, with health being defined as the absence of disease. A **disease** is a specific disorder characterized by a recognizable set of signs and symptoms and attributable to heredity, infection, diet, or environment. A disease is an interruption in the continuous process of health. A disease may disrupt the person's ability to function or even shorten life.

Using this definition of health, health care is the diagnosis and treatment of disease based on identification of a specific disorder and its etiology. **Etiology** is

the cause of the disease. If the cause of the disease can be removed, the person often will be cured of the disease. For example, using antibiotics to remove the cause of a disease will cure an infection caused by bacteria. Etiologies of diseases include the following:

- Biological agents, such as viruses, bacteria, fungi, rickettsia, protozoa, and helminths
- Chemical agents, such as metals, poisons, and strong irritants
- Physical agents, such as heat, cold, radiation, and electricity
- Stress
- Genetically transmitted defects
- Wear and tear on the body

However, the paradigm of treating the disease by removing the etiology only works for certain diseases. Function may be irreversibly altered before the etiology is removed. Thus, not all diseases can be cured.

An acute condition is one with a sudden onset and usually a short duration. If the disease cannot be cured, it may become chronic. A chronic disease is one that lasts for an extended time, often for the person's lifetime. The definition of a chronic disease frequently specifies that it lasts 6 months or longer. Chronic diseases can have periods of remission in which symptoms disappear or are minimal and periods of exacerbation in which symptoms reappear or become worse.

Chronic illness makes us less comfortable with a definition of health as an absence of disease. People with chronic illnesses may define themselves across a continuum of health from very poor health to even excellent health. The definition of health becomes less a matter of "Do I have a disease?" and more a matter of, "How well can I function?" People with arthritis, muscular dystrophy, psoriasis, and even heart disease may believe themselves to be healthy and only describe themselves as ill during an exacerbation of the disease. That is why **illness** refers to the personal experience of feeling unhealthy, caused by changes in a person's state of well-being and social function.

Health as a Continuum

If health is not merely the absence of disease, then perhaps we should think of health as a continuum. A **health-illness continuum** ranges from high-level wellness—an optimal state of mental and physical well-being—to premature death (Fig. 24–2). In the center of the continuum is a neutral state in which the person cannot be considered either healthy or ill. From the neutral state to the limits of the continuum exist wide variations in levels of health and illness. Every person exists at some point on the continuum and may move back and forth between the two extremes. A person at any point on the continuum can be focused in the direction of wellness (Ryan & Travis, 1988).

Thinking of health as existing on a continuum has several advantages. For one, the health-illness continuum recognizes that few people are in an optimal

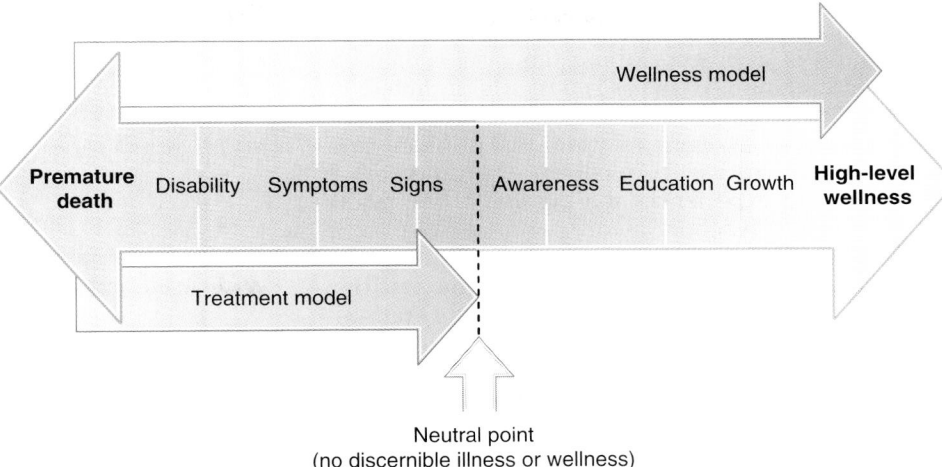

Figure 24–2. Health as a continuum. (Redrawn from Ryan, R.S., & Travis, J.W. [1988]. Wellness workbook. Berkeley, CA: Ten Speed Press.)

state of health, thus providing the philosophy of optimal health as a goal and health care as a way of helping people move toward this goal. For another, the continuum discounts the notion that disease and health are dichotomous terms.

The health-illness continuum recognizes that more than one factor is necessary to determine a person's state of health. A person with arthritis who walks 3 miles a day, eats a well-balanced diet, and has a positive outlook on life may be closer to optimal health on the continuum than a person with no identifiable illness but with a sedentary lifestyle, a junk-food diet, a lack of energy, and a fear of the world.

The health-illness continuum makes room for health within illness. **Health within illness** is an event that can expand human potential by providing an opportunity for personal growth and well-being despite having an illness. The outcome of an illness is that the person becomes stronger as a human being, even though the disease may not be cured. Many people who suffer from chronic illness or life-threatening acute illness can develop a heightened sense of self and personal potential, can feel greater spiritual inner peace, and can discover new meaning and purpose in life.

Health as Wellness and Well-Being

Health as high-level wellness includes both positive physiological function and a sense of well-being. **Well-being** is a subjective perception of a good and satisfactory existence in which the individual has a positive experience of personal abilities, harmony, and vitality. Like illness, well-being is a relative, changing state experienced in the course of everyday living.

Wellness is a state of optimal health or optimal physical and social functioning. Wellness includes optimal physical function, successful and satisfying relationships with others, emotional stability, managing feelings comfortably, intellectual growth, and a spiritual element that gives meaning and purpose to life

(Fig. 24–3). Additionally, several assumptions underlie the concept of wellness to give it meaning as a framework for health care (Ryan & Travis, 1988).

Individuals possess their own optimal level of functioning, which represents the best state of well-being that is possible for them. Each person sets individual goals that are compatible with their body build, age, and physical state. Not everyone can jog 5 miles a day, nor would they enjoy the benefits associated with long-distance jogging.

Wellness is a choice that cannot be passively achieved. To achieve optimal health, the person must choose to engage in behaviors associated with health. Positive health actions are necessary to achieve wellness. The person purposefully engages in actions to attain and maintain health. These actions can be in re-

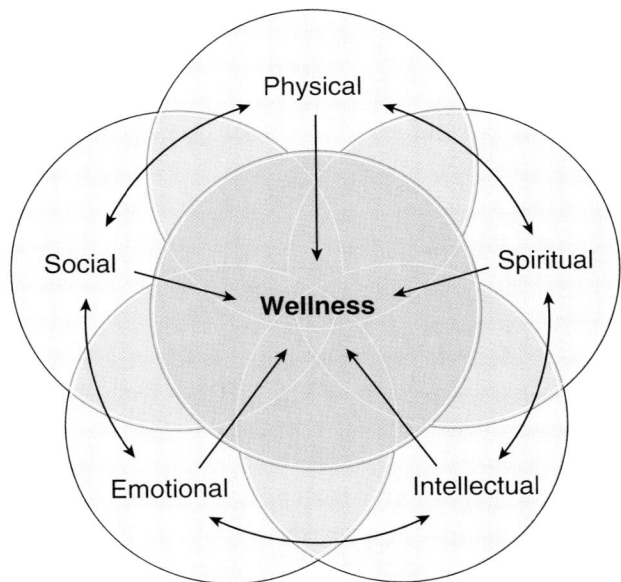

Figure 24–3. Dimensions of wellness.

sponse to internal drives, stressors, or bodily functions, or they can be in response to environmental risk factors that threaten health and well-being.

Wellness is a process; thus, the achievement of wellness is ongoing. Wellness is not a finite state to be achieved in the future with the here-and-now being atime of constant struggle to attain this utopian state. Rather, the process itself is wellness when the person recognizes and experiences the possibility for health and happiness in each moment.

Wellness is an efficient channeling of energy received from the environment, transformed within you, and sent on to affect the world outside. Wellness is the integration of body, mind, and spirit, the appreciation that everything you do, think, feel, and believe has an impact on your state of health. Wellness is holding yourself in high esteem. Accepting yourself as a worthwhile person and recognizing the value in your personal attributes is necessary for high-level wellness. High-level wellness is associated with a good feeling about yourself in relationship to other people.

Knowledge of the environment in which wellness is achieved is necessary to understand wellness. Dunn (1959) uses a grid to depict a concept of wellness (Fig. 24–4). The horizontal axis is the continuum from peak wellness to death. The vertical axis is the environment, from very favorable to very unfavorable. The four quadrants in the grid represent the interactions of the state of wellness with the environment.

- *High-level wellness in a favorable environment.* This quadrant represents a person who is in an optimal state of health. The environment supports the person's efforts to achieve high-level wellness.
- *Emergent high-level wellness in an unfavorable environment.* This person has the knowledge, motivation, and physical stamina to achieve high-level wellness. Nonsupportive environmental factors could be demanding role responsibilities, a lack of financial resources, an unclean water supply, or an unsafe environment. High-level wellness is possible but would require more planning and effort.
- *Protected poor health in a favorable environment.* This person has one or more health problems but is able to manage them because the environment is supportive. The person has access to high-quality medical care, nursing services, and social services. Financial resources allow the person to engage home maintenance services as needed.
- *Poor health in an unfavorable environment.* This person has one or more health problems—such as old age, diabetes, and obesity—and an environment unfavorable to wellness. For example, the person might live in a rural farming community without medical services. She may lack health insurance to pay for medicine. And her diabetes may frequently be uncontrolled, making complications likely.

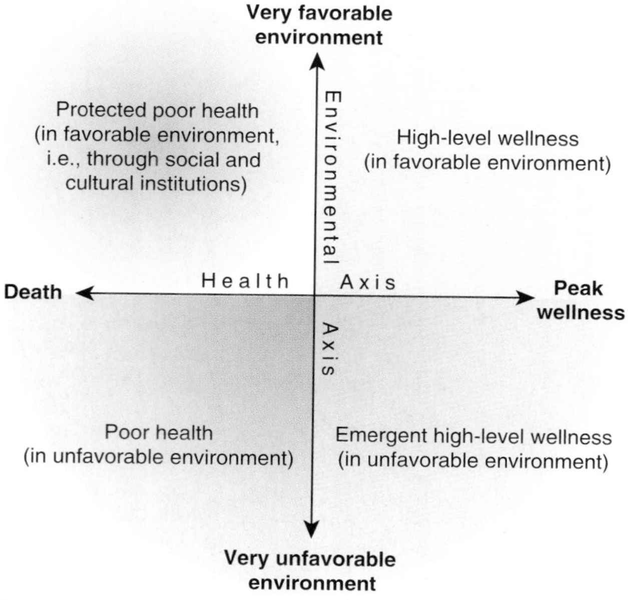

Figure 24–4. Dunn's concept of well-being. (Redrawn from Dunn, H.L. [1959]. High-level wellness for man and society. American Journal of Public Health, 49[6], 786–792.)

BOX 24–3

THE POPULATION HEALTH APPROACH

A population health approach differs from traditional medical and health care thinking in two main ways.

- Population health strategies address the entire range of factors that determine health. Traditional health care focuses on risks and clinical factors related to particular diseases.
- Population health strategies are designed to affect the entire population. Traditional health care deals with one person at a time, usually after the person has either a health problem or a significant risk of developing one.

From Health Canada. (1994). Strategies for population health: Investigating the health of Canadians for the Meeting of the Ministers of Health. Halifax, Nova Scotia. September 14–15, 1994.

Health in Populations

Health in a community is defined by the parameters of population health (Box 24–3). **Population health** considers health problems encountered as a result of being a part of a group and focuses intervention on the population rather than on the individual. A population can be a subgroup within a community, such as teenage mothers in the local high school, or a larger group, such as men at risk for heart disease.

Today, key partners inside and outside governments are pursuing strategic actions to foster and improve health by addressing the full range of factors known to influence population health. These factors of population health include living and working conditions, economic well-being, and a personal sense of control over and skills for coping with the challenges and stresses of everyday living. Healthy lifestyles and the availability of health services are also taken into account.

Adopting these broad determinants of health as the foundation for planning and action will significantly enhance the possibility of improving population health. Because most determinants of health fall partly or wholly outside its purview, the health care sector of a society cannot act alone. Therefore, collaboration of social services, sanitation services, environmental control, and other sectors is the key to a healthy society. Having a common framework for action based on broad determinants of health would mean that concerted efforts could be made by all sectors to address factors known to influence health (Health Canada, 1994).

A population health perspective does not exclude consideration of individual needs and responsibility. Population health reflects the individual perspective that "health is a positive state of being that includes physical fitness, mental (or emotional) stability, and social and spiritual ease. It is not a constant or absolute entity but rather an ever-changing and evolving state in which people actively strive to achieve the highest level of functioning that is possible for them" (DuGas & Knor, 1995).

Achieving this definition must include individual responsibility and a willingness to consider health as a way of living rather than as a goal to be attained. Specifically, "health is the extent to which an individual or group is able, on the one hand, to develop aspirations and satisfy needs; and on the other hand, to change or cope with the environment. Health is therefore seen as a resource for everyday life, not the objective of living; it is seen as a positive concept emphasizing social and personal resources, as well as physical capacities" (British Columbia Ministry of Health and Ministry Responsible for Seniors, 1993).

FACTORS AFFECTING HEALTH

Planning for health care must consider multiple factors that affect health. Some factors have greater impact on the types of services needed than others. The following factors are commonly considered in community health planning.

Genes

Heredity, or genetic predisposition to specific illnesses, raises known health risks. Family histories of diabetes mellitus, cancer, and coronary artery disease are examples of known genetic risk factors. The methods of managing genetically transmitted disease include case-finding and treating the manifestations of the illness. However, genetics as a cause of disease is not clear-cut. The onset of many genetically transmitted diseases requires an interplay of environmental and lifestyle factors with heredity.

Education (Knowledge)

Individual, family, and community health is affected by a variety of intellectual factors. In individuals, cognitive abilities, educational level, and past experience all play a role in shaping a person's attitude toward health care. A family's knowledge about health and illness influences its members' ability to understand disease patterns, factors involved in health and illness, and the importance of personal health practices. Likewise, the community's health status is influenced by the knowledge of its citizens. As citizens become more informed through modern communication and technology, more and more communities are calling for improved health standards and practices.

Social Network

Social networks have a profound influence on the health status of individuals, families, and communities. The organization of the community and health care system can determine how clients can access and obtain health care. Recreational facilities, churches, and social organizations are part of the community social network that affect health and health status. You, along with other individuals, families, and communities, need to work toward shared values and collective actions that will ensure equitable health practices and treatment for all citizens.

Health Care

Good health depends on equitable access to all necessary and appropriate health services. These consist of prevention and health promotion services, services to reduce pain and suffering and restore health, and services to enhance quality of life for those with chronic diseases and limitations. For example, adequate perinatal care can result in healthier babies.

Personal Habits

In recent years, lifestyle factors have received major attention for their influence on health. Lifestyle includes diet, exercise, stress level, health practices, coping skills, education, work, interpersonal relationships, and cultural practices. It is the sum of a person's life experiences.

Family health practices play an important role in the health of individuals and communities. Families can promote a positive perception of health by providing a supportive environment, by promoting positive health practices, by appropriate use of health services, and by seeking safety and security for family members.

Cultural factors influence individual beliefs and values. Established customs influence entry into the health care system and personal health practices. In Canada, aboriginal communities face poor housing conditions, low incomes, and, given the long history of external control, more significant impediments to community action. Furthermore, most illnesses occur much more frequently among aboriginal peoples, and their health status indicators are worse than the country's average (National Forum on Health, 1996c). The United States faces similar challenges. In 1989, a study on health education practices of African-Americans showed that most did not have access to health education as a means of primary prevention (Airhihenbuwa, 1989).

Income (Economic Status)

Factors such as income, layoffs, the cost of housing, the cost of health services, community design, education and training, social services, and public policy can all affect health status. In fact, these economic factors affect individual, family, and community health status in many ways. Thus, economic factors must be addressed if citizens are to achieve improved health.

Physical Environment

Physical environmental factors contribute to the health status of individuals, families, and communities. The quality of one's work life, safety and security factors, and environmental ecosystem issues are examples of the many possible environmental factors that can influence health. It is important for you to assess the client's physical environment, recognize possible risk factors, and work with other health disciplines and team members to address the health risks identified.

ASSESSMENT

The public forum for the citizens of Delta continues. Participants have searched for a definition of health that applies to their community. They now have a better understanding of the many related factors that contribute to a definition of health. They are ready to begin the process of assessing the health needs of the community, diagnosing problems, setting goals, and planning strategies to improve the health of individuals, families, and communities.

The Delta planning group is concerned with health primarily from the broad perspective of the needs of the community. A health assessment of an individual, family, or community shares a common definition of health but requires different data. Notice the differences in data used for assessment for the dimensions of health for individuals, families, and communities.

Individual Health

Assessment of individual health includes physical, social, emotional, intellectual, and spiritual dimensions. Specific individual health assessment is addressed throughout this book and may include characteristics of individual health such as these:

- Coping skills
- Capacity for making healthy lifestyle decisions
- Physical, mental, social, and emotional limitations
- Education and training
- Quality of work life

- Positive, supportive, interpersonal relationships and social networks.

Family Health

Assessment of family health includes physical, social, emotional, intellectual, and spiritual dimensions. Family strengths and problems are identified to provide a basis and direction for further assessment of individual family members (Fig. 24–5).

Your nursing care plan for family health may address many factors that relate to family health. Those factors may belong to such broad characteristics as these:

- Positive, supportive interpersonal family relationships
- Consequences of family employment opportunities
- Consequences of family level of poverty
- Consequences of lower status occupations
- Impact of job loss
- Safety and security issues
- Access to and appropriate use of health care service

The many other factors that relate to family health and function are addressed in other areas in this text.

Community Health

Assessment of community health includes physical, social, emotional, intellectual, and spiritual dimensions.

Community health assessment commonly uses statistics on populations and uses data to compare community needs with available services. Some examples include mortality and morbidity studies, annual health reports from multiple agencies, and health inventories and resource reports. Traditional methods of

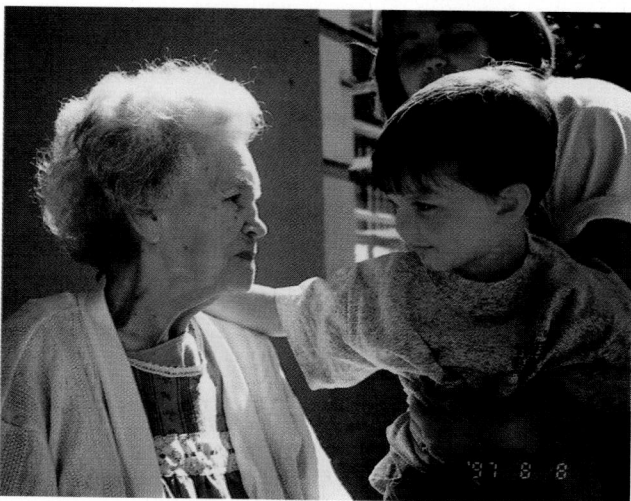

Figure 24–5. Family strength is seen in the contribution of a great-grandmother to the emotional development of a child. (Courtesy of David A. Zerr.)

measuring the health of a community have centered on mortality (death rate), longevity (life expectancy), and morbidity (illness).

An example of a community working together to assess the current social planning practices of its area can be found in the work program set up by the Corporation of Delta. Participants defined social planning at the community level as "a local, democratic system of planning and taking action toward community social needs and interests in support of community well-being."

When assessing community health, your plan may address broad social issues of community health, such as the following:

- A safe environment
- Affordable housing
- Community design
- Social services and public policy
- Cost-effective health services
- Preventive health practices
- Joint action for minority and cultural health issues

Community health is complex and specific to the community involved. No one pattern of community health can be understood without knowing the multitude of relevant environmental, social, and economic factors that affect it.

Focused Assessment for Health-Seeking Behaviors

Health-seeking behaviors is observed in individuals, families, and communities. *Health-seeking behaviors* is a diagnostic category too broad to be useful in clinical practice without specifying the health-seeking behavior (Jenny, 1995).

The key element of *Health-seeking behaviors* is choice. The individual, family, or community expresses the desire to seek a higher level of wellness, or you may observe behaviors that indicate a motivation to attain a higher level of wellness. Additional defining characteristics include the following:

- Expressed or observed desire for increased control of health practices
- Expression of concern about the effects of current environmental conditions on health status
- Stated or observed unfamiliarity with wellness community resources
- Demonstrated or observed lack of knowledge about health promotion behaviors

You will need to look for specific indicators of health-seeking behaviors in individuals, families, and communities to recognize opportunities to support health promotion activities and provide teaching (Box 24–4).

DIAGNOSIS

NANDA recognizes the need for both wellness nursing diagnoses and risk nursing diagnoses for individuals,

families, and communities. Wellness nursing diagnoses describe human responses to levels of wellness in an individual, family, or community that have a potential for enhancement to a higher state (NANDA, 1999). Risk nursing diagnoses describe human responses to health conditions/life processes that may develop in a vulnerable individual, family, or community.

Nursing diagnoses can occur along the entire health-illness continuum. The individual, family, or community can be described as having a deficiency, dysfunction, or decrease in health behaviors that creates risk for diminished health. Additionally, the individual, family, or community can be recognized as having a potential for enhancing a state of wellness. The client—whether individual, family, or community—starts from a state of wellness and has the desire to increase that level of wellness.

PLANNING

Participants of the public forum can now move on to identify their community's health priorities. The goal of this community-planning group is to meet the identified needs of individuals and families within the group as well as the needs of the community as a whole. Planning will include identifying community resources to meet the health needs of individuals, families, and the community.

A statement of health goals flows from the perception of health. An understanding of related factors that contribute to the concept of health provides the assumptions that underlie health goals. Explicit goals provide guidelines for implementation. Thus, planning includes designing interventions that can realistically be expected to achieve the goals.

INTERVENTION

Designing interventions to improve health requires both health promotion and preventive health care. Although, from a philosophical perspective, these two concepts are different, they are not mutually exclusive. As mentioned earlier, health promotion is the advancement of health through the encouragement of activities that enhance the wellness of individuals, families, and communities. **Preventive health care** is the recognition of the risk for disease and actions taken to reduce that risk.

Interventions to Promote Health

If the 21st century becomes the era of health promotion, health will be viewed as a part of everyday living and health care an essential dimension to enhance the quality of life (Epp, 1986). Health in the context of health promotion is a dynamic rather than a static state in which individuals and communities strive to maintain or regain a positive state of physical and psychological being. It is a basic force in daily life, influenced by circumstances, beliefs, culture, and the social, economic, and physical environment. Health

---

BOX 24–4

EXAMPLES OF HEALTH-SEEKING BEHAVIORS

Individuals

- Having periodic physical examinations.
- Seeking counseling for weight loss.
- Requesting a health evaluation before starting an exercise program.
- Using a seat belt.
- Using a bicycle helmet.
- Using sunscreen.
- Using condoms.
- Joining a support group to help break an addictive behavior pattern, such as the use of nicotine, alcohol, or illicit drugs.
- Participating in recreational, social, and cultural community activities.

Families

- Obtaining a family membership at a fitness center.
- Seeking family therapy to manage addictive behavior in a teenager.
- Making a commitment to reduce the incidence of colds and flu in the family.
- Asking for assistance in managing the care of an elderly family member.
- Expressing a need for information about caring for a new infant.
- Expressing a need for information about making the home safe for all family members, especially children and older adults.

- Seeking opportunities to enhance an employment situation.
- Working with the community to address problems of low-income families, single-parent families, and gender-gap inequities in the labor force.

Communities

- Petitioning of the city council by a neighborhood association for a new park in the area.
- Organizing a group of concerned citizens to form a health clinic in a neighborhood with poor access to health care.
- Seeking volunteers for a community action group to reduce violence in the public schools.
- Creating a public outcry to an incidence of hepatitis in the community and organizing a petition for better testing of community water supplies.
- Attending a public hearing to discuss the provision of health services by schools.
- Forming a committee in a community action group to study the need for affordable housing for disadvantaged groups.
- Meeting to explore the possibilities of providing an education program to young parents about the importance of prenatal care and parenting skills.

---

promotion is the process of enabling people to be responsible for improving their health in keeping with its personal meaning (Epp, 1986).

Designing Health Promotion Activities

Health promotion is often described as educational techniques to help people take control of their lives and their health. However, it is more properly described as including educational, political, organizational, regulatory, and environmental supports for actions and conditions of living conducive to the health of individuals, families, and communities. Health promotion includes modifying the individual and collective lifestyle, modifying environments to support health, strengthening community action, reordering health services, and using public policy to enhance health. The activities that can be labeled as health promotion recognize the interrelationship of the person and the environmental, biological, social, and political determinants of health. The expected outcomes perhaps better define health promotion than the methods used to achieve the outcomes.

The outcomes for health promotion have little to do with the absence of disease. Health is expected to result in an improved quality of life. Quality living is in part being able to do what you want to do, do it well, and derive a sense of satisfaction from the effort. It is described in terms of effective functioning in areas of life that are important to each person. Through improved health, people can have the opportunity to maintain vigor and stamina throughout their lifespan. Additionally, better health will contribute to an increase in both individual and social productivity.

The outcomes for health promotion are described in practical, situation-specific results. For an occupational health effort, the expected outcomes include increased worker satisfaction, increased productivity, and a lower cost of employee health care. In a school setting, the expected outcomes are decreased absence from school, improved learning, increased motivation, and increased self-esteem.

The paradigm for health promotion recognizes the potential impact of the self-care movement that has been occurring in the last quarter of the 20th century. An activity can be labeled health promotion if it provides people with tools or knowledge to take control of their own health. The paradigm describes self-reliance, person-centered activities, and client participation.

The paradigm for health promotion, by its very nature, must include decisions about who is responsible for decision-making in primary health care. The philosophy of health promotion places the responsibility for health on the individual and family rather than on the professional. However, if the individual is solely responsible for his own health, there is danger of "blaming the victim," that is, ignoring the biological, social, political, and environmental determinants of health.

Considering these broad determinants of health, society at large becomes responsible for the health of its members. The question is then raised whether health promotion is a responsibility of the public or private sector. If it is society's responsibility, and the public sector assumes some or all of the responsibility, should the decision-making and program support lie with the local, state, or national government? To the extent that health is a national resource serving a common national interest, perhaps the responsibility is best placed in the federal government. To the extent that health needs reflect local conditions and interests, the responsibility may be best achieved at the local and state level.

Health promotion is expected to provide the means to revolutionize public health as a means to manage chronic illness the same way infection control practices revolutionized public health in the first half of the 20th century.

Primary Health Care

Primary health care focuses on prevention and health promotion but with a much broader perspective than just medical and nursing care. **Primary health care** means all care necessary to people's lives and health, including health education, nutrition, sanitation, maternal and child health care, immunizations, prevention, and control of endemic disease (WHO, 1978).

Primary health care is related to the common term *primary care* as it is used when referring to a primary care physician, but primary health care is broader in scope (Kerr & MacPhail, 1996). Primary medical care refers to care provided at the point at which a client first enters the health care system. It is the first contact for the provision of coordinated care for a wide range of health concerns within a sustained relationship with a health care provider. If the range of concerns truly encompasses a comprehensive view of health care, it can be labeled primary health care.

In the definition of primary health care created by WHO (Box 24–5), there are five principles:

- Equitable accessibility of health services to all populations
- Maximum individual and community involvement in the planning and operation of health services

---

BOX 24–5

WORLD HEALTH ORGANIZATION DEFINITION OF PRIMARY HEALTH CARE

Primary health care is "essential health care based on practical, scientifically sound and socially acceptable methods and technology made universally accessible to individuals and families in the community through their full participation and at a cost that community and country can afford to maintain at every stage of their development in the spirit of self-reliance and self-determination. It forms an integral part both of the country's health system, of which it is the central function and main focus, and of the overall social and economic development of the community. It is the first level of contact of the individual, the family, and the community with the national health system bringing health care as close as possible to where the people live and work, and constitutes the first element of a continuing health care process."

From World Health Organization. (1978). Primary health care: Report on the international conference on primary health care, p. 21, Alma Ata, USSR, 6–12 September 1978. Geneva: Author.

- Increased emphasis on services that are preventive and promotive rather than only curative
- Use of appropriate technology
- Integration of health development with social and economic development (Stewart, 1995)

The essence of the WHO definition integrates many of the associated factors. It combines a focus on individuals and families with a focus on the health of a defined population within a community. Primary health care is delivered by a variety of health professionals and providers working collaboratively with clients to maintain health, support wellness, and treat illness. Full participation of clients and accountability to clients and the community for high-quality comprehensive services are essential features of primary health care.

The above definitions indicate the important shift from a "medical" focus to a "health" focus in health care. The WHO definition identifies the multidisciplinary nature of the primary health contact, the collaborative nature of relationships between consumers and health care workers, and the accountability of consumer and community to strive for a high level of health.

The need for changes to primary care is fundamental to a reform of the health care system in both the United States and Canada. Nursing as a profession has the expertise to play a vital role in this change. Emerging roles and expanded nursing functions are part of this reform.

Interventions to Prevent Illness

Health promotion and illness prevention can be best understood in terms of health activities on the primary, secondary, and tertiary levels.

Levels of Preventive Care

Primary prevention consists of actions that are considered true prevention because they precede disease or dysfunction and are applied to clients considered physically and emotionally healthy to protect them from health problems. Activities aim to decrease the probability of specific illnesses or dysfunction. They may include health education programs, immunizations, and physical and nutritional fitness activities. Primary prevention can be applied to an individual or to a general population, or it can focus on individuals at risk for developing specific diseases. An example is a public health nurse providing health education programs in high schools to inform teenagers about sexually transmitted diseases.

Secondary prevention consists of actions that focus on the early diagnosis and prompt treatment of people with health problems or illnesses and who are at risk for developing complications or worsening conditions. Activities are directed at diagnosis and prompt intervention to reduce the severity of the disease and to enable the client to return to normal function as quickly as possible. Secondary prevention includes nursing care delivered at home, at a hospital, or at a nursing center for screening techniques and treatment of early stages of disease. An example is a public health nurse who carries out screening tests for postpartum depression on mothers attending well-baby clinics.

Tertiary prevention involves minimizing the effects of a permanent, irreversible disease or disability through interventions directed at preventing complication and deterioration. Activities are directed at rehabilitation rather than diagnosis and treatment. Care at this level aims to help the client achieve as high a level of functioning as possible, despite the limitations caused by illness or impairment. The term *preventive* is applied to this level of care because it involves prevention of further disability or reduced functioning. An example includes a nurse working in a geriatric care center who refers a diabetic client to a foot-care education program.

Methods of Prevention

The concept of disease prevention is based on identifying risk factors and using those factors to identify persons at risk for a specific disease. The value of prevention is a reduction in morbidity or mortality rates for the specific disease. However, not all diseases can be prevented. Hence, prevention is often aimed at early detection of the disease to prolong life and reduce suffering.

The decision to implement widespread prevention strategies needs to consider multiple factors: the prevalence of the disease, whether the disease can be prevented, the degree of devastation resulting from the effects of the disease, and the availability of treatment options that can eradicate the disease or prolong the client's life.

Another consideration is the availability and accuracy of methods to screen for risk factors and for the disease. If prevention demands major lifestyle changes or requires costly, risky, toxic, or unpleasant preventive measures, the benefits of prevention may not outweigh the risks. Additionally, screening tests need to have an acceptable margin of error. That is, the tests should produce a low number of false-positive or false-negative results. False-positive results can cause unnecessary worry and sometimes unnecessary procedures. False-negative results give a false sense of security that the disease is not present.

Preventive measures can be difficult to administer. Without clear cost savings, reimbursement for prevention may not be available. Additionally, a well-coordinated system of health care delivery is needed to ensure optimum use of money available for prevention.

Disease prevention is derived only in part from the hard sciences. Clinical interventions should address personal health practices and engage the client in joint decision-making. Although a one-to-one relationship with a clinician gives the client and clinician the opportunity to selectively make choices about screening tests, some problems may be more effectively prevented through prevention strategies at the community level. Examples include sexually transmitted diseases, AIDS, teenage pregnancies, and child abuse. Chapter 25 discusses the methods of promoting lifestyle changes, and Chapter 59 discusses working with groups of clients in the community.

EVALUATION

After much discussion and debate, the workshop participants arrived at eight health priority/action statements for Delta: (1) promote a perception of health for individuals, families, and community; (2) pursue a process to gather and analyze health data; (3) promote collaborative planning and coordination of health promotion decisions and strategies; (4) promote education on health issues and community involvement with the issues identified; (5) make an effort to break down established stereotypes that hinder health promotion, such as multicultural issues, aboriginal issues, and youth issues; (6) foster initiatives that address child and youth health issues; (7) foster initiatives that address women's health issues; and (8) promote efforts to provide adequate resources for preventive health initiatives.

The last step for the workshop participants is to work toward measurable outcomes for the health priorities identified. The hour is late, and participants have exhausted their energies with the identification of health priority/action statements. They agree to draft action plans for each of the eight statements. Plans are made for the next meeting, when future steps in the quest to develop health goals for the citizens of Delta will be addressed.

The case situation that appears throughout this chapter provides the community context that illus-

THE STATE OF NURSING SCIENCE
NEEDS AND CONCERNS OF CLIENTS WITH CANCER AND THEIR CAREGIVERS IN RURAL AREAS

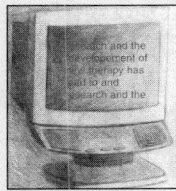

What Are the Issues?

Cancer is increasingly considered a chronic illness that takes a heavy toll on both clients and caregivers. To learn how to provide better care for families, researchers are interested in identifying the needs and concerns of cancer clients and their caregivers. They also want to know if there are differences in these needs and concerns between men and women, as well as between clients and caregivers. There is also interest in whether people with cancer who live in rural settings have different needs and concerns from those who live in urban settings.

What Research Has Been Conducted?

To address these questions, Burman and Weinert (1997) developed a 14-item survey that asked clients with cancer and their caregivers to rank some of their concerns. The concerns covered in the survey occupied four categories: interpersonal relationships, self-image, occupational issues, and relationships with health care personnel. The researchers gathered responses to this survey from 498 clients and caregivers from rural areas of Montana. All but one of their subjects were white, so their findings cannot be generalized to people from other ethnic backgrounds.

The researchers found that clients with cancer ranked a relationship concern—the fear that other people felt about talking with them—as the most important concern. This concern was less often noted by the caregivers. Men with cancer ranked threats to job security second among their concerns, whereas women ranked a self-image concern—hair loss—in second place.

Women caregivers also ranked a relationship concern—feeling alone—as their most important concern. Men caregivers ranked lack of sufficient information as their most important concern. Caregivers went on to rank interpersonal concerns next, including feeling alone (for men) and the fear that other people felt about talking with the clients (for women). Women clients and caregivers more often identified lack of support from and lack of understanding by spouses than did the men in the sample.

Researchers Silveira and Winstead-Fry (1997) had already studied these questions among a population of clients and caregivers in an urban setting. They then sought to replicate the study by asking the same questions of a new sample of people in rural Vermont. As they did in the urban study, these researchers used two research instruments, called the "Client Needs Scale" and the "Caregiver Needs Scale," to examine health sta-

tus, performance abilities, activities of daily living, and the needs of both clients and caregivers in a population of clients with cancer. Both research instruments included items related to personal care, activities of daily living, relationships with health care workers, and interpersonal relationships.

The researchers found that people in rural settings identified additional needs not identified by people in urban areas. They related to physical care, such as knowing when to call the physician and being well organized. Caregivers in this rural population identified additional needs related to how to provide personal care and related to support and communication.

What Has the Research Concluded?

Burman and Weinert (1997) concluded that there are some gender differences in the needs and concerns of both clients and caregivers. Women emphasize relationship concerns more than men. However, lack of information was an important concern for all groups and could be addressed by nurses in a variety of settings.

Silveira and Winstead-Fry (1997) found that the needs and concerns of cancer clients in rural settings are very similar to those of cancer clients living in urban areas. They therefore suggest that nurses who care for clients in rural settings may be able to use the findings from studies conducted in urban settings.

Both research teams caution that individual assessments are needed so that care can be tailored to meet the priorities of each family.

What Is the Future of Research in This Area?

Burman and Weinert (1997) recommend that people in other rural areas be studied. They also suggest that better research instruments be developed to assess the needs and concerns of clients and caregivers. Silveira and Winstead-Fry (1997) recommend studying the needs and concerns of cancer clients and their caregivers over time to see whether the needs and concerns change as the illness changes. Additional work is also needed to determine whether the findings of these research teams hold true for other populations.

References

Burman, M.E., & Weinert, C. (1997). Concerns of rural men and women experiencing cancer. *Oncology Nursing Forum, 24,* 1593–1600.
Silveira, J.M., & Winstead-Fry, P. (1997). The needs of patients with cancer and their caregivers in rural areas. *Oncology Nursing Forum, 24,* 71–76.

trates the significance of health promotion. The importance of a perception of health for establishing goals and actions for individuals, families, and communities emerged as the top health priority in the workshop scenario.

To evaluate health goals fully, those goals must be explicit, and they must provide specific implementation guidelines and evaluation criteria. For example, consider the goal of improving nutrition by reducing saturated fat intake. During the planning process for a community, you might establish as an expected outcome that community members would reduce their fat intake by reading food labels properly. As one step of the evaluation process for this outcome, you could demonstrate by survey that foods available in the community's grocery stores have fat content listed on their labels. If the survey finds that foods are not clearly labeled with fat content, then your expected outcomes will need revision.

The concept of health perception relates to all health disciplines and to the many factors and determinants of health. For this reason, a plan of action specific to nursing may not be appropriate. The plans developed may need to be broad and multidisciplinary in scope. As a result, the plan will help to develop a perception of health for the individual, family, and community.

KEY PRINCIPLES

- Because we are all citizens of the world, health cannot be viewed only from an individual or local perspective.
- Health is more than the absence of disease.
- Health exists on a continuum.
- Wellness includes positive physiological function and a sense of well-being.
- Population health considers health problems encountered by being a part of a group and focuses intervention on the population rather than on the individual.
- An individual's health is affected by many personal, family, and community factors.
- Families are the primary unit of health.
- Community health studies have revealed that health is also affected by changing conditions in communities.
- Influences from internal and genetic factors and from external sources affect health.
- Assessment of individual health includes physical, social, emotional, intellectual, and spiritual dimensions.
- Family health assessment requires gathering health data on each member of the family and on the function of the family as a whole.
- Community assessment uses statistics on population data, statistics on the use of services, and data that compare community needs with available services.

- The nursing diagnosis *Health-seeking behaviors* addresses the desire or need for positive health action by individuals.
- Primary health care consists of all care necessary to people's lives and health, including health education, nutrition, sanitation, maternal and child health care, immunizations, prevention, and control of endemic disease.
- Nurses carry out preventive health care and health promotion in a multitude of ways each day of nursing practice.

BIBLIOGRAPHY

*Airhihenbuwa, C. (1989). Health education for African Americans: A neglected task. *Health Education, 20*(5), 9–14.

British Columbia Ministry of Health and Ministry Responsible for Seniors. (1993). *New directions for a healthy British Columbia.* Victoria, BC: Author.

British Columbia Provincial Health Officer. (1996). *A report on the health of British Columbians: Provincial health officer's annual report 1995.* Victoria, BC: Ministry of Health and Ministry Responsible for Seniors.

Corporation of Delta. (1996). *Social planning work program file no. 96–10.* Delta: Author.

Dorval, M., & Stewart, C. (1997). *Personal communication.* January 15, 1997.

DuGas, B.W., & Knor, E.R. (1995). *Nursing foundations: A Canadian perspective.* Scarborough, ON: Appleton & Lange Canada.

*Dunn, H.L. (1959). High level wellness for man and society. *American Journal of Public Health, 49*(6), 786–792.

*Epp, J. (1986). *Achieving health for all: A framework for health promotion.* Ottawa: Ministry of Supply and Services (Cat. No. H39102/1986E).

Friedemann, M.L. (1995). *The framework of systemic organization: A conceptual approach to families and nursing.* Thousand Oaks, CA: Sage.

*Gordon, M. (1994). *Nursing diagnosis: process and application.* St. Louis: Mosby-Year Book.

*Government of Ontario. Ontario Minister of Health. (1992). *Ontario Health Survey 1990.* Toronto: Author.

Griffith, J.K. (1996). *The religious aspects of nursing care.* Vancouver, BC: Author.

*Hartrick, G., Lindsey, A.E., & Hills, M. (1994). Family nursing assessment: Meeting the challenge of health promotion. *Journal of Advanced Nursing, 20,* 85–91.

*Health and Welfare Canada, (1992). *Canada Health Act Annual Report 1991–1992.* Ottawa: Ministry of Supply and Services. Cat. HI-4/1992.

*Health and Welfare Canada. (1987). *The active health report: Perspectives on Canada's health promotion survey 1985.* Ottawa: Ministry of Supply and Services Canada, 9.

*Health Canada. (1994). *Strategies for population health: Investigating the health of Canadians for the meeting of the ministers of health.* Halifax, Nova Scotia, September 14–15, 1994.

Jenny, J. (1995). Advancing the science of nursing. In M.J. Rantz, & P. LeMone (Eds.), *Classification of nursing diagnosis: Proceedings of the eleventh conference, North American Nursing Diagnosis Association.* Glendale, CA: CINAHL Information Systems.

Kellner, F. (1997). *Personal communication,* January 17, 1997.

Kerr, J.R., & MacPhail, J. (1996). *Canadian nursing: Issues and perspectives* (3rd ed.). St. Louis: Mosby.

Maiese, D.R., & Fox, C.E. (1998). Laying the foundation for healthy people 2010: The first year of consultation. *Public Health Reports, 113,* 92–95. Can be accessed at http://web.health.gov/healthy-people/2010article.htm.

*Asterisk indicates a classic or definitive work on this subject.

National Forum on Health. (1995a). *Let's talk about our health and health care (Cat. No. H21–126/1995E).* Ottawa: Ministry of Supply and Services Canada.

National Forum on Health. (1995b). *Reporting: A one-year report on the national forum on health.* Ottawa: Ministry of Supply and Services Canada.

National Forum on Health. (1996). *Advancing the dialogue on health and health care: A consultation document (Cat. No. H21-126/4-1996).* Ministry of Supply and Services Canada.

North American Nursing Diagnosis Association. (1999). *NANDA nursing diagnoses: Definitions and classification 1999–2000.* Philadelphia: Author.

Papenfus, H., & Bryan, A.A. (1998). Nurses' involvement in interdisciplinary team evaluations: Incorporating the family perspective into child assessment. *Journal of School Health, 68*(5), 184–189.

Province of British Columbia. Office of the Provincial Health Officer. (1995). *Health goals for British Columbia: Identifying priorities for a healthy population, a draft for discussion.* Victoria, BC: Author.

Putting health in the patient's hands. (1998, January 21). *The Globe and Mail,* p. A2.

*Registered Nurses Association of British Columbia. (1994). *Creating the new health care: A nursing perspective (Pub. No. 49).* Vancouver: Author.

Ryan, R.S., & Travis, J.W. (1988). *Wellness workbook.* Berkeley, CA: Ten Speed Press.

Savoi, I., & Pastore, M.T. (1997). *Personal communication,* January 27, 1997.

Stewart, C. (1997). *Personal communication,* January 15, 1997.

Stewart, M.J. (Ed.). (1995). *Community nursing: Promoting Canadians' health.* Toronto: Saunders Canada.

Sutherland, R. (1996). *Will nurses call the shots? A look at the delivery of health care twenty years from now.* Ottawa: Tri-Graphic.

United States Department of Health, Education, and Welfare. (1995). *Healthy people 2000: 1995 report and progress.* Washington, D.C: Author.

*United States Public Health Service. (1990). *Healthy people 2000: National health promotion and disease prevention objectives.* Washington, D.C.: Government Printing Office.

*World Health Organization. (1978). *Primary health care: Report on the international conference on primary health care.* Alma Ata, USSR, 6–12 September 1978. Geneva: Author.

*World Health Organization. (1981). Global strategy for health for all by the year 2000. *Health for All Series,* (3), 15.

*Wright, L.M., & Leahey, M. (1994). *Nurses and families: A guide to family assessment and intervention.* Philadelphia: F.A. Davis.

25

Health Maintenance: Lifestyle Management

Doris Holeman and Dee M. Baldwin

Key Terms

action stage
contemplation stage
counseling
emic dimension
etic dimension
lifestyle
maintenance stage
perceived barriers
perceived benefits

perceived severity
perceived susceptibility
precontemplation stage
preparation stage
referral
self-efficacy
social support
termination stage

LEARNING OBJECTIVES

After studying this chapter, you should be able to:

1. **Describe world views of health and health care and models of behavioral change that underlie decision-making about lifestyle changes to manage a therapeutic regimen.**
2. **Describe factors affecting behavioral change.**
3. **Assess the client who is experiencing problems in maintaining health when a therapeutic regimen requires alterations in lifestyle.**
4. **Write diagnoses for clients who need to manage a therapeutic regimen to maintain health.**
5. **Plan nursing interventions that would assist the client to effectively manage the lifestyle changes needed to implement a therapeutic regimen.**
6. **Evaluate the behavioral outcomes of lifestyle changes made to maintain health through a therapeutic regimen.**

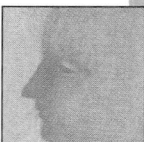

Mr. Oscar Kitchen is a 69-year-old African-American man who keeps house for himself. He is a widower. His only living relatives are distant cousins living in another state. He receives a monthly Social Security check and a small retirement check from employment as a janitor in a public school.

Six weeks ago, Mr. Kitchen reluctantly went to a primary health care clinic when he became short of breath. The nurse assessed Mr. Kitchen and determined that he had an irregular pulse and pitting edema of the lower extremities. The doctor prescribed medication for his heart and a diuretic. After the first week of medication, Mr. Kitchen felt better and decided to stop the medication. He missed his follow-up clinic appointment.

Two weeks ago, Mr. Kitchen once again became short of breath. He awakened soon after going to bed and was unable to breathe when lying in the supine position. He slept very little during the night. Mr. Kitchen returned to the clinic the next morning.

The nurse discovered that Mr. Kitchen had discontinued medications on several occasions, and that he continues to smoke. The nurse makes the diagnosis *Ineffective management of therapeutic regimen: individuals* related to (1) knowledge deficit regarding current diagnosis, medications, and consequences of failure to comply with treatment and (2) unwillingness to modify or change an unhealthy lifestyle.

HEALTH BEHAVIORS
NURSING DIAGNOSES

Ineffective Management of Therapeutic Regimen: Individuals: A pattern of regulating and integrating into daily living a program for the treatment of illness and the sequelae of illness that is unsatisfactory for meeting specific health goals.

Noncompliance (Specify): The extent to which a person's and/or caregiver's behavior coincides or fails to coincide with a health-promoting or therapeutic plan agreed on by the person (and/or family, and/or community) and health care professional. In the presence of an agreed-upon, health-promoting or therapeutic plan, a person's or caregiver's behavior may be fully, partially, or nonadherent and may lead to clinically effective, partially effective, or ineffective outcomes.

Ineffective Management of Therapeutic Regimen: Families: A pattern of regulating and integrating into family processes a program for treatment of illness and the sequelae of illness that is unsatisfactory for meeting specific health goals.

Ineffective Management of Therapeutic Regimen: Community: A pattern of regulating and integrating into community processes programs for the treatment of illness and the sequelae of illness that are unsatisfactory for meeting health-related goals.

Effective Management of Therapeutic Regimen: Individual: A pattern of regulating and integrating into daily living a program for the treatment of illness and its sequelae that is satisfactory for meeting specific health goals.

Decisional Conflict (Specify): The state of uncertainty about the course of action to be taken when choice among competing actions involves risk, loss, or challenge to personal life values.

From North American Nursing Diagnosis Association. (1999). NANDA nursing diagnoses: Definitions and classification 1999–2000. Philadelphia: Author.

CONCEPTS OF BEHAVIORAL CHANGE

A person's **lifestyle** is a behavior or group of behaviors, chosen by the person, that may have a positive or a negative influence on health. In other words, lifestyle choices and behavioral patterns influence one's health and longevity. A healthy lifestyle is evident when one avoids poor health habits, such as smoking and overeating, engages in good habits, such as achieving adequate nutrition and rest, and effectively manages a therapeutic regimen prescribed by a physician (Fig. 25–1).

Lifestyle is connected to the incidence of heart disease, diabetes, and other chronic illnesses. Pender (1996) believes that healthy lifestyles are the foundation for preventing chronic diseases, and that preventive and health-promoting behaviors are components of a healthy lifestyle. Although health promotion and primary and secondary disease prevention activities will not replace sophisticated medical care, these methods offer the best hope for achieving improvement in life expectancy and maintenance of health into old age.

Acute or chronic disease may demand changes in a person's lifestyle and behavioral patterns to manage the disease. For an acute illness, those changes are only temporary. For a chronic illness, permanent lifestyle changes are the only avenue to successful living with the illness.

However, getting a client to change well-established health and lifestyle habits is easier said than done. The development of health habits begins in early childhood; once developed, these habits become lifelong fixtures, difficult to change. To understand some of the complexities involved in helping clients change lifestyle behaviors, you will need to reconsider the definitions of health in conjunction with theories about behavioral changes.

In Chapter 24, you learned about definitions of health from the perspective of the individual, the family, and the community. Thus, you will rightly conclude that health can be defined from multiple perspectives. Furthermore, a person's definition of health stems in part from his personal world view. This is true for the health care provider's definition as well. When client and provider have differing world views, the result may be misunderstandings and differences in the selection of expected outcomes for health promotion and prevention (Spector, 1991).

Tripp-Reimer (1984) conceptualized health as two-dimensional, having an etic dimension and an emic dimension. The **etic dimension** refers to the objective

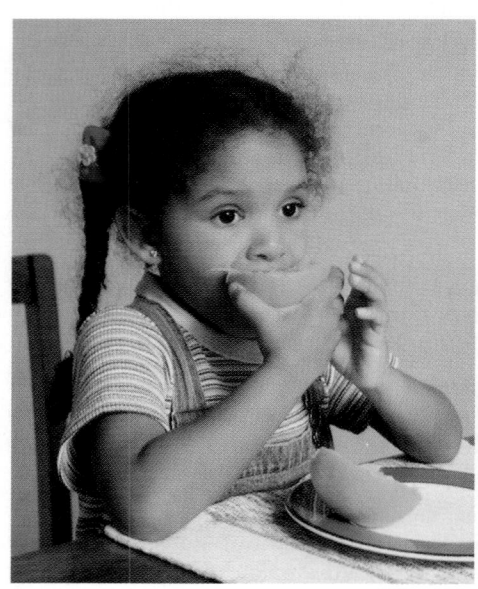

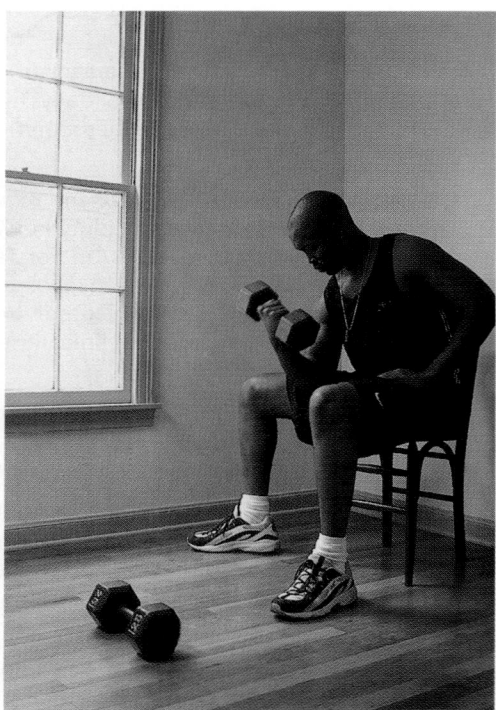

Figure 25–1. Lifestyle patterns associated with health include good nutrition and exercise, among others.

interpretation of health by a scientifically trained practitioner. The **emic dimension** refers to an individual's or social group's subjective perception and experiences related to health. Understanding health from the sometimes opposing perspectives of client and provider is critical to the development of health services.

To effectively help others, health care professionals must first understand the impact of their own beliefs about health on the health practices of their clients. This means understanding the health and quality-of-life perspective of the client. Hartsock (1983) suggests that a person's identity, role assignment, health, and opportunities in life are greatly influenced by such factors as gender, skin color, age, income, and place of origin. Additionally, health-related quality of life is not only defined by the signs and symptoms of disease or its effects on survival, but also by functional status, opportunity, and one's perception of relative well-being (Woolf, Jonas, & Lawrence, 1996).

World Views of Health and Health Care

Culture refers to the learned, shared, transmitted values, beliefs, norms, and lifeways of a particular group that guides their thinking, decisions, and actions in patterned ways (Leininger, 1991, p. 47). These ways of living, or lifestyles, determine a person's understanding of health and health practices. They also affect the person's view of illness. The experience of that illness is determined in part by how illness is defined by one's culture and how illness is defined by the individual or sick person (Spector, 1991).

All cultures have concepts of health and illness. They also have theories of disease causation, although these may differ widely from group to group (Clark,

1996). These concepts and theories include an explanatory model of illness that defines the nature of illness, its treatment, and the type of relationships that should occur between client and health care provider. Additionally, ethnic groups with different cultural histories have different approaches to reality, socialization, and health practices.

Ideas and beliefs related to health and illness are intricate parts of a culture's world view. To understand the link between culture, health, and illness, it can be helpful to divide culture groups into Western and Nonwestern practices (Table 25–1). Cultures with a Western world view include European-Americans (primarily men) and minorities with a high degree of acculturation. Cultures with a Nonwestern world view include Native Americans, Mexican-Americans, African-Americans, Vietnamese-Americans, Chinese-Americans, Japanese-Americans, and many European-American women.

A client's world view is important because ideas related to health and illness originate from everyday experiences. Klienman, Eisenberg, and Good (1978) suggest that 70% to 90% of health care is provided by family, social networks, and the community. They suggest that most people seek advice from family, friends, or lay sources before seeking professional advice. Clark (1996) suggests that there are two domains of health care: the folk, or generic, form and the scientific, or professional, form (Table 25–2).

The folk medicine system classifies illnesses into two parts: natural and unnatural. "This division of illnesses or diseases into natural and unnatural phenomena is common among persons from Haiti, Trinidad, and Mexico and among Mexican-Americans, African-Americans, and some southern White Americans"

TABLE 25–1
Comparison of Nonwestern and Western World Views

Nonwestern	Western
Emphasizes group cooperation	Emphasizes individual competition
Values achievement as it reflects group	Values achievement for the individual
Values harmony with nature	Values mastery and control of nature
Sees time as relative	Adheres to rigid time schedule
Accepts affective expression	Limits affective expression
Embraces extended family	Prefers nuclear family
Thinks holistically	Thinks dualistically
Religion permeates culture	Holds religion distinct from other parts of culture
Accepts world views of other cultures	Feels own world view is superior
Emphasizes social orientation	Emphasizes task orientation

Adapted from Anderson, A. (1988). Cognitive styles and multicultural populations. Journal of Teacher Education, 39(1), 2–9.

(Giger & Davidhizar, 1995, p. 118). Illnesses treated by folk medicine tend to be described as chronic, nonincapacitating maladies, and those believed to be caused by supernatural agents (Clark, 1996). Natural illnesses in the folk medicine system relate to events that have to do with the world as God made it or as God intended it (Giger & Davidhizar, 1995). Unnatural illnesses relate to events that cause disharmony with nature. Therefore, unnatural illnesses may be viewed as forces of evil or as events that interrupt the plan intended by God (Giger & Davidhizar, 1995).

Although Western medicine offers a bio-psycho-socio-cultural (spiritual) approach to explain illness, it also focuses on cure and prevention. Folk medicine focuses on personal data and experiences rather than on scientific persuasion (Giger & Davidhizar, 1995). Health care is provided in dyads (nurse-client or physician-client relationships), whereas in the folk medicine system, people tend to seek health care from multiperson health care networks, including relatives and nonrelatives (Giger & Davidhizar, 1995).

Clark (1996) suggests that many similarities exist between folk and scientific health care systems. One such similarity is the way people initially approach a health problem. According to Kavanagh and Kennedy (1992), "virtually no one runs for professional help at the first hint of a symptom. Traditional and folk remedies, most of them as benign as herbal tea, might be used and a homemade diagnosis and etiology tentatively constructed. The next resort may be to popular or over-the-counter resources, which may or may not be associated with allopathic medicine. Finally, if relief is not in sight, professional consult is likely to be undertaken" (pp. 19–20).

Additionally, a person's culturally acquired world view can be modified by social and economic conditions, with the economically disadvantaged adopting lifeways that may be more a product of poverty than culture. However, despite the shared characteristics of

TABLE 25–2
Similarities and Differences Between Folk and Scientific Health Care Systems

Similarities	Differences	
	Folk Health System	*Scientific Health System*
• Employ similar diagnostic techniques including observation and listening.	Takes into account the religious and social	Focuses primarily on the personal implications of disease
• Use verbal and nonverbal communication.		
• Engage in naming of illnesses and creation of positive expectations.	Makes no definite distinction between mental and physical illness	Makes a definite distinction between mental and physical illness
• Employ suggestion, interpretation, emotional support, and manipulation of the environment as therapeutic modalities.	Oriented to the community	Oriented to the individual
• Use medicinal substances and employ some form of laying on of hands in the care of the sick.	Takes place in familiar surroundings	Takes place in unfamiliar surroundings
• Based on asymmetric relationships between experts and laypersons.	Emphasizes humanistic care	Emphasizes impersonal care
• Provide an explanation of disease, a rationale for treatment, and a rationale for social and moral norms.	Emphasizes familiar, practical, and concrete	Emphasizes abstract concepts
	Provides holistic care	Provides fragmented care
	Emphasizes caring	Emphasizes curing
	Stresses prevention	Stresses diagnosis and treatment
	Emphasizes cultural support	Does not emphasize cultural support
	Is of moderate cost	Is of high cost

From Clark, M. (1996). Nursing in the community (2nd ed.). Stamford, CT: Appleton & Lange.

the economically disadvantaged among minorities, it is incorrect to assume that common approaches are to be used for improving the health status of various ethnic minorities.

Models of Behavioral Change

In addition to using culturally specific lifestyle knowledge to promote health, you need to incorporate theories of behavioral change to understand, explain, and predict health-related behaviors. However, these models were not developed as culturally specific models. Therefore, keep in mind that any one model may not be fully applicable to explain the behaviors and belief systems of a specific cultural group.

Theory of Reasoned Action

The theory of reasoned action is a human behavior framework designed to explain a person's intention to perform a behavior. The theory is based on the assumption that people are reasonable and, in deciding which actions to take, systematically process and use the information available to them (Fishbein & Middlestadt, 1989). The theory further assumes that behavior is under voluntary control and that barriers to performance of the intended behavior do not exist (Pender, 1996).

The theory of reasoned action does not rely solely on facts and logic. It also considers the relations between beliefs, attitudes, and intention in determining behavior (Fishbein & Middlestadt, 1989). To change or reinforce a given intention, the person must change or strengthen the attitude toward performing that behavior.

The theory further holds that a behavioral intention is determined both by attitudes toward the specific behavior and by subjective norms (what others think) regarding the behavior. Thus, people intend to perform a behavior when they evaluate that behavior positively and when they believe significant others think they should perform it. Compelling as it is, the theory of reasoned action is not sufficient to explain health behaviors.

Remember Mr. Kitchen? A reasonable person would associate shortness of breath with smoking, be able to see the decrease in leg swelling caused by the medication, and take the actions necessary to improve his health. Why do you think Mr. Kitchen has stopped taking his medication and continued to smoke?

Transtheoretical Model for Behavioral Change

The transtheoretical model for behavioral change adds stages of behavioral change that could help explain behaviors across all theories of behavioral change. According to Prochaska and colleagues (1994), people must change their behavior to make major reductions in risks for chronic disease. Six stages of behavioral change are described: precontemplation, contemplation, preparation, action, maintenance, and termina-

tion. People move through these stages as they think and act on reducing risky behaviors. Assessing a client's stage can help you determine appropriate interventions to help the person change a risky behavior (Prochaska et al., 1994).

In the **precontemplation stage,** the person does not intend to change a high-risk behavior in the foreseeable future (the next 6 months), primarily because he is unaware of the long-term consequences of the behavior. Furthermore, the person may feel demoralized about his inability to change and defensive because of social pressures to change (Prochaska et al., 1994). Although unconvinced of the need for change, the person may agree to make changes under pressure from family and friends. These changes are usually minimal and last only as long as pressure continues to be applied.

In the **contemplation stage,** the person intends to change within the next 6 months. However, despite this good intention, the person usually stays in this stage for at least 2 years. He tells himself that he is going to change, but he keeps putting it off. The person is ambivalent about changing and usually substitutes thinking for acting (Prochaska et al., 1994).

In the **preparation stage,** the person intends to take action in the very near future, usually within the next month. This stage has both intention and action. The person usually develops a plan of action and may take small steps toward behavioral change. Furthermore, the person evaluates the advantages and the disadvantages of the risk behavior and decides that the disadvantages outweigh the advantages (Prochaska et al., 1994).

In the **action stage,** the person changes risky behaviors and the context of the behavior (environment, experience) and makes significant efforts to reach goals. This is the busiest but most risky stage because of the chance for relapse. The person is considered to be in the action stage if the behavior is changed for 1 day to 6 months. This stage offers the most external recognition because others become aware of the effort that the person is making toward the change.

The **maintenance stage** takes place during the 6 months after the person changes the high-risk behavior. This stage is characterized by a period of continuing change, with fewer mechanisms needed to prevent relapse. However, the time frame set for continuous maintenance is 5 years. Prochaska and others (1994) discovered that people must continuously abstain from the high-risk behavior for 5 years to prevent the fear of relapse. For example, they found that, even after 12 months of continuous abstinence from smoking, 37% of people will return to regular smoking. After 5 years of continuous abstinence, only 7% will return to regular smoking.

In the **termination stage,** the person is no longer tempted to engage in old behavior. He has confidence in no longer being tempted by previous situations.

Most people go through some or all of these stages several times before conquering an addiction, despite professional help. Movement through the stages occurs in a spiral pattern as the person moves backward into previous stages and forward through later stages. The upward and forward spiral movement toward elimination of the behavior occurs as the person learns from previous experience. The greater the number of successes the person has over time in this spiral movement, the greater the possibility of sustained change.

When the nurse expresses her concern to Mr. Kitchen, he pats her on the hand and says, "Don't you worry none, the good Lord will take care of me." Which of these stages describe Mr. Kitchen's frame of mind concerning his health behaviors? Are any of these stages relevant?

Health Belief Model

The health belief model is a health protection model that provides a framework to explain why some people take specific actions to avoid or treat illness, whereas others fail to protect themselves (Lancaster, Onega, & Forness, 1996; Pender, 1996). The model has been used to predict and explain health behavior based on the value-expectancy theory and Lewin's cognitive theory.

Lewin is a cognitive theorist who conceptualized that certain aspects of a person's life space has negative, positive, or neutral values. He believed that disease has a negative value and, as a result, exerts a force to move the person toward health behaviors. He also believed that behavior is a function of the subjective value of an outcome and of the subjective expectation that a particular action will achieve that outcome (Rosenstock, 1974).

The health belief model states that the probability that the person will take appropriate health care actions depends on the person's value of health, perceptions about disease, and perceived threat of disease. Additionally, perceptions about the medical team and therapy plans, past experience, contact with risk factors, level of participation in regular health care, life aspirations, and factors in the environment motivate action.

Four components of the health belief model have been identified: perceived susceptibility, perceived severity, perceived benefits, and perceived barriers (Rosenstock, 1974). People will take action to ward off, to screen for, or to control ill health if they regard themselves as susceptible to the condition, if they believe it to have potentially serious consequences, if they believe that actions available to them would reduce either their susceptibility to or the severity of the condition. If they also believe that the anticipated barriers to (or costs of) taking the action are outweighed by its benefits action is more likely.

Perceived susceptibility refers to a person's subjective perception of the risk of contracting a health condition. For example, with cigarette smoking, the person might not perceive any risk of getting lung cancer. **Perceived severity** refers to the perceived seriousness of contracting an illness or leaving it untreated. In cigarette smoking, the person might not perceive that

serious personal harm will occur as a result of smoking. **Perceived benefits** refers to the person's perceptions and beliefs about the effectiveness of the recommended actions in preventing the health threat. **Perceived barriers** refers to perceived negative aspects of a health action or the perceived impediments to undertaking the recommended behaviors (Rosenstock, 1974). Key components of the health belief model can be found in Box 25–1.

Self-efficacy is a central concept in the health belief model. **Self-efficacy** is defined as the conviction that one can successfully execute the behavior required to produce the outcomes (Rosenstock, 1974, p. 40). Bandura (1977) believes that efficacy expectancies differ from outcome expectancies, in that efficacy expectancies refer to one's capacity to perform the behavior, whereas outcome expectancies refer to beliefs about what will happen as a result of engaging in the behavior. For example, for a person to quit smoking, he must believe that cessation will benefit his health (outcome expectation) and also that he is capable of quitting (efficacy expectation). Pender (1996) agrees that self-efficacy is the judgment held by the individual that he has the capability to accomplish a certain level of performance in carrying out a specific behavior. According to Bandura (1977), self-efficacy judgments are based on four major sources of information: the individual's own performance accomplishments, vicari-

---

BOX 25–1

KEY COMPONENTS OF THE HEALTH BELIEF MODEL

Threat

- Perceived susceptibility to an illness (or acceptance of a diagnosis).
- Perceived seriousness of the condition.

Outcome Expectations

- Perceived benefits of specified action.
- Perceived barriers to taking that action.

Efficacy Expectations

- Conviction about one's ability to carry out a recommended action (self-efficacy).

Sociodemographic factors—such as education, age, sex, race, ethnicity, and income—are believed to influence behavior indirectly by affecting perceived threat, outcome expectations, and efficacy expectations.

From Rosenstock, I. (1974). Historical origins of the health belief model. Health Education Monograph, 2(4), 328–335.

ous observation on the performance of others, the influence of external persuasion and social influence, and states of emotional arousal. A person's success with coping in a variety of high-risk situations increases his sense of self-efficacy and decreases the probability of relapse.

Health Promotion Model

The health promotion model, developed by Pender, describes the multidimensional nature of a person's interactions with the environment in the pursuit of health. This model integrates nursing and behavioral science perspectives with factors influencing health behaviors (Pender, 1996, p. 51). Unlike the health belief model, the health promotion model does not rely on "personal threats." The model uses constructs from the value-expectancy theory and social cognitive theory.

Value-expectancy theory suggests that behavior is rational and economical. This means that people will not waste their time and resources on investments that have little value to them (Pender, 1996). Furthermore, people will not invest in a goal if they perceive that the goal is impossible to achieve. The motivational significance of the expectancy of successfully changing behavior is based on the person having some past experiences with success. In other words, the person must have some confidence in his achievement of the goal.

Social cognitive theory focuses on the person's beliefs interacting with environmental influences (Pender, 1996). Behavior is not solely driven by inner forces or automatically shaped by external stimuli. Rather, there is an interaction between cognitive factors, personal factors, and environmental events.

Beliefs about oneself formed through self-observation and self-reflective thought have the potential for influencing behavior. These beliefs, according to Pender, include self-attribution, self-evaluation, and self-efficacy. Perceived self-efficacy "is a judgment of one's ability to carry out a particular course of action. The greater the perceived self-efficacy, the more persistent individuals will be in achieving the behavior outcome" (Pender, 1996).

FACTORS AFFECTING BEHAVIORAL CHANGE

In helping a client make behavioral changes to manage health, you need to understand the possible areas that can influence the relationship with the client. Some area are under the control of the nurse and the client; others are not.

Communication

Impaired verbal skills or language differences prevent a client from expressing health needs or communicating effectively with health care professionals. Comprehension and meaning vary among cultures. Words and their meanings carry different nuances and significance, depending on a person's culture, values, and beliefs. Language barriers, whether from foreign languages or varying dialects of the same language, can result in anxiety, fear, and frustration for people who need to communicate, especially when health care is required. Because communication involves body language along with verbal language, the meaning of body position and expression can further facilitate or impede communication. A person's values regarding what personal thoughts and feelings are appropriate to share with others also affect communication.

A client's inability to provide a nurse or physician with accurate assessment data may result in erroneous or ineffective treatment of illness or disease. Likewise, a client's ability to communicate with health care providers can improve the treatment of illness—and the client's satisfaction with treatment.

Cognition and Perception

Cognition is the systematic way in which a person thinks, reasons, and uses language. Perception of information includes the sensing and interpretation of stimuli from the external and internal environment. The person's cognitive-perceptual functioning provides information on his ability to understand and follow directions, retain information, make decisions, solve problems, and use language appropriately. Cognitive-perceptual impairments include limitations of the senses, such as blindness or deafness, or brain dysfunction, such as memory loss or confusion. These impairments may reduce the level of knowledge a person acquires about a health condition or prescribed treatment.

Inability to make deliberate and thoughtful judgments can create a delay in seeking professional assistance. Signs and symptoms may be ignored or disregarded by the client as being relevant to the onset or exacerbation of disease. Health education or discharge instructions may be misinterpreted, not assimilated and remembered, or not followed, resulting in inadequate health maintenance or an exacerbation of disease.

Age and Developmental Level

The age and developmental level of the client influence his health beliefs and practices. A person's health status can be significantly altered by unachieved developmental tasks. Lack of education about nutrition, safety, fitness, or health-protecting practices during childhood or adolescence can have a significant impact on adult health. An inability to meet basic human needs at various developmental stages may result in the development of a distorted value system or a lack of motivation for self-care.

Age and developmental level also may have a significant impact on the person's ability to manage and maintain health. Although infants and children rely on parents and guardians for the management of health, school-aged children can be assisted in the management of some self-care activities to promote and maintain health. Common problems in older adults may also affect health maintenance. For example, loss of teeth may preclude proper nutrition, arthritis may affect the ability to exercise, and slowed cognitive processes may affect safety practices.

Developmental level plays a significant role in cognitive and perceptual abilities. The ability to problem-solve and conceptualize is marked by developmental level. As the adult reaches maturity, decline in visual acuity, hearing, touch, and taste begin, and this decline continues through the later years.

Age increases susceptibility to certain illnesses. For example, the risk of cardiovascular disease increases with age for both sexes. The risks of birth defects and complications of pregnancy increase among pregnant women over age 35. Age risk factors are often associated with other risk factors, such as family history and personal habits. For example, a man at age 60 who has smoked for 40 or more years is at greater risk of developing lung cancer than a man at age 30 who has smoked for 10 years.

Lifestyle and Habits

Lifestyle and health are closely related. Therefore, changes in one usually create changes in the other. Lifestyle and personal health habits are learned through the developmental process. The family plays a critical role in the developmental process of health-promoting and health-protective behaviors.

Health-related decisions regarding diet and leisure activities affect all family members. The health practices of children and adolescents are greatly influenced by the examples set by adults within the family. Those behaviors that are most satisfying are retained and reinforced and largely determine their potential for health maintenance. Inappropriate health habits, such as overeating, lack of exercise, use of alcohol and tobacco, and ineffective coping patterns are often established in early childhood and adolescence, and carried through adulthood.

Health practices and behaviors can have positive or negative effects on health. Practices with potential negative effects are risk factors. These practices include overeating or poor nutrition, insufficient rest and sleep, and poor personal hygiene. Other habits that put a person at risk for illness include smoking, alcohol or drug abuse, and activities involving a threat of injury, such as skydiving, mountain climbing, or bungee-jumping. Some habits are risk factors for specific diseases. For example, excessive sunbathing increases the risk of skin cancer; being overweight increases the risk of cardiovascular disease.

Economic Resources

Economic factors can affect a client's level of health by increasing the risk of developing disease, by influenc-

ing how or at what point the client enters the health care system, or by limiting compliance with a prescribed treatment plan.

People who have health insurance are more likely to seek health care at the onset of symptoms, and they seek health care more frequently than people who have no insurance. People who have no health insurance may feel forced to fill basic needs, such as food, rather than obtaining health care. Plus, access to health care facilities frequently requires transportation, which may be unaffordable or unavailable to low-income people.

Even when good health care is available, the poor do not generally avail themselves of this important resource to the extent that white-collar, middle-class people do. The poor and the working class tend not to put a high priority on minor conditions. And although prevention can help avoid the cost and anxiety of treatment, as described in the Cost of Care chart, low-income people tend to seek medical treatment only at a relatively late stage in an illness. A person's compliance with a treatment plan designed to maintain or improve health is also affected by economic status. A person who has a high utility bill, a large family, and low income tends to give higher priority to food and shelter than to costly drugs or treatments or expensive foods for special diets.

Crowded living conditions contribute to an increased incidence of illness and disease because of the close proximity of people, the sharing of utensils and belongings, poor sanitation, and other poor health habits. Other factors affecting health maintenance include isolation, language or communication difficulties, seasonal work occupations, and migration patterns.

Compared with the poor population, middle-class people work in more protected jobs, are better educated, and are more likely to seek treatment for minor illnesses. Members of the upper income group live longer and tend to make effective use of the health care system in promoting and maintaining health.

Cultural Values and Beliefs

Cultural background influences individual beliefs, values, and customs. It influences entry into the health care system and personal health practices, as suggested in the Cross-Cultural Care chart. The range of health definitions, practices, and beliefs about prevention manifested by members of the various ethnic groups is infinite. Also, there are variations in health definitions, beliefs, and practices within a given ethnic group.

A*ction* A*lert!*
The basic needs of all human beings, regardless of cultural background, are the same. How a person seeks to meet these needs is influenced by culture. Cultural and ethnic factors are often inter-related with psychological, social, and economic factors.

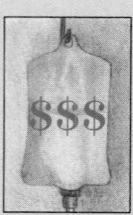

THE COST OF CARE
COLON CANCER SCREENING

In the United States alone, about 109,000 new cases of colon cancer are diagnosed each year. Of these, about 64,000 will be fatal, a number that accounts for about 10% of all cancer deaths each year. Encouraging clients to participate in screening programs for early detection of colon cancer can help to reduce such deaths—and the costs associated with treating colon cancer. However, the screening program itself incurs considerable costs. At least according to one study, it may be possible to lower even these costs safely (Getzen, 1997).

The test used most often to screen for colon cancer is the guaiac test. It uses guaiac as a reagent to detect occult blood in the client's stool. If the results are positive, they raise the suspicion of colon cancer. However, blood in the stool does not always result from colon cancer, which means that, in a certain percentage of people, positive results can stem from a bleeding ulcer, consumption of certain foods, even random error. Nevertheless, each person who has a positive result from a stool guaiac test must have a follow-up barium enema to check for colon cancer. Plus, the American Cancer Society recommends six guaiac tests as a complete screening for colon cancer, with any one positive test raising suspicion of cancer.

Among a group of 100,000 people, about 720 of them will have asymptomatic colon cancer. If the entire group has a stool guaiac test, the initial test will show positive results for about 90% of those who have colon cancer (648 people) and about another 20% of the group for unrelated reasons. So the initial test (at $4 per person) would return positive results in about 20,648 people. Each person must then have a follow-up barium enema, at about $100 each. Thus, following up on false-positive results accounts for more than 80% of the $2,464,800 cost of the initial screening test. Overall, the program has so far cost $3,803 per case of colon cancer found.

The second stool guaiac test would cost $1 per person and would detect 90% of the remaining undiagnosed cancers (64.8 cases) and another group of people with false-positive result. At $1.7 million, the total cost for the

second test is less than the initial test. However, the number of colon cancer cases detected is far lower. Considering the cumulative cost of the first two tests, the average cost per case detected has grown to $5,852. More importantly, the marginal cost of cancer detection with the second test is much higher, at $26,335 per additional case found ($1.7 million in additional costs divided by 64.8 additional cases). The marginal cost is "the increase in total costs caused by the production of one more unit of output" (Getzen, 1997, p. 453).

The third, fourth, fifth, and sixth tests would cost $1 per person and would each pick up 90% of the cancers not yet diagnosed. These additional tests are finding very few new cases of colon cancer, but are still generating substantial numbers of false-positive results. According to Getzen, "Since 5 tests will have uncovered almost all (719.9928 out of 720) of the cancer, the additional cases of cancer detected by the sixth test is almost negligibly small, .0065—but the sixth stool guaiac will account for 100,000 tests and another 6,554 false positives, so that the marginal cost per case detected for the sixth stool guaiac is $755,400 divided by .0065, an almost astronomical $116,574,074 per additional case found" (Getzen, 1997, p. 33).

Discussion

This study demonstrates the obvious benefits of screening tests for colon cancer. It also suggests that undergoing fewer than six tests may produce equal, or nearly equal, benefits at a considerably lower cost. The study also illustrates that the marginal cost can differ from the actual cost. And the study points out that the direct cost (screening tests) may be much less that the indirect cost (barium enemas to rule out cancer among false-positive tests) of the screening program.

Reference

Getzen, T.E. (1997). *Health economics: Fundamentals and flow of funds.* New York: John Wiley & Sons, Inc.

The spiritual dimensions of values and beliefs are a vital force that integrates all other dimensions of human beings—physical, mental, psychological, and social. The spiritual dimension helps one find meaning in life, suffering, pain, illness, and death. Religious participation can influence lifestyle, attitudes, and feelings about illness that may conflict with interventions to promote, maintain, or restore health. These conflicts often are revealed when clients enumerate the course of an illness, refuse recommended medical intervention, or refuse to comply with other treatment modalities for spiritual reasons.

Roles and Relationships

Social relationships within the family, social group, work setting, and the community at large are significant to one's well-being. An inability to engage in satisfying relationships or to feel comfortable in social interactions may lead to social isolation. Social isolation prevents the seeking of preventive health services and the formation of positive support systems. Conflicting role expectations within the family, social group, and work setting produce stress. Communication patterns, decision-making, perceived power and authority, feel-

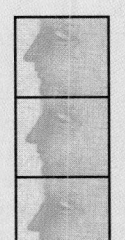

CROSS-CULTURAL CARE
CARING FOR AN AFRICAN-AMERICAN CLIENT

Oscar Kitchen is an African-American man who ascribes to the traditional definition of health held by many African-Americans. Like those of many other cultures, African-Americans have a unique way of classifying illness that aids in diagnosis and treatment. Likewise, many beliefs and values held by African-Americans can influence health behaviors and lifestyle. Some of these beliefs include the following:

- Health as harmony with nature, feeling good (no pain), ability to engage in activities of daily living and go to work.
- Illness as feeling bad, inability to work or engage in activities of daily living, and disharmony of mind, body, and spirit.
- Prayer and a well-balanced diet as helpful in avoiding illness and recovering from illness.
- Group orientation.
- Spirituality as an influence on perception of health and illness.
- Close personal space.
- Strong family and kinship ties.
- Family resources as a source of support rather than outside assistance.
- Health values and beliefs vary with age, socioeconomic status, and location (rural/urban).
- Dietary pattern reflects many cultures.
- Home remedies accepted for their effectiveness, decreased cost, and lack of segregation and racism that can be found in formal health care.
- Distrust of "the system."

Mr. Kitchen's nurse, Ms. Emanuel, shows an effective way to meet the client's needs while considering his cultural beliefs and values in this conversation.

Ms. Emanuel: Mr. Kitchen, how are you feeling today?

Mr Kitchen: I'm feeling alright, just a little short of breath.

Ms. Emanuel: How long have you been a little short of breath?

Mr. Kitchen: It just started late yesterday evening. I was feeling fine until then.

Ms. Emanuel: Did you take your medication yesterday?

Mr. Kitchen: No, I didn't take it. I didn't need to take it. I had been feeling alright for the last few days. It seemed to have gotten rid of the problem so I didn't need to keep taking it.

Ms. Emanuel: Mr. Kitchen, did you forget your last appointment? You didn't call to cancel it.

Mr. Kitchen: No, I didn't forget. I just didn't figure that I had to come back since I was feeling alright. I had been able to work in my garden and do other things I needed to do.

Ms. Emanuel: Mr. Kitchen, I need to talk with you about your medications after I finish examining you. It's important that you understand why you are taking each medication and how each works to keep you feeling good and to prevent your shortness of breath. It's important that you take your medications each day until the doctor tells you to stop. If you don't take your medication each day, you will continue to have shortness of breath.

Mr. Kitchen: Well, I guess if I have to. Lord knows, I don't want to take all of this stuff.

Critical Thinking Questions

- What reasons can you give for Mr. Kitchen's minimizing his "shortness of breath" even though it caused him to sleep very little the night before?
- Which part of Ms. Emanuel's conversation indicated that she was taking beliefs and values of the African-American culture into consideration?
- Which part of Mr. Kitchen's conversation indicates that he is at risk for *Ineffective management of therapeutic regimen?*

ings of self-worth, and perceived support will have an impact on health maintenance.

Coping and Stress Tolerance

Stress can affect health and well-being in any of the adaptive modes: physiological, psychological, spiritual, developmental, and social. In the physical dimension, stress can threaten a person's homeostasis. In the emotional dimension, stress can lead to negative or counterproductive feelings or greatly threaten the way a person normally perceives and solves problems. In

the social dimension, stress can threaten a person's relationship with others, the support he receives from others, and his sense of belonging. In the spiritual dimension, stress can threaten a person's general outlook on life and attitude toward a supreme being. In essence, stress can affect how a person satisfies all his basic human needs.

Workplace and Environmental Conditions

The environment has many influences on health and illness. The physical environment in which a person works or lives can increase the likelihood that certain illnesses will occur. Industrial workers exposed to certain chemicals are more likely to develop certain kinds of cancer and other diseases. In some work environments, high noise levels or increased emotional stress may be prevalent. Environmental pollution, high crime rates, or overcrowding can lead to stresses that make people more susceptible to disease.

ASSESSMENT

A thorough assessment of health, attitudes, cultural beliefs, and health practices is critical to developing an effective health promotion plan for your clients (Pender, 1996). You will collect information about nutrition, elimination, rest and sleep, activity and exercise, and hygiene. Patterns of psychological health can be determined by assessing coping, interactions, and self-concept. Sociocultural health can be assessed through cultural practices, recreation, and significant relationships. Religious beliefs and values are determinants of spiritual health.

General Assessment of Health Promotion

The health history may be the most important part of the database. Cues from the nursing history can alert you to traits that increase the client's vulnerability to a certain condition or disease. In addition to the health history, you can identify the client's risk factors by using health-risk appraisal tools.

Health Practices

Pender (1996) describes several components of health assessment that focus on wellness for the individual client: physical fitness evaluation, health risk appraisal, social support systems, and lifestyle assessment.

Physical fitness evaluation is an important part of personal health status and a critical part of assessment. Pender suggests that physical fitness is divided into skill-related physical fitness and health-related physical fitness. "Skill-related fitness is defined by those qualities that contribute to successful athletic performance: agility, speed, power, and reaction time. Health-related fitness includes qualities found to contribute to one's general health, including cardiorespiratory endurance, muscular strength and endurance, body composition, and flexibility" (p. 118). Health-related fitness also includes qualities that contribute to a person's general well-being.

Health-risk appraisal is also part of assessment data that provides clients with essential information about health threats from hereditary factors, lifestyle, and family history (Pender, 1996). Categories of risk factors include: genetics, age, biological characteristics, personal health habits, lifestyle, and environment.

The health risk appraisal only provides an average indication of risk. Additionally, a client must know his own health experience and what improvements he could make in his mortality profile if he adopted more positive behaviors of other groups (Pender, 1996).

Social support systems are important in enhancing successful coping and promoting comfortable and effective living. These factors reduce stress and improve health and well-being (Pender, 1996). **Social support** can be defined as the subjective feeling of belonging, or being accepted, loved, esteemed, valued, and needed for oneself, not for what one can do for others (p. 257). Although all people need some type of social support, the amount and type of social support may vary based on the person's age and situation. Types of social support that have been clearly documented in the literature include emotional support, informational support, family support, and instrumental support, which includes assistance with specific tasks (Pender, 1996).

Obtaining assessment data related to cultural beliefs and attitudes is also important to facilitating the health and well-being of your clients. Clark (1996, p. 282) suggests the use of the following four basic principles when collecting data related to culture:

- View all cultures in the context in which they developed.
- Examine underlying premises for culturally determined beliefs and behaviors.
- Interpret the meaning and purpose of behavior in the context of the specific culture.
- Recognize the potential for intercultural variation.

Lifestyle assessment is closely related to assessment of cultural beliefs and attitudes. Aspects of lifestyle that you should assess include life events, dietary patterns, and health habits (Clark, 1996). "The desired outcomes of health assessment are to: (1) identify health assets, (2) identify health-related lifestyle strengths, (3) determine key health-related beliefs, (4) identify health beliefs and health behaviors that put the client at risk, and (5) determine how the client wants to change to improve the quality of life" (Pender, 1996, p. 116).

A*ction* A*lert!*
The total risk for developing any disease increases with the number of risk factors present and the intensity of each risk factor. Risk appraisal is based on the experience of the current referent group (personal risk age) and the prediction of improvement in their mortality profile if they were to adopt more positive health-promoting behaviors.

Illness Practices

A person experiencing a health problem may have prescribed adjustments in many aspects of day-to-day living to maintain health. These changes may be for treatments to restore optimal health, for prevention of health problems, or for early detection of health problems. Your assessment should include identifying factors and cues that would indicate ineffective management.

THE STATE OF NURSING SCIENCE

HEALTH PROMOTION PRACTICES OF AFRICAN-AMERICAN WOMEN

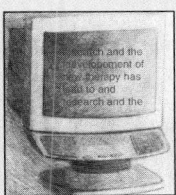

What Are the Issues?

African-American women are at higher risk than others for poor health outcomes related to cancer, heart disease, and diabetes. In particular, African-American women have higher mortality rates from breast cancer because of delayed diagnosis. Efforts to understand factors related to these outcomes include examining both health beliefs and health promotion practices.

What Research Has Been Conducted?

Using the Health Belief Model to identify variables to measure, researchers Martin and Panicucci (1996) surveyed a group of 40 African-American women from a local church to learn about the beliefs of these women about the importance of, and adherence to, 20 health behaviors. The researchers asked the women whether they performed each of the health behaviors and then asked them to rate how important the behavior was in maintaining good health.

The women reported high levels of adherence to 17 of the 20 health behaviors, including such behaviors as controlling intake of fat, cholesterol, salt, and alcohol, and avoiding stress and home accidents. However, the women reported low levels of adherence to four health behaviors: dental care, regular exercise, seatbelt use, and use of smoke detectors.

The researchers also measured each woman's assessment of her current health status as well as her belief in her ability to control her future health. The women reported their current health status as better than most, but their scores for control of future health status were lower, perhaps related to belief that future health lies in the control of God rather than the individual.

Two major health practices not examined in the study by Martin and Panicucci (1997) were breast self-examination and mammography to screen for breast cancer. These health practices are important because early detection of breast cancer increases survival rates. Using the Health Belief Model to guide their study, Champion and Scott (1997) therefore revised an assessment tool to measure African-American women's beliefs about, and compliance with, mammography and breast self-examination. The tool was designed to measure a woman's beliefs about her susceptibility to breast cancer, the benefits of both mammography and breast self-examination, barriers to obtaining a mammogram or performing breast self-examination, and confidence in performing breast self-examination. The researchers believed that it was important that the tool be sensitive to the special needs of low-income African-American women, so they added new items to the barriers scale that were important to these women, including fear of rude professionals and issues of transportation and child care.

Champion and Menon (1997) used this revised tool to try to predict compliance with mammography recommendations, proficiency in breast self-examination, and frequency of breast self-examination among low-income African-American women. The researchers found that women who had a regular physician were more likely to obtain mammograms and to perform breast self-examination. The women who reported facing significant barriers to obtaining mammograms were less likely to obtain them. Having a regular physician who suggested having a mammogram made it more likely that the women would actually obtain a mammogram. The women who rated themselves as confident in their breast self-examination skills, who faced less formidable barriers to obtaining a mammogram, who understood the benefits of mammography, who were knowledgeable about breast cancer, and who had a regular physician were more likely to perform breast self-examination frequently.

What Has the Research Concluded?

The African-American women in these studies were aware of and practiced many health-promoting behaviors. For some health-promoting behaviors, such as taking steps to control high blood pressure, using seatbelts, and using smoke detectors, the perceived importance of the behavior in maintaining health was a good predictor of whether the women would actually practice them. In the special case of mammography and breast self-examination, however, perceived barriers were the best predictor. The researchers concluded that education might have an impact in overcoming these barriers, such as fear, time constraints, embarrassment, and the perception that other problems are more important.

What Is the Future of Research in This Area?

Understanding the barriers to care that low-income African-American women face is a necessary first step in the development of new strategies to increase health-promoting behaviors among these women. Now, research is needed on the effectiveness of interventions to increase health behaviors among these women. Research is also needed on the impact of managed-care systems on provider-patient relationships. That is because these studies have identified good relationships with health care providers as important in encouraging low-income African-American women to engage in health-promoting behaviors such as mammography

(continued)

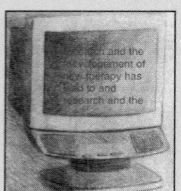

THE STATE OF NURSING SCIENCE
HEALTH PROMOTION PRACTICES OF AFRICAN-AMERICAN WOMEN (continued)

and breast self-examination. Additional attention is needed to develop effective ways of promoting health behaviors that these women perform with low frequency, such as dental care and seatbelt use. Champion and Menon (1997) also recommend studying additional samples of African-American women to see whether similar patterns of predictors are present in other samples.

References

Champion, V. & Menon, U. (1997). Predicting mammography and breast self-examination in African-American women. *Cancer Nursing, 20,* 315–322.

Champion, V.L. & Scott, R.S. (1997). Reliability and validity of breast cancer screening belief scales in African-American women. *Nursing Research, 46,* 331–337.

Martin, J.C. & Panicucci, C.L. (1996). Health-related practices and priorities: The health behaviors and beliefs of community-living black older women. *Journal of Gerontological Nursing, 22*(4), 41–48.

Factors that should be considered in the management of a therapeutic regimen include the following:

- The client's knowledge of the disease, including severity and prognosis
- Disease history and previous treatment patterns (including the number of previous admissions for acute care)
- Previous history of accessing health care resources
- Treatment and preventive measures
- Pattern of adhering to prescribed therapeutic regimen
- Factors that prevent full implementation or adherence to recommended therapeutic regimen
- Missing knowledge or information that prevents the comprehension of recommended treatment program and subsequent implementation
- The extent to which adherence to the treatment program has altered the person's life and relationships

Additionally, attention should focus on health care resources, presence of sensory deficit, and expressed feelings regarding illnesses or disease process.

KNOWLEDGE OF DISEASE

Knowledge of the disease process deals with the client's understanding of the onset of symptoms, causes and consequences of the current condition, and level of health knowledge. Solicit the following information from the client: how this illness affects his present health, his personal ideas about the cause of the symptoms, factors that aggravate or alleviate the symptoms, how the present illness affects the performance of activities of daily living, and the types of health promotion and illness prevention activities he has engaged in since he last had similar symptoms.

DISEASE HISTORY

The length of the disease process and the frequency with which the person has presented for acute treatment for exacerbation of symptoms are cues to the extent to which the client has been able to manage his therapeutic regimen and health maintenance. Soliciting and recording this information in the client's own words will give vital clues when clustered with data collected during the assessment of cognitive-perceptual abilities.

HISTORY OF ACCESSING HEALTH CARE RESOURCES

A person's perception of health and illness, culture and spiritual beliefs, roles, relationships, and support systems are among the many factors that will influence his use of health care resources. Each person has his own definition of health. A person may define his health as being "good" even though he has hypertension or symptoms of a respiratory infection. The extent to which these altered states dictate a need for action will influence the person's decision to seek health care or engage in health maintenance practices.

The attitudes and behaviors of significant others in the family, social groups, work, or community have a direct impact on the person's beliefs and actions. When significant others express apathy or distrust in a particular treatment regimen or health promotion practices, the person may have difficulty with or reservations about making decisions to adhere to the regimen. The family's sociocultural beliefs influence not only how a client perceives illness, but also from whom assistance is sought and what types of treatment will be considered most advantageous.

Focused Assessment for Ineffective Management of Therapeutic Regimen

Defining Characteristics

Several subjective factors may emerge from the health history that may suggest that the client is ineffectively managing a therapeutic regimen. The most important defining characteristic is the person's or family member's verbal expression of a desire to adhere to the therapeutic program. Additionally, the client may report difficulty in carrying out proposed activities or in

CONSIDERING THE ALTERNATIVES
ACUPUNCTURE AND TRADITIONAL CHINESE MEDICINE

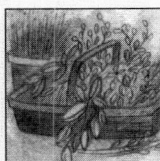 Traditional Chinese medicine, also called Oriental medicine, is a system of medical practice and philosophy with ancient roots predating the Hippocratic works in the West. The earliest known work in the field of traditional Chinese medicine that survives and is still read today, the *Nei Jing,* or *Emperor's Classic of Internal Medicine,* is a compilation of knowledge and theories about disease and acupuncture that dates from the third century BC. An earlier work, written about 400 BC, mentions acupuncture having been practiced as early as 581 BC (Lu, 1978).

Traditional Chinese medicine includes the techniques of acupuncture, moxibustion (the burning of the herb mugwort *[Artemesia vulgaris]* on or near acupuncture points), cupping, and herbal medicine, as well as related exercise and dietary practices, massage, and even manipulative techniques. As with other medical systems, traditional Chinese medicine grew out of, and was influenced by, the religious and philosophical environment of its home country. Over the centuries, many additional theories, techniques, and schools of thought about traditional Chinese medicine have developed, giving this alternative therapy a rich heritage.

Foundational to traditional Chinese medicine is the theory of yin and yang. This theory posits that two opposing but complementary forces—yin and yang—exist in the universe. These two forces are said to be in constant dynamic flux but normally remain in balance. For example, the opposing yet complementary actions of the sympathetic and parasympathetic divisions of the autonomic nervous system can be viewed as having a yin and yang relationship. Adherents to traditional Chinese medicine believe that imbalance in these forces in the body gives rise to symptoms. Diagnosing and correcting imbalances, which leads to restoration of health, is the essence of traditional Chinese medicine.

Once developed, the theories and practices of traditional Chinese medicine spread throughout the Orient. Today, they are commonly used by people in most other parts of the world. In China today, there are many schools and hospitals in which traditional Chinese medicine is taught and practiced. Some hospitals have both modern and traditional wings. Patients commonly choose modern methods for acute problems and traditional Chinese methods for chronic problems. Some receive a combination of both treatment methods.

Acupuncture is the best known component of traditional Chinese medicine in the West. Early European traders and missionaries, as well as Asians traveling to Europe, brought the knowledge and practice of acupuncture to Europe in the 17th and 18th centuries. In the United States, some physicians recommended the use of acupuncture even in the early 19th century, and Asian immigrants brought the practices of traditional Chinese medicine with them to America.

Acupuncture involves the careful insertion of fine-gauge needles, generally now made of stainless steel, into the skin and muscles at a variety of locations on the body to alleviate symptoms. Other styles of acupuncture have evolved as well. Some styles, like the Japanese, use finer-gauge needles that the patient barely feels. A Korean method uses points on the hand to treat the whole body.

Proponents of acupuncture attribute its effect to the influence of the needles on the client's *qi* (pronounced "chee"). *Qi* is said to be a form of energy and functional activity that flows continuously through an intricate network of invisible channels on and in the human body. A lack of, or an obstruction to, this flow of *qi* may be both cause and effect of disease or imbalance. Acupuncture needles, moxibustion, and acupressure massage on the acupuncture points are ways for the practitioner to manipulate the flow of *qi,* improving flow where inadequate and removing obstructions to flow where it is stagnated. Again, the idea of balance is critical. For example, to treat a headache, an acupuncturist may insert needles into the client's feet.

Today, acupuncture is one of the most popular of all complementary and alternative therapies. Americans make 9 to 12 million visits to acupuncturists each year, according to the Food and Drug Administration. As of 1998, there were approximately 10,000 acupuncturists in the United States, and that number was expected to double by the year 2000 (Office of Alternative Medicine, 1998).

Some physicians and more scientifically minded practitioners believe that the theoretical basis of traditional Chinese medicine is not necessary to explain its effect and that the traditional theoretical basis may provide a false explanation. Instead, they believe that the effects of acupuncture involve neuromuscular anatomy (Ulett, 1992). On the other hand, many traditionally trained practitioners feel the best results are obtained using the traditional diagnostic and treatment methods of traditional Chinese medicine.

Modern research has found that a number of events take place when needles, such as those used in acupuncture, are inserted into the body. Endorphin levels increase, and some hormone levels change. Some research has shown a blocking of acupuncture effects when nerve conduction is blocked (Melzack, 1989).

At a conference sponsored by the National Institutes of Health in 1997, research was presented showing that acupuncture "is an effective treatment for nausea caused by cancer chemotherapy drugs, surgical anes-

(continued)

ACUPUNCTURE AND TRADITIONAL CHINESE MEDICINE (continued)

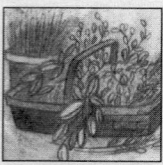

thesia and pregnancy; and for pain resulting from surgery and a variety of musculoskeletal conditions" (National Institutes of Health, 1997). Preliminary research on the efficacy of acupuncture in other conditions has indicated possible benefits, but further research is needed. One difficulty with this research is that acupuncture treatment is difficult to standardize even for people with the same biomedical diagnosis; traditional Chinese medical diagnoses may vary among people with the same Western medical diagnosis, and acupuncture treatment may differ as well.

An interesting use of acupuncture is in the treatment of drug addiction. This use grew out of the discovery in Hong Kong in the 1960s that people addicted to controlled substances who were given electrical ear acupuncture for surgical analgesia did not experience symptoms of drug withdrawal (Wen & Teo, 1975). As a result of these findings, a drug treatment center in New York City began using a five-point ear acupuncture treatment, eventually without the electrical stimulation. The center found that acupuncture is an effective adjunct in the treatment of drug and alcohol addiction. The technique is now used in many areas of the world. In the United States, it is even used as a treatment modality in many court-mandated drug treatment programs (Smith & Khan, 1988).

Chinese herbal medicine is a complex system that employs hundreds of substances (herbal, animal, and mineral) and hundreds of formulas, many dating from the works of ancient practitioners. Formulas may include as few as two to as many as dozens of herbs and are administered as teas, powdered extracts, and pills. Until the 1800s, traditional Chinese medicine was the sole medical system in China and much of the Orient. It is

therefore no wonder that traditional Chinese herbal formulas and acupuncture treatment protocols exist for most of the illnesses known and experienced by humankind.

Research has shown a variety of effects from the various herbs and formulas used in traditional Chinese medicine. Some specific research on Chinese herbs is examined in the "Considering the Alternatives" chart in Chapter 40.

Resources

Publications that can expand and keep your knowledge of complementary and alternative medicine current:

Beinfeld, H. & Korngold, E. (1991). *Between heaven and earth: A guide to Chinese medicine.* New York: Ballantine Books.
Kaptchuk, T. (1983). *The web that has no weaver: Understanding Chinese medicine.* New York: Congdon & Weed.

References

Lu, H.C. (1978). *A complete translation of the Yellow Emperor's Classic of Internal Medicine and the Difficult Classic.* Vancouver: Oriental Heritage.
Melzack, R. (1989). Folk medicine and the sensory modulation of pain. In P. Wall & R. Melzack (Eds.), *Textbook of pain* (2nd ed.) (pp. 897–905). London: Churchill Livingstone.
National Institutes of Health. (1997). Acupuncture. *NIH consensus statement Nov. 3–5, 15*(5), 1–34.
Office of Alternative Medicine. (1998). Acupuncture effective for certain medical conditions, panel says. *Complementary & Alternative Medicine at the NIH, Volume V, Number 1.* Silver Springs, MD: Office of Alternative Medicine Clearinghouse.
Smith, M.O. & Khan, I. (1988). An acupuncture programme for the treatment of drug-addicted persons. *Bulletin on Narcotics, 40*(1), 35–41.
Ulett, G.A. (1992). *Beyond yin and yang: How acupuncture really works.* St. Louis: Warren H. Green.
Wen, H. & Teo, S.W. (1975). Experience in the treatment of drug addiction by electro-acupuncture. *Modern Medicine Asia, 11*(6), 23–24.

making choices to incorporate the activities of the regimen into daily living. Or the client may report making no attempt to incorporate these activities into patterns of daily living.

The reasons may reflect the person's lifestyle, work patterns, or roles and relationships. The exacerbation of symptoms is an objective characteristic in making this diagnosis. Expression of failure to seek out health care and related support, to make needed appointments, or to keep appointments would be additional defining characteristics.

Related Factors

Related factors contributing to the diagnosis of *Ineffective management of therapeutic regimen: individuals* in-

clude many of the factors affecting behavioral change. Additional ineffective management can be related to aspects of the treatment regimen, to the health care system, and to personal factors.

Factors related to treatment include the complexity of the therapeutic regimen, side effects of therapy, the financial cost of the regimen, and the complexity of the health care delivery system. Therapeutic regimens may be complex for several reasons. Modern advances in medicine and technological advancements have resulted in the development of many useful devices for managing health problems; however, they can create confusion for the clients who must use them. Many electronic devices are used in the home to assist the client in monitoring the status of health problems, such as blood sugar level, blood pressure, urinalysis, and so on. The client's cognitive-perceptual level must be assessed to detect cognitive or sensory deficits that may contribute to the complexity of the therapeutic regimen.

Access to care is a factor in the health care system. Some clients enter the system easily through physician's offices, clinics, or hospital emergency rooms. Other clients experience difficulties in entering the system because of confusion or unfamiliarity with the various agencies or because of low income status. Some geographical locations, such as rural communities, still lack adequate health care resources.

Fragmentation of services is a second factor within the system. Specialization and technological advancement throughout the health care system has led to fragmentation in the provision of care. During the course of an illness, a person may be seen by several health care providers that treat, prescribe, and initiate a health maintenance program that requires different follow-up visits. This process may overwhelm the client and family and lead to failure to initiate any health maintenance activities at all.

Personal factors also affect a client's adherence to a therapeutic regimen. Decisional conflict is reflected in the client's statement that he is unable to make choices even when information is appropriate. Family conflict or excessive demands made on the client or family can lead to failure to incorporate the planned program into activities of daily living. The client's unrealistic expectations of family members can produce conflict or role strain, which can lead to a breakdown in communication and problem-solving abilities, as well as anger.

You must give some attention to the premise that a person's health beliefs, locus of control, and self-efficacy influence motivation, learning, and the capacity for behavioral changes needed to manage a therapeutic regimen and maintain health. By assessing the client's health beliefs, you can determine the extent to which the client's ineffective management of a therapeutic regimen relates to his mistrust of the regimen, his feeling that the health problem is not serious, or his belief that he is not susceptible to disease. Assess his level of self-efficacy by investigating the amount of personal confidence the client has about initiating proposed activities and reaching desired outcomes. Remember that the perceived value of the proposed therapeutic program will influence the client's willingness to follow it. If he believes an activity will be very effective in preventing the development of a health problem, he will be more likely to perform it. Additionally, the perceived benefits of the activities, when weighed against the adverse reactions and the cost, should be considered as causative factors.

What questions would you ask Mr. Kitchen to determine his problems with adhering to his therapeutic regimen? Do you think knowledge is a factor? Cost? The need to change his usual pattern of living? His beliefs about health?

Focused Assessment for Related Nursing Diagnoses

Altered Health Maintenance

Altered health maintenance includes a large category of possible problems in managing health care. The client may have to make major lifestyle changes in diet, exercise, medications, sleep, and stress reduction. Assessment has already been described. This diagnosis suggests the need for comprehensive planning in multiple areas.

Health-Seeking Behaviors

The health-seeking client does not necessarily have a medical diagnosis. Perhaps the person has been to the physician with complaints of fatigue, stress, forgetfulness, and poor concentration. The physician finds no treatable medical problems and the client seeks services to improve his overall health. You would assess his general health status and health practices, along with his lifestyle, beliefs about health, and resources for improving health.

Knowledge Deficit

The client who needs knowledge to improve or maintain health could be a person with a new medical diagnosis, a person being discharged from the hospital after surgery, or the mother of a new baby. Assess the client's level of knowledge, what the client wants to know, what the client needs to know, and the client's ability to understand the information.

Noncompliance

Assessment of noncompliance is a two-part task. First, assess whether or not the person is in compliance with a medication or treatment regimen. Compliance is determined by measuring the blood level of a medication, by counting the remaining pills in a bottle, by having the client come to the clinic for medication, or sometimes by assessing for the therapeutic effects. Compliance issues arise particularly for communicable diseases, such as tuberculosis, where noncompliance may be a public health threat. Second, assess the reason for noncompliance. Noncompliance can occur because the person chooses not to follow the treatment regimen, because the person does not understand the regimen, or for other less obvious reasons.

Decisional Conflict

When a client has a choice about treatment or even a choice not to accept treatment, assess for decisional conflict. Listen for signs of uncertainty about any aspect of the treatment. Allow the client to freely express concerns about the treatment or its consequences. Delay in making a decision is often the result of conflict. Signs of anxiety may be the only evidence of decisional conflict.

DIAGNOSIS

When the objective of care is primarily that the client learns behaviors to improve health maintenance, you will cluster data to help select a diagnosis from the list of health maintenance diagnoses. The list includes *Health-seeking behaviors, Altered health maintenance, Noncompliance, Knowledge deficit, Decisional conflict,* and *Ineffective management of therapeutic regimen.*

The diagnosis *Health-seeking behaviors* is appropriate when a person is in a state of wellness but is seeking ways to achieve a higher level of wellness. A person of normal weight, for example, may wish to improve his physical fitness and stamina and may verbalize his unfamiliarity with community resources or his lack of knowledge about how to achieve this goal.

Altered health maintenance is appropriate for a person who expresses a desire to change an unhealthy lifestyle, such as dissatisfaction with work, a lack of exercise, tobacco use, obesity, excessive alcohol use, or insufficient social support (Carpenito, 1995). This diagnosis can also be used for a client who must alter health maintenance activities to manage an illness.

The diagnosis *Noncompliance* is reserved for a person who has adequate knowledge and the cognitive-perceptual ability to perform preventive activities or treatments to restore or maintain health but makes an informed decision to not adhere to the recommended treatment plan. In this case, the health history or diagnostic tests may reveal exacerbation of symptoms or development of complications.

Knowledge deficit is best used when the client lacks knowledge about the relationship between an unhealthy behavior or habit and the development of community resources to assist in changing an unhealthy habit. Use this diagnosis when the knowledge

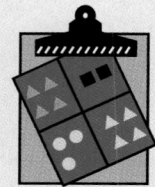

CLUSTERING DATA TO MAKE A NURSING DIAGNOSIS
HEALTH BEHAVIORS

Data Cluster	Diagnosis
An 83-year-old diabetic man lives by himself and prepares his own food when he is feeling well. He feels that family members have abandoned him because they are busy with their own families and jobs. He self-administers insulin when he thinks about it or is feeling "bad."	Ineffective management of therapeutic regimen related to feelings of abandonment and isolation.
A 20-year-old woman has a history of obesity since childhood. She desperately wants to be thin to please her boyfriend. She smokes two packs of cigarettes per day to decrease appetite. She eats a lot of fried and spicy foods and goes on "crash" diets to lose weight quickly. She frequently states, "I can't ever seem to lose weight."	Altered health maintenance related to poor self-esteem interfering with health care regimen.
A 42-year-old woman has four children and works part-time outside the home. She feels no need for exercise because she is always chasing the kids around. She loves to bake desserts for her family. She would like to regain her pre-pregnancy figure but states that she "isn't ready to diet or exercise."	Ineffective management of therapeutic regimen related to altered self-concept and resistance to adopting healthy behaviors at this time.
A 50-year-old man is head of a household that includes his spouse, two children, and his aging mother. He has just been informed that he will be let go from his job because the company must show a profit. He immediately made plans to change the family's lifestyle and health care standards because there will be no health insurance. He feels particularly bad because his mother and children will suffer from the lack of money to purchase food and medicines.	Altered health maintenance related to unexpected change in financial status.

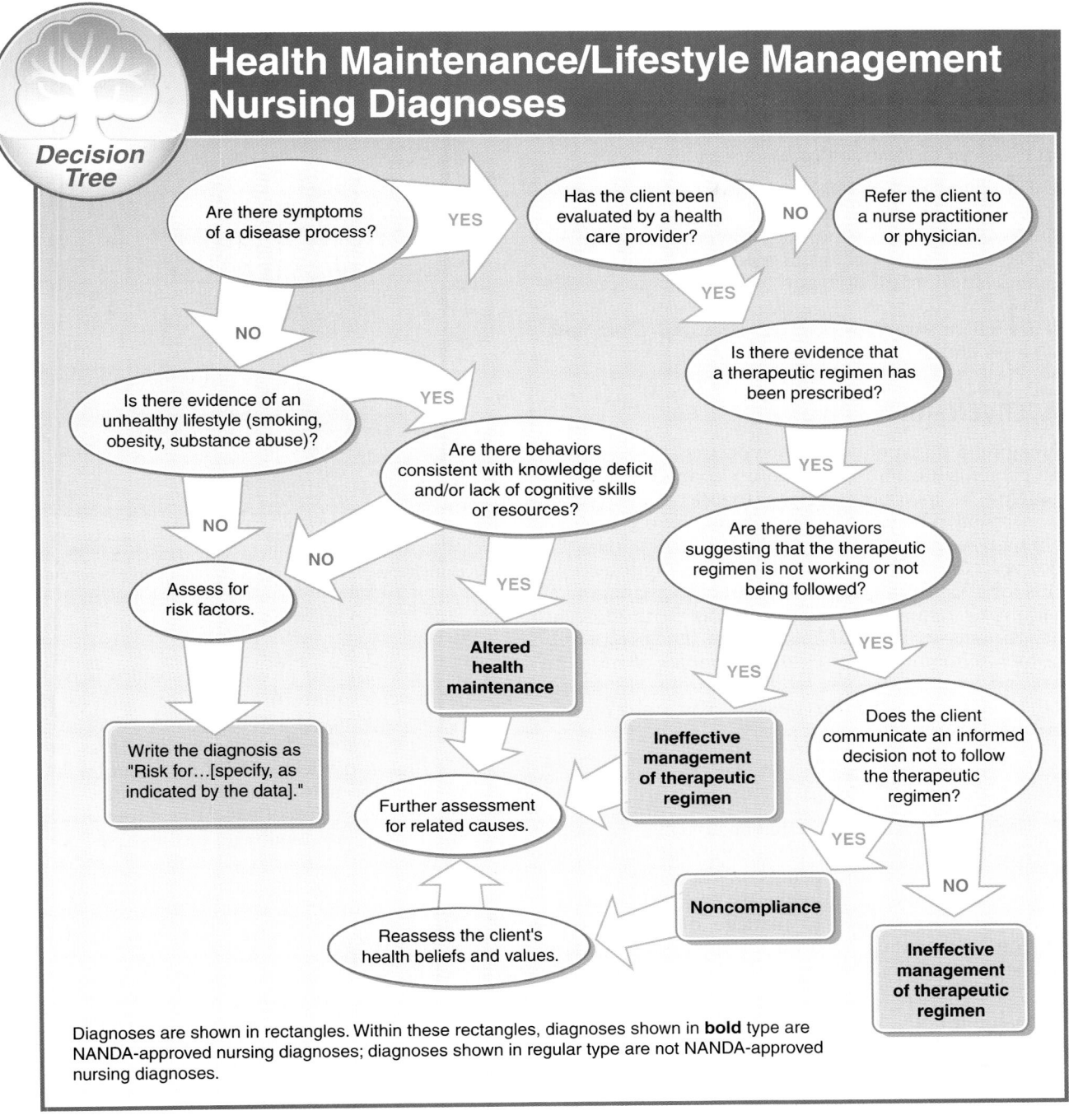

Health Maintenance/Lifestyle Management Nursing Diagnoses

Decision Tree

Are there symptoms of a disease process? — YES → Has the client been evaluated by a health care provider? — NO → Refer the client to a nurse practitioner or physician.

YES ↓

Is there evidence that a therapeutic regimen has been prescribed?

NO ↓

Is there evidence of an unhealthy lifestyle (smoking, obesity, substance abuse)? — YES → Are there behaviors consistent with knowledge deficit and/or lack of cognitive skills or resources?

YES ↓

Are there behaviors suggesting that the therapeutic regimen is not working or not being followed?

NO ↓

Assess for risk factors.

Altered health maintenance

Ineffective management of therapeutic regimen

Does the client communicate an informed decision not to follow the therapeutic regimen?

Write the diagnosis as "Risk for…[specify, as indicated by the data]."

Further assessment for related causes.

Noncompliance

YES

NO ↓

Ineffective management of therapeutic regimen

Reassess the client's health beliefs and values.

Diagnoses are shown in rectangles. Within these rectangles, diagnoses shown in **bold** type are NANDA-approved nursing diagnoses; diagnoses shown in regular type are not NANDA-approved nursing diagnoses.

deficiency is the direct cause or a potential cause of a problem.

Ineffective management of therapeutic regimen: individuals is an inappropriate diagnosis when a person is faced with a complex regimen to follow or has compromised functioning that impedes successful management. The diagnosis *Risk for ineffective therapeutic management regimen: individuals* would be appropriate in those circumstances.

Use care to differentiate among *Ineffective manage-*

ment of therapeutic regimen, Noncompliance, and *Altered health maintenance,* as shown in the accompanying Decision Tree.

Which of the diagnoses described above would you use for Mr. Kitchen? Consider whether he lacks knowledge, whether he is unsuccessful in his efforts, or whether he has chosen not to comply with the therapeutic regimen. Do you believe Mr. Kitchen has made an informed decision not to follow the therapeutic regimen?

PLANNING

The overall expected outcome for intervention to help the client manage a therapeutic regimen is that the client achieves the desired goals of the treatment plan. Outcomes related to successful movement toward achievement of treatment goals are the following:

- The client makes effective choices in integrating the treatment plan into activities of daily living and actively participates in the regimen as prescribed.
- The client seeks help as needed from family members, support groups, and/or health care providers.
- The client expresses positive ways of dealing with stress and conflict.

INTERVENTION

Managing a therapeutic regimen occurs in the context of a person's lifestyle. It can require changing patterns of living or incorporating therapeutic management into present patterns of living. It also involves overcoming physical and psychological barriers to compliance with the therapeutic regimen. Nursing interventions for clients who are having difficulty managing a therapeutic regimen include assistance with lifestyle changes and with specific aspects of the therapeutic regimen. Nursing care uses the principles of motivation and supportive care while providing the client with education, behavior modification, motivation, and therapeutic relationships.

Interventions to Motivate Health Behaviors

Motivating clients toward more effective management of the therapeutic regimen is based on increasing the client's self-efficacy and beliefs in the value of the therapeutic regimen. Consequently, you will want to design activities needed to manage the therapeutic regimen so that they produce minimal conflict with the client's lifestyle and value system.

Increasing Knowledge Level

Although knowledge is not sufficient to produce motivation, it remains a key issue in increasing self-efficacy. The goal is to provide knowledge that will be essential in making informed decisions regarding lifestyles and health promotion practices. The purpose of health education is to facilitate client decision-making regarding personal health behaviors, use of health resources, and general health issues. Teaching a client to plan meals is one example of how to educate the client. Health education is the primary intervention for the promotion and maintenance of health in individuals, families, groups, and communities (Fig. 25–2).

Knowledge helps the client recognize susceptibility to an illness or the consequences of an illness along with the potential severity of the consequences. The individualized educational plan must be focused on

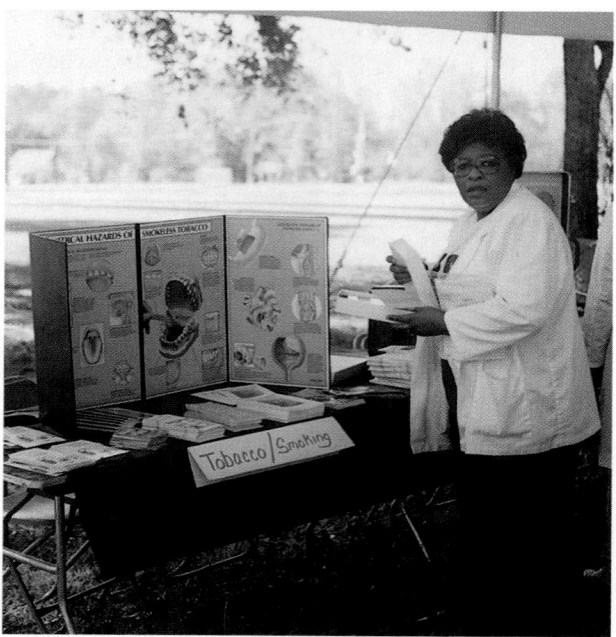

Figure 25–2. Health education is the primary intervention for promoting and maintaining health in individuals, families, groups, and communities. This nurse is participating in a community health fair to educate participants in the far-reaching physical changes caused by cigarette-smoking.

increasing awareness of the relationships between the client's specific unhealthy lifestyles (such as tobacco use, poor nutritional habits, excessive alcohol use, drug misuse or abuse, lack of exercise, stress, irresponsible sexual activities, and environmental hazards) and the development of health problems. The Teaching for Wellness chart offers an example of a way to increase a client's knowledge, in this case about how to lose weight.

Knowledge helps the client weigh benefits against risks. The risks involved with health care regimens are side effects, inconveniences, changes in lifestyle, and possibly criticism from family, friends, or coworkers. Benefits can include prolonged life, better quality of life, reduced symptoms, and a return to former activities.

Knowledge contributes to feelings of control. For clients with an internal locus of control, participation in the decision-making process is important. Even when the physician needs to be the primary decision-maker, understanding how health care providers are making decisions contributes to a feeling of participating in the decision-making process. For clients with an external locus of control, knowledge may help them recognize factors that can be internally controlled, thus increasing self-efficacy.

Clarifying Values

Values and beliefs play a role in the decision and motivation to follow a health care regimen. *Values clarification* is a self-discovery process that allows a person to find answers to situations or arrive at freely chosen

Teaching for WELLNESS

HELPING A CLIENT LOSE WEIGHT

Purpose: To support the client's motivation to lose weight through recognition of risk factors and a simple regimen.

Rationale: Overweight and poor nutrition are risk factors for such chronic diseases as heart disease, certain cancers, diabetes, arthritis, and osteoporosis. Most people who are overweight know that excessive consumption of fat and calories can lead to poor health. Teaching should support the client's maintenance of a healthy diet and exercise program.

Expected Outcome: The client will develop a plan to lose weight.

Client Instructions

1. In planning for weight loss, make nutritional adequacy your top priority. Most people cannot maintain nutritional adequacy on less than 1,200 calories a day, so you should plan to consume no less than that. To maintain weight, most adults need 2,200 and 2,500 calories per day, although older adults need less.

2. Keep in mind that you will experience a healthier, more successful weight loss with a small energy deficit that provides an adequate intake than with a large energy deficit that creates feelings of starvation and deprivation. These feelings can lead to an irresistible urge to binge.

3. Keep meals small and avoid long periods without food.

4. Choose a diet with plenty of vegetables, fruits, and grain products.

5. Drink plenty of fluids between meals.

6. Avoid foods that are greasy, fried, or highly spiced.

7. Weight loss alone can lower your cholesterol level, decrease your blood pressure, increase your energy level, and lessen joint pain. However, a regular exercise program will enhance these benefits as well as promote self-esteem, reduce the risk of heart disease, and encourage the loss of extra pounds.

8. If you are over 35, have heart trouble, or are taking medicine for high blood pressure, see a doctor before you start a physical exercise program.

9. Initiate your exercise program slowly and build up your activity level gradually.

10. Exercise at least for 20 minutes four times a week.

11. Listen to your body. Pay attention to warning signals, such as sudden dizziness, cold sweats, fainting, or pressure in the chest.

---

values. This process allows the person to determine what choices to make when faced with alternatives. The primary goal is to help the client sort out feelings and clarify meanings by listening to the client's comments and the reason for them.

In relation to lifestyle management, this involves helping the client develop self-awareness related to attitudes and beliefs held regarding smoking, overeating, or other unhealthy lifestyle habits. Help the client identify and examine all available alternatives when faced with choices regarding an unhealthy lifestyle. Guide the client through an examination of consequences associated with each choice to help promote informed decision-making. The goal is to get the client to the point of accepting primary responsibility for making healthy lifestyle choices.

Action Alert!
Accept the client's choice or point of view, even if it appears to be self-destructive, such as a decision to continue smoking. Confrontation is not beneficial and may actually be detrimental to further cooperation and goal achievement.

Recall that Mr. Kitchen continues to smoke despite his problems with edema and shortness of breath. Although Mr. Kitchen would benefit from a smoking cessation class, the nurse should also recognize that he may be depressed and lonely. Because his wife managed his health care, he may also lack the knowledge to follow through on his care. It may be difficult for him to relate to the clinic staff, and he may believe it is acceptable to stop medications if he feels better.

The clinic staff might try a follow-up telephone call a week before Mr. Kitchen's scheduled appointment to determine how the therapeutic regimen is progressing. Can you think of other ways to help Mr. Kitchen?

Engaging Participation

Active participation in learning typically increases learning and motivation. **Counseling** is a method of communication that actively involves the client in the recognition of personal risk factors and management of necessary behavioral changes (Fig. 25–3). Counseling is different from education in that it involves guiding the client through decision-making rather than merely ensuring that he has the knowledge to make a decision.

During counseling, the client is the major role-player in identifying and clarifying the problem to be solved. This involves engaging the client in a dialogue to identify the problem and examine factors that con-

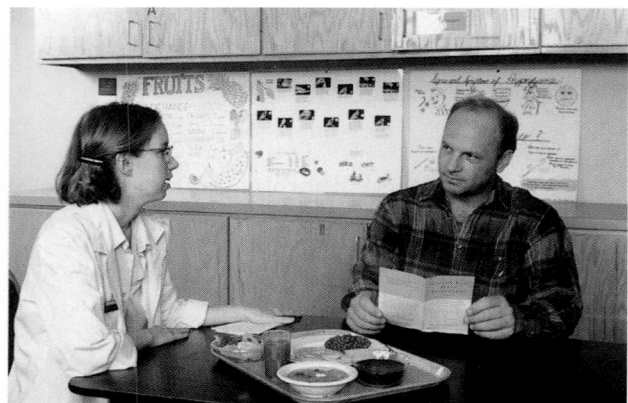

Figure 25–3. Counseling is a method of communication that helps clients recognize personal risk factors and manage necessary behavioral changes.

tribute to the problem and those that may enhance or block its resolution. When counseling, do not tell the client what to do to solve the problem but instead assist and guide the problem-solving or decision-making process.

Because many people lack the knowledge or skills to approach a problem systematically, teaching and counseling can be combined to help the client solve the dilemma successfully. If the health history reveals that the client is at risk for a sexually transmitted disease, health education would involve providing didactic information to help the person avoid infection. Counseling would involve greater interaction with the client and would entail helping him identify his risk for the infection and develop a plan to reduce the risk. Counseling should be tailored to the individual risk factors, needs, and abilities of each client.

Anticipating Problems

Anticipate problems the client may have in managing the therapeutic regimen. If the client is illiterate, has poor eyesight, has decreased mobility, or has decreased manual dexterity, you can help plan for alternative methods of managing the therapeutic regimen. You can also anticipate side effects of medication and help plan ways to manage them.

Providing Reinforcing Factors

Help the client find motivation from life goals, or desirable activities. Playing with grandchildren, traveling to Europe, attending a child's graduation from college, or caring for an elderly parent are among the important activities of life that can motivate a person to work toward better health. If the client does not have motivating factors, you can help him set personal goals that will serve as a reward for effective management of the therapeutic regimen. Rewards can be achieving a major long-term goal or engaging in small daily or weekly pleasures.

Interventions to Provide Supportive Care

Changing lifestyle behaviors to manage a therapeutic regimen can be a complex problem. Although the client may initially have strong motivation and expect to be able to make the changes, continued support from family and health care providers is often necessary to sustain the changes.

Establishing a Therapeutic Relationship

The single most influential factor in increasing the client's participation in effective management of a therapeutic regimen is the relationship with the health care provider. Give the client individual attention by providing information in a face-to-face, two-way communication with the client.

Probe for the client's level of understanding and perspective of the problem. A common and sometimes mistaken practice in providing information to the client is to wait for the client to ask questions. The assumption is that the client may not want to know everything and will ask the questions that are of the most concern. However, the client may not know what to ask and may not have enough information even to form the questions. Only after you have learned how the client perceives the problem can you offer information that deals with the client's often unspoken concerns.

Guiding the Client Through the Health System

A major focus of nursing care is to promote, provide, and assist the client in receiving the health care necessary to achieve and maintain health. Lifestyle behavioral changes may require the client to seek services from several health care agencies. Getting to and through these systems can prove to be unmanageable for many clients. Plus, the client may encounter constraints that impede or prevent him from using health care services.

Helping the client identify services available to assist in meeting desired goals should be the initial step. Determine the client's eligibility, as well as the fees involved and methods of payment, to help make sure that services are available and affordable. Identify constraints that may be involved, such as lack of transportation, cultural beliefs, and the ability to communicate. As much as possible, prepare the client to make the best use of services available.

The initial step is to help the client recognize the need for these services. A client who is in denial will not see the need for or benefit of services. When the client has acknowledged and accepted the problem, then discuss the services that are available. Give the client necessary information about the agencies involved to help ease his entry into the system.

Planning for Discharge

As defined in Chapter 12, *discharge planning* is the preparation for moving a client from one level of care

A PATIENT'S VIEW

NURSES NEED TO BE AWARE THAT PATIENTS DEPEND ON THEM TO COME IN CLOSER THAN MOST DOCTORS WILL

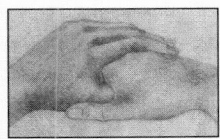 Eight years ago I was dying, hospitalized with *Pneumocystis carinii* pneumonia. I was 36 years old and alone with my secret: HIV/AIDS. I had lived with that secret for 2 years, fearing discovery by my family, my company, the government. Disclosing my diagnosis would also mean disclosing that I am gay to my coworkers. Feeling that it was a death sentence anyway, I didn't seek treatment until I got really sick.

Today, I am healthy, perhaps not the way some people would define "healthy," but I am living, not dying. New drugs and new connections to the community have made all the difference. All my fears of disclosure proved to be unfounded. My family, my friends, my coworkers have all been totally supportive, even though some of them had never known a gay or HIV-positive man before. And though I live alone, every area of my life is filled with support.

Four years ago all my medication options were exhausted. I was very weak and preparing to die when 3TC became available. It was effective in my case and was followed by the first protease inhibitor, which made me even healthier. But just as important as the drugs was reaching out to the HIV/AIDS community for support. That gave my whole life a new direction. I had been fairly closeted before I got sick. When my health began to improve, I saw it as a second chance. After discussions with my sister, I walked into an HIV/AIDS support group, and it's proved to be one of the most important things I ever did.

My support group is sponsored by a church, but you don't have to be a church member to belong to the group. There are 10 of us, and we have two co-facilitators, but it's mostly peer support, both emotional and spiritual, and it's an education. We exchange information about our counts, T-cells, viral loads, and about treatment—what's working, what's not, what's new on the horizon in terms of drug treatment. This weekly infusion of friendship and camaraderie and knowledge sustains me.

Living with AIDS gives new meaning to "continuing education." Survival means continuing to learn about your disease and about treatment options. Fortunately, we have resources like Project Inform in San Francisco.[1] I can't tell you how many times I've called their hotline. The AIDS community has taught me to be a fully informed participant in treatment decisions, a partner with my doctor and with my nurse practitioner. You need to have health professionals you get along with and feel close to. I see my doctor once a month, and when my counts are going in the wrong direction or the

symptoms or the side effects are getting worse, we talk about what the options are. I worry about using up all my options before something new comes along.

Right now I'm taking 18 to 20 pills a day, some to prevent opportunistic infections, some to control the virus, some to help with side effects of the other medications. Fortunately, the pills I'm on now can be taken with food, so that makes it easier. But included with these medications is a liquid that tastes so horrible I have to drink maple syrup before and after to coat my tastebuds. Most of the medications have side effects. The most serious for me are chronic diarrhea and severe neuropathy (numbness) in my feet and fingers. Right now I'm taking Norontin, an antiseizure drug, to counteract the neuropathy. Unfortunately, there's nothing to counteract the chronic, uncontrollable diarrhea and fatigue, so those are just things I have to live with. Orchestrating the many medications I take on a daily basis is almost a full-time job.

These symptoms make it impossible to work even part-time so I'm on disability. When I'm feeling well enough, I volunteer in the AIDS community. For example, I provided support for a fellow who was in the Interleukin 2 trial at the National Institutes of Health and needed a weekly caregiver once a month for a year. He wanted to stay alive for his daughter who also has HIV, and my support helped him get the treatment he needed.

Nurses have been some of my greatest supporters, not just when I was hospitalized but afterward. Maybe I'm just lucky, but I've never encountered homophobia among nurses. When I went home after pneumocystis, I needed nightly infusions for 2 weeks. My Korean nurse had never met a gay man before, but she couldn't have been more supportive and understanding. She would bring me home-cooked Korean food and spend time with me. We exchanged cards and letters for a long time afterward.

My nurse practitioner is the one I'm closest to—I look forward to seeing her every month. Nurses need to be aware that patients depend on them to come in closer than most doctors will, and that this helps not only physically but mentally and emotionally as well. One of the most important things nurses do is teach—providing practical information about HIV-friendly doctors and about resources such as Project Inform and resources in the community. Just a list of phone numbers can make a huge difference, especially when you're alone and afraid. The Consolidated Omnibus Reconciliation Act of 1985 guarantees the right to insurance for 18 months after separation from a COBRA employer.

(continued)

A PATIENT'S VIEW

NURSES NEED TO BE AWARE THAT PATIENTS DEPEND ON THEM TO COME IN CLOSER THAN MOST DOCTORS WILL (continued)

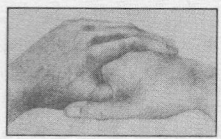

I try to be upbeat, and the support I get from my group and from other friends makes that possible most of the time. But it's easy to get very depressed. I've lost many close friends to this disease. And you live in a world of needles, pills, and paperwork: every month, 8 vials of blood drawn, 12 prescriptions refilled. Some of my medications are covered through a state insurance plan, but many are not. I lost my health insurance when I left work. After 18 months on COBRA, I had to go on Medicare. Fortunately, I had a long-term disability policy so that enables me to scrape by financially.

I'm living, not dying. And I'm grateful for a second chance to get things right, to accept myself for who I am, and to see that acceptance reflected in the eyes of others.

[1]Project Inform Hotline is staffed by trained volunteers, many of them HIV-positive. 1-800-822-7422 (national); 1-800-334-7422 (California). Call 10 AM–4 PM Monday–Friday; 10 AM–1 PM Saturday (Pacific Time).

to another within or outside the current health care agency. It is a systematic process of preparing clients and family members to manage therapeutic regimens and to engage in health maintenance activities once they leave the hospital or other health care delivery system. The objectives of discharge planning are to do the following:

- Make sure that there will be no interruption in the implementation of the therapeutic regimen.
- Provide adequate teaching and instruction or additional demonstrations of procedures to manage the therapeutic regimen.
- Identify or familiarize the client and family with appropriate resources to ensure continuity of care.

The client and his family should be actively involved in the planning process and in all decision-making. Goals to manage the therapeutic regimen should be set between the client, nurse, and family.

Although discharge planning should begin at the time of admission to allow for adequate teaching and preparation, an assessment of the needs of the client and family should be made immediately before discharge to determine additional services and teaching needs. Since most clients stay fewer days in the hospital than they once did, the scope and complexity of the discharge planning may be increased. Different clients have a differing complexity of needs as well. For example, a client being discharged from a substance abuse treatment center would require a more complex discharge plan than a middle-aged client being discharged from an emergency department with a fractured wrist. The substance abuser will require additional community resources, such as substance abuse counselors, a support group, and family members to assist in managing the treatment plan and the related lifestyle changes needed to remain free of drugs.

During your predischarge assessment, pay attention to any statements that could indicate a potential for ineffective management of health or a health plan, such as an unwillingness or an inability to modify personal habits and integrate necessary treatments into the lifestyle. Failure to adhere to a treatment plan while hospitalized (such as refusal to take medication, walk, or follow dietary modification) would suggest a potential for ineffective management of therapeutic regimen after discharge.

Referring to Health Services

Referral is a process designed to provide the client with access to health care and supportive services that are not available from the sending institution. The referral process begins after assessment data reveal a need for additional services. Referrals are made for many reasons. A client with chronic obstructive pulmonary disorder who continues to smoke, for example, may be referred to a smoking cessation class. When altered nutritional intake appears to be a family problem, the family may be referred to a nutritionist. An adolescent who shows evidence of anorexia nervosa may be referred to a clinical psychologist or physician. If the assessment data indicate that the client has not completed immunizations for his age group, the client should be referred to the local health department.

As in discharge planning, the client and family should be involved in the decision for referral. This is important in facilitating the client's follow-through. If the referral is recognized by the client as being insignificant, the client probably will not follow through.

Several factors must be taken into consideration when planning for referral. The referred source must be acceptable to the client and it must be specific to the needs of the client. Some clients will not use services that are perceived as "charity" or "demoralizing." For example, a client who is overweight may perceive different implications if referred to "Overeaters Anonymous" instead of "Weight Watchers." Also, the client must be eligible for the services. Services that are designed for Medicare or Medicaid clients will not provide services to people who do not meet the appropriate criteria.

To be effective in making referrals, you will need to know about resources in the client's community, including the location of services, name and telephone number of a contact person, types of services provided, eligibility criteria, operating hours, and a general overview of fees required. When making a referral, give the client all necessary information. Call ahead to make the appointment if you think it will encourage the client to follow through.

Promoting Social Support

An assessment of social support involves an analysis of the client's social network to ascertain actual and potential sources of social support, the client's perception of social support, and the specific helping behaviors that would be of assistance to the client. Help the client make this assessment and develop the social support structure to facilitate lifestyle behavioral changes or incorporate a therapeutic regimen into daily life. Help the client clarify his expectations of support persons and the type of support he needs. Encourage open communication of needs among family members, goal setting, and identification of strategies to be implemented to achieve goals.

Action Alert!
Assess current actions of significant others and how they are received by the client. When significant others try to be helpful, does the client perceive them as being helpful? Also assess whether significant others are withdrawn or too protective.

In addition to family and friends, a support group may be helpful with smoking cessation, adjusting dietary habits, or participating in an exercise program. Social support can be provided through groups. Group sessions provide an opportunity for clients to share the experiences of others in changing behaviors.

EVALUATION

Evaluation involves reassessing the client to determine whether all outcomes were achieved. The outcomes will have been achieved if the client reports participation in activities to increase knowledge of health promotion. Participation in these activities could entail attending classes at the local health center or health department; seeking health information through the media, such as newspaper or television; and building knowledge of preventable diseases and related risk factors.

Additionally, the client may express a desire to achieve optimal health by participating in health screening clinics or learning to perform self-examinations (Fig. 25–4). Reducing the number of risk factors or being successful in integrating the treatment plan into daily life indicates that the client has achieved the outcomes for effective management of therapeutic regimen. The client should be reassessed for the establishment of new goals.

If no noticeable change occurs in unhealthy behaviors within a reasonable period, or if the client returns

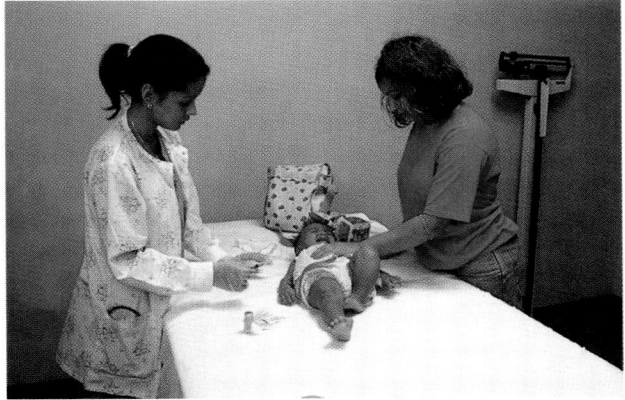

Figure 25–4. Health screening is a primary strategy used to promote health. The young mother at right understands the importance of health screening in achieving optimal health for her child. During a routine screening visit, the nurse at left has identified the need to update the child's immunizations.

with an exacerbation of symptoms, reassess the client to determine what prevented his progress. For example, a client that has successfully followed a reduced-calorie nutritional program may not show a weight loss during the first week because of medications that have fluid retention properties or other physiological alterations.

KEY PRINCIPLES

- Understanding health from the sometimes opposing perspectives of the client and provider is critical to the development of health services and nursing interventions.
- Concepts that differ across cultures include an explanatory model of illness that defines the nature of illness, its treatment, and the type of relationships that should occur between client and health care provider.
- There are two domains of health care: the folk, or generic, form and the scientific form.
- The theory of reasoned action is based on the assumption that people are reasonable and, in deciding what action to take, systematically process and use the information available to them.
- The transtheoretical model of behavioral change is useful across all theories to plan interventions that are appropriate to the stage of change: precontemplation, contemplation, preparation, action, maintenance, and termination.
- In the health belief model, behavior is a function of the subjective value of an outcome and of the subjective expectation that a particular action will achieve that outcome.
- The health promotion model uses concepts from the health belief model but decreases the focus on threats as an avenue to behavioral change.
- Factors affecting behavioral change affect the relationship with the health care provider. They in-

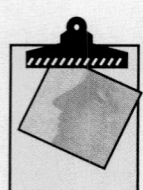

NURSING CARE PLANNING
A CLIENT WITH HEART FAILURE

Mr. Oscar Kitchen is a 69-year-old black male who is being seen in a primary health care center. This is his second visit, where he has presented with shortness of breath and edema of the lower limbs. The doctor has told him to stay on the same medication for his heart and a diuretic. With proper instructions, he believes Mr. Kitchen can manage the therapeutic regimen at home.

Physician's Orders

Admitting diagnosis: Chronic heart failure	Lasix 20 mg PO daily every morning
Digoxin 0.125 mg PO daily every morning	Low Na diet
Hygroton 25 mg PO daily every morning	Return to clinic in 2 weeks

Nursing Assessment

BP 160/98, pulse 98, respiration 32 and labored. Ht. 5' 11.5", weight 220 lb. 3+ pitting of lower extremities. Widower of 3 months. Wife previously assisted in management of health care regimen. No close relatives living near. Very little interaction with neighbors. Smokes two packs of cigarettes each day. Has smoked for 55 years.

NURSING CARE PLAN

Nursing Diagnosis	Expected Outcomes	Interventions	Evaluation (Initial Response to Intervention)
Ineffective management of therapeutic regimen: individuals, related to the following: (A) knowledge deficit regarding current diagnosis, medications, and consequences of failure to comply with treatment and	The client will demonstrate the potential for effective management of therapeutic regimen as evidenced by: Shows willingness to learn about his illness and participate in treatment	Determine client's understanding of his illness. Start with information he provides and explain chronic heart failure in very simple terms.	Mr. Kitchen agrees he would like to get rid of the swelling in his legs and will take his water pill and elevate his legs twice a day for 20 minutes. He stated, "I guess when you get old your heart just gives out."
	Makes a schedule of planned times to take medications that work best for him	Explain purpose of medications and consequences if medications are not taken.	Client says that he can remember to take medications.

clude communication, cognition and perception, age and developmental level, life style and habits, economic resources, cultural values and beliefs, roles and relationships, coping and stress tolerance, and workplace and environmental conditions.

- Lack of education about nutrition, safety, fitness, or health-protecting practices during early childhood or adolescence can have a significant impact on adult health.
- Wellness assessment focuses on physical fitness evaluation, health risk appraisal, social support systems, and lifestyle assessment.
- Assessment for behavioral change requires assessing the client's level of knowledge.

- Assessment for *Ineffective management of therapeutic regimen* often relies on indirect cues suggesting that the client needs to improve the management of the therapeutic regimen.
- The health care system can be a related factor for *Ineffective management of therapeutic regimen.*
- Educational interventions aimed at improving behavior can reduce at-risk behaviors.
- Motivation, locus of control, health perception, and one's sense of self-efficacy affect participation in activities to promote or maintain health.
- Nursing interventions for *Altered health maintenance* would include activities to help the client promote and maintain health through education, health screening, and counseling.

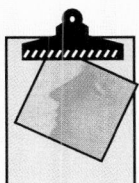

NURSING CARE PLANNING
A CLIENT WITH HEART FAILURE *(continued)*

NURSING CARE PLAN

Nursing Diagnosis	Expected Outcomes	Interventions	Evaluation (Initial Response to Intervention)
	Statements reflecting an understanding of the implications of not following the prescribed treatment	Determine the reasons why Mr. Kitchen does not take his medication.	Client says "That's the pill that makes me pass my water so often. I can't take it. It's hard on an old man to go to the bathroom so often."
	Statements reflecting an understanding of the effect of sodium on his condition	Assess dietary pattern and methods of preparing food. Explain the effect of eating foods high in sodium. Help client identify low-sodium foods he likes.	Mr. Kitchen says, "I can't cook foods like that. The 'missus' always took care of the cooking. She's gone now. The lady next door brings me something to eat every now and then."
(B) unhealthy lifestyle (smoking)	Statements indicating an interest in identifying resources for smoking cessation	*Help Mr. Kitchen find a support group for smoking cessation that has members with similar values and interests.*	Mr. Kitchen agrees to go to a smoking cessation group with his friend, but he is not yet committed to smoking cessation.
	Lists several ways to gradually reduce the number of cigarettes smoked	Help client identify ways to reduce the number of cigarettes smoked per day.	Mr. Kitchen states, "I have cut back. I only smoke after meals now."

Italicized interventions indicate culturally specific care.

Critical Thinking Questions
1. Which is the priority nursing intervention? What is the rationale for your choice?
2. Can you think of other ways the nurse could have incorporated Mr. Kitchen's culture into his care? How would you change your approach if the client was of Hispanic origin or Vietnamese origin?
3. How could the client be motivated to change behavior and accept responsibility for a more healthy lifestyle?

- Nursing interventions for *Ineffective management of therapeutic regimen* include client teaching about the current illness and treatment regimen, supporting the client's well-being through stress-management skills, and promoting health management choices through values clarification.
- Although knowledge is not sufficient to produce motivation, it remains a key issue in increasing self-efficacy.
- Knowledge helps the client recognize susceptibility to an illness or the consequences of an illness along with the potential severity of the consequences.
- Values clarification is a self-discovery process that allows the person to make choices when faced with alternatives.

- Active participation in learning is expected to increase learning and motivation.
- Anticipation of problems is an effective teaching tool for complex health care regimens.
- The single most influential factor in increasing the client's participation in effective management of a therapeutic regimen is the relationship with the health care provider.
- The objectives of discharge planning are to ensure that there will be no interruption in implementation, to provide adequate teaching, and to familiarize the client with appropriate resources.
- Social support is a key element in health promotion activities.

BIBLIOGRAPHY

*Amber, R.W. & Moriarty, D.G. (1988). *Healthier people: The Carter Center of Emory University health risk appraisal program guides and documentation.* Atlanta: The Carter Center of Atlanta University.

*Anderson, A. (1988). Cognitive styles and multicultural populations. *Journal of Teacher Education, 39*(1), 2–9.

*Bandura, A. (1977). Self-efficacy: Toward a unifying theory of behavioral change. *Psychological Review, 84,* 191–215.

*Becker, D., Hill, D., Jackson, J., Levine, D., Stillman, F., Weiss, S. (1992). Health behavior research in minority populations: Access, design and implementation. PHS, UHHS: National Heart, Lung and Blood Institute. *NIH Publication No. 92-2965.* Washington, DC: National Institutes of Health.

Carpenito, L.J. (1995). *Nursing diagnosis: Application to clinical practice.* Philadelphia: J.B. Lippincott Co.

*Centers for Disease Control (1984). *CDC health risk appraisal user manual.* Pub. No. 746-011/15233. Atlanta, GA: CDC Division of Health Education; U.S. Government Printing Office

Clark, M. (1996). *Nursing in the community* (2nd ed.). Stamford, CT: Appleton & Lange.

Cookfair, J. (1996). *Nursing care in the community* (2nd ed.). Boston, MA: Mosby.

*Fishbein, M. & Middlestadt, S. (1989). Using the theory of reasoned action as a framework for understanding and changing AIDs-related behaviors. In V. Mays, G. Albee, & S. Schneider (Eds), *Primary prevention of AIDS: Psychological approaches* (pp. 93–110). Newbury Park, CA: Sage.

*Frank-Stromborg, M. (1992). *Instruments for clinical nursing research.* Boston, MA: Jones & Bartlett.

Getzen, T.E. (1997). *Health economics: Fundamentals and flow of funds.* New York: John Wiley & Sons, Inc.

Giger, J.N. & Davidhizar, R.E. (1995). *Transcultural nursing: Assessment and Intervention* (2nd ed.). St. Louis, MO: Mosby.

*Green, L.W. & Kreuter, M.W. (1992). CDC's planned approach to community health as an application or PRECEDE and an inspiration for PROCEED. *Journal of Health Education, 23*(3), 140–147.

*Hartsock, N. (1983). The feminist standpoint: Developing the ground for a specifically feminist historical materialism. In S. Harding & M.B. Hintikka (Eds), *Discovering reality: Feminist perspectives on epistemology, metaphysics, methodology, and philosophy of science* (pp. 283–310). Boston, MA: D. Reidel Publishing Company.

*Asterisk indicates a classic or definitive work on this subject.

*Kavanagh, K.H. & Kennedy, P.H. (1992). *Promoting cultural diversity: Strategies for health care professionals.* Newbury Park, CA: Sage.

*Klienman, A., Eisenberg, L., & Good, B. (1978). Culture, illness, and care. *Annals of Internal Medicine, 88,* 251–258.

Kulbok, P.A., Laffrey, S.C., & Goeppinger, J. (1996). Community health promotion: A multilevel framework for practice. In M. Stanhope & J. Lancaster (Eds.), *Community health nursing: Promoting health of aggregates, families, and individuals* (4th ed.). St Louis, MO: Mosby.

Lancaster, J., Onega, L., & Forness, D. (1996). In M. Stanhope & J. Lancaster (Eds.), *Community health nursing: Promoting health of aggregates, families, and individuals* (4th ed.). St. Louis, MO: Mosby.

*Leininger, M.M. (1991). *Culture care diversity & universality: A theory of nursing.* New York: National League for Nursing Press.

*Leininger, M.M. (1970). *Nursing and anthropology: Two worlds to blend.* New York: John Wiley & Sons, Inc.

North American Nursing Diagnosis Association. (1999). *NANDA Nursing diagnoses: Definitions and classification 1999–2000.* Philadelphia: Author.

Pender, N.J. (1996). *Health promotion in nursing practice* (3rd ed.). Stamford, CT: Appleton & Lange.

*Prochaska, J.O., Velicer, W.F., Rossi, J.S., Goldstein, M.G., Marcus, B.H., Rakowski, W., Fiore, C., Harlow, L.L., Redding, C.A., Rosenbloom, D., & Rossi, S.R. (1994). Stages of change and decisional balance for 12 problem behaviors. *Health Psychology, 13*(1), 39–46.

*Rosenstock, J. (1974). Historical origins of the health belief model. *Health Education Monograph, 2*(4), 328–335.

*Spector, R. (1991). *Cultural diversity in health and illness* (3rd ed.). Norwalk, CT: Appleton & Lange: .

Stanhope, M. & Lancaster, J. (1996). *Community health nursing: Promoting health of aggregates, families, and individuals* (4th ed.). St. Louis, MO: Mosby.

*Thomas, S. (1992). The health of the black community in the twenty-first century: A futuristic perspective. In R.L. Braithwaite & S.E. Taylor (Eds.), *Health issues in the black community.* San Francisco: Jossey-Bass Publishers.

*Tripp-Reimer, T. (1984). Reconceptualizing the concept of health: Integrating emic and etic perspectives. *Research, Nursing & Health, 7,* 101–109.

*Walker, S.N., Sechrist, K.R., & Pender, N.J. (1987). The health-promoting lifestyle profile: Development and psychometric characteristics. *Nursing Research, 36*(2), 76–81.

Woolf, S., Jonas, S., & Lawrence, R. (1996). *Health promotion and disease prevention in clinical practice.* Baltimore, MD: Williams & Wilkins.

26

Health Maintenance: Medication Management

Mary Ann Hogan

Key Terms

adverse effect
anaphylaxis
antagonistic effect
biotransformation
chemical name
controlled substance
generic name
hypersensitivity reaction
idiosyncratic response
intradermal route
intramuscular route
intravenous route
loading dose

official name
parenteral route
pharmacokinetics
prescription
side effect
subcutaneous route
synergistic effect
target organ
teratogenic potential
therapeutic effect
topical route
toxic effect
trade name

LEARNING OBJECTIVES

After studying this chapter, you should be able to:

1. **Discuss important concepts related to safe and effective medication management.**

2. **Describe a variety of factors that influence drug actions in individual clients.**

3. **Explain how to assess a client who is receiving medication therapy.**

4. **Formulate appropriate nursing diagnosis statements for a client receiving medications.**

5. **Plan appropriate expected outcomes for a client taking medications.**

6. **Incorporate safe and effective nursing interventions for a client receiving medications.**

7. **Evaluate the effectiveness of medication therapy on goals formulated to improve a client's health.**

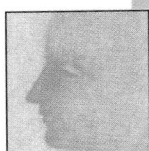

Daniel Connell is a 62-year-old Irish-American. He is married and lives at home with his wife. He came to the emergency department (ED) after experiencing chest pain while carrying an air conditioner up two flights of stairs to the attic. Upon arrival at the ED, his pulse was 96, blood pressure was 166/96, respirations were 22, and oral temperature was 98.8°F. Mr. Connell described the chest pain as a "pressure," and gave it a rating of 6 on a 0–10 pain scale. The pain did not worsen with inspiration. It was relieved in the ED with nitroglycerin.

Results of serum laboratory studies and electrocardiogram showed that Mr. Connell did not have a myocardial infarction (heart attack). By taking a more thorough history, the ED nurse learns that Mr. Connell has hypertension but has not been taking prescribed medications. His dietary intake is high in sodium, and he does not exercise regularly. Knowing that Mr. Connell is not doing what is necessary to control his health problems, the nurse considers the diagnosis of *Altered health maintenance.* The nurse also considers other nursing diagnoses that may apply to Mr. Connell's situation, such as *Ineffective management of therapeutic regimen* and *Noncompliance* (see the Nursing Diagnoses chart).

MEDICATION ADMINISTRATION NURSING DIAGNOSES

Altered Health Maintenance: Inability to identify, manage, and/or seek out help to maintain health.

Ineffective Management of Therapeutic Regimen: A pattern of regulating and integrating into daily living a program for treatment of illness and the sequelae of illness that is unsatisfactory for meeting specific health goals.

Noncompliance: The extent to which a person's and/or caregiver's behavior coincides or fails to coincide with a health-promoting or therapeutic plan agreed upon by the person (and/or family, and/or community) and health care professional. In the presence of an agreed-upon, health-promoting or therapeutic plan, person's or caregiver's behavior may be fully, partially, or nonadherent and may lead to clinically effective, partially effective, or ineffective outcomes.

North American Nursing Diagnosis Association. (1999). NANDA nursing diagnoses: Definitions and classification 1999–2000. Philadelphia: Author.

CONCEPTS OF MEDICATION MANAGEMENT

Medication administration is a critically important part of the nurse's role. Many clients take medication as part of the therapeutic regimen for health problems. This chapter examines what the client needs to know, and what you need to know, about medication therapy.

Drug Names and Forms

The terms *drug* and *medication* are often used interchangeably, although technically they differ. A *drug* is a chemical substance that alters the function of an organism and may or may not have a therapeutic effect. A *medication* is a drug that is being used for an intended therapeutic effect. Most drugs or medications can be called by several different names. The **chemical name** is of interest to pharmacists and precisely describes the chemical and molecular structure of a medication. This name is often long and complex. For example, the chemical name for acetaminophen (Tylenol) is *N*-acetyl-*para*-aminophenol.

The **generic name** or *nonproprietary name* is the name assigned to a drug when it is first manufactured. This name is assigned by the United States Adopted Names Council. Subsequent manufacturers of the drug then use the same generic name. The **official name** is the name assigned by the Food and Drug Administration (FDA) after approval of a drug and is often the same as the generic name. The official name for a drug refers to how it is listed in the *United States Pharmacopeia* (USP) and *National Formulary* (NF), two publications officially approved by the FDA.

The **trade name,** also known as the brand name or *proprietary name,* is a copyrighted name given by a specific manufacturer to a medication it produces. Because several manufacturers may produce the same medication, that medication may have several trade names in addition to the generic name. It is important that you be familiar with both the generic and the trade names of medications. This may be difficult because of the sheer number of trade names on the market and because generic names are often complex or foreign. For example, acetylsalicylic acid is the generic name for Bayer Aspirin, which has other trade names, including Ecotrin and Empirin.

Prescription and Nonprescription Medications

Medications are grouped into two categories, commonly called prescription medications or nonprescription (also called over-the-counter, or OTC). A **prescription** is an order for a medication that contains the client's name, medication name, dose, route, frequency, amount of the medication to be dispensed, number of refills allowed (if any), and the physician's signature. The physician must sign the prescription and indicate whether a generic brand may be substituted. Prescription drugs should be used under the supervision of a health care provider. Inappropriate use could cause harm or result in abuse.

In some states, revised nurse practice acts have allowed selected groups of advanced practice nurses to write prescriptions. Prescriptive privileges are limited to certified nurse practitioners, nurse anesthetists, nurse midwives, and clinical nurse specialists who work in collaboration with a physician.

A*ction* A*lert!*
Know which groups of health care providers have legal authority to write prescriptions in the state in which you are practicing nursing.

A *nonprescription medication* or *OTC medication* can be purchased without a prescription and can be used to enhance personal health (e.g., vitamins) or to treat common health problems (such as constipation or diarrhea). Nurses and pharmacists have an important role in teaching clients about possible interactive effects between medications.

Classification

Medications with similar characteristics may be classified together according to therapeutic effect (bronchodilators), the symptoms relieved (antianxiety agents), or the clinical actions and composition (narcotic analgesics). Classifications have characteristics in common that can help you understand medications. Some medications have more than one classification, so it is important to understand the drug's purpose for each client.

Drug Forms

Medications are manufactured in a variety of forms to make it more useful or easily administered. Some examples of drug forms include tablets, suspensions, suppositories, and ointments (Table 26–1). The form of a drug guides its route of administration. One form should not be interchanged with another without a specific physician order because the rate of absorption or bioavailability may differ among forms or even among brand names.

Legislation and Standards

Because medications have a great impact on the health and well-being of clients, their manufacture and use is highly regulated. This protects clients from harm and provides a common set of guidelines for personnel in the pharmaceutical and health care industries. All drugs produced in the United States and Canada must meet legal standards for quality control. Health care personnel rely on these standards for providing safe, effective medication therapy.

Pure Food and Drug Act of 1906

In the United States, the Pure Food and Drug Act of 1906 first set standards for the quality and purity of drugs. This Act empowered the FDA to monitor drug standards, such as chemical composition, quality, purity, strength, and form. The standards further required that drugs be adequately packaged and labeled. The United States standards have been updated over time with various pieces of legislation. Current standards have been broadened to include drug safety and effectiveness. State laws may be even stricter than federal standards.

In Canada, similar legislation and standards have been enacted. Refer to a pharmacology textbook for detailed information about key drug legislation in both countries.

Food and Drug Administration

The FDA is the official government agency responsible for determining that drug manufacturers maintain the standards set by law. Its scope of authority spans several areas, including drug testing, approval of drugs for use, and control of drug sale and distribution. It also specifies whether an individual medication is classified as prescription or nonprescription.

If a pharmaceutical company wishes to produce a new drug, it submits a written proposal to the FDA. Controlled studies, known as clinical trials, are then undertaken in four phases to test the drug. If it meets

TABLE 26–1
Common Forms for Drug Preparations

Preparation	General Description
Capsule	Powder or gel form of drug encased in a hard or soft outer casing that dissolves in the stomach
Caplet	A tablet coated with gelatin that dissolves in the stomach
Elixir	Drug dissolved in a clear liquid containing water, varying amounts of alcohol, and a sweetening agent or flavor
Emulsion	Drug in which one liquid is spread by means of small droplets through another liquid
Enteric-coated tablet	A tablet coated with a substance that blocks drug absorption until the tablet reaches the small intestine
Extract	A highly concentrated form of drug made when the active portion is removed from the other drug components
Liniment	Drug combined with alcohol, soap, or oil that is applied to the skin
Lotion	Drug that is dissolved in liquid and applied to the skin
Lozenge or troche	Drug in a flavored or sweet base that is released as the base dissolves in the mouth
Ointment	Semisolid form of a drug that is applied to and absorbed by the skin
Paste	Semisolid form of a drug that is applied to and absorbed by the skin, thicker than an ointment
Patch (transdermal)	Drug encased in a manufactured material that allows continuous drug absorption through the skin at a steady rate
Pill	Drug in powder form mixed in a cohesive material
Powder or granules	A finely ground form of a drug
Solution	Drug that has been dissolved in a liquid, commonly water
Suppository	Drug mixed in a firm base that melts easily when inserted into the rectum, vagina, or urethra
Suspension	Undissolved particles or powder placed in a liquid that must be shaken vigorously before use
Syrup	Drug dissolved in a solution containing water and sugar
Tablet	Solid drug that is compressed or molded into a particular shape and may be swallowed whole, chewed, or placed in the cheek or under the tongue, depending on its purpose
Tincture	A type of solution in which a drug is dissolved in alcohol or a water-alcohol base

required standards, it may be approved for use. This rigorous process explains why drugs that are available in some countries may not be authorized for use in the United States.

Controlled Substances

Control of narcotics and other selected drugs is an important element of drug legislation in both the United States and Canada. **Controlled substances** are drugs that affect the mind or behavior, may be habit forming, and have a high potential for abuse. They include narcotics, barbiturates, and illegal drugs. Controlled drugs are assigned to a specific category ranging from Schedule I to Schedule V. Their distribution and use is either highly regulated or prohibited (Table 26–2).

The Drug Enforcement Agency (DEA) is empowered to enforce narcotic laws. Violations may result in fines, imprisonment, or loss of your nursing license. Health care facilities have detailed policies and procedures for storage, distribution, and record-keeping of controlled substances. Sample guidelines for controlled substance administration by nurses are outlined in Box 26–1. Adherence to these guidelines ensures that your behavior is within the law.

Institutional Policies

Hospitals, extended-care facilities, home health agencies, and other health care facilities have policies and procedures for medication administration that are unique to that facility. You have an obligation to be aware of and comply with your facility's policies and procedures.

Institutional policies must be congruent with the Nurse Practice Act for the state in which the facility is located. The Nurse Practice Act for that state includes specific regulations about the nurse's role in medication administration. It is your legal and professional responsibility to understand the legal foundations of your nursing practice.

Sources of Information

Printed Materials

General information about many medications and their classifications is found in pharmacology texts and other printed references. Several have been written with nurses as the primary audience. There are also several drug references published in handbook form for easy use.

Detailed information about medications can be found in sources such as *American Hospital Formulary Service Drug Information (AHFS DI), Physician's Desk Reference (PDR),* and the *United States Pharmacopeia Drug Information: Drug Information for the Health Care Professional (USP DI).* Most health care institutions use one of these as the facility's official drug reference book. The *AHFS DI* and *PDR* are updated annually; the *USP DI* is updated bimonthly. Canadian publications include the *Canadian Formulary (CF)* and the *Compendium of Pharmaceuticals and Specialties (CPS).*

People

Certain key people are also good sources of drug information. Other experienced nurses and advanced practice nurses are knowledgeable and available to answer your questions during everyday nursing practice. The physician who prescribes a medication can explain why it was ordered for a particular client and its expected action or benefit.

However, pharmacists are a primary source for medication information. Larger institutions, such as hospitals, commonly employ pharmacists who are readily available on-site. Smaller facilities, such as extended-care facilities, usually have a contract with a

TABLE 26–2
Controlled Substance Schedule

Schedule	Explanation	Examples
I	Not accepted for medical use because of their high abuse potential	• Heroin. • LSD. • Marijuana.
II	Have acceptable medical uses but also have a high potential for abuse or physical or psychological dependency	• Amphetamines. • Codeine. • Meperidine (Demerol). • Methadone. • Morphine. • Oxycodone. • Propoxyphene.
III	Have acceptable medical uses and a potential for abuse or dependence that is less than schedule II drugs	• Some codeine preparations.
IV	Have acceptable medical uses with limited risk of abuse or dependence	• Benzodiazepines. • Non-narcotic analgesics. • Phenobarbital.
V	Have medically acceptable uses with minimal risk for abuse or dependence	• Opioid-containing antidiarrheals. • Opioid-containing cough remedies.

BOX 26–1

NARCOTIC ADMINISTRATION AND CONTROL GUIDELINES

- Place all narcotics in the facility-approved double-locked storage area.
- Count narcotics according to facility policy at the beginning and end of each work shift. Have an off-going and an on-coming nurse sign that the count is correct.
- Follow facility protocols for reporting discrepancies in the narcotics count.
- Obtain a key from the designated RN or LPN to gain entry to the narcotics cabinet or use your assigned code if you have a computerized storage system.
- Make an entry in the narcotic inventory when removing a narcotic unless your computerized system does so automatically. This ensures an ongoing record of the number of drugs used and remaining.
- When you sign out a narcotic, record the client's name, the date, the time of administration, the drug name, and the dose needed. Make sure to sign the record. If you have a computerized system, your entry code will serve as your signature.
- Have a second nurse witness the disposal of a partial dose of narcotic. Both of you should sign the record or use your entry codes as your signatures.

specific pharmacy. These pharmacists are generally available by telephone. Pharmacists employed in local pharmacies are yet another source of information and are the resource most often tapped by consumers.

Pharmaceutical sales representatives often have detailed information about medications produced by a specific company, and they are often eager to share information. Keep in mind, however, that their primary objective is sales, not education. Thus, they may readily present the positive aspects of a product while being less vocal about negative ones. They are best used for information about a product's benefits and how to use it for maximum effect.

Computer-Based Resources

Computer-based resources are now also available for drug reference. Use caution when selecting Internet sites, however, because there is no guarantee about the accuracy of information posted on a web site. Some facilities have computer-based resources for medication information available within the facility. An example of this type of resource is *Micromedex,* which provides information about a drug, its dosing, and interdrug reactions for health professionals, as well as aftercare instructions that can be given to clients.

Drug Actions

Mechanism of Action

The mechanism of action is the physiological change caused by the medication and that results in the body's response to the medication. This change alters either the chemistry of the cell environment or the cell itself. It can either increase or decrease the function of the cell.

Many medications exert a therapeutic effect by interacting with cell receptor sites that have a similar chemical shape. When a medication is linked to the receptor site, similar to a lock and key, a chain of physiological events occurs that ends with the intended therapeutic effect. Because the "shape" of some cell receptor sites may be unique to a certain type of tissue, some medications exert an effect only on that tissue. Others have more systemic or widespread effects. When a medication has a specific effect on one type of body tissue, the tissue is said to be the **target organ** for that medication. An example is a diuretic, which targets the kidneys. The route of administration also helps determine whether a medication exerts a more local or systemic effect. For example, a topical medication is more likely to exert a local effect on skin, whereas an intravenous (IV) medication rapidly exerts a systemic effect.

Therapeutic Effect

The **therapeutic effect** is the intended effect or action of the medication. The therapeutic action or effect of a drug is accomplished when a drug interacts with cell mechanisms, producing a change in cellular function. Effective drug therapy helps to cure or control disease (antibiotics), relieve pain or other aggravating symptoms (analgesics or decongestants), prevent disease (immunizations), or promote health (vitamin or mineral supplements). Every drug has at least one therapeutic effect, and some drugs have several. For example, acetaminophen is an analgesic, but it also reduces fever (antipyretic).

Side Effects

Side effects are effects of a medication that are not intended or planned but may occur as a result of use. Side effects can range from mildly unpleasant to harmful. Although all side effects cannot be avoided, teaching methods to reduce common side effects may help the client tolerate the medication, as outlined in the Teaching for Wellness chart.

Adverse Effects

An **adverse effect** is a medication side effect that is potentially harmful to a client. Adverse effects can occur even when taking normal drug doses.

Toxic effects are serious adverse effects of medications that may even threaten life. Some examples are a low heart rate with a cardiac glycoside or wheezing or rash with an antibiotic. Make sure to inform your cli-

Teaching for WELLNESS

AVOIDING COMMON SIDE EFFECTS OF MEDICATION THERAPY

Purpose: To help the client remain free of the most common side effects of a variety of medications.

Rationale: Most medications have a number of side effects listed in the product literature. The use of general health-promoting behaviors can be helpful in preventing or reducing the incidence of these side effects.

Expected Outcome: The client will remain free of common medication side effects or will have less severe side effects if they occur.

Client Instructions

Constipation
Many groups of medications slow the action of the gastrointestinal tract, such as narcotic analgesics, antispasmodics, and iron supplements. The following are helpful hints about actions you can take to decrease your risk of getting constipated while taking these medications:

- Drink plenty of fluids unless contraindicated by another health problem. Try to drink 2 to 3 quarts of fluid a day. Because foods also contain fluid, you will probably obtain a sufficient fluid intake by drinking 6 to 8 glasses of water each day in addition to the normal diet.
- Try to walk or do some other activity that moves and stretches the abdominal muscles each day. This movement "massages" the intestines and increases bowel activity.
- Increase the amount of fiber in your diet. Eat plenty of fruits and vegetables, and include whole grains whenever possible instead of refined carbohydrates.

Sedation
Many medications also cause drowsiness, such as decongestants, some cough preparations, narcotics, and antianxiety agents. Although you may not be able to prevent this side effect, you can modify your activities to reduce the risk of injury while taking these medications. Some suggestions include the following:

- Do not drive or do any other activity that requires concentration for at least the first few hours after taking the medication. Resume these activities only after the drowsiness has worn off.
- Make sure travel paths are sufficiently lighted at night, such as the hallway leading to the bathroom, to prevent falls caused by sedation or reduced vision. Remove scatter rugs or other objects that increase the risk of falls.
- If your take the medication once a day, do so at bedtime, if possible, to minimize the risks associated with sedation.
- Do not drink alcohol or take any other drugs with a sedative effect while taking this medication. Consult with your physician with specific questions for individualized advice.

Dizziness
Because of their effects on blood vessels, many medications taken for cardiovascular problems tend to make you dizzy or lightheaded when you sit up or stand up. The most common ones are antihypertensives and diuretics. If you are taking one of these medications, try to do the following (especially within the first few hours after taking a dose):

- Sit or stand up slowly when rising from the bed or chair.
- Avoid extremely warm environments because they can aggravate the problem by dilating your blood vessels.
- Do not drink alcohol while taking the medication because alcohol dilates blood vessels.
- If you take an antihypertensive medication once a day, do so at night to reduce your dizziness or lightheadedness. If you are taking a diuretic, however, continue to take it in the morning. Taking it at night would interfere with your sleep by making you get up to urinate.

ents about important adverse effects and which ones should prompt a call to the primary care provider.

A toxic effect occasionally results from a single ingestion of a large amount of a drug such as an overdose. When this occurs, the drug must be inactivated or removed from the body to prevent organ damage or death. This is done using activated charcoal in the gastrointestinal (GI) tract (to bind the incompletely absorbed drug) or hemodialysis (for drugs already absorbed or those that cannot be cleared via the GI tract). Other drugs known as *antidotes* may be used to reverse the toxic effect.

Action **A**lert!
If a client is exhibiting toxic effects of a medication, do not administer the next scheduled dose. Immediately report signs and symptoms of toxicity to the physician.

ALLERGIC RESPONSES
An allergic response is an antigen-antibody response to a medication. Although this can occur with the first administration, it requires previous exposure to the antigen to develop antibodies. The allergic response could be triggered by the drug itself, a preservative, or a metabolite.

A **hypersensitivity reaction** is a mild allergic reaction to a drug. Symptoms vary according to the drug and the client, but they typically include skin manifestations, such as rash, urticaria, and pruritus. Headache, rhinitis, or nausea and vomiting may also occur.

Anaphylaxis is a life-threatening allergic reaction that requires immediate intervention to prevent possible death. It is a medical emergency. Symptoms typically are cardiovascular and include dyspnea, wheezing, stridor, tachycardia, and hypotension. They are caused by bronchoconstriction, laryngeal edema, and widespread vasodilatation. Treatment includes supportive care and administration of epinephrine, bronchodilators, antihistamines, and corticosteroids to reduce the allergic response.

A*ction* A*lert!*
If a client begins to exhibit signs of anaphylaxis after receiving a medication, maintain the client's airway and call for help immediately.

Because allergic responses can be serious, carefully question clients about a history of drug allergy. For drugs that are commonly known to be antigenic, such as penicillin, also inquire about a family history of drug allergy. Inquire not only about the drug but about the nature of the allergic response. This information helps determine whether the client could safely receive the drug if given with another drug (such as an antihistamine) or whether it must not be used at all. All clients with a history of drug allergy should wear or carry identification that notes the drug allergy. They should also be taught to inform all future caregivers about the allergy.

IDIOSYNCRATIC RESPONSES
An **idiosyncratic response** is an unexplained and unpredictable response to a medication. It may be a suboptimal response, an exaggerated response, or an abnormal type of response. For example, some medications that normally produce drowsiness cause excitability in children. Idiosyncratic responses may be listed in the drug literature as rare types of adverse effects. Because these are so unpredictable, clients warrant skilled and conscientious nursing assessment.

DRUG TOLERANCE
Drug tolerance refers to the diminishing therapeutic effect of the same dosage of a drug over time, a trend that requires increasing drug dosages to achieve the same therapeutic effect. Tolerance occurs as the body becomes accustomed to a drug from prolonged use. A classic example involves pain medication. Over time, a client taking a narcotic analgesic for chronic pain may require larger doses to control the pain, even if there is no drug addiction. Carefully monitor the degree of symptom relief from a specific dose of a medication, especially if it will be used on a long-term basis.

Drug Interactions

Drug interactions can be either synergistic or antagonistic. A **synergistic effect** occurs when one drug enhances or increases the effect of another drug. This may be accidental or done purposefully by the prescriber. An **antagonistic effect** occurs when one drug reduces or negates the effect of another. Antagonistic effects can also be accidental or purposeful. A client who takes multiple medications (called polypharmacy) is more likely to experience accidental drug interactions, so review the medication regimen carefully.

Other substances, such as alcohol or sodium, can also enhance or interfere with drug action. Teach clients about the effects of these substances on prescribed medications. The recent resurgence of interest in "natural" or "herbal" remedies provides yet another area for assessment. It is likely that interactions between drugs and these alternative remedies will become an increasingly popular area of research.

Pharmacokinetics

The term **pharmacokinetics** refers to a drug's activity from the time it enters the body until it leaves. This process has four parts: absorption, distribution, metabolism, and excretion. All health care professionals responsible for managing client medications should understand these processes.

ABSORPTION
Absorption refers to the transference of drug molecules from the point of entry in the body into the bloodstream. Most medications are absorbed systemically to exert their effects. Drug absorption is influenced by many factors, including route of administration, drug dosage and form, and conditions at the absorption site.

The route of administration has a direct impact on the extent and speed of medication absorption and is related to the physical structure of the tissues. The IV route is fastest because the medication is injected directly into the bloodstream. Medications are also absorbed rapidly through mucous membranes of the mouth, nose, and respiratory tract because these tissues are highly vascular. Injected medications are absorbed fairly rapidly, but their action also depends on conditions at the injection site. Absorption from the oral route can be affected by dose form and conditions in the GI tract. The topical route has the slowest absorption rate because the skin is a natural barrier.

The dosage and form of a medication commonly affect its absorption. Higher-than-average doses may be purposefully ordered when giving a **loading dose,** which is an initial medication dose that exceeds the maintenance or therapeutic dose. A loading dose may be ordered when the client has not recently received the medication and must rapidly achieve a therapeutic serum level. Examples of drugs commonly initiated with loading doses are digitalis and aminophylline. The loading dose is followed by therapeutic doses, and serum drug levels may be periodically monitored.

The form of the medication and conditions in the GI tract greatly affect absorption. Liquid forms, such as solutions or suspensions, are absorbed more quickly than solid forms, such as capsules or tablets. Extended-release products gradually release medication for absorption over a period of time. They can usually be recognized by letters at the end of the medication name, such as ER (extended release), SR (sustained release), SA (sustained action), or XL (extended length). Enteric-coated drugs are coated to prevent them from dissolving until they reach the alkaline environment of the small intestine; usually a drug is enteric coated because it would otherwise irritate the stomach lining. Most drugs are absorbed in the small intestine because of the numerous villi there.

Medications are often administered in relation to meals. Most are absorbed better when taken between meals. Selected medications are given with food to decrease the irritating effect on the stomach. Be sure to read drug reference material to determine whether a medication should be given with food or between meals (1 hour before or 2 hours after a meal).

Medications not given via the GI tract are greatly affected by conditions at the site of absorption, especially the blood supply to the area. Muscles have a rich supply of blood, making the intramuscular (IM) route the second choice after the IV route when rapid absorption is desired. The subcutaneous (SC or SQ) route is slower than the IM route and is a better choice when you need slower absorption. Local site conditions that interfere with parenteral drug absorption include bruising, scarring, and edema. Local circulatory impairments may also impede absorption.

DISTRIBUTION

The process of drug distribution begins with absorption of a drug into the circulation and ends with its arrival at the site of action. The degree and speed of distribution are affected by the health and makeup of the client as well as chemical and physical properties of the medication.

Various circulatory dynamics affect medication distribution. The more blood vessels supplying a tissue, the better the distribution, and vice versa. Blood vessel tone also affects distribution. Vasoconstriction reduces drug distribution, whereas vasodilatation enhances it. Thus, distribution of a drug to target tissues

may be poorer in clients with poor circulatory status or with edema.

The body also has physiological barriers to certain medications. The blood-brain barrier permits transport of lipid-bound medications while preventing transport of many water-soluble drugs. This has important implications when prescribing medications meant to affect the brain. The placental barrier also inhibits transport of some drugs, but is less selective than the blood-brain barrier. Physicians ordering drug therapy for a pregnant client carefully consider this variable when selecting a medication. This decision is crucial because many medications have a high **teratogenic potential,** which is the possibility that a medication will harm a developing fetus. Medications, therefore, are classified by the FDA with a Pregnancy Category to reflect teratogenicity (Table 26–3).

Most medications are partially bound to proteins such as albumin in the bloodstream, making that portion inactive and unable to be used by the tissues. The therapeutic effects are exerted by the active, unbound, or "free" portions. Clients with low albumin levels have greater circulation of the "active" drug and require decreased dosages. Low albumin levels are typically found in infants, older adults, and those with poor nutrition or liver disease.

METABOLISM

Drug metabolism, or **biotransformation,** is the process of inactivating and breaking down a medication. Enzymes chemically alter a drug's structure, converting it to a less potent substance.

Most drug metabolism occurs in the liver, which has microsomes that trigger the enzymatic breakdown of drugs. The liver can oxidize and transform many substances before they reach the body tissues, called a *first-pass effect.* However, liver function can decrease with age or disease, allowing active drug to accumulate in the body. For this reason, infants, the elderly, and those with cirrhosis or other liver diseases experience the same effect even with reduced medication doses. Standard doses would place them at risk for drug toxicity.

Less frequent sites of drug metabolism are the kidneys, lungs, blood, and intestines. Pathology in these

TABLE 26–3

FDA Pregnancy Categories Used to Assess Fetal Risk

Risk Category	Risk Level	Interpretation
A	No risk	Study results have not shown evidence of fetal harm from use of this medication.
B	Little or no risk	Results of animal studies show no risk, but no well-controlled studies have been performed in pregnant women.
C	Uncertain risk	Results of animal studies indicate that there is risk to the fetus, but no well-controlled studies have been performed in pregnant women. The risks and benefits of using the drug must be assessed.
D	Proven risk	The risks and benefits of using the drug must be assessed and should be considered in the event of life-threatening situations.
X	Proven risk	This drug should be avoided during pregnancy because the risks outweigh any benefits.

areas also requires reduced drug doses to prevent toxicity. Know the sites of metabolism for the medications you give, and monitor the client for intended and adverse drug effects.

EXCRETION

Excretion is the movement of a drug from the site of metabolism back into the circulation and its transport to the site of exit from the body. The route of excretion is determined by the chemical properties of the drug. The kidneys are responsible for excreting most drugs. Other organs of excretion are the lungs, exocrine glands, and intestinal tract.

The nephrons of the kidneys secrete unwanted substances into the urine in the presence of an adequate glomerular filtration rate. Most medications undergo metabolism before excretion; others are eliminated in their original form. It is important to know how a drug is excreted to anticipate its effectiveness. For example, when a client has a urinary tract infection, the drug of choice is one that is excreted relatively unchanged in the urine. Otherwise, the drug will not effectively treat the infection.

Proper fluid intake is generally beneficial to aid excretion, except when the client retains fluid, such as with renal failure or heart failure. A medication dose may be reduced if the client has renal disease that impairs drug excretion.

The lungs, sweat glands, mammary glands, and GI tract excrete drugs to a lesser degree. The lungs excrete volatile gases such as alcohol, nitrous oxide, and ether. The sweat glands help excrete lipid-soluble drugs. Because the mammary glands excrete drugs, women who are breast-feeding should use medications only on the advice of a physician. This decision is made after carefully weighing the benefits to the mother and the risks to the infant. The GI tract eliminates medications in bile. The rate of medication excretion by this route can be slowed or accelerated by the same conditions that cause constipation or diarrhea, respectively.

Impaired clearance through any of the routes of excretion could result in drug toxicity. Review the results of periodically drawn serum laboratory studies, such as liver enzymes, blood urea nitrogen, and creatinine. The latter two monitor the function of the liver and kidneys, respectively.

Blood Level

To be effective, the active component of a medication must be present in the blood within a therapeutic range. The therapeutic range is the blood level that effectively treats a health problem without creating toxic effects. At a therapeutic range the medication is in different phases of being absorbed, distributed, metabolized, and excreted.

The blood (or serum) level of a medication is the amount circulating in the bloodstream at a given point in time. The peak serum concentration of a drug usually occurs just as the last bit of the most recently administered dose is being absorbed. After this has been

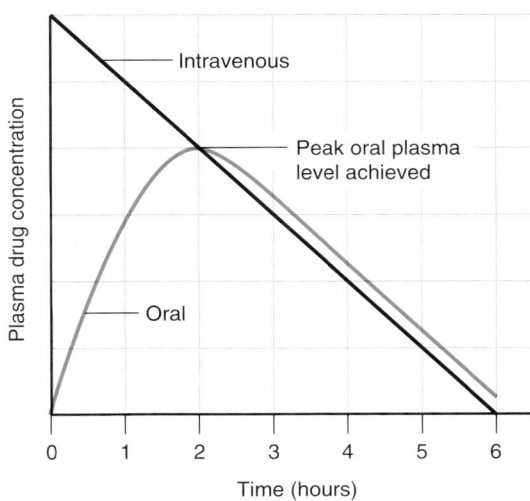

Figure 26–1. The blood level of an oral drug typically peaks about 2 hours after ingestion and then tapers steadily, whereas a drug given by the IV route reaches its peak almost immediately and tapers steadily.

achieved, absorption stops and only distribution, metabolism, and excretion continue. The serum level then falls progressively until the next dose begins to be absorbed.

The route of drug administration also influences the blood level. For example, the level of an oral drug typically peaks about 2 hours after ingestion and then tapers steadily (Fig. 26–1). Medications given by the IV route reach their peak almost immediately and taper steadily from there. In general, therapeutic drug levels are easier to maintain with IV administration because you can avoid the pronounced peaks and valleys of oral administration.

Action alert!
Monitor the results of serum drug levels, and report values that are outside the therapeutic range immediately. Assess the client for signs and symptoms of toxicity if results are high.

HALF-LIFE

Every drug has a half-life, which is the amount of time needed by the body to lower by one-half the drug's serum concentration through metabolism and excretion. A drug's half-life helps determine how frequently it should be given. Drugs with a long half-life may be given less frequently, whereas drugs with a short half-life require more frequent administration.

ONSET, PEAK, AND DURATION

Onset, peak, and duration are terms frequently used by health care personnel to describe the anticipated effects of a drug. The onset is the amount of time needed after administration of a drug to produce the desired effect. The peak action represents the amount of time needed for a drug to reach the highest concentration for effectiveness. The duration is the span of time during which the serum drug concentration is high enough to produce the intended effect.

PLATEAU

The term *plateau* refers to the serum concentration or level of a drug that has been reached and sustained with a series of fixed doses. When the plateau is achieved and maintained, the client should receive the optimal therapeutic benefit.

Systems of Delivery

Nurse-Administered Medications

When a client is admitted to a hospital or extended-care facility, the responsibility for medication administration usually shifts from the client to the nurse. You will typically be expected to obtain a medication history on admission, review current medication orders, and consult with the physician about discrepancies. Anticipate that new medications may be ordered to treat the current health problem. Realize also that medications routinely taken at home are sometimes not reordered in the hospital. This may be intentional, as in the case of digitalis toxicity. However, nurses share the responsibility for ensuring that the client receives medication for ongoing health problems as well as those ordered for the current problem. Consult with the physician whenever discrepancies are noted.

Once admitted to a health-care facility, most clients receive medications only when you provide them. In other words, you assume responsibility for obtaining the correct medication, dispensing the correct dose and form, and recording the administration in the client record. Use extreme caution to avoid errors, which can be harmful to the client, distressing to you, and costly to the institution.

Prepare medications for administration in an environment that is conducive to safety and accuracy. Plan to work alone to avoid errors that could result from interruptions and distractions. Make sure you have adequate lighting in the work area to promote accuracy.

Also, maintain the security of medications that are being dispensed. Do not leave medications unattended after beginning their preparation. If you must leave the area briefly, place medications in a locked drawer, cart, or cabinet until you return. The medication cart or storage area should always be locked whenever you are not present.

A*ction* A*lert!*
Lock the medication cart after use. Do not leave medications unattended on top of a cart during or after preparation.

Client-Administered Medications

Sometimes a client administers his own medications after admission to a health care facility. This decision is made after considering the reliability of the client, the nature and purpose of the medication, and whether client independence should be promoted. A few examples of clients who can benefit from self-administration are the young, alert postpartum woman who requires analgesics, the diabetic who regularly takes insulin and knows how to administer it, and the elderly client who takes inhalation medications at home.

General guidelines should be followed when allowing a client to self-administer medications. First, the client should be alert and reliable. The client should also be able to tell you when he has administered a medication (so you can document it) or reliably record self-medication on a special form placed at the bedside. This form becomes part of the medical record upon discharge. The client should not keep any medications at the bedside other than those permitted for self-administration.

Components and Processing of Medication Orders

Medication orders must be legally entered in the medical record. When a physician or advanced practice nurse enters an order for a medication, it must in-

TABLE 26–4
Components of a Drug Order

Component	Explanation
Date and time of order	Includes month, day, and year. Also includes time of day on orders for inpatients (written on order sheet instead of prescription pad). Time of day indicates AM or PM if military time is not used. Time of order is especially important for drugs with automatic stop times.
Name of medication	Should be clearly and precisely written. Most facilities use generic names, but sometimes both generic and trade names are identified. Prescription orders state the trade name if no interchange is permitted.
Dose of medication	Lists exact amount of the drug ordered.
Route of administration	Lists exact route by which to give the drug. This is very important because many medications can be given by more than one route.
Frequency of administration	May specify the number of times per day (such as qid for four times a day) or may state the number of hours between doses (such as q6h for every 6 hours) depending on the drug and its purpose.
Signature of prescriber	Required by law. An unsigned prescription will not be filled in a pharmacy, and you should not implement an unsigned drug order. For a narcotic prescription, the prescriber's DEA number must be provided in addition to the signature.

DEA, Drug Enforcement Agency.

TABLE 26–5
Abbreviations Commonly Used in Medication Orders

Abbreviation	Meaning
ac	Before meals
ad lib	As desired
ASAP	As soon as possible
BID	Twice daily
c̄	With
cap	Capsule
d/c	Discontinue
elix	Elixir
gtt	Drop
hs	Hour of sleep, bedtime
ID	Intradermal
IM	Intramuscular
IV	Intravenous
IVP	IV push
IVPB	IV piggyback
KVO	Keep vein open
OD	Right eye
OS	Left eye
OU	Both eyes
pc	After meals
po	By mouth, oral
pr	Per rectum
PRN	When needed, as necessary
q	Every
qd	Every day
qh	Every hour
q3h	Every 3 hours
QID	Four times a day
QOD	Every other day
qs	Quantity sufficient
Rx	Take
s̄	Without
SC	Subcutaneous
SL	Sublingual
STAT	Immediately
supp	Suppository
susp	Suspension
TID	Three times a day
tab	Tablet

clude the date and time of the order; medication name, dose, route, and frequency; and the signature of the prescriber (Table 26–4). A complete order not only fulfills the legal standard but also gives sufficient direction to the pharmacist, the nurse, and the client.

Once a drug order has been entered, it must be communicated to others. Ideally the pharmacist has direct access to the physician's order entry without transcription. Your legal responsibility includes accurate interpretation of the order and administration of the medicine. Note any special conditions or parameters for administration, such as holding an antihypertensive medication for a systolic blood pressure less than 100 mm Hg. If handwritten orders are illegible or

you are not sure what an abbreviation means, you must clarify the order (Table 26–5). It is not prudent to interpret illegible orders, and you could be held accountable for drug administration errors based on faulty interpretation.

Verbal or telephone orders may be given in emergency or unusual situations. Facility policy usually dictates whether and under what conditions you may take either of these types of orders. (Nursing students generally cannot take verbal or telephone orders.) When verbal or telephone orders are allowed, record the date and time of the order, as well as the drug, dose, route, and frequency. Write "T.O." or "V.O." to indicate a telephone or verbal order, respectively, and write the name of the ordering physician after the medication order. Record your own signature, followed by R.N. Verbal and telephone orders must be co-signed by the physician within a specified time, usually 24 hours or less. To prevent communication errors, repeat back the information to the prescribing physician after taking a verbal or telephone order. These types of orders pose the greatest liability for you and the physician. At no time should you administer a medication without an order.

It is your ethical and legal responsibility to question a medication order if you have any questions about an order. You could place yourself in legal jeopardy if an error should have been noted, based on your education and experience. If the physician does not respond appropriately to your inquiry, report the problem, following your facility's chain of command to prevent the medication error. If you believe the client could be harmed by the medication as ordered, you should withhold the medication, document this on the medication administration record, and document the rationale on the nursing progress notes.

Types of Orders

Several types of medication orders exist, and it is critically important to understand which type of order is being carried out. The type of order used depends on the goal of the medication therapy.

Standing Orders

A standing order indicates that a medication should be given on a routine basis. It may be written for a specified number of days, or it may carry no time limit. If there is no limit, the order is followed until another order is specifically written to discontinue it. Facility policy sometimes dictates when standing orders are no longer in effect. For example, narcotic analgesics often have a "stop date" that is 3 to 7 days after the original order date. In many institutions, any previously written medication orders are canceled when the client goes to surgery, is transferred to another facility, or is discharged. In these circumstances, new orders must be written because the client's status may have changed and the old orders may no longer be appropriate. Facility policy may also dictate how frequently standing orders must be reviewed.

A special type of standing order may be found in specialty nursing units, such as cardiac care or maternity units. In these areas, a standardized set of written orders is activated or followed when special circumstances occur. These orders follow medically safe protocols, are time-saving for the nurse, and are potentially life-saving for the client. Once activated, these medications are charted just as any other medication would be.

PRN Orders

A PRN order is an order for a medication that is given as needed. The label derives from the Latin *pro re nata,* meaning "as necessary." It lists the minimum amount of time that must elapse between doses and may also specify the symptoms it is used to treat. This type of drug order allows you to use discretion in administering a medication. It also requires that you have good assessment skills, noting both the situation and clinical condition of the client. One example of a PRN order is *droperidol 2.5 mg IV q6h PRN for nausea or vomiting.* This tells you that it may be given for nausea or vomiting, provided the client has not received a dose for at least 6 hours. Another example is *meperidine (Demerol) 75 to 100 mg IM q4h PRN for pain.* This example illustrates that at times you may be allowed to use discretion in determining the dose.

Single Orders

A single order is a medication order carried out one time only. It identifies the drug, dose route, and time for administration. Preoperative and preprocedure orders are commonly written as one-time orders. Another example is *nafcillin 2 g IVPB on call to OR.* This order states to infuse a specific antibiotic attached to a mainline IV when the client is called to the operating room.

STAT Orders

A STAT order is one that is implemented immediately. These orders are frequently given during emergency or near-emergency situations. An example is impending cardiac or respiratory arrest. STAT orders are more likely to be given as verbal or telephone orders. Most institutions have policies and guidelines stating the time period within which a STAT order must be completed.

Medication Distribution Systems

Medication distribution systems are designed to promote safety and accuracy, conserve time and money, and promote client self-care. Within a facility, a single system is used and the efforts of all personnel and support structures work together to provide streamlined delivery.

Unit-Dose System

The most commonly used system today is the unit-dose system. A unit dose is a single dose of a medication that is prepackaged and labeled by the manufacturer or pharmacist. A new supply of unit doses for each client is delivered to the nursing unit every 24 hours. You then take a single dose of each medication to the bedside at the appropriate time.

Computer-Controlled Dispensing Systems

The most recently developed unit-dose system is the computer-controlled dispensing system. Access to the system is menu-driven and resembles (conceptually at least) a small automated teller machine. The unit contains medications stored in specific containers that are labeled and coded in the machine. The computer is programmed with the number of unit doses stocked for each medication. You access the system using a personal identification code. After you remove a drug, the computer records the transaction in its memory and charges the drug to the client. This system is time-saving for you and is cost-effective because of better inventory control.

Routes of Administration
Oral Routes

Oral or PO (from Latin *per oris*) means given by mouth. There are actually three oral routes for medication administration: the oral, sublingual, and buccal routes.

ORAL. A medication given by the oral route is placed in the mouth and swallowed. A client with a nasogastric tube connected to suction cannot receive oral medications. Confused clients or those who are unwilling to swallow should be carefully assessed to determine if this route is appropriate. Clients with an impaired or absent swallow reflex cannot use this route but may have a feeding tube in place. Instead, medications may be given by nasogastric, gastrostomy, or jejunostomy tube and are called enteral medications. A client who is on NPO (nothing by mouth) status may not receive oral medications unless the order specifically states *NPO with meds.*

SUBLINGUAL. A medication given by the sublingual route is placed under the tongue and allowed to dissolve. The medication is quickly absorbed through the mucous membranes into the systemic circulation. Tell the client not to swallow a tablet ordered for sublingual use because it will not be effective. The client should avoid eating, swallowing liquids, or smoking while the tablet is dissolving. An example is nitroglycerin, which is used to treat chest pain.

BUCCAL. A tablet or lozenge given by the buccal route is placed against the mucous membranes of the mouth, between the cheek and the gums, near the molars. The drug dissolves and acts either locally on mucosa or systemically after being absorbed from saliva swallowed into the stomach. Teach clients using this route to alternate cheeks to minimize mucosal irritation and to avoid swallowing liquids while the medication is dissolving.

Parenteral Routes

A **parenteral route** is one that is outside the GI tract. Parenteral medications are given by injection into a body tissue using sterile technique. The four routinely used parenteral routes are intradermal, subcutaneous, intramuscular, and intravenous. These routes provide for faster drug action but are associated with risks of discomfort, infection, and even bleeding in some clients. Other less frequently used parenteral routes are the epidural and intrathecal routes. These routes are initiated by physicians or advanced practice nurses.

INTRADERMAL. The **intradermal** (ID) **route** involves injection into the dermis layer of the skin. It is commonly used to test for allergic reactions to a substance planted in the dermis. Other ID injections include purified protein derivative for tuberculosis and skin testing for mumps and *Candida.*

SUBCUTANEOUS. The **subcutaneous** (SC or SQ) **route** involves injection into subcutaneous tissue just under the dermis. It is commonly used by nurses and by clients self-administering insulin and for small amounts of medication that do not need to be rapidly absorbed.

INTRAMUSCULAR. The **intramuscular** (IM) **route** involves injection into muscle tissue, specifically the body of a muscle. Medications are absorbed quickly, making this a popular route when faster absorption is needed. It is frequently used to administer narcotic analgesics, antiemetics, and some antibiotics.

INTRAVENOUS. The **intravenous route** involves injection of a medication into a vein. This route provides the most rapid effect, with distribution throughout the body in a few minutes. For this reason, smaller drug doses are needed when using this route. A disadvantage is that the route is potentially dangerous because drugs given incorrectly cannot be retrieved. Antibiotics, histamine receptor antagonists, and selected pain medications are examples of medications commonly given by the IV route. This route is also used for patient-controlled analgesia (see Chapter 42).

Topical Route

The **topical route** is used to deliver a medication directly to a body site, such as the skin, eyes, ears, nose, throat, vagina, or rectum. A skin preparation may be applied by manually spreading it over a specific area, applying a patch, placing the drug in a medicated dressing, soaking the area in solution, or using a medicated bath.

Topical drugs often have a local effect, although some are absorbed systemically as well. There is a direct correlation between the length of exposure to a topical application and the amount absorbed. A previous dose is removed before the next dose is applied.

Suppositories as a drug form are often used for insertion into the rectum or vagina. Drops may be instilled into the eyes, nose, or ears. Irrigations may be ordered for the eye, ear, bladder, rectum, or vagina. Medications can also be sprayed into the nose or throat, or throat gargles may be used.

Inhalation Route

Inhalation is used to bring medications into the respiratory tract via the nose or throat. Most medications given by this route exert local effects on the bronchial mucosa. They are administered via metered-dose inhaler, nebulizer, or turbo-inhaler (see Chapter 39).

Clients may also receive inhaled medications via an endotracheal tube or tracheostomy, such as anesthetic gases and some emergency resuscitative drugs. This route allows for rapid systemic absorption because the lungs have a very large and highly vascular surface area.

A nasal inhaler may be used to administer certain medications. The most common example is the use of a decongestant nasal spray to constrict nasal blood vessels and relieve cold symptoms. Another type of nasal medication uses a nasal canister with a thin tube attached. The tube is inserted into the nares and is either squeezed or blown into to deliver a dose of medication. An example is desmopressin, which is used to treat diabetes insipidus.

FACTORS AFFECTING DRUG ACTIONS

A number of client-related factors can influence the action of a medication. These include diet, environmental influences, developmental factors, cultural and religious factors, socioeconomic conditions, psychological influences, and physiological considerations.

Dietary Factors

A client's overall nutritional state can either positively or negatively affect medication actions in the body. Recall that cells manufacture proteins and enzymes. Because most drugs bind with proteins, sufficient protein intake is needed for adequate drug distribution. Both proteins and enzymes are also needed for proper drug metabolism.

Specific foods can trigger drug-food interactions that either increase or decrease the drug's effectiveness. The diet may have to be changed somewhat to manage these nutrients. For example, liver or green leafy vegetables rich in vitamin K should be limited or maintained at a steady level when taking warfarin because they antagonize the drug's action. Clients who take potassium-wasting diuretics should take in extra servings of high-potassium foods.

Fluid balance also influences drug effects. Sufficient body fluid is necessary to carry drugs to their site of action and to excrete them after use. Thus, dehydration can limit the transport of drugs and their metabolites, reducing the effectiveness of drug therapy.

Environmental Factors

Physical agents in the environment can directly affect a client's response to a medication. Heat and cold produce vasodilatation and vasoconstriction, which in turn alter drug distribution or even its effects (e.g., an-

THE STATE OF NURSING SCIENCE

HELPING OLDER ADULTS TAKE MEDICATIONS EFFECTIVELY

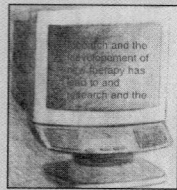

What Are the Issues?

Older adults take many medications to manage their health problems. Finding the most effective way to help them manage their medications safely is of interest to nurses, who are often the ones responsible for teaching older adults. Short-term outcomes related to knowledge and compliance are often used as indicators of the effectiveness of educational interventions.

What Research Has Been Conducted?

Hayes (1998) studied the effects of two types of medication instruction given to older adults in community hospital emergency departments. The types of instruction were the traditional method (a nurse reviewing preprinted materials with the client before discharge) and an experimental method involving the generation of individualized computer-generated instructions that focused on specific information about how to take the medication, major side effects, and when to call the physician. The information in the experimental method was developed at a fifth-grade reading level and printed in large type. Part of the intervention included teaching by the nurse in a quiet environment. The researcher collected data on client knowledge of medications through telephone interviews. Older adults who received instruction that was individualized for them based on principles of teaching older adults scored significantly higher than those people who received traditional teaching.

Martens (1998) used a qualitative approach to study medication discharge education in people with cardiovascular disease. She conducted in-depth interviews with 122 older adults, their families, and their nurses. The interviews took place in person or over the telephone after discharge from the hospital. Martens then summarized the themes that emerged from the interviews and observations—a common way of presenting qualitative data. According to Martens, medication discharge education

- "is both a structured and unstructured process" (p. 344). Martens found that in addition to information provided just before discharge, nurses instructed clients and family members about medications throughout hospitalization.
- "is an interdisciplinary process that is disjointed, uncoordinated, and largely driven by accreditation requirements" (p. 34). This theme was most evident in an institution in which the documentation system had been designed to meet accreditation standards. Martens found that not knowing what medications would be prescribed until discharge limited the amount of time nurses had to help clients incorporate medication administration into their self-care routines.
- "frequently involves family members of older hospitalized adults" (p. 345). Martens viewed the presence of family members as positive.
- "is most effective when delivered in both [an] oral and [a] written format" (p. 345). Interaction with

(continued)

tihypertensives). Advise clients to dress appropriately for the weather and to avoid temperature extremes. Ionizing radiation, such as sunlight, can affect enzyme activity in the body, altering drug actions. Many medications have photosensitivity as a side effect, so warn clients to avoid prolonged exposure or to use a strong sunscreen when outdoors.

Developmental Factors

A client's age significantly influences medication actions. Infants have immature function of the renal, hepatic, and GI systems. They also lack certain metabolic enzymes needed for proper drug metabolism. Finally, they have relatively more body water and less body mass. These factors cause the infant's system to be highly responsive to medications.

Older adults can also have an altered response to medications because of changes that occur with the aging process. Absorption, metabolism, and excretion are reduced by slowed or decreased organ function.

Drug distribution is altered by decreased size, protein-binding sites, body water, and lean muscle mass. Each of these factors increases the risk for drug toxicity. Older adults also face a higher risk of adverse effects from polypharmacy or from taking their medications incorrectly. They can benefit from an increased amount of individualized teaching, as discussed in the State of Nursing Science chart.

Cultural/Religious Factors

Cultural and religious beliefs can influence a client's thoughts about whether a medication will help and whether he should comply with therapy. A client who subscribes to Western beliefs about health and illness typically expects to receive medication as part of the total treatment plan for a health problem. A client who does not subscribe to Western beliefs may be more likely to use alternative healing methods, such as herbal therapy, talismans, and spiritual advisors or healers. These therapies may complement or interfere

HELPING OLDER ADULTS TAKE MEDICATIONS EFFECTIVELY (continued)

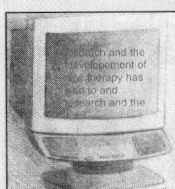

nurses allowed patients to ask questions for clarification, and the written material was useful for future reference. Written material included handouts specific to the medications as well as discharge summaries. The readability of some of the written materials was a problem for some people.

- "is delivered in varying depths and does not routinely correspond to patient/family information deficits" (p. 346). The lack of individualized instruction meant that people had to seek out information from other sources to help them apply the information to meet their needs.

Additional themes indicated that people who asked questions, were taking new medications, or were taking anticoagulants received more thorough instruction than did other clients (p. 346). Clients also valued nurses who took time to make sure they understood the information about their medications.

What Has the Research Concluded?

Hayes (1998) concluded that educational interventions designed with the special needs of older adults in mind are an effective way of communicating information. Martens' (1998) study illustrated the complex nature of educational interventions. She also identified problems in communication among staff and the need to individualize instruction.

The findings from these two studies confirm those of Wendt (1998), who reviewed a number of studies that tested interventions to help community-dwelling older

adults take their medications. These studies supported using a combination of teaching and written materials along with follow-up as the most effective method of preparing older adults to take their medications. The follow-up could be telephone calls or a written schedule for use at home.

What Is the Future of Research in This Area?

Hayes recommends studying the use of individualized instruction geared toward older adults in a variety of settings. It would also be important to see whether the effects of educational interventions are long-lasting. Martens (1998) recommends studying people from different ethnic backgrounds to see how their experience with medication education differs. Wendt (1998) suggests studies to support the memories of older adults to help them take their medications as scheduled. Other avenues of study include learning why older adults change their medication schedules and what the effects of such changes are on their health status.

References

Hayes, K.S. (1998). Randomized trial of geragogy-based medication instruction in the emergency department. *Nursing Research, 47*(4), 211–218.

Martens, K.H. (1998). An ethnographic study of the process of medication discharge education (MDE). *Journal of Advanced Nursing, 27,* 341–348.

Wendt, D.A. (1998). Evaluation of medication management interventions for the elderly. *Home Healthcare Nurse, 16*(9), 613–617.

with the actions of prescribed medications, depending on specific circumstances. At the same time, these remedies often provide a psychological benefit, which is also therapeutic. Assess for these factors in a culturally sensitive fashion to build a sufficient database for evaluating drug effectiveness. Become familiar with the basic beliefs and health practices of clients of other cultures to help you to communicate medication information more effectively (Box 26–2).

Socioeconomic Factors

Socioeconomic factors play an indirect role in influencing drug actions. Financially disadvantaged clients may not seek care for a health problem as quickly as those with adequate finances or health insurance. When a disadvantaged client does seek treatment, the medication regimen may be more complex because the health problem was not identified at an early stage. The client may be unable to afford continued medica-

tion therapy after the initial episode resolves. Thus, he may not refill prescriptions or he may take partial doses to help the medication "last longer."

Psychological Factors

Psychological factors can influence whether a client chooses to take a medication and whether the drug is ultimately effective. These factors include client's attitude toward medication use, meaning of medication use, motivation, secondary gain, and the behavior of the nurse administering the medication. Chapter 25 discusses factors affecting compliance with a health care regimen.

Physiological Factors

GENETIC DIFFERENCES. Genetic factors can influence the manner in which the body uses, metabolizes,

BOX 26–2

COMMUNICATING EFFECTIVELY WITH CLIENTS OF OTHER CULTURES ABOUT MEDICATION THERAPY

- Become informed about the health practices and beliefs of cultural groups in your community. Be aware that diversity may exist within subgroups of a larger cultural group.
- Encourage clients of other cultures to communicate their concerns and ask questions related to medication therapy.
- Provide printed or audiovisual medication information in the client's language if possible.
- Question the client directly about the use of remedies prescribed by a healer within the culture. These remedies may have an interactive effect with prescribed medication therapy.
- Watch for atypical drug responses or unexpected side effects in clients in certain cultural groups. Cultural influences such as diet, complementary therapies, or even genetic factors can precipitate unusual responses to medication therapy.

or reacts to a drug. Deficiencies in natural body enzymes used to biotransform drugs may be responsible for these events. This helps to explain why allergies to penicillin, for example, can run in families.

GENDER DIFFERENCES. Men and women have different amounts of body fat, body water, and muscle mass. They also have different circulating levels of male and female hormones. These factors influence drug actions by affecting one or more of the pharmacokinetic processes. Much clinical drug research is done with male subjects, so drug effects on women may be unexpected from time to time.

HEIGHT AND WEIGHT. Height and weight are important factors affecting drug actions. Standard drug doses are published for average-sized adults, who range in age from 18 to 65 and weigh about 150 pounds. Overweight adults may require an increased dose to achieve therapeutic results. Drug doses for infants and children are calculated according to body weight or body surface area. Record height and weight at the hospital admission or during the intake process in an ambulatory care setting. This provides a ready reference for the physician to determine drug dosages.

DISEASES. Diseases that adversely affect any one of the pharmacokinetic processes ultimately affect drug action. For example, impaired GI function may reduce absorption. Heart failure or other edema-causing conditions may impair drug distribution. Liver or renal disease limits drug metabolism and excretion, putting the client at risk for toxic effects.

ASSESSMENT

A client receiving medication therapy deserves a thorough and multifaceted assessment. This helps determine both the need for medication and the client's likelihood of response. The assessment process is twofold and includes general assessment and focused assessment.

Mr. Connell was diagnosed with hypertension (high blood pressure) 5 years ago. At that time, atenolol (Tenormin, a beta-adrenergic blocking agent) was prescribed. Within a few months, furosemide (Lasix, a diuretic) was added because his blood pressure was not effectively reduced. This regimen was effective, and he continued with therapy for a little over a year. At that time, he felt quite well and decided that he did not need the medication any longer. He has not seen a physician in more than 3 years. The Cross-Cultural Care Chart provides information useful to the nurse working with Mr. Connell and adds to the assessment database gathered thus far.

General Assessment for Medication Administration

Health History

A client's health history provides information about existing health problems being managed with medications and illnesses or organ dysfunction that may increase the risk of toxicity or other adverse drug effects. Note any significant surgical procedures performed in the past. If a hormone-secreting organ has been removed, such as ovaries or thyroid, the client may take hormone replacement therapy. These medications should be continued during inpatient care.

HISTORY OF ALLERGIES

Information about drug allergies is critically important to assess when a client is being treated for the first time. Even if the client has an existing medical record from previous admissions or visits, verify allergies at each encounter. Assess the following factors whenever possible: drug, dose and route, number of times taken before allergy symptoms occurred, and onset and nature of the reaction. Assess for both drug and food allergies because some foods contain ingredients that are also found in medications. For example, clients who are allergic to shellfish cannot receive injectable radiocontrast dye during diagnostic studies because both contain iodine. Some vaccines are made from substances in chick embryos and should not be given to a client allergic to eggs.

Record allergies in large print on the cover of the client's medical record. If handwritten physician order forms are used, place an allergy sticker on each new blank order page as it is inserted into the chart. You may also find allergy notations in nursing admission notes, physician history and physical notes, and medication administration records. On admission, put a bracelet listing all pertinent allergies on the client's wrist and leave it in place until discharge.

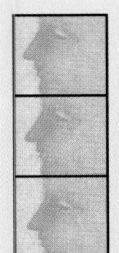

CROSS-CULTURAL CARE
CARING FOR AN IRISH-AMERICAN CLIENT

Daniel Connell, the client whose story we've been following through this chapter, is of Irish-American descent. His family came to Boston, Massachusetts in the late 1800s. Wilson (1997) describes the values that Americans of Irish descent, like Mr. Connell, tend to hold. Although there are always individual differences among clients, Irish-Americans as a group tend to

- Believe and expect that life is a difficult process.
- Understate their symptoms when ill and delay seeking health care until symptoms are severe or cannot be ignored.
- Be stoic and resist expressing emotions associated with illness or pain.
- Use facial expressions to communicate nonverbally rather than more expressive gestures, such as hand and arm movements.
- Use traditional home remedies to treat minor illnesses but seek out a traditional health care provider if these fail or if a larger health problem emerges.

The following client interview between Mr. Connell and Amy, his nurse, illustrates how cultural beliefs and behavior can be evidenced in a nurse-client interaction:

Amy: Can you tell me a little more about what led you to stop taking your blood pressure medications?

Mr. Connell: Well *(brow furrowed, thoughtful)* I remember that I didn't have those headaches anymore, and I got tired of having to go to the bathroom all the time. I figured that since I felt better, I should just get on with it!

Amy: Are you doing anything else to keep your blood pressure down, such as changing your diet or doing some exercise?

Mr. Connell: My wife, she's a good one. She started using less salt while she was cooking, and I have to say the pot roasts don't taste the same. But I've gotten used to it, and I try not to use the salt shaker too much. I started walking when they told me I had high blood pressure, but I fell off the bandwagon on that one. I guess my best exercise comes from working around the house and mowing the lawn.

Amy: Would you say that you have a stressful job, Mr. Connell?

Mr. Connell: I've been working as a truck dispatcher for a big trucking company for more years than I care to admit! Things do get crazy there from time to time. It can't be helped though, that's just the way it is. When the going gets rough, my motto is "Just grin and bear it!" Tomorrow is another day.

Critical Thinking Questions

- How do Mr. Connell's beliefs about health affect his behavior?
- To what degree does Mr. Connell's behavior resemble that of others in his culture?
- What cultural characteristics should the nurse keep in mind in developing a plan of care for Mr. Connell?

Reference

Wilson, S. (1997). Irish Americans. In L. Purnell & B. Paulanka (Eds.), *Transcultural health care: A culturally competent approach.* Philadelphia: F.A. Davis.

Action Alert!
Always check for an allergy bracelet before giving medication to a client. If a bracelet falls off or becomes illegible, replace it at once.

MEDICATION HISTORY
On admission, document the name of each drug the client routinely takes, the dose, the route (usually oral), and the time of the last dose. Document whether any medications have been brought to the hospital and their disposition (e.g., sent home or stored on the nursing unit). Question the client about his use of prescription medications, OTC medications, and herbal or other alternative therapies, as discussed in the Considering the Alternatives chart. Many clients will not mention OTC medications or herbal therapies unless specifically asked. Assess the dose and frequency of use.

DIET HISTORY
Because most medications are administered orally, assess the client's usual dietary intake, food preferences, and meal patterns. Several medications are better absorbed when taken either with or without food. Adjust the medication schedule accordingly. This may be more difficult than it seems because most facilities have policies and procedures governing routine medication administration times for standard drug therapy.

KNOWLEDGE OF DRUG THERAPY
Increased knowledge of drug therapy should positively influence compliance. Assess the client's knowledge of the following:

- What the drug is being taken for
- How and when it should be taken
- If any doses have been skipped and why

CONSIDERING THE ALTERNATIVES

HOMEOPATHY

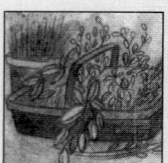

Homeopathy is a system of medical treatment founded and developed by Samuel Hahnemann in the late 1700s. Hahnemann was a distinguished physician who became dissatisfied with the medical remedies and practices of his time. In fact, his dissatisfaction was such that he nearly gave up practicing medicine, devoting himself for a time to the translation of foreign medical works into German. Finding himself in disagreement with a Scottish physician's work on the treatment of malaria with quinine, Hahnemann experimented on himself by taking quinine. He found that quinine produced in him symptoms similar to those of malaria. This experiment stimulated his development of homeopathic theory, and was the first of a series of so-called provings by Hahnemann—the testing of substances in healthy subjects—which led to the formulation of homeopathic remedies with such names as *Galphimia glauca* and arnica (Blackie, 1978).

Homeopathy, from the Greek words *homoios* (meaning *like*) and *pathos* (meaning *suffering*), asserts that an illness can be treated by administration of remedies that would produce a similar constellation of symptoms when taken by a healthy person. Thus, the idea of *similia similibus curentur:* "like will be cured by like." Homeopathic remedies are thought by homeopaths to gain strength when they are taken to higher and higher dilutions. Thus, many homeopathic remedies are diluted to the point that none of the original material, whether plant, mineral, animal or chemical, can be found in the remedy when analyzed. Originally, lower and lower doses were used to find the amount that could produce a therapeutic response with the least toxicity. This was important in Hahnemann's time because many of the medicines in common use, and those that he was testing in healthy people, were somewhat toxic.

Over the years following Hahnemann's early work, the practice of homeopathy spread and the number of remedies increased. Homeopathic historians claim that thousands if not millions of people around the world have benefitted from homeopathic treatment. They also claim that homeopathic treatments have been successful in epidemics of typhoid, yellow fever, and cholera (Blackie, 1978; Inglis, 1965).

By the late 1800s, homeopathic medical colleges had been established in the United States and many physicians practiced homeopathy. However, in the early 1900s, the standards of medical training changed. After Pasteur's work and the ascendancy of the germ theory of disease causation, the American Medical Association, which frowned on homeopathy, gained greater influence on the medical curriculum. Homeopathy gradually became relegated to postgraduate training.

Today, homeopathic practice remains widespread. Forty percent of French and Dutch, 37% of British, and 20% of German physicians practice homeopathy. Hundreds of thousands of Americans use homeopathic remedies yearly (Wagner, 1997). Homeopathy is popular in India as well, a legacy of British occupation. In parts of Europe and the Americas, lay homeopaths as well as physicians prescribe treatment. The remedies are commonly available in health food and drug stores in Europe and the United States.

Whether homeopathy is effective is controversial. Advocates and detractors debate this point. A recent journal exchange between two physicians took place, with conflicting titles: "Homeopathy Should Be Integrated Into Mainstream Medicine" and "Homeopathy Does Not Work" (Jacobs, 1995; Sampson, 1995). Critics of homeopathy claim that research has not shown homeopathy to be effective in treating disease. Although advo-

(continued)

- Any side effects experienced
- Other specific information unique to the drug

Inadequate knowledge in any of these areas should guide you to develop a teaching plan using the nursing process. If the client cannot learn the necessary information, obtain assistance from others (family or friends), who then become the focus of your teaching.

Physical Examination

CURRENT CONDITION

Use your knowledge of the client's ongoing condition or health status to assess whether current orders for drug therapy are sufficient and appropriate. Depend-

ing on changes in physical assessment data, new medications may be ordered and existing medications may be placed on hold, undergo a change in route, or be discontinued. Assess each client carefully, and report changes in condition to the physician or other person responsible for ordering medication therapy.

Be aware of any specific parameters to assess before giving a medication. For example, you may withhold a dose of some cardiac medications if the client's pulse rate is less than 60. In contrast, you may implement a medication order based on client assessment. For example, you may administer a PRN medication for nausea, pain, or high blood pressure if the client's condition warrants.

HOMEOPATHY (continued)

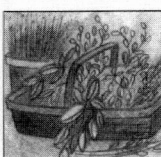

cates of homeopathy claim that research has shown effects beyond placebo effects, critics contend that such research has been of poor quality (Wagner, 1997). Yet new studies continue to appear, many of them supporting the effectiveness of homeopathy in such conditions as depression and pollinosis (Davidson, Morrison, Shore, Davidson, & Bedayn, 1997; Wiesenauer & Ludtke, 1996).

A recent usage survey showed that of 77 patients who used homeopathic treatment for a variety of disorders (most of them chronic, including respiratory, gastrointestinal, and female reproductive problems), most were satisfied with the treatment and stated that they would use homeopathy again (Goldstein & Glik, 1998). The researchers acknowledge, however, that a number of factors contribute to satisfaction with a therapy and that prior expectation may have been as important as the treatment itself for these patients. Patients liked both the noninvasive, "natural" approach offered by homeopathy and the extensive interactions that they experienced with homeopathic practitioners. The contrast of these particulars with many aspects of modern medical care may serve to remind us of what we already know: A therapy's effectiveness comes from much more than the remedy or medicine given.

A great difficulty in using double-blind, placebo-controlled studies in researching homeopathy is that homeopathic prescribing is said to be highly individualized, depending on the specific symptoms reported by the patient, not the name of the diagnosed disease. Thus, simply giving 20 patients with common colds the same remedy would not account for the actual variations in their symptoms. But critics often contend that the therapeutic effect of homeopathy may stem more from the lengthy interview done in history-taking than from the remedy itself.

These issues will be further debated and researched in the coming years while people continue taking homeopathic remedies. A recent essay in the *Journal of the American Medical Association* by a medical student showed growing interest in the use of homeopathy as possibly "another tool in the bag" of physicians (Johnson, 1998).

Resources

Publications that can expand and keep your knowledge of complementary and alternative medicine current:
Homeopathic Educational Services, 2124 Kittredge St., Berkeley, CA 94704; 800-359-9051; *www.homeopathic.com.*

References

Blackie, M.G. (1978). *The patient, not the cure.* Santa Barbara, CA: Woodbridge Press.
Davidson, J.R.T., Morrison, R.M., Shore, J., Davidson, R.T., & Bedayn, G. (1997). Homeopathic treatment of depression and anxiety. *Alternative Therapies in Health and Medicine, 3*(1), 46–49.
Goldstein, M.S., & Glik, D. (1998). Use and satisfaction with homeopathy in a patient population. *Alternative Therapies in Health and Medicine, 4*(2), 60–65.
Inglis, B. (1965). *The case for unorthodox medicine.* New York: G.P. Putnam.
Jacobs, J. (1995). Homeopathy should be integrated into mainstream medicine. *Alternative Therapies in Health and Medicine, 1*(4), 48–53.
Johnson, M.A. (1998). Homeopathy: Another tool in the bag. *JAMA, 279*(9), 707.
Sampson, W. (1995). Homeopathy does not work. *Alternative Therapies in Health and Medicine, 1*(4), 48–52.
Wagner, M. (1997). Is homeopathy "new science" or "new age"? *The Scientific Review of Alternative Medicine, 1*(1), 7–12.
Wiesenauer, M., & Ludtke, R. (1996). A meta-analysis of the homeopathic treatment of pollinosis with *Galphimia glauca. Forschende Komplementarmedizin, 3,* 230–234.

PERCEPTION AND COORDINATION

Assess whether the client has any difficulty with perception or coordination. Sensory or perceptual deficits usually relate to vision or hearing. Problems in coordination could result from muscle weakness or paralysis or from reduced sensation in the hands or fingertips. Clients with these problems could have difficulty reaching medication cabinets, opening medication packages or bottles, splitting scored tablets, or self-administering injections.

This may not be a problem when you administer the client's drugs, but it becomes a significant problem when the client prepares for discharge. An example is a client with poor vision newly started on insulin therapy who cannot see syringe markings. Another is a client with myasthenia gravis who cannot coordinate or control muscle movements. In cases such as these, assess whether family members, friends, or close neighbors can assist. If not, the client may require the services of a home health agency.

Focused Assessment for Altered Health Maintenance

Defining Characteristics

Assess the extent to which a client understands the need for the medication, the instructions for administration, and the need for a temporary or permanent change in lifestyle. Although seemingly simple, for some clients it may be complex. For example, a client given an antibiotic for infection must generally take it for 5 to 10 days, depending on the antibiotic. Although taking this medication is a temporary change in lifestyle, you must assess whether the client understands that it must be taken exactly as prescribed for the full amount of time ordered, even if symptoms disappear. Otherwise, the infection could recur and the client's condition could be worse than when originally diagnosed.

Assess the client's motivation to comply with the instructions. Motivation is often displayed as reviewing instructions and asking questions. The client's motivation for health may be directly related to motivation to take medication. Also, note any evidence of failure to comply with other aspects of the health care regimen.

Additionally assess the client's willingness and ability to take responsibility for self-care.

Related Factors

In general, related factors are those that increase the likelihood that a nursing diagnosis will apply, although they may not have a cause-and-effect relationship. Examples of assessing and responding to related factors for *Altered health maintenance* include the following:

- *Misinterpretation of medication-related information.* A client who inadequately understood previous instructions has *Altered health maintenance,* despite prior teaching. Assess the current level of understanding to plan remedial teaching.
- *Lack of motivation.* A client who has no interest in managing medication therapy may not pay attention to instructions or follow them even if properly understood. Try to assess why the client is not interested so you can develop a teaching strategy with an effective counterplan.
- *Inability to take responsibility for medications.* Sometimes clients cannot take their own medications. A young child or a client who is not ready to learn because of anxiety are two examples. In situations such as these, assess whether other people close to the client could be taught about medication therapy.
- *Cognitive impairment.* Assess the client's ability to take in and retain information. A client who has a disorder that impairs cognitive function, such as a cerebrovascular accident (stroke), closed head injury, or dementia, may not be able to respond adequately to medication teaching. For example, a cognitively impaired client may be unable to remember to take a medication at specified times. This client may benefit from a 7-day medication dispenser, which can be prefilled by a family member or home health nurse. If needed, the teaching plan is again directed to others.

- *Physical impairment.* Some clients are physically unable to administer their own medications. They may be unable to open a pill bottle or manipulate a syringe. They may be paralyzed or have some limitation that prevents mobility in the environment. Assess whether environmental changes are likely to enable the client to take medications. Determine also whether special adaptive devices, such as syringe holders or pill boxes, could help the client become independent. Some clients with physical impairments must have their medications administered by others.
- *Inadequate communication skills.* A client who cannot comprehend directions will have difficulty taking in and retaining medication information. Examples include a client with a language barrier or receptive aphasia (inability to understand the spoken word). When working with such clients, obtain an interpreter or give the instructions to someone who will be assisting the client after discharge.
- *Impaired support systems.* Assess whether the client has another person to turn to if problems arise in taking or obtaining medications. Clients with no support systems are more likely to have difficulty with their medication therapy. Remember that this could also involve assistance for follow-up laboratory work needed with some medications (e.g., the prothrombin time for warfarin therapy). Home health assistance may be required.
- *Lack of resources.* Assess whether the client can physically obtain the medication and has insurance or other financial resources to pay for it. Some medications are quite expensive, and the client may stop taking them because of cost. Others may have no transportation to a pharmacy. Determine whether the client could benefit from referral to a social worker for financial matters or whether resources are available to deliver medication refills to the client.

If medication therapy is to be effective, the client must be able to obtain the medication, store it properly, take it as directed, watch for expected drug effects, and notice and report important side effects. Difficulties in any of these areas leads you to consider *Altered health maintenance* as a nursing diagnosis.

Focused Assessment for Related Nursing Diagnoses

The issues and problems that could arise during medication therapy are so broad that several other nursing diagnoses could be relevant. Assess for factors indicating that the following nursing diagnoses are applicable, and see the data clustering chart for examples of data groups based on specific client assessments.

Constipation or Diarrhea

Assess for *Constipation* or *Diarrhea* caused by medication therapy. Many medications affect the GI tract. For

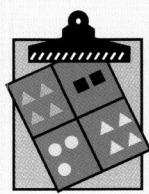

CLUSTERING DATA TO MAKE A NURSING DIAGNOSIS
MEDICATION THERAPY

Data Cluster	Nursing Diagnosis
A client with a newly prescribed medication does not know what effects to expect or how to use the medication properly, but she has expressed an interest in learning about it.	*Altered health maintenance* related to insufficient knowledge of medication use and effects.
The client has been changed from an oral hypoglycemic drug to insulin therapy. She is elderly and has arthritis in her hands and fingers. Although she expresses interest in managing her insulin therapy, she is unable to draw up the insulin or manipulate the syringe.	*Ineffective management of therapeutic regimen: individuals,* related to poor manual dexterity secondary to inflammation of joints.
An elderly client has not refilled the prescription he needs because he says he cannot afford the medication and has no transportation to local pharmacy.	*Noncompliance* related to medication therapy secondary to financial and physical barriers.

example, narcotics frequently cause constipation, whereas antibiotics may cause diarrhea. Determine the client's usual pattern of bowel elimination, and question the client about recent changes in bowel habits. Analyze these changes in relation to the onset and timing of medications. The focus of nursing care is reducing or eliminating the disturbance.

Altered Sexuality Patterns

Some drugs have side effects that affect the libido. Assess for *Altered sexuality patterns* in a candid yet sensitive manner. Examples of drugs that decrease libido are antidepressants, antihistamines, antihypertensives, and sedatives and tranquilizers (chronic use). Other drugs increase libido, such as testosterone, sedatives (low-dose), and tranquilizers. The focus of your nursing care is teaching the client about these side effects.

Sleep Pattern Disturbance

Some drugs cause drowsiness as a side effect; others cause excitability. For example, sedatives and hypnotics cause drowsiness. Yet with prolonged use, they can interrupt normal sleep cycles sufficiently so that the client has daytime somnolence with night-time wakefulness. Other drugs, such as nervous system stimulants, prevent the client from falling asleep. Assess for *Sleep pattern disturbance* and its effects on the client. Analyze whether the timing of medications could be changed to allow more normal sleep, and implement these changes whenever possible. The focus of your nursing care is otherwise directed at reducing interfering stimuli, such as noise, temperature, a full bladder, pain, fear, or stress.

Risk for Injury

A possible diagnosis is *Risk for injury* from drug side effects that negatively affect either mobility or sensorium. Clients with reduced mobility may be at risk for falls from a decreased ability to move purposefully in the environment. Clients with altered sensorium may harm themselves either by falling or by climbing out of bed over the side rails or foot of the bed. Drugs that could cause these effects include sedatives, vasodilators, diuretics, hypoglycemics, antihypertensives, and psychotropics. Assess the client's risk of injury and put precautionary measures in place, such as a call bell, ambulation aids, night light, and clutter-free environment.

Risk for Infection

Assess the client taking medications for the diagnosis *Risk for infection.* This could occur as a result of antibiotic therapy due to superinfection, which is an overgrowth of pathogens normally kept in balance by the organisms killed by the antibiotic. Assess for signs of superinfection, such as oral lesions (thrush), diarrhea *(Clostridium difficile),* or vaginal itching (yeast infection). Report these signs and symptoms to the physician so that the new infections may be treated.

Risk for infection also may be appropriate for clients taking medications that depress the immune system. Examples include clients with cancer who receive chemotherapy or radiation therapy and clients taking immunosuppressant drugs after organ transplant. Monitor vigilantly these clients' vital signs (especially temperature), white blood cell counts, and other signs and symptoms of infection. Remember that infection can occur in immunosuppressed clients when the white blood cell count is too low, not only when elevated. Report signs and symptoms of infection immediately.

Sensory/Perceptual Alterations

A few drug groups, mostly sedatives and tranquilizers, can reduce or change the perception of incoming stimuli. Assess the client for such indicators as disorientation, restlessness, blurred vision, and sometimes auditory or visual hallucinations. The diagnosis *Sensory/perceptual alterations* may be caused by toxic drug effects (such as hearing loss from ototoxity with aminoglycosides). Check the drug literature for adverse neurological effects and report them if noted. Institute a plan to reorient the client as needed, and take measures to maintain client safety.

Altered Nutrition

A number of medications cause GI side effects, such as anorexia or GI discomfort, in addition to the constipation and diarrhea previously discussed. Assess for these symptoms, which could impair the client's appetite, leading to the diagnosis *Altered nutrition.* Teach clients about the proper timing of medications in relation to meals to reduce the incidence of this problem. Report abdominal discomfort that the client cannot tolerate (such as severe abdominal pain caused by erythromycin). The physician may change to a drug with fewer GI side effects.

Ineffective Management of Therapeutic Regimen

Assess the client's ability to understand and follow the drug regimen. Sometimes clients who are labeled as noncompliant actually have barriers to effective self-administration. These barriers can stem from lack of comprehension, family conflicts, mistrust of the health care team, or a complex medication regimen.

Each of these factors requires a different approach on your part. For example, the elderly and those with multiple health problems are most likely to have complex medication schedules. Develop calendars, charts, or other visual reminders for use as needed. Some clients benefit from using prefilled weekly or monthly medication boxes to prevent them from taking the wrong medication or dose. At times, you may enlist the help of family, friends, or home health agency to ensure that the client receives correct medications.

Impaired Swallowing

Watch the client swallow and ask if he can feel medications in his mouth. If needed, assess the function of cranial nerves IX and X. Use *Impaired swallowing* as a nursing diagnosis if the client has an impaired gag reflex, if food remains in his mouth after he swallows, or if he coughs when swallowing medications, liquids, or food (see Chapter 30).

The focus of care is to give medication in a form that the client can manage. This sometimes involves crushing medications and giving them with a soft food such as applesauce. Remember not to crush enteric-coated tablets or time-release capsules. Sometimes you may need to ask the physician to change the form of a medication from solid to liquid. At other times, the route should be changed from oral to enteral. A client who cannot swallow medications is at risk for aspiration, which could lead to pneumonia.

DIAGNOSIS

A useful approach for selecting nursing diagnoses may be to think about the goal of care for a particular client. For example, consider an otherwise healthy 68-year-old female who has been hospitalized with a myocardial infarction. The client is diagnosed concurrently with hypertension and shows early signs of heart failure. The client is started on daily oral doses of furosemide (a diuretic) and metoprolol (an antihypertensive, antianginal). Nitroglycerin sublingual tablets (antianginal) are prescribed for PRN use. The client is scheduled for discharge within 24 hours and says that she doesn't understand how these medications will help her. The most logical nursing diagnosis with the information given is *Altered health maintenance.* These medications are newly ordered for this client, who was healthy before admission. A sample nursing diagnostic statement could be *Altered health maintenance related to insufficient knowledge of newly prescribed medications.* The goal of care is to return the client to independent living, and the client requires the usual information about medication therapy prior to discharge.

If this client had mild dementia and could not retain information, you might select *Ineffective management of therapeutic regimen.* A sample nursing diagnostic statement might be *Ineffective management of therapeutic regimen related to cognitive impairment.* The goal of care in this case would be to put safeguards in place to ensure that the client receives both of her daily medications and the PRN nitroglycerin as well.

If an oriented client experienced orthostatic hypotension from the vasodilating effect of metoprolol and fluid loss from furosemide, you might select the nursing diagnosis *Risk for injury.* A sample nursing diagnostic statement could be *Risk for injury related to orthostatic hypotension secondary to medication effect.* The goal of care in this instance would be to keep the client from injuring herself or experiencing falls during periods of dizziness and hypotension. The focus of care would be to teach the client to change position slowly, avoid concurrent use of alcohol, and other standard measures outlined in pharmacology references.

Even if medication use is not the driving force in formulating a nursing diagnosis, administration of medications may be included in the nursing interventions listed for other nursing diagnoses. A client with emphysema may have a nursing diagnosis of *Activity intolerance.* Teaching proper use of bronchodilators may be part of the plan of care for that nursing diagnosis.

In conclusion, clinical diagnostic reasoning is a complex process that becomes easier with time and practice. Assess each client carefully, and cluster the data to form possible alternative nursing diagnoses. Select the one that has the best "fit" with the goal or intended outcome of care. You will find that *Altered health maintenance* is often appropriate for use with the client receiving medication therapy.

PLANNING

During the planning phase of the nursing process, establish the expected outcomes or goals for the selected nursing diagnosis. Next, write the specific nursing interventions that will help the client achieve the identified outcomes. Some sample expected outcomes for the client receiving medication therapy with a nursing diagnosis of *Altered health maintenance* follow:

- Verbalizes an understanding of purposes, actions, and adverse effects of medications
- Relates an intention to comply with medication therapy
- Correctly self-administers medications
- States proper information about drug procurement, storage, and handling
- States an appropriate plan for medical follow-up for monitoring of medications

These expected outcomes could apply to the client being discharged from nursing care in any setting, including a hospital, extended-care facility, or home health agency. The expected outcomes may be modified or made more specific depending on individual client need. For example, the client who is learning to self-inject insulin may need additional intermediate goals to assist in meeting these expected outcomes. The goals developed for a specific client drive the selection of nursing interventions, which are then implemented to provide quality nursing care.

Mr. Connell will be discharged to his home from the ED. His wife has been quietly waiting with him during his evaluation. The diagnosis of myocardial infarction has been ruled out, but he has been diagnosed with hypertension and stable angina. He is being restarted on atenolol and furosemide and is being given a prescription for nitroglycerin for PRN use to relieve chest pain. As the nurse preparing Mr. Connell for discharge, what is your nursing diagnosis? What are your goals? What would you teach him about his medications? What factors should you assess about his home environment and lifestyle? What specific topics would you include in your teaching, and why? How would you modify your teaching because Mrs. Connell is present?

INTERVENTION

Interventions to Address Altered Health Maintenance

The interventions that help a client meet the expected outcomes for *Altered health maintenance* are driven by the goals established for the client. They often include the following steps:

- Explain the medication's purpose and action in clear and simple terms. Provide instruction in an unhurried manner to allow the client time to process information and ask questions.
- Describe key side effects, and stress the ones the client should report immediately.
- Determine the client's ability to obtain the medication after discharge and to take it correctly. Make referrals as needed to ensure that the client has the assistance required.
- Instruct selected clients to carry an identification card or wear a bracelet identifying the medications being used.
- Give written materials and encourage questions, both at the time of teaching and later.

The Teaching for Self-Care Chart summarizes other important teaching that will enable clients to manage a medication regimen effectively.

Interventions to Provide Safe and Effective Medication Therapy

Measuring the Dose

To correctly administer medications, you must be able to accurately calculate and measure the drug dose. Computation errors, such as incorrect placement of a decimal or addition of an extra zero, could be harmful or possibly lethal to the client. Inability to draw up a medication to the correct calibration unit on a syringe could have equally disastrous consequences. To ensure accuracy in drug calculation and measurement, become comfortable working with the three systems of weight and volume measurement currently in use. These systems are the metric, apothecary, and household systems. In the United States and Canada, the metric system is the primary system used. Because the United States has not formally adopted the metric system as the official standard of measurement, some drugs are ordered using the apothecary system. When a client is given a prescription for home use, the order is often written using household measures for convenience.

METRIC SYSTEM
The metric system is a logical, easy-to-understand measurement system based on units of 10. Movement from one metric unit to another can be done by multiplying or dividing by 10. The decimal point moves to the right when multiplying, and to the left when dividing.

There are three basic units of measurement in the metric system. These are the meter (measuring length), the liter (measuring volume), and the gram (measuring weight). Volume and weight measurements are the ones most commonly computed as part of medication therapy (Fig. 26–2).

Teaching for SELF-CARE

SELF-ADMINISTERING MEDICATIONS EFFECTIVELY

Purpose: To obtain optimal effects from medication therapy with a minimum of unanticipated effects.

Rationale. Being informed about the purpose and proper use of medications is likely to enhance a client's compliance with therapy. It also decreases the overall cost of managing a health problem by helping to minimize the number and severity of exacerbations.

Expected Outcome: The client will demonstrate proper use and handling of medications and will adhere to the medication regimen.

Client Instructions

- Take all medications according to the directions on the package.
- Finish all prescriptions given for short-term use (such as antibiotics). Do not stop taking prescription medication unless you are told to do so by the prescriber.
- Follow any guidelines given about follow-up blood work, measurement of vital signs or weight, or visits to the physician. Some medications must be monitored periodically to make sure you have the correct level in your bloodstream. In other cases, the physician may need to examine you to determine whether the medication is effective.
- Follow any guidelines given about foods, alcohol, or over-the-counter drugs to be used or avoided while taking the medication. This will help the medication to work most effectively and will reduce the risk of food or drug interactions.

- Obtain all medications from the same pharmacy so that the pharmacist will be familiar with your total medication regimen. This will enable the pharmacist to give you the most complete and thorough advice about taking your medications.
- Call the prescriber if you feel that the medication is causing adverse effects.
- Store medications properly to maintain their potency. Keep them in a cool, dry place, out of direct sunlight and out of the research of children.
- If needed, use some form of reminder system to help you to remember to take medications as directed. Use a calendar, pill box, or paper clock if these would be helpful. Ask your nurse or physician to help you decide which method would be best for you.
- Do not change brand names of a medication without checking first with the prescriber. Sometimes different brand names have different added ingredients, and the real strength of the medication (bioavailability) may vary slightly from brand to brand.
- Keep all medications in their original containers. Check the expiration dates regularly, and obtain a new supply before the expiration date arrives so that medications exert the full intended effect.
- Do not take medications that have been prescribed for another person, and do not give another person a medication that was prescribed for you.

APOTHECARY SYSTEM

The apothecary system is familiar to most people in the United States and Canada, even if it is not the most widely used system for drug measurement. It originated in colonial England and is based on the weight of a single grain of wheat. The basic unit for weight, then, is called the grain (gr.). In this system, Roman numerals are used to denote numbers that are equal to or larger than 1 (gr. X = 10 grains). Fractions are used to express weights that are less than 1 (gr. ¼). Progressions or increases in weight are labeled dram, ounce, and pound.

The basic unit of measure in the apothecary system is the minim, which is the approximate amount of water that weighs a grain. Progressions or increases in volume from the level of the minim are labeled fluid dram, fluid ounce, pint, quart, and gallon. Abbreviations are often made using special symbols, which can be confusing because they resemble other abbreviations. For example, grains and grams are often confused with each other, and the symbol for dram resembles the number 3. Cohen (1993) reports that these

confusions have led to serious medication errors. Fortunately, these symbols are rarely used today.

HOUSEHOLD MEASUREMENTS

The household system of measurement is familiar to most people. The basic units of measure for weight are the ounce and the pound. The basic units of measure for volume are the teaspoon (tsp.), tablespoon (tbsp.), ounce (oz.), pint (pt.), quart (qt.), and gallon (gal.). There is some overlap between the apothecary and household measurement systems.

The household system is the least precise because household utensils used to measure liquids, such as cups and teaspoons, vary in size. Scales (if they are used in the household) may not be well calibrated. Many times, however, the convenience and familiarity of these systems warrants their use in the home, especially if complete dosage accuracy is not essential. For example, OTC drugs such as cough syrups and antacids are often measured this way. Table 26–6 compares approximate equivalent measurements using each of the three systems.

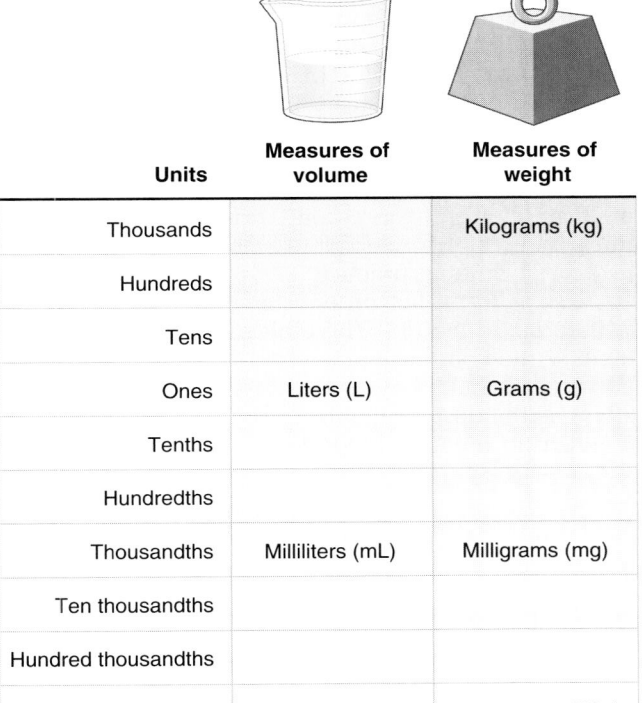

Units	Measures of volume	Measures of weight
Thousands		Kilograms (kg)
Hundreds		
Tens		
Ones	Liters (L)	Grams (g)
Tenths		
Hundredths		
Thousandths	Milliliters (mL)	Milligrams (mg)
Ten thousandths		
Hundred thousandths		
Millionths	Microliters (mL)	Micrograms (mg)

Figure 26–2. Measures of volume and weight in the metric system.

SOLUTIONS

Solutions contain a specific amount of either a liquid or solid substance dissolved in a known amount of liquid. You will use solutions frequently in clinical practice for procedures such as injections, infusions, and irrigations. Carefully check the concentration of any solution before using it. The concentration is best described as the amount of solute per unit of solvent (such as mg/mL or g/mL) and is sometimes expressed as a percentage. Common examples include IV solutions containing 5% dextrose in water or an irrigating solution of 0.9% sodium chloride. Occasionally, solutions are expressed as a proportion, such as 1:1,000 solution, which has 1 g of a solid dissolved in 1,000 mL of a liquid.

CONVERTING MEASUREMENT UNITS

Nurses routinely convert drug doses from one form of measurement to another. The most obvious example is when a dose of a narcotic analgesic is ordered in grains and the drug is supplied in milligrams. You must correctly convert between the apothecary and metric systems to administer the correct dose to the client. Other examples of common conversions include recording ounces of fluid intake as milliliters and body weight as kilograms instead of pounds.

CONVERSION WITHIN A SYSTEM. Making conversions within a system is relatively easy. Within the metric system, either multiply or divide by 10 or one of its

TABLE 26–6

Approximate Equivalents Among Metric, Apothecary, and Household Measurement Systems

Measure	Metric	Apothecary	Household
Volume			
	5 mL	1 fluid dram	1 teaspoon
	10 mL	2 fluid drams	2 teaspoons
	15 mL	4 fluid drams	1 tablespoon
	30 mL	1 fluid ounce	1 ounce
	60 mL	2 fluid ounces	1 wine glass
	120 mL	4 fluid ounces	1 teacup
	240 mL	8 fluid ounces	1 tumbler
	500 mL	1 pint	1 pint
	1000 mL	1 quart	1 quart
	4000 mL	1 gallon	1 gallon
Weight			
	1 mg	1/60 grain	
	4 mg	1/15 grain	
	10 mg	1/6 grain	
	15 mg	1/4 grain	
	30 mg	1/2 grain	
	60 mg	1 grain	
	1 g	15 grains	
	4 g	1 dram	
	30 g	1 ounce	1 ounce
	500 g	1.1 pound	1.1 pound
	1000 g (1 kg)	2.2 pounds	2.2 pounds

multiples. To convert grams to kilograms, divide the number of grams by 1,000 by moving the decimal point three places to the left (for example, 480 g = 0.480 kg). To convert grams to milligrams, multiply the number of milligrams by 1,000 by moving the decimal point three places to the right (for example, 0.75 g = 750 mg).

Within the apothecary system, use or memorize a conversion table. This enables you to know, for example, that there are 32 ounces in a quart and 64 ounces in a half gallon. Because this system is used so frequently in the United States, you will often make these conversions by memory.

CONVERSION BETWEEN SYSTEMS. In clinical practice, it is common to convert between the metric and apothecary systems to calculate drug doses. It is also common to convert from either of these systems to the household system for ease in client teaching. Begin the conversion process by comparing the ordered measurement with what is available. You must identify the equivalent needed to make the conversion. For example, say a surgeon has ordered *morphine sulfate gr. ⅙ IM q 3 to 4 h PRN for pain.* The unit dose of morphine is labeled 10 mg/mL. To calculate the dose, you must convert the grains to mg. Recall that there are 60 mg in a grain. Set up the conversion as follows:

$$60 \text{ mg/grain} \times \tfrac{1}{6} \text{ grain} = 10 \text{ mg}$$

When calculated correctly, you then know that one unit dose of the narcotic must be used for the injection. Review a pharmacological math text for ready access to multiple examples and sample problems for converting from one unit of measure to another.

DOSAGE CALCULATIONS

Standard mathematical formulas or calculations are available to solve many problems in calculating drug dosages. Some involve using ratio and proportion, whereas two other identical and commonly used ones are the following:

$$\frac{\text{Dose ordered}}{\text{Dose on hand}} \times \text{Amount on hand} = \frac{\text{Amount to}}{\text{administer}}$$

or

$$\frac{\text{Desired}}{\text{Have}} \times \text{Quantity} = \text{Dose}$$

The dose that is "ordered" or "desired" is the amount of drug prescribed by the physician. It is the precise amount that the client should receive. The dose that is on hand (or the "have") is the drug measurement (weight or volume) available from the pharmacy. The dose on hand can be determined by reading the label. It states the amount of drug present in each tablet or capsule or in a certain volume of liquid. The "amount on hand" or "quantity" is the actual unit that contains the dose on hand. This could be "1 tablet" if the medication is a solid, or it could be "5 mL" if the

medication is a liquid. For the most part, the "amount on hand" (quantity) is the most confusing part of the equation for nursing students. Some students repeatedly try to put the value of "1" into the equation for "amount on hand" instead of carefully reading the label and inserting the true unit.

Two sample problems help to illustrate drug dose calculations. The first is a calculation using a solid medication form; the second uses a liquid. Beyond this, you are again referred to a pharmacological math text for additional practice.

Example 1: The order states to give *diltiazem (Cardizem) 30 mg PO.* The tablets are labeled 60 mg/tablet. After comparing the order with the medication, you reason that 30 mg is the dose "desired," whereas 60 mg is the dose available, or the "have." You would then set up the calculation as shown:

$$\frac{30 \text{ mg}}{60 \text{ mg}} \times 1 \text{ tablet} = \text{No. of tablets to administer}$$

Simplify the fraction by dividing the numerator and denominator by 30 to get

$$\tfrac{1}{2} \times 1 \text{ tablet} = \tfrac{1}{2} \text{ or } 0.5 \text{ tablet to administer}$$

This example illustrates that a portion of a solid drug may be given. However, this can only be done if the tablet or pill is scored (has an indented line) to allow it to be broken easily into two equal halves. A tablet that is not scored may not be broken into a partial dose because it is highly likely that the dose of the broken pill will be inaccurate. The client could then receive either a high or low dose of the medication. Either situation is equally dangerous to the client.

Example 2: The order states to give *KCl Elixir 20 mEq PO.* The label on the bottle states a drug concentration of 40 mEq/15 mL. After comparing the order with the drug label, you reason that the 20 mEq is the dose "desired," whereas 40 mEq is the dose available, or the "have." The amount on hand or "quantity" is 15 mL. Set up the calculation as shown:

$$\frac{20 \text{ mEq}}{40 \text{ mEq}} \times 15 \text{ mL} = \text{No. of mL to administer}$$

Simplify the fraction by dividing the numerator and denominator by 20 to get

$$\tfrac{1}{2} \times 15 \text{ mL} = 7.5 \text{ mL to administer}$$

You should give 7.5 mL of liquid to deliver the 20-mEq dose. The formula for liquids applies regardless of whether the volume of fluid is greater or less than 1 mL. The important consideration is to multiply and divide correctly and to mark decimals properly to arrive at the correct answer.

Whenever you are performing drug calculations, make it a habit to perform a "common sense check" at the end of the problem. Compare the answer obtained in relation to the dose required and the amount of drug available. If the answer seems oddly high or low, recheck the answer or have another nurse check the dose before giving it to the client. Naturally, client safety is always of paramount importance.

PEDIATRIC DOSAGES

It is particularly important to calculate dosages correctly for pediatric clients because of their smaller body size and weight and possible differences in metabolism. Physicians usually calculate the safe dose when ordering the medication. Most drug references include the safe dose range for pediatric clients as well. Your additional responsibility when giving medications to pediatric clients is to recheck the client's dose to ensure that it is in the safe dose range.

One method for calculating a dose is based on the child's weight. For example, a drug may be ordered in mg/kg of body weight. Determine the client's weight in kilograms and multiply it by the number of mg/kg ordered. Your answer is the child's dose.

Regardless of the method used to calculate a pediatric dose, remember that these methods only provide the best estimate of the required dose. It is imperative to evaluate the pediatric client's response to medication as the final check of the appropriateness of a drug dosage. Note and report any adverse effects immediately so that dosage adjustments can be made if needed.

Administering the Dose

Safety and accuracy in medication administration are of paramount importance. During the course of a normal work shift, you may administer multiple medications to a large number of clients. Each time a medication is administered, there is a risk of error. Do not become lulled by habit when preparing medications. Each drug administration requires alertness and purposeful action. Use a systematic method of checking medications during preparation to prevent possible errors. The "gold standard" check system used by nurses is called the "five rights." The following paragraphs briefly discuss each of them.

RIGHT DRUG

Make sure that you have selected the right drug by comparing the drug name that is written on the container with the medication administration record (Fig. 26–3) or computer-generated list. In fact, you should check the medication label against the administration record three times while preparing the medication:

- When first taking the medication out of the container or unit-dose package
- Just before opening the medication package or pouring the dose
- Just before replacing the container in the storage area or giving a unit dose to the client

Never administer a medication prepared by someone else because you (who administers it) are respon-

sible for its effects. Take any client concerns about the drug seriously. If a client questions a drug or expresses any form of concern, stop and verify the order before administering it. In many cases, you will find that the physician has changed the order, but this last check *can* prevent an error. If the client refuses a drug, discard it if it was taken from a bulk container. Unopened unit doses may be stored again. Finally, only remove medications from packages or bottles with clearly marked labels.

RIGHT DOSE

The unit-dose drug distribution system widely used today minimizes the chance of errors in drug dose. Occasionally, however, the unit dose supplied by the pharmacy does not match the total dose ordered by the physician. In this instance, you must calculate the needed amount. For example, the client may have an order for digoxin (Lanoxin) 0.25 mg. The available supply is 0.125 mg. To give the correct dose, you must calculate that 2 tablets must be given.

At other times, a drug is ordered using one measurement system but has a label from another. Make the correct conversion to administer the correct dose. For example, the client may have an order for codeine gr. ½. The narcotic supply area has codeine 30-mg tablets available. Calculate or recall that 60 mg = 1 gr. Therefore, 30 mg must equal ½ gr. You would then know to sign out 1 tablet.

Ensure also that a correct dose is given by carefully handling a medication that will be crushed or broken. Tablets to be split are cut evenly with a sharp object into two pieces; if they are uneven, they are discarded and a new one is used. This limits the chance of underdose or overdose. Medications that are crushed should be completely removed from the crushing device, which should then be carefully cleaned before the next use.

Finally, there are instances when it is helpful to check the dose of an ordered medication with another nurse. Some nurses routinely check all insulin and heparin doses with another nurse. Many drugs have powerful effects on the body, and this check decreases the risk of dosage error.

RIGHT CLIENT

Check the client's identity before giving each medication to make sure that the correct client receives the dose. In most facilities, clients wear identification bracelets. Carefully check the client's bracelet against the medication administration record or name on the computer sheet before administering medications. Any identification bracelet that is smudged or cannot be easily read should be replaced immediately. This practice should be strictly followed even if you have come to know the client (such as in extended-care facilities).

Another widely accepted method of client identification is to ask the client to state his name. Avoid asking the client to identify himself using a question that could be answered with a nod of the head, such as,

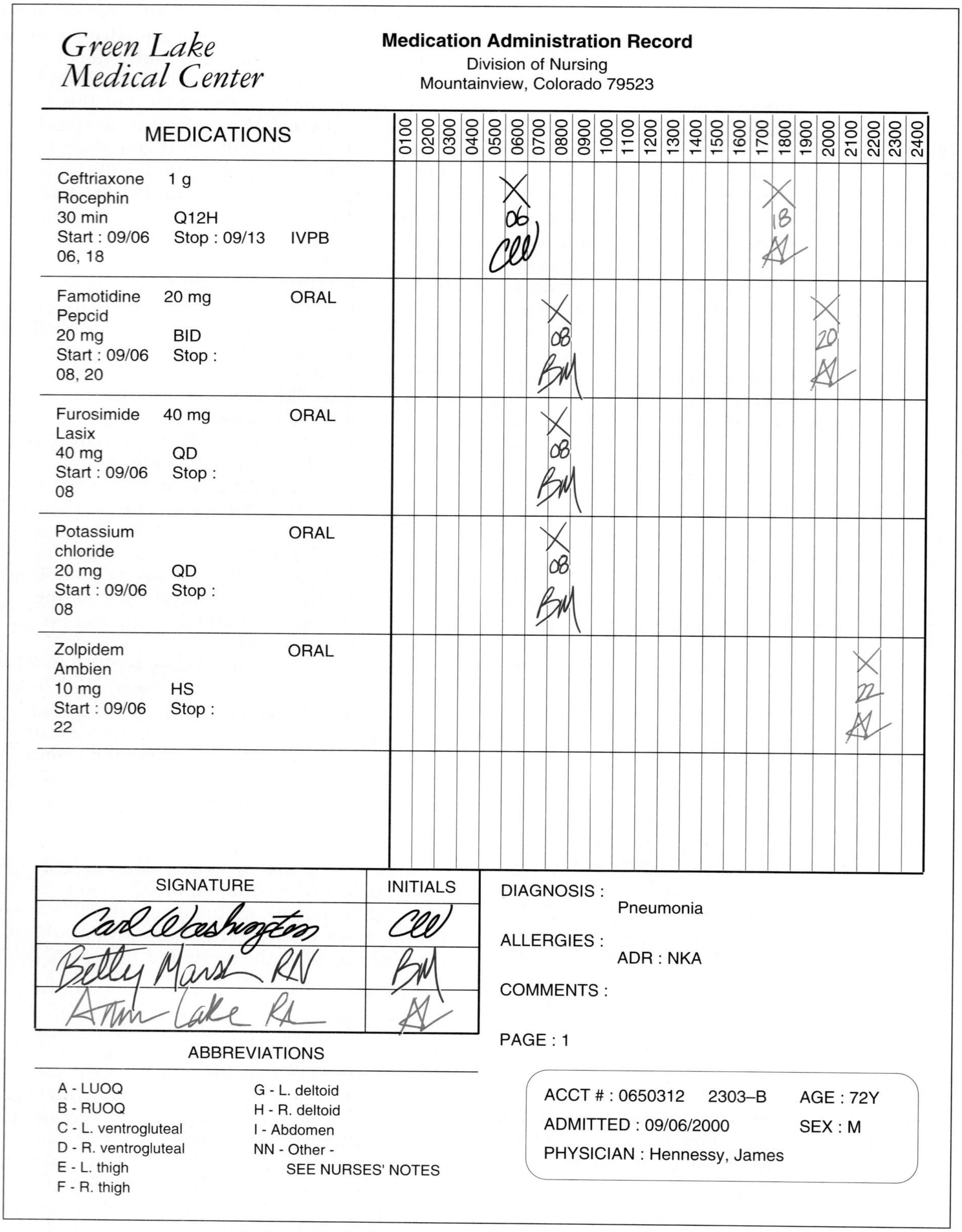

Figure 26–3. Sample medication administration record.

"Are you Mrs. Cook?" Clients who are confused or not fluent in the language used by the nurse could misunderstand and nod inappropriately.

In the home care setting, teach clients not to share their medications with others. Because both the medication and the dose are specifically ordered for that client, others cannot be expected to have the same response to the drug. In fact, it could be hazardous to the other person taking it. Include this point as part of your teaching about medication safety.

RIGHT ROUTE

Check the medication order carefully to see that the route is specified. Clarify any illegible or missing route, and question the order if you know that the medication is not usually given by the specified route.

Because drug companies manufacture drugs to be given by different routes, take care to have the correct preparation on hand. For example, oral solutions may not be injected, and parenteral medications are not administered orally. Medications manufactured for parenteral use usually state "for injection only" or something similar. Incorrectly used preparations can cause harm.

RIGHT TIME

A scheduled medication is given at specified frequencies or times. Be sure to give it at the correct time. A drug should be given within 30 minutes before or after the ordered time.

Medications that are given once daily should be given at the same time each day to maintain a therapeutic blood level. Medications that are quickly metabolized are spaced evenly around the clock for the same reason. Most health care agencies have policies indicating standard times for medication administration. For example, one institution may schedule BID medications for 8 AM and 8 PM, whereas another may choose 10 AM and 10 PM. The use of standardized times helps to decrease the number of omitted or doubled doses. It also helps to organize the nurses' work so that the entire shift is not spent administering medications to a group of clients.

Know the nature and purpose of a medication so you can ensure optimal timing. The physician will indicate the frequency for drug administration as part of the order; however, you must use critical thinking skills in scheduling the medication. For example, a medication that is ordered quater in die (QID) (four times daily) and one that is ordered every 6 hours are both given four times a day. The QID medication, however, may be given before or after meals and at bedtime, whereas the medication ordered every 6 hours must be timed so doses are spaced evenly around the clock. Question an order if the timing does not seem optimal based on concepts of pharmacokinetics and maintaining consistent serum drug levels.

The timing of PRN medications is of special concern. If a medication is ordered *q4h PRN,* you may not administer it more frequently than every 4 hours without obtaining a new order from the physician. Before administering a PRN medication, check the time the last dose was given. If more time has elapsed since the last dose than the interval specified by order, the medication may be safely given. Analgesics are commonly ordered on a PRN basis.

In the home setting, you may assist the client in planning the medication schedule within the parameters of the prescription order. Consider both drug variables and client variables, such as personal preference and the ability to remember to take the dose.

DEVELOPMENTAL CONSIDERATIONS

Both younger and older clients may have special needs with regard to medications. Assess their unique needs to facilitate safe and effective medication administration. Children under age 5 may have trouble swallowing pills, tablets, and capsules. They may require a liquid form. If a liquid form is accompanied by a special measuring device, use it in dosage preparation and clean it after use. If no liquid form is available, crush the solid form and add it to a soft food such as applesauce or pudding (Box 26–3).

BOX 26–3

HELPFUL HINTS FOR ADMINISTERING MEDICATIONS TO CHILDREN

- Hold a very young child or infant in an upright or semi-upright position with his back against your chest or abdomen. Use a dropper to place the medication between his gum and cheek. This promotes swallowing and prevents the medication from being aspirated or spit out.
- Crush pills or tablets (unless they have an enteric coating) and mix them with a small amount of soft food, such as cereal or applesauce to make them easier to swallow. Avoid using a favorite food or an essential dietary item (such as formula) so the child will not refuse the food in the future. Avoid using large volumes to ensure that the child takes the full dose.
- Use a calibrated device supplied with the medication to accurately measure liquid doses under 10 mL. If a measuring device is not provided, use a disposable syringe without the needle attached. Do not use a teaspoon to measure the dose because it may be inaccurate. A spoon may be used to actually give the medication after measuring the dose properly.
- Be honest when administering medications to children who are old enough to communicate. Tell them if the medication has an unpleasant taste or that an injection may hurt briefly. Failure to do so can damage the child's trust in you.
- Give injections quickly. Distract the child using toys or conversations as appropriate. Be prepared to briefly restrain the child if necessary. Encourage the child to look away from the site during an injection. Also encourage the child to pretend to "blow away" the pain.
- Praise the child for taking the medication, and offer rewards if they are available and appropriate, such as stickers or lollipops.
- Monitor the child carefully for side effects after medication administration. Young children especially are unable to report reactions to medications.

When giving parenteral medications to children, use proper injection sites for the client's age. For example, avoid the gluteus maximus muscle when giving an infant an IM injection because it is in close proximity to major nerves and blood vessels. Use knowledge of the child's developmental level to plan an effective approach. For instance, give a fearful toddler or preschool child a toy or blanket to hold for security. Some may cry, and you should allow them to do so. Comfort the client during and after the injection, and use rewards as appropriate.

Parents are often responsible for giving medications to children once they leave the hospital or physician's office. Teach the parents how to give the medication correctly and how to store it after use. Many times antibiotics, commonly given to children, require refrigeration. Medications are now routinely packaged in containers with child-resistant caps. Teach parents to replace the cap securely for the child's safety, and keep all medications in the original containers.

Not only do older adults commonly require smaller doses because of age-related changes, they may need some special consideration as well. Consider the following suggestions when giving medications to older clients:

- Allow sufficient time to administer medications to older clients. They may require additional explanations of the medications being given, and they may have slower reflexes and body movements.
- Offer a small amount of liquid before giving medications to ease swallowing. Administer only one or two medications at a time for the same reason.
- Encourage the client to drink an additional 5 or 6 ounces of fluid after taking all medications to ensure that they have reached the stomach and to enhance medication absorption.
- Obtain a liquid form of the medication if possible for those who have trouble swallowing. If not, crush non–enteric-coated tablets or empty the contents of capsules into soft foods or liquids. Gently massaging the laryngeal prominence or the area just under the chin stimulates swallowing.
- Teach clients to identify medications by name, not by the color of the tablet. Generic drugs could vary in color according to manufacturer, and visual changes associated with aging could make it difficult for the client to use color as a guide.
- Assess all older adults for special needs, especially in the home setting. Help diabetic clients with motor or visual problems to draw up or inject insulin. Provide prefilled medication boxes to those with memory deficits so medications are taken at the correct times.

Documenting the Dose

After administering a medication to a client, chart it immediately on the medication administration record or computerized medical record. Chart the site of a parenteral medication also. When a medication ad-ministration record is used, initial the medication in the appropriate area on the form. Write your full signature once on the bottom of the page next to your initials. When a computerized record is used, your computer code is the signature and your name is printed at the bottom of the sheet along with the computer signature when a copy is printed for the medical record.

If a client refuses a medication, or if a dose was omitted, document that the dose was not taken. It is common to chart the time and circle it to indicate a refused or missed dose. Write a follow-up note in the medical record indicating the reasons for the omission. When a computerized record is used, you may use a light-pen or mouse to select "given" or "not given." When "not given" is selected, indicate on a follow-up screen why it was omitted. Provide follow-up charting in the medical record as required by facility policy.

There are various reasons for not giving a scheduled medication. A client may refuse the dose for several reasons. A client may not think the dose is necessary, such as refusing a stool softener when he has diarrhea. A client who routinely took the medication before admission may have a medication time schedule that does not match institutional policy. (Client preferences should be respected if appropriate and possible.) At times, clients do not understand the importance of the medication, and client teaching resolves the problem.

Occasionally, a medication dose is be omitted because the client was not available at the scheduled time. This happens when the client leaves the unit for procedures such as diagnostic testing. Use facility policy and medication knowledge as guides when rescheduling these doses.

Avoiding Errors

Multiple checks and balances should be used to prevent medication errors. The physician should write legible orders that contain correct information. You should check the order during transcription and question any area of concern. The pharmacy technician and pharmacist should check the order while dispensing the medication. You should check the order again when preparing the medication for administration. Consistent use of the "five rights" of medication administration substantially reduces the likelihood of a medication error.

If a medication error does occur, it is your professional responsibility to report it. Follow facility policies and procedures for reporting and documenting the incident. Report the error to the physician and appropriate nursing management personnel. The physician will order any follow-up procedures or tests that are indicated or may prescribe an antidote.

Your highest priority after a medication error is the client's physiological status and safety. Carefully assess the drug's effects, and quickly carry out new orders given to counteract them.

Document the error carefully. Write factual information about the error in an accurate, thorough, and objective manner on the medical record. Avoid the use of judgmental words such as "error" in the documentation. Instead, chart the medication administered, the actual dose given (not the ordered dose), and any observable client effects. Document also that the physician was notified, any follow-up actions or orders that were implemented, and the client's condition after both the medication error and any corrective actions.

Most facilities require additional documentation when a medication error occurs, usually with a form called an *incident report* or *unusual occurrence report.* Document factual information about the error and corrective actions on this form as well. Complete any additional sections of the form, which may help during investigation of the incident. This report is used by the institution's risk management department. Do not document on the medical record that an incident report was filled out, and do not keep a copy of incident reports. If it becomes known that you have one, it may be subject to subpoena if the client sues for negligence. This is also why a copy of an incident report is never filed in the medical record.

Interventions Specific to Drug Route

Managing Oral Medications

The oral route is most commonly used for medication administration. Orally administered medications have a slower onset of action and a more prolonged, less potent effect. They are less expensive to manufacture, easy to administer, and do not interrupt the skin and mucous membrane barriers. This route is safe and effective provided the client can swallow adequately and has proper GI tract functioning. Clients with nausea and vomiting, impaired gag or swallow reflexes, or a decreased level of consciousness may require special consideration.

Oral medications are most frequently given in solid forms, such as tablets, capsules, and pills. Liquid forms are helpful for clients who have trouble swallowing tablets, and can be poured using a variety of aids. When pouring a dose into a calibrated measuring cup, measure the dose at the base of the meniscus (Fig. 26–4).

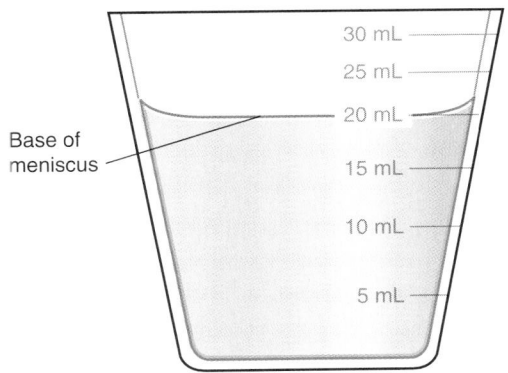

Figure 26–4. When using a calibrated measuring cup, measure the dose at the base of the meniscus.

Remember the following safety points when preparing oral medication for administration. If a medication must be removed from a bottle, make sure the label is intact and legible. Return an unlabeled bottle or one that is difficult to read to the pharmacy. Pour medications carefully to prevent unnecessary loss. If too much medication is poured, discard the excess. Never return unused medication to a container. If pouring a dose from a stock supply, do not return a solid medication to the container if it has been taken out of the cap. Do not move medications from one bottle to another because bottles can be identified by a code number or lot number assigned by the manufacturer. This number may be needed to track medications with quality control problems.

One of your key concerns when giving an oral medication is preventing aspiration. Place the client in an upright position either on his back or his side. This reduces the risk of medication accumulating at the back of the throat. Provide the client with fluid to drink, and give only one pill or tablet at a time. Allow the client enough time to swallow each medication before giving the next one. If the client begins to cough, wait until he has recovered before giving additional medications. Remain with the client until all medications have been taken. Do not leave medications at the bedside for the client to take after you leave the room. Make sure that the client drinks at least 50 or 60 mL of fluid with the last tablet to ensure that the medication does not stick in the esophagus and actually arrives in the stomach. If the client has an order for measurement of intake and output, record all fluid given with medications on this record. Specific guidelines for administering medications by the oral route are given in the accompanying procedure.

A variation of the oral route used for some clients is via an enteral tube, such as a nasogastric tube, gastrostomy tube (G-tube), or jejunostomy tube (J-tube). Important guidelines to follow when administering medications by the enteral route are given in Box 26–4.

Managing Parenteral Medications

Parenteral routes are differentiated by the angle of injection and depth of penetration. To give these medications safely, you must be familiar with the equipment, follow accepted procedures, and have manual dexterity. When preparing medications to be given by this route, keep the equipment and medication sterile.

Medications given by a parenteral route are absorbed more rapidly than those given orally. They cannot be removed or retrieved once given, making safety and accuracy key concerns.

EQUIPMENT

Needles and syringes are used to give parenteral medications. They are available in many sizes, and are selected according to the medication dose and site to be injected. All needles have a bevel (an angled end), a shaft, and a hub. All syringes have a tip, a barrel, and a plunger (Fig. 26–5).

PROCEDURE 26–1

Administering Oral Medications

TIME TO ALLOW ▼

Novice: 10 min.
Expert: 5 min.

Oral medications are administered to provide a pharmacological benefit or effect for a client. They are given carefully, using strict guidelines to prevent error.

Delegation Guidelines

At no time is it appropriate for you to delegate medication administration to a nursing assistant. Your knowledge of pharmacological agents, their administration, and ongoing patient assessment necessitate that you alone perform this procedure.

Equipment Needed

- Medication order sheet, computer-generated medication administration record, medication Kardex or cards.

- Medication cart or tray.
- Disposable medication cups (calibrated plastic or souffle).
- Glass of water, juice, or other preferred fluid.
- Drinking straw.
- Pill crushing device (as needed).
- Medications or medication cart (unit-dose system).

1 Assess the client to verify that the oral route is appropriate. Notify the physician if you find contraindications for giving medications by this route.

2 Confirm the medication order sheet against the original physician orders.
a. Clarify inconsistencies if you find any.
b. Check the client's record for allergies.
c. Determine any assessments needed (e.g., blood pressure or pulse) before the dose can be given.

3 Dispense medications one at a time, for one client at a time.
a. Unlock the drawer of the medication cart or storage area.
b. Select the correct medication and compare its label with the order sheet.
c. Calculate the dose needed.
d. Recheck the dose to be sure it is correct.
e. Place a solid medication into a disposable souffle cup.
f. For a partial dose, use a gloved hand or a cutting device to split a scored medication in half. Discard the unused half of a divided tablet.
g. If you will remove the dose from a bottle, pour the correct number of tablets into the bottle cap and then transfer them into a clean medicine cup. Do not touch the tablets with fingers, and return any extra tablets in the cap to the bottle. Use a new cup for each medication.

This method provides for aseptic preparation of medications, avoids allowing medications to touch your hands, and aids in distinguishing one medication from another.

h. For unit-dose medications, leave them in their original packaging and place them together in one cup. Do not open the wrappers until you get to the client's bedside. Keep medications that require special assessments in a separate cup.

This approach makes it easier to return refused medications to the pharmacy or to withhold medications as needed based on client assessment.

i. If you will give a liquid medication, pour it into a calibrated, disposable medication cup.
 1. Mix the medication thoroughly, and discard it if it has changed color or become cloudy.
 2. Remove the lid from the bottle or container and place it upside down.

 This position prevents contamination of the container lid.

 3. Hold the bottle so that the label is facing up, under the palm of your hand.

 This position ensures that the medication label does not become soiled or faded by spilled liquid.

 4. Hold the medication cup at eye level and use your thumbnail to mark the level of the correct dose. Pour medication into the cup until the bottom of the meniscus reaches the level of your thumbnail. Do not return any excess medication to the bottle; instead, discard it.
 5. Wipe the lip of the container with a clean paper towel before recapping.
 6. Bring a unit dose of a liquid to the bedside without opening it, unless the client needs a partial dose.

4 For medications of all types, recheck the medication and the dose after dispensing.

5 Lock the medication cart or storage area and bring the medications to the client.

6 Identify the client.
a. Read the name on client's identification bracelet.
b. Ask the client to tell you his name.

This step requires that client be alert and able to cooperate.

c. Verify the client's identity with another staff member who knows the client.

Perform this step if the client does not have an identification bracelet or is confused or unable to communicate.

7 Perform final assessments (parameters for administration, such as hold Toprol if pulse is <55) and explain the purpose of the medications to client.

8 Give the medications to the client.
a. Allow the client to choose whether to take onr or more than one medication at a time and whether to take them in a certain order.

Clients' needs and preferences should be respected if they do not threaten health or safety.

b. Recheck the accuracy of any medication that the client questions.

Doing so may help to prevent a medication error.

c. Remove unit-dose medications from their wrappers and give them to the client in a cup or in the hand according to the client's preference.

This method allows the client to see the medication, become familiar with it, or notice any discrepancies from the usual dose.

d. Offer a full glass of fluid. Have client moisten his mouth with fluid, bow his head slightly to aid swallowing, and follow the medications with an additional 60 to 100 mL.

You may need to use less fluid if the client is on fluid restriction.

e. Give liquids, chewable medications, lozenges, and sublingual or buccal medications separately from oral tablets, pills, or capsules.

f. Make sure the client has swallowed all medications by questioning the client or checking his mouth. Stay with the client until all medications have been taken.

9 Document the medication administration promptly on the client's medication administration record or computerized medication record.

10 Recheck the client when the medication has had time to take effect to assess his response to the medication.

SYRINGES. Syringes must be kept sterile with the exception of the outside barrel and the top edge of the plunger. This means that the syringe tip, barrel interior, and most of the plunger cannot be touched. The plunger moves up and down in the barrel of the syringe so that medication can be withdrawn and injected. The barrel holds the medication, and the barrel tip connects to a needle. Barrel tips may be either straight-end or luer-lock.

Most syringes used today are disposable and made of plastic. They are individually packaged to ensure sterility. They are clearly labeled with size (1 mL, 2 mL, 3 mL, 5 mL, 10 mL, 20 mL) and may be identified by their use (tuberculin, insulin). Many syringes are prepackaged with a specific size needle attached, which is also clearly labeled.

The barrel of a syringe is calibrated by volume (Fig. 26–6). For example, a tuberculin syringe can hold up to 1 mL of volume and is calibrated in units of 0.01 mL. An insulin syringe is calibrated in units. Most insulin manufactured in the United States and Canada contains 100 units per mL and is therefore called U100 insulin. An insulin syringe may hold up to either 1 mL

(most common) or 0.5 mL. Most SC and IM injections do not exceed 2 or 3 mL. A 3-mL syringe is calibrated in units of 0.1 mL. Larger syringes, such as 5 mL, 10 mL, and 20 mL, are calibrated in increments of 0.2 mL. Larger syringes may be used occasionally to draw up IV medications.

NEEDLES. Most needles used today are disposable and made of stainless steel. In selected areas, such as operating rooms, needles may be reused, but they must be resterilized after each use and inspected frequently for wear and tear.

Needles are measured by length and diameter. Lengths range from 1/4 to 5 inches (with 5/8 to 1.5 inch most common). A shorter needle is used when the client is smaller in size or when more superficial tissues are being injected (such as insulin and intradermal injections). Longer needles are used to inject deeper tissues (such as IM injections).

The angle at which the needle is injected also affects the tissue depth reached. In general, IM injections require the use of 1 to 1.5 inch needles, whereas SC injections require use of 3/8 to 5/8 inch needles. Longer needles also have longer bevels, which helps to de-

BOX 26–4

GUIDELINES FOR ADMINISTERING A MEDICATION THROUGH AN ENTERAL TUBE

- Whenever possible, obtain medications in liquid form to lessen the risk of obstructing the tube.
- Do not crush enteric-coated, extended action, sublingual, or buccal medications.
- Administer medications at room temperature rather than chilled. Also warm fluids used to flush the tube.
- Crush medications carefully; do not administer large particles or whole medications. Dissolve in warm water first.
- Put on disposable gloves. Access the tube using standard procedure. Check tube placement before administering a medication. Sit the client upright or semi-upright to reduce risk of aspiration.
- Place a waterproof pad on the bed linens under the area of the tube. Flush the tube with 15 to 60 mL of water before and after administering the medication, or flush as directed by facility policy.
- Administer medications by gravity, pouring them into an irrigation syringe with the plunger removed. Hold the syringe high enough to ensure a slow, steady flow rate. Monitor the client's tolerance of the procedure.
- Do not administer a medication through the air vent of a feeding tube.
- After the final flush, clamp the tube that was attached to suction for 20 to 30 minutes. If the client was receiving continuous tube feedings, clamp the tube for a few moments before resuming, if directed by facility policy.
- Help the client to a right side-lying position with his head elevated for at least 30 minutes after administering the medication.
- Clean up the work area, remove your gloves, and wash your hands. Document the medication and fluid intake on appropriate charting forms.

crease discomfort at the injection site. Insulin syringes are specially manufactured with a small needle attached to the syringe to meet the needs of clients who must inject themselves regularly.

The diameter of a needle is referred to as its gauge. The diameter size is inversely related to the gauge number. Gauges range from 28 (small) to 14 (large). Smaller-gauge needles are used with smaller drug volumes and produce less tissue trauma. Larger-gauge needles are used when larger volumes are injected, when the medication is viscous, or when the medication must penetrate to deeper tissues.

PREFILLED SYRINGES. Some parenteral medications are manufactured in prefilled, single-dose, disposable syringes (Fig. 26–7). These medication systems are available with a preattached needle or in a Luer format (without needle). You simply bring the prefilled syringe to the bedside, remove the needle shield, inject the medication, and dispose of the syringe. However, do not confuse this system with a unit-dose system. You may need to discard excess medication if the ordered dose is smaller than that supplied in the syringe. The purpose of prefilled syringes is to simplify and ease the injection process while decreasing the risk of needlestick injury during medication preparation. Some prefilled syringes may require you to assemble a prefilled cartridge into a holder device and then disassemble the system after use.

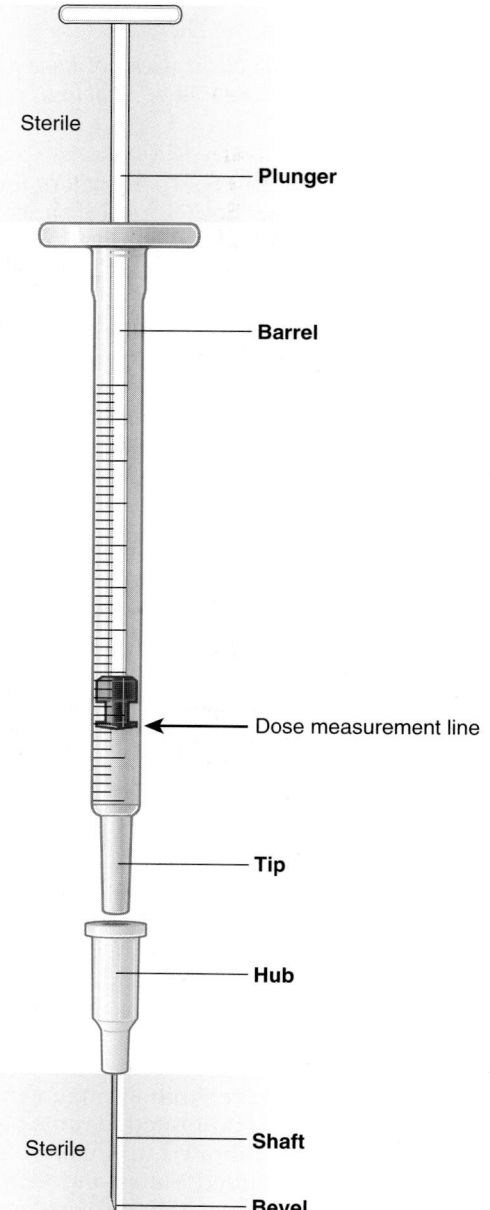

Sterile

Plunger

Barrel

Dose measurement line

Tip

Hub

Sterile

Shaft

Bevel

Figure 26–5. A needle and a syringe each have three parts.

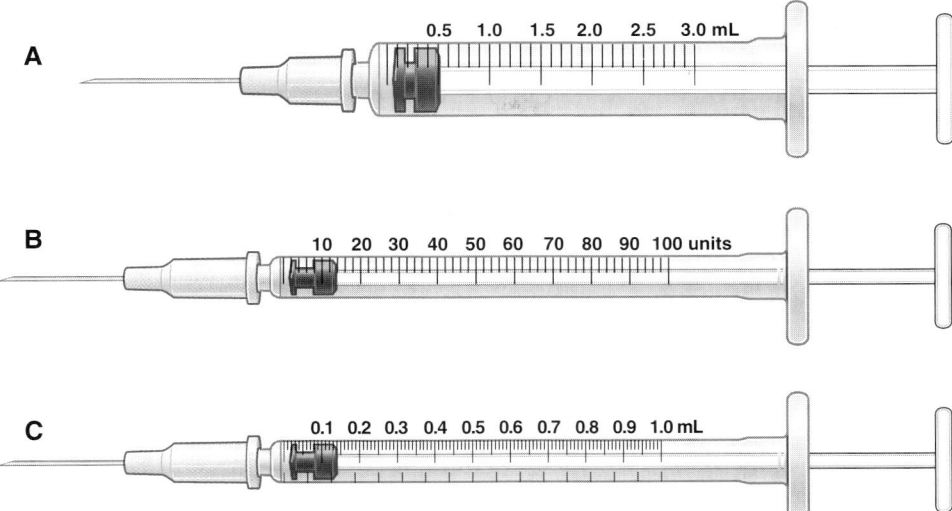

A 0.5 1.0 1.5 2.0 2.5 3.0 mL

B 10 20 30 40 50 60 70 80 90 100 units

C 0.1 0.2 0.3 0.4 0.5 0.6 0.7 0.8 0.9 1.0 mL

Figure 26–6. Three types of syringes. *A,* 3 mL; *B,* insulin, and *C,* tuberculin.

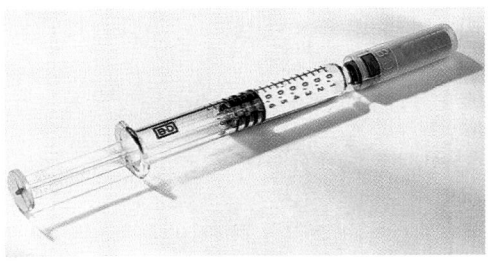

Figure 26–7. The Hypak injection system is an example of a prefilled, single-dose, disposable syringe. It consists of a cartridge holder and a prefilled medication cartilage with a needle. (Courtesy of Becton Dickinson Pharmaceutical Systems, Franklin Lakes, NJ.)

If you cannot discard a syringe immediately, encase it in a protective sheath temporarily. Some facilities use safety syringes, which have a sheath that slides down to cover the needle after use. Follow manufacturer's guidelines and facility procedures when using these devices.

Do not leave needles and syringes (even temporarily) in your pocket, on a client's meal tray, at the bedside, or in the client's bed. Do not discard them in wastebaskets, and do not place them in a rigid container that is full. Doing so places you and others at risk of needlestick injury, with possible infection from a number of pathogens, including hepatitis B and human immunodeficiency virus (HIV).

SAFE USE OF NEEDLES AND SHARPS. Preventing needlestick injuries is a vital concern in the health care industry. The Occupational Safety and Health Administration (OSHA) mandates the use of standard precautions, which includes proper handling and disposal of sharp instruments, including needles. After administering an injection, discard the syringe and needle, without recapping the needle, in a rigid container that has been specifically labeled and provided for that purpose (Fig. 26–8). The container should be leak-proof and puncture-proof. Rigid containers are kept on medication carts in all client care settings and are wall-mounted in client rooms and treatment areas in many acute care institutions.

If you must recap a needle, do so using the one-handed method. Slide the needle into the needle cover as it lies on a flat surface. Lift the syringe and twist the cover into place near the base of the needle. Never push the cap onto the needle using a finger on the end of the needle cover.

*A*ction *A*lert!
Avoid recapping needles whenever possible. If you must recap, use the one-handed method.

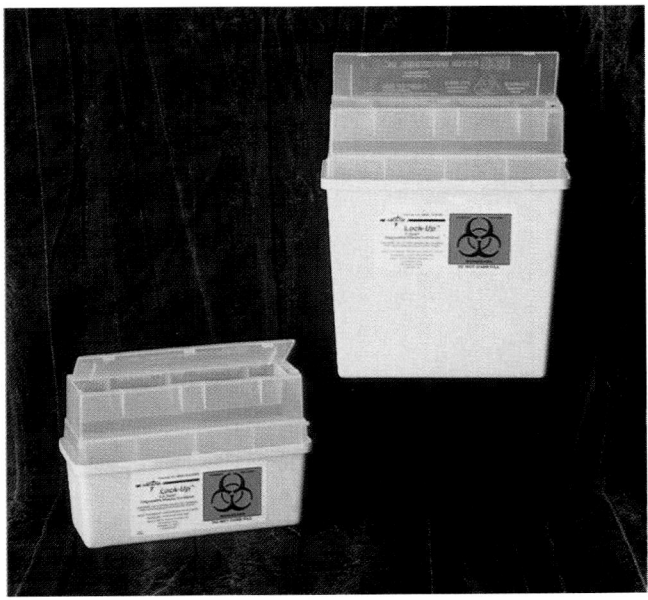

Figure 26–8. Proper use of rigid disposal containers ("sharps" containers) for used needles helps to prevent accidental needlesticks. (Courtesy of Medline Industries, Inc., Mundelein, IL.)

Withdrawing Medication From an Ampule

TIME TO ALLOW
▼
Novice:
5 min
Expert:
1 to 2 min.

Liquid medications used for injection may be supplied in ampules. You will need to withdraw the medication properly before you can administer it safely to the client.

Delegation Guidelines

The withdrawal and preparation of medication is yours alone. Consistent with the Administering Oral Medications procedure, you may not delegate this task or any of the component parts of medication preparation to a nursing assistant.

Equipment Needed

- Ampule of medication.
- Syringe and needle.
- Alcohol swab or gauze pad (2″ × 2″).
- Container for disposing of sharps

---

1 Open the ampule.

a. Tap the upper chamber of ampule quickly but lightly until all fluid drops into the lower chamber.

   This action ensures that all medication is available for use.

b. Wrap the alcohol swab or gauze pad around the neck of ampule.

   Doing so will protect your fingers from small glass fragments as you open the ampule.

c. Snap the neck of ampule so that it opens away from your body.

   This directs any fragments of glass away from you rather than toward you.

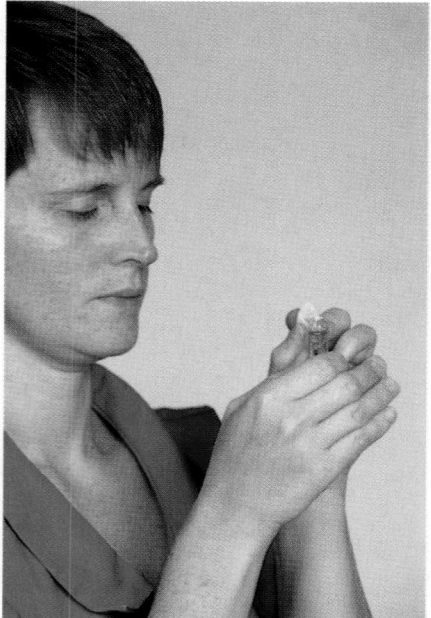

Snapping the neck of the ampule away from the body.

---

2 Place the ampule on a flat surface and withdraw medication into a syringe.

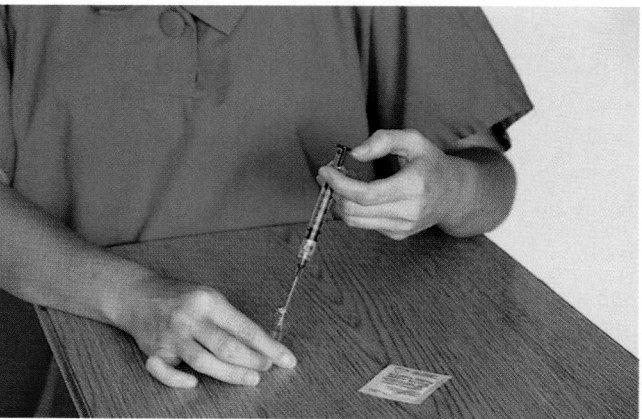

Withdrawing medication into the syringe with the ampule upright.

a. Make sure that the needle is tightly attached to the syringe and remove the needle cover. Insert the needle into the center of the opening on the ampule. Do not allow the needle tip or shaft to touch the rim of the ampule.

   This prevents contamination of the needle because the rim is considered contaminated.

b. Gently pull back on the plunger to aspirate medication into the syringe.

c. Tilt the ampule as needed to keep the needle tip below the level of medication.

   This step keeps you from withdrawing air into the syringe.

d. If air enters the syringe, do not inject it into the ampule. Instead, remove the needle from the ampule and eject the air (not fluid). Then reinsert the needle into the center of the ampule and withdraw fluid again.

These steps provide sufficient room in the syringe to withdraw the full dose needed, prevent loss of medication from excess air pressure, and ensure withdrawal of the complete dose.

3 Eject excess air or fluid as needed.

4 Recap the needle, then replace it with a new one and secure it tightly. Discard the used needle properly.

Replacing the needle prevents needle contamination and irritation of the client's tissues caused by tracking of medication through dermal and subcutaneous layers.

5 Compare the volume of fluid in the syringe with the ordered dose.

PREPARING AN INJECTION FROM AN AMPULE

An ampule is a glass container that holds a single drug dose and ranges in size from 1 mL to 10 mL or larger. The neck of the ampule is narrow and may have a colored ring indicating where it is prescored for opening. Because bits of glass or rubber sometimes found in ampules can be drawn into the syringe, some agencies require that you use a filter needle to withdraw the medication. The steps for withdrawing medication from an ampule are given in the accompanying procedure.

PREPARING AN INJECTION FROM A VIAL

A vial is a glass or plastic container with a rubber seal at the top. The seal is sterile before being opened and is protected by a soft metal or plastic cap. A vial may contain either liquid or powder medication. If a powder is used, product literature indicates the type and amount of diluent (such as sterile normal saline solution or sterile water) to use for reconstitution. Read the label carefully to determine the end concentration of the medication to avoid drawing up the wrong dose. Inject the solvent into the vial using the same technique that you would use to inject air. A powdered medication may dissolve easily or it may require you to gently roll or agitate the vial to dissolve the powder. If needed, the syringe may be removed from the vial before doing this.

Vials are labeled for a single dose or multiple doses. A single-dose vial must be discarded after one use. A multiple-dose vial may be reused but must be labeled with the date and time opened and your initials. A used vial must be discarded 30 days after being opened, even if it is not empty. Reconstituted medications in multiple-dose vials often require refrigeration after initial use. The steps for withdrawing medications from a vial are given in the accompanying procedure.

MIXING MEDICATIONS

Two medications may be mixed in one syringe if they are compatible with each other and if their total volume does not exceed the amount that may be given in one parenteral site. Most nursing units and medication texts have charts identifying compatible medications.

Consult a pharmacist if the medication is not identified or if you have any questions about compatibility.

Mixing Medications From an Ampule and a Vial

When medication from an ampule must be mixed with one from a vial, first withdraw from the vial and then from the ampule. This prevents the vial from being contaminated with medication from the ampule. It also is easier because the partially filled syringe with medication from the ampule is not used to inject air into the vial. (This recommendation assumes a multidose vial.)

Mixing Medications From Two Vials

Medications may also be mixed in one syringe by withdrawing them from two vials. Insulin is a good example. Insulin is both a protein and a hormone needed by the body to use glucose. Clients with diabetes mellitus produce either insufficient amounts of insulin or no insulin at all and many require daily insulin injections. Insulin manufactured in the United States and Canada contains 100 units (U) per milliliter (mL) of solution, and a 1-mL U100 syringe holds up to 100 U of insulin.

Several types of insulin are available that have variable onset and duration of action. Insulins are identified as long-acting, intermediate-acting, or short-acting (also known as rapid-acting). A client may require more than one type of insulin. The most common example is one in which the client needs NPH insulin (intermediate-acting) mixed with Regular insulin (short-acting) to achieve stable blood glucose levels over the course of a day (see the accompanying procedure.). Regular insulin is clear in color and may be given either SC or IV. NPH insulin is cloudy because protein has been added to slow its absorption; it may only be given SC.

A key concept to remember when mixing insulins is to withdraw them "clear to cloudy." This means that the clear (Regular, unmodified) insulin is withdrawn from the vial first, and the cloudy (NPH, modified) insulin is withdrawn second (Fig. 26–9). This technique prevents the NPH insulin from inadvertently being mixed into the regular insulin vial.

PROCEDURE 26–3

Withdrawing Medication From a Vial

TIME TO ALLOW
▼
Novice:
5 min.
Expert:
1 to 2 min.

Liquid medications used for injection may be supplied in sealed, airtight vials. You will need to add air to the vial to facilitate accurate withdrawal; otherwise a vacuum will be created by withdrawing the medication.

Delegation Guidelines

As in the previous procedures in this chapter, medication preparation is the sole responsibility of you, the RN. You may never delegate this procedure to a nursing assistant.

Equipment Needed

- Vial of medication.
- Syringe and needle.
- Alcohol swab.
- Glass disposal container.

1 Prepare the vial.
a. Remove the plastic or metal top of a new vial to expose the rubber seal.
b. Cleanse the rubber seal with an alcohol swab.
c. Check the expiration date of a previously opened vial.

Do not use the medication if the vial was opened more than 30 days ago.

2 Prepare the syringe.
a. Check for a tight connection between the needle hub and syringe barrel.

This action ensures a tight seal and a closed system.

b. Remove the needle cover.
c. Draw back on the plunger to fill the syringe with a volume of air equal to the dose of medication you will be giving.

3 Withdraw the medication.
a. Insert the needle into the center of the vial's rubber seal using gentle but firm pressure.

The center of the seal is thinner and designed for penetration.

b. Inject air from the syringe into the vial.

This step creates positive pressure inside the vial to ease medication withdrawal and prevent creation of a vacuum after removing the medication.

c. Invert the vial while holding it with the first two fingers of your nondominant hand. Use your thumb and last two fingers to brace the barrel of the syringe. Use the thumb of your dominant hand to hold the end of the syringe barrel steady. Use the fingers of your dominant hand to withdraw the plunger.

Proper hand position allows for easier medication withdrawal and prevents movement of the plunger or bending of the needle.

d. Withdraw the medication slowly and steadily while holding the vial at eye level. Keep the tip of the needle in the solution at all times. Touch only the syringe barrel and plunger tip.

This method prevents air bubbles from entering the syringe and prevents contamination of the syringe.

e. Remove excess air in the syringe by tapping the side of syringe with a finger and pushing air back into the vial. Remove additional fluid as needed to ensure the full dose.

f. Return the vial to an upright position and remove the needle by pulling back on the syringe barrel, not the plunger. Remove any excess air if present.

This ensures that the correct amount of medication remains in the syringe.

4 Recap the needle, then replace it with a new one. Secure the new needle tightly and discard the used needle properly.

5 Compare the volume of fluid in the syringe with the ordered dose.

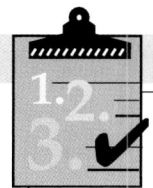

PROCEDURE 26–4

Mixing Insulins in a Single Syringe

TIME TO ALLOW

▼

Novice:
10 min.
Expert:
5 min.

Some clients require doses of short-acting (unmodified, regular) and intermediate-acting (modified, NPH) insulins at the same time. Mixing them in a single syringe requires only one injection.

Delegation Guidelines

You may not delegate the preparation of insulin to a nursing assistant. The preparation of any medication, including insulin, is your duty alone.

Equipment Needed

- Medication administration record or computerized medication order sheet.
- Insulin vials.
- Insulin syringe with attached needle.
- Alcohol swabs.

1 If the insulin is in suspension, rotate the vial between the palms of your hands.

This step mixes the solution without forming tiny air bubbles that could interfere with accurate measurement of the dose.

2 Prepare the vials.
a. Remove the metal covers if you are using new vials.
b. Wipe the rubber seals with alcohol swabs.
c. Check the expiration date.

3 Add air to both vials.
a. Remove the needle cover.
b. Draw up a volume of air equal to the dose of modified (NPH) insulin and inject it into the NPH vial without letting the needle touch the solution. Remove the needle from the vial.

   Insertion of air prevents creation of a vacuum when you withdraw the fluid.

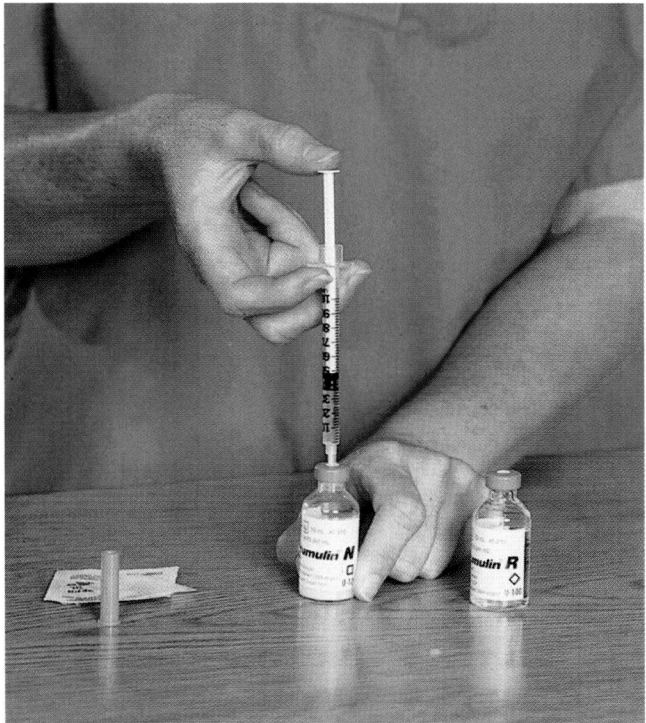

Injecting the air into the NPH vial.

c. Draw up a volume of air equal to the dose of unmodified (Regular) insulin, and inject into regular insulin vial. Do not remove the needle from this vial. *Continued*

Mixing Insulins in a Single Syringe

4 Remove insulin from the two vials.

a. Invert the vial of regular insulin and withdraw the correct dose. Make sure you draw no air bubbles into the syringe. Turn the vial upright and remove the needle from the vial.

Turning the vial upright prevents solution from leaking out of the vial.

b. Cleanse the rubber seal of the NPH insulin bottle again and insert the needle into the vial. Invert the vial and carefully withdraw the correct dose. Turn the vial upright again and remove the needle.

c. Recap the needle.

The needle is preattached to the syringe and must be brought to bedside; recapping it prevents a needlestick injury.

5 Have an RN or LPN double-check the dose. Then return the vials to their storage areas. Administer the mixed insulin dose to the client within 5 minutes of preparing it.

Double-checking verifies the correct dose. Returning the vials to storage maintains the potency of the insulin. Administering the medication within 5 minutes reduces the risk that the mixture will separate.

Site rotation is an important concept with insulin administration, and a rotation plan should be followed carefully. Warm insulin prior to use by rolling it in the palms of the hands if it was refrigerated. This also resuspends modified insulin preparations and is a better method of mixing than shaking the vials, which could cause air bubbles and foaming. Insulin can be safely stored for 1 month at room temperature but should be refrigerated if it will be kept for longer periods. In general, insulin should be stored in a cool location.

BOX 26–5

MINIMIZING THE DISCOMFORT OF INJECTIONS

- Use a needle with the smallest appropriate length and gauge.
- Make sure that the needle has a sharp bevel.
- Use anatomic landmarks to select a correct injection site and avoid unintended tissues.
- If necessary, change the position of the limb to be injected to relax the muscles at the site.
- Distract the client with conversation to relieve anxiety, but tell the client just before you insert the needle.
- If the client is very anxious, numb the site briefly with ice before administering the injection.
- Use smooth but quick hand movements when inserting the needle to minimize discomfort from tissue trauma.
- Hold the syringe steady while injecting the medication; do not rotate the syringe and needle while it is in the tissue.
- Apply gentle pressure to the injection site for about 10 seconds after withdrawing the needle unless doing so is contraindicated.

ADMINISTERING INJECTIONS

The name of the injection route identifies the tissue into which the medication is injected. The characteristics of these tissues affect the depth of injection and the rate of absorption. Before administering an injection, make sure you are familiar with the site's landmarks, the nature and viscosity of the medication, and the maximum volume that can be safely given at that site.

Incorrect administration can have serious negative effects on the client. Excess volume causes pain or discomfort and can irritate tissues. Some medications stain tissues if they are not given deeply enough or if incorrect technique is used. Failure to aspirate before injecting could result in a medication being inadvertently injected into a blood vessel. Incorrect site selection can cause damage to bones or nerves. You are liable for medications that are given incorrectly.

Receiving an injection is not a pleasant experience; however, you can reduce your clients' fear and discomfort (Box 26–5). Strategies to reduce the discomfort of injections may be particularly useful with children or clients who need multiple injections over time.

Intradermal Injections

The ID route has the slowest absorption of all parenteral routes. An advantage of this route for diagnostic testing is that the site is superficial, making it easy to determine positive reactions. Commonly used sites include the inner aspect of the forearm, the upper chest, and the upper back (Fig. 26–10). Use a site that is free

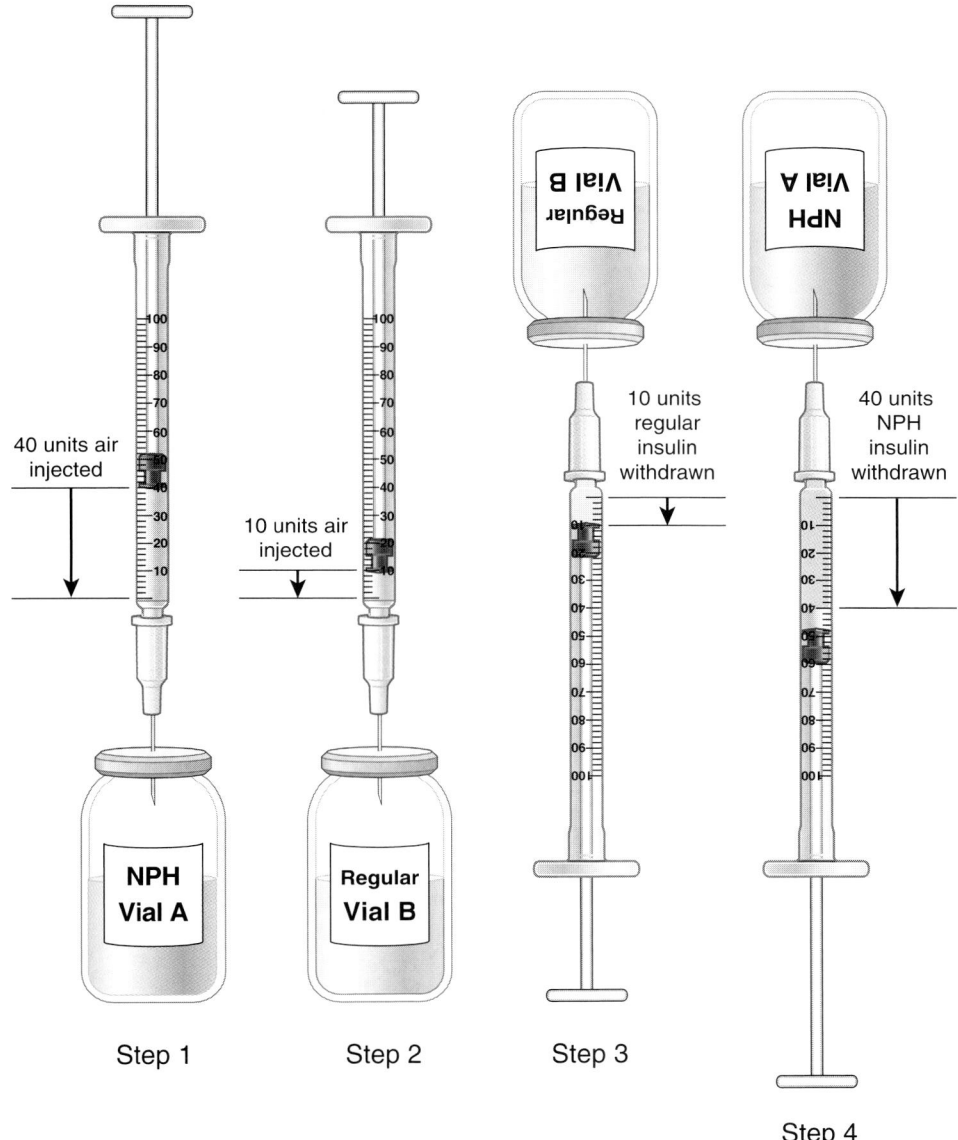

40 units air
injected

10 units air
injected

10 units
regular
insulin
withdrawn

40 units
NPH
insulin
withdrawn

NPH
Vial A

Regular
Vial B

Regular
Vial B

NPH
Vial A

Step 1   Step 2   Step 3

Step 4

Figure 26–9. Mixing two medications in one syringe.

of bruises or other lesions and is relatively hairless to allow accurate follow-up assessment. Note the date, time, and location of the injection on the medical record as well as when the test should be "read" for a reaction (usually 48 to 72 hours later). If multiple injections are given, sites should be rotated and clearly marked. If there is a reaction (a positive test result), record and report it quickly.

ID injections are administered using a tuberculin syringe, which holds up to 1 mL of medication and is calibrated in 0.1 mL and 0.01 mL. Use a small needle (25 to 27 gauge) with a short bevel that is ¼ to ½ inch long. The usual medication dose is small (0.1 to 0.01 mL). Angle the needle at 10 to 15 degrees from the skin to deposit the medication below the epidermis (Fig. 26–11). A wheal forms under the skin with proper administration. The procedure for administering intradermal injections is given in the accompanying procedure.

Subcutaneous Injections

Subcutaneous tissue is not as vascular as muscle tissue, so medication is absorbed more slowly with SC injection than with IM injection. The slower absorption rate allows for a more prolonged drug effect.

The body is well supplied with subcutaneous tissue. Common injection sites include the anterolateral upper arms, anterior thighs, and lower abdominal wall between the costal margins and the iliac crests (Fig. 26–12). Other acceptable sites are the scapular area of the back and the upper ventral or dorsal gluteal areas. Drugs commonly given by this route include heparin, insulin, and selected immunizations and analgesics.

As with any other injection, the site should be anatomically correct and free of infection, lesions, scars, or bruises. When giving injections frequently, rotate the sites to prevent local complications, such as sterile ab-

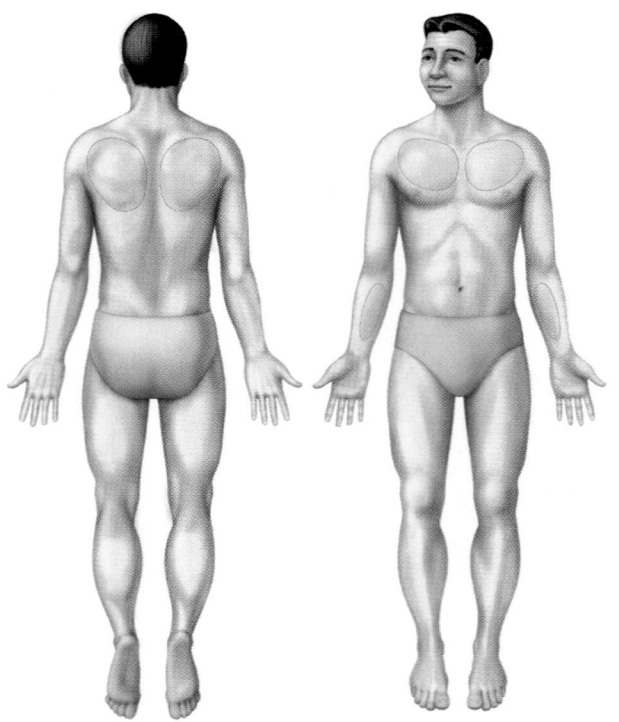

Figure 26–10. Frequently used sites for intradermal injection.

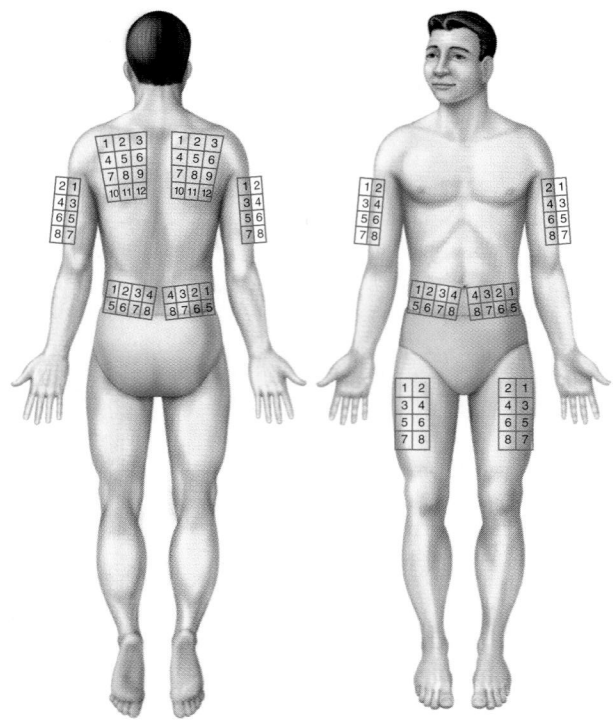

Figure 26–12. Common subcutaneous injection sites.

scesses (painful lumps), lipohypertrophy (thickening of the skin), and lipodystrophy (atrophy or dimpling of the skin). This is especially important for diabetic clients who self-inject insulin daily. Identify the site rotation plan on the client's care plan and note the sites of previously administered injections on the medication administration record. Use an injection diagram to help the client remember the site rotation pattern. Individual injection sites may be systematically rotated from one area of the body to another (site 1 in one location to site 1 in another location, for example), or the client may rotate among all sites in a given body location. Sites should be separated from each other by

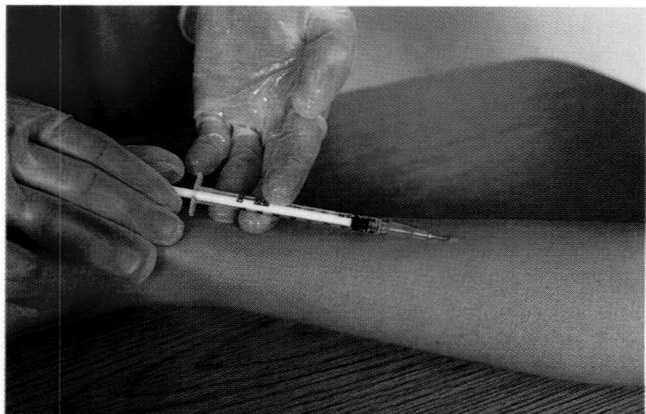

Figure 26–11. Intradermal injection. Insert the needle bevel up, with the syringe almost parallel to the skin at a 10- to 15-degree angle. As the medication is injected, a small wheal should form under the skin.

one inch. Hospitalized diabetic clients often receive insulin in the arms because this site is harder to use at home. Give heparin in the abdomen unless contraindicated by the client's condition.

The equipment used for SC injection depends on the medication to be given or the client's body size and weight. The amount of medication injected into one site is commonly 0.5 to 1.0 mL but should not exceed 1.5 mL. Insulin syringes are used to administer insulin, whereas tuberculin syringes are commonly used to administer heparin. For other medications, up to a 3-mL syringe may be used. The needle should be 25 to 29 gauge with a ⅜ to ⅝ inch needle. Within this range, use shorter needles with smaller clients and longer needles with larger ones. In most cases, you may adjust the angle of insertion according to needle length. Shorter needles (½ inch and smaller) are usually inserted at a 90-degree angle, whereas ⅝ inch needles may be inserted at a 45-degree angle or a 90-degree angle, depending on body size (Fig. 26–13). If a 1 inch needle is used, it must be inserted at a 45-degree angle. Further adjustments may be made for very small or pediatric clients according to need and facility policy. Administration techniques for SC injection are described in the accompanying procedure.

Intramuscular Injections

The IM route may be chosen when rapid absorption is desired or when the medication is irritating to SC tissue (see the accompanying procedure). There are fewer nerve endings in muscle tissue, which makes this area more comfortable when irritating substances are being injected. Nonetheless, clients can experience

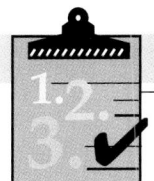

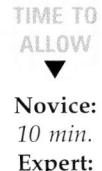

PROCEDURE 26–5

Administering an Intradermal Injection

TIME TO
ALLOW
▼
Novice:
10 min.
Expert:
5 min.

Intradermal injections are done most often to test for allergies or for diagnostic purposes. The site is evaluated within a specific time period after the injection is given.

Delegation Guidelines

You may not delegate the administration of an intradermal injection to a nursing assistant.

Equipment Needed

- Medication administration record, computerized medication order sheet, or medication Kardex or card.
- Medication vial or ampule.
- Tuberculin syringe and needle.
- Alcohol swab.
- 2 × 2 inch sterile gauze pad.
- Acetone swab if needed for oily skin.
- Disposable gloves.

1 Check the medication order and note any client allergies.

2 Withdraw medication from the vial as described in the Withdrawing Medication From a Vial procedure. Take the syringe and other supplies to client's room and place them on a clean, flat surface.

3 Prepare the client for the injection.
a. Identify the client using an identification bracelet or other accepted means.
b. Explain the procedure to the client in a calm and confident manner.
c. Don disposable gloves and open the swab(s) and gauze package using aseptic technique.
d. Provide privacy and position the client comfortably. Select and expose the injection site.

These steps reduce client tension and provide a view of the area to be used.

4 Prepare the injection site and the syringe.
a. Make sure area is free of bruises, redness, or lesions.
b. Clean the site with an alcohol swab using a circular motion, moving outward from injection site. Allow the alcohol to air dry. Use an acetone swab as well if the client's skin is oily.

Alcohol reduces number of pathogens on the skin that could be pushed into the tissues by the needle. Allowing the alcohol to dry prevents tissue irritation.

c. Remove the needle-guard or cap with your nondominant hand by pulling it straight off.

This action helps to prevent a needlestick injury.

d. Check the syringe to make sure that the volume of medication is correct and that it contains no air bubbles.

5 Inject the medication.
a. Hold the syringe in your dominant hand and spread the skin taut with your nondominant hand.

The dominant hand has better fine motor control. It is easier to inject into taut skin.

b. Insert the needle bevel-up at a 10-degree to 15-degree angle into skin for ⅛ inch or until the bevel disappears from view. The needle should be visible below the skin surface, and you should feel resistance.

This step places the needle under the epidermal layer of skin but not into subcutaneous tissue.

c. Inject the medication slowly while watching for formation of a small bleb, wheal, or blister. If none is visible, withdraw the needle slightly and continue injecting.

This procedure deposits medication into the dermis.

d. Withdraw the needle at the same angle used for insertion.

Doing so will reduce tissue trauma and client discomfort.

e. Pat the area dry using the gauze pad. Do not massage the area.

Avoiding massage prevents the medication from spreading beyond the intended injection site.

Continued

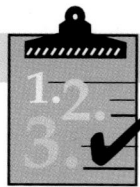

Administering an Intradermal Injection

6 Dispose of used equipment properly and clean the area.

a. Discard the needle and syringe in a rigid container without recapping the needle. Dispose of the alcohol swab, gauze, wrappers, and other used materials in a trash receptacle.

b. Position the client comfortably.

c. Remove your gloves and discard them in a proper receptacle. Wash your hands.

7 Document the procedure carefully.

a. Observe the site and the client for any immediate allergic reaction.

Anaphylaxis could occur suddenly if the client has a severe allergy to the substance you injected.

b. Use a skin pencil or a ball-point pen (according to facility policy) to circle area of the wheal.

Doing so will provide an easy way to identify the site when performing follow-up readings.

c. Document the date, time, substance, and site of the injection on the client's medication administration record. Document the date and time of follow-up observations, and inform the client and caregivers about their roles.

This will provide clear direction for caregivers responsible for interpreting test results.

---

discomfort with IM injections. For this reason, do not inject into muscles that are tender to the client or that are contracted, hard, or tense. Complications of inappropriate site selection or improper technique include abscess formation, skin sloughing and necrosis, continued site pain, nerve injury, and periostitis (inflammation of the membrane over bone).

The volume that can be safely given by the IM route varies with the client's age and the site selected. An adult can receive a maximum of 4 mL in a large muscle, such as the gluteus. Children and older adults should not receive more than 1 or 2 mL because their muscles are less developed. The deltoid should be limited to 0.5 or 1 mL, depending on client size.

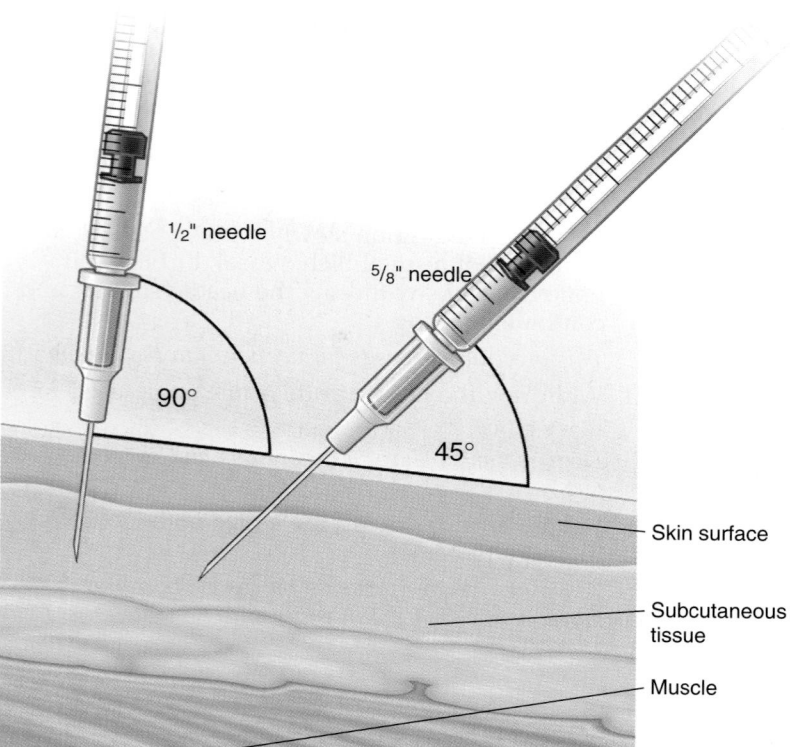

Figure 26–13. Technique for subcutaneous injection.

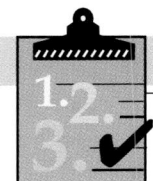

PROCEDURE 26–6

Administering a Subcutaneous Injection

TIME TO
ALLOW
▼
Novice:
10 min.
Expert:
5 min.

Subcutaneous injections are given to administer medication into subcutaneous tissue with a written physician's order. This route provides faster medication action than the oral route.

Delegation Guidelines

You may not delegate the performance or administration of subcutaneous injections to a nursing assistant.

Equipment Needed

- Medication administration record, computerized medication order sheet, or medication Kardex or card.
- Medication vial or ampule.
- Sterile, 3-mL insulin or tuberculin syringe and needle (⅝ inch or smaller).
- Two alcohol swabs.
- Disposable gloves.

---

1 Check the medication order and note any client allergies.

2 Withdraw the medication from the ampule or vial as described in the previous two procedures.

3 Take the syringe and other supplies to the client's room and place them on a clean, flat surface.

4 Prepare the client for the injection.
a. Identify the client using an identification bracelet or other accepted means.
b. Explain the procedure to client in a calm and confident manner.
c. Don disposable gloves and open an alcohol swab wrapper using aseptic technique.
d. Provide privacy and position the client comfortably. Select and expose the injection site.

   If you select the upper outer arm, place the client's arm at his side in a relaxed position. If you choose the anterior thigh, have the client sit or lie down with the leg muscle relaxed. If you choose the abdomen, have the client lie in a recumbent or semi-recumbent position. If you choose the scapula, the client may sit or lie prone or on his side. These positions give you a clear view of the area to be used.

5 Prepare the injection site and syringe.
a. Make sure the area is free of bruises, redness, or lesions.

b. Pinpoint the exact site of the injection. Clean the site with an alcohol swab using a circular motion, moving outward from injection site. Allow the alcohol to air dry. Leave swab in a clean area so you can reuse it when withdrawing the needle.
c. Remove the needle guard or cap with your nondominant hand by pulling it straight off.
d. Check the syringe to make sure that the volume of medication is correct and contains no air bubbles.

6 Inject the medication.
a. Hold the syringe in your dominant hand between your thumb and forefinger, as if holding a dart.
   The dominant hand has better fine motor control.
b. Pinch or bunch up subcutaneous tissue between the thumb and forefinger of your nondominant hand, as shown. If the client has ample subcutaneous tissue, or if you are injecting an anticoagulant drug, spread the skin taut.
   Bunching the tissue aids in needle insertion into the subcutaneous tissue. Use needle length, the amount of tissue, and tissue turgor as a guide.
c. Quickly insert the needle up to the hub at a 45-degree to 90-degree angle, depending on the length of the needle.
   This action positions the needle in subcutaneous tissue.

Continued

PROCEDURE 26–6 *(continued)*

Administering a Subcutaneous Injection

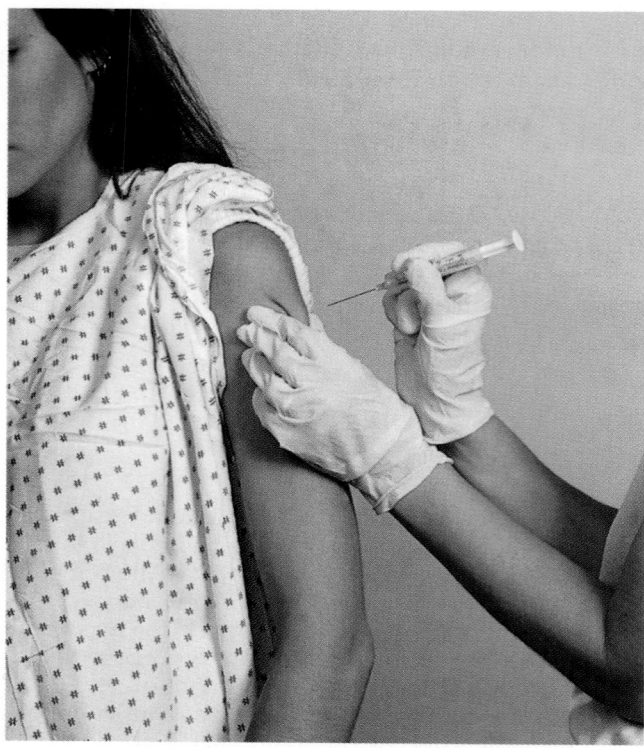

To use the deltoid, the arm should be relaxed at the side of the body.

d. Release the bunched tissue and grasp the distal end of the syringe with your nondominant hand.

Holding the syringe with your nondominant hand steadies it in the tissue, reducing movement and client discomfort.

e. Unless you are injecting insulin or heparin, aspirate for a blood return by pulling back gently on the tip of plunger with the thumb and forefinger of your dominant hand.

A blood return indicates that the needle has entered a blood vessel. Avoid aspiration with insulin or heparin because aspiration could cause local trauma.

f. If you see a blood return, remove the needle, discard the syringe, and begin the procedure again.

This prevents you from administering the medication intravenously and prevents hematoma formation from blood being injected into the tissue.

g. If you get no blood return, inject the medication slowly and steadily.

Slow, steady injection disperses the medication evenly in the tissues to enhance absorption.

h. Withdraw the needle quickly at the same angle you used for insertion. Unless you injected heparin, massage the area gently with the alcohol swab.

Massage reduces tissue trauma and client discomfort.

7 Dispose of used equipment properly.

a. Discard the needle and syringe in a rigid container without recapping the needle. Dispose of the alcohol swab, wrapper, and other used materials in a trash receptacle.

b. Position the client comfortably.

c. Remove your gloves and discard them in the proper receptacle. Wash your hands.

8 Document the procedure carefully.

a. Record the date, time, substance, and site of injection on the client's medication administration record.

b. Check on the client within 30 minutes to assess the effects of the medication.

HOME CARE CONSIDERATIONS

Subcutaneous injections commonly administered in the home include insulin, heparin, and allergy injections. Subcutaneous injections are easier for the client or family to administer than are intramuscular injections. Teach about the medication, injection technique, site rotation, and management of adverse effects.

PROCEDURE 26–7

Administering an Intramuscular Injection

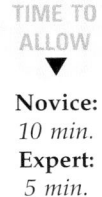

TIME TO
ALLOW
▼
Novice:
10 min.
Expert:
5 min.

Intramuscular injections are used to administer medication into muscle tissue with a written physician's order. This route provides for faster action than the oral or subcutaneous route.

Delegation Guidelines

You may not delegate the administration of an intramuscular injection to a nursing assistant.

Equipment Needed

- Medication administration record, computerized medication order sheet, or medication kardex or card.
- Medication vial or ampule.
- Sterile, 3-mL syringe and needle (1 to 2 inches, 20- to 22-gauge, long bevel).
- Two alcohol swabs.
- Disposable gloves.

1 Check the medication order and note any client allergies.

2 Withdraw the medication from the ampule or vial as described in the second and third procedures. Take the syringe and other supplies to the client's room and place them on a clean, flat surface.

3 Prepare the client for the injection.
a. Identify the client using an identification bracelet or other accepted means.
b. Explain the procedure to client in a calm and confident manner.
c. Don disposable gloves and open the alcohol swab wrapper using aseptic technique.
d. Provide privacy and position the client comfortably. Select and expose the injection site.
   If you choose the upper arm (deltoid), place the client in a sitting or lying position with the arm relaxed at the side of his body. If you choose the anterolateral thigh (vastus lateralis), place the client in a sitting or lying position with the leg muscle relaxed. If you choose the dorsogluteal location (gluteus maximus), select a side-lying position with the upper leg flexed and in front of the lower leg. You can also use a prone position with the client's toes pointed inward. If you choose the ventrogluteal location (gluteus medius), place the client in a supine position with legs relaxed or a side-lying position with hip and knee flexed. These positions reduce muscle tension and allow you to clearly see the area to be used.

4 Prepare the injection site and the syringe.

a. Make sure the area is free of bruises, redness, or lesions.
b. Pinpoint the exact site of the injection. Clean the site with an alcohol swab using a circular motion, moving outward from injection site. Allow the alcohol to air dry. Leave the swab in a clean area so you can reuse it when withdrawing the needle.
c. Remove needle guard or cap with your nondominant hand by pulling it straight off.
d. Check the syringe to make sure that the volume of medication is correct.

5 Inject the medication.
a. Hold the syringe in your dominant hand between your thumb and forefinger as if holding a dart.
b. Spread the skin taut between the thumb and forefinger of your nondominant hand, or displace the skin using a Z-track technique (see Fig. 26–20).
   Making the skin taut aids insertion of the needle into the muscle tissue.
c. Insert the needle quickly at a 90-degree angle up to the hub.
   This action positions the needle in the muscle tissue.
d. Release the skin and grasp the distal end of the syringe with your nondominant hand.
   Grasping the syringe steadies it in the tissue, thus reducing movement and client discomfort.
e. Aspirate for a blood return by pulling back gently on tip of the plunger with the thumb and forefinger of your dominant hand.
   Blood return indicates that the needle has entered a blood vessel.

Continued

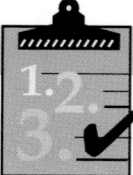

Administering an Intramuscular Injection

f. If you see a blood return, remove the needle, discard the syringe, and begin the procedure again.

Beginning again prevents the medication from being injected intravenously and the reinjection of aspirated blood.

g. If you see no blood return, inject the medication slowly and steadily, taking about 10 seconds to inject each 1 mL.

Slow, steady injection disperses the medication evenly in the tissue to enhance absorption.

h. Wait a few seconds, then withdraw the needle quickly at the same angle you used to insert it. Apply gentle pressure to the site with an alcohol swab or 2 × 2 inch gauze.

These steps allow the medication to diffuse into the muscle while reducing tissue trauma and discomfort.

6 Dispose of the used equipment.

a. Discard the needle and syringe in a rigid con-

tainer without recapping the needle. Dispose of the alcohol swab, wrapper, and other used materials in an appropriate trash receptacle.

b. Position the client comfortably. If you injected the medication into the leg muscles, encourage the client to flex and extend those muscles.

These actions promote client comfort and enhance absorption of medication from sites in the leg.

c. Remove your gloves and discard them in the proper receptacle. Wash your hands.

7 Document the procedure carefully.

a. Record the date, time, substance, and site of injection on the client's medication administration record.

b. Check on the client at an appropriate time after giving the injection (2 to 4 hours for many medications) to assess the client's response to the medication.

HOME CARE CONSIDERATIONS

The need for intramuscular injections in a homebound client is justification for a home care nurse. Intramuscular injections given in the home include iron, vitamins, antibiotics, and ketorolac tromethamine (Toradol) and other pain medications. The home care nurse must plan for the management of side effects and adverse effects. If a family caregiver is taught to administer intramuscular injections, client teaching should include recognizing and managing emergency reactions such as anaphylaxis. Teach about the medication, injection technique, site rotation, and the management of adverse effects.

Client size and drug viscosity greatly determine the appropriate needle size. The average needle used for IM injection is 21 to 23 gauge and 1 to 1.5 inch long. A 2 inch needle may be used for very large clients so the medication reaches the muscle. Give all IM injections at a 90-degree angle.

There are four common sites for giving IM injections: ventrogluteal, dorsogluteal, vastus lateralis, and deltoid. These sites are safe because they do not lie near blood vessels, nerves, or bones. The gluteus muscles are particularly large and accept medication easily (Fig. 26–14). As with SC injections, rotate sites if giving repeated injections. Identify the site rotation plan on the care plan, and chart sites used on the medication administration record.

VENTROGLUTEAL SITE. The ventrogluteal site uses the gluteus medius and minimus muscles in the area of

the hip. This is a preferred site for adults and for children and infants over 7 months old. It is particularly useful because it does not lie near major bones, blood vessels, or nerves; is relatively free of microorganisms from fecal contamination; and allows the client to lie on his back, side, or abdomen during injection.

Locate the site by placing the palm of your hand over the greater trochanter with your fingers pointed in the direction of the client's head (Fig. 26–15). Use your left hand to identify landmarks when the client is receiving the injection in the right hip and vice versa. Place your index finger on the anterior superior iliac spine and extend your middle finger dorsally to the iliac crest. Give the injection in the center of the triangle created by these fingers.

DORSOGLUTEAL SITE. The dorsogluteal site uses the gluteus maximus muscles in the buttocks and is an-

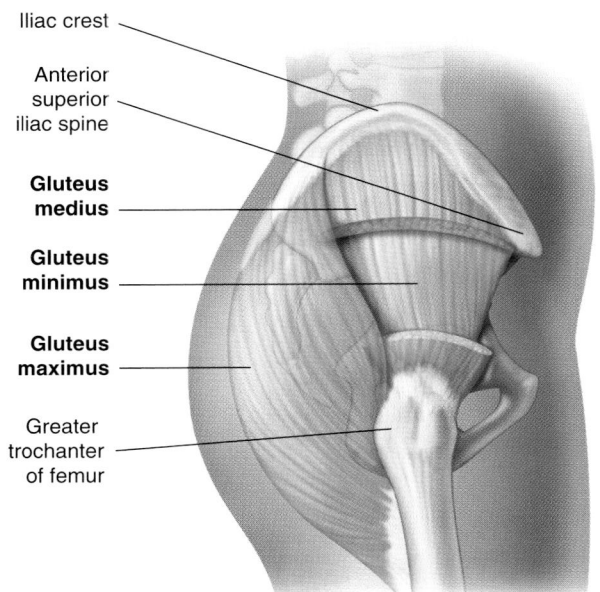

Figure 26–14. The three gluteus muscles are particularly large and accept intramuscular medication easily.

other commonly used site for IM injection. This site is recommended for adults and children over age 3 because these muscles are developed by walking. It is not recommended for infants and children under age 3 because the gluteal muscles are small and underdeveloped. This site is not the preferred site for administering IM injections, because there is a potential for injury because of the nearby location of the sciatic nerve, major blood vessels, and bone.

To expose the site, the client may lie on his side with the top leg flexed and in front of the lower leg. The client may also lie prone with the toes pointed inward. These positions reduce muscle tension and promote relaxation. The client should not stand for injection in the dorsogluteal site. Make sure you can see the area well. Have the client lower the undergarment, or move aside the hospital gown. Locate the site by drawing an imaginary line between the anatomic landmarks of the posterior superior iliac spine and the greater trochanter. Administer the injection lateral and slightly superior to the midpoint of this line (Fig. 26–16).

VASTUS LATERALIS SITE. The vastus lateralis muscle is a thick, well-developed muscle located on the anterolateral aspect of the thigh. In the adult, it extends from a handbreadth above the knee to a handbreadth below the greater trochanter. It measures in width from the midline of the top of the thigh to the midline of the lateral thigh. It is easiest to use this site by injecting the outer middle third of the thigh (Fig. 26–17). This is a preferred injection site for adults, children, and infants. It is especially useful in children

Figure 26–15. Ventrogluteal intramuscular injection site. Place the heel of your hand over the greater trochanter, with your middle finger pointed toward the iliac crest and your index finger toward the anterosuperior iliac spine. Administer the injection in the center of the triangle formed by your fingers.

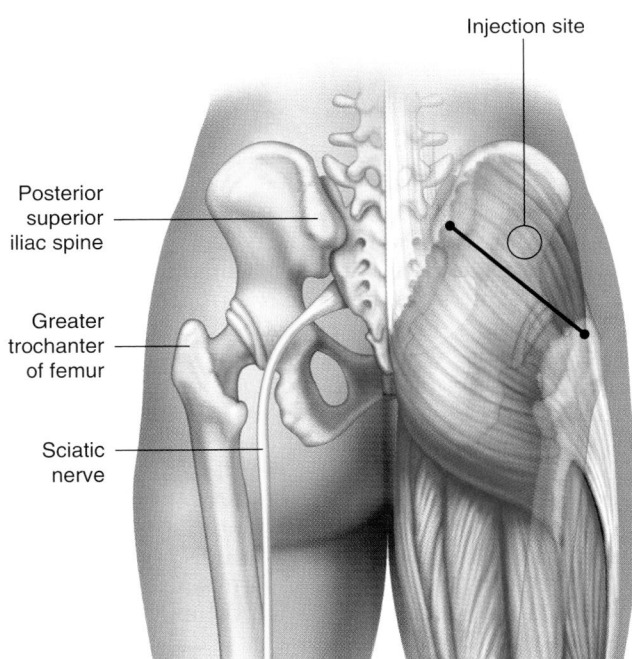

Figure 26–16. Dorsogluteal intramuscular injection site. Identify an imaginary line between the greater trochanter and the posterosuperior iliac spine. Give the injection superior and lateral to that line.

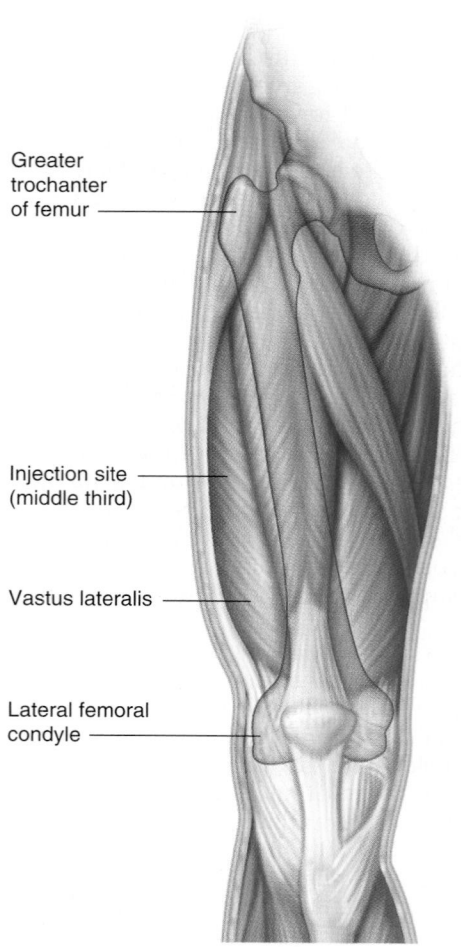

Figure 26–17. Vastus lateralis intramuscular injection site on the right thigh. Divide the thigh into thirds; give the injection in the middle third.

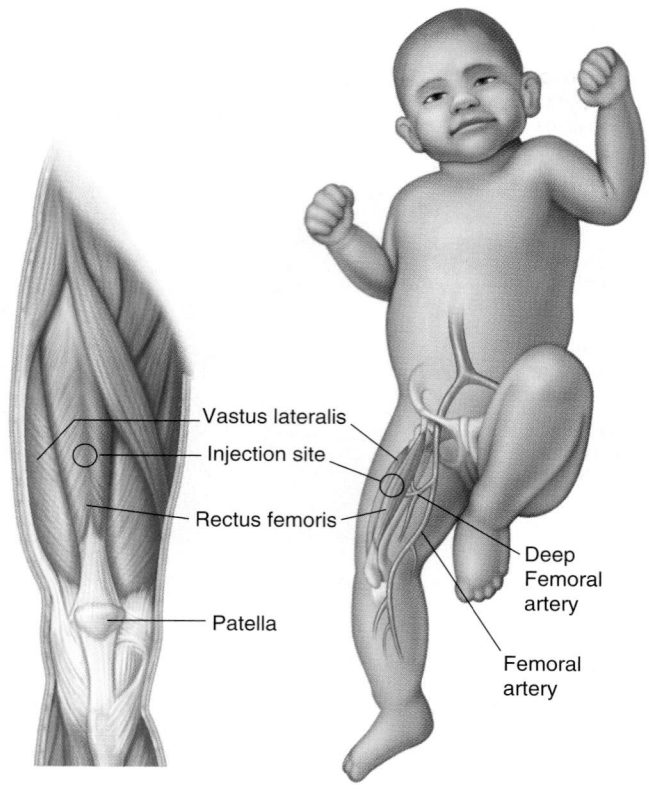

Figure 26–18. Rectus femoris intramuscular injection site on the anterior part of the thigh (used in adults only if other sites are contraindicated). In children, the site is located one-third of the distance from the patella to the greater trochanter in the center of the anterior thigh.

whose gluteal muscles are poorly developed. There are no large nerves or blood vessels in the area, and the muscle does not lie over a joint. The client may lie supine or in a sitting position during injection as long as the leg muscles are relaxed.

The rectus femoris muscle is located on the midanterior thigh and is another well-developed muscle that lies away from blood vessels and nerves (Fig. 26–18). It can safely be used in adults, children, and infants. This site is not as popular, however, because it can cause discomfort. In general, it is only used if other sites are contraindicated.

DELTOID SITE. The deltoid muscle is found on the lateral aspect of the upper arm. It is not used as often as other sites because it is a small muscle, incapable of absorbing large medication volumes. The deltoid muscle should not be used in infants and children because of its size. In adults, injected volumes should not exceed 1 mL. The client may sit or lie down during injection as long as the arm is relaxed against the body to minimize muscle tension and resistance.

Locate the site by palpating the lower edge of the acromion process. Inject the area that lies 2 to 3 finger-

breadths below the acromion process in adults. An alternative method is to locate the triangular muscle area that extends from 2.5 to 5 fingerbreadths below the acromion process (Fig. 26–19). If the site is used for a child, locate the site 1 fingerbreadth below the acromion process.

AIR-LOCK TECHNIQUE. The use of an air lock when giving IM injections is controversial. Historically, a 0.2-mL air bubble was drawn into a syringe and injected to prevent tracking of irritating medication through SC tissue when the needle was withdrawn. Although widely used in the past, recent research indicates that it should not be used when a disposable plastic syringe is used (Beyea & Nicoll, 1996). Determine and follow your employer's policies and procedures about use of air-locks.

A_ction_ A_lert!_
Do not routinely draw an air bubble into a disposable plastic syringe used for intramuscular injection.

Z-TRACK METHOD. The Z-track method for giving IM injections seals the medication within muscle tissue. It minimizes tissue irritation by preventing tracking of medication through SC tissue with needle removal after injection. Although previously used only when giving irritating or tissue-staining medications such as iron dextran (Imferon), it is now being used

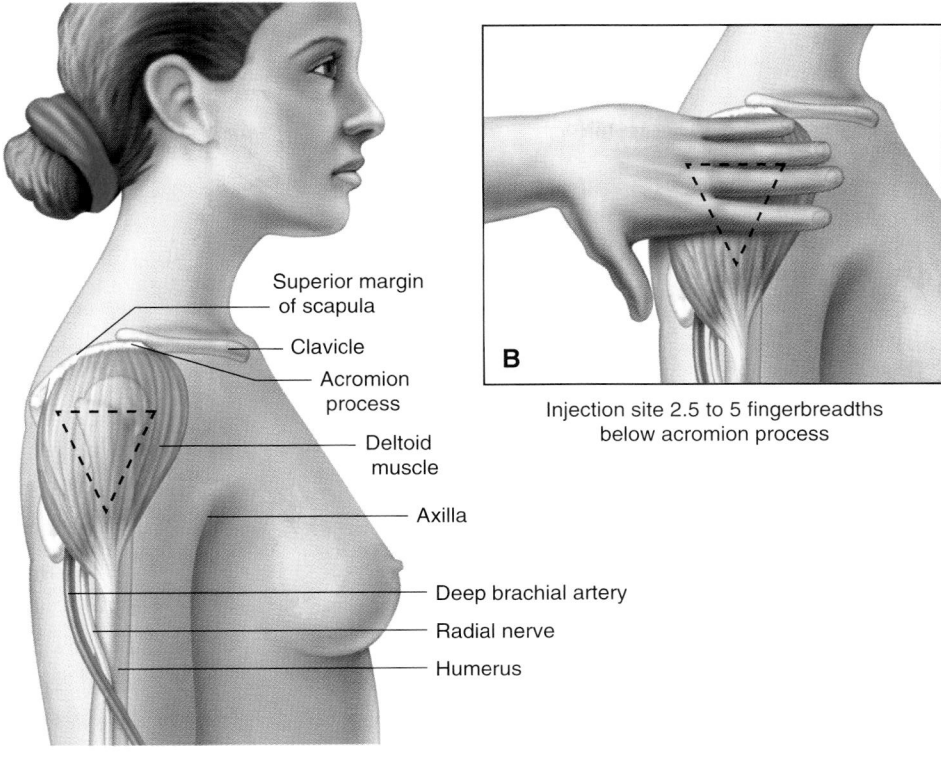

Superior margin
of scapula

Clavicle

Acromion
process

Deltoid
muscle

Axilla

Deep brachial artery

Radial nerve

Humerus

B

Injection site 2.5 to 5 fingerbreadths
below acromion process

Figure 26–19. *A,* deltoid muscle injection site in the upper arm. *B,* locate the site in the triangular area 2.5 to 3 fingerbreadths below the acromion process.

A

more frequently to minimize pain and discomfort at any IM injection site. It does not require the use of an air-lock.

Use the Z-track technique when giving injections in the ventrogluteal or dorsogluteal areas (Fig. 26–20).

After drawing up the medication, change the needle to ensure that medication is not tracked into SC tissue during needle insertion. The needle should be at least 1.5 inches long. Pull the skin and SC tissue about 1 to 1.5 inches (2.5 to 3.5 cm) to one side using your non-

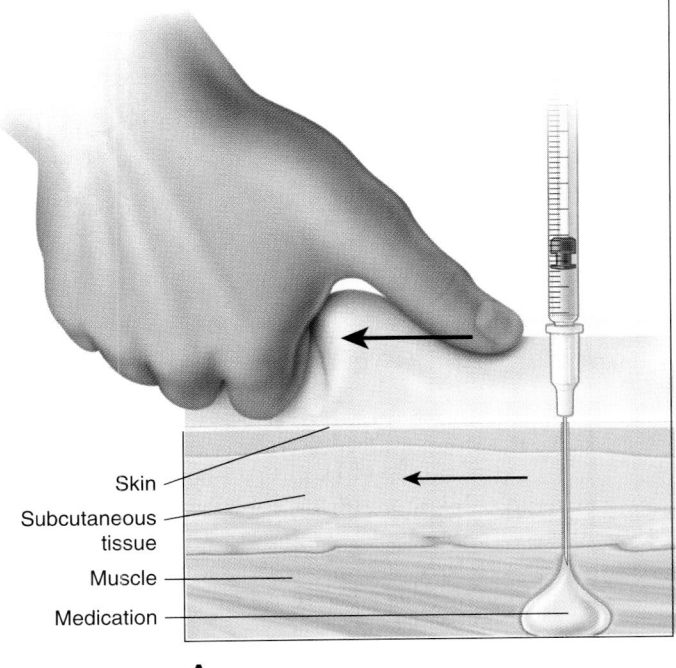

Skin

Subcutaneous
tissue

Muscle

Medication

A

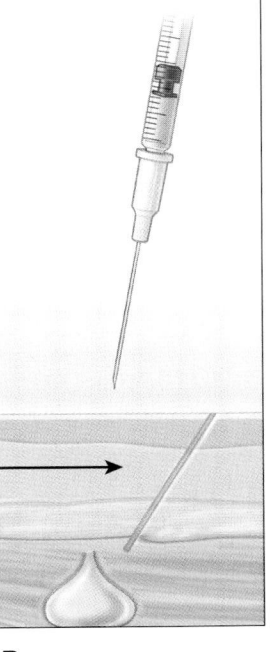

B

Figure 26–20. Intramuscular injection using the Z-track technique. *A,* pull the skin and subcutaneous tissue 1 to 1.5 inches (2.5 to 3.5 cm) to the side, and inject the medication. *B,* withdraw the needle, and release the tissue to seal the medication in the muscle.

PROCEDURE 26–8

Adding Medication to an IV Bag

TIME TO ALLOW
▼
Novice:
8 min.
Expert:
3 min.

Some medications are given to clients as part of an intravenous (IV) infusion. The pharmacy may add the medication to the IV infusion bag, or you may need to do it.

Delegation Guidelines

You may not delegate the addition of medication to an IV bag to a nursing assistant.

Equipment Needed

- Medication administration record, computerized medication order sheet, or medication kardex or card.
- Medication vial or ampule.
- IV solution.
- Medication label.
- Sterile syringe and needle of appropriate size (3 to 20 mL and 1″ to 1.5″, 19- to 21-gauge).
- Needle filter, if appropriate.
- Two alcohol swabs.
- Disposable gloves.

---

1 Check the medication order.

---

2 Withdraw the medication from the ampule or vial as described in the second and third procedures.

---

3 Inject the medication into the bag of IV solution.
a. Close the roller clamp on the tubing attached to the IV solution.

This step prevents fluid loss from the IV bag.

b. Wipe the medication port of the bag containing the IV solution.

Doing so prevents contamination of the needle by microorganisms on the outside of the port.

c. Insert the needle into the center of the medication port and inject medication from syringe into the solution bag.

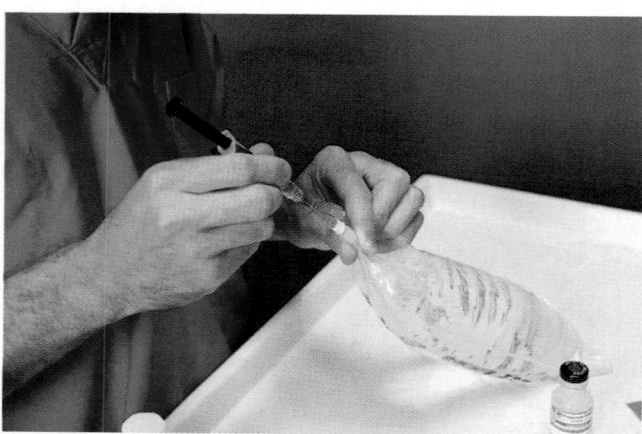

Inserting the needle into the center of the medication port.

Using the center of the port prevents accidental puncture of the sides of the port or the IV container.

d. Withdraw the needle and discard the needle and syringe, without recapping the needle, in an approved receptacle.

e. Rotate the solution bag gently but thoroughly.

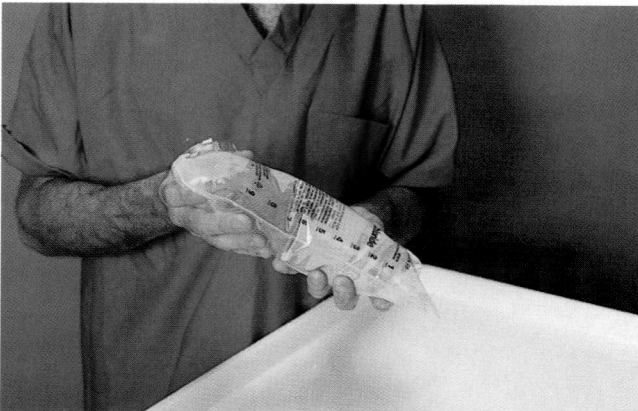

Rotating the solution bag.

Rotation distributes the medication evenly throughout the IV solution.

f. Write the name and dose of the medication, the date, the time, and your initials on a medication label. Affix the label to the IV bag without obstructing the name of the solution or the IV timetape.

The label clearly identifies what you added to the IV solution without hampering your ability to identify the solution or determine whether the IV is infusing on time.

g. Dispose of the medication container, alcohol swab, wrapper, and any other used materials in an appropriate receptacle.

This step prevents medication error and possible fluid overload.

4 Prime the tubing, bring the container to the client's room, and hang the solution bag according to standard procedure. Check the drip rate carefully. Follow all procedures needed to monitor IV therapy properly.

5 Document the date, time, IV solution used, and additive used on the client's medication administration record or other IV charting form.

HOME CARE CONSIDERATIONS

The administration of IV medications is a growing trend in home care. Clients include people with AIDS, cancer, and other serious illnesses. In home care settings today, you may administer chemotherapy, acyclovir, total parenteral nutrition, blood, and medications that were at one time administered only in a hospital setting. You will need to assess for the effects and side effects of medications, recognize serious or life-threatening reactions, and know how to respond.

dominant hand. Inject the medication as usual, withdraw the needle, and release the tissue. The tissue glides back into normal position, eliminating the needle track. Apply gentle pressure over the area, but do not massage to avoid forcing medication back into the needle track.

INTRAVENOUS MEDICATIONS

The IV route is chosen when medication effect is needed within 1 to 2 minutes or when the medication is irritating to SC or muscle tissue. Use extreme caution and follow the five rights of medication administration when using the IV route. If there is an antidote to an IV medication, it should be readily available for emergency use.

Generally, there are three possible methods for giving an IV medication. One is to add it directly to a bag or bottle of IV solution, which then infuses slowly but continuously into the client. When available, special transfer devices simplify the transfer of medication to an IV solution. See the accompanying procedure for the correct method for adding medication to an IV solution.

A second method of intermittent IV medication administration is the IV piggyback (IVPB) setup (most common) or an IV tandem setup (Fig. 26–21). The IVPB method uses gravity to determine flow rate. A roller clamp is used to adjust the flow rate of these infusions as well. The secondary solution (Table 26–7) is plugged into an intermittent IV infusion device or is added to a primary IV line using either a needle or a needleless system. Preparation and administration of an intermittent IV medication are described in the accompanying procedure.

When you need to control the infusion rate of an intermittent IV medication, use an infusion control pump. Make sure the alarm is always turned on to alert you if the line infiltrates or other problems arise. Remember that these devices are adjuncts to your care, not substitutes for your careful nursing assessment.

The third method for administering an IV medication is IV push. As with an intermittent IV infusion, you may give IV push medications through a mainline IV or an intermittent infusion device. Medications are usually injected over 1 minute or longer, according to drug literature. If an intermittent infusion device is used, flush the line with normal saline (or occasionally heparin) per facility policy to verify that the line is patent. The accompanying procedure describes how to administer an IV push medication.

Regardless of the specific method used, universal principles apply to the preparation and administration of IV medications. Be especially careful to select the correct medication and draw up the correct dose. Use proper technique when withdrawing medication from a vial or ampule, and wipe the IV port with an alcohol swab before adding the medication or entering the IV line. Label the syringe or bag according to facility policy with the medication name, dose, date, time, and your name or initials. Do not apply a label before actually adding a medication. This could lead to medication error if someone distracts you during your preparation.

Before giving an IV medication, assess the IV line for patency and for signs of phlebitis or infiltration. If found, do not use the line. Start a new IV line before proceeding. Severe tissue damage could result if irritating medications are injected into an infiltrated IV line. A vein with signs of phlebitis could be damaged further by injection of an IV medication, or the line may be resistant to flushing. Periodically assess the status of the client and the line during the infusion to

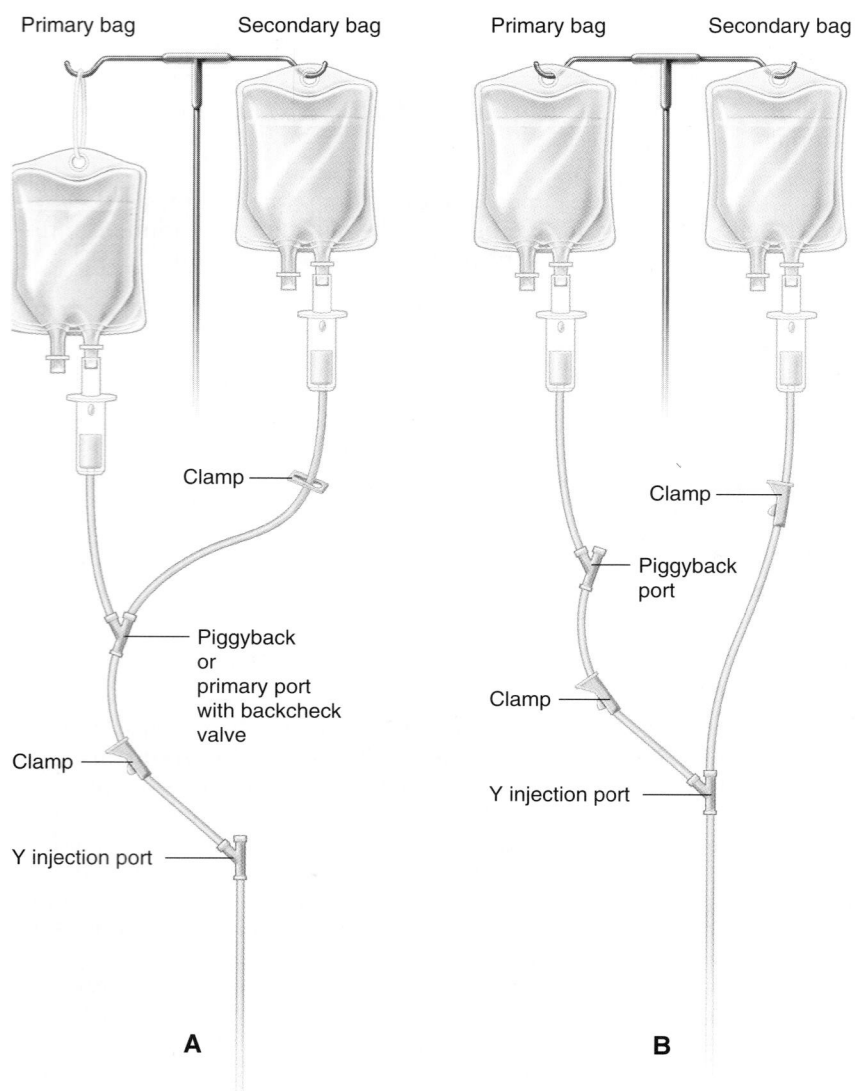

Primary bag   Secondary bag   Primary bag   Secondary bag

Clamp

Piggyback
or
primary port
with backcheck
valve

Clamp

Y injection port

Clamp

Piggyback
port

Clamp

Y injection port

A   B

Figure 26–21. Intermittent IV medication administration can be accomplished with the use of IV piggyback *(A)* or tandem *(B)* setups.

detect early signs of complications or untoward reactions.

Clients who have poor-quality veins or who require IV medication therapy for prolonged periods may undergo percutaneous insertion of a central venous catheter. Such a catheter may have multiple lumina or a single lumen. Other central venous lines are implanted surgically and are accessed using specific techniques. Such lines may be implanted in clients who need chemotherapy. Adhere to facility policies and procedures when giving IV medications through these catheters. Use strict surgical aseptic technique when accessing these lines because organisms introduced into a central line could lead rapidly to sepsis.

Managing Topical Medications

Topical medications are often used to produce an anesthetic effect, create a systemic effect, or relieve local irritation or infection. Most are given two to three times a day.

SKIN APPLICATIONS

A medication applied to the skin is manufactured in the form of a cream, lotion, ointment, powder, paste, or patch (also called a disk). Before giving a topical medication, assess the client's skin for breakdown, lesions, rashes, or erythema. The medication may be ordered to treat one of these conditions, or it may indicate that the medication should not be applied to that surface, depending on the medication and client circumstances. Use standard precautions when administering a topical drug to protect you from contact with the medication and the client's secretions. These precautions also protect the client from microorganisms on your hands.

Before giving a topical medication, cleanse the area with soap and water unless contraindicated. Use ster-

TABLE 26–7
Systems for Administering a Drug by IV Piggyback

System	Procedure
Ready-to-use Premix 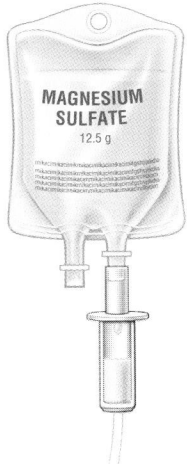	A plastic bag contains both medication and diluent. Unstable drugs may be frozen to preserve them and are thawed before use.
Minibag 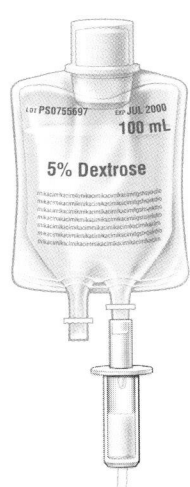	A drug is reconstituted and then added to diluent in a small plastic bag.
ADD-Vantage 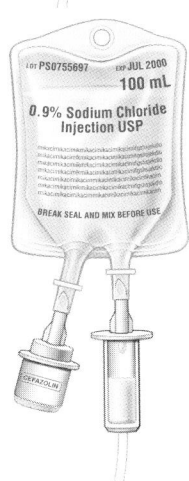	A medication vial is attached to an IV bag. You break an internal seal and mix the drug and diluent just before administration.

Table continued on following page

TABLE 26–7

Systems for Administering a Drug by IV Piggyback *Continued*

System	Procedure
Drug manufacturer's piggyback	A medication dose is prefilled in a container that must be diluted before use.

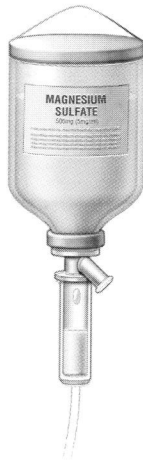

System	Procedure
Minisyringe pump	The medication is injected using a pressurized syringe plunger.

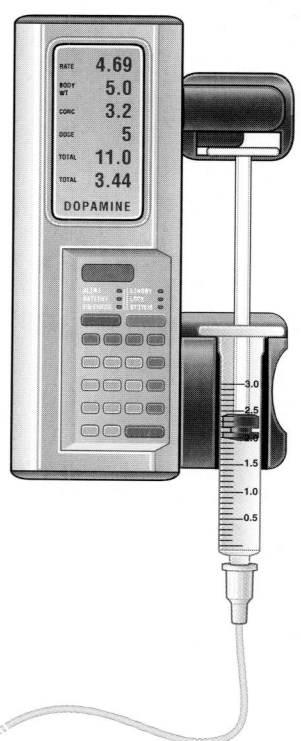

PROCEDURE 26–9

Administering an IV Medication by Intermittent Infusion

TIME TO
ALLOW
▼
Novice:
10 min.
Expert:
5 min.

An intermittent intravenous (IV) infusion is administered when a medication must be given by the IV route, but requires a longer infusion time (typically 30 to 90 minutes) than IV push provides. It is connected into a primary IV line by IVPB or tandem setup or connected to a saline lock.

Delegation Guidelines

You may not delegate the administration of IV medication by intermittent infusion to a nursing assistant.

Equipment Needed

* Medication administration record, computerized medication order sheet, or medication kardex or card.
* Medication premixed in a 50-mL to 250-mL infusion bag (usually 50 to 150 mL), clearly labeled.
* Macrodrip or microdrip tubing of appropriate length (primary tubing if attaching

to a heparin lock, secondary tubing if attaching to a primary IV line).
* Needleless IV connector or 21- to 23-gauge needle.
* Metal or plastic hook (if adding to a primary IV line) or a vial of sterile normal saline and two 3-mL syringes with attached needles (if giving medication through a heparin lock).
* Alcohol swab.
* Disposable gloves.
* Tape (optional).

---

1 Check the medication order and assess the client's allergies.

2 Prepare the medication at the medication cart or another designated area. Label the IV medication bag/bottle if the pharmacy has not done so already.

3 Administer the medication.

Administration Through an Existing IV Line (IVPB or Tandem Setup)

a. Attach secondary tubing to the IV bag or bottle that contains the medication according to standard IV therapy protocol.

Tubing may be used for 48 to 72 hours from the time of initial use in most facilities.

b. Make sure to use nonvented tubing for an IV bag and vented tubing for an IV bottle. Also make sure that the roller clamp on the tubing is closed before attaching the tubing.

c. Prime the tubing and label the IV bag with the date, time, and your initials if the bag has not been labeled yet.

d. Bring the medication administration record, IV bag with medication, needle or needleless device, alcohol swab, metal hook, gloves, and tape to client's room.

e. Identify the client using an identification bracelet or other acceptable means.

f. Assess the IV site and don gloves if your facility requires it.

g. Remove the cap from the distal end of the IV tubing and attach the needle or needleless device.

h. Wipe the IV additive port on the primary line with an alcohol swab and attach the needle or needleless device. Make sure to attach the medication above the flow regulator clamp on the primary line. Although needleless systems are typically manufactured to secure tightly to the IV port, you should tape the connection if needed for stability.

Cleaning with alcohol prevents the IV line from becoming contaminated with microorganisms from the exterior IV port. Attaching the medication above the regulator clamp allows you to regulate the flow of the IV medication.

i. Lower the primary IV solution below the level of the IV medication bag using the metal or plastic hook provided with the secondary tubing set.

The IV medication flows and the primary bag stops flowing because of the effects of gravity.

j. Regulate the drip rate of the IV medications as ordered, or set the infusion pump rate and volume.

Continued

PROCEDURE 26–9 *(continued)*

Administering an IV Medication by Intermittent Infusion

If you use a regulator clamp below the site where the IVPB is connected, the primary bag will start flowing when the IVPB is empty.

k. Come back when the medication has infused and reset the drip rate on the primary line.

   Unless readjusted, the primary line will continue to infuse at the rate set for the secondary infusion. If you use an infusion pump, the primary rate should resume once secondary medication is infused.

l. Reassess the IV site and the client's tolerance of the medication.

Administration Through a Heparin Lock (Intermittent Infusion Device)

a. Close the roller clamp and attach tubing of adequate length (70″ or longer) to the IV medication bag or bottle according to standard IV therapy protocol. Use nonvented tubing for an IV bag and vented tubing for an IV bottle. Prime the tubing.

   Closing the clamp prevents loss of the medication through the tubing. Choosing correctly vented tubing ensures that solution will flow through the tubing. Priming the tubing removes air from the system.

b. Using standard procedure, draw 3 mL of sterile normal saline solution into a 3-mL syringe (or another solution or amount according to facility policy).

   An intermittent infusion device is flushed both before and after use to ensure patency.

c. Bring the medication administration record, IV medication bag, needle or needleless device, syringe with flush, alcohol swab, gloves, and tape to client's room.

d. Identify client using an identification bracelet or other acceptable means.

e. Assess the IV site and don gloves if required by your facility.

f. Remove the cap from the distal end of the IV tubing. Attach the needle or needleless device and prime.

   Priming removes air from the system.

g. Wipe the port of the intermittent infusion device with an alcohol swab.

h. Assess the site and flush the infusion device port with sterile saline solution or another ordered solution.

i. Attach the IV medication bag to the infusion device port using the needle or needleless device. Tape the connection if needed.

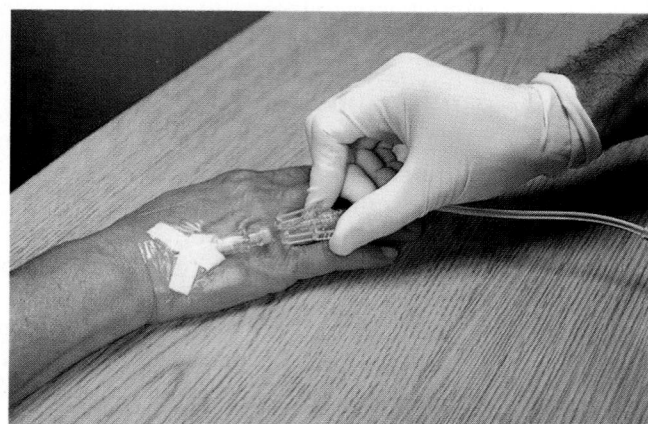

Using a needleless device, attaching the IV medication bag to the infusion device port.

j. Regulate the drip rate of the IV medication as ordered.

k. Come back when the medication has infused, close the roller clamp, and remove the tubing from the port. Recap or attach a clean needle or needleless device to the tubing according to facility policy.

   Most facilities allow IV tubing to be reused for 48 to 72 hours after the initial use, if sterility has been maintained.

l. Reassess the IV site and flush the heparin lock with a second syringe filled with the ordered flush solution (normal saline or heparin according to facility policy). Evaluate the client's response to the medication.

4 Document the date, time, and IV medication given on the client's medication administration record or computerized medication record.

PROCEDURE 26–10

Administering an IV Push Medication

TIME TO
ALLOW
▼
Novice:
10 min.
Expert:
5 min.

Push means the medication is mixed in a small amount of fluid (usually 1 to 10 mL) and administered directly into the vein (not mixed with IV fluid) over a short time (usually 1 to 5 minutes). The bolus of medication is given by the intravenous (IV) push method when the client needs an immediate effect or the medication cannot be mixed with the fluid. Product literature indicates whether a specific medication can be given using this method.

Delegation Guidelines

You may not delegate the administration of IV push medication to a nursing assistant.

Equipment Needed

* Medication administration record, computerized medication order sheet, or medication Kardex or card.
* Medication vial or ampule.
* Syringe of appropriate size for the medication dose ordered with a 21- to 23-gauge needle attached.

* Vial of sterile normal saline and two 3-mL syringes with attached needles (if using an intermittent infusion device).
* If a needleless system is used, one needleless device if injecting through a mainline IV and three devices if injecting via an intermittent infusion device
* Alcohol swabs.
* Disposable gloves.

---

1 Check the medication order and assess the client's allergies.

2 Prepare the medication at the medication cart or other designated area.

Preparing the medication before going to the bedside helps to reduce the client's anxiety.

3 Administer the medication.

Administration Through an Existing IV Line

a. Draw up the medication from an ampule or a vial as described in the second and third procedures. Recap the needle using one-handed technique. Label the syringe with the medication and dose.
b. Remove the capped needle and attach a needleless device if a needleless system is in use.
c. Bring the medication administration record, IV medication, alcohol swab, and gloves to the client's room.
d. Identify the client using an identification bracelet or other acceptable means.
e. Assess the IV site and don gloves if your facility requires it.

f. Wipe the IV additive port of the primary line with an alcohol swab. Make sure that the port being used is the port nearest to the client.

Using the closest port ensures the least resistance to the flow of medication into the client and helps to control the rate at which the medication reaches client's bloodstream.

g. Insert the needle into the port and pinch off the tubing above the injection port.

This action ensures that the medication flows into the client's vein and not upward into the IV tubing.

h. Inject the medication slowly and steadily at rate recommended by the manufacturer. Use a watch to ensure accurate timing. Assess the IV site during injection.

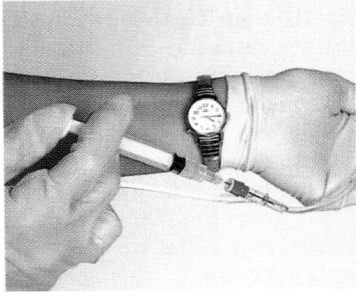

Injecting the medication slowly and steadily, using a watch to ensure accurate timing.

Continued

Administering an IV Push Medication

Overly rapid injection could be harmful to the client or cause IV infiltration. Injection that is too slow is not useful and could produce anxiety.

i. Release the tubing, remove the syringe, and assess the client's tolerance of the medication.

Administration Through an Intermittent Infusion Device (Heparin Lock)

a. Draw up sterile normal saline (or another ordered flush solution) into two syringes of 3 mL each (or another ordered volume) according to facility policy using the third procedure for drawing medication out of a vial. Label the syringes.

An intermittent infusion device is flushed with normal saline both before and after use to ensure patency.

b. Draw up the ordered medication into a syringe from an ampule or a vial as outlined in the second and third procedures. Recap the needle using one-handed technique. Label the syringe.

c. Bring the IV medication, needle or needleless devices, syringes with flush solution, alcohol swabs, and gloves to client's room.

d. Identify the client using an identification bracelet or other acceptable means.

e. Assess the IV site and don gloves if your facility requires it.

f. Wipe the port of the intermittent infusion device with an alcohol swab.

g. Insert one syringe filled with flush solution and inject it slowly into the client. Remove the syringe.

h. Wipe the port again with an alcohol swab.

i. Insert the syringe containing the medication and inject it slowly and steadily at the rate recommended by the manufacturer. Use a watch with a second-hand to ensure accurate timing. Assess the IV site during the injection. Remove the syringe.

Overly rapid injection could be harmful to the client or cause IV infiltration. Injection that is too slow is not useful and could produce anxiety.

j. Wipe the port again with another alcohol swab.

k. Insert the second syringe containing flush solution and inject it slowly into the client. Remove syringe and continue to assess the client's tolerance of the medication.

l. Dispose of supplies properly and discard syringe in rigid needle disposal container.

4 Document the date, the time, and the IV medication given on the medication administration record or computerized medication record.

---

ile procedure as indicated for cleansing an open wound. Medication does not absorb as readily if the skin has accumulated oils, dead cells, or encrustations from lesions. Body oil also reduces the adhesive properties of patches, disks, or tape. Unless there is an open wound or lesion, apply topical medications to dry skin.

Use principles of asepsis when handling topical medications. Use a tongue depressor or swab to remove creams, pastes, or ointments from the original container, such as a jar. Use a new swab or depressor to remove additional medication from the container. If the medication comes in a tube, squeeze the medication onto an applicator before use. Do not squeeze it directly onto the skin. Apply medication evenly using long, smooth strokes, moving in the direction of hair growth to prevent the medication from accumulating in hair follicles. Assess the skin within 2 to 4 hours of the application to assess the medication's effects and possible allergic reaction.

Depending on the type of application, special techniques may be used to enhance medication effective-

ness or to protect the client or nurse. Powders are usually applied to prevent friction on the skin and to promote drying. When using powder, apply it lightly and evenly, being careful not to inhale the particles.

Ointments remain in contact with skin for a long time and tend to soften the skin. Massage ointments into skin that is intact. Creams or oils are often used to treat dry or cracked skin. When applying these products to large areas, warm them in your hands before use to keep from chilling the client. Lotions protect and soothe irritated skin. Shake lotions well before use, and apply them with gauze or cotton balls if appropriate.

Pastes (such as nitroglycerin) may be applied for the purpose of systemic absorption. Remove the old dose before applying a new one, and rotate sites to avoid skin irritation. Measure these doses carefully using paper supplied by the manufacturer to avoid underdosing or overdosing.

The newest form of topical administration is the transdermal patch or disk, which allows for time-release medication absorption through the skin. This limits the number of applications needed to maintain the therapeutic effect and reduces fluctuations in circulating drug levels. A transdermal patch may be applied daily or may be left in place as long as 7 days. Examples of drugs administered by this route include nitroglycerin, estrogen, fentanyl, and scopolamine. The Teaching for Self-Care Chart outlines important guidelines for using a transdermal patch.

EYE APPLICATIONS AND IRRIGATIONS

Ophthalmic (eye) medications are available as drops, ointments, and disks. They are commonly used for diagnostic reasons or to treat problems such as glaucoma or eye infection. Although the eye is not a sterile area, conjunctival secretions protect the eye against many pathogens and eye medications are administered as a sterile procedure. Eye drops have a water base and are easily instilled. Ointments have an oily base and stay in place longer. Because of their composition, eye ointments can cause blurred vision for a period of time after application. If both an eye drop and an eye ointment are scheduled to be given at the same time, give the eye drop first.

Disks are the newest form of ocular medication and may resemble a contact lens. Disks have prolonged action and can stay in place for up to a week. They are best inserted at bedtime because they may cause temporary blurred vision after insertion.

Because the cornea is sensitive and easily damaged, eye medications are placed in the lower conjunctival sac, not directly on the eyeball. Methods for instilling eye drops, ointments, and disks are described in the accompanying procedure.

Cross-contamination is a major concern with the use of ocular medications. Follow these guidelines and teach them to clients as appropriate to decrease the risk of infection:

- Do not use eye drops prescribed for one client on another client. Teach the client not to share them with family or friends.
- Apply from the inner canthus to the outer canthus.
- Apply medication only to the affected eye.
- Avoid touching the eye with the dropper or tube. Discard and replace contaminated items.
- Discard unused solution that remains in the dropper after instillation.
- Once opened, try to keep the drug at the bedside rather than replacing it on medication cart.

At times, an eye irrigation is needed to remove secretions from an eye before giving an ophthalmic medication. It can also be done in an emergency if the eye is contaminated by caustic chemicals. In most emergency situations, the eye should be irrigated for at least 15 minutes with sterile eyewash, if available, or with copious amounts of tap water. The client should obtain professional follow-up after an emergency irrigation. The accompanying proce-

---

Teaching for SELF-CARE

USING TRANSDERMAL PATCHES

Purpose: To maintain optimal medication effect by using a transdermal patch correctly.

Rationale: Transdermal patches (also called transdermal disks) are one of the newer forms for administering selected medications. Because of their unique construction and design, the client may need focused teaching on how to use them correctly.

Expected Outcome: The client verbalizes and demonstrates correct application and removal of a transdermal patch.

Client Instructions

- Apply the patch to a hairless site on your body. Avoid sites at the ends of your arms and legs. Also avoid areas with cuts or calluses that could interfere with absorption of the medication.
- Use firm pressure when applying the patch, especially around the edges, to ensure good contact with the skin.

- If the patch loosens or falls off, apply a new one. The medication is time-released through the special backing on the patch, so you cannot overdose by replacing a loose patch.
- Do not cut or trim the patch because doing so would interfere with the timed-release absorption of the medication through the special backing.
- Because transdermal patches are waterproof, you may shower or bathe as usual.
- Do not change brands of a transdermal patch without checking first with your physician. The dosage may or may not be equivalent.
- Apply and remove the patch as directed. Some patches remain in place for 12 to 14 hours and then are removed for 10 to 12 hours to prevent tolerance from developing (such as with nitroglycerin). Others can be left in place for 3 days (such as scopolamine) or longer. Ask your physician, nurse, or pharmacist if you have questions about how to use your patch.

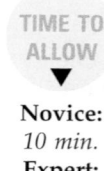

PROCEDURE 26–11

Administering an Eye Medication

TIME TO ALLOW
▼
Novice:
10 min.
Expert:
5 min.

A client with glaucoma, an eye infection, or a number of other ocular disorders will need ophthalmic (eye) medications instilled directly into the eye. Following this procedure will allow you to administer the medication without injuring sensitive eye tissue.

Delegation Guidelines

The administration of eye medications may not be delegated to a nursing assistant.

Equipment Needed

- Medication administration record, computerized medication order sheet, or medication kardex or card.
- Medication bottle, tube, or disk.
- Tissue or cotton ball.
- Warm water and facecloth, as needed.
- Disposable gloves.

---

1 Check the medication order, noting especially the eye to be treated. Note any client allergies.

2 Prepare the client for instillation of the medication.

a. Identify the client using an identification bracelet or other accepted means.

b. Explain the procedure to the client in a calm and confident manner. Help the client to sit or lie down with her head slightly hyperextended. Don gloves.

This head position assists in correct placement of the medication and minimizes drainage through the tear duct.

c. Assess the condition of the client's eye. Wash away any exudate using the facecloth and warm water, wiping from the inner canthus to the outer canthus.

This observation provides baseline assessment data to evaluate the medication's effect. Removing exudate also removes microorganisms and provides a clean surface to apply the medication.

---

3 Administer the medication.

Eyedrops

a. Remove the cap from the bottle and place it on its side. Fill the medication dropper (if used) to the prescribed amount.

This position prevents contamination of the medication's cap.

b. Place your nondominant hand on the client's cheekbone just under her eyelid and pull downward against the bony orbit to expose the lower conjunctival sac. Hold tissue or a cotton ball under the eyelid and apply slight pressure to the inner canthus.

This action exposes the lower conjunctival sac while preventing pressure and trauma to the eye. Pressing on the inner canthus blocks the tear duct temporarily and prevents the medication from leaving the eye through the duct and possibly causing systemic effects.

c. Rest your dominant hand against the client's forehead for stability and hold the medication bottle or dropper ½" to ¾" above the conjunctival sac.

Resting on the client's forehead stabilizes your hand and reduces the risk of contact between eye structures and the medication bottle, preventing trauma, infection, or both.

d. Ask the client to look up at the ceiling and, while she does, instill the prescribed number of drops into her lower conjunctival sac. If the client closes her eye or blinks, or if a drop lands on her eyelid, repeat the missed drop.

Looking up reduces stimulation of the blink reflex and thus promotes accurate delivery of the dose into the conjunctival sac.

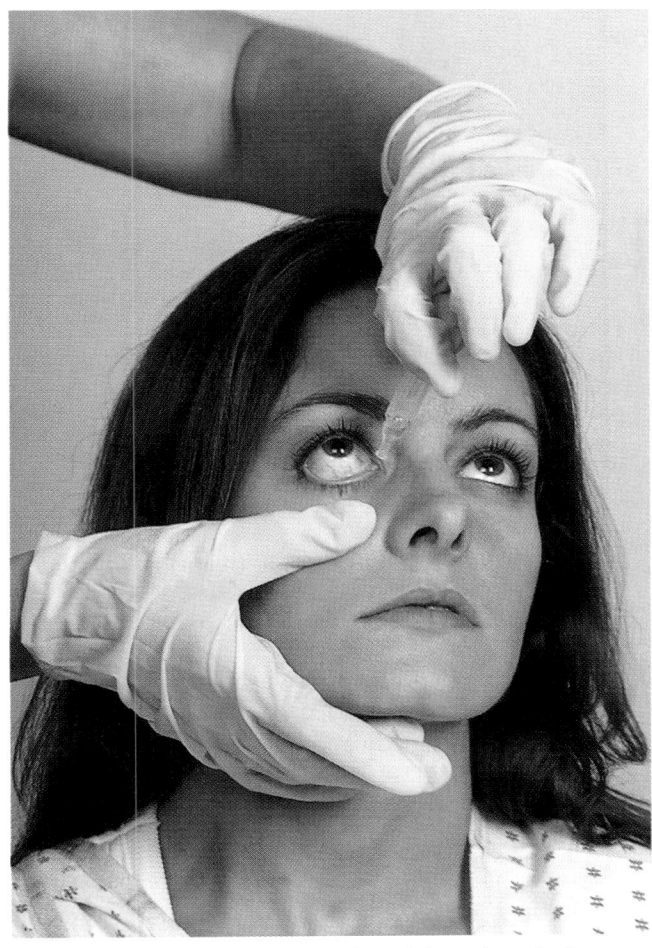

Administering the prescribed number of drops into the lower conjunctival sac.

nondominant hand, pulling lower lid downward over the bony prominence of the cheek. (For instillation in the upper lid, draw upper lid up and away from eyeball.)

c. Ask the client to look up for instillation in the lower lid or down for instillation in the upper lid.

Looking up or down reduces stimulation of the blink reflex and rotates the sensitive cornea away from the medication.

d. Apply a thin line of ointment along the inside edge of the lower or upper lid as ordered, moving from the inner canthus to the outer canthus.

e. Ask the client to gently close her eye and move it around. Apply gentle pressure over lacrimal duct for 1 minute, or ask the client to do so if she can.

Moving the eye behind the closed lid helps to distribute the medication over the conjunctiva and eyeball. Gently closing it (not squinting or squeezing) prevents loss of medication from conjunctival sac. Pressing the lacrimal duct helps to prevent systemic absorption of the medication.

Eye Ointment

a. Remove the cap from the tube and place on its side. Squeeze and discard a small bead of medication.

Placing the cap on its side helps to prevent contamination. The first bead of an ointment is considered contaminated.

b. For instillation in the lower lid, separate client's eyelids with the thumb and forefinger of your

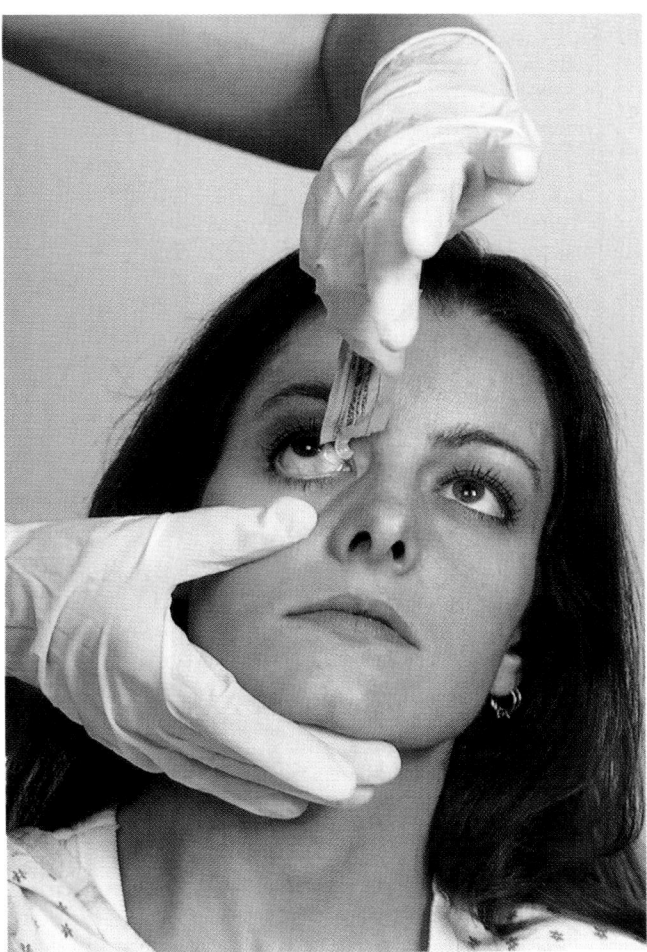

Applying a thin line of ointment along the inside edge of the eyelid.

This method ensures aseptic and even distribution of medication as well as the proper dosage.

Continued

Administering an Eye Medication

e. Ask the client to gently close her eye and move it around.

Moving the eye behind closed lids helps to distribute medication over the conjunctiva and eyeball. Gently closing it (not squinting or squeezing) prevents loss of medication from conjunctival sac.

Medicated Eye Disk

a. Open the package and press the tip of the index finger of your dominant hand against the convex part of disk.

Doing so helps the disk adhere to your fingertip.

b. Pull the client's lower eyelid away from the eye with your nondominant hand and ask the client to look up.

Looking up exposes the conjunctival sac and reduces the blink reflex.

c. Place the disk horizontally in the conjunctival sac between the iris and the lower eyelid.

d. Pull the lower eyelid out, up, and over the disk. Ask the client to blink a few times. If the disk is visible, repeat this step. Otherwise, have the client press her fingers against her closed lids, without rubbing her eyes or moving the disk.

This action ensures proper disk position.

e. If the disk falls out, rinse it with cool water and reinsert it.

Rinsing the disk reduces the risk of infection.

f. To remove a disk, pull or invert the client's lower eyelid so you can see the disk, then use the thumb and index finger of your dominant hand to pinch the disk and lift it from the conjunctival sac. If it is in the upper eye, stroke the client's closed eyelid with your fingertip, gently and in long circular motions. Ask the client to open her eye, and look for the disk in the corner of her eye. Slide the disk to her lower lid and remove it as noted earlier.

This procedure minimizes risk of trauma or infection while assisting with removal of the disk.

4 Remove your gloves and wash your hands.

5 Document the medication administration promptly on the medication administration record or computerized medication record.

---

dure describes how to perform a routine eye irrigation.

EAR INSTILLATIONS AND IRRIGATIONS

The external ear is unsterile and consists of the external auditory canal and the pinna. The middle and inner ear lie behind the tympanic membrane and are sterile areas. Because a rupture of the tympanic membrane would create an opening between these areas, sterile solutions should be used prophylactically for instillation or irrigation of the ear.

Ear instillations require special care. Warm a solution to body temperature before use if possible, but at least give it at room temperature to prevent vertigo and nausea. Avoid using excessive force when instilling medication or irrigating an ear to avoid rupturing the tympanic membrane. Do not occlude the auditory meatus during these procedures for the same reason. Assess ear drainage carefully to detect possible infection (Chapter 43).

Otic (ear) medications exert a local effect and are commonly used to soften ear wax, fight infection, relieve pain, or destroy an insect trapped in the canal. Different approaches are used when administering otic medications to adults and children because of dif-

ferences in the shape of the ear canal. Pull the pinna of an adult up and back to straighten the canal before administering ear drops or ear irrigation. In contrast, pull the pinna of an infant or young child down and back. The recommended methods for administering an ear medication are given in the accompanying procedure.

NASAL INSTILLATIONS

Medications are given by the nasal route to relieve the symptoms of sinus colds and congestion, shrink swollen mucous membranes, loosen nasal secretions, and treat nasal or sinus infection. Occasionally, medications are used for a systemic effect (such as vasopressin). Nasal medications are generally available in the form of sprays (decongestants, vasopressin) or drops (anti-infectives).

Clients have ready access to a number of OTC nasal medications, so teach them carefully about their use. Decongestants, in particular, cause rebound nasal congestion when used to excess. Teach clients how to properly administer them for maximum effect. Warn clients about other active ingredients in these products. For example, many nasal decongestants contain sympathomimetics

PROCEDURE 26–12

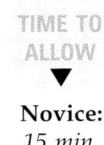

Irrigating an Eye

TIME TO ALLOW
▼
Novice:
15 min.
Expert:
8 min.

Eye irrigation is used to remove infection or other foreign matter from the eye. It can be done on a short-term ongoing basis or as a one-time order based on client need.

Delegation Guidelines

The performance of this procedure requires your expertise and skill and may not be delegated to a nursing assistant.

Equipment Needed

- Sterile irrigating solution warmed to body temperature.
- Sterile irrigation set with irrigating or bulb syringe and a sterile container.
- Emesis or curved irrigation basin.
- Waterproof pad if not supplied with irrigation set.
- Towel.
- Cotton balls.
- Disposable gloves.

---

1 Prepare the client for the irrigation.

a. Identify the client using an identification bracelet or other accepted means.

b. Explain the procedure to the client in a calm and confident manner.

c. Help the client to sit or lie with his head tilted toward the eye that will be irrigated. Place the waterproof pad under the affected side. Don gloves.

This head position enlists the aid of gravity so solution flows from inner canthus to the outer canthus without flowing through the unaffected eye.

d. Pour irrigant into the container and draw it into the syringe using aseptic technique.

e. Clean the client's eyelids and eyelashes with a cotton ball moistened with irrigant or normal saline solution. Wipe from the inner canthus to the outer canthus using a new cotton ball with each pass.

This step removes material on the lids and lashes that could be washed into the eye with irrigation.

f. Place the curved basin under the affected cheek to catch the irrigating solution as it flows from the client's eye. Ask the client to hold the basin if possible.

---

2 Irrigate the eye.

a. Use your nondominant hand to hold the client's upper lid open and expose the lower conjunctival sac.

Using the conjunctival sac reduces stimulation of the blink reflex and prevents irrigant from injuring the cornea.

b. Hold the irrigation syringe about 1″ above eye. Do not touch the eye with the syringe. Push fluid gently into the conjunctival sac, directing the flow from the inner canthus to the outer canthus.

This process uses the least amount of pressure necessary to cleanse the eye and reduces the risk of injury to the eye.

c. Repeat the irrigation until the secretions are gone or the irrigant is used up. Allow the client to close his eyes intermittently during procedure as needed.

Closed eye movements help to move secretions from the upper to the lower conjunctival area.

d. Dry the area with cotton balls, and offer the client a towel to dry his face and neck.

---

3 Remove your gloves and wash your hands.

4 Document the irrigation promptly in the client's medical record. Also record the appearance of the eye, characteristics of drainage, and the client's response to treatment.

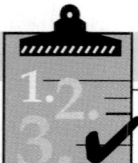

PROCEDURE 26–13

Administering an Ear Medication

TIME TO
ALLOW
▼
Novice:
8 min.
Expert:
3 min.

Ear infections are relatively common among children and are one of the most common reasons for administering a medication into the ear canal.

Delegation Guidelines

As with all medication administration procedures, you may not delegate the administration of ear medications to a nursing assistant.

Equipment Needed

- Medication administration record, computerized medication order sheet, or medication Kardex or card.
- Medication (eardrops).
- Tissue or cotton ball.
- Cotton-tipped applicator.
- Disposable gloves.

1 Check the medication order, and note any client allergies.

2 Prepare the client for instillation of the medication.
a. Identify the client using an identification bracelet or other accepted means.
b. Explain the procedure to the client in a calm and confident manner. Help the client to a side-lying position with the affected ear upward. Don gloves.

This position assists in correct placement of medication and minimizes its drainage from the ear canal.

c. Assess the condition of the ear. Gently wash away any cerumen or exudate using cotton-tipped applicators. Do not force wax or drainage into the ear canal.

This step provides baseline assessment data and cleans the area before application of the medication.

3 Administer the medication
a. Remove the cap from the bottle and place it on its side. Fill the medication dropper (if applicable) to prescribed amount.

Placing the cap on its side prevents contamination of the cap.

b. Pull the pinna up and back in an adult client or down and back in a child.

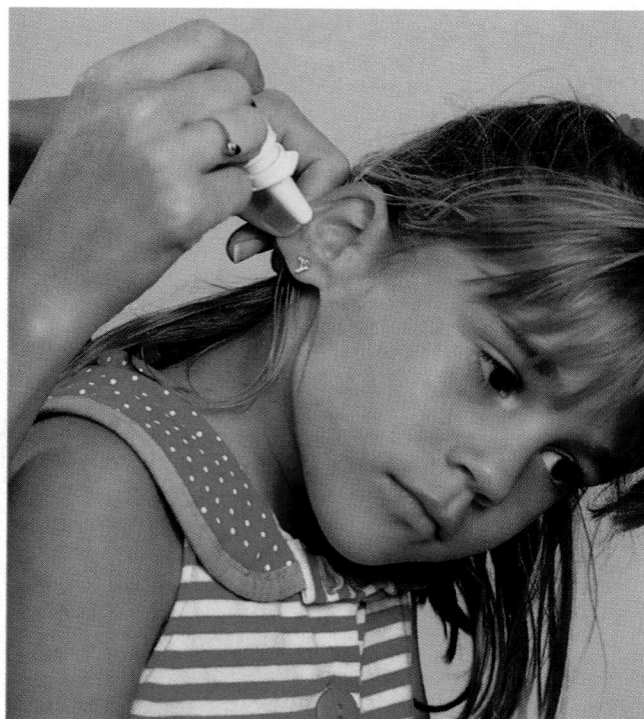

Pulling the pinna down and back.

This step straightens the ear canal.

c. Hold the dropper or bottle ½ inch above the ear canal and instill as many eardrops as ordered.

Holding the bottle above the ear canal avoids excess pressure in the canal.

d. Ask the client to maintain the side-lying position for 2 to 3 minutes. Apply gentle pressure with your finger to the tragus of the ear or ask the client to do so.

Staying in the side-lying position helps to distribute the medication. Because ear infections are painful, the client may prefer to apply the pressure herself.

e. Place a cotton ball into the outermost portion of the ear canal.

This helps to prevent medication loss when the client changes position.

4 Remove your gloves and wash your hands.

5 Document the medication administration promptly in the medication administration record or computerized medication record.

6 Check on the client in 15 minutes to remove the cotton ball from the ear, assess the client's condition, and help her to a comfortable position.

---

that exert a systemic effect and are not suitable for use with children or others who could be adversely affected. In these instances, suggest saline drops.

Use clean technique to administer a nasal medication unless the client has undergone nasal or sinus surgery; then use sterile technique. Properly position the client by tilting or hyperextending the head. The accompanying procedure describes how to give an intranasal medication.

VAGINAL INSTILLATIONS

Vaginal medications are commonly used for contraception or to treat itching, pain, or discomfort from inflammation or infection. They are supplied as gels, creams, foams, or suppositories. Keep suppositories refrigerated to prevent them from melting. Depending on the product, you will administer the medication using a gloved hand or an applicator. Allow the client to self-administer the medication if appropriate.

Before administering the medication, offer the client an opportunity to void. Administer it using standard precautions and aseptic technique as outlined in the accompanying procedure. Once the medication is in the body, it will melt and may produce drainage. For this reason, administer it at bedtime if possible. Offer the client a perineal pad to help absorb drainage. Especially when treating infection, provide meticulous perineal hygiene and assess drainage characteristics carefully.

RECTAL INSTILLATIONS

Rectal instillations are usually used to produce a local effect, such as stimulation of a bowel movement. They are used less often for systemic effects, such as relief of fever or nausea when the client cannot tolerate oral medication. Rectal medications typically come as suppositories, but they are often thinner and longer than vaginal suppositories for easier insertion. Many rectal suppositories are kept refrigerated until use.

Use standard precautions when administering a rectal suppository, and place it properly for adequate results. Do not place the suppository into a fecal mass because it will not be effective. Administer a small cleansing enema beforehand if needed. The proper method for administering a rectal suppository is described in the accompanying procedure.

Administering Inhalation Medications

Medications administered by inhalation are absorbed into the bloodstream via the alveolar epithelium in the lower respiratory tract. To be effective, a medication must be dispersed in very small droplets, such as a mist, and must be inhaled deeply. Common types of medications administered by inhalation are bronchodilators and mucolytics.

Inhalation agents are delivered either by nebulizer (or atomizer) or by metered dose inhaler (MDI). A nebulizer uses a forceful flow of oxygen or compressed air to break up liquid medication into tiny particles that can be inhaled. Teach the client to form a tight seal around the mouthpiece and to breathe through the device until the medication has been completely inhaled (often 15 to 20 minutes).

An MDI delivers a preset dose of medication when the client discharges the canister. Teach the client to form an airtight seal around the mouthpiece. Make sure that the client has manual dexterity and enough strength to push with 5 to 10 pounds of pressure. This is how much pressure the client will need to exert to depress the medication canister into the device to release a dose. It is an important consideration when working with older or debilitated clients. A turbo-inhaler is a variation of an MDI that must be assembled for use. Important teaching points for using an MDI are found in Chapter 39.

EVALUATION

Evaluation of a client's response to medication therapy is just as important as other aspects of admin-

PROCEDURE 26–14

Administering an Intranasal Medication

TIME TO
ALLOW
▼
Novice:
8 min.
Expert:
3 min.

Intranasal medications may be ordered to produce local vasoconstriction of blood vessels or for administration of medications for rapid absorption through nasal mucous membranes.

Delegation Guidelines

You may not delegate the administration of intranasal medication to a nursing assistant.

Equipment Needed

- Medication administration record, computerized medication order sheet, or medication kardex or card.
- Nasal spray or drops.
- Facial tissue.
- Disposable gloves.

1 Check the medication order, and note any client allergies.

2 Prepare the client for instillation of the medication.
a. Identify the client using an identification bracelet or other accepted means.
b. Explain the procedure to the client. Mention that the solution may cause choking, stinging, or burning as it drips into the throat. Don gloves.
c. Ask the client to blow her nose unless contraindicated because of the risk of a nosebleed or increased intracranial pressure. Assess the resulting discharge.

Blowing the nose removes secretions that could interfere with the effectiveness of the medication.

3 Administer the medication.

Administration of a Nasal Spray
a. Remove the cap from the bottle and place it on its side.

This position prevents contamination of the medication's cap.

b. Ask an adult client to tilt her head backward and support her head with your nondominant hand. Keep a child's head in an upright position.

This position allows the medication to reach nasal passages without causing the client to swallow it. Supporting the client's head reduces neck strain.

c. Hold the medication container just inside the tip of the nostril without touching nasal tissue. Ask the client to occlude the opposite nostril and inhale while you administer the spray.

Avoiding contact between the container and the nasal tissue prevents contamination of container. Occluding the opposite nostril while inhaling through the target nostril provides for maximum effectiveness of the medication.

d. Assist the client to a comfortable position.

Administration of Nasal Drops
a. Remove cap from bottle and place on its side.
b. Position the client to accommodate the intended site of action and support her head with your nondominant hand.

For the posterior pharynx, tilt the client's head backward. For the ethmoid or sphenoid sinus, either tilt the client's head back and place a pillow under one shoulder or tilt her head back over the edge of mattress while supporting the back of her head with your nondominant hand. For the frontal or maxillary sinus, assume the position just described and turn her head toward the affected side.

c. Hold the tip of the dropper just above the intended nostril and pointed toward the midline of the ethmoid bone. Do not touch the client's nasal tissue with the dropper. Ask client to breathe through her mouth, and instill the ordered number of drops.

This process provides for the greatest medication effectiveness and prevents contamination of the container.

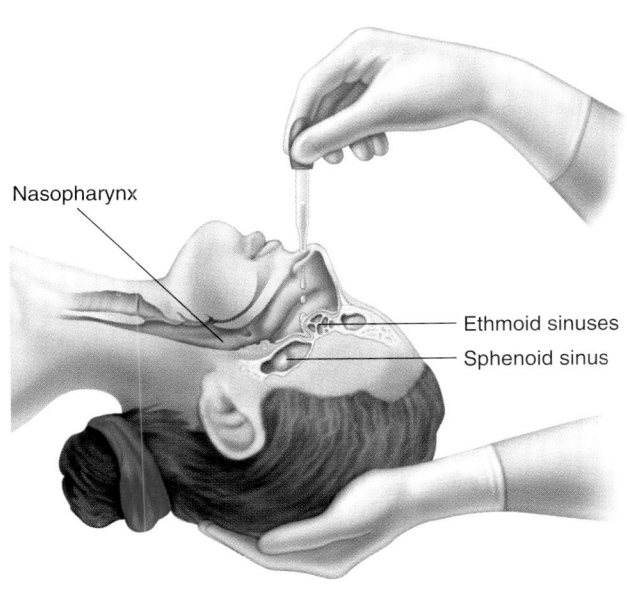

Nasopharynx

Ethmoid sinuses

Sphenoid sinus

Proper position for instillation of nasal medication.

d. Ask the client to maintain her position for 5 minutes and then help her to a comfortable position.

Maintaining her position prevents leakage of the medication from her nose and promotes absorption of the medication.

4 Remove your gloves and wash your hands.

5 Document the medication administration promptly on the medication administration record or computerized medication record.

---

istration. Reassess the client to determine whether the original symptoms have been relieved and gather objective data to further evaluate the effects of medication. For example, evaluate urine output, breath sounds, and peripheral edema to determine the effectiveness of diuretic therapy. Document and report medication effects as appropriate.

Use data from laboratory studies as an adjunct in evaluating medication effectiveness. For example, serum drug levels provide useful information about client status. Report abnormal values at once so that further adjustments can be made to the medication regimen. Finally, assess for adverse medication effects and report them promptly so corrective action may be taken.

Mr. Connell was discharged from the ED to his home with his wife. He now takes his medications regularly and has started to exercise. His job is still stressful, but he verbalizes satisfaction with his lifestyle and his health. As the nurse working in the physician's office where he is receiving follow-up care, consider the following questions:

- What measures will you use to determine the continued effectiveness of therapy?
- What suggestions can you make to further reduce his risk factors for heart disease?
- What should you teach Mr. Connell, specifically considering his Irish-American cultural beliefs and practices concerning health?

The Nursing Care Planning chart suggests a plan of care to meet this client's need for information.

KEY PRINCIPLES

- Drugs have a variety of names, including the official name, chemical name, generic name, and trade name or names. Become familiar with the generic and trade names of medications.
- A client's knowledge base for successful medication self-administration should include information about therapeutic effect, dose, side effects, adverse effects, directions for use, drug interactions, and storage and expiration.
- Drug manufacture and use is highly regulated in the United States and Canada. There are stringent controls over the distribution and use of highly addictive substances, such as narcotics.
- The nurse functions within legal guidelines when administering medications. The Nurse Practice Act in each state specifies the responsibility a nurse has in administering medications.
- Pharmacokinetics refers to the processes of absorption, distribution, metabolism, and excretion. A variety of client-related factors influence a drug's effectiveness.
- Drugs can elicit a variety of responses. Each drug may have a therapeutic effect, adverse effects, and

PROCEDURE 26–15

Administering a Vaginal Medication

TIME TO ALLOW ▼

Novice: 15 min.
Expert: 7 min.

Vaginal instillations are usually performed to treat infection. They may also be used by the client as part of a contraceptive method.

Delegation Guidelines

You may not delegate the administration of vaginal medication to a nursing assistant.

Equipment Needed

- Medication administration record, computerized medication order sheet, or medication kardex or card.
- Vaginal medication and applicator, if needed.
- Water-soluble lubricant.
- Perineal pad, if needed.
- Cotton balls or facecloth and towel for cleansing, if needed.
- Disposable tissue.
- Disposable gloves.

1 Check the medication order.

2 Prepare the client for instillation of the medication.
a. Identify client using an identification bracelet or another accepted means.
b. Explain the procedure to the client. Offer her the opportunity to void. Close the curtain or door, and help the client to a supine position with her abdomen and legs draped.

   Maintaining privacy is an important step in this type of medication administration.

c. Don gloves.
d. Inspect the client's external genitalia and provide perineal hygiene as needed.

3 Administer the medication using clean technique.

Administration of a Suppository

a. Remove the suppository from its wrapper and insert into the applicator, if used.

   Use of either a gloved finger or an applicator is acceptable.

b. Lubricate the rounded end of the suppository with water-soluble lubricant. If you will not be using an applicator, also lubricate the index finger of your gloved, dominant hand.

   Lubrication allows easier insertion by reducing friction.

c. Separate the client's labia with your nondominant hand and insert the rounded end of the suppository along the posterior vaginal wall for an entire fingerlength.

   This distance ensures complete insertion of the medication and distribution through the entire vagina.

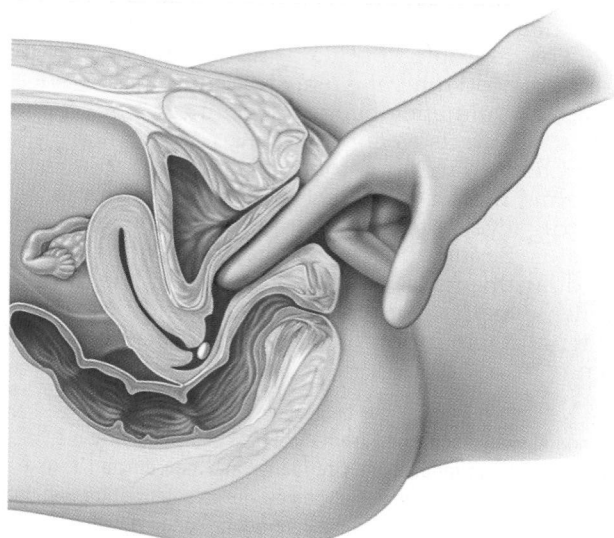

Inserting the vaginal suppository.

d. Withdraw your finger or the applicator and wipe away excess lubricant from the client's genitals.

Administration of a Foam, Jelly,
or Cream
a. Fill applicator with medication according to the package directions.
b. Separate the client's labia with your nondominant hand, point the applicator toward the client's sacrum, and use your dominant hand to insert it 2 or 3 inches into the client's vagina.
c. Depress the plunger on the applicator to push the medication out of the applicator.
d. Withdraw the applicator and place it on a tissue or paper towel. Wipe away excess medication from the client's genitals.

The applicator may contain microorganisms from the client's vagina.

4 Help the client to a comfortable position and ask her to remain supine for 5 to 10 minutes. If needed, offer her a perineal pad.

Lying still prevents loss of the medication from melting and gravity. The perineal pad absorbs excess drainage.

5 Wash the applicator with soap and water and store for future use.

6 Remove your gloves and wash your hands.

7 Document the medication administration promptly on the medication administration record or computerized medication record.

---

toxic effects. Drugs can also elicit an allergic response or idiosyncratic response in some clients. Be aware of potential responses to adequately assess the client.

- Some drugs can cause physiological or psychological dependence in the client. These are labeled as controlled substances and require special precautions for use.
- Each drug has a specific onset, peak, and duration of action. Each drug also has a specific half-life, which determines how often it must be given to maintain a therapeutic blood level.
- There are various types of drug orders. A standing order is given routinely at prescribed times. A PRN order is given as needed but cannot be given more often than specified. A single or one-time order is carried out once only. A STAT order is completed immediately.
- Numerous client-related factors affect drug actions, including dietary, environmental, developmental, cultural, socioeconomic, psychological, and physiological factors.
- Medications may be given by the oral, parenteral, topical, or inhalation routes. The route has a significant effect on the timing and duration of action. Specific procedures are followed when each of these routes is used.
- All steps of the nursing process are used when administering medications to clients.
- Consider several client factors to safely administer medications. These include health history, allergies, medication and diet histories, current condition, problems with perception and coordination, knowledge about drug therapy, and individual learning needs.
- *Altered health maintenance* is a useful nursing diag-

nosis for clients receiving medication therapy. Other nursing diagnoses may also apply. Assess each client individually to determine whether the client exhibits the defining characteristics of one or more nursing diagnoses.

- Drug doses are measured using one of three systems, including the metric, apothecary, and household systems. Familiarity with all three systems is needed to administer drugs safely.
- It is imperative to give medications correctly to protect the client's safety. Adhere to the "five rights" when giving medications. These are the right client, right drug, right dose, right route, and right time.
- The nurse is responsible for safe and accurate administration of all medications and documents administration using established policies and procedures.
- If a medication error does occur, it is your legal and ethical responsibility to report it promptly. Health care facilities have specific policies and procedures to follow if an error occurs. Client safety is the paramount concern.
- Special populations, such as children and older adults, have unique needs with regard to drug therapy. Incorporate your knowledge of these needs when giving medications to these groups.
- Standard precautions are used when administering medications. Use extreme caution when handling needles and other sharps, which can transmit pathogens (such as HIV or hepatitis) from an infected client if a needlestick injury occurs.

PROCEDURE 26–16

Administering a Rectal Medication

TIME TO ALLOW
▼

Novice:
15 min.
Expert:
7 min.

Rectal medications can be used to stimulate a bowel movement or to administer medication when the client cannot take them orally.

Delegation Guidelines

You may not delegate the administration of rectal medication to a nursing assistant.

Equipment Needed

* Medication administration record, computerized medication order sheet, or medication Kardex or card.

* Rectal medication.
* Water-soluble lubricant.
* Facecloth and towel for cleansing, if needed.
* Disposable tissue.
* Disposable gloves.

---

1 Check the medication order.

2 Prepare the client for instillation of the medication.

a. Identify the client using an identification bracelet or another accepted means.

b. Explain the procedure to client. Offer her an opportunity to void. Close the curtain or door.

c. Don gloves. Help the client to a left lateral (Sims) position with her upper leg flexed. Drape the client to expose only the anal area.

This position helps to retain the suppository and promotes relaxation of the external anal sphincter.

d. Inspect the anal area and provide perineal hygiene as needed.

3 Administer the medication using clean aseptic technique.

a. Remove the suppository from the packaging and lubricate the rounded end. Also lubricate the index finger of your gloved, dominant hand.

Lubrication eases insertion by reducing friction.

b. Instruct the client to breathe slowly and deeply through her mouth.

This form of breathing promotes relaxation of the client's rectal area and anal sphincter to prevent pain.

c. Separate the buttocks with your gloved, nondominant hand. Use your dominant hand to insert the rounded end of the suppository about 4" (10 cm) into the rectal canal along the rectal wall. Insert the suppository 2 inches (5 cm) for a child.

This distance ensures insertion of the suppository past the external and internal anal sphincters.

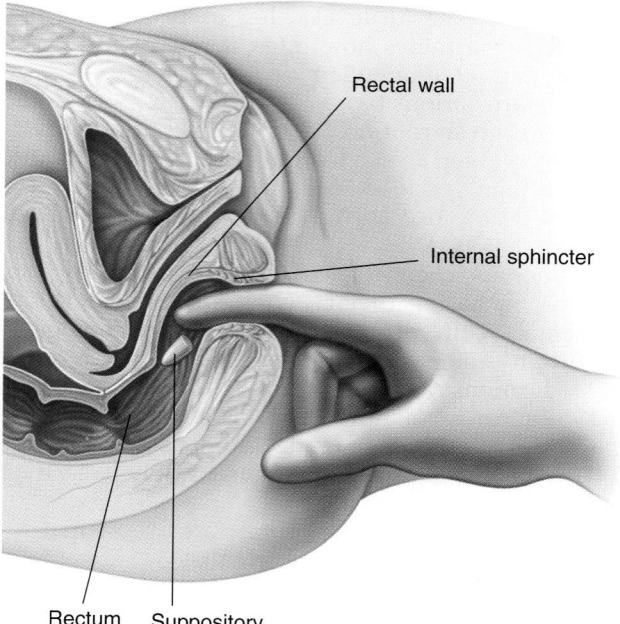

Inserting the rectal suppository.

d. Withdraw your finger and wipe away any fecal material or excess lubricant at the client's anus.

e. Ask the client to remain on her side for 5 minutes (up to 30 minutes for a laxative). Give an immobile client the call bell and ask her to call you when she feels the need for a bowel movement.

Remaining in position prevents the medication from being expelled.

4 Remove your gloves and wash your hands.

5 Return after 5 minutes to see if the suppository has been expelled.

If so, you will need to reinsert it.

6 Document the medication administration on the medication administration record or computerized medication record.

7 Return 30 minutes after administration to assess the medication's effectiveness. Assist the client as needed.

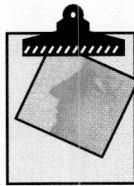

NURSING CARE PLANNING
A CLIENT BEGINNING MEDICATION THERAPY

Admission Data

Mr. Connell was admitted for a 23-hour observation following an episode of chest pain. He was taken for a cardiac catheterization and will be arriving in your unit for postcatheterization monitoring and discharge teaching.

Physician's Orders

Atenolol 50 mg PO daily.
Furosemide 20 mg PO daily.
Nitroglycerin 1/150 gr. SL PRN for chest pain, may repeat ×2.

Nursing Assessment

Before Mr. Connell goes home, he should receive initial instructions to address learning needs he has demonstrated in a variety of areas. He requires information about each of the medications ordered. He would benefit from information about exercise to slow progression of his cardiovascular disease. He could also benefit from initial information on stress management. His understanding and his wife's understanding of sodium restriction should be evaluated and reinforced. He has a definite identified need to understand the importance of continued medical supervision.

Continued

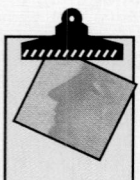

NURSING CARE PLANNING

A CLIENT BEGINNING MEDICATION THERAPY *(continued)*

NURSING CARE PLAN

Nursing Diagnosis	Expected Outcomes	Interventions	Evaluation
Altered health maintenance related to insufficient knowledge of medication therapy, follow-up care, and diet and lifestyle changes to control cardiovascular disease as evidenced by client statements and history	Client verbalizes purpose, actions, and directions for use of all ordered medications.	Give the client information about atenolol, furosemide, and nitroglycerin. Describe purpose and actions using clear and simple terms. Review directions for use of each medication (atenolol at night, furosemide in the morning, nitroglycerin at the first sign of chest pain). Describe handling and storage, especially for nitroglycerin (out of light and away from heat). Outline common side effects of each medication. Give instructions about when to call physician.	States he knows "all about atenolol and furosemide" but has never taken nitroglycerin. Reviews the printed material and asks several questions.
	Client verbalizes the benefits of aerobic exercise to diminish the risk of cardiovascular disease and states intention to begin exercise with physician approval.	Discuss the benefits of aerobic exercise on the heart, and develop a tentative plan for exercise subject to physician approval.	States he and his wife will start walking after the evening meal.
	Client and spouse list foods to be avoided that are high in sodium.	Review foods to avoid those that are naturally high in sodium. Discuss that foods from animal sources (meats, dairy products) are naturally high in sodium because of physiological saline.	Is able to list foods high in sodium but expects compliance to be difficult.
	Client verbalizes the importance of stress management as an adjunct to blood pressure control.	Begin initial teaching about the effects of stress on blood pressure. Develop an initial plan to manage stress effectively to aid in blood pressure reduction. Stress the importance of continued medical supervision, and develop a specific plan for medical follow-up.	Will visit doctor in 1 week. Has his own business and cannot reduce working hours.

Italicized interventions indicate culturally specific care.

Critical Thinking Questions
1. How would you proceed as a follow-up to Mr. Connell's statement that he knows "all about atenolol and furosemide"?
2. Do you have suggestions to help with planning for diet and exercise?

BIBLIOGRAPHY

American Hospital Formulary Service. (1996). *AHFS drug information 96.* Bethesda, MD: American Society of Hospital Pharmacists.

Anonymous. (1995). Medication review: How safe is your patient? *American Journal of Nursing, 95*(10), 44–59.

Ashby, D.A. (1997). Medication calculation skills of the medical-surgical nurse. *MEDSURG Nursing, 6*(2), 90–94.

Bailey, A., Ferguson, E., & Voss, S. (1995). Factors affecting an individual's ability to administer medication. *Home Healthcare Nurse, 13,* 57–63.

Beyea, S., & Nicoll, L. (1996). Back to basics: Administering IM injections the right way. *American Journal of Nursing, 96*(1), 34–35.

Beyea, S., & Nicoll, L. (1995). Administration of medications via the intramuscular route: An integrative review of the literature and research-based protocol for the procedure. *Applied Nursing Research, 8*(1), 23–33.

Cheek, J. (1997). Nurses and the administration of medications: Broadening the focus. *Clinical Nursing Research, 6*(3), 253–274.

*Cohen, M. (1993). Do we still need the apothecary system? *Nursing93, 23*(2), 57.

*Cohen, M., & Senders, J. (1994). 12 ways to prevent medication errors. *American Journal of Nursing, 24*(2), 34–41.

Cook, P.R. (1995). Using critical thinking skills to improve medication administration. *MEDSURG Nursing, 4*(4), 309–313.

Covington, B.P., & Trattler, M.R. (1997). Bull's eye: Finding the right target for IM injections. *Nursing97, 27*(1), 62.

Davis, N. (1995). Preventing omission errors. *American Journal of Nursing, 95*(4), 17.

Dossey, B.M., Keegan, L., Guzzetta, C.E., & Kollmeier, L.G. (1995). *Holistic nursing: A handbook for practice* (2nd ed.). Gaithersburg, MD: Aspen.

Drug information for the health care professional (17th ed.). (1997). Rockville, MD: USP Convention.

Ebersole, P., & Hess, P. (1998). *Toward healthy aging: Human needs and nursing response* (5th ed.). St. Louis: Mosby.

Hussar, D.A. (1995). Helping your patient follow his drug regimen. *Nursing95, 25*(10), 62–64.

Kee, J., & Marshall, S. (1996). *Clinical calculations* (3rd ed.). Philadelphia: W.B. Saunders.

Konick-McMahan, J. (1996). Full speed ahead—with caution. *Nursing96 26*(6), 26–31.

Lehne, R., Moore, L., Crosby, L., & Hamilton, D. (1998). *Pharmacology for nursing care* (3rd ed.). Philadelphia: W.B. Saunders.

Levins, T.T. (1996). Central IV lines: Your role. *Nursing96, 26*(4), 48–49.

Micromedex Healthcare Series: Micromedex, Inc. Engelwood, CO. Vol. 96, exp. 6/98.

Miller, D., & Miller, H. (1995). Giving meds through the tube. *RN, 58*(1), 44–48.

North American Nursing Diagnosis Association. (1999). *Nursing diagnoses: Definitions and classification 1999–2000.* Philadelphia: Author.

Phelan, G., Kramer, E.J., Grieco, A.J., & Glassman, K.S. (1996). Self-administration of medication by patients and family members during hospitalization. *Patient Education and Counseling, 27*(1), 103–112.

Pinnell, N.L. (1996). *Nursing pharmacology.* Philadelphia: W.B. Saunders.

Purnell, L., & Paulanka, B. (1998). *Transcultural health care: A culturally competent approach.* Philadelphia: F.A. Davis.

Rokosky, J.M. (1997). Misuse of metered-dose inhalers: Helping patients get it right. *Home Healthcare Nurse, 15*(1), 13–21.

Schmieding, N.J., & Waldman, R.C. (1997). Nasogastric tube feeding and medication administration: A survey of nursing practices. *Gastroenterology Nursing, 20*(4), 118–124.

Segbefia, I.L., & Mallet, L. (1997). Are your patients taking their medications correctly? *Nursing97, 27*(4), 58–60.

Seifert, C.F., Frye, J.L., Belknap, D.C., & Anderson, D.C. Jr. (1995). A nursing survey to determine the characteristics of medication administration through enteral feeding catheters. *Clinical Nursing Research, 4*(3), 290–305.

Wakefield, D.S., Wakefield, B.J., Uden-Holman, T., & Blegan, M.A. (1996). Perceived barriers in reporting medication administration errors. *Best Practices and Benchmarking in Healthcare, 1*(4), 191–197.

Whitman, M. (1995). The push is on: Delivering medications safely by IV bolus. *Nursing95, 25*(8), 52–54.

Wilson, B., & Shannon, M. (1997). *Dosage calculations: A simplified approach* (3rd ed.). Norwalk, CT: Appleton & Lange.

*Asterisk indicates a classic or definitive work on this subject.

Health Protection: Risk for Infection

Laura Bradford

Key Terms

antibiotic

antibody

antimicrobial

bacterium

differential cell count

Gram's stain

immunization

immunosuppression

infection

inflammatory response

isolation

medical asepsis

nosocomial infection

pathogen

septicemia

standard precautions

virus

LEARNING OBJECTIVES

After studying this chapter, you should be able to:

1. **Discuss the course of an infection, physiological defenses against infection, and chain of infection as they relate to infection control.**

2. **Describe the assessment of a client who has a risk for infection, an actual infection, and responses to infection.**

3. **Identify appropriate nursing diagnoses for a client with either an active infection or an increased risk for infection.**

4. **Plan for goal-directed interventions to prevent or correct the infectious process.**

5. **Identify specific interventions needed to prevent transmission of infection, manage a client with a compromised immune system, and reduce the personal risk of infection.**

6. **Evaluate the outcomes that describe progress toward the goals of health protection nursing care.**

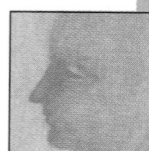

Six-month-old Luisa Martez lives at home with her parents and two siblings. Rosa is 5 years old, and Jose is 2 years old. The Martez family came to the United States from Mexico. Luisa has been developing normally for her age. She has had a runny nose for the last few days but until last night had not seemed ill.

During the night, she began vomiting. This morning, Luisa's mother noticed that Luisa seemed very sleepy and did not wake up at the usual time. Despite repeated attempts, she would not breast-feed. Additionally, her skin felt warm. When her mother took her axillary temperature, the thermometer registered 102° F. Mr. and Mrs. Martez took Luisa to the emergency room of the hospital where she had been born. She was admitted to the children's unit with a diagnosis of dehydration secondary to sepsis. In addition to being frightened, Luisa's parents were confused with the admission process. Her father speaks and understands English, but her mother speaks no English and does not appear to understand any. The nurse therefore makes plans to obtain a translator to facilitate the management of Luisa's illness, recovery, and follow-up after discharge. Because of Luisa's age and symptoms, the nurse considers the nursing diagnoses *Risk for infection* and *Altered protection.* Luisa is at increased

(continued)

risk for infection because she lives with two older siblings and has altered immunity related to her infancy and possible lack of immunizations (see the Nursing Diagnoses chart).

INFECTION NURSING DIAGNOSES

Risk for Infection: The state in which an individual is at increased risk for being invaded by pathogenic organisms.

Altered Protection: The state in which an individual experiences a decrease in the ability to guard self from internal or external threats such as illness or injury.

From North American Nursing Diagnosis Association. (1999). NANDA nursing diagnoses: Definitions and classification 1999–2000. Philadelphia: Author.

CONCEPTS OF INFECTION CONTROL

Nurses have played a major role in preventing infectious diseases since Florence Nightingale demonstrated the effectiveness of nursing care in reducing the infection rate in military hospitals during the Crimean War. Nursing management of infectious diseases encompasses the three levels of prevention. In primary prevention, nurses teach health-promotion strategies to stay well. Primary prevention includes practices in the home and in health care institutions that prevent the spread of infection. In secondary prevention, nurses monitor clients both as individuals and in groups to detect infection early, obtain prompt treatment for infection, and prevent the spread to other members of a group. In tertiary prevention, a nurse helps the client manage the medical interventions (commonly with an **antibiotic,** a drug that kills bacteria) to ensure complete recovery from the infection.

An **infection** is a clinical syndrome caused by the invasion and multiplication of a **pathogen,** a disease-producing microorganism, in body tissues. Pathogens cause local cellular injury through their metabolism, toxins, intracellular replication, or antigen-antibody response. The body responds to the invasion of causative organisms by the formation of antibodies and by a series of physiological changes known as inflammation.

Infections can be either localized or systemic. A localized infection is restricted to a well-defined or limited area of tissue. A systemic infection is one that affects the body as a whole.

Course of Infection

The clinical course of an infection varies with the causative organism, the site of infection, and the overall health status of the infected person. In general, however, the course of an infection can be described in four phases that are important to infection control in many cases.

Phases of an Infection

The *incubation period* extends from the time of a client's exposure to the organism to the appearance of the first symptoms. The length of the incubation period is sometimes helpful in diagnosing the specific causative organism. Childhood illnesses, cold viruses, and flu viruses have predictable incubation periods.

The *prodromal phase* is a period of vague, nonspecific symptoms preceding the full manifestation of the infection. The symptoms may include general malaise, low-grade fever, nausea, weakness, and general aches.

The period of *clinical illness* is the time when the symptoms are fully manifested and most clearly recognized as representing a specific infectious process. The diagnosis is made from a specific cluster of symptoms and sometimes after obtaining cultures to identify the specific organism.

The period of *convalescence* is the time following the height of the acute symptoms to the time the person experiences a return to normal health. It is common for a person recovering from an infection to complain of decreased energy or feeling tired before full recovery from an illness.

Infectious diseases can be spread from one person to another during any phase of the illness. Clients are considered to be contagious, or in a communicable phase of infection, whenever they are able to spread the infection to another person. The phases during which illnesses are communicable are variable and depend on the specific infection. With some infections, the disease may be contagious from the prodromal phase through the convalescent phase.

Socioeconomic Factors Affecting Infection

With the development of antibiotics and immunizations since the middle of the 20th century, health practitioners had hoped that the risk of infectious diseases would become a problem of historic interest only. Nonetheless, infectious diseases are an ongoing health concern.

It is important to develop awareness of clients' susceptibility to infection and be vigilant in developing plans to minimize clients' risk. It is also necessary to understand the bases for altered protection. Public health or community-based nurses, especially, should develop a heightened consciousness of manifestations of infection as well as prevent infection or decrease its spread.

All of us have experienced some sort of infection that caused minor inconvenience, such as a cold or flu virus, that required our own defense systems to overcome it. We have also probably had some sort of infection requiring an antibiotic as an adjunct to treatment. We have most likely used vaccinations to prevent an infection before an actual exposure. Each year, community-acquired infections are thought to be responsible for many school absences and lost dollars through absences from work.

Infectious diseases were once thought to be all but conquered, at least in developed countries such as the United States and Canada. Since the 1970s, however, there has been reemergence of infectious diseases with the threat of increased incidence in the near future. The most well-known of these diseases are AIDS, Ebola virus, drug-resistant tuberculosis, cyclospora, and cholera. A number of factors are thought to contribute to the emergence of new and resistant diseases.

Factors within the social structure of a society can contribute to the spread of disease. One factor is the increasing numbers of persons who are steadily becoming more economically disadvantaged. The growth of large inner-city ghettos, where public and private services are inadequate or lacking, creates conditions for the spread of infection. As the population grows, crowded living conditions become more common. Although it is easy to assume that the risk for infection could be contained in areas where risk is the greatest, a highly mobile population means that the risk can spread rapidly.

Luisa's family is large and shares a relatively small living area with the extended family. What impact would these living conditions have on her risk of infection?

The desire for a world market for goods and services has created a global economy in which individual nations are less isolated from each other. High-speed travel and migration of the world's population have increased the transmission of disease worldwide. Infectious diseases remain the leading cause of death worldwide. As populations intermingle, both evolving and new pathogens spread to produce infectious diseases where they have previously been unknown.

The potential for infectious disease to spread through the food supply is perhaps greater than it was in the recent past. Large agricultural corporations that have not paid enough attention to controls to ensure a safe food supply have come under scrutiny for the methods of mass production of food. The high demand for fresh fruits and vegetables year-round has resulted in an increase in the importation of these food items, often requiring transportation over great distances and handling at multiple points in the distribution system. The Cost of Care chart further discusses costs associated with food-borne illnesses.

At the same time, health policy in the United States has been treatment-driven, with diminishing resources going to public health. The surveillance systems for infectious diseases need to be examined to ensure that the spread of disease can be tracked. Successful early warning procedures can be implemented if reporting procedures and a national system to track infectious diseases is in place.

Infection and Health Care Institutions

The health care system itself is yet another factor in emergent infections. How antibiotics are prescribed by health care providers is a factor in the development of resistant strains of organisms. New procedures and equipment have led to an increasing variety of methods to perform invasive procedures that in turn create new problems in cleaning and sterilizing equipment. Increases in the number of organ transplants have further increased the possibility for transmission of disease. The use of **immunosuppression** therapy, medications to suppress the body's immune system, has increased because these medications are used with transplants and as new treatments for cancer. These medications prevent the transplanted organ from being rejected by the body as foreign but they also limit the ability of the body to fight infection.

The public has a right to expect that the risk for acquiring an infection during hospitalization is minimal; however, controlling infection rates in hospitals is a major problem. Even if infection is not the admitting diagnosis, hospitalized clients are at an increased risk of **nosocomial infection,** an infection acquired in the hospital, that may also be resistant to several antibiotics. It has been estimated that 5% of clients experience nosocomial infections and, of these, 25% are infected by multiple resistant organisms. An average of 4 days is added to the hospital stay for persons with nosocomial infections, costing the health care system over $2 billion annually. Twenty to forty thousand persons die each year from nosocomial infections. Up to 33% of hospital-acquired infections may be preventable.

Defenses Against Infection
Primary Defenses

The human body has a number of refined defenses against infection. The primary defenses include skin and mucous membranes, the respiratory tract, the gastrointestinal (GI) tract, and the circulatory system.

SKIN AND MUCOUS MEMBRANES
The skin and mucous membranes act as a physical barrier to prevent organisms from entering the body

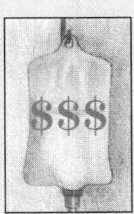

THE COST OF CARE
FOOD-BORNE INFECTIONS

Traditionally, Americans have assumed that foods bought in supermarkets are safe from disease-causing germs. However, newspaper headlines are announcing outbreaks of diarrhea from new forms of bacteria, and we have reached a new awareness of our vulnerability to infections we once relegated to third-world countries.

An incident involving contaminated lettuce was reported in the *New York Times* (January 1998) and indicates the massive extent of the problem. In this single incident, 61 people reportedly became ill and 21 were hospitalized. One of those hospitalized was a 3-year-old who was left with damaged vision despite surgery and 11 weeks in intensive care. The cost of this hospitalization alone was over $500,000, with $100,000 for drugs.

The Centers for Disease Control and Prevention (CDC, 1995) confirms that 400 to 500 food-borne disease outbreaks are reported each year. Although these outbreaks do not all result in hospitalizations, they cause time lost from work or school and they require treatment with antibiotics. These outbreaks can affect massive numbers of people. In 1996, contaminated ice cream sickened 250,000 people throughout the United States.

Discussion

These examples of food contamination demonstrate the high cost of treating just one instance of food contamination. Because of these costs and the debilitating illnesses caused by such outbreaks, the CDC has implemented several strategies involving new surveillance mechanisms and massive public education campaigns. The CDC makes the following recommendations to minimize food-borne diseases:

- Make sure food from animal sources (meat, dairy, eggs) is thoroughly cooked.
- Be careful to keep juices from raw animal foods away from other foods.
- Do not leave potentially contaminated foods at temperatures that permit bacteria to grow. In other words, avoid defrosting foods at room temperature and refrigerate leftovers promptly.

References

Belluck, P., & Drew, C. (1998). Deadly bacteria a new threat to fruit and produce in U.S. *The New York Times,* January 4, 1998.
Centers for Disease Control and Prevention. (CDC, 1995). Food and water borne bacterial diseases. March 1995 update.
Hennessey, T., Hedberg, C., Slutsker, L., White, K., Besser-Wiek, J., & Moen, M. (1996). A national outbreak of Salmonella enteritis infections from ice cream. *New England Journal of Medicine, 334,* 1281–1286.

---

through the intact dermis and epidermis. Though the skin harbors many different kinds of microorganisms, we rarely become infected from these organisms if the skin remains intact. The surface of the skin also offers **antimicrobial** properties, which is the ability to limit the spread of microorganisms. Dryness of the skin promotes desiccation of microorganisms, and the ongoing desquamation of skin cells rids the skin surface of remaining organisms. The skin surface has a low pH that provides additional protection. The low pH is due to fatty acids that occur as a byproduct of lipid conversion of normal skin flora. The mucous membranes of the urinary system, the vagina, airways, and GI tract produce mucus that traps and removes organisms. Mucous membranes also destroy bacteria through the action of macrophages and lysozymes.

RESPIRATORY SYSTEM

The respiratory tract filters and warms the air that we breathe. Hair-like structures called cilia that line the respiratory tract continuously sweep debris up and out of the respiratory tract. Cells lining the respiratory tract secrete lysozymes that can destroy certain bacteria. Macrophages engulf and destroy bacteria found in the alveoli.

GASTROINTESTINAL SYSTEM

The GI tract is a hostile environment for many microorganisms because of the pH extremes of the highly acid stomach and the highly alkaline small intestine. Nonetheless, there are bacterial colonies normally found in the colon that aid digestion and provide needed vitamins. They can also provide resistance to colonization by pathogenic organisms by competing for nutrients and by producing inhibitors in the form of proteins that limit the growth of other, possibly pathogenic, bacteria. Cells lining the digestive tract called goblet cells produce secretions that form barriers, preventing penetration by bacteria. These cells also produce enzymes that lyse or break apart bacterial cell walls.

CIRCULATORY SYSTEM

The circulatory system is essential to the inflammatory and immune response. Blood carries the components of cellular and humoral immunity and removes waste products of tissue destruction from sites of injury.

Secondary Defenses

The immune and inflammatory responses are the second line of defense against infection. The **inflammatory response** is a localized reaction to injury and is activated when there is tissue damage. The immune response is activated in the presence of foreign substances. It has various specific and nonspecific mechanisms to handle invasions of microorganisms. The very complexity of the immune response gives it enormous flexibility and effectiveness.

INFLAMMATORY RESPONSE

The inflammatory response should not be confused with infection. Inflammation can be caused by many physical, chemical, and biological agents that cause damage to tissues. The inflammatory response is the body's way of protecting and healing itself. Its purpose is to remove or destroy the invasive substance, to localize the invading organism, and to repair damage. Any type of traumatic injury including surgery initiates the inflammatory response. Redness, heat, swelling, and pain are the classic signs of an inflammatory response. Many times loss of function is included as an indicator of inflammation. The inflammatory response results from the increased permeability of blood vessels that allows for release of fluid, blood components, and blood cells into the tissue where an injury or infection has occurred.

Local tissue injury releases substances from the damaged cells that cause capillary dilatation and increased capillary permeability. Fluid that contains infection-fighting proteins from the blood then escapes through the walls of the capillaries. These proteins include nonspecific components that fight all infections. Proteins from the complement system can be activated in a series, even in the absence of antibodies. They release factors that attract phagocytic cells that engulf and lyse or destroy the invading microorganism or its toxins. Interferon is another protein released at the site of an infection that is active in fighting viral infections.

Other cells that are present in this fluid-filled space include red blood cells and white blood cells. White blood cells are of various types and have specific roles in fighting infections. Those involved in the nonspecific or innate system include polymorphonuclear leukocytes, macrophages, granulocytes, and null cells.

When the infectious organism or toxin is known to the body's immune system, additional white blood cells, the *B and T lymphocytes*, can be found at the site of infection. The B lymphocytes (B cells) are the cells responsible for production of specific antibodies or immunoglobulins. The T lymphocytes (T cells) are the cells that carry the memory of a specific infectious organism and also are the cells that kill the invading organisms. The B and T cells work together to fight infections that they recognize and, thus, require previous contact with the invading organism.

IMMUNE RESPONSE

Although inflammation is a general protective response, the immune response is specific to the antigen or foreign substance that has invaded the body. The activation of the immune response, therefore, requires that there has been a previous contact with the invading organism or antigen. Immunity is a measure of a person's ability to resist disease through formation of immunoglobulins (antibody cells that destroy antigens), development of immunologically competent cells, or a result of interferon activity in viral infections. The immune system has two closely interrelated components, the humoral and cellular immune responses.

Humoral Immunity

The humoral immune response is the antigen-antibody response that takes place in the body fluids (humors). An **antibody** (immunoglobulin) is a circulating protein that recognizes and destroys foreign invaders. Antibodies are derived from B cells in response to a substance recognized as "not self" (the antigen). Once B cells contact an antigen, in 3 days they divide into immunoglobulins, which are antibody cells that destroy antigens, and memory cells that can recognize a repeated invasion by the antigen. There are five types of immunoglobulins: IgM, IgG, IgA, IgD, and IgE. IgM is the precursor for the other immunoglobulins and is the initial response to a current infection. IgG is the delayed or secondary response and would be present if the person has had an infection in the past.

Cellular Immunity

The cellular components of immunity are derived from T and B cells. About 60 to 70% of the lymphocytes in the circulating blood are T cells. T cells have antigen-specific receptors that bind antigens to their surface. The binding of antigens causes the production of sensitized T cells that travel to the site of inflammation and bind with antigens to release chemicals (lymphokines) that attract macrophages. Because these cells help the B cell recognize an antigen, they are called helper T cells. Suppressor T cells also exist that prevent the reaction to the antigen from becoming an over-reaction or hypersensitivity. A third type of T cell actually kills cells and is most effective against viruses or protozoa.

The cellular immune response and its components provide the bases for medications to provide protection against a specific disease or disease agent. An **immunization** is a medication administered to activate an immune response before exposure to the disease agent. One inherent risk of immunization therapy is that any alteration in the immune response also escalates the possibility of infection.

Chain of Infection

The body's ability to internally protect against infection is limited; therefore, preventing infection requires

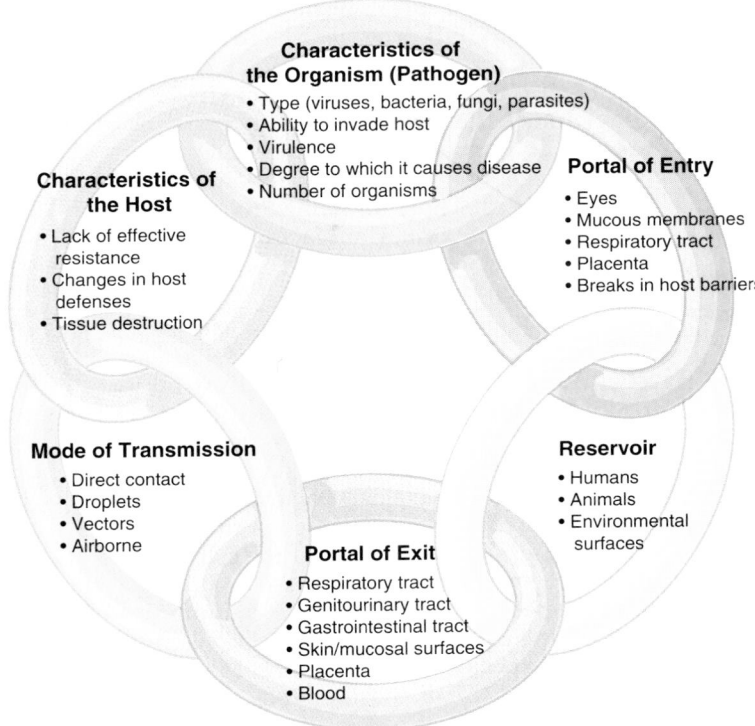

Figure 27–1. Chain of infection.

an understanding of how infectious diseases are transmitted or spread. Thinking of the elements of transmission as links in a chain is a useful, figurative way to understand the interlinking nature of these elements (Fig. 27–1). Infection can be prevented by breaking any link in the chain. The elements are the characteristics of the organism (pathogen), portal of entry, reservoir, portal of exit, mode of transmission, and characteristics of the host (client).

Characteristics of the Organism (Pathogen)

Most microorganisms that populate the internal and external surfaces of healthy people do not normally produce disease. The ability of an organism to cause disease is affected by the type of organism, its ability to invade the host (client), and the level of virulence— the power of an organism to cause disease. The number of organisms also affects their ability to cause infection, as does the susceptibility of the host. Table 27–1 lists common pathogens responsible for nosocomial infections and the usual mode of transmission for each.

TYPE
The types of microorganisms that can cause disease include viruses, bacteria, fungi, and parasites, including protozoans, helminths, and arthropods. A brief discussion of each follows.

Viruses
A **virus** is a tiny microorganism, much smaller than a bacterium, that can only replicate inside the cell of a host such as a human. The virus takes over the metabolism of the cell to make more copies of itself. The cell can then no longer function normally because of the infection. The new viral particles are released slowly through the membrane of the cell. They then continue to infect other cells but do not necessarily kill these cells. The cell remains alive but cannot carry out its normal cellular functions. Some viruses do kill the cell and release large numbers of viral particles with cell lysis. Other viruses have the characteristic of latency, which allows the cell to function normally or with some of its normal functions while the virus has integrated itself into the genetic material of the cell. At this stage of infection, the individual may not appear to be infected. It is only later, after the virus takes over the cell's machinery and begins to replicate, causing cell death, that it is apparent that the organism is infected.

Because the virus uses the host cell to reproduce, any medications used to kill them must be specific for

TABLE 27–1

Common Pathogens in Nosocomial Infections and Usual Mode of Transmission

Pathogen	Mode of Transmission
Staphylococcus	Contact
Antibiotic-resistant *Staphylococcus aureus*	Contact
Pseudomonas	Contact
Escherichia coli	Contact

the virus and not the host's metabolism. Few antiviral drugs exist. One antiviral drug is ribavirin, used against respiratory syncytial virus and some herpes viral infections. Many viral infections are eliminated because of the immune system's specific and nonspecific reactions to infection. Because the immune system "remembers" viral infections, it plays an important role in fighting specific viruses. Thus, immunization against specific viral diseases is an important factor in controlling viral infection.

Bacteria

A **bacterium** is a small, single-celled organism that can reproduce outside of cells. Bacteria cause disease by releasing deadly molecules or toxins, which can kill cells or incapacitate some cellular functions. Some bacteria cause disease by overgrowing and damaging tissues as they grow. Some very small bacteria can only grow inside of cells. They cause diseases in much the same way that viruses do, by taking over the cell's metabolism for their own functions. Again, the body's defense system for specific and nonspecific immune reactions is important in fighting these infections and can be used against specific bacterial toxins. Many antibiotics are developed to kill specific types or strains of bacteria.

Fungi

Fungi can grow as budding yeasts or as filaments when infecting individuals. Like bacteria, they can replicate very rapidly given the right growing conditions. They can also cause disease by overgrowing and damaging tissues as they grow. Unlike bacteria, their cell walls contain the substance chitin that makes them very resistant to destruction by the body's resistant mechanisms. Because their cellular metabolism is similar to ours, antibiotics successful in fighting bacteria do not harm fungi, and antibiotics that can harm fungi can also harm our cells.

Parasites

Multicellular parasites can cause disease by interfering with the nutrition of an organism. They feed off cells and tissues, depriving them of nutrition and causing tissue destruction. This can be life-threatening, depending on where the parasite is lodged and which tissues are destroyed.

VIRULENCE

Virulence is a measure of the aggressiveness of an organism in causing a disease. What sorts of features contribute to virulence? One is how well the organism adheres to the surface to be invaded. Another is the ability to penetrate the skin or mucosal surface to which it adheres. Once the microorganism has invaded the body, its ability to multiply and evade the body's natural defenses also contributes to its virulence. Much of an organism's disease-causing capability and its ability to cause tissue damage is due to the production of enzymes and toxins. Toxins are proteins or complexes of proteins, polysaccharides, and lipids that microorganisms release, causing tissue damage and/or destruction.

Portal of Entry

Organisms can enter a host through the eyes, mucosal membranes (including those of the GI and genitourinary [GU] tracts), respiratory tract, placenta, and any breaks in the host's mechanical or chemical barriers. Controlling the portal of entry involves maintaining the integrity of the protective tissues in the host.

Reservoir

Where do infections come from? A reservoir is a place where the infectious agent can survive and, possibly, multiply until it can invade a susceptible host. Three common reservoirs include humans, animals, and environmental surfaces. Reservoirs inside the hospital include clients, health care personnel and equipment, and the hospital environment. When an individual acquires a nosocomial infection, it is acquired from a reservoir in the hospital.

To grow and multiply, an organism needs a food supply and optimal conditions for growth. Many organisms grow best in a warm, moist, dark environment and need an optimal pH. Some organisms are aerobic (require oxygen); others are anaerobic (do not require oxygen). Common reservoirs in the home are improperly stored food, improperly cleaned counter surfaces where food has been prepared, and wet surfaces in bathrooms. In hospitals, the same general reservoirs are present. Additionally, the materials used to contain wound drainage create reservoirs. Hence, a bandage removed from a draining wound and discarded in a wastebasket is a good medium for the growth of organisms.

Portal of Exit

Organisms can exit a host through the respiratory tract, GU tract, GI tract, skin/mucosal surfaces, the placenta (mother to infant), and blood. Controlling the portal of exit involves management of body fluids and wastes.

Mode of Transmission

Modes of transmission are the mechanisms in which pathogens are transferred from an agent to the host. They include direct contact, droplet, vector, and airborne spread.

DIRECT CONTACT. Contact is a major mode of transmission. This can involve direct contact as in person-to-person spread. Indirect contact also contributes to infection and may involve an intermediate surface or object between the reservoir and the host, such as a dirty instrument.

DROPLET. Droplet transmission occurs when large particles produced by talking, sneezing, or coughing pass through the air from the reservoir to the host.

Droplet transmission occurs only through small distances (3 feet or less).

VECTOR. A vector is a vehicle to transmit infection from a reservoir to a host. One example of a common vector is food. Organisms can multiply in food before infecting the host, such as with *Salmonella*. Other organisms may not multiply in the food but are carried on the food, such as the hepatitis A virus.

An important mode of transmission is via a living vector, such as an insect or other arthropod. Organisms can be transmitted externally on the vector, such as on the legs of flies. Some vectors carry the organism internally, such as the malarial parasites or yellow fever virus in a mosquito.

AIRBORNE. Airborne spread of infections such as measles occurs when the causative organism can remain suspended in air for extended periods of time. The infection is acquired by breathing in the air that contains the organisms.

Characteristics of the Host

Once an organism has exited a reservoir, infection can occur in a susceptible host, a person who lacks effective resistance to the pathogen. Any changes in the natural defenses of the host increase the likelihood of infection by a pathogenic agent. Tissue destruction, either accidental or through medical/surgical intervention, accentuates the possibility of infection. Factors affecting susceptibility to infection are discussed later in this chapter.

ASSESSMENT

Focused Assessment for Risk for Infection and Altered Protection

Several risk factors make a client more susceptible to infection. These include invasive procedures, trauma, some medications, malnutrition, inadequate primary or secondary defenses, and certain chronic diseases. Assess your clients carefully for these and other factors to better anticipate which clients have an increased risk of infection. Assess the environment as well; it too can raise a client's risk.

Characteristics of the Host
PRIMARY DEFENSES
Assess the condition of the skin, respiratory tract, and GI and GU systems as the primary defenses against infection. Assess also for tissue damage and circulatory status. Assess the skin for lesions or breaks in the skin and trauma.

Any breaks in the protective barriers of the skin or membranes surrounding tissues will impair an individual's protection again infection. Trauma can break the skin barrier and may break blood vessels and tear other tissues in the area. This has several immediate results. Any infective organisms that were on the surface of the skin or membranes are now closer to the exposed tissue. The ability for the circulation to pro-

vide oxygen and remove debris is disrupted. Any immune response is also altered secondary to interrupted circulation. Finally, tissue functioning may be hampered or destroyed.

The rupture of amniotic membranes of a pregnant woman often signals the beginning of a welcomed end of pregnancy; however, the fetus now loses this defense against invasion of microorganisms in the immediate environment, including the nonsterile environment of the vagina. Thus, a prolonged break of these membranes before the birth of the child can put the infant at increased risk for infection.

Assess the amount of trauma caused by invasive procedures. The amount of altered protection depends on the amount and position of the trauma. The risk of infection due to a hangnail is considerably less than that due to a gunshot wound to the abdomen. Invasive medical procedures performed by a health care worker also can alter protection. Intravenous lines, especially central venous lines, allow exposure of the circulatory system and tissues surrounding the placement site to infection. Similarly, endotracheal intubation to provide pulmonary support alters a client's risk of infection. The procedure itself can cause trauma to the airway, but there is also altered protection from blockage of the natural mechanisms that clear the airway. Artificial suctioning further increases risk for infection by providing a vehicle for introducing pathogens into the airway. Other procedures that alter protection against infection include insertion of nasogastric tubes, other GI tubes, or urinary catheters; spinal taps; and invasive radiographic examinations. Any surgical procedure alters an individual's protection against infection.

Review the client's history for problems in the GI, respiratory, circulatory, and GU systems that can contribute to infection. Some examples are given in Box 27–1.

Assess the person's nutritional status. Malnutrition resulting from malabsorption of nutrients or poor nutrition reduces the body's ability to protect against infection as well as to repair itself after infection.

What was the impact of Luisa's unwillingness or inability to breast-feed on her hydration and nutrition?

ALTERED IMMUNITY
Review the client's history for problems that are known to alter immunity. Any alteration in the immune response can increase the risk of infection. Immunosuppression can result from any disease process that removes the secondary defenses against infection. *Leukemia* is a term for a group of infections that alter the populations of the infection-fighting white blood cells. *Lymphoma* is a cancer that can affect the lymph system, an important component of the immune response. Chronic diseases that alter the numbers of white blood cells put these people at increased risk for infection. HIV infection reduces the number of T4 cells that can function normally. Diabetes mellitus, especially of the insulin-dependent type, has also been

HOW SELECTED DISEASES AFFECT INFECTION RISK

Crohn's Disease

Crohn's disease is a genetic disease that causes chronic inflammation of the gastrointestinal (GI) tract, putting those with the disease at increased risk for infections of the GI tract. They may require hospitalization and antibiotic treatment for food poisoning, whereas someone else with a normally functioning GI tract who ate the same food would not have become ill. Other examples of chronic illnesses that increase the risk of GI infections are HIV infection and cystic fibrosis.

Cardiovascular Disease

People with cardiovascular disease may have reduced circulation and thus a poor inflammatory response in the extremities. An ingrown toenail can become severely infected, possibly leading to amputation. Diabetes, sickle cell disease, and multiple sclerosis are other chronic diseases that can result in reduced circulation and, hence, increase the risk of infection.

Asthma

Asthmatics can have chronic inflammation of their bronchial passages. Because of this alteration in the airways, what would ordinarily be a minor cold and inconvenience could lead to severe pulmonary pneumonia, requiring hospitalization. Other chronic conditions that can alter the airway and increase the risk of infection include cystic fibrosis, emphysema, smoking, and residual lung disease in premature infants.

associated with abnormal functioning of the immune system. Cirrhosis of the liver or removal of the spleen can also result in reduced functioning of the immune system.

Take a medication history. Pharmaceutical agents can alter the immune system. A common example is corticosteroid administration, which affects the functioning of white blood cells in the immune response and reduces the inflammatory response. This can be a positive effect. For example, these medications can be life-saving by reducing swelling from trauma or from allergic reactions in the airway. At the same time, however, these medications also have some negative consequences. For example, persons on corticosteroid therapy for chronic diseases such as arthritis, asthma, inflammatory bowel disease, or multiple sclerosis may experience alleviation of disease symptoms but also

do not have an inflammatory response to infection. Corticosteroids also decrease the delayed hypersensitivity response of the immune system that involves T-cell activity. Furthermore, any antibiotics used to fight infection can themselves increase the risk of infection through their effects on white blood cells and the bone marrow.

Chemotherapeutic drugs used successfully to treat some forms of cancer can attack the white cells or the bone marrow, the site of production for many of the cells in the immune system. Many chemotherapeutic drugs inhibit bone marrow activity, impairing proliferation of cells involved in the immune response. As a result, the client receiving chemotherapy will have reduced protective mechanisms and increased risk of infection due to a decrease in the number of cells that can respond to infection.

An immunosuppressed person is not only at increased risk for infection but, because of the immunosuppression, may not present with the typical signs and symptoms of infection. Increased vigilance is needed to reduce the risk of infection and to observe for signs of infection in these persons.

Finally, review the client's recent history of medical therapies. Radiation therapy, another successful treatment for cancer, can alter primary defense systems against infection, causing immunosuppression.

HEALTH PRACTICES

Assess a client's health practices for factors that contribute to the risk of infection. Contributing factors to clients with the diagnosis *Risk for infection* include contacts with infectious organisms, the environment, and personal health practices. Health practices that increase risk of infection include personal hygienic practices. Young children may not take the time or know the importance of washing their hands. Persons with impaired mental capabilities or physical limitations may not have optimal personal hygiene because of their knowledge base or physical inability to actually bathe, wash hands, and maintain a clean environment that does not promote growth of microorganisms.

What are the implications of the presence of other young children in Luisa's family on her risk of infection?

AGE

The client's age should be considered a factor in assessing the client as a susceptible host. An individual's level of immunity is age-related. A newborn infant has no antibodies of its own at the time of birth. Maternal antibodies that have crossed the placenta are the only defenses against infection at the time of birth. The infant, if breast-feeding, continues to receive antibodies from its mother in breast milk. The protective antibodies received from the mother before birth drop rapidly in the newborn period and are almost gone by 4 months of age. The infant begins to make its own antibodies but does not begin to approach adult levels until about age 2. These levels continue to rise gradually over the first 10 years of life.

The unborn fetus has multiple means to guard against infection. Although the immune response is not well developed until after birth, the mother's immunoglobulins cross the placenta and provide protection for the fetus. The placenta acts as a physical barrier between the maternal and fetal circulation. The amniotic sac that contains the fetus is an effective physical barrier to infective organisms. It is normal for the amniotic membrane to rupture at the time of delivery; however, once rupture occurs, the fetus is at increased risk for infection. If the amniotic membranes rupture more the 24 hours before delivery, there is altered protection and the fetus is at risk for infection.

After the age of 65, clients lose some of their infection-fighting abilities. Normal age-related changes can alter the protection of those over 65 years of age. The skin becomes more friable, losing some connective tissue layers, and experiences changes in the protective oils and layers of outer skin cells. Some older adults also have reduced mobility that can make minor infections more severe. For example, an upper respiratory infection can rapidly lead to pneumonia. These persons may be at increased risk for trauma due to decreased stimulus response times or to changes in the musculoskeletal system. Older persons are at higher risk for falls. Failing eyesight can also be a contributing factor. Mental changes can further contribute to altered protection. The ability to provide for personal hygiene and maintain a clean environment can become impaired, altering their protection and leading to an increased risk of infection.

HEREDITY

Heredity can play a role in *Altered protection.* Hereditary diseases may be part of the medical history; however, sometimes it is pertinent to ask about family history. Clients that lack critical components of the immune response are unable to destroy invading organisms that do not cause disease in those with normally functioning immune systems. For example, hypogammaglobulinemia is a genetic disorder that results in absent B cells, causing loss of protection against invasion by bacteria, viruses, and parasites. Clients with thymic hypoplasia (DiGeorge's syndrome) lack T cells, the main line of defense against tumors and reinfection by microorganisms. People with combined B- and T-cell deficiencies have no defense against any type of infection or tumors.

IMMUNIZATIONS

Ask about immunizations that are appropriate to the client's situation. Much of modern success in fighting infections is due to the development of immunizations that protect against a specific agent or toxin. Some common examples of immunizations include measles, mumps, rubella, polio, pertussis, hepatitis B, influenza, diphtheria, tetanus, and meningococcal vaccines. Individuals, particularly young children or older adults, who have not acquired protection with these vaccines have less resistance to infection compared with those who have received them. According to the American Academy of Pediatrics, immunizations should begin in the newborn period, with a second round occurring at 2 months of age.

If Luisa has not begun her immunizations, she would be at risk compared with infants her age who have started their immunizations.

Certain cancers can alter protection for their hosts. Persons with myeloma have defects in humoral immunity, resulting in deficiencies of antibodies. Other malignancies have an impact on cell-mediated immunity. Hodgkin's disease is an example of a malignancy that alters the ability to fight intracellular infections (including viruses and those bacteria that invade cells).

IMMUNE STATUS

Clients who are immunocompromised are more likely to experience opportunistic infections, which are those that result from overgrowth of organisms that do not normally cause disease. An example is disease from organisms that are normally present on the skin or mucosal membranes of the body. Although they generally do not cause disease and may even have protective capabilities, they can cause disease if they can reproduce in large numbers or establish colonies in tissues where they are not normally found. A reduced immune response can alter the client's protective system so that these normally nonpathogenic organisms can reproduce and cause disease.

PRESENCE OF CONGENITALLY ACQUIRED CONDITIONS

Review the history for congenitally acquired conditions. Any disease that alters the nutritional status increases the risk for infection. Physical defects present at birth can alter many of the defenses against infection. Lung disease in premature infants puts them at risk for pneumonia. Infants with cardiac defects have circulatory changes that impair their ability to deliver oxygen to tissues and remove debris and waste products, altering the tissue's ability to prevent infection. Anomalies such as spinal defects that expose internal tissues alter the protection of these tissues from possible infection.

PRESENCE OF ACQUIRED CONDITIONS

Acquired infections can alter the immune system's response to infection. These infections alter the cell-mediated immune response. Viral infections associated with decreased cell-mediated immunity include measles, mumps, varicella, influenza, Epstein-Barr virus, and rubella. Bacterial and fungal infections include tuberculosis, leprosy, syphilis, coccidiomycosis, histoplasmosis, and blastomycosis. HIV destroys the cells active in fighting infections and tumors of the immune system.

PRESENCE OF MENTAL ILLNESS

People with mental health problems may have increased risk for infection if they lack the ability or judgment to protect themselves from infection. Decreased ability to recognize or respond to illness alters their protection. Persons with dementia may be unable to protect themselves from infection. Their inability to maintain nutrition or a safe environment puts them at increased risk.

Characteristics of the Environment

Characteristics of the environment can raise the risk of infection as well and deserve careful assessment.

COMMUNITY

For clients in the community, assess the home and community environment for risk factors. Some clients are at increased risk because of contacts with infectious organisms. Visitors to foreign countries come into contact with microorganisms that are not a significant health concern in the United States. Persons living in milder climates of the United States are more at risk for mosquito vector-borne diseases. Lifestyles can put people at increased risk for some infections. IV drug abusers are at increased risk for the blood-borne infections of HIV and hepatitis B and C. People with multiple sexual contacts are at risk for sexually transmitted diseases. Homeless persons are at increased risks for airborne infections such as tuberculosis because of crowded conditions in shelters.

Environmental factors that contribute to increased risk of infection can include overcrowded living conditions, which can lead to increased contact with individuals who may have an infection. Environments that harbor pests, such as rats or roaches, raise the risk of infection because the pests harbor infectious agents. Lack of screens in mild weather can lead to increased infections caused by mosquitoes or flies.

HEALTH CARE INSTITUTIONS

Assess the health care institution's environment for risk factors. More stringent rules of cleanliness and sanitation are needed in a hospital environment because the clients as a group are at high risk for infection. Hospitalized clients may have weakened defenses to infection due to illness. They also are in close proximity to other persons who harbor infectious agents. In addition to multiple individual risk factors, hospitalized clients come into contact with antibiotic-resistant organisms not present in other places and may undergo multiple invasive procedures.

Assessing the hospital environment includes being aware of the infections that are currently present in the hospital. When a hospital has an increased incidence of nosocomial infections, especially those caused by resistant organisms, efforts at infection control should be reviewed and refined to eliminate the spread of these organisms. An example would be an outbreak of *Clostridium difficile* on a nursing unit. The department responsible for infection control may be consulted to review individual client cases and make recommendations for control on that specific nursing unit.

Focused Assessment for Infection

Localized Infection

The clinical appearance of a localized or contained infection has the four basic components of *redness* (erythema), *swelling* (edema), *pain,* and *heat.* Many times a fifth component, *loss of function,* also is present. This response occurs whether or not the body has experienced this type of infection previously. After an initial decrease of circulation to an infected area, increased permeability of blood vessel (vascular) walls allows a flow of fluid and cells into the affected tissue to aid in fighting the infection. The presence of fluid and red blood cells causes the redness, edema, and increased temperature common at the site of infection. White blood cells result in the formation of pus. These are familiar signs of infection found on the surface of the skin.

Systemic Infection

Systemic infections, those that progress to involve more than one organ system, are more difficult to treat and generally result in poorer outcomes. These infections can result from lack of treatment of a localized infection. Clients who are at increased risk for infection with decreased primary defenses or inadequate secondary defenses may experience a systemic infection.

Systemic infections are manifested by signs and symptoms that affect the entire body. These signs and symptoms define a clinical syndrome that determines the diagnosis of infection. Clients with these infections frequently can present with a general malaise, fever, myalgia, arthralgia, and nonspecific GI symptoms. Fever, though common with infections, may not always be present. If unrecognized, systemic infections can lead to dehydration, acidosis, septic shock, and possibly death within a short period.

What symptoms did Luisa exhibit that might indicate the presence of systemic infection?

Note pain of any kind: head, chest, abdominal, or in the extremities. Frequently, infants pull or rub the affected ear with acute otitis media. Increased secretions from the nose or abnormal breath sounds indicate the possibility of respiratory infection. *Luisa had a runny nose.* The GI signs and symptoms of general nausea, vomiting, abdominal cramping, and diarrhea could be additional signs of systemic infection. **Septicemia,** or infection in the bloodstream, may be accompanied by nonspecific client complaints, such as tiredness and fever, but can also include chills, sweats, myalgia, and arthralgia. Central nervous system infections can present with general malaise and fever but can also include headache and/or stiff neck. Urinary frequency, urgency, and dysuria can be presenting symptoms of a urinary tract infection, but there can also be no symptoms at all. Fever is not usually a symptom in such an infection and, if present, along with flank pain, chills, and sweats, probably indicates that pyelonephritis has developed.

Vaginal or other genital organ infections frequently cause symptoms but can result in severe infections involving the uterus and ovaries. These can lead to pelvic inflammatory disease, which can result in problems with fertility and child-bearing. Abnormal discharges (changes in color, consistency, odor), itching, and pain with intercourse can be signs of vaginal infection.

Symptoms in Immunocompromised Clients

A client who is *immunocompromised* may present with a modified clinical picture of infection. The easy-to-recognize initial symptoms of infection such as redness, swelling, heat, pain, and decreased movement can be absent in the immunocompromised client. This lack of response can delay the client's recognition of infection and, in turn, timeliness in seeking treatment. This may lead to more serious infection as well as a spread of infection from the initial site to other tissues.

Assess all clients for risk of infection, and include three major areas in your assessment. First, obtain a history and physical examination, including questions about the characteristics of the host that contribute to the person's vulnerability to infection. Second, obtain information about exposure to infection, the type of organisms to which the individual is exposed, or the characteristics of the agent of infection. This could involve ascertaining the signs of infection in other family members. Finally, examine the environment for factors that contribute to the spread of infection. This might involve questions related to the type of housing a family has.

What questions would you ask Luisa's parents to assess her risk of infection prior to the present illness?

Diagnostic Tests

Blood Cell Count

Because blood cells are important components of the immune system, a blood sample can be useful in determining whether your client has an infection or, perhaps, is at increased risk for infection. The hemoglobin and hematocrit are red blood cell measurements important for cell nutrition and repair, whereas the white blood cell count reflects the ability to fight actual infections.

HEMOGLOBIN AND HEMATOCRIT

Hemoglobin and hematocrit are measurements of the size and number of red blood cells. A decreased number or size of red blood cells would indicate anemia or blood loss. As a reflection of nutritional status and thus overall health, anemia helps define the risk for infection. Certain genetic diseases or infections can al-ter the numbers or form of red blood cells, increasing the risk of infection.

WHITE BLOOD CELL COUNT

The total white blood cell count reflects the body's response to infections. An increase in the number of white blood cells may mean active infection. A decrease in the number of white blood cells from normal indicates a reduction in infection-fighting ability. An individual's risk for infection increases proportionately with the decrease in the number of white blood cells. The cause of a decreased cell count sometimes is due to active infection. Some viral infections, specifically HIV, and some cancers cause decreases in the white blood cell count.

When evaluating a white blood cell count, look at what is called the "differential" of the white cells. The **differential cell count** breaks down the number of white cells into their different types. These include neutrophils, eosinophils, basophils, lymphocytes, and monocytes (Table 27–2). The largest group of cells are the mature or segmented neutrophils. Immature or nonfilamented neutrophils are called bands. A left shift, which is an increased number of immature neutrophils, is a possible indication of infection.

Other diagnostic tests can measure the function of the immune system. Immunoglobulin levels can be used to evaluate the integrity of the humoral immune system or B-cell function. Delayed hypersensitivity tests (skin tests) are used to test T-cell function. It is also possible to quantitatively analyze B cells and T cells, but these tests are not routinely available.

TABLE 27–2

Interpreting a Differential White Blood Cell (WBC) Count

Cell Type	Percentage of 100 Counted WBCs	Usual Reason for Increase
Neutrophil	32 to 62	Acute infections, especially localized cocci infections, such as tonsillitis or otitis media
Lymphocyte	31	Certain acute viral infections with early increase; chronic infections
Basophil	6	Infrequently increased; when elevated, most often associated with myeloproliferative disorders
Eosinophil	2.2	Allergic reactions and drug reactions
Monocyte	0 to 4	Certain bacteria, such as brucellosis, tuberculosis; protozoa, rickettsiae

Culture and Sensitivity

By determining the actual organism causing an infection, the treatment plan can be specific to the infecting organism. For this reason, cultures are an important diagnostic test. A culture of microorganisms can be grown from samples taken from a site of obvious infection such as pus draining from a wound. They can also be performed on bodily fluids that may or may not have obvious signs of infection. For example, lung secretions of an intubated client exhibiting signs of infection can be sent for culture, even if there is no obvious change in secretions. If the site of infection is not apparent in a hospitalized client, samples from various sites can be sent for culture. These can include pulmonary secretions, spinal fluid, and blood cultures. If the client has a surgical incision, a swab of the surgical site might be done even if no change in drainage is noted. Because urinary tract infections are common in the hospitalized client, urine might also be sent for culture.

Culturing of bacteria requires growing the bacteria on a medium that supports the growth. Usually within 3 to 5 days, and many times sooner, there will be enough organisms to identify the specific species of bacteria that is causing the infection. The growing bacteria can then be exposed to different antibiotics to determine which one will be most effective in fighting the infection. This is called a sensitivity test and is needed to determine the organism's resistance to a medication. Resistance is the ability of a microorganism to make genetic changes in response to environmental pressures, such as medications. Because microorganisms reproduce rapidly, they have the ability when resistant to cause new diseases, remain alive during drug treatment, or cause disease in atypical locations of the body. The sensitivity test, then, is a very important tool for telling us which medications will or will not kill the microorganism being cultured.

Various terms are used to describe drug treatment for microorganisms that are cultured. The term *antimicrobial* is a broad term and generally refers to the ability to limit the spread of microorganisms. This term, then, can also apply to soaps and other chemicals as well as medications. The term *antibiotic* typically refers to a drug that is able to kill a bacterial pathogen. Antiviral drugs are used to treat viral infections. Antifungal agents are used to treat fungal infections.

Gram's Stain

The **Gram stain** is a specific microscopic test used to obtain rapid results on a culture sent to the laboratory. Though the Gram stain specifically tests the nature of the bacterial cell walls, it can also indicate the presence of cell types, such as epithelial cells and/or polymorphonuclear leukocytes. The Gram stain divides bacteria into two basic groups based on whether the cell walls take up the stain (gram-positive) or whether they do not (gram-negative). The shape and arrangement of the bacteria are also indicated by this test. Shapes can be round (cocci), rod-like (bacilli), or spiral (spirochetes). Furthermore, the arrangement can be single, in pairs (diplococci), in chains (*Streptococcus*), clusters (*Staphylococcus*), or tetrads (*Sarcina*). This test can quickly give direction for treatment with antibiotics and determine whether any isolation procedures are recommended.

Though the Gram stain can indicate whether the infection is bacterial and narrows the number of causative organisms, culture and sensitivity testing will give a clearer indication of the most effective antimicrobial therapy. Gram's stain and sensitivity tests are useful for bacterial infections. Viral cultures are more difficult because viruses must be grown inside of cells, not just on culture media. Many times, if a virus is suspected to be the cause of an infection, the culture is sent for antibody testing and not for culturing. The presence of the viral antibody can be determined relatively rapidly, and therapy can then be started. Advances in capabilities for growing and identifying viruses may make viral culturing more commonplace in the future.

The presence of fungi can often be determined from the Gram stain if the laboratory is specifically looking for it; however, fungi grow under much different conditions in the laboratory. If a fungal infection is suspected, the sample for culture should be collected and placed in a special growth medium at the time the specimen is obtained.

In clients with an intact immune system, the inflammatory response and a complete white blood cell count are effective indicators of infection. In immunocompromised clients, however, the culture is a key element in determining whether an infection is present and in determining treatment.

Focused Assessment for Related Nursing Diagnoses

Individuals can and often do respond differently to the same medical diagnosis. The type of response can determine the outcomes for the client in terms of both a willingness to undergo treatment and the actual response to that treatment. It is important to assess the client's and family's response to the diagnosis. This response will form the basis for formulating nursing diagnoses and planning appropriate interventions. A client's culture can significantly influence the response to diagnosis and treatment as well, as suggested in the Cross-Cultural Care chart.

Altered Health Maintenance

Assess the person's health practices that are helpful in preventing the recurrence of a previous illness. A person's previous experience helps shape his or her attitude toward health maintenance. If a previous illness did little to interfere with life or caused minimal discomfort, the client may be unwilling to undertake

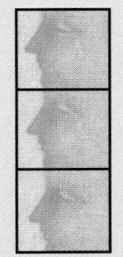

CROSS-CULTURAL CHART
CARING FOR A MEXICAN-AMERICAN CLIENT

Luisa's father came to the United States 6 years ago to find employment and lived with his brother's family for 6 months until he could send for his wife in Mexico. He is employed in a local factory, and his entire family continues to live with his brother and his family. In Mr. Martez's culture, it is not unusual for extended families to continue to live together, and this arrangement is not based on financial need.

The family's confusion with the admission process was due to lack of understanding about the infant's medical diagnosis and because of differing health practices of many Mexican-Americans. They believe that illness results from imbalance or disharmony that could be due to natural or supernatural powers. They are accustomed to using folk treatments. They may have some belief that Luisa's illness is due to the evil eye, which would require the person who gave the evil eye to touch Luisa to remove it. Luisa's extreme dehydration at the time of admission was probably due to the parents' attempt at home remedies and consultation with other family members and possibly a folk practitioner before seeking medical assistance.

Luisa's mother and father stay with Luisa throughout her hospitalization. Other family members care for their other children. Her mother is devoted to her care and follows the agreed-upon plan. The father blames the mother for Luisa's illness but supports the mother because she cares for Luisa. He is not directly involved with Luisa's care but is playful and affectionate when Luisa improves.

Luisa improves dramatically with intravenous hydration and antibiotic therapy. Her mother seems content to be able to breast-feed again. Because of their sense of not having control over their environment, adherence to an immunization schedule begun during this hospitalization will require family- and community-based support. Although every client is unique, Mexican-American clients, like those in Luisa's family, tend to

- Be tactile, communicating with touch and preferring a close personal space during interview.
- Believe in the evil eye, and in the ability of touch to dispel the devil.

- Accept pain as an expected and necessary part of life.
- Use the family as the major support system, and view the family as more important than the individual.
- View relationships with children as being more important than the marital relationship.
- Exhibit male dominance and demand allegiance from wife and children.
- Exhibit female submissiveness to husbands and devotion to children.
- Be honest and dignified.
- Be focused on relationships rather than tasks.
- Have a present-time orientation.
- Seek a harmonious relationship between social and spiritual realms.

Let's see how Luisa's nurse demonstrates cultural sensitivity to Luisa's mother:

Nurse (through translator): Your baby is very sick.

Mother (in Spanish): I'm scared.

Nurse: She doesn't have enough fluid in body. We will give her some fluid through this needle *[points to IV site].* It will make her better.

Mother: [Nods]

Nurse: You can hold her and nurse her. Here—sit in this chair and I'll help you.

Critical Thinking Questions

- What would you say to the mother if the baby is unable to nurse?
- Is this nurse being sensitive to the mother's culture? What else could she do?
- Would you use this time to teach the mother about the advisability of alternative health practices? Why or why not?

Reference

Based on information from Lassiter, S.M. (1995). *Multicultural clients: A professional handbook for health care providers and social workers.* Westport: Greenwood Press.

health maintenance practices to prevent a recurrence. If, however, the previous illness was perceived to cause extreme distress or was life-threatening, the client might take major steps to maintain health and prevent a recurrence.

Luisa's siblings had upper-respiratory infections in infancy, but they never experienced ear infections or other secondary infections. How might this family history have had an impact on the parents' response to Luisa's initial cold symptoms?

Anxiety

Assess for concerns about the risk of infection that may produce anxiety. Concerns about emerging infections and hospital-acquired infection have been publicized and may result in undue alarm. Clients whose immunity is suppressed from an illness or medical therapy need information about commonsense ways to protect themselves. Although a state of unease can accompany the diagnosis of *Risk for infection,* the knowledge of having a condition that can increase the risk of infection can add to the state of unease. The increased state of anxiety itself can reduce one's protection against infection.

Many practitioners in the health care industry believe that there is a mind/body connection that influences health and disease states. This can be a positive factor in the healing process, but it can also be detrimental in determining the outcome for an illness. Thus, clients with increased anxiety might need assistance in dealing with their unease. Different persons with the same diagnosis may behave differently—that is, some may verbalize their anxiety while others appear to have none. Interestingly, these individuals may have similar levels of anxiety. Fully evaluate your clients for anxiety beyond what their initial presentation suggests.

Fear

Fear of a diagnosis can be reality-based but also can be greater than is warranted in a particular situation. Evaluate client fears and provide a climate in which the client feels comfortable in verbalizing them. Knowledge of a particular diagnosis and usual outcomes are helpful in allaying fear of the unknown. At times, you must simply acknowledge your client's fears as being true and feel comfortable in assisting them and their families to access coping mechanisms to assist them through the illness. Your ability to assess the level of fear and help the client cope can help determine the client's outcome. Again, the mind/body connection can be very significant in the healing process.

What factors might put the Martez family at risk for fear?

Impaired Social Interaction

A person's support system is important. Many times the diagnoses of *Risk for infection* and *Altered protection* for infection require a support system in order for clients to carry out activities of daily living. Without support of friends and/or family, an infection may develop needlessly into a life-threatening situation. Homeless persons in whom active tuberculosis has been diagnosed and who are unable or unwilling to seek therapy not only endanger their own health but also that of those with whom they come in contact. Clients living alone who are unable to seek medical attention and have no one they can call for help lack a system of support not only for seeking care but also for treatment.

Assess for impaired social interaction in your initial assessment. If you determine that the client may have an impaired social situation, work with other members of the health care team such as social services to access community-based support systems for these clients.

Situational Low Self-Esteem

Self-esteem is another component of a client's mental health that plays a role in determining outcomes for the individual. Low self-esteem can be influenced by society's response to a particular illness. A diagnosis of HIV infection can carry judgment from many in society, despite public campaigns designed to eliminate these prejudices. The client, as a part of society, requires support from you to maintain a positive sense of self-worth. The infection may not even be one that is necessarily sexually transmitted (e.g., HIV can also be acquired by other means). An adult may contract chicken pox and undergo ridicule from others for having a childhood disease. Even though these examples differ in many respects, the client can have situational low self-esteem in both cases. Because this could interfere with client outcomes, it is important to assess for low self-esteem and work with the client to alleviate or eliminate it. Low self-esteem can hinder a client's healing process.

DIAGNOSIS

When a client presents with an infection, with increased risk for infection, or with altered protection against infection, evaluate the client based on a health history and physical examination that includes any sign of inflammatory response. If the risk factors are present without signs of infection, write the diagnosis as *Risk for infection related to . . . .* If the client has altered protection due to physical causes of tissue damage or to altered immune response, write the diagnosis as *Altered protection for infection related to . . . .* An active infection puts the client at increased risk for further infection. Some infections that alter the immune system of the client, such as HIV, actually result in altered protection. As another example, infants in a day care center are at increased risk for infection because of the frequent exposure to many children. If those infants have not been immunized as recommended by the American Academy of Pediatrics, they have altered protection compared with the infants with proper immunization history. The data clustering chart gives examples of client data with appropriate nursing diagnoses.

Write nursing diagnoses appropriate to the stage of the client's illness and the focus of care. Persons in whom HIV infection is initially diagnosed may need counseling about how to effectively communicate with their partners and may not need interventions based on altered health protection at this time. The focus of care for persons with HIV admitted to the hospital for *Pneumocystis carinii* pneumonia would initially be improved oxygenation. With recovery, though, the focus of care could shift to that of *Altered protection*. Be aware, though, that although the focus of care differs, some of the specific interventions may be similar.

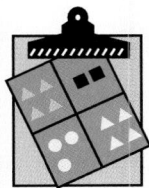

CLUSTERING DATA TO MAKE A NURSING DIAGNOSIS
HEALTH PROTECTION PROBLEMS

Data Cluster	Diagnosis
Client presents with pain, redness, swelling on leg injured during previous week. He is 86 years old and has diabetes.	*Risk for infection* secondary to poor wound healing.
60-year-old client, living by himself, is readmitted for antibiotic treatment for infected surgical incision. He lacks knowledge of wound care.	*Altered health maintenance* related to need to manage wound care.
2-year-old admitted for dehydration refusing PO foods, fluids on day 2 of hospitalization. Parents not visiting.	*Altered health maintenance* related to fear and lack of social support.
Infant at first well-baby visit 6 weeks after delivery. Infant has normal axillary temperature, respirations 40, and heart rate 100. Appears fussy in mother's arms. Mother expresses concern about the infant receiving immunization.	*Risk for infection* related to age and mother's lack of knowledge regarding immunizations.
40-year-old female receiving chemotherapy for cancer of the uterus. White blood cell count 500. Complaining of vaginal dryness and itching.	*Risk for infection* related to decreased WBC and altered vaginal mucous membranes.
25-year-old male with AIDS. Critically low T-cell count. Rents a room with no cooking facilities. Weight loss 30 pounds.	*Altered protection* related to decreased immunity and inadequate nutrition.

PLANNING

Expected Outcomes for the Client With Risk for Infection

The goal of care for the client at risk for infection is to prevent that client from getting an infection. To achieve this goal you must work to reduce risk factors. The expected outcomes are based on primary and secondary prevention strategies (i.e., elimination of those risk factors and early recognition and treatment). Sample client outcomes for the nursing diagnosis *Risk for infection* include the following. The client will

- Have intact skin and mucous membranes.
- Have containment of any infection after the initial diagnosis.
- Verbalize knowledge of measures to avoid infection.
- Avoid exposure to organisms causing nosocomial infection.
- Verbalize early signs of infection and seek appropriate treatment.
- Demonstrate no signs or symptoms of infection secondary to medical or nursing procedures.

Expected Outcomes for the Client With Altered Protection

The goal of care for the client with the diagnosis *Altered protection* is that the client will have increased ability to guard the self from internal or external threats such as illness or injury. The expected outcomes depend on the specific threat, but may include the following:

The client will

- Verbalize knowledge of how to protect the self from infection (if immunocompromised).
- Verbalize knowledge to protect the self from damage to tissue (if anticoagulated).
- Remain free of infection or injury.
- Verbalize knowledge of wound management (open wounds due to trauma or surgery).
- Show evidence of wound healing without experiencing an infection.
- Reduce the risk factors to minimize the risk of infection.
- Be able to identify an infection in its early stages when it can be treated minimally before the infection may become life-threatening.

Other goals may be formulated, knowing that it is more desirable to treat an infection with oral antibiotics (when able) rather than IV antibiotics and to treat clients at home rather than in the hospital. At times, however, clients with infections cannot be treated in the home setting. A plan of care is then developed to meet the client's needs during hospitalization.

INTERVENTION

Interventions to Prevent Transmission of Infection

Interventions to prevent the transmission of infection are discussed in two categories: hospital infection control and infection control in the home. Infection control measures used in the hospital include medical asepsis, standard precautions, and isolation precautions. The basis of infection control includes maximizing the client's primary defenses against infection by minimizing damage to the skin, respiratory tract, and GI tract. Reducing the number of pathogenic organisms in the environment also provides a more sanitary environment. Proper hand-washing is considered the single most effective way to stop the spread of microorganisms between individuals. To prevent the spread of airborne organisms, a well-ventilated environment is essential.

Implementing Medical Asepsis

Medical asepsis consists of practices designed to reduce the numbers of pathogenic microorganisms in the client's environment. The desired result is to prevent or reduce the transmission of the microorganisms from one person to another.

HAND-WASHING

The first line of defense in medical asepsis is hand-washing. For routine care situations, soap should be used. Friction or rubbing increases the amount of soil and microorganisms removed. When washing hands, wash from areas of clean to less clean. The accompanying procedure describes the correct method for hand-washing using principles of medical asepsis.

Action Alert!
The first line of defense in medical asepsis is hand-washing.

ENVIRONMENTAL CONTROLS

Minimizing the spread of infection requires the use of appropriate environmental precautions. Routine cleaning of the environment should be done daily. Any spills, especially those involving infectious materials, should be cleaned immediately to avoid spreading the infectious organisms. The use of clean materials and antimicrobial soaps for daily cleaning and cleaning between clients is important to reduce the spread of infection.

The housekeeping or environmental services department is responsible for cleaning client rooms, bathrooms, halls, waiting rooms, utility rooms, and the nurse's station. Daily cleaning of the client's room includes removing trash, wiping sinks and countertop with disinfectants, using disinfectants in the bathroom, and sweeping or vacuuming the floor. Disinfectants remove most microorganisms from surfaces, which are then considered clean. They do not prevent microorganisms from returning to these surfaces.

Nursing personnel help the client keep the room clean. The sink and bathroom are generally considered to be dirty areas. When using the sink, consider that it has been used for washing dirty hands and disposing of dirty bath water. Clean objects that come in contact with the client should not touch dirty surfaces. The bedside table and overbed table should be clean areas. It is inappropriate to place urinals, bedpans, and even potted plants on a surface that will be used for eating or storing eye glasses, hearing aids, and dentures.

For even more stringent control of microorganisms, various disinfection and sterilization methods can be used. Disinfection removes microorganisms sensitive to the disinfectant used. It does not limit reintroduction of microorganisms to the surface. Sterilization means to remove all microorganisms. The surface can be easily contaminated, however, by contact with an unsterile surface, equipment, or air currents. Table 27–3 outlines the use and limitations of various methods used to control or eliminate the growth of microbes.

TABLE 27–3
Disinfection and Sterilization Methods

Method	Use	Limitations
Steam	Kills microorganisms sensitive to heat and moisture	• Some bacterial spores seem resistant to this treatment. • Some equipment cannot withstand the high temperatures and moisture.
Gas (ethylene oxide)	Kills microorganisms on products that cannot be steam-sterilized	• Articles must be allowed to release gas by aeration before use. • Cannot use to sterilize liquids, which would absorb gas. • Is expensive and time-consuming (2 to 5 hours).
Radiation Ultraviolet light	Kills microorganisms Sensitizes microorganisms to other treatments	• Many spores are resistant, although equipment is not damaged. • May have to be used with other methods to kill additional microorganisms but does not damage equipment.

PROCEDURE 27–1

Hand-Washing

TIME TO
ALLOW
▼
Novice:
2 min.
Expert:
2 min.

Hand-washing is one of the most important ways to prevent transmission of infectious organisms. Make sure you wash your hands properly before and after contact with each client.

Delegation Guidelines

All staff members are expected to comply with proper hand-washing technique and adherence to universal precautions. Nursing assistants should follow this hand-washing procedure prior to and following any client contact.

Equipment Needed

- Sink with running water.
- Soap.
- Towel.
- Prepackaged cleansing sponge with cuticle stick, if needed.

1 Turn on the faucet so that warm water is running.

A sink operated by knee or foot pedal is preferable because your hands do not have to contact the sink surface. Warm water leaves more protective skin oils in place than hot water and is less chafing to the skin over time, when frequent hand-washings are done.

2 Wet your hands and lower arms under running water while holding your hands lower than your elbows.

This position helps microbes run off your hands rather than up your arms.

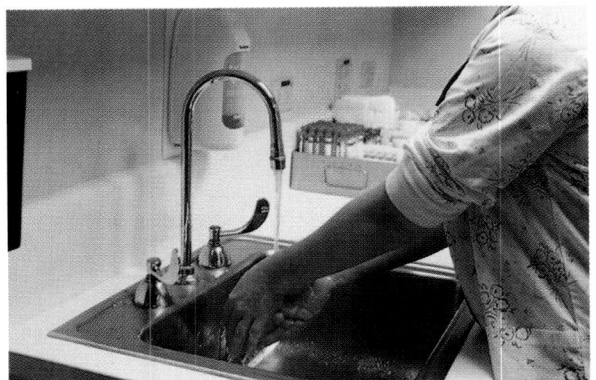

Wetting the hands while holding them lower than the elbows.

3 Using soap, thoroughly rub all surfaces of your hands, including your palms, backs of your hands, and wrists. Work the soap into a foamy lather while rubbing both hands together using circular movements.

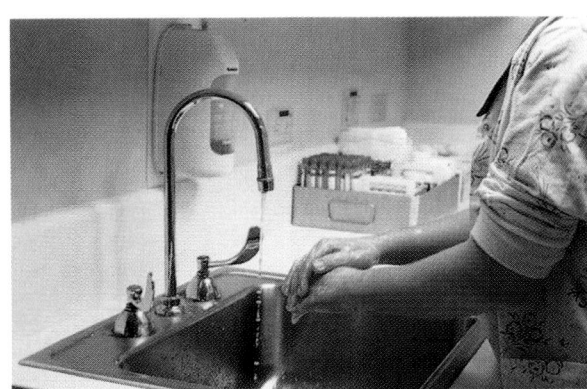

Thoroughly rubbing all surfaces of the hands with soap.

Because bar soap can provide an environment for bacterial growth if continually wet, liquid soap from a dispenser is recommended. Mechanical movements loosen and remove dirt and microorganisms.

4 Pay special attention to cleansing the following areas that can concentrate microorganisms: between the fingers, at creases and breaks in the skin, at the nail beds, and under the nails. Spend 10 to 30 seconds washing your hands.

Continued

PROCEDURE 27–1 *(continued)*

Hand-Washing

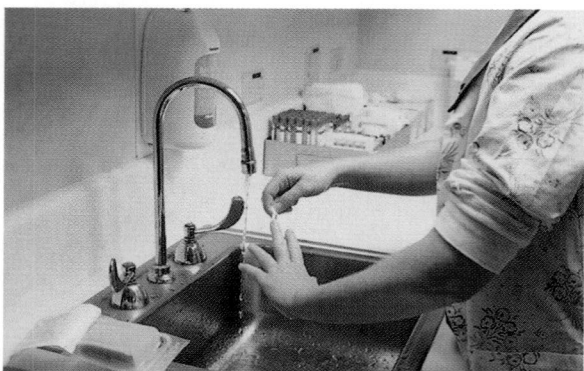

Cleaning under the fingernails.

A cuticle or orangewood stick can be used to assist in properly cleansing under the nails. The washing time may vary depending on the amount of contamination, the type of contamination, and the client's risk for infection.

5 Rinse your hands with warm running water under the faucet, allowing the water to wash down your hands and over your fingertips.

6 Dry hands thoroughly with a towel.

In some care situations, paper towels are used for drying the hands.

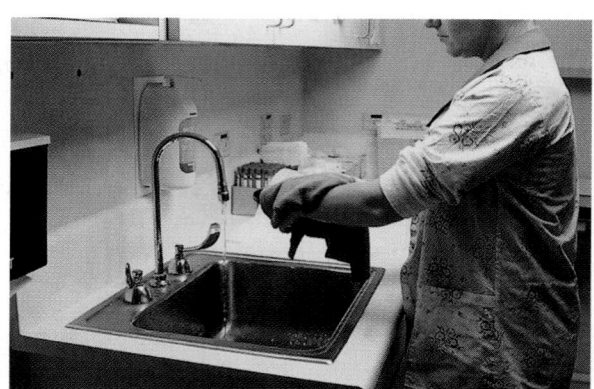

Drying the hands thoroughly with a towel.

7 If the sink is not foot-operated, turn off the faucet with the used towel, then discard the towel in the appropriate designated receptacle.

The towel acts as a barrier between your clean hand and the faucet.

HOME CARE CONSIDERATIONS

- If you work in home health care, bring bactericidal soap and paper towels with you to the client's home.
- If no running water is available in the home, you may use disposable wipes or alcohol. Be aware, however, that these can be drying to the skin if used frequently.

DISPOSING OF BODILY WASTES

Feces and urine are of course flushed through the bathroom toilet into the sewage system. If the client uses a bedpan, urinal, or bedside commode, use care to prevent spills and clean the container after disposing of urine or feces. Change any soiled linen as necessary.

PROMOTING AIR QUALITY

Designated hospital personnel monitor the institution's ventilation system to ensure that the quality of air is healthy. Maintenance of the system prevents the growth of molds that could be circulated throughout the hospital, causing disease.

EMPLOYING BARRIERS

Another component of medical asepsis is the use of barriers that can reduce the transmission of organisms from the client to the caregiver. Gloves can be used to avoid direct contact with infectious material. Gloves should never be used as a substitute for good hand-washing. A clean gown or apron can be used to protect clothing from contamination. In order to be effective, the gown or apron should be impermeable to water to prevent the soiling of clothing under the covering gown or apron.

Another technique used as part of medical asepsis is cohorting, a process in which clients with similar diagnoses are placed together to minimize the spread of their infections to clients without the same infecting organism. In intensive care or other units that have more than one bed unit per room, the beds for these clients may be grouped together in the same room.

Implementing Standard Precautions

With the awareness that any client has the potential for carrying an unknown and possibly incurable infection, the concept of universal precautions was developed a number of years ago. They included the use of hand-washing and barrier precautions to prevent the caregiver from exposure to pathogens. The practice was based on the fact that any bodily substance has the potential for harboring infectious organisms, which could be transmitted from client to caretaker and then possibly to another client.

These precautions are now generally called **standard precautions.** They are a set of actions, including hand-washing and the use of barrier precautions, designed to reduce transmission of infectious organisms. Barrier precautions include gloves, water-impermeable gowns, and eye protection if splashes are possible. Depending on the area, the care delivered, and client population served, standard precautions are tailored to fit the specific area. Standard precautions are used for all clients, not just for those with known infections. These precautions should be implemented whenever contact with potentially infectious material is anticipated. These precautions are used to protect the caregiver. Keeping the client in mind, however, remember that gloves do not replace proper hand-washing. When the task is completed, remove gloves and wash your hands using soap and friction. Change barriers between clients.

Action Alert!
Standard precautions are used for all clients, not just for those with known infections.

The government agency responsible for developing guidelines for universal or standard precautions is the Centers for Disease Control and Prevention (CDC). Box 27–2 lists common infections that are managed using standard precautions. Specific guidelines are part of standard precautions, including hand-washing; the use of gloves, masks, eyewear, face shields, and gowns; linen; client care equipment; environmental controls; and handling sharps. Box 27–3 provides specific information about each of these components.

Implementing Isolation Precautions

Historically, health care agencies developed procedures for **isolation**—that is, identification of a client who has an infection and implementation of precautions to prevent the spread of that infection. After an infecting organism was identified, guidelines were implemented specific to the organism. These guidelines were called disease-specific guidelines. That system was cumbersome because the guidelines to be used were listed according to each known organism. This system also required extensive education about the mode of transmission of the infecting organism.

Because many infections have similar modes of transmission, similar recommendations could really be used to prevent their spread. For this reason, category-specific isolation precautions were later developed. The number of different kinds of isolation was then reduced to seven, and the mechanisms for prevention were more easily implemented. Category-specific isolation procedures include the following:

- *Blood-body fluid precautions:* To prevent disease transmission by infected blood, saliva, tears, semen, vaginal secretions, urine, or fluid aspirated from body cavities.
- *Drainage-secretion precautions:* To prevent disease transmission by direct or indirect contact with drainage from body cavities or with purulent secretions.
- *Enteric precautions:* To prevent disease transmission through direct or indirect contact with feces.
- *Contact isolation:* To prevent disease transmission by close proximity or direct contact with a client. Private room is required.
- *Strict isolation:* To prevent disease transmission by air and contact with highly contagious or virulent organisms. All barriers are used when entering a private room.
- *Respiratory isolation:* To prevent disease transmission by air through droplets.
- *Tuberculosis isolation:* To prevent disease transmission of the airborne organism *Mycobacterium tuberculosis.*

Once standard precautions were implemented for all clients, the categories for isolation were able to be further reduced. Isolation for blood-borne pathogens is no longer necessary because standard precautions, when correctly implemented, already incorporate any

---

BOX 27–2

COMMON INFECTIONS MANAGED WITH STANDARD PRECAUTIONS

- Abscess with minor or limited drainage contained by a sterile dressing.
- Acquired immunodeficiency syndrome (AIDS).
- Most pneumonias, including those caused by gram-negative bacteria.
- Acute bacterial conjunctivitis, including gonococcal and chlamydial.
- Salmonella (use contact precautions if client diapered, incontinent, <6 years of age).
- Hepatitis A, B, C, E (for hepatitis A, use contact precautions if client diapered or incontinent).
- Herpes zoster (localized lesions in immune competent client).

BOX 27–3

COMPONENTS OF STANDARD PRECAUTIONS

Hand-Washing

Wash your hands before having any contact with clients and before preparing any items that will be used in client care. Wash your hands again after any contact with a client, especially after touching any blood, body fluids, secretions, excretions, and contaminated items. Even if you wore gloves, you must still wash your hands. When needed, wash your hands during the care of a client to prevent cross-contamination of body sites.

Gloves

Wear gloves to handle blood, body fluids, secretions, excretions, and contaminated items. Although blood-borne pathogens are the basis for wearing gloves, the blood does not have to be visible in the body fluids for gloves to be required. Remove the gloves immediately and wash your hands before proceeding with the next task or touching noncontaminated items, even on the same client. Change your gloves between tasks on the same client if different body sites are involved.

Mask, Eye Protection, Face Shield, Gown

Use as needed if you could be exposed to splashes or sprays of blood, body fluids, secretions, and excretions. The risk for splashes or sprays is higher in emergency departments and operating rooms; however, the risk exists in some clients in general care areas as well.

Client-Care Equipment

Handle equipment in a manner that prevents personal skin and mucous membrane exposure and cross contamination to other clients. Ensure that reusable equip-

ment is cleaned and reprocessed before using it in the care of another client.

Environment

Review hospital procedures for routine care, cleaning, and disinfection of environmental surfaces. Spills of blood and body fluid may need to be handled with special procedures.

Linen

Linen should be handled in a way that keeps it from contaminating skin, mucous membranes, and clothing. Fold soiled linen with the contamination to the inside. Hold it away from your body, place it directly in a plastic bag, tie the bag, and take it directly to the soiled linen area.

Sharp Objects

Take all possible precautions to prevent needlesticks or cuts with sharp objects (called *sharps* for short). Needles are the primary concern on a general client unit; however, scalpels and other sharp objects are sometimes used. Do not recap used needles in any manner that involves pointing the needle toward any part of your body or another person. If you must recap a needle, place the cap on a flat surface and scoop it onto the needle. After using a needle, immediately discard it in a puncture-proof container. Do not attempt to bend or break a needle before discarding it. Throw the syringe and needle away without removing the needle from the syringe.

precautions necessary for blood-borne pathogens. In addition to standard precautions, the CDC now recommends three categories of transmission-based precautions. These three categories are *airborne, droplet,* and *contact.*

Action Alert!
In addition to standard precautions, the CDC now recommends three categories of transmission-based precautions: airborne, droplet, and contact.

AIRBORNE PRECAUTIONS

Airborne precautions are used to prevent infection when the infectious organism is capable of remaining in the air for prolonged periods of time and of being transported in the air for distances greater than 3 feet. The most recognized organism in this group is the tuberculosis bacterium, although the chicken pox and

measles viruses are also included in this category. Besides standard precautions, clients with these infections should be placed in a private room with negative pressure, if possible. The room should vent directly to the outside and have a designated minimum number of air exchanges per hour. Anyone entering the room must wear a special particulate filter mask. The CDC also recommends limiting visitors and, in the cases of chicken pox and measles, limiting caretakers to those already immune.

DROPLET PRECAUTIONS

Droplet precautions refer to precautions used for organisms that can be spread through the air but are unable to remain in the air further than 3 feet. Thus, a standard mask (without a special filter) must be worn when standing within 3 feet of the client, in addition to standard precautions. Many respiratory viral infections, including influenza, require droplet precautions.

Figure 27–2 compares three different types of masks. The first is the individually fitted particulate filter mask required as part of airborne precautions. The second is a standard mask that also contains a face shield to guard against exposure to splashes (which is often used in operating rooms). The third is a standard mask that is routinely used as part of droplet precautions.

CONTACT PRECAUTIONS

Contact precautions are precautions that include standard precautions and the use of barrier precautions such as gloves and impermeable gowns. They are used for clients with diarrhea, when coming into contact with draining wounds not contained by the sterile dressing, or with clients who have acquired antibiotic-

resistant infections. An example of this type of infection is multidrug-resistant *Staphylococcus aureus* (commonly called MRSA). The goal of these precautions is to eliminate disease transmission resulting from either direct contact with the client or indirect contact through an intermediary infected object or surface that has been in contact with the client, such as instruments, linens, or dressing materials.

The CDC discusses a fourth type of isolation, known as protective isolation. This would be used for immunocompromised clients, who would have a nursing diagnosis of *Altered protection*. This type of isolation is discussed further when we look at interventions for clients with this nursing diagnosis. Table 27–4 outlines common clinical conditions that would require some form of isolation and identifies the potential pathogens for these disorders and the precautions that are warranted. The accompanying procedure describes how to

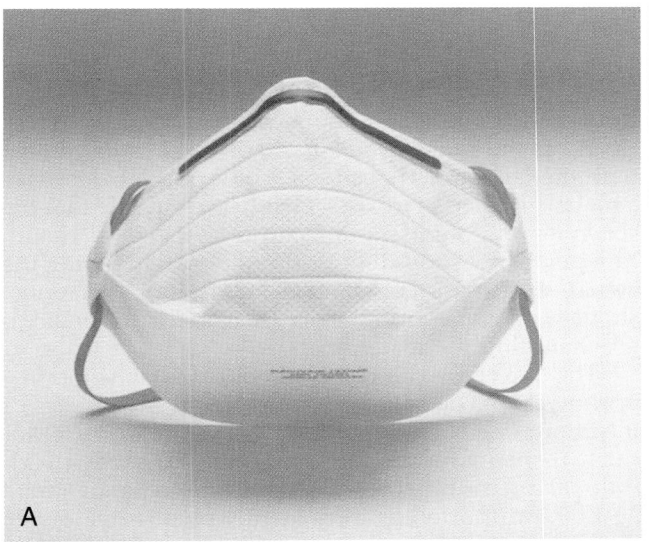

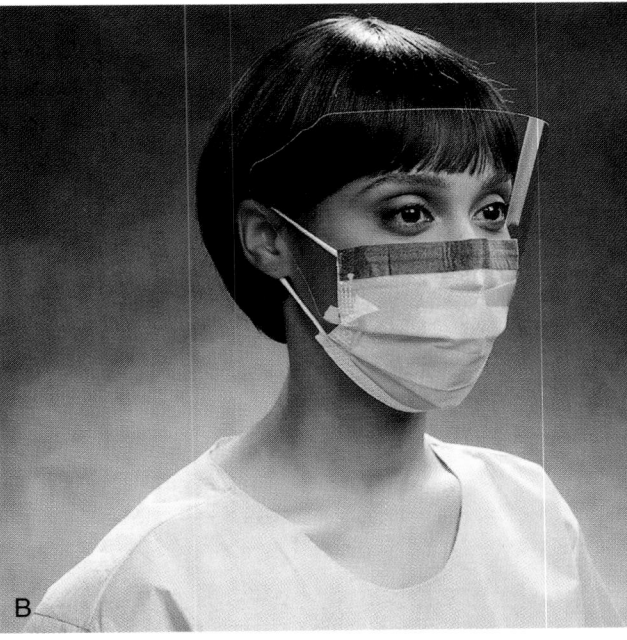

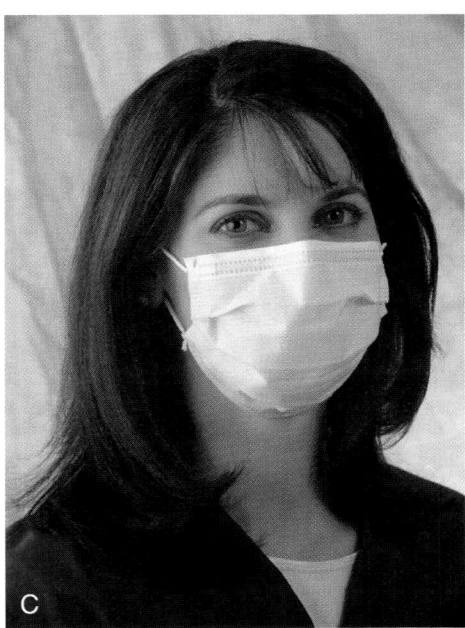

Figure 27–2. Masks used as barrier methods of infection control. *A,* Individually fitted particulate filter mask; *B,* standard mask with face shield; *C,* standard mask. (*A,* Courtesy of Uvex Safety, Smithfield, RI; *B,* Courtesy of Kimberly-Clark Corp., Roswell, GA; *C,* Courtesy of Medline Industries, Inc., Mundelein, IL.)

TABLE 27–4

Precautions for Specific Clinical Syndromes or Conditions

Clinical Syndrome or Condition	Potential Pathogens	Empirical Precautions
Diarrhea		
Acute diarrhea with a likely infectious cause in an incontinent or diapered client.	Enteric pathogens	Contact
Diarrhea in an adult with a history of recent antibiotic use.	*Clostridium difficile*	Contact
Respiratory Infections		
Cough, fever, upper-lobe pulmonary infiltrate in an HIV-negative client or a client at low risk for HIV infection.	*Mycobacterium tuberculosis*	Airborne
Cough, fever, pulmonary infiltrate in any lung location in an HIV-infected client or a client at high risk for HIV infection.	*Mycobacterium tuberculosis*	Airborne
Respiratory infections, particularly bronchiolitis and croup, in infants and young children.	Respiratory syncytial or parainfluenza virus	Contact
Risk of Multidrug-Resistant Microorganisms		
History of infection or colonization with multidrug-resistant organisms.	Resistant bacteria	Contact
Skin, wound, or urinary tract infection in a client with a recent hospital or nursing home stay in a facility where multidrug-resistant organisms are prevalent.	Resistant bacteria	Contact

appropriately don and remove gown, gloves, and mask when working with a client in isolation.

Action **A**lert!
Protective isolation should be used for clients with compromised immune systems.

Isolation rooms can be used to isolate clients with poor hygiene or those with airborne infections. They can also be used for those clients with altered protection. When available, rooms with negative pressure are useful for airborne infections such as tuberculosis, measles, or chicken pox. Negative-pressure rooms vent directly to the outside and must have air exchanges with outside air, not with air circulated from the rest of the ventilation system. Positive-pressure rooms are those rooms that prevent the air from the rest of the agency from entering the room, thereby minimizing the possibility of introducing infectious agents into the room. In order to be effective, doors to both negative- and positive-pressure rooms should be kept closed.

Before the advent of universal precautions, many health care facilities used a special cart with isolation equipment stored on it. Now, with standard precautions being the governmentally mandated standard of care, isolation carts have no particular advantage in most circumstances. Gloves, impermeable gowns, and protective eye wear are stored to be available to all staff. Whenever droplet, airborne, or protective precautions are implemented, these items must be available to all of the client's visitors. In these instances, special carts may be placed at the entrance to the client's room to facilitate these items being available to visitors.

Because standard precautions require that all bodily fluids be treated as potentially infectious, laboratory specimens are now all treated as if they are infectious. This usually requires placing the specimen container in another container, such as a bag, that is clean on the outside and has not come into contact with the laboratory specimen. The bag is labeled with a biohazard alert symbol, which tells everyone that the specimen is potentially infectious (Fig. 27–3). Health care personnel should wear gloves when handling the actual specimen containers. Laboratory personnel should use gloves and barrier precautions when actually handling the material.

The infection control methods used when transporting clients on isolation depend on the diagnosis or infection. For clients requiring just standard precautions, there are no special precautions. Those with additional precautions should have limited movement and be transported as infrequently as possible out of their room. If it becomes necessary to transport these clients from their room, it is essential to maintain precautions to minimize the risk of transmitting the infecting organism to other clients or to the environment. Additionally, clients with droplet precautions or airborne precautions should wear masks when outside of their room.

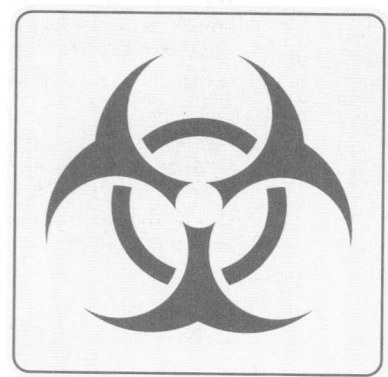

Figure 27–3. Biohazard alert symbol.

PROCEDURE 27-2

Caring for a Client in Isolation

TIME TO
ALLOW
▼
Novice:
Variable
Expert:
Variable

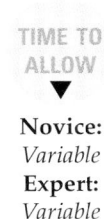

Appropriate protective equipment should be used whenever you face a risk of exposure to infectious substances. Likewise, in the case of isolation, appropriate protective equipment should be worn to protect the client from exposure to possibly infectious substances.

Delegation Guidelines

You may delegate aspects of your client's care to a nursing assistant who has received training in the performance of isolation procedures, consistent with your institution's policies and procedures.

Equipment Needed

- Gown.
- Gloves.
- Mask.
- Goggles (if risk of splash is present).
- Trash receptacle.
- Laundry receptacle (if gown is nondisposable).

Application of Barriers

1 Wash your hands.

2 Put on gown.
a. Pick up the gown by its collar and allow it to unfold.
b. Put your arms through the sleeves and pull the gown up over your shoulders.
c. Fasten the neck ties.
d. Make sure the gown laps over itself at the back and fasten the waist ties.

   Overlapping the back reduces the chance of contaminating the back of your clothing underneath the gown.

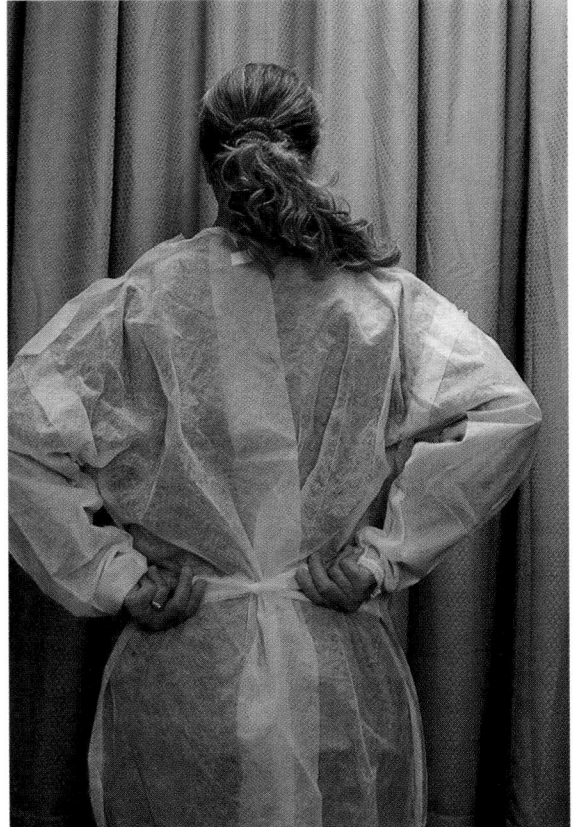

Lapping the gown over itself and fastening it with waist ties.

Continued

Caring for a Client in Isolation

3 Put on disposable gloves.

a. Pull the cuff of each glove over the edge of the gown sleeve.

This step prevents transmission of microorganisms to you from the client.

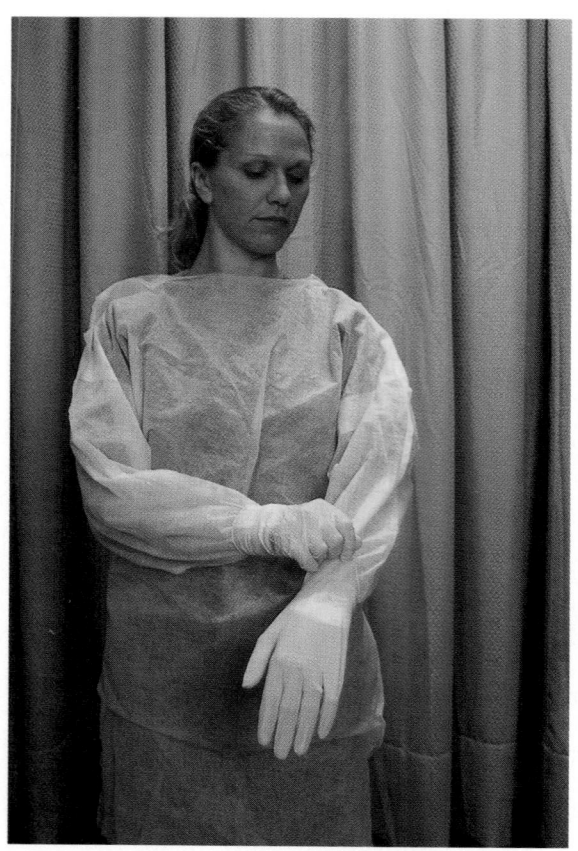

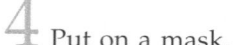
Pulling the cuff of each glove over the edge of the gown sleeve.

b. Interlace your fingers, if needed, to adjust the fit of the gloves.

4 Put on a mask.

a. Position the mask over your nose and mouth.

b. Bend the nose bar over the bridge of your nose for a snug fit.

c. Fasten the elastic bands or tie the mask securely in place if it has strings.

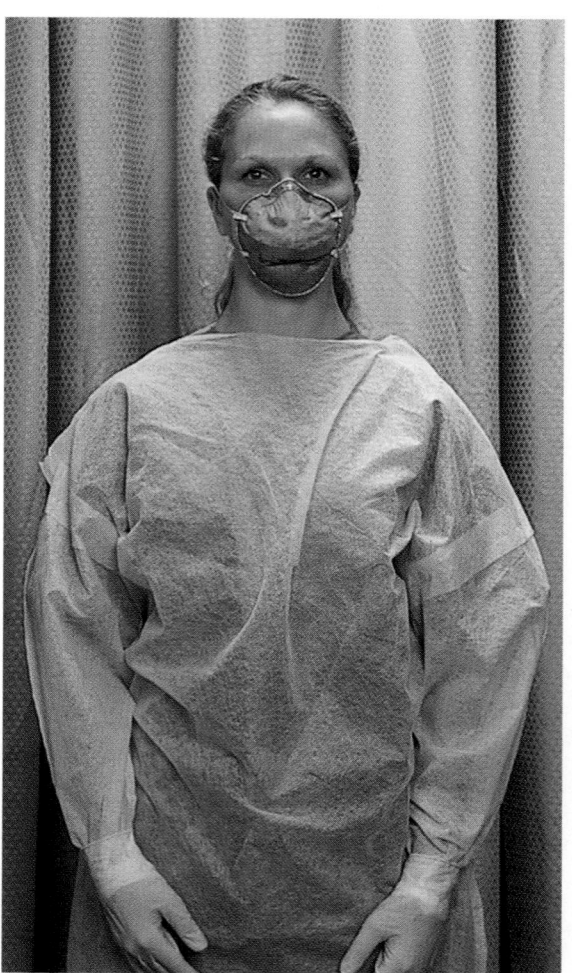
Mask positioned over the nose and mouth.

A mask reduces potential exposure to airborne droplet nuclei. Plan to change your mask every 30 minutes because its effectiveness dramatically drops after that time period.

d. Put on goggles, if indicated, after your mask is in place.

5 Administer care to client. After disposing of soiled items used in client care, tie the bag securely. If special disposal methods are used, and the bag is not prelabeled, mark the bag appropriately.

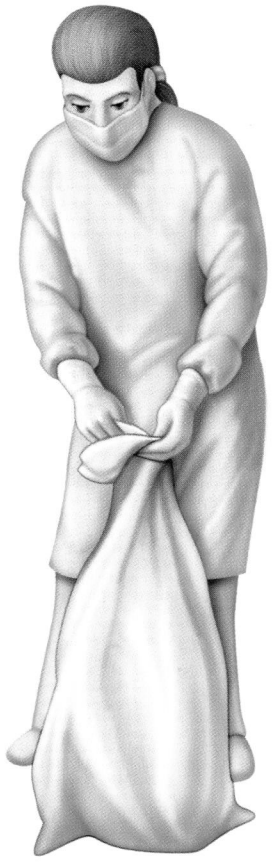

Tying the bag securely.

Removal of Barriers

1 At the door to the client's room, remove your goggles first (if used), without touching your face or hair.

Doing so prevents contamination by microorganisms on your gloves.

2 Untie your gown at the waist but do not remove it yet.

Continued

Caring for a Client in Isolation

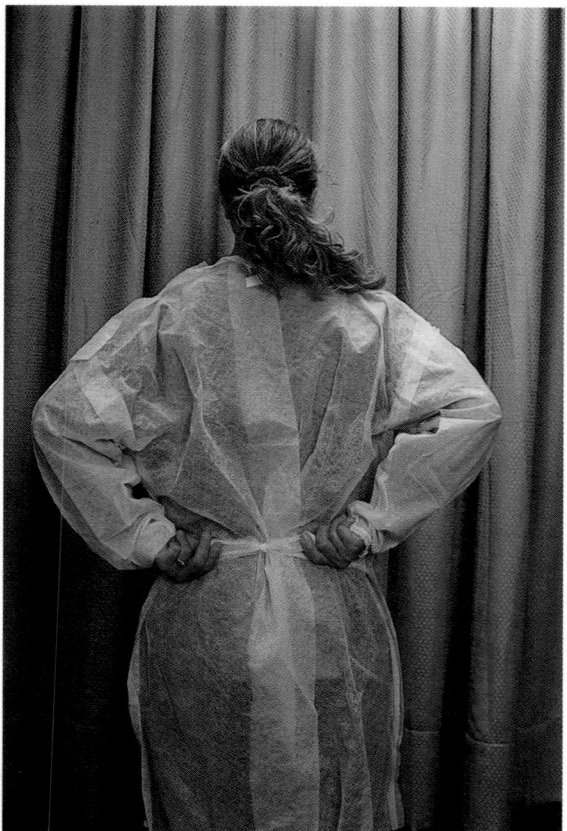

Untying the gown at the waist.

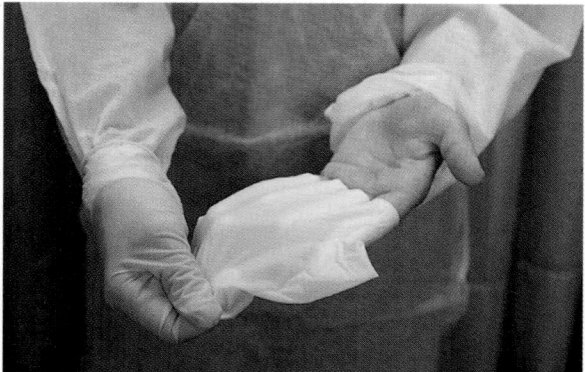

Pulling the first glove inside out.

b. Tuck an ungloved finger inside the cuff of the remaining glove.
c. Pull the second glove off inside out, and discard both gloves.

This method prevents contamination of your hands by microorganisms.

3 Remove your gloves.
a. Grasp the outside of the cuff of one glove and pull the glove inside out over your hand. Hold the removed glove in the second hand.

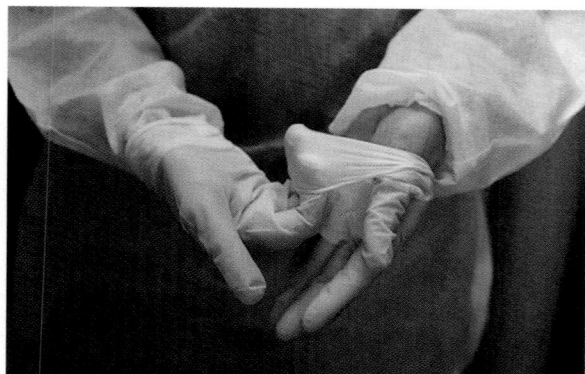

Grasping the cuff.

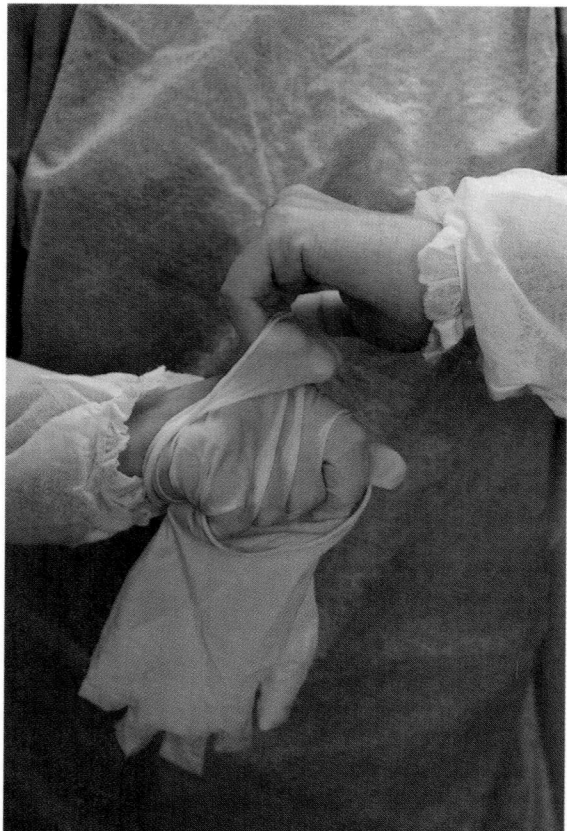

Pulling the second glove inside out.

4 Remove your gown.

a. Untie your gown at the neck and allow it to fall forward from your shoulders.

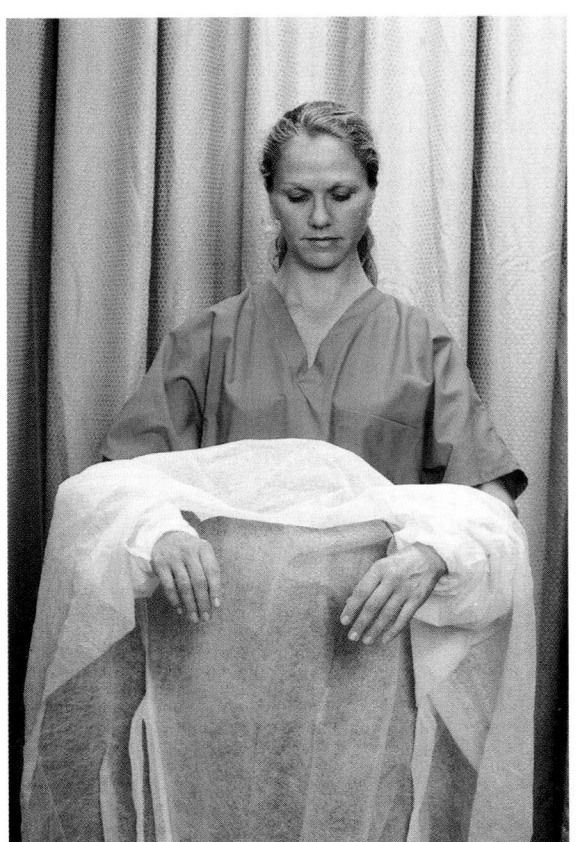

Allowing the gown to fall forward from the shoulders.

b. Slide your hands through the sleeves and remove them without touching the outside of the gown.

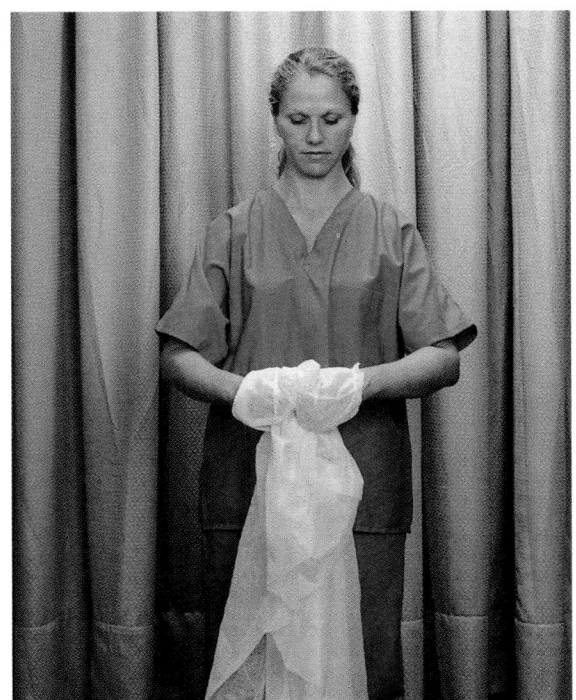

Sliding the hands through the sleeves without touching the outside of the gown.

c. Hold the gown at the inside shoulder seams and away from your body, allowing it to turn inside out. Fold the contaminated side of the gown to the inside.

d. Discard the gown in an appropriate receptacle.

5 Remove your mask.

a. Pull the elastic or untie the strings without touching the mask's outer surface.

b. Discard the mask in an appropriate receptacle.

These steps prevent contamination of your hands by microorganisms.

6. Wash your hands.

Controlling Infection in the Home

Whenever a nurse delivers care in the home, interventions must include the client's and any other resident's input into the plan of care. Because the nurse has less control over interventions to minimize the risk for infection, it is critical to get participation of both the client and others living in the household to develop needed interventions to reach the agreed-upon client outcomes. Without the participation of the entire group, outcomes will certainly be less than optimal. Many of the nursing interventions in the home revolve around education and the understanding of the residents. Because the nurse is usually there for only a prescribed period of time, the main caregivers must understand and agree to the plan. These caregivers may consist of family members or family plus home health care workers, depending on the client's situation and ability to provide self-care.

MANAGING RISK FOR INFECTION

The basics of infection control to prevent the spread of infection in the home are the same as in the hospital: good hand-washing. It is also important for the home caregiver to know how the infection is transmitted to reduce the potential for infecting others. Basic hygiene and pest control might also be issues that may require attention. Principles of good nutrition and signs and symptoms of infection are other educational issues for the nurse working in home care (Box 27–4).

> *A*ction *A*lert!
> Basic infection control in the client's home relies on the same procedure as it does in the hospital: thorough and repeated hand-washing.

The client who is discharged to home after a surgical procedure is often responsible for daily monitoring of his or her own wound status and caring for the wound until a follow-up appointment has been scheduled with the surgeon. Because an incision is a break in the skin, a first line of defense, surgical clients are at increased risk for infection by virtue of the surgery. The Teaching for Self-Care chart provides information for clients on how to manage a wound to prevent postoperative infection. Ongoing use of principles of medical asepsis also apply.

MANAGING ALTERED PROTECTION

Good hand-washing is an educational issue that can never be addressed too many times and should be reviewed periodically when caring for immunocompromised clients in the home setting. A clear understanding of what alters their protection for infection is essential to minimize their risk. Assess for situations or practices that should be changed because of the altered protection, and address these issues with the client and caregivers. The Teaching for Self-Care chart provides instructions about methods to minimize the risk of an immunocompromised client acquiring an infection in the home.

A health care worker in the home must use the same precautions to prevent the spread of infection from the client to others. Good hand-washing is still required, but unfortunately some homes may not have running water and soap as readily available resources. In these instances, although not the most desirable, you must use disposable wipes saturated with an antiseptic solution as a stop-gap measure. Use barrier precautions as you would in the health care setting if contact with potentially infectious material is possible. The barrier precautions used in the home are the same: gloves, water-impermeable gown, masks, and eye protection. If occupants of the home, other than the client, are at increased risk, they may also need to use barrier precautions. You should ensure that the necessary items are available to them and give instructions on their correct use.

Implementing Sterile Technique

Sterile technique refers to those practices that are used to prevent the introduction of microorganisms that could cause infection. This is sometimes called *surgical aseptic technique.* Sterile technique is used when there

---

BOX 27–4

TEACHING TIPS FOR PREVENTING INFECTION IN THE HOME

Food Handling

- Hand-washing is the best defense against infection.
- Wash your hands after using the bathroom and before preparing or eating food.
- When cleaning and cutting chicken, wash your hands before preparing other foods.
- Wash all fresh fruits and vegetables before eating them.
- Store leftover food in the refrigerator.
- Do not refreeze uncooked meat that has been thawed.
- Cook ground meat, chicken, and pork thoroughly.

Managing Colds and Flu

- Keep tissues handy to catch sneezes and coughs.
- Keep a waste basket close to the sick person.
- Wash your hands often to help reduce the chance of spreading a cold or the flu.

Caring for Minor Scrapes and Cuts

- Clean the wound with mild soap and water, and pat it dry.
- Cover it with a bandage if it is bleeding or likely to become contaminated.

Teaching for SELF-CARE

WOUND CARE

Purpose: To keep a wound from getting infected.

Rationale: Daily wound care will minimize the risk of infection. Looking at the wound daily will allow assessment of any beginning infection.

Expected Outcome: The client will clean the wound and experience complete healing without incurring an infection.

Client Instructions
1. Assemble the supplies you'll need, such as fresh sterile gauze, peroxide, antibiotic cream, tape, and a trash can.
2. Wash your hands.
3. Remove your old dressing and place it in the trash.
4. Look to see if the wound has any new redness, tenderness, or drainage. If it does, tell your doctor or nurse about it.
5. Using some sterile gauze moistened with peroxide, wipe your incision from the center out to an edge one time. Then throw the gauze in the trash.
6. Using a new piece of moistened sterile gauze, wipe your wound one more time from the center to the edge. Go in a different direction this time.
7. Repeat steps 5 and 6 until you have cleaned the entire wound.
8. Allow the wound to air dry.
9. Apply antibiotic cream if your doctor told you to.
10. Cover the incision with sterile gauze and tape it in place.

is a break in the first line of defense and may be indicated for selected procedures performed by the nurse or other health care personnel at the bedside, or during surgical procedures. Sterile technique as used during surgery requires extensive procedures for preventing microorganisms from entering surgical wounds. There are three areas of application of this technique: the skin, physical barriers (sterile field), and the environment.

SKIN
The skin of the client is prepared before any invasive procedure. This may involve washing first with soap to remove soil. The area is then thoroughly cleansed with an antimicrobial agent and may be referred to as a "scrub." Any hair in the area should be removed prior to cleansing with the antimicrobial cleanser.

When scrubbing and hair removal are done together, this is sometimes called a "skin prep."

Aside from surgery, sterile technique is used whenever host defenses are interrupted, such as during catheter insertion (e.g., intravenous and urinary), dressing changes of surgical wounds, or endotracheal suctioning. It should also be used during IV fluid or medication administration. Box 27–5 outlines the principles of sterile technique.

STERILE FIELD
Using sterile technique for limited procedures outside the operating room involves setting up a small sterile field with a few pieces of equipment and using sterile gloves to handle sterile equipment. The accompanying procedure describes how to apply and remove sterile gloves.

When setting up a sterile field, you may open a tray that already contains sterile materials wrapped in a drape. At other times, you may be required to use a drape to set up the sterile field and then place sterile

Teaching for SELF-CARE

PREVENTING INFECTION IN IMMUNOSUPPRESSED CLIENTS

Purpose: To prevent the client from acquiring an infection at home.

Rationale: Many infections can be prevented by modifying the home environment.

Expected Outcome: The client will continue to function at home without acquiring an infection.

Client Instructions
1. Gather as many of your friends and family as possible to learn about keeping you free from infection.
2. Wash your hands often with soap and water. This is the best means to prevent infection.
3. If you have pets, consider giving them to someone else who can care for them.
4. Have any dusting or vacuuming done when you are not in the room.
5. If you have live plants in the house, have someone else water them.
6. You may need to alter what you eat. For example, all meats should be cooked thoroughly until well done. Also, eat no thin-skinned fresh fruits or vegetables unless they are canned. This includes grapes, peaches, and apples. (Ask clients for their own examples to ensure understanding of this point.)
7. Ask your friends to visit you at another time if they feel ill.

BOX 27–5

PRINCIPLES OF STERILE TECHNIQUE

- Sterile means the absence of all microorganisms.
- The skin cannot be sterilized, but thorough cleaning can significantly reduce the number of microorganisms present.
- Sterile objects that come in contact with unsterile objects are no longer sterile.
- When a sterile field is wet, capillary action will draw microorganisms from the surface underneath a permeable drape. This is called *strikethrough*. A wet drape is not a sterile drape.
- Consider anything below the waist to be unsterile.
- Consider any part of the sterile field that falls or hangs below the top of the table to be unsterile. Waist level is the limit of a good visual field.
- Consider the edge of a sterile field and 2 inches inward as unsterile.
- Do not cough, sneeze, or talk excessively over a sterile field.
- Do not reach across a sterile field.
- Always face a sterile field. If you turn your back on a sterile field, you cannot guarantee its sterility.
- Use a sterile package immediately once it has been opened. Otherwise, it cannot be considered sterile.
- Consider a bottle of sterile liquid no longer sterile once it has been opened. If you save it to repeat a procedure, you may be performing a clean procedure, but you will not be performing a sterile procedure.
- Sterile packages have expiration dates determined by the manufacturer or the method of sterilization. Do not use packages that have passed their expiration date.
- Sterile packages are labeled as sterile. If not, consider the package unsterile.
- If there is any doubt about the sterility of an object, consider it unsterile.
- If a sterile package is wet or damaged, or if there is evidence that moisture has dried on it, consider it unsterile.

supplies onto that sterile drape. The accompanying procedures review how to prepare a sterile field using a tray wrapped in a sterile drape and how to set up a sterile field using a sterile drape.

A member of the surgical team who will work within a sterile field scrubs the hands and arms before entering the operating room to put on sterile attire. The hands and arms are first washed with soap and water to remove gross soil. Hands and arms are then washed with an antimicrobial soap using a sponge and/or scrub brush to remove as many microorganisms as possible. The soap leaves an antimicrobial residual that continues to prevent the presence of microorganisms after the washing. It should be noted, however, that the friction from use of a sponge and/or brush is the most effective component of reducing the organisms on the skin. The objective is to remove microorganisms without destroying tissue. The accompanying procedure describes how to perform a surgical hand scrub.

To maintain the area free of microorganisms, sterile gloves, gowns, and drapes are used to create a barrier between the environment (including the members of the team) and the client. To achieve an outer surface that is sterile, a gown and gloves are put on to cover the body. The technique for putting on a gown and gloves requires not touching the outer surface of the attire. After the procedure, careful removal of the gown and gloves are important to prevent contamination of the clothing under the gown. The accompanying procedure describes the process for donning a sterile gown and using closed gloving technique. The basics of setting up a sterile field in the operating room include covering the client with sterile drapes, covering work surfaces with sterile drapes, and laying out sterile instruments on the sterile field.

ENVIRONMENT

Environmental controls contribute to reducing the presence of microbes. Special areas may be set aside for special use, such as operating or procedure rooms. These rooms, when not in use, are cleaned using germicidal detergents. The area may have positive-pressure air flow to minimize the introduction of microorganisms into the air, and the ventilation system may have more frequent air exchanges to remove any introduced microbes. Any unnecessary visitors and personnel are excluded.

If a special room is not available, the designated area for a procedure can be cleaned ahead of time using a germicidal detergent. Then, traffic or other activity in the area can be curtailed during the procedure to minimize air currents from depositing microbes on the procedural area. Screens can be used to designate the area and remind personnel to avoid the area. After a sterile procedure is completed, the area is cleaned using standard precautions, followed by cleaning according to agency policy (which in turn depends on whether the area is specially designated).

Cleaning of equipment used in sterile procedures involves removing any visible soil and then disinfecting with a germicidal cleaner. Any materials used in invasive procedures that are not disposable must be sterilized after cleaning. Items are generally sterilized in autoclaves that utilize steam at high heat and pressures over a period of time. Items that could be destroyed by moisture or high heat and pressures can be gas-sterilized. Many disposable items can be bought pre-sterilized. The sterility of these item is guaranteed over a specified time period, assuming no breakage in the packaging has occurred. As a nurse, you are re-

PROCEDURE 27–3

Donning and Removing Sterile Gloves

TIME TO
ALLOW
▼
Novice:
3 min.
Expert:
1 min.

Sterile gloves should be used when performing procedures requiring surgical asepsis. This will eliminate the risk of introducing microorganisms from the caregiver to a sterile object or to the client.

Delegation Guidelines

Some of the tasks that you will delegate to your nursing assistant may require the use of sterile gloves. Nursing assistants should receive appropriate training in this skill prior to the delegation of such tasks.

Equipment Needed

- One package sterile gloves of appropriate hand size.
- Flat work surface.
- Other supplies as needed according to procedure being performed.

Donning Sterile Gloves

1 Wash your hands. Remove rings with stones or irregular surfaces.

Reduces microorganisms and the risk of puncturing the gloves with the rings.

2 Grasp the package at the tabs above the upper sealed edge. Peel down to open the outer wrapper. Discard the outer wrapper.

3 Place the inner package on a flat surface. Open the inner package at the first fold, touching the outside of the folded edge and pulling outward. Then open the next fold, pulling that edge outward without touching the inside of the package.

The package is usually labeled "up" and "down," or "left" and "right." Opening in this manner creates a sterile field. The outside of the wrapper is now contaminated. Gloves are now laid out with left glove on the left and the right glove on the right.

4 Put on the first glove.
a. Grasp the folded edge of the cuff of one glove.

   Usually, the dominant hand is gloved first.

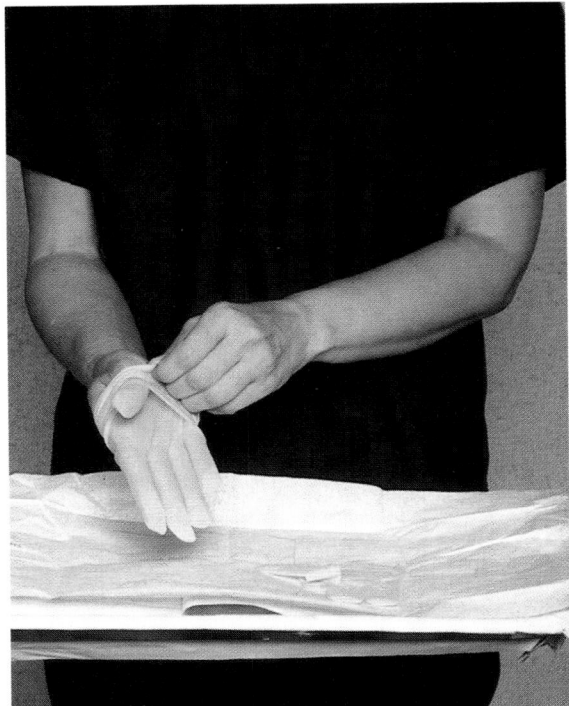

Grasping the folded edge of the cuff of one glove.

b. Lift the glove above the wrapper and away from your body.
c. Slide the opposite hand into the glove. Do not adjust the cuff or fingers now or let your ungloved hand touch the outside of the glove.

Continued

Donning and Removing Sterile Gloves

This technique maintains sterility by preventing contact of the gloves with unsterile objects, such as the hand, uniform, or other surfaces.

5 Put on the second glove.

a. Pick up the second glove by sliding your sterile gloved fingers under the edge of the cuff. Keep your gloved thumb off the cuff of the second glove.

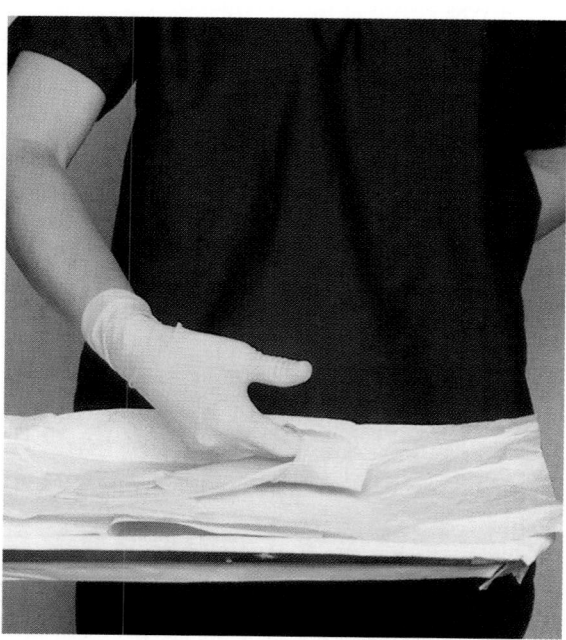

Picking up the second glove.

Prevents the gloved thumb from coming in contact with a surface that will also be touching the ungloved hand.

Removing Sterile Gloves

1 Grasp the outside of one glove near the base of the thumb and remove it by pulling it inside out.

Prevents the used and contaminated glove from coming in contact with the skin of your wrist.

2 Discard the glove or hold it in the palm of the gloved hand.

Either method is correct and depends on personal preference.

b. Slide the fingers of your opposite hand into the glove. Let go of the edge when your hand is in the glove.

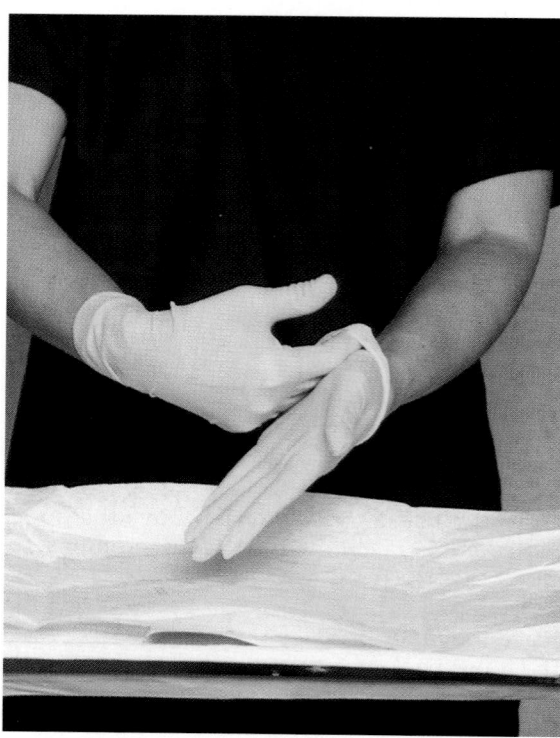

Sliding the fingers of the opposite hand into the glove.

As you slide your hand into the glove, the hand that is holding the glove should stretch the edge of the glove out to avoid touching the unsterile wrist.

b. Adjust the gloves for comfort and fit.

Your fingers are touching the outside of the glove that will remain sterile. Keep sterile surface to sterile surface. The edges of the glove touching your wrist are not sterile.

3 Slide your ungloved thumb or fingers inside the second glove and remove it by pulling it inside out also.

If you held the first glove in your hand, they are now wrapped together.

4 Discard into appropriate receptacle.

5 Wash your hands.

PROCEDURE 27–4

Preparing a Sterile Field by Opening a Tray Wrapped in a Sterile Drape

TIME TO
ALLOW
▼
Novice:
2–3 min.
Expert:
1 min.

This procedure would be used when a microorganism-free surface is needed to hold materials for dressing changes, insertion of catheters, and other procedures requiring that sterility of objects on the field be maintained.

Delegation Guidelines

You may delegate the preparation of a sterile field to a nursing assistant who has been appropriately trained in the performance of this task. You would generally not delegate the actual performance of a sterile procedure to a nursing assistant.

Equipment Needed

- Wrapped sterile package.
- Flat work surface.
- Sterile gloves and other items required to perform the intended procedure on an actual client.

1 Wash your hands.

2 Remove a commercially packaged kit from the outer wrapper.

3 Position the inner package in the center of the work surface so that the outer flap of the wrapper is facing away from you.

4 Reach around (but not over) the package to open the flap away from you. Touch the outside of the flap only.
Maintains sterility of the package.

5 Open the side flaps one at a time, in the same manner as the first, with the uppermost side flap being opened first. Remember not to let your hands cross over the sterile field.

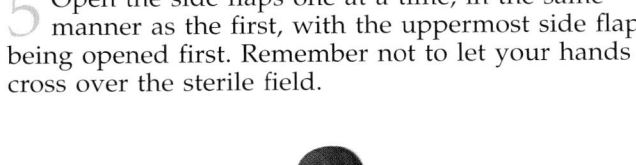

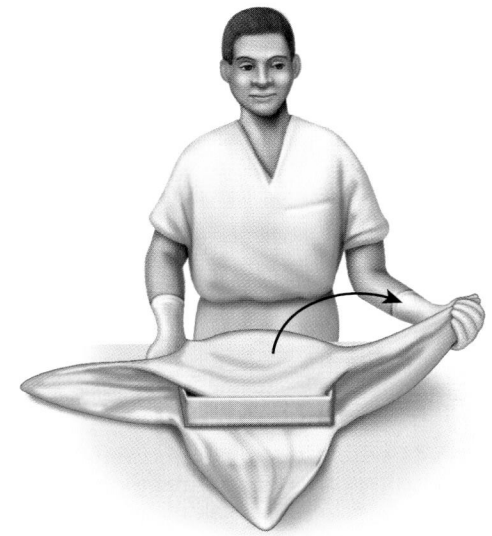

Opening the side flaps.

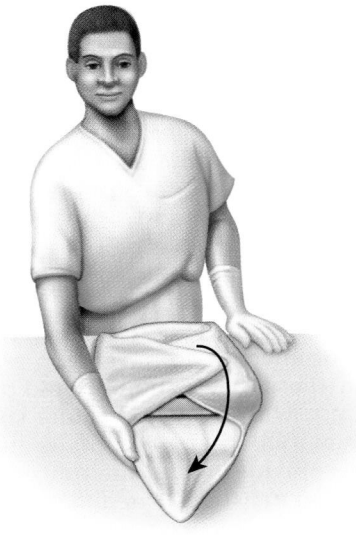

Opening the first flap away from yourself.

Continued

PROCEDURE 27–4 *(continued)*

Preparing a Sterile Field by Opening a Tray Wrapped in a Sterile Drape

6 Open the innermost flap that faces you last. Be sure to stand back sufficiently so that the flap does not touch you during opening.

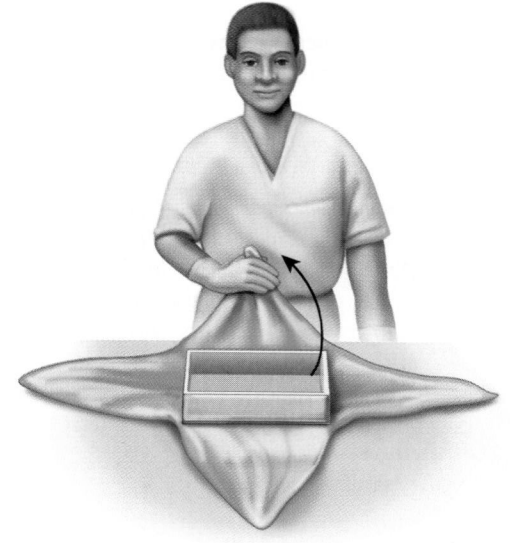

Opening the last flap toward yourself.

sponsible for ensuring that sterilized equipment is properly stored to maintain sterility for use in future procedures.

Action Alert!
You are responsible for storing sterilized equipment in a manner that maintains its sterility for future use.

Interventions to Protect Clients With Altered Immunity

Using Environmental Safeguards

Because clients with a compromised immune system have altered protection, their entire environment must be altered to minimize their risk of infection. This begins with the type of food that they are able to eat. They must not eat fresh fruits or vegetables except those with thick outer layers that are inedible. They can eat bananas but must handle the skins carefully. Oranges can be also be eaten, but again, contact with the outer part of the skin must be avoided. They should not eat fresh leafy salads but may have canned or frozen vegetables if well cooked. Fruits must also be cooked before eating, except for those mentioned. Meats should be eaten only if well done.

The physical environment should be maintained in as clean a state as possible. Not only should they avoid dusting and other chores relating to cleaning, they

should try as much as possible to avoid being in the room when these chores are done. Household pets can be perilous and are not recommended. Living plants are also not recommended, but if there are living plants in the home, they should not be watered by immunocompromised clients.

Preventing Feelings of Isolation

While in the hospital, immunocompromised clients are usually placed in isolation rooms with the door closed. If available, a room with positive-pressure ventilation to minimize air flow into the room from the rest of the hospital is recommended. Many institutions have special requirements for visitors of these clients. They may require visitors to wash their hands before entering the room, and to wear gloves, gown, and possibly a mask when inside the room to minimize the spread of normally harmless microbes to the client with altered protection. After discharge, because of the extreme risk of infection to those with an altered immune system, these clients should avoid public places, especially those with crowds. Visitors should not be allowed if they think they might have an infection.

Children with up-to-date immunizations and no signs of infection may be allowed to visit in the home. An exception is if they have recently be vaccinated with oral polio vaccine or measles, mumps, rubella, or

PROCEDURE 27–5

Preparing a Sterile Field

TIME TO
ALLOW
▼
Novice:
10 min.
Expert:
5 min.

This procedure is used when a microorganism-free surface is needed to hold materials for dressing changes, insertion of catheters, and other procedures requiring the sterility of the objects on the field.

Delegation Guidelines

You may delegate the preparation of a sterile field to a nursing assistant who has been appropriately trained in the performance of this task. You would generally not delegate the actual performance of a sterile procedure to a nursing assistant.

Equipment Needed

- Sterile drape.
- Sterile gloves.
- Sterile supplies and/or solutions as needed for the planned procedure.
- Protective barrier equipment as needed according to the planned procedure.

1 Arrange your work area. Use a clean, dry, flat, uncluttered surface at waist level.

The sterile field should be close to the client. You should position the field in a manner that allows you to work with the client and keep the field within your line of vision.

2 Ensure that supplies are sterile by checking the expiration date and for signs of dried or current moisture.

This protects the client from being touched by contaminated supplies.

Set Up a Drape

1 Prepare a sterile field or surface that is at least 2 inches larger on all sides than the area you need to work with the supplies.
a. Open the outer wrapping of a sterile cloth drape, keeping the drape itself sterile.
b. Pick up the drape by the loose corner edge and lift the drape into the air and away from your body.
c. With your other hand, grasp another corner edge and spread the drape in the air.
d. Decide which surface is to remain sterile and spread the drape on the table, with the side that will remain sterile facing up.

You can touch the edges of the drape because the edges of a sterile field are not considered sterile.

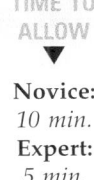

Spreading the drape on the table, with the side that will remain sterile facing up.

Add Dry Sterile Supplies
Peel-Apart Packages

1 Use both hands and grasp the edges designed to be peeled open.

2 Open the package over the sterile field so materials can fall freely from the package onto the field without touching your hands.

Continued

PROCEDURE 27–5 (continued)

Preparing a Sterile Field

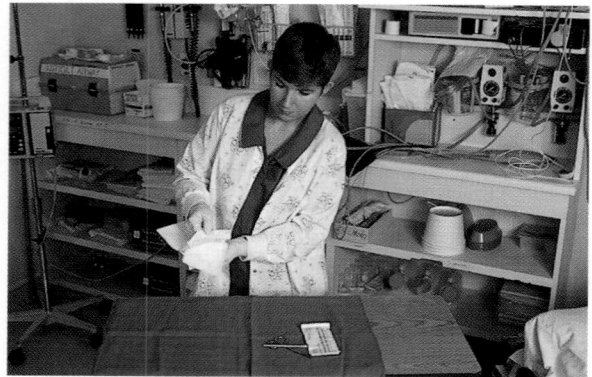

Opening the package over the sterile field.

Adding Sterile Liquids

1 Remove or loosen the cap from the bottle of liquid. Don't touch the inside of the cap or the rim of the liquid. Place the cap so the inside is face up on a flat, unsterile surface to prevent its contamination.

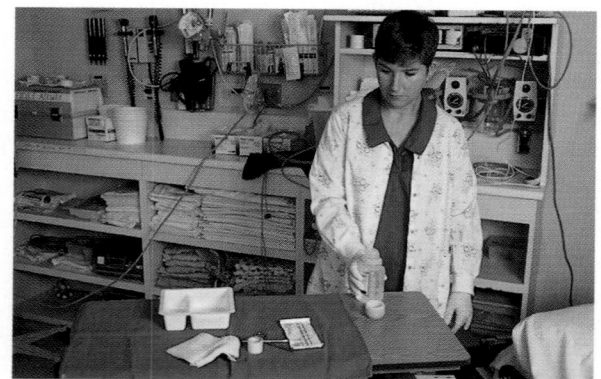

Placing the cap with the inside face up on the unsterile surface.

2 Label the bottle with the date and time.
Solutions that have been opened are considered contaminated 24 hours after opening, or earlier if according to agency policy.

3 If the container that will hold the liquid needs to be adjusted, put on one sterile glove.

4 Use the other ungloved hand to pick up the bottle of liquid so that the label is in the palm of your hand.

Wrapped Packages

1 Hold the object in one hand by the bottom or underside of the wrapping.

2 Unwrap the first corner away from you, then each side, then the last corner toward you.

3 Stabilize the corners against your wrist.
This prevents the corners from touching the sterile object.

4 Turn the object toward the sterile surface and drop it onto the field without touching the field itself.

This prevents the solution from damaging the label if fluid drips or runs down the side of the bottle.

5 Hold the bottle of solution about 10 cm (4 inches) above the container that will receive the liquid. Pour carefully to avoid spills or splashes. Do not touch the field with the lid of the bottle.

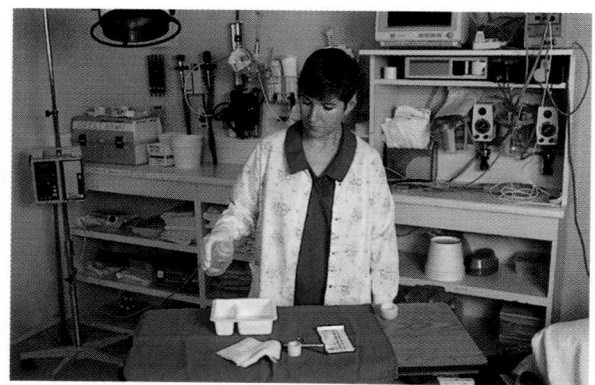

Pouring the sterile liquid.

If you get the surface of a permeable sterile field wet, it is no longer sterile. The bottle cannot touch the sterile field for the same reason.

6 Replace the lid on the bottle tightly.
Eliminates the risk of spilling the bottle during the procedure.

7 Put on the second (or both) sterile glove(s).

Performing a Surgical Hand Scrub

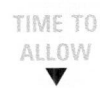

TIME TO ALLOW
▼

Novice:
Determined by agency policy
Expert:
Determined by agency policy

This procedure removes as many microorganisms from your hands as possible before entering a surgical field.

Delegation Guidelines

The scope of nursing assistant duties in a surgical arena does not generally require the completion of a surgical hand scrub. Nursing assistants may be responsible for the assembly of scrub supplies and should be familiar with this procedure for this purpose alone.

Equipment Needed

- Agency-approved antimicrobial agent.
- Surgical scrub brush (with plastic nail cleaning stick).
- Deep sink with knee or foot controls for water and soap.

1 Apply surgical attire, including shoe covers, cap or hood, face mask, and protective eyewear (possibly a mask with a face shield).

2 Open a scrub brush so that it is ready for use. Turn on the water using the control lever and adjust it to a comfortably warm temperature.

3 Wet your hands and arms, keeping your elbows flexed so that your hands remain higher than your elbows. Water will flow off your arms at the elbows.
Keeps the hands as the cleanest part of the extremities.

4 Use the plastic nail stick to clean under your nails on both hands.
Removes materials under the fingernails that could harbor a variety of microorganisms.

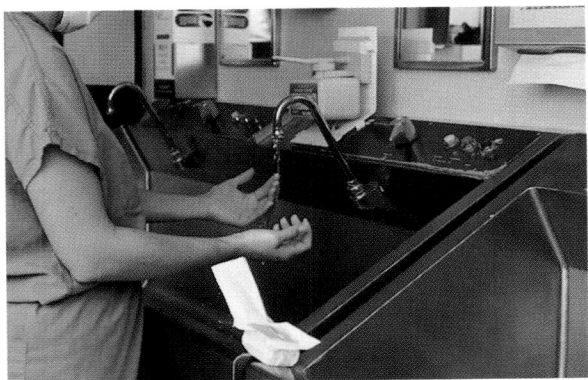

Scrub brush ready for use.

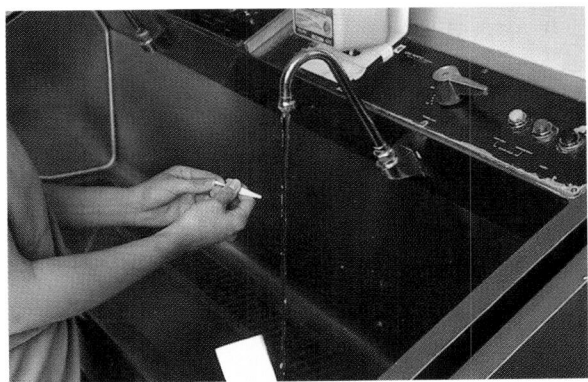

Using the plastic nail stick to clean under the fingernails.

5 Remove the scrub brush from its wrapper and wet it. Apply antimicrobial liquid if not already in the brush or according to agency policy.

Continued

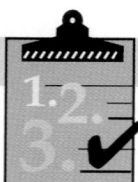

PROCEDURE 27–6 *(continued)*

Performing a Surgical Hand Scrub

6 Scrub the nails of one hand with 15 strokes. Repeat for the other hand. Scrub the palm of one hand, each side of the thumbs and fingers, and the back of the hand with 10 strokes each. Repeat for the other hand.

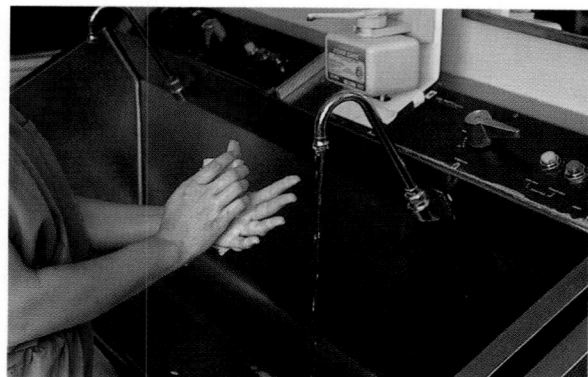

Scrubbing the palm.

Provides sufficient time for removal of microorganisms by mechanical and chemical means.

7 Divide your arms mentally into thirds. Beginning with the section nearest your hands, scrub each third with 10 strokes or by time, according to agency policy. Discard the brush.

8 Flex your arms and rinse from the fingertips to the elbow in a single smooth motion, again letting the water run off at the elbows.

Keeps the hands as the cleanest part of the extremities.

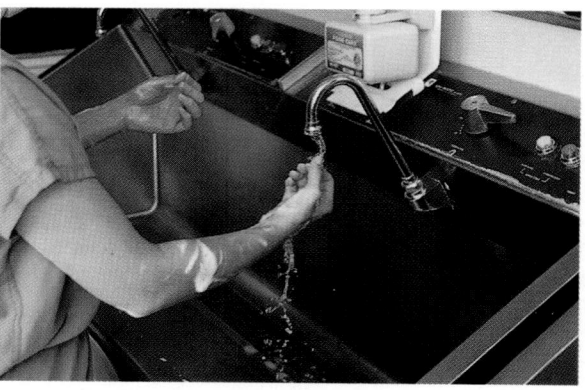

Rinsing from the fingertips to the elbow.

9 Release water control and walk backward into the operating room with your hands elevated in front of you and away from your body.

Allows you to keep cleansed hands above waist level and in your line of vision. Reduces the possibility that your hands will become contaminated.

10 Go to the sterile set-up area. Pick up a sterile towel without dripping water onto the sterile field. Using one end of the towel, dry one hand completely using a rotating motion and moving from fingers to elbow.

Dries from cleanest area (fingers) to less clean (elbows).

11 Using other end of towel, repeat with other hand and drop the towel into the designated receptacle or an assistant's hand.

---

varicella (chicken pox) inoculations; in this case they should not be allowed to visit. These vaccines are live viral preparations, and although they do not put persons with normal immune systems at risk, those with altered protection against infection can become seriously ill from shed viral particles.

To prevent a sense of isolation, encourage clients to have visitors if they have no signs of infection. Assess the support systems available to these clients once they go home. Although the numbers of visitors may be limited at any one time, visiting by the client's friends and relatives is beneficial to the client. Encourage the client to participate in activities that can be done in the home while maintaining relationships with friends and family through telephone conversations and intermittent visits.

Providing Client and Family Teaching

As a starting point for client education, recall that teaching should include any family or friends that will be involved in the client's care. Teach the client about the disease process and its underlying basis. This must include information about the change in ability to fight infections of any kind. Teach the client the basics of infection control and about the importance of keeping the environment as clean as possible, even though all germs cannot be eliminated.

PROCEDURE 27–7

Donning a Sterile Gown and Closed Gloving

TIME TO
ALLOW
▼

Novice:
Variable.
Expert:
7–10 min.

This procedure is done prior to entering a surgical (sterile) field.

Delegation Guidelines

The scope of nursing assistant duties in a surgical arena does not generally require the donning of a sterile gown and closed gloving. A nursing assistant may be responsible for the assembly of these supplies and should be familiar with this procedure for this purpose alone.

Equipment Needed

- Surgical shoe covers, cap, mask, and protective eyewear.
- One package sterile gloves of appropriate size.
- One sterile pack containing sterile gown.
- Clean, flat, dry surface for opening gown and gloves (such as a Mayo stand).

1 Don surgical attire and scrub your arms and hands as described in the Performing a Surgical Hand Scrub procedure.

2 Have the circulating nurse or other designated person open sterile gown and gloves.

Donning the Gown

1 Pick up and unfold the gown.
a. Identify the inner surface of the gown and pick up the gown beneath the neckband without touching the sterile field or the outer surface of the gown.
b. Make sure you have control of all the folded layers to avoid dangling the gown against unsterile surfaces.
c. Move away from the table, holding the gown away from your body at arm's length, and allow it to unfold from the top down. Do not let the gown touch the floor.
Maintains sterility of the gown.

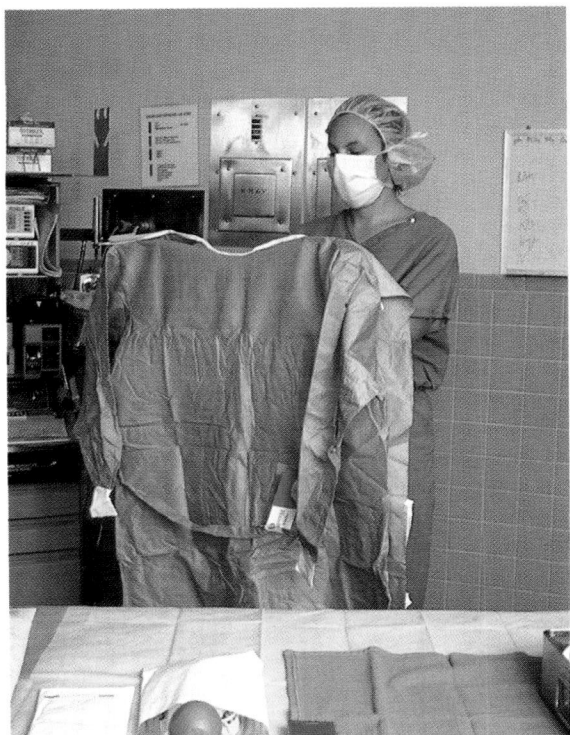

Holding the gown at arm's length and allowing it to unfold.
Continued

Donning a Sterile Gown and Closed Gloving

2 Put on the gown.

a. Hold the gown just below the neckband near the shoulders and slide both hands into the sleeves until the fingers are at the end of the cuffs but not through the cuffs.

The fingers remain covered to prepare for closed gloving.

b. Have someone tie the gown.

The gown should be lapped over itself in the back. The person tying the gown should take care to only touch the ties and not the front or sides of the gown. The front of the gown is sterile.

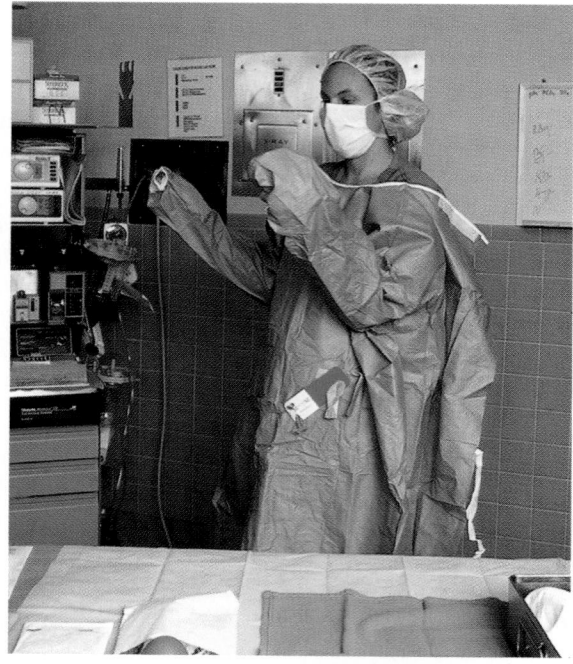

Sliding the hands into the sleeves.

Adding the Gloves

1 Apply the first glove.

a. With your hands covered by the sterile gown cuffs, open the inner sterile glove package and pick up the first glove by the cuff. The first glove goes on the dominant hand.

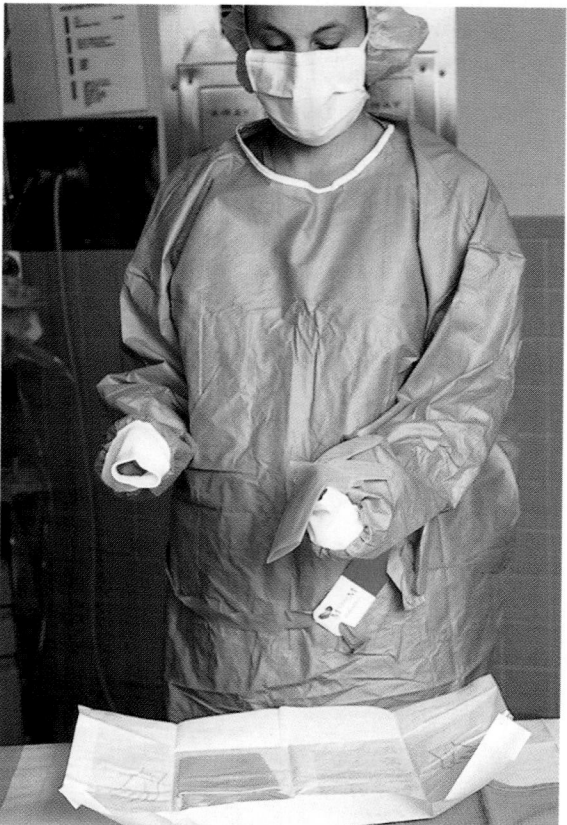

Picking up the first glove by the cuff.

b. Position the glove on the forearm so the cuff faces the hand and the fingers face the elbow.
c. Begin to put the opposite hand into the glove. Hold the cuff edge of the glove with the sleeve cover of the hand to be gloved. Grasp the back of the glove cuff with the sleeve-covered second hand and turn the cuff over the sleeve.

The fingertips of the hand you are gloving remain inside the sterile sleeve until the sleeve is covered by the sterile glove.

d. Push your fingers into the glove.

2 Apply the second glove.
a. Use your sterile hand to pick up the second glove.
b. Put the second glove in the same position as the first on the opposite forearm.

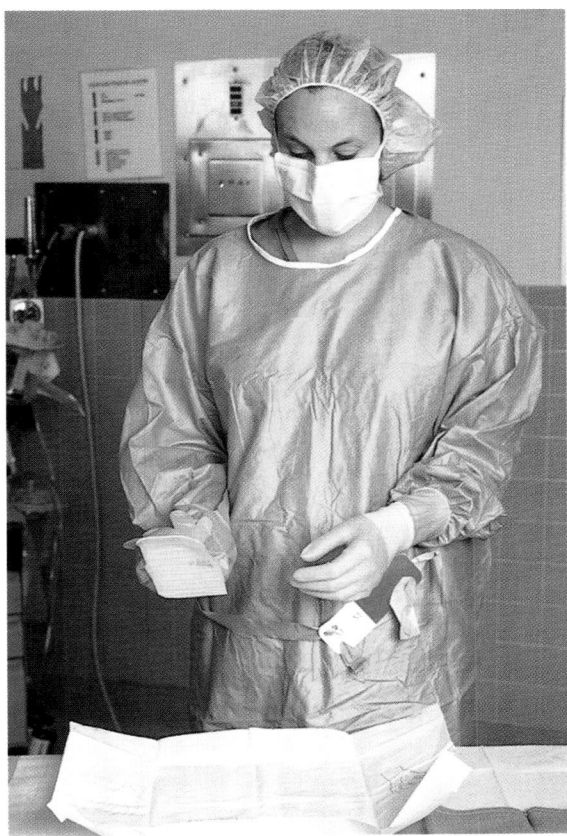

Positioning the second glove with the cuff facing the hand and the fingers facing the elbow.

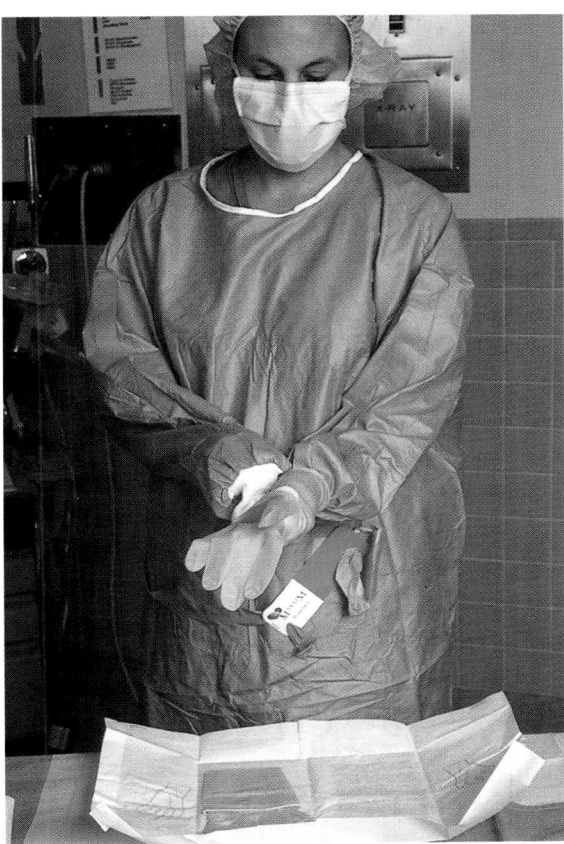

Pushing the fingers into the first glove.

Continued

Donning a Sterile Gown and Closed Gloving

c. Put on the second glove in the same manner as the first.

3 Adjust the gloves for fit and comfort.

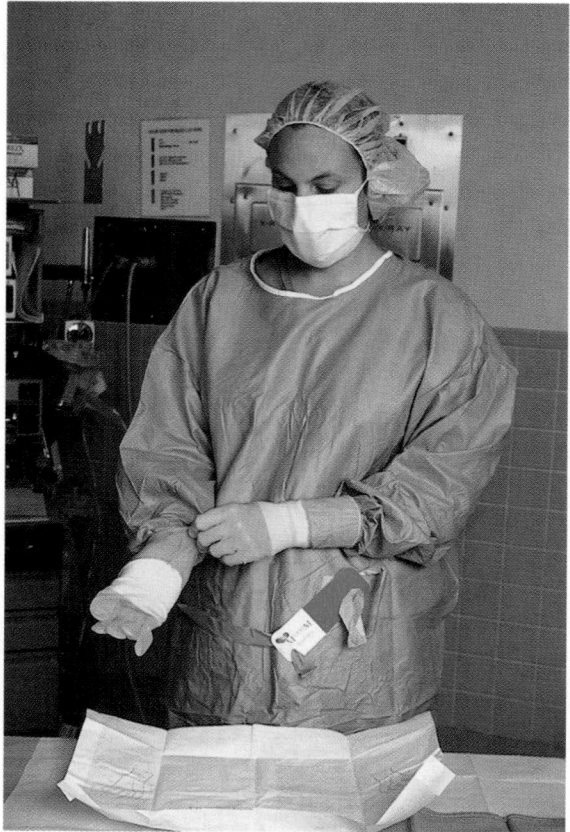

Putting on the second glove.

Other important topics for client teaching can then follow. Explain that infections that might be considered a nuisance to some will be life-threatening for the client. Teach the client about the signs and symptoms of infection to watch for, and remind the client that these may be subtle. Tell the client to report any physical changes in general health to the primary health caregiver immediately, so that the client can be evaluated as soon as possible. Subtle signs might include a change in ability to tolerate activity and quite possibly will not include fever or pain. Any rashes or skin breakdown should be reported as well. Changes in bowel habits should be noted as well as any increase in respiratory secretions. Any ear ache or continuing headache could also be an underlying symptom of infection. The timeliness of the client in reporting these subtle signs is important to reduce the risk of severe infection in the immunocompromised client.

Interventions to Reduce Your Own Risk of Infection

To reduce the risk of infection for the health care worker, strict adherence to guidelines provided by the CDC is necessary. By using hand-washing and barrier precautions when necessary, health care workers can minimize the risk for infection. Health care workers should consider the same precautions that they use for their clients to be of use when protecting themselves. Use clean technique to prevent the spread of infection to health care personnel when in contact with the client. Thoroughly wash your hands after client contact to reduce the risk of spreading the infection. If you do have a possible exposure, comply with recommended health service follow-up to minimize the potential risk. Table 27–5 provides an overview of the follow-up treatment recommended after exposure to blood-borne pathogens.

TABLE 27–5
Follow-Up for Health Care Workers Exposed to Blood-Borne Pathogens

Pathogen	Follow-Up
Unknown	• Contact should be tested for known blood-borne diseases utilizing the fast HIV screening test.
	• If contact tests positive for HIV, immediate prophylaxis with anti-HIV medications should be begun.
	• CDC recommends triple-antibiotic treatment at the site of exposure.
	• If contact does not test positive and health care worker has never undergone hepatitis B immunization, hepatitis B gamma-globulin should be administered and immunization should be started per agency protocol.
	• Health care worker should immediately be screened for the same blood-borne infections and, if negative, return for follow-up screening per agency protocol.
HIV	• If the client was positive for HIV, the health care worker should also be screened and be started on HIV prophylaxis, which could include up to three antiviral drugs.
	• The health care worker should return for follow-up screening for at least a year or according to the employing agency's recommendation.
Hepatitis B	• If the health care worker is immune, hepatitis B immunoglobulin can be offered.
	• If the health care worker is nonimmune, hepatitis B immunoglobulin will be offered and immunization begun.
Hepatitis C, D	• Health care worker can be offered immunoglobulin.
	• Initial and follow-up screening should be done according to agency guidelines.

EVALUATION

Evaluation of goal achievement of health protection involves reassessment of the client to determine that the criteria for evaluation have been met.

A discharge note for Luisa after her treatment for her dehydration secondary to effects of an upper respiratory infection might look like this:

> Infant with clear breath sounds and unlabored respirations, and without apparent nasal discharge. Tympanic temperature 98.6°F without receiving acetaminophen during the past 12 hours. Infant appears alert when awake, actively sucking at the breast, voiding freely. Intake has been PO without IV fluids for the last 12 hours. Skin turgor elastic. Infant appears free of pain without any noticeable distress when parents are present. Utilizing the translator, Mr. and Mrs. Martez accurately verbalized the instructions to continue the antibiotic until all of the medication is complete. Additionally, they have stated that they will follow up with the pediatrician at the local clinic within a week. At this appointment they will ask for information on Luisa's immunizations, request that they be updated, and request a record of all their children's immunizations.

With this note the nurse has documented that the initial diagnosis of *Altered protection* has been resolved. Additionally, the nurse, through a translator, has established new goals for the parents to attain. The nurse can assist the parents in establishing new goals with statements such as "With Luisa more like herself we need to focus on keeping her healthy and at home with her family."

If the outcomes do not progress as anticipated, a reassessment could provide information as to why. If a client who has received antibiotics for 7 days continues to show signs of inflammation and general mal-aise, the culture and sensitivity should be reassessed. This may involve reculturing the primary site of infection and/or looking for additional or new sites of infection.

Evaluation allows for continual review of the nursing care. By connecting outcomes to the interventions, nurses can evaluate the effectiveness of those interventions, as suggested in the Nursing Care Planning chart. In most instances, this requires the active participation of the clients and their families. If a client has been instructed to clean a wound two times a day and re-dress it applying antibiotic ointment and then arrives 2 days later in the emergency room with odorous, green drainage from the wound, the nurse may question the client's understanding or willingness to participate in the procedure.

KEY PRINCIPLES

- All of us are at risk for infection. There is no environment without organisms having the potential for causing disease.
- Humans have important physical and physiological mechanisms to protect ourselves from disease-causing organisms.
- Primary defenses against infections include the skin and the membrane barriers of the respiratory, GI, and GU tracts.
- Additional defenses against infection include molecules secreted by skin and membrane cells that provide additional barriers and may break down disease-causing organisms.
- Secondary defenses can be found in the immune system, which have both nonspecific disease-fighting components and very specific components in the immunoglobulin system.

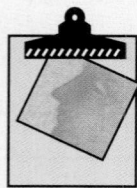

NURSING CARE PLANNING
AN INFANT WITH SEPSIS

Admission Data

Luisa is admitted through the emergency department to a general pediatric floor. The emergency room nurse telephones the following report.

Luisa is a 6-month-old Hispanic infant presenting with dehydration. Intravenous fluids have been started. Blood cultures have been drawn, as well as a CBC. Infant is lethargic. Her parents are at the bedside. She appears to have an upper respiratory infection. A CXR has been done. Her oxygen saturation is 99% on room air. She has mild intercostal and subcostal retractions. Her left ear shows redness and is fluid-filled. Throat swabs were negative for strep.

Physician's Orders

Admitting diagnosis: Dehydration, possible sepsis.
IV fluids D$_{10}$W to infuse at 25 mL/hr.
Ampicillin IV q 12 hr.
Gentamicin IV q 12 hr.

Tylenol PO 50 mg PRN q 3–4 hr for temp >100.4°F.
May breast-feed as tolerated, 20 cal/oz formula plus iron on demand when mother not available to breast-feed.

Nursing Assessment

Color pale, skin dry, with "tenting" noted, lethargic. Coarse breath sounds with mild retractions noted, rate 40/min. Heart rate regular with no murmur audible, rate = 90/min. Peripheral pulses weak but palpable, equal bilaterally. Bowel sounds active. Diaper dry (no urine output since admission). Tympanic temperature 103°F. Mother and father at bedside, quiet, appear frightened.

NURSING CARE PLAN

Nursing Diagnosis	Expected Outcomes	Interventions	Evaluation (After 24 Hours of Care)
Risk for infection related to upper respiratory congestion, age, dehydration.	Patent airway; infant with unlabored respirations; nares without discharge.	Teach parents use of bulb syringe; encourage them to suction nares PRN.	Mother uses bulb syringe to remove drainage from nose. Retractions decreased after suctioning.
	Normal hydration.	Use infusion pump to control IV fluid at 25 mL/hr.	Voiding >5 mL/kg/hr. Skin turgor elastic.
		Encourage mother to breast-feed.	Weak sucking at breast. IV fluids continued.
	Absence of fever.	Give Tylenol whenever temp. >100.4°. Evaluate effectiveness q 4 hr.	Temperature 99.6°F with last vital signs. No Tylenol for 6 hours.
	Normal tone.	*Encourage mother to interact with infant when she's awake.*	Infant alert when awake, active with handling. Absence of pain.
	Antibiotics as ordered.	Give antibiotics on time.	Infant without signs of distress when parents present.

Italicized interventions indicate culturally specific care.

Critical Thinking Questions

1. What other interventions can you think of to make the care delivered to Luisa more culturally specific?
2. What should the nurse be thinking about in order to incorporate cultural considerations in discharge planning?
3. What specific teaching would you provide to Luisa's mother to ensure that another episode such as this does not occur?

- Clients with breaks in the primary defenses have the nursing diagnosis *Risk for infection;* those with inadequate secondary defenses have *Altered protection.*
- Using the initial assessment of the client, the nurse develops plans of care to provide for the health protection of the client. The assessment includes physical findings and an evaluation of the client's mental status and social support system.
- Interventions may include education, modification of the client's physical environment, administration of antibiotics to eliminate or prevent the spread of infection, and psychosocial support.
- The outcome goals for any client are to minimize the risk of infection and to protect against further spread of infection for both the client and those caring for or associating with the client.

BIBLIOGRAPHY

Ackerly, L. (1996). Home hygiene with a baby: The new approach to advising parents. *Professional Care of Mother and Child, 6*(4), 99–102.

Ament, L.A., & Whalen, E. (1996). Sexually transmitted diseases in pregnancy: Diagnosis, impact, and intervention. *Journal of Obstetric, Gynecologic, and Neonatal Nursing, 25*(8), 657–666.

Anonymous. (1995). Proposed recommended practices for establishing and maintaining a sterile field. *Association of Operating Room Nurses Journal, 64*(4), 608–610.

Beardsley, T. (1996). Science and the citizen: Resisting resistance. *Scientific American, 274*(1), 26.

Belluck, P., & Drew, C. (1998). Deadly bacteria a new threat to fruit and produce in U.S. *The New York Times,* January 4, 1998.

Carpenter, M.T. (1996). Postoperative joint infections in rheumatoid arthritis clients on methotrexate therapy. *Orthopedics, 19*(3), 207–210.

Centers for Disease Control and Prevention. (1996). Prevention of perinatal group B streptococcal disease: A public health prospective. *Morbidity and Mortality Weekly Report. 45*(RR-7), 1–24.

Centers for Disease Control and Prevention. (1995). *Food and water borne bacterial diseases.* March 1995 update. Atlanta, GA.

Clar, R.A. (1995). Infections during the postpartum period. *Journal of Obstetric, Gynecologic, and Neonatal Nursing, 24*(6), 542–548.

Corrarino, J.E. (1998). Perinatal hepatitis B: Update and recommendations. *The American Journal of Maternal/Child Nursing, 23*(5), 246–252.

Crow, S. (1996). Prevention of intravascular infections ways and means. *Journal of Intravenous Nursing, 19*(4), 175–181.

Eliopoulos, G.M. (1995). Infections in diabetes mellitus. *Infectious Disease Clinics of North America, 9*(1), xi–xii, 1–216.

Garner, J. (1996). Guideline for isolation precautions in hospitals. *Infection Control and Hospital Epidemiology, 17,* 53–80.

Jackson, M.M. (1995). Nurses: At special risk. *Journal of Obstetric, Gynecologic, and Neonatal Nursing, 24*(6), 533–540.

Hennessey, T., Hedberg, C., Slutsker, L., White, K., Besser-Wiek, J., & Moen, M. (1996). A national outbreak of Salmonella enteritis infections from ice cream. *New England Journal of Medicine, 334,* 1281–1286.

Howser, R.L. (1995). What you need to know about corticosteroid therapy. *American Journal of Nursing, 95*(8), 44–48.

Kendig, S. (1995). Women at risk for infection: The woman who is chemically dependent. *Journal of Obstetric, Gynecologic, and Neonatal Nursing, 24*(8), 776–781.

Kontoyiannis, D.P. (1995). Infection in the organ transplant recipient: An overview. *Infectious Disease Clinics of North America, 9*(4), 811–822.

Lassiter, S.M. (1995). *Multicultural clients: A professional handbook for health care providers and social workers.* Westport: Greenwood Press.

Polinski, C. (1996). The value of the white blood cell count and differential in the prediction of neonatal sepsis. *Neonatal Network, 15*(7), 13–23.

Sale, P.G. (1995). Genitourinary infection in older women. *Journal of Obstetric, Gynecologic, and Neonatal Nursing, 24*(8), 769–775.

Shewmake, P.A. (1996). Clean versus sterile technique. *Journal of Wound Care Nursing, 23*(1), 61–62.

Shewmake, P.A. (1995). Frankly speaking. Point of view: clean vs. sterile technique. *Home Care Nurse News, 2*(5), 5–6.

Simpkins, S.M., Hench, C.P., & Chatic, G. (1996). Management of the obstetric client with tuberculosis. *Journal of Obstetric, Gynecologic, and Neonatal Nursing, 25*(4), 305–312.

Smith, C.D. (1995) Clinical issues: Cover gowns; surgical hand scrubs; smoke evacuators; operative record abbreviations; open sterile setups. *Association of Operating Room Nurses Journal, 61*(4), 753–754.

Thompson, D.G. (1995). Incorporating immunization schedules into NICU care. *Neonatal Network, 14*(3), 71–73.

Thompson, J. (1995). Clinical issues: Open sterile supplies; dress codes; eyeglass holders; insect control; sterile sleeves; compression stockings. *Association of Operating Room Nurses Journal, 62*(6), 939–940.

Ungvarski, P.J. (1997). Update on HIV infection. *American Journal of Nursing, 97*(1), 44–52.

Walter, E.A. (1995). Infection in the bone marrow transplant recipient. *Infectious Disease Clinics of North America, 9*(4), 823–847.

Weinstein, R. (1998). Nosocomial infection update. *Emerging Infectious Diseases, 4*(3), 1–7.

Wrighton, P. (1996). Incidence of infection after Cesarean section: A study. *Nursing Standard, 10*(37), 34–37.

Yoshikawa, T.T. (1996). Progress in geriatrics: Approach to fever and infection in the nursing home. *Journal of the American Geriatrics Society, 44*(1), 74–82.

Zwerneman, K.R. (1995). Research for practice: Use aseptic technique for tube feedings. *American Journal of Nursing, 95*(2), 58.

Health Protection: Risk for Injury

Beatriz Nieto

Key Terms

aspiration
burns
choking
injury
poisoning

restraint
strangulation
suffocation
trauma

LEARNING OBJECTIVES

After studying this chapter, you should be able to:

1. Discuss the epidemiology of common injuries from falls, suffocation, and poisoning.

2. Discuss the epidemiology of trauma from burns, electricity, motor vehicle accidents, and radiation.

3. Identify the behavioral, environmental, socioeconomic, developmental, cognitive, and physiological factors that affect safety.

4. Assess the client's risk for injury.

5. Distinguish between related nursing diagnoses for the client at risk for injury.

6. Plan interventions to prevent injury and promote safety in the acute care setting, the client's home, and the community.

7. Evaluate client outcomes and nursing interventions used to help the client reduce the risk of injury.

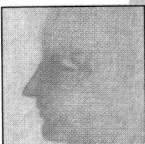

Juanita Soto is a 75-year-old widow who lives alone in a two-story house. Her sons and daughters live in distant cities and visit her whenever they can. She relies primarily on her neighbors and friends for help. Juanita has been relatively healthy most of her life and has been able to keep up her home despite the fact that, 5 years ago, she was diagnosed with rheumatoid arthritis. During the last 4 months, however, her condition has worsened. She now uses her wheelchair to get around the house, although she sometimes uses a cane to navigate the flight of stairs that leads downstairs to the washer and drier. She complains of pain and weakness in her hands and legs. At her last physician visit, she was referred to a local home health agency for evaluation of her condition and her needs.

During the initial assessment visit, the home health nurse notes that, in addition to having limited hand and leg movement, Juanita is partially blind in one eye. The nurse also notes that Juanita's home needs some repairs, especially the stairs. They are old and have no railing for support. Because of the many physical and environmental factors identified, the nurse considers the diagnosis of *Risk for injury*. He also considers related nursing diagnoses for clients with safety needs.

HEALTH AND SAFETY NURSING DIAGNOSES

Risk for injury: A state in which the inidividual is at risk of injury as a result of environmental conditions interacting with the individual's adaptive and defensive resources.

Risk for trauma: Accentuated risk of accidental tissue injury, e.g., wound, burn, fracture.

Risk for poisoning: Accentuated risk of accidental exposure to, or ingestion of, drugs or dangerous products in doses sufficient to cause poisoning.

Risk for suffocation: Accentuated risk of accidental suffocation (inadequate air available for inhalation).

Risk for aspiration: The state in which an individual is at risk for entry of gastro-intestinal secretions, oropharyngeal secretions, or solids or fluids into tracheo-bronchial passages.

From North American Nursing Diagnosis Association. (1999). NANDA Nursing diagnoses: Definitions and classification 1999–2000. Philadelphia: Author.

CONCEPTS OF SAFETY

Every person has an inherent need to be and feel safe. Feeling safe allows us to think and act with confidence. Although at birth we depend on someone else for our safety, as we mature we become responsible for our own safety. Eventually, we may even become responsible for the safety of others. Thus, safety is a need that remains with us throughout our lifetime.

Client safety is a major issue in all health care settings. Injuries, whether from environmental hazards or traumatic accidents, affect people of all ages, developmental stages, and socioeconomic groups. Injuries can result from behavioral, environmental, or physiological hazards. No matter the cause, they can have devastating effects on both the client and family. Injuries may result in pain, emotional distress, financial hardship, permanent disability, and even death.

As a nurse, you must always be aware of the potential for injury and make it a high priority to promote safety guidelines that help prevent injuries. Doing so can reduce the need for hospitalizations, reduce the risk of complications from medical treatment, reduce the hardship of long-term care, and even reduce the loss of life. Together with your clients, you can develop a plan of action to ensure the safest possible environment.

No matter what type of client you care for—a new mother, an elderly homebound client living alone, a group of clients living in a long-term care facility—you can never take their safety for granted. In fact, you should consider this issue not only with individual clients but also at the community, national, and international levels.

Epidemiology of Injury

An **injury** is clinically defined as trauma or damage to some part of the body. According to the National Cen-ter for Health Statistics (1996), accidental injuries are the fifth leading cause of death in the United States. Injury can result from physical, mechanical, biological, or chemical agents. Accidents that result most commonly in death include motor vehicle accidents and falls.

Falls

Elderly people form the group affected most often by falls, both at home and in institutional settings. Multiple falls are more common among people over age 74 and are the second leading cause of accidental death in that age group (Brady et al., 1993). When a fall occurs, morbidity, immobility, early nursing home placement, or death may result. Because of frequent occurrence and serious consequences, falls are one of the most serious problems that acute-care and long-term care facilities must manage (Hendrich, Nyhuis, Kippenbrock, & Soja, 1995).

Falls occurring in the home are a major concern and account for most reported home accidents in people age 75 and above. The pathophysiological changes that occur with aging—such as an altered gait, decreased mobility, incontinence, and confusion—place many elderly people at increased risk of falling (Hendrich, Nyhuis, Kippenbrock, & Soja, 1995).

Action Alert!
Assess elderly clients for unsteady gait, impaired memory or judgment, weakness, and a history of falls.

When older clients fall, the biggest concern is the threat of a hip fracture. Hip fracture is the primary cause of more than 200,000 hospital admissions each year. In about 8 out of 10 cases, the affected person is age 65 or over (Hendrich, Nyhuis, Kippenbrock, & Soja, 1995).

Falls tend to occur in the home when mobility and coordination are limited, when the person is in a hurry, or when the person is stressed or faced with obstacles. Stairways are commonly involved in falls at home. Factors that contribute to these falls include poor lighting, obstacles on the stairs, and poorly repaired steps. Falls that occur in the bathroom commonly involve a slippery tub or shower.

The risk for falling is significantly increased among hospitalized clients, accounting for up to 90% of all reported falls (Brady et al., 1993). Hospital falls most commonly occur in the client's room when the client is alone, trying to get to the bathroom unassisted (Hendrich, Nyhuis, Kippenbrock, & Soja, 1995). In one studied population, the use of side rails and restraints did not prevent falls because most of the clients who fell had either removed the restraint or had exited the bed safely, only to fall while walking without assistance. Polypharmacy (the use of several medications at once) was also present in all the clients who fell.

> One day when the home care nurse comes to visit with Mrs. Soto, her daughter is there. The daughter is telling Mrs. Soto that she should sell her home and come to stay with the daughter's family. Can you list the possible concerns that prompted Mrs. Soto's daughter to make this suggestion?

Suffocation

As a specific term, **suffocation** refers to a lack of oxygen caused either by airway obstruction or by oxygen starvation from insufficient atmospheric oxygen. As a general term, suffocation refers to an interruption in breathing that results in a severe lack of oxygen (asphyxia). This lack of oxygen can result specifically from aspiration, choking, or strangulation. **Aspiration** is the inspiration of foreign material into the airway. **Choking** is an internal obstruction of the airway by food or a foreign body. Critical changes in body chemistry caused by choking may quickly become life-threatening. If not immediately relieved, they may result in death. Choking can result from aspiration. **Strangulation** is constriction of the airway from an external cause.

Choking on food or objects and aspirating them into the airway as well as suffocating caused by materials that block the external airway are of special concern in young children and elderly people. Death rates from choking are especially high during the first few years of life. Each year, about 75 children under age 5 die from choking. Choking on nonfood items causes an additional 150 deaths per year. According to the World Health Organization Statistics Annual (1995), about 3,000 people died in 1994 from choking and suffocation.

In the older adult or neurologically impaired client, choking and aspiration can result from the loss or absence of protective airway reflexes. They also can occur in clients who are unconscious from drugs, alcohol, cerebrovascular accident (stroke), or cardiac arrest, or when a nonfunctioning nasogastric tube allows gastric contents to drain around the tube. Other causes that can lead to choking and aspiration in the older adult or neurologically impaired client may include ill-fitting dentures and overzealous feeding. As-

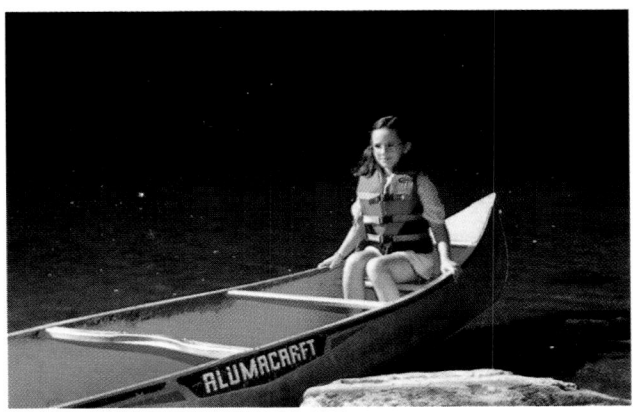

Figure 28–1. The use of a life jacket can promote water safety.

piration of stomach contents is a serious complication that may result in death.

Suffocation can result when air is blocked from outside the body, as when a child is caught in an airtight compartment from which the oxygen is gradually depleted by breathing; when airtight material, such as plastic, covers the nose and mouth; or when the chest is compressed so that breathing is impossible, as in some crushing injuries (Wilson, Baker, Teret, Shock, & Gabarino et al., 1991).

Accidental drowning, resulting in suffocation, is also of major concern. For children ages 1 to 3 years, accidental drowning is the leading cause of injury and death (Wintemute, 1992). Drowning is the third most common cause of death among adolescents (Castiglia, 1995). Children under age 1 drown most often in bathtubs. Children ages 1 to 4 years drown most often in residential swimming pools, although bathtubs, toilets, and water buckets are also common. The usual sites of adolescent drownings include lakes and other natural bodies of water. Contributing factors that may increase the risk of drowning include inadequate supervision, lack of safety devices, hazardous swimming conditions, careless boating and water sports, and the use of alcohol and drugs (Fig. 28–1).

Strangulation of a child can be caused by plastic bags, playpens, cribs, highchairs, clothing, drapery cords, drowning, or entrapment in a confined space. Other causes of strangulation, according to Jones (1993), include hanging from highchair straps and wedging of the head between crib slats, accordion-style safety gates, a bed and wall, and electrically operated car windows. In a span of 10 years, drapery cord injuries accounted for about 118 deaths in the United States (Little, 1994).

Even in the health care environment, choking, aspiration, strangulation, and suffocation can occur. Clients with neurological deficits and impaired mobility are especially vulnerable. You will need to remember that these types of accidents are preventable.

Poisoning

Poisoning is clinically defined as an adverse condition or physical state resulting from the administration of a

CAUSATIVE AGENTS IN DEATHS FROM POISONING

The following list presents suspected causative agents in 705 deaths reported to poison control centers in the United States in 1992:

- Antidepressants, such as amitriptyline, desipramine, doxepin, imipramine, and nortriptyline.
- Analgesics, such as acetaminophen, aspirin, codeine, morphine, and propoxyphene.
- Cardiovascular medications, such as digoxin and verapamil.
- Street drugs, such as cocaine, heroin, and methamphetamine.
- Sedatives and hypnotics, such as phenobarbital.
- Antiasthmatic medications, such as theophylline.
- Fumes, gases, and vapors, such as carbon monoxide and hydrogen sulfide.
- Chemicals, such as cyanide and strychnine.
- Insecticides, such as diazinon.
- Household cleaners, such as sodium hypochlorite (bleach).
- Hydrocarbons, such as butane.
- Alcohol, especially the ethanol form.
- Automotive products, such as ethylene glycol and methanol.

From Loomis, T. A., & Hayes, A. W. (1996). Loomis' Essentials of Toxicology. San Diego: Academic Press, p. 14.

the label due to poor eyesight, illiteracy, or a language barrier (Fig. 28–2).

Like most other accidents, poisoning can be prevented by proper storage, labeling, and use of chemicals and other toxic agents (Table 28–1).

Action **A**lert!
Teach clients to prevent poisonings through proper storage and labeling of containers. For hospitalized clients, triple-check all medications before administering them.

Epidemiology of Trauma

Clinically, **trauma** is defined as a physical injury or wound caused by a forceful, disruptive, or violent ac-

TABLE 28–1
Preventing Childhood Poisoning

Common Sources of Poisoning	Client Instructions to Prevent Poisoning
Medications	• Keep all medications out of the reach of children, preferably in locked cabinets. • Make sure that medication containers have childproof caps. • Store and label medications properly in their original containers. • Read medication labels carefully before administering a medication. • Do not share medications. • Use appropriate measuring devices when administering medications to ensure proper dosing. • Destroy expired medications promptly and appropriately. • Keep emergency numbers—including the local poison control center—near the phone and in plain view. • Never tell a child that a medication is candy. • Keep emergency medications (such as syrup of ipecac) in the home.
Chemicals, cleaning solutions, and other toxic substances	• Keep chemicals, cleaning solutions, and other toxic substances in locked cabinets. • Keep all such substances in their original containers with proper labels. • Maintain adequate ventilation when using chemicals and cleaning solutions. • Do not mix cleaning products, chemicals, and other such substances together.
House plants	• Keep out of reach of children. • Provide adequate supervision for young children and infants.

toxic substance. Toxic substances can produce injury or death through chemical action. They can enter the body through ingestion, inhalation, injection, application, or absorption of the noxious material. For example, accidental overdose of medications, mixing household cleaners, leaking carbon monoxide, and use of tainted street drugs can result in poisoning. There are currently more than 100,000 chemical entities to which the general population could be exposed and poisoned. Box 28–1 provides some examples. However, despite this multitude of potentially harmful chemicals, only a few have been adequately documented as causing serious health problems in humans (Loomis & Hayes, 1996).

The reasons for and types of poisonings vary with age. The people most at risk for poisoning include toddlers, young children, and adults with sensory impairment and communication barriers. Lack of adequate supervision and improper storage of toxic household substances are some of the major factors in poisonings in children. Among adolescents and adults, poisoning most often results from snake bites, recreational drugs, or suicide attempts. Poisonings among the elderly may result from medication overdose caused by mental impairment, polypharmacy, or difficulty reading

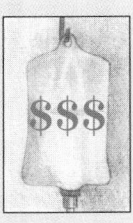

THE COST OF CARE
INJURIES

Component	Cost
Administrative expenses: Includes the administrative cost of public and private insurance, and police and legal costs.	$76.3 billion
Medical expenses: Includes physician fees, hospital charges, medicines, future medical costs, and ambulance, helicopter, and other emergency medical services.	$74.6 billion
Motor vehicle damage: Includes the value of property damage to vehicles from motor vehicle accidents.	$39.5 billion
Employer costs: Includes an estimate of the uninsured costs incurred by employers, representing the value of time lost by injured workers. It includes time spent investigating and reporting injuries and giving first aid, production slowdowns, hiring and training replacement workers, and the extra cost of overtime for noninjured workers.	$19.8 billion
Fire losses: Includes losses from both structural fires and nonstructural fires, such as those of vehicles, outside storage, crops, and timber.	$9.2 billion
Wages and productivity: Includes wages, fringe benefits, an estimate of the replacement-cost value of household services, and travel delays for motor vehicle accidents.	$222.4 billion
Total Cost	**$434.8 billion**

Information from National Safety Council. (1997). Accident facts: 1996. Washington, D.C.: Author.

tion. The impact from trauma can be profound to all those involved. Trauma is the leading cause of years of potential life lost, the fourth leading cause of death in the United States, and the cause of more than 150,000 deaths each year. Traumatic injury causes morbidity and disability and can create huge problems in lost productivity and medical costs, as shown in the Cost of Care chart. It has been estimated that each year, 57 million Americans (1 in 4) are injured seriously enough to require medical treatment.

Fires and Burns

Fire hazards can occur in all types of settings. Institutionalized clients are especially at risk for injury from fires because they may be debilitated and unable to escape without assistance. Also, the health care environment contains materials and equipment that may raise the risk of fire. They include flammable gases, such as oxygen and anesthetics, and electrical equipment, such as monitors, heating and cooling units, and respiratory equipment. Equipment that is malfunctioning or used improperly may cause sparks that could easily ignite linens, especially in an oxygen-rich environment.

Fires more commonly occur in the home setting. It has been estimated that, each year, house fires cause the deaths of about 1,200 children age 14 and under (Wilson, Baker, Teret, Shock, & Garbarino, 1991). Most house-fire deaths result from the poisoning effects of smoke inhalation rather than from burn injuries.

> Think again about Mrs. Soto. Is she at risk for injury from a fire? What would you assess about her home to determine the level of risk?

Cigarette smoking is a primary cause of fatal residential fires (Swartz, 1993). Consumption of alcohol has also been shown to increase the risk of fire injuries (Ballard, Koepsell, & Rivara, 1992). Residential fires seem to be more common during the winter months, when many families use portable heaters, fireplaces, and wood-burning stoves (Swartz, 1993).

Action Alert!
Urge clients to keep a portable heater at least 36 inches away from anything that might be flammable. Also, recommend that clients install a smoke detector with working batteries on each level of the home. Instruct clients to test the batteries weekly and to keep a multipurpose fire extinguisher on hand in case of fire (Fig. 28–3).

A **burn** is clinically defined as any injury caused by excessive exposure to electricity, chemicals, gases, radioactivity, or thermal agents. Besides fire, some of the

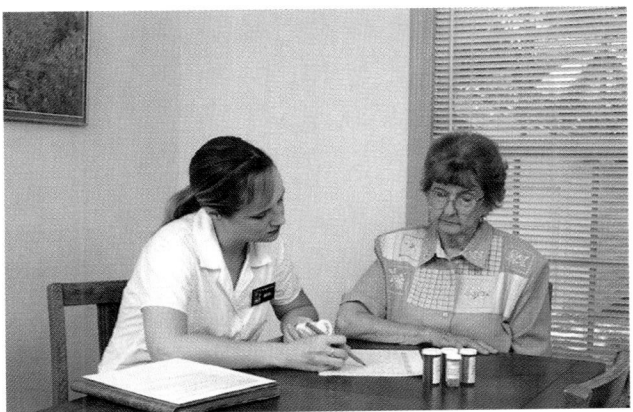

Figure 28–2. Teach a home-bound client that the proper labeling and storage of medications can help prevent accidental poisoning.

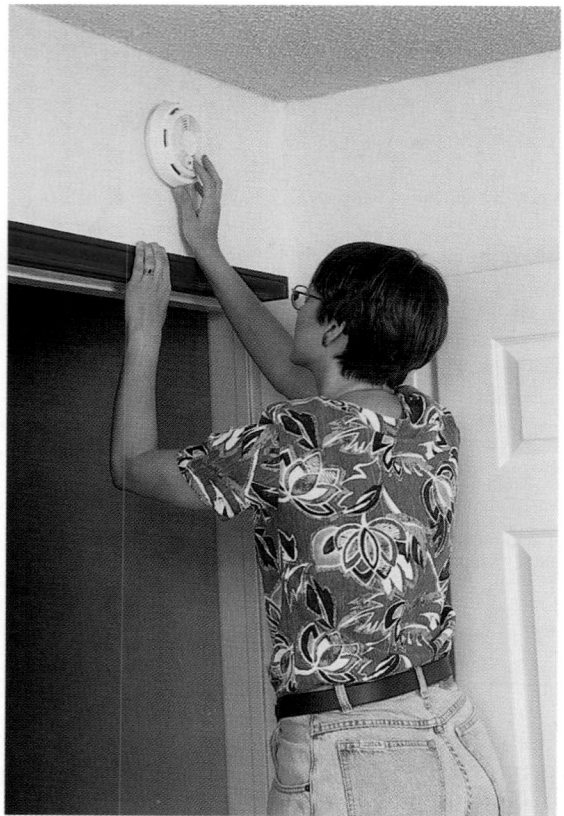

Figure 28–3. All smoke and fire detectors in the home should be installed properly and maintained with fresh batteries.

most common causes of burns in the home or health care institution include exposure to hot bath water, overly hot moist dressings, heat lamps, and other forms of equipment.

People at highest risk of burns include children age 14 and under, the handicapped, and elders with sensory impairments. Children are at risk for burns from inadequate parental supervision, misuse of matches, and exposure to hot liquids or vapors. Handicapped persons or elders with sensory impairments risk being burned from the unsafe use of space heaters, water heaters, stoves, and irons.

Electrical Shock

Injury from electrical shock can range from trivial burns to charring and destruction of the skin and underlying tissues. Hazards occurring from electrical shock are of concern both in the home and health care environment. Factors that determine the type and extent of electrical injury include the voltage involved, the type of current, the area and duration of contact, skin resistance, and the path along which the electrical current flows. Other factors include the type of clothing worn and environmental moisture (Mellen, Weedn, & Kao, 1992).

The most common type of electrical injuries are low-voltage injuries. They usually are accidental and involve electrical equipment, household appliances, or tools. Electrical shock results when current travels to the ground via the body instead of traveling through the electrical wiring. Fatalities from electrical hazards are relatively uncommon.

Motor Vehicle Accidents

Motor vehicle accidents are the leading cause of accidental death in the United States (National Center for Health Statistics, 1996). Unsafe driving practices and the use of alcohol and drugs contribute to the occurrences. Depending on the circumstances of the accident, persons at risk for sustaining injuries may include the driver, passengers, pedestrians, bicyclists, skateboarders, and so on. Children on bicycles or skateboards face an increased risk of injury when they fail to use proper safety equipment and precautions, such as wearing safety helmets and padding and following safety guidelines. Guidelines include using signals properly and not riding in traffic or near driveways (Fig. 28–4). Failure to use safety belts and infant car seats also increases the risk of injury.

Back Injuries

Back injury is a common and costly health problem that can occur in a variety of settings. It is quite common in the workplace. It often can be prevented by following guidelines such as those in the Teaching for Self-Care chart. Occupational back injury accounts for the greatest number of workers' compensation claims in the United States and Canada (Hodgson, 1996). Back injuries can have a tremendous impact on the individual, family, and society. They are the main reason for prolonged absence from work; the lost productivity creates substantial costs.

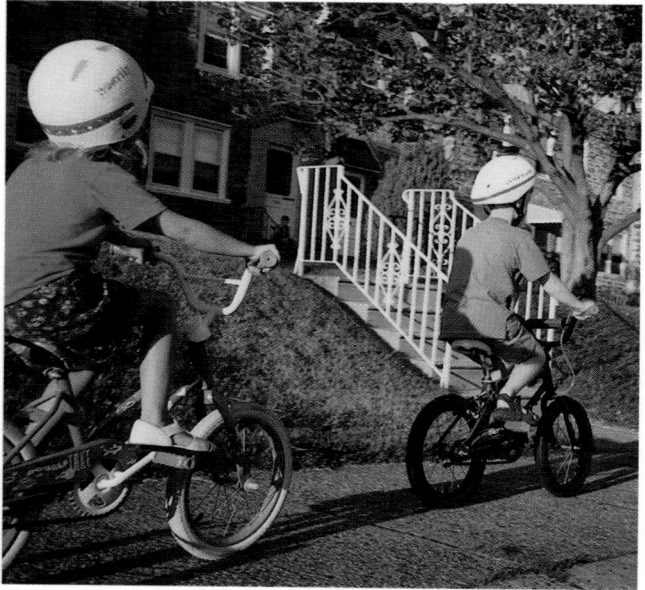

Figure 28–4. Recommend appropriate safety equipment to help prevent head injuries in school-age children.

Teaching for WELLNESS

PROTECT YOURSELF FROM JOB-RELATED BACK INJURIES

Purpose: To prevent back injuries when lifting and moving clients in the acute care setting.

Rationale: Back injuries are the most common work-related injury for health care personnel. Maintaining physical fitness, using good body mechanics, and performing thorough client assessment will help prevent back injuries.

Expected Outcome: The worker will not experience work-related back injuries.

Instructions

1. Maintain your own health. Eat a well-balanced diet, get a good night's sleep, and reduce stress in your life.
2. Maintain your level of physical fitness. Get regular exercise. Exercise for cardiovascular fitness through aerobic exercise and for muscle strength through weight-bearing exercises. Exercise 20 minutes a day to strengthen your back, leg, and abdominal muscles. Include stretching exercises before and after your exercise session.
3. Before you lift or move a client, assess the client's ability to help. Can the client move in bed, bear weight when standing, and cooperate with your instructions? How much does the client weigh? Is the range of motion sufficient to accomplish the move?
4. Assess your ability to bear the load. How much weight can you lift? Ask for assistance if necessary.
5. Arrange the environment to facilitate the move. For example, put the chair close to the bed when you are transferring a client to a chair. Move the furniture to allow you to get close to the client without twisting your back.
6. Use assistive devices to lessen your workload. A mechanical lift is suggested when the client is immobile and exceeds the weight you can lift. A gait belt is used to increase leverage and provide a firm grasp. A walker assists the client to balance and bear part of the body's weight.

Back pain and injuries can be caused by disk degeneration, obesity, postural problems, structural problems, and overstretching of the spinal supports. The consequences of injury may include prolonged pain and suffering, decreased quality of life, and a reduced potential for future earnings or job opportunities.

Certain job tasks and personal characteristics increase the probability of back injury. Job tasks include heavy lifting, repetitive lifts (especially while bending or twisting), prolonged sitting, working in a stooped or awkward position, and operating vibrating machinery (Phillips, Forrester, & Brown, 1996). Personal characteristics may include lack of job experience, obesity, smoking, alcohol consumption, job dissatisfaction, recent back injury, and lack of strength and overall physical fitness. Most back injuries probably result not from a single, stressful lifting event but rather develop gradually over time. Improper lifting techniques lead to more back injuries than any other single activity (Gustafson, 1995).

Radiation

Exposure to radiation in the form of energy, rays, or waves can lead to a variety of injuries, including radiation burns and radiation dermatitis. Radiation burns result from exposure to radiant energy in the form of sunlight, x-rays, or nuclear emissions or explosion. Exposure to ionizing radiation, as in cancer radiation therapy, can lead to an acute or chronic inflammation of skin known as radiation dermatitis. Symptoms including redness, blistering, and sloughing of the skin usually appear 3 weeks after exposure.

Exposure to radiation can occur in the community or the health care environment. Community risk increases near nuclear power plants and manufacturing industries that produce radioactive wastes. Working in proximity to microwaves and computer terminals can also increase exposure to radiation.

In the health care setting, you and other clinicians may be at risk when assisting with diagnostic procedures that use radioactive materials or caring for clients who have radioactive implants. Injury can occur if you fail to use lead shielding or follow the necessary safety procedures involving exposure time and distance from the radioactive source. Radiation can injure the skin, reproductive organs, bone marrow, gastrointestinal tract, and other parts of the body. The international radiation symbol notifies you and other health care workers of the danger of radiation injury (Fig. 28–5).

FACTORS AFFECTING SAFETY

Lifestyle Factors

A person's lifestyle can raise the risk of injury. Pertinent factors include not taking appropriate safety precautions, choosing a sedentary lifestyle, abusing chemical substances, and being unable or unwilling to provide self-care.

Lack of Safety Precautions

Careless behavior occurs when people are in highly stressful situations or have a general disregard for safety. Speeding while driving, smoking in bed, enter-

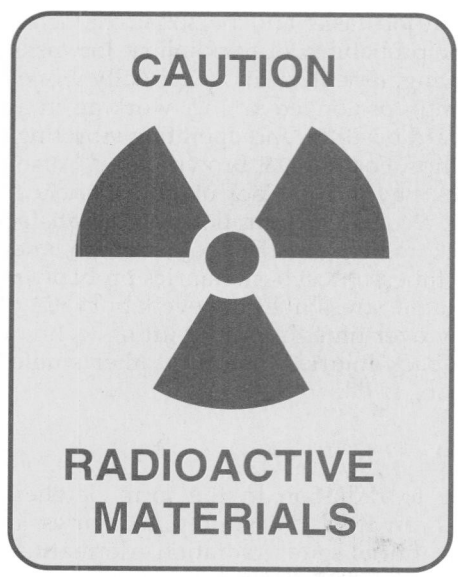

Figure 28–5. The International Radiation Symbol is commonly used in health care facilities.

ing high-crime areas at night, riding a bicycle without a helmet, and other risky behaviors invite accidents and injuries. Lack of safety precautions can affect people of all ages and walks of life. Supervision to prevent injury is important for the young child, elderly person, and mentally ill or disabled person.

Some people face a greater risk of injury because of their job or high-risk behaviors. They include people who drive or operate machinery under the influence of chemical substances, those who choose not to wear safety belts, those who exceed the posted speed limit when driving, those who work at dangerous jobs, and those who take risks and love the challenge that comes from jumping out of planes, climbing mountains, or racing cars.

Activity and Exercise

A lack of activity and exercise will negatively affect each body system and predispose the person to physiological as well as emotional hazards. Immobility increases the risk for falls and decreases the ability to flee from dangerous situations, including fires and other external hazards.

Despite the fact that activity and exercise are known to be beneficial, many people choose to live relatively inactive lives. A completely inactive lifestyle can limit a person's ability to experience and enjoy life to its fullest and will increase the risk of degenerative and chronic diseases, such as hypertension, ischemic heart disease, and diabetes.

Mrs. Soto has gradually become less active. You will need to suggest that she have her arthritis evaluated by a physician before planning a program to increase her activity. How would you approach this situation with her daughter?

Substance Abuse

The use of drugs and alcohol can affect every aspect of a person's life. Effects can encompass the loss of employment opportunities, the deterioration of personal relationships, violence, and tragic deaths. Substance abuse can reduce the person's judgment and coordination and the ability to complete typical tasks. Operating heavy equipment, driving cars, climbing ladders, or using chain saws while under the influence of alcohol are associated with a high risk for injury.

Environmental Factors

Our surroundings, no matter where we live, work, or play, are never completely hazard-free. Even when we take all the necessary precautions, there is no guarantee of our safety because we cannot be in total control of our environment. When assessing a client's environment and its potential for injury, consider the client's home, workplace, and community.

Home

The home environment contains hazards or potential hazards both inside and outside the home. Potential hazards may involve inadequate lighting, steps or handrails missing or in poor repair, cluttered stairways, and the presence of throw rugs, electrical cords, or slippery surfaces. Features that suggest a safe home environment include grab bars in the tub or shower, nonskid rugs, covered electrical plugs, and locked storage cabinets.

Work

The work environment may contain a variety of overt or covert occupational safety hazards. Potential occupational hazards may result from noise, dust, or air pollution; working at heights; working with dangerous machinery; and being exposed to toxic substances. Occupations that raise the risk of injury include those that involve exposure to radiation or high-voltage electricity or the use of heavy equipment. Farm workers, electrical linemen, construction workers, and workers in power plants are a few examples of people at increased risk of injury. Both employers and employees should be aware of potential hazards and the need for precautions, such as wearing appropriate protective apparel.

Community

Hazards that can affect the community environment include crime, landfills, busy intersections, unsafe roads or bridges, dilapidated houses, cliffs, unprotected creeks, toxic waste dumps, air pollution, water pollution, noise from nearby construction, railroad crossings, and airports. Other environmental concerns include the need for a clean water supply, an adequate sewage system, and the absence of insects and rodents. Lack of sanitation in impoverished or less developed areas increases the risk of disease and infection.

> We know that Mrs. Soto's house needs repairs, but we do not know anything about the community in which she lives. What would you assess about the community to determine Mrs. Soto's level of safety in her home?

Institution

Many potential dangers to health care workers and clients lurk within health care institutions. Many appoint safety committees, infection control committees, and hazardous waste committees to address these potential problems. For example, each institution is required to have up-to-date written policies to address such problems as chemical spills, infectious outbreaks, exposure to infectious blood and body fluids, and disposal of hazardous wastes. You must be familiar with your institution's policies and procedures to ensure your own safety and that of your clients.

Socioeconomic Factors

A frequently cited reason for ignoring safety is a lack of financial resources. Buying car seats for children and making repairs to protect the home from a faulty furnace can be expensive. A family may not have the financial means to obtain smoke detectors, fire extinguishers, or carbon monoxide detectors for their homes.

However, the cost of not preventing accidents can be devastating. When someone is injured or involved in an accident, the costs can be astonishing. They involve lost wages and productivity, medical expenses, administrative expenses, employer costs, vehicle damage, and property losses.

Developmental Factors

Each stage of human development has its own unique risks (Table 28–2). Preventing injury and promoting safety are major concerns and the responsibility of the nurse, client, family, and caregiver. The goal is to eliminate accidents in the home, community, and health care setting. Promoting awareness of potentially hazardous situations is a lifelong process that should begin early in life (Fig. 28–6) and continue throughout the life span.

Infants and toddlers are particularly vulnerable to accidents and injuries because of their limited awareness of potential dangers. The type of accident or injury sustained by this age group is closely related to normal growth and development. Because of their oral activity, mobility, and inherent curiosity, toddlers are at increased risk for lead poisoning from ingestion of paint chips, strangulation, drowning, and burns. The accompanying Teaching for Wellness chart offers tips for preventing lead poisoning.

School-age children face potential dangers as their environment expands from the home to the school.

Dangers may exist in transportation to and from school, after-school activities, participation in sports, and failure to use safety equipment, such as bike helmets and protective gear. Children should receive specific instructions from parents, teachers, and nurses regarding the safety practices they should follow while at school or play.

The risk for adolescents are motor vehicle accidents, drowning, sexually transmitted diseases, unwanted pregnancy, suicide, homicide, and drug overdose. The need for independence and peer pressure, together with high-risk behaviors common in this age group, greatly increases the risk of accidents and injury.

In adults, the risk of injury tends to result from lifestyle. Excessive use of alcohol raises the risk of motor vehicle accidents. Cigarette smoking raises the risk of cardiovascular and pulmonary diseases. Excessive levels of stress can lead to increased risk for accidents.

The physiological changes normal among older adults can increase the risk of motor vehicle accidents, burns, and falls. Older adults tend to have decreased muscle strength, restricted joint mobility, and postural changes. Nervous system changes include slower reflexes, compromised balance, and a decreased ability to attend to multiple stimuli. Vision and hearing problems are common. Also, older adults are more likely to need to urinate at night, raising the risk of falls. This is especially true if the threat of incontinence requires the person to hurry to the bathroom.

Cognitive Factors

A person's cognitive and perceptual abilities are crucial to promoting safety. The ability to acquire and interpret information is a prerequisite for judgment, orientation, and socially appropriate behaviors. Promoting safety requires a person to think clearly, recall past problems and solutions, and create solutions to current problems. To remain safe, the person must also be able to perceive impending danger. The ability to perceive danger is based primarily on knowledge or learning from past experiences.

Physiological Factors

Impaired neurological function is a major component of risk for injury. To be safe, a person must have the judgment to recognize the presence of danger and the ability to move away. Many physiological factors can raise a person's risk of injury, including poor nutrition, clotting problems, a compromised immune system, a long history of alcohol and drug abuse, a debilitating disease, difficulty swallowing, and a need for tube feedings.

ASSESSMENT

General assessment of a client's safety requires you to collect subjective data as well as objective data. Gather subjective data by interviewing the client and family

TABLE 28–2

Risk for Injury by Age Group

Age Group	Risks	Possible Causes
Developing fetus	• Maternal exposure to smoke. • Maternal use of alcohol or other drugs. • X-rays received during first trimester. • Exposure to certain pesticides.	• Mother cannot or will not assume responsibility for the safety of fetus, or she lacks the knowledge to do so. • X-ray ordered by M.D. without inquiry about possible pregnancy. • Mother lives in proximity of fields of crops where the use of pesticides may be common.
Newborn	• Falling. • Suffocating in crib. • Choking or aspiration of formula. • Burns, especially with bath water. • Injuries in automobile accidents. • Injuries in crib or playpen.	• Failure to use approved car seats, cribs, and playpens correctly. • Inappropriate supervision. • Propping bottles while feeding. • Using a microwave oven to warm formula.
Infant or toddler	• Physical trauma from falling. • Banging into objects. • Falling down stairs. • Being cut by sharp objects. • Injuries in automobile accidents. • Burns. • Poisoning. • Drowning. • Electric shock from household outlets.	• Environment not childproofed. • No gate at the top of stairs. • Obstructed passageways. • Unsafe window protection. • Improper use of car seats. • Highly flammable toys or clothing. • Pot handles facing front of stove. • Unsupervised bathing. • Unsupervised backyard swimming pool. • Unused electric outlets not blocked.
Preschool and school age	• Injuries in automobile accidents. • Injuries on playground equipment. • Choking. • Suffocation. • Obstruction of airways or ears by foreign objects. • Poisoning. • Drowning. • Electrical shock.	• History of hyperactivity; attention deficit disorder. • Experimenting with chemicals or gasoline. • Playing with matches, cigarettes, candles, or fireworks. • Improper storage of knives, guns, and ammunition. • Improper use of car seats or seat belts. • Unsupervised activities around the pool, electrical outlets, etc.
Adolescents	• Sports injuries. • Automobile accidents. • Drug or alcohol use.	• Lack of proper athletic training. • Lack of experience driving. • Failure to use or misuse of seat belts.
Older adults	• Falls. • Burns. • Pedestrian and automobile accidents.	• *Physical:* Weakness, poor vision, disturbed balance, reduced sensations, poor coordination, impaired eye-hand coordination. • *Environmental:* Slippery floors, snow or ice on walkways, unanchored rugs, no handgrips or rails in shower or bathtub, unsteady ladders or chairs, poor lighting, electrical cords in walkways, clutter or spills, unsteady or absent stair rails, inadequate method to call for assistance, cognitive or emotional disturbance.
All ages	• Fires.	• Gas leaks. • Delayed lighting of gas burners. • Unscreened fires or heaters. • Flowing clothes around open flame. • Inappropriately stored combustibles or corrosives. • Faulty wiring or frayed cords. • Smoking in bed.

about their safety needs. Gather objective data through physical examination, risk assessment tools, and environmental appraisals.

Hazard appraisal tools allow you to elicit information objectively about the client's safety. These tools may summarize data contained in the client's nursing history and physical examination, or they may allow you to obtain specific information regarding the client's behaviors or environment. For example, an adult home hazard appraisal requires an assessment of walkways and stairways (inside and outside), floors, furniture, bathrooms, kitchen, bedrooms, electrical

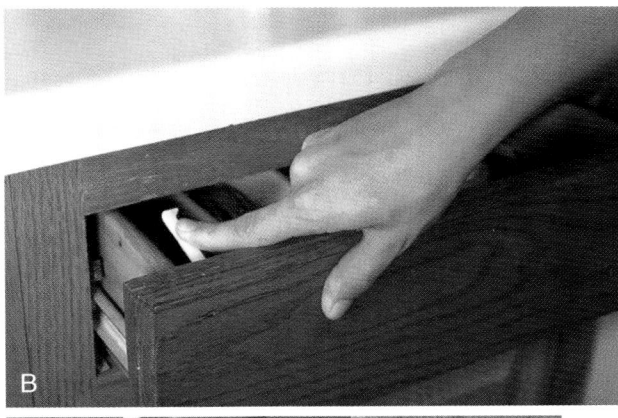

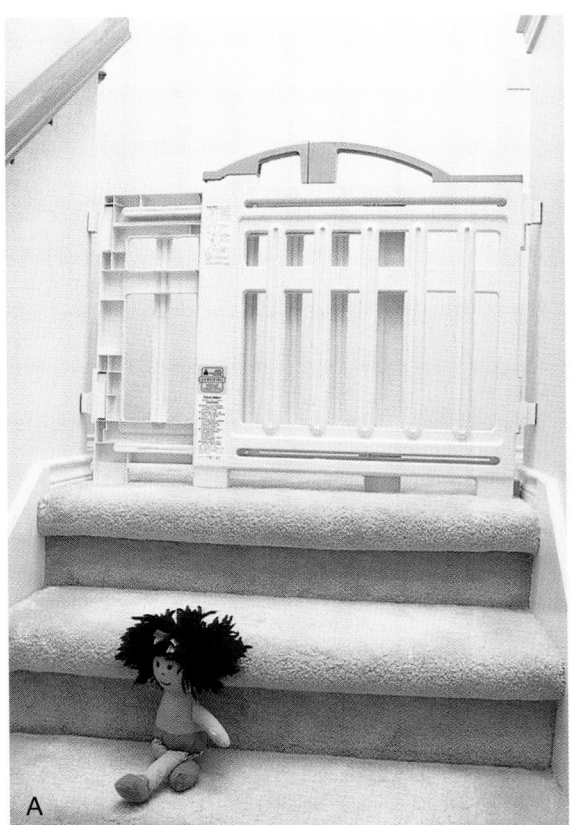

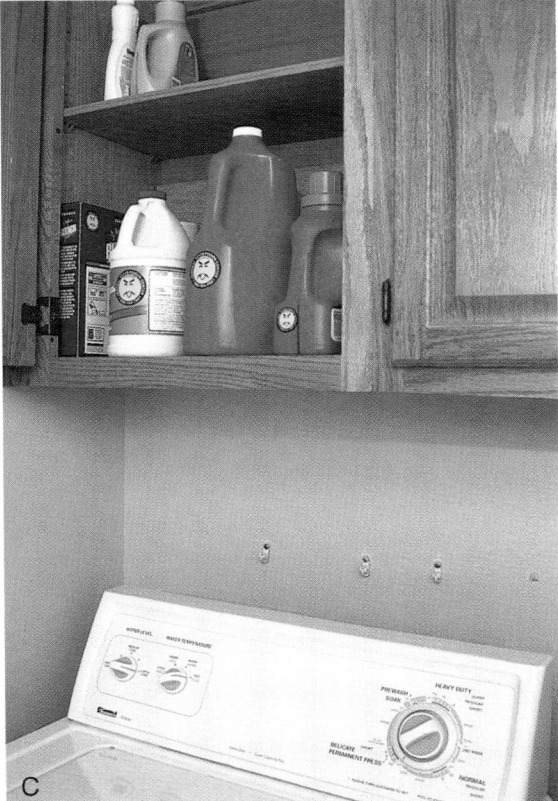

Figure 28–6. Ways to childproof a home. *A,* toddler gates on stairs and doors; *B,* childproof locks for cabinets; *C,* chemicals labeled with "Mr. Yuk" stickers and placed out of reach.

equipment and outlets, fire prevention, and the presence of toxic substances. Each category of the home hazard appraisal tool requires notation of potential hazards (Box 28–2).

Another useful hazard appraisal tool assesses the client's risk for falls. Brians, Alexander, Grota, Chen, & Dumas (1991) developed a tool that uses the following four variables to categorize the client's risk:

1. Unsteady gait, dizziness, or imbalance
2. Impaired memory or judgment
3. Weakness
4. History of falls

Many health care agencies also use tools specifically to identify a client's risk for falls (Box 28–3).

Health History

To assess the client's safety, you will begin by evaluating the client's lifestyle and health status for factors that affect safety. Take a complete health history, emphasizing areas most likely to reveal issues of safety. They include lifestyle, cardiovascular and respiratory systems, neurological function, mobility, and integument.

Lifestyle

Assess the client's lifestyle for safety risk factors. To elicit a subjective response, ask questions pertaining to the client's current safety practices or plans for man

PREVENTING LEAD POISONING

Purpose: To educate families about preventive strategies for lead poisoning.

Rationale: Lead poisoning continues to be a risk factor for very young children.

Expected Outcomes: Families will initiate action to detect and prevent ingestion of lead.

Client Instructions

Sources of Lead

- Although houses built before 1950 are the greatest threat, over 80% of houses built before 1978 contain lead-based paint.
- Although all children are at risk, those who live in dilapidated housing face the greatest danger, especially children under age 2.
- Houses in coastal towns may have been painted with paint intended for boats, which has a high lead content.
- Soil near mines, industries that use lead, and smelters can have high lead levels.
- Solder on older plumbing and brass fixtures can contain lead.
- Food grown in soil with a high lead content can contain lead.
- Ceramic tableware from some countries contains lead.
- Ethnic folk remedies, such as the Hispanic remedies *azarcon* and *greta* and the Southeast Asian remedy *pay loo lah*, may contain lead.
- Hobbies that involve working with leaded glass, artist paints, bullets, and jewelry are sources of lead.

Actions

- If you suspect a high level of lead in your home or environment, have your children tested even if they seem healthy.
- Keep your house clean; dust and dirt may contain lead.
- Do not attempt to remove lead-based paint yourself. Improper removal can increase the amount of lead in the environment.
- If you have older plumbing, have your water tested.

Information from National Lead Information Center. U.S. EPA (EPA 800-B-92-, February 1995). http://www.nsc.org; and Centers for Disease Control and Prevention, National Center for Environmental Health, Childhood Lead Poisoning Prevention. Screening young children for lead poisoning: Guidance for state and local public health officials. November 1997. http://www.cdc.gov/nceh.

BOX 28-2

HOME ASSESSMENT

To help prevent injuries in the home, assess the client's home and immediate surroundings thoroughly. Make sure your assessment includes the following areas:

- General layout of the home.
- Type of access into the home.
- Availability of adequate lighting, including night lights.
- Availability of adequate ventilation.
- Presence of uneven walkways, stairs, or pathways.
- Presence of loose steps on stairways.
- Presence or absence of railing on stairways.
- Repairs needed to make walkways, stairs, and pathways safe.
- Sturdiness and security of all stairs, stepstools, ladders, and handrails.
- Potential dangers from cluttered or obstructed hallways, stairways, and walkways.
- Presence of unanchored carpet, mats, or throw rugs.
- Types of furniture, including sharp or jutting corners, heights in relation to client, and support provided.
- Types of floors, including those in bathrooms, showers, and bathtubs.
- Presence or absence of grab bars around tubs, showers, and toilets.
- Use of or need for a raised toilet seat or bath chair in tub or shower.
- Condition of electrical appliances.
- Loose or frayed electrical cords, overloaded outlets or extension cords, and proximity of electrical cords to water.
- Presence and condition of smoke alarms and carbon monoxide detectors.
- Presence and condition of fire extinguishers and plans for an escape route to be used in case of fire.
- Appropriate disposal of expired foods and medications.
- Proper storage and labeling of medications, cleaning solutions, combustibles (such as paint thinner and gasoline) or corrosives (such as rust remover [phosphoric acid]), and other toxic substances.
- Presence of a fence around the pool.
- Presence of a reliable heating system.
- Accessibility of emergency telephone numbers, such as for the fire department, police department, ambulance, poison control center, and hospital.

DETERMINING AN ADULT CLIENT'S RISK FOR FALLS

A person may have an increased risk of falling if she has one or more of the following risk factors:

- Age 65 or over.
- A history of falling.
- Decreased mobility or difficulty walking.
- Need for assistance when getting out of bed or transferring to and from a chair.
- A history of dizziness or seizures.
- Impaired vision, hearing, or speech.
- Need for assistive devices, such as a cane, walker, wheelchair, crutches, or braces, for mobility.
- Weakness or fatigue caused by a disease process or prescribed therapy.
- Confusion, disorientation, impaired memory or judgment, or impaired cognitive function.
- Use of certain medications, such as diuretics, laxatives, or those that can alter the client's level of consciousness, including sedatives, hypnotics, tranquilizers, and analgesics.

agement of hazards. Questions could include the following:

- Do you use a seat belt in the car?
- Are your child's immunizations current?
- Has your house been childproofed?
- Do you have trouble reading warning labels or traffic signs?

Also question clients about their occupation, home environment, and habits that may put them at risk for injury. Assess the client's awareness of safety precautions and the degree to which the client implements these precautions.

Include in your assessment questions about medications the client is currently taking and any side effects she may have experienced. Cardiovascular medications, sedatives, antidepressants, and other medications that affect the central nervous system are particularly pertinent.

Cardiovascular and Respiratory Systems

Assessment of the cardiovascular and respiratory systems provides information about the client's activity tolerance. Assess changes in the client's blood pressure, pulse, and respirations with activity. Orthostatic hypotension and dizziness are factors in client safety.

Mrs. Soto's rheumatoid arthritis has kept her from remaining active, but she is determined to keep trying. How would you assess her cardiovascular status to determine her ability to tolerate an exercise program?

Neurological Function

Assessment of the neurological system can provide information about the client's mental status, sensory function, reflexes, and coordination. Level of consciousness; orientation to time, person, and place; attention span; and decision-making abilities are also included in the neurological assessment. Testing of the senses (vision, hearing, taste, and smell) should also be conducted to detect any deficits or alterations. This is important to determine the client's risk for injury during medication administration, while climbing stairs, reading warning labels, and listening for cars, smoke alarms, or other warning sounds.

Mobility

Assessment of the client's mobility is the key element of a safety assessment. Clients who experience impaired mobility because of paralysis, muscle weakness, poor balance, or poor coordination are at increased risk of injury and serious health problems. To be safe, the client needs to be able to move about freely in the environment and avoid hazards.

Integument

Ask the client about any history of accidental injuries while you inspect the skin. During a bath, inspect all areas of the client's skin for bruises, cuts, scratches, and scars. If lesions are present, document their precise location, size, color, and the client's explanation of their cause.

Physical Examination

The collection of objective data allows you to assess the client's safety function and to assess for injuries and risk factors for injuries. Examples of objective data include the client's muscle strength, joint range of motion, gait characteristics, pulse rate, results of diagnostic tests or x-rays, skin color, skin turgor, and posture. The physical assessment should focus on the neurological system, skin integrity, and mobility. Information that can be obtained from assessing these three areas can be of vital importance to the client's overall health and safety.

Focused Assessment for Risk for Injury

To assess the general category of *Risk for injury*, you need to observe the client's physical and psychological status and elements of the environment that are unsafe. Often, a combination of factors from the internal and external environments defines the client's risk.

Defining Characteristics

Internal risk factors for injury are classified as biochemical, physical, and psychological (NANDA, 1999). Biochemical factors of the neurological system include sensory, integrative, and motor dysfunction. Additionally, hypoxia affects the ability to form reasoned judgments. Immune-autoimmune dysfunction, malnutrition, and an abnormal blood profile can make even minor injuries serious. Physical factors include altered mobility and the client's developmental status, with the very young and very old being the most vulnerable. Depression and anxiety are psychological factors that affect a person's ability to reason or to be alert to environmental hazards.

External risk factors are characterized as biological, chemical, physical, and people/provider. Biological risk factors include the number and type of microorganisms present in a particular environment as well as the immunization level of the community. Chemical factors are identified as pollutants, poisons, drugs, alcohol, caffeine, nicotine, preservatives, cosmetics, dyes, nutrients, vitamins, and food types. Physical factors include the design, structure, and arrangement of the community, building, or equipment and the available mode of transportation. People/provider factors include the preventive behaviors of the health care team, staffing patterns, and the knowledge of the health care providers (NANDA, 1999).

Related Factors

LACK OF KNOWLEDGE

Knowledge is an important factor to help prevent accidents. Parents need to be especially aware of the dangers that could cause harm to their children. For example, new information has recently become available about the danger of carbon monoxide poisoning and lead content in miniblinds. Not all child car seats on the market are safe. Parents need to keep abreast of current information identifying safety features of toys, cribs, playground equipment, and household furnishings.

LACK OF SELF-CARE SKILLS

An important component for promoting physical and emotional health and well-being is self-care capability. Often, a person who has infirmities associated with age, disease, or disability will not be able to take the actions needed to prevent accidents. For example, a very young child or a frail elderly person may lack the knowledge, support, or resources to evaluate potentially hazardous situations and make the necessary changes to prevent injury. People with physical limitations may be unable to recognize a high-risk situation or take corrective actions.

LACK OF ADEQUATE SUPPORT SYSTEM

If your client is cognitively or physically impaired, assess the support system available. The client may be receiving support from a variety of sources, such as family, friends, volunteer agencies, and professional services. Determine any gaps in service that may leave the client vulnerable to injury.

Focused Assessment for Risk for Trauma

Defining Characteristics

Risk for trauma is the nursing diagnosis that indicates the presence of any factor that increases the client's risk of accidental traumatic injury, such as a wound, burn, or fracture. Internal risk factors involve the individual. They include weakness, balancing difficulties, reduced coordination of large or small muscles, lack of safety education or precautions, cognitive or emotional difficulties, poor vision, reduced temperature or tactile sensation, reduced hand-eye coordination, insufficient finances to purchase safety equipment or make repairs, and a history of previous trauma (NANDA, 1999).

External risk factors involve hazards in the client's environment that can result in fires, burns, electric shock, or accidents, particularly from falls. Falls result from slippery (such as wet or highly waxed) floors, bathtubs without hand grips or traction mats, inappropriate call-for-aid devices for the bedridden client, snow or ice on outside stairs or walkways, unanchored rugs, use of an unsteady ladder or chair for reaching, poor lighting, unanchored electric wires, clutter or spills on floors or stairs, obstructed passageways, and unsafe window protection in homes with young children.

Burns result from pot handles facing toward the front of the stove, gas leaks, overly hot bath water, experimenting with chemicals or gasoline, and children playing with matches, candles, or cigarettes. Electrical injuries result from faulty electrical plugs, overloaded electrical outlets, and frayed wires or defective appliances. Other types of traumatic injuries can result from knives stored uncovered, unsafe use of dangerous machinery, high-crime neighborhoods, and motor vehicle accidents (NANDA, 1999).

Related Factors

LACK OF KNOWLEDGE

Assess the client's knowledge of risk factors as well as knowledge and ability to make necessary repairs.

HIGH-RISK BEHAVIORS

Assess for high-risk behaviors, such as the use of alcohol or drugs while driving. Referral for an in-depth assessment may be needed to determine the best way to help the client change high-risk behaviors.

LACK OF SELF-CARE ABILITY

Assess the client's ability to remove risk factors independently. Is there a potential to improve health or make the client more independent in behaviors that reduce risk? For example, could falls be prevented by teaching the client how to use a walker?

Focused Assessment for Risk for Poisoning

Both internal and external factors are required to produce the *Risk for poisoning*. Assess the client for internal factors that make her unable or unwilling to prevent poisoning in the presence of external factors that place her at risk.

Defining Characteristics

Internal characteristics that increase the risk for poisoning include the use of multiple medications, disability, and reduced vision. Also assess the client's knowledge of poisonous substances and storage of household chemicals. For young children, the cognitively impaired, and persons with emotional difficulties, assessment should include the level of supervision and precautions taken to prevent accidents with harmful substances (NANDA, 1999).

External factors associated with the *Risk for poisoning* include having a large supply of drugs in the house, varying therapeutic margins of safety among drugs (therapeutic versus toxic level, half-life, method of uptake and degradation in body, adequacy of organ function), dangerous products within reach of children or confused persons, flaking or peeling paint or plaster around young children, use of volatile substances (such as paint) in poorly ventilated areas or without effective protection, medicines stored in unlocked cabinets, availability of illicit drugs that may be contaminated by poisonous additives, chemical contamination of food and water, and contact with heavy metals, chemicals, poisonous vegetation, atmospheric pollutants, or industrial chemicals (NANDA, 1999).

Related Factors

Factors related to an increased *Risk for poisoning* are the same as those listed above. Nursing interventions are aimed at reducing the risk that these factors create.

Focused Assessment for Risk for Suffocation

Defining Characteristics

Internal risk factors identified as defining characteristics for *Risk for suffocation* include reduced olfactory sensation, reduced motor abilities, lack of safety education and precautions, cognitive or emotional difficulties (such as altered consciousness or mentation), and the presence of disease or injury.

External risk factors associated with the *Risk for suffocation* include a pillow or propped bottle in an infant's crib, warming a vehicle in a closed garage, children playing with plastic bags or inserting small objects into their mouths or noses, discarded or unused refrigerators or freezers with doors intact, children left unattended in bathtubs or pools, household gas leaks, smoking in bed, fuel-burning heaters not vented to the outside, a low-strung clothesline, a pacifier hung around an infant's neck, and eating large mouthfuls of food (NANDA, 1999).

Related Factors

Factors related to an increased *Risk for suffocation* are the same as those listed above. Nursing interventions are aimed at reducing the risk that these factors create.

Lack of adequate supervision is a significant factor in preventing suffocation in infants and young children. To prevent suffocation in young children, hazards must be removed, and the child must be supervised. No environment can be made completely hazard-free.

Supervision is also an important factor in preventing suffocation in neurologically, cognitively, or physically impaired people. Assess the client's ability to move in bed and maintain a body position that ensures a patent airway.

Focused Assessment for Risk for Aspiration

Defining Characteristics

Aspiration is the inhalation of a foreign body or substance into the lungs. Physiologically, it occurs because the epiglottis fails to close completely. A person who does not have a gag reflex, who cannot produce a strong cough, or who is comatose has a high risk for aspiration. A tracheostomy or endotracheal tube prevents the person from coughing and from closing the epiglottis. A nasogastric tube interferes with the gag reflex and with the lower esophageal sphincter. Any condition in which the lower esophageal sphincter is incompetent can raise the risk by causing vomiting.

Related Factors

Aspiration is often associated with feedings through a nasogastric tube. It is not uncommon for these clients to have impaired swallowing. A distended stomach from any cause increases the chance of vomiting and aspiration. Lying flat in bed with a full stomach adds to the risk. Other conditions that can impair swallowing are wired jaws or oral surgery.

The outcome of aspiration can be fatal and usually depends on the degree to which the aspiration occurred. For example, massive aspiration usually causes death. A small, localized aspiration from regurgitation may result in pneumonia or respiratory distress and can lead to the development of other complications. Still more common is the type of aspiration that results from a silent regurgitation that may go unobserved.

Every precaution needs to be taken to ensure the client's safety and prevent or reduce the *Risk for aspiration*. For example, food should be appropriate for the age, developmental stage, and condition of the client. The type of feeding (tube feeding, oral feeding, or hyperalimentation, for instance) will determine the proper client positioning, the need for assistance or supervision, and the type of teaching that will be included in the client's plan of care.

Action Alert!

Aspiration is a medical emergency. Tachycardia, dyspnea, cyanosis, and hypertension may signal inhalation of a large volume of gastric contents. The client needs immediate suctioning and oxygen therapy.

Focused Assessment for Related Nursing Diagnoses

Altered Thought Processes

The nursing diagnosis *Altered thought processes* includes a high *Risk for injury*. Assess the client for impaired memory, confusion, and unusual patterns of thinking. Altered patterns of thinking can result from sleep deprivation or the use of medications that affect thinking. Therefore, assessment should include all factors that have the potential to cause *Altered thought processes*.

Impaired Home Maintenance Management

Impaired home maintenance can cause safety hazards. If the client is unable to keep the home in good repair, accidents can involve faulty furnaces, broken stairs, and other environmental hazards. Assess the client's home environment for safety hazards.

Knowledge Deficit

Lack of knowledge about health and safety practices may be the primary diagnosis, particularly with parents of young children. Assess the parents' knowledge of childhood safety, growth and development parameters, and measures for preventing accidents. Use this nursing diagnosis—*Knowledge deficit*—when the client has skills and resources needed but does not have the knowledge of health and safety practices.

Impaired Mobility

Impaired mobility always causes an increase in the *Risk for injury*. The degree of impairment and the client's knowledge of and use of safety measures should be assessed.

DIAGNOSIS

The main nursing diagnosis used to describe alterations in safety is *Risk for injury*. This diagnosis can be used for clients in the home setting, in long-term care facilities, and in the hospital or acute care setting. Depending on the safety issue involved, a diagnosis can be written to address the specific risk for an individual client. Examples include *Risk for trauma, Risk for poisoning, Risk for suffocation,* and *Risk for aspiration.*

Risk for trauma and *Risk for injury* are closely related concepts. *Risk for injury* is the broader of the two, with *Risk for trauma* being reserved for injury to tissues. *Risk for injury* is useful in an institutional setting, where you can protect clients from a broad array of risk. *Risk for trauma* is used more often in the community set-

ting, where you would be helping to prevent accidents in individuals or groups of clients. Use the major risk factors identified so far and the accompanying data clustering chart to help you select the most appropriate nursing diagnoses for a client with a safety need.

PLANNING

Planning involves identifying appropriate nursing interventions for clients who have actual or potential safety risks, as outlined in the Nursing Care Planning chart. Nursing interventions are individualized for each client and take into consideration the severity of the risk and the client's developmental stage, level of health, and lifestyle. The main goal for the diagnoses of *Risk for injury* or *Risk for trauma* is that the client will remain free from injury.

When planning care for a client with an increased *Risk for injury*, focus mainly on prevention. You can prevent injuries by helping the client identify potential hazards and measures needed to address them. Therefore, depending on the nursing diagnosis for a particular client, specific outcomes must be identified and included in the plan of care. The expected outcomes for each of the diagnoses related to altered safety may be different, depending on the cause. Expected outcomes may include the following. The client will:

- Recognize potential hazards in the immediate surroundings
- Recognize internal risk factors that increase vulnerability to injury
- Identify and apply safety measures to prevent injuries
- Demonstrate preventive measures to minimize the risk of falls, ingestion of poison, and other accidents
- Take medications correctly
- Use medical equipment correctly
- Identify potential hazards in the work environment (exposure to radiation, use of heavy equipment, and so on)
- Identify high-risk practices, such as speeding, alcohol or drug use, and smoking in bed
- Identify safety measures and practices needed to decrease the risk of fires, electrical hazards, and burns from hot water or heating pads.

INTERVENTION

When a client is at risk for an alteration in safety, nursing interventions can be instituted to help prevent hazards, trauma, or disease. Nursing interventions should be individualized for each client. They should be holistic in nature and should take into consideration all the factors that are unique to the client, including age, developmental level, health care needs, abilities, support systems, strengths, and weaknesses.

Prevention offers a main area of nursing interventions to incorporate into the client's plan of care. Preventing hazards, trauma, and illness can be done by

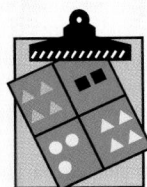

CLUSTERING DATA TO MAKE A NURSING DIAGNOSIS
INJURIES

Data Cluster	Diagnosis
85-year-old Maria Martinez lives alone, takes blood pressure medications, and has osteoarthritis. Her physician recommended a total hip replacement, but the client does not want to have surgery.	*Risk for injury* related to limited mobility, lack of assistance in the home, and possible orthostatic hypotension from blood pressure medications.
6-month-old Patrick lives with his mother in a one-room apartment. He sleeps in the bed with his mother. She pads the bed with pillows to keep him from rolling off the bed. He sleeps face down most of the time.	*Risk for suffocation* related to lack of resources for safe bedding and lack of knowledge about infant suffocation.
5-year-old Andrea lives with her great-grandmother, who takes several medications and keeps them handy on the kitchen sink. The pills include a bright red tablet and a bright green one. Andrea thinks they look like Christmas.	*Risk for poisoning* related to unsafe storage of medications.
72-year-old Millie Kendall is in the wandering stage of Alzheimer's disease. She walks constantly in the nursing home and cannot identify her room. If not monitored, she leaves the building. She was once found a half-mile from the nursing home.	*Risk for injury* related to inability to make judgments about the environment.
92-year-old Richard King lives alone and manages his own care. A corner grocery store delivers supplies to his door. After being admitted to the hospital, he wakes from naps or during the night and thinks he is at home. He has been found in the hall looking for the bathroom.	*Risk for injury* related to unfamiliar environment.

focusing on providing or promoting a safe environment, preventing falls, enhancing safety efforts, arranging ongoing surveillance measures to identify risk factors, and providing client teaching to increase awareness, knowledge, and an increased sense of physical and psychological safety and well-being.

Interventions to Promote a Safe Environment

Nursing interventions should focus on promoting a safe environment at home and in the health care institution. Promoting safety at home can be accomplished by creating a safe home environment, especially for infants, children, and the elderly. A client's safety in the hospital can be assured by creating a safe institutional environment, orienting the client to the environment, and monitoring the client carefully.

Promoting Safety at Home

When a client needs care in the home, the environment may need modifications to maintain ongoing safety.

The environment may have been safe when the client was well and able to freely move about to manage the activities of daily living and necessary maintenance and repairs. However, when a client becomes physically or mentally compromised, even on a short-term basis, home safety becomes an issue.

CREATING A SAFE HOME ENVIRONMENT
The home should be free of hazards that could result in falls. Measures to promote home safety may include using nonskid rugs or tacking down throw rugs to prevent slips and falls, installing and using grab bars in the tub or shower, installing ramps to allow for easier access, and keeping rooms, halls, and stairs free of clutter.

Safety practices to prevent burns or electrical shocks should be in place. Potential electrical hazards in the home environment include frayed cords, overloaded outlets and extension cords, use of electrical appliances near water, and lack of supervision of children near uncovered electrical outlets or electrical appliances. Covering electrical outlets when not in use, positioning pans with handles toward the back of the stove while cooking, and avoiding open-flame heaters are examples of prevention strategies.

Proper storage and labeling of bottles containing poisonous substances is essential. Have emergency telephone numbers, including the number for poison control, readily available (Fig. 28–7). Instruct the client and appropriate family members about proper medication administration. This includes information about the type of medication, dosage, reason for taking, expected effects, and possible side effects.

Encourage the client to call the poison control hotline for immediate access to information about appropriate first aid in a possible poisoning. Emetic agents should be given only after contacting the poison control center and ascertaining the guidelines for the specific poison. Although several emetic agents are available, syrup of ipecac is the most effective one to use in the home setting, especially within 30 minutes to 1 hour after ingestion of poison. Contradictions to syrup of ipecac include the ingestion of gasoline, fuel oil, paint thinner, cleaning fluid, or strychnine. Also, children under 6 months old, people with severe heart disease, and pregnant or lactating women should not use syrup of ipecac (Holdsclaw & Nykamp, 1992).

Teaching may also involve instructing the client and family in the use of safe techniques for mobility of the physically impaired client. Provide instructions on the proper use of assistive devices, such as walkers, wheelchairs, or crutches. Teach the client and family ways to prevent back injury, including proper lifting techniques, back exercises to prevent back injury, and proper use of body mechanics.

Teaching may need to address the client's lifestyle

as well. For example, the client may need to stop drinking and smoking. She and her family may need instruction on how to recognize signs and symptoms of choking and carbon monoxide poisoning and how to perform Heimlich's maneuver and cardiopulmonary resuscitation.

Safety precautions are essential for preventing injuries in elderly, mentally ill, or disabled clients. Ways to prevent injury include proper labeling of medication, assessing the home environment for potential hazards, and teaching safety measures as appropriate. Establishing an open line of communication with the client or primary caregiver is of utmost importance in enhancing and promoting the safety of all those involved.

At times you may need to refer a dependent elder to a home health agency so someone can perform a home safety assessment before the client is discharged from the hospital. If a referral is necessary, it should be done 3 days before discharge to allow appropriate planning and implementation of safety measures. Make every attempt to accommodate the client's cultural needs, as outlined in the Cross-Cultural Care chart.

PROMOTING SAFETY FOR INFANTS AND CHILDREN

Child safety is taught as part of parenting classes. Nurses may organize parenting classes for populations at risk or as part of a wellness program in a health care facility.

To promote a safe environment for infants and children, safety measures on how to childproof a home may be taught to the family. Families can employ a number of important safety measures to prevent accidents. For example, plastic bags should be stored in a cabinet out of the child's reach. Covering an infant's or child's mattress or pillow with plastic should be avoided. Crib design should follow federal safety regulations, and the mattress should be the appropriate size for the crib frame. Discourage parents from sleeping with their infant or putting the infant down to sleep with a bib, bonnet, or other snug-fitting garment tied around the infant's neck. They should be taught never to tie a pacifier around her neck. To avoid choking accidents, parents should inspect toys for removable parts and avoid feeding the infant such foods as grapes, nuts, and popcorn. When giving medication to a child, they should avoid trying to entice the child by calling it candy.

Other safety measures that can be taken to ensure a child's safety include keeping doors of large appliances, especially unused refrigerators or freezers, closed at all times. Areas around a swimming pool should be fenced, and children should be supervised and wear protective gear when swimming. Instruct parents to avoid leaving pails of water or cleaning solutions accessible to children. Tell parents to use seat belts or car seats, as appropriate for children's age and weight. Sharp objects, such as knives and other kitchen utensils, matches, and toxic substances should be kept out of children's reach.

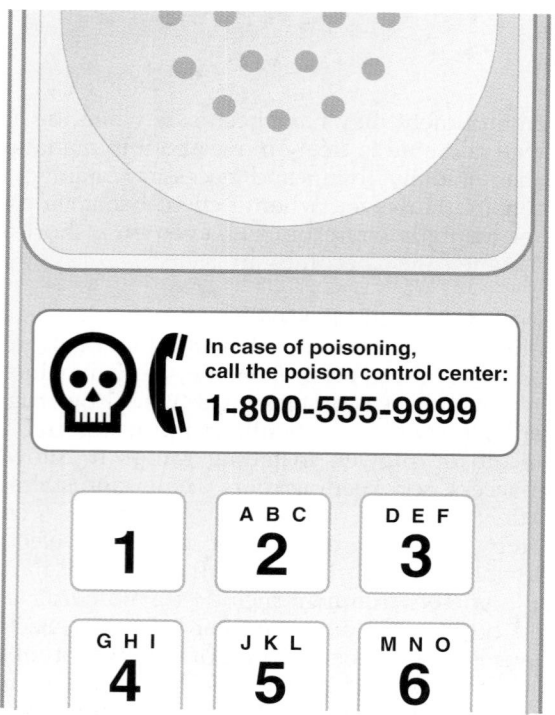

Figure 28–7. An example of a poison control label on a telephone.

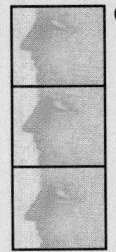

CROSS-CULTURAL CARE
CARING FOR AN ELDERLY MEXICAN-AMERICAN CLIENT

Mrs. Soto, the client described in this chapter's case study, lives in a city on the border of Texas and Mexico. She was born in Mexico and maintains close ties with family in Mexico. The following are some key facts to keep in mind when caring for Mexican-American clients:

- Mexican-Americans are the most successful of all ethnic groups in retaining their culture and language.
- In southwestern cities, Mexican-Americans often live in *barrios* (Hispanic ethnic neighborhoods), where their primary interactions are with members of their own ethnic group.
- 51% of elderly Mexican-Americans were born in Mexico.
- The elderly constitute less than 4% of the population of Mexican-Americans.
- Mexican-Americans tend not to retire; they tend to work as long as they are able.
- Mexican-American culture maintains respectful behavior toward the elderly and absolute obedience to their commands.
- Mexican-American women tend to become more outgoing and domineering as they get older.
- Elderly Mexican-Americans tend to function in the role of teacher, delineating proper conduct, relating historic events, and explaining the origin of things.
- Mexican-American grandparents are unlikely to live alone.

- Elderly Mexican-Americans are rarely placed in nursing homes by their families.

The nurse, Jim, has the following conversation with Mrs. Soto.

Jim: Have you thought about what you will do when you can no longer live by yourself?

Mrs. Soto: My daughter wants me to come live with her and her family. They think I should come now. They have their own lives, I think I would be in the way.

Jim: Have you visited their home? Do they have room for you?

Mrs. Soto: Oh yes. They have a lovely and large home. But I have family here. I want to be independent.

Critical Thinking Questions

- It is likely that Mrs. Soto will have to make some changes in her living arrangements in the near future. How can you help her make this decision?
- Based on your knowledge of her culture, how would you approach this problem?

Reference

Holmes, E. R., & Holmes L. D. (1995). *Other Cultures, Elder Years*. Thousand Oaks: Sage Publications.

As can be seen from these examples, there are many safety measures that can be emphasized to children's parents, caregivers, or family to help them promote safety and avoid accidents. Community resources are also available and can be accessed through referrals. An important aspect of promoting safety lies in getting the client and family involved in planning and implementing safety measures needed to decrease the risk of injury. Solicit involvement of the client and family through family conferences in which you help the family define mutual goals. This involvement will enhance their motivation and increases the likelihood of positive outcomes and the long-term lifestyle changes required.

Most accidents are preventable. By educating yourself, your clients, and their families, you can help reduce the risk of injury, trauma, suffocation, poisoning, and aspiration in their homes.

Providing Safety in Institutions

CREATING A SAFE INSTITUTIONAL ENVIRONMENT
The client in a health care institution is dependent on the staff to provide a safe environment, especially when the client is incapacitated by illness or disability. Therefore, safety in an institutional environment requires a team effort by nursing services, housekeeping, maintenance—indeed, every employee of the institution. Safety issues are similar to those in the home; however, a hospital has more equipment, hazardous chemicals, and a large number of people using the facility. Every employee should be trained in electrical safety and fire safety as well as in safe interactions with clients.

Stay aware of the risk for electrical injury, especially in situations that combine moisture with electrical equipment. These situations may involve spills on the floor, a leaking or disconnected intravenous line, or a client with moist skin caused by diaphoresis.

You can help prevent electrical injuries by making sure that electrical equipment stays in good working order and by using devices equipped with three-pronged grounded plugs (Fig. 28–8). The third prong of the plug is called the *ground* because it is specifically designed to carry any stray electrical current into the earth. The two regular prongs carry power to the equipment being used. However, simply having a three-pronged plug does not ensure that the plug is

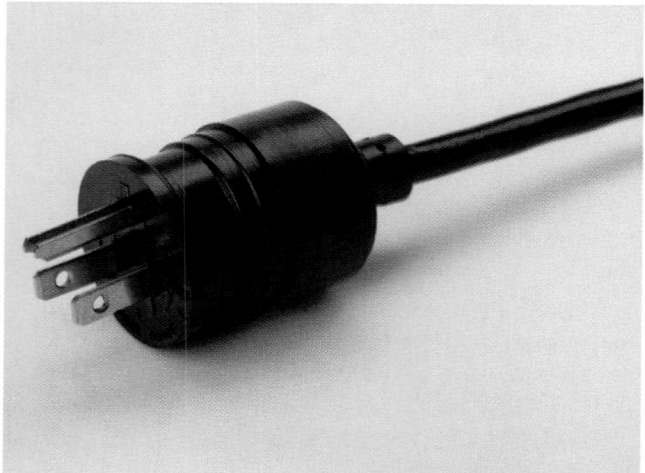

Figure 28–8. A three-pronged grounded plug, used to prevent electrical injuries. (Courtesy of Lion Electric, South Norwalk, CT.)

grounded. The grounding should be checked periodically by the maintenance department. The Teaching for Self-Care chart includes additional ideas to reduce the risk of electrical injury. Electrical shock can be prevented by identifying and correcting potential sources of danger.

Action **A**lert!
Prevent electrical shocks by using grounded equipment. Teach others to avoid the use of faulty equipment and to never overload electrical outlets or extension cords.

Although fires are uncommon in modern buildings when safety precautions are followed, fire safety programs increase the readiness to respond correctly to a fire. Any fire that arises in a health care setting requires quick actions in response. A common response plan incorporates the acronym RACE to help prioritize those actions. It stands for *rescue, alarm, confine,* and *extinguish.*

The first priority in case of fire is to rescue or remove all clients from immediate danger. The second priority is to call for help. Activate the nearest fire alarm, or report the fire to the switchboard operator, whichever is faster. The switchboard operator will page the code for a fire and its location.

The third priority is to confine the fire. Close nearby doors and windows, and turn off oxygen and electrical equipment. Close fire doors to confine the fire to an area of the building. Do not use elevators during a fire. The fourth priority is to extinguish the fire. Be sure to use the proper type of extinguisher for the type of fire involved (Box 28–4).

Also take steps to prevent back injuries—both yours and the client's. Back injuries can lead to lifelong pain, suffering, and disability. Taking care of your back is of vital importance to ensure a healthy, productive life. Many general rules and principles can be applied to home and work environments to re-

Teaching for SELF-CARE

PREVENTING ELECTRICAL SHOCKS

Purpose: To provide information about electrical safety.

Rationale: Electrical safety should be maintained in the home and institutional setting.

Expected Outcome: The client will demonstrate electrical safety practices.

Client Instructions

Equipment
- Make sure that equipment is grounded; the use of a three-prong outlet does not ensure that the outlet is grounded.
- Do not use electrical cords that are frayed or that have visible damage.
- Repair or replace all malfunctioning equipment. If you drop a piece of electrical equipment, have it tested before reusing it.
- Experiencing shocks while using equipment means that it is not safe; have it tested before continuing to use it.
- Learn about all electrical equipment that you intend to use before attempting to use it.

Electrical Outlets
- Do not overload.
- Cover outlets not currently in use, especially if small children are present.
- Install outlets with ground fault circuit interrupters near sources of water, such as bathroom and kitchen sinks.
- Never pull a plug from the socket by the cord. Grip the plug firmly and pull it straight out of the socket.

Extension Cords
- Avoid using when possible.
- Anchor extension cords to the floor using specially designed covers to prevent tripping over the cord.

duce the risk of back injuries (Butrej, 1995). Make sure to follow safety guidelines to prevent back injuries from occurring, such as using proper lifting techniques and body mechanics and engaging in appropriate exercise and activity to promote strong bones and muscles.

Action **A**lert!
Prevent back injuries from occurring. Use proper body mechanics and proper lifting and pushing techniques, and always ask for help when needed.

FIRE EXTINGUISHERS AND INDICATIONS FOR THEIR USE

Water pump extinguisher:
Use for type A fires, which involve paper, wood, or cloth.
Carbon dioxide (CO_2) extinguisher/Dry chemical extinguisher:
Use for type B fires, which involve such flammable liquids as fuel oil, cooking oil, grease, paint, solvents, and anesthetic gases, and for type C fires, which involve electrical sources.
Foam extinguisher:
Use for type B fires.
Multipurpose extinguisher:
Use for type A, B, and C fires.
Dry powder extinguisher:
Use for type D fires, which involve combustible metals and certain other metals.

ORIENTING THE CLIENT TO THE ENVIRONMENT

When a client is admitted to a hospital or nursing home, you will need to orient her to the new environment. The client and her family should know how to operate the bed and any other equipment that the client will be using. One of the most important features of the safety orientation is teaching the client how to call for help using the call light at the bedside and the emergency call light in the bathroom. If the client needs the side rails raised for safety, make a point of saying so; instruct her to call for help whenever she wants to get out of bed.

Some elderly clients, very ill clients, and clients under the influence of sedative medications may need ongoing orientation. A client with borderline dementia may function well at home but become confused in a strange environment. To maintain a client's orientation, provide information about time, person, place, and environment at regular intervals. Use clocks, calendars, even family pictures to help keep the client oriented, especially if she has an impaired awareness of time, place, or person.

PREVENTING THE INGESTION OF TOXIC SUBSTANCES

To prevent the accidental ingestion of toxic substances in the health care environment, take precautions not to leave medications or toxic solutions in the client's room. Using paper cups and containers that can be discarded immediately can prevent accidental poisonings.

MONITORING THE CLIENT

While a client is in your care, take every precaution necessary to ensure her safety. By assessing her risk for injury, you can make sound judgments about the type and frequency of monitoring needed to maintain her safety. Clients who need frequent monitoring include those with the following:

- A risk for compromised airway from muscle weakness or sedation
- Impaired mobility, especially when trying to get out of bed on their own
- Unstable (fluctuating) vital signs
- A tendency to be restless in bed, especially if medical therapy includes intravenous lines or nasogastric tubes
- Cognitive impairment, especially if it reduces cooperation with the treatment plan

Monitor a totally dependent client at least once an hour. If she has a high risk for injury, either make sure someone stays with her at all times or place her in a room close to the nurses' station, where you can monitor her frequently. A family member or private sitter can be used to provide constant surveillance.

If a client has a high risk for falls, consider using an identification system (colored tape on an arm band, a note in the chart and on the head of bed) to alert other staff members of the client's status. A device called an Ambularm can be attached to the client's leg to warn you when the client tries to get out of bed (Fig. 28–9). The device is sensitive to position changes and will sound an alarm when the client's leg goes over the side of the bed. The problem with this device is the same as with many electronic monitoring systems; when multiple false alarms occur, staff members become less sensitive to the sound and respond more slowly.

Frequent monitoring increases the likelihood of detecting risk factors if you form the habit of looking for potential hazards each time you enter the client's room. Assess the client's environment to make sure the bed stays in the low position, side rails are up, bed

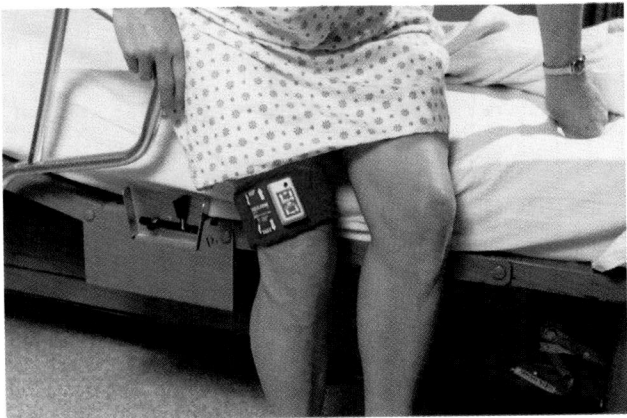

Figure 28–9. An Ambularm is a position-sensitive electronic device that is placed on the client's leg. Because it sounds a warning when the client attempts to get out of bed, it may provide a useful alternative to restraints. (Courtesy of Alert Care, Inc., Mill Valley, CA.)

wheels are locked, and items such as tissues, water, urinal, bedpan, and glasses are within the client's reach. Note the client's level of consciousness, especially if she is receiving an analgesic, a hypnotic, a sedative, or a tranquilizer.

The frequent presence of a nurse in the client's room contributes to a sense of security that may prevent the client from trying to get out of bed independently. Inform the client that you are nearby and will respond quickly to a call for help. It may be helpful to inform the client that you will return in a given period of time. However, make sure that you are indeed available when you say you will be.

> Think again of Mrs. Soto. Imagine that she is admitted to the hospital. We know she uses a wheelchair and walks with extreme difficulty. She is partially blind. How would you help her be safe in the hospital?

INFANTS AND CHILDREN IN THE HOSPITAL

In the hospital setting, all necessary precautions must be taken to keep children safe. Examples of common safety practices include the following:

- Never leave an infant unattended.
- Keep a bulb syringe readily available in case an infant's oropharynx needs to be suctioned.
- Make sure that periodic safety checks have been completed on emergency response equipment, such as suctioning devices.
- Check the infant or child's armband before giving medications; remember that young children may answer to any name.
- Keep small objects out of reach to help prevent infants and small children from putting small objects in their mouth, nose, or ears.
- Keep the side rails of the crib up, and inspect all attachments on the crib or bassinet to make sure that they are fastened securely.
- Check the temperature of bath water to prevent scalding or chilling.
- Maintain bodily contact at all times when bathing an infant or toddler; never leave a child unattended during a bath.
- Always check the temperature of food or formula before feeding an infant.
- Never microwave an infant's formula to warm it.

Interventions to Prevent Falls

Interventions to prevent falls, especially in the elderly, are of major concern. The environment should be free of potential hazards and equipped with safety devices. Certain basic safety measures should be incorporated into any prevention plan. The use of restraints can be included but only as a last resort and only under a physician's order.

Modifying the Environment

Health care environments are often crowded with equipment and people. Modifying this environment can reduce the risk of falls. For example, make sure that the ambulatory client has a clear path. Remove excess equipment or furniture. Have the client wear rubber-soled shoes or slippers for walking. Additionally, make sure that proper transfer precautions are instituted for a heavy or debilitated client in a bed or wheelchair or on a toilet. Teaching safeguards to the family can also minimize the client's risk of falls in the health care environment. Box 28–5 describes measures for preventing falls in the hospital setting.

Using Equipment Safely

Equipment used in the hospital should be in proper working order. Proper training in the use of equipment commonly used in the home or hospital (suctioning machines, monitors, and so on) should be conducted on a regular basis. Training sessions on newly acquired equipment should be presented by qualified personnel to ensure proper use of the equipment.

Equipment such as wheelchairs, beds, commode chairs, and shower chairs should have brakes that are working properly. Bed wheels should be locked, and the bed should be kept in the low position. Side rails should be kept raised when the client is in bed. Other measures include installing grab bars in the bathroom, applying safety strips in the tub or shower, and not leaving the client unattended while in the bathtub or shower (Fig. 28–10).

Using Restraints

Restraining a client is a protective measure used when the person is in danger harming herself or others. The U.S. Food and Drug Administration, which regulates medical devices, defines a **restraint** as a device (usually a wristlet, anklet, or other type of strap) intended for medical purposes that limits movement to the extent necessary for treatment, examination, or protection of the client. Restraints also can be chemical or environmental. Chemical restraints are medications used to calm the person's behavior; environmental restraints are side rails on beds, locked psychiatric units, or quiet rooms.

In the hospital or nursing home setting, the primary use of restraints is to prevent a client from falling and sustaining an injury. The client must be at high risk for falling or injury, cannot understand that risk, and has no other avenues of prevention available.

The second major reason for restraints is to prevent the client from interrupting therapy, especially when the therapy is life-sustaining. When a client is confused or sedated and therefore unable to understand the presence of an intravenous line, nasogastric tube, wound dressing, or other medical device, it is a natural human instinct to attempt to remove the irritant. The client's hands may need to be restrained to keep her from removing the therapeutic devices.

The third major reason for restraints is to prevent the client from harming herself or others. While violent or self-destructive behavior is usually associated

BOX 28–5

MEASURES TO PREVENT FALLS IN THE HOSPITAL SETTING

On admission, assess each client's risk for falls, and assign one of the following risk levels:

Low Risk: Assign this risk level if the client is alert, ambulates with a steady gait, can perform self-care activities without assistance, has no history of falls, and is cognitively intact and cooperative.

Medium Risk: Assign this risk level if the client may need some assistance or supervision when performing certain daily activities. The person may be alert and cooperative, but she may have a chronic physical ailment or a barrier that could prevent her from calling for help (a language barrier, for instance).

High Risk: Assign this risk level if the client experiences periods of confusion or denies obvious problems of ambulation or mobility. This client may refuse to call for assistance and may attempt to perform activities independently. The client may have a history of falls and noncompliance with safety measures.

General interventions for all clients:

No matter what your client's risk level, always take the following precautions to help avoid falls:

- Once your client arrives in her room, orient her to her new surroundings.
- Keep the side rails in the raised position at all times for all clients, regardless of age. Clients at low risk of falls may choose to have the side rails down during the day.

- Keep the call light, bedside table, water, glasses, and so on within the client's easy reach.
- Use a night light.
- Make sure the client has and wears footwear with nonskid soles when out of bed.
- Use restraints and bed monitors as ordered by the physician.
- Keep the client's bed in the low position at all times except during procedures.
- Teach fall prevention techniques, such as sitting up for a moment before rising from the bed.

Specific interventions for at-risk clients:

If your client has a medium risk of falling, allow her to ambulate only with assistance. Make sure her family and other visitors understand this restriction. Anticipate and meet the client's needs as much as possible. Offer assistance frequently.

If your client has a high risk of falling, try to locate her in a room close to the nurses' station. Keep the side rails raised at all times. Answer the client's call light as quickly as possible. Assess the client more frequently than usual. Maintain the client's scheduled toileting routine, and provide assistance with all activities of daily living. Encourage family members or other visitors to stay with the client.

---

with psychiatric units, general medical or surgical units have occasion to manage violent behavior. Usually, combative behavior results from confusion and fear that arises in a situation the client cannot understand. It sometimes occurs after withdrawal from certain drugs (Procedure 28–1).

The use of restraints is controversial and the subject of concern in the health care setting. Historically, it has not been uncommon to find physical restraints used in health care institutions, especially with elderly clients who interfere with medical treatments or devices, demonstrate disruptive behaviors, or face an increased risk of falls (Wilson, 1996). Psychiatric facilities have adopted policies of treating the client in the least restrictive manner possible. In 1987, the Omnibus Reconciliation Act extended this philosophy to nursing home residents, using the following language: "The client has the right to be free from any physical restraints imposed or psychoactive drug administered for purposes of discipline or convenience, and not required to treat, the resident's medical condition."

All health care facilities have well-defined written policies regarding the use of restraints. Unnecessarily restraining a person may be construed as assault or

false imprisonment. You must be able to document a clear need for a restraint and that the need is for the client's safety, not for the staff's convenience. The documentation should include that other avenues of protecting the client have been pursued. Box 28–6 lists alternatives to restraints.

It is important to emphasize that the use of restraints is generally not advocated and should be considered only as a last resort. Although the use of restraints by health care workers is usually with the best intentions, the complications of restraints can be more devastating than the absence of restraints. In spite of the belief that restraints prevent falls, some research challenges this position (Health Care Financing Administration, 1990). In fact, the use of restraints in older clients can actually increase the risk of falls because of the client's desperate struggle to free herself from the perceived bondage (Wilson, 1996). Other potential complications include the following:

- Hypostatic pneumonia from failure to turn and move in bed or from the inability to take a deep breath because of a constricting device
- Skin abrasions, edema, or pressure injuries from the use of improperly padded restraints

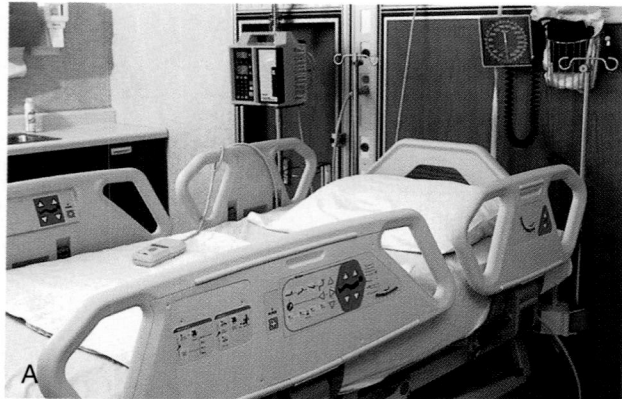

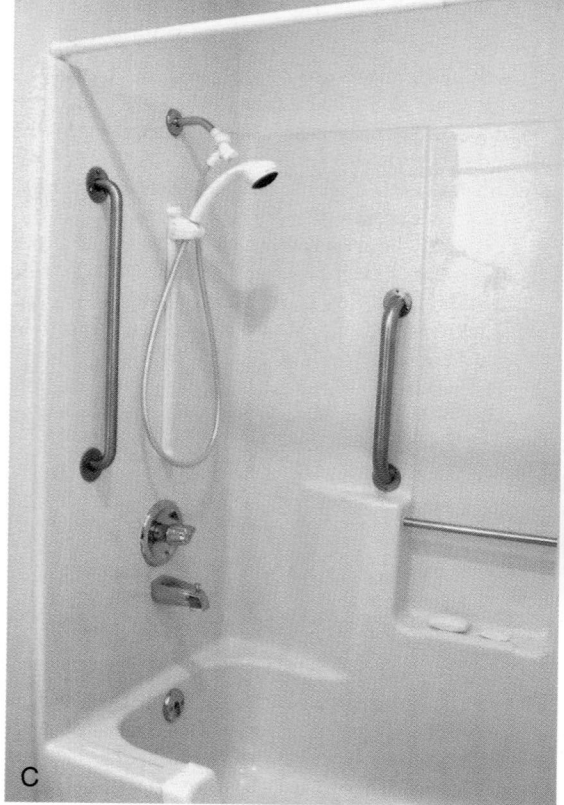

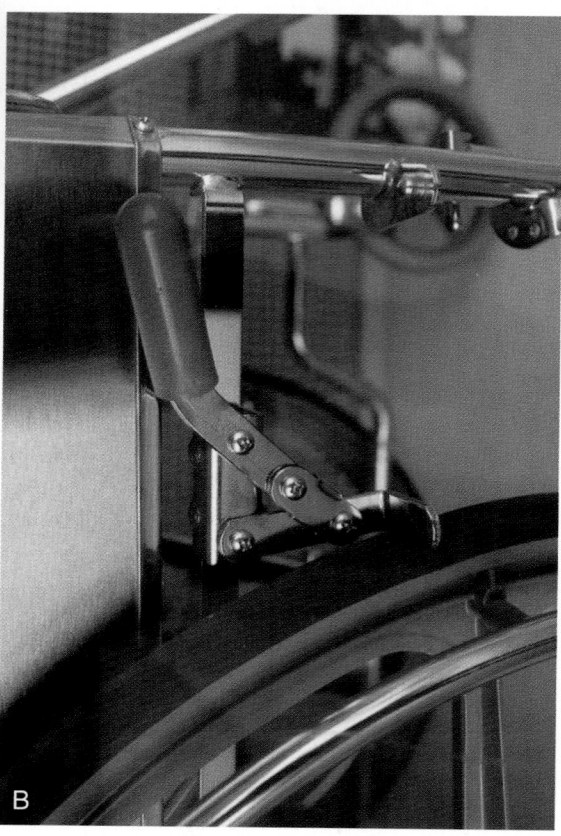

Figure 28–10. Safety devices to help prevent falls in health care institutions and in the client's home. *A,* side rails on beds; *B,* locking devices on wheeled equipment; *C,* grab bars in showers.

- Ischemia and nerve damage if the restraint is applied too tightly
- Strangulation from a vest restraint when the client slides down in bed and is unable to move or call for help
- Contractures from immobility
- Shoulder dislocation from struggling against a restraint
- Aspiration pneumonia

Side rails, stretchers, and other typical types of equipment provide the simplest and least restrictive method of restraint used in the health care environment. If the client needs traditional restraints, several types are available, such as jacket or vest restraints, belt restraints, mitt or hand restraints, and wrist or ankle restraints. Some commonly used restraints must be tied to another object, such as a chair, wheelchair, or bed. They must be tied securely enough to prevent the client from releasing them but precisely enough so that you or another staff member can release them quickly in case of an emergency.

EVALUATION

The effectiveness of nursing interventions used to promote safety and prevent injury is evaluated by comparing the expected outcomes to the goals devised during the planning phase. Nursing interventions are considered effective if the client remains free from injury.

Text continued on page 675

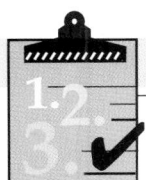

PROCEDURE 28–1

Using Protective Restraints

TIME TO
ALLOW
▼
Novice:
10 min.
Expert:
5 min.

Restraints are any devices or methods for restricting or controlling a client's behavior for the purpose of protecting the client from harm or from causing injury to others. A person can be restrained by confinement to a room or a bed or restrained by the use of drugs that decrease angry or aggressive behavior. The term *restraints* most often refers to restraining devices used to prevent the person from moving the arms or legs.

Delegation Guidelines

The decision to restrain a client may not be delegated to a nursing assistant. Physical restraint requires a physician's order. As a registered nurse, you will be able to determine whether to restrain a client when the client is deemed to be in immediate danger of causing harm to self or others and no other more appropriate means of managing the behavior exist. However, you must inform the physician and provide direction to continue the restraints. You may delegate observation of the restrained client to a nursing assistant. You may also elect to delegate supervision *or assistance with eating, toileting, and repositioning to a nursing assistant, and the reapplication of restraints in these circumstances may be delegated to a nursing assistant. However, you must provide specific criteria for observation and supervision.*

Equipment Needed

- Restraints: jacket, vest, waist, wrist, or ankle restraint
- Padding as needed

---

1 Assess need for restraints.
The client's behavior could cause her to injure herself (risk for fall, risk for suicide, risk for wandering into unsafe areas) or others. Alternatively, it could interrupt medical therapy, thus increasing the risk for complications, delaying the healing process, or causing an early death.

2 Consider alternatives to restraints.
Discuss with the physician and with the client's family.

---

3 Choose the least restrictive type of restraint.
A *jacket restraint* allows the client to turn side-to-side in the bed but prevents the client from getting out of bed or a chair. It secures both the shoulders and the waist.

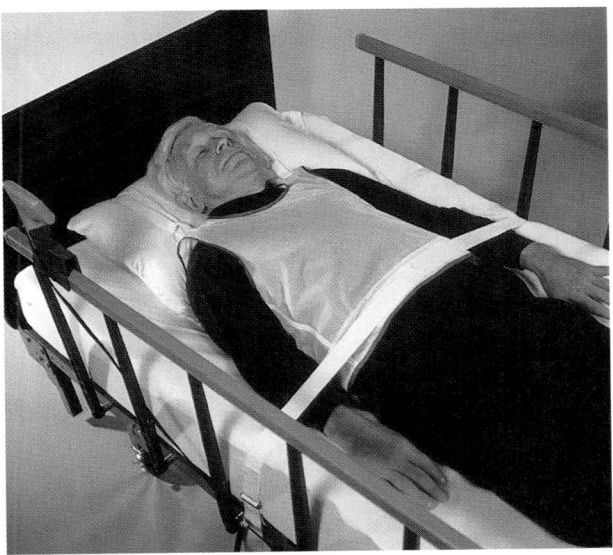

Jacket restraint. (Courtesy of Medline Industries, Mundelein, IL.)

Continued

PROCEDURE 28–1 *(continued)*

Using Protective Restraints

A *belt restraint* secures the person at the waist only. Less restrictive than a jacket, it is also not as protective. It also allows the client to turn side-to-side in bed.

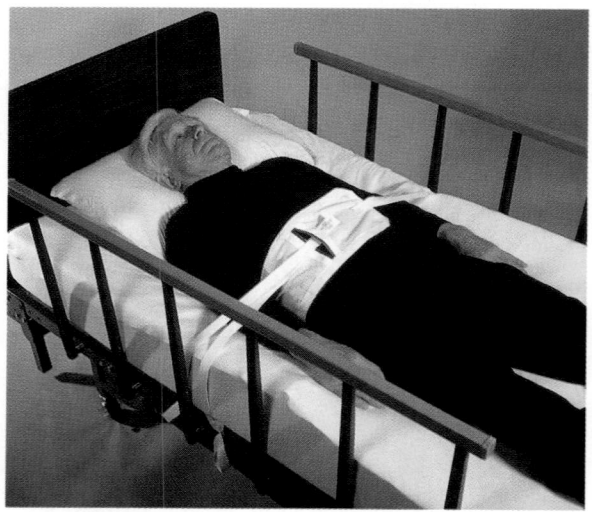

Belt restraint. (Courtesy of Medline Industries, Mundelein, IL.)

A *wrist restraint* secures one or both of the client's hands. By positioning the client's hand or hands away from tubes and dressings, it prevents the client from removing an intravenous line, a nasogastric tube, an indwelling urinary catheter, or a wound dressing. It also can prevent infiltration of an intravenous drug by immobilizing the client's arm. And it can prevent the client from striking people standing nearby.

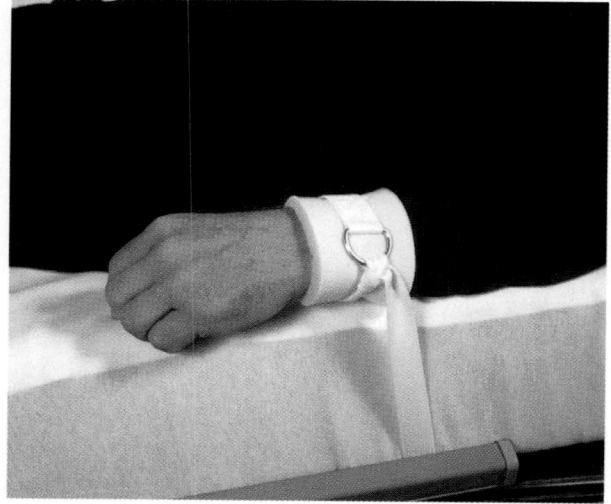

Wrist restraint. (Courtesy of Medline Industries, Mundelein, IL.)

An *ankle restraint* secures one or both ankles and prevents injury caused by thrashing about in bed. It also prevents the client from dislodging a femoral arterial line.

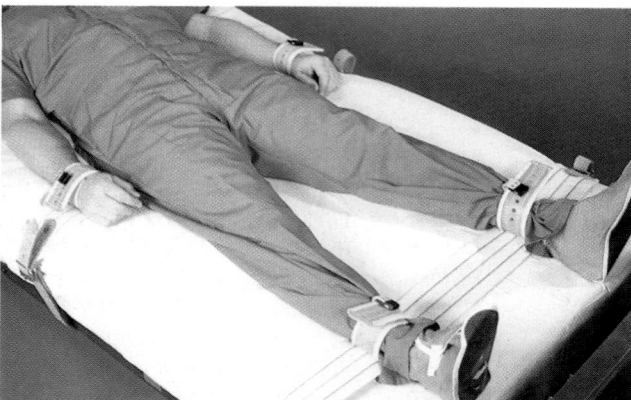

Ankle restraints. (Courtesy of Humane Restraint Co., Inc., Waunakee, WI.)

A *mitten restraint* prevents use of the hands while allowing free arm movements. It is useful for a client who is disturbed by wrist restraints but needs to be prevented from dislodging an intravenous line, indwelling urinary catheter, nasogastric tube, or wound dressing.

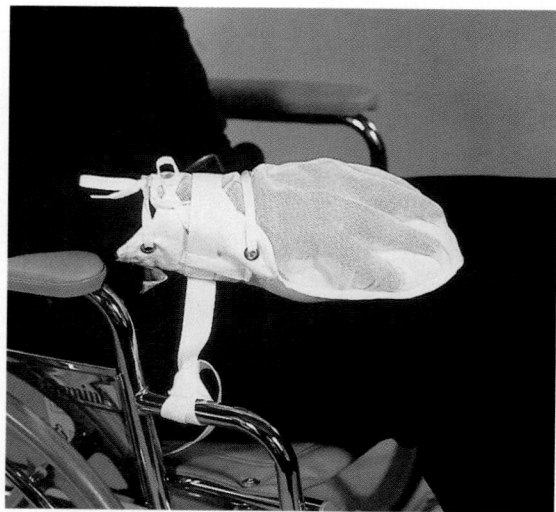

Mitten restraint. (Courtesy of Medline Industries, Mundelein, IL.)

4 Apply the restraint.
   a. Approach the client in a calm, reassuring manner. Avoid sudden or threatening movements.
   b. If the client can understand, explain the need for restraint.
   c. If the client cannot understand the need for restraint, proceed by applying it in a gentle but firm manner.
   d. Pad the skin under the restraint, especially over bony prominences.
   e. Allow room for two fingers to be inserted between the restraint and the client's limb. *Doing so will prevent circulatory constriction.*
   f. Avoid constricting the client's breathing.
   g. Allow the client freedom to turn in bed, if possible.
   h. Tie the restraint to the bed frame rather than a side rail. *The side rail can be moved, which may make the restraint too tight (and harmful to the client) or too loose (ineffective).*
   i. Tie the restraint in a location where the client cannot reach it but where an attendant can quickly and easily release it in an emergency.
   j. Use a slip knot, and never tape a restraint knot.

5 Monitor the client and intervene to prevent complications.
   a. Observe the client every 30 minutes.
   b. Check the client's skin and circulation every 30 minutes.
   c. Provide a regular schedule of toileting.
   d. Turn the client at least every 2 hours; position her for comfort.
   e. Orient the client to her environment every time you check on her.
   f. Assess the client's respirations, cough, and deep breathing every 2 hours.
   g. Reassess the need for restraints every 2 hours.
   h. Help the client with food and fluid intake as needed.

6 Document properly.
   a. Rationale or behavior that led to restraint.
   b. Type of restraint and time it was applied.
   c. Ongoing assessment and interventions to prevent complications.
   d. Time restraints are discontinued and client's response.

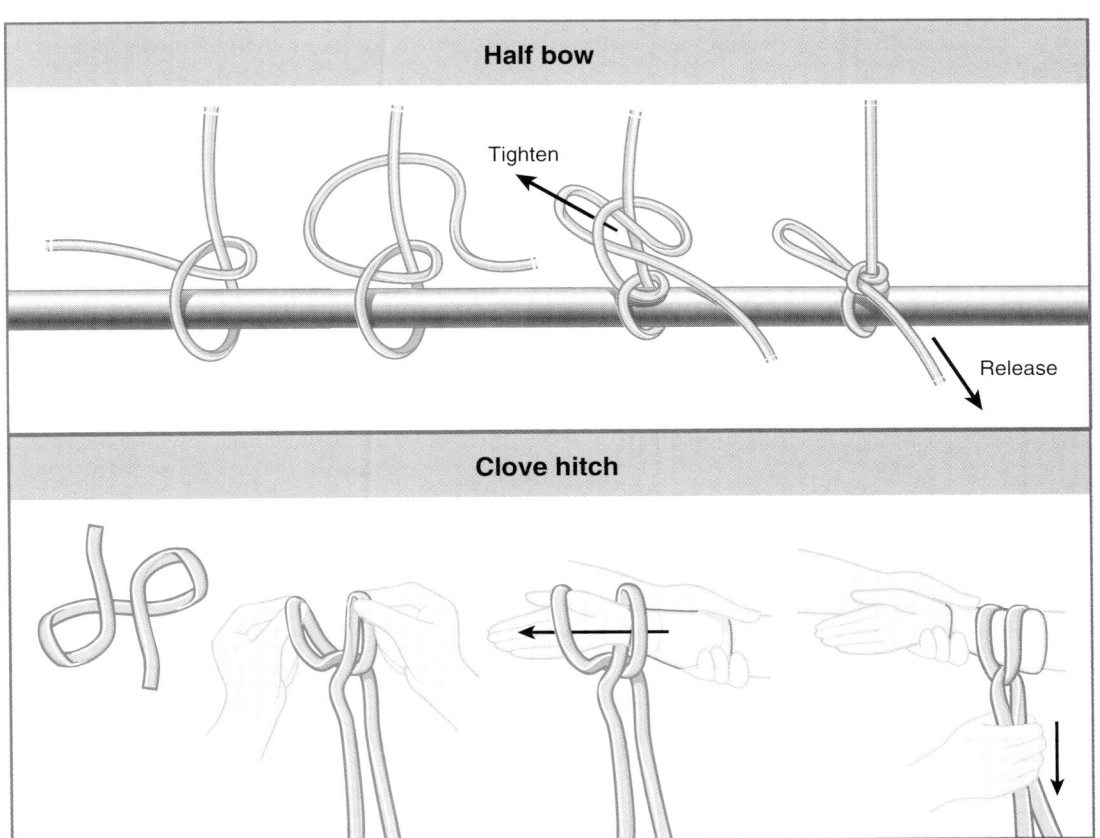

Half bow

Tighten

Release

Clove hitch

Continued

PROCEDURE 28-1 *(continued)*

Using Protective Restraints

HOME CARE CONSIDERATIONS

When the client's behavior in the home requires protection to prevent falls or otherwise keep the client from injuring himself, you should work with the family to provide the protection in the least restrictive manner. If the client needs frequent personal care, a hospital bed may help the family caregivers because of the ease of raising the bed to a working height and lowering the bed to transfer the client to a chair. If the side rails are sufficient restraint, a hospital bed is a good solution. Otherwise, placing the mattress on the floor may give the client freedom from restraints and afford protection from falling when trying to get out of bed. Also talk to the family about supervision and help them work out a schedule to ensure that the client is attended closely.

BOX 28–6

FINDING ALTERNATIVES TO RESTRAINTS

Increase monitoring frequency:

- Assign the client a room near or within view of the nurses' station.
- Perform hourly safety checks.
- Use an electronic monitoring device, such as an Ambularm, which sounds an alarm when the client's leg reaches a 45-degree angle. An ankle alarm can be used to reveal when an ambulatory client wanders off the nursing unit.
- Have family members or a sitter remain with the client.

Provide a familiar environment:

- Familiarize the client to her immediate surroundings.
- Provide continuous orientation to person, place, time, and environment. Remind the client to use her call light.
- Use colors as environmental cues.
- Allow the client to use personal belongings, such as pillow or clothing, when possible.
- Assign familiar personnel, if possible, to help the client feel secure and provide a more accurate assessment of her needs.
- Encourage the family's participation in the client's care.

Prevent the need to get out of bed unassisted:

- Promote a restful environment by minimizing noise, maintaining appropriate lighting, playing relaxing music, and so on.
- Provide comfort measures, such as pain relief and proper positioning.
- Assist with toileting on a regular schedule.

Institute safety measures:

- Use antitip devices, slanted seats, or positioning devices (such as pillows, rolled blankets, and wedge cushions) on wheelchairs to keep the client positioned safely.
- Use bed, chair, or position-sensitive alarms.
- Keep the client's bed in the low position; use half rails; or keep the side rails down.
- Increase lighting in the room; use night lights.

Change the treatment plan:

- Consult with the physician to review the need for intravenous catheters, urinary catheters, or nasogastric tubes.

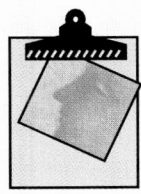

NURSING CARE PLANNING
AN ELDERLY CLIENT WITH A HEAD INJURY

Admission Data

Mrs. Juanita Soto is a 75-year-old Hispanic woman who will be discharged from the hospital in a few days and needs reevaluation by her home health nurse. Mrs. Soto had been admitted through the emergency room to the general medical nursing unit after sustaining a head contusion when she fell trying to get out of the shower. Mrs. Soto informed the nurse, "I never have hurt myself this much before. Usually, I catch myself before I fall all the way, but this time I could not. I guess I'm not as strong as I used to be. Since my husband died, I have lived by myself. My sons and daughters live far away, and I don't want to be a burden on anyone." Mrs. Soto lives alone in a two-story woodframe home.

Nursing Report to Home Health Agency

Client was admitted because of a head contusion sustained while trying to get out of the shower. Her son is present and staying with her while she is in the hospital. Client stated that this has happened before but not to this extent. States that she had been feeling weaker. Has limited movement in hands and legs and is partially blind in one eye.

Mrs. Soto is referred back to the home health agency by her physician. Her daughter had expressed concern about her mother living alone safely and being able to manage her arthritis. Because Mrs. Soto refused to leave her home, the physician requested an evaluation by the home health nurse.

Physician's Referral Request

Evaluate client's ability to perform activities of daily living and instrumental activities of daily living. Arrange for home health aide and Meals on Wheels if needed. Monitor compliance with arthritis medication and assess for side effects. Assist client to plan for two 30-minute to 60-minute rest periods during the day. Arrange for physical therapy to teach isometric and range-of-motion exercises. Home paraffin therapy before exercise, b.i.d.

Home Nursing Assessment

The home assessment revealed an older, two-story home with no safety equipment in the bathroom, some throw rugs, inadequate lighting at night, cluttered hallways, and broken stairs with no railing.

NURSING CARE PLAN

Nursing Diagnosis	Expected Outcomes	Interventions	Evaluation
Risk for injury from falling.	Avoid personal injury from falling in the home environment.	Assess the client for risk factors.	Client maintains order in her home and is familiar with environment. Basement stairs are a hazard; will have son repair stairs to basement. Not safe to cook hot meals; *will arrange Meals on Wheels with provider who caters to Hispanic food preferences. Living in her familiar community is an important value to Mrs. Soto. She has neighbors who are willing to visit frequently and perform small tasks.*

Continued

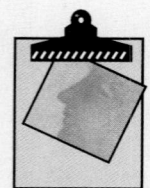

NURSING CARE PLANNING

AN ELDERLY CLIENT WITH A HEAD INJURY *(continued)*

NURSING CARE PLAN *(continued)*

Nursing Diagnosis	Expected Outcomes	Interventions	Evaluation
		Evaluate client's strength, gait, mobility, coordination, and posture. Instruct client to wear rubber or crepe-soled shoes.	Client has limited range of motion in lower extremities and sometimes uses a cane to get around. Also uses a wheelchair. Has shoes with nonskid soles.
	Identify potential hazards in the home environment.	Discuss floor plan of the home with the client and family.	Client stated that the stairs were going to be fixed by her son while he was there. Her home is about 50 years old; it has four bedrooms and two baths. The bathroom floor has tile, and she usually has throw rugs on the floor because it tends to be cold, especially during the winter months.
	Verbalizes understanding of essential safety modifications.	Make suggestions for modifications that may lead to a safer environment.	Client and her son were open to discussion regarding potential modifications.
		Explain to client and family the importance of safety at home (removal of clutter, use of night light, anchoring rugs, application of nonskid material on shower floor, installation of grab bars in bathrooms).	Client verbalized understanding of importance of safety home modifications and decided they would be able to incorporate most of the safety measures mentioned. Client verbalized concern over ability to install grab bars because of cost.
		Assess for cultural practices in the treatment of arthritis	Wears a copper bracelet. States that she prefers this to the medications that the doctor has ordered because they upset her stomach.

Italicized interventions indicate culturally specific care.

Critical Thinking Questions

1. How would you handle the subject of using a copper bracelet rather than the medications the physician has ordered?
2. How would you approach the subject of having a caretaker live with Mrs. Soto?
3. Would adult day care be helpful to this situation?

- Evaluation of safety is an ongoing process throughout the client's illness or hospital stay. You should continuously reevaluate the client's situation and determine whether new threats to safety have developed or previous ones remain. Additionally, continuous reevaluation will help you make good judgments about discontinuing unnecessary restrictions, especially the use of restraints. The evaluation phase requires frequent assessment of the client's situation to identify specific needs for support services, such as home health care, nursing home placement, or physical and occupational therapy.
- It is important to be aware of all the different categories of accidents and hazards that create the potential for risks. Also of importance is an awareness of the people most at risk, such as children and older adults, the handicapped, and the debilitated. You can make a significant difference in the lives of many individuals, especially when it concerns safety issues. Nurses are in a unique position to teach preventive measures, promote safety guidelines, and alleviate alterations in safety.

KEY PRINCIPLES

- To feel safe and to be safe in the home setting or health care facility is a basic human need.
- Nurses are in a prime position to help prevent accidents, promote safety, and alleviate alterations in safety.
- Falls, suffocation, choking, and poisoning can be categorized as general injuries.
- Traumatic injuries can result from fires, electrical shock, motor vehicle accidents, and exposure to radiation.
- Falls are the second leading cause of death in people over the age of 74 years.
- The risk for falls is significantly higher in the hospitalized elderly.
- Asphyxiation or suffocation is a leading cause of mortality during childhood.
- People most at risk for poisoning include toddlers, young children, and adults with sensory impairment.
- Cigarette smoking and the use of alcohol are common factors that can increase the risk of fire injuries.
- Factors that determine the type and extent of an electrical injury include voltage, type of current, area and duration of contact, skin resistance, and path of current flow.
- Motor vehicle accidents are the leading cause of accidental death in the United States.
- Measures to prevent back injuries may include using proper lifting techniques, the use of proper body mechanics, and proper exercise and activity to promote strong bones and muscles.
- Prevent exposure to radiation by using lead shield-

ing and by observing the increased distance/decreased time rule when caring for a client with radioactive implants.
- Factors affecting a person's risk of injury can be identified in the person's home, work, and community.
- Assessment of clients who are at risk for injury includes the collection of subjective and objective data.
- The nurse's role in home safety includes education appropriate for age and developmental status; it also includes making referrals to help the family attain and maintain safe housing.
- The nurse's role in institutional safety involves the safe use of equipment, appropriate client education, and collaboration with the housekeeping and maintenance departments to ensure a safe environment.
- Clients should be restrained only in the absence of viable alternatives and when there is clear evidence that the failure to restrain could cause harm to the client.

BIBLIOGRAPHY

*Ballard, J.E., Koepsell, T.D., & Rivara, F. (1992). Association of smoking and alcohol drinking with residential fire injuries. *American Journal of Epidemiology, 135*(1), 26–34.

Bartscherer, D.J. (1997). Syrup of ipecac: Appropriate use in the emergency department. *Journal of Emergency Nursing, 23*(3), 251–253.

*Brady, R., Chester, F.R., Pierce, L.L., Salter, J.P., Schreck, S., & Radziewicz, R. (1993). Geriatric falls: Prevention strategies for the staff. *Journal of Gerontological Nursing, 19*(9), 26–32.

Brakey, M.R. (1996). Myths and facts about patient falls. *Nursing, 26*(6), 17.

*Brians, L.K., Alexander, K., Grota, P., Chen, R.W.H., & Dumas, V. (1991). The development of the RISK tool for fall prevention, *Rehabilitation Nursing, 16*(2), 67–69.

Butrej, T. (1995). You only get one back! *The Lamp, 52*(11), 12–15.

Castiglia, P.T. (1995). Drowning. *Journal of Pediatric Health Care, 9*(3), 185–186.

Centers for Disease Control and Prevention, National Center for Environmental Health, Childhood Lead Poisoning Prevention. 1997. Screening young children for lead poisoning: Guidance for state and local public health officials. http://www.cdc.gov/nceh.

Cho, C.Y., Alessi, C.A., Cho, M., Aronow, H.U., Stuck, A.E., Rubenstein, L., & Beck, J.C. (1998). The association between chronic illness and functional change among participants in a comprehensive geriatric assessment program. *Journal of the American Geriatric Society, 46*(6), 677–682.

Gustafson, M.C. (1995). To prevent back injury, change behavior. *Occupational Health & Safety, 64*(5), 67–69.

Health Care Financing Administration. (1990). *Federal Register, 54*(21), 1.

Hendrich, A., Nyhuis, A., Kippenbrock, R., & Soja, M.E. (1995). Hospital falls: Development of a predictive model for clinical practice. *Applied Nursing Research, 8*(3), 129–139.

Hodgson, E.A. (1996). Occupational back belt use. *American Association of Occupational Health Nurses Journal, 44*(9), 438–443.

*Holdsclaw, V.A., & Nykamp, D. (1992). Treating poisonings: Focus on syrup of ipecac. *American Pharmacist, 32*(7), 31–33.

*Asterisk indicates a classic or definitive work on this subject.

*Jones, N.E. (1993). Childhood residential injuries. *American Journal of Maternal Child Nursing, 18*(3), 168–172.

Kemp, A., & Sibert, J. (1995). Preventing scalds to children [editorial]. *BMJ, 311*(7006), 643–644.

*Little, A.S. (1994). Drapery cord injury and strangulation in babies. *American Family Physician, 49*(2), 335.

Loomis, T.A., & Hayes, A.W. (1996). *Loomis' Essentials of Toxicology.* San Diego: Academic Press.

McCulloch, C.A., & Tucker, D.E. (1996). Continuous quality improvement in the care of older patients with hip fractures. *Canadian Journal Nursing Administration, 9*(4), 53–72.

*Mellen, P.F., Weedn, V.W., & Kao, G. (1992). Electrocution: A review of 155 cases with emphasis on human factors. *Journal of Forensic Sciences, 37*(4), 1016–1022.

National Center for Health Statistics. (1996). Monthly vital statistics report, *46*(1), 1016–1022.

National Lead Information Center. U.S. EPA (EPA 800-b-92, February 1995). http://www.nsc.org.

National Safety Council. (1997). *Accident facts: 1996.* Washington, D.C.: Author.

North American Nursing Diagnosis Association (1999). *NANDA nursing diagnoses: Definitions and classification 1999–2000.* Philadelphia: Author.

North American Nursing Diagnosis Association (1996). *Official communication.* Philadelphia: Author.

Northridge, M.E., Nevitt, M.C., Kelsey, J.L., & Link B. (1995). Home hazards and falls in the elderly: The role of health and functional status. *American Journal of Public Health, 85*(4), 509–515.

Phillips, J.A., Forrester, B., & Brown, K.C. (1996). Low back pain: Prevention and management. *AAOHN J, 44*(1), 40–52.

Rodriguez, J.G., Baughman, A.L., Sattin, R.W., de Vito, C.A., Ragland, D.L., Bacchelli, J., & Stevens, J.A. (1995). A standardized instrument to assess hazards for falls in the home of older persons. *Accident Analysis Preview, 27*(5), 625–631.

Sattin, R.W., Rodriguez, J.G., DeVito, C.A., & Wingo, P.A. (1998). Home environmental hazards and the risk of fall injury events among community-dwelling older persons. Study to Assess Falls Among the Elderly (SAFE) Group. *Journal of the American Geriatric Society, 46*(6), 669–676.

*Swartz, M.K. (1993). Home and holiday safety. *Journal of Pediatric Health Care, 7,* 290–291.

Walker, B.L. (1998). Preventing Falls. *RN, 61*(5), 40–42.

Wilson, E.B. (1996). Physical restraint of elderly patients in critical care. *Critical Care Nursing Clinics of North America, 8*(1), 61–70.

*Wilson, M.H., Baker, S.P., Teret, S.P., Shock, S., & Garbarino, J. (1991). *Saving children: A guide to injury prevention.* New York: Oxford University Press.

*Wintemute, G.J. (1992). Drowning in early childhood. *Pediatric Annals, 21,* 417–421.

World Health Organization. (1995). *World Health Statistic Annual: 1994.* Geneva: Author.

Nutritional-Metabolic Pattern

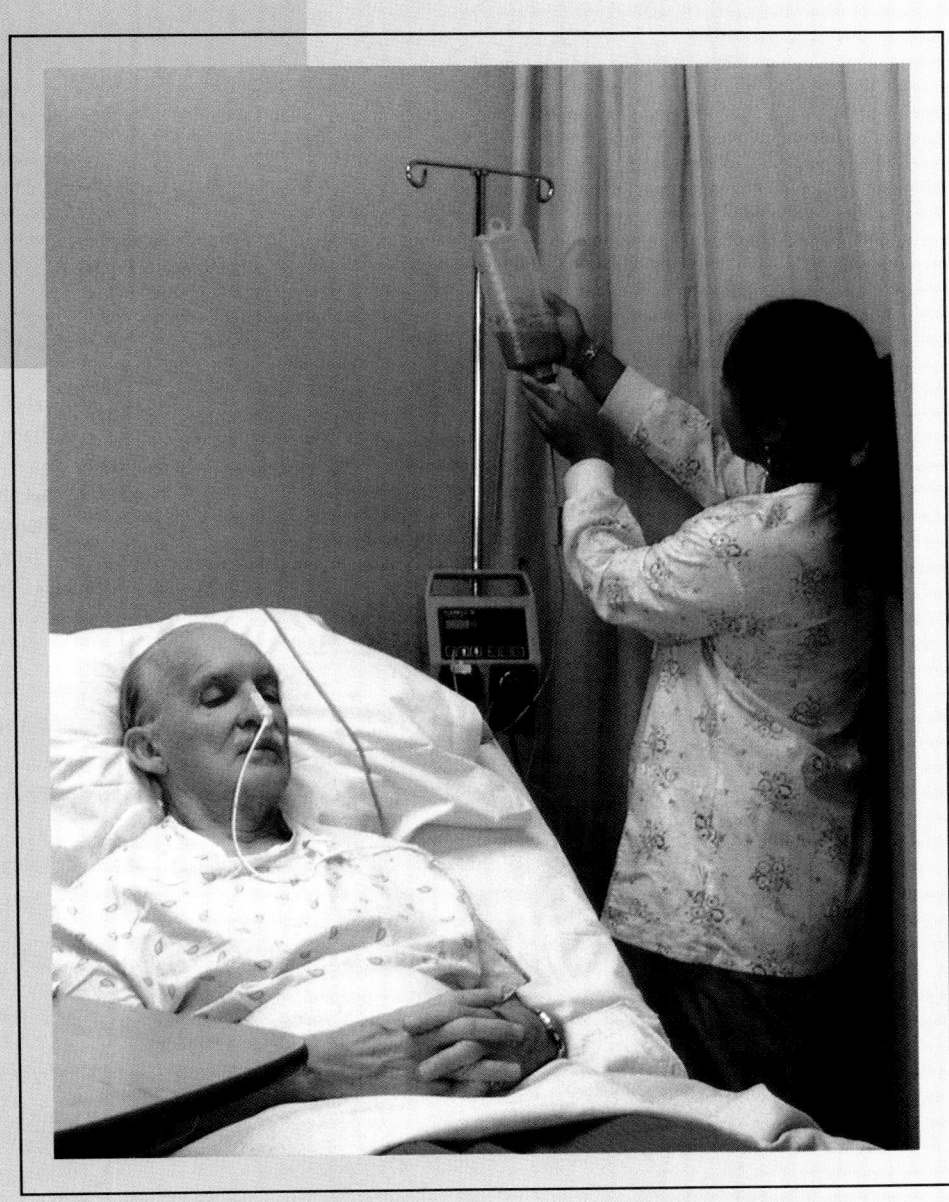

Nutrition

Brenda Leigh Yolles Smith and Katherine S. Schulz

Key Terms

amino acids
anthropometric measurements
calorie
carbohydrate
disaccharide
fiber
glycogen
metabolism
minerals
monosaccharide

nutrient
nutrition
nutritional status
polysaccharide
protein
recommended dietary
    allowance
starch
triglyceride
vitamin

LEARNING OBJECTIVES

After studying this chapter, you should be able to:

1. Describe the elements of a nutritious diet and how the body uses nutrients.
2. Distinguish among various guidelines for normal nutrition.
3. Discuss the factors that affect nutritional status, such as lifestyle, culture, economics, developmental stage, pregnancy and lactation, and psychological and physiological states.
4. Describe the assessment of a client's nutritional status.
5. Identify nursing diagnoses applicable to the client with a normal nutritional balance.
6. Plan for goal-directed interventions to promote optimal nutrition and reduce nutritional risk factors.
7. Describe specific interventions and strategies to promote optimal nutrition and reduce nutritional risk factors throughout the life span.
8. Evaluate the outcomes of nutritional interventions.

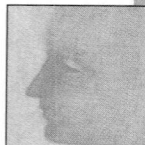

Joan, a 20-year-old, arrives in the nurse practitioner's office for a wellness examination, stating that she feels good and has "no problems." She is of "normal weight" at 115 pounds for her 60-inch (5′0″) frame. Joan says that she has never been hospitalized and has had no serious illnesses. She is an office secretary and participates in many church activities but engages in very little physical activity. Previous medical records reveal that her cholesterol was elevated at an examination 1 year ago.

Joan never eats breakfast but begins a continuous eating pattern beginning about 11:00 AM. She says that she doesn't really eat a meal at lunch but snacks continually until dinner on cookies, candy, rolls, cheese, potato chips, and other snack foods. For dinner she eats fried foods, potatoes, bread, and dessert, and she admits disliking fruits and vegetables.

The clinical evaluation reveals no abnormalities or specific alterations. The triceps skin-fold measure is within normal limits. Joan's total cholesterol is still elevated, and she wants to know how she can reduce it. In analyzing Joan's status, the nurse considers *Altered health maintenance* and *Health-seeking behaviors* from the list of possible nursing diagnoses (see accompanying chart of Nursing Diagnoses) that relate to nutrition.

**NUTRITION
NURSING DIAGNOSES**

Altered Nutrition: More Than Body Requirements: The state in which an individual is experiencing an intake of nutrients that exceeds metabolic needs

Altered Nutrition: Less Than Body Requirements: The state in which an individual is experiencing an intake of nutrients insufficient to meet metabolic needs.

Risk for Altered Nutrition: More Than Body Requirements: The state in which an individual is at risk of experiencing an intake of nutrients that exceeds metabolic needs.

Altered Health Maintenance: Inability to identify, manage, and/or seek out help to maintain health.

Health-Seeking Behaviors: A state in which an individual in stable health is actively seeking ways to alter personal health habits and/or the environment in order to move toward a higher level of health.

From North American Nursing Diagnosis Association. (1999). NANDA nursing diagnoses: Definitions & classification 1999–2000. Philadelphia: Author.

CONCEPTS OF NUTRITION

The human body constantly builds, maintains, and heals itself with the molecules it derives from food. For this reason, there is no single factor that influences a person's health more than decisions about the types and amount of food to eat. It is important for optimal health that the daily diet is balanced and high in quality. Health professionals, such as nurses, physicians, and dietitians, are key sources of information about the role of nutrition in promoting health.

Nutrition and Nutrients

Nutrition is the science of food and nutrients and of the processes by which an organism takes them in and uses them for energy to grow, maintain function, and renew itself. To the layperson, the term *nutrition* is synonymous with food or diet. The building block of the diet is a **nutrient,** which is a biochemical substance used by the body for growth, maintenance, and repair. For optimal health, the diet must be sufficient in a variety of nutrients.

Nutritional status is the condition of the body resulting from its use of essential nutrients available to it. A client's nutritional status may be good, fair, or poor, depending on her intake of dietary essentials, on the relative need for them, and on the body's ability to use them. A good nutritional status is essential for normal organ development and function; for normal reproduction, growth, and maintenance; for optimal activity and working efficiency; for resistance to infection; and for the ability to repair bodily damage or injury. Poor nutritional status exists when the body is deprived of adequate amounts of essential nutrients over an extended period of time.

Nutritional status is relative because the body's stores of some nutrients last longer than others. Additionally, at certain times, demands for particular nutrients may rise. If intake remains constant, stores of these nutrients may be depleted. This may happen, for instance, if a pregnant woman fails to increase her intake of iron, calcium, and certain vitamins.

The Gastrointestinal System

The gastrointestinal (GI) or digestive system converts food into elemental materials that build, maintain, and repair the body's cells. These materials are then absorbed through the intestinal membranes into the bloodstream for use by the body.

Structure

The organs of the GI system include the mouth, pharynx, esophagus, stomach, small intestine, and large intestine (Table 29–1). Ancillary organs that play a role in digestion include the liver, gallbladder, and pancreas. Food enters the system through the mouth, passes into the pharynx and is swallowed, and then passes through the esophagus into the stomach.

The stomach is much wider than the rest of the GI tract and has a J-shaped curve at the bottom. It holds food until the food is digested to the right consistency before allowing it to flow into the intestine. The C-shaped duodenum is the first and shortest portion of the small intestine, followed by the jejunum (the longest portion), and the narrow ileum. The ileocecal valve joins the small intestine to the large intestine, which continues to the rectum and anus.

Function

The four main functions of the GI system are digestion, absorption, metabolism, and excretion. This chapter focuses on the first three. Concepts related to excretion are discussed in Chapter 34.

TABLE 29–1
Digestive Functions of Gastrointestinal Structures

Structure	Function
Mouth	Chews food and mixes it with saliva
Salivary glands	Produce enzymes to begin the breakdown of carbohydrates
Epiglottis	Closes when food is swallowed to prevent aspiration
Esophagus	Transports food bolus from mouth to stomach
Cardiac sphincter	Protects the esophagus from regurgitation of hydrochloric acid
Stomach	Mixes food with hydrochloric acid, pepsin, and lipase to form chyme
Pyloric sphincter	Prevents backflow of alkaline intestinal contents into stomach
Liver	Secretes bile for the emulsification of fat
Gallbladder	Stores and releases bile when fat is present in food
Bile duct	Transports bile to duodenum
Pancreas	Produces trypsin, chymotrypsin, amylase, and lipase for digestion of carbohydrates, fats, and proteins
Pancreatic duct	Collects pancreatic enzymes and transports them to duodenum
Duodenum	Mixes chyme with digestive enzymes and begins nutrient absorption across numerous villi
Jejunum	The main area of digestion and absorption across a great number of villi
Ileum	Finishes digestion of chyme and absorption across a smaller number of villi, especially at distal end
Ileocecal sphincter	Slows absorption time and prevents bacteria from entering small intestine
Appendix	Function unknown
Colon	Reabsorbs water and electrolytes and prepares waste for excretion
Rectum	Stores wastes until peristalsis produces urge to defecate
Anus	Internal and external sphincters control bowel elimination

Digestion is the process by which the body changes food into elemental nutrients that can be absorbed. The process begins in the mouth, where the food is chewed and mixed with saliva. Ptyalin, the enzyme in saliva, begins the breakdown of starches into simpler sugars. The powerful peristaltic action of the stomach churns, liquefies, and mixes the food with gastric juices. Pepsin and hydrochloric acid in the stomach break down proteins into proteases, peptones, and polypeptides. Gastric lipase, which is most active in infants for milk digestion, is a weak fat-splitting enzyme secreted in the stomach.

Food exits the stomach at the pyloric sphincter and enters the small intestine, where most enzymatic digestion and virtually all absorption occur. The pancreatic enzymes—amylase, trypsin, and lipase—are secreted into the small intestine to break down carbohydrate, protein, and fats into sugars, amino acids, and fatty acids, respectively. Bile from the liver, which is concentrated and stored by the gallbladder, emulsifies fats for the action of the fat-splitting enzymes. Once digested material reaches the large intestine, it contains very few nutrients. Here, water and electrolytes are absorbed from this mass, resulting in semisolid feces.

Absorption is the passage of the end products of carbohydrate, protein, and fat digestion as well as many vitamin and mineral molecules through the intestinal wall into the body fluids and tissues. Absorption takes place through diffusion or active transport. The intestinal lining is designed for absorption because it has multiple folds and villi that yield a large surface area.

Metabolism is the process by which energy from nutrients is used by the cells or stored for later use. Individual cells convert chemical energy from molecular bonds into energy for growth, maintenance, and repair as well as for muscle contraction and nerve function. Metabolism can be either anabolic or catabolic. Anabolic processes build up substances and body tissues, whereas catabolic processes break them down. Body reserves are used when one does not eat or when the body has an increased need for nutrients.

Major Components of Food

The body's main nutrients are carbohydrates, proteins, fats, vitamins, and minerals. An adult's metabolism requires nine amino acids, one fatty acid, 13 vitamins, and 12 minerals. All of the major energy-yielding nutrients are composed of smaller units. Carbohydrates, proteins, and fats must by hydrolyzed into their smaller characteristic units before absorption.

Energy and Calories

Carbohydrates, proteins, and fats are collectively called the energy nutrients because they contribute the energy value (calories) from food. Their primary physiological function is the production of energy for health and activity. A healthy body requires not only the minimal level of energy needed for its work but also the extra energy needed for vitality and well-being.

Energy is power that can be translated into motion, overcome resistance, or effect physical change. Energy production in the body is a chemical process that indirectly involves the use of vitamins, minerals, and water. For example, iron is one of the minerals required in the long series of complex chemical reactions needed to release energy.

The human body may be likened to a machine or engine that must constantly be refueled to enable it to perform work. The fuel needed by the body for both external and internal work is, of course, food. The chemical energy available from food is converted in the body to electrical energy for impulse transmission in the brain and nervous system, to thermal energy for regulation of body temperature, and to other forms of chemical energy for the synthesis of body compounds. Chemical energy from food is also converted into mechanical energy, which allows muscles to contract and for work to be accomplished in the external environment.

Foods are frequently discussed in terms of the calories they contain. **Calorie** is the common term used to refer to the more accurate *kilocalorie* (kcal), a measure of the energy content of food. Foods themselves do not actually contain calories; rather, the potential energy of their carbohydrates, proteins, and fats is measured in calories. The calorie used in nutrition is defined as the amount of heat needed to raise the temperature of 1 kg of water 1°C. This unit (the kilocalorie) is 1,000 times larger than the calorie used in either biology or chemistry.

As the United States gradually converts to the metric system of measurement, we must replace the familiar calorie with a more precisely defined unit called the *joule*. The calorie used in nutrition has not been rigorously defined and is not directly derived from the metric system. A *joule* is defined as the energy expended when 1 kg is moved a distance of 1 meter by a force of 1 newton. One calorie equals 4.184 joules; and a calorie (kilocalorie, really) equals 4.184 kilojoules, or 4,184 joules.

Three major factors determine a human being's daily energy requirement: the *basal metabolic rate,* the degree of *physical activity,* and the *specific dynamic action* of food. The basal metabolic rate is the amount of energy needed to maintain essential body functions expressed as calories per hour per square meter of body surface. Essential body functions include respirations, circulation, peristalsis, muscle tone, body temperature, glandular activity, and the other vegetative functions of the body. For infants and children, growth is an additional factor. Energy requirements are stated in calories.

Carbohydrates

A **carbohydrate** is a simple or complex compound composed of carbon, oxygen, and hydrogen. A **monosaccharide** is a six-carbon sugar (a subunit of carbohydrates). Glucose, fructose, and galactose are examples of monosaccharides. A **disaccharide**· is a molecule that forms when two monosaccharides condense and join together to form a double sugar. Sucrose is a disaccharide formed from glucose and fructose; maltose is formed from two units of glucose; and

lactose (milk sugar) is formed from glucose and galactose. Notice that glucose is a component of all disaccharides. A **polysaccharide** is a group of monosaccharides joined together in a chain. They can be converted back to monosaccharides through a process called acid hydrolysis.

Carbohydrates are stored differently in plants and animals. **Glycogen** is the form in which carbohydrates are stored in the muscle tissue of humans and animals. When the body needs quick energy, it uses glycogen stores, which can be broken down into glucose by enzymes. **Starch** is the form in which plants store glucose. They use this energy for growth. When a plant is eaten, the plant starch is hydrolyzed by enzymes into glucose, which can then be used for energy or rearranged to form glycogen for storage. Carbohydrate as an energy source provides 4 kcal per gram.

Fiber is the structure of which plants are composed. Plant fiber includes cellulose, hemicellulose, pectins, gums, and mucilages. A diet high in fiber contains foods such as cereals (especially bran), whole wheat bread, and raw fruits and vegetables. Although most fiber begins as polysaccharides, human enzymes cannot further digest or break down the bonds between monosaccharide units of fiber. Because fiber retains water and increases the rate at which residue moves through the large intestine, people who consume sufficient fiber have fewer problems with constipation.

Other advantages of a high-fiber diet include delayed absorption of glucose and lower blood cholesterol levels. A high-fiber diet also may prevent diverticulosis from developing later in life and may decrease the risk of colon cancer. People who increase fiber in their diet should do so gradually to prevent diarrhea caused by the added bulk and water. They should also drink plenty of fluids to prevent impaction.

Protein

Protein is a compound containing polymers of *amino acids,* linked together in a chain to form polypeptide bonds. There are over 20 **amino acids,** which are compounds composed of carbon, hydrogen, oxygen, and an amino group. Amino acids can be classified as essential or nonessential depending on whether or not the body can manufacture them from other sources.

Proteins form the structure of the body and regulate body processes. Skin, hair, and eyes are made of protein, as are the enzymes needed for digestion and absorption. The antibodies that defend against disease, hormones that regulate body functions, and red and white blood cells are all made of protein. Even lipoproteins, molecules that carry fat and cholesterol in the blood, have a protein core. Proteins also help to maintain fluid, electrolyte, and acid-base balance.

Dietary proteins in the form of polypeptides are broken down by enzymes into individual amino acids called peptides. In this form, they can be absorbed through the intestinal wall and into the bloodstream.

Some dipeptides (two amino acid chains) and tripeptides (three amino acid chains) are also transported through the wall of the small intestine. Protein as an energy source provides 4 kcal per gram. When the body is storing protein (anabolism), the person is said to have a positive nitrogen balance. Conversely, when the body is breaking down protein (catabolism), it is said to be in negative nitrogen balance. Nitrogen that is released during protein catabolism is excreted through the kidneys.

Lipids

Lipids, or fats, are a family of compounds that includes *triglycerides* (fats and oils), phospholipids, and steroids. Like carbohydrates and protein, fat is also composed of carbon, oxygen, and hydrogen. A key difference, however, is that there are more carbon and hydrogen atoms in proportion to oxygen atoms, so fat molecules yield more energy: 9 kcal per gram. **Triglycerides,** each composed of three fatty acids and a glycol unit, are the chief form of fat in the diet and the main form of fat transport in the blood. Ninety-nine percent of body fat is stored in the form of triglycerides.

Enzymes and bile salts are needed to break triglycerides into smaller units (fatty acids, monoglycerides, and glycerol) for use by the body. Small units of digested fat can be absorbed through the cells of the small intestine and into the bloodstream. Larger units can be released by intestinal cells into the lymph system and enter the bloodstream at the thoracic duct.

Vitamins

A **vitamin** is an organic substance found in food that serves as a coenzyme in enzymatic reactions. Vitamins are essential nutrients required in small amounts by the body for physiological and metabolic functioning (Table 29–2). Vitamins cannot be synthesized by the body. They must be obtained from foods. No single food contains all vitamins.

Unlike the carbohydrates, proteins, and fats, vitamins are not linked together in long chains. They are individual units that release energy from food but do not add any energy themselves. Vitamins are measured in very small units, such as milligrams and micrograms.

There are 13 different vitamins. Water-soluble vitamins include the B vitamins and vitamin C. Fat-soluble vitamins include vitamins A, D, E, and K. These vitamins perform many important functions. For example, one vitamin protects the lungs from air pollution; another helps us see in dim light.

Minerals

Minerals are inorganic elements present in small amounts in virtually all body fluids and tissues (Table 29–3). There are 16 minerals essential to human nutrition. Minerals do not yield energy, and they are not metabolized. The major minerals regulate fluid, electrolyte, and acid-base balance and help form the structure of bone. They are also important in the function of muscle and nerve cells.

The major minerals include sodium, chloride, potassium, calcium, phosphorus, magnesium, and sulfur. In addition to major minerals, trace minerals are needed by the body in smaller amounts. They include iron, zinc, iodine, selenium, copper, manganese, fluoride, chromium, and molybdenum.

A balanced diet composed of a wide variety of foods is the best source of all nutrients needed for good health. Dietary vitamin and mineral supplements, if used, should only supplement nutrients obtained from a balanced diet.

FACTORS AFFECTING NUTRITIONAL STATUS

Despite an increase in public awareness, good nutrition typically ranks low on the scale of priorities when most people are making food choices. Consequently, you must fully appreciate the meanings and values associated with food because they commonly transcend its nutrient content and health impact in the minds of clients.

A person's dietary pattern is usually slow to change because food habits are deeply rooted in the past. Even among people who want to change, social pressures tend to make it difficult. Food choices have always been influenced by non-nutritional, social, and cultural factors, including religious taboos, ethnicity, gender roles, and social status. Meal preparation, for example, can reflect relatedness, obligation, self-fulfillment, creativity, or love. Mealtimes have historically been viewed as social occasions, bringing together family and friends. Nonetheless, if national nutrition statistics are an accurate indicator of emerging trends, we apparently are witnessing a dietary revolution unprecedented in the history of nutritional science.

Lifestyle Factors

Lifestyle factors are closely related to food habits. The term *food habits* refers to what people eat and the way they eat. Food habits are derived from total life experience and are very resistant to change. Strong rejections or desires for foods are learned either through role-modeling or compliance (a strong desire to please the caretaker or food distributor, usually the mother). Thus, food habits are more closely linked to associations with others and attitudes toward food than to food nutrient value.

Food habits may be influenced by beliefs about food. Historically, foods that have a higher social status, or "prestige foods," have been more likely to be accepted by consumers. For example, shoppers will buy a steak for a special occasion because it is prestigious, not necessarily because it is nutritious or tasty. Corned beef and cabbage, once considered a "poor man's food," is rarely served on a special occasion. If

TABLE 29–2
Overview of Important Vitamins

Vitamin and Its Adult RDA*	Sources	Functions	Evidence of Imbalance
Vitamin A (Retinol, retinal, retinoic acid) *RDA:* 800 to 1000 retinol equivalent	Dark-green and yellow vegetables, broccoli, carrots, winter squash, sweet potatoes, liver, egg yolks, breakfast cereals, dairy products, margarine, fortified milk, peaches, apricots, cantaloupe.	• Better vision in dim light. • Formation and maintenance of skin and mucous membranes. • Normal growth and development of bones and teeth.	*Deficiency:* Night blindness; dry, rough skin; dry eyes (xerosis); dry mucous membranes; decreased saliva secretion, leading to difficulty chewing and swallowing; impaired digestion and absorption; diarrhea; increased susceptibility to respiratory, urinary tract, and vaginal infections; impaired development of bone and teeth. *Excess:* Anorexia, nausea, vomiting, abdominal pain, diarrhea, weight loss, irritability, fatigue, portal hypertension, loss of hair, dry skin, bone pain and fragility, spleen enlargement, extensive liver damage, hydrocephalus (in infants and children).
Vitamin B₁ (Thiamine) *RDA:* 1.0 to 1.4 mg	Pork, organ meats, liver, enriched and whole-grain grains, eggs, nuts, dried peas, dried beans.	• Energy metabolism, especially of carbohydrates. • Normal nervous system functioning.	*Deficiency:* Anorexia, edema, enlarged heart, heart failure, mental confusion, peripheral paralysis, fatigue, beriberi, painful calf muscles. *Excess:* None known.
Vitamin B₂ (Riboflavin) *RDA:* 1.2 to 1.7 mg	Dairy products, milk, eggs, organ meats, enriched grains, green leafy vegetables.	• Carbohydrate, protein, and fat metabolism. • Other metabolic functions.	*Deficiency:* Reddening of the cornea, dermatitis, cheilosis, glossitis, photophobia, ariboflavinosis. *Excess:* None known.
Niacin (Nicotinic acid) *RDA:* 13 to 19 mg	Lean meat, kidney, poultry, liver, fish, enriched and whole grains, nuts, yeast, peanut butter, and dried peas and beans.	• Carbohydrate, protein, and fat metabolism.	*Deficiency:* Dermatitis, pellagra, diarrhea, dementia, death. *Excess:* Nausea, diarrhea, vomiting, hypotension, tachycardia, hypoglycemia, flushing and itching, liver damage.
Vitamin B₄ *RDA:* 2.0 to 2.2 mg	Organ meats, pork, egg yolk, potatoes, whole grain cereals, wheat germ, yeast.	• Amino acid metabolism. • Blood formation. • Maintenance of nervous tissue. • Conversion of tryptophan to niacin.	*Deficiency:* Anemia, dermatitis, cheilosis, glossitis, abnormal brain wave pattern, convulsions. *Excess:* Sensations of shock or numbness in hands or feet, difficulty walking.
Folic acid *RDA:* 400 μg	Organ meats, milk, eggs, green leafy vegetables, broccoli, asparagus, wheat germ, yeast.	• RNA and DNA synthesis. • Formation and maturation of red blood cells. • Amino acid metabolism.	*Deficiency:* Macrocytic anemia, fatigue, weakness, weight loss, pallor, diarrhea, glossitis. *Excess:* None known.

Table continued on following page

TABLE 29–2

Overview of Important Vitamins *Continued*

Vitamin and Its Adult RDA*	Sources	Functions	Evidence of Imbalance
Vitamin C (Ascorbic acid) *RDA:* 60 mg	Citrus fruits and juices, Brussels sprouts, broccoli, green peppers, strawberries, tomatoes, cabbage, greens, guava.	• Collagen formation. • Protection of other nutrients from oxidation. • Enhancement of iron absorption. • Conversion of folic acid to its active form. • Metabolism of certain amino acids.	*Deficiency:* Bleeding gums (scurvy); hemorrhage; muscle degeneration; delayed wound healing; softening of bones; soft, loose teeth; anemia; increased risk infection. *Excess:* Kidney stones, scurvy upon withdrawal, nausea, abdominal cramps, diarrhea, false-positive test for urinary glucose.
Vitamin D (Cholecalciferol, ergosterol) *RDA:* 5 to 10 μg	Sunlight, liver, egg yolks, fish-liver oils, breakfast cereals, margarine, butter, fortified milk.	• Metabolism of calcium and phosphorus. • Stimulation of calcium absorption. • Mobilization of calcium and phosphorus from bone. • Stimulation of reabsorption of calcium and phosphorus by kidney.	*Deficiency:* In infants and children, rickets, retarded bone growth, bone malformation, enlargement of ends of long bones, malformed teeth, tooth decay; in adults, osteomalacia, bone deformities, pain, easy fracture, involuntary muscle twitching and spasms. *Excess:* Excessive calcification of bones, kidney stones, nausea, vomiting, headache, weakness, weight loss, constipation, polyurea, polydipsia, mental and physical growth retardation (in children), failure to thrive (in children), drowsiness and coma in severe cases.
Vitamin E (Tocopherol) *RDA:* 8 to 10 mg	Vegetable oils, wheat germ, whole-grain products.	• Protection of vitamin A and polyunsaturated fatty acids from oxidation. • Maintenance of cell membrane integrity. • Heme synthesis.	*Deficiency:* Increased hemolysis of red blood cells and macrocytic anemia in premature infants. *Excess:* With large doses, possible depression, fatigue, diarrhea, cramps, blurred vision, headaches, interference with normal blood clotting and vitamin A metabolism.
Vitamin K *RDA:* 70 to 140 μg	Dark-green leafy vegetables, vegetables of the cabbage family. Also produced by gut bacteria in the intestines.	• Synthesis of certain proteins needed for blood clotting.	*Deficiency:* Hemorrhagic disease of the newborn, delayed blood clotting. *Excess:* Hemolytic anemia and liver damage with synthetic vitamin K.

*Others include vitamin B_{22} (cobalamin), 3.0 μg; pantothenic acid, 4 to 7 mg; and biotin, 100 μg to 200 μg.

TABLE 29–3
Overview of Important Minerals

Mineral and Its Adult RDA*	Sources	Functions	Evidence of Imbalance
Macrominerals			
Calcium *RDA:* 800 mg	Milk and dairy products, canned fish with bones, green leafy vegetables.	• Bone and tooth formation. • Blood clotting. • Nerve transmission. • Muscle contraction. • Cell membrane permeability. • Activation of certain enzymes.	*Deficiency:* Osteomalacia, osteoporosis, tetany (intermittent, tonic contractions of the extremities, muscular cramps, uncontrolled seizures, possible convulsions). *Excess:* Nausea, abdominal pain, vomiting, constipation, anorexia, polydipsia, polyuria, calcium kidney stones, excessive calcification of bones and soft tissues, possible coma and death.
Phosphorus *RDA:* 800 mg	Milk and milk products, meat, poultry, fish, eggs, dried peas, dried beans, nuts, soft drinks, processed foods.	• Bone and tooth formation. • Acid-base balance. • Energy and metabolism. • Cell membrane structure. • Component of nucleic acids. • Regulation of hormones and coenzymes. • Fat absorption and transport. • Glucose absorption.	*Deficiency:* Anorexia, weakness, circumoral paresthesia, hyperventilation. *Excess:* Symptoms of hypocalcemic tetany.
Magnesium *RDA:* 350 mg	Green leafy vegetables, nuts, dried peas, dried beans, grains, seafood, cocoa, chocolate.	• Bone and tooth formation. • Smooth muscle relaxation. • Carbohydrate metabolism. • Protein synthesis. • Hormonal activity. • Cell reproduction and growth.	*Deficiency:* Increased neuromuscular and central nervous system (CNS) irritability, loss of muscular control, tremors, disorientation, tetany, convulsions. *Excess:* CNS depression, hypotension, coma.
Sodium *RDA:* 1,100 to 3,300 mg	Salt, sodium-containing preservatives and additives, processed foods, canned meats and vegetables, condiments, pickled foods, ham, soft water, foods prepared in brine solutions, milk, meat, carrots, celery, beets, spinach.	• Fluid balance. • Acid-base balance. • Muscular irritability. • Cell permeability. • Nerve impulse transmission.	*Deficiency:* Cold and clammy skin, decreased skin turgor, apprehension, confusion; irritability, anxiety, hypotension, tachycardia, headache, tremors, seizures, abdominal cramps, nausea, vomiting, diarrhea. *Excess:* Edema; weight gain; hot, flushed, dry skin; dry, red tongue; intense thirst; restless agitation; oliguria or anuria.

Table continued on following page

dietary changes can be associated with a high-status category, they are more likely to be accepted.

A fast-paced lifestyle is consistent with increased consumption of snack foods and fast foods. The onset of the American snack phenomenon and of drive-through fast-food restaurants represents an apparently irreversible social change. A striking aspect of the fast food revolution is that the top food chains in the United States offer an extremely limited variety of food choices. Consumption of french fries, pickles, catsup, beef, fish, and chicken have increased tremendously in recent decades.

The increased dietary fat, decreased complex carbohydrate, and increased simple-sugar components of the fast food diet is clearly contradictory to nutritional goals. In addition, the typical fast-food meal is high in calories, ranging from 900 to 1,300 kcal per meal. That represents a large percentage of a typical person's

TABLE 29–3

Overview of Important Minerals *Continued*

Mineral and Its Adult RDA*	Sources	Functions	Evidence of Imbalance
Potassium *RDA:* 1,875 to 5,625 mg	Whole grains, legumes, fruits, leafy vegetables, broccoli, sweet potatoes, potatoes, meat, tomatoes.	• Fluid balance. • Acid-base balance. • Nerve impulse transmission. • Striated skeletal and cardiac muscle activity. • Carbohydrate metabolism. • Protein synthesis. • Catalyst for many metabolic reactions.	*Deficiency:* Muscle cramps and weakness, including cardiac muscle weakness; anorexia; nausea and vomiting; mental depression or confusion; lethargy; abdominal distention; increased urine output; shallow respirations; irregular pulse. *Excess:* Irritability, anxiety, listlessness, mental confusion, nausea, diarrhea, poor respirations, GI hyperactivity, muscle weakness, numbness of the extremities, hypotension, cardiac arrhythmias, heart block, cardiac arrest.
Microminerals			
Iron *RDA:* 10 to 18 mg	Liver, lean meats, enriched and whole-grain breads and cereals.	• Oxygen transport via hemoglobin and myoglobin. • Constituent of enzyme systems.	*Deficiency:* Microcytic anemia, pallor, decreased work capacity, fatigue, weakness, spoon-shaped fingernails. *Excess:* Acute iron poisoning from accidental overdose, which leads to GI cramping, nausea, vomiting, possible shock, seizures, coma.
Iodine *RDA:* 150 mg	Iodized salt, seafood, food additives, dough conditioners, dairy disinfectants.	• Component of thyroid hormones.	*Deficiency:* Goiter. *Excess:* Acne-like skin lesions, "iodine goiter."
Zinc *RDA:* 15 mg	Oysters, liver, meats, poultry, dried peas, dried beans, nuts.	• Tissue growth, development, and healing. • Sexual maturation and reproduction. • Enzyme formation. • Immune response.	*Deficiency:* Impaired growth, sexual maturation, and immune system functioning; skin lesions; decreased sense of taste and smell. *Excess:* Anorexia, nausea, vomiting, diarrhea, muscle pain, lethargy, drowsiness, bleeding gastric ulcers, decreased serum levels of high-density lipoproteins.

*Others include copper, 2 to 3 mg; manganese, 2 to 5 mg; fluoride, 1.5 to 4 mg; chromium, 0.05 to 0.2 mg, selenium, 0.05 to 0.2 mg; molybdenum, 0.15 to 0.5 mg.

daily calories. The nutritional implications of the trend toward "fast" and "convenient" foods are a source of growing concern to many health professionals. Excessive use of these foods could have adverse long-term health effects.

Remember Joan, who was introduced at the beginning of this chapter? What aspects of her nutritional lifestyle could put her at risk for health problems later in life, even if she is healthy at the present time?

Cultural Factors

Cultural agents of society (those that promote adaptation to a culture and assimilation of its values), such as family, religion, and schools, are all very complex and inter-related. It is difficult to determine the extent to which one agent is more influential than another in determining food habits. Family, particularly parents, usually play the most significant role in determining food served and eaten.

Certain generalizations can be made about cultural influences on eating habits. The first is that most cultures will eat foods in a complex mixture with a staple, such as potatoes, rice, or pasta. These staples, sometimes called "cultural super-foods," form the basis of the meal. Second, to make the food more palatable, its flavor is augmented with spices or flavorings. Third, every cultural group tends to have its unique mixtures of foods, such as the beef bourguignon of the French or the beef Wellington of the English. The continual use of certain foods and their combinations through cultural, technological, and geographical changes shows their value to that cultural group.

Characteristic eating habits and patterns of cultures are observed among different nationalities and religious groups, as discussed in the accompanying Considering the Alternatives chart. A Jewish client might become ill after eating pork, or a Seventh-Day Adventist might become upset after drinking punch that has been made with alcohol. It is important to understand the food preferences and taboos of various cultural and religious groups to provide meals that are acceptable and promote good nutrition.

Economic Factors

The cost of an item is another determinant in food selection, with economics playing a major role in determining food habits. People living in poverty have an increased risk of malnutrition, not because they lack the knowledge to eat nutritious foods (such as fresh fish, organic fruits and vegetables, and fiber-rich breads) but because they lack the money to do so. Some people may be unable to purchase what they might "traditionally" choose to eat. For others, a diet reflecting current dietary goals may be completely unaffordable.

Another effect of culture on food preferences is that certain foods have been associated with social class. Refined sugar was once considered a luxury, but today it seems more fashionable to obtain the harder-to-get "natural" sugar. Upper-class Asians preferred polished white rice to the more nutritious unpolished variety, risking a vitamin B deficiency to remain identified with the upper class. Even in the United States, advertisements often depict obviously affluent families eating healthful cereals and obviously poorer families eating potato chips.

Geographic and economic factors have also historically contributed to the cost and availability of food. Consumption rate, availability, and affordability are inter-related. At one time, it was very rare to find artichokes or avocados from California in Midwestern supermarkets. Now they are more prevalent and far less expensive than they were 20 years ago. In parts of the United States, as another example, veal is less expensive and more readily available because of its higher consumption rate.

Developmental Factors

Infants and Children

Growth during infancy, toddlerhood, and childhood is rapid. Sufficient calorie and protein intake is important in meeting a child's nutritional needs. Because the growth process is rapid, the need for carbohydrates, fats, and other minerals and vitamins is constantly changing. As a health professional, you can support the growth process by supervising the diet.

Adolescents

Adolescents vary in their growth patterns. In general, however, their rapid physical growth requires increased calories to meet their metabolic demands. Specific nutrients also assume added importance. Calcium is important for the support of long-bone calcification, and iron is critical for maintaining increased red blood cell mass.

Vitamins A and C are necessary at this stage as well, although intake of both vitamins may be inadequate if food intake is erratic. Typically, adolescence is a time when peer group pressure often leads to increased snacking and intake of a diet based on a limited number of foods and calories.

Menstrual blood losses in pubescent girls further increase iron needs and put girls at risk for iron-deficiency anemia. Young boys may suffer from the same condition if they are growing rapidly.

Middle Adults

Maintaining health for the middle adult includes eating a well-balanced diet. Appropriate calorie intake depends on each person's body type and physical activity. An adequate nutritional program should include balanced nutrients, vitamins, adequate fiber, and sufficient water.

Older Adults

Many nutrition-related changes occur with aging, including decreases in salivation, chewing efficiency, numbers of taste buds, GI secretions, calcium absorption, renal function, glucose tolerance, and hemopoiesis. The risk of constipation tends to increase.

The rate at which these changes occur varies. However, they are common enough to influence general dietary recommendations for elderly clients. Many older adults have dietary deficiencies in protein, iron, calcium, and zinc. Individual differences may vary and depend on mobility, financial status, and socialization. Other factors that affect nutrient needs and nutritional status include chronic or acute diseases, drug use, and mental problems.

Drug-nutrient interactions are important in older adults because medications may alter nutrient needs.

DIET AND NUTRITION

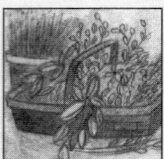 The essential role of nutrition in human health has been recognized in many cultures since antiquity. For example, it is believed that Hippocrates said, "Let your food be your medicine, and your medicine be your food." Though controversies persist about optimal diets and the role, if any, of supplements, scientific evidence supports one important message: Our health is related to what we take into our bodies.

Although the typical American diet is abundant in quantity, it may be lacking in quality. Excesses of animal proteins and fats and a lack of fresh, unprocessed foods are of concern in the typical American diet. Even when Americans do consume adequate fresh, unprocessed foods, there may be legitimate concern about the health consequences of pesticide residues left on those foods. In addition, high-calorie diets and sedentary lifestyles contribute to an increasing incidence of obesity among Americans.

An important factor in the consideration of diet is the concept of *nutrient density*. Nutrient-dense foods have a high ratio of important nutrients in relation to calories. The snack and fast foods that are so common in the American diet, which is high in fats and salt, are not dense in nutrients. To address this problem, federal dietary recommendations have been developed to encourage greater consumption of low-fat foods and fresh fruits and vegetables. Such dietary changes would likely have cancer-preventing effects (World Cancer Research Fund, 1997).

Researchers who have examined diets in other parts of the world have come to the conclusion that certain traditional diets are beneficial. Studies in China have shown that "the closer people get to a plant-based diet, the healthier they are, the lower the rates of cancer, heart disease, osteoporosis, diabetes, etc." (Center for Medical Consumers, 1997). The Chinese population that these researchers studied consumed, on average, about one-tenth the animal protein found in the typical American diet.

Other researchers have looked at the relationship of fats to health and have concluded that the type of fat consumed may be as important as the quantity. The Mediterranean diet primarily uses olive oil, a monounsaturated fat, and is also high in legumes, whole grains, fish, nuts, and low-fat dairy foods. This diet has long been recognized as a very healthy one. Not surprisingly, Mediterranean countries have lower rates of heart disease, certain cancers, and osteoporosis than the United

States, even though the fat intake is comparable. As one researcher summarized: "[People] should eat lower on the food chain—that means less animal products and more fruit, vegetables, beans, and whole grains. If people do that, they will lower their intake of saturated fat. When fat is added, monounsaturated oils should be emphasized" (Center for Medical Consumers, 1998).

Other researchers have focused on omega-3 and omega-6 fats and the ratio between them. Omega-3 fats are found in cold-water fish, flaxseed oil and meal, and perilla oil (commonly found in Japan) and in lesser amounts in beans, eggs, lamb, and pork. Omega-6 fats are found in whole grains, seeds, and nuts and thus the oils made from them. A high ratio of omega-6 oils to omega-3 oils may increase the rates of certain diseases. The traditional Japanese diet had a ratio of 2.8 omega-6 oils to 1 omega-3 oil in 1955. In Japan today, the ratio approaches 5:1. Researchers speculate that concurrent increases in the rates of cancer, heart disease, allergies, and lung disease in Japan may be related to this dietary change and others. Given those changes, it is alarming that in the Western world the ratio of omega-6 to omega-3 fats may be 10 to 30 times higher than in Japan (Felix, 1997). High intake of omega-3 oils may be the reason why Eskimos, who have traditionally consumed a primarily fish-based diet, typically have low serum triglycerides and total cholesterol and high levels of high-density-lipoprotein cholesterol—findings that have been associated with a reduced incidence of cardiovascular disease and some cancers (Garrison & Somer, 1990).

Studies using vegetarian or near-vegetarian diets as part of treatment programs have shown reductions in, and even reversals of, coronary artery disease and improvements in 5-year survival rates from melanoma, the most deadly form of skin cancer (Gar Hildenbrand, Hildenbrand, Bradford, & Cavin, 1995; Ornish, 1990).

What about the use of dietary supplements, such as vitamins and minerals? Nutritionists debate this issue (Garrison & Somer, 1990). Some assert that adequate amounts of vitamins and minerals can be obtained from a well-balanced modern diet. Others believe that, practically speaking, many people do not eat a well-balanced diet and could thus benefit from dietary supplements. In support of the latter assertion, a number of studies have shown that the American diet is deficient in nutrient intake. These deficiencies are exacerbated, especially in women, by reduced-calorie diets adopted for weight loss. Many practitioners of comple-

(continued)

CONSIDERING THE ALTERNATIVES

DIET AND NUTRITION (continued)

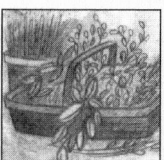

mentary and alternative therapies believe that supplements can improve health, prevent disease, and help to remedy particular problems.

Beneficial effects from many individual nutrients have been found. Vitamin B_1 (thiamin) has been shown effective for moderate to severe dysmenorrhea (Gokhale, 1996). Vitamin E appears to decrease the risk of prostate cancer as well the risk of some other cancers ("Vitamin E reduces," 1998). Numerous studies have shown that calcium may have beneficial effects on bone in postmenopausal women (Murray, 1998), although other studies dispute these findings and indicate possible risks (Center for Medical Consumers, 1997). Supplemental omega-3 fatty acid and gamma-linolenic acid (GLA) have been shown to reduce the severity, frequency, and duration of migraine headaches (Nootbar, 1997). These are just a few of the many benefits of dietary supplements that have been researched.

But vitamin and mineral supplementation is not without risks. A number of vitamins, such as D, A, and B_6 and some minerals can be toxic when taken in very high doses. Also, supplements of one mineral may lead to decreased absorption of others. The manufacture and sale of supplements is a huge industry; although some advertising may be based on research, the conclusions reached may have more to do with boosting sales than with sound scientific study. Professionals and consumers alike need to be as well informed as possible about research on vitamins and minerals.

A provocative area of research in diet and nutrition, which also relates to weight control and other problems, is that of food allergy testing. Food allergy tests expose the subject's blood constituents to food antigens and then record the reactions. One study found that people who eliminated foods from their diet to which they had reacted positively in allergy tests were better able to lose weight and reported fewer troubling symptoms (Kaats, Pullins, & Parkev, 1996). Other researchers have implicated food allergy or sensitivity in headaches, arthritis, irritable bowel syndrome, and a number of other disorders. Elimination of those foods led to improvements in a significant percentage of cases (Solomon, 1992).

A related area of interest is what is known as *leaky gut syndrome*, a condition of increased intestinal permeability, which leads to absorption of larger food particles than normal and possibly microorganisms or their components. A number of conditions may be linked to leaky gut, including arthritis, autoimmune problems, and skin disorders. Leaky gut is also associated with inflam-

matory bowel disease (Murray, 1997) and may be increased by certain medications, such as nonsteroidal anti-inflammatory drugs such as aspirin and ibuprofen.

Resources

Publications that can expand your knowledge of CAM and keep it current:

Galland, L. (1997). *The four pillars of healing.* New York: Random House.

Garrison, R.H., Jr., & Somer, E. (1990). *The nutrition desk reference* (2nd ed.). New Canaan, CT: Keats.

Goodwin, J.S., & Tangum, M.R. (1998). Battling quackery: Attitudes about micronutrient supplements in American academic medicine. *Archives of Internal Medicine, 158,* 2187–2191.

"Healthfacts," Center for Medical Consumers, 237 Thompson Street, New York, NY 10012-1090.

References

Center for Medical Consumers. (1997). Americans don't need more calcium, they need less animal protein. *HealthFacts, 22*(10), 4–5.

Center for Medical Consumers. (1998). Dietary fat reconsidered. *HealthFacts, 23*(3), 1–2.

Felix, C. (1997). *The Felix letter: A commentary on nutrition.* (94/95), 4–8.

Gar Hildenbrand, G.L., Hildenbrand, C., Bradford, K., & Cavin, S.W. (1995). Five-year survival rates of melanoma patients treated by diet therapy after the manner of Gerson: A retrospective review. *Alternative Therapies in Health and Medicine, 1*(4), 29–37.

Garrison, R.H., Jr., & Somer, E. (1990). *The nutrition desk reference* (2nd ed). New Canaan, CT: Keats.

Gokhale, L.B. (1996). Curative treatment of primary (spasmodic) dysmenorrhoea. *Indian Journal of Medical Research, 103,* 227–231.

Kaats, G.R., Pullin, D., & Parker, L.K. (1996). The short term efficacy of the ALCAT test of food sensitivities of facilitate changes in body composition and self-reported disease symptoms: A randomized controlled study. *The Bariatrician,* Spring 1996, 18–23.

Murray, M. (1998). Calcium vs. osteoporosis in postmenopausal women. *Natural Medicine Journal, 1*(1), 16–17.

Murray, M. (1997). Chronic candidiasis: A natural approach. *American Journal of Natural Medicine, 4*(4), 13–14.

Nootbar, W.W. (1997). Prophylactic treatment of migraine with gamma-linolenic and alpha-linolenic acids. *Cephalalgia, 17,* 127–130.

Ornish, D. (1990). *Dr. Dean Ornish's program for reversing heart disease.* New York: Ballantine.

Solomon, B.A. (1992). The ALCAT test—a guide and barometer in the therapy of environmental and food sensitivities. *Environmental Medicine, 9,* 54–59.

Vitamin E reduces prostate cancer risk (March 18, 1998). *Fort Myers News Press,* p. 1.

World Cancer Research Fund, American Institute for Cancer Research (1997). *Food, nutrition and prevention of cancer: A global perspective* (Summary). Washington, D.C.: Author.

The timing of food ingestion in relation to medication administration is another important consideration, particularly among clients who take several drugs. Many older adults take three or more medications each day. Institutionalized older adults may take as many as 10 each day.

Pregnant and Lactating Women

Pregnancy and lactation increase a woman's need for calories and fluid. Further, physiological changes occur during pregnancy that can alter body status. For example, increased intravascular volume can cause a "pseudo-anemic" condition. The overall increase in blood volume and total body fluid can also cause fluid retention and edema, which may be treated in part with diet.

Psychological Factors

People eat for many reasons, only one of which is hunger. Emotional states—such as boredom, anger, depression, or loneliness—can influence the quality and quantity of a person's intake. Emotions can overpower subtle physiological cues that regulate hunger and can result in undereating or overeating, depending on the person. Emotions can also influence poor eating habits.

Food is often used as reward or punishment. We can offer food to express love and approval or withhold it to express disapproval. In the United States, it is acceptable to give children candy, cookies, or ice cream when they are good. Adults may continue this symbolism established in childhood by rewarding themselves with a special food or by going out to dinner if they have been especially good or have worked hard.

Good eating behavior continues when it is positively reinforced. Reinforcement may be physiological, as when hunger is eliminated. Eating may also be situational, such as eating at the same time each day, when arriving at Grandma's house, or when guests come to visit.

Children sometimes rebel against their parents through food. The daughter who develops anorexia nervosa (see Chapter 30) or the son who feels unloved and tends to overeat at mealtime is communicating with us.

> A*ction* A*lert!*
> Recognize anorexia nervosa or overeating as possible attempts to cope with frustration, anger, aggression, depression, or unmet needs for affection. Become aware of the behavior exhibited and try to understand the meaning of that behavior in relation to food.

Physiological Factors

Healthy body functioning promotes optimal digestion and absorption of food. Healthy teeth and gums or well-fitting dentures are important for chewing, which is needed to break up food for digestion. The GI system must function well for optimal use of ingested nutrients. Normal production of insulin and digestive enzymes is also important for food use.

Physical factors can affect a person's ability to buy, transport, cook, and eat food. Physical mobility and energy are needed for shopping, cooking, and eating. When a person physically cannot complete such tasks, assistance may be needed to ensure adequate nutrition.

ASSESSMENT

Most people could benefit from an assessment of their nutritional status and dietary patterns. The three purposes of a nutritional assessment are to identify clients who need further nutritional assessment, to establish baseline values for evaluating the efficacy of nutritional regimens, and to provide a system for early recognition of increased health risk caused by nutritional factors.

General Assessment of Nutritional Status

Assessment of a client's nutritional status involves measuring both the degree to which the physiological need for nutrients is being met and the degree of balance between nutrient intake and nutrient expenditure. Because nutritional status has an effect on well-being, growth, performance, and resistance to disease, a thorough and accurate nutritional assessment is important. The components of a nutritional assessment include the health history (including diet history), evaluation of food intake, and physical examination.

Health History

If a client has a severe problem or an unusual eating pattern, you should refer her to a registered dietitian who is trained to evaluate nutritional states and to provide recommendations and sample meal plans for the client. The registered dietitian can be an excellent consultant for you and resource for your clients if you work in home health. You would then reinforce the information provided by the dietitian.

To take a diet history, collect and analyze data about the type and amount of food the client eats. It can be difficult and frustrating to accurately record and evaluate dietary intake for several reasons. First, it is difficult to record a client's food intake without influencing it. When people are watched, questioned about what they eat, or asked to write down what they eat, eating patterns tend to change. The extent of change depends on how well the client understands the dietary history or to what extent she is influenced by what she thinks you want to see or hear.

Second, many people simply cannot remember the types or amounts of food eaten. Third, it can be difficult to accurately evaluate the nutrient composition of food unless the specific ingredients are known. Carefully reading food labels on manufactured foods can be helpful. Food labels are required by law to list, among other things, the calories and specific nutrients in each product. Be aware that methods of cooking can greatly affect nutrient values. Even the area in which a fruit or vegetable is grown can affect its nutrient content.

24-HOUR RECALL

The most popular and easiest method for obtaining data about a client's intake is the *24-hour recall.* The person completes a questionnaire or is interviewed by you, a dietitian, or a nutritionist experienced in dietary interviewing. The client is asked to recall everything eaten the previous day or within the last 24 hours. When performing this test, keep in mind that it has three significant sources of error:

- The client may not be able to recall accurately the amounts of food eaten.
- The previous day's intake may not represent the usual intake.
- The client may not tell the truth for a variety of reasons, including possible embarrassment.

Clients have a tendency to underestimate intake as the portion size increases and overestimate intake as the portion size decreases. Foods that are least likely to be accurately reported are sauces, gravies, fruits, and snack items.

When conducting an interview for a 24-hour recall, compare an actual day (the previous day is best) with a typical day. Be objective, and use open-ended questions, such as *When did you get up? What was the first thing that you ate? What did you drink?* and *What time did you eat next?* This type of questioning may elicit information on snacks and unusual patterns of eating. It is less likely to encourage incorrect information because it avoids giving clients clues about what answers are considered appropriate. To foster accurate reporting, do not react negatively to any response from the client.

FOOD FREQUENCY QUESTIONNAIRE

To help overcome some of the inherent weaknesses in the 24-hour recall method, a *food frequency questionnaire* may also be completed. Using this tool, you can collect information about how many times per day, week, or month a client eats particular foods. This information can help validate the accuracy of the 24-hour recall data and clarify the client's real food consumption pattern. The food frequency questionnaire may be general, containing questions concerning all foods, or selective, containing questions about suspected deficient or excessive foods in the diet.

FOOD DIARY

A *food diary* is a written record of food intake maintained for a specified period of time, usually 3 to 7 days. The time frame depends on the purpose, the nutrients being assessed, and the interest level of the client. This type of assessment may also be used to determine food allergies. Consider carefully the days chosen to observe intake. Food consumption on weekends and holidays

is usually different from that of weekdays. A combination of weekday and weekend recordings often reflects a more accurate picture. In the hospital setting, you may be required to keep track of food intake on a calorie count sheet kept at the bedside.

For best results, client teaching must be clear. For each day the food diary is kept, ask the client to record the names of foods eaten, the way food was prepared, and (if indicated) the time and place the food was eaten. A legitimate concern with the food diary is that the client may change eating patterns on the days of the recording. Encourage clients to eat the foods and amounts that are normal for them on these days. Again, a nonjudgmental manner helps.

When a very accurate record of food consumption is required, the *weighed intake record* is best. Teach the client to weigh all food consumed during the recording and to correct for food waste (food served but not eaten). Because this method is tedious, the client must be well-motivated to achieve accurate results. Risks are that the client will try to find shortcuts in preparation to make the weighing less time-consuming and that the client's eating patterns may change. The weighed intake method is most frequently used in controlled laboratory studies.

HOUSEHOLD FOOD CONSUMPTION

This method involves visiting a household periodically and recording the amounts and types of food purchased for that household and the disappearance of that food. The food unaccounted for is assumed to have been eaten by the family. Household food consumption is most commonly used in large population surveys. It is not a good evaluation of individual intake because it does not record food waste or food consumed by each household member. It is helpful, however, in trying to gain insight into the nutritional situation in a community.

Food in the household can be compared with the income of the household, the food available in the marketplace, and other factors. For example, farming communities may have rich supplies of grains and vegetables but lack access to imported or specialty foods. Foods available in the market may also be limited for some inner-city dwellers, such as the frail elderly, who may have to shop at a corner market that does not carry items such as soy milk, salt-free crackers, or fresh fruits and vegetables.

EVALUATION OF FOOD INTAKE

There are basically two methods by which food intake information is evaluated for adequacy. These are the food group method and the nutrient composition method.

Food Group Method

The simplest and fastest way to evaluate food intake data is to determine how many servings from each of the six food groups were consumed during the recorded day. The number of servings from each group is then compared with the number of servings suggested in the food guide pyramid (Fig. 29–1). It becomes more difficult to use this method if the diet has many food mixtures or unusual cultural foods that do not fit into one of the food groups. For many people, however, gross deficiencies of protein and a number of vitamins can be detected using this method.

Vitamin deficiencies can often be linked to deficiencies in specific food groups. Intake of folic acid and vitamins A and C is most variable because they are not widely present in foods, except for particular fruits and vegetables. Intake of these nutrients is frequently seasonal, with higher intake in the summer and fall when fresh fruits and vegetables are abundant and cheaper.

Riboflavin, calcium, and vitamin D intake largely depends on the intake of milk and milk products. Daily intake of protein, thiamine, niacin, phosphorus, iron, and vitamins E, B_6, and B_{12} is more consistent because these nutrients are present in a wide variety of foods.

Use the food group method to determine the degree to which Joan, our case study client, is taking in a nutritionally balanced diet.

Nutrient Composition Method

Dietary intake can be evaluated more accurately by calculating the amounts of a nutrient in each food consumed. This analysis can be done manually or by computer. The nutrient values for foods can be obtained from several nutrition publications, nutrition labels, and food manufacturers' information on a food's nutrient composition. After recording the nutrient composition for individual foods, you can determine composition of the total diet.

Once the nutrient composition of the diet is determined, the amount of an individual nutrient can then be compared with the **recommended dietary allowance** (RDA). The RDA is the level of a nutrient that is adequate to meet the needs of almost all healthy people as determined by the Food and Nutrition Board of the National Research Council. Although the RDA is frequently used to evaluate the components of a person's diet, this is theoretically an improper use. RDAs are set at a level slightly above average requirements so they can include everyone in the population who might have an increased need for a particular vitamin or mineral. Because the RDAs include this "safety factor," they are probably higher than a typical person needs. Nutrition textbooks typically contain published tables of RDAs for fat- and water-soluble vitamins and minerals according to age group, height, and weight.

Energy and protein intake should be evaluated on the basis of body weight or, in the case of an underweight or overweight person, on the basis of height. This increases the usefulness of the RDA in individual assessment, especially with children, who at any particular age may differ greatly in size.

RDAs are not meant to be applied to sick people, whose requirements may be very different from those of healthy people. At present, however, there are no established nutrient requirements for various disease states. With these limitations in mind, you can use nutrient RDAs as a general evaluation of the dietary intake of clients who are ill.

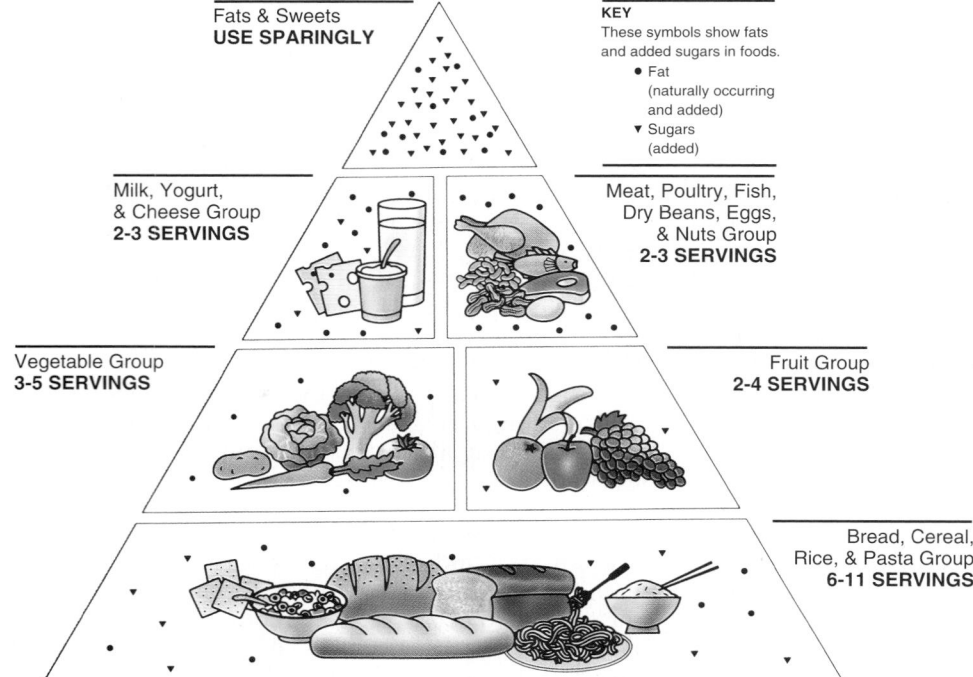

Figure 29–1. Food Guide Pyramid. (U.S. Department of Agriculture and U.S. Department of Health and Human Services.)

Physical Examination

CLINICAL SIGNS OF NUTRITIONAL STATUS

A thorough physical examination will reveal physical signs of nutritional deficiencies. Vitamin and mineral deficiencies can be manifested by clinical signs and symptoms, as previously illustrated in Tables 29–2 and 29–3.

ANTHROPOMETRIC MEASUREMENTS

Anthropometric measurements are measurements of physical characteristics of the body (such as height and weight) as well as the amount of muscle or fat tissue in the body.

Height-Weight Tables

Various tables are available that list average heights and desirable weights for infants, children, males, and females. All suggest approximate weights for healthy adults. Charts listing desirable weights for adults according to frame size are also available. These charts, often produced by insurance companies, list the weight for each inch of height that is associated with the lowest morbidity and mortality. These charts are commonly found in nutrition textbooks.

Another frequently-used height/weight figure is the Usual Weight. In an older adult, the Usual Weight might be more indicative of nutritional health than a figure based on the optimal height/weight tables.

Remember that these tables are guides and should be used for screening purposes. To obtain a quick ballpark figure useful for basic screening, use the following:

- A male of 5'0" should weigh about 106 pounds. Add 6 pounds for each additional inch.
- A female of 5'0" should weigh about 100 pounds. Add 5 pounds for each additional inch.

Being either underweight or overweight may be associated with increased risk of morbidity and mortality.

A disadvantage of height/weight tables is that they group all adults together without considering age. Insurance tables have also been criticized as under-representing lower socioeconomic classes.

Body Mass Index

Because of the disadvantages of height/weight methods, many health professionals prefer to use a mathematical standard called body mass index (BMI). You determine a person's BMI using this formula:

BMI = weight (kg) divided by height (meters)

A result above 27 indicates obesity, a result of 24 to 27 indicates excess weight in women, and result of 24 to 25 indicates excess weight in men.

Body Composition

Various body compartments (fat stores or lean tissue) can be affected by over- or under-nutrition. To esti-

mate the degree to which these compartments are affected, use fat-fold measurements and midarm muscle circumference.

About half the body's fat is located directly beneath the skin. Consequently, skin thickness reflects total body fat. The fat-fold measure may be useful when performed by a trained person following a standard procedure using reliable calipers. The most easily accessible area is the triceps fat fold, making it the most practical in clinical settings (Fig. 29–2A).

The midarm muscle circumference is an indicator of lean tissue stores (Fig. 29–2B). It can be derived by

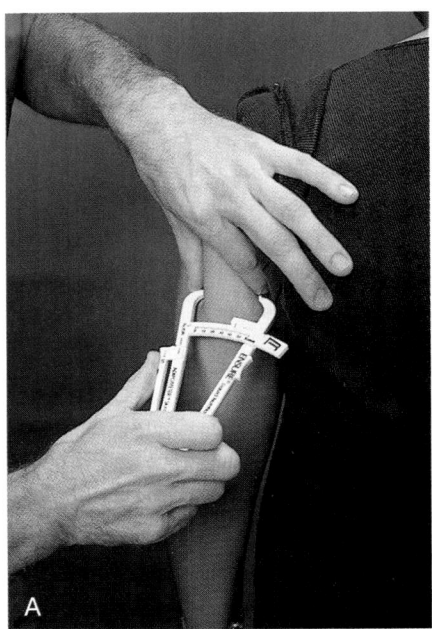

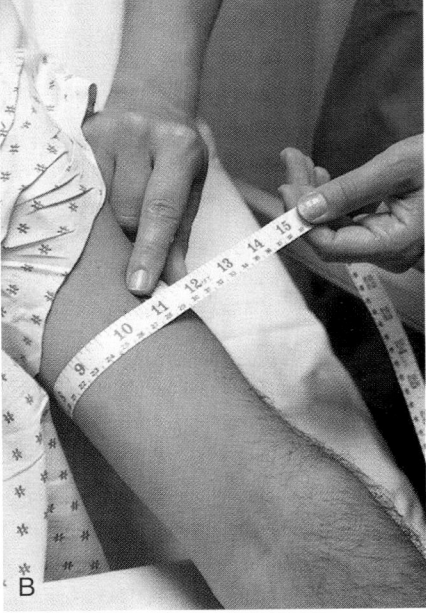

Figure 29–2. Anthropometric measurements. *A,* Using calipers to measure triceps fat-fold; *B,* Measuring midarm muscle circumference.

taking the mid-arm circumference and the triceps fat fold using the following equation:

$$\text{Mid-arm muscle circumference} = \text{Mid-arm}$$
$$\text{circumference (cm)} - [0.314 \times \text{triceps fat-fold}$$
$$\text{(mm)}], \text{where } 0.314 \text{ is the conversion factor}$$

The 50th percentile value for mid-arm muscle circumference is 281 for middle-aged men and 222 for middle-aged women.

Joan's triceps fat-fold measure is within normal limits. Remember also that her clinical evaluation revealed no specific abnormalities. What does this tell you about the impact of her eating habits to this point?

Diagnostic Tests

The most common laboratory indices of nutritional status are serum pre-albumin, albumin, transferrin, lymphocyte count, hemoglobin, hematocrit, and urine specific gravity.

Albumin, pre-albumin, and *lymphocyte count* are indicators of protein intake, whereas *transferrin* reflects protein and iron stores.

Hematocrit measures the percentage of whole blood that is composed of red blood cells. An increase or decrease in either red blood cell count or plasma volume affects the hematocrit. Conditions that increase red blood cell production increase the hematocrit, whereas anemia can lower both hemoglobin and hematocrit. Extracellular fluid volume deficit may increase hematocrit, whereas fluid volume excess decreases it.

With normal fluid intake, *urine-specific gravity* is usually 1.010 to 1.020. Concentrated urine has a higher specific gravity, and dilute urine has a lower specific gravity. These findings correlate with hypovolemia and hypervolemia, respectively.

Focused Assessment for Risk for Altered Nutrition: Less Than Body Requirements

Some populations at risk for nutritional deficiencies are the elderly, adolescents, children, pregnant women, and infants. In the well client, nutritional deficiencies may not be severe enough to produce actual signs and symptoms of deficiency; however, general fatigue, irritability, frequent colds or flu, and symptoms of stress may result from a diet that is deficient in one or more nutrients.

A*ction* A*lert!*
Be alert to the presence of fatigue, irritability, frequent colds and flu, and stress-related symptoms as cues to the possibility of mild nutritional deficiency.

Assess the client's dietary pattern for risk factors, such as overuse of snack foods, using fast-foods as a main dietary source, use of processed foods, and cooking methods that destroy nutrients. Determine if the client eats a balanced diet. Assess the client's lifestyle for related factors as well. The nutritional deficiency may be related to lack of money, knowledge, or time to prepare food.

Focused Assessment for Risk for Altered Nutrition: More Than Body Requirements

Risk factors for *Risk for altered nutrition: more than body requirements* include the following:

- Reported use of solid food as a major food source before 5 months of age
- Concentrated food intake at the end of the day
- Reported or observed obesity in one or both parents
- Reported or observed higher baseline weight at the beginning of each pregnancy
- Rapid transition across growth percentiles in infants or children
- Pairing food with other activities
- Observed use of food as reward or comfort measure
- Eating in response to internal cues other than hunger, such as anxiety
- Eating in response to external cues, such as time of day or social situation
- Dysfunctional eating patterns

Although Joan is not overweight, why might the nursing diagnosis *Risk for altered nutrition: more than body requirements* be appropriate? Joan has indicated an interest in reducing her elevated cholesterol level. What other nursing diagnosis might be appropriate for her?

DIAGNOSIS

There are several options in the NANDA nursing diagnosis system for addressing nutritional problems. Diagnostic labels are needed for the well client who seeks a higher level of wellness, the client who has risk factors for nutritional problems, and the client who actually has a deficit or excess in one or more nutrients.

The diagnosis *Health-seeking behaviors: nutrition* can used for a client who is well but seeks an optimal state of physical and mental well-being. The goals of *Health-seeking behaviors* suggest the need for health promotion activities, one of which is proper nutrition.

The diagnosis *Altered nutrition: less than body requirements* indicates that the client has nutritional deficiencies. The diagnosis *Altered nutrition: more than body requirements* indicates obesity or a diet that is high in nutrients such as fat, carbohydrates, or sodium.

Altered health maintenance suggests that factors have changed the way health is maintained, such as an illness that requires management, inadequate control of disease risk factors, or a lack of knowledge and skills needed to maintain health. The need for information about the nutritional content of food, eating habits, or cooking falls into this category.

PLANNING

Planning for clients includes using assessment data to identify nutritional needs. Guidance, supervision, and education may be needed to help improve the client's nutritional knowledge. Direct nursing care may be also be part of the plan. Sample expected outcomes for a client who has received nutrition education include the following:

- Client will plan meals using the food pyramid guide.
- Client will implement shopping and cooking methods for economical food preparation, such as using beans and legumes as a protein source, using powdered milk for cooking, and making soups or stews with leftover food.
- Client will eat the bulk of calories early in the day.
- Client will eat only when seated at the dining table, not in front of the television or while performing other activities.
- Client will increase activity level by using stairs instead of elevators, parking the car in more remote parking spots, and taking a daily walk.

INTERVENTION

If we are to succeed in our efforts to promote wellness, prevent disease, and improve quality of life, we must do so cooperatively. You must be willing to work with educators, researchers, industrial and political leaders, and informed consumers to continue to develop assertive strategies to improve nutrition. There is an ever-expanding body of knowledge about nutrition being generated by research done at numerous government and private agencies and at industrial and academic institutions. Thus, there are many valuable and reliable sources of information that you can use to develop nutrition-oriented wellness programs.

Interventions to Promote a Healthy Diet

Knowledge of the nutritional value of foods and their relationship to wellness is essential but is clearly not enough to induce clients to consume appropriate foods. Otherwise, health professionals themselves would be by far the slimmest, best-exercised, optimally nourished group in the nation! What can be done, then, to actually get clients to change their nutritional patterns?

One key is educating and encouraging the population from infancy. Health professionals too often encounter adolescents and adults who have well-established eating patterns that are far from ideal. You, as a nurse working with clients at varying points in the life span, are in a unique position to assess cultural, economic, and environmental factors influencing their food choices. This information is crucial to successful dietary intervention.

Nutrition education is a broad area; however, most nutritional counseling takes place in acute or long-term care facilities and community-based clinics. Most nutrition education begins with assessment of dietary intake. A broad knowledge of food, nutrition, pathophysiology, and biochemistry is important in analyzing food habits and making recommendations for improved or modified eating behaviors. As in all types of teaching and counseling, you must develop instructional objectives, devise evaluation tools, assess the learner's knowledge, screen and organize information needs, select education materials, implement the teaching, and critique and revise your instruction. It is also essential for you to keep the learner's needs in the forefront and work to maintain rapport with the client.

To successfully educate clients, you must include information about the types and the amounts of foods to eat. To maintain an appropriate body weight and prevent obesity, food intake and physical activity must be balanced. The need for calories can be calculated from the resting energy expenditure (REE), which is calculated as 15.3 times body weight (kg) plus 679 (for men ages 18 to 30); and 11.6 times body weight (kg) plus 879 (for men ages 30 to 60).

For women ages 18 to 30, the formula is 14.7 times body weight (kg) plus 496. For women ages 30 to 60, it is 8.7 times body weight (kg) plus 829. Very light physical activity requires 1.5 times the REE, light physical activity uses 2.5 REE, moderate physical activity burns 5.0 REE, and heavy physical activity requires 7.0 REE.

Using Recommended Dietary Allowances

The RDA is the level of intake of essential nutrients considered, on the basis of available scientific knowledge, to be adequate to meet the known nutritional needs of practically all healthy persons. Nutrient requirements during illness may be higher than the RDA, depending on the nature of the illness. Requirements are also known to be higher when the body is under stress or recovering from trauma, infection, or surgery.

To optimize nutrition for relatively healthy clients, teach them to read nutrition labels that appear on manufactured foods, in accordance with the Nutrition Labeling and Education Act of 1990. These labels, titled "Nutrition Facts," contain information about the percentage of Daily Value that a specific product has for fat, cholesterol, sodium, carbohydrate, protein, vitamins, and minerals. The Reference Daily Intakes (RDI) are based on RDA. Another type of labeling is the Reference Daily Values (RDV), which is identified for important nutrients for which an RDA has not yet been established.

Developing Healthy Dietary Patterns

A healthy diet is based on the food guide pyramid, developed in 1992 by the U.S. Department of Agriculture. The design of the pyramid conveys the three essential elements of a healthy diet: proportion, moderation, and variety. Proportion is the relative amount of food to choose from each major food group.

Moderation pertains to sparing use of fats, oils, and sugars. And variety emphasizes the importance of eating a selection of foods from each of the major groups every day. Appropriate daily selections of a variety of foods according to the Food Guide Pyramid should provide one with the RDA for all necessary nutrients.

The base of the pyramid is the foundation of a healthy diet. You and your clients should eat six or more servings of complex carbohydrate foods daily. This group is a source of fiber, vegetable protein, and B vitamins. Whole grains supply more nutrients and fiber than processed grains. A diet high in complex carbohydrates from plant sources is associated with a lower incidence of atherosclerotic disease and some forms of cancer. High-fiber foods, especially cruciferous vegetables (broccoli, cabbage, cauliflower, Brussels sprouts), protect against colorectal cancer.

The second level of the pyramid includes fruits and vegetables. These are significant sources of vitamins A, C, and K, folate, niacin, and riboflavin. You and your clients should eat five or more servings of these daily. Fresh fruits and vegetables have a higher vitamin content than when cooked by boiling. To cook vegetables, use a minimum amount of water and cook only until tender. Steaming preserves the vitamin content.

The third level is primarily the animal foods. Protein should be consumed in moderate amounts. The RDA for both genders is 0.8 g/kg per day. Most Americans eat more than this amount of protein. Most protein should come from plant sources rather than animal sources. Remember, however, that animal proteins are the only source of vitamin B_{12}, the best source of readily absorbable iron, and a good source of zinc.

The small top point of the pyramid suggests that fats, oils, and sweets should make up the smallest part of the diet. To reduce cholesterol and fat intake, limit meat, fish, and poultry to 3 to 6 ounces in cooked weight daily. Ground beef is the single largest source of dietary fat in the United States, with half the calories coming from fat even in low-fat ground beef. One egg yolk contains more than two-thirds of the RDI of cholesterol. The skin of poultry contains most of its fat. More than 70% of the energy content of cheese comes from fat.

Using General Nutrition Recommendations

Various government agencies and programs in the United States and Canada provide nutritional guidelines for consumers. These include recommendations for nutrient intake, food guides, menu plans, and sample diets. Teaching these recommendations can help a client to establish her own goals for improved nutrition; however, knowledge of the recommendations is not usually sufficient to change a dietary pattern.

The importance of dietary habits in preventing disease and maintaining health is becoming more apparent. Diet has been associated with heart disease, stroke, and cancer, the three major causes of death in the United States. Fortunately, the incidence of heart disease and stroke has declined in recent years, possibly because of improved dietary habits. As a result of the increased evidence of relationships between diet and chronic diseases, changes in the American diet are being promoted by dietitians, nutritionists, and several organizations, such as the American Heart Association, the American Cancer Society, and the U.S. Department of Agriculture in conjunction with the U.S. Department of Health and Human Services. Nutritional guidelines published in Canada are similar to the U.S. Daily Food Guide.

Fat intake should be 30% or less of caloric intake. Saturated fat intake should be less than 10% of calories, and the intake of cholesterol should be less than 300 mg daily. Polyunsaturated fats have a cholesterol-lowering effect, and vegetable oils containing polyunsaturated fats are the best source of vitamin E. Hydrogenated vegetable oil has a cholesterol-elevating effect.

Although not all persons are sensitive to salt, a limited use of salt may help prevent high blood pressure. Total daily salt (sodium chloride) should be limited to 6 g or less. For people who are sensitive to salt, it should be restricted to 4.5 g or less. Most Americans eat more than 6 g of salt (2,400 mg sodium) per day. Additionally, eating large quantities of foods pickled or preserved in salt is associated with cancer of the stomach.

*A*ction *A*lert!
Advise salt-sensitive clients to restrict their salt intake to 4.5 g per day or less. Most Americans consume more than 6 g of salt per day.

Calcium-containing foods (such as dairy products and dark leafy vegetables) promote bone growth just before the onset of puberty and during adolescence. They also protect against osteoporosis later in life. The RDA for calcium is 800 mg for adult men and nonpregnant adult women. The best sources of calcium are milk and milk products. Calcium in dietary supplements is often present in the poorly-soluble forms of phosphate or carbonate, which are not well-absorbed.

Alcohol consumption should be avoided. Some studies have shown that small amounts of daily alcohol may reduce the risk of coronary disease; however, there are better ways to reduce this risk. If you or your clients must drink, keep the amount to less than one ounce of pure alcohol each day. The "proof" identified on the bottle represents twice the percentage of alcohol it contains; in other words, 80 proof means 40% alcohol.

Dietary supplements are unnecessary when a balanced diet is eaten that contains the recommended servings of the basic food groups. Although a single multivitamin with 100% of the RDA is not known to be harmful, it has also not been proven to be decidedly beneficial for the vast majority of people.

Fluoride intake is recommended to prevent tooth decay, particularly when consumed before permanent teeth erupt. This benefit persists throughout life as long as fluoride intake continues. Some communities have sufficient fluoride in the water supply, making supplements unnecessary.

How would you use the food guide pyramid in teaching Joan how to improve her diet?

Interventions for Special Populations

Promoting Nutrition During Pregnancy

The recommendations for dietary management during pregnancy emphasize an increase in total calories, protein, vitamins, and minerals. Poor nutrition is a factor in excessive maternal weight gain, pre-eclampsia, postpartum infections, and an increased incidence of premature babies, low-birth-weight babies, anomalies, developmental disabilities, and stillbirths.

Although the mother's preconception nutrition also affects the outcome of pregnancy, most nutritional care begins during the first trimester of pregnancy. Three well-planned meals, plus one or more snacks, provide the RDA for all nutrients with the possible exception of iron and folacin (folic acid). Daily supplementation of 30 to 60 mg of ferrous iron and 400 μg of folacin are recommended. Prenatal vitamin-mineral supplements are commonly prescribed but unnecessary unless the woman is at high nutritional risk. Depending on preferences and tolerance, adequate calcium and zinc may be difficult to achieve and may require supplementation as well.

Adequate calories and weight gain are necessary throughout pregnancy. For women entering pregnancy at or near their ideal body weight, a total weight gain of 25 to 35 pounds over the course of the pregnancy is recommended at a rate of 2 to 4 pounds in the first trimester and 0.75 to 1 pound per week thereafter. Underweight women should gain the amount they are underweight plus a normal pregnancy gain of 25 pounds. Women whose weight is 120 to 130% of their ideal body weight are encouraged to gain about 20 pounds, whereas those whose weight is more than 135% of the ideal body weight are urged to gain 15 to 16 or 18 to 20 pounds, depending on the source. Most authorities discourage dieting for weight loss during pregnancy. Instead, the emphasis is on high-quality food choices to meet nutrient needs.

A*ction* A*lert!*
Teach pregnant women the importance of appropriate weight gain during pregnancy. Advise them that pregnancy is not the time for dieting for weight loss.

All pregnant women should be counseled about avoiding potentially harmful substances during pregnancy. They should avoid smoking, alcohol, and caffeine. Finally, they should avoid nonprescription drugs, pica, saccharin and other artificial sweeteners, and all fad-diet products or regimens.

Promoting Nutrition in Infants

Breast milk or iron-fortified formula is the only source of nourishment needed for the first 4 to 6 months after birth. The infant is ready to start solid food when his birth weight has doubled and he can control head movements and sit up with support.

Vitamin and mineral recommendations are based on the contents of human milk. Daily water requirements are usually met with breast milk or infant formula, except when the weather is hot or the infant has diarrhea or vomiting. Supplemental water is needed at these times to prevent dehydration.

A*ction* A*lert!*
Watch for signs of dehydration in infants with persistent diarrhea or vomiting. With persistent diarrhea or vomiting, severe dehydration can develop quickly in infants.

Promoting Nutrition in Children

Children need adequate calories, protein, water, vitamins, and minerals. Meals should be selected using food from the food guide pyramid for children. Children 1 to 2 years old require smaller servings, more frequent snacks, and three cups of whole milk each day (Table 29–4). A good rule of thumb is 1 to 2 tablespoons of a food group with each meal or snack. When planning a child's meals, the caretaker should select from a variety of foods from each food group. Serving sizes increase with age.

Each year a child grows 2 to 3 inches and gains about 5 pounds. A standard gain-growth chart reflects the child's nutritional health. Weight gain out of proportion to height may reflect overeating or inactivity. If the child's weight-to-height ratio drops below the normal curve, it may indicate malnutrition. By periodically measuring weight-to-height, the child's progress on the standard growth curve can be plotted over time.

Promoting Nutrition in Adolescents

Growth rate increases with the onset of adolescence. In girls, the growth spurt begins around age 10 and peaks at age 12. Boys begin their growth spurt around age 12, and it peaks at age 14. Body composition in girls include a higher percentage of fat tissue. Boys' growth spurt includes a higher proportion of lean body mass, such as muscle and bone.

Two minerals of special concern include iron in girls as they begin menstruation and calcium in both boys and girls for bone growth and optimal bone mass. Adequate calcium remains one of the best protectors against age-related bone loss and fractures.

Promoting Nutrition in Older Adults

The diet for older adults addresses the nutritional needs of the elderly for foods with less energy but higher nutrient density. The diet promotes adequate protein, vitamin, and mineral consumption while restricting foods low in nutrient density and high in calories. It provides the RDA for all nutrients when a variety of foods are selected and consumed in appropriate quantities. The diet should also correct for possible nutrient deficits and physiological changes common in the older adult. The diet should be further modified for clients with particular diseases or conditions.

TABLE 29–4
Child's Daily Food Plan

Food Group	Servings per Day	Average Size of Serving		
		Age 1 to 3	*Age 4 to 6*	*Age 7 to 10*
Bread and cereals (whole-grain or enriched)[a]	6 or more	½ slice	1 slice	1 slice
Vegetables[b]	3 or more	2 to 4 tablespoons or ½ cup juice	¼ to ½ cup or ½ cup juice	½ to 1 cup
Fruits[b]	2 or more	2 to 4 tablespoons or ½ cup juice	¼ to ½ cup or ½ cup of juice	½ to 1 cup
Meat and meat alternatives[c]	2 or more	½ ounce	1 to 2 ounce	2 to 3 ounces
Milk and milk products[d]	3 to 4	¼ to ½ cup	¾ cup	¾ to 1 cup

[a]1 slice bread = ¼ cup dry cereal, ½ cup cooked cereal, or ½ cup potato, rice, or noodles.
[b]Sources of vitamin C (weekly) include citrus fruits, berries, tomatoes, broccoli, cabbage, and cantaloupe. Sources of vitamin A (3 to 4 times weekly) include spinach, carrots, squash, and cantaloupe.
[c]1 ounce of meat, fish, or poultry = 1 egg, 1 frankfurter, 2 tablespoons peanut butter, or ½ cup cooked legumes.
[d]½ cup milk = ½ cup cottage cheese, pudding, or yogurt; ¼ ounce cheese; or 2 tablespoons dried milk.
Adapted from Queen, P.M., & Henry, R.R. (1987). Growth and nutrient requirements of children. In R.J. Grand, L. Sutphen, & W.H. Dietz, Jr. (Eds.), Pediatric nutrition: Theory and Practice (p 347). Boston: Butterworths.

Nutrition education for older adults requires careful planning because common techniques may not be appropriate. Group discussion, as opposed to lecture, is often more beneficial in teaching normal nutrition. Counseling on *very* strict diet modifications, such as the diabetic diet and fat-restricted diet for heart disease, may be less appropriate because of decreased learning ability and resistance to changing life-long eating habits. These diets may be more successful for the younger client and have not been proven as effective for those age 65 and older. The diabetic diet in the elderly may be effectively taught as a normal diet, restricting simple sugars, establishing regular meal times, and distributing foods consistently among meals.

Action Alert!
Teach elderly diabetics to eat a normal diet while restricting simple sugars, establishing regular meal times, and distributing foods consistently among meals.

Improved nutrition at home may also reduce hospitalization rates for older adults and decrease the number entering hospitals with signs of malnutrition. A dietitian can provide you with valuable information about feeding programs for older adults, low-cost nutritious foods, foods with a longer shelf-life and minimal preparation, and programs that provide shopping assistance.

EVALUATION

Education is not complete until learning has been evaluated. Formal and informational tools may be used to measure learning against established objectives. Using evaluation helps to identify whether the client needs further dietary teaching or clarification.

To some degree, demonstrating successful learning at evaluation reinforces new behaviors, which is the goal of nutrition education.

KEY PRINCIPLES

- Good nutritional status is essential for normal organ development and function, for optimal activity and working efficiency, for resistance to infection, and for the ability to repair bodily damage or injury.
- The four functions of the GI system are digestion, absorption, metabolism, and excretion.
- Carbohydrates, proteins, fat, vitamins, minerals, and water are essential nutrients.
- Factors that affect nutrition include lifestyle, culture, economics, developmental stage, and psychological and physiological state.
- General assessment of nutritional status includes a complete health history, diet history, evaluation of food intake, and physical examination.
- The nursing diagnosis *Health-seeking behaviors: nutrition* may be used to promote optimal nutrition for the well client.
- The nursing diagnosis *Altered health maintenance* may be used to reduce nutritional risk factors for clients with alterations in health.
- Planning for expected outcomes should focus on individual client needs and sound dietary principles.
- The nurse's role in nutritional intervention includes teaching and counseling about appropriate dietary modifications.
- Evaluation is necessary to review and improve or change dietary or nutritional plans.

BIBLIOGRAPHY

Alabaster, O., Blumberg, J., Stampfer, M.J., & Stavir, B. (1995). Antioxidants. *Patient Care, 29*(18), 436–438.

Anderson, J., Denke, M., Foreyt, J., & Smith, B. (1995). Cutting dietary fats: Advice that really works. *Patient Care, 29*(2), 16–32.

Bernshaw, N.J. (1998). Breastfeeding as the norm. *Journal of Human Lactation, 14*(1), 14.

Burnham, P. (1997) Nutrition: A healthy degree of success. *Nursing Times, 93*(21), 71, 74.

Cerrato, P. (1997). Pharmacology in practice: Vitamins and minerals. *RN, 60*(11), 52–56.

DiGuiseppi, C., Atkins, D., & Woolf, D. (1996). *Guide to clinical preventive services.* Baltimore: Williams & Wilkins.

Dudek, S.G. (1995). *Nutrition handbook for nursing practice* (2nd ed.). Philadelphia: J.B. Lippincott.

Futterman, L.G., & Lemberg, L. (1999). The use of antioxidants in retarding atherosclerosis: Fact or fiction? *American Journal of Critical Care, 8*(2), 130–133.

*Food and Nutrition Board, Subcommittee on the Tenth Edition of the RDAs. (1989). *Recommended dietary allowances* (10th ed.). Washington, D.C.: National Academy Press.

Gallo, A. (1996). Building strong bones in childhood and adolescence: Reducing the risk of fractures in later life. *Pediatric Nursing, 22*(5), 369–374, 422.

*Georges, J.M., & Heitkemper, M.M. (1994). Dietary fiber and distressing gastrointestinal symptoms in midlife women. *Nursing Research, 43*(6), 357–361.

Gillis, A.J. (1997). The adolescent lifestyle questionnaire: Development and psychometric testing. *Canadian Journal of Nursing Research, 29*(1), 29–46.

Heitkemper, M., & Jarrett, M. (1997). Research issues in nutrition support. *Nursing Clinics of North America, 32*(4), 755–768.

Herbert, V., & Subak-Sharpe, G. (1995). *Total nutrition.* New York: St. Martin's Press.

---

*Asterisk indicates a classic or definitive work on this subject.

Houston, D.K, Johnson, M.A., Nozza, R.J., Gunter, E.W., et al. (1999). Age-related hearing loss, vitamin B_{12}, and folate in elderly women. *American Journal of Clinical Nutrition, 69*(3), 564–571.

Johnson, R.M., Kaiser, F.E., Kerstetter, J.E, & Rueben, D.B. (1995). Nutritional support for the elderly. *Patient Care, 29*(18), 46–68.

Kramer, L. (1995). Implementing new dietary guidelines of the national cholesterol education program. *AACN Clinical Issues, Advanced Practice in Acute and Critical Care, 6*(3), 418–431, 495–496.

Loftus-Hills, A., & Duff, L. (1997). Implementation of nutrition standards for older adults. *Nursing Standards, 11*(44), 33–37.

Lutz, C.A., & Przytulski, K.R. (1997). *Nutrition and diet therapy* (2nd ed.). Philadelphia: F.A. Davis.

McLennan, C.L., & Hartz, D.J. (1998). Use of a pediatric diet history form to create individualized, consistent carbohydrate meal plans. *Diabetes Educator, 24*(4), 459–460, 463–464.

Meydani, M., Lipman, R.D., Han, S.N., Wu, D., et al. (1998). The effect of long-term dietary supplementation with antioxidants. *Annals of the New York Academy of Science, 854,* Nov. 20, 352–360.

Perry, L. (1997). Nutrition: A hard nut to crack. An exploration of the knowledge, attitudes and activities of qualified nurses in relation to nutritional nursing care. *Journal of Clinical Nursing, 6*(4), 315–324.

Phaneuf, C. (1996). Screening elders for nutritional deficits. *American Journal of Nursing, 96*(3), 58–60.

*Queen, P.M. & Henry, R.R. (1987). Growth and nutrient requirements of children. In R.J. Grand, L. Sutphen, and W.H. Dietz, Jr. (Eds.), *Pediatric nutrition: Theory and practice* (p 347). Boston: Butterworths.

*Schulz, K. (Ed.). (1993). *Memphis District Dietetic Association diet manual.* Memphis: MDDA.

*U.S. Department of Agriculture (1992). *USDA's food guide pyramid.* USDA human nutritional information service, Pub. No. 249. Washington, D.C.: U.S. Government Printing Office.

Whitney, E., & Rolfes, S. (1996). *Understanding nutrition* (7th ed.). St. Paul, MN: West.

Wynn, M., & Wynn, A. (1998). The danger of B_{12} deficiency in the elderly. *Nutritional Health, 12*(4), 215–226.

Yen, P.K. (1998). Stopping heart disease with diet. *Geriatric Nursing, 19*(1), 50–51.

Nutritional Deficiency

Nancy Spector

Nancy Spector

Key Terms

anorexia
catabolism
deglutition
dysphagia

enteral nutrition
malnutrition
parenteral nutrition
resting energy expenditure

LEARNING OBJECTIVES

After studying this chapter, you should be able to:

1. Describe the physiology of malnutrition and starvation.
2. Discuss factors affecting nutritional deficits.
3. Assess clients experiencing severe nutritional deficits.
4. Formulate nursing diagnoses for nutritional deficits.
5. Plan for goal-directed interventions for clients with nutritional deficits.
6. Employ a variety of interventions to facilitate optimal nutrition for clients.
7. Evaluate the achievement of measurable outcomes for clients with nutritional deficits.

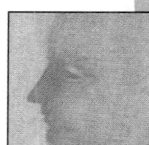

Mrs. Rosalie Goldman is a 54-year-old lawyer whose parents came to the United States from Russia in the early 1900s. She has had surgery for cancer of the breast and now is receiving outpatient chemotherapy. Because of her treatments, she experiences early satiety and anorexia and says that food does not have much taste. Mrs. Goldman is 5'4" tall and her usual weight is 140 pounds. Currently she weighs 115 pounds. Her serum albumin level is 2.7 g/100 mL.

The clinic nurse is concerned with Mrs. Goldman's weight loss and considers her a risk for malnutrition. She makes the diagnosis of *Altered nutrition: less than body requirements* (see chart on Altered Nutrition Nursing Diagnoses).

ALTERED NUTRITION NURSING DIAGNOSES

Altered Nutrition: Less Than Body Requirements: The state in which an individual is experiencing an intake of nutrients insufficient to meet metabolic needs.

Altered Nutrition: More Than Body Requirements: The state in which an individual is experiencing an intake of nutrients that exceeds metabolic needs.

Impaired Swallowing: Abnormal functioning of the swallowing mechanism associated with deficits in oral, pharyngeal, or esophageal structure or function.

Risk for Aspiration: The state in which an individual is at risk for entry of gastrointestinal secretions, oropharyngeal secretions, or solids or fluids into the tracheobronchial passages.

From North American Nursing Diagnosis Association. (1999). NANDA nursing diagnoses: Definitions & classification 1999–2000. Philadelphia: Author.

CONCEPTS OF NUTRITIONAL PROBLEMS

As a nurse, you will observe nutritional problems in clients in all care settings, from their homes to rehabilitation settings to clinics to hospitals. Collectively, nutritional problems create a condition known as **malnutrition,** which is any disorder of nutrition caused by imbalanced, insufficient, or excessive diet or from impaired absorption or metabolism of nutrients. To care for clients with malnutrition, you will need a sound understanding of inadequate and excessive nutrition and the many factors that affect nutritional status.

Nutritional deprivation results from inadequate intake from nausea and vomiting, difficulty swallowing, or inability to obtain food. It can also result from problems that raise energy needs, such as infection, trauma, stress, or surgery.

Extreme malnutrition can lead to death through starvation. Starvation is the physiological response to chronic food deprivation. During starvation, the body attempts to reduce its energy use by lowering voluntary activity and the basal metabolic rate (BMR). Next, endogenous fuels are used as the source of energy. When nutrient intake fails to meet the body's energy expenditure (energy needs), the body resorts to breaking down muscle and lean body mass. This phenomenon, called **catabolism,** yields glucose from protein breakdown in a process called glyconeogenesis. Catabolism results in a negative nitrogen balance. Figure 30–1 summarizes the metabolic changes that occur when the body uses endogenous fuels to meet energy needs. After 10 to 14 days of starvation, the body uses fat rather than glucose for energy. The liver makes ketone bodies for use as fuel by most tissues, including the brain.

If clients have been starving for a period of time, the urine will be positive for ketones and the nitrogen balance will be negative. Because of decreased protein intake, the blood urea nitrogen (BUN) and creatinine values will fall, reflecting fewer products of protein breakdown. In nonobese adults, fat (the body's main

stored fuel) is depleted in about 1 to 2 months. Protein can supply about 2 weeks of calories; however, this protein breakdown affects the body (Zaloga, 1994).

Protein-calorie malnutrition in hospitalized clients

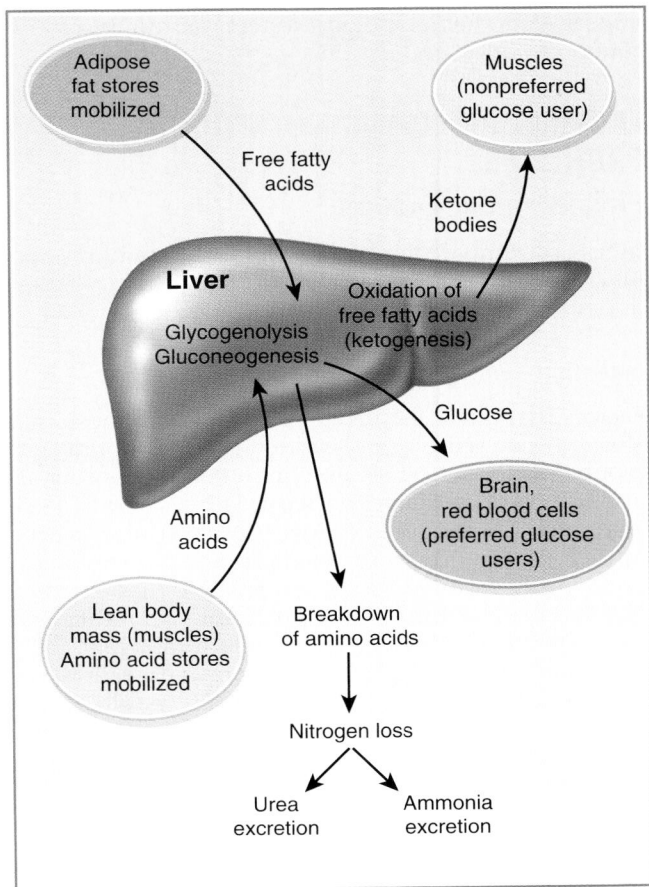

Figure 30–1. Metabolic changes that occur when the body uses endogenous fuels to meet energy needs. (Modified from Lemoyne, M., & Jeejeebhoy, K. N. [1985]. Total parenteral nutrition in the critically ill patient. Chest, 89[4], 568.)

ranges from 40 to 70% and results from inadequate assessment and nutritional support (Stein, 1994). It can be from inadequate calories, proteins, or both.

Marasmus is a condition of starvation that results from deficient caloric intake. It is a chronic condition that develops over months or years and is characterized by severe fat and muscle loss. Clients appear starved and weigh less than 80% of their ideal body weight (IBW) but have a normal serum albumin level. Fortunately, they respond fairly well to therapy as long as they are not refed too quickly.

Kwashiorkor is a condition of starvation, usually in young children after weaning, caused by decreased protein intake; symptoms can develop in a few weeks. A client with kwashiorkor may appear well-nourished but is at tremendous risk. The serum albumin level falls below 2.8 g/dL, leading to significant edema. Wounds heal more slowly, and the client risks infection from decreased immunity. The mortality rate is high because of altered immune status and poorer response to refeeding than with marasmus.

Vitamin and mineral deficiencies can also result from decreased intake or increased loss (as with diarrhea or vomiting). Table 30–1 summarizes manifestations of the major deficiencies. Vitamin and mineral deficiencies commonly affect the skin, peripheral nervous system, hematopoietic system, immunity, calcification of bones, and vision.

FACTORS AFFECTING NUTRITIONAL PROBLEMS

Physiological Factors

Illness can impair the body's ability to maintain normal nutrition by affecting ingestion, digestion, absorption, or metabolism.

Ingestion

Factors that affect the ingestion of food are those that affect the appetite and disorders of the mouth and esophagus that affect swallowing. If an illness such as upper respiratory infection reduces the sense of taste and smell, the appetite is lost. Anorexia also can be caused by liver disease, medications, psychological problems, acquired immunodeficiency syndrome (AIDS), or gastrointestinal problems. Vomiting impairs intake and causes loss of certain minerals.

Swallowing, or **deglutition,** refers to the reflex passage of food, fluids, or both from the mouth to the stomach (Fig. 30–2). It is initiated by voluntary action and is controlled by the central nervous system. The term **dysphagia** refers to difficulty in swallowing.

Involuntary control of swallowing is coordinated from the swallowing center in the reticular formation of the medulla and the lower pons in the brain. The process uses cranial nerves V, IX, X, and XII. After food is propelled to the back of the throat with the tongue and palate muscles, an involuntary wave of pharyngeal muscle contraction pushes food into the esophagus. Meanwhile, the glottis and epiglottis move to close off the trachea and suspend breathing. When this mechanism malfunctions, food is aspirated into the lungs.

Muscle tension at the upper esophageal (hypopharyngeal) sphincter and the lower esophageal sphincter normally keep these sphincters tightly closed except during swallowing, when they relax to allow food to move into the stomach by peristalsis. Increased pressure in the lower esophageal sphincter can cause dysphagia. Decreased pressure can cause reflux of acidic stomach contents back into the esophagus. Pressure in the lower esophageal sphincter is increased by parasympathetic drugs and gastrin. It is decreased by anticholinergics, cigarettes, fatty foods, alcohol, and certain digestive substances, such as cholecystokinin and secretin.

Several factors may hinder swallowing. Damage to the cranial nerves that innervate the tongue and pharynx may interfere with initiation of the swallowing reflex, effective chewing, and pushing food back into the pharynx and esophagus. The discomfort of an inflamed throat, obstruction, and decreased muscular contraction of the esophagus also can impede swallowing.

Clients often have problems swallowing because of decreased alertness or partial paralysis to the tongue, mouth, or throat. Examples of difficulties include drooling, inability to form a seal around a cup or a straw, uncoordinated tongue movements, and pocketing of food in the mouth. All of these problems raise the risk of aspiration.

Aspiration occurs when the client cannot protect the airway. This may result from difficulty swallowing, a decreased level of consciousness, seizures, impaired gag or cough reflexes, or a compromised immune system. Weakness of muscles in the soft palate, pharynx, and upper esophagus hinder the cough reflex.

Digestion and Absorption

Certain diseases alter the digestive process and impair food absorption. Inflammatory bowel disease, diarrhea, and cystic fibrosis decrease the client's ability to use nutrients. Additionally, in diarrhea, the intestinal villi do not produce enough lactase to absorb lactose.

Metabolism

Liver diseases also affect food metabolism. Vitamins normally stored in the liver may be deficient. Liver disease impairs protein metabolism because the liver cannot transform ammonia to urea.

Infection causes hypermetabolism and catabolism, requiring added calories. Infection may also cause anorexia and electrolyte imbalances. Infection also can lead to anemia because the body stores iron to deprive the bacteria of iron.

When calculating energy needs from predictive equations for clients who have infections, be sure to

TABLE 30–1
Manifestations of Major Nutritional Deficiencies

Nutritional Deficiency	Disease	Manifestation
Calcium	None (linked to rickets)	• Osteoporosis. • Tetany. • Hypertension (possibly).
Folate (a salt of folic acid)	None	• Anemia. • Glossitis or slick tongue. • Gastrointestinal disturbances.
Iron	None	• Anemia, pallor, fatigue. • Poor tolerance to cold. • Pica.
Protein	Kwashiorkor	• Onset of manifestations within weeks. • Well-nourished appearance but edema and easily plucked hair. • Albumin level 2.8 or below. • Total lymphocyte count 1,500/mm^3 or below. • Poor healing, skin breakdown, increased infections.
Protein and calories	Marasmus	• Onset of manifestations over months or years. • Weight 80% of ideal or less. • Starvation. • Good response to therapy.
Vitamin A	None	• Night blindness. • Skin lesions. • Scaly skin (also called fish skin, toad skin, or goose flesh).
Vitamin B$_1$ (thiamine)	Beriberi	• In wet beriberi, edema, low urine output, increased pulse, and jugular venous distention. • In dry beriberi, no edema, trouble walking, neuropathy, foot drop, and Wernicke-Korsakoff syndrome (decreased memory, disorientation, nystagmus, ataxia).
Vitamin B$_2$ (riboflavin)	None	• Impaired vision. • Cheilosis. • Angular stomatitis. • Glossitis.
Vitamin B$_3$ (niacin)	Pellagra	• Dementia. • Dermatitis. • Diarrhea. • Glossitis.
Vitamin B$_{12}$ (cobalamin)	Pernicious anemia	• Anemia. • Sore tongue. • Progressive neuropathy and other neurological changes, such as loss of memory.
Vitamin C	Scurvy	• Anemia. • Petechiae. • Gingivitis. • Failure of wounds to heal. • Impacted hair follicles and corkscrew hairs.
Vitamin D (calciferol)	Rickets	• Sweating and restlessness. • Bowed legs, pigeon breast, pot belly. • Rachitic rosary (beading of the ribs).
Vitamin K	None	• Increased bleeding, such as ecchymoses and petechiae.

consider body temperature. Fever increases metabolic needs by 7% for each degree Fahrenheit and 13% for each degree Centigrade. Clients with massive trauma or burns have very high calorie needs.

Developmental Factors

Throughout the life cycle, a complex balance exists between the anabolism of growth and the catabolism of aging. Energy expenditure and nutrient requirements are higher early in the life cycle, are stable throughout the middle years, and decline with aging. Specifically, metabolism peaks during the first 5 years and then rises again during puberty. After age 20, the BMR declines steadily. During pregnancy, BMR increases by about 13%. Exercise, activity, and even nursing procedures such as dressing changes can increase a client's energy needs significantly (Spector, 1993).

1.

ORAL PHASE (VOLUNTARY)

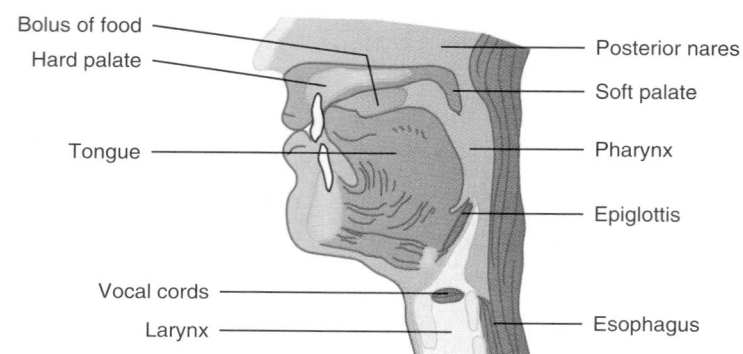

Bolus of food
Hard palate
Tongue
Posterior nares
Soft palate
Pharynx
Epiglottis
Vocal cords
Larynx
Esophagus

2.

PHARYNGEAL PHASE (INVOLUNTARY)

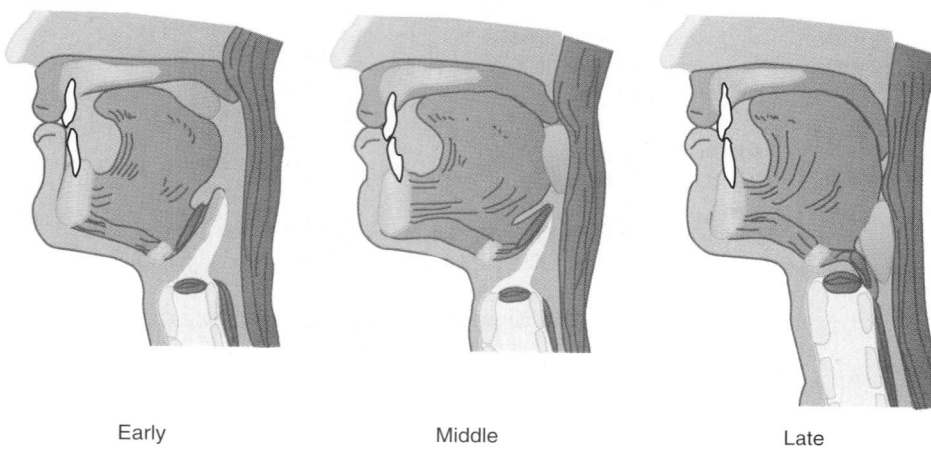

Early   Middle   Late

3.

ESOPHAGEAL PHASE (INVOLUNTARY)

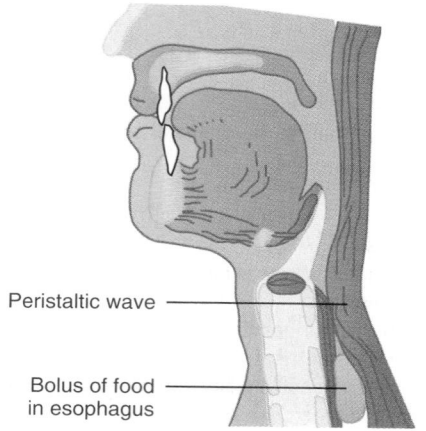

Peristaltic wave

Bolus of food
in esophagus

Figure 30–2. Mechanics of swallowing. *1,* In the oral phase, food is pushed to the back of the pharynx. *2,* In the pharyngeal phase, food is pushed down the pharynx into the esophagus. Respirations cease, and the glottis is closed during this phase. *3,* In the esophageal phase, relaxation of the upper esophageal sphincter allows a peristaltic wave to move the bolus of food down the esophagus. (Black, J. M., & Matassarin-Jacobs, E. [1997]. Medical-surgical nursing: Clinical management for continuity of care [5th ed.]. Philadelphia: W.B. Saunders.)

Infants and Children

Low-birth-weight infants are at risk for undernutrition and need close monitoring. These newborns weigh less than 2,500 g (5.5 pounds) and are classified as small for gestational age (retarded intrauterine growth rate) or premature (shortened length of gestation). Premature infants may be given tube feedings because the suck-swallow reflex does not develop until 34 weeks of gestation (Marian, 1993). These infants also have fewer nutritional reserves because fetal nutrient stores are deposited in the last 3 months of pregnancy.

Infants or children may need extra nourishment if they experience hypermetabolism or decreased growth. Trauma, burns, and failure to thrive are examples of conditions that need special nutritional support.

Adolescents

Eating disorders are common during adolescence, a time of emotional and physical turmoil. Adolescents gain 20% of adult height and 50% of adult weight during this time. They are also developing a sense of self and may feel uncomfortable about their changing bodies. In a society that favors slimness, these factors all encourage the development of eating disorders. About 20 million people in the United States suffer from eating disorders, about 90% of whom are female (Whitney, Cataldo, & Rolfes, 1994). There has been a significant increase in these disorders in Western countries since the 1950s, especially in females aged 15 to 24 (Shils, Olson, & Shike, 1994).

Older Adults

In general, aging causes an increased proportion of connective tissue and a loss of functioning cells. No one knows exactly why this happens, but one theory states that free radicals attack the cells and impair energy production in mitochondria. Antioxidant nutrients (such as vitamin C, vitamin E, and selenium) may reduce free radical damage to tissues.

Some nutritional deficits may be linked with aging. For example, deficiencies of calcium, iron, zinc, thiamine, vitamin B_{12}, and folate are common in the older adult and may be secondary to problems with chewing, swallowing, and digesting foods. Reduced secretion of gastric hydrochloric acid limits absorption of calcium, iron, and vitamin B_{12}.

About half of clients aged 65 and older wear dentures, which can also affect nutritional intake (Davis & Sherer, 1994). Dentures may be ill-fitting, creating problems with chewing and limiting intake of nutritious foods. Finally, many older adults take multiple prescription and over-the-counter drugs, increasing the risk of potentially dangerous drug-nutrient interactions. Be especially aware of the possibility of poor nutrition in older adults, as discussed in the State of Nursing Science chart.

ASSESSMENT

General Assessment for Nutritional Problems

Nutritional assessment and screening can identify cues to nutritional problems (see Box 30-1 on Cues to Possible Nutritional Problems). Chapter 29 covers general assessment for nutrition status. When the client is identified as having a nutrition problem, assessment focuses on the etiology, severity, and factors affecting the problem.

The results of routine and specialized laboratory tests can provide valuable cues to the client's nutritional status (Table 30–2). However, no single laboratory test is available to diagnose nutritional problems. A physician will probably order serum studies if the client has unintentionally lost 10% of her weight in the last 6 months or has evidence of a nutritional deficiency.

For example, creatinine and BUN levels rise with kidney disease. If the creatinine level is normal, the BUN level provides useful information on protein status. If the serum creatinine level is high, the BUN alone will not give reliable information about nutrition. In this case, rely on the ratio of BUN to serum creatinine. Serum albumin levels are frequently measured, but albumin has a 21-day half-life. To determine nutritional repletion, look to substances with shorter half-lives, such as prealbumin or transferrin.

Laboratory tests are rarely done to measure vitamin deficiencies. Instead, use the nutritional history, physical examination, and anthropometric measurements. Electrolyte levels are commonly measured, and they can provide information about nutritional problems as well.

Swallowing and aspiration may be evaluated using videofluoroscopy, a procedure also known as a video swallow esophagography, a modified barium swallow, or a swallow study. The client swallows barium, which is observed passing through the oropharynx during swallowing. This study is done in the radiology department and exposes the client to a minimal amount of radiation (Ellpern, 1997).

Focused Assessment for Altered Nutrition: Less Than Body Requirements

While loss of weight is the most commonly identified cue to nutritional deficiency, more subtle cues need to be considered. Cluster various cues to make this diagnosis.

BOX 30–1

CUES TO POSSIBLE NUTRITIONAL PROBLEMS

- Anorexia.
- Artificial airway.
- Diarrhea.
- Increased metabolic need.
- Compromised immune system.
- Less-than-normal nutrient consumption.
- Low socioeconomic status.
- Malabsorptive condition.
- Polypharmacy.
- Greater-than-normal nutrient consumption.
- Muscle weaknesses in pharynx, soft palate, or esophagus.
- Psychological disturbance (low self-esteem, depression).
- Reduced level of consciousness.
- Nausea and vomiting.

Defining Characteristics

The chief complaint for clients with nutritional problems may include any of the following: weight changes, inability to swallow or eat, fatigue, skin lesions, or other physical findings. Take a detailed history for these clients, making sure to include the following elements:

- Body weight 20% or more under ideal. Assess for weight changes in the last 6 months. Ask about the client's *usual weight* and find out whether she thinks her current weight differs from her usual weight. Abnormal weight gain can indicate either fluid gain or obesity. Involuntary weight loss can indicate disease or malnutrition and can be a grave sign.
- Changes in appetite: anorexia, early satiety, lack of interest in food, aversion to food, loss of taste
- Symptoms, such as an inability to eat independently
- Nutritional supplements taken
- Medications taken, including prescribed and over-the-counter. Obtain a history of other health problems and use of prescription and over-the-counter medications as well.
- Difficulty swallowing, chewing; obstructed esophagus or pharynx

---

STATE OF NURSING SCIENCE
POOR NUTRITION IN OLDER ADULTS

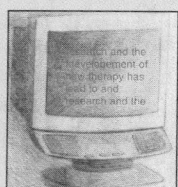

WHAT ARE THE ISSUES?

Adequate nutrition is necessary for performing daily activities as well as for defending against disease and injury. However, older adults have an increased risk of inadequate nutrition and, consequently, an increased risk of impaired activity and illness. Nurses are in an excellent position to identify older adults who are at risk. This is the first step toward providing alternative means for ensuring that nutritional needs are met.

WHAT RESEARCH HAS BEEN CONDUCTED?

McCormack (1997) reviewed the literature on the nutritional status of older adults in community settings, primarily in Great Britain. Factors related to poor nutrition in older adults included the following:

- Physiological changes due to aging, including decreased taste and chewing difficulties.
- Medical problems that interfered with self-care, such as stroke and dementia.
- Drug interactions that reduced appetite.
- Lack of resources to buy food.
- Social isolation, with depression.

Elmstahl, Persson, Andren, & Blabolil (1997) studied the impact on client survival of the nutritional intake of clients after 6 months of confinement in nursing homes. The researchers found that higher energy intake was related to a decreased risk of mortality (p. 853). They stressed the importance of identifying people at nutritional risk so that early intervention could be implemented.

Zylstra, Beerman, Hillers, & Mitchell (1995), a group of dietitians, used a self-report tool from the Nutrition Screening Initiative to assess for nutritional risk factors in a group of older adults who participated in a meal program. The tool considers such risk factors as meal frequency, food type, use of alcohol, financial resources, ability to prepare meals, weight loss or gain, oral health,

use of medications, and concurrent illness. People who score high on the scale are considered at increased risk for nutritional problems. The instrument is meant to be a screening tool, and people with high scores are referred for individual assessment and intervention. The researchers found that the people served by a meal program were more likely to be at nutritional risk if they had low incomes and were members of a minority group.

WHAT HAS THE RESEARCH CONCLUDED?

Regular screening for nutritional risk is an effective way to identify older adults who might benefit from interventions to supplement their intake. Self-report tools such as those developed by the Nutrition Screening Initiative can identify older adults who could benefit from individual assessment and intervention. Physical factors are not all to consider when trying to determine who is at nutritional risk. Psychosocial factors also play an important role.

WHAT IS THE FUTURE OF RESEARCH IN THIS AREA?

Research is needed on ways to reach older adults who are at risk for nutritional problems. Once these people are identified, interventions that take into account their individual preferences should be examined for effectiveness. Collaboration among disciplines—such as nursing, dietetics, and medicine—is needed to ensure effective screening, referral, and intervention.

References

Elmstahl, S., Persson, M., Andren, M., & Blabolil, V. (1997). Malnutrition in geriatric patients: A neglected problem? *Journal of Advanced Nursing, 26,* 851–855.

McCormack, P. (1997). Undernutrition in the elderly population living at home in the community: A review of the literature. *Journal of Advanced Nursing, 26,* 856–863.

Zylstra, R.C.E., Beerman, K., Hillers, V., & Mitchell, M. (1995). Who's at risk in Washington state? Demographic characteristics affect nutritional risk behaviors in elderly meal participants. *Journal of the American Dietetic Association, 95*(3), 358–360.

TABLE 30–2
Implications of Laboratory Tests for Nutritional Status

Laboratory Test	Normal Range of Values	Possible Nutritional Implications of Abnormal Values
Blood urea nitrogen	8–23 mg/dL	If decreased, low protein intake
Hematocrit	Female: 34–44% Male: 39–49%	If decreased, anemia (deficiency of iron, pyridoxine, folate, vitamin B_{12}, protein)
Hemoglobin	Female: 12–15 g/dL Male: 14–17 g/dL	If decreased, anemia (deficiency of iron, pyridoxine, folate, vitamin B_{12}, protein)
Ratio of blood urea nitrogen to serum creatinine	12 or above	If 8 or below, poor protein intake
Serum albumin	3.5–5.5 g/dL	If decreased, compromised protein status (levels under 2.8 are associated with edema and possible kwashiorkor)
Serum creatinine	0.6–1.6 mg/dL	If decreased, muscle wasting
Total lymphocyte count	1,500/mm³ or above	If decreased, not specific for any particular nutritional deficiency, but correlates best with protein deficit

- Pale conjunctiva
- Gastrointestinal symptoms, such as abdominal cramping, abdominal pain with or without pathology, hyperactive bowel sounds, diarrhea or steatorrhea, nausea, vomiting, constipation
- Misconceptions, lack or information, or misinformation
- A perceived inability to ingest food
- Reports or evidence of lack of food or inadequate intake
- Condition of skin, teeth, and mucous membranes: rashes, scaling, bleeding, poor wound healing, capillary fragility, pale or ulcerated mucous membranes, depapillation of the tongue, bleeding, gum disease, cracks in the mouth, and dental caries; a sore or inflamed mouth or an altered taste sensation
- Hair condition, such as brittleness and how easily it can be plucked
- Fingernail condition, including ridges, clubbing, and brittleness
- Neck characteristics, including enlarged lymph nodes, enlarged thyroid
- Musculoskeletal condition, such as bone deformities and muscle wasting, muscle weakness, decreased muscle tone
- Central nervous system function, including difficulty walking and peripheral neuritis
- Other medical conditions: liver, specifically any enlargement on palpation; heart condition, such as cardiomegaly; kidney disease; diabetes; cancer; or AIDS

Related Factors

The defining characteristics give cues to the etiology or other related factors. Additional related factors may include the following:

- Economic factors in obtaining food
- Misconceptions, lack of information, or misinformation
- Inadequate caregivers or support systems

Focused Assessment for Impaired Swallowing

Defining Characteristics

Defining characteristics for the diagnosis *Impaired swallowing* may arise in any of the three phases of swallowing and include the following:

- Pharyngeal phase: Altered head positions, inadequate laryngeal elevation, refusal of food, unexplained fevers, delayed swallowing, recurrent pulmonary infections, a gurgly voice, nasal reflux, choking, coughing, gagging, multiple swallows, abnormal swallow study results
- Esophageal phase: Heartburn or epigastric pain, acidic-smelling breath, unexplained irritability at mealtime, vomitus on pillow, repetitive swallowing or ruminating, wet burps, bruxism, nighttime coughing or awakening, observed difficulty swallowing, hyperextension of head during or after meals, abnormal swallow study, painful swallowing, limiting or refusing food, complaints of "something stuck," vomiting (including blood)
- Oral phase: Lack of tongue action to form a bolus; weak sucking in an infant; incomplete lip closure; food pushed out or falls out of mouth; slow bolus formation; premature entry of bolus; nasal reflux; inability to clear the mouth; long meals with little consumption; coughing, choking, or gagging before swallowing; abnormal swallow study results; lack of chewing; pooling, drooling, or excessive saliva formation

Related Factors

Factors related to the diagnosis *Impaired swallowing* may include the following:

- Weakness or tiredness
- Decreased or lack of motivation
- Severe anxiety

- Neuromuscular or musculoskeletal impairment
- Perceptual or cognitive impairment
- Pain or discomfort
- Environmental barriers

Focused Assessment for Related Nursing Diagnoses

Noncompliance may be diagnosed if clients do not follow nutritional advice. Obese clients may have trouble following the prescribed dietary regimen. People with eating disorders see themselves in a distorted way and have a hard time thinking normally about food and weight. A related nursing diagnosis to consider would be *Ineffective management of therapeutic regimen.*

Clients who are not receiving sufficient fluid may be at risk for dehydration. Consider the diagnosis *Fluid volume deficit.* This is of special concern for the elderly or those with swallowing difficulty, anorexia, or eating disorders.

Use the diagnosis *Impaired skin integrity* for a client with nutritional problems that result in skin problems. They may stem from a low serum albumin and decreased protein. The client may also have edema, making her more prone to skin breakdown. Dehydration causes dry skin and mucous membranes. Another related nursing diagnosis to consider is *Altered oral mucous membrane.*

Use the diagnosis *Diarrhea* for a client with nutritional problems caused by diarrhea, which leads to a loss of fluids and decreased absorption of nutrients. Diarrhea is a common complication of enteral feedings given to clients with nutritional problems.

The diagnosis *Fatigue* may be appropriate when a client receives insufficient nutrients for metabolism and energy production and, as a consequence, feels fatigue. Fatigue can also be a risk factor for both impaired swallowing and aspiration.

DIAGNOSIS

It is relatively easy to distinguish *Altered nutrition: less than body requirements* from *Altered nutrition: more than body requirements.* It may be more difficult to distinguish among *Altered nutrition: less than body requirements, Impaired swallowing,* and *Risk for aspiration.* If the client has a swallowing disorder but also has reduced intake, use the *Altered nutrition* diagnosis until the nutritional state has stabilized. This allows you to focus your care on improving the client's nutritional state.

Remember that impaired swallowing increases the risk of aspiration. Focus your efforts first on preventing aspiration, since aspiration can be life-threatening. Review data from the history and physical examination to find cues to an increased risk for aspiration. If you cannot make a definitive diagnosis of *Risk for aspiration,* then focus on impaired swallowing. Remember that interventions to improve swallowing also help to prevent aspiration.

Make the diagnosis that best focuses on nursing care. For example, if a client with anorexia nervosa is acutely ill in the emergency room, use *Altered nutrition: less than body requirements* until the acute episode resolves. If she has life-threatening fluid and electrolyte imbalances, use *Fluid volume deficit.* As treatment continues and the client gets psychological help, focus on *Self-esteem disturbance* or *Body image disturbance.* The data clustering chart shows how to select nursing diagnoses according to client data.

PLANNING

Planning involves setting general goals and specific outcome criteria with the client. Write the outcome criteria so they are objective and measurable; thus, you can evaluate whether or not they are achieved. For example, "weight gain of 3 pounds" is objective and easy to measure, while "client looks better" is subjective and difficult to measure. Devise a plan for the client to use during the hospital or clinic stay, but also begin discharge planning for the client upon admission.

The clinic nurse sets goals with Mrs. Goldman and her daughter to prevent further nutritional deterioration and to gain 2 pounds per month. The nurse assesses Mrs. Goldman's food preferences and notes that she maintains a kosher diet. What foods would you recommend including in Mrs. Goldman's diet? How would you encourage Mrs. Goldman to monitor her progress toward her nutritional goals?

Expected Outcomes for the Client With Altered Nutrition: Less Than Body Requirements

Goals for the diagnosis *Altered nutrition: less than body requirements* focus on an improved nutritional state. Weight gain is a good outcome criterion for this nursing diagnosis.

Generally, if the client gains at least 2 pounds a month, the plan is considered successful; however, this rate is individual with each client. In some clients, such as those with eating disorders, the initial plan may be simply to avoid further weight loss. A maximum of 1.5 kg/week can be expected from intensive parenteral nutrition. A weight gain of more than 1 pound per day indicates fluid retention rather than an increase in lean muscle mass.

Action Alert!
A weight gain of more than 1 pound per day means that the gain results from fluid and not from lean body mass.

Laboratory test results may also be used to determine the plan's success. However, make sure to interpret albumin levels cautiously because they take about 3 weeks to reflect results of refeeding. Prealbumin or transferrin levels are better short-term indicators.

If pretreatment physical assessment findings are

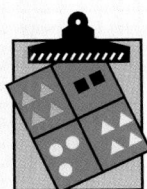

CLUSTERING DATA TO MAKE A NURSING DIAGNOSIS
NUTRITIONAL PROBLEMS

Data Cluster	Diagnosis
A 27-year-old client presents with a weight 120% of normal; has been overweight since age 10; preoperative for gall bladder surgery and referred for weight loss.	*Altered nutrition: more than body requirements* related to unknown etiology.
A 45-year-old client is 120% above his ideal body weight; has been coming to the weight-control clinic for 6 months and continues to gain weight. Refuses to exercise and to keep a food diary.	*Noncompliance* with weight control program related to lack of motivation.
A 14-year-old bulimic client comes to the emergency department with a weight of 55 pounds, height of 5'2", blood pressure of 70/20, pulse of 124, respiratory rate of 30, decreased skin turgor, weakness, and thirst.	*Fluid volume deficit* related to frequent vomiting without sufficient fluid replacement.
A 76-year-old man has had a stroke and is comatose. He is receiving nasogastric feedings and has developed pneumonia.	*Risk for aspiration* related to esophageal reflux and pharyngeal muscle weakness.
A 52-year-old woman receiving chemotherapy for cancer has developed stomatitis, early satiety, anorexia, and decreased taste. Her serum albumin is 2.7 and she has had recent unintentional weight loss.	*Altered nutrition: less than body requirements* related to stomatitis, early satiety, anorexia, and decreased taste.
An 81-year-old client with Parkinson's disease is drooling and pocketing food. Recently he has lost 5 pounds unintentionally. His lungs are clear, and he is ambulatory and alert.	*Impaired swallowing* related to muscle rigidity.

consistent with nutritional deficiency, then cite improvement in these as outcome criteria. For example,

- Wound begins to heal
- Edema resolves
- Petechiae disappear

Expected Outcomes for the Client With Impaired Swallowing

The client should be able to maintain a stable weight, show no signs of dehydration, and report no difficulty swallowing. Outcome criteria indicating normal hydration are

- Good skin turgor
- Normal vital signs (no hypotension, tachycardia, or fever)
- Skin and mucous membranes moist, not dry
- No complaints of thirst
- Normal hematocrit (not elevated)

INTERVENTION

Interventions for nutritional problems in any setting requires a team approach. New hospital standards require performance-based interdisciplinary delivery of nutritional support, so it is likely that nutritional support teams will continue (Standards for nutrition support nurses, 1996; Standards for nutrition support: hospitalized patients, 1995).

Interventions to Increase Nutrient Intake

Make sure that your client is comfortable during meals. A client who is fatigued, immobilized, or paralyzed will need assistance. Until the client can eat independently, feed him and teach the family or caregiver about feeding (Fig. 30–3). When an adult requires feeding, maintain the client's dignity. Feed her in an unhurried manner, and converse pleasantly with her. If the client is blind, describe the food and caution her about hot foods. Allow time for her to

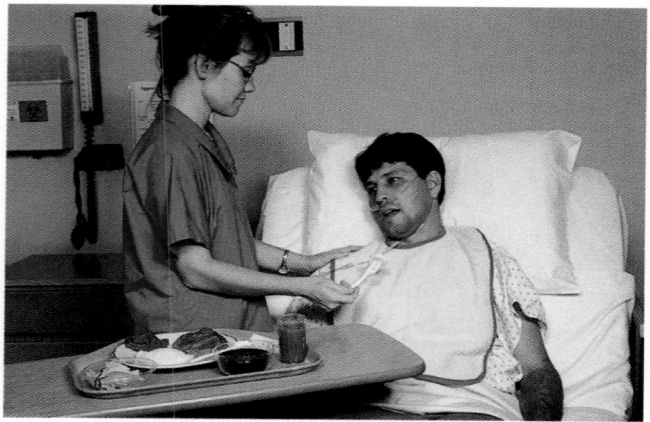

Figure 30–3. Until clients can eat independently, feed them, and teach the family or caregiver about feeding.

chew and enjoy the food. Studies show that clients eat more food if you switch from one food to another during feeding (Davis & Sherer, 1994).

Consider food preferences and serve food in an attractive manner to improve intake. Young children generally like their food bland, while the elderly (with diminished taste) prefer food that is seasoned. Fresh herbs are a good choice. Assess the older client's ability to chew, and puree the food as needed if his teeth are in poor condition.

Often, an evaluation team will recommend treatment for complex feeding problems. The team works to improve the client's hand-to-mouth coordination, vision, or ability to suck, chew, swallow, or grasp. Special feeding equipment may be used, including weighted utensils, two-handed cups, and unbreakable dishes with suction cups. Battery-powered machines are also available (Whitney, Cataldo, & Rolfes, 1994).

Enriching the Insufficient Diet

The diet should be the primary source of good nutrition, but sometimes the diet is insufficient. Pregnant women need extra folic acid, calcium, and iron. Clients with osteoporosis need extra calcium and magnesium, and many chronically ill clients require multiple vitamin or mineral supplements.

Some clients cannot eat enough at mealtime and begin to lose weight. To remedy this, give supplemental feedings to increase calories and nutrients. The extra food should be nutritious and something the client enjoys. Generally, six small meals are preferable to three larger ones.

With Mrs. Goldman, you would encourage small, supplemental meals. Which types of food would you consider offering her?

Liquid foods are less filling and easier for debilitated people to handle. Milkshakes, puddings, and instant breakfast drinks can be recommended. Adding powdered milk, yogurt, or tofu to foods provides extra protein, while adding sugar or corn syrup provides calories. Sweet additives increase the solution's osmo-

lality but also increase the risk of gastrointestinal distress. Commercial supplements can add protein, fat, carbohydrate, and calories (Whitney, Cataldo, & Rolfes, 1994).

Managing Therapeutic Diets

In the hospital setting the physician prescribes the diet. The diet may meet therapeutic needs or be based on the client's ability to tolerate food.

Hospitalized clients may be on *NPO (nothing per os, or nothing by mouth)* status to prevent complications from diagnostic tests, surgery, trauma, or acute illness. Intravenous fluids are prescribed, often with 5% dextrose, to prevent dehydration, not provide nutrition. One thousand milliliters of a 5% dextrose solution yields only *170 kcal* per liter. Most healthy people can tolerate a few days of NPO status but should receive enteral nutrition if the need persists longer than 5 days; infants and children should receive it even sooner.

When a diet order is resumed, clients are often started on a *clear liquid diet,* which contains liquids that are thin and without pulp. Examples of clear liquids include apple juice, ginger ale, gelatin, decaffeinated coffee, tea, broth, fruit ices, or popsicles. This diet is temporary and provides about 400 to 500 kcal, 5 to 10 g of protein, 100 to 120 g of carbohydrate, no fat, and very few vitamins and minerals (Mahan & Escott-Stump, 2000).

The client may then progress to a full liquid diet, including milkshakes, all juices, gruels, blenderized foods, custards, puddings, and eggnog. This diet contains as much as 1,500 calories and has more nutrients than a clear liquid diet. With careful planning and the addition of fiber, it can be used indefinitely.

A *soft diet* is sometimes used as a transition to a general diet or for clients who have difficulty eating. This diet is low in fiber and is devoid of brans, grains, strong vegetables (such as cabbage), and raw fruits or vegetables. However, institutions sometimes differ in their definition of a soft diet, and the trend is to define it more liberally, allowing more whole-grain products, cereals, and vegetables (Mahan & Escott-Stump, 2000).

DIABETES. Diabetics should eat three meals per day, with snacks in the late afternoon and before bedtime to coincide with peak action times of insulin. The diet should be well-balanced and avoid concentrated sweets. A dietitian will develop the dietary prescription based on a physician's order.

Action Alert!
Urge a diabetic client to immediately report any illness that prevents her from eating.

AIDS AND CANCER. Clients with AIDS and cancer may have cachexia, a syndrome of anorexia; anemia; fatigue; and muscle wasting. They may have a decreased sense of taste (which may respond to zinc supplements). They also tend to eat better in the morning and tolerate small, frequent feedings during the day.

Encourage foods that contain protein, especially milk shakes, poultry, and eggs, but remember that these clients may have an aversion to red meats. Immunosuppression may lead to a sore mouth and throat, as well as to xerostomia—mouth dryness caused by insufficient saliva. Encourage fluids, limit spicy or acidic foods, and emphasize good oral hygiene.

HEART DISEASE. Clients with heart disease require a diet low in saturated fat, cholesterol, and salt. Foods to be avoided include butter, whole milk, eggs, red meat, and cheese. Skim milk, poultry, fish, and fresh fruits and vegetables are encouraged, along with foods high in soluble fiber, such as apples, citrus fruits, oats, and barley.

A 2-g sodium diet (moderate restriction) is common for clients with hypertension. Teach clients on this diet not to add salt while cooking or at the table and to avoid foods high in sodium, such as canned, prepared, and processed foods. Encourage hypertensive clients to increase the amount of calcium and potassium in their diet.

KIDNEY DISEASE. Therapeutic dietary management of kidney disease depends on the type and stage of disease. Protein is generally restricted as the disease advances. Fluid, sodium, potassium and phosphorus are restricted because the kidneys cannot maintain an adequate fluid and electrolyte balance. Vitamin D and calcium levels may be low, causing fractures and bone softening. Administer vitamin D and calcium supplements as ordered. With less erythropoietin to stimulate production of red blood cells, iron supplements are needed to treat anemia.

LIVER DISEASE. Therapeutic nutrition is also important in treating liver disease. Protein intake should be normal to maintain nitrogen balance; however, if the client has impending liver failure, protein is restricted. When the liver fails, ammonia (a byproduct of protein metabolism) does not convert to urea and ammonia levels rise to toxic levels in the blood. The diet for these clients should provide adequate kilocalories and carbohydrates, as well as vitamins normally stored in the liver (especially vitamin K, thiamine, pyridoxine, vitamin B_{12}, folate, and niacin). Sodium and fluid may be restricted because the liver no longer breaks down aldosterone.

Providing Enteral Feedings

When a client cannot eat sufficient nutrients to sustain life and health, enteral feedings may be initiated. While **enteral nutrition** can refer to any form of nutrition delivered to the gastrointestinal tract (orally or by tube), it generally is used to mean tube feedings. Feeding a client through a tube inserted into the gastrointestinal tract can help to keep it functioning normally. Table 30–3 identifies clinical situations in which such artificial nutrition may be necessary.

FEEDING TUBES AND ROUTES OF ACCESS
A feeding tube may be inserted through the nose and placed in the stomach, duodenum, or jejunum. These

are known as nasogastric, nasoduodenal, or nasojejunal tubes, respectively. The tube can also be inserted surgically into the esophagus, stomach, or jejunum. These are known as esophagostomy, gastrostomy, and jejunostomy tubes, respectively (Fig. 30–4A). When endoscopy is used to insert the tube, it is referred to as a percutaneous endoscopic gastrostomy (PEG) or percutaneous endoscopic jejunostomy (PEJ) tube (Fig. 30–4B). PEG and PEJ often use low-profile tubes because they are comfortable underneath clothing. Figure 30–5 provides some examples of low-profile gastrostomy tubes.

The choice of enteral nutrition support depends on the client's status, the anticipated length of use, the cost, and the availability of a person experienced in placing the feeding tube, as discussed in the accompanying Decision Tree. The gastric site is preferred to the jejunal site because the stomach has a larger reservoir. However, the jejunal site may be used if the client has significant esophageal reflux, a history or risk of aspiration, or a dysfunctional stomach from gastric surgery or gastritis (Duh, 1996). Also, function returns to the small intestine faster than to the stomach after stress or trauma.

Endoscopic feeding tube placement is less invasive and less expensive than surgical placement. Surgical placement is done under general or local anesthesia using a laparoscopy or open laparotomy.

Tube feedings are usually initiated with a nasogastric tube. A pliable, small-bore tube is used because it causes less discomfort and less interference with the lower esophageal sphincter than a large-bore tube. To place a feeding tube, follow the relevant procedure in Chapter 31, with the modifications shown in this chapter in the Box 30-2 on Placement of a Feeding Tube.

The definitive way to make sure a tube has reached the stomach is by x-ray. The next most reliable indica-

TABLE 30–3
Clinical Situations in Which Artifical Nutrition May Be Necessary

Situation	Possible Cause
Inability to ingest food	• Cancer of the mouth, tongue, esophagus. • Facial trauma. • Unconsciousness. • Severe stomatitis. • Impaired swallowing. • Muscle weakness in mouth or esophagus.
Inability to digest or absorb food	• Pancreatitis. • Cancer of the stomach. • Crohn's disease or ulcerative colitis. • Biliary disease.
Inability to meet nutritional needs	• Increased resting energy expenditure from major trauma or surgery, burns, or severe infection. • Anorexia nervosa or bulimia nervosa.

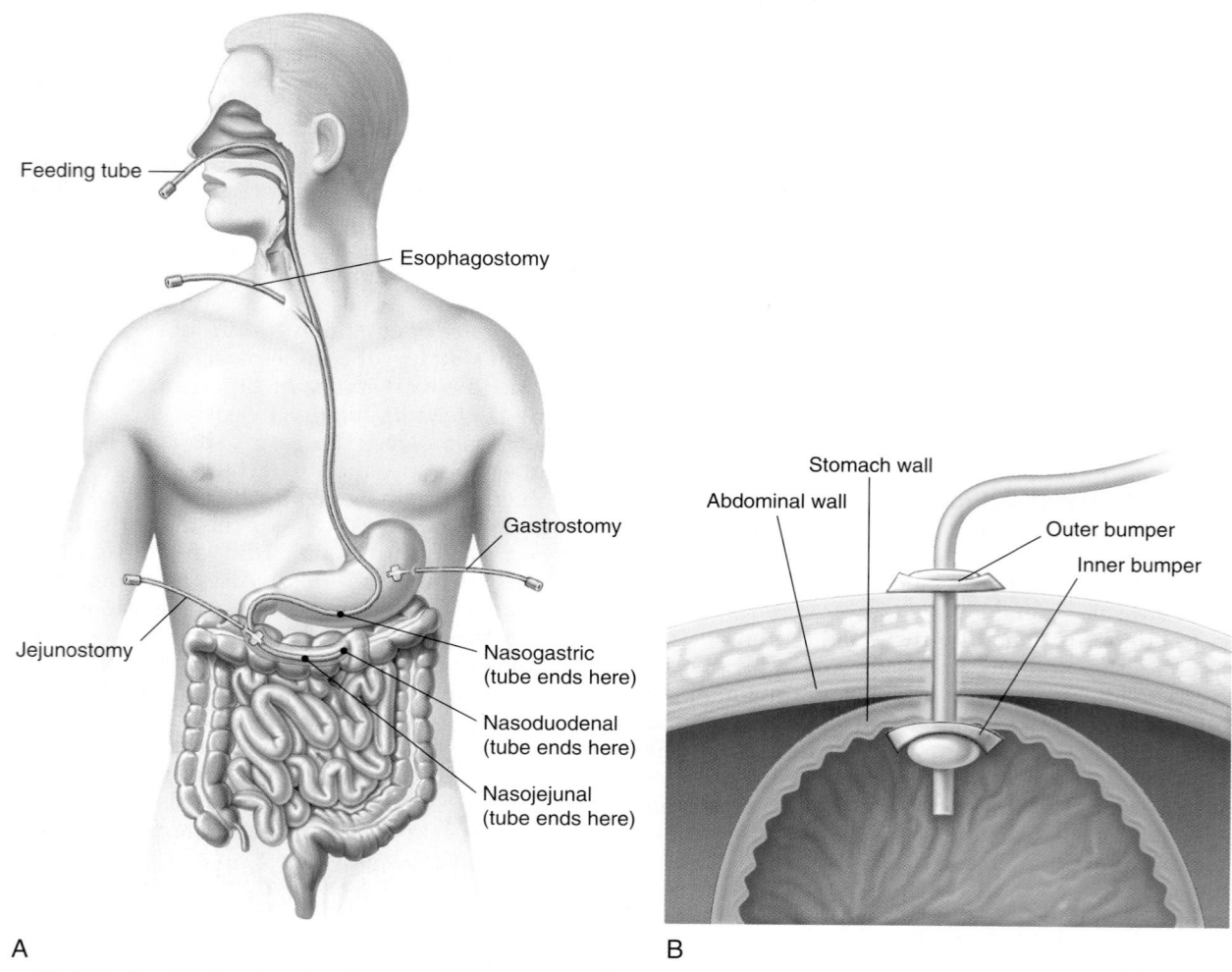

Figure 30–4. Feeding tubes and routes of access. *A,* Nasogastric and surgically placed feeding tubes. *B,* Percutaneous endoscopic gastrostomy tube.

tor is checking the pH of the fluid withdrawn through the tube. If the pH is less than 5.0, the tube is most likely in the stomach (Welch, 1996). With duodenal tube placement, you should note a pH change of the fluid from less than 5.0 to more than 6.0, along with a change of color from green to golden.

The disadvantages of using pH for confirming placement are twofold. First, the flexible, small-bore tubes sometimes collapse during aspiration of gastric contents, preventing removal of the fluid. Second, other factors can affect gastric pH, such as acid-inhibiting agents, aging, pernicious anemia, AIDS, and intestinal bile reflux. Welch (1996) advocates dipping the end of the tube into a glass of water when the feeding tube has been advanced to the 25-cm mark. If the water bubbles, it should be removed and attempted again because the tube may be in the lungs.

You can also instill 60 mL of air into the tube (in short bursts) and listen with a stethoscope over the left upper quadrant for air sounds; however, Metheny (1993) reports that the sounds are spread throughout

the thorax. Welch (1996) states that, when used with the other criteria, this method can be useful. Aspirating at least 40 mL of the air is also used to verify stomach placement. If more than 10 mL of air cannot be removed, the tube is probably still in the esophagus.

In summary, more than one method should be used to check enteral tube placement. Metheny (1996) reports consulting on several tragic malpractice cases of inadvertent respiratory placement of an enteral tube in which only auscultation was used to confirm tube placement.

Action Alert!
When placing a feeding tube, the definitive method of confirming gastric placement is an x-ray. Auscultation and obtaining the pH of gastric contents do not eliminate the need for an abdominal x-ray.

TYPES OF ENTERAL FORMULAS
Enteral formulas can be made by blenderizing regular foods or using commercially prepared formulas. Blenderized formulas should be refrigerated and hung

only long enough to be infused. Baby foods can also be used for clients who will receive tube feedings indefinitely. Polymeric feedings are milk-based or lactose-free and are similar to oral supplements. They contain whole protein, long-chain fatty acids, and complex carbohydrates, and they require an intact intestine for digestion. Elemental or hydrolyzed formulas contain short-chain peptides or amino acids for easy digestion, as well as short-chain fatty acids and simple carbohydrates. These feedings are partially digested and are used for clients with abnormal bowel function. Specialty feedings are designed for use in specific disease situations. For example, diabetic formulas have a lower sugar content. The latter two types of formulas are more costly than polymeric ones.

The components of formulas can vary but usually provide about 1.0 kcal/mL along with recommended amounts of vitamins and minerals. Many formulas now have fiber added to maintain normal gastrointestinal function. The osmolarity of the formula is another variable. Hyperosmolar (e.g., hydrolyzed) formulas pull water into the gastrointestinal tract and can cause diarrhea. Standard formulas provide 80 to 85% of the client's water needs, so tube-fed clients who do not have another source of fluid require additional water to meet their physiological needs.

ADMINISTRATION OF ENTERAL FEEDINGS

Initiate tube feedings slowly, especially if the client has not eaten for a period of time. Monitor the serum phosphorus level for a drop after the metabolism begins to rise. The administration of feedings through various types of tubes at different time intervals is described in the procedure on Administering an Enteral Feeding. Continuous feedings are given over 24 hours. Intermittent feedings deliver no more than 250 mL of feeding over 30 minutes periodically during the day. Bolus feedings of up to 400 mL of formula are given by the nurse or client within about 10 or 15 minutes (Whitney, Cataldo, & Rolfes, 1994). Because the small intestine tolerates bolus feedings poorly, the duodenum and jejunum require continuous feedings (Clevenger & Rodriguez, 1995).

The disadvantages of bolus or intermittent feedings include diarrhea and an increased resting energy expenditure. The diarrhea results from an osmotic effect and is more common in the elderly. The resting energy expenditure increases by 5 to 10% daily because of the fluctuation in fuel reserves with periodic feeding; it does not occur with continuous feedings. Disadvantages of continuous feedings include clogging of the tube and a lower serum protein synthesis. Clogging generally results from a slow feeding rate through a small-bore tube. Decreased protein syn-

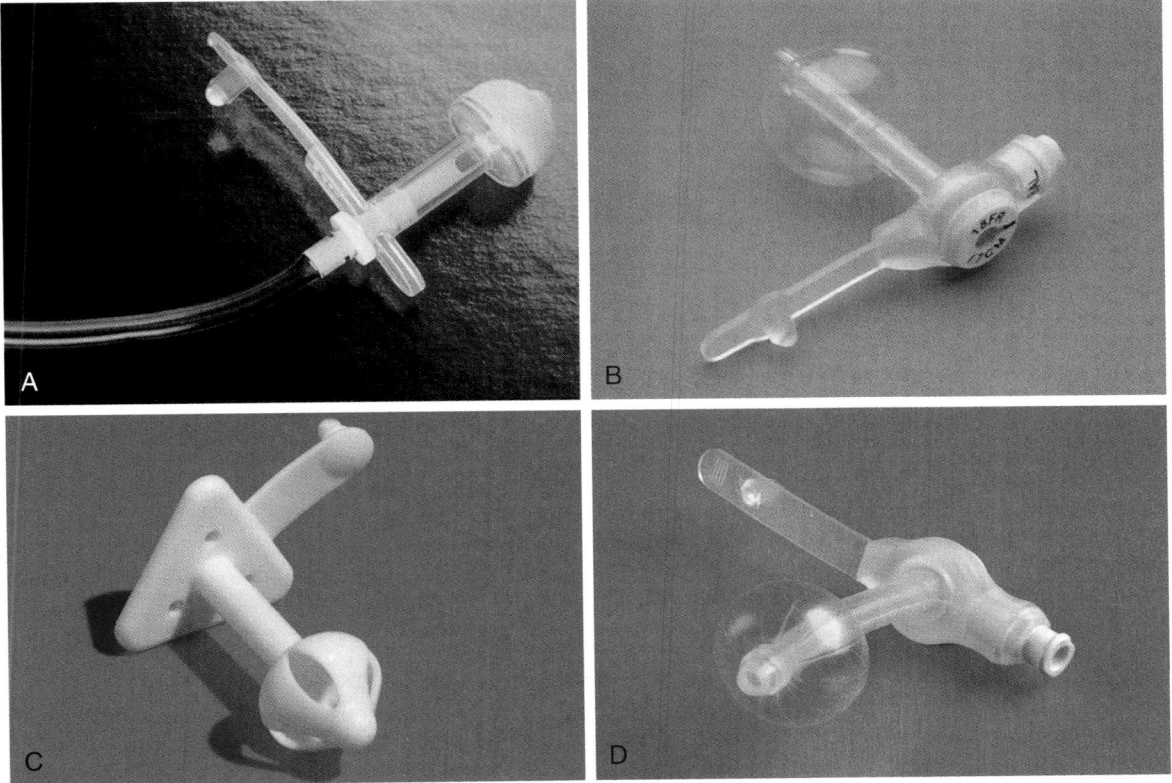

Figure 30–5. Examples of low-profile gastrostomy tubes. *A*, Bard Button; *B*, Ballard Mic-Key; *C*, Ross Stomate; *D*, Ross Hide-A-Port. (*A*, courtesy of C. R. Bard, Inc., Billerica, MA; *B*, courtesy of Ballard Medical Products, Draper, UT; *C* and *D* used with permission of Ross Products Division, Abbott Laboratories, Inc., Columbus, OH 43216.)

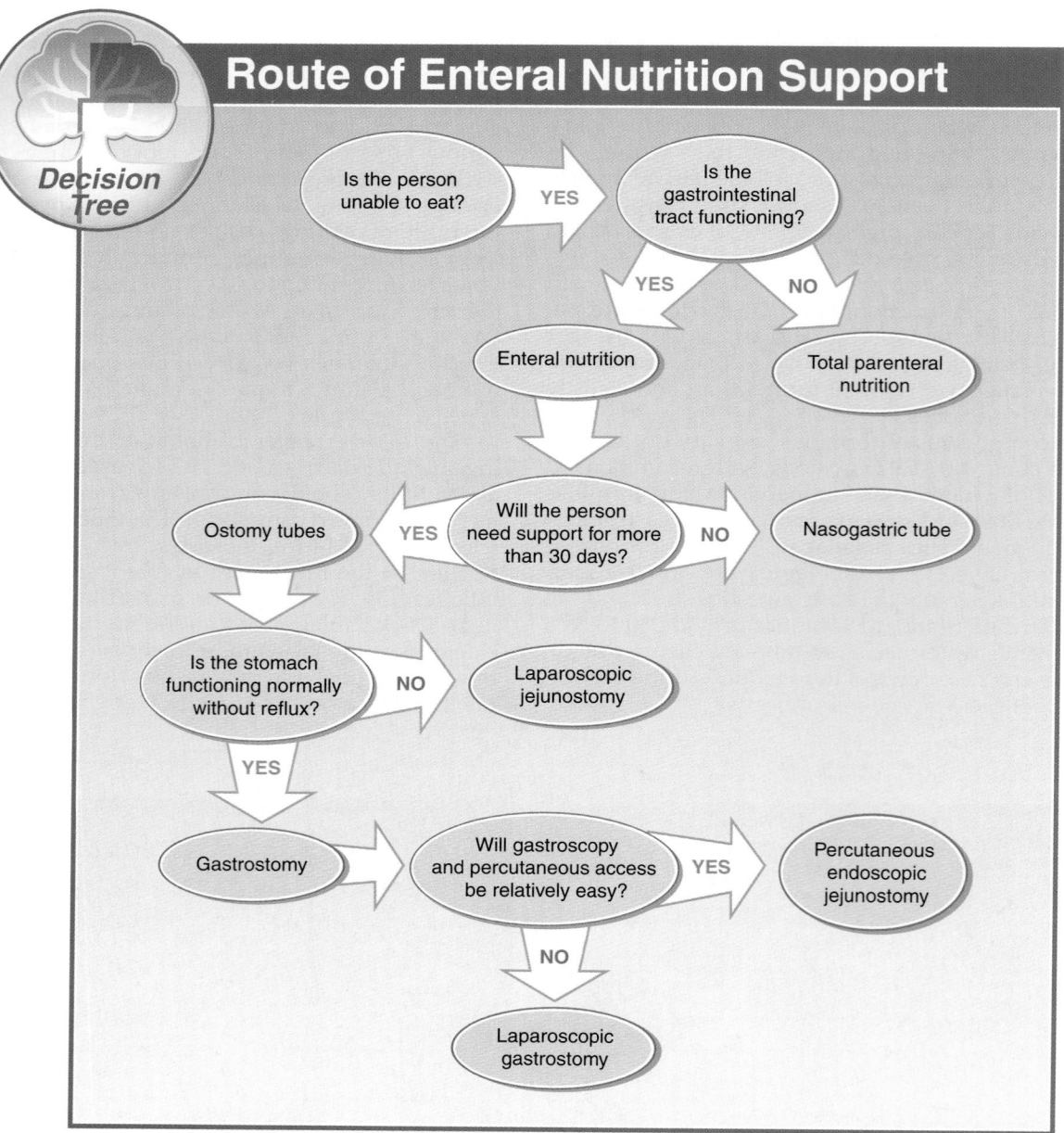

Route of Enteral Nutrition Support

Decision Tree

- Is the person unable to eat? — **YES** → Is the gastrointestinal tract functioning?
  - **YES** → Enteral nutrition
  - **NO** → Total parenteral nutrition
- Enteral nutrition → Will the person need support for more than 30 days?
  - **YES** → Ostomy tubes
  - **NO** → Nasogastric tube
- Ostomy tubes → Is the stomach functioning normally without reflux?
  - **NO** → Laparoscopic jejunostomy
  - **YES** → Gastrostomy
- Gastrostomy → Will gastroscopy and percutaneous access be relatively easy?
  - **YES** → Percutaneous endoscopic jejunostomy
  - **NO** → Laparoscopic gastrostomy

Modified from Duh, Q. Y. (1996). Decision tree for route of enteral nutrition support: Placement techniques. Current issues in enteral nutrition support: Report of the first Ross Conference on Enteral Devices, pp. 9–16. Columbus, OH: Ross Products Division, Abbott Laboratories. Used with permission of Ross Products Division, Abbott Laboratories, Columbus, OH 43216. Copyright 1996, Ross Products Division, Abbott Laboratories.

thesis occurs because continuous feedings increase insulin and glycogen levels, favoring the use of protein for fuel rather than tissue storage (DeLegge, 1996). Bolus and intermittent feeding methods are more natural and allow greater client mobility. Seriously ill clients are often fed continuously, with a goal of intermittent or bolus feedings.

Regardless of the method used, always ensure correct tube placement and the presence of bowel sounds before giving a feeding. Raise the head of the bed as much as the client can tolerate and keep it elevated for 30 minutes after a bolus or intermittent feeding.

When administering enteral feedings using a feed-

ing bag, use good hand-washing technique to prevent bacterial contamination. Results of a nursing study by Kohn (1991) indicated that bags should be changed every 24 hours. Identify on the bag the date and time it was hung.

COMPLICATIONS OF ENTERAL FEEDINGS

It is very important to monitor any client receiving tube feedings to prevent or minimize complications (see Box 30–3 on Monitoring Clients Receiving Tube Feedings). As discussed previously, the most dreaded complication of tube feedings is aspiration. To minimize it, follow the procedures described for confirm-

BOX 30–2

MODIFICATIONS FOR PLACEMENT OF A FEEDING TUBE

A feeding tube can be a small-bore tube designed for administration of enteral formula feedings. Feedings can be given through a Levin-type nasogastric tube, but a small-bore flexible feeding tube reduces discomfort and trauma and can thus be safely used for a longer time. To place a feeding tube, follow Procedure 31–1, with the following modifications.

Equipment

- No. 6–10 French feeding tube with or without guidewire.
- 60-mL Luer-Lok or irrigation-tip syringe, as indicated, to fit the specific tube.
- Cup of tap water.
- Water-soluble lubricant.
- pH strips.
- Clean gloves.

Measuring

Measuring for gastric placement is the same as for any nasogastric tube. To place the tube in the client's duodenum, you will need at least 75 cm of tube to reach the ligament of Treitz.

Lubrication

Use water-soluble lubricant or moisten the surface with water. For some tubes, follow the manufacturer's directions to insert 10 mL of water into tube with a syringe to activate the lubricant.

Using a Guidewire

A guidewire is provided with small-bore feeding tubes to make the tube rigid during insertion. After you become experienced with tube placement, you may be able to place a tube without a guidewire. If you will be using a guidewire, insert it into the tube, make sure it fits, and make sure you can remove it easily. The guidewire must be secure to prevent damage to the gastrointestinal tract.

Checking for Placement

Check for placement with the guidewire in place. Use more than one method to check for placement.

Removing the Guidewire

Remove the guidewire only after the placement of the tube is confirmed. Never reinsert a guidewire after removing it unless the tube is specifically designed for reinsertion of the guidewire. Reinserting a guidewire could puncture the tube and injure the client.

Using a Topical Anesthetic

If you used a topical anesthetic on the client's throat, test for the return of the client's gag reflex with a tongue blade when finished. The use of a topical anesthetic may be contraindicated when a client has dysphagia.

Documentation

Document the time you inserted the tube; the type of tube inserted; the amount, color, consistency, and pH of secretions; the amount of water instilled; and the client's response.

Home Care

Pediatric tubes should be replaced every 2 to 6 weeks and adult tubes every 6 weeks to 3 months. Health care agencies establish differing protocols. Teach the family as follows:

- The teeth need to be brushed even though the client is taking nothing by mouth. Clean the nostrils daily and inspect for irritation or incrustations. The tape or fixator device on the nose should be changed a minimum of every 5 days. Inspect for any allergic response to the adhesive.
- Some clients can take small amounts of soft foods and swallow around the tube. The tube feeding supplements the diet.
- Maintain tube patency. Flush with water at regular intervals. Always flush before and after medications.
- If the tube becomes clogged, use a 20-mL or larger syringe half filled with water. Attempt to flush in and out. Flushing with a clear diet carbonated beverage instead of water may help unclog the tube. Keep in mind that it is possible to exert enough pressure to puncture the tube. Use caution.

ing tube placement. Check residual volume before giving the feeding, or at least every 4 hours. If the residuals are greater than 150 mL (or 10 to 20% over the hourly flow rate), withhold the feeding. Assess the client's respiratory status at least every shift and note any changes. If a blue dye is added to the feedings and the client's respiratory secretions become blue, stop

the feedings immediately because aspiration has occurred.

To prevent clogging of a feeding tube, flush the tube with water before and after giving all feedings and medications. Flush also when adding new formula or at least every 4 hours (even when not in use) to avoid obstruction. Record the amount of water used

Administering an Enteral Feeding

TIME TO ALLOW

▼

Novice:
15–25 min.
Expert:
10–15 min.

Enteral feedings can be administered into the stomach, duodenum, or jejunum through a tube inserted in the client's nose or a tube implanted in the abdominal wall (gastrostomy or jejunostomy tubes). These feedings are administered on a specific time schedule specified in the physician's order to provide nutrition to a client who cannot eat or swallow.

Delegation Guidelines

The assessment of the client and the administration of enteral nutrition via gastric, duodenal, or jejunal tube require the expertise of the RN. The gathering and assembly of the necessary equipment and the preparation of the tube feeding formula may be delegated to a nursing assistant who has received special training in the performance of this task. You are then responsible for initiating the infusion of the enteral nutrition along with evaluating the client's response. Institutions vary in their approach to the nursing assistant role in delivering enteral nutrition; some allow nursing assistants to deliver tube feeding via the bolus method only. It is essential that your actions are in compliance with your institution's policies and procedures regarding delegation of this task.

Equipment Needed

- 60-mL syringe.
- Cup of water.
- Stethoscope.
- Clean gloves.
- Feeding pump and IV pole if feeding will be continuous.
- pH tape.
- Prescribed formula.
- Adapter for gastrostomy or jejunostomy tube, if needed.
- 4″ × 4″ gauze pads (possibly pre-cut), nonallergenic tape, and soap to clean and dress a gastrostomy or jejunostomy tube site.

---

1 Make sure the client is comfortable and the room is private, and raise the head of bed 30 to 45 degrees.

These steps help the procedure go smoothly and reduce the risk of aspiration.

---

2 Assess the client.
a. Listen to bowel sounds.
b. Observe for abdominal distention or distress.

Distention and absence of bowel sounds may indicate paralytic ileus.

c. Inquire about diarrhea.

Diarrhea is not always a reaction to the tube feeding; always assess for the cause.

If you detect any of these problems, report them and confirm that you should still give the feeding.

---

3 Prepare for the feeding.
a. Make sure the formula is at room temperature and within its expiration date.

Cold formula can cause cramping.

b. Confirm placement and check for residual. With the tube clamped, insert a syringe into the end of the tube, unclamp the tube, and aspirate residual fluid in the client's stomach. For a small-bore tube, use a 10-mL syringe. For a large-bore tube, use a 60-mL syringe.

If the client has more than 150 mL of fluid in her stomach, withhold the feeding. Remember that a jejunostomy tube typically has the smallest residual volume.

c. Test the pH of the gastric fluid.

---

4 Flush with water. Remove the plunger from the irrigating syringe, and insert the barrel into the end of the tube. The barrel is then used as a funnel to pour the water through. For small-bore tubes, the water is injected slowly with a syringe.

Flushing with water helps keep the tube patent and prevents stomach acid from clumping the formula.

---

5 To give a bolus feeding with a syringe, follow these steps.
a. Using the barrel of the syringe as a funnel, add formula until it nearly fills the syringe.

Feedings flow by gravity and may take up to 15 minutes.

b. When the syringe is almost empty, refill it with formula until the total amount has been instilled.

By refilling the syringe before it empties, you avoid instilling air into the tube. Do not force feedings by using the plunger because the client will be at increased risk for aspiration, diarrhea, and bloating.

c. Instill 50 mL water after the feeding is complete.

Instilling water helps to avoid clogging in the tube.

d. Clamp the tube.
e. Remove the syringe, wash it with tap water, and store it for future use.
f. Cover the end of the tube with clean gauze.

6 To give an intermittent feeding with a bag and tubing, follow these steps.
a. After instilling water into the tube as explained above, clamp the tube and attach the feeding tube.
b. Fill the feeding bag with the prescribed amount of formula and prime the tubing.
c. Hang the feeding bag on an IV stand.
d. Unclamp the feeding tube.
e. Regulate the flow so the formula is instilled over 20 minutes.
f. When formula has finished flowing, clamp the tube and remove the feeding bag. Instill 50 mL water into the feeding tube.
g. Wash out the feeding bag with tap water and store it for future use.

> *Hints: change the bag and tubing every 24 hours, or according to agency policy, to avoid bacterial contamination.*
>
> *Fresh formula should be hung after 4 to 8 hours. Consult agency policy.*

h. When hanging a new feeding bag, label it with the time, the date, and your initials.

7 To give a continuous feeding, follow the steps listed above but use an infusion pump to regulate the flow of formula.

The infusion pump ensures a regular rate.

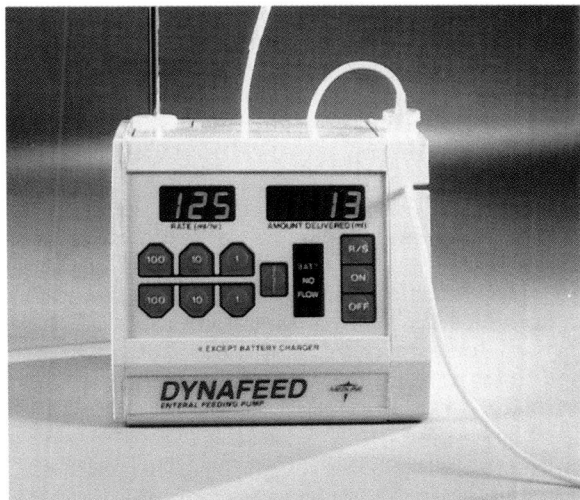

Feeding infusion pump. (Courtesy of Medline Industries, Inc., Mundelein, IL.)

a. Thread the tubing from the feeding bag through infusion pump.

> *Read manufacturer's pump instructions because they vary.*

b. Set the infusion pump at the prescribed rate.

8 If you need to give a medication through a nasogastric tube, make sure it is available in liquid form or can be finely crushed if necessary.

Medication that is not crushed finely enough could clog the tube.

9 If necessary, clean and dress the entrance site of a gastrostomy or jejunostomy tube.

Most clients do not require a dressing over the site. If leaking gastric acid is a problem, a duoderm dressing will protect the skin.

a. Use clean technique to clean the entrance site unless the client is in the immediate postoperative period. Use soap and water to remove all leakage of gastric contents and crusty drainage. Dry the area well.

> *Using careful cleaning technique and teaching the client thoroughly about these long-term feeding tubes can help avoid problems and the need for surgical replacement.*

b. Observe for and report any unusual drainage (thick, green, yellow, or foul-smelling), redness, puffiness, or pain at the site.
c. To dress the site, use a pre-cut 4" × 4" gauze pad or make a cut to the middle of the pad. Place the pad around the tube so the tube protrudes from the middle of the pad and use nonallergenic tape to affix the pad in place.

10 Monitor the client.
a. Make sure the tube is taped securely to the client's nose and pinned safely to her gown when you finish with the feeding.
b. Assess the client for gastric distress, distention, cramping, and diarrhea.

11 Tidy the client's environment and discard any used materials. Discard your gloves and wash your hands.

12 Document the amount and type of feeding delivered on an intake and output sheet, the time of the feeding, your assessment findings, residual gastric contents and its pH, and the client's daily weight.

Teach family caregivers to administer feedings. Include feeding technique, cleaning and storing equipment, preventing and managing complications, skin care, and monitoring nutritional status.

BOX 30–3

MONITORING CLIENTS RECEIVING TUBE FEEDINGS

- Measure residual gastric contents every 4 hours. If the amount is greater than half the feeding given in the last 4 hours, stop the feeding, assess the abdomen, and consult the physician.
- Weigh the client daily to detect fluid retention; weekly to detect actual weight gain.
- Assess for signs of edema daily.
- Assess for signs of dehydration daily.
- Obtain fingerstick glucose readings daily.
- Assess intake and output daily.
- Record stool output daily.
- Assess calorie, protein, fat, mineral, and vitamin intake twice weekly.
- Check serum electrolytes, serum phosphorus, blood urea nitrogen, creatinine, and complete blood count two or three times weekly (by physician's order).
- Obtain a chemistry profile weekly (by physician's order).
- Check nitrogen balance weekly (optional).

to flush the tube on the client's intake and output record. If the client is on fluid restriction, consult with the nutrition support team about methods to keep the tube patent. Medications given through the tube should be in liquid form if at all possible. Even finely crushed medications clog small-bore nasoenteric tubes. If the medication is not available in liquid form, dissolve the finely crushed pill in warm water. Enteric-coated tablets should not be given through enteric tubes because crushing the pills circumvents the coating.

If the tube does occlude, various methods can be used to reopen it. Flushing with very warm water is currently the most acceptable method (Brennan & Heximer, 1998). Pancreatic enzyme or sodium bicarbonate crushed in 5 mL of water may be helpful (Davis and Sherer, 1994). Some sources suggest the use of meat tenderizer, cola, or cranberry juice, but others discourage their use. The best treatment is prevention with adequate flushing.

Diarrhea can result from hyperosmolar feedings, medications, or bacterial contamination of the feeding. Assess the cause of diarrhea carefully rather than simply stopping the feeding, decreasing the rate, or diluting the formula. Send a stool specimen and evaluate all medications, especially laxatives, and those containing sorbito-elixirs or magnesium.

If the feeding itself is causing the diarrhea, the rate can be lowered, although doing so also lowers calorie intake. Once the problem is resolved, the rate should be gradually increased as tolerated. The formula could also be changed to one that is more elemental or has a lower osmolality (Ireton-Jones, Hennessy, & Orr, 1996). Antidiarrheal medication can be given while the cause is treated.

Other complications can occur during enteral nutrition. These may include infection at the ostomy site, nausea and vomiting, hyperglycemia, and tube dislodgment. Continually assess the skin around the gastrostomy or jejunostomy site for infection. If the client is nauseated, stop the feeding and report the finding. Nausea and vomiting can stem from contaminated formula or feeding bag or from completely unrelated factors. Perform fingerstick glucose readings daily. If the tube becomes dislodged or clogged beyond repair, it must be replaced.

HOME ENTERAL NUTRITION

Shortened hospital lengths of stay have escalated the numbers of clients receiving enteral nutrition at home (Ireton-Jones, Hennessy, & Orr, 1996). Adequate home care, professional and family support, and teaching are needed for this to be effective. The Teaching for Self-Care chart describes how to teach a family caregiver to provide home enteral nutrition.

General training for caregivers should include stoma assessment and monitoring of devices. Analysis of associated costs should be ongoing. For example, could the client use syringe feeding rather than an infusion pump and feeding bags? Will future nursing research show that feeding tube bags used in the home can be safely changed less frequently than every 24 hours?

Parenteral Nutrition

Parenteral nutrition is the provision of total nutrition through a central or peripheral intravenous catheter. When a central vein (such as the subclavian) is used, this procedure is known as total parenteral nutrition (TPN), hyperalimentation, or central venous nutrition. Sometimes parenteral nutrition is given in a smaller peripheral vein in an extremity. It is then called peripheral parenteral nutrition (PPN). This peripheral approach is being used more widely, and some authors recommend it for most hospitalized clients who need parenteral nutrition for less than 14 days (Payne-James & Khawaja, 1993). Parenteral nutrition is indicated for any client who does not have a functional gastrointestinal tract for an extended period of time.

ADMINISTRATION OF PARENTERAL NUTRITION

Most clients receive continuous parenteral nutrition; however, some clients in the home setting receive cyclic feedings on a 12- to 18-hour cycle to increase their quality of life. Often, they receive feedings at night so that they can be mobile during the day.

Initiate parenteral nutrition slowly to avoid the refeeding syndrome. A suggested regimen is to start the feedings at 42 mL/hour or 1,000 mL/day and then increase slowly over a 2- to 3-day period. Watch for

Teaching for SELF-CARE

HOME ENTERAL NUTRITION

Purpose: To teach a client or family member to deliver feedings through a gastrostomy tube and to care for the tube properly.

Rationale: Proper feeding and tube maintenance will allow the client to remain comfortably at home.

Expected Outcome: The client or a family member will be able to successfully feed the client through a gastrostomy tube and will prevent infection at the entrance site.

Client Instructions

Giving a Feeding

1. If your feeding formula is refrigerated, allow it to come to room temperature before using it, because cold feeding formula can cause cramping.
2. Wash your hands and put on clean gloves.
3. If your doctor wants you to, check for residual gastric contents before delivering a feeding. To do so, insert a syringe into the tube, unclamp the tube, and use the plunger to remove and measure the volume of gastric secretions. If you have too much residual contents, you may have to withhold the feeding for a while.
4. Measure the prescribed amount of feeding formula.
5. After removing the plunger from a 60-mL syringe, insert the syringe into the end of the tube.
6. Unclamp the tube.
7. Pour enough of the formula into the syringe to nearly fill the syringe. If you unclamp the tube before inserting the syringe, gastric contents may leak out.

8. When the syringe is still about a quarter full, refill it with formula. Refilling before the syringe is empty will prevent air from entering the tube.
9. After instilling all of the formula, flush the syringe and tube with about 60 mL of water.
10. Before removing the syringe from the tube, clamp the tube. Clamping the tube keeps gastric contents from leaking out.
11. Expect this entire process to take about 15 minutes.
12. Wash the syringe after each feeding and change syringes daily.
13. Store the formula according to the package directions.

Caring for the Gastrostomy Site

1. To clean the area where the tube enters your skin, use a washcloth or a 4″ × 4″ gauze pad. Wet it with warm, soapy water and clean around the site. Rinse with clear water and dry thoroughly with a soft towel.
2. Usually, a gastrostomy tube needs no dressing. If your doctor tells you to use one, use a pre-cut 4″ × 4″ gauze pad or use scissors to cut to the middle of the pad. Slide the slit in the pad over the tube so the tube protrudes from the middle of the pad. Affix the pad in place with nonallergenic tape.
3. Tell your doctor right away if you notice redness, swelling, abnormal drainage (thick, foul-smelling, yellow or green), or pain at the tube's entrance site. Also report any abdominal pain, bloating, cramping, or diarrhea.

---

changes in serum glucose, potassium, magnesium, and calcium levels caused by increased cellular metabolism of these nutrients. Assess for both cellular dehydration and signs of heart failure, because the hyperosmolar serum attracts water from cells. See Box 30-4 containing recommendations for Monitoring a Client Receiving Parenteral Nutrition.

The accompanying procedure describes Administering Parenteral Nutrition Through a Central Line. Ongoing site care is especially important because the client is at risk for infection at the site and in the bloodstream (sepsis). Sepsis is a life-threatening complication with a high mortality rate.

Change the client's central catheter dressing at least every 72 hours, more often if facility policy dictates or if the dressing is wet or no longer occlusive. There is controversy over the correct technique for this dressing change, but generally it includes the use of sterile technique (including sterile gloves and masks) in the hospital setting to avoid nosocomial infection.

In the home, the client can use clean technique when changing his own dressing. Most hospitals use transparent polyurethane dressings. The catheter site is scrubbed with an antiseptic, such as povidone-iodine. Some clinicians use an antiseptic ointment at the site as well, but current recommendations from the Centers for Disease Control and Prevention are not to use such an ointment. If used with a transparent dressing, the amount should be small because the dressings are designed to adhere to the skin and promote visualization of the site (Collins et al., 1996).

COMPOSITION OF PARENTERAL NUTRITION
Various combinations of protein, fat emulsions, and carbohydrates are used to meet clients' energy needs. The dextrose concentration of parenteral nutrition given through a central vein can vary from 5 to 70%. Ireton-Jones, Lawson-Braxton, and England (1996) recommend that 5% or 10% dextrose be given to clients via PPN.

BOX 30–4

MONITORING A CLIENT RECEIVING PARENTERAL NUTRITION

To monitor the nutritional status of a client receiving parenteral nutrition, make sure to complete the following steps. You may need to measure some values more frequently than shown here until the client stabilizes.

Growth Variables

- Weigh the client daily.
- Measure an infant's head circumference weekly.
- Measure an infant's length weekly.

Metabolic Variables

- Assess for signs of edema or dehydration daily.
- Obtain fingerstick glucose levels daily.
- Assess intake and output daily.
- Assess calorie, fat, protein, carbohydrate, vitamin, and mineral intake twice weekly.
- Check serum sodium, potassium, chloride, CO_2, phosphorus, blood urea nitrogen, creatinine, and triglycerides twice weekly.
- Assess complete blood count, prothrombin time, albumin, calcium, magnesium, copper, zinc, and liver function tests weekly.
- Obtain a urinalysis weekly.
- Check nitrogen balance weekly (optional).

Protein is given in ranges from 3 to 15%. Fat emulsions of 10% and 20% are given to avoid fatty acid deficiency. An all-in-one mixture includes lipids, protein, and carbohydrate and helps to reduce solution osmolarity. Nutrition given through a central vein often includes the carbohydrate and protein in one bag and the fat emulsion in another. Vitamin and mineral contents are slightly lower than the recommended daily amount because they do not undergo digestive processes. The client's fluid needs are calculated and factored into the solution requirements. The osmolality of PPN should be kept to a minimum (Payne-James & Khawaja, 1993).

COMPLICATIONS OF PARENTERAL NUTRITION

Refeeding syndrome is an important complication of parenteral nutrition. Assess for a drop in serum phosphorus level, which can cause a weakened diaphragm and respiratory failure. Hyperosmolar fluids can cause extracellular fluid overload and pulmonary edema or heart failure. Listen to the client's lungs for crackles and watch her urine output carefully. If her urine output increases significantly, the flow rate may be too fast or erratic. Use an infusion pump to deliver the

TPN, and do not try to "catch up" if the infusion has fallen behind.

Obtain fingerstick glucose levels at least daily because hyperglycemia can result from high glucose loads. Insulin is sometimes added to the solution or given on a sliding scale as needed. TPN should be discontinued slowly because the client could experience rebound hypoglycemia if it is abruptly stopped.

Infection is a major complication of parenteral nutrition. One of the first signs of sepsis is glucose intolerance (Davis & Sherer, 1994). Others include fever or hypothermia, shaking chills, hypotension, and tachycardia. A significant advantage of PPN is that infection, if it occurs, is local rather than systemic. These signs can include pain, redness, edema, and warmth at the site.

Some clients react to lipid emulsions. Adverse reactions include fever, chills, vomiting, and pain in the chest or back. A milder symptom is an itchy skin rash (Davis & Sherer, 1994). Alert the nutrition support team if these reactions occur. Lipid overload is accompanied by increased triglyceride levels, an enlarged liver, and altered liver function test results. Lipid emulsions are usually discontinued if these reactions occur.

HOME PARENTERAL NUTRITION

About 40,000 people are currently receiving home parenteral nutrition (Ireton-Jones, Hennessy, & Howard, 1995). Box 30-5 provides information about Home Care for Clients Receiving Parenteral Nutrition. This therapy is often quite successful with proper professional support.

Interventions to Manage Impaired Swallowing

Positioning the Client

The position that best facilitates swallowing is 90-degree flexion at the hips and 45-degree flexion at the neck. Sit the client as upright as possible and have him remain there for at least 30 minutes after eating.

If he has partial paralysis (as from a stroke), rotate his chin toward the weaker side to improve swallowing. Encourage neck flexion to enhance the pharyngeal phase of swallowing and facilitate closure of the glottis. Place food in the unaffected side of his mouth for optimal control.

You can also enhance the swallowing reflex by using an ice collar or by brushing the client's neck with a small brush, such as a small paint brush, just before he eats. Place food behind the client's front teeth and instruct him to tilt his head back to swallow (Price & Dilorio, 1990).

Encouraging Appropriate Foods

Certain foods are easier to swallow than others (Table 30–4). Thin liquids are the most difficult for clients with dysphagia to handle. Liquids require greater oral coordination and finer motor movements of the swal-

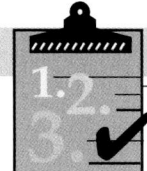

PROCEDURE 30–2

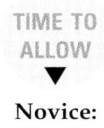

TIME TO
ALLOW
▼
Novice:
20 min.
Expert:
10 min.

Administering Parenteral Nutrition Through a Central Line

Parenteral nutrition is administered to provide fluids and balanced nutrition to a client who cannot eat and who cannot receive such nutrition in her gastrointestinal tract. Total parenteral nutrition is infused into either a central or a peripheral vein according to a physician's order. This procedure describes using a central line.

Delegation Guidelines

The assembly of the necessary equipment to perform this procedure may be delegated to a nursing assistant. The verification of the solution with the physician's order, preparation of the tubing and catheter, and initiation of the infusion are your responsibility and may not be delegated.

Equipment Needed

- Prescribed infusion.
- IV tubing with extension tubing.
- 0.22-µm filter (or 1.2-µm filter if solution contains lipids or albumin).
- Alcohol sponges.
- Infusion pump.
- Sterile dressing package.
- Labels.
- Clean gloves.
- Sterile gloves.

1 Confirm the physician's order and check it against the listed ingredients.

Parenteral nutrition usually requires special physician orders that are written daily, specifying all ingredients and the rate of infusion.

2 Check the solution.
a. Remove the solution from the refrigerator at least 1 hour before using it.
b. Observe the solution for cloudiness, turbidity, particles, or cracks in the container.
c. If the solution has a brown layer, return it to the pharmacy because the lipid emulsion has separated from the solution.

3 Assess the client.
a. Know client's potassium, phosphorus, and glucose values.

Glucose and electrolyte values can change dramatically on parenteral nutrition.

b. Look for any signs of inflammation or swelling at the infusion site.
c. Assess the client's frame of mind and, to ease any fears, reassure her that the procedure is not painful.

Clients associate eating with positive feelings and may be upset by not being able to eat.

4 Prepare the tubing in the infusion pump.
a. Connect tubing, extension tubing, and filter.

Place the filter close to the client.

b. If the tubing does not have Luer-Lok connections, tape all connections.

Accidental separation of IV tubing could cause air embolism or infection.

c. Prime the tubing and clamp it.
d. Thread the tubing through infusion pump.
e. Time and date the IV tubing.

The tubing should be changed every 24 to 72 hours, according to your facility's policy.

5 Prepare the central line catheter.
a. Flush the catheter, according to your facility's policy, with saline.
b. Put on sterile gloves.

Asepsis at the site prevents infection.

c. Clean the catheter cap with alcohol.
d. Using aseptic technique, insert the needle into the injection cap.
e. Unclamp the tubing.

Continued

PROCEDURE 30-2 *(continued)*

Administering Parenteral Nutrition Through a Central Line

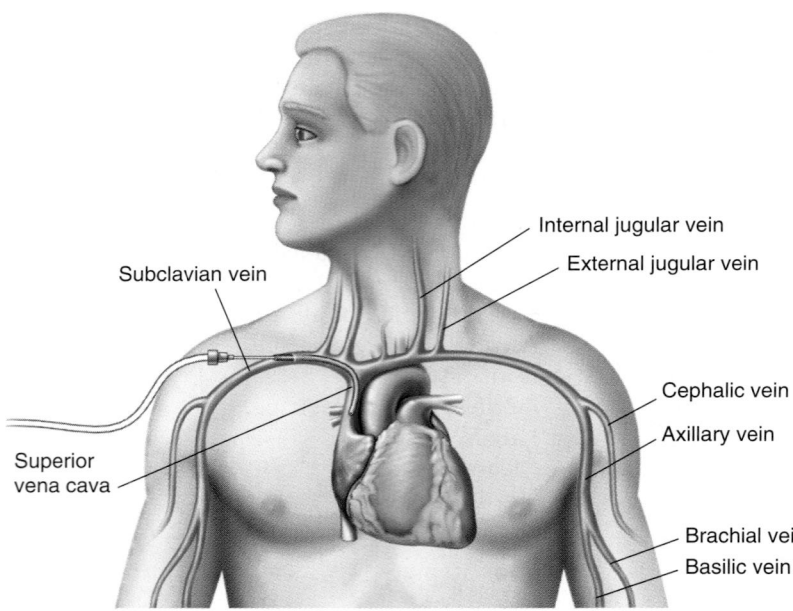

Infusion site for parenteral nutrition through a central line.

6 Set the infusion pump at the prescribed rate. Start the flow slowly and monitor the rate carefully.

7 Do not use a single-lumen central line to infuse blood or draw blood. Also, if possible, avoid giving any IV medication during parenteral nutrition. Before adding a piggy-back medication to parenteral nutrition, check with the pharmacist to make sure it is compatible. Never add a medication to parenteral nutrition solution.

8 Monitor and document the client's vital signs, laboratory values (including electrolytes), vital signs, glucose levels, daily weight, urine output, and catheter site. Use sterile technique for dressing changes.

Continued assessment is essential because extravasation of the solution can cause tissue necrosis.

9 Document the type of solution used, the time and date the bag was hung, the client's response, and the amount of solution added on the intake and output sheet.

HINT

If for any reason you must remove the gummed rubber cap from the central line, *be absolutely sure* the catheter is clamped or the client is performing the Valsava maneuver. Otherwise, the negative intrathoracic pressure can draw air into the vein.

lowing muscles. Dysphagic clients should never "wash food down" with liquids. Fluids for clients with dysphagia must be met with fluids that are thickened with potato flakes, corn starch, fruit, or commercial products.

Flavorful foods that are either warm or cold stimulate the swallowing reflex better than bland, lukewarm foods. The flavoring also stimulates the flow of saliva. Sauces and gravies are good choices because they are flavorful and lubricate food. Fragmented foods, such as corn kernels, peas, rice, and ground meat, are easily aspirated and should be moistened. Moist pastas, casseroles, and egg dishes are good choices for dysphagic clients.

HOME CARE FOR CLIENTS RECEIVING PARENTERAL NUTRITION

Assess

- Confirm the physician's order. (Will the parenteral nutrition be given only at night or also during the day? For what length of time will the client need it?)
- Does the client have a support system, such as family?
- What motivation level do the client and family have?
- Can client and family understand the complexities of parenteral nutrition?
- Do the client and family have adequate financial resources to maintain safe, accurate therapy? (Consult a social worker about solving financial problems.)
- Is the client mobile? (If so, consider suggesting that the client wear a lightweight vest with large pockets to hold parenteral nutrition supplies if feedings will occur during the day.)
- What safety problems are present in the client's home?
- Does the client have access to nursing services or a hospital?

Teach

- Find a quiet space where the client and family can concentrate.
- Include family in all teaching sessions.
- Because the material is complex and important, begin with simple content and use drawings or models as needed. For example, use a teddy bear with a central line site to show procedures.

- Make sure to fully teach the following concepts:
  Strict hand-washing techniques.
  How to hang solution.
  Setting the feeding rate (operating an infusion pump).
  Cleaning the site and changing the dressing.
  Flushing the catheter.
  Taking fingerstick glucose readings, if needed.
  Which problems to report, such as redness, swelling, drainage, or pain at the site; fever; inability to flush catheter; shortness of breath; increased urinary output; hyperglycemia; chest pain.
- When teaching procedures, avoid placing time limits on the client or family members because manual dexterity can vary from client to client.
- Provide written handouts with specific directions, important adverse responses, and actions to take.
- Provide client with list of phone numbers for reporting problems.

Evaluate

- Ask the client (and family) to give you a return demonstration of cleaning the site, changing the dressing, and hanging the solution.
- Have the client or a family member keep a record of amount of parenteral nutrition taken in a 24-hour period and any abnormal responses or symptoms that develop.

TABLE 30–4

Comparing Easy-to-Swallow and Hard-to-Swallow Foods

Easy to Swallow	Hard to Swallow
Warm or cold foods	Lukewarm foods
Flavorful foods (salted or mildly sweetened)	Bland foods
Thickened liquids	Thin liquids and milk
Sauces and gravies	Foods that fall apart (such as peas or rice)
	Pureed foods, which do not stimulate swallowing
Moist pastas, casseroles, egg dishes	Slippery foods, sticky or bulky foods
Blenderized soups	Foods with combination of textures, such as chunky soups

Milk seems to stimulate thick mucus production and should be used cautiously with clients who have excessive phlegm or drooling. The client can drink milk if it is followed by thickened liquids to flush the throat (Mahan & Escott-Stump, 2000).

Pureed foods are not tolerated as well as textured foods because they fail to stimulate swallowing. Sticky foods (such as peanut butter) or bulky foods (such as raw fruits and vegetables) are also more difficult to swallow and should be avoided. Foods with a combination of textures should also be avoided because they are difficult to control. These include chunky soups, although blenderized soups are good.

Interventions to Reduce the Risk for Aspiration

Many interventions for *Risk for aspiration* have already been discussed, since two major risks for aspiration are impaired swallowing and enteral feedings. Carefully monitor clients because silent aspiration can pro-

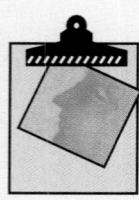

NURSING CARE PLANNING
A CLIENT WITH INADEQUATE NUTRITIONAL INTAKE DURING CHEMOTHERAPY

Outpatient Clinic Data

Mrs. Goldman is halfway through her 6 months of chemotherapy. She uses prochlorperazine (Compazine) for nausea for 3 days after her treatments, has experienced a 25-pound weight loss, and has signs of depression.

Physician's Orders

Assist with diet planning to maintain ideal body weight.

Nursing Assessment

Client is 54 years old, is 5'4" tall, and weighs 115 pounds. Adheres to a kosher diet. Reports weighing 140 pounds before chemotherapy; weight/IBW = 95%; energy needs from Harris-Benedict equation plus 10% for activity = 2000 calories; serum albumin 3.0 g/dl; hemoglobin 11.5 g/dl & hematocrit 32%; client describes feeling fatigued and has decreased interest in eating. Client is concerned about recent weight loss.

NURSING CARE PLAN

Nursing Diagnosis	Expected Outcomes	Interventions	Evaluation (After 1 Month of Care)
Altered nutrition: Less than body requirements	Weight gain of at least 2 pounds in 1 month.	Offer choices of good-tasting protein supplements to be taken between meals.	Weight has increased by 1 pound. Reports that supplement is nauseating.
	Eats at least 2,000 calories.	Have client keep a calorie diary; consider suggesting zinc for increasing taste.	Client reports that she has been eating better and has kept a record of her food intake. Eating 1,500 calories.
	Decreased fatigue in 1 month.	Establish a contract with client to engage in one pleasurable activity a day. Limit rest periods to one or two per day.	Has increased number of pleasurable activities. Takes an afternoon nap. Otherwise engages in light activities. Reports that fatigue has improved.
	Increase in hemoglobin and hematocrit by 1 month.	Include a source of iron in diet. *Select culturally agreeable foods.*	Hemoglobin and hematocrit show moderate increase after 1 month.
	Increase in albumin by 3 weeks.	*Select high-protein foods that are culturally agreeable.*	Albumin has begun to slowly increase by 3 weeks.

Italicized interventions indicate culturally specific care.

Critical Thinking Questions

1. How frequently does Mrs. Goldman need follow-up once her nutritional status stabilizes?
2. Who is the most desirable member of the health care team to provide this follow-up?
3. What further dietary teaching might be needed if current interventions are not successful?

duce only subtle cues (see the defining characteristics for aspiration). To check the swallowing reflex, put 3 mL of water on the client's tongue. The swallow reflex should be initiated within 1 second. If it is delayed or absent after three attempts, have the client evaluated (Thelan, Urden, Lough, & Stacy, 1998). Also assess the client's bowel sounds and check for abdominal distention that could indicate increased gastric residual volume. Keep the client's head positioned at a 30-degree angle. If the client's head cannot be elevated, place the client in a right lateral position to facilitate gastric emptying.

Also, suction oral secretions to keep the oropharynx patent. Treat nausea to prevent vomiting. The physician may order gastric secretion inhibitors to decrease gastric acidity and limit chemical burns to the lungs (Thelan, Urden, Lough, & Stacy, 1998).

EVALUATION

During evaluation, determine if the plan and interventions were successful in achieving the established goals, as outlined in the Nursing Care Planning chart. If the outcome criteria are specific and measurable, simply indicate whether the criteria were met. At times, they may not be met because of unrealistic time frames or intervening variables. If so, revise the plan with new outcome criteria and interventions, and re-evaluate the client.

With Mrs. Goldman, the outcome criteria were a weight of 117 pounds by 1 month and a serum albumin of 3.0 g/dL by 1 month. One month later, Mrs. Goldman weighs 116 pounds, and her serum albumin is 2.8 g/dL. The criteria were not quite met, although the change is in the right direction. How would you write an evaluation statement for Mrs. Goldman? How might you revise the interventions? What intervening variables might have interfered with Mrs. Goldman's reaching her goal?

Remember, evaluation is an assessment of whether the outcome criteria were or were not met. It is not a statement of what you expected to happen, but rather what actually happened.

KEY PRINCIPLES

- Nutrition inadequate to meet the body's needs results from energy needs that exceed the amount taken in and may have many physical and psychological causes.
- Impaired swallowing typically results from neuromuscular problems or a decreased level of consciousness.
- The risk for aspiration is high in clients who receive tube feedings, are intubated, or have decreased consciousness or impaired swallowing.
- There is no single marker for nutritional problems. To detect it, you must review the collected assessment data. Unintentional loss of 10% of body weight within a 6-month period is a red flag for *Altered nutrition: less than body requirements*.
- Impaired swallowing can be definitively diagnosed with evidence of aspiration.
- Refeeding of malnourished clients must be done carefully to prevent serious metabolic complications.
- Enteral feeding is a major risk factor for aspiration.
- When making a differential diagnosis for nutritional problems, choose the diagnosis that will best focus care on the client's most immediate needs.
- Interventions for nutritional problems require a team approach, whether carried out in the client's home or in the clinic, hospital, or other health care setting.
- Parenteral and enteral nutritional support include specialized nursing procedures important for clients with *Altered nutrition: less than body requirements*.
- Interventions for *Impaired swallowing* focus on providing foods and techniques that will encourage the swallow reflex and preventing aspiration.
- When evaluating outcome criteria for *Altered nutrition: less than body requirements*, expect a weight gain of at least 2 pounds a month; a weight gain of 1 pound per day or more indicates a fluid gain.

BIBLIOGRAPHY

Bak, L., Heard, K.A., & Kearney, G.P. (1996). Tube feeding your diabetic patient safely. *American Journal of Nursing, 96*(12), 47.

Billon, W. (1995). *Clinical nutrition case studies* (2nd ed.). Minneapolis: West.

Brennan, K. (1998). Going with the flow. *Nursing 98,* April, 54–55.

Carr, P., Freund, K., & Somani, S. (Eds.). (1995). *The medical care of women.* Philadelphia: W.B. Saunders.

Clevenger, F., & Rodriguez, D. (1995). Decision-making for enteral feeding administration: The why behind where and how. *Nutrition in Clinical Practice, 10*(3), 104–113.

Collins, E., Lawson, L., Lau, M., Barder, L., et al. (1996). Care of central venous catheters for total parenteral nutrition. *Nutrition in Clinical Practice, 11*(3), 109–115.

*Davis, J., & Sherer, K. (1994). *Applied nutrition and diet therapy for nurses* (2nd Ed.). Philadelphia: W.B. Saunders.

DeLegge, M. (1996). Continuous vs intermittent feedings: Slow and steady or fast and furious? *Current issues in enteral nutrition support: Report of the first Ross conference on enteral devices* (pp 50–53). Columbus, OH: Ross Products Division, Abbott Laboratories.

Duh, Q. (1996). Decision tree for route of enteral nutrition support: Placement techniques. *Current issues in enteral nutrition support: Report of the first Ross conference on enteral devices* (pp 9–16). Columbus, OH: Ross Products Division, Abbott Laboratories.

Ellett, M.L., Maahs, J., & Farsee, S. (1998). Prevalence of feeding tube placement errors and associated risk factors in children. *The American Journal of Maternal/Child Nursing, 23*(5), 234.

Ellpern, E. (1997). Pulmonary aspiration in adults. *Nutrition in Clinical Practice, 12*(1), 5–13.

Ireton-Jones, C., & Francis, C. (1995). Obesity: Nutrition support practice and application to critical care. *Nutrition in Clinical Practice, 10*(4), 144–149.

*Asterisk indicates a classic or definitive work on this subject.

Ireton-Jones, C., Hennessy, K., & Howard, K. (1995). Multidisciplinary clinical care of the home parenteral nutrition patient. *Infusion, 1*(8), 21–30.

Ireton-Jones, C., Hennessy, K., & Orr, M. (1996). Care of patients receiving home enteral nutrition. *Infusion, 2*(6), 30–43.

Ireton-Jones, C., Lawson-Braxton, D., & England, L. (1996). Peripheral parenteral nutrition: The other alternative for nutrition support. *Infusion, 2*(1), 44–48.

*Kohn, C. (1991). The relationship between enteral formula contamination and length of enteral delivery set usage. *Journal of Parenteral and Enteral Nutrition, 15*(5), 567–571.

Mackin, D. (1997). How to Manage PICCs. *American Journal of Nursing, 97*(9), 27.

Mahan, K., & Escott-Stump, S. (2000). *Krause's food, nutrition, & diet therapy* (10th ed.). Philadelphia: W.B. Saunders.

*Marian, M. (1993). Pediatric nutrition support. *Nutrition in Clinical Practice, 8*(5), 199–209.

*Metheny, N. (1993). Minimizing respiratory complications of nasoenteric tube feedings: State of the science. *Heart and Lung, 22,* 213–223.

Metheny, N. (1996). Verification of feeding tube placement. *Current issues in enteral nutrition support: Report of the first Ross conference on enteral devices* (pp 34–41). Columbus, OH: Ross Products Division, Abbott Laboratories.

*Metheny, N., Reed, L., Wiersema, L., McSweeney, M., Wehrle, M.A., and Clark, J. (1993). Effectiveness of pH measurements in predicting tube placement: An update. *Nursing Research, 42,* 324–331.

Metheny, N., Wehrle, M.A., Wiersema, L., & Clark, J. (1998). Testing tube placement: Auscultation vs. pH method, *American Journal of Nursing, 98*(5), 37.

Ottery, F. (1996). Nutritional screening & assessment in home care. *Infusion, 2*(12), 36–45.

Payne-James, J.J., and Khawajor, H.T. (1993). First choice for total parenteral nutrition: The peripheral route. *Journal of Parenteral Enteral Nursing, 17*(5), 468–478.

*Price, M., & Dilorio, C. (1990). Swallowing: A practice guide. *American Journal of Nursing, 907*(7), 42.

Schwartz, D., & Dominguez-Gasson, L. (1997). Aspiration in a patient receiving enteral nutrition. *Nutrition in Clinical Practice, 12*(1), 14–19.

*Shils, M., Olson, J., & Shike, M. (Eds.). (1994). *Modern nutrition in health and disease* (8th ed., Vols. 1–2). Philadelphia: Lea & Febiger.

*Spector, N. (1993). *Use of indirect calorimetry to predict sepsis in a critically ill sepsis sample.* Unpublished doctoral dissertation, Rush University, Chicago.

Springhouse Corporation. (1996). *Nursing procedures* (2nd ed.). Springhouse, PA: Author.

Standards for nutrition support: Hospitalized patients. (1995). *Nutrition in Clinical Practice, 10*(6), 208–218.

Standards for nutrition support nurses. (1996). *Nutrition in Clinical Practice, 11*(3), 127–134.

Stein, J.H. (Ed.). (1994). *Internal medicine* (4th. ed.). St. Louis: Mosby.

Thelan, L., Urden, L., Lough, M., & Stacy, K. (1998). *Textbook of critical care nursing: Diagnosis and management* (3rd ed.). St. Louis: Mosby.

Wesley, J. (1995). Nutrition support teams: Past, present, and futures. *Nutrition in Clinical Practice, 10*(6), 219–228.

Welch, S. (1996). Certification of staff nurses to insert enteral feeding tubes using a research-based procedure. *Nutrition in Clinical Practice, 11*(1), 21–27.

*Whitney, E., Cataldo, C., & Rolfes, S. (1994). *Understanding normal and clinical nutrition* (4th ed.). Minneapolis: West.

Woolf, S., Jonas, S., & Lawrence, R. (Eds.). (1996). *Health promotion and disease prevention in clinical practice.* Baltimore: Williams & Wilkins.

*Zaloga, G.P. (1994). *Nutrition in critical care.* St. Louis: Mosby.

31

Fluid and Electrolyte Balance

Bernie White

Key Terms

active transport
anion
cation
colloid
colloid osmotic pressure
diffusion
electrolyte
filtration
hydrostatic pressure
hypertonic
hypotonic

isotonic
metabolic acidosis
metabolic alkalosis
milliequivalent
milliosmole
nonelectrolyte
osmolality
osmolarity
osmosis
third spacing

LEARNING OBJECTIVES

After studying this chapter, you should be able to:

1. Describe the normal physiology of fluid balance, including fluid compartments, functions of body fluids, and types of electrolytes.

2. Identify 10 mechanisms that contribute to the regulation of fluid and electrolyte balance.

3. Discuss five common problems related to fluid balance.

4. Discuss the factors affecting fluid balance, including physiological problems and medical and nursing therapies.

5. Describe the general assessment of a client's fluid balance.

6. Describe the focused assessment of clients at risk for fluid problems, the manifestations of actual fluid problems, and client responses to fluid problems.

7. Diagnose the problems of clients with fluid imbalances that are within the domain of nursing.

8. Plan and carry out goal-directed interventions to prevent or correct fluid and electrolyte imbalances.

9. Evaluate outcomes in terms of progress or lack of progress toward the goals of fluid balance with revision of the care plan as appropriate.

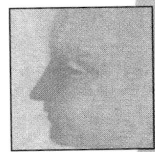

Elli Thompson, an 81-year-old African-American female, has lived independently in her own home since her husband died 4 years ago. She has one daughter who lives 500 miles away and two sons, one within 10 miles and one within 100 miles. She has adequate financial support for a modest lifestyle. She has Medicare, but she cannot afford supplemental insurance. She has been very involved in her church and community but lately has developed arthritic joint changes and visual changes that interfere with this activity as well as with her ability to drive, cook, and maintain her usual standard of hygiene.

Her physician prescribed an antiarthritic, an analgesic, and an ophthalmic medication. Mrs. Thompson has found these medications helpful, but she still has problems meeting her everyday needs. She still tries to make three meals for herself, even though cooking has become difficult. The inconvenience has led her to choose foods other than the ethnic foods she so dearly loves. In addition, she becomes

(continued)

so full with smaller amounts of food that she has stopped drinking in order to make room for the food. Her fatigue has also resulted in fewer trips to the kitchen for more fluids.

Mrs. Thompson's son Gerald stopped by for a visit and noticed that his mother looked thin and listless. He consulted with the rest of the family and decided that Mrs. Thompson should schedule an office visit. Mrs. Thompson's physician, Dr. Kline, found her to be severely dehydrated. He believed that her lack of energy and change in self-care and social activity were related to the dehydration. Mrs. Thompson also said that her medication "makes me tired."

Dr. Kline recommended a change in her prescription and a home visit from a nurse from the Visiting Nurses' Association. Mrs. Thompson and her family were very agreeable to this approach. The visiting nurse's evaluation supported the diagnosis of *Fluid volume deficit*. The challenge was to help Mrs. Thompson overcome this current problem as well as help her prevent it in the near future.

Mrs. Thompson progressed well. She met most of the goals that she and her nurse, Judy Carson, had agreed on within the allotted number of visits prescribed by Dr. Kline. Therefore, Judy told Mrs. Thompson, neither she nor the home health aide would be seeing her any longer. To increase Mrs. Thompson's ability to detect problems in the early stages, Judy reviewed with her a written list of signs and symptoms that should be reported to Dr. Kline.

Mrs. Thompson was on her own again, with support from her family and friends. But she was so concerned about not getting in "this shape" again that she forced herself to drink fluids almost continuously. A week later, Gerald stopped by to check on his mother. This time, she looked puffy and was having trouble breathing. Gerald become alarmed and immediately called Dr. Kline, who admitted Mrs. Thompson to the hospital with a diagnosis of acute congestive heart failure.

Although Mrs. Thompson's treatment for fluid volume deficit was very appropriate, as with many elderly people, she had a compromised myocardium that could not adapt to the increased fluid intake and the stress of the illness. Mrs. Thompson's myocardium began to show signs of pump failure. She presented with manifestations of both right and left ventricular failure. This syndrome is an example of *Fluid volume excess*.

FLUID IMBALANCE NURSING DIAGNOSES

Risk for Fluid Volume Deficit: The state in which an individual is at risk for experiencing vascular, cellular, or intracellular dehydration.

Fluid Volume Deficit: The state in which an individual experiences decreased intravascular, interstitial, and/or intracellular fluid. This refers to dehydration, water loss alone without change in sodium.

Fluid Volume Excess: The state in which an individual experiences increased isotonic fluid retention.

From North American Nursing Diagnosis Association (1999). NANDA nursing diagnoses: Definition and classification 1999–2000. Philadelphia: Author.

Although elderly people like Mrs. Thompson represent the fastest growing segment of the American population—and the segment most often endangered by fluid imbalance—they are not the only group prone to fluid imbalances. Consider the otherwise healthy child who becomes dehydrated from vomiting or diarrhea. Or consider the pregnant woman who suddenly develops abnormal swelling in her legs, feet, and elsewhere, or the middle-aged man who chronically consumes too much alcohol; he develops skin changes, bloating of the face, and an increasingly large abdomen. These are only a few examples of situations that lead to fluid imbalance.

It is critical that you have the knowledge and skills you need to care for any client who develops a fluid imbalance. Understanding the concepts of fluid balance will help you in planning and administering care appropriately.

CONCEPTS OF FLUID BALANCE

Water is not found in its pure state in the body but instead is the medium in which all chemical products of nutrition, metabolism, and excretion are found. The term *fluid* is used to mean water and the components it contains. Chemical compounds are the principal components of most body fluids. An **electrolyte** is any compound that, when dissolved in water, separates into electrically charged particles, which are called *ions.* Positively charged ions are called **cations;** negatively charged ions are called **anions.**

The most common compound that becomes an electrolyte in solution is table salt, or sodium chloride (NaCl). Important cations in body metabolism are sodium (Na^+), potassium (K^+), calcium (Ca^+), magnesium (Mg^{2+}), and hydrogen (H^+). Important anions are chloride (Cl^-), bicarbonate (HCO_3^-), sulfate (SO_4^{2-}), and proteinate. **Nonelectrolytes** are substances that do not ionize, and thus do not carry an electrical charge. Glucose is an example of a nonelectrolyte compound in body fluids.

Fluid balance is dependent on the chemical and physical properties of electrolytes and plasma proteins. Therefore, from a practice perspective, one cannot address fluid deficit or fluid overload in isolation from electrolytes and proteins because they are so inter-related. In other words, when a client has problems of fluid balance, you will also have to assess the client's electrolyte and protein status. Therefore, this chapter will also present an overview of major electrolytes as they relate to the person's risk or actual state of illness.

There are many fundamental physiological concepts that you must understand to anticipate a fluid imbalance or understand the nature of fluid deficit or fluid excess. These include the storage of fluids in different compartments, the shifting of fluid between compartments, the functions of body fluids, the role of electrolytes, the regulation of fluids, and common problems of fluid distribution.

Fluid Compartments

Fluids exist in several compartments in the body. Although fluid is in a continual state of exchange between each compartment, the amount of fluid and the relative components in each compartment remain relatively constant.

Body fluid is in a state of balance when the following occurs:

- Its water and electrolyte components are present in the proper proportions.
- Fluids are distributed normally between compartments.
- Lost body water and electrolytes are replaced.
- Excess water and electrolytes are eliminated.

For the body's cells to function normally, the composition of body fluids must remain constant and the distribution among compartments must remain nor-

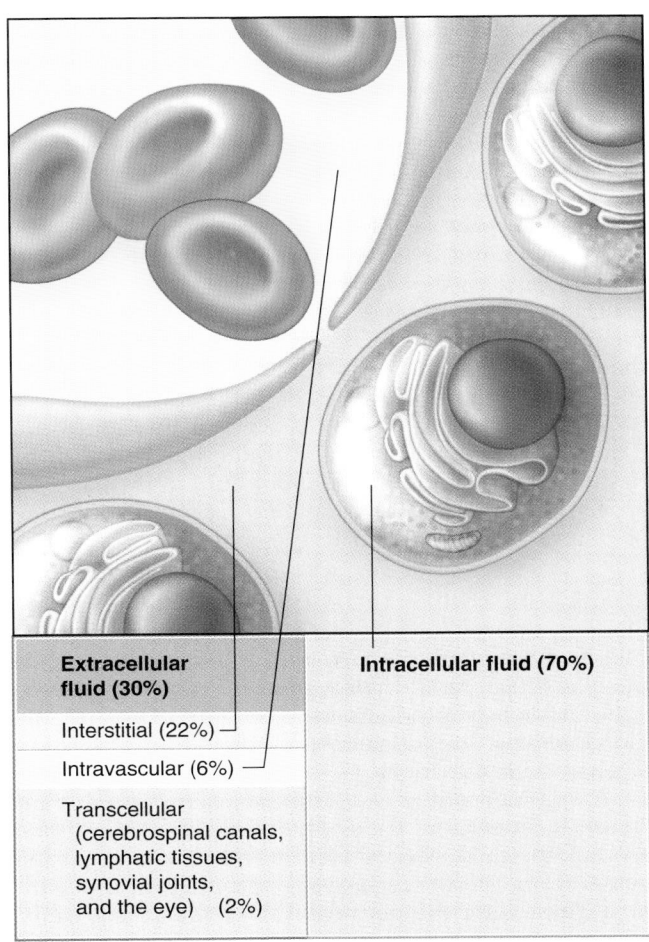

Figure 31–1. Fluid compartments. In the average adult, 50 to 60% of the body weight is from fluid, 70% of which is intracellular and 30% extracellular. The extracellular compartments are further divided into approximately 6% intravascular, 22% interstitial, and 2% transcellular.

mal. Homeostasis depends on the relationship of the components within the intracellular and extracellular fluid compartments (Fig. 31–1).

Intracellular Fluid Compartment

Intracellular fluids provide cells with the internal aqueous medium necessary for their chemical functions. About 70% of the body's fluid exists in the intracellular spaces. Therefore, anything that affects fluid loss at the cellular level has significant implications for the entire body.

Extracellular Fluid Compartment

Extracellular fluids are found outside the body cells and serve as the body's transportation system. They carry water, electrolytes, nutrients, and oxygen to the cells and remove the waste products of cellular metabolism. About 30% of the body's fluid exists in the extracellular compartment, which includes intravascular, interstitial, and transcellular divisions.

In figure:

Extracellular fluid (30%)

Interstitial (22%) —
Intravascular (6%) —
Transcellular
(cerebrospinal canals,
lymphatic tissues,
synovial joints,
and the eye)   (2%)

Intracellular fluid (70%)

INTRAVASCULAR FLUIDS

The term *intravascular* refers to the space within the arteries, veins, and capillaries. As you recall, the major function of these vessels is to carry blood. Blood consists of the fluid known as *plasma* and the cells carried in that plasma. Plasma contains **colloids** (macromolecules that are too large to pass though a cell membrane and do not readily dissolve into a solution, such as proteins) and byproducts of cellular function and metabolism.

Having too little blood (fluid) in this space affects the nutrient and oxygen supply to all tissues. Tissues that have a high demand for oxygen and nutrients, such as the brain, heart, and kidneys, are compromised first. Having too much fluid in this space can damage the intimal lining of the blood vessels and the tissues. Changes in the volume of fluid in the vascular space trigger a series of compensatory neuroendocrine responses discussed later in the chapter.

INTERSTITIAL FLUIDS

Fluid is everywhere in the body, even between the cells and vascular compartments, in spaces known as the *interstitial spaces.* Interstitial fluid transports nutrients and waste products between the cells and the blood vessels. Too much or too little fluid in this space affects bodily functions.

A sprained ankle is a familiar example of an increase in interstitial fluid. The swelling of the tissue around the ankle bones results from damage to the vessel walls and the release of byproducts of tissue injury. These alter the permeability of the vessel walls, allowing excess fluid to seep into the interstitial spaces. Excess fluid in the interstitial spaces is called *edema.*

TRANSCELLULAR FLUIDS

Transcellular fluids are found in spaces in the cerebrospinal canals in the brain and in the lymph tissues, synovial joints, and eyes. Although these fluids contribute only about 2% of the total fluid volume in the body, even small changes in fluid volume in these compartments can have a major impact on the health of these organs.

If Mrs. Thompson, from our case study, was eating three meals a day, why didn't the food sustain her? Is drinking water and other fluids really that important?

Functions of Body Fluids

The body needs at least 1,500 mL of water every day in addition to water that comes from the foods we eat (about 700 mL) and the oxidation of food (about 300 mL). Why does the body need so much fluid?

The answer is partly because fluid makes up about 50 to 60% of the normal adult's weight. As we have seen, it functions to transport nutrients and wastes to and from cells and acts as a solvent for electrolytes and nonelectrolytes. Fluids also play a role in maintaining body temperature, facilitating digestion and elimination, and lubricating joints and other body tissues.

Electrolytes

As noted earlier, electrolytes are ionized substances that perform their functions within a fluid environment. The electrolytes that are most plentiful inside the cells are potassium, magnesium, phosphate, and protein. Sodium, calcium, chloride, hydrogen, and bicarbonate are the most plentiful electrolytes in the extracellular fluid. Electrolytes exert a major influence on the movement of water between compartments, enzyme reactions, neuromuscular activity, and acid-base regulation. The specific functions of protein, hydrogen, and bicarbonate and other electrolytes affecting acid-base balance will be discussed later.

It is through complex regulatory systems that the body maintains electrical neutrality. This means that the number of negative ions (anions) is equal to the number of positive ions (cations) in the body. Table 31–1 provides a more thorough listing of functions and regulators of the sodium, potassium, calcium, magnesium, chloride, and phosphate ions.

An example of fluid and electrolyte relationships occurs daily when a person eats. Besides the water, proteins, fats, and carbohydrates that are being ingested, minerals are being consumed as well, including sodium, potassium, calcium, magnesium, chloride, phosphate, and others. When these minerals are consumed, they ionize and become electrolytes. For example, table salt (NaCl) separates into Na^+ and Cl^- when it dissolves in the body fluid.

Extracellular and intracellular fluids contain the same electrolytes but in different amounts. For example, about 98% of the body's potassium is found in the intracellular compartment, compared with 2% in the extracellular compartment. In contrast, 99% of the sodium is found in the extracellular compartment with the remaining 1% in the intracellular compartment.

Sodium

The osmotic role of sodium is essential to maintaining the proper amount of water in and between compartments. Vascular volume, which affects blood pressure, is a direct response to the level of sodium. Sodium is also critical to nerve impulse conduction because of its effect on the electrical potential of cells. The sodium-potassium pump is an active transport mechanism that promotes the opening of sodium and potassium channels during different phases of the impulse propagation. In **active transport,** molecules move from an area of lower concentration to an area of higher concentration through an expenditure of energy. These changes in sodium and potassium are critical to nerve conduction. Without them, the cells would die.

TABLE 31–1
Electrolyte Functions and Regulators

Electrolyte	Normal Plasma Levels (mEq/L)	Functions	Regulation
Sodium (Na^+)	135–145	• Maintains blood volume. • Controls water shifting between compartments. • Major cation involved in sodium-potassium pump necessary for nerve impulses. • Interacts with calcium to maintain muscle contraction. • Major cation in bicarbonate and phosphate acid-base buffer system.	Renin-angiotensin-aldosterone system
Potassium (K^+)	3.5–5.0	• Affects osmolality. • Major cation involved in sodium-potassium pump necessary for transmission of nerve impulses. • Promotes nerve impulses, especially in heart and skeletal muscles. • Assists in conversion of carbohydrates to energy and amino acids into proteins. • Promotes glycogen storage in liver. • Assists maintenance of acid-base balance through cellular exchange with hydrogen.	Renin-angiotensin-aldosterone system
Calcium (Ca^{2+})	4.5–5.5	• Nonionized form promotes strong bones and teeth. • Promotes blood coagulation. • Promotes nerve impulse conduction, decreases neuromuscular irritability. • Strengthens and thickens cell membrane. • Assists in absorption and utilization of vitamin B_{12}. • Activates enzymes for many chemical reactions. • Inhibits cell membrane permeability to sodium. • Activates actin-myosin muscle contraction.	Parathormone • Increases calcium resorption from bone. • Increases calcium reabsorption by inhibiting phosphate reabsorption from kidney tubules. • Increases calcium absorption from gastrointestinal tract.
Magnesium (Mg^{2+})	1.5–2.5	• Promotes metabolism of carbohydrates, fats, and proteins. • Activates many enzymes (B_{12} metabolism). • Promotes regulation of Ca, PO_4, K. • Promotes transmission of nerve impulses, muscle contraction, and heart function. • Powers sodium-potassium pump. • Promotes conversion of adenosine triphosphate (ATP) to adenosine diphosphate (ADP) for energy release. • Inhibits smooth muscle contraction.	Parathormone • Increases or decreases magnesium reabsorption in kidney tubules relative to body need.
Chloride (Cl^-)	98–106	• Regulates extracellular fluid volume. • Promotes acid-base balance through exchange with bicarbonate in red blood cells (chloride shift). • Promotes protein digestion through hydrochloric (HCl) acid; acid pH required for activation of protease.	
Phosphate (HPO_4^-)	1.2–3.0	• Nonionized form promotes bone and teeth rigidity. • Promotes acid-base balance through phosphate buffer system. • Necessary for ATP production.	Parathormone • Increases phosphate resorption from bone. • Inhibits phosphate reabsorption in kidney tubules. • Increases phosphate absorption in gastrointestinal tract as needed.

Potassium

Potassium plays a key role in maintaining the sodium-potassium pump and thus transmission of nerve impulses. Potassium balance is critical to the normal function of all cells, but especially those of the cardiac and skeletal muscles.

Calcium

Calcium plays a primary role in the formation of healthy bones and teeth. It promotes normal blood coagulation and is critical to nerve conduction. The slow calcium channels open after the more rapid sodium and potassium channels to maintain the electrical potential necessary for the propagation of the nerve impulse across the cell membrane.

Magnesium

Although magnesium is of low concentration, it also is critical to the function of many body systems through its effect on over 300 enzyme systems. It promotes the release of a phosphate bond (conversion of adenosine triphosphate [ATP] to adenosine diphosphate [ADP]), which provides the energy source for the sodium-potassium pump. Therefore, any change in any of these four ions can make the cell more or less responsive to stimuli. The degree and acuteness of the imbalances, as well as the client's adaptive mechanisms, determine the client's responses.

Chloride

Since chloride is the major anion associated with sodium, its role in osmolality and nerve conduction is also critical. Chloride also plays a key role in the process of digestion because it is the anion link in the formation of hydrochloric acid.

Phosphate

Phosphate works with calcium to promote the integrity of bone and teeth. It is an integral part of ATP and ADP, which maintain our energy sources for all cell functions.

Movement of Fluids and Electrolytes

To maintain homeostasis, fluid shifts constantly between compartments, exchanging nutrients and waste products. For example, nutrients from ingested food are transported from the bloodstream to the cells so that the byproducts of food can be used to build new cells. The waste products from the digestion of these nutrients are then transported from the cells to the bloodstream for removal from the body. Water is the medium that allows the transport of essential particles to the cells and waste products from the cells.

The factors that regulate the shifting of water between compartments are discussed below. Under-standing the normal mechanisms of fluid transport will enhance your ability to identify potential or actual fluid and electrolyte problems. Remember that fluid movement depends on the *relationship* between each of these factors, not on one factor alone.

Osmosis

The cell wall is a semipermeable membrane that selectively allows water and smaller particles to pass through it. Larger particles, such as proteins and glucose, are transported by more complex processes. The movement of fluid between compartments is influenced by a transport mechanism called osmosis as well as the pressure forces that were discussed earlier. **Osmosis** is the movement of water through a semipermeable membrane from an area containing a lesser concentration of particles to area of greater concentration of particles.

Osmolality and osmolarity are expressions of the osmotic force of a solution. Osmotic force can be illustrated by considering ordinary table salt, sodium chloride (NaCl), as a gargle for a sore throat. The salt particles in the water create an osmotic force that draws fluid from the tissues and reduces swelling (Fig. 31–2). The force from the dissolved particles (such as salt) in a solvent (such as water) can be represented as **milliosmoles**, the number of dissolved particles needed to produce one unit of force. **Osmolality** refers to the number of milliosmoles per kilogram of water. The term **osmolarity** is similar but refers to the measurement of milliosmoles per liter of solution. The term *osmolality* is used to describe body fluids, whereas the term *osmolarity* is used more often in reference to solutions measured by volume, such as an intravenous (IV) fluid.

To illustrate osmolality even further, consider a client receiving a hypotonic IV solution and another receiving an isotonic solution, both given at a fairly rapid rate. An **isotonic** solution has an osmotic pressure equal to that of plasma. A **hypotonic** solution has an osmotic pressure less than that of plasma. A **hypertonic** solution has an osmotic pressure greater than that of plasma. Whenever there is a difference in osmolality between the cell and the plasma, fluid shifting is likely to occur.

Diffusion

Diffusion refers to the passive process by which molecules move through a cell membrane from an area of higher concentration to an area of lower concentration without an expenditure of energy. For example, gases such as carbon dioxide and oxygen diffuse across the respiratory membrane into the pulmonary capillaries from the area of higher to lower concentration. Electrolytes move passively from an area of higher concentration to an area of lower concentration, such as from the small bowel at the end of digestion into the blood stream.

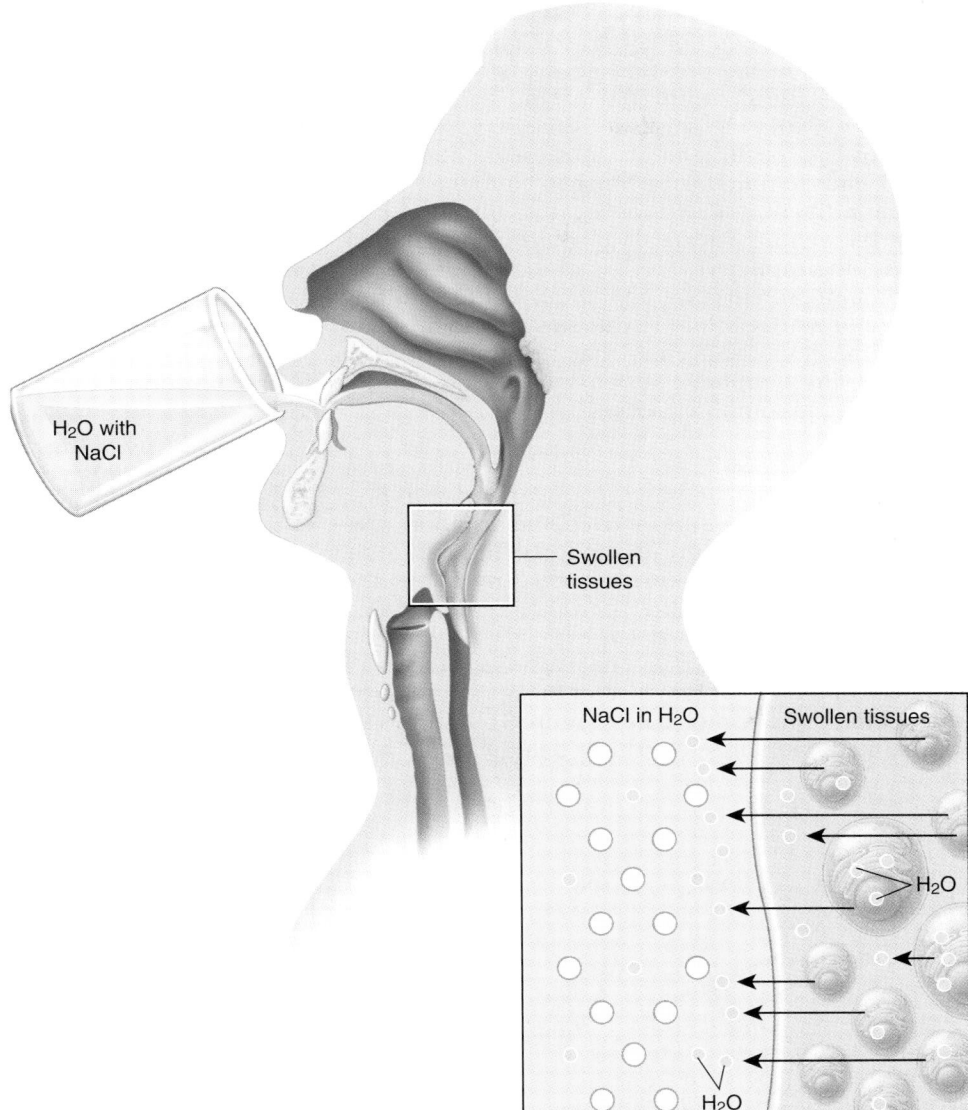

Figure 31–2. Osmosis. When a client uses a saline solution as a gargle for swollen tonsils, the gargle provides a feeling of comfort. This is because of the process of osmosis. The excess water in the swollen tonsils moves from the area of lesser concentration of particles (in the swollen cells) to the extracellular spaces that now have a higher concentration because of the added sodium.

Active Transport

In contrast, when an electrolyte moves against a concentration gradient, from an area of lower concentration to an area of higher concentration, energy is required. This active process of molecules moving against a concentration gradient is known as active transport. This is the process necessary to maintain the sodium-potassium pump. This pump is critical to the maintenance of an electrical impulse, such as in the heart. It is the active movement of sodium from inside the cell to the outside of the cell by this pump that results in a negativity on the inside of the cell.

This electrical difference between the outside and inside of the membrane results in a resting potential, so that the cell can respond to an impulse. When it does so, the response is called an action potential because the cell is no longer in a state of rest, but is in a state of action.

Filtration

Filtration pressure is the sum of (1) the forces tending to move water and dissolved substances out of the blood vessels and (2) the opposing forces. **Hydrostatic pressure** is the pressure exerted by the weight of fluid within a compartment. **Colloid osmotic pressure** is the osmotic pressure exerted by large molecules, such as proteins. Arterial hydrostatic pressure is greater than colloid osmotic pressure. The increased hydrostatic pressure "pushes" fluids out of the arterial end of the capillary into the interstitial compartments for cellular nourishment. Colloid osmotic pressure tends to hold fluid within a compartment. The difference between hydrostatic pressure and colloid pressure is +10 mm Hg at the arterial end of the capillary. The process by which water and certain smaller particles pass through a semipermeable membrane, assisted by hydrostatic and filtration pressures, is known as **filtration.**

In the venous end of the capillary, the pulling force of the colloids draws fluids into the capillaries. Note the difference in the pressure gradients between venous hydrostatic pressure and colloid osmotic pressure. It is −10 mm Hg; this is the filtration pressure. In other words, a positive filtration pressure at the arterial end leads to fluid being "pushed" into the interstitial compartment, whereas a negative filtration pressure at the venous end leads to fluid being "pulled" back into the capillary.

Although proteins play a vital role in fluid shifting, they cannot manage fluid homeostasis by themselves. Besides the essential factors that have already been discussed, the lymphatic system plays a life-sustaining role in this complex process.

HYDROSTATIC PRESSURE

The balance of fluids within the capillaries depends on both hydrostatic pressure and colloid osmotic pressure. Hydrostatic pressure acts to force fluid out of the semipermeable capillary membrane. Any factor that affects blood pressure in the arterial or venous system or the flow of blood through the capillary network can affect hydrostatic pressure. This includes blood volume, size of the vessel lumen, and the opposing forces from all the osmotic molecules. Figure 31–3 shows the approximate pressures found in a healthy adult. Note

that the pressure at the arterial end of the capillary is about 32 mm Hg.

COLLOID OSMOTIC PRESSURE

As explained earlier, osmosis is the movement of water across a semipermeable membrane from an area of lower solute concentration to an area of higher solute concentration. Colloid osmotic pressure is the osmotic force created by colloids, which are large molecules such as proteins. It functions to draw fluid into the capillary or interstitial space.

Proteins are the only dissolved substances that do not readily diffuse through the capillary membrane. Thus, they exert a greater osmotic force than smaller molecules. The term *oncotic pressure* is used interchangeably with the term *colloid pressure,* but they both refer specifically to the osmotic force of protein, its superior ability to pull in water.

Proteins found in the plasma include albumin, globulin, and fibrinogen. Albumin has the greatest influence on the "pulling" pressure in the capillary. It constitutes 50% of the plasma proteins but is responsible for 80% of the colloid osmotic pressure in plasma.

Colloid osmotic pressure is the major force opposing hydrostatic pressure in the capillary. It maintains a relatively constant value of 22 mm Hg. It is this opposition that affects how much fluid filters from the arterial end of the capillary to the interstitial spaces and the cell itself. On the arterial end of the capillary, hydrostatic pressure exceeds colloid osmotic pressure, and fluid moves into the interstitial compartment.

In a healthy person, the interstitial compartment contains electrolytes and some proteins that have leaked through the capillary membrane; thus, it has its own colloid osmotic pressure. However, the concentration of proteins is always greater in the plasma compartment than in the interstitial compartment. Therefore, on the venous end of the capillary, the hydrostatic pressure is less than the colloid osmotic pressure (about 12 mm Hg), and the fluid is "pulled" back into the venous capillary by the osmotic force of protein. This process of fluid being pulled back into the capillary is known as *reabsorption.*

When a person has a deficiency in protein, more of the fluid stays in the interstitial spaces. This abnormality, called edema, will be discussed later in the chapter.

Regulation of Fluid Balance

Thirst

Why do you drink fluids? Is it because of habit or socialization, or are you thirsty? All of these factors probably affect your fluid intake. Western culture emphasizes the provision of beverages at social activities and in the home. Health publications remind us continually to drink plenty of fluids each day. But although habit and culture certainly influence our fluid consumption, our internal thirst mechanism is also a powerful stimulant that encourages us to drink.

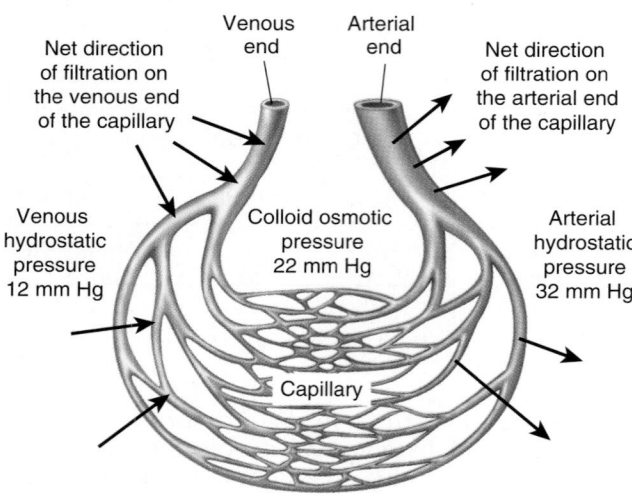

Figure 31–3. Filtration. Complex factors affect the movement of water and nutrients among the plasma, interstitium, and cellular spaces. Two critical factors are hydrostatic pressure and colloid osmotic pressure. On the arterial end of the capillary, the hydrostatic pressure (approximately 32 mm Hg) is greater than the colloid osmotic pressure (approximately 22 mm Hg). This +10 difference is known as filtration pressure and results in the movement of fluid from the arterial end of the capillary into the interstitium; this process is called filtration. On the venous end, the hydrostatic pressure (approximately 12 mm Hg) is less than the colloid osmotic pressure, approximately a −10 difference in filtration pressure. This pulling pressure results in reabsorption of the fluid back into the venous end of the capillary. The lymphatic tissues transport any remaining fluid or proteins to the right atrium.

The thirst center is located in the hypothalamus. The stimulation or inhibition of the thirst response depends on changes in local plasma osmolality. For example, when the osmolality of the blood flowing around the lateral preoptic cells of the hypothalamus becomes more concentrated, the cells sense this change and trigger the thirst response. Situations that promote increased osmolality include a decrease in fluid intake, excessive fluid loss, or an excessive sodium intake either orally or intravenously. On the other hand, a high intake of fluids, fluid retention, a low sodium intake, and excessive IV infusion of hypotonic solutions inhibit the thirst mechanism.

To return to our case study, why didn't Mrs. Thompson's thirst mechanism stimulate her to drink more? Recall that Mrs. Thompson is 81 years old. Like all elderly persons, she has a decrease in thirst as a normal consequence of aging. This will be addressed later in the chapter.

Lymphatic System

The lymphatic system performs the essential role of "sponging up" excess fluid that is not reabsorbed into the capillaries. The lymphatic ducts also release any protein "leaked" into the subclavian veins, which in turn empty into the right atrium of the heart. When the lymphatic system is not functioning properly, fluid excess occurs in the interstitial compartments. Severe lymphatic dysfunction can lead to localized tissue ischemia and cell death. It also can lead to systemic sepsis caused by metabolites from necrotic tissue.

Neuroendocrine System

Another very powerful regulator of fluid intake is the neuroendocrine system. It regulates body fluid volume by producing and secreting hormones that stimulate or inhibit osmotic receptors in the carotid arteries and aortic arch. These receptors are very sensitive to blood volume. It also uses specialized nerve endings in the walls of the large blood vessels and atria to respond to changes in intravascular fluid volume.

HORMONES

One of the most influential hormones affecting fluid balance is the antidiuretic hormone (ADH). This hormone opposes ("anti") fluid loss ("diuresis"). ADH is produced by the hypothalamus and stored in the vesicles in the posterior pituitary gland. The osmolality of extracellular fluid as it passes through the hypothalamus is the major stimulant or inhibitor of the secretion of antidiuretic hormone.

The osmolality of Mrs. Thompson's plasma was increased when she was in a state of fluid deficit. It makes sense, then, that her body, in an attempt to compensate, promoted a decrease in water loss. Increased secretion of ADH caused the pores in the distal and collecting tubules of her kidney nephrons to become larger. This resulted in increased reabsorption of the water back into the capillaries and a decrease in urinary output (oliguria).

Aldosterone is another hormone with a major effect on fluid balance. Although low sodium levels, high potassium levels, and the release of adrenocorticotropic hormone (ACTH) affect the release of aldosterone, the major stimulant for its release is the hormone angiotensin II. This hormone is produced whenever renin, a proteolytic enzyme synthesized and stored in juxtaglomerular cells of the kidney, is secreted in response to decreased kidney blood flow. Angiotensin in turn stimulates the release of aldosterone from the adrenal cortex. Unlike antidiuretic hormone, aldosterone has only an indirect effect on water. Instead, when it is released, aldosterone promotes the reabsorption of sodium and the excretion of potassium in the distal and collecting tubules of the kidney. Sodium reabsorption results in the passive reabsorption of water.

When fluid excess is present, the opposite occurs: aldosterone secretion is decreased, resulting in sodium and water excretion and potassium retention. Note that when one cation (sodium) is retained, another (potassium) is excreted. This is one of the ways in which the delicate balance of electrical neutrality is maintained. Also recall that cation changes result in changes in the movement of anions. Usually, the chloride ion passively accompanies its leader, the sodium ion, to its destination.

Thyroid hormones (thyroxine [T_4] and triiodothyronine [T_3]) affect fluid volume by influencing cardiac output. An increase in thyroid hormones causes an increase in cardiac output, which in turn increases glomerular filtrate and thus urinary output. A decrease in these hormones has the opposite effect.

The cardiovascular system also plays a role in fluid balance through the release of atrial natriuretic peptides whenever the atrial cells are overloaded with fluid. Any condition that causes fluid overload, vasoconstriction, or direct cardiac damage stimulates an increase in the release of atrial natriuretic peptides. Their release has an effect opposite to that of the renin-angiotensin-aldosterone system. It causes dilation of the arterioles and venules, sodium excretion (natriuresis), and diuresis.

BARORECEPTORS

Have you ever felt your heart pounding after a stressful event? If someone took your blood pressure at that time it would be much higher than normal. However, this rise in blood pressure does not cause a problem in a healthy person because of the "minute-to-minute" control of the blood pressure by baroreceptors. These receptors are specialized nerve endings in the walls of the large veins and arteries and in the atria of the heart. They respond to the slightest changes in pressure inside the blood vessels and relay this information to the vasomotor centers in the medulla. Anything that affects the relationship of the size of the blood vessels or the volume inside the blood vessels affects these receptors.

Now that you have an understanding of the major compensatory responses that a person experiences when fluid is lost, you can transfer this knowledge to the opposite scenario, fluid excess. When a person consumes too much fluid, baroreceptors and the hypothalamus sense a decrease in osmolality. This causes a decrease in antidiuretic hormone, an increase in urinary output, and inhibition of the thirst mechanism. The increased volume reaching the kidney will inhibit the release of renin and aldosterone, thus decreasing reabsorption of sodium. This mechanism also promotes diuresis.

Gastrointestinal System

Besides the fluid absorbed from dietary intake, the gastrointestinal (GI) tract produces about 7 to 9 L of glandular and tissue secretions per day. All but about 100 mL of this fluid is reabsorbed. About every 90 minutes, a volume of blood equivalent to the total body plasma level (about 3,000 mL in a person who weighs 70 kg) passes through the intestinal mucosa. The GI fluid contains many nutrients, including electrolytes. Understanding the relationship between fluid balance and normal GI function is essential to anticipating fluid and electrolyte imbalances in a state of altered GI function.

Renal System

The renal system works interdependently with the neuroendocrine system to regulate the volume of extracellular fluid. Recall that the kidney is the target organ for antidiuretic hormone and aldosterone. Antidiuretic hormone (through the regulation of water) and aldosterone (through the regulation of water, sodium, and potassium) play a major role in fluid and electrolyte homeostasis.

The kidney also affects many other electrolytes, including calcium, magnesium, phosphate, hydrogen, chloride, and bicarbonate. The renal nephrons regulate electrolyte balance by secreting excess ions into the tubules, where they are later excreted as urine. When a deficit occurs, electrolytes are reabsorbed from the renal tubules back into the capillary network surrounding the tubules of the nephron.

Problems of Fluid Balance

These regulators of fluid balance are important to consider when a client is at risk for or has an actual fluid volume deficit or excess. Compare the following definitions to get a clearer picture of the basic concepts related to fluid imbalance.

Fluid Volume Deficit

Fluid volume deficit refers to a state of hypovolemia, or dehydration, in either the extracellular fluid (intravascular or interstitial) compartment or the intracellular fluid compartment. The defining characteristic is a direct or indirect result of a rapid change in fluid output or a lack of intake without compensation by fluid shifts or other homeostatic mechanisms.

Fluid Volume Excess

Fluid volume excess refers to a state of hypervolemia, or water intoxication, in the vascular compartment, the presence of edema in the interstitial compartment, or excess fluid in the intracellular spaces. The defining characteristic is a direct or indirect result of an increase in fluid intake or decrease in excretion without compensation by intercompartmental fluid shifts or other regulatory mechanisms.

Electrolyte Imbalance

An *electrolyte imbalance* means that a person has either a deficit or an excess of one or more electrolytes. Table 31–2 lists the risk factors and manifestations of common imbalances of sodium, potassium, calcium, magnesium, and phosphorus. Note the similarity of some manifestations, as well as the manifestations that are unique to each ion. A client often has more than one electrolyte imbalance, as well as an accompanying fluid imbalance.

Metabolic Acidosis

Normal cellular function depends on the maintenance of hydrogen ion concentration within very narrow limits. The normal range of pH (a negative logarithm used to express the H ion concentration) is 7.35 to 7.45. Cellular function is seriously affected when pH drops to 7.20 or lower or rises to 7.50 or higher. Ranges outside of 6.80 and 7.80 are usually incompatible with life. In a healthy state, four systems interactively maintain this narrow margin: cellular buffer systems, the lungs, the kidneys, and the three chemical buffers systems. Figure 31–4 illustrates acid-base balance.

Respiratory acidosis or alkalosis is secondary to an imbalance in volatile acids, such as carbonic acid. These are discussed in Chapter 39. Metabolic abnormalities are secondary to imbalances in nonvolatile acids or in the amount of alkali and are often more difficult to diagnose.

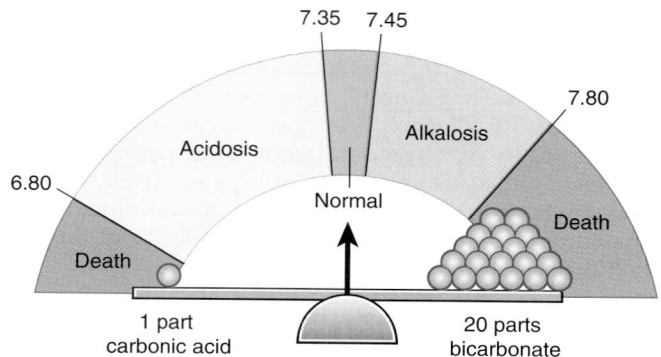

Figure 31–4. Acid-base balance. In the healthy state, a ratio of 1 part carbonic acid to 20 parts bicarbonate provides a normal plasma pH between 7.35 and 7.45. Any deviation to the left of 7.35 results in an acidotic state. Any deviation to the right of 7.45 results in an alkalotic state. Death usually results if the pH goes below 6.80 or above 7.80.

TABLE 31–2
Common Electrolyte Imbalances: Risk Factors and Manifestations

Imbalance	Risk Factors	Manifestations
Hyponatremia • Sodium <135 mEq/L • Chloride <98 mEq/L • Plasma osmolality <285 mOsm/kg	Low-salt diet, especially when taking diuretics at same time.	*General:* fatigue, weight loss *Musculoskeletal:* weakness *Cardiac:* orthostatic hypotension; rapid, thready, weak pulse; peripheral vein filling takes more than 5 seconds *Respiratory:* tachypnea *Gastrointestinal:* nausea, vomiting, diarrhea *Renal:* oliguria, anuria *Neurological:* hypothermia, decreased thirst, confusion, stupor, seizures
Hypernatremia • Sodium >145 mEq/L	• Increased intake, especially in renal disease. • Excessive IV saline solutions. • Increased retention from cardiac disease, renal disease, liver disease, Cushing's disease, hyperaldosteronism. • Conditions in which water loss exceeds sodium loss, such as diabetes mellitus, diabetes insipidus, hyperventilation, hypertonic feedings, diaphoresis, decreased water intake.	*General:* fatigue, pitting edema, puffy eyelids, ascites, weight gain *Musculoskeletal:* weakness *Cardiac:* rapid, bounding pulse; third heart sound; hypertension; peripheral vein emptying takes more than 5 seconds; neck vein distention *Respiratory:* dyspnea, crackles, pulmonary edema, pleural effusion *Gastrointestinal:* anorexia, nausea, vomiting *Renal:* oliguria, anuria *Neurological:* fever, restlessness, confusion
Hypokalemia • Potassium <3.5 mEq/L	• Certain medications, such as diuretics and laxatives.	*General:* malaise, fatigue, alkalosis *Musculoskeletal:* weakness *Cardiac:* hypotension; arrhythmias; cardiac arrest; peaked P waves, depressed S–T segments, and flattened T and U waves on electrocardiogram (ECG) *Respiratory:* shallow breathing, apnea, respiratory arrest *Gastrointestinal:* anorexia, nausea, vomiting, distention, paralytic ileus *Neurological:* dysphasia, lethargy, disorientation, irritability, hyporeflexia, paresthesias, tetany, seizures
Hyperkalemia • Potassium >5.0 mEq/L	• Increased oral or IV intake, especially in renal disease; stored blood. • Decreased output, as from taking angiotensin-converting enzyme inhibitor with potassium-rich salt substitutes or potassium-sparing diuretics, renal failure, postoperative oliguria, Addison's disease. • Excessive cellular loss, as from metabolic or respiratory acidosis (except diabetic acidosis) or during the first 3 days after a severe burn or cellular trauma.	*General:* restlessness, acidosis *Musculoskeletal:* severe weakness *Cardiac:* hypotension; arrhythmias; cardiac arrest; depressed P waves, wide QRS complexes, depressed S–T segments, and tall, tented T waves on ECG *Respiratory:* dyspnea *Gastrointestinal:* nausea, colic, diarrhea *Renal:* oliguria, anuria *Neurological:* restlessness, paresthesias, dysphasia, seizures
Hypocalcemia • Calcium <4.5 mEq/L	• Certain medications, such as diuretics and laxatives.	*General:* bleeding *Musculoskeletal:* muscle cramps, pathological fractures *Cardiac:* hypotension; palpitations; arrhythmias; prolonged QT intervals on ECG *Respiratory:* laryngospasm, stridor *Neurological:* paresthesias, positive Trousseau's and Chvostek's signs, diplopia, tetany, seizures

Table continued on following page

TABLE 31–2

Common Electrolyte Imbalances: Risk Factors and Manifestations *Continued*

Imbalance	Risk Factors	Manifestations
Hypercalcemia • Calcium >5.5 mEq/L • Phosphate decreased	• Excessive intake of milk, calcium-based medications, or vitamin D. • Increased loss from bone due to immobilization, cancer (bone, lung, breast, leukemia), multiple fractures, hyperparathyroidism. • Decreased opposition, from Addison's disease, hypophosphatemia. • Decreased binding, from acidosis. • Decreased loss, from thiazide diuretics.	*General:* dehydration, polydipsia *Musculoskeletal:* weak, relaxed muscles; osteoporosis; osteomalacia; bone pain; pathological fractures *Cardiac:* dysrhythmia, cardiac arrest, short QT intervals on ECG *Gastrointestinal:* nausea, vomiting, constipation *Renal:* polyuria, calculi, renal colic, flank pain *Neurological:* confusion, lethargy
Hypomagnesemia • Magnesium <1.5 mEq/L	• Certain medications, such as diuretics.	*General:* refractory hypokalemia, hypocalcemia, or both *Musculoskeletal:* weakness *Cardiac:* tachycardia, arrhythmias *Neurological:* nystagmus, diplopia, disorientation, tremors, hyperactive reflexes, tetany, seizures
Hypermagnesemia • Magnesium >2.5 mEq/L	• Certain medications, such as magnesium antacids.	*General:* flushing *Musculoskeletal:* weakness, dysarthria *Cardiac:* hypotension, arrhythmias, cardiac arrest *Respiratory:* bradypnea, apnea, respiratory arrest *Gastrointestinal:* nausea, vomiting *Neurological:* thirst, hyporeflexia, lethargy, coma
Hypophosphatemia • Phosphate <1.2 mEq/L	• Certain medications, such as aluminum antacids and diuretics.	*General:* fatigue *Musculoskeletal:* weakness, bone pain, pathological fractures *Cardiac:* decreased cardiac function *Neurological:* confusion, seizures
Hyperphosphatemia • Phosphate >3.0 mEq/L • Calcium decreased	• Certain medications, such as phosphate antacids and sodium phosphate enemas.	*Cardiac:* tachycardia *Gastrointestinal:* anorexia, nausea, vomiting *Neurological:* hyperreflexia, tetany

ECG, electrocardiogram.

Metabolic acidosis is a pathological condition caused by an increase in noncarbonic acids or a decrease in bicarbonate in the extracellular fluid, or both. Any pathology that results in altered tissue perfusion and the accumulation of lactic acid leads to lactic acidosis, a type of metabolic acidosis. Because the kidney is the primary organ responsible for the excretion of acids and the reabsorption of bicarbonate, any state of severe renal insufficiency leads to metabolic acidosis.

Any pathology that leads to a deficit of sodium, phosphate, or protein impairs the base component of the chemical buffer systems, resulting in excess hydrogen. A decrease in hemoglobin or chloride can also increase the risk for metabolic acidosis by altering the following process: Most dissolved carbon dioxide from tissue cell metabolism diffuses into the red blood cells, combines with water to form carbonic acid, and dissociates into hydrogen and bicarbonate. The bicarbonate shifts across the plasma membrane in exchange for chloride. The hydrogen combines with hemoglobin and thus is buffered.

An increase in potassium ions also increases the risk of metabolic acidosis. Whenever plasma potassium rises, the protective cellular buffer attempts to decrease the risk of hyperkalemia by exchanging potassium for hydrogen across the cell membrane. Thus, potassium enters the cell in exchange for hydrogen, which enters the plasma.

The most common manifestations of metabolic acidosis are neurological (headache, lethargy), GI (anorexia, nausea, vomiting, diarrhea), cardiovascular (arrhythmias), and respiratory. The client may develop deep, rapid respirations (Kussmaul's respirations) as her body attempts to blow off carbonic acid. Severe acidosis can lead to coma and death.

Metabolic Alkalosis

In contrast, when the pH rises above 7.45, the client has **metabolic alkalosis.** This is a pathological condition caused by an increase in bicarbonate or a decrease in acid in the extracellular fluid, or both. Any pathology or situation that leads to excessive vomiting (and loss of hydrochloric acid) or diarrhea (and excessive loss of the bicarbonate ion) increases the risk for metabolic alkalosis. Potassium deficiency, regardless of cause, promotes the shifting of hydrogen into cells and potassium into plasma—thus metabolic alkalosis. An overingestion of bicarbonate (as in antacids), especially in the presence of renal insufficiency, can result in metabolic alkalosis.

Common manifestations of metabolic alkalosis include generalized weakness, muscle cramps, neurological problems (hyperactive reflexes, tetany, confusion, convulsions), cardiac arrhythmias, and respiratory changes. As in metabolic acidosis, the respiratory system attempts to compensate. In this state, however, the respirations become slow and shallow in an attempt to conserve carbonic acid.

FACTORS AFFECTING FLUID BALANCE

Many variables influence a client's risk of fluid, electrolyte, and acid-base imbalance, including lifestyle, environment, developmental stage, physiological state, and treatments. Table 31–3 lists the many etiologies of fluid deficit and fluid excess and the contributing factors for each variable.

Lifestyle Factors

Nutrition

An alteration in the intake of fluids increases risk. Although the majority of fluid intake comes from water or other liquids, the importance of the water obtained from foods should not be underestimated (Fig. 31–5). The water byproduct of food oxidation in the cell also contributes to our fluid balance, but to a lesser degree. The amounts listed in the illustration are for a healthy, relatively inactive person exposed to a temperate climate. People require at least 1,500 mL of fluid daily to maintain essential cellular functions. The usual recommendation for fluid intake is 8 to 10 glasses of fluid daily (about 2,000 to 2,400 mL).

Now it makes sense that Mrs. Thompson became ill when she stopped drinking an adequate amount of fluid.

In a healthy person, the body compensates for excess fluid, sodium, or both by increasing excretion. However, if the person has cardiac, renal, or liver disease, excess intake only prompts the retention of more fluid. Excess fluid compromises the exchange of nutrients and wastes across the cell-plasma membrane.

Hypoproteinemia, or decreased protein in the plasma, either from decreased intake or increased loss, will result in decreased intravascular oncotic pressure. This will ultimately result in hypotension because of the decrease in reabsorption at the venous end of the capillary.

Exercise

A client who has a risk of fluid deficit does not present with the actual signs and symptoms of an imbalance. However, recognizable risk factors can lead you to believe that the person has a high probability of developing a fluid deficit. Exercise, especially in a hot, humid environment, is one such risk factor.

In fact, a water loss of only 1.2% has been found to impair thermoregulation. A fluid loss of only 2% can cause increased heart rates, increased body temperature, and decreased plasma volume. It is not just one factor but the relationship of the temperature and humidity that determines a person's response. A temperature as low as 62°F with a 97% humidity and as high as 92°F with a 50% humidity has caused fatal heat strokes in high school football players (Maughan, 1992).

Stress

Regardless of whether a stressor stems from a physiological, psychological, environmental, or other cause,

Fluid intake		Fluid output	
Ingested water	1200-1500 mL	Kidneys	1500 mL
Ingested food	800-1100 mL	Insensible loss through skin	600-800 mL
Metabolic oxidation	300 mL	Insensible loss through lungs	400-600 mL
		Gastrointestinal tract	100 mL
TOTAL	2600-3000 mL	TOTAL	2600-3000 mL

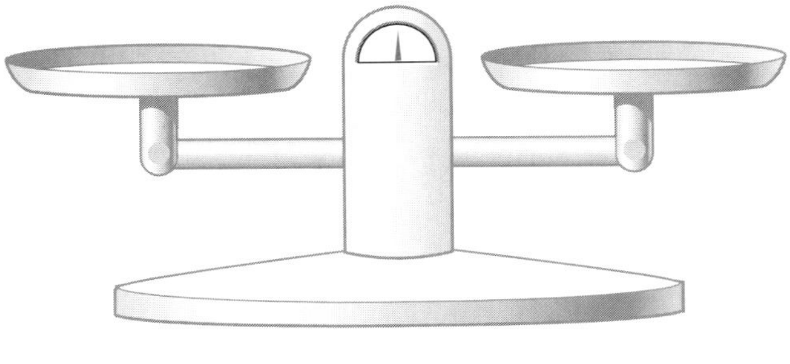

Figure 31–5. Sources of fluid intake and fluid output. In health, fluid intake and fluid output are approximately equal. Fluid output includes both sensible loss and insensible loss. *Sensible fluid loss* is fluid loss that is easily perceived, such as through urination. *Insensible fluid loss* is fluid loss that is not easily perceived, such as through normal respiration.

TABLE 31–3

Risk Factors for Fluid Volume Imbalance

Risk Factor	Contributing Factors
Fluid Volume Deficit	

Lifespan

Children	• Decreased ability to concentrate urine (immature kidneys). • Higher metabolic rate. • Greater body surface area relative to weight. • Hormonal and growth demands. • Compensatory responses less stable. • Fevers higher and last longer.
Pregnancy	• Increased need for fluid (fetal and supportive tissue changes).
Elderly	• Decreased thirst mechanism, even in healthy elderly. • Decreased ability to concentrate urine.
Weight extremes	• Fatty tissue contains less fluid. • Excess fluid may be in compartments outside the blood vessels, making it unavailable. • Thirst may be an indicator of plasma deficit. • Women have larger proportion of fat tissue.

Altered intake

Decreased thirst	• Elderly population. • Hypo-osmolality of the plasma inhibits thirst. • Decreased level of consciousness impairs perception of thirst.
Pain	• Alters desire or perception of thirst.
Dysphagia	• Increases time required for fluid intake. • Makes swallowing more difficult. • Requires thickened fluids.
Decreased access	• Lack of transportation, limited finances, ill health.

Increased gastrointestinal (GI) loss

Diarrhea, vomiting, GI suctioning, ileostomy, fistula	• Rapid movement of fluid through GI tract decreases absorption of water, nutrients, and electrolytes. • Massive amounts of fluid can be lost via these sources regardless of etiology.
Hypertonic feedings (osmolarity >300 mOsm/kg)	• Increased osmolarity of feeding pulls water into bowel, which can cause diarrhea and dehydration.
Lactose-based feedings	• Lactose intolerance is common and may cause diarrhea.
Medications	• Many medications cause GI side effects, including anorexia, nausea, vomiting, and diarrhea. • Many elixirs are made with sorbitol, which can cause osmotic diarrhea.

Increased urinary loss

Decreased antidiuretic hormone	• May result from hypo-osmolality of extracellular fluid, increased blood volume, exposure to cold, acute alcohol ingestion, carbon monoxide poisoning.
Hyperglycemia	• Causes osmotic diuresis.
Diuretic phase of renal failure	• Excess fluid lost through urine.
Medications	• Diuretics are a common cause.

Increased integumentary loss

Environmental	• Temperatures above 30°C (86°F) and humidity above 50%.
Fever	• Insensible water loss, can be large amounts.
Wounds/burns	• Loss of fluid, protein, electrolytes. • Damage to capillary membrane with direct fluid loss and secondary fluid loss due to loss of protein.

Increased respiratory loss

Hyperventilation	• Increased loss of water through expired air.

Other losses

Hemorrhage	• Increased loss of fluid, nutrients, electrolytes.
Addison's disease	• Decreased sodium retention, thus decreased water reabsorption.
Third spacing	• Abnormal amounts of fluid accumulation in compartments that normally have minimal fluid decreases availability of fluids needed to maintain blood volume and cellular function.

TABLE 31–3
Risk Factors for Fluid Volume Imbalance *Continued*

Risk Factor	Contributing Factors
Fluid Volume Excess	
Excessive intake	
Excess fluid	• Increased oral or IV volume.
	• Electrolyte-free infusion, such as dextrose 5% in water.
Excess sodium	• Increased sodium promotes water reabsorption.
Decreased excretion	
Renal disease	• Kidney cannot excrete excess fluid.
Increased antidiuretic hormone	• More chronic disease in elderly.
	• Increase in osmolality of extracellular fluid (water loss, sodium gain), reduced blood volume, pain, stress (emotional and physiological), medications (such as morphine, barbiturates, general anesthetics).
	• Excessive stress activates hypothalamic center, causing release of both antidiuretic hormone and adrenocorticotropic hormone.
Increased capillary permeability	
Sepsis, inflammatory processes, major trauma and burns, acid-base imbalance	• Increased capillary permeability allows more fluid to leak into the interstitial spaces, causing fluid excess or edema.
Hypoproteinemia	
Decreased intake or increased loss	• Any state of decreased protein, regardless of etiology, results in a decrease in capillary colloid osmotic pressure that impairs reabsorption. Excess fluid is left in the interstitial spaces, causing edema.

the body's response will vary with the client's perception of the seriousness of the stressor, the actual degree of physical damage, and the body's ability to adapt to the insult. Any stressor activates the general adaptation system, which results in hypothalamic releasing factors that stimulate the anterior pituitary to release adrenocortical hormone and then target the adrenal cortex.

Cortisols and aldosterone released from the adrenal cortex play a major role in improving tissue perfusion through increasing blood volume. Cortisols improve vascular volume through healing of the damaged capillary membranes, which decreases capillary leaking, and through increased sodium retention. Aldosterone has an even stronger influence on sodium retention. Both promote the loss of potassium. If the stressor results in marked hypokalemia, metabolic alkalosis may result. To maintain electroneutrality, when the potassium moves out of the cell into the plasma, the hydrogen ion moves from the plasma into the cell, increasing the risk for metabolic alkalosis.

Environmental Factors

As noted above, risk for fluid loss can be a life-threatening risk. It is not just limited to periods of exercise. Any time the body is exposed to a relatively high temperature, whether in the work or home setting, the risk is just as high. Common examples include the city maintenance crew and the person mowing a lawn on a hot day or a humid day or, especially, a day that is both hot and humid.

Intolerance to environmental toxins can lead to fluid and electrolyte loss through vomiting, diarrhea, or both. Trauma leading to fluid and electrolyte losses can occur anywhere. Anyone driving a vehicle or operating dangerous equipment or handling dangerous products is at increased risk as well.

Developmental Factors

Everyone is at risk for fluid and electrolyte imbalance, but the very young and the elderly are at greatest risk because of their varying water distribution (Table 31–4).

Infants and Children

The younger the child, the greater the risk for fluid deficit. This is partly because the highest growth rate, or period of greatest metabolic activity after fetal de-

TABLE 31–4
Proportion of Body Water by Age

Age	Percent of Body Weight
Neonate	77
6 months	72
2–16 years	60
20–39 years	59 (female) to 60 (male)
40–59 years	47 (female) to 55 (male)
65 years and older	45 to 50

velopment, is during infancy. Infants and children also have immature kidneys with a decreased ability to concentrate urine. Plus, an increased body surface area compared with weight leads to increased fluid loss through the skin. Compensatory mechanisms are also less efficient.

Adolescents and Middle-Aged Adults

Adolescents have an increased risk for fluid deficit due to an increase in hormonal activity and increased loss with exercise-related activities. Teenagers who become pregnant further compromise their health because of the increased demands of the fetus during a time when their own bodies have an increased need.

Middle-aged adults are the age group least at risk for fluid imbalance. Developmentally, however, the demands of work-related activities and family rearing can increase the risk for self-care deficit.

Older Adults

The older adult is more at risk for fluid imbalances because of the increased incidence of chronic diseases. Fluid deficit, or dehydration, is the most common fluid and electrolyte problem in the elderly population. Even healthy elderly people have a decreased thirst mechanism. The aged kidney also has a decreased ability to concentrate urine. Lack of access to food purchasing due to financial, health, transportation, or other barriers also decreases intake. The older adult usually takes more medications, over-the-counter or prescribed, than any other age group. The most common side effects of most of these medications are nausea, vomiting, and diarrhea.

Referring to the case study, Mrs. Thompson was drinking less. She also was losing fluid by four routes. Increased perspiration, diarrhea, vomiting, and, to a lesser extent, rapid respiration each contributed to the dehydration she experienced.

Remember that in the early phases of Mrs. Thompson's fluid deficit, her body compensated. Recall that thirst was not a compensatory mechanism for Mrs. Thompson because of her advanced age. Mrs. Thompson's manifestations of oliguria, constipation, and dry skin were expected responses to her body's need to conserve fluid. As her regulatory systems could no longer compensate, she became very ill.

Physiological Factors

The most common physiological factors that increase the risk for fluid, electrolyte, and acid-base problems are pathologies, stressors, or treatments that affect the cardiovascular, respiratory, gastrointestinal (GI), renal, and integumentary systems. Trauma can affect any one or a combination of these systems.

Uncommon, but just as serious, is the fluid deficit risk raised by conditions that alter the function of the adrenal gland. Hypoaldosteronism can lead to severe sodium deficit and, thus, fluid loss. Hyperaldosteronism and Cushing's syndrome both increase the risk for

fluid retention secondary to sodium retention. Certain cancers also increase the risk for fluid overload secondary to the increased secretion of antidiuretic hormone (also called vasopressin) from the tumor cells. They include some lymphomas and bronchogenic, pancreatic, and prostatic cancers.

Cardiovascular Problems

Cardiovascular diseases can lead to a state of weakness or inability to access fluids and food products so that a deficit results. More common, however, is fluid overload caused by heart disease. When the left ventricle cannot contract efficiently, the buildup of fluid pressure has a retrograde effect, causing an increase in left atrial pressure followed by increased pulmonary pressure, which leads to pulmonary congestion.

The most critical consequence of left ventricular failure is pulmonary edema. This can lead to a subsequent increase in right ventricular pressure, followed by systemic fluid overload. Excess fluid or sodium intake in a person who has cardiac or renal dysfunction will only further exacerbate the fluid overload.

Respiratory Problems

Any situation or pathology that increases the respiratory rate also increases the amount of fluid lost in expired air.

Gastrointestinal Problems

Many GI problems, including vomiting, diarrhea, ileostomies, and fistulas, lead to fluid loss. Prescribed therapies such as gastric or bowel suction also increase fluid loss. Decreased fluid intake, as in dysphagia, is a common factor in dehydration. The most common GI pathology that causes fluid overload is liver disease.

Renal Problems

End-stage renal disease is usually characterized by polyuric, oliguric, and anuric phases. During the polyuric phase, a client is at risk for fluid volume deficit. In the oliguric and anuric phases, fluid overload predominates because of the excessive retention of fluid.

Integumentary Problems

Loss of the protective skin barrier results in increased fluid loss. The blisters that accompany partial-thickness burns are filled with fluid that is no longer available to the body. This process by which fluid moves into an area that makes it physiologically unavailable is known as **third spacing**. Other examples of third spacing include the movement of fluid into the peritoneal space (ascites), the pericardial space (pericardial effusion), and the pleural space (pleural effusion).

Protein loss from burn wounds into the interstitial spaces results in decreased plasma colloid osmotic pressure. The etiology of the resulting edema is twofold: impaired reabsorption of water into the capillaries and increased interstitial oncotic pressure. Hypoproteinemia is a common example of how an extracellular fluid deficit (plasma) can exist at the same time as an extracellular fluid excess (interstitium).

Trauma

As with burns, tissue damage from any type of trauma can lead to fluid loss. Metabolites released by cell damage trigger the inflammatory process, which in turn stimulates the release of byproducts that increase capillary permeability. Increasing permeability allows more fluid to shift from plasma into the interstitial space. This extra interstitial fluid is not available for maintaining body functions, and it alters gas and nutrient exchange in the involved tissues.

Protein loss from traumatized tissues is also a consequence of increased capillary permeability and has the same manifestations as in burn trauma. Sepsis, a possible complication of trauma, promotes increased capillary permeability and more fluid, electrolyte, and protein loss.

A client with head trauma may develop either fluid deficit or fluid excess. Head trauma can result in diabetes insipidus or syndrome of inappropriate antidiuretic hormone (SIADH). Diabetes insipidus manifests with polyuria (2 to 15 L of urine daily), which can lead to severe fluid deficits. SIADH results in an obligatory increase in antidiuretic hormone, a secondary decrease in urinary output, and thus a risk for fluid overload.

Clinical Factors

Many interventions can increase a client's risk for fluid imbalance. They include surgery, chemotherapy, medications, suctioning, and long-term use of intravenous (IV) therapy.

Surgery

Clients are at risk in both the preoperative and the postoperative phases of surgery. The longer the client has had nothing by mouth or has had a decreased intake or increased loss before surgery, the greater the risk of intraoperative and postoperative complications. For example, a client who receives a series of cathartics or enemas before surgery faces a higher risk of morbidity and mortality after surgery because of the fluid and electrolyte losses (Incalzi et al., 1992). Excessive blood loss during or after surgery can also cause a fluid volume deficit.

Infection is still one of the most common postoperative complications. The fever, diaphoresis, and tachypnea that accompany infection increase fluid loss.

Chemotherapy

Many chemotherapeutic drugs have a high incidence of GI cell damage, leading to frequent complications of stomatitis, anorexia, taste changes, nausea, and vomiting. These effects promote a fluid deficit through a decreased intake or an increased loss.

Fluid volume excess is also a risk with chemotherapeutic drugs that increase release of antidiuretic hormone. They include vincristine, cyclophosphamide, vinblastine, cisplatin, and oxytocin (Held, 1995).

Medications

Medications that cause fluid loss (such as diuretics) and adverse effects that result in fluid loss (such as vomiting and diarrhea) are common causes of fluid deficit. For example, elixirs that contain sorbitol are commonly ordered for clients with GI tubes. Sorbitol can cause diarrhea in some people (Edes et al., 1990).

Medications such as insulin and oral hypoglycemics are commonly used to control the hyperglycemia of diabetes mellitus. Hyperglycemia, regardless of the cause, increases fluid loss secondary to the osmotic effect of the glucose molecule in the renal tubules.

General anesthetics, barbiturates, and some narcotics (such as morphine) increase the secretion of antidiuretic hormone, which increases the risk for fluid excess. Glucocorticoids and mineralocorticoids increase sodium retention and, consequently, water retention. Taken to excess, any medication that contains sodium, such as an over-the-counter antacid, increases the risk of water retention. Some medications increase the secretion of antidiuretic hormone and thus increase fluid retention. They include carbamazepine, many narcotics (including morphine), and several barbiturates.

Gastrointestinal Intubation

Gastrointestinal intubation is performed for one of two reasons: to empty the stomach contents or to provide an alternative route for nutrients. When a nasogastric tube is placed for purposes of gastric emptying (decompression), it increases the client's risk for fluid deficit. After insertion, you will need to monitor the client for fluid and electrolyte deficit and metabolic alkalosis (Procedures 31–1 and 31–2).

The second most common use for a nasogastric tube is to provide a route for foods or fluids for a client who cannot take them by mouth. Diarrhea resulting in fluid deficit is a common complication of tube feedings. The two most common sources of diarrhea secondary to tube feedings are the use of hypertonic feedings and a rapid delivery rate. The increased osmolality of hypertonic feedings promotes fluid shifting into the small bowel, which can result in diarrhea and dehydration. Likewise, the client may not tolerate a rapid delivery of a feeding and may develop diarrhea. Giving water boluses with hypertonic feedings and either giving feedings slowly or diluting them will decrease these risks.

Intravenous Therapy

Many clients receive IV therapy as part of their treatment. If the amount of fluid that the client is receiving is not adequate to meet maintenance and replacement

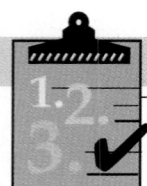

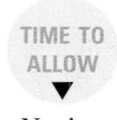

PROCEDURE 31–1

Inserting and Maintaining a Nasogastric Tube

TIME TO ALLOW
▼
Novice:
20 minutes
Expert:
5 minutes

Decompression relieves pressure by removing gas and fluids from the stomach. It can be used to prevent nausea, vomiting, and gastric distention when gastrointestinal tract motility is slow or absent, when the client has a bowel obstruction, or when the client has a fresh abdominal suture line that must be protected.

Delegation Guidelines

The complex assessment and potential risks associated with the insertion and maintenance of nasogastric tubes dictate that this procedure may not be delegated to a nursing assistant. However, you may delegate the gathering and assembly of the necessary equipment, along with the measurement, recording, and testing of nasogastric drainage. The temporary discontinuation of suction for purposes of toileting or ambulation may be appropriate for delegation under RN supervision. Reconnection of the nasogastric tube to the suction device necessitates RN verification of the suction pressure settings.

Equipment Needed

- Single-lumen or double-lumen nasogastric tube.
- Water-soluble lubricant or water to be used as lubricant.
- Portable suction machine or wall suction outlet.
- Collection device, short tubing to attach collection device to suction, and long tubing to attach suction to distal end of nasogastric tube.
- Five-in-one connector to connect nasogastric tube to suction tubing.
- Clean gloves.
- Tongue blade and penlight.
- Glass of water with a straw.
- Towel or drape to place across the client's chest.
- Emesis basin.
- 50- or 60-mL cone-tipped syringe.
- Specified dressing for securing tube to nose (tape, H-shaped occlusive dressing, or clear, 2″ × 2″ occlusive dressing).
- Safety pin and rubber band.

1 Prepare the equipment.
  a. Arrange all equipment on a small table or bedside stand.
  b. Prepare the dressing needed to secure the tube to the client's nose.

   If using tape, tear a 3-inch strip of 1-inch tape and make a 1½-inch horizontal tear up to the center of this strip. If using a clear occlusive dressing, open the package.

  c. Check the suction apparatus.

   Attach the collection device to the suction apparatus and the tubing. Make sure the lid is on the canister tightly and turn on the suction to confirm a pressure of 80 to 100 mm Hg.

2 Prepare the client.
  a. Place the client in a position that enhances his ability to assist you by swallowing.

Usually, high Fowler's position (head of the bed elevated 60 to 90 degrees) is the best position to allow the client to bring his head forward to swallow. If this position is contraindicated or the client is unconscious, it may be necessary to keep him in a recumbent position.

  b. Explain each step of the procedure as you perform it.

   Talking through the procedure as the tube is passed helps a conscious person anticipate and cooperate with the procedure.

  c. Determine which of the client's nostrils is most open.

   Occlude one of the client's nostrils and listen while he breathes through the other nostril. Repeat the process on the opposite side to compare openness. Also inspect the nose for septal deviation, and ask the client about any history of a broken nose.

3 Pass the tube.
   a. Find the proper length for the nasogastric tube by measuring from the client's nose to the earlobe and then to the xiphoid process.

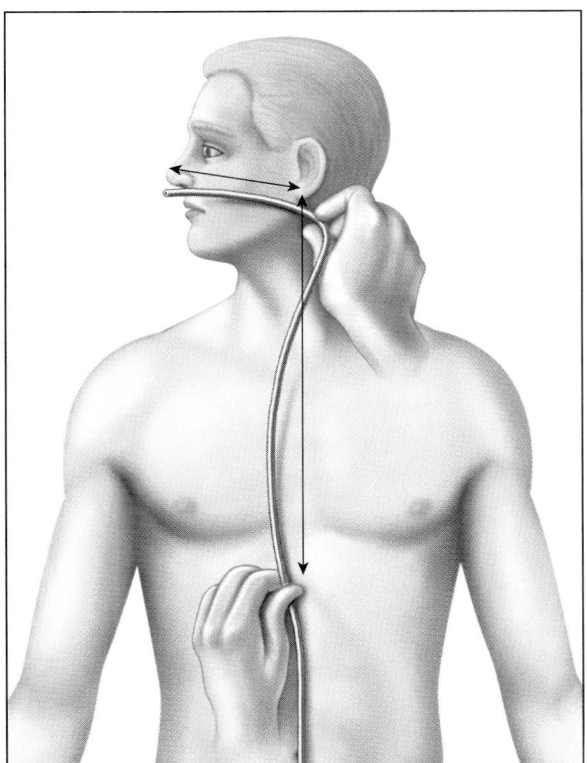

Measuring the insertion length of the nasogastric tube.

   b. Mark the length of tube to be passed with a small piece of tape, and then lubricate the final 3 inches at the tip of the tube.
   c. Insert the tube through the client's most patent nostril and pass it through to the nasopharynx.

   Have the client tilt the head slightly forward while holding the water glass in one hand. Grasp the lubricated tube with your dominant hand about 6 inches from the end. Place your forefinger on the top and your thumb on the bottom. When you reach the posterior part of the nostril, press your thumb and forefinger together to bend the tube, thus facilitating advancement past the sharp curvature of the nasopharynx.

   d. Once you clear the client's epiglottis, advance the tube until you reach the tape marker, indicating that the tube has reached the stomach.

The client's epiglottis must be closed as the tube passes to prevent the tube from entering the trachea. Ask the client to sip water through the straw and, each time he swallows, advance the tube. If he cannot swallow, have him hold his breath to close the epiglottis. If he is unconscious, watch his respirations. If the client begins coughing or becomes cyanotic at any time, remove the tube immediately. If he gags or vomits, stop advancing the tube but leave it in place if possible. Give him an emesis basin, if appropriate, and allow him to rest for a moment.

4 Connect the tube to suction and ensure client safety.
   a. Verify tube placement in the stomach.

   Attach the cone-shaped syringe to the tubing and aspirate for gastric secretions. If no gastric secretions appear, advance the tube 2 more inches and repeat the test.

   b. Use the five-in-one connector to attach the distal end of the tube to the tubing marked "to patient" on the lid of the suction collection device.
   c. Tape the tube to the client's nose using the method specified by your facility.

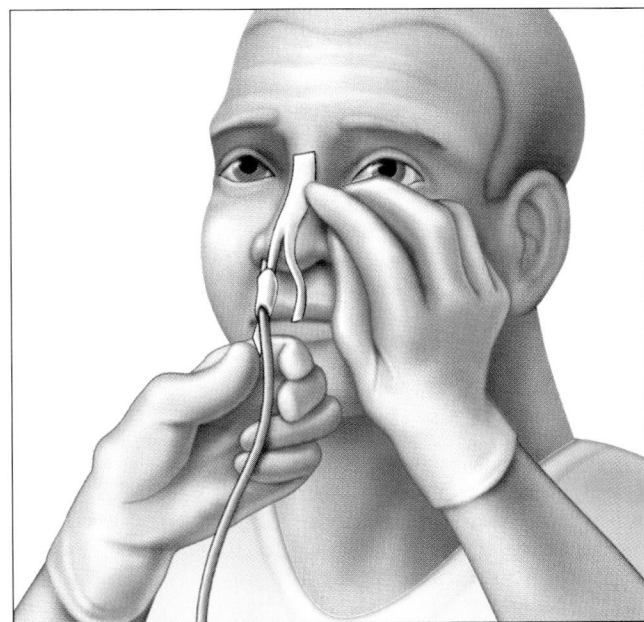

Taping the nasogastric tube to decrease trauma to the nares.

By leaving some slack in the tube when you affix it to the gown, you can prevent accidental pulling on the tube when the client turns his head.

Continued

Inserting and Maintaining a Nasogastric Tube

d. Set the suction control at the prescribed level.

Usually, you will use low intermittent suction (80–120 mm Hg). Only with a double-lumen tube can you safely use high suction (>120 mm Hg). This is because the second lumen allows constant air exchange and thus prevents gastric tissue trauma from the high suction pressure. The second lumen must be kept clear of secretions to decrease this risk. If you notice secretions in the second lumen, instill about 10 to 20 cc of air into it to displace the secretions.

5 Finish.

a. Document the reason for the nasogastric tube, your collaboration with the physician, the actual procedure, and the client's responses.

Documentation is essential to validate care and provide data for future comparison and follow-up.

b. Provide comfort care for the client's nose and mouth at least every 8 hours and as needed.

Use a clean cotton-tipped swab and water-soluble lubricant to clean the client's nostril. Assess the amount and characteristics of his nasogastric drainage as you provide care. Avoid alcohol-based mouth care agents for oral care because they tend to promote dryness.

6 Monitor.

a. Inspect the client's abdomen and auscultate bowel sounds at least every 8 hours.

To decrease the possibility of mistaking suction sounds for bowel sounds, pinch the suction tubing as you auscultate the client's abdomen.

b. Monitor and document the amount and characteristics of the client's nasogastric output, manifestations of fluid volume deficit, low electrolyte levels (especially sodium, potassium, calcium, chloride, and magnesium), or plasma levels that suggest fluid volume deficit (elevated sodium, blood urea nitrogen, and hematocrit).

c. Notify the physician if the client's nasogastric output exceeds 100 mL/hour, if total output exceeds total intake, or if he has new or worsening signs of fluid volume deficit.

Signs of fluid volume deficit include hypotension, a pulse of more than 20 beats/minute above the client's baseline when resting, urine production of less than 30 mL/hour for 2 consecutive hours or more, seizures, confusion, sudden behavioral changes, and abnormal electrolyte levels.

d. If the client's nasogastric tube stops draining well, first assess the equipment for function errors. If this is not the problem, consult a physician for an irrigation order.

Irrigate the tube using a 50- or 60-mL cone-shaped syringe with 30 to 60 mL of normal saline. Repeat as necessary. Normal saline is the only acceptable irrigating solution because its isotonicity will not further compromise the client's fluid and electrolyte balance. Make sure to compute the difference in the amount of irrigant instilled and the amount removed; subtract or add that figure to the client's 8-hour nasogastric drainage total.

---

needs, she has a risk for fluid deficit. For example, a client who is receiving IV therapy over several days with no other source of intake is at risk for fluid deficit as well as electrolyte deficit. Fluids, sodium, and potassium are required on a daily basis to maintain homeostasis. When a client has been 3 or more days without food through the oral or gastric route, an IV approach is chosen to provide these nutrients.

When an IV route is used to provide carbohydrates, proteins, fats, and other electrolytes, it is known as total parenteral nutrition. You will need to monitor the client for hyperglycemia and secondary polyuria because of the risk for osmotic diuresis from the high glucose levels in the solution. Frequent monitoring with Chemstrip glucose readings and administration of regular insulin on a sliding scale will prevent this syndrome.

ASSESSMENT

General Assessment of Fluid Balance

Perform a general health history to gather baseline data that will help you screen for specific risk factors. Also, focus your physical assessment on systems that are related to the fluid imbalance.

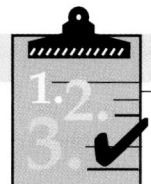

PROCEDURE 31–2

Removing a Nasogastric Tube

This procedure is used to discontinue gastric decompression therapy.

TIME TO
ALLOW
▼
Novice:
10 minutes
Expert:
5 minutes

Delegation Guidelines

The necessity for assessment prior to discontinuation of a nasogastric tube, the risk of aspiration associated with tube removal, and the short nature of this procedure suggest that this procedure not be delegated to a nursing assistant.

Equipment Needed

- Clean gloves.
- Towel.
- Emesis basin.
- Plastic bag.
- 50- or 60-mL syringe.

1 Prepare the client.
  a. Before removing the tube, assess for the presence of bowel sounds.

  Do not remove the tube if bowel sounds are absent.

  b. Explain the removal procedure to the client, place the emesis basin and opened plastic bag on a nearby table, don clean gloves, and place the towel across the client's upper chest.
  c. Turn off the suction machine and disconnect the nasogastric tube from the suction tubing.
  d. Unpin the nasogastric tube from the client's gown.
  e. Instill 20 cc of air into the nasogastric tube to displace secretions back into the client's stomach.

  Doing so decreases the client's risk of aspiration.

  f. Loosen the tape on the client's nose while holding the distal end of the nasogastric tube.

2 Remove the tube. Instruct the client to hold her breath, and then pull the tube out in one quick, steady motion.

3 Finish.
  a. Assist with or provide skin and mouth care.
  b. Document the presence of bowel sounds, the tube removal procedure, and the client's response.
  c. Continue to monitor the client for return of bowel dysfunction.

Health History

Because fluid and electrolyte imbalances affect so many systems, a complete history and physical examination are necessary. The health history begins with the gathering of more data about the client's chief complaint. When the problem is one related to fluid and electrolyte deficit, the client's chief complaint is usually related to one of the following: nausea, vomiting, diarrhea, anorexia, increasing fatigue and weakness, weight loss, fever, blood loss, excess urine output, or a change in mental status. Or the client's chief complaint may be a condition or traumatic injury, such as a burn, in which manifestations of a fluid and electrolyte imbalance might be hidden by the more obvious problem of the injury itself.

When the problem is one related to fluid and electrolyte excess, the client's chief complaint is usually related to one of the following: weight gain, cough, dyspnea, cardiac palpitations, pitting edema, or mental status changes.

Whatever the chief complaint, it is important to find out the characteristics of the client's symptoms, including the onset, location and radiation if applicable, frequency, severity, associated signs and symptoms, aggravating or alleviating factors, and the client's previous history or treatment of this problem.

Also, find out the client's past history of illnesses, hospitalizations, surgeries, trauma, allergies, current or recent medication, and currency of immunizations. Obtain an obstetrical history if applicable. Collect data related to family history and psychosocial history and then complete the review of systems. If the client's condition is acute, collect data pertinent to the immediate problem and intervene quickly. When possible, obtain additional history from family members or old records and complete the history when the client's condition stabilizes.

Physical Examination

A full head-to-toe physical examination may be necessary for an accurate diagnosis. Again, if the client's condition is critical, collect only the data needed for safe and immediate intervention. Besides the initial physical examination, an accurate diagnosis of fluid and electrolyte imbalances often requires monitoring of the client's intake and output, weight trends, edema levels, diagnostic tests, and ongoing physical assessments.

STANDARD CLINICAL MEASUREMENTS

A basic understanding of standard measurements related to fluid balance is essential to assessing and evaluating a client's fluid status. Volume is commonly measured in liters, milliliters, and cubic centimeters. For all practical purposes, the milliliter and the cubic centimeter are equivalent. Oral fluid measurements are usually expressed as cubic centimeters (cc), whereas intravenous (IV) solutions are expressed as liters (L) or milliliters (mL).

Weight is commonly measured in grams (g) and milligrams (mg). One gram equals 1,000 milligrams. Protein is expressed on a laboratory printout as grams per 100 mL of fluid. The normal plasma protein is 6 g/100 mL.

The **milliequivalent (mEq),** one-thousandth of a chemical equivalent, is the measurement used to express the chemical activity or chemical combining power of an ion. Although electrolytes have variable milligram weights, the weight has no relationship to its chemical combining power. One mEq of any electrolyte is chemically equal to 1 mEq of any other electrolyte. Chemical neutrality, an equal number of milliequivalents of cations and anions, must be present for normal neuromuscular excitability to exist.

WEIGHING THE CLIENT

When the accuracy of intake and output measurements is uncertain, or when the client has generalized body edema, weighing is the preferred method for determining fluid loss or gain. One pound, or 2.2 kilograms, is equal to 1 L of fluid loss or gain.

Because interventions are based on the data obtained from weight assessments, standardization is very important. Standardization includes weighing the client at the same time of day, with the same amount of clothing on, and on the same scale. When any of these standards are unavoidably changed, the documentation should reflect this change.

MEASURING INTAKE AND OUTPUT

You do not need to measure intake and output (I&O) for all clients because it is not always cost-efficient. Rather, this assessment is commonly seen in the acute care setting, where clients are at higher acuity levels and at greater risk for complications. In chronic care settings, measurements of I&O become important only when the client actually presents with manifestations of fluid volume deficit or excess.

Most clients in a chronic care setting are elderly. Since dehydration is the most common fluid imbalance in this group, prevention is the key. Giving fluids frequently throughout the day and early evening usually prevents this problem. However, if a client develops an actual deficit with signs of altered tissue perfusion, it is time to start tracking her I&O. Also monitor

I&O for any client at risk for or experiencing an actual fluid volume deficit or excess. This includes all settings, even the home.

When the problem is fluid overload, it is more accurate to assess the specific systems involved than to measure I&O. Be alert for progressive worsening and response to prescribed interventions. For example, if the client's primary problem is pulmonary congestion, an increase in crackles would indicate a worsening condition. In contrast, a decrease in crackles is an expected response to independent or dependent nursing interventions.

Remember to measure I&O from all sources. Intake includes fluids taken orally, by tube, or by IV. Fluid output also includes all sources, such as urine, diarrhea, vomitus, suction, wound drainage, diaphoresis, hyperventilation, or other drainage. Two other factors should also be considered. **Insensible fluid loss** is fluid lost through means imperceptible to the senses, such as through normal breathing and through the skin. **Sensible fluid loss** is fluid lost through means perceptible to the senses, such as through hyperventilation or diaphoresis.

In situations such as critical care or neonatal care, it may be necessary to compare the weight of the clean product (e.g., linens, pads) with the weight of the soiled product. The difference in grams is equal to the output in milliliters.

To perform an I&O measurement accurately, use the appropriate measurement device for the quantity being measured (such as a medicine cup for amounts less than 30 mL, or a graduated cylinder to measure 100 to 1,000 mL for larger amounts). Other tools required include appropriate documentation forms, such as an I&O form (Fig. 31–6).

It is essential to document and communicate the amount of IV fluid that is left hanging for the next shift to count. This is known as the "credit." For example, if a client receives 1,000 mL IV every 8 hours and had 600 mL from the current bag and 400 mL from the previous IV bag, the credit for the next shift, from the current 1,000 mL bag, is 400 mL. If you use a pump form of delivery, you may just clear the 8 hour intake of feeding or IV fluid and leave the next shift with a starting base of 0 instead of a credit.

Other essential tools include appropriate elimination collection devices (fracture pan or regular bedpan, specimen collection devices for toilet or commode, or urinal) and clean disposable gloves. Some fluid collection devices have graduations marked on the container. It is acceptable to use these if the measurement can be made accurately.

Adaptation to the home setting includes teaching the client and family how to keep a diary of fluid intake and output. Suggest a simple notebook with a column for the client's sources of intake, a column for measured output, a column for date and time (if appropriate), and a column for other essential data (such as a description of drainage). Graduated measuring cups normally used for cooking purposes will facilitate accuracy. Other supplies—such as a graduated

Elkins Park Medical Center

Intake and Output Record

Date:		2200 – 0600		0600 – 1400		1400 – 2200	
Intake	Oral						
	Tube feeding						
	Intravenous	Intake	Credit	Intake	Credit	Intake	Credit
	Primary						
	Secondary						
	Blood products						
	TPN						
	Other						
Output	Urine						
	Gastric						
	Emesis						
	Suction						
	Stool						
	Other						
Total 24° Intake =				**Total 24° Output =**			

Figure 31–6. I&O form. A standard I&O form should include all of the common sources of intake and output to provide cues to the caregiver. Compare the trend of the total intake and output with weight changes.

cylinder, specimen pan, bedpan, or urinal—may need to be purchased at a local pharmacy or medical supply outlet.

Tools include more than equipment: knowledge is also essential. For example, you must know which clients should be placed on I&O monitoring. Although collaboration with the physician is vital, measurement of I&O is an independent nursing function. This requires knowledge of who is at risk for or has an actual fluid imbalance, as well as appropriate assessment skills.

Your assessment should include the client's and family's willingness and readiness to learn and their level of understanding of the importance of I&O monitoring. It also includes assessing functional abilities, financial resources and barriers, and developmental, cultural, and religious variables. Collaborate closely with the social worker to maximize care that is constrained by financial barriers, such as purchasing a bedside commode or other equipment.

Referring to the case study, Mrs. Thompson was very willing to learn but was not capable of cooking or shopping for herself due to extreme fatigue and weakness. Developmentally, her decreased thirst mechanism interfered with her perception of fluid need. Culturally, she didn't like the prepared food items available at the local grocery store. However, because she raised her children with the strong African-American value of family bonding, she had them as a resource. Daily, one of the children assisted her with monitoring of I&O, grocery shopping, and provision of many of her favorite ethnic food dishes.

ASSESSING EDEMA

Edema scales vary among different institutions. If your facility has an edema scale, all personnel should use that scale to promote continuity in communication and evaluation of client responses. If no scale is available, measure the level of pitting edema by assessing the residual indentation left by pressing your finger into the area for 5 seconds. Document the site, the depth of the tissue indentation in millimeters or centimeters, and the time needed for the tissue to spring back.

Assessment for pitting edema works well with small, localized edematous areas, such as the sacrum, feet, ankles, or tibia. In situations where the edema is more pronounced, however, such as when it involves the entire leg, thigh, or abdomen, you will need a more objective assessment. Because consistency is important, mark the site you are measuring with a marker. Use a centimeter tape to measure the circumference of the leg, thigh, or abdomen. Document the measurement and compare against earlier data for changes. When a client has generalized body edema, called anasarca, weighing is more accurate.

Diagnostic Tests

The plasma levels most commonly used to assist in the diagnosis of dehydration or fluid volume deficit are plasma sodium, plasma and urine osmolality, hematocrit, and blood urea nitrogen (BUN). The sodium ion is used as a direct measure of osmolality because it is the major ion in extracellular fluid. Plasma sodium, osmolality, hematocrit, and BUN levels are elevated in fluid volume deficit. Urine osmolality is also increased secondary to the release of antidiuretic hormone and aldosterone. The kidney still excretes an obligatory amount of urine to rid the body of waste products of metabolism; this is about 30 mL of urine per hour.

Urine osmolality is measured and reported by the laboratory. Less commonly, you may be asked to test specific gravity using a test tube and a floating urinometer. If you test urine specific gravity on the unit, obtain enough urine to half fill the test tube, spin the urinometer inside the test tube, and read the level of the calibrated mark on the urinometer as it is spinning. Normal specific gravity is 1.003 to 1.030.

Osmolality measurement is often ordered when the concentrating ability of the kidney is being evaluated. This function is significant because, if the kidney cannot concentrate urine, the client loses more fluid and develops a fluid volume deficit. Remember that, in the body, it is the *relationship* of the solute (such as sodium, protein, glucose, or urea) to the solvent (water) that determines the body's response, not the level itself.

Decreased BUN, decreased hematocrit, decreased plasma sodium, and decreased plasma osmolality are classic laboratory findings in fluid volume excess. These diagnostic studies represent the relationship of the solvent (water) to the solute in the plasma. In fluid volume excess, the proportion of water exceeds the normal amount found in the vascular compartment. Therefore, the sodium, urea, and red blood cells appear to be decreased when actually they are just diluted.

When plasma levels tend toward the unexpected or the client presents with manifestations that suggest a specific pathology for a fluid volume deficit or excess, the physician will order other plasma studies or diagnostic tests. For example, creatinine levels can help evaluate renal dysfunction, liver function studies can reveal liver pathology, and glucose studies can show glucose intolerance.

Plasma levels are accurate indicators of potassium, sodium, and chloride levels. However, since potassium is primarily an intracellular ion, small deficits in the plasma level are very reflective of a decrease in total body potassium. Indeed, a level of 3.4 mEq/L, a deficit of only 0.1 mEq/L, requires potassium replacement. Alternately, the plasma level of sodium, which is predominantly extracellular, gives a much more accurate presentation of total body sodium levels. A client rarely needs replacement if sodium levels exceed 125 mEq/L.

The plasma calcium level helps identify imbalances but can become a false indicator if the client has abnormal albumin levels, an acid-base imbalance, or hypoparathyroidism. Since 99% of the calcium in plasma is bound to albumin and only 0.5% is free (ionized), the amount of albumin has an inverse relationship to the level of functional ionized calcium. For example, when a client has a protein deficit, less calcium is bound, resulting in an increase in free calcium. The plasma level (the bound version) may appear normal, when in reality the ionized calcium is higher. The reverse is true when a client has an excess protein intake. The client presents with signs of hypocalcemia because of the excess binding of the calcium to the protein, which leaves less free, ionized calcium.

Alkalosis and acidosis also affect the calcium binding and result in similar manifestations. For example, in alkalosis, more calcium is bound and thus less is ionized. So the client presents with signs of hypocalcemia. In acidosis, less calcium is bound, leaving more free ionized calcium. The client presents with signs of hypercalcemia. In any client with critical calcium regulation, a plasma ionized calcium test should be performed to discover the true functional level of calcium.

Magnesium plasma levels are not commonly ordered because they have not proved accurate as indicators of cellular levels. Assessment of tendon reflexes has been suggested as a more accurate indicator of magnesium imbalance than plasma levels. Many authorities suggest that the presence of normal (+2/4) reflexes ensures that body levels of magnesium are normal (Altura et al., 1994).

Another diagnostic indicator of magnesium imbalance is refractory hypokalemia or hypocalcemia. This syndrome refers to a condition in which the manifestations of hypokalemia or hypocalcemia fail to improve even with K or Ca replacement. In many clinical cases in which refractory hypokalemia or hypocalcemia has existed, magnesium supplementation has reversed this syndrome (Altura et al., 1994).

Since the cardiac conduction system is so sensitive to electrolyte imbalance, an electrocardiogram (ECG) is a helpful diagnostic test. The more serious and acute the imbalance, the more grave the changes on the ECG.

Arterial blood gases are essential to properly diagnose acid-base imbalances. If only oxygenation data are necessary, an oxygenation saturation level can easily be obtained through pulse oximetry.

Focused Assessment for Fluid Volume Deficit

Fluid deficit is a common problem. Data collection and analysis will help determine its presence and seriousness. Many pathologies and situations increase the risk for or result in fluid deficit. Recognizing and intervening in high-risk situations or in early phases of fluid deficit are very important to the client's outcome.

Defining Characteristics

The official definition for *Fluid volume deficit* does not differentiate between vascular, interstitial, and intracellular dehydration. Although all compartments are interactive, the cellular compartments are the last ones to be affected by a fluid deficit. This is because the body's homeostatic mechanisms attempt to correct the deficit. Therefore, early recognition and intervention targeted at reversing extracellular fluid deficit will help prevent intracellular dehydration.

EXTRACELLULAR

Defining characteristics for extracellular fluid deficit include muscle weakness, decreased skin turgor, dry mucous membranes, furrowed tongue, soft and sunken eyeballs, tachycardia, a weak pulse, a peripheral vein-filling time greater than 5 seconds, orthostatic hypotension (systolic blood pressure falls more than 25 mm Hg, diastolic pressure falls more than 20 mm Hg, and pulse increases more than 30 beats/minute when the client stands up), narrow pulse pressure, decreased central venous pressure, flattened neck veins in the supine position, weight loss unless masked by third spacing, oliguria, and a decrease in the number and moisture of stools. Muscle weakness results primarily from the altered relationship of fluid to sodium. The decreased plasma volume is responsible for the compensatory increase in pulse rate, orthostatic hypotension, prolonged peripheral vein filling, decreased central venous pressure, flattened neck veins, and compensatory conservation of fluid by the bowel and kidneys.

Note the age-related manifestations of extracellular fluid volume deficit in Box 31–1. None of the manifestations by themselves increase morbidity or mortality as long as compensatory mechanisms or planned interventions reverse the deficit. However, cerebral manifestations indicate an involvement in the intracellular tissues that could result in irreversible cerebral tissue damage.

> *A*ction *A*lert!
> Notify the physician if a client experiences a rapid, unexpected weight loss (more than 3 lb/day); vomiting or diarrhea that lasts more than 24 hours in a child, a pregnant woman, an elderly person, or a person with chronic disease; unexplained tachycardia greater than 120 beats/minute; other atypical cardiac irregularities, such as premature beats or palpitations; blood pressure more than 20 mm Hg below the client's baseline; or signs of intracellular fluid volume deficit.

INTRACELLULAR

Intracellular dehydration is much more serious than extracellular dehydration because of the potential dysfunction of mitochondrial formation of adenosine triphosphate (ATP); ATP is critical to all cell function and transport. Defining characteristics include fever, thirst, and central nervous system changes. Shrinkage of cerebral cells stimulates osmoreceptors in the hypothalamus, which triggers the thirst mechanism. The fluid imbalance also disrupts cortical functioning. Early cerebral manifestations include restlessness, headache, irritability, and a feeling of apprehension. As the fluid deficit progresses, confusion occurs, followed by seizures and, in severe deficit, coma.

Because compensatory mechanisms are so protective, intracellular fluid volume is maintained except in sudden or severe fluid losses or when there is a loss of

---

---

the body's homeostatic ability to compensate for this loss.

> *A*ction *A*lert!
> Notify the physician if the client experiences a fever over 38.3°C (101°F) or a change in mental status, such as a headache (new, unrelenting, or increasing in severity), confusion, or such behavioral changes as irritability, seizures, or deterioration in level of consciousness.

Related Factors

Many underlying pathological and situational factors can cause fluid volume deficit. Excessive output from the urinary system, gastrointestinal (GI) tract, skin, or respiratory system can result in extracellular followed by intracellular deficit if not corrected. Decreased intake, whether from lack of access to fluids, financial constraints, pathologies impairing intake, fatigue, weakness, or the decreased thirst mechanism found in the elderly, is the other major contributory factor to fluid deficit. If excess output and insufficient intake coexist, the client is at an even higher risk for more serious consequences. The following four major variables determine how critical these manifestations are:

- The acuteness of the loss
- The severity of the loss
- The client's age and state of health
- The degree to which the client's compensatory mechanisms or therapeutic interventions combat the deficit

Focused Assessment for Fluid Volume Excess

Defining Characteristics

Again, the official definition of *Fluid volume excess* does not differentiate between extracellular and intracellular excess. Because the cell is the last compartment to undergo shifting (unless the excess is very acute or massive), it is important to be able to differentiate between extracellular and intracellular changes.

EXTRACELLULAR

Box 31–2 provides a list of defining characteristics common in a client with extracellular fluid excess. The excess fluid can be localized to a small area of the body and have little or no effect on overall body function. It can be localized to a specific compartment and cause alterations to specific tissues. Or it can be generalized

throughout the body and cause major system dysfunction. An example of extracellular fluid excess at the local level is an ankle sprain. As the fluid accumulates around the joint, joint function is compromised.

If generalized manifestations of extracellular excess are present, they are secondary to fluid accumulation either throughout the body or in large body spaces, such as in the peritoneum. This is called ascites. As excess fluid accumulates, it interferes with the exchange of nutrients and waste products between the cells and plasma spaces. A buildup of waste products leads to feelings of generalized weakness and fatigue, as well as manifestations of tissue dysfunction.

An example of localized tissue edema that can have systemic effects is pulmonary fluid overload or pulmonary edema. In pulmonary overload, manifestations are related to fluid in the alveoli of the lungs, which reduces exchange of oxygen and carbon dioxide. The fluid pressure in the lungs may also lead to shifting of fluid into the pleural spaces, a condition called pleural effusion. This complication decreases the ability of the lungs to expand during inhalation, and thus can compromise the body's oxygen status even further.

As with any altered health state, the body attempts to compensate. The cardiac signs of bounding pulse, increased blood pressure, and gallop rhythm are all related to the increased volume of fluid in the heart and blood vessels. The bounding pulse and tachycardia are

---

BOX 31–2

CHARACTERISTICS OF EXTRACELLULAR FLUID EXCESS

Generalized

- Weakness and fatigue.
- Body edema (anasarca).
- Pitting or nonpitting edema in dependent areas, such as legs and sacrum.
- Ascites.
- Sudden weight gain of more than 2 lb/week (1 L of fluid = 2.2 lb or 1 kg).
- Peripheral venous distention.
- Peripheral vein emptying takes more than 5 seconds.
- Jugular venous distention (distended neck veins with client sitting at 45 degrees or higher).
- Bulging fontanels in an infant.

Pulmonary

- Progressive worsening of dyspnea, from dyspnea on exertion to orthopnea to dyspnea at rest.
- Increased respiratory rate.
- Respiratory rhythm may become irregular or apneic.
- Crackles present from fluid congestion in alveoli.
- Possible pulmonary edema from severe fluid congestion in alveoli secondary to left ventricular failure.

- Possible pleural effusion with audible pleural rub from fluid congestion in pleural spaces.

Cardiac

- Tachycardia.
- Bounding pulse.
- Hypertension (systolic blood pressure >140 mm Hg or diastolic >90 mm Hg).
- Possible pericardial effusion with audible pericardial rub from fluid congestion in pericardium.
- Third heart sound (sometimes called an S_3 gallop) from left ventricular fluid overload.

Gastrointestinal

- Anorexia, nausea, and vomiting.

Renal

- Increased output if kidney can compensate.
- Decreased output if kidney damage is part of etiology.

examples of the cardiovascular system's attempt to increase cardiac output through increasing the volume of blood ejected with each heart beat (stroke volume) and increasing the rate. The same phenomenon of effusion in the lungs can occur in the pericardial spaces when the heart suffers from increased fluid overload. As with pleural effusion, pericardial effusion not only compromises cardiac function further but also affects tissue perfusion to the other body systems.

The renal response to fluid overload varies. The decreased osmolality will result in a decrease in ADH. If the kidneys are healthy, this will lead to an increase in urinary output. However, if the kidneys are part of the etiology of the fluid overload, polyuria followed by oliguria and then anuria will occur as the renal function diminishes.

Action Alert!
Notify the physician if the client has a rapid weight gain (more than 2 lb/day); a new onset of severe pulmonary difficulty (respiratory rate greater than 30; irregular or apneic rhythm, marked increase in crackles or bronchial breath sounds, pleural friction rub); new onset or increased severity of cardiac manifestations (pericardial friction rub, arrhythmia, more than 5 premature beats/minute, a rate less than 50 or greater than 120 beats/minute, an S_3 gallop); or a change in urinary output (marked diuresis without taking a diuretic, output less than 20 mL/hour for 2 or more consecutive hours).

INTRACELLULAR
Recall that, in a healthy person, protective mechanisms provide a very delicate balance between intracellular and extracellular fluid compartments. However, many conditions can overpower these protective mechanisms, resulting in abnormal fluid shifting into the intracellular spaces. Since brain cells are very sensitive to minimal changes in fluid balance, the early manifestations of intracellular shifting are cerebral.

Action Alert!
Notify the physician if the client shows a change in mental status or cerebral perfusion, such as a new, unrelenting, or worsening headache, confusion, lethargy, irritability, restlessness, or seizures.

The key variable that indicates the need to collaborate with the physician is *change*. This reinforces the importance of thorough and accurate communication and documentation between caregivers. Without this critical communication, client outcomes may be compromised.

Related Factors

Several variables are related to the risk for fluid volume excess. Any increase in fluid intake, sodium intake, or both, especially in the presence of altered excretion, places a person at risk for fluid volume excess. Pathologies that result in increased capillary permeability or protein loss also increase this risk. The same four variables that influence a person's response to

fluid volume deficit also influence her response to fluid volume excess.

Focused Assessment for Associated Problems

The North American Nursing Diagnosis Association (NANDA) began the process of identifying and classifying nursing knowledge in 1973 using a Nursing Diagnosis classification system that focuses on a problem, response, or risk for a problem that nurses can diagnose and treat. However, there are many problems that are not addressed by the NANDA taxonomy that require nursing interventions. These include problems in which the interventions require both nursing and other disciplines in a collaborative effort. Electrolyte and acid-base imbalances are examples of collaborative problems.

Electrolyte Imbalances

Because fluid imbalance rarely exists without electrolyte imbalance, you will need a basic knowledge of electrolyte homeostasis to be able to identify risk factors and intervene early.

CONTROL MECHANISMS
Because of the interactive relationship of water and electrolytes, assessment involves the collection of data that are used to evaluate this relationship. Abnormalities in one or more of the normal control mechanisms commonly cause fluid and electrolyte imbalances.

Assessment of fluid balance through careful monitoring of intake and output and weight provides an early indication of imbalances, as well as providing data for evaluating major regulators, such as the kidney, gastrointestinal (GI) system, lungs, and skin. Excess losses through urine, vomiting, suction, diarrhea, tachypnea, and wounds require early intervention, especially in young, aged, and compromised clients. Anticipate the risk for imbalance in clients who have a pathology or receive medications or treatments that affect the thirst mechanism, thyroid hormones, antidiuretic hormone, aldosterone, baroreceptor responses, and renal or GI regulation of fluids and electrolytes.

In addition to plasma and urine osmolality studies, plasma and urine electrolyte studies, thyroid hormone levels, and renin-angiotensin levels provide data sometimes necessary for an accurate differential diagnosis.

RELATED FACTORS
The same major variables that affect a client's response to fluid imbalance affect her response to electrolyte imbalance. The more severe and sudden the onset of fluid or electrolyte loss or gain, the less the regulatory systems can compensate for the change. The very young and the elderly are even more at risk when sudden or severe imbalances occur due to the greater inefficiency of the regulatory systems.

Pre-existing health abnormalities, especially those that affect regulatory systems—such as the brain, kidney, heart, or bowel—will only increase the client's risk for fluid and electrolyte imbalance. Anticipation of these risks through careful assessment is the key to early intervention and prevention of serious outcomes.

Metabolic Acidosis

Nurses assess for the manifestations of metabolic acidosis in clients who are at high risk. These include clients with end-stage renal disease or bicarbonate loss from severe diarrhea and anyone with hypoxia or hyperglycemia. Neurologic assessments identify early signs of metabolic acidosis, such as headaches and a decreased level of consciousness. Apical pulse assessment detects early cardiac arrhythmias secondary to hypoxia and acidosis. Monitoring for high plasma glucose levels, urinary ketones, fruity-smelling breath, and hyperpnea in clients at risk for improper fat metabolism (such as a client with diabetes mellitus or malnutrition) will provide early indicators of metabolic acidosis. Nausea, vomiting, and diarrhea are early indicators of GI involvement. The diarrhea is secondary to increasing potassium levels. As metabolic acidosis progresses, life-threatening cardiac arrhythmias, extreme muscle weakness, and coma ensue.

Arterial blood gas levels will show a pH below 7.35, a decreased bicarbonate level, and variable oxygen and carbon dioxide levels. If the client has a healthy respiratory system, a compensatory increase in respiratory rate and depth will lower the carbon dioxide level in an attempt to reduce the acidotic state. If the acidosis is secondary to hypoxia, the partial pressure of oxygen will be decreased. Plasma potassium levels are higher due to movement of hydrogen into the cell in exchange for potassium. This is a cellular compensatory mechanism to reduce the acidosis. An exception to hyperkalemia occurs in diabetic ketoacidosis due to the loss of potassium that accompanies the osmotic diuresis from hyperglycemia.

Metabolic Alkalosis

Anticipate metabolic alkalosis in clients who have consumed excessive bicarbonate products, lost excessive potassium and hydrochloric acid from vomiting or gastric suction, or lost excessive hydrogen, chloride, and potassium from diuretics or other medications.

Alkalosis has a stimulating effect on the neurological system. Early manifestations include irritability, disorientation, muscle twitching, and paresthesias. Apical pulse assessment will reveal arrhythmias as evidence of early cardiac involvement. Bowel assessment will indicate a hypotonic peristalsis as the potassium level decreases.

The diagnostic findings are the opposite of those found in metabolic acidosis: a pH above 7.45, an increase in plasma bicarbonate, and a decrease in plasma potassium. In addition, a healthy respiratory system attempts to compensate through slow, shallow respirations. The increased retention of carbonic acid results in an increase in the partial pressure of carbon dioxide.

If the alkalotic state progresses, tetany, convulsions, paralytic ileus, and life-threatening arrhythmias occur.

A_{ction} $A_{lert!}$
Notify the physician if the client has an electrolyte or acid-base imbalance (especially if preoperative), a high risk for imbalance, low or borderline plasma levels, a urine output that decreases to less than 30 mL/hour when the client receives intravenous (IV) potassium, a marked change in bowel sounds in a high-risk client, a new onset of atypical cardiac irregularities or palpitations, or a new onset of confusion or other alteration in behavior.

As noted earlier, many manifestations are common to more than one imbalance. Table 31–5 lists many of these commonalities.

Focused Assessment for Related Nursing Diagnoses

Clients may have one or many varied responses to fluid imbalances. The most common are discussed here. To help make appropriate nursing diagnoses, you can cluster these and other responses into a data set specific for your client.

Fatigue

A client who has fatigue experiences an overwhelming sense of exhaustion and decreased capacity for physical and mental activity. It is a common response to both fluid deficit and fluid excess. This is because fluid imbalance alters cellular metabolism, which affects the production of energy and the metabolism of nutrients and waste products.

Anxiety

A client with anxiety experiences an uneasy feeling from an unidentifiable source. It often coexists with fluid deficit and excess. Fluid deficit that is accompanied by compensatory sympathetic responses (tachycardia, hypertension, diaphoresis, a feeling of tension, and hormonal stimulation) can lead to a sense of anxiety. Many conditions that lead to fluid volume excess also lead to anxiety. This is a result of the uncertainty that accompanies the disease itself or from the pathology that alters the stability of the neuroendocrine transmission.

Altered Health Maintenance

Fatigue and anxiety may lead to a diagnosis of *Altered health maintenance* because the client who lacks energy or feels anxious has difficulty caring for even basic needs, let alone the increased demands of the illness.

TABLE 31–5
Diagnostic Clues to Fluid and Electrolyte Imbalances

Diagnostic Clue	Possible Imbalance	Diagnostic Clue	Possible Imbalance
Thirst	• Decreased blood volume resulting in hypertonic extracellular fluid.	Central nervous system stimulation	• Fluid volume deficit or excess. • Hyponatremia or hypernatremia. • Hypokalemia or hyperkalemia. • Hypocalcemia. • Hypomagnesemia. • Hypophosphatemia or hyperphosphatemia. • Alkalosis.
Weakness, fatigue	• Fluid volume deficit or excess. • Potassium deficit. • Protein deficit.		
Nausea	• Fluid volume deficit or excess. • Hyponatremia. • Hypokalemia or hyperkalemia. • Hypercalcemia. • Hypermagnesemia. • Hyperphosphatemia. • Alkalosis.	Central nervous system depression	• Fluid volume deficit or excess. • Hyponatremia. • Hypercalcemia. • Hypermagnesemia. • Acidosis.
Hypotension	• Fluid volume deficit. • Hyponatremia. • Hypokalemia or hyperkalemia. • Hypermagnesemia. • Hypoproteinemia.	Paresthesias (tingling or numbness) in fingers or extremities	• Fluid volume excess. • Hypokalemia or hyperkalemia. • Hypocalcemia. • Hypomagnesemia. • Alkalosis.
Hypertension	• Fluid volume excess. • Hypernatremia. • Hypomagnesemia.	Muscle cramps	• Hypocalcemia.
Hyperthermia	• Intracellular fluid deficit.	Bone pain	• Hypocalcemia or hypercalcemia. • Hypophosphatemia.
Hypothermia	• Extracellular fluid excess or deficit.	Swelling	• Fluid volume excess. • Hypernatremia. • Hypoproteinemia.
Bounding pulse	• Fluid volume excess. • Hypernatremia.		
Thready, weak pulse	• Fluid volume deficit. • Hyponatremia.	Weight changes Acute weight loss	• Fluid volume deficit. • Hyponatremia.
Tachycardia	• Fluid volume deficit. • Hypomagnesemia or hypermagnesemia. • Hyperphosphatemia. • Alkalosis or acidosis.	Chronic weight loss Weight gain	• Hypoproteinemia. • Fluid volume excess. • Hypernatremia.
Bradycardia	• Hyperkalemia. • Hypercalcemia. • Hypermagnesemia.	Changes in urinary pattern Oliguria Polyuria	• Fluid volume deficit. • Fluid volume excess.
Dysrhythmias	• Hypokalemia or hyperkalemia. • Hypocalcemia or hypercalcemia. • Hypomagnesemia or hypermagnesemia. • Alkalosis or acidosis.	Changes in bowel pattern Constipation	• Fluid volume deficit. • Hypokalemia. • Hypercalcemia.
Kussmaul's (deep, rapid) respirations	• Respiratory alkalosis. • Compensatory response to metabolic acidosis.	Diarrhea	• Hyponatremia. • Hyperkalemia.
Shallow, slow respirations	• Respiratory acidosis. • Compensatory response to metabolic alkalosis. • Severe hypokalemia or hyperkalemia from respiratory muscle weakness.		

Altered Nutrition

It is not unusual for a client with a fluid imbalance to also have a diagnosis of *Altered nutrition: less than body requirements*. Fluid is a major component of overall nutritional needs. As the fluid deficit or excess worsens, the client's appetite and level of fatigue also worsen. This further contributes to a decreased nutrient intake.

Impaired Skin Integrity

Fluid deficit and excess can lead to an impaired skin integrity because of the relationship of fluids to cellu-

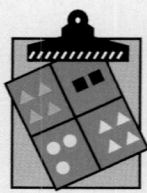

CLUSTERING DATA TO MAKE A NURSING DIAGNOSIS
PROBLEMS OF FLUID BALANCE

Data Cluster	Diagnosis
A 9-month-old child has been vomiting for 24 hours. Even a sip of water does not stay down. The mother has noticed a decrease in the number of times the child's diaper is changed.	Fluid volume deficit related to vomiting, inability to take fluids, and secondary effects of decreased urine output
A 25-year-old man has had violent emesis and diarrhea for 2 days. He is weak and has dry mucous membranes. He states he is thirsty.	Fluid volume deficit related to protracted emesis and diarrhea
An 80-year-old female arrived in the emergency department struggling for breath with audible gurgling sounds. She has crackles and rhonchi throughout the lung fields. She is in high Fowler's position, appears ashen, and has distended jugular veins. Her blood pressure is 220/110. Her family states that she did not refill her prescriptions last week.	Fluid volume excess related to the body retaining fluid secondary to the client's stopping her medication regimen
A 50-year-old man severely decreased his intake of fruits and vegetables in an attempt to lose 25 pounds in 3 weeks on a fad diet. He is also taking a prescription diuretic (furosemide) every day. As part of the diet, he started exercising and developed painful cramps in his calves.	Hypokalemia related to changes in nutritional and exercise habits secondary to a weight-loss diet

lar function. Skin cells require transport of nutrients to and waste products from the cells, both of which are altered in fluid volume deficit or excess. The impaired nutrient and waste exchange impairs cell growth and repair, thus increasing the risk for cellular breakdown in both types of imbalance.

Altered Tissue Perfusion

Both fluid deficit and fluid excess impair the transport of nutrients and the removal of waste products from all cells. Each grouping of tissues has specific functions. Therefore, the manifestations are specific to the specialized functions of those tissues. If enough of the tissue is impaired, it can lead to altered tissue perfusion in that system.

Impaired Gas Exchange

Fluid volume deficit can lead to impaired gas exchange when there is a decreased volume of blood available to transport respiratory gases. Fluid volume excess interferes with the diffusion of oxygen and carbon dioxide between the capillaries and cells.

Constipation

An inadequate amount of fluid can lead to constipation. This is because fluid helps provide volume to the stool, promoting easier transit through the bowel. Although each part of the gastrointestinal (GI) system plays a role in digestion, the large intestine, or colon, plays a major role in the formation of stool volume.

Altered Oral Mucous Membrane

A client with a fluid volume deficit may develop an altered oral mucous membrane because of cellular dehydration in the mouth. This may manifest as dry, cracked lips, bleeding gums, stomatitis (inflammation of the mucous membranes), vesicles, edema, oral pain, decreased salivation, a coated tongue, or halitosis (offensive breath). Another more serious type of oral lesion is leukoplakia, which is a collection of premalignant white patches.

Fluid volume excess can be localized to the oral cavity or be the result of systemic overload. When the oral tissues are swollen, the cells can break down into open lesions or ulcers that may become infected.

Sleep Pattern Disturbance

A client with a fluid volume deficit may have trouble sleeping because of anxiety or other physical problems—such as nausea, impaired gas exchange, incontinence, or diarrhea—that may accompany the fluid imbalance. A client with fluid excess may have trouble finding a comfortable position to sleep, may have pain from the edematous site, or may have difficulty breathing, any of which can result in a diagnosis of *Sleep pattern disturbance.*

The neurons in the brain are very sensitive to fluid changes, whether the alteration is one of deficit or excess. Any change in fluid status alters the chemical function and transmission of nerve impulses.

Action Alert!
Notify the physician when the client's fatigue and anxiety interfere with activities of daily living and role functions, when illness persists more than 48 hours or cerebral or cardiac manifestations are present, when an unplanned lack of food intake leads to an unwarranted weight loss greater than 5 lb, when a wound will not heal with basic cleansing and time, when a wound infection develops, or when decreased tissue perfusion becomes progressively worse. In the feet, for example, you might notice that edema continues to increase, the feet are growing cooler, and pulses are barely palpable. Cerebral effects might include atypical confusion. Also notify the physician if the client develops a new productive cough accompanied by increasing dyspnea especially at rest, constipation that lasts more than 3 days and does not respond to typical remedies, mouth sores that do not heal normally, or sleep pattern disturbances or altered thought processes that persist after a few weeks of treatment.

DIAGNOSIS

When a client presents with a fluid, electrolyte, or acid-base problem—or a risk for one—the nurse uses the health history, physical assessment, and findings from the diagnostic tests to determine whether there is an imbalance or risk for imbalance. When the data support the presence of dehydration, the diagnosis is written as *Fluid volume deficit.* When the data support a risk for fluid loss, as in a client with gastric suction, the diagnosis could be written as *Risk for fluid volume deficit related to increased fluid loss via gastric suction.* If the data support a state of fluid overload, the diagnosis of *Fluid volume excess* is appropriate.

When fluid excess is not present but the data support a risk for it, use the *Risk for* construction. For example, in a client with a recent myocardial infarction, the diagnosis could be written as *Risk for fluid volume excess related to decreased myocardial contractility secondary to myocardial infarction.* Prevention and early detection of these imbalances influence the level of health alteration in the client. This is especially important in clients with fewer adaptive mechanisms, such as the young and elderly, and those with chronic diseases.

Collaborative statements are written in a very similar manner. The electrolyte that is in or at risk for a state of imbalance becomes the focus in the diagnostic statement. An example is *Hypokalemia related to loss of potassium secondary to diarrhea.* If the data do not support an actual imbalance but a risk for one, use *Risk for hypokalemia related to diarrhea.* Each of the other electrolyte collaborative problems is written in this manner by merely substituting the specific electrolyte.

Acid-base imbalances are also collaborative problems. These too, are written in the same format as for the electrolyte imbalances. For example, *Metabolic acidosis related to increased formation or retention of hydrogen and increased loss of bicarbonate secondary to renal failure.* The *Risk for* statements are also written in the same format: *Risk for metabolic alkalosis related to hydrogen movement into the cell secondary to state of hypokalemia.*

Note that in each of the above examples, it is the *related to* or etiology component of the diagnostic statement that individualizes the problem. The etiology is derived from the data.

PLANNING

Planning is an essential part of the care delivery. The expected outcomes must be specific to the etiology of the nursing diagnosis. The goal for a client with a fluid imbalance is to improve the existing deficit or excess. If it is not an actual problem but a risk, the goal is to reduce any risk factors that can be controlled. An example of a goal statement is *Client will improve fluid volume deficit as evidenced by . . .* or *Client will improve risk for fluid volume deficit as evidenced by . . . .* A listing of expected outcomes that are specific to the etiology follows the goal statement.

Expected Outcomes for the Client With Fluid Volume Deficit

Each expected outcome for fluid volume deficit focuses on measurable data that indicate an improvement in the client's fluid deficit. Some examples include the following:

- Increase in fluid intake to at least 1,500 mL/24 h (unless contraindicated)
- Mucous membranes moist
- Absence of tongue furrows
- Absence of tenting when skin turgor assessed
- Neck veins full in a supine position
- Absence of orthostatic hypotension
- Presence of full-volume peripheral pulsations ($\frac{2}{3}$ or $\frac{3}{4}$ scale)
- Plasma osmolality, hematocrit, sodium, and urine specific gravity within normal limits
- Client relates the need for, amount, and type of increased fluid intake during periods of excess loss

Again, the expected outcomes are specific to the etiology. If knowledge deficit is part of the etiology, then *relates the need for . . .* is an example of how to write an outcome criterion focusing on lack of knowledge.

The acuteness and severity of the deficit also influence the focus of the expected outcomes. In very acute states, the expected outcomes address the return to a hemodynamic state in the most critical tissues of the

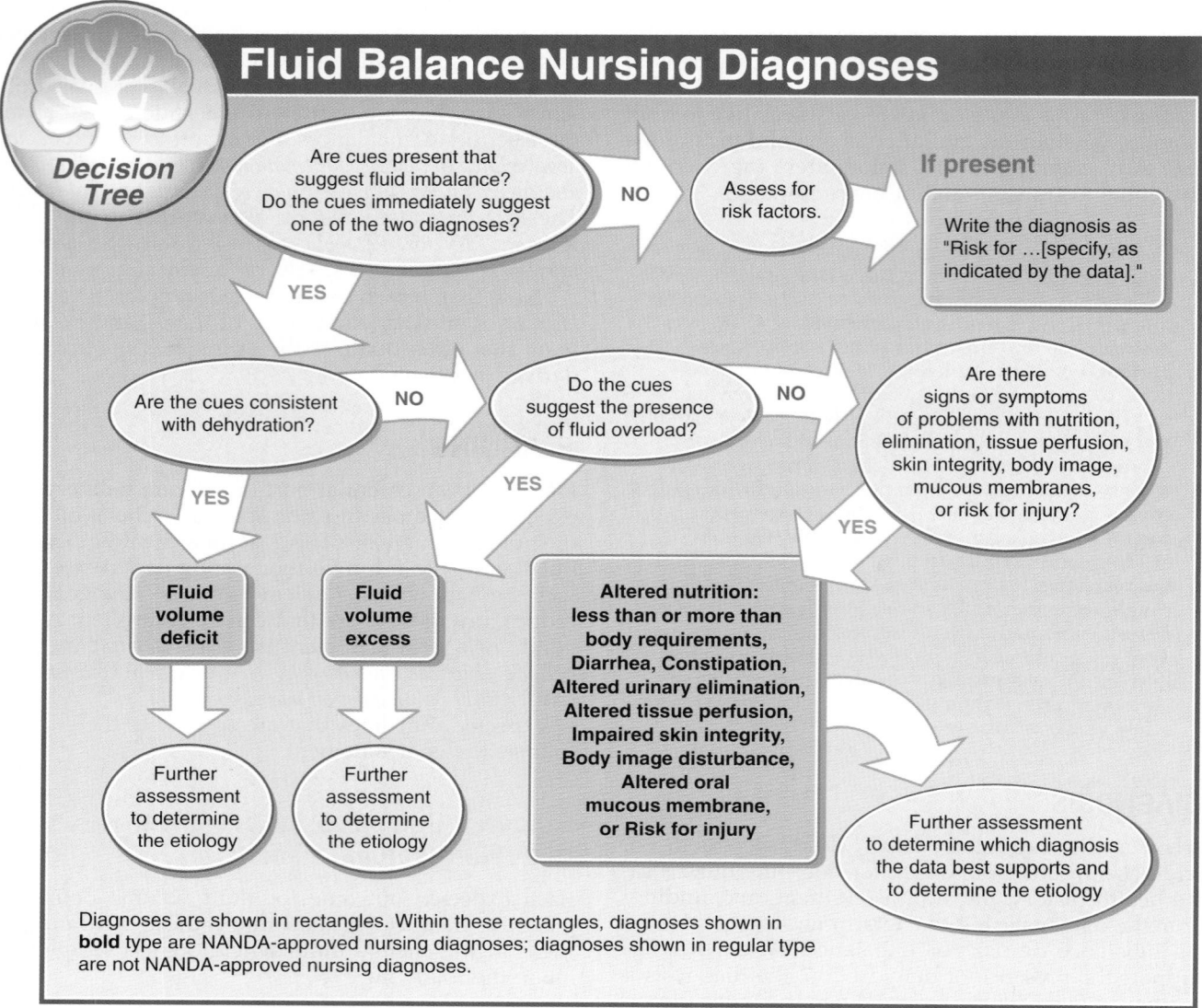

Fluid Balance Nursing Diagnoses

Decision Tree

Are cues present that suggest fluid imbalance? Do the cues immediately suggest one of the two diagnoses?

NO → Assess for risk factors. → **If present** → Write the diagnosis as "Risk for ...[specify, as indicated by the data]."

YES ↓

Are the cues consistent with dehydration? — NO → Do the cues suggest the presence of fluid overload? — NO → Are there signs or symptoms of problems with nutrition, elimination, tissue perfusion, skin integrity, body image, mucous membranes, or risk for injury?

YES ↓ (dehydration)

Fluid volume deficit → Further assessment to determine the etiology

YES ↓ (fluid overload)

Fluid volume excess → Further assessment to determine the etiology

YES ↓

Altered nutrition: less than or more than body requirements, Diarrhea, Constipation, Altered urinary elimination, Altered tissue perfusion, Impaired skin integrity, Body image disturbance, Altered oral mucous membrane, or Risk for injury

→ Further assessment to determine which diagnosis the data best supports and to determine the etiology

Diagnoses are shown in rectangles. Within these rectangles, diagnoses shown in **bold** type are NANDA-approved nursing diagnoses; diagnoses shown in regular type are not NANDA-approved nursing diagnoses.

---

brain, heart, and kidney. Examples of expected outcomes in this situation include the following:

- Absence of confusion, lethargy, hallucinations, seizures
- Decrease in myocardial arrhythmias
- Increase in blood pressure to within normal range
- Increase in pulse volume (⅔ or ¾ scale)
- Increase in urinary output with decrease in urine osmolality to within normal limits

Expected Outcomes for the Client With Fluid Volume Excess

Expected outcomes for fluid volume excess also focus on measurable data that indicate an improvement in the state of fluid overload. Some examples include the following:

- Decrease in peripheral edema, as from 3+ to 2+
- Weight loss in an amount specific to the aggressiveness of the treatment

- Decreasing fatigue and weakness
- Decreasing dyspnea
- Absence of jugular venous distention at 45-degree elevation
- Plasma osmolality, hematocrit, sodium level, and urine specific gravity within normal limits
- Client reporting knowledge of foods and fluids limited on low-sodium diet
- Client reporting correct technique and importance of weighing herself

The etiology again directs the choice of outcome criteria. The last two examples would be indicative of a client who had a knowledge deficit of behaviors specific to diet and weighing.

Examples of outcome criteria that are more specific to acute fluid overload again relate to the following manifestations of involvement of the brain, heart, and kidney:

- Absence of confusion, lethargy, hallucinations, seizures

- Decrease in myocardial arrhythmias
- Absence of bounding blood pressure and pulse
- Decrease in pulmonary crackles
- Improvement in blood pressure, pulse, respiratory response to activity
- Increase in urine osmolality to within normal limits

Expected Outcomes for the Client With Associated Problems

Because the planning for electrolyte and acid-base problems involves collaboration with other disciplines, the goal statement is written differently. The expected outcomes are preceded by the phrase: *The nurse will monitor the client for . . .* instead of *Client will improve . . . .* Goals and expected outcomes related to electrolyte and acid-base deficits also require focusing on the specific data obtained from the client assessment. Examples of hypokalemia and metabolic alkalosis are as follows. With a diagnosis of hypokalemia, the nurse will monitor the client for the following:

- Potassium level greater than 3.5 mEq/L
- Decrease in cardiac arrhythmias (less than 5 premature beats/minute)
- Absence of U wave on electrocardiogram (ECG)
- Improved bowel sounds, active in all four quadrants.

With a diagnosis of metabolic alkalosis, the nurse will monitor the client for the following:

- Plasma pH between 7.35 and 7.45
- Plasma bicarbonate between 23 and 26 mEq/L
- Improved level of consciousness with no seizures
- Respirations deep and regular at 16 to 20/minute
- Less than 5 premature beats/minute

Examples of goals and outcome criteria specific to electrolyte and acid-base excess are as follows. With a diagnosis of hyperkalemia, the nurse will monitor the client for the following:

- Plasma potassium level less than 5.0 mEq/L
- Less than 5 premature beats/minute
- Absence of tented T waves on ECG
- Decrease in number of diarrheal stools

With a diagnosis of metabolic acidosis, the nurse will monitor the client for the following:

- Plasma pH between 7.35 and 7.45
- Plasma bicarbonate between 23 and 26 mEq/L
- Improved level of consciousness, absence of coma, improved signs of orientation
- Respirations deep and regular at 16 to 20/minute
- Less than 5 premature beats/minute

INTERVENTION

Interventions to Reduce the Risk of Fluid Volume Deficit

There are three main categories of interventions to consider in reducing a client's risk for fluid volume deficit: teaching the client about fluid needs, preventing excessive fluid deficits, and restoring lost fluids.

Teaching the Client About Fluid Needs

Health teaching is a primary nursing intervention to support fluid needs in well clients. This includes information to support fluid needs when the body is in a resting state as well as in a state of activity. Remind clients to increase their fluid intake during hot weather, when working or exercising in the heat, during periods of heightened stress, and during pregnancy.

For normal cellular function, a well adult needs 2 to 2½ L of water daily, school-aged children need 100 to 110 mL/kg/day, toddlers need 120 to 135 mL/kg/day, and infants need 70 to 100 mL/kg/day (Newmark & Nugent, 1993). This amount will change when illness or other factors alter normal body functions.

Changing the fluid intake must be within the client's capabilities. Clients confined to bed, or those extremely weakened or fatigued, and those confined by treatments may need assistance. Collaborate with the dietitian, the physician, the client, and her family to achieve a level of intake that maximizes the client's state of health. The accompanying self-care instructions can help your clients reduce their risk of fluid volume deficit.

Preventing Excessive Fluid Deficits

The second major intervention is to prevent excessive fluid deficits related to increased activity levels, medication use, or hypertonic feedings. Fluid needs during exercise can be met in most circumstances by following the recommendations in the Teaching for Wellness chart. Even clients who take medications to promote water loss need to have the recommended daily amount of water unless the physician has prescribed otherwise.

When a hypertonic feeding reaches the small bowel, it increases the risk of fluid shifting into the bowel from the other compartments in an attempt to offset the state of hypertonicity. These shifts can result in fluid deficit in those compartments, as well as diarrhea, which further compromises the state of fluid deficit.

Fluid loss with hypertonic feedings can be avoided by providing fluid to equal 1 mL/kilocalorie (kcal). Calculate the difference between the kilocalories in the feeding and the volume of liquid, and give the difference in water boluses divided over 24 hours. For example, for a client receiving 2,160 kcal in 1,440 mL of feeding over 24 hours, the difference of 720 can be divided by 6 (1 bolus every 4 hours). Giving an additional 120 mL of water every 4 hours will not only keep the tube from plugging but also provide the additional water needed to prevent the dehydration that can result from hypertonic feedings.

Restoring Lost Fluids

The third major intervention is to restore fluid lost during mild illnesses to prevent actual fluid deficit.

Taking 30 to 100 mL of fluid every hour during illness can prevent a fluid deficit from occurring. Choose fluids that are preferred by the client, contain electrolytes, and are nonacidic. Cool fluids are better tolerated and absorbed faster from the stomach. Placing the fluids within the client's reach and in nonspilling cups or with covers and straws will improve access for the more debilitated client. Thickened liquids are safer for the client with dysphagia.

Interventions to Increase Fluid Volume

There are four major categories of interventions to increase fluid volume: restoring fluid balance, prevent-

ing further loss, instituting rehabilitative care, and administering intravenous (IV) therapy.

Restoring Fluid Balance

The normal maintenance fluid is not enough when a person is experiencing an actual moderate to severe fluid loss. The physician's directive to "force fluids" usually means to provide twice the amount of recommended daily intake, or 3,000 mL. You will then need to calculate the client's fluid intake per shift. Usually, the goal for the day shift is to give three-fifths of the total fluid prescription; the evening shift and night shift often divide the remaining amount. For example, if the prescription is for 3,000 mL/24 h, the day shift attempts to achieve an intake of 1,800 mL, the evening shift 800 mL, and the night shift 400 mL. The client at home may find it useful to plan the intake around three meals and three periods between meals. The client needing 3,000 mL would thus drink two 8-ounce glasses of fluid with each meal. Alternatively, for a period of 16 waking hours, the client could choose to drink 12 ounces every 2 hours. Careful measurement and documentation of intake and output (I&O) and weights are critical to the evaluation of the client's progress toward the goal of improved fluid balance.

If the fluid loss is related to exercise, follow these guidelines:

- Gradually rehydrate an alert adolescent or adult (cold water, 1 to 2 L over 2 to 4 hours).
- Rehydrate the unconscious client with IV fluids (dextrose 5% in normal saline) up to 800 mL/h depending on pre-existing contraindications.
- If the client is hyperthermic, lower her body temperature by moving her to a shady area and applying ice packs to her neck, axilla, and groin. Establish evaporative surfaces through sponge baths with towel drying of skin and changing washcloths frequently. Promote heat loss through convection by using a fan. Administer niacin, if prescribed, to promote a cutaneous flush. Monitor I&O, vital signs, and fluid status hourly (Maughan, 1992).
- Remember that thirst is not a reliable indicator of the need for fluid replacement. Two percent to 3% of body weight can be lost before thirst is stimulated. Replacing fluids only until thirst is relieved can result in one-half to two-thirds of the lost fluid lost not being replaced (Reherer, 1994).

Preventing Further Loss

The second major intervention is to provide supportive care to prevent further fluid loss. In addition to fluid replacement, interventions should be individualized to the etiology of the fluid loss. For example, when diarrhea or vomiting is present, antidiarrheal or antiemetic medications are appropriate. When loss is secondary to diaphoresis, choose appropriate interventions such as controlling fevers with medications that fight the etiology of the fever and giving prescribed antipyretics and removing excess bed linens.

Teaching for WELLNESS

PREVENTING EXERCISE-RELATED FLUID VOLUME DEFICIT

Purpose: To maintain hydration during exercise.

Rationale: The type and length of exercise, age of the client, weather, and fluid status before exercise can influence fluid balance.

Expected Outcome: The client will understand and respond to the relationship between fluids and exercise.

Client Instructions

- Avoid rapid replacement of fluids because it only overflows to the gastrointestinal tract and kidneys.
- Drink 8 ounces of cold water 15 minutes before exercise. Cold water lowers the gastrointestinal temperature faster.
- Drink 8 to 12 ounces of fluid (5 ounces for a child) for each 20 to 30 minutes of exercise. Another rule of thumb is to drink a pint of water for each pound of weight lost during exercise.
- Cold water is the preferred fluid for replacement for loss secondary to exercise. Sports drinks have no advantage over water in maintaining plasma volume or electrolyte concentrations. They also do not improve intestinal absorption. However, their carbohydrate content may enhance performance.

- Take breaks during strenuous exercise, especially in hot or humid conditions.
- Avoid diuretics. If your physician has prescribed one for you, ask about its safety during exercise.
- Avoid wearing excess clothing during exercise because it reduces evaporation. If possible, wear one layer of absorbent clothing, expose as much skin as possible, and replace wet garments with dry ones.
- Follow your physician's conditioning recommendations. For example, start an exercise program with a few minutes daily. Over time, increase to 30 minutes of aerobic exercise at least three times weekly.
- Use extra caution if you are obese because obesity impairs the sweating mechanism.
- Use extra caution with children because they have a less efficient thermoregulation response, decreased sweat output, and a slower rate of acclimatization.
- Use extra caution if you take medications that impair thermoregulation, such as thyroid hormones, amphetamines, haloperidol, antihistamines, anticholinergics, phenothiazines, and benztropine.

Adapted from Maughan, R.J. (1992). Fluid balance and exercise. *International Journal of Sports Medicine, 13,* S132–S135.

Instituting Rehabilitative Care

The third intervention is to provide and recommend rehabilitative care to maximize client and family potential. Teach the client and family the importance of replacing lost fluids, maintaining nutrition, monitoring weight changes, and reporting significant concerns to the physician. The Teaching for Self-Care chart helps clients and families decide when to call a physician. Also, emphasize safety precautions if weakness or orthostatic hypotension is a problem. Safety precautions include changing positioning slowly, using assistive devices as appropriate, and removing scatter rugs or other objects that increase the risk of falls.

Administering Intravenous Therapy

Many routes are available for fluid intake: oral, tube (nasogastric, gastric, duodenal, or jejunal tubes), or parenteral (subcutaneous or IV). The oral route is the most preferred, common, and cost-efficient. Recall from our earlier discussion that maintaining a balance in body fluid is dependent on the total amount of fluid intake from pure water as well as from other fluids and food products. When fluid homeostasis cannot be maintained through the oral route, alternative methods must be initiated to ensure cellular function. For

more information on fluid given via an artificial tube, see Chapter 30.

When a client's homeostatic fluid needs cannot be met through an oral route or tube, or replacement is needed more quickly than either of these two routes can offer, IV therapy is the method of choice. Examples of clients requiring IV therapy include those who receive nothing by mouth, those unable to ingest oral fluids (possibly because of nausea, vomiting, or mental status changes), and those unable to absorb nutrients because of a dysfunctional bowel. Intravenous therapy is also used to deliver medications that would be destroyed by gastric enzymes, when rapid medication response is necessary, or when higher plasma levels are necessary. Clients with life-threatening situations from loss of plasma volume (such as hemorrhage, shock, and severe burns) also require IV therapy.

As with any medication, nurses have the responsibility of following the six Rs (right client, right drug, right dose, right time, right route, and right documentation). Table 31–6 lists common IV fluids, their purpose, and specific nursing implications.

Accurate IV administration requires many skills. These include the preparatory phase for starting an IV line, the actual starting of an IV infusion, regulating the flow rate, administering IV medications, and discontinuing the IV infusion (Procedures 31–3 and 31–4). Cost savings is another essential component of IV therapy, as outlined in the Cost of Care chart on page 768.

EQUIPMENT

Selection of the proper equipment is essential for the safe administration of IV therapy (Fig. 31–7). All solutions and connecting tubing must remain sterile to decrease the risk of infection. To begin, compare the solution to the physician's order to ensure accuracy. Choose the type of tubing appropriate to the site, the type of solution, and the type of delivery. For example, basic solutions including 5% dextrose or saline solutions can be given by gravity flow in a peripheral vein; therefore, gravity tubing is sufficient. The size of the drip factor in gravity tubing varies between microdrip (60 drops/mL) and macrodrip (10, 12, or 15 drops/mL).

Microdrip tubing has less risk of flowing in too rapidly if the IV needle or catheter changes positions in the client's vein. Also, amounts less than 30 mL/hour have to be given by microdrip or on a pump. Use macrodrip tubing when a solution needs to infuse rapidly. Any solution that has potassium chloride in it or any other medication that carries a high risk or needs

precise delivery requires an infusion pump. Solutions given through a central vein (subclavian or jugular) also require an infusion pump to decrease the risk of air embolus. Many IV pumps have specialized tubing. Other solutions, such as many blood products and total parenteral nutrition, require an IV pump as well as filter tubing.

The type of pump also varies. Most pumps are volume-specific. The most commonly used pumps deliver 1 mL or more per hour, but there are also micropumps that deliver less than 1 mL/hour. Specialized tubing is required for some medications, such as nitroglycerin, that can be absorbed by the tubing. Specialized tubing with chambers called burretrols is also available and used with children and critically ill clients to precisely deliver small amounts of fluid or medication. Extension tubing is also available to increase mobility and facilitate position changes.

Often, you will need to "piggyback" a prescribed medication into the client's main IV line. The type of piggyback tubing is manufacturer-specific. Several manufacturers have created needleless IV equipment to decrease the risk of needle sticks.

In addition to the right solution, tubing, and pump if necessary, you will also need additional equipment if you are starting an IV line. After assessing the client's veins, choose the correct needle or catheter, and a tourniquet, gloves, dressing, and site preparation agents (alcohol and povidone-iodine [Betadine]) required by agency policy. The size of the needle or catheter is specific to the type of IV therapy. For example, a 23- to 25-gauge needle or 20- to 22-gauge catheter is sufficient for most IV therapy. Larger sizes, such as a 19-gauge needle, 20-gauge catheter, or larger, are required if you will be giving blood products or hyperosmotic solutions, or if the client is being prepared for surgery.

SOLUTIONS

Many types of intravenous (IV) solutions are available. Solutions are categorized by the *osmolarity*, or number of milliosmoles per liter of solution or, more importantly, by their *osmolality*, how they affect the other fluids they are being compared with. Solutions come in three levels of osmolality: isotonic, hypertonic, and hypotonic. To review, an *isotonic* solution is one that has an osmotic pressure very similar to that of the solution or fluid with which it is being compared and thus does not affect fluid shifting. A *hypertonic* solution is one that has more osmotic pressure than the one with which it is being compared. A *hypotonic* solution is one that has less osmotic pressure than the one with which it is being compared.

Both the *hypertonic* and *hypotonic* solutions increase the risk of fluid shifting between compartments. IV solutions that are hypertonic increase the risk for fluid shifting into the plasma and fluid excess because of the increased osmotic *pull*. *Hypotonic* IV fluids increase the risk of fluid shifting from the plasma to the interstitial compartments and cells because of the decreasing osmolality in the plasma. This concept is discussed

Text continued on page 769

TABLE 31–6
Understanding Intravenous Solutions

IV Fluid	Purpose	Nursing Implications
Dextrose solutions Hypotonic (<250 mEq/L), such as dextrose 5% in water (D_5W)	• Adds water. • Adds enough calories to prevent ketosis (170 calories/L).	• Risk for hyponatremia and hypokalemia if excess. • Need other nutrient source if used for long-term therapy.
Hypertonic (>375 mEq/L), such as dextrose 10% to 50% in water	• Used in total parenteral nutrition.	• Risk for phlebitis and hyperglycemia. • Monitor infusion site and glucose levels. • Client may need sliding scale of regular insulin.
Saline solutions Hypotonic, such as 5% dextrose in 0.2 normal saline or 5% dextrose in 0.45 normal saline	• Adds water (amount varies with flow rate and excretion rate). • Adds sodium. • Adds calories.	• Risk for hyponatremia and fluid volume excess.
Isotonic (310 mEq/L), such as 5% dextrose in 0.9 normal saline	• Adds saline in normal physiological amounts. • Expands extracellular fluid without changing osmolality. • Used to prime an IV catheter before use and flush it afterward, as indicated.	• Risk for fluid volume excess.
Hypertonic, such as 3% to 5% normal saline	• Reverses severe sodium deficit.	• Risk for hypernatremia, extracellular fluid excess, pulmonary edema, phlebitis. • Give slowly to prevent cellular dehydration.
Potassium-containing solutions 20 to 80 mEq/L	• Potassium maintenance.	• Risk for hyperkalemia, especially if client has oliguria. • Agitate IV bag to prevent potassium bolus, which can cause cardiac arrest. • Phlebitis is more likely in a small vein.
	• Potassium replacement. >80 mEq/day	• Risk for hyperkalemia, especially if client has oliguria. • Agitate IV bag to prevent potassium bolus, which can cause cardiac arrest. • Phlebitis is more likely in a small vein. • Keep client on cardiac monitoring.
Ringer's solutions Ringer's (isotonic) Lactated Ringer's	• Replaces fluids, sodium, potassium, calcium, and chloride. • Same as Ringer's except provides lactate-precursor bicarbonate. • Used for metabolic acidosis (except lactic acidosis).	• Risk for fluid volume excess. • Risk for fluid volume excess.
Total parenteral nutrition Hypertonic	• Provides carbohydrates, amino acids, lipids, vitamins, electrolytes. • Provides energy and nutrients for cellular function and repair.	• Give via a central IV line. • Can give via a peripheral line if tonicity is decreased. • Monitor client's glucose levels.
Blood products Red blood cells	• Used for symptomatic anemia because increases oxygen-carrying capacity of blood. • Provides volume expansion.	• Follow procedural guidelines exactly for validating product, assessing client, and administering product. • Use of acetaminophen as a premedication may mask a fever response, which may be the only early warning of anaphylaxis.
Plasma Platelets	• Provides volume expansion. • Given to client with idiopathic or therapy-induced thrombocytopenia.	• Same as above. • Same as above.
Albumin	• Provides volume expansion. • Reverses protein malnutrition.	• Same as above.
Irradiated leukocytes	• Given to client with severe leukopenia or possible need for bone marrow or stem cell transplant	• Same as above.
Antihemophilic factors	• Reverses hemophilia.	• Same as above.

Initiating Peripheral Intravenous Therapy

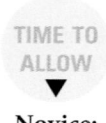

TIME TO ALLOW
▼
Novice:
20 minutes
Expert:
10 minutes

Peripheral IV therapy is the administration of fluid, electrolytes, or nutrients through a needle or cannula inserted into a vein in the arm. Fluid therapy is initiated by inserting the needle or cannula into a vein and connecting it to tubing through which the fluid is administered. The term *peripheral* **distinguishes this form of IV therapy from central venous therapy. Central venous therapy is administered through a catheter in the subclavian vein, jugular vein, vena cava, or right atrium.**

Delegation Guidelines

Initiating IV therapy may not be delegated to a nursing assistant.

Equipment Needed

- Tourniquet.
- Warm moist pack with warm moist towel, plastic bag, and tape.
- IV catheter or needle.
- IV extension tubing, if appropriate.
- IV pole for gravity infusion or infusion pump, if needed.

- IV lock, if needed, prefilled with saline solution.
- 3-mL syringe with Luer-Lok end, pre-filled with saline; needle or needleless adapter.
- IV bag with appropriate tubing attached, preprimed.
- Alcohol or povidone-iodine (Betadine) to prepare the site.
- IV dressing.
- Tape.
- Clean gloves.

1 Prepare for IV therapy.
  a. Validate the physician's order, verify the six Rs, investigate any client allergies, check for incompatibility between solutions or IV medications, and read your facility's procedure manual for specific instructions.

  The six Rs include the right client, right medication, right rate, right time, right route, and right documentation. If you determine that solutions or medications may be incompatible, you may need to start an IV line at a second site unless an existing IV access device has more than one port.

  b. Explain the procedure to the client.
  c. Obtain an IV strip and mark it. Place the strip on the IV bag.

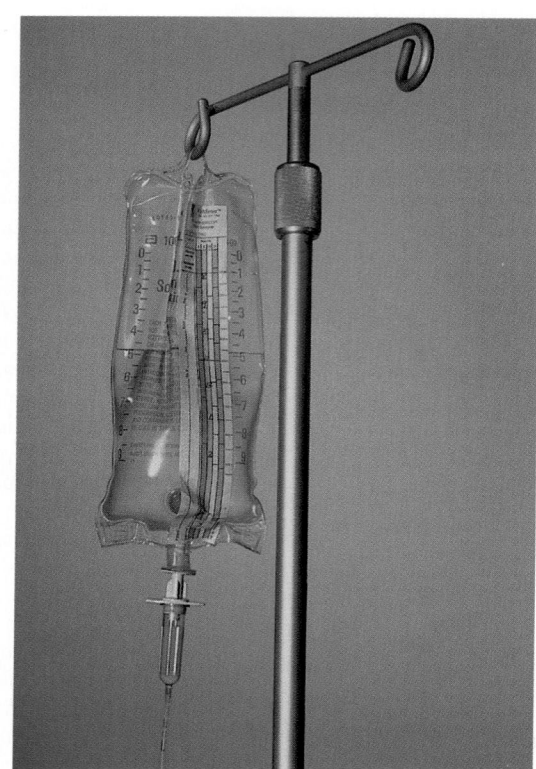

An IV strip on an IV bag.

d. Using the appropriate tubing, close the roller regulator clamp. Then remove the protective covers on the IV injection port and on the IV spike, keeping both sites sterile. Now spike the IV port.

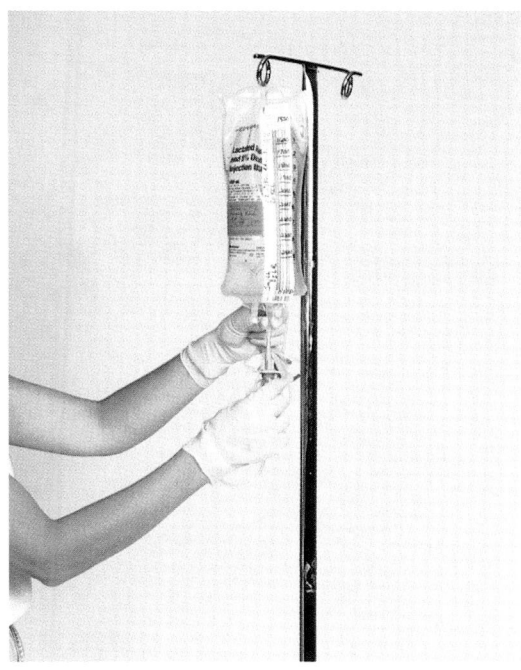

Spiking the IV port.

e. Prime the IV chamber and tubing.

Prime the chamber one-third to one-half full by pressing it between your thumb and index finger. Prime the tubing on a gravity system by opening the roller clamp and allowing the IV fluid to completely displace the air in the tubing. Then close the roller clamp. If using a pump, follow the manufacturer's guidelines to prime the IV tubing. **Never purge the air from the tubing while it is connected to a client's vein.** *Doing so could cause an air embolus and tissue necrosis.*

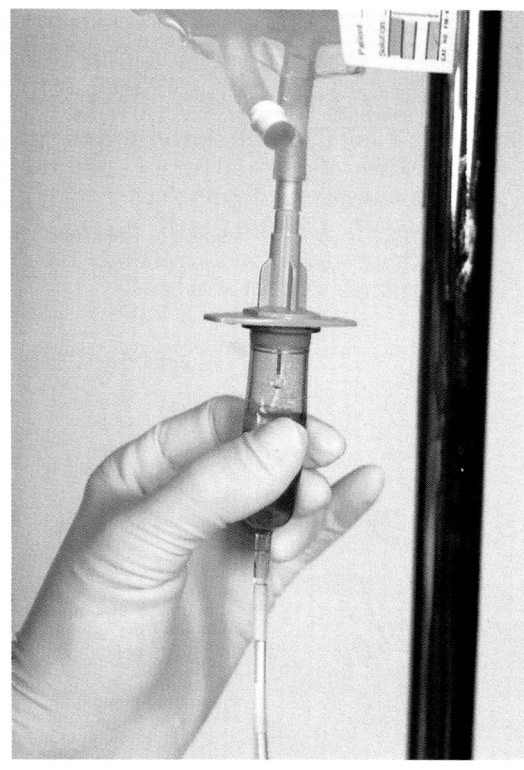

Priming the IV chamber and tubing.

2 Start an IV line.

a. If the client has no IV line in place or an existing line is not appropriate for your current needs, start a new line.

For example, although a 22-gauge or occasionally a 25-gauge catheter is adequate for most solutions, you will need to use a 20-gauge catheter or 19-gauge needle or larger if you are preparing a client for surgery or administering blood products.

b. Don clean gloves and assess the client for an appropriate site to start a new IV line.

Always use the most distal vein possible. Also, avoid using an arm that has had previous lymphatic problems or has been affected by surgery (such as mastectomy) or a fistula.

Continued

PROCEDURE 31–3 *(continued)*

Initiating Peripheral Intravenous Therapy

c. To find a suitable vein, lower the client's arm to below heart level and apply a tourniquet at least 6 inches above the projected site.

If the veins are difficult to see or the client is elderly, apply a warm, moist pack over the site for 5 to 10 minutes and reassess.

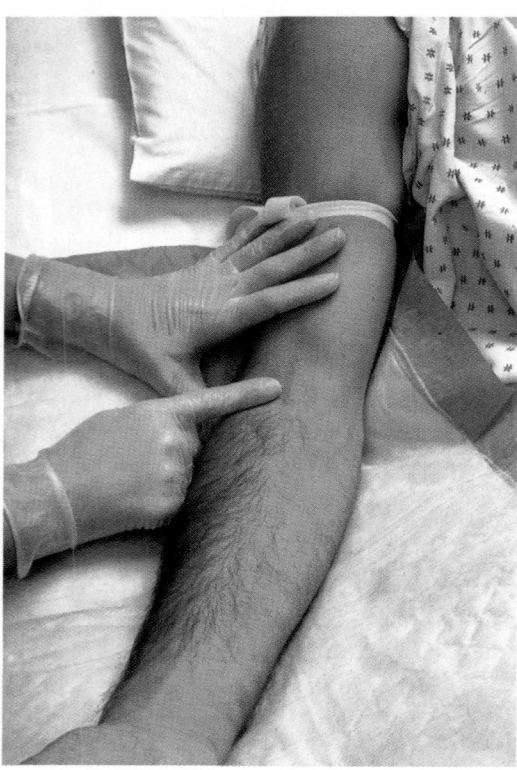

Finding a suitable vein.

d. Cleanse the site as directed by your facility's procedure manual.

Using alcohol or Betadine, start at the point of needle insertion and wipe in an enlarging spiral until you have cleaned a 3-inch circle around the site. Or, if your facility specifies, use two pledgets. Prepare the site for 30 seconds with the first one by applying friction and multidirectional cleansing

around the hair follicles. Then use the second sterile pledget in the circular method described above.

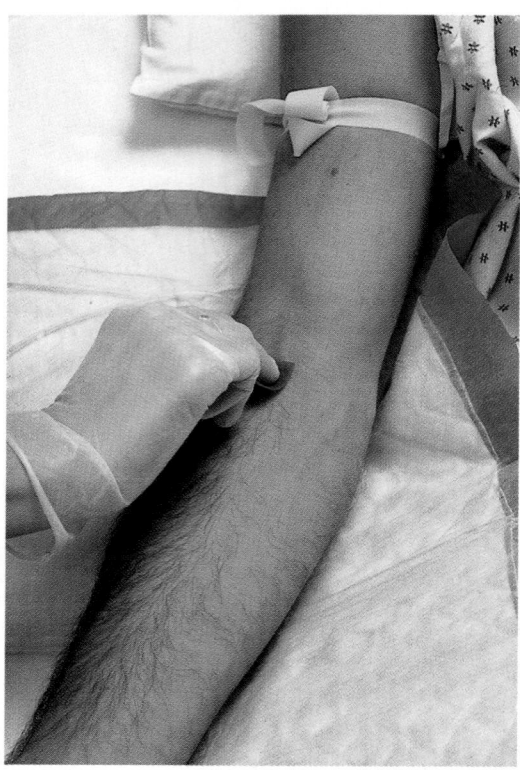

Cleansing the site.

e. Remove the needle or catheter from its protective cover and, with your dominant hand, hold it bevel-up at a 30-degree angle to the skin, either directly over or parallel to the vein.

The direct approach usually works better for a larger vein, whereas the indirect approach often works better for a smaller vein. To prevent the vein from wandering, use your nondominant hand to stabilize the vein from above or below the targeted entry site.

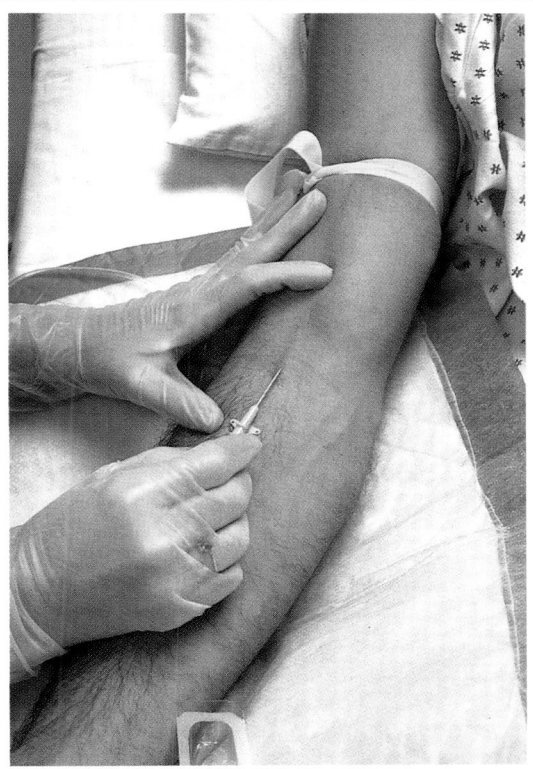

Preparing to insert the needle.

f. Pierce through the skin with one quick motion. As you do, decrease the angle of the needle or catheter to 15 degrees. Continue advancing toward the vein until you see blood return in the catheter or tubing. Then advance a catheter about another ¼ inch to make sure it is well into the vein. If inserting a needle, continue to advance it until the entire needle is within the vein.

If you are inserting a catheter, use one hand to advance the catheter and the other to stabilize the needle guidewire. Do not readvance the needle guidewire once you have begun to remove it. When the entire catheter has been threaded, remove the remaining part of the needle guidewire.

g. Attach the IV tubing immediately to prevent blood loss. Label the IV tubing.

h. Attach a saline lock device. Prime the lock with saline before accessing the vein. Then you can immediately attach the lock when you have entered the vein.

Access the IV port with the prefilled syringe. Aspirate to validate blood return, and inject the saline into the vein. If no swelling occurs, proceed to dressing the site. If swelling occurs, remove the needle or catheter. Keep in mind that some types of needleless systems require the use of the

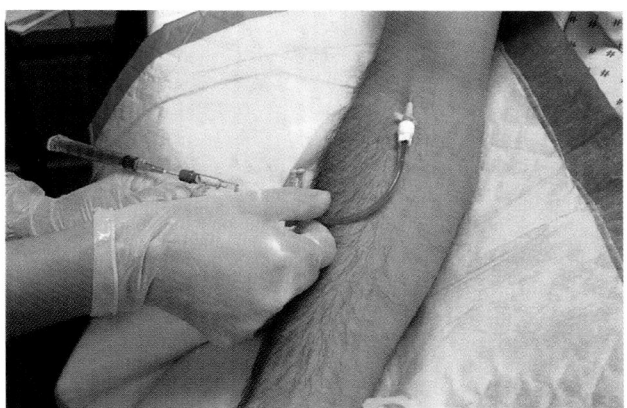

Flushing the IV tubing.

needleless device to access. Others require you to attach the prefilled syringe to the distal end of the tubing until flushing has validated correct placement. Then you place the needleless cap. Follow the manufacturer's recommendations.

3 Dress the IV site following your facility's procedural guidelines.
   a. Transparent dressing
   b. Butterfly tape and gauze 2″ × 2″
   c. Other

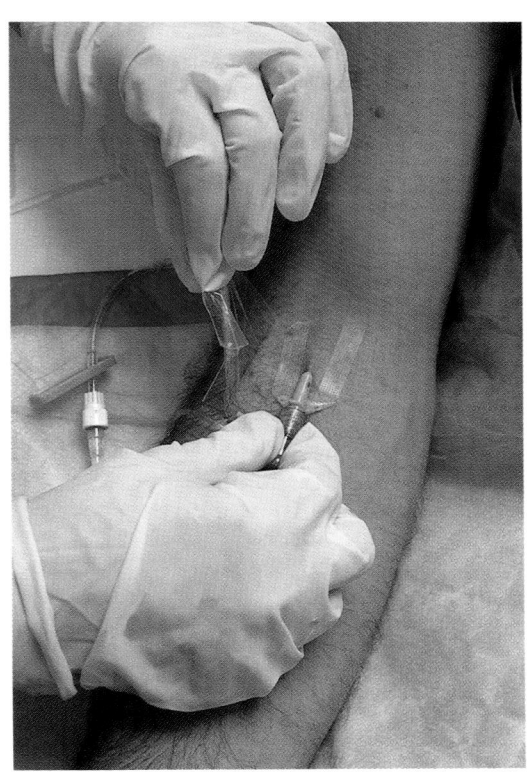

Dressing the IV site.

Continued

Initiating Peripheral Intravenous Therapy

Use an armboard to stabilize the IV site only as a last resort. Armboards increase the risk of altered tissue perfusion.

4 Regulate the infusion.

Regulate the flow of the infusion as ordered. Use the following formula to help calculate the flow rate:

$$\frac{\text{amount of solution} \times \text{gtt/mL (tubing factor)}}{\text{time in minutes}}$$

For example, imagine that the physician ordered 1000 mL D$_5$W/0.25NS to be given over 8 hours. The tubing drop (gtt) factor is 15 gtt/mL. The resulting formula is as follows:

$$\frac{1{,}000 \text{ mL} \times 15 \text{ gtt/mL}}{8 \times 60 \text{ minute}} = \frac{15{,}000 \text{ gtt}}{480 \text{ minute}}$$

$$= 31.25 \text{ gtt/minute (31 gtt/minute)}$$

You can also use the two-step method, as follows:

$$\frac{1{,}000 \text{ mL}}{8 \text{ hours}} = 125 \text{ mL/hour and}$$

$$\frac{125 \text{ mL} \times 15 \text{ gtt/mL}}{60 \text{ minutes}} = 31.25 \text{ gtt/minute (31 gtt)}$$

In other words, when the physician orders 1,000 mL of IV fluid in 8 hours, you will be giving 125 mL/hour. Using IV tubing with a drop factor of 15 gtt/mL means that, to give 125 mL/hour, you will need about 31 drops/minute in the IV chamber. This is about 8 drops every 15 seconds.

Use the second hand on your watch to achieve precise measurement of drops/minute. Keep in mind that movement of the client's arm or a change in arm position can alter gravity drip rates. Also, changing the height of the bag will alter gravity pressure.

5 Monitor and maintain the ongoing drip rate.

You can provide ongoing monitoring by counting the drip rate each hour and by placing a time strip on the side of the IV bag. To manage precise delivery or delivery at a keep-vein-open rate, use an infusion pump. Also use an infusion pump when an IV infusion contains additives caustic to interstitial tissues, when a change in delivery rate increases the risk of dangerous adverse effects, and when the client has an increased risk of air embolus (as with a central line).

HOME CARE CONSIDERATIONS

Intravenous therapy in the home is usually intermittent therapy performed by the nurse. If the medication or fluid therapy is ongoing over days, weeks, or months, it is usually administered through a central venous access route. However, peripheral intravenous sites are also used. The nurse may go to the home, perform a venipuncture, and complete the administration of fluids or medications before leaving the home. However, the nurse may initiate the therapy and teach the family to monitor and maintain the therapy until it is complete. Nurses may need to teach the family to maintain the venous access site and prevent infection. Teaching may include the following:

- Signs and symptoms of infiltration.
- Troubleshooting an IV pump.
- Discontinuing the infusion and removing the IV cannula.
- Observing for side effects.
- Cleaning and dressing the site.
- When to call the nurse.
- When to call the doctor.

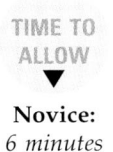

PROCEDURE 31–4

Discontinuing Peripheral Intravenous Therapy

TIME TO ALLOW
▼

Novice:
6 minutes
Expert:
3 minutes

To discontinue peripheral IV therapy, the nurse removes the needle or cannula from the vein and takes precautions to prevent hematoma or infection.

Delegation Guidelines

Peripheral IV catheter discontinuation may be delegated to a nursing assistant who has received training in this skill.

Equipment Needed

- Alcohol swab or cotton ball.
- Band-Aid.
- Clean gloves.
- Tourniquet, if required by your facility.

1 Prepare to discontinue IV therapy. Before discontinuing an IV line, validate the order to do so.
Validation is not necessary if phlebitis or infiltration is present.

2 Don clean gloves.

3 Remove the tape and dressing covering the insertion site.
Remove tape from the skin, not necessarily from the catheter.

4 Remove the catheter.
a. Stabilize the catheter.
   Stabilization prevents unnecessary trauma from an accidental removal.
b. Hold the alcohol swab or cotton ball over the IV insertion site but do not apply pressure.
   Premature pressure can cause discomfort and injure the vein.

c. Slide the catheter out of the vein and promptly apply pressure to the site.
   Apply pressure for 1 to 2 minutes or until the vein no longer leaks blood. Removing pressure prematurely will result in continued bleeding and a bruise.
d. Apply a bandage (Band-Aid) to the site.

---

further under Potential Complications. The primary functions and implications of the most common IV solutions are listed in Table 31–6.

SITES

Sites for IV therapy are categorized as peripheral or central (Fig. 31–8). Any IV line that is inserted into the subclavian or jugular vein or into a peripheral vein and threaded past the axillary line (a peripherally inserted central catheter, also called a PICC line) is considered a central line. The subclavian veins are accessed more often than the jugular veins, especially for long-term therapy, because of the increased risk of phlebitis, catheter displacement, disconnection, and client discomfort associated with an IV placement in the neck area. All other IV sites are considered peripheral IV sites. The most common site for peripheral IV therapy is in the arms. The purpose and duration of the IV therapy, the type of solution, and the age and physical condition of the client are factors that determine the most appropriate IV site.

Avoid starting an IV over a joint to decrease the need for joint immobilization. Avoid the small, thin-walled veins in the hand if possible. This site is more painful and at greater risk for infiltration and limits the client's hand mobility. Also avoid the veins in the legs since their decreased flow rate increases the risk for thrombus or embolus formation. The most recommended site is the most distal site in the forearm above the wrist area. This allows for later venipunctures in more proximal veins. Sites that are compromised by venous or lymphatic flow changes should be avoided. These include veins on the same arm a mastectomy or lymphatic resection has been performed, arms with fistulas or shunts, or those with varicosities or history of phlebitis or thrombosis.

BASELINE ASSESSMENT

To make an accurate evaluation of your client's response to IV therapy, it is important that a baseline head-to-toe assessment be done before the IV therapy is initiated. Repeat the assessment every 8 hours and compare data. Clients with risk factors for overload may need to be assessed more frequently than every 8 hours.

A baseline assessment includes vital signs, level of

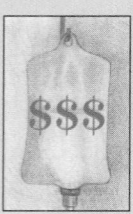

THE COST OF CARE
COST-SAVING ALTERNATIVES IN INTRAVENOUS THERAPY

The cost of health care includes prevention and treatment as well as conservation of resources. Some cost-saving alternatives in IV therapy include the following:

- Promote self-care and family involvement whenever possible, including positive health behaviors, such as fluid maintenance and replacement to decrease the need for IV therapy.
- Use primary prevention strategies to anticipate and prevent complications that could create a need for IV therapy.
- Use gravity flow instead of an IV pump when possible.
- Change IV tubing every 72 hours instead of every 48 hours.
- Use retrograde flushing of primary solution through piggyback tubing.
- Collaborate with other caregivers to avoid duplication.

consciousness, mucous membranes for color and moisture, jugular venous distention, heart sounds, lung sounds, abdominal assessment, peripheral pulses, and urinary output. If the client experiences any changes in status, such as changes in level of consciousness, marked changes in vital signs, shortness of breath, chest pain, or feeling like "something is wrong," initiate a thorough assessment immediately. Consult the physician about your findings.

POTENTIAL COMPLICATIONS
Phlebitis is an inflammation of the intimal layer of the vein. The earliest manifestation of phlebitis is the client's report of tenderness when you palpate over the vein. As the inflammation progresses, redness and warmth will develop along the vein distal to the end of the IV catheter or needle. The catheter or needle should be removed when tenderness is first present to decrease the risk of clot formation in the vein. If the client still requires IV therapy, an alternative site will need to be selected.

Infiltration means that the IV fluid has leaked through the venous wall into the interstitial tissue surrounding that vein. The area may feel hard or cold and probably will be painful. It is possible to still get blood return when you aspirate via the tubing with a syringe, even though the site is infiltrated. If there is swelling distal to the IV site that was not there when the IV infusion was initiated, you must remove the catheter or needle even if you can get blood return. The longer the infiltration continues, the more that

fluid will accumulate and put pressure on the surrounding nerve endings, causing discomfort.

Infiltrated fluid is not functionally useful when it is in the interstitial tissues. Also, if the IV infusion contains medication that is caustic to tissues, it is even more critical that the infusion be discontinued immediately when infiltration is first noted. If this occurs, notify the physician of the infiltration. Depending on the medication, the physician will prescribe an antidote to be given subcutaneously in the infiltrated tissue. Use your procedure manual for further guidance. Table 31–7 lists the common data and nursing interventions for other IV complications, including circulatory overload, infection, air embolism, and allergic reactions. The most common risk factors for circulatory overload include the administration of hypertonic solutions, rapid IV administration, and the presence of renal insufficiency.

SITE CARE
Peripheral
Review your facility's procedure manual for specific guidelines for peripheral IV site care. Studies of peripheral IV infection rates have prompted most facilities to require changing of the peripheral IV site every 72 hours. The type of IV dressing will dictate whether the dressing requires changing more frequently. For example, if an occlusive, transparent dressing has been applied at the time of catheter insertion and the dressing remains intact and dry, it does not usually require changing, since it will be removed when the IV catheter site is changed. However, if the dressing is not occlusive (gauze, for example), it will need to be changed every 24 hours so that you can perform an accurate site assessment. Many facilities require that a gauze dressing be used if a client is neutropenic because a neutrophil count below 1,000/mm^3 increases the risk for bacterial infection. Gauze dressing decreases moisture retention and daily changes increase the frequency of inspection and site care (Treston-Aurand, Olmsted, Allen-Bridson, & Craig, 1997).

Whenever you change a dressing or change or start an IV line, you will cleanse the IV site with an antimicrobial substance. Tincture of iodine (1 to 2%), 70% alcohol, and chlorhexidine are the solutions recommended for IV site preparation. Agency policy dictates the type and order of cleansing. All cleansing is done in a circular motion starting at the IV insertion site and moving outward in a 2- to 3-inch circular motion. Let the antimicrobial agent dry before inserting the IV needle or catheter. Place the date and your initials on the IV dressing.

Central
Many variables influence the physician's choice for the type of intravenous (IV) access device. Among these are cost, ease of surgical placement, infection rates, length of therapy, client choice when possible, quality of vascular tissue, and urgency of placement. Commonly used types include the Swan-Ganz (or introducer) catheter, triple-lumen catheter, tunneled cath-

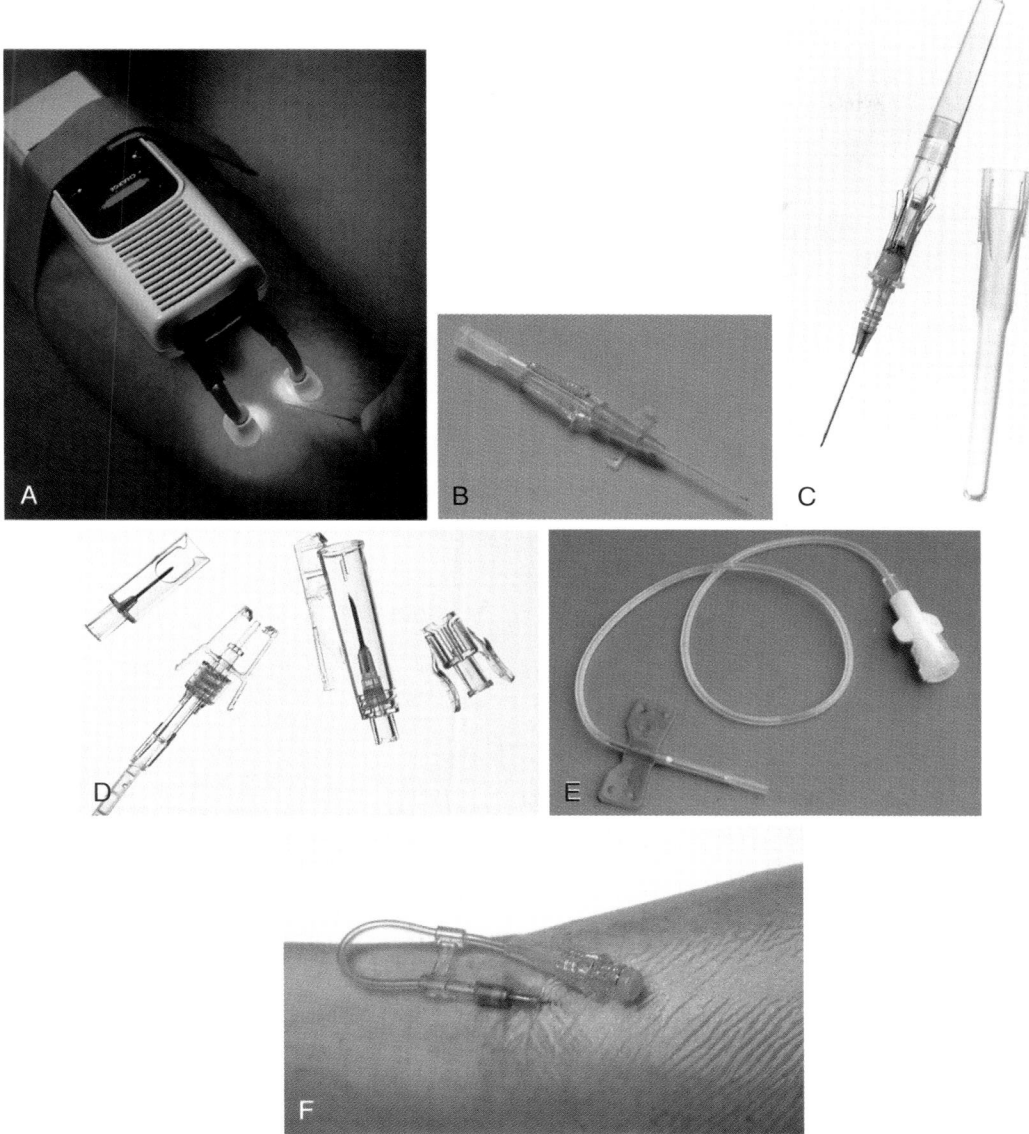

Figure 31–7. Examples of equipment used in IV therapy. *A,* Vein finder (Venoscope); *B,* over-the-needle IV catheter; *C,* Insyte Autoguard IV cannula; *D,* two types of protected needles with locking covers and two types of needleless lever locks; *E,* butterfly infusion set; *F,* saline lock with transparent dressing. (*A* courtesy of Applied Biotech Products, Inc., Lafayette, LA: *B* courtesy of Becton Dickinson, Sandy, UT; *E* courtesy of Medline Industries, Inc., Mundelein, IL.)

Illustration continued on following page

eter (such as Groshong or Hickman, implanted port (such as a Mediport, Infusaport, or Port-a-Cath), and a PICC line. Figure 31–9 illustrates a tunneled and an implanted central catheter.

Regardless of the type of central line used, you are responsible for following the manufacturer's and the facility's procedural guidelines for care and flushing protocols. For example, a normal saline flush maintains patency in a Groshong catheter and in some implanted ports, whereas heparin is recommended for a PICC line and many other types of central lines. The amount of flushing solution varies with the length and diameter of the catheter and the procedure. For instance, you may need as little as 1 to 3 mL of flush to

keep a line open but as much as 10 to 20 mL of saline solution to cleanse the line after a blood draw. If heparin is recommended, it is always the last solution in the flushing sequence because its only purpose is to prevent coagulation in the catheter system.

Follow your agency's procedure manual for changing a dressing on a central line (Procedure 31–5). The frequency of dressing changes for central lines is similar to that for peripheral dressings. When a client is neutropenic, daily dressing changes with varying types of gauze may be mandated. Otherwise, change the dressing every 72 hours. Sterile technique is required with all IV dressing changes, and a mask is also recommended when changing central line dressings.

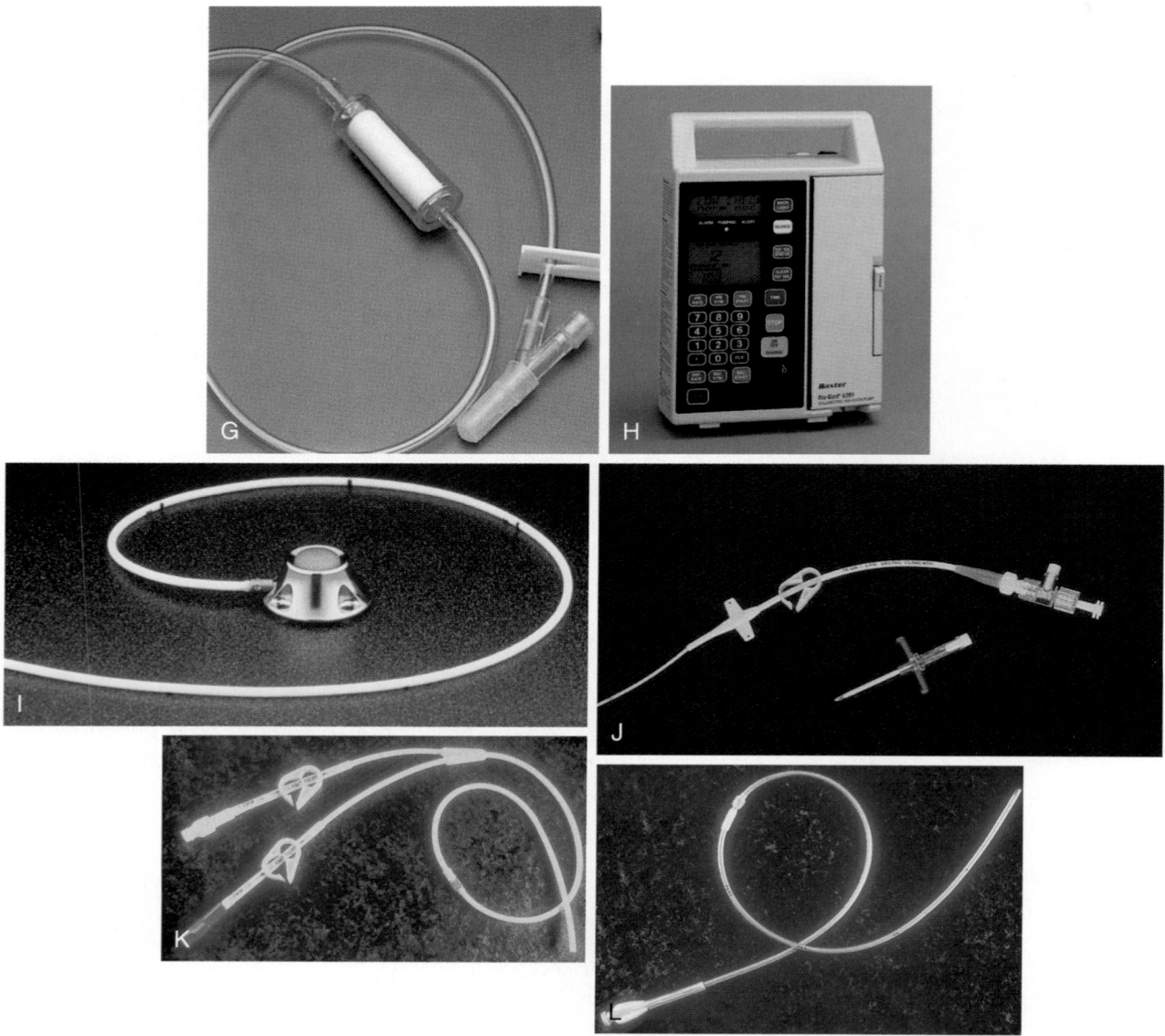

Figure 31-7 *Continued. G,* in-line IV filter (Millipore IV Express); *H,* IV pump (Flo-Gard Volumetric); *I,* implantable vascular access device (PORT-A-CATH); *J,* peripherally inserted central catheter, or PICC (CliniCath); *K,* Hickman catheter; *L,* Groshong catheter. (*G* courtesy of Millipore Corporation, Bedford, MA; *H* courtesy of Baxter Healthcare Corporation, Deerfield, IL; *I* and *J* courtesy of SIMS Deltec, Inc., St. Paul, MN; *K* and *L* courtesy of Bard Access Systems, Inc., Salt Lake City, UT.)

Sterile technique may be adapted to clean technique in the home setting if the client is not neutropenic.

Interventions to Decrease Fluid Volume

There are three primary interventions related to decreasing fluid volume: restoring fluid balance, preventing complications, and instituting rehabilitative care.

Restoring Fluid Balance

Limit the client's fluid and sodium intake. You will need to instruct the client and her family about the rationale for fluid and dietary restrictions to ensure compliance.

Administer prescribed medications. Diuretics are often ordered to help rid the body of excess fluid. Another focus of drug therapy is to correct the etiology of the fluid excess. If the overload is from an ineffective myocardial pump, the physician may prescribe an inotropic drug to enhance myocardial contractility or a medication to decrease myocardial workload, such as a calcium channel blocker or angiotensin-converting enzyme (ACE) inhibitor.

If capillary permeability is the etiology, in addition to treating the underlying sepsis, acid-base imbalance, or other factors, the physician will prescribe corticosteroids to promote healing of the membrane. If protein deficit is present, the source of this deficit is investigated and corrected if possible and additional protein is given if appropriate. The etiologies of fluid volume excess are quite numerous.

Preventing Complications

To prevent complications, provide appropriate supportive care. Monitor and record intake and output (I&O) and weigh the client daily. Compare your findings with previous documentation. Maintain the cli-

ent's nutritional needs, consulting with a dietitian if necessary. To decrease the client's feeling of mucosal dryness that accompanies the intervention of fluid restriction, you can encourage the family to bring hard candies or lozenges, provide ice chips, and give or assist with oral care frequently (up to hourly if necessary).

Performing a thorough head-to-toe assessment, to determine how a client is responding to the interven-

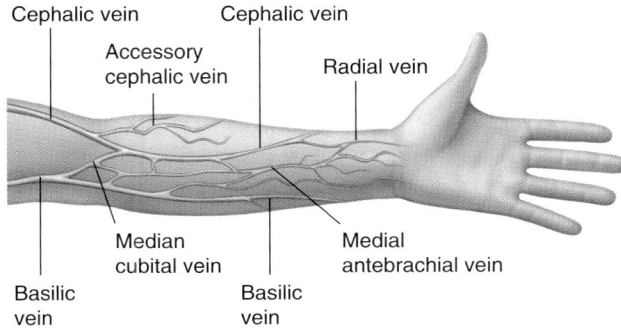
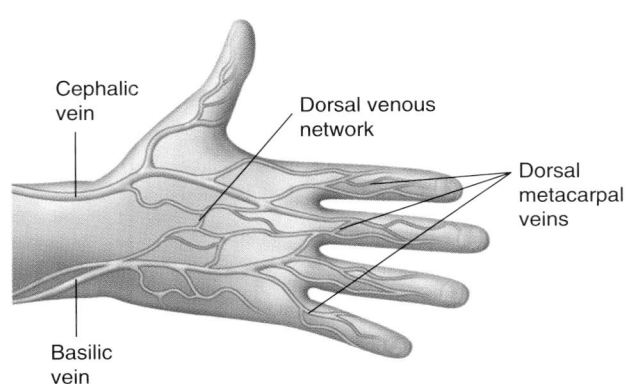
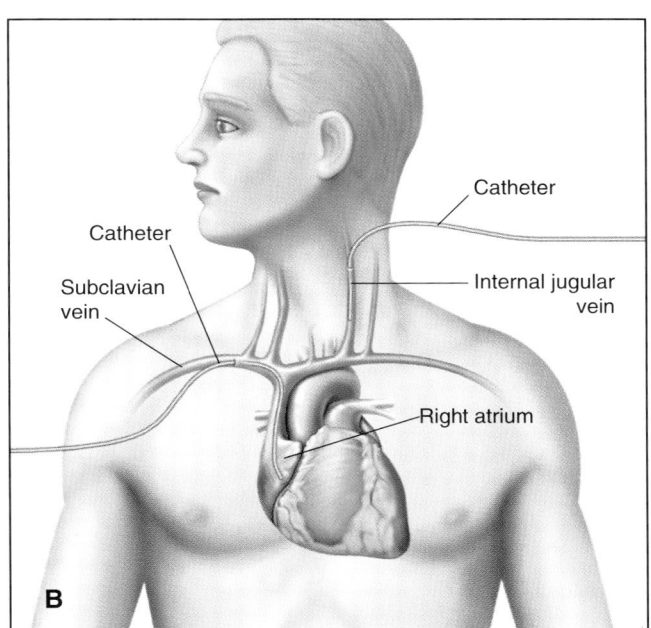
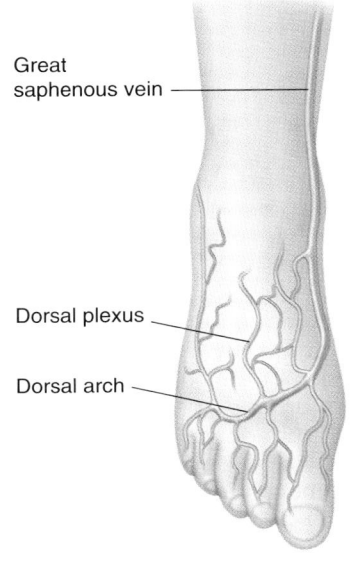

Figure 31–8. IV sites. *A,* Peripheral sites. Sites on the inner arm are preferred. Sites on the dorsum of the hand are often used, but the use of these sites increases the risk of vascular trauma and pain. Sites on the dorsum of the foot should be used only as a last resort because they are associated with an increased risk of thrombi. *B,* Central sites: subclavian vein and internal jugular vein.

TABLE 31–7

Managing Complications of Intravenous Therapy

Complication	Assessment Findings	Interventions	Prevention
Infiltration	• Site is edematous, blanched, painful, cold. • Fluid will not flow by gravity despite confirmed patency of line (blood backflow when bag lowered below site).	• Discontinue infusion. • Restart in opposite arm. • Elevate arm if edema is severe. • Warm, moist pack may be comforting.	• Tape IV catheter securely in place and protect it from being pulled. • Avoid joints when placing catheter.
Phlebitis	• Heat, pain, redness, and edema develop into a streak running along the course of the vein.	• Discontinue infusion. • Avoid massage because it might dislodge clots. • Warm, moist pack may be comforting.	• Dilute irritating medications. • Use smallest-gauge catheter appropriate. • Change site every 3 days or as specified.
Infection	• Same as for phlebitis. • Possible discharge at site. • Possible fever and sepsis.	• Physician will order blood cultures and start antibiotic therapy. • Client may be treated in intensive care unit because sepsis is life-threatening.	• Use strict sterile technique for all IV care. • Change dressing every 24 hours.
Air embolism	• Decreased blood pressure. • Cyanosis. • Tachycardia. • Jugular vein distention. • Loss of consciousness.	• Immediately turn client on left side with head down. • Administer oxygen and monitor vital signs. • Notify physician.	• Remove air from tubing before connecting to catheter (small air bubbles will not be harmful). • Have client perform Valsalva maneuver or place head below heart level while changing tubing on central line.
Allergic reaction	• Minor reaction produces rash, redness, itching. • Major reaction can cause coughing, dyspnea, swollen tongue, cyanosis, unconsciousness, death.	• Discontinue infusion and notify physician. • Client may need epinephrine, corticosteroids, oxygen, or mechanical ventilation.	• Assess client for history of allergies. • Monitor closely.
Circulatory overload	• In pulmonary edema, findings include dyspnea; cough; cyanosis; frothy, pink sputum; jugular vein distention. • Other findings include ascites, weight gain, edema.	• Slow infusion and notify physician. • Verify correct fluid and rate of administration. • Diuretics and sodium restriction may be indicated.	• Take precautions to ensure correct fluid and rate of administration. • Monitor client's intake and output.

tions, is essential to secondary prevention. The frequency of the assessments varies with the acuteness of the fluid overload. Assessments may be needed as often as hourly in a critical-care setting, every 8 hours when the condition has stabilized, or weekly or monthly in a chronic-care or home setting.

Fluid retention impairs tissue perfusion. The interventions for altered tissue perfusion are specific to the organ or system that is involved. Although the goal is to promote optimal perfusion of all body tissues, fluid overload in the heart, lungs, liver, kidneys, and brain must be treated immediately to avoid life-threatening complications.

One of the systems that is often affected by fluid retention is the skin. One of the most common interventions to decrease the risk for impaired skin integrity is pressure relief. Repositioning the client every 2

hours or more as necessary may be enough to decrease the pressure on these tissues. However, if this is not enough, consult the physician about ordering a pressure-reducing mattress or bed. If the edema is localized to an extremity, elevation of that limb will promote venous return and thus decrease swelling. Passive or active range-of-motion exercises five or more times to each joint twice a day will also promote venous return and maintain joint function.

If fluid retention has involved the pulmonary system, elevate the head of the bed to the level necessary for the client's comfort and optimal diaphragmatic excursion. The more pulmonary fluid the client has, the higher the head of the bed will need to be. A client with severe pulmonary fluid overload often needs a 90-degree headrest with arms supported on pillows on a bedside table. Elevating the client's head will also

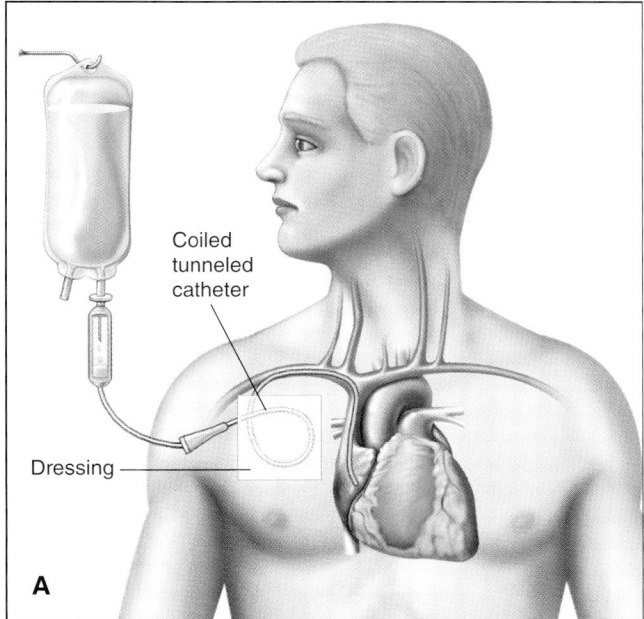

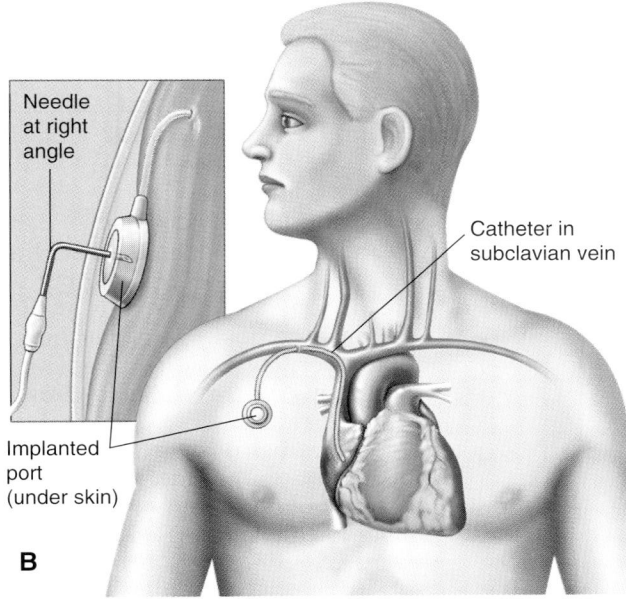

Figure 31–9. *A,* Placement of a tunneled central venous catheter; *B,* an implanted central port. The distal ends of both the tunneled central catheter and the implanted port are in the subclavian vein.

decrease venous return to the right side of the heart and thus decrease cardiac workload. The greater the amount of fluid overload, the more aggressive the interventions need to be. Minimal fluid overload can often be managed with deep breathing, incentive spirometry, repositioning, mild diuretics, inotropics, and calcium channel blockers or ACE inhibitors.

Fluid retention is always a risk with a postoperative client who has received a general anesthetic. Administer fluids cautiously in early postoperative or post-traumatic stress periods. Increased antidiuretic

hormone during this period can cause fluid overload. The presence of or increase in crackles is an early sign of pulmonary fluid and should alert you that fluids are being given faster than the body can tolerate them. An increase in urinary output is an early sign of the end of this phase.

Instituting Rehabilitative Care

Self-care is a major component of rehabilitation from fluid volume excess. Promote self-care by teaching the client and family about restricting fluid and table salt, reading food labels, avoiding products high in sodium, keeping a diary of weights, balancing activity and rest, and calling the physician whenever significant health changes occur.

Additional interventions for fluid balance maintenance include the following:

- Control delivery of fluid by using IV and feeding pumps when appropriate.
- Monitor laboratory results specific to fluid and electrolyte homeostasis, such as blood urea nitrogen (BUN), creatinine, hemoglobin, hematocrit, urine or plasma osmolality, and plasma electrolytes.
- Monitor responses to prescribed medications, including expected and unexpected responses.
- Provide referrals to assist with lifestyle changes and financial constraints as appropriate, such as social services, dietitian counseling, home health care nursing services, and home health aide.
- Evaluate fluid balance in relationship to output and compare data with the client's other presenting data.
- Provide client and family teaching.

Interventions to Balance Electrolyte Levels

When caring for a client who has an electrolyte imbalance, your goal is to decrease the risk for serious consequences. With electrolyte deficits, the goals of the interventions include replacing the lost nutrient, decreasing the rate of nutrient loss, or both. With electrolyte excess, the goals of the interventions focus on limiting intake, increasing loss, or both.

General Interventions

Nutrition is a key intervention in most electrolyte imbalances. Consult with a dietitian for information on specific foods to include or exclude in therapeutic diets specific to each imbalance. Give your client a written handout listing these food items. Keep in mind that dietary changes are among the most difficult for clients to make. Providing resources such as the names of local dietitians or nutrition support groups may help the client with this behavioral change.

Providing practical examples of how to "eat healthier" can also be helpful. For example, you can suggest that the client use fresh lemon on foods and salads instead of prepared sauces. Or, when dining out, the client could request that food be prepared

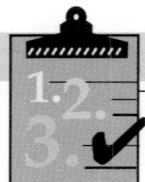

Changing the Dressing on a Central Line

TIME TO ALLOW
▼
Novice:
20 minutes
Expert:
10 minutes

A central venous access line is cleaned and dressed with meticulous care to prevent infection from entering the line. The old dressing is removed, the site cleaned, and the new dressing applied using sterile technique. Infection in the bloodstream (septicemia) is a life-threatening complication.

Delegation Guidelines

The indications for RN assessment and the potential risks associated with improper care of a central line suggest that this procedure not be delegated to a nursing assistant.

Equipment Needed

- Facemask.
- Clean gloves.
- Sterile gloves.
- Three swabs or sticks of povidone-iodine (Betadine).
- Three swabs or sticks of alcohol.
- Sterile, occlusive transparent dressing.
- Huber needle (½-inch to 1½-inch needle with extension tubing) if the client has an implanted port.
- Sterile syringe with saline solution to flush the extension tubing.
- Cap for saline or heparin lock.
- Plastic bag.
- Black pen or marker.
- Bedside table or flat surface for setting up a sterile field.

1 Prepare to change the dressing. Explain the procedure to the client.

Remember that a client with a port that is not accessed does not require a dressing.

2 Remove the soiled dressing.
  a. Don the facemask, wash your hands, and don the clean gloves.
  b. Remove the old dressing with your dominant hand while stabilizing the central line device with two fingers of the nondominant hand.
     Be careful not to touch the catheter entry site.
  c. Holding the old dressing in your dominant hand, use your nondominant hand to pull the glove on your dominant hand off over the the old dressing. Remove the other glove and discard them both in the plastic bag.
     If the client has an implanted port, just loosen the dressing from the skin. Stabilize the port under the skin by pressing on either side of the Huber needle with two fingers of your nondominant hand. Grasp the Huber needle firmly with two fingers of your dominant hand and pull the needle straight out. Place the needle in a sharps box.
  d. Wash your hands.

3 Clean the site.
  a. Set up a sterile field. If a kit is available, don sterile gloves and then tear open the Betadine and alcohol swabs. Check the dressing but do not remove its backing yet. If no kit is available, open the package of sterile gloves but do not don them yet. The inside of the package will become your sterile field. Now, tear open Betadine and alcohol swabs and place them on the corner of the sterile field. Open the outer packaging of the dressing and drop the dressing on the center of the sterile field. If a Huber needle is necessary, open its package and preflush the extension tubing with saline. Touching only the distal end of the tubing, place the Huber needle on the sterile field while keeping the attached syringe at the margin of the sterile field. Open the plastic bag, make a cuffed edge, and set it to the side of your sterile field. Now, don the sterile gloves.

     To do so, grasp the first glove on the top inside of the cuff (so the place you grasped will be against the skin of your arm) and pull the glove over your dominant hand. Now use the sterile gloved hand to grasp the second glove under the cuff and pull it onto your nondominant hand.

b. Using the elbow of your nondominant arm, hold the packaging of the alcohol swab in place as you grasp the swab with your dominant hand.

c. Starting at the site of IV access, use a circular motion moving outward in a 3-inch circle to cleanse the site. Discard the swab in the plastic bag and cleanse the site in the same manner with the other two alcohol swabs.

d. After the alcohol has evaporated (about 15 seconds), repeat the above cleansing motion with the three Betadine swabs.

   Allowing the alcohol and Betadine to mix when the alcohol is still wet can cause skin irritation and alter the bacteriostatic properties.

e. For an implanted port, grasp the Huber needle firmly in your dominant hand. Stabilize the port with two fingers of your nondominant hand. Insert the Huber needle through the center of the port until you can feel the stainless steel back of the port. Using your nondominant hand, grasp the prefilled saline syringe and aspirate. You should get a blood return. Flush the line with the recommended amount of saline followed by heparin if required.

If you do not get a blood return, try instilling 2 mL of saline and then aspirate again. If the catheter is resting against the wall of the vessel, it may prevent backflow. If you still get no blood return, pull back on the needle slightly. If still unsuccessful, have the client cough (away from the catheter site) and change positions. If you still cannot confirm accurate placement, ask the physician for an order for a chest x-ray before giving fluids or medications through this access site.

4 Dress the site.

a. If gauze is recommended, apply it over the cleansed site and tape it according to policy. If a transparent dressing is being used, remove the backing and, holding the edges of the dressing taut, place it over the site so the IV access device is in the center of the dressing. Use the fingers of one hand to smooth the dressing from the center outward to make a tight seal.

b. Use a marker or label to show the date and time of the dressing change. Add your initials as well.

HOME CARE CONSIDERATIONS

If the client or a family member will perform dressing changes at home, teach them how to use clean technique unless the client is neutropenic. In that case, sterile technique is required. If the site has no dressing, teach the client or family member to cleanse the site with soap and water and to place a Band-Aid over the entry site using tape to support the tunneled catheter.

without salt and cooked by grilling, baking, or broiling. The client may also wish to carry along a seasoning that fits the prescribed diet. Also teach the client or food buyer the importance of reading the entire nutritional label for levels of sodium, potassium, and other nutrients. Bold print is often misleading.

When teaching about dietary restrictions, it is very important that the "cook" and other family members be involved. The more support the client has, the more successful the behavioral change will be. Finally, be very clear as to whether the dietary restriction is a temporary change or a lifelong change.

In a client at high risk for malnutrition, especially a client unable to consume nutrients orally, the physician may prescribe a nutritional supplement that contains all of the above electrolytes as well as some trace electrolytes. This may be delivered by gastric or intestinal tube for a person with long-term nutritional

needs or by the IV route in the form of total parenteral nutrition for someone with short-term needs.

Whether the client is experiencing a deficit or an excess, the promptness of the intervention will depend on two key factors: the severity of the imbalance and the presenting manifestations. The following nursing interventions are appropriate to all electrolyte imbalances.

- Monitor the client's liver, kidney, and bowel function. Normal medication processing and excretion depend on the interactive function of these systems. Dysfunction in any of these systems can lead to toxicity, which often includes fluid and electrolyte imbalances.
- Monitor the client's level of plasma electrolytes, especially when giving medications that either affect or are affected by electrolyte levels.

- Assess the client's vital signs. Frequency varies with the severity of the alteration. You may need to assess vital signs as often as every 15 minutes when the electrolyte level is critical, or once a week or month in a more chronic situation.
- Assess an apical pulse for a full minute whenever the peripheral pulse is irregular. Remember that many electrolytes affect the rate and rhythm of the cardiac cells: these include sodium, potassium, magnesium, and calcium.
- If the client is on a cardiac monitor, watch for arrhythmias and other changes.
- Monitor intake and output (I&O) every hour in an acutely ill client. Teach the client and family to monitor and compare weight trends at least weekly for a stable "at home" client.
- Assess peripheral vein filling and emptying time. Normally, veins take less than 5 seconds to empty or fill.
- Because weakness is a common manifestation of many electrolyte imbalances, remember to initiate fall precautions when appropriate, such as removing obstacles from the environment, providing mobility support, and so on.
- Teach clients and families about the importance of consuming foods within the prescribed diet. Encourage intake of a well-rounded diet when possible. Encourage intake of foods that replace nutrients that are lost secondary to an illness or other condition. For a state of electrolyte excess, avoid foods high in that electrolyte.
- Teach clients to follow pharmaceutical recommendations for electrolyte replacement, and to avoid taking more than the recommended daily vitamin-mineral supplement without consultation with a physician. Tell the client to avoid other over-the-counter medications unless approved by a physician, because many of these drugs can alter fluid and electrolyte balance.
- Irrigate nasogastric tubes with normal saline only; if ice chips are ordered, use sparingly.
- When "enemas till clear" are prescribed, give no more than three in a row. Hypotonic solutions can alter fluid and electrolyte status. Consult the physician before proceeding.

Interventions for Sodium Imbalance

Hyponatremia is one of the more common electrolyte imbalances. The client's response to hyponatremia varies with the cause, rate of loss, and type of associated fluid imbalance. A client can present with a sodium level of 120 mEq/L and be asymptomatic if the imbalance developed slowly. The same level, if due to an acute loss, can cause life-threatening manifestations.

The client's amount of body water also affects response. Sodium deficit can occur in the presence of decreased, normal, or increased body water. However, one of the most common types of hyponatremia is due to fluid overload. When this is the etiology, fluid re-

striction is the intervention of choice. Fluid restriction is very difficult for any client to abide by. You can help the client understand the importance of this intervention as well as provide suggestions that will increase compliance. Ice chips, lozenges, frequent mouth care, and small, frequent sips of fluids will provide comfort.

If the hyponatremia is truly due to a sodium deficit, then the physician will prescribe additional sodium either orally, by tube, or in intravenous (IV) form. If the level is 125 mEq/L or greater, diet supplementation and interventions to decrease the loss are the usual treatment. Other common interventions include prescriptions to improve the function of the organs that are causing the problem, such as digitalis and diuretics for cardiac overload.

Interventions for Potassium Imbalance

Potassium imbalance can be very dangerous. Because potassium is predominantly an intracellular ion, the plasma level is only an indirect reflection of the cellular level. Minor plasma imbalances can indicate serious risk for cellular imbalance. Although many systems are affected by a potassium imbalance, the cardiovascular system is most critically affected. A low serum potassium level increases the automaticity in the cardiac cells, which in turn increases the risk of dysrhythmia. The risk of digitalis toxicity is also increased. Therefore, you should consult the physician before giving digitalis derivatives when potassium is low, when the plasma digitalis level is high, or when the client has bradycardia (pulse less than 60/minute).

Physicians usually prefer to be notified of the bradycardia and often will prescribe the continuance of digitalis as long as the apical pulse is above 50. This is because the client is at a greater risk from the complications of an ineffective myocardial pump without the digitalis.

If dietary replacement is insufficient, oral potassium supplements are usually prescribed. If the level is critical, then the more rapid IV replacement route is chosen.

Oral potassium should be given with food because it is a gastrointestinal (GI) irritant. Intravenous potassium can *only* be given in diluted form; direct IV potassium has been known to cause cardiac arrest. The maintenance dose is 40 to 80 mEq/day. If the potassium level is critically low or the client has serious cardiac arrhythmia, up to 10 mEq/hour can be given in as little as 125 mL of solution, but the client must be on a cardiac monitor during this infusion. An IV pump will ensure a safer delivery of IV potassium. Potassium is a venous irritant; if the client experiences pain at the IV site, the infusion rate may need to be slowed or the potassium diluted further. Potassium is very toxic to interstitial tissues; if infiltration occurs, stop the IV infusion immediately and notify the physician. Since potassium is excreted primarily via the kidneys, it is essential to monitor urinary output. If the output is borderline (about 30 mL/hour), outputs must be monitored hourly. If the urine output drops to less than 30 mL/hour for at least 2 consecutive hours, notify the physician.

Hyperkalemia can be a medical emergency. If the potassium level has caused significant cardiac conduction changes, the physician may order IV glucose and insulin to promote immediate, but temporary, shifting of the potassium from the plasma into the cells. To ensure excretion of potassium from the body, a cation exchange resin (such as sodium KayExalate in oral or rectal form) may be ordered or, if time permits, peritoneal or hemodialysis may be done to remove excess potassium from the body.

Interventions for Calcium Imbalance

Calcium imbalance is less common than sodium and potassium imbalances. Therefore, as a cost-conscious effort, the physician tests this level only when a client is at high risk for imbalance or has manifestations that suggest an imbalance. You play an active role in helping the physician identify such clients.

Calcium must be taken with vitamin D to promote absorption. High-phosphate products (such as milk and carbonated beverages) promote calcium loss. Therefore, it is important to teach clients to avoid these products if the hypocalcemia is due to hypoparathyroidism. When a client has normal parathyroid functioning, parathormone is able to manage the high phosphate levels in milk products, and the client is then able to receive the full calcium benefit from the calcium in the milk product.

The bone softening that accompanies calcium deficit or excess can result in a fracture with minimal strain. Teach clients the importance of weight-bearing activities to decrease calcium bone loss. Calcium deficit also increases the client's risk for bleeding; teach clients to report signs of bleeding. If hypercalcemia is present, strain or teach the client to strain urine to identify the presence of renal calculi. Teach the client that forcing fluids will decrease this risk. Also help the client understand the role of prescription medications for hypercalcemia. These include saline IV infusions, diuretics (nonthiazides), etidronate disodium (Didronel), phosphates, and corticosteroids.

Interventions for Magnesium Imbalance

When a magnesium deficit exists, increasing dietary intake is seldom sufficient. Usually an oral replacement is given unless the situation requires a more aggressive IV approach. The oral magnesium is often given in the form of magnesium-containing antacid. The parenteral form is usually magnesium sulfate. IV magnesium must be diluted in a nonsaline solution. Monitoring for blood pressure improvement and monitoring the ECG for decreased dysrhythmia are top priorities. Providing safety and seizure precautions for any client who is confused or at risk for seizure is also imperative. Assessing the return of the deep tendon reflexes provides an indication that magnesium balance has been restored.

Interventions for Phosphate Imbalance

Phosphate imbalances are rare. A deficit is treated by oral or IV replacement. A phosphate excess is treated with calcium or aluminum supplements.

EVALUATION

The time frame for evaluating fluid or electrolyte imbalance, whether deficit or excess, varies with the urgency of the imbalance. For example, if the client is experiencing a life-threatening arrhythmia, cardiac monitoring with narrow alarm parameters will be continuous. Neurological manifestations that indicate a worsening condition also require continuous evaluation. As the client stabilizes, however, the frequency of evaluation decreases. Hourly assessments are followed by assessments every 4 hours, progressing to every 8 hours. In extended care facilities and in the home, clients may require evaluation of risk or actual imbalances on only a weekly or monthly basis.

If the client is not improving, collect data to help evaluate the reason that outcomes are not being achieved. There are many possible variables, including barriers such as nausea or lack of access to food or fluids, another etiology or underlying pathology that is not responding to the current treatment, or perhaps a lack of compliance with the prescribed treatments for other reasons.

If a client has an actual fluid and electrolyte imbalance, compare the current manifestations with those present on the last assessment. The desired outcome is an improvement in any of the signs or symptoms discussed in this chapter. Obviously, improvement of manifestations involving life-sustaining tissues is the highest priority. However, even a fluid imbalance at a local level, such as severe edema in an extremity, could pose a threat to the life of that tissue. Naturally, life-threatening signs and symptoms require aggressive intervention. Care plan revision is indicated if the client's responses indicate that she no longer has a risk or an actual problem, that she is not improving, that she is not improving at the desired or expected rate, or that her condition is worsening. See the accompanying Nursing Care Planning chart for more information.

KEY PRINCIPLES

- Fluid and electrolyte imbalances are fairly common and often overlooked.
- Fluid and electrolyte imbalances rarely occur in isolation. It is the relationship of the solute to the solvent that determines the client's response, not the level of the deficit by itself.
- The most common fluid imbalance is dehydration, which occurs most often in the very young and in the elderly.

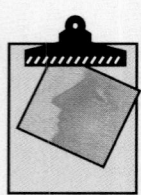

NURSING CARE PLANNING
A CLIENT WITH FLUID VOLUME DEFICIT

Admission Data

Mrs. Thompson was examined by her physician's nurse in the outpatient clinic. The nurse reported the following data to Dr. Kline:

Nursing Assessment

Color pale, skin dry, oral mucous membranes dry with tongue furrows, weight 110 pounds (decrease of 10 pounds in 2 weeks), blood pressure 116/50, pulse 110 and weak, respirations 24 (usually 142/70, 80, 16). Appears restless and is unable to remember when she last ate. Reports extreme fatigue and weakness over the last several weeks, states stools have been hard and infrequent.

Dr. Kline examined Mrs. Thompson and wrote the following on her chart:

Physician's Progress Note

Diagnosis: Dehydration secondary to decreased intake, extreme weakness, and fatigue. Early signs of ECF deficit with minimal signs of intracellular affect (confusion). In no acute distress at this time. Believe she can be managed at home due to supportive family who will assist in monitoring and care delivery. Visiting Nurse three times a week for 2 weeks. Hospitalization for IV therapy only if signs worsen.

Office Care

The office nurse completed teaching with Mrs. Thompson and her son Gerald. While consulting with Mrs. Thompson, especially about her ethnic preferences, a grocery list was compiled. The nurse also reinforced the importance of Gerald's daily visits until his mother became stable. She also gave them a list of signs and symptoms that meant that Dr. Kline's office must be notified. Later, the office nurse contacted the Visiting Nursing Agency and gave Judy Carson, RN, Mrs. Thompson's nurse, a full report with the following orders:

Initial visit today to include the following:

- Home baseline assessment.
- Instruct Mrs. Thompson and her family on schedule for oral fluid replacement.
- Plan to include increasing fluid intake to 1500 mL per day; stopping 3 hours before bedtime.
- Plan to include increasing food intake to 6 small meals per day.
- Validate understanding of teaching.

Additional orders:

- Contact Meals on Wheels about meal supplementation.
- Evaluate progress every 2 days for 2 weeks.

NURSING CARE PLAN

Nursing Diagnosis	Expected Outcomes	Interventions	Evaluation (Home Visit, 48 Hours Later)
Fluid volume deficit related to decreased intake, inability to shop and cook for self secondary to extreme weakness and fatigue	Oral mucous membranes moist; no tongue furrows.	Assess oral mucous membranes and tongue.	Tongue furrows absent, but oral mucous membranes remain dry.
	Weight increased by 1 pound.	Weigh with approximate amount of clothing had on when made initial visit.	Weight gain of 1 pound.
	Oriented to person, time, and place.	Assess orientation to person, place, and time.	Able to state name, home address, and month.
	Vital signs improved: BP, systolic >120 Pulse <100 Respirations <20	Assess vital signs.	BP 118/70, P 96, R 20.

Continued

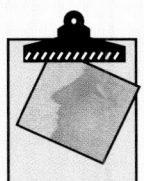

NURSING CARE PLANNING
A CLIENT WITH FLUID VOLUME DEFICIT *(continued)*

NURSING CARE PLAN

Nursing Diagnosis	Expected Outcomes	Interventions	Evaluation (Home Visit, 48 Hours Later)
	Reports of softer stools at least once since doctor's visit.	Question about stool characteristics since office visit.	Stated one stool, moderate amount, still somewhat hard.
	Reports of taking 60 mL fluids/hour, 6 small meals/day	Assess fluid and diet history since office visit.	Diary of fluid/food intake: Day I: 1,000 mL, 4 meals. Day II: 1,200 mL, 4 meals but one bigger; daughter-in-law, Sue, made favorite ethnic dish.
	Reports of more strength; improvement in self-care activities	Evaluate her ADL since office visit as well as level of fatigue and weakness.	Able to serve self breakfast, heat up meals from Meals on Wheels; too tired to cook at supper; Gerald fixed supper; Sue helped her with bath each night. Required nap morning and afternoon.

Critical Thinking Questions

1. Mrs. Thompson has made progress toward the expected outcomes but has not achieved them. When the family expresses concern about this and asks you if you think she should come to live with them or be placed in a residential home, how would you answer and why?
2. Referring to the original case study, review the changes that occurred 1 week later. What signs and symptoms was Mrs. Thompson having now? Why? What other signs and symptoms indicate fluid volume excess? Which ones are the most serious and why?

- Seventy percent of the body fluid is in the intracellular spaces. Therefore, acute or severe loss can have serious consequences for cellular functioning.
- Fluid shifting occurs between the extracellular compartments first, unless the loss or excess is acute or severe. Regardless, cellular fluid shifting occurs last after the extracellular compensatory mechanisms have been exhausted.
- The most common electrolyte imbalance is hyponatremia. It is more common in the elderly population, especially in those on low salt diets who are taking diuretics.
- Nurses must anticipate imbalances in high-risk clients: the very young, the elderly, those experiencing pregnancy, especially teenage pregnancy; and those with acute or chronic illnesses.
- Thorough history and physical assessments including diagnostics are necessary for making an accurate differential diagnosis.
- The outcomes of the imbalance depend on the acuteness and severity of the condition, age and health state of the client, and the degree to which the client's compensatory mechanisms or therapeutic interventions combat the imbalance.
- The nurse has many roles, including teaching the clients and their families positive health behaviors, promoting nutritional maintenance and replacement, collaborating with the physician for early detection of imbalances and poor responses to treatment, and collaboration with the dietitian in the promotion of positive nutritional outcomes.
- Through individualization of interventions and mutual goal setting with the clients and their families, nurses can facilitate optimal health outcomes.
- Nurses are in a key position to influence cost-effectiveness and cost-efficiency through utilization of appropriate resources, delegation of appropriate interventions, promotion of primary and secondary prevention, and ongoing care plan evaluation and revision.

BIBLIOGRAPHY

*Altura, B.M., Brodsky, M.A., Elin, R.J., Gums, J.G., Resnick, L.M., & Seelig, M.S. (1994). Magnesium therapy: Coming of age. *Patient Care, 28*(2), 79–94.

*Batcheller, J. (1994). Syndrome of inappropriate antidiuretic hormone secretion. *Critical Care Nursing Clinics of North America, 6*(4), 687–692.

Bergeron, M.F., Armstrong, L.E., & Maresh, C.M. (1995). Fluid and electrolyte losses during tennis in the heat. *Clinics in Sports Medicine, 14*(1), 23–32.

Bove, L.A. (1996). Restoring electrolyte balance: Sodium & chloride. *RN, 96*(1), 25–28.

*Constants, T., Delarue, J., Rivol, M., Theret, V., & Lamisse, F. (1994). Effects of nutrition education on calcium intake in the elderly. *Journal of the American Dietetic Association, 94*(4), 447–448.

Crow, S., Salisbury, J., Crosby, R., & Mitchell J. (1997). Serum electrolytes as markers of vomiting in bulimia nervosa. *International Journal of Eating Disorders, 21*(1), 95–98.

*Cullin, L. (1992). Interventions related to fluid and electrolyte balance. *Nursing Clinics of North America, 27*(2), 569–597.

*Edes, T., Walk, B.E., & Austin, J.L. (1990). Diarrhea in tube-fed patients: Feeding formula not necessarily the cause. *American Journal of Medicine, 88*(2), 91–93.

Gisolfi, C., Summers, R., Schedl, H., & Bleiler, T. (1995). Effect of sodium concentration in a carbohydrate-electrolyte solution on intestinal absorption. *Medical Science Sports Exercise, 27*(10), 1414–1420.

*Hall, J.K. (1994). Caring for corpses or killing patients? *Nursing Management, 25*(10), 81–89.

Held, J.L. (1995). Cancer care: Correcting fluid and electrolyte imbalances. *Nursing, 25*(4), 71.

*Hoot-Martin, J., & Larsen, P.D. (1994). Dehydration in the elderly surgical patient. *AORN, 60*(4), 666–671.

*Incalzi, R.A., Gemma, A., Capparella, O., Terranova, L., Sanguinetti, C., & Carbonin, P.U. (1992). Post-operative electrolyte imbalance: Its incidence and prognostic implications for elderly orthopaedic patients. *Age and Ageing, 22*, 325–331.

*Innerarity, S.A. (1992). Hyperkalemic emergencies. *Critical Care Nursing Quarterly, 14*(4), 32–39.

*Kaplan, M. (1994). Hypercalcemia of malignancy: A review of advances in pathophysiology. *Oncology Nursing Forum, 21*(6), 1039–1046.

Kaufmann, M. (1996). Preventing dehydration in the elderly. *Provider, 9*, 65–66.

*Kelso, L.A. (1992). Fluid and electrolyte disturbances in hepatic failure. *AACN, 3*(3), 681–685.

King, P.A. (1995). Oncologic emergencies: Assessment, identification, and interventions in the emergency department. *Journal of Emergency Nursing, 21*(3), 214–217.

Kubena, K., & McMurray, D. (1996). Nutrition and the immune system: A review of nutrient-nutrient interactions. *Journal of American Diet Association, 96*(11), 1156–1164.

*Maughan, R.J. (1992). Fluid balance and exercise. *International Journal of Sports Medicine, 13*, S132–S135.

McConnell, E.A. (1995). What's wrong with this patient? Assessing altered level of consciousness. *Nursing, 25*(6), 66–67.

*Mendyka, B.E. (1992). Fluid and electrolyte disorders caused by diuretic therapy. *AACN, 3*(3), 672–680.

Miller, C.A. (1995). *Nursing care of older adults: Theory and practice* (2nd ed.). Philadelphia: JB Lippincott Co.

Miller, K. (1996). Diabetes insipidus. *ANNA Journal, 23*(3), 285–292.

Mulloy, A.L., & Caruana, R.J. (1995). Hyponatremic emergencies. *Medical Clinics of North America, 79*(1), 155–169.

*Newmark K., & Nugent, P. (1993). Milk-alkali syndrome. *Postgraduate Medicine, 93*(6), 149–156.

O'Donnell, M.E. (1995). Assessing fluid and electrolyte balance in elders. *American Journal of Nursing, 95*(11), 41–45.

Okun, J.P. (1995). Clinical pathology rounds: Severe hypernatremia. *Laboratory Medicine, 26*(8), 507–509.

Perez, A. (1995). Hyperkalemia. *RN, 95*(11), 33–36.

*Porth, C., & Erickson, M. (1992). Physiology of thirst and drinking: Implication for nursing practice. *Heart & Lung, 21*(3), 273–282.

*Radke, K.J. (1994). The aging kidney: Structure, function, and nursing practice implications. *ANNA Journal, 21*(4), 181–190.

Reber, P.M., & Heath, H. (1995). Hypocalcemic emergencies. *Medical Clinics of North America, 79*(1), 93–107.

*Reherer, N.J. (1994). The maintenance of fluid balance during exercise. *International Journal of Sports Medicine, 15*(3), 122–125.

Sansevero, A. (1997). Dehydration in the elderly: Strategies for prevention and management. *The Nurse Practitioner, 22*(4), 41–70.

*Seshadri, V., & Meyer-Tettambel, O.M. (1993). Electrolyte and drug management in nutritional support. *Critical Care Nursing Clinics of North America, 5*(1), 31–36.

Simmons-Holcomb, S. (1997). Understanding the ins & outs of diuretic therapy. *RN, 97*(2), 34–40.

Smith, S.A. (1997). Controversies in hydrating the terminally ill patient. *Journal of Intravenous Nursing, 20*(4), 193–199.

Smith, S.A. (1995). Patient-induced dehydration: Can it ever be therapeutic? *Oncology Nursing Forum, 22*(10), 1487–1497.

Stark, J. (1997). Dialysis choices. *RN, 97*(2), 41–46.

*Sutcliffe, J. (1994). Dehydration: Burden or benefit to the dying patient? *Journal of Advanced Nursing, 19*, 71–76.

*Terry, J. (1994). The major electrolytes: Sodium, potassium, and chloride. *Journal of Intravenous Nursing, 17*(5), 240–247.

Treston-Aurand, J., Olmsted R., Allen-Bridson, K., & Craig, C. (1997). Impact of dressing materials on central venous catheter infection rates. *Journal of Intravenous Nursing 20*(4), 201–204.

Urine chemistry: Monitoring fluid and electrolytes. *Nursing, 86*(4), 24j, 24l.

Vonfolio, L.G. (1995). Back to basics: Would you hang these IV solutions? *American Journal of Nursing, 95*(6), 37–39.

Wong, P., & Warren, A. (1995). Electrolytes in cardiac patients. *Nursing Standard, 9*(35), 52–53.

Wood, N. (1992). Reader offers strategies for identification and treatment of dilutional hyponatremia. *Nurse Practitioner, 17*(10), 9–10, 16.

Worobec, F., & Brown, M. (1997). Hypodermoclysis therapy. *Journal of Gerontological Nursing, 23* (6), 23–28.

Zerwekh, J. (1997). Do dying patients really need IV fluids? *AJN, 97*(3), 26–30.

*Asterisk indicates a classic or definitive work on this subject.

32

Skin Integrity and Wound Healing

Elizabeth Abrahams

Key Terms

abrasion
blanchable erythema
débridement
dehiscence
eschar
epithelialization
evisceration
exudate

fistula
friction injury
hematoma
hemorrhage
laceration
reactive hyperemia
shearing force
wound

LEARNING OBJECTIVES

After studying this chapter, you should be able to:

1. Describe skin disruptions, wound healing, and problems of wound healing.
2. Discuss the staging of pressure ulcers.
3. Explain the effect of lifestyle, age, and illness on skin integrity and wound healing.
4. Assess the client who has *Risk for impaired skin integrity* or an actual impairment of skin integrity
5. Distinguish among the various nursing diagnoses for clients with alterations in skin integrity.
6. Plan for goal-directed interventions to prevent *Impaired skin integrity* or promote wound healing.
7. Evaluate the outcomes of interventions for *Impaired skin integrity.*

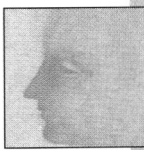

Violetta Jacan is a 72-year-old woman who has been living alone in an apartment since her husband died 3 years ago. Her daughter lives nearby. One morning while getting out of the shower, Mrs. Jacan fell onto the bathroom floor and fractured her right hip. Unable to get to the phone to call for help, she lay on the floor until her daughter checked in on her late the next day. On admission to the emergency department, Mrs. Jacan is diagnosed with a broken hip. She also has reddened areas on her sacrum and heels.

Once Mrs. Jacan arrives on the surgical unit, the nurse prepares her for hip surgery and begins to plan for her postoperative skin care needs. She notes that Mrs. Jacan is elderly and shows the beginning of pressure ulcer formation. She also considers that the client will have a hip incision and limited mobility during the postoperative period. Because all of these factors put Mrs. Jacan at risk for skin breakdown, the nurse considers the diagnoses *Risk for impaired skin integrity, Impaired skin integrity,* and *Impaired tissue integrity.*

SKIN INTEGRITY NURSING DIAGNOSES

Risk for Impaired Skin Integrity: A state in which the individual's skin is at risk of being adversely altered.

Impaired Skin Integrity: A state in which an individual has altered epidermis and/or dermis.

Impaired Tissue Integrity: A state in which an individual experiences damage to mucous membrane, corneal, integumentary, or subcutaneous tissues. It is a state in which an individual has altered body tissue.

From North American Nursing Diagnosis Association. (1999). Nursing diagnoses: Definitions and classification 1999–2000. Philadelphia: Author.

CONCEPTS OF SKIN INTEGRITY AND WOUND HEALING

Throughout your nursing career and in all of the health care settings in which you practice, you will be concerned with your clients' skin care needs. In all cases, you will seek to prevent disruptions in skin integrity. For clients who already have such disruptions, you will seek to promote healing. Some of your clients will have minor skin disruptions, such as an abrasion or a tape blister. Some disruptions will be major, such as a deep pressure ulcer or a wound from major abdominal surgery. Throughout this range, skin care is an integral part of the overall nursing care plan in virtually all settings.

Skin Disruptions

Protection is the primary function of the skin. Skin protects from many forms of trauma including mechanical, thermal, chemical, and radiant. The epidermis serves as a tough mechanical layer that protects against bacteria, foreign material, other organisms, and chemicals. When the skin is disrupted, a route is created for the loss of body fluids, and the risk for infection is great.

Skin Lesions

A lesion is any pathological or traumatic discontinuity of tissue or loss of function of a part. This definition includes wounds, sores, ulcers, tumors, cataracts, and any other tissue damage. It is often used to refer to a visible local abnormality in the skin. Skin lesions may or may not be related to the client's medical condition. Lesions can be caused by mechanical injuries, pathological changes, allergies, or bites. To determine the etiology of common skin lesions you should be able to distinguish between primary and secondary lesions. A **primary lesion** is the first lesion to appear on the skin in response to a causative agent and usually has a recognizable structure. Figure 32–1 identifies and describes 10 types of primary lesions. Changes can occur in primary lesions and can result in **secondary lesions.** These

changes are caused by several factors and occur in the epidermal layer. Many factors cause these lesions, including scratching, rubbing, medications, client's medical condition, or disease process. Figure 32–2 illustrates secondary lesions.

Wounds

A wound is a type of lesion. A **wound** is a disruption of normal anatomic structure and function that results from bodily injury or a pathological process that may begin internally or externally to the involved organ or organs (Lazarus et al., 1994).

Wounds can be classified by cause and descriptors of the wound. It is important to be able to identify the cause of the wound and describe it accurately to the health care team.

The cause of a wound may be intentional or unintentional. An intentional wound results from a surgical procedure or treatment (such as intravenous therapy). Unintentional wounds result from accidental injury or trauma, animal bites, violence, or health care. The cause of the wound is closely related to the amount of tissue damage that has occurred.

Wounds are classified as open or closed. In an open wound, the skin has been broken and a range of soft tissue damage is present. A surgical wound can be intentionally left open or be open as a complication of healing.

Wounds are classified based on the severity and nature of the injury. Superficial wounds involve the surface layers of the skin or the body. *Deep* may refer to the deep layers of the skin or deep within a body cavity, penetrating internal body organs. Severity also has to do with the amount of tissue damage. Tissue damage results both from the break in the skin and from trauma to surrounding tissue. It may also result from damage to the blood supply to the site of injury.

Wounds are classified based on the risk for infection. A clean wound was created with a clean instrument and contains little or no debris; a dirty wound was created with a grossly contaminated instrument and may contain dirt and other debris. The surgical wound is the cleanest of all wounds.

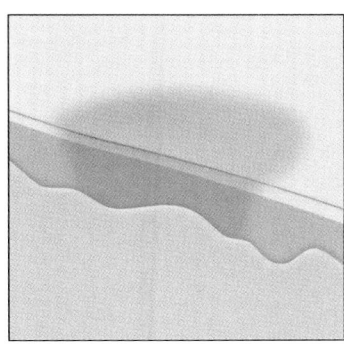

Macule
Skin color change without elevation, i.e., flat (freckles or petechiae). Described as a "patch" if greater than 1 cm (e.g.,vitiligo).

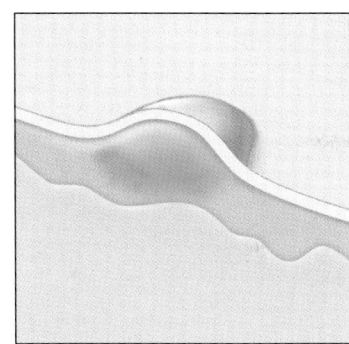

Papule
Elevated, solid lesion of less than 1 cm, varying in color (e.g., warts or elevated nevi [moles]).

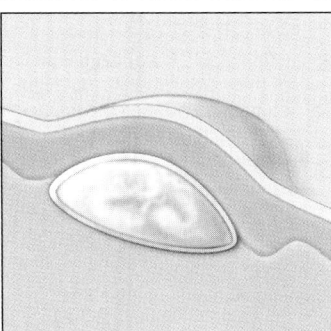

Cyst
Elevated, thick-walled lesion containing fluid or semisolid matter.

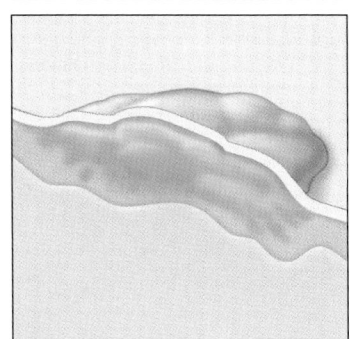

Plaque
Raised flat lesion formed from merging papules or nodules.

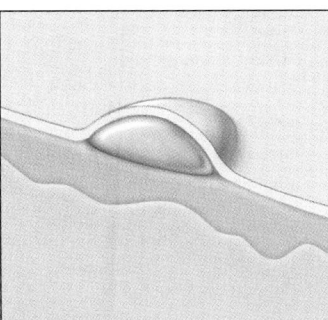

Vesicle
Elevated, sharply defined lesion containing serous fluid. Usually less than 1 cm (e.g., blister, chickenpox, or herpes simplex).

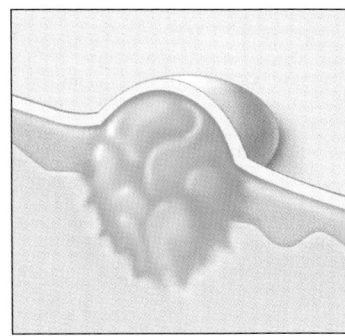

Nodule
Larger than a papule. A raised, solid lesion extending deeper into the dermis.

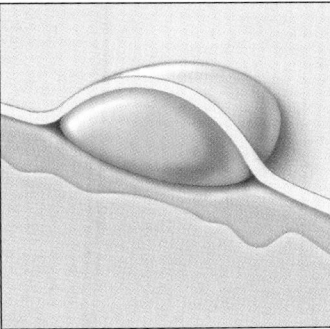

Bulla (plural, *bullae*)
Large, elevated, fluid-filled lesion greater than 1 cm (e.g., second-degree burn).

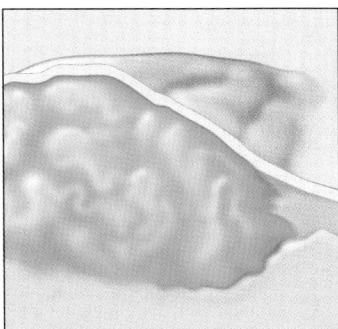

Tumor
Larger than a nodule. An elevated, firm lesion that may or may not be easily demarcated.

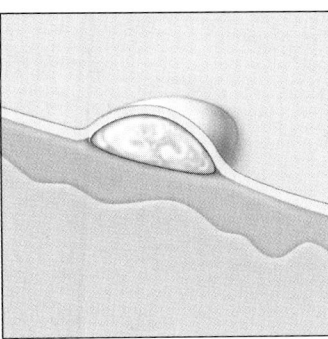

Pustule
Elevated lesion less than 1 cm containing purulent material. Lesions larger than 1 cm are described as boils, abscesses, or furuncles (e.g., acne or impetigo).

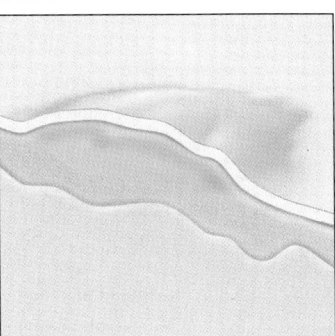

Wheal (hive)
Fleeting skin elevation that is irregularly shaped because of edema (e.g., mosquito bite or urticaria).

Figure 32–1. Primary skin lesions. (Descriptions modified from Black, J. M., & Matassarin-Jacobs, E. [1997]. Medical-surgical nursing: Clinical management for continuity of care [5th ed.]. Philadelphia: W.B. Saunders.)

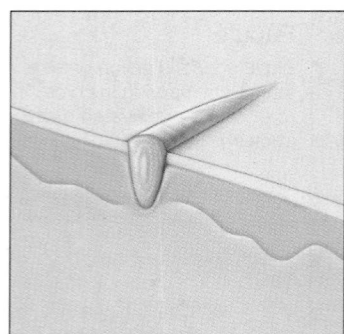

Scar
Mark left on the skin after healing. Replacement of destroyed tissue by fibrous tissue.

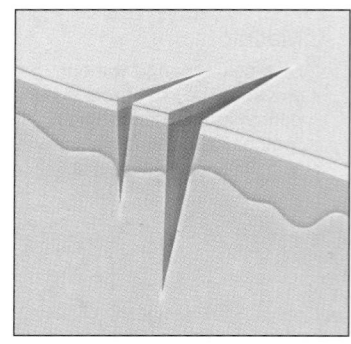

Fissure
Deep linear split through the epidermis into the dermis (e.g., tinea pedis).

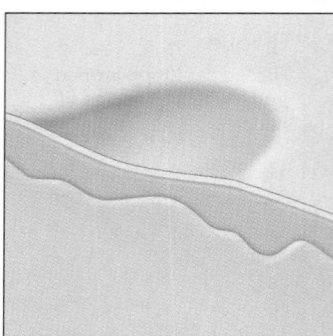

Atrophy
Wasting of the epidermis in which the skin appears thin and transparent, or of the dermis in which there is a depressed area (e.g., arterial insufficiency).

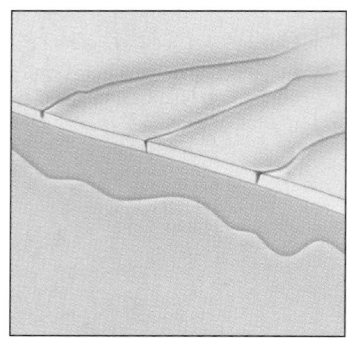

Excoriation
Superficial, linear abrasion of the epidermis. Visible sign of itching caused by rubbing or scratching (e.g., atopic dermatitis).

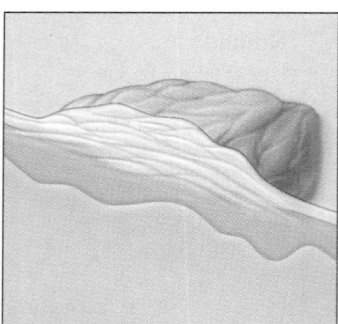

Lichenification
Epidermal thickening resulting in elevated plaque with accentuated skin markings. Usually results from repeated injury through rubbing or scratching (e.g., chronic atopic dermatitis).

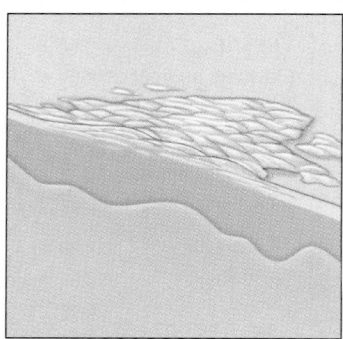

Scale
Dried fragments of sloughed epidermal cells, irregular in shape and size and white, tan, yellow, or silver in color (e.g., dandruff, dry skin, or psoriasis).

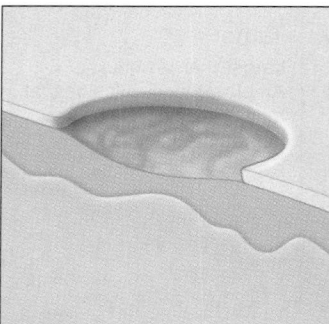

Erosion
A moist, demarcated, depressed area due to the loss of partial- or full- thickness epidermis. Basal layer of epidermis remains intact (e.g., ruptured chickenpox vesicle).

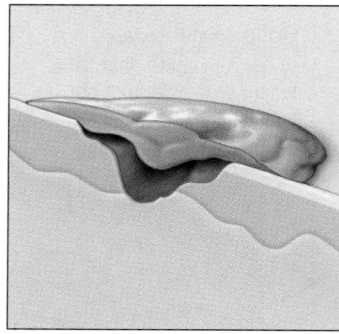

Crust
Dried serum, sebum, blood, or pus on the skin surface, producing a temporary barrier to the environment (e.g., impetigo).

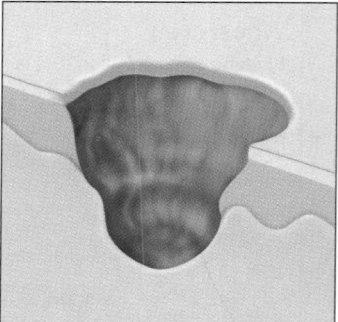

Ulcer
Irregularly shaped, exudative, depressed lesion in which the entire epidermis and the upper layer of the dermis are lost. Results from trauma and tissue destruction (e.g., stasis ulcer).

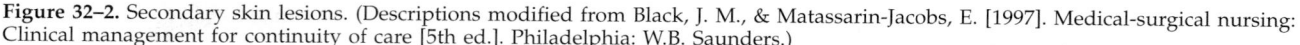

Figure 32–2. Secondary skin lesions. (Descriptions modified from Black, J. M., & Matassarin-Jacobs, E. [1997]. Medical-surgical nursing: Clinical management for continuity of care [5th ed.]. Philadelphia: W.B. Saunders.)

Table 32–1 summarizes terms used to classify wounds based on a description of the wound and possible causes.

Most wounds have several characteristics. The surgical incision is created under sterile conditions, tissue damage is minimized, and healthy wound edges are approximated so that new tissue can grow and connect the tissue with minimal scarring. Wounds resulting from trauma are created under "dirty" conditions, tissue damage is variable, the wound edges may not be easily approximated, and scarring is more likely. Healing for a open traumatic wound may be impeded by damage to the soft tissue surrounding the open wound.

A chronic wound is a wound that has an insidious onset and heals slowly or is resistant to healing. Pressure ulcers are an example of a chronic wound in which the wound is open, increasing the risk for infection; blood flow to the wound bed is impaired, resulting in the presence of necrotic tissue; and a large amount of scar tissue will be needed to fill the wound bed for healing to occur. The etiology of pressure ulcers is discussed in Chapter 38.

Chronic wounds are often classified by a description of the wound. Descriptors include color of the wound bed and characteristics of drainage.

The red-yellow-black (RYB) classification system is based on wound bed color. Use this system in conjunction with other wound classification criteria. Based on the wound healing process, the RYB system identifies the wound on a continuum of wound healing. Generally, red wounds are healing wounds. However, a red wound may be in one of several different stages of the healing process, such as the inflammatory, regeneration, or remodeling phase. A yellow wound bed indicates that the wound is not yet ready to heal because it has fibrous slough or exudate that must be cleansed and removed. A black wound bed indicates the presence of **eschar,** a thick, leathery, necrotic, devitalized tissue (Bergstrom et al., 1994). Such tissue must be removed for the wound to heal (Krasner, 1995).

Another important characteristic by which you can classify and describe a wound is its drainage. Wound drainage, or **exudate,** refers to the fluid and cells that have escaped from blood vessels during the inflammatory response and are left in the surrounding tissues. Wound exudate varies with the type of tissue involved, the amount of inflammation, and the presence or absence of bacteria or other microorganisms.

Types of wound exudate include serous, sanguineous, serosanguineous, and purulent. Serous drainage is clear and watery plasma. Sanguineous (from the Latin word for blood) drainage is bright red. Serosanguineous drainage, a mixture of serous and sanguineous drainage, consists of plasma and red blood cells and is pale red and watery. Drainage from a surgical wound is initially sanguineous. Over several days, it changes to serosanguineous and then serous. Purulent drainage is pus, a protein-rich liquid product of the liquefaction of necrotic tissue. It is made up of cells and cellular debris and is usually caused by an infection. It is thick and yellow, green, tan, or brown.

Wound Healing

The human body has the ability to heal itself and uses many processes to aid skin and wound healing and promote the restoration of function and structure. The skin performs wound healing through a complex physiological process.

Phases of Wound Healing

The inflammatory phase, the first phase of wound healing, begins at the time of tissue injury and lasts 3 to 4 days. The cardinal signs of inflammation are edema, erythema, heat, and pain at the wound site. Hemostasis, the control of bleeding, is the process by which injured blood vessels constrict and platelets accumulate to stop the bleeding. The blood clots that subsequently develop in the wound area form a fibrin matrix, which acts as a structure or framework for fur-

TABLE 32–1
Types of Wounds

Type	Description	Possible Cause
Open	Disruption or break in skin	Penetration by sharp object or instrument (such as knife, scalpel, bullet)
Closed	No disruption or break in skin	Trauma caused by blow with blunt object
Clean	Wound free of infectious organisms	Surgical incision not entering or affected by secretions from respiratory, gastrointestinal, or genitourinary tracts
Contaminated	Wound with microorganisms	Penetration of skin by dirt, bacteria
Penetrating	Wound with break through epidermis, dermis, and underlying tissues; may enter organs	Penetration by object or instrument (usually accidental)
Abrasion	Superficial injury caused by rubbing or scraping of skin against another surface	Friction injury resulting from fall or rubbing against bed linens
Laceration	Open wound with jagged edges	Penetration of skin by sharp object
Contusion	Closed wound; may be swollen, discolored, and painful	Blunt trauma, such as being hit by object

ther cellular repair. A scab forms on the wound surface, promoting homeostasis and helping to prevent wound contamination. Histamine is secreted by mast cells and damaged tissues, leading to capillary dilation with an increase in the supply of blood and other nutrients to the wound. Cell migration occurs when leukocytes (neutrophils) move into the wound and begin to ingest bacteria and wound debris. Monocytes change into macrophages and clean the wound bed of cellular debris and dead cells through phagocytosis. This process rids cellular debris from the site and prepares the wound bed for healing.

Monocytes continue cleaning the wound and stimulate the formation of fibroblasts (connective tissue cells). The fibrin network of the clot provides a structure to aid the formation of fibrous bridges as well as epithelial cells that move from wound edges to create an epithelial layer.

The proliferative, or reconstruction, phase of healing lasts 4 to 21 days. During this phase, collagen fills the wound bed, new blood vessels develop (angiogenesis), and granulation tissue forms. Granulation tissue is formed by fibroblasts and has a bright red granular appearance. Also, the wound closes by **epithelialization,** a process in which epithelial cells grow to cover the wound bed. By day 5, the wound has filled with highly vascular fibroblastic connective tissue. By day 7, the surface epithelium has a normal thickness and the subepithelial layers are bridged. Progressive collagen accumulation during the second week results in the basic structure of the scar. Bright red, the scar does not achieve its full tensile strength for a long time.

The final stage of wound healing is the maturation, or remodeling, phase. Although much maturation occurs by 3 to 4 weeks, the scar may not achieve maximum strength for up to 2 years. This phase is characterized by reorganization of the collagen fibers, wound remodeling, and maturation of the tissues to approximate the skin's original strength. Although the wound is considered fully healed, the tissue will always be at risk for breakdown because the wound's tensile strength never exceeds 80% of its preinjury strength (Haas, 1995).

Types of Wound Healing

Most acute wounds and surgical wounds close by primary intention (Fig. 32–3). The clinician brings together (approximates) the wound edges or margins without **hematoma** (an accumulation of bloody fluid beneath tissue), debris, or exudate, and secures them using sutures, staples, or tape. The wound bed then fills in with granulation tissue, and the scar is usually thin and flat. Primary intention occurs in the first 14 days after the injury. Wounds that have healed through primary intention have a lower risk of infection, involve little tissue loss, and heal with minimal scarring. Healing by primary intention takes a predictable course through the stages of inflammation, proliferation, and maturation.

In contrast, healing by secondary intention is prolonged (Fig. 32–4). When the skin or wound edges

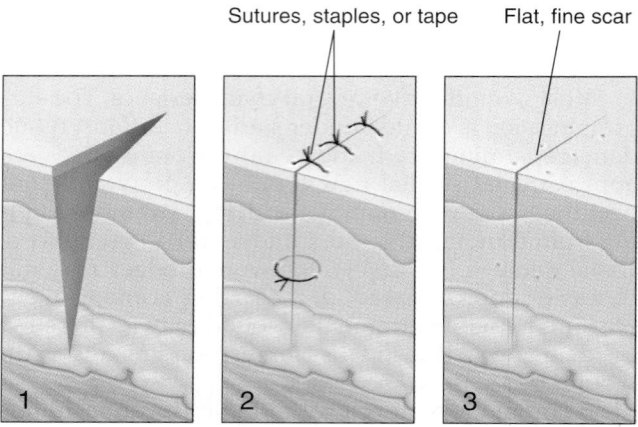

Sutures, staples, or tape   Flat, fine scar

Figure 32–3. Wound healing by primary intention.

cannot be approximated, as in a pressure ulcer or a wound that is large or infected, the wound must be filled with new tissue and all dead (necrotic) and infectious tissue must be removed. The wound fills mostly with granulation tissue, but some tissue regeneration occurs at the wound margins. As granulation tissue fills the wound, epithelialization proceeds from the margins. Wound contraction plays a greater role in healing by secondary intention, reducing the size of the final surface scar. Secondary intention generally involves greater tissue loss, a higher risk for infection, and a prolonged healing time.

Tertiary intention, or delayed primary closure, occurs in wounds that may be contaminated, infected, or draining exudate (Fig. 32–5). These wounds may be left open intentionally for 3 to 5 days to let healing begin by allowing the contaminated or infected matter or exudate to drain out. Once the infection clears, the wound is closed with sutures, staples, or tape.

Pressure Ulcers

The Agency for Health Care Policy and Research (AHCPR) (Bergstrom et al., 1994) defines a **pressure ulcer** as any lesion caused by unrelieved pressure that leads to damage of underlying tissues. Typically, a

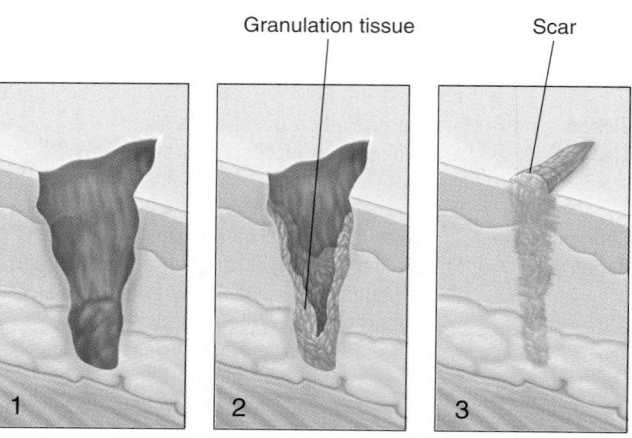

Granulation tissue   Scar

Figure 32–4. Wound healing by secondary intention.

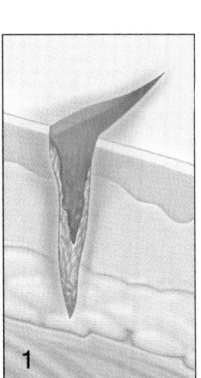 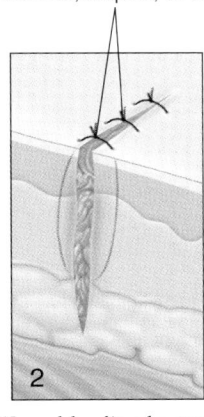 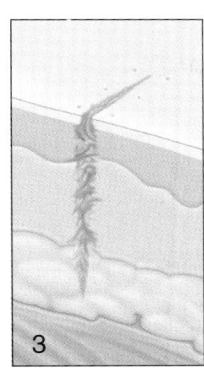

Sutures, staples, or tape

Figure 32–5. Wound healing by tertiary intention.

pressure ulcer is located over a bony prominence or an area that sustains prolonged pressure. Alternatively, Margolis (1995) defined a pressure ulcer as a disruption of the skin's normal anatomic structure and function caused by an external force associated with a bony prominence that does not heal in an orderly fashion. Pressure ulcers occur mainly in persons who are chairbound, bedbound, or incontinent, have difficulty feeding themselves, or have an altered level of con-

sciousness. Pressure ulcers are sometimes called decubitus ulcers, pressure sores, or bed sores. However, the Wound, Ostomy, and Continence Society considers *pressure ulcer* the correct term.

The economic impact of pressure ulcers is significant, both for hospitals and for long-term-care facilities, as described in the Cost of Care chart. According to one estimate, the total national cost of pressure ulcer treatment exceeds $1.3 billion per year (Miller & Delozier, 1994). This high cost is but another reason to consider maintenance of skin integrity a high priority.

Two clinical practice guidelines developed by the AHCPR address pressure ulcers. The first, *Pressure Ulcers in Adults: Prediction and Prevention Guidelines #3* (Bergstrom, Allman, & Carlson, 1992), lists strategies for identifying clients at risk and describes preventive strategies and treatment guidelines. The other guideline, *Treatment of Pressure Ulcers #15* (Bergstrom et al., 1994), focuses on treating adults with pressure ulcers. Developed after an extensive literature review, these clinical practice guidelines are supported by clinical research and expert opinion. This chapter discusses pressure ulcers in reference to these practice guidelines as well as other current nursing literature.

The AHCPR identifies four stages of pressure ulcers (Fig. 32–6), consistent with those identified by the

---

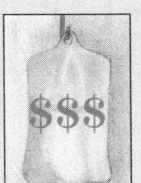

THE COST OF CARE
WOUND CARE

The cost of wound care involves much more than simply the cost of dressings. In general, wound care involves direct costs and indirect costs, as listed below. The direct costs of wound care include the following:

• Primary wound dressing.
• Secondary dressing.
• Other materials needed (normal saline, tape, underpads).
• Caregiver time (assessment, positioning, dressing changes).
• Consultations.
• Diagnostics.
• Equipment (specialty beds and mattresses).
• Pharmacy.

The indirect costs of wound care include the following:

• Extra inpatient days.
• Client days lost from work.
• Treating complications.
• Costs of waste of disposal of used wound care materials.
• Litigation costs.

Discussion

Reducing and preventing infection play a significant role in reducing the cost of wound care (Hermans & Bolton, 1996). Indeed, spending money to prevent pressure ulcers can save much more money by avoiding the need to treat pressure ulcers, which usually are difficult to resolve.

Additionally, research into new products has identified less costly treatments than the traditional methods. For example, research was conducted on the use of moist gauze versus a hydrocolloid dressing in treating pressure ulcers. Results indicated that the hydrocolloid dressing was more cost-effective; the dressing was less expensive and saved 29 minutes of nursing time. (Collwell, Foreman, & Trotter, 1993).

References

Collwell, J.C., Foreman, M.D., & Trotter, J.P. (1993). A comparison of the efficacy and cost effectiveness of 2 methods of managing pressure ulcers. *Decubitus, 6*(4), 28–35.
Hermans, M.H., & Bolton, L.L. (1996). The influence of dressings on the costs of wound treatment. *Dermatology Nursing, 8*(2), 93–100.
International Committee on Wound Management. (1995). An overview of economic model of cost effective wound care. *Advances in Wound Care, 8*(5), 46.

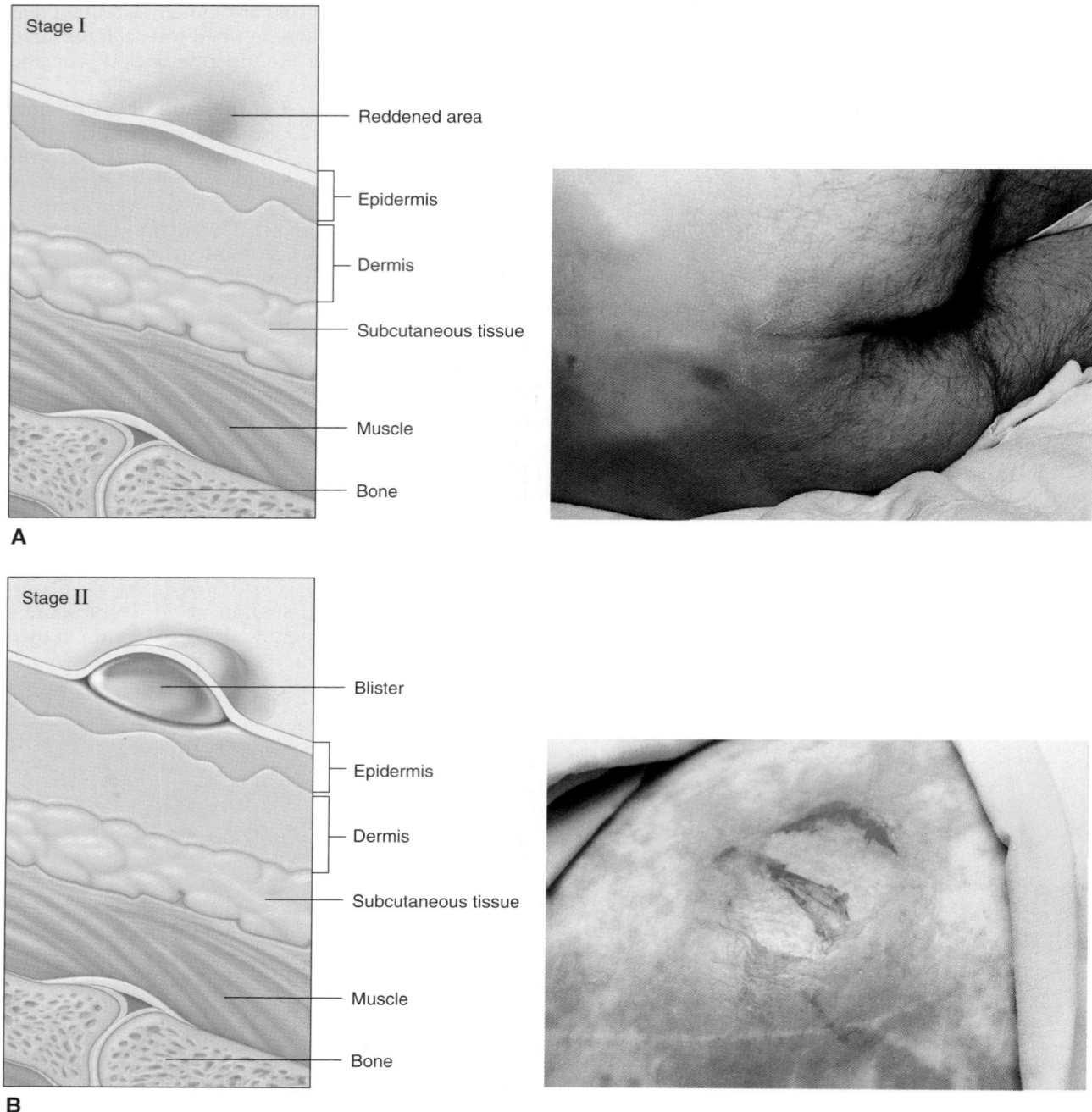

Figure 32–6. Stages of development of pressure ulcers. *A,* stage I; *B,* stage II. (From Ignatavicius, D. D., Workman, M. L., & Mishler, M. A. [1999]. Medical-surgical nursing across the health care continuum [3rd ed.]. Philadelphia: W.B. Saunders.)

National Pressure Ulcer Advisory Panel (NPUAP) (Margolis, 1995).

- *Stage I: Nonblanchable erythema of intact skin, the heralding lesion of skin ulceration.* In dark-skinned individuals, skin discoloration, warmth, edema, induration, or hardness also may be indicators. Do not confuse this stage with reactive hyperemia. **Blanchable erythema** refers to a reddened area that turns white or pale temporarily when finger pressure is

applied. A normal reactive hyperemic response results in blanchable erythema over a pressure site (Bergstrom et al., 1994). This concept is important to understand when staging pressure ulcers.

- *Stage II: Partial-thickness skin loss involving the epidermis, dermis, or both.* The ulcer is superficial and looks like an **abrasion,** which is a superficial injury caused by rubbing or scraping the skin against another surface. A stage II ulcer also may look like a blister or shallow crater.

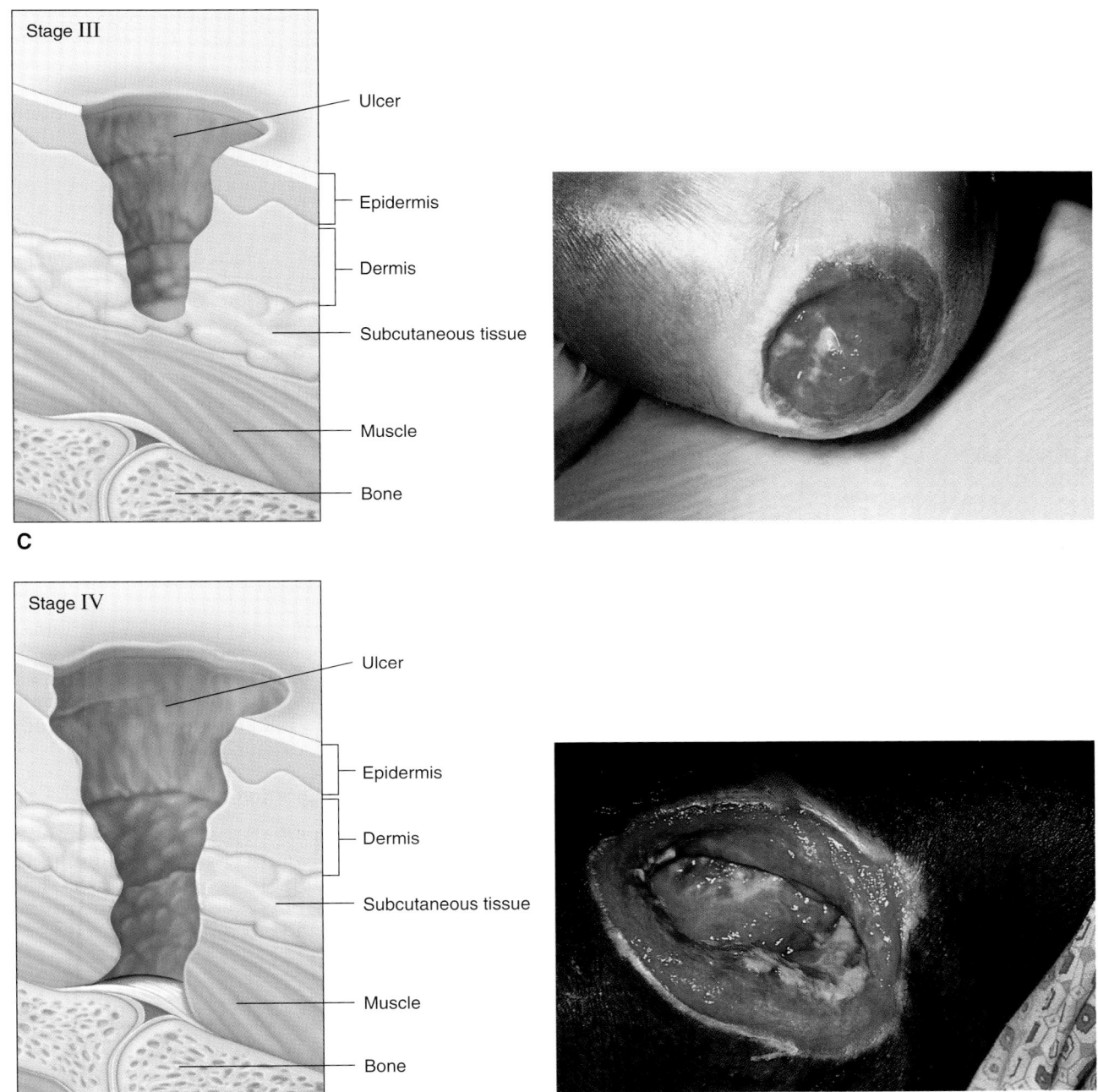

Figure 32–6 *Continued. C,* stage III; *D,* stage IV. (From Ignatavicius, D. D., Workman, M. L., & Mishler, M. A. [1999]. Medical-surgical nursing across the health care continuum [3rd ed.]. Philadelphia: W.B. Saunders.)

- *Stage III: Full-thickness skin loss involving damage to or necrosis of subcutaneous tissue that may extend to, but not through, the underlying fascia.* The ulcer looks like a deep crater with or without undermining of adjacent tissues.
- *Stage IV: Full-thickness skin loss with extensive destruction, tissue necrosis, or damage to muscle, bone, or supporting structures.* Undermining and sinus tracts also may be developed.

Be aware that this sequential staging system is somewhat controversial. According to the NPUAP, pressure ulcer staging is appropriate only for defining the maximum depth of tissue involvement. When using a sequential staging system, remember that pressure ulcers do not progress from Stage I to Stage IV (Margolis, 1995). Also beware of using reverse staging (also called downstaging) to describe a healing pressure ulcer. For example, if a client has a Stage IV pressure ulcer that has healed and now looks like a Stage II ulcer, you should identify it as a healing Stage IV ulcer instead of a Stage II ulcer.

Problems of Wound Healing

Many factors affect wound healing (Box 32–1). Local factors can affect the wound site itself, whereas a systemic condition may affect overall healing. Complications—such as infection, hemorrhage, fistulas, dehiscence, and evisceration—can occur during wound healing.

Infection

Wound infections most commonly occur within 36 to 48 hours after surgery. Usually, the symptoms of infection arise 5 to 7 days after surgery. Postoperative monitoring must include assessment for signs and symptoms of infection, such as fever, wound drainage, swelling, and tenderness. Increased drainage, drainage of another color, erythema at the wound perimeter, an elevated white blood cell count, and general malaise may indicate wound infection.

An infected wound must be cleansed of the infecting organism and cellular debris so that healing can begin. Factors that can predispose a client to wound infection include obesity, a debilitating condition, advanced age, a long and complicated operative procedure, other medical conditions, corticosteroid use, radiation therapy, and wound dehiscence and evisceration.

Hemorrhage

Hemorrhage, or bleeding from the wound bed or site, can occur in the immediate postoperative or initial postinjury period. Normally, hemostasis occurs quickly and clotting begins. However, hemorrhage may occur if a blood vessel continues to bleed or the client has poor clotting function. Causes of hemorrhage include a surgical drain, a loose surgical suture, and infection. Internal hemorrhage can occur with no external evidence of bleeding. To assess for internal hemorrhage, check for distention or swelling of the affected area, a change in the amount or type of drainage from a drain, and signs and symptoms of hypovolemic shock (elevated heart rate and decreased blood pressure).

Hemorrhage is easily detected as bloody drainage on the surgical dressing, especially if the dressing becomes saturated rapidly. However, be sure to assess not just the dressing but the area around the dressing and posterior to the wound site. For instance, if your client has an incision and dressing on the anterior part of the neck, check the posterior neck region for drainage. A hematoma, a collection of blood in a space in tissues, may form during the early postoperative period. To detect a hematoma, assess for hard painful swelling around the incision site. Assess all surgical wounds closely during the first 24 to 48 hours postoperatively.

Fistula

A **fistula** is an abnormal passage between two internal organs or between an organ and the external skin surface. The fistula forms because healing tissue layers do not close. A fistula may result from an abscess or infection, traumatic injury, inflammatory process (radiation), or a disease process such as cancer.

Dehiscence and Evisceration

Dehiscence refers to partial or total separation of the wound edges (Fig. 32–7). **Evisceration** is the protrusion of an internal organ (such as a bowel loop) through the incision. Wound eviscerations are medical emergencies. If one of these complications occurs, con-

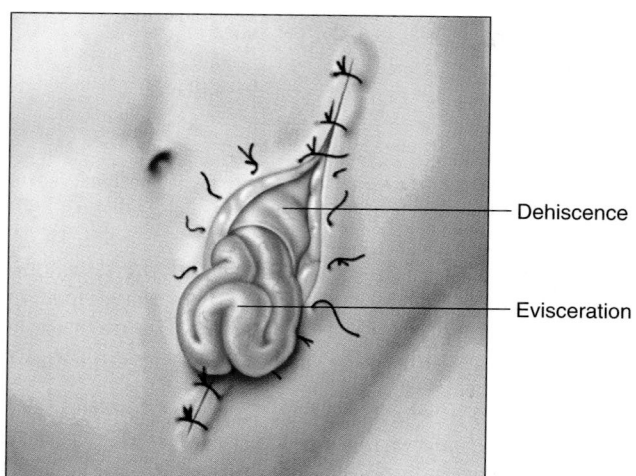

Figure 32–7. Wound dehiscence is the opening of the edges of a surgical wound. Evisceration is the protrusion of internal organs through the incision.

RESPONDING TO WOUND EVISCERATION

If your client's wound eviscerates, you will need to respond swiftly and accurately as outlined here.

1. Stay calm. Projecting a calm and confident manner will help keep the client and her family calm as well.
2. Ask a colleague to obtain supplies and to notify a physician while you stay with the client.
3. Help the client into semi-Fowler's position with her knees slightly gatched. This position will ease pressure on the wound, prevent further tearing of the wound edges, and reduce the risk of further evisceration.
4. Cover the protruding intestine with a sterile dressing moistened with sterile normal saline solution to help prevent wound contamination and keep the abdominal contents moist. If no sterile dressing is available, use clean towels or dressings.
5. Monitor the client closely and assess her vital signs and pulse oximetry readings. Frequent monitoring will help you detect impending shock.
6. Establish intravenous access to provide fluids and prepare the client for surgery as ordered. The client will most likely need surgery to repair the wound and will not be permitted oral intake.
7. Continue to provide emotional support to client and her family. Wound evisceration can be extremely frightening. A calm, supportive approach can help the client through this emergency.

tact the physician immediately. Box 32–2 describes your role in caring for a client with wound evisceration.

FACTORS AFFECTING SKIN INTEGRITY AND WOUND HEALING

Several factors affect skin integrity and potential for wound healing. They include lifestyle, developmental, physiological, and environmental factors.

Lifestyle Factors

Lifestyle factors that affect skin integrity include personal hygiene, nutrition and fluid status, activity and exercise level, smoking, and substance abuse.

PERSONAL HYGIENE. People with poor hygiene may have an increased risk for a wound infection or skin disorder. Routine skin cleansing removes bacteria, sweat, and other substances that may cause skin problems.

NUTRITION AND FLUID STATUS. Malnutrition with deficiencies of protein and vitamins A and C can impair wound healing. In a severely underweight or emaciated client, cells cannot transport oxygen and nutrients to the tissues to aid wound healing. Conversely, obesity is a risk factor for poor wound healing because adipose tissue has a poor blood supply and less resistance to infection.

ACTIVITY AND EXERCISE. Active people who get adequate exercise tend to experience fewer skin problems. On the other hand, immobilization (such as from advanced age or spinal cord injury) increases the risk for skin breakdown and other skin problems. Clients who cannot change position independently also have a greater risk for pressure ulcer formation.

SMOKING. Smoking constricts blood vessels and reduces the blood's oxygen-carrying capacity, resulting in decreased tissue oxygenation. Smoking also increases platelet aggregation, which in turn may cause hypercoagulability with decreased tissue perfusion to the skin or a wound.

SUBSTANCE ABUSE. People who abuse substances, such as alcohol or illicit drugs, often have poor nutrition, which can lead to poor wound healing and skin care.

Developmental Factors

Skin problems can occur at any time of life, from infancy to advanced age. However, infants and children heal faster than older adults. Elderly persons may be less mobile and have fragile skin that tends to heal more slowly than that of younger adults.

Physiological Factors

Such factors as advanced age, immunosuppression, incontinence, hypoxemia, diabetes, infections, neurological impairments, medical-surgical procedures, and medications can affect wound healing.

AGE. Age plays an important role in wound healing. As a person ages, the wound healing phase can be prolonged because of decreased initial inflammatory responses. Changes in the vascular, immune, and respiratory systems can also impair wound healing.

IMMUNOSUPPRESSION. Immunosuppressed persons may have a slowed inflammatory response, slowed re-epithelialization, and a decrease in leukocytic activity.

INCONTINENCE. Bowel and bladder incontinence can affect and delay wound healing because contact with stool or urine can contaminate a wound, prolonging healing and providing a medium for bacterial growth and subsequent infection.

HYPOXEMIA. Poor or impaired blood flow to a wound and surrounding tissues impairs wound healing. Decreased tissue oxygenation impairs collagen synthesis and epithelialization.

DIABETES. Diabetic clients may have small-blood-vessel disease, which can impair tissue oxygenation and tissue perfusion. Hyperglycemia inhibits leukocytic activity, can delay the formation of granulation tissue, and provides an ideal environment for the growth of yeast and fungi.

INFECTION. Wound infections cause a prolonged inflammatory response and delayed wound healing. Wounds cannot heal when infection is present.

NEUROLOGICAL IMPAIRMENT. Clients with neurological impairments, such as spinal cord injury, dementia, or diabetic neuropathy, are at greater risk for *Impaired skin integrity*. These people may not be able to care for themselves and, because they may lack sensation, cannot feel pressure or irritation to the skin. Clients with a change in level of consciousness (such as comatose clients or intensive care clients who are sedated) also cannot protect themselves from factors that can lead to skin breakdown.

PROCEDURES. Medical and surgical procedures, such as operative incisions, intravenous therapy, venipuncture, and radiation therapy, can raise the risk of *Impaired skin integrity*. Orthopedic clients who undergo traction to immobilize a fractured extremity or who have casts to repair fractures are at increased risk for skin breakdown. Friction and pressure from medical devices, such as casts, cervical collars, oxygen tubing around the nose and ears, and nasogastric tubes can also cause skin breakdown.

MEDICATIONS. Drugs—such as steroids, anti-inflammatory medications, and chemotherapy—can alter protein synthesis, cellular growth, and the inflammatory phase of wound healing.

Environmental Factors

Environmental factors that can affect skin integrity include moisture from incontinence, perspiration, emesis, wound drainage, friction from bed linens, and skin dryness. Skin may become easily macerated (wet and softened) if exposed to moisture for a prolonged period. Friction and shear from wrinkled bed linens can lead to pressure ulcers unless appropriate prevention strategies are implemented.

Even general environmental factors can affect a client's ability to relax and heal, as described in the accompanying Cross-Cultural Care chart.

ASSESSMENT

Collecting client data is the first step in nursing assessment. Using the data you collected during assessment allows you to develop a plan of care for the client. The two primary skin integrity diagnoses are *Risk for impaired skin integrity* and *Impaired skin integrity*.

General Assessment of Skin Integrity and Wound Healing

A thorough skin assessment is an important part of the physical examination, especially if the client was treated for or has risk factors for *Impaired skin integrity*.

You should identify risk factors and assess the skin of all clients routinely, especially those who need long-term care.

Health History

When obtaining the health history, use a holistic perspective. Consider the client's medical history, history of present illness, surgical history, current and past medications, nutritional state, mobility level, circulatory status, continence status, and presence of current infection. Perform a psychosocial assessment that includes the client's age, marital status, occupation, living arrangements, financial status, insurance coverage, cultural beliefs, and spirituality. Also assess the client's learning potential to determine her learning needs.

Physical Examination

If your client has *Impaired skin integrity* or a risk for impaired integrity, be sure to conduct a thorough physical examination. Assess height, weight, activity level, muscle mass, circulatory function, and respiratory function.

During a physical examination, you may notice a wide variety of lesions on your client's skin. Some are harmless variations; others are evidence of a disease process. If your client has a wound, assess it carefully.

Diagnostic Tests

Several diagnostic studies help identify skin or wound infection, poor oxygenation, and general nutrition status—factors that can affect skin integrity and wound healing. Use these laboratory values to assess the client's hydration status, identify possible infections, and help you formulate nursing diagnoses and develop the nursing plan of care.

COMPLETE BLOOD COUNT. The complete blood count reveals the blood's oxygen-carrying capacity and may suggest an infection. For instance, the hemoglobin (Hgb) level indicates the blood's oxygen-carrying capacity and an elevated white blood cell count may suggest a systemic or local infection.

ERYTHROCYTE SEDIMENTATION RATE. The sedimentation rate can help assess the client's inflammatory, infectious, and necrotic processes.

PRE-ALBUMIN AND ALBUMIN LEVELS. Abnormally low pre-albumin and albumin levels indicate poor nutritional status, which, in turn, slows wound healing.

RADIOLOGICAL STUDIES. If the client has a suspected infection and has a wound over a bony prominence (such as the sacrum or heel), a physician will typically order radiological studies to rule out osteomyelitis. Standard x-rays or a bone scan can be used to detect infection.

Focused Assessment for Risk for Impaired Skin Integrity

Assessing your client's risk for developing pressure ulcers is an important nursing role. To help determine your client's risk, you can use a systematic risk assess-

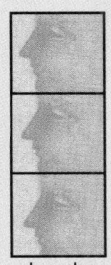

CROSS-CULTURAL CARE
CARING FOR A FILIPINO CLIENT

Mrs. Jacan is of Filipino descent and came to America at age 18 after World War II. She and her parents fled the country after the war and settled in the Washington D.C. area. Mrs. Jacan lives in close proximity to her daughter, who checks in on her frequently. Postoperatively, Mrs. Jacan was quiet and cooperative but not progressing well in her physical therapy. She tried to maintain a harmonious relationship with the nursing and physical therapy staff but felt that she had little privacy in a semiprivate room and little quiet time for herself. Leininger (1995) identified a number of values that Americans with a Filipino background, like Mrs. Jacan, tend to exhibit. Although every client is unique, many Filipino clients tend to hold the following values:

- Showing respect for others and deferring to authority.
- Maintaining smooth and harmonious relationships with others, especially family.
- Maintaining a deep sense of loyalty, mutual respect, and obligation to each other.
- Preserving social relationships and maintaining a sense of self-esteem.
- Giving to others when they need assistance.
- Eating fish, rice, vegetables and other "hot-cold" foods.
- Involving and facilitating extended family in nursing care activities.
- Privacy and quiet periods of time as essential to recovery.
- Pain as gift from God.

Sarah, Mrs. Jacan's nurse, demonstrated cultural sensitivity when talking with her:

Sarah: Good morning, Mrs. Jacan. How are you this morning?

Mrs. Jacan: Oh, I guess I'm okay.

Sarah: (Sensing the hesitancy of her answer, Sarah followed up on her response) You're just okay? You were doing so well yesterday. Is there something different today?

Mrs. Jacan: Well, I don't want to be a bother *(whispering)*. It's not that I don't like my roommate, but it seems as if so many people are always walking in here. I just can't seem to get any peace and quiet.

Sarah: Maybe we could switch you to a private room where you could get a little more privacy and rest. Let me check into it for you.

Mrs. Jacan: Well, you're the boss and I don't want to go against you. Maybe we should call my daughter and tell her about this.

Critical Thinking Questions

- Why was Mrs. Jacan so worried about offending her roommate by switching to a private room?
- Why is it important for Sarah to call Mrs. Jacan's daughter to inform her of the plan to switch her to a private room?
- Why does Mrs. Jacan need so much privacy and quiet? Once Sarah has moved her to the private room, what can she do to ensure that Mrs. Jacan will receive the needed quiet periods?

Reference

Leininger, M. (1995). *Transcultural nursing: Concepts, theories, research and practices.* New York: McGraw-Hill.

ment tool. Such tools include the Norton Scale, the Gosnell Scale, and the Knoll Assessment Tool. One of the most commonly used is the Braden Scale for Predicting Pressure Sore Risk (Fig. 32–8). It is based on risk factors for clients in a nursing home population.

Using the Braden scale, you assess your client in six areas: sensory perception, moisture, activity, mobility, nutrition, friction, and shear. The client's total score may range from 6 to 23. The lower the score, the higher is the client's risk for pressure ulcer development. The Braden Scale is highly reliable for identifying clients at risk for pressure ulcer development (Bergstrom et al., 1987; Braden & Bergstrom, 1989).

Risk factors common to *Risk for impaired skin integrity* may be internal or external. External factors include the following:

- Radiation
- Physical immobilization

- Mechanical factors, such as shear, pressure, and restraints
- Hypothermia or hyperthermia
- Exposure to moisture, including excretions, secretions, and humidity
- Exposure to chemical substances
- Young or old age

Internal factors include the following:

- Medications
- Skeletal prominence
- Immunological problems
- Developmental or psychogenetic factors
- Altered sensation, circulation, metabolism, skin turgor, nutrition, or pigmentation

Using a conceptual framework called the "web of causation" helps in understanding the development of a pressure ulcer (Fig. 32–9). This framework demon-

BRADEN SCALE
For Predicting Pressure Sore Risk

Patient's Name _____ Evaluator's Name _____ Date of Assessment

	1	2	3	4
SENSORY PERCEPTION ability to respond meaningfully to pressure-related discomfort	**1. Completely Limited** Unresponsive (does not moan, flinch, or grasp) to painful stimuli, due to diminished level of consciousness or sedation. OR limited ability to feel pain over most of body.	**2. Very Limited** Responds only to painful stimuli. Cannot communicate discomfort except by moaning or restlessness OR has a sensory impairment which limits the ability to feel pain or discomfort over ½ of body.	**3. Slightly Limited** Responds to verbal commands, but cannot always communicate discomfort or the need to be turned. OR has some sensory impairment which limits ability to feel pain or discomfort in 1 or 2 extremities.	**4. No Impairment** Responds to verbal commands. Has no sensory deficit which would limit ability to feel or voice pain or discomfort..
MOISTURE degree to which skin is exposed to moisture	**1. Constantly Moist** Skin is kept moist almost constantly by perspiration, urine, etc. Dampness is detected every time patient is moved or turned.	**2. Very Moist** Skin is often, but not always moist. Linen must be changed at least once a shift.	**3. Occasionally Moist:** Skin is occasionally moist, requiring an extra linen change approximately once a day.	**4. Rarely Moist** Skin is usually dry, linen only requires changing at routine intervals.
ACTIVITY degree of physical activity	**1. Bedfast** Confined to bed.	**2. Chairfast** Ability to walk severely limited or non-existent. Cannot bear own weight and/or must be assisted into chair or wheelchair.	**3. Walks Occasionally** Walks occasionally during day, but for very short distances, with or without assistance. Spends majority of each shift in bed or chair	**4. Walks Frequently** Walks outside room at least twice a day and inside room at least once every two hours during waking hours
MOBILITY ability to change and control body position	**1. Completely Immobile** Does not make even slight changes in body or extremity position without assistance	**2. Very Limited** Makes occasional slight changes in body or extremity position but unable to make frequent or significant changes independently.	**3. Slightly Limited** Makes frequent though slight changes in body or extremity position independently.	**4. No Limitation** Makes major and frequent changes in position without assistance.
NUTRITION usual food intake pattern	**1. Very Poor** Never eats a complete meal. Rarely eats more than ⅓ of any food offered. Eats 2 servings or less of protein (meat or dairy products) per day. Takes fluids poorly. Does not take a liquid dietary supplement OR is NPO and/or maintained on clear liquids or IV's for more than 5 days.	**2. Probably Inadequate** Rarely eats a complete meal and generally eats only about ½ of any food offered. Protein intake includes only 3 servings of meat or dairy products per day. Occasionally will take a dietary supplement. OR receives less than optimum amount of liquid diet or tube feeding	**3. Adequate** Eats over half of most meals. Eats a total of 4 servings of protein (meat, dairy products) per day. Occasionally will refuse a meal, but will usually take a supplement when offered OR is on a tube feeding or TPN regimen which probably meets most of nutritional needs	**4. Excellent** Eats most of every meal. Never refuses a meal. Usually eats a total of 4 or more servings of meat and dairy products. Occasionally eats between meals. Does not require supplementation.
FRICTION & SHEAR	**1. Problem** Requires moderate to maximum assistance in moving. Complete lifting without sliding against sheets is impossible. Frequently slides down in bed or chair, requiring frequent repositioning with maximum assistance. Spasticity, contractures or agitation leads to almost constant friction	**2. Potential Problem** Moves feebly or requires minimum assistance. During a move skin probably slides to some extent against sheets, chair, restraints or other devices. Maintains relatively good position in chair or bed most of the time but occasionally slides down.	**3. No Apparent Problem** Moves in bed and in chair independently and has sufficient muscle strength to lift up completely during move. Maintains good position in bed or chair.	
				Total Score

© Copyright Barbara Braden and Nancy Bergstrom, 1988

Figure 32–8. Braden scale for predicting pressure sore risk. (Barbara Braden and Nancy Bergstrom, 1988.)

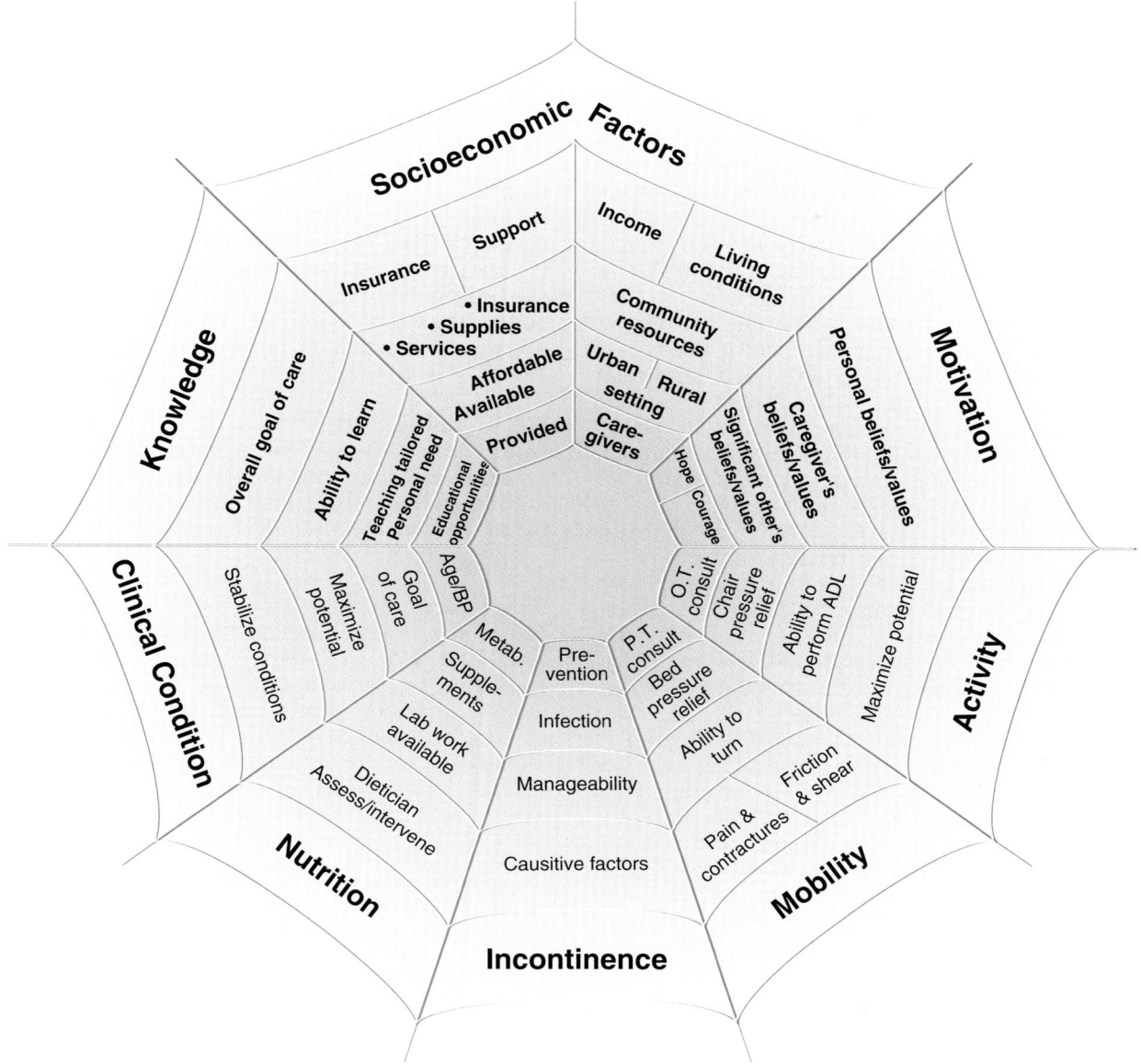

Figure 32–9. The web of causation of pressure ulcer development. (Redrawn with permission from Barbara Oot-Giromini, RN, MS, CETN, Binghamton, NY.)

strates the complex interrelationships of the factors affecting the skin. It considers many factors, including the client's clinical condition, nutrition, incontinence, mobility, activity, motivation, socioeconomic factors, and knowledge.

Focused Assessment for Impaired Skin Integrity

Defining Characteristics

Defining characteristics for *Impaired skin integrity* include invasion of body structures, disruption of the epidermis, and destruction of the dermis. When assessing a client's wound, you must document many

characteristics of the wound and the surrounding area, including those described here.

LOCATION
Always document the exact anatomic location of a wound. For example, write "client has 4 cm abdominal incision in the right lower quadrant" or "pressure ulcer on left lateral malleolus."

SIZE
When measuring the wound, determine its length, width, and depth, in centimeters (cm) unless directed otherwise. Accurate wound measurement is important to developing an appropriate treatment plan and to aid evaluation of skin and wound healing.

To properly define a pressure ulcer, measure the length, width, and depth of the affected area. Use the concept of the face of a clock to help define landmarks and areas of the wound or impaired skin area. Measure wound length from head to toe (with 12 o'clock representing the client's head and 6 o'clock representing the feet). Measure the width of the wound from side to side (3 o'clock to 9 o'clock). Also assess wound depth by measuring how far the wound proceeds below the skin surface. Be sure to check for tunneling (a sinus tract or tunnel) or undermining of the wound or pressure ulcer.

You can use one of various measuring instruments to measure and assess a wound. One of the easiest methods involves using a cotton-tipped applicator and a centimeter rule (Fig. 32–10). Another common method employs a tape measure or ruler. In the client's chart, record the wound length and width in centimeters, the measurement method you used, and the client's position at the time of measurement.

The advantages of the ruler method are that it is easy, quick, inexpensive, and reliably reproduced by the same person and other people (van Rÿswÿk, 1996). Disadvantages are that it may be difficult to decide which dimension to measure if the wound is irregular, that you may tend to overestimate the wound size, and that reliability tends to decline as the wound increases in size.

Another way to measure a wound is to trace it. Hold a disposable acetate sheet, a measuring guide, or a plastic bag over the wound and trace the edges with a fine-tip permanent marker. Also write the date, the client's name or number, your name, and location markers (such as head and toes) on the tracing. Calculate the wound area and document the area, the method of obtaining and calculating the measurement, and the client's position at the time of the measurement. Also place the tracing itself in the client's chart.

The advantages of this method are that it is easy, quick, and reliably reproduced by the same person and other people, especially for a large wound. Wound tracings can be a valuable addition to the client's medical record, and they allow easy monitoring of changes in the wound. The expense incurred by this method depends on the materials you use. Disadvan-

tages of this method are that it may be difficult to see the margins of the wound while tracing it and that the accuracy of the tracing declines in smaller wounds. If your transparency does not contain a grid, you will need to copy the tracing to grid paper to calculate the size of the wound.

COLOR
Document the color of the wound bed. A red wound bed is ready for healing and consists of viable tissue. A yellow wound bed indicates fibrinous slough, old tissue, or exudate that must be removed for healing to occur. Black tissue indicates eschar, a thick, leathery necrotic tissue that is not viable (Bergstrom et al., 1994).

SURROUNDING SKIN
Note the condition of the wound edges or margins. Assess the skin around the wound for redness or induration, temperature, moisture, color, and odor. Erythema around the wound edges may indicate underlying infection.

DRAINAGE
Assess any wound drainage for color, amount, consistency, and odor. Describe the drainage as serous, sanguineous, or serosanguineous. Be aware that the wound location, depth, and extent determine the amount of drainage. Noting drainage color can help identify the type of organism that may be infecting the wound. A foul, fecal, musty, or strong odor from a wound may indicate wound infection.

*A*ction *A*lert!
Be careful when documenting drainage and infection. Yellow drainage from a wound does not always mean the wound is infected. Slough from the wound bed can be yellow and consist of wound debris, old white blood cells, and macrophages.

TEMPERATURE
Be sure to assess the temperature of the wound. Increased warmth of the wound bed or surrounding tissues may indicate pressure ulcer formation or an infection. To assess temperature, palpate the wound and surrounding tissues.

PAIN
Always assess for pain at the wound site. Absence of pain may indicate nerve impairment or involvement. Although pain at the wound site indicates intact nerves, severe pain may indicate infection and underlying tissue involvement.

WOUND CLOSURES
Surgical wounds and incisions are usually closed with sutures or stainless steel staples. Suture material may be silk, nylon, cotton, linen, wire, or Dacron (polyester). When suturing, the physician sews the inner tissue layers together, usually with a suture material that is absorbed by the body during healing. Usually, skin sutures are left in the incision for 7 to 10 days.

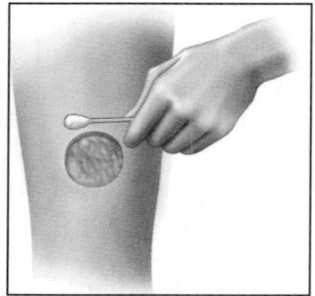
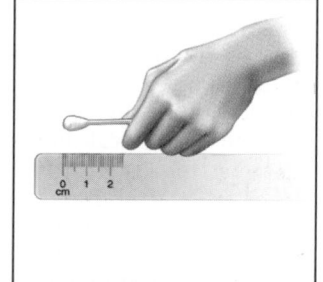

Figure 32–10. An easy method for measuring a wound using a cotton swab and centimeter rule.

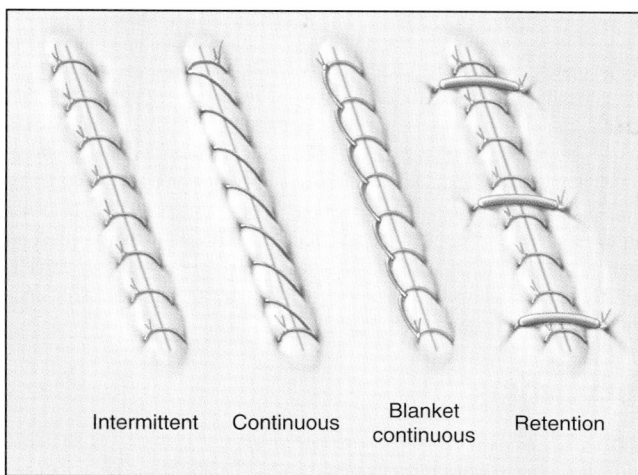

Figure 32–11. Types of sutures.

Several different suturing methods can be used (Fig. 32–11). They include intermittent suturing (in which each stitch is knotted) and continuous suturing (in which one thread is used to create several stitches and is tied only at the beginning and the end). Retention sutures (large sutures covered by rubber tubing, which prevents further skin disruption) are used for large abdominal incisions in which additional support is needed (such as in obese clients), if swelling is substantial, or when the sutures must be left in place for a prolonged period.

Stainless steel staples are commonly used to approximate incision edges (Fig. 32–12). Staples have advantages over sutures. For instance, they are stronger and less irritating to the skin, and the final scar is more cosmetically acceptable. Steri-Strips (small, thin strips of tape) can be used for smaller incisions (Fig. 32–13). These strips may minimize incisional irritation, swelling, and scar formation.

Postoperative assessment of the surgical wound should include inspection of the skin around the staples for redness, irritation, or excessive swelling. These signs may indicate a wound infection or overly

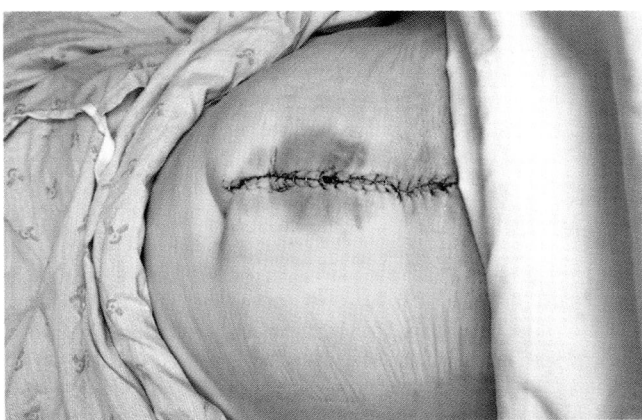

Figure 32–12. Staples in an incision line.

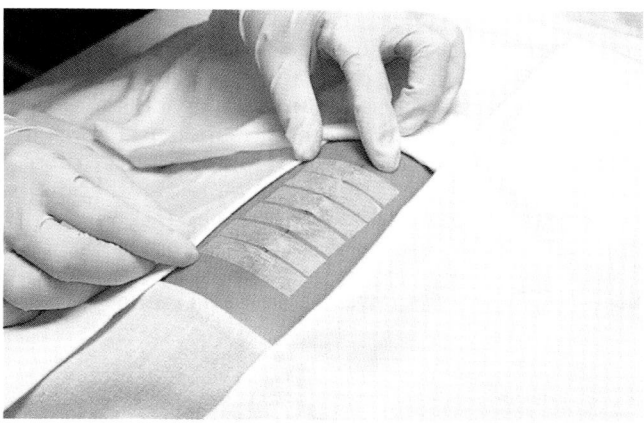

Figure 32–13. Steri-Strips.

tight wound closure, which ultimately can lead to wound edge separation.

Related Factors

Factors related to the diagnosis *Impaired skin integrity* may be either internal or external. External factors include the following:

- Extreme heat or cold
- Chemical substances
- Mechanical factors, such as shear, pressure, or restraints
- Physical immobilization
- Moisture and humidity
- Medications
- Radiation
- Diminished circulation

Internal factors include the following:

- Altered metabolism
- Skeletal prominence
- Immunological deficit
- Altered sensation, circulation, turgor, pigmentation, or nutritional state (such as obesity or emaciation)

Keep in mind that proper wound healing requires adequate perfusion. Altered circulation may lead to poor tissue oxygenation and subsequent ulceration. Decreased arterial circulation causes ulcers because the tissues fail to receive enough oxygenated blood. These ulcers most commonly appear on the bony prominences of the ankle and toes. Chronic diminished circulation produces atrophic changes, including hair loss and thin, shiny skin. Also, pulses may be absent or weak. Venous stasis ulcers, caused by poor venous return, are associated with varicose veins and thrombophlebitis. With venous stasis ulcers, arterial pulses are present but venous blood is not returning to the heart. The chronic skin changes of dark pigmentation and stasis dermatitis are usually present.

Chemical irritation can result from urinary or fecal incontinence, gastric secretions, and harsh products that can cause skin irritation and breakdown. To help prevent chemical irritation, make sure the client's plan of care includes measures to protect the epidermis from contact with these irritants.

Radiation is the least common mechanism of skin injury. Excluding occupational radiation accidents, the most common type of radiation injury results from radiation therapy. The skin is vulnerable to radiation injury because the cells of the basal layer are continually and rapidly dividing. Signs of injury develop 2 to 3 days after radiation exposure and peak in 2 to 3 weeks. When the skin is severely affected, ulceration may develop.

Focused Assessment for Related Nursing Diagnoses

Risk for Infection

The client with a pressure ulcer or postoperative surgical incision is at risk for infection. The skin opening creates an entrance site for microorganisms to enter the wound.

Impaired Tissue Integrity

Assess the tissues surrounding the client's wound for further skin breakdown or interruption. A client may have impaired tissue integrity even without skin breakdown on the surface. Palpate the area around the incision or pressure ulcer to assess for bogginess or hardened tissue.

Impaired Physical Mobility

Assess for other conditions that may lead to impaired physical mobility. For instance, a client with visual or neurological impairment may be at risk for *Impaired skin integrity.* Clients with a neurological deficit such as spinal cord injury or multiple sclerosis may be unable to feel pressure and other skin sensations or to reposition themselves to decrease the risk of pressure ulcer formation.

Body Image Disturbance

Clients suffering from *Impaired skin integrity* may have a disturbance in their body image. Large surgical wounds or pressure ulcers can make the client feel self-conscious and apprehensive about appearance. Take measures to help the client maintain a positive body image (see Chapter 46).

Hopelessness

Clients with *Impaired skin integrity* may feel a sense of hopelessness. Most surgical incisions follow a predictable course of healing. However, chronic wounds, especially pressure ulcers, can take months to heal. The client may begin to feel that the wound will never heal. Encouraging the client to focus on wound healing stages and to participate in wound care may help ease feelings of hopelessness.

Altered Nutrition: Less Than Body Requirements

The client with *Impaired skin integrity* needs adequate nutrition for wound healing. Depending on the client's medical condition, alternative feeding methods may be necessary. For instance, a client with a large abdominal wound who cannot receive oral intake may require total parenteral nutrition. A client with a poor appetite may need nutritional supplements and a daily multivitamin supplement. Vitamins C, A, and B complex, and iron, copper, and zinc are especially important for wound healing.

DIAGNOSIS

The diagnoses *Risk for impaired skin integrity, Impaired skin integrity,* and *Impaired tissue integrity* are interrelated. *Impaired tissue integrity* encompasses the broad category of skin, tissue, and other mucous membrane disorders. *Risk for impaired skin integrity* applies to a client with a medical, surgical, developmental, or mobility problem that could affect skin health. *Impaired skin integrity* results from skin injury caused by moisture, pressure, friction, shear, and other factors.

Be sure to take a thorough assessment, including a complete health history, physical examination, and evaluation of mobility and nutritional status to determine whether the client has a nursing diagnosis of *Risk for impaired skin integrity* or *Impaired skin integrity.* If the client has risk factors without signs or symptoms of skin impairment, assign a nursing diagnosis of *Risk for impaired skin integrity,* as suggested by the accompanying decision tree. Typical candidates for this nursing diagnosis include clients who are bedbound with poor nutrition and those with an altered level of consciousness. In contrast, a client who is being treated for pressure ulcers has a nursing diagnosis of *Impaired skin integrity.* The accompanying Decision Tree can be helpful in developing the client's plan of care.

Assigning an appropriate nursing diagnosis depends on the assessment data you collect. In some cases, another nursing diagnosis may be more suitable. For example, for a client recovering from a total hip replacement, you might choose *Impaired physical mobility* because it addresses skin integrity as well as mobility problems. *Risk for infection* may be appropriate for the postsurgical appendectomy client with an abdominal incision. The data clustering chart provides examples of ways to formulate appropriate nursing diagnoses.

PLANNING

After choosing appropriate nursing diagnoses, you must develop a plan of care based on the diagnoses. When planning care, assign priorities to the nursing diagnoses, select appropriate nursing interventions to achieve expected outcomes (client-centered goals), and document the nursing diagnoses, outcomes, interventions, and evaluations on the plan of care. For a cli-

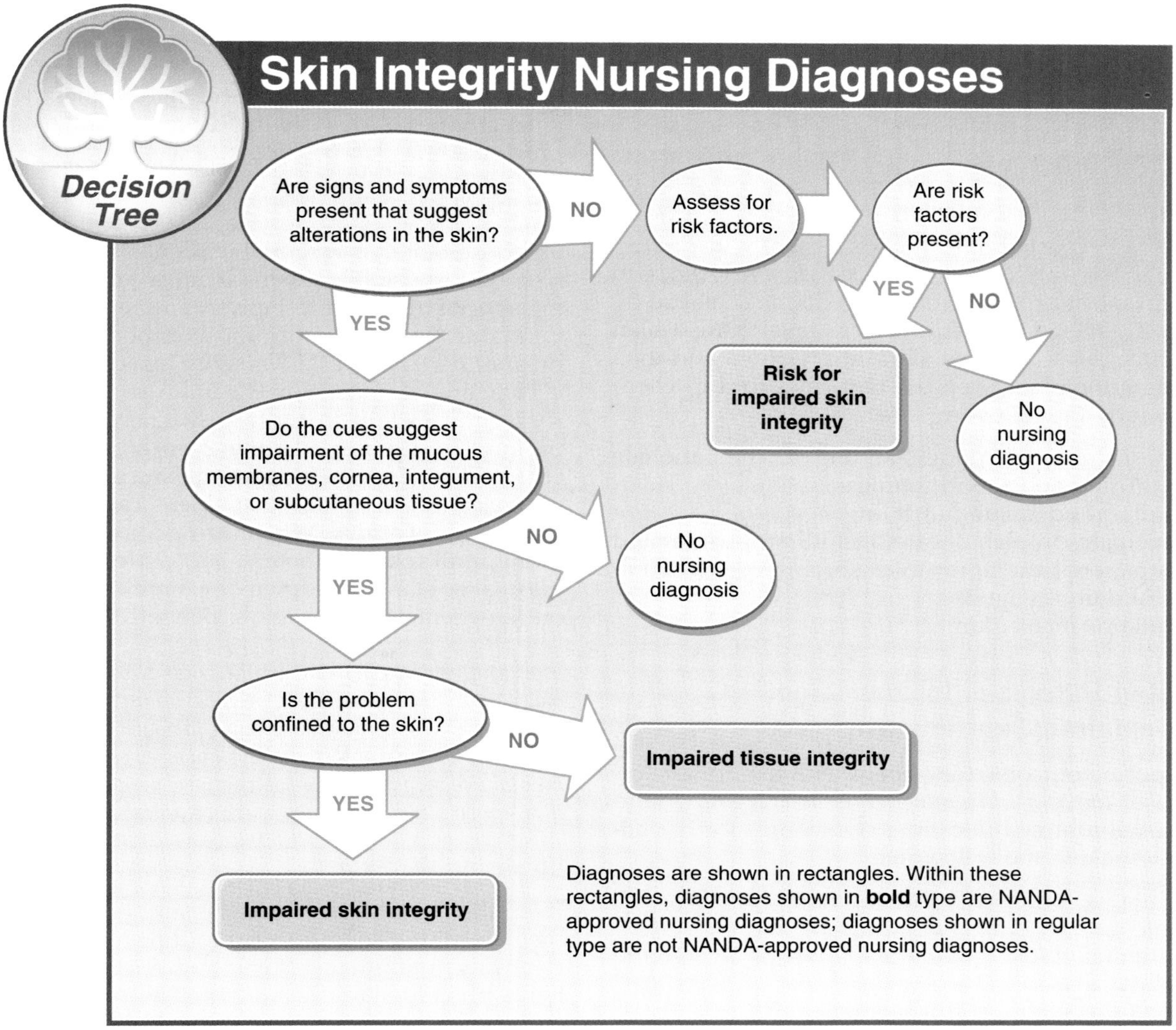

Skin Integrity Nursing Diagnoses

Decision Tree

Are signs and symptoms present that suggest alterations in the skin?

— NO → Assess for risk factors. → Are risk factors present?

— YES ↓ (from first question)

Do the cues suggest impairment of the mucous membranes, cornea, integument, or subcutaneous tissue?

— NO → No nursing diagnosis

— YES ↓

Is the problem confined to the skin?

— NO → **Impaired tissue integrity**

— YES ↓

Impaired skin integrity

Are risk factors present? — YES → **Risk for impaired skin integrity**

Are risk factors present? — NO → No nursing diagnosis

Diagnoses are shown in rectangles. Within these rectangles, diagnoses shown in **bold** type are NANDA-approved nursing diagnoses; diagnoses shown in regular type are not NANDA-approved nursing diagnoses.

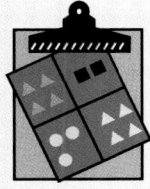

CLUSTERING DATA TO MAKE A NURSING DIAGNOSIS
SKIN PROBLEMS

Data Cluster	Diagnosis
A single 44-year-old female on the third postoperative day is very concerned about the large abdominal incision created during her hysterectomy and worries about her future cosmetic appearance.	*Body image disturbance* related to large abdominal incision secondary to hysterectomy
An 18-year-old male injured while body surfing at the beach sustained a C4 fracture and now is quadriplegic.	*Risk for impaired skin integrity* related to impaired physical mobility
A 72-year-old female in a motor vehicle accident needs balanced suspended traction for a fracture of her right femur. Has a stage II pressure ulcer measuring 2×3 cm on left buttock.	*Impaired skin integrity* related to bedrest and traction

ent who is bedbound after a motor vehicle accident, the goal is to prevent skin breakdown and pressure ulcer formation. For a client with a pressure ulcer, the goal is to achieve timely healing of the pressure ulcer.

Expected Outcomes for the Client With Risk for Impaired Skin Integrity

The overall expected outcome for a client with a nursing diagnosis of *Risk for impaired skin integrity* is to maintain intact skin. This outcome can be achieved by identifying the client's risk factors, developing a plan with strategies to prevent skin interruption, and then evaluating the plan. Expected outcomes for this client may include the following:

- Demonstrates an understanding of the rationale for turning and repositioning
- Maintains adequate nutrition
- Participates in plan of care, including physical and occupational therapies to maintain normal activities of daily living
- Maintains intact skin

Expected Outcomes for the Client With Impaired Skin Integrity

The expected outcome for a client with the nursing diagnosis of *Impaired skin integrity* is to achieve wound healing without complications. Outcomes for the client may include the following:

- Maintains a normal temperature or baseline vital signs
- Maintains nutritional intake to support wound healing
- Maintains adequate fluid intake
- Performs activities of daily living
- Can perform wound care and dressing changes as instructed
- Can state the signs and symptoms of infection
- Can verbalize discharge instructions for wound care

INTERVENTION

Interventions for a client with *Impaired skin integrity* are developed by the multidisciplinary team, including the nurse, physician, physical and occupational therapists, and dietitian, as well as the client and family. A valuable resource to medical and nursing staff is the certified enterostomal therapist nurse. This specially trained wound, ostomy, and incontinence nurse can assist in selecting dressings and support surfaces, planning and implementing care, and evaluating the plan of care.

Interventions to Reduce the Risk for Impaired Skin Integrity

Preventing pressure ulcer development and promoting wound healing are the responsibility of the multi-

disciplinary team members. Several strategies should be used to prevent skin impairments: monitoring the client, cleansing the skin, providing nutrition, repositioning the client, and encouraging the client to maintain activities of daily living. Client teaching can help prevent some skin problems as well.

Monitoring the Client

Skin assessment is essential in identifying the client at risk. Perform skin assessment at least once a day, paying special attention to bony prominences.

Naturally, one of the most important aspects of preventing *Impaired skin integrity* is recognizing which clients are at risk (Box 32–3). Also consider environmental factors in the at-risk client. For instance, prolonged supine positioning on a stretcher in the emergency department, skin moisture caused by diaphoresis, and wrinkled bed linens can put a client's skin integrity at risk. When caring for a surgical client, monitor all tubes, catheters, and drains because these may cause skin breakdown or exert excessive pressure on the client's skin (Leigh & Bennett, 1994).

After Mrs. Jacan's hip surgery, the nurse assesses her skin. Because Mrs. Jacan had pressure ulcer formation preoperatively, the nurse is aware of the importance of ongoing skin assessment, especially because of Mrs. Jacan's *Impaired physical mobility* and *Risk for infection* during the postoperative period. To what areas of Mrs. Jacan's skin should the nurse pay most attention?

Cleansing the Skin

Keep the client's skin clean. Be sure it is cleansed immediately after soiling and at routine intervals. During cleansing, minimizing force and friction to the skin helps prevent skin breakdown. Try to reduce the client's exposure to moisture caused by incontinence, perspiration, and wound drainage (Bergstrom, Allman, & Carlson, 1992). Keep in mind that prolonged

---

BOX 32–3

CONDITIONS THAT INCREASE THE RISK OF IMPAIRED SKIN INTEGRITY

- Advanced age.
- Altered level of consciousness.
- Chronic conditions.
- Dehydration.
- Diabetes.
- Fractures.
- Immobility.
- Impaired circulation.
- Impaired nutrition.
- Incontinence.
- Multisystem trauma.
- Obesity.
- Paralysis.

exposure to moisture may cause skin maceration or breakdown.

Action Alert!
Do not use hot water and soap to cleanse the client's skin. Tailor the plan for skin cleansing based on the client's preferences and skin care needs (Bergstrom, Allman, & Carlson, 1992).

To minimize dry skin, apply topical moisturizing agents and maintain adequate skin hydration. Keep in mind that although the client may find a gentle massage relaxing and soothing, caution must be used when applying creams and lotions to high-risk or reddened skin areas.

Action Alert!
Avoid massaging over bony prominences because the pressure may increase the risk of pressure ulcer formation (Bergstrom, Allman, & Carlson, 1992).

Providing Nutrition

Promoting nutrition and a well-balanced diet can help prevent skin breakdown and pressure ulcer development (see Chapter 38).

Positioning the Client

Positioning the client at risk for skin breakdown is one of your major roles. You can use various strategies to position the client and reduce the risk of skin breakdown, including the following:

*   Reposition high-risk clients at least every 2 hours.
*   Use positioning devices such as pillows to keep bony prominences from touching one another.
*   Raise the client's heels completely off the bed.

Action Alert!
Do not use doughnut devices to relieve pressure on the client's heels. Instead, suspend the heels off the bed to prevent pressure ulcers on the heels (Bergstrom, Allman, & Carlson, 1992).

*   Avoid placing the client's body weight directly on the trochanter when she is in a side-lying position. Instead, position the client at a 30-degree angle to reduce pressure on both the trochanter and the sacrum (Fig. 32–14).
*   Keep the head of the bed as low as the client can tolerate.
*   When moving the client, use proper positioning, transferring, and turning techniques to minimize friction and shear. For example, use assistive devices such as a trapeze or the bed linens. Consider using lubricants (such creams and cornstarch), protective films (such a transparent dressing), and protective dressings to help reduce friction.
*   For a client at risk for pressure ulcer development, use a pressure-reducing mattress such as a static air, gel, or water mattress.
*   Avoid prolonged sitting in a chair or wheelchair by repositioning the client at least every hour.
*   Develop a written plan of care for positioning and turning.

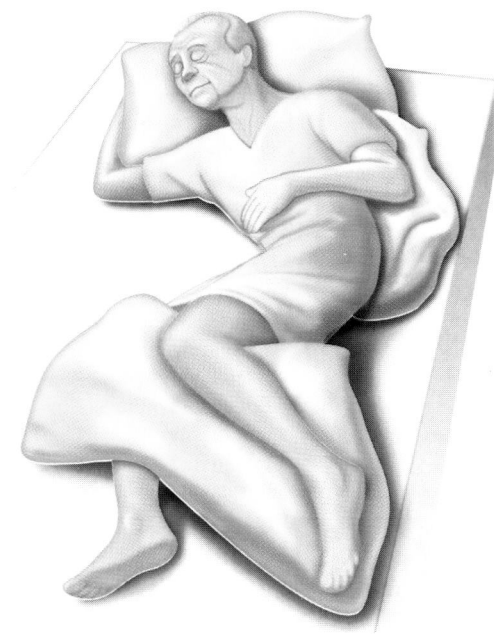

Figure 32–14. Position the client on his or her side at a 30-degree angle to prevent pressure on the trochanter and sacrum. To keep the client in this position, provide support with pillows, as shown.

Encouraging the Client to Maintain Activities of Daily Living

Other interventions to reduce the risk of *Impaired skin integrity* include maintaining the client's current activity level and promoting mobility and range of motion. A physical therapist can assist with measures to maintain the client's mobility as well as passive and active range-of-motion exercises. An occupational therapist can assist with strategies for maintaining the client's daily activities. These strategies should be incorporated into a plan of care tailored to the client's specific needs and overall goals.

Be sure to monitor and document all interventions to reduce the risk of *Impaired skin integrity* as well as the outcomes of these interventions. A written plan of care that specifies each intervention and necessary supplies should be available to the multidisciplinary team to ensure continuity of care (Bergstrom, Allman, & Carlson, 1992).

Client Teaching

Teach the client about skin care and explain the risk factors for pressure ulcer development. Helping the client understand how skin impairment occurs can promote compliance with the plan of care. Be sure to provide instruction on proper positioning, nutritional support, and other prevention strategies to help the client avoid pressure ulcers. Customize your teaching to meet the needs of both the client and family or home caregiver.

Explain the intended outcomes or goals, the duration of treatment, strategies to prevent pressure ulcer

TABLE 32–2
Nutrients and Their Roles in Wound Healing

Nutrient	Role in Wound Healing
Carbohydrates, fats, and calories	Energy for wound regeneration and repair
Copper	Cross-linking of collagen fibers
Iron	Oxygen transport
Protein	Collagen synthesis, epidermal proliferation, and immune response
Vitamin A	Collagen synthesis, epidermal proliferation, and immune response
Vitamin B complex	Protein synthesis and cross-linking of collagen fibers
Vitamin C	Collagen synthesis and capillary wall integrity
Zinc	Collagen synthesis and immune response

recurrence, and the value of participating in self-care. For example, give the client the following instructions:

- Cleanse your skin gently using gentle soaps and mild cleansers.
- Use warm water, not hot, to avoid drying your skin.
- Apply lotions, creams, or moisturizers daily or as needed to keep your skin smooth and soft.
- If sitting for a prolonged period, change positions at least every 2 hours by shifting your weight to relieve pressure areas.

Interventions to Promote Skin Healing

Skin care and wound care have changed dramatically over the past 30 years. Extensive research has led to new wound care treatment protocols and products. However, wound healing cannot be approached solely from a procedural perspective. Instead, the treatment plan must take the client's entire condition into consideration. Physical condition, nutritional status, and treatment methods all affect the healing process (Maklebust, 1996).

Providing Adequate Nutrition

Adequate nutrition is essential for the client with *Impaired skin integrity* (Haas, 1995). Malnutrition inhibits wound healing and may increase the risk for wound infection (Table 32–2). Commonly, a client with *Impaired skin integrity* needs assistance in meeting daily nutritional requirements. Wound healing depends on the availability of adequate protein, vitamins, and minerals. Postoperative clients and elderly, debilitated clients with pressure ulcers require particularly close nutritional monitoring.

Improving a client's nutritional status requires a multidisciplinary effort. Assess the client's intake and help the client meet nutritional needs, as outlined in the accompanying decision tree. One way to help the

client choose nutritious meals is to help her fill out a menu. Also consult a dietitian, as appropriate, to help determine the client's minimal caloric intake required to promote wound healing. The dietitian may request a calorie count to monitor the client's intake and determine whether nutritional requirements are being met. Commonly, the client requires dietary supplementation, such as multivitamins or liquid supplements. A client who cannot take nutrition orally may require enteral or parenteral feedings.

Postoperatively, Mrs. Jacan has little appetite and is not getting adequate nutrition. What effect might Mrs. Jacan's nutrition have on wound healing and development of pressure ulcers? Although Mrs. Jacan tries some nutritional milkshakes, she just cannot eat the solid food on her tray. Keeping in mind Mrs. Jacan's admission history, what foods might the nurse want to include in her diet? How might the nurse involve Mrs. Jacan's daughter in promoting good nutrition for her mother?

Cleansing the Wound

For a wound to heal, the wound bed must be clean and free of infection. To promote healthy granulation tissue, bacteria, devitalized tissue, and exudate must be removed. To cleanse a wound, you will need a wound cleansing solution and a mechanical way to apply the solution to the wound. Numerous wound cleansing solutions or antiseptics are available. However, the benefits of a clean wound must be weighed against the potential trauma to the wound bed that

TABLE 32–3
Irrigation Pressures by Device

Device	Irrigation Pressure (psi)
Spray Bottle-Ultra Klenz (Carrington Laboratories, Inc.)	1.2
Bulb Syringe (Davol Inc., Cranston, RI)	2.0
Piston Irrigation Syringe (60-mL) with catheter tip (Premium Plastics, Inc., Chicago, IL)	4.2
Saline Squeeze Bottle (250-mL) with irrigation cap (Baxter Healthcare Corp., Deerfield, IL)	4.5
Water Pik at lowest setting (#1) (Teledyne Water Pik, Fort Collins, CO)	6.0
Irrijet DS with tip (Ackrad Laboratories, Inc., Cranford, NJ)	7.6
35-mL syringe with 19-gauge needle or angiocatheter	8.0
Water Pik at middle setting (#3) (Teledyne Water Pik, Fort Collins, CO)	42
Water Pik at highest setting (#5) (Teledyne Water Pik, Fort Collins, CO)	>50
Pressurized Cannister-Dey wash (Dey Laboratories, Inc., Napa, CA)	>50

From Beltram, K.A., Thacker, J.G., & Rodeheaver, G.T. Impact pressures generated by commercial wound irrigation devices. (Unpublished research report). Charlottesville, VA, University of Virginia Health Sciences Center.

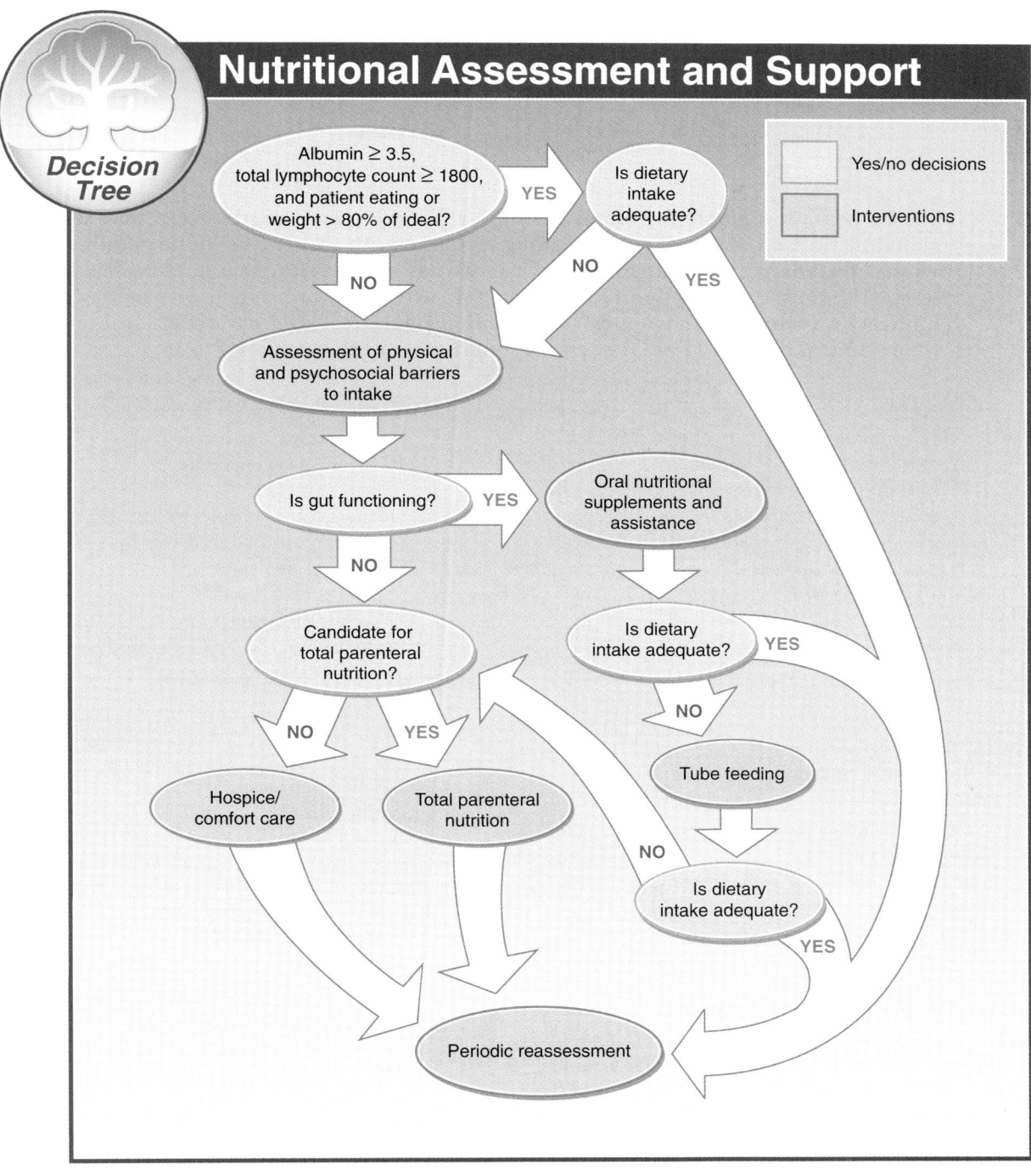

Nutritional Assessment and Support

Decision Tree

could result from cleansing (Bergstrom et al., 1994). Use caution when applying these products. Povidone-iodine, acetic acid, sodium hypochlorite, and hydrogen peroxide are toxic to fibroblasts (Lineaweaver et al., 1985). Dakin's solution and some commercial wound cleansers have also been found to be cytotoxic. Rodeheaver (1989) offers a general rule regarding wound cleansing: "Put nothing into a wound that you would not put in your eye."

Normal saline solution is the preferred cleansing agent because it is physiologically compatible, will not

harm tissue, and adequately cleanses most tissues (Bergstrom et al., 1994). Irrigate wounds with a device that provides 4 to 15 pounds of pressure per square inch (Table 32–3). Using adequate irrigation pressure enhances wound cleansing without damaging the tissues (Bergstrom et al., 1994). One of the easiest ways to irrigate a wound is to use a 35-mL syringe with a 19-gauge needle or angiocatheter. This method provides enough force to remove eschar, bacteria, and other debris (Stevenson et al., 1976). Procedure 32–1 outlines the steps of wound irrigation.

PROCEDURE 32–1

Irrigating a Wound

TIME TO ALLOW
▼
Novice:
15 minutes
Expert:
7 minutes

Wound irrigation promotes wound healing by removing exudate, drainage, pus, and slough. Irrigation is a method of cleaning a wound with a gentle flow of a solution. It washes the wound without wiping delicate tissues with a fabric that might cause damage to newly forming granulation tissue. Irrigation also has the advantage of penetrating tunnels or fissures in the wound. The irrigation solution should not be harmful to the tissues and should be injected at a psi (pounds per square inch) of 4 to 15.

Delegation Guidelines

You may not delegate wound irrigation to a nursing assistant. The complex nature of this type of wound requires your ongoing assessment and careful attention to irrigation technique. The nursing assistant may help with assembling the necessary equipment and positioning the client for your performance of wound care.

Equipment Needed

- Irrigation kit or sterile basin.
- 18- or 19-gauge needle.
- 35-mL syringe.
- Sterile normal saline 150 to 500 mL or other irrigant ordered by physician.
- Clean gloves.
- Sterile gloves.
- Waterproof underpad.
- Protective eyewear (if needed).

1 Prepare for the procedure.

a. Check the wound care order and the specific order for irrigant.

Wound irrigations are prescribed by a physician or a clinical nurse specialist.

b. Premedicate the client for pain if you anticipate discomfort.

c. Wash your hands and don protective eyewear and a gown if you anticipate splashing during the irrigation procedure.

Following these steps maintains standard precautions.

d. Place the underpad and/or clean basin to catch the irrigant fluid when it drains from the wound.

e. Decide whether the procedure should be clean or sterile. Set up a clean or sterile field by opening the irrigation tray. Add new sterile dressings to the field or open packages where sterile dressings can be accessed once you have donned your sterile gloves.

f. Pour irrigant into the sterile basin.

2 Remove the old dressing using clean gloves.

a. Remove the outer layer. If the dressing is stuck to delicate granulation tissue, moisten it for easier removal.

b. Remove any packing from the wound.

Dispose of the dressing according to hospital policy for standard precautions for blood and body fluids.

3 Irrigate the wound.

a. Don sterile gloves.

b. Fill the syringe with irrigant. With the tip of the needle about 2 inches from the wound bed, flush with slow continuous pressure. Repeat as needed. Irrigate the wound thoroughly.

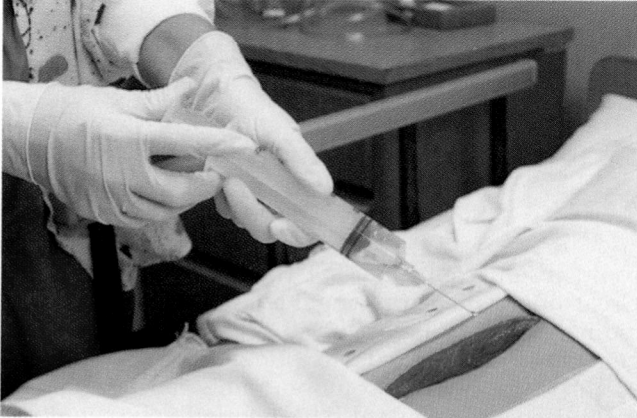

Flushing the wound with slow continuous pressure.

4 Redress the wound.
a. Wet-to-moist packing with a dry outer dressing is often used in conjunction with wound irrigations.

Redressing the wound with an appropriate dressing promotes healing.

b. Dispose of used supplies according to standard precautions. If hospital policy dictates that a wound irrigation be a clean procedure, the irrigation kit can be reused for 24 hours. The open bottle of normal saline is good for 24 hours.

5 Document the client's tolerance of the wound irrigation and dressing change, as well as a description of the wound bed.

Documentation of client tolerance and the appearance of the wound bed facilitates communication of the client's condition and allows ongoing assessment of the client plan of care.

Commonly, a physician will order that an incision be cleansed. When cleansing around an incision or drain, always wipe from the cleanest area to the dirtiest (Fig. 32–15). Remember that, generally, the wound is cleaner than the surrounding skin. To apply the "clean to dirty" rule, start cleaning from the incision and wipe outward. To cleanse around a drain, wipe in a circular direction, changing swabs with each concentric circle.

Maintaining a Moist Wound Bed

It was once thought that wounds should be kept dry, and wound care focused on that goal. However, Winter (1962) found that far from inhibiting wound healing, moisture enhances wound re-epithelialization, helping the wound heal faster and with less scar tissue. Winter found that the scab that forms when a wound is kept dry does not allow the movement of epidermal cells in the healing process.

Dressing the Wound

Most surgical wounds heal by primary intention and move through the three healing phases described earlier in the chapter. Optimal dressings should absorb drainage and provide an aseptic environment, which provides a barrier against further trauma to the site (Aronovitch, 1995). To support the "moist wound" concept, numerous wound care products, including transparent films, hydrocolloid dressings, hydrogels, and foams, have been developed (Table 32–4). Before selecting a dressing, identify its intended purpose. Dressings serve many purposes. For instance, a dressing can do the following:

* Protect the wound from contamination
* Guard the wound from injury
* Provide compression
* Allow medication application
* Absorb drainage
* Débride necrotic tissue

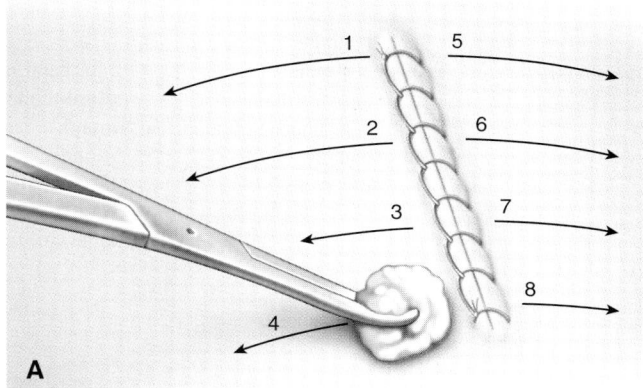

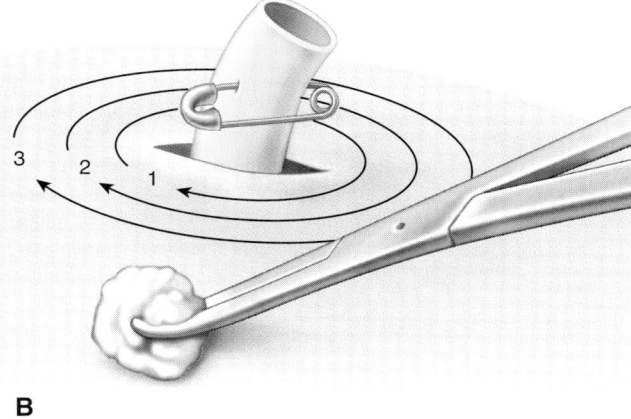

Figure 32–15. Cleaning a surgical wound. *A,* Start at the incision and clean outward. *B,* Start at the drain site, and clean around the drain in a circular fashion. Use a clean, new sterile swab for each stroke to prevent contamination of the wound.

TABLE 32–4

Common Wound Care Products

Product	Action	Indication	Advantages	Disadvantages
Gauze dressing	Wound débridement	• Prevent trauma and infection. • Wick exudate away from wound. • Provide a moist environment for healing (when moistened).	• Moderately absorptive. • Cost-effective. • Universally available. • Can be combined with other dressings. • Can be packed into wounds.	• May require frequent changes. • May adhere to wound bed and débride healthy tissue.
Transparent film	Provides a moist environment that promotes granulation tissue and autolysis of necrotic tissue, allowing oxygen and water vapor to escape while remaining impermeable to bacteria and contaminants	• Superficial wound. • Partial-thickness wound. • Wound with sloughing or necrosis. • Wound with little or no exudate.	• Retains moisture. • Impermeable to bacteria and other contamination. • Promotes autolysis. • Allows visualization of wound.	• Not recommended for infected wounds or those with heavy exudate. • May be difficult to apply. • May not stay in place in high-friction area or if exudate is heavy.
Hydrocolloid dressing	Provides a moist environment that allows a clean wound to granulate and a necrotic wound to débride autolytically	• Superficial or partial-thickness wound. • Wound with necrosis or sloughing. • Wound with light to moderate exudate.	• Impermeable to bacteria and other contaminants. • Promotes débridement. • Self-adhesive and molds well. • May be left in place for 3 to 5 days, minimizing skin trauma and disruption of healing. • May be used under compression.	• Not recommended for sinus tracts, infection, fragile skin, exposed bone or tendon, or wounds with heavy exudate. • May become dislodged if wound produces heavy exudate. • May curl at edges.
Hydrogel dressing	Water- or glycerin-based amorphous gel, impregnated gauze, or sheet dressing used to maintain a moist wound	• Partial- and full-thickness wound. • Deep wound with light exudate. • Wound with necrosis or sloughing.	• Soothes and reduces pain. • Rehydrates wound. • Promotes débridement. • Is easily removed.	• Not recommended for wounds with heavy exudate. • May be difficult to secure. • Becomes dehydrated easily.
Alginate dressing	Interacts with exudate to form a soft gel that keeps the environment moist	• Partial- or full-thickness wound with moderate to heavy exudate. • Wound with tunneling or sinus tracts. • Wound with necrotic tissue and exudate. • Infected or noninfected.	• Can absorb up to 20 times its weight in exudate. • Forms a gel over wound. • Promotes débridement. • Fills in dead space.	• Not recommended for wounds with dry eschar or light exudate. • May dry out wound bed. • Requires secondary dressings.
Composite dressing (combination of two or more products)	Combines moisture retention with absorption	• Partial- or full-thickness wound with moderate to heavy exudate and with healthy tissue. • Necrotic tissue or mixed wounds.	• May promote débridement. • May be used on infected wounds. • Easy to apply and remove.	• Not recommended for wounds with minimal or no exudate.

TABLE 32–4
Common Wound Care Products *Continued*

Product	Action	Indication	Advantages	Disadvantages
Exudate absorber	Conforms to wound surface, eliminates dead space, and absorbs exudate while maintaining a moist environment	• Full-thickness wound with moderate to heavy exudate. • Wound that requires packing and absorption. • Wound with necrotic tissue.	• Absorbs at least 5 times its weight in exudate. • Fills in dead space. • Promotes débridement. • Easy to apply.	• Not recommended for wounds with light exudate or dry eschar. • May rehydrate wound bed. • Requires secondary dressings.
Foam	Creates a moist environment and can be removed without trauma	• Partial- or full-thickness wound with minimal to heavy exudate. • To absorb drainage around tubes.	• Nonadherent. • Will not injure surrounding skin. • Easy to apply and remove.	• Not recommended for wounds with no exudate. • May macerate surrounding unprotected skin.

Data from Hess, C.T. (1998). Nurse's clinical guide to wound care. (2nd ed.). Springhouse, PA: Springhouse.

Always match the dressing or wound care product to the wound characteristics. Hess (1995) suggests asking yourself a series of questions when selecting a dressing:

• Will the dressing protect the wound from secondary infection?
• Will it provide a moist wound healing environment?
• Can the dressing be removed without causing wound trauma?
• Will the dressing remove drainage and wound debris?
• Is the dressing free of particulates and toxic products?

Sometimes you may have difficulty determining which type of dressing to apply. Table 32–5 suggests specific dressings for each stage of a pressure ulcer.

Action Alert!
Always check the physician's dressing orders for the specific site, method, dressing type, frequency of dressing changes, and time frame to evaluate healing.

Sterile dry dressings are most commonly used for closed surgical incisions. These dressings protect the incision and absorb drainage or exudate. The initial postoperative dressing is usually left in place for 24 to 48 hours. Remove the dressing correctly, as described in Procedure 32–2. And remember that repeatedly applying and removing a dressing can further impair your client's skin integrity. Montgomery straps are a good choice for clients who need frequent dressing changes or have sensitive skin (Fig. 32–16). These straps reduce irritation to the skin from repeated dressing changes.

Occasionally, a dressing will stick to the wound bed. To loosen the dressing without disturbing the new granulation tissue, moisten it with normal saline

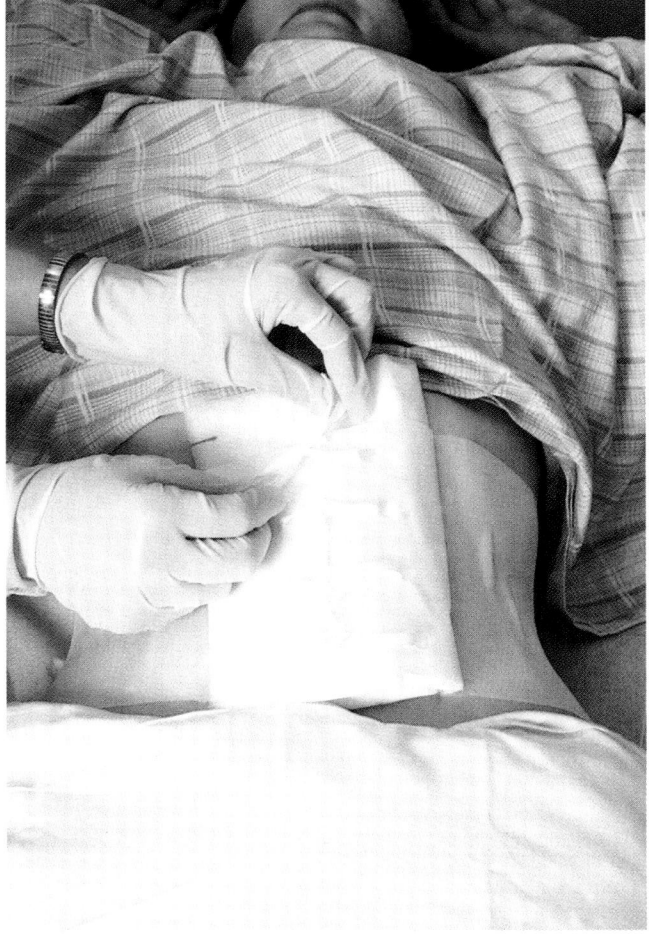
Figure 32–16. Montgomery straps are useful for clients with sensitive skin who cannot tolerate tape or those clients who require frequent dressing changes.

TABLE 32–5
Choosing the Right Dressing for a Pressure Ulcer

Pressure Ulcer Stage	Dressing Options
Stage I pressure ulcers	• Hydrocolloids. • Lubricating sprays. • Moisturizing lotions. • Skin sealants. • Transparent films.
Stage II pressure ulcers with light exudate or drainage	• Collagen. • Composites. • Foams. • Hydrocolloids. • Hydrogel wafers. • Moist impregnated gauzes. • Specialty absorptives. • Transparent films.
Stage II pressure ulcers with moderate exudate or drainage	• Alginates. • Collagen. • Composites. • Foam (covers). • Hydrogel wafers. • Moist impregnated gauzes. • Specialty absorptives.
Stage III pressure ulcers with light-to-moderate exudate or drainage; no necrosis	• Collagen. • Foam (fillers). • Hydrocolloids (pastes, fillers). • Hydrogels (amorphous, gauze). • Moist impregnated packing gauzes. • Wound fillers.
Stage III pressure ulcers with moderate-to-heavy exudate or drainage; necrosis present; tunneling or undermining present	• Alginats. • Collagen. • Débriding agents. • Foams (fillers). • Moist impregnated gauzes. • Wound fillers.
Stage IV pressure ulcers with light-to-moderate exudate or drainage; no necrosis present	• Collagen. • Foams (fillers). • Hydrocolloids. • Hydrogels (amorphous, gauze). • Moist impregnated packing gauzes. • Wound fillers.
Stage IV pressure ulcers with moderate-to-heavy exudate or drainage; necrosis present; tunneling or undermining present	• Alginates. • Collagen. • Débriding agents. • Foams (fillers). • Moist impregnated gauzes. • Wound fillers.

Adapted from Hess, C.T. (1998). Nurse's clinical guide to wound care (2nd ed.). Springhouse, PA: Springhouse.

solution. This makes the dressing easier to remove and minimizes disruption of the wound bed.

Some surgeons prefer to change the first postoperative dressing themselves, so check your institu-tion's policy on initial postoperative dressing changes.

Dressings are secured in place by tape, other bandages, or binders, as described in Procedure 32–3. To determine the best method for securing the bandage, assess the wound (including its size), the client's activity level, and the frequency of ordered dressing changes.

Generally, open surgical wounds are managed by keeping the wound clean, moist, free of necrotic tissue, and protected with dressings. When caring for an open surgical wound, follow those principles for providing pressure ulcer care.

Keep in mind that all pressure ulcers are colonized with bacteria; on occasion, you may need to culture a wound to assess the bacteria growing in it (Procedure 32–4). The AHCPR recommends effective wound cleansing to minimize wound colonization. When culturing a wound, do not use swab cultures because they detect only surface colonization. The Centers for Disease and Control and Prevention (CDC) recommend obtaining fluid through needle aspiration or through tissue ulcer biopsy.

Topical antibiotics can be used on a clean ulcer that is not healing. Local pressure ulcer infections do not require systemic antibiotics (Bergstrom et al., 1994).

Action **A**lert!
A pungent, foul, fecal, or musty odor coming from a wound or pressure ulcer suggests infection. Check with the physician about obtaining a wound culture.

Draining the Wound

Drains are placed in wounds before the surgical incision is closed to prevent fluid from collecting between the surfaces of the wound. When fluid collects in pockets in a wound, it holds the wound surfaces apart, thus preventing the surfaces from growing together to heal the wound. Drains commonly are left in place for 3 to 7 days, depending on the type of incision and the surgeon's preference. Common drains include the Penrose, Hemovac, and Jackson-Pratt. A Penrose drain is a small pliable flat latex tube placed in the wound to promote drainage (Fig. 32–17A). Although sometimes sutured in, this drain may simply be placed in the wound. Therefore, use caution when changing a dressing with a Penrose drain in place to avoid dislodging it. Hemovac and Jackson-Pratt drains are closed drainage systems that perform self-suction and collection of drainage. Both are opened to air, compressed, and held compressed while closed, thus creating a vacuum. A Jackson-Pratt drain (Fig. 32–17B) has a bulb and a Hemovac drain (Fig. 32–17C) has a cartridge, either of which creates its own suction. As the bulb or cartridge fills with drainage, less suction is placed on the wound.

Your responsibilities in caring for a drain include

• Maintaining its patency
• Emptying fluid from the drain, usually once a shift when intake and output are measured

PROCEDURE 32-2

Removing a Dressing

TIME TO
ALLOW
▼
Novice:
10 minutes
Expert:
5 minutes

Removal of a dressing allows for direct observation of the client's wound and replacement of the contaminated dressing with a clean (or sterile) dressing. The physician will order the frequency of dressing changes.

Delegation Guidelines

A nursing assistant may be helpful in assisting you in the general performance of wound care. The assembly of necessary equipment and removal of a dressing may be delegated to a nursing assistant who has received specific training in this procedure. You are then responsible
for your direct assessment of the dressing and the wound, as described.

Equipment Needed

- Clean gloves.
- Red trash bag.

1 Wash hands and apply gloves.
Washing your hands and applying gloves decreases the risk of spreading infection.

2 Gently begin to remove old dressing by pulling the tape toward the dressing and parallel to the skin. Simultaneously apply pressure to the client's skin at the edge of the tape to prevent the skin from being pulled with the tape.

Applying pressure to the client's skin while pulling off the dressing will reduce the chance of causing further skin breakdown and can reduce the client's pain. If the tape has been in place for several days, use of an acetone-free adhesive remover may help you remove the tape. Do not use acetone if the skin is irritated or broken.

3 Observe the removed dressing for drainage, especially noting the amount, color, and odor (if any) of the drainage.
Thorough assessment of the dressing can assist with evaluation of the client's treatment plan.

4 Dispose of the dressing according to your facility's policy and government regulations.
If the dressing is heavily soiled with body fluids or bloody drainage, dispose of it in a red trash bag.

5 Document the odor, color, amount, and consistency of the drainage. Describe the appearance of the wound.

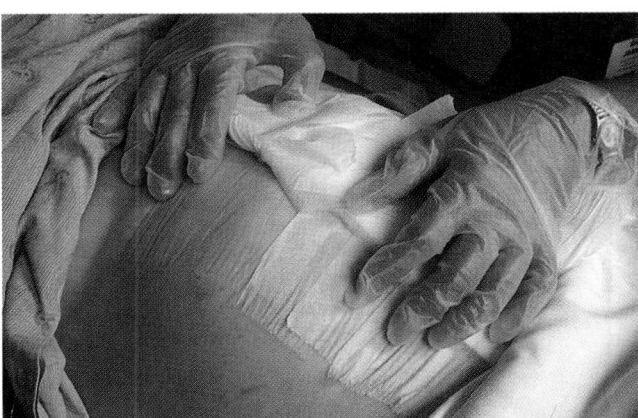

Applying pressure to skin at the edge of the tape. (Modified from Bergstrom, N., Bennett, M.A., Carlson, C.E., et al. Treatment of Pressure Ulcers. [1994]. *Clinical Practice Guideline No. 15.* Rockville, MD: US Department of Health and Human Services, Public Health Service, Agency for Health Care Policy and Research, Publication No. 95-0652.)

HOME CARE CONSIDERATIONS

For a nondraining surgical wound, before sutures or staples are removed, the client may wish to use a light dressing to protect the wound under clothes. Clothes should fit loosely and comfortably over the wound without binding. A dressing is not essential, however.

PROCEDURE 32–3

Dressing a Simple Wound

TIME TO
ALLOW
▼
Novice:
10 minutes
Expert:
5 minutes

Wounds are covered with dressings to protect them from contamination and injury, to provide compression, to absorb drainage, to débride necrotic tissue, and to apply medication. A simple nondraining wound is covered for protection and in most cases the dressing is optional.

Delegation Guidelines

Institutional policy regarding delegation of this procedure may vary widely. In many institutions, the performance of simple, clean dressing changes may be delegated to nursing assistants who have received specialized training in this skill. However, application of new postoperative dressings should not be delegated, nor should dressing changes to open wounds that are known to contain fistulas, that contain draining sinus tracts, or that require packing. The ongoing assessment of the wound and the effectiveness of the dressing technique lie with you; you may therefore determine not to delegate this procedure. A nursing assistant may assemble the necessary equipment and assist in positioning the client for the dressing change.

Equipment Needed

- Clean gloves.
- Type of dressing ordered by the physician.
- Tape, bandages, or binders needed to secure the dressing in place.

1 Answer any questions client may have.

Allowing the client to ask questions sets the stage for the client to provide self-care at home. If the client or a caregiver will be changing dressings at home, practicing in the hospital will be helpful.

2 Confirm the dressing change order.

Dressing changes are commonly ordered by a physician, so you will need to verify the specific order.

3 Assemble the supplies needed for the dressing change.

4 Wash your hands and apply gloves.

Dressing changes should be done in sterile fashion.

5 Remove the dressing from its package and apply it to the center of the wound. The dressing change is sterile as long as the surface of the dressing placed next to the client is sterile. The wound and 1 inch beyond should be covered with the dressing.

A sterile field may be used to hold all dressings, or individual packages may be opened and left in their original packaging.

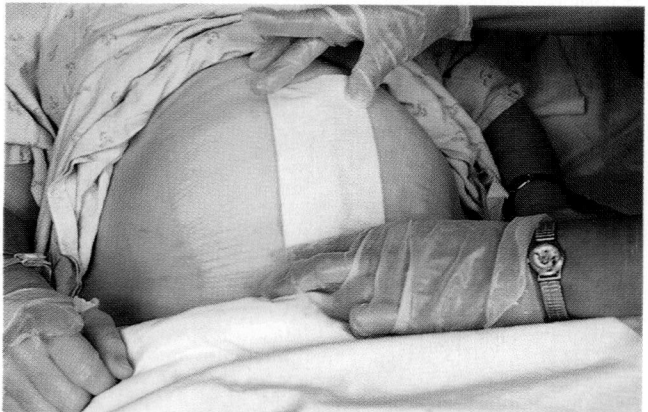

Applying the dressing to the center of the wound.

6 Secure the edges of the dressing to the client's skin with tape.

Use the least amount of tape necessary to hold the dressing in place.

7 If the dressing will be changed frequently or the client has sensitive or impaired skin, consider using Montgomery straps rather than tape.

Montgomery straps will allow you to change the dressing repeatedly without having to pull tape from the client's skin each time.

If the client or family will need to change a dressing at home, ensure that they have the necessary clean or sterile supplies. An array of sterile dressing supplies can generally be purchased at a pharmacy. If special dressings are needed, determine whether the hospital can supply the needed items on discharge.

- Maintaining accurate measurements of wound drainage
- Maintaining the dressing around the drain
- Checking the wound for signs that drainage is incomplete
- Describing the drainage

Débriding the Wound

Débridement is the removal of dirt, foreign matter, and dead or devitalized tissue from a wound. Moist, devitalized tissue supports the growth of organisms. Thus, removing this tissue promotes wound healing. Débridement methods include sharp, mechanical, enzymatic, and autolytic. Always use the method most appropriate to the client's condition and care goals (Bergstrom et al., 1994).

SHARP DÉBRIDEMENT. Sharp débridement is the removal of necrotic tissue using a scalpel, scissors, or laser. This method is rapid and efficient but should be performed only by persons skilled at and specially trained to perform this technique. Check your state's nurse practice act for details (Bergstrom, Allman, & Carlson, 1992).

MECHANICAL DÉBRIDEMENT. Mechanical débridement removes dead tissue by applying a mechanical force, such as scrubbing, whirlpool therapy, or a wet-to-moist dressing. The latter is a gauze dressing that is applied wet and removed after it has partially dried (Procedure 32–5). As the dressing dries in the wound, the gauze adheres to the wound bed. Removing the dressing removes necrotic tissue. Be aware that mechanical débridement is nonselective and can lead to removal of healthy as well as dead tissue (Maklebust, 1996).

ENZYMATIC DÉBRIDEMENT. Enzymatic débridement is a form of chemical débridement in which enzymes are used to break down necrotic tissue without targeting viable tissue. This method must be monitored closely because it can cause erythema around the wound perimeter (Maklebust, 1996).

AUTOLYTIC DÉBRIDEMENT. Autolytic débridement uses the body's ability to digest devitalized tissue. It is most often performed by applying a moisture-retentive dressing (such as a hydrocolloid dressing) to the wound bed (Procedure 32–6). The dressing creates an occlusive seal and then macrophages and neutrophils eliminate the necrotic tissue. Using an occlusive dressing does not promote infection. In fact, such a dressing has many benefits, including less pain at rest, during ambulation, and during dressing changes (Field & Kerstein, 1994).

Action Alert!
Hydrocolloid dressings should not be used for immunocompromised clients.

The accompanying decision tree summarizes the treatment of pressure ulcers.

Removing Sutures and Staples

Sutures and staples are typically removed 7 to 10 days after surgery according to the physician's order. The physician may order only a certain number of sutures or staples to be removed. For instance, removing every other suture may allow continued wound healing. Check your institution's policy to find out which personnel are permitted to remove sutures.

Before removing sutures, determine the type of sutures in place. Interrupted sutures are individually tied, whereas continuous sutures are a series of sutures with one thread. When removing sutures, never pull suture material that has been on the skin surface through the incision. Doing so may transmit microorganisms into the incision and lead to infection. Use suture scissors designed specifically for suture removal. Cut the suture material as close to the skin as possible and pull the suture material through the other side of the incision (Fig. 32–18).

To remove staples, obtain a staple remover and insert the two lower prongs of the staple remover beneath the staple and the middle upper prong on top of

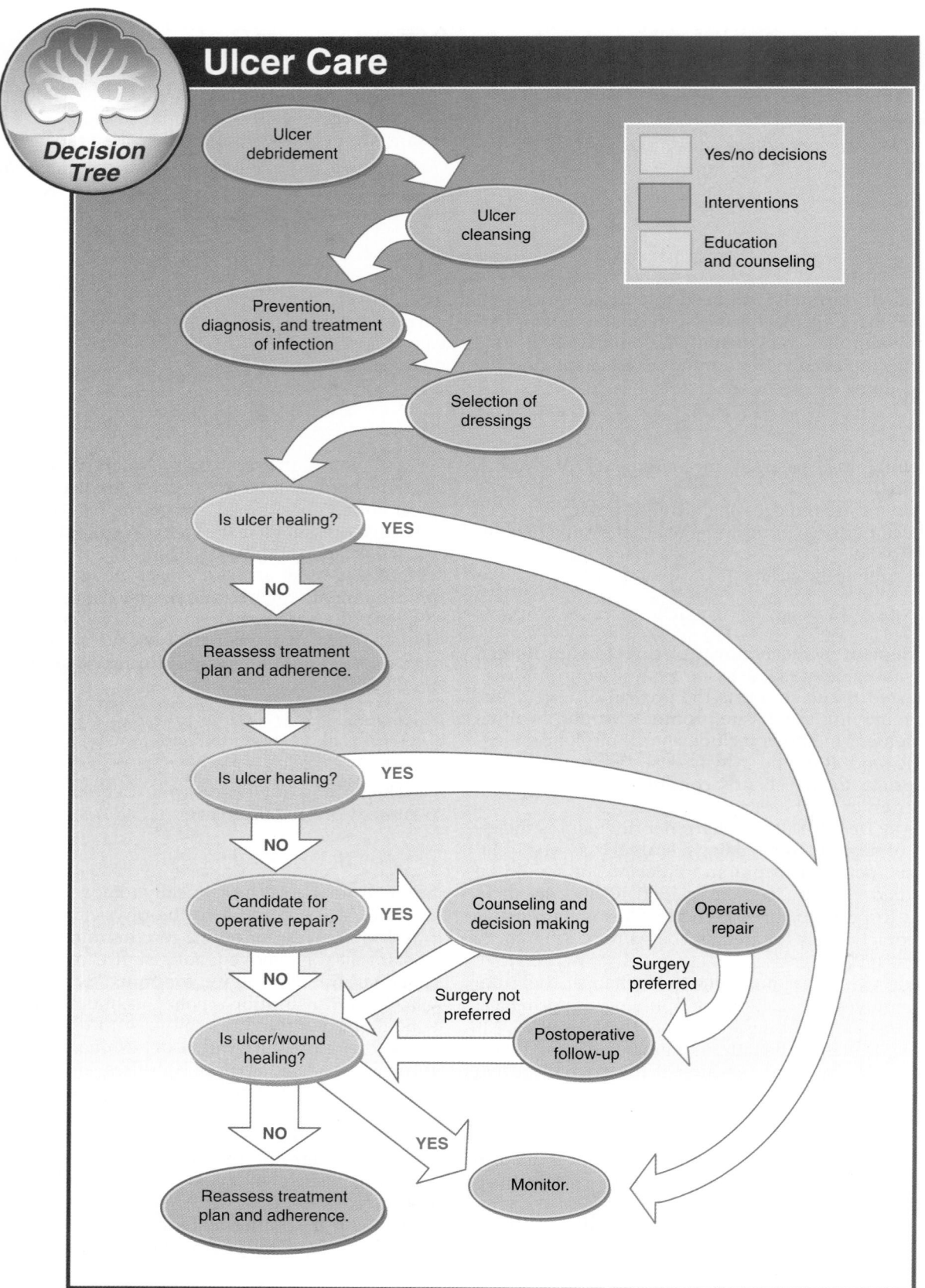

Ulcer Care

Decision Tree

Ulcer debridement

Ulcer cleansing

Prevention, diagnosis, and treatment of infection

Selection of dressings

Yes/no decisions
Interventions
Education and counseling

Is ulcer healing? — YES
NO
Reassess treatment plan and adherence.
Is ulcer healing? — YES
NO
Candidate for operative repair? — YES → Counseling and decision making → Operative repair
NO
Surgery preferred
Surgery not preferred
Postoperative follow-up
Is ulcer/wound healing?
NO — YES → Monitor.
Reassess treatment plan and adherence.

(Modified from Bergstrom, N., Bennett, M. A., Carlson, C. E., et al. Treatment of Pressure Ulcers. [1994]. Clinical Practice Guideline No. 15. Rockville, MD: US Department of Health and Human Services, Public Health Service, Agency for Health Care Policy and Research, Publication No. 95-0652.)

PROCEDURE 32–4

Culturing a Wound

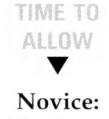

TIME TO
ALLOW
▼

Novice:
15 minutes
Expert
5 minutes

Wounds are cultured to determine the type of bacteria that may be present in them. Swab cultures are used to detect surface colonization.

Delegation Guidelines

The sterile nature of this procedure generally precludes the delegation of wound culturing. However, nursing assistants in specialized burn and wound care units, having received specialty training, may perform wound cultures under your direct supervision.

Equipment Needed

- 18- or 19-gauge needle.
- 35-mL syringe.
- Normal saline solution.
- Sterile swab.
- Sterile culture tube.
- Gloves.

1 Rinse or irrigate wound thoroughly with sterile normal saline before obtaining a culture.
Cleansing the wound before culturing it will remove any surface bacteria.

2 Swab the entire wound bed using a zig-zag technique starting at the top of the wound and proceeding to the bottom of the wound.
Using this technique will cover the entire wound bed.

3 Place the swab in the culture tube and send it to the laboratory. Prompt delivery of the swab and specimen will facilitate prompt testing of the swab.

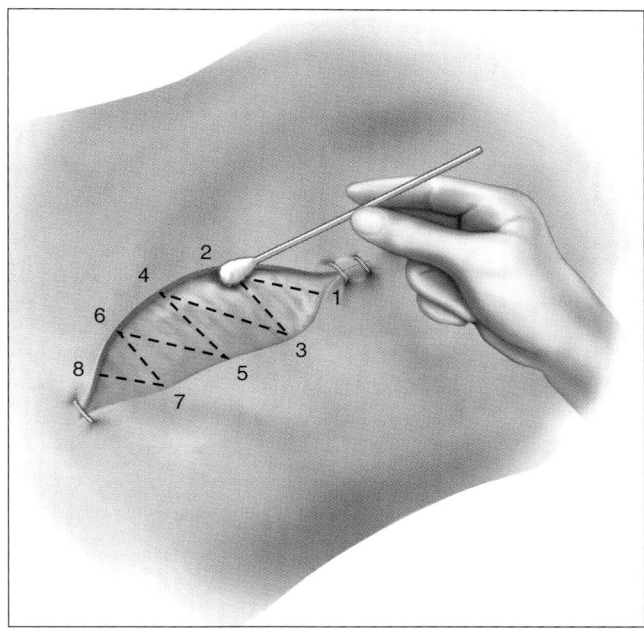

Swabbing the wound bed in a zigzag pattern.

Note: Swab cultures generally should not be used because they detect only surface bacteria, and a diagnosis should not be based solely on a swab culture. The Centers for Disease Control and Prevention recommends that you obtain fluid through needle aspiration or tissue ulcer biopsy.

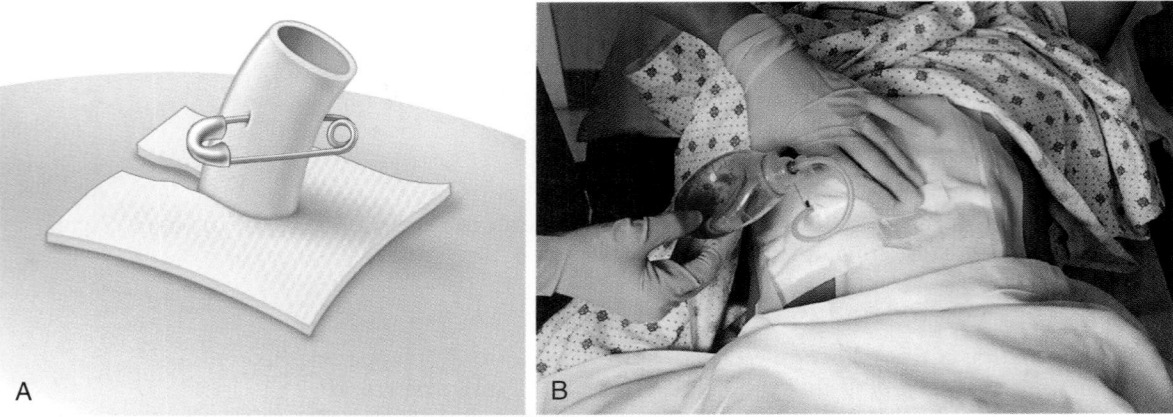

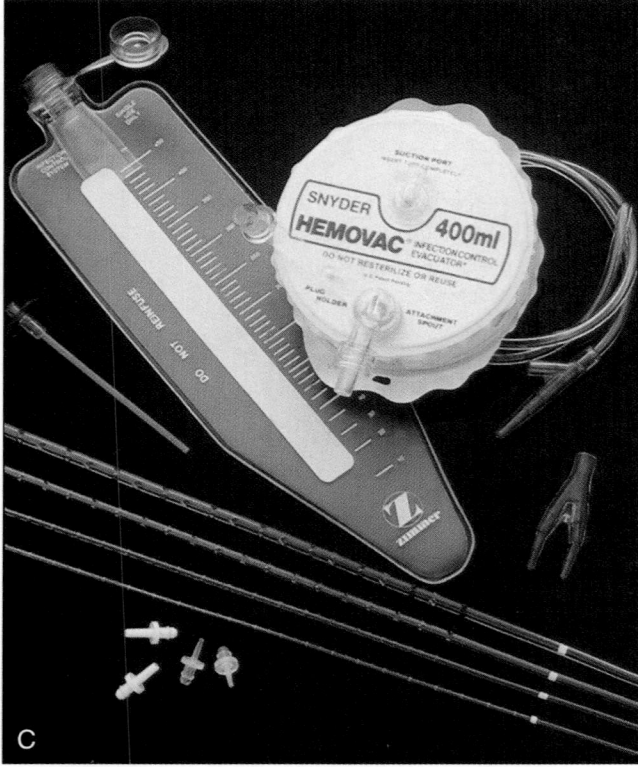

Figure 32–17. Common drainage systems. *A*, Penrose drain; *B*, Jackson-Pratt drain (shown in use on a client); *C*, Hemovac drain. (*C*, courtesy of Zimmer, Inc., Warsaw, IN.)

the staple. Then squeeze the staple remover closed. The staple should separate from the skin (Fig. 32–19). Avoid pulling the skin with the staple as it is removed. While the staple should be removed with a smooth steady hand, quickly squeezing the staple remover will cause less dragging of the skin. It is common practice to spray the wound edges with tincture of benzoin and apply Steri-Strips at 1-inch intervals across the wound. The client is taught that she can shower with Steri-Strips in place and discontinue use of Steri-Strips when they fall off.

Applying Heat and Cold

Applying heat and cold can create therapeutic local and systemic effects. For example, cold constricts blood vessels, while heat dilates them. Cold decreases

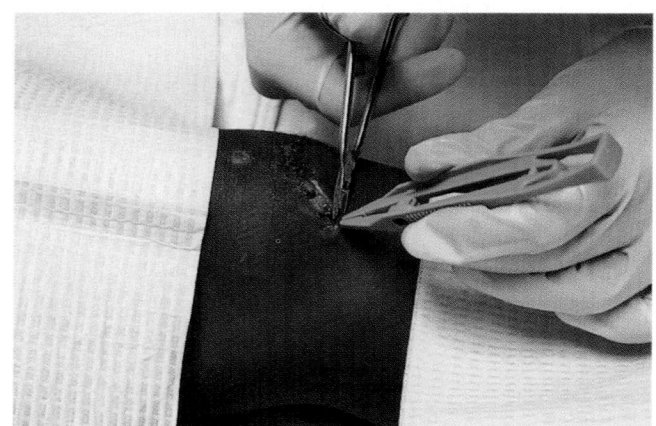

Figure 32–18. Removing sutures.

PROCEDURE 32–5

Applying a Wet-to-Moist Dressing

TIME TO ALLOW
▼
Novice:
15 minutes
Expert:
5 minutes

The purpose of a wet-to-moist dressing is to mechanically débride a wound. This type of gauze dressing is applied wet and removed moist. As the dressing changes from wet to moist in the wound, the gauze adheres to the wound bed. Thus, removal of the dressing removes necrotic tissue as well. The dressing should not be allowed to become dry, because this type of débridement is nonselective and can result in the removal of healthy tissue as well as dead tissue.

Delegation Guidelines

The nature of a wound requiring a wet-to-dry or wet-to-moist dressing change is such that you would not want to delegate the treatment to a nursing assistant. The assessment, sterile procedure, and intervention of mechanical débridement requires your expertise. Within a burn or wound care unit, some unlicensed personnel receive specialized training to perform such dressing changes; these are generally the exception. Assembly of the necessary equipment and supplies, along with positioning the client for the dressing change, may be delegated to a nursing assistant.

Equipment Needed

- Sterile gauze dressing or type ordered by physician.
- Sterile dressing to cover wet dressing per physician order.
- Tape or Montgomery straps.
- Sterile normal saline or other solution as ordered by physician.
- Sterile gloves.
- Sterile cotton swabs.

1 Confirm the physician's dressing order and assemble the needed supplies.

2 Use sterile normal saline solution (or another ordered solution) to dampen the dressing that will be placed into the wound.
Wetting the dressing will promote a moist healing environment.

3 Don sterile gloves and twist the wet dressing so it remains wet but is not dripping. Open the dressing fully and fluff it open.
The dressing should be damp to moderately wet.

4 Gently place the dressing into the wound. Do not pack the wound tightly.
Packing the dressing tightly will block air from entering the wound and will keep the dressing from drying out.

5 Cover the damp dressing with a dry sterile dressing and secure it with tape. If the client is allergic to tape, has sensitive skin, or needs repeated dressing changes, consider using Montgomery straps to affix the top dressing.

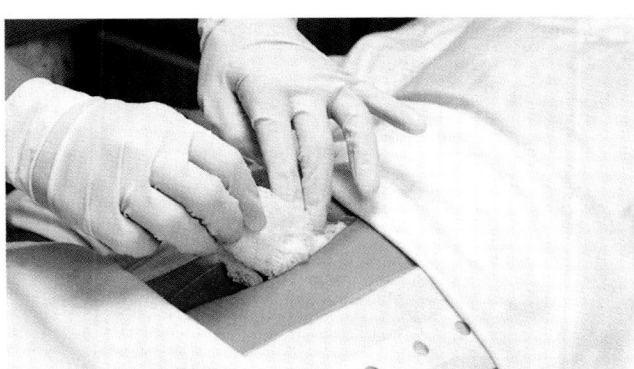
Packing the wound.

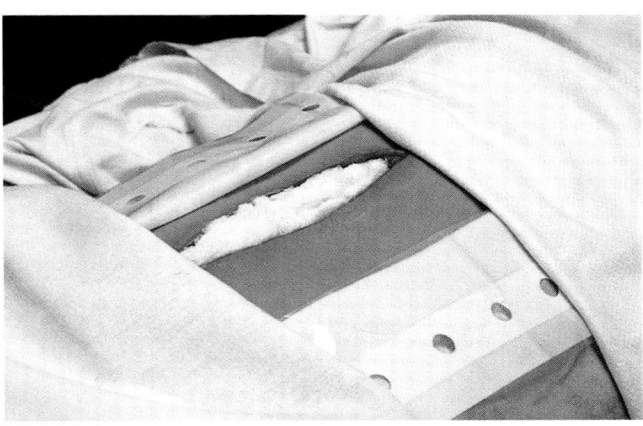
Packed wound with the wound edges free.

Applying a Hydrocolloid Dressing

TIME TO ALLOW
▼
Novice:
15 minutes
Expert:
5 minutes

Hydrocolloid dressing is a type of autolytic débridement. This type of dressing causes an occlusive seal, then uses the body's own macrophages and neutrophils to eliminate necrotic tissue. Instead of drying out a wound, this treatment aims at maintaining the moisture in a wound bed.

Delegation Guidelines

The application of a hydrocolloid dressing requires your assessment and expertise and should not be delegated to a nursing assistant. However, assembly of the necessary equipment and supplies may be delegated to a nursing assistant. You may also need the help of a nursing assistant in positioning a client for dressing application.

Equipment Needed

- Sterile gauze dressing or other dressing according to physician's order.
- Sterile normal saline or other solution as ordered by physician.
- Sterile gloves.
- Sterile cotton swabs.
- Hydrocolloid dressing; size will depend on the size of the wound.
- Hypoallergenic tape.

1 Clean the wound by irrigating it or lightly swabbing it with a gauze dressing soaked in sterile normal saline solution.
The wound bed must be cleansed and debris removed before you apply the hydrocolloid dressing.

2 Select a hydrocolloid dressing of an appropriate size. It should extend past the wound margins by at least 1 inch.
If the dressing is too small, it will not adhere to the wound bed and, consequently, will not function properly.

3 Apply the dressing from one side of the wound to the other side. Use hand pressure to hold the dressing in place for a minimum of 1 minute.
Applying pressure and warmth with your hands will make the dressing adhere better to the wound.

4 Depending on the location of the wound and hydrocolloid dressing used, you may need to place hypoallergenic tape around the edges of the dressing to secure it.
Applying tape will help prevent the edges of the dressing from rolling back.

5 Leave the dressing in place for 5 to 7 days. Remove the dressing if it is leaking or peeling off and apply another one.
Leaving the dressing in place will allow moist wound healing to occur.

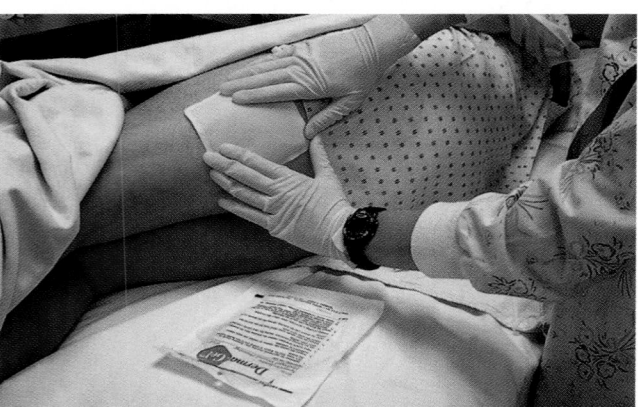

Applying a hydrocolloid dressing. Apply pressure with your hands over the dressing for at least 1 minute to ensure good adherence of the dressing.

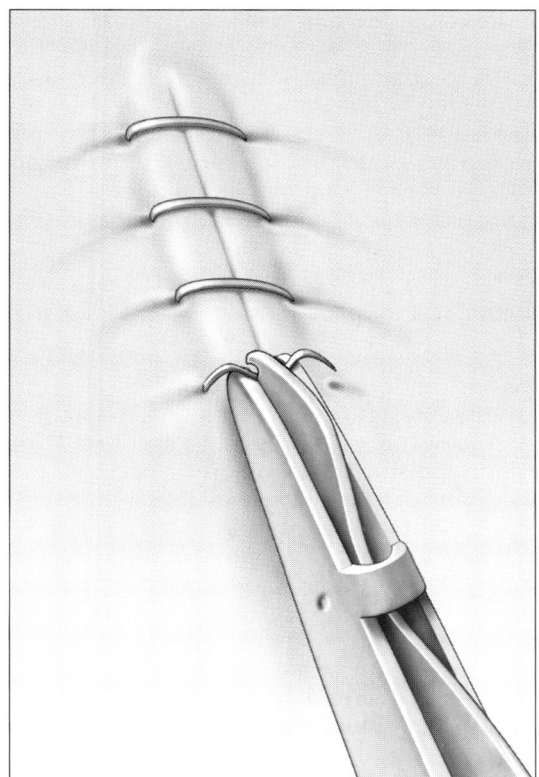

Figure 32–19. Removing staples.

capillary permeability, while heat increases it. Cold decreases cellular metabolism, while heat increases it. Cold provides local anesthetic effects, while heat provides local sedative effects. And both therapies produce muscle relaxation.

HEAT THERAPIES. Heat can be applied in a variety of dry or moist methods. One method for applying either dry or moist heat is with a disposable Aquathermia pad (Kpad). Its water-filled tubes are heated by a small electrical unit. Aquathermia pads are moldable and can be used on limbs (Fig. 32–20).

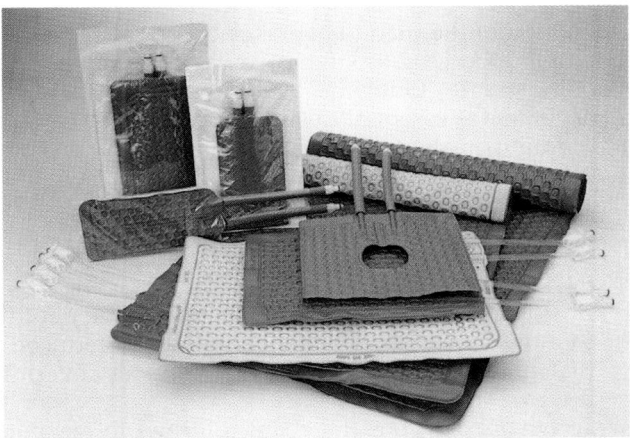

Figure 32–20. Aquathermia pads. (Courtesy of Zimmer, Inc., Warsaw, IN.)

Another method for applying constant, even heat is with a heating pad molded to the client's body. Use care when applying a heating pad because it can cause serious burns if set too high. Some institutions allow the use of heating pads only with preset limits to prevent burns.

Action Alert!
Avoid using heat therapy immediately after surgery to prevent bleeding into the incision or wound bed.

COLD THERAPIES. Cold decreases pain and inflammation and can reduce bleeding. To apply cold therapy, you can use a compress, an ice pack, or an ice bag. Compresses are moist, cool dressings. Cold packs come in a variety of shapes and are activated by striking or twisting the pack (Fig. 32–21). To prepare an ice bag, you can place crushed ice into a small or large plastic bag depending on the size of the area you need to cover. For a small area, such as a finger, consider filling a glove with ice. For a larger area, such as a fractured ankle, fill a plastic bag. Always cover an ice bag before placing it on a client's skin to avoid a cold injury.

Action Alert!
Do not use heat or cold therapies for a client with neurological impairment, impaired mental status, or impaired circulation.

Bandaging the Wound

Bandages and binders are used to secure dressings in difficult-to-secure areas (such as the elbow) or provide

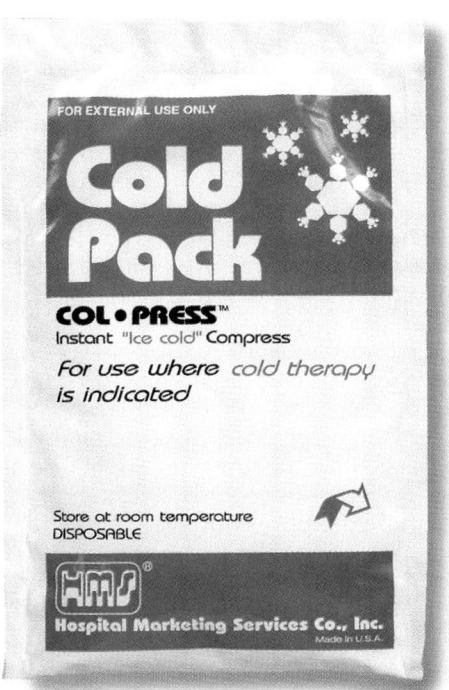

Figure 32–21. Cold pack. (Courtesy of Hospital Marketing Services, Inc., Naugatuck, CT.)

support to a wound. They may also be used for other purposes, such as to

- Apply pressure (for example, after central line removal or postoperative incision)
- Immobilize a body part (as an elastic bandage wrapped around a sprained wrist)
- Maintain splint placement (as in an elastic bandage placed over an ankle splint)

When applying a bandage or binder, be sure to follow assessment strategies that should be performed before application:

- Inspect the area for swelling, wounds, and wound drainage.
- Assess the client for pain and provide prescribed medication as appropriate.
- Assess the client's ability to apply the bandage.
- Assess the client's ability to perform activities of daily living with the bandage in place.
- Assess circulatory function in the bandaged area.

Several types and sizes of bandages are available. Woven or gauze dressings, the most common type, are considered the gold standard in dressing supplies. These inexpensive bandages provide support to other bandages, allow air circulation to the skin, and can be used on many different body parts, including extremities. Gauze also wicks away moisture and exudate from the skin, preventing maceration, and can assist in débridement. This type of dressing is used in wound packing.

Nonwoven dressings are made of synthetic fibers (most often rayon or polyester). These dressings are soft and most often are used for skin preparation and cleansing. They are not ideal for absorbing drainage (Aronovitch, 1995). Elasticized bandages are used to provide support or pressure to a specific area.

Choose a dressing type and size based on the area to be bandaged. Generally, a narrow bandage is suitable for smaller areas (such as a hand or wrist), whereas a larger bandage is more suitable for a leg. Applying a bandage of the wrong width may cause constriction or excessive pressure on the skin.

Five basic methods or turns can be used to start a bandage, wrap it evenly, and secure the dressing (Fig. 32–22). Circular turns are used to anchor the beginning and end of the bandage. Spiral turns are used to bandage extremities by ascending up the extremity. Each turn overlaps the previous turn by half or a third.

Spiral reverse turns are used to bandage oblong body parts (such as the forearm, thigh, or calf). Recurrent turns are used to cover distal body parts (for instance, a stump, skull, or finger). The bandage is first secured with two circular turns and then folded back on itself and brought to cover the distal end. Again, each turn covers the affected body part and overlaps the previous turn by half or a third. The figure-eight turn is most often used to bandage joints because it allows mobility after application. Apply this bandage over the joint in a figure-eight motion above and below the joint.

Binders are used to provide support and protection to larger areas, such as the abdomen or chest (Fig. 32–23). A Velcro attachment secures the binder to the client. Apply the binder snugly to provide support, but not so snugly that it creates excessive compression. T-binders are used to provide support for dressings in the perineal area. Use a single T-binder for a female client and a double T-binder for a male client (Fig. 32–24).

Positioning and Support Surfaces

Support surfaces are therapeutic devices used to control pressure and protect bony prominences. These devices serve many functions, including relieving pressure, reducing pressure, reducing shear and friction, controlling moisture, and inhibiting bacterial growth. Many support surfaces are available in various sizes and shapes for use on beds and in chairs (Fig. 32–25). They should be used in conjunction with meticulous turning and repositioning and proper wound care to enhance the healing of pressure ulcers and help prevent new ulcers.

Be aware that no single support surface eliminates the effects of pressure on the skin. Assess your client carefully to determine the most appropriate support surface, as shown in the accompanying decision tree.

Keep in mind that *pressure-relieving* devices reduce the interface pressure between the body and the support surface below 32 mm Hg (the capillary closing pressure). *Pressure-reducing* devices also reduce the interface pressure—but not below the capillary closing pressure. Support surface therapy must be tailored to the client's individual needs. Foam overlays that are 3 to 4 inches thick may also help reduce pressure. Support surface characteristics and cost are important factors to consider. Static air overlays—mattresses that are blown up—also serve to reduce pressure. Low-air-loss beds can benefit a client who needs moisture control and prevention of maceration and friction (Hess, 1995).

EVALUATION

Evaluation of the plan of care is in an ongoing part of the nursing process, as suggested in the Nursing Care Planning chart. Outcome measurement in wound management is essential to evaluating the plan of care and wound healing. To measure outcomes, consider questions such as the following (Bolton, Rijswijk, & Shaffer, 1996):

- By what percentage has a client's wound decreased in size?
- By how much has a wound been reduced in depth?
- By how much has the client's pain been reduced?
- By what percentage has necrotic tissue covering the wound been reduced?
- To what extent has the client returned to her normal activities?
- Was the client's wound kept free of infection?

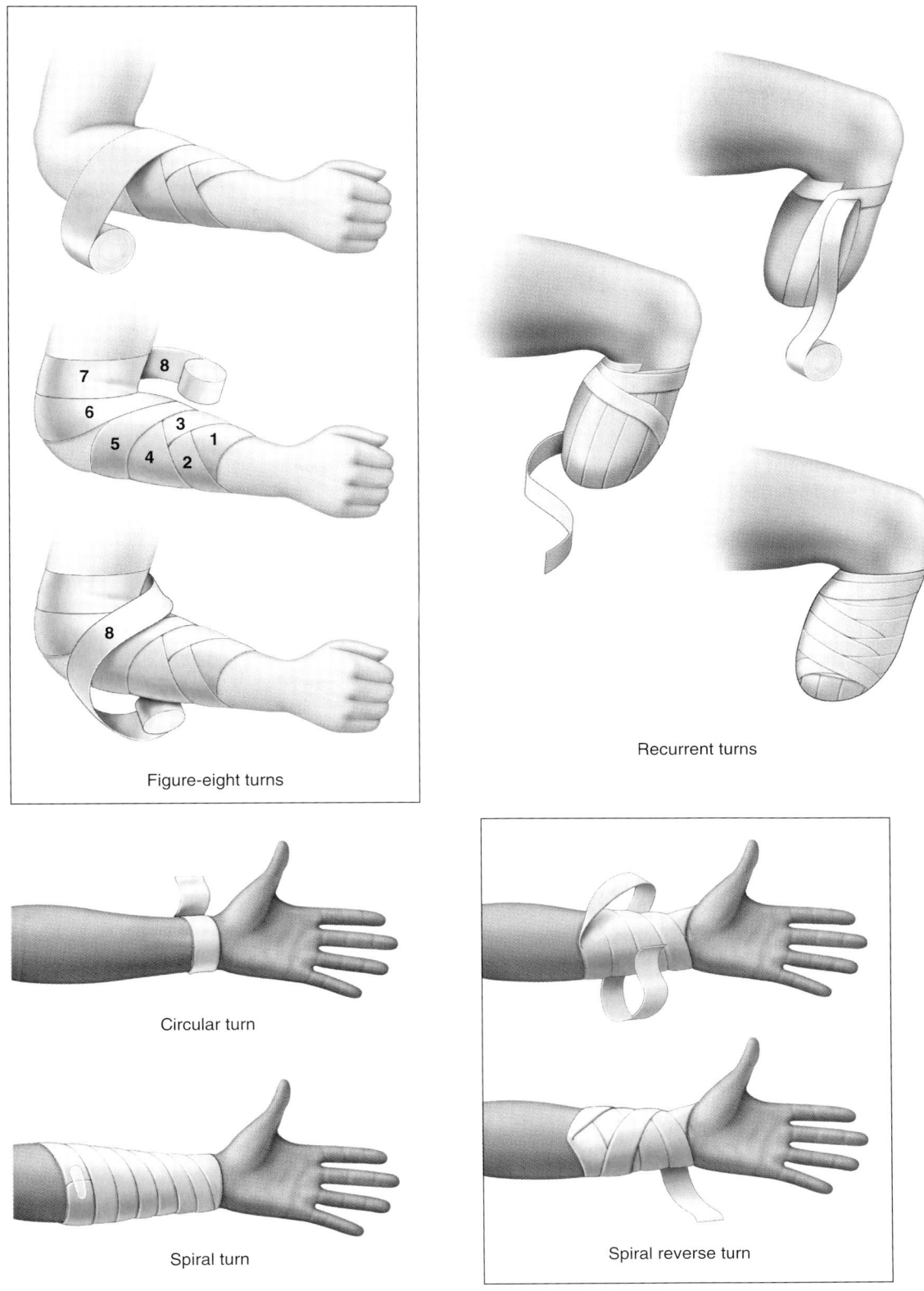

Figure-eight turns

Recurrent turns

Circular turn

Spiral turn

Spiral reverse turn

Figure 32–22. Methods of bandage application.

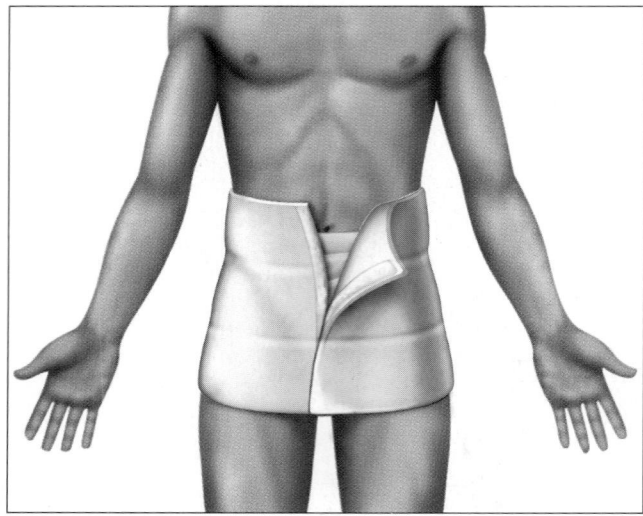

Figure 32–23. Abdominal binder.

Naturally, in the largest sense, the desired outcome is that the client have an intact integumentary system that serves its normal functions. If the client has *Impaired skin integrity,* the expected outcome is wound healing without infection and further prevention of *Impaired skin integrity.*

KEY PRINCIPLES

- The functions of the skin are protection, sensation, thermoregulation, and excretion.
- There are four stages of pressure ulcers.
- Wounds can be classified into different categories. Intentional wounds are those caused by surgical procedures or treatments (operations, intravenous therapy). Unintentional wounds are accidental in cause (abrasion or laceration from a fall).
- The "web of causation" is a conceptual framework that can be used to understand the development of pressure ulcers.
- Although not all pressure wounds can be prevented, the nurse plays an important role in the care of the client in assessing for risk, providing care to a surgical wound, or participating in the treatment of a pressure ulcer.
- A multidisciplinary effort is required to maintain and facilitate intact skin of clients. Members of the multidisciplinary team include physicians, nurses, rehabilitation therapists, enterostomal therapists, social workers, and home care providers.
- The skin diagnoses are *Risk for Impaired skin integrity, Impaired skin integrity,* and *Impaired tissue integrity.*
- The goals of wound healing include keeping the wound and wound bed clean, moist, and free from infection.
- Moisture was once thought to be harmful in the wound healing process. Through research, we now know that moisture facilitates wound healing.
- Appropriate nursing interventions include positioning the client correctly to decrease pressure to bony prominences.
- When the client has an impairment of skin integrity, the expected outcome is wound healing without infection and further prevention of *Impaired skin integrity.*

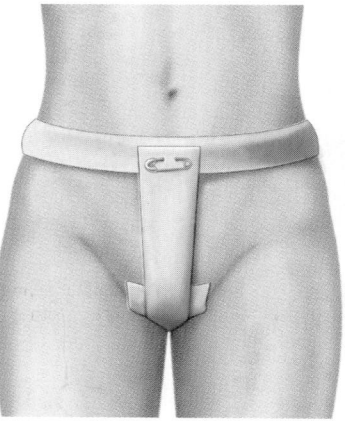
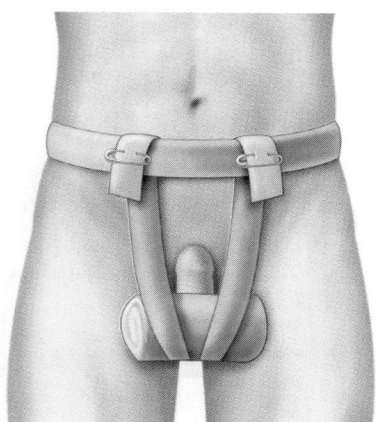

Figure 32–24. Female and male T-binders.

Female

Male

CHAPTER 32 **Skin Integrity and Wound Healing** 823

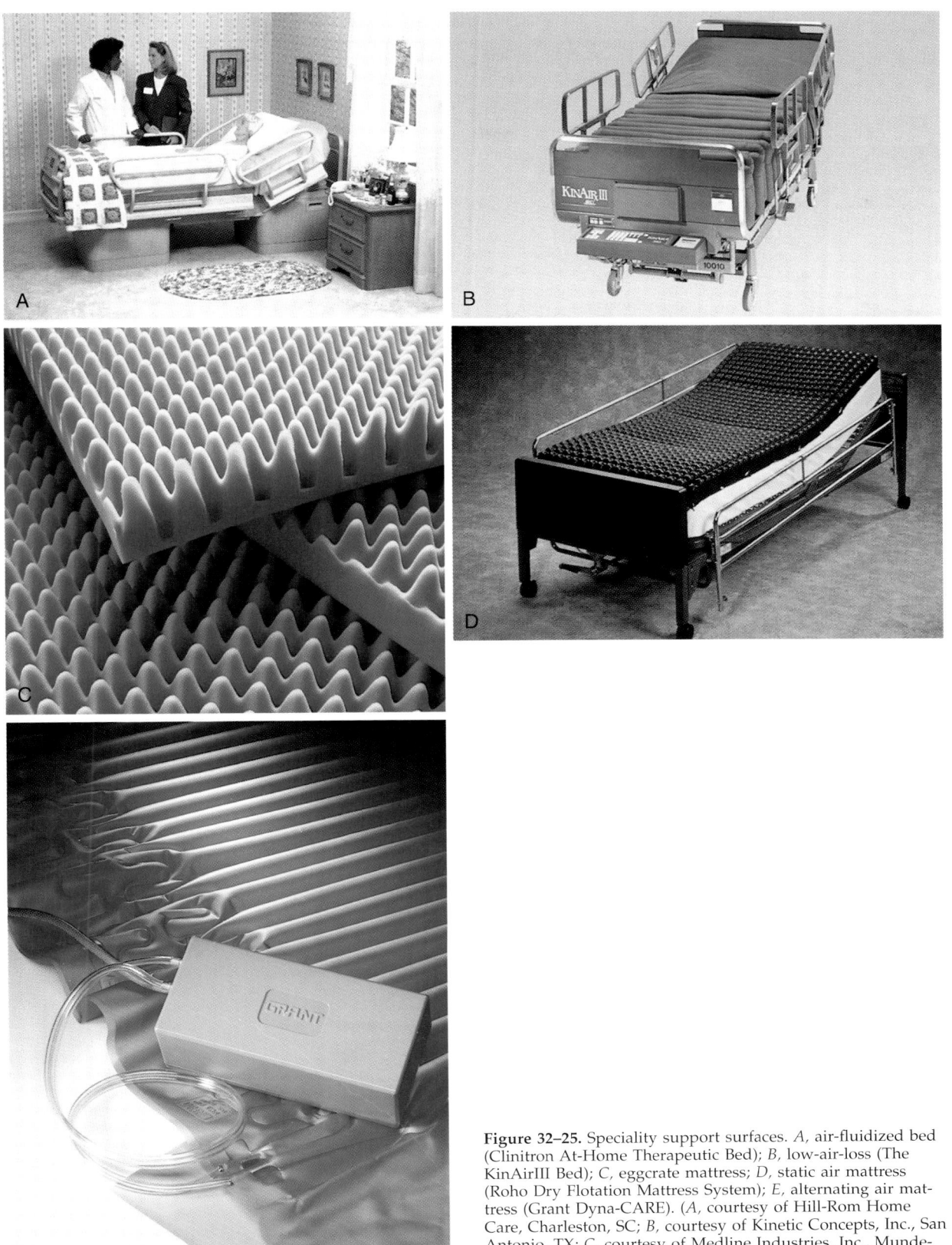

Figure 32–25. Speciality support surfaces. *A,* air-fluidized bed (Clinitron At-Home Therapeutic Bed); *B,* low-air-loss (The KinAirIII Bed); *C,* eggcrate mattress; *D,* static air mattress (Roho Dry Flotation Mattress System); *E,* alternating air mattress (Grant Dyna-CARE). (*A,* courtesy of Hill-Rom Home Care, Charleston, SC; *B,* courtesy of Kinetic Concepts, Inc., San Antonio, TX; *C,* courtesy of Medline Industries, Inc., Mundelein, IL; *D,* courtesy of Roho Incorporated, Belleville, IL; *E,* courtesy of Grant Airmass Corporation, Stamford, CT.)

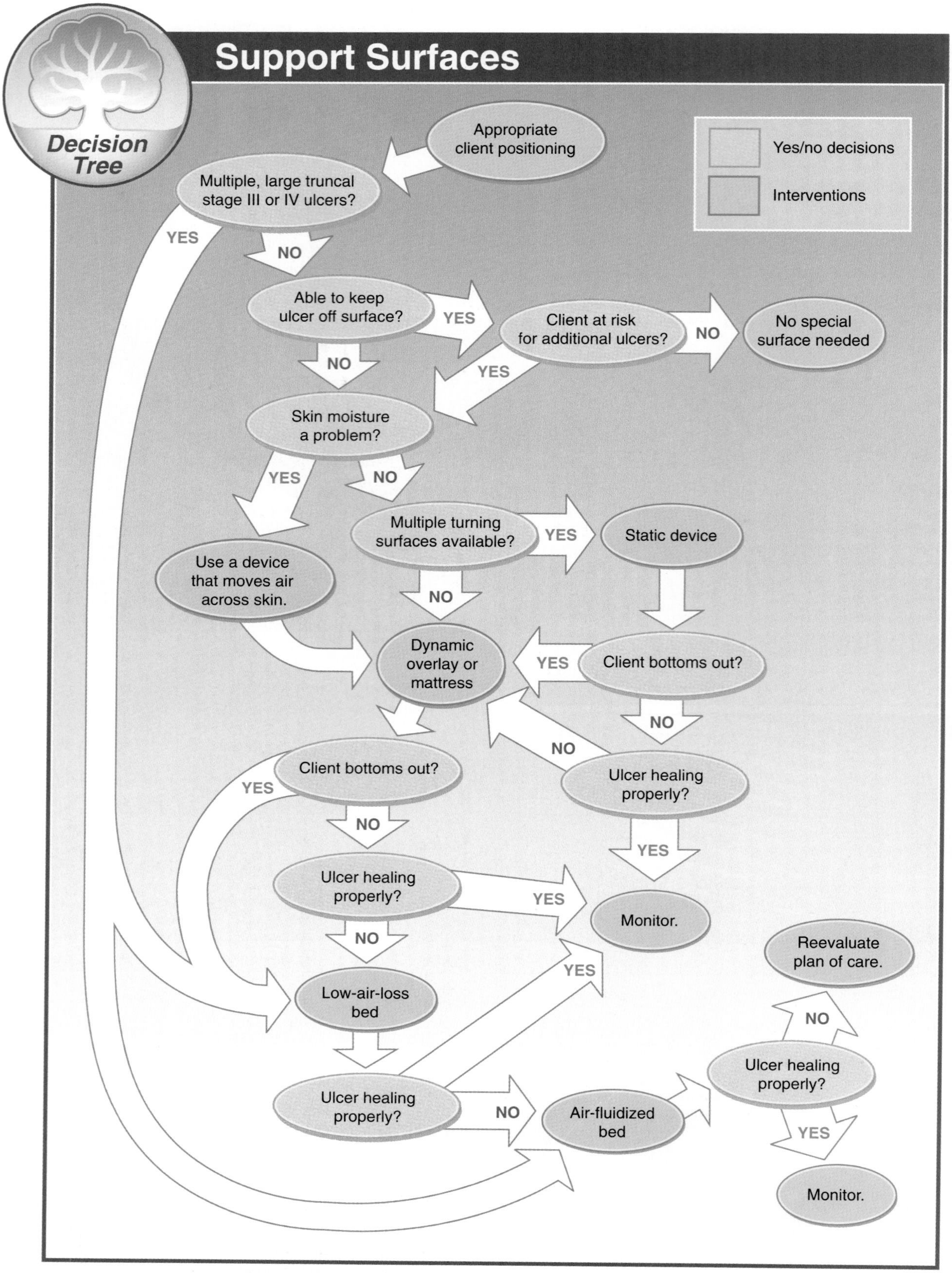

Support Surfaces

Decision Tree

Yes/no decisions

Interventions

Appropriate client positioning

Multiple, large truncal stage III or IV ulcers?

YES

NO

Able to keep ulcer off surface?

YES → Client at risk for additional ulcers? → NO → No special surface needed

YES

NO

Skin moisture a problem?

YES → Use a device that moves air across skin.

NO

Multiple turning surfaces available?

YES → Static device

NO

Dynamic overlay or mattress

Static device → Client bottoms out?

YES → Dynamic overlay or mattress

NO → Ulcer healing properly?

YES → Monitor.

Client bottoms out?

NO

YES

Ulcer healing properly?

YES → Monitor.

NO

Low-air-loss bed

Ulcer healing properly?

NO → Air-fluidized bed → Ulcer healing properly?

YES

Air-fluidized bed

Ulcer healing properly?

NO → Reevaluate plan of care.

YES → Monitor.

(Modified from Bergstrom, N., Bennett, M. A., Carlson, C. E., et al. Treatment of Pressure Ulcers. [1994]. Clinical Practice Guideline No. 15. Rockville, MD: US Department of Health and Human Services, Public Health Service, Agency for Health Care Policy and Research, Publication No. 95-0652.)

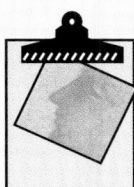

NURSING CARE PLANNING
A CLIENT WITH A HIP FRACTURE

Admission Data

Mrs. Jacan was admitted through the emergency department to an orthopedic unit where she was prepared for surgery. Phone report from the postanesthesia recovery unit is as follows:

72-year-old female who fell at home in the bathroom 2 days earlier sustained a right femoral neck fracture. She lay on the bathroom floor for 2 days before being discovered by her daughter and had a reddened area to her sacrum and bilateral heels. Underwent pinning of right hip.

Physician's Orders
Turn every 2 hours to unaffected side only
Keep heels elevated off bed at all times
Out of bed (OOB) bid with physical therapy starting tomorrow

Nursing Assessment
Quiet, cooperative elderly female post hip surgery with stage II pressure ulcer formation on sacrum and bilateral heels. Right hip dressing intact, no drainage on dressing. Slow to progress in physical therapy as well as positioning in bed due to postoperative pain.

NURSING CARE PLAN

Nursing Diagnosis	Expected Outcomes	Interventions	Evaluation (After 24 Hours of Care)
Impaired skin integrity related to surgical incision and stage II pressure ulcers on sacrum and heels	Right hip incision will heal with primary intention and free from infection	Change dressing per physician order maintaining sterile technique Assess for drainage from right hip incision	Right hip dressing clean, dry, and intact Dressing changed qd by RN using sterile technique
	Dressing to sacrum and heels will prevent further breakdown and will promote wound healing	Apply hydrocolloid dressing to sacrum and bilateral heels	Hydrocolloid dressing intact, no drainage
	Pain rated as less than 5 on scale of 0–10	Teach client pain scale (0 = no pain, 10 = worst pain ever) Medicate with small dose of narcotic to relieve pain	Client able to describe pain using pain scale Rates pain a 3 on scale
	No further skin breakdown	Turn and reposition q2h Apply air mattress to bed Explain importance of repositioning and OOB *Instruct family on proper methods to reposition client safely and comfortably*	Client turned and repositioned q2h with nursing staff and family Hydrocolloid dressing intact No further breakdown noted
	Diet meets nutritional requirement	Provide meals for client that meet her cultural requirement Obtain dietary consult	*Client's daughter bringing in food that mother likes, client tolerating 90% of meals* Ingesting plenty of liquids to stay hydrated
	Minimize anxiety	Soft assuring touches by nursing staff Hold client's hand when explaining new procedure or activity	Client calm and cooperative *Daughter reports minimal anxiety*

Italicized interventions indicate culturally specific care.

Continued

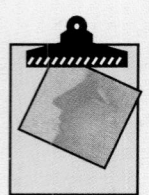

NURSING CARE PLANNING
A CLIENT WITH A HIP FRACTURE *(continued)*

Critical Thinking Questions

1. Before falling at her home, Mrs. Jacan was living independently. Her daughter is concerned about her mother's future ability to care for herself. Mrs. Jacan's daughter asks you about nursing home placement for her mother. How would you respond to her?
2. Mrs. Jacan's daughter thinks that she can care for her mother at her house and would like to take her home with her. Which members of the multidisciplinary team would you consult regarding the appropriateness of this plan? What information would you teach the client and her daughter?
3. Mrs. Jacan prefers to lie only on her back while in bed. What rationale would you give her daughter for the need to reposition and turn her mother to her side?

BIBLIOGRAPHY

Aronovitch, S. (1995). The best dressing sponge. *Nursing95,* 52–54.

Beltram, K.A., Thacker, J.G., & Rodeheaver, G.T. *Impact pressures generated by commercial wound irrigation devices.* (Unpublished research report). Charlottesville, VA, University of Virginia Health Science Center.

*Bergstrom, N., Allman, R.M., & Carlson, C.E. (1992). Pressure ulcers in adults: Prediction and prevention. *Clinical Practice Guideline No 3.* Rockville, MD: Agency for Health Care Policy and Research, Public Health Service. U.S. Department of Health and Human Services. AHCPR Publication No. 92-0047.

*Bergstrom, N., Bennett, M.A., Carlson, C.E., et al. (1994). Treatment of Pressure Ulcers. *Practice Guideline No. 15.* Rockville, MD: U.S. Department of Health and Human Services, Public Health Service, Agency for Health Care Policy and Research. Publication No. 95-0652.

Bolton, L.L., van Rijswijk, L.A., & Shaffer, F.A. (1996). Quality wound care equals cost effective wound care. *Nursing Management, 27*(7), 30–37.

*Braden, B.J. (1989). Clinical utility of the Braden scale for predicting pressure sore risk. *Decubitus, 2*(3), 44–46, 50–51.

Casey, G. (1998) Three steps to effective wound care. *Nursing Standard, (Aug 26–Sep 1) 12*(49), 43–44.

Cave, P. (1998). Nursing knowledge: The role of Plato in wound care. *Nursing Standard, (Dec 2–8) 13*(11), 40–3.

Collwell, J.C., Foreman, M.D., & Trotter, J.P. (1993). A comparison of the efficacy and cost effectiveness of 2 methods of managing pressure ulcers. *Decubitus, 6*(4), 28–35.

*Field, C.K., & Kerstein, M.D. (1994). Overview of wound healing in a moist environment. *American Journal of Surgery, 167,*(1A) Supp, 2s–6s.

Fowler, E. (1998). Wound infection: A nurse's perspective. *Ostomy Wound Management, 44*(8), 44–52.

*Guarlnik, J.M., Harris, T.B., White, L.R., & Cornoni-Huntley, J.C. (1988). Occurrence and predictors of pressure sores in the national health and nutrition exam survey follow-up. *Journal of the American Geriatric Society, 36*(9), 801–812.

Haas, A. (1995). Wound healing. *Dermatology Nursing, 7*(1), 28–74.

Hermans, M.H., & Bolton, L.L. (1996). The influence of dressings on the costs of wound treatment. *Dermatology Nursing, 8*(2), 93–100.

Hess, C.T. (1995). *Wound care: Nurses clinical guide.* Springhouse, PA: Springhouse Corporation.

Hess, C.T. (1998). Treating an arterial ulcer. *Nursing98, 28*(11), 12.

Hess, C.T. (1999). Assessing an external fistula. *Nursing99, 29*(1), 14.

*Hill, M.J. (1994). *Skin Disorders.* St. Louis: Mosby.

International Committee on Wound Management (ICWM). (1995). An overview of economic model of cost effective wound care. *Advances in Wound Care, 8*(5), 46.

Kalailieff, D. (1998). Vacuum-assisted closure: Wound care technology for the new millennium. *Perspectives, 22*(3), 28–29.

Krasner, D. (1995a). Minimizing factors that impair wound healing: A nursing approach. *Ostomy/Wound Management, 41*(1), 22–30.

Krasner, D. (1995b). Wound Care: How to use the red yellow black system. *American Journal of Nursing, 95*(5), 44–47.

*Lazarus, G.S., Cooper D.M., & Knighton, D.R. (1994). Definitions and guidelines for assessment of wounds and evaluation of healing. *Archives of Dermatology 130*(4), 489–493.

*Leigh, I.H., & Bennett, G. (1994). Pressure ulcers: Prevalence, etiology, and treatment modalities–A review. *American Journal of Surgery, 167*(1A), 25s–29s.

Leininger, M. (1996). *Transcultural nursing: Concepts, theories, research and practices* (2nd Ed.). New York: McGraw-Hill.

Lineaweaver, W., Howard, R., Saucy, D., McMorris, S., Freeman, J., Crain, C., Robertson, J., & Rumley, T. (1985). Topical antimicrobial toxicity *Archives Surgery, 120*(3), 267–270.

Maklebust, J. (1996). Using wound care products to promote a healing environment. *Critical Care Nursing Clinics of North America, 8*(2), 141–158.

Maklebust, J., & Sieggreen, M. (1996). *Pressure ulcers: Guidelines for prevention and nursing management.* Springhouse, PA: Springhouse Corporation.

Margolis, D.J. (1995). Definition of a pressure ulcer. NPUAP Proceedings. *Advances in Wound Care, 7*(4), 28.

*Miller, H., & Delozier, J. (1994). Cost implications of the pressure ulcer treatment guidelines. *Center for Health Policy Studies,* Contr 282-9-0070, 17. Sponsored by the Agency for Health Care Policy and Research.

North American Nursing Diagnosis Association. (1999). *Nursing diagnoses: Definitions and classification 1999–2000.* Philadelphia: Author.

*Ponder, R.B. & Krasner, D. (1993). Gauzes and related dressings. *Ostomy/Wound Management, 39*(5), 48–60.

van Rijswijk, L.V. (1996). The fundamentals of wound assessment. *Ostomy/Wound Management, 42*(7), 40–42, 44, 46.

*Rodeheaver, G. (1989). Controversies in topical wound management. *WOUND: A Compendium of Clinical Research and Practice, 1*(1), 19–27.

*Stevenson, T.R., Thacker, J.G., Rodeheaver, G.T., Bacchetta, C., Edgarton, M.T., & Edlich, R.F. (1976). Cleansing the traumatic wound by high pressure irrigation. *JACEP, 5*(1), 17–21.

*Turner, T. (1989). The development of wound management products. *Wounds, 1,* 155–171.

*Winter, G.D. (1962). Formation of the scab and the rate of epithelization of superficial wound in the skin of the young domestic pig. *Nature, 93,* 293–294.

*Wysocki, A.B., & Bryant, R. (1994). Skin. In R. Bryant (Ed.): *Acute and chronic wounds: Nursing management.* St. Louis: Mosby.

*Asterisk indicates a classic or definitive work on this subject.

Body Temperature

Richard Henker

Key Terms

fever
heat exhaustion
heat stroke
hyperthermia

hypothermia
malaise
pyrogen
set-point

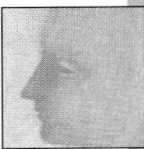

LEARNING OBJECTIVES

After studying this chapter, you should be able to:

1. Describe fever, hyperthermia, and hypothermia.
2. Identify characteristics of clients with fever, hyperthermia, or hypothermia.
3. Describe the assessment of the client with fever, hyperthermia, or hypothermia.
4. Write a nursing diagnosis for the person with fever, hyperthermia, or hypothermia.
5. Plan for nursing interventions for clients experiencing fever, hyperthermia, or hypothermia.
6. Evaluate the effectiveness of interventions for clients with fever, hyperthermia, or hypothermia.

Andrew Stephen is a 64-year-old African-American male transferred to the cardiac telemetry unit 36 hours after having coronary artery bypass surgery. His vital signs after transfer include a heart rate of 120 beats per minute, a temperature of 38.9°C (102°F), a blood pressure of 140/82, and a respiratory rate of 16. Mr. Stephen is complaining of feeling cold and has asked for additional blankets. The nurse's physical examination indicates decreased breath sounds on the left posterior side of his chest. The most likely cause of Mr. Stephen's fever is atelectasis. Less likely causes are wound infection, respiratory infection, or urinary tract infection. Treatment of fever in Mr. Stephen may include administration of an antipyretic to decrease core body temperature. Considerations when treating fever in Mr. Stephen include the facts that an elevated body temperature contributes to host defense and that an elevated body temperature increases metabolic demands. The report regarding Mr. Stephen's cardiac function is important to consider in treating Mr. Stephen. If he has diminished cardiac function, his fever should be treated to decrease the demands on his heart. The nurse makes a diagnosis of fever.

THERMOREGULATION NURSING DIAGNOSES

Risk for Altered Body Temperature: The state in which the individual is at risk for failure to maintain body temperature within normal range.

Hyperthermia: The state in which an individual's body temperature is elevated above normal range.

Fever: A regulated rise in body temperature that is mediated by a rise in temperature set-point.

Hypothermia: The state in which an individual's body temperature is reduced below normal range.

Definition of fever from Cooper, K. E., Cranston, W. I., & Snell, E. S. (1964). Temperature regulation during fever in man. Clinical Science, 27, 345–356. Other definitions from North American Nursing Diagnosis Association (1999). NANDA nursing diagnoses: Definitions and classification 1999–2000, Philadelphia: Author.

The management of fever presents significant problems to the nurse in managing the responses of the client and in providing education to the public about evaluating and making decisions about the meaning of a fever. Fever, resulting from infection or inflammation, is the most common change in body temperature requiring nursing care. Understanding fever is enhanced by a brief introduction to problems in thermoregulation.

CONCEPTS OF THERMOREGULATION

This section will describe concepts important to the understanding of nursing care of the client with alterations in thermoregulation. It helps to understand that body temperature is the balance between heat production and heat loss (Fig. 33–1).

Heat production and conservation

Heat production
• Basal metabolism
• Muscle contraction
• Increased metabolic rate

Heat conservation
• Shivering
• Vasoconstriction

Heat loss

• Evaporation (sweating)

• Conduction (contact with cold surfaces)

• Radiation (vasodilation of blood vessels in the skin)

• Convection (contact with air currents)

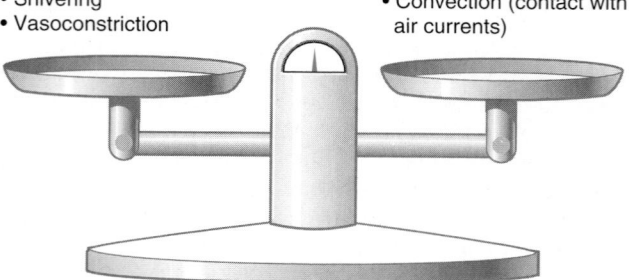

Figure 33–1. Body temperature is the balance between the production of heat and the loss of heat.

Physiology of Thermoregulation

The thermoregulatory system consists of a sensory component, a control center, and effector mechanisms. Most temperature sensation occurs in the skin. The face and hands have the greatest concentration of thermoreceptors for hot and cold sensation (Hensel, 1981). Deeper structures, such as the abdominal organs, are also thought to have the ability to sense temperature, but this claim is not well proven (Hensel, 1981). The hypothalamus and other structures in the brain and spinal cord sense temperature. Again, a combination of sensory neuron activity from the periphery and the central nervous system provide sensory input.

Once control centers have interpreted the sensory signals, they activate effector mechanisms that raise or lower the body's temperature. Effector mechanisms activated when body temperature is above the person's **set-point**—the temperature that thermoregulatory mechanisms attempt to maintain—include sweating and dilation of the blood vessels in the skin. These actions promote heat loss into the surrounding environment by the mechanisms of evaporation, conduction, radiation, and convection (Fig. 33–2). Effector mechanisms activated when body temperature is below set-point include shivering and constriction of the blood vessels in the skin. Shivering generates heat by causing muscle contraction, which increases metabolic rate 100 to 200% (Horvath, Spurr, Hutt, & Hamilton, 1956). Vasoconstriction of the skin decreases heat loss by radiation, convection, and conduction.

Definitions of Thermoregulatory States

Regulated Rise in Temperature

Fever is a regulated rise in body temperature that is mediated by a rise in temperature set-point (Cabanac & Massonett, 1974; Cooper, Cranston & Snell, 1964). Mediators released in response to a pathophysiological process, such as infection or inflammation, facilitate the rise in temperature set-point in the central ner-

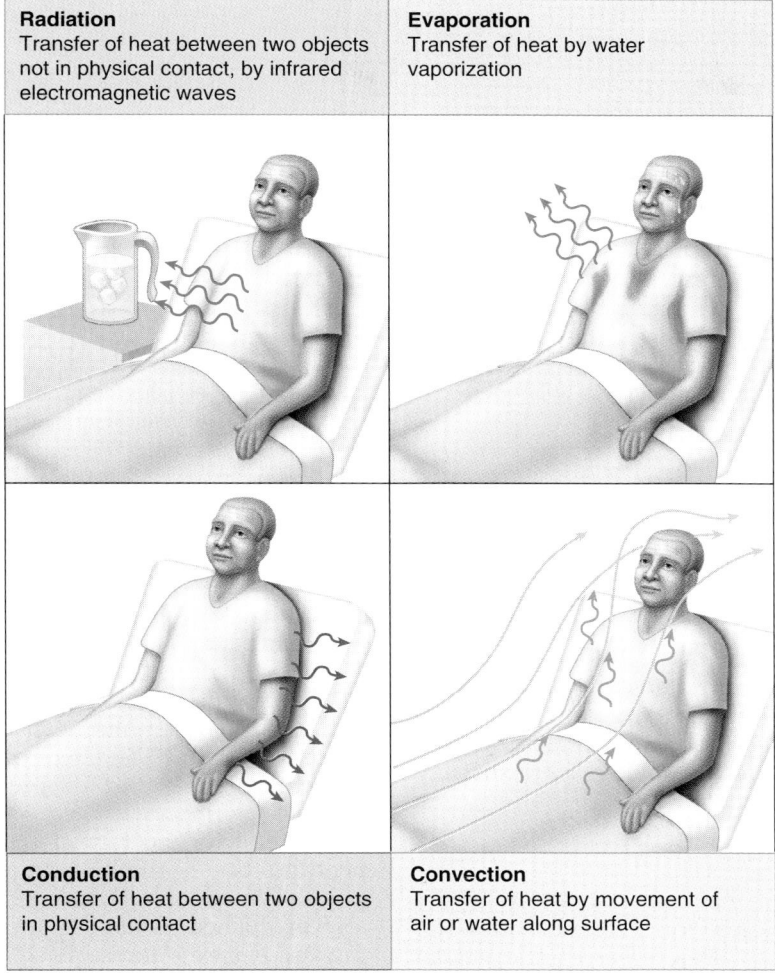

Radiation	Evaporation
Transfer of heat between two objects not in physical contact, by infrared electromagnetic waves	Transfer of heat by water vaporization
Conduction	**Convection**
Transfer of heat between two objects in physical contact	Transfer of heat by movement of air or water along surface

Figure 33–2. Mechanisms of heat loss.

vous system. Physiological effector mechanisms are activated by the central nervous system in an attempt to attain this new elevated temperature set-point.

Fever is a host defense response that frequently occurs in hospitalized people; 30% of clients admitted to the hospital develop a fever during their stay. Therefore, you are likely to encounter this phenomenon while caring for clients in an acute care setting (Bor et al., 1988; McGowan et al., 1987). In outpatient and home settings, you will be responsible for providing information to clients and families to help them evaluate and manage a fever.

Fever can be caused by a wide variety of processes, including infection, inflammation, autoimmune diseases, vascular diseases, neoplasia, and drug reactions. The most frequent causes of fever are infection and inflammation.

Nonregulated Changes in Temperature

Although the term hyperthermia means elevated temperature, the term is generally used to refer to extremes of temperature elevation. Thus, specifically, **hyperthermia** is a nonregulated elevation in body temperature related to an imbalance between heat gain and heat loss. In contrast to fever, the temperature set-point during hyperthermia is not elevated. Instead, the problem is an imbalance between heat loss and heat gain. The problem may be neurological damage that prevents the control of body temperature.

The most common example of hyperthermia is **heat stroke,** which is an extreme elevation of body temperature, usually above 40.6°C (105°F), resulting in altered central nervous system function and shock. Heat stroke results from failure of the temperature-regulating capacity of the body, caused by prolonged exposure to sun or high temperature. Heat loss cannot keep up with heat gain; therefore, the body temperature increases.

Hypothermia is a state in which body temperature is reduced below normal. It too is a problem of imbalance between heat gain and heat loss. In this case, heat production cannot keep up with heat loss; therefore, body temperature decreases. For example, hypothermia occurs when a person falls through the ice of a lake and loses heat rapidly in the cold water.

TABLE 33–1

Comparison of Fever and Hyperthermia

Characteristic	Fever	Hyperthermia
Etiology	Infection or inflammation	Elevated environmental temperature, physical activity, impaired heat loss
Temperature Range	Usually less than 40.6°C (105°F)	In severe cases such as heat stroke 40.6°C (105°F)
Mechanism	Host defense response	Loss of ability to thermoregulate
Manifestations	Increased heart rate, chills, sleepiness, anorexia	Decreased level of consciousness, increased heart rate, decreased blood pressure, tissue injury
Nursing Interventions	Monitor temperature frequently, provide fluids, prevent shivering, change linen to keep client dry, administer antipyretics as ordered, obtain blood cultures as ordered	Remove from warm environment and actively cool the client in more severe cases, monitor temperature and other vital signs frequently, prepare for insertion of IV line to provide fluids, monitor urine output

Fever

Differentiating between fever and hyperthermia is important in terms of diagnosing and treating a rise in body temperature (Table 33–1). Fever is often associated with infection and requires additional diagnostic evaluation based on localizing signs and symptoms. If the fever is treated, medications to reduce the fever attempt to decrease the elevation in temperature set-point. Other therapies are not related to decreasing set-point but promoting heat loss.

Pyrogens

A **pyrogen** is any agent that causes or stimulates a fever. The initial stimulus for fever is often an exogenous pyrogen. The word *exogenous* indicates an outside stimulus that is introduced into the body. Exogenous pyrogens include bacteria, viruses, fungi, allergens, incompatible blood products, and foreign substances. Exogenous pyrogens stimulate the production of *endogenous* pyrogens, internal stimuli that act directly on the hypothalamus. Some of the endogenous pyrogens that are produced in response to exogenous pyrogens include hormone-like chemical messengers called cytokines. Endogenous pyrogens are produced by monocytes, macrophages, neutrophils, and eosinophils. Endogenous pyrogens may result from inflammatory reactions, such as those that occur in tissue damage, cell necrosis, rejection of transplanted tissues, malignancy, and antigen-antibody reactions.

Phases of a Fever

There are three phases of fever: initiation, plateau, and defervescence (Fig. 33–3). Thermoregulation during these phases involves activation of the effector mechanisms discussed earlier as well as initiation of behavioral and experiential responses.

During the initiation phase of fever, pyrogens act on the hypothalamus to reset the temperature set-point higher than body temperature. Activation of effector mechanisms, such as shivering and decreased

blood flow to the skin, increases body temperature to attempt to reach the set-point. Additionally, the feverish client exhibits behaviors to decrease heat loss, such as putting skin surfaces together in a fetal position and increasing insulation by adding blankets or clothing. The client will feel cold and may have chills.

During the plateau phase of fever, the body temperature has risen and is maintained at this new elevated set-point. The client may feel quite warm because of this elevation in core body temperature.

During the defervescence phase of fever, the body's effector mechanisms are activated to promote heat loss due to the lowering of the temperature set-point. The client will feel warm and may sweat and appear flushed. Behaviors include shedding of clothing and blankets and requests for ice and fluids. Fever may resolve by a rapid return to normal over a period of a few hours (resolution by crisis) or resolve slowly (resolution by lysis).

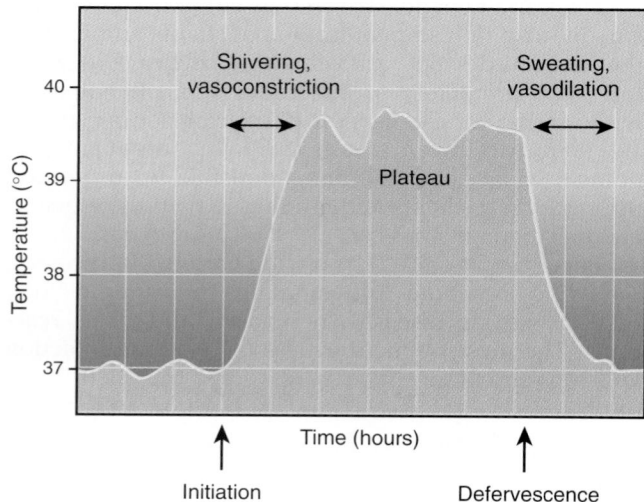

Figure 33–3. The three phases of fever: initiation, plateau, and defervescence.

Fever Patterns

The pattern of the rise and fall of body temperature is occasionally useful for the diagnosis of a particular causative organism. *Continuous or sustained fever* is sometimes seen with drug fever. *Remittent fever* is defined as an elevation and fall in temperature each day, with the baseline temperature remaining above normal for the entire day. Malaria is one example of a disorder that causes remittent fever. *Intermittent fever* is defined as an elevation and fall in temperature to baseline each day. Some forms of sepsis (fever and toxicity due to microbial disease may result in septic shock and death) may present with intermittent fever, although this finding is not necessarily helpful in determining the causative organism. With many infections, fever is most likely to be elevated in the late afternoon.

Physiological Responses

Associated physiological responses that occur during fever include increased cardiovascular demands and altered metabolism and immune system function. Cardiovascular responses related to fever include increased heart rate and increased cardiac output. Metabolic rate during fever increases 10% per 1.0°C (1.8°F) elevation in body temperature; if the client shivers, the rise in metabolic rate is approximately 100 to 200% above baseline. Other changes in metabolism include the production of acute-phase proteins that assist with host defense. Effects of fever on immune system function have not been determined fully. Drug reaction fevers are not accompanied by the signs of increased metabolic need.

Recall Mr. Stephen, the client in the case study. His fever is in the initiation phase. What behaviors would Mr. Stephen display next?

Action Alert!

Observe for fever that occurs without associated changes or an increase in heart rate—the cause may be a drug reaction.

Additional behavioral responses that occur as part of fever include malaise, anorexia, drowsiness, and altered sleep patterns. **Malaise,** a feeling of indisposition, is thought to be an adaptive response that decreases most daily activities, thereby maintaining energy stores for fever generation (Hart, 1988). Changes in sleep that have been identified in animal studies include an increase in total sleep time and an increase in the amount of slow-wave sleep (Krueger, Walter, Dinarello, Wolff, & Chedid, 1984).

Because Mr. Stephen has had cardiac surgery, his caregivers should be concerned about the effect of fever on the workload of his heart. What changes in vital signs might be attributed to his fever?

Hyperthermia

A person who develops hyperthermia does so either by generating too much heat, as during sports activities in hot weather, or by failing to lose heat while in a warm environment (e.g., elderly, children).

Sweating is an effective mechanism of heat loss, unless the environment is humid. Increased water saturation in the air prevents evaporation of sweat from the skin, thus decreasing heat loss. Therefore, hyperthermia is more likely to occur in humid environments. The amount of fluid loss attributed to sweating has been reported to average 1.8 L/hr in marathon runners (Pugh, Corbett, & Johnson, 1967). Fluid balance always needs to be monitored in clients at risk for hyperthermia. Maintenance of fluid balance is necessary to maintain perfusion of body systems and perfusion of the skin. Inadequate hydration will reduce blood flow to the skin, thus reducing heat loss.

Increased blood flow to the skin in response to temperature elevation may be impaired in the elderly and some clients with autonomic nervous system dysfunction, such as those with diabetes (Khan, Spence, & Belch, 1992). The autonomic nervous system controls vasoconstriction and vasodilation in the skin. Problems with nervous system control of blood flow to the skin predispose clients to hyperthermia.

Another population at risk for hyperthermia consists of clients with central nervous system injury, such as head injury, cerebrovascular accident (stroke), or subarachnoid hemorrhage. Hyperthermia in this group is thought to result from interference with thermoregulation in the central nervous system (Goodman & Knochel, 1991).

Heat exhaustion is a rise in body temperature that is usually related to inadequate fluid and electrolyte replacement during physical activity (Knochel, 1989). Physiological responses associated with heat exhaustion from physical exertion include an increase in cardiac output, release of antidiuretic hormone, increased production of aldosterone, and increased release of norepinephrine. Serum sodium levels usually increase because of the loss of body water in sweat, which has a low concentration of sodium.

In heat stroke, in which the body temperature exceeds 40.6°C (105°F), the client develops alterations in central nervous system function, such as confusion or a coma (Knochel, 1989). Physiological responses associated with heat stroke include dry skin, hypotension, seizures, vomiting, and diarrhea (Hales, 1997).

Hypothermia

Accidental hypothermia occurs due to decreased heat production, increased heat loss, or impaired thermoregulation. Hypothermia is often associated with clinical conditions or factors that predispose clients to a decrease in core body temperature.

In a study evaluating circumstances related to hypothermia (temperature 32.2°C [91.9°F] or lower), conditions present in the 73 clients who died included serious illness, systemic infection, trauma, immersion, frostbite, and overdose (Danzl et al., 1987). Another common finding in hypothermic clients is the incidence of high alcohol intake. Alcohol ingestion affects thermoregulation in a number of different ways. It provides a false sense of warmth, inhibits shivering, and vasodilates the skin, thus promoting heat loss (Granberg, 1991a). Alcohol also impairs judgment and decisions, raising the person's risk of making inappropriate decisions about exposure.

Hypothermia that occurs in hospitalized clients may be related to treatment (intentional) related to decreasing the metabolic rate. This might occur in clients with head injuries. Or hypothermia may be associated with therapies implemented in the hospital. Medications, particularly anesthetic agents, inhibit shivering and vasoconstriction, therefore promoting heat loss. In the operating room, anesthetics not only contribute to heat loss, but surgical incisions contribute significantly to evaporative heat loss. Hypothermia is also associated with rapid infusion of large volumes of fluid, known as fluid resuscitation. Body temperature has been found to decrease in trauma clients after admission to the emergency department (Bernardo, Henker, Bove, & Sereika, 1996). This decrease in body temperature is thought to be partially due to fluid resuscitation.

Classification of hypothermia and physiological responses are based on the level of body temperature. Mild hypothermia is a temperature between 35°C and 32°C (95°F and 89.6°F); moderate hypothermia is a temperature between 32°C and 28°C (89.6°F and 82.4°F); and severe hypothermia is a temperature below 28°C (82.4°F) (Granberg, 1991b). Physiological responses associated with hypothermia affect the cardiovascular, respiratory, renal, nervous, and endocrine systems (Box 33–1).

FACTORS AFFECTING THERMOREGULATION

Factors That Place Clients at Risk for Fever

Clients most likely to develop acute fever are those at risk for infection or inflammation. The most likely cause of infection in febrile hospitalized clients is bacteria (Bor et al., 1988). The most likely site of infection is the respiratory system.

Immunosuppressed people are at particular risk for fever because of their high incidence of infection. An immunosuppressed person is still able to generate a fever (Donowitz, 1996). Examples of causes of immunosuppression include neoplasms, infection with human immunodeficiency virus, and medications received after an organ transplant.

Factors That Place Clients at Risk for Hyperthermia

There are two classifications of hyperthermia: classic and exertional. Classic heat stroke is most likely to occur in people who have problems with thermoregulation, such as children, the elderly, or people with chronic diseases. Additional risk factors include alcoholism, an urban residence, poverty, the use of major tranquilizers, and living on higher floors of multistory buildings.

Risk factors such as chronic disease, alcohol, and the use of tranquilizers also affect a person's ability to thermoregulate. Urban residence and living on the higher floors of a building expose a person to greater amounts of environmental heat. People with classic heat stroke typically have problems with limited abilities to lose heat.

Exertional heat stroke occurs in people who have been physically active in hot, humid conditions. Examples of people at risk for exertional hyperthermia are marathon runners, football players, and military recruits. Heat gain is more of a problem in people with exertional heat stroke. Heat stroke is more common in the humid Southern climates. Heat-related deaths occur in prolonged periods of high temperature and humidity.

Factors That Place Clients at Risk for Hypothermia

People at risk for hypothermia have an altered ability to thermoregulate or excessive exposure to a cold environment. Altered thermoregulation occurs in the elderly and in people who have diseases that alter auto-

---

BOX 33–1

PHYSIOLOGICAL RESPONSES TO HYPOTHERMIA

Central Nervous System

Apathy
Poor judgment
Paradoxical undressing
Dilated pupils

Cardiovascular System

Decreased heart rate at temperatures <32°C (89.6°F)
Decreased cardiac output at temperatures <32°C
Ventricular fibrillation at temperatures <28°C (82.4°F)

Renal System

Cold diuresis
Decreased glomerular filtration rate at temperatures <32°C

Endocrine

Increased aldosterone
Increased T_4 and T_3

From Granberg, P. (1991b). Human physiology under cold exposure. Arctic Medical Research, 50(Suppl. 6), 23–27.

nomic nervous system function, such as diabetes mellitus. Decreased ability to vasoconstrict in response to cold in these people will inappropriately promote heat loss. Children are at risk for hypothermia due to the high ratio of body surface to mass. This high ratio promotes rapid heat loss, placing children at increased risk for hypothermia.

ASSESSMENT

Temperature is measured as part of the vital signs during a general health screening or when the client presents with evidence suggesting a fever or is at risk for developing a fever. The accompanying Data Clustering chart shows examples of data used to support thermoregulatory nursing diagnoses.

Focused Assessment for Fever

Most hospitalized clients are at risk for an elevated temperature. Inflammation and infection commonly affect the hospitalized client. (See Chapter 27 for a discussion of *Risk for infection.*)

Defining Characteristics

The definition of fever is an elevation of set-point manifested as a rise in body temperature and usually associated with chills. Acute fever is considered a temperature rise greater than 37.8°C (100°F), but circadian variation must be taken into consideration when assessing fever. A temperature of 37.8°C at 5:00 AM is more of a rise above normal than a temperature of 37.8°C at 6:00 PM in a client with a normal circadian rhythm.

Chronic fever or fever of unknown origin is defined as fever of 3 weeks' duration with evaluation by a medical team for 1 week. Chronic fever is most likely to occur in people with neoplasia, autoimmune disease, and vascular disease.

Fever is often associated with a rise in heart rate and cardiac output. In a person with an increased body temperature, who does not also have an increased heart rate, fever may result from a drug reaction. A person with underlying cardiac problems may not tolerate the additional cardiovascular stress associated with fever.

Another consequence of fever is a change in the metabolic absorption and distribution of medications in the gastrointestinal tract. Acid secretion decreases and transit time decreases, altering the absorption of medications (Sarwari & Mackowiak, 1996). The increase in cardiac output that occurs with fever alters the distribution of medications.

In some clients, fever may not be present during infection. A phenomenon termed afebrile bacteremia has been reported in the elderly (Gleckman & Hibert, 1982). Because fever does not develop as readily in the elderly, diagnosis of infection may be delayed, leading to serious consequences. Fever is also a poor indicator of infection in clients receiving nonsteroidal anti-inflammatory medications for conditions such as rheumatoid arthritis.

Related Factors

Fever is related to a variety of etiologies, including infection, inflammation, neoplasia, autoimmune disease, vascular disease, drug reaction, and miscellaneous causes (Box 33–2).

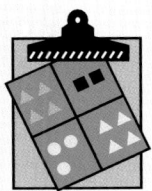

CLUSTERING DATA TO MAKE A NURSING DIAGNOSIS
PROBLEMS OF BODY TEMPERATURE

Data Cluster	Diagnosis
A mother calls the pediatrician's office, concerned that her 4-year-old has a temperature of 37.5°C (99.6°F). The child is active, does not appear ill, and does not have any gastrointestinal symptoms or respiratory symptoms. Further assessment reveals that the child has a sunburn after swimming yesterday.	Low-grade fever related to inflammation.
A 90-year-old female is admitted to the hospital with a temperature of 40.6°C (105°F). The city is experiencing a heat wave, and the woman lives in a high-rise apartment without air conditioning or adequate ventilation. She has no signs of infection.	Hyperthermia related to environmental conditions.
A first-day postsurgical client has a temperature of 39°C (102.2°F). Respirations are 10, breath sounds diminished, and the person is unable to cough.	Fever related to postoperative hypoventilation.

BOX 33–2

SOME OF THE POSSIBLE ETIOLOGIES OF FEVER

Inflammation

Pancreatitis
Cholecystitis
Burns
Trauma

Infection

Bacterial
Viral
Parasitic
Fungal

Drug Fever
Neoplastic Disease
Vascular Occlusion

Myocardial infarction
Stroke
Thrombophlebitis

THE COST OF CARE
TEMPERATURE MONITORING

The cost of electronic thermometers and tympanic membrane thermometers is often related to the number of disposable covers that are used in a year. If a health care agency purchases a large enough number of disposable covers, the device is often provided at no cost to the health care agency.

Mercury thermometers are inexpensive to purchase and can be reused after sterilization. However, one of the costs that needs to be taken into consideration with mercury thermometers is the cost of mercury disposal following accidental breakage of one of these thermometers. Mercury is considered a toxic substance that must be disposed of properly.

One advantage of chemical indicator thermometers is that they are disposable. Disposing of the thermometer after one use eliminates the risk of transmitting infection, which may occur with electronic thermometers or tympanic membrane thermometers. Although there is some cost associated with the purchase of these disposable thermometers, the cost may be outweighed by savings from the prevention of infection.

Diagnostic Tests

Temperature Measurement

A thermometer is the instrument used to measure body temperature. Thermometers measure temperatures via many routes: oral, rectal, axillary, and tympanic membrane. The most common type of thermometer used today is an electronic device, although glass thermometers may still be used on occasion. See Chapter 9 for a Procedure that covers measuring body temperature.

Blood Cultures

One of the frequently ordered diagnostic procedures in a febrile client is a blood culture. Blood cultures can indicate to the clinician the etiology of a fever. Most blood cultures are used to identify bacteria in the blood (bacteremia), but they can also be used to identify viruses in the blood (viremia). It is important to realize that in bacterial pneumonia, urinary tract infection, and wound infection, bacteria may not be present in the blood even though the client has developed an infectious process.

Blood cultures are ordered when body temperature reaches a specific threshold. This threshold varies, depending on characteristics of the client and practitioner preference. Blood cultures are sometimes drawn at lower temperature levels in immunosuppressed clients because of the likelihood of a life-threatening infection.

When drawing blood cultures from a client, the blood should not be drawn through an intravascular device, such as a central line or intravenous catheter. Blood cultures should be drawn from a peripheral site to prevent contamination of the culture (Bryant & Strand, 1987). Drawing blood cultures through the intravascular device may be appropriate, however, if you are trying to determine whether the device itself is the source of the infection.

Action Alert!
If a blood culture is ordered at the same time as an antibiotic, draw the blood culture before giving the antibiotic. Administration of an antibiotic will alter the results.

Assessment of Responses

Responses associated with fever that need to be monitored include increased cardiac demand (such as increased heart rate), increased metabolic rate, altered drug metabolism, and altered comfort. Treatment will be based on the client's ability to tolerate fever and the discomfort associated with fever. Table 33–2 summarizes decision-making in the assessment of temperature for different age groups.

Focused Assessment for Hyperthermia

Hyperthermia includes heat exhaustion and heat stroke. At both of these levels of hyperthermia, heat gain occurs at a greater rate than heat loss. Heat exhaustion is defined as a body temperature greater than normal but less than 40.6°C (105°F). Heat stroke is a

TABLE 33–2
Decision-Making in Assessing Temperature for Different Age Groups

Age	Assessment Data	Decision Considerations
Infant	• Infants have immature thermoregulation. • A temperature of 38° C (>100.4° F) in the first 12 months of life is considered significant. • Convulsions and delirium may occur.	• Protect from environmental changes; keep dry and appropriately clothed. • The parent is often advised to see the primary care provider. • Tympanic or axillary site is preferred. • Risk for febrile convulsions begins at 6 months. Febrile convulsions generally occur as the temperature is elevating
Child	• Risk for febrile convulsions and delirium lasts up to 6 years. • May experience temperature elevation after exercise.	• Educate parents about the risk for convulsions and appropriate actions. • Tell the child experiencing hallucinations that the image is not real and will go away when the fever is down. • Temperature regulation is still labile.
Adult	• 37.1° C to 38.2° C (98.8° F to 100.6° F) low grade. • >38.2° C (>100.6° F) significant fever. • >40.5° C (>104.9° F) hyperpyrexia.	• Older adults may have decreased sensitivity to temperature changes.
Older Adult	• Body temperature drops to an average of 36° C (96.8° F) in the older adult.	• Confusion may be a sign of impending infection with fever.

body temperature greater than 40.6°C (Goodman & Knochel, 1991).

Defining Characteristics

Heat exhaustion is more severe than simple heat-related symptoms that can be relieved by resting in a cool environment and replacing fluids. Symptoms associated with heat exhaustion include weakness, fatigue, headache, giddiness, anorexia, nausea, vomiting, diarrhea, and skeletal muscle cramps. Heat stroke is a severe and sometimes fatal condition. It is characterized by hot, dry skin; the absence of sweating; and neurological manifestations.

A person with exertional heat stroke still produces sweat. Manifestations associated with heat stroke include central nervous system alterations, acute renal failure, liver damage, cardiovascular abnormalities, and electrolyte imbalance (Hales, 1997). Neurological manifestations that occur with heat stroke include coma, seizures, and confusion. Sinus tachycardia and hypotension are common. Electrolyte abnormalities include increased serum sodium and decreased serum potassium levels. Potassium is initially decreased because the person has a metabolic acidosis. The Teaching for Self-Care chart lists teaching points to help parents prevent or manage febrile convulsions in their small children.

Related Factors

AGE. Several factors contribute to an increased risk for heat exhaustion or heat stroke in the elderly. In the elderly, the size, number, and activity of the sweat glands diminish, making the body less efficient at losing excess heat. Also, decreased mobility may affect an elderly client's ability to get water. And elderly clients also have decreased thirst sensation. If an elderly client has diminished cognitive capacities, this will also affect decision-making related to heat exposure and water intake. Table 33–3 lists other factors that can affect thermoregulation.

SOCIOECONOMIC CONDITIONS. Prevention of heat stroke is a public health issue, particularly in crowded urban areas where it is difficult to maintain cool, well ventilated housing. In conditions of prolonged heat and humidity, ventilation and air conditioning become important. The cost of electricity and air conditioning units may be prohibitive for the poor.

OCCUPATION. Heat-related illness, a concern for an occupational health nurse, may occur where a significant number of employees work in conditions of extreme heat. Laborers who do heavy physical work in the hot sun or in metal foundries, mines, or closed shops are vulnerable. Regular breaks, ventilation, lightweight clothing, and plenty of liquids may be helpful in preventing heat-related problems.

MEDICATIONS. Hyperthermia can also occur as a side effect of medications. Malignant hyperthermia can occur in response to general anesthetic agents, such as halothane (Wlody, 1991). This increase in body temperature is due to a genetic abnormality that causes muscle rigidity, leading to a rise in body temperature. Neuroleptic malignant syndrome can occur in clients receiving Haldol (haloperidol) or phenothiazines. Haloperidol impairs thirst, leading to dehydration that contributes to hyperthermia (Hooper, Herren & Goldwasser, 1989).

Other medications can make the person vulnerable to heat stroke. Diuretics reduce the amount of total

Teaching for SELF-CARE

MANAGING FEBRILE CONVULSIONS

Purpose: To provide parents of small children information about febrile convulsions.

Rationale: Febrile convulsions in children can be especially frightening to parents. They might feel helpless and panic in such situations. Knowing what to do can help them handle febrile convulsions with a measure of confidence.

Expected Outcome: Parents will feel confident that febrile convulsions can be prevented or safely managed.

Client Instructions

General Information
- Febrile convulsions are associated with a fever of 38.9°C to 40°C (102°F to 104°F).
- They occur as early as 3 months of age and as late as 7 years of age; 95% of febrile convulsions occur before the age of 5 years, and they are most likely to occur before the age of 24 months.
- Febrile convulsions occur in only 3 to 4% of children, but the risk is greater if the child has had a previous febrile convulsion.
- The child's EEG remains normal during a febrile convulsion; the child will have little of the confusion that occurs after other types of convulsions; and most importantly, febrile convulsions do not cause brain damage.
- The height of the child's fever does not seem to trig-

ger febrile convulsions as much as a sudden spike in body temperature.
- You can treat your child at home with the specific dosage of medication that the physician prescribes.
- When the child has a fever, dress her in lightweight clothing; infants should be dressed only in diapers.
- Febrile convulsions occur mostly at night, when parents are not aware of temperature elevations until the temperature is quite high.
- If your child has had one episode of a high fever, try to prevent a second high fever in order to reduce the risk of febrile convulsions.
- Whenever the child has a high fever, make sure you take him to the doctor.

Treatment of Febrile Convulsions
- Remain calm, and protect the child from injury.
- Following the convulsion, put a cool cloth to the child's head, and call the physician to determine where the child can be checked (physician's office, emergency department).
- Do not put the child in a tub of cold water; extreme cooling is a shock to the nervous system.
- Do not use alcohol to cool the child; it will be absorbed by the skin, and the fumes are toxic.
- Do not give the child any medications by mouth.
- Do not use an oral thermometer to measure the child's body temperature.

body fluid. Beta-blockers, phenothiazines, and anticholinergics decrease the ability to sweat.

Assessment of Responses

In addition to treating the manifestations of hyperthermia, you will be involved in assessing and managing complications. Complications associated with hyperthermia include altered perfusion of the central nervous system, altered perfusion of the kidneys, and breakdown of muscle. Clients with a family history of malignant hyperthermia may have anxiety before surgical procedures. Clients with neuroleptic malignant syndrome will often have decreased thirst that contributes to the development of hyperthermia. Nursing diagnoses that may be appropriate are *Anxiety, Fluid volume deficit, Confusion,* and *Altered tissue perfusion.*

Focused Assessment for Hypothermia

In clients with hypothermia, heat gain is at a lower rate than heat loss. Because of the higher heat loss, body temperature decreases. The accompanying Teaching for Wellness chart offers information to help clients prevent both hypothermia and hyperthermia.

Defining Characteristics

Hypothermia has been categorized as mild (35°C to 32°C [95°F to 89.6°F), moderate (32°C to 28°C [89.6°F to 82.4°F]), and severe (less than 28°C [82.4°F]) (Granberg, 1991b). Levels of hypothermia are associated with pathophysiological responses. Life-threatening sequelae, such as ventricular fibrillation, are associated with severe hypothermia. Level of consciousness will be diminished in the severely hypothermic clients as well.

Manifestations associated with hypothermia depend on temperature level (see Box 33–1). Shivering caused by hypothermia will become progressively more intense to the point where the hypothermic person will have trouble performing voluntary motor functions. Level of consciousness will also decrease as body temperature decreases. Hyporeflexia occurs with severe hypothermia.

Initially during hypothermia, cold diuresis occurs due to peripheral vasoconstriction (Jolly & Ghezzi, 1992). Cold diuresis is increased urine production due to a smaller vascular compartment. Subsequently, the hematocrit level will increase because of the fluid loss. As body temperature decreases, cold diuresis slows,

TABLE 33–3
Factors Affecting Thermoregulation

Factor	Effect
Age	Children have a greater body-surface-to-mass ratio, and children also have a higher metabolic rate. Elderly clients have a lower average body temperature.
Percent Body Fat	Increased body fat prevents heat loss. This can be beneficial in cold environments or detrimental in warm environments.
Gender	Women have changes in body temperature that are related to menstrual cycle.
Chronic Illness	Some chronic illnesses, such as diabetes mellitus and renal failure, interfere with thermoregulation.
Medications	Neuroleptic medications affect thermoregulation by impairing thirst. Fever may not occur in clients taking nonsteroidal anti-inflammatory agents.
Environment	Living areas that have poor ventilation due to windows that cannot be opened or materials that hold heat, such as concrete, may impact thermoregulation in clients.
Occupation	Work that requires exposure to cold environments or physical labor in warm humid environment affects thermoregulation.
Recreation	Activities such as running, football, etc. generate heat and may be of concern in warm, humid environments.

renal blood flow decreases, and urine output decreases.

Cardiovascular responses also depend on temperature level. Sinus tachycardia occurs with mild hypothermia. Sinus bradycardia occurs with moderate and severe hypothermia. Ventricular fibrillation can occur when body temperature is at 28°C (82.4°F) (Jolly & Ghezzi, 1992). The major concern with hypothermia is preventing cardiovascular compromise because of ventricular arrhythmias.

Related Factors

EXPOSURE. People exposed to the cold—such as hikers, hunters, and others who spend time outdoors—are at risk for hypothermia, particularly if some unforeseen injury occurs and the person is a distance from assistance. Heat loss in people accidentally submerged in cold water occurs at a much faster rate than exposure to air. Therefore, death will occur rapidly in a person exposed to very cold water. In the southern United States, a case of hypothermia is rare;

in Northern regions, emergency departments are well-equipped to manage the condition.

MEDICAL PROCEDURES. Hypothermia is also a consequence of procedures performed in the hospital. Clients undergoing surgery and clients receiving fluid resuscitation may be hypothermic after these procedures.

Diagnostic Tests

Thermometers normally used in clinical practice do not provide a scale low enough to assess hypothermia. A thermometer with a lower range should be available, particularly in emergency departments, for accurate assessment of body temperature in the client with hypothermia.

DIAGNOSIS

An elevation in body temperature is due to either hyperthermia or fever. To differentiate fever from hyperthermia, it is useful to consider client history and setting. It is most difficult in clients admitted to the hospital with neurological injury. The elevation in temperature could be due to the underlying injury or to an infectious process. You need to assess for signs of infection to make the final determination.

Determination of the cause of fever can be difficult because of the many possible etiologies. Identification of the cause of fever requires examining for localizing signs, such as increased sputum production, abdominal pain, or cloudy urine. Without localizing signs, identification of the cause of fever is more difficult and may be classified as fever of unknown origin.

The age and other demographic data about the client may be useful in knowing what questions to ask when you are looking for the cause of an elevated body temperature. As an example, assessment for causes of fever in children is illustrated in the accompanying decision tree. A pattern of body temperature change during fever in some cases is related to particular diseases. For example, continuous fever, an elevation of temperature over days, is related to bacterial pneumonia. Remittent fever, an elevation in temperature with a decrease in temperature to above normal each day, is associated with malaria (Cunha, 1996).

One of the clues that an elevation in body temperature is drug fever is no change in heart rate with the rise in body temperature. Generally during fever, there is an associated elevation in heart rate; during drug fever, this may not occur.

PLANNING
Expected Outcomes for the Client With Fever

Fever is a component of host defense and should be treated only in clients who cannot tolerate physiological or experiential stress caused by the fever. In clients unable to tolerate the additional stress of fever, body

Screening Fever* in Children

Decision Tree

Is the child's temperature 39°C (102°F) or above? — **YES** → Call the physician immediately. Convulsions may occur.

Does the child have a rash? — **YES** → Assess for exposure to measles, rubella, or chickenpox. If the rash consists of purple spots, contact a physician immediately.

* A fever is defined as a temperature of 38°C (100°F) or above associated with a flushed appearance, irritability, or drowsiness.

NO ↓

Does the child have stomach pain? — **YES** → Many causes of stomach pain in children are benign. However, if the child has pain so severe that the child screams with pain, it may be a sign of an acute abdomen, such as seen in appendicitis. Refer to a physician.

NO ↓

Does the child have diarrhea? — **YES** → The child probably has gastroenteritis. Simple gastroenteritis usually resolves in 24-48 hr. If child has severe water loss and signs of dehydration, refer to a physician.

NO ↓

Is the child coughing? — **YES** → Is the child having difficulty breathing? — **YES** → Call the physician. The child may have pneumonia.

NO ↓ (coughing)   **NO** ↓ (difficulty breathing)

Does the child have a sore throat or hoarseness? — **YES** → The child probably has an upper respiratory infection. If the child has green or yellow discharge, refer to a physician.

NO ↓

Does the child have a runny nose? — **YES** → Has the child had contact with a contagious disease, such as measles?
— **YES** → The child probably has an early-stage infection. Refer to a physician.
— **NO** → The child probably has a feverish cold. Refer to a physician.

NO ↓

Does the child have swelling and tenderness between the ear and the angle of the jaw? — **YES** → The child may have mumps. Refer to a physician.

NO ↓

Does the child seem very ill? Does the child have two or more of the following symptoms:
• Vomiting? • Headache? • Neck stiffness? — **YES** → Call a physician. The child may have meningitis.

NO ↓

If the child's temperature remains elevated for more than 6 hours, call a physician.

Teaching for WELLNESS

PREVENTING HYPOTHERMIA AND HYPERTHERMIA

Purpose: To prevent an unbalanced state of heat loss and heat gain.

Rationale: Factors such as climate, individual activity, age, fluid status, and finances may impact thermoregulation negatively.

Expected Outcome: The client will maintain a balanced state of thermoregulation.

Client Instructions to Prevent Hypothermia

- In cold weather, dress warmly, keep the environment warm, and drink warm fluids.
- Wear a cap to prevent heat loss through the head; children and older people in particular need to conserve body heat in cold weather.
- In extremely cold climates, wear a muffler or a long scarf to protect your face, gloves or mittens to protect your hands and fingers, and insulated boots to protect your feet. All of these articles of clothing prevent exposure to extreme cold that can cause frostbite.
- If necessary, seek help from local community agencies that can help you pay your utility bills to keep your home warm.

Client Instructions to Prevent Hyperthermia

- In warm, humid weather, dress lightly, keep the environment cool with air conditioning if possible, circulate air with fans, and drink cool fluids.
- Avoid exercising in hot, humid weather (indoors or outdoors).
- Use a swimming pool or sprinkler on hot, humid days.
- If you need to, seek help from local community agencies that can help you pay your utility bills and that may help you obtain an air conditioner.
- Recognize that heat stroke may manifest itself with hot, dry skin, the absence of sweating, vomiting, diarrhea, and seizures.
- Recognize that heat exhaustion may manifest itself with weakness, fatigue, headache, giddiness, loss of appetite, nausea, vomiting, diarrhea, and muscle cramps.
- If you or someone you know has been exposed to extreme heat or cold, seek medical attention promptly.

temperature will be brought within normal range using therapies that do not induce shivering. Therefore, the goal may be to reduce the fever or to make the client comfortable. Sometimes the goal is to teach the client self-care. Possible outcomes may include the following. The client will:

- Maintain a body temperature that is normal for the client
- Maintain dry skin, clothes, and linens
- Maintain comfort
- Maintain fluid intake sufficient to prevent dehydration
- Demonstrate the correct method for measuring a temperature
- Identify when a nurse or physician should be consulted for a fever

Expected Outcomes for the Client With Hyperthermia

Body temperature will be brought to within normal limits to prevent complications related to hyperthermia, such as muscle breakdown. Ideally, there will be no neurological deficits present after cooling. Fluid balance as assessed by serum sodium and urine output will be within normal limits. Precipitating causes

of hyperthermia will be evaluated to determine etiology to prevent future episodes of hyperthermia.

When the diagnosis is *Risk for hyperthermia,* the goal is to prevent heat-related problems. The outcomes may include the following. The client will:

- Modify the environment to prevent hyperthermia, such as by repairing an air conditioning unit or increasing ventilation with fans or open windows
- Identify appropriate dress for a hot, humid environment
- Identify precautions to take when exercising or working in a hot environment

Expected Outcomes for the Client With Hypothermia

The goal in hypothermia is to bring temperature to a normal level without complications. Therapies should be monitored closely to prevent the afterdrop that may occur during peripheral warming. Possible outcomes may include the following. The client will:

- Have minimal or no tissue necrosis
- Return to a normal sinus rhythm
- Have urinary output within normal limits
- Have blood pressure and pulse within normal limits

When the diagnosis is *Risk for hypothermia,* the goal is prevention. The possible outcomes may include the following. The client will:

- Recall safety precautions for walking or skating on frozen ponds
- Demonstrate appropriate dress for cold weather
- Modify the environment to maintain heat in the home, such as by repairing the furnace, seeking public assistance for utility bills, or insulating the home
- Implement a plan for checking on the welfare of elders in the family

INTERVENTION

Interventions to Monitor Temperature

Temperature is monitored as part of routine vital signs. The scheduling of routine vital signs varies for an outpatient clinic, a general nursing unit in a hospital, a long-term care facility, or the client's home. On a general hospital unit, the routine depends on institution policy; it may specify two, three, or four times a day. For the low-risk client, twice a day has a high probability of detecting a rise in temperature.

Frequency of monitoring must be adjusted based on the client's risk for changes in body temperature.

For Mr. Stephen, what schedule of vital signs would be appropriate, given his postoperative status and present vital signs?

A*ction* A*lert!*
The temperature of clients at risk for infection should be measured every 4 hours. If temperature is monitored every 8 hours, a febrile episode may occur between temperature measurements.

If the client has an elevated temperature, monitoring every 4 hours is usually sufficient. However, you should be aware of signs of possible fever and take the client's temperature more often if needed. Clients with severe alterations in thermoregulation, such as hyperthermia or hypothermia, should be monitored as often as every 15 minutes.

Temperature is reported in either centigrade or Fahrenheit units; both units continue to be used clinically. The temperature should be recorded according to the agency's charting format.

Interventions to Manage a Fever

Because fever is considered a host defense response, treatment is somewhat controversial (Kluger, 1986; Vaughn, Veale, & Cooper, 1980). Decisions to treat fever should be based on the benefits of host defense associated with fever versus the ability of the host to tolerate the cardiopulmonary demands created by the fever.

Covering the Client

The first sign of the onset of fever may be a chill. The client complains of being cold and requests additional covering. The temperature may be collected as a baseline measurement, but the temperature is not elevated until the chill phase has passed. Chills last from 10 to 30 minutes. Cover the person with a light blanket, but avoid heavy covering. Covers will aid in the body's attempt to maintain heat and may actually increase the impending elevation of temperature.

Administering Antipyretics

The two classes of interventions used for treating fever include antipyretics and physical cooling. Antipyretics are medications that are effective against fever and include acetaminophen, aspirin, and other nonsteroidal anti-inflammatory medications. Aspirin and other salicylates are effective for treating fever because they act directly on the hypothalamus to decrease temperature set-point.

For example, because treating a fever masks the symptoms of an illness, it is important to know if the absence of fever is a sign of recovery or simply a result of the use of an antipyretic. Knowing the half-life of the medication will help. The half-life of acetaminophen, one of the more commonly used antipyretics, is 2 hours. It will influence temperature for about 4 to 6 hours (Gilman, Rall, Nies, & Taylor, 1990).

Acetaminophen, unlike other antipyretic agents, inhibits cyclo-oxygenase production only in the central nervous system. Treatment with an antipyretic agent, such as aspirin or acetaminophen, is relatively safe. However, serious effects can occur in high-risk clients. One of the side effects of acetaminophen is hepatic toxicity. This usually occurs only when acetaminophen is taken in very large doses (Gilman, Rall, Nies, & Taylor, 1990) or when the person has pre-existing liver disease. Common side effects of aspirin include bruising of the skin as a result of its anticoagulant effect and tinnitus (ringing in the ears).

A*ction* A*lert!*
Teach clients to avoid overdose of acetaminophen, especially if they have a history of liver disease. Persons with a history of gastrointestinal bleeding or who are taking an anticoagulant medication should avoid aspirin and the ibuprofens. Aspirin is contraindicated in children and teenagers with chickenpox or flu due to the risk of developing Reye's syndrome.

Acetaminophen can be administered either orally as tablets or elixir or rectally as a suppository. One of the problems with administration of acetaminophen to acutely ill people is variable absorption. A study evaluating acetaminophen administration found drug levels to be lower when acetaminophen was given by nasogastric tube 3 hours after surgery compared with oral administration before surgery (Elfant et al., 1995). This effect was attributed to decreased gastric emptying that occurred after surgery and not clamping the nasogastric tube for a long enough time (i.e., more than 30 minutes). Only the more commonly used anti-pyretics, such as acetaminophen, are available as preparations that can be administered via the nasogastric tube.

Providing Physical Cooling

Methods used for cooling include cooling blankets, ice packs, fans, and tepid baths. Physical cooling does not alter the set-point; therefore, use of these interventions to decrease temperature is controversial. Methods of physical cooling decrease body temperature by increasing the temperature difference between the skin and the environment. Subsequently, the difference between the skin and the core of the body increases heat loss.

Cooling blankets can be set at various temperatures to promote conductive heat loss. Fans promote convective heat loss by moving air closest to the skin away from the client. Air that is closer to the skin is warmed by the body. When the fan moves this air away, colder air moves next to the skin, increasing the difference between the skin and air temperature. Tepid baths used on febrile clients promote evaporative heat loss. Heat can be lost through evaporation of water on the skin in a manner similar to sweating. One of the more recent innovations in cooling is the use of a convective cooling blanket. This system blows cool air by the client to increase convective heat loss. This system is very similar to mechanisms of heat loss. Remember, however, that cooling systems that blow air by a client who has a wound infection may promote movement of infectious agents into the air.

Action Alert!
The decrease in skin blood flow caused by cooling measures increases vascular resistance and may increase the work of the heart. The decreased skin blood flow may also lead to skin breakdown, particularly if the cooling blanket is placed under the client.

Another consequence of using physical cooling is shivering. Because physical cooling does not affect the set-point, the thermoregulatory response to cooling will be to maintain the current body temperature. This increase in metabolic rate may add stress to the client who is already physiologically compromised.

Providing Nutrition and Fluids

Anorexia (loss of appetite) is often associated with fever. In an otherwise healthy person, not eating for a short time will not change the course of the illness or result in nutritional deficits. If the person is compromised, however, maintaining nutrition is important. Assess the likelihood of the person tolerating food. Decreased bowel sounds, a distended abdomen, or nausea would suggest the person may not tolerate eating. As soon as the person is able, provide a well-balanced diet that includes proteins, minerals, and vitamins. Carbohydrates may be the food of choice because they are easily digested and provide energy.

Action Alert!
Maintaining fluid volume is essential for maintaining the balance between heat loss and heat gain. Inadequate circulating blood volume impairs an individual's ability to eliminate heat due to less blood transferring heat to the skin.

Dehydration often contributes to the development of hyperthermia. Clients with fever often lose fluid due to sweating that occurs when the set-point decreases. They sweat to decrease body temperature to attain this lower set-point. Fluid replacement should take these losses into consideration.

Providing Comfort and Rest

Treatment of fever often affects client comfort. If fever is treated with antipyretics on a regular schedule, the client will avoid the cycle of chills and defervescence. Treatment with antipyretics on a less frequent schedule leads to defervescence when the antipyretics are administered and chills when the effects of antipyretics end. This may be more uncomfortable than not being treated for fever at all.

Interventions to Manage Hyperthermia

The treatment of hyperthermia is considerably different than treatment of fever because hyperthermia is not a rise in set-point but an alteration in thermoregulation. Appropriate treatment of hyperthermia depends on the etiology, but the goal of therapy in most cases is to promote heat loss. Therefore, physical cooling measures that promote heat loss are the standard treatment.

Methods of physical cooling for individuals with hyperthermia include warm air spray, cooling blankets, ice packs, iced gastric lavage, and convective cooling blankets. Warm air spray is an effective means for heat loss because the water sprayed on the client promotes heat loss by evaporation, and the blowing of the air on the client promotes convective heat loss. Although the person is hyperthermic, the warmth of the spray prevents vasoconstriction of the skin, which would impair heat loss. Warm air spray systems can be seen on the sidelines of football games in warm, humid environments. They are being used in an attempt to prevent hyperthermia in football players.

Cooling blankets increase the gradient between core and shell temperature by cooling the skin temperature. However, cold applied to the skin also causes vasoconstriction of the vessels in the skin, decreasing heat loss (Henker, 1993). Methods that avoid cooling the skin, such as iced saline gastric lavage, do not directly stimulate vasoconstriction in the skin and may be more effective at decreasing body temperature.

Managing Malignant Hyperthermia

Malignant hyperthermia is an autosomal dominant genetic disorder that affects calcium levels within the skeletal muscle. Treatment of malignant hyperthermia due to general anesthesia focuses on decreasing heat production.

Action Alert!
Increased calcium levels in the skeletal muscle in response to general anesthetic agents such as halothane lead to skeletal muscle hyperactivity. The skeletal muscle hyperactivity increases body temperature to life-threatening levels.

Treatment of malignant hyperthermia is based on decreasing heat production by the skeletal muscle. The medication that is most effective in treating malignant hyperthermia is dantrolene. Dantrolene decreases the calcium available for excitation in the skeletal muscle cells. Physical cooling measures are also applied to promote heat loss and decrease body temperature.

Managing Neuroleptic Malignant Syndrome

Treatment of neuroleptic malignant syndrome is similar to that for malignant hyperthermia, although the underlying mechanisms causing neuroleptic malignant syndrome are not well understood. Treatment of neuroleptic malignant syndrome includes administration of dantrolene, physical cooling, and hydration. Dehydration is thought to be a contributing factor because many neuroleptic medications inhibit thirst. Decreased fluid volume will impair the person's ability to lose heat because less heat can be transferred to the skin through the blood.

Interventions to Manage Hypothermia

Treatment of hypothermia varies according to the level of body temperature. Passive warming methods—such as blankets and increased ambient temperature—will be used to decrease heat loss if the hypothermia is mild. Active warming methods may be incorporated in more severe cases.

Peripheral methods of active warming, such as warm blankets and radiant warmers, will have more of an effect on the shell of the person. Central methods of warming are more invasive and include administration of warmed intravenous fluid. If hypothermia is severe, active methods such as extracorporeal warming of blood by means of a device similar to a cardiac bypass machine may be utilized to warm the client. Other invasive methods of warming include instillation of warm fluid into the peritoneum.

Action Alert!
One of the consequences that may occur during peripheral rewarming is a decrease in body temperature termed afterdrop. As warming of the skin increases skin blood flow, the blood becomes cooler than usual because of the coldness of the peripheral tissues. Blood returning to the core will then decrease core temperature (Giesbrecht & Bristow, 1997; Henker, 1993). Therefore, during attempts to warm a client peripherally, one of the consequences may be an even lower core temperature.

Hypothermia not only occurs in outlying settings, but may also occur in hospitalized clients after surgery.

EVALUATION

To evaluate the care provided for a client with an altered body temperature, ask yourself the following four questions. First, was the client's comfort maintained? Second, was his body temperature controlled in a timely manner? Third, does he have any residual effects? Fourth, are appropriate measures in place to prevent future occurrences?

Fever is uncomfortable and commonly produces a feeling of drowsiness. Appropriate care includes relieving the discomfort and providing a quiet environment to allow the client to rest. Usually, fever is relatively easy to control. Evaluation data include the client's level of satisfaction with his care. Evaluation of prevention measures includes the effectiveness of teaching the client to avoid infections.

In hyperthermia, evaluation includes assessment for residual effects. If a hypothermia blanket was used, the client's skin should be inspected for damage. The client's neurological status should also be assessed to determine that no neurological damage has occurred.

The hypothermic client should be assessed for comfort during the course of treatment. In severe hypothermic states, skin damage and sloughing of tissue can occur. Inspect the skin carefully, especially the toes, finger, and earlobes, for damage from frostbite.

KEY PRINCIPLES

- Fever is a regulated rise in temperature mediated by a rise in temperature set-point.
- Fever is a host defense response and may have a beneficial effect; therefore, treatment of fever is controversial.
- The etiology of a fever can be a wide variety of processes, including infection, inflammation, autoimmune disease, vascular disease, neoplasia, and drug reaction.
- A chill may be the first sign of a fever; the temperature rises after the onset of the chill.
- Hyperthermia is a nonregulated rise in body temperature that occurs when a person is unable to lose sufficient heat or is generating more heat than can be lost.
- Hypothermia is often associated with clinical conditions or factors that predispose clients to a decrease in core body temperature, such as severe illness, trauma, immersion, and frostbite.
- Temperature should be monitored frequently enough to detect elevations in temperature.
- Fever is treated with antipyretics to lower the set-point or with physical cooling to increase the temperature difference between the environment and the skin. Although the most common antipyretics

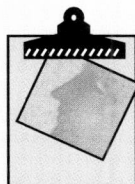

NURSING CARE PLANNING
A CLIENT WITH A WOUND INFECTION AND FEVER

Admission Data

On the 12th postoperative day, Mr. Stephen was visited at home by a friend who is a registered nurse. She took his temperature: 39°C (102.2°F). Further assessment revealed the following about Mr. Stephen: feeling hot for 2 days, with no chills for 24 hours; malaise; lack of appetite; unwilling to drink adequate fluids even though the mucous membranes are dry; lung sounds are clear, blood pressure is 138/84, pulse 130, and respirations 20. The incisions were healing except one suture line that was oozing a foul-smelling butter-yellow discharge that was enough to saturate a 2 × 4 in about 2 hours.

The nurse suggested to the family that the physician should be notified. The family asked the nurse to call the physician and report her observations.

Following the report of client status to the physician, the client was transported to the hospital for admission.

Physician's Orders

Admitting diagnosis: wound infection
Vital signs every 4 hours
Acetaminophen 650 mg PO or rectally every 4 hours, now and prn if temperatures over 39°C (102.2°F)
Culture and sensitivity of wound
IV of 1,000 mL D₅W/1/2NS at 100 mL/hr

Cefoxitin sodium (Mefoxin) 2 gm every 8 hours IV
Dressing change as needed
Fluids of choice at 240 mL/hr while awake
Diet as tolerated
Up ad lib
Laxative of choice

Nursing Assessment

Color pale, diaphoretic, vital signs: BP 136/82, T 39°C (102.2°F), P 126, R 20. Reports feeling weak and tired. Incision draining thick, yellow, foul-smelling drainage, edges are red and not approximated distally for about 1 inch. Mucous membranes dry, lips cracked, skin flushed and warm to touch. Sleeping, easily aroused.

NURSING CARE PLAN

Nursing Diagnosis	Expected Outcomes	Interventions	Evaluation (After 24 Hours of Care)
Fever related to postoperative wound infection.	Temperature will return to client's normal range.	Provide comfort without heavy linens/blankets.	Temperature ranges from 37.5°C (99.5°F) to 38°C (100.4°F). Continue interventions.
		Offer fluids every hour: 240 mL while awake.	
		Keep room cool.	
		Give medications as needed.	
		Monitor temperature status.	

Critical Thinking Questions

1. What factors related to aging might be contributing to the client's impaired immune status?
2. What differences in treatment would there be if the client were a 3-year-old child?
3. What part of the ordered treatment could be carried out in the home?

(aspirin and acetaminophen) are relatively safe medications, serious side effects can occur in high-risk clients.

• When a client has a fever, management should include nutrition, fluid and electrolytes, and physical comfort measures.

BIBLIOGRAPHY

Bernardo, L., Henker, R., Bove, M., & Sereika, S. (1997). The effect of administered crystalloid fluid temperature on aural temperature in moderately and severely injured children. *Journal of Emergency Nursing, 23*(2), 105–111.

*Bor, D.H., Makadon, H.J., Friedland, G., Dasse, P., Komaroff, A.L., & Aronon, M.D. (1988). Fever in hospitalized medical clients: Characteristics and significance. *American Journal of Medicine, 3,* 119–125.

Boulant, J.A., Chow, A.R., & Griffin, J.D. (1997). Determinants of hypothalamic neuronal thermosensitivity. *Annals of New York Academy of Sciences, 813,* 133–138.

*Bryant, J.K., & Strand, C.L. (1987). Reliability of blood cultures collected from intravascular catheter versus venipuncture. *American Journal of Clinical Pathology, 88,* 113–116.

*Cabanac, M., & Massonnet, B. (1974). Temperature regulation during fever: Change of set point or change of gain? *Journal of Physiology, 238,* 561–568.

*Caruso, C.C., Hadley, B.J., Shukla, R., Frame, P., & Khoury, J. (1992). Cooling effects and comfort of four cooling blanket temperatures in humans with fever. *Nursing Research, 41*(2), 68–72.

*Cooper, K.E., Cranston, W.I., & Snell, E.S. (1964). Temperature regulation during fever in man. *Clinical Science, 27,* 345–356.

Cunha, B.A. (1996). The clinical significance of fever patterns. *Infectious Disease Clinics of North America, 10*(1), 33–44.

*Danzl, D.F., Pozos, R.S., Auerbach, P.S., Glazer, S., Goetz, W., Johnson, E., Jui, J., Lilja, P., Marx, J.A., Miller, J., Mills, W., Nowak, R., Shields, R., Vicario, S., Wayne, M. (1987). Multicenter hypothermia survey. *Annals of Emergency Medicine, 16*(9), 1042.

Donowitz, G.R. (1996). Fever in the compromised host. *Infectious Disease Clinics of North America, 10*(1), 129–148.

Elfant, A.B., Levine, S.M., Peikin, S.R., Cencora, B., Mendez, L., Pello, J.J., Atabek, U.M., Alexander, J.B., Spence, R.K., & Cambishion, R.C. (1995). Bioavailability of medication delivered via nasogastric tube is decreased in the immediate postoperative period. *American Journal of Surgery, 169,* 430–432.

Erickson, R.S., Meyer, L.T., & Moser Woo, T. (1996). Accuracy of chemical dot thermometers in critically ill adults and young children. *Image, 28*(1), 23–28.

Giesbrecht, G.G., & Bristow, G.K. (1997). Recent advances in hypothermia research. *Annals of New York Academy of Science, 813,* 663–675.

Gilman, A., Rall, T. W., Nies, A. S., & Taylor, P. (1990). *The Pharmacological Basis of Therapeutics.* New York: McGraw-Hill.

*Gleckman, R., & Hibert, D. (1982). Afebrile bacteremia: A phenomenon in geriatric clients. *Journal of the American Medical Association, 248*(12), 1478–1481.

*Goodman, E.L. & Knochel, J.P. (1991). Heat stroke and other forms of hyperthermia. In P. Mackowiak (Ed.), *Fever basic mechanisms and management* (pp. 267–287). New York: Raven Press.

*Granberg, P. (1991a). Alcohol and cold. *Arctic Medical Research, 50*(Suppl. 6), 43–47.

*Granberg, P. (1991b). Human physiology under cold exposure. *Arctic Medical Research, 50*(Suppl. 6), 23–27.

Grossman, D., Keen, M.F., Singer, M., & Asher, M. (1995). Current nursing practices in fever management. *Journal of MedSurg Nursing, 4*(3), 193–198.

Hales, J.R.S. (1997). Hyperthermia and heat illness: Pathophysiological implications for avoidance and treatment. *Annals of New York Academy of Science, 813,* 534–544.

*Hart, B.L. (1988). Biological basis of the behavior of sick animals. *Neuroscience and Biobehavioral Reviews, 12,* 123–137.

*Henker, R.A. (1993). Human responses to an alternating versus a continuous pattern of total body cooling. *Unpublished Dissertation.*

*Henker, R., & Coyne, C. (1995). Comparison of peripheral temperature measurements with core temperature. *AACN Clinical Issues, 6*(1), 21–30.

*Henker, R., Kramer, D., & Rogers, S. (1997). Fever. *AACN Clinical Issues, 8*(3), 351–367

*Hensel, H. (1981). *Thermoreception and temperature regulation.* London: Academic Press.

*Hooper, J.F., Herren, C.K., & Goldwasser, H. (1989). Neuroleptic malignant syndrome: Recognizing an unrecognized killer. *Journal of Psychosocial Nursing, 27*(7), 13–15.

*Horvath, S.M., Spurr, G.B., Hutt, B.K., & Hamilton, L.H. (1956). Metabolic cost of shivering. *Journal of Applied Physiology, 8*(6), 595–602.

*Jolly, B.T., & Ghezzi, K.T. (1992). Accidental hypothermia. *Emergency Medicine Clinics of North America, 10*(2), 311–327.

*Khan, F., Spence, V.A., & Belch, J.J.F. (1992). Cutaneous vascular responses and thermoregulation in relation to age. *Clinical Science, 82,* 521–528.

Khogali, M. (1997). Heat illness alert program. *Annals New York Academy of Science, 813,* 526–533.

*Kluger, M. J. (1986). Is fever beneficial? *Yale Journal of Biology and Medicine, 59,* 89–95.

Krochel J.P. (1989). Heat stroke and related heat stress disorders. *Dis Mon 35*(5), 301–377.

*Krueger, J.M., Walter, J., Dinarello, C.A., Wolff, S.M., & Chedid, L. (1984). Sleep-promoting effects of endogenous pyrogen (interleukin-1). *American Journal of Physiology, 246,* R994–999.

McGowan, J.E. Jr., Rose, R.C., Jacobs, N.F., Schaberg, D.R., & Haley, R.W. (1987). Fever in hospitalized patients: With special reference to the medical service. *American Journal of Medicine, 82*(3), 580–586.

*Mravinac, C., Dracup, K., & Clochesy, J. (1989). Urinary bladder and rectal temperature monitoring during clinical hypothermia. *Nursing Research, 38*(2), 73–76.

North American Nursing Diagnosis Association (1999). *NANDA nursing diagnoses: Definitions and classification 1999–2000.* Philadelphia: Author.

*Pugh, C.E., Corbett, J.L., & Johnson, R.H. (1967). Rectal temperatures, weight losses, and sweat rates in marathon running. *Journal of Applied Physiology, 23*(3), 347–352.

Sanford, M.M. (1997). Rewarming cardiac surgical clients: warm water vs. warm air. *American Journal of Critical Care, 6*(1), 39–45.

Sarwari, A.R., & Mackowiak, P.A. (1996). The pharmacologic consequences of fever. *Infectious Disease Clinics of North America, 10*(1), 21–32.

*Steele, R.W., Tanaka, P.T., Lara, T.P., & Bass, J.W. (1970). Evaluation of sponging and/or oral antipyretic therapy to reduce fever. *Journal of Pediatrics, 77*(5), 824–829.

Vaughn, L.K., Veale, W.L., & Cooper, K.E. (1980). Antipyresis: Its effect on mortality rate of bacterially infected rabbits. *Brain Research Bulletin, 5*(1), 69–73.

Wlody, G.S. (1991). Malignant hyperthermia. *Critical Care Nursing Clinics of North America, 3*(1), 129–134.

*Asterisk indicates a classic or definitive work on this subject.

Elimination Pattern

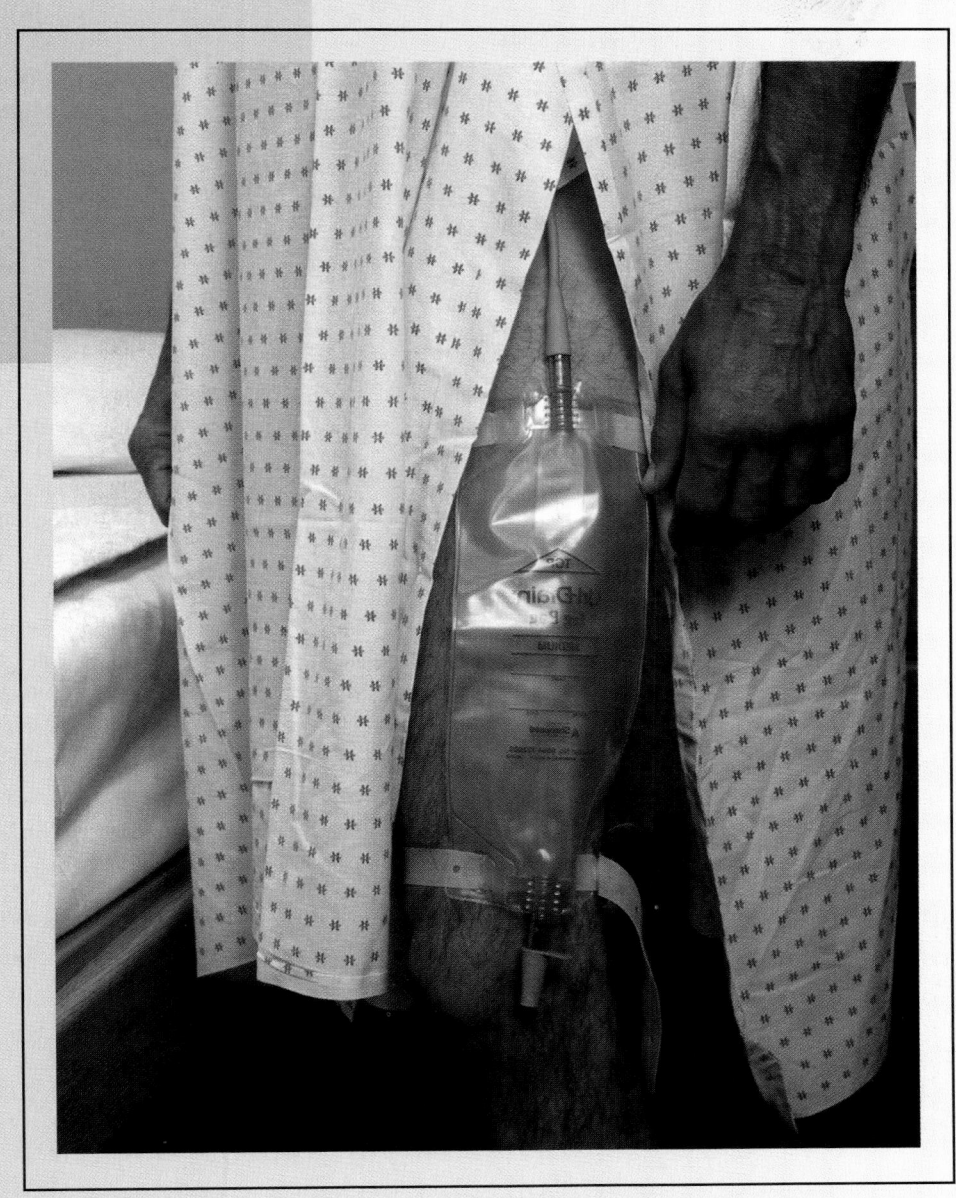

34

Bowel Elimination

Jeanette Marie Daly

Key Terms

bowel incontinence	guaiac test
cathartic	ileostomy
colostomy	laxative
constipation	occult blood
diarrhea	ostomy
fecal impaction	paralytic ileus
feces	peristalsis
flatus	steatorrhea
flatulence	stoma

LEARNING OBJECTIVES

After studying this chapter, you should be able to:

1. Describe the structure and function of the lower gastrointestinal tract.

2. Discuss problems of bowel elimination, including constipation, diarrhea, and bowel incontinence.

3. Explain the effect on bowel elimination of the client's diet and exercise, personal habits, cultural background, age, and physiological and psychosocial factors.

4. Assess the client for manifestations of and responses to problems of bowel elimination.

5. Distinguish among the variety of nursing diagnoses for problems of bowel elimination.

6. Plan for goal-directed interventions to prevent or correct problems of bowel elimination.

7. Evaluate the outcomes that describe progress toward the goals of bowel elimination.

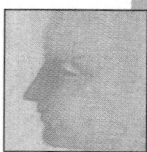

Ninety-two-year-old John Daly lives in a private room in a long-term care facility. He lived alone in his apartment in independent living as long as he could, but because of bone cancer and declining functional abilities, he moved to the long-term care facility. Dr. Daly is a retired neurosurgeon. He knows the consequences of immobility and decreased dietary intake and the side effects of pain medications. He called the nurse to report lower abdominal pain and difficulty having a bowel movement that morning. He reported that he had a small bowel movement the day before, but it was not his usual pattern. Questioning the client further, the nurse ascertained that Dr. Daly's usual pattern of elimination was daily after intake of a high-fiber breakfast. When his routine was regular, the stool was usually firm and soft. The nurse considers the diagnosis of *Constipation*.

LOWER GASTROINTESTINAL **NURSING DIAGNOSES**

Constipation: A decrease in a person's normal frequency of defecation accompanied by difficult or incomplete passage of stool and/or passage of excessively hard, dry stool.

Perceived constipation: The state in which an individual makes a self-diagnosis of constipation and ensures a daily bowel movement through abuse of laxatives, enemas, and suppositories.

Diarrhea: Passage of loose, unformed stool.

Bowel incontinence: A change in normal bowel habits characterized by involuntary passage of stool.

Risk for constipation: At risk for a decrease in a person's normal frequency of defecation accompanied by difficult or incomplete passage of stool and/or passage of excessively hard, dry stool.

From North American Nursing Diagnosis Association. (1999). Nursing diagnoses: Definitions and classification 1999–2000. Philadelphia: Author.

CONCEPTS OF BOWEL ELIMINATION

As a nurse, your role in helping a client with bowel elimination involves both independent and dependent actions. You may be responsible for assessing the client's bowel status, helping him maintain a normal bowel pattern, collecting stool specimens, performing diagnostic tests, and intervening in collaboration with the physician to meet the client's bowel elimination needs.

A number of bowel elimination needs can be met through independent nursing measures that do not require a physician's order. The nurse can initiate them after appropriate assessment and application of relevant scientific principles. Nursing diagnoses relevant to the lower gastrointestinal (GI) system that have been approved by the North American Nursing Diagnosis Association (NANDA) include *Constipation, Perceived constipation, Diarrhea, Bowel incontinence,* and *Risk for constipation.*

Structure and Function of the Lower Gastrointestinal Tract

To understand and successfully treat bowel elimination problems, you will need to understand the structure and function of the GI tract. Naturally, a change in any aspect of the GI tract can affect a client's elimination process.

Organs of Bowel Elimination

The GI tract, also called alimentary canal, is a hollow, muscular tube that extends from the mouth to the anus (Fig. 34–1). Food is broken down in the stomach into a semiliquid mass called chyme, which is more easily absorbed than solid food. Chyme leaves the stomach and enters the small intestine, which has three sections: duodenum, jejunum, and ileum. In the

ileum, chyme mixes with digestive enzymes to prepare the nutrients for absorption. Unabsorbed chyme enters the large intestine through the ileocecal valve in a semiliquid state. The large intestine, or colon, begins at the ileocecal valve and is the primary organ of bowel elimination. The four segments of the colon are the ascending, the transverse, the descending, and the sigmoid portions (Fig. 34–2).

Formation of Feces

The colon absorbs water, sodium, and chloride while passing waste materials out of the body. These processes require a number of ancillary organs and anatomic structures, chemical substances, and physiological processes. As digested, unabsorbed food travels through the colon, it changes from a liquid to a solid as the colon absorbs water from it.

Feces refers to body waste discharged from the intestine. This waste is also called stool, excreta, or excrement. It moves through the large intestine propelled by peristalsis and segmental contractions (Fig. 34–3). **Peristalsis** refers to the rhythmic smooth muscle contractions of the intestinal wall that propel the intestinal contents forward. Although the force may propel intestinal contents in either direction, movement in the GI tract is usually toward the anus. In segmental contractions, circular muscles in a segment of the colon mix the contents of the colon.

In addition to constant peristalsis, periods of mass peristalsis occur two or three times a day, usually following meals and facilitated by the gastrocolic reflex. The gastrocolic reflex occurs when the bolus of food enters the stomach and stimulates peristalsis throughout the entire GI tract. The duodenocolic reflex acts in a similar but less forceful manner. The gastrocolic and duodenocolic reflexes are strongest when a person eats following a period of fasting—at breakfast after a night's sleep, for instance.

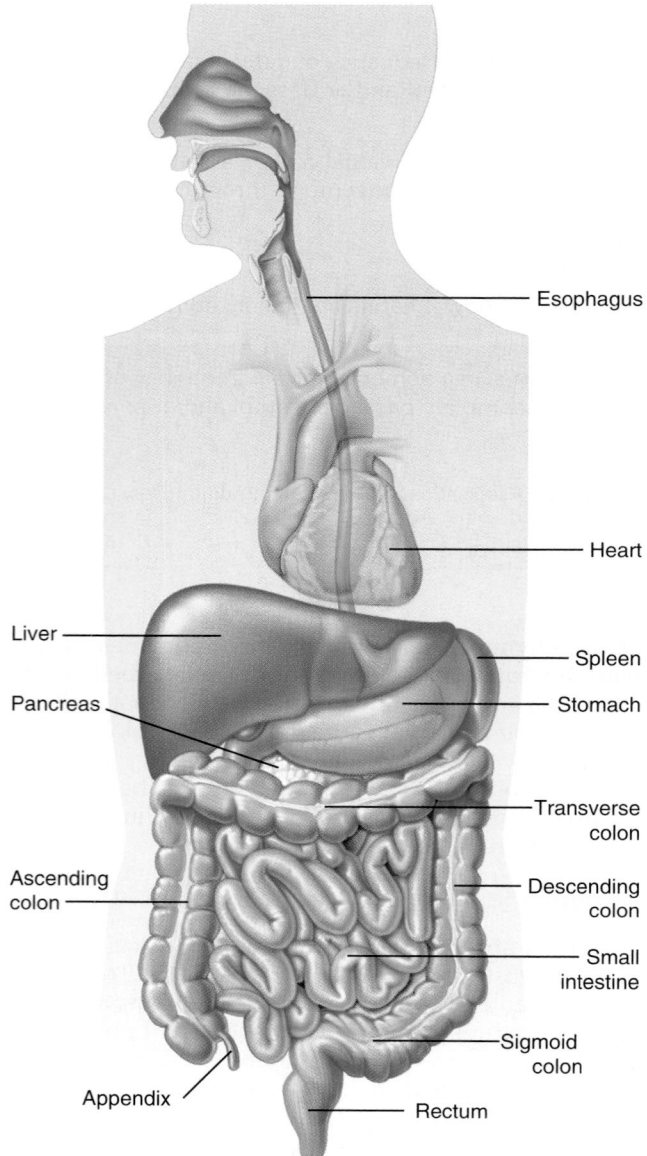

Figure 34–1. Organs of the gastrointestinal tract. (The heart is shown for reference.)

Labels on figure:
- Esophagus
- Heart
- Liver
- Spleen
- Pancreas
- Stomach
- Transverse colon
- Ascending colon
- Descending colon
- Small intestine
- Sigmoid colon
- Appendix
- Rectum

Eventually, fecal material enters the sigmoid colon, where it stays until it is eliminated from the body. The time required for food to move through the entire GI tract, called transit time, is affected by such factors as rate of motility, amount of residue, and the presence or absence of irritating substances in the colon. However, it usually takes from 8 to 15 hours for the contents to travel from the stomach to the sigmoid colon.

Another substance that the GI tract removes is **flatus,** which is the gas normally found in the GI tract and passed through the anus. Flatus is formed partly from the fermentation processes in the bowel and partly from air taken in through the mouth.

Defecation

To complete passage from the body, feces and flatus move through the rectum, anal canal, and anus. This process is referred to as defecation, or "having a bowel movement," and is under both voluntary and involuntary control. Defecation is initiated by reflexes mediated by local enteric nerves and by the parasympathetic nerve center in the sacral segments of the spinal cord.

The rectum usually remains empty until just before and during defecation. When the fecal mass or flatus moves from the sigmoid colon into the rectum, the defecation reflex begins. Feces enter the rectum either from an involuntary mass propulsive movement in the colon or from a voluntary increase in intra-abdominal pressure caused by contraction of the abdominal muscles and forced expiration with a closed glottis. This straining or bearing-down action is called *Valsalva's maneuver.* It forces the diaphragm downward, thus increasing pressure. Rectal distention then causes increased intrarectal pressure and the urge to evacuate the bowel. Voluntarily forcing feces into the rectum to stimulate the defecation reflex is less efficient than the involuntary mass propulsive movement.

The anal canal has two sphincters, as shown earlier in Figure 34–2. The internal sphincter is made up of smooth muscle and is innervated through the autonomic nervous system. Distension of the rectum causes this sphincter to relax and allow passage of the feces. The external anal sphincter consists of striated muscle and is under voluntary control in most healthy people. When the internal sphincter is being stimulated to relax by descending feces, the external sphincter is stimulated as well. However, the person can voluntarily constrict the external sphincter to delay defecation. In that case, stool remains in the rectum until the defecation reflex is again stimulated.

Problems of Bowel Elimination

Bowel elimination is a basic human need susceptible to a number of problems. Common bowel elimination problems include constipation, fecal impaction, diarrhea, bowel incontinence, and flatulence.

Constipation

Constipation is a condition in which feces are abnormally hard and dry and evacuation is abnormally infrequent. Discomfort created by constipation typically interferes with the client's daily activities and sense of well-being. The term constipation is used in various ways to include any or all of the following: character of stool, frequency of defecation, time required for passage of the stool through the intestinal tract (intestinal transit time), and difficulty expelling rectal contents through the anal sphincter.

Based on the popularity of over-the-counter aids for elimination, we know that constipation is a com-

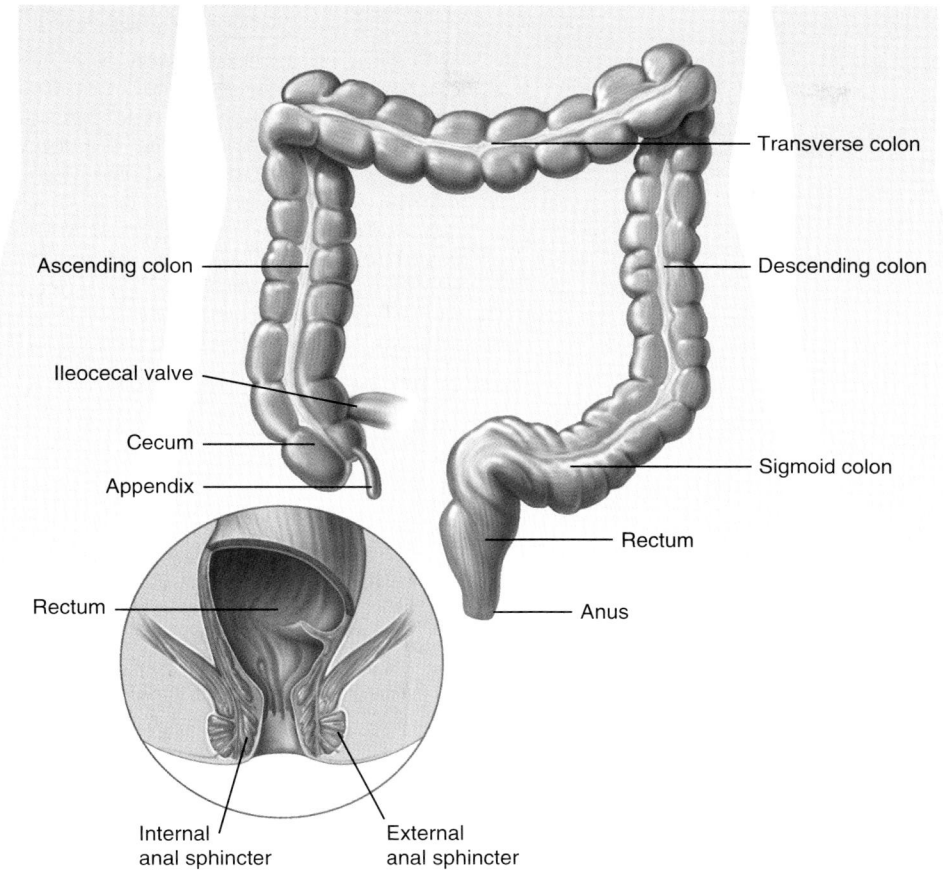

Figure 34–2. The four segments of the large intestine: ascending, transverse, descending, and sigmoid. The inset shows the detailed anatomy of the rectum.

mon worry. In fact, many people claim to be constipated if they have not had a bowel movement for a day or so.

Constipation is a major complaint among elderly people; about 30% use laxatives at least once a week.

Besides being uncomfortable, constipation can be hazardous. The hazard results from the Valsalva maneuver employed by the constipated person in an effort to pass feces. This action can cause angina pectoris (chest pain) or even cardiac arrest if the person has underlying cardiac disease. It may also be detrimental to a person with head injuries (by increasing intracranial pressure), respiratory disease (by increasing intrathoracic pressure), or thromboembolic disorders (by causing thrombi to dislodge). Exhaling through the mouth during straining reduces the chance of increasing intrathoracic pressure. The best precaution, however, is to avoid constipation.

Straining to pass a stool is detrimental in other ways. Over time, it may contribute to the development of hemorrhoids. If the person has had recent bowel surgery, straining might disrupt the suture line. As a precaution, most clients are given enemas preoperatively to eliminate the need for a bowel movement for several days after surgery.

What evidence do you see in this description to suggest that *Constipation* is the correct diagnosis for Dr. Daly?

Fecal Impaction

A **fecal impaction** is a collection of putty-like or hardened feces in the rectum or sigmoid colon that prevents the passage of a normal stool and becomes more and more hardened as the colon continues to absorb water from it. As the fecal mass moves down from the sigmoid colon, additional fecal material may be added to it. Eventually, the mass becomes so hard and large that it cannot pass through the anal canal.

Diarrhea

Diarrhea is the rapid movement of fecal matter through the intestine, resulting in poor absorption of water, nutrients, and electrolytes and producing abnormally frequent evacuation of watery stools. As with constipation, some people consider the frequency of defecation as part of the definition, but stool consistency is the primary component.

In general, diarrhea indicates increased intestinal motility, which causes gastrointestinal (GI) contents to

Mass peristalsis

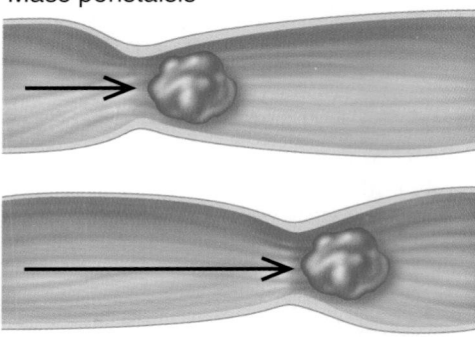

Segmental contractions

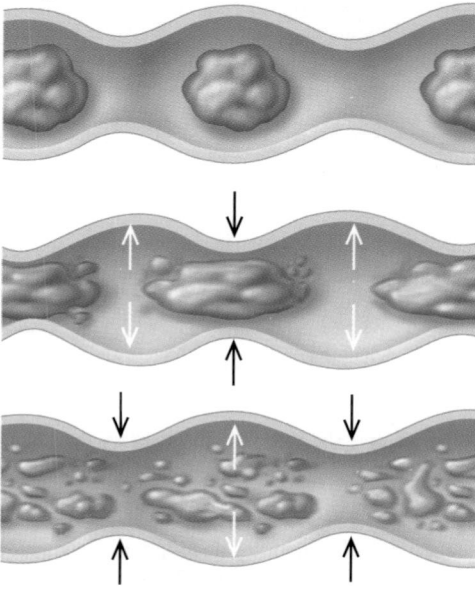

Figure 34–3. Movement of feces through the large intestine by mass peristalsis and segmental contractions.

move rapidly through the tract. Because of the rapid transit time, normal amounts of water are not removed from the feces. In addition, irritation of the mucosal walls may stimulate increased secretions, which add moisture to the fecal mass. Therefore, when the feces reach the rectum and anus, they are still liquid.

Bowel Incontinence

Bowel incontinence is the inability to voluntarily control the passage of feces and gas. Bowel evacuation usually occurs voluntarily in response to defecation reflex stimulation. Lack of control is accepted during infancy and toddlerhood. However, following toilet training, continence is the norm and any deviation meets with both personal and social disapproval. Incontinence causes great embarrassment for the person, whose life is often arranged to conceal the problem from other people.

Flatulence

A certain amount of gas occurs normally in the GI tract—usually about 150 mL. Some of it is swallowed, some of it is produced by fermentation in the intestine, and some of it comes from diffusion of gases from the bloodstream. **Flatulence** refers to the presence of abnormal amounts of gas in the GI tract, causing abdominal distention and discomfort. Belching is the expulsion of gas from the upper GI tract and has its origin as swallowed air. Flatulence is expelled from the lower GI tract. Because it may be painful, noisy, and malodorous, flatulence can be distressing to the client.

FACTORS AFFECTING BOWEL ELIMINATION

The bowel elimination process can be affected by many factors, such as a person's lifestyle, culture, and development. Physiological and psychological factors can influence the bowel elimination process as well.

As you read about the factors affecting bowel elimination, can you relate the information to Dr. Daly? What factors may have influenced his bowel elimination problem?

Lifestyle Factors

The client's lifestyle affects bowel elimination through personal habits surrounding elimination, fluid intake, diet, and exercise. Healthy bowel function is maintained through regular patterns of elimination.

Personal Habits

Personal habits of bowel elimination are important to health. As discussed later, the bowel can be trained to evacuate at a certain time. If this pattern is followed, and all other variables remain constant, the bowel continues to empty regularly. On the other hand, if a person continually ignores the urge to defecate, no rhythmic pattern is established. Travel, which usually disrupts a person's normal schedule, often leads to constipation and sometimes to diarrhea.

Along with timing, many people have other established habits related to bowel elimination, such as drinking warm or cold water, eating prunes, having a cup of coffee, or reading. Continuing these activities may trigger conscious mental stimulation of the defecation reflex.

Nutrition and Fluids

Diet strongly influences bowel habits. Fiber, or indigestible dietary residue, provides bulk in fecal material. Bulk assists peristalsis and increases stimulation of the defecation reflex. A low-fiber, high-carbohydrate diet tends to diminish the reflex. Reduction of overall intake also directly reduces the amount of bulk present. Gas-producing foods may stimulate peristalsis by distending the intestinal walls.

How the GI tract reacts to a particular food depends on the individual (Box 34–1). For instance, chocolate has no effect on many people, but causes constipation in some and diarrhea in others. Likewise, milk and milk products constipate some people and cause diarrhea in others. Various foods also can adversely affect defecation patterns and act as irritants. Irritants, such as spicy foods, within the GI tract usually stimulate peristalsis by local reflex stimulation.

The amount of water in the fecal mass affects stool consistency. The less the water content, the harder the mass, and the more difficult it is to pass the mass through the anus. If the person is fluid depleted, more fluid is absorbed from the GI tract to maintain adequate hydration. Thus, dehydration can result in constipation.

Exercise

Muscle tone affects not only the activity of the intestinal musculature itself, but also the ability of the supporting skeletal muscles to aid the process of defecation. Weak or atrophied muscles in the abdomen or pelvic floor are ineffective in increasing intra-abdominal pressure or assisting the anus to control defecation. This inadequate musculature may result from lack of exercise, immobility, neurological impairment, or multiple pregnancies.

Cultural Factors

Cultural teachings significantly influence a person's defecation habits. In Western society, we are taught strict rules about when and under what conditions defecation can take place. Failure to follow these rules results in social censure and even isolation. Defecation is a private matter and people go to great lengths to ensure this privacy. Many people avoid any discussion of bowel activity. Therefore, some people feel highly anxious when forced to seek out a health professional regarding problems with bowel elimination. Even more dangerous, some people with such problems avoid seeking professional help altogether because they are too embarrassed. Although people in some cultures tend to be very bowel conscious, not all

---

BOX 34–1

FOODS THAT ALTER GASTROINTESTINAL FUNCTION

Foods That May Cause Gas

- Beans.
- Beer.
- Cabbage family vegetables.
- Carbonated beverages.
- Cucumbers.
- Dairy products.
- Onions.
- Radishes.

Foods That Cause Odor

- Asparagus (urinary).
- Beans.
- Cabbage family.
- Cheese.
- Eggs.
- Fish.
- Garlic.
- Onions.

Foods That Thicken Stool

- Applesauce.
- Bananas.
- Bread.
- Cheese.
- High-fiber foods.
- Marshmallows.
- Pasta.

- Peanut butter.
- Rice.
- Tapioca.

Foods That Loosen Stool

- Alcohol.
- Beans.
- Beer.
- Chocolate.
- Coffee.
- Fried foods.
- Prune or grape juice.
- Raw fruits and vegetables.
- Spicy foods.
- Spinach.

Foods That May Block an Ileostomy

- Celery.
- Coconut.
- Coleslaw.
- Mushrooms.
- Corn.
- Nuts.
- Popcorn.
- Raisins.
- Raw vegetables and fruits.
- Seeds.
- Stringy meats.

people will be embarrassed or reluctant to discuss bowel habits. Assess the client's lifeways for information pertinent to bowel elimination, as suggested in the Cross-Cultural Care chart.

Developmental Factors

Age plays a role in establishing bowel patterns. Before a child acquires bowel control through toilet training, defecation occurs whenever stool stimulates the rectum. In infancy, the stomach is small and secretes less digestive enzymes. Rapid peristalsis propels food quickly through the gastrointestinal (GI) system, and, because the neuromuscular system is not developed, the infant cannot control defecation.

Bowel elimination usually is not a problem in the adolescent unless the person has a health problem. However, adolescents can experience changes in bowel habits associated with growth and irregular patterns of eating and sleeping. During adolescence,

the large intestine grows rapidly. At the same time, adolescents tend to eat more. Adolescent eating habits vary from very good to poor, with the person's self-concept influencing the intake.

Among elderly people, vulnerability to GI disturbances rises. Cancer occurs more frequently, and motor and neurological disturbances are more prevalent. In addition, diverticulosis (an outpouching in the intestinal wall) occurs almost exclusively after age 40.

Nutritional intake commonly changes in the elderly as well. Inadequate dentition impairs mastication, allowing food to enter the GI tract not adequately chewed. Further, the amount of digestive enzymes in saliva and gastric acids in the stomach declines, reducing the ability to break down foods. Along with upper-GI changes, the lower GI tract develops deficiencies in proteins, vitamins, and minerals. A muscular decline occurs as well, and the internal and external sphincters may not be controlled normally. In addition, slowing of nerve impulses to the rectum may

---

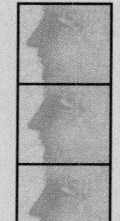

CROSS-CULTURAL CARE
CARING FOR A RURAL CLIENT OF ENGLISH DESCENT

As many rural Americans did, Dr. Daly lived on a farm when he was a boy. He recounts memories of tending a garden, keeping beehives, and raising chickens, cows, pigs, ducks, and other livestock. All of the family's meals were cooked at home, and Dr. Daly's mother commonly used home remedies and medications made from plants to treat illness and injuries. Laxatives were not a choice for constipation problems, but instead a high-fiber diet was provided.

Dr. Daly's family believed in living from the land and using all of its products as fully as possible. Additionally, Dr. Daly may have been exposed to the following traditionally Anglo-Saxon beliefs:

- Strength in individualism and self-reliance.
- Competition and achievement.
- Health is achievable through science.
- Helping others is more likely in times of crisis.
- Better life through technology.

He also may have embraced the following values commonly held by farming families:

- The best things are those that we work for.
- God gave man dominion over the earth and the responsibility to care for the earth.
- "She did not send me to Sunday School but instead went with me."
- A person has a right to own property, a responsibility to work, and an obligation to take care of his property for his own sake and the sake of his children and the community.
- A person should do his best to take care of himself and not be a burden to others.

- It is possible to love wealth too much, but a greater danger is to be careless of it.

See how the following conversation between Dr. Daly and his nurse, Janet, respects his cultural upbringing and educational level.

Janet: [Responding to the call light] Can I do something to help you?

Dr. Daly: I am having a great deal of pain in my lower abdomen, but I am afraid to take any more morphine because I haven't had a bowel movement.

Janet: Why don't you lie down and show me where the pain is located?

Dr. Daly: [Lies down on the bed and indicates left lower abdomen]

Janet: [Palpating his abdomen] Dr. Daly, I can feel a fecal mass here. I think you are badly constipated. What would you like to try?

Critical Thinking Questions

- Would you have handled this situation differently?
- Has the nurse given culturally competent care in this situation?

References

Fish, C. (1995). *In good hands: The keeping of a family farm.* New York: Farrar, Straus & Giroux.
Leininger, M.M. (1991). *Culture care diversity and universality: A theory of nursing.* New York: National League for Nursing Press.

cause some people to be less conscious of the need to defecate.

Physiological Factors

Bowel elimination problems can be caused by such physiological factors as motor and sensory disturbances, intestinal pathologies, pregnancy, medications, surgical procedures, and diagnostic procedures.

Motor and Sensory Disturbances

Motor or sensory disturbances may result from spinal cord injury, head injury, cerebrovascular accident (stroke), neurological disease, or any condition that causes immobility or otherwise interferes with motor/sensory function. Immobility hinders the person's ability to respond to the urge to defecate. For instance, the person who is unable to walk to the bathroom or reach a call bell to summon help may (1) suppress the urge to defecate, which could eventually lead to constipation; or (2) suffer fecal incontinence.

Intestinal Pathologies

Pathological conditions in the intestine itself can alter defecation. For example, bowel obstruction caused by a tumor or adhesion can delay the passage of stool. Inflammatory processes, such as colitis, usually increase motility. Constipation may be secondary to something more serious that should be referred to a physician. Signs and symptoms that may indicate referral are a change in bowel habits and rectal bleeding. Encourage clients to obtain routine screening tests for colon and rectal cancer, as outlined in the Teaching for Wellness chart, as appropriate.

Pregnancy

Pregnancy itself and medications taken during pregnancy can influence a woman's normal bowel elimination pattern. As the fetus grows, pressure may be exerted on the rectum, slowing the passage of feces through the intestine. Exertion for defecation can cause other elimination problems, such as hemorrhoids. Iron and vitamin supplements prescribed for many women during pregnancy are constipating, which can cause additional problems.

Medications

Medications administered for bowel regulation or for other purposes may cause constipation and diarrhea. A drug given to prevent constipation may cause diarrhea, and vice versa. The overuse of laxatives can lead to physiological and psychological dependence on them. Additionally, diarrhea or constipation is a side effect of many medications.

Surgical Procedures

Surgical procedures commonly result in constipation. They do so for several reasons. For one, direct handling of the bowel during the procedure can tempo-

Teaching for WELLNESS

SCREENING FOR COLON CANCER

Goal: To provide the client information about screening for colon cancer.

Rationale: The client is more likely to take preventive action if given information about recommendations for screening.

Expected Outcome: The client will verbalize information about the recommendations for screening for colon cancer.

Client Instructions

Keep in mind the following risk factors, which can place you at higher risk for colon cancer:

- Age over 50.
- A family history of polyps or colorectal cancer.
- A history of inflammatory bowel disease, such as ulcerative colitis or Crohn's disease.
- Living in an urban area.
- A diet high in fat and low in fiber.

Notify your health care provider if you notice any of the following warning signs of colon cancer:

- Change in bowel habits.
- Rectal bleeding.

Ask your health care provider about the following recommended screening tests:

- Digital rectal examination every year after age 40.
- Guaiac test for occult blood every year after age 50.
- Proctoscopy every 3 to 5 years after age 50, after two annual examinations show no evidence of colon cancer.

rarily stop peristalsis; when the absence of peristalsis persists beyond 3 days, the condition is called **paralytic ileus.** For another, any procedure involving the perineal area, such as rectal or gynecological surgery, can affect defecation patterns through the effects of postoperative edema and discomfort. Operative and postoperative medications can contribute to constipation as well.

Bowel function also can be altered permanently by surgical intervention. Fecal diversion involves channeling intestinal contents out of the body at a site other than the anus. The surgical procedure used to create an opening through the abdominal wall and into the intestine is called an **ostomy** procedure. An **ileostomy** is a surgical procedure involving the creation of an opening between the ileum and the abdominal wall. Water is not reabsorbed until feces reaches the colon, so the feces that leave the ileostomy will be liquid. A **colostomy** is a surgical procedure involving the creation of an opening between the colon and the abdominal wall. Feces from this area of the colon will be semisolid or solid, depending on the segment of the colon that is resected. Each of these surgical procedures establishes a **stoma,** which is the opening between the abdominal wall and intestine through which fecal material passes.

An ileostomy may be performed because of cancer, a congenital defect, or trauma. However, the most frequent reason stems from ulcerative colitis or regional ileitis (Crohn's disease). Because of the placement of the stoma in the small intestine, the flow of fecal material in most cases is constant and cannot be regulated. Surgical techniques do exist in which a continent ileostomy is formed by creating an internal pouch with a nipple valve that can be emptied with a catheter at the person's convenience.

A colostomy may be performed because of trauma, intestinal obstruction, birth defect, or cancer. It may involve the ascending (rarely), transverse, descending, or sigmoid portions of the colon. The farther down the intestine the stoma is placed, the better are the chances of regulating the bowel. Some people develop such reliable bowel control that they wear no fecal collection bag and only a small dressing to protect the stoma from irritation by clothing. However, most people with ostomies wear a collection pouch or bag that is changed periodically (Fig. 34–4).

Psychosocial Factors

The weight of clinical evidence seems to suggest a relationship between bowel elimination patterns and emotions, although it is not clear whether a person's emotional state affects his defecation pattern or vice versa. We know that several disease processes that cause diarrhea, gaseous distension, and ulcer formation have psychological elements.

By slowing all bodily activities, mental depression can contribute to constipation. Indeed, it may be the client's chief complaint. In contrast, agitation and nervousness can cause diarrhea, usually in the form of frequent small stools without a large-volume fluid loss. When a client develops a GI problem, carefully assess whether a psychological concern exists as well.

ASSESSMENT

The need for assessment of bowel elimination problems commonly arises after a client reports a problem.

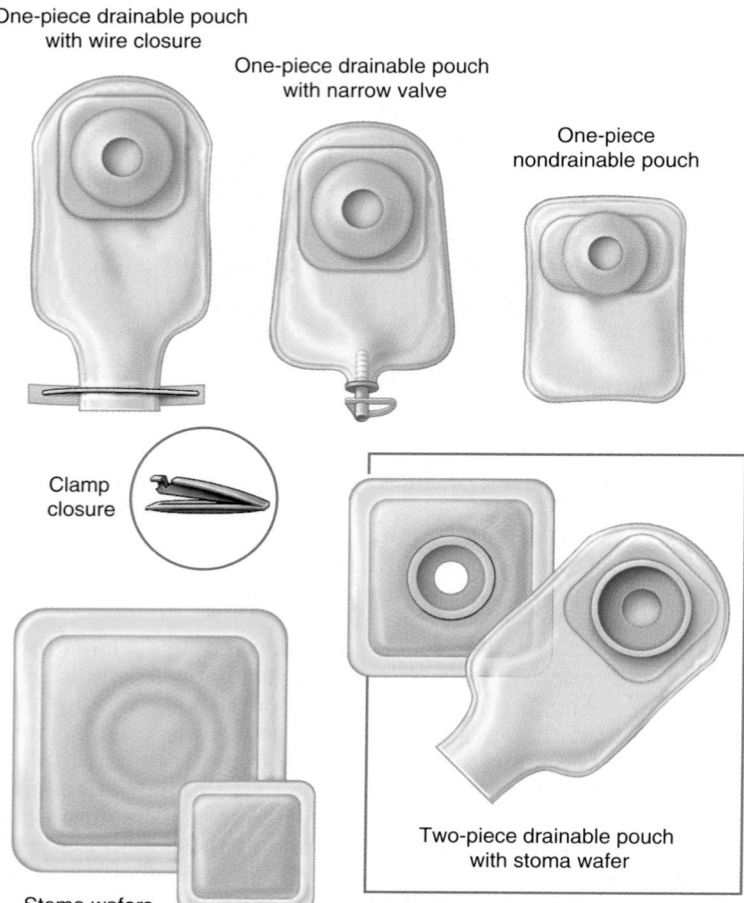

Figure 34–4. Examples of ostomy pouches, closures, and stoma wafers.

However, it should also be a routine part of any health assessment because bowel elimination is frequently disrupted by illness or treatment.

General Assessment of Bowel Elimination

The general assessment of bowel elimination should include a history pertinent to bowel elimination, a physical assessment of the abdomen, observation of feces, and review of diagnostic tests.

Health History

The health history should include questions regarding the client's normal elimination pattern, information about lifestyle (such as exercise and fluid and food intake), and any psychological or physiological alterations pertinent to bowel elimination. The following are pertinent historical questions:

- What is your normal bowel elimination pattern, including time of day and frequency?
- What do your feces look like, including amount, color, consistency, constituents, frequency, odor, and shape.
- What medications do you take?
- How often do you use laxatives or bowel elimination aids?
- Have you noticed any changes in your bowel elimination pattern?
- Has your use of bowel elimination aids changed recently?
- What is your normal dietary intake for a day? Has it changed recently?
- What is your normal fluid intake for a day? Has it changed recently?
- What kind of exercise or physical activity do you get? Has it changed recently?
- Have you had any surgery pertinent to bowel elimination?
- How is your current emotional state? Is it different from your normal?

What questions would you ask Dr. Daly to determine the best course of action to assist with his bowel elimination problem?

Physical Examination

Physical assessment of the bowel system should include inspection, auscultation, percussion, and palpation of the abdomen. It also should include inspection and palpation of the anus. With the client in the supine position, inspect the abdomen for peristalsis, contour, symmetry, and masses. Auscultate the client's bowel sounds, noting their frequency and character. Use percussion to elicit tympany or dullness, which indicate the presence of gas, fluid, and feces in the GI tract. Use palpation to assess for areas of tenderness or masses in the abdomen. Inspect and palpate the anus to assess for lumps, ulcers, inflammation, rashes, or excoriations.

Evaluate the client for abdominal distention and "gas pains." Ask about the duration of any problem, abdominal cramps, dietary and medication intake, and anxiety, stress, or systemic disease that might contribute to the problem.

Diagnostic Tests

In addition to the history and physical examination, several diagnostic tests help locate and identify problems with bowel elimination. They include observation of fecal characteristics and laboratory analysis of feces, x-ray examination of the bowel, and direct endoscopic visualization of the bowel.

Stool Analysis

SPECIMEN COLLECTION

Stool specimens are collected in a sterile or clean bedpan or any functional receptacle, depending on the test. If the client uses a toilet, place a receptacle under the seat. If he collects the specimen at home, the client can drape a piece of plastic wrap over the toilet seat so it droops in the middle to catch the feces. After depositing the specimen, the client then finishes the collection process by bringing the corners and edges of the wrap together and twisting them to form a sealed package.

To perform a test on the specimen, you will probably use a tongue blade to transfer a portion of it to a smaller, covered specimen container. If you see blood or mucus in the total sample, be sure to include it in the final specimen. Avoid mixing urine with the specimen.

If the client cannot produce any feces, gently pass a rectal swab beyond the internal sphincter and rotate it carefully to collect fecal material. Then place the specimen in a suitable container for transport to the laboratory.

When collecting stool specimens, make sure you maintain the conditions needed for accurate test results. For example, you will collect specimens for culture in a sterile container and either send them to the laboratory immediately or place them in an appropriate medium to avoid bacterial overgrowth. A specimen to be tested for ova and parasites should be examined immediately because the organisms die if they cool below body temperature. On the other hand, you can refrigerate specimens not needing microscopic examination if you are unable to deliver them to the laboratory right away.

Action **A**lert!
Always make sure stool specimens are free of oil, barium, and bismuth.

To check for pinworms, you will need to collect a specimen from the anal region itself. To do so, press the sticky side of a strip of nonfrosted cellophane tape over and around the client's anus. Remove it immediately, place it on a glass slide, and send it to the laboratory for examination. Because the female worm deposits eggs on the perianal area during the night, you will want to collect the specimen early in the morning, before the person has bathed or had a bowel movement.

CHARACTERISTICS OF FECES

Fecal material is composed of food residues, bacteria, some white blood cells, epithelial cells, intestinal secretions, and water. Assessing frequency, amount, color, consistency, shape, and odor can help to identify gastrointestinal (GI) problems (Table 34–1).

The normal brown color of stool is produced by bile pigments. Absence of bile causes the stool to be white, gray, or clay-colored and may indicate biliary obstruction or lack of bile production (acholia). Light-colored stools also can result from barium or antacid ingestion. A gray stool mixed with observable fat and mucus is called **steatorrhea** and results from the malabsorption of fat. In infants, the first stools (called meconium) are normally black and tarry from ingested amniotic fluid, epithelial cells, and bile.

The consistency of stool is a reflection of its water content. Stools can be liquid, unformed, soft, or hard. An abnormal consistency indicates constipation or diarrhea.

The shape of the stool normally resembles that of the rectum. An abnormal finding would be that of a consistently narrowed, pencil-shaped stool, which indicates obstruction of the distal portion of the large intestine, as might occur with carcinoma.

The odor of the stool is characteristically pungent and is produced by bacterial flora and by some foods and medications. Blood or infection in the GI tract causes detectable noxious changes in the normal odor.

LABORATORY ANALYSIS OF FECES

In the laboratory, stool specimens can be examined for bile or bilirubin, blood, micro-organisms, ova, and parasites. Bacteria are detected through cultures. Microscopic examination may reveal meat fibers and fat, indicating a malabsorption syndrome.

TABLE 34–1
Characteristics of Feces

Characteristic	Normal	Abnormal	Possible Cause
Amount	150 g (varies with diet)		
Color	Adult: brown Infant: yellow	Black or tarry	• Iron ingestion. • Bismuth ingestion. • Charcoal ingestion.
		Black and tarry (melena)	• Upper GI bleeding.
		Pale	• Malabsorption of fat. • Diet high in milk and low in meat.
		Red	• Lower GI bleeding. • Ingestion of beets. • Ingestion of pyrvinium pamoate, an antiparasite agent. • Hemorrhoids, if the red is smeared on the surface of feces.
		Red-orange	• Ingestion of rifampin, an antibiotic.
		Green or orange	• Large amounts of ingested chlorophyll. • Intestinal infection.
		White or clay-colored	• Absence of bile.
Consistency	Formed, soft	Liquid	• Diarrhea. • Increased intestinal motility.
		Hard	• Constipation.
Constituents	Cells lining intestinal mucosa, dead bacteria, bile pigment, fat, protein, undigested food, water	Blood	• GI bleeding.
		Fat	• Malabsorption.
		Foreign objects	• Accidental ingestion.
		Mucus	• Inflammatory condition.
		Pus	• Bacterial infection.
Odor	Pungent (affected by client's own bacterial flora)	Noxious change	• Blood in feces. • Infection.
Shape	Appearance of diameter of rectum, about 2.5 cm (1 inch) for adults	Narrow, pencil-shaped, or string-like	• Obstructive condition.

Testing Feces for Occult Blood

TIME TO ALLOW

▼

Novice:
5 min.
Expert:
5 min.

The Hemoccult test is one of many commercial products used as a screening test for blood in the feces that is not visible to the naked eye. The test is used to detect gastrointestinal bleeding and to screen for colorectal cancer. Testing three separate specimens reduces the incidence of false-negative results. Restricting red meat for 2 to 3 days before the test reduces false-positive results.

Delegation Guidelines

The test for occult blood is a simple test that may be delegated to a nursing assistant. Review of the instructions for collecting the specimen and test performance can ensure uniform test results.

Equipment Needed

- Hemoccult test slide folder
- Clean gloves
- Wooden applicator
- Hemoccult developing solution

1 Instruct the client about the purpose of the test and have him defecate into the collection container. Tell him to avoid urinating in the container.
Urine may contaminate the stool sample. If the client has to urinate, he can do so before collecting the stool sample.

2 Put on clean gloves.
Clean gloves help to prevent transmission of microorganisms from the client's feces.

3 With the applicator, obtain a small specimen of feces and smear a thin layer in the first box of the cardboard Hemoccult slide. While obtaining the specimen, observe and document its characteristics.
A small specimen is sufficient to perform the test accurately.

4 With the opposite tip of the applicator, obtain a second specimen of feces from another location and smear it thinly in the second box of the cardboard Hemoccult slide.
Using the opposite end of the applicator prevents contamination of the second sample with the first. Consider the test result positive if both samples are positive for occult blood.

5 Close the cardboard Hemoccult slide cover and turn it over to the reverse side. Open the cardboard flap on the reverse side and apply two drops of Hemoccult developing solution to the guaiac paper.
Apply the exact amount of solution specified to ensure the accuracy of the test.

Continued

A chemical test used to detect **occult blood** in feces (an amount too small to be seen without a microscope) may be your responsibility. You will perform the actual test, which is called a **guaiac test,** as outlined in Procedure 34–1.

Besides supplying information about a current bowel disorder, this test also can be used as a screening procedure for colorectal cancer. The American Cancer Society recommends that people over age 50 have annual guaiac tests.

X-Ray Examination of Bowel

X-ray examination reveals the location and contour of the bowel and supporting structures as well as the presence and distribution of fecal material and gas in the bowel. A flat plate x-ray of the abdomen is taken without contrast material and therefore requires no special preparation. It shows shadows, fluid levels, and gas.

Another common diagnostic test is the barium x-ray, usually called a "lower GI series." Barium is a contrast medium that outlines the bowel. Be aware, however, that the barium enema can produce an anaphylactic reaction in a very small number of people, about 1 in 750,000 examinations. Following a barium x-ray, large doses of laxative are administered to ensure its complete evacuation. Barium left in the colon can cause impaction (a stool mass too large and hard to pass through the anus) and even obstruction.

Testing Feces for Occult Blood

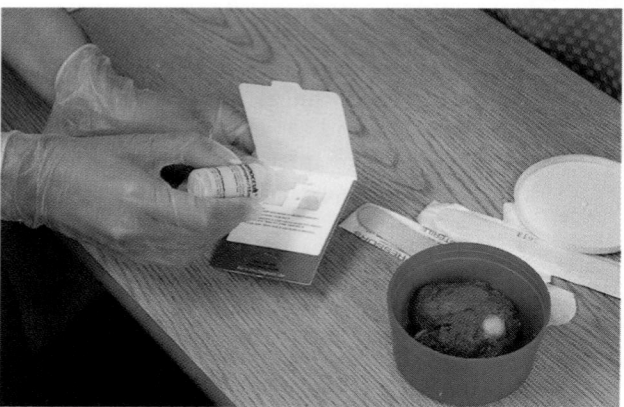

Applying Hemoccult developing solution to the guaiac paper.

6 As soon as you apply the developing solution, start keeping track of the time. If you notice a bluish discoloration on the guaiac paper 30 to 60 seconds after applying the solution, the sample contained occult blood.

Consider the result significant if both samples show a positive result.

7 Dispose of the Hemoccult slide in a hazardous waste container, discard your gloves, and wash your hands.

Standard precautions dictate that human excrement be treated as hazardous waste.

8 Document the characteristics of the client's feces and the results of the guaiac test in the client's chart.

Charting both objective findings and test results gives a complete picture of the specimen.

HOME CARE CONSIDERATIONS

Clients are often taught to collect a specimen for screening for occult blood in the home. Supply the person with the Hemoccult slide and a tongue blade. Provide instructions for use. Instruct the client to refrigerate the sample if time elapses between collecting the specimen and testing the specimen, such as when the specimen must be transported to a laboratory for testing. Have the client return the slide to the clinic for testing.

Action **A**lert!
Anaphylactic reactions can occur with barium enema administration. Be prepared to administer an antidote if necessary.

Direct Visualization of Bowel

A fiberoptic endoscope inserted through the anus and advanced through the bowel allows direct visualization of the lower GI tract. The physician may perform a proctoscopy, sigmoidoscopy, or colonoscopy, depending on the area of the colon to be examined. The endoscopes used to observe the bowel are hollow tubes through which the examiner can see GI structures. They also allow suction and collection of tissue for biopsy.

Before an endoscopy procedure, explain the test to the client to allay his anxiety. Also, make sure that bowel preparation is complete. The success of these procedures depends on adequate bowel preparation. In fact, if the person's bowel has not been thoroughly cleansed, feces can obscure the fiberoptic examination. Typically, preparation begins 24 to 48 hours before the procedure and includes dietary and fluid restrictions, laxatives or purgatives, enemas, or a combination.

A common method of emptying the bowel uses a solution called GoLYTELY (pronounced "go-lightly"). GoLYTELY cleanses the bowel without causing the excretion or absorption of fluid and electrolytes by the body that often occurs with traditional purgatives and enemas. This method is safer for people with congestive heart disease, chronic obstructive pulmonary disease, or controlled renal failure. The solution is consumed cold at a rate of 1.2 to 1.8 L per hour. The client soon develops diarrhea and, within 2 to 4 hours, the rectal output is clear. Because the solution works so quickly, make sure the client has ready access to toilet facilities.

Throughout the endoscopic procedure, provide emotional support. Before the procedure, administer a relaxant medication, as prescribed. Then help the client into a jack-knife or knee-chest position. Assess the client throughout the procedure because of the awkward position and the effects of the medication. Monitor his vital signs regularly during the procedure. Assist the physician with equipment and specimens, as necessary.

After the procedure, continue to monitor the client's vital signs. Inspect often for fresh anal bleeding, which may indicate continued oozing at a biopsy site. Severe abdominal pain could indicate a bowel perforation.

A*ction* A*lert!*
Monitor for circulatory and respiratory problems during endoscopy examination.

Focused Assessment for Constipation

Assessment for constipation is initiated from a client complaint or your observation that the client has been 3 days without a bowel movement. Assess for signs and symptoms and the probable cause.

Defining Characteristics

The client usually recognizes or suspects constipation when the frequency of bowel movements is less than usual and the abdomen feels full and distended. Additionally, the client may report a feeling of fullness or pressure in the rectum, straining at stool, abdominal pain, appetite impairment, back pain, headache, interference with daily living, and the use of laxatives. Sometimes the fecal mass can be palpated in the abdomen (NANDA, 1999). Hard, dry stool confirms the diagnosis of constipation.

Clients sometimes complain of constipation when digestive signs are absent. The diagnosis of *Perceived constipation* should be made only after ruling out actual constipation. Perceived constipation is common among elderly people who have health practices ingrained from the knowledge of another era. Defining characteristics for perceived constipation are psychological: the "expectation of a daily bowel movement with the resulting overuse of laxatives, enemas, and suppositories; expected passage of stool at same time every day" (NANDA, 1999).

Related Factors

To select appropriate nursing actions, you need to identify the causes specific to each client. Common causes include a lack of established bowel pattern; inadequate diet, fluids, and exercise; emotional depression; and weak pelvic floor muscles. Inconvenience also is frequently a factor. When the urge to defecate is repeatedly ignored, stool remaining in the rectum continues to lose water and stops stimulating normal reflexes.

Immobilizing a person for any reason decreases the intensity of colonic propulsion and heightens the risk of constipation. Intestinal pathological conditions, including neoplasm, stricture, hernia, megacolon (excessive dilation or stretching of the colon), diverticular disease, and painful anal lesions, all interfere with normal expulsion of the feces. Constipation frequently accompanies pregnancy, both because of hormonal changes and because of external pressure on the intestine.

Numerous medications contribute to constipation, such as analgesics (especially narcotics), anesthetics, anticholinergics, some antihypertensives, tricyclic antidepressants, calcium- and aluminum-containing antacids, iron supplements, and monoamine oxidase inhibitors, which slow neural transmission and thereby slow peristalsis. Overuse of laxatives, suppositories, and enemas contribute to the problem primarily through the resulting loss of intrinsic innervation and atrophy of the smooth muscle necessary for defecation.

Focused Assessment for Diarrhea

As with any condition, assess the person before deciding on the appropriate intervention. Question the client carefully about the frequency and characteristics of the stool. Ask the client to describe the nature of the diarrhea. Diarrhea may involve frequent, small stools, or it may represent the loss of a large volume of water. In that case, the person may become dehydrated and deficient in important electrolytes.

Also ask questions that will help determine the cause of the diarrhea. Ask about the duration of the problem, recent exposure to infected people, recent travel, dietary and medication intake, and the existence of anxiety, stress, or systemic disease that might contribute to a change in elimination patterns.

Defining Characteristics

Symptoms associated with diarrhea include abdominal pain or cramping and hyperactive bowel sounds. The stool is described as loose, liquid, or unformed. Accompanying symptoms may include distention, flatus, nausea and vomiting, bleeding, anorexia, urgency, fever, malaise, and symptoms of fluid imbalance. Severe diarrhea can lead to significant fluid and electrolyte imbalance, since the body does not reabsorb water, potassium, and sodium. There is also malabsorption of other nutrients. Diarrhea is usually alkaline, because it con-

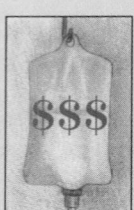

THE COST OF CARE
LAXATIVE USE

In one Midwestern community, there is a 48-bed long-term-care facility licensed for intermediate care. On one particular day, a tabulation of laxative use was completed on the 45 residents of the facility.

The tabulation found that 10 residents (22%) were not currently using laxatives. Laxatives prescribed for the other 35 residents ranged from one laxative to five laxatives. Docusate (Colace) was ordered daily for five residents, twice a day for nine residents, and three times a day for one resident. A natural fiber laxative was ordered daily for five residents, twice a day for one resident, and three times a day for one resident. Sorbitol was ordered daily for two residents, and bisacodyl (Dulcolax) tablets daily were ordered for one resident.

In addition to the daily prescribed laxatives, p.r.n. laxative medications had been ordered for some residents. Milk of magnesia had been ordered p.r.n. for 25 residents (56%), bisacodyl suppositories had been ordered p.r.n. for five residents, glycerin suppositories had been ordered p.r.n. for three residents, and one resident had had an order for a Fleet enema p.r.n.

The cost of just two of the laxatives used as prescribed daily were as follows: 26 Colace = $2.10, sorbitol (2 doses) = $1.01. If 5% of the population of North America is living in nursing homes, and 80% of those people are taking laxatives at the rate of the residents at this nursing home, how much is the use of laxatives costing in North America alone?

tains digestive enzymes. It causes skin breakdown if it comes into prolonged or frequent contact with the skin. This problem is exacerbated by frequent wiping with toilet paper.

Related Factors

The causes of diarrhea are numerous and different for acute and chronic diarrhea. *Acute diarrhea* may be caused by emotional states, especially anxiety; infectious organisms, such as bacteria, viruses, and parasites; alterations in diet, such as increased greasy or spicy foods, or food to which the person is allergic; and medications, such as iron supplements, thyroid agents, magnesium-containing antacids, antibiotics, lactulose, cimetidine, antihypertensives, colchicine, digitalis, and laxatives. A wide variety of laxatives may be used in varying dosages and to varying effects, as mentioned in the Cost of Care chart.

Causes of *chronic diarrhea* have been identified as lactose-containing or hyperosmolar nutritional supplements; sorbitol and mannitol (ingredients); such diseases as hyperthyroidism, diabetes mellitus, adrenal insufficiency, hyperparathyroidism, inflammatory bowel diseases, and cancer of the colon; GI surgery; radiation enterocolitis; laxative abuse; alcohol abuse; and chemotherapeutic agents.

Focused Assessment for Bowel Incontinence

The risk for bowel incontinence is associated with physical and mental disabilities. An elderly person with decreased mobility, cognitive impairment, or both is the most likely to have bowel incontinence. Developmentally disabled people with physical handicaps and mental retardation are the second largest group in whom incontinence is seen.

> A*ction* A*lert!*
> Usually, a client will report a problem with bowel incontinence. However, make sure to investigate any fecal odor that arises near a person or a source of soiled clothes or linens, especially if the affected person is physically or mentally disabled or is a small child.

As with any condition, assess the person before deciding on the appropriate intervention. Determine the frequency and involuntary nature of the stool, the duration of the problem, and the presence of abdominal cramps.

Defining Characteristics

The defining characteristic for bowel incontinence is "involuntary passage of stool" (NANDA, 1999). This involuntary passage of stool can occur at any age and in any health care setting.

Related Factors

Related factors for bowel incontinence are "gastrointestinal disorders, neuromuscular disorders, colostomy, loss of rectal sphincter control, and impaired cognition" (NANDA, 1999). Causes of fecal incontinence are both physical and psychological. Physical causes include anything that interferes with the integrity of sphincter function. Thus hemorrhoids, tumors, lacerations, rectal prolapse, fistulas, and loss of sensory innervation may lead to incontinence. People with explosive diarrhea may find the urge to defecate too overwhelming to control.

Psychologically, incontinence may be the result of an emotional state, as well as being itself the cause of various emotional problems. Encopresis is the socially inappropriate passage of a stool when no physical reason exists to account for the behavior. It is believed to occur because of an emotional disturbance or delay in the maturation process. Sometimes a formerly continent child or adult becomes incontinent as a means to gain attention or to express anger.

Probably the most important consequence of incontinence is the loss of self-respect, which is intensified by the reactions of significant others in the person's environment, including nurses, physicians, friends, and relatives. Also, incontinence causes skin irritation and breakdown, and soiling of clothes and linen.

Focused Assessment for Flatulence

Flatulence has defining characteristics of a bloated feeling, abdominal distention, cramping pains, and excessive passage of gas from the mouth (eructation) or from the anus (flatus). Respiratory distress may also occur if the distended abdomen pushes against the diaphragm. Abdominal percussion produces a tympanic sound.

Probably the most common predisposing factor in flatulence is excessive air swallowing, which results from chewing gum, drinking carbonated beverages, eating rapidly, or sucking through straws. Anxiety and postnasal drip can also lead to excessive air swallowing.

Other causes of gaseous distention include constipation; slowed intestinal motility, as may occur after abdominal surgery; bowel obstruction; medications that decrease peristalsis; decreased physical activity; and such foods as beans, cabbage, radishes, onions, cauliflower, and cucumbers.

Focused Assessment for Fecal Impaction

Impaction consists of hardened feces that a person cannot pass voluntarily or involuntarily. Probably the most common predisposing factor is immobility. Other predisposing factors are nutritional intake, abuse of laxatives, and poor fluid intake.

> A*ction* A*lert!*
> Assess for fecal impaction when there is a continuous seeping of loose feces.

Suspect a fecal impaction when the client has abdominal distention, small amounts of liquid stool, and the absence of a bowel movement. However, a fecal impaction can be present even if the client has had small regular bowel movements that have not emptied the colon. The impaction is confirmed by palpation, the presence of hardened stool in the rectum, or x-ray confirmation. Inquire about the date of the client's last known bowel movement, any previous impaction problems, dietary and medication intake, and the existence of immobility that might contribute to the problem. Previous bowel surgery, decreased bowel sounds, immobility, and chronic use of suppositories are risk factors. It is usually associated with decreased mental status.

Often the first symptom of a fecal impaction is the inability to pass a normal stool. However, probably the most definitive symptom is the seepage of liquid stool from the anus. Liquefaction provides the only way that fecal material can get around the impaction. Usually the liquid appears in small amounts, which helps to differentiate it from diarrhea. However, bacterial action on the fecal mass sometimes causes the production of copious amounts of liquid stool. Also, the seepage of stool is usually uncontrolled, since the anal sphincters have become less competent, secondary to prolonged stimulation of the defecation reflex by the hardened mass. Other symptoms indicating impaction include an almost continuous urge to defecate, rectal pain, abdominal fullness, nausea and vomiting, shortness of breath, hypertension, and abdominal distention.

Confirm the presence of an impaction by performing a digital rectal examination. This examination is completed by wearing a glove and liberally lubricating the forefinger, then inserting the forefinger through the anus into the rectum. If you feel a hard fecal mass, an impaction probably exists. If you do not feel a mass but symptoms are present, the mass may be higher up in the colon, out of reach.

Focused Assessment for Related Nursing Diagnoses

Body Image Disturbance

Body image disturbance may be present in the client who has had a fecal diversion procedure, such as an ileostomy or a colostomy. The presence of an ostomy is an actual change in body image and may result in the client being reluctant to learn to manage the ostomy care. Bowel incontinence also can produce a body image disturbance because it represents a socially unacceptable activity. Embarrassment is often a major factor in managing incontinence.

Altered Health Maintenance

Altered health maintenance is present any time a client has to change his lifestyle to manage a bowel elimination problem. The client with an ostomy obviously has to change his methods of self-care for bowel elimination. However, any client who is required to change his diet, take medications, or alter his usual pattern of activity and exercise will have to manage the effect of those changes on bowel elimination.

Many times, elderly clients have the nursing diagnosis *Altered health maintenance* because they cannot identify and manage a bowel elimination problem. For example, a client may be homebound with very poor nutritional intake. Mobility has declined over time and, as a result, the usual routine of a daily bowel movement after a high-fiber diet is gone. The visiting nurse becomes involved with the client and identifies the nursing diagnosis *Altered health maintenance* not only for bowel elimination but for dietary intake and hygiene needs.

Risk for Impaired Skin Integrity

A risk for impaired skin integrity is present when the client has bowel incontinence. The contents of the colon are alkaline compared to the skin and, therefore, highly irritable to the skin. The risk for impaired skin integrity is especially high when other risk factors for *Impaired skin integrity* exist.

Toileting Self-Care Deficit

The inability to independently meet the needs associated with toileting activities is highly associated with bowel elimination problems. The client may be unable to independently perform toileting activities because of immobility, lack of full range of motion, weakness, or intolerance for activity.

DIAGNOSIS

The choice of using a "risk for" diagnosis is based on the philosophy of early detection and prevention of health problems. For example, a postoperative client is at risk for constipation. Once the diagnosis is actual, it could be written as *Constipation related to immobility and anesthesia.* The accompanying Decision Tree offers more information.

Nursing diagnoses are made with thought to the focus of care and interventions that are appropriate to the client. Examples of various nursing diagnoses that are pertinent to bowel elimination are: *Diarrhea related to excessive use of laxatives, Bowel incontinence related to cognitive impairment, Perceived constipation related to impaired thought process,* or *Bowel incontinence related to effects of medication.* Clustering

appropriate data can help to arrive at the most appropriate nursing diagnoses, as shown in the accompanying chart.

PLANNING

After performing a thorough bowel history and assessment, you will plan care to address the nursing diagnoses. During the planning phase of the nursing process, nursing interventions are identified to assist the client in achieving outcomes for problem resolution.

Expected Outcomes for the Client With Constipation

The goal for a diagnosis of *Constipation* is that the client resume a normal bowel elimination pattern. Most of the time, a positive outcome is inferred from observation of frequency and the client's subjective experience and report that bowel elimination is normal. Box 34–2 lists the definition and indicators for Bowel Elimination Outcome.

If the problem is a direct result of an acute illness, such as a postoperative client who had no bowel elimi-

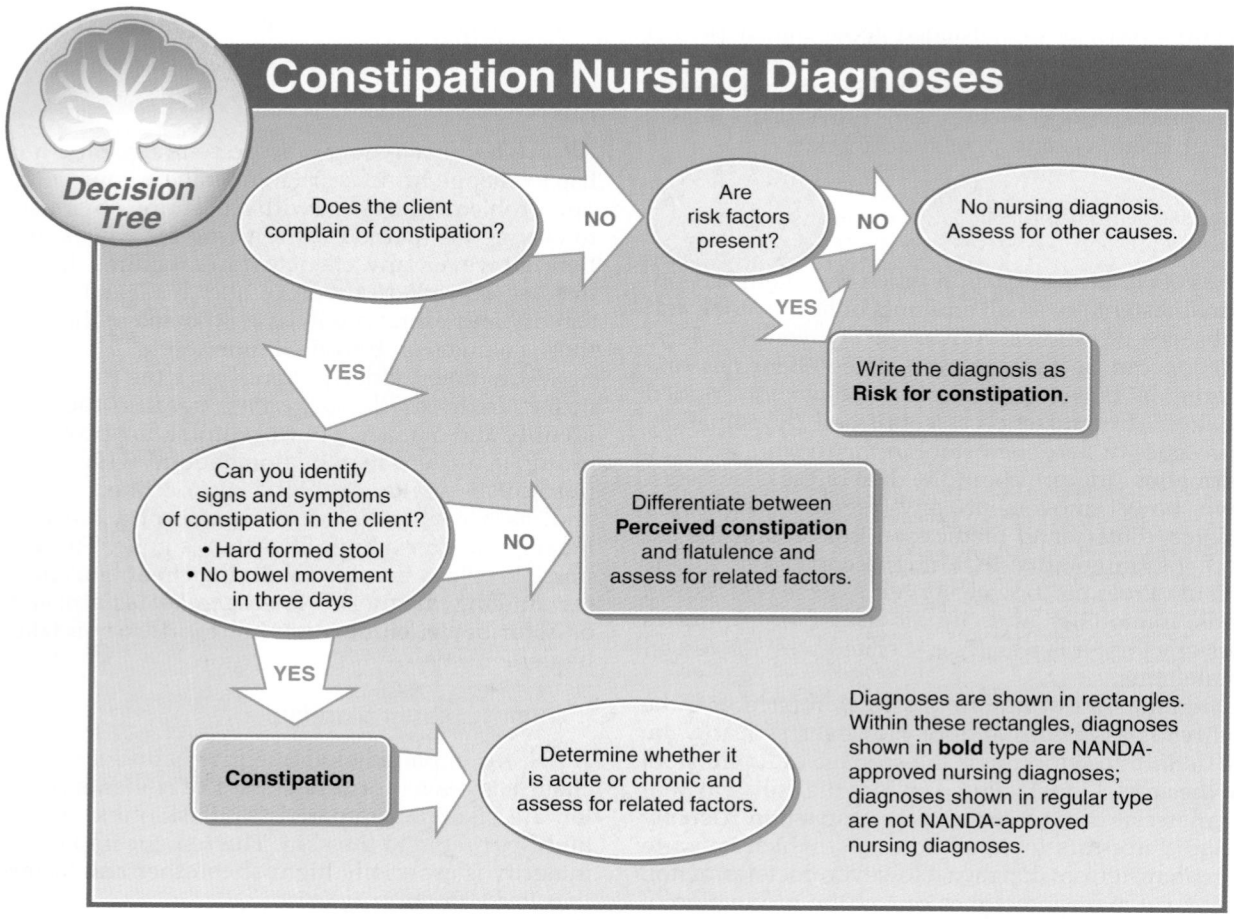

Constipation Nursing Diagnoses

Decision Tree

Does the client complain of constipation? — NO → Are risk factors present? — NO → No nursing diagnosis. Assess for other causes.

YES ↓ (from risk factors) → Write the diagnosis as **Risk for constipation**.

YES ↓ (from complain of constipation)

Can you identify signs and symptoms of constipation in the client?
• Hard formed stool
• No bowel movement in three days
— NO → Differentiate between **Perceived constipation** and flatulence and assess for related factors.

YES ↓

Constipation → Determine whether it is acute or chronic and assess for related factors.

Diagnoses are shown in rectangles. Within these rectangles, diagnoses shown in **bold** type are NANDA-approved nursing diagnoses; diagnoses shown in regular type are not NANDA-approved nursing diagnoses.

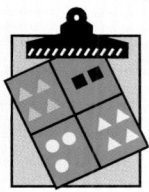

CLUSTERING DATA TO MAKE A NURSING DIAGNOSIS
BOWEL ELIMINATION PROBLEMS

Data Cluster	Diagnosis
An 84-year-old ambulatory woman with Alzheimer's disease has an incontinent bowel movement every morning after breakfast. She cannot find her room in the nursing home; it is not clear if she feels the urge to defecate.	*Bowel incontinence* related to impaired cognition
The 3rd day after gallbladder surgery, a 50-year-old women calls the doctor's office complaining of abdominal distention and cramping. She reports that she has not had a bowel movement since the surgery. She has been taking acetaminophen with codeine for pain.	*Constipation* related to decreased physical activity and use of pain medication
A 70-year-old woman has been admitted to the hospital with leukemia. She tells you that she must have milk of magnesia every morning before breakfast. She reports that her stool is unformed and a small amount.	*Perceived constipation* related to inappropriate health belief
After returning home from traveling in a foreign country, parents report that their 18-month-old infant has developed loose stools that have occurred about seven times a day for more than 2 days.	*Diarrhea* related to infectious processes
A 47-year-old male had abdominal exploratory surgery. On the 2nd postoperative day, he complained of abdominal cramping and gas pains.	*Flatulence* related to surgery
A resident of a long-term-care facility has been unable to ambulate or move herself for about 2 years. She recently began losing weight, about 2 to 3 pounds per month, because she was refusing her meals. She also began refusing to take her laxatives on a regular basis. A nurse's aide reported to the charge nurse that she was constantly cleaning up loose, seeping stool for this resident.	*Fecal impaction* related to decreased mobility, decreased nutritional intake, and refusal of laxative medications

nation for 76 hours after surgery, the outcome of normal bowel elimination by discharge from the hospital is usually sufficient. However, if the problem can be expected to return, that is, the client is at continued risk or the problem is the result of chronic illness, the outcomes need to include evidence that the person is prepared to manage the risk.

The outcomes may include the following:

- Listing foods with high-fiber content
- Explaining the importance of exercise in relation to the GI system
- Stating types of laxatives available
- Identifying side effects and contraindications of bowel laxatives
- Administering appropriate laxatives to maintain normal bowel elimination

Expected Outcomes for the Client With Diarrhea

The expected outcome for the diagnosis *Diarrhea* is also that the client resume a normal bowel elimination pattern. No evidence of diarrhea will be present, as manifested by a soft, medium-sized to large bowel movement every day or every few days, as is the client's routine. The client with diarrhea should be evaluated for risk for reoccurrence. The outcomes may include the following:

- The client will be clean and dry.
- The client will avoid foods that contribute to diarrhea.
- The client will note the frequency and amount of diarrhea.

BOX 34–2

DEFINITION AND INDICATORS FOR BOWEL ELIMINATION OUTCOME

Definition

Ability of the gastrointestinal tract to form and evacuate stool effectively.

Indicators

- Elimination pattern in expected range.
- Stool color within normal limits.
- Stool amount for diet.
- Stool soft and formed.
- Constipation not present.
- Diarrhea not present.
- Ease of stool passage.
- Comfort of stool passage.
- Visible peristalsis not present.
- Painful abdominal cramps not present.
- Bloating not present.
- Bowel sounds.
- Sphincter tone.
- Rectal tone.
- Fat in stool within normal limit.
- Intestinal motility.
- Defecation urge.
- Fat in stool within normal limit.
- Stool free of blood.
- Stool free of mucus.

From Johnson, M., & Maas, M. (Eds.). (1997). Nursing outcomes classification (NOC). St. Louis: Mosby-Year Book.

Expected Outcomes for the Client With Bowel Incontinence

The expected outcome for a diagnosis of *Bowel incontinence* depends on the illness that has caused the problem. If the bowel incontinence is a permanent problem, the appropriate outcome is that the client's skin integrity will remain intact. If the bowel incontinence is not permanent or can be minimized by intervention, then an outcome for a client could be that bowel elimination will occur daily with digital stimulation.

INTERVENTION

Interventions to Promote Healthful Elimination

Helping clients to attain and maintain healthy defecation habits is a goal you can meet through learning and teaching activities; supporting normal bowel habits through adjustments in diet, fluids, exercise, and positioning; and providing for relaxation and privacy.

Teaching About Bowel Needs and Care

Even clients whom you assume to be knowledgeable may have misconceptions about defecation. For example, many people incorrectly believe that it is necessary to defecate every day. If they fail to have a daily bowel movement, they may then use laxatives, suppositories, or enemas to induce one. As described later, continued use of such measures begins a cycle that may lead to physical dependence. Because there are many other misunderstandings about defecation, you must give clients accurate information about this normal body function. With appropriate teaching, a client who needs intervention is more likely to be compliant.

TOILET HABITS

Many factors influence the timing of bowel movements, such as availability of a bathroom and the demands of personal and professional responsibilities. Consequently, you will need to assess each client's daily routine before planning a bowel program. However, keep in mind that, although defecation can occur at any time, it is best to encourage bowel movements during stimulation of the gastrocolic reflex. As described earlier, this reflex is usually strongest after breakfast. Therefore, attempts to have a bowel movement at this time are likely to be the most successful.

Frequency of bowel movements varies from person to person. The normal range for an adult is from three times per week to three times per day. Infants often have three to five stools per day, but for adults and older children, passing stools more than three times a day or less than once a week may indicate a problem. Because many people worry needlessly about the frequency of their bowel movements, emphasize to your clients that the frequency of bowel movements varies among individuals. Stress that it is not necessary to have a bowel movement every day.

Action Alert!
Stress that the frequency of bowel movements is individualized, and that it is not necessary to have a bowel movement every day.

The amount of stool varies according to the amount and type of food ingested, fluid intake, and frequency of bowel evacuation. It is normally about 150 g per day. Because much fecal material is not dietary in origin, the person with no oral intake still passes stool. Also, it may take several days for food to move through the entire gastrointestinal (GI) tract. The colon therefore is not empty even if the person has not eaten for several days. Inform people of these facts to motivate them to take measures to prevent constipation.

Help people select a time during the day when they can take time to attend to bowel needs. As indicated, timing depends on lifestyle and daily activities. Once decided, encourage people to make this habit a daily routine. If the time selected is inappropriate, alter it until a suitable one is found. People who have little routine in their lives are a particular challenge.

In addition, hospitalization often alters established routines. During this time, determine the client's normal routine, and then help him to maintain it.

DIET

Dietary fiber is one of the most important elements in maintaining normal bowel function. Dietary fiber increases the weight and water content of feces. It also speeds the progress of feces through the GI tract. Fiber may be soluble or insoluble. The digestive system cannot break down insoluble fiber from a plant. Likewise, it does not break down in water, but rather retains water. Water retained by fiber softens the stool and promotes regularity. Thus, supplementing diets with bran, whole grain cereals, nuts, and raw fruits and vegetables is effective in promoting normal bowel elimination.

A high-fiber diet can also prevent diverticular disease. A diverticulum is an outpouching of the colon wall that results from weakened muscles in the intestinal wall. This condition can cause problems if the diverticula fill with feces. Perforation, ulceration, and infection can also develop. Diverticular disease is commonly asymptomatic when the client eats a high-fiber diet.

The National Cancer Institute recommends a daily intake of 25 to 35 g of fiber. To increase a client's consumption of fiber, add high-fiber foods slowly to allow time for the GI tract to adapt. Large amounts of dietary fiber added abruptly can cause abdominal cramps, gaseous distention, and diarrhea. The client's fiber consumption should include both insoluble and soluble fiber. It should come from foods rather than from supplements, which may not contain needed vitamins and minerals.

In addition to adding fiber, help the client identify and avoid foods that disrupt his bowel function. If there are several suspect foods, urge the client to eliminate all of them from his diet and then add them back, one at a time. Tell the client to wait for several days, longer if necessary, between each introduction, to see which foods cause the problem.

FLUIDS

Hydration helps maintain normal bowel function by keeping stools soft. Although experts recommend differing amounts of fluid to maintain adequate hydration, most consider about 1,200 to 1,500 mL per day to be a reasonable minimum for adults. A client with significant fluid replacement needs (such as from increased sweating caused by activity or fever) should consume more. Immobility also requires increased fluid intake because one of the normal aids to defecation—exercise—is limited. However, before increasing a client's fluid intake, make sure that the person has no contraindications, such as cardiac disease, renal disease, or head injury.

Although the amount of fluid intake is critical, the type of fluids consumed may also be important. For example, milk constipates some people. Prune juice is a natural laxative for most people. Other fruit juices,

such as apricot, lemonade, cranberry, and orange, can also stimulate bowel activity.

EXERCISE

Encourage and assist clients, as necessary, to take part in daily physical activity, because exercise improves muscle tone and strengthens the muscles used in defecation. Walking, for example, is an excellent body toner.

Also, teach exercises specifically designed to strengthen the abdominal and pelvic floor muscles. Probably the most effective are isometric exercises in which the client contracts or tightens muscles as strongly as possible for about 10 seconds, and then relaxes them. Instruct the client to repeat each exercise five to 10 times, four times a day. Remember that isometric exercises raise blood pressure and may cause coronary ischemia (deficient blood flow to the cardiac muscle) in a client with cardiac disease. Therefore, you may need to consult a physician about the client's health status before instituting an exercise program.

USE OF LAXATIVES

Laxatives are short-acting medications that cause defecation. They should not be used on a routine basis by healthy people. For clients who cannot defecate because of such bowel elimination problems as constipation and fecal impaction, laxatives are used to aid in the bowel elimination process.

Positioning the Client

Proper positioning for elimination promotes comfort and aids defecation in several ways. For one, it makes use of the force of gravity. For another, good positioning facilitates contraction of the abdominal muscles, thereby increasing intra-abdominal pressure. Since squatting is the best position for defecation, position the client as near to this posture as possible. The commode and toilet promote this position naturally. You can increase external pressure on the abdomen by having the client lean forward.

If the person is short, place a footstool or other appropriate device under his feet at the toilet to increase hip flexion. Exercise caution, however, with a client who has had hip surgery, especially total hip replacement. This client must avoid flexing the hips beyond 90 degrees to prevent dislocation of the prosthesis. Some clients can use the toilet only with the aid of a device that raises the seat height to decrease hip flexion. Instruct these clients not to lean forward.

If the client must use a bedpan, raise the head of the bed into a high-Fowler position, if not otherwise contraindicated. If head elevation is contraindicated, use a fracture bedpan instead.

Promoting Relaxation and Privacy

Relaxation is critical to normal bowel function. Probably the most important factor in achieving relaxation is privacy. When the client feels that the odors and

THE STATE OF NURSING SCIENCE

UNDERSTANDING AND MANAGING BOWEL ELIMINATION CHANGES

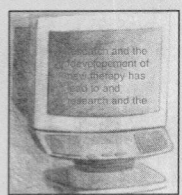

What Are the Issues?

Bowel elimination patterns are a very individual aspect of daily living. The normal pattern for some people may be to have a bowel movement once every 3 days, while others are concerned if they do not have a bowel movement at least once a day. Nevertheless, most people have a bowel movement every day. However, events ranging from travel to surgery can disrupt a person's usual bowel elimination pattern.

Part of a holistic nursing assessment is to determine a person's usual bowel elimination pattern and offer preventive measures during times of stress and change that may alter bowel function. Nurses are interested in what factors interfere with normal bowel function, the frequency of constipation as a problem for hospitalized clients, and interventions for reducing the frequency of constipation in various client groups.

What Research Has Been Conducted?

Ross (1995) compared changes in bowel patterns of middle-aged and older adults during hospitalization for medical conditions. Several instruments were used to collect data, including a guided interview to ascertain the client's usual bowel elimination pattern, recording of client-reported changes in bowel elimination, nursing assessment of bowel movement frequency and cognitive status, and researcher assessment of functional status and severity of illness. The researchers used the data to develop a model that could help predict who would develop changes in their bowel elimination pattern during hospitalization.

Ouellet et al. (1996) examined the effect of dietary fiber in the form of bran cereal on the bowel patterns of adults admitted to the hospital for joint surgery. Subjects in the experimental group were given a bran muffin the night before surgery and a combination bran cereal postoperatively once they tolerated a full liquid diet. Subjects in the control group received a low-fiber muffin the night before surgery and a low-fiber cereal postoperatively once they tolerated a full liquid diet. All subjects drank a minimum of six glasses of water per day in the postoperative period. Researchers visited subjects twice a day for data collection and to remind them to drink water.

What Has the Research Concluded?

In Ross' study of bowel elimination patterns during hospitalization, the researcher found that older women experienced the most change in bowel elimination patterns during hospitalization, and older adults experienced the most severe changes in their bowel elimination patterns (Ross, 1995). There were seven episodes of impaction in the sample of older adults. Constipation was the most common change that the subjects experienced. The factors that best predicted who would have a change in bowel elimination patterns were decreased function and cognitive status, female gender, and severity of illness.

Ouellet et al. (1996) found that subjects who received the bran cereal intervention were less likely to require other interventions such as laxatives and enemas. During the course of the study, the researchers learned that people tolerated commercial cereal preparations better than plain bran as the fiber source. This is important for future studies that want to look at increasing dietary fiber as an intervention.

What is the Future of Research in This Area?

Ross (1995) recommends studies on the effects of other factors, such as medications and diet and activity changes, on the bowel elimination patterns of hospitalized adults. Once nurses know who is at risk for developing changes in bowel elimination patterns, interventions such as increased activity and dietary changes can be tested for their impact on the prevention of such problems as constipation.

Current studies of the use of fiber in the diet suggest that they may prevent constipation, although other studies that rely on self-report do not consistently support these results (Towers et al., 1994). More research using other instruments is needed to enable researchers to evaluate the preventive effect of dietary and activity interventions with specific populations. Such studies should include cost comparisons of various methods of constipation and impaction management as well as patient outcomes.

References

Ouellet, L.L., Turner, T.R., Pond, S., et al. (1996). Dietary fiber and laxation in postop orthopedic patients. *Clinical Nursing Research, 5*(4), 428–440.

Ross, D.G. (1995). Altered bowel elimination patterns among hospitalized elderly and middle-aged persons: Quantitative results. *Orthopaedic Nursing, 14*(1), 25–31.

Towers, A.L., Burgio, K.L., Locher, J.L., et al. (1994). Constipation in the elderly: Influence of dietary, psychological, and physiological factors. *Journal of the American Geriatrics Society, 42,* 701–706.

sounds that naturally accompany this body function may be communicated to others, he may become anxious. Anxiety causes tension in the voluntary musculature, which in turn can suppress defecation. Provide as private an environment as possible to facilitate normal defecation.

For example, if the client is using the bathroom, make sure that other people know the room is occupied. This is especially important when the bathroom has two doors opening into adjacent rooms. If the client must use a bedpan or commode in the room, pull the bed curtains around the bed, ask all visitors or staff to leave the room, open the window if appropriate, and turn on the television or radio. Use room deodorizers to reduce odors.

Make sure that the client has a way to call you when he is finished or needs help. In addition to providing a call light, assure the client that there is no hurry. Communicate this fact by your actions as well as your words. For example, avoid interrupting the client simply to see if he has finished. On the other hand, do keep careful watch on any client who is at risk for accidents, such as fainting or falling. In fact, fainting in bathrooms is a rather frequent occurrence. Bathrooms are notoriously warm and stuffy and, when a weakened person strains to have a bowel movement, his cardiovascular system may not be able to maintain sufficient blood flow to the brain.

Some clients may need pain relief before trying to defecate. If you must administer a narcotic pain reliever, time its administration carefully because these drugs depress central nervous system function. Time the administration so that the client can attempt defecation when pain has been relieved, but before drowsiness and sleep set in.

Interventions to Manage Constipation

The treatment of typical constipation requires all the preventive measures mentioned: learning and teaching activities; changes in diet, fluid intake, and exercise; and development of healthy bowel habits.

Sometimes, additional intervention is needed. Box 34–3 lists the definition and practice activities for managing constipation and impaction.

Administering Medications

Laxatives and **cathartics** are medications used to induce emptying of the bowel. The two terms are often used interchangeably, although cathartics have a stronger action than laxatives. Laxatives come in four categories: bulk-forming, lubricant, saline, and stimulant. Besides these oral medications, laxatives are also available as medicated suppositories. When inserted into the rectum, they stimulate defecation.

Bulk-forming laxatives are the most natural and least irritating laxative preparations and are frequently used to wean laxative-dependent people from medication misuse. They use synthetic or natural poly-

---

BOX 34–3

DEFINITION AND PRACTICE ACTIVITIES FOR MANAGING CONSTIPATION AND IMPACTION

Definition

Prevention and alleviation of constipation and impaction.

Activities

- Monitor for signs and symptoms of constipation.
- Monitor for signs and symptoms of impaction.
- Monitor bowel movements, including frequency, consistency, shape, volume, and color, as appropriate.
- Monitor bowel sounds.
- Consult with physician about a decrease or increase in frequency of bowel sounds.
- Monitor for signs and symptoms of bowel rupture or peritonitis.
- Explain etiology of problem and rationale for actions to client.
- Identify factors that may cause or contribute to constipation, such as medications, bedrest, diet.
- Encourage increased fluid intake unless contraindicated.

- Evaluate client's medication profile for gastrointestinal side effects.
- Instruct client or family to record color, volume, frequency, and consistency of client's stools.
- Teach client or family how to keep a food diary.
- Instruct client or family on high-fiber diet, as appropriate.
- Instruct client or family on appropriate use of laxatives.
- Instruct client or family on the relationship of diet, exercise, and fluid intake to constipation and impaction.
- Evaluate recorded intake for nutritional content.
- Consult physician if signs and symptoms of constipation or impaction persist.
- Administer laxative or enema as appropriate.
- Inform client of procedure for manual removal of stool, if necessary.
- Remove fecal impaction manually, if necessary.
- Administer enema or irrigation, as appropriate.
- Weigh client regularly.

From McCloskey, J.C., & Bulechek, G. (1996). Nursing interventions classification (2nd ed.). St. Louis: Mosby-Year Book.

saccharides and cellulose derivatives to absorb water and add bulk. This increased volume stretches the intestinal wall, thus stimulating peristalsis. Common examples are bran, psyllium, karaya gum, agar, and methylcellulose. Mix bulk-forming agents with water and follow the dose with additional fluid to make sure that it has been cleared from the esophagus. Results usually occur in 12 to 24 hours, but they may take up to 72 hours. Encourage high fluid intake to improve the action of the laxative and to avoid GI tract obstruction.

Lubricant laxatives include mineral oil and the docusates. They coat the outside of the fecal mass, making it slippery and inhibiting fluid absorption from it. Mineral oil is a classic example of a lubricant laxative. It is not very palatable, but you can mask the oily aftertaste by mixing it with orange juice or root beer. Administer mineral oil when the client's stomach is empty to keep it from interfering with the absorption of fat-soluble vitamins. Watch carefully if the client has trouble swallowing, because mineral oil aspiration can cause pneumonia. The docusates act as wetting and dispersing agents. Common examples are Dialose, Colace, Doxidan, and Surfak. Poloxamer 188, a nonionic surfactant, is a stool softener.

Saline laxatives, or osmotic agents, contain poorly absorbed salts and sugars, which, through osmotic activity, draw water into the intestine to increase bulk and lubricate feces. These drugs usually act within 1 to 3 hours. Many are purgatives that empty the bowel completely. Magnesium sulfate (Epsom salts), magnesium hydroxide (milk of magnesia), magnesium citrate, and lactulose are osmotic agents. Lactulose causes a severe osmotic reaction and, unless dosed carefully, causes intestinal rumbling, colic, and flatulence. Because of the salts used and the severity of their action, osmotic agents are usually contraindicated in people with renal, cardiac, or inflammatory bowel disease.

Stimulants (also called irritants) increase peristalsis by stimulating sensory nerve endings of the colonic epithelium or by directly irritating the GI mucosa. In addition, some (such as bisacodyl) may increase GI secretory activity, thus producing bulkier feces. Examples of stimulants include cascara, castor oil, senna, glycerin, and bisacodyl. Be aware that these medications are transmitted through breast milk, causing diarrhea in the nursing infant.

Laxatives are one of the most widely used and misused over-the-counter drugs. Most laxative abuse results from advertising that supports the public's misconceptions about the need for a daily bowel movement. In addition to teaching clients about the proper use of laxatives, warn them never to take these drugs in the presence of undiagnosed abdominal pain or cramps, nausea or vomiting, or diarrhea. These symptoms may indicate appendicitis, inflammatory bowel disease, or obstruction.

A*ction* A*lert!*
Daily laxative administration is detrimental to normal bowel elimination.

Suppositories are semisolid, cone-shaped, or oval-shaped masses that melt at body temperature. To stimulate defecation, medicated suppositories are inserted into the rectum, where they release their active ingredients as they melt. Many types of suppositories are refrigerated because it is easier to insert a cold, firm suppository than a warm, soft one.

The suppositories used most often are glycerin and bisacodyl. Each acts as a local irritant to stimulate GI mucosal secretion. Fecal softeners may also be given by suppository to moisten and lubricate the fecal mass. After administering the suppository, cleanse the client's anal area to remove excess lubricant. Instruct the client to retain the suppository as long as possible—at least 20 to 30 minutes. If appropriate, teach the client how to self-administer the suppository.

Administering Enemas

An enema involves the instillation of fluid into the rectum to stimulate defecation. This treatment is commonly administered in the home by people who have had no formal instruction in the procedure. Indeed, some people use a daily enema to prevent constipation. Consequently, most people consider enemas to be a harmless, necessary treatment for constipation. This is a misconception. To achieve the safest and most effective results, it is necessary to understand and apply the scientific principles underlying enema administration.

PURPOSE

Enemas are given for several purposes. The *cleansing enema* is used to treat constipation or fecal impaction, to clean out the bowel before diagnostic procedures or surgery, and to help establish regular bowel function during a bowel training program. A *retention enema* is retained in the bowel over a prolonged period. It is usually administered to lubricate or soften a hard fecal mass with oil, thus facilitating its expulsion through the anus. Less frequently, a retention enema is used to administer medications, to protect and soothe the mucous membrane of the intestine, to destroy intestinal parasites (anthelmintic), to relieve distention (carminative), or to administer fluids and nutrition (nutritive). Another kind of enema, the *return flow enema,* relieves gaseous distention. It is sometimes called a Harris flush and is described later, in the discussion of flatulence.

Enemas stimulate peristalsis through bowel distention, irritation of the mucosal wall, or both. Bowel distention results from filling the colon with fluid, either via a large-volume enema, which injects large amounts of fluid into the colon from an external source, or via a small-volume enema, which draws internal fluid into the bowel.

The concepts of osmosis and concentration gradient are important to an understanding of how some enemas work. Briefly, osmosis is the movement of water through a semipermeable membrane to equalize the concentration of particles on both sides of the membrane. Although water continuously flows back and forth across the membrane, the major net flow of water is toward the solution with a higher concentration of molecules.

TYPES OF ENEMAS

A cleansing enema may use a hypotonic, isotonic, or hypertonic solution. Hypotonic solutions (such as tap water) have a lower osmotic pressure than the fluid in the interstitial tissues, so the net flow of water is out of the bowel into the tissues. The net flow occurs slowly, however, and defecation is usually stimulated before any appreciable fluid is absorbed into the body. Significant absorption can occur if the client is fluid depleted or receives multiple enemas. Isotonic solutions (such as normal saline solution) produce equal concentrations on both sides of the semipermeable membrane. Consequently, no net water flow occurs. Hypertonic solutions are of higher concentration than the interstitial fluid. Thus, the net water flow is into the colon, leading to distention. Hypertonic solutions draw water into the colon, which stimulates the defecation reflex.

Hypotonic and isotonic enema solutions are used for large-volume enemas (500–750 mL) that result in immediate colonic emptying. The large volumes, however, may present a danger to people with weakened colon walls. In addition, these enemas often require special preparation and equipment. Conversely, hypertonic small-volume enemas (120–250 mL) are available commercially and are easier to administer. A commonly used over-the-counter product is the prepackaged enema, such as the Fleet brand (Fig. 34–5). These commercially packaged enemas are available as normal saline enemas or mineral oil enemas. People who have problems with sodium retention should avoid using hypertonic solutions.

One common enema additive is Castile soap. Added to either tap water or saline solution, it causes mucosal irritation. Other enema solutions, such as milk and molasses, vegetable oils, hydrogen peroxide, and champagne are reported in the literature. However, these types are rarely used. Various medicated and nutritive formulas, such as sucralfate enemas, are also used, depending on the person's needs.

Procedure 34–2 describes the techniques for preparing and administering a large-volume enema. Use these methods for enemas of any volume, but make any necessary changes when preparing the solution.

Administration of a hypertonic enema requires several variations in the procedure for an enema, mainly because the solution comes prepackaged and ready to inject. You do not need to warm the solution, but make sure that it is at room temperature to prevent intestinal cramps. The client may be in any position to receive this enema; however, the left lateral position with right leg flexed is recommended to distribute the solution throughout the colon.

To administer a commercially prepared hypertonic enema, remove the cap and insert the prelubricated tip into the client's rectum. Squeeze the collapsible reservoir steadily until the solution is gone. Have the client retain the solution until the urge to defecate is very strong. Clients can be taught to self-administer a hypertonic enema, and they may be asked to administer one at home before x-ray studies or proctological examinations.

Administration of a retention enema is similar to administration of a hypertonic enema, except that the solution must be retained over a prolonged period, usually for at least an hour. Some enemas (such as medicated or nutritive enemas) are never evacuated. The method of solution preparation depends on what type of solution has been ordered. A smaller administration tip is used (usually a No. 14 to No. 20 French catheter for adults) to avoid stretching the sphincter, thereby diminishing stimulation of the defecation reflex. Make sure you elevate the reservoir only high enough to allow the solution to run slowly into the rectum. Administration under higher pressure distends the rectum, causing defecation. Finally, protect the bed linen in case the client cannot retain the fluid.

COMPLICATIONS

Enema administration is not without its hazards. Complications include fluid and electrolyte imbalances, tissue trauma, vagal nerve stimulation, and dependence. Fluid imbalances usually occur because of the tonicity of the enema solution. Remember that the body absorbs water from hypotonic solutions. Use caution when administering enemas to people who are susceptible to fluid imbalance (such as infants or clients with decompensated cardiac or kidney reserve). Water intoxication can occur. Symptoms of this

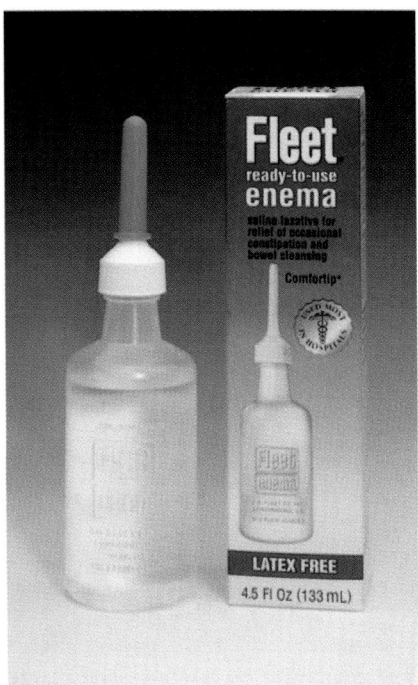

Figure 34–5. A Fleet enema. (Courtesy of C.B. Fleet Company, Inc., Lynchburg, VA.)

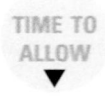

Preparing and Administering a Large-Volume Enema

TIME TO ALLOW
▼
Novice:
15 min.
Expert:
10 min.

A large-volume enema is defined as the administration of 500 to 1,000 mL of fluid to stimulate the colon to empty. It is unpleasant at best, may have some hazardous consequences for the client, and is seldom used in the health care environment. A large-volume enema is useful when rapid cleansing or evacuation of the bowel is needed. It may also be useful when the gentler forms of bowel cleansing are not effective.

Delegation Guidelines

An enema requires a physician's order. Administration of a large-volume enema may be delegated to a nursing assistant. First, however, you must assess the client for risk factors associated with receipt of an enema and instruct the nursing assistant in safety precautions. If the client has diverticular disease or other disorder of the colon, you may instruct the nursing assistant to use a smaller volume of solution or choose to administer the enema yourself.

Equipment Needed

- Enema solution container
- 36 inches of tubing with rectal tip (adult, No. 22 to No. 30 French; child, No. 12 to No. 18 French)
- Solution: tap water with 1 teaspoon mild liquid soap without additives; tap water; or normal saline
- Water-soluble lubricating jelly
- Clean gloves
- Waterproof pad
- Bedside commode or bed pan

Normal saline solution is the safest option for an enema solution, and tap water requires the least preparation. If the client has severe constipation or needs a thorough cleansing of the bowel, soap suds may be most useful because they irritate the colonic mucosa.

1 Set up the equipment and close the door or draw the curtain. Position the client on his left (or most comfortable) side. Drape him so only his buttocks are exposed. If you expect that the client will be unable to retain the enema solution, position him on a bedpan or commode instead.

Positioning the client on his left side allows gravity to help the enema solution flow into the rectum. Exposing only his buttocks will help to give the client a sense of privacy. Allowing him to face the door may help as well.

2 Make sure the enema solution is lukewarm, about 40.5°C (105°F). Coat the tip of the enema tube with water-soluble lubricant and gently insert it 2 to 3 inches into the client's rectum.

If the client has hemorrhoids, consider using extra lubricant. Insert the tip gently, with a twisting motion, to pass the hemorrhoids.

3 Allow 500 to 750 mL of the enema solution to flow slowly into the client's rectum, over about 10 minutes. The enema bag should be approximately 18 inches above the rectum.

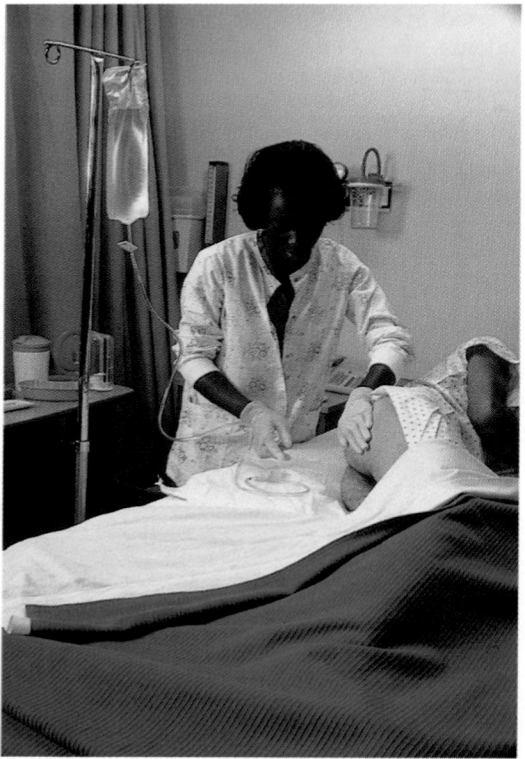

Positioning and equipment for administering a large-volume enema.

Keep the flow rate slow enough to prevent cramping and an uncontrollable urge to evacuate the bowel. If the client develops an uncontrollable urge, stop the flow until the urge passes.

4 Encourage the client to retain the solution in the bowel for up to 15 minutes.

With a large-volume enema, most clients will need to expel the solution quickly.

5 Help the client to the toilet or assist him with the bedpan or commode, as needed.

If the client has mobility problems, you may be able to place him more quickly on a bedpan than on the toilet. However, the best position for bowel evacuation is on the toilet or bedside commode.

6 After bowel evacuation, cleanse the client's perianal skin, control odors, and make the client comfortable.

Cleanse the skin thoroughly and gently. Controlling odors promptly can help to minimize the client's embarrassment.

7 If the physician has ordered enemas until clear, you may need to administer up to three large-volume enemas as described here. If three enemas fail to produce clear results, consult the physician.

Remember that a large-volume enema may produce more than one bowel movement. Allow time between enemas for maximum results.

HOME CARE CONSIDERATIONS

Enemas should not be used with any frequency in the home setting. Teach the family that cleansing enemas and laxatives should not be used any more often than once every 3 days. Once the bowel is thoroughly cleansed, the client may not need another bowel movement for 3 days. If the client is in the habit of managing constipation with enemas, help family caregivers with an overall bowel management program designed to reduce the need for enemas.

condition include weakness, dizziness, pallor, sweating, and respiratory difficulties. Signs of congestive heart failure or cerebral edema may also be present. On the other hand, hypertonic solutions draw fluid from the interstitial tissues and can lead to fluid depletion, especially in children and other people susceptible to dehydration.

Electrolyte imbalances also occur. Usually, normal saline is the safest enema solution because of its isotonicity. However, in clients who have problems with sodium retention (such as those with congestive heart failure or cirrhosis of the liver), the body absorbs sodium, which leads to fluid retention. Therefore, these clients should not receive saline solutions. Depending on the contents of the enema solution used, other electrolyte imbalances may also occur, such as hypokalemia, hypocalcemia, or hyperphosphatemia.

Action Alert!
Avoid giving an enema to a person with inflammatory bowel disease.

Enemas can also cause tissue trauma. The four major sources of trauma are the administration tip, solution delivered under high pressure, a soapsuds solution, and increased peristalsis. If the enema tip has any chips or broken areas, it may lacerate or abrade the rectal mucosa. High fluid pressures can rupture the in-

testinal wall without causing pain at the time of perforation. In fact, the first indication of rupture may be signs of peritonitis (inflammation of the peritoneum). Do not use a bulb syringe to administer an enema, because you will not be able to control the pressure. Tissue trauma from peristalsis can occur in clients with inflammatory bowel diseases. Increased bowel motility enhances cramping, bleeding, and so on.

Although the use of soapsuds enemas is questionable, they are still sometimes ordered. As stated, the soapsuds solution chemically irritates the mucosa. This irritation commonly leads to rectal inflammation and colitis, sometimes lasting up to 3 weeks after administration. The higher the concentration of soap in the solution, the greater the chance of inflammation. Thus, the practice of swirling a bar of soap or soap pieces in the enema reservoir is extremely dangerous, since it is impossible to determine the concentration. A soapsuds solution is somewhat safer if you use standardized packages of soap.

As is true of laxatives and suppositories, people can develop physical and psychological dependence on enemas. The underlying mechanism is the same: the enema cleans the bowel so that it takes 2 or more days for enough fecal mass to collect again to stimulate defecation. In the meantime, the person becomes anxious because he has not had a bowel movement. Thus, he self-administers another enema. Gradually,

TABLE 34–2
Agents Used to Relieve Constipation

Type	Action	Examples
Laxatives		
Bulk-forming	Increases the fluid, gaseous, or solid bulk in the intestines and absorbs water into the intestine	• Methylcellulose. • Hydrolose. • Psyllium (Metamucil).
Lubricant	Softens and delays the drying of feces	• Mineral oil. • Docusate sodium (Colace, Dialose).
Saline	Draws water into the intestine to increase bulk and lubricate feces	• Magnesium sulfate (Epsom salts). • Magnesium hydroxide (milk of magnesia). • Magnesium citrate.
Stimulant	Irritates the intestinal mucosa, increasing peristalsis	• Bisacodyl (Dulcolax). • Castor oil. • Cascara sagrada.
Enemas		
Hypertonic	Distends colon and irritates mucosa	• Sodium phosphate. • Fleet enema.
Hypotonic	Distends colon, stimulates peristalsis, and softens feces	• Tap water.
Isotonic	Distends colon, stimulate peristalsis, and softens feces	• Normal saline solution.
Soap	Irritates mucosa and distends colon	• Castile soap.
Oil	Lubricates the feces and the colonic mucosa	• Mineral oil. • Olive oil. • Cottonseed oil.

the bowel becomes less sensitive to normal defecation reflex stimuli, and the person becomes physically dependent on bowel aids. Table 34–2 summarizes agents used to relieve constipation.

Removing an Impaction

The goal of treatment for a fecal impaction is removal of the mass from the rectum. Oral laxatives or cathartics may be used to moisten and lubricate the fecal mass, although their action may be too slow. A program of enemas may be instituted, starting with the administration of an oil retention enema and followed by a volume cleansing enema. These two enemas may need to be repeated.

If the fecal mass is extremely large or the enemas are ineffective in expelling it, you will have to remove the impaction digitally. To do this, insert a gloved, heavily lubricated finger into the client's rectum (Fig. 34–6). Remove pieces of the mass manually with a bedpan close at hand. Even though you can use a topical anesthetic agent such as lidocaine, this intervention is uncomfortable and embarrassing for the person. Gentleness may help, but prevention is the best treatment. Occasionally, a fecal impaction must be removed surgically.

Interventions to Alleviate Diarrhea

The usual intervention for diarrhea is to inhibit peristalsis. However, because this action may slow the expulsion of pathogenic organisms or irritants, it may actually prolong the problem. Consequently, treatment may first involve removing the precipitating fac-

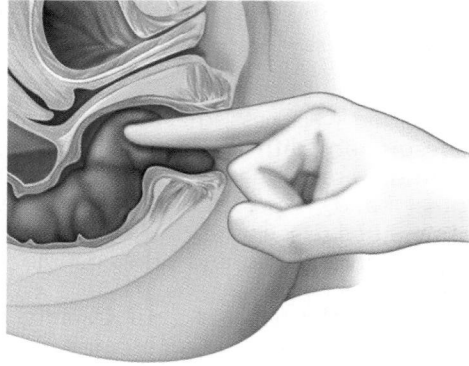

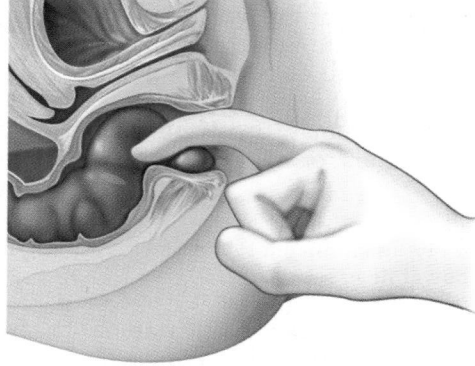

Figure 34–6. Digital removal of a fecal impaction.

BOX 34–4

DEFINITION AND PRACTICE ACTIVITIES FOR MANAGING DIARRHEA

Definition

Prevention and alleviation of diarrhea.

Activities

- Obtain stool for culture and sensitivity, if diarrhea continues.
- Evaluate client's medication profile for gastrointestinal side effects.
- Teach client appropriate use of antidiarrheal medications.
- Instruct client or family to record color, volume, frequency, and consistency of client's stools.
- Evaluate recorded intake for nutritional content.
- Encourage frequent, small feedings, adding bulk gradually.
- Teach client to eliminate gas-forming and spicy foods from diet.
- Suggest a trial elimination of foods containing lactose.
- Identify factors that may cause or contribute to diarrhea, such as medications, bacteria, and tube feedings.
- Monitor for signs and symptoms of diarrhea.

- Instruct client to notify staff about each episode of diarrhea.
- Observe skin turgor regularly.
- Monitor skin in perianal area for irritation and ulceration.
- Measure volume of bowel output.
- Weigh client regularly.
- Notify physician of an increase in frequency or pitch of bowel sounds.
- Consult physician if signs and symptoms of diarrhea persist.
- Instruct client or family in low-fiber, high-protein, high-calorie diet, as appropriate.
- Instruct client or family in avoidance of laxatives.
- Teach client or family how to keep a food diary.
- Teach client stress-reduction techniques, as appropriate.
- Assist client in performing stress-reduction techniques.
- Monitor safe food preparation.
- Perform actions to rest the bowel, such as NPO status (nothing by mouth) or liquid diet.

From McCloskey, J.C., & Bulechek, G. (1996). Nursing interventions classification (2nd ed.). St. Louis: Mosby-Year Book.

tors, then stopping the diarrhea itself. For example, a client with a GI infection typically receives antibiotics and possibly antidiarrheals. Box 34–4 lists the definition and practice activities for managing diarrhea.

Administering Medications

Commonly used antidiarrheal drugs, such as kaolin and pectin, may be used. These medications bind and remove irritants from the GI tract and form a soothing, protective coating on the mucosa. In severe diarrhea, the physician may prescribe opiates (such as paregoric or codeine) or anticholinergic drugs (such as diphenoxylate/atropine sulfate [Lomotil]) to inhibit peristalsis. As stated, antibiotics can be used to eliminate the cause of the diarrhea. Normal intestinal bacterial flora can be re-established by giving the client yogurt, buttermilk, or bacillus-containing medications such as Bacid or Lactinex.

Limiting Food Intake

Good nutrition is important during episodes of diarrhea. Diet modification maybe necessary to counteract the decreased absorption. For mild to moderate diarrhea, short-term therapy involves decreasing or eliminating food intake to reduce stimulation of peristalsis. For severe diarrhea, dietary modification may include a diet low in residue and high in calories and vitamins. Food may also be withheld or restricted to clear liquids,

followed by a soft diet in frequent small amounts. Raw fruits, vegetables, whole grains, and concentrated sweets would be avoided and added to the diet later.

Restoring Fluids and Electrolytes

Fluid and electrolyte losses are a common complication of diarrhea. Infants and debilitated clients are especially susceptible to this complication. In fact, age is a significant factor when a person has diarrhea. A young infant can soon have a serious depletion of electrolytes, water, and nutrients unless the disorder is promptly corrected. Fluids and electrolytes must be replaced by either oral or parenteral (intravenous) therapy. Emphasize to the client that decreasing fluid intake will not stop the diarrhea.

Using a Bedpan

Many clients need to use a bedpan for elimination, including those restricted to bedrest because of a fracture, recent surgery, or other illness. A client receiving an enema or who has diarrhea may need to use a bedpan as well.

Bedpans come in two styles: a regular bedpan and a fracture bedpan. The regular and fracture bedpans shown in Figure 34–7 are made of metal or plastic. Fracture bedpans were developed for clients with fractures of the lower limbs who could not elevate easily to have a regular bedpan placed. Because of the ease of

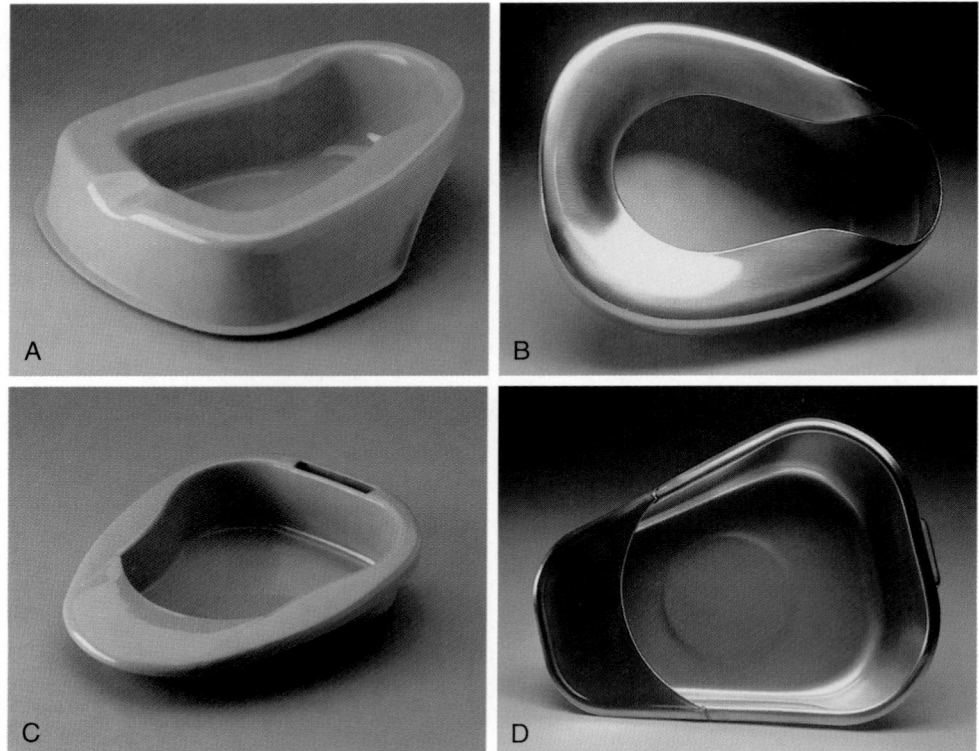

Figure 34–7. Types of bedpans. *A,* regular bedpan—plastic; *B,* regular bedpan—metal; *C,* fracture bedpan—plastic; *D,* fracture bedpan—metal. (*A* and *C,* courtesy of Bemis Health Care, Inc., Sheboygan Falls, WI; *B* and *D,* courtesy of Vollrath Group, Inc., Gallaway, TN.)

use of the fracture bedpans, it is becoming a common practice to use fracture bedpans with all clients. A metal bedpan of any style is cold; if possible warm it before use by running warm water over its edges. This is not necessary for plastic bedpans.

You can place a bedpan by having the client lift his hips and sliding it under him. Or you can have him roll onto his side, place the bedpan against his buttocks, and have him roll back onto his back. You will need to judge the best method for placing a bedpan for each client. Either way, the closed lip end of the bedpan should be placed under the buttocks, making sure that it is positioned to collect the waste (Fig. 34–8).

Preventing Skin Breakdown

Skin care is especially important for the client with diarrhea. Provide the client with soft material for wiping after each stool to help reduce the irritation. Also, washing the client's perianal area with soap and water

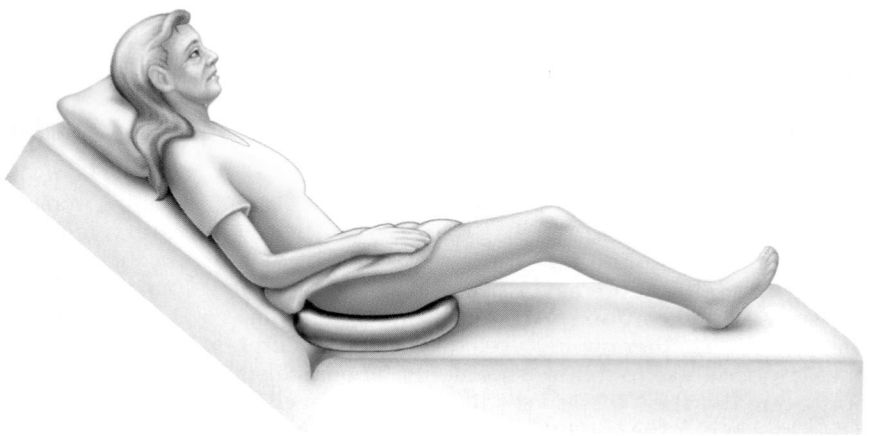

Figure 34–8. Proper client position on a bedpan.

BOX 34–5

DEFINITION AND PRACTICE ACTIVITIES FOR BOWEL INCONTINENCE CARE

Definition

Promotion of bowel continence and maintenance of perianal skin integrity.

Activities

- Determine physical or psychological cause of fecal incontinence.
- Explain to client etiology of problem and rationale for actions.
- Determine goals of bowel management program with client or family.
- Discuss procedures and expected outcomes with client.
- Instruct client or family to record fecal output, as appropriate.

- Wash client's perianal area with soap and water and dry it thoroughly after each bowel movement.
- Use nonionic detergent preparation, such as Peri-Wash, for cleansing, as appropriate.
- Use powder and creams on perianal area with caution.
- Keep bed and clothing clean.
- Implement bowel training program, as appropriate.
- Monitor for adequate bowel evacuation.
- Monitor diet and fluid requirements.
- Monitor for side effects of medication administration.
- Use rectal pouch, as appropriate.
- Empty rectal pouch, as needed.
- Place client on incontinence pads, as appropriate.
- Provide protective pants, as needed.

From McCloskey, J.C., & Bulechek, G. (1996). Nursing interventions classification (2nd ed.). St. Louis: Mosby-Year Book.

after each stool reduces the time that irritating diarrhea stays in contact with the skin.

Ensuring Privacy

The frequency and urgency of bowel movements causes fatigue and embarrassment. Therefore, make sure that the client has quick and easy access to the bathroom, commode, or bedpan. Place the call bell nearby at all times. Provide for privacy and odor control.

Interventions to Restore Bowel Continence

Interventions for bowel incontinence include promoting continence through bowel training and maintenance of skin integrity. Caring for the skin of an incontinent person may be a time-consuming task. The main goal is to prevent prolonged contact between the skin and fecal material, which leads to excoriation and breakdown. Box 34–5 lists the definition and practice activities for bowel incontinence care.

Maintaining Skin Integrity

Washing the perianal area with soap and water and drying it thoroughly after each stool keeps the skin in good condition and controls fecal odor. Nonionic detergent preparations (such as Peri-Wash) are even more effective than regular soap. Use powders and creams with caution because they may contribute to skin breakdown.

Application of a rectal incontinence pouch for a client with bowel incontinence protects the skin and the bed linens (Fig. 34–9). The rectal pouch has a circular

paper adhesive backing that adheres to the perianal skin. An attached plastic bag collects the feces. The adhesive opening can be altered in size to facilitate individual fitting. Perianal hair should be shaved to allow a tight fit of the adhesive back.

If a rectal pouch is not in use, the bed and clothing of the incontinent person must be kept clean. When using plastic or rubber sheeting to protect bed linens, make sure that it does not contact the skin, thus caus-

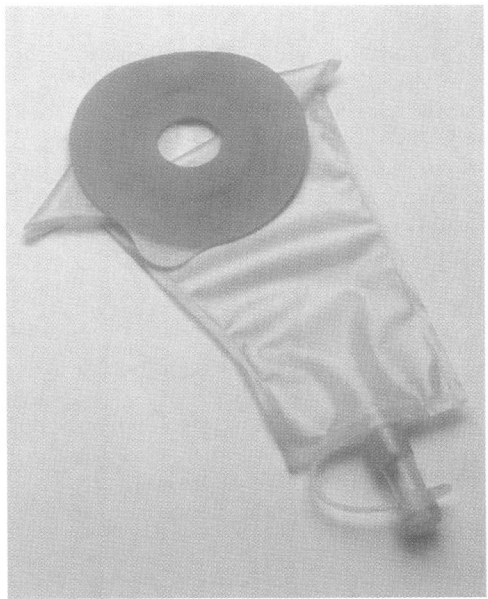

Figure 34–9. A rectal incontinence pouch. (Reproduced with permission of Hollister Incorporated, Libertyville, IL.)

ing irritation. A client with severe incontinence may need to wear waterproof undergarments to protect clothing. Adult-size disposable briefs are available with cellulose padding to draw fluid away from the skin by capillary action. However, diapers make the person feel infantile and appear to give "permission" to be incontinent. Avoid using them whenever possible. The best way to reduce the physiological and psychological effects of incontinence is to re-establish bowel control.

Providing Bowel Training

Bowel training programs are effective for regaining bowel control. They require time, patience, and commitment from nurses and the client, but the results are well worth the effort. Box 34–6 lists the definitions and practice activities for bowel training.

First, assess and diagnose the factors causing the incontinence. Then, discuss bowel training with the

---

BOX 34–6

DEFINITION AND PRACTICE ACTIVITIES FOR BOWEL TRAINING

Definition

Assisting the client to train the bowel to evacuate at specific intervals.

Activities

- Plan a bowel program with the client and appropriate others.
- Consult with physician and client regarding use of suppositories.
- Teach client or family the principles of bowel training.
- Instruct client about which foods are high in bulk.
- Provide foods high in bulk or those identified as helpful by the client.
- Ensure adequate fluid intake.
- Ensure adequate exercise.
- Initiate an uninterrupted, consistent time for defecation.
- Ensure privacy.
- Administer suppository, as appropriate.
- Perform digital rectal dilatation, as necessary.
- Teach the client digital rectal dilatation, as appropriate.
- Evaluate client's bowel status regularly.
- Modify bowel program, as needed.

From McCloskey, J.C., & Bulechek, G. (1996). Nursing interventions classification (2nd ed.). St. Louis: Mosby-Year Book.

---

client and significant others. Together, decide on a routine for bowel elimination. Base the routine on the person's previous bowel habits and on alterations in bowel habits that have resulted from illness or trauma. In addition, note when the client is most likely to be incontinent during the day.

All bowel training programs include independent nursing measures used to aid normal defecation: diet, fluids, exercise, and maintenance of defecation patterns. Probably the most crucial element of the program is timing. The schedule for defecation should be carefully determined and then strictly followed. If possible, position the client on the commode or toilet at the designated time to take advantage of gravity.

Bowel programming is individualized, although there are many common factors. Habit training, control of diarrhea, and biofeedback are possible strategies for bowel programming. Most programs include stool softeners to facilitate passage of feces. This intervention is especially important for clients with spinal cord injuries or extreme debilitation because they frequently cannot bear down. Suppositories may be used every 1 to 3 days to stimulate evacuation. In people with spinal cord injuries, the suppository is usually followed in 20 to 30 minutes by digital stimulation of the anal sphincter to augment stimulation of the defecation reflex. In some programs, enemas are used in place of the suppositories. Suppository or enema administration is usually discontinued as soon as bowel elimination can be maintained without them.

Modify the training program as needed until a successful routine is found. Generally, a person is kept on a particular program for at least 3 days before it is changed. This period allows you to be sure that changes are indeed necessary.

Other methods of treating incontinence are available. For example, biofeedback therapy works for some people. This method helps the client modify the incontinence using feedback from instruments. Surgical intervention to create new tissue sphincters has been tried. And electrical stimulation of sphincter control has also been successful in some cases.

Interventions to Reduce Flatulence

The goal of therapy is to remove gas from the GI tract. The most effective and natural way to expel the flatus is by exercise. Exercise stimulates peristalsis, which speeds the transit time of the gas through the colon. Walking is the best method but, if this is not possible, moving around in bed will help. Prevention is also important. Teach clients to avoid situations and substances that cause flatulence. Box 34–7 lists the definition and practice activities for reducing flatulence.

If simple, natural methods fail, you may need to use a rectal tube to allow gas to escape from the body. To insert a rectal tube into an adult, lubricate a No. 22 to No. 32 French rubber or plastic rectal tube and insert it about 10 cm (4 inches) into the rectum. Place the

BOX 34–7

DEFINITION AND PRACTICE ACTIVITIES FOR REDUCING FLATULENCE

Definition

Prevention of flatus formation and facilitation of passage of excessive gas.

Activities

- Teach client how flatus is produced and review methods for alleviation.
- Teach client to avoid situations that cause excessive air swallowing, such as chewing gum, drinking carbonated beverages, eating rapidly, sucking through straws, chewing with an open mouth, or talking with a full mouth.
- Teach client to avoid foods that cause flatulence, such as beans, cabbage, radishes, onions, cauliflower, and cucumbers.
- Monitor client for a bloated feeling, abdominal dis-

tension, cramping pains, and excessive passage of gas from the mouth or anus.
- Monitor bowel sounds.
- Monitor vital signs.
- Provide for adequate exercise, such as ambulation.
- Insert lubricated nasogastric tube or rectal tube into the rectum, as appropriate. Tape it in place and insert the distal end of the tube into a receptacle.
- Administer a laxative, suppository, or enema, as appropriate.
- Monitor side effects of medication administration.
- Limit oral intake, if lower gastrointestinal system is inactive.
- Position client on left side with knees flexed, as appropriate.
- Offer antiflatulence medications, as appropriate.

From McCloskey, J.C., & Bulechek, G. (1996). Nursing interventions classification (2nd ed.). St. Louis: Mosby-Year Book.

distal end of the tube into a collecting receptacle to catch any feces that may be expelled. Tape the tube in place and leave it there for 20 minutes or less. Longer periods may cause sphincter damage. Reinsert the tube every 2 or 3 hours if necessary.

A return-flow enema (Harris flush) also relieves flatulence, although this intervention is controversial because it can cause intestinal trauma. In this procedure, the rectum is alternately filled and drained to move flatus by stimulating peristalsis. Prepare the client, the equipment, and the solution (tap water or saline) as shown earlier in Procedure 34–2. After inserting the rectal tube, infuse about 200 to 300 mL of fluid into the colon. Then lower the solution container 45 cm (18 inches) below the level of the anus to allow the solution and flatus to drain back into the reservoir. Expelled gas bubbles up through the solution in the container. When the return flow ceases, raise the reservoir 45 cm above the anus and allow 200 to 300 mL to flow in. Repeat this process until the returned gas is minimal.

Several medications may help to relieve flatulence. Simethicone-containing medications cause gas bubbles to coalesce, making them easier to expel. Some physicians order neostigmine to be given intramuscularly about 20 minutes before a rectal tube or return flow enema is administered. Neostigmine increases gastrointestinal (GI) motility and facilitates downward movement of the gas. However, this practice is controversial because of the drug's numerous side effects, such as dizziness, severe abdominal cramping, respiratory depression, and nausea and vomiting. If postnasal drip

causes excessive air swallowing, a decongestant or antihistamine may eliminate the problem.

Interventions to Manage Fecal Diversions

As with any condition, fecal diversions must be assessed to detect problems and determine appropriate nursing interventions. Physiological problems vary depending on whether the type of ostomy is an ileostomy or colostomy (Fig. 34–10).

The major problems with ileostomies are obstruction, diarrhea, and skin irritation. Obstruction is prevented by chewing food thoroughly, and can usually be relieved by massaging the abdomen around the stoma or by gentle lavage (washing out) of the stoma with a catheter. Diarrhea is treated as described earlier. The person with an ileostomy is particularly susceptible to fluid and electrolyte imbalances. Therefore, diarrhea must be quickly controlled.

Skin irritation is best treated by preventive measures, such as proper fitting and fixation of the collection bag. If irritation does occur, the skin must be kept clean and dry, and a protective skin barrier should be used between the pouch faceplate and the skin. Use topical medications to treat severe irritation.

Emptying and Changing the Ostomy Pouch or Bag

Except for continent ileostomies, ostomies continually drain fecal material. After surgery, and after the stoma heals, the client is fitted with a reusable ostomy pouch or bag. (A client with a colostomy usually wears an os-

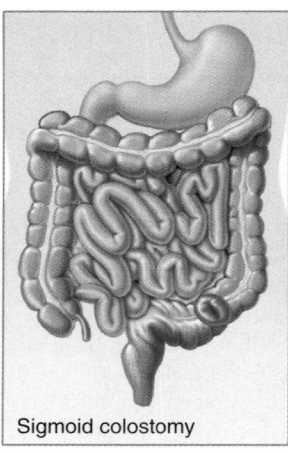
Sigmoid colostomy

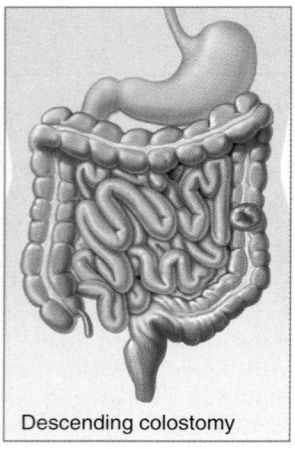
Descending colostomy

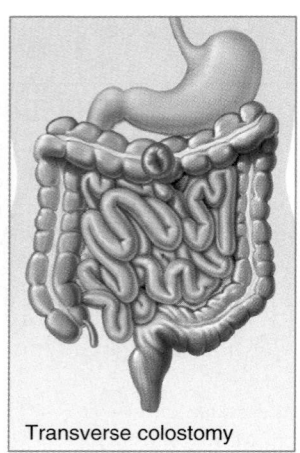
Transverse colostomy

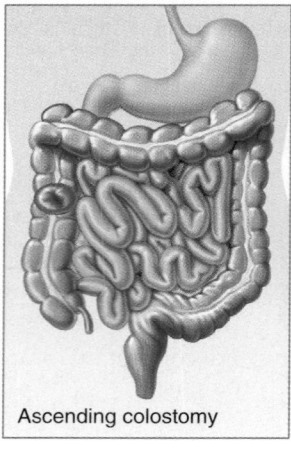
Ascending colostomy

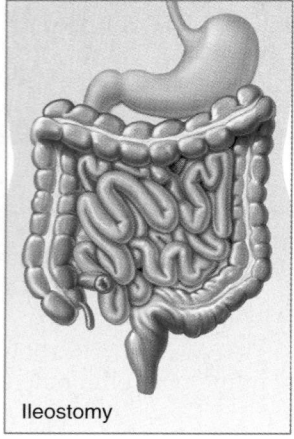
Ileostomy

Figure 34–10. Locations of ileostomies and colostomies.

tomy pouch rather than an ostomy bag). Regardless of whether the client has a continent ileostomy or a colostomy, however, the ostomy pouch or bag must be emptied at regular intervals.

The client empties the pouch or bag whenever necessary (typically at the time of urination) through an opening at the bottom. To do so, the client removes the clamp from the end of the pouch or bag, places the end into the toilet, and lets the pouch or bag drain (Fig. 34–11). Once the pouch or bag is

empty, the client replaces the clamp on the end until it needs emptying again.

In addition to emptying an ostomy pouch or bag, the appliance needs to be changed when it is loose, or about every 3 days (Fig. 34–12). When an ostomy bag needs to be changed, the old pouch and stoma wafer are removed. The stoma and skin are washed with warm water and soap. To replace the appliance, the stoma is first measured to ensure a proper fit. Once the size of the stoma has been measured, the stoma wafer is then cut to the proper size. If the client is very active, a special skin prep is applied to the skin as a protectant. Next, an adhesive paste is applied. The backing material is removed from the stoma wafer, and the center hole of the stoma wafer is placed over the stoma with light pressure applied to ensure adherence to the skin. The ostomy pouch or bag is then snapped onto the ring of the stoma wafer. The ostomy pouch or bag may be closed or open at the end, depending on the location of the stoma and the client's preference.

Irrigating the Bowel

A colostomy can function adequately without irrigation, but irrigation helps to avoid fecal spillage during the day. Most clients are taught to care for their stomas

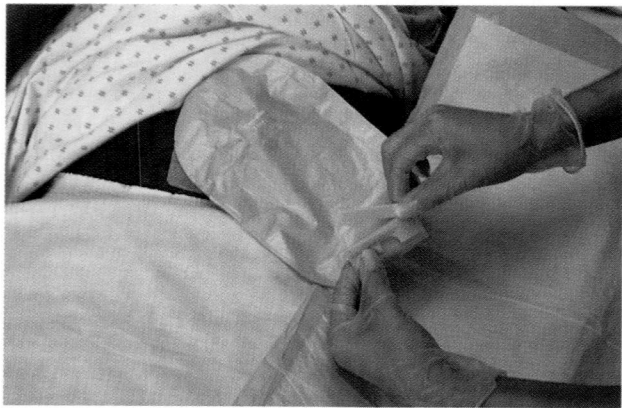

Figure 34–11. Emptying an ostomy pouch or bag.

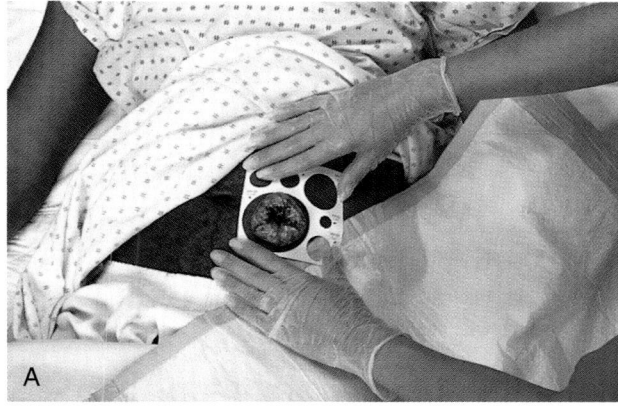

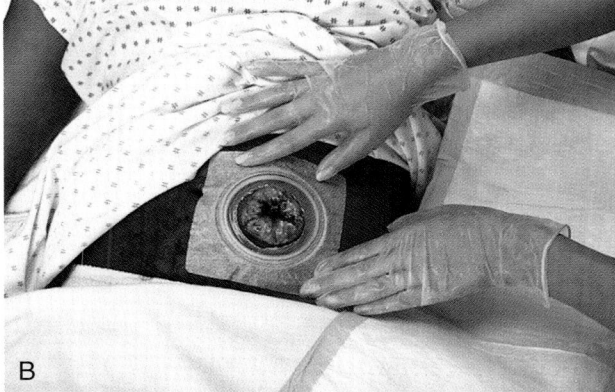

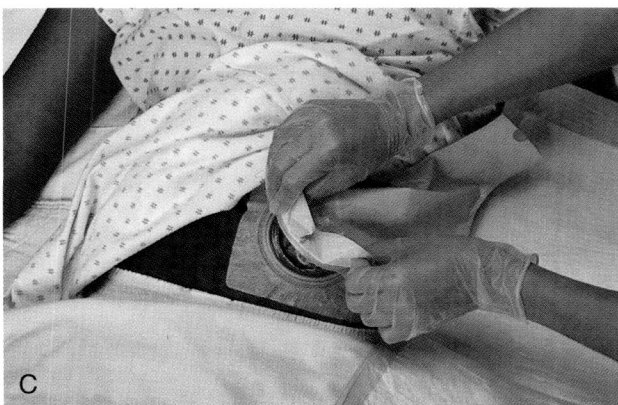

Figure 34–12. Changing an ostomy pouch or bag. *A,* measure the stoma size to ensure a proper fit. *B,* place the center hole of the stoma wafer over the stoma. *C,* snap the ostomy pouch or bag onto the ring of the stoma wafer.

and irrigate the bowel if necessary. If a client with a stoma comes into the hospital, he may continue his own care if able. If not, you may temporarily assume these tasks.

Irrigation of a colostomy is very similar to administration of a normal saline enema. The major differences are the insertion site and the client's inability to control the expulsion of solution and fecal material. Consequently, some variation in equipment and technique is necessary. An irrigation sleeve channels the expelled contents into the toilet or bedpan. It is a

plastic tunnel that fits around the stoma and is held in place by a belt around the waist (Fig. 34–13). The irrigating solution and enema equipment are prepared as for a volume enema. Cone-shaped irrigation tips are preferred to catheters because they reduce the danger of bowel perforation. The nipple cone also seals off the stoma so that the irrigating fluid cannot leak. Make sure of the location of the stoma before inserting the cone. If using a catheter, gently insert it about 7.5 to 10 cm (3 to 4 inches) and infuse the enema.

When you are ready to remove the administration tip, be sure the irrigating sleeve is well in front of the stoma, since the initial drainage may gush out. Close the top of the sleeve with clips, and allow most of the content to be expelled. This usually takes about 10 to 15 minutes. Control odor by occasionally rinsing the sleeve with water and flushing the toilet. When the client is sure that the irrigation returns have finished, the irrigation sleeve may be removed, peristomal skin cleaned, and either a clean pouch or dressing applied.

Teaching the Client Ostomy Self-Care

A client with an ostomy should be taught to live independently and care for his ostomy needs on his own, if possible. Changing the ostomy pouch or bag is the first step in learning and is the same as the procedure outlined above. If the client will be irrigating the colostomy, the irrigation procedure needs to be taught. Odor control and medication use are other topics of concern, as outlined in the accompanying Teaching for Self-Care chart.

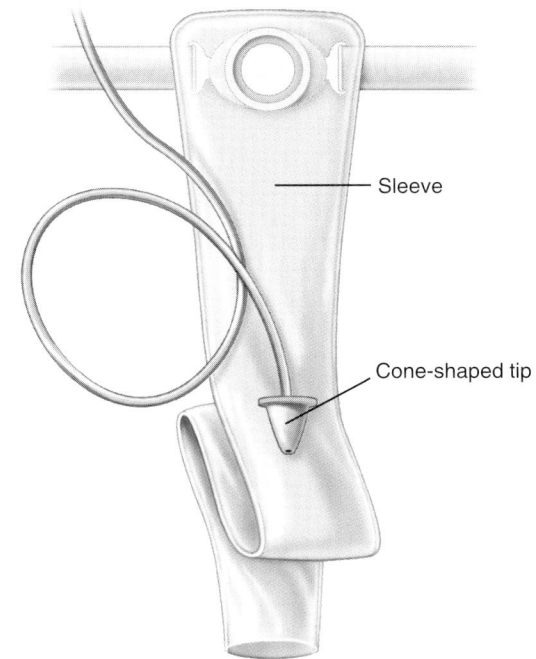

Sleeve

Cone-shaped tip

Figure 34–13. Sleeve and cone-shaped tip for colostomy irrigation.

Teaching for SELF-CARE

OSTOMY CARE

Goal: To make the client independent in the management of bowel elimination in the presence of an ostomy.

Rationale: Self-care skills are needed to promote health and return the client to his usual lifestyle.

Expected Outcome: The client will demonstrate the ability to manage bowel elimination through an ostomy, prevent complications, and manage lifestyle changes.

Client Instructions

Maintain a regular bowel elimination pattern by following these steps:

- Plan for daily elimination at a time most consistent with the your urge to defecate.
- Keep in mind that regular patterns of meals and activity may be helpful.

Maintain the necessary supplies:

- Skin barriers.
- Ostomy pouches.
- A pouch belt, if needed.
- Clamps or closing devices.
- Hypoallergenic tape.
- Towel and washclothes.
- A mild skin cleanser.

Use a pouching system to collect waste from the bowel:

- Ensure a proper fit of the pouch to prevent leaks and protect your skin.
- Measure the stoma diameter and prepare a skin barrier/pouch with each pouch change. The opening should be no more than ⅛ inch larger than your stoma. Measure the stoma weekly for at least 8 weeks or until the stoma has stopped shrinking.
- Apply the skin barrier first. Then ensure that there are no wrinkles in the barrier. Apply the pouch to the barrier.
- Center and apply the pouch. Practice applying the pouch while sitting and standing.
- Change the appliance any time it leaks or is not intact.
- To remove the ostomy appliance, support the skin of your abdomen and gently loosen the seal.
- Cleanse the skin around the stoma. Waste from an ileostomy is especially irritating to the skin.
- Use a mild soap and carefully dry the area with a clean cloth or towel.

Empty the pouch when necessary:

- Choose an ostomy pouch with an open end or a closed end. An open-ended pouch is best for liquid wastes, and the bag can be emptied without changing it.
- Use a clamp that you can manage easily, given your eyesight and manual dexterity.
- Empty the pouch when it is one-third full.
- To close the pouch, fold the tail up once around the bar of the clamp and fasten the clamp.
- If you have a urinary diversion, use a night drainage system to prevent the pouch from overfilling while you are asleep.

Keep in mind the following lifestyle tips:

- Avoid foods that cause odor and gas.
- Do whatever you need to to avoid constipation.
- Treat diarrhea promptly.
- Check periodically to make sure that your ostomy is not blocked.
- Drink six to eight glasses of water daily, 10 to 12 if you have an ileostomy.
- Exercise regularly, especially to strengthen abdominal muscles.
- You can bathe and shower with or without the pouch.
- You can swim with the pouch, but use waterproof tape around edges of the pouch in a picture-frame fashion.
- You can continue to wear your normal wardrobe after an ostomy. No change in clothing is necessary.

Manage skin irritation:

- Assess for irregularities in the skin that might cause leaks.
- Use a skin barrier to protect the skin.
- Use a skin barrier paste, if needed, to fill in any abdominal creases or irregular contours.
- Change pouching systems to maintain or create a well-functioning appliance.
- Add an ostomy belt, if needed.
- Notify your health care provider if you detect the following signs and symptoms of a candida (yeast) infection: itching, burning, pain around the stoma, redness of the skin, or whiteheads (pustules).
- Apply an antifungal powder or spray, such as Mycostatin, to the skin around the stoma.

Follow a dietary plan:

- Follow a well-balanced diet.
- Watch for foods that cause gas or changes in the consistency of your stool.
- Avoid foods that tend to block your stoma.

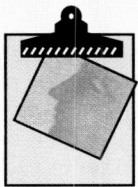

NURSING CARE PLANNING
A CLIENT WITH CONSTIPATION

Admission Data

Dr. Daly reported that, yesterday, he consumed only one-fourth of his usual intake of prune juice and bran flakes for breakfast. He consumed only half of his other two meals because of severe pain from bone cancer. He reported that he was concerned about increasing his morphine for fear of falling and other side effects.

   Because Dr. Daly is having difficulty with his bowel elimination this morning, the nurse realizes that his nursing diagnosis of *Constipation* may lead to impaction.

Physician's Orders

Diet as desired
Laxative of choice

Nursing Assessment

Dr. Daly has not had his usual bowel movement in 3 days, his bowel sounds are hypoactive, and a fecal mass can be palpated in his lower abdomen. Therefore, the nurse considers the possibility of an impaction.

NURSING CARE PLAN

Nursing Diagnosis	Expected Outcomes	Interventions	Evaluation (After 24 Hours of Care)
Constipation related to decreased mobility and morphine use	**Bowel elimination:** • Elimination pattern in expected range. • Stool soft and formed.	**Bowel management:** • Note date of last bowel movement (BM). • Monitor BM frequency, consistency, shape, volume, and color.	• Laxative administered *at client's request.* Large, hard, formed BM today.
	• Constipation not present.	• Monitor bowel sounds. • Report diminished bowel sounds.	
	• Ease of stool passage.	• Monitor for signs and symptoms of constipation and impaction.	• Passage was difficult.
	• Comfort of stool passage.	• Teach about alternative foods that help in promoting bowel regularity. • Instruct in foods that are high in fiber. • Give warm liquids after meals as appropriate. • Evaluate medication profile for GI side effects. • *Allow client choices in bowel management.*	• *Dr. Daly chooses to continue his usual routine.*

Italicized interventions indicate culturally specific care.

Critical Thinking Questions

1. How would you prevent further constipation in Dr. Daly?
2. Is reducing the dose of morphine an acceptable method of preventing constipation in this client?
3. The client prefers to use fiber as a means of managing constipation. What would you say to him about continuing to use this method?

For the ostomate who wears a pouch, odor control can be a problem. Careful washing, pouch deodorizers, and medications are possible solutions. The client should also avoid gas-forming foods. Cabbage, cauliflower, onions, and turnips often increase fecal odor. Yogurt, buttermilk, parsley, and green leafy vegetables may reduce fecal odor. Odor control, which can be very distressing, can be managed by the following:

- Carefully washing the appliance after use
- Placing a deodorizing agent in the pouch
- Using internal medications, such as bismuth subgallate
- Ingesting yogurt, buttermilk, parsley, or orange juice
- Placing a few drops of Dispatch in the collection receptacle to mask the odor while emptying the pouch

Review of the new ostomate's medication regimen can help eliminate contraindicated medications. Diuretics, laxatives, enteric-coated medications, and sustained-release oral medications are usually not administered for the ileostomate and some colostomates.

EVALUATION

Evaluation of nursing care for the management of bowel elimination problems involves making decisions about the expected time frame for the intervention to be successful, ongoing monitoring, and measuring the parameters of the outcome criteria. Decision-making is centered around whether the problem is acute or chronic. Look for data that suggest the problem is improving, the client is participating in care, and the problem is resolving.

Evaluation of the effectiveness of interventions for constipation is based on ongoing assessment to determine that the problem is resolving. When the problem is constipation, the client should have a bowel movement usually within 24 hours of the onset of treatment. Collect data to determine that the signs and symptoms of constipation are not persistent. When the problem is chronic, data are collected over time to determine that the client establishes a regular pattern of elimination without the signs and symptoms of constipation. See the Nursing Care Planning chart.

The evaluation of the effectiveness of interventions for diarrhea requires ongoing monitoring to determine that the diarrhea is resolving, usually within the first 24 hours. Monitor for signs of dehydration and electrolyte loss. Intake and output measurements should be taken. The time frame for diarrhea resolution is directly related to the cause of the diarrhea. For example, some viral infections may have a natural course of 24 to 48 hours. On the other hand, a client with inflammatory bowel disease will have outcome criteria that suggest the problem is controlled rather than cured.

For the problem of fecal impaction, the initial outcome criterion is that the client will have the impaction removed. Long-term goals are set to prevent the problem from recurring. The client's bowel management program must be modified on an ongoing basis.

For the problem of bowel incontinence, the time frame for evaluation depends on the cause of the problem. If the cause is a medication combined with weakness from an acute illness, the problem can often be resolved quickly. If the problem is a permanent change in mental status combined with immobility, management will be ongoing. It may take several weeks to determine the best schedule of toileting to prevent bowel incontinence.

KEY PRINCIPLES

- The lower GI tract is the main organ system responsible for the elimination of the body's solid waste. It consists of the ascending, transverse, descending, and sigmoid portions of the colon, and the rectum.
- Physiological and psychosocial factors have a strong influence on the act of defecation.
- Assessment of bowel elimination needs includes noting the history of psychological and physiological factors affecting elimination; completing a physical assessment of the abdomen and observing fecal characteristics; and noting the outcome of diagnostic tests completed by x-ray examination, direct visualization, and laboratory analysis.
- The current NANDA list of nursing diagnoses relevant to bowel elimination needs includes *Bowel incontinence, Constipation, Perceived constipation,* and *Diarrhea.*
- The nurse does not order diagnostic tests but, along with assessment findings, does use the results in diagnosing nursing problems.
- Interventions to treat constipation would meet the goals of regular bowel elimination pattern.
- Interventions to treat diarrhea would meet the goals of no loose stools and a return of regular bowel elimination pattern.
- Interventions to treat bowel incontinence would meet the goals of maintaining skin integrity and promoting normal bowel elimination.
- Evaluation of outcomes should show that the fecal contents and bowel movements are as near to normal as possible for the client, or that the client has adapted successfully to elimination changes.

BIBLIOGRAPHY

Benton, J.M., O'Hara, P.A., Chen, H., Harper, D.W., & Johnston, S.F. (1997). Changing bowel hygiene practice successfully: A program to reduce laxative use in a chronic care hospital. *Geriatric Nursing, 18*(1)12–17.

*Blair, G.K., Djonlic, K., Fraser, G.C., Arnold, W.D., Murphy, J.J., & Irwin, B. (1992). The bowel management tube: An effective

---

*Asterisk indicates a classic or definitive work on this subject.

means for controlling fecal incontinence. *Journal of Pediatric Surgery, 27*(10), 1269–1272.

Block, K.L. (1997). The rest of the story about diet and cancer. *Bottom Line Health, 11*(10), 3–4.

Bohm, B., Milsom, J.W., & Fazio, V.W. (1995). Postoperative intestinal motility following conventional and laparoscopic intestinal surgery. *Archives of Surgery, 130*(4), 415–419.

Brown, E.W. (1995). An inexpensive and painful alternative to colonoscopy. *Medical Update, XIX*(2), 1, 4.

Camberg, L.C. (1996). Palliative care: How do you manage "other" distressing symptoms? *Geriatrics, 51*(10), 13–14.

Cockburn, J., Thomas, R.J., McLaughlin, S.J., & Reading D. (1995). Acceptance of screening for colorectal cancer by flexible sigmoidoscopy. *Journal of Medical Screening, 2*(2), 79–83.

Day, R.A., & Monsma, M. (1995). Fruitlax: Management of constipation in children with disabilities. *Clinical Nursing Research, 4*(3), 306–322.

Dean, O.E. (1995). When analgesia leads to constipation. *Nursing95, 25*(1), 31.

Doughty, D. (1996). A physiologic approach to bowel training. *Journal of Wound, Ostomy, and Continence Nursing, 23*(1), 46–56.

Gallands, L. (1997). How to be healthy. *Bottom Line Personal, 18*(24), 11–12.

*Gleeson, R.M. (1990). Bowel continence for the child with a neurogenic bowel. *Rehabilitation Nursing, 15*(6), 319–321.

Hall, G.R., Karstens, M., Rakel B., Swanson, E., & Davidson, A. (1995). Managing constipation using a research-based protocol. *MEDSURGNursing, 4*(1), 11–20.

Heitkemper, M., Levy, R.L., Jarrell, M., & Bond, E.F. (1995). Interventions for irritable bowel syndrome: A nursing model. *Gastroenterology Nursing, 18*(6), 224–30.

Held, J.L. (1995). Preventing and treating constipation. *Nursing 95, 25*(3), 26–27.

Helzlsouer, K. (1997). Is breakfast bran really GRRRREEAAT? *The Johns Hopkins Medical Letter, 9*(10), 1–2.

Johnson, M., & Mass, M. (Eds.) (1997). *Nursing outcomes classification (NOC).* St. Louis: Mosby-Year Book.

*Kovach, T. (1992). Managing geriatric chronic constipation. *Home Healthcare Nurse, 10*(5). 57–58.

McCloskey, J.C., & Bulechek, G.M. (Eds.). (1996). *Nursing interventions classification (NIC)* (2nd Ed.). St. Louis: Mosby-Year Book.

Maestri-Banks, A., & Burns, D. (1996). Assessing constipation. *Nursing Times, 92*(21), 28–30.

Moore, L., Shannon, M.L., Richard, P., & Vacca, G.R. (1995). Investigation of rocking as a postoperative intervention to promote gastrointestinal motility. *Gastroenterology Nursing, 18*(3), 87–91.

Moore, T. (1996). Describing and analyzing constipation in acute care. *Journal of Nursing Care Quality, 10*(3), 68–74.

North American Nursing Diagnosis Association. (1999). *Nursing Diagnoses: Definitions & Classification 1999–2000.* Philadelphia: Author.

O'Connor, T. (1995). How much does your patient drink? *International Journal of Nursing Practice, 1*(1), 65–66.

*Olszewski, L.M. (1991). The use of wheat bran to prevent constipation in orthopedic patients. *Orthopeadic Nursing, 10*(3), 8.

Reese, J.L., Means, M.E., Hanrahan, K., Clearman, B., Colwill. M., & Dawson, C. (1996). Diarrhea associated with nasogastric feedings. *Oncology Nursing Forum, 23*(1), 59–68.

*Venn, M.R., Taft, L., Carpenter, B., & Applebaugh, G. (1992). The influence of timing and suppository use on efficiency and effectiveness of bowel training after a stroke. *Rehabilitation Nursing, 17*(3), 116–120.

Wadle, K. (1991). Diarrhea. In M. Maas, K.C. Buckwalter, & M. Hardy (Eds.). *Nursing diagnosis and interventions for the elderly.* Redwood City, CA: Addison-Wesley.

Wright, P.S., & Thomas, S.L. (1995). Constipation and diarrhea: The neglected symptoms. *Seminars in Oncology Nursing, 11*(4), 289–297.

*Yakabowich, M. (1990). Prescribe with care: The role of laxatives in treatment of constipation. *Journal of Gerontological Nursing, 16*(7), 4–11.

35

Urinary Elimination

Helen Harkreader

Key Terms

anuria

bacteriuria

diuresis

dysuria

enuresis

hematuria

Kegel exercises

micturition

nocturia

oliguria

polyuria

reflex incontinence

stress incontinence

total incontinence

urge incontinence

urinalysis

urinary frequency

urinary hesitancy

urinary incontinence

urinary retention

urinary urgency

urination

void

LEARNING OBJECTIVES

After studying this chapter, you should be able to:

1. Describe the normal structure and function of the urinary system.
2. Identify common problems of urinary elimination.
3. Discuss factors affecting urinary elimination.
4. Assess urinary function and identify a client experiencing urinary elimination problems.
5. Diagnose problems of urinary elimination that can be managed with nursing care.
6. Plan goal-directed nursing interventions for managing problems in urinary elimination.
7. Implement basic nursing care for a client experiencing problems with urinary elimination.
8. Use expected outcomes as aids in evaluating care for a person experiencing problems with urinary elimination.

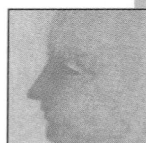

Fatami Shireem is a 60-year-old West Indian Hindu American who had a vaginal hysterectomy 2 days ago. She has an indwelling (Foley) catheter that is scheduled to be removed this morning. Her three daughters are present in the room; in the evening, several more family members are usually present. Although Mrs. Shireem has lived in the United States for 30 years, she speaks English with an accent and retains strong ties with the culture of her homeland. This is her first hospitalization.

The nurse knows that Mrs. Shireem will most likely need assistance in re-establishing a normal pattern of urinary elimination after removal of the catheter, and she considers the diagnosis of *Risk for urinary retention*. She also is concerned with providing privacy for the client during this highly personal aspect of nursing care.

URINARY ELIMINATION NURSING DIAGNOSES

Altered Urinary Elimination: The state in which the individual experiences a disturbance in urine elimination.

Stress Incontinence: The state in which an individual experiences a loss of urine of less than 50 mL occurring with increased abdominal pressure.

Reflex Urinary Incontinence: The state in which an individual experiences an involuntary loss of urine, occurring at somewhat predictable intervals when a specific bladder volume is reached.

Urge Incontinence: The state in which an individual experiences involuntary passage of urine occurring soon after a strong sense of urgency to void.

Functional Urinary Incontinence: The state in which an individual experiences an involuntary, unpredictable passage of urine.

Total Incontinence: The state in which an individual experiences a continuous and unpredictable loss of urine.

Risk for Urinary Urge Incontinence: Risk for involuntary loss of urine associated with a sudden, strong sensation or urinary urgency.

Urinary Retention: The state in which the individual experiences incomplete emptying of the bladder.

From North American Nursing Diagnosis Association (1999). NANDA nursing diagnoses: Definitions and classification 1999–2000. Philadelphia: Author.

CONCEPTS OF URINARY ELIMINATION

As a nurse, you will assess urinary elimination in a wide variety of clients to determine their health practices and to identify any urinary problems they may be having. For example, your client may be an outpatient who needs teaching to manage urinary dysfunction; the family of a homebound, disabled, incontinent person; or an older adult who has undergone a surgical procedure for cancer of the bladder. Additionally, community health nurses are involved with screening and health teaching to manage urinary elimination. Nursing diagnoses involve either incontinence or retention, but you also will assist clients with problems associated with infection, obstruction, and urinary diversion.

Normal urination depends on the production of urine, adequate function of the lower urinary tract, cognitive function, physical mobility, and access to toilet facilities. Personal habits and health practices may enhance or impede normal urinary elimination. Some urinary problems are associated with particular age groups.

Structure and Function of the Urinary System

The structures of the urinary system are the kidneys, ureters, bladder, and urethra (Fig. 35–1). The kidneys filter the blood to remove waste products from the body and to regulate water, electrolyte, and acid-base

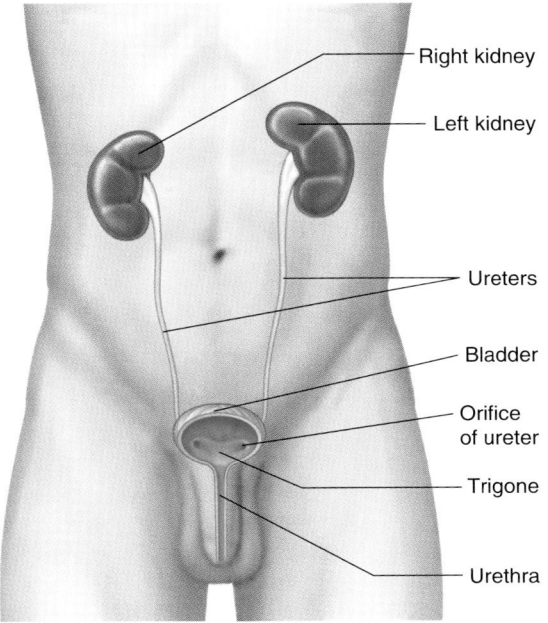

Figure 35–1. Structures of the urinary system.

balance. As a result, they produce urine. The ureters are two small muscular tubes that carry the urine from the kidneys to the bladder, where the urine remains until the bladder fills enough to produce an urge to urinate. Then urine is allowed to pass out of the body through the urethra.

Kidneys

The two bean-shaped kidneys are anatomically located for maximum protection of these vital organs. They are retroperitoneal, positioned on the upper, posterior wall of the abdomen outside the peritoneal cavity. They are protected posteriorly by the 11th and 12th ribs and anteriorly by the abdominal cavity.

The kidneys form and excrete urine through a process of filtering the blood and concentrating waste products for excretion. The waste products are urea (from metabolism of amino acids), creatinine (from muscle creatine), uric acid (from nucleic acids), the products of hemoglobin breakdown (such as bilirubin), and metabolites of various hormones (Guyton & Hall, 1996).

The kidneys also control the electrolyte composition of the blood and body fluids. Sodium and potassium are two important electrolytes controlled by the kidney. However, although the kidney excretes or conserves sodium in response to blood levels of sodium, it is a poor conservator of potassium. Most of the potassium that passes through the kidney is excreted. The kidney maintains the proper acid-base balance primarily by excreting or conserving bicarbonate ions and by excreting acids produced by the metabolism of proteins.

Adequate blood flow and oxygen are essential to renal function. Although each kidney is only about the size of an orange and weighs only about 150 g, the kidneys together receive a blood flow equal to about 21% of the cardiac output. The kidneys play a role in maintaining this blood flow through their ability to control arterial pressure. One mechanism by which the kidneys control arterial pressure is through the excretion of water and sodium. Another is through the excretion of renin from the juxtaglomerular cells. Renin contributes to the formation of vasoactive substances such as angiotensin II. The kidney is also self-protective through the production of erythropoietin in response to hypoxia, which in turn stimulates the production of red blood cells.

Action Alert!
Monitor urinary output as an indicator of renal function, especially when cardiac output is diminished, such as when the client is in a state of shock.

The nephron is the functional unit of the kidney and consists of a glomerulus and a tubule system. The glomerulus filters water, electrolytes, and waste products from the plasma, and the tubule system controls reabsorption to maintain a balance of electrolytes, buffers, and acids in the body. Glucose and amino acids are completely reabsorbed by the tubules. Many electrolytes are selectively reabsorbed, depending on the body's need. Waste products, such as creatinine, are almost completely excreted with little reabsorption. Once urine enters the pelvis of the kidney, it passes unchanged through the ureters to the bladder. Urine is about 95% water. In the renal nephron shown in Figure 35–2, notice the glomeru-

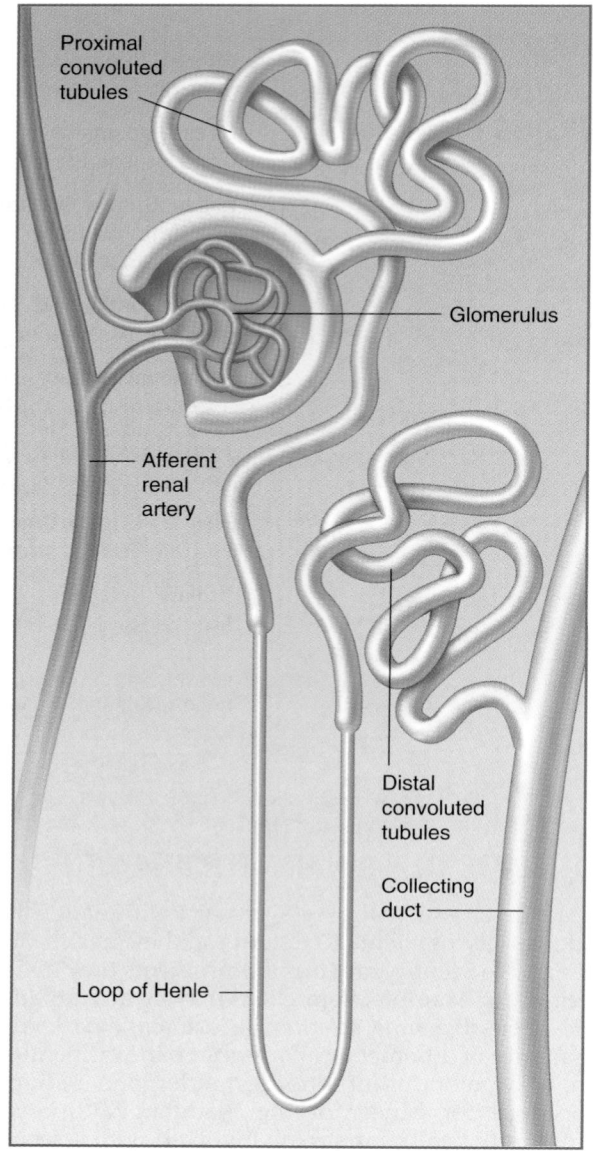

Figure 35–2. The renal nephron is a complex system consisting of the glomerulus, where the arterial blood is filtered, and the convoluted tubules and loop of Henle, where reabsorption controls acid-base and electrolyte balance.

lus, where the arterial blood is filtered, and the system of tubules that controls the resorption of water and electrolytes.

Ureters

The ureters are smooth, muscular tubes of small diameter that connect the kidneys to the bladder. Urine is propelled through the ureters by peristaltic waves. These peristaltic contractions are enhanced by parasympathetic stimulation and inhibited by sympathetic stimulation. The ureters are well supplied with nerve endings, and obstruction usually results in severe pain.

Bladder

The urinary bladder is a body cavity composed primarily of a smooth muscle known as the detrusor muscle. The mucosal surface of the detrusor lies in folds, or rugae, that allow for expansion of the bladder. The trigone muscle is a triangle-shaped muscle at the base of the posterior side of the bladder. The apex of the trigone is in the bladder neck at the posterior opening of the urethra. The ureters enter the bladder through the detrusor at the upper angles of the trigone.

Each ureter enters the bladder obliquely through the detrusor muscle and passes 1 to 2 cm through the detrusor before entering the body of the bladder at the upper trigone angle. The placement of the ureters through the detrusor muscle creates a vesicoureteral valve. The tone of the detrusor muscle collapses the ureter and prevents backflow of the urine into the ureters and renal pelvis. Incompetence of this valve allows urine reflux, or backward flow, into the renal pelvis, thus creating pressure on the nephrons. Excessive or prolonged pressure could cause renal damage.

The funnel-shaped bladder neck at the base of the bladder is 2 to 3 cm long and is composed of detrusor muscle and elastic tissue that forms the internal sphincter for the urethra. The internal sphincter prevents urine from entering the urethra until a critical pressure is reached.

The bladder is innervated by both sensory and motor nerves. The sensory fibers detect stretch in the bladder wall, especially in the posterior urethra. A conscious desire to urinate occurs when the bladder has filled, producing tension above a threshold level in the bladder wall. Bladder contractions occur as a reflex arc at the level of the second and third sacral vertebrae. The motor fibers are primarily parasympathetic, which contracts the detrusor and relaxes the trigone, thus aiding voiding. Sympathetic stimulation relaxes the detrusor and contracts the trigone muscle, thus inhibiting voiding.

Action Alert!
If a client is taking anticholinergic drugs, which inhibit the parasympathetic nervous system, you should observe for difficulty in voiding.

Urethra

The urethra is a small tubular structure that drains urine from the bladder to the outside of the body. Its mucous membrane is continuous with that of the bladder. Contraction of the detrusor muscle increases pressure in the bladder to produce the urge to urinate and to aid emptying of the bladder. The urge to urinate is experienced when pressure in the bladder overcomes the internal sphincter and urine enters the urethra.

The urethra also has an external sphincter composed of voluntary skeletal muscle in the floor of the pelvis. It can be contracted consciously to prevent urination. Urination requires relaxation of the external sphincter. When the person is ready to urinate, the external sphincter is consciously relaxed and the abdominal muscles are contracted to assist in **micturition,** the process of emptying the bladder.

The urethra in females is about 3 cm (1.5 inches) long. It curves obliquely downward and forward. In males, the urethra is about 20 cm (8 to 9 inches) long. It has a double curve when the penis is flaccid and a single curve when the penis is erect. The male urethra also serves as a passageway for semen to exit the body. The male prostate gland lies at the neck of the bladder, about 1.5 inches from where the ureters enter the bladder, and it surrounds the urethra. Figure 35–3 illustrates the male and female genitourinary tracts.

Physiology of Urination

Urination is the term commonly used for the act of micturition. **Void** is a term synonymous with micturition and urination that you will hear most often in clinical settings. Clients may or may not be familiar with these terms and may instead use slang or vernacular expressions to refer to urination.

As the bladder fills, waves of contractions begin. They occur every 5 to 60 seconds. With each contraction, the pressure rises and the person may feel an urge to void. At this point, however, voiding can easily be delayed. If a person waits less than a minute, the urge usually passes. When the bladder reaches a volume of 300 to 400 mL of urine, pressure rises rapidly and the urge to void becomes strong. Keep in mind, however, that bladder size is an important component of the urge to void. For example, very young and very old people may have small bladders. The urge to void may be strong when the bladder reaches only about 150 mL.

The cerebral cortex exerts final control over voiding. Normally, all the urine is emptied from the bladder, but 5 to 10 mL may remain.

Problems With Urinary Elimination

As a nurse, you will encounter clients with various problems of urinary elimination, such as dysuria, altered amounts of urine, enuresis, incontinence, retention, urinary tract infection, obstruction, or diversion.

Dysuria

Dysuria refers to difficult or painful urination. It may be accompanied by frequency, hesitancy, or urgency of urination. **Urinary frequency** refers to urination that occurs at shorter-than-usual intervals without an increase in daily urine output. **Urinary hesitancy** refers to a delay in starting the urine stream, commonly with a decreased force of the stream. **Urinary urgency** is a sudden, forceful urge to urinate. Further assessment is needed to determine the cause of these problems.

Often, dysuria is related to irritation, inflammation, or obstruction of the lower urinary tract, where sensory nerve endings are plentiful. Pain immediately before voiding may be related to an irritated or distended bladder. Pain at the start of the stream indi-

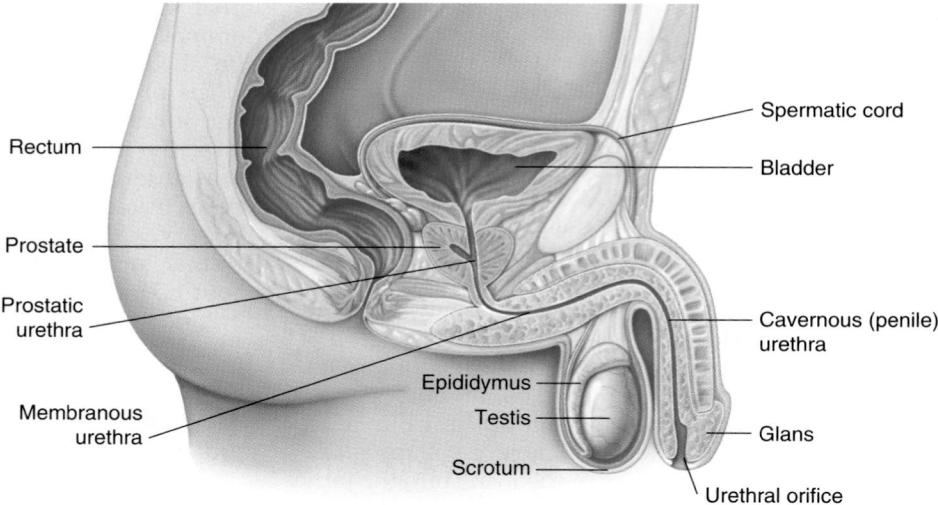

A

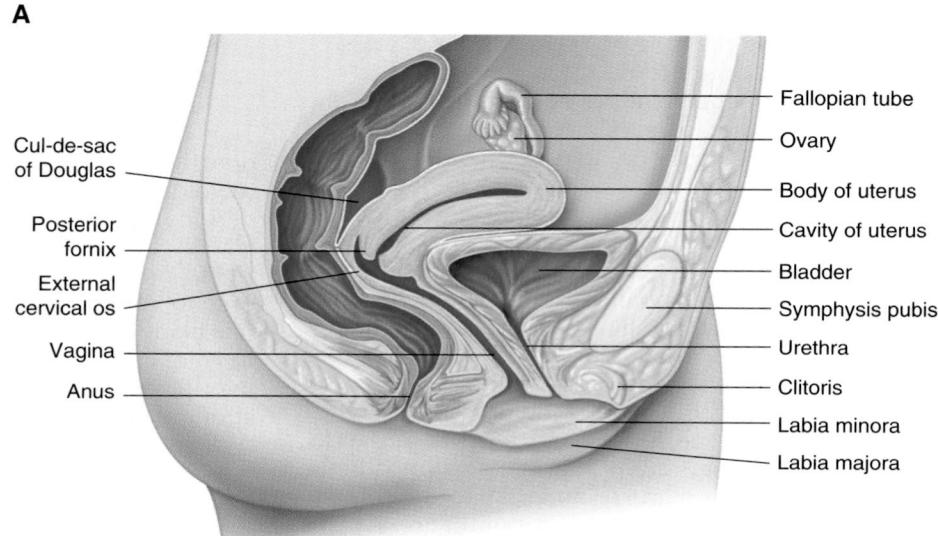

B

Figure 35–3. *A* and *B*, the male and female genitourinary tract. In the female, the bladder is anterior and inferior to the uterus. The urethra opens immediately anterior to the vagina.

cates an irritated bladder neck. Pain at the end of voiding is usually associated with bladder spasms.

Action Alert!
Ask questions to determine the specific timing and nature of pain associated with dysuria.

Altered Amount

The amount of urine varies normally with the amount of fluid ingested and the amount lost through the skin, lungs, and bowels. However, altered amounts of urine can also indicate health problems. **Oliguria** is a diminished, scanty amount of urine. It can result from dehydration, a lower-than-normal volume of body water that in turn reduces urine output. Production of less than 30 mL of urine per hour may reflect a blood flow that is inadequate to maintain renal function. This can result in permanent kidney damage.

Anuria is the absence of urine, usually clinically defined as less than 100 mL in 24 hours. It occurs in renal failure, shock, or dehydration.

Polyuria is a large amount of urine usually associated with diabetes mellitus or diabetes insipidus. Diabetes insipidus results from failure of the pituitary gland to secrete the antidiuretic hormone. It is sometimes seen with head injuries. A person who produces more than 1,500 mL of urine in 24 hours may have polyuria, although you must always consider urine output in relation to the client's intake of fluids. Diabetes mellitus is a disturbance in the utilization of glucose secondary to inadequate production of insulin.

Enuresis

Enuresis is recurrent involuntary urination that occurs during sleep. Bed-wetting during sleep is not considered a problem until a child has reached the age when bladder control can reasonably be expected. For example, only about 30% of 4-year-olds and 7% of 8-year-olds wet the bed during sleep.

However, bed-wetting without a functional disorder does occur in a small percentage of older children, even as late as adolescence. Functional nocturnal enuresis typically runs in families and is sometimes associated with Stage IV sleep, a small bladder capacity, allergy attacks, and urinary tract infections. It may be related to the maturity of the brain and the production of antidiuretic hormone during the night. All children without underlying medical problems grow out of enuresis.

Action Alert!
If parents have concerns about a child's enuresis, provide information and instructions about whether to see a physician for an evaluation. Although only a small number of children have physical problems underlying enuresis, a thorough physical examination is important to rule out underlying causes.

Urinary Incontinence

Urinary incontinence is the involuntary passage of urine. It can be transient (acute) or persistent (chronic). Transient incontinence may develop from a medical or surgical condition and resolves when the underlying cause is removed. Persistent incontinence continues over time and may become worse. However, it is often treatable.

Persistent incontinence is highly associated with the cognitive and physical impairments associated with advanced age. Identifying the specific type of persistent incontinence experienced by a client (stress, urge, overflow, reflex, and functional) may be useful in selecting interventions, but incontinence commonly results from a mix of problems and may respond only to a comprehensive treatment approach.

Urinary incontinence affects about 13 million Americans. The prevalence of incontinence increases with age, but it should not be considered a normal part of the aging process. The reported incidence of incontinence in the noninstitutionalized elderly ranges from 15% to 35%. For institutionalized or homebound elderly, the incidence exceeds 50% (AHCPR, 1996).

Incontinence is strongly associated with factors leading to institutionalization, such as dementia and immobility. In the noninstitutionalized, incontinence interferes with excursions outside the home, social interactions, and sexual activity. It may threaten self-esteem and independent living. Often, minor incontinence is managed independently to the person's satisfaction and never reported to a health care provider. Correctable causes of incontinence include infection, cystocele, rectocele, vaginitis, and uterine prolapse.

Urinary Retention

Urinary retention is the inability to pass all or part of the urine that has accumulated in the bladder. It should not be confused with failure of the kidneys to produce urine. The person may or may not detect this fullness in the bladder. Urinary retention is common in older men because of the increased incidence of benign prostatic hypertrophy, which can partially or totally obstruct urine outflow.

Think about Mrs. Shireem, the client introduced at the beginning of the chapter. Can you think of any reason she might have urinary obstruction after a vaginal hysterectomy?

Urinary Tract Infection

A urinary tract infection can occur in any portion of the urinary tract. The infection is termed cystitis if it affects the bladder, urethritis if it affects the urethra, and ureteritis if it affects the ureters. Pyelonephritis is an infection of the kidney. Urinary tract infections are more common in women than men.

Urinary Obstruction

Stones, or calculi, can block or partially block the kidneys, ureters, or bladder. You may hear the condition called urolithiasis. Most renal calculi are composed of calcium, but they may also contain oxalate, uric acid, and cystine. Additionally, obstruction can occur from strictures, tumors, or edema.

Urinary Diversion

Urine can be diverted from its normal pathway, either by congenital malformation or by surgical creation. Hypospadias, in which the urethra opens on the underside of the penis or inside the vagina, is an example of a congenital malformation.

Various types of urinary diversions can be created surgically to treat cancer, a birth defect, an obstruction, or a neurogenic dysfunctional bladder (Fig. 35–4). Although the principles of care for urinary diversions are similar, understanding the nature of the following surgical procedures may help you anticipate normal findings in the function of the diversion.

- An *ileal conduit* connects the distal ureters to a resected portion of the terminal ileum, which is used to form a stoma, or opening, onto the surface of the abdomen.
- A *Kock pouch* is a special type of ileal conduit in which a surgeon uses a segment of ileum to create a pouch for holding urine. Nipple valves created from intussuscepted portions of the ileal segment help keep the pouch continent. The client drains the pouch by inserting a catheter through the stoma.
- A *ureterosigmoidostomy* procedure connects the ureters to the sigmoid colon, which allows urine to drain through the colon. The procedure (not shown in Figure 35–4) is a variation of the Kock pouch procedure.
- In a *cutaneous ureterostomy,* the distal end of the ureter is brought to the surface of the skin to create a stoma.
- In a *vesicostomy* (also called cystostomy), an opening is made directly into the bladder.

Unless the client has a Kock pouch, she will need to attach a bag to the skin around the stoma to collect urine as it drains from the stoma. The client must be taught to manage drainage from the stoma, to care for

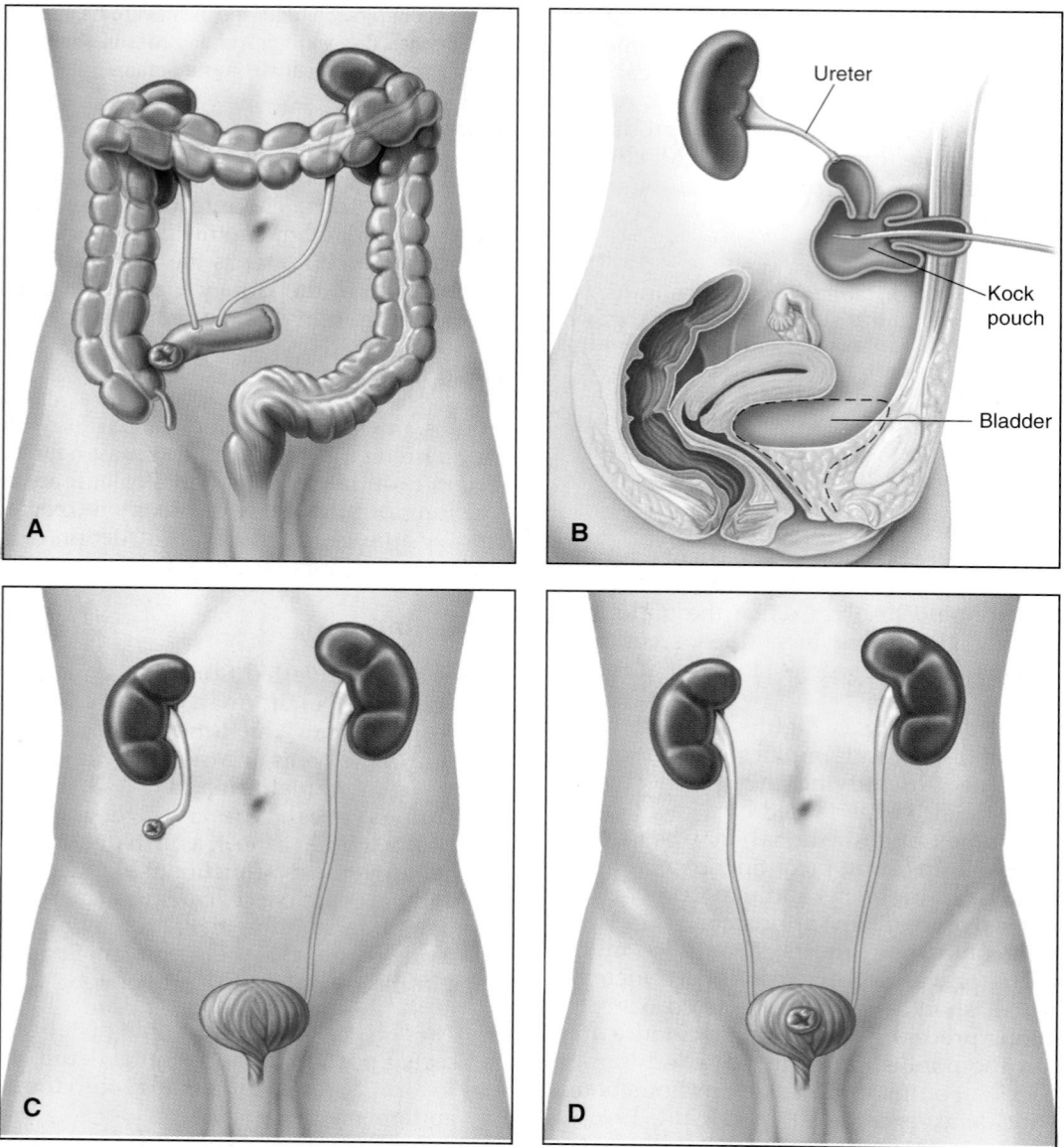

Figure 35–4. Types of urinary diversions. *A*, ileal conduit; *B*, Kock pouch; *C*, cutaneous ureterostomy; *D*, vesicostomy.

the skin, to recognize signs and symptoms of abnormal function, and to manage the feelings associated with a change in body image.

FACTORS AFFECTING URINARY ELIMINATION

Most people do not give much thought or planning to maintaining a normal pattern of urinary elimination. Voiding typically occurs five or six times daily, although the actual number may vary widely with the volume of fluid intake, the size of the person's bladder, and the availability of toilet facilities.

Urinary output has diurnal variation. The action of antidiuretic hormone and decreased renal blood flow in the recumbent position decrease the volume of urine produced at night. However, some people need to urinate at night, possibly because of a small bladder capacity, increased fluid intake before bed, habit, or certain health problems. **Nocturia** is the term used for nighttime urination. Many factors can affect urination, both at night and during the day.

Lifestyle Factors

Nutrition and Fluids

The amount of urine produced in a 24-hour period is directly related to the amount of fluid consumed in the same period. The kidneys function to maintain a balance of body water by excreting excess fluids that the body does not need. Six to eight glasses (1,200 to 2,000 mL) of water daily is the recommended amount to maintain optimal renal function. Because fluid is also lost through perspiration and respiration, any activity that increases these functions also increases the body's need for water. Diarrhea and vomiting may lead to excessive loss of fluids from the gastrointestinal tract.

The water lost through perspiration and respiration is balanced by the water taken in through foods. Foods contain varying amounts of water. Fruits, especially watermelon, will add to the fluid intake and increase the production of urine. **Diuresis** is the increased secretion of urine. Watermelon may actually have a diuretic effect. Drinks with caffeine (coffee, tea, some carbonated beverages) and alcoholic beverages (especially beer) cause diuresis and increase the urge to urinate. Artichokes may have some diuretic effect. Foods high in sodium encourage fluid retention.

Psychosocial

Privacy is probably the most important psychosocial issue. Most people consider urination to be a private matter. Some people will have difficulty initiating urination in the presence of others. Both men and women may have difficulty voiding in the presence of a person of the opposite sex.

Stressful life events can interfere with complete emptying of the bladder or cause a person to urinate more frequently even though the amount is small. The urge to urinate can occur in response to fear, nervousness, cold, wind, running water, or other stimuli.

Activity and Exercise

The periurethral striated muscle or external sphincter is part of the pelvic floor muscles. The tone of the muscles of the pelvic floor can affect the person's ability to maintain voluntary control over urination.

Developmental Factors

Childhood

Given an average intake of fluid, a 6-month-old infant produces about 500 mL of urine, an amount that increases gradually until about age 14, when the average adult volume of 1,500 mL is produced.

Old Age

Aging is associated with a gradual decrease in the number of nephrons. After age 40, nephrons decrease in number until around age 80, when a person may have 40% fewer functioning nephrons.

The weight and size of the kidneys decrease with age as well. Interstitial tissue increases, the number of glomeruli decrease, and the membranes thicken. However, old age and renal failure are not synonymous; adequate renal function is possible with a loss of 70% of the normal number of nephrons (Guyton & Hall, 1996). Under conditions of good health, renal function is not compromised, but the elderly are more vulnerable to renal failure that may occur secondary to serious illness.

As a person ages, bladder capacity decreases, involuntary contractions increase, and the antidiuretic hormone is less active at night. Thus, the older adult voids more frequently. Up to 70% have nocturia, and some older adults need to urinate more than once during the night (Ouslander, 1993).

Physiological Factors

Hormonal Changes

For some women from puberty throughout the childbearing years, the period preceding menses is marked by fluid retention and weight gain. There may be a temporary decrease in urinary output from extrarenal causes, but it has no significance in terms of normal urinary function.

Pregnancy may also be a period of fluid retention, commonly relieved by reducing sodium in the diet. Pregnant women frequently complain of frequent urination, especially during the first and last trimester.

With the onset of menopause, the incidence of incontinence increases. It continues to increase as age advances. This results largely from a decrease of estrogen, which causes relaxation of the pelvic floor muscles and atrophic changes in the urethra. In some cases, the changes are associated with multiple births.

What risk factors for incontinence does Mrs. Shireem have?

Cognitive Impairment

Because urination is cognitively controlled, a person with cognitive impairment is vulnerable to uncontrolled urination. Cognition is one of the reasons for lack of control over urination in Alzheimer's disease. Any neurologically damaged client could have a problem with the control of urination.

Neuromuscular Disease

A person with a spinal cord injury may or may not have damage to the nerves that innervate the bladder and, thus, may or may not have difficulty controlling urination. A client with Alzheimer's disease may initially have incontinence because he forgets to go to the bathroom or forgets where the bathroom is located. Eventually, however, he will have no neurological control over his bladder. A client with multiple sclerosis has intermittent control over bladder function. The detrusor loses tone and the person may find it difficult to relax the external sphincter to begin the urine stream.

Impaired Mobility

Physical mobility is necessary to move to a toilet and to do so in a timely manner. If a person is physically compromised and otherwise cognitively intact, episodes of uncontrolled urination will be particularly embarrassing.

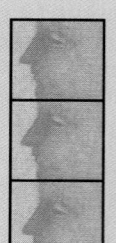

CROSS-CULTURAL CARE
CARING FOR A WEST INDIAN HINDU AMERICAN

Fatami Shireem is a 60-year-old woman who emigrated from India to the United States with her family as an adult. She belongs to the Hindu religion, which evolved over 4,000 years, represents no single creed or founder, and has diverse, spiritually based health practices and customs. Formal religious organization is minimal and there is no religious hierarchy. Mrs. Shireem married a West Indian Hindu American whom she chose, but it was important that her parents approved of her choice. She alternates between traditional Indian dress and American style dress. Although every client is unique, many West Indian Hindu people hold certain unifying beliefs, such as the following:

- Awe, respect, or reverence for life.
- Belief in reincarnation (transmigration of the soul at the time of death into another body).
- Belief in dharma, or moral responsibility, as in law, religion, virtue, morality, custom; dharma requires the pursuit of Nirvana as defined by the priests.
- A divine mandate to separate people by castes, in which those of a lower caste can advance to a higher caste in the next life by fulfilling moral obligations in the present life.
- Use of the Hindi language to maintain cultural unity, especially for older West Indian Hindu people; younger people often adapt to the use of English.
- The social status of women being below that of men (with a female client, a greeting should be first addressed to the husband).
- Avoidance of direct eye contact between a man and any woman other than his wife.
- Avoidance of hand-shaking as a greeting between a man and any woman other than his wife.
- A family orientation, in which the entire family may gather at a client's bedside, in part to help guard the client's personal space and to increase her feelings of control.
- A preference for being stoic rather than praying for recovery because praying for recovery is the lowest form of prayer.
- Requirement for a daily bath as a religious duty.

- The importance of the mother-in-law in making health care decisions.
- Soft-spoken manner.
- Vegetarian diet.

The conversation excerpted below between Mrs. Shireem and her nurse, Janine, shows deference to the client's cultural background:

Janine: Has your doctor given you instructions about when you can resume sexual relations with your husband?

Mrs. Shireem: He said I should wait until I've had a check-up in about 6 weeks. I wish he would explain it to my husband.

Janine: Do you think your husband will have trouble understanding?

Mrs. Shireem: I just don't want him to think that I'm avoiding him.

Janine: I'm sure your doctor will be glad to talk to him. Are you comfortable mentioning this to the doctor or would you like for me to tell him your concern.

Mrs. Shireem: Could you tell him? I am kind of embarrassed about it.

Janine: I'll let him know when he makes rounds.

Critical Thinking Questions

- Did the nurse do a good job of responding to Mrs. Shireem's concern? Would you have done anything differently?
- Assuming the nurse is a woman and the physician is a man, is it likely that Mr. Shireem will accept the restrictions on sexual activity better if the explanation comes from the physician?
- What additional teaching might the nurse consider concerning sexual activity?

Reference

Giger, J.N., & Davidhizar, R.E. (1996). *Transcultural nursing: Assessment and intervention.* St Louis: Mosby.

ASSESSMENT
General Assessment of Urinary Elimination
Health History

Begin the nursing history with a review of the client's pattern of urinary elimination. Begin by asking the person to describe the duration and frequency or urination, and the characteristics of urine. Most people void every 3 to 4 hours. However, the normal range varies widely depending on personal habits that have trained the bladder to accommodate more or less urine. If the person reports increases in the amount of urine, consider diabetes and the use of diuretics. Decreases in the amount may be associated with dehydration or renal failure. Ask about any difficulties with voiding, unusual color or odor to the urine, and variations in amount. Remember that anticholinergic drugs can decrease the ability to empty the bladder.

Ask about any history of difficulty with urination or medical problems that have affected urination. Chronic illness, such as multiple sclerosis or diabetes mellitus, may impair bladder function. If the client reports incontinence, ask if it is associated with coughing, sneezing, or other activities that contract the abdominal muscles. Try to estimate the amount of incontinent urine by asking how many absorbent pads the person needs a day. It may be useful to learn the frequency, timing, and amount of urination other than during incontinent episodes as well. If the client reports urinary retention or difficulty starting the flow of urine, ask about associated symptoms and events.

To investigate the client's past medical history, ask about a family history of incontinence, injury to the urinary tract, surgery, pelvic radiation therapy, trauma, onset of illness, and use of medications. Ask about a history of previous urinary tract problems, renal failure, calculi, or urinary tract infections. Has there been a history of genitourinary surgery?

Your history pertaining to the presenting problem should include at least the following topics:

- Signs and symptoms involving the urinary tract, such as nocturia, dysuria, hesitancy, a poor or interrupted urine stream, straining, hematuria, suprapubic or perineal pain, urgency, frequency, enuresis, dribbling, bladder distention, incontinence, and large residual urine volumes.
- Fluid intake pattern, including caffeine-containing or other diuretic fluids.
- Alterations in bowel habits or sexual function.
- Previous treatments for urinary tract infections, and their apparent effects.
- Expectations for outcomes of treatment.
- A bladder record.
- Amount and types of pads, briefs, and protective devices used.
- The client's mental status.
- The client's mobility status, living environment, and social factors, especially in the elderly.

Assess for the presence of pain. Kidney pain is dull, aching, and steady, located at or below the posterior costal margin (flank pain). Ureteral pain begins in the costovertebral angle and radiates anteriorly into the lower abdomen, groin, and perineum. It is often a severe, colicky pain. Bladder pain may be felt over the symphysis pubis. Urethral pain can usually be pinpointed as pressure or burning with urination.

Physical Examination

Perform a thorough physical examination to detect conditions that have a potential effect on urinary elimination. Because the production of urine is a reflection of total health status, many problems can affect the urinary system. The assessment may include collecting a sample of urine for urinalysis.

Assess the client's skin. You are primarily looking for signs of dehydration or edema. Edema contributes to nocturia and nocturnal urinary incontinence because the fluid shifts when the person assumes a recumbent position to sleep, improving blood flow to the kidneys and increasing urine production. Dehydration is associated with oliguria and concentrated urine.

Assess for neuromuscular problems that may affect the person's ability to empty the bladder or control urination. Mobility, cognition, and manual dexterity are related to toileting skills among frail and functionally impaired clients.

Assess the abdomen for separation of the abdominal muscles, enlarged organs, masses, inflammation, and the collection of fluid. Changes in the ability to increase intra-abdominal pressure or the function of the detrusor muscle may be a factor in emptying the bladder.

Assess for urinary retention by palpating the bladder to determine whether it is distended above the symphysis pubis. When the bladder is filled to about 150 mL, palpation of the bladder may produce the urge to urinate. Remember, however, that an adult's bladder may contain 500 to 700 mL before it is distended enough to be palpated over the symphysis pubis. If you cannot feel the distended bladder but the client reports discomfort or an urge to urinate during palpation, the bladder most likely does contain urine. Percussion of the abdomen reveals a dull sound over a full bladder.

Ask about bowel elimination and feel for a mass that indicates the presence of feces. Pressure from a fecal impaction may be a factor in urinary incontinence.

The physical examination may include inspection of the perineum. Observe for inflammation, edema, and abnormal discharge. It is normal to find an accumulation of smegma—a white, cheesy discharge from sebaceous glands.

Although rectal examination is not routinely performed by nurses, in some settings it may be part of the nurse's examination. Rectal examination allows you to test for perineal sensation, sphincter tone (both resting and active), fecal impaction, or a rectal mass, and to evaluate the consistency and contour of the prostate gland in men. The pelvic examination in women is used to assess for genital atrophy, pelvic organ prolapse (cystocele, rectocele, uterine prolapse), pelvic masses, paravaginal muscle tone, and other abnormalities.

Diagnostic Tests

Diagnostic tests for urinary disorders involve blood studies to determine renal function, radiological and imaging studies, and direct examination of the urine. When diagnostic testing involves examination of the urine, the nurse often has the responsibility for collecting urine specimens and making observations about the characteristics of the urine.

Urinalysis

Urinalysis is a physical, chemical, and microscopic examination of the urine (Table 35–1). It is performed to screen for urinary tract disorders, renal disorders, and

TABLE 35–1
Normal Values for Urinalysis

Characteristic	Normal Value
Color	Yellow
Clarity	Clear
Specific gravity	1.003–1.030
pH	4.5–7.8
Protein	Negative
Bilirubin	Negative
Urobilinogen	Normal in small amounts
Glucose	Negative
Ketones	Negative
Occult blood	Negative
Red blood cells	No more than three (males) to five (females) per high-power field
White blood cells	No more than five per high-power field
Bacteria	Negative
Leukocyte esterase	Negative
Casts	No more than four hyaline casts per low-power field
Crystals	Few

other medical conditions that produce changes in the urine. It is economical, produces rapid results, and usually is noninvasive. Although it is usually performed by a laboratory technician, some analysis of urine can be done with simple procedures not requiring a laboratory.

URINE CHARACTERISTICS

Urine is primarily water, but it also contains varying amounts of the waste products urea, creatinine, ammonia, and purine bodies. Sodium and potassium are the principal electrolytes excreted by the kidneys. The excretion of phosphoric acid, sulfuric acid, uric acid, hippuric acid, and ammonia along with the bicarbonate ion help regulate the acid-base balance of the body. The bicarbonate ion is a buffer that can take on hydrogen ions.

Color

Urine is normally pale, straw-colored, and clear. Changes in the color of urine may have diagnostic significance.

- Amber-colored urine results from the concentration of urine caused by decreased fluid intake or excretion of water. Urine darkens as it stands outside the body.
- Dark amber urine can also mean bilirubin in the urine. Bilirubin is the pigment of bile and is normally excreted by the liver. When the liver or gallbladder is diseased, bilirubin levels rise in the blood and bilirubin is excreted in urine.
- Blood appears in various shades of red in urine. It may be occult (not visible to the naked eye) or it may cause the urine to become pink tinged or frankly bloody. Remember, however, that red urine

is not always caused by blood. Foods can turn the urine red as well, including rhubarb, beets, blackberries, and red food dyes.

- Bright yellow urine comes from large amounts of carotene in the diet or vitamin therapy. Medications can also change the color of urine.

Clarity

Freshly voided urine should be clear. Cloudiness indicates the presence of bacteria (a condition called **bacteriuria**), inflammation, or the presence of sperm or prostate fluid. Urine can also become cloudy when it stands.

Odor

Freshly voided urine is aromatic. When it stands, it develops a characteristic pungent odor of ammonia because it quickly becomes contaminated with bacteria. The odor of urine may be affected by foods. A sweet, fruity odor is associated with ketone bodies produced by diabetic ketoacidosis.

ACID-BASE BALANCE

The body's acid-base balance is reflected by its pH, a measure of hydrogen ion concentration. The normal pH range for urine is 4.5 to 7.8, depending on the body's need for excretion of acids. Abnormal pH measures can indicate systemic acid-base imbalances. Some foods and medications can change urine pH. A diet high in meats, eggs, cheese, whole grains, plums, prunes, and cranberries may decrease pH (more acidic). Vegetables, citrus fruits, and milk increase pH (more alkaline). You can readily measure urine pH by using a multi-agent dipstick and comparing it to a standardized color chart after waiting a specified period.

SPECIFIC GRAVITY

Specific gravity is a measure of the concentration of dissolved solids in urine, thus gauging the ability of the kidneys to concentrate and excrete urine. Urine specific gravity normally ranges from 1.003 to 1.030. If the client's kidneys are functioning normally, specific gravity indicates fluid status; in other words, dehydration raises the specific gravity and overhydration lowers it.

A urinometer is used to measure specific gravity. It consists of a test tube and a device that floats in the urine in the test tube. The test tube must be filled with a sufficient volume of urine to allow the urinometer to float freely. The glass float is calibrated to display the specific gravity of the urine when you read across the bottom of the meniscus formed by the urine. The urinometer is a simple device that can be used at the bedside if frequent specific gravity measurement is needed. Figure 35–5 illustrates its use.

PROTEINS AND GLUCOSE

Proteins and glucose are large molecules and are normally not excreted by the kidneys. Laboratory findings should be negative for glucosuria (glucose in the urine) and proteinuria (protein in the urine). In people who have diabetes, glucose spills into the urine when the

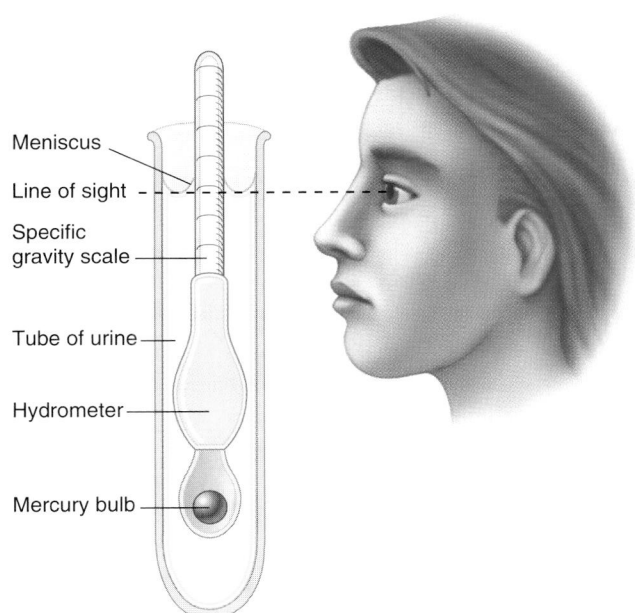

Figure 35–5. A urinometer measures the specific gravity of urine. The bulb must float freely in the urine, and the base of the meniscus must be read at eye level.

Labels (top to bottom): Meniscus; Line of sight; Specific gravity scale; Tube of urine; Hydrometer; Mercury bulb

blood glucose levels become too high. If cells are deprived of glucose long enough, the body metabolizes fat to provide energy, a process that also produces ketones. Ketones in the urine indicate impending ketoacidosis. Glucose sticks can be used for screening in healthy populations but are not sufficiently sensitive for monitoring type I diabetics. The presence of protein in the urine indicates glomerular disease.

BILIRUBIN AND UROBILINOGEN
Bilirubin normally does not appear in urine, and urobilinogen normally appears only in small amounts. If the biliary tract becomes obstructed, the bilirubin level rises in the blood and eventually spills into the urine. Urine urobilinogen levels rise in liver disease.

LEUKOCYTE ESTERASE
If leukocyte esterase appears in urine, it indicates lysed or intact neutrophils—an indirect indication of bacteria in the urine. This test should be combined with the nitrite dipstick to avoid false-positive results. Reagent strips should be used with the first voided specimen in the morning. Use only a clean-catch or mid-stream specimen to avoid the presence of leukocytes from vaginal contamination.

BLOOD
Blood in the urine is never a normal finding. **Hematuria** is the presence of blood in the urine. Blood at the start of urination indicates the urethra as the source. Blood at the end of urination indicates pathology of the bladder neck, posterior urethra, or prostate. Blood throughout urination indicates pathology above the bladder neck. Usually, dark blood comes from the upper urinary tract and bright red blood comes from the bladder neck or urethra. Occult blood is detected using reagent strips dipped into the urine specimen and compared to the color chart on the bottle of reagent strips.

Urine Culture

A culture can be grown from a sample of urine to determine the specific organism causing a urinary tract infection and to monitor the number of organisms in the urine. The urine and urinary tract are sterile except for normal flora in the distal urethra and urinary meatus.

As with any culture, the specimen should be collected in a manner that prevents contamination from other sources of bacteria. A clean specimen caught in midstream or a specimen from a catheterization procedure is needed. Culture results with no growth are available after 24 hours. Positive cultures require 24 to 48 hours to complete.

When the organism is identified, a sensitivity test is usually performed to determine which antibiotics will be effective against the specific organism. The results will report a list of antibiotics to which the organism is sensitive and to which it is resistant. The physician may then modify the prescription if a change in antibiotic is warranted.

Collecting Urine Specimens

Depending on the test planned for the specimen, you may collect a urine specimen in either a clean or a sterile container. Figure 35–6 shows commonly used containers for collecting and measuring urine. When a bedpan, urinal, or specimen hat is used, warn the client that the specimen will need to be free of feces or toilet paper. To measure the urine, it must be poured into a calibrated measuring device. The calibrations on the urinal or specimen hat are accurate only for estimation purposes.

If you will be evaluating urine for bacteria, you will need to use a sterile container to avoid contaminating the specimen. Or you will need to obtain the specimen from the client's indwelling urinary catheter or instruct her in obtaining a clean-catch, mid-stream specimen.

MIDSTREAM URINE COLLECTION
Instruct the client to wash her hands before collecting the specimen. A female client should spread the labia and clean the perineum, vulva, and urinary meatus with three soapy sponges or wipes using one front-to-back stroke for each sponge (Fig. 35–7A). Tell her to discard each sponge after using it for one stroke. She should wipe each side of the labia and down the center over the meatus. Ideally, the labia should stay separated until the urine is collected.

A male client should clean the urinary meatus with three soapy sponges (Fig. 35–7B). If uncircumcised, he should retract the foreskin and clean the glans penis. The minimum recommended amount for a urine specimen is 15 mL.

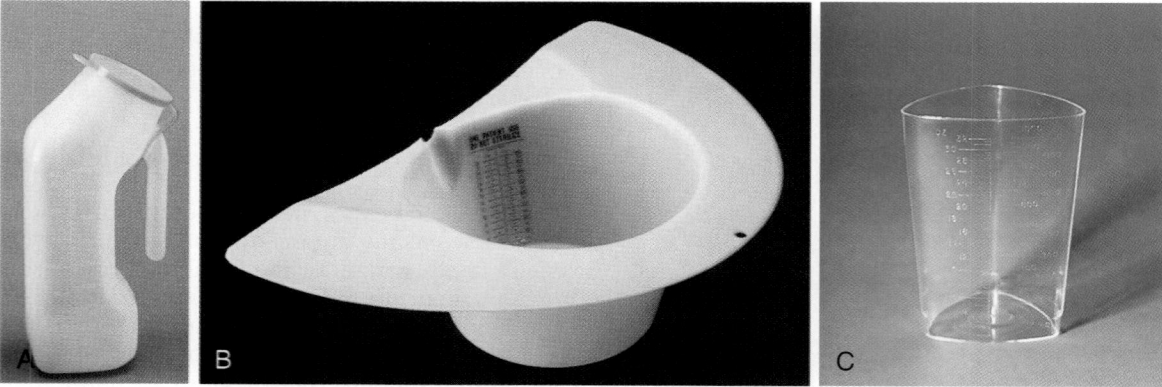

Figure 35–6. In addition to bedpans, illustrated in Chapter 34, devices for collecting and measuring urine include: *A*, a urinal, which is curved to allow placement parallel to the body when the client is recumbent; *B*, a specimen hat, which fits onto the rim of a toilet under the seat, thus allowing the client to sit to void; and *C*, a calibrated urine measuring device. (*A*, courtesy of Bemis Healthcare, Inc., Sheboygan Falls, WI; *B*, courtesy of Kendall Healthcare Co., Mansfield, MA.)

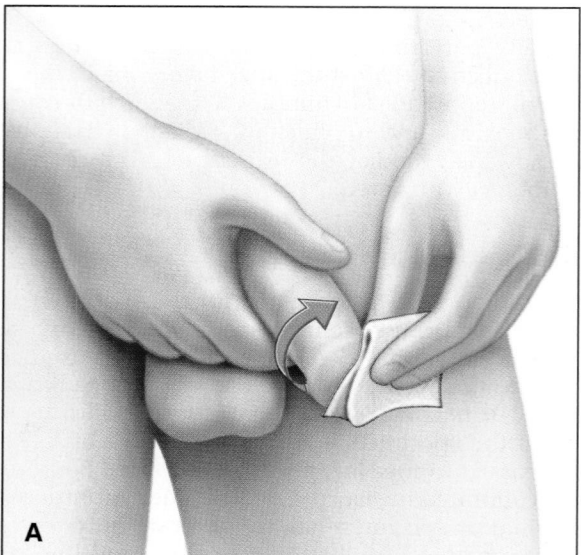

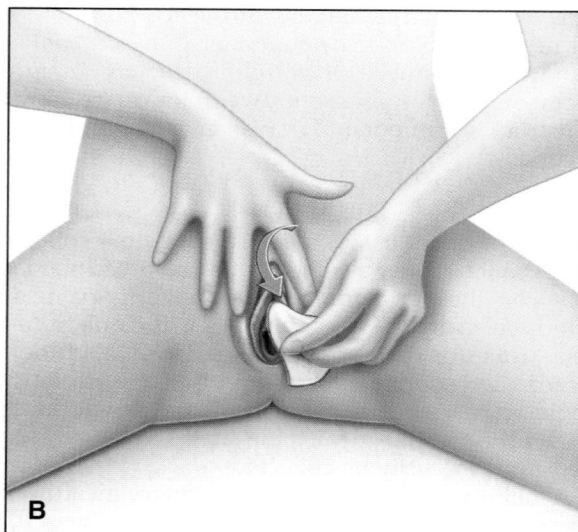

Figure 35–7. Cleaning the urinary meatus for collection of a midstream urine specimen. *A*, instruct male clients to clean in a circular motion around the urinary meatus. *B*, instruct female clients to clean the meatus from front to back.

CATHETERIZATION

If the client already has a catheter in place, you can obtain a urine specimen from a port located on the proximal end of the collecting tubing. Clean the port with alcohol and insert a needle to collect at least 4 mL of urine that is fresh from the bladder. (Inserting the needle directly into the catheter is a less desirable method of collection.) You may need to clamp the tubing below the port for 10 to 30 minutes to allow urine to collect in the catheter (Procedure 35–1).

Sometimes you may need to catheterize a patient to collect a urine specimen. A small-diameter catheter attached to a collection bag is recommended because it has the advantage of being a closed system. The catheter is inserted using sterile technique and urine fills the bag. As soon as the specimen is collected in the bag, the catheter is removed.

URINE COLLECTION FROM INFANTS AND YOUNG CHILDREN

Infants and young children who cannot cooperate with collection of a mid-stream urine specimen will require a special device to collect the specimen. A disposable plastic bag with adhesive attachment is available to collect urine. The bag is attached to the external genitalia and the child voids directly into the bag (Fig. 35–8).

TWENTY-FOUR-HOUR COLLECTION

Collection of all the urine produced in 24 hours is necessary to test for the excretion of creatinine, total urine protein, or electrolytes because the excretion rate of these substances is not constant over a 24-hour period. At the start of the collection period, the first voided specimen is discarded. At the end of 24 hours, the last voided specimen is saved. Thus, all the urine produced in a 24-hour period is collected. The end of the test may vary by 15 to 30 minutes from exactly 24 hours, but the time should be noted precisely on the laboratory request.

The collected urine is stored in a large container in the client's bathroom until the 24-hour period has ended. Depending on the substance being tested, the

PROCEDURE 35-1

Collecting Urine From an Indwelling (Foley) Catheter

TIME TO ALLOW
▼
Novice:
6 minutes
Expert:
3 minutes

If your patient has an indwelling urinary catheter, you can obtain a sterile urine specimen directly from the catheter's closed drainage system.

Delegation Guidelines

The collection of urine from an indwelling catheter is a simple, low-risk procedure that you may delegate to a nursing assistant who is trained in this collection technique.

Equipment Needed

- Alcohol wipes
- 10 mL syringe with attached needle
- Sterile container
- Marking pen

1 Clean the collection port with an alcohol wipe.

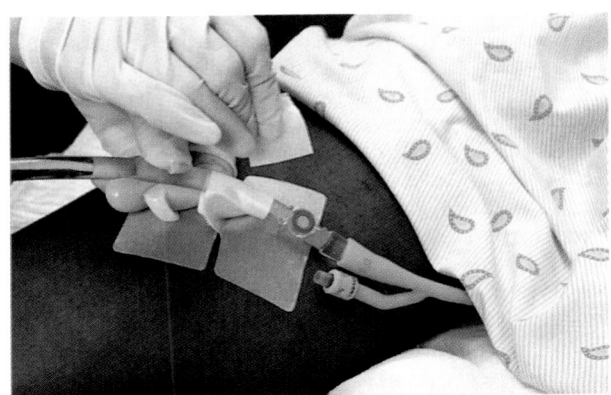

Cleaning the collection port.

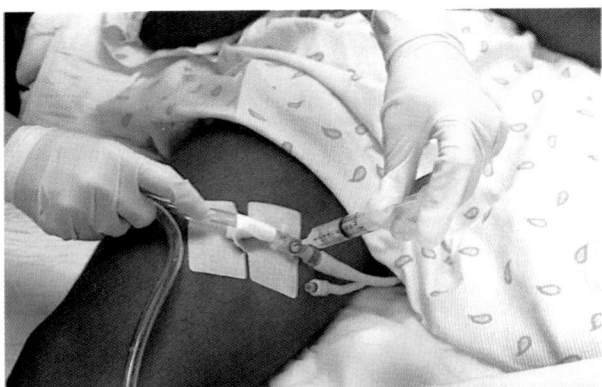

Inserting the needle and withdrawing urine.

2 Using a 10 mL syringe and attached needle, insert the needle into the port and withdraw 10 mL of urine.

3 Inject the urine into a sterile container.

4 Label the container with the client's name and the date and time of collection. Immediately send the container to the laboratory.

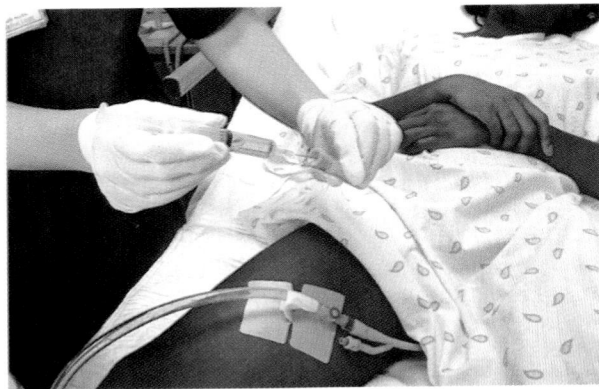

Injecting the urine into a sterile container.

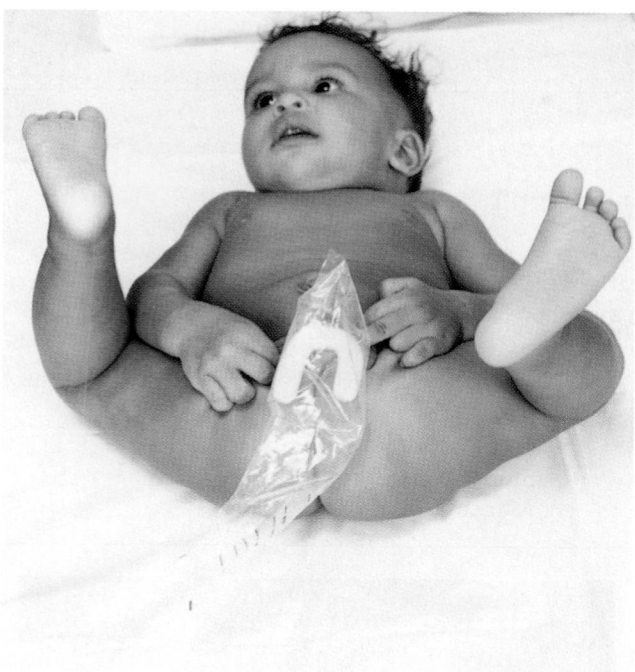

Figure 35–8. To collect a urine specimen from an infant or toddler who is not toilet-trained, apply an adhesive pouch over the perineum.

container may have a preservative added to it, or it may be iced. The client, the family, and all staff members who care for the client should be carefully instructed to save all of the client's urine in the appropriate container. If a specimen is accidentally discarded, the collection procedure will have to be restarted. Make sure the client and family know that the specimen must not be contaminated with toilet paper or feces.

Blood Chemistry

CREATININE
Creatine is an intermediate product of protein metabolism that is synthesized in the liver, kidneys, and pancreas and is stored in muscle tissue. Creatinine is the end product of the metabolism of creatine. The kidneys filter creatinine from the blood. When renal function is impaired, the serum creatinine level rises. Thus, serum creatinine levels can be used to evaluate renal function and to estimate the effectiveness of glomerular filtration.

Creatinine can also be measured in the urine. Creatinine clearance measures the total amount of creatinine excreted in the urine. The meaning of the results is improved by simultaneous measurement of serum creatinine. Urine is collected in an iced or refrigerated container for a 24-hour period as described above. The client should avoid excessive intake of meat the day before the test and should drink adequate fluids before and during the collection period. At the end of the test, the specimen should be promptly transported to the laboratory.

BLOOD UREA NITROGEN
Urea nitrogen is the major nitrogenous end product of protein and amino acid catabolism. It is manufactured in the liver and excreted by the kidneys. Dehydration and overhydration affect the excretion of urea nitrogen. Increased dietary protein, increased catabolism, and muscle-wasting diseases will increase blood urea nitrogen, as will prerenal (decreased blood flow), intrarenal (damage to renal parenchyma), or post-renal (obstruction to outflow of urine) kidney failure. Therefore, the test is less specific than serum creatinine in the diagnosis of renal failure.

ELECTROLYTES
Abnormal excretion of sodium, chloride, potassium, and calcium may indicate renal disease or other problems. The test results must be considered together with related symptoms and diagnostic tests.

Cystoscopy

Cystoscopy is a procedure using a metal or fiberoptic endoscope passed through the urethra for direct visualization of the bladder. The procedure is performed in a urologist's office or in an operating room under local, spinal, or general anesthesia. A sedative is sometimes administered before the procedure and a local anesthetic is applied to the urethra. The tranquilizer diazepam (Valium) or a short-acting anesthetic that produces a twilight sleep, such as midazolam (Versed), is used. The procedure may be used to dilate strictures, implant radium, or place a ureteral stent. A common reason for cystoscopy is the diagnosis of painless hematuria.

Following the test, you will monitor the client's recovery from anesthesia and the client's ability to void normally. The client may need medication for pain or bladder spasm. Some burning with urination and blood-tinged urine are normal for the first three voids. Warm tub baths or sitz baths may help relieve the discomfort. Prophylactic antibiotics are sometimes prescribed for 1 to 3 days. Drinking extra fluids may help the client begin to void normally and relieve some of the discomfort.

The outpatient client should be instructed to report the following problems:

- Persistent, painless hematuria; bright red urine; blood clots in the urine.
- Inability to urinate within 8 hours despite a full bladder and the urge to urinate.
- Signs of infection, such as flank or abdominal pain, chills, fever, or cloudy urine (an indication of pus).

Urodynamic Tests

Urodynamic tests measure the function of the bladder and urethra by measuring the flow rate of urine passing through the urethra. They produce a graphic record of pressures in the bladder and urethra during voiding. They also show variations in the volume of urine and allow visualization of the bladder with contrast media during voiding. Information obtained from this test is used to evaluate the client for vesicoureteral reflux (backflow of urine into the ureter) and for problems associated with residual urine and incontinence.

Imaging

Computed tomography and magnetic resonance imaging are used to evaluate urinary lesions. Bladder tumors can be detected and evaluated. Malignant tumors can be distinguished from benign growths. If contrast media will be used, make sure to question the client about any allergies to shellfish or iodine, or any reactions to dye or contrast material used in previous x-rays. Sedatives are used to assist children under age 3 with the prolonged period of immobilization.

Focused Assessment for Urinary Incontinence

Defining Characteristics

For a client who has evidence of incontinence, ask questions to determine the nature of the problem. The type of incontinence and the extent of the problem are factors in determining the appropriate interventions (Box 35–1).

STRESS INCONTINENCE
Stress incontinence is a reported or observed dribbling with increased abdominal pressure. The client may report dribbling of urine with coughing, sneezing, laughing, bending, lifting, sudden exposure to cold air, and climbing stairs. Urgency and frequency may be associated with stress incontinence. The client may wear a sanitary pad for protection.

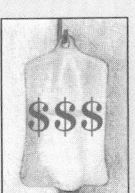

THE COST OF CARE
MEASURING RESIDUAL URINE

When a client needs to be checked for residual urine, noninvasive ultrasonography may offer the best approach. The test is brief, is performed at the bedside, and accurately reflects residual urine volume. In addition, it can reduce costs in two ways. First, the cost of the ultrasonographic test is less than the cost of repeated catheterization. Second, the reduced number of invasive catheterizations reduces the client's risk of urinary tract infections and the added costs (and discomfort) they impose.

Reference

Chan, H. (1993). Noninvasive bladder volume measurement. *Journal of Neuroscience Nursing, 25*(5), 309–312.

DIAGNOSTIC CUES FOR URINARY INCONTINENCE

Assess a client for urinary incontinence if

- She has a wet bed or wet undergarments.
- She has an odor of urine.
- She reports incontinence.
- She is in a high-risk group for incontinence, such as women after menopause, the elderly, or neurologically impaired.

Assess a client for urinary retention if

- She complains that her bladder feels full but she cannot void.
- She complains of difficulty starting the urine stream.
- She has risk factors for acute retention and has not voided in 6 to 8 hours.
- She is in a high-risk group for retention, such as past pelvic surgery, difficulty voiding, or use of anticholinergics.

URGE INCONTINENCE
Urge incontinence is a reported or observed sudden desire to urinate and immediate seeking of toileting facilities. If you are helping such a client to the toilet, you may notice that her clothing becomes wet by the time the toilet has been reached. Urge incontinence is associated with a sudden, overwhelming urge to urinate that cannot be controlled long enough to reach a toilet. Urination occurs frequently and in small amounts. Uncontrollable contractions of the detrusor muscle may be the cause.

FUNCTIONAL URINARY INCONTINENCE
If a client has been evaluated for causes of incontinence and no abnormalities have been found in the urinary tract, the problem is described as **functional urinary incontinence.** Usually, it is associated with cognitive impairment. Functional urinary incontinence occurs as unpredictable, involuntary passage of urine in the presence of normal bladder and urethral function. The person is cognitively unaware of the need to urinate, perhaps because of dementia, depression, or neurological damage.

REFLEX URINARY INCONTINENCE
Reflex urinary incontinence is unexpected voiding without awareness of the need to void and is specific to the client with a spinal cord injury. It is associated with neurological damage to the spinal cord above the level of the third sacral vertebra. The person is unaware that the bladder is full and voids in response to the spinal reflex. It is sometimes possible to predict the voiding pattern.

TOTAL INCONTINENCE

Total incontinence is the inability to control urination, usually in immobile cognitively impaired persons, in which the undergarments or bed is almost continually wet. The person is unaware of cues to a full bladder and may be unaware of the incontinence. The incontinence is either continual or unpredictable.

Related Factors

INCOMPETENT OR DECREASED MUSCLE FUNCTION
The muscles involved in urinary elimination must have good tone and be functional for urination to proceed normally. The periurethral striated muscle (external sphincter) is part of the pelvic floor muscles. The tone of the muscles of the pelvic floor can affect the person's ability to maintain voluntary control over urination.

Stress incontinence is associated with weakness of the pelvic floor muscles, postmenopausal atrophic changes of the urethra, cystocele, and rectocele. The muscles of the pelvic floor may be weak secondary to obesity, aging, childbirth, and recent substantial weight loss.

Decreased bladder capacity results in increased difficulty in holding the urine. Decreased bladder muscle tone can occur secondary to habitual frequency of urination or any other reason that causes the bladder size to never be challenged. An incompetent bladder outlet can occur secondary to congenital urinary tract anomalies.

BLADDER INFECTION OR IRRITATION
Infection or inflammation can cause urge incontinence. Stasis or pooling of urine contributes to bacterial growth. The client who is on bedrest or with bladder outlet obstruction is at risk for stasis of urine that can lead to urinary tract infection. Symptoms of urinary tract infections include pain or burning on urination, frequency, and sometimes blood in the urine. Trauma to the urethra causes pain and edema that can interfere with voiding. Urethritis can be caused by vaginal infections, use of harsh soaps, or bubble baths. Other causes of irritation are glucosuria and cancer.

IMPAIRED ABILITY TO RECOGNIZE BLADDER CUES
Neurological injury or disease can affect the person's ability to recognize the need to urinate or to control urination. Injury, tumor, or infection of the spinal cord or brain may be the underlying cause. A cerebrovascular accident (stroke) can make the person cognitively unaware of the need to urinate. Multiple sclerosis and other demyelinating diseases can make the person unable to recognize the need to urinate. Diabetic neuropathy that affects the smooth muscle of the bladder can result in the inability to control the bladder.

Decreased attention to bladder cues can result in incontinence. The person may ignore the urge to urinate secondary to depression, confusion, or an inability to communicate needs.

TREATMENTS
Clients may experience incontinence following surgery. An example is a transurethral resection of the prostate that may affect the bladder sphincter. Transient incontinence or retention may occur following a cystoscopy or a procedure requiring general or spinal anesthesia. Drugs that affect urinary elimination include antihistamines, epinephrine, anticholinergics, sedatives, immunosuppressants, diuretics, tranquilizers, and muscle relaxants. Clients who have indwelling catheters removed may temporarily experience problems of retention as well.

ENVIRONMENTAL BARRIERS
A major feature of incontinence for the elderly is having to walk a distance to the toilet, poor lighting, unfamiliar surroundings, or a bed that is too high or has side rails. These barriers can make getting to the bathroom difficult. Inability to access the bathroom on time can be secondary to caffeine, alcohol, or impaired mobility.

Focused Assessment for Urinary Retention
Defining Characteristics

A client with urinary retention typically complains of an inability to void despite a feeling of bladder fullness. A post-void residual of less than 50 mL is considered normal; more than 100 mL or residual urine indicates inadequate emptying. Overflow incontinence occurs when the person cannot empty the bladder. When the bladder reaches a critical volume, urine passes involuntarily to relieve the distention.

> **Action Alert!**
> Monitor the voiding patterns of any client at risk for urinary retention. The client who voids frequently in small amounts should be assessed for urinary retention.

Related Factors

Post-surgical clients are at risk because of the use of anticholinergic drugs with anesthesia. Clients who had surgery in the pelvic region, particularly gynecological surgery or procedures involving the bladder, are at risk of urethral obstruction from edema or blood clots. Discomfort associated with surgery in the pelvic region may make the person reluctant to void. Clients who have had hip surgery have limited mobility, pain, and edema that may lessen their control over urination.

The primary reason for retention is bladder outlet obstruction caused by an enlarged prostate, stricture, or edema. It can also be secondary to fecal impaction or chronic constipation. When the bladder or bladder neck bleeds, blood clots can obstruct the urethra. Calculi in the urinary tract are more likely to obstruct the ureters than the bladder outlet.

Obstruction is a second leading cause of urinary retention. Men over age 50 have a high risk of benign prostatic hypertrophy. Because the prostate gland encircles the urethra, the incidence of retention is high in this group. Tumors, bladder stones, and blood clots are other causes of obstruction.

Focused Assessment for Related Nursing Diagnoses

Self-Esteem Disturbance

Ask the client to describe the problems caused by the incontinence. Urinary elimination problems are embarrassing to many people because managing the problem involves discussing private body functions with a health care provider. Incontinence is particularly disturbing because the adult learned in early childhood the importance of controlling urination. Most people are concerned about controlling the odor of urine or having their clothes wet and soiled with urine. People with urinary diversions who must wear a collection bag have a need to conceal the bag and manage the odor.

Risk for Infection

Assess for factors that increase the risk for urinary tract infections. Ask what the client does to prevent urinary tract infections. Usually, they can be easily managed with low-cost antibiotics. For a person with allergies to the usual antibiotics, more expensive alternatives are required. The client who must manage an indwelling catheter, intermittent catheterization, or urinary diversion on a long-term basis must also consider the possibility of developing resistant strains of the organism causing the infection. The best course of action is to prevent the infection, as described in the Teaching for Wellness Chart.

Social Isolation

Ask if the urinary problem interferes with socialization. The initial response to urinary incontinence, urinary diversion, or the need for self-catheterization is to avoid social situations that would require modifications in the management of elimination or where odor could become an embarrassing problem. The client needs to become familiar with modifications that can help to maintain a normal pattern of social interaction.

Self-Care Deficit

Ask whether the person requires any assistance in managing urination. The presence of an indwelling catheter or a urinary diversion requires a different approach to managing urinary elimination. The diagno-

---

Teaching for WELLNESS

METHODS TO PREVENT URINARY TRACT INFECTIONS

Purpose: To minimize the risk of urinary tract infections.

Rationale: By following certain recommendations, clients can reduce the chance of developing a urinary tract infection.

Expected Outcome: The client will avoid urinary tract infections.

Client Instructions

For Women:
- Maintain perineal hygiene by wiping from front to back after defecating.
- Wear cotton-crotch rather than synthetic-crotch underpants because synthetic fabrics tend to increase perineal moisture.
- Do not wear tight slacks or pantyhose.
- Do not wear a damp swimsuit for extended periods of time.
- Avoid the use of bubble bath, perfumed soaps, feminine hygiene sprays, or hexachlorophene.
- Urinate before and after intercourse.
- If you need a lubricant during intercourse, use a water-soluble lubricant.

- Women who use diaphragms are twice as likely to contract urinary tract infections as women who do not use diaphragms. Check with your physician if you use a diaphragm and are experiencing frequent urinary tract infections.

For Men and Women:
- Take showers instead of baths because bacteria in the bath water can gain access to the urethra.
- Immediately obtain treatment if you develop symptoms of a urinary tract infection, such as painful urination, increased urgency or frequency of urination, fever, and malaise.
- Take medications prescribed to treat a urinary tract infection exactly as ordered. Take all of the prescription, even if you feel better before the prescription is finished.
- If you have a cardiac condition that causes frequent urination, learn to tell the difference between that condition and the frequency associated with a urinary tract infection.

sis of *Self-care deficit* is appropriate until the person has learned the necessary self-care practices.

Impaired Skin Integrity

Careful assessment of the skin is a high priority. If the client has a problem with incontinence, inspect the skin or ask about irritation or maceration of the skin. Urinary incontinence is highly associated with skin breakdown and the formation of pressure ulcers. An incontinent client requires special care to prevent irritation or maceration of the skin.

DIAGNOSIS

The diagnosis of *Altered urinary elimination* may be used when you know that a client has a problem with urinary elimination but you have not yet narrowed the focus to a precise problem. Some nurses prefer to use this general diagnosis when the problem is related to a medical procedure, such as a stent, or to the potential complications from a medical procedure. An alternate method is to simply write the diagnosis as *Poten-*

tial complication: (name the complication) or as *Risk for* (name the complication). The Data Clustering chart shows examples of specific diagnoses.

Incontinence should be evaluated to distinguish the type of incontinence so that you can plan interventions appropriate to the specific problem. Usually, you can identify the type of incontinence without specialized testing. The use of an incontinence diagnosis ideally should be accompanied by a plan to restore continence. Many times, incontinence responds to treatments that are within the practice of nursing. Indeed, because the least invasive methods are tried first, the management of incontinence often falls to a nurse.

The absence of urine requires that you differentiate renal failure from the inability to urinate. If your client has not voided for 8 hours, you will need to decide whether the evidence points to a failure to produce urine or to the retention of urine in the bladder. Often, the client's history will give you some idea of what problems to anticipate. The nursing diagnosis in renal failure is *Fluid volume excess* and is discussed in Chapter 31.

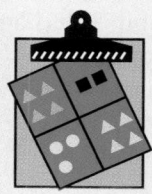

CLUSTERING DATA TO MAKE A NURSING DIAGNOSIS
URINARY ELIMINATION PROBLEMS

Data Cluster	Diagnosis
A 60-year-old male client complains of frequent dribbling and a feeling of bladder fullness even after he urinates.	Urinary retention related to possible enlarged prostate.
A 25-year-old woman with multiple sclerosis has occasional episodes of difficulty in urinating. She has made several trips to the emergency room to have a catheter inserted.	Urinary retention related to episodic neuromuscular dysfunction.
A 20-year-old has come to a clinic for premarital sexual counseling. She has no previous experience with sexual intercourse.	Risk for infection related to being in a high-risk group for urinary tract infection.
A 50-year-old menopausal woman has recently been experiencing incontinence when she sneezes, laughs, or suddenly encounters cold air.	Stress incontinence related to changes in pelvic floor muscles secondary to hormonal changes.
A 75-year-old woman had a total hip replacement yesterday. She has called for the bedpan, but each time she has called too late and has urinated in bed. She did not previously have a problem with incontinence.	Incontinence related to immobility.
A 90-year-old female with Stage 4 Alzheimer's disease continuously dribbles urine, has no apparent recognition of her urination, does not have a bladder infection, and does not have residual urine.	Functional urinary incontinence related to cognitive and neuromuscular limitations.

PLANNING

To obtain a complete picture of the effects of nursing care, outcomes include measuring the expectation that the client will take the desired action, the client's ability to take the desired action, measurement of progress, and the actual result of the actions taken. For this reason, outcomes may include measurements in the following areas: motivation, knowledge, taking action, sustaining consistent action, and obtaining and measuring results.

For example, expected outcomes for a client with incontinence will be affected by the following client variables:

- Is the client mentally able to participate in the treatment plan?
- Does the client have the knowledge needed to make choices about managing incontinence?
- Does the client have the motivation to follow a systematic daily regimen for an extended period of time?

Some clients may only be able to reduce the number of incontinent episodes, using incontinence aids to manage the remaining episodes. Other clients may be satisfied with managing infrequent, small-volume incontinence with incontinence aids. Therefore, the goal will be learning to manage incontinence with protective pads. Naturally, goals may vary for each client and each situation.

Expected Outcomes for the Client With Stress or Urge Incontinence

Expected outcomes for a client with *Stress incontinence* or *Urge incontinence* could include the following: The client will

- Manage small-volume, infrequent episodes of incontinence with incontinence aids.
- Seek medical evaluation for incontinence.
- Recognize the signs of bladder infection.
- List measures to prevent urinary tract infection.
- Verbalize knowledge of possible medical and surgical treatments for incontinence.
- Make a commitment to a management regimen.
- Report extended periods between urination to increase the bladder capacity.
- Correctly perform Kegel exercises.

Expected Outcomes for the Client With Functional Urinary Incontinence

Functional urinary incontinence is frequently associated with the elderly or disabled person who is physically or mentally unable to toilet without assistance. A caregiver is usually involved in managing the incontinence. Expected outcomes for a client with *Functional incontinence* could include the following: The client will

- Not be embarrassed by the need for assistance to manage toileting.
- Be treated with compassion and understanding.
- Initiate or ask for assistance to toilet.
- Be assisted to the toilet before incontinence occurs.
- Have no skin breakdown.
- Remain clean and dry.
- Have no odor of urine.
- Have a reduced number of episodes of incontinence over a 24-hour period.

Expected Outcomes for the Client With Reflex Urinary Incontinence

Expected outcomes for the client with *Reflex urinary incontinence* include the following: The client will

- Develop a method of controlling urination.
- Remain dry and odor-free.
- Maintain intact skin.

Expected Outcomes for the Client With Urinary Retention

Expected outcomes for a client with *Urinary retention* could include the following: When retention with overflow incontinence is the result of a neurogenic bladder, the client will

- Express motivation to perform self-catheterization.
- Master self-catheterization.
- Maintain clean technique.
- Have no urinary tract infections.

For other causes of *Urinary retention*, the expected outcomes could include the following: The client will

- Establish a normal pattern of voiding without residual urine.
- Void within 8 hours of removal of an indwelling (Foley) catheter.
- Report no discomfort with voiding.
- Recognize the signs of bladder distention.

INTERVENTION

Interventions to Promote Urinary Continence

Many interventions are available to help control urinary incontinence, as summarized here and in Table 35–2.

Establishing Continence

PELVIC MUSCLE EXERCISES
Kegel exercises are exercises performed to strengthen the pelvic and vaginal muscles to help control stress

TABLE 35–2

Interventions for Urinary Incontinence

Intervention	Application
Basic evaluation	• Obtain history, physical examination, post-void residual volume, and urinalysis on all clients with urinary incontinence. • After basic evaluation and initial treatment, clients who fail or are not appropriate for treatment based on presumptive diagnosis should undergo further evaluation.
Routine or scheduled toileting	• Offer to incontinent clients on a consistent schedule. • This technique is recommended for clients who cannot participate in independent toileting.
Habit training	• Use for clients in whom a natural voiding pattern can be determined.
Prompted voiding	• Recommended for clients who can learn to recognize some degree of bladder fullness or the need to void, or who can ask for assistance or respond when prompted to toilet. • Clients who are candidates for prompted voiding may not have sufficient cognitive ability to participate in other, more complex behavioral therapies.
Bladder training	• Use to manage urge incontinence, mixed incontinence, and stress incontinence.
Exercises to strengthen pelvic muscles	• Use to decrease the incidence of urinary incontinence. • Pelvic muscle exercises are strongly recommended for women with stress incontinence, men and women with urge incontinence who also receive bladder training, and men who develop urinary incontinence after prostatectomy. • Pelvic muscle rehabilitation and bladder inhibition using biofeedback therapy are recommended for clients with stress incontinence, urge incontinence, and mixed incontinence.
Vaginal weight training	• Recommended for premenopausal women who have stress incontinence.
Pelvic floor electrical stimulation	• Used to decrease incontinence in women with stress incontinence. • May be useful for urge and mixed incontinence.
Medications	• Alpha-adrenergic agonists are the first line of therapy when not contraindicated. • Estrogen is recommended as adjunct therapy in conjunction with alpha-adrenergic agonist. • Anticholinergic agents (especially oxybutynin) and tricyclic antidepressants are reportedly useful for detrusor instability. However, tricyclic antidepressants produce adverse effects, especially in the elderly.
Surgery	• May be used as first-line treatment for some clients with stress incontinence; used uncommonly for urge incontinence. • Surgery to relieve the obstruction is used for overflow incontinence.

From Urinary Incontinence Guideline Panel (1992). Urinary incontinence in adults. AHCPR Publication Nos. 92-0038 and 92-0041. Rockville, MD: Agency for Health Care Policy and Research.

incontinence in women. They are named after Dr. Arnold H. Kegel, a gynecologist who first developed them. Performed correctly, Kegel exercises can reduce or eliminate incontinence in approximately 60% of cognitively intact, cooperative women (AHCPR, 1996). The exercises are described in the accompanying Teaching for Wellness chart. Although used primarily for stress incontinence, they sometimes can be beneficial for reducing urge incontinence.

Performing the exercises correctly depends on the woman's ability to selectively contract the muscles of the pelvic floor. The initial tendency is to contract the abdominal muscles or the muscles of the buttocks. The correct muscle can be located by starting the stream of urine, then contracting the muscles to stop the flow. Another method is to place one finger in the vagina and contract the pelvic floor muscles around the finger. Biofeedback training is useful for some women to become familiar with the contraction of the correct muscle. A vaginal or rectal probe may be used to provide visual feedback when the correct muscle has been contracted. Two-thirds of women will need some practice to find the correct muscle.

BLADDER RETRAINING

For the person with urge incontinence associated with a small bladder capacity, training is designed to increase the bladder capacity by having the client adopt a gradually lengthening voiding schedule. Strategies to control the urge to urinate are practiced.

Training is different for the cognitively competent person than it is for the cognitively impaired person. A bladder diary may be useful in selecting the most useful protocol for training. A daily record is kept of the time of urination, whether the person was incontinent, whether the accident involved a small or large amount, and associated events or the reason for the accident. For the cognitively impaired person, a scheduled toileting regimen may be successful. The person's voiding pattern should be recorded for several days to determine whether a pattern exists. Electronic devices to monitor for wetness are sometimes useful in establishing the pattern. People often need to urinate on arising in the morning, after meals, and at bedtime. However, for some older clients, the schedule may need to be as frequent as every 2 hours. Patience is required. Over time, the regimen becomes habitual and incontinence will improve. Success is partially related to a consistent daily schedule of meals and fluid intake.

For a person with some ability to recognize the need to urinate, a schedule of prompted voiding may be successful, as described later in the chapter.

Maintaining Dry and Intact Skin

EXTERNAL CATHETERS

External catheters are devices that can be attached to the skin to collect urine. External collecting devices for women are not widely available and have tended to leak and cause skin abrasions. Condom catheters are used successfully for men, however. The condom is a heavy rubber sheath that fits over the penis and is secured with a soft, flexible band (Procedure 35–2). The end of the condom has a drainage tube molded into the condom and is connected to a bedside drainage bag or leg bag (Fig. 35–9).

The risk of urinary tract infection is reduced with an external catheter. The advantages of using a condom catheter are keeping the skin dry and controlling odor. The disadvantages are the difficulty in securing the catheter adequately to control leakage of urine and to keep the catheter in place without causing edema to the penis and excoriation to the skin. The catheter should be removed at least daily to inspect the skin.

Complications include abrasion, dermatitis, ischemia, necrosis, edema, and maceration of the penis. The incidence of urinary tract infection is less than with an indwelling catheter but is still a factor in using condom catheters. An alternative to a condom catheter for men is a retracted penis pouch (Fig. 35–10). This device is sometimes successful if the man has a retracted penis that cannot support a condom catheter.

Action **A**lert!
Avoid constricting the penis with a condom catheter because doing so will cause edema. Remove the condom and inspect the skin daily.

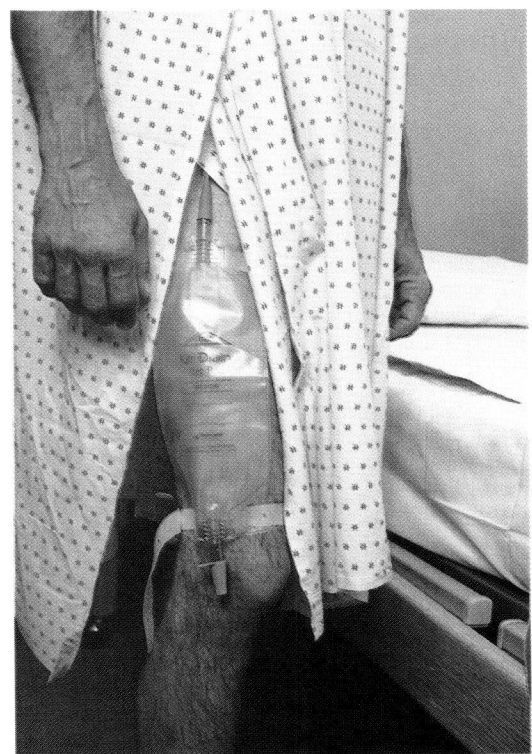

Figure 35–9. For the ambulatory client with an indwelling catheter, a drainage bag can be attached to the leg and hidden by the client's clothes.

Applying a Condom Catheter

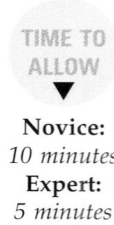

TIME TO
ALLOW
▼
Novice:
10 minutes
Expert:
5 minutes

The purpose of applying a condom catheter is to control incontinence in a male client without the risk of urinary tract infection and with greater comfort to the client than an indwelling catheter.

Delegation Guidelines

The application of a condom catheter is a noninvasive procedure that you may delegate to a nursing assistant who has received specific instruction in this skill. Instruction should include safety and skin care considerations.

Equipment Needed

- Commercially packaged condom catheter
- Soap and water
- Disposable gloves
- Drainage bag and tubing

1 Position the client on his back and drape him so only his penis is exposed.

2 Clean his genitals with soap and water and dry thoroughly.

3 Apply skin-protecting cream packaged with the catheter to the client's penis. Allow it to dry.

4 Wrap the adhesive spirally around the shaft of the penis.

Be careful not to apply the adhesive too tightly. Severe edema can result if the adhesive strip constricts the shaft of the penis, and the client will develop pain and difficulty urinating.

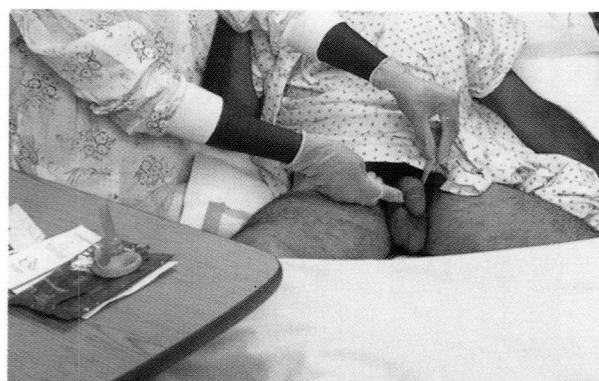

Wrapping the adhesive spirally around the penis.

5 Place the rolled condom over the client's glans penis and unroll the condom over the adhesive liner and the shaft of the penis.

If the client is uncircumcised, make sure his foreskin remains in place over the glans penis as you unroll the

condom. If retracted, the foreskin may be tight enough to constrict the penis and cause edema of the glans penis.

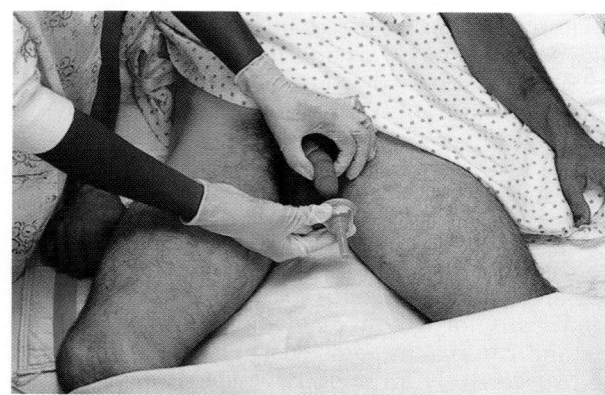

Placing the rolled condom over the client's glans penis.

6 Attach the catheter to a collecting system and tape the tubing to the client's leg.

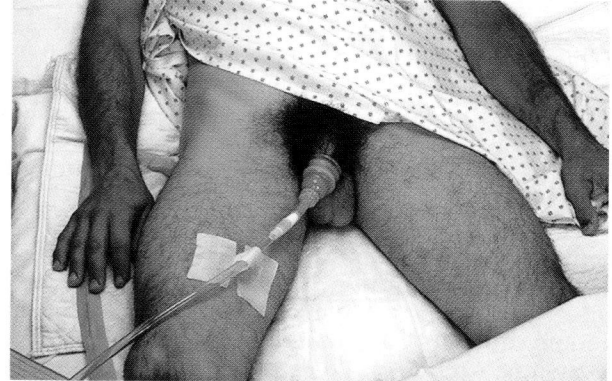

Catheter attached to a collecting system and taped to the client's leg.

7 Observe the client's penis after applying the condom catheter to detect such problems as urine leakage, edema, and changes in skin color.

Teach family caregivers to apply the catheter. Skin care is essential. The family should remove the condom and clean the skin daily.

ABSORBENT PRODUCTS

Protective garments and absorbent products are highly useful in managing urinary incontinence. Both washable and disposable products may be used. Cost, absorbency, and skin protection should be considered in selecting a product. Underpads may be the most convenient when the client is in bed. Adult diapers (briefs) allow protection when the client is moving from bed to chair or using a wheelchair. For a female client with incontinence of small amounts of urine, a feminine protection pad may be sufficient. Many people adopt this intervention on their own rather than consulting a health care professional about minor incontinence, as described in the State of Nursing Science chart.

Disposable products are widely used for institutional care, often because the cost of laundry makes the disposable products less expensive. The protective lining in disposable products may have some benefit in pulling moisture away from the skin, but the client should have the pad changed immediately after voiding.

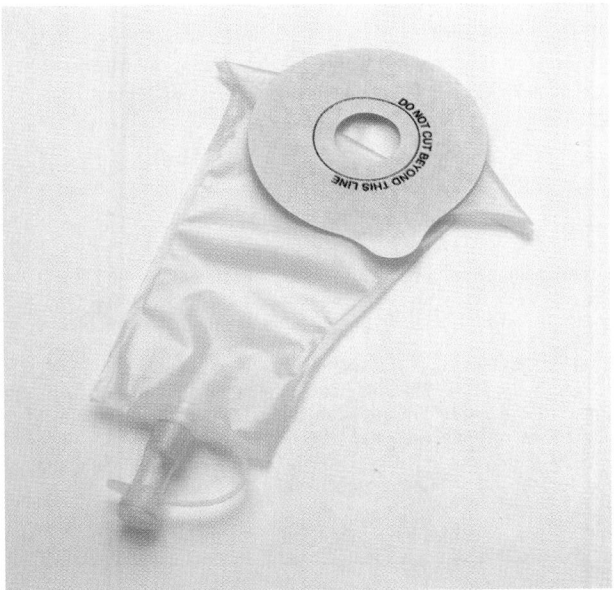

Figure 35–10. A retracted penis pouch is available as an alternative to a condom catheter for a male client with a retracted penis. (Reproduced with permission of Hollister Incorporated, Libertyville, IL.)

Urine that has remained for a period of time has a characteristic foul odor that is associated with poor nursing care and is unpleasant to the client, family, and staff. Besides the problem of odor, the skin can quickly develop a rash or excoriation from prolonged wetness, and the client becomes more vulnerable to pressure ulcers.

Managing Bowel Elimination

Urinary incontinence can be reduced by preventing constipation. Hydration therapy is an important component of preventing constipation, so reducing fluid intake is not recommended for the management of urinary incontinence.

Establishing Continence in the Cognitively Impaired

SCHEDULED TOILETING AND PROMPTED VOIDING

Prompted voiding and regularly scheduled toileting are effective for preventing urinary accidents in some clients who are homebound or need long-term care. In a prompted voiding program, the client should be checked on an hourly basis, offered the opportunity to void, and have her protective pad changed if wet (Box 35–2). The time can be extended as the caregiver becomes familiar with the person's pattern. Colling,

---

BOX 35–2

THE STEPS OF PROMPTED VOIDING

To perform prompted voiding, follow these steps:

1. At scheduled times (usually every 2 hours), ask the client whether she feels wet or dry.
2. Check to see whether she is wet or dry.
3. If the client correctly identified being dry, give her positive feedback.
4. Ask the client if she would like to use the toilet.
5. If she responds positively, assist her to the toilet as needed. If she responds negatively, encourage her to try using the toilet. Never force a client to toilet.
6. Give positive feedback for appropriate toileting; never give negative feedback.

THE STATE OF NURSING SCIENCE

MANAGING URINARY INCONTINENCE IN ELDERLY ADULTS LIVING IN THE COMMUNITY

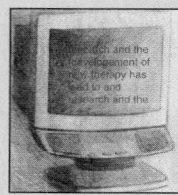

What Are the Issues?

Most people who experience urinary incontinence try various methods of controlling their symptoms on their own rather than seeking immediate professional treatment. Methods include using pads, restricting fluid intake, staying close to bathroom facilities, and using pelvic muscle exercises. Because management of progressive incontinence commonly requires admission to long-term care facilities, nurse-researchers are interested in finding effective ways to help people cure their incontinence or manage their symptoms more effectively.

What Research Has Been Conducted?

Finding out what people do on their own to manage incontinence is a good place to start in helping them manage their symptoms. Engberg and colleagues (1995) therefore interviewed 147 women who lived at home and who reported having some form of urinary incontinence. The researchers were interested in what methods the women used to control their incontinence. They also asked about the effectiveness of those methods and how satisfied the women were with them.

Most women in the study had a mixed type of incontinence, with symptoms occurring seven or fewer times per week. The most common behaviors used to control symptoms were staying close to the bathroom, voiding more often, and wearing a protective garment. Other common behaviors included restricting fluid intake and performing pelvic muscle exercises. Most of the women studied were satisfied with their methods and thought they were effective in controlling symptoms.

In 1997, Engberg and coworkers tested a treatment approach to controlling incontinence in 124 homebound elderly adults. Subjects who were not cognitively impaired received biofeedback-assisted pelvic floor muscle training and 8 weeks of follow-up. The biofeedback helped them to isolate the muscles that they were contracting to increase urethral pressure. Once the subjects experienced the sensation of effective muscle contractions, researchers had them perform up to 45 muscle-contraction exercises per day. During follow-up sessions, a nurse would coach the person to improve the effectiveness of the exercises through such means as changes in position or timing.

Caregivers of people with cognitive impairment were taught how to oversee prompted voiding. This intervention involves asking the person every 2 hours whether she is wet or dry. If the client is dry, the caregiver praises her for staying dry for 2 hours. The client is then asked if she needs to go to the bathroom. If the answer is positive, the caregiver provides any needed assistance. The prompted voiding schedule is used throughout the day and evening.

All people who were studied, whether cognitively impaired or not, received instruction in additional methods of controlling incontinence, including changes in the environment.

What Has the Research Concluded?

The 1995 study by Engberg and colleagues supported previous research that found most people using self-care to control their symptoms. With high levels of satisfaction in self-care methods, people may delay seeking medical or surgical evaluation that could lead to a cure or to better management of their symptoms.

In their 1997 study, Engberg and colleagues were able to use an individualized urinary incontinence protocol for homebound elders based on cognitive status. The researchers did not report outcome data on how incontinence symptoms changed after the use of the protocol.

What Is the Future of Research in This Area?

As our population ages and more people develop urinary incontinence, they will need to know what options they have for managing symptoms so they will not interfere with activities of daily living. For example, the need to ensure easy access to bathroom facilities can be limiting to older adults with urge incontinence. It is especially important to develop cost effective approaches to incontinence management. Also, for such interventions to work, clients must be willing to use them. Testing interventions in the home environment is an excellent means of making sure that such interventions are clinically useful.

References

Engberg, S.J., McDowell, B.J., Burgio, K.L., Watson, J.E., & Beele, S. (1995). Self-care behaviors of older women with urinary incontinence. *Journal of Gerontological Nursing, 21*(8), 7–14.

Engberg, S., McDowell, B.J., Weber, E., Brodak, I., Donovan, N., & Engberg, R. (1997). Assessment and management of urinary incontinence among homebound older adults: A clinical trial protocol. *Advanced Practice Nursing Quarterly, 3*(2), 48–56.

Ouslander, and Hadley (1992) used an electronic monitoring device to determine a pattern of wetness and constructed an individualized toileting schedule. Clients were given positive reinforcement for successful toileting. Incontinence was decreased for 86% of the clients. Clients with greater mental impairment had higher failure rates.

PATTERNED URGE RESPONSE TRAINING

In this intervention, you help the client develop strategies to control the urge to urinate. For example, if she feels the urge to urinate, tell her to stop, take a slow, deep breath, and relax. Instruct her to quickly squeeze the muscles of her pelvic floor three or four times without holding the squeeze. Tell her to wait for the urge to pass, and then to walk slowly to the bathroom. To help her succeed with this intervention, warn her to avoid beverages that contain caffeine, such as coffee and colas.

ENVIRONMENTAL MODIFICATIONS

To maximize the success of interventions for incontinence, toilet facilities should be familiar to the client. A clear path should be available. A new client in an institutional setting may need to be assisted to the toilet until the facilities become familiar, especially if the client has poor vision or is easily confused by the new surroundings. The toilet seat should be at a proper height. A grab bar may increase the client's safety and ease of sitting on the toilet. In semiprivate rooms, lack of privacy becomes an issue that may make the person delay urination and increase the chances of incontinence.

Interventions to Relieve or Prevent Urinary Retention

Promoting Urination

FLUID MANAGEMENT

Maintaining the recommended intake of 1,500 to 2,000 mL (six to eight glasses) of water daily will assist the bladder to fill and stimulate the urge to urinate. Water lost through profuse perspiration should be replaced in addition to the usual amount. Water is preferred to fluids that contain sodium, sugar, or caffeine. Adequate fluid intake will flush the bladder and urethra of bacteria and help prevent urinary tract infections, as suggested in the accompanying Nursing Care Planning chart.

ENHANCING THE STIMULUS TO VOID

For the client who is having difficulty urinating, you may need to provide assistance to stimulate urination. The post-surgical client may have initial difficulty urinating, especially if the procedure involved the use of an indwelling catheter or manipulation of the bladder. Provide privacy to help the person stay comfortable and relaxed. Allow adequate time and avoid making the person feel a need to hurry.

You will aid urination by helping the person to the position usually used for voiding. For example, a man may be more able to void in a standing position rather than sitting on a toilet or lying in bed. A man with prostatic hypertrophy may not be able to use a urinal lying in bed. A woman may be better able to void when sitting on a toilet rather than lying in bed. If a woman cannot walk to the bathroom, consider using a bedside commode.

If the client cannot get out of bed or the medical treatment requires bedrest, offer a bedpan or urinal. To the extent possible, help a female client sit up in bed on the bedpan to promote the natural position for urination. It may be helpful to warm the bedpan by filling it with warm water, emptying it, and drying it thoroughly before offering it to the client. Using a small amount of talcum powder on the rim helps prevent the bedpan from sticking to the skin as it slides under the buttocks.

If the client cannot raise the buttocks enough to place the bedpan in the correct position, turn the client to the side, place the bed pan in the correct position, and turn the client back onto the bedpan. As you turn the client, push down on the side of the bedpan to help it stay under the buttocks. As an alternative, use a fracture pan, which was specially designed for clients who have fractured bones and cannot raise the buttocks. The client simply raises one leg and the small end of the pan is placed in the angle between the buttocks and the bed. It is not necessary for the client to raise the hips to slide the pan under the buttocks.

Some clients have difficulty with the initial voiding after an indwelling catheter is removed or after having surgery in the pelvic region. The problem can be the result of edema, irritation, or tenderness. It is exacerbated by feeling tension about being able to urinate or about the possibility of pain when urinating. You can try methods to help the person relax, such as relaxation breathing techniques. Running water in a nearby sink may stimulate urination. Using a spray of warm water over the perineum may relax the perineum and help start the stream of urine. The client's sitting in a warm sitz bath can also be helpful. If the client's urine must be measured, however, you will not be able to use a method that mixes the urine with water.

Remember Mrs. Shireem from the introductory story? On the second day after surgery, she can walk to the bathroom. What methods would you think are the most appropriate to help her urinate for the first time?

Using Catheters

A urinary catheter is a tube inserted into the bladder to drain urine. Urinary catheters can be used to prevent incontinence, to avoid the inconvenience of a bedpan in a client confined to bed, to collect urine specimens, and to drain urine from a person unable to void. The primary purpose of a urinary catheter is to prevent urinary retention.

CATHETERIZATION

Catheterization refers to inserting a tube into the bladder through the urethra for the purpose of draining

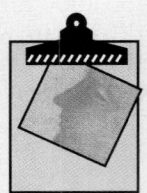

NURSING CARE PLANNING
A POSTOPERATIVE CLIENT AT RISK FOR URINARY TRACT INFECTION

Nursing History

Mrs. Shireem is in the second postoperative day following a vaginal hysterectomy. She has no history of difficulty with urination.

Physician's Orders

Clear liquids; advance diet as tolerated
Activity as tolerated
Demerol 50–100 mg q4h prn for pain
Vicodin i or ii prn for pain
Tylenol 650 mg prn for temperature over 38.8°C (102°F).

$D_5/\frac{1}{2}$ NS @ 100 mL/hr
Discontinue intravenous fluid when able to take fluids by mouth.
Discontinue Foley catheter
Laxative of choice

Nursing Assessment

(Morning change-of-shift report) The physician removed the vaginal pack this morning. Client's vital signs are within normal limits. Her temperature is 37.2°C (99°F). She was able to eat a soft diet for breakfast, including 600 mL of fluids. She was out of bed for two brief periods yesterday. Her pain has been controlled with 75 mg of Demerol used every 4 to 6 hours since surgery, but she took two Vicodin this morning. Skin turgor is brisk.

NURSING CARE PLAN

Nursing Diagnosis	Expected Outcomes	Interventions	Evaluation (After 24 Hours of Care)
Risk for urinary retention	The client will resume a normal pattern of voiding within 12 hours after Foley is removed.	Avoid trauma when removing Foley. Clean perineum and pat dry.	Foley easily removed without pain. Client states she has some irritation at the meatus.
	Will maintain fluid intake of 3,000 mL over 24 hours	Engage daughters to assist mother with fluid intake and monitor intake and output.	Intake 2,800 mL; output 2,500. Initially voided at 1-hour intervals, but now goes 4 to 6 hours and voids about 300 mL. Daughters accurately recorded intake and output. Provided client with cranberry juice to relieve irritation.
	Will void 300 mL of urine four to six times a day	Assess voiding pattern. Assess for urgency, frequency, burning, feeling of bladder fullness. Instruct client to void when she first feels the urge. If she has difficulty starting the flow of urine, suggest running water or rinsing the perineum with a spray of warm water.	No complaints of urgency, frequency, burning, feeling of bladder fullness. Voided a small amount three times, then resumed a normal pattern of urination.

Italicized interventions indicate culturally specific care.

Critical Thinking Questions

1. Mrs. Shireem has resumed a normal pattern of voiding. Would she still be vulnerable to urinary tract infections after discharge? Why?
2. What would you teach about preventing urinary tract infections after discharge?
3. What signs and symptoms of urinary tract infection should she report to her physician?

urine from the bladder. It may have various indications (Box 35–3). For one-time relief of retention, the catheter is passed, urine is drained, and the catheter is removed. Sometimes referred to as straight catheterization or in-and-out catheterization, intermittent catheterization is also used by clients who need self-catheterization.

When a problem is expected to persist, an indwelling (Foley) catheter is used. This type of catheter has two or three lumens. One lumen drains urine, the second allows inflation of a balloon in the client's bladder, and a third can be used to irrigate the bladder with fluids or medications (Fig. 35–11).

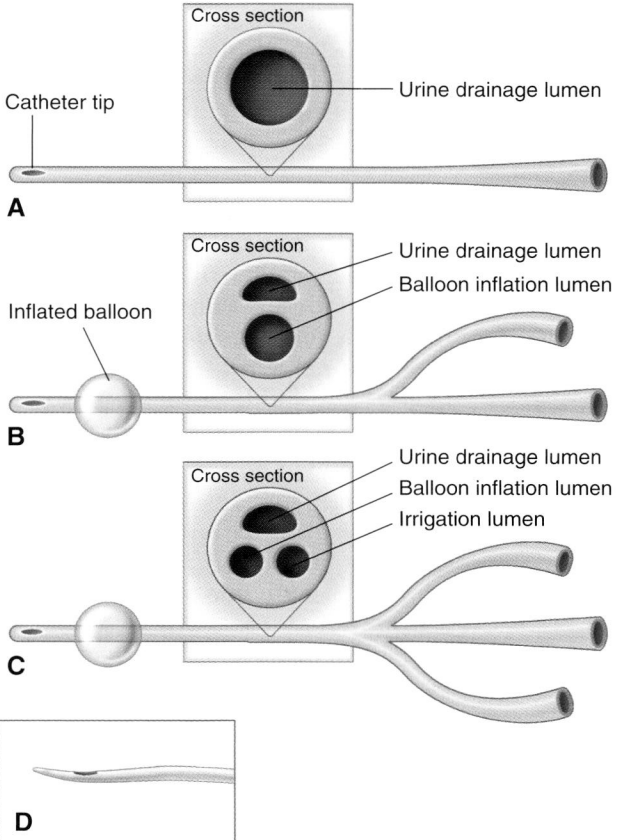

Figure 35–11. Types of catheters. *A*, a straight catheter is inserted to drain the bladder and is then immediately removed; *B*, an indwelling (Foley) catheter has a second lumen used to inflate a balloon that holds the catheter in place in the bladder; *C*, a triple-lumen indwelling catheter has a third lumen for instillation of fluid into the bladder for irrigation; *D*, a Coudé tip.

BOX 35–3

INDICATIONS FOR CATHETERIZATION

Short-Term Indwelling Catheterization

- After surgical procedures known to interfere with normal urination, such as bladder surgery, pelvic surgery, some types of hip surgery.
- When the client's kidney function must be monitored, as when renal function is compromised or the client has a critical illness and a high risk of shock.
- After surgical procedures involving the urinary tract, when a catheter can help prevent obstruction from blood clots.
- When an orthopedic client cannot be safely turned and repositioned.
- When frequent moving causes pain.

Intermittent Catheterization

- For relief of discomfort from an overdistended bladder when the client cannot initiate urination.
- When obtaining a sterile urine specimen for culture.
- When assessing residual urine volume after the client voids.
- For long-term management of urination in spinal cord injuries, multiple sclerosis, or other causes of incompetent bladder.

Long-Term Catheterization

- For irreversible incontinence, when skin rash, ulcers, or wound management is negatively affected by urine on the skin.
- For a terminally ill client (especially one in severe pain) whose comfort is improved by minimizing the amount of turning and cleaning needed.
- For irreversible, severe urinary retention, especially when the client develops frequent urinary tract infections.

Action **A**lert!
Check an indwelling catheter regularly for patency to prevent urinary retention. Catheters can be obstructed by crusts formed with long-term use, blood clots when bleeding is present, or kinking and incorrect positioning of the tube.

Indwelling catheters are used for short-term problems that will benefit from catheterization to relieve or prevent urinary retention that cannot be corrected medically or surgically, that cannot be managed practically by intermittent catheterization and, occasionally, to manage the incontinent client. A client with chronic retention may benefit from a catheter if bothered by persistent overflow incontinence, symptomatic urinary tract infections, or an increased risk of renal dysfunction. If an incontinent client has pressure ulcers, skin lesions, or surgical wounds that are being contaminated by urine, an indwelling catheter may be beneficial as well. Indwelling catheters are sometimes used for short-term management of elimination in the severely ill, in clients undergoing major surgery, and in the terminally ill (Procedure 35–3).

PROCEDURE 35–3

Inserting an Indwelling Catheter

TIME TO
ALLOW
▼
Novice:
20 minutes
Expert:
10 minutes

Unlike a straight catheterization, in which you insert a urinary catheter, drain urine, and remove the catheter right away, an indwelling catheter remains in the client's bladder to provide continuous urine drainage. An inflated balloon holds the catheter in place in the urinary bladder. Besides providing continuous urine drainage, an indwelling catheter can be used to prevent bladder distension, obtain sterile urine specimens, and irrigate the bladder with fluids or medications.

Delegation Guidelines

The assessment and complexities of sterile technique suggest that the insertion of an indwelling catheter not be delegated to a nursing assistant. This is particularly true in an acute care setting, where the risk for nosocomial infection exists, or in a client in whom difficulty passing a catheter may be anticipated. In a long-term care setting, it may be appropriate to consider delegation of this procedure following a careful assessment.

Equipment Needed

- Bottom drape
- Gloves
- Fenestrated drape
- Catheter, connecting tubing, and collection bag
- Prefilled syringe
- Antiseptic cleaning solution
- Cotton balls
- Forceps
- Water soluble lubricant
- Gooseneck lamp or flashlight, especially for a female client

1 Select a catheter of appropriate size and material, with a balloon of appropriate size.

Catheters range from size 6 French (the smallest) to size 24 French (the largest). For a child, you probably will use a size 8 to 10 French. Most adult women need a size 14 to 16 French. Most men need a size 16 to 18 French. A client who has had an indwelling catheter for a long time will need a larger catheter to prevent urine leakage from the stretched urethra.

For short-term catheterization, you probably will use a plastic catheter. It can be inserted easily when well lubricated but may be less comfortable because it is stiff and inflexible. For catheterization lasting up to 3 weeks, you may use a latex or rubber catheter, which is softer than plastic. For catheterization lasting 4 to 6 weeks, you may use a polyvinylchloride catheter, which softens at body temperatures. For catheterization lasting 2 to 3 months, you may use a silicone or Teflon catheter, on which secretions are less likely to adhere and form crusts that could irritate the urethra or obstruct the catheter.

Pediatric catheters usually come with a 3 mL balloon; adult catheters have either a 5 mL or a 30 mL balloon. You may need to use the 30 mL balloon if the client has had an indwelling catheter for a long time or if he has had a transurethral resection of the prostate. The larger balloon is thought to provide some hemostasis at the neck of the bladder after prostate resection.

2 Position the client for catheterization.

a. If the client is female, have her lie in a supine position with her knees flexed and separated.

This position allows access to the urinary meatus and typically is comfortable for the client. If she cannot hold her knees open, ask a colleague to hold them for you; do not spread the client's knees if doing so causes her pain. If the client cannot lie on her back or open her knees, place her in Sims' position with her upper leg flexed at the hip and knee.

b. If the client is male, have him lie in a supine position.

3 Drape the client for privacy.

a. If the client is female, expose only her labia. To do so, place one corner of a sheet between her legs so that two corners cover her legs and the remaining corner covers her abdomen. Leave the drape fully in place over the client's labia until you are ready to perform the catheterization. At that time, you can then lift the corner of the drape that covers her labia and fold it back.

b. If the client is male, use his gown or a bath blanket to cover his upper body down to his penis. Use a bed sheet to cover his lower body up to his penis.

Draping should make the client feel covered and as private as possible, but should be simple and not add significantly to the length of the procedure.

4 Establish a sterile field.

a. Open the prepackaged catheter tray and place it in a convenient location. If your patient is female, consider placing the opened tray on the bed near her perineum. If your client is male, consider placing the opened tray on an overbed table.

b. Place the bottom drape adjacent to a female client's buttocks. Hold the drape only by a corner, allow it to fall open, and place it under her buttocks, still touching only the corners. Place the drape so it overlaps the outer wrapper of the open catheter tray. This will form a continuous sterile field from the tray to the client's buttocks.

This procedure is not practical for females who are likely to move their legs during the catheterization procedure.

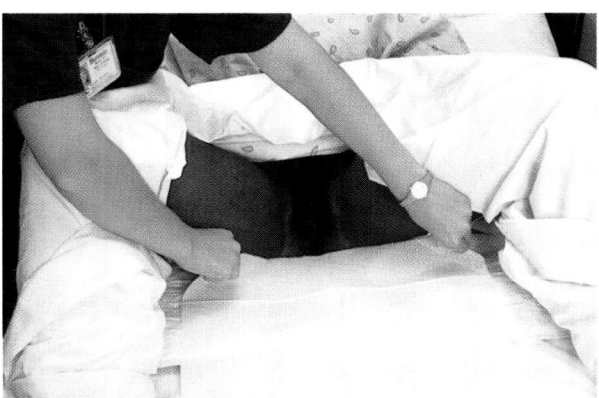

Placing the bottom drape. Touch only the corners to avoid contamination. (The edge of a sterile field is never considered to be sterile.)

c. Put on sterile gloves. If you wish, or according to your facility's policy, use a fenestrated drape to create a sterile field that encircles a female client's labia or a male client's penis.

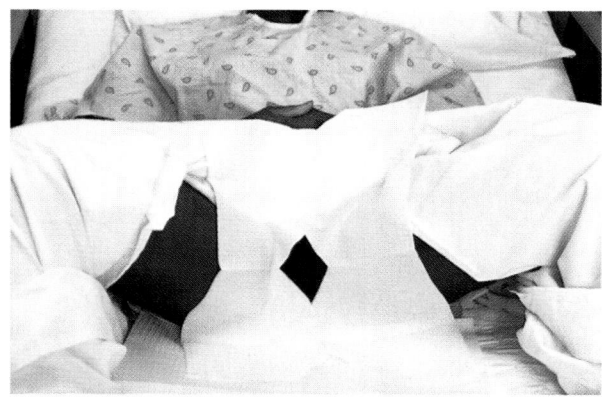

Fenestrated top drape in place.

d. Inflate the catheter balloon to test it for leaks.

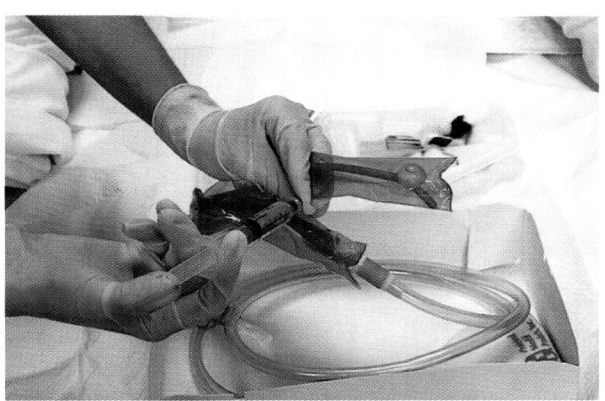

Testing the catheter balloon for leaks.

5 Clean the area around the urinary meatus

a. Pour antiseptic on all three cotton balls.

b. If the client is female, spread her labia with your nondominant hand while using forceps to hold a cotton ball in your dominant hand.

Remember that the hand used to spread the labia is no longer sterile.

Continued

Inserting an Indwelling Catheter

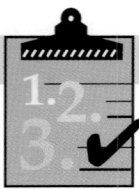

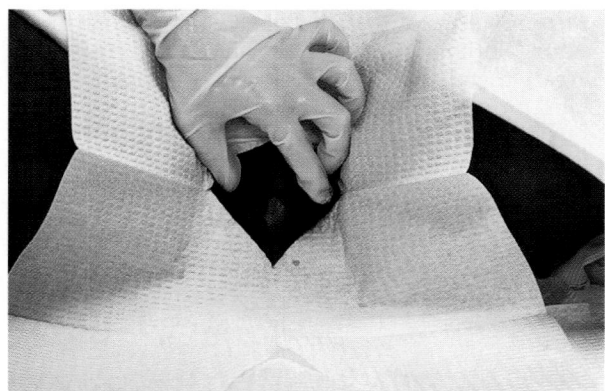

Spreading the labia.

c. With the first cotton ball, clean to the right of the client's urinary meatus. Make one stroke from top to bottom and discard the cotton ball. With the second cotton ball, clean to the left of the client's urinary meatus, again making one stroke from top to bottom before discarding the cotton ball. With the third cotton ball, clean down the middle of the client's perineum, directly over the urinary meatus. Then discard the cotton ball. Keep the client's labia spread until the catheter is inserted.

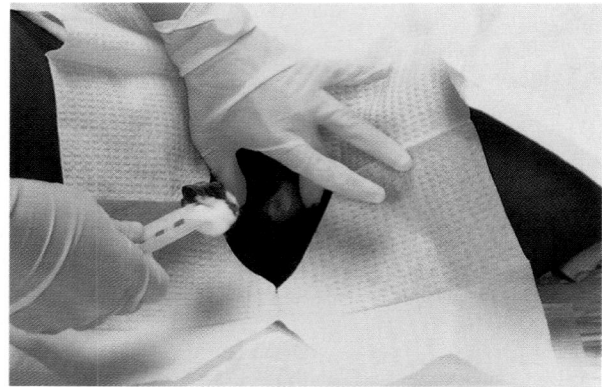

Cleaning the labia and meatus from top to bottom.

d. If the client is male, use at least two cotton balls soaked in antiseptic. Use the first to clean around the glans penis. Use the second to clean over the meatus. Make sure to retract the foreskin if the client has not been circumcised.

Remember to replace the foreskin to avoid edema of the glans penis.

6 Lubricate and insert the catheter.
a. Holding the catheter 2.5 to 5 cm (1 to 2 inches)

from its tip, lubricate it and insert it into the urinary meatus. If the client is male, use your nondominant hand to hold his penis perpendicular to his body, using your fingers to gently encircle and stabilize the shaft.

If you meet resistance when inserting a catheter, do not force it. Instead, have the client take a deep breath as you twist the catheter while trying to pass it. Often this method will allow the catheter to slide in easily. If it does not, try using a catheter with a Coudé tip; it is smaller and curved to help the catheter pass an obstruction, such as prostatic hypertrophy.

b. Insert the catheter until urine begins to flow.

The catheter should enter a female client by 5 to 7.6 cm (2 to 3 inches) or a male client by 15.2 to 20.3 cm (6 to 8 inches).

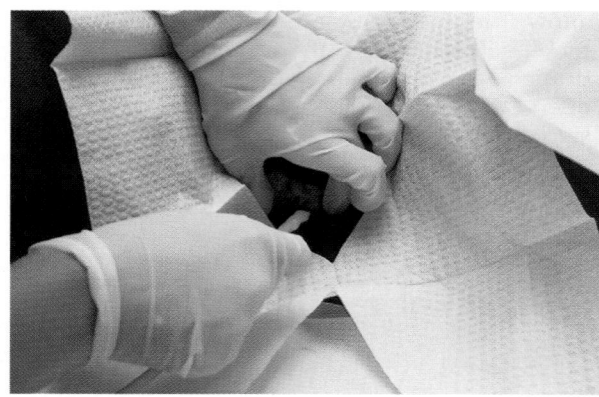

Inserting the catheter.

c. After urine begins to flow, insert the catheter 2.5 cm (1 inch) more.

Doing so will ensure that the balloon is in the bladder, not the urethra.

7 Inflate the balloon. If the syringe has been previously attached to the pigtail, simply inject 5 mL of water (30 mL if the catheter has a 30 mL balloon).

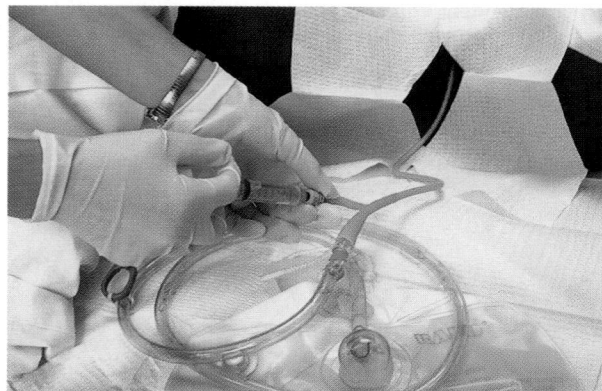

Inflating the balloon.

8 Tape catheter to the inner aspect of the thigh.

9 Establish the drainage system.
a. If the client will use a leg bag to collect urine, attach the catheter to the inner thigh.

Allow enough slack in the catheter tubing to avoid tugging on the catheter when the client's leg moves.

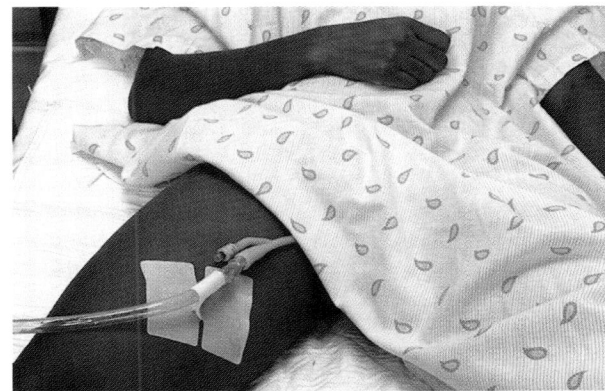

Catheter taped to the inner thigh.

b. If the client will use gravity drainage, attach the bag to the bed frame below the level of the client's bladder.

In a hospital bed, the bag and tubing should go under the side rails in a position that allows for straight gravity drainage and does not interfere with the operation of the side rails.

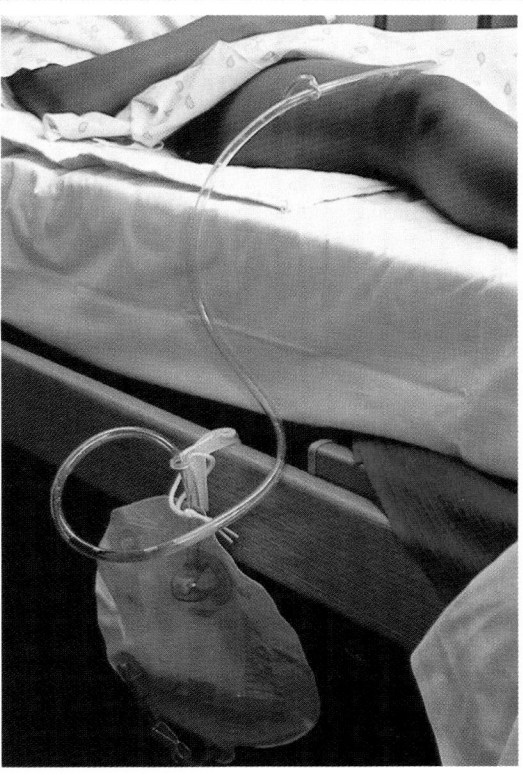

Bag attached to bed frame for gravity drainage.

10 Complete the procedure
a. Discard all trash.
b. Make the client comfortable.
c. Document the time the catheter was inserted, the amount and characteristics of urine that drained from the bladder, and the size of the catheter and balloon.

HOME CARE CONSIDERATIONS

In the home setting, you will need to be creative in positioning yourself, setting up the sterile field, and establishing adequate lighting to insert the catheter. Provide perineal hygiene before catheterizing. Teach any family caregivers about maintenance of the catheter.

Action **A**lert!
Maintaining straight, gravity drainage from an indwelling catheter will prevent backflow of possibly contaminated urine into the bladder.

Urinary catheterization carries a high risk of urinary tract infection and should be avoided unless the potential benefits outweigh the potential risks. After a single catheterization (not indwelling), 1% of ambulatory clients will develop infection. With an open drainage system, all clients will develop an infection in 4 days. If a closed system is used with a triple-lumen catheter to provide access for irrigation with neomycin and polymixin B, most clients will avoid infection for 10 days (Stein, 1994, p. 1963).

Suprapubic catheters are sometimes placed to reduce the incidence of infection. A puncture wound is made through the abdominal wall into the bladder and a catheter is inserted (Fig. 35–12). The incidence of infection is less than with a typical indwelling catheter because the abdominal skin has a lower bacterial count than the urethra.

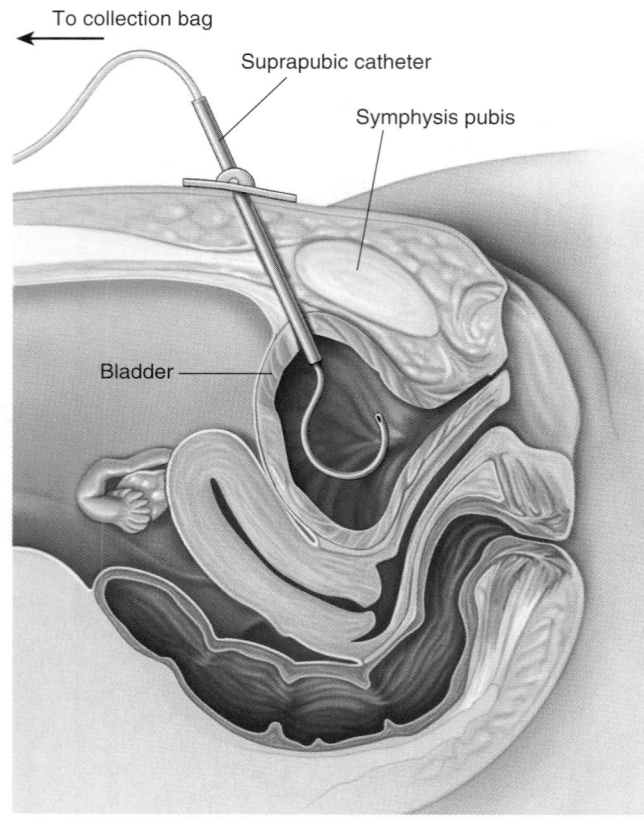

Figure 35–12. A suprapubic catheter is surgically placed through a puncture wound to drain urine until the client can void normally through the urethra.

MANAGING URETHRAL CATHETERS
Maintaining Comfort
The client with an indwelling catheter should be physically and mentally comfortable. Probably the greatest discomfort for most people is embarrassment and invasion of privacy.

Maintaining a Patent Catheter
The catheter should be taped to the leg (women) or abdomen (men) to prevent it from pulling on the urethra and to ensure the free flow of urine. Disposable anchoring devices are available, but nonallergenic tape can be used as well. Keep enough slack in the catheter to allow the client to move about without the catheter pulling on the urethra. Taping a male catheter laterally to the side or to the abdomen more naturally follows the normal anatomic direction of the male urethra and avoids the possibility of abscess formation at the penoscrotal junction.

When the client is in bed, the connecting tubing can be placed under the leg or over the leg. Under-the-leg placement may use gravity more effectively for drainage, but the tubing is made of hard plastic and may cause discomfort or pressure on the skin. Coil any excess tubing on the bed to prevent stagnation of urine in dangling loops of tubing. Keep the drainage bag below the level of the bladder, even when moving the person in and out of bed or to a stretcher. Urine in the collection tubing is not sterile and, because bacteria growing in the collection bag could travel up the tubing, urine should not be allowed to flow back into the bladder.

Relieving Bladder Spasms
Bladder spasms are involuntary, sudden, violent contractions of the muscles of the bladder that can be prolonged and painful. Spasms can occur as a side effect of catheterization or secondary to surgery on the bladder or urethra. Even though the client has a catheter, the urge to urinate is often strong.

Sometimes the spasms can be alleviated by manipulating the catheter to move the balloon away from the neck of the bladder. Increasing fluid intake may be helpful as well. Anticholinergic medications may be prescribed to reduce bladder tone and relieve the spasm. Narcotics will relieve the pain.

Re-establishing Urination After Catheterization
Because of the high incidence of infection, an indwelling catheter should be removed as soon as possible. The criteria may be that the person is able to ambulate to the bathroom, the edema has subsided, or the initial inflammatory stage of healing of a surgical wound has passed.

To remove the catheter, select a syringe appropriate to the amount of water in the balloon (usually 5 mL), insert the syringe into the pigtail used to inflate the balloon, aspirate the water from the balloon, and pinch and withdraw the catheter (Fig. 35–13). The client may feel a pulling sensation as the catheter is removed. For clients who have urethral irritation, the procedure may be momentarily uncomfortable. Having the client take a deep breath and removing the catheter slowly is helpful. A small amount of urine may escape, so it is useful to have a towel under the catheter as it comes out. Measure the urine in the bag and discard the bag. Removing a catheter is a clean procedure employing standard precautions.

Following removal of the catheter, monitor the client for the return of a normal pattern of urination. The client should drink extra liquid to fill the bladder and relieve irritation. Most people void after 2 to 4 hours. Sometimes, measures to help the person relax and ini-

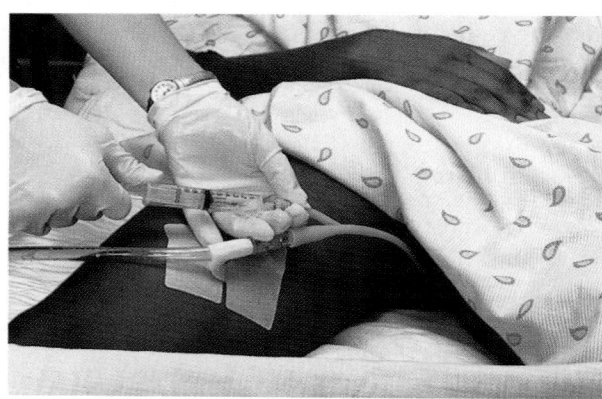

Figure 35–13. To remove an indwelling catheter, attach a 10-mL syringe (without a needle) to the pigtail port, and withdraw the normal saline from the catheter balloon.

tiate the stream are needed for the first voiding. The maximum time to the first voiding should be 6 to 8 hours. If the bladder becomes overdistended, it may be more difficult to void the first time. If the client has had surgery on the bladder or urethra, the urine should be monitored for diminishing amounts of blood.

For a client who has had an indwelling catheter for a prolonged period of time, training or reconditioning of the bladder before removing the catheter may be helpful. The bladder tone and capacity may have diminished. To do so, clamp the catheter, allow time for the bladder to fill, and then drain the bladder. When the client can tolerate having the catheter clamped for 4-hour periods, the catheter can be removed.

Single and Intermittent Catheterization

Single catheterization refers to the practice of inserting a catheter, draining the bladder, and removing the catheter. If the client is unable to void, the catheter can be inserted again when the bladder needs to be emptied. Intermittent catheterization is performed to check for residual urine, to manage long-term lack of control over urination, and to collect urine specimens.

Intermittent catheterization may be prescribed by a physician after a surgical procedure that produces a high risk of urinary retention. The order is often written as "catheterize prn" or "in and out catheter prn." You must make judgements about the need for catheterization and the frequency of catheterization. This judgement is based on the client's report of fullness, the interval since the last voiding, and an examination for bladder distention. Before inserting the catheter, have the client attempt to urinate. Then immediately insert the catheter. Because the client has just emptied the bladder, the amount of urine remaining in the bladder represents retention and is referred to as residual urine.

Intermittent self-catheterization is a procedure that can be taught to clients who are unable to spontaneously empty the bladder and have chronic urinary retention with overflow incontinence. These clients are usually relatively young, cognitively intact victims of spinal cord injury with permanent paralysis from the waist down. The procedure may also be used for a client with an underactive or a partially obstructed bladder. It is easier for a male to perform self-catheterization than for a female to perform it.

Before teaching self-catheterization, determine the reason that the client needs the procedure. A client with a neurogenic bladder will be able to perform the procedure differently than a client who is paraplegic. Also assess the client's ability and motivation to learn. The client may need a period of adjustment before deciding to master self-catheterization. Assess the client's usual health practices to determine the likelihood of safe management of the procedure.

If the client's immune system is not impaired, you most likely will teach self-catheterization as a clean procedure, as described in the accompanying Teaching for Self-Care chart. Clean technique has not been shown to result in a higher incidence of urinary tract infection than sterile technique (Webber-Jones, 1991; Wyndaele & Maes, 1990). Long-term use of intermittent catheterization may be preferable to indwelling catheterization from the standpoint of preventing infections and the formation of stones.

Teaching the Use of Urinary Catheters at Home

If necessary, the client and family will need to know how to manage a catheter safely at home, as outlined in the accompanying Teaching for Self-Care chart. The client and family caregivers should understand the functions and purpose of the catheter. Preventing urinary tract infection is probably the most important concept to teach. Clean technique and adequate fluid intake should be included in teaching. The caregiver should have the knowledge to monitor for the signs and symptoms of urinary tract infections.

Interventions to Irrigate the Bladder

Surgery on the bladder or prostate may result in bleeding into the bladder. That is why, when a client has had surgery on the bladder or a transurethral resection of the prostate, the indwelling catheter will need to be irrigated to maintain its patency by preventing the formation of blood clots or removing those that do form.

Irrigation can be accomplished using a closed-bladder irrigation system or by opening the system and using an irrigation syringe attached to the indwelling catheter. Because the urine and bladder are normally free of bacteria, either method should be used with sterile technique.

> **A**ction **A**lert!
> In high-risk populations, such as hospitalized clients, you will need to maintain sterile techniques for catheterization or irrigation of a catheter.

A closed irrigation system uses a three-lumen indwelling catheter (Fig. 35–14). The advantage of this closed irrigation system is a reduced risk of infection. The disadvantage is that the client is attached to multiple tubes and the bag of irrigation fluid. The physician's order usually specifies irrigation of the bladder to maintain patency. The fluid can be run continuously through the bladder or instilled intermittently. You will use a sliding clamp to regulate the flow of irrigant to keep the urine pink. If the urine becomes burgundy or red, you will need to increase the flow rate of the irrigant. If the urine stops flowing, the catheter may need to be irrigated with an irrigation syringe to apply more force to remove clots. Preventing clots is preferable to irrigating forcefully because forceful irrigation increases the risk of bleeding.

The catheter also may be irrigated to remove sediment, to reduce the number of microorganisms in the bladder, and to instill medications. When catheters are used for the long-term management of urinary incontinence, sediment is formed from minerals excreted in the urine, and it may solidify in and around the catheter. Keep in mind that irrigation for the purpose of removing sediment is controversial because it increases the chance of urinary tract infection.

Teaching for SELF-CARE

SELF-CATHETERIZATION

Purpose: To help client manage bladder elimination and establish skills for independent living.

Rationale: By learning to self-catheterize, the client can increase independence and, consequently, self-esteem.

Expected Outcome: The client will be able to self-catheterize successfully to minimize incontinence and the risk of urinary tract infection.

Client Instructions

Establishing a Schedule for Catheterization
- Together with your health care providers, determine an optimal schedule for self-catheterization. It will depend in part on how often you experience incontinence, which may relate directly to your bladder capacity and fluid intake. Consider your work and social schedules as well.
- Seek to maintain a routine catheterization schedule, such as three or four times daily or after a certain number of hours have passed. Some people need self-catheterization every 4 hours.

Performing Catheterization
- Plan to drain the urine into a receptacle or directly into the toilet. If you drain it into a receptacle, you may want to have a towel on hand to catch any spills.
- Assume a position that allows access to your urinary meatus. If necessary, if you are female, you can use a mirror to locate the meatus. Many women locate it by feel.
- Clean your urinary meatus with warm, soapy water and rinse.

- If you are male, retract your foreskin, if necessary, and hold your penis erect or at a right angle to your body. If you are female, spread your labia.
- Holding the catheter about ½ inch from the tip, insert it into your urinary meatus. This should not hurt, and you should feel no resistance. The first time you perform self-catheterization, you may feel some pressure as your urethra stretches.
- Advance the catheter until urine begins to flow (about 2 to 3 inches for a woman and 6 to 8 inches for a man). Then advance the catheter 1 to 2 inches farther to make sure it is in your bladder.
- When the urine has stopped flowing, lean forward and use your abdominal muscles to remove any residual urine.

Maintaining Safety Measures
- Wash your hands vigorously before and after self-catheterization.
- Clean the catheter with warm, soapy water and rinse it thoroughly after each use.
- After cleaning, either boil the catheter in water for 20 minutes or soak it in half-strength vinegar and rinse it before its next use, as prescribed.
- Once the catheter is clean and dry, store it in a clean plastic bag or towel.
- Immediately report any signs and symptoms of urinary tract infection to your doctor, such as burning or pain on urination, increased incontinence, malodorous or cloudy urine, or swelling or redness at your urinary meatus.

Interventions to Manage a Urinary Diversion

In the initial postoperative period, you will monitor the client for postoperative complications. This involves tracking the flow of urine and watching for signs of peritonitis, hemorrhage, and a decrease in vital signs. The newly created stoma may have a stent to maintain its patency. If urine leaks from the operative site into the peritoneum, the client will report pain and you will note abdominal distention, guarding, and tenderness.

The goal for the client is to learn to manage life with a urinary diversion. If the person does not have a continent stoma, an appliance will be attached to the skin around the stoma and urine will drain into a bag either at the site or attached to the client's leg. The person with a continent stoma must learn self-catheterization.

Because of the absence of the normal protective mechanisms of the urinary tract, a urinary diversion is prone to infection. So the person must learn to maintain clean technique and must know the signs and symptoms of infection. The skin around the stoma must remain dry and must be monitored for irritation.

Interventions to Manage Urinary Tract Infections

Urinary tract infections usually are treated with specific or nonspecific antibiotics. When a client has a urinary tract infection, increased fluid intake keeps urine dilute and promotes rapid reduction of the bacterial count in the urinary tract. On the other hand, it can hinder therapy by producing increased urine output, thus lowering urinary concentrations of antimicrobial agents. Therefore, the client should drink six to eight glasses of fluid per day but should not force fluids when taking most urinary antibiotics. Encourage clients to void when they feel the urge.

Changing the pH of urine has been recommended as an adjunct to therapy. Lowering the pH enhances

Teaching for SELF-CARE

MAINTAINING AN INDWELLING (FOLEY) CATHETER AT HOME

Purpose: To maintain the function of the catheter, maximize comfort, and prevent complications from the use of an indwelling catheter.

Rationale: Regular cleaning and maintenance will prevent complications.

Expected Outcome: The client will not experience a urinary tract infection as a result of the use of an indwelling catheter.

Client Instructions

Care of the Catheter
- Cleanse the area around the catheter's exit site with mild soap and water. Some people prefer to clean the area around the catheter while showering. Afterward, rinse thoroughly. If you are not bathing in the shower, use a squeeze bottle filled with warm water to rinse the area while sitting on the toilet. Do not soak in the bathtub.
- Use nonallergenic tape to secure the catheter to your thigh. Allow enough slack in the tube to avoid pulling on the catheter when you move in bed or walk.
- Keep the drainage bag below your bladder at all times.
- Avoid using powders and sprays on your perineal area.
- Call your doctor if your temperature goes above 38.3°C (101°F).

Care of the Drainage Bag
- Empty the drainage bag often.
- To drain urine, open the port at the bottom of the bag and allow the urine to drain into the toilet or into a receptacle that you can easily empty into the toilet. When urine stops flowing, reclamp the drainage tube.

- If you use a receptacle, rinse it after emptying it to prevent odor and bacterial growth.

Removing the Catheter
- If your physician prescribes it, schedule an appointment to check for residual urine in your bladder.
- Before you leave the hospital, review the instructions for removing the catheter.
- As instructed, remove the catheter 2 hours before your office visit. To do so, first wash your hands thoroughly with soap and warm water.
- Sit on the toilet. Insert a 10 mL syringe (without a needle) into the pigtail on the catheter and withdraw all the water from the pigtail. It should be about 5 mL.
- Gently pull the catheter out of your urinary meatus. It should slide out easily.
- Drink 32 ounces of water, and urinate when you feel the urge. If you have trouble starting your urine stream, try running water or rinsing your perineum with warm water from a squeeze bottle. Do not panic if you are unable to urinate.
- At the doctor's office, you will be asked to urinate and your urine will be measured. You will then have a catheter inserted to check for residual urine. If you have more than 3 ounces of residual urine, the indwelling catheter will need to remain in place.
- If you are not ready to have the catheter out, you will be given another appointment and will repeat the same procedure. It is not uncommon to need the catheter for an additional period of time. It does not mean that anything is wrong.
- If you have any questions, always feel free to ask a doctor or nurse.

the antibacterial activity of urine by increasing the concentration of organic acids normally found in urine. The pH of urine also affects the activity of some chemotherapeutic agents. The activity of methenamine mandelate, methenamine hippurate, and nitrofurantoin (all urinary antibacterials) is increased at a low urinary pH, whereas aminoglycoside antibiotics are more effective at an alkaline pH.

Acidification can be achieved by the use of ascorbic acid or methionine, by a modification of the diet, and by restricting milk, sodium bicarbonate, and fruit juices (except for cranberry juice). However, urinary acidification can be difficult to achieve and can cause precipitation of urate stones. Lowering the pH of the urine with a special diet or with ordered medications is advised. For the client with frequent urinary tract infections, preventive measures should be taught.

EVALUATION

Evaluation of urinary tract problems should be specific to the nature of the problem. Ask yourself if the problem is resolvable or if the problem is expected to be ongoing. Examine the outcomes, the methods to achieve the outcomes, and the client's level of satisfaction with care.

Urinary incontinence in immobile, neurologically impaired elderly clients often cannot be resolved. Evaluation seeks to ensure that the client is clean, dry, and comfortable. Equally important is determining that the skin remains intact. The diet should be free of foods or fluids that irritate the bladder. The client should be well hydrated, and the environment should be free of the odor of stale urine. Measures to prevent

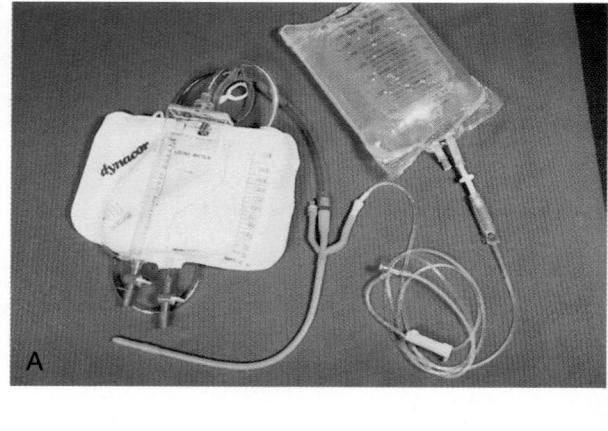
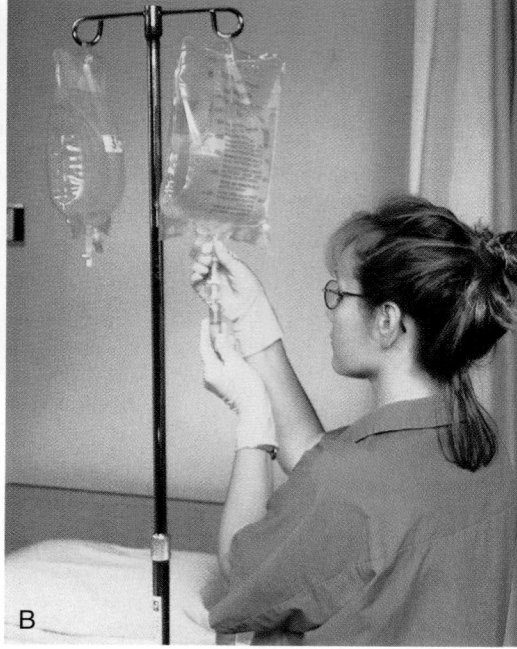

Figure 35–14. Closed bladder irrigation. *A*, the setup for closed bladder irrigation consists of a three-way indwelling catheter, a bag of irrigant with tubing, and a gravity drainage system. *B*, the irrigant is hung on an IV pole and is regulated with a sliding clamp on the tubing.

and detect urinary tract infection should be in place. If the client develops a urinary tract infection, ask what measures should be added to prevent future occurrences.

Urinary incontinence in many cases can be resolved with exercises or other treatment methods. If the problem is not resolved, evaluation includes asking whether the client has been given all available options and whether the client is satisfied with the level of resolution. Management may be considered successful if the number of episodes or the severity of each episode is reduced. Consider the client's ability to participate in the treatment regimen and the level of participation observed.

Evaluation also includes examining nursing care. Were the methods of teaching appropriate to the client's ability to learn and to the client's value system? Was the immobile client checked for dryness at sufficiently frequent intervals to detect incontinence? How frequently was the client offered a bedpan or assisted to the toilet? What measures were used to control odor? If odor is present, additional measures should be included in the care plan. Was the client offered a sufficient amount of appropriate fluids? Were measures included to ensure the client's privacy and avoid embarrassment over incontinence?

Evaluation of the care of the client with a urinary diversion considers the same parameters for skin care, diet, fluids, odor control, privacy, and embarrassment. However, a major part of the evaluation examines the client's level of self-care and whether the care is managed in a manner that minimally disrupts the client's preferred lifestyle.

KEY PRINCIPLES

- Understanding problems of urinary dysfunction includes an understanding of the structure and function of the kidneys, ureters, bladder, and urethra.
- Examination of urine provides information relevant to the function of the urinary tract and to the general health and function of the body.
- Substances in the urine are a result of the filtration, reabsorption, and secretion functions of the kidney as an organ of homeostatic balance.
- Dysuria can result from obstruction, infection, neurological injury, or decreased muscle tone.
- Low urine volumes can result from dehydration, hypotension, antidiuretic hormone, renal failure, or urinary retention.
- The diagnosis of *Altered urinary elimination* requires differentiation between stress, urge, reflex, functional, overflow, and total incontinence.
- Urinary tract infection is not a nursing diagnosis because the nurse cannot prescribe definitive therapy, but the nurse can treat the risk for urinary tract infection by instituting measures to prevent the problem and to educate the client about healthy practices.
- A nurse can assist a client in avoiding urinary tract infections by teaching about hygiene, fluid intake, and measures to change the pH of the urine.
- The bladder is a sterile body cavity but is at risk for

infection because the entrance to the bladder is in close proximity to the anus. Women have higher risk than men because of the short urethra.

- The concept of cleaning the perineum from clean to dirty, front to back, is key to preventing urinary tract infection, especially in women.
- The bladder feels full when it contains an average of 300 mL, after which it is emptied completely with each voiding.
- An indwelling catheter should be the treatment of last resort for urinary incontinence.
- Urinary tract infections are highly associated with the use of indwelling catheters.
- Incontinence often results from a correctable cause. A medical evaluation may be appropriate before deciding on nursing care to manage incontinence.

BIBLIOGRAPHY

Agency for Health Care Policy and Research (1996). *Urinary incontinence in adults: Acute and chronic management. Clinical practice guideline No. 2.* AHCPR Publication No. 96-0682. Rockville, MD: Author. Available at: http://text.nhm.nih.gov.

*Bristall, S.L. (1989). The mythical danger of rapid urinary drainage. *American Journal of Nursing, 89*(3), 344–345.

*Burgio, L.D., McCormick, K.A., Scheve, A.S., Engel, B.T., Hawkins, A., & Leahy, E. (1994). The effects of changing prompted voiding schedules in the treatment of incontinence in nursing home residents. *Journal of the American Geriatric Society, 42*(3):315–320.

Catanzaro, J. (1996). Managing incontinence: An update. *RN, 59*(10), 38–39, 41–44.

*Chan, H. (1993). Noninvasive bladder volume measurement. *Journal Neuroscience Nursing. 25*(5), 309–312.

*Charbonneau-Smith, R. (1993). No-touch catheterization and infection rates in selected spinal cord injured population. *Rehabilitation Nursing, 18*(5), 296–299, 305.

Colling, J. (1996). Noninvasive techniques to manage urinary incontinence among care-dependent persons. *Journal of Wound, Ostomy, and Continence Nursing 23*(6), 302–308.

Colling, J., Ouslander, J., Hadley, B.J., Eisch, J., & Campbell, E. (1992). The effects of patterned urge response toileting (PURT) on urinary incontinence among nursing home residents. *Journal of the American Geriatric Society, 40*(2), 135–141.

DiBattiste, J.M. (1997). Uses of a Kock pouch. *American Journal of Nursing, 97*(12), 17.

*Dille, C.M., & Kirchhoff, K.T. (1993). Decontamination of vinyl urinary drainage bags with bleach. *Rehabilitation Nursing, 18*(5), 292–295.

Duffield, P. (1996). Managing urinary tract infections. Part 1: diagnosing and treating adults. *American Journal of Nursing, 96*(9), 16B–16D.

Duffield, P. (1997). Urinary tract infections in the elderly: A common complication of aging. *Advance for Nurse Practitioners, 1*(5), 30–32.

Ebersole, P.R. (1998). Continence care pioneers: Thelma Wells, RN, PhD, FAAN, FRCN, and Joyce Colling, RN, PhD, FAAN. *Geriatric Nursing, 19*(2), 103–105.

Epps, C.K. (1996). The delicate business of ostomy care. *RN, 59*(11), 32–36.

Foster, P. (1998). Behavioral treatment of urinary incontinence: A complementary approach. *Ostomy and Wound Management, 44*(6), 62–66, 68, 70.

*Garvin, G. (1994). Caring for children with ostomies. *Nursing Clinics of North America, 29*(4), 645–654.

Gibbons, G. (1996). Assessing and managing incontinence in women. *Community Nurse, 2*(5), 34–36.

Gray, M. (1998). Ostomy care? Show me the data! *Journal of Wound, Ostomy, and Continence Nursing, 25*(1), 2–4.

Guyton, A.C., & Hall, J.E. (1996). *Textbook of medical physiology* (9th ed.). Philadelphia: W.B. Saunders Co.

Haus, E. (1998). Urinary tract infections in the homebound elderly. *Home Healthcare Nurse, 16*(5), 323–327.

Huston, C.J., & Boelman, R. (1995). Emergency, autonomic dysreflexia. *American Journal of Nursing, 95*(6), 55.

Jackson, B., & Hicks, L.E. (1997). Effect of cranberry juice on urinary pH in older adults. *Home Healthcare Nurse, 15*(3), 199–202.

Jaramillo, O., Elizondo, J., Jones, P., Cordero, J., & Wang, J. (1997). Practical guidelines for developing a hospital-based wound and ostomy clinic. *Ostomy and Wound Management, 43*(4), 28–32, 34–36, 38–39.

*Jirovec, M.M. (1991). Effect of individualized prompted toileting on incontinence in nursing home residents. *Applied Nursing Research, 4*(4), 188–191.

Krissovich, M., & Safran, R. (1997). Urinary incontinence in adults. *Lippincott's Primary Care Practitioner, 1*(4), 361–381.

Lilley, L.L., & Guanci, R. (1996). Sulfa drug reaction. *American Journal of Nursing, 96*(1), 14.

Marchiondo, K. (1998). A new look at urinary tract infection. *American Journal of Nursing, 98*(3), 34–38.

McKinney, B.C. (1995). Cut your patients' risk of nosocomial UTI. *RN, 58*(11), 20–23.

Mitchel, J.V. (1998). A clinical pathway for ostomy care in the home: Process and development. *Journal of Wound, Ostomy, and Continence Nursing, 25*(4), 200–205.

Mogus, M. (1997). Pelvic floor surgery? *RN, 60*(4), 36–41.

*Moore, K.M., Kelm, M., Sinclair, O., & Cadrain, G. (1993). Bacteria in intermittent catheterization users: The effects of sterile versus clean reused catheters. *Rehabilitation Nursing, 18,* 306–309.

Nazarko, L. (1996). In search of relief. *Nursing Times, 92*(32), 68, 70.

Ouslander, J., Schnelle, J., Simmons, S., Bates-Jensen, B., & Zeitlin, M. (1993). The dark side of incontinence: Nighttime incontinence in nursing home residents. *Journal of the American Geriatric Society, 41*(4), 371–376.

Pinkowski, P.S. (1996). Urinary incontinence in the long-term care facility. *Journal of Wound, Ostomy, and Continence Nursing, 23*(6), 309–313.

*Rainville, N.C. (1994). The current nursing procedure for intermittent urinary catheterization in rehabilitation facilities. *Rehabilitation Nursing, 19*(6), 330–333.

Ramos, L., & Glosson, A. (1996). Teaching ostomy care to a patient who is blind. *Journal of Wound, Ostomy, and Continence Nursing, 23*(4), 235–236.

*Resnick, B. (1993). Retraining the bladder after catheterization. *American Journal of Nursing, 93*(11), 46–49.

Rogers, J. (1998). Promoting continence: The child with special needs. *Nursing Standards, 12*(34), 47–52.

Savage, C. (1998). Information for patients having bladder augmentation. *Nursing Times, 94*(30), 52–53.

*Schnelle, J.F., Adamson, G.M., Cruise, P.A., al-Samarrai N., Sarbaugh, F.C., Uman, G., & Ouslander, J.G. (1997). Skin disorders and moisture in incontinent nursing home residents: Intervention implications. *Journal of the American Geriatric Society, 45*(10), 1182–1188.

Schnelle, J.F., Cruise, P.A., Alessi, C.A., al-Samarrai, N., & Ouslander, J.G. (1998). Individualizing nighttime incontinence care in nursing home residents. *Nursing Research 47*(4), 197–204.

Schnelle, J.F., Ouslander, J.G., Simmons, S.F., Alessi, C.A., & Gravel, M.D. (1993). Nighttime sleep and bed mobility among incontinent nursing home residents. *Journal of the American Geriatric Society, 41*(9), 903–909.

Scura, K.W., & Whipple, B. (1997). How to provide better care for the postmenopausal woman. *American Journal of Nursing, 97*(4), 36–43.

Semple, M., & Elley, K. (1998) Practical procedures for nurses. Catheter specimen of urine. *Nursing Times, 94*(30), suppl 1–2.

*Skoner, M. (1994). Self-management of urinary incontinence among women 31 to 50 years of age. *Rehabilitation Nursing, 19*(6), 339–343, 347.

---

* Asterisk indicates a classic or definitive work on this subject.

*Stark, J. (1994). Interpreting BUN/creatinine levels: It's not as simple as you think. *Nursing94, 24*(9), 58–61.

*Stein, J.H. (Ed.) (1994). *Internal Medicine.* St. Louis: Mosby.

*Talbot, L.A. (1994). Coping with urinary incontinence: Development and testing of a scale. *Nursing Diagnosis, 5*(30), 127–132.

*Thayer, D. (1994). How to assess and control urinary incontinence. *American Journal of Nursing, 94*(10), 42–47.

Torres, S.A., Holley, J.A., Ando, J., DeVera, J., Harris, P., & Giles, A. (1998). Maximizing care outcomes of a patient with impaired bladder function: A P.I. project in a rehabilitation unit. *Journal of Nursing Care Quality, 12*(6), 64–69.

*Urinary Incontinence Guideline Panel (1992a). *Urinary incontinence in adults: Clinical practice guideline.* AHCPR Publication No. 92-0038. Rockville, MD: Agency for Healthcare Policy and Research.

*Urinary Incontinence Guideline Panel (1992b). *Urinary incontinence in adults: Quick reference guide for clinicians.* AHCPR Publication No. 92-0041. Rockville, MD: Agency for Healthcare Policy and Research.

Walton, J.C., & Miller, J.M. (1998). Evaluating physical and behavioral changes in older adults. *Medical-Surgical Nursing, 7*(2), 85–90.

*Warlemtom, R. (1992). Implementation of a urinary continence program. *Journal of Gerontological Nursing, 18,* 31–37.

*Webber-Jones, J. (1991) Performing clean, intermittent self-catheterization. *Nursing91, 21*(8), 56–59.

Wells, M. (1998). Coping with common catheter care problems. *Community Nurse, 4*(3), 22–24.

*Winslow, E.H. (1993). Myth of the clean catch. *American Journal of Nursing, 93*(8), 20.

*Wyndaele, J. J., & Maes, D. (1990). Clean intermittent self-catheterization: a 12-year follow-up. *Journal of Urology, 143,* 906–908.

Activity-Exercise Pattern

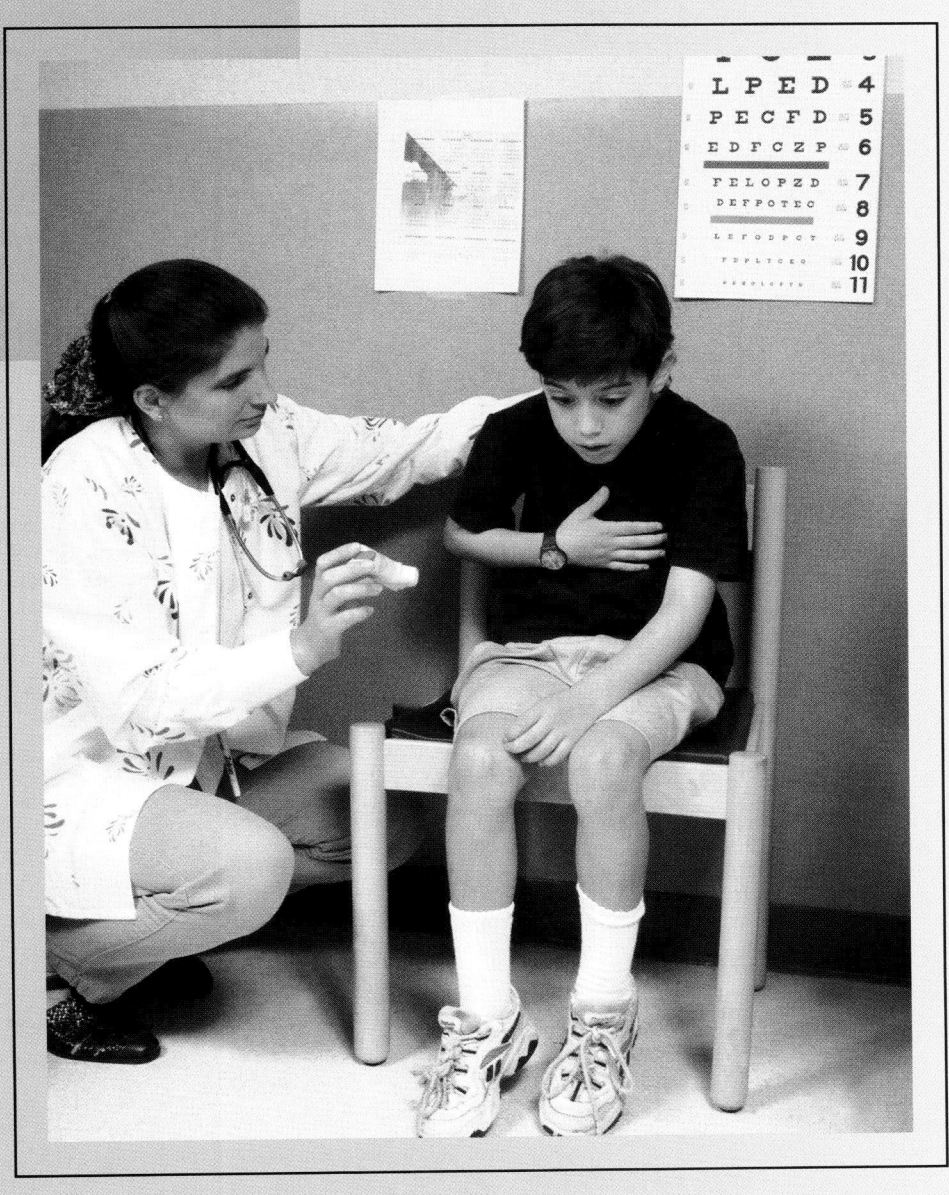

36

Hygiene

Rachel A. Taylor

Key Terms

alopecia	*gingivitis*
caries	*perineum*
cerumen	*plaque*
dentures	*tartar*

LEARNING OBJECTIVES

After studying this chapter, you should be able to:

1. Describe the structure and function of the skin, hair, nails, and oral cavity.

2. Discuss some problems of personal hygiene.

3. Describe some cultural, developmental, socioeconomic, physical, and psychosocial factors affecting hygiene.

4. Discuss assessment of the client who is at risk for or shows manifestations of self-care deficit for managing personal hygiene related to physical, psychological, or cognitive impairment.

5. Differentiate among a variety of nursing diagnoses related to the client's bathing and hygiene.

6. Plan client-centered outcomes to assist the client with meeting personal hygiene needs.

7. Describe nursing interventions to promote hygiene of the skin, mouth, and hair.

8. Evaluate outcomes of nursing care as being helpful in assisting the client to meet self-care needs for personal hygiene.

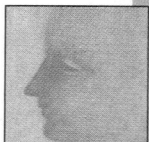

Joy Wilson, age 78, resides with her daughter and son-in-law. Mrs. Wilson is of African-American ancestry. She was admitted to the hospital 2 weeks ago after a sudden onset of weakness, nausea, and resulting left hemiplegia. A stroke (cerebrovascular accident) was diagnosed. Her hospital stay is ending, and she is being prepared for discharge to her daughter's home. Her progress in physical therapy has been only fair. Her left side is dominant, so she is being required to master and adapt motor skills completely foreign to her. She has a great desire to learn to care for herself but she is weak and is able to tolerate only minimal activity before becoming extremely fatigued. Her cognitive status is slightly impaired because of short-term memory deficit as well as some emotional lability. Her frustration at not being able to care for her hygiene needs is evidenced by tears and anger when she cannot achieve a goal.

Mrs. Wilson's daughter is devoted to her mother and desires to provide home care. Both mother and daughter are opposed to consideration of nursing home placement at this time. Her daughter is eager to learn to care for her mother and asks pertinent questions that reflect interest in her mother's welfare. Although she plans to be the primary caregiver for Mrs. Wilson, she will use community resources to assist her in giving the best possible care. Because of Mrs. Wilson's related problems of cognitive

(continued)

impairment, exercise intolerance, and frustration with her altered state of wellness, the nurse assesses that in addition to *Bathing/hygiene self-care deficit,* there are related nursing diagnoses that must be addressed (see the Nursing Diagnoses chart).

HYGIENE NURSING DIAGNOSES

Bathing/Hygiene Self-Care Deficit: Impaired ability to perform or complete bathing/hygiene activities for oneself.

Impaired Skin Integrity: A state in which an individual has altered epidermis and/or dermis.

Altered Oral Mucous Membrane: Disruptions of the lips and soft tissue of the oral cavity.

Ineffective Individual Coping: Inability to form a valid appraisal of the stressors, inadequate choices of practiced responses, and/or inability to use available resources.

Powerlessness: Perception that one's own action will not significantly affect an outcome; a perceived lack of control over a current situation or immediate happening.

From North American Nursing Diagnosis Association. (1999). NANDA nursing diagnoses: Definitions and classification, 1999–2000. Philadelphia: Author.

CONCEPTS OF PERSONAL HYGIENE

Personal hygiene consists of those activities which an individual undertakes in order to maintain body cleanliness and freedom from disease; namely, bathing, oral hygiene, and hair care. These activities are considered to be independent functions that are usually maintained daily. For that reason, they are called activities of daily living (ADLs). Usually acquired in early childhood, these skills and abilities become an integral part of adult behavior. Self-care is the ability to meet hygiene needs without the assistance of another person. It is essential to both physical and psychological well-being that hygiene needs be adequately met. If the body is not kept clean, the skin will be compromised and the body will be threatened by infection or disease. The individual's self-esteem and body image are also enhanced by the cleanliness of the body.

When illness or injury prevents the client from meeting all of the hygiene needs, it is the responsibility of the caregiver to assist with meeting these needs. The ultimate aim of nursing care is to assist the client to be as independent as possible and to teach toward resumption of self-care abilities to the extent that physical and mental capacities will allow.

Skin

The skin is an organ with highly specialized functions that are essential for human survival. Without skin, adaptation to the environment would be impossible because the intricate functions of this vital organ serve to maintain biological integrity and homeostasis.

The surface area of the skin makes it one of the larger organs in the body. In the average size adult, this surface covers approximately 20 square feet, or 3,000 square inches.

Strata of the Skin

The skin is composed structurally of two portions (Fig. 36–1). The outer portion, the epidermis, is composed of stratified squamous epithelium and contains four kinds of cells. The largest number of these cells are the keratinocytes, which produce keratin, a substance that protects skin and underlying tissues and plays a part in immune function. A second type of cell in the epidermis is the melanocyte, which is located at the base of the epidermis. The melanocyte produces melanin, one of the pigments responsible for skin color. Melanin also assumes a protective function by absorbing ultraviolet light rays, thereby lessening their harmful effects on the skin. The other types of cells in the epidermis are the nonpigmented granular dendrocytes, which are made up of two distinct cell types, Langerhans' cells and Granstein cells. These cells interact with T cells to assist in the immune process.

The second layer of skin is the dermis, which is composed of connective tissue containing collagenous and elastic fibers. Numerous blood vessels, nerves, glands, and hair follicles are embedded in this stratum of skin.

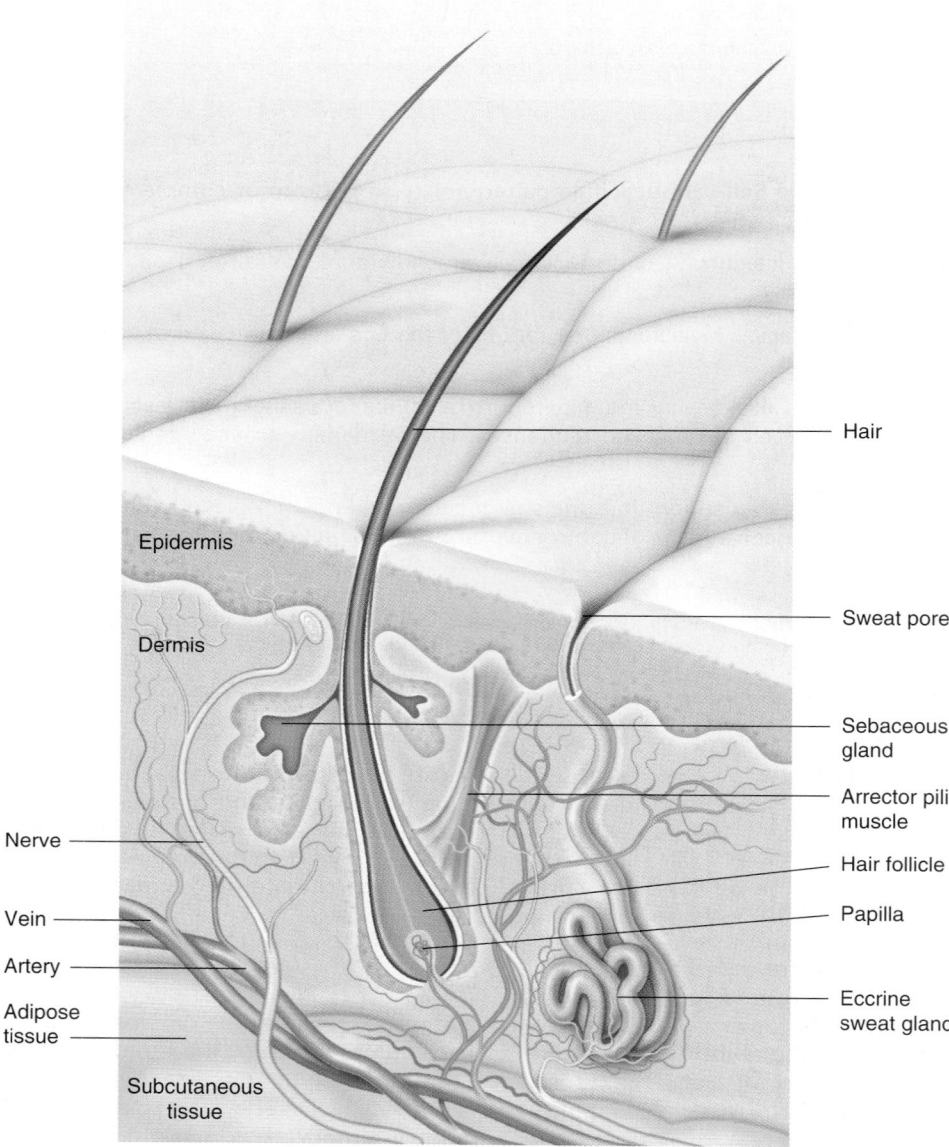

Epidermis

Dermis

Nerve

Vein

Artery

Adipose
tissue

Subcutaneous
tissue

Hair

Sweat pore

Sebaceous
gland

Arrector pili
muscle

Hair follicle

Papilla

Eccrine
sweat gland

Figure 36–1. Anatomy of the
skin.

The third layer, the innermost layer of skin under-neath the dermis, is the subcutaneous tissue, also known as the superficial fascia or the hypodermis. This subcutaneous layer consists of areolar and adipose tissue and provides support and blood supply to the dermis. The strata that make up the skin are all connected by fibers that extend all the way from the dermis to the underlying tissues and organs.

Glands of the Skin

Three kinds of glands are associated with the skin. They are the sebaceous glands, sudoriferous glands, and ceruminous glands. Most sebaceous glands are connected to hair follicles. The secreting portions of the glands lie within the dermis. These glands, which

are associated with hairs, open into the necks of the hair follicles. Those that are not associated with hair follicles open directly onto the surface of the skin (lips, glans penis, labia minora, and tarsal glands of the eyelids). They are absent in the palms and soles. Their size and shape vary throughout the body. They are small in most areas of the trunk and extremities and larger in the skin of the breasts, face, neck, and upper chest.

The sebaceous glands secrete an oily substance called sebum, which is made up of a mixture of fats, cholesterol, proteins, and inorganic salts. Sebum serves to protect hair from drying and forms a protective film on the skin that prevents excessive evaporation of water. It also helps to keep the skin soft and supple and inhibits the growth of certain bacteria on the skin.

Sudoriferous, or sweat, glands are identified according to their structure and function. Apocrine sweat glands are simple, branched tubular glands that are distributed primarily in the skin of the axilla, pubic region, and pigmented areas (areolae) of the breasts. The secretory portion of the gland is located in the dermis, and the excretory duct opens into hair follicles. Apocrine glands begin to function at puberty and produce a more viscous secretion than eccrine sweat glands.

Eccrine sweat glands are more numerous than apocrine sweat glands and are simple coiled tubular glands. They are distributed throughout the skin except for the margins of the lips, nail beds, glans penis, clitoris, labia minora, and eardrums. They are most numerous in the skin of the palms and soles, and their density can be as high as 3,000 per square inch in the palms. This is easily observed in the peculiar wetness of palms when a person is under stress or anxiety. The secretory portion of the gland is located in the subcutaneous layer, and the excretory duct projects upward through the dermis and epidermis to terminate at a pore on the surface of the epidermis. Eccrine sweat glands function throughout life and produce a secretion that is more watery than that of the apocrine glands. Through perspiration, small amounts of waste products are excreted through the skin.

Ceruminous glands secrete a thick, heavily pigmented oily substance called cerumen. **Cerumen** is a waxy secretion of the glands of the external acoustic meatus; it is commonly known as ear wax. This substance is found most often in the external ear canal.

Functions of the Skin

The skin is the body's first line of defense, and that principle is of paramount importance in the consideration of a client's hygiene needs. Normally, the skin hosts a large contingent of resident bacteria that serve a useful function. On intact skin, these resident organisms prevent excess growth of fungi. Sebum, a product of the sebaceous glands, is secreted into the hair follicles. Sebum has antibacterial and antifungal properties. Normal skin acidity also inhibits growth of pathogenic organisms.

The skin assists in regulating body temperature through production of perspiration by the sudoriferous glands, which help to lower body temperature. Perspiration, or sweat, is a mixture of water, salts (mostly sodium chloride), urea, uric acid, amino acids, ammonia, sugar, lactic acid, and ascorbic acid. Its principal function is to help regulate body temperature by way of evaporation of water in perspiration, which carries off large quantities of heat energy from the body surface.

The skin helps screen out harmful ultraviolet (UV) rays from the sun, but it also lets in some necessary UV rays that convert a chemical in the skin called 7-dehydrocholesterol into vitamin D, which is vital to the normal growth of bones and teeth. A lack of UV light and vitamin D impairs the absorption of calcium from the intestine into the bloodstream.

The skin is an important sensory organ containing sensory receptors that respond to heat, cold, touch, pressure, and pain. Skin offers protection through its many nerve endings, which warn of environmental sources of harm such as hot coals or sharp blades. The nerve endings can also help in sensing the outside world so that physiological adjustments can be made to maintain homeostasis.

Hair

Because it arises from the skin, hair is considered to be an appendage of the skin. In the human, hair covers the entire body with the exception of the palms, soles, lips, tip of penis, inner lips of vulva, and nipples. The hair consists of two major parts: the shaft or the portion protruding from the skin, and the root, which is embedded in the skin. The root contains a matrix of epithelial cells called the bulb. The bulb itself is contained within the hair follicle, which is composed of three sheaths: an inner epithelial sheath, an outer epithelial sheath, and a connective tissue sheath.

About halfway up the length of the hair follicle is an oil gland, which is located between the follicle and the arrector pili muscle. When this muscle contracts, it pulls the follicle and its hair upright, elevating the skin above the follicle and producing what is commonly called goose-flesh.

Rate of hair growth appears to depend on several factors, of which age, seasonal changes, and hair texture are prominent. Rate of hair growth slows with advancing age. Hair grows faster at night than during the day and faster in warm weather than in cold. Location of the hair is also a determining factor. Scalp hairs may last 3 to 5 years, whereas eyebrow and eyelash hairs may last only 10 weeks. Coarse black hairs grow faster than fine blonde hair. Human hair follicles have a growing and resting phase. Scalp hairs usually grow about 0.4 mm a day and last from 3 to 5 years. After the hair is shed, the follicle rests for 3 to 4 months. Eyebrow hair has a longer resting phase than growing phase (growing for 1 to 2 months and then resting for 3 to 4 months). Eyelashes have an even shorter growing phase. Baldness is not a problem because 80 to 90% of hairs are always in the growing stage at the same time. The average scalp contains about 125,000 hairs.

Although the human does not have the need for a protective covering of hair as do many other mammals, hair does serve some protective functions in humans. Scalp hair serves to insulate against cold air and external heat from the sun. Most hair follicles are associated with sebaceous glands, and some sweat gland ducts open into hair follicles. Therefore, the scalp becomes moist and oily in a hot environment.

Hair also serves to protect through providing a cushion for the cranium. Also, the eyebrows are cushions for protecting the eyes. Eyelashes serve to screen the entry of foreign particles or objects. Nostril hairs serve as catchers of dust particles and foreign matter that are present in the surrounding air and that are constantly being inhaled.

Nails

The nails are composed of hard keratinized cells of the epidermis. These cells form a clear, solid covering over the dorsal surfaces of the terminal surfaces of the fingers and toes. Each nail consists of three basic parts: the nail body, which is the visible portion; the free edge, which projects beyond the tip of the digit; and the nail root, which is hidden in the proximal nail groove.

Most of the nail body is pink because of the underlying vascular system. The whitish semilunar area of the proximal end of the body is called the lunula. It appears white because the vascular tissue underneath does not show through because of the thick stratum in the area. The eponychium (or cuticle) is a narrow band of epidermis that extends from the margin of the nail bed (lateral border), adhering to it. It occupies the proximal border of the nail and consists of stratum corneum.

The epithelium of the proximal part of the nail bed is known as the nail matrix. Its function is to bring about the growth of nails. Essentially, growth occurs by the transformation of superficial cells of the matrix into nail cells. In the process, the outer harder layer is pushed forward over the stratum germinativum. The average growth in the length of fingernails is about 1 mm (0.04 inch) per week. The growth rate is somewhat slower in toenails. Functionally, nails help with grasping and manipulating small objects in various ways. They also provide protection against trauma to the ends of the digits.

Oral Cavity

The oral cavity is composed of the teeth, the tongue, and the oral mucosa. Eruption of deciduous teeth (baby teeth) begins at approximately 6 months of age. These deciduous teeth are lost in childhood and are replaced by a set of 32 permanent teeth (16 in each jaw) composed of four incisors, two canines, four premolars, and six molars (see Chapter 20). All teeth consist of three parts: a root embedded in a socket (alveolus) in the alveolar process of the jaw bone; a crown projecting upward from the gum; and a neck between the root and the crown, which is surrounded by the gum (Fig. 36–2).

Each tooth is composed of dentin, enamel, cementum, and pulp. The dentin is the sensitive portion surrounding the pulp cavity and forms the bulk of the tooth. The enamel is the white covering of the tooth. The cementum is the bone-like covering of the neck and root. The pulp is the soft core of connective tissue that contains the nerves and blood vessels of the tooth.

The teeth are held in their sockets by connective tissue called periodontal ligaments. These collagenous

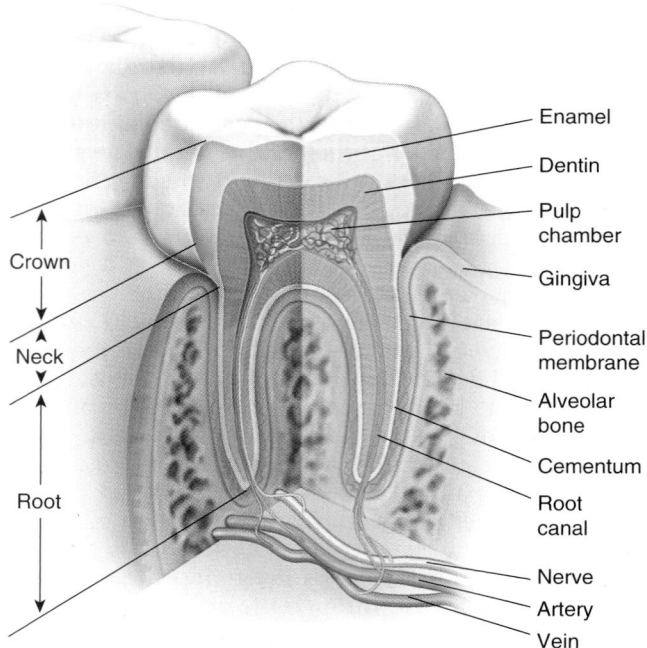

Figure 36–2. Anatomy of a tooth.

fibers of each ligament extend from the alveolar bone into the cement of each tooth, allowing for some tooth movement during the process of chewing.

The mouth and teeth play vital roles in the mastication (chewing) and digestion of food, which begins in the mouth as food is mixed with saliva for food breakdown and for further digestion. The muscles in the cheeks aid in chewing. The tongue has taste buds for discerning different tastes of food and helps mix saliva with food. The tongue also aids in swallowing by moving the food toward the pharynx. Phonation (the forming of words) is also a function of the tongue.

Problems of Personal Hygiene

Problems of the Oral Cavity

Table 36–1 lists some common problems of the oral cavity. Halitosis may be an early indicator of either poor oral hygiene or some systemic disorder. An offensive breath odor caused by inadequate oral hygiene can be alleviated with cleansing of the teeth and oral mucosa. If the origin of the halitosis is systemic, oral hygiene will not remove the odor.

Dental **caries** is a destructive process causing decalcification of the tooth enamel and leading to continued destruction of the enamel and dentin with resulting cavitation of the tooth. When the enamel barrier is breached, cavities develop. Dental caries is a disease of the calcified structure of the tooth. The agent responsible for dental caries is dental plaque. Dental **plaque** is a soft, thin film of food debris, mucin, and dead epithelial cells that is deposited on the teeth and provides a medium for the growth of bacteria. Freshly deposited plaque is transparent unless stained brown by tobacco or coffee or tea. When old dental plaque is present, the teeth appear dull with a dingy, yellowish cast.

Cavity formation results from bacterial enzymes combining with the dental plaque, fermenting the dietary carbohydrates and organic acids. These acids initiate the decalcification of tooth enamel. Once the bacteria have gained access to the tissue substance of the tooth, the next step is the development of caries.

Plaque and food remaining in the mouth produce an environment that is conducive to cavity formation. Dental plaque can be removed by brushing and flossing. Food remnants left trapped between the teeth set the stage for the beginning of decay and periodontal disease. When dental plaque remains on teeth, it becomes hardened (calcified) and forms calculus or tartar. **Tartar** is a yellowish film of calcium phosphate, carbonate, food particles, and other organic matter deposited on the teeth by saliva. Calculus must be removed with dental instruments.

Sound nutrition provides some resistance to dental decay. Dietary needs vary with such factors as age and general physical condition. Moderation in diet is important because both deficiencies and excesses can decrease resistance to decay. The use of a nonabrasive dentifrice (toothpaste or toothpowder) containing fluoride and the consumption of whole-grain foods that contain phosphorus inhibit caries. Dietary fats provide a barrier to acid penetration by forming an oily film on the surface of the tooth.

The gum is also known as the gingiva. It is the firm connective tissue covered with mucous membrane that surrounds the alveolar processes of the teeth.

Gingivitis is an inflammation of the gums usually manifested by the primary symptom of bleeding of the gums. It is an early stage of periodontal disease. Gingivitis may result from waste products and toxins from organisms in the mouth, which may cause initial injury. Then, when plaque and bacteria accumulate, they form calculus, which contains more microorganisms and causes further gingivitis. Others at increased risk for gingivitis include people who breathe through their mouths, diabetics, people who use orthodontic supplies (e.g., braces), and people experiencing hormonal fluctuations (adolescents, pregnant women, and those taking oral contraceptives).

Chronic gingivitis causes the inflammation to spread and destroy the underlying bone, causing periodontitis. In an advanced stage of periodontal disease, the periodontium atrophies so that the gums appear to have receded completely away from the tooth. Without adequate supporting structure, the tooth becomes very loosely attached or falls out.

A large number of young people have dental caries and mouth and gum disease. During pregnancy the increased circulating levels of hormones cause gingival hypertrophy, which can increase the incidence of periodontal disease if good oral hygiene is not consistently practiced. Periodontal disease is common among young adults. It is often precipitated by emotional stress, which aggravates the inflammatory process.

Many elderly people have few permanent teeth left and have partial or full dentures. **Dentures** are a complement of teeth, either natural or artificial, ordinarily used to designate an artificial replacement for the natural teeth. Half the people over age 65 years have no teeth. With age, the gums tend to recede and to develop a brownish pigmentation along the tooth edge. Salivation decreases and many older people complain of a dry mouth. Tooth loss is not inevitable.

Alterations in the oral mucosa may result from several causes. The mucosa should be moist and pink without ulceration or dryness or bleeding. Dryness of the lips and mucosa may occur in the client who is dehydrated or who is breathing through the mouth. Cli-

TABLE 36–1
Common Problems of the Oral Cavity

Problem	Description	Nursing Implications
Halitosis	Offensive odor of breath	Provide regular oral hygiene or teach client; assess for cause of halitosis.
Caries	Teeth may be dark in carious areas; may be painful.	Advise client to seek dental intervention.
Gingivitis	Gums may be pale and spongy; bleeding may occur with brushing and flossing or may occur spontaneously.	Provide regular oral care or teach client; dental intervention may be necessary.
Periodontal disease	Gums may bleed easily; teeth may be loose.	Advise client to seek dental care.
Stomatitis	Inflammation of oral mucosa; occurs in clients who are in a state of immunosuppression.	Rinse and cleanse mouth at least every 2 hours and after eating; local anesthetic rinses may provide some comfort.
Dryness	Lips and oral mucosa dry and cracked and may bleed; noted in clients who are dehydrated, who are on oxygen therapy, or who are mouth breathers.	Increase fluid intake as appropriate; apply water-based lubricants or petrolatum jelly to lips.

TABLE 36–2

Common Problems of the Skin

Problem	Description	Nursing Implication
Abrasion	Broken skin that may be weeping or bleeding; may be noted on elbows, heels, sacrum, and other areas that are subject to rubbing motions.	Remove source of irritation. Prevent secondary infection; keep wound clean; avoid wearing rings or jewelry when caring for client; lift client when moving rather than pulling across the bed (shearing factor).
Acne	Oversecretion of sebum, which enlarges the gland and plugs the pore with pus; often occurs on face, chest, and back; most common in adolescence.	Prevent secondary infection; instruct client to avoid squeezing and causing additional trauma to tissue; treatment may vary depending on severity of the problem; encourage meticulous skin cleanliness.
Dryness	Flaking and rough skin (generalized or patchy)	Prone to infection if the skin cracks; skin should be kept lubricated; reduce frequent bathing; hot showers or tub baths; rinse skin thoroughly because soap residue promotes dryness; avoid irritating soaps and alcohol-based lotions; encourage increased fluid intake.
Dermatitis	Inflammation of skin with itching, redness, and blisters; may be allergic reaction to external chemical irritants (fabrics, solutions, plants) or internal (foods or medications).	Identify and remove source of irritation if possible; provide comfort for client with treatment for itching; discourage scratching to prevent breaking of skin and secondary infection.

ents receiving oxygen therapy are prone to this because oxygen tends to dry out the mucosa.

Irritated, reddened, or excoriated mucosa may also result from ill-fitting dentures. Clients who have experienced rapid weight loss or who have sustained significant changes in facial features may have dentures that are loose, which may cause irritation and pain when eating. Stomatitis is a common problem with certain clients. This condition is an inflammation of the oral mucosa and may occur in clients who are receiving drugs that cause decreased salivation with resultant mouth dryness, those whose oral hygiene is poor, those who are in treatment with chemotherapy or radiotherapy for cancer, and those who have an immune deficiency.

Problems of the Skin

Skin types, textures, and conditions are governed by many factors. Overall health status, age, nutritional status, and activity level may play a big part in determining the client's skin condition. Infants have skin that is delicate and sensitive because it has yet to be exposed to the environmental influences that alter skin texture. Because of this delicacy of skin, infants cannot usually tolerate harsh soaps and extremes of water temperature. Their skin is particularly prone to trauma in the form of abrasions, which are breaks in the skin that may lead to infection.

Adolescents are prone to development of enlarged sebaceous glands of the face because of accumulated sebum, which may take the form of blackheads, pimples, or boils. At puberty, the sebaceous glands, under the influence of androgens (male hormones), grow in size and increase production of sebum. Although testosterone, a male hormone, appears to be the most potent circulating androgen for sebaceous cell stimulation, adrenal and ovarian androgens can stimulate sebaceous secretions as well.

Acne occurs predominantly in sebaceous follicles that are rapidly colonized by bacteria that thrive in the lipid-rich sebum. When this occurs, the cyst or sac of connective tissue cells can destroy and displace epidermal cells, resulting in permanent scarring, a condition called cystic acne. Cystic acne may be treated by a synthetic form of vitamin A called isotretinoin (Accutane). However, it must not be used by females who are pregnant or who intend to become pregnant while undergoing treatment. Major fetal abnormalities have been traced to isotretinoin. This drug may also cause serious side effects in those who take it and should be used only if less toxic forms of therapy have failed.

Dry skin is a problem common to aging. Older adults cannot tolerate harsh soaps because of their delicate skin. Skin of older people is also prone to breakdown. Abrasions may be slow to heal or may become infected.

Skin rashes or dermatitis are common skin problems. They may be due to an allergic or nonallergic contact. It is important to identify the source irritant and to prevent secondary infection from scratching with resultant destruction of the body's first line of defense, the intact skin. Table 36–2 lists some common problems associated with the skin and the cause and the treatment for those problems.

Problems of the Hair

Normal hair loss in an adult scalp is about 70 to 100 hairs per day. The rate of growth and the replacement cycle may be altered by illness, diet, and other factors. High fever, major illness, major surgery, blood loss, or severe emotional stress may increase the rate of shedding and may result in **alopecia,** which is loss of hair and baldness. Rapid weight-loss diets with severe caloric restriction or protein restriction may also increase hair loss. Certain drugs and radiation therapy are also factors in increasing hair loss.

Dandruff is a chronic, diffuse scaling of the epidermis of the scalp. It is characterized by itching and flaking of whitish scales, which are annoying and embarrassing.

Infestation with lice is called pediculosis. Lice may be found on any part of the body that has hair. Lice may be found in the hair of the head, eyebrows, eyelashes, and beard (pediculosis capitis), on the body (pediculosis corporis), and in the pubic hair (pediculosis pubis). Head lice and pubic lice attach their eggs (nits) to the hair shaft with a sticky substance that makes them hard to remove. They may be visible to the naked eye or seen through a magnifying glass as shiny ovals. They may look to the naked eye like dandruff. They live on the skin, and their bites cause itching. Inflamed sores may be visible along the hairline. Body lice suck blood from the skin and live in clothing, making them hard to detect. Scratching and hemorrhagic lesions of the skin are clues that should alert the caregiver to the possibility of infestation. Table 36–3 lists common problems of the hair.

Problems of the Nails and Feet

Care of the nails is vital to good hygiene. The accumulation of dirt and debris around the cuticle and underneath the fingernail is a potential source of infection, especially if the nail should become torn. Hangnails, ragged cuticles, and long untrimmed nails are hazardous to the client in many ways. Confused clients sometimes injure themselves by scratching or otherwise abrading the skin. Dirty fingernails open the avenue to infection.

The nails are greatly affected by aging and disease. Increased brittleness and angulation between the nail and the nail bed and changes in the thickness or texture of the nails can indicate illness. Clubbing of the nails or marked curvature and lines in the nails may be indicative of serious health problems. The toenails are vital for good ambulation. Assessment of the client as to gait may point toward sore feet, ingrown toenails, corns, and calluses, which are uncomfortable but not life-threatening. However, in a client with circulatory impairment or diabetes, an ingrown toenail may be a source of serious problems. Fungal infections of the nails are a common problem of the aged, primarily due to dehydrated epidermal cells and decreased sebaceous gland secretion. If nails are thickened and yellow, this may indicate a fungal infection.

The diabetic client is at high risk for infection from breaks in skin integrity and may have decreased sensation to pain because of peripheral neuropathies. Diabetes is associated with changes in microcirculation in peripheral tissues. Edema may be present because of renal disease or congestive heart failure or other conditions that interfere with blood flow to surrounding tissues. Table 36–4 lists common problems of the nails and feet.

FACTORS AFFECTING PERSONAL HYGIENE

Self-care practices vary among individuals, groups, and cultures. It is a mistake to assume that all clients will adhere to similar practices of hygiene or that everyone has similar beliefs about hygiene and methods of practicing it. Variations in hygiene practices may be due to cultural or religious factors, developmental factors, socioeconomic factors, physiological factors, or psychosocial factors.

Cultural/Religious Factors

Culture is an important influence on hygiene practices. Cultural and social norms as well as the teachings of family create different perspectives on cleanliness and hygiene. The common bathing rituals and the application of preparations to the skin may vary widely among groups. In some cultures, bathing is done daily or even more often. In other cultural groups, bathing may not occur daily because it is not

TABLE 36–3
Common Problems of the Hair

Problem	Description	Nursing Implication
Alopecia	Absence of body hair; may be sudden onset of patchy scalp and beard hair loss without any inflammation and usually reversible or sudden loss of all scalp hair or total loss of all body hair including scalp and face.	Be aware of client's history and treatment to know if condition is likely to be reversible (chemotherapy) or irreversible; recognize significance of hair to client's self-esteem and body image.
Dandruff	A scaly collection of dried sebum and flakes of dried skin on the scalp; characterized by itching of the scalp.	Daily brushing and shampooing; medicated shampoos may help; instruct client to avoid scratching scalp.
Pediculosis	Infestation with lice; characterized by itching and scratching.	Removal of nits (eggs) from hair shaft; bathing and shampooing with topical medication; careful treatment of clothing and bed linens to prevent reinfestation with lice.

TABLE 36–4
Common Problems of the Feet and Nails

Problem	Description	Nursing Implications
Athlete's foot	Fungal infection of the foot characterized by weeping, itching, excoriated lesions, usually located between the toes.	Medicated antifungal medications may be used; regular washing and drying of feet is important; instruct client to wear white cotton socks during treatment to prevent potential infection from dyes in colored socks and to alternate shoes each day.
Corn/callus	A hardened area on the foot, usually caused by pressure or friction.	Instruct client to avoid attempting to remove by cutting; use pumice stone to soften; encourage wearing of well-fitting shoes.
Fungal infection of nails	Nails may be yellow or black and thickened.	Observe for signs of side effects of treatment regimen, which consists of oral antifungal medication.

deemed necessary or for reasons such as the reduced availability of an adequate water supply or provisions for bathing. Some groups apply oils and other preparations to the skin and hair. Shaving of leg and axillary hair, which is practiced by most women in the United States, is not necessarily a standard of hygiene practice by all women of the world, particularly in some parts of Europe. It is important to understand these individual differences in caring for clients of diverse ethnic and cultural backgrounds. Some personal hygiene practices may seem foreign or strange, but their significance to the client should be respected.

Religious rituals may also influence the client's hygiene habits. Some religions have prohibitions against the exposure of body parts, the cutting and care of hair, and bathing during menses or immediately after delivery of a child. In some groups, it is forbidden for a male to attend to the hygiene needs of a female. Respect for differences must be accompanied by knowledge of the beliefs and practices that vary from the traditional Western cultural standards, as suggested by the Cross-Cultural Care chart.

Developmental Factors

Developmental considerations affect hygiene practices. The age of the individual usually dictates the expectation of what that person should be able to achieve in self-care. However, the interventions should be in accordance with the identified needs and abilities, whether or not they are congruent with chronological age and stage of development.

There is a need for independence in self-care that is manifested early in childhood as the child takes pride in grooming, dressing, and caring for hygiene needs. The loss of this ability in adulthood can be stressful even if the loss is temporary.

Self-concept and the feeling of being in control of the body are threatened by the loss of self-care abilities. Being bathed and dressed by a caregiver is often equated with regression to an infantile state. For some individuals, this feeling of "being a baby" is not ac-

ceptable, particularly if the need for independence is very strong in the individual. A sense of powerlessness may result from this loss. It is important to be sensitive to the client's emotional needs when providing hygiene care.

Newborns and Infants

The infant is totally dependent on the caregiver to meet self-care needs. Crying, when in need of feeding and diapering, is the only action the infant can take in the interest of self-care. Bathing, dressing, and grooming are the total responsibility of the caregiver. Frequency of urine and stool elimination may vary, but infants usually urinate about 20 times a day (250 to 500 mL per day). Stools may vary according to amount and consistency but may be soft or liquid and may occur frequently. Meticulous cleaning is essential because the infant's tender skin is susceptible to breaking. The skin should be kept as dry and clean as possible. Infants should never be left in wet or soiled diapers for extended periods of time. The infant's skin and mucous membranes are easily injured and are susceptible to injury and infection.

Action Alert!
Remind parents that they need to take special care to avoid injury and infection to their children's skin.

Toddlers and Preschoolers

During the toddler/preschool years, the child develops gross and fine motor skills so that some independent grooming and toileting are possible. Bowel and bladder control is usually achieved by the age of 3 years even though some assistance may still be needed with wiping after toileting. Night-time dryness may not be complete until the age of 5. The preschooler is usually eager to help with dressing and derives great satisfaction with learning to master buttons and zippers.

Toddlers and preschoolers may regress in times of illness or stress and resume infantile behaviors in relation to toileting and self-care. Bed-wetting may occur again during this period of stress. This is the infant's primary means of coping and securing the comfort and security that is needed at this time of crisis. Skills previously learned will be regained when the child no longer needs to use the coping mechanism.

School-Aged Children and Adolescents

The school-aged child may be independent in self-care activities related to personal hygiene but may need adult supervision on occasion to see that skin care and oral hygiene are being done completely and correctly. As the child approaches adolescence, assistance with

---

CROSS-CULTURAL CARE
CARING FOR AN AFRICAN-AMERICAN CLIENT

Mrs. Wilson, the client discussed in this chapter, is of African-American ancestry. She grew up in the Deep South as the daughter of sharecroppers who struggled to feed and clothe their large family of 10 children. Mrs. Wilson is the fifth child and the only surviving sibling. She has never lived more than 50 miles from the place of her birth.

Poverty was a reality of her early life, but she says that the difficulties were made bearable by the intensity of love within the family, and she feels that this has been a blessing in her life. She has been a widow for 10 years. Her daughter is her only child, and two granddaughters live nearby.

Several characteristics have been identified in African Americans that demonstrate their values, beliefs, and world views. Attribution of specific characteristics to population groups is not without risks and is not intended to stereotype individuals. African Americans may tend to value the following:

- Having a strong will to survive.
- Being steeped in a particular culture and tradition.
- Showing adaptive behavior.
- Showing strong belief in self-reliance.
- Avoiding self-blame for failures.
- Having major concern for health and ability to maintain activities of daily living.
- Tending to overestimate health status.
- Seeing trouble as a "cross one must bear."
- Believing that avoidance of worry and tension is the same as problem-solving.
- Relying on kinship and family networks to cope with health concerns.

Let's see how the nurse (Jean) talks with Mrs. Wilson:

Jean: Good morning, Mrs. Wilson. I hear that you are going home in a few days. How do you feel about that?

Mrs. Wilson: The Lord has blessed me to be able to go to my home. I am so thankful that this stroke didn't kill me. Two of my sisters had strokes and they died right away. One brother had a stroke, but he didn't die. He was paralyzed and never could do anything for himself after that. He just lived in a wheelchair and a bed until he died. He couldn't even feed himself. I felt so sad to see him like that. I just hope I get my strength back so I

don't have to stay in a bed all the time or just sit and look at the TV.

Jean: It sounds like you are a little bit worried about how things will turn out for you.

Mrs. Wilson: I really am. I feel so bad that I can't help my daughter in the house any more. I have been able to help with the cooking and that takes a weight off her with me living there, but now I'm going to be a burden to her. I can't do anything *(starts to cry).*

Jean: It sounds like being able to help is really important to you. I bet you have always taken care of yourself.

Mrs. Wilson: Oh yes, I have always taken care of myself and others too. I just love helping people. When my daughter was a baby, I could work all day, take care of her at night and get right up and go back to work in the morning. I can't do that now. My weakness is really showing, isn't it?

Jean: Well, you do have a problem with a little weakness in your left side, but it seems that doing things for yourself is the most important thing for you right now.

Mrs. Wilson: It really is. I can't even dress myself, can't zip a zipper or button a button. I just want to get back to being myself. I don't want anybody to have to wash my face or brush my teeth. I just want to take care of myself.

Critical Thinking Questions

- Did Mrs. Wilson show strong indication of the cultural characteristics of the need for self-reliance?
- Did Jean really hear what Mrs. Wilson was saying? Were her responses appropriate to the context of the discussion?
- If Jean had ignored Mrs. Wilson's expression of concern for lack of independence, what do you think Mrs. Wilson would have done?
- Why is self-reliance so important to Mrs. Wilson in light of very real limitations?

Based on information in Harel, Z., McKinney, E.A., & Williams, M. (Eds.). (1990). Black aged: Understanding diversity and service needs. Newbury Park, CA: Sage.

self-care is no longer necessary, but because of the many physical changes that are occurring, a different kind of assistance and supervision and teaching may be needed. This is a time when hormonal changes bring about the emergence of axillary and pubic hair in both sexes and facial hair in males. The skin may become more oily because of the increased activity of the sebaceous glands. Skin problems such as acne may occur during this period and can be a source of great distress to the adolescent who is becoming increasingly aware of the importance of good grooming in being attractive to the opposite sex and accepted by their peers. The sweat glands also become functional during adolescence, and the presence of body odor becomes an incentive for daily bathing and shampooing and for wearing clean clothes.

Adults and Older Adults

During early and middle adult life, self-care is usually an independent function unless some temporary or permanent physical or mental impairment prevents the individual from performing self-care. Patterns of hygiene practices are well established by this time in order to meet the individual's goals for personal appearance and health.

Developmental considerations related to aging may affect the hygiene practices of clients. This is particularly true in the elderly because the aging process may limit some agility and endurance and therefore the ability to perform safely and capably some of the functions that make up good hygiene. Some elderly adults who were previously meticulous in their grooming may be noted by family members to be less attentive or even totally negligent in bathing and changing clothing. This may be due to either mental or physical changes and requires attention from the caregiver because the client is no longer able to meet hygiene needs independently.

As physiological changes occur with aging, some of the hygiene needs and practices must change accordingly. For example, the skin becomes thinner and less elastic and tends to break more readily. Because less oil is being produced, the skin becomes drier. The appearance of the skin also changes with wrinkling and discoloration in the form of age spots, which occur particularly on the face and the dorsal surface of the hands. Skin carcinomas are also prominent in aging skin.

The hair changes. It becomes thinner and grows more slowly. Baldness in both men and women may occur. Hair color changes as the pigment in the hair is lost. Gray or white hair is common. The oral mucosa changes, and with the decreased production of saliva, it becomes drier. The teeth in the presence of periodontal disease may become loose or may even be lost. Many older adults wear dentures.

Care of the nails may be difficult. Nails become thickened and harder to maintain. The older adult may have both decreased visual acuity and agility and may have difficulty with this psychomotor task. The feet of the older client are of special concern because many older adults cannot see well enough to inspect their feet or care for the feet. Decreased circulation in the extremities due to reduced peripheral blood flow from arteriosclerosis or poor circulation puts them at risk.

Action Alert!
Special care must be taken to prevent trauma or infection in the feet of older adults due to decreased circulation in the extremities.

Many older adults, especially diabetics, use the skills of a podiatrist because of the danger inherent in accidentally traumatizing the feet with manicure tools. Some hospitals and nursing homes prohibit foot care by nurses and require clients to secure the services of a podiatrist because the danger caused by inadvertent foot trauma is so great.

Older adults frequently have to use at least one or more of the assistive tools to support sensory function. Hearing aids, glasses, and artificial eyes are common. The care of these devices may be a problem for the older adult who has lost some visual and hearing acuity as well as psychomotor skill. Even so, having the means to enhance quality of life and safety for the older person is worth any difficulty encountered.

Socioeconomic Factors

Socioeconomic factors influence personal hygiene habits and practices in a number of ways. Financial resources to purchase the necessary tools for hygiene may be limited. An environment that is depressed and unclean does not encourage the individual toward meticulous hygiene. Bathing may assume low priority in an environment with inadequate heat or a lack of privacy for hygiene practices. When a significant amount of physical and emotional energy is required to meet daily subsistence needs for food and shelter, grooming and hygiene may be neglected. This is not to imply that the individual no longer values them. It is simply because the basic human needs for physical survival become paramount. An example of this may be seen in the homeless person who is hospitalized and the comfort that is derived from being in a warm and comfortable environment where hygiene needs can be met.

Physiological Factors

The state of health is a major influence in the practice of self-care. Regardless of the motivation to maintain good hygiene or the desire to do so, the client may be so ill or weak that there is insufficient energy to perform self-care activities.

Physical Illness

Clients may be paralyzed or weakened by loss of physical mobility from a cerebrovascular accident, a neuromuscular disorder, a spinal cord injury, or another catastrophic event. The degree of assistance needed may vary depending on the nature of the neuromuscular involvement and which muscle groups are affected. Muscular movements are classified as either fine motor movement involving precise movements, such as applying toothpaste to a toothbrush, or gross motor movement involving the coordination of large muscle groups. An example of coordinating large muscle groups is the ability to get in and out of the bathtub or on and off the toilet. An intact nervous system is essential for the performance of these tasks. To perform these activities, the pathways from brain to muscle and the muscle fibers themselves must be open and able to give and receive the message. Neuromuscular diseases may affect any level of this pathway.

A*ction* A*lert!*
Clients may need help with applying toothpaste or getting in and out of the bathtub or on and off the toilet because of changes in their nervous system.

Conservation of energy is another factor in self-care. Sometimes clients are placed on enforced bed rest or limited activity by their physicians in order to conserve energy. Certain pathological conditions that are particularly prone to influence one's energy level are cardiovascular and respiratory diseases in which there is inadequate removal of waste products from cellular metabolism, so that fatigue is a prominent symptom of the disease.

Pain is a factor that affects the ability to perform self-care. Some clients are in such a severe state of pain that they cannot care for themselves. Simple movements, particularly of painful joints, prevent self-care.

Cognitive dysfunction may vary in degree from the client's simply needing assistance to the client who is so impaired that total care is needed. It is important to accurately assess the client's potential for self-care because it is important for the client to maintain as much independence as possible. It is also important not to expect too much from a client who is too impaired to meet self-care needs.

Sensorimotor deficits, such as blindness or deafness, may prevent the client from self-care. Help may be needed to learn how to eat or get to the bathroom. Hearing-impaired clients may not be able to follow instructions.

Medical or Surgical Procedures

Medical or surgical procedures may alter the client's ability to perform self-care. An acutely ill client with a medical or surgical diagnosis usually needs a great deal of help with care. Not only is there impairment by the medical or surgical problem but there may be associated weakness or pain from the treatment or from medications.

Frequently, narcotics or sedatives are given in sufficient doses to make the client drowsy or sedated and unable to perform self-care. There may be associated problems, such as fluid and electrolyte imbalances, hypoxia or hypovolemia, IVs, other monitoring equipment, central lines, oxygen, and catheters, which encumber the client and decrease mobility. In addition, a general anesthetic will cause weakness.

Psychosocial Factors

Mental Illness

Emotional disturbances may cause disruptions in the ability to perform self-care. The client who is actively psychotic will need assistance because she is out of touch with reality and pays little heed to the need for hygiene. Sometimes an alteration in grooming may be an early indicator of mental illness. Depression can slow a person down because she has no psychic energy and therefore no physical energy. Poor grooming, lack of interest in appearance, or inappropriate dressing may reflect the need for assistance.

Stress

The stress often associated with physical illness may cause the client to need help with self-care, even if it is only in the form of a reminder or encouragement that a bath or shampoo might help. If the client is dealing with the stress of a serious diagnosis for herself or a loved one, it is important to encourage the highly stressed client to participate in hygiene activities.

Knowledge Level

Take into account the knowledge level of the client in regard to hygiene. Practices, such as bathing frequently, shampooing, and good oral care including flossing and brushing, are usually taught by significant others during childhood. These teachings are not always incorporated into the client's behavior. These experiences can still be used by the caregiver for health teaching about the value of good hygiene.

Health teaching may be done informally as it is pointed out to the client that there are ways in which overall health might be improved through specific actions. If family members are present with the client during hospitalization, health teaching is essential if they are to care for the client at home after hospitalization. They need to know principles of aseptic technique as well as specific procedures that will be necessary at home. All of these can be incorporated into teaching and are most easily taught while care is being given.

Territoriality

Caring for the most intimate needs of ill persons requires that you operate within the personal space of each client. Each client has a sense of "space" in which they feel comfortable. This space not only includes the physical area surrounding the person but also the emotional possession of the body and personal self-knowledge. Optimal territorial space needed by most persons in Western culture is 86 to 108 square feet. In hospitals and institutions, some research has shown that 60 square feet should be the minimum for multi-occupancy rooms and 80 square feet for private rooms.

Intrusion into this personal space or territory without permission often causes discomfort. Nursing has implicit permission from society to move into an individual's space as necessary in order to give care. This is a rare opportunity not offered other disciplines and should be considered a privilege. It is important to be aware, however, that some clients may be uncomfortable with this physical and emotional closeness. Awareness of this discomfort helps one to assess the client's comfort level so that care can be taken to reduce discomfort and anxiety.

Privacy in an institutional setting is difficult to achieve at times. Respect for the client's privacy is important in preserving dignity and feeling of worth. Careful draping and screening during care, avoidance of intrusion when the client has visitors or is talking on the telephone, and knocking before entering the room show concern for the client's right to privacy. Respect for the client's personal space can be enhanced by providing privacy when sensitive matters are to be discussed.

Institutions tend to be very depersonalizing. In a hospital, one of the first events that a client encounters is the removal of clothing and personal belongings. Providing an identified space for personal belongings and encouraging the inclusion of personal and familiar objects in the client's hospital environment will help to make it the client's space. The importance of creating this environment may be observed as family members bring items from home and in other ways attempt to create a space that is psychologically comforting to the client. Pictures, cards, and flowers are used, not only to bring a cheerful look to the client's room, but also to make that space unique for the client. It is a way of defining who that person is as an individual.

ASSESSMENT

General Assessment of Personal Hygiene

Hygiene depends on the client's physical and emotional ability to perform bathing, hair care, and oral care. An accurate assessment allows you and the client to mutually determine how much assistance is needed and to what extent the client can participate. If the client has a deficit in self-care ability, it may range from total inability to participate in any self-care activities to a partial deficit in that the client may be able to assist in hygiene activities, even though participation may be of a very limited degree. If you presuppose lack of ability, when some ability may be present, it can further reinforce a client's sense of dependence and helplessness.

*A*ction *A*lert!
If you expect the client to perform hygiene when physical or emotional resources are severely limited, it may lead to frustration or anxiety in the client.

Health History

The health history is important in that it will give you information on which to base current self-care status. Why was the client admitted for home care services, to an acute care facility, or to a skilled nursing facility? How long has this problem existed? Is it new or long-standing? What was lifestyle prior to event? What is history of illness? What was previous activity level? What are hygiene habits? The health history provides information about the client's present and past health and illness experiences. The health history interview should include a review of functional health patterns, questioning the status and change of patterns. When did the ability to manage ADLs change? Is this a recent change or has it been coming over time? Is the alteration in functional ability of sudden or slow onset?

Note the client's physical status. Observe for the presence of pain or discomfort and whether this is aggravated by movement. Assess the intactness of the client's sensory apparatus (vision and hearing). Determine the ability to follow your directions. An assessment of cognitive function will provide you with clues as to how to approach the client and how to proceed. Note the presence of neuromuscular weakness or neuromuscular impairment (tics, spasticity, rigidity, palsy, paralysis). If the client's mobility is severely impaired, it may necessitate the involvement of more than one caregiver. An assessment of the client's energy level is important so that care can be provided while minimizing the client's expenditure of energy.

Assess for factors that place the client at risk for *Self-care deficit* in hygiene. Risk factors include developmental stage, current health status, mobility, cognitive status, emotional status, and medical plan of care.

Be aware of the client's age. The very young and the very old have special needs for assistance. Young infants have no capacity to perform self-care, whereas the aged may have some need for dependency on caregivers when self-care abilities are affected by physical or psychological impairments.

Mobility may be a risk factor if there is any impairment due to neuromuscular weakness or sensory deficits. Some clients may have limited mobility due to the weakness of one or more extremities.

The client's ability to recognize the need for hygiene measures and the ability to implement this knowledge are necessary to prevent a deficit in self-care. A cognitively impaired individual may not be able to focus well enough to plan the essential steps necessary for hygiene or to carry them out.

*A*ction *A*lert!
Careful assessment of clients' cognitive status is essential because they may appear to be well-oriented and capable of doing self-care, but on more careful assessment, short-term memory loss or other deficits may be apparent.

The client who is very stressed or emotionally unstable may outwardly appear to have self-care skills, but because of the intense focus on the emotional stressor, the client may simply not have enough energy to carry out a plan for hygiene.

The medical plan of care may put the client at risk for self-care deficit. Therapeutic management of illness or trauma, surgical or medical procedures that cause weakness, or pain or nausea may necessitate bed rest and interfere with the client's ability to do self-care activities.

Action Alert!
You need to anticipate what is forthcoming for the client in the way of treatment so as to anticipate the risk for *Self-care deficit.*

Subjective assessment data arise from interaction with the client and the family. Functional pattern assessment provides valuable information as to the client's perceived self-care abilities and difficulties and feelings about the adequacy of those abilities. The assessment may include the normal routine for bathing, grooming, and toileting and personal satisfaction with this routine. Ask the client what causes problems with hygiene and what has been done to deal with these problems. What does the client want to happen? Is the client satisfied with the current state of daily self-care activities? What are the client's goals and expectations? Is there is hope for improvement in self-care status? What level of dependence on family caregivers is necessary?

Focused Assessment for Bathing/Hygiene Self-Care Deficit

Defining Characteristics

Defining characteristics for bathing/hygiene self-care deficits are the inability to wash body or body parts, inability to obtain water or regulate temperature or flow of water, or inability to sit or stand while bathing (North American Nursing Diagnosis Association, 1999). These manifestations in conjunction with clinical evidence of musculoskeletal or perceptual/cognitive impairment and the client's inability to maintain hygiene at a satisfactory level validate the diagnosis of self-care deficits that require nursing intervention.

Illness or functional limitations may necessitate assistance with personal hygiene. In some cases, when the client is unable to perform any self-care measures for hygiene, a caregiver must assume responsibility for total care of the individual's hygiene needs. Total hygiene care consists of bathing, skin care, oral care, hair care, perineal care, back massage, shaving, changing the bed linens, and changing client's gown or pajamas.

Related Factors

The most common related factors are impaired physical mobility, activity intolerance, pain, depression, severe anxiety, alteration in sensory perception, or cognitive impairment. *Impaired physical mobility* may be due to acute or chronic illness, trauma, psychological impairment, or the need to conserve energy as with bed rest or reduced activity. *Activity intolerance* occurs when the physical or psychological demands of the activity are more than the client can tolerate without manifestations of distress, which may take the form of dyspnea, muscle weakness, fatigue, or tachycardia.

Focused Assessment for Related Nursing Diagnoses

Impaired Skin Integrity

Impaired skin integrity is a problem with the client who cannot manage self-care/hygiene.

During the client's bath is a good time to assess the skin. Your assessment should include the color and temperature, particularly in the extremities. Especially note areas that are different from other areas (cooler, warmer, paler, pinker), texture as to dryness or oiliness, any lesions or impaired integrity, any rectal bleeding, and pain or sensitivity in any area as it is bathed or moved. You can observe the client's sense of touch (temperature of water, pressure with rubbing), limitation of motion, or stiffness or pain during range of motion (ROM) exercises and emotional state and ability to communicate.

Altered Oral Mucous Membrane

The client may not be able to manage oral hygiene because of a number of factors. Persons who have altered states of consciousness are unable to meet self-care needs for oral care. Others have mobility impairment so that it is difficult or impossible to get to the sink or bathroom and to manipulate toothbrush or dental floss (e.g., a client with arthritic hands may have difficulty in picking up and holding small items).

Powerlessness

The client who is dependent on others for activities of daily living may experience powerlessness. Assess the client's behavior for attempts at establishing control. The client who is demanding and manipulative may be feeling out of control. On the other hand, powerlessness may be expressed as apathy or fastidiousness.

DIAGNOSIS

You use physical assessment data base and observation to determine the appropriate nursing diagnoses. When the client presents with a self-care deficit problem, it may be total or partial. If it is total, it includes deficits in feeding, bathing/hygiene, dressing/grooming, and toileting. If it is partial, one or more deficits may be present. The client may have a diagnosis of "Risk for" if the potential is there for loss of self-care ability. Nursing diagnoses are those accepted by the North American Nursing Diagnosis Association

(NANDA), and they cover all problems and potential problems relating to all body systems. The data clustering chart demonstrates how to cluster data to create a nursing diagnosis.

PLANNING

Planning for outcomes should be a collaborative effort between you, the client, and, when appropriate, the client's family. Setting mutually acceptable and attainable goals is essential in moving the client on a continuum toward some degree of independence.

Expected Outcome for the Client With Self-Care Deficit

Planning to help the client meet hygiene needs when there is a self-care deficit is essential. For the client who has a total self-care deficit, the goal is to provide hygiene measures that will prevent complications. For the client with partial self-care deficit, the goal is to assist the client as needed and to encourage as much independence as possible. The goal is always to encourage independence and to return the client to a state of independent self-care. Take the following factors into account when planning:

- The client's general physical condition and functional status
- Individual specific hygiene requirements
- Personal preferences and wishes

Expected Outcomes for Client and Family With Self-Care Deficit

Planning with the client and family is important because the desired outcomes may vary with the client's level of illness or with priorities that are different than those you believe to be necessary for the client. Expected outcomes for the client and family with self-care deficit might be the following:

- Client's self-care needs are met.
- Complications are avoided and minimized.
- Client and family members carry out self-care program daily.
- Client and family communicate feelings and concerns.
- Client and family identify resources to help cope with problems after discharge.

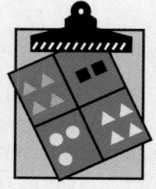

CLUSTERING DATA TO MAKE A NURSING DIAGNOSIS
SELF-CARE PROBLEMS

Data Cluster	Diagnosis
65-year-old poorly nourished neurasthenic woman who was diagnosed with Alzheimer's disease 5 years ago. She has shown rapid deterioration and now is unable to care for any of her basic hygiene needs.	*Self-care deficit* related to loss of memory and neuromuscular function.
Young adult male, age 30, has metastatic brain tumor secondary to progressive bronchogenic carcinoma. He is totally blind in his right eye. He also has right hemiplegia and is very limited in his self-care abilities.	*Self-care deficit* related to decreased visual and motor ability.
55-year-old woman with history of chronic obstructive pulmonary disease who is now in acute congestive heart failure. She has extreme dyspnea, and she is able to ambulate only to the bathroom and back to recliner.	*Self-care deficit* related to activity intolerance.
40-year-old female who has had severe rheumatoid arthritis for 20 years. She has severe limitations of lower extremities as well as the upper ones. She has difficulty grasping objects because of the malformation of hands and fingers.	*Self-care deficit* related to limited range of motion (ROM).
20-year-old man hospitalized after motor vehicle accident, fx pelvis. Fx left tibia and fibula. He refuses to move because of the intense pain caused by any movement.	*Self-care deficit* related to pain and limited mobility from fractures.

BOX 36-1

GUIDELINES FOR BATHING CLIENTS

- Promote safety and prevent falls.
- Assess psychological and physical needs.
- Determine self-care abilities and limitations.
- Encourage self-help except when contraindicated.
- Allow as much control and involvement as possible; let the client make some choices.
- Provide privacy and warmth at time of bathing; cover and drape sufficiently.
- Use good body mechanics for yourself by keeping a wide base of support, keeping back straight, and using leg and abdominal muscles to move and lift clients.

Mrs. Wilson, the subject of our case study, is ready for discharge after 2 weeks of hospitalization following a cerebrovascular accident. What expected outcomes might be appropriate for her and her family?

INTERVENTION

Interventions to Promote Skin Hygiene

Bathing the Client

Bathing is an important intervention to promote hygiene. Choice of the method of bathing depends on your judgment as well as the medical plan of care in regard to the client's activity level and mental and physical capabilities to perform self-care (see Box 36-1 on guidelines for bathing). Consider the client's preferences for type of bath and time of day for bathing to allow her some degree of control. This may not always be possible because of the client's condition and other factors.

Bathing may be accomplished with a bed bath, a tub or shower, or the client's bathing at a sink or lavatory. Bed baths are less commonly used than in the past as recognition of the need for mobility assumes precedence over bed rest. Assistive devices such as shower chairs, which can be rolled into the shower and lifting devices such as the Hoyer lift, which can lift a client in and out of a tub, allow tub and shower bathing for clients who previously would have received bed baths.

Action **A**lert!
The benefits of bathing in a tub or shower for the client are so significant that, if that option is available, you should use it even though it may be more difficult and time consuming. The physical and emotional state of the client will be enhanced so that it will be worth the effort.

Some of the goals of hygiene care are

- Comfort and relaxation, which help to relax tense muscles and allow the client to feel refreshed

- Stimulation of circulation through friction and massage circulation
- Cleanliness, which removes body waste products and secretions

Bathing a client is a time of close contact that provides you with an opportunity to not only assess the client's physical and mental status but to communicate with the client. The client may feel that she has your undivided attention for a concentrated period of time and so may feel free to express concerns that otherwise would not be expressed. It is a time to provide special skin care and teach the client and family about skin care, as outlined in the Teaching for Wellness chart.

Several types of baths can be used, depending on the client's need (Table 36-5). Baths may be for cleans-

Teaching for WELLNESS

SKIN CARE

Purpose: To teach client about skin care.

Rationale: Dry skin is susceptible to breaking as well as being uncomfortable with itching and roughness.

Expected Outcomes: Client will follow prescribed regimen for skin to alleviate dryness.

Client Instructions
- Sometimes your skin can become dry because you haven't taken in enough fluids. Make sure you drink 8 glasses of water a day. Avoid dehydrating fluids, such as sodas and caffeine-containing drinks. These are not substitutes for water.
- Bathing can dry your skin as well. Use a gentle bath lotion or mild soap. No soap is sometimes the best answer.
- Too-frequent bathing may dry the skin. It may be wise to reduce baths from daily to every other day or even twice a week. When bathing, don't use hot water. Use warm water instead.
- Using bath oils or lubricants immediately after bathing will prevent immediate loss of moisture.
- Also pay attention to the way your linens and clothing are being laundered. Harsh detergents and bleaches are irritating to already dry skin. Use mild nondetergent cleaning products rather than harsh detergents. Avoid perfumed fabric softeners.
- Dry skin tends to itch, and you may want to rub or scratch it. Try not to do this because you can hurt your skin. Also avoid rubbing your skin roughly with a towel after bathing. Patting dry is much less harmful to the skin.

TABLE 36-5
Types of Therapeutic Baths

Type of Bath	Purpose
Sitz bath	To decrease pain and inflammation after rectal or perineal surgery or for pain relief from hemorrhoids. Water should be warm to client's comfort level.
Hot-water bath	To relieve muscle spasm and muscle tension. Water should be deep enough for immersion. Warm to client's comfort level.
Warm-water bath	To relax and soothe. Client's comfort will dictate water temperature. Caution client about time limits for soaking (20 minutes) because of vasodilation.
Cool-water bath	To decrease fever and to reduce muscle tension. Avoid chilling. Water should be cool but not cold.
Oatmeal or Aveeno	To soothe irritated skin. Softens and lubricates dry scaly skin. Place 3 cups cooked oatmeal in a cheesecloth bag and place in tub of water.
Corn starch	To soothe skin irritation. Dissolve 1 pound of cornstarch in cold water, then add boiling water until mixture is thick and add to tub water.

ing or for therapeutic measures related to some skin problem.

BATHING THE CLIENT IN BED
The accompanying procedure, Giving the Client a Bed Bath, provides detailed steps in bathing a client in bed. The bed bath is given for the purpose of providing cleanliness for a client who is unable to be out of bed and who is unable to care for hygiene needs because of physical or mental limitations. It is indicated primarily for clients with restricted mobility (people with casts, traction, or back problems), those who have heart and respiratory problems and thus limited exercise tolerance, or those who are at the first postoperative day and thus may be too weak to get out of bed to bathe.

Various methods are

- Complete bed bath, giving the complete bath without any assistance from the client
- Partial bed bath, assisting with key areas such as axilla, back, and perineal care
- Self-help, giving the client help with hard-to-reach areas, such as the back, legs, and feet

A bed bath may be a bag bath or a towel bath. The client is covered with a warm towel saturated with a quick-drying solution, such as Septi-Soft. As the body is cleaned with the solution, the solution dries immediately. An advantage of this type of bath is that it is brief (10 minutes) and can be used for the client who is easily fatigued and who has limited tolerance for any activity. The oil in the solution softens the skin, and clients report a refreshed feeling from this kind of bath.

PROVIDING PERINEAL CARE
Cleaning the genitalia is usually a part of the bath. Perineal care for female and male clients is described in the accompanying procedure, Providing Perineal Care. If the client is unable to maintain adequate perineal care, this part of the care is your responsibility. Perineal care for women involves washing the labia majora and the labia minora, the inner thighs, the perineum, and the anal area. The **perineum** is the pelvic floor and associated structures occupying the pelvic outlet, bounded anteriorly by the symphysis pubis, laterally by the ischial tuberosities, and posteriorly by the coccyx. For men, perineal care involves cleaning the upper inner thighs, penis, and scrotum. In uncircumcised men, the foreskin must be retracted and the glans penis washed. In both sexes, the perianal area is cleaned last with the client in a side-lying position. Professional behavior will help to reduce anxiety and embarrassment in the client. It is essential to wear gloves for this procedure because of the intimate contact with body fluids and exudates and because any open wounds or sores on your hands are avenues for transmission of infections. Clients may receive perineal care while sitting on the bedpan or toilet.

Clients at risk for skin breakdown, who may have particular needs for meticulous and frequent perineal care, include clients with indwelling catheters, postpartum clients, clients with perineal, rectal, or lower urinary tract surgery, and incontinent clients.

ASSISTING THE CLIENT WITH A SHOWER OR TUB BATH
Assess the client to determine the degree of independence to allow the client in bathing. Safety becomes a priority because injuries due to falls in bathtub or shower are common and often have serious consequences. Assess the client for dizziness; weakness in extremities; hypotension; any sensory impairment, particularly visual; mental capacity; degree of judgment; and clarity of thought in determining the client's ability to bathe independently. You may determine that the client can be left alone for bathing, or you may plan to remain with the client during the bath.

The accompanying procedure, Helping the Client With a Tub Bath or Shower, gives the procedure for assisting a client with a tub or shower bath. The client may be transported to the tub or shower in a wheelchair, on a stretcher, or in a rolling shower chair. If the person is ambulating, nonskid slippers should be worn. If a wheelchair or rolling shower chair is used, safety precautions such as belt restraints may be used to prevent falling from the chair. Shower chairs are made of metal or plastic so they can be rolled into the shower. A hand-held shower nozzle allows the client or caregiver to direct the flow of water.

Dressings and casts need not always be deterrents to bathing in a tub or shower. Improvised covers and plastic wrap taped over a cast or dressing can afford the person freedom to bathe as desired without damage to cast or dressing.

Text continued on page 947

PROCEDURE 36–1

Giving the Client a Bed Bath

The bed bath is given for the purpose of providing for the cleanliness and comfort of a client who is unable to be out of bed because of physical or mental limitations. The client who is unable to perform any of the bath is given a complete bed bath. Most clients can perform some of the bath and in most circumstances should be encouraged to do so. The bed bath is an opportunity to perform range of motion (ROM) and skin assessment.

Standard precautions are followed for all bath procedures. In standard precautions, the nurse wears clean gloves for any contact with blood, body fluids, secretions, excretions, and contaminated items. Put on clean gloves just before touching mucous membranes and nonintact skin. Change gloves between tasks and procedures on the same client after contact with material that may contain a high concentration of microorganisms. Remove gloves promptly after use, before touching noncontaminated items and environmental surfaces, and before going to another client, and wash hands immediately to avoid transfer of microorganisms to other clients or environments (Hospital Infection Control Advisory Committee, 1999).*

Delegation Guidelines

Once you have assessed your client, as outlined below, you may delegate the performance of a bed bath to a nursing assistant. Remember that although the nursing assistant may be instructed to observe for changes in the client's skin, such as irritation or discoloration, you alone maintain the professional responsibility for assessment and appropriate action based on your assessment. You are responsible for re-establishing any disruption in IV infusions or drainage devices at the completion of the bath.

Equipment Needed

- Wash basin.
- Soap or cleansing lotion.
- Two towels and two wash cloths.
- Clean gown or pajamas.
- Powder, deodorant, skin lotion.
- Oral care items.
- Hair care items.
- Shaving items.
- Clean gloves (essential for perineal and oral care; otherwise as needed).

---

1 Check physician's orders for activity and any special positioning needs or contraindications. Assess for ability to participate in the bath even if on a limited scale. Evaluate client's need for teaching relative to skin care and plan to incorporate teaching into the procedure. Assess for presence of IV lines, catheters, tubes, casts, and dressings. Assess client's ROM.

Cleansing of skin and teaching about skin care and ROM can be smoothly integrated so that time and energy are conserved for you and client. If assessment indicates that the bath can be done more efficiently or safely with two people, it is advisable to secure this help. Allowing the client to participate in the bath provides a source of exercise and ROM as well as providing for enhancement of self-worth and feelings of independence.

2 Prepare the environment.
a. Wash your hands and apply gloves if needed.

Change gloves after oral care, perineal care, or washing nonintact skin.

Some agencies adopt a policy of using gloves for the bath without regard to assessing for intact skin. Other agencies leave it to the nurse's judgment.

b. Gather equipment and take to the bedside. Have all necessary supplies and equipment ready for use.

Having necessary supplies readily at hand enhances organization and efficiency in bathing the client.

c. Raise bed to comfortable working height, ensure privacy by closing door or curtains, and regulate temperature of the room for comfort.

Application of principles of body mechanics allows you to work comfortably and efficiently without muscle strain. Privacy and comfort are prerequisites for making the bed bath a positive experience for the client. The side rails should always be up on the side of the bed opposite to where you are working.

Continued

Giving the Client a Bed Bath

d. Place articles on overbed table, within easy reach.

Organization of supplies conserves energy and increases efficiency of movement. Having supplies within reach also promotes client's safety because it eliminates the necessity for your turning away from the client or moving away from the bedside to reach for supplies.

3 Prepare the client.

a. Assist client to use bedpan, commode, or urinal.

Bathing, turning, and placement of extremities in warm water may stimulate the need to void.

b. Place bath blanket over the client covering the top linen.

The bath blanket is warmer and more absorbent than a sheet. If a bath blanket is not available, the top sheet may be used to cover the client.

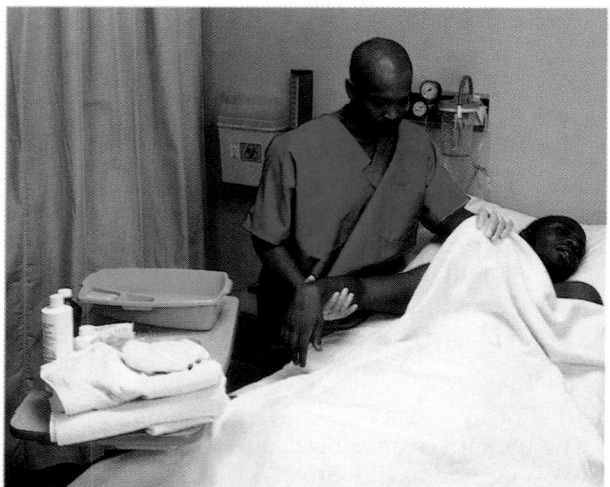

Placing the bath blanket over the client, covering the top linen.

c. Loosen top linen at the foot of the bed and remove from under the bath blanket. To do so, ask the client to grasp the top of the bath blanket. If client is unable to grasp the blanket, grip it with one hand while removing the linen with the other. The client remains covered with the bath blanket while the soiled sheet is pulled out. Refold any linen that is to be reused and place on a chair. Place dirty linen in a laundry hamper or laundry bag.

d. Place bath towel under head. Remove pillow if the client can tolerate it. If removal of pillow causes any discomfort, leave it in place and place the towel over the pillow.

Removal of the pillow allows for better access to the back of the neck and skin surfaces. It also prevents the pillow from becoming damp while the face and neck are being washed.

e. Help client move to the side of the bed nearest you. Be sure that the side rail on opposite side of bed is in raised position.

Having the client close to you lowers your center of gravity and enhances efficiency of movement and energy as well as protecting you from stretching back muscles.

f. Remove client's gown or pajamas. If an IV is in place, remove the arm without the IV first; then, on arm with IV, slide the sleeve down, lower the IV, and slide the IV through the sleeve opening. Rehang IV and assess rate of flow.

4 Wash the client's face and neck.

In general, bathe from head to toe (cleanest to dirtiest). Wash, rinse, and dry before moving to the next area.

a. Fill washbasin ⅓ to ½ full of warm water. Test the temperature of the water with a bath thermometer or with your wrist. It should be comfortably warm, between 114.8°F and 109.4°F (43°C to 46°C).

If the pan is too full, the basin is difficult to handle and spilling is likely. Too little water cools very quickly and is not sufficient for adequate bathing and rinsing.

b. Put on clean gloves if there is possibility of exposure to body fluids during the bath.

Standard precautions should be maintained when any exposure to body fluids is anticipated.

c. Make a mitt with the washcloth. Use either the triangular or the rectangular method of folding.
   Place your hand in the center of the washcloth.

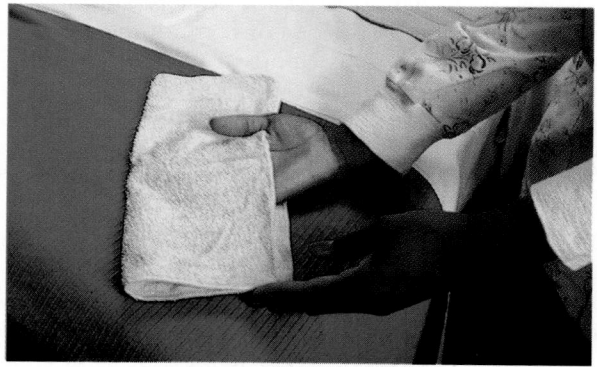

Folding the edges of the washcloth over the hand to make a mitt (rectangular method).

   Fold the edges over hand.
   Tuck the edges in to make a mitt.

Using the mitt prevents the loose ends of the washcloth from dragging across the client's skin and chilling or irritating the skin.

d. Wash and dry client's face using clear water.

Soap is sometimes drying to the skin, especially in older people. Many people do not want soap on their face. Ask client for preference before using soap.

e. Wash the client's eyes with clear water.
    With one corner of the mitt, begin washing the eye at the inner canthus and work toward the outside.

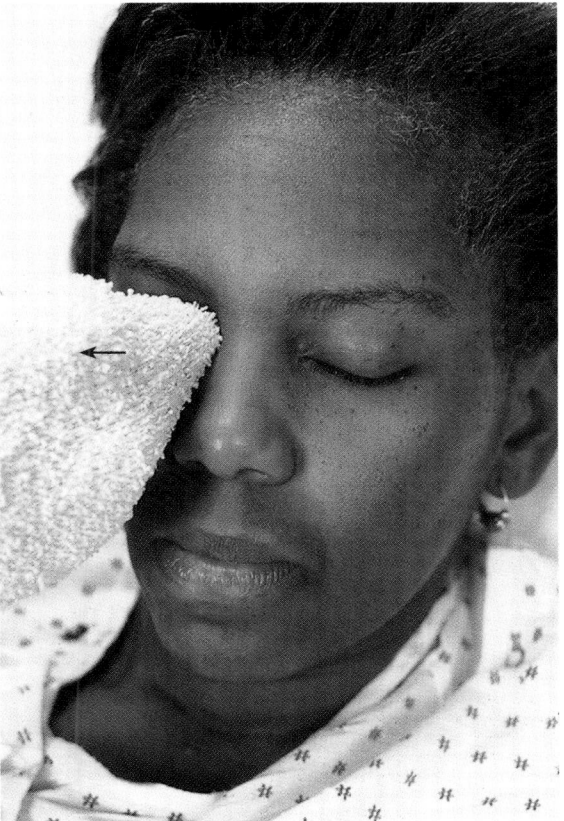

Washing the eye from the inner canthus outward.

Change the placement of your hand in the mitt and repeat with the other eye. Dry thoroughly. If crusted secretions are present, place warm washcloth or cotton ball over the eye until secretions are moist enough to be easily removed.

Using different points on the washcloth prevents cross-contamination of the eyes if there is any infection. Infectious secretions are prevented from entering the lacrimal ducts. Moistening dried secretions prevents trauma to the eye on removal of the secretions.

f. Wash forehead, cheeks, nose, and perioral areas.
g. Wash the postauricular area. Clean the anterior and posterior ear with the tip of the washcloth.
h. Wash the front and back of the neck.
i. Remove the towel from beneath client's neck.

5 Wash the client's arms.

As you move down the body you can wash larger areas at a time. Wash small to moderately sized sections of the body at a time. The size of the area is determined by the likelihood of the person experiencing the discomfort of chilling.

a. Place a towel lengthwise under upper arm and axilla. Wash the upper surface of the arm. Use long firm strokes, proceeding from distal to proximal areas.

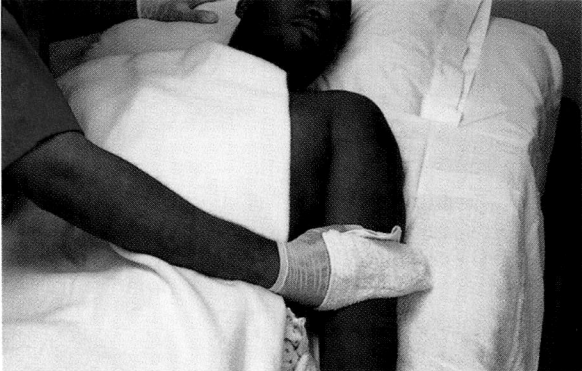

Washing the client's arm.

b. Grasp the client's wrist firmly and elevate the arm to wash the lower surface of the arm.
c. Wash the axilla.

Elevating the arm helps with ROM whereas distal-to-proximal stroking aids venous return. Extremities should be grasped at the joint rather than by the body of the muscle when they are being elevated. Gripping the muscle body may cause great discomfort.

d. Wash the client's hands. Support wrist joint and immerse the hand in warm water. Allow it to soak for a few minutes. Do ROM with the client's fingers. Dry the hand thoroughly. Nails may be cleaned now or after the bath. Apply lotion if desired.

Moving the joints provides ROM. Soaking the hand is relaxing and pleasant for the client. It also softens the cuticle and makes it easier to clean the nails by loosening any dirt under the nails.

Continued

PROCEDURE 36–1 *(continued)*

Giving the Client a Bed Bath

6 Wash the client's chest.
a. Fold the bath blanket down to the umbilicus.
b. For a female client, cover her chest with a towel. Then lift up one side to wash her chest. Dry under the breasts and in any skin folds. Bath powder or cornstarch may be used in small amounts under the breasts if desired. Assess breasts and teach breast self-examination if appropriate. Palpate for axillary node enlargement.

Keeping the client covered protects privacy and prevents unnecessary exposure. Powder or cornstarch serves to absorb perspiration and helps to prevent skin breakdown in body folds, but large quantities of powder under breasts and in skin folds tend to clump.

7 Wash the client's abdomen.
a. Expose only areas being washed. Keep remaining areas covered with a towel. Fold the bath blanket down to symphysis pubis.
b. Use firm strokes to wash the abdomen from side to side, including the umbilicus.

Firm strokes decrease the sensation of tickling, which some people have on light abdominal touching.

c. Observe for signs of distention or visible peristalsis.
d. Re-cover the client with the bath blanket.

8 Wash the client's legs.
a. Expose one leg at a time. Keep the other leg covered with the bath blanket. Keep the rest of the body covered. Remove bath blanket from the farthest leg first.
b. Use firm distal-to-proximal strokes.

Distal-to-proximal stroking stimulates circulation and promotes venous return.

c. Place the client's foot in the basin for a few minutes to soak. Do ROM with the toes. Inspect the feet and nails. When flexing the leg, grasp and support the heel while cradling the calf.

Although it is not essential, soaking the feet can be comforting, especially if the client has been in bed for several days. Soaking aids circulation and softens nails and calluses. Supporting the extremity at the joint prevents discomfort that is initiated by grasping the body of a muscle.

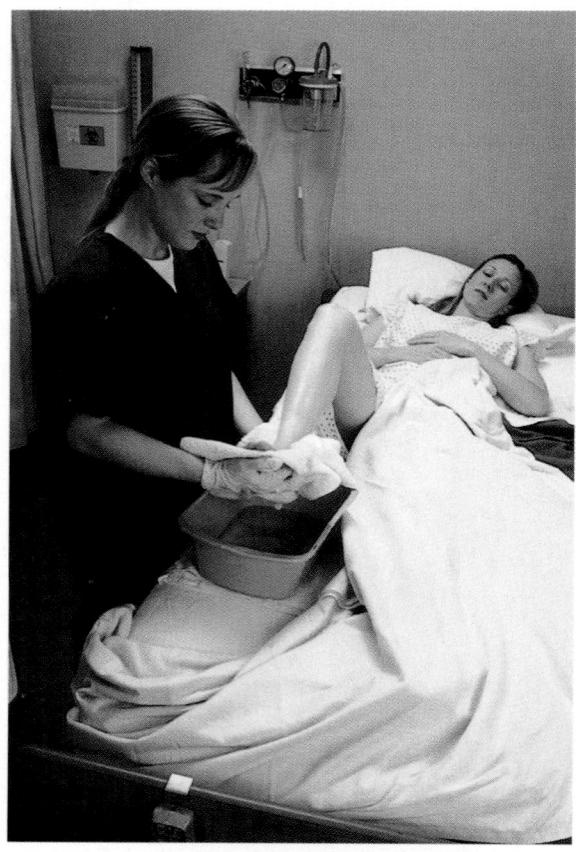

Drying the feet thoroughly.

d. Dry the feet thoroughly, especially between the toes.
e. Repeat this process for the other leg.

If flexing the leg causes pain, this may be suggestive of a positive Homans sign, which should be reported to the physician immediately.

9 Provide perineal care.
a. Change the bath water.
b. Place the client in a supine position. If the client is able to wash genitalia without assistance, place a basin of warm water, washcloth, and towel within reach and provide privacy. If the client cannot wash the perineal area, drape the area with bath blanket so that only genitalia is exposed.
c. Wash the perineal area, as explained in the Providing Perineal Care procedure.

10 Wash the back, buttocks, and perianal area.
a. Place the client in side-lying position.
b. Place a towel lengthwise along the client's back and buttocks.

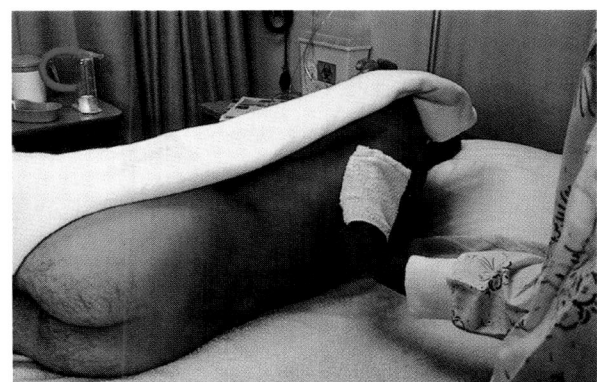

Washing the back and buttocks.

c. Wash, rinse, and dry the client's back and buttocks.

The perianal area is considered the dirtiest area of the body and is bathed last in order to prevent microor-ganisms from being transferred to cleaner parts of the body.

d. A back massage with powder or lotion may be done at this time or it may be done at the completion of the bath.

11 Help the client don a clean gown or pajamas.
a. While the client is still on one side, place one arm in the sleeve of the gown.
b. Turn the client to the back and place the other arm in the sleeve.

12 Assist with hair care.

13 Assist with oral care, as explained in the Providing Oral Hygiene procedure.

14 Make the bed with clean linens, as explained in the procedures on making beds.

15 Leave client's environment clean and uncluttered.

16 Document significant observations and assessment findings.

HOME CARE CONSIDERATIONS

Giving a bed bath in the home follows the same general guidelines for body mechanics, cleaning from clean to dirty, maintaining physical comfort, and working efficiently. However, the typical home environment requires some modification to meet these guidelines. If the client will need a bed bath on a long-term basis, obtaining a hospital bed may be a helpful solution. Some modifications to teach the family caregiver include the following:

• Place a work table at the bedside.
• Sit on the side of the bed instead of bending over.
• Use a minimum amount of soap.
• Use a no-rinse cleansing product.
• Give a complete bath only every 3 days with axillary and perineal care in between.
• Check and massage skin daily.

*Information from Hospital Infection Control Advisory Committee. (1999). *Part II: Recommendations for isolation precautions in hospitals.* Atlanta: Centers for Disease Control and Prevention. Available at http://www.cdc.gov/ncidod/hip/isolat/ispoart2.htm. Accessed May 6, 1999.

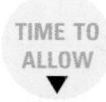

Providing Perineal Care

TIME TO ALLOW
▼
Novice:
15 min.
Expert:
5 min.

Perineal care is the cleansing of the external genitalia, perineum, and surrounding skin. It is usually part of the bath but is sometimes needed more frequently and is done as a separate procedure. See Procedure 36–1 for standard precautions guidelines.

Delegation Guidelines

You may delegate the performance of perineal care to the nursing assistant who has received specific training in the performance of this task. You remain responsible and accountable for assessing your client's perineum.

Equipment Needed

- Bedpan.
- Two towels.
- Two wash cloths.
- Soap.
- Cotton balls.
- Warm water or prescribed solution.
- Waterproof pad.
- Toilet tissue.
- Bath blanket.
- Clean gloves (required).

For a Female Client

1 Prepare for the procedure.
a. Organize necessary equipment. Don clean gloves.
b. Place a protective pad or towel underneath the client before placing on bedpan if doing perineal care in bed.

Perineal care may be done with the client on a bedpan or sitting on toilet or commode chair.

c. Place in a comfortable position on bedpan, toilet, or commode chair. Client may also sit on bedpan in a semi-Fowler position if dorsal recumbent position is not possible.

Adapting position to the client's needs ensures a more positive outcome of the procedure.

d. If care is to be given in bed, ask client to bend her knees and separate her legs.
e. Drape her with a bath blanket. Cover the client's legs and wrap the corners of the bath blanket around the client's feet so her legs are covered. Leave a flap of drape covering the perineum until you are ready to begin the procedure.

Privacy and respect for the client's dignity is essential, with as little exposure as possible.

2 Clean the perineum.
a. Pour warm water or prescribed solution over the perineum.
b. Separate the labia with one hand to expose the urethral and vaginal openings.
c. With your free hand, wipe from front to back in a downward motion with water and soap, wash cloth, or cotton balls. Use a new cloth or cotton ball for each downward stroke.

Wiping in this manner prevents cross-contamination of areas.

d. Wash the external labia. Turn the client to a side-lying position and wash her anal area.
e. Pat dry with a second towel.

3 Make the client comfortable.
a. Remove equipment and cover the client.
b. Position client for comfort.

For a Male Client

1 Prepare for the procedure.
a. Organize necessary equipment.
b. Cover the client with a bath blanket. Expose him only as needed to clean the genitalia.

Avoiding unnecessary exposure respects the client's need for privacy.

2 Clean the perineum.
a. If the client is uncircumcised, retract the foreskin to remove smegma.

Smegma is a cheesy-like substance secreted by the sebaceous glands. It collects under the foreskin.

b. Hold the shaft of the penis firmly but gently with one hand. With the other hand, begin washing at the tip of the penis. Using a circular motion, clean from the center to the outside.

c. Wash down the shaft toward the scrotum. Do not repeat washing an area without changing to a clean area on the washcloth.

d. After washing the penis, replace the foreskin if necessary.

e. Wash around the scrotum.

3 Make the client comfortable.

a. Remove equipment.

b. Cover client and position for comfort.

HOME CARE CONSIDERATIONS

For the client who is unable to provide self-care at home, perineal care should be done daily to prevent unpleasant body odor and for comfort. If the client has a Foley catheter, daily perineal care will help prevent urinary tract infection. Gentle cleansing with soap and water is all that is required. Teach the family how to turn and position the client to work efficiently.

ASSISTING THE CLIENT WITH A SINK BATH

Sometimes the client is well enough to sit up in a chair and bathe at the sink or can sit on the side of the bed with the bath basin positioned on the overbed table. Provide privacy by closing the door and using a drape or sheet for cover and warmth. Wash the back, legs, and feet as necessary. If necessary, provide perineal care. Because the client bathes in a seated position, it is wise to stay close in case assistance is needed or the client becomes weak or dizzy. If the client is bathing at the sink or in a chair, you may use this opportunity to change the bed linens. If the client is sitting on the side of the bed, you may use this time to prepare for mouth or hair care.

Bedmaking

In the hospital setting, the changing of bed linens is usually considered to be part of the routine of morning care and is done in conjunction with the bath and grooming. At other times, linens are changed as needed when they become wet or soiled. In the home setting, the changing of linens may not be done every day, but care should always be taken to smooth the linens and remove crumbs and foreign objects to ensure comfort and safety for the client.

In bedmaking, you must incorporate a variety of skills to make the procedure safe, efficient, and coordinated. The use of good body mechanics is important for protection of your back. Keep your center of gravity close to a wide base of support. Keep the bed at a working height that is comfortable for you so that there is no need to stretch or twist to reach the bed or the client. Use your strong leg and arm muscles in order to protect weak back muscles.

The type of bedmaking required depends in large measure on the condition and needs of the client. If the client is able to be out of bed, the bed should be made at this time. The accompanying procedure, Making an Occupied Bed, provides detailed steps in making an occupied bed.

Preparation for bedmaking is important for the sake of efficiency. Clean linen should be stacked on a chair in the reverse order of use so that each item is accessible as needed. Soiled linens should be placed in a hamper as soon as they are removed. Soiled linen should never be placed on the floor. It should be held away from the uniform at arm's length until it can be placed in the hamper. Neither clean linen nor soiled linen should be shaken because this readily disperses organisms into the air. Do not place soiled linens on the overbed table. This is not only unclean but aesthetically unpleasing because this is the table from which the client eats.

A different type of linen arrangement is needed for the client returning from surgery. Consider the needs of the client and prepare the room accordingly. The bed is made as with any unoccupied bed with a few exceptions. The accompanying procedure describes the steps in preparing a surgical bed (and an unoccupied bed). The purpose of this linen arrangement is that when the client returns from the operating room, an easy transfer from stretcher to bed can be made and the top covers can quickly be put in place. The bed should be in high position, and the room should be cleared of any clutter so that there is no obstruction to transfer of the client. Knowing what to anticipate as a result of the surgical procedure is important. If you anticipate that the client will need assistance with turning and moving, place a draw sheet on the bed for use as a lift sheet. Add extra precautions such as incontinent pads if you anticipate drainage, bleeding, or incontinence.

Text continued on page 953

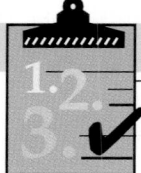

Helping the Client With a Tub Bath or Shower

TIME TO ALLOW
▼
Novice: *30 min.*
Expert: *15 min.*

Clients are assisted with a tub bath or shower when they are able to bathe themselves and there is no contraindication to bathing in a tub or shower. The client should be carefully monitored because the change in temperature and exertion can precipitate weakness or dizziness. Clients who have had medical or surgical treatments in a hospital setting need orders from a physician. Follow standard precautions.

Delegation Guidelines

The nursing assistant may help with the performance of a tub bath or shower. In addition to instruction regarding bathing, the nursing assistant should receive safety and mobility training to appropriately assist your client with this task. You remain responsible for the assessment of your client's independence, skin, gait, mobility, and response to this activity.

Equipment Needed

- Bath towel.
- Two wash cloths.
- Soap or bath lotion.
- Skin care products (deodorant, talcum powder, lotion).
- Clean gown or pajamas.
- Clean gloves (if indicated).

1 Assess the client's capacity for self-care. Assess tolerance for activity, cognitive state, and musculoskeletal function.

An assessment of the client's ability prior to initiating the bath procedure is critical in order to maintain the client's safety and comfort.

2 Make sure that the bathroom is prepared and that tub or shower is clean. Place a disposable bath mat or towel on the floor by tub or shower. Adjust the room temperature so the client is not chilled during bath.

Cleanliness and safety are primary responsibilities in caring for the client.

3 Put on clean gloves.

4 Assess the client's ability to access bathroom. Transport her in a wheelchair or shower chair if the client cannot safely ambulate without assistance. Accompany her to the bathroom.

5 Keep the client covered with a bath blanket while preparing the water.

Chilling occurs quickly when skin is uncovered. Keeping the client covered conserves body heat, preventing chilling.

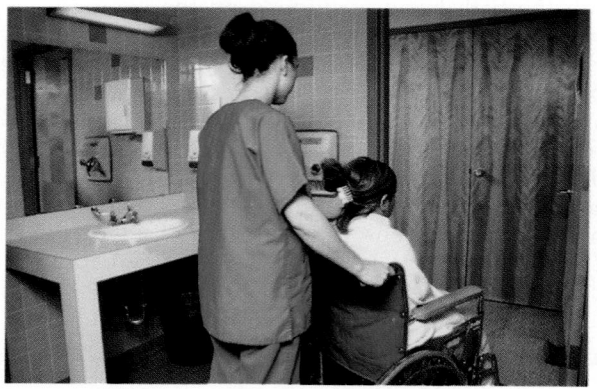

Keeping the client covered with a bath blanket during transport to the bathroom.

6 Provide privacy for the client by placing an "occupied" sign on the door.

Bathroom doors are not locked for safety reasons because clients may sometimes need unexpected assistance. The need for privacy while bathing is basic to human dignity, and provision for privacy demonstrates respect for the person.

7 Test the water temperature before the client gets into tub or shower. Adjust the temperature until it is comfortable. Fill the bathtub no more than half full of warm water (105°F). Caution client not to adjust temperature without assistance.

Testing the temperature before entering the water prevents burns. Attempts to adjust the water temperature without assistance can result in scalding.

8 Provide assistance for client while client is entering tub or shower.

Falls in the tub or shower are common accidents and must be prevented by safety measures.

9 Assess whether the client can safely bathe without assistance. If the client can remain unattended, show her how to use the call signal and the safety bars in the tub or shower. The client may wish to sit in shower chair to conserve energy while bathing. Place all bath supplies within easy reach.

Falls in the tub or shower often occur when client is reaching for an object, such as soap or towel. Placing everything within easy reach prevents need for reaching.

10 If the client can be safely left to bathe unattended, check every 10 to 15 minutes to determine if she needs help.

11 If client is not able to bathe independently, remain with her at all times. Assist as needed with bathing.

Encourage the client to do as much of the bathing as possible. This encourages independence as well as motor function.

12 Wash any areas that the client is unable to reach, such as the back and legs. Assist a female client with shaving her legs or axillae if desired.

13 Watch closely for signs of dizziness or weakness while client is in the tub or shower and immediately on exiting tub or shower.

Vasodilation and pooling of blood in extremities occurs with prolonged exposure to warm water. This may manifest as dizziness, weakness, or faintness.

14 Help the client out of the tub or shower. Assist with drying.

15 Assist with grooming and dressing in clean pajamas or gown.

16 Help the client return to her room.

17 Assess the client's tolerance for the procedure (level of fatigue, musculoskeletal strength, and sensorium).

18 Leave the bathroom clean. Discard soiled linen. Clean the tub or shower according to agency policy.

19 Document the client's response to the activity.

HOME CARE CONSIDERATIONS

The home care client who can get in the tub or shower will have some concerns about mobility and will need modifications for safety. Be sure the bathroom is equipped with grab bars and that a steady stool or shower chair is available. The bathtub should have a nonskid surface. The bath mat should be nonskid and the floor should not be slippery when wet. For showers in a chair, it may be helpful to install a long hose-type shower head.

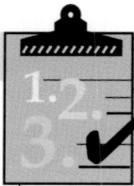

PROCEDURE 36–4

Making an Occupied Bed

TIME TO
ALLOW
▼
Novice:
20 min.
Expert:
10 min.

If the client cannot be out of bed, the linens are changed at the end of the bed bath. This can be accomplished by turning the client to one side, making half the bed, turning the client to the other side, and making the other half of the bed. In an acute care facility, bed linens are changed daily for the client's comfort and to eliminate a reservoir for the growth of microorganisms. When linens become wet or soiled they are changed more frequently. In the home setting, linens are not changed daily but should be changed when wet or soiled.

Delegation Guidelines

Once you have assessed your client's ability to be turned and positioned in a side-lying fashion, you may delegate the performance of an occupied bed change to the nursing assistant. Clients with neurological or orthopedic injuries may have special positioning restrictions that require your direct supervision and assistance with the performance of this task. The nursing assistant should receive specific instruction in the performance of this task, including safety, patient comfort, and infection control in the basic training program.

Equipment Needed

- Top sheet, bottom sheet, draw sheet (optional).
- Bedspread (change if soiled).
- Blanket (if needed; change if soiled).
- Mattress pad (change if soiled).
- Pillowcases.
- Waterproof pads.

---

1 Organize the environment and position the client to expose half the bed.

a. Wash your hands.
b. Close the door or curtain for privacy.
c. Fold a full-size sheet to be used as a draw sheet.
d. Lower the rail on the nearest side of the bed. Be sure that the side rail on the opposite side is up and locked.

   This ensures safety as client rolls to side of bed. Upright side rails also allow the client something to grasp to help in turning.

e. Position the bed at a comfortable working height. Move the client toward the near side of the bed.

   Having the bed at waist height and the client at side of bed allows use of correct body mechanics by lowering center of gravity and avoiding stretching of lower back muscles.

f. Loosen the top linens.
g. Remove spread, top sheet, and blanket in one movement, at the same time pulling the bath blanket over the client. If top linens are to be reused, fold and place them in a chair.

   Linens should always be folded and not fluffed in the air. It is important to prevent the spread of microorganisms.

h. Place any linen that is not to be reused in laundry hamper or linen bag. Avoid contact with your uniform. Hold at arm's length while removing from bed to linen hamper.

   The spread of microorganisms from soiled linen to uniform to other clients is prevented by avoiding contact with linen.

i. Loosen bottom sheet on near side of bed. Have the client roll to opposite side of bed. Adjust pillow under head.
j. Lower the bed position to flat if the client can tolerate it. If the client cannot breathe when lying flat, adjust the bed to as near flat as possible.

   The flatter the surface of the bed, the more efficiently the sheets can be tucked under the mattress.

---

2 Make half the bed from top to bottom.

a. Fan-fold the dirty bottom sheet and draw sheet, and tuck them under the client's back and buttocks as tightly as possible. This allows space for you to place clean linens, and it moves dirty linen close to other side of bed for easy removal.

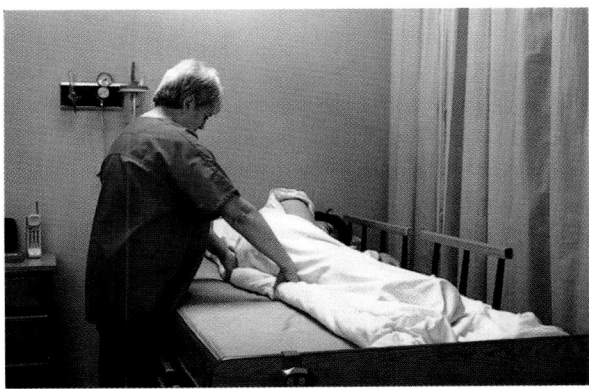

Fan-folding the dirty bottom sheet and draw sheet and tucking them under the client's back and buttocks.

b. Place the clean bottom sheet on bed. Start with the bottom edge even with foot end of bed, with the center fold in the middle of the bed. Unfold to the top and allow the extra length to hang over the top.

c. Fan-fold the top layer to the middle of the bed.

   Make the roll of linens as flat as possible. The client will need to roll over the linens gathered in the middle of the bed.

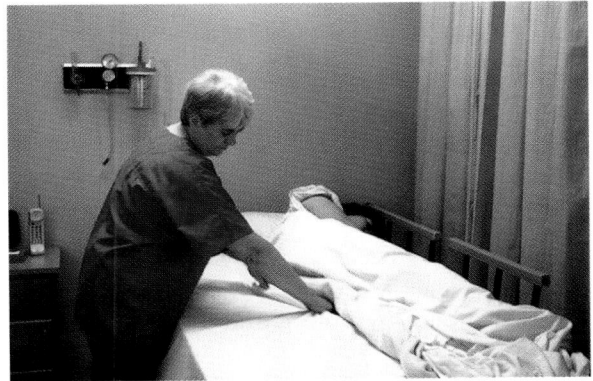

Fan-folding the top layer to the middle of the bed.

d. If contour sheets are to be used, fit the elastic edges under top and bottom corners of mattress. If regular sheets are used, make a mitered corner. Tuck the top of the sheet well under the mattress at the head of the bed.

   To make a mitered corner, lay a triangular fold of sheet on the bed.

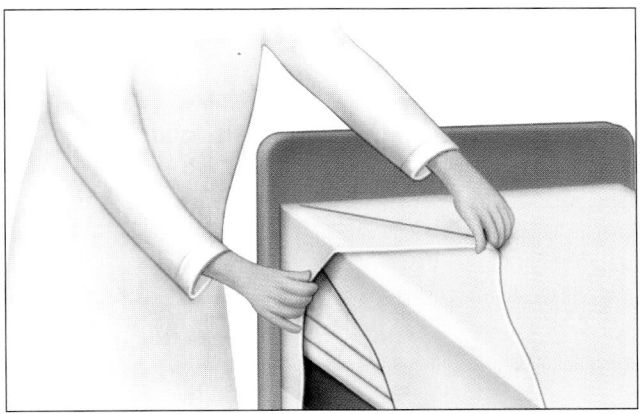

Laying a triangular fold of sheet on the bed.

Tuck the end of the sheet under the mattress.

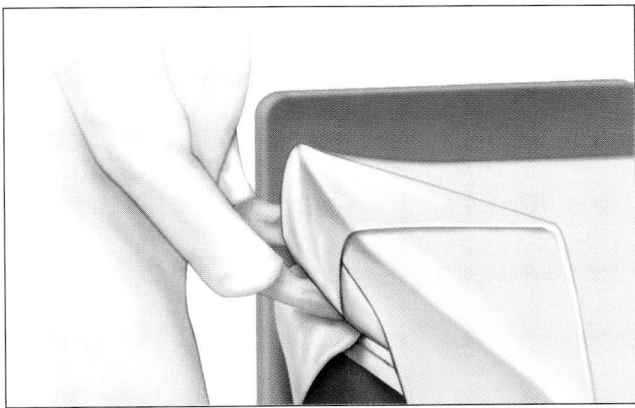

Tucking the end of the sheet under the mattress.

Pull the triangular fold over the side of the mattress.

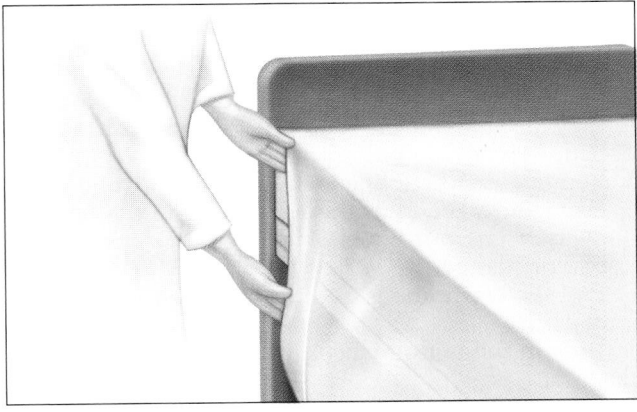

Pulling the triangular fold over the side of the mattress.

Continued

Making an Occupied Bed

Tuck the triangular fold under the mattress.

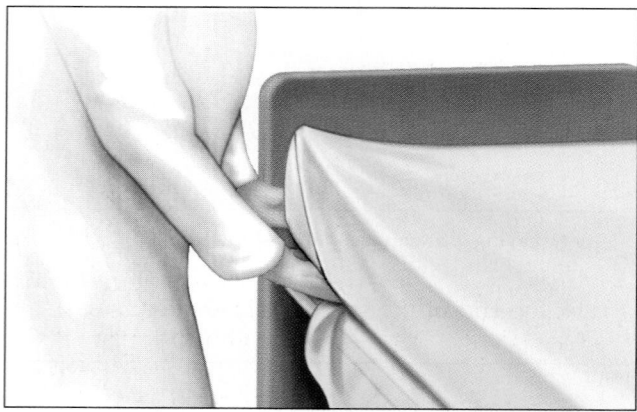

Tucking the triangular fold under the mattress.

Tuck the sheet well under the mattress, working from top to bottom.

3 Place a draw sheet on top of bottom sheet. The folded edge is placed at the top of the client's shoulders.

The draw sheet should cover the bed from the client's shoulders to below the hips.

a. Place the center fold along the center of the bed.
b. Fan-fold the top layer toward the client.
c. Tuck the excess under the mattress along with the bottom sheet.
d. Smooth out the wrinkles as much as possible.
e. If an incontinence pad is used, fan-fold and place it on top of the linens near the client's back.

4 Make the second half of the bed.
a. Help the client turn onto the clean sheets. Raise the side rail and move to opposite side of the bed. Lower side rail on that side.
b. Remove the dirty linens, folding toward the center or one end of the bed. Holding the linens away from your body, place them in dirty linen bag or hamper.
c. Pull the clean linens over the exposed half of the bed.
d. Tuck in the bottom sheet.

As you work from top to bottom, pull the linens tight and tuck one section at a time.

e. Tuck the draw sheet, moving from the middle, to the top, to the bottom.

5 Put on the top sheet and spread.
a. Help the client move back to the center of the bed.
b. Place the top sheet over client with the seam side up. The center crease should be at the center of the bed. Unfold the sheet from head to toe.
c. Have the client grasp the top sheet while you pull the soiled sheet or bath blanket from under the clean sheet.
d. Place the blanket and spread evenly over the top sheet. Be sure that they are even on both sides.
e. Make mitered corners at the foot of bed with the top sheet, blanket, and spread together.
f. Pull the top sheet, blanket, and spread into a tent over the client's toes.

Pleating removes pressure of bed covers on client's toes.

g. Cuff the spread, blanket, and top sheet at head of bed. Be sure that there is adequate sheet at head of bed to cover the client's shoulders.

6 Change the pillow case.
a. Grasp the closed end of a clean pillow case at the center point.
b. With the other hand, hold the open end of the case.
c. Invert the case over your hand and forearm (at the closed end) by pulling the open end of case back toward the closed end. Maintain your grasp at the closed end.

7 Return the bed to its low position. Place the call light within the client's reach.

8 Position the client for comfort.

9 Wash your hands and document your care.

Help the family make modifications for ease in bedmaking. Both sides of the bed should be accessible. The client may be using a double bed. To move the client from one side to the other, the family caregiver can get on the bed on the knees. A turn sheet can be used to slide the client across the bed without risking damage to the skin. Teach the family about the importance of a wrinkle-free bed. If soiling is a problem, instruct the family about options for protecting the mattress. A heavy-duty lawn and leaf bag can be used to cover the mattress. Any plastic that is used should be covered with a mattress pad to prevent excess perspiration.

Interventions to Promote Oral Hygiene

The client who is unable to provide for oral hygiene is host to potentially serious problems that are preventable. Assessment of the client's physical status will determine the degree of assistance needed with oral hygiene. The arthritic client may find it difficult to grasp a small toothbrush handle, so it may be helpful to use an electric toothbrush, which tends to have a bigger handle, or to pad the handle of the toothbrush to make it bigger and easier to hold. The blind client may need assistance with knowing where basin, water, and mouthwash are located. The mentally impaired client may need assistance because of a short attention span or an inability to focus on the required components of the task.

The performance of oral hygiene presents an excellent opportunity for teaching. Inadequate oral hygiene may occur for lack of knowledge of oral hygiene practices, poor nutritional habits, inadequate oral hygiene practices, or painful oral lesions that serve as reasons for the neglect. Information relative to drug interactions, nutrition, and the need for periodic dental assessment can easily be incorporated into the demonstration of correct oral hygiene measures. The accompanying Teaching for Wellness Chart suggests some information to teach the client about oral hygiene.

Assisting the Conscious Client

If the client is unable to go to the sink for oral care, it is still possible to provide oral hygiene. The accompanying procedure, Providing Oral Hygiene, describes the steps in assisting clients with oral care.

Clients with dry mouths or lips may need frequent mouth care, sometimes as often as every 2 hours, to preserve the integrity of the oral mucosa. Dry lips and mucosa tend to crack and fissure, and this leads to infection and other problems. Rinsing the mouth with water, saline solution, or mouthwash can be helpful for these clients. Mouthwashes come in several varie-

ties. Bactericidal mouthwashes should be used with caution because they tend to destroy the normal bacterial flora of the mouth, resulting in overgrowth of fungus. Avoid commercial mouthwashes that contain high concentrations of alcohol, which can increase mouth dryness. Saline solution is soothing for some patients. Some patients have stomatitis from radiation

---

Teaching for WELLNESS

ORAL HYGIENE

Purpose: To teach client the importance of good oral hygiene and need for preventive dentistry.

Rationale: Regular oral hygiene and dental assessments serve as preventive measures in the incidence of dental pathology.

Expected Outcomes: The client will perform oral hygiene after each meal, floss daily, and visit the dentist every 6 months for supervision.

Client Instructions
- Brush your teeth thoroughly at least twice a day.
- Floss your teeth once a day.
- Remember that good dental health contributes to your overall well-being.
- Keep in mind that recent studies seem to suggest a relationship between gum disease and heart disease.
- Visit your dentist regularly for preventive care and cleaning. Doing so will not only prevent painful dental problems but also is more cost-effective in the long run.
- Certain foods are best for oral health, such as raw fruits and vegetables. Others are not good for oral health, such as sugary drinks and candy. Try to avoid the latter.

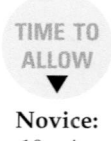

PROCEDURE 36–5

Making an Unoccupied Bed and a Surgical Bed

TIME TO ALLOW
▼
Novice:
10 min.
Expert:
5 min.

In an acute care facility bed linens are changed daily for the client's comfort and to eliminate a reservoir for the growth of microorganisms. When linens become wet or soiled they are changed more frequently. In the home setting, linens are not changed daily, but should be changed when wet or soiled. Bed linens are changed when the client is out of bed.

A surgical bed is made for the client who is returning from the operating room on a stretcher. It is an *open bed* as described in making an unoccupied bed. However, the sheets are fan-folded top to bottom to receive the client from a stretcher.

Delegation Guidelines

You may delegate the full performance of this task to a nursing assistant.

Equipment Needed

- Top sheet, bottom sheet, draw sheet (optional).
- Bedspread, blanket.
- Waterproof pad (if needed).

Making an Unoccupied Bed

1 Organize the environment.
a. Wash your hands.
b. Raise the bed to a comfortable working height.
c. Lower the side rails.

2 Remove soiled linens. Fold soiled surface inward and place in hamper.
a. Remove the bedspread and blanket. Fold and put them in a chair if they will be reused. If they are soiled, place them in laundry hamper or linen bag. Remove the pillow from its pillow case.
b. When handling soiled linens, always hold them away from your body.
This prevents the spread of microorganisms from person to person.

3 Make one side of the bed at a time. Then move to the other side.
This conserves time, energy, and movement and contributes to the smoothness of the sheets.

a. If the bottom sheet is a contour sheet, place the elastic bands under the top and bottom corners of the mattress. Tuck along the sides. If the bottom sheet is not contour, unfold it lengthwise and place the vertical crease at the center of the bed. Unfold it toward the opposite side of mattress. Make the bottom edge even with the bottom edge of the mattress. Smooth any wrinkles out of bottom sheet. Make a mitered corner at the head of the bed as explained in the procedure Making an Occupied Bed.

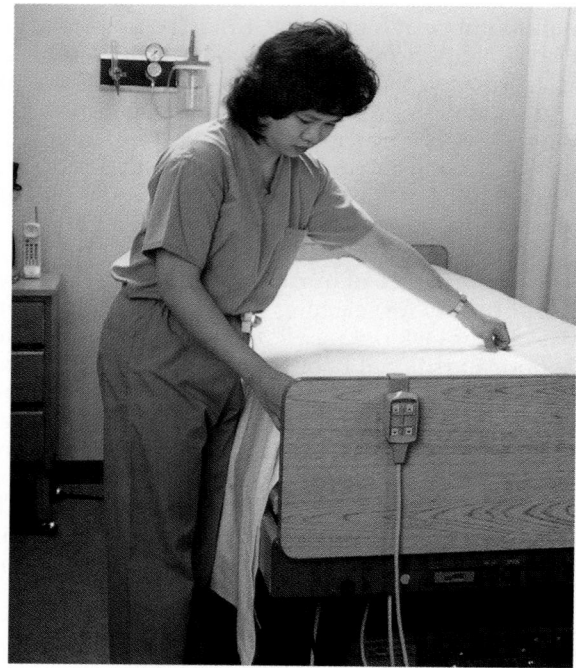
Centering the bottom sheet.

b. Tuck the side in along the mattress.
c. If the client needs a draw sheet, center the draw sheet on the bed and unfold toward the opposite side. Tuck under the mattress. If a pull (turn) sheet is needed, fold draw sheet in halves (full sheet is folded into four layers), creating a strong sheet to turn and move the client in bed. If absorbent pad is needed, position at center of bed on top of draw sheet.

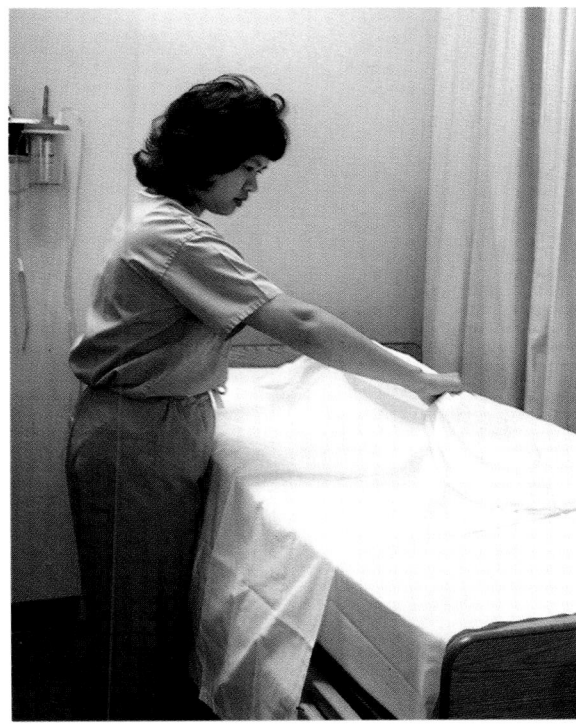

Centering the draw sheet and unfolding toward the opposite side.

d. Move to the other side of the bed. Remove the soiled linen. Fold the soiled side in. Hold the bundle of linen away from your body and place in a linen bag or hamper.
e. Pull the linen to your side. Tuck the top of the sheet at the head of the bed. Make a mitered corner at the head of the bed. If a draw sheet is used, pull and tuck it along with the bottom sheet.

4 Place top sheet, blanket, and spread over bed.
a. Leave a cuff at the top of the spread.
b. Miter the corners all together at foot of bed.

5 Prepare the bed for the client to return.
a. Make a toe pleat.

Making a Surgical Bed

1 Make the bed as above in steps 1 to 4.

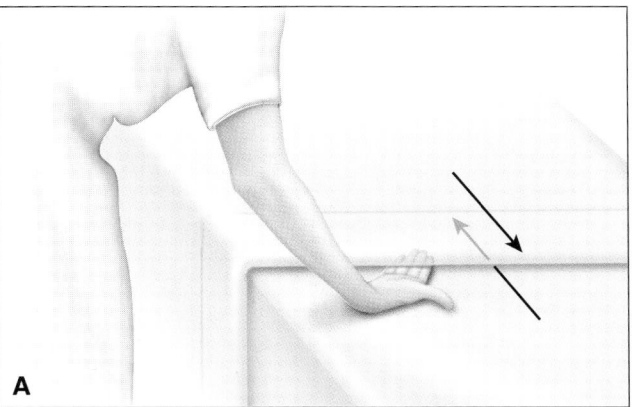

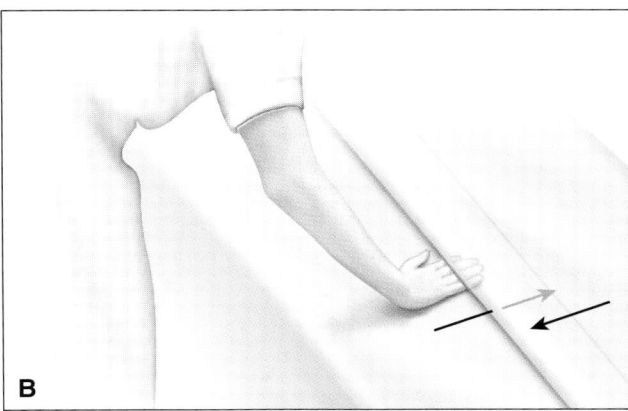

Making a toe pleat. *A,* vertical toe pleat; *B,* horizontal toe pleat.

b. Fan-fold the linen to the foot of the bed to create an *open bed.*
c. Change the pillowcase.
d. Return the bed to its low position.
e. Position the call light.
f. Dispose of soiled linens.

6 Wash your hands and document your care.

2 Fold the bottom and top corners on the near side to the opposite side, making a triangle.

Continued

PROCEDURE 36–5 (continued)

Making an Unoccupied Bed and a Surgical Bed

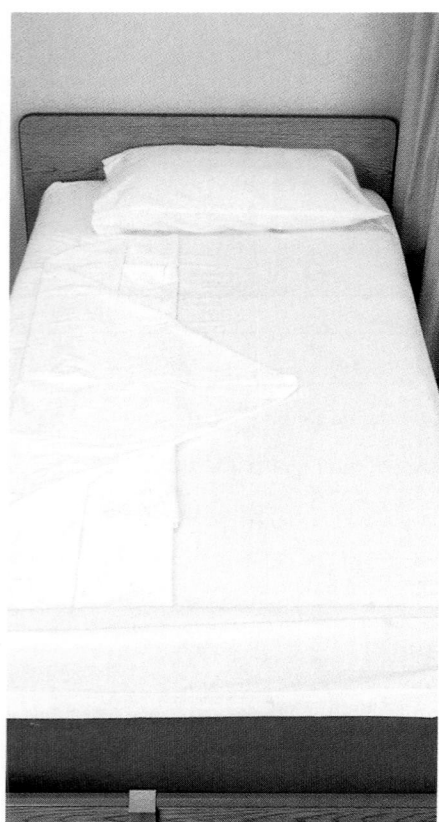

Triangle of sheet on surgical bed.

3 Pick up the center point of the triangle and fan-fold the linen to the side of the bed.

4 Leave the bed in high position.

5 Change the pillowcase and leave the pillow at the foot of the bed or on a chair to be accessible for placement under the client's head after the client is transferred to the bed.

6 Move all objects away from bedside area to leave room for the stretcher.

---

or chemotherapy, which leads to mouth ulcerations that are extremely painful. Anesthetic solutions maybe soothing for them.

A dilute solution of hydrogen peroxide and water is good for removing debris and microorganisms from the tongue and mouth. By removing debris, hydrogen peroxide reduces halitosis. Half-strength peroxide is comforting to clients who have stomatitis. It should be used four times a day. Prolonged use of hydrogen peroxide can cause sponginess of the gums and decalcification of tooth surfaces, and this substance should be used with caution.

Assisting the Unconscious Client

Oral care for the unconscious client is critical for the person's well-being. Clients who have altered sensorium levels are often mouth breathers, which accentuates the problems related to the mouth and makes frequent oral care essential.

The comatose client can receive adequate oral hygiene with the use of a minimal amount of liquid. Po-

sition the client flat in side-lying position to prevent aspiration. Position the back of the head on a pillow so that the face tips forward and fluid will flow out of the mouth, not back into the throat. Swallowing and gag reflexes may not be intact; therefore, it is important to be very careful to prevent aspiration. It is important to have oral suction at hand.

Once the client is safely positioned, the usual manner of brushing can be used to clean the teeth. It will be necessary to find a means to keep the mouth open. An easy way is to tape tongue blades together and cover them with gauze taped in place. Never place your fingers in the mouth of a person with altered level of consciousness. Human bites are very painful and potentially dangerous. After brushing the teeth and cleaning the tongue, apply a water-soluble lubricant, lip balm, or petroleum jelly to the lips.

Assisting With Denture Care

Care of dentures becomes your responsibility when the client is unable to care for the dentures. Dentures

PROCEDURE 36–6

Providing Oral Hygiene

TIME TO
ALLOW
▼
Novice:
10 min.
Expert:
5 min.

Oral hygiene is provided to maintain the integrity of the client's teeth, gums, mucous membranes, and lips. Oral hygiene ideally means brushing the client's teeth or cleaning the dentures per the client's usual routine. Moistened toothettes can be used for comfort and moisture in between brushing.

Delegation Guidelines

Generally, you may delegate the performance of providing oral hygiene to a nursing assistant. Knowledge of the client's oral anatomy and any necessary precautions related to the performance of this task are your responsibility. A client having undergone an oropharyngeal procedure or known to have a bleeding disorder should have a careful assessment by you, prior to your considering delegation of this task.

Equipment Needed

* Soft-bristle toothbrush long enough to reach the back teeth.

* Toothpaste of client's choice.
* Cup of water.
* Emesis basin or sink.
* Dental floss, regular or fine, waxed or unwaxed.
* Tissues.
* Towel.
* Mouthwash, if desired.
* For an unconscious client, petroleum jelly, sponge swab (if desired instead of a toothbrush), bulb syringe or suction catheter, padded tongue blade.

1 Prepare for the procedure.
a. Assess the client's ability to participate in procedure.
b. Wash your hands and don clean gloves.
c. Position the client either in high or semi-Fowler's position or in a lateral side-lying position. These positions decrease the possibility of aspiration and choking.

2 Place a towel under the client's chin and over the upper chest.
This prevents soiling of the bed linens or the client's gown or pajamas.

3 Moisten the toothbrush with small amount of water and apply toothpaste.

4 Either give the toothbrush to the client for brushing or brush the client's teeth if necessary.
a. Ask the client to open her mouth wide and hold an emesis basin under the client's chin.
b. Position the toothbrush at 45-degree angle to the gum line.

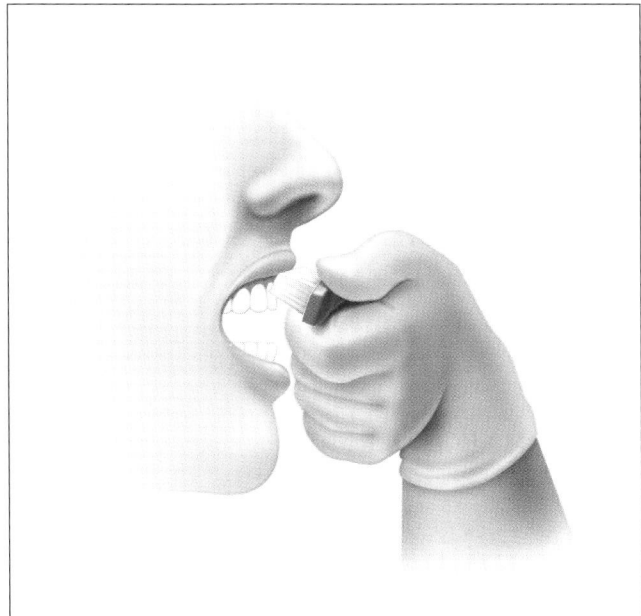

Positioning the toothbrush at a 45-degree angle to the gum line.

c. Directing the bristles of the toothbrush toward the gum line, brush from the gum line to the crown of each tooth, making sure to clean all surfaces.

Continued

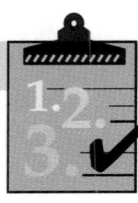

Providing Oral Hygiene

Brushing action removes food particles from gum line and stimulates the gums.

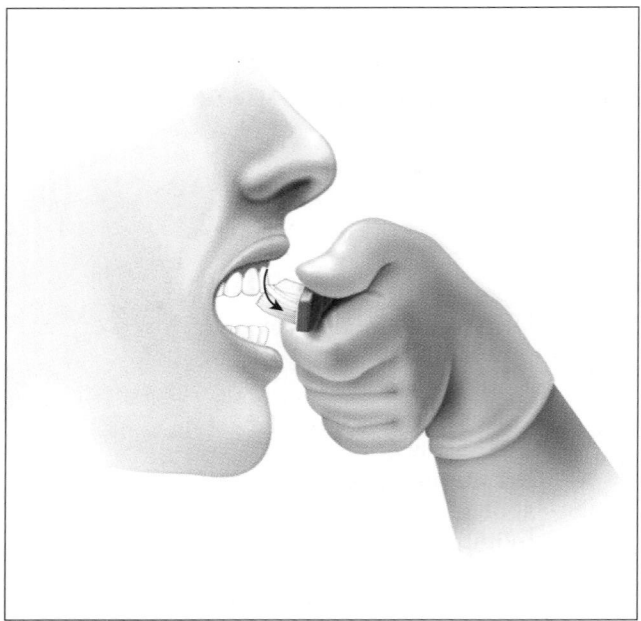

Brushing from the gum line to the crown of the tooth.

d. Using back-and-forth strokes, clean the biting surfaces of the teeth.
e. Gently brush the client's tongue. Do not stimulate the gag reflex by reaching the back surface of tongue.

Bacteria, oral secretions, and food particles accumulate on the tongue and must be removed.

f. Have the client rinse her mouth with water and expectorate into the emesis basin.

5 Have the client rinse with mouthwash if desired. A solution of half-strength hydrogen peroxide may serve to remove extremely heavy coating on the tongue. Ask the client to hold the solution in her mouth for 10 to 15 seconds before expectorating. This can be repeated at hourly intervals if needed.

For an Unconscious Client

1 Prepare for the procedure.
a. Wash your hands and don clean gloves.
b. Place the client in a side-lying position.

The lateral position allows for gravity drainage of fluid and decreases the chance of aspiration. A full lateral position may be preferred for the completely unconscious client.

c. Place the bulb syringe or suctioning equipment nearby for when the client needs to be suctioned.

6 Remove the tooth-brushing equipment.

7 Floss the client's teeth.
Flossing removes plaque and food particles that collect between teeth and below the gum line that brushing cannot reach.

a. Cut a 10-inch piece of floss. Wind the ends of the floss around the middle finger of each of your hands.
b. Holding the floss tightly to provide tension, start with the back lower teeth and floss up and down around the lower teeth from one side of the mouth to the other. Use a sawing motion between the teeth.

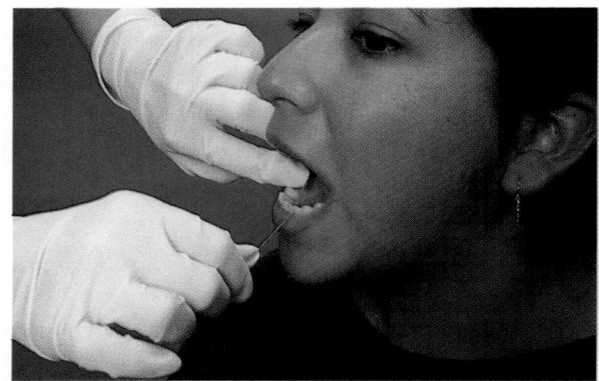

Flossing, using a "sawing" motion.

c. Cut a fresh piece of floss and repeat the procedure on the upper teeth, moving from one side to the other.
d. Ask the client to rinse her mouth and expectorate into the emesis basin.
e. Dry the client's mouth and help her to a comfortable position.

8 Remove all equipment and make the client comfortable.

d. Place a towel or waterproof pad under the client's chin. Place an emesis basin under his chin as well.

2 Clean the client's teeth and mouth.
a. Use a padded tongue blade to open the client's mouth.

Never attempt to open an unconscious client's mouth

with the fingers. Oral stimulation often causes the biting-down reflex, and serious injuries can occur.

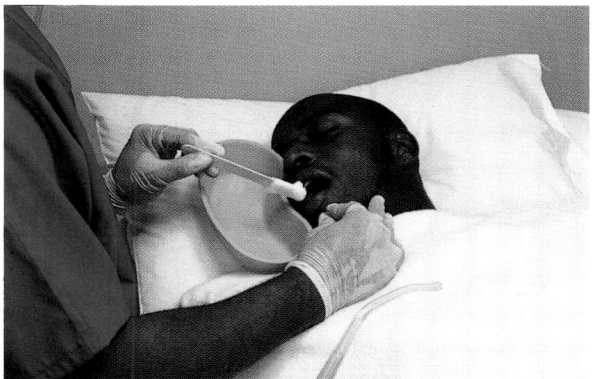

Using a padded tongue blade to open the client's mouth.

b. Swab the inside of the mouth, tongue, and teeth with a moist, padded tongue blade.
c. Brush the client's teeth as directed above. A toothbrush or sponge swab may be used.

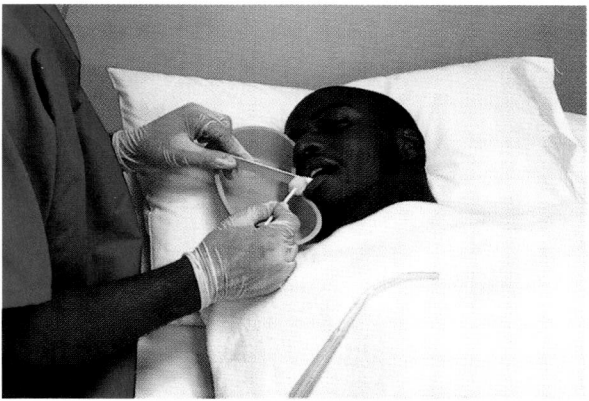

Brushing the client's teeth with a sponge-tipped swab.

d. Rinse the client's mouth using a very small amount of water that can be suctioned readily from his mouth.
e. Lubricate client's lips with petroleum jelly. *Petroleum jelly may be applied as often as necessary to prevent drying and cracking of the lips.*

3 Remove your equipment and document your care.

4 Leave the client dry and comfortable.

For Dentures

1 Prepare for the procedure.
a. Ask the client to remove her dentures. If this is not possible, place a gauze square on the front of the denture. Grasping the front teeth between your thumb and forefinger, pull down gently until the suction that holds the upper dentures in place is loosened. Loosen lower dentures by lifting up and out.
Use of the gauze square prevents your fingers from slipping. Dentures are slippery. Hold the dentures firmly until they are secured in a basin or denture cup.

2 Clean the dentures according to client's usual routine or the instructions on your cleaning product.
It is usually acceptable to clean with any gentle toothpaste.

a. Soak in a denture cleanser. If unavailable, use warm (not hot) water and a gauze square or toothbrush to clean.
Place wash cloth in sink while you are cleaning the dentures and work close to the bottom of the sink in case you drop them.
b. Brush the dentures with a soft-bristle brush.
c. Rinse under warm water.

Continued

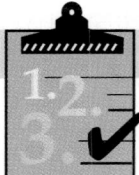

PROCEDURE 36–6 *(continued)*

Providing Oral Hygiene

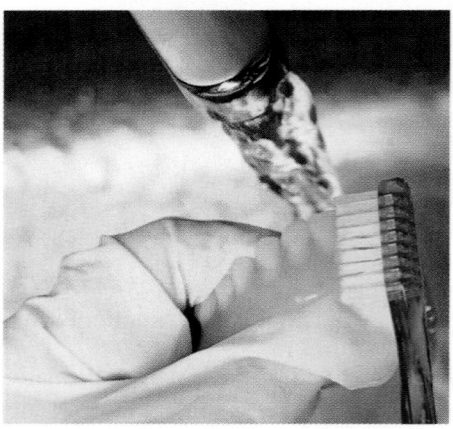

Brushing the dentures with a soft-bristle brush.

3 Help the client replace the denture.
If you need to put the dentures in, start with the molars and use one edge at a 45-degree angle to open the mouth, then turn to a 90-degree angle and stretch the lips to insert the other side.

4 Use denture adhesive according to the package directions if the client desires.

5 Clean your work area and make the client comfortable. Document your care.

HOME CARE CONSIDERATIONS

Teach the family the importance of daily oral hygiene. Help them develop methods to prevent choking and aspiration.

---

are expensive, and it is important that you treat them carefully and with respect.

Clients should be encouraged to wear their dentures at all times. Dentures should be cleaned after each meal. This helps with speech, eating, and appearance. If they are removed at night, they should be placed in a denture cup covered with water. While the dentures are out of the mouth, assess the oral cavity. Improperly fitting dentures can cause irritation and sometimes make the client vulnerable to cancer of the mouth. Rinse dentures and help the client rinse the mouth with water or mouthwash before replacing the dentures. If rinsing and spitting is not possible, clean the mouth with gauze. If dentures are not to be returned to the client's mouth, they must be stored in a water solution. Assess dentures for breaks, cracks, or food debris.

Assisting With Flossing

Flossing as an adjunct to brushing is essential to removing dental plaque and food debris trapped between the teeth that cannot be removed with the toothbrush. Many people do not floss; therefore, instruction may be necessary while demonstrating. Dental floss comes in waxed and unwaxed textures. Unwaxed is easier to use because it is thinner, slides between teeth more easily, and is more absorbent than waxed floss. After flossing, rinse vigorously to remove debris that has come loose in the mouth.

Interventions for Grooming

Caring for Normal Hair

Grooming includes caring for normal hair. The appearance of the hair is important because it influences one's self-image and makes one feel better. Clients with a bathing/hygiene self-care deficit are unable to groom or clean their hair. The scalp perspires, oil is secreted, and dirt collects along the hair shaft. Hair care involves daily brushing and combing to remove dead cells and dirt and shampooing to clean the hair shafts and the scalp. Hair care should be a part of daily care, and shampooing should be done at least once a week.

When brushing the hair, assess for the presence of scalp lesions and abrasions, dandruff, and the overall quality of hair. The hair itself is an excellent measure of general health. Dull, lifeless hair may indicate problems with nutrition as well as self-care deficit. Shiny, healthy hair is usually a valid measure of overall health.

Combing and brushing the hair may be done by the caregiver if the client is unable to do so. However, if the person is able to handle comb and brush, these activities should be encouraged because they facilitate ROM of upper extremities. If the client is able to sit up in bed or a chair, this facilitates styling. It is important to learn about caring for hair of various racial and gender groups. Asking the client or family member about grooming preferences and methods will be helpful in providing care that is in keeping with the client's usual routine. Some people prefer oils or other substances to be applied to their hair. Women who are confined to bed for long periods of time may prefer hair to be braided so that tangling does not become a problem, particularly if the hair is long.

Caring for Hair With Special Needs

EXCESSIVELY MATTED OR TANGLED HAIR
Very curly hair requires some additional care and handling, such as a wide-toothed comb. African-American clients may prefer to use a large pick comb to prevent damage to the hair (Fig. 36–3). An effective way to work with very curly hair is to divide it into small sections and comb and brush to break up tangles. Using a wide-toothed comb or pick, gently lift hair and smooth it out evenly. Work from the tip of the hair, then from the middle to the tip, then from the scalp to the tip. Be very gentle because some people have extremely sensitive scalps and this can be an uncomfortable procedure if done roughly and with haste. Patience and adequate time are essential. For corn-rowing, make small rows of braids close to the scalp in the client's choice of design. This type of braid is left in the hair for a longer period of time. If hair is tangled, hold hair above the tangle to reduce discomfort. Use short, gentle strokes. Work out the tangle from the end of the hair shafts toward the scalp. Work on a small amount of tangle at a time. Working on large tangles results in broken ends and damaged hair shafts. A small amount of vinegar or alcohol may be applied to the hair to make combing of the tangles easier. Style the hair to prevent further tangling.

If the hair is very matted and tangled, the first impulse is to cut the snarled parts rather than trying to remove the matted hair. This is not acceptable unless the person agrees to having the hair cut. Hair may sometimes be matted with blood in addition to the tangles. First, work with water and alcohol and hydrogen peroxide. Then, divide the hair into sections and clean each section at a time. When combing and brushing, be careful to prevent injury to the scalp. Brushes and combs with sharp bristles and teeth should be avoided because they are potentially harmful. Combs and brushes should be cleaned after each use by soaking them in a solution of ammonia or by washing them with hot water and soap.

BRAIDING THE HAIR
Comb or brush the hair. Before braiding, remove tangles, especially those close to the scalp. Section the hair to equal the number of desired braids. Divide each section into three equal strands. Begin the braid so that the base will not be in a pressure area of the head. If the braid is directly at the base of the scalp, it may be uncomfortable for the client who is bedridden. Weave each of the three strands, alternately placing the right strand over the middle strand, then the left strand over the middle one. Work with smooth motions as you move strands from one hand to the other. Keep the strands in your hands at all times. If the tension is released, the strands become loose and you will need to begin braiding again. Continue until the ends of the strands are reached. Fasten the ends of the braid with a barrette or covered elastic to prevent the braid from coming loose. Avoid use of rubber bands because they damage the hair shaft.

DANDRUFF
Dandruff is usually associated with excessive flaking of the scalp. Brush dry patches loose from the scalp and work them toward the end of the hair. Shampooing every day helps to reduce dandruff in some people; others require a medicated dandruff shampoo. Some conditioners (e.g., petroleum jelly or various oils) may help decrease itching and flaking.

PEDICULOSIS
Pediculosis is infestation with lice and is associated with poor hygiene, crowded living conditions, and exposure to others with lice. Pediculosis capitis refers to infestation of the head, eyebrows, eyelashes, and beard. Pediculosis corporis (scabies) refers to infestation of the body. Pediculosis pubis refers to infestation of the perineal area.

Lice live on the skin, attaching their eggs (nits) to hair, and must be removed. Itching and scratching are a response to lice. Lice nits are difficult to remove because the nits are attached to the hair by an adhesive substance. Pediculosis corporis can be treated with complete bathing, application of topical medication, and washing linen and clothing in very hot water. To treat pediculosis capitis, vigorously massage the hair and scalp with gamma benzene hexachloride (Kwell). Pediculosis pubis may be more resistant to treatment because of the heavy hair growth. Apply the medication to the involved area and leave it on for 12 to 24 hours. Then bathe the client with soap and water. When lice are discovered, remove and bag clothing and linen to prevent spreading. Assure the person that

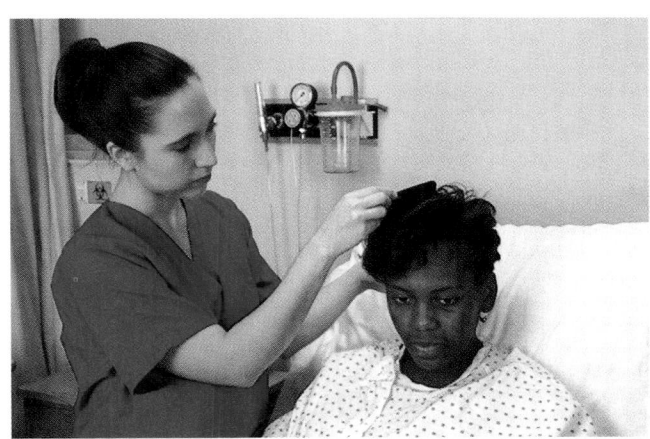

Figure 36–3. Combing the hair of an African-American client.

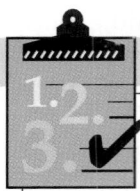

PROCEDURE 36–7

Shampooing the Client in Bed

TIME TO
ALLOW
▼
Novice:
20 min.
Expert:
10 min.

When a client has undergone a prolonged hospitalization or an emergency admission, the hair may need to be shampooed for cleanliness and comfort. The clients most in need of a hair shampoo are those who have been in a motor vehicle accident or lack hygiene facilities, such as the homeless.

Delegation Guidelines

You may delegate the performance of shampooing to a nursing assistant. The requisite skills should be a component of the nursing assistant's basic training program. Special precautions may be necessary for the client with a scalp laceration or glass fragments in the hair after a traumatic injury. You should supervise the application of medicated shampoo for the removal of parasites from the hair and scalp.

Equipment Needed

- Shampoo/conditioner.
- Two bath towels.
- Wash cloth.
- Bath blanket.
- Comb/brush.
- Shampoo board or inflatable basin.
- Water pitcher.
- Waste basket or bucket.
- Waterproof pads.

---

1 Prepare for the procedure.

a. Place waterproof pads under client's head and shoulders.

   This helps keep the bed dry.

b. Remove pins, clips, or barrettes from client's hair. Undo braids and brush the hair thoroughly.

   Brushing the hair before wetting it reduces tangling and allows for even distribution of shampoo.

c. Place the bed in its flat position.

d. Place a shampoo board or inflated basin under the client's head.

   Pad as needed to absorb water leaks.

e. Drape one towel over the client's shoulders. If using a board, place a folded wash cloth to pad the rim where the client's neck touches the board.

   The towel prevents the client from becoming damp and provides neck support for comfort.

f. Uncover the client's upper body by folding the linens down to waist level. Place a bath blanket over her chest.

g. Place a wash cloth over the client's eyes.

   The client's eyes should be protected from irritation from shampoo accidentally getting into the eyes.

h. Place a receptacle in position to catch water.

   The water receptacle should be a level lower than the client's head so that water will run away from the head and face. It may need to be emptied several times.

2 Shampoo the client's hair.

a. Using a water pitcher, pour water over the hair until it is thoroughly wet. The water should be comfortably warm (110°F).

   Water that is too hot may burn the client, and water that is too cold is uncomfortable and chilling.

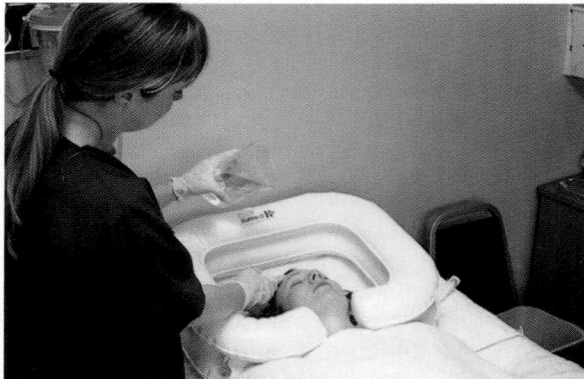

Pouring warm water over the client's hair.

b. Apply a small amount of shampoo. Using your fingertips, gently work it into a lather over the entire scalp. Work from the hairline to the neckline.

   Massage is beneficial to scalp circulation as well as aiding in the cleansing effect of shampoo throughout the hair.

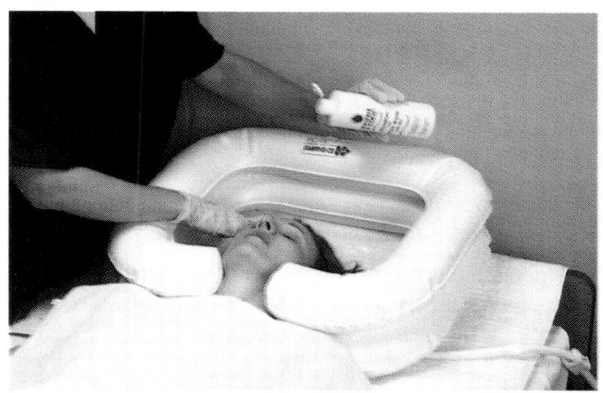

Applying shampoo.

3 Rinse the hair with warm water and reapply shampoo if needed. Repeat until hair is "squeaky clean" when hair shafts are rubbed.

Thorough rinsing is important because shampoo residue is irritating to the scalp and dulls the hair luster.

4 Apply a small amount of conditioner if desired.
Conditioner serves as a "detangler" and makes hair easier to comb.

5 Make a turban by wrapping a towel around the client's head. Pat or towel dry until the hair is free of excess moisture.

6 Change the client's gown and linens if they are wet.

7 Dry and style the client's hair.

8 Help the client to assume a comfortable position.

9 Remove all equipment and leave environment clean.

HINTS

- If hair dryer is used to dry hair, avoid the hot setting.
- Use electrical equipment only after shampoo trough and water have been removed.
- Special care should be taken with an African-American client's hair. It tangles easily, so after shampooing it should be combed while wet. Mineral oil or petroleum jelly can be applied if the hair seems dry. This will make braiding and styling easier.

HOME CARE CONSIDERATIONS

Cleansing sprays can be used for short-term use. However, the long-term care client will need to have the hair shampooed periodically. Obtaining a shampoo board may be the easiest option. However, the same can be accomplished by repositioning the client crosswise on a double bed with the head at the edge of the bed. Use plastic garbage bags to protect the bed and to fashion a drainage system to a pan sitting by the bed. Use a minimum amount of water.

lice infestation does not necessarily mean that they are unclean. Explain what must be done to treat the problem and prevent reinfestation. The person may need emotional support. If crab lice (pediculosis pubis) are found, emphasize the need for treatment of sexual partners to prevent reinfestation.

Shampooing the Client's Hair

Shampooing may be done in a variety of ways even if the client is confined to bed. Unless there are contraindications related to the medical condition, the client may be shampooed in bed, at the sink in a chair, or at the sink on a stretcher (see the Shampooing the Client in Bed procedure).

It is helpful to know how to improvise if the client is to be shampooed in bed or at the sink. The one item that is necessary is a "trough." This is an item that may be available in the hospital or home. If no plastic trough is available, you can easily make one from plastic and newspaper or from a rubber sheet and newspaper. Form a trough with raised edges, place the flat portion on the bed, and make a run-off channel that will drain into a waste receptacle.

Shaving the Client

Shaving is an important grooming measure for men. Most men shave daily and do not feel well groomed when facial stubble is present. If the client is unable to shave himself, determine his preferences for shaving soap, colognes, and aftershave lotions (see the procedure, Shaving the Client).

Interventions for Nail and Foot Care

Nail care is part of personal hygiene and usually includes trimming nails, cleaning under nails, and thoroughly rinsing and drying skin of the hands and feet, especially between the fingers and toes. Filing of nails may be safer than clipping or cutting. Some agencies do not permit you to clip the nails of clients. Families are required to provide a podiatrist for the client or one is supplied by the agency. Check agency policy in this regard. Clients with peripheral vascular disease or diabetes are particularly prone to injury and nail care must be done with extreme caution since even a minor cut or abrasion on the foot can lead to serious complications, even gangrene, with resultant amputation. The accompanying procedure describes the details of foot and nail care.

Problems with nail and foot care usually occur because of neglect or abuse. Improper trimming of nails and cuticles, frequent exposure to chemicals, trauma, ill-fitting shoes, and inadequate hygiene can cause problems. Be sure to trim fingernails with the finger tips and cut straight across to prevent the nails from breaking (Fig. 36–4).

Some general physical problems, such as diabetes, obesity, and peripheral vascular disease, make a person more prone to nail and foot problems. Poor circulation and altered metabolic function can lead to skin breakdown and infection and alter nail growth and

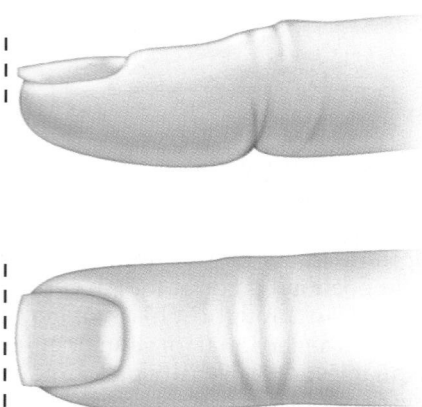

Figure 36–4. Fingernails should be trimmed, even the fingertips, and cut straight across to prevent the nails from breaking.

texture. Nails easily grow into soft tissue around them, causing pain, tissue trauma, and infection. Aging also brings about changes in the nails, and elderly people often have thick, discolored nails that must be trimmed by a podiatrist. Feet are more susceptible to trauma and prone to infection than other parts of the body. The dark, often moist environment of shoes promotes the growth of bacteria and enhances the chance of infection. Dirty socks or stockings and poorly ventilated shoes also create an environment that encourages bacterial and fungal growth (see the nail and foot care procedure).

Interventions for Ear Care

Unless the client has an ear infection, the ears require minimal care. The external auricles can be cleaned with a wash cloth, and excess cerumen can be removed with the tip of a wash cloth. Clients should be instructed to avoid insertion of objects such as Q-tips and bobby-pins to remove cerumen because they may cause trauma to the ear by traumatizing the ear canal or rupturing the tympanic membrane. The ear should be assessed for signs of inflammation, drainage, or external lesions and evidence of discomfort.

PROCEDURE 36–8

Shaving the Client

TIME TO
ALLOW
▼
Novice:
15 min.
Expert:
10 min.

Shaving the face is an important grooming measure for men. Most men shave daily and do not feel well groomed when facial stubble is present. Clients who are taking anticoagulants should use electric razors because of the prolonged clotting time.

Delegation Guidelines

The nursing assistant may be assigned to perform or assist with shaving your client. Special precautions may be necessary if the client has undergone a craniofacial procedure. It is your responsibility to assess the safety of shaving the client in this situation. You may choose to shave this client yourself.

Equipment Needed

- Safety razor or electric razor.
- Three towels.
- Soap or shaving cream.
- Aftershave lotion.

1 Prepare for the procedure.
a. Place the client in a sitting position, either in bed or in a chair.
b. If using a safety razor, apply a warm, wet towel to the client's face before beginning to shave.
   This softens the beard.
c. Apply a thick layer of soap or shaving cream to the client's face.

2 Shave with even strokes in the direction of hair growth.
This decreases irritation and prevents ingrown hairs. If the skin is not taut, use your opposite hand to hold the skin motionless while you shave.

3 Use a damp wash cloth to remove excess shaving cream. Inspect for areas that may have been missed. Apply aftershave lotion if desired.

4 Clean the area, make the client comfortable, and document your care.

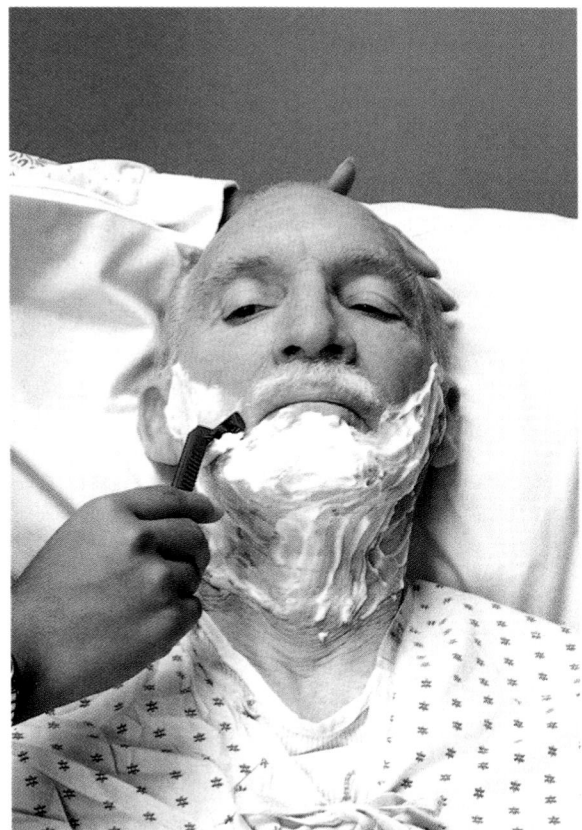

Shaving in the direction of hair growth.

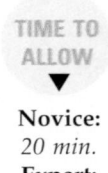

Performing Foot and Nail Care

TIME TO ALLOW
▼
Novice:
20 min.
Expert:
10 min.

Foot and nail care are given to clients to prevent infection and soft tissue trauma from ingrown or jagged nails and to eliminate odors. The elderly and the diabetic client are the most likely to need special attention to their feet.

Delegation Guidelines

Once you have assessed your client's feet you may choose to delegate routine foot care. Special consideration may be appropriate for your clients with diabetes or vascular insufficiency. You may deem it more appropriate to perform the nail maintenance part of foot care yourself in such cases because of the risk of injury if improperly performed by the nursing assistant.

Equipment Needed

- Nail clippers, file.
- Orange stick/cotton-tipped applicator.
- Waterproof pad.
- Wash cloth.
- Towels.
- Washbasin.
- Soap.
- Lotion.

1 Prepare for the procedure.
a. Wash your hands. Don gloves if necessary.
b. Help the client to sit in a chair if possible. If the client cannot sit in a chair, elevate the head of the bed.
c. Fill a basin half full of warm water (105°F).
d. Test the temperature with bath thermometer or by inserting your elbow.

Clients with impaired circulatory status can be burned if water is too hot. Peripheral sensations may be diminished so that pain is not felt.

e. Place a waterproof pad under the basin.

2 Place the client's foot or hand in the basin. Wash with soap and allow to soak for about 10 minutes.

Warm water serves to soften nails and skin, loosen debris under the nails, and comfort the client.

3 Rinse the foot or hand thoroughly with the wash cloth, remove from the basin, and place on a towel.

4 Dry the foot or hand thoroughly but gently, being especially careful to dry between the digits.

Moist skin between the digits tends to encourage maceration of tissue. Harsh rubbing may damage tissues.

5 Empty the basin, refill with warm water, and repeat with the other foot or hand.

6 While the second foot or hand is soaking, provide nail care for the first hand or foot.
a. Carefully clean under the nails with cotton-tipped applicator. Use an orange stick to remove debris. Push the cuticle back with the orange stick. Be careful to avoid injury to skin under the nail rim.
b. Beginning with the large toe or thumb, clip the nails straight across. Clip small sections at a time, starting with one edge and working across. File and shape each nail with an emery board or nail file.

Trimming nails straight across prevents splitting and the development of ingrown nails. Filing removes rough edges that might produce trauma and injury.

c. After completing the manicure or pedicure, apply lotion to the client's feet or hands. Powder may be dusted between the digits.
d. Repeat the procedure with the other hand and foot.

7 Help the client to a comfortable position, remove all equipment, wash your hands, and document care.

HOME CARE CONSIDERATIONS

Ongoing nail and foot care is especially important for the home care client. For problem feet, a clinical nurse specialist or a podiatrist may be consulted to develop a plan for care.

Interventions for Eye Care

Some clients are unable to maintain their own eye care for a variety of reasons. Those clients who have undergone surgery or who are critically ill or comatose may have lost the blink reflex, which serves to protect the eye from trauma. Assess the eyelids first. Are they encrusted with dried exudate? Are they edematous? Are they inflamed with styes or pustules? Are the lacrimal ducts functioning normally, neither too dry nor tearing excessively? Assess the sclera (white portion of the eye). It should be white, without redness or jaundice. The conjunctivae should be pink and moist and not reddened. Pupils should be equal, round, and reactive to light and accommodation, not constricted or dilated, and eye movements should be coordinated.

If the eyes are draining or if there is crusted exudate, the eyes must be gently cleaned with care to avoid transferring infection from one eye to the other.

Eyeglasses need to be cleaned at least once daily. Cleaning may be done with warm water and a mild soap. If the lenses are plastic, it is wise to clean them with an appropriate cleaning solution made especially for plastic lenses. Be careful in drying and wiping lenses, especially plastic lenses, because they scratch easily. Dry with a soft nonabrasive cloth or chamois skin. Eyeglasses should be labeled with client's name and put in a safe place.

Contact lenses come in two varieties: hard and soft lenses. Hard lenses are worn during waking hours and must be removed while sleeping. Some soft lenses may be worn for extended periods of time and may be worn while sleeping.

An unconscious client may require frequent eye care, as often as every 4 hours. Eyes must be kept clean, moist, and protected from the drying effects of the air. If the corneal reflex is lost or decreased, the eye has lost a vital protective mechanism. This reflex is the automatic closing of the eyes in response to a sudden movement of an object toward the eye. In the unconscious client, the eyes may remain open and become dried from the air. Dry eyes can lead to corneal ulceration and possible vision loss. It may be necessary to provide artificial tears or moisture through instillation of liquid tear solution or normal saline into the eyes or the conjunctival sac. If the eyes remain completely or partially open, it may be necessary to gently close them and cover them with a protective shield or patch.

EVALUATION

Evaluation of the achievement of self-care outcomes involves determining that the expected outcomes have been met. Safety is an essential outcome. Evaluate both the client and the environment for safety before you leave the room (Fig. 36–5).

The expected outcome for Mrs. Wilson's *Bathing/hygiene self-care deficit* is that Mrs. Wilson maintains a satisfactory appearance and that hygiene needs are met. Direct observation will allow

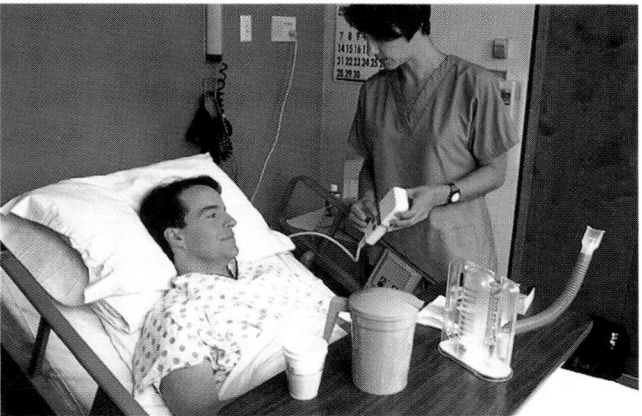

Figure 36–5. A minimum standard of safety is an accessible call light and the knowledge to use it.

you to infer a positive outcome. Mrs. Wilson is well-groomed and clean. Her skin and hair are clean and odor-free. The oral mucosa is intact with no signs of gingivitis or irritation. Subjectively, she indicates a feeling of comfort and well-being and demonstrates a positive feeling about herself as indicated in verbal interaction. The outcomes may include the following:

• Maintains skin clean and intact
• Maintains intact oral mucosa without gingivitis or caries
• Has clean hair without scalp lesions or abrasions
• States confidence in caregiver's ability to provide safe care at home
• Actively participates in physical therapy activities

If Mrs. Wilson does not have a self-care deficit/hygiene in a particular aspect of hygiene but one is likely to develop in the future because of aging changes compounded by residual deficits from her cerebrovascular accident, she and her daughter will need to learn how to manage the aspects of care that may change in the future. What outcomes might be appropriate?

In the example given, you have documented that the client has resolved difficulty with initiating and implementing oral hygiene, one aspect of the self-care regimen. As goals are met, new ones can be established so that the client can emerge from the experience not only with the resumption of previously acquired skills but with new goals. For Mrs. Wilson, new goals are to pay closer attention to oral hygiene and to pursue regular dental assessments that had not previously been done.

If the outcomes are not achieved or the client is not making sufficient progress toward achievement of the goals within the expected time, reassessment may reveal an explanation for lack of progress. For example, if Mrs. Wilson continues to have halitosis even after adequate brushing and rinsing, assessment for other causes of the odor is necessary.

Refer to the Nursing Care Planning chart for an example of the application of the nursing process to Mrs. Wilson.

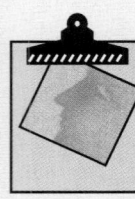

NURSING CARE PLANNING
A CLIENT WITH A STROKE

Admission Data

Mrs. Wilson was admitted to the unit from the Emergency Department. Her daughter and son-in-law accompanied her. She appeared slightly listless and lethargic and allowed her daughter to answer all the questions. Her daughter stated that when Mrs. Wilson awoke after an afternoon nap, she was slightly disoriented and nauseated and had marked left hemiplegia. Her physician advised immediate hospitalization and she was brought to the hospital in an ambulance.

Physician's Admission Orders

Admit to Neurology.
Dx: Cerebrovascular accident.
Regular diet.
Skull x-ray stat.
MRI in AM.

Vital signs QID.
Up in chair TID with assistance.
Physical therapy consult.
Tylenol Gr X PRN for headache.
Milk of magnesia 30 mL PRN constipation.

Nursing Assessment (6 Days After Admission)

Vital signs: BP 170/86, pulse 76, respirations 14, temperature 98.6°F. Skin moist and warm with good turgor. Appetite good but requires assistance with feeding because she is left-handed. Alert and oriented ×3. Responds appropriately to questions. Has some short-term memory deficit. Affect somewhat flat. Speaks in a monotone. Cries easily, especially when frustrated by inability to use left side. Speech clear; no slurring, hesitancy, or stammering. Bowel and bladder control intact; no incontinence. No difficulty swallowing.

NURSING CARE PLAN

Nursing Diagnosis	Expected Outcomes	Interventions	Evaluation (After 1 Week of Care)
Bathing/hygiene self-care deficit	Skin dry and clean	Bathe daily. *Encourage her to use right hand.* Prevent fatigue by allowing her to rest at intervals.	Used right hand to wash face. Asked for rest period after bath. Assisted with washing of upper body.
	Hair is clean and free of dandruff.	Shampoo every week.	Used right hand to brush hair. Asked for shampoo.
	Oral mucosa is clean; teeth and gums clean; no halitosis.	*Assist with brushing by putting paste on brush and guiding hand.*	Attempted to brush teeth without assistance.

Italicized interventions indicate culturally specific care.

Critical Thinking Questions

1. On day 2, Mrs. Wilson says, "Leave me alone. I am just too tired to bathe. I just want to rest." How would you respond?
2. Mrs. Wilson's daughter says that she wants to care for her mother at home, but she is unsure as to whether she can manage all the care. How would you advise her in regard to the availability of community resources and their accessibility?
3. On day 4, Mrs. Wilson was incontinent of urine for the first time since hospitalization. She says that she just "waited too long" because she knew the nurses were busy and she didn't "want to bother anyone." How would you respond to this comment?

KEY PRINCIPLES

- Self-care and hygiene are important to disease prevention and health promotion.
- *Self-care deficit* may be related to physical or mental factors or a combination of both.
- *Self-care deficit* usually includes both a deficit for bathing and one for dressing/grooming and toileting.
- *Self-care deficit* may be partial or total, requiring either total or assisted nursing care. Alterations in functional ability may occur suddenly or over time.
- Inability to bathe oneself, to dress and groom oneself, or to toilet oneself is validation of *Self-care deficit*.
- Interventions can meet the needs of the client for skin care, hair care, and oral care.
- Interventions can focus on prevention of complications from the inability to maintain adequate hygiene.
- Interventions can meet the needs of the client for positive self-image and self-concept.
- Interventions can meet the needs of the client for comfort.
- Evaluation of the achievement of self-care outcomes involves determining that the expected outcomes have been met.

BIBLIOGRAPHY

Adams, R. (1996). Qualified nurses lack adequate knowledge related to oral health, resulting in inadequate oral care of patients in medical wards. *Journal of Advanced Nursing, 24*(3), 552–560.

Anderson, M.A., & Helms, L.B. (1998). Extended care referral after hospital discharge. *Research in Nursing and Health, 21,* 385–394.

Anthony, D. (1996). The treatment of decubitus ulcers: A century of misinformation in the textbooks. *Journal of Advanced Nursing, 24*(2), 309–316.

Ayello, E.A. (1996). Keeping pressure ulcers in check. *Nursing '96, 26*(10), 62–63.

Baker F., Smith L., & Stead L. (1999). Washing a patient's hair in bed. *Nursing Times, 95*(5, Suppl.), 1–2.

Baker F., & Smith L. (1999). Giving a blanket bath—1. *Nursing Times, 95*(3, Suppl.), 1–2.

Blair, C.E., Lewis, R., Vieweg, V., & Tucker, R. (1996). Group and single-subject evaluation of a programme to promote self-care in elderly nursing home residents. *Journal of Advanced Nursing, 24*(6), 1207–1213.

Brubaker, B.H. (1996). Self-care in nursing home residents. *Journal of Gerontological Nursing, 22*(7), 22–29.

Carpenito, L.J. (1997). *Nursing diagnosis: Application to clinical practice.* Philadelphia: J.B. Lippincott.

Cirolia, B. (1996). Understanding edema: When fluid balance fails. *Nursing '96, 26*(2), 66–70.

Cox, H.C., Hinz, M.D., Lubno, M.A., Newfield, S.A., Ridenhour, N.A., Slater, M.M., & Sridaromount, K.L. (1997). *Clinical applications of nursing diagnosis: Adult, child, women's, psychiatric, gerontic, and home health considerations* (3rd ed.). Philadelphia: F.A. Davis.

Hardy, M.A. (1996). What can you do about your patient's dry skin? *Journal of Gerontological Nursing, 22*(5), 10–17.

*Harel, Z., McKinney, E.A., & Williams, M. (Eds.). (1990). *Black aged: Understanding diversity and service needs.* Newbury Park, CA: Sage.

Kirkevold, M. (1997). The role of nursing in the rehabilitation of acute stroke patients: Toward a unified theoretical perspective. *Advances in Nursing Science, 19*(4), 55–64.

North American Nursing Diagnosis Association. (1999). *NANDA nursing diagnoses: Definitions & classification, 1999–2000.* Philadelphia: Author.

Pearson, L.S. (1996). A comparison of the ability of foam swabs and toothbrushes to remove dental plaque: Implications for nursing practice. *Journal of Advanced Nursing, 23*(1), 62–69.

Senol M., & Fireman P. (1999). Body odor in dermatologic diagnosis. *Cutis, 63*(2), 107–111.

Skewes, S.M. (1996). Skin care rituals that do more harm than good. *American Journal of Nursing, 96*(10), 33–35.

Smith, S.F., Duell, D.J., & Martin, B.C. (1996). *Clinical nursing skills: Basic to advanced skills* (4th ed.). Stamford, CT: Appleton & Lange.

Whittle, H., & Goldenberg, D. (1996). Functional health status and instrumental activities of daily living performance in noninstitutionalized elderly people. *Journal of Advanced Nursing, 23*(2), 220–227.

---

*Asterisk indicates a classic or definitive work on this subject.

37

Physical Mobility

Donna D. Ignatavicius

Key Terms

flaccid	*PQRST model*
hemiparesis	*proprioception*
hemiplegia	*quadriparesis*
isometric exercise	*quadriplegia*
isotonic exercise	*range-of-motion exercises*
kyphosis	*spastic*
paraparesis	*synovium*
paraplegia	

LEARNING OBJECTIVES

After studying this chapter, you should be able to:

1. **Describe the concepts of the structure and function of the musculoskeletal system pertaining to mobility.**
2. **Discuss factors affecting mobility.**
3. **Describe the assessment of a client with impaired mobility.**
4. **Identify appropriate nursing diagnoses for clients with mobility problems.**
5. **Identify expected outcomes for permanent and temporary mobility problems.**
6. **Intervene to assist a client to restore or improve mobility.**
7. **Evaluate nursing care for the nursing diagnoses** *Impaired physical mobility* **and** *Activity intolerance.*

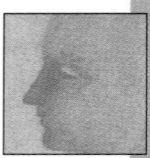

Kristina Lasauskas has been in an assisted living facility since her husband died 5 years ago. Last year she had a stroke, which left her weak on the right side. She ambulates independently with a cane. This morning her neighbor found her on the floor, and subsequent examination found that she had fractured her hip. She was admitted to the hospital for emergency surgery to repair the hip.

Following surgery, the nurse assesses her to identify nursing diagnoses and subsequent interventions. Because the client has previous right-sided weakness and has had surgery on her left hip, the nurse assesses for *Impaired physical mobility* and *Activity intolerance.* The nurse also expects the client to have *Pain.*

MOBILITY NURSING DIAGNOSES

Impaired Physical Mobility: A limitation in independent, purposeful physical movement of the body or of one of the extremities.

Activity Intolerance: A state in which an individual has insufficient physiological or psychological energy to endure or complete required or desired daily activities.

From North American Nursing Diagnosis Association. (1999). NANDA nursing diagnoses: Definitions and classification 1999–2000. Philadelphia: Author.

CONCEPTS OF PHYSICAL MOBILITY

No matter which health care setting you choose to practice in, you will care for clients with varying limitations in physical mobility. These limitations commonly result from musculoskeletal or neurological injury, disease, or surgery. However, any severe illness or injury may affect a client's physical mobility. For example, congestive heart failure can cause severe fatigue. Complications of long-term impaired mobility, regardless of cause, can lead to serious or life-threatening conditions, such as pneumonia. You will need to understand the structure and function of the musculoskeletal system to assist the client with problems associated with mobility.

Structure of the Musculoskeletal System

As a body system, the musculoskeletal system is second in size only to the integumentary system. It includes bones, joints, skeletal muscles, and other soft tissues.

Bones

Bone is a highly vascular and dynamic body tissue. Throughout childhood until puberty, bone tissue growth is influenced by many hormones and other substances in the body. Growth hormone, secreted by the anterior lobe of the pituitary gland, determines bone structure formed before puberty. As an adult, the parathyroid hormone, estrogens, and glucocorticoids work together to ensure a balance in calcium, phosphorus, and vitamin D. Over 99% of the body's calcium and 90% of the body's phosphorus are stored in a total of 206 bones.

From puberty through young adulthood, the amount of bone formation (osteoblastic activity) is greater than the amount of bone resorption, or destruction (osteoclastic activity). Beginning at about 35 years, osteoclastic activity becomes greater than osteoblastic activity. The resulting decreased bone mass predisposes middle-aged and older adults to bone injury.

Besides forming the skeletal framework for the body and storing vital minerals, bone assists in movement of joints and produces blood cells in its red marrow. Long bones that bear weight, such as the femur, manufacture more blood cells than short bones, such as the phalanges (fingers and toes). Some of the flat bones, especially the sternum and part of the pelvis, also contain blood-forming cells. These sites are commonly used for bone marrow aspiration and analysis to determine the body's ability to produce blood cells.

Joints

A joint is the point of articulation between two or more bones and usually allows voluntary movement. The most common type of joint is the freely movable synovial, or diarthrodial joint (Fig. 37–1). The surface of each bone end of a synovial joint is covered with articular cartilage and attached by ligaments. The **synovium** (synovial membrane) is the inner layer of the articular capsule surrounding a freely movable joint. It is loosely attached to the external fibrous capsule and it

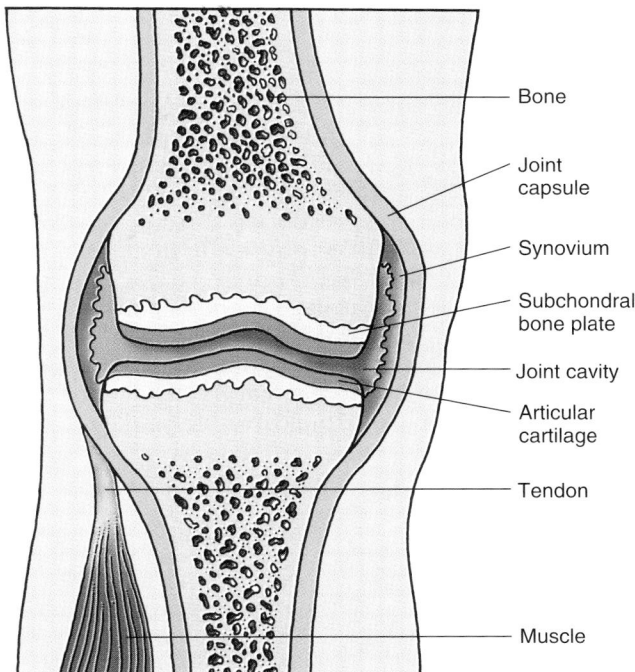

Figure 37–1. Structure of a synovial joint. (From Ignatavicius, D.D., Workman, M.L., & Mishler, M.A. [1999]. Medical-surgical nursing across the health care continuum [3rd ed.]. Philadelphia: W.B. Saunders.)

Bone
Joint capsule
Synovium
Subchondral bone plate
Joint cavity
Articular cartilage
Tendon
Muscle

secretes a thick fluid to lubricate the joint and absorb shock.

As adults age, deterioration of cartilage causes pain and possible inflammation. Arthritis, or joint inflammation and degeneration, results from "wear and tear" and can limit mobility.

Some joints are not movable. Joints in the adult skull, for example, are not movable. They are called synarthrodial joints. In the normal newborn infant, however, the cranial bones are separated by fibrous tissue (sutures) in which growth occurs.

Other joints are slightly movable and are called amphiarthrodial joints. Joints within the pelvis must be slightly movable to allow for childbirth. Joints between the ribs and sternum are slightly movable to allow the chest to expand with respiration.

Skeletal Muscles

Unlike the smooth, or nonstriated, muscles in organs and the muscle in the heart, skeletal muscles are voluntarily controlled by the central and peripheral nervous systems. Skeletal muscles are surrounded by dense, fibrous tissue called fascia. Small bundles of muscle tissue, blood vessels, and peripheral nerves make up compartments in the extremities, especially the distal part of each extremity.

During the aging process, muscle fibers decrease in size and number, even when the muscles are regularly exercised. Exercise helps keep the intact fibers from atrophy, which is a decrease in the size of a normally developed tissue or organ as a result of inactivity or diminished function. Muscle atrophy causes weakness that can limit physical mobility.

Soft Tissues

Adjacent fibrous tissues, such as tendons and ligaments, support skeletal muscles and bones. Tendons attach muscles to bone (Fig. 37–2); ligaments attach bones to bones at joints. Both of these soft tissue types are prone to injury, especially as a result of contact sports, such as football, or physically demanding activities, such as tennis and skiing.

In addition to the cartilage on bone ends of synovial joints, cartilage is located in the rib-sternum junctions (costal cartilage), nasal septum and trachea (hyaline cartilage), and external ear (yellow cartilage). Cartilage is flexible tissue but can withstand enormous tension.

Function of the Musculoskeletal System

Together with the nervous system, the musculoskeletal system enables us to move in a coordinated manner. Muscles are grouped according to the type of movement they allow. For example, *flexors* allow a joint or an extremity to flex or bend; *extensors* allow the joint or extremity to extend or straighten out. The elbow is an example of a synovial joint that can flex and extend. These movements are discussed later under range-of-motion (ROM) exercises.

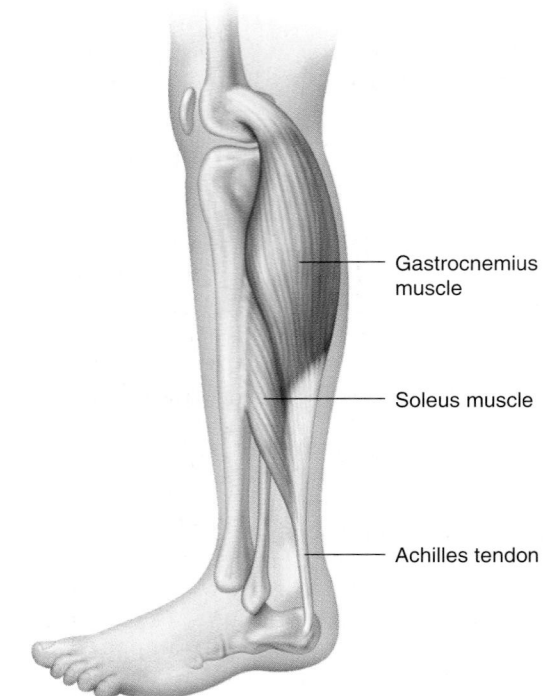

Figure 37–2. Tendons attach to muscles and bone.

Regulation of Movement

Movement is regulated by the central and peripheral nervous systems. The primary *motor area* (the motor "strip"), located in the frontal lobe of the cerebrum, is responsible for voluntary muscle contraction of muscle groups. Adjacent to the motor area is the *premotor area*, which directs new movements or movements that have been changed. Motor neurons and premotor neurons, also referred to as upper motor neurons, synapse with the corticospinal tract nerve fibers and descend into the spinal cord. At the level of the medulla, these fibers cross to the opposite side of the body. Therefore, the left motor area in the brain controls the right side of the body, and vice versa.

As the nerve fibers descend into the spinal cord, some synapse with peripheral nerves that supply the head, trunk, and limbs (lower motor neurons). Others synapse with interneurons in the cord. The peripheral nerves contain motor, sensory, and sometimes autonomic fibers. The motor fibers stimulate muscles to contract. Special chemicals called neurotransmitters, such as acetylcholine, facilitate muscle contraction. After muscle contraction, the muscle then relaxes because certain enzymes destroy the neurotransmitters after muscle contraction.

Proprioception

Proprioception is sensation pertaining to stimuli originating from within the body regarding spatial position and muscular activity or to the sensory receptors that they activate. It is our awareness of body position, posture, and movement. Small receptor cells in skeletal muscle, subcutaneous tissue, and the inner ear respond to stimuli within the body, like pressure or muscle stretch, promoting this awareness. For example, we know if we're standing or sitting, even if our eyes are closed. In a sense, proprioception is a protective function, enabling us to be aware of our bodies without actually seeing them.

Body Mechanics

Body mechanics describes the use of the body in movement and at rest. Improper use can cause fatigue and injury, such as back strain. Back injury among health care workers and others who perform physical activities is a common and costly health problem that commonly results from poor body mechanics. Health care workers must use proper body mechanics to prevent injury, maintain balance, and conserve energy.

COMPONENTS. The *center of gravity,* located within the pelvis, is the point where the body's mass is centered. The body maintains optimal balance and alignment when the *line of gravity* (an imaginary line) passes through the center of gravity. The base of support for the body includes the feet and the distance between the feet.

PRINCIPLES. While sitting, standing, or lying, the body can easily maintain alignment. However, when lifting, pushing, or pulling an object, the center and line of gravity shift, possibly causing poor body alignment and injury from loss of balance or stress on soft tissues.

Large muscle groups in the legs and arms should perform the work required to lift an object. As seen in Figure 37–3, the proper use of these muscles prevents back stress and strain. The back must remain straight during lifting, pulling, or pushing. Moving the feet farther apart broadens the base of support and keeps the body balanced during physical activity. Twisting the body should also be avoided. Pivoting on the ball of one foot keeps the back straight. Table 37–1 summarizes key principles of proper body mechanics.

Body Alignment

When the body is not moving, alignment is also important. When in a standing, sitting, or lying position, the body should be aligned so that the line of gravity passes through the center of gravity and work is done by the longer and stronger muscles. Poor positioning changes the center and line of gravity, causing muscle fatigue and stress. When sitting, standing, or walking, good posture allows the least amount of stress on muscles, joints, and soft tissues because the line of gravity passes perfectly through the center of gravity.

CHILDREN. When an infant sits, the thoracic spine appears curved or convex due to weak chest and truncal muscles. As the muscles strengthen and the child begins to walk, the back straightens. Normal toddlers and preschool children may actually appear to have an increased lumbar concavity because they have protuberant abdomens. Adolescents who grow quickly may slouch forward, producing a round-shouldered appearance.

ADULTS. Good posture for adults means that the head is held erect, the shoulders are back, and the vertebral column is held straight. Poor posture can result in back discomfort from excessive strain. As adults age, especially postmenopausal women, vertebral bone mass decreases and the thoracic spine becomes more convex, or curved.

GAIT. The manner in which we walk is referred to as gait. As a person ages, the long, smooth steps often shorten and become less steady. This change is particularly obvious for elderly women who have decreased vertebral bone mass. The normal, automatic gait has two phases—the stance phase and the swing phase (Fig. 37–4). The *stance phase* includes the heel strike through the push-off action of the first foot. An abnormality in the stance phase is called an antalgic gait. The *swing phase* includes the action of the second foot from acceleration through decelera-

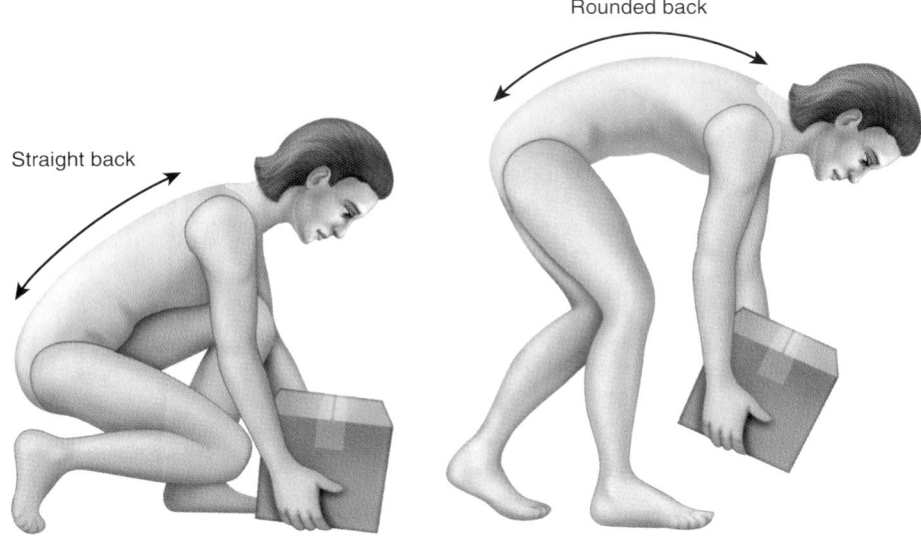

Figure 37–3. Lifting an object using proper (left) and improper (right) body mechanics.

TABLE 37-1
Principles and Benefits of Proper Body Mechanics

Principle	Benefit
• Pull, push, or roll objects rather than lifting them. • Pulling is usually easier than pushing, so pull clients toward you rather than pushing them.	Reduces the workload
• Lower the head of the bed to move a client up in bed.	Decreases opposition from gravity and decreases friction and shear
• Size up your load to determine whether you need help. • Keep your back straight when moving an object. • Use the longest and strongest muscles of your legs and arms rather than the weaker muscles of your back. • Rock your body to use the weight of your body to enhance the force of your arm muscles. • Move your body as a unit; avoid twisting, stretching, or reaching.	Prevents muscle strain
• Lower your center of gravity by bending your knees. • Widen your base of support by moving your feet apart. • Maintain your center of gravity (your pelvis) over your base of support. To support a client, stand close; carry an object close to your body.	Maintains stability

tion. An abnormality in this phase is called a lurch. Pain, muscle weakness, and limb shortening are common causes of abnormal gait.

FACTORS AFFECTING MOBILITY

Many factors can affect a person's mobility, including lifestyle, the environment, physical development, and pathophysiological conditions.

Lifestyle Factors

Some recreational activities place people at a high risk for injury to the musculoskeletal system. For example, physically demanding sports such as skiing, football, and tennis can result in fractures or soft tissue damage. Failure to adequately train or physically prepare for these activities contributes to injuries. Carelessness and taking unnecessary risks also cause accidents, which in some cases are fatal.

STANCE PHASE

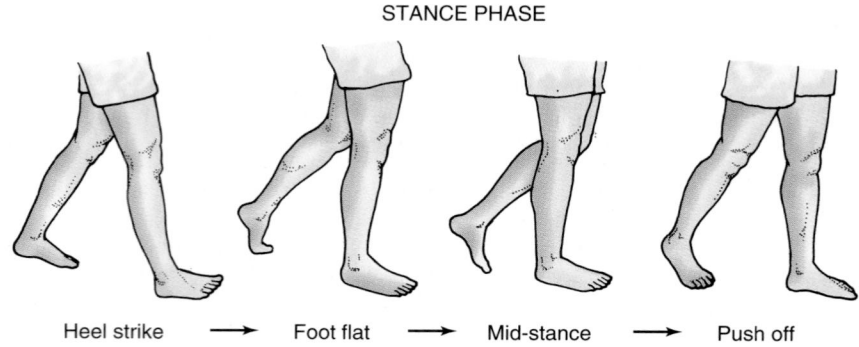

Heel strike   ⟶   Foot flat   ⟶   Mid-stance   ⟶   Push off

SWING PHASE

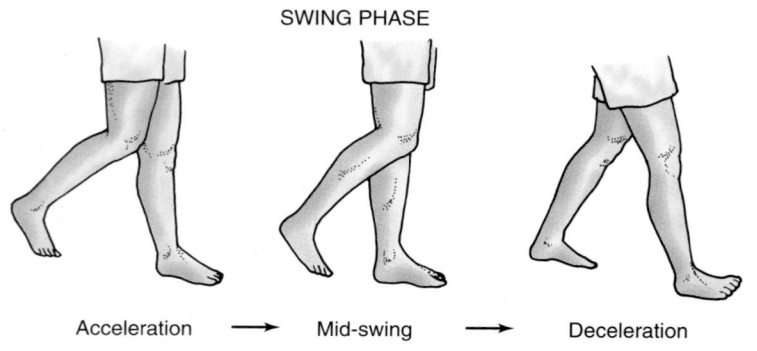

Acceleration   ⟶   Mid-swing   ⟶   Deceleration

Figure 37-4. Normal phases of gait. (From Ignatavicius, D.D., Workman, M.L., & Mishler, M.A. [1999]. Medical-surgical nursing across the health care continuum [3rd ed.]. Philadelphia: W.B. Saunders.)

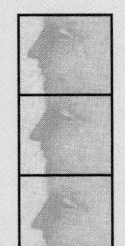

CROSS-CULTURAL CARE
CARING FOR A LITHUANIAN-AMERICAN WOMAN

Mrs. Lasauskas is a Lithuanian-American who came to the United States when she was 30 years old with her husband and two small children. The family lived with relatives in Boston, where her husband worked as a janitor while he learned English. He then received a position as a college professor. Kristina is a devout Catholic and has enjoyed being visited by the young priest from her parish. Her daughter lives nearby and visits her mother daily and sometimes brings the great-grandchildren to play games with "Nana." Although each person is an individual and customs vary, some Lithuanian-Americans may share the following values:

- Closeness among extended family.
- Religious beliefs and prayers (Roman Catholic).
- The importance of education.
- Hard work and industriousness.
- Thriftiness and good use of material resources.
- Endurance, persistence, and suffering with economic hardships.
- Charity to others.
- Helping in times of need.
- Hospitality to others.
- Sharing with others.
- Flexibility.
- Cooperation with others.
- Praying with others.
- Using subtle humor.

The nurse, Josephine, has the following conversation with Mrs. Lasauskas' daughter:

Josephine: Your mother doesn't seem motivated to try to do things for herself. I'm worried about her mood.

The daughter: Yes, I am too. Mother has always been so independent and her faith has been such an important part of her life. She wouldn't talk to the priest when he came yesterday.

Josephine: Do you know what's wrong?

The daughter: I think she's convinced that she won't walk again. And maybe she's right. All I know to do is be there for her. She was always there for us.

Josephine: Maybe we can get her to do some small things for herself to help her know that she's not completely helpless.

The daughter: That's a good idea. Let's try it.

Critical Thinking Questions

- Is the nurse's approach a good idea based on the description of cultural values?
- Why is the nurse trying to enlist the daughter's help to formulate a plan?
- How would you approach Mrs. Lasauskas?

Reference

Leininger, M.M. (1991). *Culture care diversity and universality: A theory of nursing.* New York: National League for Nursing Press.

Diet can affect mobility. For example, a diet that is low in calcium, protein, and other vital nutrients prevents bone growth and development in children and contributes to bone loss in older adults. The resulting "brittle" bones are prone to deformity and fracture. Regular exercise helps build strong bones and muscle tissue. Assess the client's cultural beliefs regarding diet and other lifestyle considerations to determine whether any factors might affect your client's mobility. The Cross-Cultural Care chart offers one example.

Environmental Factors

Environmental factors can lead to accidents or injury either in the workplace or at home. You can be instrumental in teaching clients about ways to prevent musculoskeletal injury.

Workplace

In the United States, the Occupational Safety and Health Administration (OSHA) establishes standards for workplace safety. The purpose of OSHA is to protect workers from injuries and accidents. The three major causes of worker injury are repetitive motion, poor body mechanics, and accidents.

When a worker performs the same activity repeatedly over a period of time, repetitive motion injuries can occur. For example, workers who use computers are at risk for carpal tunnel syndrome. The median nerve in the wrist becomes inflamed and entrapped, leading to pain, tingling, and decreased function of the hand. Preventive measures such as a wrist support bar on the keyboard and adjusting the height of the chair and computer station can help minimize the risk of carpal tunnel syndrome.

The use of poor body mechanics in the workplace can also cause musculoskeletal injury. Back supports are commonly required for workers who lift objects as part of their jobs. Classes on proper body mechanics, often provided by occupational health nurses, help workers protect themselves from back and other work-related injuries. Construction workers have the most back injuries of all employees; nurses are second in the number of job-related back injuries.

Accidents in the workplace can cause trauma and possibly lead to death. The workplace building and equipment should be safe and periodically inspected for continued safety. Most accidents can be prevented.

Home

Accidents from environmental hazards also occur in the home. Because OSHA has no jurisdiction in private residences, the homeowner must ensure that the home structure and equipment are safe. For the elderly, reducing environmental hazards is especially important for preventing falls (see Chapter 28).

Developmental Factors

Most age groups are at risk for decreased mobility, especially children, young adults, and older adults.

Children

Infants may be born with congenital musculoskeletal deformities that decrease their ability to crawl or walk. Abnormal fixed positions of the feet, such as metatarsus varus (pigeon toe), metatarsus valgus (duck walk, toeing out), and clubfoot (twisted foot), are deformities that can worsen and delay physical development if not corrected.

Congenital dysplasia of the hip is one of the most common musculoskeletal malformations. The femoral head is partially displaced from the pelvic acetabulum. If this condition is not diagnosed until after the child walks, the child will have a limp. If both hips are affected, the child will have a waddling gait.

A small number of infants are born without complete extremities, causing marked problems with learning to sit, crawl, and walk. If present, toes or fingers may be webbed, ultimately resulting in decreased function.

Congenital spinal deformities may also occur (Fig. 37–5). The most common is scoliosis, a lateral deviation of the spine that is typically diagnosed in preadolescent and adolescent children. If not corrected, this deformity can also affect the cardiopulmonary system.

Young Adults

The highest incidence of musculoskeletal injuries is among young men between ages 18 and 25. Young men often take risks, such as reckless driving without a seat belt or operating a motorcycle without a helmet. Alcohol or drug consumption increases the risk of these activities.

Older Adults

Aging typically results in muscle weakness and atrophy, decreased coordination and balance, and loss of bone tissue. These physiological changes decrease mobility but should not prevent the individual from independent function. Staying active and exercising help keep intact muscle fibers strong and promote coordination and balance.

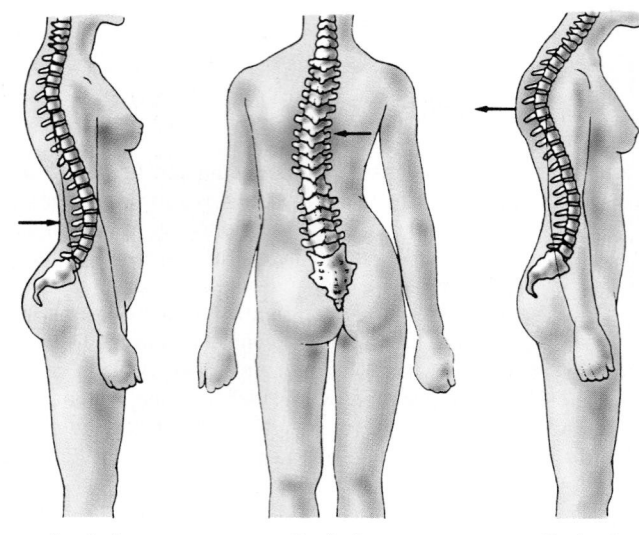

Lordosis   Scoliosis   Kyphosis

Figure 37–5. Common congenital spinal deformities. (From Ignatavicius, D.D., Workman, M.L., & Mishler, M.A. [1999]. Medical-surgical nursing across the health care continuum [3rd ed.]. Philadelphia: W.B. Saunders.)

As discussed earlier, after the age of 35, bone breakdown exceeds bone formation. After menopause in women, bone mass decreases (osteoporosis), possibly causing painful fractures of the wrist, vertebral column, and hip. Men have large amounts of testosterone that continue to build bone until about age 80. After 80, men also have a high risk of hip fractures. Measures to prevent or slow bone loss include calcium supplements, exercise, and precautions to prevent falls.

Physiological Factors

Many acute and chronic health problems can decrease mobility; this discussion is limited to common problems affecting the musculoskeletal and nervous systems.

Musculoskeletal Problems

Musculoskeletal health problems can be divided into inflammatory, degenerative, traumatic, and congenital problems. Rheumatoid arthritis is one of the most common inflammatory problems affecting people at any age and potentially causing joint deformity and chronic pain. This systemic disease also affects major body organs and must be treated aggressively to slow its progress. Degenerative joint disease, sometimes referred to as osteoarthritis, is an example of a degenerative process that is seen most typically in older adults, but also commonly affects athletes and obese individuals.

Trauma often results in bone fractures or dislocations and soft tissue damage. Fractures occur in any age group, but heal more readily in infants and young children. A young, healthy adult heals in 4 to 6 weeks; young children heal in 1 to 2 weeks, and older adults may take up to 3 months for bone healing.

Neurological Problems

Damage to the brain or spinal cord is a leading cause of immobility. Depending on the level of injury, the person will be weak (paresis) or paralyzed (plegia). When injured at the cerebral or cervical spine level, the client may experience **quadriplegia**—an abnormal condition characterized by paralysis of the arms, legs, and trunk below the level of an associated injury to the spinal cord. Or the client might experience **quadriparesis,** which is a numbness or other abnormal or impaired sensation in all four limbs and the trunk. Lower level spinal injuries result in **paraplegia**—paralysis characterized by motor or sensory loss in the legs and trunk. Or the client might experience **paraparesis,** which is a numbness or other abnormal or impaired sensation in the legs and trunk.

Middle-aged and older adults are at risk for degenerative or thrombotic neurological health problems. Parkinson's disease is a common degenerative, progressive process in which the client eventually becomes completely immobile. Cerebrovascular accidents (strokes) are the most costly disability. Part of the brain becomes damaged (infarcted) as a result of hypoxia due to a thrombus (stationary blood clot), embolus (dislodged blood clot), or hemorrhage. The typical client with a stroke has **hemiplegia**—paralysis of one side of the body, or **hemiparesis**—a numbness or other abnormal or impaired sensation experienced on only one side of the body and that limits mobility and activities of daily living (ADLs).

Recall the case study, in which Kristina Laskauskas had a previous stroke that left her with hemiparesis. What concerns should you have about her postoperative rehabilitation program? Might she be at risk for another stroke?

ASSESSMENT

General Assessment of Physical Mobility

Health problems that impair mobility may affect any body system. The intent of this section is to collect data related to the musculoskeletal system.

Health History

The health history elicits information about the client's chief complaint, risk of musculoskeletal health problem, previous or current treatment plan, and current condition.

CHIEF COMPLAINT

The most common complaints associated with musculoskeletal health problems are pain, muscle weakness, and inflammation. Pain may be acute or chronic, and may be assessed using the following **PQRST model:**

P What was the *provoking incident* that caused the pain, if any?
Q What is the *quality* of the pain? Is it burning, throbbing, stabbing?
R Where is the *region* of pain? Does it *radiate?* Does anything *relieve* the pain?
S How *severe* is the pain?
T What is the *timing* of the pain? When does it occur and how long does it last?

Also assess any history of muscle weakness or inflammation:

- Have you experienced muscle weakness or fatigue? If so, when does it occur?
- Do you find that you drop items or stumble at times when walking?
- Have you noticed any redness or excessive warmth around your joints or over muscles?
- Have you been unable to carry out any usual daily activity? Have you had to restrict some of your usual activities?

RISK FOR MUSCULOSKELETAL HEALTH PROBLEMS

Determine which factors place the client at risk for a musculoskeletal health problem, such as age, environment (both work and home), lifestyle, and personal and family history of musculoskeletal problems. Some health problems tend to recur. A complete history of previous problems and how they were managed could be very important in assisting with the diagnosis and management of the current condition, as suggested in the Considering the Alternatives chart.

Ask the client about treatments that she may have received or is receiving that could contribute to the current health problem, such as:

- Have you had any surgery? If so, what and when? (Previous surgery could cause nerve or muscle weakness.)
- What medications are you taking, both prescription and over-the-counter? (Some medications have side effects that cause weakness, lowered blood pressure, or muscle atrophy. Other medications may be given to prevent musculoskeletal problems, such as calcium and alendronate [Fosamax], to prevent or treat osteoporosis.)
- Are you currently under a physician's care? If so, what for and how is it being treated?

Physical Examination

The musculoskeletal physical examination includes assessment of body alignment, gait, joints, and skeletal muscles. For clients who experience musculoskeletal trauma or surgery, you frequently monitor neurovascular function as well.

BODY ALIGNMENT

If possible, observe the client's posture and positioning while sitting, lying, and standing. Assess for scoliosis and kyphosis. In scoliosis, the vertebral column deviates laterally. In children or adolescents, it may result from habit (functional), muscle weakness, contractures, or a tilted pelvis. Have the client bend forward at the waist. If the deviation disappears when the cli-

CONSIDERING THE ALTERNATIVES
CHIROPRACTIC

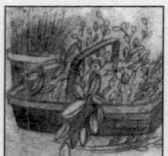 Chiropractic is a system of physical manipulation of the spine and other joints. Along with osteopathy (originally a similar system of physical adjustment), chiropractic grew out of the folk tradition of bone-setting, generally practiced by lay practitioners, some of whom became very well known for their abilities (Inglis, 1965). Chiropractic, from the Greek *cheir* (hand) and *praktikos* (practitioner), was developed as a therapeutic technique by Daniel Palmer in the late 1890s.

Chiropractic theory holds that "subluxations" in the spine, a form of structural abnormality, cause nerve irritation that in turn causes pain and can impede the function of organs related to those nerves. Subluxation as a concept is considered to be "the classic chiropractic lesion . . . some combination of structural abnormality and consequential alteration of function" (Plaugher & Lopes, 1993, pp. 5–6).

"Adjustments" made by a chiropractor are intended to correct the subluxation and thus alleviate the problem by restoring proper nerve function. There is debate within the chiropractic profession as to the exact definition of a subluxation. The medical profession has tended to denigrate the concept entirely. However, while subluxation may not be conclusively defined, research exists to substantiate the value of chiropractic treatment.

There is a common-sense aspect to chiropractic, that proper spinal alignment (and thus proper body alignment) will decrease stress and strain on muscles, connective tissues, and joints. Maintaining proper alignment allows for optimal nerve and circulatory function, enhancing overall health. In many respects, this idea parallels that of Chinese medicine's concept of *qi* circulation, the proper flow of which is said by adherents to be essential for health.

The history of chiropractic is remarkable for the virulence with which its practitioners were attacked by organized medicine. Palmer himself and thousands of others were prosecuted for practicing medicine without licenses. But so vigorous were the attacks on chiropractors that public sympathy was aroused. In California in 1922, chiropractic licensure was established by public referendum. This bill had been defeated in the prior election, but won after three quarters of the chiropractors in the state had been jailed (Inglis, 1965). Over the years, more and more states licensed chiropractors. Insurance began covering chiropractic care, and public acceptance and use of the practice increased dramatically.

Chiropractic care is now widely covered by insurance programs, including worker's compensation insurance. According to the Office of Alternative Medicine of the National Institutes of Health, "Chiropractic is the third-largest doctorate health care profession in the United States, with approximately 1 in 15 Americans seeing chiropractors yearly." Testament to the widespread interest in chiropractic, the Office of Alternative Medicine has established the Center for Chiropractic Research as its 11th research site ("Chiropractic Consortium," 1998).

Many chiropractors have long maintained their ability to treat a variety of organic and visceral disorders, as well as skeletal problems. Over time, visits to chiropractors for treatment of visceral disorders has declined (Plaugher & Lopes, 1993, p. 356). Nevertheless, interest in optimizing homeostatic function through achieving proper spinal alignment and nervous system function remains strong. This may be an important area where chiropractic treatment could complement other medical practices.

There are a number of types of chiropractic, and different schools emphasize different approaches and techniques. Some techniques focus on adjustment of the first cervical vertebra. Others advocate adjustment of the entire spine and pelvis as needed. Still others focus adjustments on the cranium and sacrum. The different styles also vary in terms of degree of force used in adjusting.

(continued)

ent bends forward, the problem is functional. If it does not disappear, the problem may require treatment.

Kyphosis is an abnormal condition of the vertebral column characterized by increased convexity in the thoracic spine when viewed from the side. It is common in middle-aged and elderly clients. The client's shoulders are slouched and the vertebral bones are very prominent. Check to ensure that this problem is not interfering with breathing.

GAIT
Observe the client while ambulating if the client can walk. Note the stance and swing phases, looking for limps or other abnormalities in gait. If the extremities are not the same lengths, the client will walk with a limp. Ask the client if she has a congenital abnormality or if surgery was performed on one or both extremities.

JOINTS
The best method for assessing joints is to use a head-to-toe approach, beginning with joints of the head and neck and progressing to the lower extremities. Inspect, palpate, and put through its range of motion every movable joint. Inspect the joints for proper alignment, symmetry, redness, and swelling. Then, palpate each

CONSIDERING THE ALTERNATIVES

CHIROPRACTIC (continued)

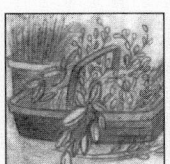

Chiropractors often use x-ray films to attempt to pinpoint problem areas in the spine.

Along with the growth of chiropractic has been a trend within the profession to increase its scientific basis. The quality of much of the research on chiropractic has not been good, and few controlled trials have been performed (Shekelle, 1994; Assendelft et al., 1996). However, a number of studies support the use of chiropractic. One study showed manipulative therapy to be slightly superior to physical therapy for persistent back and neck pain (Koes et al., 1992). Another, comparing treatment of acute low back pain by primary care physicians, orthopedists, and chiropractors, found the highest degree of satisfaction with chiropractic treatment, although recovery times were similar (Carey et al., 1995).

Yet another study published in the same year and following up on an earlier report confirmed that chiropractic treatment was more effective than outpatient hospital-based physical therapy for treatment of low back pain, with greater long-term benefit and better client satisfaction (Meade et al., 1995). Another 1995 study, based on RAND Foundation research, found that one-third of people with low back pain chose chiropractic care. It also found that chiropractors retained a greater percentage of people who sought care for subsequent painful episodes, indicating—again—greater satisfaction among users of chiropractic care (Shekelle, Markovich, & Louie, 1995). Nonetheless, the need for more scientific research on chiropractic is highlighted by certain chiropractors who make great claims not supported even by the literature they cite (McGregor, 1993).

The dramatic growth of the chiropractic profession, stimulated by the growing use of chiropractic care by the public, attests to chiropractic's efficacy as a health care modality. Further scientific evidence will not only support this use but allow better, and perhaps expanded, use of chiropractic care.

Resources

Publications that can expand and keep your knowledge of complementary and alternative medicine current:
Redwood, D. (Ed) (1997). *Contemporary chiropractic.* New York: Churchill Livingstone.

References

Assendelft, W.J., Koes, B.W., van der Heijden, G.J., & Bouter, L.M. (1996). The effectiveness of chiropractic for treatment of low back pain: An update and attempt at statistical pooling. *Journal of Manipulative and Physiological Therapeutics, 19,* 499–507.

Carey, T., Garrett, J., Jackman, A., McLaughlin, C., Fryer, J., Smucker, D. & the North Carolina Back Pain Project (1995). The outcomes and costs of care for acute low back pain among patients seen by primary care practitioners, chiropractors, and orthopedic surgeons. *New England Journal of Medicine, 333,* 913–917.

Chiropractic consortium becomes OAM's 11th research center. (Spring, 1998). *Complementary & Alternative Medicine at the NIH, V*(2), 3.

Inglis, B. (1965). *The case for unorthodox medicine.* New York: Putnam.

Koes, B.W., Bouter, L.M., van Mameren, H., Essers, A.H., Verstegen, G.M., Hofhuizen, D.M., Houben, J.P., & Knipschild, P.G. (1992). Randomised clinical trial of manipulative therapy and physiotherapy for persistent back and neck complaints: Results of one year follow up. *British Medical Journal, 304,* 601–605.

McGregor, M. (1993). Chiropractic magazines. *Journal of Manipulative and Physiological Therapeutics, 16,* 4–6.

Meade, T.W., Dyer, S., Browne, W., & Frank, A.O. (1995). Randomized comparison of chiropractic and hospital outpatient management for low back pain: Results from extended follow-up. *British Medical Journal, 311,* 349–351.

Plaugher, G., & Lopes, M. (Eds.) (1993). *Textbook of clinical chiropractic: A specific biomechanical approach.* Baltimore: Williams & Wilkins.

Shekelle, P.G. (1994). Spine update: Spinal manipulation. *Spine, 19,* 858–861.

Shekelle, P.G., Markovich, M., & Louie, R. (1995). Factors associated with choosing a chiropractor for episodes of back pain care. *Medical Care, 33,* 842–885.

joint for tenderness and masses. Finally, put each joint through its range of motion to determine function and listen for *crepitus,* a continuous grating sound caused by deterioration of the joint.

Assessing the extremities is particularly important because the client needs full use of these joints for performing ADLs. For example, the client who has shoulder limitations and pain may not be able to comb her hair. The client with hand deformities due to arthritis may have trouble cutting up food or opening food containers.

Ask the client to move each joint through its range of motion. The normal ROM for each joint is illustrated in Table 37–2. As long as the client can perform ADLs, a slight limitation of ROM is acceptable, especially for older adults.

SKELETAL MUSCLES

Skeletal muscles can be examined at the same time as joints. Observe each major muscle group for symmetry in size, shape, tone, and strength. Palpate the muscle and ask the client to demonstrate strength by squeezing your hand or a sphygmomanometer. The latter method provides a numerical score that can be used later for comparison. To check for movement against resistance, ask the client to move

Text continued on page 984

TABLE 37–2
Reviewing Range of Motion

Area of Body	Motion		Range (Degrees)
Neck	Flexion, extension, hyperextension		45 - 45 - 50
	Lateral flexion		40 - 40
	Rotation		70 to right, 70 to left
Shoulder	Flexion, extension, hyperextension		180, 180, up to 50
	Abduction, adduction	Abduction Adduction	180, 50 across midline

TABLE 37–2
Reviewing Range of Motion *Continued*

Area of Body	Motion		Range (Degrees)
	Circumduction		360
	External rotation, internal rotation		90 - 90
Elbow	Flexion, extension		160 - 160
	Rotation for supination, rotation for pronation		hand moves 180
Wrist	Flexion, extension, hyperextension		90 - 90 - 70

Table continued on following page

TABLE 37–2
Reviewing Range of Motion *Continued*

Area of Body	Motion		Range (Degrees)
	Ulnar flexion (adduction), radial flexion (abduction)		30 - 50—up to 30
Hand and fingers	Flexion, extension, hyperextension		90, 90, 15
	Abduction, adduction		spreads to 90
	Opposition of thumb		thumb touches each finger
Hip	Flexion, extension, hyperextension		90 to 120, 90 to 120, 30 to 50
	Abduction, adduction		30 to 50, 30 to 50

TABLE 37–2
Reviewing Range of Motion *Continued*

Area of Body	Motion		Range (Degrees)
	Circumduction		foot makes small circle
	External rotation, internal rotation		moves foot 90
Knee	Flexion, extension		120 - 130
Ankle	Extension, flexion		20 to 30 - 45 to 50
	Eversion, inversion		10 to 20 - 10 to 20

Table continued on following page

TABLE 37–2
Reviewing Range of Motion *Continued*

Area of Body	Motion		Range (Degrees)
Foot and toes	Flexion, extension		30 to 60, 30 to 60
	Abduction, adduction		15 or less, 15 or less

Flexion: bending at a joint in the natural direction of movement.
Extension: moving from the flexed position to a neutral or straight position.
Hyperextension: moving beyond a straight or neutral position.
Rotation: pivoting a body part on its axis.
Abduction: movement of a limb in a direction away from the midline of the body.
Adduction: movement of a limb in a direction toward the midline of the body.
Circumduction: a combination of movements that causes a body part to move in a circle.
External rotation: rotation from a joint in the direction away from the midline of the body.
Internal rotation: rotation from a joint in the direction toward the midline of the body.
Supination: rotation of the palm of the hand upward or in the anterior direction.
Pronation: rotation of the palm of the hand downward or in the posterior direction.
Opposition: the relationship of the thumb and fingers for the purpose of grasping objects.
Eversion: movement of the ankle to turn the sole of the foot laterally (away from the midline).
Inversion: movement of the ankle to turn the sole of the foot medially (toward the midline).
Dorsal flexion: flexion of the ankle in the direction of the dorsal surface.
Plantar flexion: flexion of the ankle in the direction of the plantar surface.

an extremity while you are trying to prevent that movement.

Physical and occupational therapists perform more detailed assessments of muscle strength using various scales. Table 37–3 describes Lovett's Scale for determining muscle strength. Using this scale, the therapist assesses each muscle and scores it as a rating out of a possible 5. For example, if a muscle is rated as a 3/5, the client has fair strength, can complete ROM, but cannot move against resistance. If available, review the client's muscle strength evaluation to help determine how much assistance you might need when getting the client out of bed or ambulating.

NEUROVASCULAR FUNCTION

In the extremities, especially the legs, sheaths of inelastic fascia (compartments) partition blood vessel, nerve, and muscle tissue. The pressure in the compartments is normally less than capillary pressure. External devices, such as casts and bulky dressings, can

compress the compartments, causing extensive tissue damage. Excessive tissue fluid from severe burns, insect bites, or infiltration of intravenous fluids can also increase compartmental pressure. If this pressure is not relieved, ischemic tissue necrosis can result in 4 to 8 hours, known as *compartment syndrome.*

Your major responsibility is frequent monitoring of neurovascular function, or CMS (circulation, movement, sensation) assessment. Check for skin color, temperature, movement, sensation, pulses, capillary refill, and pain. Always compare the affected limb with the unaffected one. Table 37–4 describes assessment of neurovascular assessment, including the normal, expected findings.

*A*ction *A*lert!
Increased pain on passive motion when compared with active motion, or loss of sensation in the web space between the great and second toes (or between the thumb and second finger on the hand), indicates early compartment syndrome. Notify the physician immediately!

TABLE 37–3
Lovett's Scale of Muscle Strength

Rating	Description
5	Normal: ROM unimpaired against gravity with full resistance
4	Good: Can complete ROM against gravity with some resistance
3	Fair: Can complete ROM against gravity
2	Poor: Can complete ROM with gravity eliminated
1	Trace: No joint motion and slight evidence of muscle contractility
0	Zero: No evidence of muscle contractility

ROM, range of motion.
From Ignatavicius, D.D., Workman, M.L., & Mishler, M.A. (Eds.). (1999). Medical-surgical nursing across the health care continuum (3rd ed.). Philadelphia: W.B. Saunders.

When the client is in late-stage compartment syndrome and damage is not reversible, the six "Ps" may be present, including the following:

- Pain not relieved
- Paresthesias
- Pallor
- Pulselessness
- Paralysis
- Palpated tense tissue

Do not wait until these signs and symptoms are present. The earlier that compartment syndrome is treated, the better the prognosis. Compartment syndrome may require amputation of the limb if the neurovascular compromise is not promptly assessed and managed.

Postoperatively, Mrs. Lasauskas has a physician's order to perform "CMS checks" every 4 hours. Why is this client at risk for neurovascular compromise?

Diagnostic Tests

Diagnostic tests are commonly performed to determine the nature and extent of musculoskeletal health problems that may interfere with mobility.

Radiographs, or x-rays, are used to detect bone density, swelling, alignment, and continuity. Joint structure can also be visualized, but soft tissues are not always clearly differentiated. Remind the client that she needs to remain still during the procedure, although the table may feel cold and hard.

The computed tomography (CT) scan provides a better picture of soft tissues and less dense bone than standard x-rays, especially of the vertebral column. It is also used to identify problems of the central nervous system, such as strokes and tumors. The test may be performed with or without use of a contrast medium to enhance the views. If a contrast medium is going to

TABLE 37–4
Assessing Neurovascular Status

Characteristic	Assessment Technique	Normal Findings
Skin color	Inspect the area distal to the injury.	No change in pigmentation compared with other parts of the body
Skin temperature	Palpate the area distal to the injury (the dorsum of the hands is most sensitive to temperature).	The skin is warm.
Movement	Ask the client to move the affected area or the area distal to the injury (active motion).	The client can move without discomfort.
	Move the area distal to the injury (passive motion).	No difference in comfort compared with active movement.
Sensation	Ask the client if numbness or tingling is present (paresthesia).	No numbness or tingling. No difference in sensation in the affected and unaffected extremities.
	Palpate with a safety pin or paper clip, especially the web space between the first and second toes or the web space between the thumb and forefinger.	Loss of sensation in these areas indicates perineal nerve or median nerve damage.
Pulses	Palpate the pulses distal to the injury.	Pulses are strong and easily palpated; no difference in the affected and unaffected extremities.
Capillary refill	Press the nail beds distal to the injury until blanching occurs (or the skin near the nail blanches if nails are thick and brittle).	Blood returns (return to usual color) within 3 seconds (5 seconds for elderly clients).
Pain	Ask the client about the location, nature, and frequency of pain.	Pain is usually localized and is often described as stabbing or throbbing.

From Ignatavicius, D.D., Workman, M.L., & Mishler, M.A. (Eds.) (1999). Medical-surgical nursing across the health care continuum (3rd ed.). Philadelphia: W.B. Saunders.

be used, check that the client has had nothing by mouth (NPO status) for at least 4 hours and that she is not allergic to iodine or seafood.

Magnetic resonance imaging (MRI) is often more accurate than either the standard x-ray or CT scan for detecting soft tissue damage. The image is produced by the interaction of radio waves and magnetic fields. Like the CT scan, a contrast medium may be used to enhance the view. Ask the client to remove any metal objects, such as clothing with metal fasteners. Metal joint implants are safe, but pacemakers are not.

An arthrogram is an enhanced x-ray of a joint following the injection of contrast medium. The test is performed most commonly on knees and shoulders. Ask the client about allergies to iodine and seafood. Instruct the client that joint swelling caused by the injection fluid will diminish within a day or two. If the joint injury is not severe, usual activities can typically be resumed within 12 to 24 hours.

A myelogram is an x-ray of the vertebral spine following injection of a contrast medium into the lumbar subarachnoid space. The spinal cord, vertebral bones, intervertebral disks, and surrounding soft tissues can be visualized. The client will be asked to take a fetal position or to sit and bend at the waist to open the lumbar intervertebral space before injection.

If a cervical myelogram is done, the client bends the neck forward. The injection site is locally anesthetized. After the contrast medium is injected, the client is moved into various positions while x-rays are taken. After the test, the client must be properly positioned to prevent cerebrospinal fluid leakage and subsequent headaches.

Action Alert!
The client must remain flat or in a semi-Fowler's position for at least 4 to 8 hours to prevent spinal headache or meningeal irritation. Check the injection site for cerebrospinal fluid leak. Also frequently monitor the level of consciousness, ability to move and feel the limbs, and ability to void spontaneously.

An arthrocentesis may be performed for diagnostic or treatment purposes. A sample of synovial fluid from the affected joint is withdrawn and sent to the laboratory for pathological analysis. Clients with rheumatoid arthritis usually have copious synovial fluid that contains antibodies and white blood cells that are characteristic of inflammatory disease. If the joint swells excessively, some of the fluid can be removed to alleviate discomfort. Instruct the client that this test is usually done in the physician's office, clinic, or bedside. The injection site is locally anesthetized before the larger aspirating needle is inserted. After the aspiration, apply pressure until fluid leakage subsides.

In a healthy person, calcium and phosphorus have an inverse relationship, meaning that when the serum calcium level decreases, phosphorus increases and vice versa. Bone disease and parathyroid dysfunction can cause alterations in this relationship.

Alkaline phosphatase is an enzyme that tends to increase when bone or the liver is damaged. Increases

in serum levels reflect an increase in osteoblastic (bone-building) activity.

When skeletal muscles are damaged or diseased, serum muscle enzymes typically increase, including skeletal muscle creatine kinase, lactate dehydrogenase, aspartate aminotransferase, and aldolase. Muscle trauma, polymyositis, and muscular dystrophy commonly cause increased serum muscle enzymes.

Focused Assessment for Impaired Physical Mobility

Nursing assessment includes interpreting data to help you select meaningful interventions. A client has *Impaired physical mobility* when she experiences limited ability to physically move. If the client has a prolonged impairment, complications of immobility that are potentially life-threatening may occur (see Chapter 38).

Defining Characteristics

Defining characteristics for the nursing diagnosis *Impaired physical mobility* include the following:

- Postural instability while performing ADLs
- Limited ability to perform gross or fine motor skills, uncoordinated or jerky movements, limited range of motion, or difficulty turning
- Decreased reaction time
- Slowed movement or movement-induced shortness of breath or tremor
- Gait changes (such as decreased walk speed, difficulty initiating gain, small steps, shuffles feet, exaggerated lateral postural sway)
- Substitutions for movement (such as increased attention to other's activity, controlling behavior, focus on pre-illness/disability activity)

A client's inability to move includes bed mobility, transfers from the bed to chair, and ambulation. Assessing a client's ability to move and perform ADLs is referred to as a *functional assessment.* Several functional assessment tools can be used to determine a client's functional level. A very simple classification system is often used to designate the functional status. This system rates the client's functional ability from a 0, completely independent, to a 4, dependent and does not participate in activity.

Some clients may be able to move but are reluctant to move because of pain or discomfort, fear of falling, or fear that they will dislodge or disrupt equipment that is being used in their care, such as intravenous therapy. Reassure the client that the pain can be controlled and should not be tolerated. If equipment and lines are the concern, secure them so they will not become dislodged, kink, or disconnect.

Diseases such as arthritis and trauma such as fractures limit ROM in synovial joints, which affects the client's ability to move and perform ADLs. ROM is also limited in clients with contractures.

Prolonged immobility can cause muscle atrophy that leads to further impairment in mobility. Neuro-

A PATIENT'S VIEW

MY RIGHT LEG WAS GONE . . . MY LEFT LEG AND ARM WERE SHREDDED BY SHRAPNEL . . .

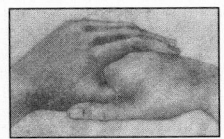 Growing up, I always went to church with my folks—you might say I cut my teeth on the back of a church pew—but I hadn't been a born-again believer until we were sailing toward Okinawa. I was 19 years old when the Navy shipped me out. As our commander explained, "You come back from this war in one or two ways: in a pine box or all shot up." Either way, I figured, it was time to put my trust in God, and I was right.

As a medic tending the wounded, I saw the ravages of World War II up close. One day I was treating three or four wounded men in a trench when an enemy mortar shell scored a direct hit. My right leg was gone; my left leg and arm were shredded by shrapnel, which also tore through my spine. If the shrapnel hadn't seared the arteries in my legs, I would have bled to death then and there. My first thought was, There go my dreams: college, a career in professional basketball, marriage, everything I'd hoped for. I was right about basketball but wrong about everything else.

The first year at home was the hardest, like a dark tunnel, wondering what the future had in store, wanting to be as independent as possible, so much to learn. Fortunately, I had nurses and therapists who took time to get to know me before prescribing just how I should achieve maximum independence. They listened. They understood my disability and the limits it imposed. They tried to get me to do as much as possible for myself but didn't push me too hard or too fast. You need to go at your own speed in learning about assisted living. Each person is different. I'm living proof that with the right care and therapy, the body can rebuild itself marvelously.

Once I was through with rehabilitation, I wanted to work but I couldn't get a job. No one wanted to hire people with handicaps; they wanted us out of sight. "We can't insure you," they said. So I just turned my life over to the Lord, and that made all the difference.

The beautiful black-haired girl I was engaged to still wanted to marry me, disabilities and all. We've been together 53 years now. She's the greatest thing that ever happened to me. With her love and support, I completed a 2-year business college course in accounting and worked as an accountant for a trucking company until 1948, when the poor circulation in my legs and my spinal problems made it impossible to work at a desk job.

From day one, the VA (Veterans Administration) system has done wonders for me, both in the hospital and out. Whatever I needed for assisted living—wheelchairs, prosthetic legs—they've provided. With the support of the VA, I designed my own house with everything on one level and totally accessible. The sidewalks are 48 inches wide so I can go outside, work in the garden, or do projects in my woodworking shop. I've made furniture, cabinets, you name it, I've made it.

Fifty years with a disability have taught me a lot. Probably the most important lesson is that attitude is everything. How you perceive and respond to your situation has a tremendous influence on your life—your physical, emotional, and spiritual well-being. I believe that God's good plan for our lives is never frustrated by the nature or magnitude of circumstances. Instead, our problems, painful as they might be, can actually contribute to vigor and life. We can allow our circumstances, with their fears, conflicts, and confusion, to control us or we can submit to the gracious and powerful sovereignty of God. It's our choice, and how we choose can make the difference between surmounting our problems and succumbing to them. I know I made the right choice for me and I've had a wonderful life: marriage to the woman I love, two sons, eight grandchildren, and, just last week, our first great grandson. Because I've been so blessed, I enjoy giving to others, especially people who are just learning to live with disabilities. Until 2 years ago, I did chaplaincy work in nursing homes and hospitals.

Now cancer is part of my life. I'm a survivor of bladder cancer, and, 2 years ago, I was diagnosed with kidney cancer. One kidney had to be removed and I have only about 30% function in the other kidney. When that fails, it's the end. Dialysis would be fatal because of the blood clots in my left leg. Recently, I learned I also have prostate cancer, but right now I'm feeling good and in no pain. The doctors can't understand why I'm still here, but I know it's just not my time. I think there's something left for me to do.

---

muscular diseases, such as Parkinson's disease, muscular dystrophy, and amyotrophic lateral sclerosis, are also characterized by muscle atrophy and subsequent decreased muscle strength. Clients with these disorders often experience respiratory failure because of muscle fatigue.

Spinal cord injuries disrupt nervous system communication between the brain and peripheral muscles. A cervical or high thoracic injury (quadriplegia) spares the lower motor neurons such that reflex activity remains intact. The skeletal muscles below the injury are **spastic,** that is, they contract by reflex activity rather than by central nervous system control.

Injuries that occur in the lower thoracic or lumbosacral spine may result in paraplegia. The lower motor neurons, or reflex arcs, are damaged and the client's muscles are **flaccid**—the state of being weak, soft, and flabby, lacking normal muscle tone, or having no ability to contract. Flaccid muscles tend to atrophy and decrease mass more quickly than spastic muscles.

Related Factors

Factors related to the diagnosis *Impaired physical mobility* include the following:

- Medications
- Prescribed movement restrictions or lack of knowledge about the value of physical activity
- Discomfort, intolerance to activity, reluctance to initiate movement, limited cardiovascular endurance, or decreased strength and endurance
- Body mass index above 75th age-appropriate percentile
- Sensoriperceptual, neuromuscular, or musculoskeletal impairments; cognitive impairment; pain
- Depression, anxiety, lack of physical or social environmental supports
- Decreased muscle strength, control, and/or mass; joint stiffness or contractures
- Sedentary lifestyle, disuse, or deconditioning
- Selective or generalized malnutrition, altered cellular metabolism
- Loss of integrity of bone structures
- Developmental delay
- Cultural beliefs regarding age-appropriate activity

Many chronic diseases, such as coronary artery disease, chronic respiratory disorders, terminal cancer, and neuromuscular diseases, can cause decreased muscle strength and endurance. Assess muscle strength using the Lovett scale or suggest a physical therapy evaluation to assess individual muscle groups. Consider the effect that fatigue could be having on your client, as discussed in the State of Nursing Science chart.

Acute or chronic pain may prevent a person from moving a part or all of the body. Assess the type, nature, duration, and location of pain as discussed in Chapter 42. Repositioning the client, providing massage, or enhancing imagery may help relieve pain and promote mobility. For more severe pain, administer a prescribed analgesic and evaluate its effectiveness.

*A*ction *A*lert!
For clients who cannot verbalize complaints of pain, especially the elderly who have dementia or delirium, use nonverbal cues to assess their pain level, such as moaning, crying, or restlessness. Anticipate the need for pain relief interventions, including medication.

Neuromuscular or musculoskeletal impairments may be acute and reversible or chronic and disabling. In addition to the chronic spinal cord injuries, stroke, and neuromuscular diseases described earlier, clients may experience acute problems that temporarily decrease mobility. Fractures or other soft tissue injuries are common examples of acute musculoskeletal impairments. When these injuries heal, the client usually returns to baseline activity level.

Clients with late-stage dementia, as in Alzheimer's disease, experience *Impaired physical mobility* and usually die as a result of complications of immobility. The client forgets how to perform ADLs and how to ambulate.

In the case study, Mrs. Lasauskas had been living independently in an assisted living residence. Why might you expect her to be confused immediately after surgery? Did surgery cause her to become demented?

Focused Assessment for Activity Intolerance

Activity intolerance results when a client has insufficient physiological or psychological energy to endure or complete a desired activity. It is evidenced when the client reports fatigue or weakness, experiences abnormal vital signs or electrocardiographic (ECG) changes, or has exertional discomfort or dyspnea during or after the activity. If a client has *Activity intolerance*, health care professionals tend to document that the client did not "tolerate" the activity. If the client was able to tolerate the activity without the fatigue or abnormal vital signs and ECG changes, the documentation is usually summarized as "tolerated well."

*A*ction *A*lert!
The term "tolerated well" is a vague judgment. If you are absolutely sure that the client has no fatigue or weakness, and experiences no abnormal vital signs or ECG changes during an activity, then you can use the term.

Defining Characteristics

Before you ask a client to perform any activity, ask if she is tired or weak. Fatigue or weakness can result from a number of causes, including pain, hypoxia, fluid and electrolyte imbalances, and decreased muscle tone and strength. If she is willing to perform or participate in the activity, observe the client for increased fatigue or weakness and discontinue the activity if necessary.

Monitor the client's vital signs and observe for ECG changes for clients in monitored beds. Clients with coronary artery disease or respiratory disease are particularly likely to experience changes in heart rate or ECG recording while performing ADLs or following a physical therapy plan of care.

Clients experiencing pain may have increased discomfort during activity. Evaluate the change in the client's pain level and discontinue the activity if indicated. Clients with respiratory or coronary artery disease may experience exertional dyspnea during activity. Assess the client before, during, and after the activity for changes in breathing pattern or rate.

Related Factors

Prolonged immobility due to chronic disease or severe injury leads to generalized weakness and subsequent

THE STATE OF NURSING SCIENCE
HOW CLIENTS EXPERIENCE FATIGUE

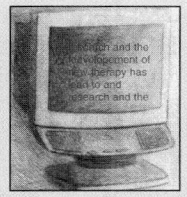

What Are the Issues?

Fatigue is a common symptom. It can be a component of many chronic illnesses, as well as a side effect of treatment. Because nurses are responsible for helping to manage fatigue, and because fatigue is a subjective experience, it is important for nurses to understand more about it. How does it present itself? How does it change over time? What is the individual variation in the experience of fatigue? Are there other symptoms associated with but different from fatigue? How does fatigue change as the illness or treatment changes? What do clients do when they feel fatigued?

What Research Has Been Conducted?

To begin to address these sorts of questions, Messias and colleagues (1997) analyzed information collected from relatively healthy outpatients undergoing chemotherapy who were part of another study. A benefit of this approach was that the detailed and spontaneous descriptions of fatigue provided by clients in response to open-ended questions meant that fatigue was important to them. On the other hand, this research method did not allow the researchers to ask specific questions or to use quantitative tools for measuring fatigue. Researchers had to depend on the information originally collected.

Varvaro and colleagues (1996) used several measurement tools to study the type, degree, patterns, and management of fatigue in women who had experienced myocardial infarction. They also examined the relationships between fatigue and measures of well-being.

What Has the Research Concluded?

These studies found that although fatigue is a common experience in clients undergoing chemotherapy and recovering from acute myocardial infarction, it is a very individualized experience for each client. Among those studied, clients chose many different words to describe their experience, and those word choices may have reflected subtle differences in the degree of fatigue experienced by each client. For example, words used by the people undergoing chemotherapy in the study by Messias and colleagues (1997) included *tired*, *worn out*, *slumpish*, *wiped out*, and *drained*. The clients described

such states as affecting their general well-being and body image, attributing the fatigue to their disease and treatment.

Clients described their emotional reactions to the experience of fatigue in negative terms. In general, the experience was disabling. The strategies that subjects used to cope with fatigue included rest, pacing their activities, and adjusting expectations.

In the study by Varvaro and colleagues (1996), the women studied (most of whom were interviewed in the sixth week of recovery from myocardial infarction) reported fatigue lasting weeks or months that was generalized and moderate. To cope with the fatigue, these women primarily rested and paced their activities. Among these women, the researchers found significant relationships between levels of fatigue and measures of well-being.

What Is the Future of Research in This Area?

Nurses are interested in finding ways to help people cope with their illnesses and treatments. The frequency of fatigue as a client experience therefore warrants additional attention. The use of measurement tools that take into account the range of individual experience may help capture the differences among individuals, as well as changes in the experience over time. Ideally, such research would include assessment of fatigue levels prior to the beginning of treatment.

Research is also needed to test the effectiveness of interventions to relieve fatigue, as well as to determine the effects of preparing people for the experience. To prepare people for the experience, researchers would also need to gather data on changes in role function of clients and family members in response to fatigue, as well as the response of employers to the often chronic nature of fatigue for clients with cancer and following myocardial infarction.

References

Messias, D.K., Yeager, K.A., Dibble, S.L., & Dodd, M.J. (1997). Patients' perspectives of fatigue while undergoing chemotherapy. *Oncology Nursing Forum, 24,* 43–48.
Varvaro, F.F., Sereika, S.M., Zullo, T.G., & Robertson, R.J. (1996). Fatigue in women with myocardial infarction. *Health Care for Women International, 17,* 593–602.

Activity intolerance. These clients need to be out of bed and moved as much as possible. Assess changes in muscle tone and joint ROM.

All body tissues require oxygen. When an oxygen deficit occurs or the demand for oxygen exceeds available oxygen, fatigue develops and vital signs change. If the oxygen deficit is severe, ECG changes can occur. For clients with cardiovascular or respiratory problems, use a pulse oximeter to check for oxygen saturation before, during, and after activity. Arterial blood gases provide additional information about the partial pressure of arterial oxygen (see Chapter 39).

Focused Assessment for Related Nursing Diagnoses

Clients with *Impaired physical mobility* and *Activity intolerance* often have additional nursing diagnoses. Assess the client comprehensively.

Clients who cannot bathe, dress, groom, toilet, or feed themselves have one or more self-care deficits. The nursing diagnosis *Self-care deficit* may be appropriate for these clients. Clients experiencing neurological, neuromuscular, or musculoskeletal health problems are often unable to move and therefore cannot perform ADLs independently. Perform functional assessments periodically to determine the client's progress in achieving independence, if possible. Do your best to consider each client's situation with an open mind, no matter how difficult her circumstances.

Clients who cannot move are at a high risk for pressure ulcers, especially over bony prominences, and the nursing diagnosis *Risk for impaired skin integrity* may apply. Thin, emaciated, and poorly nourished clients are at the highest risk of any group. Assess the skin for reddened areas. Assess nutritional status, especially laboratory indicators such as serum albumin, pre-albumin, and transferrin. When these indicators are decreased, the client has inadequate protein stores to prevent or heal tissue breakdown.

Mrs. Lasauskas is a petite woman, weighing 102 pounds. What preventive measures should you use for Mrs. Lasauskas to help prevent skin breakdown after her surgery?

Exercise, hydration, and fiber are necessary to prevent *Constipation*. Clients who are immobile cannot exercise and often have an inadequate intake of food and water. Assess intake, especially fiber content. Elderly clients are particularly prone to decreased peristalsis and constipation. Monitor bowel habits and the consistency of stools.

The inactive client is at risk for deterioration of all body systems, sometimes referred to as disuse syndrome or complications of immobility. For these clients, the diagnosis *Risk for disuse syndrome* may apply. Assess every body system for possible complications or risk of complications. Chapter 38 discusses disuse syndrome in detail.

The client with *Impaired physical mobility* is at *Risk for injury* from falls and fractures as a result of osteoporosis. Anemia often contributes to the risk. Additionally, the person is at risk for thromboembolic complications.

As described earlier, clients with musculoskeletal trauma or conditions that increase peripheral compartment pressure are at high risk for neurovascular compromise, and the nursing diagnosis *Risk for peripheral neurovascular dysfunction* may apply. Monitor clients frequently for this potentially lethal complication.

Musculoskeletal injury, surgery, or disease can be very painful, so you will need to assess acute pain in a client with injury or surgery, such as a fracture or surgery to repair a fracture. For these clients, the nursing diagnosis *Pain* may apply. Clients with such chronic joint diseases as degenerative or rheumatoid arthritis experience chronic pain, which is often difficult to control. For these clients, the diagnosis *Chronic pain* may apply.

Clients who have chronic musculoskeletal, neuromuscular, or neurological health problems may feel hopeless when they are unable to move or care for themselves. They depend on others for care and often feel like they are a burden to their families and significant others. This sense of hopelessness can result in clinical depression or suicide. Assess the client's response to illness and identify clients at risk for *Hopelessness*.

DIAGNOSIS

When you care for a client with musculoskeletal, neuromuscular, or neurological problems, analyze the assessment data to identify the common nursing diagnoses that will guide your care. If clients are at risk for any of the diagnoses, add "Risk for" at the beginning of the diagnosis; for example, *Risk for activity intolerance*.

Also identify the related factors for actual nursing diagnoses and the risk factors for potential diagnoses. For instance, clients with back injury have *Pain related to muscle spasms*. But they may also be at *Risk for impaired physical mobility* related to pain, depending on how severe the back injury is.

Clients who have had a stroke usually have an actual nursing diagnosis of *Impaired physical mobility* related to hemiparesis or hemiplegia, but are at *Risk for activity intolerance* related to generalized weakness. The related factors or risk factors help guide nursing interventions.

Adolescents who have suffered a spinal cord injury have *Impaired physical mobility*. However, they may also have *Hopelessness, Self-care deficit, Risk for injury, Risk for impaired skin integrity,* and *Risk for disuse syndrome*.

The accompanying chart shows examples of clustering data to arrive at appropriate nursing diagnoses.

PLANNING

Once the nursing diagnoses have been determined, think about what outcomes can be expected for the client. To the extent possible, outcomes should be individualized, measurable, and realistic. For the client with *Impaired physical mobility,* the overall goal is to improve mobility and prevent complications of immobility. For the client who has *Activity intolerance,* the goal is to improve endurance and tolerance to activities.

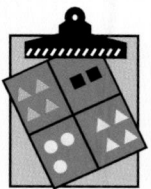

CLUSTERING DATA TO MAKE A NURSING DIAGNOSIS
MOBILITY PROBLEMS

Data Cluster	Diagnosis
An elderly woman who fell, resulting in a fractured hip; history of previous stroke with hemiparesis; cries out when moved; degenerative arthritis in both knees	*Impaired physical mobility* related to muscle weakness, severe pain, and joint degeneration
A 12-year-old girl with rheumatoid arthritis; uses a walker to ambulate short distances but relies on wheelchair most of the time; becomes very fatigued when walking; takes two to three naps each day	*Activity intolerance* related to generalized weakness and fatigue
An elderly woman with acute vertebral compression fractures; complains of severe pain when moved; heart rate 120 and weak, blood pressure 180/90	*Pain* related to muscle spasm and nerve impairment

Expected Outcomes for the Client With Impaired Physical Mobility

Improvement in mobility depends on several factors. First, try to determine whether the mobility deficit is permanent or temporary. A severed spinal cord results in permanent paralysis below the level of injury. Therefore, expecting the client to walk is not likely. However, expecting the client to be able to ambulate in a wheelchair may be very realistic. The client with a total knee replacement is expected to walk with a walker or cane within a few days after surgery. The client's physical mobility impairment is temporary.

Second, look at the causes or related factors that could be managed or resolved. For example, if the client cannot move because of pain and discomfort, then interventions directed at pain relief should improve physical mobility.

Third, assess the client's willingness to participate in the treatment plan. If exercises are expected to increase muscle strength and endurance, the client has to be willing and able to exercise as prescribed.

The outcomes that might be expected for the client with a permanent impairment in mobility may include the following:

- Ambulates independently in a wheelchair
- Transfers independently from the bed to chair and vice versa using a sliding board
- Performs ADLs independently using assistive or adaptive devices
- Maintains intact skin, especially over bony prominences
- Drinks at least 2,000 mL of fluid per day to prevent constipation and renal or urinary calculi
- Demonstrates passive and active ROM exercise techniques.

Possible expected outcomes for a client with a temporary or less severe impairment in mobility may include the following:

- Ambulates independently in home using a walker, crutches, or cane
- Maintains optimal joint function
- Performs ADLs independently
- States that pain is reduced or relieved.

Each of these long-term outcomes can be broken into progressive stages. For example, for the postoperative client with a total knee replacement, a realistic intermediate outcome is that the client is expected to walk in the hospital room using a walker. By discharge from the rehabilitation program several weeks later, the client is expected to walk up and down stairs using the walker or cane.

Expected Outcomes for the Client With Activity Intolerance

The major expected outcome for *Activity intolerance* is that the client tolerates activity without evidence of fatigue or weakness, abnormal vital signs, ECG changes, or exertional discomfort or dyspnea.

INTERVENTION

Interventions to promote mobility and improve activity intolerance are inter-related. Mobility skills cannot improve unless the client can tolerate the interventions that are directed toward building tolerance. Therefore, interventions for *Activity intolerance* are discussed first.

You will collaborate with members of the interdisciplinary team, including rehabilitation nurses, physical therapists (PT), occupational therapists (OT), and physicians, when planning and implementing these interventions. The rehabilitation team is discussed in Chapter 56.

Regardless of whether your client is treated by a PT or OT, you are still responsible for carrying out interventions that help the client achieve the health care team's expected outcomes.

Interventions to Improve Activity Tolerance

Interventions for improving activity tolerance center around building muscle mass and strength while managing other causes of activity intolerance, such as pain and discomfort.

Building Muscle Mass and Strength

A structured, consistent exercise program is started as soon as the client is medically stable. Several types of exercise may be used to build muscle mass and strength, including isometric, isotonic, and isokinetic exercises.

Isometric exercise (Fig. 37–6A) is a form of active exercise that increases muscle tension by applying pressure against stable resistance. Isometric contractions can be accomplished by opposing different muscles in the same person. There is no joint movement and the length of the muscle remains unchanged, but the tone and strength are maintained or increased. They are also called static or setting exercises. Ask the client to tighten certain muscle groups without moving the adjacent joints. These exercises are particularly helpful for strengthening leg, hip, and abdominal muscles. Clients who have lower extremity musculoskeletal surgery, such as hip and knee replacements, are taught how to do "quad setting" exercises. Ask the client to tighten the quadriceps muscles and hold for a few seconds. Then repeat this exercise about 10 times in a set at least twice a day.

Isometric exercises also have the advantage of increasing heart rate and cardiac output, but blood flow to other parts of the body is not increased. In addition, these exercises are not helpful in preventing contractures because joints do not move.

Isotonic exercise (Fig. 37–6B) is a form of active exercise in which the muscle contracts and moves. There is no significant change in the resistance, so the force of the contraction remains constant. Isotonic exercise has the advantage of increasing cardiopulmonary function and blood flow, preventing contractures, and building muscle mass and strength. These dynamic exercises involve muscle contraction and shortening of muscle. Examples of isotonic exercises performed in a hospital are straight leg raises following hip or knee surgery. Swimming, walking, and cycling are also examples of isotonic exercises that can be done by the client independently to continue the physical conditioning of muscles. These exercises are sometimes referred to as *isokinetic* (Fig. 37–6C) because they are dynamic exercises performed at a constant velocity.

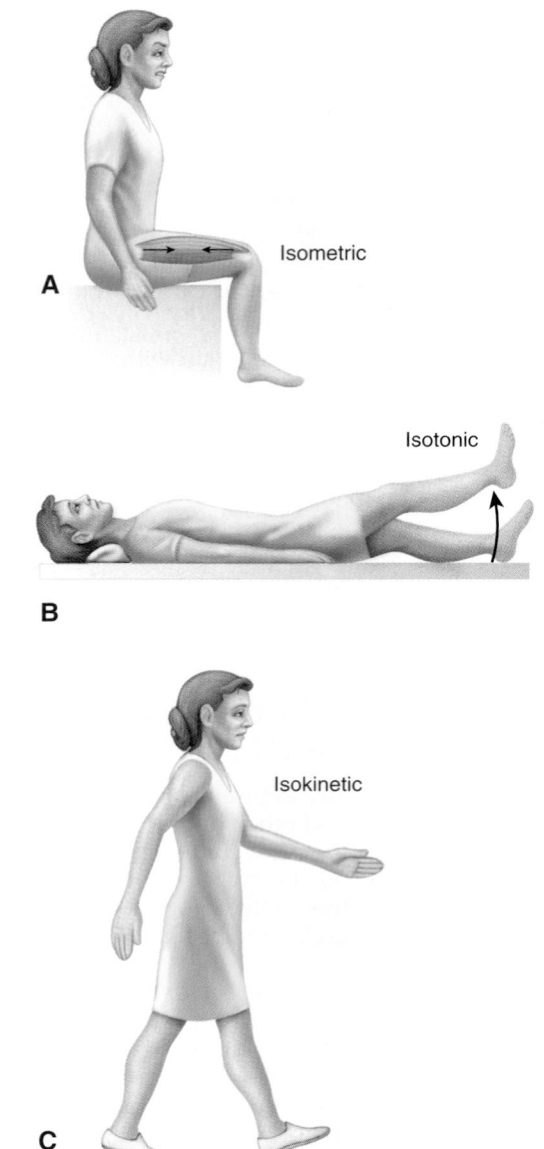

Figure 37–6. Three types of exercise: A, isometric; B, isotonic; C, isokinetic.

Mobilizing the Client Progressively

When a client experiences an acute musculoskeletal or neurological health problem, recovery may be gradual. Being confined to bed for more than a day can cause generalized weakness. Anesthesia during surgery also causes weakness and fatigue, sometimes for several weeks after surgery. Infections and other illnesses also deplete the client's energy.

Therefore, you will want to slowly build the client's activity tolerance level. For instance, before the client gets out of bed for the first time, you will want her to sit on the bed with legs dangling on the side. The client may be able to tolerate only this simple activity the first time. Once the client can tolerate dangling, help the client transfer from the bed to the chair. Each time the client gets out of bed, increase the activity, so that eventually the client can walk a few steps.

Action Alert!
Monitor the client for vital sign changes, fatigue, and exertional discomfort or dyspnea before, during, and after each activity. If the client's heart is monitored, look for ECG changes. Discontinue the activity immediately if any of these changes occur and notify the physician.

Controlling Pain and Discomfort

If the client is experiencing pain before, during, or after the activity, she will most likely be reluctant to increase activity level or even perform the same activity again. Before the client gets out of bed or goes for therapy, administer pain medication or provide other appropriate pain relief measures. Check with your physical therapy department, however, because heavy sedation could prevent client participation in the treatment plan. In some instances, physical therapists do not want clients to have medication because pain is used as an indicator that the client needs to discontinue treatment for that session.

Interventions to Promote Mobility

You and the therapist are responsible for promoting mobility, including ADLs. The goal is that the client will be independent at home or at another facility to which the client will be transferred. Maintaining or improving joint mobility helps with transfer and ambulation skills.

Maintaining Joint Mobility

Range-of-motion exercises include any body action (active or passive) involving the muscles, joints, and natural directional movements, such as abduction, extension, flexion, pronation, and rotation. They are the most important interventions to promote and maintain joint mobility. ROM exercises are isotonic exercises in which the client or health care provider moves each synovial joint through its complete range of motion (see Table 37–2). When the client can perform the exercises, they are termed active. When you or the physical therapist performs the exercises on the client's joints, they are termed passive. These exercises also prevent contractures and help build activity tolerance.

If the client can move, teach her how to perform active ROM exercises. The client can move each joint through its range of motion several times a day independently. If the client cannot move or exercise her own joints, perform passive ROM exercises for each joint as described in Procedure 37–1. If the client can assist you, the ROM exercises are called active-assistive.

Action Alert!
When putting a joint through its range of motion, follow these important guidelines:

Position the bed at an appropriate height to maintain good body mechanics.

Support the limb being moved above and below the joint.
Do not force the joint into any position.
Move the body part smoothly and slowly, observing the client for discomfort.

Assisting With Movement

If the client is strong enough, teach her how to get out of bed independently, as described in the Teaching for Self-Care chart.

Transferring the Client

If the client cannot transfer independently, you will need to assist. Always remember to use good body mechanics (discussed earlier) and size up your load. If the client cannot help with the transfer, use at least two people to move her. If the client is obese or has multiple pieces of equipment, seek help with the transfer as well.

TRANSFERRING FROM BED TO CHAIR
A client may need assistance transferring from the bed to a regular chair, wheelchair, or bedside commode. Transfer belts provide extra security and the safest way to perform a transfer. Procedure 37–2 describes how to help a client from a bed to a chair with or without a transfer belt. This procedure assumes that the client is strong enough to help you with the transfer.

For clients who are totally immobile and unable to assist with the transfer, two people are needed, as described in Procedure 37–3. One nurse lifts the upper portion of the body while the other lifts the legs and hips. Be sure to lock the brakes on both the bed and wheelchair before the client is transferred. Also, position the client in the chair in proper alignment using pillows and bath blankets for support. Be sure that the client's feet are supported by the foot rests and that all necessary items are within reach, including the call light.

Another option for transferring an immobile client is using a mechanical, hydraulic lift. Although designed to be used by one person, you will need an assistant for safety. The lift requires a one- or two-piece sling that is placed under the client. The sling is hooked into the lift device and the client is moved into position over a chair before lowering. As seen in Procedure 37–4, the sling remains under the client at all times.

The physician wants Mrs. Lasauskas out of bed in a chair on the first full postoperative day. Given her weakness, hemiparesis, and pain, what transfer technique would you use? How many people should be used to transfer her?

TRANSFERRING FROM BED TO STRETCHER
Transferring a client from the bed to a stretcher requires at least two people. Transfers are easiest when a turning sheet or drawsheet is placed under the client. First, adjust the height of the client's bed to be even with the height of the stretcher. Ensure that the wheels on both the bed and stretcher are locked. Then

Text continued on page 1001

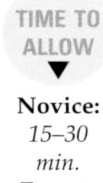

PROCEDURE 37–1

Performing Range-of-Motion Exercises

TIME TO ALLOW
▼
Novice: 15–30 min.
Expert: 15–30 min.

Range-of-motion (ROM) exercises are performed to maintain joint flexibility and movement in the client who is unable to move or is confined to bed. It has the added benefit of stimulating circulation and relaxing the body. It may be full ROM, which includes all the joints, or ROM for selected joints. Range of motion will not maintain or improve strength. You need to be familiar with the normal range of motion for each joint.

Delegation Guidelines

Following your assessment of your client's functional status and joint mobility, you may delegate the performance of range of motion exercises to a nursing assistant who has received special training in the performance of this skill. Provide special instructions outlining those ob-servations and findings that should be brought to your immediate attention.

Equipment Needed

- Bath blanket to cover the body other than the part being exercised.
- Pillows for positioning.

1 Explain the procedure to the client and assess the client's ability to assist with the exercises.

If the client can assist or can perform the exercises independently, active-assistive or active ROM can be performed rather than passive ROM.

2 If moving the joints of the entire body through their range of motion, use a head-to-toe approach (see Table 37–2).

This approach helps to organize the intervention so that all joints are moved through their range of motion.

3 Support the client's body part by cradling or cupping above and below the joint being moved.

Supporting the joint prevents injury and stress on the joint and also promotes client comfort.

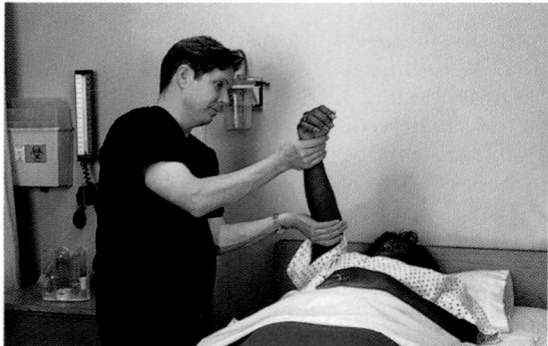

Supporting the body part above and below the joint being moved.

4 Put the joint through its complete ROM, but do not force it beyond where it will move comfortably.

Complete ROM of each joint is more beneficial in preventing contractures and building muscle tone.

5 Throughout the exercises, observe the client for tolerance, including pulse rate and discomfort, if any. Do not exercise to the point of producing pain.

If the client cannot tolerate the exercises, discontinue them immediately.

1. Use slow, smooth movements.
2. Move joint only to the point where you feel resistance. Stop if you reach the point of pain.
3. Assess for fatigue.
4. Finish with the joint in good alignment.
5. Check physician's instructions about the number of sets and repetitions. A typical protocol is four sets daily, with five repetitions for each joint.

ROM exercises should be taught to family caregivers as part of the routine care for a client who has mobility limitations. The family may need help to make ROM part of all activities rather than trying to make room in a crowded schedule for several ROM sessions.

Teaching for SELF-CARE

GETTING OUT OF BED INDEPENDENTLY

Purpose: To promote client independence in transfer skills

Rationale: Promoting independence in mobility increases self-esteem and maintains muscle tone and endurance.

Expected Outcome: The client will transfer from bed to chair independently.

Client Instructions

1. If you have an electric bed, put the bed in its lowest position.
2. Raise the head of the bed.
3. Turn onto your side. (If you're stronger on one side than the other, turn toward the stronger side.)
4. Push against the mattress with either your elbows or hands to raise your upper body off the bed.

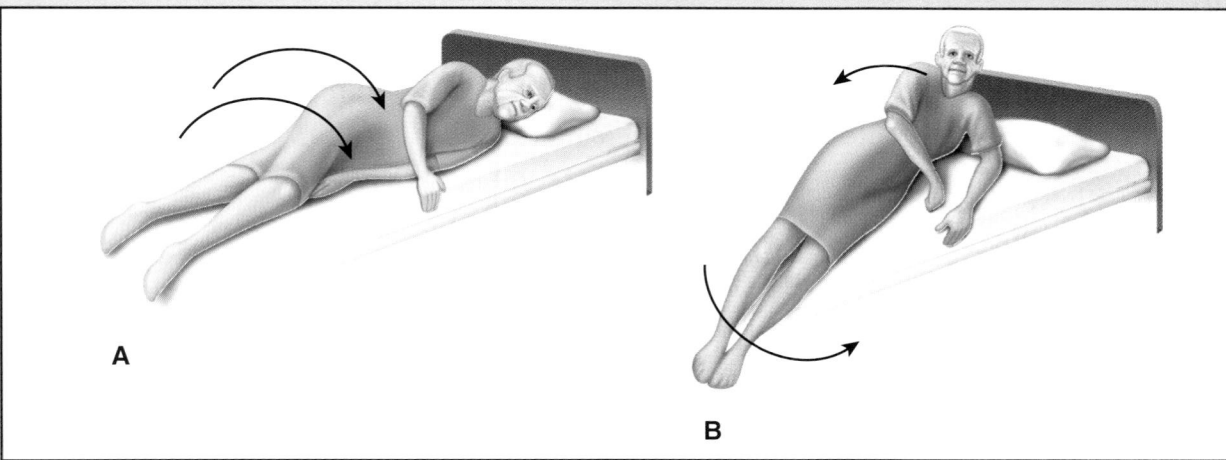

A

B

5. Once you're in a sitting position, let your legs dangle for a moment over the side of the bed. This will help you get your balance and make sure you aren't dizzy.
6. If you aren't dizzy, go ahead and stand up.

Hint: If the client is too weak to push up from the bed, set up an overhead frame and trapeze for the client to pull on. Clients with lower-extremity trauma or surgery, including amputations, especially benefit from this device.

PROCEDURE 37–2

Helping a Client Get Out of Bed

TIME TO
ALLOW
▼
Novice:
15 min.
Expert:
10 min.

You can help a client get out of bed with or without a transfer belt. A transfer belt is a woven canvas belt about 2½ to 3 inches wide and 6 feet long. It is fastened around the client's waist and secured with a locking device. The belt is used to maintain control of the client when you help her stand, transfer to a chair, or walk. Transferring with a belt is safer and avoids pulling on the arm and shoulder joints.

Delegation Guidelines

Once you have assessed the client's ability to stand safely, you may delegate assistance with bed-to-chair transfer to the nursing assistant. The nursing assistant should receive specific instruction in body mechanics and safety concerns related to patient mobility. Instruct the nursing assistant to report any client complaints of dizzi- *ness or observation of unsteady gait or imbalance to you.*

Equipment Needed

- Transfer belt.
- Supportive shoes with rubber soles.
- A bathrobe.

Without a Transfer Belt

1 Place the bed in its lowest position and raise the head of the bed.

Having the bed in the lowest position is safest in case the client falls. The client can sit up more easily if the head of the bed is up.

2 Place a chair or wheelchair at a 45-degree angle to the bed. Plan for the client to get out of bed on her strongest side.

Having the client get out of bed on the strong side helps prevent loss of balance and possible falls.

3 Using good body mechanics, help the client to a full sitting position while swinging the client's legs over the edge of the bed in a single, smooth motion. Support the client's upper body as she comes to the sitting position.

Moving the client's legs reduces friction or shearing from the sheets while increasing the force of the movement. Supporting the client's upper body keeps her from falling backward.

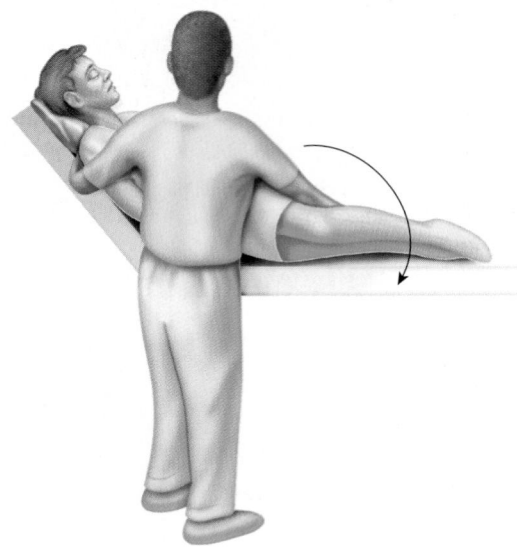

Assisting the client to a full sitting position.

4 Support the client in a sitting position on the side of the bed with her feet dangling.

Moving from a lying to sitting position can cause postural hypotension, which can lead to dizziness and a subsequent fall unless the client has time to gather equilibrium.

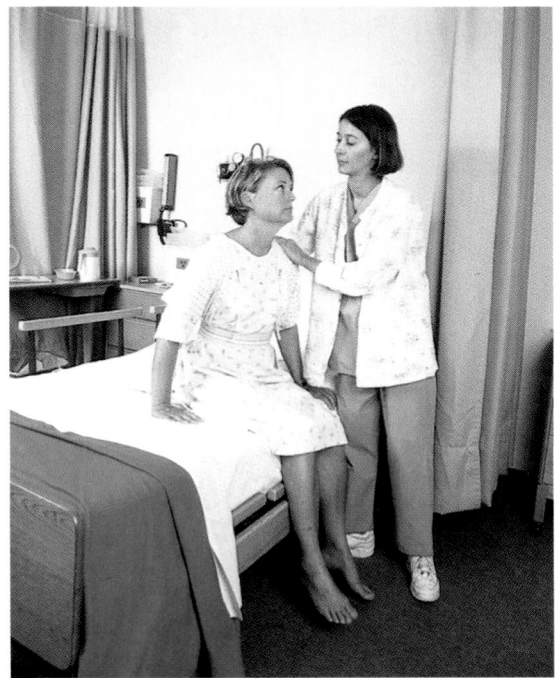

Supporting the client in a sitting position.

5 If she is able, have the client place her hands on your shoulders or on the mattress on either side of her body.

When you help the client stand, she can assist you by balancing against your shoulders while using the leg muscles to stand or by pushing off the mattress with the hands.

6 Place your hands under the client's arms. Place your knees in front of the client's knees and help her rise to a standing position.

Keeping your knees against the client's knees prevents them from buckling, thus reducing the risk of a fall. Avoid axillary pressure.

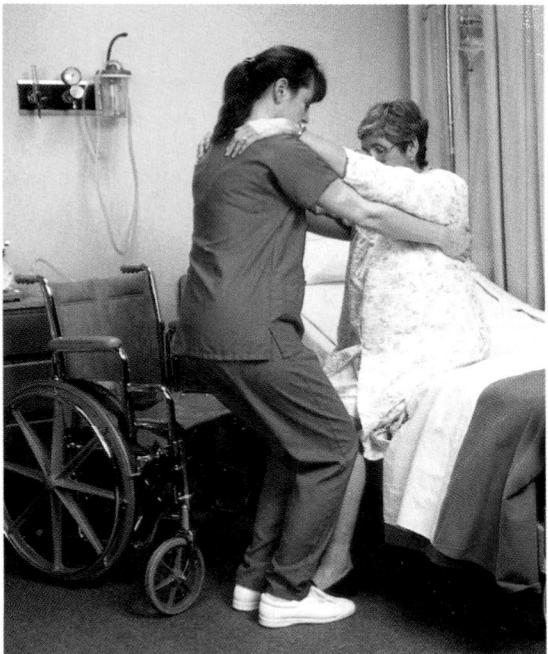

Helping the client to a standing position.

7 Pivot with the client toward the chair or wheelchair, being careful not to dislodge equipment or lines.

Pivoting prevents twisting your spine and causing injury.

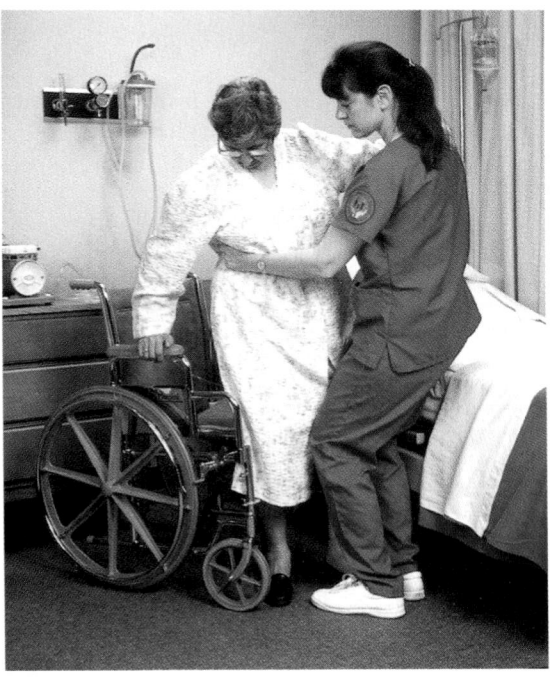

Pivoting and turning the client toward the wheelchair.

Continued

PROCEDURE 37–2 *(continued)*

Helping a Client Get Out of Bed

8 Using good body mechanics, lower the client into the chair or wheelchair slowly and reposition her in proper body alignment. Make her as comfortable as possible.

Moving slowly helps prevent dizziness or other discomfort.

With a Transfer Belt

1 Place a transfer/gait belt around the client's waist.

The transfer belt allows you to guide the client and offer support during the transfer.

2 Standing in front of the client, grasp the transfer belt on both sides of the client toward the back. Assess whether the client has the strength to stand. When the client is ready, help her to a standing position by rolling your body and arms upward, pulling the client with the transfer belt.

Favoring the client's weaker side helps prevent falls because most clients drift toward or lose balance on their weaker side.

3 Pivot the client toward the chair and lower her slowly into it. Ideally, the client will take two or three small steps to get into position to sit.

Pivoting prevents twisting of your spine.

4 Have the client reach for the armrests, if available, while lowering into the chair.

Holding onto the armrests provides additional support for the client.

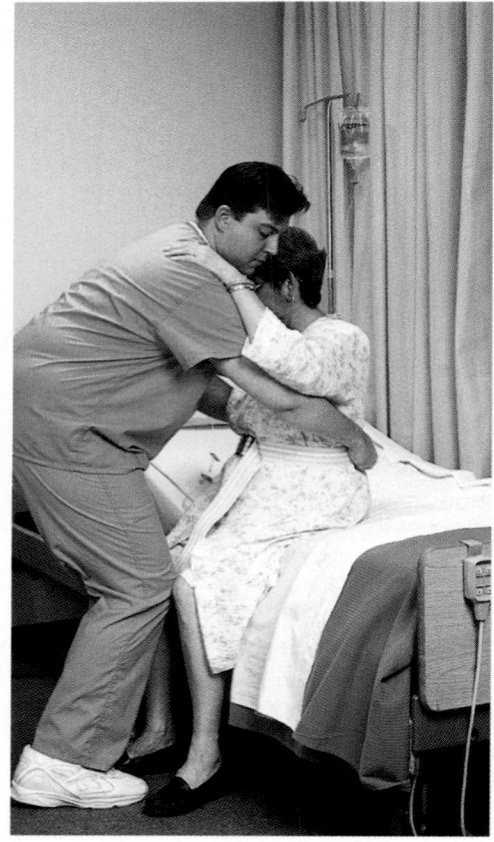

Grasping the transfer belt to assist the client to a standing position.

HOME CARE CONSIDERATIONS

Teach family caregivers how to use good body mechanics to prevent back injuries when transferring the client. Most caregivers can be easily taught how to use a transfer belt. If the family cannot transfer the client to a chair, they can rent a mechanical lift or a geriatric chair. The chair reclines and the feet can be elevated. It also has a tray that fastens on the front for meals and other activities.

PROCEDURE 37-3

Transferring an Immobile Client From Bed to Wheelchair

TIME TO
ALLOW
▼
Novice:
15 min.
Expert:
10 min.

An immobile client who cannot bear weight on her feet and legs can be moved to a wheelchair using a two- or three-person lift.

Delegation Guidelines

The transfer of an immobile client from bed to wheelchair, and back to bed, may be delegated to a nursing assistant who has received training in body mechanics and safety techniques. Two nursing assistants, having received this training, may perform this task without you present.

Equipment Needed

* Wheelchair with locking wheels, removable armrest, and movable leg and feet supports.
* Bath blanket to cover the chair and wrap around the client's shoulders.

1 Obtain an assistant before transferring the client.
At least two people are needed to lift an immobile client to prevent back injury and maintain the client's safety. Assess the client's weight and make sure you can lift that weight safely.

2 Place the chair parallel to the bed before transferring the client.
A parallel position makes the transfer into the chair easier.

3 Pull the bed out from the wall, if necessary, so one nurse can get behind the client's shoulders and upper body from the other side of the bed. Meanwhile, you will be lifting the client's hips and legs.

4 In unison and using good body mechanics, you and your colleague should lift the client's shoulders and legs.
This technique distributes the weight among two people and, therefore, prevents injury. A turning sheet will make the lifting easier.

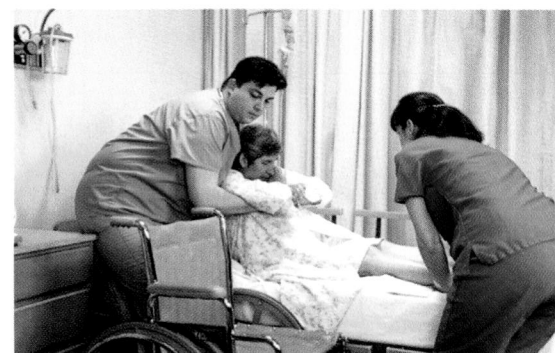
Lifting the client from the shoulders and legs.

5 Lower the client into the chair and position her in good body alignment using pillows and other devices as needed.
Proper body alignment promotes optimal function and prevents discomfort.

HOME CARE CONSIDERATIONS

Consider the age and physical condition of the caregiver before teaching this transfer technique. If no strong males are present in the home, help the caregiver arrange for assistance with transfers. As an alternative, consider a mechanical lift.

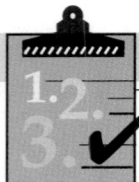

PROCEDURE 37–4

Using a Mechanical Lift

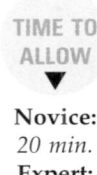

TIME TO
ALLOW
▼
Novice:
20 min.
Expert:
15 min.

A mechanical lift uses a hydraulic pump or electric motor to hoist a sling. With the sling around the client, the lift can raise the client off the bed and swing her into position above a chair. The lift is then lowered and the client is slowly rolled into the chair. Possible disadvantages of a mechanical lift are the insecurity the client feels while suspended in the air and the training required to properly use the lift.

Delegation Guidelines

The use of a mechanical lift for client transfer may be delegated to a nursing assistant who has received training in body mechanics, safety, and the use of this piece of equipment. You should place special emphasis on the client's perception of the experience of being suspended in the air as well as protection of the skin from injury when

reviewing the key aspects of this skill with your assistant.

Equipment Needed
- Mechanical lift.
- Bedside chair or wheelchair.
- Bath blanket.

1 Obtain a functioning lift and move it into the client's room.

Make sure that the lift works correctly and safely to prevent accidents. Practice before you take it into the client's room.

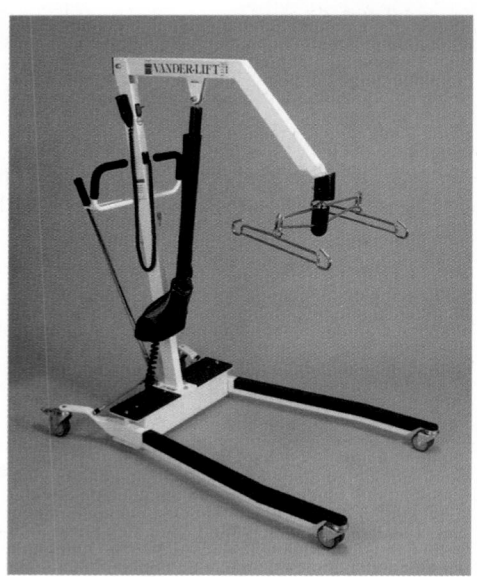

Mechanical lift. (Courtesy of Vancare, Inc., Aurora, NE.)

2 Place the bed in its lowest position and place the one- or two-piece sling under the client. Make sure the sling supports the client's shoulders and buttocks. Have the client cross her arms across her chest.

If the sling is not positioned correctly, the client may fall. Take care not to injure the client's skin with the metal attachments when placing the sling under her.

3 Securely connect the sling hooks to the lift. Raise the lift to elevate the client enough to clear the bed.

If the client is not completely off of the bed, shearing or friction of the skin can result.

4 Move the lift until it is aligned with the chair, lock the wheels, release the pressure valve, and lower the client slowly into the chair. Remove the sling from the lift and store it in a corner out of the way of traffic.

Correct alignment with the chair prevents the client from falling or other injury.

5 Keep the sling under the client, but position the client into proper body alignment.

The sling remains under the client until it is used again to return the client to bed.

HOME CARE CONSIDERATIONS

Teach family caregivers how to use the mechanical lift and help them practice until they are proficient and feel secure before trying to move the client.

move the client to the edge of the bed closest to the stretcher. Pull the turning sheet and lift the client onto the stretcher in unison. Place a pillow under the client's head, pull up the stretcher side rails, fasten the strap around the client, and push the stretcher from the head.

Supporting the Ambulating Client

Some clients cannot ambulate independently and require human or mechanical assistance. The transfer belt serves as the gait or walking belt that you can hold during ambulation. If the client is weaker on one side than the other, stand on the weaker side. The client can also push a portable intravenous pole and use it as an extra support if needed (Procedure 37–5).

If the client starts to fall or faint, support the client and ease her to the floor. Make the client as comfortable as possible and stay with her until help arrives.

Compensating for Physical Impairments

When human assistance is not available or the client is ready to learn to ambulate independently, assistive devices may be used. If available, a physical therapist will do the initial teaching, but you will need to reinforce the techniques that were taught. Walkers, canes, crutches, and wheelchairs allow independence in ambulation.

USING A WALKER

A walker provides better support than either a cane or crutches (Fig. 37–7). They are used most often for older adults who have decreased muscle strength. The standard walker can be adjusted for the client's height so that the hand bar is just below the client's waist and the elbows are slightly flexed. The standard walker is used for clients who can bear partial weight and must be picked up to be used correctly. Exercises to strengthen the arms are important. For clients who have insufficient arm strength, roller walkers with two or four wheels can be substituted. Some roller walkers have a seat where the client can sit when fatigued.

When teaching a client how to use a walker, place a gait belt around her and help her to a standing position. Tell the client to place both hands on the walker. If the client has severe arthritis in the hands, platforms for resting the arms can be used instead of handgrips. Teach the client to lift the walker and move it about 1 to 2 feet forward, depending on the client's comfort level and strength. While resting on the walker, ask the client to take one or two small steps and check balance. Repeat this procedure while ambulating. You should grasp the gait belt until the client is strong enough to ambulate independently with the walker.

USING A CANE

A variety of canes are available for ambulation, depending on the amount of support the client needs. The quadripod ("quad") and hemi-cane provide the most support (Fig. 37–8). They are used most often for

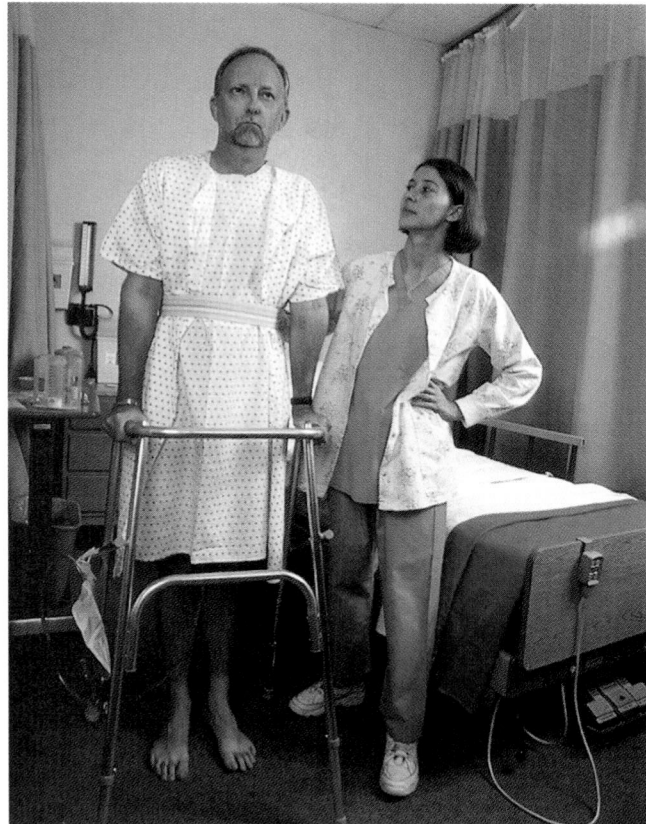

Figure 37–7. Client using a walker.

clients who have had strokes. The straight cane provides the least support. All canes should have rubber tips on the end to prevent slipping.

When teaching the client how to use a cane, again use a gait belt and help the client to a standing position. Have the client place the cane in the hand of the strongest side of the body. Have the client move the cane forward about a foot, then move the weaker leg one step forward. Then have the client move the stronger leg forward and check her balance.

Like walkers, canes may be used on a temporary or permanent basis. Some clients learn to ambulate using a walker, but then progress to a series of canes as needed.

USING CRUTCHES

For most clients, crutches are used as a temporary measure until they regain full mobility. However, for clients with permanent disability, they may be needed on a permanent basis. Axillary crutches are used most often when temporary support is needed. Lofstrand crutches are used most often for permanent needs (Fig. 37–9). Before use, the client should be measured carefully for adjustments to prevent axillary nerve damage or muscle strain. Each crutch end should have a rubber tip to prevent slipping.

Arm strength needs to be assessed. If needed, the client performs exercises to prepare for the demands of crutch walking. The basic crutch stance is called the

Supporting the Ambulating Client

TIME TO
ALLOW
▼
Novice:
20 min.
Expert:
10 min.

The first time a client gets out of bed after anesthesia, prolonged illness, or bedrest you will assist with ambulation to ensure the client's safety. It is better to be overly cautious in deciding which clients need assistance than to risk a fall.

Delegation Guidelines

You may delegate assisting the client with ambulation, following your initial assessment of the client's functional status and the client's risk factors for falling. The nursing assistant should receive training in body mechanics, safety, and assisting with mobility.

Equipment Needed

- Comfortable, supportive shoes with rubber soles.
- Bathrobe.

1 Apply a gait belt (also called a transfer or walking belt) around the client's waist and help the client to a standing position as outlined in Procedure 37–2.

2 Stand at the client's side and slightly behind her, and walk with the client while holding onto the back of the belt.

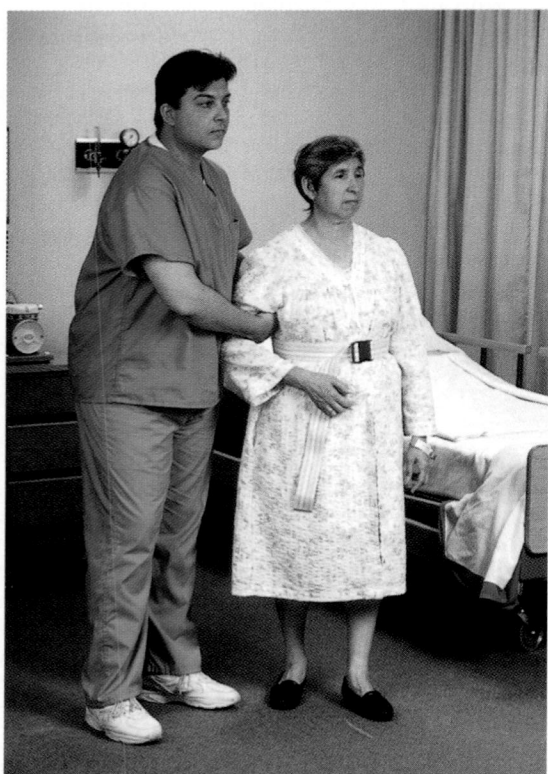

Standing at the client's side while holding onto the back of the transfer belt.

By holding onto the gait belt while the client is walking, you provide support for the client and you gain some control over ambulation.

3 If the client has an intravenous pole, ask her to push the pole while walking.

If the client has an intravous line, she will need a portable rolling pole. It can be used as additional support. However, caution the client that the pole rolls freely and should not be used to support her weight.

4 If the client is weaker on one side than the other, walk on her weak side while grasping the belt.

The client will tend to lean and could fall toward the weaker side of her body.

5 If the client is especially weak or this is her first time ambulating, ask another person to walk with you to support the client. If necessary, have another assistant follow with a wheelchair in case the client becomes too weak to stand.

An additional person helps by supporting the client from the opposite side or by moving portable equipment that must go with the client.

6 If the client starts to fall, do not try to prevent the fall by supporting her weight with your own body. Rather, help her to fall safely, without injury to her or to you.

7 As the client starts to fall, move your feet so your stronger leg is somewhat behind you.

This action forms a solid base of support for you and allows you to bear most of the weight on your strongest leg.

8 At the same time, use the transfer belt to pull the client toward you, allowing her to slide against you, supported, as you ease her onto the floor.

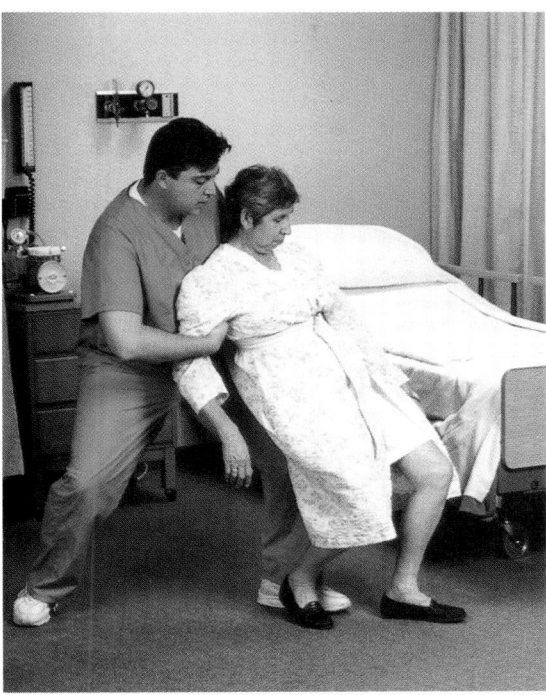

Supporting the client and easing her to the floor.

9 Stay with the client until help arrives. Assess her for injury before trying to move her. Even a minor fall can result in a fractured hip for an older adult, especially one who has osteoporosis. You may need to use a three-person lift to a stretcher rather than having the client try to stand. Have the client evaluated by a physician.

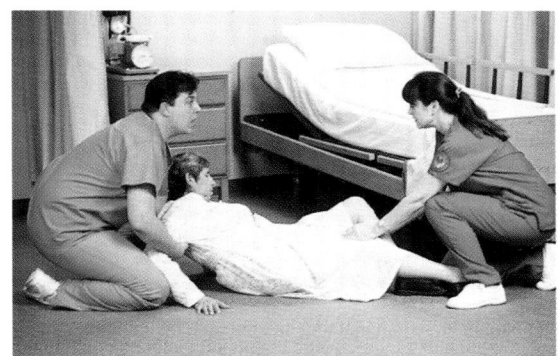

Staying with the client until help arrives.

10 Document the events leading up to the fall, your client assessment, notification of the physician, and any action taken.

HOME CARE CONSIDERATIONS

Help the family caregivers assess their home environment for hazards—such as throw rugs, slick floors, or obstructed pathways—before getting her out of bed to walk. A chair should be available that is sturdy, comfortable, and easily accessible. A high-backed chair is preferable to support the client's neck in anatomic alignment.

tripod, or triangle, position. It provides a broad base of support. Several gaits can be used for ambulating, depending on the injury and the client's weight-bearing status. The four-point gait provides the most support, but requires coordination to maneuver. The three-point gait requires that the client be able to bear full weight on the unaffected leg. The two-point gait is the quickest and requires at least partial weight-bearing ability for both legs. Procedure 37–6 describes these gaits and how to manage stairs and sitting.

Swing-to or swing-through gaits are used for clients who are paralyzed in both legs. Teach the client to move both crutches ahead together by about 2 feet, then lift the body and swing to or past the crutches, whichever is most comfortable and balanced.

USING A WHEELCHAIR

For some clients, walking is no longer possible. Clients with complete spinal cord injuries, advanced multiple sclerosis, cerebral palsy, or muscular dystrophy are often confined to a wheelchair. These clients ambulate in their wheelchairs using their arms or other part of the body to propel the chair. Some use electric wheelchairs that can be advanced by a hand control or with a slight head movement.

Clients who are confined to wheelchairs are at risk for skin breakdown and other complications of immobility previously described. Teach the client and family or significant others to inspect skin every day and perform wheelchair push-ups if possible to decrease pressure on the ischial tuberosities. Push-ups also build

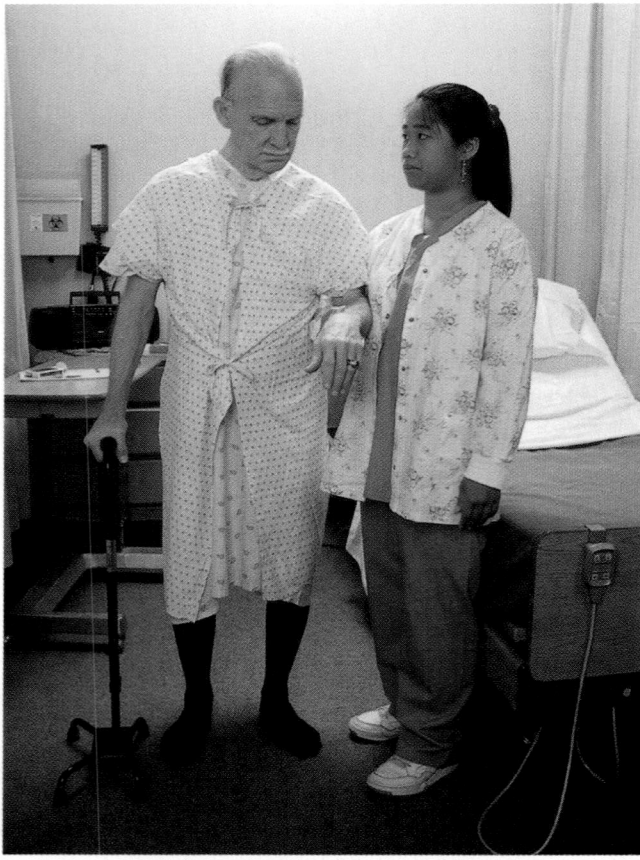

Figure 37–8. Client using a "quad" cane.

arm strength, which is essential for propelling a manual wheelchair.

As a result of the federal Americans with Disabilities Act, all public places are wheelchair accessible. Ramps, handicapped toilets, and designated parking spaces have allowed wheelchair-bound people access to places they were previously not able to visit.

EVALUATION

Evaluation involves determining whether expected outcomes have been met. If they have not been met, the plan may need modification.

In our case study, Mrs. Laskauskas required rehabilitation for her fractured hip repair. By the fifth postoperative day, she was discharged to the hospital's transitional care unit (TCU). She was able to transfer from her bed to a chair and walk about 15 feet using a walker. Beyond that distance, she became dyspneic and tired. The plan for her continued rehabilitation in the TCU is to increase her ambulation distance and continue to build her tolerance for activity so that she can return to her assisted living apartment. In this example, the client has progressed slowly, but is able to ambulate with a walker independently for a short distance. The intermediate expected outcomes were met, but the long-term outcomes still need to be achieved before she can be discharged back into the community. The accompanying nursing care plan illustrates Mrs.

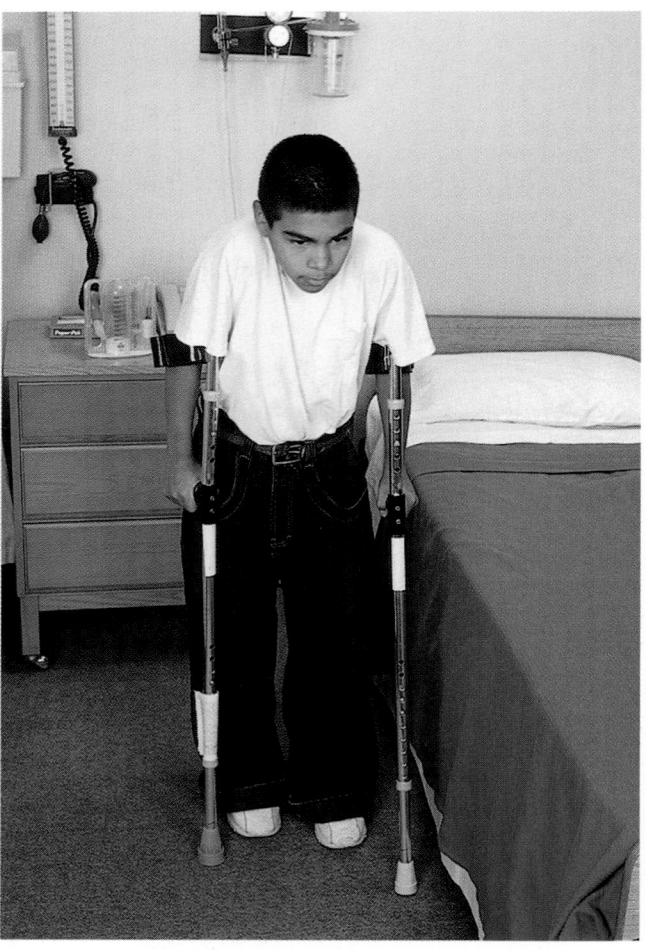

Figure 37–9. Client using Lofstrand crutches.

Lasauskas' care after surgery, when she is ready to get out of bed for the first time.

KEY PRINCIPLES

- Factors affecting mobility include lifestyle, environment, growth and development, and pathophysiological factors, especially musculoskeletal and neurological health problems.
- *Impaired physical mobility* occurs when the client experiences limited ability to move within the physical environment.
- *Activity intolerance* results when a client has insufficient physiological or psychological energy to endure or complete a desired activity.
- Physical examination of a client with impaired physical mobility includes assessment of body alignment, gait, joints, skeletal muscles, and neurovascular function.
- Diagnostic tests help you select appropriate nursing diagnoses for clients with musculoskeletal health problems.

Text continued on page 1010

PROCEDURE 37–6

Walking With Crutches

TIME TO
ALLOW
▼
Novice:
*20–30
min.*
Expert:
*20–30
min.*

Crutches are usually used for clients with orthopedic injuries who are unable to bear weight on one or both legs. Using crutches properly requires good upper body strength and balance.

Delegation Guidelines

The evaluation of the need for crutches and instruction in the use of crutches may not be delegated to a nursing assistant. Assessment and instruction for crutch-walking are the domain of a licensed professional, such as you or a physical therapist. Once a client has been instructed and successfully demonstrates crutch walking, you may assign or delegate a nursing assistant to accompany the client, much as you would do with ambulation.

Equipment Needed

- Crutches with rubber tips.
- Supportive shoes with rubber soles.

---

1 Inspect the prescribed crutch or crutches to make sure that the rubber tips are in place.

Rubber tips prevent slipping and therefore promote safety.

---

2 Reinforce the importance of arm exercises, such as flexing and extending the arms, body lifts, and squeezing a rubber ball.

Arm muscles need to be toned to use crutches. Upper body strength is required.

---

3 Check that crutches are the correct length.
a. First, have the client stand.
b. Next, with the crutch tips and the client in the basic crutch stance (tripod position) check the distance between her axilla and the top of the crutch. It should be at least three finger widths or 1 to 2 inches (2.5 to 5 cm).

If the crutches are not the correct length, the client could sustain axillary nerve damage.

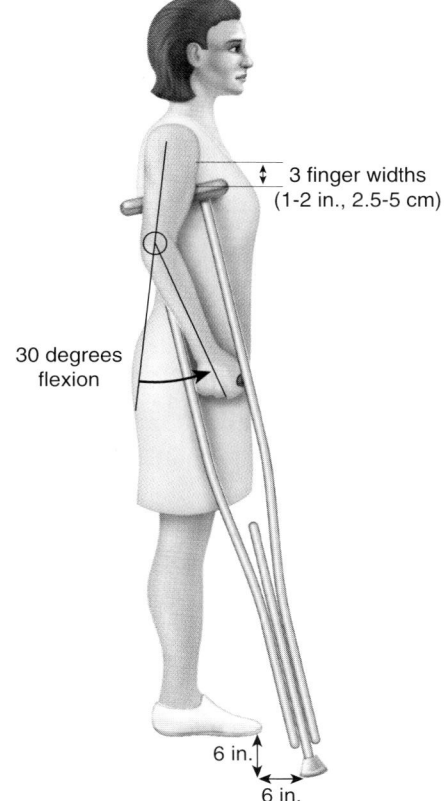

3 finger widths
(1-2 in., 2.5-5 cm)

30 degrees
flexion

6 in.

6 in.

Measuring crutch length.

Continued

Walking With Crutches

4 Teach the client how to balance using the tripod (triangle) position by placing the crutches 6 inches (15 cm) in front of the feet and out laterally about the same distance.

The tripod position provides a wide base of support and balance to prevent falls.

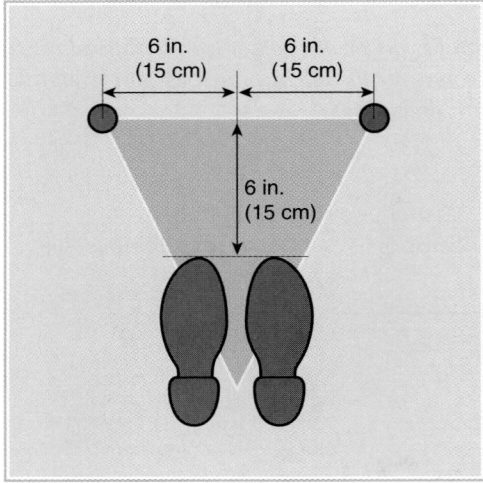

Basic crutch stance, tripod position.

5 Check with the physician or physical therapist to determine which gait the client needs, a four-point, three-point, or two-point gait.

a. For a four-point gait, have the client follow this series of steps:
- Move the right crutch forward about 6 inches (15 cm).
- Move the left foot forward.
- Move the left crutch forward.
- Move the right foot forward.

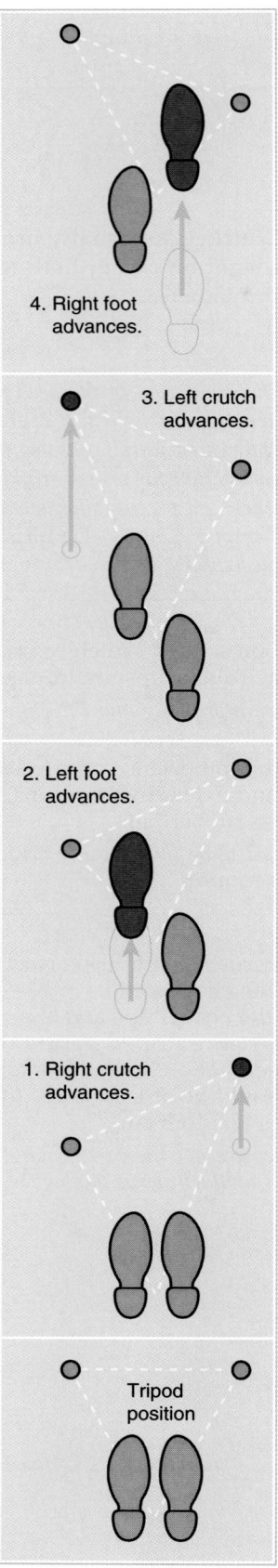

4. Right foot advances.

3. Left crutch advances.

2. Left foot advances.

1. Right crutch advances.

Tripod position

Four-point gait.

b. For a three-point gait, have the client follow this series of steps:
   - Move both crutches and the weakest leg forward.
   - Move the stronger leg forward.

c. For a two-point gait, have the client follow this series of steps:
   - Move the left crutch and the right foot forward at the same time.
   - Move the right crutch and the left foot forward at the same time.

The type of injury and the client's balance determine which gait will be recommended.

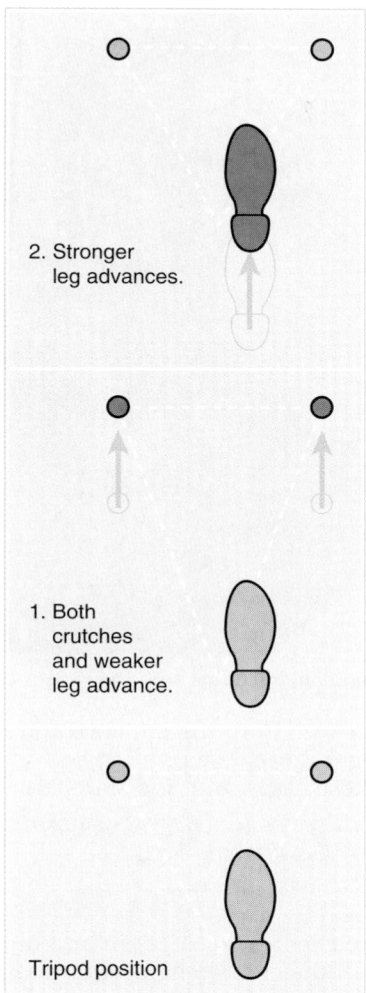

Three-point gait.

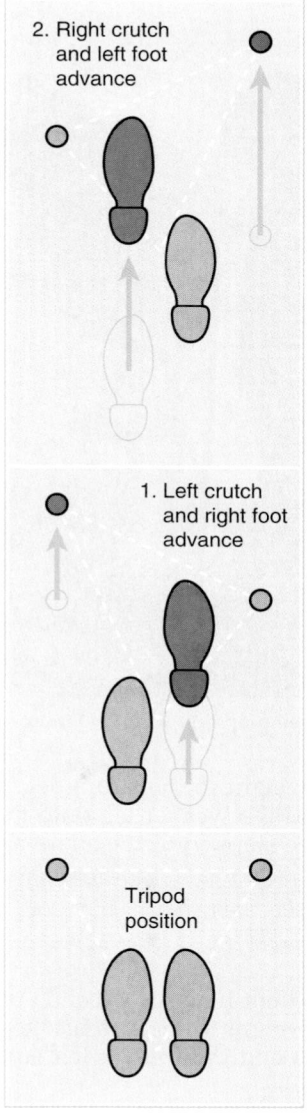

Two-point gait.

Continued

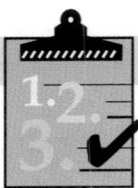

Walking With Crutches

6 Teach the client how to ascend stairs:
a. Step up first with the stronger leg.

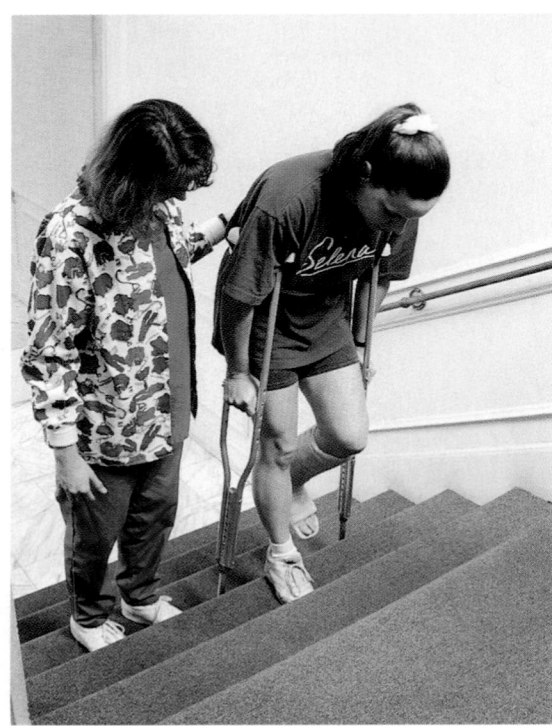

Stepping up first with the stronger leg.

b. Shift your weight to the strong leg and move the crutches and the weaker leg onto the same step.
c. Repeat these steps until the stairs are negotiated.

The weaker or affected leg is always supported by the crutches using this method.

7 Teach the client how to descend stairs:
a. Shift your weight to the stronger leg and move the crutches and the weaker leg onto the lower step.

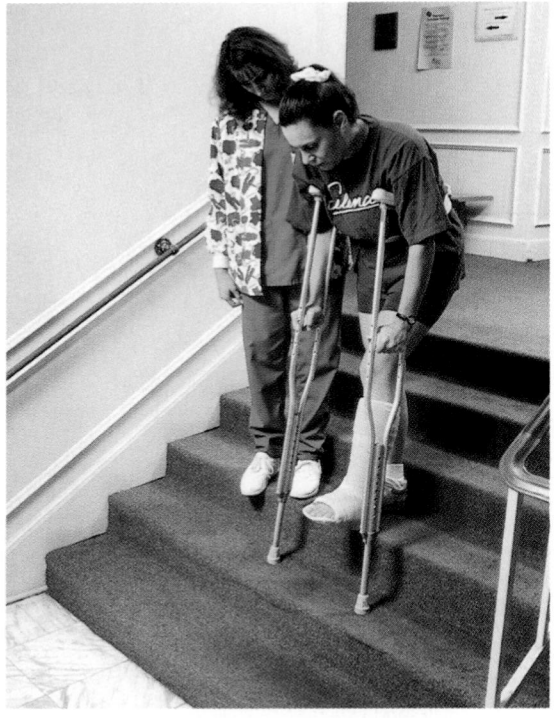

Stepping down first with the weaker leg.

b. Shift your weight to the crutches and move the strong leg onto that step.
c. Repeat these steps until the stairs are negotiated.

The weaker or affected leg is always supported by the crutches using this method.

8 Teach the client how to get in and out of a chair:
a. Stand with the chair behind you, making sure that the back of your strongest leg is against the chair.
b. Transfer your crutches to your weaker side and hold them by the hand bar.
c. Grasp the arm of the chair with the hand on your strong side, then lean forward and flex your hips and knees while lowering yourself into the chair.
d. To get out of the chair, move to the edge of the chair.
e. Hold both crutches by the hand bar using the hand on your weaker side. Hold the arm of the chair with the hand on your stronger side.
f. Push down on the crutches and the armrest to push yourself out of the chair.

This technique supports the weaker leg and provides the best balance for the client.

HOME CARE CONSIDERATIONS

Help the client do a safety check of the home environment for slippery floors, loose throw rugs, or obstructions in walkways. If the client will need to use stairs, it is preferable to have a hand rail.

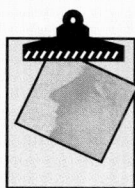

NURSING CARE PLANNING
A CLIENT WITH A FRACTURED HIP

Admission Data

Mrs. Kristina Lasauskas is an 80-year-old woman admitted for a fractured left hip. She was taken from the emergency room to the operating room, where she had an open reduction and internal fixation.

Physician's Orders

D₅ in ½ NS @ 75 mL per hour
Up in a chair tid as tolerated
ROM qid

Laxative of choice
Regular diet, encourage fluids
Plan for discharge to rehabilitation center

Nursing Assessment

In morning report the following information was provided. Mrs. Lasauskas is 3 days post-op for open reduction and internal fixation of the left hip. Her vital signs are stable. She has an I.V. of 5% dextrose in ½ NS running at 75 cc per hour. She has not been out of bed because she is partially paralyzed on her right side. She will get up for the first time today. Physical therapy is doing range of motion twice a day and the nurses are doing it twice a day. The client is depressed and feels she will never walk again.

NURSING CARE PLAN

Nursing Diagnosis	Expected Outcomes	Interventions	Evaluation
Impaired physical mobility related to right-sided weakness and healing fracture of left hip	The client will maintain full ROM.	Full active/passive range of motion by physical therapy 0800, 1300; by nursing 0500, 0900. *Use client's history of self-determination to motivate.*	Has full ROM in upper extremities. Can perform active ROM. Performs active ROM on right leg. Straight leg raising to a 30-degree angle. Can raise left leg by bending knee to 30 degrees hip flexion.
	Increase upper body strength. Tolerate sitting in a chair.	Use 3-pound weights to exercise arms during ROM; *have great grandchildren bring colored weights and make a game of exercising.* Pivot to chair 1000, 1500, 1900, increasing to 30 minutes as tolerated.	Exercises arms with 3-pound weights. Tolerates flexion at elbow. Raises weight over her head. Tires right arm. Can stand and pivot to chair with assistance.
	Perform resistance exercises to right leg and ROM to left leg. Stand at bedside with partial weight-bearing to left hip.	Use light resistance for ROM to right leg.	Can raise right leg against light resistance of nurse's hand on knee. Puts left leg on floor for balance when standing. Minimal if any weight-bearing.

Italicized interventions indicate culturally specific care.

Critical Thinking Questions

1. Estimate Mrs. Lasauskas's potential for rehabilitation on a scale of 1 to 10, with 10 meaning she will be able to walk as well as she did before she fell.
2. List the criteria you used to make the decision in Question #1.
3. Mrs. Lasauskas refuses to do active ROM with her arms. How would you motivate her?

- Functional assessment includes determining a client's ability to move and perform activities of daily living.
- Assessment of the client with *Impaired physical mobility* should be holistic and include assessment of all functional health patterns for emotional as well as physiological responses, including hopelessness and pain or chronic pain.
- Expected outcomes for clients with musculoskeletal problems are that the client will experience improved mobility and tolerance to activities.
- Interventions for improving activity tolerance focus on building muscle mass and strength, progressive mobilization, and controlling pain and discomfort.
- Interventions for improving mobility include maintaining joint mobility, assisting with movement, and compensating for physical impairments.
- Evaluation of outcomes for clients with musculoskeletal problems involves promoting ambulation, including wheelchair ambulation, preventing complications of immobility, and building activity tolerance.

BIBLIOGRAPHY

Badley, E.M. (1995). The impact of disabling arthritis. *Arthritis Care Research, 8*(4), 221–228.

Boss, B.J., Pecanty, L., McFarland, S.M., & Sasser, L. (1995). Self-care competence among persons with spinal cord injury. *SCI Nursing, 12*(2), 48–53.

Donohue, K.M., Wineman, N.M., & O'Brien, R.A. (1996). Are alternative long-term-care programs needed for adults with chronic progressive disability? *Journal of Neuroscience Nursing, 28*(6), 373–380.

Edwards, P.A. (1996). Health promotion through fitness for adolescents and young adults following spinal cord injury. *SCI Nursing, 13*(3), 69–73.

Evans, R.W. (1997). The role of the neuropsychologist in life care planning for brain-injured populations. *The Journal of Care Management, 3*(5), 46–47, 49.

Galindo-Ciocon, D., Ciocon, J.O., & Galindo, D. (1995). Functional impairment among elderly women with osteoporotic vertebral fractures. *Rehabilitation Nursing, 20*(2), 79–83.

*Granger, C.V., & Gresham, G.E. (1984). *Functional assessment in rehabilitation medicine.* Baltimore: Williams & Wilkins.

Hamilton, L., & Lyon, P.S. (1995). A nursing-driven program to preserve and restore functional ability in hospitalized elderly patients. *Journal of Nursing Administration, 25*(4), 30–37.

Herbert, P., Rochman, D.L., & McAlary, P.W. (1998). Dealing with pain. *Case Review, 4*(6), 16–19.

Hickey, J.V. (1996). *The clinical practice of neurological and neurosurgical nursing* (4th ed.). Philadelphia: J.B. Lippincott.

Huntt, D.C., & Growick, B.S. (1997). Managed care for people with disabilities. *Journal of Rehabilitation,* July/August/September, 10–14.

Ignatavicius, D.D., Workman, M.L., & Mishler, M.A. (1999). *Medical-surgical nursing across the health care continuum* (3rd ed.). Philadelphia: W.B. Saunders.

Leininger, M.M. (1991). *Culture care diversity and universality: A theory of nursing.* New York: National League for Nursing Press.

McCaffery, M., & Ferrell, B.R. (1999). Opioids and pain management. *Nursing99, 29*(3), 48–52.

Neal, L.J. (1995). The rehabilitation nurse in the home care setting: Treating wounds as a disability. *Rehabilitation Nursing, 20*(5), 261–264.

North American Nursing Diagnosis Association. (1999). *NANDA nursing diagnoses: Definitions and classification 1999–2000.* Philadelphia: Author.

Somervill, B.A. (1997). Transitional and subacute care. *Case Review, 3*(3), 61–63.

Wojner, A.W. (1996). Optimizing ischemic stroke outcomes: An interdisciplinary approach to rehabilitation in acute care. *Critical Care Quarterly, 19*(2), 47–61.

*Asterisk indicates a classic or definitive work on this subject.

CHAPTER 38

Disuse Syndrome

Judy Sweeney

Key Terms

atrophy

bedrest

contracture

deep vein thrombosis

disuse

excoriation

footdrop

friction injury

hypostatic pneumonia

immobility

inactivity

interface pressure

maceration

orthostatic hypotension

osteoporosis

pressure ulcer

pulmonary embolus

renal calculi

shear

trochanter roll

wrist drop

LEARNING OBJECTIVES

After studying this chapter, you should be able to:

1. **Describe the physiological concepts underlying the diagnosis of *Risk for disuse syndrome*.**

2. **Discuss the factors that may lead to immobility and disuse.**

3. **Assess a client who is at risk for complications from disuse.**

4. **Diagnose the client at risk for disuse complications.**

5. **Plan for goal-directed interventions to prevent complications of disuse.**

6. **Describe interventions needed to prevent complications of disuse.**

7. **Evaluate outcomes that describe progress toward managing immobility and preventing disuse.**

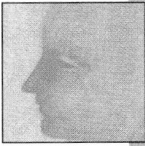

Mr. Jackson is a 48-year-old African-American male who presents to the emergency room following an injury on the job. The physician diagnoses a compound fracture of the left tibia and a fractured left clavicle. He is taken to the operating room where the bone fragments are pinned and a stabilizing device applied. His arm is placed in a sling. After 24 hours Mr. Jackson is sent home with instructions to keep the left leg elevated at all times, apply an ice pack to the left knee for 20 minutes every 4 hours, and to bear no weight on the leg. He is to return to the orthopedic clinic in 1 week. It will be at least 3 months before he will be able to return to the heavy construction work he has done since he was 16 years old. He is likely to lose strength and endurance in addition to atrophy of the limb. Additionally, he is at risk for cardiovascular deconditioning, respiratory infection, urinary tract infection, depression, and skin breakdown. The nurse makes the diagnosis of *Risk for disuse syndrome.*

DISUSE
NURSING DIAGNOSES

Risk for disuse syndrome: A state in which an individual is at risk for deterioration of body systems as the result of prescribed or unavoidable musculoskeletal inactivity.

From North American Nursing Diagnosis Association. (1999). NANDA nursing diagnoses: Definitions and classification 1999–2000. Philadelphia: Author.

Activity and movement develop and maintain the normal functioning of all body systems. In contrast, prolonged inactivity causes physical and mental deterioration. You will care for clients who are inactive from immobility, prescribed bedrest, critical illness, neurological damage, trauma, or pain. Through astute assessment and aggressive interventions you can prevent many of the complications of disuse.

CONCEPTS OF INACTIVITY AND IMMOBILITY

Disuse means to cease or decrease use of organs or body parts, to restrict activities, or to be immobile. Complications of disuse occur in every body system. Disuse can affect a single body part or multiple interrelated body systems. Complications of disuse occur if the client has a prescribed or an unavoidable period of inactivity or immobility. Preventing complications of disuse will decrease suffering and the cost of health care.

Immobility is the inability to move the whole body or a body part. It occurs in clients who are paralyzed or unconscious or who have neuromuscular diseases or orthopedic conditions. Many frail older adults have fewer spontaneous movements secondary to neurological or musculoskeletal problems. The immobile client is totally dependent on the nurse for maintaining safety and body functions.

Bedrest is a prescribed or self-imposed restriction to bed for therapeutic reasons. Complete bedrest is seldom prescribed because of the potential complications of immobility. However, critically ill clients, some orthopedic clients, and clients with severe limitation of movement may be confined to bed. The client with prescribed bedrest ranges from being able to move about freely in bed to requiring a lot of effort to move to needing assistance to move.

Inactivity and immobility have a cyclic relationship with the development of complications. For example, when a client remains inactive, the joints begin to get stiff, and the muscles get weak. The client is less able to participate in activities of daily living and experiences an increased risk of immobility. Eventually, the client develops skin breakdown and respiratory and cardiovascular deconditioning. The longer the person is immobile, the higher the risk of complications of disuse. Preventing the complications of immobility requires support of all body systems to break the cycle of disuse.

Psychosocial Effects of Inactivity and Immobility

Initially, most people welcome a brief relief from the activities of daily living with a quiet rest period. However, long-term or permanent inactivity or immobilization can alter that feeling. Often, the client loses motivation or interest in participating in daily living. Losing contact with friends and work can result in loneliness and social isolation. The client who is forced to rely on others for help feels powerless. Loss of self-esteem is associated with the absence of social roles as caregiver, parent, or breadwinner.

Behavior changes in response to a prescribed or unavoidable restriction in activity. Acting out negative feelings in the form of irritation, anger, or aggression can result from feelings of dissatisfaction and frustration. Additionally, inactivity can increase mental confusion as a consequence of sensory deprivation. The person is less able to concentrate and focus on learning, memory may be impaired, and problem-solving abilities decline.

Resting in bed 24 hours a day also interferes with the normal circadian rhythm and pattern of sleep. When the client sleeps during the day, the quality of the sleep is not the same as it is during the night. However, having slept during the day, the client may be unable to sleep through the night. The psychological manifestations of sleep deprivation may be present.

Mr. Jackson is the primary financial support for his family. He has good health insurance but does not have sick leave. What psychosocial manifestations would you predict for him?

Musculoskeletal Effects of Inactivity and Immobility

The strength of bones, strength and tone of muscles, and mobility of joints are maintained through active use. Much as the trained athlete becomes deconditioned when not in training, the client who is inactive experiences deterioration of bones, muscles, and joints.

To maintain their mass and strength, muscles must move against resistance. **Atrophy** is a decrease in the size of a normally developed tissue or organ as a result of inactivity or diminished function. When muscles atrophy, they lose size and strength. After about 24 to 36 hours of inactivity, muscles begin to lose their contractile strength. Already, they have begun the process of atrophy.

When a person is immobile, the body breaks down muscle mass to obtain energy, which can result in a negative nitrogen balance. The strength and endurance lost with a brief period of immobility can take several weeks to regain. The client becomes more susceptible to ambulation problems and injury by falling.

Thinking again about Mr. Jackson, what problems might he experience when he is able to return to work?

After about 5 days of immobility, fibrotic cells and calcium deposit in joints, causing them to become stiff and lose their full range of motion. Reduced range of motion can also be caused by fibrosis of tissues that support the joint or muscles. A joint losing its ability to move and becoming fixated is called ankylosis. Contractures also limit joint movement.

A **contracture** is the abnormal shortening of muscle fibers or their associated connective tissue, resulting in resistance to stretching and eventually to flexion and, thereby, resulting in permanent fixation. It also can result from loss of normal skin elasticity, as in scar formation. Fibrosis occurs in the muscle or the structures supporting the muscle, causing it to become stiff. A reversible contracture is a shortening of a muscle, which can be corrected by exercise. In a nonreversible contracture the muscle or tendon becomes permanently fixed or frozen and can be corrected only by surgical intervention.

Although any joint can become contracted, the wrists and ankles are common—and commonly overlooked—locations. These contractures are particularly disabling when they occur. **Footdrop** is a contracture deformity in which the muscles of the anterior foot lengthen. At the same time, the muscles of plantar flexion and the Achilles tendon shorten, resulting in plantar flexion of the foot (Fig. 38–1A). Footdrop can result from the weight of gravity on weakened foot muscles or from damage to the peroneal nerve. **Wrist drop** is a contracture of the wrist in the flexed position (Fig. 38–1B). Contractures also commonly occur in the elbows, knees, hips, and hands. Contractures of the neck result in kyphosis.

Contractures are flexion abnormalities resulting from the longer and stronger flexor and adductor muscles overcoming the weaker opposing muscles. Additionally, the client assumes the most comfortable or resting position for a joint that is often in the flexed position.

A client with a contracture loses functional ability in the affected muscles and joints. For example, a client with a contracture of the wrist or elbow may be unable to hold a spoon or a comb. Other activities of daily living will be affected as well. Footdrop is a crippling deformity that prevents the person from walking.

If Mr. Jackson keeps his arm in a sling for a month, what changes would you expect? If he asks you about exercises for his shoulder, what would you tell him?

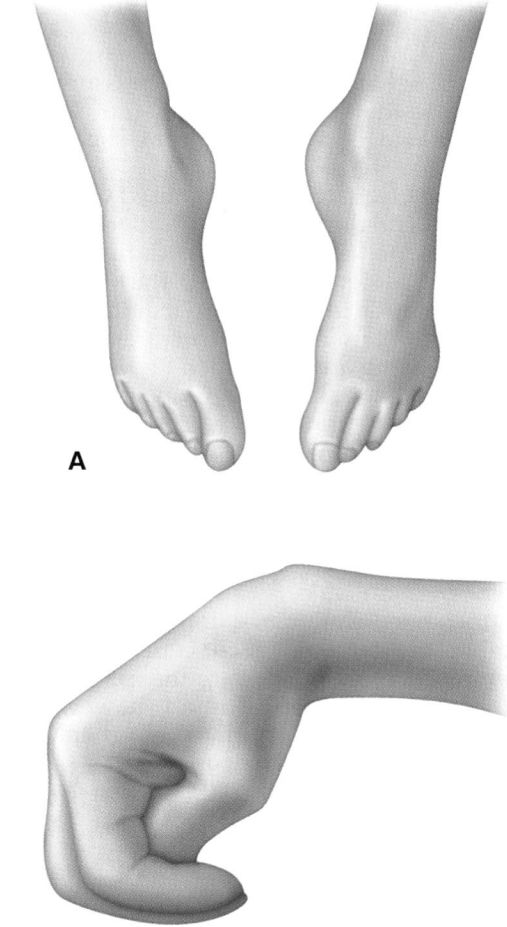

A

B

Figure 38–1. Two common contractures resulting from immobility. *A,* footdrop involves plantar flexion, inversion of the ankle, and flexion of the toes; *B,* Wrist drop involves flexion of the wrist and fingers and opposition of the thumb. (*B* redrawn from Bolander, V.B. [1994]. *Sorensen and Luckmann's basic nursing* [3rd ed.]. Philadelphia: W.B. Saunders Co.)

Osteoporosis is a condition in which there is a decreased mass per unit volume of normally mineralized bone, primarily from a loss of calcium, that makes bones brittle and porous. Osteoporosis can occur when functional stress on bones declines. Functional stress is essential to the continuous reformation of bone. Osteoblasts are continually building bone matrix while osteoclasts are continually breaking down bone matrix. Reformation maintains the tensile strength of bones. Without the stress of weight-bearing, osteoblastic activity slows, and osteoporosis occurs.

Within about 2 or 3 days of decreased muscle activity and weight-bearing, osteoblastic activity slows and interrupts bone reformation. Osteoclastic activity (breakdown) continues, releasing large amounts of calcium from the bone matrix into the blood. The extra calcium is excreted by the kidneys or deposited in the muscles and joints. The bones become brittle and porous, and they fracture easily.

Integumentary Effects of Inactivity and Immobility

Damage to the skin from prolonged pressure on bony prominences is the major complication of immobility. Additional damage can result from shear, friction, maceration, and infection.

A **pressure ulcer** is any lesion caused by unrelieved pressure that leads to damage of underlying tissues. When pressure on the skin exceeds capillary pressure, blood flow to the skin is impaired. The supply of oxygen and nutrients is insufficient to maintain the viability of the skin and underlying structures. The cells die and slough, leaving an open crater. Pressure ulcers can range from reddened skin to large, open, deep wounds. Poor nutrition and continued pressure lead to poor wound healing and wound infections. A pressure ulcer can develop in a single day.

The most affected areas are the tissues overlying bony prominence (Fig. 38–2). The area over the coccyx is probably the most common site of pressure ulcers. However, pressure ulcers also develop over the greater trochanter, shoulder, elbow, back of the skull, heels, ankle, and ear. For a client confined to a wheelchair, the most common sites are the ischial tuberosities and the coccyx. Keep in mind, however, that a pressure ulcer can develop anywhere there is sufficient pressure for a sufficient period.

For an ulcer to occur, the amount of pressure in the capillaries needs to exceed that of the arterioles (capillary closing pressure of about 35 mm Hg), and the duration of pressure must be long and unrelieved. **Interface pressure** is pressure created in tissues that are compressed between the bones and a support surface by the weight of the body. As the client lies in bed or sits quietly in a chair, interface pressure exerted on the tissues by the external surface of the bed or chair interrupts blood flow through the vessels and impairs the delivery of oxygen and nutrients to the cells.

Although the development of pressure ulcers has a sole cause (prolonged, unrelieved pressure), additional factors increase the risk of developing a pressure injury. A client who is unable to move independently in bed because of cognitive or musculoskeletal limitations is at high risk. Chronic illness, such as renal failure, diabetes, and anemia, further exacerbates the risk. Frail or edematous skin is more likely to sustain damage. Dehydration and hypoproteinemia also decrease the skin's tolerance to injury.

The term pressure ulcer accounts for a large proportion of skin injuries that result from bedrest. Treating these injuries is costly, as described in the accompanying Cost of Care chart, and often difficult. Prevention is always the treatment of choice.

Supine

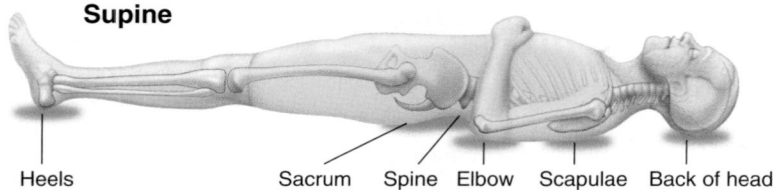

Heels   Sacrum   Spine   Elbow   Scapulae   Back of head

Side-lying

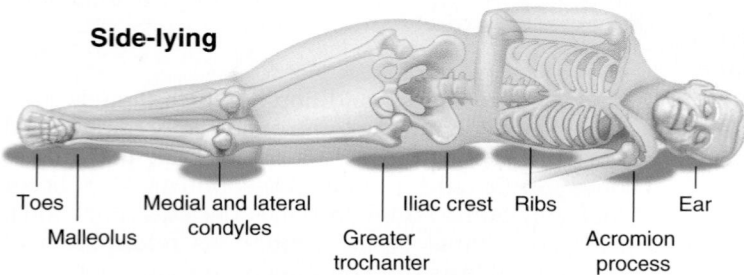

Toes   Medial and lateral   Iliac crest   Ribs   Ear
Malleolus   condyles   Greater   Acromion
                           trochanter   process

Prone

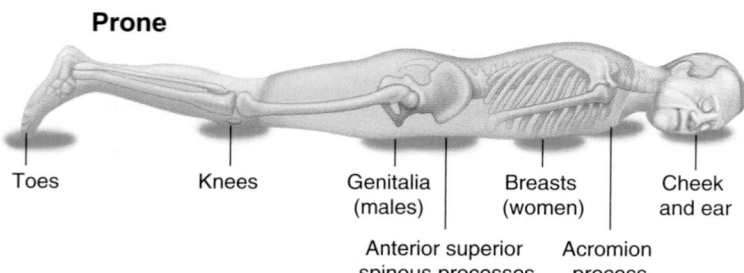

Toes   Knees   Genitalia   Breasts   Cheek
                             (males)   (women)   and ear

              Anterior superior   Acromion
              spinous processes   process

Figure 38–2. Bony prominences subject to pressure, ischemia, necrosis, and ulceration in the supine, side-lying, and prone positions.

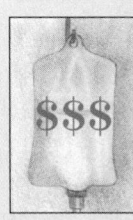

THE COST OF CARE
ILLNESS PREVENTION

In the United States, an important national goal is to control the cost of health care. Many experts believe the best way to do that is by paying to prevent illness rather than by paying to treat illness. Many studies have shown that treatment is more costly than prevention. Indeed, it is estimated that $6.5 billion is spent each year on the treatment of pressure ulcers alone.

Preventing the complications of disease will help to keep clients out of the hospital and allow an earlier release for those who do need hospitalization. Both results will decrease the financial burden of medical care. And both results depend at least in part on your participation in a commitment to prevention.

References

Carroll, P. (1995). Bed selection: Help the patient rest easily. *RN, 58*(5), 44–50.
Zerwekh, J., & Claborn, J.C. (1994). *Nursing today: Transition and trends.* Philadelphia: W.B. Saunders Co.

If Mr. Jackson wears a brace on his knee, how could you help him prevent pressure points?

Shear is a mechanical force that acts on a skin area in a direction parallel to the body's surface. Shear injuries are a serious form of pressure injury resulting in necrosis and ulceration, usually over the coccyx. They result from improper positioning, usually when the client slides down in bed (Fig. 38–3). When that happens, blood vessels in the two sacral tissue layers are stretched and torn, which disrupts the blood supply to the cells and causes skin breakdown. Shearing forces cause deep ulcers. Although they may appear small on the skin surface, considerable necrosis may be present in the underlying tissues.

Injuries can occur to the superficial layers of the skin. In a **friction injury,** the epidermal layer of skin is rubbed off, possibly from a restraint, a dressing, or a tube. Friction injury commonly affects the elbows, which can become irritated as the client moves around in bed. An **excoriation** is an injury to the epidermis caused by abrasion, scratching, a burn, or chemicals, such as sweat, wound drainage, feces, or urine coming in contact with skin. Maceration increases the risk of damage by decreasing the skin's ability to resist trauma. **Maceration** is a softening of the epidermis caused by prolonged contact with moisture, such as from a wet sheet or diaper.

Once the skin's first line of defense is broken, microorganisms can freely invade an ulcer or lesion, causing an infection. Infections slow wound healing and carry the risk of the serious complication of septicemia. As well, the absence of circulation decreases the oxygen, immune response, and nutrients that are necessary for healing.

Cardiovascular Effects of Inactivity and Immobility

When a client is on bedrest, the demands of the cells for oxygen initially decrease. However, the cardiovascular workload may actually increase. Additionally, without exercise, cardiac deconditioning begins. These changes in the cardiovascular system lead to decreased energy and further inactivity.

Additionally, it is harder for the client to change positions and perform the activities of daily living when restricted to bed. Often, during the "work" of moving in bed or using a bedpan, the client will use Valsalva's maneuver, that is, hold the breath and increase the intrathoracic pressure by straining against a closed glottis. When a breath is taken, the intrathoracic pressure drops, and blood flow suddenly increases to the right heart, causing an increased workload. Reflex bradycardia occurs, which can cause a heart attack in vulnerable persons.

Unlike arteries, in which blood is pumped forward by the heart, the veins rely on the "squeezing" action of calf muscles to move the venous blood along. In a bedridden client, decreased calf muscle activity and increased external pressure from the bed gradually allow blood to pool in the distal veins. This stasis of blood contributes to three problems: orthostatic hypotension, edema, and thrombus formation.

Orthostatic hypotension is a drop in systolic blood pressure of 20 mm Hg or more and a drop in diastolic blood pressure of 10 mm Hg or more for 1 or 2 minutes after a client stands up. It is also called postural hypotension, and it commonly results from immobility.

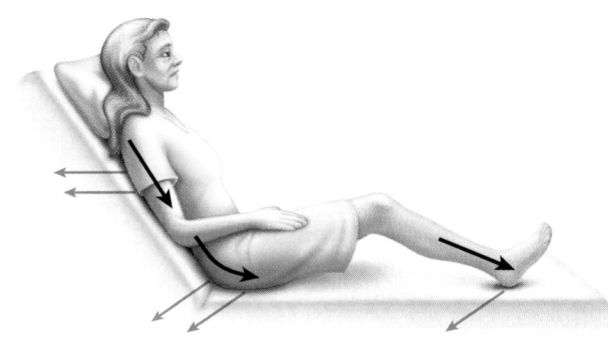

Figure 38–3. Shearing forces pull tissue layers in opposite directions. Tissue near the bone slides downward and forward, whereas the skin tends to be held upward and back by friction from the sheets.

In the supine position (lying flat on the back), blood pools in the legs, and venous return and cardiac output decrease. When the client sits or stands up, blood pressure can drop rapidly. Prolonged supine positioning also decreases the sensitivity of baroreceptors in the aortic arch to positional blood pressure changes. These receptors become sluggish and less responsive in stimulating the sympathetic nervous system to maintain normal blood pressure with changes in positions. Dehydration can also contribute to this problem by decreasing the blood volume.

Low blood pressure and orthostatic hypotension increase the client's risk of falling. Signs and symptoms of orthostatic hypotension include dizziness, feeling faint, or feeling lightheaded. Orthostatic hypotension is present in about 20% of people over age 65 and in at least 30% of people over age 75.

Stasis of blood in the legs and sacral area increases hydrostatic pressure on the walls of the veins. As the veins dilate in response, the valves open and allow backflow of blood down the veins. Also, this increase in hydrostatic fluid pressure "pushes" more fluid out of the veins into the interstitial spaces as edema. Edema constricts blood flow to the tissues and cells, decreasing their oxygen supply.

Stasis of venous blood, viscosity of the blood, and injury to vessel walls predispose the client to thrombus formation in the legs. **Deep vein thrombosis** is the condition caused when a blood clot (thrombus) develops in the lumen of a deep leg vein, such as the tibial, popliteal, femoral, or iliac vein. Superficial vein thrombosis is a clot in a superficial vessel.

Deep vein thrombosis can develop when slowed blood flow allows platelets and increased levels of calcium (from the bones) to settle out and come in contact with the intimal lining of the vessel. This activates the clotting process and forms blood clots along the vessel wall, particularly if the walls are damaged or if the vessels are tortuous. Dehydration contributes to thrombus formation by causing the blood to become more viscous.

Signs of deep vein thrombosis are calf tenderness, calf pain with passive dorsiflexion of the foot (Homans' sign), edema that causes one calf to increase in diameter, and slight warmth of the involved leg. The major risk created by deep vein thrombosis is a **pulmonary embolism,** which results when a piece of a deep vein thrombus breaks free, floats in the bloodstream to the pulmonary circulation, and lodges in a pulmonary blood vessel. As a result, blood flow and oxygen are prevented from reaching the area of lung tissue served by the blocked vessel.

Signs and symptoms of pulmonary embolism include the sudden onset of dyspnea, a cough, sudden chest pain, hemoptysis, tachycardia over 100 beats per minute, and tachypnea over 20 breaths per minute. A pulmonary embolus can be life-threatening and requires immediate emergency action.

Respiratory Effects of Inactivity and Immobility

The lungs function at their best in the upright position. The recumbent position compromises respiratory function and predisposes the client to respiratory complications, such as hypoventilation, atelectasis, stasis of secretions, and altered gas exchange.

Initially, bedrest decreases the body's metabolic need for oxygen. The respiratory rate slows, and the depth becomes shallow. Eventually, immobility causes the respiratory muscles to weaken, which decreases the bellows effect of the bony structures of the chest. Pressure of the mattress against the thorax decreases the respiratory movement of the chest as well. As well, the abdominal contents pushing against the diaphragm decreases the diaphragm's effectiveness in contracting and expanding the lungs.

Immobility also compromises the client's ability to cough—the normal mechanism for moving secretions out of the lungs. With a diminished cough effort, secretions accumulate and block the airways. Dehydration causes the secretions to become thick and tenacious, making them even more difficult to mobilize. Gravity contributes to the stagnation of secretions in the dependent areas of the lungs.

Hypostatic pneumonia is an inflammation of the lungs, caused by stasis of secretions, that becomes a medium for bacterial growth. Signs of pneumonia are thickened yellow sputum, crackles, wheezes, fever, and an increased respiratory rate.

Gastrointestinal Effects of Inactivity and Immobility

Immobility or inactivity slows the basal metabolic rate, slows gastrointestinal motility, and decreases nutrient absorption. These effects are manifested as anorexia, constipation, increased storage of fat and carbohydrates, and negative nitrogen balance.

A client confined to bed may experience a loss of appetite (anorexia) because the metabolic rate slows with rest, thus reducing calorie requirements. With inadequate intake of nutrients, the client feels tired and prefers to sit quietly, becoming more and more inactive. If the client does not eat, muscle and subcutaneous tissue are broken down for energy needs. Changes in the client's nutritional status affect endurance and muscle strength. Loss of energy and tiredness lead to further inactivity and immobility.

Anorexia combined with muscle atrophy can produce a negative nitrogen balance when nitrogen secretion exceeds nitrogen intake. The body begins to break down fat for energy, and the client begins to lose adipose tissue and overall weight. The client may become malnourished, and the skin may become dry and cracked.

Cells cannot be synthesized by bone marrow in the absence of protein. Without enough white blood cells (leukocytes), there is an increased susceptibility to infections. The immune system is less effective in these clients. The red blood cells also decrease, which leads to generalized fatigue, anemia, and poor wound healing. The skin, nails, and hair are also affected and become dull, dry, and brittle. The client loses subcutaneous fat and, thereby, the ability to effectively conserve heat and protect bony prominences.

Fluid intake may also be affected if the client on bedrest is unable to obtain and drink water. A decrease in fluid results in dehydration, which causes constipation, decreased blood volume (decreased cardiac output and orthostatic hypotension), decreased tissue perfusion (skin ulceration and poor wound healing), decreased urine output (oliguria and stasis of urine), and stasis of respiratory secretions.

Hypomotility is decreased peristalsis from lack of stimulation of the gastrocolic reflex. Bowel sounds are faint and slowed. With slowed peristalsis, the transient time of food through the gastrointestinal tract is lengthened, allowing for more water to be absorbed. Thus, constipation and flatulence often accompany bedrest.

For the 1st week after his injury, Mr. Jackson is expected to be either in bed or sitting down with his leg elevated. Do you think constipation could be a problem for him?

Genitourinary Effects of Inactivity and Immobility

Immobility diminishes the function of the kidneys and bladder and results in an increased incidence of urinary stasis, retention, renal calculi, and urinary tract infections. Urinary tract infections are the most prevalent iatrogenic infections in bedridden clients.

The client may also be unable to empty the bladder completely because of the inability to assume a normal voiding position while in bed. The male client with enlargement of the prostate may be unable to urinate in the recumbent position. Retention of urine results in residual urine remaining stagnant in the bladder for a long period. Residual urine leads to bladder distention, reflux of urine to the kidneys, growth of bacteria, and urinary tract infections.

Placing a client in the supine position can prevent urine from draining from the renal pelvis into the ureters. This allows urine to fill up and accumulate in the kidneys and become static. Residual urine becomes an excellent medium for bacteria growth.

Alkaline urine and inadequate personal hygiene further predispose the immobile client to urinary tract infections. The end products of metabolism in an inactive client are generally alkaline because of the decreased muscle activity. The high pH of the urine promotes bacteria growth. Additionally, personal hygiene and perineal care are difficult for the bedridden client. The accumulation of micro-organisms outside the urethra from the anal area encourages bacteria to invade the bladder. Reflux of urine back into the ureters can spread micro-organisms from the bladder into the kidneys. Signs of a urinary tract infection are dysuria (pain or burning sensation on voiding), urgency, frequency, fever, and voiding small amounts.

Stasis of urine and infection increase the risk for calculi (stones or lithiasis) to form in the kidneys, renal pelvis, or urinary bladder. **Renal calculi** are stones formed in the kidney when the excretion rate of calcium or other minerals is high, as when osteoclastic activity releases calcium from the bones during immobility. Calculi can occur after only 1 or 2 weeks of inactivity.

FACTORS AFFECTING ACTIVITY AND MOBILITY

An optimal level of activity may be altered by a myriad of factors affecting the client's ability or desire for mobility. These factors place a client at risk for the complications of disuse.

Pain

The immediate response to pain is to keep quiet. The pain of a broken arm causes the person to immobilize the involved limb. For example, postoperative or cancer pain prevents the client from getting up in bed and freely moving around.

Mr. Jackson, the client in our case study, may limit his activity because of pain. However, his cultural values may influence his response to pain, as described in the Cross-Cultural Care chart.

Therapeutic or Prescribed Inactivity

Although complete bedrest is seldom prescribed, rest aids healing for a variety of problems. For example, rest reduces the workload to allow the heart to heal. Immobilization allows a broken bone, skin, or nerve tissue to regenerate and grow together.

Change in Level of Consciousness

A client who is in a coma or unconscious remains unmoving in bed. An automobile accident that causes a head injury may leave the client immobile. The person who experiences a cerebrovascular accident (stroke) may be unable to move.

Change in Musculoskeletal Functioning

Musculoskeletal disorders often limit mobility. Although paralysis is the most obvious cause, amputation, arthritis, and Parkinson's disease are common causes of impaired mobility. Muscular dystrophy and multiple sclerosis cause the muscles to lose their ability to function.

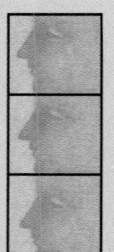

CROSS-CULTURAL CARE
CARING FOR A SOUTHERN AFRICAN-AMERICAN MAN

Mr. Jackson is a 48-year-old African-American man. He is the head of his household and proud to be its breadwinner. He is active in his job as a construction worker, but he gets no other exercise. He eats a Southern diet of eggs, ham, and buttered grits every morning. His wife does all the cooking in the household. Mr. Jackson is slightly overweight but powerfully built.

When Mr. Jackson leaves the hospital, his wife and extended family will take care of him. His wife will "do" everything for him, encouraging him to rest. Although every client is unique, many Southern African-Americans have a tendency to value:

- Matriarchal family structure.
- Male role as decision-maker.
- Large, extended families.
- Strong tradition of religion.

Let's see how this telephone conversation between Mrs. Jackson and her husband's nurse Judy demonstrates sensitivity to their cultural values.

Judy: How can I help you?

Mrs. Jackson: I'm worried about my husband. He won't follow the doctor's orders. He's supposed to stay off his left leg, but he is up all the time. Says he needs to get something or other. What can I do?

Judy: Can you be more specific. How many times has he been up in the last 4 hours?

Mrs. Jackson: Let me see. He got up to go to the bathroom, and then he was in the kitchen getting a drink.

Judy: Is he bearing weight on his leg?

Mrs. Jackson: Yes, he can't use crutches because of his shoulder. He hops around and sometimes puts weight on his injured leg.

Judy: The bones are pinned. Brief partial weight is OK. Why don't you put the things you think he might need next to his chair or bed? Maybe that will help keep him resting.

Critical Thinking Questions

- How did Judy respond to culturally specific needs in the way she handled the phone call with Mrs. Jackson?
- If you were handling the call, would you have asked to speak to Mr. Jackson? Why or why not?

Emotional or Psychological Disturbances

A depressed client may lack the emotional energy to participate in activities of daily living, even to the extent of fixing a meal or getting dressed for the day. Extreme fear may prevent a client from leaving the room or even the house for days.

Chronic Illnesses

Illnesses that cause physiological changes in the body can affect the person's ability or energy to move. Either from fatigue or physical inability, the client remains inactive for a period. For example, anemia from blood loss or renal failure decreases the oxygen-carrying capacity of the blood, and the person experiences severe fatigue.

ASSESSMENT

General Assessment of Activity and Mobility

There are two purposes in assessing the immobile client. One is to detect the risk of complication of immobility. The other is to determine how much assistance the client will need to manage the activities of daily living and prevent complications. Whether the client is in the hospital or at home, risk for complications of immobility should be identified and treated early.

Health History

Assessment begins with gathering data about the client's ability and motivation to be active. You should do the following:

1. Note any medical or surgical conditions that would preclude movement before you attempt to move the client or ask the client to move.
2. Assess for pain that may be limiting movement.
3. Assess the person's ability to understand and follow your instructions for self-care while in bed.
4. Assess any risk factors affecting movement.
5. Assess for *Risk for disuse syndrome.*
6. Determine the client's previous level of functioning to set appropriate goals for care.

The following client questions may be helpful if the client is able to answer questions. Alternatively, you may have some access to information in the medical records and from a family member.

- Describe your usual activities. Are you limited in your exercise or leisure activities because of fatigue, muscle weakness, joint changes, or breathing problems?

- Describe your usual health practices. Nutrition? Elimination? Exercise?
- Have your noticed any sores on your skin? Do you bruise or injure easily?
- Do you have a history of cardiac, gastrointestinal, respiratory, urinary, or skin problems?

When Mr. Jackson returns for his 1-week clinic visit, you ask him all of these questions. What problems would you anticipate in helping him maintain his activities of daily living?

Physical Examination

Assess the client's ability to move in bed. Sometimes you can observe the person moving and make a judgment about how much assistance is needed. Other times you may have to ask the client to move his arms and legs, squeeze your hands, hold a glass, or perform another activity. You can observe the speed of movement, strength, and coordination. As you perform a complete physical examination, you are assessing the person's ability to move. This is one of the reasons your daily assessment in the hospital or assessment in the home setting includes a physical examination.

Focus especially on the musculoskeletal system, including the client's ability to move in bed, his muscle strength, and his muscle tone. Check the range of motion in each joint. Assess the skin carefully; this step is a key element of the physical examination for clients with mobility problems. Examine the skin for lesions and frailty.

Focused Assessment for Risk for Disuse Syndrome

Defining Characteristics

Risk for disuse syndrome is defined as the presence of risk factors. The primary risk factor is immobility. In considering this diagnosis, you will want to assess whether your client is at minimal risk, moderate risk, or high risk for disuse syndrome, as shown in the accompanying decision tree.

Two important criteria for assessing degree of risk include the client's level of inactivity and duration of inactivity. Additionally, the client may experience a combination, such as being maximally inactive for a short, minimal duration. Assessment parameters and interventions should reflect the most aggressive category.

LEVEL OF INACTIVITY

The level of inactivity can be categorized as minimal, moderate, or maximal. A client with minimal inactivity can move about freely within the confines of prescribed rest (in bed or a chair) or in a wheelchair. A client with moderate inactivity can move in the bed or chair but moves slowly, infrequently, or with assistance. A client with maximal inactivity does not move or is incapable of moving in the bed or chair.

DURATION OF INACTIVITY

Duration can also be categorized as minimal, moderate, or maximal. A minimal duration is short and measured in hours. Moderate duration typically means inactivity that lasts for days. Maximal duration typically means inactivity that lasts for weeks, months, or years.

Related Factors

The primary related factors for *Risk for disuse syndrome* are the client's level of inactivity and the duration of inactivity. However, other related factors contribute to the risk as well. If the client has one or more of these factors, you will need to increase the frequency of your assessments and the aggressiveness of the interventions to prevent the complications of disuse syndrome. To help remember these risk factors, use the mnemonic ABCDE, which stands for age, body weight, chronic illness, discomfort, and environment.

Using this method of risk assessment, how would you assess Mr. Jackson's risk for disuse problems?

AGE

Age-related changes occur in all systems, making them more prone to deterioration caused by disuse. For example, an older adult's skin may become dry, fragile, and more easily damaged by shear or pressure. Additionally, the frail elderly adult may be undernourished as a result of not eating balanced meals because of difficulty obtaining or preparing food.

BODY WEIGHT

The decreased defenses of a malnourished client raise the risk of complications from disuse. Reduced levels of red blood cells (anemia) decrease the oxygen available to the tissues, as well as causing generalized fatigue. Reduced levels of white blood cells (leukopenia) decrease the immune system's ability to fight off infections. Breakdown may occur because the skin is less resistant to pressure and shearing forces. Ulcers form more easily in elderly people because of the loss of subcutaneous fat.

The weight of an obese client places excessive pressure on bony prominences and may raise the risk of pressure ulcers. Joint changes stem from the increased weight as well, making mobility difficult. The overweight client experiences increased efforts to breathe, which may cause respiratory changes.

CHRONIC ILLNESS

Many chronic illnesses can increase the risk of complications from disuse. For example, diseases (such as renal failure, cancer, and diabetes) that interfere with metabolic processes increase the risk for disuse complications. Diseases (such as heart disease, respiratory disease, and anemia) that interfere with the transport of oxygen must also be considered. Neurological problems must be added to the list because they commonly decrease mobility.

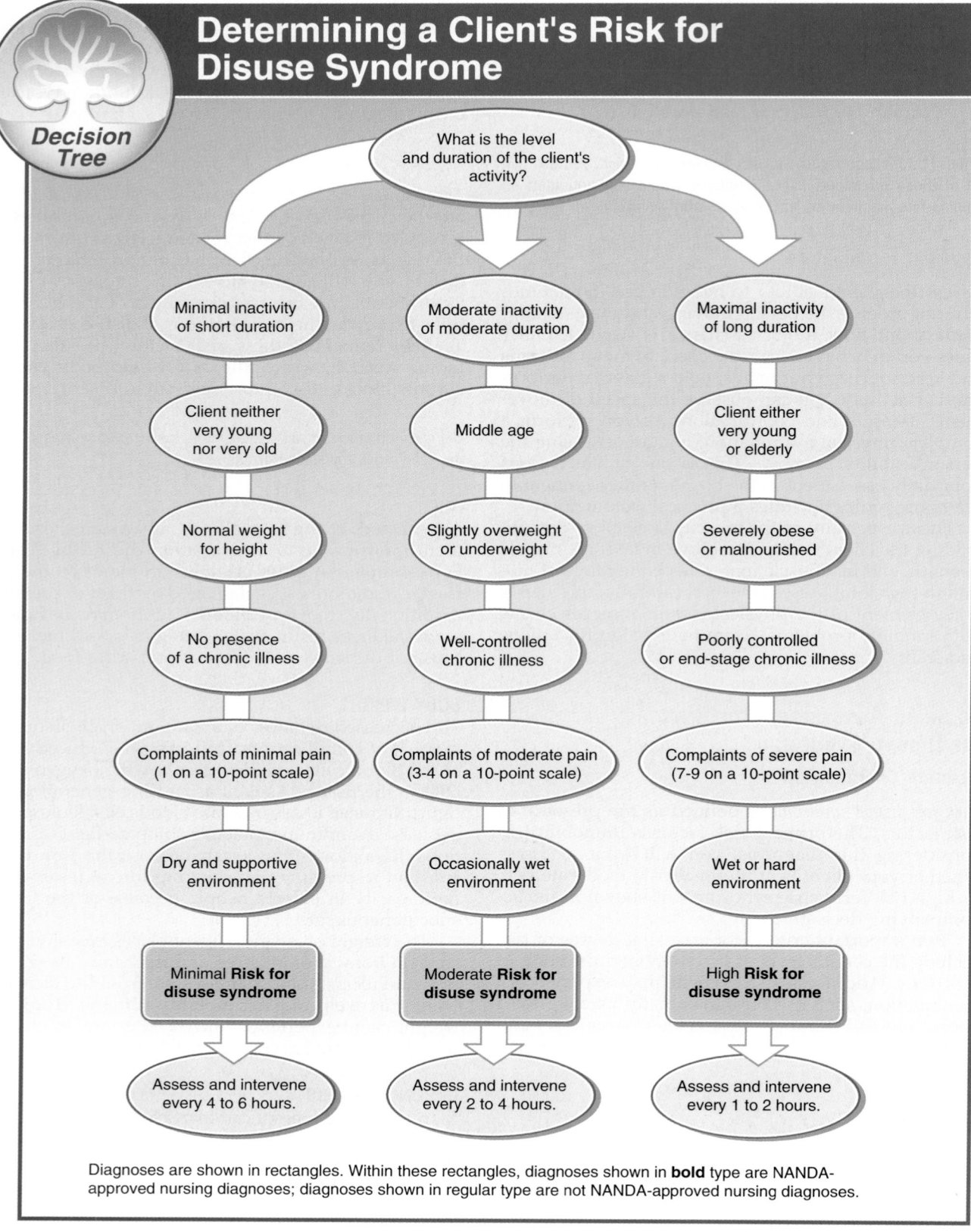

Decision Tree

Determining a Client's Risk for Disuse Syndrome

What is the level and duration of the client's activity?

Minimal inactivity of short duration	Moderate inactivity of moderate duration	Maximal inactivity of long duration
Client neither very young nor very old	Middle age	Client either very young or elderly
Normal weight for height	Slightly overweight or underweight	Severely obese or malnourished
No presence of a chronic illness	Well-controlled chronic illness	Poorly controlled or end-stage chronic illness
Complaints of minimal pain (1 on a 10-point scale)	Complaints of moderate pain (3-4 on a 10-point scale)	Complaints of severe pain (7-9 on a 10-point scale)
Dry and supportive environment	Occasionally wet environment	Wet or hard environment
Minimal **Risk for disuse syndrome**	Moderate **Risk for disuse syndrome**	High **Risk for disuse syndrome**
Assess and intervene every 4 to 6 hours.	Assess and intervene every 2 to 4 hours.	Assess and intervene every 1 to 2 hours.

Diagnoses are shown in rectangles. Within these rectangles, diagnoses shown in **bold** type are NANDA-approved nursing diagnoses; diagnoses shown in regular type are not NANDA-approved nursing diagnoses.

DISCOMFORT

A client in pain typically will be reluctant to move and instead prefer to lie quietly in bed. This compounds the risk of disuse by creating further inactivity. Adequate pain relief can help to offset the effects of this risk factor, especially if relief is attained before a scheduled activity.

ENVIRONMENT

Wrinkled sheets or pillows increase the risk of skin breakdown and ulceration by causing uneven pressure on the skin. Excoriation of the skin occurs when the client is exposed to wound drainage, urine, or feces for long periods. The enzymes and altered pH of the drainage irritate and chemically burn the skin. Constant contact with a bed made wet by perspiration causes maceration of the skin. Hard surfaces increase the interface pressure, causing the skin to become ischemic and necrotic.

Mr. Jackson has moderate inactivity of moderate duration, middle age, normal to slightly increased body weight, no chronic illnesses, minimal discomfort, and low environment risk. These characteristics yield a moderate *Risk of disuse syndrome.* How often should he receive assessment and intervention?

Focused Assessment for Related Nursing Diagnoses

Powerlessness

A client who is confined to bed, paralyzed, or in traction for a broken bone is helpless. All of this person's needs must be met by a nurse or caregiver. Merely needing to use the bathroom or bedpan requires assistance. The client is unable even to get a glass of water to drink. This feeling of loss of control over the basic functions of life can be frustrating and embarrassing.

Risk for Altered Nutrition: Less Than Body Requirements

With a lack of activity, decreased energy, slowed peristalsis, and abdominal distension, an immobilized client often fails to eat an adequate diet. The client complains of not being hungry or of being full too fast. The person may eat only 20 or 30% of the diet. Fluid intake is decreased.

Risk for Fluid Volume Deficit

The inability to obtain fluids or the decreased desire to drink can result in fluid deficits and electrolyte imbalances. A client confined to bed relies on you or another caregiver to provide adequate fluid (see Chapter 31).

Impaired Physical Mobility

Assess the degree to which the client can become mobile. The best prevention for disuse syndrome is to maintain activity (see Chapter 37).

Impaired Skin Integrity

Assess for skin breakdown. A thorough assessment of the skin should be done daily with the bath and change of linen. Additionally, assess the skin each time you change the client's position. Chapter 32 describes pressure ulcers and their treatment.

DIAGNOSIS

The diagnosis of *Risk for disuse syndrome* is a comprehensive way of intervening to prevent deterioration from inactivity. You must differentiate the diagnosis *Risk for disuse syndrome* from *Impaired physical mobility* and *Activity intolerance.* Nursing interventions for *Impaired physical mobility* are directed at increasing the client's ability to move about. Interventions for *Activity intolerance* are focused on the client's endurance in performing activities. However, because immobility and lack of endurance are risk factors for disuse, these two diagnoses are often written as the "related to" phrase.

With inactivity and immobility, the client's list of problems or potential problems may be long. Instead of writing multiple diagnoses to accommodate this list, the diagnosis *Risk for disuse syndrome* ensures a comprehensive approach.

Mr. Jackson would have the nursing diagnosis *Risk for disuse syndrome related to prescribed rest secondary to left knee injury and left clavicle break.*

PLANNING

Whether a client's period of inactivity is short-term or long-term, the expected outcome goal is to prevent complications from inactivity and immobility. The primary prevention strategy is to maintain activity. Expected outcomes for *Risk for disuse syndrome* are as follows. The client will

- Participate in decision-making about his own care
- Have intact skin and mucous membranes
- Maintain full range of motion of joints
- Maintain optimum cardiac and respiratory function
- Maintain optimum patterns of elimination
- Maintain orientation to person, place, and time
- Consume calories and nutrients to meet energy requirements and promote healing
- Maintain contact with the outer world consistent with physical ability

INTERVENTION

The most important nursing intervention to prevent the complications of disuse syndrome is to keep the client as active and mobile as possible.

Interventions to Prevent Musculoskeletal Disuse

You should position and move the client in bed to maintain maximum function of the joints, stimulate circulation, maximize respiration, and prevent skin breakdown.

Maintaining Readiness for Activity

Activity is a priority in preventing the complications of disuse. Make sure that the activity is appropriate to the client's condition and age. Working as a team with the physician, physical therapist, and others, you will implement a plan of progressive activity that may include some or all of the following interventions. If the client has pain, remember to provide pain relief before engaging in these or any activities.

- Perform passive, assisted, or active range-of-motion exercises for all joints in sets of 5 to 10 three times daily. Active range of motion, in which the client moves his limbs rather than having them moved, provides the best level of activity for both muscles and joints.
- A passive range-of-motion machine (Figure 38–4) is prescribed after orthopedic knee or hip surgery to maintain continuous joint motion. Maintain the device at the prescribed speed and degree of joint flexion. Use of continuous passive motion not only maintains range of motion, it actually reduces postsurgical pain.
- Perform range-of-motion exercises against resistance. Foot, ankle, and leg exercises can be done every 1 or 2 hours and before changing from a lying position to a sitting position. These exercises include range of motion for the ankles and toes and pushing the feet against a footboard or the end of bed for about 1 or 2 minutes. A footboard is a board placed at the foot of the bed,

perpendicular to the mattress, to prevent the feet from plantar flexion in the supine or Fowler's position.

- Encourage other isometric exercises. Tell the client to tighten his muscles while in bed or in a chair, especially the abdominal muscles used for bowel elimination and the gluteal and quadriceps muscles used for ambulation. Kegel exercises strengthen the perineum muscles. Teach the client to tighten, hold, and release the perineal muscles 10 times, three times daily. This can be done also during voiding. Remember that isometric exercises help maintain muscle strength but not joint integrity.
- Encourage the client to perform activities of daily living independently, such as the self-care activities of bathing and combing hair. Encourage the client to move independently in bed using the side rails or trapeze.
- With a physician's order, get the client out of bed. While he stands, have the client begin to shift his weight back and forth, rocking on both feet. Have him walk to a chair and sit three times daily. Encourage the client to be in the chair as long as he can tolerate sitting. An initial goal would be 30 to 45 minutes. As possible, have him ambulate with assistance or with an assistive device (such as a walker, cane, or quad cane) four times daily or as much as possible. As the client progresses, encourage him to be up most of the day with ad lib activity.

Action Alert!
Prevent the complications of disuse with an aggressive intervention of progressive activity.

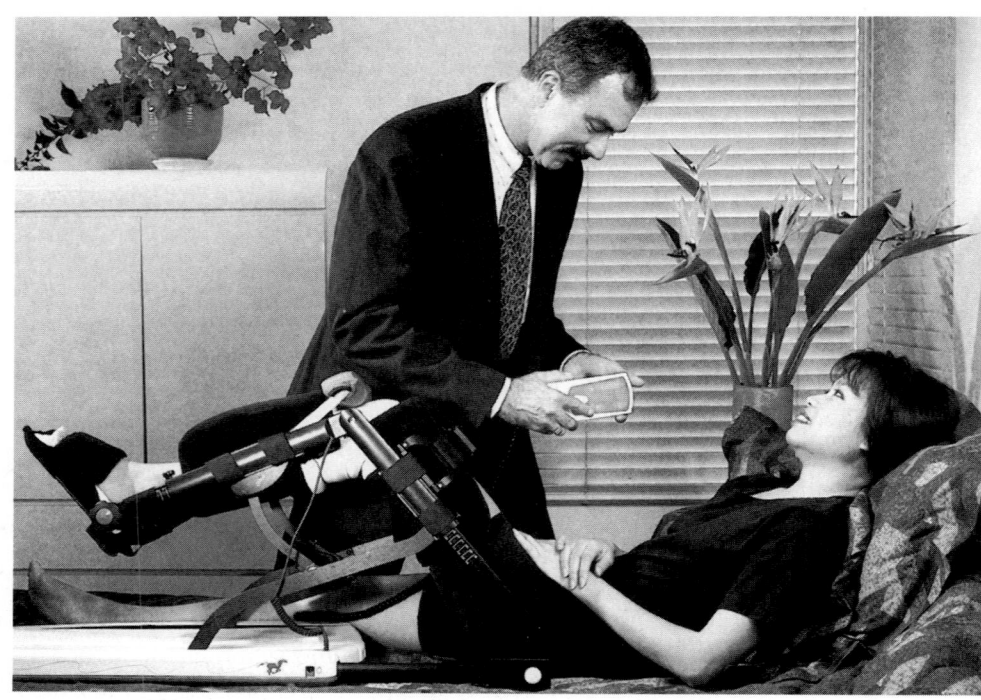

Figure 38–4. A passive range-of-motion, or continuous passive motion, device. (Courtesy of Orthologic, Tempe, AZ.)

Maintaining Body Alignment

While in a bed, chair, or wheelchair (or while walking), the client should be positioned in good body alignment. When positioning a client who is unable to move, position joints in anatomic or functional alignment. Provide support above and below the joint. Alternate positions frequently with side-lying, Sims', semisupine, supine, Fowler's, or prone (Box 38–1).

A*ction* A*lert!*
Perform range-of-motion exercises on each joint to prevent contractures in the client who is immobile. Inactive muscles will contract and become inflexible. The joints will become fixed in a flexed position, making activities of daily living almost impossible to perform.

Change the client's position every 1 to 2 hours throughout the day and night. Make sure that all joints are positioned in extension (neutral) or in a functional position whenever possible and that you have taken proper precautions (Table 38–1). If a joint is in flexion for a period of time, perform active or passive range-of-motion exercises before the next position change. Use positioning devices such as foam boots or high-top tennis shoes, footboards, hand mitts, hand rolls or supports, eggcrate pads, overbed cradles, trochanter rolls, wrist splints, and heel protectors to keep joints in alignment while the client is in bed (Table 38–2).

When the client is sitting in a chair, his head should be up, and the shoulders should be back. The arms should be supported to prevent pulling on the shoulders. Make sure that the feet are resting comfortably on the floor or are elevated on a footstool. When the client walks, he should do so with his head up and facing forward, shoulders back, and feet forward.

Interventions to Prevent Skin Breakdown

Skin care is governed by culture, education, socioeconomic status, religion, and individual preference. You should respect the client's desires while trying to prevent skin complications caused by disuse.

Increasing Circulation

Dilation of blood vessels improves the circulation of oxygen and nutrients to cells in the skin.

Increase the temperature in the room to a comfortable level. Use a bath blanket when bathing the client, and keep the bath water between 105° and 110° F to prevent chilling and vasoconstriction. Gently massage the skin, but avoid areas that are reddened or those over bony prominences. Use long, firm strokes, and move from distal to proximal areas during the bath. Elevate the client's arms on pillows. If the client cannot brush his own hair, offer to do so twice a day. If the client is cold, offer extra blankets, socks, and other warm clothing. Encourage the client to perform his own activities of daily living to increase blood circulation.

Decreasing Micro-organisms

Removing dead skin cells decreases the growth and accumulation of micro-organisms, which can help to prevent skin irritation and infection. Body odor is also reduced. Use mild soap for bathing the client's skin, perineum, and hair. Most clients need to be bathed every day and any time they become soiled. Elderly clients may need only a partial bath of the back and perineum.

If a client is bedridden, a bed bath is indicated. The client can still participate in the bath, however, by performing it as independently as possible. Avoid the use of powder because it holds moisture and may cause pulmonary damage after being inhaled.

Removing Excess Moisture

To help keep the skin dry, make sure that bed linens are breathable cotton, not plastic. Dry the client's skin well after bathing, particularly in areas where the skin folds over on itself, such as at the axillae, under the breasts, and in the perineal area. Change the client's bed linens immediately if they become wet from diaphoresis (sweating) or incontinence. Position the client to allow air to circulate to the axilla and perineal areas.

Remember that, although dry skin discourages the growth of micro-organisms, overly dry skin can crack open and form lesions. To help the skin from becoming too dry, use a moisturizing lotion after baths. Do not use soap every day for bathing. Do not use alcohol on the skin because it has a drying effect and can crack the skin.

While Mr. Jackson's arm is immobilized, his axilla becomes chafed from perspiration. What suggestions would you give him to prevent this problem?

Decreasing Friction and Excoriation

Friction and excoriation can alter the skin's function as a protective barrier. To decrease the risk of friction and excoriation, gently pat the client's skin dry rather than rubbing with a towel after baths. Use a soft washcloth and soft towels during the bath. Linens should be soft and smooth as well.

Use a turning sheet (also called a draw sheet) or trapeze when moving the client in bed. Lift the client, rather than dragging him, when moving him in bed. Use extra help to move the client if needed (Procedure 38–1).

Use protective ointment around wounds or on the client's perineum, as needed. According to the physician's order, change the client's wound dressings frequently. Take care when removing the tape. Place a drainage bag on wounds as needed. Check casts, braces, traction, restraints, and splints for irritation.

Preventing Shear

Placing the head of the bed in a low or flat position reduces the gravitational pull and helps keep the client

BOX 38–1

COMMON CLIENT POSITIONS

Lateral, Semiprone, and Semisupine Positions

In the lateral (side-lying) position, the trunk is at a right angle to the bed. To increase the base of support and comfort, one or both legs are bent, and both arms are extended in front of the body. Because the body weight is borne on the shoulders and hips, the semiprone or the semisupine position is preferred.

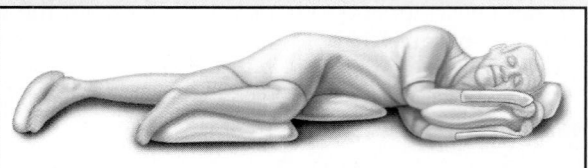

Lateral (side-lying) position.

In the semiprone position (the Sims' or forward side-lying position), the trunk is rotated 15 to 30 degrees forward from the lateral position, with the superior arm and leg supported in front of the body to form part of the base of support.

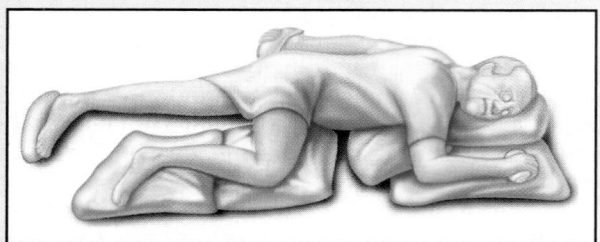

Semiprone (Sims' or forward side-lying) position.

In the semisupine position (the modified lateral or oblique position), the trunk is rotated 15 to 30 degrees from supine, with the superior arm and leg supported in a comfortable position. The semiprone and semisupine positions minimize pressure on prominences of the shoulder and hip.

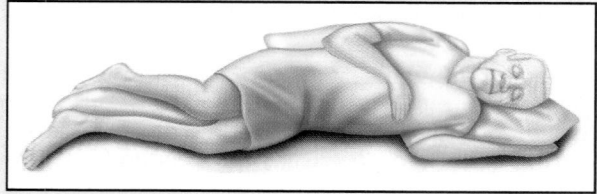

Semisupine (modified lateral or oblique) position, which can be used as a substitute for the side-lying position and results in less pressure on the trochanter area.

Supine and Fowler's Positions

Both the supine and Fowler's positions are back-lying positions. Supine is a horizontal position, and Fowler's is a sitting position. The supine position prevents lordosis or kyphosis.

In high Fowler's position, the head of the client's bed is elevated to 90 degrees. In semi-Fowler's position, it is elevated to 45 degrees. In low Fowler's position, it is el-

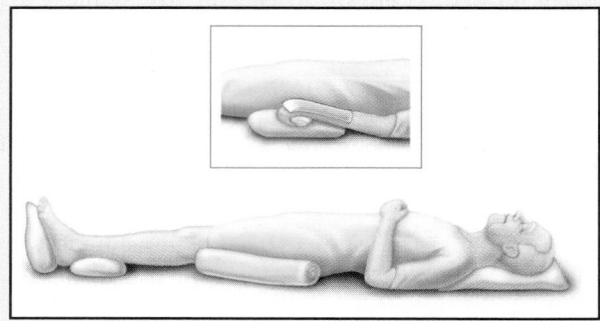

Supine position, including the use of the footboard, trochanter roll, and lumbar support. The inset shows correct positioning of the client's arm, which is elevated and has a wrist support.

evated about 30 degrees. Usually, the client's knees are bent slightly.

Fowler's position concentrates body weight on the sacrum and creates shearing force. Reducing the angle and the time in the position are preventive measures. Prevent hip and knee contractures by instructing the client to shift positions and perform range-of-motion exercises.

Prone Position

In the prone position, the client lies front down with his face turned to the side and one or both arms turned up, as shown. This position may be contraindicated in the presence of abdominal distention or wounds.

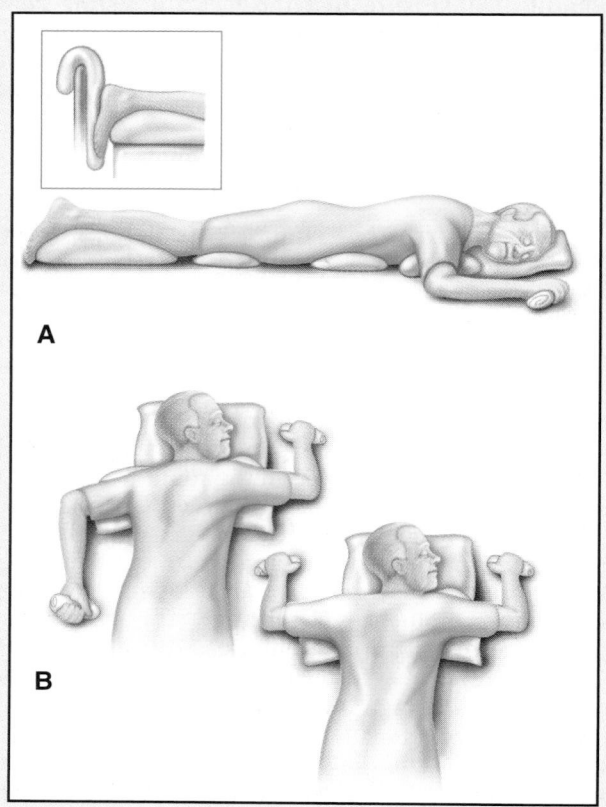

A

B

Prone position. The client's arms and shoulders may be positioned in internal or external rotation.

TABLE 38-1

Precautions for Proper Positioning

Lateral Position, Semiprone Position, Semisupine Position	Supine Position, Fowler's Position	Prone Position
Head and Neck		
• Prevent forward flexion of head, neck, and cervical spine.	• Prevent forward flexion of head, neck, and cervical spine.	• Prevent hyperextension, lateral bending, and pressure on cheek and ear.
• Prevent lateral bending of head, neck, and cervical spine.	• Prevent lateral bending of head, neck, and cervical spine.	
	• Avoid pressure on back of head.	
Shoulders		
• Avoid direct pressure on acromion process.	• Prevent forward flexion.	• Prevent forward flexion of neck.
• Prevent adduction of shoulders.	• Avoid pressure on scapulae.	• Avoid skin-to-skin contact at axillae.
• Avoid skin-to-skin contact at axillae.	• Avoid skin-to-skin contact at axillae by abducting shoulders slightly.	
Breasts and Male Genitalia		
	• Prevent skin-to-skin contact in presence of moisture.	• Avoid abdominal pressure.
Elbows and Wrists		
• Prevent flexion or hyperextension.	• Prevent flexion.	• Prevent flexion by positioning elbows in extension.
• Avoid pressure on thorax and ribs from upper arms.	• Prevent edema.	
• Avoid pressure on lateral condyle of humerus.	• Avoid pressure on elbow.	
• Prevent edema.		
Fingers and Thumb		
• Prevent flexion and opposition of fingers and thumb.	• Prevent flexion and opposition of fingers and thumb.	• Prevent flexion and opposition of fingers and thumb.
Spine		
• Prevent lateral bending.	• Prevent flexion of lumbar spine.	• Prevent hyperextension of lumbar spine by using a firm mattress or lumbar support.
• Prevent rotation.	• Prevent lateral bending (shoulders and hips in alignment).	
	• Avoid pressure on lumbar-sacral area.	
Hips and Knees		
• Prevent adduction, flexion, and internal rotation of upper leg.	• Prevent adduction, flexion, and internal rotation of upper legs.	• Prevent internal rotation.
• Avoid pressure on iliac crest.	• Avoid prolonged flexion.	• Avoid pressure on patella and anterior iliac spine.
• Avoid skin-to-skin contact at perineum.	• Avoid skin-to-skin contact at perineum.	• Avoid skin-to-skin contact at perineum.
	• Avoid compression of popliteal artery.	
Ankles and Toes		
• Prevent inversion and plantar flexion of upper foot.	• Prevent plantar flexion.	• Prevent plantar flexion.
• Avoid pressure on ankle of lower foot.	• Avoid pressure on toes and heels.	• Avoid pressure on toes.

from sliding down in the bed. As a result, it prevents shearing of the skin on the client's lower back. Lifting the client (rather than dragging) and using a turning sheet helps to prevent shear injuries as well. As needed, ask for help when turning or moving a client (see Procedure 38–1). Also, limit the time the client spends in Fowler's position to 30 to 60 minutes. During that time, use a footboard, and support the client's arms on pillows.

Decreasing Pressure

To relieve pressure, turn the client to a new position every 1 to 2 hours. To ensure pressure relief, follow a 24-hour turning schedule (side to back to side to supine). Encourage a client who can sit in a chair to shift his position every 15 minutes or to do push-ups on the arms of the chair.

Text continued on page 1034

TABLE 38–2
Positioning Devices

Device	Description
Foam boots or high-top tennis shoes 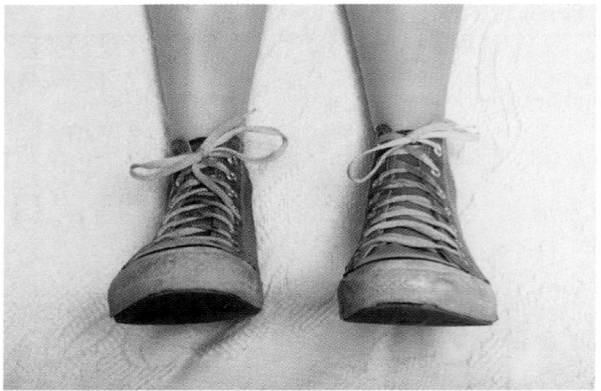	Foam boot or high-top tennis shoe to keep the ankle in dorsiflexion.
Footboard 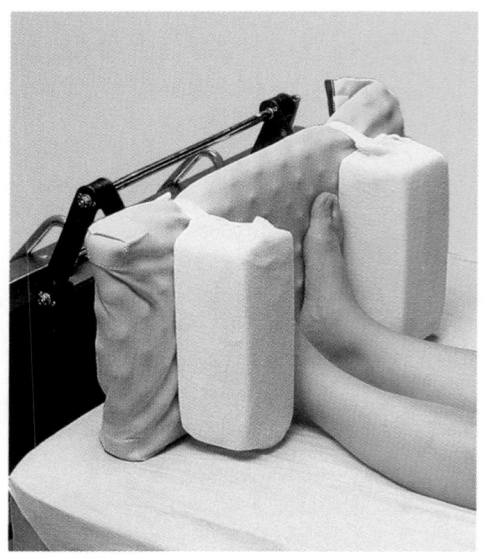 (Courtesy of J.T. Posey Co., Arcadia, CA.)	Board placed at the end of bed, perpendicular to the mattress, to prevent the feet from assuming plantar flexion in the supine or Fowler's position. May be used for isometric exercises of the foot and leg to prevent deep vein thrombosis.
Hand mitt 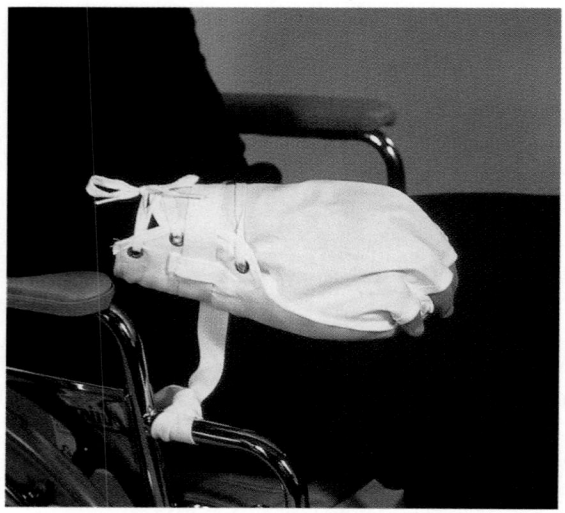 (Courtesy of Medline Industries, Inc., Mundelein, IL.)	Mitten that slides over the fingers to keep the fingers from flexion and the thumb from opposition.

TABLE 38–2 *(Continued)*
Positioning Devices

Device	Description
Hand roll/support	Roll of cloth or manufactured hand grip placed in the palm of the hand used to keep the fingers from flexion and the thumb from opposition.

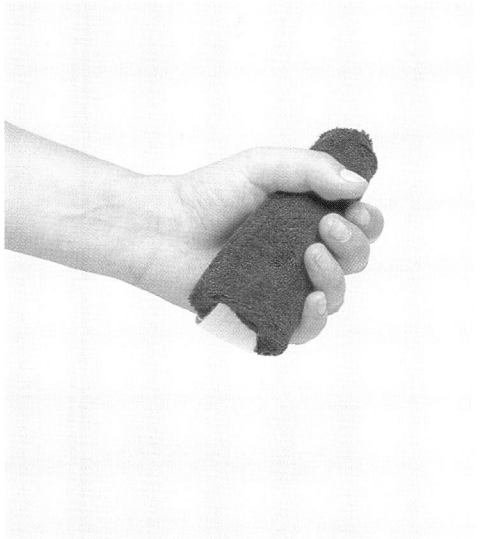

(Courtesy of J.T. Posey Co., Arcadia, CA.)

Eggcrate pad	Pad made of sheepskin or eggcrate foam that is placed on the mattress and used to reduce pressure.

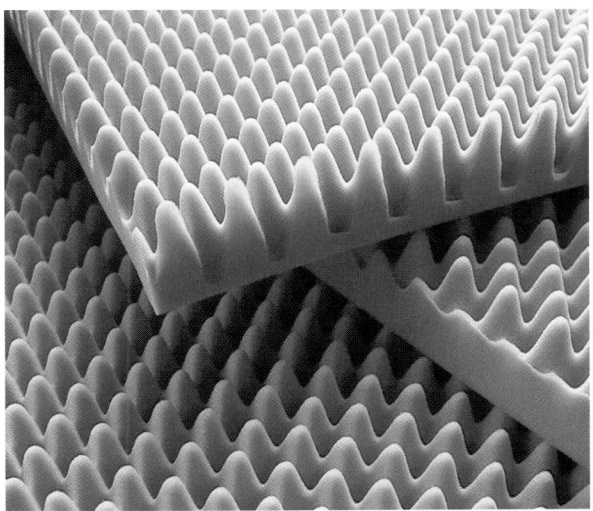

(Courtesy of Medline Industries, Inc., Mundelein, IL.)

Overbed cradle	Device placed at the end of the bed to raise the top sheet and thus prevent pressure ulcers on the toes and plantar flexion of the ankles.

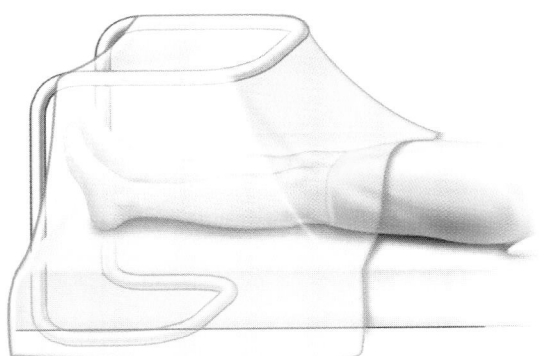

Table continued on following page

TABLE 38–2 *(Continued)*
Positioning Devices

Device	Description
Trochanter roll	Sheet placed halfway under a client's hip and rolled snugly against the hip to prevent external rotation of the trochanter (hip joint).

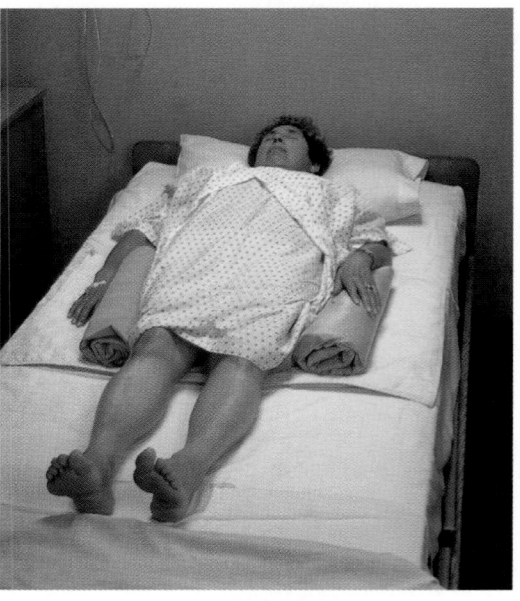

| Wrist splint | Support placed on the client's wrist to prevent flexion. |

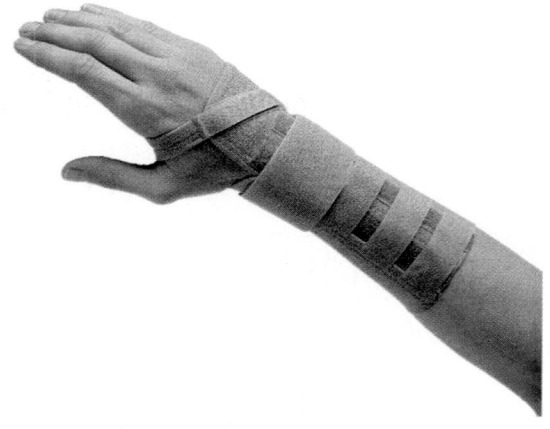

(Courtesy of North Coast Medical, Inc., San José, CA.)

| Heel protectors | Sheepskin or other padded device to prevent skin breakdown at the heels. |

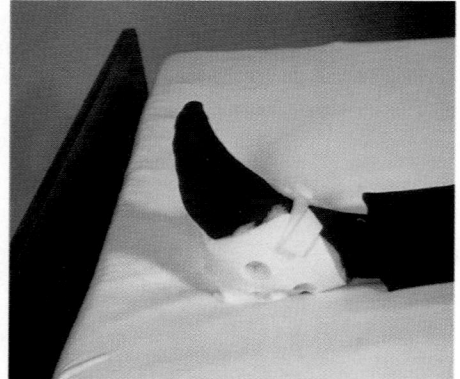

(Courtesy of Medline Industries, Inc., Mundelein, IL.)

Turning and Moving a Client in Bed

TIME TO
ALLOW
▼

Turning
Novice:
10 minutes
Expert:
5 minutes
**Moving
up in bed**
Novice:
10 minutes
Expert:
5 minutes
**Transfer-
ring to a
stretcher**
Novice:
10 minutes
Expert:
5 minutes

Especially for a client with a *Risk for disuse syndrome,* you will need to pay special attention to proper turning and positioning. Often, you will perform these activities on a schedule tailored to the client's condition and needs. Each time, you must follow appropriate steps to avoid injuring your client or yourself. This procedure describes proper methods for turning a client in bed (alone or with another nurse), moving a client up in bed (alone or with another nurse), and transferring a client from bed to stretcher.

Delegation Guidelines

The routine positioning and repositioning of a client in bed may be delegated to a nursing assistant. For clients with mobility or positioning restrictions, however, you must first assess the client and then determine the appropriateness of delegation based on risk to the client. For a client requiring multiple personnel for turning and moving, you may perform the procedure together with multiple nursing assistants.

Equipment Needed

- Turning sheet.
- Pillows or wedges for positioning.
- Trapeze.
- Transfer board.

Before turning or moving a client in bed or transferring him to a stretcher, lock the bed's wheels and assess the client's condition.

a. Can the client assist with turning, moving, or transferring?

b. Do any joints have contractures or need special handling?

c. Can the client tolerate having the head of the bed lowered briefly?

d. Can you turn or move the client alone, or will you need help from colleagues?

Turning or moving a client alone requires that you be sure you can manage the client's weight. If the procedure requires two or three nurses, one should take charge of the procedure.

Turning a Client Alone

1 Lower the head of the bed and the knee gatch until the bed is flat.

You will be better able to handle the client's weight on a flat surface. Also, the flat position allows you to avoid moving uphill against gravity.

2 Move the client to one side of the bed.

This allows room to turn the client to the opposite side.

a. First, slide your arms under the client's shoulders and back, and move the client's upper body to one side of the bed.

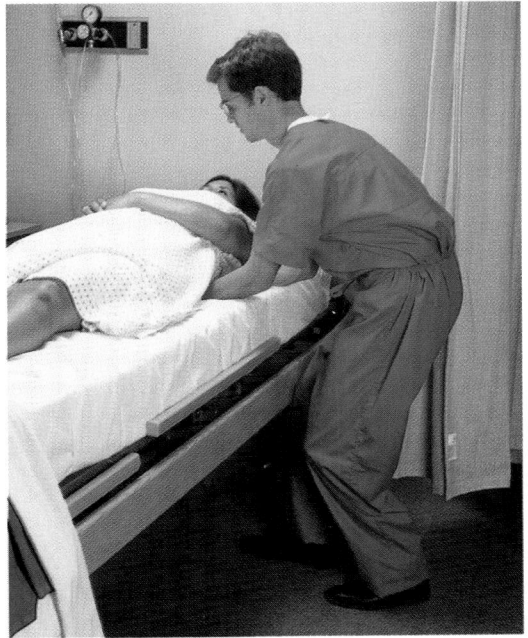

Sliding the arms under the client's shoulders and back.

Continued

Turning and Moving a Client in Bed

b. Then, slide your arms under the client's hips, and slide the hips to the side.

c. Finally, move the client's feet and legs to the side of the bed.

---

3 Cross the client's arms across the chest, and cross the legs at the ankle. Position a pillow or wedge at the head or foot of the bed to be used behind the client's back after turning.

Crossing the client's arms and legs helps the body turn as a unit.

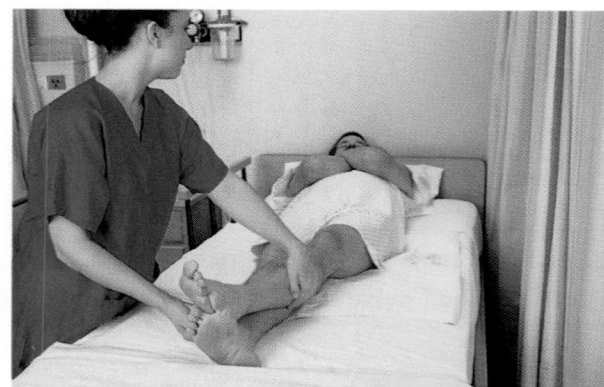

Crossing the client's arms and legs.

---

4 Place one hand on the client's shoulder and the other hand on the client's hip, and roll the client toward you.

Pulling is easier than pushing.

---

5 Turn the client far enough forward so you can release one hand and position a pillow or wedge behind the client's back.

---

6 You may need to go to the opposite side of the bed and pull the client's hips toward the center of the bed to make the position more stable. Check the position according to Table 38–1.

Turning a Client With Another Nurse

1 With the bed in a flat position, move the client to one side of the bed.

This allows room to turn the client to the opposite side.

a. If the client is on a turning sheet (a sheet that extends from the shoulders to below the hips), stand on opposite sides of the bed so that each nurse can grasp the top and bottom of the sheet.

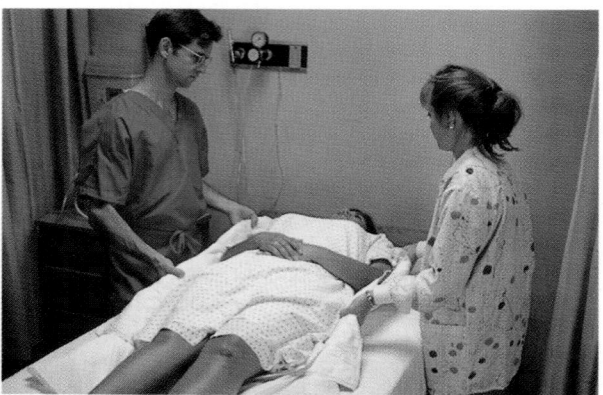

Two nurses grasping the top and bottom of a turning sheet.

b. If the client is not on a turning sheet, both nurses should stand on the same side of the bed. One nurse should slide her arms under the client's shoulders while the other slides her arms under the client's hips. On the count of three, both nurses should slide the client to one side of the bed.

When turning a client, make sure you stand with your knees somewhat bent and your feet spread so you have a wide base of support.

---

2 Bend the client's knee on the opposite side to which you will be turning. Fold the client's arms over the chest. One nurse is positioned on each side of the bed.

---

3 Turn the client.

a. If you do not have a turning sheet, the nurse positioned on the side of the bed toward which the

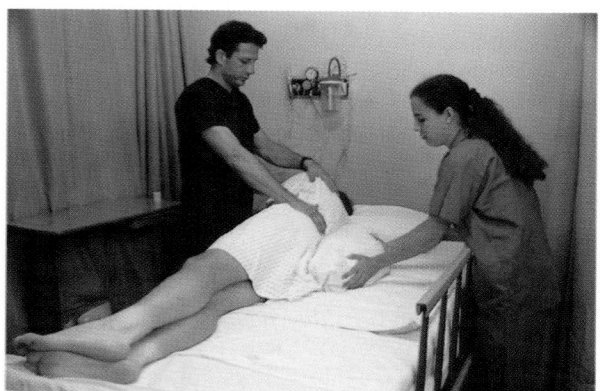

Placing a pillow at the client's back.

client will turn should place one hand on the client's shoulder and one hand on the client's hip. He then pulls the shoulder and hip toward himself. At the same time, the nurse on the opposite side of the bed slides her hands under the client's bottom hip, pulls the hip toward her, and places a pillow at the client's back.
b. If you have a turning sheet, use it to pull the client's hips and shoulders in the direction of the turn.

4 Place a pillow between the client's legs.
The pillow at the back supports the client in the side-lying position. The pillow between the legs maintains alignment of the spine and prevents skin-to-skin contact.

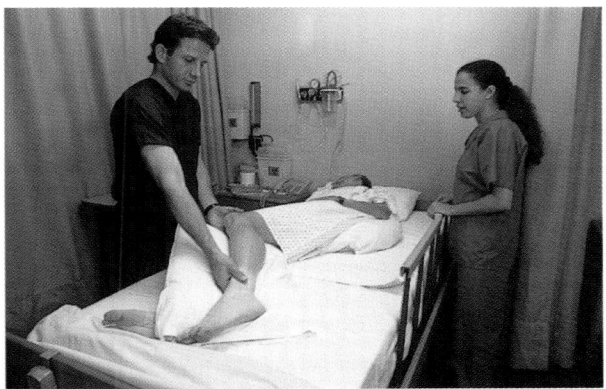
Placing a pillow between the client's legs.

5 Check the client's position against Table 38–1 to make sure that the client is properly positioned.

6 If the client's condition demands that you maintain anatomic alignment of the spine during turns, you may need three nurses working together to turn the body and head as a unit. The spine is kept straight as the client is turned.

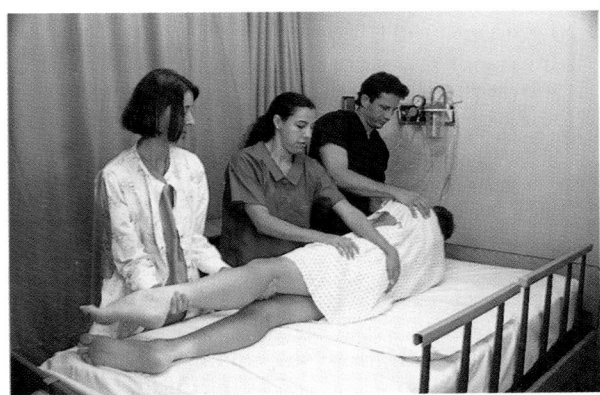
Keeping the spine straight as the client is turned.

7 After turning a client, make sure to document that the client was turned. Also document the position assumed.
Proper documentation helps to maintain continuity of care. The next nurses to work with the client will know what positions have been used and the amount of time in the position.

Moving a Client up in Bed

1 Before moving a client up in bed, determine whether you can do it alone or whether you need help from another nurse. If you can do it alone, determine whether to stand at the side of the bed or the head of the bed.
If the client is very light in weight, you can assist from the side of the bed. For heavier clients, position yourself at the head of the bed.

a. For one nurse to move the client up in bed from the side of the bed, have the client bend her knees and place her feet flat on the bed so she can push. Place one hand under the client's back and one under the thighs, close to the hips. Tell the client to push with her legs on a count of three. When she does, slide the client up toward the head of the bed.

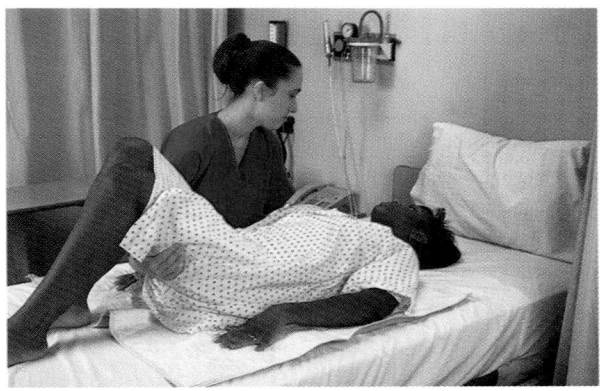
One nurse assisting a client to move up in bed from the side of the bed.

b. For one nurse to move the client from the head of the bed, start by removing the headboard from the bed. Place the bed in a slight Trendelenburg position (head lower than the feet). Slide your hands under the client's shoulders, and pull the client toward you. If possible, use a turning sheet to perform this maneuver.

Continued

PROCEDURE 38–1 *(continued)*

Turning and Moving a Client in Bed

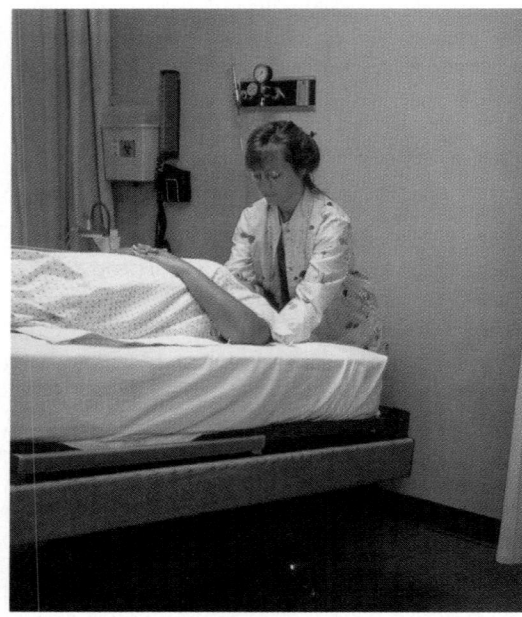

One nurse assisting a client to move up in bed from the head of the bed, using the force of gravity created by a slight Trendelenburg position.

2 If the client has good upper body strength, use a trapeze to move her up in bed.
a. Place a trapeze over the bed.
b. Have the client bend her knees and place her feet flat on the bed so she can push.
c. Have the client hold onto the trapeze and pull with her arms to lift her hips slightly off the bed.
d. With hips lifted, have the client push with her legs to move up in bed.
e. You may assist by placing your hands under the client's thighs, close to the hips.

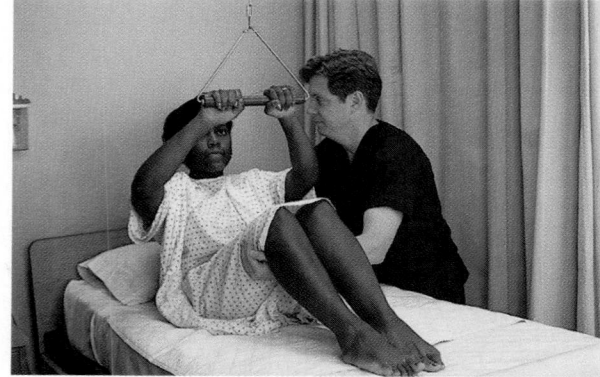

One nurse assisting a client to move up in bed using a trapeze.

3 If the client is too heavy to move her by yourself, solicit help from a colleague.
a. Stand on opposite sides of the client's bed.
b. With the client's knees bent and feet flat on the bed, each nurse grasps the turn sheet with one hand at the level of the shoulders and the other hand at the level of the hips.
c. On the count of three, the client pushes with his legs as the two nurses slide his torso up in bed.

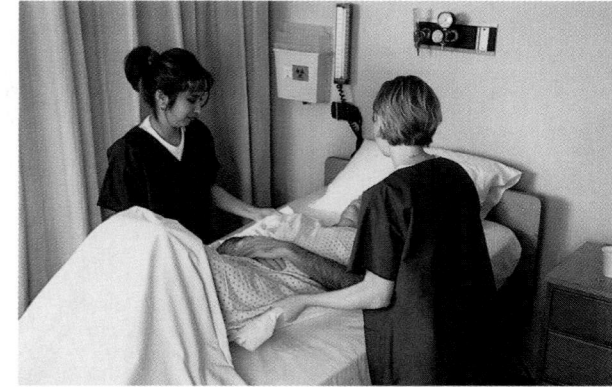

Two nurses assisting a client to move up in bed.

4 After moving the client up, raise the head of the bed, and check the position against Table 38–2.

5 Document that the client was repositioned and the position assumed.

Moving a Client From a Bed to a Stretcher

1 If a client is unable to move from the bed to a stretcher on his own, you will need to move him.
a. At least two nurses should be positioned on each side of the stretcher.
b. If the client is unconscious, a fifth nurse should stand at the top of the stretcher to support the client's head, and a sixth should stand at the bottom to support the client's feet.
   Make sure the wheels are locked on both the bed and the stretcher. Position the bed and stretcher next to each other without any gaps in between.

2 Use a sheet to make the transfer easier.
a. Untuck the sheet from the client's bed.
b. Have one nurse grasp the sheet under the client's shoulders while another on the same side grasps

it at the client's hips and legs. The nurses on the opposite side of the bed should do the same.

c. On a count of three, the nurses on the stretcher side should lift and pull the client onto the stretcher. The nurses on the opposite side of the bed provide minimal assistance because it is more difficult to push than pull.

3 As an alternative, use a transfer board.
a. Two nurses standing on the same side of the bed turn the client away from the stretcher.
b. Place the transfer board where the client was lying, and turn the client back onto the board.

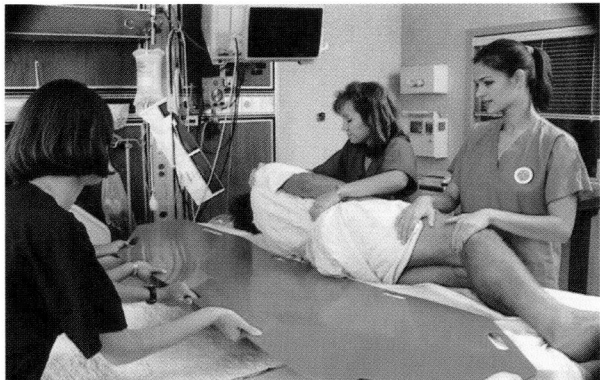

Placing the transfer board where the client was lying.

c. Pull the board onto the stretcher with the client on it.
d. Turn the client again to remove the board.

4 Raise the side rails on the outside of the stretcher, then move between the bed and stretcher and raise the remaining side rails.

5 If the stretcher cannot be positioned adjacent to the bed, but can be positioned at a right angle to the bed, use a three-person lift to transfer the client.
a. Position three nurses on the same side of the bed.
b. One nurse slides her hands and arms under the client's head and shoulders. The second slides his hands under the client's back and buttocks, and the third one slides her hands under the legs and thighs. On the count of three, the nurses simultaneously lift the client.

In this procedure, each nurse bears only a third of the client's weight.

c. The three nurses then walk as a unit to rotate and carry the client to the stretcher.

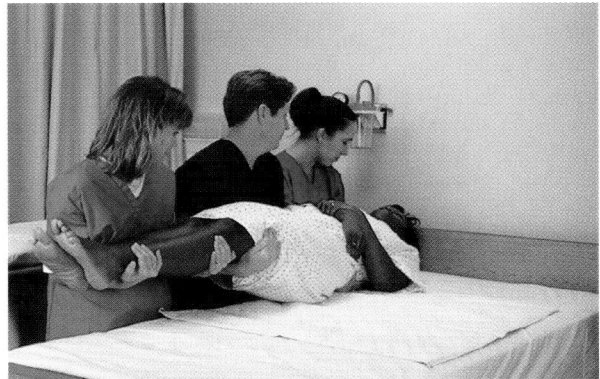

Moving a client from a stretcher to a bed using a three-person lift.

6 Cover the client with a sheet. Supply a pillow, and raise the head of the stretcher if needed for the client's comfort. Fasten a safety strap over the client. It can be fastened loosely if the client is fully alert. Put side rails up.

HOME CARE CONSIDERATIONS

Work closely with family caregivers to teach methods of turning and methods of preventing back strain in the caregiver. The family must understand the importance of a regular schedule of turning, even through the night. A single caregiver is not sufficient to provide care around the clock to a family member who is unable to turn and move in bed. All family members must understand the importance of skin integrity and agree to participate in maintaining it. Families must also understand that pressure ulcers can form in a chair or wheelchair; the client must periodically shift weight to relieve pressure.

*A*ction *A*lert!
Turn the client on bedrest every 1 to 2 hours, keep the bed dry and wrinkle-free, and keep the client dry to help prevent pressure ulcers.

If needed, have the client set a timer so he remembers to shift his weight. Remember that standard mattresses exert considerable pressure against the skin. As needed, use a special mattress to reduce the pressure, such as an eggcrate, foam, sheepskin, gel, flotation, or waterbed. Keep the bed linens and pillows free of wrinkles.

Interventions to Maintain Circulatory Function

Interventions are needed to maintain the circulatory status and prevent complications.

Decreasing Edema Formation

Unless contraindicated, the client's legs should be elevated to counteract gravity and assist with venous return. This position can prevent dependent edema formation and can reduce edema if present. Keep the client's legs at heart level while he is in bed. Place his feet on a footstool while he sits in a chair. Elevate his arms to prevent edema formation or decrease edema in his hands.

Decreasing Blood Stasis

Elastic antiembolism stockings and sequential compression devices can be used to apply external pressure on the client's legs to prevent blood from pooling in the veins. These devices, with the assistance of the calf muscles, "milk" venous blood back up to the heart. They decrease blood stasis and prevent the formation of thrombi and edema.

Antiembolism stockings are elasticized stockings that provide varying degrees of pressures at different areas of the leg. To provide the optimum amount of pressure, the stockings should fit properly and be free of wrinkles. You should periodically inspect the feet for evidence of poor circulation and remove the stockings two to three times daily to inspect the skin (Procedure 38–2).

Leg exercises can supplement the effect of antiembolism stockings in preventing venous stasis. One exercise that can be done by most clients is to flex and extend the foot five times per hour. A second exercise is to bend the knee and draw the foot up to the thigh, then extend the leg again. A third exercise is to raise the leg off the bed, one leg at a time. These exercises can be active or passive.

Sequential compression devices are plastic sleeves that are wrapped around the client's legs. The sleeves have air tubes that are inflated in sequence from the bottom of the leg to the top, helping to move venous blood out of the leg veins and toward the heart (Procedure 38–3). Once the client can ambulate, the device is discontinued.

Avoiding Compression of Leg Vessels

Avoiding compression of leg veins maintains blood flow and prevents venous stasis. To avoid compressing the leg vessels, teach the client not to cross his legs at the knee, either while in bed or sitting in a chair. Also teach the client to avoid tight knee socks or garters.

Also, do not routinely use the knee gatch on the client's bed or pillows behind the client's knees because they could put pressure on the popliteal artery at the back of the knee. If you use pillows under the client's legs, use them to support the entire length of the leg, not just under the knee. Assess the client's antiembolism stockings frequently to make sure they have not rolled down.

Encouraging Correct Breathing

Pressure changes in the thorax during inspiration pulls blood into the inferior vena cava, thus promoting venous return. If the client holds his breath and bears down, blood is unable to return to the heart and can cause decreased blood pressure and cardiac disturbances. When the client moves in bed, instruct him to breathe out through his mouth rather than holding his breath. He can also use an overbed frame, a trapeze, or the bed's side rails when changing positions or moving in bed.

Preventing Orthostatic Hypotension

Providing the client with a planned program of gradual adjustment to vertical positioning reconditions the baroreceptors and helps in stabilizing blood pressure. Have the client perform foot and leg exercises for 1 to 2 minutes before beginning any position change. If he has been lying flat for a long time, elevate the head of the bed for 15 minutes three times daily for a few days before sitting the client up or getting him out of bed. When you do sit him up, let his feet dangle over the edge of the bed for a few minutes until he is not dizzy or lightheaded before standing.

*A*ction *A*lert!
If a client is experiencing orthostatic hypotension, return him to the sitting position, and take his blood pressure. Do not leave the client because he may fall. The dizziness, fainting, and lightheadedness experienced on standing usually resolve within a few minutes.

If the client experiences severe hypotension after a prolonged time in the supine position, a physical therapist may need to use a tilt table for position changes.

Interventions to Maintain Respiratory Function

Without enough oxygen, the client does not have the endurance to be active. Interventions aim to maximize respiratory function by encouraging lung expansion and mobilizing secretions.

PROCEDURE 38–2

Applying Antiembolism Stockings

TIME TO
ALLOW
▼
Novice
20 minutes
Expert:
10 minutes

Antiembolism stockings increase venous return, decrease venous stasis, and decrease dependent edema by applying external pressure to the lower legs. They are used to prevent deep vein thrombosis.

Delegation Guidelines

The application and maintenance of antiembolism stockings may be delegated to a nursing assistant who has been properly trained in this skill. Periodic removal of the stockings and inspection of the skin may be delegated to the nursing assistant, with specific attention to findings that necessitate immediate RN notification.

Equipment Needed

- Measuring tape.
- Calf-length or thigh-length antiembolism stockings of correct size.

1 Place client supine in bed with his legs horizontal for 15 minutes.

This prevents blood from pooling in the legs.

2 Measure the client's legs to determine the correct stocking size.
a. If the client will wear calf-length stockings, measure calf circumference and the distance from the foot to the knee.
b. If the client will wear thigh-length stockings, measure calf and thigh circumference and the distance from the foot to the thigh.

Determining the correct size ensures that the client will receive firm support but no restriction of the circulation.

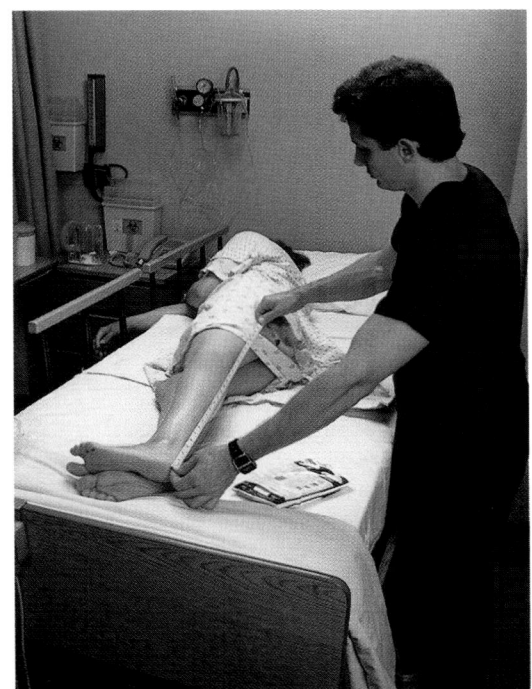

Measuring foot-to-thigh distance.

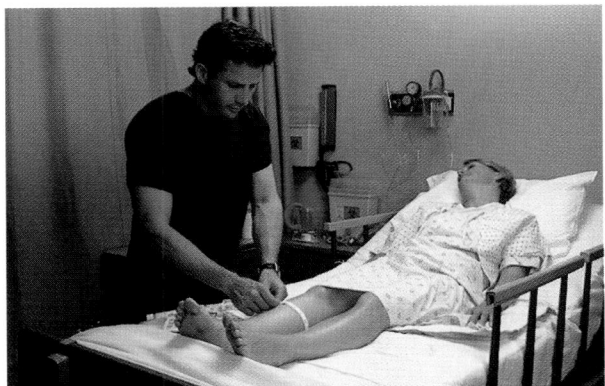

Measuring calf circumference.

Continued

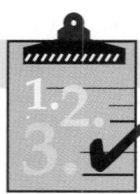

Applying Antiembolism Stockings

3 Place a stocking on the client's foot.

a. Gather or roll the stocking approximately to the ankle.

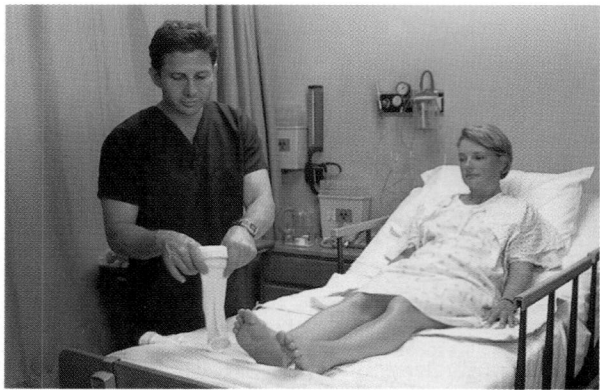

Gathering the stocking to the ankle.

b. Slide it on the foot and ankle.

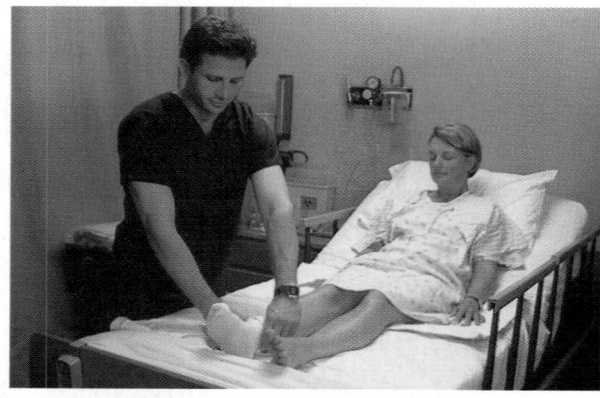

Sliding the stocking onto the foot and ankle.

c. Make sure the hole is on the bottom of the client's foot.

Gathering the stocking allows easier application over the foot. The hole allows you to check circulation in the client's toes.

4 Pull the stocking firmly up the client's leg, smoothing wrinkles as you work.

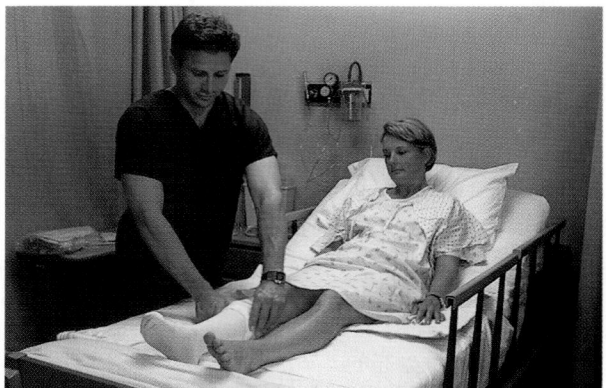

Pulling the stocking firmly up the leg.

5 Check the client's toes for pressure.

Pull the stocking away from the toes to release pressure on them.

6 As an alternative, turn the stocking inside-out down to the ankle. Turn it right-side out as you work the stocking up the leg. Avoid leaving tight bands that could restrict the circulation as you work the stocking over the ankle and up the leg.

7 Repeat with the other leg.

8 Assess the client to make sure the stockings are functioning properly.

a. Make sure the stockings have no wrinkles

Wrinkles can cause uneven pressure and ulcerations.

b. Prevent the stockings from rolling down.

Rolls create a tourniquet effect that decreases arterial blood flow and impedes venous return.

c. Remove the stockings at bath times and before bed to provide skin care and a more complete assessment.

Assess the skin for temperature, color, capillary refill, pulses, redness, irritation, or lesions. Ask whether the client feels any tingling or numbness.

9 Document the size and length of the stockings, the time they were applied, the condition of the client's skin, any client complaints, and times the stockings were removed and reapplied.

HOME CARE CONSIDERATIONS

For clients at risk for thrombophlebitis, antiembolism stockings should be worn at home. Suggest that the client keep two pair on hand so she can wash one pair (in mild soap, by hand) while wearing the other pair.

PROCEDURE 38–3

Using a Sequential Compression Device

TIME TO
ALLOW
▼
Novice:
15 minutes
Expert:
*7.5
minutes*

A sequential compression device creates waves of external pressure that move from distal to proximal areas of the legs. By doing so, the device enhances venous return, decreases venous stasis, and prevents deep vein thrombosis. Typically, you will use a sequential compression device with a bedridden client who is at high risk for thrombosis.

Delegation Guidelines

The application and maintenance of a sequential compression device may be delegated to a nursing assistant who has been properly trained in this skill. Periodic removal of the device to promote mobility or inspection of the skin may be delegated to the nursing assistant, with specific attention to findings that necessitate immediate RN notification.

Equipment Needed

- Antiembolism stockings of the correct size.
- Tape measure.
- Sequential compression sleeves.
- Compression controller.

---

1 Place the client in a supine position with her legs horizontal.
This keeps blood from pooling in the legs.

2 Apply antiembolism stockings.
Antiembolism stockings protect the legs from overheating and sustaining skin damage. Cotton also absorbs excess moisture from the skin, helping to prevent maceration.

3 Measure the circumference of the client's upper thigh.
This ensures that the device is the correct size.

4 Open the inflatable sleeve on the flat bed, cotton-side up, and place the client's leg on the sleeve.

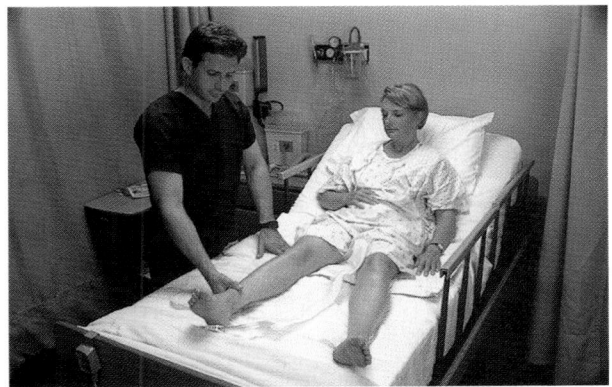

Placing the client's leg on the sleeve.

Avoid positioning the sleeve so it places direct pressure on the popliteal artery. Also, avoid positioning it in a manner that could cause skin breakdown on the client's ankle.

5 Wrap the sleeve snugly around the client's leg, beginning with the side that does not contain tubes. Fasten the sleeve closed with the Velcro fasteners.

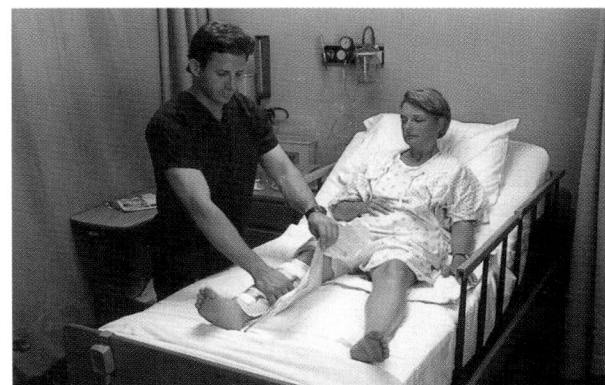

Wrapping the sleeve snugly around the client's leg.

Make sure you can fit two fingers between the sleeve and the client's skin. If the sleeve is too loose, it will function less effectively. If it is too tight, it could cause skin breakdown, compression of the arteries, and neurological changes.

6 Connect the tubing on the sleeve to the compression controller.

Continued

PROCEDURE 38–3 *(continued)*

Using a Sequential Compression Device

7 Follow the physician's orders in setting the controller to the correct amount and time of compression. After turning it on, observe to make sure the unit is working properly.

8 Remove the client's antiembolism stockings three times daily, and perform skin care during this time.

Assess for skin breakdown and pressure ulcers. Examine the toes for arterial changes, such as coolness, pallor, and decreased capillary refill. Ask whether the client feels tingling or numbness.

9 Document the date and time the sleeves were applied or removed. Also, document your assessment findings.

Encouraging Lung Expansion

To help maximize your client's lung expansion, elevate the head of the bed to 45 or 90 degrees (Fowler's or high Fowler's position). Support the client's arms on pillows. Remind the client to perform deep breathing 10 times every 2 hours while awake. If necessary, have the client use an incentive spirometer 10 times every 2 hours while awake. Reposition the bedridden client every 2 hours. With a physician's order, begin progressive activity and ambulation as soon as possible.

Mobilizing Secretions

Thin, watery secretions are easier to expectorate than thick, sticky sputum. Drinking 2,000 to 3,000 mL of fluid daily can help keep secretions more liquid. A forceful cough is the most effective method for removing sputum. For a more effective cough, the client can be taught cascade coughing or huff coughing. Coughing should be done five times every 2 hours.

Regular position changes can help to mobilize secretions as well by using the pull of gravity. Turn the client every 1 to 2 hours. Also, perform chest physiotherapy and postural drainage two or more times daily. Humidify the client's inspired air. As needed, obtain an order for aerosol therapy and a liquefying inhaler medication.

EVALUATION

Risk for disuse syndrome is the nursing diagnosis used to keep the body systems healthy if the client's activity status is suddenly altered. Interventions are implemented to prevent the complications of disuse from occurring, as suggested in the accompanying Nursing Care Planning chart. For a more specific and complete list of interventions for each of the nursing diagnosis and collaborative problems, consult the appropriate chapter in this book.

Evaluation of outcomes should be done on a daily basis. Because this a "Risk" diagnosis, achievement of the health outcomes occurs if no problems develop. If the outcome is not met because a problem does occur, add the appropriate nursing diagnosis. For example, if the client experiences deterioration of the psychosocial system, the appropriate additional nursing diagnosis might be *Anxiety, Altered role performance, Self-care deficit, Powerlessness, Self-esteem disturbance, Sensory/ perceptual alterations,* or *Diversional activity deficit.*

If the client experiences deterioration of nutrition and metabolism, you might add *Altered nutrition: Less than body requirements, Risk for infection,* or *Risk for fluid volume imbalance.* If the client experiences deterioration of the skin you might add *Impaired skin integrity, Risk for infection,* or *Impaired tissue integrity.* If the client experiences deterioration of the musculoskeletal system, you might add *Impaired physical mobility, Activity intolerance, Self-care deficit,* or *Risk for injury.* If the client experiences deterioration of the cardiovascular system, you might add *Altered tissue perfusion, Activity intolerance,* or the collaborative problems orthostatic hypotension, deep vein thrombosis, pulmonary embolism, or decreased cardiac output.

If the client experiences deterioration of the respiratory system, you might add *Ineffective breathing pattern, Ineffective airway clearance, Impaired gas exchange,* or the collaborative problems atelectasis or pneumonia. If the client experiences deterioration of the gastrointestinal system, you might add *Constipation* or *Incontinence.* And if the client experiences deterioration of the genitourinary system, you might add *Altered urinary elimination, Bowel incontinence,* or *Risk for infection.*

KEY PRINCIPLES

- Disuse syndrome refers to clients at risk for deterioration of body systems from inactivity and immobility.
- Short periods of rest are beneficial.
- Prolonged inactivity causes behavioral changes of anger, hostility, loneliness, and social isolation.

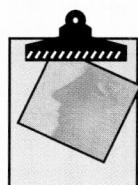

NURSING CARE PLANNING
A CLIENT WITH WORK-RELATED INJURIES

Admission Data

Mr. Jackson is a 48-year-old African-American male who presents to the emergency room following an injury on the job. The emergency department physician diagnoses a compound fracture of the left tibia and a fractured left clavicle. Mr. Jackson is taken to the operating room where the bone fragments are pinned and a stabilizing device applied. Mr. Jackson is sent home to rest, elevate the left leg, and apply an ice pack to his knee. He has a sling to prevent him from moving his left arm. He is to return to the orthopedic clinic in 1 week.

Physician's Orders	Apply ice pack to left knee for 20 minutes every 4 hours.	Fill prescription for pain medication.
	No weight bearing on left leg.	Do not use left arm and keep in sling at all times (including sleeping) except for bathing.
	Return to clinic in 1 week.	Elevate left leg 90% of the time.

Nursing Assessment

Vital signs were temperature 98.4°F, pulse 88, respirations 16, BP 136/86. All WNL for him. He appears in minimal distress. C/o pain in his left knee (4 out of 10-point pain scale) and in his left shoulder (8 of 10). Toes pink, good capillary refill, and movement. Unable to perform ROM on his left shoulder.

NURSING CARE PLAN

Nursing Diagnosis	Expected Outcomes	Interventions	Evaluation (At Home After 24 Hours of Care)
Risk for disuse syndrome related to prescribed rest secondary to left knee injury and left clavicle break	Muscles will remain strong, without contractures.	Encourage right arm and leg exercises against resistance three times daily.	No evidence of muscle changes in upper or lower extremities.
	Unaffected joints will have full ROM.	Encourage full ROM for right arm and leg at least three times daily. Keep left shoulder immobilized.	Mr. Jackson has full ROM in right arm and leg. Left shoulder is immobilized with sling. Pain is 3 on a scale of 10. Left knee is still slightly swollen but not red. Movement is painful (2 of 10) on flexion and limited.
	Skin will be free of irritation, redness, ulceration, or edema. *Black skin needs to be palpated for increased heat over bony prominences.*	Inspect skin under sling, around pins, back, and sacrum twice daily. Teach client to shift weight every 15 minutes while sitting in the chair. Support arm on a pillow while sitting in chair.	No evidence of skin irritation. No edema present in hands or ankles. States that he does shift his weight every 15 minutes or so while in a chair.

Italicized interventions indicates culturally specific care.

Critical Thinking Questions	1.	What other discharge instructions should have been given to Mr. and Mrs. Jackson? Does he need a home health referral?
	2.	Mrs. Jackson calls the clinic stating that Mr. Jackson has a fever, feels warm, and is not feeling well. What do you tell her? Should he come to the clinic or be sent to the hospital? Can Mrs. Jackson drive him safely?
	3.	What other nursing interventions should be done for Mr. Jackson to prevent the complications of immobility?

- Independence in performing activities of daily living is lost during immobility.
- Muscle is broken down for energy in states of decreased protein intake.
- Malnutrition causes a decrease in red blood cells, causing anemia, and a decrease in white blood cells, causing infection.
- Lack of activity leads rapidly to muscle weakness and atrophy.
- Bone decalcification causes weak bones and increased serum levels of calcium.
- Immobilization of joints leads to stiffness and limited movement.
- Skin breakdown occurs with increased pressure, shear, friction, excoriation, and maceration.
- Loss of skin integrity allows micro-organisms to invade and produce infection.
- Stasis of blood in dependent limbs leads to edema and thrombus formation.
- The development of deep vein thrombosis and subsequent pulmonary embolism can lead to client's death.
- Sudden changes in a client's position can cause blood pressure to drop sharply, a condition known as orthostatic hypotension.
- Hypoventilation and stasis of respiratory secretions can lead to atelectasis and hypostatic pneumonia.
- Hypomotility of the gastrointestinal tract causes abdominal distension, discomfort, constipation, and flatulence.
- Difficulty in voiding leads to urinary retention, residual urine, and urinary tract infections.
- The best treatment for complications from disuse is prevention.
- Increased activity and exercise can prevent most of the complications of disuse.
- When positioning a client who is unable to move, position joint in anatomic alignment or functional alignment. Provide support above and below the joint.

BIBLIOGRAPHY

Aronovitch, S. (1995). Select the best dressing sponge. *Nursing95, 25*(7), 52–54.

Ayello, E.A. (1996). Keeping pressure ulcers in check. *Nursing96, 26*(10), 62–63.

*Barnes, H.R. (1993). Alternating transparent and hydrocolloid dressings. *Nursing93, 23*(3), 59–61.

*Bright, L.D., & Georgi, S. (1994). Protect your patient from DVT. *American Journal of Nursing, 94*(12), 28–32.

Chinn, P.L. (1996). Environment, health, and nursing. (editorial). *Advances in Nursing Science, 18*(4).

*Flanagan, M. (1993). Predicting pressure sore risk. *Journal of Wound Care, 2*(4), 215–218.

Hangartner, T.N. (1995). Osteoporosis due to disuse. *Physical Medicine and Rehabilitation Clinics of North America, 6*(3), 579–594.

Hess, C.T. (1998). Keeping tabs on a pressure ulcer. *Nursing98, 28*(1), 18.

Hess, C.T. (1998). Treating a stage 3 pressure ulcer. *Nursing98, 28*(2), 20.

Hunter, S.M., Langemo, D.K., Olson, B., Hanson, D., Cathcart-Silberberg, T., et al. (1995). The effectiveness of skin care protocols for pressure ulcers. *Rehabilitation Nursing, 20*(5), 250–255.

Metzler, D.J., & Harr, J. (1996). Positioning your patient properly. *American Journal of Nursing, 96*(3), 33–37.

*Olson, E.V. (1967). The hazards of immobility. *American Journal of Nursing, 67*(4), 779–796.

*Rondorf-Klym, L.M., & Langemo, D. (1993). Relationship between body weight, body position, support surface, and tissue interface pressure at the sacrum. *Decubitus, 6*(1), 22–25.

Skewes, S.M. (1996). Skin care rituals that do more harm than good. *American Journal of Nursing, 96*(10), 33–35.

*Skewes, S.M. Spotting pressure ulcers in patients with dark skin. *Nursing96, 26*(6), 24q–24r.

St. Pierre, B.A., & Flaskerud, J.H. (1995). Clinical nursing implications for the recovery of atrophied skeletal muscle following bed rest. *Rehabilitation Nursing, 20*(6), 314–317.

*Topp, R., Mikesky, A., & Bawel, K. (1994). Developing a strength training program for older adults: Planning, programming, and potential outcomes. *Rehabilitation Nursing, 19*(5), 266–273.

Von Rueden, K.T., & Harris, J.R. (1995). Pulmonary dysfunction related to immobility in the trauma patient. *AACN Clinical Issues, 6*(2), 212–228.

Walker, D. (1996). Back to basics: Choosing the correct wound dressing. *American Journal of Nursing, 96*(9), 35–39.

*Winslow, E.H. (1994). Mattresses that spell pressure R-E-L-I-E-F. *American Journal of Nursing, 94*(9), 48.

*Asterisk indicates a classic or definitive work on this subject.

Respiratory Function

Helen Harkreader

Key Terms

bronchospasm
chest percussion
chest physiotherapy
cough
cyanosis
diaphragmatic (abdominal)
  breathing
dyspnea
endotracheal tube
hemoptysis
hypercapnia
hyperventilation

hypoventilation
hypoxemia
hypoxia
incentive spirometer
postural drainage
pulse oximeter
pursed-lip breathing
respiration
sputum
ventilation
vibration

LEARNING OBJECTIVES

After studying this chapter, you should be able to:

1. Describe the physiological concepts underlying the respiratory nursing diagnoses.
2. Discuss the most common lifestyle, environmental, developmental, and physiological factors affecting respiration, as well as contributing pathologies.
3. Assess the client who has risk for experiencing a respiratory problem and the client's responses to the respiratory problem.
4. Diagnose the client's respiratory needs that are amenable to nursing care.
5. Plan for goal-directed interventions to prevent or correct the respiratory diagnoses.
6. Describe and practice key interventions for respiratory care, including positioning, suctioning, providing supplemental oxygen, and maintaining a patent airway.
7. Evaluate the outcomes that describe progress toward the goals of respiratory nursing care.

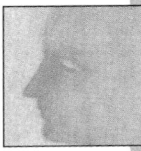

Eighty-eight-year-old Anna Wilheim lives alone since her sister died last year. She called her daughter this morning to say that she did not feel well. Because Mrs. Wilheim had assured her daughter that there was no cause for concern, it was noon before the daughter arrived. Mrs. Wilheim had a temperature of 38.9°C (102°F), was pale, cold, and weak. She complained of pain with breathing. Her daughter called the doctor and drove her to the emergency room. She was admitted to the hospital with a diagnosis of pneumonia. Both the daughter and Mrs. Wilheim were frightened.

The nurse makes plans to assist Mrs. Wilheim to manage the effects of her illness and support her recovery. Because Mrs. Wilheim is having difficulty breathing, the nurse considers the diagnosis of *Ineffective breathing pattern*. Because pneumonia is likely to increase the secretions in her lungs and could interfere with the oxygenation of her blood, the nurse also assesses for *Ineffective airway clearance* and *Impaired gas exchange*. The Nursing Diagnoses chart defines these three NANDA nursing diagnoses.

RESPIRATORY NURSING DIAGNOSES

Ineffective breathing pattern: A state in which the rate, depth, timing, rhythm, or chest/abdominal wall excursion during inspiration, expiration, or both, does not maintain optimum ventilation for the individual.

Ineffective airway clearance: A state in which an individual is unable to clear secretions or obstructions from the respiratory tract.

Impaired gas exchange: A state in which the individual experiences an excess or deficit in oxygenation and/or carbon dioxide elimination at the alveolar-capillary membrane (specify: hypercapnia or hypoxemia).

From North American Nursing Diagnosis Association. (1999). NANDA nursing diagnoses: Definitions and classification 1999–2000. Philadelphia: Author.

CONCEPTS OF RESPIRATION

Nurses encounter clients with respiratory problems in virtually every area of practice and virtually every practice setting. Nursing care of clients with respiratory problems may range from prevention of the spread of the common cold in a school setting to sustaining the life of a client in respiratory failure in the intensive care unit. Respiratory problems are potential or actual problems in the majority of clients admitted to hospitals and nursing homes. Public health and community health nurses screen for respiratory problems and plan community programs for the prevention of respiratory disease. A respiratory diagnosis may be related to a medical diagnosis of respiratory disease or it may be present as a complication of a medical or surgical condition. Regardless of the area of practice or the practice setting, many of these client situations can be described using one, two, or three of the respiratory nursing diagnoses.

Physiology of Breathing

As we begin to consider the physiology of breathing, it is important to differentiate two important concepts: respiration and breathing. The term **respiration** refers to two processes. The first is the exchange of oxygen and carbon dioxide between the atmosphere and the cells of the body. The second process is actually a series of metabolic activities by which living cells break down carbohydrates, amino acids, and fats to produce energy in the form of adenosine triphosphate. The term *breathing* refers strictly to **ventilation**—the process of exchanging air between the ambient air and the lungs. The term *pulmonary ventilation* refers to the total exchange of air, whereas the term *alveolar ventilation* refers to the effective ventilation of the alveoli.

Air enters the body through the nose or the mouth. The nose is designed to warm and moisten the air as well as to filter debris from the air. The air then passes through the pharynx and trachea before entering the bronchi. The right and left bronchi divide into smaller bronchioles, which in turn branch into millions of tiny air sacs called alveoli. Each alveolus is surrounded by a capillary bed. Gas exchange occurs where the capillary meets the alveolus.

Figure 39–1 illustrates gas exchange in the alveoli. The alveolar wall and the capillary membrane are only a single cell thick. Exchange of oxygen and carbon dioxide between the alveolus and capillary bed depends on contact between oxygen-laden air in the alveoli and hemoglobin-rich blood in the capillary. The thickness of the capillary membrane is therefore critical to the rate of gas exchange.

Ventilation

Ventilation refers to the cycle of inspiration and expiration of air into and out of the lungs. Air moves into the lungs when the atmospherical pressure is greater than the pressure in the air passages. Two things happen simultaneously to create this pressure gradient:

- The size of the chest cavity is enlarged (expanded) by elevation of the ribs and movement of the diaphragm. The diaphragm moves downward when it contracts, thus creating more intrathoracic space.
- As the chest wall expands, it pulls away from the lungs, creating negative pressure, which draws the lungs open. As the lungs are pulled open, negative pressure is created in the airways inside the lungs, and the air is drawn into the lungs.

Figure 39–2 illustrates chest wall expansion during inspiration. The chest wall and the lungs must remain intact (no air allowed in the pleural space) for the negative pressure to be created.

Inspiration is a more active process than expiration, because in inspiration the diaphragm contracts, moving downward, and the intercostal muscles contract to elevate the ribs. When the intercostal muscles and the diaphragm relax, the chest cavity becomes smaller and air passively leaves the lungs.

Muscles of Respiration

The primary muscle of respiration is the *diaphragm*. When the diaphragm is relaxed, it assumes a dome shape that ascends into the thorax. As we have seen,

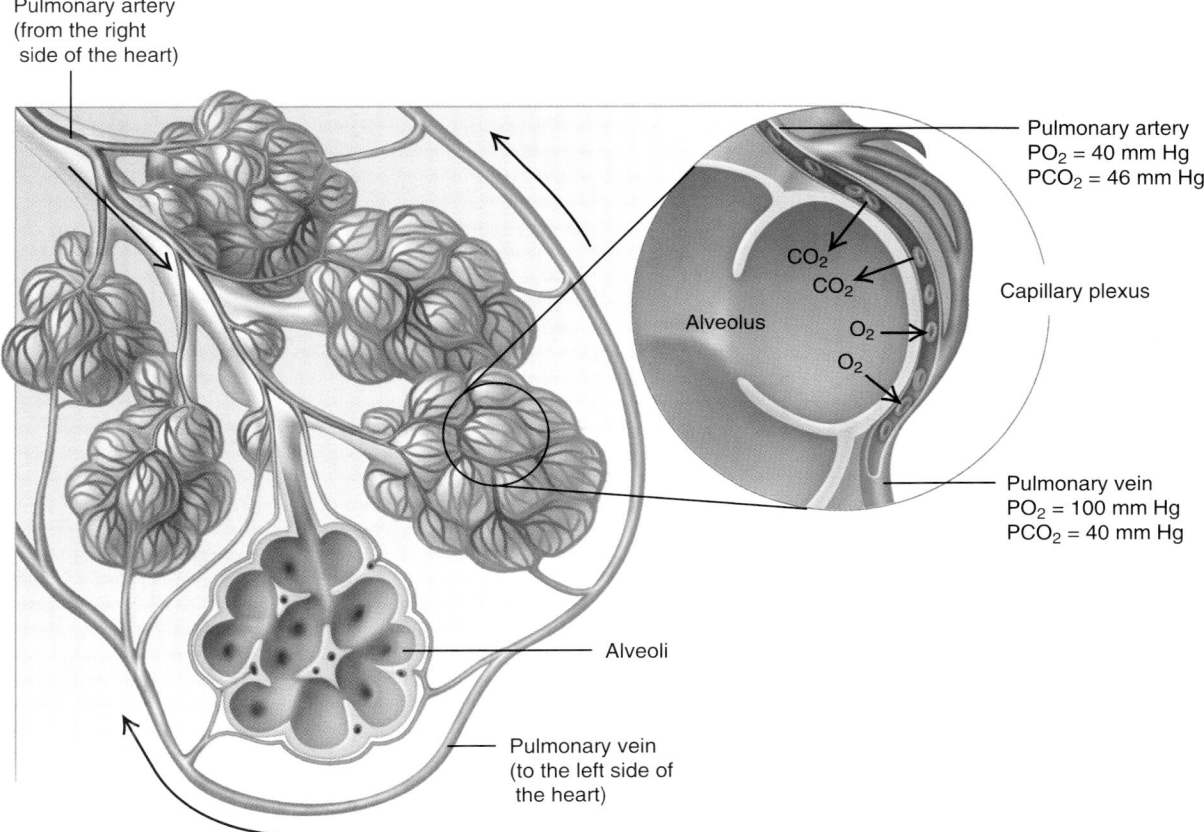

Pulmonary artery
(from the right
side of the heart)

Pulmonary artery
$PO_2 = 40$ mm Hg
$PCO_2 = 46$ mm Hg

CO_2
CO_2

Capillary plexus

Alveolus

O_2
O_2

Pulmonary vein
$PO_2 = 100$ mm Hg
$PCO_2 = 40$ mm Hg

Alveoli

Pulmonary vein
(to the left side of
the heart)

Figure 39–1. Millions of alveoli interface with the capillary bed, providing a tremendous surface for gas exchange. Rapid diffusion of oxygen and carbon dioxide saturates the blood with oxygen and removes excess carbon dioxide.

when the diaphragm contracts, it flattens along the lower border of the ribs. Again, relaxation of the diaphragm is associated with exhalation, and contraction of the diaphragm is associated with inhalation.

The additional muscles that assist the diaphragm are called the *accessory muscles of respiration.* Three important sets of accessory muscles are the sternocleidomastoid, the scaleni, and the intercostals. During inspiration, the *sternocleidomastoid* muscle raises the sternum, the *scaleni* muscles elevate the first two ribs, and the external *intercostal* muscles elevate the remaining ribs. During quiet respiration, these inspiratory muscles exert little observable activity. The muscles that assist expiration are the internal intercostal muscles and the abdominal muscles. The expiratory muscles become more active during forceful expiration.

Compliance and Elasticity

Normal ventilation depends on compliance and elastic recoil of the lung tissue. *Compliance* is a measure of the distensibility of the lungs—the degree to which the lungs can stretch. *Elastic recoil* is the tendency of the lungs to return to a nonstretched state. This rebound effect contributes to expiration.

Surface Tension

In the lungs, elastic recoil is produced by elastic fibers in lung tissue and by the surface tension of the fluid that lines the alveoli. This surface tension causes a continuous tendency of the alveoli to collapse. Surface tension is the attraction between the molecules on the surface of a fluid. If you observe various fluids in a glass, you will notice that some have a convex surface (upward curve) created by surface tension. Fluids with less surface tension have a concave surface (downward curve). *Surfactant,* a lipoprotein mixture secreted by the alveolar epithelium, acts like a detergent to reduce the surface tension and hold the alveoli open. Stretching of the alveoli through periodic deep breaths, known as sighing, stimulates the production of surfactant. For this reason, periodical sighing is an essential physiological mechanism to maintain open alveoli. Surfactant is absent or diminished in premature newborns.

Airway Resistance

The work of breathing is directly related to the amount of *airway resistance*, which is the amount of opposition to airflow within the air passages. Airway resistance is

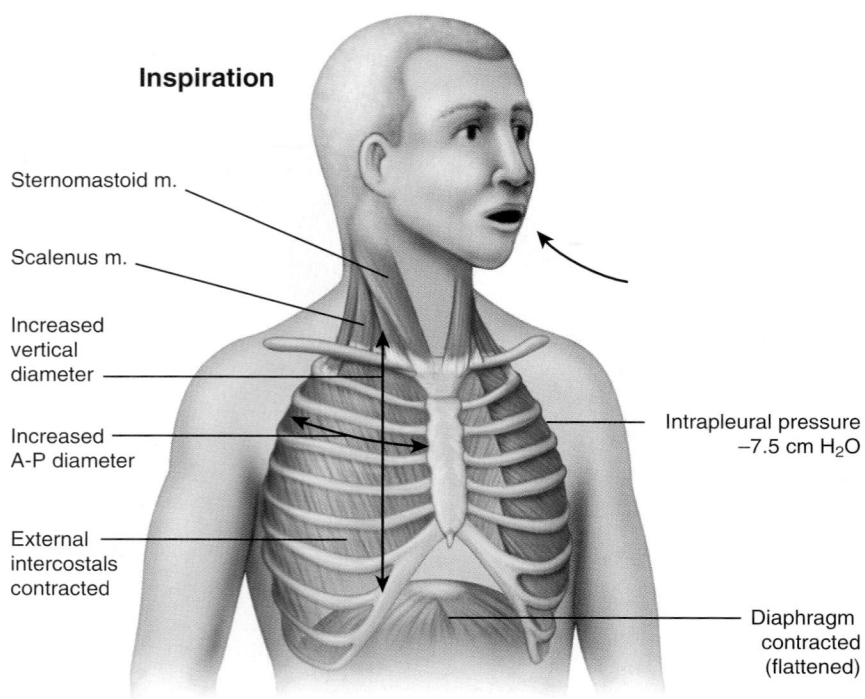

Inspiration

Sternomastoid m.

Scalenus m.

Increased vertical diameter

Increased A-P diameter

External intercostals contracted

Intrapleural pressure −7.5 cm H_2O

Diaphragm contracted (flattened)

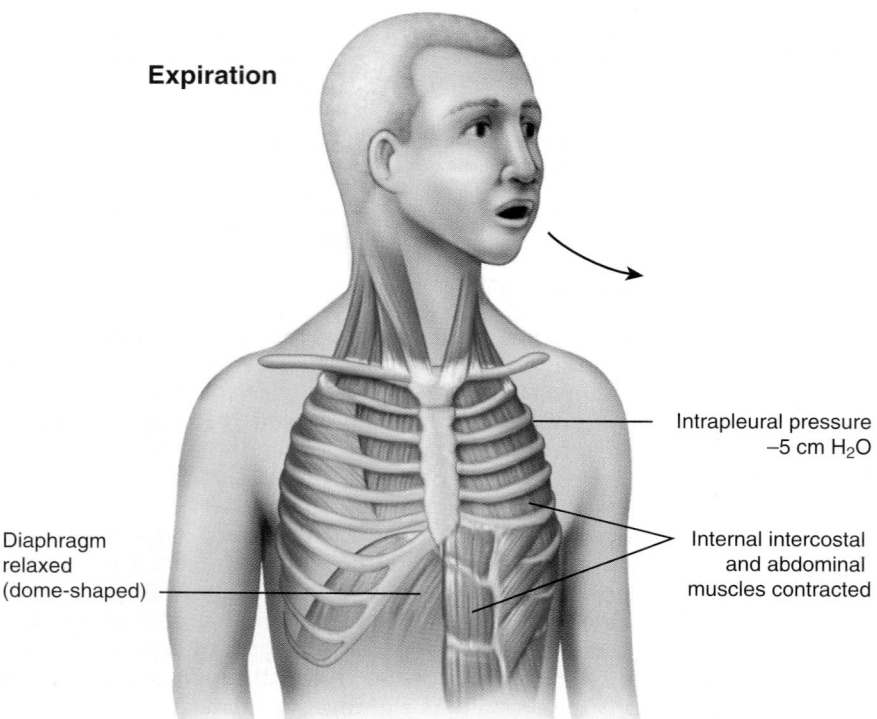

Expiration

Diaphragm relaxed (dome-shaped)

Intrapleural pressure −5 cm H_2O

Internal intercostal and abdominal muscles contracted

Figure 39–2. During inspiration, the diaphragm and the external intercostal muscles contract to increase the intrathoracic space, decreasing the intrapleural pressure to −7.5 cm H_2O, which expands the lungs. During expiration, the diaphragm relaxes, and the internal intercostal and abdominal muscles contract to reduce the size of the thoracic cavity. A negative intrapleural pressure of −5 cm H_2O holds the lungs in a somewhat inflated position.

determined by the diameter and the length of the airways. It is normally low; however, any obstruction in the respiratory passages, whether a foreign body, a mass, or mucus, narrows the diameter and increases airway resistance. Contraction of the smooth muscles of the bronchi also decreases the diameter.

Dead Space

Dead space is any surface of the airways that contains air but does not participate in gas exchange. On inspiration, a tidal volume of 500 mL of air (in the adult) fills the nose, pharynx, trachea, bronchi, bronchioles, and alveoli. However, only the air that reaches the alveoli is available for gas exchange. The remaining air is said to occupy dead space. Therefore, the volume of air that enters the alveoli with each breath is equal to the inhaled air minus the dead space volume. Normal dead space volume in the average adult is approximately 150 mL.

Control of Respiration

Ventilation is controlled by a combination of neurological and chemical mechanisms. Neurological control is in the respiratory centers in the pons and medulla of the brain stem. Several groups of neurons exert different influences on respiration. The medullary rhythmicity area controls the rhythmicity of inspiration and expiration. The apneustic and pneumotaxic areas of the medulla smooth the pattern of respiration into a short inspiration and a longer expiration. These respiratory control centers respond to changes in carbon dioxide (CO_2) and oxygen (O_2) in the blood but are more sensitive to carbon dioxide. Increased carbon dioxide can increase ventilation sevenfold. Additionally, chemoreceptors, present primarily in the aortic arch and the carotid artery, respond to changes in CO_2 and O_2 but are more sensitive to oxygen deficit. Together these neurological and chemical mechanisms control ventilation almost exactly to the demands of the body.

Pulmonary Symbols

Symbols are used in respiratory care as a shorthand method of representing the parameters of ventilatory function. Table 39–1 lists common symbols used in respiratory care.

Physiology of Airway Clearance

The ability to maintain clean, clear airways is an important defense mechanism of the body. Because the lungs are open to polluted atmospherical air, foreign matter and micro-organisms are a constant threat. The design of the respiratory tract protects the body from invasion.

Respiratory Defense Mechanisms

UPPER AIRWAYS
The upper airways are designed to maintain an internal environment essentially free of micro-organisms or foreign matter. As air enters the nose, the upper airways begin the defensive function of the respiratory system. The hairs of the anterior nostrils and the mucus remove large foreign particles from the air. The irregular surface of the turbinates, septum, and pharynx creates obstruction to the passage of smaller particles that escaped the hairs and remained suspended in the air. Figure 39–3 illustrates the structural upper airway defenses.

The upper airways are lined with a mucous membrane that protects the lungs by cleaning, moisturiz-

TABLE 39–1

Common Symbols Used in Respiratory Care

Symbol	Interpretation
A	Alveolar
a	Arterial
CO_2	Carbon dioxide
O_2	Oxygen
V	Ventilation
V_T	Tidal volume
$\dot{V}/\dot{Q}$	Ventilation/perfusion ratio
VC	Vital capacity
FEV_1	Forced expiratory volume/time
SaO_2	Percentage hemoglobin oxygen saturation
PAO_2	Partial pressure of alveolar oxygen
PaO_2	Partial pressure of arterial oxygen
$PaCO_2$	Partial pressure of arterial carbon dioxide
pH	Hydrogen ion concentration, acidity or alkalinity
FIO_2	Fraction of inspired oxygen, expressed in decimal form (0.40 = 40% oxygen)

ing, and warming the air. The upper airways are lined with a mucous membrane that secretes mucopolysaccharides that trap the foreign particles. Its ciliated epithelium, extending from the nose to the bronchioles, propels the mucus into the pharynx, where it can be expelled from the body or swallowed. The mucus also humidifies the air. Finally, the high vascularity of the mucous membrane contributes to warming of the inspired air.

The sneeze reflex provides added protection against larger particles and more irritating substances. A *sneeze* is stimulated by irritation to the nasal passageway caused by foreign bodies, chemicals, or temperature extremes. During a sneeze, the uvula is depressed, allowing a large volume of air to be forced through the nose and mouth, thus clearing the offending substance. Increased pressure is created in the lungs by taking a deep breath and holding the breath immediately before the sneeze.

LOWER AIRWAYS
The *glottis* is the opening at the top of the larynx between the resting vocal folds. It divides the upper from the lower respiratory tract. The glottis is open with inspiration, but when we speak, the vocal folds come together, temporarily eliminating the glottis. When we swallow, the epiglottis tips downward to seal off the glottis. This reflex sometimes fails when we try to talk and swallow food or fluids at the same time. However, if foreign particles do pass the glottis, additional protection exists: cilia propel the particles upward, phagocytes engulf the particles, and the cough reflex produces a forceful exhalation to expel the irritating matter.

The cleaning and moisturizing activity of the upper airways continues in the lower respiratory tract. A ciliated epithelium interspersed with mucus-secreting cells lines the lungs down to the level of the bronchi-

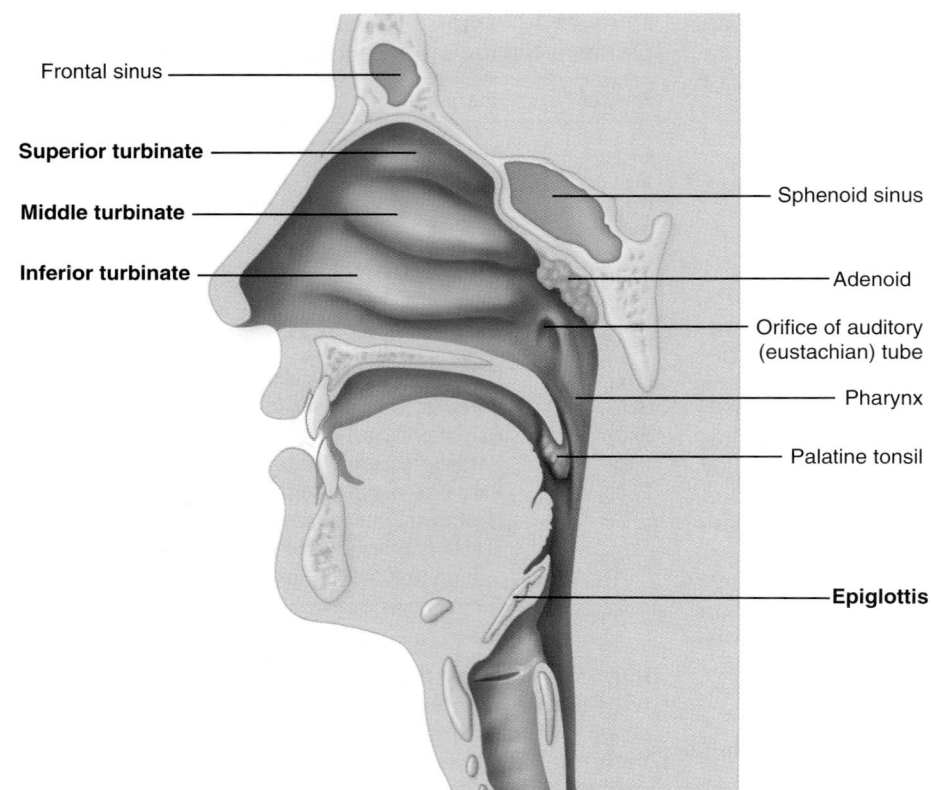

Frontal sinus

Superior turbinate

Middle turbinate

Inferior turbinate

Sphenoid sinus

Adenoid

Orifice of auditory (eustachian) tube

Pharynx

Palatine tonsil

Epiglottis

Figure 39–3. Upper airway defense mechanisms. The irregular turbinates trap debris that would otherwise fall into the pharynx. The epiglottis protects foreign matter from entering the lower respiratory tract.

oles. Thus, the air reaches the alveoli essentially clean, 100% humidified, and at body temperature (Guyton & Hall, 1996).

The cough reflex is the last line of defense. A **cough** (a sudden, audible, forceful expulsion of air from the lungs, usually an involuntary, reflexive action in response to an irritant) is stimulated when foreign particles or infection irritate the airways. Further down, a cough control center exists in the carina where the bronchi bifurcates into the right and left primary bronchi. If the irritating substance passes the bronchi, the bronchioles and alveoli, which are particularly sensitive to chemical stimulation, will trigger a cough.

The automatic sequence of events in a cough is triggered in the medulla. The person simultaneously takes a deep breath, closes the vocal cords to trap the large volume of air in the lungs, and contracts the abdominal muscles and other accessory muscles of respiration to increase the pressure in the lungs. When the pressure in the lungs rises to an uncomfortable level, the vocal cords and epiglottis are forced open, and the air, with a velocity equivalent to a speeding car, expels foreign particles. The cough reflex is weak or absent in a person with central nervous system depression, such as occurs in comatose clients or in clients on high doses of narcotics for pain management.

Threats to Airway Defenses

The natural defense mechanisms of the airways are vulnerable to damage or destruction from a variety of

causes. Box 39–1 lists threats to normal airway clearance. Physical damage that destroys or inflames respiratory cilia or mucus-secreting cells renders these defense mechanisms ineffective. Such damage can be caused by a sudden overwhelming assault or persistent irritants. Although respiratory defense depends on a moist mucous membrane, an overproduction of mucus threatens the ability of the respiratory tract to clear the airways.

Physiology of Gas Exchange

The exchange of carbon dioxide and oxygen depends on adequate ventilation, which requires not only the movement of air, but a clear air passage. Inefficient patterns of breathing or obstruction of airways can be severe enough to impair gas exchange. *Impaired gas exchange* results in **hypoxemia** (deficient oxygenation of the blood) or **hypercapnia** (high carbon dioxide level in the blood, usually resulting from failure of the lungs to remove carbon dioxide), or both.

Diffusion

Gas exchange depends on efficient transport of oxygen and carbon dioxide across the alveolocapillary membrane by the process of diffusion. Diffusion is a passive process by which molecules move through a cell membrane from an area of higher concentration to an area of lower concentration without the expenditure of energy. For oxygen and carbon dioxide to dif-

BOX 39–1

THREATS TO NORMAL AIRWAY CLEARANCE

Chronic persistent irritation

- Air pollution.
- Cigarette smoking.

Acute traumatic injury

- Endotracheal suction.
- Aspiration of vomitus or other foreign body.
- Endoscopic examination.
- Endotracheal or tracheostomy tubes.

Other

- Dehydration.
- Extreme heat or cold.
- Medications that depress the cough reflex.
- Pathology that causes increased mucus, irritation, edema.

fuse across the semipermeable alveolocapillary membrane, there must be both adequate ventilation and adequate blood flow. Oxygen-rich air must reach the alveoli as unoxygenated blood flows into the capillary bed.

Diffusion is also affected by the relative concentration of the gases, the thickness of the membrane, and the surface area of the alveoli. Carbon dioxide is highly concentrated in the blood entering the capillary bed. It crosses the alveolocapillary membrane into the alveoli where the carbon dioxide concentration is lower. Similarly, since the partial pressure of oxygen is greater in the alveoli than in the pulmonary capillaries, oxygen readily diffuses across the membrane from the air sacs into the blood. The thin alveolocapillary membrane and the extremely large surface area across the capillary bed allows rapid, efficient diffusion.

Ventilation/Perfusion Ratio

As we have seen, for optimal transport of oxygen and carbon dioxide, the amount of blood flow *(perfusion)* must be matched to the amount of airflow *(ventilation)*. The upright position is the anatomic position of the body that is optimal for ventilation and perfusion matching. In fact, the overall ventilation/perfusion ratio in the normal upright lung is 0.9, or slightly less than 1:1. This ratio occurs because ventilation is at the maximum in the apices of the lungs and perfusion is at the maximum in the bases of the lung. This phenomenon reflects the relative weights of air and blood in response to gravity. Any condition that upsets this balance may result in a mismatch of ventilation to perfu-

sion and in a less than optimal exchange of oxygen and carbon dioxide.

Oxygen-Carrying Capacity of the Blood

Additionally, gas exchange is dependent on the presence of hemoglobin. Ninety-seven percent of oxygen is carried by hemoglobin in the red blood cells; the remaining 3% of oxygen is dissolved in plasma. The hemoglobin combines with the oxygen to form oxyhemoglobin. Oxygenation of tissues is dependent on the perfusion of oxygen-rich blood to those tissues (see Chapter 40).

FACTORS AFFECTING RESPIRATION

A number of factors affect a person's respiratory function. They include lifestyle factors, environmental factors, developmental factors, and physiological factors.

Lifestyle Factors

Lifestyle factors that affect respiratory function include smoking and the person's general state of health.

Smoking

The primary lifestyle factor affecting respiration is smoking. Inhaling tobacco or marijuana smoke from cigarettes, pipes, or cigars is a chronic irritant to the lungs. Irritation causes increased mucus production. Smokers have varying degrees of reduced ciliary function, bronchoconstriction, and decreased compliance and elasticity. Smoking increases the heart and respiratory rate, constricts blood vessels, and increases blood pressure. Smoking is highly associated with emphysema and lung cancer as well as other respiratory diseases. Seventy-eight to 90% of lung cancers occur in people who smoke (National Cancer Institute, 1996).

Smoking is a potential hazard to nonsmokers. Passive smoke in the home has been linked to the incidence of respiratory symptoms, episodes in asthmatics, and acute lower respiratory tract infections in school children. Breathing in children can be affected through frequent exposure in the homes of friends, in restaurants, and in crowded housing situations that are common among those in low socioeconomic groups.

Nicotine is a highly addictive substance. Once a person starts smoking, quitting is not easy. In addition to the addiction to nicotine, other barriers to quitting include the following:

- Strong link to habits.
- Other smokers in personal environment.
- Facing stressful situations without a cigarette.

The best defense against the effects of inhaled smoke from tobacco products is to never start smoking in the first place. Adolescents are the highest risk group for starting to smoke. Most people who smoke started as adolescents, often around the age of 12. The Teaching for Wellness chart provides some guidelines for helping a client stop smoking.

General Health

Exercise and proper nutrition are important to respiratory function. Aerobic exercise increases maximal exercise ventilation (the most that the person can actually breathe). It also increases the ratio of maximal exercise ventilation to maximal *voluntary* ventilation (the most that the person *typically* breathes during exercise). As the ratio of possible ventilation to voluntary respiration increases, the person experiences less dyspnea with exercise. Endurance training improves the efficiency of breathing even in the elderly. Besides general health benefits from nutrition, nutrition is directly related to obesity, which decreases the ventilatory capacity and increases the work of breathing.

Environmental Factors

Risk for respiratory disease is highly associated with the quality of the air that we breathe. Air pollution increases the incidence of respiratory disease and the exacerbation of respiratory diseases. Additional hazards can occur in the work place or home.

Workplace Exposure

The risk for respiratory disease from environmental exposure can be associated with a specific occupation or avocational activities. Acute respiratory injury can occur from exposure to sulfuric acid, ammonia, or hydrochloric acid. Fungal diseases may be associated with a particular occupation, such as "farmer's lung disease" in Midwestern farmers. Often the damage done by environmental exposure does not manifest itself in signs and symptoms for years after the exposure has occurred. The person who has been exposed to asbestos, dust from grinding heavy metals, or caustic chemicals may have no evidence of the disease, but the stress of anesthesia or serious illness may precipitate symptoms. Thus, a history of exposure is an essential component of assessment of risk for respiratory complications.

Home Exposure

Besides the presence of tobacco smoke, other hazards exist in the home. For people who have allergies, allergens in the home can precipitate asthma attacks. The use of strong chemicals for cleaning, paint fumes, insecticides, and sources of carbon monoxide should be monitored.

Developmental Factors

Risk for respiratory disease is present throughout the life span, with the very young and the very old being the most vulnerable. Exposure to specific respiratory risk factors is related to the age of the person, however.

Infants and Children

Respiratory risk factors in infants and children generally are confined to exposure to common upper respiratory infections. Preschool children who attend day care centers are more likely to be exposed to respiratory infections than children raised at home. School-aged children are likely to pick up colds and flu viruses from classmates. Fortunately, respiratory infections in infants and young children are usually not serious, and most children are able to recover quickly without complications.

Certain respiratory conditions are potentially more serious in infants and children. Pneumonia is always a serious infection, but it is especially dangerous in babies under the age of 1 year. It can be fatal for premature infants, especially when surfactant production has not sufficiently developed (hyaline membrane disease).

Other than infections, reactive airway disease (asthma) is the most common respiratory condition in infants and children. It appears as early as 6 months of age, ranges from mild to severe, and can be fatal. The incidence of asthma is on the rise from multiple allergens. One example of an allergen that has been investigated is the presence of dead roaches in low-income housing.

Adolescents and Middle Adults

The most prominent risk factor in adolescents and adults is smoking. Most people who smoke start smoking in adolescence, and the age of starting to smoke is younger than in previous generations. Inhaling substances to get "high," like glue or paint, can cause damage to the lungs. For adults, respiratory risk include smoking and occupational exposure as described above.

Older Adults

As a person ages, a decreasing amount of surfactant is produced in the lungs and there is a decrease in compliance, elasticity, and total lung capacity. In addition, the rib cage is less mobile. These physiological changes increase the risk for respiratory dysfunction by reducing the reserve capacity to compensate for increased need for oxygen. Among older adults, exercise tolerance may be compromised by inactivity. The elderly client who is immobilized has a high risk for developing the respiratory complications associated with any illness that requires bedrest. Thus we can see that age alone does not produce respiratory dysfunction but does increase the risk.

Physiological Factors

Normal Physiological Variations

Respiration varies to meet the demands of the body for oxygen and elimination of carbon dioxide at different levels of activity. An increased rate and depth of

Teaching for WELLNESS

HELPING A CLIENT STOP SMOKING

Purpose: To support the client's motivation to stop smoking

Rationale: Most people who smoke know that smoking is bad for their health, and many have tried to quit at least once, often multiple times. Teaching should support the client's instinctive drive for health.

Expected Outcome: The client will develop a plan to stop smoking.

Client Instructions

Nicotine is a highly addictive substance. While addiction is the primary reason people smoke, smoking is also associated with relaxation, pleasurable activities, relief of boredom, and coping with stress.

Nicotine Replacement
While nothing delivers nicotine as effectively as a cigarette, about 30% of people receiving nicotine replacement along with support and counseling are able to quit smoking. Nicotine replacement is available as gums, patches, and nasal sprays. Gums and nasal sprays may work better for people who have trouble controlling the immediate urge to smoke, because these forms get nicotine into the bloodstream faster than patches. Nasal sprays have the fastest absorption. However, some people will be more successful with the constant nicotine levels provided by the patches, which keep the craving for nicotine under control. People with gum disease or dentures also may prefer the patches.

Some side effects are associated with the use of nicotine gums, sprays, and patches. Some of these side effects are unique to each form of nicotine replacement; other side effects are related to the nicotine itself. The most common problem with nicotine gum is using the product incorrectly. The gum should be chewed by biting one or two times and "parking" it between the cheek and gums. If it is rapidly chewed and the nicotine is swallowed, it causes nausea. The nasal spray can irritate the nose, causing a hot, peppery feeling and sneezing. The patch can irritate the skin. Patches that provide 24 hours of nicotine coverage have been associated with sleep disturbances and strange dreams.

Tips for Helping People Quit Smoking
Most people know that smoking is harmful to health, that it is sometimes offensive to others, and that it is costly. However, because some smokers will use any excuse for not quitting ("My doctor has never told me I should quit."), health professionals should use every

opportunity to reinforce the wisdom of quitting. Consider the following gentle reinforcers:

- [As part of discharge instructions for a respiratory client:] "And of course you know you need to quit smoking."
- "I would like to see you quit smoking."
- "Have you thought about quitting?"
- "How can I help you quit smoking?"
- "What methods have you tried to quit smoking?"

The common theme in these statements is that each one places the control with the client and does not make a negative value judgment of the person.

When a client indicates the need for suggestions as to how to stop smoking, assess the client's smoking behavior and offer specific suggestions:

- If smoking is strongly associated with specific activities, then it may help to change the person's routine. For example, if the strongest urge to smoke comes with morning coffee when the person has just gotten out of bed, suggest a change in routine. On arising, the client might take a bath, brush her teeth, and eat a light breakfast in a different location (on the patio, or in the dining room, rather than in front of the morning news on the couch).
- If smoking is associated with social activities, especially seeking company in a bar or tavern, joining a support group may be a good suggestion. The support group provides an avenue for social interaction that reinforces the client's desire to quit smoking. Eventually, however, the person has to learn to control the urge to smoke in a variety of social situations where others are smoking.
- Increased exercise is an important suggestion. An exercise program may confirm the negative effects of cigarettes, it will give the client something to do rather than smoking, and it will help reverse the cardiovascular and respiratory effects of smoking, thus shortening the time before the client begins to feel a tangible benefit from quitting.
- If the person reports smoking as a response to stress, learning relaxation techniques and coping skills may help.
- Help the smoker find rewards for quitting: reduction of lines in the face, clearer skin, improved taste and smell, reduced stains on the hands and teeth, easier housecleaning, reduced cough, and reduced incidence of respiratory illness. Sometimes living to see grandchildren grown is a motivating force.

breathing is especially noticed with exercise because exercise increases the demand for oxygen and generates carbon dioxide as a byproduct of metabolism. At rest, breathing becomes slower and quieter.

Body position also affects respiration. As a person assumes different positions throughout the day, ventilation and perfusion shift to maintain the optimal ratio. When a person sits slumped in a comfortable chair, the lungs cannot fully expand, but the oxygen demand is low. When the carbon dioxide level reaches a certain point, the person will sigh or shift position to establish a better balance of ventilation and perfusion. Turning and moving during sleep accomplishes the same physiological purpose.

Respiration changes to compensate for changes in body size and shape. When a person gains weight or is pregnant, the metabolic demand for oxygen increases. In the 9th month of pregnancy, the uterus may displace the diaphragm enough that the woman becomes short of breath with usual activities or lying down in some positions in bed. Severe obesity is associated with shortness of breath with moderate activity and a preference for sleeping with the upper torso elevated. The severely obese person has an increased risk for respiratory infection.

Respiratory Disorders

Physiological factors affecting ventilation generally fall in one of two categories. The problem is either restrictive to lung expansion or obstructive to the movement of air into and out of the lungs. Restriction to chest wall expansion can be from muscle dysfunction, nerve dysfunction, skeletal abnormalities, decreased intrathoracic space, or changes in lung compliance. Obstructive disorders produce difficult breathing because reduction in the size of the airway increases airway resistance.

Restrictive airway disease is any pathology that decreases the ability to expand the lungs. Paralysis, muscle weakness, and fatigue limit changes in the size of the thoracic cavity. Chest wall abnormalities can restrict expansion, particularly when the problem produces pain. Examples of chest wall abnormalities include fractured ribs and thoracic surgery. Expansion can also be impaired by hemothorax (blood in the pleural space) or pneumothorax (air in the pleural space). The lungs cannot expand because the space in the thorax is diminished and the lungs are atelectatic (collapsed). Fibrotic changes in the lungs decrease expansion because compliance is decreased. Pulmonary fibrosis is the formation of scar tissue (fibers) as a sequel to any inflammation or irritation.

Restriction to expansion can be from factors other than respiratory disease. Bedrest restricts lung expansion, as does a cast, brace, or rib binder used to treat orthopedic injuries. Abdominal distention, whether from pregnancy, abdominal surgery, or ascites (fluid in the abdominal cavity), inhibits movement of the diaphragm, thus restricting expansion of the lungs. Some examples of restrictive disorders are shown in Box 39–2.

Airway obstruction can be from mucus, inflammation or infection, a tumor, a foreign body, or constriction of the bronchi. Infection or inflammation causes swelling and increased production of **sputum,** the mucus secreted from the lungs, bronchi, and trachea. A tumor or foreign body can partially or totally occlude an airway. Bronchoconstriction is caused by contraction of the smooth muscles of the bronchi or bronchioles in response to an irritant or allergen. Some examples of obstructive disorders are shown in Box 39–2.

ASSESSMENT
General Assessment of Respiration

As a nurse, you will perform a respiratory assessment as part of a general health screening, as a baseline review of a client just admitted to a hospital or clinic, or in response to cues to possible respiratory problems. The general health screening focuses on risk factors for respiratory disease and evidence of any current problems. For the client being admitted to the hospital, you will be looking for evidence that the client has a risk for the development of a respiratory complication or for the manifestations of respiratory disease. When a cue, such as a cough or shortness of breath, prompts the assessment, you will conduct a focused assessment to determine the nature and extent of the problem.

Regardless of the circumstances, the assessment begins with reviewing available data. Because nurses encounter clients at various stages of wellness and illness, the type and amount of data will vary. Pertinent cues to the risk for respiratory problems in the database would include history of cardiovascular or respiratory disorder, advanced age, anticipated use of anesthetics or narcotics, obesity, inability to cooperate with instructions, and immobility.

When assessing respiratory status, you need to be able to determine whether immediate, definitive action is needed. Cues to significant respiratory problems may suggest the need for emergency response to prevent or treat respiratory arrest. You can reduce the need to treat respiratory complications or even respiratory failure by taking preventive action early in the client's illness.

Health History
CHIEF COMPLAINT
The assessment begins with the chief complaint. Respiratory complaints are difficulty breathing, cough, and pain. Identify the subjective findings by asking the questions necessary to analyze the symptom, such as the following:

- Are you having any difficulty breathing?
- When did it start? How long have you had the problem?
- Is it worse with activity? How much or what kind of activity?
- Is there anything that seems to relieve your difficult breathing?

BOX 39–2

COMMON RESPIRATORY DISORDERS

Restrictive Disorders

Atelectasis—A collapsed or airless state of the lung or a portion of a lung caused by obstruction, hypoventilation, restriction to expansion, or absence of surfactant. May be a whole lung, a lobe, a lobule, or diffuse microatelectasis (scattered microscopic areas of collapse that cumulatively represent significant nonfunctional lung tissue).

Pleural effusion—Accumulation of fluid in the space between the membrane encasing the lung and that lining of the thorax, usually from an inflammatory process secondary to pneumonia, malignancy, or trauma.

Hemothorax—Bleeding into the pleural space secondary to trauma to the chest. May occur in a motor vehicle accident, fall, or following thoracic surgery.

Pneumothorax—Air from the lung leaking into the pleural space or from atmospheric air entering the pleural space through a traumatic opening in the chest wall. Spontaneous pneumothorax can occur at high altitudes in depressurized airplane cabins.

Pneumoconiosis—A group of fibrotic lung diseases caused by prolonged inhalation of dust particles, usually from industrial dust like silica, asbestos; eventually develops a chronic obstructive component.

Obstructive Disorders

Pneumonia—Inflammation of the lung with consolidation and exudation. May be infectious (viral, bacterial, fungal) or inflammatory (aspiration of vomitus, chemicals, gases, oily substances, or foreign bodies). The airways are reduced by consolidation and filling with edema, exudate, and sputum.

Asthma—An inflammatory response that constricts the bronchi and causes edema and increased production of sputum. Asthma can be caused by an allergic response to allergens, such as pollen, dust, smoke, and animal dander, or secondary to chronic infections or heart disease. Marked by recurrent attacks of dyspnea, with wheezing due to spasmodic constriction of the bronchi and increased production of sputum.

Emphysema—Pathological accumulation of air in tissues or organs, usually refers to pulmonary emphysema where air (carbon dioxide) accumulates in the alveoli because of loss of elasticity. Fatigue and dyspnea are the most prominent symptoms.

Tuberculosis—An infectious, inflammatory, reportable disease that is chronic in nature and commonly affects the lungs, although it may occur in almost any part of the body. The causative agent is *Mycobacterium tuberculosis*.

Lung cancer—Malignant growths of the lung tissue. Early symptoms are vague or may not appear at all. The earliest and most common symptom is a dry, hacking cough.

- Have you tried anything to manage the problem? Medications? Breathing moist air?
- Any pain associated with breathing? Describe the pain. Where is the pain?
- Do you have a cough? Is it productive? Describe the sputum. Color? Amount? Is the cough nonproductive? Hacking? Does it occur at a particular time of day? Does it disturb sleep?

RISK FOR RESPIRATORY DISEASE

When the client's problems have not been identified, begin a screening history by assessing for factors that place the client at risk for specific respiratory disorders. Risk factors include age, environment, lifestyle, family history, and history of respiratory problems.

AGE. Note the client's age. The very young and the very old have the highest risk for respiratory complication. Ask about recent exposure to respiratory infections.

ENVIRONMENT. Ask about the client's home and work environment. Take an occupational history and a history of travel, particularly to foreign countries, where exposure to uncommon diseases may have occurred.

LIFESTYLE. Assess for lifestyle factors that contribute to respiratory disorders. Respiratory assessment should include a complete history of smoking behaviors. Smoking is not only associated with lung cancer and emphysema, but increases the risk for the person who is having anesthesia. The smoking history is calculated by multiplying the number of packs per day by the number of years the person has smoked and is expressed as pack years. For example, someone who has smoked 1½ packs a day for 20 years has smoked 30 pack years. If you ask about the use of tobacco products rather than smoking, the client may be prompted to give information about cigars and smokeless tobacco. Additionally, any history of smoking should include marijuana use, because marijuana is even more harmful to the lungs than is tobacco.

FAMILY HISTORY. Taking a family history is important because of the possibility of genetically or environmentally transmitted disease. Asthma is an example of a respiratory disease that tends to run in

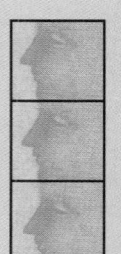

CROSS-CULTURAL CARE
CARING FOR A GERMAN-AMERICAN CLIENT

Anna Wilheim, the client whose story we've been following through the chapter, is of German descent. Her family came to Texas in the 1800s through the port of Galveston and settled in central Texas. Leininger (1991) identified a number of values that Americans of German descent, like Mrs. Wilheim, tend to exhibit. Although every client is unique, many German-Americans have a tendency to value the following:

- Being orderly, keeping things in the proper place, performing well, being well organized.
- Being clean and neat.
- Providing direct help to others, giving explicit assistance, getting into action.
- Watching the details, following the rules, being punctual.
- Protecting others against harm and outsiders.
- Controlling oneself and others.
- Eating the proper foods and getting rest and fresh air.
- Stoicism, not complaining, maintaining a "grin and bear it" attitude toward discomfort.
- Acting on the belief that the scientific approach will solve problems.

Let's see how Greg, Mrs. Wilheim's nurse, demonstrated sensitivity to Mrs. Wilheim's cultural values:

Greg: Good morning, Mrs. Wilheim. How are you feeling today?

Mrs. Wilheim: I'm doing fine for an old lady.

Greg: [Observing that her respiratory rate seems slightly elevated] Are you having any shortness of breath?

Mrs. Wilheim: No, I'm fine. I do need to get outside where I can breathe some fresh air. I would feel better then.

Greg: Feeling a little cooped up?

Mrs. Wilheim: Yes, don't you have a sun porch? Hospitals should have a sun porch. It's a beautiful day out, and the fresh air and sunshine would do me good.

Greg: I'll tell you what, Mrs. Wilheim. How about letting me listen to your lungs for a moment? Then we'll see about getting some fresh air.

Mrs. Wilheim: What does my daughter Greta say? She would know what to do.

Greg: Your daughter's not here yet, Mrs. Wilheim. But I think it's important for me to listen to your lungs now, before we make any decisions about going outside. How about letting me take a listen? If everything's clear, I'll ask Dr. Wilbraham if it's OK for you to go outside, and I'll send Greta to you just as soon as she gets here.

Mrs. Wilheim: Do whatever you think best.

Critical Thinking Questions

- Why might Mrs. Wilheim have said that she was "fine" even though her respiratory rate appeared elevated?
- What might have happened if Greg hadn't taken the German-American cultural value of stoicism into account when assessing Mrs. Wilheim's responses?
- Why might Mrs Wilheim have valued Greta's opinion over Greg's?
- Did Mrs. Wilheim exhibit the German-American cultural characteristic of "following the rules"?

Reference

Leininger, M. (1991). *Culture care diversity and universality: A theory of nursing.* New York: National League for Nursing Press.

families and may have a genetic component. Additionally, family history may suggest the need to screen for infectious diseases like tuberculosis that can be contacted by exposure within the family. Family history may also suggest the need to screen for cystic fibrosis or ciliary defects.

HISTORY OF RESPIRATORY PROBLEMS. Ask if the client has a history of respiratory problems, especially asthma and emphysema. Particularly, ask about a history of tuberculosis.

PHYSICIAN'S TREATMENT PLAN
Knowledge of the physician's diagnostic and treatment plan will guide the assessment. Interventions that have a risk for respiratory complications include the use of sedatives and narcotics, diagnostic procedures in which an instrument is passed into the gastrointestinal tract or airways, bedrest, and intravenous fluids. Any surgical procedure requiring general or spinal anesthesia has a risk of respiratory complications.

CURRENT CONDITION
Observe the client's general condition. The person may be described as in excellent or good health, debilitated, or having a high stress level. The general nutritional status may have an impact. It may be sufficient to note that the person appears well developed and well nourished, obese, or undernourished. A history of chronic illness may reveal risk factors. Fatigue and the severity of the current illness can add to the risk. Assess the level of consciousness.

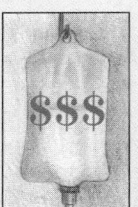

THE COST OF CARE
TUBERCULOSIS SCREENING

The cost of health care includes the cost of prevention as well as the cost of treatment. For an individual, it should theoretically be cheaper to prevent disease than to treat it. For a population, however, determining the cost-effectiveness of prevention strategies is complex. The following research summary presents some of those complexities.

A community-based survey of the prevalence of tuberculosis in Canada used tuberculin skin tests to screen 7,669 people for exposure to tuberculosis. Of these 7,669 people, 782 (called "tuberculin reactors") tested positive, indicating that they had been exposed to the disease. Of the 525 tuberculin reactors who reported for follow-up, 404 qualified to receive preventive therapy according to the American Thoracic Society's guidelines for preventive therapy, but only 293 were prescribed therapy by their physicians (prophylactic isoniazid therapy for at least 6 months), and only 140 completed their therapy. Of the 140 people who completed their therapy, the therapy was effective in approximately 119.

In Canadian dollars, the cost of the screening program alone was approximately $43,714. If the cost of the screening program is divided by 782 (the number of tuberculin reactors), then the screening could be thought of as costing approximately $56 for each positive result. However, follow-up and preventive therapy cost an additional $116,960. The total cost of screening plus follow-up was therefore $160,674. If this cost is divided by the number of people for whom the therapy was effective (119), the entire program of screening plus follow-up can be thought of as costing approximately $1345 per positive result.

Discussion

This study is one example of studies that demonstrate that the cost of tuberculosis screening is high in terms of the number of cases actually prevented. The high cost of mass screening is one reason why public health officials recommend that tuberculin skin testing be reserved for people at high risk of developing tuberculosis. These people include the following:

- Those infected with HIV.
- Close contacts of people with known or suspected tuberculosis (including health care workers).
- People with medical risk factors associated with tuberculosis.
- Immigrants from countries with a high prevalence of tuberculosis (i.e., most countries in Africa, Asia, and Latin America).
- Medically underserved low-income populations (including high-risk racial or ethnic minority populations), alcoholics, injection drug users, and residents of long-term care facilities, including correctional institutions, mental institutions, and nursing homes.

Although, like many studies, this study found the cost of tuberculosis prevention to be high, it did not consider what costs might have been incurred had the 119 potential cases of tuberculosis not been prevented and had the tuberculosis spread to the family and friends of these people.

Reference

Adhikari, N., & Menzies, R. (1995). Community-based tuberculin screening in Montreal: A cost-outcome description. *American Journal of Public Health, 85*(6), 786–790.

Physical Examination

The physical examination focuses on assessing for abnormal respiratory findings, the effects on vital signs, and signs of oxygen deficit in all body systems. The following help identify objective findings:

ORIENTATION, LEVEL OF CONSCIOUSNESS, AND BEHAVIOR. A sudden or gradual change in the person's level of consciousness or behavior can indicate that the person is not getting enough oxygen.

VITAL SIGNS. An increase or decrease in pulse, respiration, and blood pressure indicates that the client is compensating for an oxygen deficit or can no longer compensate for the deficit.

SKIN AND MUCOUS MEMBRANES. Check for color, warmth, turgor, and moisture. Cold, pale, clammy (moist) skin is a compensatory mechanism for oxygen deficit. Decreased skin turgor indicates dehydration.

BREATHING PATTERN. Check breathing for unusually quiet, labored, noisy, shallow breathing, shortness of breath, and dyspnea.

LUNG AUSCULTATION. Listen for crackles, diminished sounds, rhonchi, and wheezes. Adventitious sounds help identify the cause of the change in breathing pattern.

ABDOMINAL ASSESSMENT. Listen to bowel sounds. Assess for abdominal distention. Diminished bowel sounds and distention may be associated with oxygen deficit.

URINE OUTPUT. Check the amount and concentration. If the client has a Foley catheter directly, observe the urine. Otherwise ask when the person last urinated and have her describe the amount and color. Diminished urinary output is associated with insufficient oxygenated blood flow to the kidneys.

Recall the case of Mrs. Wilheim, introduced at the beginning of the chapter. The nursing assessment for Mrs. Wilheim on admission to the emergency room was as follows:

> 88-year-old white female in acute respiratory distress. Temperature 38.9°C (102°F), P 100, R 36, BP 106/70. Diminished breath sounds left lower base. Wheezes and rhonchi left lower lobe. Fremitus present. Oxygen saturation 87%. Oxygen started per face mask at 6 L. Oxygen saturation 91%. Skin pale, diaphoretic. Skin turgor sluggish. Complaining of feeling cold. Denies pain. Oriented to person, place, and time. Extremely weak and frightened. Abdomen soft, flat. Hypoactive bowel sounds. Foley catheter inserted. Returned 200 mL concentrated urine. Daughter at bedside. Blood drawn for electrolytes, CBC, chest x-ray, and blood cultures.

Diagnostic Tests

Review the client's chart and correlate your clinical findings with any available diagnostic data. The physician uses the tests to make a medical diagnosis, whereas you will use the tests to assist in making nursing diagnoses and decisions about nursing interventions.

Complete Blood Count

A *complete blood count* provides information about the oxygen-carrying capacity of the blood expressed as a red blood cell (RBC) count, an hematocrit index (the volume percentage of RBCs in the total plasma), and a hemoglobin concentration. The white blood cell count provides clues to the presence of the infection that may be the primary cause of the respiratory problem or secondary to the problem.

Chest X-Ray

Chest x-rays provide basic diagnostic information about chest disorders and are used for health screening. Pneumonia, pneumothorax, atelectasis, fractured ribs, foreign bodies, and tumors can be distinguished on x-ray. Follow-up chest x-ray may be used to monitor the progress of the disease. Chest x-ray is used to screen for tuberculosis when the client has a positive tuberculin skin test. To prepare the client for a chest x-ray, have the client remove clothing and jewelry from the waist up and don a hospital gown. Advise the client that the quality of the x-ray will depend on the client's ability to take a deep breath and hold it. A portable chest x-ray can be taken with the client in a high Fowler position. You may need to assist with placing the x-ray film behind the client, but then you will need to leave the room to avoid exposure to radiation.

Mrs. Wilheim's chest x-ray shows pneumonia in the left lower lobe. Notice that she had pain with breathing when her daughter found her. Can you correlate the location of her pain with her chest x-ray? How do you think an 88-year-old woman would feel about having pneumonia?

Pulmonary Function Tests

Pulmonary function tests measure lung volumes associated with the mechanics of breathing when the client performs a series of respiratory maneuvers. The volumes are recorded using a spirometer (an instrument for measuring air taken into and expelled from the lungs). Pulmonary function tests may be simple measurements performed at the bedside, in the home, or in a clinic. The full scope of pulmonary function tests requires more sophisticated equipment available only in a pulmonary function laboratory.

The expected lung capacity and volumes are calculated for each client using a formula that includes height, weight, sex, and age. Results are reported as a percentage of the expected value. Table 39–2 describes basic measurements of pulmonary function and illustrates the relationships of lung volumes and capacities. The tests used for bedside monitoring are tidal volume and vital capacity.

Arterial Blood Gases

Arterial blood gases are measured to determine the partial pressure of oxygen and carbon dioxide as an indicator of respiratory function. Full interpretation of arterial blood gases is an advanced skill, but it is possible to quickly learn a beginning level of interpretation.

An arterial blood draw is an invasive procedure performed only by respiratory therapists and specially trained nurses. Arteries are deep under the surface of the skin and are located adjacent to nerves; therefore, insertion of the needle is highly painful. Use of a heparinized syringe prevents the blood from clotting before the test can be run. A glass syringe may be selected because the plunger will move easily, allowing the pressure of the arterial blood to fill the syringe. The needle must be occluded after drawing the blood to prevent the escape of the blood gases; the blood is chilled, especially if the laboratory is a distance from the bedside.

Subcutaneous bleeding is a likely complication even after the needle has been withdrawn. Uninterrupted pressure is applied to the artery for a minimum of 5 minutes to prevent a hematoma from forming.

Blood gas results provide information about oxygenation. The normal value of the arterial partial pressure of oxygen (PaO_2) is based on room air; therefore, it can be interpreted only with knowledge of the amount of oxygen the person is breathing. The percentage saturation is the percentage of hemoglobin saturated with oxygen. If the client is on oxygen therapy, the liter flow and delivery device are written on the report. The physician may order the blood gases to be drawn on room air if the client can tolerate having the oxygen removed. It takes about 30 minutes for the arterial oxygen level to become stable on room air.

TABLE 39–2
Basic Measurements of Pulmonary Function

Measurement	Description
Measurement of Lung Volume	
Tidal volume (V_T)	Volume of air inhaled and exhaled with each quiet respiration
Residual volume (RV)	Volume of air remaining in the lungs after a maximum exhalation
Measurement of Lung Capacity	
Total lung capacity (TLC)	Volume of air in lungs after maximal inhalation
Vital capacity (VC)	Volume of air that can be exhaled after a maximal inhalation
Functional residual volume (FRV)	Volume of air remaining in the lungs at the end of normal expiration
Inspiratory capacity (IC)	Largest volume of air that can be inspired in one breath from the resting expiratory level
Measurements Related to the Mechanics of Breathing	
Forced vital capacity (FVC)	Volume of air forcefully (with maximum effort) exhaled after a maximum inhalation
Forced expiratory volume in 1 second (FEV_1)	Amount of air expelled from the lungs during the 1st second of the FVC

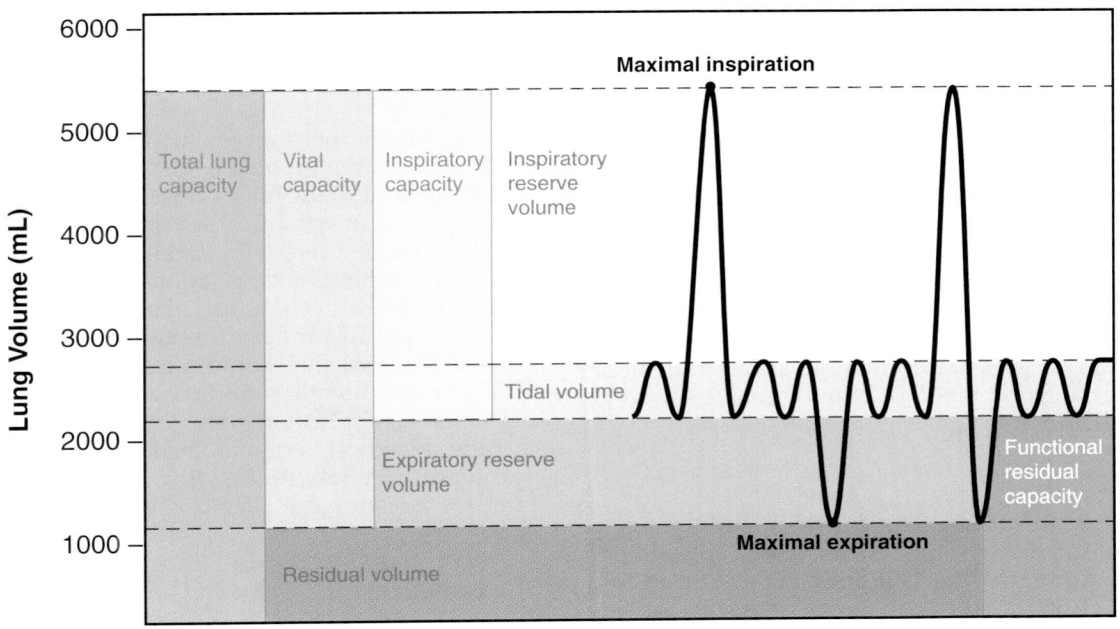

Spirographic representation of the relationship of lung volumes and capacities. Notice that the lungs always have a residual volume of approximately 1,000 mL and a vital capacity far in excess of the tidal volume.

Blood gas results also provide information about acid-base balance. The arterial partial pressure of carbon dioxide ($PaCO_2$) is directly correlated with the pH or acidity of the blood. The respiratory system helps maintain the acid-base balance of the body by controlling the carbon dioxide level in the blood. If the carbon dioxide level is high, indicating acidosis, and the pH is normal, the kidneys have compensated for the acidosis by retaining the bicarbonate ion as a buffer. Renal compensation is observed by an elevation of the bicarbonate level ($H_2CO_3^-$) in the reported blood gases. Acidosis or alkalosis can result from metabolic problems, so it is important to distinguish pH changes as having a metabolic or respiratory cause.

Pulse Oximetry

Pulse oximetry is a method of measuring the oxygen saturation of hemoglobin in the blood. It can be used at the hospital bedside, in the home, or in a clinic. A sensing device is clipped to a finger or earlobe. Within this device, a photoelectrical detector records the amount of light transmitted or reflected by deoxygenated versus oxygenated hemoglobin. Figure 39–4 shows placement of a finger sensor.

Pulse oximetry is a useful clinical tool for monitoring oxygen level. Arterial saturation measured with the pulse oximeter is reliable because it has a close correlation with the saturations obtained from the blood

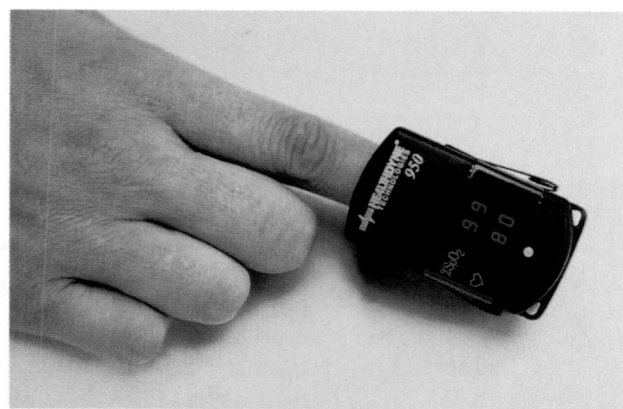

Figure 39–4. A pulse oximeter. Before you attach the sensor, clean the client's finger with an alcohol wipe, and remove any nail polish or artificial nails. (Courtesy of Respironics, Pittsburgh, PA.)

gases when the saturation is above 70%. A saturation of 90% is the critical value for oxygenation to support life. Arterial blood does not develop any significant degree of desaturation until the PaO_2 falls below 60; therefore, when the percentage of saturation falls below 90, the PaO_2 may be below 60.

Pulse oximetry is a helpful tool but should be used only in conjunction with other assessment data. Hypotension, vasoconstriction, hypothermia, reduced blood flow, and movement of the finger can interfere with the measurement. Because pulse oximetry does not provide as much information as arterial blood gases, arterial blood is still drawn for analysis in some situations (Ehrhardt & Graham, 1990).

Sputum Culture

Sputum culture means to grow micro-organisms from sputum. When the client has a productive cough, sputum may be collected for a culture and sensitivity test. It takes 24 to 72 hours to grow a culture of the organisms in laboratory conditions. The organism is then identified and tested for sensitivity to a list of antibiotics. In the meantime, the physician makes a judgment of the most likely causative organism based on the presenting signs and symptoms and starts an antibiotic. A gram stain may be done to narrow the choice of antibiotic within a few hours. Often an appropriate antibiotic has been chosen and the infection is resolving by the time the culture and sensitivity report is available. If the antibiotic needs to be changed, then no further time is lost identifying an appropriate antibiotic.

Any sputum specimen is best collected early in the morning when the sputum has collected in the lungs during the night. For the client who cannot cough deeply enough to obtain sputum rather than pharyngeal mucus, endotracheal suctioning is sometimes requested. Use of a sterile container will prevent cross-contamination. The specimen is sent to the laboratory within 30 minutes of collection.

Throat Cultures

Throat culture means to grow a culture from material swabbed from the throat. The most common use of a *throat culture* is to evaluate a possible streptococcal infection. Because infections with β-hemolytic streptococcus can result in rheumatic fever or acute glomerulonephritis, permanent damage to the heart or kidneys can occur. A Gram stain may be used to aid in promptly beginning appropriate therapy. Throat cultures can screen for asymptomatic carriers of organisms.

To obtain a specimen for culture, tilt the head to expose the tonsillar surfaces and with a sterile cotton-tipped applicator swab the area from side to side, including any inflamed or purulent sites (Fig. 39–5). Return the swab to the culture tube. To ensure that the swab is not cross-contaminated by your hands, touch only the cap and the outside of the culture tube, not the swab. Break the ampule of fluid in the bottom of the tube and send it directly to the lab.

Bronchoscopy

Bronchoscopy is the direct visualization of the larynx, trachea, and large bronchi using a flexible, fiberoptical scope passed into the lungs. It is used to visually guide the physician in obtaining specimens of secretions or tissue for biopsy, removing foreign bodies and mucus plugs, or implanting medications for treating tumors.

Following bronchoscopy, the client is positioned for maximum respiratory function (usually in a semi-Fowler position) and monitored for complications. Vital signs and breath sounds are helpful in detecting problems. Complications are usually minor but may include bleeding, edema, *bronchospasm,* aspiration, and temporary hoarseness. Box 39–3 provides guidelines for assisting the client experiencing a bronchoscopy.

Thoracentesis

In a *thoracentesis,* the physician punctures the chest wall and enters the pleural space. When pleural effusion or blood in the pleural space has been demonstrated on chest x-ray, thoracentesis drains the fluid and relieves the respiratory distress. Thoracentesis may also be used to obtain a specimen for diagnostic studies. The fluid is examined for abnormal cells, white blood cells, red blood cells, glucose, and micro-organisms. Box 39–3 describes the steps for assisting the client undergoing a thoracentesis and shows the most common position for a thoracentesis.

Focused Assessment for Ineffective Breathing Pattern

Because oxygenation is a high-priority problem, you will need to recognize problems and intervene before the person has an oxygen deficit or before the deficit becomes critical. Keep in mind that the diagnoses are closely inter-related.

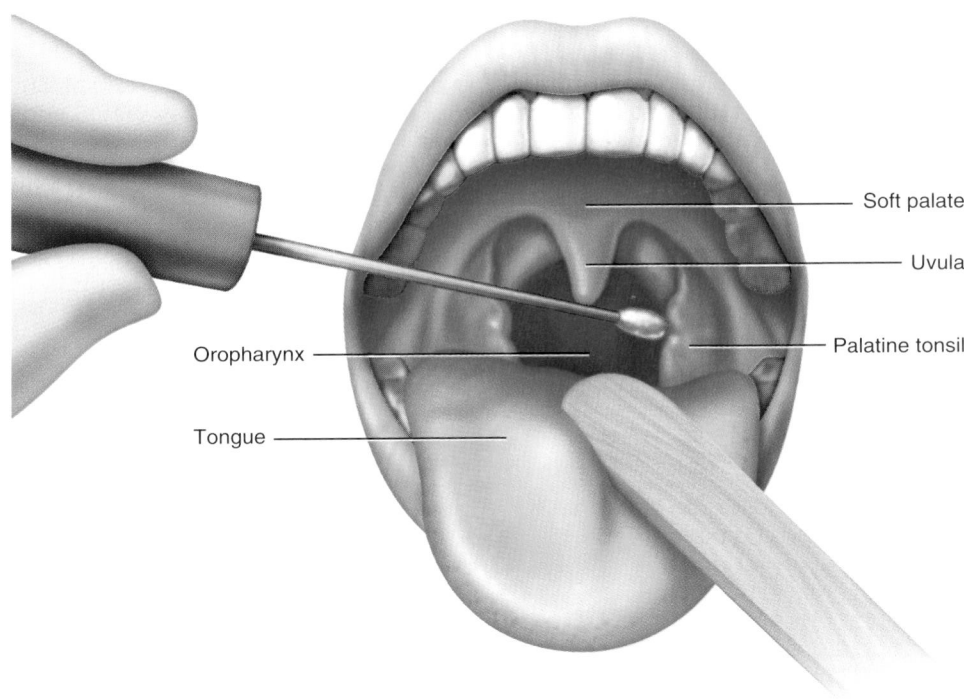

Soft palate

Uvula

Oropharynx

Palatine tonsil

Tongue

Figure 39–5. To collect a specimen for a throat culture, depress the tongue with an applicator, and swab the tonsillar area. Work quickly to prevent gagging.

BOX 39–3

ASSISTING WITH BRONCHOSCOPY AND THORACENTESIS

Bronchoscopy

1. Bronchoscopy is an invasive procedure requiring informed consent and performed by a physician.
2. Keep the client NPO for 4–6 hours before the procedure. Have the client remove any dentures.
3. Administer an analgesic or sedative, if ordered, 30 minutes before the procedure.
4. The physician will apply a local anesthetic to the throat. Keep in mind that the gag and swallowing reflexes will be impaired while the effects of the anesthetic are present.
5. Withhold fluids and food until the swallowing reflex has returned.
6. After the procedure, provide warm saline gargles to relieve a sore throat.
7. Observe for hemoptysis, atelectasis, and bronchitis, which are complications of bronchoscopy.

Thoracentesis

1. Thoracentesis is an invasive procedure requiring informed consent and performed by a physician under sterile conditions.
2. Take baseline vital signs before the procedure. The client may have a drop in blood pressure, especially when a large volume of fluid is withdrawn.
3. Advise the client that a local anesthetic will be injected subcutaneously, but that the client will feel pressure from insertion of a large-bore needle.
4. Position the client on the side of the bed, with the arms folded and supported by an over-bed table at nipple height.

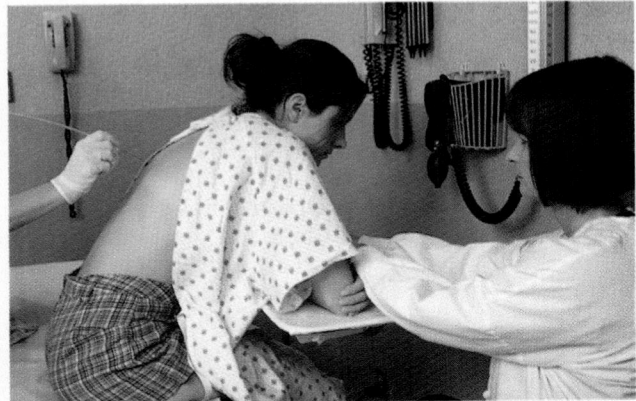

The most common position for a thoracentesis. Gravity allows the fluid to accumulate in the lower thoracic cavity. The spine is slightly curved. The needle must enter the fluid to avoid puncturing the lungs.

5. Assist the client to remain still during the puncture to help prevent damage to lung tissue.
6. If a large amount of fluid is removed from the lungs, observe the client for hemodynamic changes. Take the client's vital signs.
7. Assess the client for atelectasis and pneumothorax.
8. Keep the specimen-filled test tubes upright. Label them and send them to the laboratory.

Breathing patterns can vary in rate, depth, timing, rhythm, and chest wall and abdominal excursion during inspiration, expiration, or both. Abnormal breathing patterns are those that produce less than optimal ventilation for the individual. *Ineffective airway clearance* describes a client who has difficulty maintaining a clear airway. The airway may be obstructed with secretions, edema, a foreign body, or a tumor or because it has collapsed. *Impaired gas exchange* is a defect in the ability to oxygenate the blood or eliminate carbon dioxide from the blood, or both.

Defining Characteristics

HYPOVENTILATION

When a client is not breathing well, assess for hypoventilation. **Hypoventilation** is a decrease in the rate and depth of breathing, clinically defined as $PaCO_2$ greater than 45 mm Hg. Assessment of the breathing pattern includes rate of breathing, depth of breathing, breath sounds, and sometimes the relationship of inspiration to expiration.

Assess the rate, rhythm, and depth of respiration. The normal pattern of breathing includes inspiration lasting about 2 seconds and expiration lasting about 3 seconds at a rate of 11 to 24 cycles per minute. Normal tidal volume, the amount of air inhaled and exhaled with each breath, is 500 mL. The rhythm should be regular with periodic sighing. The rate that is considered normal varies across the life span. Normal tidal volume is based on age, sex, and body size.

The presence of hypoventilation is inferred at a respiratory rate less than 10 per minute, a depth of respiration that diminishes breath sound, or as a combination of both. Although a rate of less than 10 is generally considered a critical level, the client's base line rate and associated symptoms should be considered. Rapid, shallow breathing reflects hypoventilation at the alveolar level because the person is not inflating as much as the lower two-thirds of the lung. Auscultation for breath sounds reveals absent or diminished sounds in the bases.

To be clinically significant, hypoventilation must produce a change in minute ventilation. Minute ventilation is the total amount of air that enters the respiratory passages in 1 minute and is calculated as a product of tidal volume and respiratory rate. At a respiratory rate of 12, the minute ventilation would be 500 mL multiplied by 12 or 6 L.

However, even if you could measure the total volume of air moving into and out of the lungs, it would not be sufficient information to decide whether adequate ventilation is occurring throughout the lung fields. Diminished breath sounds are most frequently detected in the bases of the lungs when the person is not taking deep enough breaths to fill the alveoli. Breath sounds could also be diminished to a specific area because of a mucous plug, edema, bronchial constriction, or other obstruction to airflow. Table 39–3 describes the interpretation and management of abnormal breath sounds.

Oxygen deficit and carbon dioxide retention are closely associated with hypoventilation. From a physiological perspective, hypoventilation is defined as a pattern of breathing producing a $PaCO_2$ of more than 45 mm Hg. This definition is sometimes referred to as alveolar hypoventilation. The carbon dioxide level, rather than the oxygen level, is used as the definition because the respiratory control center is more sensitive to carbon dioxide.

*A*ction *A*lert!
Rapid, shallow breathing is a definitive sign of hypoventilation. Institute measures to increase ventilation and assess for oxygen deficit.

HYPERVENTILATION

Hyperventilation is an increase in the rate and depth of breathing, clinically defined as $PaCO_2$ less than 35 mm Hg. Under normal conditions, the physiological respiratory control mechanisms return rapid respiration to normal. In some circumstances, however, rapid deep-breathing continues to a point that causes a change in the blood gases. Alveolar hyperventilation is defined as deep, rapid respirations sufficient to lower the $PaCO_2$ and produce respiratory alkalosis. From a physiological perspective, hyperventilation is defined as a pattern of breathing producing a $PaCO_2$ less than 35 mm Hg. The signs and symptoms of alkalosis are feeling lightheaded, muscle twitching, numbness, tetany, and, in severe cases, convulsions.

*A*ction *A*lert!
The client who has rapid, deep respirations and complains of numbness and tingling in the fingers is in a state of alkalosis and needs definitive treatment to slow the respiration.

Respirations are increased by metabolic need, exercise, fever, acidosis, hypoxemia, or hypercapnia. Hyperventilation can result from any metabolic disease that causes acidosis (increased acids in the blood). The body attempts to reduce the acid by elimination of carbon dioxide.

DYSPNEA

Rather than being a specific pattern of breathing, **dyspnea** is the subjective sensation of difficulty in breathing and is usually associated with increased rate of breathing. The client reports dyspnea when the work of breathing necessary to meet metabolic demands reaches conscious awareness. Dyspnea is important to consider in a discussion of breathing patterns because it is more closely related to the ventilatory component of pulmonary function than to the gas exchange component. Dyspnea may be acute or chronic. Table 39–3 describes the recognition and management of abnormal breath sounds that may be associated with dyspnea.

With normal pulmonary function, the increased work of breathing with exercise will produce dyspnea. Dyspnea becomes a symptom when the level of activity necessary to produce dyspnea is a level of activity that would not usually produce dyspnea in a given individual. Dyspnea is an important diagnostic cue for

TABLE 39–3
Interpreting and Managing Abnormal Breath Sounds

Abnormal Sound	Etiology	Management
Diminished or absent	Hypoventilation, atelectasis, consolidation of lung tissue	Bronchial hygiene, coughing, deep-breathing, position changes, ambulation
Abnormal location of bronchial or bronchovesicular sounds	Consolidation or compressed lung tissue	Provide rest to decrease oxygen need. Assist to cough and deep-breathe until definitive medical therapy re-establishes ventilation.
Crackles (fine): a discontinuous fine crackling sound at the middle or end of inspiration; the sound of alveoli popping open	Atelectasis, mucus in small airways, fluid overload, left ventricular heart failure, or interstitial fibrosis	Diuretics, fluid restriction, a low-sodium diet, or treatment for heart failure
Crackles (coarse): a discontinuous, bubbling sound (sometimes called coarse rales or bubbling rhonchi)	Mucus in the bronchioles	Bronchial hygiene; hydration to loosen mucus; may clear with coughing
Rhonchi: a continuous sonorous or sibilant sound, like air through a hollow tube	A sound in the larger airways (bronchi), produced by vibration of narrowed airways; narrowing could result from edema, bronchospasm, or mucus	Measures to open the airways such as administration of bronchodilators, coughing, or humidification
Wheezes: continuous, high-pitched musical sounds	Bronchoconstriction or bronchospasm, or other obstruction	Bronchodilators; diuretics if the airways are narrowed by edema
Pleural friction rub: the grating, rubbing sound of two inflamed surfaces rubbing together	Inflammation of the pleura	Treatment for the underlying inflammatory process, possibly antibiotics; disappearance may indicate the development of pleural effusion

the respiratory nursing diagnoses and for the nursing diagnoses *Activity intolerance* (see Chapter 37) and *Decreased cardiac output* (see Chapter 40).

Dyspnea can be acute or chronic difficulty in breathing. Signs of acute dyspnea are increased rate and depth of breathing, struggling to breathe, use of accessory muscles of respiration, flared nostrils in infants, and, in severe distress, paradoxical respirations. The person may need to sit up to breathe. Assess for pain and gather information about the pain if present. Chronic dyspnea is evidenced by hypertrophy of accessory muscles, sitting in a forward position with the hands supported on the knees (three-point position), and pursed-lip breathing.

Although dyspnea can occur with or without hypoxemia, the assessment of dyspnea should include assessing for signs and symptoms of diminished tissue oxygenation. Hypoxemia occurs when the compensatory mechanisms that produce dyspnea fail to provide enough oxygen.

Related Factors

FACTORS RELATED TO HYPOVENTILATION
IMMOBILITY. Bedrest or immobility compromises the ventilation/perfusion ratio, decreases the tidal volume, and decreases the total lung capacity. The part of the lung resting against the bed cannot fully expand. Ventilation is best in the upper portion of the lungs. Secretions become stagnant in the lower airways where the alveoli may not be filled by the diminished volume of inspired air.

PAIN. Pain or discomfort will prevent the client from taking a deep breath. Pain in the abdomen or thorax causes the client to splint the chest and decrease expansion of the lungs. The presence of abdominal distention, whether from surgery or disease, should prompt assessment of respiratory status. High or lengthy abdominal incisions may compromise respiratory function. Obesity, pregnancy, and severe *ascites* (lymphatic fluid accumulation in the abdomen secondary to cirrhosis of the liver) can compromise respiratory function by exerting pressure on the diaphragm.

MEDICATIONS. On the other hand, the measures to treat pain carry risk of respiratory depression. Narcotics and anesthetic agents are the most prominent among the central nervous system depressants causing hypoventilation. The first dose, a high dose, an elderly client, or the presence of liver disease or respiratory disease demand close monitoring of the client during administration of central nervous system depressants. *Obtundation* describes the client rendered insensitive to painful stimuli by reducing the level of consciousness with a narcotic or anesthetic.

MUSCLE OR NERVE DYSFUNCTION. Muscle or nerve damage may compromise respiratory function. High spinal cord injuries result in paralysis of accessory muscles of respiration or may even affect the medulla to depress respiration. Muscle-weakening diseases such as multiple sclerosis, Guillain-Barré syndrome, and myasthenia gravis result in hypoventilation.

RESTRICTIONS TO EXPANSION. Trauma to the chest or abdomen should be a cue for assessment. Chest wall damage, hemothorax (blood in the pleural space), pneumothorax (air in the pleural space), kyphoscoliosis, or fractured ribs can be the cause of hypoventilation. The client is not able to fully expand the lungs or may have a significant portion of the lungs that is collapsed (atelectatic).

FATIGUE. The client may be so physically overwhelmed by an illness that decreased energy and fatigue contribute to hypoventilation. This phenomenon is seen in the critically ill, especially when the person has had a prolonged episode of difficulty in breathing.

FACTORS RELATED TO HYPERVENTILATION

Hyperventilation may be in response to severe anxiety, fear, or metabolic disease. Other causes should be ruled out before deciding that anxiety is the cause. Acidosis resulting from metabolic disease like renal failure or diabetes can be the underlying cause of hyperventilation. Metabolic acidosis means that excess acids have been produced through a metabolic process. The respiratory system attempts to compensate for the excess acid by eliminating carbonic acid in the form of carbon dioxide. Lactic acid produced by the skeletal muscles during exercise contributes to the increase in respiration with exercise. Head injury, salicylate overdose, and hypoxemia result in increased respiration.

FACTORS RELATED TO DYSPNEA

The underlying causes of dyspnea are a variety of neurological, respiratory, metabolic, and cardiac conditions. Dyspnea can be caused by obstructed or restricted breathing. Obstructed breathing is discussed under *Ineffective airway clearance* below.

Focused Assessment for Ineffective Airway Clearance

Defining Characteristics

You may be prompted to assess for clear airways when the person complains of dyspnea, has a change in rate or depth of respiration, complains of feeling "congested," has a cough, or complains of pain. Because the client is not taking deep breaths, fluid may accumulate in the airways. When the fluid remains stagnant, infection may develop, resulting in hypostatic pneumonia. A fever may be present before infection occurs and is a cue that should prompt respiratory assessment. Therefore, risk factors for hypoventilation also apply to *Ineffective airway clearance*. Additionally, any respiratory disease that results in increased production of sputum carries the risk of *Ineffective airway clearance*.

The most obvious signs of failure to clear the airways are the audible signs of obstructive breathing. *Stridor* is a shrill, harsh sound, especially the respiratory sound heard during inspiration in laryngeal obstruction. While stridor indicates a narrowing of the larynx or trachea, secretions are probably retained below the obstruction. *Wet respirations* refers to an audible, bubbling sound with inspiration and expiration.

Audible wheezing also indicates obstructive breathing that is resulting in the retention of secretions.

When the respirations are quiet, you can detect *Ineffective airway clearance* using a stethoscope to auscultate the lung fields.

Action **A**lert!
Rhonchi indicate the retention of secretions that can be coughed out. Have the client cough and take deep breaths to reduce rhonchi and an associated fever.

A cough is an attempt to clear the airway; therefore, it is a cardinal sign of *Ineffective airway clearance*. A wet- or loose-sounding cough suggests mucus retention. A dry, hacking cough generally indicates airway irritation, but it may result from an obstructive disorder. Sometimes a cough is the only sign of asthma (constricted airways) observable without a stethoscope. A harsh, barky cough suggests upper airway obstruction secondary to subglottic inflammation, especially edema, as in bronchitis. A cough that results in the expectoration of sputum is described as *productive*. A productive cough that does not clear rhonchi, or clears the rhonchi for only a short period of time, is appropriately described as *Ineffective airway clearance*. Absence of a cough reflex is highly associated with *Ineffective airway clearance*.

Related Factors

SPUTUM ABNORMALITIES

Pathology of the lungs carries the risk of *Ineffective airway clearance*, especially when excess sputum is produced. As defined earlier, sputum is the mucus secreted from the lungs, bronchi, and trachea. Interventions are directed at reducing the amount of sputum or helping the client manage expectoration of sputum.

The characteristics of the sputum should be monitored. As sputum is removed from the lungs by ciliary action, the lung is cleared of dead cells and debris. When an infection is present, sputum also contains micro-organisms and white blood cells. The volume of the sputum and the tenacity of the sputum are directly related to the ability to clear the airway. The normal daily production of approximately 100 mL of sputum cannot be coughed out. Foreign matter that irritates the respiratory passage increases the production of sputum and stimulates a cough. Detailed observations of sputum help you assess the problem and monitor the course of illness.

ABNORMAL QUANTITY. The *quantity of sputum* can be measured as the frequency of the productive cough or directly measured as milliliters produced in a 24-hour period. Clients are more likely to describe the volume of sputum using the more familiar terms of teaspoons, tablespoons, or cups. Intensive care nurses may describe the quantity based on the frequency of the need for suctioning. A reduction in the quantity of sputum indicates progress or, in the case of chronic respiratory disease when excess sputum is always present, may be the desired outcome.

ABNORMAL COLOR. The *color of sputum* should be clear or somewhat white. Purulent (yellow or green) mucus indicates infection (e.g., lung abscess or pneumonia). Mucopurulent sputum contains both the increased mucus from an airway disease (e.g., bronchitis, bronchiectasis) and the pus from infection. Blood-streaked sputum indicates airway irritation that can result from excessive coughing with rupture of pulmonary capillaries from high intravascular pressures. Pink, watery, frothy sputum is typical of an acute episode of pulmonary edema. Rusty sputum is from blood that has been in the airways for a period of time. Pneumococcal pneumonia characteristically produces rusty sputum.

HEMOPTYSIS. Hemoptysis is defined as coughing and spitting up blood as a result of bleeding from any part of the lower respiratory tract. It may indicate a potentially life-threatening bleeding problem, cardiopulmonary disease, or irritation of the mucous membrane as occurs with frequent endotracheal suctioning. On the other hand, an overdose of an anticoagulant can result in hemoptysis. A small amount (5 to 10 mL) of frankly bloody sputum may be present in tuberculosis, lung cancer, or pulmonary embolism. Large amounts (60 mL or more) is more likely to be chest trauma with rupture of a larger blood vessel.

ABNORMAL CONSISTENCY. The *consistency of sputum* may help diagnose the client's problem. Thick, tenacious sputum is difficult to cough out. Lack of moisture causes it to stick to the alveoli and the surfaces of airways and predisposes the person to mucus retention. Thick, tenacious sputum is often associated with chronic obstructive pulmonary disease (COPD) or may be caused by dehydration. Thin, watery sputum is associated with allergic responses.

ABNORMAL ODOR. The *odor of the sputum* is an important observation. Normal sputum is odorless. Sputum may have a sweet, foul, or decomposed stench. The odor of sputum may be detected as *halitosis*. Other causes for halitosis (bad breath) are poor oral hygiene, infection in the mouth, or dental caries. A sweet odor to the breath is a reason to suspect diabetic ketoacidosis.

FATIGUE OR DECREASED ENERGY

When the client's energy level is a related factor, nursing interventions are directed at conserving energy. The prescription for bedrest in the client who is weak or fatigued is sufficient reason to assess for *Ineffective airway clearance*. The client's energy need is a factor in the decision to treat a cough. Recovery is compromised in the client who lacks the energy to cough out sputum or even to take deep breaths. On the other hand, coughing is tiring and may need to be treated to conserve the client's energy. Energy needed for other activities of getting well must be balanced against the need to cough.

ALTERED LEVEL OF CONSCIOUSNESS. When *Ineffective airway clearance* is related to a decreased level of consciousness, more aggressive nursing intervention may be necessary to maintain a clear airway. Both the respiratory control center and the bronchial cough reflex can be suppressed from a neurological cause. A client in a coma, or unconscious from anesthesia or narcotics, does not have a cough reflex. At a higher level of consciousness, the client may be unable to consciously produce a cough but retains the cough reflex and will cough when the epiglottis is stimulated with a suction catheter. A decreased level of consciousness is also associated with the inability to spontaneously reposition the self in bed. Stagnation of secretions is further exacerbated by a reduction in the sighing mechanism.

PAIN. Pain can contribute to *Ineffective airway clearance;* therefore, pain management may be helpful in maintaining respiratory function. Chest wall or abdominal pain is aggravated by coughing or even by deep-breathing. The client attempts to control the pain by splinting the chest and fails to take the deep breaths necessary to clear the airways and prevent atelectasis. Additionally, pain is exhausting, depleting the client's energy store and psychological reserves needed for recovery.

Focused Assessment for Impaired Gas Exchange
Defining Characteristics

Any factor that predisposes a client to altered respiratory function can be a risk factor for *Impaired gas exchange*. High-risk clients include the client who is postsurgical, has sustained severe trauma, is seriously ill, or has severe respiratory disease. Hypoventilation and *Ineffective airway clearance* are primary risk factors both for the retention of carbon dioxide and for inadequate oxygenation.

HYPOXEMIA
As indicated, hypoxemia refers to low oxygen levels in the blood. **Hypoxia** refers to inadequate oxygenation at the level of body tissues. Hypoxemia is the usual cause of hypoxia. Hypoxemia is definitively diagnosed with arterial blood gases or pulse oximetry or is inferred from signs and symptoms of hypoxia. Holistic assessment is well illustrated in the examination for hypoxemia because every body system is affected.

Recognize any sign or symptom of hypoxia as a cue to thoroughly assess respiratory status, particularly when the client has multiple predisposing factors. It is easy to think of hypoxemia when the client has multiple signs of oxygen deficiency, but if you are aware of the client's risk, you will consider subtle cues.

A*ction* A*lert!*
Restlessness in a semiconscious or unconscious client suggests the need for a thorough assessment for any indication that an oxygen deficit may exist. Call the respiratory therapy department for a pulse oximeter if your nursing unit does not have one.

CHANGES IN MENTAL STATUS. The mental status of the client may be the first cue to diagnosis. Restlessness is the earliest and most often missed sign of hypoxia. A diminishing level of consciousness may progress from difficulty concentrating to confusion, lethargy, and finally coma. The elderly client who becomes restless and confused after surgery should be assessed for hypoxemia.

CHANGES IN VITAL SIGNS. Vital signs change to compensate for hypoxemia. The respiratory rate is initially elevated as a compensatory response to hypoxemia and then may drop as the level of oxygen becomes insufficient to support life. The blood pressure and heart rate will initially increase and then drop. A narrow pulse pressure (difference between the diastolic and systolic pressures) is a warning sign that may be quickly followed by shock. If the client is on a heart monitor, heart block or bradycardia (slow rate) may be seen.

CHANGES IN THE SKIN. **Cyanosis** is a blue color to the skin that results from the concentration of deoxygenated hemoglobin close to the surface of the skin. It is usually a late sign of hypoxemia. Cyanosis may be absent when the skin is vasoconstricted or if the hemoglobin level is low. Cyanosis may be present without hypoxemia if there is an abnormal elevation of red blood cells (polycythemia vera). Cyanosis is most frequently seen as central cyanosis, that is, in the earlobes, mucous membranes of the mouth, or circumorally (around the mouth). A pale skin color is associated with the compensatory mechanism of peripheral vasoconstriction that occurs in the physiological stress response, which shunts blood away from the skin to the vital organs.

CHANGES IN GASTROINTESTINAL FUNCTION. Gastrointestinal symptoms are not of immediate concern in identifying hypoxemia but may be considered as secondary symptoms or complications. The gastrointestinal tract slows either from the physiological stress response or from the lack of oxygen. Constipation, abdominal distention, and even paralytic ileus may occur.

CHANGES IN RENAL FUNCTION. Lack of oxygen to the kidney may be from hypoxemia or from decreased renal blood flow secondary to shock or congestive heart failure. Renal function is assessed by the volume of urinary output. A Foley catheter may be ordered to assist in assessing renal function. Less than 30 mL per hour of urine output suggests renal failure. Blood urea nitrogen (BUN) and blood creatinine levels may be ordered by the physician to determine the effect on the kidneys.

HYPERCAPNIA

Hypercapnia, the retention of carbon dioxide, is synonymous with acidosis from a respiratory cause. In the body fluids, carbon dioxide combines with water to become carbonic acid; therefore, the pH immediately drops (respiratory acidosis) when the client hypoventilates or stops breathing. Diminished breath sounds and confusion are cues that alert you to consider the diagnosis.

Hypercapnia is defined as a $PaCO_2$ greater than 45 mm Hg. Clinical signs and symptoms occur in the cardiac, respiratory, and neurological systems. However, the signs and symptoms are not definitive for hypercapnia; therefore, the signs and symptoms must be accompanied by a reason to believe carbon dioxide retention has occurred. The cardiovascular signs are increased pulse rate, increased blood pressure, bounding pulse, and palpitations. Cardiac arrhythmias can result from potassium depletion. The respiratory response to hypercapnia is an increased respiratory rate often resulting in a complaint of dyspnea. With persistently elevated levels of carbon dioxide, cerebral edema can cause headache, dizziness, and a feeling of pressure in the head. The client may have lethargy, disorientation, and confusion, and be uncooperative. The end result can be convulsions and coma.

Related Factors

FACTORS RELATED TO HYPOXEMIA

The related factors or etiology are those risk factors that, if left untreated, will result in hypoxemia. Refer to the sections on *Ineffective breathing pattern* and *Ineffective airway clearance*. The client's care is managed as a collaborative problem because the physician must order the definitive treatment to restore oxygenation and to remove the underlying cause. Table 39–4 describes the causes of hypoxemia.

FACTORS RELATED TO HYPERCAPNIA

Hypercapnia is associated with hypoxemia caused by hypoventilation, apnea, and trapping of air in the alveoli. It is not associated with hypoxemia from other causes. The client with CAL is prone to retention of carbon dioxide and may live with chronic hypercapnia.

Focused Assessment for Respiratory Failure

Recognizing the client who should be closely observed to prevent respiratory arrest or respiratory failure requires synthesis of information about the client. Seldom does one factor suggest the need for close monitoring. The severity of the pathology, the client's general condition, the client's medical or surgical treatment (especially medications), and the client's age all must be considered together. However, even in an otherwise healthy person, a history of allergies may suggest the need to monitor for an anaphylactic reaction that could result in obstructive edema of the airway.

It is crucial that a nurse recognize impending respiratory failure and sudden respiratory arrest. Respiratory failure is a term used to indicate that the respiratory system is unable to exchange enough oxygen and carbon dioxide to sustain life. More technically speaking, *respiratory failure* is a PaO_2 of less than 60 mm Hg or a $PaCO_2$ of greater than 55 mm Hg. *Respiratory arrest* means the absence of spontaneous ven-

TABLE 39–4
Causes of Hypoxemia

Cause	Example
Inadequate inspiration of oxygen	Airway obstructed with secretions, foreign objects, or tumors; high altitude
Hypoventilation	Impaired ventilation due to disease, injury, medications, or anesthesia
Impaired diffusion	Interstitial lung disease, pulmonary edema, destruction of lung tissue
Impaired perfusion and transport	Anemia, decreased cardiac output, hemorrhage, pulmonary emboli
Altered uptake of oxygen by the tissues	Fever, carbon monoxide poisoning, cyanide poisoning, blood transfusion

tilation. It will result from mechanical obstruction of the airway or from respiratory failure. See Table 39–5 for guidelines for the recognition and management of airway obstruction. Prevention of respiratory failure is a priority in any client with hypoxemia, especially when the person's condition is deteriorating.

The client who cannot exchange air may have no respiratory movement or may have exaggerated chest wall movement with no discernible air movement felt at the nose or mouth. Respiration can often be started by establishing a patent airway. Lack of a patent air-way from upper airway obstruction is a life-threatening emergency. Airway obstruction is defined as any significant interruption in airflow through the nose, mouth, pharynx, or larynx. A partial obstruction may be obvious or the client may have vague symptoms. Unexplained or persistent symptoms warrant evaluation even if the symptoms are vague.

Respiratory failure is also an emergency but is more difficult to identify. Observe for signs of progressive deterioration in the client's condition to anticipate and prevent respiratory failure. Because signs of hypoxia are often subtle, an emergency can exist before the signs are detected. To prevent death, respiratory failure must be identified before it is complete.

The related factors are the same as the respiratory problems previously discussed. The *severity of the condition* and *fatigue* are predictive factors. The client who is severely ill and has been struggling to breathe for a prolonged time finally becomes exhausted with the work of breathing and is at risk for respiratory failure. Additionally, decreased ventilatory drive, edema, and laryngospasm are especially important.

In particular, consider a decreased ventilatory drive from narcotics, sedatives, anesthetics, and tranquilizers in the client who has multiple risk factors. The client with CAL is vulnerable to decreased ventilatory drive when oxygen is administered. The client who is heavily sedated (*obtunded*) may have relaxation of the muscles of the throat and neck that allow the tongue to drop into the back of the throat and obstruct the airway.

TABLE 39–5
Recognition and Management of Airway Obstruction

Etiology	Recognition	Management
Loss of control of the tongue and cricopharyngeal muscles	Noisy, snoring inspiratory sound (partial obstruction) Marked inspiratory effort without ventilation; forceful contraction of the thorax and neck muscles (complete obstruction)	Place the client in a side-lying position with the neck extended. Insert an oral airway. If respiration is not established, initiate the emergency response system.
Retention of mucus	A wet, gurgling noise with respiration or with cough	Assist the client to cough, or suction the client.
Paralysis, edema, or other obstruction of the vocal cords, larynx, or epiglottis; foreign object	Stridor, inability to produce sound, hoarseness, restlessness, dyspnea, anxiety, respiratory effort without moving air	Call the physician for STAT orders: high Fowler's position, oxygen, and vasoconstrictive or anti-inflammatory drugs. Prepare for emergency endotracheal intubation or tracheostomy. The Heimlich maneuver may remove a large foreign object from the upper airway.
Aspiration of stomach contents	Evidence of vomitus in or around the mouth, odor of vomitus, dyspnea, cyanosis, respiratory distress, diminished breath sounds, coarse rales or bubbling rhonchi, crackles	Suction STAT; call the physician for STAT orders as above. Monitor closely.

Edema is part of the inflammatory response and therefore can be caused by any condition that produces inflammation. *Laryngeal edema* can result from burns, smoke inhalation, or anaphylactic reaction to allergens. Even the client with tracheobronchitis should be observed for severe laryngeal edema. Additionally, any irritation to the larynx can cause *laryngospasm* that tightens the throat and obstructs the airway.

Focused Assessment for Related Nursing Diagnoses

Anxiety

Anxiety is an expected response to *Ineffective breathing pattern,* whether that pattern is hypoventilation, hyperventilation, or dyspnea. It is also commonly seen in clients with *Ineffective airway clearance,* especially when caused by asthma, anaphylactic shock, and other conditions of rapid onset. If the client's dyspnea, wheeze, or cough is severe, the level of anxiety can reach panic. Because anxiety can further increase the difficulty in breathing, you must assist the client to constructively manage both the respiratory symptoms and the anxiety.

Anxiety may be the underlying cause of hyperventilation rather than a response. This response is outside the parameters of a normal anxiety response and requires prompt intervention directed toward controlling anxiety (see Chapter 47).

Hopelessness

The client with chronic respiratory disease has no hope for recovery. The best that can be expected is to adapt and to live well with the disease. The ability to live with hope in the face of an incurable illness may be further diminished each time the client is admitted to the hospital for treatment of yet another exacerbation, complication, or episode.

Additionally, for the client with severe chronic respiratory disease, situational depression is not an unexpected response, and you must be alert to the possibility of depression in these clients. Living with chronic breathlessness and fatigue severe enough to interfere with activities of daily living prohibits the client from gainful employment, an active social life, and even the small pleasures of daily living. Complex, time-consuming daily routines for self-care use up the client's small amount of energy.

Altered Thought Processes

Chronic hypoxemia reduces the ability to concentrate and may even produce delusions and hallucinations. While it has not been objectively demonstrated, the hallucinations and confusion that occur after open heart surgery or other major surgery, particularly in the elderly, may result from an undetected episode of hypoxemia. At the least, hypoxemia may be a contributing factor. These symptoms may be obvious to you

and the client's family or may go undetected because the client is reluctant to describe abnormal thoughts and feelings.

Powerlessness

The sensation of not being able to breathe, especially if the client is too weak to describe the sensation, is the ultimate feeling of helplessness, of having no control over the body. Although an acute episode of *Ineffective breathing pattern* temporarily produces a situation of powerlessness, this feeling is not expected to last beyond the immediate situation. But for the chronic respiratory client, the powerlessness evoked by the acute episode may continue and be compounded by the feelings generated by recurrent episodes.

Altered Health Maintenance

As a client recovers from any episode of illness, give extra attention to the need for health maintenance. The client with a single, isolated episode of respiratory disease that resolves without complications or residual effects does not necessarily need interventions to maintain health beyond the period of convalescence. For example, a healthy 30-year-old man who develops a postoperative fever from hypoventilation, is treated with antibiotics and respiratory therapy, and spends one extra day in the hospital probably has minimal need for interventions for *Altered health maintenance* on discharge. However, if the same man has frequent episodes of asthma, requiring constant adjustment of his lifestyle and medication regimen, he will need assistance to manage the problem of *Altered health maintenance* (see Chapter 25).

Altered Nutrition

The client with a respiratory problem may need assistance with maintaining nutrition for a number of reasons. First, the physiological stress response to illness suppresses the appetite at a time when energy reserves are already depleted and proper nutrition is especially important. Second, the client with a respiratory problem may find it difficult to breathe while trying to eat. Finally, if the gastrointestinal tract has slowed, the resulting abdominal distention often produces a sensation of fullness that further suppresses the desire to eat.

Fluid Volume Deficit

The client with respiratory problems is at risk for dehydration (a deficit in body water) resulting from an increased insensible water loss from hyperventilation or the diaphoresis associated with an infection. Oxygen therapy compounds the problem because oxygen is drying to the mucous membrane. Also, with an oxygen mask, taking fluids is as difficult as eating. Just when the clients needs more fluids, they are less likely to remember or to have the energy to obtain fluids.

Mrs. Wilheim is started on an intravenous solution of D5/¼NS at 100 mL per hour. Does this therapy meet her needs for fluid? How much fluid should she have in addition to the intravenous fluids? Would you anticipate having difficulty meeting her fluid needs?

Fatigue

Because the work of breathing is increased, fatigue often accompanies prolonged ineffective breathing patterns. The fatigue may also result from the illness that underlies the ineffective breathing pattern. Overwhelming, debilitating fatigue is a major finding in chronic respiratory disease. For the client with chronic obstructive pulmonary disease (COPD), fatigue is one of the major contributors to *Activity intolerance* (see Chapter 37).

Constipation

If gastrointestinal function has slowed and dehydration is present, constipation is a likely problem. The risk is increased in the client who does not have the energy for defecation. The exertion required can cause the client to postpone having a bowel movement, thus increasing the likelihood of *Constipation* (see Chapter 34).

DIAGNOSIS

The choice of diagnosis is based on a philosophy of early detection and prevention of health problems. For example, a post-operative client is at risk for hypostatic pneumonia. The diagnosis could be written as *Risk for ineffective breathing pattern: Hypoventilation* related to postanesthesia recovery, narcotic side effects, and immobility. If the client develops hypoventilation with no signs of retention of secretions, the diagnosis would be *Ineffective breathing pattern: Hypoventilation.* If secretions are present, the diagnosis is *Ineffective airway clearance,* and if signs of hypoxemia are present, the diagnosis is *Impaired gas exchange.* See the decision tree for making a nursing diagnosis.

The nursing diagnosis is made with thought to the focus of care and interventions that are appropriate to

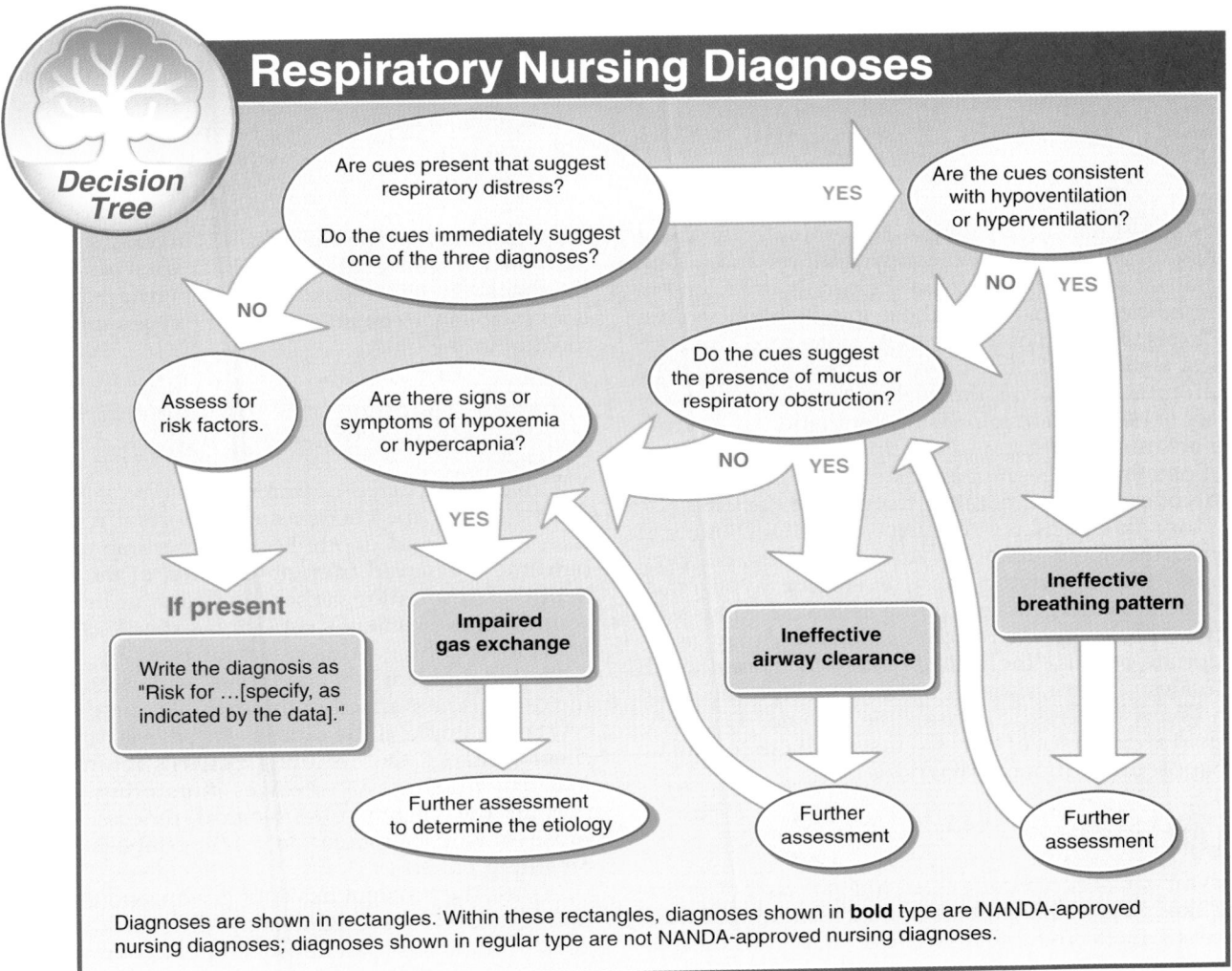

Respiratory Nursing Diagnoses

Decision Tree

Are cues present that suggest respiratory distress?

Do the cues immediately suggest one of the three diagnoses?

YES — Are the cues consistent with hypoventilation or hyperventilation?

NO

Assess for risk factors.

Are there signs or symptoms of hypoxemia or hypercapnia?

Do the cues suggest the presence of mucus or respiratory obstruction?

NO / YES

YES

NO / YES

If present

Write the diagnosis as "Risk for …[specify, as indicated by the data]."

Impaired gas exchange

Ineffective airway clearance

Ineffective breathing pattern

Further assessment to determine the etiology

Further assessment

Further assessment

Diagnoses are shown in rectangles. Within these rectangles, diagnoses shown in **bold** type are NANDA-approved nursing diagnoses; diagnoses shown in regular type are not NANDA-approved nursing diagnoses.

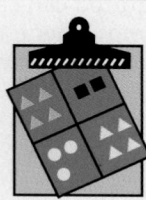

CLUSTERING DATA TO MAKE A NURSING DIAGNOSIS
RESPIRATORY PROBLEMS

Data Cluster	Diagnosis
First post-operative day, respiratory rate 30, shallow, lungs clear, elevated BP and pulse, no spontaneous cough, taking narcotics q4h for pain	*Ineffective breathing pattern:* Hypoventilation related to fatigue, use of narcotics, and residual effects of anesthesia
10-year-old asthmatic boy, needs cromolyn sodium for exercise tolerance to play soccer, refuses medication, does not want to be different from peers. Has dropped out of the team after getting "benched" because of an asthma attack	*Altered health maintenance* related to self-esteem interfering with health care regimen
History of COPD, tachypnea, barrel chest, hypertrophy of accessory muscles; unable to prepare own meals because of dyspnea; refuses Meals on Wheels or residential care facility	*Activity intolerance* related to increased work of breathing
Admitted to hospital following a motor vehicle accident with three fractured ribs and multiple contusions; vomited and aspirated; oxygen saturation 85%	*Impaired gas exchange* related to inflammation in the lungs, decreased lung expansion
First postoperative day, midline abdominal incision, splinting chest, refuses to turn, coarse crackles throughout lung fields; temperature 38.8°C (102°F).	*Ineffective airway clearance* related to pain, inability to cough

the stage of the client's illness. For example, the client with COPD lives with a low oxygen level and a high carbon dioxide level. Oxygen therapy is used only in selected cases, particularly those in which oxygen can be expected to increase activity tolerance. In such cases, a diagnosis of *Impaired gas exchange* would be appropriate. However, the goals of treatment are more likely to be aimed at improving ventilation by altering the breathing pattern and clearing the airway.

Sometimes other nursing diagnoses may depict the goals of care more accurately than any of the three respiratory diagnoses. For the client with COPD living at home, the focus may be *Activity intolerance,* even though the underlying cause is chronic hypoxemia. For the nonemergent care of the asthmatic child, a diagnosis of *Risk for altered health maintenance* may be appropriate because the child is likely to ignore health activities. *Powerlessness* is appropriate for the child who feels helpless to control the asthma. The chart provides examples of how to cluster data to formulate an appropriate nursing diagnosis

PLANNING

As you can see, planning is an integral part of selecting the nursing diagnosis. For the client who has difficult or ineffective breathing, the goal is to improve the breathing. For the client who is unable to maintain clear airways, the goal is to establish clear airways. For the client who has hypoxemia or hypercapnia, the goal is to establish acceptable levels of oxygen and carbon dioxide in the blood.

Expected Outcomes for the Client With Ineffective Breathing Pattern

The overall expected outcome for *Ineffective breathing pattern* is that the client resumes normal respiratory rate, rhythm, and depth. Most of the time a positive outcome is inferred from observation of the rate and depth of respiration, absence of diminished breath sounds, and the client's subjective experience of comfortable breathing. This outcome is easily achieved when the problem is related to an acute situation and the cause is eliminated in the natural course of recovery. For example, if the cause is anesthesia, then as the client recovers, the breathing patterns return to normal. The nursing care involves monitoring and supporting the client's physiological processes. If the cause is bedrest, ambulation will re-establish a normal breathing pattern.

When the problem has a longer duration, intermediate outcomes are used to show progress toward the goal. In some cases, an improved tidal volume or vital capacity measured with bedside spirometry is an intermediate outcome.

For the goals of increasing ventilation by stimulation or by opening airways, the outcome is an observation of increased depth of respiration and auscultation of increased breath sounds. Measuring depth is a subjective judgment: it is dependent on your having observed or auscultated the lungs before the interventions.

Improving the efficiency of respiration and managing energy requirements are long-term goals that may result in an improved quality of life for the client with chronic disease. The measures are usually a subjective report from the client that dyspnea has decreased and activity tolerance has improved. Quality of life is only measurable through the subjective report of the client.

If the problem is a direct result of an acute illness, such as hypoventilation in the postoperative client during the first 24 hours after surgery, the outcome of normal respiration by discharge from the hospital is usually sufficient. However, if the problem can be expected to return, that is, the client is at continued risk or the problem is the result of a chronic illness, the outcomes need to include evidence that the person is prepared to manage the risk.

The client with a respiratory infection should be evaluated for risk for recurrence. The outcomes may include the following:

- Demonstrates understanding of benefits of flu and pneumonia vaccines.
- States that she will contact an appropriate agency for assistance in weatherproofing home.
- Has made an appointment with Meals on Wheels.
- States daughter will provide transportation to doctor's appointment next Thursday.

Expected Outcomes for the Client With Ineffective Airway Clearance

The expected outcome for *Ineffective airway clearance* is that the client demonstrates no evidence of airway obstruction or secretion retention as indicated by normal breath sounds. Wheezing, crackles, or rhonchi have disappeared.

A short-term outcome is that the client coughs out sputum without fatigue and vital signs return to normal in 10 minutes. A long-term plan would include the outcome that the client demonstrates regular use of a regimen for maintaining airway clearance.

Expected Outcomes for the Client With Impaired Gas Exchange

The expected outcome for *Impaired gas exchange* is that the client has normal arterial blood gases or shows no evidence of hypoxia or hypercapnia on room air, or both. An intermediate outcome would be that while on oxygen therapy, the client has an oxygen saturation of greater than 95% by pulse oximeter.

Expected Outcomes for the Client With Respiratory Failure

The expected nursing outcome for *Respiratory failure* is that the client is able to breath unassisted by an artificial airway or ventilatory support. The short-term outcomes include that the client has a patent airway and breath sounds throughout the lung fields. Normal blood gases would be included in the criteria for adequate ventilatory support.

INTERVENTION

The choice of interventions for the respiratory client is derived through a team approach that includes the physician, respiratory therapist, nurse, and dietitian. Many of the interventions that provide definitive therapy are within the medical treatment plan. Respiratory therapy includes a broad range of respiratory interventions, and in many institutions the respiratory therapist provides many of these interventions. Today's respiratory care practitioners graduate from American Medical Association–accredited programs. They are either certified respiratory therapy technicians or registered respiratory therapists. A person with the registered respiratory therapist credential has passed an advanced national registry test and is the most qualified individual to practice respiratory therapy. Respiratory therapists also provide home care for persons with chronic illness. The active role of the respiratory therapist in the hospital or home setting, however, does not relieve you of responsibility for the client's respiratory needs.

Interventions to Change the Breathing Pattern

Intervening when the client has an ineffective breathing pattern is based on the related or etiological factor. At the same time there are general goals that can be applied to the care of any person with an ineffective breathing pattern.

Positioning for Maximum Respiratory Function

Positioning implies both the position and the frequency of position changes. Maximal chest expansion is possible and the ventilation/perfusion ratio is optimal in the upright unsupported position. Lying down limits lung expansion in the dependent portion (subordinate part) of the lung, but, at the same time, helps increase ventilation in the nondependent portion of the lung. Perfusion is greatest in the dependent lung. Turning and repositioning redistributes pulmonary blood and airflow, thus compensating for the recumbent position to maintain function throughout the lungs.

The client should be positioned for maximum ventilatory function. Because it is natural to shift positions based on respiratory need, a client who is having difficulty breathing should be allowed to assume the most comfortable position. On the other hand, a weak or debilitated client may not be able to reposition herself. When the client is having difficulty breathing, the first thing to do is raise the head of the bed. Positioning is particularly important in the client with obesity, abdominal distention, and ascites. Elevating the head of the bed in these clients will allow gravity to eliminate the impediment of the abdominal organs on the lungs (Burns, Egolff, Ryan, Carpenter, & Burns, 1994).

A second factor to consider in positioning the client is stagnation of secretions. Drainage of secretions is improved by positioning to allow drainage of all the lobes of the lung over time. For most clients, this is accomplished by turning every 2 hours. Others may need postural drainage. Postural drainage is discussed in detail under a separate heading. Box 39–4 lists possible benefits to be gained from positioning.

In positioning the client, the client's ability to tolerate changing position and different positions should be considered. The best positioning regimen for respiratory function will be determined for the individual client and evaluated based on data indicating respiratory function. The person who is positioned to increase drainage and expectoration may tire from the coughing induced by the drainage of mucus and may need to be repositioned. The person who seeks the position of maximum comfort for pain relief may need to be encouraged to periodically change positions to increase drainage and improve ventilation. For the critically ill client, vital signs may help assess the person's ability to tolerate the repositioning (Yeaw, 1992).

Again consider the case of Mrs. Wilheim. As soon as she arrives on the unit, the nurse elevates Mrs. Wilheim's head 30 degrees. Mrs. Wilheim thanks the nurse, saying that she is more comfortable with her head elevated and is grateful for the nurse's help.

BOX 39–4

POSSIBLE RESPIRATORY BENEFITS TO BE GAINED FROM POSITIONING

- The cough reflex may be activated by positioning the client on the right side to encourage sputum to come in contact with the cough control center in the right bronchi at the carina.
- Positioning on a painful affected side may help reduce the pain.
- Positioning with the good lung up may increase ventilatory compensation for pathology.
- Positioning on the unaffected side allows drainage of the area of pathology.
- The Sims position, with the jaw falling forward, is useful for maintaining a patent airway.
- Frequent repositioning will help accomplish multiple purposes.

You notice that her skin is thin and fragile. How will you plan for preventing skin breakdown?

Stimulating Respiration

Stimulating respiration means increasing the client's rate and depth of breathing to meet the needs of respiratory function. It opens alveoli and distributes the airflow throughout the lungs.

AMBULATION

Ambulation is an effective, noninvasive, inexpensive method of stimulating respiration. While walking, the client is in the optimal physiological position to breathe. Additionally, respiration is stimulated by the client's increased metabolic need (Guyton & Hall, 1996). Be careful to confine ambulation to the limits of the client's tolerance (see Chapter 37).

INCENTIVE SPIROMETRY

An **incentive spirometer** is a device that provides a visual goal for and measurement of inspiration, thus encouraging the client to execute and sustain maximal inspiration. Achieving and sustaining a maximal inspiration opens airways, reduces atelectasis, and stimulates coughing. The client benefits from active participation in recovery by developing a feeling of control over the recovery process.

For any of the available incentive spirometers, the goal is to achieve and maintain a maximal inspiration. Correct use requires a slow, voluntary, deep breath. When full or maximal inhalation is reached, the breath is held for at least 3 seconds. This sequence is repeated up to 10 to 20 times per hour; the client is usually started with five repetitions per session. Incentive exercises are most effective when used every hour while the person is awake. Each device has a means of setting an inspiratory goal derived from a formula based on height, weight, and sex. Visual reinforcement is provided by lights, balls rising in a column, or other indicators of success. While the client initially will need instruction and supervision, most people learn the skill quickly. However, occasionally watch the client performing incentive spirometry to ensure that the client continues to use the device correctly.

Incentive spirometer therapy is often used postoperatively or when physical mobility is limited. It is most effectively used when people are alert, cooperative, coordinated, and motivated, and have sufficient strength to generate an inspiratory flow rate that will produce a deep breath and activate the indicator on the incentive device. Repetitions of the deep breaths must be slow to avoid overbreathing, which will lead to dizziness and tremors as a result of sudden hypocapnia. The Teaching for Self-Care chart provides guidelines for teaching the client to use an incentive spirometer.

MEDICATIONS

Naloxone (Narcan) is used to stimulate respirations in the client whose respirations have been severely de-

Teaching for SELF-CARE

USING AN INCENTIVE SPIROMETER

Purpose: To prevent or treat atelectasis and mobilize secretions.

Rationale: Through visual validation of the volume of inspiration the client is motivated to gradually increase the maximal inspiration. Sustained maximal inspiration forces the alveoli open and allow the secretions to drain.

Expected Outcome: The client will gradually increase the volume of inspiration to reach a predetermined volume based on age, sex, and body size.

Client Instructions

1. Sit up straight.
2. Breathe out normally and hold the spirometer upright. Holding the spirometer upright is important for correct function and for ease of airflow.
3. Position the mouthpiece between your teeth and seal your lips around the mouthpiece.
4. Take a slow, deep breath. Rapid, forceful inhalation can collapse your airways.
5. Continue inhaling until the indicator on the device reaches the pre-set goal. The initial goal is based on your gender, size, and medical condition.
6. When you reach the goal, hold your breath for 2 to 6 seconds. This is your sustained maximal inspiration. Holding your breath at this point opens your alveoli and stimulates the production of surfactant.

7. Exhale slowly. This prevents discomfort and airway collapse.
8. Repeat steps 1 through 7 five to 10 times. Repeat this treatment every hour.

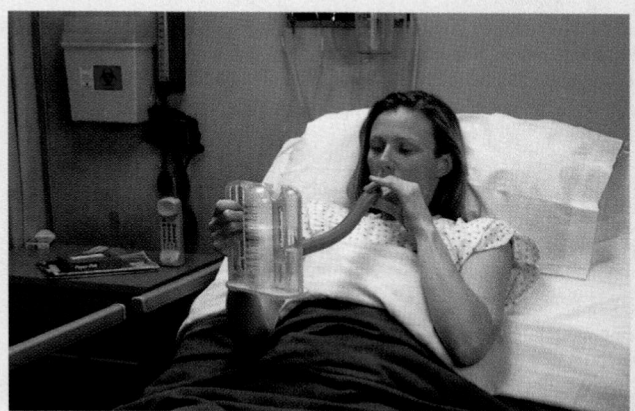

Use of the volume-oriented incentive spirometer. The client inhales slowly. The ball should stay in the "best" area as the client inhales. The incentive indicator is set, based on the client's height, weight, age, and sex. The postoperative client may have ½ to ⅓ the capacity of a preoperative client.

A review of the literature that establishes a research basis for these recommendations is found in Titler, M.G., & Jones, G.A. (1992). Airway management. In G.M. Bulechek & J.C. McCloskey (Eds.), Nursing interventions: Essential nursing treatments. Philadelphia: W.B. Saunders Co.

---

pressed by narcotics. The physician's guideline for administering naloxone is usually to administer as necessary (p.r.n.) for respiration rates of 10 per minute or below. Before deciding that naloxone is needed, attempt to arouse the client and instruct her to take deep breaths. If the client does not improve, that is, if the respirations remain fewer than 10 per minute, administer naloxone. If the client does not have a prescription for naloxone, immediately consult the physician.

Intravenous naloxone will immediately reverse the narcotic and result in a deep inspiration. However, the pain-relieving effects of the narcotic are also reversed, so the client may be in pain.

A*ction* A*lert!*
When a narcotic has depressed the client's respirations to less than 10 per minute, the situation may be life-threatening. Administer naloxone as ordered to reverse the effects of the narcotic.

Opening the Airways

When airway obstruction is caused by *bronchoconstriction*, bronchodilators are used to dilate the bronchi by relaxing smooth muscles. Airway constriction in asthma or emphysema that responds to bronchodilators is called "reversible airway disease." Bronchodilatation is achieved by sympathomimetic drugs, beta$_2$-agonists, and theophylline. These medications have varying degrees of the side effects of tachycardia, palpitations, nervousness, excitability, and irritability.

Bronchodilators can be administered orally, intravenously, by nebulizer, or by a *metered-dose inhaler* (delivers a single dose of medication for inhalation). The oral dose provides a sustained blood level over a long period for the client who has frequent symptoms. The intravenous route is used for an asthma attack that continues despite more conservative treatment. Topical application by inhalation of a small volume of nebulized medication reduces side effects and is used for the occasional intermittent attack. The metered-dose inhaler is actually the most common type of small-volume nebulizer. The Teaching for Self-Care chart shows how to teach clients to use a metered-dose inhaler. When a metered-dose inhaler is not effective to reverse an acute asthma attack, a nebulizer driven by compressed air (commonly called a hand-held nebulizer) may be more effective in penetrating the airways. It is used for topical administration of bronchodilators, anti-inflammatory agents, and antiallergenic medications. See Table 39–6 for examples of respiratory medications.

Remember Mrs. Wilheim. Do you think the inflammation from her pneumonia could produce wheezes in her chest? What problems would you anticipate in teaching her to use a hand-held nebulizer?

Improving the Efficiency of Respiration

In clients with chronic airflow limitation from emphysema, loss of elasticity causes air to become trapped in the alveoli. Breathing exercises can be effective in strengthening these clients' accessory muscles of respiration and increasing the use of the diaphragm for efficient exhalation of trapped air (Ingersoll, 1989). The two most common breathing techniques are pursed-lip breathing and diaphragmatic breathing.

PURSED-LIP BREATHING

Pursed-lip breathing is a technique of mouth breathing that creates slight resistance to exhalation by contracting the lips to reduce the size of the opening, thus maintaining an even reduction of intrathoracic pressure during exhalation. This technique helps prevent the airway collapse that can occur when the functional residual volume rapidly falls below a critical volume during exhalation. By exhaling slowly through slightly pursed lips, the client prolongs expiration and creates resistance that maintains pulmonary pressure to keep the airways open. The Teaching for Self-Care chart describes how to teach pursed-lip breathing.

Once the client has learned pursed-lip breathing, the technique can be used with activities on the borderline of the person's exercise tolerance. Although objective signs of improvement in ventilation have been difficult to demonstrate, individual clients report good results. Some chronic respiratory clients will naturally employ this technique without instruction. An added benefit of teaching the technique may be relaxation and a sense of control over a body function that is out of control.

TABLE 39–6
Examples of Respiratory Medications

Medication	Action	Side Effects	Nursing Implications
Bronchodilators		All of these medications have sympathetic nervous system side effects, such as tremors, anxiety, insomnia, headache, palpitations, and elevated blood pressure.	Monitor vital signs.
Epinephrine	Epinephrine is for emergency use.		Teach the client to take only as prescribed to avoid overdose.
Isoproterenol (Isuprel)	Isoproterenol is an adrenergic agent.		Teach the client that bothersome side effects may decrease with continued use.
Metaproterenol (Alupent)	Metaproterenol is a later-generation agent (similar to isoproterenol) designed to reduce side effects.		Side effects are less common with metered-dose inhalers.
Theophylline (aminophylline)	Theophylline is the prototype for the group. Aminophylline is used for continuous IV administration in status asthmaticus.		
Corticosteroids	Anti-inflammatory	Fluid retention, hypertension, mood swings, weight gain, gastritis, hyperglycemia Warning: Prolonged use can suppress adrenal function.	Local application by metered-dose inhaler reduces the side effects and the danger of adrenal suppression. Warn diabetic clients that they may need to adjust their insulin.
Antihistamines	Reduces allergic response	Drowsiness, dry mouth, constipation, blurred vision, urinary retention	Use only with the advice of a physician in asthma; drying effects may increase airway constriction.
Cromolyn sodium (Intal)	Reduces allergic response. Prevents asthma attacks.	Cough, sore throat, dry mouth	Not used to control acute asthma attacks. Takes 2 weeks to become effective.

USING A METERED-DOSE INHALER

Purpose: To deliver a specific dose of aerosolized medication to be inhaled into the lungs for a local effect.

Rationale: Inhaled medications are easily deposited on the oral mucous membranes without reaching the lungs if a metered-dose inhaler is not used properly.

Expected Outcome: The client will correctly use an administration technique that results in the medication reaching the lungs.

Client Instructions

1. Insert the medicine canister into the inhaler unit and remove the cover from the mouthpiece. Shake the unit gently according to the manufacturer's recommendations.

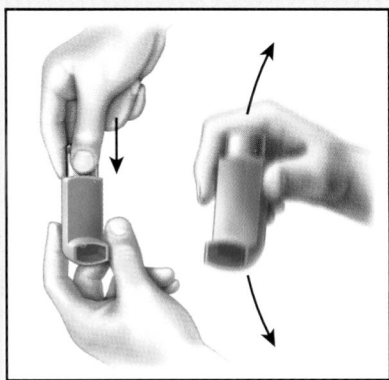

2. Hold the inhaler ready for inspiration. Exhale slowly. (Do not breathe into the inhaler; that could clog the inhaler valve.)

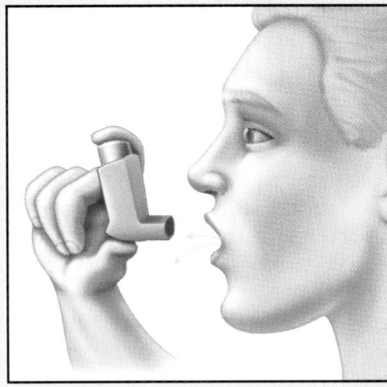

3. Place the mouthpiece into your mouth and seal it with your lips. Tilt your head slightly back and keep your tongue away from the mouth of the inhaler.

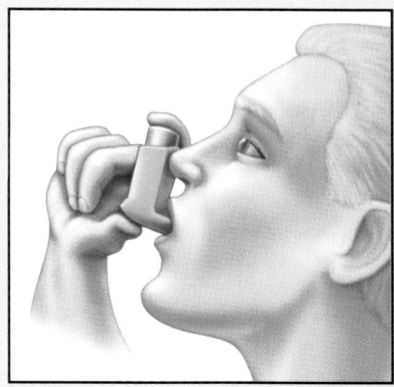

4. Press the top of the canister at the same time as you breathe in through your mouth.

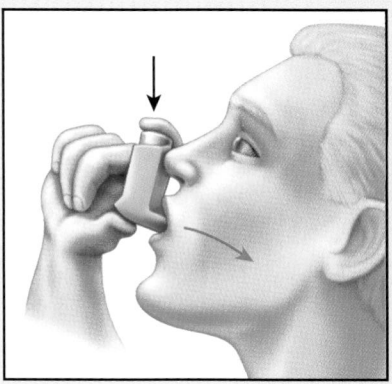

5. Remove the inhaler. Hold your breath for 2 to 3 seconds, then breathe out slowly through pursed lips.

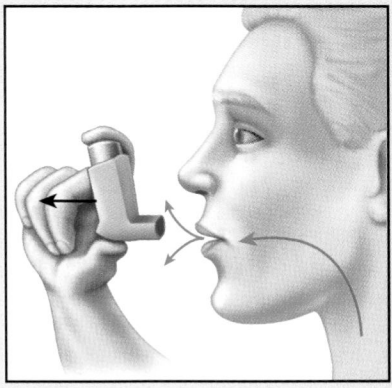

Keep the cap in place between uses to prevent dirt from getting into the inhaler. To clean the inhaler, remove the metal canister and rinse the holder in warm water. Dry the holder thoroughly before using it again.

Teaching for SELF-CARE

PURSED-LIP BREATHING

Purpose: To obtain control of breathing and reduce feelings of panic and dyspnea through training the muscles to prolong exhalation and increase airway pressure during exhalation.

Rationale: The client with chronic airflow limitation traps air in the lower airways because of increased airway resistance on exhalation. Prolonging expiration decreases air trapping. Maintaining airway pressure by creating resistance to expiration prevents airway collapse.

Expected Outcome: The client will be able to consciously reduce the rate of breathing and prolong expiration.

Client Instructions

1. Inhale slowly through your nose, keeping your mouth closed. Count "one and two." Pause briefly.
2. Exhale through pursed lips as if gently blowing a candle flame. Count "one, two, three, four." Allow adequate time to empty your lungs and reduce air trapping. Exhalation should take at least twice as long as inhalation.

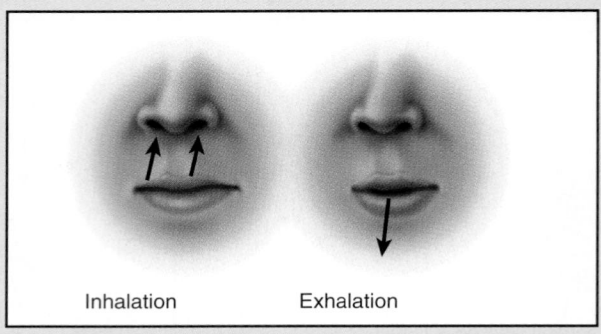

Inhalation   Exhalation

Pursed-lip breathing. The client should inhale through the nose and exhale through slightly pursed lips.

DIAPHRAGMATIC OR ABDOMINAL BREATHING

Diaphragmatic (abdominal) breathing, defined as breathing in which the majority of ventilatory work is accomplished by the diaphragm and abdominal muscles. It is deliberate use of the diaphragm and abdominal muscles to control breathing, strengthen the accessory muscles of respiration, and provide the client with chronic respiratory disease with a technique to reduce the high functional residual volume associated with air trapping. First, the client is made aware of the sensations associated with the use of abdominal muscles; then the client learns to use the abdominal muscles to complete the expiratory cycle by contracting the abdominal muscles at the end of expiration. The technique is then used to gain control over dyspneic episodes. Relaxation and a sense of control may contribute to the effectiveness of this technique. The Teaching for Self-Care chart provides guidelines for teaching diaphragmatic breathing.

Additional techniques are aimed at more efficient respirations. General body conditioning and strengthening of respiratory muscles have some usefulness in pulmonary rehabilitation. Severe skeletal muscle deconditioning, commonly associated with chronic respiratory disease, increases the work of breathing (O'Donnell, Webb, & McGuire, 1993). An incentive spirometer resistive breathing device is used to increase respiratory muscle strength and increase exercise tolerance.

Reducing Anxiety

A key to treating the anxiety of acute respiratory distress is to recognize that the client's anxiety is a normal compensatory response to difficulty in breathing. Any verbal or nonverbal suggestion that you believe the client is over-reacting can be perceived as a lack of understanding or as a belief that the client is "overly emotional." A positive nurse-client relationship will be jeopardized.

A second key to treatment is to remove the cause of the anxiety—in this case, the difficulty in breathing. No other possible cause is pertinent at the moment. You can gain the client's trust by acting swiftly and assuredly to help the client gain control over respiration. Another effective intervention is reassurance that the client is not in immediate danger. Tell the client that she is in a safe place where help will be provided.

Teaching for SELF-CARE

DIAPHRAGMATIC BREATHING

Purpose: To reduce the respiratory rate, increase tidal volume, and reduce functional residual capacity.

Rationale: The diaphragm is dome shaped and does 80% of the work of breathing. In chronic lung disease, the diaphragm becomes weak and flattened from disease. Conscious use of the diaphragm will strengthen it.

Expected Outcome: The client will be able to consciously use the diaphragm during respiration.

Client Instructions

1. Assume a comfortable resting position.
2. Place one hand over your upper abdomen so that you will be able to feel the movement of your diaphragm.
3. Place the other hand on your upper chest so that you will be able to feel the movement of your accessory muscles.

4. Exhale through pursed lips. Feel the inward motion of your abdominal muscles.
5. Inhale. During inhalation, your abdomen should expand outward.
6. Avoid overbreathing, which may lead to lightheadedness.
7. Repeat this exercise five to six times. Practice several times a day, until the exercise is comfortable and relaxing. Use the technique both to help you relax and to alleviate shortness of breath.

Once the client is comfortable with abdominal breathing, teach him or her to experience the contraction of the lower rib cage and the abdominal muscles at the end of respiration, to push excess residual volume from the lungs. This exercise can be used during periods of dyspnea to gain control over breathing or with activity to increase exercise tolerance.

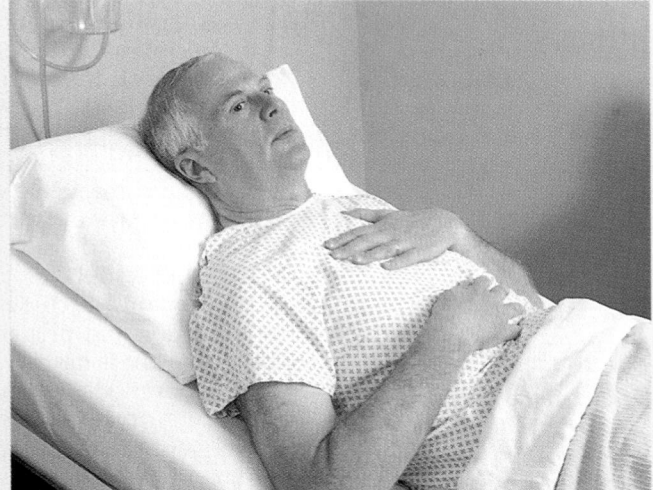

Diaphragmatic breathing is practiced best in a relaxed semirecumbent or recumbent position. Some people require little practice, but others may need several sessions of practice to learn the technique. (From Monahan, F.D., & Neighbors, M. [1998]. Medical-surgical nursing: Foundations for clinical practice (2nd ed.). Philadelphia: W.B. Saunders Co.)

Once the acute episode has passed, techniques to prevent and control anxiety can be taught (Gift, Moore, & Soeken, 1992). For the chronic respiratory client or the client with multiple acute episodes, reducing the general level of anxiety and learning to control episodes of anxiety can be useful in managing respiratory disease and improving the quality of life. Carrieri-Kohlman, Douglas, Gormley, and Stulbarg (1993) suggest a program of desensitization and guided mastery to assist clients in the management of dyspnea.

Mrs. Wilheim's anxiety level is high. She knew several people who died of pneumonia in the 1930s, including one of her sisters. Mrs. Wilheim's daughter assumes responsibility for the care of her mother and provides direct practical care to help her feel more comfortable. The daughter also takes responsibility for interacting with the health care team. How would you work with

Mrs. Wilheim and her daughter to manage Mrs. Wilheim's anxiety?

Managing Energy Requirements

NUTRITION

Whether the condition is acute or chronic, nutrition intake should, at a minimum, meet the daily requirements for nutrients. In acute illness, more than the minimum daily requirements are needed to meet the increased metabolic demand associated with fever or prostration. However, the severely ill person may not be able to tolerate a normal diet. Small, frequent meals may be helpful in meeting nutritional needs. The foods should be easily digested, easily chewed and swallowed, and palatable to the client.

For the chronic respiratory client who has lost excessive weight, improved nutrition can restore strength and endurance to respiratory and skeletal muscles. This effect is difficult to achieve and maintain, especially in the home, because the problems of activity intolerance, meal preparation, and chronic hypoxemia are closely inter-related. Increased intake of calories for energy is more important than added protein because loss of lean body mass is not usually the problem.

Mrs. Wilheim's daughter expresses concern over how much her mother is eating. Making sure her mother eats properly is her major concern. How would you meet the daughter's need while minimizing the risk of abdominal distention that normal food intake poses for Mrs. Wilheim?

ACTIVITY AND REST

The client with respiratory problems needs activity to stimulate respiratory function and needs rest to conserve energy or reduce the metabolic demand. In the hospitalized client, the physician's treatment plan may have specific guidelines for activity or simply call for activity as tolerated. You must make a judgment about the client's needs. Useful parameters may include changes in vital signs and the client's report of fatigue or dyspnea. In planning for activity, consider other scheduled treatments and procedures. Activity as simple as a bedbath can adversely affect oxygen saturation (Atkins, Hapshe, & Riegal, 1994).

The chronic respiratory client living at home may need assistance with planning a schedule or with modification of activities to incorporate efficient work habits and conserve energy. Teaching may include the following:

- Prioritize activities. Only schedule part of the day. Plan to accomplish the most important activity on a list. Allow time for rest periods.
- Arrange needed items conveniently. For example, have the coffee pot and all supplies close to the sink. Keep a stool handy to sit at the sink. Keep items needed for paying bills in one location to avoid having to gather supplies to sit down to take care of personal business.
- Simplify everyday life. Uncluttered surfaces are easier to clean. It is easier to find needed items in uncluttered drawers and cabinets. Place most often used items within easy reach in closets and shelves.
- Work at a steady pace. As many tasks can be accomplished by working at a steady pace as when hurrying, and it will reduce the energy requirements.
- Save energy by rolling, pushing, or pulling rather than lifting. A small cart to carry items around the house or yard may be helpful.

Mrs. Wilheim remains on bedrest with bathroom privileges for the first 48 to 72 hours. While on bedrest, she asks many questions about the bedside stand, lights, and bed controls and continually reviews the location of her glasses, tissues, wastebasket, call button, and personal articles. What do you think is the meaning of her behavior? How can you help her?

ENVIRONMENTAL CONTROL

Pollutants or allergens in the environment may exacerbate respiratory disease. The client may need to be advised to avoid persons with respiratory infections or areas where smoking is permitted. If the problem in the home environment is severe, the client may need to make some modifications. Carpeted floors can harbor allergens. Installing special air filters, damp dusting of the furniture, discarding feather pillows, or even giving away a pet are among the changes that may be needed. The client's personal preferences and values should be considered and changes recommended only if a real benefit can be anticipated. It is sometimes helpful to wear a mask for activities outside the house where the environment cannot be controlled.

INFECTION CONTROL

Infection control includes both protecting the client from infection and preventing the spread of infection when the client is already infected. Always apply universal precautions when working with the person with respiratory disorders. Wear clean gloves if the client has a productive cough or when working with equipment that has been contaminated with the client's sputum. Teach the client to cover the mouth when coughing and provide a convenient container for disposing of tissues. Wash your hands after each contact with the client. Use all necessary attire including gown and mask, as needed, to protect yourself from contact with airborne respiratory secretions. When working with clients who have a history of copious secretions or those receiving aggressive respiratory interventions, such as coughing or airway suctioning, you may need to wear goggles.

To avoid infection, the client must practice good health habits. A balance of rest and activity, avoiding exposure to extremes of cold or heat, and balanced nutrition are important. Visitors should be screened, and anyone who might expose the person to infection should be asked to leave. A clean environment and personal hygiene will reduce the number of microorganisms to which the client is exposed.

The threat of infection is one of the primary hazards of home respiratory therapy care. Respiratory equipment harbors bacteria; the *Pseudomonas* organism is a major problem. The client needs to be taught hand-washing and cleaning protocols for caring for any equipment being used. Mold growth is also a problem, especially since mold spores are a common allergen. Even though the equipment appears to be clean, periodic cultures may be taken to verify that pathogenic organisms are not present.

Managing Primary Hyperventilation

The treatment for hyperventilation that is not from a metabolic or respiratory cause is rebreathing carbon dioxide. Special equipment is available that can be used with a mask to allow the client to rebreathe carbon dioxide until the carbon dioxide level is brought within normal limits. However, a brown paper bag held over the nose and mouth is less expensive and just as effective.

Re-Expanding Collapsed Lungs

Atelectasis occurs with any event causing air or fluid to enter the pleural space. Trauma to the chest wall can result in a *hemothorax* or *pneumothorax.* Inflammation of the pleurae from pneumonia or cancer can result in a *pleural effusion* (exudation or transudation of fluid into the pleural space).

A physician inserts a chest tube to remove the trapped fluid or air. The lung can then re-expand. In some cases, the client may continue to bleed or have an air leak from the lungs. If the fluid or air is expected to continue to enter the pleural cavity, the chest tube is left in place until the lung has re-expanded and it is confirmed that no further problem exists. Placing a chest tube may be done as an emergency procedure or a planned procedure, depending on the severity of the compromise to ventilation.

Nurses assist with the placement of chest tubes and manage the tube after insertion. Management includes maintaining the placement of the tube, maintaining the patency of the tube, and maintaining the drainage system. The tube is easily dislodged because it is held in place only by the mushroom end of the tube and the occlusive dressing at the tube site. The tube must remain patent to drain the fluid or air. Box 39–5 provides guidelines for managing chest tubes.

Chest tube drainage systems use a tube submerged in water, where atmospheric pressure provides the pressure necessary to counter the negative intrapleural pressure and the water seal prevents air from entering the intrapleural space. The system can use a one-, two-, or three-bottle system. The disposable system is essentially a three-bottle system.

The one-bottle system is the simplest system, with the bottle serving to provide both the underwater seal and the drainage collection receptacle. The drainage tubing is connected to a tube that goes through the sealed top of the bottle and is submerged in the water. The water prevents air from entering the connecting tubing, where it could be drawn into the pleural space. The system must be airtight. Connections are some-

times taped to ensure that no air leaking occurs. The one-bottle system is appropriate for cases in which the amount of drainage is expected to be small and to readily drain from the intrapleural space. When air is being removed from the lungs it can be seen to bubble in the water seal.

The two-bottle system adds a separate bottle for drainage when larger amounts of drainage are expected. Typically, drainage does not enter the water seal bottle, but if the drainage bottle fills, it could overflow into the water seal bottle. Usually the chest tube would be briefly clamped and the drainage bottle changed before overflow occurs.

The three-bottle system adds a bottle, which is attached to suction to provide negative pressure when more rapid chest drainage is desired. The third bottle is open to the atmosphere with an under-water sealed tube so atmospheric air is drawn into the water and bubbles through the water. The suction pressure is determined by the length of the tube that is under water. Pressure is measured in centimeters of the tube that is under water.

Glass bottles for chest tube drainage are hazardous and have given way to the disposable systems. Because the collection system must be lower than the client's chest at all time, glass bottles sitting on the floor are vulnerable to breakage. Air would then be immediately drawn into the client's pleural space and the lung would be collapsed. The disposable systems are economic and convenient. A one-bottle chest tube suction device that is mounted on a three-point stand is also commonly used.

Interventions to Clear the Airways
Assisting the Client to Cough

As a common symptom of respiratory disease, a cough serves a protective function to clear the airway of irritants and secretions or to protect the client from aspiration of irritating or foreign substances. In general, coughing is encouraged as a means of clearing the airways. In the absence of the cough reflex, in the presence of a weakened condition or abnormal lung function, the client may need assistance to clear the airways by coughing.

Assisting the client to effectively clear the airways by coughing out sputum begins before the client attempts to cough. Other interventions to promote movement of secretions may be implemented in preparation for coughing. The secretions must be mobile; that is, non-sticky and liquid. The client must be able to manage deep inspirations before the cough to increase the lung volume and widen the airways, allowing air to get behind mucus and propel it upward. Forceful contraction of the expiratory muscles is needed to expel air at a velocity sufficient to move the mucus. The client must be able to assume a posture that will allow effective use of the abdominal muscles and maximum expansion of the chest. The Teaching for Self-Care chart provides guidelines for teaching an effective cough.

BOX 39–5

MANAGING A CLOSED CHEST TUBE DRAINAGE SYSTEM

Understand the Function of the Components of the System

Closed chest tube drainage systems are designed to maintain negative pressure to assist drainage and to prevent air from entering the pleural space.

The system consists of three main components. The first component, called the *suction control chamber,* is a column of water that acts as a suction control. The level of the water (10–20 cm), rather than the amount of suction from the vacuum source, determines the amount of negative pressure created to facilitate drainage. The opening to the atmosphere prevents the buildup of nega-

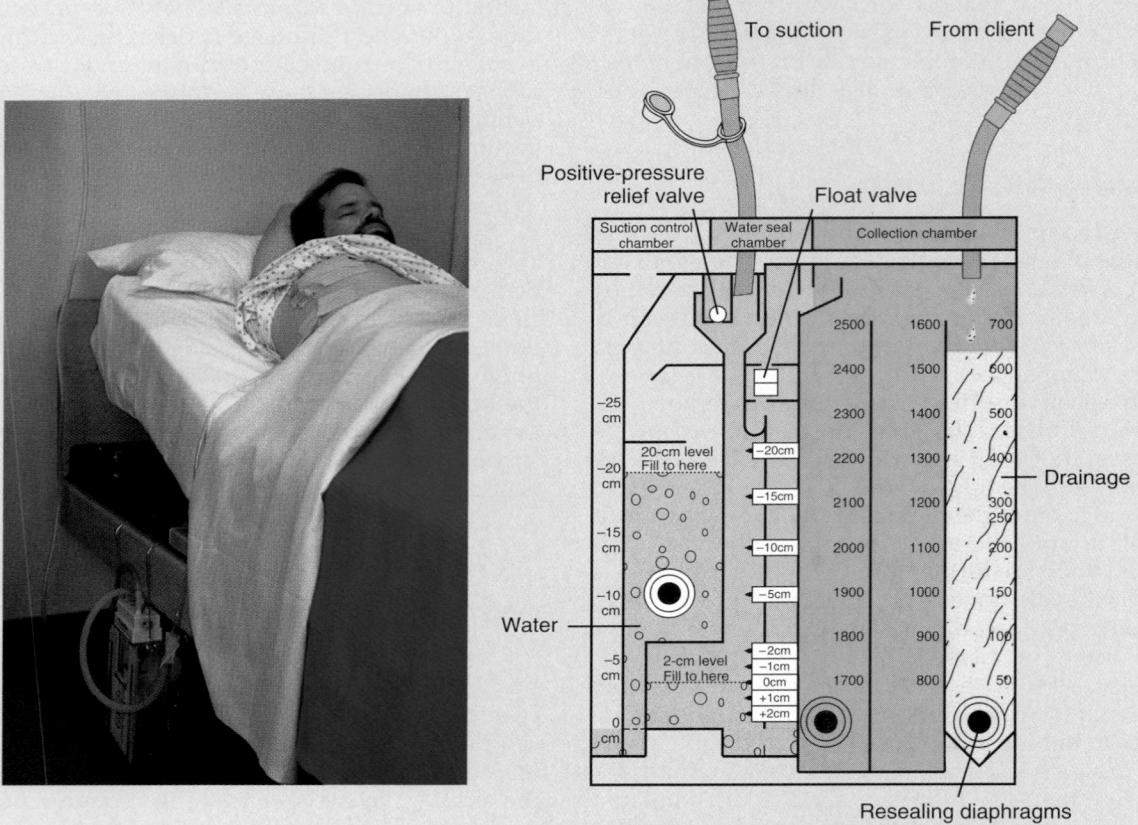

A chest tube attached to a typical drainage device. The chest tube is positioned in the lower thoracic cavity to drain serous fluid or blood. Notice the occlusive pressure dressing at the insertion site.

Continued

The sudden forceful change in pressure that accompanies a cough can have a deleterious effect, especially for the client with anatomic pulmonary disease (diseases that cause a structural change in the alveoli). In rare instances, already weakened alveoli may rupture, causing pneumothorax. A more common though less observable occurrence is collapse of small airways. Clients with anatomic pulmonary diseases like emphysema may benefit from learning a *controlled cough,* or "huff" technique. The client produces a cough by taking small breaths and, with the glottis partially open, coughs two to four times until all the

air is exhaled. This process may need to be repeated two to three times before the sputum is actually expectorated.

Suctioning the Airways

If the client is unable to effectively cough sputum from the airways, the airways can be cleared by *oral* or *endotracheal* (into and beyond the trachea) suctioning. Suctioning is a traumatic experience for most clients and should be implemented as a measure of last resort. The benefits should be weighed against the risk of

BOX 39–5

MANAGING A CLOSED CHEST TUBE DRAINAGE SYSTEM (continued)

tive pressure in the system. If bubbling occurs in this chamber, this is an indication that the suction is too high, because the suction has overcome atmospheric pressure. The second component is a dual-compartment *water seal chamber*. One compartment is open to the drainage chamber, and the other compartment is open to a second water seal barrier. The water seal (2 cm) prevents air from entering the chest tube. The third component is a three-compartment *collection chamber*. It holds up to 3000 mL of drainage. Connecting tubing is attached from the chest tube to the collection chamber. The collection chamber is open to the dual-compartment water seal chamber.

Nursing Responsibilities

MAINTAIN THE INTEGRITY OF THE SYSTEM

Maintain the Patency of the Tube. Observe for drainage. Assess the client's breath sounds. Absence of breath sounds indicates collapsed lung.

Maintain the Occlusive Dressing. The dressing should remain intact.

Maintain the Water Seal. The water seal must be maintained at all times by avoiding movements that would disturb the water seal, keeping the system upright, and keeping the system below the level of the chest. The tubing should be positioned to maintain a straight line of drainage from the chest to the collection system.

Maintain Suction. Suction is regulated by the balance between atmospheric pressure and the height of the column of water. The atmospheric air vent must remain open. Suction pressure of 10 mm Hg to 20 mmHg is sufficient to create subatmospheric pressure.

Observe for Air Leaks. Bubbling occurs in the water seal chamber when air is present in the pleural space and is being removed from the chest. When bubbling continues beyond a reasonable time for removing the

trapped air, you should consider a possible air leak from the lungs or from the system. Air leaks occur in the system when the connections are not tight. To check for air leaks in the system, use a padded Kelly clamp. Briefly clamp the chest tube as it comes out of the chest wall. If the bubbling stops, the air is coming from the chest. If the bubbling does not stop, move the clamp to below the connection. If the bubbling stops now, air is leaking into the connection. If the bubbling continues now, the leak is at the connection of the connecting tubing to the water seal system.

Monitor the Client's Response to Treatment

Respiratory Function. Audible breath sounds throughout the lung fields indicates ventilation. When the chest tube is inserted to relieve atelectasis caused by pneumothorax or hemothorax, the client should experience immediate relief of respiratory distress. Signs of tension pneumothorax: severe respiratory distress, absence of breath sounds on affected side, hyperresonance on affected side, mediastinal shift to affected side, tracheal shift to affected side, hypotension, tachycardia.

Character of Drainage. A chest injury or chest surgery may result in air in the pleural space. Bubbles occur in the drainage compartment until the air is removed. An air leak in the lungs will result in bubbles until the leak is sealed. Bloody drainage from a healing wound will change to the straw color of serous drainage in 24 to 48 hours. Continued bloody drainage indicates continued bleeding.

Amount of Drainage. Measure the amount of drainage each shift. Because the system must remain intact, do not empty the drainage. Mark the level of drainage on the apparatus and subtract the previous level of drainage.

possible complications. Table 39–7 lists indications for suctioning.

Oral suctioning refers to suctioning the mouth and oropharynx. Several types of suctioning tips are available. A Yankauer tip is the least traumatic for oral suctioning, but a whistle tip may also be used (Fig. 39–6). Oral suctioning may be helpful when the client is coughing up sputum but cannot get it beyond the oropharynx or when an artificial airway impedes removal of mucus from the oropharynx. Suctioning the oropharynx will sometimes stimulate a cough. It is used

when swallowing is impaired and aspiration of accumulated oral secretions is a danger. It carries a low risk for complications.

Endotracheal suctioning is accomplished using a whistle-tip catheter attached to a suctioning device. Entering the trachea and branches of the bronchi with minimal trauma to the client requires skill and knowledge of the anatomy of the airways. Since endotracheal suctioning is irritating to the airways, it can actually increase the production of mucus and exacerbate the problems of airway clearance rather than re-

Teaching for SELF-CARE

EFFECTIVE COUGHING

Purpose: To maintain clear airways.

Rationale: The natural cough mechanism may be suppressed by medications, fatigue, or pathological changes in the respiratory tract.

Expected Outcome: The client will produce an effective cough.

Client Instructions

1. Take three slow, relaxed deep breaths. This will open your alveoli and get air behind the mucus in your respiratory tract.
2. On the last breath, hold your breath for 2 to 3 seconds. Holding your breath increases the pressure in your chest to produce a more forceful cough.
3. Contract your abdominal muscles and force the air out through your mouth. This contraction produces the forceful exhalation recognized as a cough.

Hints:

*   Splinting an abdominal incision with a pillow or soft blanket will protect the client from pain caused by uncontrolled movement of the abdomen.
*   Having the client sit upright and lean slightly forward will help produce the increased airway pressure that is needed to produce an effective cough.
*   Have facial tissues and a waste receptacle close at hand.

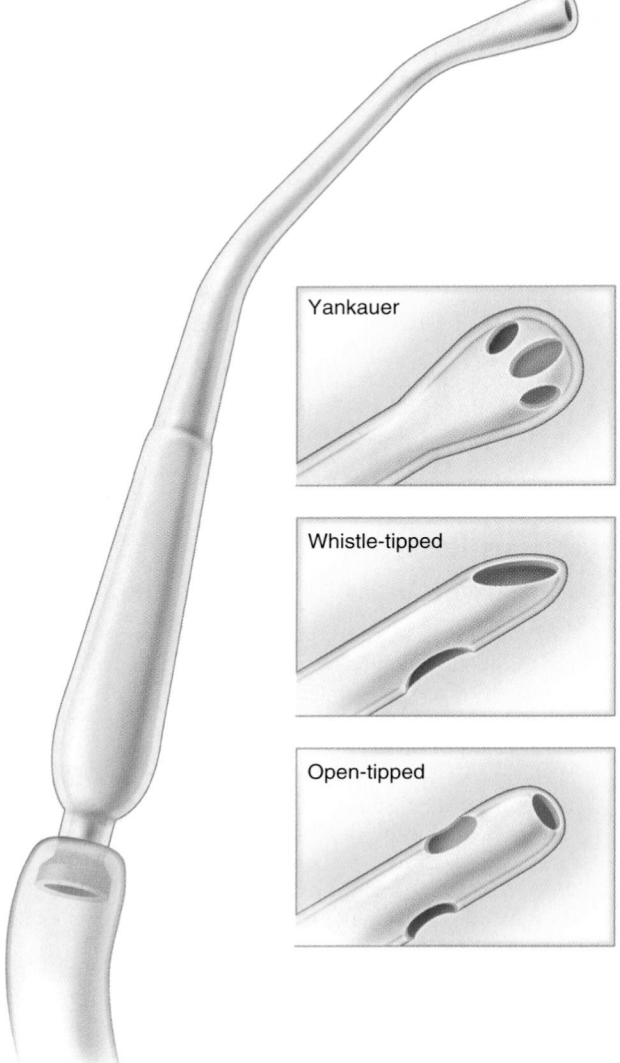

Yankauer

Whistle-tipped

Open-tipped

Figure 39–6. Types of suction catheter tips: Yankauer tip, whistle tip, and open tip.

TABLE 39–7
Indications for Suctioning

Assessment	Indications for Suctioning
Visual	Rapid, shallow breathing or difficult, labored breathing suggests need for further assessment.
Auditory	Moist, noisy, or gurgling sounds associated with breathing are definitive if the client cannot cough.
Tactile (fremitus)	Placing a hand flat over the client's chest wall detects vibrations of loose secretions; a more likely finding in an infant.
Auscultation	Coarse crackles (bubbling rhonchi); a loose, continuous, low-pitched rattling sound that disappears after suctioning or coughing

ducing the volume of mucus. Capillary bleeding can further complicate the situation. Procedure 39–1 provides guidelines for endotracheal suctioning. Table 39–8 identifies common complications of suctioning and strategies for prevention.

SUCTIONING ROUTE

The principle to be followed in clearing the airways is to use the least invasive procedure necessary to produce the desired result. If a cough can be produced by entering the trachea, the sputum can be quickly suctioned without trauma to the lower airways. If no cough is stimulated, the catheter is passed to the carina and an attempt is made to enter both the right and left bronchi. The right bronchus is anatomically easier to enter because the angle is small as it branches off the main bronchi. The left bronchi can sometimes be en-

PROCEDURE 39–1

Endotracheal Suctioning

TIME TO ALLOW
▼
Novice:
10 min.
Expert:
5 min.

The purpose is to remove secretions, thus relieving airway obstruction. This procedure is traumatic to the airways and requires attention to safety to prevent complications.

Delegation Guidelines

Assessment of the need for airway clearance may not be delegated to a nursing assistant. The potential risks associated with airway clearance by suctioning dictate that this task not be delegated to a nursing assistant in the hospital setting. The assembly of equipment and assistance with suctioning may be delegated to a second person. In this circumstance, the nursing assistant receives direct, immediate supervision. The nursing assistant must receive specialized instruction and demonstrate ongoing competence in the performance of this skill. In long-term care settings, it may be appropriate to delegate clearance of artificial airways to a nursing assistant who has received appropriate training and supervision.

Equipment Needed

- Portable or wall suction unit
- Sterile suction kit
  or
  Sterile gloves
  Sterile suction catheter with Y port (thumb control port)
  Sterile normal saline
  Sterile cup for normal saline
- Option: clean supplies
- Towel or waterproof pad

1 Recognize the need for suctioning.

Accurate assessment ensures suctioning when needed and prevents unnecessary suctioning.

    a. Wet, gurgling respirations without the strength to cough productively; or
    b. Auscultation of bubbling rhonchi in the tracheobronchial tree; or
    c. The presence of a nasotracheal or tracheostomy tube.

2 Gather the necessary equipment.

3 Determine whether to use a sterile or clean procedure.

The choice of using a sterile or clean procedure depends on the client's risk for infection, especially the risk for nosocomial infection. The lungs are not sterile; however, suctioning bypasses normal respiratory defense mechanisms and therefore places the client at risk for infection. Also, the client who needs suctioning is often critically ill. Sterile technique prevents the entry of any microorganism into the lungs at a time when the client is most vulnerable to infection. On the other hand, clients with permanent tracheostomies or who are on mechanical ventilators at home also need suctioning. There, clean rather than sterile procedures are often used. Clean technique is less expensive and therefore can be used over a longer period.

4 Get the client's cooperation.

Suctioning will be less traumatic if the client is able to cooperate. When a client needs to be suctioned, the explanation should be brief and to the point. If the client is unable to cooperate fully, a second person may be needed to restrain the client's hands.

5 Set up the equipment.

You should be ready to suction the client immediately once the client is preoxygenated.

    a. Turn on the suction. Use a vacuum pressure of 80 to 120 mm Hg with wall suction (60–100 mm Hg for an infant; 80–115 mm Hg for a child).
    b. Open the sterile saline; place the cap inverted on a clean surface.
    c. Open the suction kit.
    d. Pick up the container for the saline, squeeze to open it, and set it aside; keep the inside sterile. Pour water or saline into the container.
    e. Put on one sterile glove. Open the sterile cup and pour the saline solution into it with your nonsterile hand. Then put on the other glove.
    f. Pick up the sterile catheter with your sterile dominant hand and the unsterile suction connecting tubing with your nondominant hand.

Continued

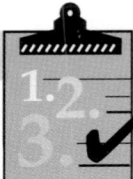

PROCEDURE 39–1 *(continued)*

Endotracheal Suctioning

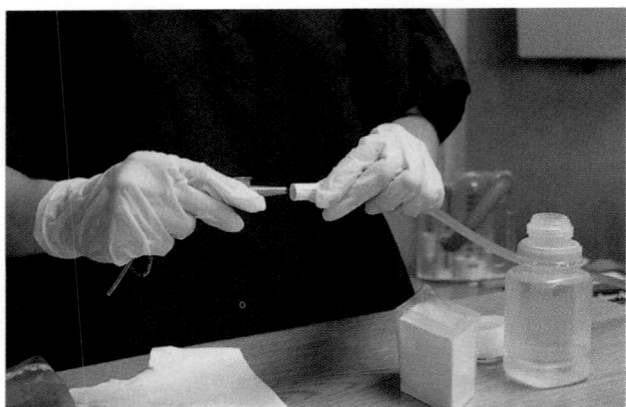

Connecting the sterile suction catheter to the unsterile connecting tubing that leads to the suction unit.

Connect the two, keeping your dominant hand and the catheter sterile. The nondominant hand becomes unsterile when it is used to attach the unsterile connecting tubing to the suction catheter.

6 When you are ready to suction, have an assistant hyperinflate the lungs with 100% oxygen.

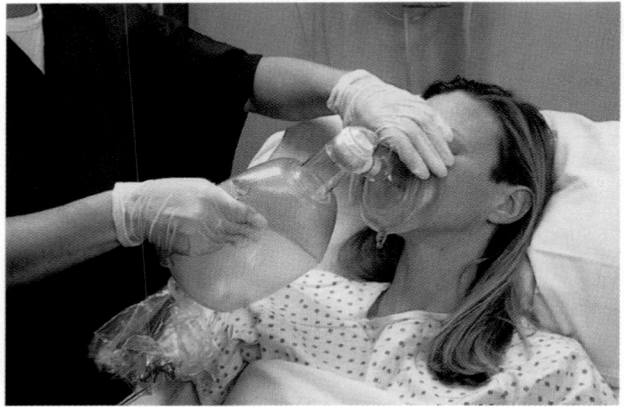

Hyperinflating the lungs with an Ambu bag.

Preoxygenation will temporarily increase the PaO₂ and reduce the risk of hypoxemia during suctioning.

   a. If the client does not have an artificial airway, have the client take several deep breaths.
   b. If the client has an endotracheal tube or tracheostomy, use an Ambu bag to give two to three deep breaths. You have to make a clinical judgment about whether or not to increase the oxygen supply.

7 Pass the catheter through the nose into the oropharynx. Watch the client's respiration and pass the catheter into the trachea when the person inhales. Or, pass the catheter directly into the endotracheal or tracheostomy tube. Leave the Y port open while passing the catheter. Pass the catheter until you meet resistance, then close the Y port to apply suction. When you enter the trachea, start counting; you should be out of the trachea by the time you reach 10.

Suctioning only while withdrawing the catheter will reduce the degree of trauma to the tracheobronchial tree. Time is a factor in reducing the oxygen deficit with suctioning.

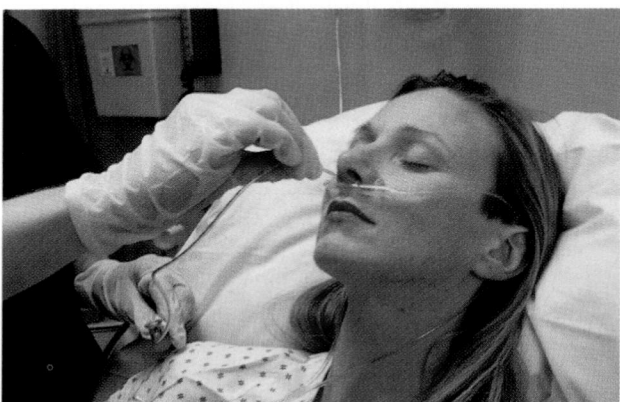

Passing the suction catheter through the nose as the client takes a breath.

8 Hyperinflate the lungs to reoxygenate the client.
Hyperinflation helps the client restore oxygenation and regain control of breathing.

   a. Client-initiated: If the client is able or is not intubated, have the client take several slow, deep breaths.
   b. Nurse-initiated: Use an Ambu bag attached to an endotracheal tube or tracheostomy tube, or use a face mask if the client is not intubated.

9 Assess the results; repeat if needed. Do not withdraw the catheter from the client's nose until you are sure you will not pass the catheter into the trachea again. Clear the catheter by suctioning the normal saline or water before repeating the procedure. Assess the amount and characteristics of the

sputum; assess for decreased rhonchi. Suctioning is effective if the rhonchi have cleared or diminished.

Limiting suction prevents excessive trauma from suctioning. The generally accepted practice is to limit suctioning

to three times with the same catheter in a single session of suctioning. Clearing the catheter allows you to better assess the sputum with each suctioning.

HINTS

1. Having the client in a semi-Fowler position facilitates passing the catheter and may help the client cough, if a cough reflex is stimulated.
2. If you stimulate a cough reflex when entering the oropharynx or trachea, you can stop passing the catheter and suction the sputum that the client has coughed up into the trachea. You will have accomplished your goal of clearing the airway without having to pass a catheter deep into the tracheobronchial tree.
3. It is helpful for a second person to hyperinflate the lungs, especially when you are inexperienced.
4. Rotate the catheter as you withdraw it, to clear all sides of the airway.
5. Use standard precautions when contact with sputum is likely, especially if blood is present in the sputum. Masks and goggles may be necessary.

HOME CARE CONSIDERATIONS

When a client requires suctioning in the home, it is usually suctioning through a tracheostomy. Some clients learn to suction themselves; however, the procedure is most often performed by family caregivers. The caregiver will need support from the nurse to learn to perform the procedure. Ideally, the caregiver will have an opportunity to practice the procedure before the client is discharged from the hospital. A home care nurse can then follow up with a home visit to help modify the technique for the home, to plan for the cleaning and storage of supplies, to obtain supplies, and to reinforce the essential elements of technique. The caregiver will need to be taught to recognize the need for suctioning and to evaluate the results. Some caregivers can learn to use a stethoscope to listen to the lungs.

tered successfully by having the client hyperextend the neck, turning the head to the right. Successful suctioning is confirmed by auscultation of the lungs.

CLIENT POSITIONING
Position the client to maximize the normal physiological functions in the conscious client and to prevent aspiration in the unconscious client. If the client can tolerate a semi-Fowler or high Fowler position, airway clearance will be more effective when a reflexive cough is produced when the catheter enters the posterior pharynx or trachea. Administer suction as the client coughs up the secretions; this technique clears the airway with minimal trauma. The unconscious client may be protected from aspiration by use of the lateral position to allow drainage from the mouth by gravity. However, the airway is less accessible for suctioning when the client is in the lateral position. Turning con-

sumes time if the client is not already in the lateral position.

STERILE VERSUS CLEAN TECHNIQUE
Although *sterile* means the absence of any micro-organisms, and the airways are not sterile, the airways past the glottis are considered to be sterile. Even though the lungs have protective mechanisms against micro-organisms, the principle of preventing infection by not introducing any organisms into a body cavity would suggest the use of sterile technique. Furthermore, the action of suctioning traumatizes the epithelium of the airways, providing a portal for entry of micro-organisms.

Hospital protocol generally includes the use of sterile technique for endotracheal suctioning and clean technique for oropharyngeal suctioning or nasopharyngeal suctioning. If both pharyngeal suctioning and

TABLE 39–8

Etiology and Prevention of Complications of Suctioning

Complication	Etiology	Prevention
Hypoxemia and atelectasis	Suction removes oxygen-laden air.	The PaO$_2$ can be significantly raised by increasing the FIO$_2$. Preoxygenate the client with 100% oxygen and hyperventilate the client at 1½ of the tidal volume. For the client without an artificial airway, you can accomplish this by increasing the liter flow of oxygen and having the client take deep breaths. Hyperinflation and oxygenation after suction are expected to restore the oxygen level and open the alveoli. Avoid vacuum pressure greater than 80 to 120 mm Hg for the adult.
Mucosal trauma	The plastic catheter can damage the mucosa.	Lubricate the catheter. Twist rather than push past minor resistance. Stop when you meet resistance. Apply suction only when withdrawing catheter, and use intermittent suction. If bleeding occurs and frequent suctioning is necessary, consider using a nasal airway.
Vagal stimulation	Suctioning stimulates the parasympathetic vagus nerve, which supplies both the trachea and the heart.	Vagal stimulation slows the heart rate. Bradycardia, ventricular arrhythmias, or cardiac arrest may occur. Suction only when needed and use preoxygenation and hyperventilation.
Increased mean arterial pressure	Associated with hyperinflation	Hyperinflation by changing the ventilator settings to 1½ times the tidal volume is less likely to increase the mean arterial pressure than is the use of a manual resuscitation bag. This is particularly important for clients with new vascular grafts or with increased intracranial pressure.
Paroxysmal coughing	Irritation of the cough control center at the carina	While stimulating a cough may prevent the need for deeper suctioning in some clients, the uncontrolled cough of others can collapse airways and irritate the tracheobronchial tree, stimulating bronchospasm. Suction only as necessary and maintain oxygenation.

endotracheal suctioning are required, you may change catheters after pharyngeal suctioning and before endotracheal suctioning or may first suction endotracheally. Sterile technique is believed to have benefits that outweigh the cost in a situation where the risk of nosocomial infection is high.

For the homebound client who requires frequent suctioning on a long-term basis, the cost of sterile technique may outweigh the benefits. Teach family caregivers proper suctioning technique and how to maintain a clean environment. Also, family members may have difficulty maintaining sterile technique. Provide sterile suctioning catheters but explain that the catheters can be reused. Between uses, catheters are immersed in an antiseptic solution of boric acid and 0.4 to 0.5% sodium hypochlorite (Dakin's solution) or washed in warm soapy water. The catheter is rinsed thoroughly before it is introduced into the trachea. Clean rather than sterile gloves reduce the cost of equipment.

SUCTIONING FREQUENCY

Suction as often as needed to maintain a clear airway without damaging the epithelial lining of the airways. Limiting suctioning to three passes of the catheter for each session of suctioning and 1 to 2 hours between sessions may help reduce trauma and the concurrent increase in mucus production. Bedside judgment must be made to balance the two goals.

OXYGENATION

Suctioning removes not only mucus, but also oxygen-laden air from the airways. The resulting hypoxemia can be life-threatening. Hypoxemia may be prevented by increasing the inspired oxygen concentration to the highest possible safe percentage of oxygen and hyperinflating the lungs with manual or spontaneous breaths before and after suctioning (Jacobsen, 1993). The best levels of oxygenation and hyperinflation are achieved with 100% oxygen delivered by a self-inflating resuscitation bag (Ambu bag). Monitor the rate and rhythm of the pulse and respiration to detect adverse effects.

Choose the method of oxygenation appropriate for each individual client. The client who is able to take deep breaths and does not have other risk factors for oxygen deficit may tolerate suctioning with only deep breaths of room air. The homebound client who is otherwise stable also can usually tolerate suction without supplemental oxygen. The intensive care client is almost always preoxygenated with 100% oxygen before and after suctioning. However, the presence of chronic airflow limitation (CAL) makes administration of 100% oxygen risky.

HYDRATION OF SECRETIONS

Thick, tenacious sputum is not easily removed by suctioning. Applying the principle of employing the least harmful treatment that will produce the best results, the client's secretions are best hydrated by adequate fluid intake. However, if the client continues to have tenacious sputum, normal saline can be instilled immediately before passing the suction catheter (Ackerman, 1993). This technique is easily managed in the client with a *tracheostomy* (an opening directly into the trachea, made by a surgical incision) or an endotracheal tube (ET tube), but it may irritate the airways and increase bronchospasm.

VACUUM PRESSURE CONTROL

The maximum pressure setting on the vacuum suction device should be the lowest pressure required to remove secretions. The gauges on wall-mounted suction units in a piped-in vacuum system are calibrated in mm Hg vacuum pressure. The safe range for vacuum pressures for adults is 80 to 120 mm Hg. If the catheter is too small or the secretions are too thick, excessive vacuum pressure may be reached, that is, higher than safe limits. Use a larger catheter and step up measures to reduce the tenacity of the secretions.

CATHETER SELECTION

A suction catheter is selected that will cause the least trauma, minimize occlusion of the airway, and be large enough to remove the secretions. Suction catheters are rubber or plastic tubes approximately 18 inches long ending in a whistle tip. The whistle tip is a smooth, rounded, nontraumatic, sealed end with one or more openings on the side. The vents are spaced 1½ to 2 inches on alternate sides of the catheter. This prevents the collapse of the catheter if it becomes occluded or if high vacuum pressures are created. The vents also help reduce mucosal trauma by reducing the pull of the catheter against the mucosa.

You must be able to control the vacuum pressure, turning it off or on. To allow control of suction, the catheters are designed with a Y-port, which is attached to the connecting tubing. The port can be occluded by your thumb to close the system and produce a vacuum. This feature allows you to enter the trachea without suction on and to apply the suction as the catheter is withdrawn. Entering without suction reduces trauma by allowing the catheter to easily pass through the airway.

Liquefying and Mobilizing Sputum

EXPECTORANTS

Expectorants are used to loosen or liquefy the mucus so it can be coughed out more easily. Iodinated glycerol (Organidin), supersaturated solution of potassium iodide (SSKI), and guaifenesin are thought to stimulate sputum clearance. Guaifenesin is available both over the counter and by prescription. It is available as a single ingredient or in combination, frequently with the antitussive dextromethorphan. If the client is using over-the-counter medications, you may need to teach the difference between antitussives and expectorants. Difficult generic names should be provided in written form. The client should be questioned about allergies to iodine before using one of the iodinated compounds.

Guaifenesin and SSKI stimulate sputum clearance but also increase the production of mucus. The overall effectiveness of expectorants has not been clearly defined in careful clinical studies. Clients often report increased ability to cough out sputum.

MUCOLYTICS

Mucolytics are medications that alter the viscosity of the mucus so that it is more easily expectorated. Oral mucolytics or expectorants are more effective than topically applied agents. Acetylcysteine (Mucomyst), a once popular mucolytic, is irritating to the tracheobronchial tree and has not been proven to be effective in randomized studies but continues to be used on a limited basis. It is administered through a nebulizer. Bronchodilators are recommended in conjunction with mucolytics because the incidence of bronchospasm is high.

COUGH SUPPRESSANTS

Antitussives, or cough suppressants, are antithetical to the goal of expectoration of sputum. They are given only for symptomatic relief. It is reasonable to suppress a dry, hacking, nonproductive cough or a cough that is increasing fatigue or disturbing the sleep. A productive cough is a means of clearing the airways but might be treated with cough suppressant when the cough is tiring or is severe enough to cause concern about the complications of rib fracture or pneumothorax.

HUMIDITY

The viscosity of sputum may be directly related to the client's general level of hydration. Assess the client for dehydration and institute measures to treat or prevent it (see Chapter 31). Systemic hydration is thought to be the most effective means of maintaining moist airways.

Topical hydration of airways may be accomplished by increasing the humidity of the inspired air using room humidifiers and by creating an aerosol. The goal is to provide air with sufficient moisture and of a particle size to carry the moisture to the small airways. Results vary, however, and some practitioners do not believe it is effective.

A *humidifier* is a mechanical device that adds water vapor to the air. Humidification equipment may deliver water at room temperature, heated to body temperature, or slightly above body temperature. Heated air is able to carry more moisture. An *impeller humidifier* produces larger particles of water that may be too large to penetrate deeply into the tracheobronchial tree. Room humidifiers, used in many homes for upper respiratory infections, are the most common examples of impellers. Safe use includes careful cleaning between uses to prevent growth of molds and bacteria. Other, more complex forms of humidification are used with mechanical ventilators.

An *aerosol* is a fine suspension of a liquid or powder carried on a stream of gas. Aerosols may be large in volume (for hydration) or may be produced in small amounts, such as dry aerosols that deliver medications topically into the airway (see section on bronchodilators). To enter the tracheobronchial tree, a particle of liquid produced by an aerosol generator must be 1 to 3 μm in size. Large volume aerosols can potentially run on a continuous basis. These devices deliver a dense, large volume of water on a large volume of gas (compressed air or oxygen). The large volume of gas plus the dense aerosol significantly helps to hydrate the tracheobronchial tree. Large volume aerosols are administered via an aerosol face tent, face mask, or tracheostomy tent.

All methods of topical hydration carry a risk of contamination because all devices include a water reservoir. Sterile solutions are used in nebulizers because the warm, moist environment can grow organisms that can be trapped in the particles of moisture and carried to the lungs. Hospitals have protocols for changing equipment regularly to provide sterile mask and tubing.

CHEST PHYSIOTHERAPY

Chest physiotherapy, abbreviated CPT or chest PT, is an approach to mobilizing and draining secretions from gravity-dependent areas of the lung that uses a combination of postural drainage, chest percussion, and vibration. When hydration, aerosol medication, deep breathing, and coughing are not sufficient to clear the airways, chest physiotherapy may be added.

Because secretions are more likely to be retained in gravity-dependent parts of the lungs, chest physiotherapy relies on positioning the person to use gravity to drain the various lobes of the lungs. **Postural drainage** is a technique in which the client assumes one or more positions that will facilitate the drainage of secretions from the bronchial airways. It is accomplished by placing the client in positions that allow gravity to facilitate drainage of mucus out of the lobes of the lungs and bronchopulmonary segments and into the larger bronchi (Fig. 39–7). When secretions reach the upper airways, they may be coughed up spontaneously or removed by tracheobronchial suctioning. Nine or more positions are required to drain all the areas of the lungs. However, the specific location of the pathology may suggest the position that will be the most effective.

It is not clear that postural drainage has more benefit than incentive spirometry, deep-breathing, and coughing for most clients with COPD, pneumonia, or postoperative atelectasis. If routine measures are not producing the desired results, postural drainage may be given an empiric trial and discontinued if there is no beneficial response. Clients with COPD and cystic fibrosis who benefit from postural drainage may continue the treatment on a long-term basis at home.

*A*ction *A*lert!
Scheduling of chest physiotherapy treatments may affect the results. Try to schedule chest physiotherapy as follows: in the early morning, when secretions

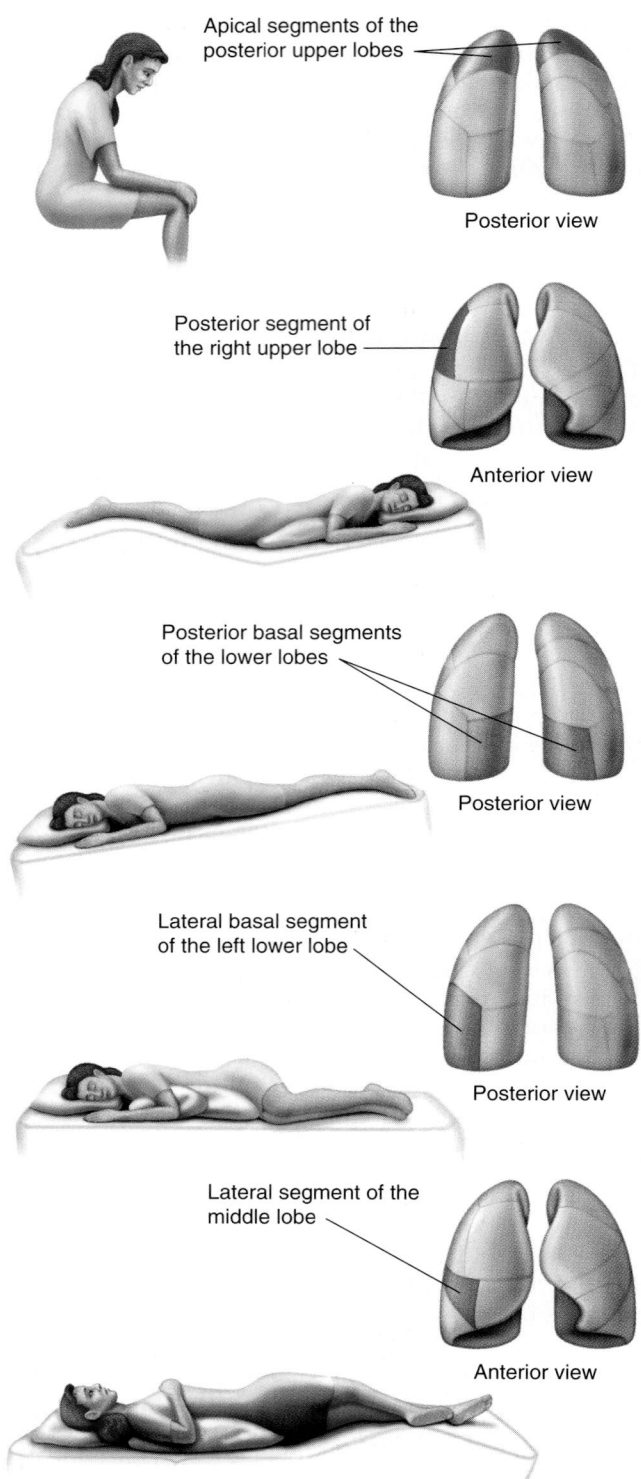

Figure 39–7. Examples of positions for postural drainage based on the area of the lung to be drained.

have accumulated during the night; 1 hour before meals or 2 hours after meals, to avoid aspiration; at bedtime, to clear the lungs and allow sleep free of coughing; at an appropriate time interval after administration of a bronchodilator when the medication has taken effect.

Percussion and vibration are added to postural drainage to increase the velocity of mucus movement up the tracheobronchial tree. **Chest percussion** is defined as using cupped hands to rhythmically clap on the chest wall over various segments of the lungs to mobilize secretions. It is performed immediately over the portion of the lung where secretions are retained (Fig. 39–8*A*). Cupping the hands in a manner to produce a hollow sound on impact with the chest prevents discomfort to the client. **Vibration** is a technique of chest physiotherapy whereby the chest wall is set in motion by oscillating movements of the hands or a vibrator for the purpose of mobilizing secretions (Fig 39–8*B*). Vibration theoretically increases the air currents to aid in removing trapped air and mucus.

Clients for chest physiotherapy should be carefully selected. Clients with heart problems, pneumonia, or CAL should be observed for hypoxemia. Rupture of a blood vessel or an abscess can rapidly obstruct the airway. Clients with osteoporosis or on long-term steroid therapy have fragile bones and can fracture a rib.

A*ction* A*lert!*
Some clients become dyspneic or hypoxic with postural drainage. Monitor the client carefully and discontinue the treatment if problems occur.

Reducing Sputum Production

CORTICOSTEROIDS
Both anti-inflammatory and antiallergenic effects may be achieved with corticosteroids. Aerosolized corticosteroids are available as nasal sprays used to prevent allergic rhinitis or oral inhalers to prevent asthma attacks. Two weeks of use is required before results are experienced. During acute bronchospasm, corticosteroids must be administered systemically (orally or intravenously). Inhalation of steroids may cause an overgrowth of *Candida albicans* in the mouth; therefore, the mouth should be rinsed after each administration.

A*ction* A*lert!*
If a client is on corticosteroids, ask questions about the length of use. Long-term use of corticosteroids can suppress production of corticosteroids by the adrenal gland. Check the physician's orders for supplemental corticosteroids to be given to manage the stress of acute illness or of surgery.

CROMOLYN SODIUM
Cromolyn sodium has both anti-inflammatory and antiallergenic effects. It is used to prevent allergic responses in the airway by preventing the rupture of mast cells and the release of bronchoconstrictive chemicals in the lungs. It is not a steroid, nor is it a drug used during acute bronchospastic episodes. It is most effective in asthmatic children and young adults but must be used for 2 weeks before it is effective.

ANTIHISTAMINES
Antihistamines provide symptomatic relief of rhinitis. The combination with decongestants is sometimes helpful. Newer antihistamines have less of a sedative side effect. Some antihistamines are more effective after several days of therapy. Because antihistamines have drying effects, asthmatic clients should seek the advice of a physician before using these drugs.

ANTIBIOTICS
A broad-spectrum antibiotic is ordered when there is evidence that a respiratory infection is caused by a

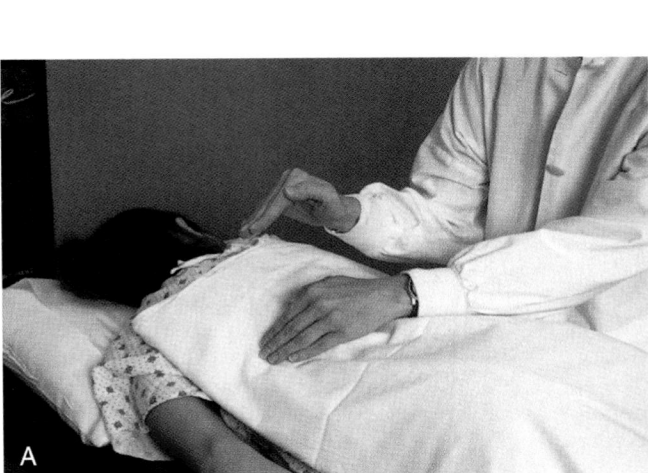
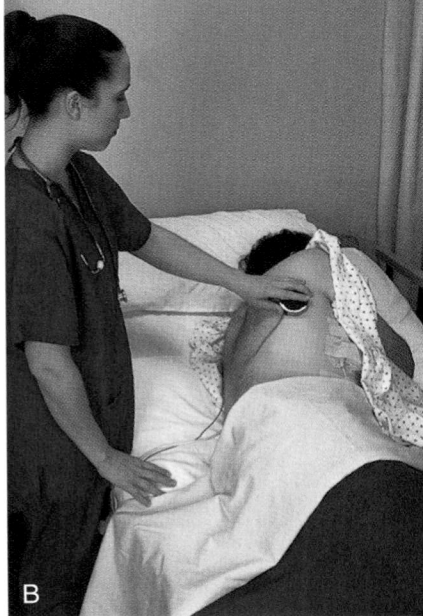

Figure 39–8. *A,* percussion is performed with "cupped" hands. The chest is protected with a towel while the hands rhythmically clap the chest wall. Using the wrist to control the motion ensures a gentle clapping motion. *B,* use of a vibrator for chest percussion.

bacteria or when there is high risk for developing an infection. Occasionally, antibiotics are aerosolized to treat pulmonary infections, but topical administration is generally less effective than systemically administered antibiotics. In the home setting, oral antibiotics may be used to treat infection and avert hospitalization. Prophylactic use of antibiotics in the home setting is sometimes prescribed for chronic respiratory clients but is controversial.

VASOCONSTRICTORS

Vasoconstrictors are used as decongestants of the respiratory mucosa. Because they are frequently sympathomimetic drugs, side effects of sympathetic stimulation occur. Pseudoephedrine is an example commonly found in over-the-counter cold remedies. Topically administered nasal sprays should only be used for a limited course of symptomatic relief. Development of rebound congestion after 2 to 3 days of therapy may lead the client to prolonged use.

Interventions to Improve Gas Exchange

Providing Supplemental Oxygen

Oxygen therapy may be prescribed for one of three goals: to maintain the arterial blood oxygen level, to reduce the work of breathing, or to reduce the myocardial workload. For the client with a serious acute illness that results in desaturation because of hypoventilation or a ventilation/perfusion abnormality, the goal is to maintain the arterial blood oxygen level until the cause of the hypoxemia can be corrected. For the chronic respiratory client who has exertional dyspnea directly related to hypoxemia, the goal is to reduce the work of breathing and increase activity tolerance. For the client who has a heart problem (myocardial infarction, heart failure) the goal may be to reduce the myocardial workload. For any specific client, these three benefits will often overlap.

Oxygen is a potentially toxic substance and is prescribed by a physician. You will participate in the decision-making process by reporting to the physician findings that indicate a change in the client's condition or the failure to respond to the prescribed oxygen therapy. The goal of oxygen therapy is to achieve an optimal arterial oxygen tension by giving the lowest possible, most effective dose of oxygen while avoiding its toxic effects.

$\mathbf{A}ction\ \mathbf{A}lert!$
Oxygen deficit is life-threatening. Notify the physician at the earliest sign of hypoxia.

Oxygen is given to keep arterial PaO_2 in the normal range of 80 to 100 mm Hg. Oxygen administration should not cause the arterial $PaCO_2$ to rise above 45 mm Hg. Different criteria may be used for a person with COPD who lives with chronically low oxygen and high carbon dioxide levels. In chronic lung disease, the normal drive to breathe from a high carbon dioxide level is suppressed, therefore the only drive to breathe is from a low oxygen level. When oxygen is needed to decrease the work of breathing and increase activity tolerance, low doses are used to avoid bringing the oxygen up to a normal level. Procedure 39–2 provides guidelines for administration of oxygen.

$\mathbf{A}ction\ \mathbf{A}lert!$
Always ask if the client has COPD before starting oxygen in amounts greater than 2 L/min. Be prepared to recognize the clinical appearance of a client with COPD.

Prolonged exposure to oxygen in high concentrations can cause structural damage to the lung tissue, which can be fatal. Oxygen toxicity is most often seen in the adult or neonatal intensive care unit. Although the exact relationship of long-term high concentrations of oxygen and blindness in premature infants is not clear, oxygen dosage is monitored closely as a preventive measure.

OXYGEN DELIVERY SYSTEMS

Oxygen delivery devices are divided into two broad categories: high-flow oxygen systems and low-flow oxygen systems. A high-flow system delivers a flow of gas that exceeds the volume of air required for the person's minute ventilation. Low-flow systems deliver oxygen at variable liter flows designed to supplement the inspired room air to provide airflow equal to the minute ventilation. Because the oxygen is imprecisely mixed with room air, oxygen percentages delivered by low-flow systems are not as consistent as the percentages in high-flow systems.

In a low-flow system, the percentage of oxygen delivered to the tracheobronchial tree is determined by the person's respiratory rate, the tidal volume, and the pattern of ventilation (deep, fast, shallow, irregular). The high-flow system provides a flow rate and reservoir capacity adequate to meet total inspired-air needs. The amount of oxygen to be delivered is ordered as liters of 100% oxygen per minute (LPM), percentage of oxygen in inspired air, or fraction of inspired oxygen (FIO_2). FIO_2 is the preferred method.

The choice of oxygen delivery device and liter flow depends on the client's condition. The principle is to provide the lowest percentage of oxygen that will maintain arterial oxygen saturation within normal range. Arterial blood quickly desaturates below 60 to 70 mm Hg, so the partial pressure of oxygen should be kept above 70. Anything higher is unnecessary. Clinical judgment is needed to decide that the client's condition suggests that a higher FIO_2 may be needed to achieve oxygen saturation. Once the client is stabilized on the prescribed FIO_2, arterial blood gases or pulse oximetry may be used to confirm that the desired results are being achieved. Consideration is also given to selecting a device that the client will find tolerable for continuous use. For guidelines on administering oxygen see Procedure 39–2.

LOW-FLOW SYSTEMS. Low-flow systems include a nasal cannula, an oxygen mask, or an oxygen mask with reservoir. The nasal cannula is the most com-

PROCEDURE 39–2

Administering Oxygen

TIME TO
ALLOW
▼
Novice:
10 min.
Expert:
5 min.

The administration of oxygen requires a physician's prescription. In an emergency, however, a nurse or respiratory therapist can make a decision to initiate oxygen therapy without a physician's order. In many hospitals, oxygen therapy is initiated by the respiratory therapy department. The respiratory therapist and the nurse work together to monitor the effects of oxygen therapy and to maintain safe, effective administration of oxygen.

Delegation Guidelines

The decision to initiate oxygen therapy may not be delegated to a nursing assistant. The gathering and assembly of equipment, along with administration of oxygen, may be delegated to a nursing assistant. In this case, specific instructions must be provided to help the nursing assistant monitor the client: measuring and recording vital signs, observing for evidence of breathing difficulties, noting respiratory rate and depth, color of lips and nail beds, and presence of restlessness or irritability. Be sure to provide parameters for immediate RN notification.

Equipment Needed

- Nasal cannula, simple face mask, nonrebreathing mask, or partial rebreathing mask
- Oxygen tubing
- Humidifier
- Sterile distilled water
- Oxygen flowmeter
- Oxygen source
- No-smoking sign

1 Assemble the necessary equipment. Check the physician's order for the delivery device and liter flow.

Supplemental oxygen is considered to be a drug and normally requires a physician's prescription. In emergency circumstances, however, you are legally permitted to decide to start oxygen.

a. No-smoking sign. Also, remove all smoking materials from the room.

Oxygen is not combustible but is necessary to support combustion. Fire from a small spark spreads rapidly in the presence of an oxygen source. A posted sign alerts personnel and visitors to the use of oxygen.

b. Humidification device

Humidity prevents drying of the mucous membranes from dry oxygen gas. An amount greater than 2 L or for administration longer than 24 hours requires humidification. The use of sterile water for humidification reduces the possibility of growth of organisms in the oxygen delivery system. The use of distilled water prevents the accumulation of mineral deposits in equipment. Limiting the use of humidity to occasions in which the benefit is clearly demonstrated is cost-effective.

c. Nasal cannula

*Flow: 1–6 LPM
Percent delivered: Range 22% at 1 LPM to 40% at 6 LPM. The exact amount varies with the minute ventilation.*

A nasal cannula is the most commonly used device. It is used when a low liter flow is required or sufficient. It is relatively comfortable and allows the client to eat or drink. However, it is easily dislodged, and it requires patent nasal passages. It is also not comfortable at higher liter flow.

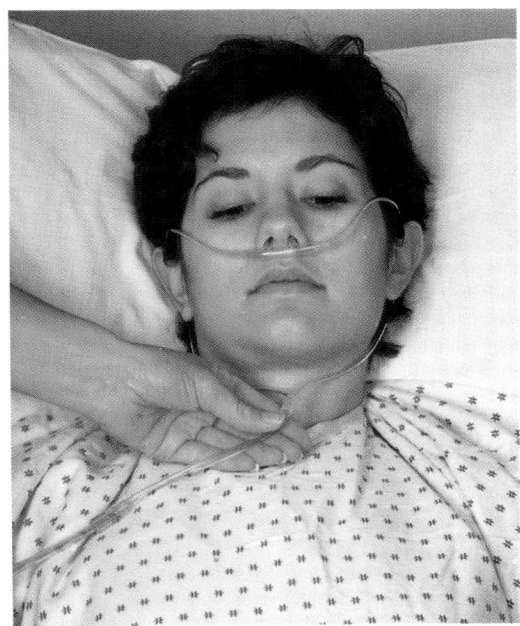

Nasal cannula.

Continued

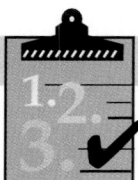

Administering Oxygen

d. Simple face mask

Flow: 6–12 LPM

Percent delivered: Range 40% at 6 LPM to 65% at 12 LPM. The exact amount varies with the minute ventilation.

Caution: Must not be used at flow rates under 6 LPM A face mask makes it difficult for the client to eat or drink. It may also cause a feeling of confinement or claustrophobia. Use with caution in a client in danger of airway obstruction or aspiration.

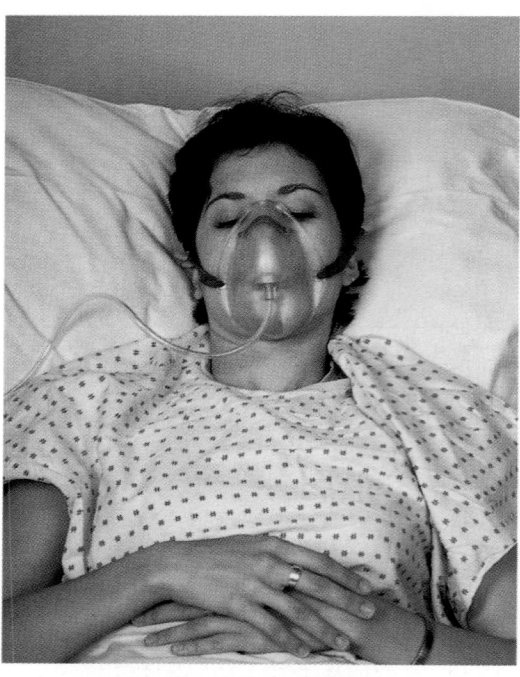

Simple face mask.

e. Face mask with a nonrebreathing oxygen reservoir bag

Flow: As required to keep the reservoir bag inflated at least one-third full during inspiration; varies from 6 to 15 LPM

Percent delivered: Range 60% to 90%. A higher percentage requires a well-fitting mask.

Useful for short-term administration of high concentrations of oxygen

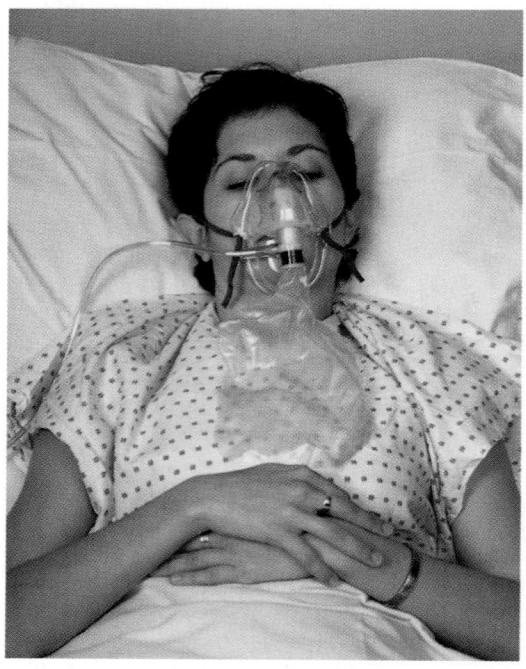

Face mask with a nonrebreathing oxygen reservoir bag.

f. Venturi mask

Flow: As recommended by the manufacturer
Percent delivered: Precisely provides 24, 28, 31, . . .
or 50% oxygen
Humidification is not used with a Venturi mask
because it interferes with efficient air entrainment.
Because a high liter flow is required and the mask is
specialized, the system is expensive and is used when
clear benefits are clearly expected to outweigh the
costs.

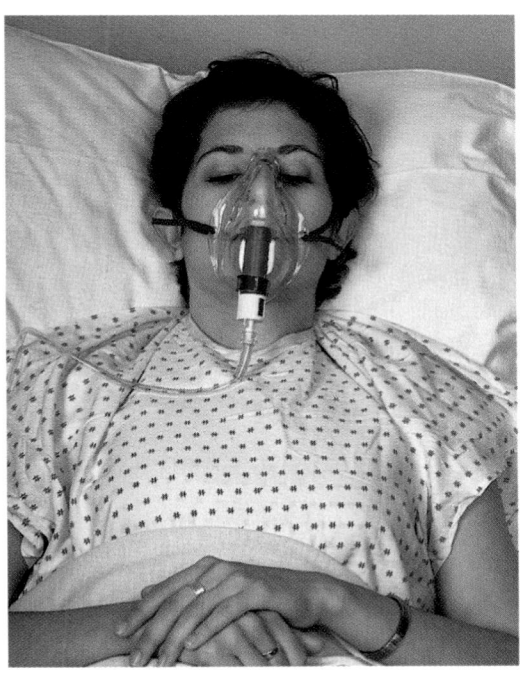

Venturi mask.

g. Face tent

Delivers an imprecise amount of oxygen. Can be used
with compressed air for humidification only. However,
this high humidity is sometimes associated with in-
creased airway resistance.

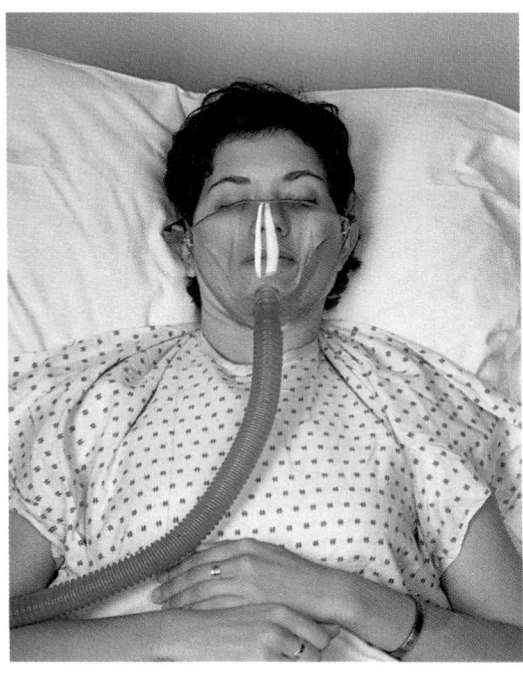

Face tent.

2 Set up the system. Insert the flowmeter into the oxygen source. Attach the connecting tube and delivery device. Add extra connecting tubing if needed. Check the function of the system after establishing the oxygen flow. Observe for bubbling in the water.

The client's movement is limited by the length of the tubing. This step flushes the system with oxygen and ensures client safety.

3 Place the delivery device on the client and make the client comfortable. Relieve the client's concerns about the need for oxygen. Adjust the strap comfortably around the client's head and prevent pressure behind the ears. Use a water-soluble lubricant to relieve irritation to the external nares.

Explanations about the need for oxygen should convey in a balanced way the importance of ensuring continuous oxygen use against the client's concern that the situation may be life-threatening.

4 Frequently assess the client and the delivery system. Check the liter flow, the humidity, and the position of the device. Monitor for signs and symptoms of oxygen deficit.

This assessment provides information for rapid response if therapy is not effective.

Continued

PROCEDURE 39–2 *(continued)*

Administering Oxygen

HINTS

1. Observe the skin under the elastic band on the cannula or mask. Skin breakdown is common behind the ears. Padding with a gauze pad or cotton ball may increase comfort and prevent skin breakdown.
2. If the client can be out of bed, use extension tubing to allow the person to move to a chair.
3. If the client can ambulate or go to the bathroom, a portable oxygen unit can be used to maintain oxygen therapy. Remember that getting out of bed increases the oxygen need. A pulse oximeter can be used to monitor the effects of activity on oxygenation.

HOME CARE CONSIDERATIONS

If a client needs oxygen in the home, a medical supply company will deliver the oxygen to the home and set up the equipment. A respiratory therapist is often sent to provide the initial teaching. The nurse's role is to reinforce teaching and monitor the effectiveness of the therapy. Because of the high risk for infection with oxygen equipment, monitoring the frequency of cleaning and the technique for cleaning the equipment is important.

---

monly used oxygen delivery device. It is relatively comfortable and does not interfere with talking or eating. Because the tubing is secured in place by an elastic band placed over the ears and behind the head or by tubing looped behind the ears, you should ensure that prolonged pressure does not cause skin damage. The nasal cannula can be used even if the client is breathing through the mouth. The oropharynx and nasopharynx are natural reservoirs for the 100% oxygen flow. When the client inhales through the nose or the mouth, this accumulated oxygen is drawn into the lungs. Because the nasal cannula can cause the discomfort of dry nasal passages at higher liter flows, it is usually used when a low FIO_2 is indicated.

The simple face mask is shaped to fit snugly over the nose and mouth. The sides of the mask have holes to allow the exhaled carbon dioxide to escape from the mask and decrease rebreathing of carbon dioxide. Because of the hole and because the mask does not fit to totally occlude airflow, the oxygen is mixed with room air. The simple face mask is used when the client needs a higher FIO_2 than provided by a nasal cannula to correct hypoxemia. If the mask is removed for meals, the client may need a nasal cannula while eating.

Mrs. Wilheim's oxygen therapy was started with a face mask in the emergency department. Her oxygen saturation was low, and she appeared quite ill. Now, however, you realize that the oxygen mask is frightening to Mrs. Wilheim; she even says that she knows she must be really sick if she needs oxygen. How can you help Mrs. Wilheim? What criteria would you use to request that the physician change the order to a nasal cannula?

To achieve an even higher FIO_2, an oxygen reservoir is added to the face mask. The highest FIO_2 is achieved with the non-rebreathing mask. The bag fills with 100% oxygen from the wall outlet to provide a tidal volume of 100% oxygen. The air holes on the sides of the mask are equipped with a one-way valve to allow escape of exhaled air and to prevent the entrance of room air with inhalation. While most of the tidal volume is supplied from the reservoir, the system does allow some entrance of room air so the mask with reservoir bag never delivers 100% oxygen. If the bag collapses by more than half its volume with each breath, an adequate tidal volume of oxygen-rich air will not be maintained and the client could suffocate.

A variation of the mask with reservoir bag is the partial rebreathing mask. Part of the exhaled volume enters the reservoir bag. This air is assumed to be mostly from the dead space, and thus is oxygen-rich because it has not entered the alveoli where diffusion occurs. The partial rebreathing bag supplies an FIO_2 higher than the simple face mask, but not as high as the non-rebreathing reservoir bag. The partial rebreathing bag has limited usefulness.

HIGH-FLOW SYSTEM. The mask with a Venturi device is the only true high-flow system. A higher liter flow is needed to achieve the same FIO_2 as with a nasal cannula or simple face mask. The Venturi device creates a pressure drop that draws room air in precise amounts to create the desired FIO_2. The fact that small amounts of oxygen can be delivered precisely has been beneficial in treating the client with chronic respiratory disease.

HUMIDIFICATION

Oxygen is a dry gas. Prolonged exposure to the drying effects of oxygen may cause irritation and damage to oral, nasal, and pharyngeal mucous membranes. Oxygen is humidified to prevent irritation and drying of the airways and to maintain an optimal environment for the normal function of the cilia. As mentioned previously, humidification is the addition of water vapor to a dry gas.

Bubble-diffusion humidifiers are most often used with oxygen. Oxygen is bubbled through water to allow molecules of water vapor to be mixed with the oxygen. When oxygen is delivered at a low liter flow for a short time (usually less than 24 hours), the client can usually tolerate oxygen without humidity. Figure 39–9 shows two types of bubble-diffusion humidifiers.

Oxygen humidifiers have limited ability to humidify the inhaled gas. If both oxygen and high humidity are needed, an open face tent can be used. The face tent is loose-fitting, forming a semicircle around the face. With a properly working face tent, a cloud of vaporized water is seen around the person's face. Condensation accumulates in the large tube that delivers

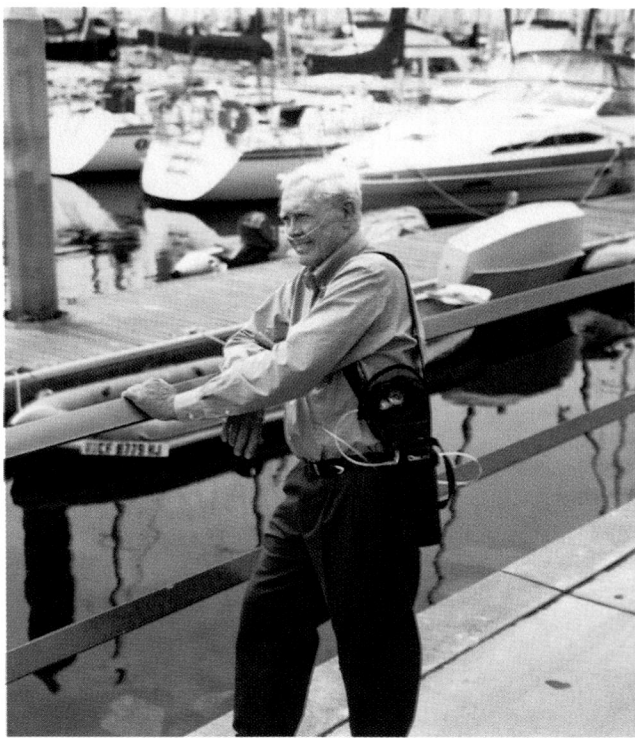

Figure 39–10. Portable oxygen systems such as the one worn by this client can enhance the quality of life for clients with chronic respiratory disease. (Courtesy of Chad Therapeutics, Inc., Chatsworth, CA.)

the oxygen and humidity and must be periodically emptied. The water vapor can be either cool or warm. Warm mist carries a larger volume of water, but cool mist is considered to be equally effective in hydrating secretions. The face tent delivers a highly variable amount of oxygen and is not appropriate when the FIO_2 needs to be carefully controlled.

HOME OXYGEN SYSTEMS

The advent of portable (home) oxygen systems has provided selected clients who have chronic respiratory disease with increased exercise tolerance, improved length and quality of life, and reduced hospitalizations (Fig. 39–10). Exercise tolerance and the quality of life are closely related. Oxygen therapy may allow the person to manage activities of daily living, walk a block, or attend a family gathering. Exercise is needed to increase the overall fitness of skeletal muscles, particularly accessory muscles of respiration, which further increases activity tolerance. Oxygen therapy may also improve sleep. Oxygen during sleep is needed if the client has nocturnal hypoxemia. In some clients, improved health and an overall sense of well-being may be a factor in prolonging life. In clients with hypoxemia at rest, continuous oxygen (24 hours a day) is more effective than intermittent use at improving survival time and reducing neuropsychiatric symptoms.

Three methods of oxygen administration suitable

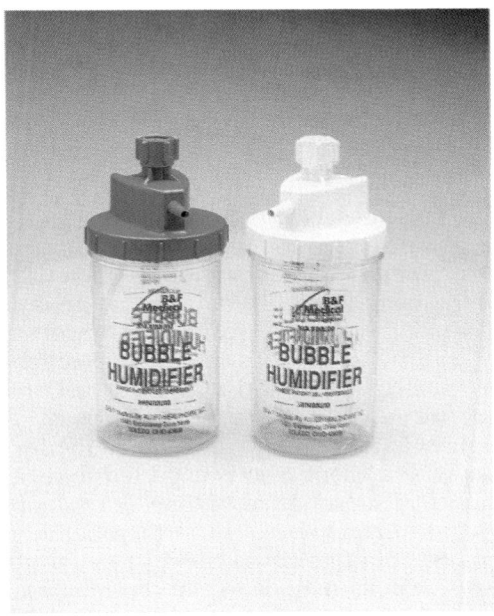

Figure 39–9. Bubble diffusion humidifiers. Oxygen is blown through sterile distilled water in these humidifiers to add moisture to the inspired gas. (Courtesy of Allied Health Care, St Louis, MO.)

for home use are liquid systems, portable cylinders of gaseous oxygen, and oxygen concentrators. Liquid portable oxygen systems are the most versatile and are suitable for people who wish to remain active. Liquid oxygen systems are composed of three parts: a reservoir of liquid oxygen (contained in a Thermos-like container), a flow meter, and a humidifier. One disadvantage of most liquid oxygen tank systems is that the client's movement is limited by the length of the oxygen tubing. A portable unit for ambulatory use can be filled with oxygen from the liquid system tank. When filled, the portable unit weighs approximately 9 lb. It may be carried with a shoulder strap or pulled in a cart. Home oxygen may also be supplied by small portable cylinders of gaseous oxygen, which can be wheeled about on a cart. Oxygen concentrators are used when stationary, low-flow oxygen is appropriate. Rather than requiring an oxygen source, room air is concentrated into a higher percentage of oxygen. Liter flow rates are generally limited to 2 to 3 LPM. Medicare has very stringent guidelines for reimbursement for home oxygen. Documentation that demonstrates a clear benefit is important.

ADJUNCTIVE NURSING MEASURES

When a client requires oxygen, nursing measures are an adjunct to oxygen therapy. You will employ these measures to increase ventilation, to reduce the body's need for oxygen, and to clear the airways. Position the client for maximum ventilation. While activity can increase ventilation, it also can increase the metabolic need for oxygen. You will work with the client to maintain the delicate balance between rest and activity. Measures to reduce anxiety, discomfort, and pain are equally important in reducing the demand for oxygen. Based on the chest assessment, you may assist the client with coughing and deep-breathing. If the client is unable to cough to clear the chest, suctioning may be needed. When the client can tolerate it, incentive spirometry or chest physiotherapy may be prescribed.

Interventions to Treat Respiratory Failure

Whether the situation is one of an acute obstructed airway or a decline in respiratory function, respiratory failure is an emergency. You must swiftly establish an airway and support the client's breathing to prevent death.

Maintaining a Patent Airway

Sudden respiratory arrest is treated by establishing an airway and providing ventilation mouth-to-mouth or with a manual breathing bag (commonly referred to by the trademark name Ambu). When the primary problem is an airway, establishing an airway is often sufficient to re-establish breathing. (See Chapter 58 for the procedure for cardiopulmonary resuscitation [CPR].) If the client continues to be unable to breathe without assistance, mechanical ventilation may needed.

Action Alert!
Be prepared for the need for CPR. Airway obstruction is an emergency. Assessment and definitive action take place in the same instant. (1) Activate the emergency response system. (2) Lift the client's chin. This action may establish an airway and prevent the need for CPR. Hint: Calling for the resuscitation team when you do not need it is better than not calling for the team when you do need it!

Time is often a crucial factor in the prevention of serious and sometimes lethal side effects of a poorly functioning airway. In the case of a totally obstructed airway, an open airway must be established in fewer than 4 minutes to prevent brain damage or death. A partially obstructed airway can cause hypoxemia and may result in irreversible brain damage. Ideally, airway obstruction is corrected before total occlusion occurs.

OROPHARYNGEAL AIRWAY

An *oropharyngeal* airway (Fig 39–11A) is a curved rubber or plastic piece that is inserted into the mouth over the posterior tongue and maintains a patent airway through the pharynx. The purpose of oropharyngeal airways is to hold the tongue forward. The distal end of the airway is positioned in the mouth between the posterior pharynx and the back of the tongue.

To insert an oral airway, follow this procedure: With the airway turned on its side, slide the airway along the top of the tongue until the tip of the airway reaches the posterior portion of the tongue. Rotate the airway to follow the natural curve of the tongue as it enters the oropharynx. The rotating motion assists in opening the throat to allow correct position of the airway. The curved end will hold the tongue forward. If the airway is the correct size, the flat end clears the lips and serves as a "bite block" between the front teeth.

Action Alert!
When the airway is compromised, work quickly to insert an oral airway.

Oropharyngeal airways are used for unconscious and semiconscious clients. When the client is conscious enough to have a gag reflex, an airway may cause vomiting with aspiration, which is a life-threatening complication. Remove the airway immediately if gagging occurs. Turning an unconscious or semiconscious person into a side-lying position allows the jaw to fall forward and may effectively maintain an open airway without an artificial airway.

Oropharyngeal airways are generally for short-term use with a client who is expected to regain consciousness in a short period of time. For example, oral airways are frequently placed in the operating room and remain in place until the client has recovered from anesthesia. Mucus may collect in the mouth and can be aspirated into the lungs; therefore, the client may need to be suctioned or placed in a side-lying position for drainage, or both. If the client begins to cough and gag on the airway, you will need to remove it.

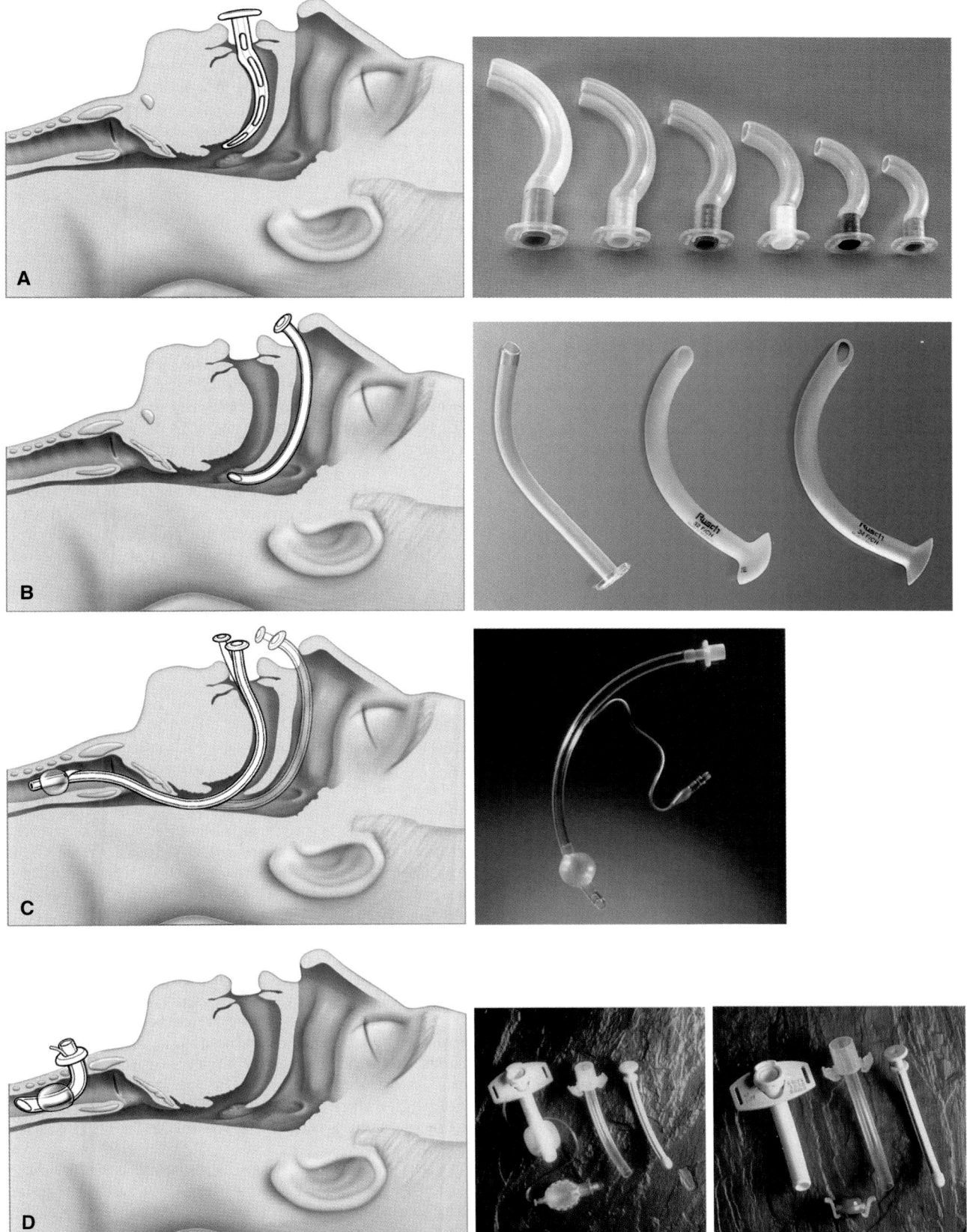

Figure 39–11. Types of airways. *A,* oropharyngeal airway; *B,* nasal trumpet airway; *C,* endotracheal airway; *D,* tracheostomy tube (left, cuffed; center, cuffed; right, uncuffed). (Photos in *A* and *B* courtesy of Rusch, Inc., Duluth, GA; photo in part *C* courtesy of Mallinckrodt, Inc., St Louis, MO; photos in part *D* courtesy of Mallinckrodt, Inc./Shiley Tracheostomy Products, St Louis, MO.)

Oral airways are also used when the client's condition is deteriorating and the airway is becoming obstructed, because with loss of consciousness the muscles of the throat relax and allow the tongue to occlude the airway. Try lifting the jaw or chin. If lifting the chin establishes airflow, an oral airway will maintain an open airway.

NASAL TRUMPET AIRWAY

Nasal trumpet airways (Fig. 39–11*B*) are cuffless tubes made of soft rubber or plastic and passed through a nostril into the nasopharynx. When inserted into the nares, the tube acts as a guide for the insertion of a suction catheter. The nasal trumpet airway is most commonly used in the clients who require frequent nasotracheal suctioning and are developing epistaxis from the traumatic insertion of the suction catheter through the nose.

A nasal trumpet airway extends into the pharynx and is positioned at the base of the tongue. The tongue is separated from the posterior pharyngeal wall, preventing obstruction from the tongue "falling" into the pharynx. The proximal end (nearest the nostrils) of a nasal airway is flared and fits against the external nares. Insertion of a large safety pin through the flared end stops the airway from slipping further into the nose or larynx. Nasal airways are more appropriate and comfortable for conscious and semiconscious clients than are oropharyngeal airways.

Select an airway that is slightly smaller than the nares and slightly larger than the suction catheter to be used. Using a penlight, observe the nose for septal deviation that may make one side of the nares more open. Lubricate the airway with a water-soluble lubricant jelly containing a local anesthetic. Petroleum-based lubricants are not acceptable because of the danger of aspiration into the lungs. Insert the tube gently, but firmly, following the contour of the nasopharyngeal passageway.

ENDOTRACHEAL AIRWAY

An **endotracheal tube** (ET tube; Fig. 39–11*C*) is a catheter passed through the nose or mouth into the trachea for the purpose of establishing an airway. Most endotracheal tubes are made of disposable polyvinyl chloride or other synthetic material. A ballooned cuff that is molded into the plastic can be inflated to occlude the main bronchus so air passes only through the endotracheal tube. The client can then be ventilated using an Ambu bag or placed on a ventilator.

Endotracheal tubes can be passed through the nose or the mouth. In an emergency, or when the nares cannot accommodate the tube, or when the practitioner prefers the oral route, it is passed through the mouth. Passing an endotracheal tube requires special training and practice under supervision. A laryngoscope is used to open the airway and visualize the glottis. The scope then acts as a guide for passing the tube. Air is immediately injected into the balloon by way of a pig tail attached to the cuff. The Ambu bag fits directly to the endotracheal tube and respiration is immediately established. The whole procedure is completed in seconds, rapidly establishing respiration in the client who is not breathing. Endotracheal tubes are also placed in the operating room, especially when muscle paralysis is needed during the surgical procedure. An endotracheal tube can be left in place for up to 3 weeks only if the cuff pressure is carefully monitored to prevent tissue necrosis at the site of the cuff. If mechanical ventilation is needed for an extended period of time, a tracheostomy may be performed.

TRACHEOSTOMY

As we have said, a tracheostomy is an opening made directly into the trachea by surgical incision. It is performed when there is obstruction above the trachea or when the client is in respiratory failure and may benefit from reduced airway resistance (length of airway) and dead space. A tracheostomy has the advantages over an endotracheal tube of improved airway suctioning and client comfort. If the need for a tracheostomy is prolonged, the client with a tracheostomy tube can eat soft, well-chewed foods in small bites.

Tracheostomy tubes are inserted through the surgical incision into the trachea. Most tracheotomies are not performed as emergency procedures but under more controlled conditions for the purpose of maintaining long-term mechanical ventilation. A tracheostomy would be performed as an emergency in a case such as that of a burn victim with severe upper airway edema that prevents passing an endotracheal tube. While the tracheostomy wound is fresh and pathology is present in the lungs, the risk of infection is high.

Tracheostomy tubes (Fig. 39–11*D*) are disposable and made from a polyvinyl chloride or other synthetic material that does not react with human tissue. Steel or silver tracheostomy tubes are rarely used.

Caring for a client with an artificial airway makes use of the nursing diagnosis of *Ineffective airway clearance*. The tube is a foreign object in the airway and increases the production of mucus. In addition, the client is unable to cough to clear the airway. Frequent respiratory assessment and suctioning are required. As the client gains strength and can get in the upright position, it is possible to produce a cough that will clear the tracheostomy tube of mucus. Mouth care is important because it helps the client manage the accumulation of mucus and may prevent infections that could enter the lower airways. The humidifying function of the upper airways is absent; therefore, humidification of inspired air is essential. Because mucus accumulates around the tracheostomy tube, frequent cleaning of the site is needed to prevent infection, especially when the wound is fresh (Procedure 39–3).

The nursing diagnosis of *Impaired verbal communication* is pertinent because the client with a tracheostomy cannot speak unless equipped with a special tracheostomy tube that is designed to allow speech. These tubes have a one-way valve that closes with exhalation and directs the air across the larynx. The Communitrach is another type of tracheostomy tube

Cleaning a Tracheostomy

TIME TO
ALLOW
▼
Novice:
20 min.
Expert:
10 min.

A tracheostomy is an artificial opening into the trachea that bypasses the normal defense mechanisms of the upper respiratory tract. Therefore, cleaning the surrounding skin protects the lower respiratory tract from the entrance of bacteria. Additionally, when the tracheostomy is a fresh wound, cleaning is especially important to prevent wound infection. Cleaning methods should protect the respiratory tract from the entrance of foreign substances or objects.

Delegation Guidelines

Care of a new tracheostomy is not generally delegated to a nursing assistant because of the risks associated with inconsistent or improper technique. New tracheostomies are generally present in acute and critically ill clients. However, for clients with long-term, stable tracheostomies, you may be able to delegate tracheostomy care to a nursing assistant who has received appropriate training.

Equipment Needed

- Tracheostomy care kit
  or

4×4 gauze
Cotton-tipped applicators
Tracheostomy dressing
Basin
Small bottle brush or pipe cleaner
Twill tape or tracheostomy ties
- Scissors
- Gloves
- Hydrogen peroxide
- Normal saline
(Supplies should be clean or sterile, depending on whether the procedure will be clean or sterile.)

1 Decide whether the procedure should be clean or sterile.

When the wound is less than 48 hours old and/or the client is at high risk for respiratory infection, sterile technique is recommended.

2 Gather the appropriate equipment.

3 Prepare the client for the procedure. Suction the tracheostomy or have the patient cough. Remove any dressing that is present.

You can use sterile gloves to suction the tracheostomy and then remove the dressing without changing gloves. A dressing is recommended only if irritated skin needs protection.

4 Select a clear area to set up the equipment, in reach of the client's tracheostomy. Set up a sterile field; the outer wrapper of the kit forms the sterile field. Don sterile gloves. Pour hydrogen peroxide into one basin and normal saline into the other.

If the client is on a ventilator, you will need to work quickly and immediately replace the inner cannula because it is needed to attach to the ventilator.

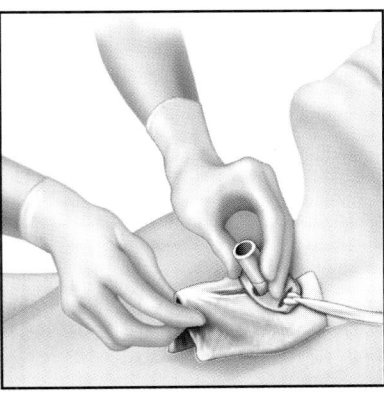

Removing the tracheostomy dressing.

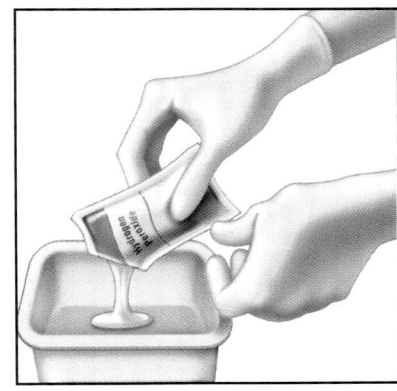

Pouring hydrogen peroxide into a basin.

Continued

Cleaning a Tracheostomy

5 Unlock and remove the inner cannula. Twist the inner cannula and pull it out following the curve of the tracheostomy tube. Avoid moving the outer tube. Place the inner cannula in the hydrogen peroxide.

Avoid irritating the wound. The cotton-tipped applicators can be dipped in hydrogen peroxide to clean small crevices of the tracheostomy tube. Absolutely do not get hydrogen peroxide into the trachea.

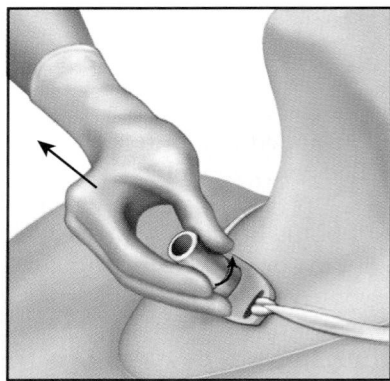

Removing the inner cannula.

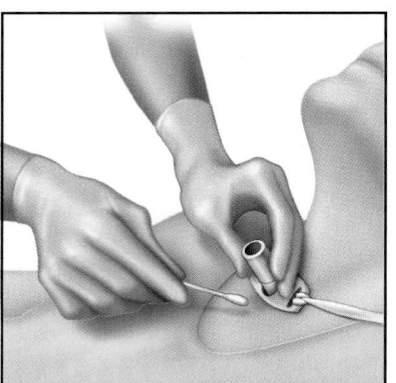

Cleaning the tracheostomy site.

6 Clean the inner cannula inside and out with a brush or pipe cleaner. Frequent cleaning with normal saline prevents encrusted secretions that require more vigorous cleaning. Rinse the cannula in normal saline. Replace and lock the inner cannula.

Rinsing in normal saline prevents hydrogen peroxide from entering the tracheostomy.

8 Change the tracheostomy ties and apply a dressing, if necessary. When the tracheostomy ties are removed, the tube can easily be dislodged, and the airway will quickly close. Use a helper to hold the tracheostomy tube while you remove and replace the ties. The ties should be tight enough that only one finger can be slipped under the tie.

This technique prevents the tracheostomy tube from being dislodged.

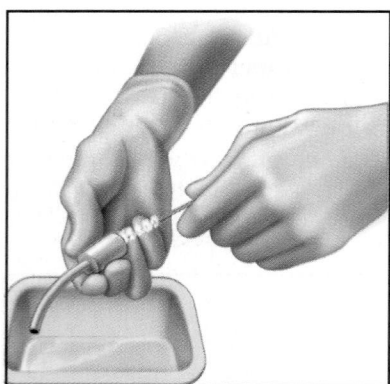

Cleaning the inner cannula with a brush.

7 Clean the tracheostomy site. Use normal saline to clean the skin, hydrogen peroxide to clean the external tube. Use gentle pats or strokes. Use either gauze or cotton-tipped applicators, depending on the amount of secretions.

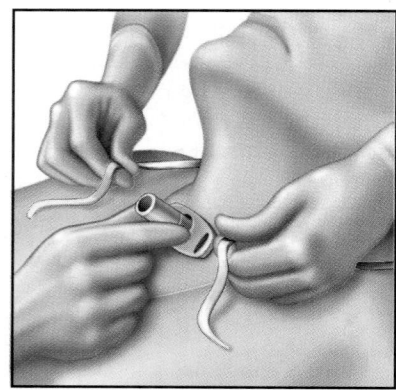

Changing the tracheostomy ties with the help of an assistant.

9 Evaluate the results of the procedure. Is the skin clean, dry, and free of inflammation? Is the tube clean and dry? Is the client comfortable?

1. Avoid moving the tracheostomy tube to prevent discomfort to the client and irritation to the trachea.
2. Having an assistant helps the procedure go smoothly. The assistant helps with preoxygenation and holding the tracheostomy tube in place while the ties are changed.
3. Gauze should not be cut to use for a tracheostomy dressing. Frayed, loose ends could enter the tracheostomy.
4. When tying the tube to secure it in the opening, one tie should be longer than the other. Tie the knot to the side of the neck to prevent the client from lying on the knot. Pad the knot, if needed, to prevent pressure.
5. Tracheostomy care is done as often as needed to maintain a clean, dry area. In the hospital, the frequency is usually once a shift. In the home, daily care may be sufficient. Ties are changed daily or more frequently if wet or soiled.

with an airflow tube that allows the air to be directed over the larynx when the tracheostomy is covered, thus allowing speech.

For a small group of clients, a tracheostomy becomes permanent. The home care nurse manages clients with long-term or permanent tracheostomies. Much of the care focuses on teaching the family or other caregiver to manage the client's care and to be prepared to manage emergencies, should any arise. It is also important to plan for assisting the client and family to maintain the quality of life while living with a chronic illness that easily becomes the focus of all the activities in the home (see Chapter 60).

EVALUATION

Evaluation of the achievement of health outcomes involves reassessing the client to determine that the criteria for evaluation have been met.

The nursing note for Mrs. Wilheim when she is ready for discharge following treatment for respiratory infection might look like the following:

Lungs clear to auscultation. Breath sounds throughout. Temperature 37°C (98.6°F), P 66, R 14, BP 124/84. No cough. Has verbalized instructions to continue antibiotics at home until the prescription has been completely taken. Will report signs and symptoms of recurrent infection to the physician. Is able to ambulate the length of the hall. Daughter will assist with eating a balanced diet. Home health nurse will follow up and work with daughter to determine need for protected living.

Notice in the above example that the nurse has documented that the respiratory problem has resolved and that she worked with the client to establish new

goals. The goals are to maintain health during recovery and to report recurring signs and symptoms.

The nurse helps the client establish new goals through statements like, "Now that your lungs are clearing, we need to concentrate on being more active and think about going home from the hospital."

If the outcomes are not achieved or the client is not improving within the expected time, reassessment may reveal a reasonable explanation for the lack of progress. For example, a post-surgical client who continues to have fever on the 4th post-operative day, but whose post-operative crackles have cleared, should be assessed for other causes of the fever.

Process evaluation helps connect the outcomes to the nursing care. Connecting outcomes to the interventions requires examining all the process elements that could affect the outcomes. For example, if a client had a physician's order for an incentive spirometer, but only used it the two times you actually stayed in the room to provide support, then the outcome of breath sounds throughout the lung fields cannot be attributed to the incentive spirometer. Refer to the care plan for an example of the application of the nursing process to Mrs. Wilheim.

KEY PRINCIPLES

- Factors affecting respiration, including smoking, environmental exposure, age, and cardiovascular disease, suggest the need for more intensive monitoring for respiratory complications.
- The nurse does not order diagnostic tests but does use the results in diagnosing nursing problems.

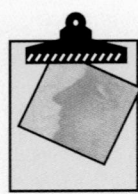

NURSING CARE PLANNING
A CLIENT WITH PNEUMONIA

Admission Data

Mrs. Wilheim is admitted through the emergency department to a general medical nursing unit. The emergency department nurse phones the following report:

Mrs. Wilheim is an 88-year-old white female in respiratory distress. We have started oxygen and taken a chest x-ray. Looks as though she has pneumonia. Her oxygen saturation was 85% before we started the oxygen at 4 L by face mask. If she is doing alright, she can try a nasal cannula. The saturation is up to 95%, but you will probably need to monitor her. Dr. Anderson is coming up to write orders.

Physician's Orders	Admitting diagnosis: pneumonia Oxygen per NC @ 4 L Pulse oximeter Sputum for culture and sensitivity IV D$_5$/1/4 NS at 100 mL/h Keflin 500 mg IV q6h	Darvocet i or ii q4h p.r.n. pain Tylenol gr 10 temperature over 38.8°C (102°F) Laxative of choice Diet as tolerated Bedrest with BRP as tolerated
Nursing Assessment	Color pale, skin moist, oxygen saturation 93%, complains of pain in lower left chest with inspiration, diminished breath sounds left lower lobe, wet rhonchi over bronchi, temperature 38.3°C (101°F), pulse 100, respiration 30, BP 118/70. Reports no appetite, appears frightened, moving from wheelchair to bed results in dyspnea.	

NURSING CARE PLAN

Nursing Diagnosis	Expected Outcomes	Interventions	Evaluation (After 24 Hours of Care)
Impaired gas exchange related to excess secretions, weakness, pain secondary to pneumonia	Lungs clear to auscultation	Encourage deep breaths q2h.	Diminished breath sounds over left lower lobe. Rhonchi diminishing, clear with coughing.
	Effective cough	Observe coughing behavior; assess sputum; assist with coughing.	Cough nonproductive and tiring. Antitussive given.
	Oxygen saturation >95% on room air	Maintain oxygen therapy with all activity.	Oxygen saturation 97% on 4 L per NC
	Rate and depth of respiration within normal limits	Monitor respiration with activity and reduce activity if needed.	Sat in chair 20 minutes; respiration 16, P 88, BP 130/90.

Continued

- *Ineffective breathing patterns* are generally hypoventilation, hyperventilation, or dyspnea. A high priority goal of care is to prevent hypoxemia.
- *Ineffective airway clearance* results from failure of the normal respiratory defense mechanisms or is secondary to hypoventilation. The presence of coarse crackles or rhonchi is sufficient to diagnose *Ineffective airway clearance*.
- *Impaired gas exchange* can be the end result of *Ineffective breathing pattern* or *Ineffective airway clearance* or can result from poor perfusion or damage to the alveolar membrane.

- Definitive evidence of *Impaired gas exchange* is abnormal arterial blood gases, but the diagnosis can be inferred from signs of hypoxemia.
- Assessment for nursing diagnoses related to respiratory diagnoses includes assessment of all the functional patterns for emotional responses, such as anxiety and hopelessness as well as physiological problems, such as fluid volume deficit.
- Because the nursing diagnosis is chosen based on the goal of nursing care, respiratory diagnoses are more commonly used in the acute care setting where the care is associated with physician-

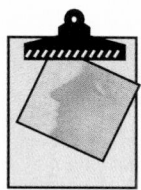

NURSING CARE PLANNING
A CLIENT WITH PNEUMONIA *(continued)*

NURSING CARE PLAN

Nursing Diagnosis	Expected Outcomes	Interventions	Evaluation (After 24 Hours of Care)
	Absence of pain	Offer Darvocet q4h. Observe for effects on respiration, cough mechanism.	Refuses pain medication, even though appears uncomfortable.
	Absence of anxiety	Explain care to client, *more detailed explanations to daughter.* Reassure that recovery is expected.	*Relies on daughter to make decisions. States that "God will take me when it's time to go."*
	Diet meets nutritional requirements	Provide six small feedings of easily digestible foods of choice.	Ate oatmeal with 4 oz. milk for breakfast. States she is not hungry. *Daughter will bring dish from home for lunch.*
	Ambulates length of hall qid	Reposition q2h. Allow use of bedside commode if oxygen saturation >95%.	Turns self in bed. Uses bedside commode. Up in chair 20 minutes. Vital signs and oxygen saturation WNL.

Italicized interventions indicate culturally specific care.

Critical Thinking Questions

1. Because Mrs. Wilheim lived alone and she was hesitant to call for help, her treatment was delayed. Her daughter asks if you think she needs to move to a protected living situation. How would you respond to the daughter?
2. When Mrs. Wilheim is almost ready for discharge, the nurse begins preparing the discharge teaching plan. What criteria should be used to determine whether Mrs. Wilheim is ready for discharge? What information should be included in the teaching plan? Consider activity restrictions, knowledge of signs and symptoms, diet, medications, and follow-up health care. What possible factors would suggest the need for a home health referral?
3. On the third day after admission, the night nurse reports that Mrs. Wilheim has slept through the night and that her vital signs are stable. While conducting the morning assessment, you find that Mrs Wilheim's vital signs are T 37.8°C (100°F), R 30 and shallow, P 100, BP 108/68. Her skin is pale, cold, and clammy. She has diminished breath sounds and bilateral rales. What action would you take? What additional data would you collect?

initiated interventions aimed directly at managing the respiratory status.
- The outcomes for respiratory diagnoses are a normal breathing pattern, clear lung fields, and normal arterial oxygen and carbon dioxide levels or evidence that the client is making a behavioral change that is expected to improve the respiratory status.
- Interventions to change the pattern of breathing would meet the goals of maximum respiratory function, stimulating respiration, decreasing airway resistance, improving the efficiency of respira-

tion, reducing anxiety, and managing energy requirements.
- Interventions to treat *Ineffective airway clearance* would meet the goals of liquefying and mobilizing secretions and reducing the production of sputum.
- Interventions for *Impaired gas exchange* would meet the goals of compensating for *Impaired gas exchange,* maintaining a patent airway, and providing ventilatory support.
- Evaluation of outcomes for respiratory nursing diagnoses includes evidence that the respiratory sta-

tus has improved and that the client has a commitment to changing behaviors to prevent future problems.

BIBLIOGRAPHY

*Ackerman, M. (1993). The effect of saline lavage prior to suctioning. *American Journal of Critical Care, 2*(4), 326–330.

Adhikari, N., & Menzies, R. (1995). Community-based tuberculin screening in Montreal: A cost-outcome description. *American Journal of Public Health, 85*(6), 786–789.

*Ahrens, T. (1993). Changing perspectives in the assessment of oxygenation. *Critical Care Nurse, 93*(4), 78–83.

*Atkins, P., Hapshe, E., & Riegal, B. (1994). Effects of a bedbath on mixed venous oxygen saturation and heart rate in coronary artery bypass graft patients. *American Journal of Critical Care, 3*(2), 107–115.

Bates, T.D. (1996). Pharmacology update. Asthma medications: A quick review. *Journal of School Nursing, 12*(2), 28, 30–32.

Berry, J.K., Vitalo, C.A., Larson, J.L., Patel, M., & Kim, M.J. (1996) Respiratory muscle strength in older adults. *Nursing Research, 45*(3), 154–159.

*Boutotte, J. (1993). T. B. the second time around. *Nursing93, 23*(5), 42–50.

Brock, E.T., & Shucard, D.W. (1994). Sleep apnea. *American Family Physician, 49*(2), 385–394.

Burns, S., Egolff, B., Ryan, B., Carpenter, R., & Burns, J. (1994). Effect of body position on spontaneous respiratory rate and tidal volume in patients with obesity, abdominal distention, and ascites. *American Journal of Critical Care, 3*(2), 102–106.

Burns, S.M., Spilman, M., Wilmoth, D., Carpenter, R., Turrentine, B., et al. (1998). Are frequent inner cannula changes necessary?: A pilot study. *Heart and Lung, 27*(1), 58–62.

*Carlson-Catalano, J., Lunney, M., Paradiso, C., Bruno, J., Luise, B.K., et al. (1998). Clinical validation of ineffective breathing pattern, ineffective airway clearance, and impaired gas exchange. Image: *Journal of Nursing Scholarship, 30*(3), 243–248.

*Carrieri-Kohlman, V., Douglas, M.K., Gormley, J.M., & Stulbarg, M.S. (1993). Desensitization and guided mastery: Treatment approaches for the management of dyspnea. *Heart and Lung, 22*(3), 226–234.

Chitila, W.C., Hall, J.B., & Manthous, C.A. (1995). The effect of pulmonary secretions on respiratory mechanics in intubated patients. *Respiratory Care, 40*(10), 1048–1051.

Cornook, M.A. (1996a). Making sense of arterial blood gases and their interpretation. *Nursing Times, 92*(6), 30–31.

Cornook, M.A. (1996b). Dressing up for a change: Chest tube insertion site. *Nursing96, 26*(7), 44–46.

Crowe, J.M., & Bradley, C.A. (1997). The effectiveness of incentive spirometry with physical therapy for high-risk patients after coronary artery bypass surgery. *Physical Therapist, 77*(3), 260–268.

*Ehrhardt, B., & Graham, M. (1990). Pulse oximetry—an easy to check oxygen saturation. *Nursing90, 20*(3), 50–54.

Elpern, E.H., & Girzadas, A.M. (1993). Tuberculosis update: New challenges of an old disease. *MEDSURG Nursing, 2*(3), 176–183.

Faria, S.H., & Taylor, L.J. (1997). Interpretation of arterial blood gases by nurses. *Journal of Vascular Nursing, 15*(4), 128–130.

*Fedson, D. (1992). Clinical practice and public policy for influenza and pneumococcal vaccination of the elderly. *Clinics in Geriatric Medicine, 8*(1), 183–189.

Field, D. (1997) Every breath you take. *Nursing Times, 93*(26), 28–30.

Fritz, D.J. (1997). Fine tune your physical assessment of the lungs and respiratory system. *Home Care Provider, 2*(6), 299–302.

Gift, A.G. (1996). Applications in research. A mother's smoking behavior during pregnancy affects the fetus. *Perspectives in Respiratory Nursing, 7*(1), 6, 11.

*Gift, A.G., Moore, T., & Soeken, K. (1992). Relaxation to reduce dyspnea and anxiety in COPD patients. *Nursing Research, 41*(4), 242–246.

Gordon, P.A., Norton, J.M., Guerra, J.M., & Perdue, S.T. (1997). Positioning of chest tubes: Effects on pressure and drainage. *American Journal of Critical Care, 6*(1), 33–38.

Graydon, J.E., & Ross, E. (1995). Influence of symptoms, lung function, mood, and social support on level of functioning of patients with COPD. *Research in Nursing and Health, 18*(6), 525–533.

Guyton, A.C., & Hall, J.E. (1996). *Textbook of Medical Physiology.* Philadelphia: W.B. Saunders Co.

Haas, C.F., & Weg, J.G. (1996). Exogenous surfactant therapy: An update. *Respiratory Care, 41*(5) 397–415.

Hall, J. (1996). Evaluating asthma inhaler technique. *Professional Nurse, 11*(11), 725, 728–729.

Hanson, M.J.S. (1997). The theory of planned behavior applied to cigarette smoking in African-American, Puerto Rican, and non-Hispanic white teenage females. *Nursing Research, 46*(3), 155–162.

*Ingersoll, G. (1989). Respiratory muscle fatigue research: Implications for clinical practice. *Applied Nursing Research, 2*(1), 6–15.

*Jacobsen, A. (1993). Prone to oxygenate. {Working Smart.} *American Journal of Critical Care, 93*(8), 20.

Jones, S. (1997). Oxygen therapy. *Community Nurse, 3*(2), 23–24.

Kirton, C.A. (1996). Assessing breath sounds. *Nursing96, 20*(6), 50–51.

Klinnert, M.D., McQuaid, E.L., & Gavin, L.A. (1997). Assessing the family asthma management system. *Journal of Asthma, 34*(1), 77–88.

Lareau, S.C. (1993). Respiratory problems. In D.L. Carnevali & M. Patrick (Eds.), *Nursing management for the elderly* (3rd ed., pp. 625–657). Philadelphia: J.B. Lippincott Co.

Lazzara, D. (1996). Why is the Heimlich chest drain valve making a comeback? *Nursing96, 26*(12), 50–53.

*Lehrer, S. (1993). *Understanding Lung Sounds* (2nd ed.). Philadelphia: W.B. Saunders Co.

Leidy, N.K., & Traver, G.A. (1996). Adjustment and social behavior in older adults with chronic obstructive pulmonary disease: The family's perspective. *Journal of Advanced Nursing, 23*(2), 252–259.

National Cancer Institute (1999). PDQ Screening and Prevention: Health Professionals. cancernet.nci.nih.gov.

*O'Donnell, D.E., Webb, K.A., & McGuire, M.A. (1993). COPD: Benefits of exercise training. *Geriatrics, 48*(1), 59–69.

O'Hanlon-Nichols, T. (1996). Clinical savvy. Commonly asked questions about chest tubes. *American Journal of Nursing, 96*(5), 60–64.

Provine, B. (1996). Consultation: Education about tracheostomy care. *Perspectives in Respiratory Nursing, 7*(2), 6.

Sabot, J.S., Sabah, D., Kite-Powell, D., & Houston, S. (1995). Pulmonary outcomes come of age. *The Journal for Respiratory Care Practitioners, 8*(6), 23–24, 26, 101.

Sheahan, S.L., & Wilson, S.M. (1997). Smoking cessation for pregnant women and their partners: A pilot study. *Journal of the American Academy of Nurse Practitioners, 9*(7), 323–326.

Sidhu, A. (1997). Limitations in predicting pO$_2$ from sO$_2$ measured by pulse oximetry. *Neonatal Intensive Care, 10*(3), 16–18.

Somerson, S.J., Husted, C.W., Somerson, S.W., & Sicilia, M.R. (1996). Mastering emergency airway management. *American Journal of Nursing, 96*(5), 24–31.

*Springfield, Y. (1993). Acidosis, alkalosis, and ABG's. *American Journal of Nursing, 93*(11), 43–44.

*Stiesmeyer, J. (1993). A four-step approach to pulmonary assessment. *American Journal of Nursing, 93*(8), 22–25.

Thomas, J., et al. (1995). To vibrate or not to vibrate: Usefulness of the mechanical vibrator for clearing bronchial secretions. *Physiotherapy-Canada, 47*(2), 120–125.

Toder, D.S., & McBride, J.T. (1997). Home care of children dependent on respiratory technology. *Pediatric Reviews, 18*(8), 273–280.

Torrance, C., & Elley, K. (1997). Practical procedures for nurses: Respiration technique and observation. *Nursing Times, 4*(93), 44, Supplement 1–2.

*Winslow, E. (1993). Open and closed debate on hyperoxygenation. (Working Smart). *American Journal of Nursing, 93*(9), 16.

*Yeaw, E. (1992). How position affects oxygenation: Good Lung down? *American Journal of Nursing, 93*(3), 26–29.

---

*Asterisk indicates a classic or definitive work on this subject.

Cardiovascular Function

Eileen Klein

Key Terms

afterload
antidiuretic hormone
atherosclerosis
baroreceptors
cardiac output
claudication
diastole
dysrhythmia
edema

inotropic agent
ischemia
necrosis
preload
stroke volume
systole
tachycardia
viscosity

LEARNING OBJECTIVES

After studying this chapter, you should be able to:

1. **Describe the anatomic and physiological concepts underlying the three tissue perfusion diagnoses.**

2. **Discuss some common problems of cardiovascular function.**

3. **Identify the lifestyle, developmental, physiological, and psychological factors affecting tissue perfusion and cardiac function.**

4. **Explain how to assess the client at risk for problems of tissue perfusion or cardiac function, how to detect the manifestations of an actual problem, and how to recognize the client's responses to problems.**

5. **Differentiate among nursing diagnoses used for clients with cardiovascular problems amenable to nursing care.**

6. **Plan for goal-directed interventions to prevent or correct problems of tissue perfusion and cardiac function.**

7. **Evaluate the outcomes of cardiac nursing care and interventions to ensure tissue perfusion.**

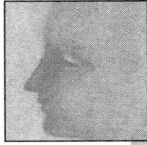

Mr. John Yoder, a 74-year-old Amish carpenter, experienced chest pain and lightheadedness while moving lumber in his workshop. A neighbor brought Mr. Yoder and his family to the hospital. Mr. Yoder is admitted to the hospital's coronary step-down unit for observation. He is accompanied by his wife and son. The admitting diagnosis is angina pectoris.

The initial nursing assessment reveals a moderately anxious man who is currently experiencing dull chest pain (7 on a 0–10 pain scale) that radiates to his left arm. The client's skin is pale. He has the following vital signs: blood pressure 150/92; apical pulse regular at 94 beats per minute; respirations 24 per minute. Admitting orders include bed rest, nitroglycerin for chest pain, and a scheduled cardiac catheterization in the morning.

After making Mr. Yoder comfortable, the nurse initiates the nursing care plan for this client. Based on Mr. Yoder's presenting signs and symptoms, the nurse identifies *Altered cardiopulmonary tissue perfusion* as a priority nursing diagnosis. Because altered cardiopulmonary tissue perfusion can adversely affect the function of the heart muscle, the nurse also assesses for *Decreased cardiac output*.

CARDIOVASCULAR
NURSING DIAGNOSES

Altered Tissue Perfusion: The state in which an individual experiences a decrease in nutrition and oxygenation at the cellular level due to a deficit in capillary blood supply.

Decreased Cardiac Output: A state in which the blood pumped by the heart is inadequate to meet the metabolic demands of the body.

Risk for Peripheral Neurovascular Dysfunction: A state in which an individual is at risk of experiencing a disruption in circulation, sensation, or motion of an extremity.

From North American Nursing Diagnosis Association. (1999). NANDA nursing diagnoses: Definitions and classification 1999–2000. Philadelphia: Author.

CONCEPTS OF TISSUE PERFUSION AND CARDIAC FUNCTION

All body tissues need oxygen and nutrients to survive. These needs are met by the cardiovascular system, which includes the heart and a complex system of blood vessels. The heart pumps blood, and the interconnected blood vessels carry it to all parts of the body. By doing so, the cardiovascular system delivers oxygen and nutrients to all parts of the body while removing the waste products of metabolism.

Cardiovascular disease accounts for 43% of deaths in the United States. Heath care costs for treatment and lost productivity equal about $151 billion each year (Anderson & Rosen, 1996). Because of the high incidence of cardiovascular disease, nurses regularly care for clients with problems of tissue perfusion or impaired cardiac function—or an increased risk for them.

Clients experience changes in tissue perfusion that range from acute, life-threatening problems, such as heart attacks, to chronic conditions, such as peripheral vascular diseases that linger for many years and adversely affect quality of life. Care of clients with circulatory problems is delivered in a variety of health care settings, from hospitals to outpatient sites to clients' homes. Nurses provide direct interventions, implement screening programs, and institute preventive teaching.

Although all cells require oxygen, demands for oxygen vary among different body tissues. Varying oxygen needs, as well as the degree to which tissue perfusion is impaired, determine the specific interventions indicated for individual clients. Relatively minor decreases in tissue perfusion can alter the function of the affected organ or body system. A major decrease in blood supply produces tissue **ischemia** (a decreased supply of oxygenated blood to tissues) and **necrosis** (localized death of tissues caused by disease, oxygen deficit, or injury).

Medical intervention is required to correct circulatory problems, and the collaborative role of the nurse in the care of clients with these problems is crucial. Continuous assessment and monitoring allow for early detection of potential complications in clients at risk. Early detection and prompt intervention for problems of tissue perfusion and cardiac dysfunction are critical for optimal client outcomes.

Nursing diagnoses applicable to clients with circulatory problems vary, depending on the area of the body affected. Three common nursing diagnoses related to circulation are *Altered tissue perfusion, Decreased cardiac output* and, in certain circumstances, *Risk for peripheral neurovascular dysfunction*. These diagnoses will be examined in this chapter. Remember that decreased circulation impacts multiple body systems. When caring for clients with circulatory problems, you will need to be prepared to evaluate skin integrity, respiratory status, and kidney function in addition to data about circulatory function.

The Cardiovascular System

Primary factors essential for circulation of blood throughout the body are a functioning heart to pump the blood and patent systemic blood vessels to transport blood to and from the tissues.

Heart

The heart is a muscular organ that acts as a pump to create the force to cause the blood to flow throughout the vascular system. It consists of four chambers: two atria and two ventricles. The thin-walled atria contract simultaneously to force blood into the ventricles. Then the heavily muscled ventricles contract to propel blood to the lungs and the general circulation. The right atrium and ventricle transport blood to the lungs. The left atrium and ventricle pump blood to the rest of the body. Figure 40–1 depicts the internal anatomy of the heart.

Blood flow through the heart results from a combination of a pressure gradient, contractions of the heart muscle, and a system of valves (Fig. 40–2). Blood flows into the right atrium from the vena cava because of pressure differences between the vena cava and the atrium. Contraction of the right atrium increases atrial pressure and opens the tricuspid valve, allowing

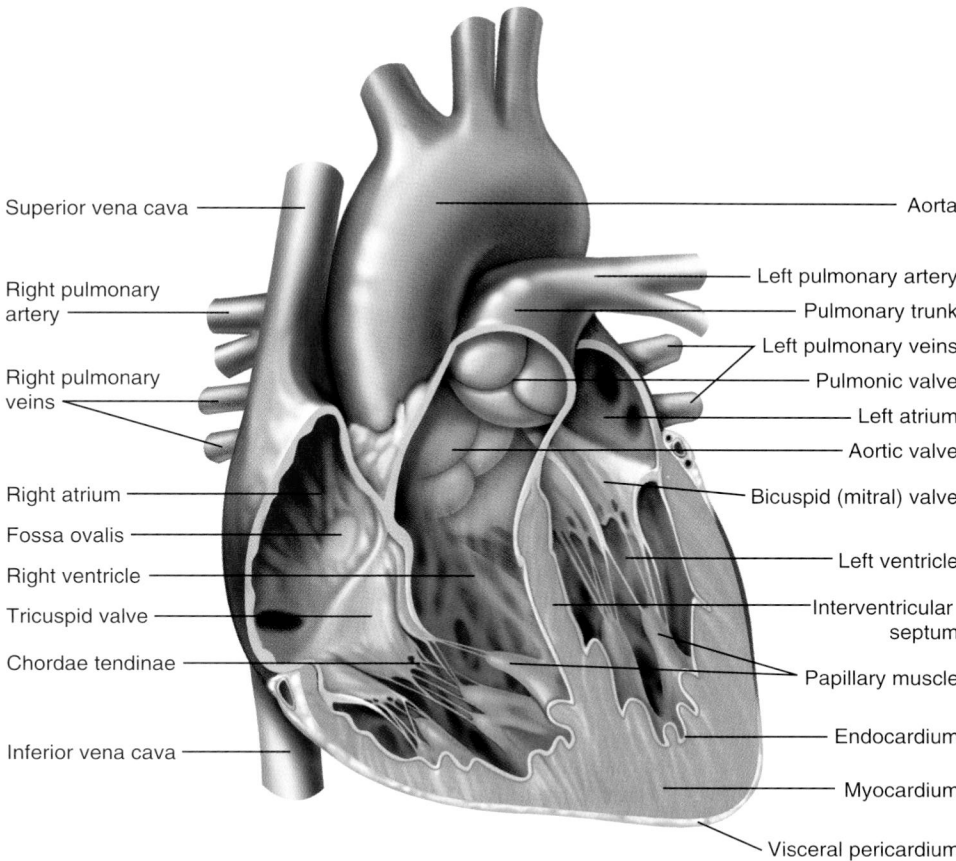

Superior vena cava

Right pulmonary artery

Right pulmonary veins

Right atrium

Fossa ovalis

Right ventricle

Tricuspid valve

Chordae tendinae

Inferior vena cava

Aorta

Left pulmonary artery

Pulmonary trunk

Left pulmonary veins

Pulmonic valve

Left atrium

Aortic valve

Bicuspid (mitral) valve

Left ventricle

Interventricular septum

Papillary muscle

Endocardium

Myocardium

Visceral pericardium

Figure 40–1. Internal anatomy of the heart.

blood to flow into the right ventricle. When the right ventricular pressure is great enough to exert pressure on the tricuspid valve, it closes, and the pulmonic valve opens, allowing blood to flow into the pulmonary artery and the lungs.

From the lungs, blood flows through the pulmonary veins to the left atrium. When the left atrium is full, it contracts, causing the mitral valve to open and blood flows into the left ventricle. Contraction of the left ventricle increases pressure in the ventricle, closes the mitral valve, and opens the aortic valve. Because of

the thick, strong, muscular wall of the left ventricle, blood entering the aorta is under high pressure.

The time from the beginning of one ventricular contraction to the beginning of the next ventricular contraction is called the cardiac cycle. Because the ventricles perform the work of pumping blood out of the heart, the events of the cardiac cycle are identified in relation to the contraction and relaxation of the ventricles. **Systole** refers to the contraction of the ventricles, and **diastole** refers to the relaxation of the ventricles.

Figure 40–2. Dynamics of blood flow through the heart. *A,* during diastole, blood enters the right atrium from the venae cavae and the left atrium and from the pulmonary artery; from there it passively flows into the ventricles. *B,* at the end of diastole, the atria contract (a movement called atrial systole), completing filling of the ventricles. *C,* during systole, ventricular contraction propels blood into the lungs and aorta.

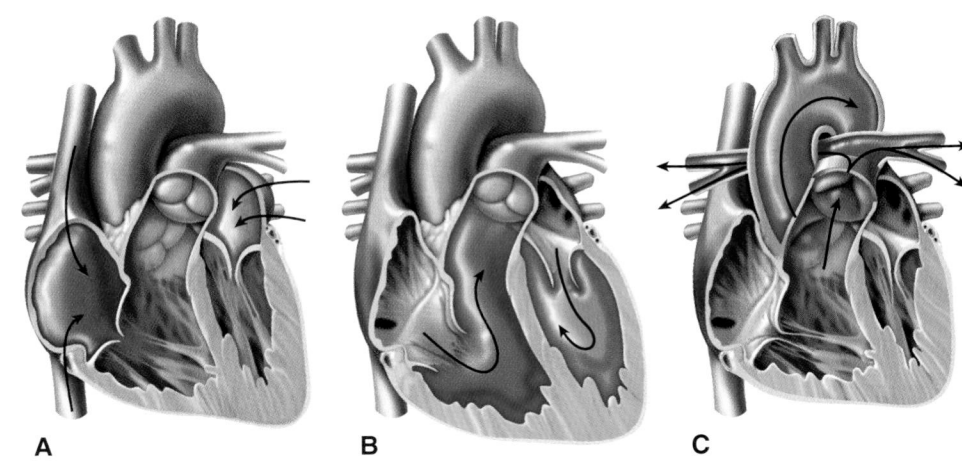

A   **B**   **C**

Blood Vessels

The systemic circulation consists of a network of blood vessels that begin and end at the heart. This vast vascular network is composed of three types of vessels: arteries (including arterioles), which carry oxygenated blood away from the heart; tiny capillaries, where the exchange between the blood and tissues occurs; and veins (including venules), which transport oxygen-depleted blood back to the heart. Blood flow within the circulatory system is determined, to some extent, by the unique anatomic characteristics of each of the vessels (Fig. 40–3).

ARTERIES

Arteries carry blood away from the heart. These blood vessels are exposed to fluctuating pressures from the pulsing force of heart contractions. A thick middle layer of muscle and elastic tissue in the arteries, called the *tunica media,* enables arteries to expand and contract in response to these constant pressure changes. The walls of arteries are composed primarily of smooth muscle, which contracts and relaxes to regulate the diameter of vessels.

VEINS

Thin-walled veins return blood to the heart in a relatively passive manner. Because of their relatively thin tunica media and large lumina, veins can distend to accommodate a large amount of blood. In fact, up to 64% of the total blood supply of the body can be held within the venous system (Guyton & Hall, 1996). The

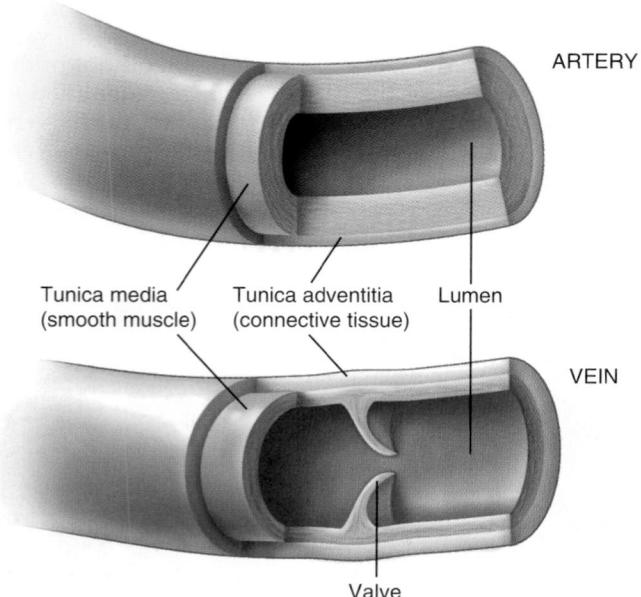

Figure 40–3. Comparison of an artery and a vein. Arteries have a thicker elastic tunica media, which means that they have more smooth muscle to control the diameter of the vessel (and thus control blood pressure). Veins are very distensible. Venous blood flow relies on one-way valves and the action of skeletal muscle.

tunica adventitia, or outer layer of the wall of veins, is composed of a thick layer of collagen tissue that provides protection and support.

The walls of veins have little smooth muscle to contract and to help propel blood back to the heart. However, contraction of leg and abdominal muscles assists venous blood return. One-way valves inside the veins prevent the backward flow of blood in the venous system. When those valves function ineffectively, however, blood stagnates in the venous system. Varicose veins can result from incompetent valves and subsequent distention of the venous system.

CAPILLARIES

Capillaries connect the arterial system to the venous system and allow the exchange of nutrients and wastes between the blood and the tissues. This exchange is possible because capillaries are the smallest vessels of the circulatory system. They consist of a single layer of epithelial cells.

Capillaries range from 4 to 9 μm in diameter, a figure similar to the diameter of a single red blood cell (Guyton & Hall, 1996). The small diameter of capillaries and the proximity of blood cells to the porous epithelium facilitates the exchange of substances between the blood and the tissues.

To summarize, blood leaves the left ventricle via the aorta and travels through a series of smaller and smaller arteries to tissue capillaries. Blood returns to the heart via increasingly larger veins. Figure 40–4 shows a schematic view of the systemic circulation.

Blood Components

All cellular components develop from mother cells, known as a stem cells, which subsequently differentiate, or specialize, into red cells, white cells, and platelets. Red blood cells transport oxygen to tissues in the molecule called oxyhemoglobin, which forms when oxygen and hemoglobin combine.

White blood cells fight infection and maintain the body's immune function. Platelets, also known as thrombocytes, are essential for coagulation or clotting of the blood. Plasma is the fluid component of the blood that carries the cellular elements, electrolytes, protein, glucose, fats, bilirubin, and gases.

Regulation of Tissue Perfusion

The body precisely regulates the amount of blood it sends to various tissues, based on their changing metabolic needs. Three elements—blood viscosity, a pressure gradient, and vascular resistance—form the primary factors in the control of tissue perfusion.

Viscosity of Blood

Viscosity is the relative ability of a fluid to flow. It results from the thickness of the fluid. Highly viscous blood flow encounters more resistance while moving through blood vessels. Because increased resistance slows blood through the vascular system, tissue per-

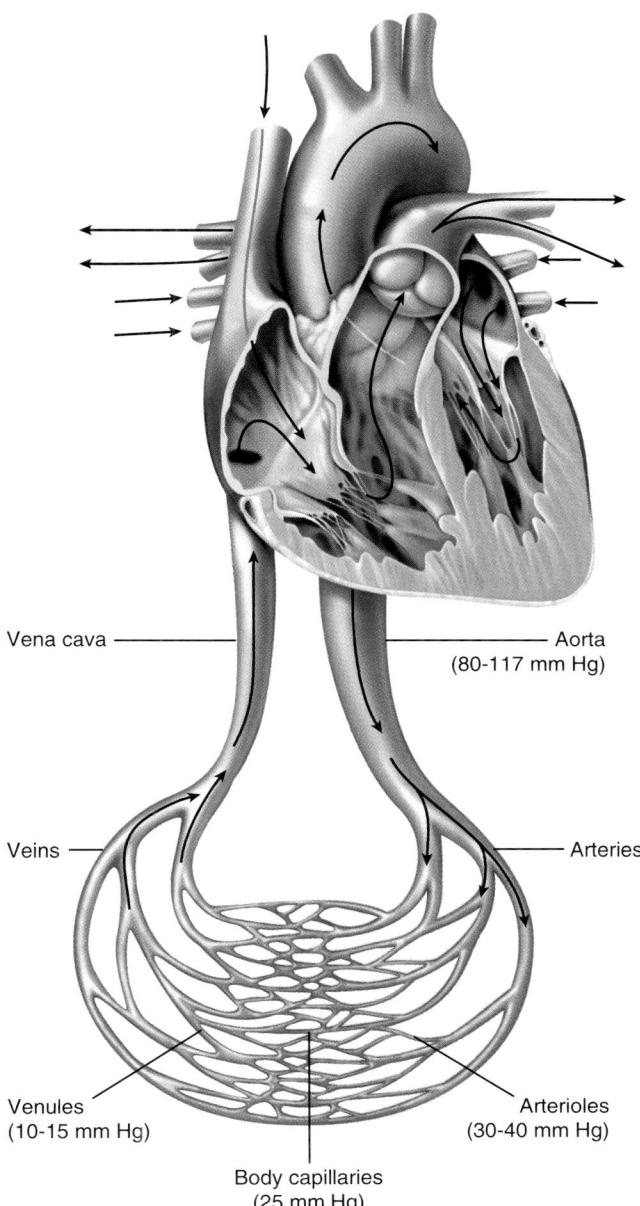

Vena cava

Aorta
(80-117 mm Hg)

Veins

Arteries

Venules
(10-15 mm Hg)

Arterioles
(30-40 mm Hg)

Body capillaries
(25 mm Hg)

Figure 40–4. The systemic circulation. Oxygenated blood exits the left ventricle via the aorta. Exchange of oxygen and carbon dioxide occurs in the systemic tissue capillaries. Veins return deoxygenated blood to the right atrium.

fusion is less efficient. Underlying health problems predispose clients to increased blood viscosity. For example, dehydration decreases the plasma components of blood, which increases viscosity.

Pressure Gradient

Blood flows from areas of higher pressure to areas of lower pressure. Contractions of the heart produce a strong pulsating force that moves blood through the circulatory system. Because the left side of the heart is larger and stronger, arteries closest to the left side of the heart have the highest pressures. As blood flows from arteries to arterioles to capillaries to veins, pressure in the vessels decreases. Pressure differences between arteries and veins help move blood through the circulation, much like fluid flowing downhill.

Vascular Resistance

Forces that slow the movement of blood are known collectively as vascular resistance. Viscous blood, constricted arteries, vessel lumina narrowed by fatty deposits, and bends or turns in the vessels are examples of factors that slow the movement of blood. Sluggish blood flow decreases tissue perfusion and increases the client's risk of developing blood clots.

Control of Blood Pressure

Adequate blood pressure is needed to maintain tissue perfusion. An increase in blood pressure causes blood to circulate more rapidly, whereas a decrease in blood pressure slows blood flow and decreases tissue perfusion. Pressure receptors, the autonomic nervous system, and hormones play important roles in controlling blood flow and blood pressure.

Control by Pressure Receptors

Baroreceptors are specialized cells located in the aorta and carotid arteries that detect pressure changes in the vascular system. Higher pressure in the arteries causes the vessel walls to stretch, triggering high-pressure receptors; lower pressure results in less stretch. Low-pressure receptors in the right side of the heart and the pulmonary artery detect reduced pressure in the vascular system. Both types of receptors send messages to the autonomic nervous system that help the body adjust to changes in pressure and thus maintain a constant flow of blood and a stable blood pressure.

Autonomic Nervous System Controls

The autonomic nervous system is composed of sympathetic and parasympathetic branches. Stimulation of the sympathetic branch of the autonomic nervous system causes an immediate increase in the strength and rate of the heart's contractions, which, in turn, increases the amount of blood pumped by the heart as well as the pressure in the circulatory system. When the parasympathetic branch of the autonomic nervous system is stimulated, heart rate slows, and blood pressure falls.

Hormonal Controls

Hormones secreted by the endocrine system control blood flow by changing the diameter of blood vessels. For example, the adrenal medulla releases neurotransmitters—epinephrine and norepinephrine—when the sympathetic nervous system is stimulated. These hormones constrict blood vessels, causing a temporary increase in blood pressure. Acetylcholine, a neurotransmitter released by stimulation of the parasympathetic branch of the nervous system, slows cardiac function.

Long-acting hormonal compensatory mechanisms also play a role in tissue perfusion. For example, the renin-angiotensin-aldosterone system helps keep the volume and pressure in the circulatory system constant (Fig. 40–5). When the juxtaglomerular cells of the kidneys detect a drop in blood pressure, the enzyme renin is released. Renin, in turn, facilitates the formation of angiotensin II, which is a powerful vasoconstrictor. The resulting vasoconstriction increases blood pressure. In the final step of the cascade, aldosterone is released from the adrenal cortex. This hormone stimulates the kidney to retain sodium and water, which increases plasma volume and circulating blood volume. Expansion of circulating blood volume raises blood pressure. When the kidneys detect a rise in blood pressure, renin secretion decreases, and the cascade is no longer activated; therefore, blood pressure subsequently decreases.

A second hormonal compensatory mechanism involves **antidiuretic hormone (ADH),** also called vaso-

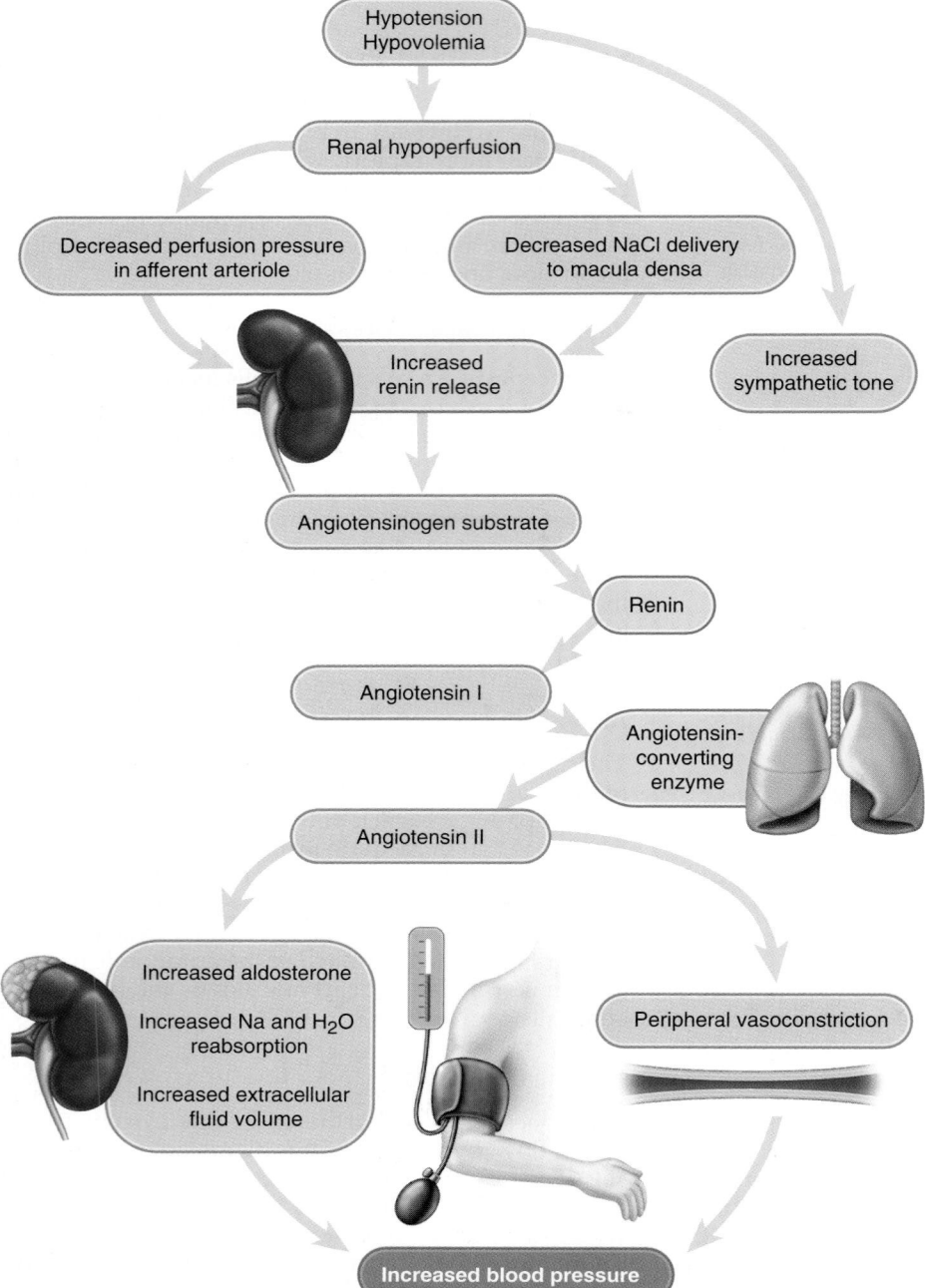

Figure 40–5. The renin-angiotensin-aldosterone system, which controls arterial blood pressure. The kidneys play a key role in the control of arterial blood pressure by initiating this chain of reactions in response to decreased renal blood flow.

pressin. ADH is produced by the hypothalamus and is secreted by the posterior pituitary gland when the sympathetic nervous system is stimulated by physiological stress. It prompts the kidneys to retain water, thereby increasing circulating blood volume and maintaining blood pressure.

Regulation of Cardiac Output

Cardiac output is the amount of blood pumped by the ventricles in 1 minute. The average cardiac output for an adult is 5 to 6 L/min. Cardiac output is highly variable, however, because it changes to meet metabolic needs. Cardiac output is calculated by using the following equation: cardiac output = stroke volume × heart rate

Stroke Volume

Stroke volume is the amount of blood ejected from the heart with each contraction. Normal stroke volume for an adult is about 70 mL. Distensibility (the stretch of the heart's muscle fibers), contractility, and resistance to blood flow affect stroke volume.

Preload, the amount of blood in the left ventricle immediately before contraction, is the main force that stretches cardiac muscle fibers. Imagine preload as the force needed to blow up a balloon. As air fills the balloon, the balloon stretches to accommodate more air. Heart muscle fibers are like a rubber band. The more they are stretched, the more forcefully they recoil. Stronger recoil produces greater stroke volume. This phenomenon is known as *Starling's Law.*

The strength of the myocardial contraction is a second major determinant of stroke volume. Hormones (such as epinephrine and norepinephrine) and sympathetic stimulation increase contractility. Chemical imbalances, myocardial ischemia, and parasympathetic stimulation decrease contractility and stroke volume.

Afterload is the final determinant of stroke volume. It is the pressure against which the left ventricle pumps—in other words, aortic diastolic pressure. Higher aortic pressure forces the heart to work harder, and less blood is ejected from the ventricles with each contraction. Afterload is like trying to open a door against a wind; the stronger the wind, the more difficult it is to open the door. In the heart, the door corresponds to the aortic valve, and the wind is the pressure in the aorta.

Heart Rate

A person's heart rate equals the number of times the heart contracts each minute. There is a direct relationship between heart rate and cardiac output. As heart rate increases, cardiac output increases—up to a point. However, if the heart beats fast enough to have a rhythm called **tachycardia** (a heart rate above 100 beats per minute), ventricular filling time shortens, and stroke volume falls. The autonomic nervous system and some hormones alter heart rate.

Regulation of Peripheral Neurovascular Function

All cells, including nerve cells, require oxygen to survive and to function properly. The circulatory system transports oxygen-rich red blood cells to all body tissues. Interruption or obstruction of blood flow to nerves produces ischemia of the nerve, with loss of neurological function. Prolonged obstruction causes permanent nerve damage.

FACTORS AFFECTING TISSUE PERFUSION AND CARDIAC FUNCTION

The development of problems involving tissue perfusion and cardiovascular function is usually a complex process with multiple factors. Heredity, lifestyle, psychological factors, and underlying health problems all influence circulatory function.

Lifestyle Factors

In recent years, lifestyle choices and their relationship to circulation have been the focus of intense scrutiny. Diet, exercise, and smoking have direct effects on circulation. Insurance companies are paying more attention to lifestyle behaviors. Some insurers reward healthy behaviors, such as regular exercise and optimal body weight, with lower insurance premiums. More and more people are experimenting with herbal and other alternative forms of medicine, as described in the Considering the Alternatives chart. Behaviors thought to pose health risks, such as smoking, can increase insurance costs.

Nutrition and Fluids

Nutrients, particularly protein and iron, are essential for the formation of blood cells. Diets with inadequate protein are deficient in amino acids needed to build red and white blood cells. Also, if protein intake falls, serum protein levels fall, and the ability to keep fluid in the vascular system is impaired.

Iron is needed to manufacture oxygen-carrying hemoglobin molecules. Iron-deficiency anemia develops when the diet lacks adequate iron. Anemia reduces delivery of oxygen to the tissues.

Fat intake also influences circulatory function. Excessive intake of such high-fat foods as red meat, animal fats, and some dairy products raises blood (serum) cholesterol levels. Hypercholesterolemia (high blood cholesterol) is a major risk factor for atherosclerosis.

Fluid balance also affects circulation. Clients on fluid restrictions or those with excessive fluid losses, as from diarrhea or vomiting, have the potential to become dehydrated and thus develop more viscous blood. Viscous blood clots more readily and can block blood vessels.

CONSIDERING THE ALTERNATIVES

HERBAL MEDICINE

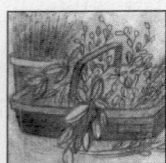 Herbs were probably the first medicines used by human beings. Early humans most likely observed the effects of herbs on other humans as well as on animals. From those observations, people learned that certain herbs produced certain predictable results. These observations led to experimentation with herbs as remedies. In fact, the Old Testament and many other ancient books attest to the use of herbs in healing. Later, extraction of plant constituents led to the development of drugs. To this day, pharmaceutical companies search the world for plants that may yield active ingredients useful in medicine. Today, roughly half of all prescriptions in the Western world are for medicines derived from plants (De Smet, 1997).

Herbs have been and still are used as medicines by people all over the world. In fact, in developing countries, they remain a mainstay of health care. Developed countries have seen a recent resurgence of interest in the use of herbs. Many people in developed countries now see herbs as an alternative to drugs and as a practical means of self-care. More and more scientific research is elucidating the usefulness of herbs. And traditions of professional herbal practice, some with thousands of years of history, still exist.

A useful distinction when discussing herbal medicine is between the use of herbs solely on the basis of their reputed activity and their use as part of a theoretical diagnostic and treatment system.

Consider the example of echinacea. Like many herbs, primarily from the European or Western herbal traditions, echinacea became popular in developed countries in the 1990s. This herb, originally used by Native Americans, was the most widely used herb in America in the 1800s, primarily for treating infections. Today, echinacea has made a comeback on the basis of its reputed activity, and it is widely promoted and used on the basis of its anti-infective and possible immune-stimulating properties. Contemporary European research has shown positive effects of echinacea in the symptomatic treatment of flu and other upper respiratory tract infections as well as of lower urinary tract infections (Ogletree & Fischer, 1997).

A recent study (Melchart, D., et al., 1998) showed a lack of effect using an echinacea extract to prevent upper respiratory infections. However, this study has been criticized for using too low a dosage (Murray, 1999).

In contrast, herbs are also used as part of theoretical diagnostic and treatment *systems* such as Ayurveda and traditional Chinese medicine, both ancient traditions with elaborate diagnostic and treatment protocols. These systems use herbs in a context that practitioners deem appropriate based on each client's constitution and presenting symptoms. In these systems, each herb is known by its properties, such as whether it is warming or cooling, and whether it raises or lowers energy in the body. In these systems, herbs are generally given in formulas of three to occasionally dozens of herbs. Also in these systems, the match between the client and the prescription is considered critical in order to avoid untoward effects and to increase efficacy.

A great deal of research has been and continues to be done on Chinese herbs. For example, a recent issue of *The Journal of Chinese Medicine* presented abstracts of Asian research on the use of the herb ginseng in the treatment of impotence; its apparent ability to reduce the incidence of tumors in regular users; and the beneficial effects of various formulas of this herb for the treatment of rheumatoid arthritis, impotence, male sterility, senile memory loss, neonatal hyperbilirubinemia, diabetic neuropathy, and heart failure, among other conditions (News; Abstracts, 1988).

A Japanese study that examined the use of a traditional Chinese herb formula in treating uterine myomas resulted in decreases in the size of these tumors and decreases in symptoms of hypermenorrhea and dysmenorrhea in more than half the clients treated (Sakamoto Yashino, Shirahata, Shimodairo, & Okamoto, 1992). Another traditional Chinese formula was studied in England for the treatment of the allergic skin disorder eczema (atopic dermatitis). Results showed significantly less redness, damage, and itching of the skin while clients used the formula (Sheehan et al., 1992).

Another recent study (Bensoussan, 1998) showed improvements in symptoms of irritable bowel syndrome in patients taking Chinese medicinal herb formulas versus placebo.

Other herbs from the West have shown promise in clinical studies. St. John's Wort *(Hypericum perforatum)* has been shown in trials with more than 3,000 people to be effective for the treatment of mild to moderate depression. St. John's Wort has been found to be superior to a placebo in the treatment of depression and appears to be comparable in its effects to pharmaceutical antidepressants. Further studies are examining its effects with long-term use and its effectiveness for severe depression (Upton, 1997).

(continued)

HERBAL MEDICINE (continued)

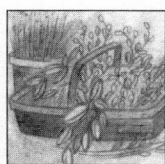

The seed of *Ginkgo biloba,* an ancient tree, has long been used in Asian cooking and medicine. The leaf extract of this tree has also been studied and used in Europe for the treatment of cerebral dysfunction, marked by such symptoms as poor memory, dizziness, tinnitus, and headaches, all stemming from insufficient cerebral blood flow. Some studies have shown promise in the use of this herb in the treatment of intermittent claudication, a circulatory disorder in which insufficient blood flow to and from the legs results in cramping (Kleijnen & Knipschild, 1992).

Stinging nettles *(Urtica dioica)* was shown in one study to have mild beneficial effects in treating seasonal allergic rhinitis (Mittman, 1990). It has recently been shown to be sufficiently beneficial when combined with anti-inflammatory medication so that clients were able to decrease their dosage of the anti-inflammatory drug (Nettle Leaf Enhances, 1998).

Another interesting study compared the use of dried horse chestnut seed extract with use of a placebo and leg compression stockings to treat clients with edema resulting from chronic venous insufficiency. The researchers concluded that use of dried horse chestnut seed extract was an acceptable alternative to the use of compression stockings and commented that oral medication tends to have higher compliance rates than the use of compression stockings (Diehm, Trampisch, Lange, & Schmidt, 1996).

With the tremendous amount of information that exists in the field of herbal medicine, and with the dramatic claims of its proponents, it is important to pay close attention to the quality of the research, the quality of the products, and the sources of both. Claims are often made based on hearsay, wild extrapolations from research, or unverified folk usage. Also, as with any medication, what works for one person may not work for another. This is where the more individualized approach of Ayurveda and Chinese medicine bear further scrutiny, perhaps even in terms of the use of pharmaceutical medications. Particular attention must also be paid to the effects of various herbs on various diseases and the interactions that may occur between herbs and pharmaceutical medications (Miller, 1998; O'Hara, 1998). The bottom line is that herbs used as medicine should be approached with the respect and caution that medicines deserve.

Resources

Publications that can expand and keep your knowledge of complementary and alternative medicine current:

Foster, S., & Yue Chongxi. (1992). *Herbal emissaries: Bringing Chinese herbs to the West.* Rochester, VT: Healing Arts Press.

HerbalGram, the Journal of the American Botanical Council and the Herb Research Foundation. P.O. Box 201660, Austin, TX 78720; (512) 331-8868.

Tyler, V. (1993). *The honest herbal* (3rd ed.). New York: Pharmaceutical Products Press.

Tyler, V. (1994). *Herbs of choice: The therapeutic use of phytomedicinals.* New York: Pharmaceutical Products Press.

References

Bensoussan, A., Talley, N.J., Hing, M., Menzies, R., Quo, A., & Ngu, M. (1998). Treatment of irritable bowel syndrome with Chinese herbal medicine. *JAMA, 280,* 1585–1589.

De Smet, P. (1997). The role of plant-derived drugs and herbal medicines in health care. *Drugs 54,* 801–840.

Diehm, G., Trampisch, J.J., Lange, S., & Schmidt, C. (1996). Comparison of leg compression stocking and oral horse-chestnut seed extract therapy in patients with chronic venous insufficiency. *The Lancet, 347,* 292–294.

Kleijnen, J., & Knipschild, P. (1992). Ginkgo biloba. *The Lancet, 340,* 1136–1139.

Melchart, D., Walther, E., Linde, K., Brandmaier, R., & Lersch, C. (1998). *Archives of Family Medicine, 7,* 541–545.

Miller, L.G. (1998). Herbal medicinals: Selected clinical considerations focusing on known or potential drug-herb interventions. *Archives of Internal Medicine, 158,* 2200–2211.

Mittman, P. (1990). Randomized, double-blind study of freeze-dried *Urtica dioica* in the treatment of allergic rhinitis. *Planta Medica, 56,* 44–47.

Murray, M. (1999). Echinacea tinctures shown to be ineffective. *Natural Medicine Journal, 2*(2):21.

Nettle leaf enhances effectiveness of anti-inflammatory drug (1998). *HerbalGram, 42,* 16–17.

News; Abstracts. (1988). *The Journal of Chinese Medicine, 56* (January).

Ogletree, R.L., & Fischer, R.G. (1997). *Physician's and pharmacist's guide to the top 10 scientifically proven natural products* (2nd ed.). Missouri: Natural Source Digest.

O'Hara, M.A., Kiefer, D., Farrell, K., & Kemper, K. (1998). A review of 12 commonly used medicinal herbs. *Archives of Family Medicine, 7,* 523–536.

Pittler, M.H., & Ernst, E. (1998). Horse-chestnut seed extract for chronic venous insufficiency. *Archives of Dermatology, 134,* 1356–1360.

Sakamoto, S., Yoshino, H., Shirahata, Y., Shimodairo, K., & Okamoto, R. (1992). Pharmacotherapeutic effects of kuei-chi-fuling-wan (keishi-bukuryo-san) on human uterine myomas. *American Journal of Chinese Medicine, XX,* 313–317.

Sheehan, M.P., Rustin, M.H.A., Atherton, D.J., Buckley, C., Harris, D.J., Brostoff, J., Ostlere, L., & Dawson, A. (1992). Efficacy of traditional Chinese herbal therapy in adult atopic dermatitis. *The Lancet, 340,* 13–17.

Upton, R. (Ed.) (1997). St. John's Wort, *Hypericum perforatum,* quality control, analytical and therapeutic monograph. Santa Cruz, CA: American Herbal Pharmacopoeia and Therapeutic Compendium.

Activity and Exercise

Clients with chronic health problems sometimes must lead more sedentary lives or may be immobile. Many clients without such health problems lead sedentary lives as well. For whatever reason, decreased activity slows venous blood return to the heart.

Changes in activity can be long- or short-term. For example, heart problems, severe anemia, and debilitating neuromuscular diseases produce long-standing fatigue. On the other hand, travelers on long trips or clients with bone fractures may experience temporary episodes of less dynamic circulation because of activity restrictions. Stagnation of blood in the veins contributes to clot formation.

Smoking

Smoking is a major risk factor that damages circulation in several ways and doubles the risk of heart disease (Anderson & Rosen, 1996). Nicotine produces vasoconstriction, which restricts blood flow to tissues, lowers the oxygen-carrying capacity of hemoglobin, and causes cellular changes in the intimal lining of arteries. In addition, nicotine lowers blood levels of beneficial, high-density lipoproteins and elevates levels of harmful, low-density lipoproteins; these serum changes hasten the atherosclerotic process. Finally, smoking enhances the detrimental effects of other cardiovascular risk factors, such as blood sugar and cholesterol levels; this is known as a synergistic effect. Box 40–1 summarizes research findings on the synergistic effects of smoking.

Substance Abuse

Substance abuse poses unique hazards to the cardiovascular system. Cocaine and amphetamines are stimulants that increase heart rate and oxygen demand. Large amounts of cocaine ultimately have an

---

BOX 40–1

THE EFFECTS OF SMOKING ON OTHER RISK FACTORS

Frati, Iniestra, and Ariza (1996) studied the effects of smoking on serum glucose, lipids, blood pressure, and pulse. Smokers were found to have higher glucose levels than nonsmokers. Smokers were also found to have higher levels of cholesterol, triglycerides, and low-density lipoproteins. Of particular interest was the fact that smoking after eating further increased serum cholesterol levels. Resting heart rates and blood pressures were also found to be higher overall in smokers.

---

anesthetic effect on myocardial cells, which decreases cardiac output and produces hypotension (Jackson, 1997).

In contrast, sedatives and opiates depress the central nervous system, causing respiratory depression and hypotension. The availability and delivery of oxygen to body tissues then decline.

Developmental Factors

Age is an important developmental factor that affects circulation in several ways. The primary effect of age relates to the development of atherosclerosis, which has long been known to increase with age. Also, some elderly clients also experience activity-limiting physical changes associated with aging.

Recently, attention has shifted to circulatory risk factors for children. The Bogalusa Heart Study (Bao et al., 1997) examined more than 200 children whose parents had coronary artery disease. Children with a positive family history were found to have obesity, hypercholesterolemia, and elevated blood sugar at younger ages than children without a family history of cardiovascular disease. Because these risk factors correlate with more rapid development of atherosclerosis, the researchers postulate that the overall risk of cardiovascular disease is increased in children with positive family histories.

Although family history is a risk factor that cannot be modified, early interventions with at-risk children may help to slow the atherosclerotic process. Significantly, the particular risk factors detected by this study—namely obesity, hypercholesterolemia, and elevated blood sugars—can be modified by weight control and dietary interventions. Researchers continue to follow this population of high-risk children to further evaluate the relationship between age, risk factors, and coronary artery disease.

Certainly, food intake affects the weight, blood sugar, and cholesterol levels of children at all ages. A study involving 55 high schools looked at the types of foods offered in school. Although food served by schools is regulated by federal guidelines and must comply with the Healthy Meals for Americans Act, alternative foods are available to students in vending machines, school stores, and snack bars. Story, Hayes, and Kalina (1996) found that the majority of foods sold via alternative sources were high in fat, sugar, and calories. Table 40–1 identifies common foods available in high school stores and vending machines. Healthy options, such as fresh fruit, fruit juices, and pretzels, were less readily available and often more expensive. This study raises interesting questions about food availability and nutritional choices for children.

Physiological Factors

Physiological factors also affect circulatory status. In addition to gender and weight, physical circumstances

TABLE 40–1

Foods Available in High School Stores and Vending Machines

Type of Food	Percent of Schools Offering
Beverages	
Juice-based drinks	88
Carbonated drinks	81
Fruit juice	77
Skim or 2% milk	6
Snacks	
Cheese puffs	54
Chips	54
Pretzels	27
Granola bars	27
Fruit	8
Desserts	
Candy bars	60
Cookies	58
Pies	23

such as pregnancy, health problems, and medications produce circulatory changes.

Gender

Although cardiovascular disease is the leading cause of death in the United States, gender differences create unique risk factors. For example, men are more likely than women to have earlier heart attacks. Estrogen levels in premenopausal females maintain the elasticity of blood vessels and keep serum cholesterol levels low. However, women have a poorer prognosis for recovery and experience more complications once they develop coronary disease.

Peripheral vascular disease also affects men and women differently. Women have an increased incidence of the peripheral vascular disease *Raynaud's disease,* which involves vasospasms, and men are more likely to have *Buerger's disease,* an occlusive vascular condition.

Weight

Obesity stresses the cardiovascular system. Excess adipose tissue requires the development of more blood vessels to nourish the tissue. Additional blood vessels lengthen the circulatory network and are associated with hypertension, a condition in which blood pressure is persistently higher than 140/90 mm Hg. Also, the heaviness of adipose tissue resting on blood vessels can compress the vessels.

Pregnancy

The growing fetus and amniotic fluid during pregnancy place considerable pressure on pelvic veins, which flatten easily because of their thin walls. This results in slowed venous return and pooling of blood in the veins of the lower extremities.

Problems of Cardiovascular Function

Cardiovascular dysfunction stems from problems within the heart or blood vessels that can alter tissue perfusion, cardiac output, or peripheral neurovascular function. Diminished heart contractility or blood flow through the chambers of the heart decreases pumping efficiency. Restricted flow through systemic blood vessels lessens perfusion to vital organs.

DISORDERS OF TISSUE PERFUSION

Patent blood vessels are essential for the delivery of blood to tissues. Conditions that decrease the lumina of blood vessels limit the ability of vessels to carry sufficient blood to meet tissue needs.

Atherosclerosis is a pathological condition in which fat and plaque form deposits on the intimal (inner) surface of the arteries (Fig. 40–6). It is the most common disorder that affects the size of blood vessel lumina. These deposits pose a twofold risk to tissue perfusion. First, fat and plaque narrow the lumen of the artery, which decreases the available space through which the blood must pass—like clogging a pipe. Second, plaque deposits create a rough spot on the normally smooth inner surface of the blood vessel. This roughness creates turbulent blood flow in the area. Platelets, the blood cells responsible for clotting, adhere to the rough area and further narrow the vessel lumen. The danger is that pieces of plaque will break off, lodge in smaller blood vessels, and thus obstruct blood flow.

Atherosclerosis particularly targets heart, brain, kidneys, and peripheral vessels. Diminished function in one or more of the target organs is a consequence of long-standing atherosclerosis. Accompanying health problems, such as hypertension, kidney failure, and diabetes mellitus, speed the development of atherosclerosis. A cerebrovascular accident is a condition in which a blood vessel in the brain is occluded by an embolus, a thrombus, or cerebrovascular hemorrhage, which results in ischemia or death in the brain tissues normally perfused by the damaged vessel.

DISORDERS OF CARDIAC OUTPUT

Some illnesses and medical treatments put clients at risk for a decrease in cardiac output, which is a way of saying the heart becomes ineffective as a pump. When caring for clients with any of the following conditions, be sure to monitor for a decrease in cardiac output:

- *Angina pectoris* is chest pain resulting from inadequate oxygen supply to the heart muscle, caused by partially occluded coronary arteries.
- *Myocardial infarction* is necrosis of heart muscle resulting from complete occlusion of a coronary artery.
- **Dysrhythmias** are abnormalities of heart rate or rhythm. Dysrhythmias may shorten the time avail-

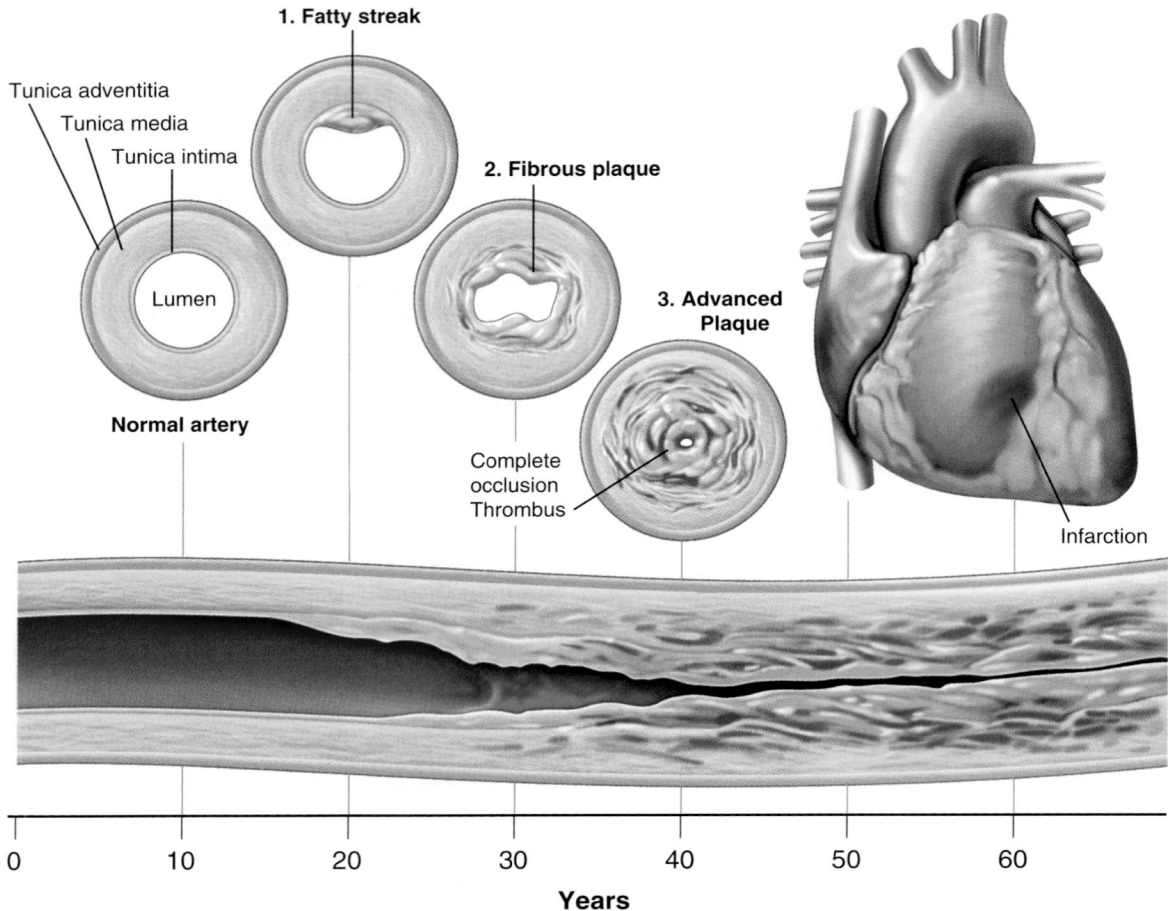

Figure 40–6. Formation of an atherosclerotic plaque. *1*, cholesterol deposits cause fatty streaks. *2*, fibrin infiltrates the fatty streaks, forming a fibrous plaque. *3*, platelets aggregate on the irregular endothelial surface, producing what is called a complicated lesion or an advanced plaque. Total vessel occlusion blocks blood flow, eventually killing the tissue cells normally supplied by the blocked vessel. This killing of tissue cells is called infarction.

able for the heart to fill with blood. Shortened filling time decreases stroke volume and cardiac output.
- *Bacterial and viral infections* can attack the heart, causing inflammation and scarring of the heart, valves, and pericardial sac. Scarring restricts blood flow through the heart and decreases contractility.
- *Congestive heart failure* is a condition in which the heart has failed as a pump (resulting in a decrease in cardiac output). Swelling of the feet and legs is a prominent symptom of right-sided heart failure. Fluid in the lungs is a prominent symptom of left-sided heart failure.

PERIPHERAL NEUROVASCULAR DYSFUNCTION
Conditions that disrupt circulation to an extremity raise the risk of neurovascular damage. Lack of circulation destroys nerves and impairs motor function in the involved extremity. Failure to detect early signs of neurovascular dysfunction can lead to permanent damage. This is a common cause of litigation in the United States.

Examples of situations that can obstruct blood flow include severe tissue edema; excessive pressure on blood vessels from a cast, splint, or tourniquet; clots or occlusions within blood vessels; and trauma to blood vessels, as from invasive procedures involving the vascular system.

Psychological Factors

Emotional stress burdens the circulatory system as well. Stress increases the heart rate and blood pressure which, in turn, raise the body's oxygen demands.

Many diseases that affect tissue perfusion and cardiovascular function are chronic. The affected person may have to contend with long-term health care issues, changes in quality of life, and complex medication regimens. Living with chronic health care problems requires constant adjustments by clients as their level of wellness fluctuates.

You will need to establish a trusting relationship with long-term clients, assess their motivation, and monitor their compliance. Depression and discouragement can lessen compliance, and you can be instrumental in recognizing these problems. You can also assist with problem-solving as a client's condition changes. Typically, nurses provide the client's main source of information and motivation to make life changes and maintain them, as one client described in A Patient's View.

ASSESSMENT

A thorough cardiovascular assessment includes a complete history and physical examination. However, ongoing assessment focuses on known problems or potential problems.

General Assessment of Tissue Perfusion and Cardiac Function

You will include some component of cardiovascular assessment for all clients. The prevalence of cardiovascular disease, the value of early detection, and the po-

tential for complications make cardiovascular data an essential component of every assessment. Assessment data include both general and specific observations about circulatory status. Overall appearance, condition of the skin, and activity tolerance give general cues about cardiac function. Data about heart sounds, peripheral pulses, and pain provide more specific information about cardiac function.

Health History

The health history consists of the duration of the client's chief complaint, past history, and lifestyle data. These categories of information create a detailed picture of the client's immediate needs as well as the impact of the problem on daily life.

CHIEF COMPLAINT
Chief complaints related to cardiovascular function range from dramatic to subtle. These include chest pain, palpitations, dyspnea, cough, fatigue, weight

---

A PATIENT'S VIEW
"NURSES DO THE REAL CARING"

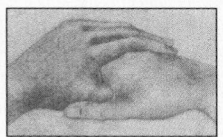 To celebrate my 65th birthday, I planned a 2-month walking tour with friends across my native England. Tickets, passport, and hotel reservations were at the ready when a routine doctor's appointment abruptly changed my destination.

A stress test on Tuesday led to an angiogram on Friday. Looking at the x-ray images, I knew England would have to wait. Bypass surgery was scheduled for the following week.

I'm a tall, skinny fellow who eats a reasonably good diet, has annual physical checkups at a world-class medical center, and, since my divorce 4 years ago, takes long, early-morning walks. But a 10-year history of angina (unrelieved by angioplasty) and a family history of heart disease have made me cautious about my health. My father died of a heart attack at 61; my brother also has a heart problem. I never really felt sick, but if I was active after eating or walked in the cold, the pains were always there. Thus the routine exam that derailed my long-awaited vacation.

Although disappointed about the change in plans, I spent a pleasant weekend in hospital, telephoning and writing friends. I felt completely comfortable about the surgery, trusting my doctor and the surgeon he recommended, who explained the operation very carefully and thoroughly. That trust proved to be well-founded because at no point did things go wrong.

The hours between the chilly wait outside the OR and

the tangle of tubes in the ICU are forever lost to me. I only remember the extraordinarily attentive care of the ICU nurses and my own curiosity about what was happening. About the 2nd day, most of the tubes were removed, and soon I was in a regular room. Almost immediately, the nurses got me out of bed and had me walking down the hall (staggering might better describe it), pushing my IV pole. My three incisions—chest, left arm, and right leg (the latter two where veins were removed for grafting to the cardiac vessels)—were held together with amazing adhesive patches. No external stitches.

It took 9 days in hospital to adjust my various medications. Infection developed in the arm incision but was quickly cleaned out and cleared up. Nurse practitioners briefed me on how to care for the chest incision at home as well as on tips on medications, diet, and lifestyle changes to aid the healing process. They were outstanding. You could tell they'd been in "the heart business" for years. They were also skilled in pain control. I don't remember any intense pain—just difficulty in finding a comfortable position to sleep.

The nursing care varied from good to excellent. Everyone was terribly nice but the experienced nurses had a different energy level than the younger ones and a more intense focus on you and what they were doing. They were more attentive to the little details that matter: being quiet when quiet is needed, turning out the lights at night, being right on time with medications. They were strong, direct, and definite. When they drew

(continued)

A PATIENT'S VIEW
"NURSES DO THE REAL CARING" (continued)

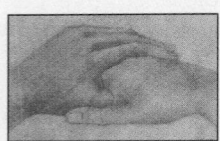

blood, plunk! The needle was in. You *knew* they knew what they were doing.

It also helped me to be in a Catholic hospital, even though I'm an Episcopalian. They don't throw religion at you— but a heartfelt spirit of giving and caring seemed to support everything that took place. The nurses impressed me most. They do the real caring. But there were amazingly good young doctors, too: gentle, considerate, very focused on me. Having faith myself, and a generally positive outlook on life—and being visited by friends from church—it was all a huge help.

My recovery was blessed by the kindness of friends and the presence of my 30-year-old daughter, who flew in from England. She and I spent 6 hours talking with nurses and other hospital people about diet do's and don'ts. She took notes. When we left the hospital, I insisted on walking out, so she pushed the wheelchair beside me. Friends drove me to their air-conditioned home where I would begin my 2-month recuperation.

The next morning, I awoke feeling restored, had breakfast, and from that point on, my recovery has been a beautiful, serene experience. It's the closest I've ever been to my daughter. She supervised my medication regimen, got me out and walking, observed my swallowing and breathing habits, took wonderful care of me. My friends gave me a bedroom with a view, lots of attention, and nutritious, delicious food.

After 4 weeks of pampering, I returned home, troubled only by long periods of interrupted sleep. That problem seems to have resolved, and my eight or nine pills are now down to four. Morning walks are still a must. While I was hospitalized, one of the Mended Heart people visited me, a volunteer who had heart surgery some time ago. I plan to go to their meetings and to volunteer to talk with other heart surgery patients.

My 2-month "vacation" has now ended; I'm revving up again but with some major changes. Next week I fly to Chicago for a 2-day workshop. The following week, I do another workshop there but, instead of flying back to Washington for 2 days and then flying back to Chicago, I'll just stay in Chicago and relax.

My career has been up and down. I bailed out of the corporate world in 1975 and have been a management consultant ever since, doing team-building work all over the world—places like West Africa and Haiti— with high temperatures and stress levels to match. I used to take on too much work. Now, I've begun to share more of my work with colleagues.

I used to rush through meals, doing 10 other things while eating. Now I cook intelligent, well-balanced meals and take time to savor them. I'm also taking more time to enjoy my photography hobby. Even as a member of two galleries, I'm still amazed and gratified that someone would pay for one of my photographs.

More than anything, this experience has shown me the value of peace and quiet, friends, and family. How fortunate I am. I can't imagine what it would have been like without that support. Though England still beckons, I cherish the insights gained on this unexpected journey.

---

gain, edema, syncope, and extremity pain. Because the systemic effects of cardiovascular disease can produce a wide array of signs and symptoms, clear identification of the chief complaint can help you prioritize your client's needs. Consider using the following mnemonic (HEART) to guide your assessment of cardiovascular problems:

H—Have the client describe the specific location, onset, and duration of the problem.
E—Explore associated signs and symptoms.
A—Ask about activities that worsen or ease the problem.
R—Rate the severity of discomfort or incapacity.
T—Talk about treatments or interventions that were used to alleviate the problem and their effectiveness.

Ask the client about medications, both prescription and nonprescription, used as treatment for cardiovascular conditions. Keep in mind that some over-the-counter medications interact with prescription medications. For example, aspirin and warfarin, an oral anticoagulant, have blood-thinning effects.

Clients who inadvertently take both drugs have a dangerous risk of bleeding. Similarly, antihistamines and appetite suppressants are contraindicated for clients with hypertension because they cause vasoconstriction. What you find out in the client's medication history may help to focus your data collection during the physical examination portion of the assessment.

HISTORY

The past health history of the client and his family can help to identify genetic tendencies and other risk factors. Assess for the following conditions in the client's past history because they are associated with the development of cardiovascular disease:

- Hypertension
- Rheumatic fever
- Elevated blood cholesterol and lipids
- Bleeding tendencies
- Peripheral vascular disease
- Myocardial infarction
- Heart failure

Also assess for noncardiac conditions known to influence cardiovascular function. For example, anemia produces tissue perfusion deficits, and diabetes and renal disease accelerate the development of atherosclerosis.

LIFESTYLE
Assess for lifestyle behaviors, such as smoking, diet, and exercise. Nicotine, alcohol, and recreational drugs have detrimental effects on the heart and blood vessels. Ask the client about the frequency and the amount of use for each of these substances.

Also gather a diet history. Identify food preferences, portion size, snacks, and methods of food preparation. Note the intake of foods high in fat, which raise serum cholesterol and lipid levels. Also note high-sodium foods, because they contribute to hypertension.

Investigate the client's exercise habits, because exercise is beneficial for circulation. Ask about the frequency, duration, intensity, and type of exercise he gets. Also discuss how well the client tolerates exercise.

Finally, explore the client's perceived stress level. Ask about his occupation, hobbies, and recreational activities. Identify coping strategies and support systems.

Physical Examination
Use data gathered in the history to focus your physical examination. Although the heart and blood vessels are the primary components of the examination, attention to all body systems is important because of the potential systemic effects of circulatory problems.

INSPECT THE CHEST
First, inspect the client's chest for symmetry and the presence of any pulsations. Some people have a small, nickel-sized pulsation visible near the apex of the heart. The pulsation is known as the *point of maximum intensity*. It is normally located at the fifth intercostal space left of the midclavicular line. Other visible pulsations are not usually normal. Describe the size and location of all pulsations.

ASSESS VITAL SIGNS
Vital signs provide baseline data about cardiac function. Document the arm you use for taking the reading, and note the client's position during the measurement. Take orthostatic blood pressure readings (in the lying, sitting, and standing position) for any client who takes an antihypertensive medication or complains of dizziness. Notify the physician if the client's pressure readings drop by more than 15 mm Hg during position changes.

AUSCULTATE HEART SOUNDS
Auscultate heart sounds at the aortic, pulmonic, tricuspid, and mitral areas and at Erb's point. Note the heart rate and rhythm. Report heart rates below 60 and above 110 beats per minute to the physician. Also

report any irregularities. If the client has an irregular apical heart rate, check the apical-radial pulse for differences in rate. Finally, listen for other heart sounds, such as murmurs. Document the location of any unusual heart sounds.

ASSESS PERIPHERAL CIRCULATION
Examine the carotid arteries and jugular veins in the neck. Gently palpate the carotid arteries, one at a time, for discernible vibrations called thrills. Auscultate each carotid artery for a *bruit,* which is an audible swishing sound. Normally, carotid arteries are silent. A bruit or a thrill indicates narrowing of the artery.

Action **A**lert!
Assess one carotid artery at a time. Bilateral palpation of the carotid arteries can cause bradycardia in susceptible clients.

Next, place the client in a 30- to 45-degree Fowler's position to examine the jugular veins. Distention of the jugular veins is a sign of heart failure or circulatory overload. To measure jugular vein distention (Fig. 40–7), document the highest level of the fluid wave.

Finally, palpate and grade the client's brachial, radial, femoral, popliteal, dorsalis pedis, and posterior tibial pulses. Palpate pulses on bilateral extremities simultaneously to detect subtle changes in pulses from side to side. Normal peripheral pulses are equal and symmetrical.

While assessing the pulses, make note of the skin's color, temperature, and texture. Look for hair distribution, skin discoloration, or ulcerations. Note the presence and severity of any peripheral edema by pressing your fingertips into edematous areas (Fig. 40–8). Note the depth of the indentation produced and the time needed for the indentation to disappear. Check for pain in the calf when you dorsiflex the client's foot. Pain indicates a positive Homans sign, which suggests deep vein thrombosis. Last of all, check capillary refill of the extremities.

Diagnostic Tests
Diagnostic tests provide valuable information about the function of the circulatory system. Some diagnostic tests are used to screen high-risk populations. Periodic laboratory or diagnostic tests track clients' positive and negative responses to treatment and guide modifications in therapeutic regimens.

Complete Blood Count
A complete blood count provides preliminary data about circulation. The red blood cell, hemoglobin, and hematocrit components of the complete blood count indicate the oxygen-carrying capacity of the blood. Data from this test can reveal circulatory problems that result from the body's inability to deliver blood, as opposed to delivery of blood that is deficient in oxygen.

The complete blood count also includes the total number of platelets. Clients with low platelet levels

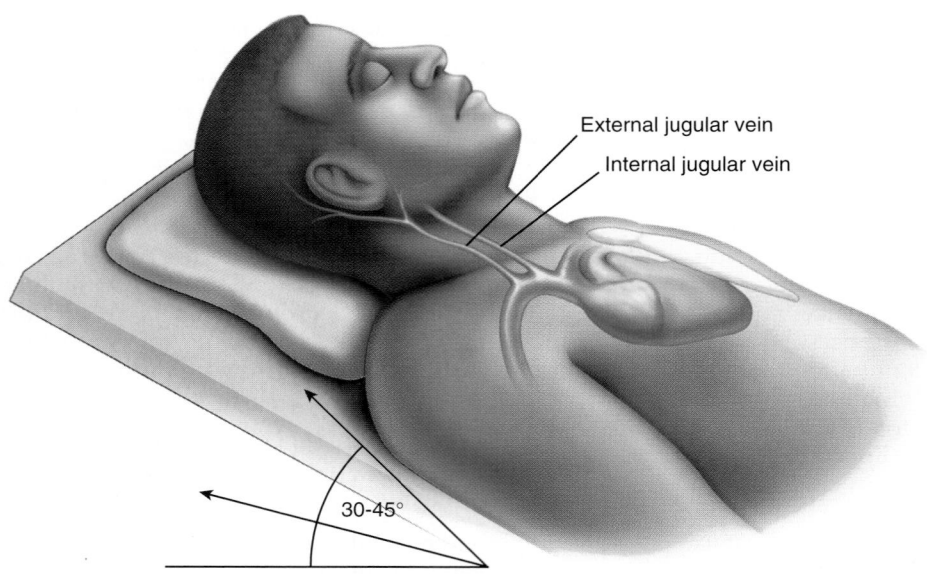

External jugular vein

Internal jugular vein

30-45°

Figure 40–7. Measurement of jugular vein distention.

are more likely to bleed, whereas those with elevated platelet counts are at risk for hypercoagulability.

Coagulation Studies

Coagulation studies, such as the prothrombin time and partial thromboplastin time, provide specific data about the body's ability to form blood clots. Pathophysiological conditions and some medications alter coagulation abilities and times. Inadequate clotting increases the risk of hemorrhage. On the other hand, clotting within blood vessels obstructs blood flow. Both of these conditions have the potential to dramatically alter circulation and tissue perfusion. The primary use of prothrombin time in cardiovascular disease is to monitor the therapeutic effects of warfarin. The primary use of partial thromboplastin time is to monitor the therapeutic effects of heparin.

Lipid Profile

Cholesterol, triglycerides, and lipids are fatty substances found in the blood. Lipids are further subdivided by laboratory analysis according to density and percentages of high-density, low-density, and very-low-density lipoproteins. Collectively, the measurement of these substances constitutes a lipid profile.

The lipid profile is used to assess risk for atherosclerosis and vascular disease. Elevations of cholesterol, triglyceride, and low-density and very-low-density lipid levels are associated with atherosclerosis. Conversely, high-density lipoproteins protect blood vessels against the development of atherosclerosis and cardiovascular disease.

The ratio of cholesterol to high-density lipoproteins is also calculated. High ratios increase the risk of atherosclerosis.

Electrocardiogram

The electrocardiogram is a graphic recording of heart rate, rhythm, and electrical conduction. By examining the pattern of the electrical wave through the atria and ventricles, information is gathered about the efficiency of the heart as a pump, tissues that are unable to transmit a normal electrical wave, and the rate and rhythm of the heart.

Angiography

The anatomic status of blood vessels is evaluated by angiography. An iodine-based contrast dye injected into a blood vessel traces blood flow and provides information about the diameter and patency of vessels. Narrowed or obstructed vessels impede the delivery of blood to tissues.

Before angiography, assess the client for allergies to medications and foods high in iodine, such as shellfish. Nausea, vomiting, difficulty breathing, tachycardia, and chest pain during the angiogram indicate an allergic reaction to the dye. Report any of these findings to the physician immediately.

*A*ction *A*lert!
Maintain a patent airway if an allergic reaction occurs.

Angiograms are invasive procedures of the circulatory system. Monitor the client's peripheral circulation before and especially after the procedure. Adequate circulation is evidenced by strong, equal peripheral pulses; warm, pink skin; and the absence of numbness, tingling, or pain. Inform the physician of any abnormal circulatory findings.

This common test can provoke considerable anxiety for a client whose cardiovascular function is already threatened. Thus, it is all the more important that you spend time teaching the client about the test and helping to relieve his anxiety in addition to providing ordered treatments.

*A*ction *A*lert!
Immediately report pain, pallor, pulselessness, or paresthesia of the client's extremity following angiography.

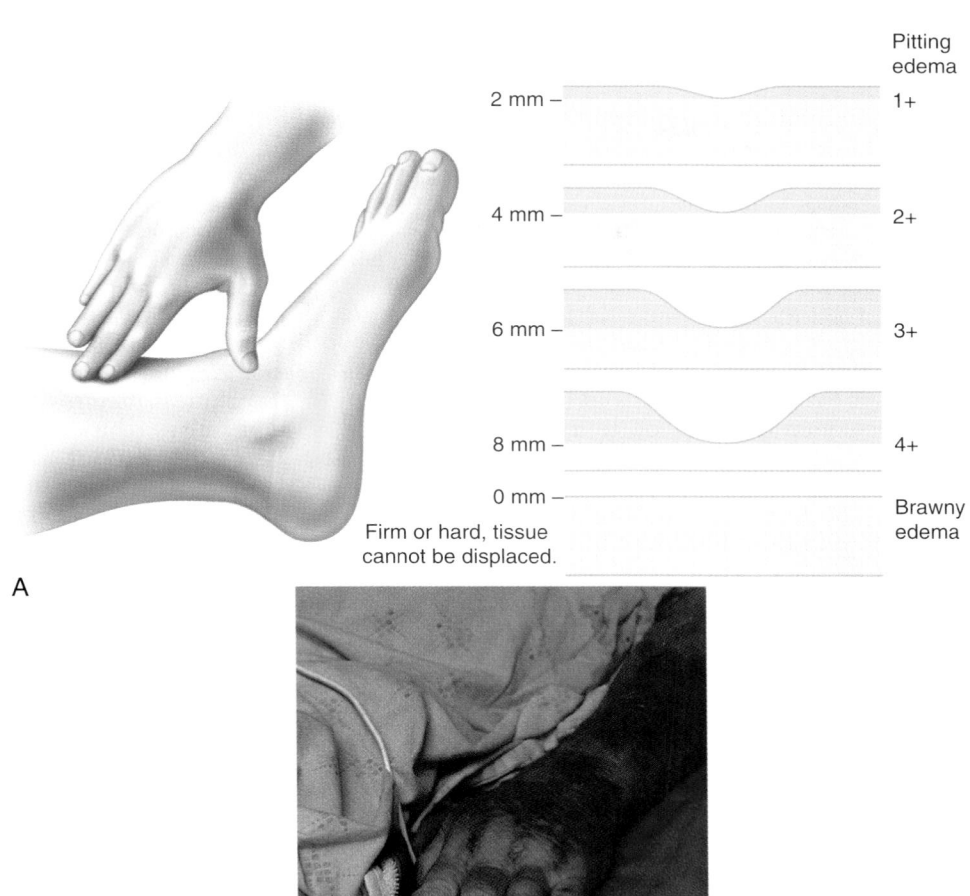

Pitting
edema

2 mm —   1+

4 mm —   2+

6 mm —   3+

8 mm —   4+

0 mm —   Brawny
                                          edema
Firm or hard, tissue
cannot be displaced.

A

B

Figure 40–8. Pitting edema. *A,* assessment and grading. Pressing on the surface of edematous tissue leaves an indentation that does not immediately rebound once the pressure is released. Pitting edema is graded by the depth of the indentation. *B,* a clinical example of pitting edema.

Doppler Blood Flow Studies

Doppler studies use sound waves to evaluate the patency of peripheral blood vessels. Diminished blood flow as well as clots in the vessels are detected by the Doppler ultrasound probe. This noninvasive test poses few risks for clients.

Focused Assessment for Altered Tissue Perfusion

Impaired blood flow to an organ reduces the delivery of oxygen and nutrients needed by that organ to function effectively. Pain and impaired organ function are cues to a state of *Altered tissue perfusion.* Whenever possible, focus any diagnosis of *Altered tissue perfusion* by specifying the area of the body affected: cerebral, renal, cardiopulmonary, gastrointestinal, or peripheral (NANDA, 1998). Use the client history and current

clinical manifestations to identify specific areas of compromised perfusion.

Defining Characteristics

Defining characteristics for *Altered tissue perfusion* are related to the area of the body affected. For example, Mr. Yoder, the client introduced at the beginning of this chapter, has *Altered cardiopulmonary tissue perfusion.* Mr. Yoder's admitting diagnosis is angina pectoris. Angina results from a coronary blood supply inadequate to meet myocardial metabolic needs.

In Mr. Yoder's situation, chest pain is the primary manifestation of his cardiopulmonary perfusion problem. Myocardial oxygen deprivation impairs the heart's pumping efficiency, which in turn limits oxygen delivery to other parts of the body. This produces other manifestations of *Altered tissue perfusion,* such as pale, clammy skin and lightheadedness. Based on his signs and symptoms, which other areas of Mr. Yoder's body are also experiencing tissue perfusion deficits?

A client with decreased perfusion in peripheral tissues will have different signs and symptoms than Mr. Yoder. Peripheral perfusion problems can involve either arteries or veins; the client's signs and symptoms will offer clues to the vessels involved (Table 40–2). Arterial perfusion alterations are the more serious of the two. Defining characteristics of decreased arterial perfusion include decreased or absent pulses, skin that is pale and cool, numbness and tingling of the extremity, claudication, and slow capillary refill. **Claudication** refers to cramp-like pains in the calves caused by poor circulation of the blood to the leg muscles.

Venous occlusion, inflammation of a vein (phlebitis), or prolonged immobility can impair the return of blood to the heart. The resulting venous congestion produces redness, swelling, and warmth in the involved extremity.

Related Factors

Atherosclerosis is the primary physical cause of *Altered tissue perfusion* because it narrows the blood vessels. Eventually, blood flow distal to the obstruction is blocked, and occlusion results. Occlusion can occur in blood vessels throughout the body. Myocardial infarction, cerebral vascular accident, and deep vein thrombosis are examples of occlusive events.

Edema can compress blood vessels. **Edema** (an abnormal accumulation of fluid in the interstitial spaces of tissues, commonly known as swelling) that occurs in areas with limited space for expansion is especially risky. Four factors that contribute to edema formation are disruptions of hydrostatic pressure, oncotic pressure, capillary permeability, and lymph drainage (see Chapter 31).

Focused Assessment for Decreased Cardiac Output

Pathological conditions that directly affect the heart can reduce the heart's pumping ability, which can result in inadequate tissue perfusion. Therefore, assessment of cardiac output is assessment of the whole circulatory system.

Defining Characteristics

The major defining characteristics of *Decreased cardiac output* are signs that the cardiac system is trying to compensate, specifically by means of an increased pulse and a drop in blood pressure. Tachycardia (a heart rate over 100 beats per minute) is a short-term compensatory mechanism to restore stroke volume. When this compensatory mechanism fails, hypotension develops.

Clinical manifestations include decreased peripheral pulses, chest pain, dysrhythmias, and cyanosis. As cardiac output decreases, the heart becomes congested with blood that it cannot expel. Congested blood within the heart increases hydrostatic pressure. Eventually, fluid pools in the form of edema of the lungs or the lower extremities. Signs include dyspnea, fatigue, jugular vein distention, and peripheral edema.

Other defining characteristics of *Decreased cardiac output* relate to impaired blood supply to the vital organs. The brain is especially vulnerable to decreases in blood supply. Restlessness, dizziness, and syncope (fainting) are common manifestations of cerebral hypoxia. Because kidney function depends on adequate blood pressure, urine output drops as a consequence of decreases in cardiac output. Additionally, because the body shunts blood to vital organs during periods of decreases in cardiac output, the client's skin will become cold and clammy, cyanosis will appear, and capillary refill will be slow.

Related Factors

Underlying cardiovascular disease is the primary factor that affects cardiac output. Disturbances in heart rhythm, medications that decrease contractility, heart surgery, and shock also adversely affect cardiac output. Heart conditions that decrease heart rate or stroke volume result in decreases in cardiac output. Bradycardia, heart failure, myocardial infarction, and cardiogenic shock are examples of problems originating

TABLE 40–2

Comparison of Peripheral Arterial and Venous Circulatory Dysfunction

Dysfunction	Arterial	Venous
Pain	Intermittent and related to activity	Constant aching
Pulses	Decreased or absent	Unchanged
Capillary refill	Less than 3 seconds	Unchanged
Skin color	Pale	Red
Skin temperature	Cool	Warm
Skin appearance	Shiny, with hair loss	Patchy brown discoloration
Edema	Absent	Present
Sensory/motor function	Impaired	Unchanged
Ulcers	Pale ulcer base with even edge	Red ulcer base with uneven edge
Healing	Delayed	Delayed

in the heart. In these situations, the heart is unable to pump effectively.

Additionally, cardiac output is reduced secondary to decreased circulating blood volume. Hemorrhage, burns, or severe dehydration produce hypovolemia (low vascular volume) due to a loss of blood cells or plasma from the vascular space. Although the heart initially functions properly, stroke volume and cardiac output fall rapidly because of decreased venous return.

Focused Assessment for Risk for Peripheral Neurovascular Dysfunction

Neurovascular dysfunction is a preventable complication for most clients. Vigilance on your part is the primary preventive action, starting with identification of clients at risk for neurovascular dysfunction. Frequent assessment will help you detect circulatory compromise promptly and intervene appropriately to relieve pressure on vessels and nerves.

Defining Characteristics

The defining characteristics of peripheral neurovascular dysfunction vary with the type of vessel that is occluded. Usually, arterial occlusions present a picture of oxygen deficit, whereas venous occlusions are characterized by venous engorgement.

ARTERIAL OCCLUSION. Manifestations of arterial occlusion include decreased pulses, pallor, cool skin, slow capillary refill, numbness, tingling, burning, decreased movement of the affected limb, and pain in the affected limb. These signs indicate oxygen deprivation in the tissues and nerves of the involved extremity.

VENOUS OCCLUSION. Occlusion of a vein prevents blood from returning to the heart. Venous engorgement in the extremity produces warm skin, red skin, edema, and slow capillary refill in the affected area.

Related Factors

Situations in which pressure is exerted on blood vessels and nerves, particularly pressure in body areas with limited capacity for expansion, constitute risks for peripheral neurovascular dysfunction. Hemorrhage into a muscle or joint, edema secondary to trauma or surgery, or a severe burn increases pressure due to local accumulation of blood or fluid. Burns that encircle an extremity are especially dangerous because the circular pattern of edema acts like a tourniquet to block blood flow distal to the injury.

Therapeutic treatments also pose risks for clients. Edema under newly applied casts, an elastic bandage or tourniquet that is applied too tightly, extensive infiltration of intravenous fluids, or misaligned traction leads to neurovascular damage, if undetected.

Focused Assessment for Shock

Shock is a life-threatening circulatory collapse that results from a severe volume deficit, cardiac pump failure, or redistribution of blood. In shock, the heart cannot pump sufficient blood to vital organs. Early manifestations of shock include tachycardia and hypotension, but malfunctions of the heart, brain, and kidney quickly develop. Shock is a medical emergency that requires prompt intervention to prevent permanent damage to vital organs.

Early detection of shock is essential because it is a progressive condition that develops in four stages (Fig. 40–9).

Fortunately, shock responds well to treatment in the early stages. Nurses, because of their frequent client contact and ongoing assessment, are instrumental in preventing shock and its devastating consequences. Because of the physiological complexity of shock, the physician and nurse work collaboratively to care for affected clients.

Defining Characteristics

Shock is characterized by signs of impaired tissue perfusion. Changes in vital signs, neurologic status, skin, and renal function are evident in roughly the following order:

- *Tachycardia.* In the initial stage of shock, slight tachycardia is the only manifestation. As shock progresses, tachycardia worsens.
- *Hypotension.* When the body can no longer maintain cardiac output by increasing the heart rate, blood pressure falls. Decreases in both systolic and diastolic blood pressure eventually occur.
- *Weakened peripheral pulses.* The heart's inability to deliver blood to peripheral areas of the body progressively weakens peripheral pulses.
- *Changes in neurological status.* Brain cells are very sensitive to oxygen deprivation. Cerebral hypoxia, in early shock, causes restlessness, agitation, and confusion. As shock progresses, the client becomes progressively less alert.
- *Skin changes.* Because blood is shunted away from the skin and sent to vital organs such as the heart and lungs, the client will develop pale, cold, clammy skin characteristic of shock.
- *Decreased urine output.* Hypotension decreases kidney filtration, reducing urine output to less than 30 mL/h.

Related Factors

As mentioned earlier, heart failure, loss of blood volume, and extensive peripheral vasodilation are critical events that lead to shock. Each of these events triggers shock by altering a component of circulation.

CARDIOGENIC SHOCK. Heart failure occurs when contractility or stroke volume falls. When heart failure results in shock it is called cardiogenic shock.

HYPOVOLEMIC SHOCK. Loss of blood or plasma decreases the circulating blood volume, which results in hypovolemic shock. Hemorrhage, severe burns, and extensive vomiting or diarrhea can trigger hypovolemia.

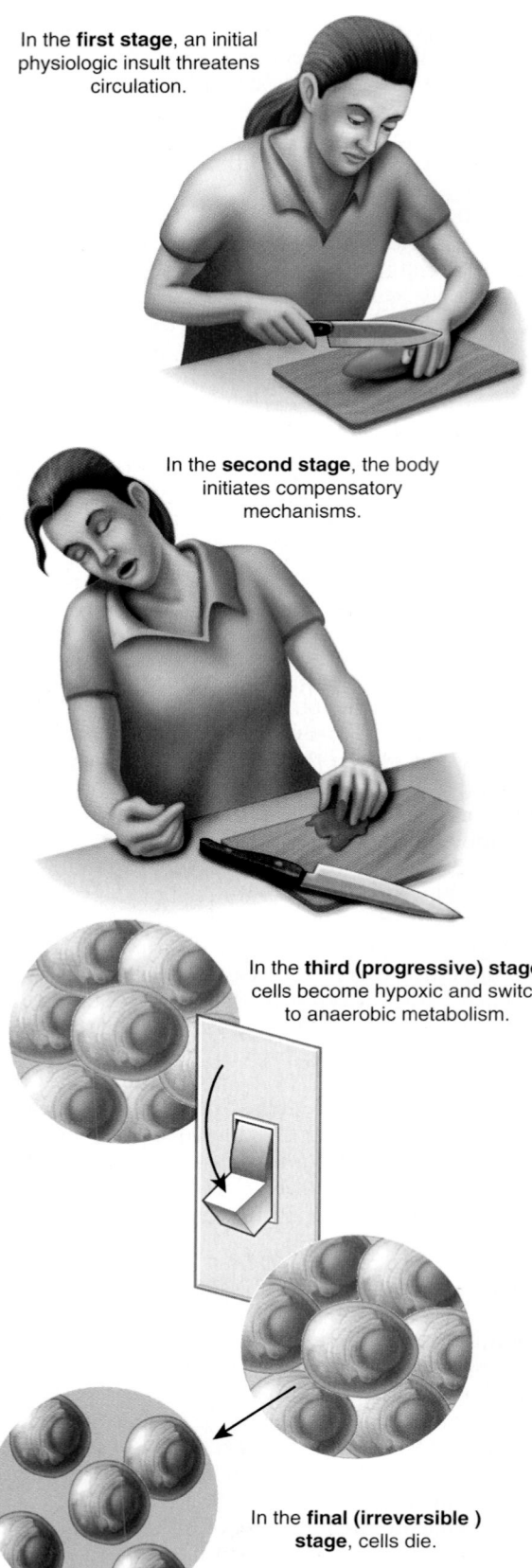

In the **first stage**, an initial physiologic insult threatens circulation.

In the **second stage**, the body initiates compensatory mechanisms.

In the **third (progressive) stage**, cells become hypoxic and switch to anaerobic metabolism.

In the **final (irreversible)** **stage**, cells die.

Figure 40–9. The four stages of shock.

DISTRIBUTIVE SHOCK. Massive peripheral vasodilation that traps blood in the peripheral microcirculation can result in shock. Although the actual circulating blood volume is unchanged, vasodilation produces a relative state of hypovolemia. Severe allergic reactions, neurological injury, and blood-borne infections from gram-negative organisms are examples of conditions that can cause distributive shock.

Focused Assessment for Related Nursing Diagnoses

Problems of tissue perfusion and cardiac dysfunction lead to other problems as well. You will need to prioritize client needs and plan interventions to address problems associated with circulatory dysfunction. The following are nursing diagnoses commonly associated with cardiovascular dysfunction.

Pain

Pain commonly accompanies decreases in circulation. As compensatory mechanisms for inadequate circulation fail, body tissues adapt by switching from aerobic to anaerobic metabolism. The byproduct of anaerobic metabolism is lactic acid. When it accumulates in the tissues, lactic acid irritates nerve endings and produces pain.

The location of pain caused by decreased circulation depends on the area of the body deprived of blood and oxygen.

For example, Mr. Yoder, the client introduced at the beginning of the chapter, experienced chest pain from inadequate circulation to the myocardial muscle.

Another example is a client with a newly applied cast who develops swelling of the casted extremity. In this situation, pain in the fractured limb is the expected finding. Restoration of circulation is a priority to prevent damage to tissues and nerves.

Anxiety

Anxiety is a common response both to pain and to the effects of decreased circulation. It also may result from cerebral hypoxia. As mentioned earlier, the brain requires a constant source of oxygenated blood to function properly.

Risk for Impaired Skin Integrity

When circulation is impaired, blood is shunted away from nonessential organs to improve perfusion to vital organs. Diversion of blood from the skin decreases the delivery of nutrients and removal of metabolic waste. Vasoconstriction, which accompanies blood shunting, produces cold, clammy, mottled skin. Chronic circulatory impairment puts clients at risk for pressure sores and delayed tissue healing. For example, clients with arterial or venous insufficiency of the lower extremities are likely to develop ulcers and necrotic areas on the legs.

Altered Health Maintenance

Clients with cardiovascular problems are frequently advised to change their lifestyle. Assess the client's lifestyle as well as the knowledge and motivation needed to make the changes.

Activity Intolerance

Assess the client with cardiovascular problems for problems in tolerating activities that are essential or desirable for the client. Muscles with inadequate blood supply fatigue quickly, especially activity that increases their demand for oxygen.

DIAGNOSIS

Altered tissue perfusion, as a nursing diagnosis, addresses a variety of client situations characterized by

diminished circulation. Generally, the consequences of tissue perfusion deficits involve decreased or lost organ function. Internal organs, such as the heart, brain, and kidneys, as well as peripheral extremities are common targets of perfusion deficits.

Altered tissue perfusion and *Decreased cardiac output* are closely related, as suggested by the accompanying Decision Tree. A delicate balance is necessary to maintain circulation. Pathophysiological change in either of these vital components impacts the other.

Mr. Yoder provides a good example of the interrelatedness of these two nursing diagnoses. Mr. Yoder has coronary artery disease, which narrows the blood vessels that nourish the myocardial muscle. Because of these narrowed vessel lumina, less blood passes through the coronary arteries, creating a perfusion deficit to the heart muscle. When Mr. Yoder's activity increases, as when he works in his carpenter shop, his myocardium has an increased demand for oxygen that the narrowed coronary arteries cannot meet. An imbalance of supply and demand develops that eventually results in chest pain. If Mr. Yoder stops his activity, the oxygen

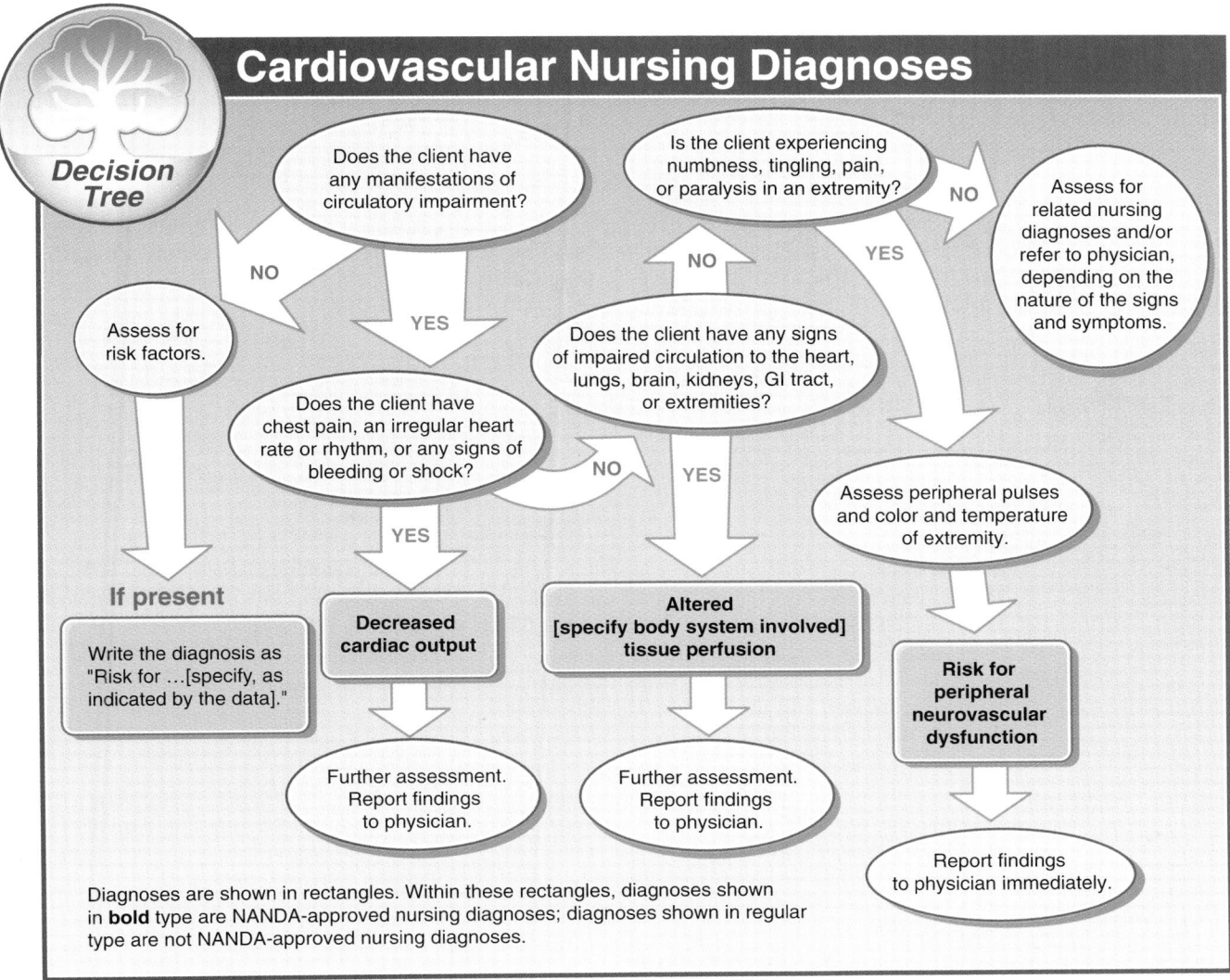

demand falls, and his chest pain ceases. However, if his circulatory system cannot meet his heart's oxygen demand for too long a time, myocardial cells will die. Mr. Yoder will have a myocardial infarction.

The final nursing diagnosis discussed in this chapter, *Risk for peripheral neurovascular dysfunction*, focuses on a smaller cluster of client situations in which circulation to an extremity is jeopardized. Generally, burns, constricting treatment devices, invasive vascular procedures, and occlusive events constitute threats that warrant selection of this nursing diagnosis.

Careful assessment and consideration of underlying health problems will help you to prioritize between *Altered tissue perfusion* and *Decreased cardiac output* for individual clients. Goals and interventions that aim to correct the underlying cause of the problem produce the best client outcomes. The data clustering chart gives examples of how to identify the appropriate nursing diagnosis.

PLANNING

Expected outcomes for clients with cardiovascular problems are different for acute and chronic problems. This section focuses on acute care when interventions are frequently aimed at early detection and prevention. Interventions for acute circulatory diagnoses include assessment, monitoring changes in circulatory status, support of circulation, and implementation of medical therapies. Early recognition of impending complications is crucial for successful client outcomes.

However, you must consider multiple factors even when planning care for acute client problems. In addition to physiological factors, you will identify aspects unique to each client. Explore the client's living arrangements, transportation, finances, support systems, and cultural background to help formulate a holistic plan of care that addresses individual client needs.

Consider the special needs of Mr. Yoder, the client introduced at the beginning of this chapter. Mr. Yoder's Amish beliefs and lifestyle must be incorporated into the plan for his care. The general cultural needs of Amish clients are summarized in the Cross-Cultural Care chart.

Expected Outcomes for the Client With Altered Tissue Perfusion

The goal for acute *Altered tissue perfusion* is the prevention of permanent tissue damage or even death. Rapid assessment and intervention mean the difference between positive and negative client outcomes. The goals for chronic perfusion problems include improving circulation and adaptation to the problem. The role of the nurse in managing a chronic perfusion alteration is to detect subtle signs of circulatory deterioration, teach clients, foster compliance with the treatment regimen, and provide emotional support.

You will evaluate the effects of interventions to maintain or improve tissue perfusion by assessing the client's circulatory status. Examine his overall circulation as well as the target organs specifically at risk. Expected outcomes that demonstrate adequate tissue perfusion include the following:

- Blood pressure within normal limits for the client
- Palpable peripheral pulses of equal strength and quality
- Skin warm and dry

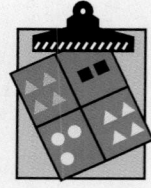

CLUSTERING DATA TO MAKE A NURSING DIAGNOSIS
CARDIOVASCULAR PROBLEMS

Data Cluster	Diagnosis
A 15-year-old client fractured his arm while playing soccer. A cast has been applied to the arm, and the client has just arrived in the nursing unit.	*Risk for peripheral neurovascular dysfunction* related to tissue trauma and edema formation.
An elderly client is admitted with a myocardial infarction. Two hours after admission, the client becomes confused and disoriented. Her blood pressure has dropped to 90/50 mm Hg, and her pulse has increased to 120 beats per minute.	*Decreased cardiac output* related to impaired myocardial contractility.
A 48-year-old man is admitted with complaints of periodic leg cramps. Assessment reveals very diminished pulses and pale, shiny skin on his lower extremities. He has no hair on his shins. The client reports a 20-year history of high blood pressure and diabetes mellitus.	*Altered peripheral tissue perfusion* related to diminished blood flow to the lower extremities. Secondary to the effects of hypertension and diabetes

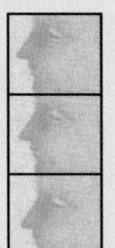

CROSS-CULTURAL CARE
CARING FOR AN AMISH CLIENT

Mr. Yoder is an elderly gentleman of Amish descent. He still follows the Old Order Amish beliefs and practices of his parents. Mr. Yoder turned over the management of the farm to his sons 5 years ago. He currently works as a cabinetmaker in his carpenter shop in the family barn. Mr. Yoder, his wife, their three sons, and their families all live close by on the farm. Within Amish communities, strict as well as more moderate practices exist. It is important to clarify individual practices of Amish clients. Leininger (1991) and Brewer & Bonalumi (1995) identified the following beliefs and practices as being common to the Old Order Amish:

- Maintain a culture distinct and separate from non-Amish, whom they refer to as "English."
- Reject materialism and worldliness.
- Value living simply; may choose to avoid technology, such as electricity and cars.
- Avoid vanity; dress in handmade, unadorned clothing.
- Highly value responsibility, generosity, and helping others.
- Often work as farmers, builders, quilters, and homemakers.
- Use traditional health care and alternative health care, such as healers, herbs, and massage.
- Believe that health is a gift from God, but that clean living and a balanced diet help to maintain it.
- May choose not to have health insurance.

The following conversation between Mr. Yoder and his nurse, Jim, demonstrates culture sensitivity to Mr. Yoder.

Jim: Hello, Mr. Yoder. I wanted to check and see how you're feeling since you took that nitroglycerin pill.

Mr. Yoder: My chest pain is completely gone; I'm feeling much better. I wonder if I will be able to go home soon.

Jim: The doctor has scheduled some tests for you tomorrow.

Mr. Yoder: Yes, the doctor said I would have a heart test. Do you know what time?

Jim: The cardiac catheterization is scheduled for 10 AM.

Mr. Yoder: My family wants to be here with me for the test.

Jim: Would you like me to contact your family?

Mr. Yoder: Yes. You'll have to call my English neighbors. We don't have a phone at home, but they will get the message to my family. The doctor said my wife could bring me some herbal tea from home. Would you please remind her?

Jim: I'll be glad to get both messages to your family. Do you need anything else before I go to make the call?

Critical Thinking Questions

- Why is it important for Mr. Yoder's family to be with him tomorrow?
- What important issues should the nurse explore with the family?
- Is the herbal tea necessary for Mr. Yoder?

- Capillary refill in less than 3 seconds
- Absence of pain
- Mental status within normal limits for the client
- Urine output at least 30 mL/h

Accurate evaluation of tissue perfusion also requires close attention to affected body systems. For example, if you suspect a cerebral perfusion deficit, you would expand the data you gather related to the client's neurological system. If renal perfusion is a concern, you would pay extra attention to urine output and fluid balance.

Expected Outcomes for the Client With Decreased Cardiac Output

The goals for *Decreased cardiac output* are to reduce the cardiac workload, to use prescribed medications effectively to restore or maintain cardiac output, and to control salt and water retention. Short-term or intermediate goals are used to measure progress. Expected

outcomes that indicate adequate cardiac output include the following:

- Blood pressure within normal limits for the client
- Absence of abnormal heart sounds
- Lungs clear to auscultation
- Absence of peripheral or dependent edema
- Mental status within normal limits for the client
- Urine output at least 30 mL/h
- Absence of fatigue and weakness

Expected Outcomes for the Client With Risk for Peripheral Neurovascular Dysfunction

Risk for peripheral neurovascular dysfunction is a narrowly focused diagnosis that addresses impaired circulation to an extremity. Interrupted blood flow or pressure that compresses vessels damages nerves. Immediate intervention is essential to achieve the goal of preserving neurovascular function. Expected outcomes that indicate adequate neurovascular function include the following:

- Palpable peripheral pulses
- Skin warm and pink
- Capillary refill in less than 3 seconds
- Absence of pallor, pain, paresthesia, or paralysis of the extremity.

INTERVENTION

Nurses intervene to maximize cardiovascular function and tissue perfusion. Nurses intervene both in prevention and supporting the client during medical treatment.

Interventions to Maximize Tissue Perfusion

A functional circulatory system depends on patent blood vessels. Nursing actions that maintain open blood vessels and dynamic blood flow maximize circulation.

Modifying Risk Factors

Preventing problems of tissue perfusion is a primary nursing goal; therefore, you will spend time teaching clients how to reduce their risk factors for cardiovascular disease. Although genetic tendencies contribute to the development of atherosclerosis, risk factor modification slows the atherosclerotic process and protects the circulatory system. Clients of all ages benefit from preventive teaching about diet, cholesterol control, weight management, exercise, and controlling concurrent health problems that contribute to atherosclerosis.

DIET

A diet low in cholesterol and saturated fat benefits clients by decreasing the amount of fats available to form atherosclerotic deposits. The Teaching for Wellness chart gives tips for helping clients decrease their dietary fat intake.

Another benefit of a low-cholesterol diet is better maintenance of optimum body weight. Fats provide 9 calories per gram, whereas carbohydrates and proteins provide only 4 calories per gram. Thus, diets high in fat are also high in calories. Excess fat intake is stored as adipose tissue. Box 40–2 summarizes the estimated cost-benefits of a low-fat diet.

EXERCISE

Exercise enhances circulatory health in several ways. It helps control weight by increasing caloric expenditure. It also increases the proportion of high-density lipoproteins in the blood; these lipoproteins protect blood vessels. Finally, it stimulates the development of collateral circulation and new blood vessels that supplement tissue perfusion. The Teaching for Wellness chart describes exercise guidelines for cardiovascular fitness.

CONCURRENT HEALTH PROBLEMS

Underlying health problems, such as hypertension and diabetes mellitus, accelerate atherosclerosis. Teach clients about the relationships between these conditions and circulation, and encourage them to comply

Teaching for WELLNESS

DECREASING DIETARY FAT INTAKE

Changing ingrained food habits is difficult for most clients. To foster success, identify food preferences, patterns of eating, and commonly used food preparation methods. Stress the value of making small changes in the diet initially; then build on the client's success. Help the client, or the person who prepares the food, to adapt favorite recipes.

Purpose: To educate clients about dietary sources of cholesterol and saturated fat.

Rationale: A lower fat intake helps decrease the risk of atherosclerosis.

Expected Outcome: The client will be able to select low-fat food options.

Client Instructions

Certain foods are high in fat and cholesterol; these substances contribute to the formation of fatty deposits inside blood vessels that can eventually lead to heart and circulatory problems.

Tips to Lower Fat Intake
- Avoid visible fats, such as butter and oils, especially coconut oil.
- Use vegetable oil sprays rather than bottled oil when cooking.
- Limit red meats and processed food such as hot dogs and luncheon meats.
- Use skim or 2% milk rather than whole milk.
- Substitute egg whites for whole eggs if possible when baking.
- Limit dairy products made with whole milk or cream, such as cheese and ice cream.
- Remove the skin from poultry before cooking it.
- Eat desserts, such as cakes, pies, and candy, sparingly.

BOX 40–2

ESTIMATED COST BENEFIT OF LOW-FAT DIETS

A review of data from the National Health Interview Survey found that 44 million people in the United States, with no symptoms of cardiovascular disease, had elevated serum cholesterol levels. An estimated 3 million of these people are projected to develop heart disease within the next 10 years. Research has demonstrated that decreasing saturated fat intake by 1% ultimately lowers serum cholesterol by three points. The researchers projected that approximately $13 billion in health care costs could be saved in the next 10 years if high-risk individuals would decrease dietary intake of fat by 1% (Oster & Thompson, 1996).

with treatment regimens. Careful management and consistent follow-up care keep these problems under better control and may delay the development of circulatory complications.

Preventing Vasoconstriction

Even moderate degrees of vasoconstriction can compromise circulation for clients with already narrowed blood vessels. Improper positioning, cold temperatures, nicotine, and emotional stress are common causes of vasoconstriction.

POSITIONING

Compression of blood vessels slows and can even obstruct circulation. To help prevent the effects of vessel compression, change your client's position frequently, and limit prolonged sitting. Instruct affected clients not to cross their legs for long periods while in bed. Do not place pillows behind a client's knees, and do not use the knee gatch on his bed.

Position facilitates circulation. However, optimal positioning depends on the nature of the client's health problem. For a client with arterial insufficiency, place the legs in a dependent position in order to enhance arterial blood flow. Elevate the legs of a client with venous insufficiency because this position uses gravity to improve venous return. Because veins have little elastic tissue, they are very distensible. Elastic stockings provide external support for veins and minimize venous pooling. Active range of motion and ambulation also assist venous return. Muscular contractions of the legs during activity compress veins and drive blood back to the heart.

COLD TEMPERATURES

Peripheral vasoconstriction is a normal physiological response to conserve body heat. However, some underlying circulatory dysfunctions produce more pronounced and prolonged vasoconstriction. For example, Raynaud's disease causes severe arterial spasms when the limbs are exposed to cold temperatures. Teach affected clients to dress warmly, wear mittens, and layer clothing to minimize vasoconstrictive episodes.

NICOTINE

Nicotine also causes vasoconstriction. Teach a client with circulatory problems about the effects of nicotine on blood vessels and urge him to stop smoking. Health care providers have tried a variety of smoking cessation strategies. Cromwell, Bartosch, Fiore, Hasselblad, and Baker (1997) found that intense counseling combined with the use of a nicotine patch yielded the best results. The second best cessation strategy was intensive counseling combined with nicotine gum. The researchers estimated that an average of $10,000 in medical costs could be saved for each smoker who successfully quits.

To maximize a client's success with smoking cessation, inform him of the range of available options. Help him select the support option that will be most effective for him and refer him to support groups. Both the American Heart Association and the American Cancer Society sponsor community programs.

Teaching for WELLNESS

GUIDELINES FOR EXERCISE

Purpose: To help the client recognize the cardiovascular benefits of regular exercise.

Rationale: Aerobic exercise stimulates circulation, helps the formation of collateral blood vessels, and increases high-density lipoproteins.

Expected Outcome: The client will develop and implement an exercise plan.

Client Instructions

- Exercise promotes circulatory health. To be beneficial, it should be done regularly and energetically.
- Check with your physician before beginning any exercise program.
- Ask your physician to establish your target heart rate.
- Select activities that produce rhythmic contractions of large muscles; walking, biking, swimming, and rowing are examples of good choices.
- Participate in exercise three to five times a week.
- Engage in exercise for at least 20 to 30 minutes per session.
- Check your pulse to see that you maintain your target heart rate for 20 minutes.

EMOTIONAL STRESS

Emotional stress activates the fight-or-flight response, in which vasoconstriction diverts blood to essential body systems. Teach your client how to reduce stress through deep breathing, progressive relaxation, and imagery.

Be sure to provide all clients with the information they need to maintain their cardiovascular health, including the instructions listed in the Teaching for Self-Care chart.

Administering Medications

For high-risk clients, anticoagulant therapy may prevent occlusion of arteries. You will monitor the client and provide education about medications. Antiplatelet aggregates, anticoagulants, and vasodilators are medications that improve circulation or prevent complications in clients at risk. Antiplatelet aggregates, such as acetylsalicylic acid (aspirin) and ticlopidine (Ticlid), reduce the stickiness or adhesiveness of platelets. Clot formation decreases when platelets are less adhesive.

Anticoagulants act directly to increase coagulation time by interrupting a step in the clotting cascade. Examples of anticoagulant medications are warfarin (Coumadin) and heparin. A client who takes an anticoagulant is at risk for bleeding. Observe his gums, skin, urine, and stool carefully for signs of visible bleeding. Using chemical reagents such as Hemoccult and Hemastix, body secretions or excretions can be tested for hidden (occult) blood. Institute safety precautions for all clients who receive anticoagulants. Encourage use of a soft-bristle tooth brush and electric razor to prevent injuries and bleeding. Monitor serum prothrombin time or partial thromboplastin time, as appropriate. Report current coagulation results to the physician before administering an anticoagulant.

Action Alert!
Frequently assess clients on anticoagulation therapy for signs of bleeding.

Additionally, some clients with impaired circulation receive vasodilating medications. These medications enlarge the lumina of blood vessels to deliver a greater volume of blood to the tissues. These medications produce vasodilation by various pharmacological actions. Table 40–3 reviews vasodilating medications and nursing responsibilities.

Preventing Surgical Complications

All postoperative clients are at risk for developing deep vein thrombosis, which is a blood clot in the deep veins of the legs. Positioning during a surgical procedure and decreased activity afterward slow circulation. Stagnation of blood in the lower extremities favors clot formation. Frequent changes of position and early ambulation help to prevent deep vein thrombosis.

A client with severe circulatory diseases unresponsive to medications and other treatments may require surgery to restore circulation and improve tissue perfusion. These procedures include the removal of obstructions and bypassing of diseased vessels.

Interventions to Improve Cardiac Output

Cardiac output changes based on tissue needs for oxygen. Therefore, a primary nursing goal for clients with *Decreased cardiac output* is to lessen the need for oxygen at the tissue level. Interventions that decrease oxygen demand ease the heart's workload.

Promoting Rest

Rest is an excellent strategy for conserving a client's energy and decreasing oxygen demand. Remember that physical and emotional rest are needed because both types of activity boost oxygen demand. Even normal activities, such as turning in bed and coughing, affect cardiac output and oxygen demand for clients with limited cardiac reserves. In one study, oxygen consumption increased 20 to 30% when critically ill clients were turned to the side. Clients who turned without assistance used even more oxygen (Jesurum, 1997).

Schedule frequent, uninterrupted rest periods for these clients. Help them with activities of daily living. Space activities such as eating, bathing, and ambulating so clients have rest periods in between. Monitor pulse, blood pressure, respirations, and skin color before and after activities to evaluate each client's activity tolerance. Place necessary items, such as water and the call light, within easy reach in order to conserve the client's energy.

Action Alert!
Assess vital signs before, during, and after activity. Terminate any activity that provokes hypotension, tachycardia, dyspnea, or chest pain.

A quiet environment promotes rest. Conversely, loud noises, frequent interruptions, and numerous visitors can exhaust clients. Do your best to limit external stimuli to promote a restful environment for a client with impaired cardiovascular function. Involve

---

Teaching for SELF-CARE

MAINTAINING CARDIOVASCULAR HEALTH

- Exercise regularly.
- Keep weight within normal limits.
- Eat a balanced diet; avoid fatty foods.
- Have your blood pressure, blood sugar, and cholesterol levels checked by your physician.
- Do not smoke.
- Take time to relax.

TABLE 40–3
Vasodilating Medications

Medication	Action	Side Effects	Nursing Responsibilities
Nitrates • Nitroglycerin (Nitro-Bid, Transderm-Nitro). • Isosorbide dinitrate (Isordil).	Relax vascular smooth muscles and decrease venous return and preload.	• Headache. • Flushing. • Hypotension.	• Monitor client's blood pressure, especially with position changes. • Report dizziness, headaches. • Instruct the client to avoid alcohol.
Calcium Channel Blockers • Verapamil (Calan). • Nifedipine (Procardia). • Amlodipine besylate (Norvasc). • Diltiazem (Cardizem).	Slow movement of calcium into vascular smooth muscle cells.	• Hypotension. • Dizziness. • Constipation. • Peripheral edema.	• Monitor vital signs. • Encourage intake of fluids and fiber. • Assess client for edema. • Instruct client that medication interacts with digoxin and some gastrointestinal medications. • Advise client to notify all physicians about all current medications.
Beta-Adrenergic Blockers • Propranolol (Inderal). • Metoprolol (Lopressor, Toprol XL). • Atenolol (Tenormin). • Labetalol (Normodyne).	Compete for norepinephrine binding sites, thus blocking sympathetic nervous system stimulation.	• Fatigue. • Hypotension. • Bradycardia. • Insomnia. • Depression.	• Monitor client's blood pressure and pulse. • Report other health problems, such as heart failure or asthma, to physician before giving a beta-adrenergic blocker. • Instruct client to consult with physician before exercising.

the client when identifying interventions that contribute to a restful environment. For example, some clients prefer a darkened room for a nap, and others find music relaxing.

Positioning to Improve Cardiac Output

Dilation of the heart with congested blood stretches myocardial fibers beyond the limits of optimum elastic recoil, which further diminishes cardiac contractility. Positioning eases cardiac workload and helps prevent complications. Placing the client in a semi- to high-Fowler's position decreases venous return and preload by pooling blood in the lower extremities. Lowering preload decreases the risk of heart congestion and the development of heart failure. Elevating the head of the bed also optimizes chest expansion and oxygen intake, which in turn reduce dyspnea and shortness of breath associated with heart failure.

Avoiding Valsalva's Maneuver

Teach cardiac clients to avoid Valsalva's maneuver. Instruct them not to hold their breath while moving or turning in bed. Assist clients with position changes by lowering the head of the bed before turning and by helping with the turn.

Bearing down during bowel movements also induces Valsalva's maneuver, especially if the client is constipated. Assess the frequency and consistency of each client's bowel movements. Encourage fluid intake to keep stools soft. Offer foods that increase gastrointestinal motility, such as fruits and fruit juices. Gather input from clients about successful strategies used at home to relieve constipation. Administer stool softeners as ordered.

Avoiding Stimulants

Teach clients to avoid stimulants because these substances increase heart rate and oxygen demand. Some over-the-counter medications, such as appetite suppressants and cold medications, contain stimulants. Advise clients to check with their physician before using these types of medications. Instruct clients to avoid dietary stimulants as well, such as coffee, tea, and chocolate. Offer appropriate dietary substitutes such as decaffeinated beverages and fruits.

Maintaining Fluid Balance

A normal fluid balance prevents circulatory overload, which a weakened heart may be unable to accommodate. Assess your client's fluid status routinely by monitoring intake, output, and daily weights. Assess the client's breath sounds, jugular vein distention, and dependent areas (such as the ankles) for pitting edema. Prompt detection and treatment of fluid overload prevents the life-threatening complication of pulmonary edema.

Action Alert!
Monitor for a sudden onset of dyspnea, feelings of suffocation, cyanosis, gurgling respirations, and frothy sputum. Elevate the head of the bed and notify the physician immediately. Report dyspnea, shortness of breath, and lung crackles immediately.

Fluid and sodium restriction are used to correct fluid overload, along with a low-sodium diet. See Box 40–3 for foods high in sodium. Some clients need more aggressive treatment to maintain their fluid balance. Diuretics, such as furosemide (Lasix), increase urine output and remove excess fluid from the body. Weighing the client daily evaluates the effectiveness of diuretic medication. Diuretic therapy can cause electrolyte imbalances, especially involving potassium. Monitor the client's electrolyte levels and report abnormal laboratory data to the physician.

Administering Medications

Medications are a cornerstone in the treatment of cardiovascular problems. They are used to enhance cardiac output as well as to manage complications associated with *Decreased cardiac output*.

INOTROPIC MEDICATIONS
Inotropic agents are medications that increase the contractility of the heart muscle, thereby increasing cardiac output. Digoxin (Lanoxin) is a commonly used inotropic medication. Assess the client's apical heart rate and rhythm for a full minute before administering this drug. Report pulse rates below 60 or above 110 beats per minute to the physician before giving it. The medication dose may need to be adjusted. Also, check the client's serum potassium level; low potassium levels predispose the client to digitalis toxicity. Review the client's serum digitalis level, if ordered, and report a level outside of the normal therapeutic range to the physician.

BOX 40–3

FOODS HIGH IN SODIUM: THE SIX S's

The following types of foods are high in sodium:

- Soups.
- Sauces.
- Salty snacks.
- Smoked meat or fish.
- Sauerkraut and other pickled food.
- Seasonings.

Dudek, S. G. (1997). Nutrition handbook for nursing practice (3rd ed.). Philadelphia: J. B. Lippincott Co.

ANTIDYSRHYTHMIC MEDICATIONS
Hypoxic myocardial muscle is prone to develop a **dysrhythmia,** which is an abnormality of heart rate or rhythm. Dysrhythmias pose a serious threat because they further impair cardiac output.

Assess the apical pulse for regularity. If you detect a dysrhythmia, note the frequency of the irregularity and the client's blood pressure, apical-radial pulse, and skin color. Report hypotension, apical-radial pulse deficit, and pale, moist skin to the physician. Antidysrhythmic medications and other treatments may be needed to correct rhythm disturbances.

ANTIHYPERTENSIVE MEDICATIONS
Medications that lower blood pressure, such as nitrates (nitroglycerin), captopril (Capoten), and nifedipine (Procardia), ease the workload of the heart and improve cardiac output. Dilation of vessels allows for greater blood flow, and a lower blood pressure decreases afterload, thus enabling the heart to eject blood with less effort.

Carefully monitor the blood pressure of any client receiving an antihypertensive medication. Evaluate his response to the medication by checking for orthostatic hypotension—decreases in blood pressure when the client changes from lying to sitting to standing positions. If dizziness or lightheadedness occur, take safety precautions to prevent falls. Instruct the client to call for help before getting out of bed. Teach him to change positions slowly and to sit on the side of the bed for a few minutes before standing.

Increasing Oxygen Supply

Clients with impaired cardiac output deliver less oxygen-rich blood to tissues. Some pathophysiological causes of decreases in cardiac output are irreversible and others take time to correct. In either instance, interventions may involve strategies to enhance available oxygen. Increasing the oxygen supply helps the client perfuse tissues more easily.

ADMINISTERING OXYGEN
Clients with *Decreased cardiac output* require a careful balance between oxygen demand and supply. Administration of oxygen by nasal cannula increases the supply side of the supply-and-demand equation. Supplemental oxygen increases the oxygen available for use by the circulatory system. Nursing responsibilities for clients receiving oxygen therapy are addressed in Chapter 39.

AVOIDING SMOKING
Smoking is contraindicated in all situations where circulation is less than optimal because nicotine causes vasoconstriction. The reduced diameter of blood vessels during vasoconstriction lessens the amount of oxygenated blood that can be delivered to body tissues. Teach clients the physiological effects of nicotine and the relationship between smoking and cardiovas-

cular disease. Provide emotional support to clients who are trying to quit smoking.

POSITIONING TO FACILITATE BREATHING

Positioning optimizes chest expansion and enhances respiratory effectiveness. Elevating the head of the bed facilitates respirations by shifting the abdominal organs downward in the abdominal cavity and providing maximum space for chest expansion. This position enables the client to breathe deeply and more effectively.

Interventions to Prevent Peripheral Neurovascular Dysfunction

Neurovascular dysfunction is a complication that is largely preventable. You can foster prevention by identifying clients at risk and detecting signs and symptoms as early as possible.

Careful assessment is the cornerstone to preventing neurovascular dysfunction. Follow hospital protocol for the frequency of neurovascular assessment after designated procedures, such as cast application or angiography. Use professional judgment to institute more frequent assessments if the client's condition warrants them.

Assess the involved extremity for color, temperature, pulses, numbness, tingling, and pain. Objective findings—such as pale, cold skin and decreased or absent pulses—require immediate intervention. Numbness, tingling, and pain are subjective symptoms of impaired circulation and nerve irritation. Instruct the client to report any of these sensations promptly.

If the client's condition permits, elevate the extremity to decrease edema, which exerts pressure on nerves and blood vessels. Encourage the client to move the fingers and toes of the involved extremity to enhance venous return and reduce edema. Notify the physician promptly whenever you detect abnormal neurovascular findings. The client may need medical interventions, such as cutting a cast or evacuating accumulated blood from a body compartment.

> A*ction* A*lert!*
> Immediately report absence of pulse, pallor, pain, paresthesia, and paralysis.

Interventions to Manage Shock

Shock is a complication of serious circulatory dysfunction. It has a number of distinctive clinical manifestations (Table 40–4). For a client at risk for shock, assess vital signs as often as every 15 minutes. Check for tachycardia and hypotension. Monitor changes in skin color, mental status, and urine output. Detection of shock in the early stage improves the client's prognosis.

Clients who develop shock have complex physiological needs; most clients are transferred to an intensive care unit, where a physician directs their care. The

TABLE 40–4
Manifestations of Shock

Parameter	Alterations in Shock
Pulse	Rapid, weak, and thready
Respirations	Rapid and shallow
Blood pressure	Systolic blood pressure below 90 mm Hg
Level of consciousness	Restlessness progressing to lethargy
Skin	Pale, cool, and clammy
Urine output	Less than 20 mL/hour
Thirst	Increased

nurse works closely with the physician to implement the plan of care and respond promptly to changes in the client's status.

Maintaining Oxygenation

Oxygenation of tissues is essential for survival of clients in shock. A patent airway and supplemental oxygen help correct oxygen deficits at the tissue level. Clients who can breathe on their own receive oxygen via a nasal cannula or mask. Clients who cannot breathe spontaneously require placement of an endotracheal tube and mechanical ventilation.

Positioning for Shock

Positioning the client in shock depends in part on what caused the shock. For example, in hypovolemic shock, you will elevate the client's feet about 15 to 20 inches above the level of the heart. This position uses gravity to increase venous return, thus helping to maintain stroke volume. In cardiogenic shock, the client cannot expel blood effectively from the heart. Thus, your priority is to decrease venous return to minimize heart congestion. You will place the client in a semi- to high-Fowler's position. The physician will give specific orders regarding position for clients in shock.

Maintaining Circulating Blood Volume

Fluid replacement during shock also depends on the underlying cause of the problem. Blood, packed red blood cells, volume expanders, and intravenous solutions are used to restore circulating blood volume for the client in hypovolemic shock. Procedure 40–1 outlines the steps needed to administer blood safely and accurately. Monitor your client closely for transfusion reactions during blood transfusions.

> A*ction* A*lert!*
> Monitor the client for chills, rash, dyspnea, chest pain, itching, or changes in vital signs during a transfusion. Stop the transfusion immediately if any signs of a reaction occur. Maintain the client's intravenous line, and stay with the client. Notify the physician immediately.

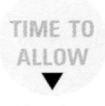

Administering Blood

TIME TO
ALLOW
▼

Novice:
20 min.
Expert:
15 min.

Blood and blood products are administered to increase the circulating blood volume following blood loss from surgery, trauma, or other causes of hemorrhage. Packed red blood cells are administered in severe anemia. Fresh frozen plasma is administered to provide clotting factors to help control bleeding in clients with hemophilia. You must be absolutely certain to follow hospital policy to ensure that the blood has been properly typed and crossmatched for the specific client. Additionally, you must be fully knowledgeable about transfusion reactions and the management of these reactions.

Delegation Guidelines

Some aspects of monitoring a client during a blood transfusion may be delegated to a nursing assistant. The nursing assistant may measure and record vital signs. However, you must provide specific parameters for immediate RN notification. The responsibility for ongoing monitoring and assessment, throughout the transfusion, is yours.

Equipment Needed

- Y-type IV tubing with blood filter
- 250- to 500-mL bag 0.9% normal saline
- IV site with 18-gauge catheter
- Signed consent form (if required by agency)
- Arm band on client for identification
- Type and crossmatch identification on client arm band
- Properly labeled and identified blood or blood products
- Clean gloves

---

1 Check the physician's order to verify the type of blood product and number of units to be administered.

A physician's order is legally required for the administration of blood products.

2 Verify that the blood is crossmatched and ready in the blood bank.

Blood must be administered within 20 minutes after leaving the blood bank because it provides an excellent medium for bacterial growth. If blood stays at room temperature for a prolonged period, it raises the client's risk of infection.

3 Ask the client about allergies and any previous reactions to blood transfusion.

This step identifies clients at risk for possible transfusion reactions.

4 Follow your institution's procedures for consent forms.

Most institutions require informed consent before blood can be administered.

5 Assess and document the client's blood pressure, pulse, respiration, and temperature on the transfusion record.

Baseline vital signs are required before transfusion. Deviations in vital signs during the transfusion indicate an adverse reaction to the blood.

---

6 Assemble the necessary equipment.

7 Obtain the blood from the blood bank.

8 Together with another registered nurse, compare the blood and crossmatch slip from the blood bank. Also compare the data with the client's identification band. Verify and document that the following data match:
Client's name
Client's identification number
Blood type
Donor number on blood container
Expiration date of blood

The correct blood product must be administered to the correct client to prevent a transfusion reaction.

9 Don gloves.

Standard precautions mandate gloves in situations in which you could be exposed to blood or body fluids.

10 Prime the Y tubing by following these steps:
Close all clamps on the Y tubing.
Insert one spike of the Y tubing into the bag of normal saline solution.
Open the clamp, and prime the arm of the Y tubing, drip chamber, and tubing below the chamber.

Clamp the tubing.

Gently rotate the unit of blood.

Insert the second spike of the Y tubing into the port on the unit of blood.

Open the clamp, and prime the arm of the Y tubing to the drip chamber.

Close the clamp.

---

11 If the client does not have an IV line in place, perform a venipuncture with an 18- or 19-gauge catheter.

IV catheters smaller than 18- or 19-gauge will damage blood cells and slow the transfusion rate.

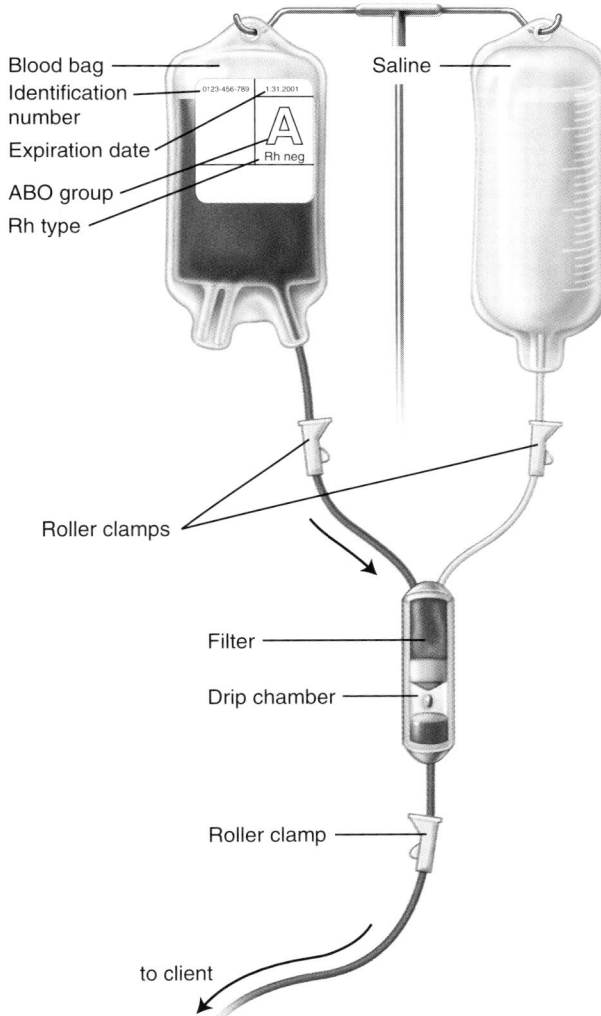

Blood bag

Identification number

Expiration date

ABO group

Rh type

0123-456-789 1-31-2001

A

Rh neg

Saline

Roller clamps

Filter

Drip chamber

Roller clamp

to client

Setup for blood administration.

---

12 Open the clamp on the normal saline and infuse about 50 mL of saline at a slow rate.

This step verifies patency of the IV line before starting the transfusion.

---

13 Close the clamp on the normal saline solution.

---

14 Open the clamp on the blood, and infuse at a keep-open rate for 15 minutes. Stay with the client throughout this time.

Most transfusion reactions occur within the first 15 minutes of the infusion.

---

15 Monitor the client's vital signs, and watch for signs of a transfusion reaction according to your institution's protocol.

Signs of a transfusion reaction include chills, flushing, headache, rash, chest or back pain, nausea, fever, tachycardia, respiratory distress, and hypotension.

---

16 If the client has no adverse reactions after 15 minutes, infuse the blood at the prescribed rate.

---

17 Continue to monitor the client's vital signs and responses according to your institution's protocol.

Most institutions require assessment of vital signs every 15 minutes for the first hour and every 30 minutes thereafter until the transfusion is complete. Ongoing assessment is needed to detect a delayed transfusion reaction.

---

18 When the transfusion is complete, flush the IV line with normal saline solution.

---

19 Complete the transfusion record and return the designated portion of the form to the blood bank with the empty blood bag.

This step verifies the client's identity and the blood product that was transfused.

---

20 Place the designated portion of the transfusion record in the client's chart.

---

21 Document the following aspects of the transfusion procedure in the client's chart:

Date

Time transfusion started

Type and identification number of blood product

Time transfusion ended

Client's response to transfusion

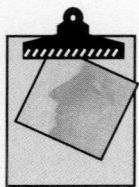

NURSING CARE PLANNING
A CLIENT WITH ANGINA PECTORIS

Admission Data

Mr. Yoder is admitted with chest pain. On arrival in the nursing unit, he reports dull chest pain radiating to the left arm. He rates his pain as 7 on a scale of 0 to 10. The admitting diagnosis is unstable angina pectoris.

Physician's Orders

Bedrest with bathroom privileges
Oxygen 3 L/min per nasal cannula
Stat ECG
Insert saline lock
Nitroglycerin gr 1/150 sublingual as needed for chest pain up to 3 doses
Morphine 10 mg IV for chest pain unrelieved by nitroglycerin

Vital signs q 2 hours
Cardiac monitor
Soft diet
Draw complete blood count, coagulation studies, and lipid profile in AM
Schedule for cardiac catheterization in AM

Nursing Assessment

Mr. Yoder is lying quietly in bed and appears anxious. His wife is at the bedside. Initial vital signs are blood pressure 150/92 left arm lying; apical pulse regular at 92 beats per minute; respirations regular at 24 per minute. Skin is pale.

NURSING CARE PLAN

Nursing Diagnosis	Expected Outcomes	Interventions	Evaluation
Altered cardiopulmonary tissue perfusion related to imbalance in oxygen supply and demand.	• Absence of chest pain. • Vital signs within normal limit for client.	• Assess for presence, absence, or change in chest pain. • Administer nitroglycerin sublingual as needed. • Give morphine for chest pain unrelieved by nitroglycerin. • Administer oxygen 3 L/min. • Semi-Fowler's position. • Bedrest with bathroom privileges.	• Chest pain on admission relieved by nitroglycerin sublingual times 1. • No subsequent episodes of chest pain.
Anxiety related to acute change in health status and unknown prognosis.	• Client verbalizes decreased anxiety. • Client resting quietly in bed.	• Quiet environment. • *Assess prior coping strategies.* • *Identify support systems.*	• Client reports decreased anxiety; resting quietly. • Client says deep breathing and reading a book are relaxing to him. • Client states wife is his primary support.
Knowledge deficit related to no previous experience with cardiac catheterization.	• Client is able to state purpose and general procedure to expect during cardiac catheterization.	• Instruct client about cardiac catheterization procedure.	• Client is able to describe basic cardiac catheterization procedure and state purpose of test is to evaluate his coronary arteries.

Italicized interventions indicate culturally specific care.

Critical Thinking Questions

1. How would you help Mrs. Yoder with her anxiety while Mr. Yoder is having his cardiac catheterization?
2. Mr. Yoder will probably need an angioplasty to treat his angina. Mrs. Yoder believes that he will not be able to work again, even though the physician has not said this. How would you help Mrs. Yoder?
3. The nurse from the cardiac catheterization laboratory tells you to get ready because Mr. Yoder is returning to his room. How frequently do you think you should take his vital signs?

A client in cardiogenic shock requires very cautious fluid replacement. He will receive care in the intensive care unit, where advanced hemodynamic monitoring devices are used to evaluate his tolerance for fluid replacement and to monitor for fluid overload.

Preventing Complications

For a client in shock, it is important to continuously monitor circulatory status and tissue perfusion. You must be able to quickly recognize progression of shock and deteriorating organ function. Promptly report all changes in the client's vital signs, skin color, mental status, respiratory function, and urine output.

EVALUATION

On the third day after admission, Mr. Yoder gets the news that his cardiac catheterization shows moderate atherosclerosis of the coronary arteries. His serum cholesterol and lipid profile are elevated. Mr. Yoder is to be discharged. He is to start taking an antianginal medication and restrict his activity until he sees his physician for follow-up care in 1 week. In addition, Mr. Yoder is to begin a low-cholesterol diet.

Evaluation and documentation of a client's status involves comparing current data with the outcome criteria previously established. A sample of nursing documentation at the time of discharge for Mr. Yoder might include the following:

Denies chest pain at rest. Skin warm and dry. All peripheral pulses strong and equal bilaterally. Vital signs at rest BP 132/82, P 78 and regular, R 18. Ambulated 75 feet in hall. Vital signs after ambulation BP 138/88, P 82 and regular, R 20 and unlabored. Denies chest pain with activity. Verbalizes medication regimen, "I will take the Procardia in the morning and at night. If I have chest pain, I will rest and put a nitroglycerin tablet under my tongue. I can take up to three nitroglycerin pills at 5-minute intervals. Then, if I still have chest pain, I need to go to the emergency room." The client and his wife demonstrate comprehension of the low-cholesterol diet by selecting low-fat foods from sample menus. Client states that he will restrict activity to walking to the barn and back for next week. Clinic appointment scheduled for next week; son will transport.

These data identify that Mr. Yoder is no longer experiencing the chest pain that initially brought him to the hospital. His current level of activity tolerance is documented as well as his post-discharge activity restriction. Safety precautions for home management of chest pain and medication regimen are documented. The dietary risk factor modification plan is identified. Because the client's wife is the primary cook, Mrs. Yoder was included in dietary teaching. Peripheral circulation is specifically addressed because Mr. Yoder had a cardiac catheterization 1 day before discharge. The Nursing Care Planning chart outlines common client needs and nursing actions.

KEY PRINCIPLES

- Circulation is essential for life and optimal function of all body systems.
- Age, genetic predisposition, underlying health problems, and medications can affect circulation.
- Risk-factor modification enhances circulatory health and delays the development of cardiovascular complications.
- Changes in the effectiveness of the heart as a pump, the integrity of blood vessels, or the dynamics of blood flow produce both acute, life-threatening and chronic, long-term manifestations.
- The heart, brain, and kidneys are especially vulnerable to decreased blood supply.
- *Decreased cardiac output* occurs when the heart pumps ineffectively; this threatens blood delivery to body tissues.
- *Altered tissue perfusion* results when blood vessels are narrowed by atherosclerosis, vasoconstriction, or obstruction.
- *Risk for neurovascular dysfunction* exists when the nerves are deprived of oxygen.
- Vital signs, peripheral pulses, skin color, level of consciousness, and urine output provide clues about cardiovascular function.
- Early detection and prompt intervention to restore circulation improve client outcomes.
- The health care team works collaboratively to provide acute and long-term care for clients with cardiovascular dysfunction.

BIBLIOGRAPHY

Ackley, B.J., & Ladwig, G. (1997). *Nursing diagnosis handbook: A guide to planning care* (3rd ed.). St. Louis: Mosby.

Adam, J.K.(1996). Coronary risk factor modification in women after coronary artery bypass surgery. *Nursing Research, 45*(5), 260–265.

Allen, C.V. (1997). *Nursing process in collaborative practice* (2nd ed.). Stamford, CN: Appleton & Lange.

Anderson, A., & Rosen, P.B. (1996a). Toxic emergencies. *Emergency, 97*(4), 42–46.

Anderson, A., & Rosen, P.B. (1996b). *Cardiovascular statistics.* Dallas: American Heart Association.

Ashton, K.C. (1997). Preceived learning needs of men and women after myocardial infarction. *Journal of Cardiovascular Nursing, 12*(1), 95–100.

*Bao, W., Srinivasan, S.R., Valdex, R., Greenlund, K.J., Wattigney, W.A., & Berenson, G.S. (1997). Longitudinal changes in cardiovascular risk from childhood to young adulthood in offspring of parents with coronary artery disease. *Journal of the American Medical Association, 278*(21), 1749–1754.

Bhambhani, Y.N. (1995). Prediction of stroke volume during upper and lower body exercise in men and women. *Archives of Physical Medicine & Rehabilitation, 76*(8), 713–718.

Bosely, C. (1995). Assessing cardiac output. *Nursing 95, 25*(9), 43–5.

Brewer, J.A., & Bonalumi, N.M. (1995). Cultural diversity in the

*Asterisk indicates a classic or definitive work on this subject.

emergency department: Health care beliefs and practices among Pennsylvania Amish. *Emergency Nursing, 21*(6), 494–497.

Carson, M.A. (1996). The impact of a relaxation technique on the lipid profile. *Nursing Research, 45*(5), 271–276.

*Cromwell, J., Bartosch, W.J., Fiore, M.C., Hasselblad, V., & Baker, T. (1997). Cost-effectiveness of the clinical practice recommendations in AHCPR guideline for smoking. *Journal of the American Medical Association, 278*(21), 1759–1776.

Doenges, M.E., Moorhouse, M.F., & Geissler, A.C. (1997). *Nursing care plans* (4th ed.). Philadelphia: F.A. Davis.

Dudek, S.G. (1997). *Nutrition handbook for nursing practice* (3rd ed.). Philadelphia: J.B. Lippincott.

Dunbar, S.B., & Farr, L. (1996). Temporal patterns of heart rate and blood pressure in elders. *Nursing Research, 45*(1), 43–49.

Fischbach, F. (1996). *A manual of laboratory and diagnostic tests* (5th ed.). Philadelphia: J.B. Lippincott.

Fleury, J., Thomas, T., & Ratledge, K. (1997). Promoting wellness in individuals with coronary heart disease. *Journal of Cardiovascular Nursing, 11*(3), 26–39.

Frati, A.C., Iniestra, F., & Ariza, C.R. (1996). Acute effects of cigarette smoking on glucose tolerance and other cardiovascular risk factors. *Diabetes Care, 19*(2), 112–117.

Guyton, A.C., & Hall, J.E. (1996). *Textbook of medical physiology* (9th ed.). Philadelphia: W.B. Saunders Co.

Hinojosa, R., & Steelman, V. (1995). Intraoperative music therapy: Effect on anxiety and blood pressure. *Plastic Surgical Nursing, 15*(4), 228–231.

Jackson, L.D. (1997). Different presentations of cocaine intoxication: Four case studies. *Journal of Emergency Nursing, 23*(3), 232–234.

*Jesurum, J. (1997). Tissue oxygenation and routine nursing procedures in critically ill patients. *Journal of Cardiovascular Nursing, 11*(4), 12–27.

*Leininger, M.M. (Ed.). (1991). *Cultural care diversity and universality: A theory of nursing.* New York: National League for Nursing Press.

Marieb, E.N., & Branstrom, M.J. (1995). Nursing assessment and documentation: Hospital not liable for nurses' failure to document vital signs in the chart. *Legal Eagle-Eye: Newsletter for the Nursing Profession, 3*(4), 8.

Marieb, E.N., & Branstrom, M.J. (1996). *A.D.A.M. interactive physiology—cardiovascular system* (Version 1.1). (Computer software). Atlanta: A.D.A.M. Software.

North American Nursing Diagnosis Association. (1998). *NANDA nursing diagnoses: Definitions and classification 1999–2000.* Philadelphia: Author.

Oster, G., & Thompson, D. (1996). Estimated effects of reducing dietary saturated fat intake on the incidence of and costs of coronary heart disease in the United States. *Journal of the American Dietetic Association, 96*(2), 127–131.

Place, B. (1996). Inotrope therapy. *Nursing Times, 92*(35), 55–57.

Ramsey, J.D., & Tisdale, L.A. (1995). Use of ventricular stroke volume work index and ventricular function curves in assessing myocardial contractility. *Critical Care Nurse, 15*(1), 61–67.

Roper, M. (1996). Back to basics: Assessing orthostatic vital signs. *American Journal of Nursing, 96*(8), 43–46.

Sommers, M.S. (1995). Missed injuries. *AACN Clinical Issues, 6*(2), 187–195.

Story, M., Hayes, M., & Kalina, B. (1996). Availability of foods in high schools: Is there cause for concern? *Journal of the American Dietetic Association, 96*(2), 123–126.

Swan, L. (1995). The neurophysiological bases of vital signs: A review with clinical considerations. *Neurology Report, 19*(3), 12–16.

Thomas, D.O. (1996). Assessing children: It's different. *RN, 59*(4), 38–44.

Tonstad, S., & Silvertsen, M. (1997). Dietary adherence in children with familial hypercholesterolemia. *American Journal of Clinical Nutrition, 65*(4), 1018–1026.

Sleep-Rest Pattern

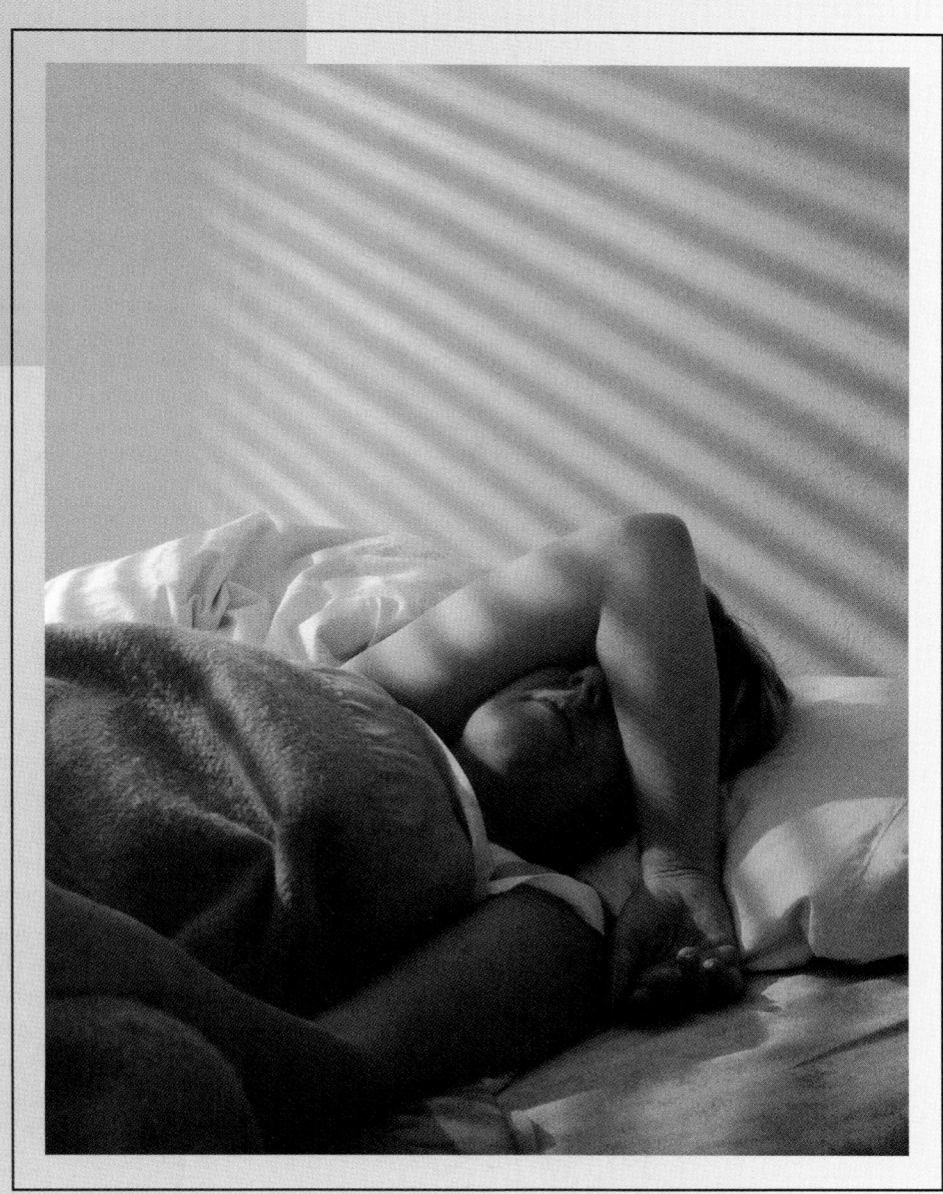

Sleep and Rest

Gwyneth Lymberis

Key Terms

bruxism

circadian rhythm

dyssomnia

hypersomnia

hypnotic

insomnia

multiple sleep latency test

narcolepsy

nightmare

non–rapid eye movement sleep

obstructive sleep apnea

parasomnia

polysomnography

rapid eye movement sleep

rest

restless legs syndrome

sedative

sleep

sleep deprivation

sleep enuresis

sleep terrors

slow-wave sleep

somnambulism

sundowning

LEARNING OBJECTIVES

After studying this chapter, you should be able to:

1. Describe the physiological concepts underlying normal rest and sleep.

2. Distinguish between dyssomnias and parasomnias and give examples of each.

3. Discuss the lifestyle, environmental, developmental, and physiological factors that affect rest and sleep.

4. Describe the general assessment of rest and sleep, including the sleep diary.

5. Assess clients for risk of sleep problems, manifestations of actual sleep problems, and responses to sleep problems.

6. Distinguish between related diagnoses for problems of rest and sleep that are amenable to nursing care.

7. Plan for goal-directed interventions that address sleep pattern disturbances and meet rest needs.

8. Evaluate outcomes of nursing care for clients with sleep pattern disturbances.

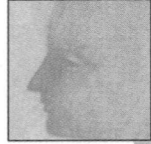

Emma Weiss, a 48-year-old single female, arrives at your health maintenance organization complaining of tension headaches and exhaustion over the past 3 months. She has been calling daily for the past week in an attempt to see the nurse practitioner as soon as possible. Deep circles under her eyes and frequent yawning confirm her statement that she is tired and unable to remember when she last had a good night's sleep. Ms. Weiss feels that her symptoms are closely linked to a recent job promotion, which requires longer work hours. She is also enrolled in a master's degree program at a local university, and she is anxious about her upcoming midterm examinations. Her attempts to alleviate insomnia with a glass of wine at bedtime have not helped. Even her mother's chicken soup eaten as a bedtime snack has not been successful. Ms. Weiss is worried that her fatigue is beginning to affect her job performance and wants to speak with the nurse practitioner about the possibility of a sleeping pill prescription. Because the client has identified sleep as her priority, the nurse considers the diagnosis of *Sleep pattern disturbance*. However, Ms. Weiss displays signs of physical and mental exhaustion, so the nurse also assesses the client for *Fatigue*. The Nursing Diagnoses chart defines these two NANDA nursing diagnoses.

SLEEP AND REST
NURSING DIAGNOSES

Sleep Pattern Disturbance: Disruption of sleep that causes discomfort or interferes with desired lifestyle.

Fatigue: An overwhelming sustained sense of exhaustion and decreased capacity for physical and mental work.

From North American Nursing Diagnosis Association. (1999). NANDA nursing diagnoses: Definitions and classification 1999–2000. Philadelphia: Author.

CONCEPTS OF REST AND SLEEP

Rest and sleep are needed to achieve and maintain optimal health. The robust, young adult usually sleeps through the night and rests more or less, depending on daily energy expenditure. When illness strikes, more metabolic energy is expended. The resultant accelerated metabolic rate often leads to increased rest and sleep needs. Furthermore, illness may disrupt normal, well-established sleep patterns. Measures to restore these patterns may be necessary.

To become an "expert" on sleep and rest in both the hospital and the community, you must understand the concepts of normal rest and sleep and be able to recognize deviations from these norms. This theoretical background, coupled with the nursing process, will help you identify and effectively treat clients who have sleep pattern disturbances and/or fatigue.

Normal Rest

Our waking activity is not usually continuous. Periods of activity normally alternate with periods of rest. A person at **rest** is in a state of being physically and mentally relaxed while being awake and alert. Mental rest, sometimes described as "peace of mind," implies serenity and freedom from worries. To experience such psychic rest, the person must feel secure and anxiety-free. Mental rest does not necessarily imply the absence of mental or physical activity. The homemaker who enjoys working in her garden or the schoolchild who enjoys drawing are both engaging in mentally restful activities, and yet they are physically or mentally active.

Unlike mental rest, physical rest always implies decreased movement; the person is stationary or inactive. In healthy people, heightened physical activity is usually followed by short periods of physical rest. Chronically or acutely ill clients reduce physical activity in response to fatigue, but their rest needs are usually greater than those of healthy people. Other factors that may influence the need for physical rest include medications, conditioning, and age.

When assessing client rest needs, health care professionals often focus solely on physical activity. Physical rest, however, does not necessarily imply mental rest. The depressed client who feels too sad to get out of bed may be mentally drained. As this ex-

ample illustrates, it is important to address both the physical and mental components of rest.

The need for rest is highly individualized. Some people seem to have higher energy levels and require little or no rest between activities. They enjoy "keeping busy." Just as each person's need for rest is unique, individual perceptions of what constitutes a restful activity are also subjective. Whereas one person may find knitting restful, someone else may think it is boring, tedious, or a waste of time.

Normal Sleep

Sleep is a reversible behavioral state in which perceptions of and responses to environmental stimuli are decreased, and the body is relatively quiet (Carskadon & Dement, 1994). It is a regularly occurring event in which a quieted mind and body do not respond to most external stimuli.

This lack of responsiveness to external input differentiates sleep from rest. The person at rest is aware of what is going on in the immediate environment, whereas the sleeper is not. For example, the person relaxing in front of the television will hear a phone ringing in the next room, whereas the sleeper in the deepest stages of sleep will not.

Sleep is one of many biorhythms. *Biorhythms* are rhythmic biological clocks that occur at regular intervals in all living creatures. These rhythms are classified on the basis of the time it takes to complete their cycle. Examples include sleep-wake cycles, serum cortisol levels, and body temperature fluctuations. The **circadian rhythm** is one of the most familiar patterns; it is a biorhythmic pattern that is regularly repeated at 24-hour intervals. The word *circadian* comes from the Latin *circa dies* meaning "about a day." Within this circadian context, sleep can be viewed as part of a cyclic change in level of consciousness embedded in a sleep-wake rhythm. For most people, sleep occurs as a single 7- to 8-hour event once every 24 hours. As we shall see, sleep also has *ultradian rhythms*. These are cycles completed in minutes or hours.

States of sleep and wakefulness are created and maintained by the central nervous system (CNS), which prompts changes in endocrine, cardiovascular, and respiratory function. Although sleep and wakefulness are two distinct states, it is sometimes difficult to differentiate them clinically. A client lying still with his eyes closed may be resting but awake, whereas another client sitting in a chair with a book open on her lap may be asleep. Additionally, clinical differentiation between sleep and coma is sometimes challenging. Given the proper stimulus, a sleeper can usually be awakened. The comatose client, however, can be awakened by neither painful nor noxious stimuli. When attempts to distinguish among coma, sleep, and wakefulness are inconclusive, an electroencephalogram (EEG) may be used. The EEG traces electrophysiological differences between these states. As we shall see, sleep is a highly active neurophysiological process, and brain oxygen consumption does not fall below normal levels. In coma, oxygen consumption is below normal and ultimately affects the brain's electrical activity; the EEG voltage of a person in irreversible coma is minimal or absent (Kelly, 1991).

Sleep can thus be defined by both clinical and laboratory measures. It should be noted, however, that laboratory tests such as the EEG are often unavailable to the practicing clinician.

Action Alert!
A client who does not arouse to painful or noxious stimuli may be in a coma. Take the client's vital signs, and report your findings to the physician immediately.

REM and NREM Sleep

In the 1950s, researchers first identified two ultradian forms of sleep: rapid eye movement (REM) sleep, with its characteristic rapidly rolling eye movements, and non–rapid eye movement (NREM) sleep (Table 41–1). Further research has shown that these two states are as different from one another as sleep is from wakefulness.

REM sleep can be described as a state in which a highly active brain functions in an immobilized body. It is also known as paradoxical sleep because the EEG tracings are similar to those seen in the waking state. As one of two distinct sleep states, REM sleep is characterized by high brain activity (EEG activation), loss of muscle tone, dreaming, variable arousability, and potential physiological instability. This sleep state accounts for about 25% of total sleep time.

The cerebral metabolic rate is increased, and blood flow to the brain nearly doubles. The heightened brain activity is accompanied by decreased motor activity whereby deep tendon reflexes may be absent and muscles are relaxed. Blood pressure, heart rate, and cardiac output all increase and may begin to fluctuate. Vital sign variability can be particularly detrimental to a client who already has compromised function, such as the cardiac or asthmatic client.

In contrast to REM sleep, **NREM sleep** can be viewed as a state in which a quiet brain functions in an active body. NREM sleep accounts for about 75% of total sleep time. This sleep state can be further divided into the following four stages, which are defined by EEG tracings and arousal thresholds:

* Stage 1, the lightest sleep, heralds the transition from wakefulness to sleep. EEG tracings show low-voltage, nonsynchronous brain activity, and the sleeper is easily awakened (the arousal threshold is low).
* In stage 2, brain waves begin to fire more synchronously, and the arousal threshold increases.
* Stage 3 marks the beginning of bursts of delta or **slow-wave sleep.** Also called deep sleep, slow-wave sleep is characterized by high-voltage EEG activity and a high arousal threshold, which can make it difficult to arouse the sleeper.
* Stage 4 represents the deepest sleep, when resistance to external arousal is greatest. Almost continuous, high-voltage, slow-wave patterns appear on the EEG.

Characteristic physiological changes accompany NREM sleep. The metabolic rate slows, and regional cerebral blood flow decreases. In addition, blood pressure, temperature, pulse, and respiration are decreased. The body moves, especially during transitions from one stage to another.

Normal Sleep Cycles

Normal adult sleep occurs in four to five cycles each night (Fig. 41–1). Each cycle lasts about 90 minutes and has both NREM and REM phases. Typically, sleep begins with light, stage 1 sleep and descends through

TABLE 41–1
Characteristics of REM Sleep and NREM Sleep

Characteristics	REM Sleep	NREM Sleep
Synonyms	Active or paradoxical sleep	Slow-wave or delta sleep (stages 3 and 4)
Eye movements	Episodic bursts of rapid eye movements	Slow rolling or no eye movements
Vital signs	Variable; may be increased	Blood pressure, temperature, and heart rate decreased during stages 3 and 4
Muscle tone	Large-muscle immobility	Occasional whole body jerk or movement; in slow-wave sleep, muscles are more relaxed
Manifestations of deprivation	Lack of alertness; apathy, irritability, confusion, disorientation, delusions, hallucinations	Fatigue, restlessness, decreased pain tolerance, anxiety, increased illness, increased cortisol secretion, increased immunosuppression, delayed healing

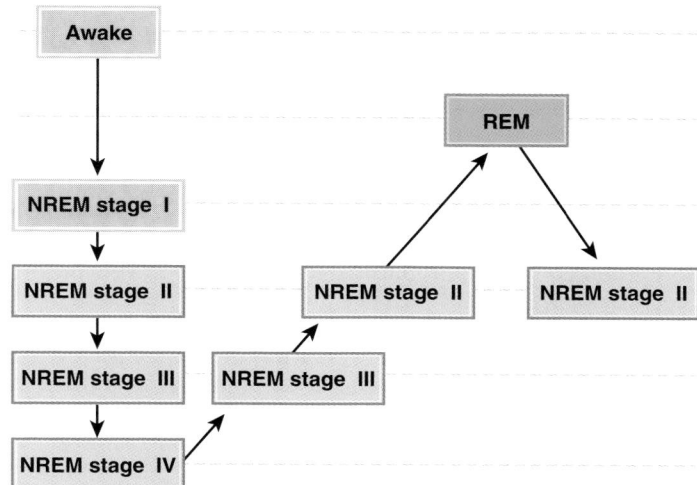

Figure 41–1. A normal adult sleep cycle. The stages are typically repeated 4 to 5 times during a night's sleep.

stages 2 and 3 to stage 4. After a few minutes in stage 4, there is an ascent back through stages 3 or 2, followed by REM activity. From REM sleep, the sleeper re-enters stage 2, NREM sleep. The transition from REM back to NREM marks the end of the first cycle. In uninterrupted sleep, this sequencing is repeated for three or four more cycles until the hour of awakening. The normal adult sleeps an average of 7 to 8 hours, but the normal range varies from 5 to 10 hours.

Although the order of these sleep stages normally remains relatively fixed, the actual time spent in each stage varies. In general, slow-wave sleep predominates during the first third of the night, and REM sleep time increases as each cycle is repeated. Thus, frequent awakenings during the first few hours of sleep are more likely to result in total NREM sleep being shortened. Later awakenings more commonly abbreviate REM sleep.

Functions of Sleep

The exact function of sleep is still a mystery. It is much easier to explain what sleep is than why it occurs. The two most widely accepted theories about sleep function are energy conservation and restoration.

ENERGY CONSERVATION

Proponents of the conservation theory argue that sleep is an extension of homeostasis. High energy use during the day must be balanced by decreased energy use at night. The body's metabolic fluctuations offer support for this theory. At night, particularly during slow-wave sleep, the metabolic rate decreases by 5 to 25%. This dip may represent the body's attempt to conserve energy.

Further evidence for the conservation theory can be found in developmental sleep pattern changes. The amount of slow-wave sleep declines with age. This decline may parallel the decreasing cerebral and body metabolism over the life span. Because energy requirements decrease with age, the need to conserve energy also declines.

RESTORATION

The most widely accepted view of sleep function is that it serves as a period of restoration and recuperation. It is thought that REM sleep promotes emotional healing and brain restoration and growth, whereas NREM sleep (especially stages 3 and 4) fosters physical growth and healing. Proponents of the restoration theory argue that sleep provides the perfect opportunity for maximum protein synthesis: energy levels and anabolic growth hormone are high while the catabolic hormones, cortisol and epinephrine, are low.

Although the exact purpose of sleep remains unknown, most researchers agree that sleep is essential for normal function, that the need for sleep varies in length from person to person, and that sleep requirements increase during stress or illness. In hospital environments, these facts are often de-emphasized; active client care is deemed more important than letting the client sleep (Southwell & Wistow, 1995).

Regulation of Sleep

Three processes regulate sleep: homeostatic mechanisms, circadian rhythms, and ultradian rhythms. Of these regulators, homeostatic mechanisms are perhaps the least well understood. Researchers believe that a complex network of neurons passing through the medulla, pons, midbrain, thalamus, hypothalamus, and basal forebrain maintains homeostatic balance between sleep and wakefulness.

The mechanisms controlling the circadian nature of sleep are better understood. The body's internal clock is set for a 25-hour day (Kryger, Roth, & Carskadon, 1994). Environmental triggers called synchronizers or *zeitgebers* adjust this clock to a 24-hour solar day. The most powerful zeitgeber is each day's pattern of light and darkness.

Melatonin, the "hormone of darkness," regulates the circadian phases of sleep. Other zeitgebers that may influence sleep-wake patterns include daily routines and social events. As we shall see, these regulators can sometimes desynchronize, as may occur in jet lag or shift changes at work. The result is a disruption in circadian sleep-wake patterns.

The ultradian process, a regulatory process within sleep itself, is represented by the two sleep states previously discussed, REM and NREM sleep.

Sleep Pathologies

It is estimated that 1 in 7 Americans has a chronic sleep-wake disorder (Shapiro & Dement, 1993). The sleep disorders or pathologies are classified on the basis of their epidemiology (Box 41–1). The International Classification of Sleep Disorders identifies three major sleep disorder categories: the dyssomnias, the parasomnias, and medical-psychiatric sleep disorders.

Dyssomnias

A **dyssomnia** is any sleep disturbance that involves the amount, quality, or timing of sleep. The dyssomnias are further subdivided into three major groups: the intrinsic sleep disorders, the extrinsic sleep disorders, and the circadian rhythm sleep disorders.

BOX 41–1

SLEEP DISORDER CLASSIFICATIONS

Dyssomnias

- *Intrinsic Sleep Disorders,* including insomnia, narcolepsy, sleep apnea, restless legs syndrome, and periodic limb movements.
- *Extrinsic Sleep Disorders,* including inadequate sleep hygiene and environmental sleep disorders.
- *Circadian Rhythm Disorders,* including shift-work sleep disorders and jet lag disorder.

Parasomnias

- *Arousal Disorders,* including sleepwalking and sleep terrors.
- *Parasomnias Associated with REM sleep,* including nightmares.
- *Other Parasomnias,* including bruxism and sleep enuresis.

Sleep Disorders Associated With Medical or Psychiatric Illness

- *Mental Disorders,* including psychoses, mood disorders, panic disorders, and alcoholism.
- *Neurologic Disorders,* including dementia, Parkinsonism, familial insomnia, and sleep-related epilepsy.
- *Other Medical Disorders,* including asthma, chronic obstructive pulmonary disease, sleep-related gastroesophageal reflux, and peptic ulcer disease.

INTRINSIC SLEEP DISORDERS

In intrinsic sleep disorders, the sleep disturbance arises from within the body; the primary cause of these disorders is an internal pathophysiological process rather than an external event. Insomnia, narcolepsy, obstructive sleep apnea, and restless legs syndrome are examples of such disorders.

Insomnia

Insomnia is characterized by difficulty initiating or maintaining sleep. It is by far the most common dyssomnia; about one-third of the population suffers from it at some point during their lives, and 10% of those who suffer from it consider it serious (Thorpy & Brunton, 1994).

Insomnia is characterized by the subjective sense that sleep quality is poor and inadequate. The sleeper will complain of difficulty initiating sleep, sleeping too lightly, easily disrupted sleep with many spontaneous arousals, or early-morning awakenings. Short-term insomnia is usually self-limiting and can often be traced to acute stress or lifestyle changes, such as disruption of the sleep schedule, unfamiliar environments, or environments not conducive to sleep.

If not resolved within 2 weeks, such transient sleep disruptions are considered chronic insomnias. Long-term or chronic insomnia is more difficult to cure because of its self-perpetuating nature.

Insomnia can lead to symptoms of sleep deprivation. **Sleep deprivation** is the state that results from a person not getting enough sleep. Awakenings during the first few hours of sleep usually result in total NREM sleep time being shortened. Such deprivation has been linked to decreased tissue repair, increased anxiety, high serum cortisol levels, decreased pain thresholds, a depressed immune response, delayed healing, gastrointestinal (GI) upset, headache, vertigo, and ataxia (Chuman, 1983). Later awakenings more commonly shorten REM sleep. Lack of REM sleep causes decreased alertness and psychological disturbances, such as anxiety, apathy, irritability, confusion, and disturbed or aggressive behavior (Evans & French, 1995; Hodgson, 1991).

Although deprivation of both NREM and REM sleep may have serious consequences, NREM stage 3 and 4 sleep takes priority over all other sleep stages during the rebound sleep of sleep-deprived people. Only two-thirds of the lost REM is recovered, whereas almost all of Stage 3 and 4 sleep is reclaimed (Evans & French, 1995).

Insomnia from NREM and REM sleep deprivation can occur if total sleep time is decreased or sleep is frequently interrupted. Horne (1983) first demonstrated that fragmented sleep can lead to symptoms of sleep deprivation even if the total sleep time exceeds 8 hours. Deprivation occurs because, after each awakening, the sleeper returns to stage 1 rather than to the stage from which she was aroused. Thus, research has shown that sleep continuity is at least as important as amount of sleep. Researchers continue to study the effects of interrupted or unsatisfactory sleep, especially among people with chronic diseases, as discussed in the State of Nursing Science chart.

Narcolepsy

Narcolepsy is a striking hypersomnia characterized by abnormal sleep tendencies as well as by pathologi-

cal REM sleep, manifested as excessive daytime sleepiness, disturbed nighttime sleep, cataplexy, sleep paralysis, and hypnagogic hallucinations. Narcolepsy is classified as a **hypersomnia,** which is a sleep disorder characterized by excessive sleepiness. By an unknown mechanism, the CNS loses control of REM sleep.

THE STATE OF NURSING SCIENCE
THE IMPACT OF ILLNESS ON SLEEP

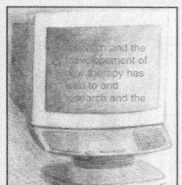

What Are the Issues?

Sleep is a part of everyone's life. It restores the body and influences how people feel when they are awake. Nurses assess for sleep pattern disturbances in their clients in an effort to improve the quality and quantity of sleep, particularly in people with chronic illnesses, many of whom are at greater risk for sleep pattern disturbances.

What Research Has Been Conducted?

Nokes and Kendrew (1996) surveyed 53 men and 2 women infected with the human immunodeficiency virus (HIV) to assess the quality of their sleep, their levels of anxiety, the severity of their symptoms, and the manner in which they became infected with HIV. The researchers sought to understand whether the method of contracting HIV correlated in any way with quality of sleep.

Redeker, Mason, Wykpisz, and Glica (1996) studied changes over time in the sleep patterns of women who had undergone heart surgery. Participants wore wrist sensors at home that allowed researchers to calculate the total amount of sleep and number of awakenings each woman experienced during four 1-week periods. This objective method of assessing sleep patterns at home allowed the researchers to record sleep patterns relatively free from interference.

What Has the Research Concluded?

Nokes and Kendrew (1996) found that the people with HIV whom they studied frequently experienced sleep pattern disturbances that interfered with daily living. About 30% of the participants reported that their sleep quality was "bad" or "very bad." Most had trouble getting to sleep and got less than 7 hours of sleep. More than one-third of the people studied reported using sleeping medications within the week before the study. For most of the participants, poor sleep affected their ability to function during the day. People who contracted HIV through drug use reported poorer sleep quality than other subjects.

In contrast to the people with HIV, the women who were recovering from heart surgery experienced an improvement in their sleep over the course of the 6-month

study. Their most disrupted sleep occurred during the first postoperative days. The participants also reported having slept more during the day and evening than at night, possibly because of medications taken during the day. The participants were able to sleep for longer periods at night when they napped less during the day.

The researchers noted that the women varied greatly in the length and quality of their sleep. However, because the age of the subjects ranged from 43 to 83 years, the researchers suggested that some of this variation may have been normal and age-related. A key nursing role before surgery and other procedures is helping to prepare clients for how their lives might change after the procedure. This study suggests that information about how sleep patterns may gradually return to normal after cardiac surgery could become a reassuring part of preoperative teaching.

What Is the Future of Research in This Area?

The researchers who studied sleep in HIV-infected people recommended that people who are in various stages of HIV disease be studied to see whether the severity of their symptoms influences the quality of their sleep. Research studies that help nurses understand the factors that influence the quality of sleep may help in the development of interventions that can improve sleep in HIV-infected people. Also unexplored by researchers are differences in sleep quality between HIV-infected men and women.

Postoperative care for people who have undergone heart surgery includes frequent monitoring and intervention. The researchers who studied sleep in women after heart surgery suggested examining how and when these interruptions influence sleep quality. They also postulated that postoperative medications could have an adverse impact on the quality of sleep and suggested that future research examine that relationship.

References

Nokes, K.M., & Kendrew, J. (1996). Sleep quality in people with HIV disease. *Journal of the Association of Nurses in AIDS Care,* 7(3), 43–50.
Redeker, N.S., Mason, D.J., Wykpisz, E., & Glica, B. (1996). Sleep patterns in women after coronary artery bypass surgery. *Applied Nursing Research, 9*(3), 115–122.

Sudden *daytime sleep attacks,* the most obvious symptom of narcolepsy, usually last 20 to 30 minutes and are episodes of REM sleep. *Cataplexy* results from the abrupt bilateral loss of muscle tone and paralysis of voluntary muscles. Narcoleptics may also experience *hypnagogic hallucinations.* These are vivid, bizarre, dream-like experiences that last from 1 to 15 minutes. *Sleep paralysis,* or the inability to move during the onset of sleep or awakening, is another common symptom.

Obstructive Sleep Apnea

Obstructive sleep apnea, another primary dyssomnia with serious consequences, is a sleep disorder manifested by periodic cessation of airflow at the nose and mouth during inspiration, which arouses the person from sleep. Sleep apnea occurs in 1 to 4% of the population, with increased incidence in middle and old age. The airway obstruction is commonly created when the back of the throat is sucked closed or narrowed as the sleeper inhales (Fig. 41–2). This airway collapse results from a sleep-induced loss of upper airway muscle tone. Typical symptoms include loud snoring followed by silence, during which the sleeper struggles

to breathe against a blocked airway. After a number of seconds, decreased oxygen levels cause the sleeper to awaken, usually with a loud snort. In adults, flailing arms and legs or a total body spasm may accompany the snort. Restlessness and bedwetting may be observed in children.

Treatment may involve the surgical resection of the palatopharynx or the use of continuous positive airway pressure (CPAP). Surgery removes portions of the airway that may be impeding airflow during sleep. The CPAP mask, worn over the nose during sleep, helps keep the sleeper's upper airway patent by maintaining continuous positive pressures during ventilation. Children with obstructive apnea caused by enlarged adenoids or tonsils benefit from an adenotonsillectomy.

Restless Legs Syndrome

Restless legs syndrome is an intrinsic sleep disorder characterized by intense, abnormal, lower extremity sensations and irresistible leg movements that delay sleep onset; the sleeper describes an uncomfortable deep creeping, crawling sensation in the calf or thigh muscles that leads to an irresistible urge to move the legs when sitting or lying down.

EXTRINSIC SLEEP DISORDERS

Extrinsic sleep disorders are caused by problems outside the body. External factors create the sleep disturbance, and if they are removed, the sleep disturbance will resolve. The environment and drugs constitute the two major contributors to such disorders. They will be discussed at length later in the chapter.

CIRCADIAN RHYTHM SLEEP DISORDERS

Circadian sleep disorders are characterized by a mismatch between the person's sleep schedule and normal circadian sleep patterns. Such persons cannot sleep when sleep is wanted, needed, or expected. Additionally, they may be sleepy at undesirable times. The two most common transient circadian rhythm disorders are shift-work sleep disorder and time zone change (jet lag) syndrome.

Some employees, such as nurses and firefighters, must periodically change the shift during which they work. For these workers, short-term sleeping medications may be necessary during adjustment to shift rotations. However, these drugs only partially solve the problem. Although they promote sleep, they do not reset circadian clocks. Thus, shift workers who change to another work schedule must ultimately reset their internal clocks to maintain their work performance and sleep at appropriate times. Shift rotation in a forward direction (nights, mornings, then evenings) rather than a backward direction (evenings, mornings, then nights) facilitates circadian realignment. In Europe, companies with shift workers are switching to "rapidly rotating" systems, during which employees rotate two morning shifts, two evening shifts, two night shifts, followed by two days off. It is argued that such shift changes allow the circadian system to retain its natural daily orientation (Monk, 1994).

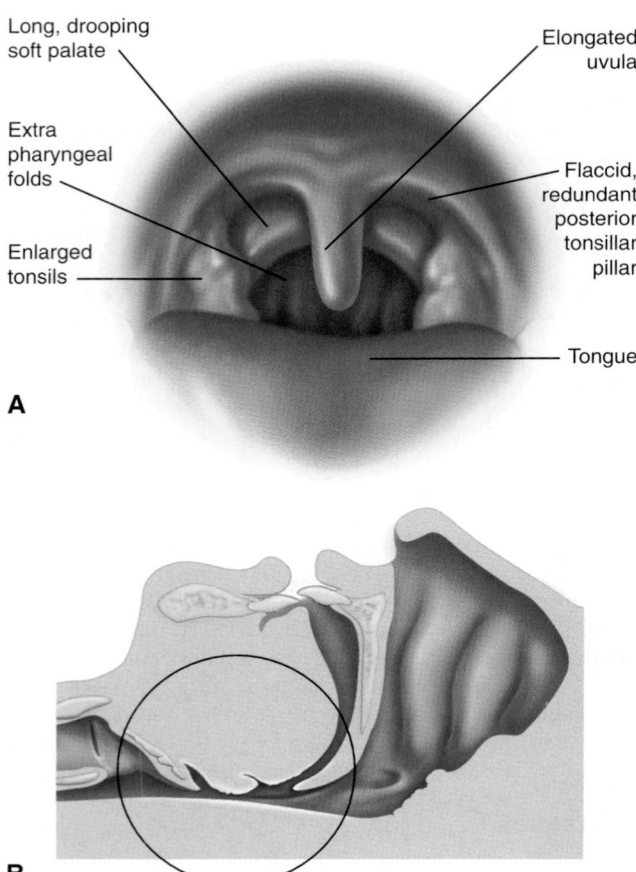

Long, drooping soft palate

Extra pharyngeal folds

Enlarged tonsils

Elongated uvula

Flaccid, redundant posterior tonsillar pillar

Tongue

A

B

Figure 41–2. Anatomy of obstructive sleep apnea. *A,* the collapsible anatomic structures that can obstruct the airway. *B,* obstruction of the upper airway as the sleeper inhales. (Redrawn from Shemwell, A., & Wilson, P. [1994]. Rest and respiration during obstructive sleep apnoea. Nursing Times, 90[19], 31.)

The term *jet lag* describes a constellation of symptoms that develops as the result of rapid travel across several time zones. Symptoms include malaise, headache, loss of appetite, irregular bowel movements, difficulty concentrating, fatigue during the new daytime, and an inability to sleep well at night. The symptoms reflect the circadian system's failure to rapidly adjust to sudden shifts. Although both physical cues (nighttime and daylight) and social cues (mealtimes and noise) encourage adaptation to the new circadian system, readjustment may still take several days, particularly if the person has taken an eastward flight.

Parasomnias

In contrast to the dyssomnias, **parasomnias** are not difficulties with sleep itself, but rather with abnormal movements and behaviors that occur during sleep. Examples include somnambulism, sleep terrors, sleep enuresis, nightmares, and bruxism. These events are undesirable, acute, episodic, physical phenomena that occur during sleep or are worsened by it.

Somnambulism and sleep terrors are most prevalent in children. Because they occur during deep sleep, however, they are frequently not remembered in the morning. **Somnambulism** is a slow-wave sleep parasomnia associated with stereotypical "sleepwalking" behaviors. The sleeper may sit up with glassy eyes, make body movements, get up, and walk around. Somnambulists often avoid or "look through" anyone who attempts to talk to them. Although visual intake and coordination of the CNS is maintained to some extent during sleepwalking, safety is an important consideration.

By contrast, **sleep terrors** (also known as night terrors) occur during slow-wave sleep and are characterized by arousal, agitation, and signs of sympathetic nervous system activity, such as dilated pupils, sweating, tachypnea, and tachycardia. Sleep terrors may be frightening to watch, but they pose little danger to the sleeper. They are marked by 10 to 20 minutes of partial awakening accompanied by thrashing, kicking, rolling movements, and garbled speech; the sleeper often looks terrified and screams. If left alone, the adult or child afflicted with sleep terrors will return to a resting state. Highly correlated with times of stress, sleep terrors will usually resolve spontaneously within a few months of onset.

Sleep terrors must be differentiated from **nightmares,** which are vivid or frightening dreams that occur during REM sleep, awaken the sleeper, and can be vividly recalled. Nightmares often correlate with increased stress, depression, painful life events, insecurity, anxiety, guilt, fever, or abrupt discontinuation of drugs that affect REM sleep (Driver & Shapiro, 1993).

Sleep enuresis, another parasomnia, is defined as bedwetting during sleep. Sleepers typically awaken to find themselves in urine-soaked bedclothes. It results from incomplete toilet training in children.

About 1 to 3% of adults and 70% of mentally retarded clients of all ages also suffer from this disorder. Treatment may include low doses of tricyclic antidepressants, behavioral techniques (such as bladder training or the use of a pad and buzzer), and fluid restriction in the evening.

Bruxism is a parasomnia characterized by violent, repetitive grinding of the teeth that occurs during the lighter stages of sleep or during partial arousals. It produces a loud and unpleasant sound that commonly awakens the bed partner or even someone sleeping 10 or 20 feet away. Episodes last 4 to 5 seconds, sometimes longer. Damaged teeth and jaw pain may result. The afflicted sleeper may be treated with a rubber mouth guard over the teeth at night.

FACTORS AFFECTING REST AND SLEEP
Lifestyle Factors

Lifestyle issues—such as nutrition, exercise, smoking, and disruptions in daily routines—may influence sleep and rest patterns. Because these issues are the most subject to change, they are particularly significant for clients who wish to modify their sleep and rest patterns.

Nutrition

Sleep pattern disturbances may be linked to diet. Hunger or excess food consumption near bedtime can lead to delayed sleep onset, increased arousals, or both. In addition, intake of caffeine and alcohol may influence sleep. Excess caffeine consumption (in tea, coffee, chocolate, cocoa, and cola) may be detrimental. Because it has such a long half-life, caffeine taken late in the day may increase insomnia and nighttime arousals. Alcohol, a brain sedative, shortens sleep onset. However, it disturbs sleep patterns late at night because its rapid metabolism causes a rebound arousal. It may also cause early morning awakenings secondary to a full bladder.

Although the biochemical effects of diet on sleep need more study, it is known that adherence to routine habits enhances sleep. Therefore, to the extent possible, hospitalized clients should be allowed to eat and drink the bedtime snacks they would normally ingest at home.

Exercise

The person who exercises during the day is more likely to sleep well at night (Fig. 41–3). Increased physical activity increases both REM and NREM sleep. Moderate fatigue, brought on by exercise, is thought to promote restful sleep. Apparently, increased exercise increases fatigue, which, in turn, produces a soporific effect. However, activity must be carefully timed. Exercise within 2 hours of retiring can lead to difficulty getting to sleep.

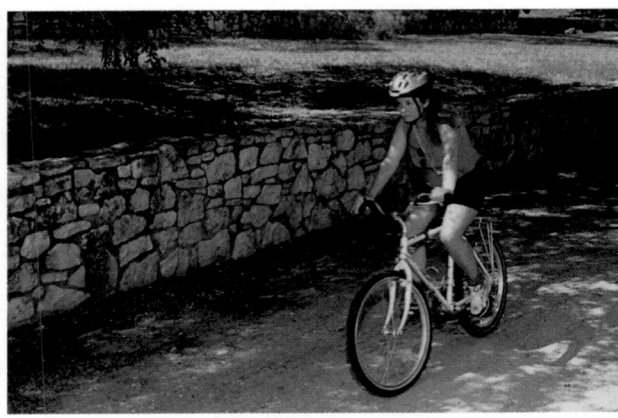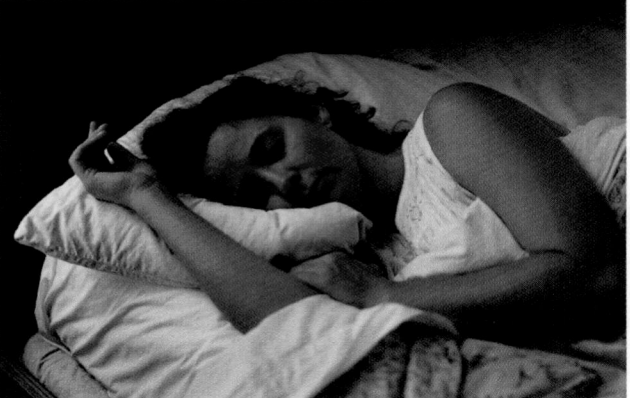

Figure 41-3. The person who exercises during the day is more likely to sleep well at night.

Smoking

High levels of nicotine cause feelings of arousal and agitation. As the half-life of nicotine is 1 to 2 hours, the person who smokes more than one cigarette within an hour of bedtime may delay sleep onset. The average smoker sleeps ½ hour less than the average non-smoker (Stradling, 1993).

Long-term smoking can eventually contribute to a need for increased physical rest. Permanent lung damage caused by chronic smoke inhalation commonly leads to hypoxia. Hypoxia, in turn, is associated with increased fatigue and a need to intersperse activities with rest.

Lifestyle Disruptions

People who have a regular sleep-wake pattern are more likely to report beneficial sleep and better performance during the day than people with variable sleep patterns. It may be that adhering to a fixed sleep schedule is more important than the actual number of hours slept. Anticipated and unanticipated lifestyle modifications can disturb a fixed sleep pattern. A work schedule change, the birth of a baby, out-of-town visitors, or a move to a culture with different meal and sleep times are just a few examples of such potential lifestyle disruptions.

Environmental Factors

A familiar, comfortable environment is most conducive to sleep induction and maintenance. People become habituated to certain sights, sounds, lights, and temperatures, and the absence of these or the presence of novel disruptions can disrupt sleep.

Hospitalization

The hospital, an unfamiliar setting to most clients, can wreak havoc with normal sleep patterns. Strange, loud noises, bright lights, uncomfortable beds and temperatures, restraints in uncomfortable positions, lack of privacy, lack of control, anxiety or personal worry, separation from loved ones, and sleep deprivation can

lead to sleep problems. Noises are particularly bothersome. In fact, hospitalized clients find noise so intrusive that they often cite it as the major reason for taking hypnotics while in the hospital (Halfens, Lendfers, & Cox, 1991).

The acute care setting, in which clients are monitored around the clock, can be conducive to relaxation and sleep if clients feel protected. However, clients may be frightened by the fact that they require such intensive observation and their fears may contribute to difficulty falling asleep.

Nowhere are sleep stressors more acute than in intensive care units (ICU). An early, groundbreaking study by Walker (1972) showed that cardiotomy clients were disturbed about 14 times per hour in the immediate postoperative period. The author concluded that critical care nurses tended to provide continual care with no regard to the time of day. This oversight can have significant, adverse consequences. *ICU psychosis* is a well-documented iatrogenic complication strongly correlated with REM sleep deprivation in ICUs. This syndrome is characterized by restlessness, loss of reality perception, transient paranoia, hallucinations, and delusions. It occurs after 3 to 5 days in a critical care unit and typically disappears after transfer to another unit.

Temperature

Body and ambient temperature influence sleep-wake patterns. An excessively cold environment will cause frequent awakenings. Fever and a higher environmental temperature are also associated with an increased number of awakenings, as well as increased total waking time and decreased slow-wave sleep and REM sleep (Closs, 1988). Such findings suggest that regulation of body and ambient temperatures is an important component of managing sleep pattern disturbances.

Client Perception of the Environment

Most people are accustomed to their home sleep environment. The familiar ambiance provides comfort and security. Without this supportive environment, a person may not be able to relax, and insomnia may result. Many sleepers experience difficulty sleeping in a strange bed. City dwellers may find the darkness and quiet of the country disconcerting and perceive the early morning crowing of the rooster as an unwelcome alarm clock. By contrast, rural travelers may be overstimulated by the urban environment.

Developmental Factors

To accurately diagnose sleep pattern disturbances, you must first be able to recognize normal, developmental changes in sleep architecture (Fig. 41–4).

In general, sleep patterns stabilize during the 1st year of life. Normal newborns sleep an average of 16 to 17 hours per day. However, they often alternate between REM sleep and wakefulness, skipping stages 1 through 4 of NREM. This phenomenon shortens the duration of each sleep period. Their sleep cycle is also shorter, lasting about 40 to 50 minutes instead of 90. If sleep is a time of growth, it is not surprising that newborns spend so much of their time sleeping; their body weight doubles in the first 6 months. By 6 weeks of age, infants are awake more during the day than at night, but more than half will still not be sleeping through the night. At the end of the 1st year, most children are sleeping through the night and nap only once a day. However, sleep needs are individual. As long as infants are active during waking periods and growing normally, they are probably getting enough sleep.

The sleep-wake cycle is fully developed by age 2, and the REM sleep pattern during preschool years is similar to that of an adult. Infants and toddlers seldom have primary sleep disorders. The most common sleep problems at this age are a difficulty learning to sleep alone, difficulty with bedtime routines, and transitions from wake to sleep (Johnson, Wise, & Jimmerson, 1995).

As children mature, they spend fewer hours sleeping but a greater portion of their sleep time in slow-wave sleep. Infants spend only 50% of their sleep time in deep sleep, whereas older children spend 80% of their sleep time in deep sleep. Although sleep needs by this age are individualized, most school-aged children require an average of 8 to 10 hours of sleep. During growth spurts, sleep needs may increase. As noted, parasomnias are more common in children and usually first occur before age 10 (Driver & Shapiro, 1993).

During adolescence, total sleep time increases. Teenagers' rapid physical growth, tendency toward overexertion, and overall increased activity levels contribute to fatigue and increased sleep needs. Their increased need for sleep, coupled with their tendency to stay up late, often makes it difficult for teenagers to get up in the morning. These symptoms overlap with those of *delayed sleep phase syndrome,* a common and underdiagnosed circadian rhythm disturbance in this age group. The internal clocks that regulate the sleep-wake cycles in some teenagers are thought to be exceptionally long. The net result is a sleep cycle shift that causes sleep onset insomnia and difficulty with

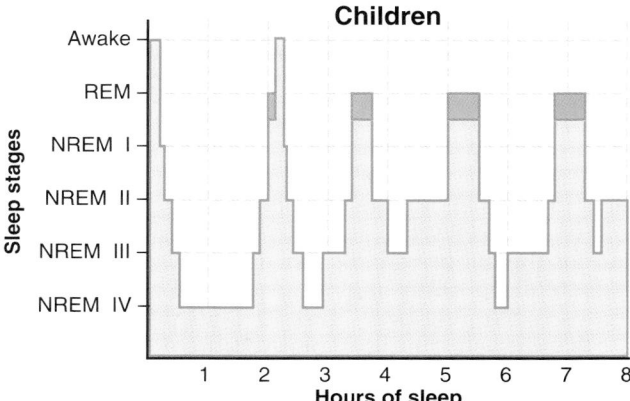

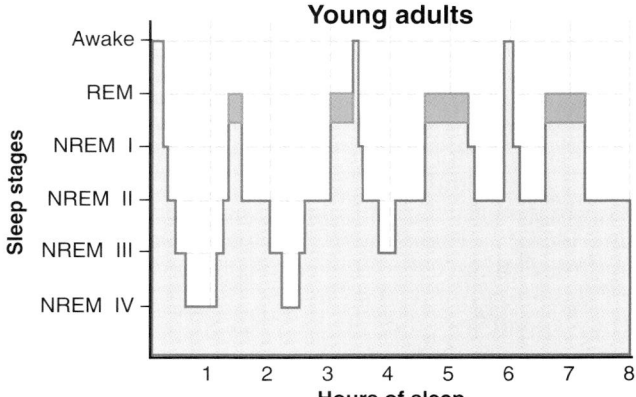

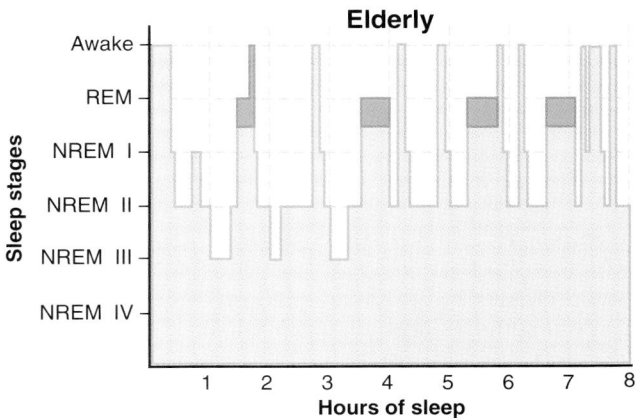

Figure 41–4. Sleep architecture over the lifespan. The amount of slow-wave sleep decreases with age, and the number of awakenings increases with age. (Redrawn from Kales, A., et al. [1968]. Sleep and dreams: Recent research on clinical aspects. Annals of Internal Medicine, 68(5), 1078–1104.)

early morning rising. The adolescent may be unable to fall asleep until 2:00 or 3:00 AM but may then sleep soundly and feel refreshed if allowed to sleep for 7 to 8 hours.

Slow-wave sleep declines after adolescence. In fact, it decreases by nearly 40% during the teen years and continues to decline in a linear fashion until age 60, after which there is little remaining delta sleep (Closs,

1988). For the majority of young adult and middle-aged males, other stages of sleep stabilize. Among their female counterparts, however, sleep changes are often triggered by hormonal fluctuations.

Pregnant women, for example, have an increased need for sleep during the first trimester of pregnancy. Typical symptoms include naps during the day and sleeping "hard" at night (Richardson, 1996). By the end of pregnancy, the woman's increased body size, as well as the unborn child's size and movement, make it hard to sleep. Sleep may be disturbed also by nightmares concerning body integrity and safety.

Another shift in hormones occurs at midlife with the onset of menopause. Complaints of sleep disturbances occur at this time. Such disturbances may be an early harbinger of decreasing estrogen levels. Changes in both estrogen and progesterone levels have been shown to influence many sleep modulators, including norepinephrine, dopamine, acetylcholine, and serotonin (Vliet, 1995).

When men and women enter senescence, they are at greater risk for sleep disturbances as a result of normal aging. Studies have shown that the healthy elderly generally spend more time in bed, spend less time asleep, awaken more often and for longer periods of time, and have less efficient sleep time. That is, they are spending more time in bed but less time asleep. They spend less time in REM sleep and slow-wave sleep and are more likely to nap (Vitiello, 1997). The net effect of all these physiological changes is that, by age 65, most people awaken at least 12 times a night and only spend 30 minutes in deep sleep (Carey, 1996). In addition, aging increases the risk of developing a primary sleep disorder or a sleep disorder secondary to chronic medical and psychiatric illnesses.

Physiological Factors

Genetics

Narcolepsy is one of the few sleep disorders with a demonstrated genetic link. Roughly 5 to 10% of narcoleptic clients have an affected first-degree relative. Some insomnias and somnambulism also seem to be familial, although no genetic links have been conclusively established.

Sleep Position

Poor sleepers spend more time on their backs and change positions more frequently than do good sleepers. There is also an increased incidence of sleep apnea associated with people who sleep on their backs (Closs, 1988).

Therapeutic regimens sometimes require that clients assume uncomfortable positions. For example, a client with a right hip replacement may not be able to lie on either side initially. At least one study suggests that health care workers may overlook positioning problems. Whereas clients frequently cited pain and having difficulty finding a comfortable position as reasons for not being able to sleep, nurses identified pain as a problem but were less aware of client concerns about positioning (Beyerman, 1987).

Pain

Unrelieved pain often contributes to sleep difficulties, perhaps because of heightened fear and anxiety experienced during the quiet of the night. Pain actually presents a twofold problem. First, it is an obstacle to falling and staying asleep. Second, sleep deprivation decreases the pain threshold; that is, the patient is less able to tolerate the pain when it occurs. Thus, more aggressive pain management will often alleviate symptoms of both pain and insomnia.

Medications

Because any drug may affect sleep patterns, it is important to take a thorough drug history when assessing clients for sleep problems.

For the insomniac, a hypnotic, or "sleeping pill," may be ordered. A **hypnotic** is a drug that acts on the CNS to shorten sleep onset, reduce nighttime wakefulness, or decrease anxiety when insomnia is associated with increased anxiety. There are several different classes of hypnotics, including sedatives, anesthetics, analgesics, and intoxicants. A **sedative** is a drug that exerts a soothing, tranquilizing effect on the CNS, resulting in a shortened sleep onset and the alleviation of anxiety. Sedatives are the hypnotics used most frequently to alleviate insomnia.

Classified as both sedatives and anxiolytics (anxiety-reducing drugs), the benzodiazepines are the most frequently prescribed hypnotics. This drug family includes triazolam, lorazepam, temazepam, flurazepam, and diazepam (Table 41–2). Barbiturates are no longer used for insomnia because of their high potential for abuse. Although benzodiazepines are less likely to be abused than barbiturates, they can cause psychological and physical dependence. Their abrupt discontinuation can lead to withdrawal symptoms. Withdrawal increases insomnia for 1 to 2 weeks, but it may take up to 2 months for the drug-associated insomnia to resolve completely. In addition, benzodiazepines, especially diazepam and flurazepam, are associated with global cognitive impairment (Grad, 1995). To avoid such symptoms, insomniacs should take these medications for short intervals and only if absolutely necessary.

In addition to the benzodiazepines, zolpidem and chloral hydrate are two nonbenzodiazepines commonly used as hypnotics. Zolpidem is as effective as a benzodiazepine in treating acute and chronic insomnia. Additionally, it is less likely to change sleep architecture and to cause adverse psychomotor or cognitive effects. However, it carries the same theoretical risk of dependence as the benzodiazepines. Chloral hydrate, one of the oldest hypnotics, is usually well tolerated by the elderly. However, it can also produce tolerance and drug dependence. Other frequently associated side effects are nausea, vomiting, flatulence, and an unpleasant taste (Kuhn, 1998).

TABLE 41–2
The Benzodiazepine Sedative-Hypnotics

Drug Name	Half-Life	Dose	Possible Effects
Triazolam (Halcion)	1.6–5.4 hrs (short-acting)	0.125–0.25 mg	• Rebound insomnia (early morning awakening), especially in high doses in the elderly. • Amnesia, confusion, daytime anxiety, memory changes. • Daytime alertness after use.
Lorazepam (Ativan)	10–20 hrs (intermediate)	1–4 mg	• Morning sedation, lethargy. • Memory changes, anger. • Mild paradoxical excitation during first 2 weeks of treatment.
Temazepam (Restoril)	10–20 hrs (intermediate)	15–30 mg	• Sleep-onset insomnia may continue. • Rebound insomnia with discontinuation. • Daytime alertness after use.
Clonazepam (Klonopin)	18–50 hrs (long-acting)	0.75–16 mg	• Useful in treatment of restless legs syndrome. • Possible daytime sedation and poor coordination.
Flurazepam (Dalmane)	50–240 hrs (long-acting)	15–30 mg	• Possible daytime sedation and poor coordination. • Suppresses daytime anxiety. • Relative lack of withdrawal effects.

*A*ction *A*lert!
Hypnotic and sedative drugs are contraindicated for clients with breathing disorders. Sleeping medications can severely exacerbate respiratory problems.

The hormone melatonin also has hypnotic effects. This drug can be easily purchased over-the-counter. Unfortunately, because it is not yet regulated by any government agency, its purity cannot be ensured. Long touted as a remedy for a wide variety of sleep problems, melatonin has only recently undergone controlled clinical studies. These studies cite convincing evidence that melatonin may be useful in the treatment of jet lag and delayed sleep phase syndrome, as well as insomnia in the elderly and in neurologically impaired children. However, more data are needed to define the parameters of use and the optimal dosage. The National Sleep Foundation states that the long-term use of melatonin is not justified for any sleep disorder at this time (Cupp, 1997).

Spices and herbs thought to have sedative properties include almonds, chamomile, catamount, fennel, ginseng, hops, indian hemp, lettuce, lime, marjoram, may blossom, melissa oats, orange blossom, passion flower, rosemary, willow, and valerian. Most of these substances have not been scientifically investigated. Valerian is the exception. In some studies it has been shown to improve the quality of subjective sleep (Idzikowski & Shapiro, 1993). Nondrug forms of alternative medicine may aid sleep as well, such as massage and therapeutic touch, described in the Considering the Alternatives chart.

Psychiatric Disorders

Ninety percent of clients with mood disorders complain of disturbed sleep. Depression, a common mood disorder, is most often associated with difficulty falling asleep and early morning awakening. However, 20% of depressed clients will complain of constant exhaustion and sleeping too much (Jamieson & Becker, 1992).

Sleep problems commonly occur in people who have anxiety or panic attacks. Prolonged sleep onset and decreased stage 4 and REM sleep mark these disorders. The hospitalized client may be particularly susceptible to anxiety. The stress of radiation and chemotherapy, end-stage symptoms, or a life-threatening illness can trigger anxiety.

If fatigue cannot be explained by any of the foregoing medical or psychiatric conditions, then a diagnosis of *chronic fatigue syndrome* may be considered. Chronic fatigue syndrome is a long-standing fatigue (6 months or more) accompanied by persistent flu-like symptoms. The afflicted person will typically present with pharyngitis, fever, and lymphadenopathy. Currently, there is no consensus in the medical community about the etiology of this disorder, and the course of the illness is unpredictable, with exacerbations and remissions (Houde & Kempfe-Leacher, 1997).

ASSESSMENT

Guided by a theoretical knowledge of normal and abnormal sleep-rest patterns, you can apply the nursing process to better identify individual clients who have or are at risk for developing these problems. A culturally sensitive assessment forms the critical first step in the nursing process.

The Cross-Cultural Care chart offers tips that relate to Ms. Weiss, the client described at the beginning of the chapter.

If your assessment is patchy or incomplete, sleep problems may remain unrecognized and unaddressed. Assessment must include a sleep history and a physical examination. The sleep history should help diagnose specific problems accurately. Physical assessment may yield nonspecific findings of fatigue or sleep problems.

CONSIDERING THE ALTERNATIVES

MASSAGE AND THERAPEUTIC TOUCH

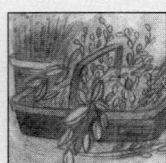 Massage is perhaps humankind's oldest attempt at healing, from the instinctive rubbing of a sore muscle to reaching out to soothe another's hurt. Massage has traditionally been a part of nursing training, generally used as part of evening (or "HS") care, and is exemplified by the back rub. It remains part of the nursing curriculum and is included in this text.

In recent years, however, nursing has become more technologically oriented. Nurses are spending more and more time with machines. Direct patient-care tasks are frequently being delegated to others. And nurses are becoming busier in general. Because of these trends, the use of massage by nurse has tended to fall by the wayside. In many hospitals, the evening back rub is now a thing of the past.

Paradoxically, however, even as massage has fallen into disuse among many nurses, there has been a proliferation of massage techniques, schools, and therapists in society at large. Many nurses have worked to keep massage a part of nursing practice, and many others have tried to reintroduce it into areas where it is no longer a part of nursing practice. Along with these trends, researchers are studying the effects of massage and publishing results that support its benefits.

Many types of massage are practiced today, and there are several different types of licenses and certifications for massage therapists. Swedish massage is well known as a full-body technique using oil as a lubricant on the skin. Oriental massage, such as acupressure and shiatsu, are techniques of traditional Chinese medicine (see Chapter 25). In China, some traditional doctors practice massage as a specialty for treating a variety of problems. Massage is a recommended modality for the treatment of infants and children in Chinese medicine (Jiming, Xinming, & Junqi, 1990). Interestingly, a focus of research on massage in the United States has been on infant massage. This research has shown many benefits of massage for premature, HIV infected, and drug-affected babies, including improvement in appetite, weight gain, decreased stress behavior, and, in some cases, shorter hospitalizations (Knaster, 1998; Wheeden, Scafidi, Field, & Ifonson, 1993; Scafidi, Field, & Schanberg, 1993). Other types of massage include sports massage (now used by many professional sports teams), deep tissue massage, and reflexology, to name just a few.

Research has shown many interesting effects of massage. For example, research has shown increases in microcirculation and beta-endorphin levels (Kaada & Tor-

steinbo, 1989) and in immunoglobulin A in saliva (Groer, Mozingo, Droppleman, & Davis, 1994), which may help explain some of the apparent benefits of massage in relation to pain control and immune function, respectively. Research has also identified positive benefits of massage in clinical trials for back and neck complaints (Koes, Bouter, van Mameren, & Essers, 1992) and chronic tension headache (Puustjarvi, Airaksinen, & Pontinen, 1990). Benefits of massage have even been shown with autistic children. Currently, many other conditions are being investigated in ongoing studies of massage therapy (Knaster, 1998).

Many hospitals across the United States have begun hiring licensed massage therapists (LMT) and starting hospital-based massage programs. Some of these programs were pioneered by nurses who became LMTs after becoming RNs. Today, there may be hundreds of such programs in the United States, and some are studying the therapeutic effects of massage in different conditions.

In the United States, at least a dozen states accept massage as a nursing intervention if the nurse has been properly trained. And the National Federation of Specialty Nursing Organizations recognizes massage as a nursing specialty (Mower, 1997).

For many nurses, close contact, including touch, is important to their concept of caring for clients. While attempting to keep massage within their practice can be challenging to nurses, involvement in hospital massage programs and advancing their knowledge through additional training in massage can expand the ability of nurses to maintain this form of client contact.

At least one nursing school in Japan, affiliated with an acupuncture school, includes techniques for Oriental massage in its training. The school's president believes that massage is especially useful for prevention and treatment of bedsores and enhancing circulation (S. Goto, personal communication, May 8, 1998).

A practice that is related to but different from massage and that has been associated with nursing since the 1970s, is therapeutic touch. According to Olson and colleagues (1997), "Therapeutic touch is a specific nursing intervention designed to decrease anxiety and improve one's sense of relaxation and well-being. It is a conscious intention to help another, by using focused attention and patterned movements of the hands in a method first described by Krieger." Therapeutic touch is actually not a massage technique, because the practitioner's hands do not touch the client but instead hover over the patient a few inches above the skin to manipulate what

(continued)

MASSAGE AND THERAPEUTIC TOUCH (continued)

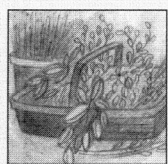

practitioners refer to as the client's energy field. The technique was initially developed by Dolores Krieger, Ph.D., RN, and colleagues, and taught at the graduate level at New York University. Today, "therapeutic touch, as a nursing intervention, is being taught to nurses through many colleges and universities, and by the National League for Nursing through its continuing education videotape series . . . . It is completely within the mainstream of modern nursing practice" (Scheiber, 1997). According to Krieger, therapeutic touch is "a dual process. One aspect involves helping and healing the person who is ill, the other concerns what happens within the therapist." She describes the process of therapeutic touch as one of centering: "The centering I'm talking about is an in-turning in the sense of trying to find the center of your own consciousness" (Horrigan, 1998).

Although proponents of therapeutic touch claim that research provides evidence supporting its use, many critics contend that the research is of poor quality and design (Scheiber, 1997; Ulett, 1997). A study of the ability of therapeutic touch practitioners to perceive a "human energy field"—a perception that practitioners require in order to practice the technique—failed to show evidence of this ability. Rosa, Rosa, Sarner, & Barrett, (1998) cite this finding as proof "that the claims of TT are groundless and that further professional use is unjustified." However, the results instead may simply fuel the ongoing controversy about therapeutic touch (Rosa, Rosa, Sarner, & Barrett, 1998; Neie, 1998). George Ulett, a physician and a critic of therapeutic touch, is insightful about its appeal to nurses: "TT appeals to nurses who have a long tradition of healing characterized by loving care, genuine concern and an expressed intent to heal their patients . . . . Economics have changed the nurse's role to technologist and dispenser of medicines. Part of the popularity of TT may be due to its once again giving nurses a more active role on the treatment team." Further research is needed to settle some of the issues surrounding therapeutic touch. The enthusiasm of many of its practitioners and of many patients who have received it is certainly grounds for careful examination.

Resources

Publications that can expand your knowledge of complementary and alternative medicine and keep it current:
"The Hospital-Based Massage Network Newsletter" (focusing on massage therapists working in hospitals), 5 Old Town

Square, Suite 205, Fort Collins, CO 80524, 970-407-9232. Sample issue: $6; $28 yearly (4 issues).
Nurse Healers Professional Associates, Inc., 1211 Locust St., Philadelphia, PA 19107, 215-545-8079 (information about therapeutic touch).
Massage Magazine, 1315 W. Mallon Ave., Spokane, WA 99201, 800-533-4263.
Massage Therapy Journal, American Massage Therapy Association, 820 Davis St., Suite 110, Evanston, IL 60201, 847-864-0123.
National Association of Nurse Massage Therapists, P.O. Box 904, Carrboro, NC 27510, 888-805-7879, mailbox #125; e-mail: nanmt1@aol.com; Internet: http://www.mindspring.com/~csanks.

References

Groer, M., Mozingo, J., Droppleman, P., & Davis, M. (1994). Measures of salivary secretory immunoglobulin A and state anxiety after a nursing back rub. *Applied Nursing Research, 7*(1), 2–6.

Horrigan, B. (1998). Dolores Krieger, RN, PhD, Healing with therapeutic touch. (Interview). *Alternative Therapies in Health and Medicine, 4*(1), 86–92.

Jiming, C., Xinming, S., & Junqi, C. (1990). *Essentials of traditional Chinese pediatrics.* Beijing: Foreign Languages Press.

Kaada, B., & Torsteinbo, O. (1989). Increase of plasma beta-endorphins in connective tissue massage. *General Pharmacology, 20*(4), 487–489.

Knaster, M. (1998). Tiffany Field provides proof positive, scientifically. *Massage Therapy Journal, 37*(1), 84–88.

Koes, B.W., Bouter, L.M., van Mameren, H., & Essers, A.H. (1992). The effectiveness of manual therapy, physiotherapy, and treatment by the general practitioner for nonspecific back and neck complaints. *Spine, 17*(1), 28–35.

Mower, M.B. (1997, September/October). Massage returns to nursing. *Massage Magazine,* 46–55.

Neie, G. (1998, June 1). The truth about touch. [Letter to the editor]. *NurseWeek, 11*(11), 5.

Olson, M., Sneed, N., La Via, M., Virella, G., Bonadonna, R., & Michel, Y. (1997). Stress-induced immunosuppression and therapeutic touch. *Alternative Therapies in Health and Medicine, 3*(1), 68–74.

Puustjarvi, K., Airaksinen, O., & Pontinen, P.J. (1990). The effects of massage in patients with chronic tension headache. *Acupuncture and Electrotherapeutics Research, 15*(2), 159–162.

Rosa, L. (1998, June 1). The truth about touch. [Letter to the editor]. *NurseWeek, 11*(11), 5.

Rosa, L., Rosa, E., Sarner, L., & Barrett, S. (1998). A close look at therapeutic touch. *JAMA, 279*(13), 1005–1010.

Scafidi, F.A., Field, T., & Schanberg, S.M. (1993). Factors that predict which preterm infants benefit most from massage therapy. *Journal of Developmental and Behavioral Pediatrics, 14*(3), 176–80.

Scheiber, B. (1997). Therapeutic touch: Evaluating the "growing body of evidence" claim. *The Scientific Review of Alternative Medicine, 1*(1), 13–15.

Ulett, G. (1997). Therapeutic touch: Tracing back to Mesmer. *The Scientific Review of Alternative Medicine, 1*(1), 16–18.

Wheeden, A., Scafidi, F.A., Field, T., Ifonson, G. (1993). Massage effects on cocaine-exposed preterm neonates. *Journal of Developmental and Behavioral Pediatrics, 14*(3), 318–22.

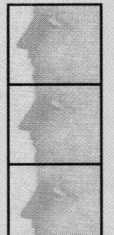

CROSS-CULTURAL CARE
CARING FOR A POLISH-AMERICAN JEWISH CLIENT

Ms. Weiss, the client whose story we have been following through the chapter, is an American-born Jew who lives in Manhattan. Her parents are Polish holocaust survivors who came to New York in 1944 and settled in Brooklyn. Although every client is unique, Jewish Americans from Poland tend to value the following:

- Open expression of feelings
- Getting the most direct and best help
- Being persistent and persuasive
- Achieving financial and educational success
- Solicitous maternal nurturing, such as overfeeding, permissiveness, and overprotection
- Educational and intellectual achievements
- Jewish values
- Observing certain precautions to prevent illness, such as not going out with wet hair, getting enough rest, staying in bed when not feeling well
- Home treatment for insomnia: a glass of wine

By the client's account, her sleepless nights are rooted in the stresses of school and job. Her ambitious work and school schedule reflects a heritage that prizes financial and educational success as well as intellectual achievements. Ms. Weiss' home remedies for her insomnia suggest that she has been taught additional Jewish values: that illness may result from lack of rest and that drinking wine at bedtime may help insomnia. The fact that her mother still regularly cooks for her even though she is living in a separate dwelling reveals a typically strong nurturing maternal tie. Finally, Ms. Weiss' culture is also reflected in her problem-solving approach; she persistently contacted the HMO until she obtained an appointment with the nurse practitioner. By availing herself of such services, she is attempting to obtain the most direct, readily available help.

Let's see how Susan, Ms. Weiss' nurse, demonstrated sensitivity to her client's cultural norms.

Susan: It sounds like your life is pretty stressful right now.

Ms. Weiss: Yes, it is. Between work and school, I am at my wit's end. To top it off, I can't get enough sleep. I'm beginning to feel as if life is too much. *[Ms. Wiess begins to cry.]*

Susan: [Hands Ms. Weiss some facial tissues and gives her a big hug. After a few minutes, she resumes the conversation.] I'm sorry you're having such a difficult time. Although your life is stressful right now, I can teach you ways to get a better night's sleep. Feeling well rested may help you to better manage your other problems and avoid getting sick. Let's talk about progressive muscle relaxation first.

Ms. Weiss: Muscle relaxation may be all very well and good, but I think that sleeping pills may be a more expedient method to begin with.

Susan: Have you ever heard of progressive muscle relaxation?

Ms. Weiss: No . . . but don't sleeping pills help you relax?

Susan: Actually, one of the best cures for insomnia is a relaxed body and mind. Progressive muscle relaxation helps your body relax. There are several studies that document the adverse effects of sleeping medications. Others have shown that muscle relaxation and cognitive strategies are very effective in treating insomnia. If you're interested, I'll be glad to give you copies of these studies at your next scheduled appointment."

Ms. Weiss: I would like that very much. I'm willing to try and learn about progressive muscle relaxation since, as you suggest, it is one of the best treatments.

Critical Thinking Questions

- What maternal nurturing did Susan use to foster the client's comfort and security?
- How did Susan use her understanding of Ms. Weiss' cultural patterns to teach effectively?
- Did Susan show a lack of cultural sensitivity when fielding Ms. Weiss' questions about sleeping pills? Justify your answer.

References

Leininger, M. (1991). *Culture care diversity and universality: A theory of nursing.* New York: National League for Nursing Press.
Spector, R.E. (1991). *Cultural diversity in health and illness* (3rd ed.). Norwalk, CT: Appleton & Lange.

Portions of chart from Spector, R.E. (1991). Cultural diversity in health and illness (3rd ed.). Norwalk, CT: Appleton & Lange.

General Assessment of Sleep and Rest
Sleep History

Because most data about sleep pattern disturbances are subjective, the nursing history serves as the primary source of information about sleep problems. To obtain such a history, conduct an interview that identifies normal sleep-wake patterns, bedtime routines, and risk factors that contribute to sleep disturbances. To screen for sleep problems, ask the following questions (Cohen, Ferrans, Vizgirda, Kundle, & Cloninger, 1996):

- What time do you usually go to bed?
- Do you have any bedtime routines?
- How long does it take you to get to sleep?
- How easy or difficult is it for you to fall asleep?
- Do you awaken at night? If so, how often, and what is it that most frequently awakens you?
- What do you do when you awaken in the middle of the night?
- How would you describe your sleep?
- Is your sleep restless or restful?
- What time do you awaken in the morning?
- When you awaken, do feel refreshed or tired?
- Is the number of hours you sleep at night about right for you?

- Do you nap during the day? If so, how many naps do you take?
- How long is your usual nap?
- Does your bed partner ever complain about your sleep behaviors?
- Do you regularly take any over-the-counter or prescription drugs?

A weekly sleep diary may provide additional clues about sleep disorders and sleep pattern disturbances (Fig. 41–5). Instruct the client to record the following information:

- Changes in sleep-wake patterns
- The number and duration of awakenings
- Sensations just before and during sleep
- The emotional content of dreams

SLEEP DIARY

Name: _____ Remember to complete this diary each morning approximately 15-20 minutes after awakening.

Fill in date under each day   YESTERDAY: THIS MORNING:

	When I went to sleep last night I felt (circle one)	I went to bed at: (time)	I fell asleep in: (minutes)	During the night, I awoke at: (time)	And stayed awake for: (minutes)	During the night I awoke at: (time)	I slept a total of: (hours)	When I got up this morning, I felt: (circle one)	Overall, my sleep last night was: (circle one)	I use an alarm (yes/no)
Monday	–2 –1 0 +1 +2			— — — — — —	— — — — — —			–2 –1 0 +1 +2	–2 –1 0 +1 +2	
Tuesday	–2 –1 0 +1 +2			— — — — — —	— — — — — —			–2 –1 0 +1 +2	–2 –1 0 +1 +2	
Wednesday	–2 –1 0 +1 +2			— — — — — —	— — — — — —			–2 –1 0 +1 +2	–2 –1 0 +1 +2	
Thursday	–2 –1 0 +1 +2			— — — — — —	— — — — — —			–2 –1 0 +1 +2	–2 –1 0 +1 +2	
Friday	–2 –1 0 +1 +2			— — — — — —	— — — — — —			–2 –1 0 +1 +2	–2 –1 0 +1 +2	
Saturday	–2 –1 0 +1 +2			— — — — — —	— — — — — —			–2 –1 0 +1 +2	–2 –1 0 +1 +2	
Sunday	–2 –1 0 +1 +2			— — —	— — —			–2 –1 0 +1 +2	–2 –1 0 +1 +2	

Figure 41–5. A sleep diary. Clients use such diaries to document difficulty falling asleep, interrupted sleep, awakening earlier or later than desired, and not feeling well rested. (Recreated from Berrios, G.E., & Shapiro, C.M. [1993]. ABC of sleep disorders: "I don't get enough sleep, doctor." British Medical Journal, 306(6892), 843–846.)

- Alterations in diet, weight, lifestyle
- Alcohol intake
- Menstruation
- Sexual habits
- Consumption of sleeping pills and other drugs
- Daytime work performance
- Conditions under which the client is unable to fall asleep (Berrios & Shapiro, 1993).

If chronic fatigue syndrome is suspected, question the client also about complaints of impaired memory and concentration, muscle pain, multijoint pain without inflammation, headache, depression, and anxiety. In addition, a thorough description of the fatigue is important, including the nature of the fatigue and the impact of fatigue on the client's lifestyle.

Physical Examination

Behavioral manifestations of insufficient or unsatisfactory sleep include agitation, disorientation, mood alterations, restlessness, memory loss, difficulty concentrating, a decreased attention span, lethargy, and apathy. The client also may have mild, fleeting nystagmus (constant involuntary movement of the eyeballs), ptosis (drooping of the eyelids), thickened speech, dark circles under the eyes, frequent yawning, muscle tremors, and a lack of coordination.

Some physical findings in fatigued clients overlap with those found in clients with sleep pattern disturbances. They too may demonstrate memory loss and an inability to concentrate. In addition, fatigued clients often suffer from activity intolerance, manifested as an increased heart rate, blood pressure, and respirations in response to minimal exertion. Their movements may be slow and deliberate, reflecting an attempt to conserve energy. These clients appear lethargic and disinterested in their surroundings.

Recall the case of Emma Weiss. The nursing assessment for Ms. Weiss during her visit to the health maintenance organization was as follows:

Client is a 48-year-old, white, Jewish female with complaints of transient situational insomnia for 3 months. Wants sleeping pills. Self-medication with chicken soup and/or a glass of wine at bedtime unsuccessful in controlling symptoms. Client reports increasing cigarette consumption in response to stress of school and work. Now smokes one PPD compared with one-half PPD 3 months ago, and she smokes from the minute she awakens until the moment she gets into bed. Drinks up to 10 cups of coffee a day to "stay awake at work." Feels that mood swings and irritability secondary to sleep deprivation are affecting relationships with coworkers. Notes decreased ability to focus on details of work. Reports usual HS is 11:00 PM. For the past 2½ months, cannot fall asleep for at least 2 hours after retiring. Awakens four to five times during the night because of nightmares and once or twice due to nocturia. Sometimes tries to nap during lunch hour. Yawns frequently. Fine intentional tremor present. Eyes have deep circles. BP 120/80, HR 104, RR 24, T 98.6° Fahrenheit, orally.

Ms. Weiss' blood pressure, pulse, and respirations are slightly higher than normal. Can you suggest possible reasons for these elevations? Consider what action(s) you might take to validate your hypotheses about the cause of these elevated vital signs.

Diagnostic Tests

People with long-standing unresolved sleep problems may be referred for formal sleep studies. **Polysomnography** is the continuous measurement and recording of physiological activity during sleep by using electroencephalogram (EEG), electro-oculogram (EOG), electrocardiogram (ECG), and electromyogram (EMG) tracings to monitor brain activity, eye movements, heart rate and rhythm, and muscle movements. Polysomnography is usually performed during an overnight stay in a sleep laboratory; synchronized recordings of electrical activity in the brain, muscles, eyes, and heart are taken (Fig. 41–6).

An EEG quantifies the brain's electrical activity by means of electrodes placed on the scalp. It monitors all stages of REM and NREM sleep. The EOG measures electrical activity associated with eye movements, helping to identify periods of REM sleep. In the EMG, electrodes are placed on the anterior tibialis and submental muscles (under the chin) to detect muscular electrical activity. An ECG reveals any cardiac arrhythmias that may occur. Analysis of data collected from polysomnography can help diagnose dyssomnias and parasomnias as well as pathologies that might cause disturbed sleep.

The **multiple sleep latency test** is a direct, objective measure of sleepiness used to evaluate excessive somnolence and daytime sleepiness. Another formal sleep study, it is a well-validated instrument designed to quantify daytime sleepiness. The client is given four to five 20-minute nap opportunities at 2-hour intervals. If sleep occurs in less than 7 minutes for three or more tests, an abnormal level of sleepiness is indicated. This test can help establish a definite diagnosis for narcolepsy because narcoleptics will have sleep-onset REM episodes in addition to rapid sleep onset. For the test to be valid, the client must be instructed to discontinue all drugs that are known to affect sleep at least 2 weeks before the day of the test. The client should not take alcohol or caffeine on the day of the test and must discontinue smoking and strenuous activity at least 30 minutes before the test.

Wrist actigraphs are a relatively new means of measuring outpatient clients' sleep in their homes. A transducer is worn on the wrist so that all wrist movements can be recorded during sleep. Increased movement signals restlessness and therefore lighter sleep.

Based on her sleep history and physical findings, is Ms. Weiss a candidate for these diagnostic tests? Justify your answer.

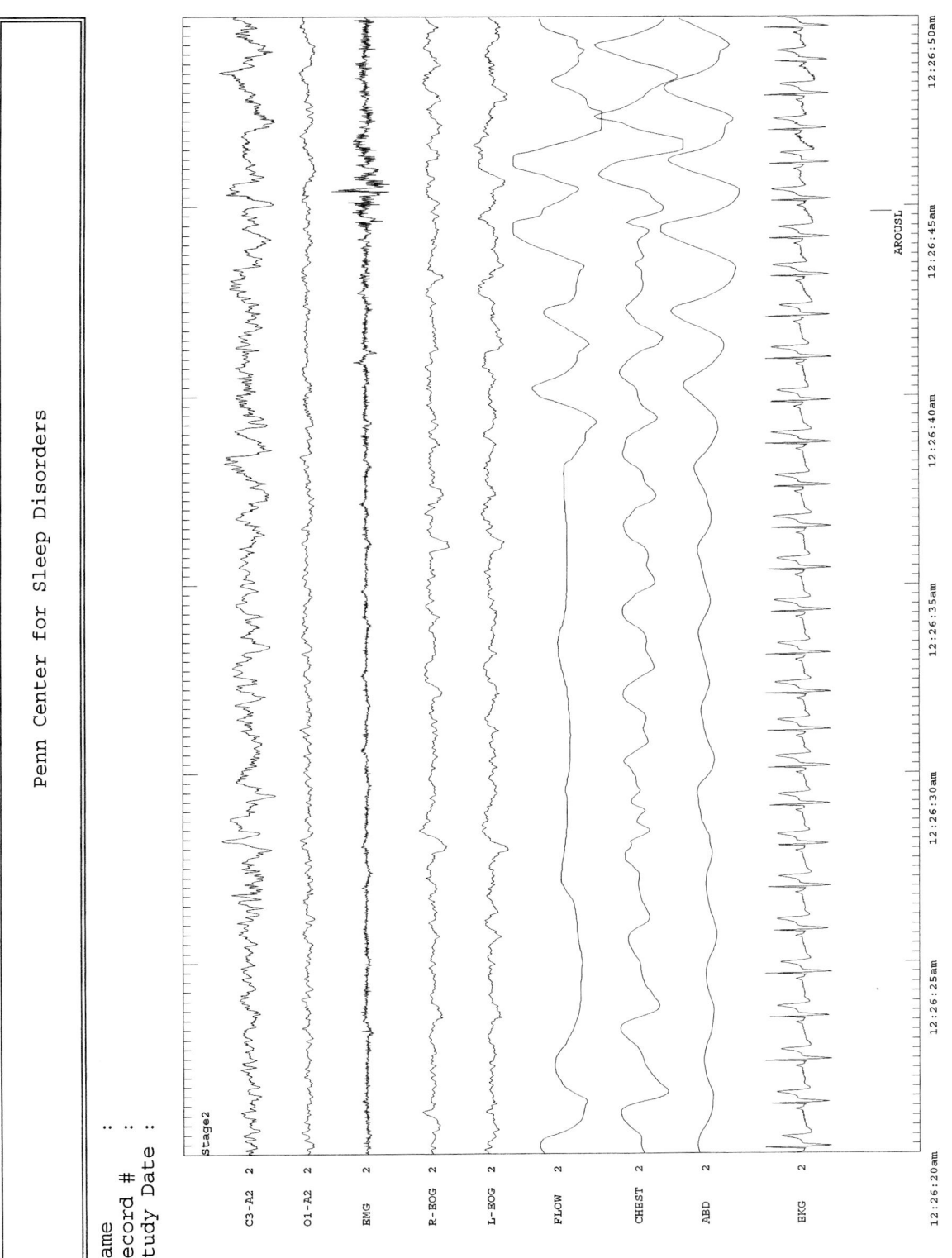

Penn Center for Sleep Disorders

Name   :
Record #   :
Study Date :

Stage2

C3-A2   2

O1-A2   2

EMG   2

R-EOG   2

L-EOG   2

FLOW   2

CHEST   2

ABD   2

EKG   2

AROUSL

12:26:20am   12:26:25am   12:26:30am   12:26:35am   12:26:40am   12:26:45am   12:26:50am

Figure 41-6. Polysomnography. Continuous electro-oculography, electromyography, electrocardiography, and electroencephalography tracings are recorded while the client sleeps. The tracings are then reviewed for evidence of sleep disorders. (PSG tracing courtesy of the University of Pennsylvania Center for Sleep Disorders, Philadelphia, PA.)

Focused Assessment for Sleep Pattern Disturbance and Fatigue

Defining Characteristics of Sleep Pattern Disturbance

A *Sleep pattern disturbance* is a temporary disruption or disturbance in the client's usual sleep patterns that a nurse can prevent or treat independently (NANDA, 1998). Clients with such disturbances typically present with at least one of four critical defining characteristics: difficulty falling asleep, interrupted sleep, awakening earlier or later than desired, and not feeling well-rested. Data clusters help identify these defining characteristics.

When a client complains of sleeplessness, increased restlessness, an inability to relax, and racing thoughts at bedtime, it typically indicates difficulty

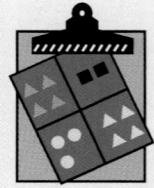

CLUSTERING DATA TO MAKE A NURSING DIAGNOSIS
SLEEP PROBLEMS

Data Cluster	Diagnosis
76-year-old admitted to the hospital from nursing home with a diagnosis of urosepsis. History of nocturnal confusion and wanderings. Awakens 3–4 times with nocturia since onset of urinary tract problems	*Risk for injury* related to nocturnal confusion and nocturia
60-year-old hospitalized for gastroesophageal reflux. Awakened for the following interventions during the night: 12 midnight and 1:00 AM for IV medication administration; 2:00 AM for vital sign check and 6:00 AM for hygiene measures. Sleep also interrupted at 3:30 AM by ringing phone and nurses' conversation about phone call. In addition, heartburn disturbed sleep at 3:00 AM Client complains of feeling poorly rested the following morning	*Sleep pattern disturbance* related to pain and frequent awakenings
40-year old factory worker with a 1-year history of narcolepsy, fired from several jobs after repeatedly falling asleep. Admits to "heavy drinking" after being fired.	*Ineffective individual coping* related to changes in arousal secondary to narcolepsy
A 50-year-old 1 week after open-heart surgery refuses to perform AM care or ambulate as instructed. Complains of inability to sleep at night in such a strange and noisy environment. Reports an average of 0–1 hour of sleep per night.	*Self-care deficit* related to lack of motivation secondary to sleep deprivation
69-year-old with GI bleeding and multiple complications has been in ICU for 4 days. Requires NG tube suctioning, cardiac and arterial monitoring, multiple medication pump delivery systems, and a ventilator. Staff keep lights on at all times to monitor the client more closely. Client has become increasingly irritable and confused about where he is and how long he has been there. He constantly pulls at the IV tubing, the NG tube, and ventilator attachments.	*Risk for altered thought processes* (ICU syndrome) related to sensory overload and sleep deprivation
64-year-old spouse of a stroke victim confides to the nurse that she is at wit's end with caring for her husband. Feels she could handle daytime caregiver activities if able to get a good night's sleep. Awakens 10–12 times a night from her husband's loud snoring and snorting.	(Wife) *Risk for ineffective family coping* related to stress associated with spouse's care (Husband) *Impaired gas exchange* related to sleep apnea

falling asleep. Problems falling asleep may also be linked to a change in one's normal sleep schedule.

A client may describe interrupted sleep as awakening at night and being unable to go back to sleep. Excessively rumpled bedding may indicate that increased restlessness has caused brief but unremembered arousals. The client's bed partner may describe frequent leg twitching, jerks, or kicks during the night. If obstructive sleep apnea is causing the interrupted sleep, the partner may mention loud snoring, gasping, or choking.

Action Alert!
When a client or bed partner complains of pauses, gasps, choking, or loud respirations during sleep, the client should be referred to a physician for evaluation of possible sleep apnea.

A cue that the client is awakening earlier than desired might be the statement, "I woke at 4:00 AM and tossed and turned until the alarm went off." Alternatively, the client awakening later than desired might complain, "I just can't seem to drag myself out of bed to get to work on time."

The client who does not feel well-rested may complain of feeling exhausted or fatigued from lack of sleep. This client may doze frequently and need frequent naps or increased caffeine to stay alert during the day. Excessive daytime sleepiness due to a sleep pattern disturbance is most frequently associated with sleep deprivation. Sleep deprivation and other sleep problems that result in excessive sleepiness must be differentiated from the excessive sleepiness associated with narcolepsy. The narcoleptic frequently falls asleep while doing tedious tasks, while driving, or during a conversation.

Action Alert!
The statement "I can fall asleep anytime" can be a sign of trouble. Consider referring a client who makes such statements to a physician for further evaluation for narcolepsy.

Defining Characteristics of Fatigue

Fatigue is an overwhelming sustained sense of exhaustion and decreased capacity for physical and mental work (NANDA, 1999). It is characterized by an incessant and overwhelming lack of energy and an inability to maintain usual routines. Manifestations of physical and mental fatigue differ. Clients often describe physical fatigue as feeling tired, exhausted, or weak. They may also complain of muscle aches, no energy, and a need to lie down to recover. Symptoms of mental fatigue include poor concentration, poor memory, little interest, feelings of sadness, or an inability to get out of bed.

Although fatigue can be a symptom of excessive physical activity and emotional stress, it can also be attributed to lack of sleep. In essence, fatigue is nature's warning that rest or sleep is needed. However, chronic fatigue is abnormal and commonly associated with illness.

Based on information collected in the nursing interview with Ms. Weiss, is she experiencing fatigue, a sleep pattern disturbance, or both? Justify your answer.

Related Factors

As implied in earlier discussions, a sleep pattern disturbance is influenced by changes in internal sensory input and external stimuli. Internal alterations include such variables as hormones, neurotransmitters, illness, and psychological stress. External events, such as environmental changes and social cues, may also create sleep pattern disturbances.

Fatigue may be experienced after increased or decreased metabolic demands, overwhelming psychological or emotional demands, increased energy needs to carry out activities of daily living, demanding role or social interactions, states of discomfort, and changes in body chemistry (as from medications, drug withdrawal, and chemotherapy).

Focused Assessment for Related Nursing Diagnoses

Risk for Injury

A client with a primary sleep disorder is at high risk for injury. Two-thirds of narcoleptics have fallen asleep while driving, and 80% have fallen asleep while at work (Aldrich, 1992). Several studies have found a twofold to sevenfold increase in traffic accidents among people with sleep apnea (Shapiro & Dement, 1993).

Even people who do not suffer from a primary sleep disorder may be at risk for motor vehicle accidents during vulnerable periods of the sleep-wake cycle. Most people are sleepiest and least alert between 2:00 AM and 7:00 AM, and between 2:00 PM and 5:00 PM. Research into accidents and performance failures within a 24-hour period show a pattern that correlates very closely with these sleep-vulnerable periods (Shapiro & Dement, 1993).

Accidents in the home can also occur during periods of arousal from sleep. If a person needs intermittent medication at night, for example, she is at risk for falling when getting out of bed to take the medication. Likewise, clients with nocturia or incontinence may be injured in their efforts to reach the bathroom. A client with dementia may become confused or disoriented and try to climb out of bed. If the side rails are up, the person may fall and become injured.

Because sleep deprivation increases the risk for accidents and Ms. Weiss is sleep-deprived, what safety issues need to be addressed with her?

Self-Care Deficit

The sleep-deprived or fatigued client may experience a *Self-care deficit,* an inability to carry out activities of daily living. The tasks most influenced by inadequate sleep are those that require prolonged concentration or

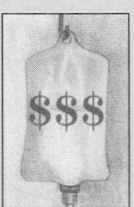

THE COST OF CARE
UNTIMELY SLEEPING

Falling asleep at inopportune times costs billions of dollars in accidents per year. Research has demonstrated that in every work situation in which vigilance is necessary, accident probability correlates positively with the biological tendency to fall asleep. Thus, the majority of work-related accidents occur from midnight to 6:00 AM and 1:00 to 3:00 PM, when humans are most sleep-prone.

Nowhere is this trend better documented than in the trucking industry, where long hauls during peak sleep times place truck drivers at increased risk for accidents. An estimated 57% of the 4,800 annual truck-related fatal accidents result from what sleep specialists would describe as "sleepiness." Since the mean cost of a fatal crash is 2.7 million dollars, the estimated annual expense of sleep-associated fatal trucking accidents alone is over 7 billion dollars!

Discussion

These grim statistics suggest a need to focus public attention on the hazards of sleep-based fatigue. They also point to the necessity of developing a wiser public policy concerning sleep and sleep disorders.

Reference

Mitler, M., Dinges, D.F., & Dement, W.C. (1994). Sleep medicine, public policy and public health. In M.H., Kryger, T., Roth, & W.C. Dement, (Eds.), *Principles and practice of sleep medicine* (2nd ed.). Philadelphia: W.B. Saunders Co.

vigilance, such as cooking, shopping, and driving (Foreman & Wykle, 1995). Performance worsens as the time between the morning awakening and the task performance lengthens. For hospitalized clients, the psychological effects of sleep deprivation may influence recovery. The lack of motivation or cooperation may impede progression to independent self-care and can result in noncompliance with the treatment regimen.

Ineffective Individual Coping/Ineffective Family Coping

Ineffective individual coping may easily result from some sleep disturbances. For example, narcolepsy and sleep apnea can impair job performance and cause problems in interpersonal relationships. These additional stressors may make it even more difficult to deal with the primary illness. The family may be adversely affected by such sleep disorders, especially if family members think that daytime sleepiness can be voluntarily controlled.

Likewise, sleep deprivation can lead to a decreased ability to cope in any number of stressful situations. For example, parenting frequently leads to chronic sleep deprivation. Coping with a newborn's nocturnal awakenings, dealing with a colicky baby, or working outside the home while trying to raise a family can lead to a chronic lack of sleep. Family coping can also be strained by childhood parasomnias. Sleepwalking and night terrors can be very frightening to parents, and nocturnal enuresis can be a major nuisance. Parents may develop symptoms of sleep pattern disturbance as they attempt to cope with their child's nocturnal arousals.

Parenting is not the sole source of sleep deprivation and ineffective coping. For the working adult, a demanding job or shift rotations may limit the number of hours available for sleep. Illness can take its toll as well. Chronic pain, cardiovascular disease, pulmonary disorders, neurological problems, endocrine imbalance, renal disease, and cancer may impinge on sleep cycles, further taxing the client's ability to cope with these health problems. Finally, family caregivers may suffer from exhaustion, sleep deprivation, and an inability to cope. In all cases, chronic sleep deprivation may lead to ineffective and dangerous self-treatment programs, such as abuse of hypnotics or alcohol.

What are some key elements in Ms. Weiss' story that suggest she is having difficulty coping?

Altered Thought Processes

A client suffering from sleep deprivation may experience *Altered thought processes* because sleep deprivation can cause an inability to sustain one's thoughts, increased anxiety, and visual or auditory hallucinations. Such changes may translate into an inability to concentrate, suspiciousness, and inaccurate interpretations of the environment. This phenomenon is well documented in *ICU psychosis*, which has been previously discussed.

DIAGNOSIS

Sleep pattern disturbances are distinct from the diseases of sleep, called sleep pathologies, which are treated by a physician. Although nurses are not expected to diagnose these sleep pathologies, they do collaborate with other members of the health care team to manage them. This management includes monitoring and reporting signs and symptoms that suggest the presence of or a change in a sleep pathology; teaching clients about medications, equipment, and procedures necessary to manage the disorder; and treating any sleep pattern disturbances that may arise as the result of a sleep pathology.

Clues that you gather during the nursing history and physical examination will help you differentiate sleep pattern disturbances from sleep pathologies, fatigue, and other related nursing diagnoses that may mimic or share common features with these problems.

To use the nursing diagnosis *Sleep pattern disturbance* accurately, you must determine if the sleep pattern is the problem or if it is an etiologic factor contributing to another problem. For instance, pain and anxiety may contribute to sleep pattern disturbances, but they are also sometimes nursing problems themselves.

Likewise, for a client with symptoms of physical or mental exhaustion, you must decide if the fatigue is a symptom of a sleep pattern disturbance or if it is actually a discrete nursing problem.

If *Fatigue* has been ruled out, and you have ascertained that the client has a sleep problem, you must differentiate sleep pattern disturbances from primary and secondary sleep disorders.

Sometimes *Sleep pattern disturbance* and *Fatigue* may be accurate diagnoses, but they do not focus on key elements of care as well as other nursing diagnoses might. For example, cardiac clients often have increased rest needs and fatigue as a result of chronic hypoxia. However, if the cardiac client is undergoing rehabilitation, *Activity intolerance* rather than *Fatigue* better focuses on the goals of therapy.

PLANNING

If the identified problem has been difficulty falling asleep, then the client's report of rapid sleep onset is the expected outcome. Additional relevant client behaviors that support this outcome include the following:

- Demonstrates use of bedtime routines
- Exercises 20 to 30 minutes three to four times a week
- Keeps a sleep diary for at least 1 week
- Discontinues use of any prescription or over-the-counter medications that might interfere with sleep onset (such as analgesics that contain caffeine, CNS stimulants, etc.)
- Recites the purpose, dose, schedule, and side effects of hypnotics used

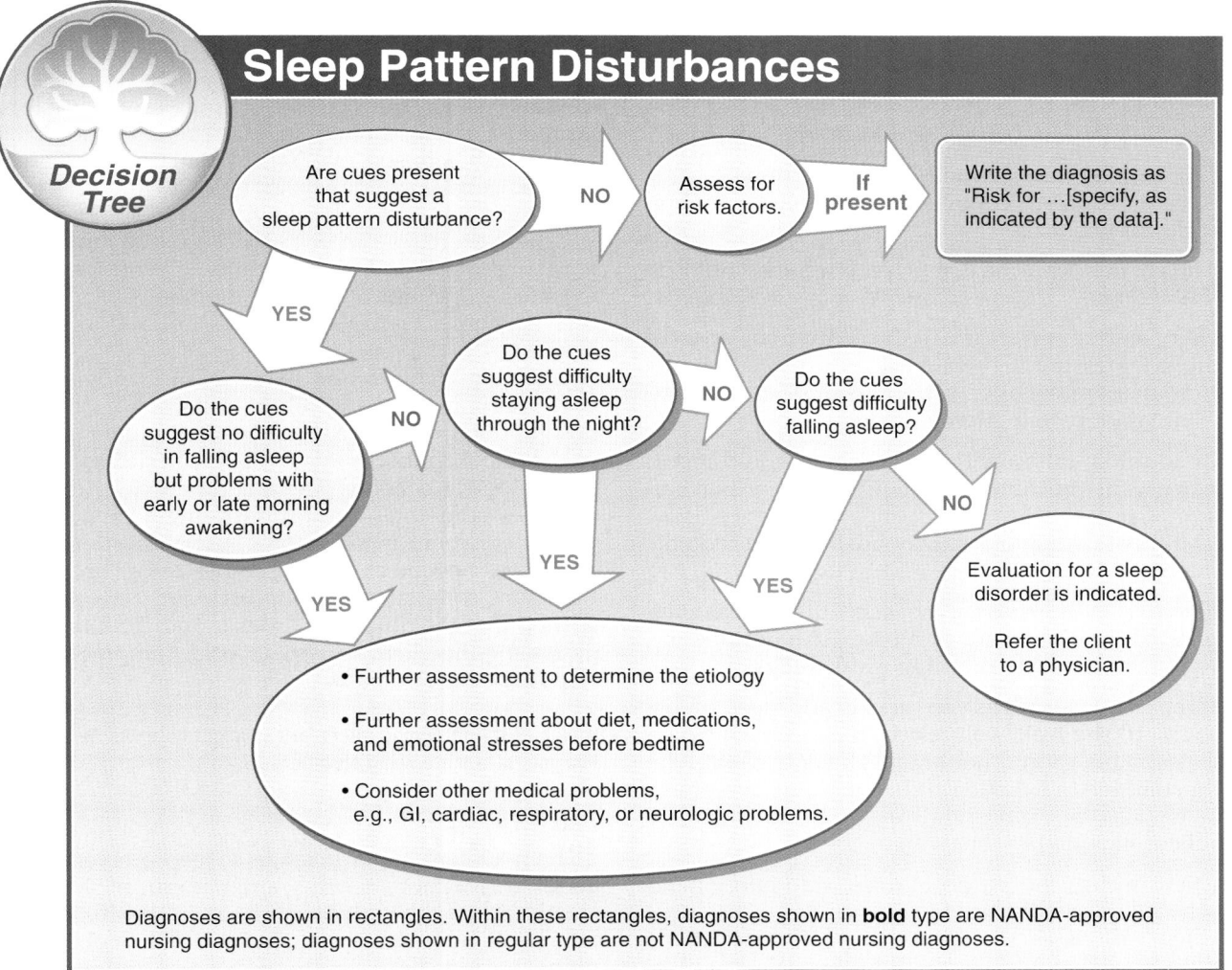

Sleep Pattern Disturbances

Decision Tree

Are cues present that suggest a sleep pattern disturbance? — **NO** → Assess for risk factors. — **If present** → Write the diagnosis as "Risk for …[specify, as indicated by the data]."

YES ↓

Do the cues suggest no difficulty in falling asleep but problems with early or late morning awakening? — **NO** → Do the cues suggest difficulty staying asleep through the night? — **NO** → Do the cues suggest difficulty falling asleep? — **NO** → Evaluation for a sleep disorder is indicated. Refer the client to a physician.

YES (from early/late morning awakening)
YES (from difficulty staying asleep)
YES (from difficulty falling asleep)

↓

- Further assessment to determine the etiology
- Further assessment about diet, medications, and emotional stresses before bedtime
- Consider other medical problems, e.g., GI, cardiac, respiratory, or neurologic problems.

Diagnoses are shown in rectangles. Within these rectangles, diagnoses shown in **bold** type are NANDA-approved nursing diagnoses; diagnoses shown in regular type are not NANDA-approved nursing diagnoses.

Which of these behavioral outcomes might be appropriate for Ms. Weiss? Justify your answer.

For problems with interrupted sleep, successful management should result in client behaviors to decrease factors that interfere with sleep. Possible outcomes include:

- Client does not eat heavy or fat-filled foods just before going to sleep.
- Client eliminates sources of sleep disruption in the home environment (purchases heavy drapes to darken sleep area, for example, or uses white noise or ear plugs to eliminate excess noise).
- Client avoids alcohol for at least 5 hours before going to sleep.

Are any of these behavioral outcomes appropriate for Ms. Weiss? Justify your answer.

If sleep has been interrupted by concomitant medical problems, then expected behaviors would be those that suggest better management of responses to such problems. For example, the client with pain would be expected to do the following:

- Report that pain has decreased to an acceptable level, using a pain scale from 0 to 10 to describe what is acceptable
- Take analgesics as needed 30 to 60 minutes before going to bed

The client with nocturia would do the following:

- Discontinue fluids 2 hours before bedtime
- Keep a bedpan or commode at the bedside for episodes of nocturia

The client with obstructive sleep apnea would do the following:

- Demonstrate correct use of the continuous positive airway pressure (CPAP) mask
- Eliminate intake of CNS depressants
- Maintain a patent airway during sleep

In addition, this client's bed partner would report a decrease in the number of snoring, snorting episodes.

The client with depression or anxiety would do the following:

- Describe the purpose, dose, schedule, and side effects of antidepressant or anxiolytic medications
- Report fewer early morning awakenings

If the client can fall asleep quickly and sleep undisturbed until she feels well rested, then excessive daytime sleepiness should not occur. The only client who might continue to experience such daytime symptoms is the narcoleptic. Appropriate expected outcomes for this client include the following:

- Client recites the purpose, dose, side effects, and schedule of medications.
- Client discusses the illness and its implications with employer and significant other(s).

- Client takes daytime naps, when needed, to maintain alertness.
- Client reports decreased number of sleep attacks, hypnagogic hallucinations, and cataplexy.

Given Ms. Weiss' sleep history, what statements would be appropriate subjective measures that her sleep has improved? What objective parameters could serve as sleep improvement outcome criteria?

INTERVENTION

To better plan and implement strategies that promote sleep among hospitalized clients, you must consider factors that clients find disruptive and those they find conducive to sleep. In a study by Reimer (1987), clients identified the following sleep-promoting factors: staying up later than lights out, back rubs, sleeping medications, position changes, supportive communication, snacks or drinks, turning the lights down, and ensuring quiet. The interventions described below focus on meeting these client-identified needs.

Interventions to Promote Sleep Onset

Helping the Client Relax

A client with insomnia has increased sympathetic nervous system tone. Relaxation may help decrease this tone and, hence, promote sleep. Progressive muscle relaxation and deep breathing have proven beneficial in insomniacs (Johnson, 1991). The client can be taught to tense and relax voluntary muscles in the feet, legs, back, stomach, arms, shoulders, neck, face, and eyes.

These exercises can be practiced for 20 minutes after going to bed and at other times of protracted waking during the night. In adults, hot baths taken in the early evening may also promote relaxation (Carey, 1996).

Position changes and extra pillows provide support and comfort. In addition, a back rub—the purposeful manipulation of back, neck, shoulder, and upper buttock muscles—provides physiological and psychological benefits. The accompanying Procedure provides guidelines for administering a back rub.

For the client who has pain, premedicate with analgesics as needed about 30 minutes before bedtime. If the client complains of constant pain, consider suggesting that the physician order round-the-clock analgesics for the client. Warm or cold compresses may also help alleviate pain.

Which of the foregoing interventions might help Ms. Weiss meet her goal of a more rapid sleep onset?

Teaching Behavioral Strategies

To help a client better manage a sleep problem, teach about the function, benefits, and patterns of sleep. You should also work with the client to establish a regular, reliable 24-hour sleep-wake pattern. The Bootzin technique involves behavioral modification strategies that

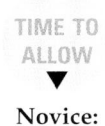

PROCEDURE 41-1

Back Massage

TIME TO
ALLOW
▼
Novice:
20 min.
Expert:
20 min.

A therapeutic massage is given for the purpose of relaxing tense muscles, relieving muscle spasms, inducing rest or sleep, or stimulating circulation to maintain skin integrity. It may be given as part of a bed bath, as part of a bedtime ritual, or at any time when the client needs a period of quiet rest.

Delegation Guidelines

Back massage may be delegated to a nursing assistant following RN assessment of the appropriateness of massage for the individual client and possible contraindications, such as skin impairment, wounds, and position intolerance. The nursing assistant should receive training in massage techniques and be instructed to observe skin integrity, especially overlying bony structures.

Equipment Needed

- Soft towel
- Body lotion of client's choice

---

1 Decide if the client needs or can tolerate a back massage.

Back massage promotes relaxation and comfort, which can help induce sleep. Rib or vertebral fractures, burns, or open wounds may be contraindications.

---

2 Prepare the environment for the procedure.
a. Adjust the light and temperature, and eliminate any unnecessary noises.
b. Close the door or curtain.

Bright lights, noise, and lack of privacy can increase muscle tension or make the client feel ill at ease.

---

3 Prepare the client for the procedure.
a. Raise the bed to a comfortable working height.
b. Lower the side rail and help the client into a prone or semiprone position. The client's position should be relaxed and comfortable.
c. Expose the client's back, shoulders, upper arms, and sacral area, covering the rest of her body with the extra blanket.

A raised bed and proper client positioning help ensure proper body mechanics while you apply pressure to the client's back muscles.

---

4 Administer the back rub.
a. Type of stroke
  Effleurage–Long, smooth stroke sliding over the skin; relaxing and soothing.
  Petrissage–Kneading of skin and underlying muscles; induces relaxation in tight or tense muscles and promotes circulation.

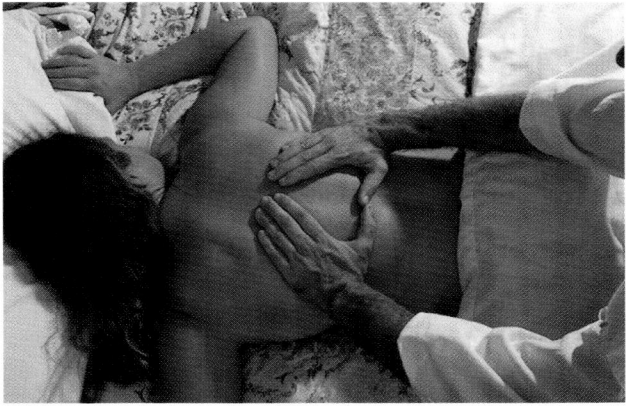

Friction: small circular strokes moving down both sides of the vertebral column.

  Tapotement–Rhythmic percussion or tapping; used particularly over tense muscles; should be done gently.
  Friction–Use of small circular strokes where movement of the hands also moves the underlying tissue.
b. Pattern of stroke
  1. Begin with effleurage. Start in the small of the back, using both hands (one on each side, close to the vertebral column), and stroke gently but firmly to the shoulders. Leave the hands on the skin and return to the small of the back, tracing the lateral aspects of the back. *This technique begins the relaxation process and allows you to assess for tension in particular muscles.* Repeat 8–10 times.
  2. Focus on the neck and shoulders. Use friction strokes at the base of the skull. Knead the shoulder (trapezius) muscles. Repeat 8–10 times.

Continued

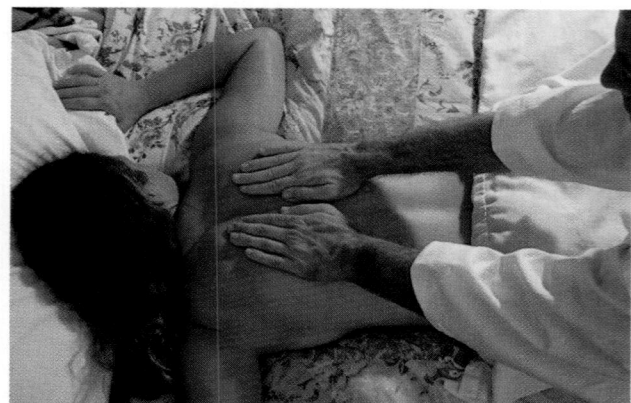

Effleurage: long, smooth strokes from the small of the back to the shoulders.

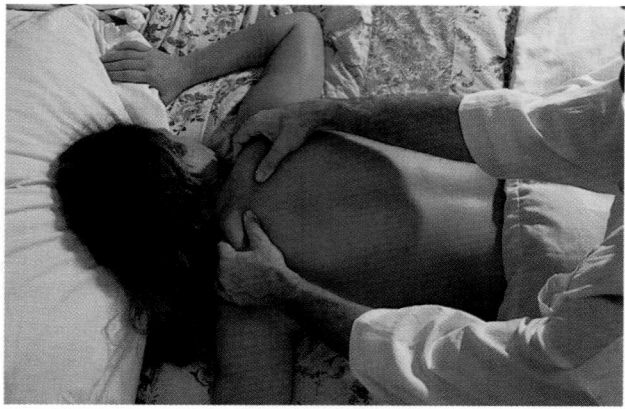

Petrissage: kneading the shoulder muscles.

3. Focus on the muscles, moving down both sides of the vertebral column. Use circular friction strokes. Repeat 3–5 circles in each area, ending with the lumbar region. *Concentrate on areas of tension.*
4. Focus on the small of the back. Use effleurage from the center of the spine and out in all directions.
5. Repeat steps 2 to 4 with tapotement if desired.
6. Use effleurage from side to side. Start at the top, and move down the back. Repeat 1–3 times.
7. Finish with effleurage as in step 1. *This is the most relaxing stroke and will induce sleep in some clients if the massage has been well done.* As a final step, gradually slow the strokes and decrease the pressure until your hands are no longer touching the client.

Gentle firm pressure applied to all muscle groups facilitates muscle relaxation. Kneading increases circulation to the back muscles.

5 Wipe off the extra lotion and help the client put on her gown or pajamas, if needed.

Some clients find wet lotion too irritating and bedclothes too confining.

6 Lower the bed and raise the side rails, if necessary, before you leave the bedside.

Safety is an important consideration. Restraints can sometimes cause more injury than less restrictive interventions.

7 Make sure that client has no pain or, if the client has chronic pain, that the pain level is acceptable.

Client discomfort can interfere with sleep onset and maintenance.

8 Provide bedside equipment or medications if needed.

A client with nocturia may need a bedside commode, for example, and a client with angina may need medications at the bedside.

HINTS

1. Use prewarmed lotion. You can warm it by placing it in a basin of warm water for a few minutes before giving the back massage.
2. While massaging, keep continuous contact with the client's skin. Most clients find this contact soothing and are less likely to be startled by your hand movements.
3. Consider the client's cultural norms and personal preferences. For example, administer a modified massage if the client does not wish to disrobe during the procedure.

HOME CARE CONSIDERATIONS

Just like a nurse in an institutional setting, a busy family caregiver may find that giving a massage is one activity that is tempting to skip. However, if a massage helps prevent pressure ulcers or helps the client sleep through the night, it may be worthwhile. Encourage the family to use the time as a means of maintaining a bond with the client through a pleasurable activity. Teach skin assessment techniques as part of the massage.

Teaching for WELLNESS

THE BOOTZIN TECHNIQUE

Purpose: To improve sleep hygiene through behavioral modification techniques.

Rationale: Sleep onset insomnia is often related to poor sleep hygiene habits.

Expected Outcome: The client will fall asleep within 20 minutes after going to bed.

Client Instructions

- Go to bed only when you are sleepy.
- Use the bed only for sleeping and sex. Do not read, eat, or watch television in bed.
- If you cannot go to sleep after 30 minutes, get up and go to another room. Stay up until you are really sleepy, then return to bed. If sleep does not come easily, get out of bed again. The goal is to associate the bed not with frustration and sleeplessness, but with falling asleep easily and quickly.
- Repeat previous as often as necessary throughout the night.
- Set the alarm and get up at the same time every morning, regardless of how much or how little you slept during the night. This helps the body acquire a constant sleep-wake rhythm.
- Do not nap during the day.

Modified from Bootzin, R.R., & Nicasso, P. (1978). Behavioral treatments for insomnia. In M. Heron, et al., (Eds.). Progress in behavior modification. New York: Academic Press.

may help meet this goal. The Teaching for Wellness chart provides guidelines for teaching these behavioral techniques.

Although the role of naps remains somewhat controversial, most clinicians agree that naps can lead to desynchronization of the circadian sleep-wake cycle and thus contribute to sleep problems.

At home, the client should maintain a regular exercise program. One study showed that exercise helped to induce deep sleep and growth hormone production in a group of elderly clients (Carey, 1996). Even though 20 to 30 minutes of exercise three to four times a week is helpful, you should discourage the client from exercising within 2 hours of sleep because such physical exertion increases mental activity and physical functioning (Cohen & Merritt, 1992). Encourage an elderly client who cannot exercise to engage in a stimulating daytime schedule and increased social interaction. Such activities tend to decrease napping, which can interfere with nighttime sleep.

Bedtime routines have proven effective in shortening sleep-onset time and nocturnal awakenings in children and the elderly (Johnson, 1991; Johnson, Wise &

Jimmerson, 1995). Hygiene measures, prayer, light snacks, reading, or listening to music may be part of such rituals. Listening through headsets to quiet, non-vocal music and tapes with meditative prayers or messages from loved ones all help (Knapp, 1993). If the client has an established routine, you should honor it to the extent possible. For the client who has not yet recognized the importance of a bedtime ritual, identify and offer suggestions for activities that can be used at bedtime to enhance sleep.

While such behavioral techniques may be successful in alleviating insomnia, they cannot be expected to compensate for lack of discipline or an overtaxing daytime lifestyle. Some insomniacs may need to learn more about time, people, and stress management than about sleep management.

Which of the preceding intervention strategies would be appropriate for Ms. Weiss? What should you counsel her about naps?

Teaching Cognitive Strategies

Because insomnia is often precipitated by reflection or intrusive thoughts, you can help insomniacs by teaching them strategies to forestall such cognition. Remind the client that reflective thoughts may occur at bedtime only because bedtime is often the first opportunity to review the day's events. Teach her to prevent such bedtime ruminations by setting aside 20 minutes in the early evening after dinner to reflect on the day's events and consider achievements relative to objectives. Once problem areas and loose ends have been identified, she should schedule time to deal with the issues but do no actual work that evening.

Administering Medications

A client taking a hypnotic needs to be monitored and taught about the potential side effects, as outlined in Table 41–2. Some of these drugs affect memory; thus, more verbal and written reinforcements may be necessary. In addition, safety is an important issue in the sedated or less coordinated client.

Action **A**lert!
Monitor the sleep of an elderly client taking a hypnotic very closely! If she tries to get out of bed, she is likely to fall and injure herself.

Instruct the client to take her sleeping medication shortly before going to bed. Remember that many clients take their medication hours after retiring, when they have finally become frustrated by an inability to sleep. Consequently, their sleep will be out of phase with their normal sleep-wake circadian pattern, and they may experience increased daytime residual effects (Farney & Walker, 1995).

Do you think the nurse practitioner should give Ms. Weiss a prescription for hypnotics on the first visit? Justify your answer.

Preparing the Environment for Sleep

The sleep environment should be dark, uncluttered, comfortable, and as free of noise as possible. To darken the room, pull down window shades, and draw heavy drapes closed. In addition, shut the client's door, and dim the lights. Check equipment and door hinges regularly to decrease noise from these sources. Telephones and intercom systems should be equipped with flashing lights for nighttime use. If her condition permits, try to place the client away from the nurses' station and housekeeping closets. If needed, provide the client with earplugs or cotton balls to dampen excessive environmental noise.

In addition, when nursing units are being built or remodeled, toilets should be soundproofed and windows double-glazed. Floor coverings, such as carpets, can also decrease noise. Heating-system controls should be installed so that nurses can regulate ambient temperatures to meet client needs.

Institutions should make noise or disturbance audits part of ongoing nursing quality assurance. They should also provide in-service education about normal sleep patterns and primary and secondary sleep disorders to evening- and night-shift nurses.

In the intensive care unit, with its heavy reliance on equipment and intensive monitoring, noise is a particularly acute problem. When intravenous controllers and ventilator alarms are routed away from the bed at night, sleep pattern disturbances may be reduced. Prepare needles and syringes away from the bedside, and turn suction and oxygen off after use if they are unnecessary. You should also consider the meaning of noise to each individual. If you explain the necessity and significance of unfamiliar sounds, the client is less likely to perceive the noise as a threat.

Do you have all the information you need to counsel Ms. Weiss about how to make her home environment more conducive to sleep? What other data might be helpful?

Interventions to Facilitate Uninterrupted Sleep

Promoting Dietary Changes

Because diet may play a role in sleep induction and maintenance, counsel clients about specific dietary measures. Instruct clients to avoid alcohol, nicotine, and caffeine, because all of these substances have been associated with an increased frequency of arousals. A light bedtime snack may be helpful. Some clients respond well to foods high in tryptophan, such as bananas and milk. Spicy foods should be avoided because they can cause gastrointentinal (GI) discomfort and increased awakenings. Heavy meals and too much liquid in the evening can also lead to increased arousals from digestive actions and bladder distention (Cohen & Merritt, 1992).

What dietary changes would you encourage Ms. Weiss to make?

Scheduling Nighttime Care

Traditional hospital routines violate many chronobiologic findings about human activity and rest cycles. Most people have an early-morning deep sleep cycle

associated with a low body temperature, yet they are often awakened at this period while in the hospital. They also experience a postprandial dip in energy and alertness between 1:00 and 3:00 PM, a period when therapy is often scheduled. To the extent possible, hospital routines should be adapted to more closely parallel client circadian rhythms.

Minimize the number of times you awaken clients during the night, and be certain that the benefits of the intervention outweigh those of undisturbed sleep. Consolidate tasks to avoid unnecessary nighttime interruptions. Make sure that daytime turning schedules are modified at night. Most people turn spontaneously 30 to 40 times during a typical night's sleep. If you observe the client turning adequately, do not use prompted turning. In addition, post a "Do Not Disturb" sign on the client's door to alert family members and caregivers to check at the nurses' station before entering (Fig. 41–7). Finally, report and chart the amount of a client's uninterrupted sleep per shift to help the oncoming nurse better plan client care.

To minimize the effects of arousals when they do occur, anticipate each client's nocturnal needs. For a client with angina or asthma, intervention may mean placing nitroglycerin or bronchodilators within easy reach at the bedside. Help the client with nocturia or a chronic disabling condition by putting a commode at the bedside.

Managing Parasomnias

Parasomnias, which typically occur in children, may result in interrupted sleep. By collaborating with par-

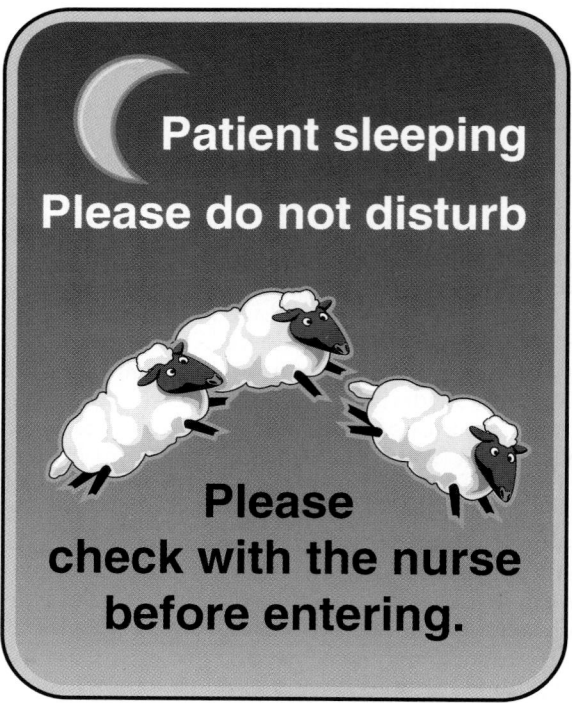

Figure 41–7. A "Do Not Disturb" sign posted on a client's door can discourage unnecessary awakenings.

ents and physicians to better manage these disorders, you can help promote undisturbed sleep.

Enuresis is a common parasomnia that may distress both the parents and the child. Provide parents with reassurance that the symptoms usually resolve with age, as the child gains better bladder control. Explaining to children that they have different sleep patterns than adults and do not always sense the need to urinate may help alleviate some of the shame and guilt associated with the disorder. You may also provide instructions about bladder training and encourage the parents to restrict fluids before bedtime.

Teach parents of children who sleepwalk or experience night terrors about safety. For the sleepwalker, stair guards, bars on the upstairs windows, and combination locks on outside doors need to be installed. The child with sleep terrors may need to be restrained during an episode, and breakable objects must be placed out of reach. Parents should not attempt to awaken the child. Teach parents of children with either problem about the importance of maintaining the child's routines and ensuring that the child gets enough sleep to prevent an exacerbation of the symptoms. Additionally, the child with sleep terrors may need to be referred for psychotherapy and hypnosis.

If a child has nightmares, teach parents that the child needs comfort and reassurance. Environmental triggers, such as horror stories at bedtime, should be avoided. Recurrent nightmares, a parasomnia seen in both children and adults, may resolve if you help clients verbalize their feelings and resolve their psychic conflicts. If such interventions fail to solve the problem, the client may require psychotherapy and medications that suppress REM sleep.

Bruxism, another parasomnia highly correlated with stress, can be treated with biofeedback. If a rubber mouth guard is prescribed to protect the teeth at night, you may need to instruct the client about proper cleaning, maintenance, and insertion.

Managing Dyssomnias

Interrupted sleep also marks two primary sleep disorders: sleep apnea and narcolepsy. As with the parasomnias, you will be involved in the collaborative management of these disorders.

A client with sleep apnea may have little trouble falling asleep but may be awakened up to 100 times a night by apnea episodes. Clients who require nightly, nasal CPAP to manage their symptoms are fitted with a nasal mask to deliver it. CPAP pressure is set to meet individualized needs (Fig. 41–8).

Teach the client undergoing this treatment about the operation, long-term use, and maintenance of the device. She also needs to know that the underlying disease will recur if the apparatus is not used, even for short periods. Nasal stuffiness, one of the most common side effects of CPAP, can be managed with nasal sprays. The sleep partner and the client may need earplugs or background white noise to obliterate CPAP sounds. Teach the client to avoid sleeping in the supine position. Encourage her to use pillows to help el-

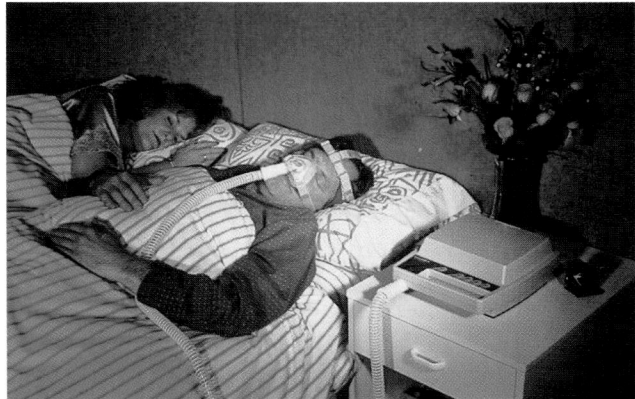

Figure 41–8. A client with obstructive sleep apnea wearing a CPAP mask. The CPAP mask provides positive pressure to maintain an open airway. (Courtesy of ResMed, San Diego, CA.)

evate her head. Alternatively, tell her to put a tennis ball in a pocket in the back of a nightshirt to prevent her from lying on her back. An obese client with obstructive sleep apnea should be given a weight-reduction diet.

If a client with obstructive sleep apnea fails to respond to CPAP treatments, a uvulopalatopharyngoplasty may be necessary. This surgery corrects the apnea by removing tissue from the soft palate, uvula, and pharynx to increase the diameter of the upper airway. Provide preoperative instruction to a client undergoing such surgery.

Narcolepsy, the other dyssomnia that causes marked sleep pattern disturbances, is characterized by excessive daytime sleepiness. Treatment of these daytime sleep attacks with psychostimulants often leads to insomnia and interrupted sleep. Such drugs can also cause irritability, habituation, addiction, psychosis, and insomnia. Remind the client to take her last medication in the late afternoon or early evening to minimize the risk of delayed sleep onset and interrupted sleep. In addition, instruct the client to discontinue any psychostimulants 1 day per week to decrease the risk of medication tolerance. Tricyclic antidepressants help alleviate the narcoleptic symptoms of cataplexy and hypnagogic hallucinations, but tolerance to these drugs may also develop. Therefore, the client may need to take a "vacation" from the drugs. Remind her to taper doses because abrupt discontinuation can lead to withdrawal symptoms.

In addition to medication instructions, counsel a narcoleptic about lifestyle changes. Instruct the client that relaxation and the avoidance of intrinsic stimulation just before scheduled sleep may help extend nighttime sleep. Encourage her to follow a healthy diet and to avoid alcohol and sedatives, both of which may increase daytime drowsiness. Even a well-managed narcoleptic may need additional daytime sleep, and she may benefit from 10- to 60-minute naps.

Teach the client that the benefits of short naps usually last 2 hours, enough time for the client to engage in activities that require more alertness. You should also assess both leisure and employment activity safety. The client may benefit from vocational counseling. To avoid cataplexy symptoms, the client will need to look for a stimulating work environment where the chances of monotony are minimal. You may also need to educate an employer about the disorder and suggest marital counseling and child care issues.

Managing Symptoms That Disturb Sleep

Both GI and respiratory disorders may interrupt sleep. Nursing interventions directed at improving symptoms can help the client maintain unbroken sleep. Teach a client with gastroesophageal reflux to sleep propped up by pillows. This position will help prevent regurgitation of gastric contents. Giving the client with ulcers an antiulcer medication at bedtime will help decrease nocturnal acid secretion and promote more rapid healing of ulcers.

Better management of this condition should also lead to fewer nocturnal awakenings from burning gastric pain. Make sure the client keeps GI and respiratory medications within easy reach at night. Extra pillows may also help the client with dyspnea. Oxygen therapy may be required for a client with hypoxia, which worsens during REM sleep, causing restlessness and arousals.

Managing Bedtime Agitation

Any dementia may severely disrupt sleep. In fact, a reduced ability to sleep typically accompanies the cognitive decline. **Sundowning** is a sleep disruption involving the nocturnal exacerbation of disruptive behaviors and agitation associated with clients who have dementia. An exact definition of sundowning remains elusive. The behaviors are apparently caused by, or at least strongly correlated with, darkness (Bliwise, 1994). The agitated behaviors may be triggered when some event during the day, such as a holiday outing with the family, breaks a person's comfortable routine (Myers, 1996). To manage the agitation, try to distract and calm the client by playing soft music or turning on the television. Rocking in a rocking chair can also be soothing and have a sedative effect. Physical restraints usually make the agitation worse. You may want to institute a "floor bed" program by placing the client's mattress on the floor to avoid restraints and eliminate the risk of the client falling out of bed. The client may also benefit from phototherapy. In one study, institutionalized clients with dementia who were daily exposed to sunlight experienced decreased night waking hours, decreased daytime sleeping hours, increased uninterrupted nighttime sleep, increased mean sleep hours, and decreased daytime sleepiness (Castor, Woods, & Pigott, 1991).

Interventions to Prevent Early or Late Awakenings

The client most susceptible to early or late awakenings is the one with a disturbed circadian rhythm, as from jet lag, shift work, or clinical depression.

To minimize the effects of jet lag, teach the client to adapt to the destination's time zone a few days before the trip. She should eat lightly and avoid alcohol on the flight, reset her wristwatch on the plane, and adapt to the destination's circadian clock on arrival, even if it seems awkward or difficult at first.

Like the client who is adjusting to jet lag, the shift worker must make circadian phase shifts as well. Very bright lights in the nocturnal work place and complete darkness for the 8-hour sleep period at home will expedite the process of circadian realignment (Monk, 1994). If possible, shift workers should be encouraged to make such modifications in their environment. Help your client adapt to shift work by teaching her how to manipulate zeitgebers to her advantage and by organizing self-help networks. You may also refer the client and family for counseling, if indicated.

Early-morning awakenings are a classic sign of depression. In addition, a depressed client may be taking a tricyclic antidepressant, monoamine oxidase inhibitor, or selective serotonin re-uptake inhibitor. Teach the client about medication doses, frequency, and side effects.

Interventions to Promote Rest

Remind the client who has an increased need for physical rest that she will benefit from prioritizing and pacing her activities. She should also alternate activity with frequent rest periods. Naps may be helpful if they do not disrupt her usual sleep patterns. Teach the client how to conserve energy while engaging in activities. She should sit as much as possible when engaged in relatively sedentary activities, such as food preparation and taking a shower. Environmental modifications that may help the client conserve energy include replacing steps with ramps, installing grab bars, and raising chairs by 3 to 4 inches. For other energy conservation measures, see Chapter 39.

If the client needs rest but is bored by inactivity, encourage her to participate in hobbies that do not require high energy expenditures, such as reading, writing, knitting, carving, model-building, or playing a musical instrument.

If the client complains of mental exhaustion, you may want to teach her relaxation techniques, such as meditation or guided imagery. Such strategies are helpful in quieting the mind and promoting relaxation.

In the case of chronic fatigue syndrome, teaching health promotion activities is critical. You must remind the client to maintain a consistent pattern of rest and sleep, followed by a gradual return to normal activity. Be specific about the rest schedule. Focusing on the need for planned rest will gradually weaken the link between symptoms and activity, and the client will be more eager to engage in activities. Clients with chronic fatigue syndrome are sometimes treated with low doses of antidepressants; you will need to give instructions about these medications.

EVALUATION

Ultimately, nursing interventions directed at alleviating sleep pattern disturbances or fatigue share a common goal: to promote a client's sense of being well rested. Until researchers can identify and quantify events that must occur during sleep for a client to feel well rested, evaluation must be made primarily on the basis of client reports.

Let us return to Ms. Weiss. A nursing note for this client after her visit might look like this:

> Agreed to try the Bootzin technique. Plans to purchase and listen to relaxation audiotapes at bedtime. States that she will limit coffee to three cups per day, taken before 5:00 PM. Will consider cutting back on cigarette consumption after her midterm. Will keep a sleep diary, to be reviewed with RN on return to clinic in 1 month. RN will also monitor vital signs, effectiveness of behavioral modification techniques, and dietary changes at that time. If measures to improve sleep prove unsuccessful, will refer client to nurse practitioner for possible short-term hypnotic prescription.

Refer to the accompanying care plan for an example of an application of the nursing process to Ms. Weiss.

Notice that the nurse documents that the sleeping problem has been addressed and that she has worked with the client to develop new goals. The goals are to use Bootzin's strategies and audiotapes for sleep induction, to make dietary modifications that will promote sleep onset, and to monitor progress toward meeting those goals through use of a sleep diary.

These are goals in progress; full evaluation of the client's ability to meet these goals must be deferred until her next clinic visit. If outcomes are not achieved, or the client has not improved by her next scheduled visit, you would reassess the client to identify possible explanations for her lack of progress. For example, if Ms. Weiss has not been able to incorporate the Bootzin technique into her sleep routine, you would ask her about specific difficulties she encountered and review her sleep diary. Based on her response and any significant findings in the diary, you might want to give her written instructions about the technique, refer her for more intensive counseling services, or teach her additional stress reduction techniques, such as meditation and guided imagery.

As the case study illustrates, your evaluation of care should focus on individual client needs. If the plan to improve the client's sleep is not successful after appropriate modifications have been attempted, then the physician may want to consider the next step: referral to a sleep clinic. These sleep disorder centers are often successful in diagnosing and treating severe or less common sleep problems. The American Sleep Disorders Association or the National Sleep Foundation should have a complete listing of local facilities.

KEY PRINCIPLES

- Rest is a state of mental and physical quiet. Lack of rest can lead to fatigue.
- Sleep is a cyclic event lasting about 8 hours and occurs once every 24 hours.
- Sleep can be subdivided into two categories: REM sleep and NREM sleep.
- During REM sleep, the brain is very active, but the body is quiet, and vital signs fluctuate. In adults, REM sleep lengthens progressively as the night progresses.
- In adults, NREM sleep predominates during the first third of the night. This sleep can be further divided into stages 1 to 4, with stages 3 and 4 representing the deepest or slow-wave sleep. During NREM sleep, the brain's metabolic rate slows, and vital signs are decreased, although the body remains active.
- Sleep induction and arousal are regulated by a complex interplay of neurotransmitters. In addition, zeitgebers (circadian synchronizers) help keep the body's internal 25-hour sleep-wake cycle adjusted to a 24-hour solar clock.
- Sleep disorders fall into one of three major categories: dyssomnias, parasomnias, and other medical or psychiatric illnesses.
- Dyssomnias (disorders of initiating and maintaining sleep or excessive sleepiness), include intrinsic disorders (insomnia, narcolepsy, obstructive sleep apnea, and restless legs syndrome), extrinsic disorders (drugs and the environment), and circadian disorders (jet lag and shift work changes).
- Parasomnias, or episodic, undesirable phenomena that occur during sleep, include somnambulism, sleep terrors, nightmares, sleep enuresis, and bruxism.
- Lifestyle factors, environmental factors, developmental factors, and physiological factors can all affect sleep and rest patterns. These variables must be considered when assessing, diagnosing, and treating sleep pattern disturbances or fatigue.
- When assessing a client for sleep or rest problems, a thorough sleep history is critical. Nonspecific physical findings may be used to confirm subjective findings. Diagnostic tests, such as polysomnography or the multiple sleep latency test, may be needed for a client with long-standing, unresolved sleep problems.
- Sleep pattern disturbances are sleep problems that nurses can treat independently. These problems may result from sleep disorders, other medical or psychiatric disorders, pain, positioning, medications, diet, lifestyle disruptions, or changes in environment.
- Sleep pattern disturbances are defined as difficulty falling asleep, interrupted sleep, awakening earlier or later than desired, and not feeling well rested.
- Fatigue can be described as an overwhelming sus-

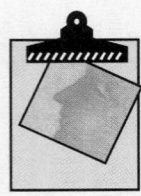

NURSING CARE PLANNING
A CLIENT WITH SITUATIONAL INSOMNIA

Admission Data

A 48-year-old white female with transient situational insomnia for past 3 months. Attributes symptoms to stress of new job and to enrollment in graduate school courses. Usually retires at midnight. Takes her about 2 hours to fall asleep. Describes herself as a light sleeper but number of arousals have increased in the past 2½ months. Now awakens two to three times because of nightmares and once or twice due to nocturia. Awakens to alarm at 6:30 AM. Often feels "exhausted" on arising. Thinks mood swings and irritability secondary to sleep deprivation are affecting relationships with coworkers. Notes decreased ability to focus on details of work. Rarely naps. Tried eating chicken soup and/or drinking a glass of wine at bedtime to alleviate symptoms, but these remedies did not help. Does not take any OTC or prescription drugs regularly. Drinks up to 10 cups of coffee a day, including two cups in the afternoon and one cup after dinner. Over the last 3 months, has increased cigarette consumption to one pack per day. Smokes until bedtime. Wants sleeping pills.

Nurse Practitioner's Orders	Counsel for sleep disturbance.
Nursing Assessment	Yawns frequently. Fine intentional tremors present. Eyes have deep circles. BP 130/90, HR 106, RR 25, afebrile.

NURSING CARE PLAN

Nursing Diagnosis	Expected Outcomes	Interventions	Evaluation (During Return Visit to Clinic)
Sleep pattern disturbance related to stress and ineffective coping mechanisms	Will substitute glass of milk for alcohol at bedtime	• Teach about rebound insomnia associated with alcohol and about sleep-inducing properties of foods high in tryptophan, such as milk.	Reported drinking milk at bedtime
	Will report falling asleep within 30 minutes of going to bed at night	• Teach about: 1. Progressive muscle relaxation. 2. Bootzin's technique. 3. Importance of reviewing the day's events several hours before retiring. 4. How to establish a daily bedtime routine. • Discourage smoking after supper. • Discourage coffee consumption after noon.	Stopped drinking coffee after lunch but still unable to cut back on cigarettes. Sleep onset shortened to 1 hour after retiring.

tained sense of exhaustion and decreased capacity for physical and mental work.

- *Sleep pattern disturbance* and *Fatigue* may increase a client's *Risk for injury* and contribute to *Self-care deficit, Ineffective individual coping* and *Ineffective family coping,* and *Altered thought processes.*
- Expected outcomes of interventions to correct *Sleep pattern disturbance* include client reports of rapid sleep onset, uninterrupted sleep, a satisfactory amount of sleep, and daytime alertness.
- Expected outcomes of interventions to promote rest include reports of feeling well rested and having an increased ability to engage in progressively more demanding activity.

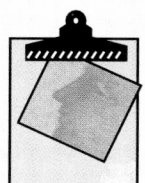

NURSING CARE PLANNING
A CLIENT WITH SITUATIONAL INSOMNIA *(continued)*

NURSING CARE PLAN

Nursing Diagnosis	Expected Outcomes	Interventions	Evaluation (During Return Visit to Clinic)
	Will walk briskly for 30 minutes at least four times a week.	• Teach about the importance of daily exercise to promote sleep induction. • Encourage exercise as part of ADLs, such as walking partway to work.	Made an appointment with the nurse practitioner to discuss exercise program and need for pre-exercise testing, if any
	Will report 8 hours of uninterrupted sleep	• Teach to stop drinking beverages at least 2 hours before bedtime. • Refer to nurse practitioner for possible hypnotic prescription if current measures to induce and maintain sleep fail.	No further awakenings for nocturia
	Will report decreased anxiety	• *Discuss possibility of decreasing the number of credits taken while adjusting to new job role.* • Reassure client that insomnia is transient. • *Review past successful coping strategies that could be used in present situation.* • Refer for psychotherapy if needed.	Spoke with boss about prioritizing and delegating. Averaging only one nightmare every other night.

Italicized interventions indicate culturally sensitive care.

Critical Thinking Questions
1. Can you think of any other measures that might be helpful for Ms. Weiss?
2. After reviewing the evaluation data, do you think that Ms. Weiss needs further follow-up?
3. What criteria would you use to decide whether a referral for psychotherapy would be useful?

• Interventions that help meet the goal of sleep induction include relaxation and comfort measures, behavioral and cognitive measures, encouraging regular exercise and bedtime routines, and creating an environment conducive to sleep.
• Most measures that promote sleep onset also facilitate sleep maintenance. In addition, instruction about diet and drugs and appropriate interventions for specific sleep disorders can help most clients meet the goal of sleep maintenance.
• Interventions to help clients cope with jet lag, shift-work adjustment, and depression will assist them in achieving the goal of awakening at a desired time.

- Interventions that promote rest, relaxation, and energy conservation will help alleviate fatigue.

BIBLIOGRAPHY

*Aldrich, M.S. (1992). Narcolepsy. *Neurology, 42*(Suppl. 6), 34–43.

*Berrios, G.E., & Shapiro, C.M. (1993). ABC of sleep disorders: "I don't get enough sleep, doctor." *British Medical Journal, 306*(6881), 843–846.

*Beyerman, K. (1987). Etiologies of sleep pattern disturbance. In A.M. McLane (Ed.), *Classification of nursing diagnoses: Proceedings of the seventh NANDA conference* (pp. 193–198). St. Louis: C.V. Mosby.

*Bliwise, D. (1994). What is sundowning? *Journal of the American Geriatrics Society, 42*(9), 1009–1011.

Carey, B. (1996). The slumber solution. *Health* (July/August), 70–75.

*Carskadon, M.A., & Dement, W.C. (1994). Normal sleep: An overview. In M. Kryger, T. Roth, & W.C. Dement (Eds.), *Principles and practice of sleep medicine* (2nd ed.). Philadelphia: W.B. Saunders Co.

*Castor, D., Woods, D., & Pigott, K. (1991). Effect of sunlight on the sleep patterns of the elderly. *Journal of the American Academy of Physician Assistants, 4*, 321–326.

*Chuman, M.A. (1983). The neurological basis of sleep. *Heart & Lung, 12*(2), 177–181.

Clark, A.J., Flowers, J., Boots, L., & Shettar, S. (1995). Sleep disturbance in mid-life women. *Journal of Advanced Nursing, 22*(3), 562–568.

*Closs, S.J. (1988). Assessment of sleep in hospital patients: A review of methods. *Journal of Advanced Nursing, 13*(4), 501–510.

Cohen, F.L., Ferrans, C.E., Vizgirda, V., Kundle, V., & Cloninger, L. (1996). Sleep in men and women infected with human immunodeficiency virus. *Holistic Nursing Practice, 10*(4), 33–43.

*Cohen, F.L., & Merritt, S.L. (1992). Sleep promotion. In G. Bulechek & J. McCloskey (Eds.), *Nursing interventions: Essential nursing treatments* (2nd ed.). Philadelphia: W.B. Saunders Co.

Cupp, M.J. (1997). Melatonin. *American Family Physician, 56*(5), 142–1425.

*Driver, H.S., & Shapiro, C.M. (1993). ABC of sleep disorders: Parasomnias. *British Medical Journal, 306*(6882), 921–924.

Evans, J.C., & French, D.G. (1995). Sleep and healing in intensive care settings. *Dimensions of Critical Care Nursing, 14*(4), 189–199.

Floyd, J.A. (1995). Another look at napping in older adults. *Geriatric Nursing, 16*(3), 136–138.

Foreman, M.D., & Wykle, M. (1995). Nursing standard-of-practice protocol: Sleep disturbances in elderly patients. *Geriatric Nursing, 16*(5), 238–243.

Grad, R. (1995). Benzodiazepines for insomnia in community-dwelling elderly: A review of benefit and risk. *The Journal of Family Practice, 41*(5), 473–481.

*Halfens, R.J.B., Lendfers, M.L., & Cox, K. (1991). Sleep medications in Dutch hospitals. *Journal of Advanced Nursing, 16*(12), 1422–1427.

*Hodgson, L.A. (1991). Why do we need sleep? Relating theory to nursing practice. *Journal of Advanced Nursing, 16*(12), 1503–1510.

Houde, S. C., & Kempfe-Leacher, R. (1997). Chronic fatigue syndrome: An update for clinicians in primary care. *The Nurse Practitioner, 22*(7), 30–48.

*Idzikowski, C., & Shapiro, C.M. (1993). ABC of sleep disorders: Nonpsychotropic drugs and sleep. *British Medical Journal, 306*(6885), 1118–1120.

*Jamieson, A.O., & Becker, P.M. (1992). Management of the 10 most common sleep disorders. *American Family Physician, 45*(3), 1262–1268.

Johnson, A., Wise, M.S., & Jimmerson, K.R. (1995). The nurse practitioner's role in a pediatric sleep clinic. *Journal of Pediatric Health Care 9*(4), 162–166.

*Johnson, J.E. (1991). A comparative study of the bedtime routines and sleep of older adults. *Journal of Community Health Nursing, 8*(3), 129–136.

*Kelly, D. (1991). Disorders of sleep and consciousness. In E.R. Kandel, J.H. Schwartz, & T.M. Jessell (Eds.), *Principles of neural science* (3rd ed.). New York: Elsevier.

Kendler, B.S. (1997). Melatonin: Media hype or therapeutic breakthrough? *The Nurse Practitioner, 22*(2), 66–72.

*Knapp, M. (1993). Clinical outlook: Night shift—the restorative sleep specialists. *Journal of Gerontological Nursing, 19*(5), 38–42.

*Kryger, M.H., Roth, T., & Carskadon, M. (1994). Circadian rhythm in humans: An overview. In M. Kryger, T. Roth, & W.C. Dement (Eds.), *Principles and practice of sleep medicine* (2nd ed.). Philadelphia: W.B. Saunders Co.

Kupfer, D.J., & Reynolds, C.F. (1997). Management of insomnia. *The New England Journal of Medicine, 336*(5), 341–346.

Leininger, M. (Ed.). (1991). *Culture care diversity and universality: A theory of nursing.* New York: National League for Nursing Press.

*Monk, T.H. (1994). Shift work. In M. Kryger, T. Roth, & W.C. Dement (Eds.), *Principles and practice of sleep medicine* (2nd ed.). Philadelphia: W.B. Saunders Co.

Mornhinweg, G., & Volignier, R. (1996). Rest. *Holistic Nursing Practice, 10*(4), 54–60.

Myers, D.L. (1996). Remedies beyond counting sheep. *Provider, 22*(2), 62–64.

North American Nursing Diagnosis Association. (1999). *NANDA nursing diagnoses: Definitions and classification 1999–2000.* Philadelphia: Author.

Penev, P.D., & Zee, P.C. (1997). Melatonin: A clinical perspective. *Annals of Neurology, 42*(4), 545–553.

*Reimer, M. (1987). Sleep pattern disturbance: Nursing interventions perceived by patients and their nurses as facilitating nocturnal sleep. In A.M. McLane (Ed.), *Classification of nursing diagnoses: Proceedings of the seventh NANDA conference.* St. Louis: C.V. Mosby.

Renaud, M. (1996). Neonatal sleep patterns: Implications for nursing. *Holistic Nursing Practice, 10*(4), 27–32.

Richardson, P. (1996). Sleep in pregnancy. *Holistic Nursing Practice, 10*(4), 20–26.

Rivkees, S. (1997). Developing circadian rhythmicity. *Pediatric Clinics of North America, 44*(2), 467–487.

*Shapiro, C.M., & Dement, W.C. (1993). ABC of sleep disorders: Impact and epidemiology of sleep disorders. *British Medical Journal, 306*(6892), 1604–1607.

Southwell, M.T., & Wistow, G. (1995). Sleep in hospitals at night: Are patients' needs being met? *Journal of Advanced Nursing, 21*(6), 1101–1109.

*Spector, R.E. (1991). *Cultural diversity in health and illness* (3rd ed.). Norwalk, CT: Appleton & Lange.

*Stradling, J.R. (1993). ABC of sleep disorders: Recreational drugs and sleep. *British Medical Journal, 306*(6877), 573–575.

*Thorpy, M.J., & Brunton, S.A. (1994). Sleep disorders: Simple or complex? *Hospital Practice, 29*(9), 39–45.

Vliet, E.L. (1995). *Screaming to be heard: Hormonal connections women suspect and doctors ignore.* New York: M. Evans and Co.

*Walker, B.B. (1972). The postsurgery heart patient: Amount of uninterrupted sleep and rest during the first, second and third postoperative days in a teaching hospital. *Nursing Research, 21*(2), 164–169.

*Asterisk indicates a classic or definitive work on this subject.

Cognitive-Perceptual Pattern

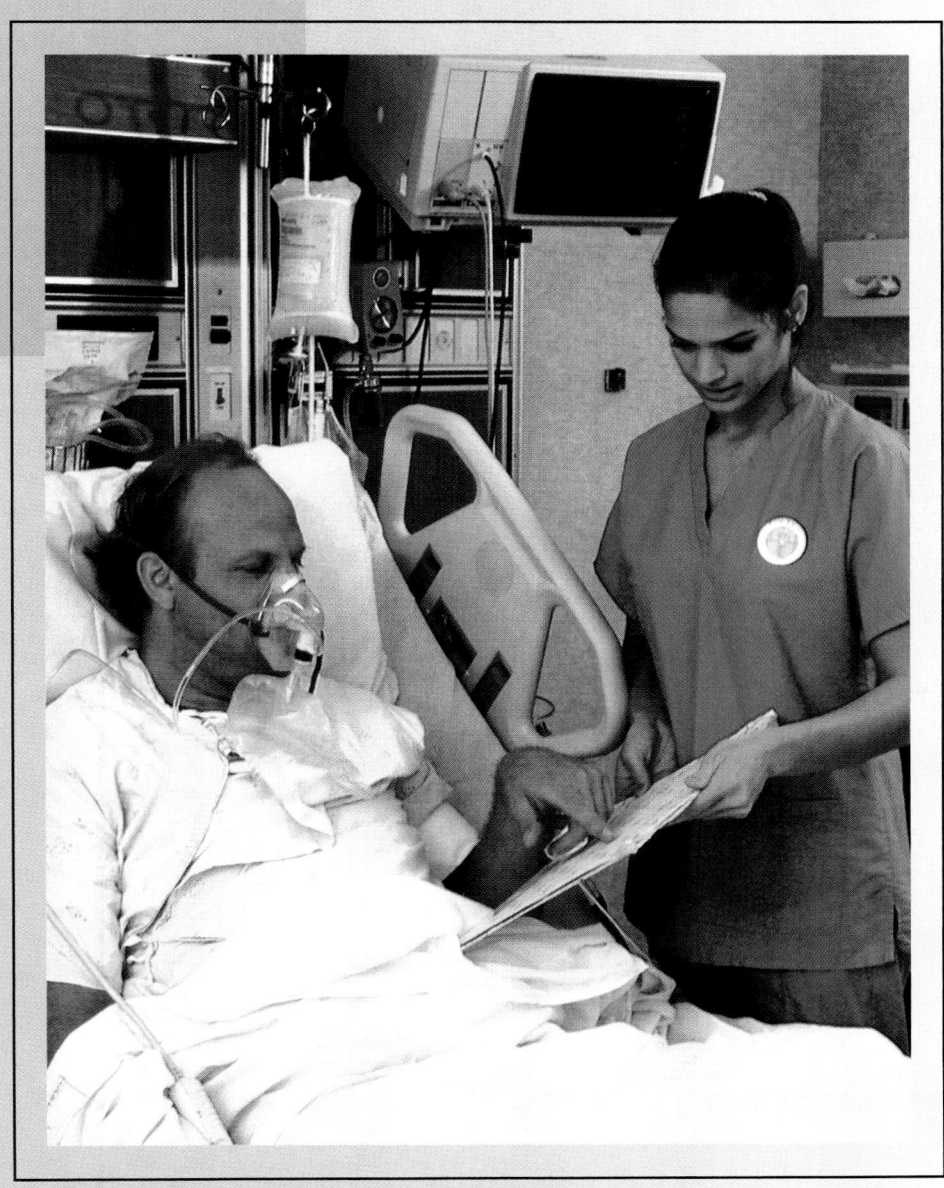

Pain

Karen Stanley

Key Terms

acute pain
adjuvant analgesic
agonist analgesic
analgesia
antagonist
atypical analgesic
breakthrough pain
chronic pain
endorphin
epidural analgesia
equianalgesia
first pass effect
gate control theory
intrathecal analgesia
mixed agonist-antagonist analgesic
modulation
neuropathic pain
nociception

nociceptive pain
nociceptor
nonopioid analgesic
opioid analgesic
opioid naive
opioid receptor
pain
pain behavior
patient-controlled analgesia
physical dependence
psychological dependence
referred pain
rescue dose
somatic pain
suffering
tolerance
visceral pain

LEARNING OBJECTIVES

After studying this chapter, you should be able to:

1. **Describe the physiological concepts supporting pain-related nursing diagnoses.**
2. **Discuss the pathophysiological, cognitive, affective, sensory, cultural, environmental, and other variables that affect the pain experience.**
3. **Assess the client at risk for or experiencing a pain problem and the client's responses to the experience.**
4. **Diagnose the client's pain management needs that will respond to nursing care.**
5. **Plan for goal-directed interventions to prevent or correct the pain diagnoses.**
6. **Describe and practice key nonpharmacological and pharmacological interventions for pain management.**
7. **Evaluate outcomes that indicate progress in providing effective pain management.**

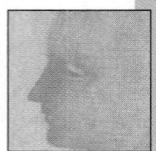

Joseph Valdez is a 54-year-old man who lives with his wife and three children. Two children are in college. The third, who is 19 years old, works. Joseph has worked for the same company since he was 18 years old. His wife, Pamela, has raised the children while working part-time. About a year ago, Joseph was diagnosed with adenocarcinoma of the stomach and underwent a partial gastrectomy. After recovering from surgery, he received chemotherapy.

He returned to work, working half days until his determination allowed him to work full-time. In recent weeks, however, he has developed abdominal pain, bloating, and malaise. He refused to see his physician until the discomfort became so severe that he could not work.

Although he has trouble standing, Joseph insisted on driving himself to the physician's office, accompanied by his wife. The physician elicited significant pain on palpation of the abdomen. He admitted Joseph to the hospital for a work-up for recurrent malignant disease.

The nurse assigned to Joseph selects *Pain* as the nursing diagnosis. However, given her knowledge of recurrent gastric carcinoma, she believes the diagnosis will be *Chronic pain.*

PAIN-RELATED NURSING DIAGNOSES

> **Chronic Pain:** An unpleasant sensory and emotional experience arising from actual or potential tissue damage or described in terms of such damage (International Association for the Study of Pain); sudden or slow onset of any intensity from mild to severe, constant or recurring without an anticipated or predictable end and a duration of greater than 6 months.
>
> **Pain:** An unpleasant sensory and emotional experience arising from actual or potential tissue damage or described in terms of such damage (International Association for the Study of Pain); sudden or slow onset of any intensity from mild to severe with an anticipated or predictable end and a duration of less than 6 months.
>
> From North American Nursing Diagnosis Association. (1999). NANDA nursing diagnoses: Definitions and classification 1999–2000. Philadelphia: Author.

CONCEPTS OF PAIN

According to the International Association for the Study of Pain (IASP), **pain** is an unpleasant sensory and emotional experience associated with actual and potential tissue damage. It sounds an alert that tissue damage has occurred or threatens to occur somewhere in the body. Often, pain is a symptom of an underlying disorder. Pain is primarily a protective mechanism, but it is also a complex biopsychosocial phenomenon.

Indeed, pain is common in many types of illnesses and can last for variable periods. Therapeutically, it functions as a diagnostic tool, an assessment variable, and a measure of response to interventions. Pain may or may not have an easily identified cause; it may occur at any time during an illness; it may not always respond to conventional interventions; and it may change in nature over time. It has several common denominators: all pain has a starting point; clients do not choose to have painful experiences; and clients must interpret and consider that experience as significant before they enter the health care system.

Clients will experience pain in the diagnostic, acute, ambulatory, home, hospice, extended, and rehabilitative settings. In general, you will find it easier to focus on a client's pain when the person is actually experiencing it. To be most successful in managing pain, however, keep in mind that it can result from many disorders and procedures.

McCaffery (1979), a pioneer nursing advocate for clients with pain, defined pain as "whatever the experiencing person says it is and existing whenever he says it does." The IASP acknowledges sensory and emotional components of pain, whereas McCaffery further qualifies the experience as individualized and based on client self-report. People with similar illnesses do not necessarily report similar pain experiences.

The incorporation of client self-report into a working definition of pain acknowledges the highly subjective nature of the experience. The client's evaluation of pain is your most important indicator of its nature and intensity. For clients unable to give a verbal self-report, such as newborns, infants, small children, comatose people, and mentally or verbally impaired people, you can assess nonverbal, behavioral signs of pain.

Pain as a Physiological Response

When the body is injured, a nociceptive response is activated. **Nociception** is the process of transmitting a pain signal from a site of tissue damage to areas of the brain where perception occurs. It involves anatomic structures and biochemical neurotransmitters. The initial tissue damage causes the release of biochemical substances (such as potassium, substance P, bradykinin, and prostaglandin) that begin or enhance the nociceptive response. An ascending system of nerve fibers carries the pain signal to the brain, and chemical substances known as neurotransmitters assist in delivering the pain message across synapses.

The Nociceptive Process

This initial injury triggers a series of events: transduction, transmission, and perception (Fig. 42–1). Transduction is the process by which a chemical, thermal, or mechanical noxious stimulus is changed into an electrical stimulus by activating nociceptors. **Nociceptors** are the primary afferent fibers that initiate the pain experience when stimulated by tissue damage. These nociceptors have the ability to encode the intensity of the painful stimulus.

Transmission involves a series of events in which the electrical impulse passes from the site of injury to the dorsal horn of the spinal cord and then to the brain. Once the signal enters the dorsal root of the spinal cord, the nerve fibers separate into groups of larger-diameter and smaller-diameter fibers. These fibers synapse with the spinothalamic tract neurons via neurotransmitters, such as substance P. Then the spinothalamic tract nerve fibers cross to the other side of the spinal column and continue upward through the

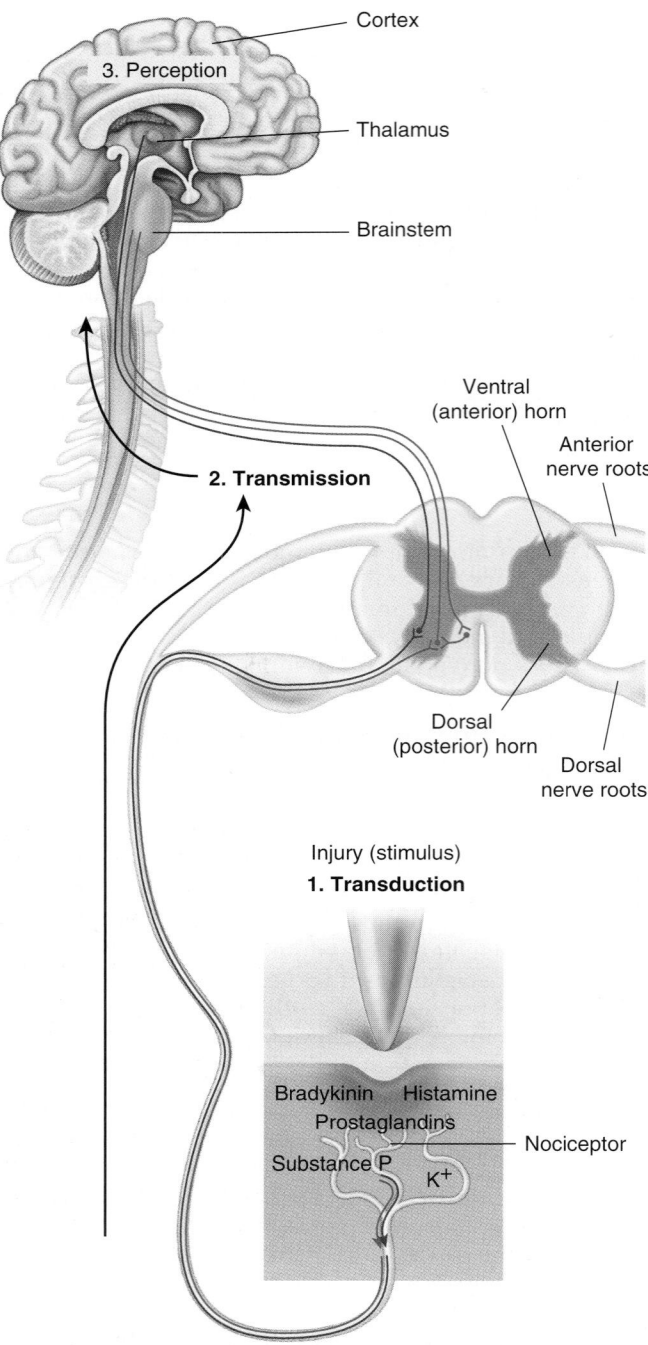

Figure 42–1. In the nociceptive process, tissue injury triggers a series of events. *1,* In *transduction,* the injured cells release brady-kinin, substance P, prostaglandins, potassium, and histamine, which stimulate the nociceptors to initiate the pain signal. *2,* In *transmission,* the pain signal is sent to the dorsal horn of the spinal cord by A or C fibers, then relayed to the thalamus. *3,* The thalamus relays the pain signal to areas in the cortex where *perception* occurs.

spinal cord, ending in the thalamus. There, the pain signal is transmitted to various areas of the cortex.

In perception, the action potential reaches cortical areas (the somatosensory projections and limbic system) that allow recognition of the pain sensation.

Nociceptive pain is pain transmitted from a site of injury to the higher brain centers along an intact nervous system. It is the most generic type of pain, such as the sensation associated with surgery, a broken bone, a cut, or a headache. Common descriptors are *aching, gnawing, pounding,* and *dull.* Types of nociceptive pain include **somatic pain, visceral pain,** and **referred pain,** as defined in Table 42–1.

Neuropathic pain is the transmission of a pain signal from the site of injury to the higher brain centers via a nervous system that has been temporarily or permanently damaged in some way. Damage may include cutting, crushing, or compression injuries, as well as viral or neurotoxic chemical exposure. These changes in the nervous system can trigger aberrant signal transmissions that alter the qualitative nature of the pain experience. *Burning, shooting,* and *electrical* are typical verbal descriptors, although the pain differs so markedly from nociceptive pain that clients may find it difficult to describe the sensation accurately. Tumor infiltration of a nerve plexus (plexopathy), neuralgia, diabetic neuropathy, and a collapsed vertebra impinging on a spinal nerve root are classic causes of neuropathic pain.

A single disorder may have components of both nociceptive and neuropathic pain. The degree of each can determine the anatomic distribution and characteristics of the pain sensation, effective intervention, and the duration of the pain.

Modulation is an internal or external restraining of the nociceptive process that inhibits transmission of the pain signal at any place along the transmission pathway. An important type of modulation is the inhibition of transmission through a descending system of nerve fibers that originate in the pons and medulla and release biochemicals, such as serotonin, norepinephrine, and noradrenergic substances. These biochemicals attach to receptors in the dorsal horn.

Certain drugs can inhibit transmission of the pain signal as well. Because transmission depends on neurons for transport and on neurotransmitters to carry the signal across the synapse, many analgesics reduce pain interfering with the production or reuptake of a neurotransmitter, or they prevent its attachment to the appropriate receptor site. Table 42–2 describes the mechanisms of drugs that modulate the nociceptive process. By doing so, they produce **analgesia,** which is a reduction in the perception or experience of pain.

Opioid Receptors

An **opioid receptor** is a portion of a nerve cell to which an opioid or opiate-like substance can bind. These receptors are located throughout the central nervous system at the spinal and supraspinal levels as well as in the periphery. The three primary receptor types, *mu,*

TABLE 42–1
Types of Pain

Pain Type	Description
Nociceptive Pain	
Somatic pain	Well-localized pain, usually from bone or spinal metastases or from injury to cutaneous or deep tissues. Described as achy, throbbing, dull.
Visceral pain	Poorly localized pain. Occurs as a result of nociceptor activation from stretching, distention, or contraction of smooth muscle walls; ischemia of the visceral wall; irritation or inflammation; or torsion or traction on mesenteric attachment organs. Described as squeezing, pressure, cramping, distention, deep stretching.
Referred pain	Pain experienced at a site distant from the injured tissue. Visceral pain is often referred to skin, muscle, and bone. Deep referred pain demonstrates a segmental pattern to sclerotomes (bones supplied by a single spinal segment) and myotomes (muscles supplied by a single spinal segment), whereas superficial referred pain is often felt in a dermatomal distribution (skin supplied by a single spinal segment) related to the affected viscera. Varied descriptors used.
Neuropathic Pain	
Paresthesia	An abnormal sensation, whether spontaneous or evoked.
Dysesthesia	An unpleasant abnormal sensation, whether spontaneous or evoked.
Allodynia	Pain from a stimulus that does not normally provoke pain (e.g., touching skin with a wisp of cotton; contact with clothing or bed linens).
Hypoalgesia	Diminished pain in response to a normally painful stimulus.
Hyperalgesia	Painful syndrome characterized by an abnormally painful reaction to a stimulus, especially a repetitive stimulus, as well as an increased threshold; explosive onset and greatly exaggerated severity.

International Association for the Study of Pain. (1994). Pain terms. A current list with definitions and notes on usage. In H. Merskey & N. Bogduk (Eds.), Classification of chronic pain: Descriptions of chronic pain syndromes and definitions of terms (2nd ed.) (pp 209–213). Seattle: IASP Press.

kappa, and *delta,* mediate analgesia, euphoria, sedation, respiratory depression, physical dependence, tolerance, and decreased gastrointestinal (GI) motility via their interaction with an **opioid analgesic.** This is a morphine-like drug that attaches to an opioid receptor and produces analgesia by blocking substance P. When the opioid locks into the receptor, substance P cannot be released, and analgesia occurs. The strength of the bond between the opioid analgesic and the receptor determines the efficacy and duration of the analgesic effect. A **nonopioid analgesic** is a drug that provides analgesia at the peripheral level by a mechanism other than the opioid receptor sites.

The *mu* receptor mediates analgesia for most common opioid-agonist analgesics, including codeine, fen-tanyl, hydrocodone, hydromorphone, levorphanol, meperidine, methadone, morphine, and oxycodone. The *kappa* receptor mediates analgesia and sedation but rarely affects respiratory drive or causes physical dependence. The *delta* receptor primarily mediates analgesia. An **agonist analgesic** is an opioid that stimulates activity at an opioid receptor to produce analgesia. It may also trigger physical dependence, tolerance, decreased GI motility, euphoria, sedation, and respiratory depression.

An **antagonist** blocks activity at *mu* and *kappa* opioid receptors by displacing opioid analgesics that are currently attached. The most common antagonist drug—naloxone (Narcan)—is used to counteract the life-threatening side effects of the agonist opioids at-

TABLE 42–2
Mechanisms by Which Drugs Relieve Pain

Drug Type	Mechanism of Pain Relief
Nonsteroidal anti-inflammatory drugs (NSAIDs)	Traumatized cells release prostaglandins that sensitize primary afferent fibers; NSAIDs inhibit prostaglandin synthesis and interrupt the pain signal at the peripheral level
Opioids (systemic and intraspinal)	Bind to opioid receptors in the dorsal horn, inhibit release of neurotransmitters (such as substance P), and interfere with the relay of the pain signal across the neuronal synapse
Membrane stabilizers, anesthetics, and anticonvulsants	Block ion channels (exchange of potassium and sodium), preventing generation of the pain signal; primarily indicated for neuropathic pain
Antidepressants	Inhibit reuptake of serotonin, a neurotransmitter, into neuronal fibers, which makes less serotonin available to relay the pain signal across the synapse; primarily indicated for neuropathic pain
Noradrenergic agonists	Attach to alpha$_2$ noradrenergic receptors in the dorsal horn of the spinal cord and modulate ascending pain signal

tached to the *mu* receptor sites and the agonist-antagonist opioids attached to the *kappa* sites. The **mixed agonist-antagonist analgesics** (such as butorphanol, buprenorphine, nalbuphine, and pentazocine) are formulations that attach to both the *kappa* and *mu* receptor sites. They provide analgesia at the *kappa* receptor site (agonist activity) but can simultaneously block activity (antagonist activity) at the *mu* receptor site if given after the client receives a morphine-like drug.

The **endorphins** are a group of internally secreted opiate-like substances released by a signal from the cerebral cortex. They attach to opioid receptors and block transmission of the pain signal. Multiple factors affect their release, such as brief pain or stress, physical exercise, massive trauma, some types of acupuncture, some types of transcutaneous electrical nerve stimulation (TENS) units, and sexual activity. Factors that reduce their circulating levels include prolonged pain, recurrent stress, and prolonged use of opioids or alcohol. They seem to have the most benefit for moderate types of pain.

Tolerance, Physical Dependence, and Psychological Dependence

The *mu* receptors mediate tolerance and physical dependence. Both are frequently mistaken for addiction.

Tolerance is an involuntary physiological phenomenon that occurs after repeated exposure to an opioid analgesic; it involves a decreased-level pain relief despite a stable or escalating opioid dosage. It does not occur with short-term use of opioids and is more likely to occur with chronic opioid use for malignant pain. Usually, the client complains of a decreased duration of relief and then a decreased degree of relief. It is not a sign of psychological dependence.

Physical dependence is an involuntary physiological phenomenon that occurs after repeated exposure to an opioid analgesic. The client develops withdrawal symptoms if the opioid is abruptly withdrawn or an opioid antagonist is administered. Physical dependence occurs only after repeated opioid administration and usually produces mild, unrecognizable withdrawal symptoms. If opioid exposure is significant and of long duration, a tapering dose of opioid therapy may be necessary. Withdrawal symptoms are not a sign of psychological dependence but rather of mismanagement of the tapering process.

Psychological dependence (addiction) is a chronic disorder demonstrated by overwhelming involvement with obtaining and using a drug for its mind-altering effects. This kind of dependence can cause great physical, psychological, and social harm to the user. Active, compulsive, drug-seeking and a tendency to relapse even after physical withdrawal subsides are primary behaviors. Quality of life is never improved by use of the drug.

Psychological dependence should be differentiated from pseudoaddiction. **Pseudoaddiction** refers to a syndrome of abnormal behavior that develops as a direct consequence of inadequate pain management. It is manifested by behaviors that mimic dependency, namely an overwhelming and compulsive interest in obtaining and using opioid medications. The client may request medication frequently, ask for specific medications by name, and demonstrate behaviors to convince you that pain is both real and severe. These behaviors can develop when the client receives analgesics on an as-needed (p.r.n.) basis rather than on a schedule, when pain is continuous, and when the drug or schedule is inadequate to manage the total pain needs.

Very rarely does the use of opioid therapy during an illness cause psychological dependence. The majority of clients who derive pain relief from opioids typically experience improved function and better quality of life without harmful consequences.

Action Alert!
Tolerance and physical dependence are involuntary, physiological behaviors and should not be confused with psychological dependence (addiction).

Gate Control Theory

In 1965 Melzack and Wall proposed the gate control theory of pain. The **gate control theory** hypothesizes an alteration in the transmission of the ascending pain signal by a spinal gating mechanism located in the dorsal horn; the pain signal may be inhibited or facilitated by multiple variables. The gating mechanism allows activity in large-diameter fibers to inhibit transmission (close the gate), and small-diameter fibers tended to facilitate transmission (open the gate). These large-diameter, rapidly conducting fibers could activate cognitive processes that would subsequently modulate the pain experience via descending fibers.

The theory's emphasis on a restraint mechanism in the dorsal horn and the important role of the brain in modulating the pain experience revolutionized treatment approaches. Attention to psychological factors, such as past experience, attention, and other cognitive activities, led to a multidisciplinary approach to pain management that integrated physiological and psychosocial variables for clients with chronic pain (Fig. 42–2).

The Pain Experience

In 1968 Melzack and Casey proposed three major dimensions of the pain experience: sensory-discriminative, cognitive-evaluative, and motivational-affective. As this framework factored in cognitive and emotional variables, additional physiological structures had to be incorporated into the total pain experience. Somatosensory projections, the limbic system, brain centers that mediated visual and vestibular mechanisms, and cognitive processes were identified as contributors to the overall pain experience.

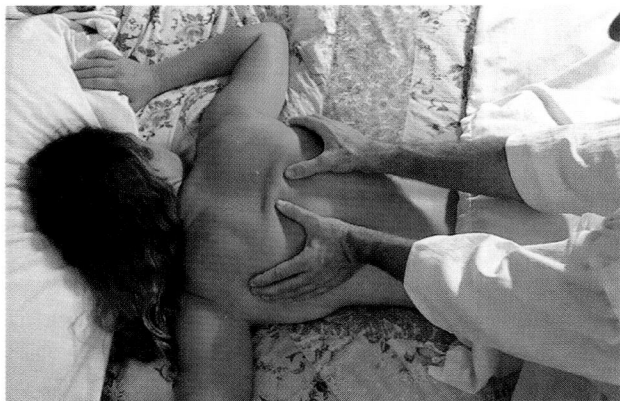

Figure 42–2. The gate control theory provided a basis for a multidisciplinary approach to pain management that integrated physiological and psychological variables.

Sensory Dimensions

The physical sensation of pain can alert a person that tissue injury has occurred. It can serve a useful, diagnostic purpose and trigger a medical plan of care. You can use the client's description of pain and its location to help diagnose his medical problem. However helpful the pain might be for these purposes, it remains an unpleasant experience for most clients and may take on more importance than its etiology.

Cognitive Dimensions

It is impossible to separate the physical sensation of pain from coexisting intellectual and emotional processes. When a client's attention is focused on pain, the pain is usually perceived to be more intense in nature. Educating a client about what to expect during a painful procedure decreases the pain's intensity and controls pain behaviors.

A **pain behavior** is anything a person says or does that infers the presence of pain. Behavioral expressions of pain are learned from others. Children are particularly susceptible to this kind of learning experience and will imitate the people who are important to them.

The meaning of pain also affects its intensity, its emotional impact on the client, and sometimes the client's response to medical and nursing interventions. A serious or life-threatening illness that causes the pain can trigger a "why me?" response as the client searches for meaning. If the client believes that the disease and subsequent pain are a well-deserved punishment from a higher being, are inevitable, or are a predetermined learning experience, the person may deny the painful state or fail to comply with analgesic therapy.

Pain can threaten beliefs about control and self-image, largely because most people fear a loss of independence. The feeling that pain cannot be controlled can produce extreme anxiety and a sense of helplessness. Conversely, for some clients, pain may produce significant secondary gain. It can elicit attention and assistance. For those with chronic, malignant pain, pain may serve as a valuable reminder that they are still alive.

Affective Dimensions

Affective or emotional factors can aggravate and be aggravated by the pain experience. Anxiety, fear, apprehension, and depression are affected by the perception of pain.

Anticipatory anxiety can intensify pain and affect pain behaviors. Many report feeling pain before the procedure begins. If the client has repeated experiences of unrelieved pain, the result is a cumulative sense of fear and anxiety.

Pain can also deplete a person's energy. When a client's emotional resources are low, the response to pain is more intense. The most inconsequential of stressors can trigger pain disproportionate to the circumstances. Whereas pain is the actual physical sensation of discomfort, **suffering** is the unpleasant emotional response to pain.

Characteristics of Acute and Chronic Pain

Generic definitions of nociceptive and neuropathic pain are not comprehensive enough to describe the pain experience. Although it is essential to qualify the nature of pain, the chronicity of the experience is what determines the quality of the client's life.

It is clinically useful to distinguish the experience of pain based on duration. **Acute pain** is short-term, self-limited pain with a probable duration of less than 6 months. **Chronic pain** is long-term, constant or recurring pain without an anticipated or predictable end and a duration of more than 6 months. It may be both permanent and permanently disabling. Acute pain has more limited implications than chronic pain (Table 42–3). Acute pain may absorb a person's physical and emotional energy for a brief time, but the knowledge that it will disappear as the tissue heals provides the person a certain amount of security and comfort. Chronic pain can quickly deplete a person's physical and emotional resources, immobilize the person, lead to physical disability and subsequent loss of employment, significantly impact daily activities, interrupt sleeping habits, and interfere with interpersonal relationships. As the pain experience becomes more complex and seemingly endless, the impact on the client becomes more extensive.

FACTORS AFFECTING PAIN

Given that pain can be such a complex phenomenon, it is impossible to separate or isolate its impact on any part of the client's experience of living. It can color the most trivial of everyday affairs as well as the most profound existential issues. Thus, the duration or intensity of pain a person is willing to endure is a unique response influenced by many physiological and psychological issues.

TABLE 42–3
Comparing Acute and Chronic Pain

Acute Pain	Chronic Pain
Precipitating event with well-defined pattern of onset	Occurrence may not be associated with an identified injury or event
Warning signal that tissue damage has occurred	No useful purpose after diagnosis is made
Evidence of tissue damage	May not have identifiable cause
Short-term (6 months or less), then pain resolves and normal function returns	Long-term (longer than 6 months and possibly permanent)
Signs and symptoms reflect hyperactivity of the autonomic nervous system (increased heart rate, blood pressure, respiratory rate, diaphoresis)	Signs and symptoms of acute pain no longer present, indicating adaptation of the autonomic nervous system
Behavioral manifestations including groaning, grimacing, guarding, wincing, crying, restlessness, anxiety	Behavioral manifestations include a blank or normal facial expression, sleeping or resting, and a focus on activities that distract from the pain
Client reports pain	Client may not mention pain unless asked
Pain usually responds to commonly prescribed medical and nursing interventions	May be difficult to treat, unresponsive to conventional modalities, and ultimately disabling

Physiological Factors

A client may have coexisting morbidities that affect the pain experience. Take, for example, a person with osteoarthritis who falls and breaks an arm. The pain experience is not new, but the additive pain may decrease the person's ability to tolerate what has been an acceptable norm of discomfort.

Gastrointestinal, renal, or hepatic dysfunction may influence the selection of appropriate analgesics. An opioid analgesic is metabolized by the liver and cleared by the kidneys and may be contraindicated in certain instances of hepatic or renal dysfunction. The nonopioid analgesics, in particular the nonsteroidal anti-inflammatory drugs (NSAIDs), interfere with prostaglandin synthesis and can damage the GI mucosa and interfere with renal function. Clients with a history of GI problems or any level of renal dysfunction may not be able to receive these medications.

Psychological Factors

The dimensions of the human personality, such as a predisposition to respond in a certain way to a given set of circumstances, can influence how a client adapts to or deals with a painful process. Because threat and stress are part of the pain experience, the response to pain is usually consistent with the person's response to any other stressful event. If there are concurrent stressors, the addition of pain may produce a more intense response than might otherwise occur.

Developmental Factors

There is no doubt that the client's developmental stage markedly affects cognitive and behavioral manifestations of the pain experience. Pain behaviors vary in infancy, childhood, and adolescence, and clinical assessment and interventions are based on the client's ability to understand the circumstances and their language skills.

However, developmental factors can occur at any age. The confused or demented adult or the client with severe learning disabilities may be at greater risk for inadequate assessment and intervention. When communication of pain is disrupted by complicating factors, the client's inability to communicate may be both frightening and frustrating.

Social and Environmental Factors

The social environment is intricately linked to the pain experience. The way others respond to pain will affect how the client responds. The presence of a strong emotional support system or assistance from others in performing daily tasks may make the pain experience more tolerable. Conversely, the demands of daily life coupled with a lack of understanding or sympathy from others can worsen the pain experience. If the client lives a relatively isolated life, the absence of support may make the pain less tolerable.

A person's ability to perform activities of daily living and to participate in meaningful leisure activities can markedly affect the pain experience. A client accustomed to physical activity at work, at home, or during leisure time may aggravate a painful condition by refusing to change a behavior even when he understands its potential harm. The perception of self as active and strong may be more appealing and emotionally nurturing than acceptance of any kind of disability.

Cultural Factors

Culture can mold a client's beliefs about pain, the meaning of pain, expected pain behaviors, and the way the pain is treated medically. Cultural orientation functions as an experiential filter and a grid for decision-making, thus distinctly influencing the pain experience, as discussed in the Cross-Cultural Care chart.

More importantly, cultural background can influence thoughts and attitudes about pain relief. For example, many people believe that older people experience less pain because of a changing pain threshold. Another common myth is that pain is a normal part of aging. The fact is that pain in the elderly is the same as for any other population.

Gender can influence response to pain. Studies suggest that female clients are less likely than male clients to receive adequate analgesia. Health care providers believe that gender affects sensitivity to pain, pain tolerance, pain distress, and exaggeration of the pain experience. Intervention typically occurs earlier for males because their pain is more often attributed to physiological causes. In fact, where poor psychological adjustment to pain is concerned, there is no numerical difference in females versus males.

Many nurses also have biases based on the cause of a client's pain or doubts about the client's self-report of pain. Clients particularly at risk for inadequate pain management include those with sickle cell disease, acquired immunodeficiency syndrome (AIDS), and substance abuse.

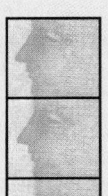

CROSS-CULTURAL CARE
CARING FOR A MEXICAN-AMERICAN CLIENT

Joseph Valdez, the client who presented with possible recurrent gastric carcinoma, is of Mexican descent. He was born in Mexico City and immigrated to the United States with his parents when he was 14 years old. He became fluent in English very quickly, but his parents continued to speak Spanish, settled into a Spanish-speaking neighborhood, and continued their previous customs. Joe married a classmate from high school who had been born and raised in the United States. This concerned his family for fear he would drift away from their customs. Diversity in the Mexican-American population about health beliefs and practices is dependent on the amount of time spent in the United States and the degree of affinity to traditional Mexican culture. Traditional beliefs include the following:

- Avoidance of direct eye contact with health care providers because they are seen as authority figures or of a higher class.
- Showing respect when the provider enters the room.
- Use of silence to show lack of agreement with the plan of care.
- Keeping the most sensitive issues inside the family.
- Discussion of particularly sensitive issues with those of the same gender.
- Protecting the client from knowledge about the seriousness of the illness.
- Strong belief in the mind-body connection and concern that worry will worsen health status.
- Traditional belief that health is controlled by environment, by fate, and by the will of God.
- Involvement of family members in activities of daily living.
- Belief that self-care may adversely affect recovery.
- Avoidance of complaints about pain because they show weakness and loss of self-respect.
- Respect for inner control and self-endurance.
- Embarrassment and secrecy about depression because it is seen as a sign of mental illness and weakness.

Anna, Joe's primary care nurse, approached him respectfully:

Anna: Hello, Mr. Valdez. How are you this morning?

Mr. Valdez: I'm very well, thank you.

Anna: [Observing that Joe's movements are guarded, that he is very still in the bed, and that he is breathing carefully and not very deeply] Are you having any pain right now?

Mr. Valdez: A little, but it's nothing I can't handle.

Anna: So, you're having just a small bit of pain?

Mr. Valdez: Yeah, it's not much.

Anna: I've noticed that you're not breathing as easily as you could. Sometimes even the smallest amount of pain will interfere with breathing. Your doctor has ordered a mild pain medicine for you. I would like to give it to you and see if it eases your discomfort and your breathing.

Mr. Valdez: Okay, if you think it will help my breathing.

Critical Thinking Questions

- Why would Mr. Valdez minimize what must have been relatively strong pain?
- What would have been the consequences if Anna had insisted that he had real pain that must be treated immediately?
- Could Anna have done anything else to approach him in a culturally sensitive manner?

Reference

de Paula, T., Laganam, K., & Gonzalez-Ramirez, L. (1996). Mexican Americans. In J.G. Lipson, S.L. Dibble & P.A. Minarik (Eds.), Culture and nursing care: A pocket guide (pp. 203–221). San Francisco: UCSF Nursing Press.

Religious Factors

Religious beliefs can have a profound impact on the client's response to pain. Historically, there has been great significance attached to pain and suffering. The pain may be perceived as deserved retribution for prior actions or seen as atonement for past behaviors. The client's religious denomination may have belief systems that require certain behaviors (such as stoicism or acceptance) that is independent of cultural orientation.

ASSESSMENT

The nature of a client's pain experience will determine the complexity of the assessment required. Although pain is always multifaceted, it is not always complex. A client with temporary, manageable pain secondary to a known cause (e.g., surgery to repair a joint) may require no more than an assessment for pre- and post-analgesic pain to ensure adequate pain relief. Conversely, a cancer client with recurrent disease accompanied by significant pain requires a thorough assessment that includes both psychosocial and physiological data.

Pain that is chronic, intractable, or resulting from a life-threatening illness carries a far different meaning than an acute episode that will readily resolve when the tissue heals. The person as well as the pain must be assessed.

In all cases, assessment determines the appropriate treatment approach. When the disorder cannot be identified, the nature and location of the pain may serve as the basis for treatment. Ongoing assessment of pain status allows evaluation of the treatment's efficacy and determines the direction of further intervention.

General Assessment of Pain

Pain assessment may occur in the ambulatory or acute care setting, in the client's home, or in an extended care or rehabilitation facility. In some cases, the client's detailed health history may already be available for you to consult. In others, you may need to obtain it at your initial visit with the client. In either case, the goals of your assessment are to do the following:

- Determine the current nature and status of the client's pain.
- Review the history of the client's pain and its therapies.
- Explore psychosocial, religious, and cultural variables that may influence the pain experience.
- Collaborate with other health care team members to plan for and deliver effective pain relief.

Your pain assessment should focus on both subjective and objective variables. As you interpret the client's pain experience, remember to keep the following basic principles in mind:

- Because pain is a subjective experience, you must use the client's evaluation as your initial standard, even if your attitudes and life experiences make you tend to doubt or disagree with it.

Action Alert!
Failure to accept a client's self-evaluation of pain with respect can trigger an adversarial relationship between the client and the health care team.

- When you cannot rely on the spoken word to document a client's pain, you will need to rely on behavioral characteristics instead. Stay particularly alert for such behavioral clues as restlessness or agitation in a comatose client or crying in a neonate.
- The nature and duration of the pain experience can activate physiological and psychological adaptation over time. Consequently, the absence of common pain behaviors in a client with chronic pain does not negate the presence of pain.

Action Alert!
As the client with chronic pain adapts to the experience, observable signs lessen, although the pain's severity remains unchanged. Assessing a client who has chronic pain by using the acute model serves the client unfairly and produces an inaccurate nursing assessment.

Health History

To obtain a detailed history when pain is involved, it is important that you avoid any hints of symptoms or diagnoses that could affect the client's report. By allowing the client to explain his pain experience without prompting, you may obtain such a clear picture that the diagnosis can be determined primarily from reported symptoms.

Begin your assessment by addressing the details of the client's chief complaint. His pain may be new, an exacerbation of existing pain, a different type of pain than he has previously experienced, or a pain affecting a location other than what he previously reported. The pain's onset can provide etiologic clues. Its duration establishes chronicity, a detail that may offer insight into the client's behaviors. The client's description of his pain experience will help you determine whether to continue the assessment using the acute pain model or the chronic pain model.

Ask questions like the following:

- Are you having pain at the present time?
- Do you have any illnesses at present? Have you ever had pain due to this illness?
- When did the pain start? Did you do something that you normally would not do when the pain began? When it began, did it come on suddenly? Did it happen over a period of time?
- Is it persistent, or does it come and go?
- Do any other symptoms accompany the pain?
- What do you think is causing your pain right now?

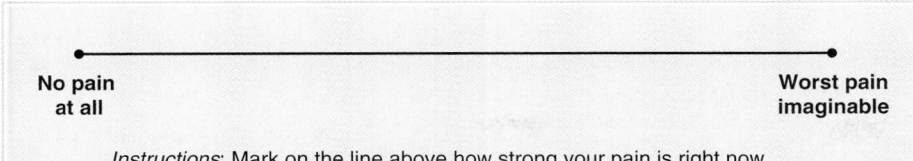

Figure 42–3. Visual analogue pain rating scale.

DIMENSIONS

As you continue to assess the client's pain, you will want to explore the dimensions of the pain. Assessing these dimensions will provide you with an overall "photograph" from the client's perspective.

LOCATION. Location is a critical variable. It is helpful to obtain this information while the pain is actually present because the accuracy of the client's report will decrease as the pain diminishes. Have the client point to the areas on his body where he feels pain. Or you could have him make marks on a simple anatomic figure. Many standard pain assessment tools include anatomic renderings for that purpose. Make sure the drawings you use include front, back, left, and right views of the whole body, and right, left, front, and back sides of the head.

When the client indicates an area of pain, inquire whether the pain is new, recurring, or worse than before. Also ask whether it stays at that location or moves.

QUALITY. Descriptive words can qualify the pain sensation and give you clues to whether the pain is nociceptive, neuropathic, or both. Words like *dull, aching, gnawing,* and *tender* tend to describe nociceptive pain. Words like *prickly, shooting, electric,* and *burning* are more likely to be used for neuropathic pain.

Clients with neuropathic pain commonly have trouble finding adequate words to describe the sensation. In that case, you may want to give the client a list of descriptors to help him describe his feelings. Many standard pain assessment tools contain descriptor words from which the client can choose. Tell him that he can choose as many words as he wants. He can also chose different words for different areas of his body.

INTENSITY. Intensity is the most subjective of the dimensional characteristics. To measure it, you will use one of several types of pain rating scales. These scales seek to make the client's subjective experience as objective as possible. Once you choose a pain rating scale for a client, continue to use the same scale throughout your ongoing assessment to keep the responses as comparable as possible over time.

Single-dimension, self-report tools include the visual analogue scale, numerical rating scale, and verbal descriptor scales. A visual analogue scale is a 10-centimeter horizontal line (Fig. 42–3). At its left endpoint is written *No pain at all.* At its right endpoint is written *Worst pain imaginable.* The client makes a mark at the point along the line that corresponds to his level of pain. Simple and quick, this scale has proven to be reliable and valid. It is abstract in nature, however, and may be difficult for some clients to use.

A numerical rating scale is also quick, simple, and easy to use. The client can point to, mark, or say the number that corresponds to the intensity of his pain (Fig. 42–4). Although the numerical scale is relatively easy for most clients to use, it may not reflect subtle changes. When using it, make sure the client can count up to the high end of the scale. The numerical rating scale tends to work best for assessing pain before and after analgesic intervention, the worst pain in a defined period of time, the least pain in a defined period of time, the intensity of continued pain, the intensity of pain that may flare up on occasion, and the amount of pain that the client can tolerate.

A verbal descriptor scale requires the client to choose one word to describe his pain (Fig. 42–5). This scale is most effective when the client can see it. Verify the client's understanding of the meaning of each word. The limited choice of words may make the assessment less accurate.

When choosing the scale to be used, consider the client's level of comprehension, eyesight, and developmental status. Collaborating with the client is always appropriate. An accurate assessment is more likely if you define the parameters each time you use a scale until the client is comfortable with it.

Regardless of the scale used, clients tend to choose the middle rather than the ends of the scale, a tendency that can alter the accuracy of your assess-

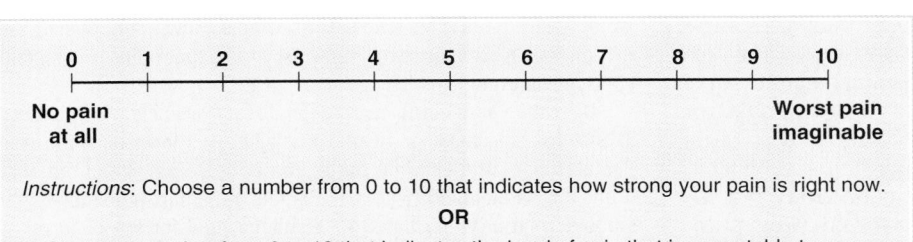

Figure 42–4. Numerical pain rating scale.

None / Annoying / Uncomfortable / Dreadful / Horrible / Agonizing

Instructions: Choose the word above that best describes how your pain feels right now.

Figure 42–5. Verbal descriptor pain rating scale.

ment. Make sure to query the client closely to clarify the level of pain that he can tolerate or considers acceptable. He may feel able to tolerate a higher level of rare or brief pain. This kind of clarification will help you set collaborative, reasonable goals with the client. Absence of pain is not always attainable. Tolerable relief, increased activity, or improved eating and sleeping habits may be more realistic goals.

AGGRAVATING AND RELIEVING VARIABLES. Ask the client what, if anything, makes the pain better or worse. Ask the client whether any specific movements or positions make the pain better or worse. Ask what he thinks works best to relieve the pain. These and similar questions may provide valuable diagnostic leads as well as direction for planning analgesic interventions.

EFFECTS OF PREVIOUS THERAPY. Assessing a client's previous treatment can eliminate repetitive interventions that are not helpful or even harmful. It can also point out interventions that the client believed *were* helpful. Have him describe both pharmacological and nonpharmacological interventions. Doing so will give you a fairly clear window into the client's past experiences.

Be sure to ask the client questions about specific interventions. For example, ask whether any nondrug interventions have relieved his pain, such as heat, cold, a TENS unit, massage, or relaxation techniques. Ask whether he has taken any pain medications and whether they relieved the pain. Ask what drug and dosage seemed to work best, what did not work, and whether any pain medications made him nauseous or produced an allergic reaction.

CURRENT ANALGESIC THERAPY. Exploring the client's current therapy can help you manage future regimens. You may find that the current regimen controls the client's pain adequately. Or you may find that the regimen needs changes to enhance analgesic efficacy.

When asking a client to name the medications he takes for pain management, also ask what amount he takes. Find out how long it takes for the pain to subside after he takes the drug. Ask whether he thinks the drug is working for him.

Also, make sure to ask what other medications the client takes, including over-the-counter ones. This allows you to assess any risks from polypharmacy and to identify **atypical analgesics,** which are drugs not primarily indicated for pain but used to treat specific types of pain. An anticonvulsant may be used to treat neuropathic pain, for example. The client may not remember that these medications are for treating pain. Also ask if anyone other than the client's doctor is helping with pain management.

EFFECTS ON ACTIVITIES OF DAILY LIVING. Chronic pain and sometimes acute pain can markedly impair activities of daily living. A thorough assessment should include questions about the impact of pain on the regular routine. For example, ask whether his pain medications cause side effects that interfere with his activities. Find out whether the client can go to work every day, whether his appetite is good, and whether he is sleeping normally at night. Ask whether he feels rested in the morning, and whether he needs to take pain medications during the night.

CULTURAL VARIABLES. Just as cultural expectations can mold the meaning of pain and the client's subsequent behaviors, so too can your lack of understanding of those expectations interfere with an accurate pain assessment. For example, if cultural norms demand stoicism even in the presence of severe pain, the client may not only deny the presence of pain but may not demonstrate any behavior that pain is a problem.

Although every client has the right to deny pain rather than acknowledge it, your tactful, skilled questions may help lead the client toward acceptance of analgesic intervention. For example, ask questions like these:

- You seem to be having difficulty moving around. Are you are hurting right now?
- It's not unusual after surgery for people to have aches or sore places. Are you having pain now?
- May I have your permission to give you the pain medicine your doctor has ordered for you? It will probably make it easier for you to breathe deeply and get up and out of bed.
- This particular illness can make people hurt and prevent them from doing things they have always done. Would you like to try the pain medicine the doctor has ordered to see if it can help you to do those things again?

Joseph Valdez was born in Mexico City and came to the United States when he was 14 years old. His English skills were limited, but through determination and hard work, he became fluent within the year. At age 16 he got a part-time job after school at a grocery store, where he met his wife-to-be, Pamela. How might this strong will affect the response to pain? Is your expectation consistent with your stereotype of Hispanics?

Over the years of their marriage, Joseph was clearly in charge of the decision-making. He did not allow his wife to work, and Pamela raised the children during the early years. When the children were in elementary school, Pamela got a part-time job so that money could be contributed to a college fund for the children.

When Joseph was diagnosed with gastric carcinoma, he suffered in silence. He did not allow anyone to accompany him to the physician's office or say anything about pain or pain medicine. He underwent surgery and adjuvant therapy without complaint. When it was clear that the cancer had recurred and he was readmitted to the hospital, the pain was such that he did agree to take some pain medicine. Even though he hurt most of the time, he did not speak of it. His brothers told him to be tough, that he could "beat this thing."

RELIGIOUS ORIENTATION. In addition to asking the client about his belief systems, appropriate assessment may include interaction with the client's family members and friends. Their comments about religious beliefs or expectations of conduct may provide important data for your assessment.

For example, ask if the client is affiliated with any religious group. Ask whether his church promotes any beliefs about pain and its meaning in life. Ask what pain means to the client.

Joseph's faith was strong. Although he was unsure that he would be healed of his cancer, he believed that God would not allow him to suffer too much. He considered the possibility that the pain was God's way of getting his attention so that he would become a better person. When he thought of this, he became more reluctant to take the pain medicine that his physician had prescribed for him. How would you respond to his beliefs?

PSYCHOSOCIAL MODIFIERS. Your assessment will be more insightful if you understand the client's personal and family dynamics and stressors. If possible, observe family interactions to obtain information the health care team can use to intervene. Pain can drain the client's energy reserves. Concurrent stressors can further reduce those reserves. To assess the client's psychosocial modifiers, consider asking questions like these:

- You seem worried right now. Is there any way I can help you? Can I put you in touch with someone who might be able to help you deal with these worrisome events?
- Pain can be such an energy-draining experience. Are there other things happening in your life that are also depleting your reserves?
- I've noticed that when you have visitors, you seem to hide your pain from them. Would you like to talk about that?
- You look tired. Is there something besides the pain that is causing your fatigue?
- Has the pain interfered with your enjoyment of others? Have you found it necessary to limit your social activities? Can you participate in family, church, and other social functions as you would like?

PSYCHOLOGICAL EVALUATION

A psychological evaluation can be useful when pain prevents a client from participating in routine activities, adversely affects his relationships with others, or causes inappropriate emotional distress. It may also be indicated for clients who use the health care system excessively or demand further assessment or treatment when none is indicated. Clients most likely to benefit from a psychological evaluation are those who are experiencing chronic, disabling pain. The purpose of the evaluation is to determine which psychological and behavioral treatment strategies are indicated.

Physical Examination

When examining a client who has pain, ask him to identify the location of the pain on his body. This allows you to evaluate the area, check for any signs of infection or damage to the tissue, and gently palpate the area to confirm the source of the discomfort. It is also important to query the client about and to palpate any pathological areas that have been documented in previous diagnostic tests. Also, assess the client's vital signs, behaviors, and physical appearance.

VITAL SIGNS

An objective assessment should include the client's blood pressure, pulse, respiratory rate, and temperature. A client in acute pain will most likely show an elevation of some vital signs. He may be sweating as well.

If you detect a change in vital signs in a client at risk for pain, it is appropriate to ask the client if he has pain. As previously mentioned, a client with chronic pain undergoes an adaptation of the autonomic nervous system and usually will not exhibit any changes in vital signs.

CLIENT BEHAVIORS

Moaning, grimacing, crying, guarding or restricting activity, or refusing to get out of bed or walk are typical behaviors for a client with acute pain. They should always elicit queries about the presence of pain.

A client with chronic pain may have adapted behaviorally and have few visible signs despite considerable pain. The person's facial expression may be without affect. Your knowledge that the client has a painful condition should elicit questions about his pain status even without behavioral cues.

PHYSICAL APPEARANCE

Pain can interfere with activities of daily living, such as grooming. A client who normally is very careful about his personal appearance may be unable to perform his normal routine because of pain. A client's focus on chronic pain can absorb available physical and emotional resources and divert the energy needed for personal hygiene and aesthetics.

Assessment of Pain in Special Populations

Infants and Children

Many outdated misconceptions interfere with the accurate assessment of pain in infants and children. These misconceptions should be recognized and dismissed. These biases include the following erroneous beliefs:

- Neonates and infants do not feel pain.
- Children are not as sensitive to pain as adults.
- Children get used to pain and tolerate it very well.
- Children do not remember pain.
- Children will tell you if they have pain.
- Children are always truthful about pain.
- A child is not in pain if he can be distracted or is sleeping.
- Parents exaggerate their child's pain.

In reality, infants may show facial grimacing, vigorous crying, generalized body movements, or chin quivering in response to pain. Physiological responses to pain among children include increases in heart rate, blood pressure, and respiratory rate; restlessness; diaphoresis; and dilation of the pupils. However, children will respond in a similar manner when they are anxious, afraid, or angry, so you cannot assume that pain has caused the problem.

Your assessment should be based on the client's developmental level. Whereas cries, screams, behavioral regression, and difficulty in comforting may be appropriate pain behaviors in toddlers, different behaviors are appropriate in preschoolers. Such behaviors include struggling against restraint, aggressiveness, striking out physically and verbally when hurt, and a low frustration level.

As with adults, it is important to obtain a pain history for a child. Wong (1995) believes that a child's statements and descriptions of pain are the most important assessment factors. Involving parents provides insight into the child's developmental level and coping strategies.

Many pain assessment tools have been developed for children, using behavioral observation or, for those able to quantify their pain in some manner, self-report. As with adult assessment tools, however, reliability and validity should be verified. The Eland Color Tools (ages 4 to 6) require that the child pick crayon colors representing pain levels (Ball and Bindler, 1995). The Poker Chip Scale (ages 4 to 18) has the client select red poker chips to indicate pain levels (Hester & Barcus, 1986). The Wong/Baker FACES Rating Scale uses picture faces with expressions that represent varying levels of pain (Fig. 42–6). The child chooses the face that best represents how she is feeling.

Older Adults

Pain is a significant problem for the older adult. Pain is very common in the frail elderly and can cloud thinking and slow body movement. It should not be accepted as a normal part of aging but rather as a sign of disease.

Other assessment barriers include the desire of older adults to present themselves as "good patients"; fears that complaints may affect quality of care; a desire to please the doctor; fear of seeming burdensome to family members; fear of tests, operations, or treat-

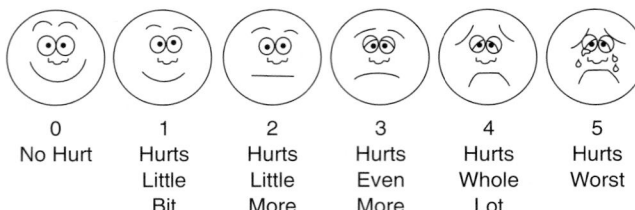

Figure 42–6. The Wong/Baker FACES Pain Rating Scale uses faces that represent varying levels of pain. Explain to the person that each face is for a person who feels happy because he has no pain (hurt) or sad because he has some or a lot of pain. **Face 0** is very happy because he doesn't hurt at all. **Face 1** hurts just a little bit. **Face 2** hurts a little more. **Face 3** hurts even more. **Face 4** hurts a whole lot. **Face 5** hurts just as much as you can imagine, although you don't have to be crying to feel this bad. Ask the person to choose the face that best describes how he is feeling. Rating scale is recommended for persons age 3 years and older. (From Wong, D.L., Hockenberry-Eaton, M., Wilson, D., Winkelstein, M.L., Ahmann, E., & DiVito-Thomas, P.A. [1999]. Whaley and Wong's nursing care of infants and children [6th ed.]. St. Louis: Mosby.)

ment costs; and fear of opioid dependence and loss of functioning.

Identifying the cause of pain may be difficult in a population at risk for memory failure, depression, sensory impairment, dementia, and confusion. The cognitively impaired older adult may minimize the presence of pain slightly, but the report is no less valid. The client may not be able to remember "past" pain, so it is important to assess the current pain status.

An observed decrease in the client's usual function may be the most sensitive indicator of pain in a frail older adult. This variable takes on added importance for those who cannot communicate their pain status or who cannot comprehend or use assessment tools. Poor appetite, depression, sleep disturbances, and anxiety may develop as well. Although overt behaviors, such as guarding and facial grimacing, may be apparent, the older adult may not exhibit any outward signs of discomfort. Thus, focused attention on slow or decreased movement is essential.

Dementia and delirium can impair the client's ability to communicate his pain status, as discussed in the accompanying State of Nursing Science chart. Consequently, you must be able to distinguish between normal and abnormal behavior. For example, someone who is generally nonverbal may blink rapidly, become agitated, or move around frequently. It may also be helpful to ask those who know the client to comment on any behavioral changes that could indicate pain.

A*ction* A*lert!*
Confusion or a marked change in behavior may be a sign of pain in the older adult.

Clients With Communication Barriers

Although neonates, infants, and some elderly clients are included in this population, the main groups at risk for impaired communication are those who speak a different language, have limited language skills, are severely emotionally disturbed, have an endotracheal tube, or have an altered level of consciousness. You should be especially alert for signs of pain in these groups.

Systematic observation for possible pain and comfort behaviors related to vocalizations, facial expressions, body movements, changes in behavior or activity, or autonomic responses is important. If a client is known to have a painful condition or undergoes a procedure known to be painful, it is appropriate to treat the pain before it occurs with a trial of analgesic. Intubated but alert clients may be offered writing materials or asked to use a pain intensity scale for assessment purposes.

Clients at Risk for Substance Abuse

Clients at particular risk for psychological dependence (addiction) include those with a history of alcoholism; a history of drug-related problems and previous treatment; loss of a job due to drug use; regular use of illicit drugs; or a history of mental illness or depression.

You must be careful to look for physiological causes for pain and be cautious in ruling them out if they are not quickly identified, even if you are convinced that the client is drug-seeking. Interviewing strategies include questioning about drug use in a matter-of-fact manner. Begin with questions about

---

THE STATE OF NURSING SCIENCE
ASSESSING PAIN IN COGNITIVELY IMPAIRED OLDER ADULTS

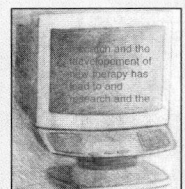

What Are the Issues?

Because pain is a subjective experience, cognitively impaired older adults may be at a disadvantage in communicating their need for nursing intervention. Current pain assessment tools rely on a person's self-report of pain according to a numerical or other graphic system. Without validation of the person's report of pain, nurses may miss opportunities to relieve suffering.

What Research Has Been Conducted?

Kaasalainen et al. (1998) studied the pain assessment and frequency of administering p.r.n. pain medications by nurses who worked with institutionalized older adults. They asked the nurses to use a standardized assessment tool to rate the pain of their patients. The researchers then examined the medication administration records to see what was available for pain management and when it was administered. Despite the availability of medications for pain, a significantly lower percentage of cognitively impaired older adults received analgesics when compared with cognitively intact older adults. Fewer cognitively impaired older adults were on scheduled analgesics prescribed by their physicians.

Parke (1998) used a qualitative approach to interview experienced nurses and nursing assistants about their assessment of cognitively impaired older adults who were thought to be in pain. She asked these nursing personnel to describe how they knew the older adults were having pain. Their descriptions indicated that experienced caregivers relied on their previous knowledge of the person to detect changes in "overt behavior, appearance, and sounds" (p 25). Some of the behaviors to which nurses paid attention were aggression, restlessness, and changes in activities of daily living. Changes in sounds included silence, complaints, and painful vo-

calizations. Facial expressions of grimacing or changes in body language were also identified as possible indicators of pain. Nurses also used information about the diagnosis and circumstances surrounding the condition of the older adults to determine whether pain was the correct assessment. They evaluated the responses to pain relief measures to infer that their assessment was correct. These nurses also employed the impressions of other team members to support their assessments.

What Has the Research Concluded?

Pain is undertreated in cognitively impaired older adults. This may be because of the lack of valid and reliable assessment tools that do not rely solely on subjective data. However, nurses with expertise in gerontological nursing are well equipped to detect patterns of pain behavior in cognitively impaired older adults, especially in those well known to them.

What Is the Future of Research in This Area?

Reliable pain assessment tools that do not rely on subjective data are needed for use with cognitively impaired older adults. Such tools may help nurses accurately assess the presence of pain in older adults and then treat the pain to relieve suffering. A potential source of information to use in creating such tools are expert nurses who have the experience to detect patterns that indicate pain in older adults.

References

Kaasalainen, S., Middleton, J., Knezacek, S., Hartley, T., Stewart, N., Ife, C., & Robinson, L. (1998). Pain and cognitive status in the institutionalized elderly. Journal of Gerontological Nursing, 24, (8), 24–31.

Parke, B. (1998). Gerontological nurses' ways of knowing: Realizing the presence of pain in cognitively impaired older adults. Journal of Gerontological Nursing, 24, (6), 21–28.

over-the-counter medications (including caffeine and cigarettes), and continue with questions about prescription medications, both current and past. Proceed to questions about alcohol and illicit substances. If you suspect drug use, ask questions that presume normal quantities used such as, "When was your last drink?" "When did you last use cocaine?" or "Do you ever mix drugs?"

Look for drug-related behaviors that suggest substance abuse. Prescription abuse, such as forging prescriptions, selling prescription drugs, or obtaining drugs from nonmedical sources, is a typical behavior. Investigate multiple episodes of prescription "loss" and misuse of prescribed medications or therapies. Also follow up on what seem to be "opioid protection strategies." These may include requests for a specific brand of analgesic, a history of therapeutic response to opioids only, reports of multiple drug allergies that severely limit the choice of analgesic given, and extreme resistance to multimodal pain therapies. Also watch for deteriorating functional and social skills and frequent missed appointments or late arrivals for appointments. Toxicology screening is essential but requires strict confidentiality.

This client population requires skill, sensitivity, compassion, and patience. By following these diagnostic and assessment practices, you will enable the multidisciplinary team to plan carefully for the client's care.

Focused Assessment for Acute Pain

The relatively short-term nature of acute pain demands that you focus your assessment on the nature and intensity of the pain, client behaviors, and response to analgesic interventions. Your assessment should be directed toward gathering an accurate picture of the client's pain and collaborating with other team members to discern the most appropriate treatment interventions.

Defining Characteristics

Defining characteristics for *Pain* include the following:

- A verbal or coded report of pain
- Observed evidence of pain, such as a facial mask, sleep disturbance, self-focus or narrowed focus, moaning, crying, restlessness, irritability, sighing, and altered appetite
- Antalgic position or gestures to counteract or avoid pain, protective behavior, guarding behavior
- Distraction behaviors, such as pacing or repetitive actions
- Autonomic evidence, such as diaphoresis, blood pressure elevation, increased respirations, increased pulse, dilated pupils, altered muscle tone
- Quiet, distracted, or withdrawn behaviors

Related Factors

Factors related to *Pain* include biological, chemical, physical, and psychological injury agents. Other re-

lated factors that you may notice include the following:

ANXIETY. It is common to become anxious when one encounters sudden or unexpected pain. The anxiety, in turn, aggravates the pain experience. If the prescribed intervention fails to relieve the discomfort, the client may develop even greater anxiety that the pain will not be relieved.

FEAR. Clients can become quite fearful in the midst of a pain experience. There are inevitable worries about the cause of the pain, whether it will eventually be gone, and whether the analgesic will be effective. Some clients fear that they will become dependent on the analgesic.

NAUSEA AND VOMITING. Many of the analgesics prescribed for acute pain can cause nausea or vomiting. Opioid analgesics act on the chemoreceptor trigger zone in the brain, causing an emetic response. NSAIDs can cause gastric mucosal irritation, another potential cause of an emetic response.

IMMOBILITY. Clients with significant pain are reluctant to move because movement exacerbates the pain. They may refuse to ambulate, breathe deeply (after abdominal surgery, for example), get out of bed, or move in any way that might make the pain more intense.

IMPAIRED VERBAL COMMUNICATION. Although this is an issue for any client unable to communicate a health problem, it is especially important for the client with pain. Because your assessment relies partially on the client's verbal report, impaired communication makes the task of selecting diagnostic and treatment methods much more difficult. It also places the client at greater risk of inadequate pain relief. Neonates, children, mentally challenged or comatose clients, or clients with a language barrier require special approaches.

Focused Assessment for Chronic Pain

Chronic pain falls into two major categories: chronic *malignant* pain, which is associated with cancer and other rapidly progressive disorders, and chronic *nonmalignant* pain, which occurs when tissue injury remains stable or is healed. These two types share similarities and differences.

Nonmalignant etiologies are more likely to produce neuropathic pain, which tends to be difficult to treat and, at times, more disabling than cancer pain. Also, the client may be less likely to report the pain because it has become a "normal" and unchanging part of life. The accompanying A Patient's View chart offers one client's personal experience.

Components of acute pain assessment are also part of chronic pain assessment; however, emotional, relational, functional, sociocultural, psychological, and economic issues are of such importance that they must be probed in order to understand the client's perception and meaning of the pain experience. Planning and treatment depend on that assessment.

Keep in mind that cancer pain can be acute if treatment cures the disease. It becomes chronic if the dis-

A PATIENT'S VIEW
"SOMETIMES IT EVEN HURTS TO BREATHE"

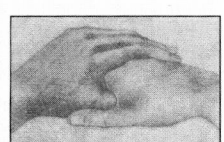

I was 19 years old when my first child was born. It was a difficult birth. The doctor tried to deliver the baby using forceps but ended up doing a cesarean. That was December 1955. The following March, I fell and hit my tailbone. In June of that year, I began to have pain in my lower back. Since then I've never been without pain, despite eight spinal operations and two spinal fusions. I'll soon be 62.

Nearly 2 years after my son was born, I became pregnant with my daughter. That was a really hard time. The pain was so intense I had to have injections in my back to give me any relief. A few months after she was born, the pain was just indescribable, not just in my back but a constant headache as well. One look at the myelogram and the surgeon told me he would operate the next day. Scar tissue—probably from the first unsuccessful attempt at forceps delivery of my son—had wrapped around and squeezed my spinal cord. The surgeon said that without that operation I would have been paralyzed. Waking up afterward, I realized that for the first time in months I didn't have a headache.

Each of the surgeries has helped to a degree, but it seems like when one spot gets fixed, another flares up. Fifteen years ago, an MRI showed that I had a disk protruding and bone spurs were pressing on a nerve. By then I'd had seven operations and didn't really want more surgery but the pain was so intense I couldn't walk, so I had no choice. Right now I'm having trouble with my upper back and sometimes it even hurts to breathe. But I've learned to live with the pain. I don't like to take pain medications, other than daily Tylenol and once in a while Darvocet. But I don't like to take any kind of narcotics. I don't want to trade off one problem for another.

Part of living with the pain is learning to relax. Lie down and let your body go limp. That eases the pain, sometimes even without medication.

Keeping busy takes my mind off the pain. I hurt worse when I sit down and do nothing. I love to cook, any kind of cooking, but especially Southern dishes and trying new recipes. I bake cookies for church events. Any excuse will do. Sometimes I have to stop and rest for a while, but then I can do more. When I'm in the kitchen, I almost never worry about anything.

It also helps to have a lot of interests. Besides cooking, I enjoy collecting things: teapots, angels, and antique glassware. Most of all, I enjoy my family—not just my children but nieces and nephews, too—and my church.

My life hasn't been easy. I had a bad marriage, and that was rough, but I've never lost hope. My family is loving and supportive. I'm still able to drive and do my own shopping. I'm still able to work, and I love my work. You can't do a good job if you don't love your work.

I do home care for the elderly. Back in the 1950s, I was trained as a nurse's aide, so I've taken care of people most of my life, including my mother when she was dying. Right now I'm caring for an 86-year-old lady who lives alone. She has to use a walker, and she needs help with her bath, but she's a very "up" person, just a dream to care for. I fix her food, see that she takes her medications, take her to get her hair done or out to dinner. It's a great job.

People in pain need understanding and compassion—tender loving care—but they also need not to feel sorry for themselves; that can make you a total invalid. My father always told us there's no such word as "can't." So I chose to be productive, to fight the pain and not give in to it. And I have a lot of faith. I pray a lot. God gives me the strength I need to go on. I feel sorry for people who don't have this kind of faith. I wouldn't trade one instant of my life for all of theirs. Love and faith and health are far more important than material things.

I can't remember a time without God in the center of my life. When I was growing up, we read the Bible at home, and my sister and I rode the bus to church every Sunday. My father taught Sunday school the last 20 years of his life. Despite my trials and tribulations, I've never lost hope. I have an inner peace that, like the Bible says, "passes all understanding," and I never feel alone. That's why I say: I'm not lucky, I'm blessed.

---

ease is metastatic or rapidly progressive and will most likely intensify as the tumor grows. Chronic cancer pain is very likely to have both nociceptive and neuropathic components and requires attention to the client's verbal descriptors. Pain secondary to a progressive malignant disease is a daily reminder of the illness and limited life expectancy.

Defining Characteristics

In general, the characteristics of chronic pain are more subtle than those of acute pain; the pain area is more difficult to pinpoint; and the intensity is harder to evaluate. The client's suffering is likely to increase over time. The long-term, possibly intractable nature of chronic pain requires a more varied assessment that, of necessity, integrates many variables, such as those discussed below.

VERBAL REPORTS. In nonmalignant chronic pain, the client's description of pain may be vague. He may have trouble pinpointing the source. He may have described the sensations to so many different health care professionals that he is weary of the effort and may provide abbreviated information that is less than helpful. Certainly, your report should document his lengthy pain experience.

In malignant pain, diagnostic assessment can usually locate the site of the primary tumor and metastases, if present, to support the client's description of pain. In addition, treatment for the tumor (such as chemotherapy, surgery, and radiation therapy) can itself cause pain. Clients with malignant disease are usually more able to describe the location and particular sensation of the pain than are clients with neuropathic pain.

OBSERVED BEHAVIORS. In nonmalignant chronic pain, the client may have a mask-like look of pain, with a dull affect and pinched eyes. His behavior may be guarded and protective, especially around the painful area. Some clients will limp or stay very still.

In malignant pain, the client's facial expressions and guarding behaviors can be similar to those of any person with chronic pain. What may differ somewhat is that a client with advanced disease or undergoing rigorous treatment may feel marked malaise and appear not only tired but also very unwell.

When Joseph would come to visit his doctor at the office, it was evident that he had a significant amount of pain. He was very cautious in his movements, sat rigidly in the chair, was extremely tense during the physical examination, and kept his face very still. He would respond that the pain was "pretty much okay" when questioned about it. His physician put him on a sustained-release analgesic preparation to be taken two times a day, telling him that although it was a pain medicine, it was also helpful for his breathing, which was becoming somewhat more difficult because of the tumor pressing against his diaphragm. Joseph reluctantly agreed to take the medicine for his "breathing."

WEIGHT CHANGES. In nonmalignant chronic pain, the client may lose weight because of a decreased focus on eating, or he may gain weight if eating becomes a substitute for more active behaviors or a form of self-soothing. Weight loss may further jeopardize the client's health by depleting energy stores and muscle mass. Increased weight can worsen the pain if weight-bearing is a contributing variable or if it interferes with prescribed therapeutic exercise or other nonpharmacological interventions.

In malignant pain, weight loss is common for many reasons: tumor growth, cancer therapies and their side effects, loss of appetite, anxiety, and depression. Some clients who receive corticosteroid medications will gain weight.

AFFECTIVE DISORDERS. Nonmalignant chronic pain can deplete the client's energy reserves very quickly, and irritability, restlessness, and depression are common. You might see emotional withdrawal when the client focuses exclusively on himself in relation to the pain experience.

In malignant pain, an existential kind of suffering may be superimposed on the pain state. The threat of loss of life and the loss of control over the disease can contribute to significant sadness and depression.

CHANGES IN SLEEPING PATTERNS. Nonmalignant chronic pain may make it difficult for the client to find a comfortable position at night, may disturb sleep many times during the night, or may prevent sleep altogether. Clients may describe "walking the floor" at night or getting up to watch television if the pain prevents sleep. Sleeping habits may shift to a series of short naps spaced over the 24-hour period.

As the art and science of palliative medicine grow, the increasing emphasis on excellence in symptom management allows clients with malignant chronic pain greater access to opioid analgesics, anxiolytic agents, and sleeping medications. As a result, a client with cancer may be able to sleep relatively well at night, despite the presence of significant pain-producing disease.

DISRUPTED SOCIAL RELATIONSHIPS AND ACTIVITIES. Both nonmalignant and malignant chronic pain can disrupt previously established social relationships with family members and friends. Socializing may take energy the client feels he no longer has, or depression may reduce his ability to be with others. An inability to be involved in previous activities, whether social or more functional in nature, is a common occurrence.

A client with malignant pain caused by cancer may find that friends and relatives avoid him. The reasons are varied. Most people "do not know what to say." Some may fear disease transmission. Other are extremely uncomfortable being around someone with a life-threatening illness. Conversely, clients may not want visitors as the level of fatigue rises.

Related Factors

Factors related to *Chronic pain* include chronic physical or psychosocial disability, fatigue, misconceptions about pain and its treatment, and a low tolerance for pain.

CHRONIC PHYSICAL DISABILITY. Intractable pain—malignant or nonmalignant—can cause permanent disability. The client may no longer be able to work, may work in a limited capacity, or may have to find employment that does not aggravate the illness.

A client with malignant pain but controlled disease may be able to continue employment and activities of daily living with minor modifications. As the disease advances, the ability to work or pursue activities of daily living will decline.

CHRONIC PSYCHOSOCIAL DISABILITY. Chronic, disabling pain—malignant or nonmalignant—also affects the client at an existential level. It is difficult for others to understand how life-changing such pain can be. The client may not be able to verbalize the unappreciated need to grieve for a formerly healthy self. The client's self-esteem, if grounded in his ability to be productive and function in multiple capacities, may be shattered. He may feel ashamed and inadequate that he is not strong enough to endure the discomfort. Ultimately, if the pain is unrelenting and severe, atypical and dysfunctional behaviors may appear.

A client in the terminal phase of an illness may withdraw from others, even those who are emotionally close to the person. Some clients turn away from everyone as they face their final days.

FATIGUE. Pain depletes energy, and dealing with it on a chronic basis can absorb the client's physical and emotional resources. The fatigue may be compounded by the illness itself or interventions used to treat it.

MISCONCEPTIONS ABOUT PAIN AND TREATMENT. Clients with chronic nonmalignant pain are rarely treated with one modality and are best served by a multidisciplinary team. As a result, many clients are confused about which intervention is helping them and whether to seek others to assist in their care. Difficulty in accepting a diagnosis of intractable pain often results in "selective listening." The client may continue to believe that the pain will one day be gone. If you cannot articulate the source of the pain, the client may continue to hope that the problem can be solved once the cause is known.

The management of malignant cancer pain can be extremely effective in most cases if clients comply with the prescribed regimen. There may be "selective listening" in this client population as well, however, and many people who require substantial doses of opioid analgesics to relieve pain will refuse to comply with the regimen because they fear addiction. Others may choose to "forget" the discomfort because the pain is a constant reminder of their illness and prognosis.

LOW TOLERANCE FOR PAIN. Many clients with nonmalignant pain have suffered significant and unrelenting pain for so long that their ability to cope with any more or any new pain is impaired. As the pain takes its toll and emotions rise close to the surface, the slightest amount of new or extra pain may produce a disproportionate emotional response.

In malignant pain, the emotional burden of the cancer diagnosis superimposed on significant pain, whether relatively new or long-standing, can trigger a strong emotional response. Anxiety, helplessness, depression, and loss of control deplete the client's ability to tolerate any more pain. Many clients feel that it is not only unjust that they have cancer, but also that pain adds indignity and punishment.

Focused Assessment for Related Nursing Diagnoses

Constipation

Many types of acute and chronic pain require the use of opioid analgesics for effective management. Constipation is a common side effects of opioids. Although clients may become tolerant of other opioid side effects, they never develop tolerance of the constipating effects.

Contributing factors for the person in pain may include decreased activity, additional disorders, decreased liquid and oral intake, stress, or grief. A client with acute pain may require temporary intervention for constipation, but the problem will be resolved when opioid therapy is discontinued if there is no other contributing factor. A client with chronic malig-

nant pain may be not only on significant doses of opioid analgesics but may also have limited oral intake. An aggressive bowel regimen will usually always be necessary for clients on chronic or substantial opioid therapy.

Joseph did comply with the analgesic regimen for his "breathing" and became increasingly constipated. The nurse prescribed a bowel regimen, expecting that he would have a bowel movement at least every 3 days. Joseph did not follow the bowel regimen, however, and went for 10 days without a bowel movement. He did not tell his wife but did discuss the matter with his brothers. They could see his distended abdomen, and he even mentioned that it "hurt a little bit." One of his brothers went to the drugstore and bought over-the-counter enemas for him. Joseph managed to remove the impaction himself and used two small enemas to clear out his lower bowel. He started at that time on the stool softeners that had been prescribed for him. He never told his wife. Can you think of a teaching approach that might have prevented this problem?

Activity Intolerance

One of the primary effects of pain is an instinctive response to be still and wait until the pain abates. Both acute and chronic pain can trigger varying degrees of intolerance to movement. The client quickly learns what activities to avoid. A client with acute pain understands its time-limited nature and may take analgesics to reduce pain enough to allow some activity. As the tissue heals, activity naturally increases.

In chronic pain, however, clients who begin to consistently decrease their activity levels will become weaker and even less tolerant of activity. Sleep disorders, fatigue, and deconditioning all contribute to the inability to perform as they did before the chronic pain began.

Altered Role Performance

Role performance and role expectations are influenced by social forces, cultural norms, and values. Because performance defines who and what a person is, any disruption can have a significant impact on the sense of self.

Acute pain can cause a temporary disruption in the ability to perform activities of daily living and work at full capacity. Some clients may need to use sick leave as they recover from an injury or surgical procedure. Others may be allowed to continue their jobs in a different capacity until wellness returns. Role expectations may be set aside temporarily because others understand that the person will return to prior functional levels.

Chronic pain can dramatically alter the ability to work, to perform activities of daily living, and to interact with others. Because a person's sense of self is closely tied to the ability to perform as expected, low self-esteem is not uncommon in the client who has become even partially disabled. Failure to meet role expectations can threaten life goals, alienate others, and produce extreme stress.

Hopelessness

The term chronic conjures up words such as *interminable* and *forever*. A client who discovers that he may live with disabling or severe pain for a long time, possibly forever, can be overwhelmed by this knowledge. Intertwined are feelings of helplessness, loss of control, and depression. The client with recurrent malignant disease, unresponsive to further therapies, suffers the loss of time in which to complete the business of life.

Hopelessness affects physical, psychological, and spiritual health. Clients may become very passive, withdraw from others, demonstrate a decreased affect, refuse to solve problems or make decisions, and lose their spiritual beliefs.

Ineffective Individual Coping

A person's ability to cope is reflected in his day-to-day management of his affairs. While he may at times feel burdened by extra work, temporary crises or problems, the woes of a friend or family member, or changing careers, the average person can use "reserve" physical and emotional resources to deal with and adjust to changing circumstances.

Problems with health can severely reduce a person's coping resources. When illness and its symptoms (such as pain) become chronic, those resources may become so depleted that the client no longer knows how to function effectively. Pessimism, increased anxiety, general unhappiness, self-focus, and defensive behaviors are common. Clients may become unproductive and dependent on others. Pain, even though very real and deserving of attention, becomes the excuse for every change in the client's behavior. Support systems may be lost as others turn away from this person they no longer seem to know or like.

Caregiver Role Strain

As families become more geographically separated and people with chronic illnesses live longer, traditional support systems such as neighborhoods, churches, and social clubs are less prominent in people's lives. It is not uncommon for a client with a chronic illness to rely primarily on a very limited circle of family and friends.

Clients with chronic pain can be extremely demanding, irritable, often angry, and at times very unpleasant. Caring for such a person, with or without a constellation of accompanying symptoms, can be demanding, exhausting, and depressing and can socially isolate the caregiver. Caregivers may find themselves becoming defensive, irritable, and angry, which triggers feelings of guilt. They may become ill as they deal with the needs of the client for whom they are caring.

Pamela Valdez did not know what to do. Joseph was becoming increasingly withdrawn and quiet and never told her how he felt about his illness. He muttered that he was "okay" when she asked him about his pain. He did not play with his children as he once had and rarely paid any attention to them. He went to work every day and, when he came home exhausted, he would sit down in front of the television set and not speak to anyone. How could you help Pamela cope?

The caregiver may not feel competent to provide the kind of care required. Clients with chronic malignant pain who are in the terminal phase of illness often require an array of pain medications and other interventions to manage symptoms. They may be on multiple medications that must be given on schedule at varied times of the day and night. They may have ambulatory infusion pumps for intravenous or intraspinal opioid delivery. Or they may need some kind of medical device, such as an oxygen delivery system, a nasogastric suction pump, a nasogastric feeding device, or an indwelling urinary catheter. Managing these complex needs can be overwhelming for the layperson.

Ineffective Management of Therapeutic Regimen: Individuals

Acute pain rarely requires a difficult or multifaceted regimen. The short-term nature of the pain and limited interventions can generally be managed by the client or caregiver. Issues may arise if the client or caregiver fears taking or administering opioid analgesics or if the primary caregiver is forgetful. Even for short-term pain management, provide education to client and family about medications, dosages, schedules, side effects, and the expected outcomes of treatment.

The management of chronic pain requires more complex strategies. Multiple nonpharmacological and pharmacological modalities may be involved. Clients must be motivated and disciplined to devote their energy to adhere to a complex regimen. Feelings of helplessness, hopelessness, and depression as well as lack of confidence in the outcomes may predispose the client to miss appointments or be uncooperative or noncompliant with interventions.

The management of chronic malignant pain may require multiple types of typical and atypical analgesics. It may seem to the client and caregiver that every day must be focused on taking the medication at the proper time. Additionally, fears of opioid addiction may affect both client and caregiver as they struggle to balance this fear with adequate analgesia. If the pain requires complex medical equipment for delivery of the opioid analgesic, clients and caregivers may give up on this intervention as too bothersome or burdensome.

DIAGNOSIS

When a client has a risk for pain or has pain as a primary or secondary diagnosis, you will base the nursing diagnosis on assessment factors that include the health history, results of diagnostic tests, current vital signs, physical assessment, client self-report of the pain state, anticipated interventions (such as surgery), and an understanding of the expected course of the client's illness. These factors will determine whether *Pain* or *Chronic pain* is the more appropriate nursing diagnosis, as you can see in the data clustering chart.

Pain or *Chronic pain* can be a primary diagnosis or a related factor. Because pain is a common symptom for many treatable and untreatable illnesses, you must distinguish whether it is the primary or secondary focus. Even though pain is always worthy of intervention, you may select another diagnosis and provide analgesic treatment as an intervention for managing the primary diagnosis.

Take, for example, the client who has a total hip replacement. Significant pain will be present during the postoperative period. However, to recover fully by participating in a rehabilitative regimen, the client must be comfortable enough to ambulate and perform the proper range-of-motion exercises. In this instance, the nursing diagnosis would be *Activity intolerance related to pain.*

Conversely, a client admitted to the hospital with intractable pain secondary to breast cancer metastatic to the bone would have a primary nursing diagnosis of *Chronic pain.* If the primary disease is no longer amenable to curative intervention, pain, which has been a symptom of the primary disease, now becomes the primary illness and the focus of aggressive intervention.

PLANNING

Developing a plan of care for a client who risks pain or has pain requires collaboration with the client and family. The plan will be driven by the nature of the pain, the underlying disorder, cultural and social variables that influence the client, the chronicity of the pain experience, and any other confounding variables that require consideration and integration into the plan of care.

Expected Outcomes for the Client at Risk for Pain

A client may be at risk for *Pain* if he faces a surgical or diagnostic procedure known to cause pain. Your goals

---

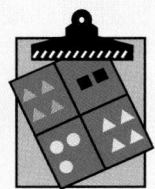

CLUSTERING DATA TO MAKE A NURSING DIAGNOSIS
PAIN

Data Cluster	Diagnosis
27-year-old male admitted to hospital via the emergency department following a motorcycle accident with fractured leg, 2 fractured ribs, multiple contusions. Repeatedly complains of pain and asks for "anything to make this pain better."	*Pain* related to extensive tissue damage from multiple trauma and anxiety
Client has history of osteoporosis and steroid use for respiratory disease. Admitted to hospital for hip replacement. Does not want to participate in physical therapy because of hip pain.	*Impaired physical mobility* related to postsurgical tissue trauma, anxiety, and low tolerance for pain
38-year-old woman with recurrent breast cancer metastatic to multiple skeletal sites. Rates pain consistently as an 8 (scale 0–10) despite maximizing current analgesic regimen.	*Chronic pain* related to malignant disease progression
35-year-old man injured in industrial accident. Chronic, intractable back pain has forced him to go on disability. He can no longer help around the house as he did before, and he does not want his buddies to see him in a disabled state.	*Body image disturbance* related to functional loss secondary to pain
Elderly client with severe, escalating pain secondary to metastatic prostate cancer. Disease has progressed despite continued active therapy. Physician referred him to hospice for palliative care. Client believes that the pain will never get better because it is "punishment from God for bad things I've done."	*Hopelessness* related to disease progression, increased pain, and psychological stress

should be to prepare the client for the experience and to plan interventions. Client education should include a clear explanation of the expected nature and duration of the pain and planned treatment strategies. Expected outcomes include decreased anxiety before the procedure and verbalization that the client understands the planned interventions.

Expected Outcomes for the Client With Acute Pain

The goal for a client with *Pain* is to provide relief using pharmacological and nonpharmacological interventions. Client education should focus on the rationale for and description of the plan of care. Expected outcomes include decreased anxiety, client verbalization of planned analgesic interventions, decreased verbal complaints and behaviors that indicate unrelieved pain, and a decreased need for analgesic interventions as the tissue heals. Usually, the outcome is positive. Pain that is undertreated may result in chronic pain, so it is essential that the pain be controlled.

Expected Outcomes for the Client With Chronic Pain

Desired outcomes for a client with *Chronic pain* (malignant or nonmalignant) are to set realistic goals with the client and his family, to reduce pain to a level that the client can tolerate, to actively involve the client or caregiver in the treatment regimen, and to maximize the client's quality of life. It is imperative that the client understand the rationale for nonpharmacological and pharmacological interventions and be able to verbalize the treatment plan. An additional outcome for the client with chronic nonmalignant pain would be to improve the level of functioning or return the client to a prior level of functioning.

For the client with chronic malignant pain, additional outcomes would be to dispel myths about the use of opioid analgesics, to enable the client to function as appropriate for a person with malignant disease at any place on the illness continuum, and to provide the psychosocial support needed by the client and family to cope with chronic pain caused by a terminal illness.

INTERVENTION

Interventions to Manage Acute Pain

Acute pain from surgery, diagnostic procedures, burns, and trauma is underestimated and undertreated. Clinical surveys document that intramuscular injections on a p.r.n. basis are inadequate for about half of postoperative clients, yet this continues to be a commonly prescribed and very uncomfortable intervention. Assessment should be frequent, with a focus on the efficacy of the prescribed intervention.

Management Principles

SELECTING ANALGESICS

If the client's pain is mild to moderate, nonopioid analgesics may be effective. They provide analgesia at the peripheral level by physiological mechanisms independent of the opioid receptor sites. Acetaminophen, aspirin, and NSAIDs are likely choices. If the client cannot tolerate anything by mouth, another route is chosen. Nonpharmacological methods may provide relief.

If the pain is moderate to severe, an oral or parenteral opioid analgesic is indicated, possibly in combination with an NSAID. Dosage, schedule, incidence and intensity of side effects, and treatment settings are important variables to be considered. Morphine, meperidine, and hydromorphone are typical parenteral opioids used to manage moderate-to-severe pain. Meperidine is used for only a limited time and in moderate dosages. Many effective oral analgesics are available, as well as transdermal, sublingual, and rectal formulations.

TITRATING THE DOSAGE

A loading dose is the initial analgesic dose adequate to reduce pain to the client's self-defined level of comfort. Failure to provide an adequate loading dose for severe pain will delay pain relief even though the client may receive several p.r.n. or scheduled doses. Delivery of a loading dose may be accomplished by giving small, frequent doses until the client reports relief or becomes drowsy or by administering a single dose that provides relief.

Continue analgesic dosing until the pain is consistently relieved. If the client requests pain medication before the next dosage is scheduled, the dosage is inadequate or the scheduled interval inappropriate. A client who has previously received opioid analgesics or who has a history of prior or concurrent substance abuse may require higher initial and maintenance doses.

CHOOSING A SCHEDULE

The administration schedule should be based on the known half-life of the drug. Because each analgesic has a limited period of effectiveness, scheduling is driven by the duration of analgesia. When the analgesic is scheduled to keep the client comfortable between doses, anxiety is decreased. If the pain is expected to last for a time, the drug should be given on a scheduled basis during that time. A preventive approach provides effective analgesia and energy to devote to restorative activity. As the tissue heals and pain decreases, p.r.n. dosing is acceptable.

A major barrier to the proper prescribing of opioid analgesics for acute and chronic pain is fear of respiratory depression. An appropriate dose and schedule rarely cause respiratory depression. Monitoring the sedative level and decreasing the opioid dosage if the client is excessively drowsy prevent any life-threatening side effects. If the respiratory rate is moderately affected (around 8 to 10 breaths a minute) or the client is excessively drowsy, withhold the opioid, and reduce subsequent dosages. If the respiratory rate is significantly affected (fewer than 8 breaths a minute), 0.4 mg of Narcan diluted in normal saline to equal 10 mL may be slowly pushed intravenously until an adequate respiratory rate returns but pain relief remains intact.

A*ction* A*lert!*
Administration of significant doses of Narcan in the presence of respiratory depression restores respiratory function but also removes the opioid analgesic from receptor sites, causing significant pain. Dilute Narcan with normal saline, and titrate only to produce a respiratory effect.

IDENTIFYING THE APPROPRIATE ROUTE
The immediacy of the need for analgesic relief should determine the route. Outside of spinal analgesia, the intravenous route produces the most rapid onset of action. Moderate-to-severe pain responds favorably to intravenous opioids, making it the preferred route if intravenous access is available. Oral opioids may be used before discharge to make sure they provide adequate relief. Oral and intramuscular (IM) routes have a significant lag time to peak effect. The IM route also has the disadvantages of wide fluctuations in absorption and client discomfort.

There are multiple opioid preparations other than oral that can circumvent nothing-by-mouth status, intractable nausea and vomiting, inability to swallow, and obstruction of the small bowel. Opioid preparations are available as transdermal patches, rectal suppositories, parenteral solutions, and preservative-free parenteral solutions for intraspinal use.

When changing the route of administration, use equianalgesic conversion data. **Equianalgesia** is the dosage that provides the same amount of pain relief independent of the drug or the route. Oral analgesics are absorbed from the small bowel via the portal circulatory system and travel to the liver, where they undergo significant metabolism. This **first pass effect** refers to the partial metabolism of opioid analgesics by the liver before they reach the systemic circulation, thereby resulting in a decrease in opioid availability (dosage). Because the first pass effect decreases the available oral opioid dosage, oral dosages are greater than comparable parenteral dosages. Table 42–4 lists equianalgesic dosages for commonly prescribed opioids.

TREATING PROCEDURAL PAIN
Although procedural pain is usually short-term, it still requires adequate treatment. Describe the procedure to the client and family, and describe what can be done to minimize discomfort. The expected discomfort should be treated as a significant event that may require the use of local anesthetics, sedatives, opioid analgesics, or some combination of these drugs. Children may benefit from the parents' presence

TABLE 42–4
Equianalgesic Chart for Commonly Prescribed Opioids

Drug	Parenteral Dosage	Oral Dosage
Codeine	130 mg	200 mg
Fentanyl (Sublimaze)	100 μg	NA
Hydromorphone (Dilaudid)	2 mg	7.5 mg
Levorphanol (Levo-Dromoran)	2 mg	4 mg
Meperidine (Demerol)	100 mg	300 mg
Methadone (Dolophine)	10 mg	20 mg
Morphine*	10 mg	30 mg
Oxycodone (OxyIR, OxyContin)	NA	15 mg

*Morphine is the "gold standard" opioid with which all other opioids are compared.

during the procedure. The goal is comfort. Clients on concurrent opioid therapy will require more medication than those who are **opioid naive;** that is, who have had no or minimal exposure to opioid analgesics.

PLANNING ACROSS THE CONTINUUM OF CARE
As clients spend less time in the health care system, pre-discharge assessment for the adequacy of analgesia becomes ever more important. Clients must be prepared to manage their discomfort at home or in an outpatient setting. An analgesic plan should be implemented 24 hours before discharge to assess the efficacy of the drug and route.

The intensity of the client's pain determines the approach. If the client has been managed in the acute care setting with parenteral opioids and is to be discharged on oral medications, you will need to convert the parenteral analgesic requirement to an equianalgesic oral dosage. Box 42–1 demonstrates a common equianalgesic conversion.

Although oral medications are the simplest to manage, the client may require parenteral opioids subcutaneously or intravenously, using an ambulatory infusion device. The client and family will need the following:

* Instructions on pump management
* Visits by a home health nurse to check that the device is working and that analgesia is adequate
* Reinforcement of previous client and family teaching

Clinical Accountabilities

Because you will have more contact with the client than any other health professional, an effective pain management strategy requires that you have excellent assessment, intervention, and advocacy skills. Evaluation of treatment results based on your knowledge of the drug, dosage, duration of effect, and side effects positions you to serve the client well and to collabo-

EQUIANALGESIC CONVERSION PROBLEM

Equianalgesic Data

10 mg of parenteral morphine is equianalgesic of 30 mg of oral morphine

Current Analgesic Regimen

Client has required 4 mg of parenteral morphine an hour while hospitalized for trauma from a motorcycle accident. This dosage is expected to be required for 2 more weeks as he participates in the rehabilitative process.

Conversion From Parenteral to Oral Route Before Discharge

Step 1: 24 hours × 4 mg = 96 mg parenteral morphine in 24 hours
Step 2: 96 × 3 (equianalgesic conversion ratio) = 288 mg oral morphine in 24 hours
Step 3: 288 ÷ 2 (twice daily dosing) = 145 mg of sustained release morphine every 12 hours until transition to prn dosing

rate with other members of the health team. Table 42–5 outlines your clinical accountabilities in managing a client with acute pain.

Interventions to Manage Chronic Pain

Chronic pain has been defined, at its simplest level, as lasting more than 6 months, but it cannot be explained by duration alone. It is a complex problem that affects significant numbers of people and interferes markedly with their quality of life. The sensation of discomfort ceases to serve a useful purpose for diagnostic reasons and becomes a symbol of injury and disability.

Chronic nonmalignant pain requires a multidisciplinary approach that addresses physiological, psychological, emotional, social, and economic variables. It is not uncommon for clients to experience social isolation, financial loss, altered self-image, and a continuous search for relief. The pain may be such that the client's life is dominated by that one experience and its profound effects on physical and mental health.

A*ction* A*lert!*
Depression does not cause pain, but unrelieved pain can cause depression.

Client assessment may require a psychological evaluation in addition to the more generic components of pain assessment. Physical capabilities, a pain history, role appraisal, a self-esteem and social evaluation and, most importantly, the client's description of the total experience will help the clinical team to make an appropriate and useful evaluation.

When you encounter a client with chronic pain, especially from a long-standing problem, barriers can arise. Most likely you have had limited experience with this client population, and misunderstandings are not uncommon. It is difficult to visualize the cause of chronic pain, and you may tend to view the client as a malingerer or drug seeker. The fact that the pain may not be readily amenable to a multitude of interventions can frustrate the health team and further separate the client from those providing the interventions.

A*ction* A*lert!*
The amount of pathology is not necessarily proportional to the degree of pain.

Management Principles

DEVELOPING A THERAPEUTIC RELATIONSHIP
A trusting relationship results from listening carefully to the client, without judgment. Acknowledging the existence of pain may markedly reduce client anxiety and establish the foundation for a therapeutic relationship. Although you should not promise to absolutely relieve the pain, it is nevertheless comforting for the client to see concern and a willingness to mutually attempt to address the problem.

PARTNERING WITH THE CLIENT AND FAMILY
The pain belongs to the client and family as well as to the multidisciplinary team. Any solution requires that all persons involved be equal partners in the process. The client and family members will be involved in assessment, planning, intervention, and evaluation. They must be empowered to manage the pain with the clinical team as partners and facilitators. Realistic goals might include improved function, a decrease in pain, and improved quality of life.

INVOLVING A MULTIDISCIPLINARY TEAM
The multifaceted nature of chronic pain requires the involvement of a diverse group of health professionals who collaborate to provide the therapies needed for pain relief and improved function. You may provide this client's care alongside physicians, physical therapists, occupational therapists, dietitians, psychologists, and other professionals. Each member of the team must have a clear understanding of the treatment plan and be accountable for supporting or discouraging specific client behaviors.

USING MULTIPLE MODES OF THERAPY
Although management of acute pain is primarily pharmacological, the basis of chronic pain management is nonpharmacological. Medications are adjunctive rather than primary components of the treatment

plan. Nonpharmacological therapies vary depending on the underlying disorder, but multiple types of intervention generally serve the client well.

Nonpharmacological therapies include both cognitive-behavioral and physical interventions. Client and family education, relaxation, and distraction techniques; imagery; biofeedback; and music therapy may be used. Yoga, meditation, and other stress-reducing activities may be chosen (Fig. 42–7). Skilled practitioners may assist with hypnosis in selected cases.

Physical agents may include moist or dry heat, diathermy, ultrasound, cold packs, massage, physical therapy, exercise, and transcutaneous electrical nerve stimulation (TENS) units. TENS works in selected cases by modulating the transmission of painful stimuli. Alternatives to conventional therapies may include therapeutic touch, meridian tracing (light massage at points along specific pathways of the body), acupressure, and reflexology.

More invasive treatments may be indicated such as sympathetic nerve blocks, intravenous or subcutane-ous administration of local anesthetics, and neurosurgical procedures. Less invasive is acupuncture, an old Eastern therapy that is receiving attention from Western medicine.

Pharmacological management of chronic nonmalignant pain remains controversial. A first-line approach typically includes such nonopioids as aspirin, acetaminophen, and NSAIDs. Certain clients may benefit markedly from an opioid. Intractable pain that is unrelieved by other modalities and medications deserves a trial course of opioid analgesics. Criteria for opioid use include a stable dosage, increased or improved function, improved analgesic relief, and improved quality of life.

When opioid therapy is used, it is important that it provides pain relief without reinforcing dependency on the medication. The role of opioids in relieving chronic nonmalignant pain, while controversial, nevertheless has demonstrated markedly good effect without harm in multiple client populations. Long-acting opioids, either oral or transdermal, may be cho-

TABLE 42–5
Management of Acute Pain

Clinical Accountability	Elements
Assess at appropriate intervals	• Have the client rate the pain intensity before and at an appropriate time after the analgesic is administered. • Consistently use the same rating scale, making sure the client understands its use. • Ensure adequate pain relief. • Monitor for analgesic side effects.
Cultivate knowledge of pharmacology	• Understand equianalgesic conversion. • Know the efficacy, onset of action, appropriateness of analgesic routes. • Be familiar with the expected duration of effect of commonly used analgesics.
Advocate for the client	• Treat the client respectfully and appropriately if he reports inadequate analgesia. Do not say that nothing else can be done, that the medication should have worked, or that he must endure the pain. • Assure the client you will communicate with the physician immediately. In the interim, maximize the existing ordered analgesics. • Report the client's status to the physician and other appropriate team members immediately. • Provide an articulate, concise pain assessment based on the client's self-report. Include location, intensity, qualitative descriptors, and response to ordered analgesics, including drug, dosage, route, duration of relief, and side effects. • When requesting changes, identify that a particular drug or dosage has been maximized. If necessary, make suggestions for alternative therapy, including drug, route, dosage, and schedule. • Refer to reference or research articles when appropriate. • Address biases and misconceptions of other clinical team members.
Administer ordered analgesics skillfully	• If more than one drug or route is ordered, select the most effective one for the client's situation. • If there are dosage or titration parameters, use those orders to benefit the client. • Promptly treat analgesic side effects.
Educate the client and family	• Help client and family to become knowledgeable consumers and effective self-advocates. • Prepare the preoperative client for the location and type of pain, assessment tools that will be used, and expected pain management techniques. • Provide instruction on the importance of preventive intervention, such as asking for or taking the prescribed analgesic when the pain is still mild to moderate in intensity.
Document pertinent data	• Drug, dosage, route administered. • Pain intensity before and at an appropriate time after analgesic is administered. • Efficacy of nonpharmacological interventions. • Rationale for changes in analgesic regimen.

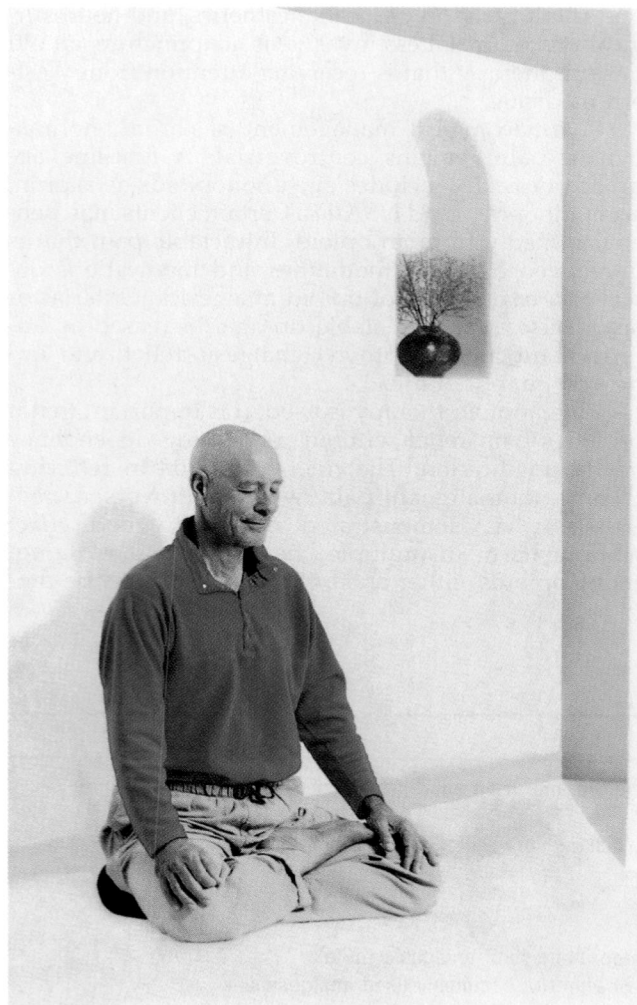

Figure 42–7. Yoga is one nonpharmacological approach to pain relief that some clients find helpful.

sen as they minimize the focus on taking an analgesic preparation.

Clinical Accountabilities

It is clear that chronic pain management requires a multidisciplinary, multimodal approach. You are a vital and integral part of the health care team. Table 42–6 describes appropriate clinical accountabilities for managing chronic pain, both for you and for other members of the team.

Interventions to Manage Cancer Pain

Pain is one of the most feared consequences of cancer, and it has historically been undertreated. Many clients have known people with cancer who died in pain. Current efforts focus on educating consumers and health professionals and on influencing legislative bodies and regulatory agencies to remove barriers to the appropriate prescribing of opioid analgesics. Unrelieved cancer pain triggers frequent use of the health

care system, unscheduled readmissions, and high costs for management of pain, as described in the Cost of Care chart.

Cancer pain results from tumor progression, related disorders, and interventions such as chemotherapy, radiation therapy, and surgery. Nearly 75% of clients with advanced cancer have pain; almost half describe it as moderate to severe. The management of cancer pain generally involves multiple treatment options. A combination of nonpharmacological, pharmacological, surgical, neurosurgical, radiologic, anesthetic, and psychological interventions may be indicated.

The primary cancer treatment modalities do not generally provide complete pain relief. Surgical and neurosurgical procedures may be used to debulk the tumor, relieve spinal cord compression, stabilize bony structures, and destroy nerve pathways that transmit the pain signal. Chemotherapy can shrink the tumor and relieve pressure on adjoining tissue and nerves. A short course of radiation therapy can relieve pain from tumor metastases to the bone or alleviate painful nerve compression or infiltration by a tumor.

Anesthetic interventions include temporary and permanent neural blockades and intraspinal catheter placement. Neurosurgical procedures may also be indicated for the rare few for whom less invasive methods have been unsuccessful.

Most cancer pain is relieved pharmacologically. The World Health Organization has formulated an analgesic ladder using nonopioid, opioid, and adjuvant analgesics alone or in combination to treat cancer pain (Fig. 42–8). An **adjuvant analgesic** is any medication that may increase analgesic efficacy, thus allowing for a smaller opioid dosage. This escalating pharmacological approach begins with nonopioids and advances to the highly effective opioid analgesics as the pain increases in intensity.

Management Principles

Many of these principles may be used in the management of acute pain, but the long-term, more complex, and significant degrees of cancer pain require a more intensive approach. The most important principle is to use opioid analgesics in dosages that control the pain adequately.

SELECTING ANALGESICS

Begin with the mildest agents that control the pain, using a multidrug approach. Even though a stepped approach is recommended, clients may have enough pain to make opioid therapy the initial treatment of choice. Nonopioids and adjuvant analgesics may be used as well and allow a smaller opioid dosage with fewer side effects.

Most NSAIDs affect platelet aggregation, the gastric mucosa, and the renal system. Combining them increases the risk for gastric and renal toxicity. Acetaminophen, an exception, may be given safely with the NSAIDs.

When the nonopioid/mild opioid combination becomes ineffective at the maximum recommended daily dosage (for example, eight Vicodin tablets in 24 hours contain the 4,000-mg maximum daily dose of acetaminophen), proceed to a more potent opioid.

Use the agonist opioids as first-line agents, such as oxycodone, hydrocodone, codeine, morphine, methadone, hydromorphone, and fentanyl. Meperidine is not recommended for chronic use because its active metabolite, normeperidine, accumulates and causes central nervous system excitatory effects. Unmanageable side effects require the choice of an alternative opioid. Agonist-antagonist opioids are unsuitable for pain requiring significant and chronic dosages.

Atypical analgesics—pharmacological preparations used for analgesia that are not primarily indicated for the management of pain (such as antidepressants and anticonvulsants)—may be useful for clients with neuropathic pain unresponsive or partially responsive to opioid therapy.

Action **A**lert!
The use of placebos for the control of cancer pain is unethical. The administration of a nonanalgesic substance for one that the client believes to be analgesic forces the clinician into deceitful behavior.

TITRATING AND SCHEDULING THE DOSAGE
Scheduled dosing is the standard for chronic cancer pain. The administration schedule is based on the analgesic's duration of effect. Maintaining consistent serum (blood) levels of the analgesic provides a baseline of consistent pain relief but does not preclude the need for treating breakthrough pain. **Breakthrough pain** is defined as intermittent episodes of pain that occur despite continued use of an analgesic. Breakthrough pain is treated with **rescue dosing,** which involves giving as-needed doses of an immediate-release analgesic in response to breakthrough pain and in addition to the scheduled analgesic dosage.

Scheduled dosing is best accomplished by sustained release products (every 8 to 12 hours, every 24

TABLE 42–6
Management of Chronic Pain

Clinical Accountability	Elements
Foster a therapeutic relationship	• Listen to the client. • Be sensitive to complaints of pain and its effect on activities and emotions. • Ask permission to include significant others in discussion of the issues.
Recognize and respond to the complexity of the pain experience	• Remember that chronicity reduces or eliminates physiological evidence of pain; use a chronic pain assessment model. • Appreciate that persistent pain produces decreased functioning. • Prolonged discomfort can cause depression and despair. Make sure they are treated. • Identify the impact of physical limitations on lifestyle and role relationships.
Include family and significant others in the plan of care	• Assess the family's and significant others' contributions to the client's pain status, including role expectations, reinforcement of pain behaviors, and supportive behaviors. • Involve all significant others in assessment, planning, treatment, and evaluation phases.
Identify cause of pain	• Participate in the diagnostic work-up, remembering that pain may persist after disorder is eliminated. • Consider preexisting medical problems and medication regimens. • Educate the client and family about the purpose of all diagnostic interventions, including any psychological testing.
Set goals that improve quality of life	• Minimize pain, anxiety, depression • Maximize functional level.
Help client develop realistic expectations	• Be clear that elimination of pain may not be possible, but relief may be feasible. • Outline in a forthright manner that activities may not be fully resumed. • Explore how adaptation to a revised self or new role or identity can be accomplished.
Empower client	• Use cognitive restructuring to give the client as much control as possible. • Continually reinforce that client ownership of the pain experience is key to pacing activities, setting boundaries, and obtaining pain relief.
Use multimodality, multidisciplinary approach	• Employ nonpharmacological and pharmacological interventions. • Provide a consistent approach from all health team members, with effective and clear communication among those members. • Include psychological intervention, when appropriate, and social services for financial and social issues.
Use prophylactic approach	• Medicate on a scheduled basis, preferably using long-acting analgesics to break the pain cycle. • Dispel fears of addiction. Use nonopioids, opioids, and adjunctive medications to relieve pain, then establish a long-term plan. • Educate the client about self-directed pain-relief interventions.

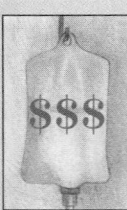

THE COST OF CARE

UNRELIEVED CANCER PAIN

Health care costs for unrelieved pain are becoming increasingly visible. As health care systems scrutinize admissions to the acute care setting, unrelieved or intractable pain is increasingly found. The oncology client population is at high risk for significant pain throughout the illness. Most will require aggressive use of opioids by a skilled practitioner. As care shifts to the outpatient setting, the family or a hired caregiver typically takes responsibility for the analgesic regimen. If the clinical team fails to manage the client effectively, visits to the emergency department and admissions to the hospital become the client's and caregivers' only solution to a miserable and frightening health problem.

A National Cancer Institute–designated Clinical Cancer Center in the western United States looked at readmissions for uncontrolled pain. The average length of stay was 12 days. Using an average daily cost of $1,666 for each of 255 clients admitted with uncontrolled pain, the annual total exceeded $5 million. Subsequent interventions to improve pain management included training of pain resource nurses, making pain a focus in the continuous quality improvement process, assessing knowledge and attitudes of the medical and nursing staff, and the implementation of a supportive care service.

Two years after implementation of this problem, 121 clients had been admitted for uncontrolled pain during the previous year, with an average length of stay of 11.8 days. The cost was just under $2.5 million.

Discussion

This study highlights the incredible cost of unrelieved pain. Not only must we consider the tremendous toll of suffering on the client and family but also the significant drain on health care resources. In a society struggling to contain expenditures for health care, it is clear that a multifaceted approach is essential, including the following:

- Curriculum changes in medical and nursing schools to include pain management.
- Continuing education for physicians and nurses currently practicing.
- Individual and institutional accountability for pain management.
- Removal of regulatory barriers that impede the proper prescribing of opioid analgesics.
- Consumer education concerning the right of the individual to good pain management.

Reference

Grant, M., Ferrell, B.R., Rivera, L.M., & Lee, J. (1995). Unscheduled readmissions for uncontrolled symptoms. *Nursing Clinics of North America, 30,* (4), 673–682.

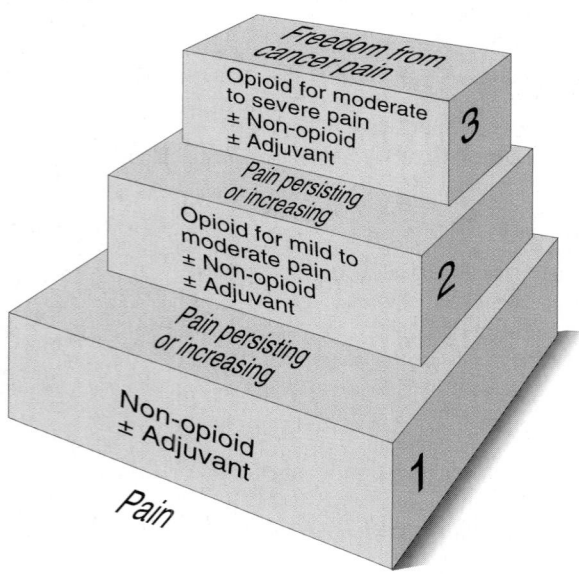

Figure 42–8. The World Health Organization analgesic ladder. (Reproduced by permission of WHO, from Cancer pain relief [2nd ed.]. Geneva: World Health Organization, 1996.)

hours, or every 72 hours). Rescue dosing requires immediate-release preparations with a short half-life. If possible, use the same analgesic for both scheduled and rescue dosing.

Joseph reluctantly agreed to take a sustained-release morphine twice a day (b.i.d.). The physician also prescribed an immediate-release sublingual morphine tablet every 2 hours as needed for breakthrough pain. Although Joseph did have breakthrough pain, he rarely used the sublingual tablets. When the physician questioned him about his need for the analgesics, Joseph replied that he did have extra pain "sometimes" but did not want to use the sublingual tablets. His physician cautiously titrated the sustained-release analgesic upward at each visit. Joseph was compliant with the twice-daily dosing. He did, however, need to take six tablets b.i.d.

Rescue dosing can be used alone when the analgesic dose is uncertain, during initial titration of opioids with a long half-life (such as methadone), or during therapy that may decrease the analgesic dose needed for pain relief (such as radiation therapy for bone metastases).

Frequent rescue dosing requires a change in the scheduled dose. The 24-hour cumulative sums of the scheduled and rescue doses should be added to determine the new 24-hour scheduled dose. This dosage is divided by the number of times in 24 hours that the drug will be given. For example, assume the client's scheduled dose is 800 mg of sustained-release oral morphine every 8 hours (2,400 mg in 24 hours) plus 10 rescue doses of 30 mg of sublingual morphine each (300 mg). That equals 2,700 mg of morphine in 24 hours. The new scheduled dose would be 2,700 divided by 3, or 900 mg of sustained-release morphine every 8 hours.

Taper the opioid analgesic if a client needs a significant decrease in dosage. Chronic opioid exposure produces physical dependence, and sudden cessation will produce signs and symptoms of withdrawal, such as agitation, tremors, insomnia, fear, autonomic nervous system hyperexcitability, and increased pain.

Action Alert!
Cancer pain is chronic in nature and requires, with rare exception, both scheduled and rescue dosing.

IDENTIFYING THE APPROPRIATE ROUTE
The appropriate route is based on physiological needs, client comfort and preference, and caregiver capacity. It is frequently necessary to change the route as the illness progresses. Choose the route that provides prompt relief. Severe, escalating pain requires intravenous administration with rapid onset of action. Intravenous opioids may be given by intermittent dosing, continuous infusion, or a combination of the two. Patient-controlled analgesia (PCA) has been used effectively to titrate the analgesic dose to desired effect.

Joseph's pain became less responsive even with ten sustained-release morphine tablets b.i.d. His physician talked to him privately and told him that the pain was not going to get better and would most likely get worse. He recommended a peripherally inserted central catheter (PICC) and the use of an ambulatory infusion pump to deliver a continuous dosage of morphine, with the capability of rescue dosing when Joseph had breakthrough pain. Joseph thought about it for a few days and agreed, hoping that the increased pain relief would allow him to continue working. The pump was small and, after the PICC line was inserted, the nurse instructed Joseph how best to place it so that it would not interfere with his job. Do you think the nurse and physician should support Joseph's decision to continue working?

IM and subcutaneous injections are painful and provide inconsistent absorption. However, low-volume continuous subcutaneous infusions may be very effective when intravenous access is unavailable or impractical. The epidural or intrathecal route may be appropriate for specified clients when less invasive measures have provided inadequate pain relief.

MANAGING SIDE EFFECTS
Carefully monitor the client when you begin giving opioid therapy. Respiratory depression can occur in opioid-naive clients and those with pulmonary disease, but it is uncommon with careful titration. Naloxone (Narcan) is not recommended to reverse non–life threatening effects, such as confusion or sedation. Hypersensitivity (allergic) reactions are rare. Opioid use routinely causes constipation, and clients do not develop tolerance to this side effect. A prophylactic bowel regimen is recommended.

Clinical Accountabilities

The management of cancer pain requires diligent assessment, a significant pharmacological knowledge base, comfort with the liberal use of opioid analgesics, and ease in the use of multiple administrative routes. The nurse's role incorporates knowledge, skill, compassion, and advocacy to ensure client safety and comfort. Table 42–7 summarizes clinical responsibilities in managing the client with cancer pain.

Interventions to Manage Pain in the Older Adult

The principles of acute and chronic pain management generally apply to the older population with slight modifications. Polypharmacy, side effects of typical analgesics, comorbidities, declining renal and hepatic function, less lean body mass, and decreasing mental faculties are variables that must be factored into the pain management equation.

Management Principles

PHARMACOLOGICAL INTERVENTIONS
The use of analgesics in general is not impaired by normal aging, but the older adult is at greater risk for analgesic toxicity. Physiological variables may cause slower metabolism of analgesics, thus increasing their potential for producing harmful side effects.

Nonopioid analgesics, acetaminophen, and NSAIDs are used to provide relatively safe and effective relief for mild-to-moderate pain, generally at a decreased dosage. Opioids can be used for moderate-to-severe pain but are more likely to cause side effects. Constipation, nausea, vomiting, alterations in cognition, and severe agitation may occur. These side effects can be treated and do not contraindicate the use of opioids for significant pain. As is true with the nonopioid analgesics, an older adult may need smaller opioid dosages than a younger person.

NONPHARMACOLOGICAL INTERVENTIONS
Pain can be lessened by common nonpharmacological remedies. Physical and occupational therapists can provide practical advice on ways to reduce physical pain as the older adult goes about the activities of daily living.

The older adult is also at risk for emotional problems associated with pain. Older adults who seek emotional support and education seem to hurt less. Adequate analgesia depends, in part, on the family's and caregiver's understanding of the client's illness

TABLE 42–7
Management of Cancer Pain

Clinical Accountability	Elements
Understand basic pain management strategies	• Principles of drug selection and dosing. • Equianalgesic conversion methods. • Advantages and disadvantages of varied administrative routes. • Nonopioid, opioid, atypical analgesic side effect management.
Assess pain systematically	• Evaluate effectiveness after each dose until pain is well controlled. • Base assessment on client's report. • Consistently use same rating scale. • Reassess when client's pain has changed or is escalating.
Advocate for the client	• Communicate with the physician when relief is inadequate. • Provide articulate, concise assessment. • Offer suggestions for dosage or medication alternatives if appropriate. • Continue collaboration with the physician until the client is comfortable. • Question the use of placebos.
Ensure appropriate analgesic intervention	• Choose appropriate analgesic when more than one is ordered. • Ensure that a multidrug approach is used when appropriate. • Monitor ordered analgesics for incompatibility.
Clarify questionable orders	• Chronic use of meperidine or an agonist-antagonist opioid. • Scheduled or rescue analgesics not ordered. • Scheduled analgesic does not provide adequate relief because of ordered interval. • Frequent rescue dosing is necessary to maintain adequate pain control. • Conversion to alternative route or drug is not based on equianalgesic conversion principles, resulting in inappropriate dosage. • Route of chronic opioid administration is intramuscular. • Ordered route is or becomes inadequate or inappropriate. • An opioid antagonist is ordered to counteract non–life-threatening sedation.
Anticipate and manage side effects	• Bowel regimen titrated to effect for all clients on chronic opioid dosing. • Prophylactic antiemetics during initial opioid therapy. • Monitor for central nervous toxicity as opioid dosage escalates.
Educate client and family	• Right to and benefits of adequate analgesia. • Client's role in assessment. • Analgesic side effects and their management. • Misconceptions and fears about physical dependence, tolerance, and psychological dependence. • Contractual agreement for opioid use in clients with history of substance abuse.
Documentation	• Nature, location, and intensity of pain. • Consistent report of results of ordered interventions. • Rationale for changes in analgesic regimen.

and treatment, supportive and encouraging attitudes, and communication of the client's worth independent of functional status.

Clinical Accountabilities

Your role in responding to the older adult with pain, while grounded in generic analgesic principles, does incorporate some behaviors specific to this special population. Table 42–8 summarizes your accountabilities of pain management in the older adult.

Interventions to Manage Pain in Clients With a History of Substance Abuse

Clients with a history of substance abuse do experience pain and have the right to effective analgesia. Un-

dertreatment is common in this client population as clinicians try to balance their responsibilities to the client with their ethical concerns. Common barriers to adequate management include reluctance to believe the client's self-reported pain status, reluctance to prescribe opioids or other controlled substances, difficulty in identifying common maladaptive behaviors, moral disapproval of client behaviors, and difficulty in successfully treating these clients.

The plan of care for clients with a substance abuse disorder must include management of acute intoxication and efforts to prevent or minimize withdrawal, followed by establishing an effective analgesic regimen. Problematic behavior must be addressed, and realistic goals must be established. The cause of the pain must be understood in order to intervene successfully. This process occurs within the context of the client's history—whether the substance abuse is current or occurred in the distant past with ongoing participation in a recovery program. The client's relationship with medications differs markedly if the abuse is current or in the distant past.

Analgesics

General principles of acute and chronic pain management apply to this client population. For chronic pain, scheduled and rescue dosing are appropriate. The client's sense of control may be enhanced when you provide information about the medication, dosage, and schedule. Opioids may be used when they are appropriate for the type of pain the client is experiencing. Withholding analgesics from chemically dependent clients who have pain does not increase or decrease recovery from addictive behaviors.

Communication Strategies

Effective communication among clinical team members is essential to ensure consistency and maintain therapeutic direction. The coordinator of care should be identified as soon as possible to keep the team focused and goal-directed. The client deserves a clear understanding of the frequency of assessment, treatment goals, and who will be prescribing the analgesics. It is very important to limit negotiations about medications and dosages. Regular team meetings should occur to promote planning, discuss differences of opinion about interventions, and collaboratively set limits and identify boundaries.

> A*ction* A*lert!*
> Setting limits is in the best interest of the client. Never use pain relief as a bargaining tool.

Use of a written contractual agreement can help make the treatment plan explicit. Components of the contractual agreement might include goals of treatment, treatment plan, client and staff expectations, consequences of noncompliance, the staff responsible for the client's care, reevaluation intervals, and consent for random urine screens.

Outpatient treatment requires additional considerations. There must be policies regarding the replacement of lost or stolen medications, unsanctioned dose escalation, and early refill requests. Clear expectations must be articulated about follow-up appointments; whom to call about medications, analgesic relief, and side effects; and the limited quantity of prescription medications.

The best intentions of the multidisciplinary team may not guarantee success. The client may refuse treatment or fail to comply with the prescribed regimen. The focus must still remain on effective pain management for all clients regardless of one person's dysfunctional behavior.

Interventions Involving Opioid Infusion Devices

Management of pain may incorporate the use of PCA or intraspinal analgesia at some point during the illness. These approaches to opioid administration are used in multiple settings.

Patient-Controlled Analgesia

Patient-controlled analgesia (PCA) is a drug-delivery approach that uses an external infusion pump to deliver an opioid dose on a "client demand" basis (Fig. 42–9). This intermittent dosing is driven by the client's need for analgesic relief and the pump's preprogrammed instructions to deliver an identified dosage at specified intervals. The infusion pump's program cannot be overridden by the client. Most pumps also

---

TABLE 42–8
Management of Pain in the Older Adult

Clinical Accountability	Elements
Set aside misconceptions	• Understand that pain in the older adult is a sign of disease or impending dysfunction. • Be sensitive to the underreporting of pain, the "good patient" presentation, and the fear of "becoming a burden" to one's family.
Assess systematically	• Pursue decreased function, slowness of movement as signs of pain. • Be vigilant in assessing for acute pain; it may present in the older adult as atypical or referred pain. • Distinguish between dementia and delirium; search for subtle signs of behavior that are abnormal for that client. • Watch for any behavior change in the confused older client because it may result from pain.
Intervene appropriately	• Respect client's past experience of "tried and true" remedies. • Maximize relief and improve function through pharmacological and nonpharmacological means. • Manage opioid therapy by adequately treating both the pain and opioid side effects. • Treat anxiety or depression (commonly associated with chronic pain)
Maximize relief and function	• Respect the older adult's expectations, and support them to the extent possible. • Provide individualized treatment, differentiating between the well and the frail elderly. • Investigate ways the older adult may contribute to the family and others.

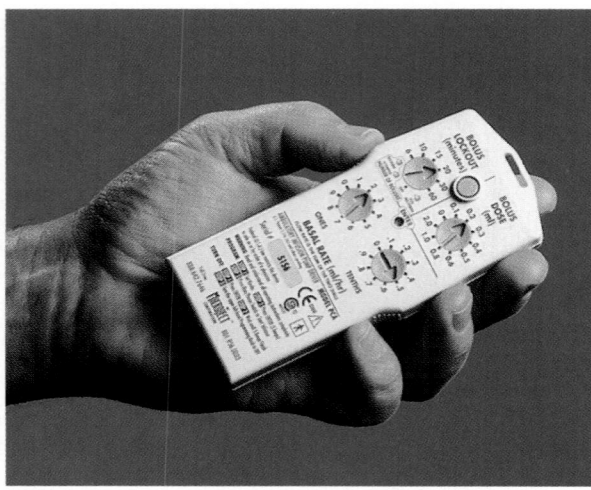

Figure 42–9. A patient-controlled analgesia device. (Courtesy of Microject Corporation, Salt Lake City, UT.)

have the capacity to deliver a continuous or background infusion as well.

PCA was developed to manage postoperative pain. These clients had been commonly managed with *as-needed* IM injections of an opioid, usually in combination with an antiemetic. This approach was problematic because it created a significant delay in pain relief caused by the multistep process from the client's recognition of discomfort to the actual administration of medication. It also created large swings in serum levels of opioid secondary to the *as-needed* administration approach, which resulted in over- and undermedication.

Extensive clinical experience with PCA devices has demonstrated that they provide:

- Improved pain relief with smaller opioid dosages
- The ability to finely titrate the opioid dosage, with decreased potential for overdosing
- A decreased delay in receiving analgesic relief at the time of need
- Decreased dependency on nursing personnel
- Earlier activity with improved pulmonary status
- Decreased client anxiety secondary to inadequate pain relief

CLIENT SELECTION

Clients selected for PCA are those who require repeated parenteral opioid doses for moderate-to-severe pain, those who can understand and follow the instructions, and those willing to use this type of therapy. PCA is not appropriate for clients unable to understand the mechanics of its usage or those with insufficient dexterity to self-administer a dose of analgesic.

There continues to be some controversy about the use of PCA in clients with a history of substance abuse. The issue is not one of the need for pain relief but rather a reluctance to place responsibility for opioid dosing in the hands of the client. This issue should be evaluated by the clinical team before the actual time of need.

USING A PCA INFUSION PUMP

PCA can be delivered by many routes. Although initially developed for intravenous use, subcutaneous and intraspinal administrations are growing more common. These allow the client increased access to this modality across care settings.

Intravenous and epidural PCA have been used very effectively in the immediate postoperative period. A client undergoing major thoracic surgery, for instance, may benefit markedly from epidural administration. Adequate analgesia can shorten the client's stay in the intensive care unit and maximize his pulmonary function. A client undergoing less invasive surgery does as well with the intravenous route. Indwelling intravenous access provides a rapid onset of action and precludes the further discomfort of an intravenous injection. Analgesics commonly used include morphine, hydromorphone, and meperidine.

The efficacy and practicality of PCA in managing postoperative pain has extended its usage to other client groups in the inpatient setting. Moderate-to-severe pain that decreases in intensity as tissue heals lends itself to this dosing method. For example, clients with burns or trauma pain respond well to this management approach.

On-demand dosing, alone or in combination with continuous infusion, may be used very effectively for analgesic relief. When on-demand dosing is used as single therapy, the pump is typically programmed to provide a modest amount of opioid at intervals of 5 to 15 minutes. A continuous or background infusion typically runs as well. When the client feels a need for pain relief, he self-administers a dose using the PCA device.

If the client tries to administer another dose before the programmed time goes by, the device will not deliver it. Once the programmed time has elapsed, the device will once again deliver a dose of the opioid.

When on-demand dosing is used concurrently with a continuous or background infusion of opioid, the continuous opioid dosage is generally inadequate to manage the client's total analgesic need. This combined approach allows the client to titrate the remainder of needed analgesic relief with the on-demand dosing.

Both approaches provide clients the ability to titrate the final opioid dosage based on their analgesic needs. As with any other method, it is appropriate and essential to assess the client's response. Dosages may be titrated upward or downward, depending on the level of pain relief obtained.

Clients with chronic pain are also well served by this approach. The on-demand capacity allows rapid titration and determination of the overall analgesic dosage required in a 24-hour period. Chronic cancer pain with episodes of breakthrough pain that is severe, increasing rapidly, or has not responded to less invasive approaches can be effectively managed with

PCA. In these circumstances, the intravenous route with its rapid onset of action is the most efficient and effective way to control the pain and titrate the dosage.

Once the client is maintained on a stable opioid dose with both continuous and on-demand dosing, the clinical team can make an informed decision about the client's discharge needs. Alternatives include the following:

- Converting the parenteral dosage to an equianalgesic oral dosage.
- Establishing stable intravenous access for a client who needs substantial opioid dosages and discharging him with an intravenous ambulatory PCA device.
- Converting the intravenous route to subcutaneous PCA. This route requires adequate subcutaneous tissue to handle up to 2 to 3 mL. If analgesic requirements are significant, an opioid must be chosen that is available in a highly concentrated formulation.

Experience in the acute care setting has provided the experience necessary to transfer this method of therapy to the outpatient setting. Home health and hospice programs now routinely service clients who have PCA pumps. Although permanent or long-term indwelling intravenous access devices would support the intravenous route for ambulatory use, subcutaneous administration is more practical in the home setting and is the route of choice for those without reliable intravenous access. Reliability and ease of access by a layperson render it both sensible and dependable.

Joseph continued his PCA therapy with some success. The shoulder strap and carrying bag for the pump allowed him to conceal the system under his jacket when he went to work, and he had the nurse titrate his dosage upward when he needed to use frequent bolus doses. He did allow his wife to help him with the dressing changes because he could not manage it alone. When he could, he preferred to have the office nurse do the dressing change. Do you think the office nurse should accommodate his wishes?

Intraspinal Analgesia

Intraspinal analgesia involves the placement of a catheter to deliver medication to the epidural or intrathecal space. This invasive therapy can be temporary or permanent. Temporary catheters are used for short-term postoperative pain relief and to evaluate the efficacy of intraspinal analgesia before placing a permanent catheter. Permanent catheter placement is used for clients unresponsive to less invasive analgesic methods.

EPIDURAL ANALGESIA
In **epidural analgesia,** a catheter is placed between the spinal vertebrae and the dura mater to allow the diffusion of an analgesic drug across the dura mater into the cerebrospinal fluid. There, the drug binds with opioid receptors in the dorsal horn of the spinal cord.

Epidural analgesia can be used to manage acute and chronic pain. Indications include the following:

- Short-term pain relief via a temporary catheter for postoperative pain and pain from multiple trauma
- Postoperative pain conditions where mobility and full lung expansion immediately after surgery are especially important
- Chronic cancer pain that does not respond to conventional opioid intervention

Epidural analgesia may be produced by intermittent injections, continuous infusions, or a combination of the two. Patient-controlled epidural analgesia may be used to deliver both continuous and intermittent dosing and is generally reserved for the management of chronic malignant pain.

Benefits of epidural analgesia for the management of acute pain include improved respiratory function, earlier mobilization and return of bowel function after surgery, and heightened alertness. Benefits for the client with cancer pain include improved pain management at a significantly lower opioid dose and the relief of dose-limiting or unmanageable side effects from conventional therapy. Identified risks for both client populations include respiratory depression, catheter tip migration, epidural abscess formation, and epidural hematomas. The accompanying Teaching for Self-Care chart identifies client instructions for changing the dressing on a permanent epidural catheter.

Joseph's pain has been escalating despite consistent upward titration of his parenteral morphine infusion. He reluctantly rates it to be a 7 on a scale of 0 to 10, although he reports that the pain is not too bad. He says the pain in his abdomen sometimes seems to "shoot" down his leg. He refuses to move in any way that might aggravate the pain and is found to hold his upper abdomen when he does move. He is now unable to work. When in bed, he is very still and sits upright in a rigid position. The morphine infusion has been increased to 300 mg per hour with a 100-mg bolus allowed every 15 minutes p.r.n. He uses at least two boluses every hour. Joseph is developing significant muscle twitching, a side effect of high parenteral opioid dosing. Treatment with anticonvulsants and benzodiazepines has not controlled the twitching, and it is increasing in severity. His physician decides to place an epidural catheter to improve analgesia and minimize the toxicities of treatment.

INTRATHECAL ANALGESIA
In **intrathecal analgesia,** a catheter is placed in the subarachnoid space between the dura mater and the spinal cord to allow immediate drug diffusion into the cerebrospinal fluid. There, the drug binds with opioid receptors in the dorsal horn of the spinal cord. Intrathecal opioid therapy provides the most rapid onset of analgesic relief.

Intrathecal therapy is traditionally reserved for chronic pain unrelieved by less invasive methods. Selection criteria for cancer pain clients include inadequate pain relief despite escalating doses delivered via conventional routes, intolerable or unmanageable side effects from systemic opioids, and a life expectancy greater than 3 months. Client selection criteria

CHANGING THE DRESSING ON A PERMANENT EPIDURAL CATHETER

Purpose: To prevent infection during epidural analgesia.

Rationale: By teaching the client and caregiver to maintain proper technique when cleaning and handling an epidural catheter and its exit site, you will reduce the risk of infection and the consequent need to remove the catheter.

Expected Outcome: The client will remain free of infection at the catheter exit site, the tunneled area, and the epidural space, thus ensuring continued analgesia.

Client Instructions

1. Assemble the required supplies as they appear on the list I have given you.
2. Clean a work surface, and cover it with paper towels.
3. Wash your hands with warm, soapy water. Rinse them well, and dry them with a clean paper towel.
4. Open the supplies, being careful not to touch any sterile supplies or the inside surfaces of their wrappers.
5. Remove the old dressing, starting at the top and working your way downward. Be careful not to pull on the catheter. Discard the old dressing into a plastic bag.
6. Wash your hands again.
7. Look closely at the exit site and the skin around it. If it is hot or red or fluid is oozing from it, notify your nurse or doctor after completing this procedure.
8. Take one of the povidone-iodine swab sticks in your dominant hand, and clean the exit site. Starting at the center, wipe the skin in a circular motion, working outward 2 to 3 inches from the catheter. *Never touch the exit site with a swab that has touched skin other than at the site itself.*

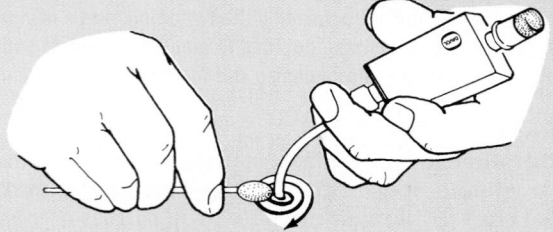

Wiping the skin in a circular motion. (Illustration from Bard Access Systems. [1993]. DuPen long-term epidural catheter: Use and maintenance. Salt Lake City: UT: Bard Access Systems.)

9. Use a second swab stick to clean the exit site one more time with the same circular motion.
10. Use a third swab stick to clean the catheter itself. Use an upward motion from the exit site to clean about 2 inches of the catheter. Leave the iodine solution on the skin and the catheter, and allow it to completely air-dry. This may take 1 to 3 minutes.
11. Place the precut sterile gauze dressing around the catheter.

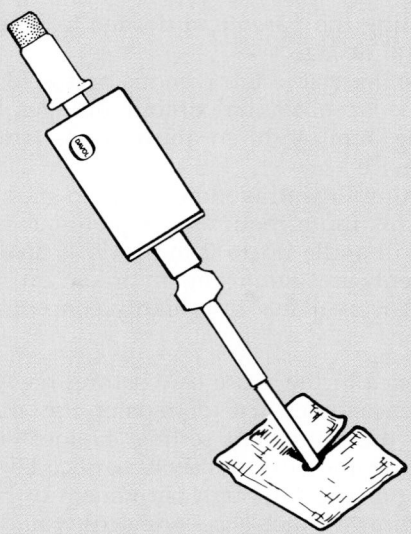

Placing the precut sterile gauze dressing around the cather. (Illustration from Bard Access Systems. [1993]. DuPen long-term epidural catheter: Use and maintenance. Salt Lake City: UT: Bard Access Systems.)

12. Place a 3″ × 3″ sterile gauze dressing over the precut dressing and catheter, and tape it in place.

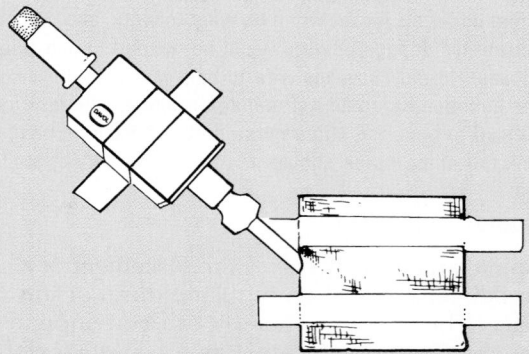

3″ × 3″ sterile gauze dressing taped over the precut dressing and catheter. (Illustration from Bard Access Systems. [1993]. DuPen long-term epidural catheter: Use and maintenance. Salt Lake City: UT: Bard Access Systems.)

13. Make sure the catheter is not kinked or pinched. You may want to tape the catheter to your skin or to the dressing to avoid extra "tug" on the catheter exit site as you move about.

for chronic nonmalignant pain are more controversial and less straightforward. They include therapy of last resort, a baseline neurologic examination to identify the causes(s) of pain, and psychometric testing and psychological evaluation documenting that pain is not primarily of psychological origin.

A "closed" system is typically used to minimize the risk of infection. The system includes a tunneled catheter attached to an surgically implanted infusion pump. The pump is programmed percutaneously via computer, and the pump's drug reservoir is accessed percutaneously. A positive response to a trial of epidural or intrathecal infusion therapy should be documented before the catheter and pump are placed.

SELECTING INTRASPINAL ANALGESICS

Preservative-free opioids (such as morphine, hydromorphone, fentanyl, and sufentanil), local anesthetics (such as bupivacaine), and alpha$_2$-adrenoreceptor agonists (such as clonidine) are currently used singly or in combination to provide intraspinal analgesia. Opioids are used in significantly decreased dosages because of the proximity of the opioid to the receptors in the spinal cord. This altered dosage decreases the incidence of central nervous system side effects because very little opioid ascends to the higher brain centers or is absorbed systemically via the blood supply in the epidural space.

Opioids may be used in combination with a local anesthetic when there is a prominent neuropathic component to the pain or when the client has unstable bone pain. Use of local anesthetics may decrease the amount of opioid required. Alpha$_2$-adrenoreceptor agonists provide spinal analgesia that is not reversed by naloxone. This therapy seems to be most effective in clients whose pain is primarily neuropathic in origin.

There are fewer side effects with intraspinal analgesia versus conventional opioid therapy because of the relatively low drug dosages required. Nevertheless, opioid side effects may include gastrointestinal distress (including nausea, vomiting, or constipation), urinary retention, pruritus on the face or palate, and drowsiness or sedation. Local anesthetics and alpha$_2$-adrenoreceptor agonists have differing side-effect profiles.

Intraspinal therapy is becoming more commonplace in the acute care and ambulatory settings. These clients are no longer relegated to intensive care units alone. Medical/surgical units and home health and hospice agencies now routinely care for this client population. Appropriate care requires a different knowledge base and skilled clinicians to direct and administer therapy.

EVALUATION

To evaluate a client's health outcomes secondary to assessment, planning, and intervention, you will need to reassess the client to ensure that his goals have been met. The hospice nursing note for Mr. Valdez after his hospitalization for epidural catheter placement is described in the accompanying nursing care planning chart and might look like this:

Epidural exit site without signs of infection. Somewhat tender to palpation; no warmth, exudate, or swelling. Tunneled track without signs of redness or swelling. Posterior incision site dry, no discharge, sutures intact. Temperature 98.6° F. Respiratory rate 12. Alert and oriented. Rates pain in abdomen to be 3 on a scale of 0 to 10. Epidural morphine at 3 mg/h in 0.15% bupivacaine solution. PCA bolus dose of 1 mg every hour p.r.n. used times three in past 24 hours when client bent over. No complaints of nausea, constipation, itching, or numbness in lower extremities. Client reports

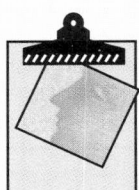

NURSING CARE PLANNING
A CLIENT WITH UNCONTROLLED PAIN

Admission Data

Mr. Valdez is admitted to the oncology unit for epidural catheter placement. The nurse who will be caring for him understands that he has unrelieved and severe pain and will have a permanent epidural catheter placed. Dr. Terry is on the way to the unit to write orders.

Physician's Orders

Admitting diagnosis: uncontrolled pain secondary to adenocarcinoma of the stomach
Morphine 300 mg/h via PICC line. Bolus dose 100 mg every 15 min p.r.n. May increase continuous infusion by 100 mg/h if client uses 2 bolus doses/h times 4 hours.*
Acetaminophen 650 mg for temperature >101°F
Valium 10 mg po every 4 hours p.r.n. for muscle twitching
Elavil 50 mg hs

Lactulose 60 cm^3 qid
Activity as tolerated
Diet as tolerated
PT, PTT, CBC with differential, stat
ECG stat
Chest x-ray stat
Consent for permanent epidural catheter placement
NPO after midnight

Continued

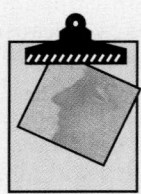

NURSING CARE PLANNING
A CLIENT WITH UNCONTROLLED PAIN *(continued)*

Nursing Assessment

Color pale, diaphoretic. Reports pain to be 7 on a 0–10 scale, primarily in abdominal area but shoots down leg unexpectedly. Guarding, reduced movement, and wincing when turning in bed. BP 130/90, pulse 100, respiratory rate 14, temperature 98.6°F. Morphine is infusing via PICC line at 300 mg/h with a 100-mg bolus allowed every 15 minutes p.r.n. He has used 2 bolus doses in the hour since admission.

NURSING CARE PLAN

Nursing diagnosis	Expected Outcomes	Interventions	Evaluation (After 24 Hours of Care)
Chronic pain	Pain rating decreased to 4 (scale of 0–10)	Assess pain level and titrate intravenous analgesics preoperatively and epidural analgesics postoperatively per physician orders	Preoperative: pain rating of 7. Postoperative: pain rating of 3 after 24 hours.
	Decreased anxiety	*Explain procedure to client in the presence of the family so family can learn without client feeling dependent on them.* Provide reassurance that analgesia is the goal.	Preoperative: anxiety unrelieved. Ativan 0.5 mg PO q 6 hr given. Postoperative: anxiety controlled with Ativan 1.0 mg PO q 6 hr.
	Adequate bowel function	Assess bowel function and administer laxatives as ordered.	Client had two effective bowel movements before surgery and one movement 36 hours after surgery.
	Increased activity with ability to ambulate	Provide bedside commode and urinal before surgery. Encourage and help client to ambulate after surgery as pain level decreases.	Client stayed in bed before surgery. Walked in room with help 4 hours after surgery. Walked in hallway with help 12 hours after surgery. Went to bathroom without help 18 hours after surgery.

Italicized interventions indicate culturally specific care.

*This dose of morphine is in excess of the usual dose for acute pain and would be lethal in the client who has not developed tolerance.

Critical Thinking Questions

1. Given that Mr. Valdez has reluctantly admitted his pain to be at an intensity of 7 and has even demonstrated some behavioral indications that his pain is severe, how will you assess him once the epidural catheter is placed?
2. During the immediate postoperative period, Mr. Valdez's pain is controlled remarkably well as the epidural analgesics are titrated upward. During the night before his morning discharge, he begins to complain of severe pain in his abdomen. What would you look for to explain this sudden change in comfort level?
3. Compare the dose of intravenous morphine for Mr. Valdez with the usual dose given for a client who is morphine-naive. What precautions would you take the first time a client receives morphine or other parenteral opioids?
4. Mr. Valdez is neither inclined to ask his wife for help nor to rely on her for assistance with his care. He would rather not have the care than have someone provide it for him. How will you educate Mr. and Mrs. Valdez regarding epidural catheter care, understanding that Mrs. Valdez must also learn the proper techniques?

that he and wife have been out to dinner and a movie on two occasions and that he walks around the house during the day and goes to the table for meals. Client and wife verbalize and demonstrate proper technique for catheter site care and infusion pump maintenance.

The nursing note reflects assessment of postsurgical sequelae (catheter placement), signs of infection, analgesic status, functional level, and client/family education. The postoperative goals of decreasing the side effects of opioid therapy, maintaining adequate analgesia, increasing physical mobility, and improving the quality of life have been achieved.

KEY PRINCIPLES

- Pain can be a complex, biopsychosocial phenomenon with sensory, affective, and cognitive dimensions. The client and the pain experience may be woven together, making it difficult to separate them into distinct entities.
- The client's self-report of the pain experience is a standard of the assessment process.
- Transmission of the pain signal from the site of injury to the higher brain centers where the sensation is recognized involves multiple anatomic structures and biochemical neurotransmitters. The pain signal may be modulated at various steps along this pathway.
- Tolerance and physical dependence are involuntary, physiological occurrences. They are distinct from psychological dependence (addiction) and should not be considered addiction.
- Psychological dependence (addiction) rarely occurs when clients are using opioid analgesics for the relief of pain. Fears of opioid addiction are exceptionally disproportionate to the reality and are a major barrier to the adequate relief of pain.
- Acute and chronic pain are markedly different experiences. The acute pain model is characterized by increased activity of the autonomic nervous system (increased blood pressure, pulse, respiratory rate, diaphoresis) and typical pain behaviors such as crying, moaning, and grimacing. In chronic pain, the client adapts physiologically and psychologically to the pain experience. Changes in vital signs and behavioral clues may not be evident. Assessing a client with chronic pain using the acute model is inadequate and misleading.
- Pain assessment in a client unable to communicate requires particular attention to behavioral clues that indicate discomfort. Neonates, small children, elderly adults who are delirious or confused, and comatose clients are especially at risk.
- Neonates, children, and older adults experience pain in the same way the younger adult population does. Painful states deserve equal attention.
- Acute pain is short-term and generally resolves when the tissue heals. If acute pain is treated inadequately, the client may risk chronic pain.

- Severe acute pain should be treated immediately using an analgesic with a rapid onset of action. The intravenous route provides rapid relief, and the analgesic can be given safely if administered in small increments until the client is comfortable.
- Chronic pain that is intractable, difficult to treat, or that leads to disability affects the client physically and emotionally. It is always appropriate to use a multidisciplinary approach that treats all facets of the pain experience.
- Although nonpharmacological interventions and nonopioid analgesics have been given precedence in the treatment of chronic nonmalignant pain, there is increasing evidence that opioid analgesics may be administered to subsets of this client population in a controlled, safe manner.
- Cancer pain is chronic and requires, with rare exception, both scheduled and rescue dosing using nonopioid, opioid, and atypical analgesics.
- Clinicians should include client and family education about pain and its management in the treatment plan, and they should encourage clients to be active participants in the process.

BIBLIOGRAPHY

Anand, K.J.S., & Craig, K.D. (1996). New perspectives on the definition of pain. *Pain, 67*(1), 3–6.

Ball, J., & Bindler, R. (1995). *Pediatric nursing: Caring for children.* East Norwalk, CT: Appleton & Lange.

Busbaum, A.I. (1995). Insights into the development of opioid tolerance. *Pain, 61*(3), 349–351.

*Bonica, J.J. (1990). Anatomic and physiologic basis of nociception and pain. In J.J. Bonica (Ed.), *The management of pain* (2nd ed.) (pp. 400–460). Philadelphia: Lea & Febiger.

*Carr, D.B., & Jacox, A.K. (1992). *Acute pain management: Operative or medical procedures and trauma.* (AHCPR Publication No. 92-0032). Rockville, MD: Agency for Health Care Policy and Research, Public Health Service, U.S. Department of Health and Human Services.

Cleeland, C.S., Serlin, R., Nakamura, Y., & Mendoza, T. (1997). Effects of culture and language on ratings of cancer pain and patterns of functional interference. In T.S. Jensen, J.A. Turner, & Z. Wisenfeld-Halin (Eds.), *Proceedings of the 8th World Congress on Pain* (Vol. 8) (pp 35–51). Seattle: IASP Press.

de Paula, T., Laganam, K., & Gonzalez-Ramirez, L. (1996). Mexican Americans. In J.G. Lipson, S.L. Dibble & P.A. Minarik (Eds.), *Culture and nursing care: A pocket guide* (pp 203–221). San Francisco: UCSF Nursing Press.

Ferrell, B.R., & Ferrell, B.A. (1996). *Pain in the elderly.* Seattle, WA: IASP Press.

Grant, M., Ferrell, B.R., Rivera, L.M., & Lee, J. (1995). Unscheduled readmissions for uncontrolled symptoms. *Nursing Clinics of North America, 30*(4), 673–682.

Guyton, A.C., & Hall, J.E. (1996). *Textbook of medical physiology* (9th ed). Philadelphia: W.B. Saunders Co.

*Hester, N., & Barcus, C. (1986). Assessment and management of pain in children. *Pediatrics: Nursing update.* Princeton: CPEC, Inc.

*International Association for the Study of Pain. Subcommittee on Taxonomy. (1979). Part II. Pain terms: A current list with definitions and notes on usage. *Pain, 6,* 249–252.

*Asterisk indicates a classic or definitive work on this subject.

*Jacox, A., Carr, D.B., & Payne, R. (1994). *Management of cancer pain: Clinical practice guideline.* (AHCPR Publication No. 94-0592). Rockville, MD: Agency for Health Care Policy and Research, U.S. Department of Health and Human Services.

Kaasalainen, S., Middleton, J., Knezacek, S., Hartley, T., Stewart, N., Ife, C., & Robinson, L. (1998). Pain and cognitive status in the institutionalized elderly. *Journal of Gerontological Nursing, 24*(8), 24–31.

Kingdon, R.T., Stanley, K.J., & Kizior, R.J. (1998). *Handbook for pain management.* Philadelphia: W.B. Saunders Co.

Lister, B.J. (1996). Dilemmas in the treatment of chronic pain. *American Journal of Medicine, 101*(1A), 2S–5S.

*Loeser, J.D. (1982). Concepts of pain. In M. Stanton-Hicks & R. Boas (Eds.). *Chronic low back pain.* New York: Raven Press.

*McCaffery, M. (1979). *Nursing management of the patient with pain.* New York: J.B. Lippincott.

*Melzack, R., & Casey, K.L. (1968). Sensory, motivational, and central determinants of pain. In D.R. Kenshalo (Ed.), *The skin senses* (pp. 423–439). Springfield: Charles C. Thomas.

*Melzack, R., & Wall, P.D. (1965). Pain mechanisms: A new theory. *Science, 150,* 971–979.

Miakowski, C. (1997). Women and pain. *Critical Care Nursing Clinics of North America, 9*(4), 453–457.

North American Nursing Diagnosis Association. (1999). *NANDA nursing diagnoses: Definitions and Classification 1999–2000,* Philadelphia: Author.

Parke, B. (1998). Geronotological nurses' ways of knowing: Realizing the presence of pain in cognitively impaired older adults. *Journal of Gerontological Nursing, 24*(6), 21–28.

Portenoy, R.K. (1998). *Contemporary diagnosis and management of pain in oncologic and AIDS patients.* Newton, PA: Handbooks in Health Care.

School of Nursing, University of California, San Francisco. (1996). *Culture and nursing care: A pocket guide.* J.G. Lipson, S.L. Dibble, P.A. Minarik (Eds.). UCSF Nursing Press.

Sullivan, E. (Ed.). (1995). *Nursing care of clients with substance abuse.* St. Louis: Mosby.

*Turner, J.A., & Romano, J.M. (1990). Psychologic and psychosocial evaluation. In J.J. Bonica (Ed.), *The management of pain* (2nd ed.) (pp 595–609). Philadelphia: Lea & Febiger.

Wong, D. (1995). *Nursing care of infants and children.* St. Louis, MO: Mosby.

Sensory/Perceptual Function

Delois Laverentz

Key Terms

auditory	presbycusis
chemoreceptors	presbyopia
exteroceptors	reticular activating system
gustatory	sensation
interoceptors	sensory deprivation
kinesthetic	sensory overload
olfactory	somesthetic
ototoxic	tactile
perception	visual
proprioceptors	

LEARNING OBJECTIVES

After studying this chapter, you should be able to:

1. Describe the normal physiology of sensation and perception.
2. Differentiate between sensory deficit, sensory deprivation, and sensory overload.
3. Discuss a variety of factors affecting sensory/perceptual function.
4. Describe techniques for assessing a client at risk for sensory/perceptual alterations, the manifestations of a sensory/perceptual alteration, and the client's responses to sensory/perceptual alterations.
5. Differentiate among the related diagnoses for the problems of sensory/perceptual alterations that are amenable to nursing care.
6. Plan goal-directed nursing interventions to manage sensory/perceptual alterations.
7. Evaluate outcomes for sensory/perceptual alterations to determine effectiveness of nursing care.

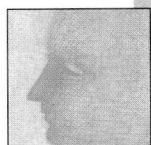

Sarah Jane Pfannenstiel is an 82-year-old widow who lives with her only daughter and son-in-law. She has been seeing an ophthalmologist for decreasing visual acuity in her left eye. She describes her vision as "trying to see through a dirty, greasy window." She has difficulty driving at night because of the glare of the headlights. She no longer enjoys reading or watching television because her left eye tears and becomes fatigued after short periods of time. She takes frequent afternoon naps because she is "bored." She is anxious and tells her daughter she is afraid of "going blind" and does not want to become a "burden" to her. The daughter reports that her mother doesn't go out socially any more because she is afraid of falling and breaking an arm or a leg.

The ophthalmologist recommends surgical removal of a cataract in her left eye. Mrs. Pfannenstiel is anxious about surgery and having someone "cutting on my eye." The nurse makes the diagnosis of *Sensory/perceptual alteration: visual.*

CONCEPTS OF SENSORY/PERCEPTUAL FUNCTION

Sensory/perceptual alterations can occur at any stage of a client's life. Nurses observe sensory deficits more commonly in older adults because of age-related changes in the sense organs. However, vision or hearing loss can occur at any age.

Nurses in every practice setting are concerned about sensory/perceptual alterations. In the neonatal intensive care unit, the nurse is concerned with preventing blindness, sensory deprivation, and sensory overload. The school nurse is concerned with identifying vision and hearing problems in school-aged children. In the acute care setting, nurses may care for clients hospitalized for a primary sensory deficit or for other health problems, such as an injury or stroke, that can alter sensory/perceptual functioning.

Clients with a primary sensory deficit are also often seen in outpatient clinics or by home health nurses. Community health nurses are concerned with screening older adults and helping them identify risks for and manifestations of sensory/perceptual alterations. Even when a sensory/perceptual alteration is not the primary reason for nurse-client contact, such a loss is important for the nurse to consider because it may interfere with the client's ability to provide self-care and maintain health and independence.

Physiology of Normal Sensory/Perceptual Functioning

Human beings depend on a continual flow of sensory stimulation from both the internal and the external environment. The process of sensory stimulation has three components: sensation, perception, and response. **Sensation** is the reception of stimulation through receptors of the nervous system. It is the registering of a sound, for example, before the sound is identified as a barking dog or a ringing phone. **Perception** is the conscious mental recognition or registration of a sensory stimulus, as, for example, when a person smells a sweet fragrance and gets a mental image of a cherry. It is the ability to receive input from the senses, interpret the information in the cerebral cortex, and correlate it in a meaningful way. A response is the action a person takes after identifying the sensation, as, for example, when a person responds to heat by pulling her hand away from the stove.

The human body has six types of **somesthetic** receptors, which pertain to sensations and sensory structures of the body as follows:

- **Visual,** for the sensation of sight.
- **Auditory,** for the sensation of hearing.
- **Gustatory,** for the sensation of taste.
- **Tactile,** for the sensation of touch.
- **Olfactory,** for the sensation of smell.
- **Kinesthetic,** for the sensation of position.

Minute by minute, these receptors take in tremendous amounts of information.

Somesthetic receptors are found in both the central and the peripheral nervous systems. Vision and hearing are carried out by the central nervous system. Taste, touch, smell, and position senses result from peripheral sensory receptors located throughout the body.

These peripheral receptors are classified according to the specific type of stimuli they transmit. **Exteroceptors** are sensory receptors located in the skin and mucous membranes and are stimulated by touch, light pressure, pain, temperature, odor, sound, and light. **Proprioceptors** are sensory receptors located chiefly in the muscle, tendons, and inner ear. They convey a sense of position movement and muscle coordination. **Interoceptors** are sensory receptors located in the viscera and blood vessels. They provide visceral information regarding pain, cramping, and fullness. **Chemoreceptors** are specialized cells adapted for excitation or stimulation by various chemicals. Taste buds and olfactory cells are chemoreceptors (Marieb, 1995).

Peripheral sensation involves not only detection of the stimulus, but also transmission of information to the central nervous system. Transmission begins when a peripheral receptor detects a stimulus and sends impulses by means of *afferent* (or *sensory*) *neurons* from peripheral nerve endings to the posterior horn in the gray matter of the spinal cord (Fig. 43–1). The impulse or sensation may then cause a reflex response, such as withdrawing a hand from a painful stimulus. For this to occur, the impulse must travel across *interneurons* to the anterior horn of the gray matter, and then back to the peripheral muscles on *efferent* (or *motor*) *neurons.* Alternatively, the spinal nerves may transmit data to the cerebral cortex, where it will be interpreted and a more complex response formulated.

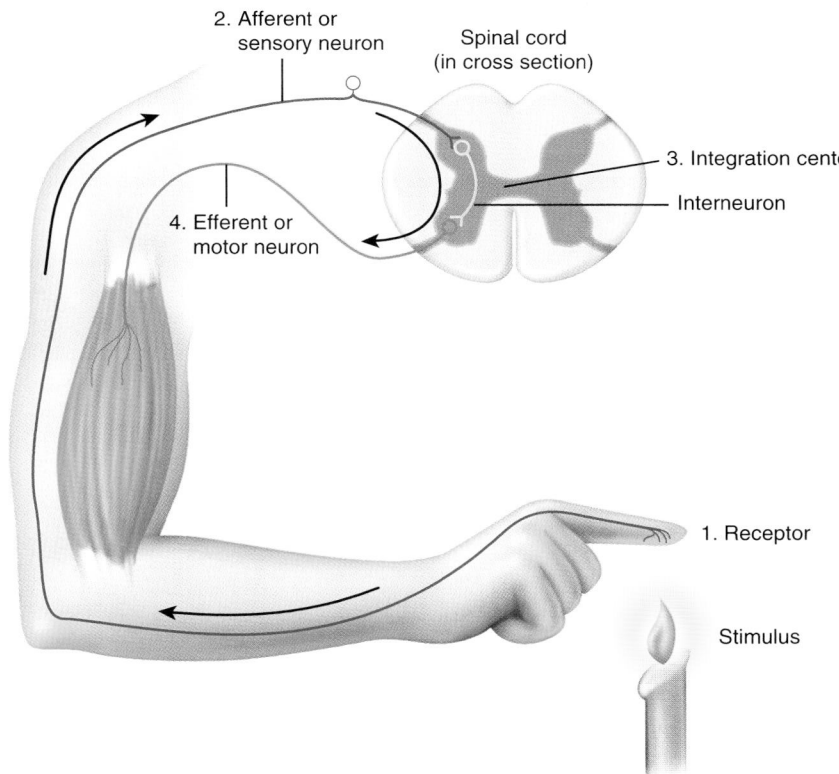

Figure 43–1. Reflex response. A sensory stimulus travels via afferent or sensory neurons to the spinal cord. The impulse enters the spinal cord at the posterior horn and travels across interneurons to the anterior horn. The impulse travels back to the peripheral muscle via the efferent or motor neuron.

The cerebral cortex must be alerted or aroused to perceive and produce a conscious act in response to stimuli. The **reticular activating system** (RAS), located in the midbrain and thalamus, keeps the brain aroused. The RAS controls the sleep-wake cycle, level of consciousness, the ability to direct attention to specific tasks, and the perception of sensory input that might alter behavior. When the RAS receives an adequate amount of sensory stimuli from the periphery, the person is aroused and alert; perception and adaptive responses occur. When the RAS receives an inadequate amount of sensory stimulation, the person may experience confusion, boredom, or drowsiness.

Sensory/Perceptual Alterations

Alterations in sensation, perception, and response may result from deficits in the sense organs, from sensory deprivation, or from sensory overload. Hearing and vision loss are the most common sensory losses.

Sensory Deficits

A *sensory deficit* is any loss in the ability to sense or perceive stimuli. It occurs in the sense organs and is not related to the amount of stimulation in the environment. A person may be born with a sensory deficit (a congenital deficit), or the deficit may be acquired suddenly or gradually. If a sensory function is lost gradually, the person may be able to compensate for the loss. If the loss occurs abruptly, however, compensation becomes much more difficult.

VISUAL

Because 85% of all information received from the environment is visual, vision impairment is a difficult experience at any age. However, most visual impairments can be corrected.

Uncorrectable visual impairments are relatively uncommon in childhood; however, 1 in 500 school-aged children is partially sighted. *Strabismus* (an abnormal position of the eye, commonly called crossed eyes) occurs in about 5% of children under age 4. If left untreated, it can result in amblyopia—vision loss in the nonfocusing eye (Thompson & Wilson, 1996). Rarely, an infant can be born blind because of maternal exposure to rubella.

Although vision loss in adults presents as a wide range of problems, presbyopia and cataracts are among the most common. **Presbyopia** is a loss of near vision in older people; it develops because the crystalline lens loses elasticity, and the ciliary muscles, which focus the lens by changing its shape, begin to weaken. A cataract results when the lens becomes opacified and cloudy.

In the United States, a person is considered legally blind when the best possible vision in the better eye is 20/200 or less, after correction with glasses. Blindness can also be caused by a constricted field of vision. Legally, a person is considered blind if the field of vision is 20 degrees or less in the better eye (Thompson & Wilson, 1996). See Box 43–1 for terms associated with blindness.

AUDITORY

Deafness can be partial or complete, and it can be conductive, sensorineural, or mixed. A *conductive loss* results from a problem in the outer and middle ear that reduces sensitivity to tones received by air conduction. A *sensorineural loss* is a weakening of sound produced in some portion of the sensorineural mechanism. Usually, it reduces bone conduction (Hegde, 1995).

Even though hearing deficits are thought to occur primarily in the elderly population, children may also have hearing impairments. Hearing loss in children is usually genetic, congenital, or a result of trauma. Children with repeated ear infections, usually before age 2, may experience conduction deafness. Other causes of hearing loss in children include meningitis, mumps, and encephalitis.

As people age, they may experience a change in their hearing acuity. Hearing of high-pitched tones commonly becomes impaired as the elderly client loses hair cells in the organ of Corti. Sound transmission may be impaired by sclerosis of the ossicles in the middle ear. Sound perception can be impaired from a loss of ganglion cells in the cochlea and a loss of neurons in the auditory cortex. These changes result in sensorineural and conductive hearing loss.

Presbycusis is a sensorineural hearing loss of high-frequency tones that occurs in the elderly and may lead to a loss of all hearing frequencies. Consonants become difficult to hear, making many spoken words difficult to discern. Cerumen impaction, which obstructs sound transmission, can cause conductive hearing loss in the older adult as well.

KINESTHETIC

Nerve fibers that conduct information about the body's position (sitting, standing, walking, on a moving bus) pass directly into the posterior columns of the spinal cord. These fibers then travel up to the medulla and synapse with secondary sensory neurons. At the secondary neurons, they cross over to the other side the medulla before continuing on to the thalamus.

Loss of position sense occurs with diseases of the posterior column, such as multiple sclerosis and vitamin B$_6$ deficiency. Tumors and vascular malformations in the vertebral column, by compressing the spinal cord, can also keep kinesthetic information from reaching somesthetic areas in the cerebellum, parietal lobe, or both.

The inner ear also plays a role in maintaining a sense of position and equilibrium. Disorders of the inner ear, such as an infection or Ménière's disease, may impair a person's sense of balance.

GUSTATORY

Taste sensations decline normally with age, but a loss of taste may also be associated with damage to the nerves, such as the facial nerve (cranial nerve VII) or the glossopharyngeal nerve (cranial nerve IX). Also, receptors in the taste buds can be damaged by chemotherapy or radiation to the head or neck. Cigarette smoking inhibits taste sensation. And because the senses of smell and taste work together to enable us to distinguish between foods, people who have permanent tracheostomies or laryngostomies have diminished taste sensations.

TACTILE

Alterations in touch can occur with certain types of damage to the spinal cord. With partial damage, touch is commonly preserved. With a complete transection of the spinal cord, all sensation is lost and the person develops paralysis and hyperactive reflexes.

BOX 43–1

TERMS ASSOCIATED WITH VISION

accommodation—use of contraction of the ciliary muscles to change the focus to an object at a different distance

ametropia—abnormal vision

astigmatism—uneven curvature of the cornea causing the person to be unable to focus horizontal and vertical rays of light on the retina at the same time

blurred vision—objects appear not to have sharp, distinct borders

color blindness—inability to detect the difference in some colors

diplopia—double vision; objects appear twice in visual field

emmetropia—the ideal optical condition of having no refractive error of vision

halos—appearance of circles of light or color around objects

hemianopia—bilateral or defective vision or blindness in half of the visual field

hyperopia or farsighted—near vision is impaired because objects at a distance of 20 feet or more are focused in back of the retina (error of refraction); distance vision is normal. Most children are born with hyperopia that disappears by age 8.

myopia or nearsighted—near vision is normal; distance vision is impaired because objects at a distance of 20 feet or more are focused in front of the retina (error of refraction). Usually appears before age 8.

photophobia—sensitivity to light

presbyopia—a decrease in the elasticity of the lens with age that impairs the ability to focus on near objects

spots—appearance of dots of various size in the visual field

OLFACTORY

The sensation of smell declines with age, nerve damage, or the presence of other odors in the nasal passages. The location of the olfactory nerve makes it vulnerable to damage from facial fractures and head injuries. Tumors or atherosclerotic changes at the base of the frontal lobe can also damage the nerve. If one of the two olfactory nerves is intact, the person will still be able to smell. If both olfactory nerves are affected, the sense of smell is permanently lost. This condition is called *anosmia.* Non-neurological factors, such as nasal congestion, sinus infection, zinc deficiency, smoking, or cocaine use, may also result in anosmia.

Sensory Deprivation

Sensory deprivation is inadequate reception or perception of environmental stimuli. The cause may be physiological, such as a sensory deficit, or it may stem from an inadequate variety or amount of stimuli in the environment. An example of inadequate variety in environmental stimuli is a radio tuned to play "elevator music" in a client's otherwise silent room. The same room without any radio at all is an example of an inadequate amount of environmental stimuli.

Data on sensory deprivation are derived from experiments involving total sensory deprivation. However, symptoms can be seen in persons who experience little variety in sensory stimulation, such as elderly people who live alone and rarely socialize (Fig. 43–2). As the sensory deprivation becomes more extreme and prolonged, the symptoms appear more severe. Persons deprived of sensory stimulation may experience central nervous system changes, such as impaired judgment, an inability to solve problems, confusion, disorientation, and even hallucinations and delusions.

Sensory Overload

A problem of increasing proportions in modern society, **sensory overload** results from excessive environmental stimuli or a level of stimuli beyond the person's ability to absorb or comprehend it. The hospital environment, for example, is filled with sights, sounds, smells, and tactile stimuli unfamiliar to most people. These stimuli place them at risk for sensory overload.

A person may be in the hospital recovering from surgery and in pain, only to find herself in a room near a busy nurse's station with a talkative roommate. Sensory overload can interfere with the person's ability to focus on the important aspects of a situation, such as learning a new skill for health care.

FACTORS AFFECTING SENSORY PERCEPTION

People need an adequate amount of sensory stimulation for normal growth and development. There is considerable variation in the amount of stimulation in-

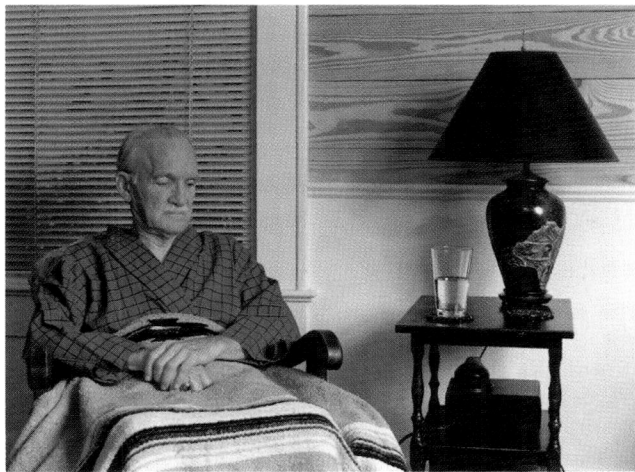

Figure 43–2. An elderly person who lives alone and has little opportunity to socialize may experience sensory deprivation.

dividuals consider optimal. Factors influencing the amount and variety of stimuli include lifestyle, environmental, developmental, socioeconomic, physiological, and psychological.

Lifestyle Factors

The amount and quality of sensory stimuli with which a person is comfortable are determined by her lifestyle. Some people are energized from the activity around them, whereas others prefer a quiet environment that promotes thinking.

Lifestyle choices, such as smoking and the use of recreational drugs, can alter a person's sensation. The senses of taste and smell are diminished by smoking. Intranasal drug abuse with cocaine or amphetamines can also alter the sense of smell. A lifestyle characterized by stress can impair a person's tolerance for sensory stimuli and the ability to correctly perceive those stimuli.

Environmental Factors

Environmental factors can affect a person's sensory/perceptual status. Chronic exposure to high levels of noise can affect a person's hearing. People who work around noisy equipment, such as farmers or factory workers, are at risk for hearing loss. Inhalation of irritants, such as chlorine fumes, can decrease the sense of smell. People who live in large cities get used to more noise and may become unaware of the high noise level.

The amount of environmental stimuli will also affect a person's response to stimuli. Exposure to excessive stimuli can result in symptoms of sensory overload, such as anxiety, confusion, disorientation, and an inability to make decisions. Too few stimuli result in sensory deprivation and a decreased response to the environment, which could lead to social isolation.

Developmental Factors

The nature and meaning of sensory stimulation changes with age. In the developing infant, sensory stimulation is needed for normal growth and development. As a person ages, there is an alteration in the perception of sensations and in the sensory organs themselves.

Infants and Children

The newborn has immature nerve pathways and cannot discriminate among sensory stimuli. Adequate stimulation is necessary for neural pathways to develop, become refined, and function adequately. Appropriate stimulation includes the following:

- Tactile and kinesthetic sensation, such as holding, rocking, and changing positions.
- Auditory sensation, such as singing and talking.
- Visual sensation, as from mobiles and bright objects.

Assessment of hearing loss in infants and children requires attentiveness to subtle signs. The first sign that alerts a parent to a possible hearing loss in an infant may be a failure to respond to loud noises. The infant may not awaken or startle at the sound of a sudden loud noise, for example. Another sign of possible hearing loss is a delay in speech development. The child may respond more to movement than to sound, be afraid of strangers, or avoid interacting with other children.

Adolescents and Middle Adults

Adolescents are at risk for hearing loss if they are exposed to chronic loud noise. Typically, in this age group, listening to loud music is a popular pastime and may lead to hearing loss.

Sensory changes related to the aging process begin in the middle adult years. Around age 40, adults begin to hold reading material farther from their eyes. When the distance exceeds the length of the arm, the person goes for an eye examination and reading glasses. Hearing changes, which also begin in the middle years, include decreased hearing acuity, speech intelligibility, pitch discrimination, and hearing threshold. There is also a reduced taste discrimination and sensitivity to odors.

Older Adults

The decline in sensory function that begins in the middle adult years becomes more apparent in the older adult years. However, loss of one sensory function may increase or sharpen the function of another sensation. For example, loss of vision may increase or sharpen the sense of hearing to compensate for the loss. Visual changes include reduced visual fields, increased glare sensitivity, impaired night vision, reduced accommodation, and reduced color discrimination.

Because Mrs. Pfannenstiel feels that she is trying to see through a dirty, greasy window, she has lost the enjoyment she used to receive from reading and watching television. She also has started to withdraw socially. What nursing concerns would you have regarding Mrs. Pfannenstiel's care? What interventions should be implemented?

The hearing changes experienced by the older adult can vary rather widely. There may be difficulty in discriminating consonants (f, s, th, and ch sounds, for example). Speech sounds may be garbled. Reception and reaction to speech may be delayed or low-pitched sounds may be heard best. The person may have trouble hearing conversations over the background noise.

Older adults should be observed for subtle cues to hearing loss. When the onset is gradual, the person may compensate for the loss and either not be aware of it or be embarrassed to admit to the hearing deficit. One of the early signs is talking louder than usual or turning up the volume on the television or radio. The person will turn her head toward the sounds.

Careful observation will sometimes reveal that the person smiles and nods but does not understand what is said, has a blank look, or does not give full attention to the person talking. Learning to lip-read may help the person compensate partially for the hearing loss. The person may have trouble following directions or ask for the directions to be repeated. Keep in mind that hearing loss can impair relationships and cause the person to withdraw from social activities.

In addition to visual and hearing changes, the older adult also can experience a loss of balance, spatial orientation, and coordination. Tactile changes develop as well, including reduced sensitivity to pain, pressure, and temperature. These changes place the older client at risk for injury.

Socioeconomic Factors

Socioeconomic factors can affect a person's ability to manage sensory/perceptual problems. If the person does not have the financial resources, she may not be able to afford the cost of health care. A person with decreased vision may not be able to afford an eye examination or eye glasses. This would affect the person's ability to see and place the person at risk for injury.

Physiological Factors

A range of physiological factors can affect sensory/perceptual functioning, such as trauma, physical illness, medications, and medical procedures.

Trauma

Traumatic injuries may result in a complete loss of sensation, decreased sensation (called hypoesthesia), or increased sensation (called hyperesthesia). Any of the six somesthetic senses can be affected by traumatic injury.

Eye trauma is a health concern for both children and adults. Penetrating eye injuries from firecrackers, slingshots, rocks, sticks, scissors, toy weapons, and other objects is a common cause of blindness in children. Adults are at risk for eye trauma when playing sports or working in an environment that contains chemicals or flying objects. In high-risk work areas, employees are required by the Occupational Safety and Health Administration (OSHA) to use protective eyewear.

Physical Illness

Pre-existing illnesses cause a variety of changes in sensory function. Disorders such as diabetes mellitus, renal failure, and vascular disease can lead to peripheral neuropathy, a disturbance or pathological change in the peripheral nervous system. Other disorders include deficiencies of the vitamins thiamine, pyridoxine, and folic acid and disorders caused by environmental exposure to heavy metals and industrial solvents. These problems cause an alteration in pain, touch, temperature, and motor function.

Clients with diabetes mellitus also have sensory alterations secondary to microvascular changes in the eye, which results in loss of vision that can lead to blindness. Stroke, multiple sclerosis, and spinal cord tumors are neurological disorders that can also cause sensory alterations.

A stroke may cause a loss of sensory function and motor function, depending on the location of the underlying vascular lesion. The person may have a loss of proprioception (coordination and balance). Visual changes may occur as well. Hemianopia results from damage to the optic tract or the occipital lobe.

Sensory alterations with multiple sclerosis include paresthesias and a diminished sensitivity to pain. Numbness, tingling, burning, or crawling sensations may develop. The sensory deficits caused by spinal cord tumors depend on the tumor's location and rate of growth. Clients may present with a slowly progressive numbness, tingling, pain, or temperature loss. They may also have a decreased sense of touch, an inability to sense vibration, and loss of position sense.

Medications

Medications can affect a person's neurosensory system. Sedatives and narcotics can alter perception of sensory stimuli. Phenytoin (Dilantin), hydralazine, isoniazid, and amitriptyline can cause peripheral neuropathy and other sensory changes. Captopril, ampicillin, tetracycline, griseofulvin, and carbamazepine can alter taste sensation. Chemotherapy and radiation therapy can affect taste sensation as well. Some medications can be **ototoxic,** having a damaging effect on cranial nerve VIII or the organs of hearing and balance. Aminoglycoside antibiotics are ototoxic. Aspirin can cause ringing in the ears.

Psychological Factors

In addition to physical causes, psychological problems—such as stress—can cause alterations in sensation and perception. The stress of an illness, hospitalization, or surgery can provide greater stimulation than the person can process without assistance. Pain and fatigue can alter mental status as well, changing the way the person perceives and reacts to stimuli.

A person's mental status affects her sensory perception. An agitated client may misinterpret a nurse's touch as aggressive rather than comforting, and may respond with aggression. A depressed person has a shaded view of the world and responds to sensory/perceptual stimuli based on this perspective. The person may misinterpret verbal and nonverbal communication because of this altered perspective.

ASSESSMENT

To detect and define problems with a client's sensory/perceptual status, start by performing a general assessment. Based on your general findings, you may then perform a focused assessment of any deficit areas.

General Assessment of Sensory/Perceptual Status

When assessing a client for sensory/perceptual alterations, obtain a complete health history and examine the client to determine the presence of or potential for sensory deficits and evidence of sensory deprivation or overload. Make sure to include the client's environment in your assessment.

Health History

Naturally, the chief complaint of a client with sensory/perceptual alterations will vary depending on the cause of the sensory deficit present. For example, a client with a hearing problem may complain that her ears are ringing. The health history will be focused toward the sensory system that has the alteration. Use questions such as those that follow to collect data for the health history.

VISION

- Describe the trouble you are having with your vision. Does it affect both eyes? When did it begin? Did it begin suddenly or gradually?
- What have you done to try to correct the problem?
- Do you have yearly eye examinations?
- Do you take eye medications? What kind? How often? For what reason do you take eye medications?
- Do you wear glasses? How often do you clean them?
- Do you wear contact lenses? Are they hard, soft, or extended wear? How do you clean your contact lenses?

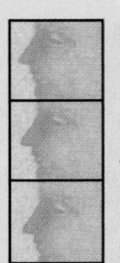

CROSS-CULTURAL CARE
CARING FOR A VOLGA GERMAN-AMERICAN CLIENT

Mrs. Pfannenstiel, the client in the case study for this chapter, is of Volga German descent. Most of these people immigrated to the United States and began farming homesteads. They worked hard to establish a better life for their families. Her family came to Central Kansas in 1870. Her daughter accompanies her to the eye doctor and is with her at the time of surgery. The Volga German-Americans tend to have the following values:

- Very strong work ethic.
- Stoic and do not like to ask for assistance.
- Skeptical of some health care practices and prefer folk treatments. Some people still use folk medicine for treatment of ear and stomach disorders.
- Close family ties.
- Strong religious values.
- Most practice the Catholic religion.

The following dialogue is between Mrs. Pfannenstiel and her nurse John. How does John demonstrate awareness of Mrs. Pfannenstiel's culture?

John: Good morning! My name is John and I will be your nurse today. I will be here when you get back from your eye surgery. How are you doing today?

Mrs. Pfannenstiel: Fine, I guess. [Daughter pats her mother's hand.]

John: [Looks questioningly at Mrs. Pfannenstiel and encourages her to expand.] Just fine?

Mrs. Pfannenstiel: I just don't like the idea of someone cutting on my eye.

John: This surgery is causing you some anxiety?

Mrs. Pfannenstiel: Yes, I wish there was some other kind of treatment [Looking at her daughter], but I guess there isn't any other treatment for this kind of eye problem.

John: This eye surgery should help your vision.

Mrs. Pfannenstiel: I am just glad my daughter is here with me. She has really helped me out since my eyesight has gotten so bad. I just don't know what I would have done without her.

Critical Care Questions

- Based on her cultural heritage, why do you think Mrs. Pfannenstiel was reluctant to consent to surgery?
- Knowing that people of Volga German culture are stoic and reluctant to ask for assistance, what will be important for John to include in postoperative nursing care and discharge planning for Mrs. Pfannenstiel?
- Since family is important to the Volga German culture, how can John utilize this information in discharge planning?

Reference

Walters, G.J. (1993). *Wir wollen deutsche bleiben: The story of the Volga Germans.* Kansas City, MO: Halcyon House.

- Do you have difficulty seeing at night?
- Do you see spots (floaters) in front of your eyes?
- Do you see rainbows or colored rings around lights or bright objects?

HEARING

- How long have you had the feeling that you do not hear well? Did the change in hearing begin suddenly or gradually?
- What types of sounds do you have trouble hearing?
- Do you have a family history of hearing loss?
- Where do you work? In your work or home environment, is there a lot of noise? If so, do you wear protective hearing devices or ear plugs? How long have you worked in this area? Has your hearing loss become a problem since working there?
- Does your hearing loss bother you? Does it keep you at home?
- Do you wear a hearing aid? How long have you worn it? Does it help?
- Do you hear noise in your ears? What does it sound like? Ringing, crackling, buzzing? When did it start?

- Are you taking any medications? Does the ringing in ears have any relationship to the start of the medications?

SENSATION

- Do you have numbness or tingling? Where is it located? Is it associated with activities? Describe how it feels.

Physical Examination

Physical examination of sensory/perceptual function includes screening for vision, hearing, position sense, taste, touch, and smell.

VISUAL

Acuity charts are used to check near and distance vision. A distance vision chart is mounted on a wall and the client reads it from 20 feet away. The Snellen alphabet chart is used most commonly and is appropriate for adults and older children. It contains 11 lines of various letters in graduated sizes. Each eye should be tested separately, and then both together. If the client wears corrective lenses, they should be worn during the test. Figure 43–3 shows a nurse screening for vision using a Snellen chart.

For children under age 4, pictures of common objects are used rather than an alphabet chart. For children ages 4 to 5 and for clients who do not speak English, the Snellen E chart is used. It consists of eight Es of graduated size facing in various directions. You can use hand gestures or ask a family member who speaks English to help explain the examination to a client who does not speak English. The client indicates the position of the E by duplicating the position with her fingers.

Near vision can be tested by asking a client to read from a newspaper, Snellen chart, or card held about 14 inches from the client's eyes. As with distance testing, each eye should be tested separately, and then both together. If the client cannot read, use a Snellen "E" chart.

Color blindness is most commonly tested by asking the client to identify patterns of colored dots on colored plates. A colorblind client will miss the patterns. Early detection allows the child to compensate for the deficit and also alerts teachers to the student's special need.

AUDITORY

There are three screening tests for hearing acuity: the whisper test, the finger-rubbing test, and the tuning fork test (which includes the Rinne and Weber tests). For the whisper test, instruct the client to cover one ear with her hand. Then stand 1 to 2 feet away from the other ear, in front of or to the side of the client. Shield

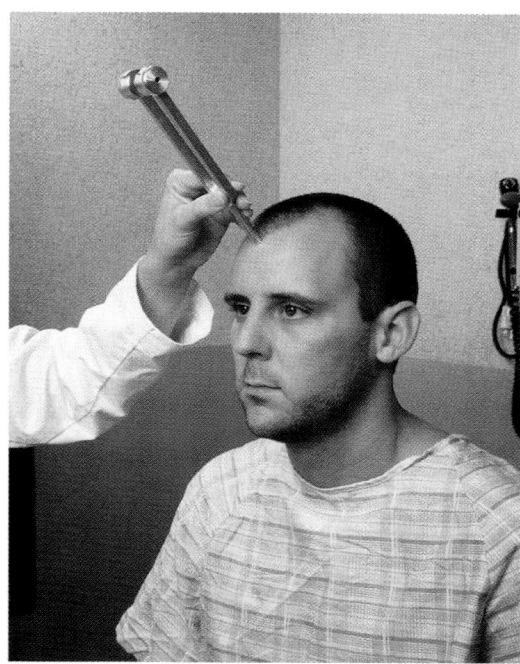

Figure 43–4. Weber's test. The nurse places a vibrating tuning fork in the middle of the client's forehead.

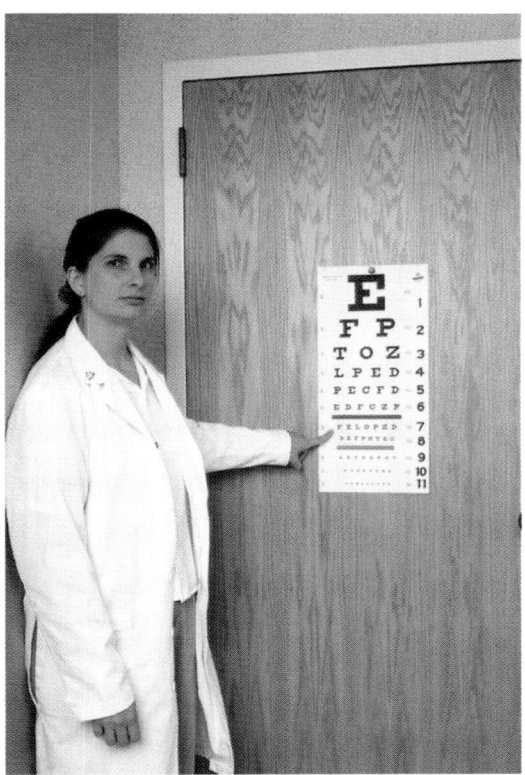

Figure 43–3. Vision screening using a Snellen chart.

your mouth and whisper monosyllabic (hat, ball, bat) or bisyllabic (baseball, overcoat, highchair) words. A client with normal hearing should be able to repeat at least half of all the words you whisper. After testing one ear, have the client cover it and test the other ear.

High-frequency sounds are evaluated by the finger-rubbing test. Hold your hands 3 to 4 inches from the client's ear and briskly rub your index finger against the your thumb. The client should be able to hear the noise produced by rubbing your fingers together. Test the other ear.

The Weber and Rinne tests are auditory screening tests used to evaluate the client for conduction or sensorineural hearing loss. These tests are done with a tuning fork with frequencies of 500 to 1,000 cycles per second.

WEBER'S TEST. The Weber test evaluates transmission of sound through the bones of the skull to the cochlea and acoustic nerve. This transmission is called bone conduction. Perform the test by placing a vibrating tuning fork at the midline of the top of the client's head, or in the middle of her forehead (Fig. 43–4).

The client should hear the resulting sound equally in both ears. If she has a conductive hearing loss, she will hear the sound more prominently in (the sound will lateralize to) the ear with the conductive loss. That is because the sound conducts directly through the bone to the ear. If the client has a sensorineural hearing loss in one ear, the sound will lateralize to the unimpaired ear because nerve damage in the impaired ear prevents hearing.

RINNE'S TEST. The Rinne test compares bone conduction to air conduction in both ears. Assess bone conduction by placing the base of a vibrating tuning fork on the client's mastoid process and noting how

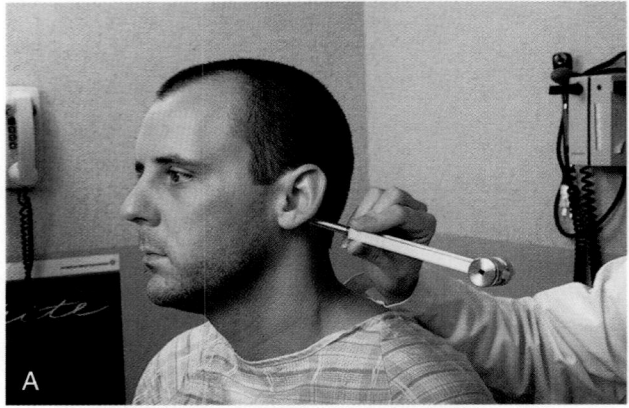

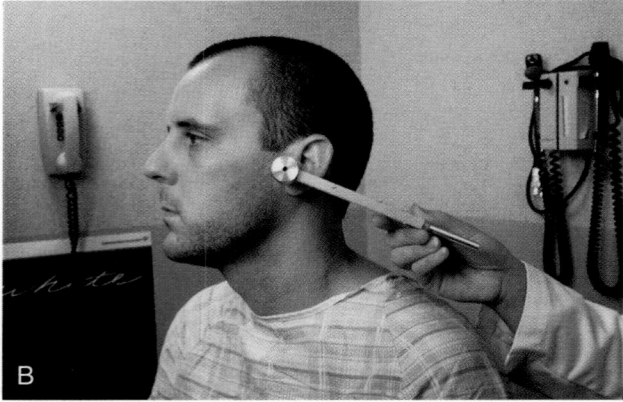

Figure 43–5. Rinne's test. A, the nurse places a vibrating tuning fork on the client's mastoid bone to assess bone conduction. B, the nurse then places the vibrating tuning fork parallel to the client's ear to assess air conduction.

many seconds pass before she can no longer hear it (Fig. 43–5). Then, test air conduction by placing the tines of a vibrating tuning fork parallel to the client's auricle, near her ear canal. Hold the tuning fork in this position until the client can no longer hear the tone. Note how many seconds the client can hear it. Repeat with the other ear.

Sound traveling through air normally remains audible twice as long as sound traveling through bone (a 2:1 ratio). Thus, sound heard for 10 seconds through bone conduction should be heard for 20 seconds through air conduction. With a conduction hearing loss, the client will report hearing sound longer through bone conduction. If she reports hearing the sound longer through air conduction, but the ratio is not the normal 2:1, the client has a sensorineural hearing loss.

KINESTHETIC

To test kinesthetic sensation, ask the client to close her eyes. Grasp the client's finger or toe and move its position 0.4 inch, or 1 cm, up or down. The client should be able to describe how the position has changed (Fig. 43–6A).

GUSTATORY

To test gustatory sense, instruct the client to stick out her tongue. Using a cotton applicator, place sugar, salt,

and lemon on the client's tongue, one at a time. The client should be able to correctly identify each taste.

SENSORY FUNCTION

Use light touch, tests of sharp and dull, and vibration to assess a client's sensory function. Test the peripheral extremities in several areas. If the sense is intact, no further evaluation is necessary. If it is impaired, move up the extremities until you reach a level or area where sensation exists.

Evaluate light touch by using a cotton wisp. Instruct the client to close her eyes, and then lightly touch the client with the wisp (Fig. 43–6 B). The client should be able to correctly identify the spot you touched. Test sharp or dull sensation using the tip of an unbent paper clip and the rounded end (Fig. 43–6 C). Again, instruct the client to close her eyes, and alternately touch the client with the sharp tip and the dull side of the paper clip. The client should be able to identify the sensation as well as the location. Test vibration sense by placing a vibrating tuning fork on a bony area, such as the wrist or ankle (Fig. 43–6 D). Ask the client to describe the sensation. The client should be able to feel the vibration. Ask the client to tell you when she no longer feels the vibration, then stop the vibration while the tuning fork is still touching the bony prominence.

OLFACTORY

Instruct the client to close her eyes, then ask her to identify common aromatic substances, such as coffee, orange, cloves, or tobacco, which are held under her nose. Test one nostril at a time. The client should be able to correctly identify the smell.

Diagnostic Tests

The physician will order specific diagnostic tests to confirm a sensory/perceptual disorder. The test ordered will be based on the potential health problem. For example, if the client presents with a chief complaint of decreased hearing, the physician will order audiometry. The results of the diagnostic tests will either be negative, or they will indicate a problem.

Slit-Lamp Examination

Microscopic examination of the anterior ocular structures is performed with a slit lamp. This instrument allows diagnosis of abnormalities in the cornea, lens, or anterior vitreous. The client places her chin in a shallow cup and leans her forehead against the device to stabilize her head. A narrow beam of light is aimed so that it brightly illuminates a narrow segment of the eye.

Corneal Staining

Corneal staining is indicated for diagnosis of corneal trauma, foreign bodies, corneal abrasions, or corneal ulcers. Fluorescein or another type of topical dye is instilled into the conjunctival sac to stain the cornea. Ir-

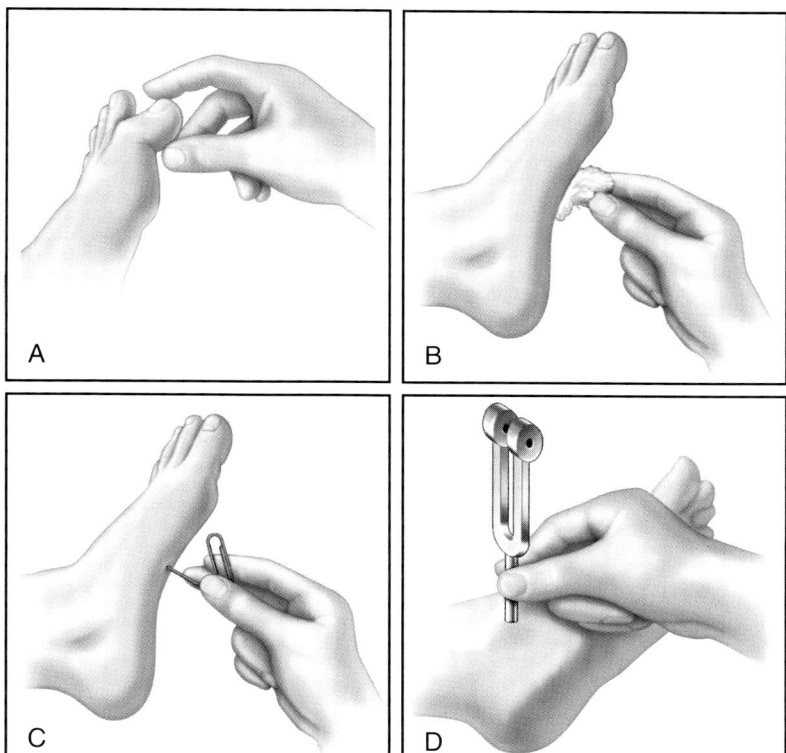

Figure 43–6. Peripheral sensory nerve testing. *A,* position sense; *B,* light touch; *C,* pain sensation; *D,* vibration sense.

regularities of the corneal surface are outlined with the dye.

Tonometry

Intraocular pressure is measured with a tonometer. Because intraocular pressure varies throughout the day, it is important to record the time of intraocular pressure reading. Elevated intraocular pressure reveals glaucoma. Tonometer readings are indicated for all clients over age 40, especially if they have a family history of glaucoma. Clients with intraocular pressure problems are taught to monitor intraocular pressure at home.

Audiometry

Audiometry is the measurement of hearing acuity by an audiologist, an expert trained in hearing and its disorders. There are two types of audiometry: pure tone audiometry and speech audiometry. The results of the audiometry can be plotted on an audiogram (Hegde, 1995).

Pure tone audiometry is performed to determine the threshold of hearing at selected frequencies (the highness or lowness of tones). The threshold is the intensity at which a tone is faintly heard at least half of the time it is presented. Pure tone audiometry is performed by either air conduction or bone conduction testing.

Air conduction testing is performed in a sound-proof booth to eliminate ambient noise. The person wears headphones that deliver sound directly to the

ear. The person raises her hand or presses a switch whenever a tone is heard. Hearing is tested at selected frequencies that are most important for speech. Each ear is tested individually.

Bone conduction testing is performed if the results of air conduction testing are abnormal. It distinguishes between conductive and sensorineural hearing loss. With this test, a bone vibrator is placed on the forehead or behind the test ear. The same procedure is followed as for air conduction testing, and tones are presented at a given frequency.

Speech audiometry determines how well the person understands speech and discriminates between speech and sounds. Two components of speech audiometry are the speech reception threshold and word discrimination. Speech reception threshold is the lowest level of hearing at which the person can understand half of the words presented. As the name implies, word discrimination tests the person's ability to understand spoken words (Hegde, 1995).

Computed Tomography

Computed tomography (CT) scanning is a radiographic diagnostic test in which a cross-sectional image is formed by the use of computers. It is helpful in diagnosing tumors, infarctions, and hemorrhage. Contrast media may be used to enhance the image, although usually not for images of the eye. The procedure must be explained to the client, and you will ascertain whether she has allergies to iodine or shellfish. If contrast media will be used, food and fluids should be withheld for 4 to 6 hours before the test. The client is instructed to lie still during the procedure.

Focused Assessment for Sensory/Perceptual Alterations: Visual

Defining Characteristics

The critical defining characteristic is impaired visual acuity. The change in visual acuity may lead to visual distortions; disorientation to person, place, and time; and alterations in the client's response to visual stimuli. Additionally, impaired visual acuity may alter the person's ability to conceptualize and problem-solve. The person may respond to the alteration with anger, apathy, anxiety, depression, or restlessness.

Related Factors

Alteration in visual acuity may result from changes in ocular structure, such as cataracts, a detached retina, glaucoma, macular degeneration, myopia, and hyperopia. Damage to the optic nerve from multiple sclerosis or a cerebrovascular accident will also affect visual acuity. Examples of three common eye disorders are cataracts, diabetic retinopathy, and retinal detachment.

Cataracts are opacities of the lens that cause gradual, painless blurring of the vision. As the cataract progresses, the milky white lens may become visible in the client's eye. Night blindness is one of the most distressing symptoms of cataracts because it interferes with night driving and seeing in darkened rooms. Bright lights are also distressing and may diminish the vision. Halo vision refers to rainbow-like, colored rings around lights or bright objects. Halos are early signs of cataracts and result from dispersion of light by abnormal opacities in the lenses.

Diabetic retinopathy refers to changes in the retina caused by diabetes. It is more likely to occur if the diabetes is poorly controlled and of long duration. It is the leading cause of vision loss in adults under age 40. Retinal edema and hemorrhage lead to gradual blurring, which can progress to blindness. Yearly eye examinations are important for early detection.

Retinal detachment is a complete or partial separation of the retina from the sclera. It is an ocular emergency that requires rapid treatment to save the client's vision. It can result from traumatic injury or disease. The onset is usually sudden and painless. The person sees bright flashes of light or floating dark spots in the affected eye. It may be described as a curtain being pulled over the eye.

Focused Assessment for Sensory/Perceptual Alterations: Auditory

Defining Characteristics

When people are unable to hear, their ability to communicate is impaired. One of the earliest assessment findings is a decrease in social interaction. This decrease may lead to increasing withdrawal from activities and, eventually, social isolation. The client may respond to changes in hearing with anger, apathy, or depression.

Related Factors

Although hearing impairment is not uncommon in an aged population, you should be alert to acute causes of hearing loss. Determine whether the client may be taking large doses of aminoglycosides to treat an infection or other medications that may affect a person's ability to hear (Table 43–1).

Hearing impairment in the elderly may be related to cerumen impaction. Risk factors for cerumen impaction include numerous hairs in the ear canal, a hearing aid, bony growths secondary to osteophyte or osteoma, and a history of repeated cerumen impaction.

Focused Assessment for Sensory/Perceptual Alterations: Kinesthetic

Defining Characteristics

You may first suspect kinesthetic alterations by observing diminished motor coordination. Closer examination may reveal an inability to identify the position or location of body parts, an inability to perceive changes in angles of joints, muscles weakness, flaccidity, rigidity, atrophy, or paralysis.

Related Factors

Alteration in position sense is primarily related to neurological conditions, such as cerebral palsy, multiple sclerosis, muscular dystrophy, spinal trauma, and spinal tumors. Surgical joint replacement can also alter the position sense, as may diseases of the inner ear.

Focused Assessment for Sensory/Perceptual Alterations: Gustatory

Defining Characteristics

A person with altered taste may present with one of the following: a complete loss of taste *(ageusia),* a distorted sense of taste *(dysgeusia),* or a partial loss of taste *(hypogeusia).* Notice the client's interest in food. Usually, a client with a loss of taste will add extra salt or other seasonings, report that the food tastes bland, or both. The decrease in taste may result in a loss of appetite or weight.

Related Factors

Changes in taste may be related to neurological, oncological, nutritional, or viral causes. The specific etiology may be unimportant in deciding how to help the person manage the problem of diminished taste. The result of altered taste can be inadequate nutrition, lack of enjoyment of food, or, in the worst case, ingestion of noxious substances or spoiled food.

TABLE 43–1
Ototoxic Drugs and Their Effects

Drug	Effects
Antibiotics	
Aminoglycosides, such as amikacin, gentamicin, kanamycin, neomycin, and vancomycin	• Can affect both the vestibular (balance) and auditory portion of cranial nerve VIII. • Most drug-induced ototoxicity is associated with aminoglycoside use.
Erythromycin	• Reversible hearing loss with high doses.
Minocycline	• Reversible vestibular toxicity. • Affects women more than men.
Diuretics	
Ethacrynic acid (Edecrin)	• High parenteral doses may cause transient or permanent hearing loss.
Furosemide (Lasix)	• Administration of other ototoxic drugs may potentiate hearing loss.
Cardiac Drugs	
Quinidine	• Tinnitis, transient hearing loss, and vertigo.
Analgesics	
Aspirin	• High doses can cause irreversible hearing loss, but usually transient • May also cause tinnitis and vertigo.
Nonsteroidal anti-inflammatory drugs, such as indomethacin (Indocin) and ibuprofen (Motrin)	• Transient hearing loss, vertigo, and tinnitis.
Antineoplastic Agents	
Bleomycin, cisplatin, dactinomycin, and mechlorethamine	• May be reversible or irreversible. • Usually causes ototoxicity when given in high doses, to people with renal impairment, or to people receiving other ototoxic drugs.

Focused Assessment for Sensory/Perceptual Alterations: Tactile

Defining Characteristics

An altered sense of touch may present as abnormal sensation *(paresthesia)*, decreased sensitivity to stimulation *(hypoesthesia)* or pain *(hypoalgesia)*, or an impaired sense of touch *(dysesthesia)*. Abnormal sensation is usually described by the client as numbness, prickling, or tingling.

Related Factors

An alteration in the sense of touch may be related to peripheral vascular disease, such as an acute arterial occlusion, arteriosclerosis obliterans, Buerger's disease, or Raynaud's disease. Clients with a metabolic disorder, such as diabetes mellitus or a vitamin B deficiency, can experience a decreased sensation related to peripheral neuropathy. Paralyzing neurological or neuromuscular diseases, such as a stroke or Guillain-Barré syndrome, will alter the person's ability to perceive touch.

Focused Assessment for Sensory/Perceptual Alterations: Olfactory

Defining Characteristics

Changes in olfaction include diminished smell *(hyposmia)* and absence of smell *(anosmia)*. Smell is important to alert the client to danger and to stimulate appetite.

Diminished smell may go unnoticed unless the person realizes that smoke or a gas leak was undetected. Sometimes it is detected secondary to weight loss.

Related Factors

An alteration in the sense of smell may be related to nasal problems, such as a nasal neoplasm, polyps, sinusitis, rhinitis, or septal fracture. Neurological disorders that cause damage to cranial nerve X, such as anterior cerebral artery occlusion, brain stem lesion, head trauma, or olfactory meningioma, can alter a person's sense of smell.

Focused Assessment for Sensory Deprivation

Because the aim of assessment for sensory deprivation is to prevent sensory deprivation, assessing the client's level of environmental stimulation is as important as assessing for signs and symptoms of sensory deprivation. Assess the amount of stimulation and its meaningfulness to the client. Determine whether the client can perceive and correctly interpret the environment.

In a situation of sensory deprivation, the usual response is to withdraw and pass the time by sleeping. Symptoms of mild depression are among the early manifestations. As time passes, the client loses track of time and decreases attention to the environment. Thoughts become less organized, and events lose significance. If sensory deprivation is severe and prolonged, symptoms appear that suggest loss of contact with reality. Hallucinations may be present, although they are usually brief and fleeting. Internal and external sensations may become confused; the client is not sure whether something happened or was just a thought. Feelings of disorientation in space and time can become overwhelming.

Sensory deprivation can be related to four causes of a reduction in stimuli:

- A reduction in the intensity, frequency, or amount of stimuli, as when the person is alone in a quiet place with little or no stimuli.
- A reduction in the meaningfulness of stimuli, as when a person is not able to understand the incoming stimuli.
- A reduction in stimuli because of impairment of the senses.
- Being removed from a familiar situation without adequate orientation to the new situation.

Focused Assessment for Sensory Overload

People who are ill, especially those who are seriously ill, are at risk for sensory overload. Factors that contribute to sensory overload include an unfamiliar routine, an environment with excessive noise or light, an altered sleep-rest pattern, and pain.

Clients experiencing sensory overload may be disorientated to time, place, and person. They may have an altered ability to think abstractly and to conceptualize and problem-solve. They may also have mood swings and exaggerated emotional responses, visual and auditory distortions, or hallucinations.

Sensory overload may occur in a variety of people. The client hospitalized in an intensive care unit following major trauma or surgery is at risk for sensory overload. The intensive care unit has many potential sources of sensory overload, such as equipment noise and alarms. The client experiencing alcohol withdrawal syndrome is also at risk for sensory overload.

Focused Assessment for Related Nursing Diagnoses

Risk for Injury

Clients with sensory deficits are at high risk for injury. Assess people with visual problems for compensatory skills to avoid danger in their path, which may cause them to stumble and fall. Assess elderly people with partial visual losses for safety in using the stove for cooking, taking medications, walking down the stairs, or driving a car. Does the hearing-impaired client have the skills to compensate for inability to hear noises that would indicate danger, such as fire alarms, sirens, horns, or oncoming vehicles? Instructions for taking medications may be misunderstood. Being able to smell odors, such as smoke or leaking gas, alerts a person to danger. A person with an alteration in touch may be unable to feel extremes of temperature, pressure, or pain. The loss of position sense places a client

at risk for injury because she may lose her balance and fall. Finally, the person with sensory overload may be so overwhelmed with stimuli that important cues to safety are ignored or missed.

Altered Nutrition: Less Than Body Requirements

Assess for the effects of altered taste and smell on nutrition. Appetite is enhanced by smell and taste, and it is important that food be flavorful. Otherwise, food is less appealing, and the appetite is diminished. Maintaining an optimal intake of a variety of nutrients becomes difficult. Often, the person will add salt and spices to improve the taste of food. If the person has heart disease, hypertension, peptic ulcers, or other health problems that require a special diet, the prescribed diet may alter appetite even more.

Impaired Verbal Communication

The process of communication involves speaking and listening. People with an auditory deficit are at risk for *Impaired verbal communication* because one of the components for communication is missing. Hearing aids are helpful but sometimes add to the problem if the level of noise produced by the hearing aid becomes more confusing than helpful. People who use hearing aids sometimes find that they need to limit the number of people in a room and delete extraneous noises like music or television. Even with a hearing aid, the person may need to be in the speaker's direct line of vision to lip-read.

Social Isolation

Assess the person with a sensory deficit for *Social isolation*. For example, a person with a hearing deficit is at risk because interacting with other people is difficult when the conversation cannot be followed. Unable to participate in the conversation, the client may withdraw and become isolated. Clients with vision loss are also at risk for social isolation. They may stay at home, where the environment is familiar. They may be reluctant to leave the house for fear of falling or being unable to find their way.

Mrs. Pfannenstiel has been reluctant to leave her daughter's home for fear of falling and breaking a bone. How might Mrs. Pfannenstiel and her daughter increase her social interactions?

Self-Care Deficit

Assess the person's ability to manage self-care. With an insidious onset of the deficit, people will automatically compensate for the loss. When the onset is sudden and severe, however, most people will need assistance with learning compensatory actions. For example, a person who has a visual deficit may find it challenging to perform her usual self-care tasks, such as bathing, feeding, dressing, and toileting. Assess the need for protective living when hearing or vision loss makes a person unsafe or unable to care for herself.

Altered Thought Processes

An alteration in the characteristics of incoming stimuli, resulting in either too much or too little stimulation, can affect a person's thought processes. The person may have a change in cognitive abilities. Assess the ability to problem-solve, think abstractly, and conceptualize. The person may experience visual or auditory distortions and hallucinations or become disoriented to person, place, or time (see Chapter 45).

DIAGNOSIS

The diagnosis of *Sensory/perceptual alteration* encompasses all of the sensory deficits, sensory overload, and sensory deprivation. The accompanying decision tree illustrates the decision-making process for *Sensory/perceptual alteration.* It is important to specify the

actual cause of the sensory/perceptual alteration. When writing the diagnostic statement, make sure to specify the sensory alteration. For example, write *Sensory/perceptual alteration: visual, related to lens opacity secondary to cataracts.*

A change in the amount of incoming stimuli may result in sensory deprivation or sensory overload. You should obtain a history and physical assessment to determine which the person is experiencing. If she is at risk rather than actually experiencing a sensory alteration, write the diagnostic statement like this: *Risk for sensory/perceptual alteration: Sensory overload related to noise from alarms and equipment in the intensive care unit.* A person with a sensory deficit is receiving less than a normal amount of stimuli. This places the person at risk for sensory deprivation. Altered thought processes may result from a change in the amount or characteristics of incoming stimuli. The accompanying chart provides further assistance in distinguishing among these related nursing diagnoses.

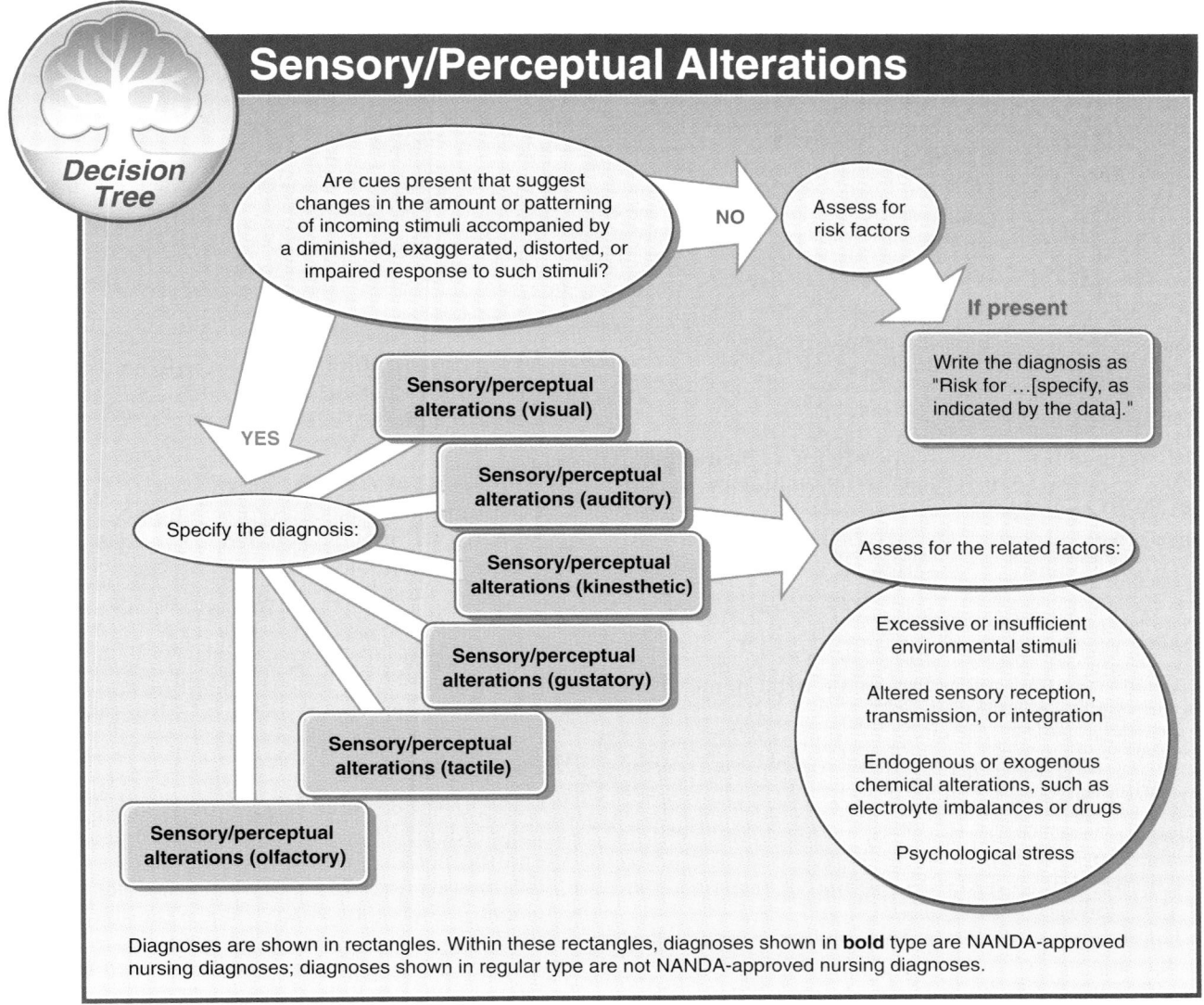

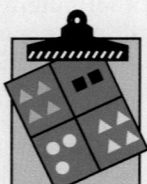

CLUSTERING DATA TO MAKE A NURSING DIAGNOSIS
SENSORY/PERCEPTUAL ALTERATIONS

Data Cluster	Diagnosis
A 76-year-old man has had progressive hearing loss over the last 6 months, has refused to participate in activities at the extended care facility, and has often been found sitting alone in his apartment.	Social isolation related to inability to communicate secondary to loss of hearing.
Forty-eight hours after admission following a motor vehicle accident, an 84-year-old woman with a fractured left femur and multiple rib fractures becomes confused and begins to pull out her indwelling urinary catheter and her intravenous line.	Altered thought processes related to a change in the environment and the amount of incoming stimuli.
On the first day after cataract surgery, the client has her left eye patched. She also has a cataract in her right eye.	Sensory/perceptual alterations: visual related to left-eye patch and cloudiness of the right lens.
A 54-year-old woman receiving chemotherapy and radiation therapy for breast cancer states that food does not taste good any more. She has lost 25 pounds in the last 3 weeks.	Altered nutrition: less than body requirements related to loss of taste sensation secondary to the effects of chemotherapy.
A 25-year-old male with a spinal cord injury has no movement or sensation below the level of the umbilicus.	Sensory/perceptual alterations: tactile related to severance of nerves in the spinal cord.
A 22-month-old has a history of repeated ear infections. The mother has noted that the child does not look toward noise and has not started to vocalize.	Sensory/perceptual alterations: auditory related to loss of hearing secondary to repeated ear infections.

PLANNING
Sensory Deficit

Preventing injury is a high priority for a client experiencing a sensory deficit. The expected outcome is that the client does not experience injury. However, because sensory deficits may take many different forms, specific outcomes are necessary. They include the following.

Visual

- Client identifies measures to alter the home environment to prevent injury.
- Client agrees to use adaptive devices.
- Client makes an appointment to have her vision evaluated.

Auditory

- Client identifies and uses alternative measures that alert danger.
- Client agrees to use adaptive devices, such as hearing aids.
- Client uses signing, gestures, lip-reading, or assistive devices to maintain communication.

- Client uses community resources to help cope with the auditory deficit.
- Client maintains social contacts.

Kinesthetic

- Client implements safety precautions.
- Skin breakdown is avoided, especially in areas around vulnerable joints.

Tactile

- Client does not experience falls or injury.
- Client does not experience skin breakdown.
- Client describes safety measures to avoid injury.

Olfactory

- Client describes how to identify noxious odors.
- Client identifies measures to maintain a safe home environment.
- Client consumes 75 to 100% of her diet.
- Client identifies ways to enhance the enjoyment of food.
- Client adheres to proper nutrition, as evidenced by her ability to maintain weight or achieve an ideal body weight.

Sensory Deprivation

The expected outcome for sensory deprivation is that the client remains oriented to person, place, and time. Short-term outcomes might include the client's using adaptive equipment as needed (such as glasses or a hearing aid), or the client's responding to environmental stimuli.

Sensory Overload

The expected outcome for sensory overload would also be that the client remains oriented to person, place, and time. Short-term outcomes might include the following:

- Client voices decreased anxiety and irritability.
- Client communicates in a lucid manner.
- Client recognizes when sensory stimuli are excessive.
- Client re-establishes routine sleep-wake cycle.
- Client demonstrates positive coping behavior when sensory situation arises.

INTERVENTION

Interventions for clients with sensory/perceptual alterations should promote adaptation to sensory deficits, provide sensory stimulation, and prevent sensory overload, as appropriate.

Interventions to Promote Adaptation for Sensory Deficits

When a hospitalized client has a vision or hearing impairment, nursing interventions are aimed at helping the person adapt to an unfamiliar environment. You will intervene to promote a safe environment, encourage self-care, facilitate communication, prevent injury, teach proper body mechanics, and promote nutrition. A client who is partially sighted or partially deaf may function well in a familiar environment but will need assistance in an unfamiliar environment. Other types of sensory/perceptual alterations will require other interventions. Some examples of interventions for various sensory/perceptual problems are described below.

Promoting a Safe Environment

Providing a safe environment for a client with a vision or hearing impairment is important. Orient the client to the room and demonstrate how to use the call light. It may take several sessions of orientation to get the client comfortably settled in the room. Remove excess furniture and equipment from the room. However, do not move furniture without letting the client know of its new location. Also, do not leave objects where the client may be walking.

Teach the visually impaired person and significant others about safe illumination, reduction of glare, and use of contrasting colors to assist with visual discrimi-

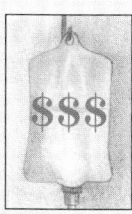

THE COST OF CARE

PREOPERATIVE TEACHING PROGRAM FOR CLIENTS UNDERGOING CATARACT SURGERY

Shortened hospital stays have necessitated alternative options for preoperative teaching. This study implemented preoperative teaching in the home within 3 to 10 days before hospital admission for cataract surgery. Eighteen patients were taught postoperative eye care, activity restrictions, application of an eye shield, instillation of eye drops, and symptoms of potential complications in their home. Eighteen control subjects received preoperative teaching in the eye clinic. Effectiveness of the teaching was measured by comparing pre-test and post-test scores regarding the content taught. The results of the study indicated that preoperative teaching in the home resulted in an increase in the subjects' post-operative scores for knowledge and skill acquisition for eye care.

Discussion

Although the cost/benefit ratio was not actually calculated, the study showed that preoperative teaching in the home increased quality of care. The increase in knowledge regarding post-operative care and skill acquisition will have a positive effect and is expected to decrease the number of post-operative complications.

Reference

Allen, M., Knight, C., Flak, C., & Strang, V. (1992). Effectiveness of a preoperative teaching programme for cataract patients. *Journal of Advanced Nursing, 17,* 303–309.

nation. Adequate lighting should be provided in all rooms during the day, and soft lighting should be provided at night. The light switch should be easily accessible. Interventions to reduce glare include avoiding glossy surfaces (such as glass and highly polished floors), using shades to provide diffuse light, wearing sunglasses or a brimmed hat when outside, and avoiding looking at headlights and other bright lights.

Contrasting colors help in visual discrimination and also promote safety. Methods to provide color contrast include marking the edges of steps with colored tape; avoiding white walls, floors, and counter tops; using smoked glass instead of clear glass; choosing objects colored black on white; and painting doorknobs a bright color.

Action Alert!
Orienting the client to her surroundings reduces the risk of injury.

Make sure that all staff are aware of the client's vision or hearing loss. Record information in the client's kardex, clinical care path, or chart cover, and post the information in the client's room. Respond to the client's call light as quickly as possible.

Glasses and contact lenses are important aids to help the partially sighted person maintain safety in an unfamiliar environment. The client should be able to easily locate these visual aids and know they are safely stored if not in use. Handle glasses carefully to prevent them from becoming misaligned or the lenses dirtied.

Occasionally the client may need you to remove or insert her contact lenses. You will need to know whether the person wears hard or soft lenses, and how long it is safe to wear them. When contact lenses are not being worn, storage guidelines appropriate for the lens type should be followed (Procedure 43–1).

Providing a safe environment for a person with a hearing impairment is important to prevent injury. Visual aids and aids to enhance hearing are helpful. Ex-amples of visual aids include a light that blinks when the doorbell or telephone rings, an alarm clock that flashes a light to awaken the person, flashing lights to warn of fires, and extra mirrors on a car to enhance vision in several directions. Aids to boost residual hearing include using telephone amplifiers and leaving the car window partly open and setting the air conditioner, heater, or radio on low so outside noises, such as sirens and other warning signals, can be heard.

Encouraging Self-Care

Usually, visually impaired clients want to be independent even in a hospital environment. Modify the environment to maximize any vision the client may have. If the client has hemianopia, place the client's personal belongings in an area of the room that maximizes the functional areas of her visual field. Approach the client from the best visual angle and remind the client to scan the environment to pick up visual cues (Table 43–2).

TABLE 43–2
Nursing Interventions to Promote Self-Care With the Visually Impaired

Self-Care Need	Nursing Interventions
Feeding	• Describe the location of utensils and food on the tray or table using the face of the clock as a reference (e.g., coffee is at 1 o'clock and dessert at 9 o'clock). • Allow client to express feelings of frustration and provide emotional support. • Place food in the person's vision if he or she has a visual field defect. • Once the client has accommodated, teach him or her to scan the area. • If perceptual deficit, choose different-colored dishes to help distinguish item (e.g., white dishes, dark linen cloth).
Bathing and hygiene	• Verbally announce yourself before entering or leaving the bathing area. • Provide privacy and inform the client of the measures taken (e.g., say "I am pulling the curtain for you to have privacy while you bathe"). • Allow ample time for client to perform bathing and hygiene. • Place bathing equipment within easy reach. • Place bathing equipment in person's field of vision if he or she has a visual field defect. Once the client has accommodated, teach him or her to scan the area. • Observe the person's ability to perform hygiene tasks of bathing, shaving, brushing teeth, and combing hair. • Provide clean clothing within easy reach. • Place call light within easy reach if person is to bathe alone. • Discuss normal aspects of bathing. Reassure the client with statements such as, "You are in the tub and the water is only 3 inches deep."
Dressing and grooming	• Allow the person to identify the most convenient location for clothing. • Encourage significant other to provide clothing that is easily managed by the client (e.g., clothing slightly larger than regular size and velcro straps may be helpful). • Adapt the environment for the person's ease of dressing. • Place clothing in the person's field of vision if he or she has a visual field defect. Once the client has accommodated, teach him or her to scan the area.
Toileting	• Place call light within easy reach. • Place toilet tissue within easy reach. • Place bedpan or urinal in person's field of vision if he or she has a visual field defect. Once the person has accommodated, teach him or her to scan the area. • Observe the person's ability to reach the bedpan or urinal. • Provide privacy. • Provide a safe, clear path to the bathroom.

From Bolander, V.B. (1994). Sorensen and Luckman's basic nursing: A psychophysiologic approach. (3rd ed.). Philadelphia: W.B. Saunders Co.

Safety is also a concern for hearing-impaired clients. Voice responses to call lights may not be effective for these clients.

Facilitating Communication

It is important to develop a means to communicate with a client with a hearing impairment to prevent social isolation. If the client has a hearing aid, encourage its use. Determine how to effectively communicate with the client through the use of gestures, written words, signing, or lip reading. Document the best way to communicate with the client in the kardex or clinical path and on the chart cover.

Interventions to facilitate communication include facing the client when speaking; enunciating the words slowly, clearly, and in a normal voice; and avoiding putting your hands to your mouth when speaking. Wearing lipstick helps to define the mouth and facilitates lip-reading. Provide sensory stimulation using tactile and visual stimuli to help compensate for the hearing loss. If the client wears a hearing aid, it is important for you to understand the proper care and usage of the device (Box 43–2). If the client is unable to insert the hearing aid, you may need to do so for her (Procedure 43–2).

Direct nursing interventions toward promoting communication to increase or maintain social interaction. When communicating with a person who can read lips, face the person and make sure you have her attention before speaking. Try not to speak too rapidly, but do not slow your rate of speech below that appropriate for normal conversation. Speak clearly and simply. Do not shout or exaggerate lip movements. Use appropriate gestures to aid in the understanding of what is being said, just as you would with a hearing person. Do not draw letters in the air or make similar gestures.

If the person has residual hearing, try lowering the pitch of your voice. This often helps in communicating with elderly people, whose hearing deficit typically involves high-pitched sounds first. Turn off the radio or television so that background noise does not interfere with the person's ability to hear.

For the profoundly deaf person who cannot read lips, supply plenty of paper and pencils for notes. Obtain a sign language interpreter as needed.

Action **A**lert!
Urge a hearing impaired client to install a smoke detector that uses a flashing light to signal a fire.

To communicate with visually impaired clients, identify yourself when you enter the client's room. Explain what you are doing and help the client anticipate your movements. Tell the client what you are going to do before you touch her.

If hearing impairment is caused by cerumen impaction, the impaction may be removed with ceruminolytic agents and lavage of the ear canal (Procedure 43–3). Teach the client the following information:

- Production of ear wax is normal.
- Do not place foreign objects, such as cotton-tipped

PRECAUTIONS FOR USING AN EXTERNAL HEARING AID

Do not store in a warm place (such as on a windowsill or in a car).
Heat can change the shape of the ear mold, which then does not fit the person's ear.
Do not twist the cord.
Do not drop.
Wash hands before handling.
Make sure battery is inserted properly and is in working order.
Take the battery out of the hearing aid when not in use for a day or longer.
Remove the hearing aid before x-ray examination or therapy to avoid damage from radiation.
Avoid using aerosol spray near the hearing aid.
Aerosol spray can clog the microphone.

applicators, into the ear canal. Bobby pins and paper clips inserted into the ear can injure the ear and increase the risk for infection.
- Clean your ears with a damp washcloth wrapped around a finger.
- Ceruminolytic agents soften ear wax and may allow for natural removal.
- See your health care professional if your hearing declines or you hear ringing, crackling, or other noise.

Action **A**lert!
Warn the client that inserting foreign objects into the ear canal may perforate the tympanic membrane or damage the ear canal.

Preventing Injury

Clients with a diminished ability to perceive the position or location of body parts are at risk for injury. The person with vertigo or dizziness, for example, is experiencing an alteration in position sense and has a potential for injury. Orthostatic hypotension (the decrease of blood pressure on standing) is the most common cause of dizziness. There are numerous contributing factors for dizziness, such as cardiac arrhythmias, dehydration, medication side effects, a prolonged recumbent position, and a sudden change in position.

The person with dizziness should be taught to change position slowly and to move from a reclining to an upright position in stages, with a few minutes between each stage. A chair, walker, cane, or other assistive device should be placed nearby to steady the person when getting out of bed. Teach the person to prevent dehydration by increasing fluid intake when excessive fluids are lost during exercise and when perspiring during hot weather.

Text continued on page 1230

Inserting and Removing Contact Lenses

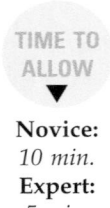

TIME TO ALLOW
▼
Novice: *10 min.*
Expert: *5 min.*

Nurses seldom need to insert or remove contact lenses. However, there are situations (such as motor-vehicle injuries) in which a client becomes unable to remove the lenses, and you may then need to do it. More often, however, you will provide assistance to a client in providing self-care for contact lenses. You should therefore become familiar with the general principles of contact lens care, including insertion and removal.

Delegation Guidelines

This procedure may not be delegated in clients who have recently undergone an eye procedure or surgery. Assisting a client with the routine insertion and removal of contact lenses may be delegated to a nursing assistant who has received training in these techniques.

Equipment Needed

- Clean gloves
- Contact lens storage container
- Products recommended by manufacturer for cleaning, disinfection, and storage
- Sterile lens disinfecting and/or enzyme solution
- Wetting solution for hard contact lenses
- Surfactant cleaner
- Rinsing solution
- Lens suction cup

Inserting a Contact Lens

1 Wash your hands.
Bacteria and debris will irritate the eye and may cause an infection. Soft contact lenses are easily damaged.

2 Remove the lens from the container and apply wetting solution to both sides.

3 Assess the lens. Check to make sure it is clean and undamaged.
If needed, clean it according to the specific type of contact lens.
Place the lens in the storage container marked for the correct eye.
Rinse the lens with sterile normal saline solution or manufacturer-recommended rinsing solution before reinserting.

4 Place the lens on the index finger of your dominant hand.
If the edges of a soft lens droop outward and downward, invert the lens.
Be sure to place each lens in the correct eye.

5 Hold the person's upper lid with the index finger of your nondominant hand and spread the upper and lower lid by slight downward pulling on the lower lid with your thumb. Have the person look straight ahead.

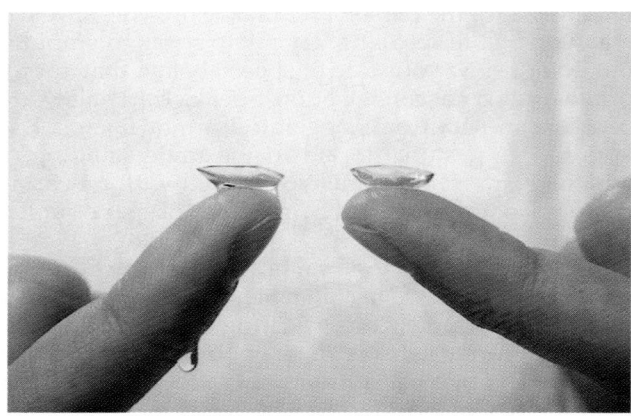

Inverted soft contact lenses.

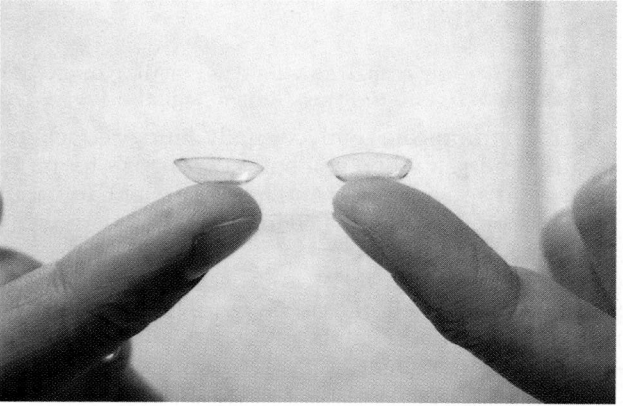

Soft contact lenses in normal orientation.

6 Place the lens over the iris.

7 Gently rub the upper lid with your finger to remove air bubbles.

Removing a Soft Contact Lens

1 Wash your hands.

2 Ask the client to look up and to the side (laterally); with your middle finger, pull down on the lid and place your index fingertip on the lower edge of the lens.

3 Move the lens medially to the white part of the eye.

4 Gently pinch the lens between your thumb and index finger, allowing air to go beneath the lens. The lens will double and can be grasped and removed.

If lens edges stick together, gently roll to separate; add normal saline as needed.

Removing a Hard Contact Lens

1 Wash your hands.

2 Pull the client's upper and lower lids apart and to the lateral side.

3 Ask the client to blink. The lens should fall into your hand.

4 An alternative method for removing a hard contact lens is to put gentle pressure on the lower edge of the lens, and then grasp the upper edge of the lens as it falls away from the eye.

5 Another method is to use a lens suction cup to lift the contact lens from the client's eye.

If the lens cannot be easily removed from an unconscious client, contact an eye care professional.

8 Ask the client to blink and determine that lens is correctly placed.

If the client feels any discomfort, remove the lens, inspect it, clean it, and insert it again.

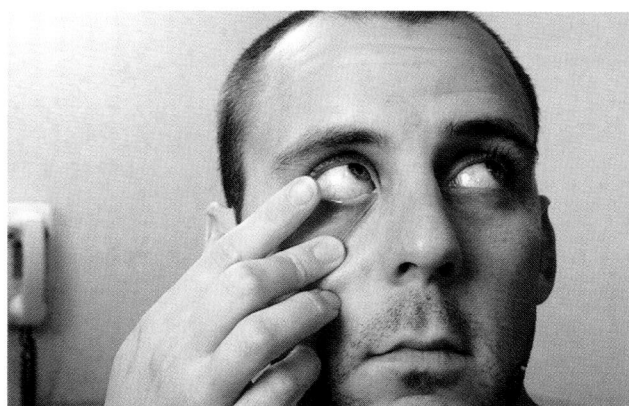

Removing a soft contact lens by pulling down on the lid and placing the fingertip on the lower edge of the lens.

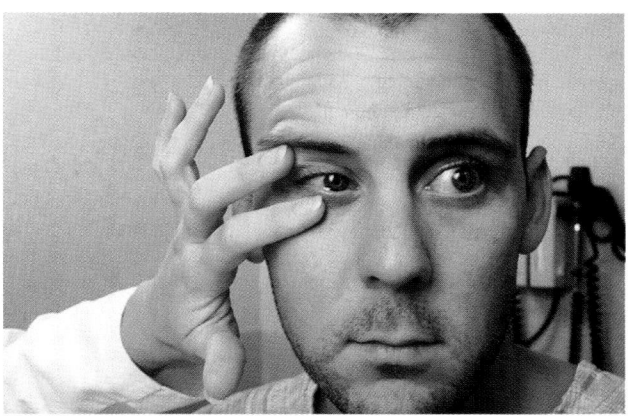

Removing a hard contact lens by pressing against its bottom edge.

HOME CARE CONSIDERATIONS

Home caregivers may need to be taught to help a client manage contact lens care. If the caregiver needs to insert and remove contact lenses, you will need to demonstrate the technique and provide support until the caregiver is comfortable with the procedure. When possible, it may be more desirable to have the client revert to wearing glasses.

PROCEDURE 43–2

Inserting a Hearing Aid

TIME TO
ALLOW
▼
Novice:
10 min.
Expert:
5 min.

Many clients over the age of 50 use hearing aids. A hearing aid is a delicate, sensitive instrument and requires careful handling and cleaning. Sometimes a client will need assistance with changing the battery or adjusting the volume. You should become familiar with hearing aids.

Delegation Guidelines

Assisting a client with the care and use of a hearing aid may be delegated to a nursing assistant. The nursing assistant should be trained in this skill.

Equipment Needed

- Soft, lint-free cotton cloth
- Cleaning solution for ear mold as recommended by manufacturer
- Mild soap and warm water to clean ear canal
- Fresh battery, if needed

1 Check that the battery is operating.

Hold the hearing aid in your hand and turn up the volume. If the batteries are working, a "feedback" whistle will be heard. Feedback is the noise resulting from the sound leaking out and going back through the microphones and becoming amplified.

2 Inspect the hearing aid.

The plastic connecting tubing, present in behind-the-ear aids, should not be cracked or broken. The ear mold should not be cracked or have a rough surface. The ear mold should be free of cerumen.

3 Turn down the volume, insert the ear mold into the ear canal, and secure the rest of the aid in place according to the design.

The ear bore or hole should be placed in the ear canal. The ear mold should precisely fit the ear. A slight twist may be needed to snugly fit the ear mold in the ear.

4 For a behind-the-ear hearing aid, secure the battery device behind the ear. Avoid kinking the connecting tubing.

5 Slowly turn up the volume while speaking to the person in a normal tone of voice. Ask the person to tell you when the volume is comfortable.

6 If feedback occurs, check for a problem.

Press on the ear mold. The ear mold may be loose and need to be replaced. Check to make sure the person's ear is not against a pillow, causing the ear mold to be dislodged.

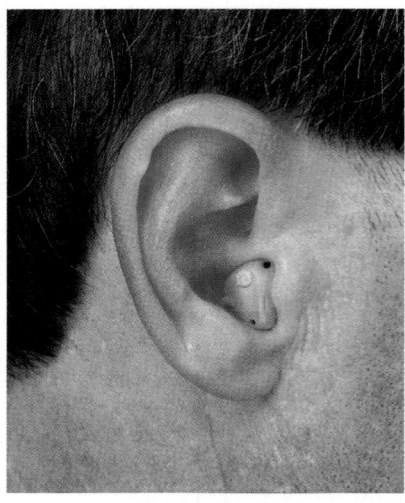

An in-the-ear hearing aid in place. (Courtesy of Dahlberg, Inc., Golden Valley, MN.)

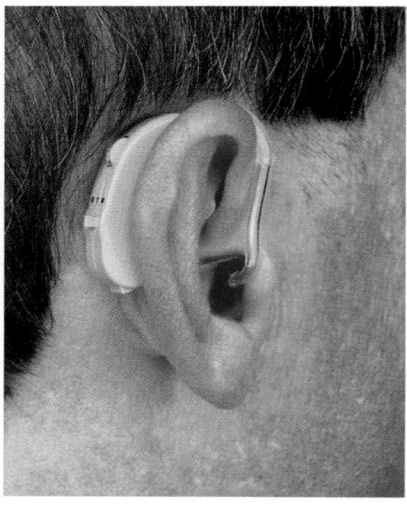

A behind-the-ear hearing aid in place. (Courtesy of Dahlberg, Inc., Golden Valley, MN.)

PROCEDURE 43-3

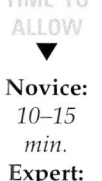

Ear Lavage/Irrigation

TIME TO
ALLOW
▼
Novice:
*10–15
min.*
Expert:
5–10 min.

Ear irrigations are generally performed for the purpose of removing a foreign body, removing accumulated cerumen, or relieving local irritation. Do not perform ear irrigation if you suspect or detect evidence of rupture of the ear drum. To prevent rupture of the ear drum, do not irrigate the ear canal under pressure.

Delegation Guidelines

The indications for RN assessment in the performance of ear lavage and the potential risk associated with improperly performed irrigation dictate that this procedure may not be delegated to a nursing assistant.

Equipment Needed

- Ear syringe
- Irrigation solution (usually water at body temperature)
- Emesis basin
- Absorbent towel or waterproof pad
- Clean gloves

1 Gather the necessary equipment.

2 Examine the ear canal with an otoscope.
Assess for an intact tympanic membrane and signs of otitis media. Irrigation is contraindicated with a tympanic membrane perforation and otitis media. However, the usual purpose is to remove cerumen, which may obstruct your vision of the ear canal.

3 Explain the procedure and instruct the client to avoid any sudden movements.
Holding still will prevent trauma from the irrigating syringe or catheter.

4 Check the temperature of the irrigant. A common irrigant is a mixture of water and hydrogen peroxide.
Water temperature should be 37°C, or about 98°F.

5 Select the irrigating device.

A 20-mL or 50-mL syringe may be used with a plastic IV catheter on the end. If a 50-mL syringe is used, caution should be exercised to avoid exerting excessive pressure, which may damage the tympanic membrane. A dental irrigation device may be used at low settings. The pulsating action of the dental irrigation device may help to break up the cerumen.

6 Cover the client's shoulder. Tip the client's head to the side that is being irrigated and ask the client to hold the emesis basin.
The head should be positioned to allow the irrigant to drain into the basin.

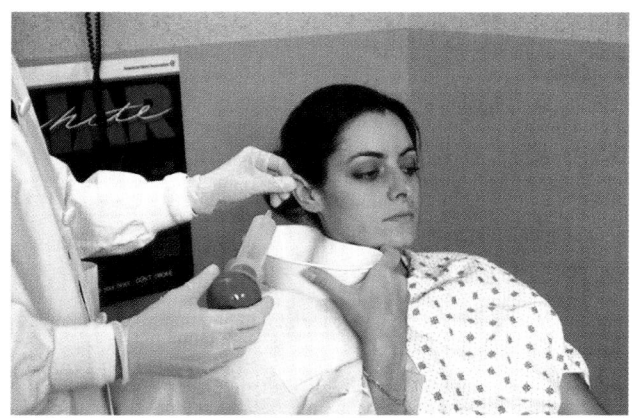

Preparation for ear irrigation.

Continued

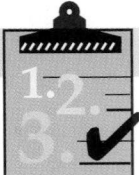

Ear Lavage/Irrigation

7 Place the tip of the irrigation device just inside the external meatus with the tip still visible.

Straighten the auditory meatus by gently drawing the pinna up and back for an adult. Pull the ear canal down and back for an infant.

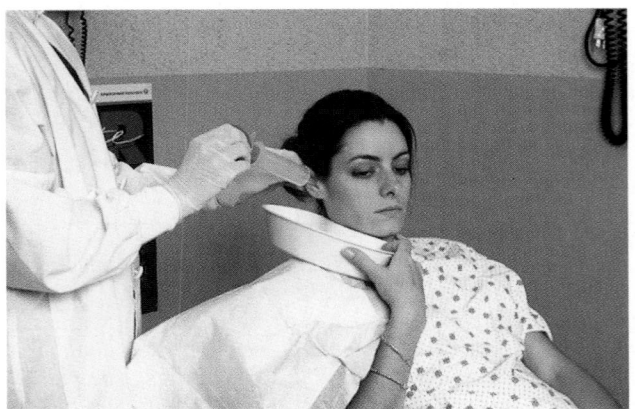

Instilling fluid for ear irrigation.

8 Direct the fluid toward the posterior wall of the ear canal.

The ear canal can be compared to the face of a clock. Fluid should be directed at 1 o'clock for the left ear and 11 o'clock for the right ear.

9 Irrigation of fluid should be steady. No more than 70 mL of solution should be used at one time.

Watch the fluid for signs of cerumen plug removal. If nausea and vomiting occur, stop the irrigation immediately.

10 Periodically examine the ear canal with an otoscope to determine patency and cerumen removal.

If cerumen does not drain out, wait 10 minutes and repeat the irrigation. If debris is not removed after a reasonable time, another method should be considered.

11 Tilt the head to drain excess fluid from the ear. Dry the ear canal gently with cotton-tipped applicator.

If cerumen cannot be removed with irrigation, the client may place mineral oil into the ear three times daily for 2 days to soften the dry cerumen. Then the irrigation may be repeated.

Teach clients with sensation deficits the following preventive measures to avoid an injury:

- Regularly observe how your hands and feet are placed.
- Inspect your skin daily, especially your feet.
- Pad the side rails of your bed and make any other appropriate environmental modifications.
- Test your bath water with a thermometer.
- Protect your hands and feet from extremely cold temperatures by wearing gloves and warm socks.

Action Alert!
Teach a client with a spinal cord injury how to shift her body weight to prevent skin breakdown.

A loss of smell can also place the person at risk for injury. Home care instructions for the client should include the following:

- Install smoke detectors and check the batteries regularly.
- If you have gas appliances, contact the utility company about measures to protect against gas leakage.
- Date all foods that spoil quickly; discard them promptly to avoid mistakenly eating spoiled food.

Promoting Nutrition

An alteration in taste and smell places the person at risk for impaired nutrition. It is important that foods be flavorful because appetite is enhanced by smell and taste. The use of spices, such as fresh garlic, onion, and lemon juice, can improve the flavor. Encourage caregivers to prepare foods the client enjoys and to serve them in an attractive manner. A variety of different colored foods presented at each meal may appeal to the client's visual sense and, thus, increase appetite. Teach the client that frequent mouth care may increase the taste sensation and improve appetite. Weigh the client weekly to detect weight loss and monitor for possible malnutrition.

Interventions to Provide Sensory Stimulation

Assist or encourage clients to use glasses, hearing aids, or other adaptive devices to help reduce sensory deprivation. Arrange the client's environment to offset any deficit.

- Encourage family to bring in personal items like photos, cards, and books.

- Provide a night-light.
- Position the client's bed for maximal visualization of the environment.
- Assist the client and family or significant other in planning short trips outside the hospital.

A*ction* A*lert!*
Monitor the environment and provide sensory stimulation for the at-risk client.
  The hospital environment particularly may be a source of sensory deprivation and sensory overload.

Reality orientation is important for the client with sensory deprivation. Reorient the client by calling her by name, introducing yourself, and orienting her to time, place, and environment. Turn on the television and radio for short periods of time based on the client's interest. Discuss the client's interests while providing care. Try to be with the client at predetermined times throughout the day to avoid isolation. Encourage family members or significant others to discuss past and present events with the client.

Interventions to Prevent Sensory Overload

Because hospitalized clients are susceptible to sensory overload, it is important to reorient the client to reality. Call her by name. Introduce yourself. Orient her to the environment, including sights, sounds and smells. And provide information about time, place, and date. Other measures to provide reality orientation include providing clocks and calendars, and placing family photos and other personal items at the bedside. Family or significant others should be encouraged to visit frequently.

Measures should be implemented to reduce environmental stimuli by reducing excessive noise and lights and keeping the environment uncluttered. Procedures and treatments should be clustered to avoid disturbing the client unnecessarily. Approach the client in a calm, gentle manner to avoid startling her. Teach the client to limit sensory overload by turning off the television or leaving or reducing a stimulating environment.

Try to stimulate a "normal" environment for the hospitalized client by dimming or turning off lights at night and keeping them on during the day. This should facilitate day/night orientation.

EVALUATION

Evaluate outcome criteria as specified in the nursing care plan to determine whether the nursing diagnosis is resolved. Remember that evaluation requires reas-

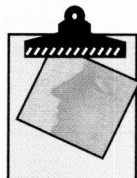

NURSING CARE PLANNING
A CLIENT RECOVERING FROM CATARACT SURGERY

Admission Data

Mrs. Pfannenstiel is admitted to same-day surgery the morning she is scheduled for removal of the cataract in her left eye. She is accompanied by her daughter and appears anxious. She repeatedly tells her daughter, "I really see okay. Maybe this surgery isn't a good idea. I don't like the idea of someone cutting on my eye."

Postoperative Physician's Orders
1. Discontinue IV when taking adequate fluids.
2. May dismiss when vital signs are stable and taking adequate fluids without nausea.
3. Please teach client regarding home care instructions.

Home Care Instructions
1. Return to the office the day after surgery with your eye patch in place.
2. Tobradex. Instill one drop four times daily in the operated eye. Begin the day after surgery.
   Ocufen. Instill one drop four times daily in the operated eye. Begin the day after surgery. Shake well before using.
3. DO NOT rub the operated eye.
4. Wear your glasses to protect the operated eye, even though the lenses will need to be changed in the glasses after surgery. The eye will not be ready for the new pair of glasses for several weeks after surgery.
5. Wear your sunglasses over your glasses for protection from wind and sunlight.
6. Tape the metal shield over the operated eye every night before going to bed. This will protect the eye while you sleep.
7. Do not resume driving your car for 1 week, and then only if your vision allows it.
8. Do not drink alcoholic beverages for 48 hours.
9. Do not do heavy work, such as moving furniture, working in the garden, mowing the grass, shoveling snow, and so on, for at least 1 week.

Continued

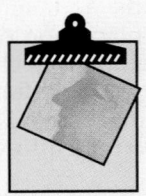

NURSING CARE PLANNING
A CLIENT RECOVERING FROM CATARACT SURGERY *(continued)*

Nursing Assessment

Upon return to her room, Mrs. Pfannenstiel's left eye is patched. She is awake and immediately recognizes her daughter. Her vital signs are stable and she denies nausea.

NURSING CARE PLAN

Nursing Diagnosis	Expected Outcomes	Interventions	Evaluation (At the Time of Discharge)
Sensory/perceptual alterations: visual related to left eye patched secondary to cataract surgery.	Implements adaptive strategies to maintain safety and comfort	Place water and personal articles in line of vision. Orient client to call light and bed controls.	Is able to independently take liquids without nausea. Calls nurse for assistance when needed.
		Provide amount of lighting that client finds most helpful.	States can see better without bright, glaring overhead lights.
		Teach daughter safety measures for discharge and modifications for home environment. *Mother and daughter should be treated as though working together for mother's safety and comfort. Tell mother that it is important to let daughter help her.*	Daughter agreed to walk on affected side; point out stairs and irregular paths. Will arrange home environment to minimize activity, to have needed items conveniently in place, have a clear path, and avoid sharp objects. Daughter will stay with mother until next physician appointment.

Italicized interventions indicate culturally specific care.

Critical Thinking Questions

1. What feelings would you anticipate in Mrs. Pfannenstiel while she has one eye covered?
2. Knowing that recovery may be more difficult for an 82-year-old woman, what measures would you employ to help Mrs. Pfannenstiel maintain a positive attitude during her recovery?
3. What kind of problems would you anticipate for Mrs. Pfannenstiel to manage while she is waiting for her eyes to have recovered enough to be fitted for new glasses?
4. How would you deal with Mrs. Pfannenstiel's unrealistic fear that she will not see again?

---

sessment of the client. A discharge nursing note for the client in this chapter's case study might look like this:

Mrs. Pfannenstiel and her daughter verbalize the following measures to prevent injury to the operated eye:

1. Wear glasses.
2. Wear sunglasses to protect your eye from wind and sunlight.
3. Tape the metal shield over your operated eye at night.
4. Do no heavy work, such as moving furniture, working in the garden, mowing the grass, or shoveling snow, for at least a week.

If the outcome criteria are not achieved, reassess the client to determine the reason for her lack of

progress. The plan of care or outcome criteria may need to be revised based on the assessment.

KEY PRINCIPLES

- Sensation and perception are processes that require sensory nerve receptors to convey stimuli to the brain, where they are perceived and interpreted. The person then responds to the stimuli.
- Sensory deficits occur when one of the senses is impaired and stimuli are not conveyed in a normal fashion to the brain.
- Sensory deprivation occurs when the brain re-

ceives too little incoming stimuli; sensory overload occurs when the brain receives too much stimuli.

- People at all points along the life span are at risk for sensory/perceptual alterations. However, elderly people are more likely to be affected.
- You can assess a client for sensory/perceptual alterations by taking the client's history, completing a physical assessment of the client's senses, noting symptoms of sensory/perceptual alterations, and noting responses to sensory deficits or sensory/perceptual alterations.
- Nursing interventions are aimed at optimizing sensory/perceptual functioning.

BIBLIOGRAPHY

*Allen, M., Knight, C., Falk, C., & Strang, V. (1992). Effectiveness of a preoperative teaching programme for cataract patients. *Journal of Advanced Nursing, 17*, 303–309.

Andrews, M.M., & Boyle, J.S. (1995). *Transcultural concepts in nursing care* (2nd ed). Philadelphia: J.B. Lippincott Co.

*Benson, C. & Lusardi, P. (1995). Neurological antecedents to patient falls. *Journal of Neuroscience Nursing, 27*(6), 331–337.

*Chen, H. (1994). Hearing in the elderly: Relation of hearing loss, loneliness, and self-esteem. *Journal of Gerontological Nursing, 20*(6), 22–28.

DeMaagd, G. (1995). High-risk drugs in the elderly population. *Geriatric Nursing: American Journal of Care for the Aging, 16*(5), 198–207.

*Erber, N.P. (1994). Communicating with elders: Effects of amplification. *Journal of Gerontological Nursing, 20*(10), 6–10.

Erber, N.P. & Heine, C. (1996). Screening receptive communication of older adults in residential care. *American Journal of Audiology, 5*(3), 38–46.

Erber, N.P., Lamb, N.L., & Lind, C. (1996). Factors that affect the use of hearing aids by older people: A new perspective. *American Journal of Audiology, 5*(2), 11–18.

Greene, A.W. & Mosher-Ashely, P.M. (1996). A residential care alternative for elderly deaf persons. *Journal of Gerontological Nursing, 23*(8), 32–36.

Grossman, D. (1996). Cultural dimensions in home health nursing. *American Journal of Nursing, 96*(7), 33–36.

*Hancock, C.K., Munjas, B., Bery, K., & Jones, J. (1994). Altered thought processes and sensory/perceptual alterations: A critique. *Nursing Diagnosis, 5*(1), 26–30.

Hegde, M.N. (1995). *Introduction to communicative disorders.* Austin, Texas: Pro-ed.

Kavanaugh, K.M. & Tate, B. (1996). Recognizing and helping older persons with vision impairments. *Geriatric Nursing: American Journal of Care for the Aging, 17*(2), 68–71.

Kelly, M. (1996). Medications and the visually impaired elderly. *Geriatric Nursing: American Journal of Care for the Aging, 17*(2), 60–62.

Kelly, M. (1995). Consequences of visual impairment on leisure activities of the elderly. *Geriatric Nursing: American Journal of Care for the Aging, 16*(6), 273–275.

Kleinschmidt, J.J., Trunnell, E.P., Reading, J.C., White, G.L., Richardson, G.E., & Ewards, M.E. (1995). The role of control in depression, anxiety, and life satisfaction among visually impaired older adults. *Journal of Health Education, 26*(1), 26–36.

*Kloosterman, N.D. (1991). Cultural care: The missing link in severe sensory alteration. *Nursing Science Quarterly, 4*(3), 119–122.

Lindeblade, D.D. & McDonald, M. (1995). Removing communication barriers for the hearing-impaired elderly. *Medsurg Nursing, 4*(5), 379–385.

*Mahoney, D.F. (1993). Cerumen impaction: Prevalence and detection in nursing homes. *Journal of Gerontolgical Nursing, 19*(4), 23–30.

*Mahoney, D.F. (1992). Hearing loss among nursing home residents. *Clinical Nursing Research, 1*(4), 317–325.

Marieb, E.N. (1995). *Human anatomy and physiology* (3rd ed). Menlo Park, California: Benjamin/Cummings Publishing.

NANDA. (1998). *Nursing diagnosis: Definitions and classifications 1999–2000.* Philadelphia: Author.

Meador, J.A. (1995). Clinical outlook. Cerumen impaction in the elderly. *Journal of Gerontological Nursing, 21*(12), 43–45.

Sander, R.L. (1995). Clinical snapshot. Glaucoma. *American Journal of Nursing, 95*(3), 34–35.

Thompson, J.M. & Wilson, S.F. (1996). Health assessment for nursing practice. St. Louis: Mosby.

*Walczak, M., Bernstein, A.L., Senzer, C.L., & Mohr, N. (1993). Elder hearing aids: Infrared listening device in a geriatric day center. *Journal of Gerontological Nursing, 19*(8), 5–9.

*Walters, G.J. (1993). *Wir wollen deutsche bleiben: The story of the Volga Germans.* Kansas City, MO: Halcyon House.

*Wilson, L.D. (1993). Sensory/perceptual alteration: Diagnosis, prediction, and intervention in the hospitalized adult. *Neuroscience Nursing, 28*(4), 747–765.

Zemlin, W.R. (1998). *Speech and hearing science: Anatomy and physiology.* Boston: Allyn and Bacon.

---

*Asterisk indicates a classic of definitive work on this subject.

Impaired Verbal Communication

Delois Laverentz

KEY TERMS

aphasia
articulation
Broca's area
communication
dysarthria
dysphagia

dysphonia
neologism
paraphasia
phonation
resonance
Wernicke's area

LEARNING OBJECTIVES

After studying this chapter, you should be able to:

1. Describe the physiological and behavioral concepts underlying impaired verbal communication.

2. Discuss the most common lifestyle, developmental, physiological, and psychological factors affecting communication.

3. Assess the client who is at risk for impaired communication, who has actual impaired communication, or who has a related nursing diagnosis.

4. Diagnose the problems of impaired communication that are amenable to nursing interventions.

5. Plan nursing interventions to prevent or correct impaired verbal communication based on client goals.

6. Implement key interventions for a client with impaired verbal communication.

7. Evaluate outcomes for impaired verbal communication to determine the effectiveness of nursing care.

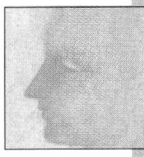

Señor Juan Martinez comes to the hospital with a persistent upper respiratory infection. His wife accompanies him. They are both from Mexico and have been in the United States for only 6 months. Neither Sr. Martinez nor his wife is fluent in English. Sr. Martinez is employed in a beef-packing plant.

  His tuberculosis skin test is positive, and he is admitted for further diagnostic work-up and placed in respiratory isolation precautions. The nurse is concerned about being able to communicate verbally with the Martinezes and uses the diagnosis of "Impaired verbal communication related to Spanish as the primary language" to alert the health care team of the need for an interpreter.

CONCEPTS OF VERBAL COMMUNICATION

In Chapter 15, we described **communication** as a complex process in which information is exchanged between two or more people. The sender and receiver of the message are unique individuals, with differing perceptions, beliefs, and interpretations of the world. Communication is effective when the message intended by the sender and the message perceived by the receiver are the same.

Communication is an essential part of human interactions, beginning at birth and continuing throughout a person's life. By sharing expressions of physical, social, and emotional needs with other people, we can fulfill those needs while establishing, nurturing, and maintaining relationships with other people. Communication is an important aspect of the nurse-client relationship.

Nurses encounter a variety of situations in which a client cannot communicate verbally. This situation commonly results from a brain injury or a cerebrovascular accident (stroke) that impairs the client's ability to understand or to express himself. Impaired communication also can result from anatomic alterations of the vocal structures or the placement of an artificial airway, such as an endotracheal tube or tracheostomy tube. Language barriers, developmental delays, and psychiatric illnesses can impair verbal communication as well. Failure to communicate is frustrating for all involved, especially the client.

Neurology of Verbal Communication

Verbal communication depends on an intact, healthy nervous system to form words and sentences and to interpret the meaning of spoken words. You can increase the effectiveness of your communication interventions by understanding the neurology of verbal communication.

Brain Centers

The parietal, occipital, and temporal lobes of the brain's dominant hemisphere are involved in the analysis, synthesis, and interpretation of somatic, visual, and auditory information and the processing of this information into coherent thoughts (Zemlin, 1998). In most people, the major speech-language and hearing areas of the brain are located in the left hemisphere (Fig. 44–1). Of these areas, Broca's area and

Wernicke's area are crucial to communication, each with its own function.

BROCA'S AREA

Located in the frontal lobe of the brain, **Broca's area** is the center of motor speech control. It is responsible for controlling the muscles of the mouth, tongue, and larynx. Muscle movements controlled and coordinated by this region are required for the production of speech (Zemlin, 1998).

WERNICKE'S AREA

Located in the temporal lobe of the brain, **Wernicke's area** helps control the content of speech and affects auditory and visual comprehension. Wernicke's area provides input to Broca's area by transmitting information via the arcuate fasciculus, a major association tract. It has an interpretive role in communication that is important for reading and auditory comprehension, spontaneous conversation, and the ability to process sensory information into coherent thoughts (Zemlin, 1998).

Cranial Nerves

Of the 12 cranial nerves, six (V, VII, IX, X, XI, and XII) are involved in speech production (Fig. 44–2). Cranial nerve V, the *trigeminal nerve,* controls the movements of the lower jaw and the tongue. The *facial nerve* (cranial nerve VII) innervates the muscles of the face (eyelids, cheeks, and lips) and affects facial expression.

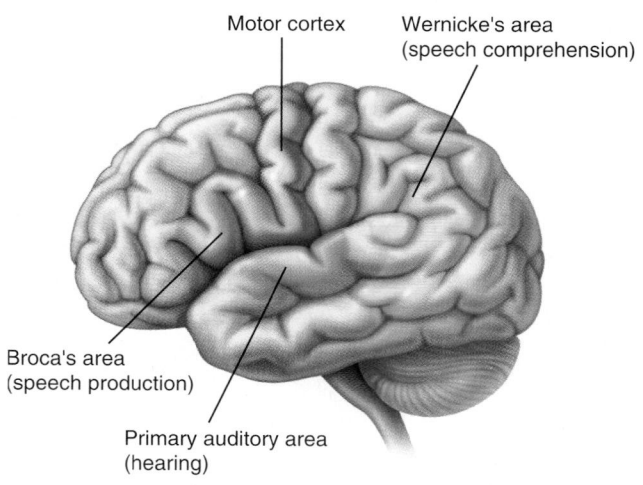

Figure 44–1. Major speech-language and hearing areas of the brain.

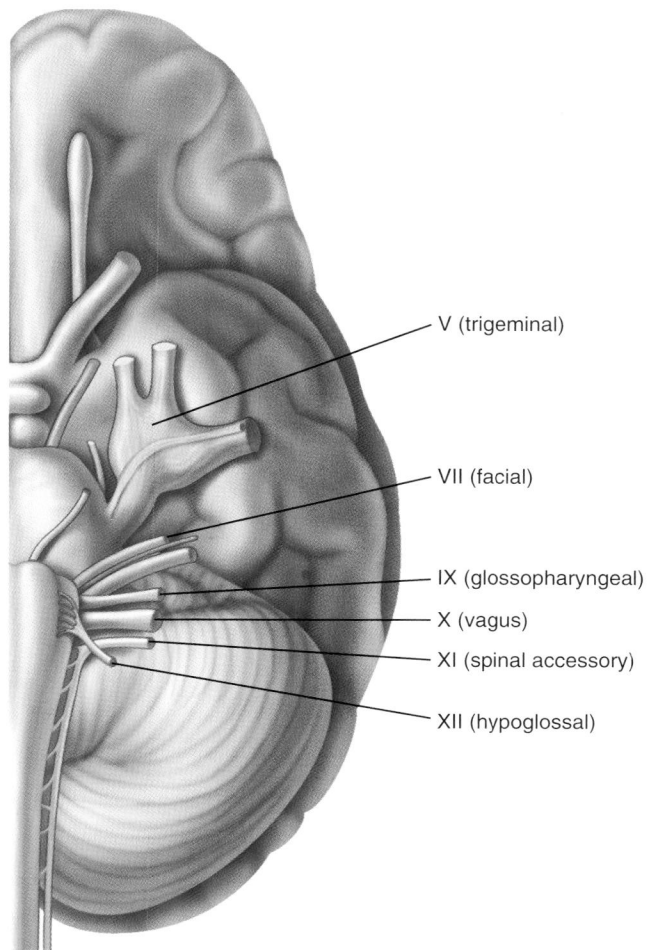

Figure 44–2. Cranial nerves involved in speech production.

V (trigeminal)

VII (facial)

IX (glossopharyngeal)

X (vagus)

XI (spinal accessory)

XII (hypoglossal)

Cranial nerve IX, the *glossopharyngeal nerve,* provides motor fibers to the pharynx and controls the movement of throat muscles. The recurrent laryngeal nerve, a branch of the *vagus nerve* (cranial nerve X), is important in speech because it stimulates the soft palate, pharynx, and larynx. If the motor portion of the vagus nerve becomes damaged, **dysphagia** (difficulty swallowing), **dysphonia** (difficulty producing vocal sounds), and **dysarthria** (impaired articulation) may result. Cranial nerve XI, the *spinal accessory nerve,* helps control the muscles of the pharynx (throat), the soft palate, and the head and shoulders. The *hypoglossal nerve* (cranial nerve XII) controls tongue movements, which are essential for **articulation,** the process of molding sounds into enunciated words and phrases. Damage to any of the cranial nerves may inhibit speech production (Hegde, 1995; Zemlin, 1998).

Sound Production in Verbal Communication

Production of speech begins with the production of sound by the lungs and larynx. The sound is modified into speech in the nasal, oral, and pharyngeal cavities through the process of articulation. These structures

also control the quality of sound by producing resonance. The structures of speech production are known as the vocal tract (Fig. 44–3).

Phonation

Phonation is the production of sound by the vibration of the vocal folds. A source of energy and a vibrating element are essential for sound production. The lower respiratory tract, especially the lung tissue, provides the primary source of energy for speech production. A smooth exhalation vibrates the vocal folds in the larynx. The vocal folds rapidly open and close to periodically interrupt the flow of air to produce vocal tone within the pharyngeal, oral, and nasal cavities (Zemlin, 1998). Thus, speech involves the intermittent release of expired air through opening and closing of the glottis, which houses the vocal folds.

The larynx functions as a sound generator or sound producer over a wide range of pitch and loudness. The intrinsic muscles of the larynx are responsible for ordinary speech production. The vocal folds, or vocal cords, are long, round bands of muscle tissue that may be lengthened or shortened, tensed or relaxed, and abducted or adducted to cause varying types of sound production (Zemlin, 1998). The length of the true vocal folds and the size of the glottis are altered by the action of the intrinsic laryngeal muscle, most of which moves the arytenoid cartilages. The arytenoid cartilages are two small cartilages (which appear to be pyramid-shaped when viewed from a posterior angle) that are capable of moving the vocal folds, which are attached to these cartilages.

Singers often describe phonation as voice registers. Registers are a series of notes with a particular quality or characteristic. They are described as high or low registers, or head or chest registers. The head register is the upper end of the scale. A stereotype of a head register is a person with a light and airy Irish brogue. The chest register is at the lower end of the scale. This is a voice that an actor or actress might to use give the voice carrying power to be heard at the back of the theater. The actor John Wayne is a classic example of the use of a chest register.

Head and chest registers are considered the normal range. Falsetto, a very high-pitched voice, is a voice register above the head register. At the other extreme, a depressed person's speech may be very low and slow.

Articulation

The vocal tract not only produces sound but refines it into intelligible speech in a process known as articulation. Movements of the vocal tract mold the sounds of speech produced by the larynx into enunciated words and phrases. Articulation is the selective modification of the voiced and unvoiced breath sounds by the tongue, teeth, and lips for the enunciation of words and sentences. It results from adjustments in the shape of the vocal tract that, in turn, change the acoustical

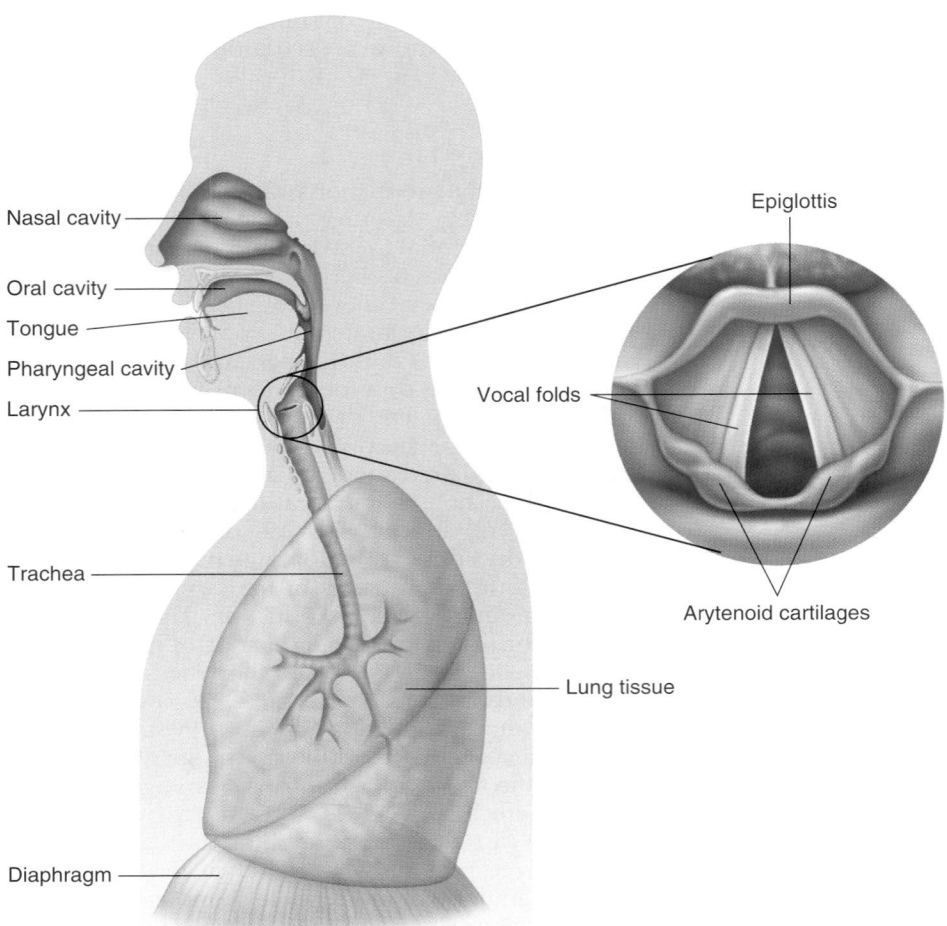

Figure 44–3. The structures of speech production (the vocal tract).

properties of the sounds. These structures are known as articulators (Zemlin, 1998).

In speaking, the muscles of the pharynx, tongue, soft palate, and lips are essential for enunciation of sounds into recognizable consonants and vowels for normal speech. Vowel sounds are initiated in the throat and are given their distinctive shapes by movements of the mouth and tongue. Consonants are formed by controlled interruptions of exhaled air.

Voice Quality

Resonance is the forced vibration of a structure that is related to a source of sound and results in changes in the quality of the sound. Although the vocal folds actually produce sounds, the quality of the voice depends on the coordinated activity of many other structures. The pharynx acts as a resonating chamber to amplify and enhance the quality of sound. The oral, nasal, and sinus cavities contribute to vocal resonance as well.

Nasality, a voice quality associated with resonance, occurs in the transmission pathway between the mouth cavity and the larynx. Nasality in the voice is

the coupling of nasal passages, the presence or absence of alternate or additional resonating nasal cavities, to the oral and pharyngeal cavities. Nasality may result from structural alterations, such as excessive adenoid tissue; pathophysiological alterations, such as damage to the brainstem or edema secondary to allergies; or an articulation problem associated with errors in articulation (Zemlin, 1998).

Vocal quality is affected by many other factors as well, such as mass, length, and tension of the vocal folds, as well as the degree of compression between the folds and the subglottal air pressure. Another factor is asymmetry of the folds. If one fold is thicker than the other, for example, they vibrate at different rates. The most common vocal qualities include breathiness, harshness, and hoarseness (Hegde, 1995).

When the vocal folds do not close completely, air leakage and friction result. The affected person will have a breathy voice. If the vocal folds do not close completely and there are irregular vibrations present at the same time, the vocal quality is known as hoarseness (Hegde, 1995). Assignment of these terms is based on individual perception and may vary from person to person.

Variety in Speech

Variety in speech refers to loudness, pitch, rate, and intonation. Variety makes verbal communication interesting and can either enhance or impede the clarity of communication.

LOUDNESS

Loudness of the voice depends on the force with which air rushes across the vocal folds. The greater the force, the stronger the vibration and the louder the sound. When a person whispers, the vocal folds do not move at all. In contrast, when a person yells, they vibrate vigorously.

PITCH

A person is able to produce laryngeal tones that can vary in range over about two octaves. Pitch is determined by changes in length and tension of the vocal folds. The more tense the vocal folds, the faster they vibrate and the higher the pitch. The glottis is wide open for deep tones and narrowed to a slit for high-pitched tones (Marieb, 1995).

Pitch varies between men and women, and it changes with age. Women have an average pitch level about one octave higher than men (Zemlin, 1998).

From birth to the onset of puberty, there is little apparent difference in pitch between boys and girls. During puberty, however, boys' vocals folds grow rapidly, while girls' vocal folds continue to grow at the same rate. This results in a lowering of the pitch by a full octave for boys (Zemlin, 1998).

RATE

Verbal communication is clear when the rate, or pace, matches the intended message. An unintended message may be conveyed if the rate is too rapid or too slow and deliberate. The rate or pace of speech may vary related to culture or geographical location.

INTONATION

Intonation, or the tone of the speaker's voice, can affect the meaning of the message. Intonation can express enthusiasm, concern, sadness, hostility, or indifference. To communicate most effectively, the message and voice tone should be congruent.

FACTORS AFFECTING VERBAL COMMUNICATION

Many factors can affect a person's ability to communicate verbally. They include lifestyle, developmental, physiological, and psychological factors.

Lifestyle Factors

Lifestyle factors can cause problems with the voice. Overuse of the voice, very dry air, bacterial infections, and inhalation of irritating chemicals can all cause laryngitis. Inflammation of the laryngeal tissues causes swelling and prevents the vocal folds from moving

---

Teaching for WELLNESS

CARE OF THE VOICE

Purpose: To prevent damage to the vocal folds.

Rationale: Most voice disorders result from vocal abuse, which can cause vocal nodules, polyps, traumatic laryngitis, vocal fold thickening, and contact ulcers. To control these disorders, the vocal abusive behaviors must be changed.

Expected Outcome: The client will establish appropriate vocal behaviors.

Client Instructions

- Do not shout.
- Stay away from noisy places.
- Relax muscle in neck and chest when you talk.
- Keep your throat moist.
- Do not smoke.
- Avoid smoke-filled, noisy, or dusty places.
- Do not drink excessive amounts of alcohol.
- Cough or sneeze as gently and softly as possible.
- Consult a speech-language pathologist about voice problem.

---

freely. Laryngitis results in hoarseness or the inability to speak above a whisper. Vocal abuse, as from cheerleading, smoking, and alcohol abuse, can lead to laryngeal cancer, which may result in loss of the vocal folds and the ability to communicate verbally. The Teaching for Wellness chart gives information about care of the voice.

Pharmacological agents, such as prescription drugs, alcohol, and illicit drugs, can interfere with communication because they inhibit or interfere with higher cortical functions. A person may experience slow, slurred speech as a result of impaired motor control of speech centers. Moderate to heavy use of drugs can cause loss of comprehension and expression by affecting the speech and motor centers of the brain. These effects may be temporary or permanent. The use of alcohol or crack cocaine by a pregnant woman may result in speech, language, voice, and fluency problems in her child.

Cultural Factors

The process of communication is universal, but the manner in which information is conveyed varies with different cultures. Nonverbal communication, such as facial expression, eye and head movement, body posture, touch, proximity, body posture, and use of silence may have different meaning to different cultures. In some cultures, head movement may mean the exact opposite of what it means in Western cultures. Elevation of an eyebrow indicates a "yes" response to Tongans, for example.

Verbal expression also varies between cultures. When a health care worker and client are of different cultures, barriers to communication can affect the client's experience and ultimately the client's health.

Action Alert!

Do not judge a client's competence by how well he uses or fails to use standard English grammar.

Socioeconomic Factors

Socioeconomic factors, such as gender and education, also affect the communication process. Even within the same cultural group, men and women communicate differently. For example, men may use language to exert influence and power, and to resist restrictions that have been imposed. Women, on the other hand, tend to use language in a relational manner to meet the needs of others and promote a sense of caring.

Communication may be difficult when people have different levels of education. A message will not be clear if the words or phrases are not part of the listener's vocabulary. Nurses communicate with clients and professionals with varying levels of education. Use of a common language is essential when communicating across varying levels of education.

Developmental Factors

At birth, most children have the physical capacity to develop speech and language. The rate of language development depends on the child's environment and may be hindered by problems in cognitive and neurological development. A stimulating environment aids language acquisition.

Remember that a child's ability to understand spoken words precedes the ability to use words. As speech development proceeds, children learn to use words correctly before they comprehend the full meaning of the words. You must understand the influence of language development and thought processes when communicating with children.

The older adult may have sensory changes in hearing and vision that affect verbal communication. Assessment of hearing and vision is especially important in communicating with the older adult.

Physiological Factors

At any age, the complicated process of language development can be disturbed by physiological factors such as illness, medications, surgery, and mechanical barriers, such as those that result from a tracheostomy.

For the developing child, disorders such as cerebral palsy, Down's syndrome, and autism have varied effects on the development of speech and language. Additionally, cleft lip and cleft palate are congenital disorders that affect speech and language development in children by preventing use of the tongue and mouth to correctly form words.

When a loss of hearing affects the child's speech and language acquisition, the child's ability to communicate will be affected. Indeed, a child who is born deaf or becomes deaf at an early age will fail to learn to speak in the usual way. The greater the loss of hearing, the more severe the impact on speech and language acquisition. Children quickly learn gestures, signs, and other modes of manual communication when hearing is impaired. Hearing loss in the adult usually does not affect speech and language, since the loss occurs after speech and language have been established.

Adult loss of language usually stems from neurological diseases. Damage to speech centers of the brain by cerebrovascular accident (stroke), multiple sclerosis, or Parkinson's disease may cause speech to be unintelligible, singsong, explosive, mechanical, or slurred. Older adults may experience progressive diseases of the nervous system.

Psychological Factors

Psychological factors that can affect a person's ability to communicate verbally include self-concept, stress, emotion, mood, and psychiatric illness.

Self-Concept

Self-concept plays a major role in communication patterns with other people. The way a person feels about himself is conveyed in his communication with others. If the person is confident and feels in control of his life, his communication will reflect this self-confidence. If the person has experienced a long series of negative interactions with other people, the person may have a negative view of the world that affects their effective communication.

Stress

Stress is part of everyday life. However, a person may communicate aggressive or defensive behaviors in response to stress, or a person may turn inward, withdraw, and become depressed. On the other hand, one way to effectively cope with a stressful event is to discuss it or communicate about it with a significant other or colleague.

Emotion and Mood

A person's emotions and mood influence the way he communicates with others and his ability to receive messages accurately. Emotions and mood can cause the message to be misinterpreted or to not be heard at all. If the person is depressed, anxious, sad, or lonely, he may not be willing to share feelings with other people.

ASSESSMENT

Assessment cues that indicate impaired verbal communication will arise as you collect baseline data during the history and physical assessment of a client. Because impaired verbal communication results from a variety of causes, the cues may be varied as well.

General Assessment of Verbal Communication

Communication skills should be assessed throughout the entire interview, health history, and physical examination. When obtaining the history and physical examination, assess the client's ability to respond to questions appropriately and communicate his needs clearly. Take note if he relies on a significant other to speak for him.

Health History

While obtaining the heath history, focus your questions to assess the client's ability to speak and comprehend the dominant language. If you see or hear cues that English is not the client's first language, the following questions may be used to elicit information about the client's verbal communication ability:

- What language is usually spoken in your home?
- How well do you speak, read, and write English?
- Is it important to observe any communication patterns in your family? (To whom should questions be directed?)
- Do you understand the meaning of common health terms?

If the client cannot speak or his speech is unintelligible, you may have to rely on his health record or an informant to obtain information about the client and his health problem. Ask how long the client has had the communication problem and whether its onset was associated with anything, such as medication use, illness, or other symptoms. Has the client tried anything to relieve the symptoms? Was it effective? Has his speech improved since the onset of the problem?

If the problem is long-term, ask whether the client has been seen by a physician or speech therapist for it. Determine whether he has received treatment for the problem. Does the client use any aids to assist speech?

The amount of information you solicit depends on whether you are evaluating the problem to establish communication with the client, to help manage another nursing problem, or to determine the best course of action to correct the problem. You may be interested primarily in determining the client's method of communication.

Physical Examination

If the client can speak, assess his speech to determine whether his communication problem is one of articu-

lation, comprehension, coherence, or voice quality. A normal voice should have inflections and sufficient volume with clear speech. Difficulty in articulation could involve thought processes or the functions of tongue and lips in forming words.

Listen for slurred speech, poorly coordinated or irregular speech, a monotone or weak voice, stuttering, whispering, and a nasal, rasping, or hoarse tone (Thompson & Wilson, 1996). Pay particular attention to tone, clarity, vocal strength, vocabulary, sentence structure, and pace. Note errors in word choice. These will give you cues to potential causes, which can facilitate diagnosis and intervention. For example, if the client's voice is hoarse or soft, it may indicate laryngitis, laryngeal cancer, or cranial nerve paralysis. A monotone voice may indicate deafness, depression, or a neurological problem. The client's vocabulary and word usage may offer clues to his level of education or a cultural or language barrier. Slow, garbled speech or hesitant, deliberate speech may indicate a neurological disorder.

The physical examination includes examination of body systems that may be related to the inability to communicate. For example, examine the client's mouth, nose, pharynx, and lungs to determine any physical cause of the impaired communication. The examination may include evaluation of the client's neurological status, hearing loss, and cognitive functioning as well.

Diagnostic Tests

Although no specific laboratory or diagnostic tests are available to assess speech or language disorders, the medical examination will include diagnostic tests aimed at detecting the underlying cause. The physician's neurological work-up may include a computed tomography scan to rule out brain tumors or lesions. Because of the potentially serious nature of the underlying causes, you have a role in providing supportive care to the client undergoing diagnosis.

Once the client's physical condition is stable, the physician may request a consult from a speech-language pathologist to assess the client's speech and language function and make recommendations to the health care team to facilitate communication. Assess the client's speech to plan appropriate interventions to facilitate communication.

Focused Assessment for Impaired Verbal Communication

Defining Characteristics

Having assessed the client's speech patterns and ability to communicate, you have already identified the defining characteristics. From the multiple factors associated with the diagnosis *Impaired verbal communication,* you can see that the defining characteristics can be grouped based on the underlying cause. Each of these groups requires further assessment.

- The client either speaks no English or speaks English as a second language.
- A child has a delay in the development of language or has developed speech problems.
- An adult or child has lost the use of language because of neurological damage.
- An adult or child has lost the ability for verbal communication secondary to medical illness or treatment (lacks the strength to speak, surgically altered vocal cords, presence of tracheostomy tube, and so on).
- The client can communicate verbally but lacks skills in communication, vocabulary, or knowledge.
- The client has psychotic thinking.

Related Factors

Impaired verbal communication may be related to a variety of factors. Related factors might include neurological injury, anatomic alterations, psychological barriers, developmental problems, or cultural differences. The related factor determines the appropriate nursing interventions.

NEUROLOGICAL INJURY

Injury to brain cells may be related to a variety of neurological conditions, such as a cerebrovascular accident (stroke); rupture of an aneurysm (weakening of an arterial wall); an arteriovenous malformation (congenital defect resulting in a tuft of arteries and veins) in the brain; or brain tumor (malignant or benign). Head trauma may also result in injury to the speech centers in the brain. Blood clots located in other parts of the body (such as the heart or lungs) may dislodge, travel to the brain, and injure brain cells by blocking their blood supply.

Depending on the area of the ischemic injury to the brain, the client may present with impaired verbal communication. He may be able to understand what is said but be unable to express himself, or he may not understand what is said. His speech may be inappropriate and meaningless. Such a client may easily become frustrated and withdrawn.

APHASIA

Aphasia is a language disorder that results from brain damage or disease that involves speech centers in the brain. It causes a variety of difficulties in formulating, expressing, and understanding language. Aphasia is classified according to the speech area affected. Assessment guidelines for aphasia are presented in Table 44–1. Paraphasia, neologism, or both may be present. **Paraphasia** is a word substitution problem of the aphasic client who speaks fluently. **Neologism** is the creation of words that are meaningless to the listener and is a common language problem of the aphasic client.

BROCA'S (EXPRESSIVE) APHASIA. Damage to the motor association area of the brain results in Broca's aphasia, also called expressive aphasia. The resulting communication problems may include difficulty with oral expression, especially spontaneous conversation. Speech is slow and monotonous, with short phrases or telegraphic speech. *Telegraphic speech* is telegram-like speech that lacks grammatical elements, such as articles, prepositions, and conjunctions. "Mommy come" for "Mommy is coming" is an example of telegraphic speech. Words may be composed of inappropriate sounds and have inappropriate meaning.

Written deficits usually parallel speech deficits. Clients with Broca's aphasia usually have weakness of the face. They may also have paresis of the right arm because damage may extend into adjacent motor areas of the brain responsible for upper extremity movement on the opposite side of the body.

People with Broca's aphasia typically retain their comprehension of written and spoken language. Usually, the affected client is aware of the deficit in his communication ability—an awareness that can lead to frustration and depression.

WERNICKE'S (RECEPTIVE) APHASIA. Damage in the auditory associations of the brain results in impaired auditory comprehension known as Wernicke's aphasia or receptive aphasia. The client speaks fluently but uses neologisms or made-up words. Paraphasias or word substitutions may be used, such as *spoot* for *spoon*. Often, the client is unaware of the deficit and may become annoyed with other people who, as far as the client knows, should be able to understand what he says. Written deficits parallel the speech deficits. The client may write many words, but they make little or no sense.

GLOBAL APHASIA. Global aphasia is the most severe form of aphasia and results from extensive damage to the dominant hemisphere (both Broca's and Wernicke's areas). Global aphasia results in both expressive and receptive aphasia. The client cannot comprehend spoken language or articulate or write words. Table 44–2 compares the different types of aphasia.

DYSARTHRIA

Dysarthria is a speech articulation problem. It results from trauma or neuromuscular disease that impairs neuromuscular control of the muscles of the face, oral cavity, and larynx. The client may have trouble manipulating his tongue, lips, soft palate, jaw, and vocal folds. You may detect this problem as slurred, labored, sluggish, weak, or hypernasal speech. The client may also have trouble chewing and swallowing. He may drool. His comprehension of language and his ability to select words and form sentences are not affected.

DYSPHONIA (APHONIA)

Dysphonia, also known as aphonia, is a disorder of voice volume, quality, or pitch. The client may be hoarse or speak in a whisper. It results from damage or disease involving the larynx or the vagus nerve (cranial nerve X). Examples include laryngitis, laryngeal tumors, and unilateral vocal cord paralysis. Voice articulation and language are unimpaired.

TABLE 44–1
Assessment Guidelines for Aphasia

Assessment Area	Assessment Steps	Rationale
Word comprehension	Ask the person to point to objects in the room or to body parts as you name them. Ask a series of questions that can be answered with "yes" or "no" or with an appropriate head movement, such as, "Are you sitting on a chair?"	Word comprehension is impaired in some but not all kinds of aphasia. Deficiencies in vision, hearing, and intellectual capacity may also affect performance.
Repetition	Ask the person to repeat items of increasing length and complexity, from monosyllabic words to sentences. Note the fluency and accuracy of the response.	Repetition is impaired in some but not all kinds of aphasia.
Naming	Ask the person to repeat items of increasing length and complexity, from monosyllabic words to sentences. Gradually increase the difficulty—from "hat" and "red" to "belt buckle" and "purple," for example. Note the fluency and accuracy of the response.	Naming is impaired in some but not all kinds of aphasia.
Reading comprehension	Write several simple commands, each on a separate piece of paper in large clear print, such as CLOSE YOUR EYES and RAISE YOUR HAND.	Failure in reading comprehension often accompanies failure in word comprehension, but each may occur independently. Keep in mind that a person's previous reading ability and educational experience affect performance.
Writing	Ask the person to make up and write a sentence about a topic, such as the room, the person's job, or his family. Note whether the sentence makes sense, has a subject and verb, and contains correctly spelled words.	Writing, like speech, is affected by some forms of aphasia. Motor impairment, such as hemiplegia, may affect performance.

Adapted from Bates, B. (1995). Physical examination and history taking (6th ed.) Philadelphia: J.B. Lippincott Co.

TABLE 44–2
Comparison of Broca's, Wernicke's, and Global Aphasia

	Broca's (Expressive) Aphasia	Wernicke's (Receptive) Aphasia	Global Aphasia
Qualities of Spontaneous Speech	• Not fluent. • Slow. The client uses few words and expends great effort to speak. • Inflection and articulation are impaired, but words are meaningful, with nouns, transitive verbs, and important adjectives. Small grammatical words are often dropped.	• Fluent, often rapid, voluble and effortless. • Inflection and articulation are good, but sentences lack meaning and words are malformed (paraphasias) or invented (neologisms). • Speech may be incomprehensible.	• Nonfluent.
Comprehension	• Fairly good.	• Impaired.	• Impaired.
Repetition	• Impaired (struggles to speak).	• Impaired due to paraphasia (e.g., saying *pink* for *sink*)	• Impaired.
Naming	• Impaired, although the client recognizes objects.	• Impaired.	• Impaired.
Oral Reading and Reading Comprehension	• Good to poor.	• Severely impaired.	• Severely impaired.
Writing	• Paucity of written output.	• Severely impaired; meaningless writing.	• Severely impaired.

Adapted from Bates, B. (1995). A guide to physical examination and history taking (6th ed.). Philadelphia: J.B. Lippincott Co.; and adapted by permission from Snyder, M. (1991). A guide to neurological and neurosurgical nursing, (2nd ed.). Albany, NY: Delmar Publishers.

TABLE 44-3
Development of Language

Age, Months	Receptive Language	Expressive Language
0–3	• Attends to voice. • Turns head or eyes. • Startles to loud sounds. • Quiets in response to voice.	• Has undifferentiated but strong cry. • Coos and gurgles. • Uses single-syllable repetition. • *g, k, h,* and *ng* appear.
3–6	• Smiles, coos, gurgles to voice. • Actively seeks sound source. • May look in response to name.	• Engages in vocal play. • Laughs. • Repetitive babbling *(gaga)* increases. • Vocalizes to removal of toys.
6–9	• May look at family member when named. • Inhibits to "no." • Begins to take interest in pictures when named. • Individual words begin to take on meaning.	• Babbles tunefully. • Sound combination increase. • Uses *m, n, b, d, t.* • Initiates sounds, such as click or kiss. • Uses nonspecific "mama," "dada."
9–12	• Will give toy on request. • Understands simple commands. • Turns head to own name. • Understands expressions such as "hot," "where is . . . ?" • Responds with gestures to "bye-bye."	• Imitating efforts increase. • Has one word with specific reference. • Accompanies vocalizations with gestures. • Jargon increases. • Imitates animal sounds.
12–18	• Follows simple one-step commands. • Understands new words weekly. • Shows increased interest in named pictures. • Differentiates environmental sounds. • Points to familiar objects and body parts when named. • Understands simple questions. • Begins to distinguish "you" from "me."	• All vowels, many consonants present. • Use of true words increases. • Jargon is sentence-like. • Names a few pictures. • Knows 10+ words. • Can imitate nonspeech sounds (cough, tongue click).

Material from D. Anderson, Ph.D., Speech Pathologist, Portland, OR, using items from a variety of developmental tests; and from Burns, C.E., Barber, N., Brady, M.A., & Dunn, A.M. (1996). Pediatric primary care: A handbook for nurse practitioners. Philadelphia: W.B. Saunders Co.

ANATOMICAL ALTERATIONS

Physical barriers—such as an endotracheal tube, tracheostomy, or tumor—commonly impair verbal communication. An endotracheal tube is a temporary physical barrier to communication used to maintain a patent airway or for alteration in breathing patterns (see Chapter 39). A tracheostomy is a temporary or permanent upper-airway diversion that results in altered speech production. A temporary tracheostomy is a surgical procedure performed to maintain a patent airway for a short period of time. A tracheostomy tube is inserted via a surgical incision into the trachea and secured.

A client who has a *total laryngectomy,* which is the surgical removal of the larynx performed primarily for laryngeal cancer, will require a permanent tracheostomy. The upper airway is diverted and separated from the pharynx and esophagus, and the trachea is brought out through the skin in the neck and sutured in place, creating a permanent stoma (opening). The client has a permanent alteration in speech production.

Action Alert!
Establish an alternate means of communication before the client receives a tracheostomy.

A client with a new tracheostomy (temporary or permanent) will not be able to communicate his needs verbally and may use hand or facial gestures as a means to communicate. This client may become anxious or frustrated by his inability to communicate, and he may become depressed and withdraw from social interactions.

PSYCHOLOGICAL ILLNESSES

A client with a psychiatric disorder may have trouble communicating with other people. During your assessment, you may notice that he has loose associations or flights of ideas that make communication difficult. He may not be able to find the right words, identify objects, name words, or speak in sentences. He may stutter or slur his words.

Clients with psychological barriers to communication may have a history of drug and alcohol abuse and

TABLE 44–3
Development of Language *(continued)*

Age, Months	Receptive Language	Expressive Language
18–24	• Follows two-step commands. • Vocabulary increases rapidly. • Enjoys simple stories. • Recognizes pronouns.	• Names some body parts. • Imitates two-word combinations. • Shows dramatic increase in vocabulary. • Speech combines jargon and words. • Names self. • Answers some questions. • Begins to combine words.
30–36	• Listens to adult conversations. • Understands preposition "under." • Can categorize items by function. • Begins to recognize colors. • Begins to take turns. • Understands contrasts such as, "big/little," "boy/girl."	• Can repeat simple phrases and sentences. • Answers questions ("wear on feet," "to bed"). • Repeats three digits. • Uses regular plurals. • Can help tell simple story.
36–42	• Understands quickly. • Understands prepositions "behind" and "in front." • Responds to simple three-part commands. • Understanding of adjectives and plurals increases. • Understands "just one."	• Understands and answers (cold, tired, hungry). • Uses mostly three- to four-word sentences. • Gives full name. • Begins rote counting. • Begins to relate events. • Asks lots of questions, some beginning prepositions ("on," "in").
42–48	• Recognizes coins. • Begins to understand future and past tenses. • Understands number concepts, such as "more than one."	• Uses prepositions. • Tells stories. • Can give function of objects. • Repeats sentences of six words and longer. • Repeats four digits. • Gives age. • Good intelligibility.
46–60	• Respond to three-action commands.	• Asks "how" questions, such as "How are you?" • Uses past and future tenses. • Can use conjunctions to string words and phrases together.

present in an alcohol-intoxicated or in a drug-overdose state. Other causes of psychiatric barriers to communication might include bipolar disorder, psychosis, or anxiety states.

DEVELOPMENTAL FACTORS

The routine well-child examination should include assessment for the development of speech and language problems. Language problems in children can be caused by cognitive, environmental, family, or cultural factors. Proper speech patterns and language are best learned in an environment rich in the use of language. Slow cognitive development is associated with language disorders. Speaking a foreign language in the home and the dominant language at school can interfere with learning both languages.

Speech disorders are also associated with physical problems, such as hearing deficits, cleft lip, cleft palate, cerebral palsy, or such psychological disorders as severe deprivation or autism. Speech problems can be idiopathic. Table 44–3 illustrates the development of language in children to help you assess a client's developmental status.

CULTURAL DIFFERENCES/LANGUAGE BARRIERS

You almost certainly will encounter clients from cultures different than your own and who speak languages different than yours. A language barrier may occur when you and the client do not speak the same language. You and the client are both fluent in your own language, but you cannot understand each other. The Cross-Cultural Care chart offers strategies for overcoming such a barrier while remaining sensitive to the client's cultural values.

When either you or the client can speak the other person's language, but not fluently, one of the risks is that you may think you understand each other when, in fact, you do not. This problem could cause you and the client to misunderstand each other over possibly crucial information.

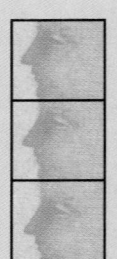

CROSS-CULTURAL CARE
CARING FOR A MEXICAN-AMERICAN CLIENT AND HIS FAMILY

Señor Martinez and his wife, the client whose story we have been following, are Mexican-Americans. They immigrated to the United States and settled in the Western part of Kansas where other Mexican-American families have found work in beef-packing plants. Mexican-Americans tend to be a close-knit, family-oriented group. Sr. Martinez and his wife live in a small house with their extended family. They speak primarily Spanish, as do most of their friends and neighbors. The Mexican-American culture is primarily Roman Catholic in its religious beliefs. This is evident in the religious items in Sr. Martinez's room. Andrews and Boyle (1995) have identified values that are important to the Mexican-American client and his family.

- Close-knit family relationships exist, in which the father is the head of the house. Other family members are subordinate to him.
- Social activities revolve around family activities.
- The primary language is Spanish.
- Touch is a common expression among members of the same sex.
- Privacy and confidentiality are valued.
- Religious practices and rituals are maintained during illness, death, or dying.
- Life events are viewed as the "will of God."
- Illness may be viewed as punishment from God.
- Folk medicine may be used.

Jane, Sr. Martinez's nurse, and the interpreter enter the room. Jane initiates teaching regarding tuberculosis. See how she shows sensitivity to Sr. Martinez's cultural values.

Jane: Good morning, Señor and Señora Martinez. This is Dominique, an interpreter. How are you this morning?

Sr. Martinez: I am fine.

Jane: I would like to talk to you about this illness you have—tuberculosis.

Sr. Martinez: Well, I know why I got sick. It is God's punishment for some bad things I did.

Jane: You believe this illness is a punishment?

Sr. Martinez: Probably.

Jane: Señor Martinez, I understand tuberculosis to be a respiratory illness caused by bacteria. Unfortunately, that means it can be passed to other people by coughing. People in close contact to with you have been exposed to this disease. Señora Martinez, this means that you and the other members of your family may have tuberculosis too. We will need to test all the members of your family. Señora Martinez, who are the other people that live in your home? *[Jane notices that Sra. Martinez looks at her husband and nods her head.]*

Sr. Martinez: We have five children living with us.

Jane: Are there any other people living in your home?

Sr. Martinez: Yes. Both of our parents and my brother and his family also live with us. They have three children.

Jane: You will all need to go to the county health department to be tested for tuberculosis. Does your family have a way to get to the Health Department?

Critical Thinking Questions

- Why does Jane inquire about the family members living in the home?
- Why might Sr. Martinez's wife defer to her husband to answer the questions?
- How does Jane respect Sr. Martinez and his wife's confidentiality and privacy?
- Did Sr. Martinez demonstrate any characteristic cultural values?

Reference

Andrews, M.M. & Boyle, J.S. (1995). *Transcultural concepts in nursing* (2nd ed). Philadelphia: J.B. Lippincott Co.

Recall the case study about Señor Martinez and his wife introduced at the beginning of the chapter. Neither Juan nor his wife is fluent in English. The nurse is concerned about their ability to understand information regarding the treatment of tuberculosis. There is a great risk for misunderstanding and lack of compliance with the health care regimen.

The client who does not speak the dominant language of the health care delivery system, or does not speak it fluently, may be anxious or become frustrated as he tries to communicate his needs to members of the health care team. The client may give responses that he thinks you want to hear. In other words, he may express the values he perceives you to have rather than his own values and beliefs. To help detect language and cultural barriers during your assessment, watch carefully for incongruities. For example, you may notice inconsistencies between verbal and nonverbal communication; the client may nod his head in agreement while his eyes reflect questioning.

Action Alert!
The risk for misunderstanding is great when the client and the nurse speak each other's languages somewhat, but not fluently. The client's level of understanding about his condition and care must be assessed carefully.

Language differences are not the only communication difficulties for the client and the nurse but also the differences in cultural expression. Cultural expression includes the nonverbal mannerisms, values, beliefs, and customs.

Focused Assessment for Related Nursing Diagnoses

Anxiety

Anxiety is a common response to an impaired ability to communicate, no matter what the cause. When a client has been able to communicate freely, the sudden loss of that ability is frightening. An alternative method to communicate must be developed to lessen the client's anxiety.

When Juan Martinez arrives on the unit, he is placed on respiratory isolation precautions. He and his wife do not understand the reason for wearing the mask in Juan's room. They become anxious, fearing something terrible has happened to Juan.

Powerlessness

Observe for the client's response to lack of control over his environment and attempts to gain control by non-verbal means. Powerlessness is not an unusual feeling for a client with *Impaired verbal communication* related to a cerebrovascular accident, a language or cultural barrier, or a tracheostomy. Refusing to eat, to cooperate with care, and to make eye contact are strategies that clients sometimes use to try to gain control in situations in which they feel powerless.

Self-Esteem Disturbance

The client with *Impaired verbal communication* related to aphasia, a tracheostomy, or a language or cultural barrier may also have *Self-esteem disturbance*. Observe the client for direct or indirect expressions of negative feelings about himself or his capabilities.

Impaired Social Interaction

Assess the client's ability to maintain social interaction. The client may become frustrated and embarrassed about his poor communication skills and decrease social interactions with his family and friends. Also assess the degree to which family and friends have the skills to maintain interactions with the client. Friends may feel uncomfortable initiating interactions and may be frustrated by their inability to communicate effectively or help the impaired person. Friends may withdraw and decrease their social interaction with the client and his significant other.

Altered Role Performance

Assess the client's ability to maintain his usual roles. This includes assessment of the degree to which the spouse or significant other is obliged to take over the client's usual roles and how that change affects the ability of the family unit to function.

DIAGNOSIS

When obtaining the client's history, assess risk factors for impaired communication and the presence of diagnostic cues that would indicate an impaired verbal communication. See the Decision Tree for making a communication nursing diagnosis.

Clients may present with other nursing diagnoses that are related to the effects of impaired communication. The client who is unable to express himself may become depressed and withdraw from social interactions. The focus of care for this client would center on the nursing diagnosis of *Impaired social interaction*. For the client with a new laryngectomy, *Anxiety* or *Powerlessness related to an inability to communicate needs* may be a concern, and the nursing care would be directed toward these diagnoses. You must be alert to diagnostic cues to accurately diagnose the situation and plan the client's care based on these assessment findings. The accompanying chart provides examples of clustering data to make appropriate nursing diagnoses.

PLANNING

After you have identified appropriate nursing diagnoses and related factors, you and the client can make a plan of care that includes short-term and long-term goals for the client with impaired verbal communication. Short-term goals include establishing an effective communication plan to meet the client's basic needs. Long-term goals include helping the client live with impaired communication or engage in speech therapy to learn to speak.

The causes of impaired communication are varied, so you will need to write expected outcomes to meet the specific needs of each client. The expected outcomes for the client with impaired communication related to injury to brain cells will depend on the client's unique deficits. An appropriate goal might be a return of speech and language to a functional level.

The client with an anatomic alteration, such as a tracheostomy or endotracheal tube, needs to learn alternative methods to communicate. This could be either a temporary or a permanent means of communication.

For a language barrier, the goal might be that the client communicates his needs through an interpreter. If the communication impairment is related to a cultural barrier, the expected outcome would be that the client expresses health beliefs and cultural practices important to him.

Other expected outcomes appropriate for impaired communication might include the following:

- Family members and friends learn techniques to promote communication.
- The client communicates needs effectively with minimum frustration.

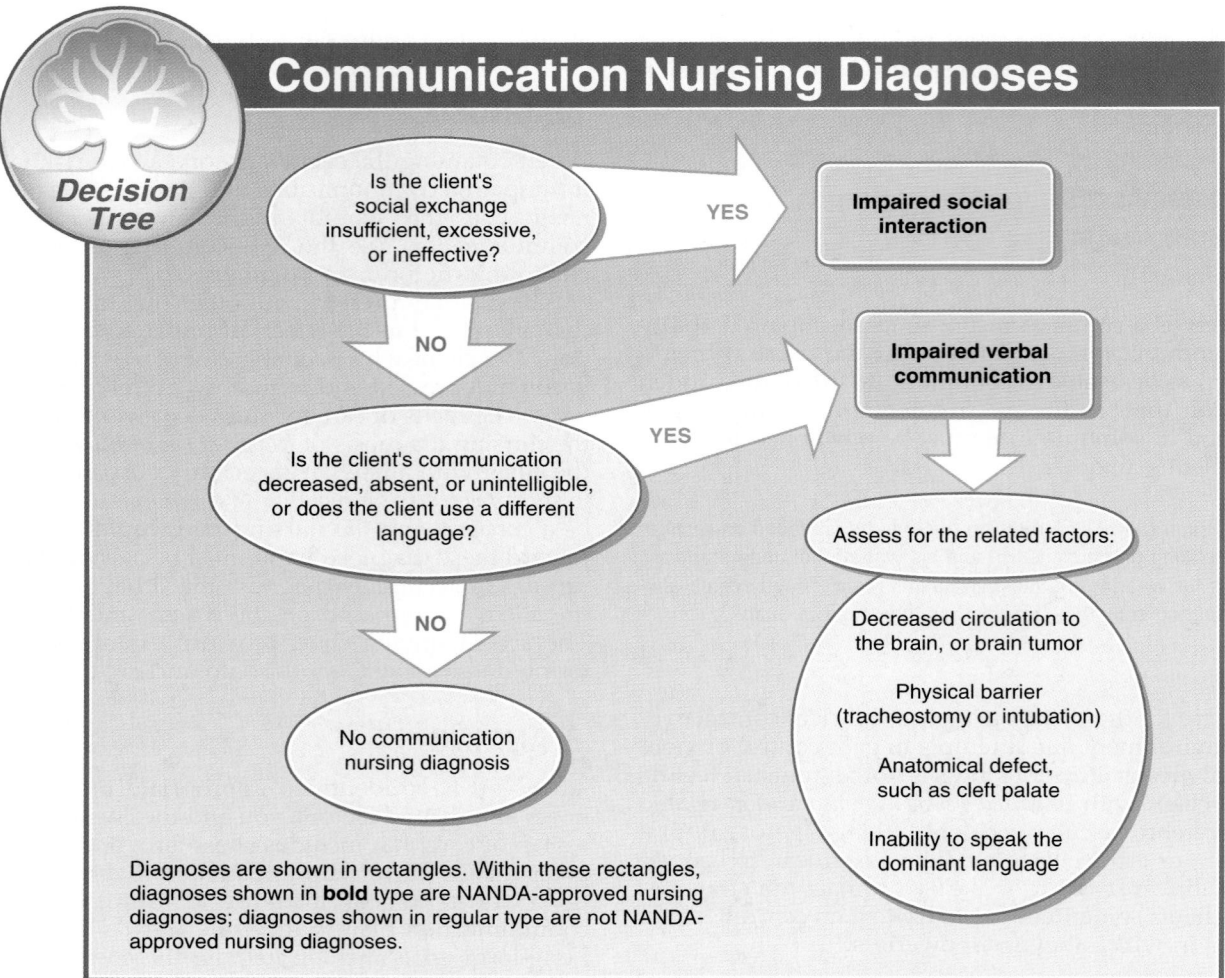

Communication Nursing Diagnoses

Decision Tree

Is the client's social exchange insufficient, excessive, or ineffective?

YES → **Impaired social interaction**

NO ↓

Is the client's communication decreased, absent, or unintelligible, or does the client use a different language?

YES → **Impaired verbal communication**

NO ↓

No communication nursing diagnosis

↓ (from Impaired verbal communication)

Assess for the related factors:

Decreased circulation to the brain, or brain tumor

Physical barrier (tracheostomy or intubation)

Anatomical defect, such as cleft palate

Inability to speak the dominant language

Diagnoses are shown in rectangles. Within these rectangles, diagnoses shown in **bold** type are NANDA-approved nursing diagnoses; diagnoses shown in regular type are not NANDA-approved nursing diagnoses.

- The client demonstrates effective use of adaptive equipment.
- The client uses appropriate resources to facilitate learning alternative forms of communication.
- The client uses alternative forms of communication.
- The client explains the relationship of causative factors, such as alcohol, to his inability to communicate.
- The client uses self-help groups and other resources to help with a psychological disorder.
- The client consistently communicates ideas to staff and family.
- The client comprehends written and verbal language.
- The client responds to verbal and auditory stimuli.
- The client uses available resources to help facilitate speech and language abilities.
- The client and his family or significant other can communicate at a satisfactory level.

INTERVENTION

Interventions for *Impaired verbal communication* will be directed to improve verbal communication and assist in resolution of the related nursing diagnosis. The following section describes some general guidelines for intervention in an area that typically requires specialized knowledge and skills.

Interventions to Promote Verbal Communication

Intervening to promote verbal communication will require an individual approach, depending on the cause of the impairment. To intervene appropriately, you will work both independently and interdependently.

Using a Team Approach

A team approach is often necessary for impaired verbal communication. Members of the team might include a speech-language pathologist, interpreter, psychiatric clinical nurse specialist, occupational therapist, physician, psychiatrist, and nurse, depending on the cause of the client's impairment.

If the client has sustained an injury to brain cells or a permanent anatomic alteration, he will need a team approach that involves a speech-language pathologist,

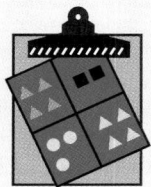

CLUSTERING DATA TO MAKE A NURSING DIAGNOSIS
IMPAIRED VERBAL COMMUNICATION

Data Cluster	Diagnosis
A 52-year-old male is first day postoperative with a new laryngectomy. His call light is on frequently. When the nurse answers, he says he doesn't need anything.	Anxiety related to inability to communicate needs.
A 66-year-old female with a new stroke has expressive aphasia. She understands what people are saying but her responses are garbled. She now lies in bed with her head turned away from the door. She has stopped trying to communicate, and, when someone tries to communicate with her, she turns her head or closes her eyes.	Impaired social interaction related to inability to respond understandably.
A Russian male is admitted following a motor vehicle accident. He speaks no English and has no relatives living nearby. None of the nurses speak Russian. His attempts to communicate are unsuccessful and he becomes frustrated.	Powerlessness related to an inability to communicate needs.
A 78-year-old male with Alzheimer's disease has trouble finding the right words when talking. He also has trouble recognizing everyday objects.	Impaired memory related to the effects of Alzheimer's disease.
A client with a history of chronic obstructive pulmonary disease is admitted in respiratory distress, which results in intubation and mechanical ventilation. The client attempts to speak to the nurse but is unable to communicate his needs.	Impaired verbal communication related to anatomical barriers.

physician, and nurse. Typically, the speech-language pathologist diagnoses the specific communication disorder. Together, the team will then develop a plan of care to help the client communicate. The speech-language pathologist helps the client relearn effective communication patterns and provides guidance and direction to the team for promoting speech and language communication.

Even though the speech-language pathologist works with the client on a daily basis you and other nurses will be with the client for extended periods of time and are responsible for his continuity of care. Always follow the speech-language pathologist's instructions when interacting with the client. Also, teach the family and significant other the recommended communication techniques to provide continuity of care.

A team approach is also used for clients with *Impaired verbal communication related to psychological and cultural barriers.* If the communication disorder is related to a cultural barrier, an interpreter may be a part of the team. For a psychological communication disorder, a psychiatrist or psychiatric clinical nurse specialist may be part of the team, as well as occupational

therapist. The nurse is responsible for coordination and ensuring that the plan is implemented and evaluated.

Sr. Martinez's nurse consults an interpreter who speaks Spanish. The interpreter facilitates communication between the client and the nurse. The nurse directs her questions to Sr. Martinez and his wife instead of to the interpreter. Through the use of the interpreter, a plan of care is developed for the client and his family. What factors would you consider in selecting a Spanish-speaking interpreter for Sr. Martinez and his family?

Providing a Supportive Atmosphere

Provide a supportive atmosphere to encourage the client to verbalize. Be aware of your verbal, *paraverbal,* and nonverbal language. *Paraverbal communication* refers to the manner in which a person speaks and includes voice tone, pitch, intonation, and body language. It is important to treat the client as an adult and not as a child or someone with poor intelligence. Assume the client can understand. Do not talk about the client in his presence. Encourage client verbalization by praising and acknowledging the client's successes.

This will help motivate the client to continue efforts at communicating.

A*ction* A*lert!*
Avoid talking down to clients with aphasia.

Listening Actively

Active listening focuses on the feelings of the person speaking as well as the nonverbal cues. As an active listener, take time to listen and focus total attention on what the client is saying. Pay attention, and keep your mind from wondering. Sit down, face the client, and maintain eye contact. Listen without making judgments. These behaviors facilitate the development of trust between the client and the nurse.

When listening, it is important to notice incongruities between the verbal, nonverbal, and paraverbal communication. For example, if the client says, "Oh, I'm fine!" but his face is tense and hands are clenched, there is incongruity between behavior and the spoken word that requires further assessment.

A*ction* A*lert!*
Listen actively; seek ways to verify that you have accurately interpreted the communication.

Helping the Client Practice Speech

Interventions to help the client practice speech will be related to the cause of the client's impaired verbal communication. A caring, gentle approach may help the client keep trying.

BROCA'S (EXPRESSIVE) APHASIA

The client with Broca's aphasia has difficulty expressing himself, and your interventions will aim to improve his speech. Delay communication when the client is tired or frustrated. In the beginning, to decrease anxiety, ask only questions that require a "yes" or "no" answer or a movement of the head.

One method of improving speech is through repeated practice of verbalization. Encourage the client to speak by use of automatic speech or imitation speech. Ask the client to say prayers or engage in social conversation, such as "Hello," "How are you?" and "I am fine."

Speech may also be facilitated by the use of special techniques, such as self-talk, parallel talk, expansion talk, and cueing. Self-talk involves talking about the activity as it is performed. Parallel talk is similar to self-talk and involves describing the activity the client is doing with you. Both self-talk and parallel-talk facilitate association of specific words with the activity.

Expansion talk is a technique that increases the complexity of verbalization by adding to the statement. However, it requires you to seek validation that you have correctly expanded the client's statement. Cueing is a technique to help the client verbalize words. Cueing may be done in several ways, such as pronouncing the first syllable of the word, showing a printed version of the word, or presenting sentence completion tasks to fill in the missing word (Dittmar, 1989). "Cue cards" are often used, and repetition greatly improves communication.

Simplifying communication while at the same time providing adequate stimulation will facilitate verbal expression. Introduce ideas one at a time using short sentences that contain simple, common words. Limit choices. Speak slowly but naturally.

Depending on the location and severity of the injury, clients with Broca's aphasia can sometimes communicate in writing. Assess the client's ability to do so.

A*ction* A*lert!*
Allow ample time for the client to respond. Do not respond for the client if the client has the ability to respond. This will increase the client's self-esteem and decrease frustration.

WERNICKE'S (RECEPTIVE) APHASIA

The client with receptive aphasia will have difficulty interpreting auditory, somatic, and visual input, which results in faulty interpretation of stimuli. Speech may be intact but inappropriate. The client may be confused and frustrated. To intervene, control the environment and limit sensory stimuli when communicating. Reducing distractions will improve comprehension.

A*ction* A*lert!*
Limiting environmental stimuli and reducing distractions may increase comprehension in the client with receptive aphasia.

Also, limit your use of adjectives, adverbs, and prepositions to increase the clarity of communication. Assess the client for clues that indicate his understanding. Reinforce appropriate responses. Alternative forms of communication—such as gestures, pictures, and communication boards—may be useful tools for some clients. A communication board allows the client to point to a picture to communicate his needs.

DYSARTHRIA

The client with dysarthria may have difficulty with speech articulation. You will need to collaborate with the speech-language pathologist to develop an effective method of communication. Many factors can affect the client's communication, such as fatigue and the rate of the conversation. If the client speaks too quickly, encourage him to slow down and use shorter phrases or single words. Ask him to repeat or rephrase what you cannot understand. Listen attentively and provide visual or verbal feedback that indicates your comprehension of the client's communication. Encourage the client to use gestures to increase comprehension.

LANGUAGE/CULTURAL BARRIERS

A speech-language pathologist can help the client to learn accent modification if his primary language is not the dominant language. This helps modify speech sounds and melodic differences that affect his intelligibility.

Developing a Communication Plan

Collaborate with family and other members of the health care team to develop a communication plan. Experiment with different methods of communication to determine which is most effective. Share the plan with the client, family, and other members of the health care team to provide continuity of care.

In communicating with clients of varying educational levels, it is important to use a common language. Assess client's knowledge by noting his response to questions, his ability to discuss health problems, and his questions. Use words and phrases congruent with his educational level to promote interest, attention, and understanding.

Providing Alternative Forms of Communication

It may be necessary to find an alternative form of communication. For example, you might teach the client to blink, nod, or tap an appropriate response to a "yes" or "no" question. Phrase questions so they can be answered with a yes or no. Consider using an assistive device, such as an alphabet board, picture board, magic slate, computerized communication device, or communication board (Fig. 44–4). However, these assistive devices may not be appropriate for a person with neuromuscular disease or with weakened or paralyzed arms. Encourage the use of gestures or pantomime.

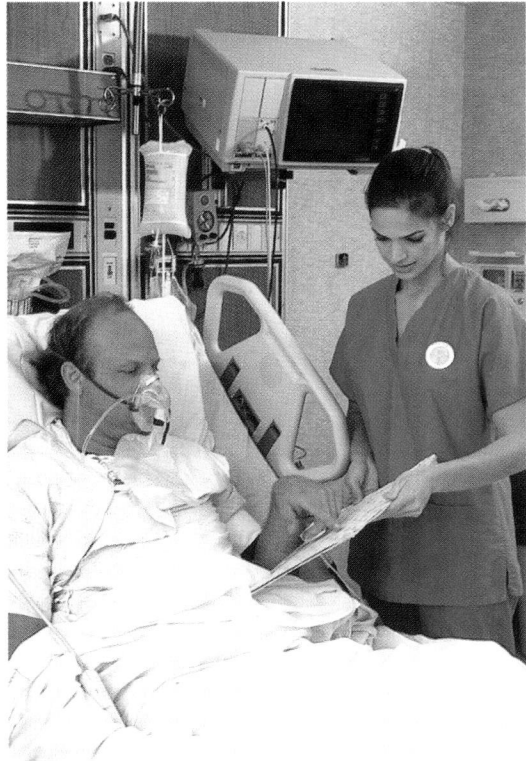

Figure 44–4. A nurse and speech-impaired client using a communication board. The client points to the picture that illustrates his need.

Before a client receives a tracheostomy, explain to the client and significant other that he will not be able to speak after surgery. Develop with the client and significant other an alternate method of communication to lessen their anxiety. Again, alternate forms of communication might include a magic slate, alphabet board, picture board, or pencil and paper. Demonstrate the chosen techniques to the client and significant other before surgery.

If the change will be long-term or permanent, a speech-language pathologist will also meet with the client before surgery to discuss long-term methods of effective speech. Esophageal speech is an effective alternative for clients with a permanent tracheostomy.

Esophageal speech is produced by eructation of swallowed air while the client articulates words with his mouth. Speech rehabilitation should begin as soon as possible after surgery. Clients who cannot master esophageal speech can use a mechanical device called an electrolarynx. If a laryngectomy has not been performed, the client may use a tracheostomy plug to facilitate communication, if tolerated.

After surgery, provide the client with a call light and answer it immediately and in person. Leave a note at the central call-light system that the client is unable to speak. Visit the client frequently. Encourage the client to communicate and allow adequate time to write words or select pictures. Do not answer questions for the client or finish their sentences.

If a laryngectomy has been done, the client should be provided with information about a laryngectomy club or support group. A visit by a laryngectomy visitor prior to surgery may be appropriate. Encourage the client and significant other to attend support meetings.

> **A**ction **A**lert!
> The laryngectomy client should be provided with a call light. Answer the call light immediately to decrease his anxiety.

Orienting the Client to Reality

The client who is experiencing impaired verbal communication may also experience confusion related to this unfamiliar state. As needed, orient the client to person, place, and time. Ask orientation questions, such as, "Do you know where you are?" and provide the information as a matter of fact. Also provide orienting information, such as, "You are in (name the health care facility) because . . . ."

Structure the client's environment and routine. Set a daily schedule. Orient the client to the schedule frequently. Provide a clock and calendar large enough to be seen by the client. Keep the clock and calendar current.

Help the client to connect words to activities or objects by cueing the client as to what he or she is doing. If the client has had a stroke, for example, have him touch named body parts on the affected side and approach him from the affected side.

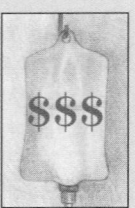

THE COST OF CARE

COMMUNICATION FOR VENTILATOR-DEPENDENT CLIENTS

Clients with neuromuscular disorders may have a tracheostomy tube and be dependent on a ventilator. If these clients have a special fenestrated tracheostomy tube, or if the cuff is deflated to divert air flow through the larynx, they can speak by manipulating the pressure and flows provided by the ventilator. Ventilator-supported speech is produced during much of the inspiratory phase and into the initial portion of the expiratory phase. Ventilator-supported speech is quite short and silent periods are quite long. These long periods of silence interfere with communication because they break up the natural rhythm of speech.

In this study, six tracheostomized people on chronic ventilator support were studied to determine whether their speech could be improved. Adjustments to each client's portable ventilator included reduced inspiratory flow and additional positive end-expiratory pressure (PEEP). These adjustments resulted in increased speaking time per ventilator cycle, increases in the number of syllables per cycle, and decreases in peak tracheal pressure for three of the six subjects. One client who did not benefit from the ventilator-adjusted speech had a substantial air leak. The speech produced was perceived to have better timing, more constant loudness, and more pleasing voice quality. The adjustments were comfortable for the subjects and gas exchange was not compromised.

Discussion

This study demonstrates improvement in communication for some ventilator-supported people without the addition of special equipment of fenestrated tracheostomy tubes. Therefore, the cost of care for this improvement is minimal. The benefits of these adjustments to speech were realized immediately and required essentially no adaptation time or practice. Simple and inexpensive adjustments that reduce inspiratory flow and add PEEP seem to be a safe intervention to improve speech for some ventilator-supported people. This study needs to be replicated with a bigger population, however, to confirm its validity.

Reference

Hoit, J.D. & Banzett, R.B. (1997). Simple adjustments can improve ventilator-supported speech. *American Journal of Speech-Language Pathology, 6*(1), 87–96.

Using an Interpreter

When you encounter a client from a culture different than your own, assess the client for a language or cultural barrier. This baseline assessment is critical because language and cultural barriers can obstruct nursing care. If you and the client do not speak the same language, the client may not understand your explanations of procedures and treatment. It also raises an ethical concern if the client cannot fully understand a consent form or completely understand the teaching related to an informed consent solicited before a test, procedure, or surgery.

If you do not speak the client's language, use an interpreter to help you communicate information about tests, procedures, and interventions. If the client does not understand why a particular intervention or treatment is necessary, he may not comply with it.

Action Alert!
When using an interpreter, always direct your questions and attention to the client, not the interpreter.

Likewise, always consider the client's cultural and health beliefs when planning and implementing nursing care. If interventions do not correspond to the client's health beliefs or culture, he may not consent to treatment or comply with it after discharge.

Interventions for Related Nursing Diagnoses

Impaired verbal communication will affect other aspects of the client and significant other's life. Nursing diagnoses related to impaired communication include *Anxiety, Powerlessness, Self-esteem disturbance, Impaired social interaction, Social isolation,* and *Altered role performance.* Interventions are directed at helping the client and significant other resolve these diagnoses—or prevent impaired verbal communication in the first place—through teaching, social services, and support.

Teaching the Client and Family

The plan to promote verbal communication is developed by the interdisciplinary team, the client, and his family. Techniques to improve communication are taught to the client and family. These techniques are reinforced until the client and family can perform them.

Referring the Client to Social Services

Referring the client to social services can facilitate a smooth transition from the acute care facility to a home situation. Social services can find assistance for services that home health care does not provide, such as housekeeping. They can also be helpful in finding financial assistance to pay for needed health care.

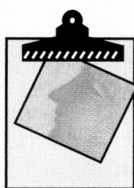

NURSING CARE PLANNING
A CLIENT WITH A LANGUAGE BARRIER

Admission Data

Sr. Martinez is admitted to the respiratory unit and placed under respiratory isolation precautions for tuberculosis. The nurse explains respiratory isolation precautions to him and his wife. As she does so, she points to pictures of the precautions on the isolation card. She then hands Sra. Martinez a mask. During the explanation, they both nod their heads and smile, but afterward they look at each other with questioning eyes. They speak to each other in Spanish and shrug their shoulders. Sra. Martinez obediently places the mask on her face.

Admitting Physician's Orders
1. Instruct client and wife regarding respiratory precautions.
2. Sputum culture for acid-fast bacillus (AFB).
3. Medications:
   Rifampin, 600 mg PO daily
   Isoniazid, 300 mg PO daily
   Pyrazinamide, 2000 mg PO daily

Nursing Assessment
When the nurse enters Sr. Martinez's room to obtain the history and physical assessment, she finds Sra. Martinez in the room without the mask. When the nurse asks why Sra. Martinez is not wearing the mask, she looks questioningly back at the nurse. The nurse begins to collect data and asks, "Do you understand English?" Both respond, "sí," and nod their heads.

The nurse continues to gather data regarding her ability to communicate with the Martinez's and asks, "Do you speak English?" The wife responds "un pequito." Further questioning leads the nurse to believe that the Martinez's understand enough English to meet their basic needs, but not enough to understand medical information. Neither the explanation for respiratory isolation precautions nor the reason for admission to the hospital was understood.

NURSING CARE PLAN

Nursing Diagnosis	Expected Outcomes	Interventions	Evaluation (After 24 Hours of Care)
Impaired verbal communication related to a cultural/language barrier	Client and wife express needs through an interpreter.	*Use a Spanish interpreter to explain isolation precautions, the disease, and the treatment plan, and to allow the client and wife to express needs and concerns. Also review the informed consent.*	Sra. Martinez agreed to wear the mask. She asked several questions about tuberculosis and the planned treatment. Sr. Martinez agreed to be treated. The interpreter translated information about isolation.
	Client and wife will verbalize satisfaction with the communication process.	*Allow adequate time for communication. Speak directly and confidentially to the client and wife.*	Sra. Martinez told the nurse, through the interpreter, that she had been frightened when they came to the hospital and that she is grateful for the interpreter and that her husband is being cared for.

Italicized interventions indicate culturally specific care.

Critical Thinking Questions
1. What feelings would you anticipate Sr. and Sra. Martinez to experience in a health care system in a foreign country where they cannot understand or speak the language?
2. How will you provide discharge teaching?
3. Write expected outcomes for communication of discharge teaching.

Promoting Social Support

The client who is experiencing social isolation or impaired social interaction because of impaired verbal communication will benefit from developing a social support network. As appropriate, refer the client and significant other to a self-help group, such as a Stroke Club, Lost Chords Society, Multiple Sclerosis Society, National Spinal Cord Injury Society, or International Society of Laryngectomies. These self-help groups provide tips and support to ease the role transition and improve the quality of relationships.

EVALUATION

Evaluation of the expected outcomes specified in the nursing care plan determines whether the nursing diagnoses have been resolved. To determine whether the expected outcome have been meet, reassess the client. Documentation in the nursing notes for the case study in this chapter might include the following:

> By discharge, Sr. Martinez and his wife verbalize an understanding of respiratory isolation precautions, treatment, and prevention of the spread of disease. Each expresses satisfaction with the care provided and with the interpreter.

In this example, the expected outcomes for *Impaired verbal communication* have been resolved. If the expected outcomes are not achieved or the client is not making progress toward achieving them, reassessment is essential to obtain additional information. The additional information may provide an explanation for the client's lack of progress. Expected outcomes may need to be rewritten to address the cause, and the plan of care may need to be revised to help meet the expected outcome.

KEY PRINCIPLES

- *Impaired verbal communication* may be related to injury to brain cells, anatomic alterations, developmental delays, psychological barriers, or language or cultural barriers.
- Aphasia results from damage to the speech centers in the brain and causes a loss of comprehension, speech production, or both.
- Broca's (expressive) aphasia causes difficulty with oral expression.
- Wernicke's (receptive) aphasia causes impaired auditory comprehension.
- Assessment of the client's responses to *Impaired verbal communication* are varied and related to psychosocial aspects of a person's life.
- No specific diagnostic test is used to assess speech or language disorders. A speech-language pathologist may assist in the diagnosis.
- A team approach is used to develop a plan of care for the client with *Impaired verbal communication*.

- Interventions for *Impaired verbal communication* related to injured brain cells would aim for a return of speech and language to a functional level and an increase in social interaction.
- Interventions related to anatomical alterations in communication patterns would aim to help the client learn alternative methods of communicating.
- Interventions for *Impaired verbal communication* related to psychological barriers would aim to help the client learn to communicate needs to family and friends.
- Interventions to meet language and cultural barriers to communication would aim to overcome those barriers through an interpreter and respectful responses to cultural differences.

BIBLIOGRAPHY

*Adkins E.R.H. (1991). Nursing care of clients with impaired communications. *Rehabilitation Nursing, 16,* 74–76.

Andrews, M.M. & Boyle, J.S. (1995). *Transcultural concepts in nursing care* (2nd ed.). Philadelphia: Lippincott-Raven Publishers.

*Barker, E. (1994). *Neuroscience nursing.* St. Louis: C.V. Mosby Company.

Bates, B. (1995). *Physical examination and history taking* (6th ed). New York: J.B. Lippincott Co.

*Buckwalter, K.C., Cusack, D., Kruckeberg, T., & Shoemaker, A. (1991). Family involvement with communication-impaired residents in long term care settings. *Applied Nursing Research, 4*(2), 77–84.

*Buckwalter, K.C., Cusack D., Sidles, E., Wadle, K., & Beaver, M. (1989). Increasing communication ability in aphasic/dysarthric patients. *Western Journal of Nursing Research, 11,* 736–747.

Burns, C.E., Barber, N., Brady, M.A., & Dunn, A.M. (1996). *Pediatric primary care: A handbook for nurse practitioners.* Philadelphia: W.B. Saunders Co.

de Carvalho, E.C. & Coler, M.S. (1995). Diagnoses of the human response pattern, communicating: A proposal for revision. *Nursing Diagnosis, 6*(4), 155–160.

*Dillard, J.P. & Wilson, B.J. (1993). Communication and affect: Thoughts feelings, and issues for the future. *Communication Research, 20,* 637–645.

*Dittmar, S.S. (1989). *Rehabilitation nursing: Process and application.* St. Louis: C.V. Mosby Co.

Erber, N.P. & Heine, C. (1996). Screening receptive communication of older adults in residential care. *American Journal of Audiology, 5*(3), 38–46.

Estes, M.E.Z. (1998). *Health assessment and physical examination.* Albany, New York: Delmar ITP.

*Geissler, E.M. (1992). Nursing diagnoses: A study of cultural relevance. *Journal of Professional Nursing, 8,* 301–307.

*Geissler, E.M. (1992). Nursing diagnoses of culturally diverse patients. *International Nursing Review, 38,* 150–152.

Grossman, D. (1996). Cultural dimensions in home health nursing. *American Journal of Nursing, 96,* 33–36.

Hall, D.S. (1996). Interactions between nurses and patients on ventilators. *American Journal of Critical Care, 5,* 293–297.

Hegde, M.N. (1995). *Introduction to communicative disorders.* Texas: Pro-ed.

Hickey, J.V. (1992). *The clinical practice of neurological and neurosurgical nursing* (3rd ed). Philadelphia: J.B. Lippincott Co.

Hoit, J.D. & Banzett, R.B. (1997). Simple adjustments can improve ventilator-supported speech. *American Journal of Speech-Language Pathology, 6*(1), 87–96.

*Asterisk indicates a classic or definitive work on this subject.

Hoit, J.D. & Shea, S.A. (1996). Speech production and speech with a phrenic nerve pacer. *American Journal of Speech-Language Pathology, 5*(2), 53–59.

Jezewski, M.A. (1995). Staying connected: The core of facilitating health care for homeless persons. *Public Health Nursing, 12*(3), 203–210.

Marieb, E.N. (1995). *Human anatomy and physiology* (3rd ed.). Redwood, CA: Benjamin/Cumming.

NANDA. (1999). *NANDA nursing diagnoses: Definitions and classification 1999–2000*. Philadelphia: Author.

Poss, R.M., Santucci, M.A., & Mull, C. (1993). Education literature for Hispanic patients. *Caring Magazine, 12*, 104–106.

Smart, J.F. & Smart, D.W. (1995). Use of translators/interpreters in rehabilitation. *Journal of Rehabilitation, 61*(2), 14–25.

Thompson, J. & Wilson, S. (1996). *Health assessment for nursing practice*. St. Louis: Mosby.

Wardd-Lonergan, J. & Nicholas, M. (1995). Drawing to communicate: A case report of an adult with global aphasia. *European Journal of Disorders of Communication, 30*, 475–491.

Zemlin, W.R. (1998). *Speech and hearing science: Anatomy and physiology* (4th ed.). Boston: Allyn and Bacon.

Confusion

Charlotte F. Young, Janet B. Moore, and Joyce Z. Thielen

Key Terms

affect

agnosia

apraxia

attention

awareness

cognition

confusion

consciousness

delirium

delusions

dementia

hallucinations

judgment

memory

orientation

pseudodementia

LEARNING OBJECTIVES

After studying this chapter, you should be able to:

1. Describe the physiological concepts underlying acute or chronic confusion.

2. Identify the lifestyle, environmental, developmental, psychological, and physiological factors affecting normal cognition.

3. Assess a client at risk for confusion, the manifestations of confusion, and client responses to confusion.

4. Diagnose the problems of a confused client that are amenable to nursing care.

5. Plan for goal-directed interventions to prevent, correct, and support a client with confusion.

6. Describe interventions designed to prevent or reduce confusion.

7. Evaluate the outcomes of nursing care for the confused client and the client's caretakers.

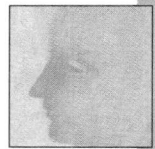

Mr. Tellis, an 83-year-old Greek man, was brought to the emergency department by ambulance with his daughter, Mary Appolos, who told the nurse that he had tried to climb out of the ambulance. He talked to the nurse in broken sentences in an incoherent manner. He could not tell the nurse where he was, where he lived, or what had happened to him. He frequently misperceived the door as a person standing nearby. He seemed agitated, terrified, and fearful of being harmed by people he believed were lurking near the door. He was unable to focus on the nurse's instructions. During one lucid moment, he looked at his daughter and said, "Oh, you take control." After saying this, he slumped into a semiconscious doze and was very difficult to arouse.

Mary told the nurse that he lived alone several blocks away from her home and had always been proud of his independence. He had never seen a family physician regularly, although he had had cataract surgery several years ago. Early the night before, Mary had talked to him on the phone. He said he was fine except that he was having "trouble with my water." Then, at about 3:00 AM, a neighbor called Mary to say that her father was "walking around the yard screaming at someone, but nobody's there." Mary came immediately to his house and called an ambulance, which brought her father to the emergency department.

Mary confided to the nurse, "It all happened so fast. He was fine. He wasn't even sick." Within an hour of Mr. Tellis's arrival, four additional family members had crowded into the emergency department requesting information about him.

(continued)

This case study identifies major clues consistent with confusion. The nurse considers the nursing diagnosis of "Acute Confusion related to unknown etiology" and begins to assess the client for acute confusion, chronic confusion, or both, as well as to rule out several other possible diagnoses.

CONFUSION
NURSING DIAGNOSES

Acute Confusion: The abrupt onset of a cluster of global, transient changes and disturbances in attention, cognition, psychomotor activity, level of consciousness, and/or sleep/wake cycle.

Chronic Confusion: An irreversible, long-standing and/or progressive deterioration of intellect and personality characterized by decreased ability to interpret environmental stimuli and decreased capacity for intellectual thought processes and manifested by disturbances of memory, orientation, and behavior.

From North American Nursing Diagnosis Association. (1999). NANDA nursing diagnoses: Definitions and classification 1999–2000. Philadelphia: Author.

CONCEPTS OF CONFUSION

The brain and central nervous system may experience changes because of a number of factors. One result of changes in the brain may be confusion. As a nurse, you may encounter confused clients in virtually any health care setting, especially acute care, long-term care, and community health care. Recognition of this disorder, initiation of treatment where possible, and administration of care and support to these clients and their families or caregivers is a concern for all professional nurses.

Before looking at the problem of confusion or altered cognition, it is important to first consider the concept of cognition and the physiology of the brain. This will allow a greater understanding of how and why confusion could occur.

Normal Cognition

Cognition, or thought, is the process of knowing and interacting with the world. It includes the concepts of awareness, attention, orientation, judgment, memory, and learning. Cognition takes place in the cerebral cortex of the brain, which is the outer layer or surface of the cerebral hemispheres. However, cognition is not exclusively a function of the brain. A person's perception of the environment is also a major factor.

Physiology of Cognition

The cerebral cortex is composed of billions of nerve cells called neurons. Neurons are the primary units of the nervous system. A neuron has three components: a cell body that contains a nucleus, dendrites, and usually a single axon (Fig. 45–1). Dendrites carry impulses toward the cell body. Axons carry nerve impulses away from the cell body. Neurons are arranged into networks that are interconnected by miles of axons and dendrites.

Neurons communicate with each other through a process called neurotransmission. Neural information passes between neurons across intercellular gaps—the spaces between neurons. These spaces are called synapses; neurotransmitters traverse them to pass electrical information from neuron to neuron. Neurotransmitters are chemical messengers manufactured in the neurons. They include acetylcholine, serotonin, dopamine, and norepinephrine. These chemicals are released from the axon, pass across the intercellular gap, and are received by the dendrite of the adjacent neuron. Each neurotransmitter fits into specific receptor cells embedded in the dendrite's membranes (Fig. 45–2).

Neurotransmitters can either excite or inhibit action. This communication between brain cells enables human activity, body functions, consciousness, intelligence, creativity, memory, and emotion. The synthesis of neurotransmitters is highly influenced by the cerebral metabolism, oxygenation, and general health of the person, as well as by diet, drug use, and other factors.

By influencing neural impulses, neurotransmitters play an important role in cognition. Interruption or disruption of cerebral metabolism or cerebral oxygenation affects neurons, transmission of neural information, and, eventually, cognition. This is often heralded by the appearance of confusion.

Components of Cognition

Cognition is not one discrete activity, but a process of inter-related steps that begins with conscious awareness and culminates in complex judgments, memory, and learning. While there seem to be no standard com-

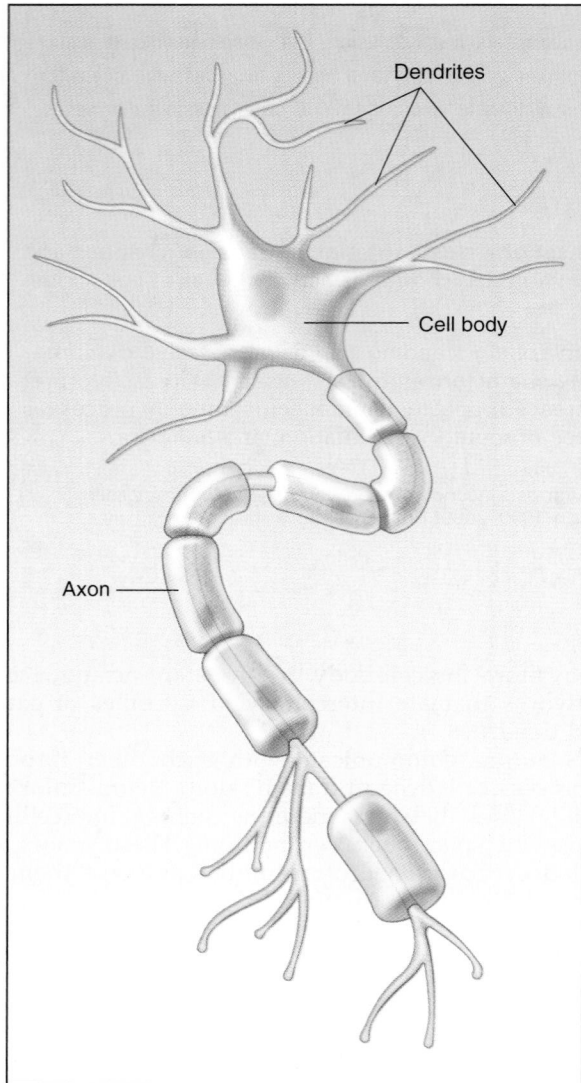

Figure 45–1. A typical neuron.

ORIENTATION

Orientation refers to an awareness of person, place, and time. An oriented client should be able to say not only who and where he is, but also what time it is.

JUDGMENT

Judgment involves the ability to make rational decisions. It includes the ability to understand facts and draw inferences from relationships. For example, if there was a fire in a wastebasket, a person with judgment could describe what to do about it.

MEMORY

Memory is the retention or storage of information learned about the world. The human brain depends on memory to recall previous information and to make decisions. For example, a person would be able to see a nurse and recall from memory not only the definition of "nurse" but also the expected role of a nurse. In addition, a person would be able to recall previous experiences with nurses. This would then enable the person to have a frame of reference with which to listen to and use the information given by the nurse. The triad of memory includes remote (long-term), recent (short-term), and new memory (or immediate recall). Immediate recall typically involves seconds or minutes. Short-term memory usually involves minutes or days. Long-term memory extends longer than several days.

LEARNING

Learning is the acquisition of knowledge, behavior, or skill through experience, practice, study, or instruction. The ability to learn does not decline with advancing age. Older adults are capable of learning, although perhaps at a slower pace than when they were younger.

ponents of cognition in the literature, the following are cited most often: awareness, attention, orientation, judgment, memory, and learning.

AWARENESS

Awareness, or **consciousness,** is the state of being awake and alert enough to react to stimuli. If a client is drowsy, shows altered alertness because of a drug, or is unconscious, you would note that he has a disorder of awareness.

ATTENTION

Attention is the ability to focus on an object or activity. It involves the ability to maintain sensitivity to important stimuli as opposed to irrelevant stimuli. Attention also includes a person's ability to select or choose to focus or shift attention at will.

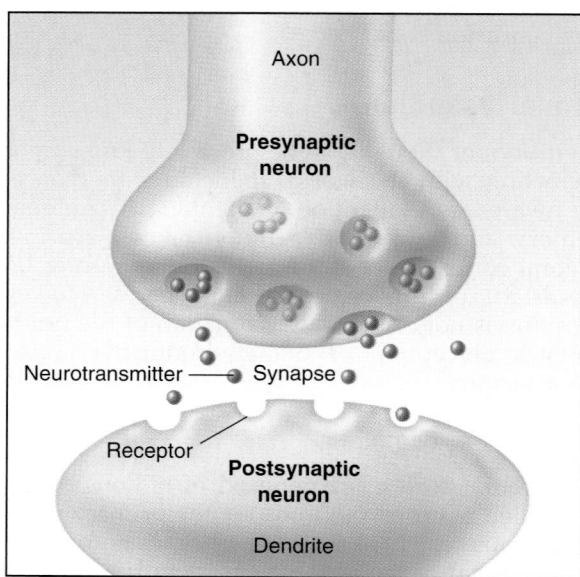

Figure 45–2. Normal neurotransmission.

Problems of Cognition

The lack of one or more of the components of cognition just described can appear as a cognitive disorder, such as confusion. **Confusion** is the "state in which the individual experiences or is at risk of experiencing a disturbance in cognition, attention, memory, and orientation of an undetermined origin or onset" (Carpenito, 1997). Confusion usually occurs when cognition is disrupted. It is not a disease, but rather a syndrome of clinically observable problems. Confusion is a profoundly important symptom of serious neurologic difficulty which, if undetected and untreated, can result in a life-threatening disorder, debilitating cognitive decline, or possible death. Despite this, recent studies confirm that confusion is often unrecognized and misdiagnosed (Simon, Jewel, & Brokel, 1997).

Confusion occurs in people of all ages, but the incidence increases with age. Since the number of elderly people is increasing quickly in the United States, confusion is likely to become an even more prevalent and important consideration in the near future. There are two major types of confusion, acute and chronic. They may appear singly or together.

The cost of treatment for clients with confusion is enormous. Health care costs related to the treatment of hospitalized elders with acute confusion are estimated to be $2 billion annually, and that figure is climbing (Inouye, 1994). The cost of chronic confusion, in particular Alzheimer's disease, is now up to $90 billion a year (Alzheimer's Disease & Related Disorders Association, 1997). The cost of care makes confusion a significant economic problem for families as well as the health care industry, as illustrated in the Cost of Care chart.

Confusion is a significant problem in all areas of practice but has special significance in long-term and acute care nursing. Not only is it often the only indicator of serious illness, particularly in the elderly, but it frequently appears at night. Thus, the evening or night nurse is the first person most likely to notice this important symptom. In addition, confusion commonly compromises the client's safety. The client may try to leave the unit, climb out of bed, or pull out intravenous lines. The client may fall or sustain other kinds of injuries. Many clients later identify the intense experience of acute confusion as traumatic.

Acute Confusion

Acute confusion is a medical emergency. It is associated with the medical diagnosis of **delirium,** which is defined as a disturbance in consciousness and a change in cognition that develops over a short period of time (American Psychiatric Association, 1994). Acute confusion or delirium is a major disorder among hospitalized elders, with occurrence rates estimated at 25% to 50%.

NATURE OF ACUTE CONFUSION

The nature of acute confusion provides important clues to its presence. Acute confusion is by nature a syndrome of observable, clinical symptoms rather than a disease. And it represents a significant change from the client's previous level of functioning. You can interview family members or caregivers to gain an idea of previous functioning. This will help establish that the client's confusion is a significant change and not a recurring symptom of some other disability.

Confusion can be a significant sign of virtually any serious disorder. It is often the only early symptom of a serious disorder in the elderly. For this reason, identification of the underlying cause or causes is imperative. Many times, confusion has multiple causes. Usually, acute confusion arises abruptly over hours or days. Usually, the syndrome is fully developed within 3 days of onset.

Action **A**lert!
Confusion that is a significant change from a client's previous level of functioning and that occurs abruptly and fluctuates throughout the day indicates possible acute confusion. Assess this client promptly and carefully!

Remember Mr. Tellis? His daughter said, "It all happened so fast. He was fine. He wasn't even sick."

The onset of symptoms depends on a number of factors, such as the type of underlying causes, the strength and number of causes, and the health and environment of the client. Symptoms of confusion, specifically alertness to stimuli, tend to fluctuate over the course of a day. Typically, the client seems to have short, lucid intervals. Then the client may become incoherent, fearful, and anxious to pull out his intravenous lines. Then, as the day progresses, he may become alert again for a short time.

Acute confusion appears four times more often in people over age 40 and is most common in people over age 70. Older adults with acute confusion are three to five times more likely to die or have a longer recuperation phase than those without acute confusion (Foreman, 1993). In addition, older adults with acute confusion are less likely to ever return to their pre-illness health status. Thus, hospitalization is longer and nursing home admission is more frequently needed after hospitalization (Levkoff, 1992). The recognition and treatment of acute confusion is an important aspect of health, not only to the client and family but also to society, which partially sponsors the expensive health care of older adults.

Acute confusion in hospitalized elderly clients tends to be a marker of poor prognosis. If acute confusion is recognized and the underlying factors treated promptly and appropriately, acute confusion usually disappears. However, if acute confusion is unrecognized and the underlying factors are left

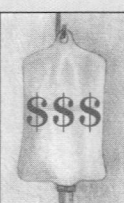

THE COST OF CARE
ALZHEIMER'S DISEASE

Alzheimer's disease is the third most costly disease in the United States, after heart disease and cancer. Indeed, the costs of diagnosis, treatment, nursing home care, and formal paid care for clients with Alzheimer's disease probably exceeds $80 billion to $100 billion a year. The average lifetime cost per client is $174,000. Federal and state governments each cover a portion of the costs, but many of the remaining costs are absorbed by clients and their families (Alzheimer's Disease and Related Disorders Assoc. Inc., 1997). Most clients stay at home as long as possible, being cared for by family and friends. The average "out of pocket" expense to keep a client at home with Alzheimer's disease is $12,500 per year. At some point, a person with Alzheimer's disease will require 24-hour care, including assistance with daily activities, such as eating, grooming, and toileting. Neither Medicare nor most private insurance covers the long-term care that most clients need. Long-term care averages about $42,000 yearly, but it can cost as much as $70,000 yearly in some areas of the country (Alzheimer's Disease and Related Disorders Assoc. Inc., 1996).

Discussion

Some families may have no choice but to care for a person with Alzheimer's disease at home. The cost of long-term care may be too prohibitive to consider, at least initially. As the disease progresses, however, the client's needs will increase and the family may have to re-evaluate the need for long-term care placement. The family may also need emotional support. Some members may feel guilty about not being able to care for their loved one at home. As a nurse, you can play an important role in counseling the family on what to look for in a nursing home. Allay fears, concerns, and misconceptions about nursing home care. Clear up myths and mistaken ideas. Educate about the positive aspects of nursing home care. Explain the unique services provided in a nursing home that specializes in the care of the memory impaired. Grove (1997) provided the following guide for families looking into nursing home placement for their loved one:

- Compile a list of local nursing homes and delete those that do not meet your family member's needs.
- Call the nursing homes and inquire about availability and cost. Ask whether they accept insurance payments. Ask which services are available. For instance, is there a special unit for clients with dementia?
- Schedule onsite meetings.
- Tour chosen facilities to get a sense of their philosophy. Ask about the care providers. Evaluate the food service. Ask any remaining questions at this time.
- Make the choice.
- Stop by unannounced to see what life is really like in the facility selected.
- As you look around the facility, check that current licenses are displayed. Look for the Department of Public Health's inspection report.

Selecting a nursing home takes time and effort. It can also be a time when nursing can support the family with this difficult decision. Take the time to discuss any concerns the client or family may have so that they understand that the choice of a nursing home is the right one.

References

Alzheimer's Disease & Related Disorders Association, Inc. (1997). IRS 229Z, *Alzheimer's Disease: Fact Sheet,* Chicago, IL: Author.
Alzheimer's Disease & Related Disorders Association, Inc. (1996). IRS 230Z, *Alzheimer's Disease: Statistics,* Chicago, IL: Author.
Grove, N. C. (1997). Helping families select a nursing home. *RN, 3,* 37–40.

untreated, a chronic condition or death is the usual result.

CHARACTERISTICS OF ACUTE CONFUSION

Symptoms of acute confusion result from temporary injury to brain tissue. Bouts of acute confusion may last from 1 to 3 weeks if the underlying etiology is identified, or it may resolve on its own. If the injury cannot be reversed, permanent brain injury can result.

The defining characteristics of acute confusion involve disorders in consciousness, attention, perception, memory, orientation, thinking, the sleep-wake cycle, and psychomotor behavior. Impairments of both consciousness and attention are hallmark characteristics of acute confusion (Box 45–1).

BOX 45–1

Characteristics of Acute Confusion

- Altered consciousness.
- Impaired attention.
- Altered perception.
- Memory loss.
- Problems of orientation.
- Impaired thinking, judgment, and language.
- Sleep/wake disorders.
- Psychomotor disturbances.

Altered Consciousness

Consciousness is significantly reduced in acute confusion. The client may be less able to respond to stimuli and may appear to be in a stupor. Or the client may become overly alert, excitable or hyperactive, and hypervigilant.

The fluctuations of consciousness that characterize acute confusion help point out the extent of the client's awareness deficit. This fluctuation is useful because it allows you to see the client in a lucid interval. Unless assessment continues over a 24-hour period, you and your colleagues may fail to notice this important symptom.

Recall the case of Mr. Tellis. He had a lucid moment where he said to his daughter, "Oh, you take control," before he slumped into a semiconscious daze and became difficult to arouse.

Impaired Attention

Impairment of attention is a major factor in acute confusion. The client's attention is usually diminished in three operations: focusing, maintaining, and shifting attention. Focusing is the ability to select important points of focus or selectively mobilize attention on some point of the client's choice. The client will be unable to focus and also unable to maintain or sustain attention. He will be highly distractible. His attention may wander. Extraneous stimuli, such as the hospital intercom or people passing in the hall, will continually distract him. Important stimuli, such as rules of safety, may be unattended and ignored.

The client's ability to shift attention is also reduced. The client may remain focused on a previous topic rather than follow a change of topics as you give instructions. These disturbances in attention prevent integration and organization of information and disrupt thinking, judgment, communication, and memory. For example, a client who cannot attend to your instructions may forget how to use the bell to call you. This client's safety and potential for injury now become important considerations.

This point was illustrated by Mr. Tellis when he was unable to focus on the nurse's instructions because of his agitated and fearful state.

*A*ction *A*lert!

If the client seems highly distractible and unable to focus attention, understand instructions, or shift attention, assess for acute confusion.

Altered Perception

Perceptual difficulties, such as illusions and hallucinations, may occur in acute confusion. The client has a reduced ability to distinguish among dreams, imagery, hallucinations, and reality. Illusions, or mistaken identification of real stimuli, are common. A coat hanging in the closet may be perceived as a person, for example. Perceptual distortions are also prevalent. For example, the client may perceive an object as too large, too small, or too misshapen to resemble real life. Stationary objects may appear to move. Objects may also be perceived as duplicating themselves or flowing into other objects.

Hallucinations are sensory reactions in the absence of real stimuli. They arise commonly in clients with acute confusion. They usually create brightly colored visual hallucinations that seem real. Clients typically see life-size, three-dimensional people or objects moving about. Although visual hallucinations are most common, some clients have auditory hallucinations as well, and hallucinations can involve all five senses.

Certain types of hallucinations are characteristic of underlying causes or related factors. For example, typhus has been connected with kinesthetic hallucinations of floating on air or falling. Acute confusion related to alcohol withdrawal (delirium tremens) is usually associated with hallucinations of animals, coffins, hearses, or ghost-like figures. Children under age 3 may hallucinate that they are being attacked by animals or snakes and react with extreme fear. Hallucinations of attacks are common and evoke a defensive response from clients of all ages. They do not, however, constitute psychosis (Box 45–2).

BOX 45–2

ACUTE CONFUSION VERSUS INTENSIVE CARE UNIT PSYCHOSIS

The term *ICU psychosis* has been used in the past as a label for acute confusion related to such factors as immobility or overstimulation and understimulation in an intensive care unit (ICU). However, the term *psychosis* should not be confused with hallucinations, perceptual distortions, or illusions experienced in acute confusion. The term *psychosis* indicates an inability to identify reality and is associated with acute anxiety rather than dysfunction of the cerebral metabolism or hypoxia.

There is a significant difference between the psychotic symptoms of acute confusion and the psychosis of a person with schizophrenia or depression. In acute confusion, the hallucinations and delusions are changeable and can be randomly related to external stimuli. Hallucinations are related to the person's perception of the environment, unattached to deep beliefs or anxiety. In contrast, the hallucinations or delusions in depression and schizophrenia may be unusual or bizarre, but they are well developed, consistent with the person's beliefs, associated with serious anxiety, and often very intricate.

Information from Crippen, D., & Ermakov, S. (1992). Stress, agitation and brain failure in critical care medicine. Critical Care Nursing Quarterly, 15(2), 52–74.

Altered perception was evident in Mr. Tellis' case. He frequently misperceived the door as a person. Further, he was walking around the yard at 3:00 AM screaming at a nonexistent person.

Memory Loss

Short-term or recent memory, as well as immediate recall, is impaired in acute confusion. The person usually suffers loss of all memory functions. He has a decreased ability to register, retain, and retrieve information. The decline of short-term memory is often associated with an impaired attention span and possible perceptual distortions of incoming stimuli. Memory simply fails to register correctly. Memory retention is also defective because it is incompletely registered.

Since acute confusion can occur in clients with chronic confusion, it is important not to rule out acute confusion based on defects in long-term memory. However, in clients with acute confusion alone, recent memory is usually more affected. The person cannot remember the routine or instructions you gave him. This often affects the person's orientation and causes fearfulness and other emotional reactions.

Problems of Orientation

Orientation to time, place, and other persons may also be affected in serious acute confusion, but rarely will a client forget his own identity. A characteristic cue of acute confusion is that clients frequently mistake unknown people as familiar. For example, the client may misidentify you as a family member.

Mr. Tellis demonstrated difficulty with orientation when he was unable to tell the nurse where he was, where he lived, or what had happened to him. If you detected these problems in a client, how would you respond?

Impaired Judgment and Language

The confused client may have a reduced ability to think sequentially, reason logically, grasp or comprehend word meaning, notice important differences and similarities of words or situations, or actively direct thinking. Thus, the person has a decreased ability to judge, reason, solve problems, plan, or think abstractly. This disturbance in cognition is reflected in language that is disordered, illogical, disjointed, and often incoherent. Conversations become extremely difficult, and safety is a major concern.

Sleep-Wake Disorders

A disrupted circadian rhythm is a classic symptom of acute confusion. Typically, the rhythm is backward; the person will stay awake at night and be less alert and need short naps during the day. The quality of sleep is also affected, and waking is commonly confused, with a dream-like quality. The person may oscillate continually between waking, dreaming, and perceiving illusions or hallucinations. Lack of sleep can distort awareness, alertness, attention, thinking, and cognition.

Psychomotor Disturbances

Psychomotor disturbances are associated with the underlying cause of confusion and usually are visible as hyperactive or hypoactive behavior. Hyperactive clients tend to be very active or hypervigilant. They may remove intravenous lines, pick at things in the air, pull at dressings, climb over side rails, call for loved ones, and have such signs as tachycardia, dilated pupils, or a flushed complexion. Hypoactive clients may seem overly fatigued and sleepy. They tend to sleep during the day and seem rather muddled or less alert than usual. Clients with confusion may also have fluctuating symptoms, presenting one clinical picture and then another.

EARLY SIGNS OF ACUTE CONFUSION IN THE ELDERLY

Matteson, Linton, and Barnes (1996) reported that early signs of acute confusion in the elderly involved forgetfulness, disorientation, fear, misperceptions, insomnia, daytime sleepiness, inattentiveness, easy distraction, and verbal complaints of feeling mixed up or fuzzy. If the factors underlying the confusion are identified and treated, improvement typically occurs in the client's overall physical condition; however, if the symptoms progress, permanent brain injury may result.

EMOTIONAL REACTIONS TO ACUTE CONFUSION

A variety of emotions ranging from panic to apathy may result from acute confusion. Commonly, these emotions change as the condition worsens. This is especially true if the person has perceptual distortions, hallucinations, or delusions. Fear and distrust of others are common. The client may try to flee or may become combative in an effort to protect himself if he has hallucinations that seem dangerous. Powerlessness and shame may arise if the person knows that he is having disorganized thinking or hallucinations. Depression, powerlessness, feelings of loss of control, anger, and fear are all common in acute confusion.

Delusions are false personal beliefs. Delusions are common in a confused person, along with attitudes that differ widely from the person's usual beliefs and attitudes. Suspiciousness, terror, and a fear of persecution or being injured by others are common emotions associated with acute confusion. Paranoid delusions and delusions of persecution may predominate the fragmented thinking already caused by partial memory and inattention. However, unlike the delusions of people with schizophrenia or mania, the delusions of a person with acute confusion are ill defined, unstable, changeable, and usually bound to external stimuli.

Many persons consider acute confusion as traumatizing in itself because of the terrifying perceptions and feelings involved. Clients with febrile conditions and acute confusion report that bright lights and noise are extremely irritating.

Some clients have after-effects from the trauma of acute confusion, such as anxiety, sleeplessness, and other symptoms of post-traumatic stress syndrome. Also, clients who recover from acute confusion but receive no education about it may be anxious that it could return without warning.

According to Crippen and Ermakov (1992), some amnesia can occur after a confused client has recovered. Indeed, some people experience only "small, random, islands of memory" about the confusing episode after they recover.

Chronic Confusion

Chronic confusion is a state in which a person experiences an irreversible, long-standing, progressive deterioration of intellect and personality (NANDA, 1999). It is usually associated with the medical diagnosis **dementia,** which involves multiple cognitive deficits including impairment of memory and judgment and resulting in a progressive decline in intellectual functioning (American Psychiatric Association, 1994). There are many forms of dementia; dementia of the Alzheimer's type is the most common.

Dementia or chronic confusion is not a single disease but a syndrome characterized by deterioration of cognition in a person who was not previously cognitively impaired. This deterioration is both acquired and progressive, and it impairs social, occupational, and functional activities (Fleming, Adams, & Peterson, 1995).

NATURE OF CHRONIC CONFUSION

Chronic confusion is characterized by a slowly progressive, permanent deterioration in cognitive ability. Symptoms progress in a stable, steady manner. Unlike acute confusion, chronic confusion typically does not involve perceptual disturbances, sleep-wake alterations, and inattention. Although chronic confusion is associated with cognitive decline, it can commonly be slowed or even halted by treating the underlying causes (Foreman, 1993).

CHARACTERISTICS OF CHRONIC CONFUSION

Characteristically, a client with chronic confusion has a loss of memory and a loss of at least one or more of the following skills: problem-solving, judgment, or planning skills; abstract thinking; and cognitive or intellectual skills (Box 45–3). There may also be a change in affect or personality, as well as disturbances of higher cortical function, such as language, motor activities, or constructional ability. There may be a progressively lowered stress threshold manifested as purposeful wandering or catastrophic behavior, such as violent, compulsive, or avoidance behaviors. As deterioration progresses, skill loss increases (American Psychiatric Association, 1994).

Memory Loss

Loss of short-term and long-term memory is the major defining characteristic of chronic confusion. Initially, the client cannot recall what happened a few moments ago. As the condition progresses, the client may be-

---

BOX 45–3

CHARACTERISTICS OF CHRONIC CONFUSION

- Loss of memory.
- Loss of problem-solving, judgment, or planning skills.
- Loss of abstract thinking, cognitive, or intellectual skills.
- Change in affect or personality.
- Disturbances of higher cortical function.
- Progressively lowered stress threshold.

---

come unable to recall his birthplace, his occupation, and so on.

Action Alert!
When a client has a loss of memory and a loss of other abilities, such as problem-solving, abstract thinking, and word recall, assess for chronic confusion.

Impaired Problem-Solving and Judgment
A person with chronic confusion gradually suffers cognitive deterioration to the point that he loses his problem-solving ability. He may not be able to judge safety issues with any degree of insight.

Loss of Abstract Thinking
Abstract thinking is indicated by a person's ability to find similarities and differences between related words and concepts. The person can define and differentiate word meanings. He can interpret proverbs and apply them to other settings. Abstract thinking deteriorates as chronic confusion progresses.

Changes in Affect or Personality
Affect, or the observable expression of feelings or emotions, changes as chronic confusion progresses, as does the client's personality. Some aspect of the personality may be accentuated, or the personality may change completely. The person's behavior may change dramatically, which is usually a source of considerable distress to the family.

Disturbances of Higher Cortical Functions
Disturbances of higher cortical functions appear as the syndrome progresses. They include aphasia, apraxia, and agnosia. Aphasia is a language disorder resulting from brain damage or disease to speech centers in the brain resulting in a variety of difficulties in formulating, expressing, and understanding language (see Chapter 44). Although the client can usually recognize the correct word if you say it, he will be unable to retrieve the word from memory. This problem can create much frustration for the client and the staff. It is important to be aware of the client's needs and develop

a method of communication that avoids undue frustration.

Apraxia is the inability to carry out motor activities despite the functional ability to perform them. For example, the client may try to put his foot into the arm of his shirt when getting dressed. **Agnosia** is the failure to recognize or identify objects despite an intact sensory ability. The client may be unable to recognize the phone or light switch because he cannot recall the object. This problem can be frustrating and frightening. Constructional ability—the ability to duplicate a design with blocks or sticks—also deteriorates because of the client's reduced ability to understand and function in a three-dimensional world.

Lowered Stress Threshold

A client with chronic confusion develops a progressively lessened ability to withstand stressful situations and adapt to environmental requirements. This lowered stress threshold tends to produce more violent, compulsive, combative, and catastrophic behaviors in response to triggers, stressful situations, or events that exceed the client's threshold.

EARLY SIGNS OF CHRONIC CONFUSION IN THE ELDERLY

Cognitive deterioration results from progressive degeneration of the cerebral cortex. Hall (1991) and Matteson and colleagues (1996) have outlined the progressive degeneration found in chronic confusion. In the first stage, the person begins to forget things and becomes concerned about possible loss of memory. Usually the person attempts to hide these deficits. In the second stage, the person loses much of his cognitive integrative functioning and becomes unable to handle money, transportation, and cooking. He may be unable to keep a job. Poor judgment and social isolation become evident.

In the third stage, the person loses much of his ability to perform activities of daily living. Wandering and combative behaviors often force the family to seek help. Combative behavior is usually very disturbing to the family, since it is a dramatic change from the client's previous behavior. By the end of the third stage, the person can no longer attend to personal hygiene, may have urinary and fecal incontinence, and may be unaware of his surroundings. The person may require placement in a protective environment.

Mobility, communication, and recognition of body parts are also affected. Nursing care will include an emphasis on protecting the client from the health hazards of immobility. Moments of lucidity and episodes of speechlessness or screaming can occur. Gradually, the client forgets how to eat. Nursing care in this stage focuses on such concerns as nutrition, skin integrity, impaired swallowing, potential for aspiration, urinary tract infections, and a risk for pneumonia. As the client deteriorates, his health needs increase and become more complex from multiple chronic illnesses, infections, and urinary and respiratory diseases. The client often dies of pneumonia.

EMOTIONAL REACTIONS TO CHRONIC CONFUSION

Early in chronic confusion, the client typically denies difficulty with memory and blames his forgetfulness on stress, feeling rushed, overwork, or a physical illness. Later, as deterioration increases, job performance may suffer and the client may lose position and functioning. At this point, anxiety, depression, and frustration may invade the person's awareness. Still, the client may attempt to counter the influence of dementia with active efforts to "be normal" (Phinney, 1998). He may try to hide defects by staying away from his usual social gatherings.

As deterioration continues, the stress threshold drops and the enormous effort needed to function with such problems as aphasia may overtax the already affected client. This may provoke what some experts call a "catastrophic reaction." The person may react with compulsive, violent, combative, hostile behavior. Sadness, frustration, fear, or simple pleasure may come and go from moment to moment.

Barriers to Identifying Confusion

Confusion has been noted and described for more than 2,500 years, but we still lack a full understanding of it. Only in 1994 did NANDA accept *Acute confusion* and *Chronic confusion* as nursing diagnoses. It is expected that by highlighting these important syndromes, the detection and possible treatment of underlying causes will proceed more quickly. Recognition of confusion, which typically leads to identification of underlying factors and provision of appropriate and speedy treatment, may help reverse the underlying disorder as well as the confusion. Even when this is impossible, treatment can usually slow the cognitive decline.

Numerous barriers make it difficult to recognize confusion. Incorrect beliefs and attitudes are major obstructions. Perhaps the most damaging belief is the myth that everyone becomes confused with age. Nothing could be farther from the truth. Confusion is a symptom of serious neurological disorder. It requires assessment and treatment. The belief that confusion is normal or should be ignored is wrong and damaging.

Lack of precise documentation is another major barrier. Overlapping terms, loosely identified symptoms, and inexact descriptions are prime reasons why confusion is often ignored or misdiagnosed. For example, if inattention is incorrectly identified as "disoriented" or hypoalertness is misidentified and documented as "drowsy," these important defining characteristics will be missed. The confusion itself may be unrecognized, undocumented, and untreated.

Lack of an appropriate and complete mental status assessment can be another barrier. A mental status examination usually will be included in your assessment of a confused client. These examinations typically identify such aspects as appearance, behavior, orientation, memory, sensorium, perception, mood, affect, thinking or intellectual functioning, the content of thought, the process of thinking, insight into difficulties, judgment, problem-solving, and abstract thinking, as discussed in the State of Nursing Science chart.

In addition, assessment of the client's orientation to time, place, and person—in the absence of further assessment—can lead to misdiagnosis because the client may seem oriented but still be confused. Early in chronic confusion, the client may not seem confused because he can rely on family or friends to aid a failing memory and obscure the full extent of his memory loss. This client may be able to hide his cognitive impairment from you during a superficial conversation; however, a full mental status assessment will reveal the problem. If you fail to fully assess the client's cognitive capacity, you may miss the underlying cues—and the opportunity to intervene while the disorder is still mild. Only after the disorder borders on debilitating will it likely come to the attention of health care personnel. Keep in mind that a full mental status assessment must encompass at least 24 hours, not just the daytime shift.

FACTORS AFFECTING NORMAL COGNITION

When the brain is deprived of oxygen, glucose, or other essential chemicals, the result may be a disruption in cognitive function. A number of factors may affect cognitive status, including lifestyle, environmental, developmental, socioeconomic, physiological, and psychological factors. They may be associated with acute confusion, chronic confusion, or both.

Lifestyle Factors

Substance Abuse

The ingestion or abuse of harmful substances, such as alcohol, barbiturates, cocaine, amphetamines, and other hallucinogens, can alter cognition.

Nutritional Deficiencies

Deficiencies of thiamine, folate, vitamin B_{12}, iron, niacin, and magnesium also may disrupt brain function. People who chronically ingest large amounts of alcohol may develop vitamin B-complex deficiencies with a resulting encephalopathy and memory loss known as Wernicke-Korsakoff syndrome.

Sleep Disruption

Cognition requires not only enough sleep but also a sleep-wake cycle that corresponds with the person's normal living environment and situation. Lack of sleep can distort awareness, alertness, attention, thinking, and cognition.

Sexually Transmitted Diseases

Infection with the human immunodeficiency virus (HIV), which causes AIDS, can lead to a syndrome called AIDS dementia complex. Usually, it is a late manifestation of HIV infection, just as neurosyphilis is a late manifestation of tertiary syphilis. HIV infection can stem from the use of contaminated needles as well as from unprotected sex.

Environmental Factors

Sensory Stimulation

People who are in unfamiliar environments, particularly when they lack sensory stimulation, may become acutely confused (Fig. 45–3). Conversely, environments with excessive stimulation—such as noise from a television, radio, intercom, and so on—may worsen confusion. Behavior problems may ensue, especially in a client with chronic confusion.

Lead Ingestion

Lead poisoning is a well-known cause of altered cognition. Lead-based paint from old housing is the most frequent source of lead poisoning in children. The ingestion of lead paint occurs during normal hand-to-mouth activity. Other sources of lead are water pipes that have been contaminated with lead solder, lead-containing pottery being used to serve or store food, and lead-contaminated soil.

This preventable pediatric problem affects young children and causes neurological and intellectual problems by shifting fluid into the interstitial spaces of the brain. As a result, intracranial pressure rises, leading to an encephalopathy that causes mental retardation, seizures, coma, and death. Even exposure to low levels of lead can lead to intellectual deficiencies that may be irreversible. These deficiencies may cause hyperactivity, impulsiveness, aggression, lethargy, irritability, and learning disabilities.

Developmental Factors

Cognitive development begins in infancy and progresses through childhood. The theory of cognitive development used most often by health care professionals was developed by Jean Piaget (see Chapter 19). It describes several stages through which children

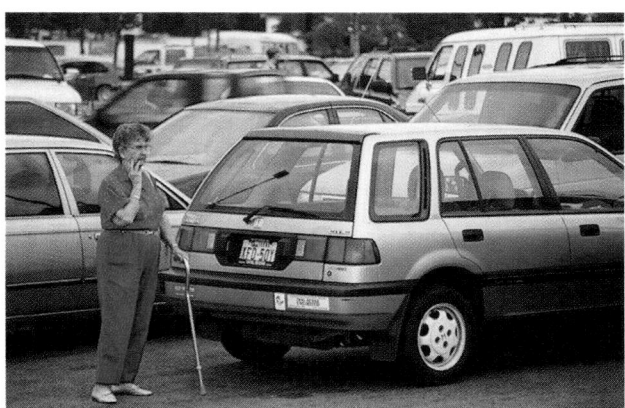

Figure 45–3. People who are in unfamiliar environments may become acutely confused.

ASSESSMENT OF CONFUSION IN THE ELDERLY

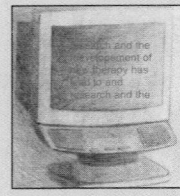

What Are the Issues?

When older adults are hospitalized for acute illnesses, they can experience confusion. Nurses often assess and document such changes in mental status using narrative descriptors such as "confused" or "disoriented to person, place, and time." Such general indicators of mental status do not allow clinicians to document subtle trends in cognitive status that may point to deterioration or improvement. To be clinically useful, assessment tools for changes in mental status should be specific, reliable, and valid, as well as easy to use.

What Research Has Been Conducted?

Several researchers have already described the clinical picture of acute confusion in older adults. Building on descriptions from earlier studies, two groups of nurse-researchers have recently developed tools to assess confusion. These tools are the NEECHAM Confusion Scale (Neelon, Champagne, Carlson, & Funk, 1996) and the Clinical Assessment of Confusion—A Checklist (Vermeersch & Hendly, 1997).

THE NEECHAM CONFUSION SCALE

The developers of the NEECHAM Confusion Scale used a holistic assessment approach that would already be familiar to nurses. They wanted a tool that took into consideration the many causes of confusion and the variety of ways in which confusion presents in older adults. They wanted a tool that was easily used by nurses in typical assessment encounters in acute-care settings. The tool that they developed is divided into three subscales: information-processing, behavior, and physiological control. For the information-processing section, the nurse rates such parameters as alertness, ability to follow commands, and orientation. In the behavior section, the nurse rates the person's appearance, motor function, and verbal skills. In the final section, physiological control, the nurse rates the person's vital signs, oxygen saturation, and urinary continence control. The result is a numeric score of 0 to 30.

Neelon and colleagues (1996) reported that the scale had a strong degree of what researchers term *internal consistency,* a measure of the reliability of the tool. They also tested how well the tool functioned when two nurses used it on the same person—its *interrater reliability*—and found it quite good. They also reported that the tool showed high levels of correlation with other measures of health status related to confusion.

In another study, Miller and colleagues (1997) evaluated the use of the NEECHAM Confusion Scale in an acute-care medical setting over a 20-week period. As part of their study, they included a 5-hour orientation program for the staff nurses that reviewed the problem of acute confusion in the older adult, as well as the use of the new tool. Their results indicated that staff nurses were able to incorporate the use of the NEECHAM Confusion Scale reliably, although use of the information was not always evident after it was documented.

CLINICAL ASSESSMENT OF CONFUSION—A CHECKLIST

Another tool developed to assess confusion in older adults is the Clinical Assessment of Confusion—A Checklist (Vermeersch & Hendly, 1997). In their 1997 study, Vermeersch and Hendly assessed the validity of a checklist of descriptors for confusion. The researchers found that the descriptors could be grouped around six factors: cognition, general behavior, motor activity, orientation, psychotic/neurotic behavior, and an ambiguous factor involving such variables as exhibiting little eye contact. The researchers asked nurses in the sample to rate assessment items that corresponded to the six factors identified in previous studies. The results provided support for the clinical validity of the checklist.

What Has the Research Concluded?

To date, the research on assessment of confusion in the elderly has determined that these two tools for identifying early signs of confusion in the hospitalized older adult are valid, reliable, and clinically useful. Whether nurses will begin to use these tools systematically will depend on institutional commitment to include them in current documentation systems. Nurses need to collaborate with other providers in using the tools as clinical indicators of acute confusion so that further diagnostic and treatment decisions can be made based on reliable and valid assessments.

What Is the Future of Research in This Area?

A major focus of future research in the assessment and treatment of acute confusion will be in finding ways to help nurses actually *use* the information that they have elicited in planning and evaluating care (Miller et al., 1997). The current research teams also plan additional work in establishing other forms of validity of these two assessment tools. In addition, Neelon et al. (1996) recommend comparing the NEECHAM scale with the other tools developed to assess confusion in the older adult. As more care is delivered in out-of-hospital settings, it will also be important to test these tools in other settings where older adults may present with acute confusion, such as the home, the emergency room, and long-term-care settings.

References

Miller, J., Neelon, V., Champagne, M., Bailey, D., Ngandu, N., Belyea, M., Jarrell, E., Montoya, L., & Williams, A. (1997). The assessment of acute confusion as part of nursing care. *Applied Nursing Research, 10,* 143–151.

Neelon, V. J., Champagne, M. T., Carlson, J. R., & Funk, S. G. (1996). The NEECHAM Confusion Scale: Construction, validation, and clinical testing. *Nursing Research, 45,* 324–330.

Vermeersch, P. E. H., & Henly, S. J. (1997). Validation of the structure for Clinical Assessment of Confusion—A Checklist. *Nursing Research, 46,* 208–213.

progress as they mature. Cognitive development is not a rigid, step-by-step process, but an individual progression.

When maladaptive cognitive responses occur during childhood, they are typically called mental disabilities or retardation. Maladaptive cognition can occur at any age, but it occurs most often in the older adult because the older brain is more susceptible to insults.

New and exciting research is being developed regarding the stages of cognitive deterioration. Matteson and colleagues (1996) have suggested the use of Piaget's theory of cognitive development as a construct to view the process of cognitive degeneration in chronic confusion.

Psychological Factors

Depression may affect cognition, particularly in the elderly. Likewise, cognitive deterioration can lead to depression in clients who understand that their cognitive ability is declining. **Pseudodementia** is a term commonly used to describe the depression that is misinterpreted as dementia.

Clients in the early stages of chronic confusion commonly experience depression. As a person becomes unable to hide his failing cognitive abilities, he may lose his job, independent living, functional abilities, his memory, his life as he previously knew it. This can flood the person with the multitude of losses already experienced as well as probable future losses.

Relatively early in the progressive decline of chronic confusion, some clients face an increased risk of suicide resulting from the twin feelings of powerlessness and hopelessness. As chronic confusion progresses to later stages and the person's memory fails, depression and the risk of suicide lessen.

Physiological Factors

Physiological factors affecting cognition are extensive. They include traumatic injury and a wide range of physical illnesses, such as febrile conditions, hypoxia, metabolic disorders, infections, and fluid and electrolyte disturbances. Cardiovascular and respiratory disorders can affect cognition as well.

Trauma

Traumatic injury to the brain may damage and change the structure of brain tissue. Specific symptoms depend on the area of the brain affected.

Physical Illness

FEBRILE CONDITIONS
Children commonly develop acute confusion if they have high fever. However, children who are acutely confused are commonly labeled by parents or staff as "uncooperative." Such negative labeling can result in the symptoms of confusion being missed entirely.

Action Alert!
When a child has a high fever, take action to reduce the fever to prevent acute confusion.

If the fever continues, the child may have a febrile seizure that can alter cognition. Febrile seizures are one of the most common neurological disorders in children 3 months to 6 years of age. A high fever that rises quickly seems to be a contributing factor. The child will have abnormal results on a neurological examination and no evidence of a pathological condition that causes seizures. Most often, a throat or ear infection is the cause of the fever.

HYPOXIA
Hypoxia, or a decrease in oxygen supply, can occur in a number of medical conditions. For example, anemia can result from a decrease in the number of red blood cells or a reduction in hemoglobin, causing mental confusion from a lack of cerebral tissue perfusion. Cardiac conditions can also lead to confusion by decreasing cardiac output and, in turn, reducing blood oxygen levels or increasing carbon dioxide levels or both.

METABOLIC DISORDERS
Metabolic disorders, such as hypothyroidism secondary to a decreased functioning of the thyroid gland, may lead to progressive cognitive impairment. Cognitive loss may not be reversible, even after thyroid hormone replacement.

INFECTIONS
Very often, an older adult with a serious infection will have no sign of fever, but will instead exhibit a change in mental status. The astute practitioner relies on past history and an understanding of age-related changes to guide assessment.

FLUID AND ELECTROLYTE DISTURBANCES
Electrolyte imbalances, specifically involving sodium, can cause mental confusion and delirium. Restoring sodium levels to normal values and preventing further fluid imbalances are the goals of intervention.

Dehydration is a serious health problem, particularly in the elderly. Conditions such as heart failure, hypertension, renal disease, infections, and diarrhea can result in confusion, disorientation, or a change in affect.

Medications

Prescription and over-the-counter (OTC) medications may be toxic, particularly to the very young and the elderly. Disruptions in cognitive function may occur from taking the wrong drug, from a drug side effect, or from drug-drug or drug-alcohol interactions. Confusion may lead to further difficulty in taking medications properly.

Neurobiological Factors

There are many types of dementia. And although the pathological conditions that cause the degeneration into chronic confusion are varied, the symptoms are similar. Following are some of the more common types of dementia.

ALZHEIMER'S DISEASE

Alzheimer's dementia is characterized by cognitive deterioration that progresses slowly over months or years. It is the most prevalent of the dementias and affects about 4 million people in the United States. The incidence and prevalence rise with age. The cause is unknown but research continues into the roles of acetylcholine (a neurotransmitter) and amyloid precursor protein. The risk of developing Alzheimer's disease rises with a family history of Alzheimer's disease and Down syndrome (Alzheimer's Disease & Related Disorders Association, 1997).

VASCULAR DEMENTIA

Vascular dementia results from multiple vascular insults to the brain. Multiple infarcts, resulting from either hemorrhage or ischemia, are associated with this cerebrovascular disorder. This type of chronic confusion progresses in a characteristically step-like fashion after each vascular insult. The client's symptoms reflect the brain areas affected.

PARKINSON'S DISEASE

Involuntary muscle movements while the person is at rest are major defining characteristics of Parkinson's disease. Language is not necessarily affected, but memory may deteriorate progressively. Postural instability caused by the tendency to become slow and rigid is another nursing consideration. Reversible delirium may be associated with medications.

HUNTINGTON'S DISEASE

Huntington's disease is a hereditary degenerative disease involving a characteristic twitching movement that increases when the client feels anxious. The chronic confusion associated with this disease is characterized by slowed thinking, poor attention span, and poor judgment. The client becomes hostile, impulsive, and easily frustrated as the stress threshold lessens and deterioration progresses.

NORMAL PRESSURE HYDROCEPHALUS

When excess fluid accumulates in the cranial cavity, the ventricles enlarge and compress the cortex. This can cause symptoms of chronic confusion. A shunt can drain the excess fluid and reverse the symptoms if inserted in time. Early onset of aphasia, ataxia, and incontinence are key characteristics of this disorder.

CREUTZFELDT-JAKOB DISEASE

Creutzfeldt-Jakob disease is an infectious form of dementia related to a slow virus. The major symptoms are muscle spasms and deterioration of cognitive abilities or chronic confusion. If this disease is suspected to be the underlying cause of a client's chronic confusion, the client must be placed on blood, secretion, and excretion precautions.

Action Alert!
A client with Creutzfeldt-Jakob disease has a communicable virus. Place the client on body substance precautions immediately.

PICK'S DISEASE

Pick's disease is characterized by the formation of Pick's cells in the frontal and temporal lobes. It is rare and usually not reversible. The major symptoms are amnesia, aphasia, and loss of inhibitions.

ASSESSMENT

General Assessment of Cognition

The cornerstone of assessment is a history, physical examination, mental status examination, functional examination, and review of present medical regimen. Assessment involves the appraisal of cognition and identification not only of the impairments but also of the strengths of the person that can be used in planning care.

Health History

A good history targets risk factors and defining characteristics that may be present. Determine the time confusion occurred, the mental status changes that occurred, possible precipitating or related factors, recent medication changes, long-term medication use, and history of substance use. Develop a history from the client's family to identify major changes in the person's characteristic behaviors and emotional function. Also check for signs of related factors, such as infection, chronic illness, depression, or previous hospitalization.

If you suspect acute confusion, review the client's medications in detail. Assess prescription and OTC medications as well as any history of long-term medication use or substance abuse. Check to see if the client is sharing medications with a spouse. Assess potential medication intoxication, especially if the client takes a sedative, hypnotic, narcotic, anticholinergic drug, or psychotropic drug.

Assess for both acute and chronic confusion. These types of confusion may exist singly or together. Identification of both types of confusion and underlying causes is necessary to plan treatment accordingly.

The assessment of mental status and cognitive functioning is important to any client with potential confusion but particularly to the elderly person. Perform a baseline assessment and then routinely reassess to detect any changes promptly and systematically. The use of a mental status questionnaire and a behavioral rating scale is recommended to provide a comprehensive assessment (Foreman, 1993).

Assessment Tools

Instruments currently used to detect acute confusion fall into several categories: mental status examinations, rating scales, clinical interviews, and psychomotor tests. All of these tests have positive and negative aspects. The most frequently used tools are mental status questionnaires and rating scales.

MENTAL STATUS EXAMINATIONS

Mental status examinations are questionnaires designed to assess various cognitive functions. You will ask questions and collect data on such components as consciousness, memory, attention, orientation, and abstract thinking. The most frequently used mental status questionnaires are Pfeiffer's Short Portable Mental Status Questionnaire (SPMSQ) and, more commonly, Folstein's Mini Mental State Exam (Fig. 45–4). These tests can help you decide whether a client does or does not have cognitive impairment, but they do not allow finer discrimination. Because these tests require the client to answer questions, you must make adaptations for clients who are deaf, blind, intubated, or otherwise unable to participate readily. For example, ask the intubated client to blink his eyes, raise his finger, or communicate the answers to you in some other designated manner (Pfeiffer, 1975; Folstein, Folstein, & McHugh, 1975).

Cultural implications must also be considered when giving a questionnaire. Some experts question the validity of these tests, since age, education, culture, and language can affect test results. It is important to recognize that any questions involving cultural issues can be misleading. For example, the new immigrant may not know answers related to U.S. history that are routinely asked in some mental status examinations. This lack of knowledge does not reflect the person's cognitive ability but simply a lack of knowledge about U.S. history.

RATING SCALES

Because much of the information needed to assess confusion is nonverbal, the use of a rating scale in addition to the mental status examination provides a more comprehensive assessment of client function. When using a rating scale, you score or rate behavior or symptoms on a predetermined scale. You simply observe the client and rate what you observed. This approach obviates the client's participation.

A number of behavioral scales have been developed to assess confusion, detect key aspects of acute confusion, differentiate between acute confusion and chronic confusion, and identify differences between confusion and depression. The most common scales are the NEECHAM Confusion Scale and the Clinical Assessment of Confusion. The NEECHAM Confusion Scale, as discussed earlier in the State of Nursing Science chart, allows rapid bedside documentation of the client's information processing defects. It allows you to document key indicators of the development of acute confusion.

The Clinical Assessment of Confusion Scale is particularly useful for differentiating between acute confusion, chronic confusion, and depression. It also helps define the severity of the client's problem. These and

several other scales are being further researched and developed.

Physical Assessment

The physical examination focuses on assessing cognitive status and identifying possible etiologies for changes in a client's cognition. It includes a head-to-toe assessment, paying particular attention to orientation, basic neurological assessment, level of consciousness, vital signs, skin turgor, lung auscultation, and elimination pattern.

Recall the case of Mr. Tellis, introduced at the beginning of the chapter. The nursing assessment and initial work-up is as follows:

83-year-old Caucasian male admitted in no acute distress. Temperature is 97.6°F, pulse 90 and regular, respirations 20, BP 140/84 lying, 130/80 sitting, and 110/70 standing. Mr. T complains of dizziness when standing for BP reading and increased sway is noted. Neurological exam: pupils equal, round, and reactive to light (PERRL), hand grasps equal and strong, moving all extremities. Able to recall name, but unable to recall place or time. Appears to be anxious at times and mentation vacillates between lucidity and confusion. Mini Mental State Exam reveals a score of 24, indicating a mild impairment. Lungs are clear to auscultation throughout all lung fields. O_2 saturation on room air is 94%. Heart sounds S_1 and S_2 heard, no irregularities noted. Skin is dry and tenting is noted over sternum and forehead. Abdomen is soft, nontender, and bowel sounds are heard in all four quadrants. Bladder percussed and palpated. Findings suggest urine retention. A #16 Foley catheter inserted and 350 mL concentrated cloudy urine are obtained. Specimen sent to lab for urinalysis and culture and sensitivity. Lower extremities reveal dry, scaly skin and dependent rubor relieved by lying down. Positive pedal, posterior tibial, and popliteal pulses. Blood drawn for CBC, electrolytes, BUN, creatinine. Family remains with client throughout assessment.

From this assessment report, can you see any clues to Mr. Tellis's confusion?

Diagnostic Tests

A number of diagnostic tests may be ordered by a physician or an advanced practice nurse to determine the cause of a client's confusion. These test results help distinguish acute from chronic confusion. Serum (blood) laboratory tests such as a complete blood count and measurement of electrolytes, blood urea nitrogen, creatinine, and glucose may be performed. A chest radiograph, computed tomography scan, electrocardiogram, and urine culture are also often part of the screen done for suspected acute or chronic confusion (Table 45–1).

Mr. Tellis's urine culture shows bacteria present in the urine greater than 100,000/mL. Remember that Mr. Tellis complained of "having trouble with my water." Can you correlate the presence of bacteria in his urine with the symptoms of confusion?

MiniMental LLC

THE ANNOTATED MINI MENTAL STATE EXAMINATION (AMMSE)

NAME OF SUBJECT _____ Age _____
NAME OF EXAMINER _____ Years of School Completed _____

Approach the patient with respect and encouragement.
Ask: "Do you have any trouble with your memory?" ☐ Yes ☐ No
"May I ask you some questions about your memory?" ☐ Yes ☐ No

Date of Examination _____

SCORE   ITEM

5 ( ) **TIME ORIENTATION**
Ask:
"What is the year _____ (1), season _____ (1),
month of the year _____ (1), date _____ (1),
day of the week _____ (1)?"

5 ( ) **PLACE ORIENTATION**
Ask:
"Where are we now? What is the state _____ (1), city _____ (1),
part of the city _____ (1), building _____ (1),
floor of the building _____ (1)?"

3 ( ) **REGISTRATION OF THREE WORDS**
Say: "Listen carefully. I am going to say three words. You say them back after I stop.
Ready? Here they are... PONY (wait 1 second), QUARTER (wait 1 second), ORANGE (wait one
second). What were those words?

_____ (1)
_____ (1)
_____ (1)

Give 1 point for each correct answer, then repeat them until the patient learns all three.

5 ( ) **SERIAL 7s AS A TEST OF ATTENTION AND CALCULATION**
Ask: "Subtract 7 from 100 and continue to subtract 7 from each subsequent remainder
until I tell you to stop. What is 100 take away 7?" _____ (1)
Say:
"Keep Going." _____ (1), _____ (1),
_____ (1), _____ (1).

3 ( ) **RECALL OF THREE WORDS**
Ask:
"What were those three words I asked you to remember?"
Give one point for each correct answer. _____ (1),
_____ (1), _____ (1).

2 ( ) **NAMING**
Ask:
"What is this?" (show pencil) _____ (1). "What is this?" (show watch) _____ (1).

For more
information or
additional copies
of this exam,
call (617) 587-4215

O V E R

---

1 ( ) **REPETITION**
Say:
"Now I am going to ask you to repeat what I say. Ready? No ifs, ands, or buts."
Now you say that." _____ (1)

3 ( ) **COMPREHENSION**
Say:
"Listen carefully because I am going to ask you to do something.
Take this paper in your left hand (1), fold it in half (1), and put it on the floor." (1)

1 ( ) **READING**
Say:
"Please read the following and do what it says, but do not say it aloud." (1)

Close your eyes

1 ( ) **WRITING**
Say:
"Please write a sentence." If patient does not respond, say: "Write about the weather." (1)

1 ( ) **DRAWING**
Say: "Please copy this design."

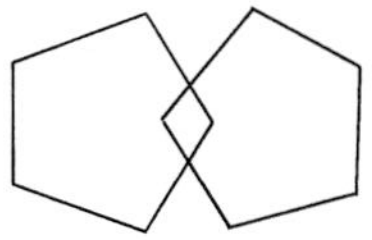

TOTAL SCORE _____ Assess level of consciousness along a continuum

Alert   Drowsy   Stupor   Coma

	YES	NO
Cooperative	☐☐☐☐☐	☐☐☐☐☐
Depressed		
Anxious		
Poor Vision		
Poor Hearing		
Native Language		

	YES	NO
Deterioration from previous level of functioning	☐☐☐☐☐	☐☐☐☐☐
Family History of Dementia		
Head Trauma		
Stroke		
Alcohol Abuse		
Thyroid Disease		

FUNCTION BY PROXY
Please record date when patient was last
able to perform the following tasks.
Ask caregiver if patient independently handles:

	YES	NO	DATE
Money/Bills	☐☐☐☐	☐	_____
Medication			_____
Transportation			_____
Telephone			_____

MiniMental LLC

Figure 45–4. Folstein's Mini Mental State Exam. (Copyright 1998, MiniMental LLC.)

TABLE 45–1

Assessing for Underlying Causes of Confusion

Area Tested	Test Used	Implications
Hematological status	• Red blood cell count. • White blood cell count. • Hematocrit level. • Hemoglobin level.	• An elevated white blood cell count is consistent with infection. • Decreased oxygen transport or acute infection may be the cause of acute confusion.
Fluid balance	• Electrolyte tests.	• Electrolyte changes are useful in determining the body's water balance, which can influence mental status.
Renal function	• Blood urea nitrogen. • Creatinine. • Urine culture.	• Because both substances are excreted in urine, changes in their levels can indicate renal dysfunction, a possible cause of confusion. • Bacteria in urine indicates infection, which can lead to confusion. • Confusion may be the only sign of urinary infection in older adults.
Cardiac function	• Electrocardiogram. • Pulse oximetry.	• An altered heart rhythm that reduces cardiac output can cause or contribute to confusion. • Reduced blood oxygen saturation may indicate cerebral hypoxia.
Respiratory function	• Chest x-ray.	• Infections (such as pneumonia), tumors, or tuberculosis may contribute to acute confusion.
Brain injury	• Computed tomography scan.	• This special x-ray technique reveals space occupying lesions (such as tumors), cerebral infarctions, or normal pressure hydrocephalus.
Metabolic function	• Serum glucose level.	• Because the brain requires a steady supply of glucose to function properly, a reduction in blood glucose may affect cognition.
Nutritional status	• Serum vitamin B_{12}. • Folic acid (folate).	• Defective B_{12} absorption may lead to pernicious anemia, degeneration in the spinal cord, and associated neurological symptoms, including confusion. • Defective folate absorption may lead to megaloblastic anemia. • This test is especially helpful for assessing an alcoholic client.
Thyroid function	• Thyroxine (T_4). • Triiodothyronine (T_3). • Thyroid stimulating hormone.	• Cognitive impairment may result from either hypothyroidism or hyperthyroidism.
Tertiary syphilis	• FTA-ABS.	• Tertiary syphilis can cause acute or chronic confusion.
HIV infection	• Enzyme-linked immunosorbent assay.	• Antibodies to human immunodeficiency virus indicate infection; AIDS leads to confusion.
Drug levels	• Alcohol • Medications, including digoxin and antiseizure medications.	• Substances abused or taken as prescribed can lead to toxicity, a possible cause of confusion.

AIDS, acquired immunodeficiency syndrome; FTA-ABS, fluorescent treponemal antibody absorption test; HIV, human immunodeficiency virus.

Focused Assessment for Acute Confusion

Many cases of acute confusion are missed or misdiagnosed by nurses and physicians. It is of vital importance to recognize acute confusion because missing this essential clinical symptom may cause the underlying pathological factors to be left untreated.

Assessment of acute confusion begins with a baseline. This will identify whether cognitive symptoms are a change from previous functioning and how abruptly the change developed. Comparing symptoms to a baseline also helps determine the client's current status.

Recall the case of Mr. Tellis. His daughter reported that his condition began suddenly. This statement suggests acute confusion and warrants further assessment. If he is found to have acute confusion, the underlying causes will need to be identified and treated.

When assessing for acute confusion, stay alert to a variety of cues. The client's inattention and inability to follow simple directions should alert you to consider a working diagnosis of *Acute confusion related to unknown etiology* and pursue further assessment. Other cues may alert you as well. For example, a heavily medicated client may suddenly become incoherent and fearful. A client in the intensive care unit may begin to hallucinate. A newly admitted client may suddenly become incoherent and complain of seeing bugs in the bed when none are present.

As discussed earlier, use a mental status examination, rating scale, or both to help differentiate between acute and chronic confusion, and between confusion and other possible conditions. In an emergent situation, in which the safety of the client or others is threatened, act to prevent injury whether or not you have a complete assessment of the client's confusion.

When possible, perform a general health screen, physical examination, and mental status examination to identify and confirm the nursing diagnosis.

ALERTNESS

When considering the client's reduced alertness or lowered ability to react to important stimuli, rule out such factors as pain, fatigue, and infection. In addition, try to differentiate between the altered alertness of acute confusion and boredom or depression. Notice whether alertness tends to lessen when stimuli are boring or meaningless. Does the client tend to doze off during boring daytime television programs or when other clients have visitors but he does not? Consider whether the client's alertness could be altered because he is focusing on the loss of a spouse or loved one.

ATTENTION SPAN

When considering the client's attention span, differentiate between anxiety and inattention. Notice whether the client is anxious and therefore unable to focus on what you are saying, or whether the client is constantly distracted by seemingly unimportant stimuli. This will help you discriminate between a lack of attention from fear or anxiety and the distractibility of acute confusion. Also notice whether redirecting the client's attention helps him maintain attention and recall the information later. If no recall is present even after redirection, proceed to assess for acute confusion.

Throughout your assessment, maintain a calm attitude and never push the client to attend and recall information if he clearly cannot. Likewise, never embarrass or "quiz" the client about what you said if he seems unable to attend. Instead, begin to develop interventions to maintain safety for a client who cannot attend to important instructions.

ORIENTATION

When considering the client's orientation, identify whether the client is oriented to time, place, and person. If he is disoriented, use environmental cues—such as a calendar or other symbolic cue—to increase his orientation. Also use casual conversation to unobtrusively assess and simultaneously provide reality orientation. These strategies help protect the self-esteem of the disoriented client during assessment. A client's orientation will not help you differentiate between acute and chronic confusion.

THINKING AND LANGUAGE

When considering the client's thinking and language, notice whether the client is having trouble finding words or difficulty understanding their meaning. This would suggest chronic confusion. Also notice whether he is thinking in a disjointed or disorganized manner and speaking incoherently. This would suggest acute confusion.

Recall that the acutely confused client's thinking is impaired. Thus, do not attempt to reason with the client or explain things in detail. If, however, the client's language is impaired but his understanding is intact, talk with the client knowing that the client can understand you. In general, communicate in a simple, clear way. Stay calm and unhurried. Do what you can to reduce distractions. And keep your session short enough to avoid fatiguing the client.

MEMORY

When considering the client's memory, assess which areas of memory may be affected: immediate, short-term, long-term, or a combination. Consider and cluster these characteristics with other data. If the client displays immediate and recent memory loss, assess further for acute confusion. If the client has difficulty with remote and present memory, assess further for chronic confusion.

Perform this assessment in an unobtrusive manner and always with an emphasis on the client's strengths. If the client can only recall very remote events, but seems to enjoy talking, use this strength of remote memory and allow the client to reminisce a short time. This could supply data as well as support client's sense of worth, dignity, and enjoyment.

SLEEP-WAKE CYCLE

When considering the client's sleep-wake cycle, differentiate between acute confusion and night-time restlessness that could stem from pain, anxiety, a medication that disrupts the normal pattern (such as a diuretic), and other possible influences on sleeping and waking.

PSYCHOMOTOR BEHAVIOR

When considering the client's psychomotor behavior, notice the type of behavior you see. For example, if the client is hyperactive or hypoactive, is it related to acute confusion or to the possible inability to coordinate motor behaviors (apraxia) that commonly arises in chronic confusion? Also differentiate between hypervigilance and agitation, a potential indicator of pain or other distress.

Defining Characteristics

Defining characteristics for a client with acute confusion include the following:

- Fluctuation in cognition
- Fluctuation in level of consciousness
- Fluctuation in psychomotor activity
- Fluctuation in sleep-wake cycle
- Hallucinations
- Increased agitation or restlessness
- Lack of motivation to initiate and/or follow through with goal-directed or purposeful behavior
- Misperceptions

Related Factors

Some of the factors commonly related to acute confusion are old age, alcohol abuse, delirium, dementia, and drug abuse. However, a wide range of disorders and conditions can be associated with this acute confusion. Indeed, several different factors may be present in a single client.

Acute confusion may be influenced by changes in cerebral metabolism, oxygenation, systemic infections, metabolic disorders (such as hypoxia, hypercarbia, and hypoglycemia), fluid or electrolyte imbalances, hepatic or renal disease, thiamine deficiency, postoperative states, hypertensive encephalopathy, postictal states, and head trauma or brain lesions (American Psychiatric Association, 1994, p. 128). Others include chronic illness, severe illness, fever, polypharmacy, and hospitalization (Foreman, 1993).

Populations at risk for acute confusion are young children, elderly persons, cognitively impaired persons, post-surgical persons, or elderly persons hospitalized for surgery or severe medical illness. Clearly, the elderly are more vulnerable to acute confusion because of altered physiology with aging and the high incidence of risk factors.

Facilitating factors contribute to the development of acute confusion, but have not been proven to actually cause acute confusion. The most common facilitating factors are sensory impairment and environmental and personal conditions (Table 45–2).

Focused Assessment for Chronic Confusion

Recall that memory loss occurs with chronic confusion. Assess the client's short-term memory, or ability to learn, by determining whether he can remember three objects after 5 minutes have passed. Assess long-term memory impairment by determining his ability to remember past personal information, such as what happened yesterday, his birthplace, his occupation, and events considered to be common knowledge. Take care to adjust for differences in the person's ability to answer questions based on sensory impairment, culture, educational level, or age.

To assess problem-solving or judgment, consider the client's ability to deal with family and staff interpersonally, to problem-solve, and to handle safety issues with insight. Ask the client what he would do if a certain event occurred, such as a fire starting in a wastebasket.

Also assess the client's ability to recognize and use written symbols, such as those you might use for orientation cues. Keep in mind that some clients are unable to read not because of chronic confusion but because of illiteracy or the size of the print.

Defining Characteristics

Chronic confusion may occur so insidiously that it is often difficult to identify. Plus, the intellectual losses can be hidden and compensated for, at least initially. At first, memory loss is mild. The client may forget where he put his keys or wallet, for example. Eventually, the loss becomes severe and extends into the client's long-term memory. Personality changes and poor judgment may occur. The client also may exhibit a loss of language abilities or aphasia.

Specific defining characteristics for chronic confusion include the following:

- Altered interpretation of or response to stimuli
- Altered personality
- Clinical evidence of organic impairment
- Impaired short-term and long-term memory
- Impaired socialization
- No change in level of consciousness
- Progressive or long-standing cognitive impairment

Related Factors

More than 60 diseases and related factors have been associated with chronic confusion, including multi-infarct dementia, Korsakoff's psychosis, head injury, Alzheimer's disease, and cerebrovascular accident. Two major processes are evident in its development:

- Primary chronic confusion results from primary pathological changes in the brain. Alzheimer's disease and vascular dementia are examples of primary dementia.
- Secondary chronic confusion results from factors outside the brain, such as metabolic and nutritional disorders and other diseases.

Focused Assessment for Related Nursing Diagnoses

Other nursing diagnoses that might be associated with acute and chronic confusion are numerous. Below are nursing diagnoses frequently used for clients with *Acute confusion* and/or *Chronic confusion.*

Impaired Environmental Interpretation Syndrome

Impaired environmental interpretation syndrome is defined as a consistent lack of orientation to person, place, time, or circumstances over more than 3 to 6 months, necessitating a protective environment (NANDA, 1999). This diagnosis is used with clients in the later stages of chronic confusion. Usually, they have irreversible dementia.

This diagnosis indicates that the client needs a protective environment because his profound chronic confusion places him at risk for injury. Initiate plans to secure a protective environment for the client. Try to maintain the client's dignity and the maximum level of independence possible. Develop a long-term plan for the client that is coordinated with family and other agencies. The client may be discharged to a secure long-term care unit for memory-impaired people.

Altered Thought Processes

Altered thought processes is defined as a state in which an individual experiences a disruption in cognitive operations and activities (NANDA, 1999). Activities such as conscious thought, reality orientation, problem-solving, judgment, and comprehension are impaired. However, this diagnosis pertains to changes caused by alterations in coping, personality, and/or mental disor-

TABLE 45-2
Common Factors Related to Acute Confusion

Because of the vast number of factors that can be related to acute confusion, this table presents categories and examples.

Category	Examples
Primary brain disturbance or impairment	Trauma Tumor
Cerebral hypoxia and/or disturbance in cerebral metabolism secondary to a medical condition	Fluid and electrolyte imbalance • Dehydration. • Acidosis or alkalosis. • Hypoglycemia or hyperglycemia. Nutritional deficiency Cardiovascular disorder • Myocardial infarction. • Arrhythmia. • Heart failure. Respiratory disorder • Chronic obstructive pulmonary disease. • Tuberculosis. • Pneumonia. Infection • Urinary tract infection. • Meningitis. Metabolic or endocrine disorder • Hypothyroidism. • Postural hypotension. • Hyperthermia or hypothermia. • Hepatic or renal failure. Rheumatoid or collagen disease
Cerebral hypoxia and/or disturbance in cerebral metabolism secondary to a treatment	Surgery (a high risk for hospitalized elderly clients)
Cerebral hypoxia and/or disturbance in cerebral metabolism secondary to a medication	Intoxication or allergy reaction to therapeutic drug use • Neuroleptic. • Narcotic. Side effects of medications • Anti-anxiety agents. • Anticholinergics. • Anti-inflammatory agents. • Atropine. • Barbiturates. • Digitalis. • Diuretics. • Lithium. • Over-the-counter cold, cough, sleeping, and some eye medications. • Phenothiazines. • Propranolol.
Chemical intoxication	Alcohol Sedative agent Hypnotic agent Heavy metal Carbon monoxide
Chemical withdrawal	Alcohol Cocaine Amphetamine Opiate Barbiturate
Contributory or facilitative factors	Pain Immobility Postoperative stress Sleep deprivation Lack of meaningful stimuli Sensory overload

Information from Judd, C. R. (1996). Delirium or dementia? Making a clinically important distinction. JAAPA, 9(4), 24–41; Foreman, M., Fletcher, K., Mion, L., Simon, L., & the NICHE Faculty (1996). Assessing cognitive function. Geriatric Nursing, 17(5), 228–232; Carpenito, L. J. [1997]. Handbook of Nursing Diagnosis (7th ed.). Philadelphia: J. B. Lippincott.

ders. Thus, it may be more clinically useful in psychiatric settings, where the client has difficulty with reality as opposed to being acutely or chronically confused.

Impaired Memory

Impaired memory is defined as the state in which an individual experiences the inability to remember or recall bits of information or behavioral skills (NANDA, 1999). The client may have deficits in recent or remote memory and may not be able to recall past or present events. Impaired memory may be related to hypoxia, anemia, fluid and electrolyte imbalances, or neurological disturbances, some of which may be reversible. This diagnosis may be used with a confused client; however, it is less useful in terms of outcomes.

Anxiety

Anxiety is a common response to confusion of all types. Anxiety develops because the client is disoriented, unable to grasp or make sense of what is happening, and usually concerned about safety. When understanding eludes the confused client, he may become severely anxious because he does not know where he is or why things are so disorganized or disturbed.

Acute confusion commonly includes frightening perceptual distortions and hallucinations. These change frequently, which tends to heighten anxiety since there seems to be no stability or logical way to understand or control the situation. When faced with frightening visions, feelings, or thoughts, the client may become terrified.

Depending on the type of confusion involved, the client may feel himself falling, confronting animals, or opposing people who would harm him. A restless, agitated client who pulls at bandages or tries to escape from visual hallucinations may experience terror and injury. Anxiety escalates as terror and unreal experiences increase (see Chapter 47).

Hopelessness

As previously stated, hopelessness is frequently seen in early chronic confusion if the person is aware of his losses, disabilities, and the expected progression of the disease. The person may begin to make strides in dealing with some disability only to develop further disabilities. Hopelessness may occur if the client assumes that there is no hope of stopping the progressive deterioration. As memory fails, hopelessness tends to disappear because the client does not remember the situation and the losses (see Chapter 48).

Powerlessness

Powerlessness is common in the chronically confused client, also in the early stages of decline. Failing memory and awareness of the progressive deterioration give the sense of loss of control. The strain to function and perform despite the deterioration commonly overwhelms the client with powerlessness and frus-

tration. Such overwhelming powerlessness and frustration also occur in clients in the later stages of chronic confusion because the stress threshold is much lower.

Powerlessness for the client who is acutely confused is often extreme. There is terror as the person feels a sense of invasion and loss of control. This is magnified in clients who have perceptual distortion and hallucinations (see Chapter 48).

Risk for Injury

Risk for injury is a major factor to consider because of the client's lack of judgment and insufficient recall of safety precautions. Acutely confused clients can pull out intravenous lines or catheters, tear or pick at bandages, climb over side rails, wander into dangerous areas, lash out at others, and harm themselves through catastrophic episodes. Frequently, clients in later stages of chronic confusion who are also depressed may harm themselves severely. Clients also may not be aware of actual hazards and may be harmed in numerous ways. In addition, a large number of confused clients are elderly and at risk for falls. An unsteady gait, failing sight or hearing, and decreased functioning may present hazards and potential injury (see Chapter 28).

Altered Nutrition

Nutrition is an essential aspect of care for the confused client, who may not eat at regular intervals or may not eat at all. The constant wandering associated with the middle stages of chronic confusion may increase the client's metabolic needs and lead to weight loss. As chronic confusion progresses, the person may forget how to feed himself and finally how to chew and swallow (see Chapter 30).

Fluid Volume Deficit

Dehydration may occur in clients who forget to replenish fluids, sweat profusely, or suffer from loss of fluid. This is a major problem in later stages of chronic confusion when clients become aphasic. The client will be unable to tell you that he is thirsty or to indicate his need for fluids. In addition, he may not be able or willing to drink fluids by himself. He must have someone else attend to his need for fluids. Attending to fluid intake and monitoring output in clients with later stages of chronic confusion is essential (see Chapter 31).

Mr. Tellis has skin tenting on his sternum and forehead, cloudy concentrated urine, and dry scaly skin on his lower legs. These indicate decreased total body water. Did you identify them as factors that could be contributing to the client's confusion? Fluid intake of 1,500 to 1,800 mL each day is necessary to ensure adequate hydration and maintain fluid balance.

Caregiver Role Strain

Most clients with chronic confusion receive care at home, at least early in the disease. Often, the caretaker goes to great lengths to keep the person at home. Family members, especially those who provide direct client care, are important to consider. The family must be considered as a unit, with needs beyond those specific to the client.

Take steps to enable family members to carry on with other roles of work, family, and society. Work to protect them from losing their financial, health, and emotional resources. Make them aware of resources available to help them care for the client. And include them in planning the client's care (see Chapters 53 and 54). The Teaching for Self Care chart gives specific suggestions to caregivers about how to provide care to a confused family member.

Other Diagnoses

As chronic confusion continues into later stages, the client's deterioration involves other systems. For example, elimination, respiratory patterns, and tissue perfusion may become essential points of focus. The last stages of chronic confusion involve numerous systems and complex nursing care.

DIAGNOSIS

Arriving at the most appropriate nursing diagnosis for a confused client primarily involves identifying the type of confusion present. The client may have acute confusion, chronic confusion, or both. If both types are present, related factors, goals, outcomes, and interven-

tions for each factor must be identified. If no etiology is found, use the nursing diagnosis *Confusion related to unknown etiology.* The accompanying data clustering chart gives examples.

Differentiating Between Acute and Chronic Confusion

Acute confusion and chronic confusion differ widely, as follows:

- Acute confusion usually occurs abruptly over a few hours or days; chronic confusion usually develops insidiously over a period of years.
- Acute confusion causes fluctuations in consciousness or alertness, often at night; chronic confusion progresses steadily with no diurnal effects.
- Acute confusion causes reduced awareness with lucid intervals; chronic confusion does not affect consciousness.
- Acute confusion reduces the client's attention; chronic confusion does not.
- Acute confusion causes disorganized thinking and incoherent language; chronic confusion typically causes aphasia.
- Acute confusion causes disturbed perception, hallucinations, frightening misperceptions, and dreams; chronic confusion causes no hallucinations until late in the course of the illness.
- Acute confusion profoundly disturbs and usually

Teaching for SELF-CARE

EFFECTIVE CAREGIVING FOR A CONFUSED CLIENT

Purpose: To help a caregiver know how to care for a confused client at home.

Rationale: Caregivers often feel isolated and unprepared to care for a confused loved one.

Expected Outcome: The caregiver will express satisfaction with her ability to manage the client's care.

Caregiver Instructions

When caring for a confused person, use the following techniques to help keep the person oriented and calm:

- Display calendars and clocks around the house and in the client's room.
- Maintain a predictable routine.
- Limit the number of visitors who come to see the client.
- Limit the number of choices given to the client.
- Use simple, clear communication.
- Avoid the use of words such as *don't* or *can't* when communicating.
- Make mealtime a pleasant experience.

- Place the client in an upright position during meals to prevent aspiration.
- Toilet the client frequently.
- If the client wants to pace, allow him to do so in a safe, secure area.
- Make sure the client carries or wears medical identification in case he wanders.
- Redirect the client if he displays inappropriate behaviors.
- Keep harmful substances (such as cleaning supplies and medicines) in a locked cabinet.
- Make use of local and national resources, including online services. Resources may include adult day care, a support group, the Alzheimer's Disease and Related Disorders Association at (800) 272-3900, and others.
- Turn the lights on at dusk to avoid the *sundown syndrome* of increased confusion and combative behavior.
- Reduce stress and obtain respite when needed.
- Avoid catastrophic behaviors.
- Take care of yourself. Laugh often and much!

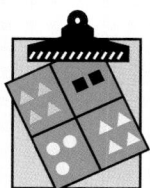

CLUSTERING DATA TO MAKE A NURSING DIAGNOSIS
CONFUSION

Data Cluster	Diagnosis
An 88-year-old female client takes multiple medications, including those with anticholinergic side effects. Exhibits symptoms of inattention and fluctuations in consciousness.	*Acute Confusion* related to disturbance in cerebral metabolism secondary to side effects of multiple drugs taken daily
A 59-year-old man with history of alcoholism sees animals in the room and insects crawling on his skin.	*Acute Confusion* related to disturbance in cerebral metabolism secondary to withdrawal from alcohol
Family reports that 79-year-old woman has loss of language ability, memory of family members, and ability to recognize body parts.	*Chronic Confusion* related to progressive degeneration of the cerebral cortex secondary to Alzheimer's disease

reverses the client's sleep cycle; chronic confusion may cause fragmented sleep but no diurnal reversal.

- Acute confusion may be associated with hyperarousal, hypoarousal, or both; chronic confusion causes no major changes in arousal.
- Acute confusion reduces immediate and recent memory; chronic confusion reduces recent and remote memory.

Differentiating Between Confusion and Depression

Confusion should be differentiated from depression because depression can be treated. Distinctive features of depression are listed below. Remember that depression can sometimes coexist with one or both types of confusion.

- Depression tends to arise with or after a significant life change, usually a loss.
- Depression tends to be worse in the morning.
- A depressed person usually seems sad or despondent and is keenly aware of feeling a major deficit in self-esteem.
- A depressed person tends to focus his attention on himself and particularly on his inabilities, which he may exaggerate.
- In depression, the person can recall small islands of memory upon which great attention is focused. The person may appear to be inattentive but can be called back to selective topics of preoccupation. Frequently, depressed clients may answer, "I don't know," or exaggerate their defects.
- Depression causes visual hallucinations infrequently.
- In the depressed person, patterns of hyperactivity or hypoactivity usually are related to the feelings being experienced at the time.

PLANNING

Expected Outcomes for the Client With Acute Confusion

The expected outcome for acute confusion is that the client is free of episodes of confusion. The etiology is identified and treated and the confusion resolves. Recurrent episodes of acute confusion are avoided by incorporating primary prevention measures into the plan of care. For example, primary prevention is incorporated by setting such goals as, "the client at risk will list medications known to influence the development of acute confusion." In this way, the client can avoid future episodes of confusion.

Expected Outcomes for the Client With Chronic Confusion

The expected outcomes for the client with chronic confusion are varied and depend on the signs and symptoms manifested. A few examples are that the client has decreased episodes of combative behavior, that he maintains the recommended body weight, that he maintains a fluid intake of 1,500 to 1,800 mL daily, and that he stays free of infection.

INTERVENTION

Numerous supportive interventions can be used to achieve these general goals and outcomes. Some of the most common interventions are highlighted in the following sections. The fundamental belief of nursing, which acknowledges every client as a person with worth and dignity, is inextricably woven into the care of the confused client. You will identify major goals, client outcomes, and interventions specifically individualized for the confused client.

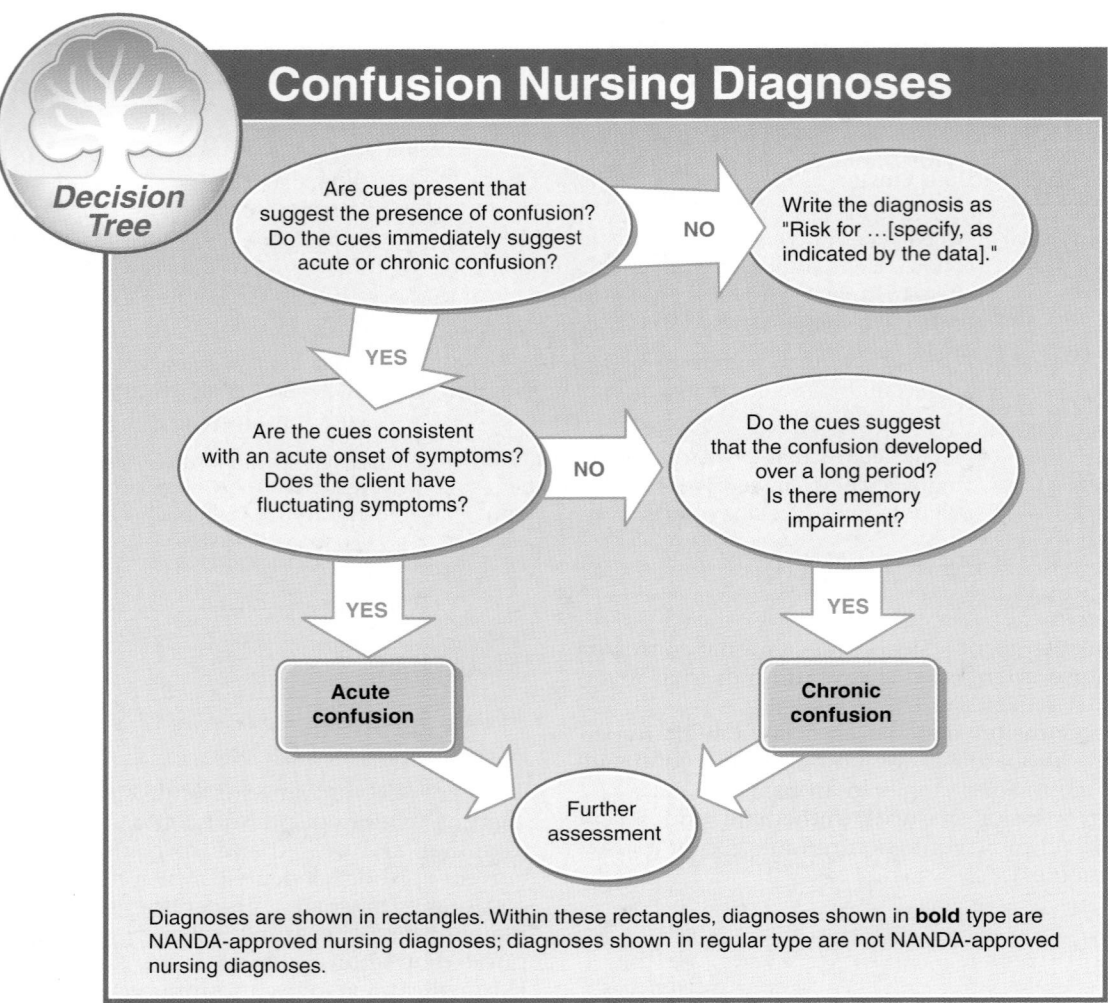

Confusion Nursing Diagnoses

Decision Tree

Are cues present that suggest the presence of confusion? Do the cues immediately suggest acute or chronic confusion? — **NO** → Write the diagnosis as "Risk for ...[specify, as indicated by the data]."

YES

Are the cues consistent with an acute onset of symptoms? Does the client have fluctuating symptoms? — **NO** → Do the cues suggest that the confusion developed over a long period? Is there memory impairment?

YES → **Acute confusion**

YES → **Chronic confusion**

Further assessment

Diagnoses are shown in rectangles. Within these rectangles, diagnoses shown in **bold** type are NANDA-approved nursing diagnoses; diagnoses shown in regular type are not NANDA-approved nursing diagnoses.

Interventions to Prevent Confusion

General goals when caring for a confused client encompass a variety of aspects, beginning with primary prevention. Interventions to prevent confusion include, among other things, education provided to health care professionals, families, and clients at high risk. Education to aid prevention might include risk factors, early warning symptoms, and preventive health maintenance procedures, such as nutrition and elimination.

Teaching the Client at High Risk

Educating nurses, health care personnel, and persons at risk about the early signs of confusion and methods to assess confusion can do much to aid its early recognition. Careful assessment as well as documentation of the client's behavior is important and should be done in a way that aids the clustering of important risk factors, defining characteristics, and data for differential diagnosis. Since many clients with confusion are elderly, consider the special needs and reactions of the elderly. For example, remember that even a slight elevation of temperature in the elderly is considered serious.

Providing Preoperative Screening and Education

Recognizing and applying interventions to eliminate postoperative confusion is imperative. Recognize such related factors as sepsis, hypothermia, or drug side effects so that treatment can begin immediately.

Preadmission education sessions for elders undergoing surgery are helpful if they identify the possibility of and the need to report unusual or strange experiences after surgery. Such preadmission education allows clients to bring early warning signs to your attention as soon as possible. You can then assess promptly and initiate appropriate treatment for acute confusion. This is especially helpful for elders undergoing cardiac surgery or surgery secondary to hip fracture, where acute confusion is common.

Monitoring Medication Use

Attention to medications and their possible side effects and interactions should be emphasized, especially for clients who are elderly (Box 45–4). Assess for the use of medications known to cause confusion at the time the client is admitted, especially with a person at risk for confusion. Note the types and numbers of medications, both prescription and OTC. In addition, monitor and identify any long-term substance use, including caffeine, nicotine, alcohol, and other drugs. Abrupt withdrawal of alcohol in a person with an established habit commonly causes acute confusion.

Minimizing Sensory Impairment

Minimize sensory impairment by making sure that the client is using all of the aids he needs for vision, hearing, and mobility. Frequently, clients are thought to be listless and hypoalert when they are merely unable to see or hear. Clients should have clean, well-fitting glasses of the proper prescription, hearing aids with working batteries, and canes or walkers that they know how to use.

Interventions to Manage Confusion

An essential nursing action is to facilitate optimal functioning to the peak of possible health. You can help the client manage his confusion by identifying strengths that may aid his achievement of goals and outcomes. Promote respect and self-esteem at all times.

Helping the Client Maintain Dignity

You can help the client maintain dignity by not equating aging with confusion. Provide care at the level the client needs while creatively taking his strengths and abilities into account. Provide comfort and a calming atmosphere in an individualized manner. Remember that confusion can make the client feel powerless or anxious; respect should be a driving force in your actions and goals.

Orientation is important for the client's sense of integrity and meaningful interpretation of the environment. When providing reality orientation, always do so in a way that promotes the client's dignity. Instead of correcting his disorientation in a way that embarrasses or frustrates him, provide information in a matter-of-fact manner or naturally and subtly as part of your conversation with him. For example, identify yourself and your reason for approaching him because doing so will provide orientation without forcing the client to constantly admit his memory deficit.

BOX 45–4

CLIENT TEACHING TIPS: ADMINISTERING MEDICATIONS SAFELY

Especially for older adults, medications and confusion may go hand in hand. This is in part because of the number of medications taken by most older people. Americans over age 65 represent about 12% of the population, but they consume about 30% of all prescription medications and 40% of all over-the-counter medications. The average older person has 12 to 17 prescriptions filled each year (Drake & Romano, 1995, p. 35).

Besides taking a larger number of drugs than younger people, older adults tend to see a larger number of doctors, go to multiple pharmacies, have some level of visual impairment, not have enough money to purchase all the medications they need, and be less able to manage the complex dosing schedules required when taking several medications at once. This combination of risk factors requires some extra effort on your part to help clients and their families manage medication regimens to achieve the best results with the lowest risk of confusion, drug interactions, and dangers.

Cover the following points when teaching clients about medication administration. And make sure to include appropriate family members and caregivers as needed.

- Make sure the client knows the names of each medication (generic as well as trade names) and the reasons for taking them.

- Explain the dose, route, and duration of each medication.
- Teach the client how to take each medication properly.
- Tell the client what to do if he misses a dose.
- Outline the possible side effects of each medication, and which side effects should prompt a call to the doctor.
- Help the client develop a written medication schedule and a method for remembering to take each medication. Use a medication calendar, for example, different-size pill containers, a multichambered medication dispensing box, or even an empty egg carton.
- Advise the client to discard expired medications.
- Warn the client against giving prescription medications to others or taking someone else's prescribed medication.
- Recommend that the client use only one pharmacy to avoid duplicating a medication and to lower the risk of drug interactions.
- Provide information on cost-saving programs if appropriate.
- If necessary, advise the client to wear or carry information that lists the medications he takes.
- Reinforce the importance of adequate hydration and nutrition for optimum pharmacokinetics.
- Educate the client about the interactions of alcohol and prescription or over-the-counter medications.

Promoting a Safe Environment

Safety is an essential aspect of intervention for the confused client. Assess any confused client for a risk for injury and then plan goals, outcomes, and interventions that relate specifically to him. Consider many factors when assessing his potential for falls and injuries, such as restless behavior, an inability to recall safety precautions, or an inability to judge dangerous situations. Plan your care appropriately to reduce risks.

Disorientation to time, place, and person requires interventions for safety as well. Restlessness and agitation can also be safety hazards. A differential diagnosis of possible pain or anxiety should be considered if the client is agitated or restless. Providing room for the client to pace or wander may be important in lowering his anxiety or restlessness.

Provide orientation cues by using bright colors or symbols to identify rooms, bathrooms, or meeting places to help prevent disorientation and increase safety. Notice what tends to orient, calm, or provide comfort to the client. For example, a religious object or picture may calm one client, while holding something comforting may calm another.

Large, uncluttered areas tend to promote safety for most confused clients. Cluttered or crowded areas tend to overstimulate. In addition, large areas are commonly needed to safely accommodate the canes, walkers, and wheelchairs clients may require for mobility.

Providing clients with freedom to move, while preventing them from wandering off the unit, crawling over side rails, or otherwise being injured will be ongoing challenges for you as a nurse. Using a bed with an alarm, a sitter, or a family member in close proximity may be helpful in providing safety. Use restraints as infrequently as possible; they commonly escalate the client's anxiety and combativeness.

Also attend to specific safety problems created by the client's medical condition. For example, if a client has lead poisoning, make sure he has no further exposure to lead. Try to identify the source of lead in his environment. Astute history taking is a valuable tool to uncover the source of lead and eradicate the problem. Interventions to prevent lead poisoning in children also include universal screening based on the guidelines set forth by the Centers for Disease Control and Prevention.

Encouraging Independence

Promote independent functioning by helping the client accomplish activities of daily living to the fullest extent possible. Provide the client with needed materials, and encourage him to do what he can independently. Then help him with the tasks that he cannot accomplish on his own. Divide activities into small steps to avoid overwhelming and frustrating the client. Provide frequent cues of tasks to be done, and give him enough time to accomplish them. Balance the benefit of allowing the client to manage some aspects of his own care against his stress threshold and capability.

Providing Appropriate Stimulation

Cookman (1996) has examined the importance of attachments to health and well-being. Attachments to people, objects, places, beliefs, and pets can all be used to maintain meaning in a client's life, especially an older client.

Meaningful stimulation is important to engage the client in living with dignity and integrity. For chronically confused clients, stimulation must be individualized and balanced with the client's capability, strengths, and interest. Try to identify objects and events that are meaningful to the client. Coordinate his emotional bonds, interests, and abilities with his activities. Make the health care environment meaningful for the client by allowing family members to bring pictures or objects that are familiar and comforting. Include beliefs that are meaningful to the client in his daily life and care. Commonly, religious beliefs and ceremonies provide significant meaning. Encourage the client's family and friends to visit and to include the client in family news and events to the extent that the client is capable of participating.

It is important to respect the client and provide him with a sense of self and integrity. Call the client by name and do not infantilize or embarrass the client in any way. Be aware of and use special objects or procedures that provide the client with an enhanced sense of self or comfort. Try to achieve a fine balance between allowing the client independence to make choices and overwhelming the client with unrealistic expectations.

Provide a routine and a consistent physical environment. Simple familiar patterns decrease stress. Limit the number of choices if this tends to overstimulate the client. Use symbols other than written signs to help the client locate bathrooms or dining rooms, especially if he has trouble reading. Also use environmental cues, such as clocks, calendars, and seasonal pictures to help maintain the client's sense of orientation to time. Use light to eradicate shadows and minimize misperceptions or perceptual distortions.

Use activities that encourage socialization and communication to promote self-esteem and meaning for the client. Use reminiscence and life review to help the client maintain a sense of worth and integrity. Activities and exercises that are nontaxing can be healthy and invigorating as well. Music therapy tends to have a soothing effect. Often, activities that involve working with the hands provide enjoyment while helping to keep the joints mobile.

Validation therapy is often used to help confused clients identify the meaning of situations. The personal meaning of each situation for the client is identified and "validated" within this therapy. Group work and group education are other ways to include the client in socialization that is motivating and empathetic.

Take care to eliminate overstimulation for both acutely and chronically confused clients. Overstimulation can overtax the client and cause frustration or disorientation. Such overstimulation may arise from competing stimuli, such as meaningless noise, the din of the intercom, an unwatched television, and traffic in the hallway. Also, try not to overstimulate the client by expecting and encouraging him to do more than he can. Such frustration can overwhelm his stress and emotional threshold. In some cases, you may need to move the client to another area to reduce stimulation and provide an opportunity for needed rest or sleep. When possible, assign the same staff members to work with the client so he can become familiar with the staff and the environment.

The client's confusion may also require other interventions to orient him to your presence or activities. For example, you may need to announce yourself when entering a room to avoid startling the client. Remember that the client may not recall why you are in his room, where he is, or why he is there. Always establish eye contact before touching the client.

Promoting Therapeutic Communication

Communication that helps promote dignity and integrity and establish a meaningful environment is especially important for clients with perceptual difficulties. Communication should be clear and simple yet respectful. Wait, and allow the client the time needed to communicate, walk, and perform activities.

Paying attention to the concern and message embedded in the client's communication will help you focus on the true meaning of the communication. If the client tends to misperceive you as a familiar person, such as a sister, you can reorient the client. However, rather than constantly correcting the client, attend to the deeper message in the client's communication. For example, you can reflect a question to the client, "Are you thinking about your sister?" Thus, without confirming the client's disorientation, you can focus on his remote memory—a strength—and allow the client to reminisce. In this way, you give the client an opportunity to talk about his deeper concern, such as missing his sister or feeling alone.

Even when a client is obviously having a hallucination, pay attention to the meaning and concern of his thoughts. This attention to the deeper meaning and concern can do much to maintain self-esteem, calm the client, and provide a more meaningful environment. For example, if the client misperceives a closet door as a dangerous person, attend not only to the need to arrange the room to prevent that misperception, but to the need to calm the client's concern about safety. Often with acute confusion, the types of hallucinations provide hints of client difficulties. One acutely confused client who hallucinated that her blood was turning to powder later expressed extreme gratitude to the nurse who assessed her for dehydration and provided appropriate intervention.

Avoiding Catastrophic Incidents

You may recall that catastrophic behaviors are combative, compulsive, violent behaviors. The chronically confused client may exhibit these behaviors in response to overwhelming stress and a lowered stress threshold. Because the threshold drops as chronic confusion progresses, catastrophic incidents become more likely as the client's confusion worsens.

Triggers are stressors that stimulate this behavior. Triggers are individualized and should be identified individually for each person. They tend to include fatigue, expectations that exceed the person's capabilities, overstimulation, and changes in routine or environment.

The Progressively Lowered Stress Threshold model is a conceptual model for the care of adults with Alzheimer's disease. It was designed by Gerdner, Buckwalter, Hall and associates (1996) to reduce stress by modifying environmental demands and promoting adaptive behavior. Catastrophic incidents and highly stimulating environments may produce stressful situations.

Avoid catastrophic incidents by preventing fatigue, overstimulation, or changes in routine or environment. Structure the environment—with soft music and consistent caregivers, for example—to ensure that the client is not stimulated into these violent, compulsive, combative outbursts. In addition, make sure that such outbursts are not precursors of further illness or actually signs and symptoms of acute confusion.

Interventions to Reduce Caregiver Role Strain

Consideration of family members and other caregivers is an essential aspect of caring for a confused client (Fig. 45–5). The strain of caring for a confused person while carrying on daily lives and attending to multiple roles can quickly exhaust financial, physical, and emotional resources. When you arrange for the care and discharge of the client, take into account not only the needs of the client, but the capabilities of the family and caretakers. Involve family members throughout the client's care.

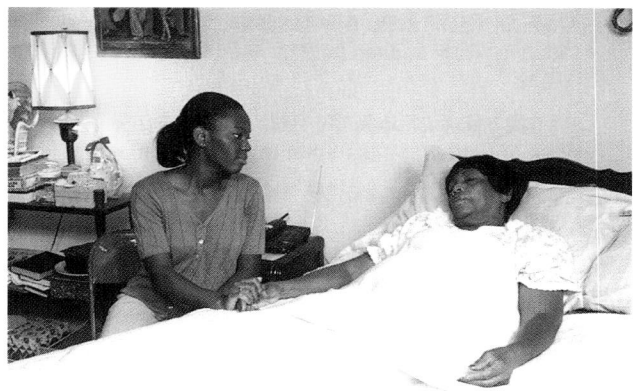

Figure 45–5. Considering the needs of supportive caregivers is an essential aspect of caring for a confused client.

Provide education, resources, information, and support for persons attempting to provide care for the client. Consider the needs and include the input from all those involved as a necessary part of discharge planning. Help family members consider their need for additional resources to prevent exhaustion. Ongoing education, input into planning, availability to answer questions, and mobilization of needed resources are important supports for families (see Chapters 53 and 54). Refer back to the Teaching for Self-Care Chart for information helpful for caregivers.

A positive attitude on your part about age and culture is important when planning home care, institutional care, or discharge for the confused client. Family members often take their cues from your expectations and attitudes. Try to understand the cultural beliefs of the client and family. Culture tends to determine how aging and confusion are viewed, how the confused person is treated, and what expectations about the client and family will be used after discharge, as suggested in the Cross-Cultural Care chart.

EVALUATION

Evaluation is done by determining whether client outcomes have been met, as shown in the accompanying Nursing Care Planning chart. A confused client may change constantly, which requires ongoing assessment. Characteristics, nursing actions, and client needs change as the client's condition changes. With acute confusion, the client develops the condition relatively abruptly. Rapid, appropriate action and continuous assessment is needed. Recognition and appropriate treatment of underlying factors can often reverse acute confusion. Nursing care of acute confusion is evaluated by the recognition, treatment, and reversal of an underlying etiology that in turn reverses the effects of confusion.

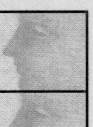

CROSS-CULTURAL CARE
CARING FOR A GREEK-AMERICAN CLIENT

Mr. Tellis, the client whose story we have been following in this chapter, is of Greek descent. He came to the United States as an adolescent in 1929 with his parents and siblings with the hope that America would offer an opportunity to build a rewarding life. He adheres to Greek cultural beliefs and has ties to a large extended family of children, brothers, sisters, and cousins. He is typical of immigrant Greeks of that time, because he has limited formal education but a strong work ethic, determination, and ethnic pride. Although every client is unique, many Greek-Americans have a tendency to hold the following views and values:

- A view of doctors and hospitals as a last resort.
- Living independently.
- Self-reliance and a sense of freedom and self-worth.
- Greater reliance on family for health care and advice than on health care professionals.
- Staying with a sick person rather than leaving him alone.

Let's see how Elizabeth, Mr. Tellis' nurse, recognizes these values and incorporates them in a conversation:

Elizabeth: Good morning Mr. Tellis. How are you feeling today?

Mr. Tellis: I'm fine, nothing wrong with me. My daughter can take me home today and take care of me. I'm strong, I just need to go to my home.

Elizabeth: I can see that you are much improved over yesterday. You are standing tall and walking with only a little assistance. Your family, your doctor, and all of your health care providers would like to understand what happened to you before you came into the hospital so that future occurrences might be avoided. Would you tell us what you were feeling before you got sick?

Mr. Tellis: I'm so ashamed because I don't remember much. I'm not losing my mind, am I? All I can say is that it started to burn when I passed my water, and it felt like I had to go all the time, but couldn't. This was going on for about a week!

Elizabeth: [Demonstrating cultural sensitivity of the social stigma of mental illness, Elizabeth tries to allay Mr. Tellis' fears of mental illness.] It must have been very frightening for you and your family to have this happen. Let me talk with your daughter and tell you about the reasons for the illness, so that future episodes might be avoided.

Critical Thinking Questions

- What cultural values does Mr. Tellis demonstrate in regard to physical illness?
- What reasons might account for the fact that Mr. Tellis' infection went unnoticed for several days?
- How does the significance of family life fit into your discharge teaching plan for Mr. Tellis?
- What community support referrals might the nurse recommend to Mr. Tellis and his family?

Reference

Tripp-Reimer, T., & Sorofman, B. (1998). Greek Americans. In L. Purnell & B. Paulanka. *Transcultural health care: A culturally competent approach.* Philadelphia: F. A. Davis.

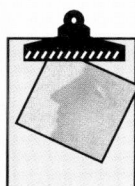

NURSING CARE PLANNING
A CONFUSED CLIENT

Admission Data

Mr. Tellis is admitted from the emergency department to a day unit until the cause of his acute confusion is established. He arrives at the unit with the following summation:

Mr. Tellis is an 83-year-old white male in no acute distress. Intravenous fluid started left antecubital, 1,000 D₅RL at 75 mL/hr due to dehydrated status. Monitor for fluid overload every hour. Preliminary urine report suggests urinary tract infection with sepsis. Ampicillin 2 g q6h started at 0900. Foley catheter in place to closely monitor output. ECG and routine chest x-ray to be done on admission to the unit as these systems seem to be uninvolved. Will be examined by attending MD upon admission to your unit. A decision to proceed with a CT scan to rule out brain pathology will be made then.

Physician's Orders	Admitting diagnosis: confusion secondary to urinary tract infection IV 1000 D₅RL at 75 mL/hr Vital signs q4h Ampicillin 2 g IVPB q6h	Intake and output q4h Repeat electrolytes and CBC 4 hours after IV has infused Chest x-ray, rule out pneumonia ECG, rule out ischemic changes

Nursing Assessment

No acute distress. Awake and alert. Denies pain, shortness of breath, or difficulty breathing. Mini-mental state exam repeated with a score of 24, same as in the emergency department. IV patent and infusing as ordered. Lungs sound clear, no jugular vein distention, and no edema to suggest fluid overload. Temperature is 97.0°F orally, but will continue to monitor frequently since elderly do not always show elevated temperature with infection. BP 140/80 lying, orthostatic BP deferred because client stated he was "dizzy" when he stood an hour ago in emergency department. Foley catheter draining concentrated urine, 350 mL. Oriented to room, call bell given to client with instruction and demonstration on how to use it. Daughter instructed to call for nurse if client becomes confused and tries getting out of bed without nurse.

NURSING CARE PLAN

Nursing Diagnosis	Expected Outcomes	Interventions	Evaluation (After 24 Hours of Care)
Acute Confusion related to disturbance in cerebral metabolism secondary to urinary tract infection as evidenced by agitation, inattention, fluctuating consciousness	Client will experience no injury	Structure the client's environment to ensure safety: • Keep side rails up when client is in bed. • Keep room and walkways uncluttered. • Assign client a room near the nurses' station. • Allow sitter or family member to stay with client (since client is unable to use call bell). • Assist client with ambulation and toileting as needed. • Monitor side effects of medications. • Keep dangerous objects out of reach.	• No injury occurs. • Family taking turns sitting with client around the clock.

Continued

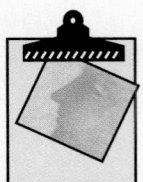

NURSING CARE PLANNING
A CONFUSED CLIENT *(continued)*

NURSING CARE PLAN *(continued)*

Nursing Diagnosis	Expected Outcomes	Interventions	Evaluation (After 24 Hours of Care)
		• Make sure client has glasses, dentures, hearing aids, and all other needed aids. • Send a staff member with client to other areas of the hospital (to tests, for example).	
	Client will experience no confusion	Provide meaningful communication to maintain reality orientation and sense of integrity and dignity: • Orient subtly and frequently, as needed. • Provide individualized attention from one nurse. • Assign the same nurses to provide client's care. • *Allow client to have personal belongings that aid orientation and calm, such as jewelry (culturally valued by Greek-Americans) pictures, etc.* • Use simple, concrete directions and a calm, quiet manner. • Provide ample time for client to process information. • Focus on client's real message and concern rather than on the confusion. Talk about what is real. • Break directions into small tasks. Provide meaningful stimuli and reduce competing meaningless stimuli: • Reduce noise, hospital intercom, loud radios, etc. • *Provide calming Greek music, photographs, familiar objects, etc.*	• Client oriented to place, time, and person. • No delusions, misperceptions, hallucinations. • Client attentive and alert. • Client able to perform all tests in neuro tool. • Memory intact except for confused episodes: "I remember everything except how it happened and how I got here."

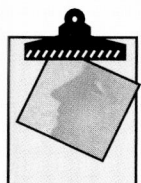

NURSING CARE PLANNING
A CONFUSED CLIENT *(continued)*

NURSING CARE PLAN *(continued)*

Nursing Diagnosis	Expected Outcomes	Interventions	Evaluation (After 24 Hours of Care)
		• Use environmental cues, such as clocks, calendars, bright colors to mark client's door and orient him to environment. *(Large picture of Greek dancer placed by family on client's door is orienting and makes him smile.)*	
		• Allow presence of familiar person if helpful.	
		• Assess interests and activity tolerance and coordinate into activity schedule.	
		• Provide good lighting to diminish shadows and possible misperception.	
	Absence of anxiety	• Explain to client and daughter (with detailed explanation to daughter) about client's condition.	• Client relies on daughter to make decisions and relaxes when daughter is there. He says, "She's the boss while I'm in the hospital."
		• Allow daughter or other family member to stay overnight with client to keep him oriented and calm.	

Italicized interventions indicate culturally specific care.

Critical Thinking Questions

1. Mr. Tellis' daughter does not understand how her father can be dehydrated when he drinks 8 cups of coffee per day. How would you explain this to her?
2. Mr. Tellis needs a reminder about how much fluid he needs to drink per day. What intervention would you put into place, in his home, to remind him?
3. What community services might be appropriate for Mr. Tellis? Who would you approach about these suggestions?

In contrast, chronic confusion gradually changes with the client's progressive deterioration. Evaluation of interventions for chronic confusion measures their ability to halt or slow deterioration, lessen catastrophic episodes, promote dignity and integrity, and enable the client to function at the height of his ability. As deterioration progresses, the needs of the client tend to increase in number and complexity. In the final stages of chronic confusion, the client needs extensive skilled nursing care. Multiple chronic illnesses are usually apparent as well. Extensive physiological and psychological issues arise. In addition, acute and chronic confusion may appear together and have multiple related factors.

KEY PRINCIPLES

- Confusion is a state in which a person experiences or is at risk of experiencing a disturbance in cognition.
- Confusion is not a disease; it is a syndrome of clinically observable phenomena.
- Confusion is profoundly important as a signal of serious neurological difficulty, which can develop into chronic illness and even death if it is undetected and underlying factors are untreated.
- There are two major types of confusion: acute and chronic. They may occur alone or together.
- *Delirium* is the medical diagnosis associated with acute confusion; *dementia* is the medical diagnosis associated with chronic confusion.
- Acute confusion is considered a medical emergency.
- Common barriers to correctly identifying confusion are incorrect beliefs and attitudes about confusion, lack of precise documentation, and mental status assessment that is incomplete or fails to use the proper assessment tools.
- A number of factors can affect cognition, including lifestyle, environmental, developmental, psychological, and physiological factors.
- Assessment of cognition includes a health history, use of assessment tools, physical examination, and diagnostic tests.
- Acute and chronic confusion can be differentiated from each other. This is important because their treatment differs.
- Confusion also must be differentiated from other disorders, such as depression.
- In acute confusion, the goals of care focus on prevention, speedy recognition, and appropriate treatment of underlying factors to reverse their effects and those of the confusion itself.
- In chronic confusion, the goals of care focus on rapid recognition, treatment, and interventions to halt or at least slow the deterioration process.
- Interventions for confusion focus on maintaining the highest level of health, promoting safety, preventing injury, promoting independence without exceeding the client's capacity, providing meaningful and appropriate stimulation and communication, and promoting dignity and integrity.
- Interventions for acute confusion relate to identifying the etiology and treating the cause.
- Interventions for chronic confusion relate to identifying triggers and structuring the environment to minimize catastrophic incidents.
- Preservation of the family unit and support of caregivers are essential focuses when working with the confused client.

BIBLIOGRAPHY

Alzheimer's Disease & Related Disorders Association, Inc. (1997). IRS 229Z, *Alzheimer's Disease: Fact Sheet,* Chicago, IL: Author.

Alzheimer's Disease & Related Disorders Association, Inc. (1996). IRS 230Z, *Alzheimer's Disease: Statistics,* Chicago, IL: Author.

American Psychiatric Association. (1994). *Diagnostic and statistical manual of mental disorders* (4th ed.). Washington, D.C.: Author.

Carpenito, L. J. (1997). *Handbook of nursing diagnosis* (7th ed.). Philadelphia: J.B. Lippincott.

Cookman, C. A. (1996). Older people and attachment to things, places, pets, and ideas. *Image: Journal of Nursing Scholarship, 28*(3), 227–231.

*Crippen, D., & Ermakov, S. (1992). Stress, agitation and brain failure in critical care medicine. *Critical Care Nursing Quarterly, 15*(2), 52–74.

DeMaagd, G. (1995). High-risk drugs in the elderly population. *Geriatric Nursing, 16*(5), 198–207.

Detwiler, C. (1997). Cognitive disorders. In B. Johnson. *Psychiatric mental health nursing.* (4th ed.) Philadelphia: Lippincott-Raven.

Drake, A., & Romano, E. (1995). How to protect your older patient from the hazards of polypharmacy. *Nursing95, 25*(6), 34–39.

Fleming, K. C., Adams, A. C., & Petersen, R. C. (1995). Dementia: Diagnosis and evaluation. *Mayo Clinic Proceedings, 70,* 1093–1107.

*Folstein, M., Folstein, S., & McHugh, P. (1975). Mini-mental state: A practical method for grading the cognitive state for the clinician. *Journal Psychiatric Research, 12,* 189–198.

*Foreman, M. D. (1993). Acute confusion in the elderly. *Annual Review of Nursing Research, 11,* 3–30.

Foreman, M., Fletcher, K., Mion, L., Simon, L., & the NICHE Faculty (1996). Assessing cognitive function. *Geriatric Nursing, 17*(5), 228–232.

Gerdner, L. A., Hall, G. R., & Buckwalter, K. L. (1996). Caregiver training for people with Alzheimer's based on a stress threshold model. *Image: Journal of Nursing Scholarship, 28*(3), 241–252.

Grove, N. C. (1997). Helping families select a nursing home. *RN, 3,* 37–40.

Hall, G. R. (1991). Altered thought processes: Dementia. In M. Maas, C. Buckwalter, & M. Hardy. (Eds.), *Nursing diagnoses and interventions for the elderly* (pp 332–347). Redwood City, CA: Addison-Wesley Nursing.

*Inouye, S. K. (1994). The dilemma of delirium: Clinical and research controversies regarding diagnosis and evaluation of delirium in hospitalized elderly medical patients. *The American Journal of Medicine, 97*(9), 278–287.

Judd, C. R. (1996). Delirium or dementia? Making a clinically important distinction. *JAAPA, 9*(4), 24–41.

Lazarou, J., Pomeranz, B., & Corey, P. (1998). Incidence of adverse reactions in hospitalized patients. *Journal of the American Medical Association, 279*(15), 1200–1204.

Levkoff, S. E., Evans, D. A, Liptzin, B., Cleary, P. D., Lipsitz, L. A., Wetle, T. T., Reilly, C H., Pilgrim, D. M., Schor, J., & Rowe, J. (1992). The occurrence and persistence of symptoms among elderly hospitalized patients. *Archives of Internal Medicine, 152*(2), 332–340.

Marcantonio, E. R., Goldman L., Mangione, C. M., et al. (1994). A clinical prediction rule for delirium after elective noncardiac surgery. *Journal of the American Medical Association, 271*(2), 134–139.

Matteson, M. A., Linton, A. D., & Barnes, S. J. (1996). Cognitive developmental approach to dementia. *Image: Journal of Nursing Scholarship, 28*(3), 233–240.

Miller, C. A. (1995). *Nursing care of older adults: Theory and practice.* (2nd ed.). Philadelphia: J.B. Lippincott.

Mentes, J. C. (1995). A nursing protocol to assess causes of delirium: Identifying delirium in nursing home residents. *Journal of Gerontological Nursing, 21*(2), 26–30.

---

*Asterisk indicates a classic or definitive work on this subject.

North American Nursing Diagnosis Association. (1999). *Nursing diagnoses: Definitions & classification (1999–2000).* Philadelphia: Author.

*Pfeiffer, E. (1975). A short portable mental status questionnaire for assessment of organic brain deficit in the elderly patient. *Journal of the American Geriatric Society, 23*(10), 433–441.

Phinney, A. (1998). Living with dementia from the patient's perspective. *Journal of Gerontological Nursing, 24*(6), 8–15.

Simon, L., Jewell, N., & Brokel, J. (1997). Management of acute delirium in hospitalized elderly: A process improvement project. *Geriatric Nursing, 18*(4), 150–154.

Tripp-Reimer, T., & Sorofman, B. (1998). Greek Americans. In L. Purnell & B. Paulanka. *Transcultural health care: A culturally competent approach.* Philadelphia: F.A. Davis.

Wilden, B., & Howling, S. (1994). Understanding delirium. *The Canadian Nurse, 90*(7), 27–30.

Wong, D. (1997). *Whaley and Wong's Essentials of Pediatric Nursing* (5th ed). St. Louis: Mosby-Year Book.

Self-Perception/ Self-Concept Pattern

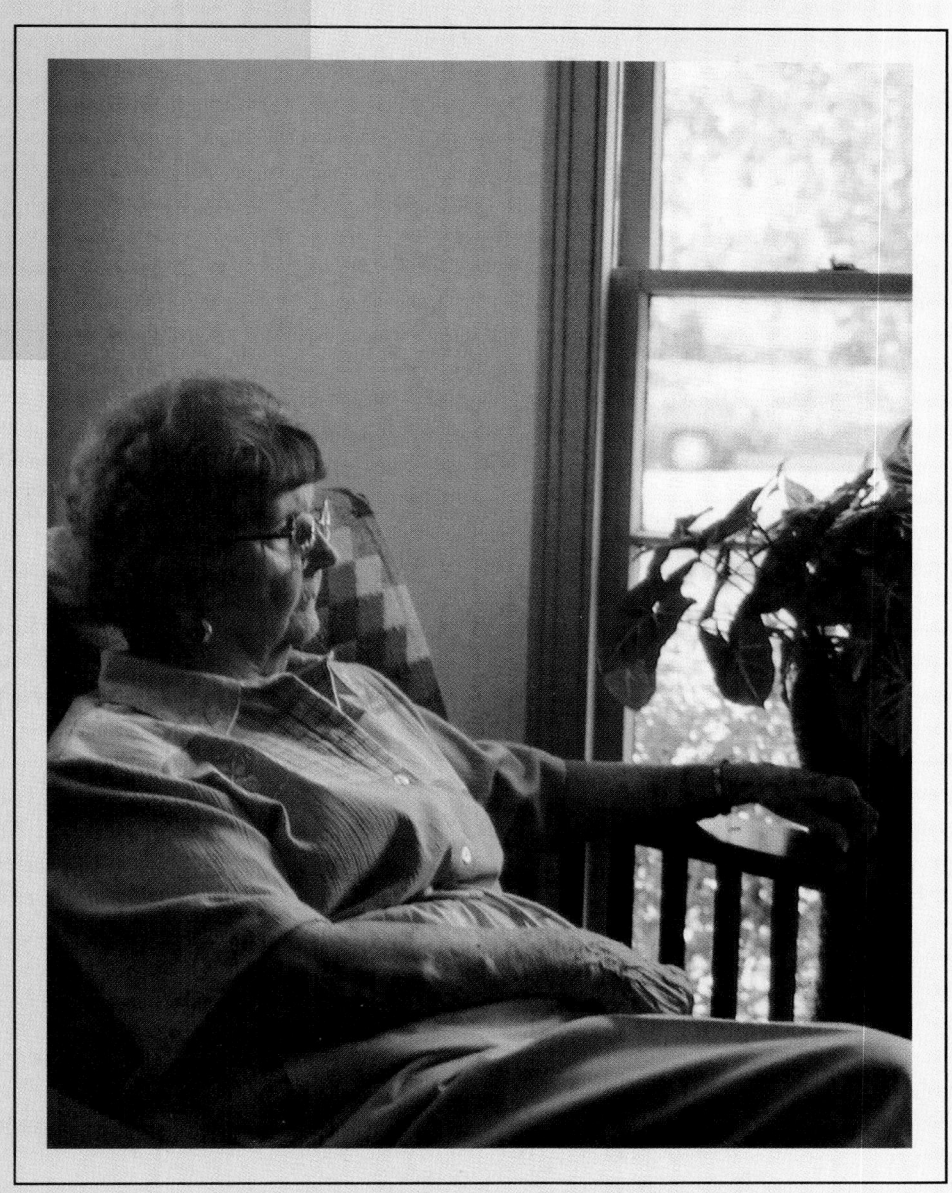

46

Self-Concept

Beverly M. Miller, Susan M. Irvin, and Shirley Eden-Kilgour

Key Terms

body image

personal identity

role performance

self-concept

self-esteem

LEARNING OBJECTIVES

After studying this chapter, you should be able to:

1. Differentiate among self-concept, self-esteem, personal identity, role performance, and body image.

2. Discuss factors affecting self-concept.

3. Assess responses of clients who may be at risk for changes in self-esteem or body image.

4. Write a nursing diagnosis and develop a care plan for a client experiencing a problem with alterations in the components of self-concept.

5. Plan for goal-directed interventions that address the identified nursing diagnoses.

6. Describe and practice key interventions for clients who are experiencing alterations in self-esteem and body image.

7. Evaluate the client's progress versus expected outcomes for alterations in self-esteem and body image.

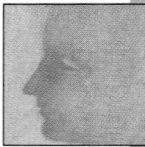

Nancy Ward, a 43-year-old Navajo woman, lives with her younger sister, Helen. Nancy's husband of 25 years died 6 months ago from complications of alcohol abuse, diabetes, and coronary artery disease. During the marriage, he was abusive and violent, especially when he was intoxicated. Nancy had been hospitalized twice for physical abuse, and she was also frequently verbally abused. Nancy weighs 285 pounds and is 5 feet 4 inches tall. She was not able to have children because of endometriosis. Two weeks ago, Nancy visited her physician for a routine mammogram. She has returned today because the results indicate a suspicious density that will require a surgical biopsy. The chance that this growth is malignant is of great concern to Nancy. The nurse plans to educate Nancy on the upcoming surgical procedure. Because of Nancy's health history, the nurse considers the diagnoses *Chronic low self-esteem* and *Body image disturbance*.

CONCEPT OF SELF

Self-concept is a relatively enduring set of attitudes and beliefs about both the physical self and the psychological self. It is the totality of ideas that a person holds about the self. Self-concept is not a static state but one that develops and changes over time. It includes the person's self-knowledge, self-expectations, and self-evaluation. Self-concept changes with life experiences and relationships that influence beliefs about the self. Self-concept guides our actions, motivations, expectations, and goals for the future.

During your career, you will work with clients who have a wide range of problems involving self-concept. A sound self-concept is important to overall health and may help determine a client's willingness to take action to improve her health status. Sometimes, a health problem itself has a negative effect on self-concept, and you will work to help a client accept a change in health status and maintain quality of life. Problems with self-concept are also a major focus for nurses who specialize in psychiatric care.

Components of Self-Concept

To fully understand self-concept, it is useful to describe the individual elements that make up the mental picture of the self. Self-concept includes four components: self-esteem, personal identity, role performance, and body image (Fig. 46–1).

Self-Esteem

The term self-esteem is often used interchangeably with the term self-concept, but "to esteem" means to regard favorably, with admiration, or respect. Therefore, **self-esteem** can be defined as the degree to which a person has a positive evaluation of self based on her perceptions of how she is viewed by others as well as on her view of herself.

There are two schools of thought about the development of self-esteem. The first is that self-esteem forms early in life, based primarily on relationships with early caregivers, and is relatively fixed throughout life. The second is that self-esteem fluctuates whenever life transitions, crises, or illnesses challenge the self-concept or alter the person's status or role (Arnold & Boggs, 1999).

For example, Nancy Ward's self-esteem was probably affected each time her husband abused her; it may be further damaged by the fear of debilitating illness or disfiguring surgery. However, we do not know what level of self-esteem was present when Nancy entered into the relationship. Do you think Nancy's self-esteem was formed in early childhood or shaped by the events of her life?

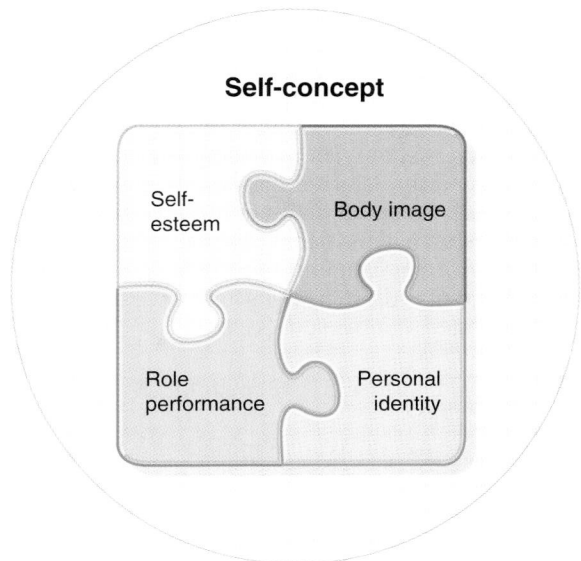

Figure 46–1. Self-concept has four interrelated components.

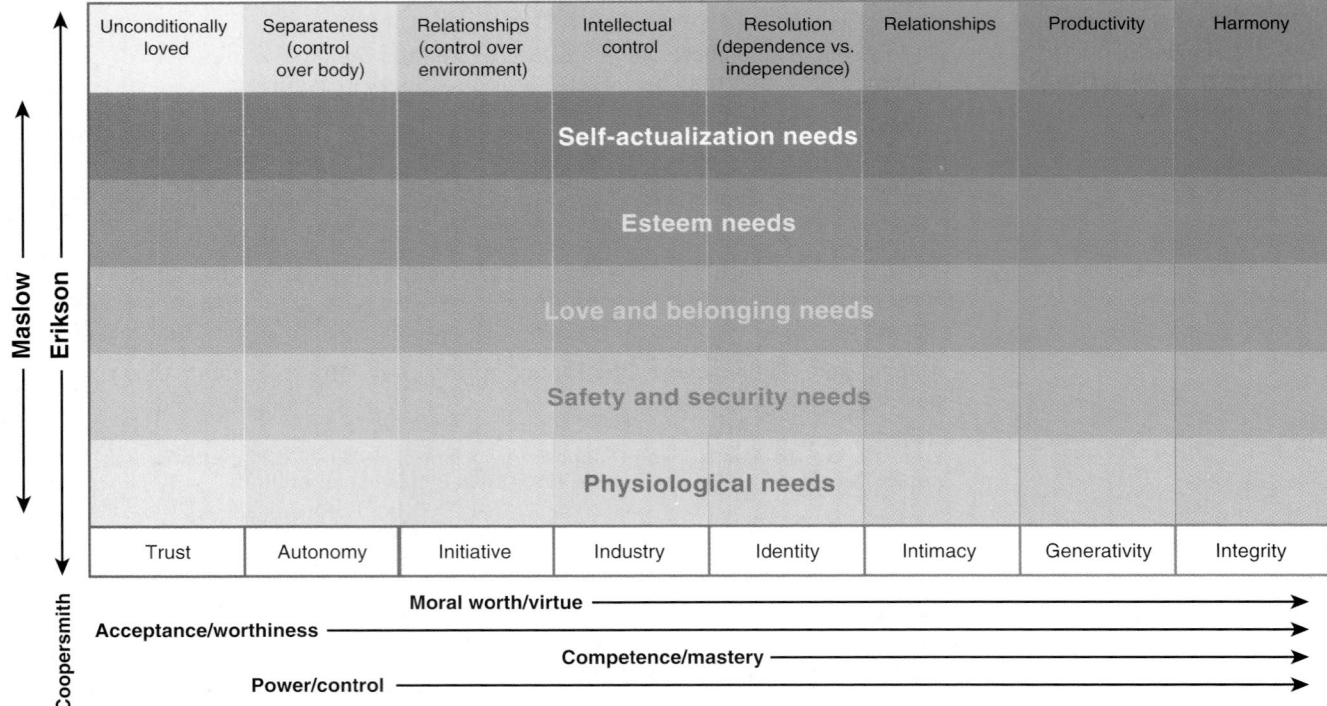

Unconditionally loved	Separateness (control over body)	Relationships (control over environment)	Intellectual control	Resolution (dependence vs. independence)	Relationships	Productivity	Harmony

Self-actualization needs

Esteem needs

Love and belonging needs

Safety and security needs

Physiological needs

| Trust | Autonomy | Initiative | Industry | Identity | Intimacy | Generativity | Integrity |

Maslow
Erikson
Coopersmith

Moral worth/virtue ⟶
Acceptance/worthiness ⟶
Competence/mastery ⟶
Power/control ⟶

Figure 46–2. Relationship between Maslow's hierarchy of basic needs, Erikson's developmental tasks, and Coopersmith's components of self-esteem. (Modified from Carson, V.B., & Arnold, E.N. [1996]. Mental health nursing: The nurse-patient journey. Philadelphia: W.B. Saunders Co.)

How do you think her past history and view of herself will affect her response to her current health situation?

Having high self-esteem entails having a high level of satisfaction with oneself. It is derived from the internal comparison of the present self to the ideal self. People who possess high self-esteem are more content, in control, confident, accountable, and capable (Vera & Wrath, 1995). Low self-esteem can result in a lack of confidence, an inability to act in one's best interest, feelings of being overwhelmed, decreased activity or energy, powerlessness, and an inability to function.

Men and women base their self-esteem on different things. Men are more likely to base their self-esteem on their personal achievements in life. Women often associate self-esteem with their social support system. Self-esteem in men is often greatly affected by having a sense of well-being, a positive outlook on life, and an ability to perform activities of daily living (ADL). Self-esteem in women is generally affected by whether they are content with their lives and have a feeling that they are needed (Anderson, S., 1995).

THEORIES OF PERSONALITY DEVELOPMENT AND SELF-ESTEEM

Theories of personality development are closely interwoven with the concepts of self and self-esteem. In this chapter we will look at two theories of personality development, those of Abraham Maslow and Erik Erikson, and see how they relate to four components of self-esteem as described by Coopersmith (1981) (Fig. 46–2).

MASLOW'S HIERARCHY OF NEEDS. Maslow (1954) described self-esteem as a requirement for reaching full personal development, which he called "self-actualization." Maslow suggested that human beings have a "hierarchy of needs," and that physiological needs form the foundation on which safety and security are built. Unless these basic, foundational needs are met, higher-level needs receive less attention and energy. According to Maslow, self-esteem develops after the need for belonging and being loved by others is met and is thus coincidental with the need for esteem from others. In other words, a positive relationship with others leads to the development of a positive self-concept or self-esteem. This theory supports the idea that self-esteem is not fixed but changes in relation to interactions with others.

ERIKSON'S EIGHT STAGES OF MAN. Erikson (1950) described the development of self-esteem in eight stages, ranging from infancy through old age. According to Erikson, in infancy the child develops *trust* through the concern of caregivers. From ages 1 to 3, the child develops *autonomy* through learning control of the body. Through developing *initiative* and *industry,* the child gradually develops broader control over the environment and finally over his own intellect. By the time the child has reached age 12, he has typically developed the ability to derive his self-esteem from what is called an "internal locus of control"—that is, from within himself rather than from outside sources. Children with an internal locus of control feel that they have the power to affect what happens to them.

According to Erikson, the adolescent develops *identity*. During this time, adolescents rebel against parents in an effort to establish their own personhood, and being accepted by peers dramatically affects self-esteem. Adolescence is also a time when a person develops her own value system and solidifies sexual identity. Adolescents continually vacillate between independence and dependence.

Erikson's last three stages of development—*intimacy, generativity,* and *integrity*—normally occur in adulthood. The tasks to be accomplished in adulthood are the forging of relationships (intimacy), productivity (generativity), and harmony with oneself and with life (integrity).

Based on Erikson's theory, self-esteem appears to be developed in childhood but could be changed throughout a lifetime of developmental struggles.

COOPERSMITH'S FOUR COMPONENTS OF SELF-ESTEEM. Coopersmith (1981) identified four important components in the development of positive self-esteem: competence/mastery, power/control, moral worth/virtue, and acceptance/worthiness (Willoughby, King, & Palatajko, 1996; Coopersmith, 1981). According to Coopersmith, it is possible to improve self-esteem by attaining or experiencing success in any of these four areas.

Competence/mastery refers to successful performance or achievement. It is marked by high levels of performance, with the level and the tasks varying depending on developmental stage. When abilities are sufficient to complete a task, competence/mastery is present. If abilities do not allow successful completion of a given task, competence is not attained. The development of *initiative* and *industry* leads to feelings of competence.

Power/control is the ability to influence and control others. Toddlers learn the concept of power and control when they begin exploring their environment. They also discover the art of manipulation of objects within the environment. Thus, power and control make their first appearance in toddlerhood. Toddlers gain an understanding that certain behaviors can bring about certain responses. Power and control over the environment continues to develop in school-aged children, further extending the concept into group behaviors in school. Initiative develops within play-groups that have leaders and followers with designated roles. Power and control begins to take on a more realistic viewpoint at this time.

Moral worth/virtue is the adherence to moral and ethical standards. The values and morals of significant others are internalized by the preschool-aged and the school-aged child. In early childhood, the child adopts behaviors through identification with the same-sex parent and a desire to please that parent. Through learning to label these and other behaviors as good or bad, moral development begins.

Acceptance/worthiness relates to the perception, attention, and affection of others. It is the amount of concern and care that a person receives from significant others. A person learns to value herself through the experience of being valued by others. In infancy, acceptance/worthiness is exemplified by the unconditional love that a parent or caregiver has for the child. Acceptance/worthiness provides toddlers with the freedom to explore further domains of their environment.

SELF-ESTEEM AND POSITIVE HEALTH PRACTICES

Studies have also shown an association between self-esteem and positive health practices. Conn, Taylor, and Hayes (1992) showed a relationship between positive self-esteem and the likelihood of practicing self-care activities after a myocardial infarction (MI). The study showed that self-esteem and social support strongly influence continued self-care activities years after the MI. Another study showed that high self-esteem predicted whether transplant clients would do well postoperatively, including having fewer symptoms of depression (Duitsman, 1993). Self-esteem is therefore associated with a better outlook on life and positive coping skills (Anderson, S., 1995).

Personal Identity

Personal identity is the organizing principle of the personality that accounts for the unity, continuity, consistency, and uniqueness of a person (Carpenito, 1999). The components of personal identity are emotional images, cognitive images, and perceptual images. *Emotional images* are those feelings about oneself that one experiences as being consistent with the self and that feel familiar and normal. *Cognitive images* are derived from thinking about oneself, which incorporates internal and external data to form a mental picture of who one is. The cognitive component involves intelligence, past experiences, educational experiences, and the process of thinking. *Perceptual images* are derived from external sensory data and translated into mental pictures of reality. Two people experiencing the same situation may interpret it in two different ways.

Role Performance

The concept of **role performance** includes the roles a person assumes or is given. It includes the actions, thoughts, and feelings associated with those roles. Roles are defined in terms of relationship to others. For example, mother, father, supervisor, teacher, and nurse are all roles. The person in the role strives to fulfill the behaviors prescribed for that role by the self, by culture, or by society. An inability to fulfill the prescribed behaviors can affect the other components of self-concept, especially self-esteem. Self-evaluation of how we perform our role behaviors contributes to self-esteem. The evaluations made by others influence it as well.

Nancy Ward, at the beginning of this chapter, probably believed that conceiving and bearing children was an integral part of a married woman's role. This may also have been her husband's opinion, as well as the belief of her culture and of society at large. Her low self-esteem was reinforced by her husband's constant negative evaluation of her abilities as a wife. How do you think this part of Nancy's history will affect her present circumstances?

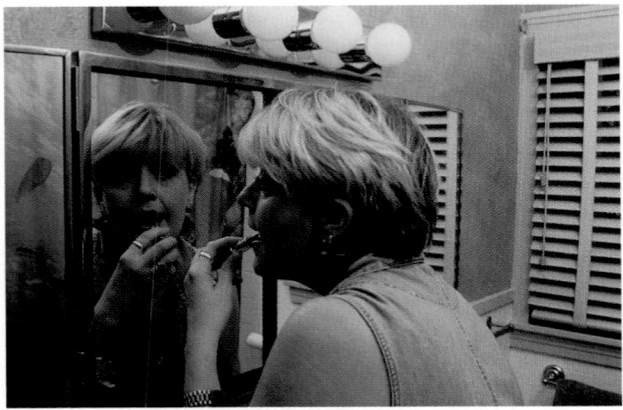

Figure 46–3. Body image is an important part of self-concept.

Body Image

Body image is a person's perception of her body (Fig. 46–3). It is the physical dimension of self-concept, or how a person perceives and evaluates the appearance and function of self. People can perceive their bodies as male or female, fat or thin, ugly or beautiful, fully functional or disabled, intact or missing some part. Body image changes with physical growth, weight gain or loss, aging, illness, accidents, and social or cultural influences. Body image is closely related to personal identity, role performance, and self-esteem. Self-evaluation of one's body, as well as the evaluations of others, contributes to self-esteem.

The significance of a person's body image varies with the value and intensity attached to that image. Body image is more important when strong emotions are attached to how the body is perceived. The social and cultural influences in American society place a high value on body image, which strongly affects people's personal perceptions.

Body image is dynamic. It develops as a person develops and can change and be changed. However, there is a certain amount of internal consistency to body image throughout life.

FACTORS AFFECTING SELF-CONCEPT

Developmental Factors

Infants to Preschoolers

Self-esteem in infants and preschoolers can be related to the type of parenting the child receives. For example, Killeen (1993) examined the relationship between parenting characteristics and the self-esteem of children and found that a child's perception of his performance correlated with his support from parents and others. Killeen also noted that a child's perception of the nonverbal aspects of parental communication had an important impact on self-esteem.

School-Aged Children

As a child leaves the preschool period and enters school, there is a threat to self-esteem when the child attempts to master the tasks of school. Problems with self-esteem often begin to appear at this time. For example, childhood obesity may lead to poor self-esteem in school-aged children.

Adolescents

Adolescence, ages 12 to 20 years, is a period of sweeping hormonal changes and rapid physiological growth. It is a very stressful period of major life transition that can threaten self-esteem. In addition, the struggle for self-esteem is part of the search for identity and the transition to adult roles and responsibilities.

Perceived rejection, a sense of unworthiness, or feelings of not being trusted are often associated with self-destructive behaviors in adolescence.

Peer relationships—positive or negative—also help to define self-concept in adolescents (Fig. 46–4). Body image for teens reflects their peer group's attitude and the desire for acceptance and sameness. Harper and Marshall (1991) identified that teenage girls report more problems with body image than boys do. Any event that causes change in a teen's body appearance can positively or negatively alter peer acceptance and thus lead to a change in body image or self-esteem. Rapid growth spurts and the emergence of acne can cause great discomfort because they perceive that those changes interfere with peer relationships. Acne can cause embarrassment, self-consciousness, and anxiety.

Many factors can contribute to, or trigger, a persistent state of low self-esteem in teens. Chronic illnesses—such as depression, chronic fatigue, and multiple sclerosis—are associated with low self-esteem. Abusive or violent relationships also can destroy positive feelings about one's capabilities or oneself. Low self-esteem in adolescents has been associated with increased cigarette smoking and substance abuse, involving cocaine, marijuana, and alcohol. However, the relationship is frequently circular rather than linear. That is, low self-esteem leads to cigarette smoking and substance abuse, and smoking and substance abuse

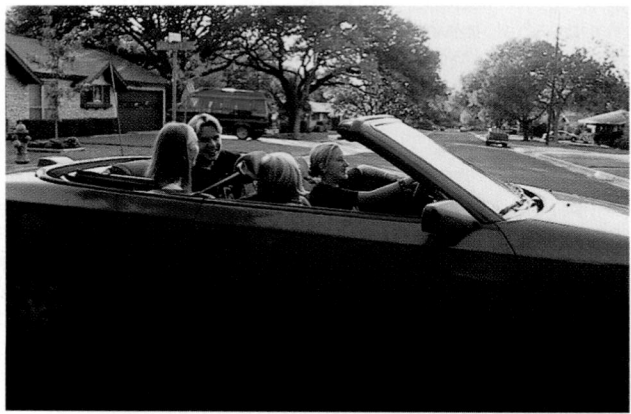

Figure 46–4. Peer relationships help define self-concept in adolescents.

lead in turn to low self-esteem (Daswell, Millor, Thompson, & Baxter, 1998).

Three specific categories relevant to self-esteem in teens include home, school, and peers. In one study, home and school were found to have a significant influence on negative self-esteem and the tendency of teens to use or abuse various substances (Young, Werch, & Bakema, 1989). Surprisingly, peers, by contrast, showed no significant influence on self-esteem among teens or on their tendency to use or abuse these substances. Prevention of substance use or abuse may therefore depend on the development of strategies to address problems in the home and school.

Young Adults

Young adults, ages 20 to 30 years, are also vulnerable to altered self-concept. This is a time of decision-making about becoming independent, furthering an education, choosing a career, deciding to marry, starting a family, deciding on a place to live, even determining a lifestyle. Decisions about all of these areas can affect self-concept, positively or negatively.

Middle Adults

In middle adulthood, according to Erickson, the task is one of caring for others (elder parents) or guiding the young (children or grandchildren). Multiple life stressors and the beginning of physical decline has a potential to alter the self-concept during this period of life.

Women today lead active lives, typically as mothers, spouses, and workers outside the home. The multiple expectations that women hold for themselves can result in feelings of overwhelming pressure and can lead to role strain or stress and possibly to illness (Napholz, 1994). How well women cope with multiple roles may also provide an indicator of how they can or will manage their overall health.

Women with high appraisal of self-worth may be better able to defend against illness than other women (O'Brien, 1993). Likewise, during stressful events or times of change positive self-esteem may help women to cope with uncertainty (Vera & Wrath, 1995). When a disease or its treatment threatens a woman's health, her security can be shaken, and her confidence can erode. This is especially true if the diagnosis can or will result in an alteration of the body. Role function disturbance or problems with interpersonal relationships may result (Anderson & Johnson, 1994).

The phenomenon of male menopause (andropause) occurs during the late 40s or early 50s. With this winding down of the reproductive period of a man's life, he may perceive a threat to his masculinity, which could lead to a disruption of a previously stable relationship. Many men begin to lose their scalp hair in middle adulthood. These phenomena may affect self-esteem and thus self-concept. Middle adulthood is also the time when men may take on the softer attributes of tenderness, caring, and assisting more with domestic tasks, such as cooking, laundry, and gardening.

Many health problems in middle age are the same for both men and women. The risk for cardiac disease equalizes in both sexes. Diseases (such as cancer and hypertension), alcohol and nicotine use, drug addictions, and accidents affect both women and men during this period.

Older Adults

The elderly have many stresses that can threaten their self-concept. Many elderly people must cope with several chronic illnesses while other changes are also occurring in their lives. Learning to live with a chronic illness can lead to depression. Other contributing factors are loss of loved ones, retirement, reduced financial resources, loss of a body part or functional ability, or reduced independence. If older adults cannot adjust to these changes, they may begin to feel powerless and exhibit negative behaviors as a mechanism of control. Elders can thus become angry, manipulative, withdrawn, self-destructive, dependent, grieved, or depressed.

Cultural and Religious Factors

Cultural and religious beliefs may contribute to a client's self-esteem, as suggested in the Cross-Cultural Care chart. For example, the prevalence of *Chronic low self-esteem* in Native Americans may impact health. Although their culture advocates a balance among body, mind, and spirit, they have the highest rate of heart disease and diabetes of any group.

Because of Nancy Ward's Native American culture, she may believe that she is in some disharmony with nature and that her illness may be the result. An interested third party, such as the medicine man, Shama, may be helpful to fully gain Nancy's participation in the health care plan. This medicine man will be interested in Nancy's spiritual and physical health, and the mutual goal will be the restoration of good health and harmony.

The average Native American usually lives to be only 45 years old. Alcohol is a big factor in the health and death of many Native Americans.

Risk factors that contribute to a lowered self-esteem in Native Americans are mistrust of the establishment (authority) and of Western health care providers. Other factors include feelings of oppression from the loss of tribal lands, high unemployment rates, lack of acceptance in the mainstream workforce, alcoholism, and a sedentary lifestyle.

Also be aware that cultural and religious influences are as diverse as the people within cultures and religions. Sensitivity and understanding are key to successful communication with all clients and family members. Remember that positive self-esteem consists of acceptance/worthiness, power/control, competence/mastery, and moral worth/virtue.

Socioeconomic Factors

Socioeconomic status has a direct relationship to self-concept. A person's position on the health/illness con-

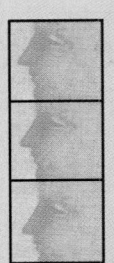

CROSS-CULTURAL CARE
CARING FOR A NAVAJO CLIENT

Nancy Ward, the client whose story we have followed throughout this chapter, is a Navajo. She and her husband left the reservation when they married. Her husband was not successful in maintaining employment off the reservation. They returned and lived most of their married life close to their families. While Navajos follow many different paths, they have a tendency to maintain the following patterns of living.

- Younger Indians often leave the reservation, voluntarily or involuntarily, to seek employment opportunities.
- The basic social unit is the nuclear family, but members live close to other families, sharing economic and social support. The Navajo family is very flexible in sharing with other families who are in need. Family may be defined in a broader context that includes kinship ties and close friends.
- The elderly are held in high esteem for their material wealth and knowledge wealth. Navajo children are expected to care for elderly grandparents and great-grandparents. Grandparents also play major roles in caring for children.
- Navajos are often initially silent and reserved when meeting strangers. Eye contact is considered disrespectful and is avoided.
- Women are expected not to achieve more than their husbands. Divorce does occur despite the strong belief in maintaining the family.
- Navajos often gather the family for consultation when a clinic or hospital visit is prolonged.

Let's see how Susan, Nancy's nurse, demonstrated sensitivity to Nancy's cultural values.

Susan: Do you expect to get the results of the biopsy today?
Nancy: I guess so.
Susan: Has your sister come with you to the clinic?
Nancy: She is in the waiting room with her children.
Susan: If you would like for her to be with you, I can find someone to watch the children while the two of you talk to the doctor.
Nancy: A friend is there. She can watch the children.
Susan: Shall I go and get your sister?
Nancy: Yes, please.

Critical Thinking Questions

- If Nancy has cancer and the physician recommends chemotherapy, how would you explain the therapy to Nancy?
- If Nancy says she will not agree to the therapy until she has talked to the tribal healer, how would you respond to her?
- Would it be better for Nancy to come to the clinic to receive her chemotherapy or have a home health nurse go to Nancy's home?

References

Bell, R. (1994). Prominence of women in Navajo healing beliefs and values. *Nursing and Health Care, 15*(5), 232–240.
Giger, J.N., & Davidhizar, R.E. (1995). *Transcultural nursing: Assessment and intervention.* St. Louis: Mosby-Year Book.
Holmes, E.R., & Holmes, L.D. (1995). *Other cultures, elder years.* Thousand Oaks, California: Sage Publications.

tinuum may be in part the result of the interrelationship of socioeconomic status, health care practices, and lifestyle. Additionally, needing public assistance may have a negative impact on self-concept.

Living conditions are an important factor in the lives of clients who must seek public assistance. Often, public housing does not supply people with much more than the basic needs. The repair and condition of government housing is sometimes poor and does not foster self-esteem. Also, illness is more common when living conditions include rodents and roaches, and illness can contribute to a negative self-concept.

Psychological Factors

Depression

Depression is associated with low self-esteem. Difficulty finding appropriate, cost-effective treatment may make matters worse, as suggested in the Cost of Care chart. Factors contributing to this prevalent problem include stress, powerlessness, helplessness, sexual bias, stereotyping, lack of control, single parenthood, multiple role conflicts, and poor educational or career status.

Stress

Stress can overwhelm a person to the point that physical and mental functioning is impaired. Self-concept is affected when a person's ability to function is reduced.

Loss

Loss is a factor that can easily lower self-esteem. Examples include the loss of a spouse, a loss or change of employment, or the episodic loss of previous good health. Even temporary losses—such as financial

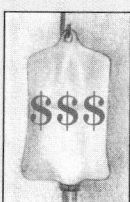

THE COST OF CARE
DEPRESSION IN THE ELDERLY

The proportion of Americans over age 65 is growing. By the year 2000, people over age 65 will number 13% of the population. By the year 2030, they will represent 21.8% of the population. That adds up to about 66 million older people, 2.5 times the number recorded in 1990. Even now, once a person reaches age 65, life expectancy extends an additional 17.3 years.

In older adults, depression is a common problem and commonly overlooked. Studies suggest that 15% of elderly people in the community are depressed and that the problem is often masked by other chronic medical conditions or medications.

Discussion

The increasing numbers of elderly and the large number who experience depression combine to create the possibility of great cost for treating depression in the future. Indeed, a 30-day hospital stay for the treatment of depression currently costs about $1,236 per day or $37,080 for the month.*

To help contain the cost of treating depression in the elderly, managed health care plans emphasize outpatient treatment rather than hospitalization or long-term psychotherapeutic interventions. Treatment commonly involves a new class of antidepressant medications called selective serotonin reuptake inhibitors. Paroxetine (Paxil) is prescribed most commonly. A 1-month supply of 20-mg tablets costs $68.39.

*1998 statistical data from Southern Health Plan, Inc. Memphis, TN.

---

problems, job layoffs, premenstrual syndrome, disharmony in relationships, children in trouble with school or law officials, career changes, incarceration, or institutionalization—may have an impact on self-concept. How these losses are accepted, and how a person moves on in life, depends greatly on the successful use of coping skills.

Research shows that people with high self-esteem are better able to employ successful coping strategies (O'Brien, 1993).

Abusive Relationships

Women who are involved in violent or abusive relationships often, understandably, have low self-esteem. Of these women, those with a weak sense of self can contribute unwittingly to the ongoing cycle of abuse. The strong, more dominant partner is rarely sensitive to the less powerful partner, and it becomes more and more difficult for the victim to resist the psychological hold of the abuser. Eventually, the victim incorporates the opinions of the dominator into her self-concept and assumes blame for the relationship.

Physiological Factors

We have said that multiple stressors can affect self-esteem. It is often a combination of the specific physical or psychosocial stressor and the associated developmental stressor that has a major impact on self-concept. The following physiological factors also have strong psychosocial components.

Fatigue

The basis of fatigue is not fully understood, but fatigue may be a factor in low self-esteem. Stress, boredom, unhappiness, and depression are related factors. Fatigue is a state in which a person lacks the energy to adequately perform the ADLs. Not only are energy levels very low, but hormonal and muscle cell activity is also decreased. Fatigue is a common complaint in both men and women, but women are more at risk, especially in the childbearing years.

A condition called chronic fatigue syndrome may be the cause of fatigue in some cases. However, the nature and existence of chronic fatigue syndrome continues to be debated. Some researchers are able to clearly define the characteristics of this elusive disorder.

Trauma

Trauma or traumatic injuries can cause a major body loss or change and may result in disfigurement that can lead to a change in body image. Even when temporary, trauma is still frightening. It forces people to become dependent, even if only for a short time, and this may affect self-esteem. Trauma may leave permanent losses or changes, such as crippling, scarring, and unrelieved acute and chronic pain, with consequent impact on self-concept. Injuries that are visible, such as facial trauma, may be even more difficult for clients to adjust to than other injuries and may have a greater impact on body image.

Chronic Illness

Coping with the burdens of chronic illness can affect one's self-concept. For example, research shows that quality of life and self-esteem are decreased in clients with chronic obstructive pulmonary disease and arthritis (Anderson, K., 1995). Likewise, Flett, Harcourt, and Alpass (1994) demonstrated that clients who have chronic leg ulcers also tend to suffer from low self-esteem, in part because of problems associated with independent functioning. During chronic illness, clients are at risk for low self-esteem because they have a sense of loss of control. In the elderly, this decreased self-esteem can lead to decreased life satisfaction, an increased incidence of depression, other physical illnesses, and medication use (Bensink, God-bey, Marshall, & Yarandle, 1992). When a person with a chronic illness must depend on a family member or other caregiver for care, this dependence can lower self-esteem (Bensink, Godbey, Marshall, & Yarandle, 1992).

Surgery

Whenever a client undergoes a surgical procedure, particularly for cancer, she is at risk for a change in body image and lowered self-esteem. Self-esteem and postoperative progress are related.

The diagnosis of cancer, especially breast cancer, has the potential to alter a woman's body image and lower her self-esteem. Not only is the diagnosis of breast cancer devastating, but the treatment can be disfiguring. Use of chemotherapy and radiation can add to the problem of an altered body image and lower self-esteem because of hair loss, including loss of the eyebrows and eyelashes.

Other surgeries can be equally disturbing to self-concept. Procedures that are related to the reproductive system can alter body image in a powerful way. Some examples include removal of the ovaries (ooph-orectomy), hysterectomy, removal of the testes (orchi-ectomy), breast surgery, circumcision, and prostate surgery. Surgery that disfigures the face, such as sur-gery for removal of skin cancers—particularly deep excisions of aggressive melanoma skin cancers—can profoundly affect body image. Procedures that drasti-cally alter lifestyle, such as a permanent tracheostomy or a colostomy, can also have a major impact on self-concept.

Disability

The disabled are at risk for a disturbance in body im-age. For example, Mona, Gardo, and Brown (1994) found that a disabled woman's self-image was directly related to the age at which the disability occurred. Women who were disabled in their younger years ap-parently were better able to master the skills needed to cope.

Body image and self-esteem can be affected by a spinal cord injury. The loss of independence and con-trol associated with spinal cord injury can lead to low-ered self-esteem, body image disturbance, loss of per-sonal identity, lessened ideal sexuality, and loss of role function.

Obesity

Being overweight elicits negative responses in people. Some people believe that obese people have poor self-esteem and are lazy, slow, and less competent than thin people. These responses may negatively affect the obese person's self-concept. Also, comparing one's ap-pearance to an unrealistic societal ideal can generate negative thoughts about oneself, resulting in feelings of shame and frustration (Vera & Wrath, 1995).

ASSESSMENT

General Assessment of Self-Concept

Health and illness affect self-concept (Fig. 46–5). As a nurse in general practice, however, you will rarely, if ever, conduct an in-depth assessment of a client's self-concept. Nurses conduct an in-depth assessment of self-concept only when the client has presented with problems that are closely associated with disturbances in self-concept and when the goals of care are likely to include working on problems in self-concept. Typi-cally, this is the case in a client with a mental health problem.

However, as you take a health history in any set-ting, you will make observations about the person's self-concept and its impact on health. For example, you may notice that the person is well groomed, at-tractively dressed, sits erect, and comfortably enters into the conversation with the nurse. The time you spend taking a health history is conducive to making these observations and to interweaving questions that help you understand the client's self-concept.

Action Alert!
Listen and observe for cues to self-concept through-out the health history.

As you take a client's health history, listen for state-ments that tell you how the client feels about herself. If you have a therapeutic relationship with the client, it may be natural to ask direct questions to elicit infor-mation about the client's self-esteem, especially in re-lation to the current situation. For example, when a woman is being scheduled for a hysterectomy or being admitted to the hospital for the procedure, you might ask how she feels about having the procedure. You can help her be more specific by making a statement of fact

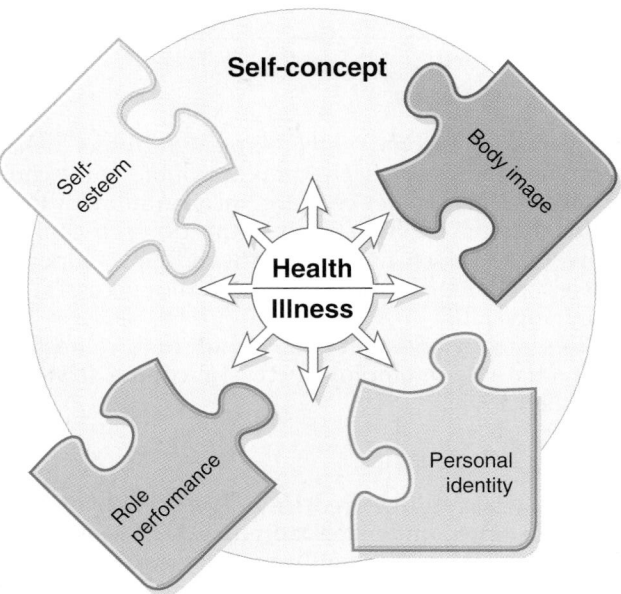

Figure 46–5. Health and illness affect self-concept.

and asking the client for a response. For example, "Some women have a sense that a hysterectomy changes their femininity or sexuality. How do you feel about that?"

When you sense that the self-concept is being affected by the health situation, you may want to follow up with questions about the impact or potential impact of changes in self-concept on the client's life. Continuing to think about the woman with a hysterectomy as an example, suppose the woman responds to you by saying, "I guess I have to accept that I'll be less interested in sex. I'm getting older, and it's natural that it's less important than it used to be." You now have the opportunity to explore the impact of the procedure on the client's perception of herself and on her relationship with her husband. You also have the opportunity to provide some health teaching.

As you listen for cues to the client's self-concept, consider the context in which the self-concept is being assessed. Are there other factors that would explain the person's behavior? In a different context, would the person display a different perception of the self? Even consider *your* influence on the client. As you ask questions and interact with the client, you want to be sure that you do not influence the client's responses. Look for evidence that in other areas of the person's life the self-concept is intact and healthy.

A*ction* A*lert!*
Validate behavioral cues. Behaviors can have many meanings.

Assess the sources of support and information the client has used in managing the feelings associated with the current situation. For example, you might ask the client about to undergo a hysterectomy whether she has discussed with her physician how soon she can engage in sexual intercourse following the hysterectomy.

Focused Assessment for Self-Esteem Disturbance

Some diagnostic cues for *Self-esteem disturbance* include not being able to deal with life events, not being able to set goals, and not being able to make decisions or to solve problems. Descriptions of oneself as a loner is a cue that suggests the need to assess for *Self-esteem disturbance.*

Defining Characteristics

The most consistent defining characteristic for *Self-esteem disturbance* is the person's affective experience of the self, manifested as any negative self-feelings. Assess the client's conversation for frequent negative comments about herself, such as referring to herself as stupid, ugly, or incompetent, or similar statements. Single, isolated negative comments about the self may not necessarily indicate low self-esteem unless they are part of a pattern of behavior. Assess further to de-

termine whether the self-negating talk is part of a pattern. Body language and tone of voice are also important when evaluating the person.

Assess the client for cues of how she behaves in relation to her own values. Values are expressed in the circumstances or behaviors that cause the person to talk about feeling ashamed or when one inappropriately blames oneself. However, failure to accept responsibility for the consequences of one's actions may also indicate low self-esteem. The person rationalizes personal failures rather than taking steps to correct the situation.

To assess a person's sense of being accepted or valued, notice the pattern of relationships with others. Clients with low self-esteem have difficulty accepting a compliment or may exaggerate negative feedback from others. The person is also frequently hypersensitive to criticism or minor rejections by others. The person who must continually seek acceptance, who is boastful, or who appears to have feelings of grandeur has not developed a positive sense of self-worth.

Observe the client's interactions with others to assess the person's feelings about his ability to influence others or to have control over his own life. A feeling of lack of control can be manifested in being reluctant to ask others for help, to engage in social activities, or to make suggestions or to offer opinions.

Assessment of feelings of competence can be determined by observing actions (Table 46–1). Low self-esteem can be manifested by a reluctance to try new things, to change jobs, or to move to a different residence. Low self-esteem can result in haphazard work or being overly concerned with details and perfection. Either of these actions can result in poor quality of work.

Related Factors

The related factors for *Self-esteem disturbance* are somewhat different if the low self-esteem is situational or chronic. *Situational low self-esteem* can be related to health care situations such as a hysterectomy, an amputation, a slow recovery from illness, or other situations that challenge a person's coping resources. *Chronic low self-esteem* may result from a more pervasive problem in unhealthy interpersonal relationships, failure to achieve developmental milestones, failure to achieve life goals, failure to live up to a personal moral code, or a sense of powerlessness (see Decision Tree).

The client's patterns of interactions with significant others are a related factor that provides direction for nursing care. If the client behaves as though his self-worth is low, others may treat him as unworthy. This treatment causes the person to behave as though he is unworthy. Low self-esteem may thus be improved by nursing interventions that help the client to interrupt this circular pattern of relating.

A second related factor that is useful in designing interventions is the client's pattern of thoughts and feelings in response to situations that produce low self-esteem. Often, the underlying situation cannot be

TABLE 46–1

Characteristics of People With High Self-Esteem Versus Low Self-Esteem

People With High Self-Esteem	People With Low Self-Esteem
Accept responsibility for their own well-being and take charge of their own lives.	Blame others for their lack of a sense of well-being and failures in life. Their behaviors are passive and obstructive.
Expect to be valued and accepted by others. They like and value others.	Expect people to be critical of them and to avoid their company. They are prone to condemn others.
Have positive perceptions of their skills, appearance, sexuality, and behaviors.	Have negative perceptions of their skills, appearance, sexuality, and behaviors.
Perform equally well when being observed as when not watched. Motivation comes primarily from within.	Perform less well when being observed. Motivation is primarily to avoid punishment.
Accept criticism, evaluate it accurately, and change behaviors if needed.	Are defensive and passive in response to criticism.
Can accept compliments easily.	Have difficulty accepting compliments.
Evaluate their performance realistically.	Have unrealistic expectations about their performance.
Are relatively comfortable relating to authority figures.	Are uncomfortable relating to authority figures.
Express general satisfaction with life.	Are dissatisfied with their lot in life.
Have a social support system that gives positive feedback and encouragement.	Have a weak social support system that reinforces resentments, fears, and vices.
Have primarily an internal locus of control.	Rely on external locus of control.

Adapted from Arnold, E., & Boggs, K. (1999). Interpersonal relationships: Professional communication skills for nurses (3rd ed.). Philadelphia: WB Saunders.

altered, but the client's perception of the situation can be redefined.

A third related factor that is useful in planning interventions is the presence of situations that strain the client's coping resources. The interventions are then directed at helping the client to develop coping skills, such as increasing the person's problem-solving ability, increasing the client's knowledge of the situation, teaching health care actions to change the situation, helping the client to reduce behaviors that increase the distress, and promoting the development of social support systems that give the client positive feedback.

Focused Assessment for Body Image Disturbance

Defining Characteristics

The nursing diagnosis *Body image disturbance* applies when a client has a change in the body and fails to accept the change, and this failure interferes with necessary health practices, abilities, or lifestyle management.

To determine whether this diagnosis applies, assess for the presence of obsessive thoughts about the loss or change, a history of attempted suicide or self-mutilation, or inappropriate increases or decreases in weight. As you conduct your assessment, be sure to observe for verbal or nonverbal cues to the client's coping.

Assess for a *Body image disturbance* whenever a client has a change in body structure or function, especially if the change is a major one. Some diagnostic cues for *Body image disturbance* include expressions of shame or embarrassment caused by a change in body

structure or function. Signs and symptoms include not wanting to look at or touch the affected body part, wanting to either hide or expose the body part, and feelings of helplessness, hopelessness, powerlessness, and vulnerability.

For this diagnosis to apply, the client must exhibit either a verbal response or a nonverbal response to an actual or perceived change in structure or function; that is, you must be able to link the cue to a change or perceived change.

Related Factors

DEVELOPMENTAL
When body image disturbance is rooted in developmental phases, interventions are aimed at providing corrective experiences. Ask the client about childhood experiences related to the development of self-concept.

PATHOPHYSIOLOGICAL
Body image disturbance may result from pathophysiological changes in the body, especially when the person has a strong emotional investment in the part of the body that has changed. For women, loss of a breast from mastectomy or the uterus from hysterectomy can have a strong emotional impact. For a man, illness that results in muscle atrophy or scarring may have the same effect.

Traumatic injuries that result in disfigurement will require the person to change the self-concept to include the changes in the body's appearance. Injuries that leave the face scarred are particularly difficult to manage. However, scars on any part of the body may have a significant impact on body image. For example,

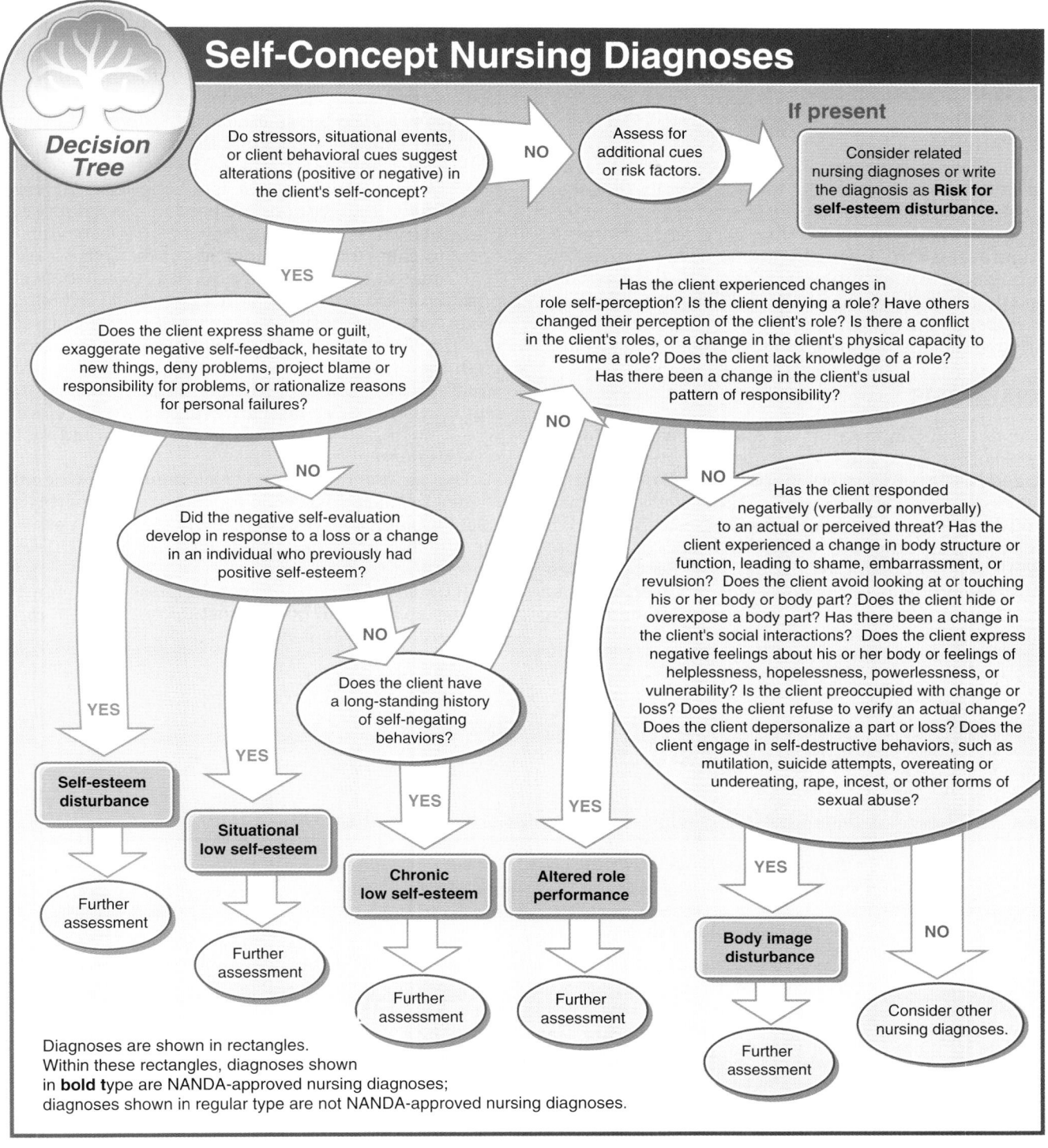

Self-Concept Nursing Diagnoses

Decision Tree

Do stressors, situational events, or client behavioral cues suggest alterations (positive or negative) in the client's self-concept?

NO → Assess for additional cues or risk factors. → **If present** Consider related nursing diagnoses or write the diagnosis as **Risk for self-esteem disturbance.**

YES

Does the client express shame or guilt, exaggerate negative self-feedback, hesitate to try new things, deny problems, project blame or responsibility for problems, or rationalize reasons for personal failures?

Has the client experienced changes in role self-perception? Is the client denying a role? Have others changed their perception of the client's role? Is there a conflict in the client's roles, or a change in the client's physical capacity to resume a role? Does the client lack knowledge of a role? Has there been a change in the client's usual pattern of responsibility?

NO

Did the negative self-evaluation develop in response to a loss or a change in an individual who previously had positive self-esteem?

NO **NO**

Has the client responded negatively (verbally or nonverbally) to an actual or perceived threat? Has the client experienced a change in body structure or function, leading to shame, embarrassment, or revulsion? Does the client avoid looking at or touching his or her body or body part? Does the client hide or overexpose a body part? Has there been a change in the client's social interactions? Does the client express negative feelings about his or her body or feelings of helplessness, hopelessness, powerlessness, or vulnerability? Is the client preoccupied with change or loss? Does the client refuse to verify an actual change? Does the client depersonalize a part or loss? Does the client engage in self-destructive behaviors, such as mutilation, suicide attempts, overeating or undereating, rape, incest, or other forms of sexual abuse?

NO

Does the client have a long-standing history of self-negating behaviors?

YES

Self-esteem disturbance → Further assessment

YES **Situational low self-esteem** → Further assessment

YES **Chronic low self-esteem** → Further assessment

YES **Altered role performance** → Further assessment

YES **Body image disturbance** → Further assessment

NO Consider other nursing diagnoses.

Diagnoses are shown in rectangles. Within these rectangles, diagnoses shown in **bold t**ype are NANDA-approved nursing diagnoses; diagnoses shown in regular type are not NANDA-approved nursing diagnoses.

a 55-year-old man who has had coronary artery bypass surgery will have characteristic scars on the chest and leg that many people will recognize.

Changes in body image may be involved even when a pathophysiological change does not affect outward appearance. Less obvious but very real changes in body image can result from the loss of function of any body organ. For example, the person with a kidney transplant may not look different but must cope with a change in body image from that of a healthy, well-functioning body to that of a body vulnerable to infection and incorporating an organ from another person.

Medical treatment, too, can affect body image. For example, chemotherapy can result in hair loss that may alter one's body image. Surgery may alter not only appearance but also function, such as in ostomy surgery, radical head/neck surgery, and amputation. Even the onset of a chronic medical condition requiring maintenance medication, such as asthma, hypertension, or diabetes, can affect body image.

SITUATIONAL

Most people have experienced events that have a negative impact on body image. Usually, however, these feelings are brief and resolve with a good night's sleep or a subsequent positive experience. However, some events are sufficiently traumatic to produce lasting effects. For example, *Body image disturbance* commonly occurs in victims of sexual abuse or rape. Rape victims, in particular, frequently report feeling dirty and that no amount of bathing will remove the feeling.

DIAGNOSIS

The five self-concept nursing diagnoses are highly interrelated. Often, intervention for any one of the five diagnoses involves intervention for one or more of the other diagnoses. For example, *Altered role performance* and *Body image disturbance* affect self-esteem. You will select the appropriate diagnosis based on the predominant feature of the problem, how the client identifies the problem, or the goals of care. Clustering data can help you arrive at the most appropriate nursing diagnoses.

When making a diagnosis that involves self-esteem, you will select among *Self-esteem disturbance, Situational low self-esteem,* and *Chronic low self-esteem.* The diagnoses *Situational low self-esteem* and *Chronic low self-esteem* are subcategories of the diagnosis *Self-esteem disturbance. Situational low self-esteem* is a temporary state caused by a significant loss or change. The goal of intervention is to prevent a long-lasting condition. *Chronic low self-esteem* is a long-term state for which more interventions are needed. The purpose of these interventions is to teach clients new behaviors in order to change their feelings about the self.

It may not be necessary to distinguish between *Situational low self-esteem* and *Chronic low self-esteem;* the broader diagnosis *Self-esteem disturbance* may suffice. If a client lacks confidence in her ability to accomplish the desired outcomes in a particular short-term situation, it is irrelevant whether the self-esteem problem is chronic or acute. However, it may be relevant when making a decision about the length and methods of intervention.

Use the diagnosis *Altered role performance* when the client's primary concern is functioning in a particular role. Problems in self-esteem, body image, or personal identity may be an underlying factor in *Altered role performance.*

Body image disturbance may be present when a client has a change in body structure or function, especially if the change is major.

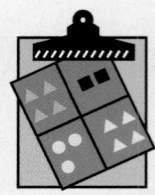

CLUSTERING DATA TO MAKE A NURSING DIAGNOSIS
PROBLEMS OF SELF-CONCEPT

Data Cluster	Diagnosis
15-year-old female with scoliosis needs to wear a brace to slow the progression of the scoliotic curve and refuses to do so. She states, "My clothes do not look right when I wear this thing."	*Body image disturbance* related to nonconformity in appearance with peers
24-year-old mother of 2-day-old infant verbalized inadequacy of her new role, stating, "My husband and I already don't have time together. I don't know how I will be able to take care of this child."	*Altered role performance* related to new role of parenting
40-year-old female was diagnosed with multiple sclerosis over a year ago. She has made a poor adjustment to her illness. She states, "I'm so tired of having to depend on someone else to do things for me. I wish I could die."	*Chronic low self-esteem* related to feelings of helplessness and hopelessness
32-year-old divorced male with custody of 3-year-old child. His ex-wife is in a drug rehabilitation program in another state. States that he does not know what to do with the child. "I have to work all day and do not have the skills to care for a child. I couldn't make my marriage work. How can I raise a child?"	*Situational low self-esteem* related to role stress secondary to divorce and change to single-parent status.

PLANNING

Because the self-concept nursing diagnoses are so closely interrelated, and because expected outcomes and interventions are so similar, we will focus our discussion on just two diagnoses as examples of how to tailor expected outcomes, interventions, and evaluation to the specific client situation: *Self-esteem disturbance* and *Body image disturbance*.

Expected Outcomes for the Client With Self-Esteem Disturbance

The goal for a client with *Self-esteem disturbance* is that the client will have improved self-esteem or perhaps develop sufficient self-esteem to accomplish a particular task. You will plan interventions to assist the person to identify the source of poor self-esteem, identify and value strengths, explore the relationship of behavior to self-appraisal, develop a positive support system, and develop coping skills. Examples of specific expected outcomes include the following:

The client will identify negative self-talk or reduce the incidence of negative self-talk.
The client will name the feelings associated with negative self-talk.
The client will identify personal strengths and positive attributes.
The client will replace negative self-talk with positive self-talk.
The client will identify how negative self-talk affects behaviors.
The client will engage in positive behaviors (name the behavior).
The client will appraise the situation in a realistic manner, without distortions.
The client will demonstrate healthy coping patterns (name the pattern desired).

When working with a client to improve self-esteem, be sure to select behavioral outcomes consistent with the client's developmental stage. When children have a sense of high self-esteem, they play in groups, may be leaders, may be better achievers, and may have positive peer relationships. They will also be better able to make independent judgments, take more initiative, and avoid troublesome situations. When adults have high self-esteem, they are more likely to be satisfied with their lives, their jobs, and their personal relationships. Adults with high self-esteem are more comfortable with themselves and need less approval from others. They better realize their own capabilities, are better able to handle criticisms and failures, and demonstrate positive coping skills.

Increased self-esteem is a long-term expected outcome for clients with *Self-esteem disturbance;* short-term or intermediate outcomes provide important milestones for the client, as demonstrated in the Nursing Care Planning chart. The short-term outcomes can be as simple as maintaining good personal hygiene and grooming. Rather than setting outcomes that sound unattainable to the client, such as demonstrating self-confidence, making decisions, or showing a belief in self and self-capabilities, you will need to help the client identify specific goals and commit to taking small steps. For example, you could encourage a client to state a short-term goal like this: "I will fill out one job application today."

Increased self-esteem has been shown to influence quality of life positively. Having the client describe what quality of life would mean to him can be helpful in establishing outcomes that will help the client to be motivated to engage in the work of increasing self-esteem.

Expected Outcomes for the Client With Body Image Disturbance

The goal for a client with *Body image disturbance* is that the client will physically and mentally adapt to the changes in body image. You will need to plan interventions to assist the client in the following four stages of adaptation:

1. Experiencing the impact of the change
2. Retreating from the situation
3. Acknowledging the meaning of the change
4. Reconstructing life psychologically and physically

To accomplish the overall goal, you will design interventions to help the client identify and express feelings, identify self-value and strengths, identify the relationship between behavior and self-appraisal, develop support systems, develop successful coping strategies, and implement new coping patterns. Expected outcomes may include the following:

The client will verbalize and demonstrate acceptance of his appearance (grooming, dressing, posture, eating patterns, presentation of self).
The client will demonstrate an interest in and willingness to resume self-care or responsibilities.
The client will discuss the impact or meaning of the change.
The client will initiate new or reestablish existing support systems.

INTERVENTION

Interventions to Increase Self-Esteem

Interventions to increase self-esteem are designed to enhance the four components of self-esteem. These interventions are summarized in Figure 46–6.

Promoting Feelings of Acceptance/Worthiness

One of the most important things you can do to help your client feel acceptance and worthiness is to establish a trusting relationship with her. Allow her to freely express herself without making judgments about her feelings or behaviors. Use touch, and maintain eye contact to help establish a relationship that

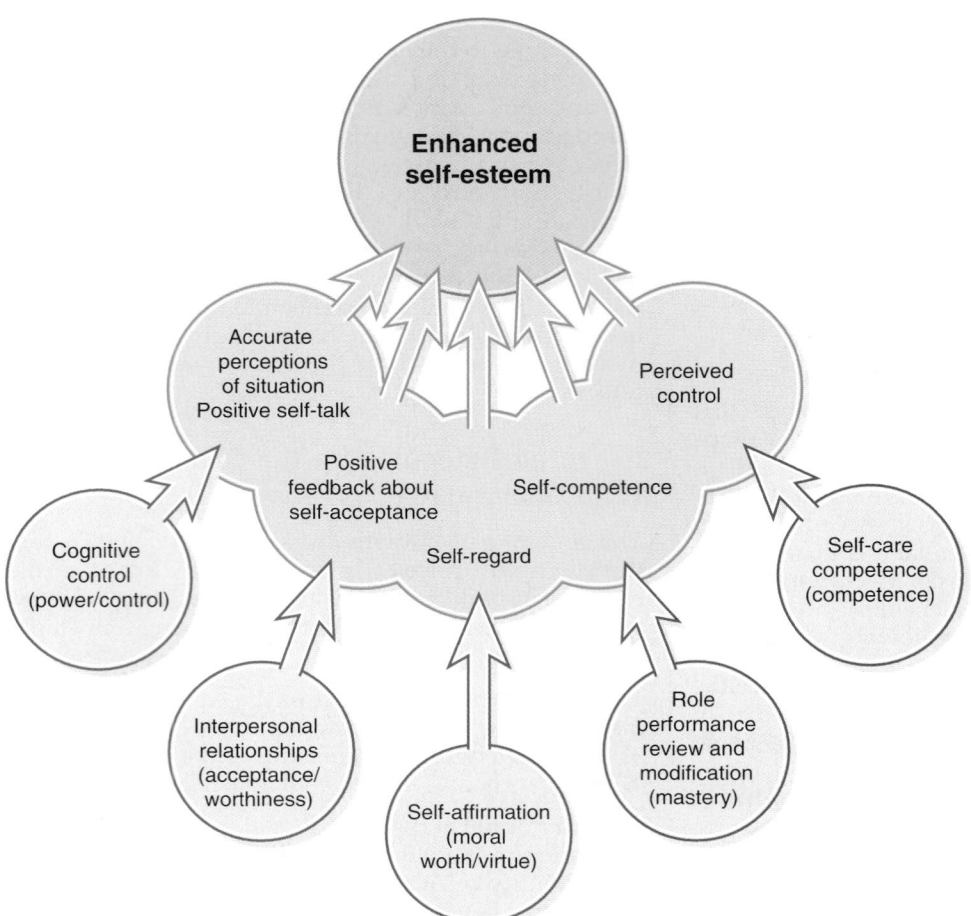

Figure 46–6. Interventions to increase self-esteem. (Redrawn from Miller, J.F. [1992]. Coping with chronic illness: Overcoming powerlessness [2nd ed.]. Philadelphia: F.A. Davis.)

enhances active listening (Fig. 46–7). If the client is angry, grieving, or fearful, offer understanding and acceptance of those feelings rather than solutions to the problem or evaluation of the reasonableness of these emotions.

*A*ction *A*lert!
To establish a trusting relationship with the client, sit at eye level, conveying a genuine interest.

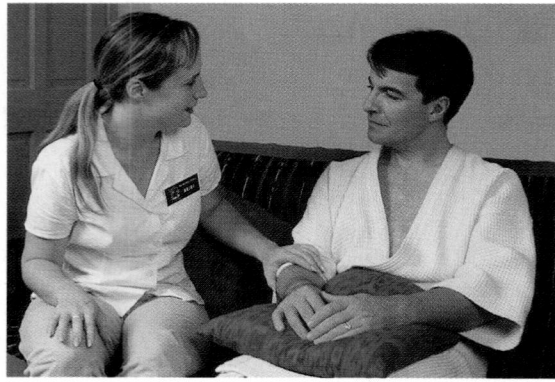

Figure 46–7. Touch and eye contact help establish a relationship that enhances active listening.

Asking the client open-ended questions may help her to open up to you. The following are some examples of open-ended questions to initiate a dialogue with the client:

How do you value yourself?
Tell me what you are most proud of about yourself.
Tell me what you like about yourself.
Name at least one of your strengths and one of you weaknesses.

Providing positive reinforcement for steps toward healthy behavior is more effective than negative reinforcement for unhealthy behaviors. High self-esteem develops in the presence of positive feedback, whether that feedback is from others or in the form of positive self-talk (Fig. 46–8).

Hospital-based nurses can provide guidance to clients suffering from *Self-esteem disturbance* by encouraging their acceptance of family members and friends. Visits or contacts with others may provide clients with a chance to share their feelings with significant others and to learn from others with similar experiences. You can also help the family to help the client by explaining the usual feelings associated with the client's illness and emphasizing that understanding the feelings is more important than trying to talk the client out of those feelings.

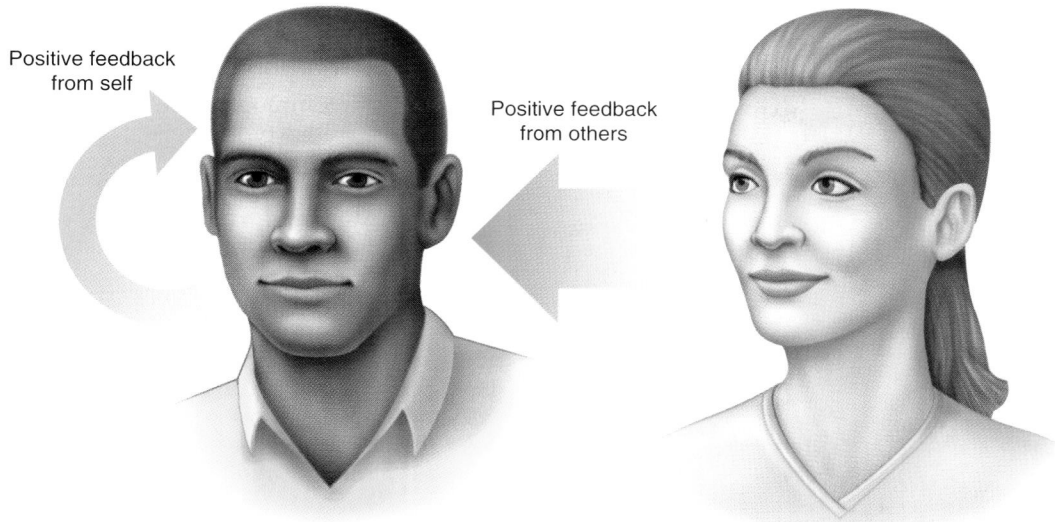

Positive feedback from self

Positive feedback from others

Figure 46–8. High self-esteem develops when a person engages in positive self-talk (positive self-feedback) and receives positive feedback from others.

Promoting a Sense of Competence/Mastery

For any client, whether a school-aged child who is crying because he is routinely excluded from a group of playmates or a 60-year-old recovering from a colostomy, mastering a skill helps develop a sense of competence. The child can learn to draw or perform gymnastics and gain the confidence to approach other children and make friends. The 60-year-old with a colostomy can learn to care for his own ostomy, and these self-care skills can promote a sense of competence (Fig. 46–9).

Promoting a Sense of Power/Control

Developing feelings of power and control is closely related to developing mastery. The diabetic can develop control over the diabetes and have the knowledge that control comes from mastery of insulin injection. The child who ignores rejection by other children and de-

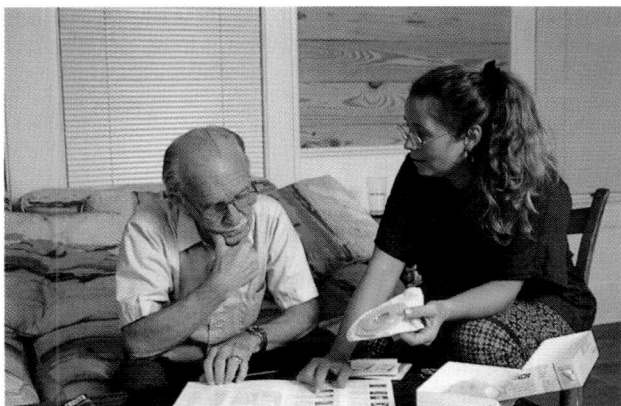

Figure 46–9. Learning self-care can help to counteract the loss of self-esteem associated with an illness.

velops skills in art or gymnastics is also taking charge of his own life and enhancing self-esteem through power and control.

Indirectly, reminiscence as a life experience or a form of therapy in the elderly may contribute to a sense of power and control. You can assist the elderly client to reminisce by listening to the stories and life events that have given meaning to the person's life. Reminiscence is useful because one of the goals in life is to come to terms with the past, often by recognizing the value that life has held. Reminiscence is thus one way to help the elderly to improve or maintain their self-esteem (Fig. 46–10).

Promoting a Sense of Moral Worth/Virtue

Values clarification is a useful tool to a sense of moral worth or virtue. A high level of self-esteem is associated with clear personal values and the ability to act in a manner consistent with those values. The first step in values clarification is to help the client identify values that underlie behavior. Approach this discussion of values with a nonjudgmental attitude. Then, help the client identify areas in which values are in conflict. Examples of value conflicts can be found in clients who state that health is a value yet behave in a manner that is not consistent with health-seeking behaviors. For example:

- A person who has sustained a severe fracture to an ankle but is not actively engaging in the exercise needed to regain mobility may have a conflicting value that states, " I deserve to rest because I have been injured."
- A mother who has had surgery returns to full-time housekeeping against her physician's advice because of a value that it is her responsibility to care for her children.

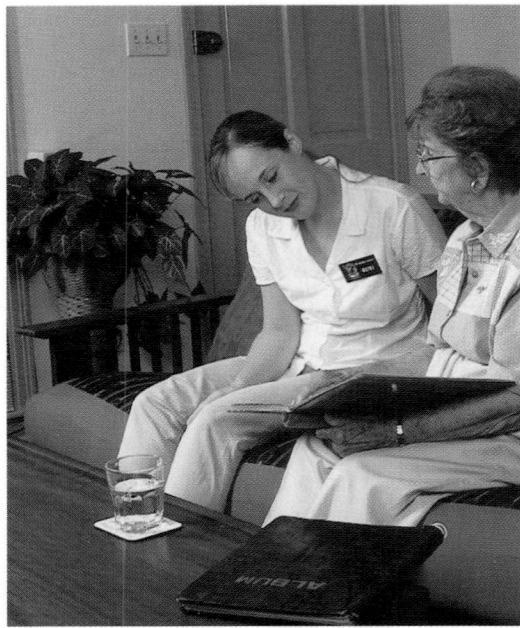

Figure 46–10. Reminiscing with the client about her family history promotes self-esteem in the elderly.

These clients need assistance to recognize and name the conflicting values and make a choice that will promote self-esteem. Consideration of the consequences of acting in accordance with each value is necessary to make a clear choice between conflicting values.

The highest level of clarity about values is acting consistently in a manner that demonstrates the value. Low self-esteem results when a person cannot or will not act in accordance with strongly held values.

Interventions to Integrate a Change in Body Image

When a client loses a body part or function, the loss activates the grieving process. The first stage of grieving is a state of shock and disbelief. The client needs time to experience the impact of the event and allow the meaning of the event to come into conscious awareness. Do not force the client to full awareness of the change in the body; rather, allow the person to proceed at a natural pace.

As the client gradually shows signs of readiness to discuss what has happened, use active listening to determine the meaning of the loss or change for the client. The meaning of the loss or change will be affected by the visibility of the loss or change, how much function has been lost, and the emotional significance of the change for the client. Amputations may take a lengthy period of adjustment because the loss of a limb is highly visible, functional loss is high, and the loss has a high emotional component. As the client begins to show readiness, encourage the client to look at the changed body part, to touch it, and to participate in care.

Action Alert!
Allow the client sufficient time to express her feelings openly and honestly.

Anger is a common phase of grieving that often sets in as the initial numbing effects of the shock are disappearing. Communicate to the client that it is acceptable to be angry. Normalize the response by suggesting that anger is a common response. Assist the person to express the anger, frustration, and resentment. Be aware of the anxiety that the client's anger may provoke in you, and learn to control this anxiety in order to continue to be present for the client. Anger can be acted out in many different ways, some of which may be harmful. Do not allow the client to cause harm to herself or others in acting out this anger.

As the client becomes exhausted with anger, feelings of helplessness and hopelessness are common. Be ready for depression to become evident. Assess for suicide tendencies, and protect the client from harming herself.

Acceptance of the loss will come gradually. With a therapeutic nurse-client relationship, you will be able to recognize teachable moments when you can provide the client with information that will help with the ultimate adjustment to the change in body image. You may be able to provide the necessary teaching yourself, or the client may need referral to specialized therapists to learn skills in self-care. Make yourself knowledgeable about the services that physical therapists, occupational therapists, enterostomal therapists, and other specialists can offer in order to be ready to help the client know what help is available and what to expect from it. Encourage clients to use these resources.

Action Alert!
Encourage clients to participate in their care to promote acceptance of the loss or change.

Assisting a client through the loss of a body part or body function is best started prior to the loss, if possible. The client who has the opportunity to plan for the loss can begin to make adjustments in advance. For example, the client who needs colon surgery that will result in the creation of a colostomy can become mentally prepared by talking to friends or acquaintances who have had the surgery. Many fears may be dispelled by knowing others who managed the problems that are the most fearful.

EVALUATION

Evaluation of clients with any of the self-concept nursing diagnoses can take several approaches. Three common approaches are the client's subjective report of progress, measurement of expected outcomes, and the use of before-and-after rating scales or instruments. Each method has advantages and disadvantages. A combination of methods may yield the best results. We now look at how these three methods can be used to evaluate changes in self-esteem and body image.

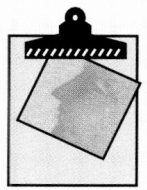

A CLIENT WITH A BREAST LUMP

Admission Data

Nancy Ward has come to the clinic to receive preoperative instructions before her breast biopsy in 2 days.

Physician's Orders
Chest x-ray
CBC

Nursing Assessment
Sister is present. Nancy seems to ignore most of the instructions but repeatedly asks how the breast will appear after the procedure. The physician has told Nancy that there will be several treatment options presented to her after the biopsy. Nancy has a friend who had a mastectomy and seems to be focusing on this possibility.

NURSING CARE PLAN

Nursing Diagnosis	Expected Outcomes	Interventions	Evaluation (End of Preoperative Visit)
Self-esteem disturbance related to the threat of loss of breast as a treatment for cancer	The client will differentiate a biopsy from a mastectomy.	Repeat the description of the biopsy several times using different words. Emphasize that the scar will be small and that no further treatment will be performed until Nancy agrees to the treatment.	The first two times the nurse repeats the description of the biopsy, Nancy asks a question like, "Yes, but how much smaller will my breast be?"
		Answer questions honestly.	Nancy does not appear to listen to the answers.
		Encourage the client to restate information about the biopsy.	Nancy's sister restates the information and says that she will tell Nancy again after they get home. *The sister asks if Nancy can wear her charm to the surgery. When the nurse says yes, Nancy looks relieved.*
	Will come for the biopsy confident that she understands what will happen to her.	Provide an opportunity for Nancy to talk about her feelings of possible loss.	Nancy does not want to talk about the possible treatments if the diagnosis is cancer.
	Will share some of her positive attributes with the nurse.	Ask Nancy about her favorite activities.	Nancy likes to babysit the children in the area. She is good at making up games for them to play.
		Notice positive features or attributes about Nancy and share these with her.	When the nurse tells Nancy she has beautiful skin, Nancy looks at her blankly.

Italicized interventions indicate culturally specific care.

Critical Thinking Questions

1. What key factors you would consider to ensure that Nancy Ward receives adequate follow-up care after the biopsy?
2. How would you use the four components of self-esteem as you plan to help Nancy accept chemotherapy?
3. Why might Nancy appear relieved upon learning that she will be able to wear her charm to surgery?

Self-Esteem

Because *Self-esteem disturbance* is a subjective experience, the response to intervention logically would be evaluated from a client's subjective report of feeling better about the self. However, several problems could occur with this method of evaluation. The client could report what the nurse wants to hear. Likewise, the client could report feeling better, but that report could be skewed by the fact that the client feels better in the presence of the nurse. A third possibility is that the client's self-esteem has improved, but troublesome behaviors (such as drug abuse) have not.

The second method of evaluation is to compare behavior with expected outcomes. The assumption with this method of evaluation is that changed behaviors indicate a change in self-esteem. Although changed behaviors are a measure of progress, they may not indicate a change in self-esteem.

The third method of evaluation—using a rating scale or instrument—is perhaps the most precise method of measuring progress in improving self-esteem. However, its effectiveness depends on the reliability and validity of the instrument. If the instrument is not sensitive to detecting the particular manifestations of self-esteem that you are trying to measure, it will not be an effective evaluation instrument. Additionally, if it relies on a subjective report, it will have the same problems as any subjective report.

Body Image

For clients with major body image changes, it may take 6 months to a year to fully integrate a change in body image. Measuring short-term goals in the form of expected outcomes is important to ensure that the client is making progress. Review the expected outcomes to ensure that they reflect movement through the phases of adaptation.

The client's subjective report of changes in body image may be less reliable than objective measures until the client has reached the stage of acceptance. While the client is in the stages of shock, disbelief, anger, and depression, progress and satisfaction are difficult for the client to recognize.

Instruments are available to measure adaptation. However, before using one of these instruments, be sure to determine whether it is appropriate for the specific population or client. To determine that, become familiar with which population the instrument was designed to evaluate and whether your particular client or population fits within that population.

KEY PRINCIPLES

- Self-concept consists of self-esteem, personal identity, role performance, and body image.
- Self-concept remains relatively enduring throughout life but can change with life experiences.

- Self-esteem is relatively fixed but can change with life transitions or crises.
- The four components of self-esteem are competency/mastery, power/control, moral worth/virtue, and acceptance/worthiness.
- Self-esteem is associated with good health practices.
- There is a difference in the way men and women tend to determine their self-esteem (men with personal achievement; women with social support systems).
- Self-esteem is developed in the child by age 12 but can be changed in adolescence and adulthood.
- Self-esteem in the preschool child is related to interactions with parents and caregivers.
- Self-esteem in the adolescent is strongly influenced by peers.
- Self-esteem may be diminished in the older adult, as a result of losses (physical, social, and mental).
- Body image is related to self-esteem.
- Body image is a critical dimension of adolescence.
- Personal identity is the ability to distinguish between self and nonself.
- Interventions for altered self-esteem are aimed at restoring competence/mastery, power/control, moral worth/virtue, or acceptance/worthiness.
- Interventions for *Body image disturbance* are aimed at helping the client through the four stages of adaptation.

BIBLIOGRAPHY

Anderson, K.L. (1995). The effect of chronic obstructive pulmonary disease on quality of life. *Research in Nursing and Health, 18*(6), 547–556.

*Anderson, M.S., & Johnson, J. (1994). Restoration of body image and self-esteem for women after cancer treatment. *Cancer Practice, 2*(5), 345–348.

Anderson, S.E.H. (1995). Personality, appraisal, and adaptational outcomes in HIV seropositive men and women. *Research in Nursing and Health, 18*(4), 303–312.

Arnold, E., & Boggs, K. (1999). *Interpersonal relationships: Professional communication skills for nurses* (3rd ed.). Philadelphia: W.B. Saunders Co.

*Bensink, G.W., Godbey, K.L., Marshall, M.J., & Yarandle, A.H. (1992). Institutionalized elderly relaxation, locus of control, self-esteem. *Journal of Gerontological Nursing, 18*(4), 30–36.

Carpenito, L.J. (1999). *Nursing diagnosis* (8th ed.). Philadelphia: JB Lippincott Co.

Carson, V.B. (2000). *Mental health nursing: The nurse-patient journey* (2nd ed.). Philadelphia: W.B. Saunders Co.

Chiverton, P.A., Wells, T.J., Brink, C.A., & Mayer R. (1996). Psychological factors associated with urinary incontinence. *Clinical Nurse Specialty, 10*(5), 229–233.

Cole, F.L., & Slocumb, E.M. (1995). Factors influencing safer sexual behaviors in heterosexual late adolescent and young adult collegiate males. *Image: The Journal of Nursing Scholarship, 27*(3), 217–223.

*Conn, V.S., Taylor, S.G., & Hayes, V. (1992). Social support, self-esteem, and self-care after myocardial infarction. *Health Values, 16*(5), 25–31.

*Asterisk indicates a classic or definitive work on this subject.

*Coopersmith, S. (1981). *The antecedents of self-esteem* (Rev. ed.). Novato, CA: Consulting Pyschologist Press.

Doswell, W.M., Millor, G.K., Thompson, H., & Braxter, B. (1998). Self-image and self-esteem in African-American preteen girls: Implications for mental health. *Issues in Mental Health Nursing, 19*(1), 71–94.

Douglass, L.G. (1997). Reciprocal support in the context of cancer: Perspectives of the patient and spouse. *Oncology Nursing Forum, 24*(9), 1529–1536.

*Duitsman, D.M. (1993). Quality of life in heart transplants. *Health Values, 17*(6), 55–61.

Eliopoulos, C. (1995). *Manual of gerontologic nursing.* St. Louis: C.V. Mosby.

*Erikson, E. (1950). Childhood and society. New York: W. W. Norton.

*Flett, R., Harcourt, B., & Alpass, F. (1994). Psychosocial aspects of chronic lower leg ulceration in the elderly. *Western Journal of Nursing Research, 16*(2), 183–192.

Forte, J.A., Franks, D.D., & Rigsby, D. (1996). Asymmetrical role-taking: Comparing battered and nonbattered women. *Social Work, 41*(1), 59–73.

Gillis, A. (1996). Teens for healthy living. *The Canadian Nurse, 92*(6), 26–30.

Guinn B., Semper, T., & Jorgensen, L. (1997). Body image perception in female Mexican-American adolescents. *Journal of School Health, 67*(3), 112–115.

Hall, L.A., Kotch, J.B., Browne, D., & Rayens, M.K. (1996). Self-esteem as a mediator of the effects of stressors and social resources on depressive symptoms in postpartum mothers. *Nursing Resource, 45*(4), 231–238.

*Harper, B.K., & Marshall, E. (1991). Adolescents' problems and their relationship to self-esteem. *Adolescence, 26*(10), 104–107.

*Killeen, M. (1993). Parent-influences on children's self-esteem in economically disadvantaged families. *Issues in Mental Health Nursing, 14*(4), 323–336.

*Klyde, B. (1994). The cultural context of Native American health issues. *Journal of American Academy of Physician Assistants, 7*(10), 700–706.

Lecomte, T. (1997). The role of self-esteem in the phychosocial adaptations of schizophrenics (French). *Canadian Journal of Community Mental Health, 16*(1), 23–38.

*Lee, K.A., Lentz, M.J., Taylor, D.L., Mitchell, E.S., & Woods, N.F. (1994). Fatigue as a response to environmental demands in women's lives. *Image: The Journal of Nursing Scholarship, 26*(2), 149–154.

Lo, G.P.H. (1996). Research forum: Perceived self-esteem in adult males with chronic obstructive airway disease. *Hong Kong Nursing Journal, 73,* 4–11.

*Maslow, A. (1954). Motivation and personality. New York: Harper & Row.

McPhee, S.J. & Schroeder, S.A. (1999). General approach to the patient; health maintenance and disease prevention; and common symptoms. In L.M. Tierney, S.J. McPhee, & M.A. Papadakais (Eds.), *Current medical diagnosis and treatment* (38th ed.). Stamford, CT: Appleton & Lange.

*Mihalopoulos, N.G. (1994). The psychologic impact of ostomy surgery on persons 50 years of age and older. *Journal of Wound, Ostomy, & Continence Care, 21*(4), 149–155.

Mona, L.R., Gardo, P.S., & Brown, R.C. (1994). Sexual self views of women with disabilities: The relationship among age-of-onset, nature of disability, and self esteem. *Sexuality and Disability, 12*(4), 261–277.

*Napholz, L. (1994). Indices of psychological well-being and sex role orientation among working women. *Health Care for Women International, 15*(4), 307–316.

North American Nursing Diagnosis Association. (1998). *NANDA nursing diagnoses: Definitions and classification 1999–2000.* Philadelphia: Author.

O'Brien, M.T. (1993). Multiple sclerosis: The relationship among self-esteem, social support, and coping behavior. *Applied Nursing Research, 6*(2), 54–63.

Overbay, J.D., & Purath, J. (1997). Self-concept and health status in elementary-school-aged children. *Issues in Comprehensive Pediatric Nursing, 20*(2), 89–101.

Polk, L.V. (1997). Toward a middle-range of resilience. *Advances in Nursing Science, 19*(3), 1–13.

Torres, R., Fernandez, F., & Maceira, D. (1995). Self-esteem and value of health as correlates of adolescent health behavior. *Adolescence, 30*(118), 403–412.

Vera, L., & Wrath, K. (1995). Feelin' groovy. *The Canadian Nurse, 91*(1), 26–30.

Warren, B.J. (1997). Depression, stressful life events, social support, and self-esteem in middle class African American women. *Archive of Psychiatric Nursing, 11*(3), 107–117.

Willoughby, C., King, G., & Palatajko, H. (1996). A therapist's guide to self-esteem. *The American Journal of Occupational Therapy, 50*(2), 124–132.

*Young, M., Werch, C., & Bakema, D. (1989). Area-specific self-esteem scales and substance abuse among elementary and middle school children. *Journal of School Health, 59*(6), 251–254.

Anxiety

Susan Lewis

Key Terms

anxiety

anxiety disorder

anxiolytics

pathological anxiety

LEARNING OBJECTIVES

After studying this chapter, you should be able to:

1. **Describe the concepts of anxiety as manifested in the health care setting.**

2. **Discuss factors affecting anxiety.**

3. **Assess the anxious client to determine the level of anxiety.**

4. **Differentiate between normal and pathological anxiety.**

5. **Plan for goal-directed interventions to prevent, reduce, or manage anxiety.**

6. **Evaluate achievement of the expected outcomes for the client who is experiencing anxiety.**

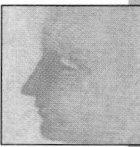

Ida Adkins is a 42-year-old woman of Appalachian descent who grew up in the mountains of West Virginia. Miss Adkins is the single parent of a 16-year-old son. They live with her parents on a small, rural hillside farm.

Miss Adkins is taken to the clinic by her mother with complaints of chest pain, shortness of breath, nausea, dizziness, numbness and tingling, palpitations, and nervousness. Her mother says that she has "a bad heart" and "even badder nerves." When the symptoms began that morning, her mother first treated Ida at home with tea from bleeding heart leaves. When that had no effect, she gave her daughter garlic to eat and two of the pills she got from the clinic the last time this happened. Ida still had "heart pains" after her mother's treatments, so they decided to come to the clinic.

In addition to nursing diagnoses related to cardiac disease, the clinic nurse assesses Miss Adkins for *Anxiety* (see Anxiety Nursing Diagnoses chart).

ANXIETY
NURSING DIAGNOSES

Anxiety: A vague, uneasy feeling of discomfort or dread, accompanied by an autonomic response; the source is often nonspecific or unknown to the individual; a feeling of apprehension caused by anticipation of danger. It is an alerting signal that warns of impending danger and enables the individual to take measures to deal with threat.

From North American Nursing Diagnosis Association. (1999). NANDA nursing diagnoses: Definitions and classification 1999–2000. Philadelphia: Author

CONCEPTS OF ANXIETY

Anxiety is a universal experience. Dating back to survival mechanisms in our prehistoric ancestors, it is an unavoidable aspect of everyday life. Anxiety is experienced as a normal part of growth, change, new experience, and finding personal identity and meaning in life (Kaplan & Sadock, 1998). Human beings experience anxiety in numerous situations and interpersonal interactions.

Anxiety is one of the most common emotions seen in health care settings. Caring for anxious clients is one of our greatest challenges as nurses. As nurses, our primary concern lies with the symptoms our clients are experiencing and how these symptoms affect their health and daily functioning.

Definition of Anxiety

Anxiety is described as a diffuse, highly uncomfortable, sometimes vague sense of apprehension or dread accompanied by one or more physical sensations. It affects a person in all domains: physiological, behavioral, cognitive, emotional, and spiritual. The anxious state can vary from edginess and uneasiness to alarm or to terror and panic.

It is caused by an interplay of factors that can be internal, external, or both. One school of thought is that physical manifestations of anxiety reflect psychological conflicts; other experts believe that biological events precede psychological conflicts. Most likely, it is a complex interaction of both psychological and physiological factors. In general, it is helpful to think of anxiety as falling into two primary categories:

- *Threat to biological integrity*—actual or anticipated hindrance to basic human needs such as food, fluid, warmth, or shelter
- *Threat to ego integrity*—unmet expectations important to identity and self-integrity, need for status, possible disapproval by significant others, inability to gain or reinforce self-respect or approval from others, and guilt or disparity between self-concept and actual behavior

Physiologically, anxiety can be explained as a sinking feeling in the pit of the stomach, tightness in the chest, a racing heart, palpitations, sweating, increased respiratory rate, shortness of breath, and a sudden urge to urinate. Behaviorally, agitation, difficulty sitting still, and tremors may be present. Cognitively, anxiety is a tense mental awareness of apprehension and a sense of impending doom or bodily danger. Emotionally, a person may be irritable, tearful, or angry. Clients may describe what they are feeling as nervousness, worry, or dread. Spiritually, a person may feel alone and as if no one understands. Socially, anxiety may interfere with the person's ability to relate to others or function in social situations.

Contacts with the health care system, such as visits to the doctor, hospital admissions, or dental appointments, evoke anxiety in almost everyone. The unfamiliar environment, anticipation of painful procedures, role changes, new rules, waiting for unknown test results, and surrendering control of one's life to caregivers can all intensify anxiety.

The effects of anxiety can be found in both normal and abnormal behavior. Ordinarily, anxiety occurs as an intermittent and transient response to stress. When it becomes so severe that it interferes with daily functioning, it is considered abnormal and pathological.

Functions of Normal Anxiety

Anxiety is a normal, expected, and temporary response to stress and may be necessary to stimulate adaptation and coping (Rosenbaum, Pollack, Otto, & Bernstein, 1997). In fact, anxiety serves several useful functions in our lives. First, it is an alerting signal that warns of potential danger and motivates us to take measures to relieve a disturbing feeling or a perceived threat. Anxiety initiates protective defense mechanisms and is a survival strategy that has life-preserving qualities and increases feelings of safety and security. The nurse who can recognize and understand anxious behavior as a protective mechanism and accepts the client's expression of anxiety can help the client to better understand what is happening and use the opportunity to teach coping strategies.

At a basic level, anxiety alerts us to a variety of threats. These include threats of bodily harm, pain, helplessness, possible punishment, or interference with social and physical needs; of separation from loved ones; of obstacles to success or status; and ultimately of threats to our sense of wholeness and harmony (Kaplan & Sadock, 1998). Anxiety provokes us to take necessary measures to defend against a threat or at least decrease its consequences—such as when we study for an examination or stop to look and listen before crossing a busy street. In addition, mild to moderate anxiety helps us to focus our attention on immediate details and may even enhance our ability to deal with anxiety-producing stimuli. For example, a mother can recognize her child's voice and cries of distress above noises made by an entire playground full of children.

A second function of anxiety is adaptation. Adaptation is self-regulation of the whole person in relation to change. It also refers to behaviors of change that occur as an individual responds to anxiety and stress. The goal of adaptation is to maintain stability, or homeostasis, during environmental change. People adapt psychologically to preserve the self and to maintain self-esteem.

Responses to Anxiety

Whether we perceive an event as stressful or dangerous depends on the nature of the event and our personal resources and coping abilities. When faced with a particular situation, we make an appraisal of the level of danger or threat and our resources to cope. Four types of response occur in situations of imminent danger, such as coming upon an attacker in a dark alley or a bear in the woods. These include fight, flight, faint, or freeze (Beck & Emery, 1985).

Physiological Aspects

Current studies of human perception have shown that before we are consciously aware of seeing or hearing a stimulus, the sensory data coming through the eyes and ears have already traveled through many stages of "selective interpretation and appraisal" (Beck & Emery, 1985). The body's physiological response to the cognitive appraisal of danger activates a chain of physiological, behavioral, cognitive, and emotional reactions designed to prepare us to face the danger and either fight or flee to safety. Human beings can experience other responses to situations of danger. Some people may become immobilized or frozen to the spot and completely unable to act. Others may actually lose consciousness or faint.

Two divisions of the autonomic nervous system (ANS) are involved in preparing the body to deal with stress or danger and then restoring homeostasis when the danger has passed. The sympathetic nervous system activates emergency resources, whereas the parasympathetic branch of the ANS induces a relaxed state.

The physiological response first identified by Hans Selye, called either the general adaptation syndrome (GAS) or the stress response, is the body's method of mobilizing its resources to defend against threats of harm (Fig. 47–1). In instances of harmful stimuli, the hypothalamus acts on the pituitary gland, causing the release of adrenocorticotropic hormone (ACTH), which stimulates the adrenal cortex to secrete glucocorticoids. In addition, the adrenal medulla is stimulated to release epinephrine (adrenaline) and norepinephrine into the bloodstream. This turbocharges body systems necessary for defense.

The parasympathetic nervous system controls many visceral functions during the normal conditions of daily living. It also returns the body to a relaxed state after the stress response: The heart rate slows, blood pressure declines, and peristalsis and other digestive processes increase again. Chapter 52 provides further discussion on the topic of stress response.

Do you recall what symptoms Ida Adkins was experiencing when she was brought to the clinic? Could those symptoms be related to the general adaptation syndrome just described?

Psychological Aspects

A core dynamic theme found at all levels of anxiety is a sense of vulnerability. Vulnerability is a feeling of helplessness, lack of control, and inadequate resources for defense when faced with threat or danger. A number of factors can contribute to a sense of helplessness and vulnerability. Feelings of shame or embarrassment can intensify this perception. Those with maladaptive personality features or poor coping skills or who tend to regress in threatening situations may feel more defenseless. Sudden onset of the threat, unavailability of significant others, feeling alone, significance of a particular illness, or having to relinquish control to others may leave us feeling unprotected and vulnerable.

Human beings can actually create or worsen their own anxiety. Negative self-talk can decrease self-confidence and set up a vicious cycle that is self-perpetuating (Fig. 47–2). Telling ourselves things like "This is awful," "This shouldn't have happened," or "I'll never be able to face anyone again" heightens the effects of anxiety. Often, an anxious person may not even be aware of such thoughts. Making clients aware of personal stresses, self-talk, and the anxiety these evoke is helpful. Just the awareness can decrease the anxiety to a great extent in many people.

One attribute of anxious thinking is its involuntary nature. We may be unaware or only partially aware of anxiety-producing thoughts and beliefs when they begin and not aware of these thought patterns until uncomfortable symptoms are noticeable. The ability to reason can be impaired, and repetitive thoughts of danger occur. Even when a person has determined that certain thoughts may not be logical, the thoughts can continue to exert pressure, and a loss of perspective occurs. There is little tolerance for uncertainty or ambiguity and a tendency to "catastrophize."

Finally, nurses should be aware of a mechanism known as self-fulfilling prophecy. People seem to bring on unwittingly the things they fear or detest the most. In fact, according to Beck and Emery (1985), "fear of an unpleasant event seems to enhance the probability of its actually happening." For example,

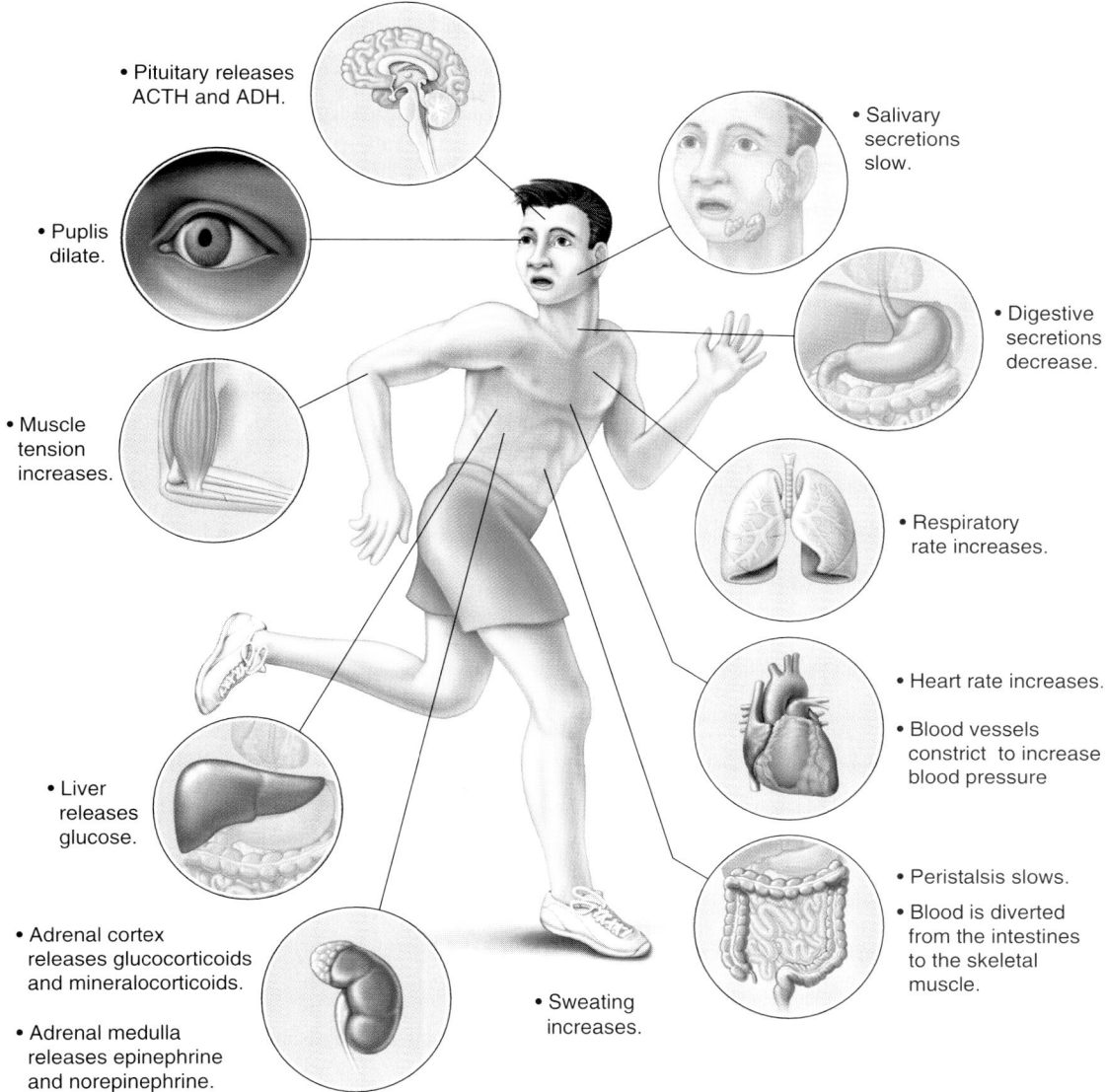

- Pituitary releases ACTH and ADH.
- Puplis dilate.
- Muscle tension increases.
- Liver releases glucose.
- Adrenal cortex releases glucocorticoids and mineralocorticoids.
- Adrenal medulla releases epinephrine and norepinephrine.
- Sweating increases.
- Salivary secretions slow.
- Digestive secretions decrease.
- Respiratory rate increases.
- Heart rate increases.
- Blood vessels constrict to increase blood pressure
- Peristalsis slows.
- Blood is diverted from the intestines to the skeletal muscle.

Figure 47–1. Physiological responses in the general adaptation syndrome.

excessive anxiety about pain in childbirth has been shown to increase the severity of perceived pain.

Levels of Anxiety

Anxiety can vary dramatically in presentation and intensity. It can range from mild tension to terror. The following list describes different levels of anxiety:

- *Mild anxiety*—The person's perceptual field is wide and acuity and alertness are enhanced. Observations are sharper. The relationship between events is clear. Symptoms such as irritability, restlessness, insomnia, repetitious questions, and seeking reassurance or attention may be noted.
- *Moderate anxiety*—The perceptual field is constricted. Alertness is intensified and concentration is focused on one specific thing. Anything irrelevant to the immediate issue is blocked from consciousness. The relationship between events

is still understandable. An increase in physiological functions and psychomotor movements occurs.
- *Severe anxiety*—The person's perceptual field is totally distorted. Details that previously served as a central focus are exaggerated and misinterpreted. Attempts to communicate may be incoherent to the listener. The client may be extremely hyperactive.
- *Panic*—Disintegration of personality organization and the ability to control thoughts and actions occurs. The client experiences profound terror and has an intense urge to escape or fight. Paralysis of functioning can occur, or the client may freeze and even lose consciousness.

Action **A**lert!
Do not leave a client alone if she is experiencing panic. At this level of anxiety, the client may harm herself.

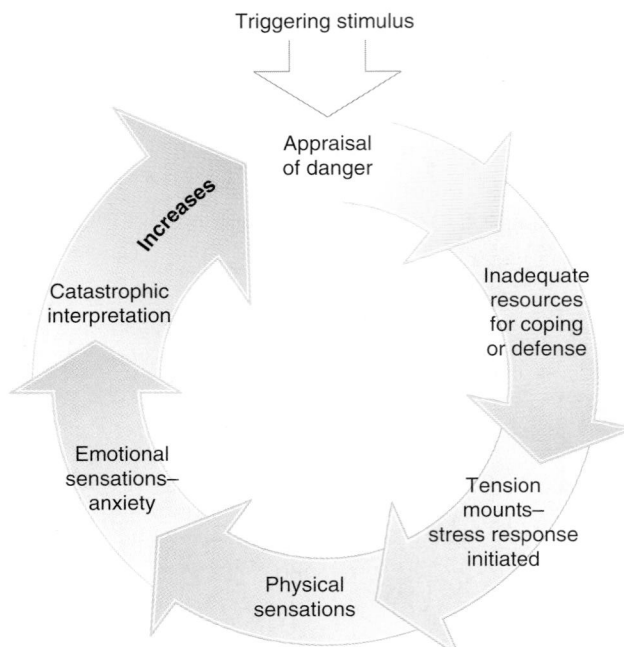

Figure 47–2. The vicious cycle of anxiety.

Effect of Anxiety on the Healing Process

Anxiety can interfere with the healing process. The symptoms of anxiety can be not only chronic and disabling in themselves but can complicate other illnesses by affecting pain perception, decreasing immune function, reducing client compliance with treatment plans, and interfering with client teaching.

Anxiety has profound effects on pain perception. It intensifies the client's appraisal of physical symptoms, making them seem more sinister and distressing. Often a client cannot distinguish anxiety from pain (Barsky, Stern, Greenberg, & Cassem, 1997). Anxiety can lower the pain threshold dramatically, causing caregivers to note marked inconsistencies between complaints of pain and objective findings. This can be misinterpreted as a dependence on pain medication.

Anxiety can also affect the immune system. Stress and anxiety have been linked to changes in the immune system. The belief is that stress impairs immunological functioning and makes a person more vulnerable if exposed to an infectious agent. It is thought that cortisol and the catecholamines, which are released under stress, have an immunosuppressive tendency (Kent & Dalgleish, 1996). The intensity and duration of anxiety, combined with the individual's coping ability and genetic makeup, affect the results.

Anxiety interferes with a client's ability to attend to stimuli and comprehend what is being said. The anxious client attends selectively to stimuli that indicate possible danger and can seem oblivious to information that indicates there is little or no danger. For example, a client who is told she has a small malignant tumor in her breast may experience so much anxiety that she may not hear the physician tell her the expected cure rate is almost 100%. The client may hear

nothing beyond the word "cancer," which in her mind may signify a certain and painful death.

Because of its impact on cognitive function, anxiety usually interferes with client teaching. An anxious client has difficulty focusing on a specific object or topic for a sustained period of time. The client's cognitive capabilities may be so burdened by coping with the perceived threat that she has little ability to handle other demands on cognitive processing.

Normal Versus Pathological Anxiety

When is anxiety considered within the range of normal experience and when is it diagnosed as pathological? Anxiety is usually considered a normal reaction if it is aroused by a realistic danger and dissipates when the danger subsides. For example, a client awaiting the results of HIV testing may be highly anxious. After hearing that the result was negative, the person feels great relief and is able to relax.

There are many occasions when anxiety is expected: infants who are separated from their parents, children going to school for the first time, adolescents going on a first date, adults contemplating aging and retirement, and anyone facing illness and hospitalization. Anxiety is a normal response to speaking in public, a musical solo, leaving for college, and getting married. Only when there is a marked discrepancy between an individual's perception of the environment and its actual characteristics is anxiety considered abnormal.

Pathological anxiety is a disproportionate anxiety response to a given stimulus by virtue of its intensity or duration (Kaplan & Sadock, 1998). If the degree of anxiety and the risk and severity of potential danger are highly disparate, and if it continues even when no objective danger exists, the response is considered abnormal. One way of assessing normal from abnormal anxiety is to note its impact on the person's ability to function. If it impedes daily living and productivity, it is pathological.

Anxiety Disorders

If anxiety is determined to be pathological and is impairing ability to function in daily life, a diagnosis of anxiety disorder is made. In **anxiety disorders,** the production of anxiety indicates a relentless, ineffective mechanism designed to compel a person to lessen the supposed danger that is triggering the anxiety response. In cases of anxiety disorder, it is not always possible to identify a trigger and in many cases the cause is thought to be related to a chemical imbalance in the body.

Anxiety disorders are fairly common in today's society. The lifetime prevalence of anxiety disorders in the United States is estimated at 10 to 15% (Kaplan & Sadock, 1998). They are diagnosed more frequently in women. This group of disorders includes a number of conditions that are categorized together because anxiety is considered to be their most common central feature (Table 47–1). Clients suspected of having an anxiety disorder should be referred for psychiatric evaluation.

FACTORS AFFECTING ANXIETY

Have you ever been surprised by the different responses people have to the same situation? Your view of an event may be totally unlike your neighbor's. This difference arises because information is not just received passively by your sensory organs. It is filtered through your own reference system and actively processed by your individual nervous system. Analysis of any piece of data is subject to variations based on what you consider important, your cognitive ability, your past life experiences, and your belief system. Other factors affecting anxiety may include lifestyle, environment, sociocultural and economic factors, developmental stage, physiological factors, and psychological factors.

Lifestyle Factors

Those who lead a healthy lifestyle are not immune to the effects of stress or to illness, but they may weather them better. A healthy diet, exercise, stress-reduction techniques, and a positive outlook can increase our health status and our resistance to stress. Many of our lifestyle habits, such as smoking, overeating, avoiding exercise, not getting enough rest, use of substances, and numerous other unhealthy habits, can affect our physical and mental health.

Environmental Factors

In the health care setting, the client is faced with a world of both internal and external dangers: threats to bodily integrity in the form of uncomfortable procedures and necessary intimacy with strangers; an atmosphere of illness, pain, suffering, and death; and separation from loved ones, friends, and familiar surroundings. Particularly in the hospital environment, we take away the client's personal possessions, require hospital clothing, and impose a new set of rules and regulations. We tell the clients when to eat, when to sleep, where they are allowed to walk, and when and whom they can visit. We take normally independent, self-determining individuals and ask them to adapt to our rules and expectations.

Sociocultural and Economic Factors

Sociocultural factors can dictate how we are expected to behave in anxious situations. In some cultures, a

TABLE 47–1
Common Anxiety Disorders

Disorder Name	Description
Panic	• A vivid, acute state of overwhelming fear with intense physiological, psychological, and behavioral symptoms. • Usually of sudden onset with increasing or frantic attempts to find safety.
Panic attack	• A sudden, discrete feeling of overpowering fright accompanied by physiological symptoms and thoughts of losing control, impending catastrophe, or death. • Usually occurs suddenly and is fairly brief.
Panic disorder	• Unexpected, recurrent episodes of intense anxiety occurring in situations that do not usually evoke anxiety.
Phobia	• A specific type of fear that is often exaggerated and incapacitating. • A main characteristic of phobias is the appraisal of high risk in a situation that is fairly safe.
Agoraphobia	• Fear and avoidance of being in places or circumstances in which help may not be readily available should some disabling or embarrassing event occur. • Some agoraphobics are unable to leave their houses or apartments.
Generalized anxiety disorder	• Unrealistic and excessive anxiety that cannot be connected with a specific trigger or situation.
Post-traumatic stress disorder (PTSD)	• An anxiety disorder associated with a traumatic event and characterized by intrusive thoughts, dramatic physiological reactivity, flashbacks, nightmares of the event, behavioral disturbances, and avoidance of stimuli associated with the trauma. • Victims of war, rape, disasters, and other major traumas can suffer from PTSD.
Obsession	• Incessant thoughts, images, or impulses that cause anxiety and that the person cannot set aside.
Compulsion	• Repetitive, stereotyped behavior that one feels compelled to carry out despite some conviction that the behavior is unrealistic. • The compulsive behavior reduces anxiety temporarily. • Common compulsions are handwashing and checking doors, windows, or appliances.
Obsessive-compulsive disorder	• An anxiety disorder marked by uncontrollable thoughts, images, or impulses and behavioral rituals that the client cannot dismiss. • Obsessions and compulsions typically occur together.
Social anxiety disorder (social phobia)	• A persistent, intense dread and avoidance of social or performance situations that evoke fear of humiliation or embarrassment.

stoic response to health problems is expected. In other cultures, emotions and feelings are expressed openly and with flair. Some cultures encourage touching, hand-holding, and hugging, whereas others may not condone personal touching at all. It is important to be aware of your client's cultural background because it has a major effect on anxiety and illness behavior (see Cross-Cultural Care chart).

Economic factors also play a major role in anxiety and illness. Our current health care system may limit available treatment options. Both public and private health insurance plans provide minimal or no coverage for mental health care—especially outpatient treatment. In our society, people with greater financial resources may have more available options. For instance, a wealthy man may be able to afford the number-one physician and hospital in the world that specialize in treatment of his specific condition. A single mother receiving welfare may be limited to the health care allowed by her medical card or state programs, and access to additional or cutting-edge treatment may not be covered.

Developmental Factors

A number of theories are used to explain the development of anxiety. Most likely there is no single factor. In all probability, it is a combination of physical, psychological, and environmental factors.

Psychoanalytic theory proposes that anxiety comes from unconscious conflicts that arose from events and situations (symbolic or real) that were threatening in infancy or childhood. These could include fears stemming from separation and loss. An individual may have problems caused by an illness, fright, or another emotionally charged event that occurred during childhood. According to this theory, the client needs to identify and deal with the unconscious conflict—for example, guilt about not living up to parents' expectations. This theory states that we all face different levels of anxiety and different conflicts at various developmental stages.

Learning theory suggests that anxiety is a learned behavior that is a conditioned response to a specific stimulus. Often the client begins to avoid the anxiety-

---

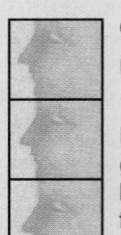

CROSS-CULTURAL CARE
CARING FOR AN APPALACHIAN CLIENT

Ida Adkins is of Appalachian descent. She grew up in rural West Virginia and has always lived within sight of her parents' home. Her family has lived in this area for 150 years. She and her husband recently divorced, and their 16-year-old son stayed to live with her. According to Purnell and Paulanka (1998), there are numerous values that Appalachian people characterize as their way of being. Although each client is unique, many people of the Appalachian culture value the following:

- The ethic of neutrality.
- Avoidance of aggression and assertiveness.
- Loyalty.
- Patroitism.
- Avoidance of dominance over others.
- Avoidance of arguments and seeking of agreement.
- Not interfering in others' lives.
- Protectiveness over personal business.
- Respect for the elderly.
- Folk healers and herb doctors.
- Medicine only when they think they need it.

Karla, a nursing student working in the clinic, tries to demonstrate cultural sensitivity during her first interaction with Ida Adkins. Let's see how she does.

Karla: Hi, Ms. Adkins. I'm Karla, a student nurse from the University. I'd like to sit with you a bit and talk about how we can help you feel better.

Ida: What you want to do?

Karla: (Observed her clutching her chest and counted a rapid respiratory rate of 30) You are breathing fast. Are you having any pain?

Ida: My head is painin' me.

Karla: What can I do to help the pain?

Ida: I need a rag to tie around my head. That is what I need.

Karla: Does that usually help when your head is paining you?

Ida: Yes.

Karla: Let me listen to your heart and check your blood pressure. Then I will go get a rag to tie around your head. Would you like to have your mother come sit with you? She is in the waiting room.

Ida: My mama takes care of me when I get sick. If she can come in—yes. You know what's best, I reckon.

Critical Thinking Questions

- What might have happened if Karla hadn't taken the Appalachian cultural value of folk healing practices into account when Ms. Adkins asked for a rag to tie around her head?
- Did Karla exhibit cultural sensitivity during her assessment of Ms. Adkins? How?

Reference

Purnell, L.D., & Paulanka, B.J. (1998) *Transcultural health care: A culturally competent approach.* Philadelphia: F.A. Davis.

provoking situation. Some of the most effective treatments for anxiety and anxiety disorders have evolved from learning theory. A man who as a child was attacked by a dog is now phobic about all dogs. A technique called desensitization may help reduce his anxiety, and fear of dogs and he could eventually enjoy petting a dog.

Physiological Factors

Researchers have determined that biochemical imbalances are implicated in anxiety and anxiety disorders. The role of neurotransmitters such as norepinephrine, serotonin, and gamma-aminobutyric acid (GABA) is being investigated. Imaging studies of brain structures and functions have identified some abnormal findings in certain areas, such as the right hemisphere, the cerebral ventricles, and the right temporal lobe. Other researchers believe anxiety involves the limbic system, thalamus, and frontal cortex as well as the neurotransmitters. It is also believed that at least some genetic component contributes to the predisposition to anxiety disorders.

Physiological processes are also found in anxiety and anxiety disorders. Physical illness, trauma, medications, and substance abuse are recognized physiological factors of anxiety.

Physical Illness

In addition to perceived danger or attack, a number of medical conditions can cause anxiety-like symptoms (Table 47–2). In fact, symptoms of anxiety may be the primary presenting complaint in an underlying medical illness. Although the medical conditions that can cause symptoms of an anxiety disorder are numerous, they probably do so through a common process, the

TABLE 47–2
Medical Conditions That Commonly Cause Anxiety

Category	Examples
Endocrine disorders	• Cushing's disease. • Addison's disease. • Hyperthyroidism. • Premenstrual syndrome.
Cardiovascular disorders	• Arrhythymias. • Myocardial infarction. • Angina.
Gastrointestinal disorders	• Colitis. • Peptic ulcer.
Infectious diseases	• Human immunodeficiency virus. • Tuberculosis.
Pulmonary disorders	• Asthma. • Pneumothorax. • Pulmonary embolus.
Neurological disorders	• Stroke. • Seizure disorder (especially temporal lobe).

noradrenergic system (Kaplan & Sadock, 1998). Of clients referred for psychiatric evaluation, up to 42% have been reported to have a medical illness causing their distress (Rosenbaum, Pollack, Otto, & Bernstein, 1997). For example, cardiac arrhythmias and mitral valve prolapse can cause symptoms that appear to be anxiety.

Trauma

Some events are considered to be inherently more stressful than others. The prevalence of psychological and somatic distress after natural disasters and serious accidents is very high (Kent & Dalgleish, 1996). The suddenness and severity of a trauma are factors that affect our reactions.

Symptoms of post-traumatic stress disorder (PTSD), such as nightmares, intrusive thoughts, insomnia, and hyper-startle response, are common after experiences such as surviving a tornado or flood, bad car accident, rape, or war-related trauma. Symptoms of PTSD have also been documented to occur after myocardial infarction, coronary artery bypass surgery, treatment of breast cancer, and surgery performed under inadequate anesthesia (Rosenbaum, Pollack, Otto, & Bernstein, 1997). Whether an event is seen as traumatic or not and whether symptoms of PTSD occur depend heavily on the meaning of the event for the person. Symptoms are more likely to occur when a traumatic event is believed to be uncontrollable and life-threatening.

Medications

Various medications can cause, exacerbate, or imitate the physical and psychological symptoms of anxiety. Because many drugs and drug classes have been implicated in anxiety states, a careful medication history is an important part of assessing the etiology of anxiety.

Substance Abuse

A great number of legal and illegal substances can cause physical symptoms of anxiety, either from intoxication or withdrawal from legal substances such as alcohol, nicotine, and caffeine or illegal substances such as cocaine. Remember that prescription medicine can be abused as well. Be sure to include questions on substance-use history in your assessment. Clients often tend to minimize their substance use, so if you suspect this is the case, information from the client's family and friends can be helpful.

Psychological Factors
Psychiatric Illness

A psychiatric history is important to note. Anxiety can be a component of almost all psychiatric disorders. Clients with a previous history of psychiatric illness or prolonged reactions to stressors may be at an increased risk for anxiety, especially when facing health problems. Those with depression, substance abuse/dependence, and personality disorders are especially vulnerable.

Stress

As nurses, we often care for clients who are under extreme stress. Health care settings, illness, surgery, and even nonoperative procedures are stressful and can trigger anxiety. The uncertainty in illness, treatment, and the health care system itself is extremely stressful. Chapter 52 describes stress more fully.

All of the stressors that affect us are not related to medical problems. Yet stressors such as marital or job problems, financial difficulties, or other personal crises can contribute to the level of stress our clients are experiencing. The number and significance of psychosocial stressors in a client's life and the ability to cope with them affect such things as the degree of disability caused by a health problem and the ability to recover. The more stressors a client experiences at one time, and the more disturbing the stressors are to the client, the greater the effect on the client's ability to adjust.

ASSESSMENT

All clients in any health care setting are vulnerable to some degree of anxiety. Although anxiety is normal and even useful, you should be aware of levels of anxiety that are not helpful and may even be harmful in some circumstances. Anxiety is usually not difficult to recognize, even when the cues are indirect, such as selective inattention, being distracted, or focusing on problems or issues unrelated to the current situation. The person who is admitted to the emergency room after a serious motor vehicle accident and is worrying about leaving the door to her house unlocked is probably highly anxious. This expression of anxiety serves a useful function of distracting the person from the reality of possible serious injuries.

General Assessment of Anxiety

Assess for anxiety by following some general guidelines. Quickly recognize and implement measures to reduce anxiety as well as plan for long-term treatment. Keep in mind that most of us experience some level of anxiety when being admitted to a hospital, facing a medical procedure, or even going to the doctor. Assess the client for the presence and intensity of anxiety. Throughout contact with a client you will continue to assess and reassess emotional status. The data are gathered from observation of the client's behavior, what she says about how she is feeling, information from family and friends, information from medical records, physical examinations, and diagnostic tests related to medical problems.

After assessing Miss Adkins' presenting symptoms, vital signs, and other physical parameters, the nurse in the clinic reviews past chart entries. She sees that Miss Adkins had a myocardial infarction about 5 years ago and has a history of psychiatric problems. The nurse notes that Miss Adkins was in the clinic 4 to 5 weeks ago with similar symptoms. Her diagnosis at that time was panic attack. What factors would you consider in determining how to proceed?

Health History

The nursing history is the arena in which the therapeutic relationship begins. Ask about the client's current life situation, personal relationships, and history of any nonspecific medical ailments or illness behavior. It is important to understand the client's frame of reference: how she reacts to and copes with stress (e.g., anger, crying, withdrawal), family history, cultural background, and belief system.

When assessing specifically for anxiety, valuable pieces of the puzzle can be gathered from the client's reported internal state, observation of the client's behavior and ability to function, reports from friends and family, and prior documented medical history. Begin by asking the client to describe thoughts and feelings. Observe the client's behavior for nonverbal clues to what the client is feeling. For example, restlessness, jumpiness, pacing in the hall, and difficulty sleeping can signal anxiety even when the client may report feeling "fine." You may use this opportunity to say to the client, "I noticed you are up walking in the halls and can't sleep. Are you worried about your surgery tomorrow?"

Help the client identify stressors and determine what fears they elicit. Use direct questions to elicit specific details. Open-ended questions can encourage elaboration and exploration of thoughts and feelings. Ask the client "What scares you the most?" or "Can you identify some ways to deal with this anxiety you are facing now?"

Anxiety may be a symptom of a medical or psychiatric problem. Critical issues to assess include medical illness that could present with anxiety-like symptoms, medication-induced anxiety, anxiety associated with use or withdrawal from substances such as alcohol or illicit drugs, and presence of a past or concurrent psychiatric disorder, such as depression or an anxiety disorder.

Talk with the client's family and friends because they are an invaluable source of information. They have known the client over a span of time and are aware of her usual behavior in both stressful and nonstressful situations. They may note reactions or symptoms of which you, the nurse, or even the client herself are not aware. For example, those close to a client may notice that she becomes more anxious at night, or a family member may tell you that her father has been getting confused at night for several weeks.

Historical data from prior health records, when available, are extremely helpful as well. Compare this information with that given by the client to develop a more complete picture. One thing to keep in mind is that the client knows best how she is feeling deep inside.

Assess the client's level of anxiety using an assessment tool such as the Sheehan Patient Rated Anxiety Scale. Alternatively, a simple way to get an idea of the client's anxiety level is to use a 10-point scale. Ask the client to rate her anxiety on a scale of 1 to 10, with 1 being totally relaxed and 10 being ready to panic and lose control. The level a client reports provides clues to the severity of the client's anxiety. If, for example, the client says "about a 7," recognize that the anxiety is bothering the client significantly.

Physical Examination

Anxiety causes a variety of symptoms in multiple functional systems and may be observed during the physical examination. Physical symptoms may be found in these domains: physical, behavioral, cognitive, and affective. Individual patterns of anxiety vary widely according to the nature of the problem and the person's frame of reference. These symptoms are both subjectively and objectively recognized.

Physical symptoms of anxiety are numerous and can be found in every major body system (see Box 47-1 on Physiological Evidence of Anxiety). These symptoms can be extremely unpleasant and range from mild to intense. Indeed, they can be so severe that clients may interpret physical symptoms as indicating a medical emergency. Severe levels of anxiety and panic can become incapacitating disorders in themselves.

Behavioral symptoms can be observed as restlessness to agitation, avoidance, impaired coordination, speech pattern and enunciation changes, freezing, fighting, or fainting. It is important to identify the source of the client's anxiety and take measures to re-

duce it; however, if the behaviors are pronounced, you may have to deal with them first before you can actually sit down and talk with the client.

Cognition can be profoundly affected by anxiety. Clients may have difficulty concentrating with an impairment in information retrieval, especially from short-term memory. They may be unable to focus on a given task or comprehend what is being said. An important consideration with clients who are very upset is their selectivity. Anxious persons are apt to select certain items in their environment and overlook others in their efforts to prove that they are justified in considering the situation frightening and responding accordingly. They will have difficulty with reasoning and decision-making. It is also important to remember this concept when talking with family or significant others who are worried about a loved one who is ill.

Anxiety's effects on thinking, perception, and learning are powerful. Anxiety can produce confusion and distortions of perception, not only of time and space but of people and the significance of events. These distortions interfere with learning ability by decreasing concentration, impairing recall, and interfering with the capacity to associate one item or idea with another (Kaplan & Sadock, 1998). Cognitive manifestations of anxiety also include a fear of losing control, self-consciousness, and even perceptual distortions to the extent of hallucinations.

Affective symptoms vary from a vague sense of uneasiness to hysteria. Irritability, crying, hostility, heightened sense of pain, constant attention-seeking, uncooperativeness, and catastrophizing are all affective or emotional manifestations of anxiety. Clients tend to describe their symptoms in psychological terms such as "I can't cope" or "I feel nervous."

BOX 47-1

PHYSIOLOGICAL EVIDENCE OF ANXIETY

- Tachycardia—palpitations.
- Dyspnea—hyperventilation.
- Dizziness—vertigo.
- Chest pain.
- Dry mouth.
- Dilated pupils.
- Itching/hives.
- Flushing or pallor.
- Nausea and vomiting.
- Changes in sleep patterns.
- Diarrhea.

- Weakness.
- Sweating.
- Cramps and abdominal pain.
- Tightness of muscles, twitching, tremors.
- Headaches.
- Urinary frequency.
- Numbness and tingling in extremities.
- Numbness around the mouth.
- Sexual dysfunction.
- Choking sensation.

Adapted from Barsky, A.J., Stern, T.A., Greenberg, D.B., & Cassem, N.H. (1997). Functional somatic symptoms and somatoform disorders. In N.H. Cassem, T.A. Stern, J.F. Rosenbaum, & M.S. Jellinek (Eds.). Massachusetts General Hospital handbook of general hospital psychiatry (4th ed., pp 173–210). St. Louis: Mosby.

Many clients attribute their symptoms to physical causes and focus their complaints on a specific body system such as the cardiovascular system. Even clients who suspect an emotional cause for their symptoms may hesitate to say so. They may believe that the health care team is concerned only with physical disorders and see emotional problems as a sign of weakness and lack of control.

Focused Assessment for Anxiety

You not only collect information about your client but you also make nursing judgments about the meaning of the information and its effect on a client's health and his or her ability to function. This helps you decide on nursing diagnoses. To focus assessment for anxiety, look at defining characteristics and related factors for the diagnosis of anxiety.

Defining Characteristics

Defining characteristics for the diagnosis *Anxiety* include the following:

- *Behavioral characteristics:* diminished productivity; scanning and vigilance; poor eye contact and glancing about; restlessness, fidgeting, or extraneous movements (such as foot shuffling and hand or arm movements); expressed concerns due to change in life events; insomnia
- *Affective characteristics:* regret or anguish; irritability, jitteriness, or overexcitement; fearfulness; feelings of being rattled or uncertain; increased wariness; focus on self; feelings of inadequacy; distress, apprehension, and anxiety
- *Objective characteristics:* trembling or hand tremors; insomnia
- *Subjective characteristics:* shakiness; worry; regret
- *Physiological (sympathetic) characteristics:* increased pulse, respirations, blood pressure, reflexes, tension; pupillary dilation; cardiovascular excitation, heart pounding, mouth dryness; increased perspiration; facial tension; anorexia; weakness; facial flushing, superficial vasoconstriction; twitching; respiratory difficulties
- *Cognitive characteristics:* blocking of thoughts; confusion, preoccupation, forgetfulness, rumination; impaired attention; decreased perceptual field; fear of unspecific consequences; tendency to blame others; difficulty concentrating; diminished ability to problem-solve; diminished learning ability; awareness of physiological symptoms

Related Factors

Factors related to the nursing diagnosis *Anxiety* include the following:

- Exposure to toxins
- Familial association or heredity
- Unmet needs

- Interpersonal transmission or contagion
- Situational or maturational crises
- Threat of death
- Threat to or change in health status, interaction patterns, role status or function, self-concept, environment, economic status
- Unconscious conflict about essential values or goals of life
- Stress
- Substance abuse

Many theorists believe that anxiety is caused by unconscious conflicts that result from actual or symbolic events and situations that threaten us as infants and children. Illness, loss, fear, or other emotionally laden events can lead to problems throughout life. Illness can produce a feeling of vulnerability in clients and cause these conflicts to become more pronounced. A related factor to anxiety may be the unconscious conflict about essential values or goals of one's life.

Self-concept is based on a belief that our capabilities will allow us to reach our goals and protect ourselves against failure and devaluation by others. Discrepancy between our expectations and actual abilities can lead to anxiety. Unmet expectations can negatively affect our identity and self-concept. Disapproval by significant others, inability to achieve goals, and loss of independence and ability to provide for ourselves change how we see ourselves and can cause intense anxiety.

Illness, disability, pain, and the possibility of death can produce intense anxiety. Most of us fear death at least to some degree. The type of death we fear, the circumstances concerning the anticipation of death, and its expected consequences vary individually. Being in a hospital, facing surgery, trauma, or serious illness make these fears very real. Loss of health, ability to function, independence, and other components important to life and identity can represent many little deaths along the way.

Like many people who suffer from panic attacks, Ida Adkins is afraid she's dying. How would you determine whether Miss Adkins is experiencing the fear of death that is typical of a panic attack from the sense of impending doom that can accompany a serious cardiac event?

Any threat, whether symbolic or actual, to a client's ability to function in roles, family, career, and other areas vital to identity poses danger to individual integrity. This can range from changes in social position to inability to control emotions. Threats to self-sufficiency, functioning of mind and body, maintenance of health status, and even survival can affect one's identity, leaving one feeling vulnerable and hopeless.

Most of us find comfort and security in familiar things and places. We generally feel safer in our own environment. A change in environment can provoke anxiety. Picture an elderly woman who must leave her home of 40 years and move to a nursing home. What might she be feeling?

From studying psychology you are aware that human beings go through various physical and emotional stages in the process of maturation. In order to progress to the next level, certain tasks must be accomplished. These tasks or stages can lead to anxiety. During adolescence we are striving to make the transition from youth to young adulthood. This can be a trying time for both the adolescent and the parent. Increasing demands and responsibilities can also create crisis. For example, a young mother who brings her new baby home from the hospital may be concerned that she cannot care for the baby properly. Any increased threat to a life situation or a client's circumstances can pose a serious risk of anxiety.

Unmet needs can also cause anxiety. These may be obvious or subtle. A client who is going home alone after surgery may worry that she cannot take care of herself. Her anxiety may decrease when she learns that a visiting nurse will check on her daily.

Focused Assessment for Related Nursing Diagnoses

Fear

Fear is an intense feeling of dread related to an identifiable source that the person can verify. The source of fear can be a threat of bodily harm or psychological harm. A primary defining characteristic for the nursing diagnosis *Fear* is the client's ability to identify the specific source of the fear. Some behaviors that may indicate fear may be refusal to leave home, refusal to risk coming in contact with the feared object or situation, symptoms of apprehension or even panic when exposed to the feared object or situation, or a tendency for flight, fight, faint, or freeze when exposed to the feared object or situation.

Fear can be related to such factors as specific phobias, being in a place from which escape may be difficult, or causing embarrassment to oneself in public. Fear can be triggered by a sudden, imminent danger of serious harm or death. Fear can be an innate or learned response. A mother who is terrified of thunderstorms may hide under the bed with her toddler and tremble. The child may also begin to fear thunderstorms. Language barriers, unfamiliar environments, or knowledge deficits can cause fear. Separation from sources of support in a potentially threatening situation, such as hospitalization, surgery, treatments, or procedures, can evoke fear. Sensory impairment, confusion, or mental illness can also contribute to *Fear*.

Powerlessness

Powerlessness is a nursing diagnosis common with clients experiencing anxiety. The client believes that she has no control over situations or events. A client who is undergoing multiple life changes or losses, who expresses feelings of insecurity or resentment over lack of control, and who shows signs and symptoms of anxiety may be given the nursing diagnosis *Powerlessness*.

Other defining characteristics include difficulty in expressing oneself directly, depression, resignation, and a passive "giving up" behavior. The client may verbally express having no control over situations, outcomes, or self-care.

Ineffective Individual Coping

Clients experience anxiety when they are unable to meet basic needs, the demands of life, or role expectations. When there is a crisis or one feels threatened and unable to cope, anxiety is experienced. However, when a client responds with maladaptive or regressive behaviors such as manipulation, anger, or denial, the nursing diagnosis is *Ineffective individual coping*. These clients have an increased risk of illness, accidents, self-destructive behavior, or violence toward others. *Ineffective individual coping* is related to illness-related loss of control over physical or mental integrity, perception or experience of a failure, loss of significant other beyond one's control and incomplete grief work, and interpersonal relationships that include consistent negative feedback.

DIAGNOSIS

Anxiety and fear have similar manifestations and are often difficult to differentiate. Clustering the available data can help, as suggested in the data clustering chart. Some experts think the distinguishing feature is their etiology. Fear is said to derive from a threat that is known, external, and definite, whereas anxiety is said to derive from an unknown internal stimulus, inappropriate to the reality of an external stimulus or concerned with a future stimulus (Rosenbaum, Pollack, Otto, & Bernstein, 1997).

The difference between anxiety and fear may lie in the intensity and duration of symptoms and in interpretation of an event by the victim. *Fear* would be the diagnosis of choice if the event occurred suddenly and was brief and vivid. Fear usually dissipates quickly once the threat is gone. From the assessment data gathered, you would choose *Anxiety* as the nursing diagnosis when the client expresses a more vague feeling of threat or an inappropriate threat that persists for a longer time span.

The nursing diagnosis *Powerlessness* is chosen for the client with apathy or passivity, dependence on others that has resulted in resentment or depressed affect, and expressions of doubt or frustration regarding ability to perform expected activities. You may see the client refuse to participate in care or decision-making.

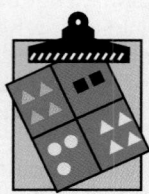

CLUSTERING DATA TO MAKE A NURSING DIAGNOSIS
ANXIETY PROBLEMS

Data Cluster	Diagnosis
A 39-year-old business executive is admitted with a myocardial infarction. "I'm scared. My father died of a heart attack when he was 40. Am I going to die?" He is restless and questions the nurse's every activity.	*Anxiety* related to change in health status and threat of death.
A 27-year-old alcoholic is admitted for substance abuse detoxification and rehabilitation. He is agitated and hyperventilating. "I don't think I'll make it through this. Will I say things I shouldn't? You won't leave me alone will you?"	*Fear* related to the unknown and withdrawal from alcohol.
A 62-year-old with metastatic liver cancer reports continuous nausea and a feeling of death being near. He is jaundiced with severe ascites. He says, "Give me enough medicine to stop this misery."	*Powerlessness* related to terminal illness and impending death.
Mother of four returns to full-time work after being out of the work force for 13 years. "I'm so tired since I've gone back to work. I can't sleep and I have constant headaches. Other women do this. Why can't I?"	*Ineffective individual coping* related to life changes and unrealistic expectations.

Ineffective individual coping is the chosen diagnosis when the client is unable to meet her basic needs and attempts to cope by using maladaptive behaviors. The client may demonstrate, denial, manipulation, or violence in response to the situation.

PLANNING

The goal of managing anxiety is not its total absence but is usually stated as anxiety at a manageable level or a level that allows the person to effectively cope with stressors. The outcomes may be indirectly related to anxiety, including behaviors that indicate trust in the health care profession, decrease in pain, or participating in managing the illness. The following expected outcomes for the anxious client are directly related to a reduced state of anxiety:

1. Experience reduction in anxiety level as evidenced by
   - Decrease in symptoms of anxiety (reduced tension, fatigue, restlessness, irritability, sweating, tremors)
   - Improved sleep, cognitive skills, mood
   - Normal vital signs (pulse, blood pressure, respirations, temperature)

2. Identify own anxiety symptoms and participate in care planning as evidenced by
   - Ability to recognize and verbalize signs and symptoms of escalating anxiety
   - Identification of stressors associated with the anxiety
   - Reporting own behaviors to nurse
   - Relating feelings and behavior
   - Verbalizing ways to intervene in anxiety escalation

3. Develops effective coping and anxiety reduction skills as evidenced by
   - Demonstrating relaxation strategies
   - Using problem-solving skills
   - Participating in decision-making related to treatment and discharge planning
   - Using available resources (e.g., chaplain)
   - Maintaining anxiety level at a tolerable level

INTERVENTION

The heart of nursing practice lies in alleviating mental and emotional suffering as well as relieving physical suffering. Caring for the highly anxious or fearful client can be challenging. Interventions to reduce anxiety will now be discussed.

Interventions to Reduce Anxiety

Many things can be done to decrease client anxiety. These range from very simple interventions to complex techniques that require specialized training. Treatment begins with recognition of the client's anxiety. The path to understanding anxiety is clarification of a client's frame of reference or belief system and her cognitive interpretation of a set of circumstances. Much of these initial data are collected in the assessment phase through the nursing interview and history; however, it continues throughout the nursing process as you gather additional information and come to know the client and her significant others better. The more you know about a client's background and point of view, the more you can understand the client's behavior.

Communicating a Sense of Caring

One of the your most powerful tools is your presence or therapeutic use of self. Communicating a sense of caring, which is the essence of nursing, through respect, listening, and being there is vital to healing. We often underestimate the profound effect of just being there for our clients. The quiet acceptance of our clients as individuals speaks abundantly about how much we value them. Clients rely on nurses to respect and protect them and to watch over them. Knowing the nurse is available if necessary reduces fear and anxiety and gives comfort.

Giving Permission

Give permission or acknowledge a client's right to her feelings. This in itself can often normalize those feelings and reduce anxiety. Everyone experiences anxiety at various times during contact with the health care system. Tell the client, "It's okay to be nervous about a spinal tap. I've never met anyone who wasn't. I will be with you during the procedure and will coach you on ways to make it easier. If you get scared or if it hurts just squeeze my hand."

Listening Actively

Another important intervention is active listening. Active listening involves more than just hearing what is being said. It involves not only listening to the words but "tuning in" to the feelings behind those words and observing nonverbal cues as well (facial expression, tone of voice, and tension level in the body). During active listening, reflect the client's feeling back to her such as "It sounds as if you are angry that your life was disrupted by a heart attack." Restate or paraphrase what has been said or use open-ended statements to encourage further exploration and clarify meaning. Encourage clients to explore the cause of their anxiety because many are able to discover the reasons for it. Once they find the cause of their anxiety, their discomfort often decreases.

Be aware of what you communicate to clients that can raise their anxiety level. Verbal and nonverbal cues communicate feeling, attitudes, and reactions. Being in a hurry or glancing at a watch are often unconscious behaviors. As your behavior can communicate positive messages, it can also decrease rapport and client trust. Through your hurried, preoccupied manners, the client can perceive an attitude of "Let's get this over with" or "I don't have time for you."

Modifying the Environment

The environment can contribute to stress and anxiety. Hospital and other health care settings are unfamiliar to most people. Many clinical areas such as intensive care units, surgical suites, and emergency rooms are designed for maximum efficiency and high-tech treatment. This may be seen by some clients and families as cold, sterile, and threatening, which can increase anxiety. Give clients simple explanations of what to expect in their particular setting to decrease anxiety. Ask family members to bring in some of the client's articles to personalize the client's space. Many surgical services departments allow comfort items such as rosary beads, bibles, small blankets, or stuffed animals to go with clients into surgery.

Noise is another environmental stressor. Studies have demonstrated that "high noise levels constrict blood vessels; increase blood pressure, pulse and respiration rates; and release extra fats into the blood stream" (Keegan, 1995). Major sources of noise are people and equipment. Nurses often become used to these noises and learn to tune them out, whereas clients do not. Turn down volume on noisy equipment. Explain noises to the client and the family. Attempt to maintain quiet in halls and client rooms during usual sleep hours.

Teaching

Education can reduce anxiety. The unknown can be terrifying. One's own imagination can make situations far worse than reality actually is. Information and knowledge empower people. Explain the reasons for diagnostic tests, treatment, and medications to help develop trust and reduce anxiety. Explain all procedures prior to doing them using a matter-of-fact and caring manner.

Acknowledge a client's right to be anxious. Take her current level of cognitive functioning into account and tailor the teaching plan to meet her needs. Initially, a client who is informed of a severe diagnosis may feel devastated and hear little else. Avoid long, involved explanations. Encourage the client to make as many decisions as possible. Do not discuss a client's diagnosis and treatment with others within the client's range of hearing. Explain alternative options because knowing there are choices helps restore the client's sense of control.

Encouraging Family Support

The presence of a family member or significant other can provide comfort and reduce anxiety for many clients. When children are ill, have a parent stay if at all possible to greatly reduce fear, anxiety, and feelings of abandonment. Encourage family and significant others that support the client to call, visit, and be involved with the client's care. However, in some cases the presence of a family member may agitate the client and increase distress. In such instances, limit visiting. Give the client and family a list of resources available to help them cope with anxiety.

Interventions to Prevent and Manage Anxiety

Administering Medications

Anxiety is a normal emotional experience. It is considered pathological only when it interferes with daily functioning. Therefore, most episodes of anxiety do not require medication or require medicine only on a short-term basis. In turn, medication does not solve all problems. Teach clients other methods of dealing with anxiety, such as relaxation and problem-solving techniques. However, if anxiety becomes disabling, medication is usually indicated.

An **anxiolytic** is an antianxiety medication used primarily to treat both acute anxiety and chronic or long-term anxiety disorders. The main class of drugs used to treat acute anxiety is the benzodiazepines. Other medications such as beta-blockers or antihistamines are sometimes used.

Long-term treatment of chronic anxiety disorders is managed with medications that are not likely to cause physical dependence. Generally, drugs such as buspirone, a newer anxiolytic, and/or the antidepressants are prescribed. Both take several weeks before full onset of therapeutic response. The client may need to be reassured or given a concomitant medication during this brief initial phase of treatment.

Action Alert!
Initiate safety measures for any client who receives an anxiolytic, especially an older adult, because most anxiolytic medications cause central nervous system depression and thus sedation.

Providing Complementary Therapies

In today's world, caregivers are discovering that complementary therapies can enhance the effects of traditional Western medicine and facilitate healing. There is no doubt that traditional Western medicine is effective in treating many physical illnesses and many mental disorders. However, it tends to overlook clients' emotional, social, cultural, and spiritual needs. Used in conjunction with traditional Western medical treatment, complementary therapies such as relaxation, spiritual support, music therapy, and touch therapies can prevent, reduce, or manage anxiety.

RELAXATION

Relaxation techniques can be extremely effective in reducing stress and anxiety. Progressive muscle relaxation is a process of alternately tensing and relaxing muscle groups in order to promote awareness of subtle degrees of tension. It is especially effective for clients with tension, anxiety, and agitation but should be used cautiously in persons with hypertension and back disorders. Progressive muscle relaxation reduces subjective feelings of anxiety and increases peak expiratory flow rates in people with asthma (Kolkmeier, 1995). This technique can be used by the nurse at the bedside, as described in the Teaching for Self-Care chart, or clients can be given taped instructions.

MUSIC THERAPY

Music therapy is defined as a behavioral science concerned with methodical use of music to promote relaxation and positive changes in emotions, behavior, and physiology (Guzetta, 1995). Nursing research has shown that soothing music of 60 beats per minute or less has a calming effect and promotes relaxation by lowering heart rate and blood pressure (Barnason, Zimmerman, & Nieveen, 1995). Musical selections without words are preferred. Classical music is often chosen, although some New Age music is designed specifically for relaxation. Music therapy has been used in the treatment of cardiovascular disease, hypertension, migraine headaches, gastrointestinal disorders, Raynaud's disease, AIDS, pain, nausea and vomiting from chemotherapy for cancer, dementia in the elderly, anxiety and stress management, and brain damage resulting from head trauma (Guzetta, 1995).

TOUCH THERAPIES

A number of techniques fall into the category of touch therapies. Healing touch is a technique recognized by the American Holistic Nurses' Association, whereas therapeutic touch, also called the Kunz-Krieger method, is recognized by the Association of Nurse Healers. Certification is available in both techniques, and both require trained practitioners.

The object of touch therapies is to "relax; soothe; stimulate; relieve physiological, mental, emotional and/or spiritual discomfort; or aid in transition of the client to a heightened plateau of being" (Dossey, 1995). The techniques involve centering (a state of deep concentration), assessing the state of the energy field, and using appropriate interventions to modulate and balance the energy field. Touch decreases the heart rate, reduces diastolic blood pressure, lowers anxiety, and relieves pain.

Teaching for SELF-CARE

PROGRESSIVE MUSCLE RELAXATION

Purpose: To promote relaxation by the release of muscle tension in all parts of the body.

Rationale: This technique can be taught and successfully used in any setting to decrease, manage, or prevent anxiety.

Expected Outcome: The client will successfully use progressive muscle relaxation that results in a decreased anxiety state.

Client Instructions

1. Find a quiet, undisturbed place for the relaxation experience and get comfortable.
2. Keep your legs and arms uncrossed.
3. Close your eyes and keep them closed throughout the exercise.
4. Become aware of your body. Take notice of any areas that feel especially tense.
5. Breathe in deeply to a count of four.
6. Hold your breath for a count of four.
7. Breathe out to a count of four.
8. Continue to breathe slowly and deeply.
9. Beginning with your feet, tense your muscles for a count of three or four. Curl your toes and point your feet. Become aware of the feeling of tension. Then relax. Become aware of the feeling of relaxation in your feet.
10. Now tense your feet by bringing them forward toward your head and spreading your toes, again for a count of three or four. Feel the tension, then relax. Feel the relaxation in your feet.
11. Now tense the calves of your legs. Feel the tension. Then relax and feel the relaxation in your calves.
12. Continue this process with all the muscle groups for the rest of the body, including thighs, buttocks, lower abdomen and pelvis, small of the back, stomach (expand it out and press it in), chest, shoulders, hands, arms, neck (bend your head forward so your chin is trying to touch your chest, then press it back into the pillow, face, forehead, and finally your entire body.
13. Relax and search inwardly for any tension. If you find any tense muscles, relax them.
14. Breathe in deeply to a count of four.
15. Hold your breath for a count of four.
16. Breathe out to a count of four.
17. Continue to breathe slowly and deeply.
18. Notice any sensations of heaviness or relaxation. Observe the changes that have taken place in your body.
19. Allow yourself to remain relaxed for a few minutes. When you feel ready, open your eyes slowly and slowly stretch.

EVALUATION

You will assess and reassess your clients for anxiety and its level of intensity. When you are sensitive to your clients' emotional needs, you can greatly reduce their suffering and promote healing. Evaluation of the attainment of outcomes previously determined will let you know whether the nursing interventions were effective or not for the anxious client. If interventions were not effective, you need to reassess the client and determine what revisions to the plan of care are needed.

Criteria being met include evaluative statements such as the following:

- The client identifies three personal stressors that induce anxiety.
- The client demonstrates progressive muscle relaxation techniques.
- The client reports a decrease in anxiety and exhibits no tremors, sweating, or restlessness.

The Nursing Care Planning chart for Ida Adkins provides an example of the application of the nursing process for the client experiencing anxiety.

KEY PRINCIPLES

- Anxiety is both a universal and a personal experience of daily life. Its purpose is to alert us to possible danger and prepare us for defense and self-preservation.
- The general adaptation syndrome is the body's method of mobilizing its resources to defend against threat or harm.
- Anxiety effects us physically, behaviorally, emotionally, cognitively, and spiritually.
- Humans exhibit four types of responses to danger: fight, flight, fainting, or freezing.
- Almost everyone who comes in contact with the health care system experiences some measure of anxiety.
- Anxiety is considered pathological when it interferes with normal daily functioning and productivity.
- The impact of anxiety may be discounted or even overlooked unless the nurse is sensitive to both the emotional and the physical needs of clients.

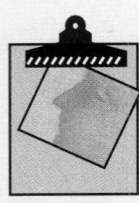

NURSING CARE PLANNING
A CLIENT WITH ANXIETY

Admission Data

Ida Adkins, a 42-year-old white, divorced female, presented to the Mountain View Clinic with complaints of chest pain, shortness of breath, nausea, dizziness, numbness and tingling, racing heart, nervousness, and a feeling of imminent doom. Her mother reports the onset approximately 1 hour prior to coming in to clinic.

At time of admission, client was afebrile, pulse 120, respirations 32, blood pressure 160/90. Pale, restless, diaphoretic, very anxious, and complaining of intermittent, nonradiating, sharp chest pain, 7 on a scale of 1–10. IV started left forearm. Gave 10 mg of morphine sulfate IV and placed on O_2 at 2 L/minute per nasal cannula. Cardiac monitor showed sinus tachycardia without ectopy.

Client's medical history includes a myocardial infarction (MI) in 1995 and a psychiatric history of panic attacks. It is significant to note that this afternoon, her 16-year-old son informed her he is unhappy with her and wants to live with his father.

At time of transport, vitals coming down toward normal limits, client rates her chest pain as a 4 on the 1–10 scale, but remains restless, slightly queasy, and fearful. Because of her history, we are sending her for admit and observation. Ambulance transport to the County Medical Center with mother in attendance.

Physician Orders

Admitting diagnosis: rule out MI.
Admit to telemetry unit—monitored bed.
Oxygen per NC at 2–6 L PRN.
Vitals qh.
Labs—CBC, electrolyte panel, cardiac enzymes/ isoenzymes, chest x-ray, and EKG upon admit and per unit protocol.
Bedrest with BRP as tolerated.
Low Na, low-fat diet.

IV D$_5$NS at 100 mL/hour.
Nitroglycerin translingual spray—1 to 2 metered doses under the tongue q 5 minutes PRN.
Morphine 10 mg IV q3h PRN pain.
Phenergan 25 mg PO q4h PRN nausea. Give rectally or parenterally if oral dose not tolerated.
Ativan 2 mg PO q4h PRN anxiety.
Notify client's psychiatrist of admission.

Nursing Assessment

Color pale, skin cool and dry. Drowsy, but arouses easily and responds appropriately to questions. Reports mild nausea. Cardiac monitor shows normal sinus rhythm at a rate of 80, respirations 20, blood pressure 140/90, temp 98.6°F. Apical heart rate 82. Says heart pain gone. Peripheral pulses palpable with immediate capillary return. Lungs clear. Abdomen soft with active bowel sounds × 4 quadrants. Mother at bedside. Awaiting laboratory work to rule out MI versus anxiety-panic attack.

Continued

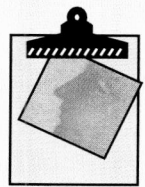

NURSING CARE PLANNING
A CLIENT WITH ANXIETY *(continued)*

NURSING CARE PLAN *(continued)*

Nursing Diagnosis	Expected Outcomes	Interventions	Evaluation (After 24 Hours of Care)
Anxiety related to threat of loss and feelings of power-lessness.	Recognize feelings of anxiety.	Encourage description of physical and emotional feelings. *Provide privacy to encourage client to talk.*	Talked about son wanting to leave.
		Allow feelings of anger, grief, sadness, fear, etc. *Allow mother to be present.*	Cried. Mother at bedside comforting client.
		Observe for verbal/nonverbal signs of anxiety.	Exhibiting mild to moderate anxiety. No further signs of severe to panic level of anxiety.
	Identify causes and con-tributing factors of anxiety.	Acknowledge client's per-ception of threat/situation.	Allowed mother to stay at bedside during the night when she said she was "so alone."
	Identify effective coping mechanisms.	Encourage to use coping mechanisms that have been successful in the past. *Allow mother to be present and provide foods of choice.*	Reports "sitting a spell with my mama and sippin' on mama's herb tea" helps calm anxiety.
		Teach relaxation tech-niques, such as progres-sive muscle relaxation.	Returned demonstration of relaxation technique.
	Report anxiety reduced to a manageable level.	Administer antianxiety medication as ordered.	Visibly relaxed with vital signs WNL. Verbalizes feeling calm and ready to go home.
		Referral to Visiting Nurse Association for home moni-toring of anxiety manage-ment and medication regimen.	Referral made and first visit scheduled with client.

Italicized interventions indicate culturally specific care.

Critical Thinking Questions

1. With a cardiac history and a known anxiety disorder, Ms. Adkins is high risk for continued admis-sions just like this one. What other information should be included in Ms. Adkins' teaching plan to prepare her for self-care at home? What are some other complementary therapies that would help Ms. Adkins with managing her anxiety? What cultural factors would you consider?
2. Ms. Adkins denies that her son will leave her because she feels it will kill her. How would you help her realize the denial and recognize the reality without causing another panic attack?

- Anxiety can also be caused by a number of medical conditions, a variety of medications, substance abuse or withdrawal, and most psychiatric disorders.
- The symptoms of anxiety are not only chronic and disabling in themselves but can complicate other illnesses by reducing client compliance with treatment plans, increasing perception of pain, and impairing the immune response.
- Anxiety can be self-perpetuating and develop into a vicious cycle without appropriate intervention.
- Symptoms of anxiety and fear are similar and may be difficult to distinguish.
- There are many interventions for management of anxiety, ranging from simple, basic techniques to complex strategies that require specialized training and certification of the practitioner.
- Evaluation of previously determined outcomes will let you know whether interventions were effective in decreasing anxiety.

BIBLIOGRAPHY

*American Psychiatric Association. (1994). *Diagnostic and statistical manual of mental disorders* (4th ed.). Washington, D.C.: American Psychiatric Association.

Anxiety Disorders Association of America. (1998). *Anxiety disorders: Social and economic costs fact sheet.* Rockville, MD: ADAA.

Barnason, S., Zimmerman, L., & Nieveen, J. (1995). The effects of music interventions on anxiety in the client after coronary artery bypass grafting. *Heart and Lung, 24*(2), 124–132.

Barsky, A.J., Stern, T.A., Greenberg, D.B., & Cassem, N.H. (1997). Functional somatic symptoms and somatoform disorders. In N.H. Cassem, T.A. Stern, J.F. Rosenbaum, & M.S. Jellinek (Eds.), *Massachusetts General Hospital handbook of general hospital psychiatry* (4th ed.) (pp 173–210). St. Louis: Mosby-Year Book, Inc.

*Beck, A.T., & Emery, G. (1985). *Anxiety disorders and phobias: A cognitive perspective.* New York: Basic Books.

Dossey, B.M. (1995). Acknowledging fear. In B.M. Dossey, L. Keegan, C.E. Guzzetta, & L.G. Kolkmeier (Eds.), *Holistic nursing: A handbook for practice* (2nd ed.) (p 483). Gaithersburg, MD: Aspen Publishers, Inc.

Dossey, B.M. (1995). Imagery: Awakening the inner healer. In B.M. Dossey, L. Keegan, C.E. Guzzetta, & L.G. Kolkmeier (Eds.), *Holistic nursing: A handbook for practice* (2nd ed.) (p 59). Gaithersburg, MD: Aspen Publishers, Inc.

Dossey, B.M. (1995). Using our healing hands. In B.M. Dossey, L. Keegan, C.E. Guzzetta, & L.G. Kolkmeier (Eds.), *Holistic nursing: A handbook for practice* (2nd ed.) (pp 537–538). Gaithersburg, MD: Aspen Publishers, Inc.

*Dossey, L. (1989). *Recovering the soul.* New York: Bantam Books.

Guzetta, C.E. (1995). Music therapy: Hearing the melody of the soul. In B.M. Dossey, L. Keegan, C.E. Guzzetta, & L.G. Kolkmeier (Eds.), *Holistic nursing: A handbook for practice* (2nd ed.) (pp 669–697). Gaithersburg, MD: Aspen Publishers, Inc.

Jones, W.A. (January 31, 1997). Role of the hospital chaplain. Personal communication, Louisville, KY.

Kaplan, H.I., & Sadock, B.J. (1998). *Synopsis of psychiatry* (6th ed.). Baltimore: Williams & Wilkins.

Keegan, L. (1995). Environment: Protecting our personal and planetary home. In B.M. Dossey, L. Keegan, C.E. Guzzetta, & L.G. Kolkmeier (Eds.), *Holistic nursing: A handbook for practice* (2nd ed.) (pp 291–311). Gaithersburg, MD: Aspen Publishers, Inc.

Kent, G., & Dalgleish, M. (1996). *Psychology and medical care* (3rd ed.). London: W.B. Saunders.

Kim, M.J., McFarland, G.K., & McLane, A.M. (1995). *Pocket guide to nursing diagnosis* (6th ed.). St. Louis: Mosby-Year Book, Inc.

Kolkmeier, L.G. (1995). Relaxation: Opening the door to change. In B.M. Dossey, L. Keegan, C.E. Guzzetta, & L.G. Kolkmeier (Eds.), *Holistic nursing: A handbook for practice* (2nd ed.) (pp 573–605). Gaithersburg, MD: Aspen Publishers, Inc.

*Krieger, D. (1986, 1979). *The therapeutic touch.* New York: Simon & Schuster.

Lawrence, M. (1995). The unconscious experience. *American Journal of Critical Care, 4*(3), 227–232.

Mentgen, J., & Bulbrook, M.J.T. (1995). *Healing touch—Level II notebook.* Lakewood, CO: Colorado Center for Healing Touch, Inc.

Messner, R.L., & Lewis, S.J. (1996). *Increasing client satisfaction: A guide for nurses.* New York: Springer Publishing Company.

Mornhinweg, G.C., & Voignier, R.R. (July/August 1995). Holistic nursing interventions. *Orthopaedic Nursing, 14*(4), 20–24.

North American Nursing Diagnosis Association. (1999). *Nursing diagnoses: Definitions & classification 1999–2000.* Philadelphia: Author.

Rosenbaum, J.F., Pollack, M.H., Otto, M.W., & Bernstein, J.G. (1997). Anxious patients. In N.H. Cassem, T.A. Stern, J.F. Rosenbaum, & M.S. Jellinek (Eds.), *Massachusetts General Hospital handbook of general hospital psychiatry* (4th ed.) (pp 173–210). St. Louis: Mosby-Year Book, Inc.

Strother, D.S. (1997). Anxiety in the medical setting. Personal communication, Louisville, KY.

Tomb, D.A. (1995). *Psychiatry* (5th ed.). Baltimore: Williams & Wilkins.

Townsend, M.C. (1997). *Nursing diagnosis in psychiatric nursing: A pocket guide for care plan construction* (4th ed.). Philadelphia: F.A. Davis.

Wilson, G.T., Nathan, P.E., O'Leary, K.D., & Clark, L.A. (1996). *Abnormal psychology: Integrating perspectives.* Boston: Allyn and Bacon.

---

*Asterisk indicates a classic or definitive work on this subject.

48

Vulnerability

Janna Lesser

Key Terms

community approach
health status
human capital
relative risk

resource availability
social integration
social status

LEARNING OBJECTIVES

After studying this chapter, you should be able to:

1. Describe the domains of the Vulnerable Populations Conceptual Model.
2. Describe how poverty, social inequality, and poor educational and vocational resources affect health problems.
3. Identify factors affecting vulnerability.
4. Describe key components of assessing a vulnerable population.
5. Describe planning for the nursing diagnoses *Hopelessness* and *Powerlessness* in vulnerable populations.
6. Describe key interventions for *Hopelessness* and *Powerlessness*.
7. Discuss the elements of evaluation for *Hopelessness* and *Powerlessness*.

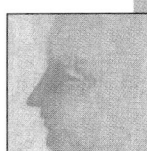

Eighteen-year-old Brenda Carter brought her 2-year-old son to the County Hospital Ambulatory Clinic for his well-child checkup. Brenda, living in poverty and alone with her son, had been unable to adapt to his developing independence:

"I take a lot of time away from him now that he's two 'cause he's got them terrible two's and it's real frustrating to be around him . . . but when he was younger, he used to be my whole life. When he was younger, it was like my face was straight on him, my focus was on him. But now, he's so bad, you know . . . ? I have to tell him 20 time before—and I won't hit him exactly when I tell him not to do it, but I'll tell him 20 times and then I'll hit him. And then he wants to hit me back."

At the clinic, Brenda described herself to her nurse as having no control over her life. "I am just stuck here with this baby with no chance to do nothing." Hopelessness had grown out of a series of abusive relationships with men and her lack of resources. Social isolation has afforded Brenda little opportunity to observe the behavior of other 2-year-old children, one way she might have learned that her son's behavior was not atypical. The nurse considers the diagnoses *Hopelessness* and *Powerlessness* (see the Nursing Diagnoses chart).

**VULNERABILITY
NURSING DIAGNOSES**

Hopelessness: A subjective state in which an individual sees limited or alternatives or personal choices available and is unable to mobilize energy on own behalf.

Powerlessness: Perception that one's own action will not significantly affect an outcome; a perceived lack of control over a current situation or immediate happening.

From North American Nursing Diagnosis Association. (1999). NANDA nursing diagnoses: Definitions and classification 1999–2000. Philadelphia: Author.

CONCEPTS OF VULNERABLE POPULATIONS

A philosophy of preventive health care requires examination of the groups who are most at risk for health problems. Risk can be approached by recognizing the presence of a single factor that is highly associated with a particular disease. For example, smoking is correlated with an increased incidence of lung cancer. However, some populations within our society are at risk for multiple health problems. Preventive health care needs to address the factors that make these populations vulnerable.

Vulnerable populations are social groups who have limited resources and consequently are at high risk for myriad health-related problems. Vulnerable social groups include the poor; persons subjected to discrimination, intolerance, subordination, and stigma; and those who are politically marginalized and disenfranchised (Flaskerud & Winslow, 1998).

The Vulnerable Populations Conceptual Model (Flaskerud & Winslow, 1998) provides a framework for understanding the relationships among the limited resource availability, the health-related risk factors,

and the health status of vulnerable populations. The major concepts, or domains, of this model are resource availability, relative risk, and health status (Fig. 48–1).

The first domain, **resource availability,** refers to the availability of socioeconomic and environmental resources. The dimensions of this domain include human capital, social integration, social status, access to health care, and quality of care. **Human capital** includes income, jobs, education, and housing. **Social integration** means having a harmonious relationship with society in which the person participates as a full member of the society. A lack of social integration is apparent when a person experiences social segregation, marginalization, discrimination, or absence of both informal and formal social supports. **Social status** is the position of an individual in relation to others in the society. It is reflected in power to control the political process and the distribution of resources. Finally, environmental resources, often lacking in the lives of vulnerable populations, include access to health care and quality of health care (Flaskerud & Winslow, 1998). A lack of socioeconomic and environmental resources is related to an increase in risk fac-

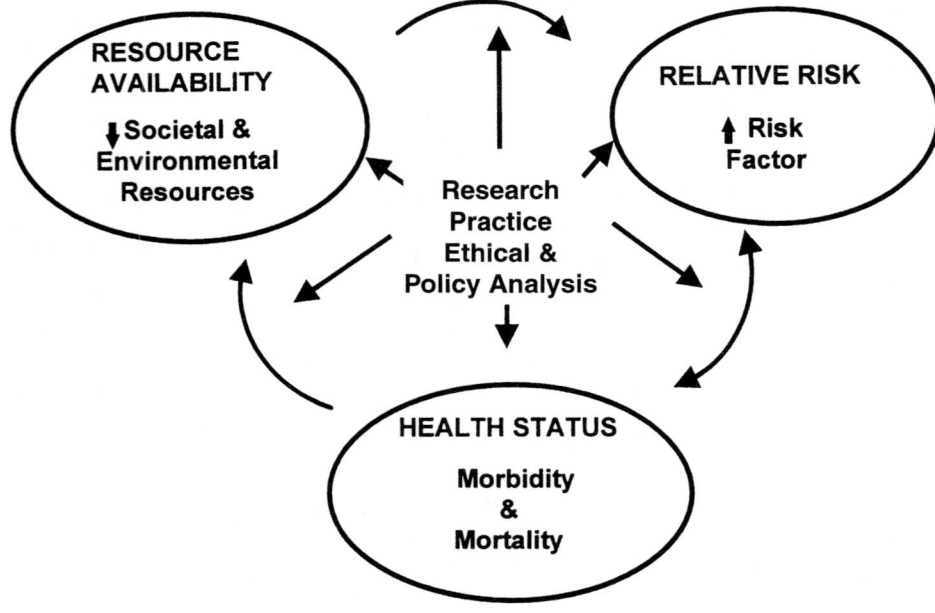

Figure 48–1. The Vulnerable Populations Conceptual Model. (From Flaskerud, J. H., & Winslow, B. J. [1998]. Conceptualizing vulnerable populations: Health-related research. Nursing Research, 47[2], 69–78.)

tors among the population who experience this lack (Flaskerud & Winslow, 1998). Research findings have shown that a lack of resources leads to an increased exposure to these risk factors.

Relative risk, the second domain of the Conceptual Model, is considered to be the ratio of the risk of poor health among populations who do not receive resources and are exposed to risk factors compared with those populations who do receive resources and are not exposed to these risk factors. The dimensions of this domain are

- Lifestyle, behaviors, and choices (e.g., dietary behavior, physical activity, sexual behaviors, and use of tobacco, alcohol, and illicit drugs);
- Use of screening procedures, immunization programs, and health promotion services (e.g., screening for cancers, tuberculosis, sexually transmitted infections [STIs] including infection with the human immunodeficiency virus [HIV], high blood pressure, prenatal care, and health education)
- Exposure to or participation in stressful life events—in particular, abuse and violence (Flaskerud & Winslow, 1998)

The dimension of **health status,** the third domain of the model, includes age- and gender-specific morbidity and mortality. Socioeconomically disadvantaged groups and those who are discriminated against, subordinated, and stigmatized are exposed to more risk factors and experience increased morbidity and premature mortality. Finally, increased morbidity and premature mortality often exacerbate socioeconomic and environmental disadvantages. Illness and death in a social group may deplete resources, resulting in a decline in human capital, social integration, social status, and access to care (Flaskerud & Winslow, 1998).

Consider the case of Brenda Carter. Apply the Vulnerable Populations Conceptual Model to her story. What aspects of her life characterize her as a member of a vulnerable population?

FACTORS AFFECTING VULNERABILITY

Vulnerable groups include the homeless, the mentally ill, the frail elderly, and the poor. Additionally vulnerable groups may be found among women and children, ethnic people of color, immigrants, gay men and lesbians, and the elderly. Childbearing adolescents, like Brenda in our case study, are a vulnerable population. Additional factors are often present that make the group vulnerable.

Socioeconomic Factors

Poverty, social inequality, and poor educational and vocational resources are just a few of the socioeconomic constraints common in vulnerable populations. These factors are tied together in a web of cause and effect, creating a maze from which there appears to be no escape. In this maze, rewards and satisfactions in

life are in the immediate here and now and are often associated with high-risk behaviors.

The effects of poverty can be illustrated as one of the major causes of teenage pregnancy (Luker, 1996). For an adolescent girl, the combination of low socioeconomic status, poor academic achievement, lack of available jobs, and resultant feelings of low self-worth may lead to pregnancy as the only reasonable alternative (Gordon, 1996). When adolescents are not afforded necessary educational and vocational resources, they may judge the consequences of unprotected sexual activity to be unimportant relative to its immediate benefit as an affirmation of adulthood (Brewster, 1994).

Lifestyle Factors

Socioeconomic factors are closely related to lifestyle. Understanding the lifestyle of vulnerable populations goes beyond the physical and social elements. It includes the values that motivate behavior, the dynamics of making choices, the mechanisms of attaining self-esteem, the effects on hope, and the nature of power in a situation wherein resources are limited.

Using our example of a pregnant adolescent, parenting may represent a hope for achieving the respect that has been missing in her past, a past in which she has been socially devalued (Lesser, Anderson, & Koniak-Griffin, 1998). Early parenthood is often deeply imbedded in the context of these young women's lives wherein they are making choices from limited options. Impoverished youth who are failing school need a positive vision for their future as well as educational and vocational resources if pregnancy is to be delayed until adulthood (Stevens-Simon, Kelly, & Singer, 1996).

Behavioral Risk Factors

Risk factors for health-related problems include the behavioral factors that can be directly related to risk. Reducing health risks in vulnerable populations must recognize the inter-relationship of multiple risk factors.

The childbearing adolescent often has multiple risk factors that reflect lifestyle and behavior choices beyond being pregnant and an adolescent. Many adolescent mothers have engaged in impulsive high-risk activities long before their pregnancies. Examples include drug and alcohol use, early initiation of sexual activity, unprotected sexual activity, multiple sexual partners, gang affiliation, and school truancy or dropout (Koniak-Griffin & Brecht, 1995).

Health-related problems of pregnant teens and adolescent mothers include both psychological and pathophysiological changes or disease states that negatively affect the lives of these young women and their children. These problems include depression and suicide attempts, parenting problems (neglect and abuse), domestic violence, poor birth outcomes (premature labor and births and low-birthweight infants), and STIs (including HIV).

Personal Factors

Taking action to change a life in which problems seem insurmountable requires both a vision of a better future and a belief that you have the power to create that future. Vulnerable populations can easily become overwhelmed by the difficulties of life so that it is impossible to envision a better future, much less implement a plan to attain that future.

Brenda's nursing diagnoses of *Hopelessness* and *Powerlessness* are common in other members of the vulnerable groups for whom nurses care, both in the community and in acute settings.

Although it is not within the scope of this chapter to discuss the many social groups that are vulnerable to health-related problems because of their general lack of resource availability and their risk factors for disease, two further examples may be helpful. Suicidal adolescents and the chronically ill elderly are two very different vulnerable social groups who experience *Hopelessness* and *Powerlessness.*

Twenty percent of adolescents will have experienced depression by age 18 (Lewinsohn et al., 1994) (Fig. 48–2). Another 60% both report depressive symptoms and experience functional impairment even though they do not meet diagnostic criteria for a depressive disorder (Harrington & Clark, 1998). In addition, 15% of deaths among adolescents in the United States are due to suicide, and depression is an important risk factor for suicide (Dorwart & Chartock, 1989). Depressive disorders evolve from both biological and contextual issues. Risk factors for depression in adolescents have been identified as the following (Allbright, 1999):

Psychopathology in parent
Dysfunction/conflict in family
Low social support
Poor peer relations
Physical illness
Loss of a parent
Poor body image

Feelings of hopelessness, low self-esteem, and powerlessness are frequently present with depression.

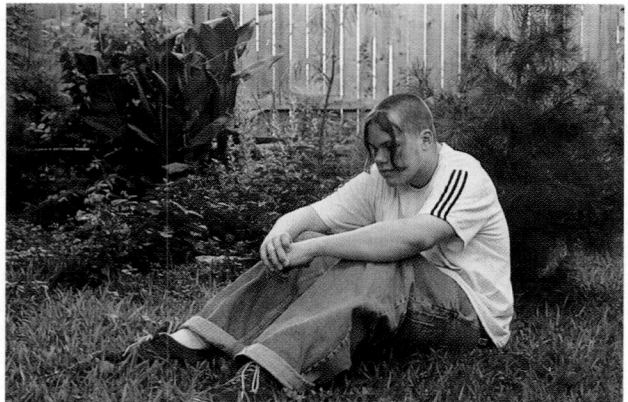

Figure 48–2. Twenty percent of adolescents will experience depression by age 18 years.

As a social group with an increased relative risk for health-related problems, the elderly are a vulnerable population (Tullmann & Chang, 1999). The elderly are more likely to be living in poverty than other adults (Matteson, Bearon, & McConnell, 1997; U.S. Department of Health and Human Services, 1991). Three factors that have been identified as associated with this poverty are inadequate retirement income, the high cost of medical care, and financial exploitation and criminal victimization (Matteson, Bearon, & McConnell, 1997). Social isolation is one of the well-known risks of the elderly that may result in increased susceptibility to illness (Harden, 1997). Thirty-one percent of the elderly persons who live in the community live alone (Matteson, 1997). Powerlessness has been identified as a significant problem and risk factor for the elderly. Reduced learning, tolerance for adverse stimuli, and task performance as well as depressive symptoms, increased stress levels, poor coping responses, and death have been linked to powerlessness (Fry, Slivinske, & Fitch, 1989).

Hope

Plato described hope as the images that man forms for himself concerning the future. It has to do both with the mental pictures of what the future might be and with the wish that it will be that way. To have hope, there must be a desire and some expectation that the desire will be fulfilled. The expectation that what is wished for will come to be does not have to be absolute; any degree of belief in the future being different, better, or meeting expectations constitutes hope.

What cues does Brenda offer that suggests that she has little hope for change in her life?

Hope exists when a person knows that certain actions will result in predictable consequences. Having inner strength and a belief that the self is efficacious in connection with the outer world comes from the self. Thus, hope is grounded in the early childhood experiences from which the self-concept develops.

However, hope exists on both a conscious and an unconscious level. On a conscious level, a person can name or describe the expectations for the future and even predict the likelihood that the expectations will be realized. On an unconscious level, hope is a life force that provides the energy to drive the individual forward.

Hope cannot exist when a person knows that no known action will result in the desired consequences. Hope comes from a belief that forces external to the self can positively influence what happens to a person, so that when the person has done everything she knows to do or is able to do, hope remains. Hope is often derived from religious faith but can be any faith in a power greater than the self.

Power

Having power means having control in direct relationship to the self, having power to control the actions of others, or having power to control the environment. The perception of personal control is the belief that through one's own actions, behaviors, or personal characteristics the person can affect outcomes. The person who feels in control perceives the ability to make decisions about one's own actions, to control a situation, and to get what is desired from life. Control has to do with preventing bad things from happening and making good things happen.

The concept of power may be viewed in terms of "power over" or "power to" (Hawks, 1991). Power over connotes an emphasis on strength, control, and competitiveness. "Power to" places more emphasis on the antecedents of power. Effective "power to" relates to formulating and achieving goals. Assisting a person with having "power to" involves developing trust, caring, knowledge, cooperation, interpersonal skills, respect for the individual's beliefs, communication skills, and decision-making.

In health maintenance and illness, the person who has a perception of power seeks knowledge and takes action to affect the outcome of the illness or to manage health. A person whose expectancy that outcomes are within the person's control will pay more attention to available information.

ASSESSMENT

The vulnerable client is assessed both as an individual and as part of a susceptible population within the community. It has become increasingly clear that a **community approach**—a nursing approach for vulnerable populations that emphasizes the provision of resources for disease prevention, treatment, and rehabilitation, with a consequent decrease in exposure to risk factors for health-related problems—is necessary for vulnerable populations. Although the nursing tradition of individualized, client-centered care is valuable and essential, nurses must look beyond the individual perspective to larger concepts of community and social responsibilities to understand the needs of vulnerable populations (Tullmann & Chang, 1999). Nurses, particularly those working in community settings (e.g., community and school-based clinics), are in a key position to be instrumental in the development and implementation of community strategies for health risk reduction.

General Assessment of Vulnerability

The complex nature of the relationship between lack of resources and the many risk factors for health-related problems makes a comprehensive evaluation necessary when nurses are making assessments of an individual who is a member of a vulnerable social group. This evaluation includes a psychological, social, and physical needs assessment.

Psychological Needs Assessment

Vulnerable populations are assessed for psychological needs that are factors in health-seeking behaviors. For example, routine psychological screening of pregnant adolescents and teen mothers includes screening for symptoms of depression, suicidal ideation, and history of suicide attempts. Other known risk factors for suicide, such as social isolation, substance use, and access to weapons, should be identified. Nurses can identify pregnant teens already suffering with depressive symptoms or suicidal ideation and assist them in seeking mental health counseling before the birth of their baby, before they experience the added stressors inherent in premature motherhood.

Action Alert!
Immediate referrals to drug treatment programs may be indicated for chemically dependent pregnant and parenting youth.

Social Needs Assessment

Social needs are concerned with the client's relationships with others. Social assessments must include screening to identify victims of previous and current violence as well as the client's perception of current family support. For example, pregnant teens and adolescent mothers often have conflict with their parents and with their partners yet still value them as an important source of support.

Social needs are also concerned with the social or environmental structures affecting the client's life. Assessment of the risk of neighborhood violence and neighborhood resources for healthy living is crucial for understanding the risks faced by vulnerable populations.

Physical Needs Assessment

Additionally, you need to assess for physical needs. Perform a thorough history and physical examination. Be aware of common medical problems in the population and include screening measures for these problems. You should also include screening for the ability to meet basic human needs such as nutrition, safety, and access to health care.

One of the most important tasks in the general health evaluation of pregnant and parenting teens is to assess their concrete needs. This includes housing needs, nutritional need, necessary supplies (e.g., diapers), educational needs, and vocational training. In order to make appropriate referrals, nurses must have extensive knowledge about available services and eligibility requirements for programs such as Medicaid, nutritional services (including a public assistance program for Women, Infants, and Children [WIC] and food stamps), child care subsidies, educational programs, and vocational programs.

Nursing diagnoses can be used to plan for individualized care, which the nurse (in the community or the hospital) can provide.

Recall the case of Brenda Carter. What concrete needs does she have that could reduce her sense of helplessness and powerlessness?

Additionally, you should assess for problems with known risk factors in the specific population. For example, early prenatal care is essential for all pregnant teens who, with proper management, can have normal pregnancies and good birth outcomes. Timely identification of problems is vital for decreasing complications of pregnancy. Besides standard prenatal and postpartum health assessments, testing for STIs (including HIV testing) must be provided. Physiological changes that occur during pregnancy, such as opening of the cervix, increase HIV risk; however, condom use during pregnancy and in young mothers is rare. Intervention programs that include skill building in the areas of sexual negotiation and condom use are imperative so that these youths can protect themselves and their unborn babies from HIV and other STIs.

Focused Assessment for Hopelessness

Defining Characteristics

Hopelessness is conveyed in the client's communication patterns, behavior, and emotional response. It may be expressed directly or indirectly.

VERBAL. Ask questions about the client's expectations for both the immediate and long-term future. Does the client have plans for the future? Does the client express a belief that the present difficult circumstances can and/or will change? Is the client able to list several alternative behaviors for managing problems, attaining goals, or otherwise coping with circumstances? Listen for verbal expressions of pessimism, of negative future expectations, and of futile efforts toward meeting desired goals. If the client does not make a direct statement about the future, the nurse could ask, "When you think of your future, say 6 months from now, how do you see yourself compared with now, and how does it make you feel?" Listen for themes of being a total failure in life, including feeling that life no longer has any meaning or purpose, a sense of loss or deprivation, and despair.

Verbal statements of hopelessness and pessimism may be very clear or require clarification to validate the meaning. Listen for themes of being incompetent, worthless, or a failure in life. Hopelessness is evident when the client describes futile efforts at problem-solving or actions that have not produced the desired results. It is often clear that the client has given up.

NONVERBAL. Hopelessness is conveyed both verbally and nonverbally (Fig. 48–3). Observe the client's appearance. Grooming, body posture, eye contact, and affect provide cues to *Hopelessness*. Nonverbally, *Hopelessness* is conveyed through affect, which is generally notably sad and often one of marked apathy. Clients experiencing *Hopelessness* actually speak very little, very seldom initiate a conversation, and usually respond to questions with few words in a monotone voice. The nonverbal defining characteristics of "turning away from speaker, shrugs in response to speaker, and minimal or poor eye contact" should be assessed

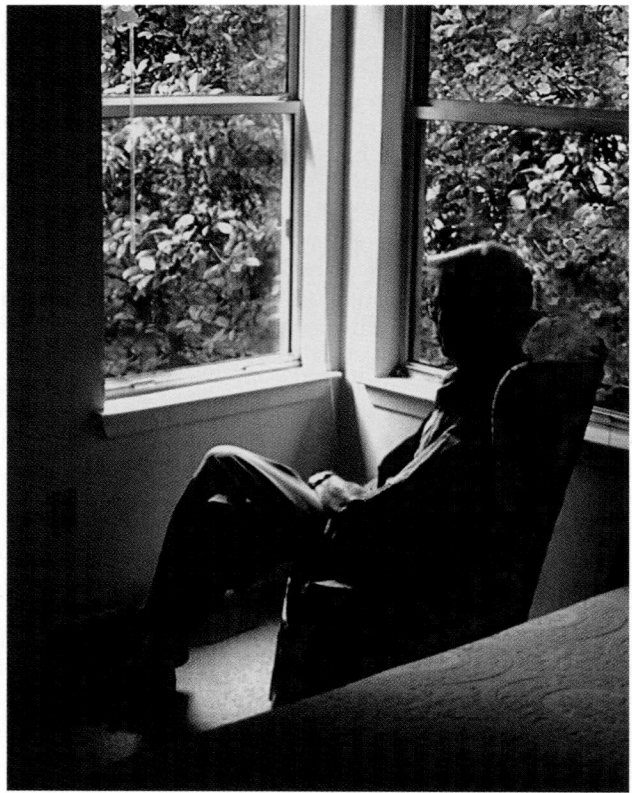

Figure 48–3. Hopelessness is conveyed verbally and nonverbally.

within the context of the client's overall communication pattern. The meaning of these behaviors needs to be validated.

SOCIAL. Additionally, defining characteristics of *Hopelessness* pertain to problems with social relationships, including perceived difficulty with interacting with others, loss of gratification from roles and relationships, impaired interpersonal relationships, perceived lack of social support, and possibly social withdrawal.

Hopelessness is also identified through need for increased sleep and lack of spontaneity. Chronic fatigue, decreased motivation, anorexia, and weight loss contribute to decreased self-care. Accompanying the noted decreased motivation the client manifests a general lack of interest or initiative.

Defining characteristics of *Hopelessness* include evidence of decreased problem-solving skills and decreased flexibility in thought processes. Thought processes are constricted so that perceptions are narrowed, with evidence of cognitive rigidity and dichotomous thinking. These cognitive characteristics limit the range of problem-solving options. This process relates to the prevalent conveyed perception of being overwhelmed by untenable situations that are perceived as affording no relief or way out. The client is unable to recognize any sources of hope.

Assess the reality of the situation. The client may be experiencing a difficult life situation perceived as unbearable with no solutions. Are there few alternatives or are alternatives available that are not apparent to the client?

AFFECTIVE. Depression is a defining characteristic of *Hopelessness.* However, not all clients who experience hopelessness are depressed. On the other hand, given the research evidence regarding hopelessness as a core characteristic of depression and the evidence of hopelessness as a predictor of suicide, both of these defining characteristics need to be considered in assessments.

Hopelessness as a psychological construct or emotional feeling is subjective, and therefore it is imperative that the diagnostic cues be validated with the client. Most important is that all of the client's nonverbal behaviors and verbal descriptions of thoughts, feelings, and behaviors must be viewed in relation to the particular cultural perspectives of the client and what hopelessness means to the client.

Related Factors

Related factors for *Hopelessness* include the following:

- Self-concept disturbance, low self-esteem
- Lack of initiative
- Self-care deficit
- Ineffective problem-solving and unrealistic goal-setting
- Failing or deteriorating physiological conditions, or prolonged pain and discomfort
- Abandonment or separation from significant others, or loss of someone or something one values in life
- Loss of belief in transcendent values/God
- Exposure to long-term physiological or psychological stress
- Inability to achieve developmental tasks (e.g., identity, integrity)

Focused Assessment for Powerlessness

Defining Characteristics

The most specific defining characteristic of *Powerlessness* is the client's verbal expression of having no control or influence over a situation, an outcome, or self-care. The client may also be observed as not participating in health care decisions. The client's affect is generally apathetic, and the overall appearance is passive.

Assess the client for participation in general health care or in decision-making when opportunities are provided and for reluctance to express feelings out of fear of alienation from caregivers. When assessing the client, the nurse needs to ask the client about usual decision-making patterns: "How would you describe your usual method of making decisions (e.g., career, health care)?" Similarly, ask questions about individual and role responsibilities. "What responsibilities did you have at school? . . . at home? . . . at work?"

Assess for indirect expressions of powerlessness such as anxiety or anger. Dependence on others may result in irritability, resentment, anger, and guilt. Additionally, the client may express discomfort or dissatisfaction with the health environment or an inability to perform previous tasks, activities, or roles. Signs of uncertainty include defending self-care practices when challenged and expressing uncertainty regarding fluctuating energy levels. On the other hand, signs of taking control in a health situation include monitoring progress and seeking information regarding care.

To assess the client's experience of control, you should ask, "How would you describe your ability (high/poor) to control or alleviate your present health situation (e.g., pregnancy, diabetes, obesity)?" "To what or whom do you attribute your ability to control (e.g., self-preventive measures, other individual[s], no control, fate)?"

Powerlessness is a subjective state, and therefore the nurse's assessment must be validated with the client. It is also imperative that all of the client's verbalizations be considered in relation to the particular ethnic and cultural perspectives on the meaning of control and influence to the client.

Related Factors

Related factors for *Powerlessness* include the following:

- Decreased self-esteem
- Lack of knowledge
- Perception of nonsupportive health care environment
- Poorly controlled chronic illness
- Perception that one has no control over the health care regimen

Focused Assessment for Related Nursing Diagnoses

People in vulnerable populations can have virtually any nursing diagnosis. Assessment of social, psychological, and physical needs leads to focused assessment for a number of problems. Frequently diagnosed problems include the following:

- *Self-esteem disturbance*
- *Ineffective parenting*
- *Social isolation*
- *Ineffective individual coping*
- *Altered nutrition: less than body requirements*
- *Risk for injury*

DIAGNOSIS

Hopelessness and *Powerlessness* are closely related concepts. A primary distinction between *Hopelessness* and *Powerlessness* rests in the concept of control.

Hope can be present even when the client feels no ability to control a situation. However, *Hopelessness* suggests that the client lacks the psychic energy to change the situation, is unable to perceive alternatives, or has alternatives that are clearly limited. The client who is experiencing *Hopelessness* may also experience *Powerlessness* in a specific situation.

When you have confirmed that the client is experiencing *Hopelessness,* the focus of intervention will be on giving the client hope and facilitating realistic positive and healthy outcomes. Outcomes will be in terms of the client's perception of herself, her interpersonal relationships, and her views of her future. Through assisting, encouraging, and teaching in areas that require changes in self-concept, self-care, interpersonal interactions, support systems, problem-solving, and developing realistic goals, you will contribute to the client's return to a healthy level of functioning.

The diagnosis of *Powerlessness* clearly deals with the need to take action, to gain control, or to gain the perception of control. When you have confirmed that the client is experiencing *Powerlessness* the focus of care will be on relieving the client's powerlessness by selecting interventions that increase the client's feelings of increased control through strategies that empower the client to achieve a healthy level of functioning. The same interventions can be used to prevent *Powerlessness.* To differentiate *Powerlessness* from other closely related diagnoses, consider the focus of care, the client's perception of the problem, and the interventions related to *Powerlessness.*

PLANNING

The goal for the client with *Hopelessness* is to experience hope. Hope may come secondary to improvement in the related factor. *Powerlessness* is perhaps more directly treated. The goal for the client with *Powerlessness* may be that the client actually gains power or gains the perception of power. Because both hope and power have to do with the ability to achieve goals, it is especially important that planning to achieve hope or power be done *with* the client. Expected outcomes for the client with *Hopelessness* and *Powerlessness* are summarized in Box 48–1.

INTERVENTION
Interventions to Restore Hope
Offering Presence

Because hope is an existential concept, instilling hope may be accomplished through the existential intervention of presence. As a nurse you cannot necessarily change the situation that has caused feelings of hopelessness. However, you can offer your presence to the client who experiences hopelessness. Through your presence you can offer the client empathy or understanding of the feelings associated with being in a desolate situation. You can offer positive regard. And sometimes you can offer physical help.

Valuing Feelings

In a therapeutic nurse-client relationship you can help the client value her own feelings and herself. Because hopelessness is closely related to the ability to achieve goals and thus related to self-assessed ability, instilling hope can happen as a byproduct of helping a person experience the self as a valued, worthwhile person.

Setting Goals

Setting goals that are realistic, achievable, and based on a well-developed personal system of values can instill hope. Whether the person is dying from cancer or

---

BOX 48–1

EXPECTED OUTCOMES FOR THE CLIENT WITH HOPELESSNESS AND POWERLESSNESS

Hopelessness

- The client identifies choices available to mobilize energy on her own behalf.
- The client has improved self-concept.
- The client takes initiative to accomplish achievable goals.
- The client participates in self-care within her capabilities.
- The client uses problem-solving strategies to accomplish achievable goals.
- The client achieves a small goal for improved health status.
- The client recognizes personal power to affect outcomes.
- The client participates in spiritual renewal activities.
- The client achieves elements of neglected developmental tasks.

Powerlessness

- The client has an increased sense of control over his life situation.
- The client verbalizes positive feelings about her abilities.
- The client engages in problem-solving.
- The client demonstrates increased self-esteem.
- The client verbalizes the knowledge needed to accomplish her goals.
- The client perceives support from the health care environment.
- The client has his chronic illness under control.
- The client demonstrates control over her health care regimen.

is a pregnant teenage girl, goals are a way of looking to the future. For the dying person the future is limited and for the pregnant teenager it is uncertain, but a plan that is achievable takes one out of the moment and connects one to the possibilities of the universe. Small accomplishments increase the belief that the present can be improved.

Recall the case of Brenda Carter. Identify three goals that the nurse might want to discuss with Brenda to reduce her sense of hopelessness and powerlessness and foster an improved relationship with her child.

Establishing Relatedness

Helping a person to have a sense of relatedness to others or helping the person in the manner of the relatedness can instill hope. Through our relationships we know ourselves as valued human beings, valued because we are important to others and because we have something to contribute to the other person. Help the client reach out to others and help others reach out to the client.

Preventing Self-Harm

When a client feels hopeless, there is a higher probability that this person will engage in self-destructive behavior. At the extreme end the person may become suicidally depressed.

> A*ction* A*lert!*
> Pay attention to hints of suicide. Take all suicide threats seriously. Do not leave the person alone. Remove anything from a hospital room that could be used to inflict self-harm. Refer the client to an appropriate therapist or psychiatrist who can help such clients to manage their feelings.

However, suicide is not the only potential for self-harm. The person who feels hopeless may engage in harmful behaviors or fail to take action to maintain health and safety. Safety may be a concern just because the person is not paying attention to the environment.

Developing Coping Mechanisms

Assess the client's methods of coping with the circumstances surrounding hopelessness. Help the person recall coping methods that have worked in the past. Some helpful coping mechanisms include the following:

- Focus on a small achievable task and away from the seemingly insurmountable problem.
- Prioritize. Accomplish essential activities. Make a list of nice-to-do activities and do one each day.
- Do something for someone else each day.
- Do something for yourself each day.

Maintaining Energy

An overwhelming fatigue often accompanies hopelessness. The very activities that might relieve the feel-

ings of hopelessness require more energy than the client has. A state of inertia sets in that is hard to overcome. Recognizing that activity is needed to overcome the inertia, you will feel tempted to recommend physical activities. However, the activities must be chosen carefully and the energy requirements must be within the energy available to the client.

Help the client maintain optimal physical health. Rest, nutrition, exercise, and vitamin supplements may be helpful. Help the client include a mentally healthy activity in each day.

Interventions to Reduce Powerlessness

Empowering Clients

To empower another individual you need to respect the individual's capacity for self-determination. Make the assumption that clients have the ability to make decisions and take action on their own behalf. Nurses cannot empower clients; only clients can empower themselves.

The client needs to be actively involved in defining both the problem and the solutions. When the nurse is the major decision-maker, dependency is the result. However, clients may either make decisions that are different from the decision the nurse might make or reject help altogether. These decisions must be accepted.

Loss of power is often associated with a sense of distrust and a feeling of alienation and an attitude of self-blame. For the empowerment process to be effective, there needs to be mutual respect, a sharing of power, and trust between the client and the nurse.

Empowerment focuses on promoting and enhancing clients' abilities to meet their own needs, make their own decisions, and to mobilize the necessary resources to feel that they are in control of their own lives. However, you can provide information and assistance to engage in empowering behaviors. Nurses can help the client to develop, obtain, and use resources that will encourage a sense of control and self-efficacy through which individuals can empower themselves.

In an ethnographic study of a group of chronically mentally ill clients, Connelly and colleagues (1993) explored empowerment involved in organizing and managing a client-run drop-in center. In this study, empowerment was defined as "a process wherein people assert control over factors that affect their lives" (p. 300). From the client's perspective, behaviors associated with empowerment were classified as choosing, participating, supporting, and negotiating.

The personal significance of empowerment varies with the individual and the level of empowerment at which the individual is currently functioning. From the client's perspective, empowerment can mean

- Identifying feelings associated with power and control
- Having knowledge

- Strengthening self-expression to express preferences, needs, values, and attitudes
- Participating in family, group, or social life or in decision-making
- Choosing among actions, friends, health care alternatives, or activities and taking responsibility for the consequences of choice
- Developing coping skills or methods of managing a problem
- Being of help to others
- Bargaining for what you want
- Expanding the spiritual self

Applying the Community Approach

As described before, the community approach to health risk reduction in vulnerable social groups is critical. This includes appropriate referrals for needed community resources and services.

For Brenda, community referrals might include educational and vocational programs, parenting and preschool programs, adolescent mother support groups, and mental health counseling for depression and history of victimization (group and individual). In addition, if Brenda is not already receiving these services, referrals should be made to WIC, Medicaid, and other financial assistance programs would be appropriate. Individualized care on which the nurse could focus would require that Brenda return to the clinic regularly (at least until she was well connected with these other services) for longer-term intervention.

Arranging for transportation, child care, and home-based interventions may be necessary to ensure that vulnerable populations are provided with necessary services. In addition, interventions must be scheduled so as not to conflict with the person's crucial daily responsibilities such as school, work, and child care.

EVALUATION

Evaluation of the interventions for *Hopelessness* and *Powerlessness* requires examination of psychological, social, and physical data. Assess for a change in the way the person thinks about the self in relation to others, the environment, and the self. Listen again for the themes in the client's conversation and compare the frequency of negative statements. Observe the client's interactions with others. Does the client wait for someone else to make decisions or take control? Does the client more frequently initiate a relationship? Assess progress in physical health and the ability to manage health problems. Is the client displaying positive coping skills?

Client satisfaction is a significant element in evaluation of these diagnoses. Does the client feel that progress is being made, that life is better, or an increased self-control? The evaluation of *Hopelessness* may mean the client has achieved acceptance of a situation that cannot be changed.

KEY PRINCIPLES

- Preventive health care must address the factors that make vulnerable populations vulnerable.
- The framework for understanding vulnerable populations recognizes the relationships among the limited resource availability, the health-related risk factors, and the health status of vulnerable populations.
- Poverty, social inequality, and poor educational and vocational resources are among the socioeconomic constraints common in vulnerable populations.
- Hope exists when a person knows that certain actions will result in predictable consequences. The perception of personal control is the belief that through one's own actions, behaviors, or personal characteristics the person can affect outcomes.
- The complex nature of the relationship between lack of resources and the many risk factors for health-related problems makes a comprehensive evaluation necessary when nurses are making assessments of an individual who is a member of a vulnerable social group.
- Hopelessness and powerlessness are closely related concepts. A primary distinction between hopelessness and powerlessness rests on the concept of control.
- Because hope is an existential concept, instilling hope may be accomplished through the existential intervention of presence.
- Instilling hope can happen as a byproduct of helping a person experience the self as a valued, worthwhile person.
- Through our relationships we know ourselves as valued human beings, valued because we are important to others and because we have something to contribute to the other person; thus hope has to do with relatedness.
- To empower another individual one needs to respect the individual's capacity for self-determination.
- To treat powerlessness, the client needs to be actively involved in defining both the problem and the solutions.
- To treat hopelessness, the client needs to be actively involved in defining both the problem and the solutions.

BIBLIOGRAPHY

Albright, A.V. (1999). Vulnerability to depression: Youth at risk. *Nursing Clinics of North America, 34*(2), 393–405.
*Brewster, K.L. (1994). Race differences in sexual activity among adolescent women: The role of neighborhood characteristics. *American Sociological Review, 59,* 408–424.

---

*Asterisk indicates a classic or definitive work on this subject.

*Connelly, J.M., Keele, B.S., Kleinbeck, S.V.M., Schneider, J.K., & Cobb, A.K. (1993). A place to be yourself: Empowerment from the client's perspective. *Image: The Journal of Nursing Scholarship, 25,* 297–303.

Davis, C.M., & Curley, C.M. (1999). Disparities of health in African Americans. *Nursing Clinics of North America, 34*(2), 345–357.

*Dorwart, T.L. & Chartock, L. (1989). Suicide: A public health perspective. In D.G. Jacobs & H.N. Brown (Eds.), *Suicide: Understanding and responding. Harvard Medical School perspectives on suicide* (pp 31–35). Madison, CT: International Universities Press,.

Flaskerud, J.H., & Kim, S. (1999). Health problems of Asian and Latino immigrants. *Nursing Clinics of North America, 34*(2), 359–380.

Flaskerud, J.H., & Winslow, B.J. (1998). Conceptualizing vulnerable populations: Health-related research. *Nursing Research, 47*(2), 69–78.

*Fry, P., Slivinske, L., & Fitch, V. (1989). Power, control and well-being of the elderly: A critical reconstruction. In P. Fry (Ed.), *Psychological perspectives of helplessness and control in the elderly* (pp 3–9). New York: Elsevier.

Gordon, C. (1996). Adolescent decision making: A broadly based theory and its application to the prevention of early pregnancy. *Adolescence, 31,* 561–584.

Harden, J.T. (1997). Nursing diagnoses related to psychosocial alterations. In M.A. Matteson, E.S. McConnell, & A.D. Linton (Eds.), *Gerontological nursing: Concepts and practice* (2nd ed.) (p 661). Philadelphia: W.B. Saunders.

Harrington, R., & Clark, A. (1998). Prevention and early intervention for depression in adolescence and early adult life. *European Archives of Psychiatry and Clinical Neuroscience, 248,* 32–45.

Hawks, J.H. (1991). Power: A concept analysis. *Journal of Advanced Nursing 16*(6), 754–762.

Koniak-Griffin, D., & Brecht, M. (1995). Linkages between sexual risk-taking, substance use, and AIDS knowledge among pregnant adolescents and young mothers. *Nursing Research, 44,* 340–346.

Lesser, J., Anderson, N., & Koniak-Griffin, D. (1998). Sometimes you don't feel ready to be an adult or a mom: The experience of adolescent pregnancy. *Journal of Child and Adolescent Psychiatric Nursing, 11,* 7–16.

Lesser, J., & Escoto-Lloyd, S. (1999). Health-related problems in a vulnerable population. *Nursing Clinics of North America, 34*(2), 289–299.

*Lewinsohn, P.M., Roberts, R.E., & Rohde, P., et al. (1994). Adolescent psychopathology: II, Psychosocial risk factors for depression. *Journal of Abnormal Child Psychology, 103,* 302–315.

Luker, K. (1996). *Dubious conception: The politics of teenage pregnancy.* Cambridge, MA: Harvard University Press.

Matteson, M.A. (1997). Psychosocial aging changes. In M.A. Matteson, E.S. McConnell, & A.D. Linton (Eds.), *Gerontological nursing: Concepts and practice* (2nd ed.). Philadelphia: W.B. Saunders.

Matteson, M.A., Bearon, L.B., & McConnell, E.S. (1997). Psychosocial problems associated with aging. In M.A. Matteson, E.S. McConnell, & A.D. Linton (Eds.), *Gerontological nursing: Concepts and practice* (2nd ed.) (p 603). Philadelphia: W.B. Saunders.

Saunders, J. (1999). Health problems of lesbian women. *Nursing Clinics of North America, 34*(2), 381–391.

Stevens-Simon, C., Kelly, L., & Singer, D. (1996). Absence of negative attitudes toward childbearing among pregnant teenagers: A risk factor for a rapid repeat pregnancy? *Archives of Pediatrics and Adolescent Medicine, 150,* 1037–1043.

Strehlow, A.J., & Amos-Jones, T. (1999). The homeless as a vulnerable population. *Nursing Clinics of North America, 34*(2), 261–274.

Tullmann, D.F., & Chang, B.L. (1999). Nursing care of the elderly as a vulnerable population. *Nursing Clinics of North America, 34*(2), 333–344.

Tyson, S., & Fleming, B. (1999). Conceptualizing battered women as a vulnerable population. *Nursing Clinics of North America, 34*(2), 301–312.

Ungvarski, P.J., & Grossman, A.H. (1999). Health problems of gay and bisexual men. *Nursing Clinics of North America, 34*(2), 313–332.

*U.S. Department of Health and Human Services. (1991). Health of older Americans. In *Health status of minorities and low income groups* (3rd ed.) Washington, D.C.: Author.

Winslow, B.W., & Carter, P. (1999). Patterns of burden in wives who care for husbands with dementia. *Nursing Clinics of North America, 34*(2), 275–287.

Role-Relationship Pattern

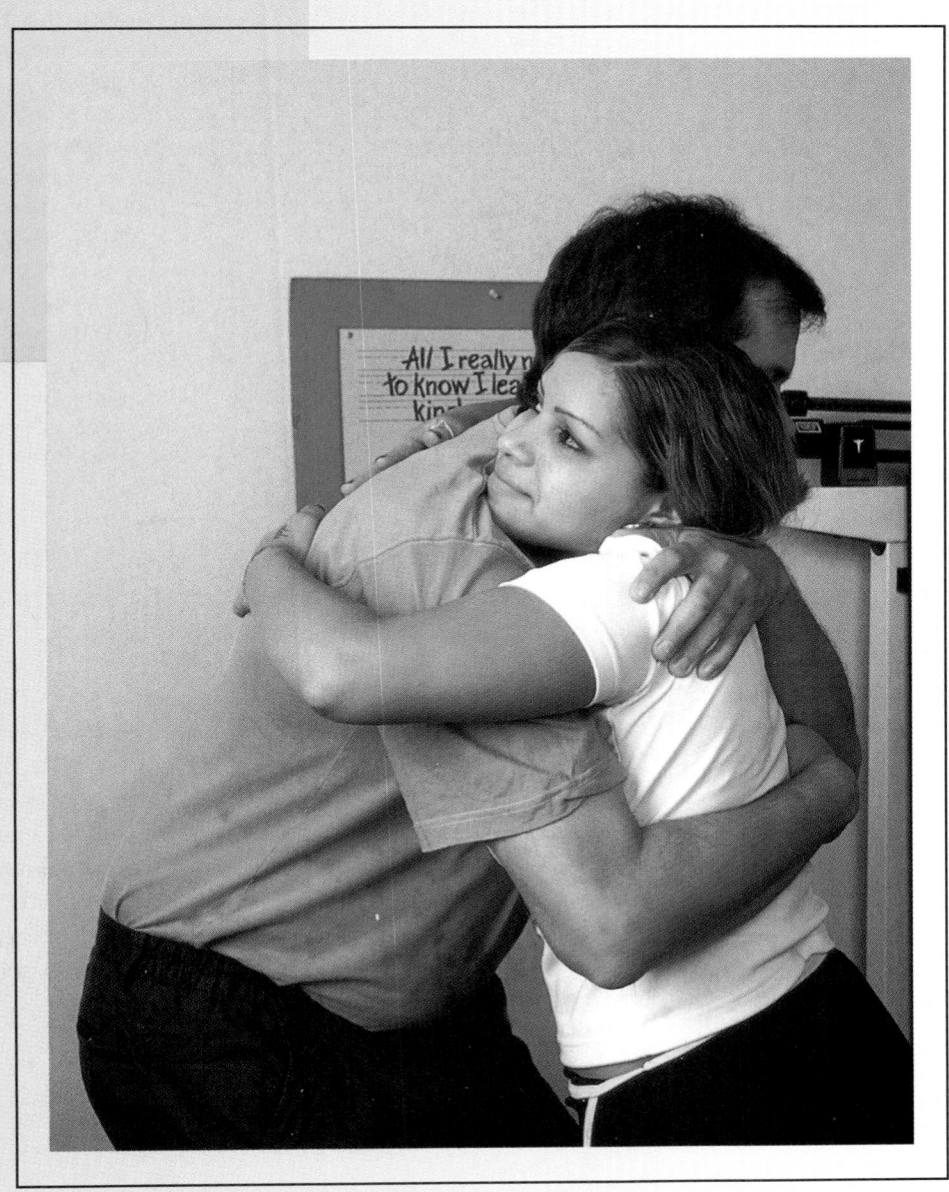

Roles and Relationships

Betty Kehl Richardson

Key Terms

learned helplessness
relocation stress syndrome
role
role conflict

role distance
role failure
role strain
role transition

LEARNING OBJECTIVES

After studying this chapter, you should be able to:

1. **Describe the concepts underlying the four relationship nursing diagnoses presented.**

2. **Identify a variety of factors affecting the health of clients' relationships.**

3. **Discuss the assessment of clients who are at risk for, or who have, one of the four relationship problems discussed in this chapter.**

4. **Differentiate among the various diagnoses for clients with relationship problems that are amenable to nursing care.**

5. **Plan for goal-directed interventions to prevent, alleviate, or correct problems of relationship.**

6. **Evaluate the outcomes that describe the degree of progress toward meeting the goals of relationship-oriented nursing care.**

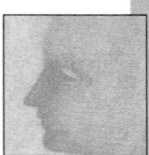

María is 22 years old and in labor with her second child. She and her older child were brought to the emergency department by ambulance from a nearby park, where passersby saw her and thought she was ill. Because she spoke only Spanish in the ambulance, a Spanish-speaking nurse talked with María when she arrived at the hospital.

The nurse determined that María was born and raised in Honduras. On a trip to the United States when she was 19, she met a man, married him against her parents' wishes, and remained in the United States. Her husband left her recently when their first child, Jesús, was 19 months old and María was 8 months pregnant with their second child. The family had been living in María's husband's car. Now she has no place to live because her husband took the car when he left.

María had been spending her days on the bus and walking to areas where she hoped to find an empty or newly constructed house where she and her child could spend the night. She has only a few dollars left and no one to turn to for help. María feels inadequate to care for herself and her children and lacks a support system. The nurse considers the diagnoses *Altered role performance* and *Social isolation*.

ROLE-RELATIONSHIP NURSING DIAGNOSES

Altered Role Performance: The patterns of behavior and self-expression do not match the environmental context, norms, and expectations.

Social Isolation: Aloneness experienced by the individual and perceived as imposed by others and as a negative or threatened state.

Impaired Social Interaction: The state in which an individual participates in an insufficient or excessive quantity or ineffective quality of social exchange.

Relocation Stress Syndrome: Physiological and/or psychosocial disturbances as a result of transfer from one environment to another.

From North American Nursing Diagnosis Association. (1999). NANDA nursing diagnoses: Definitions and classification 1999–2000. Philadelphia: Author.

CONCEPTS OF ROLES AND RELATIONSHIPS

No matter what your practice setting, you will encounter clients with problems involving their roles and relationships. For example, if you work in home health, you may encounter clients isolated because of disease; you may need to intervene to increase the client's social interaction. In the hospital, you may help a mother maintain her role with her children. This chapter introduces concepts that will help you intervene appropriately for clients with role and relationship problems, both actual and potential.

Role Performance

Role performance refers to a person's fulfillment of her roles and her current responsibilities in her life situations. A **role** is a homogeneous set of behaviors, attitudes, beliefs, principles, and values that are normatively defined and expected of a person in a given social position or status in a group. Some roles are prescribed by age, gender, or position in the family. Others are acquired, such as nurse, teacher, or executive. Still others are transitional, such as student (Carpenito, 1997; Edelman & Mandle, 1998).

Altered Role Performance

Altered role performance refers to a change in the way a person perceives or enacts a role. This change can occur when the person encounters role transition, role distance, role failure, role conflict, and role strain. Altered role performance is of interest to nurses both as a stressor in the etiology of illness and in its function in managing the effects of illness.

Role transition is a state in which a person has started to take on the behaviors of a role but has not fully developed the expected behaviors. An example is a teenager who becomes pregnant but still does not understand the responsibilities of parenthood.

Role distance, on the other hand, is a condition in which a person carries out role behaviors that differ from those expected in the person's current cultural or societal situation. A new immigrant may experience role distance when performing socially expected parenting behaviors in a foreign community.

Role failure is the absence of role behaviors or ineffective role behaviors resulting in a lack of success in a role. When a person has a physical or mental illness, is immature, or lacks support or resources, role failure may occur. An example is an operating room (OR) nurse who develops Parkinson's disease and can no longer work in the OR because she no longer has the necessary fine motor skills.

Role conflict occurs when a person has incompatible expectations for behavior within a role or between two or more roles, or when a role is incongruent with the person's beliefs and values. An example is a husband who is torn between caring for his sick wife and working.

Lastly, **role strain** is the condition in which a person feels unable to accomplish the tasks required of a role or of multiple roles. This results in feelings of frustration, tension, and overload.

Impaired Social Interaction and Social Isolation

Interaction with other people is an important factor in maintaining health and managing illness. Social isolation is the experience of aloneness, usually with the perception of its being imposed by others and viewed as a negative or threatened state. Impaired social interaction is a state in which a person engages in social exchange of insufficient or excessive quantity or insufficient quality.

Research has documented the negative results of social isolation and impaired social interaction. Blake (1995) studied quadriplegic clients who lacked social support because of self-imposed isolation. He found that they suffered from unfilled needs associated with love, belonging, self-esteem, and self-actualization.

Social support consists of interpersonal relationships and activities that supply stress-buffering benefits and resources for effectively managing stress. Although most people accept the need for social support, the exact relationship of social support to health is unclear. It may be that the stress-buffering effects of social support increase health (Thomas, 1997).

A phenomenon called learned helplessness may also influence the quality and effectiveness of social interaction. This condition is sometimes seen with frail elderly, battered, or disabled persons. **Learned helplessness** is a perception that further efforts would be useless based on the failure of previous efforts. The learning may have taken place in connection with truly uncontrollable events, but becomes generalized to the perception of all events. The person may view even temporary losses of income, relationships, health, or work as permanent, pervasive, and uncontrollable—thus confirming the sense of powerlessness and increasing feelings of insecurity. As a result, such people stop reaching out to others and become confirmed in their loneliness (Seligman, 1998).

María told the nurse that she felt unable to turn to her family in Honduras because she was sure that they would blame her for getting into this situation by marrying someone they said was "no good." Can you think of other indications that María could be experiencing learned helplessness?

Relocation Stress Syndrome

Relocation stress syndrome is a set of physiological or psychosocial disturbances (or both) caused by transferring a person from one environment to another. It could be as simple as a client being transferred from one room to another in the nursing home or as complex as relocating to the United States from Honduras.

Although moving to another room may not seem as threatening as María's relocation from Honduras, it is difficult to predict which move would prove more traumatic. In fact, a client in a nursing home may be more impaired by a move to another room. It is the meaning of the move that causes relocation stress syndrome. Factors that affect a person's adjustment to a move include previous experience, personality traits, cumulative stress, support systems in the original environment, and a lack of support systems in the new environment.

FACTORS AFFECTING ROLES AND RELATIONSHIPS

Everything we have experienced from the moment of conception to the present, along with our perception of those experiences, affects our relationships with others. Some of the factors that affect relationships are developmental, cultural, religious, socioeconomic, physiological, and psychological.

Developmental Factors

In a functional family, children are nurtured, kept secure, and encouraged to learn. Natural roles include those of child, grandchild, playmate, student, and neighbor. Parental expectations affect the roles of the children. Whereas some parents expect and encourage their children to have playmates and to fulfill the role of playmate and peer, other parents expect their children to focus more on household chores, caring for younger siblings, and fulfilling the role of helper.

In families in which one parent is emotionally or physically unavailable because of alcohol, drug abuse, or physical or mental illness, the child may have to take on the role of caretaker to one or both parents and to any siblings. When children live in an unpredictable and insecure environment, they have more difficulty mastering the task of trust versus mistrust. Not being able to place trust in others will make the attainment of close relationships difficult throughout life.

In addition to the roles of student, child, sibling, and peer, the adolescent works hard to sort out and take on the roles associated with a masculine or feminine sexual identity. Adolescents use fantasy, introjection (throwing oneself into an interest), role-playing, and projection of themselves in the role before finally internalizing the sexual identity.

Young adults become more independent from their parents and their peers, develop careers, form relationships with significant others, and possibly marry and become parents. They may continue some of the roles of childhood or adolescence, such as son or daughter or student. They also take on the new roles of sexual partner, husband or wife, worker, co-worker, wage-earner, and parent.

In middle age, or maturity, adults are concerned with productivity, creativity, giving something to society, and participating in guiding the next generation. They find themselves in changing relationships with parents, children, and significant others. For example, some will be caring for children and aging parents at the same time, while others may have adult children and parents who are healthy and independent.

The roles of the older adult vary but may include grandparent, volunteer, activist, hobbyist, and traveler. They may also include mourner, widow or widower, caretaker for ill relatives, or the sick role itself. Roles may depend largely on health and financial status. Older adults are trying to establish or maintain ego integrity and avoid despair. Threats to ego integrity include decreases in sensory acuity (vision, smell, taste, hearing) and isolation. Many factors can contribute to an older adult's risk for social isolation, including loss of friends and family, being moved by family or others to unfamiliar surroundings, having to rely on others for transportation, and dwindling resources. Older adults are especially at risk for relocation stress syndrome, particularly when they enter nursing homes and leave their belongings and old friends. Being chronically ill with physical problems increases the risk for social isolation and altered role performance (Fig. 49–1).

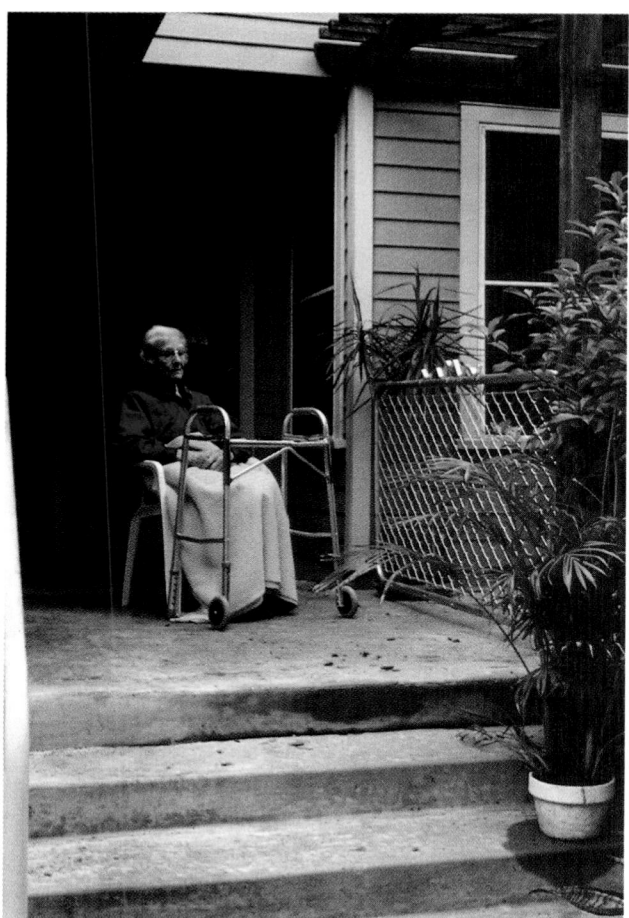

Figure 49–1. Being chronically ill with physical problems increases the risk for *Social isolation* and *Altered role performance.*

Cultural and Religious Factors

Culture helps define the various roles a person assumes and the rules for interpersonal relationships. There are many cultural groups in the United States, such as American Indian, Mexican, Haitian, and African-American, each prescribing role behaviors that have both common elements across all cultures and also culture-specific behaviors.

Role conflict can occur between the beliefs people acquire through their native culture and those acquired through the larger culture. Most people acquire values from the larger culture and subcultures such as rural, urban, drug, religion, or ethnic group. For example, the experience of growing up in a staunch Catholic family is different in many ways from growing up in a Jewish family, even in the same neighborhood.

When María arrived at the obstetrical unit with Jesús, the nurses were curious about the spot of nail polish on the child's nose. They wondered how he would adjust to the temporary separation from his mother while she was hospitalized for the birth of her second child. María continued to show great concern for her son and was thankful that she had remembered to put the nail polish on his nose. How do you think the nurses should respond to the spot?

Socioeconomic Factors

Socioeconomic factors affect the groups to which a person belongs, desired recreation activities, resources to perform a role, and the ability to achieve power or control. Poverty, for example, can make it difficult to fulfill role obligations and maintain satisfactory relationships.

Physiological Factors

The effect of trauma, physical illnesses, and medical procedures can lead to isolation, impaired social interaction, and altered role performance. Clients who are undergoing medical procedures, suffering the results of trauma, or dealing with physical illnesses often ask for more or different kinds of help from significant others, since they are unable to maintain their usual roles and responsibilities. Their significant others may provide them social support or may withdraw it, depending on the emotional or financial drain on them.

Psychological Factors

People under high stress may manage to keep their relationships intact if they have good coping mechanisms and problem-solving skills. In contrast, people who use maladaptive coping skills—such as alcohol, drugs, projection, denial, and anger—may destroy important relationships.

Mentally ill people who are not well stabilized by medication or therapy present challenges to those who are in relationships with them. Mental illness affects the way a person thinks, feels, and acts. The degree of influence varies depending on the diagnosis as well as the effectiveness of medication and other forms of treatment. Supportive relationships may lessen the likelihood of acute episodes or lessen the severity of the illness.

Role and relationship problems can worsen mental illness. In fact, loneliness and isolation may be a factor in mental illness in the homeless. Connecting the homeless to a network and providing assistance in finding jobs and shelter could be a factor in reducing the cost of care for the mentally ill, as discussed in the Cost of Care chart.

ASSESSMENT

To provide appropriate nursing care, you will need to assess clients with health problems for social isolation and clients who are socially isolated for health problems. However, you will succeed only if you can establish and then maintain a trusting relationship with each client and family.

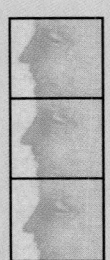

CROSS-CULTURAL CARE
CARING FOR A HONDURAN CLIENT

María is frightened when she is admitted to the emergency department in labor. One of the paramedics is carrying her 19-month-old son in his arms. The boy has a dot of red nail polish on his nose.

In the Hispanic culture, particularly in the rural areas, some members of the culture believe that an infant or small child must be protected against *mal de ojo*. They believe that if a person of power, such as an adult, looks upon a small child or infant and thinks or talks about the child without touching the child, bad things can happen to the child. The child can become sick, have bad luck, or die.

In some mountainous regions of rural Honduras, mothers dress babies and small children in red stockings, red shirts, or red head bands to reduce the risk of *mal de ojo*. Sometimes the mother will paint a spot of red on the child's nose.

In other areas of Honduras, a small bag of garlic is worn around the neck to counteract any *mal de ojo*, which can be perpetrated against adults as well as children. In some regions, water blessed by a priest is placed in a pan under the bed to counteract *mal de ojo*. Some Hispanic people in Mexico and the United States, when suspecting that a person is a victim of *mal de ojo*, will move a whole egg over the person's body. The egg is then broken and placed in water. If it cooks and an eye or face is seen in the egg, then it is certain that *mal de ojo* occurred.

The following dialogue occurs between María and Janet, the nurse:

María: Por favor! Por favor! *(Holds out her arms to the boy)*

Janet: María, you are in labor. The doctor needs to examine you. I will get a volunteer to sit here with the boy. *(Turns to a nurse's assistant and instructs him to get a translator.)*

Maria: No, señora! Por favor! *(María is clearly afraid for her son.)*

Critical Thinking Questions

- How would you help María know that her son is safe?
- Would you let the boy stay at his mother's side?

General Assessment of Roles and Relationships

You can assess a client's relationships as part of your general nursing assessment or in response to specific cues, such as a loss or change in relationships or a relocation. Less direct but equally important cues could be mood changes, a change in ability to carry out work or activities of daily living, changes in eating and sleeping habits, and client withdrawal.

Health History

As you take a health history, gather data about the client's roles and relationships and their potential effect on the client's current health status. Clarify with the client any changes in her demographic information, such as marital status, names and ages of children, type of employment, and length of time in a job.

When interviewing the client, allow enough time to encourage her to give full responses, use therapeutic communication skills, and listen closely to the responses. The following are examples of statements and questions that may solicit clues about your client's potential or actual relationship problems.

- Tell me about your important relationships.
- Describe the structure of your family or household.
- Who is the family decision-maker?
- Who does household chores?

- Has anyone in your family or circle of friends died, moved away, or stopped relating to you? Have you recently moved and lost touch with important people in your life?
- Describe a time recently when you were upset or angry with someone significant in your life.
- Have you taken on any new roles or had any changes in the roles you usually carry out?
- Have you been able to carry out your work and activities of daily living, such as bathing and personal hygiene?
- Do you feel comfortable with the amount of time you spend alone and the amount of time you spend with others?
- Are you able to take sick leave from work for this illness?
- Describe your relationships with family members. What is expected of you in the family? Do you feel that you meet your family's expectations? If you could, what would you change about your role or responsibility in the family?
- How well do you get along at work?
- What community groups do you belong to? What are your friends like? How do you spend your free time?

It may help you assess a client's problems if the client gives you permission to talk with significant others. Doing so will allow you to find out their perception of the client's problem and what goals they want the client to accomplish.

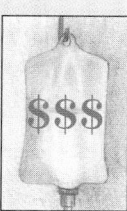

Physical Examination

During the physical examination, look for physical signs that may affect roles and relationships. Assess the client's appearance, noting grooming, dress, eye contact, posture, any physical handicaps, mannerisms, and gait. Also, assess the client's orientation to time, place, and person. Also assess the client's memory, manner of speech, and any communication problems. You will have to decide what to include in the client's physical examination based on the client's assessed needs.

Focused Assessment for Altered Role Performance

If your assessment leads you to suspect a problem in roles or relationships, consider the diagnosis *Altered role performance* and assess further to see if it is appropriate for your client.

Defining Characteristics

Defining characteristics for the diagnosis *Altered role performance* include the following:

- Altered perception of role by self or others
- Role strain, conflict, confusion, ambivalence, denial, dissatisfaction, or overload

- Inadequate external support for role enactment
- Inadequate adaptation to change or transition
- Family system conflict, uncertainty, or pessimism
- Change in usual patterns of responsibility, inadequate self-management
- Discrimination, domestic violence, harassment
- Inadequate motivation, confidence, role competency, skills, or knowledge
- Inappropriate developmental expectations
- Powerlessness, inadequate coping, anxiety, or depression
- Change in capacity to resume role
- Inadequate opportunities for role enactment.

A client with *Altered role performance* is experiencing conflict in the perception or performance of a role. The client may believe that others have changed their expectations. For example, a man who has had a heart attack says, "My wife won't let me do anything because she's afraid I'll have another heart attack."

Action **A**lert!
When working with an ill client, make sure to elicit concerns about role changes caused by illness or hospitalization.

Related Factors

Factors related to the diagnosis *Altered role performance* may be social, knowledge-based, or physiological. Social factors may include inadequate or inappropriate linkage with the health care system, job demands, youth or developmental level, conflict or domestic violence, lack of reward, poverty or inadequate support, and inadequate role socialization (expectations or responsibilities, for example). Knowledge-based factors might include inadequate role preparation or knowledge about a role, lack of opportunity for role rehearsal, unrealistic expectations, or lack of education, skills, or a role model. Physiological factors might include illness, cognitive deficits, substance abuse, mental illness, depression, low self-esteem, pain, fatigue, and altered body image.

Focused Assessment for Social Isolation

Clients at increased risk for the diagnosis *Social isolation* are those with low self-esteem, a history of being battered or homeless, depression, chronic pain, or chronic progressive illnesses.

Defining Characteristics

Defining characteristics for the diagnosis *Social isolation* may be objective or subjective. Objective characteristics may include an absence of supportive significant others, hostility, withdrawal, unwillingness to communicate, unacceptable behaviors, preoccupation with self, avoidance of eye contact, repetitive or meaningless actions, an obvious illness or disability, and a sad, dull affect.

Subjective characteristics might include expressions of feeling alone or rejected, interests or activities inappropriate for the client's age or developmental stage, no significant purpose in life, inability to meet the expectations of others, values unacceptable in the dominant cultural group, feelings of being different from others, and insecurity in public.

Related Factors

Factors related to the diagnosis *Social isolation* include the following:

- Altered mental status, physical appearance, or wellness
- Inability to engage in satisfying personal relationships
- Unaccepted social values or behaviors
- Inadequate personal resources
- Immature interests or unaccomplished developmental tasks

Focused Assessment for Impaired Social Interaction

When assessing a client for the diagnosis *Impaired social interaction,* investigate the client's perceptions of her social interactions and observe the quantity and quality of her interactions. If permitted, ask the client's family about their perceptions of the client's communication patterns.

Defining Characteristics

Defining characteristics for the diagnosis *Impaired social interaction* include the following:

- Verbalized or observed inability to receive or communicate a satisfying sense of belonging, caring, interest, or shared history
- Verbalized or observed discomfort in social situations
- Observed use of unsuccessful social interaction behaviors
- Dysfunctional interaction with peers, family, or others
- Family report of a change in the client's style or pattern of interaction

To qualify for the diagnosis *Impaired social interaction,* either the client must express discomfort in social situations or significant others must describe observations of the client's discomfort in social situations. When interactions are not mutually satisfying, they are likely to lead clients into distancing themselves from peers, family, and others. Dissatisfaction might stem from evidence that the client is unaware or not concerned with the values and feelings of others, or from using language or humor that may not be understood or appreciated by others.

Related Factors

Factors related to *Impaired social interaction* include the following:

- Deficit of knowledge or skills needed to enhance mutual satisfaction with relationship
- Communication barriers
- Therapeutic isolation or absence of available significant others or peers
- Limited physical mobility or environmental barriers
- Sociocultural dissonance
- Altered thought processes or self-concept

LACK OF SOCIAL SKILLS. Social skills are behaviors usually learned in the family of origin. Deficits in those skills can result from a lack of role models or from role models who have inadequate social skills. Some families keep secrets, do not talk openly about problems, are highly concerned with self-interests, and exhibit needy behaviors. If this type of communication pattern is learned, it will need to be unlearned. Impaired social interaction also can occur when a person does not know the rules for the behavior of a group.

COMMUNICATION BARRIERS. Communication barriers may involve a lack of common language or an inadequate medium for expressing the message. Social interaction is impaired for the deaf person who lacks an interpreter or the ability to read lips or write or sign back to others (Fig. 49–2). Another communication barrier can be found in people who have language barriers or a fear of expressing cultural beliefs in a health care setting.

HEALTH CONDITIONS. Therapeutic isolation or limited physical mobility decreases a person's opportunity for social interactions. On the other hand, significant others may lack understanding of the person's needs or may become tired of caring for the person and not having the time or energy to meet their own

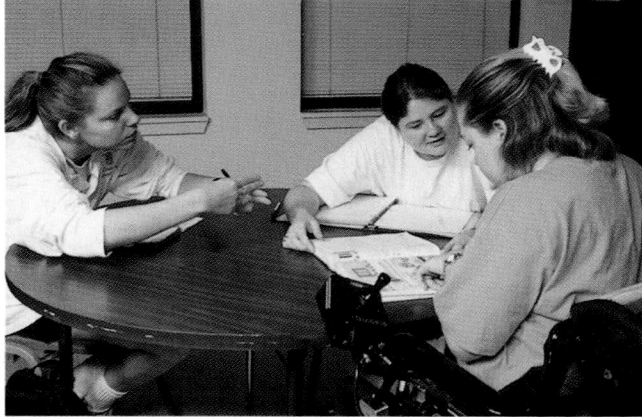

Figure 49–2. Having a severe hearing impairment can limit communication to those who can communicate through sign language.

needs. Health problems can result in psychological or physical withdrawal of significant others.

Impaired social interactions are common among persons with psychiatric illnesses. Because of the nature of symptoms associated with psychiatric illness, interactions with others become more challenging.

SELF-CONCEPT DISTURBANCE. Self-concept disturbance can result in impaired social interaction. For example, when parents tell children that no one wants to hear from them or that what they are saying is stupid, insensitive, insulting, or not appropriate, children come to see themselves as inadequate or incompetent. A child who perceives himself to be socially incompetent withdraws from social interaction or behaves in an incompetent manner consistent with what he now believes is true about himself.

Focused Assessment for Relocation Stress Syndrome

Defining Characteristics

Defining characteristics for the diagnosis *Relocation stress syndrome* include the following:

- Confusion, loneliness, depression, apprehension, anxiety, a sad affect
- Change in environment or location
- Withdrawal, vigilance, restlessness, sleep disturbance
- Verbalization of concern about relocation or unwillingness to relocate
- Lack of trust, insecurity, dependency
- Increased verbalization of needs
- Gastrointestinal disturbances, weight change, change in eating habits
- Unfavorable comparison of staff before and after relocation

To qualify for the diagnosis *Relocation stress syndrome,* the person must have been recently relocated. This is often a problem for immigrants to the United States. Baker and Arseneault (1994) studied the effects people experienced when they had a sudden emersion into a different culture. They expressed feelings of powerless, uncertainty about people's expectations, social isolation, feeling lost or bewildered, being outside society, and being different from others.

Related Factors

Factors related to the diagnosis *Relocation stress syndrome* include the following:

- Impaired psychosocial or physical health status
- Past, concurrent, and recent losses, including losses associated with the decision to move
- Moderate to high degree of environment change
- Inadequate support system
- History and types of previous transfers

- Feeling of powerlessness
- Little or no preparation for the impending move

RECENT LOSSES. Relocation is commonly associated with losses, so you will need to assess clients for past, recent, or current losses associated with their move. Loss can include a wide variety of things, such as missing people, pets, belongings, familiar surroundings, language, familiar places to do business, and many others.

MEANING OF THE RELOCATION. Whether a person experiences relocation stress syndrome depends on the meaning attached to the change. It is important to encourage clients to talk about how they feel about impending or accomplished moves and to listen closely to their responses using therapeutic communication techniques. Moves can be positive, negative, and anything in between.

OTHER FACTORS. In general, a client's adjustment to a move depends largely on the adequacy of her support system and her preparation for the move. Make sure to assess the client's preparation for the move, her previous experience with moving, and her current support system. If she has moved before, her perception of previous moves may affect her perception of the present move.

Focused Assessment for Related Nursing Diagnoses

You will want to assess a number of problems related to the four relationship diagnoses discussed in this chapter. These problems include altered nutrition, powerlessness, hopelessness, ineffective individual coping, self-care deficit, self-esteem disturbance, and sleep pattern disturbance.

Altered Nutrition

Altered nutrition, either less than or more than body requirements, is an expected response to the relationship problems discussed in this chapter. When people experience problems in their relationships, they may not eat sufficient quantities of food or a balanced diet. The reasons for this vary and include loss of appetite, preoccupation with the relationship problems, and self-punishment for not being worthy enough to deserve food.

Some people with relationship problems eat more than their body requires as an attempt to comfort themselves or to relieve a feeling of emptiness. To assess for altered nutrition, you will need to weigh your clients to determine whether their weight has changed. You can also ask them to list everything they ate and drank for the past 24 hours for additional assessment data.

Powerlessness

People in a number of societal subgroups (such as the frail elderly, chronically ill, and terminally ill) are at risk for feeling a loss of power over their physical and psychological environments. This loss of control comes with a loss of income, job, health, and significant others. You will want to assess clients for any feelings of powerlessness or feeling out of control.

Hopelessness

Byrne et al. (1994) pointed out that hope involves a relatedness with others, that "the hopeful person feels needed." Thus, the lack of relationships that occurs in social isolation or the strained relationships that occur in altered role performance tend to contribute to a feeling of hopelessness. You can assess your clients' feelings of hopelessness by asking them on a scale of 1 to 10 how hopeful they are for their future.

Ineffective Individual Coping

Many persons with relationship problems have ineffective coping skills and lack adequate problem-solving skills. To assess for ineffective coping, you can ask the client how she would approach a hypothetical problem. For example, you might say, "A friend of yours has to take an important exam and her car will not start. What would be a good way for your friend to deal with this problem?"

Self-Care Deficit

People who are having difficulty with relationships may not spend as much time on or attention to their own personal hygiene. This lack of interest and energy in caring for self may result in part from the decrease in mood and self-esteem that comes with relationship problems. Others may continue their usual good grooming or may intensify it so others will not perceive their lack of confidence in role performance and relationships.

> Action Alert!
> Remember: Not everyone with relationship problems has a self-care deficit.

Self-Esteem Disturbance

When people must face losses of income, job, health, significant others, or familiar surroundings, these losses tend to decrease the sense of self-esteem, belonging, security, and control. Any loss of relationships can be damaging to self-esteem.

Sleep Pattern Disturbance

Many people with relationship problems have sleep-pattern disturbances. Clients may be concerned about alterations in role; being isolated from others; being relocated away from familiar places, routines, and people; or not being able to interact in a socially acceptable way. They may either lack sleep or sleep excessively in an attempt to escape thinking about these problems. The sleep disturbance can also be secondary to a depressed mood caused by relationship problems.

DIAGNOSIS

The accompanying decision tree will help you decide which relationship diagnosis is the most relevant to an individual client situation. The relationship diagnoses must be differentiated from some other diagnoses as well.

For example, *Altered role performance* must be differentiated from *Altered family processes. Altered role performance* focuses mainly on change in the individual member, while *Altered family processes* focuses mainly on change in the family.

Social isolation must be differentiated from *Altered role performance*. The latter involves a person who cannot or will not perform a role, whereas the former deals with a person who is alone or thinks that she is alone and isolated from society. *Social isolation* is often a part of *Relocation stress syndrome*. You will have to choose the most appropriate diagnosis for the individual client, as discussed in the data clustering chart. The choice may change the treatment interventions or the scope of treatment interventions.

PLANNING

After assessing your client and determining that she has one of the four relationship diagnoses discussed in this chapter, you will write outcome criteria. These criteria are statements of what behaviors the client, the client's family, or both will carry out. When completed, these behaviors will demonstrate movement toward resolving the nursing diagnoses.

Expected Outcomes for the Client With Altered Role Performance

The following outcome criteria are common for clients with the diagnosis *Altered role performance.* As determined in concert with the client, the client will

- Express feelings or beliefs about roles held within a certain time frame (1 month, for example).
- Name a certain number of factors that contribute to the disturbance in role performance by a given date.
- Describe a certain number of realistic expectations for self in a given role.
- Identify behaviors needed for fulfilling a modified role expectation.
- Assume certain behaviors in a modified role by a given date.
- Design an alternative role by a given date.
- Seek assistance from selected resources inside and outside the community by a given date.

Expected Outcomes for the Client With Social Isolation

The specific outcome criteria for *Social isolation* will depend on assessed problems and identified needs.

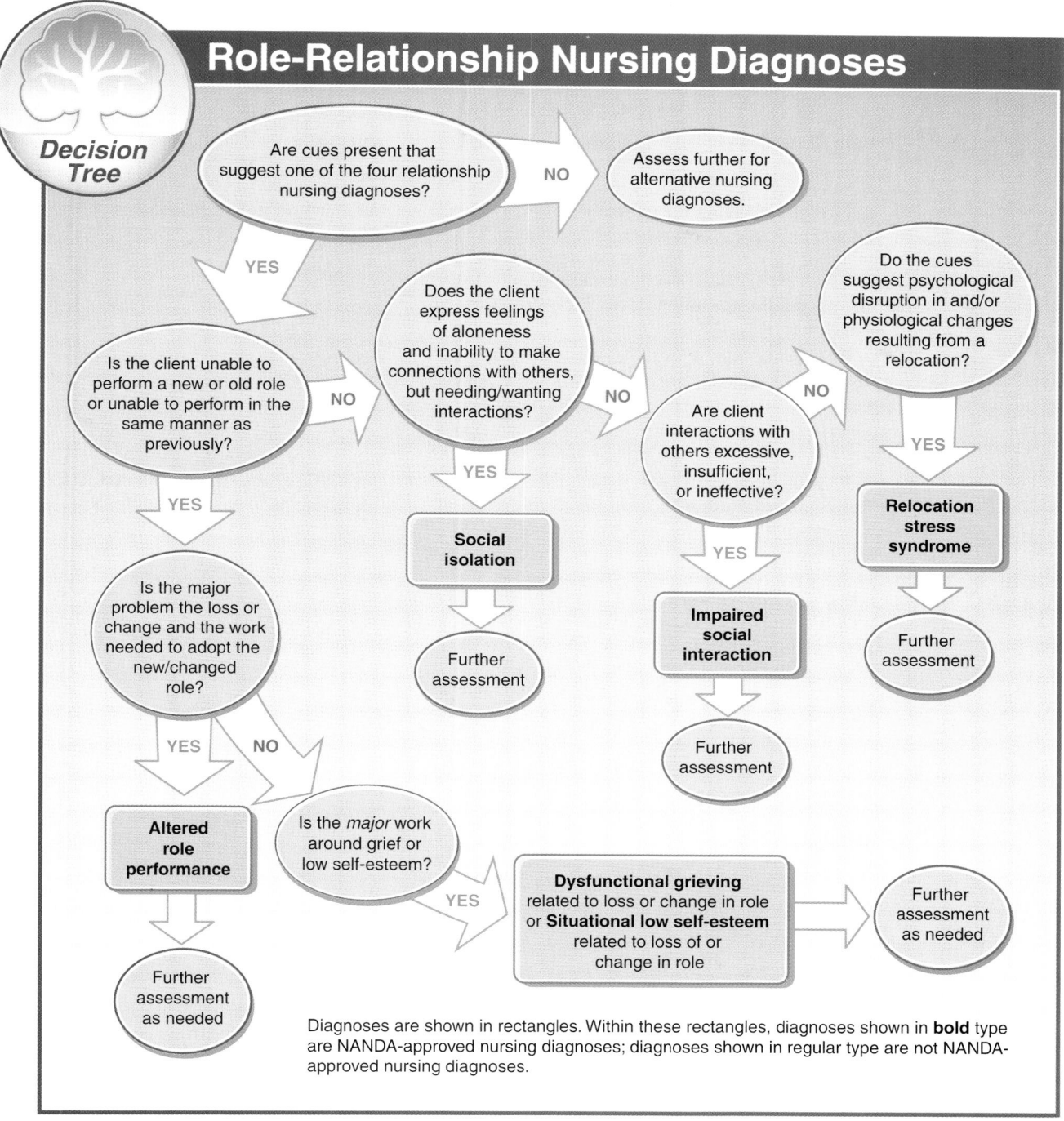

Role-Relationship Nursing Diagnoses

Decision Tree

Are cues present that suggest one of the four relationship nursing diagnoses?

→ **NO** → Assess further for alternative nursing diagnoses.

YES ↓

Is the client unable to perform a new or old role or unable to perform in the same manner as previously?

→ **NO** → Does the client express feelings of aloneness and inability to make connections with others, but needing/wanting interactions?

→ **NO** → Are client interactions with others excessive, insufficient, or ineffective?

→ **NO** → Do the cues suggest psychological disruption in and/or physiological changes resulting from a relocation?

YES ↓ (under "Is the client unable to perform...")

Is the major problem the loss or change and the work needed to adopt the new/changed role?

YES ↓ (under "Does the client express feelings...")

Social isolation

↓

Further assessment

YES ↓ (under "Are client interactions...")

Impaired social interaction

↓

Further assessment

YES ↓ (under "Do the cues suggest psychological...")

Relocation stress syndrome

↓

Further assessment

YES ↓ / **NO** ↘ (under "Is the major problem the loss...")

Altered role performance

↓

Further assessment as needed

Is the *major* work around grief or low self-esteem?

→ **YES** → **Dysfunctional grieving** related to loss or change in role or **Situational low self-esteem** related to loss of or change in role

→ Further assessment as needed

Diagnoses are shown in rectangles. Within these rectangles, diagnoses shown in **bold** type are NANDA-approved nursing diagnoses; diagnoses shown in regular type are not NANDA-approved nursing diagnoses.

Some outcomes, depending on the client's situation, could include one or more of the following:

- Name at least one other person you can talk to.
- Describe and discuss your feelings with at least one other person each day.
- Reduce your degree of social isolation by attending a support group each week, calling a friend each day, or accomplishing a similar agreed-upon goal.
- Discuss the pros and cons of adopting a pet by a given date.

María from our case study will need to develop a trusting relationship with at least one caregiver so she can talk about her feelings and develop a plan to reduce her degree of social isolation. How would you build a trusting relationship with María?

Expected Outcomes for the Client With Impaired Social Interaction

The person with *Impaired social interaction* might have one or more of the following outcome criteria, de-

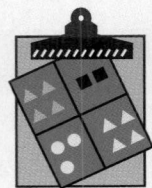

CLUSTERING DATA TO MAKE A NURSING DIAGNOSIS
ROLE-RELATIONSHIP PROBLEMS

Data Cluster	Diagnosis
A 22-year-old medical student stays awake for 3 days while studying for stressful oral examinations. The student becomes manic, profane, and sexually provocative. During medical rounds, he acts as if he knows everything needed to help the clients and the attending doctors should follow his directions.	*Altered role performance* related to stress, fatigue, and mood disturbance
A 50-year-old man with Parkinson's disease says, "I feel so ashamed. I'm so awkward and I can't talk right, so I don't talk much and I never go out. I have no friends or family any more. I fear that I'll die all alone and no one will care" (Nijhof, 1995).	*Social isolation* related to shame and decreased self-esteem
A 35-year-old woman with a diagnosis of schizoaffective disorder has been readmitted to the psychiatric hospital. In completing the nursing assessment, you learn that this client has trouble relating to her apartment complex manager, case worker, social services workers, and family. This client has a history of coping with problems with others by getting angry or running away. The client says: "No one likes me. I don't belong anywhere. My toilet doesn't flush but I can't talk to the manager. He doesn't want to talk to me. I have no way to go get my medicine."	*Impaired social interaction* related to lack of communication and coping skills
An elderly woman living alone in her home becomes progressively unable to care for herself. The children help her sell the family home and move into a long-term care facility. During the next 6 weeks, the client repeatedly says, "I don't belong here." She has difficulty sleeping, eats little at meals, cries frequently, and talks of being abandoned by the family.	*Relocation stress syndrome* related to move from family home into a long-term care facility

pending on assessment findings. As determined in concert with the client, the client will

- Engage in a certain number of planned social activities daily or weekly.
- Attend a certain number or percentage of scheduled communication classes.
- Initiate a certain number of personal interactions per day in person or on the telephone.

Expected Outcomes for the Client With Relocation Stress Syndrome

Outcome criteria vary based on the underlying situation that resulted in the diagnosis *Relocation stress syndrome* and the client's strengths, limitations, and resources. It might include the following short-term

goals based on assessment findings. As determined in concert with the client, the client will

- Identify the stressors in the new situation.
- Recognize the connection between the distressing symptoms and the relocation.
- Explore losses related to the move by a certain date.
- Identify a certain number of sources of support.
- Name a certain number of benefits of the new environment.

Examples of long-term goals for a client with *Relocation stress syndrome* are that the client will

- State that she is adjusting to the new environment.
- State that she has friends and activities that she enjoys in the new environment.

What will María's outcome criteria be? Recall that she has no home and no money. She does not speak English. While working with María on expressing feelings and concerns and verbalizing about losses, it is critical that you help her establish new resources in the United States. One outcome criterion could be that María will work with Social Services to find a home and other resources for herself and her children.

INTERVENTION

Interventions for All Relationship Diagnoses

Some interventions are common to all four of the relationship nursing diagnoses discussed in this chapter. They include building or maintaining trust and demonstrating caring.

ESTABLISHING TRUST. The importance of building trust with a client is especially pertinent when she is experiencing relationship problems. Lack of trust may be the basic unresolved issue underlying social isolation. Once you establish a trusting relationship with the client, the client will begin to interact more openly with you.

Although it is important to establish trust with every client, it is especially important for a client with impaired social interaction. Clients with *Impaired social interaction* may also have trust issues. Such a client tends to withdraw after repeated social failures. A relationship of trust helps the client come out of withdrawal and take chances again in social interactions.

To establish a trusting relationship with the client, you will need to make some small promises and keep demonstrating that you can be trusted to keep your word. Examples include being on time for appointments, listening attentively, displaying respect, and demonstrating empathy, commitment, and caring.

MUTUAL GOAL-SETTING. Goals will be individualized depending on the etiology of the diagnosis and the client's individual response. How the client identifies a problem helps in creating the goals. Also use your knowledge of the client's strengths and limitations when formulating goals. One approach is to share with the client the problems you have identified and to ask which problems she feels are most important to work on first. Another approach is to ask the client to tell you one thing that she would like to work on first. This is far less threatening than asking the client how to solve all of her problems. Plus, when the client decides on her own goals, she will be more invested in meeting them than if you have established the goals.

Even if the client is confused, try to include her in assessing her problems and formulating a plan of care. Giving the client choices is important in establishing trust and encouraging compliance with the treatment plan.

Listen carefully to what your client says. Her perceptions of her problems may be totally different from your initial impression. For example, an older person who has been admitted to a nursing home based on decisions made by family and medical personnel may define the problem as being rejected by her children.

Interventions to Improve Role Performance

Interventions specific to improving role performance center around clarifying roles, developing resources, referring for job retraining, teaching, and practicing redefined roles.

CLARIFYING ROLES. You will need to provide opportunities on a predetermined time frame (daily, biweekly, weekly) for clients to express their perception of their roles, responsibilities, and causes of altered role performance. This schedule gives them a chance to see the reality of their abilities and limitations, as well as to look at adjustments to roles or alternative roles. For example, a client may keep a daily journal in which she describes her roles.

Another task for the client is to identify how significant others' perceptions of a role differ from her own perception. Sometimes this difference in perception requires negotiation about what role behavior should take priority and what the role is to be.

DEVELOPING RESOURCES. You can help clients identify resources needed to fulfill their roles. These resources will vary and should be identified by the client and you. For example, if a client needs child care, you may help the client explore the types of child care facilities available and help narrow the list down to the most acceptable and affordable.

REFERRALS TO JOB RETRAINING. When illness or disability forces a career change, it may be appropriate for the client to receive job testing and counseling from a career counselor. An example of a resource for clients who become disabled is the state rehabilitation department.

TEACHING. You can provide clients with education about a role, model the role, or help them identify role models. In some cases, role distance can be reduced when clients obtain added knowledge and skill. You may include in your teaching strategies such activities as role clarification, exploration of role expectations, and role modeling where appropriate.

PRACTICING REDEFINED ROLES. Clients can practice roles and then share their reactions to these roles with you. Roles can be further redefined as practice reveals where clients feel successful and where they feel uncomfortable. Feedback from significant others helps clients to redefine roles as well.

Interventions to Address Social Isolation

Interventions for social isolation include exploring feelings, enhancing self-care activities, promoting involvement of family and friends, using support groups, and using pets therapeutically.

EXPLORING FEELINGS. Provide opportunities for clients to talk about their feelings (isolation, aloneness, and other feelings). Use open-ended communication techniques, such as, "Tell me about your feelings."

ENHANCING SELF-CARE. People who live alone have a tendency to neglect self-care. You can help the client maintain health through teaching behaviors that will help the person live alone more successfully and maintain good health practices. The accompanying Teaching for Self-Care chart provides some suggestions.

In addition to health practices, diversional activities may be helpful. If possible, have an activity or recreational therapist assess the client's recreational needs. Some clients may need to start with activities that include just one other person and then work up to two people and then to a small group. Build on the client strengths you identified in your assessment.

PROMOTING INVOLVEMENT WITH FAMILY AND FRIENDS. Encourage a hospitalized or homebound client to arrange or allow visits from family or significant others if this is feasible and such people are available. Explain to the family the client's need for support and how family members can help meet that need. Sometimes family members want to help but need specific, concrete suggestions.

ENCOURAGING USE OF SUPPORT GROUPS. Encourage the client to identify support needs and make use of various support systems. Examples include community support groups, religious groups, day health-care centers, and self-help groups centering around medical or mental problems.

USING PETS THERAPEUTICALLY. Pets commonly serve a therapeutic role by decreasing a client's feelings of aloneness. However, the therapeutic value of a pet must be weighed against possible problems, such as the cost of food and veterinary care and the possibility that the pet will promote allergy symptoms.

Interventions to Enhance Social Interaction

Interventions for *Impaired social interaction* include ego building, identification of strengths and weaknesses, role playing, the teaching of communication techniques, using support groups, and increasing social contact.

EGO BUILDING. Some clients are socially isolated because they have little ego strength; others start with sufficient ego strength but lose it as they become isolated because of external reasons. Praising the client appropriately and teaching self-praise for accomplishments can build ego strength. As the ego is strengthened, it is more likely that clients will attempt additional challenges in social interactions.

IDENTIFYING STRENGTHS AND LIMITATIONS. All clients have some strengths. Examples of potential strengths include being healthy, being employed, and having a sense of humor, patience, persistence, attractiveness, musical talent, and a strong interest and ability in a hobby, and having the support of family. You will need to assess the client's strengths on an ongoing basis.

Limitations can include such things as a lack of financial resources, inadequate social skills, no interest in or knowledge about self-care, impaired physical ability to carry out hygiene tasks, and fear. Whatever fears the client has, they are real to the client and must be addressed.

USING ROLE-PLAYING. Provide opportunities for the client to role-play social interactions with others. This is done through classes in some health care facilities or you may use your creativity to come up with opportunities for role-playing social interactions.

TEACHING COMMUNICATION TECHNIQUES. Help the client identify communication techniques that are not working, such as anger or blaming. Ask the client if she has had any ideas about what techniques will work better. Many clients will say that they need to count to 10 or leave a situation to calm down when they are angry and tempted to lash out at another person verbally or physically. Provide role-modeling, teaching, and practice in communication techniques that are more productive in accomplishing what the client wants.

ENCOURAGING USE OF SUPPORT GROUPS. Identify support groups that may benefit the client. If she is capable of participating, involve the client in making decisions about what types of support groups she would like to attend. If practical, have the client contact the groups and make arrangements to attend.

INCREASING SOCIAL CONTACTS. For a client who is hospitalized and isolated, plan care so that she has opportunities to interact with supportive staff, family, and friends. For clients with nonsupportive families, you and the health care team can create care plans for changing the perceptions and behaviors of the nonsupportive person or changing the client's responses to help her get her needs met. Consider increasing opportunities for communication via Internet, e-mail, writing, and telephone.

Interventions to Address Relocation Stress Syndrome

Establishing trust is an essential intervention for *Relocation stress syndrome*. Clients feel threatened or vulnerable in unknown environments, which can result in their being confused and having disorganized behavior. Because this syndrome includes withdrawal behaviors as an attempt to protect the self in an uncertain situation, establishing trust can be challenging. If possible, the client should have a consistent caregiver. Other interventions you can use include mutual goal setting, reframing perceptions, and maintaining the familiar. You will also want to utilize interventions for preventing relocation stress syndrome in clients who are at risk for this diagnosis.

REFRAMING PERCEPTIONS. If a client's perceptions are so negative that they will not serve her well, then you can begin to interject alternative ideas. For example, you can gradually suggest the positive aspects of a new location. Timing and technique are important in planting positive ideas. If your attempt to reframe comes before the client trusts you, she may reject your ideas.

Teaching for SELF-CARE

STRATEGIES FOR LIVING ALONE

Purpose: To help the client develop effective coping strategies for living alone.

Rationale: By eating a well-balanced diet, maintaining social support systems, getting an optimal amount of sleep, and keeping a positive outlook, the client may be able to extend the time during which she can live independently and also maximize her satisfaction with her living arrangement and her life.

Expected Outcome: The client will care for herself adequately and maintain satisfaction with her living arrangement.

Client Instructions

- To minimize waste and repetitive leftovers, try to buy small amounts of food or specially packaged one-person servings. Consider shopping at a store that sells some products by bulk out of large bins. That way, you can buy just the right amount of sugar, flour, beans, cereal, or other staples. Doing so will not only reduce your shopping bill but will also allow you to build more variety into your meals.

- Consider asking your butcher to cut individual-size portions of meat and to help you select tender cuts.

- Another way to maintain variety, minimize waste, and provide yourself with quick meals is to use your freezer strategically. Whenever you make bread, muffins, cookies—almost anything, really—freeze some in small portions. Consider freezing soup, spaghetti sauce, or marinade in ice cube trays; then remove the cubes and keep them frozen in plastic freezer bags. If you make something like a meatloaf, separate the mixture into four individual-sized loaves and freeze three of them uncooked. That way, you can cook one and have a reasonable amount of leftovers. Make sure to label bags and wrapped packages with the contents and date.

- To keep meals interesting and tasty, make your foods appealing to the senses. Use such flavorings as packaged herb seasoning, lemon pepper, imitation butter, dried onion flakes, minced garlic, dried parsley, and bullion cubes. (Make sure you consider the sodium content, however.) To build your seasoning collection, consider trading some of your abundant seasonings with a neighbor who has different ones. When you serve your meal, try garnishing the plate with a slice of fruit or a colorful vegetable cut decoratively.

- When you eat, set the table with a cloth or special place mat and a colorful napkin. Put a small fresh flower in water to decorate the table. Play music that you enjoy. Try inviting a friend or neighbor over for dinner on a selected night each week.

- When selecting a person to invite over for a meal, look for someone who is positive and upbeat, a problem-solver. In fact, whether you invite the person over or not, try to make contact with such a person every day just to chat.

- As possible, plan inexpensive outings, preferably in the company of a friend or neighbor. They can help boost your mood and make you feel that you are learning, developing relationships, and participating fully in life. Your local newspaper will list upcoming events. Also consider attending a group for hobbyists, people interested in a certain topic, or people simply interested in social interaction. Plan to dine out or see a movie on a regular basis. Dining out can be easy and relatively inexpensive if researched; many restaurants have early evening specials and senior citizen prices.

- Helping others can make you feel good about yourself and more satisfied with your life in addition to broadening your circle of relationships; consider doing some volunteer work. Call a nursing home, hospital, children's home, library, or other place of interest and ask about volunteer opportunities. Naturally, you will want to pick something in keeping with your interests, abilities, and need for transportation.

- A carefully selected pet can provide a valuable relationship and source of interest and responsibility. A pet may provide physical health benefits has well. Before selecting a pet, consider your interests in various types of animals, the care they require, and your physical and financial ability to provide that care.

- You will be more alert and content during the day if you can establish a satisfactory sleep schedule at night. Set up a sleep routine that you follow every night, such as a special light snack, a shower or bath, tooth brushing, and special sleeping attire. Try to use the bed only for sleeping rather than for reading, watching television, or talking on the phone.

- Take steps to help yourself think positive thoughts and take positive actions. Every day, count up the number of positive thoughts you had and positive things you said or did with others. Do something nice for someone. Try to increase your positive thoughts and behaviors every day. Positive thoughts and deeds decrease stress, increase energy, and improve relationships.

MAINTAINING THE FAMILIAR. Find out about the client's previous routines and activities and try to continue or replicate them as much as possible. Nursing homes often encourage clients to bring personal items, even furniture, to make the environment feel more like home. Pictures of family and friends help maintain the connection with a former environment as well.

PREVENTING RELOCATION STRESS. Prevention is an important aspect in minimizing the diagnosis *Relocation stress syndrome.* The relocation should be planned with the client and should begin well in advance of the actual move to give the person time to assimilate changes before moving. Some nursing homes have started planning moves with residents as much as a year in advance. It may be helpful to visit the new lo-cation, talk about it, see pictures of it, or even look at maps that help orient the client to the new environment.

EVALUATION

The evaluation of a relationship diagnosis includes looking at the outcome criteria and determining whether the client has met the short-term and long-term goals, as discussed in the Nursing Care Planning chart. If the client was to have done something a certain number of times, did she complete all of the repetitions? Did she complete any of them? The following discussion provides examples of a variety of evaluation situations.

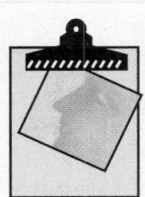

NURSING CARE PLANNING
A CLIENT WITH SOCIAL ISOLATION

Admission Data

María is admitted to the labor room area of the obstetrical unit. She is examined by the resident physician who finds her to be in active labor and ready to deliver. She delivers a baby girl within 30 minutes. The state child protective agency case worker comes to work out a temporary placement for María's 19-month-old son Jésus. After an hour in the recovery room, María is taken to the postpartum unit. She is assigned to a Spanish-speaking nurse because she speaks little English.

Physician's Orders	Routine postpartum orders Social Service consultation
Nursing Assessment	Vital signs within normal limits, breasts soft, fundus at 1/U, lochia rubra, no episiotomy, no hemorrhoids, slight abdominal cramping. Client says she is worried about her son and how he will do with strangers caring for him. Says she has no one to help her and complains of feeling all alone because her husband abandoned her and her family is in Honduras. Denies any friends or associations with groups. Expresses a desire for a friend or friends that would care about her. Says she feels down and has no money. Also says she does not know how she will survive without work skills or English skills.

NURSING CARE PLAN

Nursing Diagnosis	Expected Outcomes	Interventions	Evaluation (After 24 Hours of Care)
Social isolation related to loss of husband, separation from family and country, lack of training, and inability to communicate in English as evidenced by stating, "I feel so alone and different from everyone here. I wish I had family and friends."	Increase understanding of reasons for client feeling isolated	Assign the same nurse each day each shift whenever possible. *Establish a trusting relationship* and encourage client to talk about her feelings.	Client expressed feeling all alone and talked about how hopeless she felt to primary nurse.
	Set goals with the nurse for increasing social interactions	*Help client write (in Spanish) some goals for dealing with her isolation from others.*	Client wrote goals to contact some Spanish-speaking groups, contact her mother, and find housing.

Continued

If you set a short-term goal that the client would express her feelings and beliefs about the roles she holds, you will evaluate whether she talked about her feelings and beliefs or not. To make the goal more measurable, you could set the goal to be accomplished within a certain time frame or a certain number of times per week.

A goal for the client with *Social isolation* might be to call one friend each day. You can evaluate her progress toward this goal at the end of the week. What would your evaluation be if you found that the client made four calls during a crisis one day, but a total of three calls on the other six days? The goal was partially met because the client met the goal four out of six days. You and the client can look at what might have inter-fered with meeting the goal on the other two days. If you and the client mutually agree this is still a good goal to work on, look again to see if additional interventions are needed to help the client meet this goal.

A goal for a client with *Impaired social interaction* could be that she would stay in a reality-based conversation for 10 minutes. If your client stays in a reality-based conversation for 15 minutes, your evaluation is that your client met and exceeded the goal. You can then re-evaluate the goal and decide whether to discontinue it or to increase the number of minutes.

A goal for a client with *Relocation stress syndrome* might be to shop at a new store for groceries. If your evaluation reveals that the client shopped at two new places for groceries, the client has exceeded the goal.

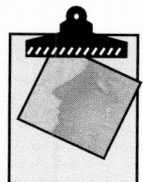

NURSING CARE PLANNING

A CLIENT WITH SOCIAL ISOLATION *(continued)*

NURSING CARE PLAN *(continued)*

Nursing Diagnosis	Expected Outcomes	Interventions	Evaluation (After 24 Hours of Care)
	Increase meaningful relationships	Identify possible support group or individuals. *Help client make calls to possible support group or individuals.*	Client contacted local Hispanic church and Hispanic Chamber of Commerce. The pastor of the Church and several women visited. Client contacted her mother by phone through funds provided by the church.
	Identify resources for housing, child care, transportation, and education	Decrease barriers to social resources. *Work through feelings about getting help from social agencies* with housing, parenting, job skills, language skills, child care, education, and transportation. Obtain list of possible resources. Refer as needed, coordinating with case worker and hospital social services.	Temporary housing is being planned through the church. The Hispanic Chamber of Commerce provided clothing and supplies for the baby.

Italicized interventions indicate culturally specific care.

Critical Thinking Questions

1. What agencies in your community might be able to help María?
2. How can you help María receive food stamps?
3. What strengths and weaknesses can you identify in María?

Do you need to set the goal higher? Probably not, but you may want to set a new but related goal, perhaps that the client will attend church on Sunday.

Returning to María, the young woman from Honduras, who has now delivered her second child, have you thought of how you would help her? The accompanying nursing care plan will give you some ideas to begin.

KEY PRINCIPLES

- Role performance includes a person's perceptions of her roles and current responsibilities in life situations.
- *Altered role performance* is a disruption in the way a client perceives her role performance. It includes role transition, role conflict, role failure, and role distance.
- Learned helplessness occurs when a person has experienced enough failure in her efforts that she comes to believe that continued efforts will also fail. Consequently, she exerts no effort.
- *Relocation stress syndrome* is a set of physiological or psychosocial disturbances (or both) created by a move from one environment to another.
- Some of the factors affecting relationships include developmental, cultural, religious, socioeconomic, psychological, and physiological.
- Interventions specific to improving role performance focus on clarifying roles, developing resources, referring for job retraining, teaching, and practicing redefined roles.
- Interventions for *Social isolation* include exploring feelings, enhancing diversional activities, promoting the involvement of family and friends, using support groups, and using pets therapeutically.
- Interactions for *Impaired social interaction* include establishing a trusting relationship and conducting mutual goal-setting.
- Interventions for *Relocation stress syndrome* include establishing trust, mutual goal-setting, reframing perceptions, and maintaining the familiar.
- The evaluation of a relationship diagnosis consists of looking at the outcome criteria and determining whether the client has met the short-term and long-term goals.

BIBLIOGRAPHY

Armer, J.M. (1996). Research brief: Degree of depersonalization as a cue in the adjustment to congregate housing by rural elders. *Geriatric Nursing, 17*(2), 79–80.

Arnault, D.S. (1998). Framework for culturally relevant psychiatric nursing. In E.N. Varcarolis (Ed.), *Foundations of psychiatric mental health nursing* (3rd ed.) Philadelphia: W.B. Saunders.

*Baker, C., & Arseneault, A.M. (1994). Resettlement without the support of an ethnocultural community. *Journal of Advanced Nursing, 20,* 1064–1072.

Bank, S.P., & Kahn, M.D. (1997). *The sibling bond.* New York: HarperCollins.

Blake, K. (1995). The social isolation of young men with quadriplegia. *Rehabilitation Nursing, 20*(1), 17–22.

Bull, M.J., & Jervis, L.L. (1997). Strategies used by chronically ill older women and their caregiving daughters in managing posthospital care. *Journal of Advanced Nursing, 25,* 541–547.

*Byrne, C., et al. (1994). The importance of relationships in fostering hope. *Journal of Psychosocial Nursing, 32*(9), 31–34.

Carpenito, L.J. (1997). *Nursing diagnosis: Application to clinical practice* (7th ed.). Philadelphia: J.B. Lippincott.

Carruth, A.K. (1996). Development and testing of the caregiver reciprocity scale. *Nursing Research, 45*(2), 92–97.

Carter, R. (1998). *When someone you love has mental illness.* New York: Random House.

Choi, N.G., & Wodarski, J.S. (1996). The relationship between social support and health status of elderly people: Does social support slow down physical and mental deterioration. *Social Work Research, 20*(1), 52–63.

Dai, Y., & Diamond, M. (1998). Filial piety: A cross-cultural comparison and its implications for the well-being of older parents. *Journal of Gerontological Nursing, 24*(3), 13–18

Dugan, J.M., Brown, A.V., & Ramsey, M.A. (1996). Health maintenance for the frail older adult: Can it improve physical and mental well being? *Journal of Advanced Nursing, 23,* 1185–1193.

Edelman, C.L., & Mandle, C.L. (1998). *Health promotion throughout the lifespan* (4th ed.). St. Louis: Mosby.

Friedman, M.M. (1998). Family role structure. In M.M. Friedman, *Family nursing* (4th ed.). Stamford, CT: Appleton & Lange, pp 293–326.

Grothaus, K.L. (1996). Family dynamics and family therapy with Mexican Americans. *Journal of Psychosocial Nursing, 34*(2), 31–37.

Hall, L.A., Sachs, B., & Rayens, M.K. (1998). Mothers' potential for child abuse: The roles of childhood abuse and social resources. *Nursing Research, 47*(2), 87–95.

Hansell, P.S., et al. (1998). The effect of a social support boosting intervention on stress, coping and social support in caregivers of children with HIV/AIDS. *Nursing Research, 47*(2), 79–86.

Johnson, R.A. (1996). The meaning of relocation among elderly religious sisters. *Western Journal of Nursing Research, 18*(2), 172–185.

Manion, P.S., & Rantz, M.J. (1995). Relocation stress syndrome: A comprehensive plan for long-term care admissions. *Geriatric Nursing, 16*(3), 108–112.

Murray, R.B. (1996). The lived experiences of homeless men. *Journal of Psychosocial Nursing, 34*(5), 18–23.

Nijhof, G. (1995). Parkinson's disease as a problem of shame in public appearance. *Sociology of Health and Illness, 17*(2), 193–205.

North American Nursing Diagnosis Association. (1999). *NANDA nursing diagnoses: Definitions & classification 1999–2000.* Philadelphia: Author.

Nypaver, J.M., Titus, M., & Brugler, C.J. (1996). Patient transfer to rehabilitation: Just another move? *Rehabilitation Nursing, 21*(2), 94–97.

Rose, L.E. (1997) Caring for caregivers: Perceptions of social support. *Journal of Psychosocial Nursing, 35*(2), 17–24.

Ryan, M.C. (1998). The relationship between loneliness, social support, and decline in function in the hospitalized elderly. *Journal of Gerontological Nursing, 24*(3), 19–27.

Seligman, M. (1998) *Learned optimism.* New York: Pocket Books.

*Selye, H. (1993). History of the stress concept. In L. Goldberger & S. Brenznitz (Eds.), *Handbook of stress: Theoretical and clinical aspects* (2nd ed.). New York: Free Press.

Sims, O.V., & Napholz, L. (1996). What are some African American working women's expressed experiences of role conflict? *Journal of Cultural Diversity, 3*(4), 116–122.

Sparks, S., & Taylor, C. (1998). *Nursing diagnosis reference manual* (4th ed.). Springhouse, PA: Springhouse.

Thomas, S.P. (1997). Distressing aspects of women's roles, vicarious stress, and health consequences. *Issues in Mental Health Nursing, 18*(6), 539–557.

*Asterisk indicates a classic or definitive work on this subject.

Loss

Janene Council Jeffery

Key Terms

anticipatory grief
bereave
code status
disenfranchised grief
dysfunctional grief
grief
grief attack
grief work

hospice
intrusive memory
loss
mourning
searching
selective attention
sense of presence
thanatology

LEARNING OBJECTIVES

After studying this chapter, you should be able to:

1. Define the concepts of loss, grief, mourning and bereavement, death, and thanatology.
2. Compare and contrast the types of loss and grieving.
3. Identify a variety of factors affecting the grief response.
4. Describe the assessment of a client or family member who is experiencing grief.
5. Describe the focused assessment of a dying client.
6. Differentiate among nursing diagnoses that describe problems associated with loss.
7. Plan for interventions to help the client and family feel understood and facilitate grief work.
8. Evaluate the outcomes of caring for a person experiencing grief.

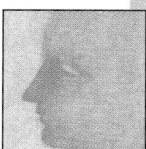

Mr. Hashimoto is a 54-year-old, first-generation Japanese-American man who holds an executive position in an international computer manufacturing company. He has been diagnosed with terminal cancer of the stomach. Until recently, the client thought he had an ulcer and had been treating his pain with meditation, prayer, and a special combination of herbs and roots prepared by the local Japanese chemist.

Four days ago, the client experienced generalized pain and vomiting. The vomitus had a fecal odor. He had his son take him to the family doctor because he was too weak to drive himself. The physician admitted him to the medical center for diagnostic tests. Statistically, the client has about 4 to 6 weeks left to live, and he understands that no aggressive treatment will cure his condition. The client's nurse knows that the consulting oncologist has been forthright with Mr. Hashimoto about his diagnosis and prognosis and makes a tentative diagnosis of *Anticipatory grieving*.

LOSS AND GRIEVING NURSING DIAGNOSES

Anticipatory Grieving: The intellectual and emotional responses and behaviors by which individuals (families, communities) work through the process of modifying self-concept based on the perception of potential loss.

Dysfunctional Grieving: Extended, unsuccessful use of intellectual and emotional responses by which individuals (families, communities) attempt to work through the process of modifying self-concept based on the perception of loss.

From North American Nursing Diagnosis Association. (1999). NANDA nursing diagnoses: Definitions and classification 1999–2000. Philadelphia: Author.

CONCEPTS OF LOSS AND GRIEF

As a nurse, you will confront loss and grief regularly in all health care settings. For some clients, loss results from changes in health and the resulting effects on lifestyle. For others, losses result from the dying process and eventual death, either of a loved one or of the client himself. You must understand the physical and psychological effects of dying and death to provide appropriate care and support to clients and family members as they work through grief and the life changes associated with loss. You must also understand how loss affects you as well, and you must learn to confront not just a client's death but your own death if you are to provide empathic care.

You may provide support to grieving, dying clients and families in settings ranging from acute care, to rehabilitation, to hospice. Currently, most people die in acute-care settings. However, nurses are becoming more involved in assisting people who choose to die in their homes or other setting where the focus is on hospice care. Hospice is a philosophical concept of providing palliative or supportive care to dying persons in which the goal of care in the last stages of life is to accentuate living and enhance the quality of life (Fig. 50–1). Hospice is not a place; rather, it is a philosophy. A person in hospice is known to be dying and receives palliative or supportive care rather than curative care. Care should be tailored to meet the specific needs of both clients and their families by using a team approach to enhance the scope of services available from the caring community.

Definitions

LOSS. Loss is the removal, change, or reduction in value of something valued or held dear and the feelings that result. Something of value, tangible or intangible, is taken away, rendered unavailable, or rendered less valuable. The loss may involve physical alterations, changes that affect public persona or self-esteem, or separation by death. A loss may be sudden and unexpected or anticipated and predicted.

Losses are encountered daily by each of us. They can be minor or major in their implications and are measurable only by the person experiencing the loss. The experience of loss must be defined broadly and with a clear understanding of the personal pain and disruption that can accompany it.

BEREAVEMENT. The term **bereave** means to rob or make desolate and is traditionally defined as being deprived through death, such as a widow who is deprived by the death of her husband. Usually, bereavement applies to immediate family members, especially those who care for the deceased near the time of death. The broader definition goes beyond the family and includes any person or group for whom the death represents a loss, such as a nation or community when natural disasters or accidents take lives. This term only means that someone has experienced a loss. It in no way conveys the extent or nature of the emotions, attitudes, or behaviors that characterize bereavement.

GRIEF. Grief includes emotional, physical, cognitive, and behavioral responses to bereavement, separation, or loss. It is a complex integration of feelings, attitudes, actions, and symptoms elicited by the body and mind at the time of a loss. The intensity of these manifestations changes over time. Grief is an individual, unique experience, not a finite set of experiences or emotions.

Grief influences all elements of a person's life and activities. Severe grief can cause physical illness, exac-

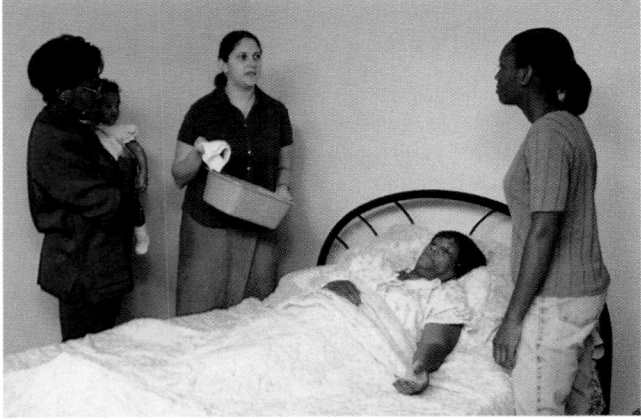

Figure 50–1. Hospice is not a place; rather it is a philosophical concept of providing palliative or supportive care to dying people.

erbate existing illness and, in extreme cases, lead to death (Steele, 1992, p. 397). Although every grieving person does not experience all grief responses, all persons in grief will encounter some of them.

MOURNING. **Mourning** is the term used to describe social and cultural acts used by a bereaved person to express thoughts and feelings of sorrow (Cooley, 1992, p. 125). It involves traditions and practices that help a person accept the reality of a loss and integrate that reality into the perception of the future (Bowlby, 1980). Mourning practices evolve, and many cultural mourning practices exist. In all cases, however, mourning honors the dead and helps manage the emptiness after death.

One common mourning practice is the wearing of black clothing to express grief for the deceased. Black bands are worn in various ways to express sorrow and respect, such as the black band on the badge of a law enforcement officer to mourn a fellow officer. A black band worn on a registered nurse's cap was instituted at the time of Florence Nightingale's death.

Acts of mourning include religious rituals, expressions of condolences, and burial practices. Mourning traditions offer mechanisms for experiencing and acknowledging grief. They are usually followed out of respect for the family and conform to cultural and societal expectations of grieving, Guidelines for the length of time to wear black clothing, to resume social activities, and to return to work have been affected by the accelerating pace of life in the United States. Mourning practices include individualizing burial sites to memorialize the deceased and comfort the family (Fig. 50–2).

DEATH. The strict definition of death has both practical and legal implications. Pronouncement of death depends on standard criteria accepted by individuals legally permitted to determine that death has occurred. Families and health care providers depend on application of consistent criteria in establishing death for purposes of discontinuing treatment or designating organ donor status. Legal implications extend to the need for accuracy in forensic investigations, probating estates, and statistical data collected by various governmental agencies.

Medical professionals, philosophers, sociologists, and lawyers agree that death occurs when the brain no longer functions. Yet, medical science has produced situations that make this simple definition difficult, if not impossible, to apply. As a result of a growing dilemma surrounding defining death, the President of the United States commissioned medical leaders to further refine and clarify a working definition of death. This definition could guide practitioners in the highly complex areas of life support, organ transplantation, and trauma. The following is a summary of the 1981 President's Commission's definition of **death** used today in the United States: "Absence of respiration and heart beat, or if mechanical means are being used to maintain these somatic activities, by the irreversible cessation or absence of all brain functions, including brain stem."

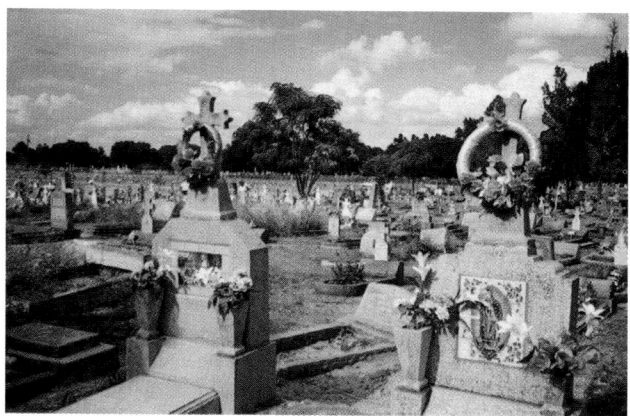

Figure 50–2. Mourning practices include individualizing burial sites to memorialize the deceased and comfort the family.

The cessation of brain function is determined through diagnostic evaluations, through determination of the cause of a coma, or through periods of observation, therapy, or both. Complications may invalidate the usual criteria and require special examinations or additional time to establish brain death when certain conditions exist, such as drug and metabolic intoxication, hypothermia, immaturity (especially children under age 2), and shock.

THANATOLOGY. **Thanatology** is the discipline of study and research that deals with death and death-related topics. This field of study examines death from the perspective of its definition, as well as attitudes, rituals, and related practices of individuals, groups, cultures, and religions. It encompasses death themes in art and literature, historical perspectives on death, mortality statistics, and factors influencing perceptions of death, dying, grief, and bereavement. It leads to a better understanding of the effects death and dying have on individuals and groups, including health care practitioners. With knowledge from this field of study, you can better assist clients, families, medical staff, and colleagues to understand death-related events and apply tools to mitigate the impact of death and facilitate grieving.

Types of Loss

Losses are categorized into two groups: those that are considered concrete or tangible and those that are psychological, symbolic, or intangible.

Tangible losses are apparent and easily recognized. Examples include death, removal of a body part, and changes in physical health. Tangible losses also include divorce, separation, property loss caused by a fire or natural disaster, relocation or job layoff, and a reduction of income.

Psychological losses are less obvious. They may be tied to personal perceptions, such as one's prestige, power, dreams, plans, ambition, confidence, security, and pride. Because these losses are less likely to be acknowledged, admitting to the accompanying feelings of loss can be difficult or embarrassing. Consequently, emotional support may be inadequate.

The death of a child from a terminal disease can easily be identified as a tangible loss for the parents. Society recognizes this loss and supports the parents' grief through various mourning practices. The symbolic or intangible losses associated with the child's death are less obvious and thus less overtly supported within mourning activities. These symbolic losses may include loss of personal and family identity and the loss of eagerly anticipated parent and grandparent roles. The symbolic loss may also include hopes and dreams for the child's success and possibly even the loss of money spent to care for the child over the course of the disease. Intangible losses often are not acknowledged at the time of the death but may be identified at birthdays, holidays, and family events. Support for the parent's grief is often minimal.

There are three specific types of losses that may be either tangible or intangible. They include

- A loss that can be recovered by replacement or substitution of a like or similar item or element
- A loss that is permanent and cannot be replaced even by remarriage or having another child
- A loss exemplified as the end of one's own physical existence

Although death is recognized as a significant and usually traumatic loss, grief can be experienced because of emotional attachments to anything lost. Loss of a job, property, marriage, or body parts is overtly recognized. Losses associated with developmental stages may be taken for granted. For example, the elderly may lose independence along with physical or mental health as they reach the latter stages of adulthood. These losses may be perceived only by the person affected because only this person recognizes the nature and magnitude of what is now missing from life. Whether apparent to others or only perceived by the heart, loss is real to those who grieve that loss.

The loss of self is recognized as the ultimate loss. People who are dying experience physical, emotional, and behavioral responses. Recognition of the end of life and the loss of contact with people and possessions held dear will precipitate many thoughts, feelings, and behaviors in the dying person. These may be components of their survivors' grief as well. The timing of grief and the feelings of the dying person and the dying person's survivors depend on the circumstances of the terminal events.

Action Alert!
The meaning of loss is individual. Be alert to the feelings associated with many kinds of loss.

Types of Grieving

Grieving is a normal human response to a loss, especially the loss of a significant person or the anticipated loss of one's own life. Both "normal" grief and "anticipatory" grief are natural responses. Appropriate nursing support can create a therapeutic environment that fosters personal growth for the bereaved. In contrast, dysfunctional grief can lead to life-long problems and breakdowns in psychological and physical health. Nursing care is especially needed to foresee such problems as they evolve and to intervene to reduce or eliminate the negative effects of grief that compromise functioning.

Normal Grieving

Significant interest in grief and grieving began in the health care literature with the work of Freud and Lindemann. In 1917, Sigmund Freud introduced the concept that grief could be normal as opposed to pathological in his classic work, *Mourning and Melancholia.* Erich Lindemann published pioneering research describing grief in 1944. By studying survivors of disasters and relatives of victims of the 1942 Coconut Grove Nightclub Fire in Boston, he described acute grief as a syndrome of psychological and somatic responses that he believed were normal after a distressing event. He proposed that appropriate interventions for "grief work" could assist in resolving the grief. His work is the single most influential work on the topic of grief symptoms.

Building on earlier works, Dr. George Engel presented a model of grief (Engel, 1964). He compared the mental trauma of grief to the physical trauma sustained with injuries. He proposed that bereavement could be tracked to a successful resolution through a series of stages just as physical healing follows a series of stages.

In 1969 Elisabeth Kübler-Ross became internationally known through the publication of her book, *On Death and Dying.* She and a team of students and practicing physicians interviewed many dying clients. From these interviews she outlined five phases displayed by persons facing death. The model was easy to remember and understand, and it gained rapid and broad acceptance. She is credited for bringing the topic of death into the open for both public and professional discussion and for promoting awareness of the needs of the dying.

Grief work is the effort by a grieving person to acknowledge the physical and psychological pain associated with bereavement and to integrate the loss into the future. It is necessary for completing normal grieving and the mourning process, thus preventing dysfunctional grieving. It uses intellectual and emotional responses to direct and guide behaviors or displays of grief. These responses help a person or group modify the self-concept, identity, and roles in life based on the reality of a loss. The significance attached to a loss will contribute to the nature of the grief work, the length of acute grief, and the outcome of grief. The concept of normal grieving includes a wide range of responses and times.

Action Alert!
Grieving over a loss is normal, and the manifestations of grief are normal even if they are not consistent with the person's usual pattern of behavior.

Anticipatory Grieving

Anticipatory grief involves the intellectual and emotional responses and behaviors by which individuals, families, and communities attempt to work through the process of modifying self-concept based on the perception of potential loss. The perception or recognition of an impending loss triggers grief responses. This preparatory grieving occurs in terminally ill clients and their families as they deal with the impending death. The extent of anticipatory grieving depends on the length of time between the understanding that a loss will occur and its actual occurrence.

As a person faces the ultimate loss—his own death—he engages in intellectual, emotional, and behavioral responses. These responses span a wide variety of reactions and thoughts. A person with a terminal illness may begin to consider a rapidly diminishing future in which his previous goals may not be achieved. The person may cognitively and emotionally address the foreseeable changes in his physical body from the terminal illness.

Family members progress through many of the same responses as the dying person. In the case of surviving relatives, however, they are faced with continuing daily life after the death of the loved one. Anticipation of such a loss can open opportunities to settle personal and family issues, confirm love and support, seek participation of the loved ones in plans for the burial, and draw families together through the pain of loss. It may be that having time prior to a loss can help lessen the pain and trauma.

> **A**ction **A**lert!
> Normal anticipatory grief includes making plans for living after an ill person dies. Do not consider it a sign of not caring about the person.

Dysfunctional Grieving

Some people have trouble dealing with grief that is unresolved over time. There is no specific time line for the completion of grief and no set series of responses that must occur for successful grieving to take place. **Dysfunctional grief** refers to the extended, unsuccessful use of intellectual and emotional responses by which individuals, families, and communities attempt to work through the process of modifying self-concept based on the perception of loss.

Sometimes people cannot reconcile their new life with the way life was before the loss. The survivor needs to acknowledge the contribution the deceased made to life and that the deceased is no longer an active part of it. This task may be daunting. The inability to make such a transition may create psychological and physiological consequences detrimental to life.

> **A**ction **A**lert!
> Be cautious in making the diagnosis of *Dysfunctional grieving*. The time needed for grieving is highly variable.

FACTORS AFFECTING THE GRIEF RESPONSE

Although grief is a highly personal response, certain aspects are common to many grieving people. These responses may vary with the person's culture, religion, values and beliefs about life and death, and practices and rituals associated with dying, death, and mourning. The Cross-Cultural Care chart offers one such example.

Developmental factors can also influence the perception and meaning given to the loss and grief responses. Children and adolescents have unique needs when handling a loss. Men and women reflect grief in differing ways, somewhat because of the difference in sex but also in the perceived roles each plays in society. Men generally display a strong, controlled reaction; women tend to be granted the allowance for weakness and emotionalism at such times. Although these reactions are clearly stereotypical, they are commonly displayed, and guilt may arise if these models are violated.

Situations associated with the nature and timing of death, and perceptions of whether the death could have been avoided, also contribute to the intensity and manifestations of grief. When a death falls outside the perceived natural order, such as a child dying before the parent, it is more difficult to accept. It is also more difficult to pursue grief work when a death is unexpected, particularly when the death involves a child or young person. If the death violates the explicit or implied mores of a society, such as suicide or some diseases, the client and survivors may be criticized or shunned while being denied needed support.

Psychosocial factors are also varied in nature and sources. Grief can be lessened by factors that link a death to feelings of fairness, rightness, and naturalness. The nature of the relationship between the deceased and the griever, and the degree of value accorded the loss by the griever, will bear significantly on the view of life and living after a loss.

Perceptions and personal integration of previous grief experiences contribute to the context within which a recent death will be placed. Indeed, cumulative grief can occur when a previous grief experience is not resolved before another loss is added to the psychological burden. The person's ability to effectively address a new loss is then compromised. The person's coping mechanisms and stress-management techniques affect the response. Nontherapeutic coping methods, such as those that use alcohol or drugs, and ineffective interpersonal relationships compromise a person's ability to engage in grief work. Depression or mental illness can complicate grief work as well. Stress will be multiplied, and existing stress management methods will be taxed even more.

Lastly, a person's physical condition influences grief. Illnesses previously in remission may return, and increased stress may yield physical manifestations. These physiological factors siphon the energy and attention needed to deal with grief. Occasionally, they may lead to life-threatening problems.

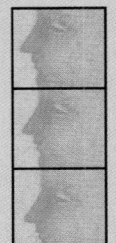

CROSS-CULTURAL CARE
CARING FOR A JAPANESE-AMERICAN CLIENT

Mr. Hashimoto is a 54-year-old, first-generation, Japanese-American. He has been a U.S. citizen for the past 23 years and currently works in corporate administration for a large computer company. His wife is 53 and has never worked outside the home. They have three children. The oldest is a 28-year-old son who is married and lives in the same town. They also have two daughters, a 24-year-old who works part-time in a laboratory and will start doctoral work in the fall and a 22-year-old who is completing the last semester of a bachelor's nursing program. Both daughters are single and living at home.

The entire family professes the Catholic faith. Mr. and Mrs. Hashimoto were raised as Buddhists and converted to Catholicism after coming to the United States. Their local parish priest is a second-generation Japanese-American and also a Buddhist convert. Although all clients are unique, many Japanese-American clients tend to value the following:

- Avoidance of physical contact or, if necessary in the health care setting, contact only after obtaining permission.
- Avoidance of direct eye contact, which is considered rude.
- Avoidance of questions that begin with, "Don't you . . ." because, to be polite, the Japanese person may say "no" three times before giving a true answer.
- The belief that a nod or smile does not necessarily mean agreement or understanding.
- Strong remnants of Buddhism in the faith practices and rituals of Christian converts.
- A view of death as a passage.
- Stoicism, especially in men.
- Restraint of public expressions of sorrow.
- Endurance of pain and suffering without complaint to show strength and avoid worrying family members.
- Clearly defined roles for husband (the breadwinner) and wife (the caretaker).
- Hospital care for the terminally ill, with daily visits from family.
- Coming home to spend the last days with family, during which the wife, daughter, or daughter-in-law will act as primary caretaker.
- Being uninformed about the true nature of a terminal illness to avoid losing strength and hope.

- The authority of the physician and dependence of the client.
- The belief in psychological interactions with deceased family members giving a greater feeling of peace with death.

Let's see how Andrew, Mr. Hashimoto's nurse, demonstrates sensitivity to the client's cultural values:

Andrew: (entering the room for a morning assessment; Andrew knows the oncologist has discussed chemotherapy to reduce the pain associated with Mr. Hashimoto's cancer) How are you today?

Mr. Hashimoto: I am fine.

Andrew: I see we are going to start you on chemotherapy today. Are you ready for that?

Mr. Hashimoto: I will do what the doctor thinks is best. Will it make me sick?

Andrew: The response is variable. It does cause some side effects, but we can give you other medications to control the side effects. I understand you plan to go home after you have received the treatments. May I talk to your wife about how to manage the side effects?

Mr. Hashimoto: She doesn't need to be concerned about me. I can manage.

Andrew: I know you want to be independent, but you may need some help. Your wife may feel better if she is able to help.

Mr. Hashimoto: Yes, you are probably right. You can talk to her.

Critical Thinking Questions

- Do you see evidence of Mr. Hashimoto's cultural values operating in this interaction?
- Was the nurse sensitive to his cultural needs?
- What could the nurse have done differently?

Based on information from Hirayama, K.K. [1990]. Death and dying in Japanese culture. In J.K. Parry [Ed.], Social work practice with the terminally ill: A transcultural perspective. Springfield, IL; Charles C Thomas; McQuay, J.E. [1995]. Cross-cultural customs and beliefs related to health crises, death, and organ donation/transplantation: A guide to assist health care professionals to understand different responses and provide cross-cultural assistance. Critical Care Nursing Clinics of North America, 7[3], 581–594; personal communication with Christine Rook, RN.

Action Alert!
Assess for nontherapeutic coping methods that will compromise a client's grief work.

ASSESSMENT

Grief is a universal human experience, but it has unique personal characteristics and varies with societal mores, the circumstances of a loss, and the value the griever associates with the loss. The responses associated with grief are extensive, complex, and personal. The differentiation of normal from abnormal grief is highly disputed; indeed, any response pattern may be normal for an individual in a given time and situation.

Erich Lindemann and Colin Murray Parkes (1972) suggest that grief is a syndrome that occurs in stages. However, grief is also nonlinear, meaning that it does not occur in a strictly predictable pattern or rigid stages. Grief has been likened to the wind that activates a pinwheel of life-changing processes. Each blade of the pinwheel catches the wind, sends it out, then lets it go until the next wind blows into life (Solari-Twadell, Bunkers, Wang, & Snyder, 1995).

General Assessment of Grieving

Normal grief reactions can be divided into three areas—recognition, reflection, and redirection—each with specific somatic, psychological, and behavioral responses (Jeffery, 1998–1999). Many responses can occur simultaneously, some recur after long periods of time, and others never arise in some people. The areas are not finite in time or type of responses displayed but progress throughout grief work. The labels of the three groups reflect the tasks encountered by the griever.

Recognition: Shock and Denial

The initial response to a loss, particularly a death, provides time to emotionally and intellectually absorb its painful reality. It has been called the "listen now, hear later" phase because it grants the griever time to buffer the truth while mobilizing coping resources to face that truth.

This initial reaction period has no clear time frame. Circumstances associated with unexpected news or anticipated news influence the time needed to recognize the reality of the events. However, many similar responses and expressions of grief have been identified at this beginning point in grief work.

Action Alert!
During the initial shock just after the death of a loved one, direct practical help in calling close family, deciding on a funeral home, and gathering the person's belongings (if in the hospital) are often needed.

SOMATIC RESPONSES
These reactions include physical symptoms, and many reflect a "panic attack" response mediated by the sympathetic nervous system. Somatic responses may include gastrointestinal symptoms, such as nausea, vomiting, abdominal cramping, a perception of hollowness in the stomach, and diarrhea.

Cardiopulmonary reactions may include tachycardia or palpitations, chest pain or tightness, dyspnea, or tachypnea. The person also may have trouble swallowing, a dry mouth, muscle weakness, tremors, dizziness or syncope, lack of energy, and increased sensitivity to noise. Reactions of diaphoresis, flushing, or cold and clammy sensations have also been reported.

PSYCHOLOGICAL RESPONSES
Initial psychological reactions serve to buffer or delay the awareness of bad news until other coping resources can be identified and mobilized. Here the concepts of shock and disbelief are most obvious. The most immediate emotional responses are often feelings of numbness, confusion, and a sense of unreality. Feelings of pain and separation generally replace the numbness when psychological awareness takes place. Anxiety, fear, and panic may be perceived along with a sense of depersonalization, isolation, or separateness from the environment. The person may sense that a part of the self has been removed or cut out and is missing. The death of a loved one may create feelings that part of the survivor also died.

A failure to comprehend events and information occurs early in many cases and may continue for some time despite an intellectual acceptance of the reality of the loss. This results from denial. Denial is a complex concept and can take various forms in differing circumstances.

Denial is both a defense mechanism and a cognitive activity. As a defense mechanism, it is primarily responsible for allowing time to assimilate and integrate new information into the cognitive realm. It is an attempt by the mind to alter a person's perception of reality. Statements of disbelief or protestations about mistaken information reflect this. Additionally, denial is an intellectual process that does not alter reality but is used to help the person cope with the undesired reality. It can take various forms. Cognitive denial is reflected in the following situations.

SELECTIVE ATTENTION. **Selective attention** is the act of choosing when and to whom a person will give attention to a loss and allow thoughts and feelings to enter the conscious mind. The person may choose to avoid talking to staff that he feels are not receptive to his concerns. Or he may avoid talking to family members in an effort to spare them emotional distress.

COMPARTMENTALIZATION. Compartmentalization is at work when a person appears to completely understand the existing circumstances yet acts in a manner that does not correlate appropriately with reality. For example, a husband may talk about taking his wife home from the hospital, as he has before, despite clear evidence that her condition is grave and prognosis poor.

DECEPTION. In deception, denial is reflected through knowingly altering facts or deliberately giving inaccurate information. Deceptive games are played and energy is wasted as efforts are expended to protect the other person. In some cultures, withholding negative medical information from dying clients is an accepted practice and is done out of respect for the emotional burdens already carried by the ill person.

TRUE DENIAL. In true denial, the person avoids recognizing reality. True denial can also arise when a person perceives reality as overwhelming. Responses may be bizarre or reflect psychotic thinking. The person may show strong self-protective efforts. For example, a mother who delivers a stillborn, full-term infant may seem to be dealing well with the unexpected event until the morning of discharge, when you find her preparing to take her new baby home from the hospital.

ANGER. Even rage is a common characteristic of grief. It occurs as the denial and disbelief are replaced with the growing awareness of reality. Anger and fear appear to be linked as the person faces a life changed by loss, especially death. The comfortable world is disrupted and security threatened.

Anger at unwanted feelings of vulnerability and powerlessness may rise to the surface. It may be displaced onto others in the environment, such as those the person holds responsible for a death or a supreme being for failure to change the outcome. Anger may be directed inward as well for perceived failures associated with the loss (Fig. 50–3).

Guilt or remorse is frequently interwoven with anger when the person takes blame for a real or imagined contribution to the death or when feelings such as relief are deemed unsuitable in the circumstances.

BEHAVIORAL RESPONSES

Behavioral responses associated with the recognition phase may include hysteria or crying, the release of anger and rage, or stoic, calm, or resigned behaviors. Cultural and societal mores commonly govern such actions. Hypoactivity or hyperactivity may also be noted, sometimes in conjunction with pointless or repetitive activity. Task-oriented activity may be helpful to the griever as he accomplishes necessary tasks associated with the loss. Critical thinking, cognitive functioning, concentration, and attention may be impaired, reducing the person's decision-making ability at a time when it is most needed. Further, hygiene, nutrition, rest, and self-care may be neglected or become an excessive focus.

The initial reaction to a loss may last a brief few minutes to several weeks. The important point is that until the reality of the loss has been acknowledged, further grief work is constrained. Responses at this stage generally reflect the griever's attempts to establish the reality in the conscious and unconscious worlds. When that task has been sufficiently addressed, further work will begin in the second broad phase of grief responses.

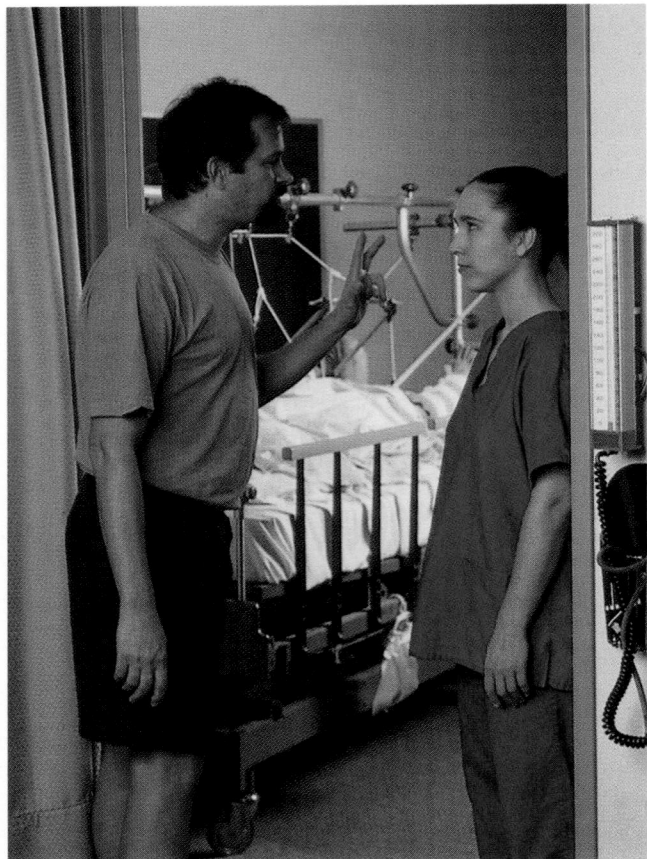

Figure 50–3. Grieving people sometimes displace anger onto others in the environment. Nurses sometimes get caught in the crossfire.

Reflection: Physical, Emotional, and Spiritual Suffering

During the second broad period of responses, grief work is focused on achieving a sense of stability after instability, control after chaos, and comfort after pain. In these responses, significant efforts are expended to return to a routine daily life without the overwhelming suffering and sorrow attached to the loss. For some this may never occur, but for many person's the pain does not lessen, it simply gets softer.

Personal growth, with resulting changes in self-concept, occurs as the person confronts, understands, and internalizes a loss. Such reconciliation of the permanency of the loss into the physical and psychological world of the griever takes place over an extended time period.

SOMATIC RESPONSES

Somatic responses can include continuing somatic distress similar to that experienced early in the grief process, such as weakness, panic attacks, and gastric distress or hollow feelings in the stomach. Depressed immune function has been observed with a correlated increase in physical illness.

Chronic diseases, such as cancer, ulcerative colitis, asthma, rheumatoid arthritis, heart failure, leukemia, and diabetes occur more often in the newly bereaved. And several studies have shown a major increase in the death rate of both sexes (especially widowers) during the first 6 months of bereavement (Steele, 1992). Complaints of fatigue are common. Eating and sleep patterns may be disturbed as well, leading to either increased or decreased activity levels.

PSYCHOLOGICAL RESPONSES

Psychological responses, after the shock dissipates, may be extensions of those begun at the initial time of grieving. This is a period when the mind comes to clearly understand that the loss is irreversible and life has changed irrevocably.

Anger resurfaces frequently and unexpectedly. Guilt can lead to remorse or regrets over past events and actions taken or not taken. The person may ruminate over the events preceding the death. Feelings of helplessness and disorganization can be precipitated by the overwhelming nature of the loss and the perceived future after that loss.

Helplessness may then slide into despair, hopelessness, and apathy as the griever succumbs to the sheer magnitude of the impact of the death. Concurrent within these feelings are elements of sadness, self-pity, loneliness, and panic or fears about the future. Clouded thinking, trouble with decision-making, and loss of confidence may still be evident at times.

The person may show emotional lability by crying spontaneously at times not clearly linked to sad events. Indeed, many grievers express surprise at the suddenness of mood swings and emotions associated with grief. These unpredictable emotional responses are a normal part of the grief process.

Keep in mind, however, that many people have feelings of relief or emancipation from burdens after a person's death. These feelings commonly stem from the end of the loved one's suffering or the release of a commitment to care for an ill person. Whatever the motivation, feelings of relief may be unacceptable to the griever or may increase feelings of guilt over this personal reaction to the death. However, especially when a lingering disease has altered life for both the client and the caregiver, feelings of relief are realistic.

Other reactions are unique to this period after the initial responses have passed. The deceased is remembered and opportunities for reminiscence affect grief in specific ways. There is sometimes an identification with the deceased, such as assuming admired traits, mannerisms, interests, goals, and opinions of the loved one. Commonly, memories become selective and filter out negative characteristics. The bereaved person may also experience a sense of presence, intrusive memories, or grief attacks.

SENSE OF PRESENCE. A **sense of presence** is a nonthreatening, comforting perception by the bereaved of the deceased's presence through one or more of the senses or in dreams, fortuitous events, or conversa-

tion. In such experiences, the griever describes the presence of the deceased as a feeling that the deceased is present in visions, in formed and unformed hallucinations, in voices and conversations, in smells and touch, in dreams and signs, or in fortuitous events (Conant, 1992). Parkes considers these events to be part of searching. In this context, **searching** refers to conscious and unconscious efforts by the bereaved to negate the reality of the loss through finding the deceased alive and well (Rando, 1984). Such events may be treated as religious experiences in which the deceased communicates a continued presence in the lives of loved ones and is safe, comfortable, and at peace.

INTRUSIVE MEMORIES. An **intrusive memory** is a vivid, realistic memory of events surrounding the death that return to the bereaved unexpectedly or unintentionally, overriding existing conscious thinking. Intrusive memories are similar to flash-back episodes. For many people, they are unwanted and disturbing. They are thought to be partially responsible for many accidents involving bereaved people who are momentarily distracted by the intrusive nature of the memories. Others find that intrusive memories and a sense of presence help to reconcile the reality of the death and internalize memories of the person (Conant, 1992 [abstract]).

GRIEF ATTACKS. A **grief attack** is an unexpected, involuntary resurgence of acute grief-related emotions and behaviors triggered by routine events and sometimes accompanied by uncontrollable crying or emotional display. An analogy to a grief attack is that of waves hitting a person standing with his back to the water at the ocean's edge. Waves come in at irregular intervals, some small enough to only flow over the feet. The person stands firm. Other waves hit higher on the legs and cause momentary wavering. Still others hit with enough force to knock the person down. The difficulty in withstanding the waves is that the person cannot see when a wave is coming or how large it will be until it hits. Triggering events for grief attacks may include special music, sights, and places shared with the deceased.

Gradually, over days and weeks, emotions become less labile. The pain of the loss never disappears, but it becomes less disruptive to daily life. Emotions may resurface at anniversaries and special holidays, but in general, emotional equilibrium is achieved and maintained.

BEHAVIORAL RESPONSES

Behaviors associated with this roller-coaster period can vary widely. Social withdrawal is common because depression and feelings of helplessness make the bereaved reluctant to engage in interpersonal activity in public. Poor hygiene may result from depression as well. Crying may continue for extended periods.

Absent-mindedness may be part of the confused and altered critical thinking processes. Seeking control over a world spinning out of control leads to questioning and efforts to clarify events associated with the loss. Searching behaviors extend beyond the emotional context, and the person may feel momentary hope when a face in a crowd resembles the deceased.

Avoidance behaviors may arise as the person tries to minimize the stress of coping with the loss. They may include smoking, drinking, or using drugs to blunt the pain, especially if the person used these forms of coping before the loss. These behaviors are physically and psychologically harmful. Overt risk-taking behaviors that threaten personal safety are infrequent but may occur. They reflect a subconscious belief that life is no longer worth living.

Personal possessions associated with the deceased are usually treasured. Belongings can be preserved by giving them special significance and honor in the home or by giving them to people special to the deceased. Honoring the memory of the deceased is then perpetuated by respecting these possessions.

Mummification is symbolic preservation of a deceased person by leaving the physical environment just as it was when the person was alive and well. This behavior is a form of denial. It differs from storing the person's belongings until a time when judgment and decision-making return to normal. A person who disperses or disposes of a deceased loved one's belongings quickly after the death may be in denial as well. This is an effort to minimize the pain of seeing or dealing with the person's belongings.

Spiritual distress is frequently present in bereavement. Long-held values and beliefs may be shaken because of the circumstances of the death. This is particularly true in the death of a child or young person, a senseless death, a violent or crime-related death, or an unusually horrific death. These can cause questioning and doubts about a supreme being and about religion.

Anger may be directed at fate or God. "Why" questions explore the unfairness of life. For many people, unanswered questions present hurdles to overcome in their grief work. Behaviors can include reluctance to return to religious rituals and ceremonies or increased efforts to place the events of the death into a spiritual context.

Serious issues regarding the spiritual elements of life, death, and grief will usually be addressed during grief work. The outcome of reviewing one's faith may be that spiritual beliefs are reinforced by the death experience. In contrast, beliefs may be undermined and abandoned for a time, possibly permanently.

Redirection, Reorganization, and Moving Forward

The third phase in grief work may last years. For some, it may never be completed. The responses reflect a griever's return to daily life in a manner that reconciles the past with the present and simultaneously looks toward the future. Realistic memories and hopeful planning are integral to successful grieving, and this final series of responses reflect a positive outcome achieved from all the previous grief work. There is optimism about a future without the loved one and willing efforts made to create that future.

SOMATIC RESPONSES
Somatic responses decline, and the person returns to the quality of health experienced before the loss. Appetite and sleep patterns return to normal. Sex drive returns to normal. Energy and strength last throughout the day. Overall health is again renewed and the person reports feeling like his old self.

PSYCHOLOGICAL RESPONSES
Although the person continues to have periods of sadness, anger, or regret, they become less frequent and less intense. Feelings of stability, hope, and personal capability begin to override negative emotions. Increasingly, the person has episodes of happiness, joy, and pleasure. Self-confidence and decision-making improve. The idealization of memories associated with the deceased decline, and the person resumes more realistic perceptions of the loved one. Grief attacks are less frequent. Overall, emotions become less intense and more balanced and realistic.

BEHAVIORAL RESPONSES
Behavioral responses mirror the person's improved emotional and physical state. Seeking behaviors diminish in frequency and realism. Decisions about the disposal of possessions are made without guilt or feelings of abandonment. The person reinvests energy into a life without the deceased and assumes new roles. The ability to look to the days ahead without the deceased is a strong indicator of successfully processing the event both intellectually and emotionally. Behaviors will communicate this accomplishment as the person returns to a routine daily lifestyle.

Focused Assessment for Anticipatory Grieving

Anticipatory grieving occurs when a person faces a potential or expected loss. Grief work before a loss is common among clients and their families when the client has a progressive or terminal disease. It has long been believed that such "preparatory grieving," as Kübler-Ross called it, results in less intense grief after the death. More recent research has cast doubt on this view, and numerous researchers have produced contradictory findings (Backer, Hannon, & Russell, 1994; Sweeting & Gilhooly, 1990). Many responses are linked with prolonged pre-death grieving, particularly in spouses and in parents of children who have extended terminal illnesses.

Defining characteristics for the diagnosis *Anticipatory grieving* may include the following:

- Potential loss of a significant object
- Expression of distress at potential loss

- Sorrow, guilt, or anger
- Denial of potential loss or the significance of the loss
- Altered communication patterns, eating habits, sleep patterns, dream patterns, activity levels, or libido
- Bargaining
- Difficulty taking on new or different roles

Anticipatory grief closely reflects normal grief in many ways and has inherent risks. Possible negative outcomes include the potential of distorting and ruining the few remaining months or weeks of a relationship. The emotional and physical pain of grief can cause an emotional distancing at a time when the dying person most needs support. In some instances, psychological detachment leads to physical and emotional withdrawal before the death occurs.

Some cultural groups believe that a critically or terminally ill client should not be told of his impending death. Families will go to great lengths to keep this information from their loved one in the belief that the knowledge will add an unnecessary burden and remove hope needed for recovery. Such events result in the illusion of uncaring and callous attitudes, which can lead to public censure and private guilt. The dying person, who is dealing with imminent death, may now have to deal with the belief that family members are not particularly concerned or aggrieved. Physical and psychological isolation can leave the person to die amid high-tech equipment and away from loved ones (Sweeting & Gilhooly, 1990).

Recognition of an impending loss can help families and friends use the remaining time to reconfirm relationships, settle issues, and build peace. However, the risks mentioned may override the positive outcomes and color the final days with negative emotions and painful memories.

Focused Assessment for Dysfunctional Grieving

Dysfunctional grieving is an extended, unsuccessful use of intellectual and emotional responses with which individuals, families, and communities attempt to work through the process of modifying self-concept based on the perception of loss. This is a possible outcome of a significant loss.

Not every person can traverse the grief experience and arrive at a comfortable emotional, physical, and spiritual assimilation of the loss. For some, the loss is perceived as so devastating that self-concept cannot be satisfactorily modified and reconciled with reality. They become overwhelmed and resort to maladaptive and unsuccessful coping strategies, further impairing their ability to function. Prolonged but unsuccessful efforts to move toward a satisfactory incorporation of the loss into their psychological and physical world ultimately will result in marked evidence of dysfunction.

Defining Characteristics

Defining characteristics for the diagnosis *Dysfunctional grieving* may include the following:

- Crying, sadness, anger, guilt, or a labile affect
- Reliving of past experiences with little or no reduction in the intensity of grief
- Expression of unresolved issues, distress at the loss
- Interference with life functioning
- Idealization of the lost object
- Difficulty in expressing loss, or denial of loss
- Alterations in eating habits, sleep patterns, dream patterns, activity level, libido, concentration, or pursuit of tasks
- Developmental regression
- Repetitive use of ineffectual behaviors in attempts to reinvest in relationships
- Prolonged interferences with life functioning
- Onset or exacerbation of somatic or psychosomatic responses

Recognition of dysfunctional grief warrants close observations for cues that may demonstrate behaviors and reactions that deviate from responses generally considered to be normal. William Worden (1991) has proposed the following four types of dysfunctional grief. Some people have two or more at once.

CHRONIC. In chronic dysfunctional grief, grief has continued for a prolonged or excessive period and does not reach a successful conclusion involving the establishment of a new and different self-concept. In this form of dysfunctional grief, the griever is unaware that the traditional period of mourning has ended and does not recognize the ongoing disruption to life.

DELAYED. Delayed dysfunctional grief is characterized by a diminished emotional response at the time of the initial loss and excessive grieving over a later, lesser loss. A correlation between two such losses is common in dysfunctional grieving.

EXAGGERATED. Exaggerated dysfunctional grief is evidenced by severe reactions, such as anxiety attacks, phobias, or irrational despair. The person has a significant interruption in daily life, illogical thinking, and an indefinite delay in restructuring a new self-concept.

MASKED. Symptoms and behaviors that the griever cannot identify as grief characterize masked dysfunctional grief. The person may develop physical symptoms experienced earlier by the deceased person, especially pain or specific somatic symptoms associated with the cause of death (Bateman et al., 1992).

General responses recognized as dysfunctional grief include a wide variety of identifiable cognitive and behavioral manifestations. Basically, the griever is trapped in a pathological stress reaction because he cannot meld the changes in his world and self with his previous environment and identity.

Related Factors

Factors related to the diagnosis *Dysfunctional grieving* include an actual or perceived loss of person, possession, job, status, home, ideals, or body parts and processes.

Factors associated with an increased risk of dysfunctional grief arise from a wide variety of issues and situations (see Box 50-1, Risk Factors for Dysfunctional Grief). Some are easily recognized and addressed in supportive ways. Others are hidden from those who could support the bereaved.

Factors that can influence a person's risk of dysfunctional grieving include how the event and the context of the event interact with the person's personality and coping style. Personality guides the conscious evaluation of the loss, the choice of coping mechanisms, the duration of each phase of grief work, and the perception of changes in self-concept that accompany grief work. Personality directly affects the adaptive completion of a mourning process.

Another factor that can influence the risk of dysfunctional grieving is the social acceptability or understanding of the loss. **Disenfranchised grief** is grief that lacks social acknowledgment, validation, and support for the bereaved (Doka, 1989). Therefore, the grief is not granted merit by society in general. It may arise in response to gay relationships, extramarital relationships, or death of an ex-spouse, for example. Social negation of grief may also arise from society's erroneous beliefs that the grief is not present or that it is inappropriate. Many believe that mentally retarded people are incapable of grieving, for example.

Yet another factor that raises the risk of dysfunctional grieving results from the attitude that grieving should occupy a rigid and restricted time frame after which the person is expected to move forward with few or no backward glances. This usually reflects the belief that grief is a sign of weakness and vulnerability and should be avoided. Risk factors for dysfunctional grief must be assessed and nursing interventions

made early to alleviate or prevent the development of dysfunctional grief.

Focused Assessment for Physical Signs of Dying

When death occurs gradually, changes take place throughout the body and are evident in major body systems (see Box 50-2, Physical Signs of Imminent Death). The changes reflect the incremental failure of each system. Assessment of these signs will help you provide appropriate information to families and determine plans of care for the terminally ill client.

DIAGNOSIS

Anticipatory grieving is a useful diagnosis when working with families and clients as they face medical tests and treatments that could change their lives. Cluster the data carefully to support your selection of this or any nursing diagnosis, as shown in the data clustering chart.

Anticipating life changes and possible death can trigger many other, more specific nursing diagnoses as well (see Box 50-3, Relevant Nursing Diagnoses for Psychosocial Support). Assess the client and family thoroughly for risk factors and current status to help differentiate between the umbrella diagnosis of *Anticipatory grieving* and other diagnostic labels.

You will use the diagnosis *Dysfunctional grieving* less frequently, but you still must assess and be vigilant about the possible development of this problem. Freud and others differentiated normal from dysfunctional grief with the following comparison. Normal grief is characterized by painful dejection, loss of interest, and inhibition of activities. Dysfunctional grief goes further and adds episodes of panic, hostility toward self, regression to narcissistic self-preoccupation, and signs of deflated self-esteem. The overwhelmed person may use maladaptive coping methods; however, the primary indicator is the inability to use coping methods that would facilitate development of a new self-concept that integrates the reality of the loss and its unique meanings.

A clear understanding of the definitions and defining characteristics of all relevant nursing diagnoses will help you use them accurately when planning care for dying patients and their families. The accompanying decision tree will help you distinguish between diagnoses that specifically address grief.

PLANNING

Planning care for a terminally ill client requires you to address widely varying responses from both client and family. You must recognize that you are really caring for two clients: the dying person and the immediate family unit. These two clients have differing needs and require separate planning. You can consider anticipatory grief and normal grief together when plan-

---

BOX 50-1

RISK FACTORS FOR DYSFUNCTIONAL GRIEF

- Highly ambivalent, narcissistic, or dependent relationships.
- Uncertain, sudden, or overcomplicated circumstances surrounding the loss.
- History of depression, low self-esteem, guilt, or previous complicated grief reactions.
- Conflict between perception of self as strong and feelings of dependency and neediness.
- Socially unspeakable, negated, or disenfranchised losses.
- History of current or past substance abuse.
- Decrease or loss of social support systems.
- Cumulative grief over multiple unresolved losses.

BOX 50–2

PHYSICAL SIGNS OF IMMINENT DEATH

Musculoskeletal System

- Loss of overall muscle tone and general weakness, including a lack of active, independent mobility and an inability to maintain positioning without support.
- Relaxed facial muscles, resulting in a sagging jaw and flaccid lips and cheeks.
- Bladder and bowel incontinence.
- Decreased gag reflex and difficulty swallowing.

Gastrointestinal System

- Anorexia.
- Dehydration, as evidenced by dry oral mucous membranes and low-grade fever.
- Decreased peristalsis, as evidenced by decreased nausea, abdominal distention, and constipation.
- Possible diarrhea.

Cardiovascular System

- Decreased peripheral circulation, in which extremities begin to appear cyanotic and mottled; they feel cool, cold, or clammy; or the client perspires and appears to be too warm.
- Poor skin turgor.

- Edema.
- Reduced rate of absorption of medications from tissues.
- Diminished kidney perfusion with decreased urine output.

Respiratory System

- Altered patterns of respiration, such as slow, labored, irregular, or Cheyne-Stokes pattern.
- Increased secretions, as evidenced by adventitious lung sounds or "death rattle."
- Irritation of tracheobronchial airway, as evidenced by hiccups, chest pain, fatigue, or exhaustion.
- Poor gas exchange, as evidenced by hypoxia, dyspnea, or cyanosis.

Neurological System

- Altered levels of alertness.
- Periods of mental cloudiness or disorientation.
- Variable pain levels.
- Possible blurred vision.
- Diminished blink reflex.
- Accumulation of secretions over eyes.
- Dry conjunctiva.
- Intact sense of hearing.

BOX 50–3

RELEVANT NURSING DIAGNOSES FOR PSYCHOSOCIAL SUPPORT

Defensive Coping

- Related to projection of blame or responsibility.
- Related to altered family dynamics.

Ineffective Individual Coping

- Related to inappropriate implementation of coping strategies.
- Related to difficulty expressing emotions (especially anger, guilt, and fear).
- Related to giving up hope and spiritual values.

Ineffective Denial

- Related to feelings of increased stress or anxiety.
- Related to fear of death, pain, loss of autonomy, separation.
- Related to feelings of omnipotence.

Social Isolation

- Related to infrequent visits by family, friends, or both.

Impaired Social Interaction

- Related to discomfort of visitors regarding terminal illness.

Spiritual Distress

- Related to challenges to belief system.
- Related to separation from faith community of support and rituals.

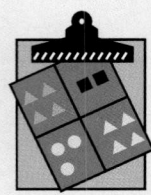

CLUSTERING DATA TO MAKE A NURSING DIAGNOSIS
LOSS AND GRIEVING

Data Cluster	Diagnosis
A 60-year-old woman has been caring for her husband for 3 years. He has terminal cancer and is hospitalized for the last time. The woman alternates between asking the doctor about further therapy, saying she wishes the suffering could be over, and making plans for life after the husband's death.	*Anticipatory grieving* related to impending loss of spouse.
A 45-year-old man has been diagnosed today with untreatable terminal lung cancer. He is quiet. When the nurse asks what the doctor said, he replies, "He said I have cancer, but I didn't really understand all of it. I guess I'll need chemotherapy."	Acute grief related to shock and confusion
A 55-year-old woman has been struggling with brain cancer for several years. She has had chemotherapy several times to reduce the size of the tumor. Currently she is going to a distant city to receive a chemotherapy implant. She says, "I don't want to die, but I have come to accept that it will happen."	Normal grief related to realization and acceptance of the inevitability of death
A young woman is hospitalized after an automobile accident in which her husband was killed. She is angry at the nursing staff for delay in receiving information about her husband's death.	Acute grief related to misdirected anger

ning supportive interventions for clients and families because of the similarity in responses.

At some point in the course of the client's disease, the goal of treatment will shift from curative to palliative. This shift must be accepted by everyone involved in planning the client's treatment. It may be difficult for both the health care team and the family, but it is crucial to recognize when further treatment becomes futile. At that point, comfort priorities become appropriate and will significantly improve the quality of the client's remaining time, both for the client and for family members.

For many dying clients, you will need to plan for the client's care daily. Be open with the client and family about care goals, and share your expected outcomes with them. Establish priorities for the dying client based on the physical manifestations of the dying process and the accompanying psychosocial needs. Make care goals realistic, accommodating of the client's and family's perspectives, and flexible as the client's condition changes.

In the past 72 hours, Mr. Hashimoto has had visits with his son to discuss financial affairs and has privately discussed with his son his view that, although he considers himself an American, he would still like to have some Buddhist rituals performed for the

benefit of the family and Japanese-American friends. The parish priest has visited the client twice and has assured the family that church members have been praying for Mr. Hashimoto and his family. He also says that he will try to accommodate any special requests they may have during this time.

Mrs. Hashimoto and both daughters have rotated their time to make sure someone has been at the bedside during the client's hospitalization. He has chosen to be treated with comfort measures only, and arrangements have been made for discharge with home health care. He is being transported by ambulance to his home today.

INTERVENTION

Nursing care of a dying client and his family demands sensitivity, creativity, and an awareness of common grief responses. Remember to consider the client's and family's cultural background as you meet these responses with appropriate interventions.

Also remember that the client's needs and the family's needs will differ, thus requiring differing interventions. Providing interventions that are tailored to both the client and the family support each one and allow you to provide excellent nursing care during the client's last days. Supportive interventions will continue for family members after the client's death.

When a grieving person does not receive appropriate support, it is much more difficult for him to achieve a healthy, satisfactory, comfortable conclusion to the loss.

Any supportive interventions, whether for physical or psychological responses or to meet ethical and legal interests, must be based on a clear understanding of the grief process. If you have a narrow view of what constitutes grief, you may have trouble designing and offering the appropriate interventions to facilitate client and family coping. Your personal attitudes about death, dying, and expressions of grief are also pivotal factors. If you are uncomfortable facing the reality of your own future death, you will find it difficult to provide support to others facing these same circumstances and issues.

Interventions for Ethical and Legal Advocacy

Medicine and client care have been tremendously influenced by technology that can extend life or prolong dying. Because of these advances, questions and concerns have arisen among health care professionals about withdrawing or withholding treatments, using heroic measures at the end of life, allocating scarce resources, and providing responsible care. Research has shown that nurses consider *do not resuscitate* (DNR) orders, client's rights, and professional practice issues the most important ethical problems being faced today (Haisfield-Wolfe, 1996; Keltner, Bourgeault, & Wahl, 1994; Corley, Selig, & Ferguson, 1993).

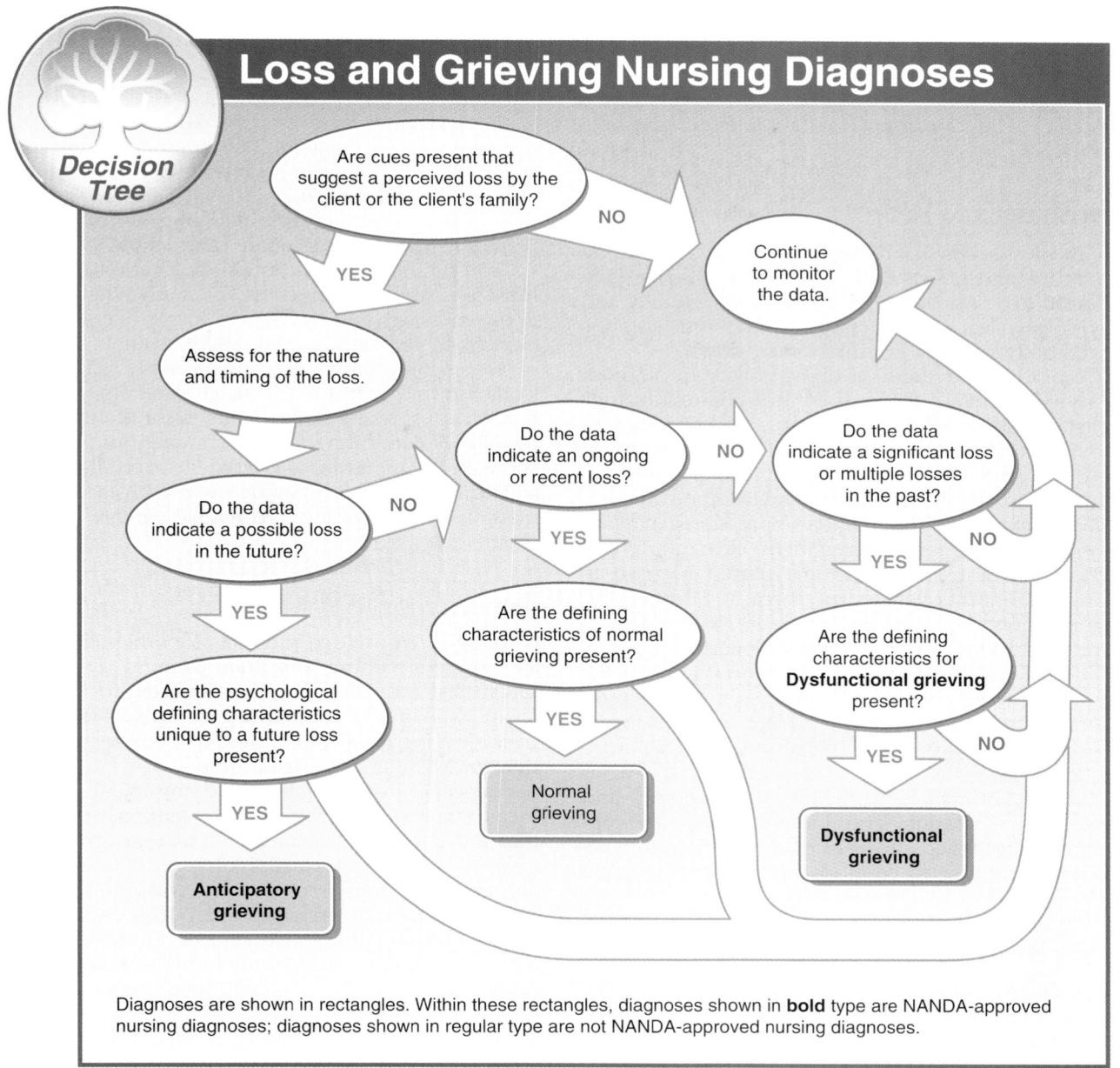

Decision Tree

Loss and Grieving Nursing Diagnoses

Are cues present that suggest a perceived loss by the client or the client's family?

NO → Continue to monitor the data.

YES ↓

Assess for the nature and timing of the loss.

↓

Do the data indicate a possible loss in the future?

NO → Do the data indicate an ongoing or recent loss?

NO → Do the data indicate a significant loss or multiple losses in the past?

YES ↓ (future loss)

Are the psychological defining characteristics unique to a future loss present?

YES ↓

Anticipatory grieving

Do the data indicate an ongoing or recent loss? — YES ↓

Are the defining characteristics of normal grieving present?

YES ↓

Normal grieving

Do the data indicate a significant loss or multiple losses in the past? — YES ↓ / NO →

Are the defining characteristics for **Dysfunctional grieving** present?

YES ↓ / NO →

Dysfunctional grieving

Diagnoses are shown in rectangles. Within these rectangles, diagnoses shown in **bold** type are NANDA-approved nursing diagnoses; diagnoses shown in regular type are not NANDA-approved nursing diagnoses.

In response to these concerns, clinical agencies are forming ethics committees to develop policies on resuscitation, advance directives, withdrawal of nutrition and fluids, and many other sensitive issues. You must be familiar with legislation, policies, standards of practice, and ethical dilemmas that influence dying clients, families, and professionals so you can offer support that is effective and within accepted legal and ethical frameworks (Edwards, 1994, 1993). For more specific information, see Chapters 2 and 3.

One major area of concern for nurses, dying clients, and their families involves resuscitation efforts if the client has a cardiac or respiratory arrest. **Code status** is a term used to identify the specific orders for a client regarding whether or not to begin resuscitative actions, and the extent of those actions, at the time of a cardiac or respiratory arrest. Interventions can range from a full code status, which indicates that all efforts should be used to resuscitate a person, to a DNR status, in which no action should be taken if an arrest occurs. An "out of hospital" DNR order is being used in some states to help guide emergency personnel who care for a dying client outside of a hospital.

Interventions to Address Physical Needs

The physical needs of a dying client depend in part on the course and effects of his particular disease. You will need to assess the client's condition routinely and provide physical care to manage these effects as the client's body systems gradually slow down.

Comfort care remains a high priority throughout the dying client's care. Pain control commonly tops the list and should involve both drug and nondrug interventions. The end of a person's life is not the time to delay or withhold narcotic analgesics out of fear of addiction. Also, avoid making judgments about the nature and extent of the client's expressions of pain. They only delay pain management. Relaxation, distraction, and anti-anxiety actions should be used to complement and enhance drug therapy. Efforts to reduce emotional tension can contribute to physical relaxation and reduce perceived pain levels.

Recently renewed interest and concerns about the comfort of dying clients have been expressed in published research findings on the subject of end-of-life issues (SUPPORT Group, 1995; McCann, Hall, & Groth-Juncker, 1994). Most studies focus on withdrawal or withholding of artificial nutrition (tube feeding) and intravenous hydration. The findings repeatedly conclude that prolonged efforts to maintain hydration actually run counter to comfort promotion (Zerwekh, 1997).

Dealing With Dehydration

The problem underlying the hydration dilemma is the emotional response to starvation and dehydration. Remember, however, that physiology changes in the dy-

ing client. Several studies have found that dehydrated dying clients rarely complain of thirst. Other studies reported that many dying people felt no thirst or only slight thirst. This level of thirst can be managed with small sips of water and by moistening the oral mucus membranes during oral care.

The advantages of dehydration in the dying client are many. Decreased urine production means less need for a bedpan, commode, urinal, or catheter. It also reduces incontinence. Decreasing gastrointestinal fluid levels decreases nausea and vomiting and reduces the need for tubes and suctioning to decompress the bowel. Respiratory secretions decline, relieving coughing and congestion. Reduced pharyngeal secretions may enhance swallowing while decreasing choking and drowning sensations.

Also, the azotemia that contributes to onset of coma is believed to provide a natural anesthesia and some measure of analgesia, possibly associated with increased production of a natural opioid. The need for narcotics and their risks and side effects can thus be reduced.

Despite what many believe, pain and suffering are not automatic sequelae of dehydration. Studies reflect a high comfort level in severely dehydrated persons nearing death. Many hospice staff believe the natural dehydration that comes with dying is not cruel but palliative and compassionate (Zerwekh, 1997).

The timing for withdrawing hydration modalities must be examined carefully. For many clients not yet in the end stage of their disease, correction of fluid and electrolyte imbalances may stabilize their condition, reverse some symptoms, and possibly prolong life. Collaborating with the physician can help you maintain an appropriate critical analysis of the timing and benefits of continuing or withdrawing fluids. Your responsibility in this arena is as client advocate and a resource to the family. Provide them with factual information, and help them converse openly with the client's physician.

Providing Comfort Measures

Nursing care provided routinely for other clients, such as complete bathing, full linen changes, and turning schedules, may need to be reprioritized for the dying client. Maximizing the dying client's comfort may mean leaving him undisturbed in a comfortable position for a longer-than-usual time.

Expected outcomes for the dying client no longer focus on skin integrity and prevention of infection through baths, linen changes, and repositioning but instead shift to fostering dignity, providing comfort, and ensuring uninterrupted time with the family.

This change in priorities for routine tasks may be difficult for you at first. Do your best to maintain a realistic sense of the client's and family's end-of-life concerns and needs. Doing so will help you alter the elements of physical care as needed and thus provide for a more individualized and humane death.

Interventions to Provide Psychosocial Support

Interventions to support the psychosocial needs of client and family stem from recognizing their feelings and emotions. Grief has a tremendous psychological impact. Keep in mind that cultural factors may influence a person's displays of emotion. Society may impose expectations on a person's displays of grief as well, possibly adding the burdens of shame and guilt to a visibly grieving person.

For you, identification of underlying emotions becomes an important assessment activity. Do not just assume that obvious behaviors and comments represent all of the feelings being experienced. Emotions can be varied and unpredictable, manifested in different ways throughout the grief period. To help the client and family navigate this period, do your best to use therapeutic communication and help them manage their denial, anger, and spiritual distress.

Promoting Therapeutic Communication

Loss, death, and grief create surprising, conflicting, confusing, often overwhelming emotions. The freedom to express these emotions and to be supported during that expression is pivotal to managing grief successfully. You will need to use therapeutic communication strategies with both the client and family members to help them cope.

COMMUNICATING WITH A DYING CLIENT

Communicating with a dying client involves personal risks. You will undoubtedly feel uncomfortable emotions and possibly unpleasant memories. You may feel inadequate to discuss your client's serious questions—questions for which you have no or only incomplete answers.

The Reverend Chuck Meyer believes that the primary mechanism for supporting dying people is to "Be there" (Meyer, 1991). Support, in this context, means allowing time when the avenues of communication are opened. When someone trusts you with personal reactions and feelings, he invites you into a private area that should be honored (see Box 50-4, Communicating With a Dying Client).

Elisabeth Kübler-Ross identifies three "languages" used by dying persons: plain English, symbolic nonverbal language, and symbolic verbal language. By plain English, she means conscious, direct articulation of thoughts, feelings, questions, and fears.

In symbolic nonverbal language, concerns, thoughts, and needs are revealed through overt behavior. Needs are communicated through frequent requests of staff, projecting anger, or asking peripheral questions. These behaviors secure attention but fail to clearly express real needs.

The clients who most need support and attention use symbolic verbal language. The meaning of the message is hidden behind symbols. For example, a client facing extensive testing for cancer may tell a story about a pet that had to be "put to sleep" after a long illness. Symbolic language can also be used when a person seeks validation of self-worth in comments like, *I don't know why you spend so much time on me. There are others who need you so much more.* Such statements may arise when the client's physical condition deteriorates and unpleasant sights and odors develop. Caregivers who are attuned to such communication techniques will be able to sense the implied fears and concerns underlying the statements.

Many factors can block your communication with a dying client and his family. If you seem emotionally detached, they may interpret your attitude as a lack of interest or a lack of empathy. Avoiding direct discussion of sensitive topics wastes opportunities for constructive exchanges and may create confusion. Misunderstanding can block communication as well; avoid using euphemisms, medical terms, analogies, and vague terms, such as *passed on* or *lost* instead of *dying* or *died.* Communication can also be blocked if the staff minimizes or overlooks pain, indignity, fear, or unresolved personal issues.

Effective communication requires that you explore beyond the obvious and seek the hidden elements of behaviors and complaints. Sensitivity, astuteness, and empathy are integral elements that enhance and improve psychosocial support.

COMMUNICATING WITH THE FAMILY

The grieving family requires many of the same communication approaches used for the client. Be sensitive to the family's emotions, behaviors, and physical reactions to loss and grief while applying nursing interventions that promote their grief work. Remember that you will have significant influence on the family. Indeed, they will see you as both a resource and an authority at this time of crisis. As such, your comments carry tremendous credibility and importance.

Choose your words carefully when talking with family members. Recognize that certain statements may be helpful, whereas others may be harmful (see Box 50-5, Facilitative and Nonfacilitative Helping Statements). Remember that families may remember your words, and the decisions your words encouraged, for years after a client's death. Your behaviors and responses will permanently color their memories of the events surrounding their loved one's death. Because of their trust in you and the important role you play in their daily life during this time, therapeutic communication is crucial.

In general, statements that diminish the uniqueness of grief and loss are perceived as not helpful. When you say something like *I understand how you feel,* you intimate that grief and loss can be reduced to a common denominator similar from one person to the next. Statements that criticize grief responses or the feelings of grievers or that dictate appropriate grief responses are also not helpful. Finally, attempts to rationalize a loss based on your priorities and alternatives

BOX 50–4

COMMUNICATING WITH A DYING CLIENT

Provide for Privacy

For a client to openly share personal, intimate feelings with you, you must provide privacy. Consider moving to the chapel, asking visitors to leave for a while, or tell the client that you will return when visitors are gone. If the client is in a semi-private room, draw the dividing curtain and sit close to the bed so the client can talk softly without worrying about being overheard.

Let the Client Set the Agenda

Allow the client to decide when, where, and to whom he will communicate. Do not try to force conversations or direct the topics of conversations. If you are doing most of the talking, you are thwarting the goals of therapeutic communication. Try not to worry that you have failed if a dying client chooses not to confide in you. Remember that not every client will find such conversations helpful. You need only convey a willingness to listen.

Avoid Cliches

Cliches, platitudes, and pat answers are patronizing and discount the uniqueness of the client's situation and the magnitude of his fears or concerns. Avoid using such phrases as *I know how you feel, Don't worry about that now,* or even *Everything will be alright.* They minimize the client's feelings, fears, and beliefs and will undermine his trust in you.

Give Accurate, Honest Answers

If you do not know an answer, say so. Then find the answer and get back to the person. Do not try to spare the client's feelings by avoiding unpleasant truths; doing so will undermine his trust in you and waste valuable communication time with game playing. Use other health care team members, such as the physician or social worker, to contribute facts to discussions as needed.

Convey Nonjudgmental Acceptance

Leave all personal opinions, judgments, and beliefs out of fact-based discussions so the client can make his own decisions. Convey your acceptance of his decisions with such phrases as *That must be important to you* or *What do you think?* Phrases that reflect your awareness of what the client is coping with might include something like *I imagine that this is hard for you.* This example does not presume to know how the person feels but acknowledges a perception of something reasonable under the circumstances. The client is then free to contradict or confirm your empathetic guess. Be alert to the client's and family's values and beliefs, and avoid talking about what you would do if you were in the client's place.

Use Open-Ended Responses

Open-ended sentences or questions offer opportunities to talk without limiting the client's responses. By using phrases such as *How do you feel about that?* or *What other things are you thinking about?*, you allow the client to direct the conversation. Closed-ended statements (such as *Are you afraid of dying?* or *Will you be able to talk to your family about this?*) restrict the client's answers.

Continued

may anger family members and harm their relationship with you. Phrases such as *You wouldn't want him to continue living in this condition* are likely to be met with clear messages that the family would indeed want to keep their loved one in any condition because they love him and do not want to lose him.

You must be mindful of the hidden messages that can be transmitted through seemingly harmless phrases. No one intends to be callous and detrimental to the grief processes. However, forgetting to convey nonjudgmental acceptance of grief can impair your relationship with a client and his family at a time when they need you the most.

Mr. Hashimoto has been at home 2 weeks and currently is being visited only twice a week by a registered nurse who performs an assessment and confers with Mrs. Hashimoto about care needs. Mrs. Hashimoto has continued her efforts to keep the household intact and has turned to her eldest daughter for advice regarding her husband's immediate care. She also provides most of his physical care while depending on her daughter for support and guidance. She does not communicate with the home health nurse but has her daughter do this instead. Can you think of anything the home health nurse can do to facilitate communication with more members of the Hashimoto family? How can the nurse determine the family's needs?

Managing Denial

Denial is a common psychological response for both client and family. Because denial is a protective function, you should support it while the impact of facts and reality comes to the client's and family's consciousness. Confronting denial directly is neither therapeutic nor effective (see Box 50-6, Guidelines for Managing Denial). It only increases anxiety and pro-

BOX 50–4

COMMUNICATING WITH A DYING CLIENT (continued)

Use closed-ended questions when you need to gather specific information; clarify a client's comments; encourage an anxious or uncommunicative client to talk; focus the client on a specific point; or move the conversation from a deep level to a more superficial one, such as when closing an interview (Rando, 1984, p. 286).

Provide Adequate Response Time

A guaranteed way to stifle communication and make your client frustrated and angry is to ask a question and not wait long enough for the answer. This gaffe also leaves you with incomplete assessment data. If you are uneasy waiting for an answer, you probably are uncomfortable with silence. You also may not be recognizing factors that naturally lengthen the dying client's response time. As the client becomes weaker and more easily fatigued, even talking can be an effort. Take time to analyze why you have trouble waiting for adequate responses, then take steps to remedy the problem.

Use Silence Effectively

Silence can be intimidating if you are unaware of its importance as a communication tool. Too many nurses try to fill periods of silence because they believe them to be an opening to speak. Unfortunately, this tactic can simply cut off or impede the client's communication. Silence can convey acceptance and support, give the client time to gather his thoughts, and prompt further discussion. An occasional nod or a single-syllable word can fill some periods of silence and convey that the client still has your attention.

On the other hand, too much silence can produce anxiety and may be interpreted as inattention or lack of interest. Maintain eye contact and sit quietly during periods of silence. Stay alert for nonverbal cues to messages behind the silence. For example, silence may precede crying. Breaking eye contact with silence may reveal the client's embarrassment or insecurity about something he just said. Sensitivity and awareness of the power of silence can help you build relationships and promote the exchange of even sensitive, intimate thoughts.

Convey Caring Through Touch

In general, clients give nurses permission to touch them in ways not offered to other acquaintances. Thus, touch offers you a special avenue by which to convey caring and acceptance.

As a person dies, he may become less physically responsive. His condition may make his friends, even his family, uncomfortable. Visitors may become less frequent. It is therefore even more meaningful when you hold his hand, stroke his back or cheek, or touch his shoulder or arm.

When touch does not cause pain and is used when providing physical care or communicating with the client, it confirms your acceptance of the client and symbolically acknowledges the difficult path he is traveling (Amenta & Bohnet, 1986, p. 135).

References

Amenta, M.O., & Bohnet, N.L. (1986). *Nursing care of the terminally ill.* Boston: Little, Brown.
Rando, T.A. (1984). *Grief, dying, and death: Clinical interventions for caregivers.* Champlain, IL: Research Press Company.

duces more denial. It can also undermine your relationship with the client and family by destroying their trust and removing you from the circle of people with whom they will confide honest feelings (Forchuk & Westwell, 1987).

Sometimes you may become frustrated and concerned that you are being manipulated while caring for client who is in denial. If so, however, you run the risk of displaying harmful judgmental attitudes and projecting blame onto the client. Do your best to recognize such feelings before they compromise your care or your relationship with the client. Use techniques known to facilitate honest communication without creating a risk of psychological harm to the client during periods of denial.

Managing Anger

The anger that arises during grief, if not addressed, can become deeply entrenched and interfere with successful grief work. It is rare for a person to have no anger during the grief process. In fact, nurses commonly bear the brunt of this anger. To keep from becoming personally distressed over misplaced anger, consider the situation from this perspective: Clients and family members who speak out in anger tend to think that your professional knowledge will keep you from taking it personally. In fact, this is a sort of compliment to your professionalism and skill.

Anger is still difficult to deal with as a caregiver, but this interpretation of being recognized as a profes-

BOX 50–5

FACILITATIVE AND NONFACILITATIVE HELPING STATEMENTS

Facilitative Helping Statements

Come be with us now.
You're being strong.
It must be hard to accept.
It's okay to be angry at God.
That must be painful for you.
You must have been close to him.
Tell me how you're feeling.
How can I be of help?
Go ahead and grieve.
People really cared for him.
I'm praying for you.

Nonfacilitative Helping Statements

He (God) had a purpose.
It's God's will.
Be thankful you have another (son, parent, child, etc).
I know how you feel.
Time makes it easier.
You shouldn't question God's will.
You have to keep on going.
You have to get on with your life.
It's inevitable.
You're not the only one who suffers.
That's over now. Let's not deal with it.
The living must go on.
She led a real life.

Adapted from Davidowitz, M., & Myrick, R.D. [1984]. Responding to the bereaved: An analysis of "helping" statements. Death Education '84, August, 8, 1–10.

sional can help decrease defensiveness that may arise in such situations. Use sound communication techniques to help clients and families manage their anger appropriately (see Box 50-7, Guidelines for Managing Anger).

Managing Spiritual Distress

A holistic view perceives each person as a balance of mind, body, and spirit. Each dimension affects and is affected by the other. The spiritual is defined as of the spirit or the soul, as distinguished from the body or material matters. Each person has this spirituality. It is different from religious affiliation or beliefs.

As a nurse, it is important for you to support your clients' spirituality. This action is grounded in your respect for each person's beliefs, values, and practices. Facilitating the expression of those beliefs is an important intervention, and it both validates your acceptance and helps the client engage coping mechanisms tied to spiritual beliefs. Members of your facility's pastoral care department are integral to this process and can draw on community-wide resources to meet specific needs in addition to those that arise within the institution (Fig. 50–4).

During the period of dying and grieving, clients and families can experience spiritual distress. You can use particular communication skills to help them cope within their own spiritual beliefs (see Box 50-8, Guidelines for Support in Spiritual Distress). Spiritual reactions to dying and death can vary widely, just as other emotions do. Many people become angry at God or a higher being because of the perceived unjustness of death. Even people who have practiced their beliefs and doctrines faithfully for a lifetime may question how God could allow such unfairness, especially in

a distressing death or one that involves a young person.

For others, death completes a cycle that is explained and justified by their faith. Death does not test their beliefs; rather, it validates their faith. One study suggested that belief in God seemed to reduce levels of depression and hopelessness, although the degree of Christian knowledge or depth of commitment to Christian beliefs did not (Austin & Lennings, 1993).

Interventions to Promote Healthy Grieving

Your interventions for a grieving person will not be strictly divided by the stage of the person's grief. In general, however, certain types of interventions do provide the most benefit at certain stages of the process.

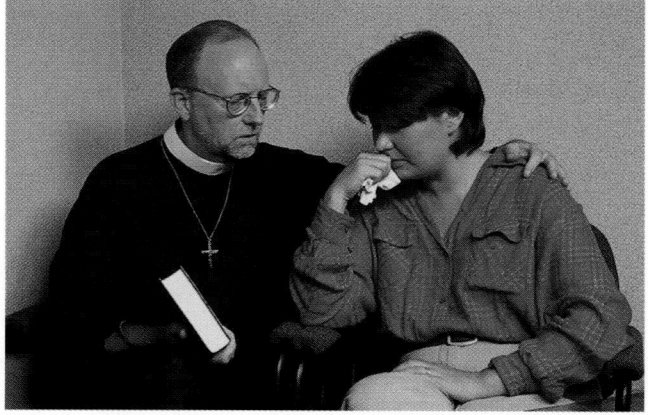

Figure 50–4. Members of the pastoral care department are integral team members in the care of people experiencing loss.

Recognition: Shock and Denial

The most important intervention during this phase of grief may be your presence. Reinforce the reality of events despite the client's denial. Remember that shock and numbness compromise the person's critical thinking, so you will need to let the person make decisions at a rate he can fully comprehend. Help to facilitate necessary decisions by clarifying the person's options and sources of assistance. Give small amounts of information at a time, and repeat the information until you know the client has understood it. Encourage questions, and be prepared to repeat answers when the person's memory is fragmented.

Allow the client to cry, and use silence supportively while the client expresses emotions or gathers his thoughts. Allow the griever to direct the course of discussions. Stay with those bereaved who are clearly shocked, dazed, hostile, or combative when faced with news of a loss. Activate appropriate resources as needed from nursing administration or the pastoral care department.

Reflection: Physical, Emotional, and Spiritual Suffering

Again, your presence is crucial. Acknowledge the client's and family's grief, and accept the validity and in-

---

BOX 50–6

GUIDELINES FOR MANAGING DENIAL

Respect Expressions of Denial

Expressions of denial help to protect a person who must adjust to unpleasant or horrifying news. Even when the person uses selective attention or deception, the goal is to protect the self or others. Respect this phase of the grief process by not challenging the person or making him "face reality."

However, do not lie to foster the denial. You must be honest; hearing the truth will not harm the grieving person. Also avoid reinforcing denial by agreeing with it. Continue to express truthful facts, and avoid perpetuating denial-induced thinking. When conversing, continue to provide reality-based information that is accurate and current. Correct misinformation in a nonconfrontational manner (Jeffery, 1998–1999, p. 13).

Use Alternative Approaches to Avoid Direct Confrontation

Using a "back door" approach can help a client focus on issues that provoke little anxiety while he processes higher-anxiety issues. Another technique derived from the assertiveness literature is called fogging or agreeing with the truth. To use this strategy, agree with the part of the denial that reflects reality. For example, say something like *It sounds like you're not sure the test results are accurate* rather than a confrontational statement, such as *The test results are accurate or your doctor wouldn't have told you they were* (Forchuk & Westwell, 1987, pp. 12–13).

Recognize and Acknowledge Hopes and Wishes

As a defense mechanism, denial reflects a desire that the truth not be true. You can validate the underlying yearning while not reinforcing the denial. Phrases such as *It would be wonderful if that happened* or *I wish it wasn't true too* leave the client's hope intact without suggesting that the hoped-for event will occur.

Encourage Discussion of Feelings, Concerns, and Fears

Talking with the client will help him process information intellectually, validate legitimate fears and concerns, and reinforce the sense of being supported during this stressful period. When talking, sit at eye level rather than standing. Doing so creates an atmosphere of conversation rather than hurried exchanges. Actively listen with undivided attention, allowing the client to do most of the talking. Remember that touch conveys attention and concern.

Provide Small Amounts of Information at a Time

Stress and denial block the conscious processing of information. Consequently, give a client smaller fragments of information at a time. These smaller amounts will be better understood and accepted. Encourage questions and open conversations to clarify and confirm facts. Encourage and facilitate decision-making, beginning with self-care and progressing to treatment choices when reality has replaced denial.

References

Forchuk, C., & Westwell, J. (1987). Denial. *Journal of Psychosocial Nursing, 25*(6), 9–13.
Jeffrey, J.C. (1998–1999, unpublished). Course guide for death and dying. Austin, TX: Austin Community College.

tensity of that grief. Continue to use touch and effective listening skills. Listen more than you talk, and ask for clarification when necessary. Make no assumptions.

Adapt your teaching strategies to accommodate any symptoms of depression. Explain any equipment being used, procedures needed, and care options. Allow family members to help with the client's care as much or as little as they desire. Foster a sense of control and collaboration about decisions. Develop plans of care with their input. Gain trust through honesty and by keeping any promises you make.

Watch for evidence of caregiver role strain and physical stressors on family members who spend a lot of time with the dying person. If possible, provide alternatives or breaks from the bedside vigil. Look beyond overt anger to determine its roots. Act as an advocate to help the client and family navigate the health care system, and facilitate physician and client or family conferences. Provide guidance and accurate information about advance directives and end-of-life decisions in understandable and nonjudgmental terms. Offer spiritual support in nonjudgmental ways as well. Meet the physical needs of the dying client, particularly comfort needs.

Redirection: Resolution and New Directions

Still, your presence is crucial. Do not abandon or neglect the client. Answer call lights and meet the person's physical needs promptly. Schedule pain medications so they are being delivered to the client at the exact administration times. Avoid the client or family needing to ask for pain medication.

Touch and talk to the dying person. Keep him informed of events and activities, particularly the approach or arrival of loved ones to the bedside. Remember that hearing seems to stay intact longer than the other senses; many clients will linger until family arrives if you tell them that family is on the way.

Avoid using euphemisms or vague terms. Instead, use clear words, such as *die* and *dead*. Act as a role model so family members will understand the importance and appropriateness of speaking to and touching the dying person. Otherwise, they may fear being intrusive or being perceived as silly.

Help family members make arrangements as necessary. Provide privacy for phone calls and, if desired, time alone with the client both before and after death. Call in clergy support when necessary. Crying with a

---

BOX 50–7

GUIDELINES FOR MANAGING ANGER

Recognize the Roots of Anger

Unresolved issues and feelings of frustration, resentment, powerlessness, confusion, fear, and guilt can be the underlying basis for anger. Such emotions may not be apparent to the person who holds them because they are integrated in complex emotional upheaval of grief. In some people, the anger is buried and unrecognizable. In others, anger displaced from past events may surface within the context of present situations. You will need to keep your focus while identifying the real issues behind a person's anger and exploring possible solutions.

Respond to the Sources of Anger, Not the Anger Itself

Confronting a client about expressions of anger places the two of you in adversarial roles and may force him to become defensive. This problem will harm the nurse-client relationship needed for therapeutic interactions to take place. Instead, use such statements as *This must be frustrating for you* or *I imagine I'd be scared if I were in your place* to convey your intuitive understanding of the real reason for the client's anger. Doing so may help the client open up rather than making him defensive and closed.

When conveying intuitive understanding, avoid statements that could patronize or presume to speak for the client. Instead, simply indicate an astute perception of what might be going on in the dynamics of grief for this client. The client should feel free to clarify the accuracy—or inaccuracy—of your perception.

Acknowledge the Emotions Behind Rhetorical Questions

Questions such as *Why me?* and *Why did God let this happen?* cannot be answered and you should not try. Simply recognize that the client is conveying frustration and anger that life is not fair, and that he is unprepared for the reality of his mortality.

Set Limits on Inappropriate or Harmful Displays of Anger

Anger that threatens the safety and welfare of clients, staff, or visitors must be addressed in an immediate and forthright manner. Acknowledge the validity of the anger but make clear that certain expressions of anger are not acceptable. Help the client redirect his energy into more beneficial outlets, such as pounding a pillow or pad, strenuous physical activity, yelling, or talking about his feelings to a sympathetic listener.

GUIDELINES FOR SUPPORT IN SPIRITUAL DISTRESS

- Provide time to listen to the person's concerns and feelings.
- Help the person explore current and past beliefs and spiritual experiences to help him put this event into perspective.
- Contact the person's usual spiritual counselor or cleric, if one exists. Encourage visits from members of the client's faith community. If the client's personal cleric is not available, solicit help from the pastoral care chaplain in your facility.
- Provide an uninterrupted few moments for silent prayer, or pray with the person if appropriate. Read from religious material if the person desires it. Make necessary arrangements for important religious rituals, such as annointing of the sick.
- Inform the client and family of available spiritual resources within the facility, such as the location of a meditation area or services held by pastoral care.
- Allow the client to continue to wear religious objects or clothing whenever possible and to keep religious mementos in view.
- At the time of death, allow the family to practice meaningful rituals. Leaving the body undisturbed for a time, saying special prayers over the body, turning the body a specific direction, or covering the body with special cloths are important rituals for some. Many of these rituals are associated with beliefs about transmigration of the soul.

(Information from McQuay, J.E. [1995]. Cross-cultural customs and beliefs related to health crises, death, and organ donation/transplantation: A guide to assist health care professionals to understand different responses and provide cross-cultural assistance. Critical Care Nursing Clinics of North America, 7[3], 581–594; Hirayama, K.K. [1990]. Death and dying in Japanese culture. In J.K. Parry [Ed.], Social work practice with the terminally ill: A transcultural perspective. Springfield, IL: Charles C Thomas.)

family is acceptable in keeping with a caring and professional image. Never allow yourself to cry so vigorously that the family must turn their energy to comforting you. Attend the funeral, if possible, when a close bond develops between you and the client or family. If you cannot attend the funeral, send a note of condolence.

Some nursing units maintain a file of client death dates with family names and addresses. Four notes are written at the time of death and signed by all the staff who interacted with the client and family. These notes are then sent at intervals beginning the week of the death and then at 3, 6, and 12 months from the death date. Family feedback has reinforced the importance of remembering and "being there" after a death.

Interventions to Maintain Yourself as a Caregiver

To maintain your function as a caregiver, you must take care of yourself physically and emotionally. Burnout is a significant risk in nursing, particularly among nurses who work frequently with dying clients. Make use of stress reduction techniques, exercise, and proper eating and sleeping patterns. Recognize and acknowledge the physical effects of the stressors of terminal care so you can care for yourself before burnout sets in. Reaffirm life and counter the repetition of death by spending time with your family and close friends.

You will need support from colleagues as well to help you deal with your grief for dying clients in your care (Fig. 50–5). The old adage, "If you can't take the heat, get out of the kitchen" has no place in the context of terminal care. Condemnation by other nurses or health care team members about attachments and feelings for clients in your care is detrimental both to you and to team dynamics.

Humor needs to be incorporated into daily activities whenever possible. However, it is inappropriate to allow the dark humor often used in health care settings to take place around clients and families. Dark humor or jokes about death can help to reduce stress for professional caregivers, but it is inappropriate and unhelpful for people outside the health care team. General humor can be therapeutic when used within appropriate limits. Some units have an area or box called the Humor Center with cartoons, fun reading, and brief humorous or whimsical stories. Laughter is healthy both physically and emotionally and should be encouraged within the professional setting.

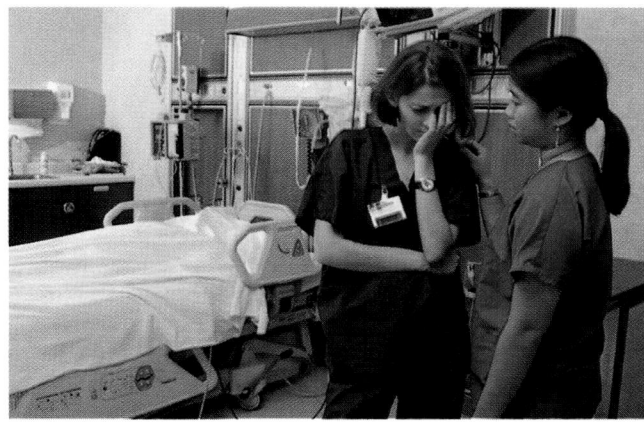

Figure 50–5. Collegial support can help nurses deal with their own grief over dying clients and their families.

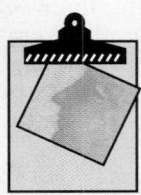

NURSING CARE PLANNING
A CLIENT WITH TERMINAL CANCER

Home Health Data

Mr. Hashimoto has resumed meditation and the use of medicinal herbs to combat nausea and pain. He has openly discussed his prognosis with his son and daughters but minimally with the home health nurse. Mrs. Hashimoto has refused to participate in these discussions, saying that she does not believe he is as sick as the doctors have told them.

The family priest has visited regularly and brought communion to Mr. Hashimoto and his wife and daughters. Further discussions have taken place between the priest and Mr. Hashimoto about his desire for cremation and the use of traditional Japanese-Buddhist mourning rituals after his death. The son has assumed the traditional family role of carrying out his father's wishes and making the necessary funeral arrangements.

Nursing Assessment

Physical: Alert, oriented ×3; skin warm, dry, and pale. Breath sounds diminished in lower lobes with crackles heard on expiration. Bowel sounds hypoactive in RUQ and RLQ; abdomen slightly distended and tender in RUQ on palpation. Last BM 2 days ago: small, formed, dark brown, Guaiac-positive. Rates pain at 2/10, refuses Demerol. Vital signs are temperature 99.8°F, pulse 104, respirations 18, and blood pressure 154/86.

Psychological: States that he can handle the discomfort, saying, "I don't want my wife to worry." His son explained his father's desires that traditional Buddhist rituals of body cleansing and purification rites be observed in preparation for the passage of death. They see this as complementary to Catholic death rituals, not counter to them.

NURSING CARE PLAN

Nursing Diagnosis	Expected Outcomes	Interventions	Evaluation (After 3 Weeks of Care)
Anticipatory grieving related to recognized terminal status	Client will discuss thoughts and feelings about impending death with family.	Encourage wife and children to talk openly about feelings and concerns. Encourage family to let go by giving the client permission to die. Facilitate expression of mutual love and respect before client's death.	Wife remains unwilling to talk about impending death. Children have had several conversations, both individually and as a group. They say that this has been helpful.

Continued

EVALUATION

Evaluation is ongoing throughout your care for a dying client and his family. They require continuous assessment and evaluation of interventions provided for physical changes, comfort, and psychological support. Compare and analyze these interventions in relation to the client goals you established, and modify the plan of care as needed. Make your nursing approaches individualized and specific. Use your evaluation to help deliver care that focuses on the person rather than on the disease process, as suggested by the accompanying Nursing Care Planning chart.

Your evaluation will also encompass nursing goals. These goals are not included in the formal plan of care, but they do help to motivate your nursing care for a terminal client and his family. Nursing goals include establishing a relationship of trust between you and the client and family. The client and family must feel that you and other nursing staff are supporting them and providing the highest quality of care possible to the dying loved one. It is imperative that you evaluate the client's and family's level of trust and confidence so you can maintain the therapeutic relationship so crucial for this arena of nursing care.

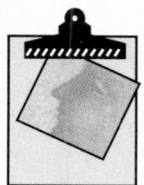

NURSING CARE PLANNING
A CLIENT WITH TERMINAL CANCER *(continued)*

NURSING CARE PLAN *(continued)*

Nursing Diagnosis	Expected Outcomes	Interventions	Evaluation (After 3 Weeks of Care)
	Client will maintain hope throughout remaining days.	Help client focus on the moment, review his assets, and maintain relationships.	Client acknowledges feelings of sadness but says that he feels positive about his life. Has had numerous visitors, which he says he enjoys.
	Client will engage in spiritual activities, both formally with the priest and informally in private.	*Offer time for prayer or meditation. Contact priest if requested. Make time in schedule for sacraments.*	Client meditates daily. Has had communion twice each week from priest and from lay eucharistic minister. Has not asked for additional visits from priest.
	Client will express concerns about family well-being after his death.	Listen openly to client's feelings and encourage expression of ideas, fears, and so on. Use therapeutic communication with open-ended questions. Allow client to select topics. Use silence to provide time for him to gather thoughts.	Client reluctant to talk to nurse about feelings. Maintains appearance of calm and peace. Open-ended sentences not successful in gaining his confidence about this topic.

Italicized interventions indicate culturally specific care.

Critical Thinking Questions

1. How would your feelings and beliefs about death affect your care for this family?
2. Mrs. Hashimoto has refused to participate in these discussions and seems to be in denial. What would your nursing interventions be for her?
3. What types of nursing interventions would indicate that you were giving culturally relevant care to this family?

KEY PRINCIPLES

- Grief is a normal response to loss, whether the loss is a person, an object, or a less tangible loss.
- The responses that are characteristic of grief are both predictable, patterned behaviors and highly individual.
- Grief has its own time and agenda based on the person involved and the loss experienced.
- Grief is neither linear nor finite. A person can express grief responses in any order, may never have some responses, and may return over and over to a response.

- Projected anger or other feelings caused by the loss of a loved one may be misdirected at nurses. Your recognition of the real source of anger is helpful both to you and to the griever.
- It is not a requirement that the dying person reach the stage of accepting death.
- Families and friends of the dying person typically need help in maintaining a relationship with the dying person and confronting the impending death.
- Care in the last hours of life is usually directed at maintaining comfort for the dying person and helping the family say good-bye.
- The most important concept in caring for a dying or grieving person is the concept of presence.

- Anticipatory grieving may or may not reduce the time and intensity of grief after a loss.
- Dysfunctional grieving indicates a person's inability to resume his life in a manner that remembers the dead person while allowing the survivor to live successfully without the person.

BIBLIOGRAPHY

*Amenta, M.O., & Bohnet, N.L. (1986). *Nursing care of the terminally ill*. Boston: Little, Brown.

*Austin, D. & Lennings, C.J. (1993). Grief and religious belief: Does belief moderate depression? *Death Studies, 17*(6), 487–496.

*Backer, B.A., Hannon, N.R., & Russell, N.A. (1994). *Death and dying: Understanding and care* (2nd ed.). Albany: Delmar.

Basile, C.M. (1998). Advance directives and advocacy in end-of-life decisions. *The Nurse Practitioner, 23*(5), 44–60.

*Bateman, A., Broderick, D., Gleason, L., Kardon, R., Flaherty, C., & Anderson, S. (1992). Dysfunctional grieving. *Journal of Psychosocial Nursing, 30*(12), 5–9.

*Bowlby, J. (1980). *Loss, sadness and depression*. New York: Basic Books.

Carpenito, L.J. (1997). *Nursing diagnosis: Application to clinical practice* (7th ed.) Philadelphia: J.B. Lippincott.

Clark, C., & Heidenreich, T. (1995). Spiritual care for the critically ill. *American Journal of Critical Care, 4*(1), 77–81.

*Conant, R. (1992). Widow's experiences of intrusive memory and "sense of presence" of the deceased after sudden and untimely death of a spouse during mid-life. Abstract from DAI V53(07), SECB PP3766. University of Massachusetts School of Professional Psychology.

*Cooley, M.E. (1992). Bereavement care: A role for nurses. *Cancer Nursing, 15*(2), 125–129.

*Corley, M.C., Selig, P., & Ferguson, C. (1993). Critical care nurse participation in ethical and work decisions. *Critical Care Nurse,* June, 120–128.

Curtin, L.L. (1996). First you suffer, then you die: Findings of a major study on dying in U.S. hospitals. *Nursing Management, 27*(5), 56–60.

Davidowitz, M., & Myrick, R.D. (1984). Responding to the bereaved: An analysis of "helping" statements. *Death Education, 8,* 1–10.

*Doka, K.J. (1989). *Disenfranchised grief: Recognizing hidden sorrow.* New York: Lexington Books.

Durham, E., & Weiss, L. (1997). How patients die. *American Journal of Nursing, 97*(12), 41–46.

*Edwards, B.S. (1994). When the family can't let go. *American Journal of Nursing, 94*(1), 52–56.

*Edwards, B.S. (1993). When the physician won't give up. *American Journal of Nursing, 93*(9), 34–37.

*Engel, G.L. (1964). Grief and grieving. *American Journal Nursing, 64*(9), 93–98.

Fanslow-Brunjes, C., Schneider, P.E., & Kimmel, L.H. (1997). Hope: Offering comfort and support for dying patients. *Nursing,* March, 54–57.

*Forchuk, C., & Westwell, J. (1987). Denial. *Journal of Psychosocial Nursing, 25*(6), 9–13.

*Freud, S. (1959). Mourning and melancholia. In S. Freud (Ed.), *Collected papers IV* (pp 288–317, 152–170). New York: Basic Books.

Goetzke, E. (1995). When your patient is in denial. *American Journal of Nursing, 95*(9), 18–21.

Hainsworth, D.S. (1996). The effect of death education on attitudes of hospital nurses toward care of the dying. *ONF, 23*(6), 963–967.

Haisfield-Wolfe, M.D. (1996). End-of-life care: Evolution of the nurse's role. *ONF, 23*(6), 931–935.

Hirayama, K.K. (1990). Death and dying in Japanese culture. In J.K. Parry (Ed.), *Social work practice with the terminally ill: A transcultural perspective.* Springfield, IL: Charles C Thomas.

Jeffery, J.C. (1998–1999, unpublished). Course guide for death and dying. Austin, TX: Austin Community College.

Johns, J.L. (1996). Advance directives and opportunities for nurses. *Image, 28*(2), 149–153.

*Kastenbaum, R.J. (1991). *Death, society, and human experience* (4th ed.). New York: Macmillan.

*Keltner, M.J., Bourgeault, I.L., & Wahl, J.A. (1994). Regulation and legislation of the dying process: Views of health care professionals. *Death Studies, 18,* 167–181.

*Kübler-Ross, E. (1969). *On death and dying.* New York: Macmillan.

LaGrand, L.E. (1998). *After death communication: Final farewells.* St. Paul, Minnesota: Llewellyn Publications.

*Lindemann, E. (1944). Symptomatology and management of acute grief. *American Journal of Psychology, 101,* 141–148.

Longaker, C. (1998). *Facing death and finding hope: A guide to the emotional and spiritual care of the dying.* New York: Doubleday.

McCann, R.M., Hall, W.J., & Groth-Juncker, A. (1994). Comfort care for terminally ill patients: The appropriate use of nutrition and hydration. *Journal of the American Medical Association, 272*(16), 1263–1266.

McFarland, G.K., & McFarland, E.A. (1997). *Nursing diagnosis & intervention: Planning for patient care.* St. Louis: Mosby.

McQuay, J.E. (1995). Cross-cultural customs and beliefs related to health crises, death, and organ donation/transplantation: A guide to assist health care professionals to understand different responses and provide cross-cultural assistance. *Critical Care Nursing Clinics of North America, 7*(3), 581–594.

*Meyer, C. (1991). *Surviving death.* Mystic, CT: Twenty-third Publications.

North American Nursing Diagnosis Association. (1999). *NANDA nursing diagnoses: Definitions & classification 1999–2000.* Philadelphia: Author.

*Omnibus Budget Reconciliation Act. (1990; OBRA-90). Patient self-determination act. *P.L.* 101–508, 4206–4751.

Ott, B.B., & Hardie, T.L. (1997). Readability of advance directive documents. *Image: Journal of Nursing Scholarship, 29*(1), 53–57.

Overbeck, B., & Overbeck, J. (1992). Dallas: *TLC Group,* Publications for Transition, Loss, and Change hawk-systems.com/web_pages/garson/helping.htm.

Parker, H.H. (1997). Untimely death: A challenge to religious faith. *The Forum: Newsletter for the Association for Death Education and Counseling,* Jan.–Feb., 9–10.

Parkman, C.A. & Calfee, B.E. (1997). Advance directives: Honoring your patient's end-of-life wishes. *Nursing,* April, 48–53.

*Parkes, C.M. (1972). *Bereavement: Studies of grief in adult life.* New York: International Universities Press.

*Parkes, C.M., & Weiss, R.S. (1983). *Recovery from bereavement.* New York: Basic Books.

*Rando, T.A. (1984). *Grief, dying, and death: Clinical interventions for caregivers.* Champaign, IL: Research Press Company.

*Ruark, J.E., & Raffin, T.A. (1988). Stanford University Medical Center Committee on Ethics. Initiating and withdrawing life support: Principles and practice in adult medicine. *New England Journal of Medicine, 318*(1), 25–30.

Smith-Stoner, M., & Frost, A.L. (1998). Coping with grief and loss: Bringing your shadow self into the light. *Nursing, 28*(2), 48–50.

Solari-Twadell, P.A., Bunkers, S.S., Wang, C., & Snyder, D. (1995). The pinwheel model of bereavement. *Image: Journal of Nursing Scholarship, 27*(4), 323–326.

*Steele, L. (1992). Risk factor profile for bereaved spouses. *Death Studies, 16,* 387–399.

Steele, R.G. & Fitch, M.I. (1996). Coping strategies of family caregivers of home hospice patients with cancer. *ONF, 23*(6), 955–960.

SUPPORT Group (1995). A controlled trial to improve care for seriously ill hospitalized patients: The study to understand prognoses and preferences for outcomes and risks of treatments (SUPPORT). *Journal of the American Medical Association, 274*(20), 1591–1598.

*Sweeting, H., & Gilhooly, M.L. (1990). Anticipatory grief: A review. *Social Science and Medicine, 30*(10), 1073–1080.

*Worden, J.W. (1991). *Grief counseling and grief therapy: A handbook for the mental health practitioner.* New York: Springer.

Zerwekh, J.V. (1997). Do dying patients really need IV fluids? *American Journal of Nursing, 97*(3), 26.

*Asterisk indicates a classic or definitive work on this subject.

UNIT

13

Sexuality- Reproductive Pattern

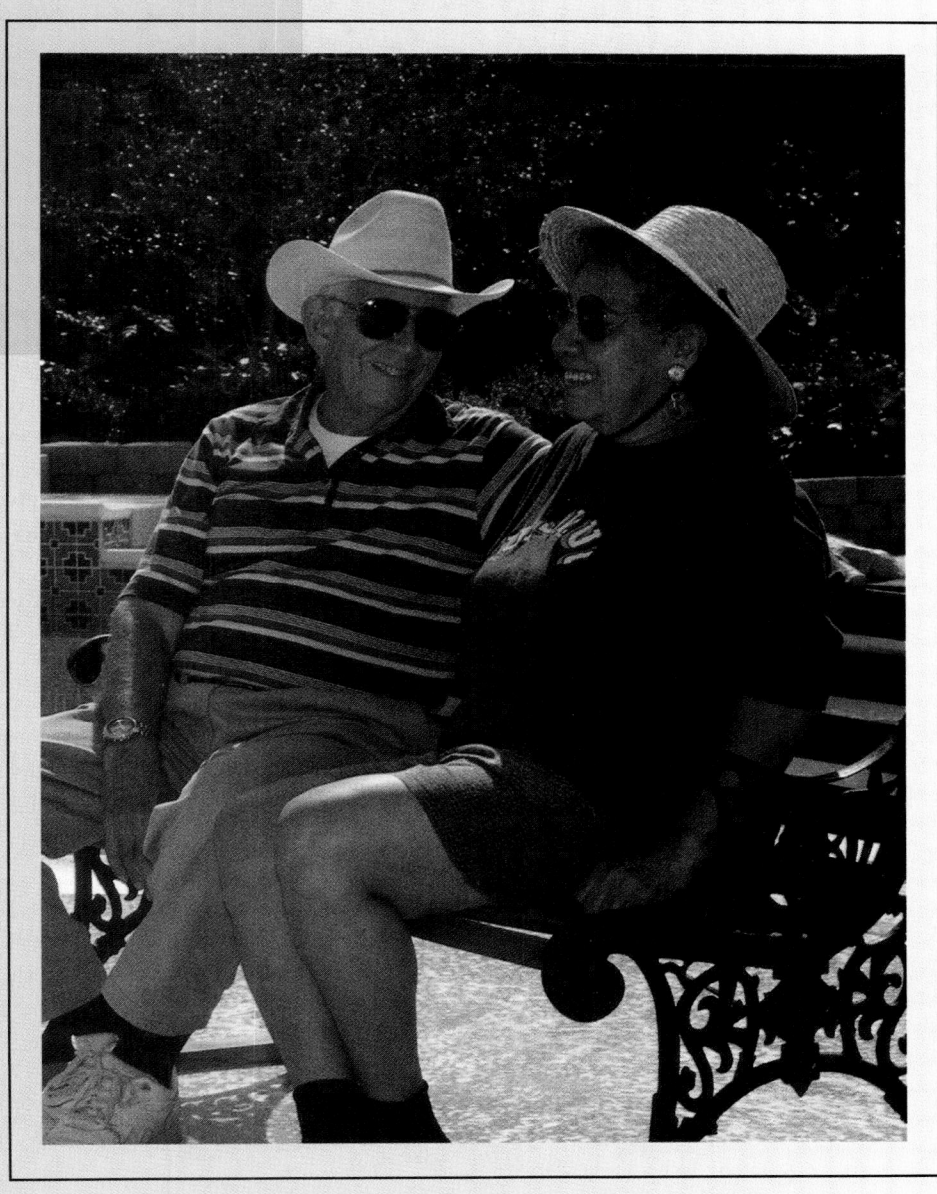

51

Sexuality and Reproductive Function

Barbara C. Rynerson

Key Terms

androgyny
arousal
bisexual
gender
gender identity
gender role
heterosexual
homophobia
homosexual

libido
orgasm
sexual desire
sexual dysfunction
sexual identity
sexual orientation
sexual patterns
sexual response cycle
sexuality

LEARNING OBJECTIVES

After studying this chapter, you should be able to:

1. Describe the biological, psychological, social, and cultural influences in the development of sexuality.
2. Discuss concepts related to sexual development.
3. Assess the client who is at risk for or is experiencing alterations in sexuality patterns or sexual dysfunction.
4. Diagnose sexual problems that are amenable to nursing care.
5. Use a standard model of care to provide goal-directed interventions to prevent or correct sexuality diagnoses.
6. Evaluate the outcomes that describe progress toward the goals of sexuality nursing care.
7. Discuss sexual health promotion across the life span.
8. Describe issues in the health care of gay men and lesbians.

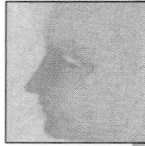

Lisa Simonelli, 46 years old, was diagnosed with breast cancer and lymph node involvement. She had a radical mastectomy 5 years ago. She has now come to the outpatient surgery clinic for a biopsy of a "growth" in her uterus. Even though her physician has indicated that the growth is probably benign, Lisa is very anxious about the outcome, and, because of her history, she is concerned about the possible need for a hysterectomy.

During the initial assessment, the nurse learns that Lisa is an Italian-American, is a practicing Catholic, has been married for 11 years to Vincent, and has no children. Lisa indicates that she and her husband have a solid relationship, but says she is concerned about their level of intimacy. Over the past 2 years, it has been declining, and the couple has not had intercourse in more than 3 months. She feels unattractive and wonders if her uterine biopsy will make intercourse impossible. Vincent refuses to talk about any of his concerns and seems indifferent to both of their sexual needs.

The nurse schedules some time to talk with Lisa before discharge to address her sexual concerns and to teach her about the effects of the biopsy and postoperative self-care. She assigns two nursing

(continued)

diagnoses. *Altered sexuality patterns* is the primary nursing diagnosis because there have been some negative changes in sexual functioning about which Lisa is concerned. *Sexual dysfunction* may also be present. How would you describe Lisa's self-image? What other factors might be contributing to the decreased intimacy she has expressed?

SEXUALITY NURSING DIAGNOSES

Altered Sexuality Patterns: The state in which an individual expresses concern regarding his or her sexuality.

Sexual Dysfunction: A state in which an individual experiences a change in sexual function that is viewed as unsatisfying, unrewarding, or inadequate.

From North American Nursing Diagnosis Association. (1999). NANDA nursing diagnoses: Definitions and classification 1999–2000. Philadelphia: Author.

CONCEPTS OF SEXUALITY

A person's sexuality is a vital component of health and is influenced by biological, psychological, social, and cultural forces. **Sexuality** is the state or quality of being sexual, including the collective characteristics that distinguish male and female. Holistically, sexuality has the following two meanings:

- Awareness and feelings of being male or female
- The pursuit of sexual pleasure, reproduction, and the need for love and personal fulfillment

Biological Sexual Development

Biological sex, or gender, is determined by chromosome structure at the moment of conception. The XX chromosome combination produces a female, and the XY combination produces a male. However, early in their development, all fetuses are dimorphic. They have basic elements of both female and male gonads and the potential to develop as either sex. Gonadal differentiation into male and female occurs in utero. The male determining factor in the Y chromosome causes testes to develop from the gonad medulla; without the male factor, ovaries develop from the gonad cortex (Bancroft, 1983).

The last stage of fetal sexual differentiation occurs when additional internal and external genital organs develop, creating obvious gender characteristics through the development of either the wolffian or the müllerian ducts. The wolffian duct system develops into the epididymis, the vas deferens, and the seminal vesicles in males. The müllerian duct develops into the fallopian tubes, the uterus, and the upper end of the vagina in the female. A combination of hormonal and genetic controls determines which one develops.

The fully developed external structures of the male include the penis and scrotum. Internal structures include the testicles, epididymis, seminal vesicles, and prostate gland (Fig. 51–1). The fully developed external structures of the female, collectively called the vulva, extend from the pubis to the perineum and include the labia majora, labia minora, clitoris, and vaginal orifice. Internal structures include the uterus, fallopian tubes, ovaries, vagina, and various glandular structures (see Fig. 51–1).

Although all reproductive organs are present at birth, they are immature and nonfunctional. Development of secondary sexual characteristics occurs through a complicated series of events that result from the action of sex hormones, produced by the ovaries and testes, on the adrenal cortex, hypothalamus, and pituitary gland in the brain.

Male spermatogenesis and female ovulation—accompanied by the production of estrogen and progesterone in the female and testosterone in the male—mark the onset of mature sexual behavior. This transition is commonly called puberty. As you know, puberty occurs during adolescence, a physiologically stressful time; not only do external bodily changes take place, but strong hormonal activity can cause the "storminess" of temperament so typically seen in teenagers. Adequate nutrition, good hygiene, exercise, and ample rest are important to maintain the body's energy during sexual development.

Psychological, Social, and Cultural Influences on Sexuality

Gender refers to a person's sex, either male or female. The terms sex and gender are used interchangeably, although the specific definitions of these terms differ. Usually, a newborn's gender is obvious at birth from the presence of either female or male external genitalia. The external genitalia reflect the internal chromosome structure. Sexual anatomy sets the stage for the gender that society believes the child to be and in which the child is raised. Gender refers to responses, meanings, and cues that are socially learned and taken

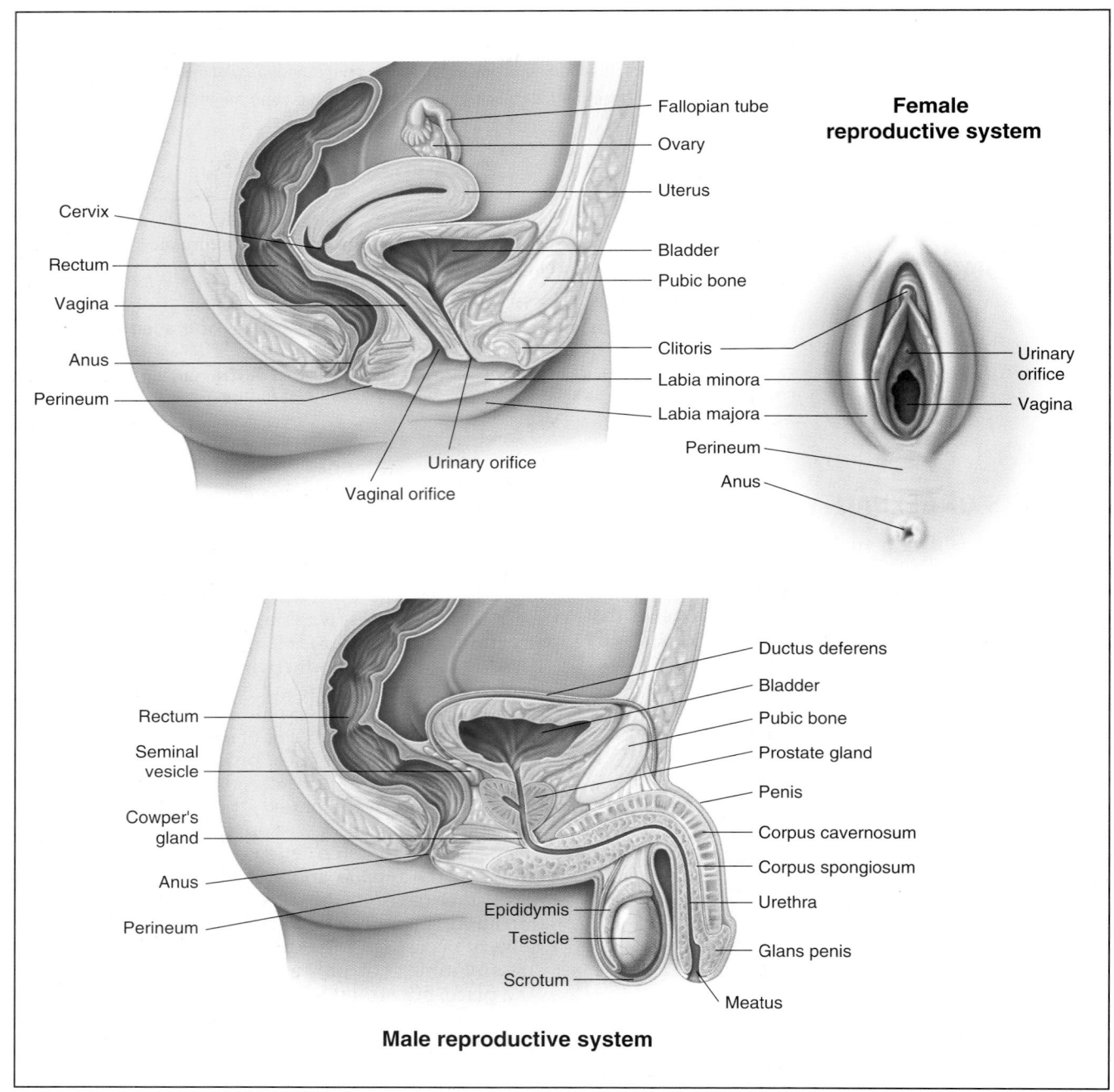

Figure 51–1. Anatomy of the male and female reproductive systems.

as reflections of society's conceptions of masculinity and femininity.

Gender identity, or **sexual identity,** is the internal belief or sense that one is male or female. This characteristic develops when a child is between 18 months and 3 years old. Psychological, social, and cultural influences shape one's gender identity and behavior. The child observes and imitates role models to learn cultural and social gender-typical behaviors and to form the basis for interactions among peers and adults.

Gender role refers to the outward appearance, behaviors, attitudes, and feelings deemed appropriate for males and females. These qualities are culturally defined as masculine, feminine, or androgynous. The contemporary concept of **androgyny,** an anthropological term, means that a person may display both male and female characteristics and may relate to both a male and female gender identity and role. In general, children learn acceptable role behaviors through praise and criticism. In Western society, however, there is increasing acceptance of a wide variety of roles and behaviors for each gender. For example, husbands are encouraged to take part in the birth experience and to help nurture and rear their children. Women can often be found engaged in work that was once thought of as "men's work."

Shively and DeCecco (1977) added a fourth concept to the three discussed above (gender, gender identity, and gender role): sexual orientation. **Sexual orientation** refers to a person's sexual attraction and feelings of erotic potential toward a partner or toward members of either gender. Types of sexual orientation include **heterosexual,** in which one is attracted to members of the opposite gender; **homosexual,** in which one is attracted to members of the same gender; and **bisexual,** in which one may be sexually attracted to members of either gender. **Sexual patterns** are a person's chosen expressions of sexuality. Because they depend to some degree on the person's psychological makeup, they may not fit precisely with the prevailing expectations of a particular culture or society.

Awareness of sexual feelings usually does not occur until adolescence, at the onset of mature sexuality; however, it is believed that sexual orientation is established in early childhood and is not changeable. At one time, homosexuality was a disorder listed in the American Psychiatric Association's *Diagnostic and Statistical Manual of Mental Disorders* and thought to be curable. In 1993, however, biologists discovered a variation on the X chromosome in 33 out of 40 pairs of brothers who were gay. This variation was thought to be the basis of their homosexual orientation. No comparable marker was found in lesbians. So far, insufficient data exist to deem that sexual orientation is or is not the result of genetic predisposition.

Most societies adhere to heterosexuality as the norm, and therefore may view homosexuality and bisexuality as deviant or not acceptable. The arbitrary ways in which sexual feelings are described as appropriate or inappropriate has been challenged by lesbian, gay, and bisexual populations to the extent that most can now live in heterosexual societies, although not yet completely openly or comfortably in many realms of their lives.

Physiological and Psychosocial Sexual Response

Basic to understanding all the facets of sexuality are concepts relating to sexual intercourse: sexual desire, arousal, and response. **Sexual desire** is a wish to participate in sexual intimacy that is activated by thoughts, fantasies, emotions, and psychological wants and needs. Sexual desire commonly precedes **arousal,** in which physical and emotional stimuli heighten desire and begin the physiological changes that mark the sexual response cycle. Arousal can result from touching, especially in erogenous body areas, from viewing provocative material, from fantasizing about a partner, and so on.

Masters and Johnson (1966) did classic studies of the bodily responses that occur during sexual arousal. They also defined four phases of the sexual response cycle: excitement, plateau, orgasm, and resolution (Table 51–1). The excitement phase results from any form of sexual stimulation that causes a person to initiate or to be receptive to sexual activity. If stimulation continues, it leads to the plateau phase, in which sexual tension continues the intense physiological changes that take place in the sexual organs. The orgasmic phase occurs when sexual tension is at its height, muscles tensed and blood vessels engorged. For a few seconds, the person experiences **orgasm,** a highly pleasurable involuntary response in which the clitoris, vagina, and uterus of the female or the penis of the male undergo repeated muscular contractions. Afterward, the person enters the resolution phase, which consists of involutional changes that return the body to the pre-excitement phase. During this phase, the female typically remains capable of continued orgasms when adequately stimulated, but the male experiences a refractory period during which restimulation is impossible.

Sexual desire and arousal are common responses and occur in many settings and circumstances. However, many problems can threaten a person's sexual experience and response, including organic problems, such as chronic illness; psychosocial problems, such as alcoholism; and situational stressors, such as the death of a spouse. A person in poor health or who takes certain prescribed or illicit drugs may not have the physical capacity for a sexual response or the emotional capacity to make the experience significant. Emotional health also influences sexual response, especially if the person is fatigued, stressed, depressed, or experiencing relationship conflicts.

In summary, sexuality encompasses a person's anatomy and physiology as well as a particular way of being male or female, feelings of being masculine or feminine, and a complete range of human experiences in biological, psychological, social, cultural, and spiritual realms (Fig. 51–2).

Sexual Health

To understand the range of experience that you might encounter regarding sexuality, the parameters of sexual health must be defined. The World Health Organization describes sexual health as the integration of somatic, emotional, intellectual, and social aspects of sexual being in ways that are enriching and that enhance personality, communication, and love (WHO, 1975). Some characteristics of being sexually healthy include the following:

- Behavior consistent with gender identity
- Knowledge about sexual phenomena
- Ability to decide about sexual behavior congruent with one's values and beliefs
- Physical and emotional ability to engage in sexual relationships and to experience pleasure in erotic stimulation with an intimate partner
- Willingness to make adjustments in sexual functioning when limitations of illness, injury, unavailability of a partner, or other situations occur

TABLE 51–1
Sexual Response Cycle

Responses in Both Sexes	Female Response	Male Response

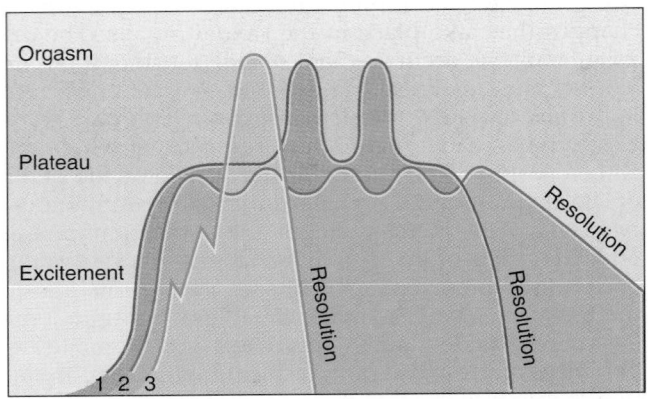

Female sexual response cycle. Pattern 1 depicts a steady progression toward plateau, followed by one or more orgasms. Pattern 2 depicts a slower progression to plateau, with peaks of pleasure but no orgasm. Pattern 3 depicts a rapid progression toward plateau, with a single orgasm.

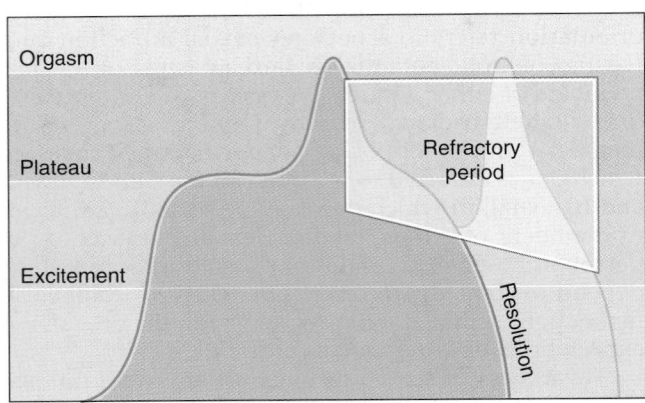

Male sexual response cycle.

Excitement

- Heart rate and blood pressure increase.
- Nipples become erect.
- Myotonia begins.

- Vaginal walls and labia thicken.
- External genital vasocongestion begins.
- Vaginal lubrication begins.
- Upper two-thirds of vagina expand.
- Cervix and uterus pull upward.
- Breasts increase in size.
- Sex flush appears.

- Penis becomes erect, increasing in length and diameter.
- Scrotal sac thickens, flattens, and elevates.

Plateau

- Heart rate and blood pressure continue to increase.
- Respirations increase.
- Myotonia becomes pronounced and grimacing occurs.

- Lower third of vagina becomes engorged.
- Uterus and cervix elevate further.
- Skin flush may appear across breasts, abdomen, or other surfaces.
- Clitoris retracts under clitoral hood.

- Head of penis enlarges slightly.
- Scrotum thickens further and tenses.
- Testes continue to elevate and enlarge.
- Two to three drops of preorgasmic fluid emerge from the head of the penis.

Orgasm

- Skin flush reaches maximal level.
- Myotonia reaches maximal level.
- Respiratory rate doubles.
- Pulse and blood pressure continue to increase.

- Clitoris remains retracted.
- Vagina and uterus undergo rhythmic muscle contractions.

- Rectal sphincter contracts.
- Internal sphincter at the bladder neck closes tightly.
- Rhythmic contractions of seminal vesicles and prostate gland eject semen and prostatic fluid through the urethra.

Resolution

- Heart rate, blood pressure, and respirations return to normal.
- Nipple erection subsides.
- Myotonia subsides.

- Vasocongestion of external genitalia and vagina decreases.
- Cervix and uterus descend and return to normal.
- Breast size decreases.
- Skin flush rapidly disappears.

- Refractory period—loss of pelvic congestion.
- Gradual loss of erection—penis returns to normal size.
- Testes and scrotum return to normal size.

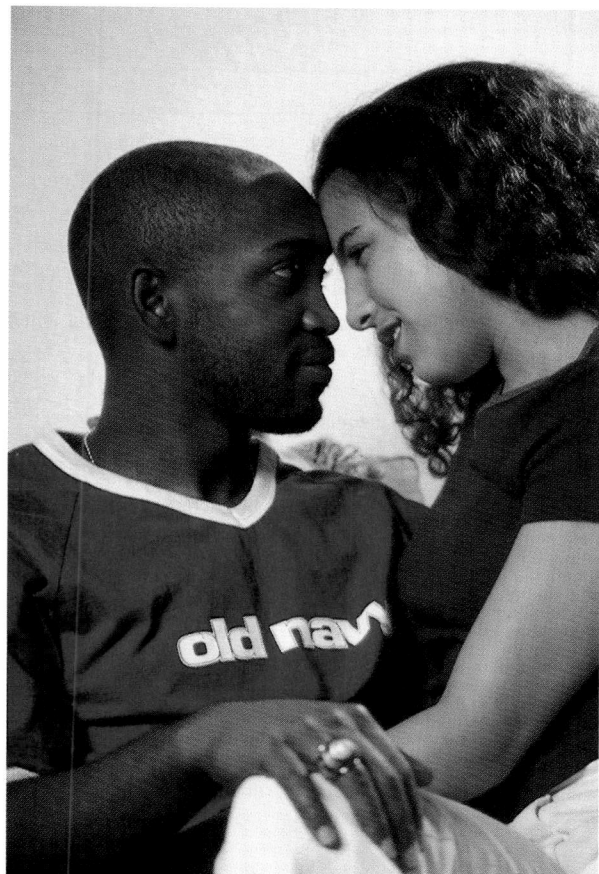

Figure 51–2. Sexuality encompasses not only a person's anatomy and physiology but his or her entire being—biological, psychological, social, cultural, and spiritual.

- Communication about sexual issues at any stage of life is without undue embarrassment, conflict, or discomfort

FACTORS AFFECTING SEXUALITY

The patterns of expressing oneself sexually can be rewarding and enriching or they can be emotionally and physically distressing. The factors that affect sexuality can be physiological, psychosocial, and developmental.

Physiological Factors

Physiological factors affecting sexuality are illness, infection, surgical procedures, and medications. Acute or chronic illnesses contribute significantly to altered sexuality patterns. Disease can affect the sexual organs directly, as in uterine or testicular cancer. Or other physical illnesses, such as diabetes, may detract from sexual expression because energy is redirected toward recovery or contending with the illness. Illness may influence a person's sense of worth, body image, attractiveness, and sexual desire (Gorman, Sultan, & Raines, 1996). Some chronic illnesses or medications

may directly interfere with or inhibit sexual arousal and response (Table 51–2).

Sexually transmitted diseases (STD) typically exert a major physiological influence on a person's sexuality. The more common STDs include chancroid, chlamydia, condylomata, genital herpes, gonorrhea, hepatitis B, human immunodeficiency virus (HIV) infection, streptococcal infection, syphilis, and trichomoniasis. These disorders cause rashes, lesions, itching, pain, and usually a desire to avoid transmission to another person through sexual contact. STDs can be transmitted through sexual intercourse; intimate oral, genital, or anal contact; or contact with the body fluids (such as blood, urine, or vaginal or penile discharge) of the infected person (Luckmann, 1997). Fear of contracting STDs inhibits participation in sexual intimacy.

Psychosocial Factors

In an otherwise physically healthy person, socialization toward embarrassment and disgust about one's genitals as well as taboos against discussing sexuality openly may have a negative effect on the patterns the person develops. Even more destructive to healthy sexual expression is exploitation through physical sexual abuse or adherence to sociocultural beliefs and myths that invoke guilt.

Culturally dictated sexual practices are very diverse, but most cultures transmit messages regarding the nature of sex and beauty, the acceptability of specific sexual behaviors, the relationship of sex and love, marital sexual behavior, homosexuality, and the appropriateness of specific sex roles (Fig. 51–3). Any diagnosis of altered sexuality patterns must consider the client's socialization and cultural context, as suggested in the Cross-Cultural Care chart.

Developmental Factors

Developmental factors that affect sexuality include the person's internal and external environments. Overall, good physical health practices aid the physical and sexual maturation of men and women. Externally, an environment that is nurturing and caring and promotes positive human interactions fosters development of healthy sexuality. A person needs to have open communication with role models to learn respect for her body and to discuss age-appropriate sexual feelings and behaviors. Every aspect of a person's life experience has the potential to influence sexual development.

ASSESSMENT

General Assessment of Sexuality

Nurse's Self-Assessment

In a study of 155 practicing registered nurses by Matocha and Waterhouse (1993), at least one-third of the nurses never assessed their clients' sexual health, discussed sexuality with clients, or taught about sexu-

TABLE 51–2
Conditions That May Alter Sexuality Patterns

Category	Example	Sexual Alterations
Pathophysiological		
Endocrine system	Diabetes	Impotence occurs primarily with uncontrolled diabetes; often improved with control of blood sugar; may interfere with orgasm in both sexes
Genitourinary system	Sexually transmitted diseases	Pain with intercourse; fear of transmitting disease
Neuromuscular and skeletal system	Parkinsonism	Interferes with male orgasm
	Arthritis	Difficulty positioning for intercourse; however, the physical activity may actually make arthritis better.
Treatment-Related		
Medications	Alpha$_1$-adrenergic blockers	These classifications are associated with alterations such as impotence, changes in libido, inhibition of ejaculation, gynecomastia, and menstrual irregularities; the incidence of alterations is usually very small. There is some thought that telling the client about the possibility of alterations increases the likelihood of their occurrence.
	Amphetamines	
	ACE inhibitors	
	Nitrates	
	Tricyclic antidepressants	
	Antihistamines	
	Beta-adrenergic blockers	
	Anticholinergics	
	Thiazide diuretics	
	Estrogen	
	H$_2$ antagonists	
	Narcotics	
	NSAIDs	
Therapeutic procedures	Perineal resection of prostate	Nerve-sparing procedure can prevent impotence.
	Irradiation of pelvis	The prevalence rate of erectile dysfunction with this procedure is 25%.
Situational		
Unprotected sex	Fear of pregnancy	Psychological barrier to enjoyment of sexual intercourse.
	Fear of sexually transmitted disease	
Maturational		
Strict religious upbringing	Guilt over sexual activity	Can inhibit sexual response or decrease enjoyment.
Negative sexual teaching	Shame regarding one's body and genitals	Interferes with sexual arousal, including erection in men and orgasm in women.

ACE, angiotensin-converting enzyme; NSAID, nonsteroidal anti-inflammatory drug.
Medication information from Drug Facts and Comparisons (1999). St Louis: Facts and Comparisons.

ality. An even smaller number routinely addressed sexuality with some or all of their clients. The nurses were more likely to include sexuality in their nursing practice if they worked in a hospital setting where sexuality was particularly relevant to their practice, if they believed they had responsibility for discussing sexual concerns, and if they felt comfortable and knowledgeable about addressing sexual concerns.

Would you feel comfortable addressing your clients' sexual concerns? Remember that your attitudes, preferences, and prejudices affect all of your interactions with clients. That is why your self-assessment is a necessary part of addressing your clients' sexuality concerns appropriately. You need to be clear about your own values and beliefs about sexuality. And you need to accept those values and beliefs without feeling that they are better or more correct than your clients'. Otherwise, you will interfere with the nurse-client interaction about the sensitive topic of sexuality. In dis-

cussing sexuality with your clients, you are asking them to disclose the most intimate aspects of their human character. That will happen successfully only if you view your clients' values and beliefs with respect.

Action **A**lert!
Your anxiety or embarrassment in discussing sexual concerns will be communicated to your client, either overtly or covertly, and will prevent you from sharing information pertinent to sexual health care.

The first step in your self-assessment about sexuality is to determine areas of comfort and discomfort with the topic. Discussing anxieties, biases, and general feelings about sexuality with a trusted colleague or peer can help you detect inappropriate nursing behaviors in the nurse-client relationship. For example, if you feel overly uncomfortable when inspecting a client's genitals, you may need to think and talk about any taboos that you learned about exposing genitals as

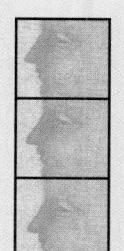

CROSS-CULTURAL CARE
CARING FOR AN ITALIAN-AMERICAN CLIENT

Lisa is an Italian-American, and, upon initial interview, the nurse learns that her family came to America four generations back. Her extended family members all live in another state (as does her husband's family). All of her family members have many traditional ethnic customs. Although all clients are unique, many Italian-Americans have a tendency to hold the following values:

- Family and the church are very important.
- Focus is on the present.
- May be fatalistic but usually are very resilient.
- Illness is caused by the "evil eye" or "curses"; severe and life-threatening illnesses are caused by more powerful sources.
- Suppressed emotions, stress, anxiety, fear, and grief can cause illness.
- Cure is in the "hands of God," although most seek explanations about care given to them.
- Value cooperation with health care providers.
- Discussions of sex and sexuality are avoided out of modesty or shame.

During the interview before Lisa's uterine biopsy, the nurse, Marla Spencer, discovered that Lisa wanted permission to talk about her problems with sexual intimacy in her marriage. See how Marla respects Lisa's cultural upbringing by giving that permission.

Marla: I'm glad to see you today. Tell me about the problems you are having. Start with what is most important for you.

Lisa: I'm not sure I can talk about my real problem. I have no one to turn to.

Marla: Go on.

Lisa: My husband and I . . . I really am nervous talking about sex in our marriage.

Marla: (Silence. Leans forward and nods her head.)

Lisa: I feel lonely and depressed. I'm not fat. I'm a good cook and fix his favorite meals. He doesn't touch me!

Marla: Doesn't touch you?

Lisa: Every week that goes by we grow farther apart. Vincent doesn't even like to kiss and hug me anymore.

Critical Thinking Questions

- What cultural behaviors might contribute to Lisa's reluctance to talk about her sexual concerns?
- How do Lisa's physical problems (past and present) contribute to her altered sexuality?
- How would Lisa react if she did not have a strong cultural and religious influence on her sexual functioning?

Reference

Spector, R.E. (1996). *Cultural Diversity in Health & Illness* (4th ed.). Stamford, CT: Appleton & Lange.

a part of your socialization. Having a general knowledge about sexuality and sexual beliefs and experiences, and obtaining information specific to a client's concerns, will help you comfortably include sexual health as a regular part of your practice.

Health History

Sexuality assessment is a legitimate aspect of holistic care and may be done as part of the client's basic history (see Chapter 8) or any time the client, either overtly or covertly, indicates concern about sexual health. You may also initiate a discussion and assessment of sexuality based on your knowledge that an illness, procedure, or medication may influence a client's sexual pleasure and functioning. Assessment may also have therapeutic value because it lets the client know that it is appropriate to discuss concerns about sexuality. This gives the client an opportunity to ask any questions she may have or to air her anxiety.

The overall personal-social history will give you knowledge about a client's sexual roles and relationships, as well as gender preference. Encouraging the

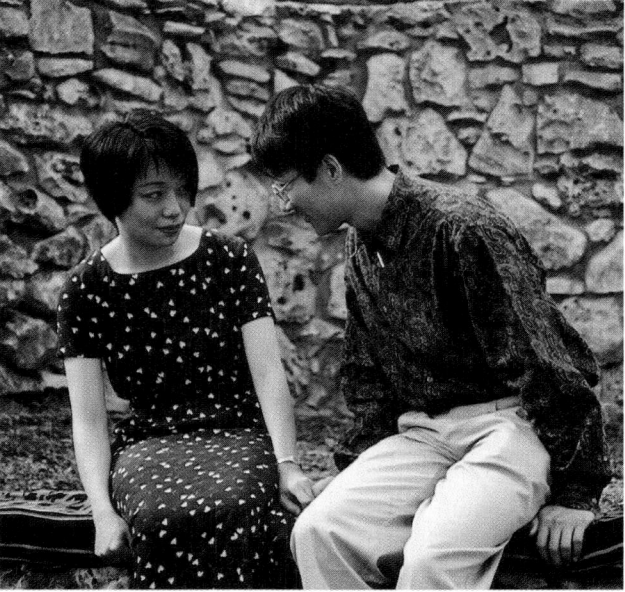

Figure 51–3. Most cultures transmit messages about sexuality.

client to elaborate on family and work roles will help you assess for typical, atypical, and more flexible, androgynous gender role behaviors. All of these assessment data, in the context of the client's developmental level, offer you a beginning framework for more formal sexual history taking or interviewing about specific sexual issues related to the client's condition.

Action Alert!
Engaging the client in a discussion about sexual issues should be carried out with sensitivity to the environment; a planned time and utmost privacy are necessary to conduct a sexual assessment.

A specific sexual assessment is initiated by gathering a sexual history. The history may be comprehensive or brief, depending on the client's needs. It should proceed from general to more specific and from comfortable to more sensitive. Make sure to use appropriate language when referring to parts of the client's anatomy, but pay attention to the client's level of knowledge. If the client uses slang terms (such as "dick" for penis), simply acknowledge the client's statement and continue on with the history. If the client has trouble responding to a specific, necessary question, allow time. If the answer is not absolutely necessary, do not press for one.

A brief sexual history may include questions such as the following:

- Do you have any concerns or issues about your sexuality or sexual response? (Remember that anything that affects the client's physical status, emotional comfort, interpersonal relationships, sociocultural mores, or moral and religious attitudes may threaten some aspect of sexuality.)
- When did the problem begin, and what were the circumstances surrounding the problem? Specifically, what prompted you to mention this problem?
- What do you think caused the problem?
- Has anything made the problem better? Worse?
- What would you like to do or have happen about the problem at this time?

A comprehensive sexual history should include details of the client's past history and current concerns (Table 51–3). While completing the history, take note of the client's nonverbal cues to help discern her attitudes or discomforts about sexuality. Watch for any reluctance to answer questions, for brief answers that are not very informative, for embarrassment or blushing, and for inappropriate acting out of a sexual nature. The client's affect—such as sadness, indifference, anger, elation—or incongruence between words and affect will give you additional information about what the client may be experiencing about sexuality issues.

Action Alert!
When taking a comprehensive sexual history, questions should be open-ended to allow the client freedom of choice in response. The nurse can ask for elaboration or clarification as necessary to understand the client's information.

Physical Examination

Physical assessment of the client's sexual anatomy is carried out by inspecting genitalia and secondary sexual characteristics (see Chapter 10). Observations that may warrant further questioning, examination, or reporting include the following:

- Deviations in genitalia or breasts
- Lesions, ulceration, infections, or unusual discharge from genitals or nipples
- Evidence of poor hygiene
- Unmet outcomes from medical or surgical interventions

While gathering data, form an opinion about the client's body image and her view of herself as a sexual being (see Chapter 46). You can infer these concepts from the manner in which the client interacts with you. Does the client use appropriate modesty in exposing the genitals for examination? Is the client overly shy and embarrassed? Too bold? Does the client hesitate to use anatomically correct terms when answering your questions? How does the client display gender identity in dress, grooming, and posture? Does the client interact with you in a manner that respects both of your sexual beings? (For example, does the client call you by name rather than by a derogatory or seductive term?) Finally, does the client practice breast or testicular self-examination? If not, provide appropriate teaching, as listed in the accompanying Teaching for Self-Care chart.

Focused Assessment for Altered Sexuality Patterns

Numerous health problems can have a biochemical effect on sexual energy and the ability to engage in sex. These conditions may affect the person's **libido,** which is the conscious or unconscious sex drive or desire to pleasure or satisfy. For example, breast cancer and all its attendant worries and stresses can negatively affect all aspects of a woman's life, including financial aspects, as discussed in the Cost of Care chart.

A vital part of your assessment of a client with altered sexuality patterns is to understand the client's sexual knowledge and attitudes. Investigate the client's sources of sexual education, formal and informal, so you can respond to negative thoughts or misconceptions that contribute to the altered sexuality patterns. Consider, for example, the nurse who discovers that her prepubertal male client is intensely embarrassed by nocturnal emissions (wet dreams). Assessment reveals that no one has told him that wet dreams are normal and will not last forever. By teaching him about hormonal changes in puberty and encouraging further discussion in an accepting, matter-of-fact manner, the nurse can reduce his concerns and promote acceptance of his developing sexuality.

TABLE 51–3
Elements of a Comprehensive Sexual History

Past History

Sexual knowledge	• From whom and how information about sexuality and sexual response was obtained.
	• Information obtained from classes or other formal learning.
	• Information about sexually transmitted diseases.
Life cycle influences on sexuality	• Influences from caretakers, role models about being male or female during formative years, development of gender or androgynous role behaviors.
	• Self-views of being male, female, gay, or lesbian.
	• Values and beliefs about sexuality from family, religion, or culture.
	• Initiation of sexual activity.
	• Sexual patterns.
	• Sexual relationships or interactions, and whether they are positive or negative.
Physical problems relating to sexuality	• Difficult menstruation or menopause.
	• Development of secondary sex characteristics.
	• Trauma, infection, or disease affecting sexual organs.
	• History of sexual abuse, including rape.

Current Concerns

Client's perception and understanding of his or her sexual health status or other physical condition affecting sexuality	• Issues related to body image or self-esteem.
	• Ways in which sexual function or response is affected.
	• Changes in sexual activity or patterns.
	• Unsatisfactory or painful intercourse.
	• Stresses influencing sexual health.
	• Potential or expected changes in sexual health or activity related to illness or injury.
	• Significance to the client of changes in sexual health or activity.
	• Client's outlook or expectations about changes in sexual health.
Sexual partners	• Inquire about single or multiple partners.
	• Specific sexual practices, including vaginal, oral, and anal intercourse.
	• Precautions client takes to practice safe sex.
Effects of client's current sexual health on significant others	• Influence of alteration in client's sexual health or function on significant other(s).
	• Anticipation of changes in significant relationship(s).
Changes in sexual function	• Changes in sexual function as a result of illness, medical treatment, surgery, emotional illness, or medications.
Client's wants and needs regarding sexual health at this time	• Thoughts about ways in which needs might get met.
	• Expected outcomes.
	• Willingness and comfort of client to discuss sexual needs with an appropriate professional, should that be warranted.

Or consider the example of a teenage girl who has unprotected sex but says she thinks little about her increased risk of pregnancy, STDs, and lowered self-esteem. While interviewing this teen, the nurse discovers that although the girl says she has had "lots" of teaching about contraception, it all was from pamphlets. The client had virtually no practical knowledge about using contraceptive devices and was uncomfortable suggesting them to her sexual partners. She felt too embarrassed to talk to peers about it, and she simply assumed that all girls her age were "doing it" (engaging in sexual intercourse). Working with a girl like this one would provide you with an excellent opportunity to explore the client's values and beliefs about sexual activity, discuss the emotional aspects of

engaging in sex without having other intimate interactions as well, and offer practical teaching about contraceptives and how to use them. Naturally, you will need to provide teaching appropriate to each client's needs to help maintain normal sexuality patterns, as discussed in the Teaching for Wellness chart.

Many of the risk factors for *Altered sexuality patterns* stem from medical-surgical conditions or the processes of aging. Most clients wonder how such factors will affect their sex lives, but few will be willing to ask you direct questions about it. Consequently, you should take the initiative to assess the client and prompt discussion about the influence of illness or aging on sexuality. Even if the client is not ready or willing to talk about it at that time, your initiative leaves

Teaching for SELF-CARE

BREAST AND TESTICULAR SELF-EXAMINATION

Purpose: To teach female clients about the monthly breast self-examination and male clients about the monthly testicular self-examination.

Rationale: Regular monthly inspection and palpation of breasts or testicles is a way to detect lumps or nodules that may prevent serious illness. The American Cancer Society recommends the following guidelines.

Expected Outcome: The client will use the breast self-examination or testicular self-examination on a monthly basis and report irregularities to a physician promptly.

Client Instruction

1. Set aside about 15 minutes on the same date each month.
2. When examining your breasts or testicles, make sure you perform a complete examination with full coverage of the area.
3. Follow the same procedure each time.
4. Use the top third of your fingers (the pads) for palpation.
5. Use adequate pressure to feel deep tissues.

Breast Self-Examination
1. Standing before a mirror with your breasts exposed, inspect your breasts with arms at your sides.

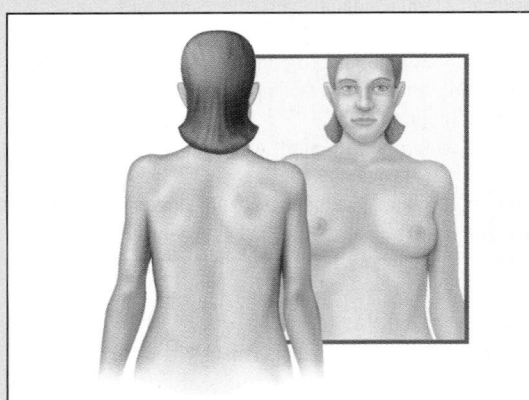

2. Raise your arms overhead and look for changes.

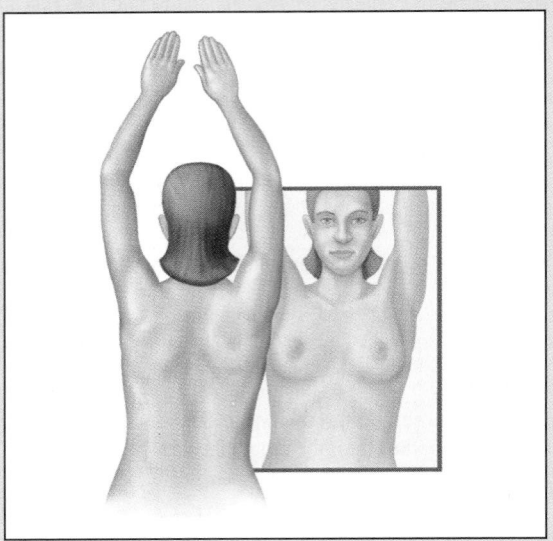

3. With your hands on your hips, flex your chest muscles and look for changes.

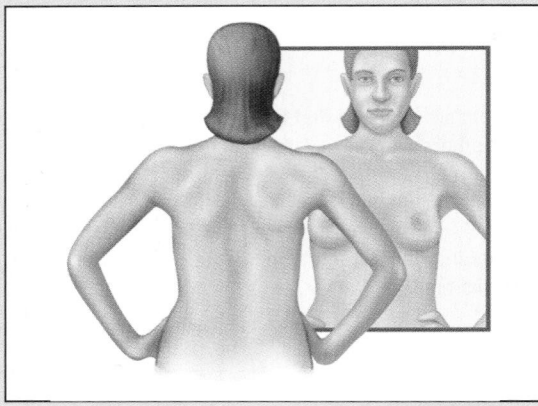

4. Gently squeeze your nipples and look for discharge.

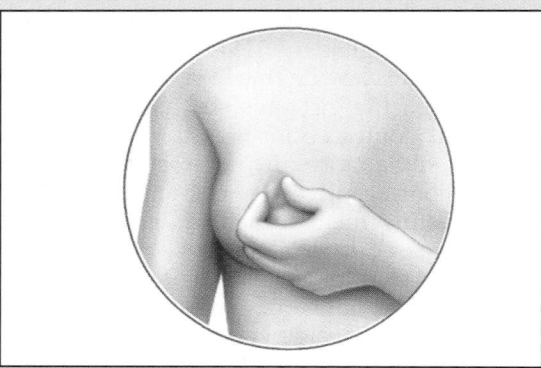

Continued

Teaching for SELF-CARE

BREAST AND TESTICULAR SELF-EXAMINATION *(continued)*

5. Palpating your breasts is easiest in the shower because your fingers will glide easily over the wet skin. With your fingers flat, move gently but firmly over every part of each breast. Use a circular motion starting with the nipple and moving outward. Alternatively, you can use a pattern of vertical parallel lines. Check for any lump, hard knot, or thickening.

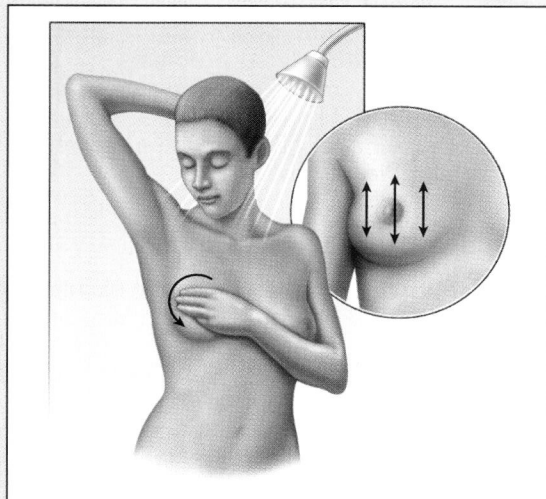

6. If you prefer to perform the examination lying down, place a pillow under your shoulder to flatten your breasts. Use the middle three fingers of your opposite hand to feel for lumps or changes in one of the same patterns described above.

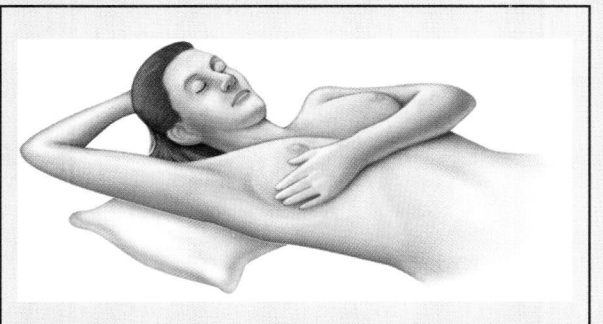

7. Examine both breasts, including your chest area and armpits.
8. If you notice any changes from one month to the next, notify your physician or nurse practitioner.

Testicular Self-Examination
1. The best time to perform this examination is right after a shower when your scrotal skin is moist and relaxed, making the testicles easy to feel.
2. Gently lift each testicle. Each one should feel like an egg, firm but not hard, and smooth with no lumps.
3. Using both hands, place your middle fingers on the underside of each testicle and your thumbs on top.
4. Gently roll the testicle between the thumb and fingers to feel for any lumps, swelling, or mass.

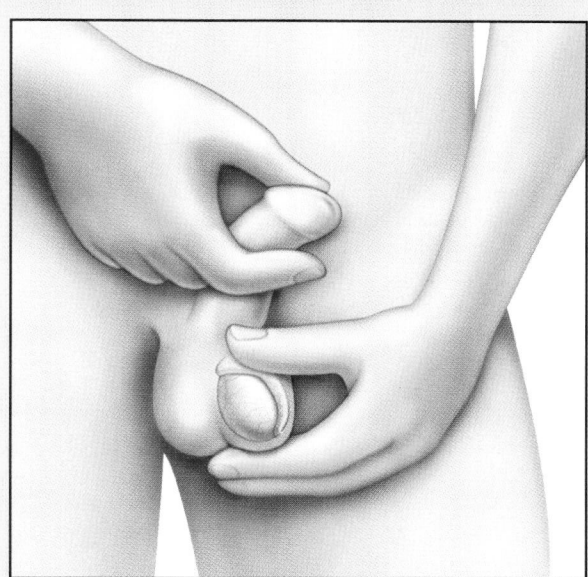

5. If you notice any changes from one month to the next, notify your physician or nurse practitioner.

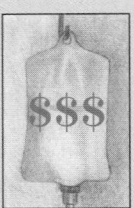

THE COST OF CARE
BREAST CANCER

Breast cancer is a highly prevalent and serious illness in women. It is the second leading cause of cancer deaths among American women (NABCO, 1998). The major risk factors for breast cancer are advancing age and a history of breast cancer in a first-degree relative (mother, sister, daughter). Each year, millions of dollars are spent in treating breast cancer: by surgery, chemotherapy, radiation, or any combination of the three. Early detection is the best way to ensure survival and to minimize costs. Following simple procedures, such as the breast self-examination, a professional breast examination, and mammography, can keep individual health care costs at a minimum. The American Cancer Society's guidelines for mammography in women who have no breast cancer history are:

- Baseline mammogram between ages 35 and 39
- Mammogram every 1 to 2 years between ages 40 and 49.
- Yearly mammogram over age 50.

A mammogram typically costs between $30 and $100. Most insurance companies will pay the full cost. In the treatment of breast cancer, many women are insisting on the most conservative treatment that has a reasonable chance of success. However, cancers that go undetected easily result in nodular or metastatic involvement and radical treatment costs are disproportionately higher. The cost of a simple, unilateral mastectomy ranges from $900 to $1300, according to Blue Cross/Blue Shield of North Carolina. These figures are based on usual, customary, and reasonable figures the medical insurers use for reimbursement to consumers or health care providers.

the client with the belief that you are ready and willing to talk about this sometimes difficult topic.

Defining Characteristics

Altered sexuality patterns is a broad nursing diagnosis that considers all physical, psychosocial, and cultural aspects of sexuality, as suggested in the accompanying Data Clustering chart. Defining characteristics include reported difficulties, limitations, or changes in sexual behaviors or activities. These may involve actual or anticipated negative changes in sexual behaviors, sexual health, sexual functioning, or sexual identity. In addition, defining characteristics may include expression of concern about inappropriate sexual verbal or nonverbal behavior, or changes in primary or secondary sexual characteristics (Carpenito, 1997).

Related Factors

Many factors may be related to alterations in sexual patterns. To assess for any of the following related factors, observe for nonverbal cues and clarify any vague or incomplete client responses during the interview. Client comments during the physical examination may also alert you to the need to inquire about additional sexual concerns, such as the following:

- Altered body function or structure due to illness or surgical interventions
- Conflicts with sexual orientation or preferences
- Fear of pregnancy or STDs
- Ineffective role models or lack of role models
- Knowledge or skill deficit about alternative responses in health-related problems
- Lack of privacy in which to engage in sexual intimacy
- Lack of significant other or impaired relationship with a significant other

Focused Assessment for Sexual Dysfunction

Sexual dysfunction implies a change or disruption in sexual health or function that the affected person views as unrewarding or inadequate (Gorman, Sultan, & Raines, 1996). Zimbler (1997) refers to sexual dysfunction as either a disruption of sexual behavior or extreme variation of sexual behavior and lists four major types: sexual desire disorders, sexual arousal disorders, orgasmic dysfunction, and sexual pain disorders (Table 51–4).

Defining Characteristics

The defining characteristics of sexual dysfunction are verbal report of an actual or perceived change in sexual function or limitation on sexual performance, often imposed by disease or therapy. Sexual dysfunction may also include a change of interest in oneself or others, value conflicts, lack of satisfaction, an altered relationship with a partner, a need for confirmation of desirability, and alterations in achieving a perceived sex role. A key nursing role is to help clients adapt to the effects of illness, as discussed in the State of Nursing Science chart.

Related Factors

Factors related to *Sexual dysfunction* are similar to those for *Altered sexuality patterns*. In fact, sexual dysfunction can alter sexuality patterns, so it may be difficult for you to differentiate between the two. Related factors for sexual dysfunction may include the following:

- Lack of information or knowledge
- Vulnerability
- Conflicting values
- Emotional or physical abuse
- Lack of privacy
- Inadequate or absent role models

Teaching for WELLNESS

MAINTAINING SEXUAL PATTERNS AFTER A MYOCARDIAL INFARCTION

Purpose: To maintain sexual health.

Rationale: Sexual health is a prerequisite for normal sexual function.

Expected Outcome: The client will achieve a preferred pattern of sexual function.

Client Instructions

1. Heart disease is a chronic illness that is laden with myths relating to sexual function. Do you believe any of the following myths?
   - Sex after a heart attack can easily cause sudden death.
   - It is best for the man to be on the bottom during sex after a heart attack.
   - Impotence and lack of sex drive always occur after a heart attack.
   - If angina occurs during sex, you should stop having sex permanently.
2. These myths are just that: myths. They are not correct. The fact is that most men and women can safely resume sex within a few weeks or as soon as

they feel ready after a heart attack or heart surgery. However, do not rush into sex just to prove yourself after a heart attack or heart surgery.
3. If you are not sure you are ready, your physician can administer an exercise test to check your physical capacity for sex.
4. You should be able to experience the same desire and arousal after your heart attack that you did before your heart attack.
5. Depression is a common response to a heart attack or heart surgery, and it may interfere with your normal level of desire temporarily.
6. Some heart medications interfere with the sex drive and sexual function. With some adaptation, however, sexual pleasure and performance need not be worrisome.
7. Feel free to discuss any concerns you have about sexuality or sexual function with me. If needed, you may want to talk with a professional sex counselor as well. The American Heart Association has excellent information to help guide you back into a fulfilling sex life.

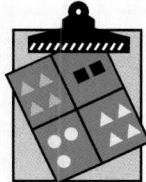

CLUSTERING DATA TO MAKE A NURSING DIAGNOSIS
PROBLEMS OF SEXUAL FUNCTION

Data Cluster	Diagnosis
A 12-year-old boy admits to his friends that he masturbates several times a week. He heard his minister say that masturbation is sinful. The boy is worried he is not normal.	*Altered sexuality patterns* related to feelings of guilt, worries about normal functioning, and need to express himself sexually through masturbation.
A 30-year-old newly married woman discovers that she does not like sex. Her mother died when she was 4 years old and she was raised by her father who was very strict with her upbringing.	*Sexual dysfunction* related to lack of sexual desire and lack of a female role model as she was developing as a young woman.
A couple in their mid-50s are thinking of separate bedrooms because sexual intercourse has become very painful for the wife. She is beginning menopause and is noticing physical changes in her body.	*Sexual dysfunction* related to painful intercourse secondary to dryness of the vagina.
A recent widower in his 60s cannot bear to look at women who speak with him at work and church. He is afraid of violating his wife's memory by interacting with any woman because he does not feel he can ever be sexually intimate again.	*Altered sexuality patterns* related to feelings of inadequacy and violation of his wife's memory through pursuing of sexual contact.

TABLE 51–4
Sexual Dysfunctions

Dysfunction	Description
Sexual Desire Alterations	
Hypoactive desire	• Deficiency or absence of desire for sexual activity.
Sexual aversion	• Aversion to and active avoidance of genital sexual contact with a partner.
Sexual Arousal Alterations	
Female	• Inability to attain or maintain sexual activity to completion.
	• May result from inadequate lubrication and swelling response in the excitement phase or from a psychological problem, medical problem, or substance abuse.
Male	• Inability to attain or maintain sexual activity to completion.
	• May result from the inability to obtain and maintain an adequate erection or from a psychological problem, medical problem, or substance abuse.
Orgasmic Alterations	
Female	• Delayed or absent orgasm following a normal sexual excitement phase.
Male	• Delayed or absent orgasm following a normal sexual excitement phase.
	• Ejaculation before the client wishes it: before, at, or shortly after penetration.
Sexual Alterations Caused by Pain	
Dyspareunia	• Genital pain associated with intercourse.
	• Occurs in both women and men.
	• May result from organic cause or traumatic event, such as rape, incest, or sexual abuse.
Vaginismus	• Involuntary contraction of the perineal muscles surrounding the outer third of the vagina upon penetration of penis, tampon, speculum, etc.

Adapted from American Psychiatric Association. (1994). Diagnostic and statistical manual of mental disorders (4th Ed.) (DSM-IV). Washington, DC: Author.

- Altered body structure or function
- Lack of a significant other
- Biopsychosocial alterations in sexuality

Focused Assessment for Related Nursing Diagnoses

Sexuality is a major part of many life processes and you will need to consider diagnoses in several other areas of nursing care. Additional nursing diagnoses that could relate to sexual concerns are in the areas of self-esteem, body image, coping, adaptation to life changes and family processes, risk for infection (STDs), mental illness (including substance use and abuse), and potential for being taken advantage of (rape or sexual abuse).

One nursing diagnosis, *Ineffective individual coping,* is illustrated in the following example. A 49-year-old male client was being assessed for psychosocial counseling in an outpatient clinic. He reported as one of his symptoms having no intercourse or any desire for sexual activity with his wife over the past year. This problem had no medical, pharmaceutical, or surgical cause. Lack of sexual desire or activity over a prolonged time is one indication of clinical depression; therefore, the client should receive a nursing diagnosis of *Sexual dysfunction* and appropriate nursing diagnoses representing responses to depression such as *Hopelessness* and *Sleep pattern disturbances.*

Another example is a divorced mother of a young child. She is in a steady relationship but finds it difficult to become more intimate with her partner because her child is anxious about her mother's intimacy with a man who is not her father. This client might receive a nursing diagnosis of *Altered family processes related to insecurity secondary to altered family structure.*

DIAGNOSIS

There is much overlap between *Altered sexuality patterns* and *Sexual dysfunction.* In the latter, the client's report of a problem is a key factor. However, interventions related to *Sexual dysfunction* are fairly complex and require the expertise of a nursing specialist (Carpenito, 1997). The generalist nurse typically will use the broader diagnostic category of *Altered sexuality patterns.*

PLANNING

Anything that affects a person's physical being, emotional comfort, sociocultural mores, or moral and ethical attitudes may threaten some aspect of sexuality and result in a diagnosis of *Altered sexuality patterns.* Planning should consider the client's category of need, such as anatomical disruptions, physiological alterations, pharmacological interference, life cycle issues, emotional alterations, or environmental influences.

THE STATE OF NURSING SCIENCE
SEXUALITY AND THE CLIENT WITH A CARDIAC CONDITION

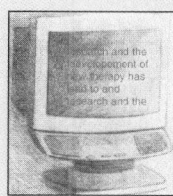

What Are the Issues?

A key role for nurses is to help clients make adaptations to the negative effects of illness and treatment. To provide effective counseling for clients in the area of sexuality, you need to understand how illnesses and their treatments affect clients and those closest to them. Many nurses hesitate to bring up the subject of sexuality. However, nursing's commitment to treating the whole person requires that this important aspect of life and relationships not be ignored.

What Research Has Been Conducted?

Sexual studies have indicated that sexuality is a major concern for people who have experienced a heart attack. However, few of these people report having received any counseling in this area. Building on this knowledge, Steinke and Patterson-Midgley (1996) conducted a pilot study to see what counseling clients received following a myocardial infarction. They were also interested in whether people of different ages, genders, and marital status were treated differently concerning counseling about sexuality.

The researchers analyzed survey information from 96 adults whose cases were being followed by a group of cardiologists. The researchers found that only one-third of the clients received sexual counseling during hospitalization, most often from cardiac rehabilitation staff and most frequently in the form of written information. The information primarily addressed when to resume sexual activity (p. 468). Many people received information on being well rested before sexual activity, on ensuring a comfortable setting for sexual activity, on warning signs to report, and on the use of medications before sexual activity (p. 469).

Jaarsma, Dracup, Walden, and Stevenson (1996) wondered whether people with advanced heart disease (heart failure) had the same concerns about sexual activity as people recovering from heart attacks. They interviewed, surveyed, and tested 62 adults with stage III and IV cardiac disease (the most serious cardiac impairment) who were being evaluated for possible heart transplantation. They measured the exercise tolerance of subjects using a 6-minute walk, ejection fractions using echocardiography, and sexual and psychological adjustment using self-report scales.

Clients reported changes in their interest in, frequency of, and problems with performance of sexual activity due to their illness. They also reported a decrease in satisfaction with sexual activity. Most of the people studied did not report problems with their spouses due to their illness. The researchers did not find any differences between men and women or younger or older clients in the area of sexual adjustment. Clients with better

performance on the 6-minute walk rated their sexual adjustment as better. This is an example of how an objective measure of the impact of a disease may be helpful in estimating changes in functional status.

What Has the Research Concluded?

Steinke and Patterson-Midgley (1996) concluded that most clients do not recall receiving any counseling related to sexual activity during hospitalization following a heart attack. The researchers also noted that the type of counseling provided fell short of offering people information on other forms of sexual expression than intercourse that could help people gradually resume sexual activity (p. 468). Married subjects were significantly more likely to receive counseling related to sexual activity than were unmarried clients. This means that the counseling needs of some clients who may engage in sexual activity go unmet. The researchers recommended that nurses address concerns about sexuality in their discussions about resuming previous activities. They offered an excellent assessment question that could be used to open the door to such a discussion: "Many people after experiencing a heart attack have concerns about resuming sexual activity. What concerns do you have?" (p. 471).

In their summary, Jaarsma and colleagues (1996) conclude that clients with advanced cardiac disease have more impairment in sexual function than people recovering from heart attacks. They recommend including the topic of sexual activity in counseling sessions with clients so that suggestions can be made for how to adapt to decreasing physical function.

What Is the Future of Research in This Area?

Future research is needed on the most effective methods of counseling people with chronic illnesses in the area of sexuality and sexual functioning. Nurses could study the experience of spouses and partners of clients with heart disease to better understand from their point of view how such changes affect their relationships. Nurses could participate in interdisciplinary research on the effects of various cardiac medications and their influence on sexual activity and interpersonal relationships. Finally, research is needed on educational interventions to help nurses increase their comfort level in addressing issues related to sexuality.

References
Jaarsma, T., Dracup, K., Walden, J., & Stevenson, L.W. (1996). Sexual function in patients with advanced heart failure. *Heart & Lung, 25*(4), 262–270.
Steinke, E., & Patterson-Midgley, P. (1996). Sexual counseling following acute myocardial infarction. *Clinical Nursing Research, 5*(4), 462–272.

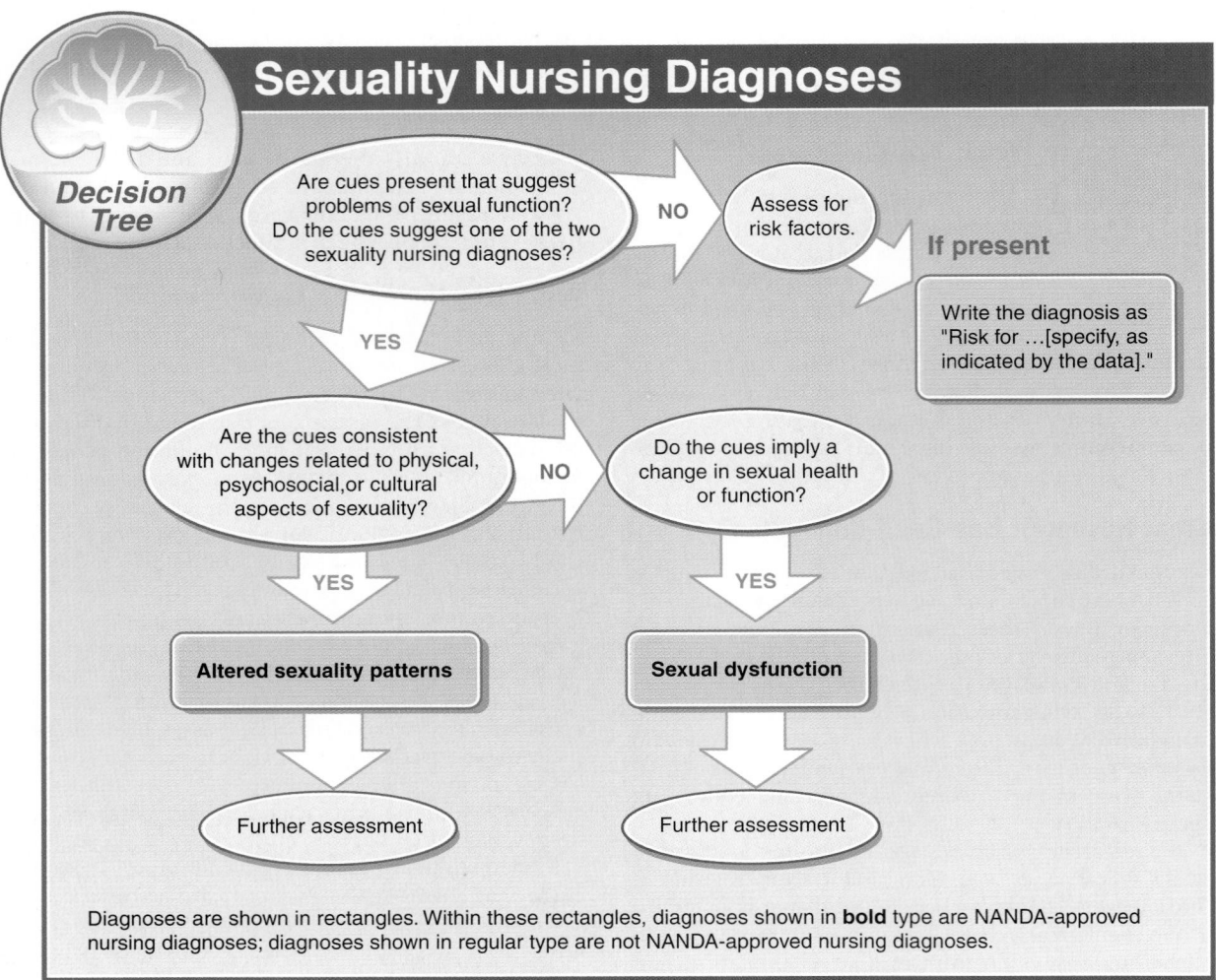

Sexuality Nursing Diagnoses

Decision Tree

Are cues present that suggest problems of sexual function? Do the cues suggest one of the two sexuality nursing diagnoses?

NO → Assess for risk factors.

If present → Write the diagnosis as "Risk for ...[specify, as indicated by the data]."

YES ↓

Are the cues consistent with changes related to physical, psychosocial, or cultural aspects of sexuality?

NO → Do the cues imply a change in sexual health or function?

YES ↓ **Altered sexuality patterns** → Further assessment

YES ↓ **Sexual dysfunction** → Further assessment

Diagnoses are shown in rectangles. Within these rectangles, diagnoses shown in **bold** type are NANDA-approved nursing diagnoses; diagnoses shown in regular type are not NANDA-approved nursing diagnoses.

Classifying the client's need will help you facilitate planning according to the client's physical skill needs or teaching and counseling needs.

In addition, your plan should consider your own level of expertise, the accuracy and depth of your information about human sexuality, awareness of your own value system, level of comfort in communicating about sexuality, and interpersonal skills. Your plan also should demonstrate your respect for the client as a sexual being by ensuring care that minimizes exposure of the client's genitals (and breasts in the female client).

Expected Outcomes for the Client With Altered Sexuality Patterns

Expected outcomes for intervening in *Altered sexuality patterns* include the following. The client will

- Discuss sexual concerns with minimal or no hesitancy.
- Express feeling less anxious about sharing private information.
- Acknowledge the nurse's professional interest and acceptance of the client's feelings.

- Restate factual information received and seek clarification of data presented.
- Identify a specific problem or problems to work on.
- Establish clear and realistic goals.
- Identify stressors that may inhibit resolution of the problem.
- Seek further treatment or counseling as needed.

Expected Outcomes for the Client With Sexual Dysfunction

If you suspect or the client reports symptoms of sexual dysfunction, your plan should include specific information that would indicate a need for referral to a professional with expertise in treating the problem. In addition, planning should include the same considerations stated for altered sexuality patterns.

It may be difficult for a client to accept referral to a "sex specialist," whether for physical care or for counseling. Be prepared to help the client understand that, while others may joke about or stigmatize the need for expert sexual care, it may offer the most effective method for reducing the emotional pain of a sexual problem. Outcomes for the client experiencing sexual dysfunction include the following. The client will

- Acknowledge that sexual concerns have been evaluated
- Display nonverbal behavior that indicates increased relaxation or less sadness about the sexual problem
- Express increased physical comfort as a result of nursing care
- State knowledge of resources available and ways to access them

INTERVENTION

Interventions for altered sexuality patterns will relate to how the client defines the problem as well as to your assessment. Engaging the client in self-care as much as possible will prevent later resistance toward improved sexual health. Asking the client what she would like to have happen here and now as well as in the future is a good place to begin. Making sure the client receives answers to all her questions is also crucial, as pointed out in A Patient's View. Interventions must also consider the client's knowledge, beliefs, and attitudes for outcomes to be successful.

The PLISSIT Model of Intervention

The PLISSIT model of intervention incorporates four progressive levels of intervention in sexual problems and is based on a behavioral approach to treatment (Annon, 1976; Matocha & Waterhouse, 1993). Each succeeding level requires increasing knowledge and clinical skills on your part. PLISSIT is an acronym that stands for Permission, Limited Information, Specific Suggestion, and Intensive Therapy.

Permission

Many clients hesitate to bring up sexual issues. Through skillful communication, however, you can give the client *permission* to discuss all of her concerns. In giving permission, you assure the client that you will give professional attention to anything she wishes to share. Permission may also involve assuring the client that she is normal. For example, a single adult woman who is not in a stable relationship may need assurance that masturbation is normal and acceptable.

In the case study, Lisa may be fearful of disclosing her personal anxieties and beliefs about sex. Assure such clients that sometimes sharing personal information is necessary to provide the best possible health care. Emphasize that you will respect her privacy.

Limited Information

Often, permission to talk about sexuality concerns will reveal that the client has negative beliefs about aspects of sexuality based on her cultural or religious upbringing. In response, you can provide factual information and appropriate resources. At this level of the model, giving *limited information* allows you to share knowledge related to the client's concerns and to answer questions directly and clearly. Do not include extraneous information that was not asked for or needed.

For example, when teaching adolescent girls about menstruation and what they might expect, you would initially refrain from overwhelming them with every detail. When conducting a seminar about HIV transmission, you would limit the discussion to relevant knowledge and research. When helping parents teach their children about sexuality, you would advise them to limit their information to what is appropriate for the child's age.

Specific Suggestion

At this level of the model, you help clients change their behavior by giving *specific suggestions*. The change in behavior should help to attain goals that are directly related to a particular problem. Once you and the client have the necessary information, and together have set clear goals, your specific suggestions may include reading appropriate literature, attending support groups *(such as a cancer survival group in Lisa's case)*, role-playing discussions a couple might have about sexuality or sexual intercourse, and referral to professional resources.

In the case study, Lisa indicates that nonsexual aspects of her relationship with her husband are good. The stress of illness and uncertainty about outcomes in a chronic or life-threatening disease may be inhibiting sexual intimacy in both partners. Perhaps providing her with increased skill in communicating her feelings, needs, and desires to her husband, as well as ways to elicit the same from him, would facilitate resolution of their altered sexuality pattern. Another intervention would be to offer to listen to the husband's thoughts or suggesting resources for him.

Few generalist nurses are prepared to intervene in detail at this level of the model and beyond. Therefore, your specific suggestion may be a referral to an expert professional, such as a nurse specialist, psychologist, marriage or sex counselor, or other mental health professional. Make sure to tell your client that counseling from an expert is a normal, natural part of treatment. Make every effort to match the client's specific problem to the specific resource.

Perhaps Lisa's husband, Vincent, is just as anxious or fearful as she is about what is happening to her. Perhaps he worries constantly about whether her cancer will recur and what her chances of survival are. If he has not heard specific medical information about Lisa's condition, start by suggesting that he talk with Lisa's physician. How else might Vincent be encouraged to share his view of their marital relationship?

Intensive Therapy

The last step in the PLISSIT model is *intensive therapy*. It is recommended for more complex and highly individualized problems of sexual health.

"BREAST CANCER SHATTERED MY LIFE"

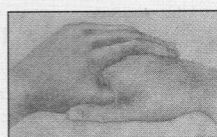 Breast cancer crashed into my life when I was 42. Noticing a lump in my left breast, I wasn't too alarmed; my small breasts were always lumpy-bumpy. But my ob/gyn froze when his fingers touched the lump. "What's this? It wasn't here at your last visit." Four hours later, I was in the surgeon's office. Two days after that, I became a one-breasted woman with a life-threatening illness.

A 3-centimeter tumor and 14 cancerous lymph nodes. Not a great prognosis. The surgeon wasn't optimistic or pessimistic. He was just what I needed—neutral and honest—so I trusted him. He didn't give me more information than I asked for. (I only ask questions if I know I can deal with the answers.) He said it was serious, one of the fastest growing types, and there was no time to waste.

Life happened at warp speed. A day and a half in the hospital after surgery. Five days later, a meeting with the oncologist. Four days after that, the first in a year of chemotherapy treatments. Then 6 weeks of radiotherapy and 6 more months of chemo.

Because I trusted my surgeon, I never hesitated or agonized over decisions about treatment. I never sought a second opinion. I just wanted the cancer out of my body and out of my life. And I wanted to know: What did I do wrong? I knew so little about breast cancer. Because I was young and had no family history of breast cancer, I thought I wasn't at risk. Sure, I had started my periods early and had my children late, but so had all of my friends and they were fine. Why was this happening to me?

At my first appointment with the oncologist, I couldn't stop crying. He pigeonholed me as "hysterical." He never gave me credit for being intelligent and he didn't listen. I was 3 months into treatment before he told me that chemo would last not 6 months but a full year!

No doctor warned me about the possibility of lymphedema. When it happened, I was told: "There's no treatment. Just learn to live with it." Living with it has meant two hospitalizations with cellulitis, repeated rounds of heavy-duty antibiotics, and continuing fear that the tiniest cut or burn will trigger another flare-up. Every day, my swollen arm and hand remind me of breast cancer.

My first post-diagnosis year, I was in treatment. My husband was in denial. He didn't go to doctor's appointments with me, which made me angry. Looking back, I realize that's the only way he could deal with it. He did look after the children on weekends and hired a babysitter for Mondays and Wednesdays. When my treatment ended, he wanted the whole thing to be over. Finished. We've worked on that issue over the years but the idea that I have cancer and could die is still horrific to him.

Our son was 5 when I was diagnosed, our daughter just 18 months. I asked the pediatrician what to tell my son. "Be factual about what's happening but don't tell him it's life-threatening. If the time comes when that's necessary, tell him then." That seems to have worked. My daughter was too young to understand, but now that she's 10, I know we need to have that conversation before many more years go by.

I never told my mother, and in 2 years of long-distance conversations, she never picked up on the fact that I was seriously ill. An alcoholic, self-centered, and unhappy, she divorced my father when I was 5. She needed help, but to her, asking for help was a sign of weakness and I grew up believing that. Instead, I intellectualized every problem, every crisis. Cancer changed that in a heartbeat. I knew I had to ask for help or die. Whether I lived 5 days, 5 months, or 5 years, I didn't want to go on living the way I had been living. I joined a breast cancer support group and started going to a shrink. The group gave me the immediate, day-to-day emotional support I needed to deal with breast cancer and the shrink helped me with long-standing issues. That combination of peer support and professional counseling has changed my life.

I had the worst possible attitude. People gave me books about the healing power of a positive attitude. I could not bear to read them; I actually threw one out the window. We need to allow people to be who they are in times of crisis, not make them feel guilty about their attitude.

I didn't consider reconstructive surgery. My small breasts and my thin body had never been a big part of my sexuality or my sense of self. And the thought of more surgery and hospitalization for something I considered cosmetic and not therapeutic seemed irrational. What if I went through all that and died anyway? I just wanted to do whatever it took to stay alive.

I had good care, but after surgery and during chemo and radiation, it was sometimes hard to understand what was happening and whether what I was feeling was something to worry about. My contacts were primarily oncologists and med techs so it was sometimes hard to get my questions answered in a timely way. Having access to a knowledgeable nurse for explanations and answers would have helped a lot. My support group was invaluable in helping to answer my questions and confirm that much of what I was going through was "normal."

Breast cancer shattered my life. Picking up the pieces and rearranging them has been an extraordinarily humbling experience. It's made me more compassionate and less patient. When I talk to women who are going through treatment, getting the same drugs I had nearly a decade ago, I get angry because so little has changed. When I look at my 10-year-old daughter, who now has a family history of breast cancer, I get furious and frightened because there's no sure way to keep it from happening to her.

Lisa's problems may need a sex therapist's expertise to be resolved. Before referring Lisa and her husband to counseling, you would assess the overall health of the couple's relationship, the extent of their knowledge, their fears, the reasons each gives for lack of sexual intimacy, what their past sexual patterns have been, and their willingness to work toward resolution, individually and as a couple.

Using the PLISSIT Model

To understand more about the PLISSIT model and how it is used, consider these examples. A 53-year-old woman who has been menopausal for 2 years is distressed about pain upon penetration during intercourse. Assessment determines that the client has no physical defect. Using the PLISSIT model, give the client permission to discuss her dilemma with her partner and together try to find more comfortable positions for intercourse. Specific suggestions would include a thorough physical assessment to determine the cause of the pain. In addition, suggesting the use of a water-soluble vaginal lubricant prior to intercourse may be helpful. Dryness is common in menopausal women and may be causing the pain.

An adolescent boy comes to the school nurse with abrasions caused by a fight in the schoolyard. While there, he says that the other boys all brag about "doing it" and ridicule him for not having sex with his girlfriend. He is not sexually active because of his religious and moral objection to sex outside of a committed relationship. Again using the PLISSIT model, give him permission to be different from his friends; stress that his sexual inactivity is just as normal as the other boys' sexual activity. Help him brainstorm assertive responses to use when other boys tease him that would not alienate or provoke them but instead would confirm his choice of abstinence.

Interventions to Resolve Sexual Dysfunction

The PLISSIT model is most appropriate to use in identifying a specific sexual dysfunction and for directing the client toward effective resources. Before referring to counseling, urge the client to have a thorough physical evaluation and diagnostic tests to rule out any physical or physiological abnormalities.

Another intervention is to recognize that anxiety or depression may accompany sexual dysfunction. Acknowledge the client's feelings, offer support that further assessment will be done, and encourage the client to follow through with referral and treatment, because many dysfunctions can effectively be relieved (Fogel, 1998). Good hygiene practices and physical care may provide the client physical comfort until further treatment begins.

Interventions to Promote Sexual Health

Educating the public on the many facets of sexual growth and development and health is an essential nursing function and an important strategy toward

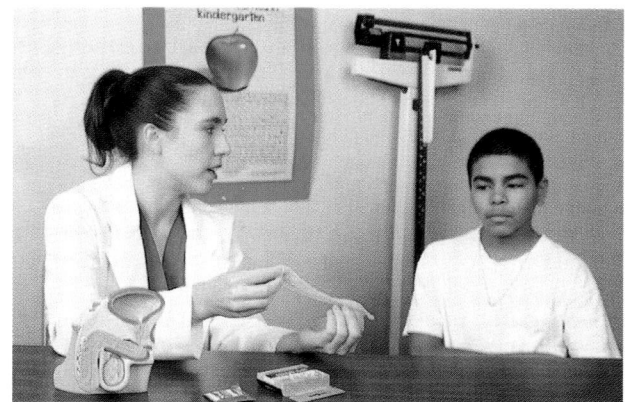

Figure 51–4. School nurses can provide sensitive counseling about sexual behavior.

promoting healthy sexuality. The astute nurse will find opportunities for discussing health issues in many arenas, such as with parents whose children are hospitalized or are in home health care, in the schools, at parent-teacher sessions, in community groups, at health fairs, and with children in hospitals and clinics (Fig. 51–4). Following are suggestions for some issues to be discussed across the life span.

Infants and Children

Sexual health begins in infancy with good hygienic practices in the care of external genitalia and protection from disease and injury. Most authors agree that there is little awareness of gender differences in infancy and early childhood. Children learn gender behaviors through interactions with adults. The ways in which children are dressed and responded to may promote gender-typical behaviors. Active display of affection by adults to both sexes promotes caring responses.

Imparting sexual values, such as respect for individual differences and expected ways of behaving toward individuals of the opposite sex, is important at an early age.

Role models that teach children to be more androgynous invite more healthy behaviors. Examples are teaching boys not to take advantage of their strength against girls (or each other) and encouraging girls to stand up for themselves and yet be fair in arguments. Developing healthy sexuality in interpersonal interactions also includes witnessing caring and loving behaviors in adults.

Early childhood is a time when gender differences may become more apparent and curiosity leads children to explore their bodies. Touching genitals is a natural part of this exploration. Encourage caretakers to allow this exploration, and discourage negative reactions to it. As language develops, children should be taught the proper words for body parts, such as vagina and penis. In working with parents or children, always answer questions truthfully and without embarrassment.

*A*ction *A*lert!
Teach children about good touch and bad touch. Encourage them to tell a parent, teacher, or other trusted adult when a touch is uncomfortable for them.

Adolescents

Adolescence is a time of establishing identity and a growing awareness of sexuality related to pubertal changes and social behaviors. The development of secondary sex characteristics tends to focus the adolescent on body image. Teaching girls about menstruation and boys about erections and wet dreams is important. Even though teaching about sexual activity should begin in childhood, reinforcing the nature of sexual intercourse and the risks involved in unprotected sex is a primary concern. Given the incidence of rape in our society, socialization about respect for the bodies of others and ways to interact in sexually appropriate ways should be a part of the education process for adolescents.

The adolescent is also in the process of affirming sexual roles and lifestyles. It is a time when nurses (and parents) might discuss personal and cultural values regarding sex and sexuality and help adolescents integrate what they have learned toward rewarding peer relationships. Role models are also important at this time of life, as is a healthy outlet for discussing sexual issues with a respected adult.

Adolescents are usually hesitant or uncomfortable talking openly about sexual issues, especially if the subject has been taboo in their families. You can be most helpful if you accept whatever the adolescent discloses, reassure the client of confidentiality (unless doing so would jeopardize the client's safety), and discuss sexual issues in a rational, nonthreatening manner.

Adults

Adult sexuality issues are multifaceted and complex. You cannot expect to be competent in all situations involving sexuality. Being sensitive and responding to specific physical, psychosocial, and relationship issues may help your clients sort out areas in which they lack information, need treatment or counseling, or desire enhancement of a relationship or sexual intimacy. Encouraging good health practices and teaching preventive activities, such as breast and testicular self-examinations, are measures that ensure continued sexual enjoyment. Knowledge about methods of birth control may be a need for adults who wish to delay or prevent pregnancy. Health care providers and other organizations provide excellent literature for the lay public on various aspects of sexuality. For example, the American Heart Association produces a pamphlet on sex and heart disease.

Older Adults

We are in an era in which people are living longer and healthier lives; sexual health is very much a part of the aging person's existence. Many older people are em-

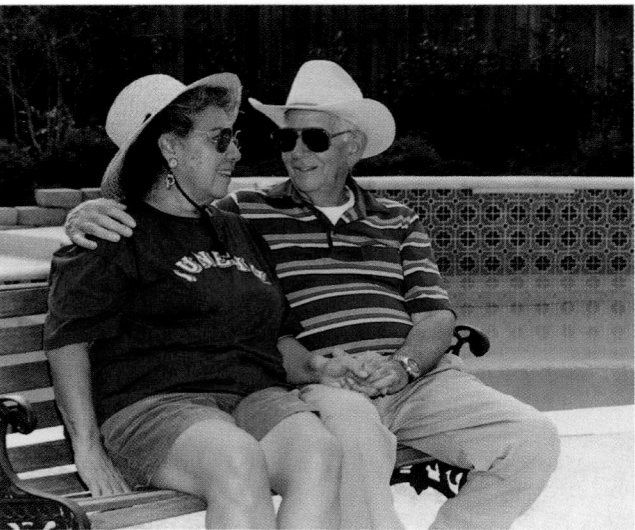

Figure 51–5. Older people express intimacy in a variety of ways.

barrassed or feel guilty discussing sexual intimacy, some of which stems from Western society's emphasis on youth and beauty. There are numerous myths surrounding older people's sexuality. Many believe older people to be asexual and not interested in or capable of sexual intercourse. In fact, most older adults who have experienced sexual intimacy throughout their lives can be just as sexually active as anyone else. As people age, some physical and hormonal changes do occur that affect sexual activity. However, based on age alone, there is no reason to not enjoy sex as long as people live.

In contrast, some older people prefer not to engage in sexual intercourse for a variety of reasons and, perhaps because of the sexual revolution, feel pressured to do so. Sexual abstinence by choice is also normal. There are many ways older people express intimacy that brings them a great deal of pleasure. You can be active in affirming whatever intimate patterns older people have chosen (Fig. 51–5).

You also can play an active role in sexual health promotion through education and consciousness raising with the elderly and the rest of society. Debunking myths, exploring attitudes and values that can inhibit sexual expression, and correcting misinformation about the aging process are appropriate topics to address. Encouraging good physical health practices is very important to sexual health in aging, and includes periodic physical check-ups, preventive measures such as exercising, and seeking medical consultation promptly when a person thinks that something adverse is happening to her body or mental state.

Interventions to Prevent Sexually Transmitted Disease

A high priority in sexual health promotion is the prevention of STDs. Recent statistics suggest that 10 to 13 million new STD cases arise each year in the United States, not counting HIV infection or acquired immunodeficiency syndrome (AIDS). Plus, the list of STDs has expanded. More than 20 disorders now qualify as STDs (Luckmann, 1997). It is also reported that women are bearing the brunt of both the risk and consequences of STDs. That is at least in part because the warm, moist vaginal environment promotes the growth of flora, and because mucosal tears during intercourse provide an entry for infection (Sharts-Hopko, 1997).

Chlamydial infection is the most prevalent STD in the United States. It is more difficult to diagnose in women than in men because it is usually asymptomatic. Untreated, chlamydial infections have serious reproductive tract consequences, which are preventable through treatment (Alexander, Treiman, & Clark, 1996). What many people do not realize is that STDs have a latent or subclinical phase in which the person is infected but asymptomatic. Thus, the disease may be transmitted without either partner knowing it exists (Tierney, McPhee, & Papadakis, 1997).

In light of this recent information and being in a society where multi-partner sexual contact is accepted, prevention would seem to be a formidable task. Publicity aimed at prevention and public education has much potential to reduce the problem. Just as you must take the initiative in assessing clients for sexual health problems, nurses also must take the initiative to speak out in appropriate public forums (such as parent-teacher meetings, health-related seminars, high school or public health fairs, and so on). Take every opportunity to do individual assessment and teaching, especially with adolescents and young, single adults, and to support social causes that promote awareness of the extent of the STD problem.

Action **A**lert!
Provide teaching about the prevention of STDs through the use of abstinence or safe sex. Be explicit when explaining that "safe sex" means that protection is always used during sexual intimacy. And explain that even "safe sex" is not as safe as abstinence.

Interventions for Lesbians and Gay Men

In the sexual health care of clients, be aware that some of your clients will be lesbians and gay men. James, Harding, and Corbett (1994) report research indicating that these clients "fear homophobia from health care providers, are anxious about the consequences of revealing their sexual orientation, are worried about breaches of confidentiality, and are concerned about having to face hostility and even physical harm" (p. 28). Discrimination against homosexuals in health care is unethical, yet it apparently exists.

Even though AIDS has raised public awareness of the existence of gay men and lesbians, many people, including nurses, still do not accept homosexuality and thus are uncomfortable or fearful about interacting with these clients. **Homophobia** is a fear of becoming homosexual through contact with lesbians and gay men or even of having close or intimate feelings toward someone of the same sex (both of which are myths).

Lesbian and bisexual women experience significant barriers to health care, partly because of homophobia and heterosexism in the health care system, but also due to finances. In general, women make less money than men and are more likely to be in jobs that have no health care benefits. If a woman identifies herself as lesbian or bisexual, attitudes of health care providers may vary from acceptance to tolerance to disapproval and even to disgust and hatred. However, if women choose not to disclose their sexual orientation, they risk being treated improperly, especially in relation to gynecological problems. In fact, lesbian and bisexual women experience similar sexual alterations and dysfunctions as heterosexual women (Eliason, 1996).

Men generally have more positive attitudes about casual sex, and therefore casual sex among gay men is more prevalent than among heterosexuals. This practice raises a number of health-related issues, including knowledge about and prevention of STDs and such medical conditions as rectal and anal infections and trauma (Eliason, 1996).

Nurses are obligated care for a homosexual client just as sensitively as for any other client. Both homosexual men and women experience a good deal of stress as a result of being an oppressed and stigmatized minority. What will facilitate more effective care is that you first examine your own beliefs, fears, and biases about homosexuality and determine to what extent, if any, they will interfere when you encounter homosexual clients. Seeking factual knowledge and exploring attitudes with peers will increase your objectivity in nursing care. Talking with lesbians or gay men who are open to such interaction can help alleviate your anxiety and assure you that, aside from their sexuality, these clients are just like your other clients.

In interviewing all your clients, it is preferable to talk about sexual practices by using the phrase "sexual partner" rather than assuming a male partner for a female client and a female partner for a male client. Viewing a client's sexual orientation as a factor in health care, not as a problem, will help you to care for homosexual clients with respect and dignity.

Nurses in a variety of practice settings have excellent opportunities to promote healthy sexuality. People of all ages and sexual orientations are likely to talk more readily with nurses about sexual issues, particularly when the nurse listens for and is comfortable with sexual themes. The caring, nonthreatening, unhurried manner in which nurses engage others in such discussions has potential to make a marked difference in the ways people view and experience themselves as sexual beings.

EVALUATION

Evaluation of nursing care for sexuality problems includes determining whether the expected outcomes have been met. Additionally, you should determine

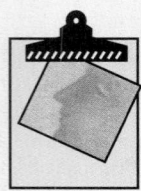

NURSING CARE PLANNING
A CLIENT WITH ALTERED SEXUALITY PATTERNS

Admission Data

Client states that she is feeling unattractive and expresses concern about the results of her biopsy. She reports there has been no intercourse with her husband for the past 3 months. She appears sad when discussing her husband's indifference to her.

Physician's Orders

Complete blood count
Sonogram, uterus
Height and weight

Chest x-ray
ECG
Preparation for uterine biopsy

Nursing Assessment

No eye contact. Fidgeting with wedding ring. States she has irregular periods and is afraid of surgery. Believes husband has stopped loving her. Does not wish to discuss problems with her spiritual advisor.

NURSING CARE PLAN

Nursing Diagnosis	Expected Outcomes	Interventions	Evaluation
Altered sexuality patterns related to loss of breast and stress of anticipated results of surgery.	Plans for sexual intimacy with mate.	Reassure Lisa that her feelings are usual following the loss of a body part. *Allow time to discuss concerns further and give permission to do so. Provide feedback on normalcy of feelings.*	Lisa reports sexual concerns on return visit. Facial expression shows relief. Shares more feelings with nurse.
		Obtain more information about comments husband and others made to her.	Describes comments and behaviors others have actually made.
	Evidence of internal locus of control.	Provide accurate information. Inform Lisa when and what results will be available to her.	Acknowledges understanding of necessary tests and time to conduct them.
		Contract for time to talk privately pre- and post-procedure.	Acknowledges difficulty in discussing sexual concerns. Agrees to talk with nurse. Agrees to talk with spouse.

Italicized interventions indicate culturally specific care.

Critical Thinking Questions
1. How should the nurse arrange for follow-up care for Lisa?
2. How might Lisa react to further suggestions for joint marital counseling?
3. How might Lisa feel a year from now? What psychological changes would be expected at that time?
4. The nurse would explain the grieving process to Lisa. When would the nurse expect that Lisa would complete the grieving process?

whether the problem has been resolved to the client's satisfaction. Particularly in the sensitive area of sexuality, the client may not have clearly identified the problem, and therefore will be left with some discomfort. Discomfort indicates that the problem has not truly been resolved. Evaluation can be based on a review of the PLISSIT model.

To evaluate the phase of *permission*, observe the client's level of comfort in discussing sexuality. Ask questions to determine whether the problem has been resolved. Questions might include: Are you satisfied with the sexual aspects of your life? Has the work we have done together helped? Has it addressed the problem as you perceived it? To evaluate the client's level of comfort with therapy and with current sexuality, nonverbal observations may be helpful. Notice the client's posture, eye contact, and ease in communicating. Have these changed from your initial contact with the client? Can the client ask questions and discuss sexual concerns freely?

To evaluate the effects of providing *limited information,* determine whether the client has understood and retained the information, whether the information has adequately addressed both spoken and unspoken questions, and whether having the information has been helpful.

To evaluate the *specific suggestions* phase of the model, ask whether the client has been able to try the suggestions and to describe the results. At this point, you would also want to know whether the client thought of other ideas that worked better than the suggestions you gave. You can use the time to reinforce positive behaviors and correct any misperceptions.

To evaluate the last phase, *intensive therapy,* ask whether the client followed up on your referral to seek more intensive therapy and whether the therapy was helpful. Because intensive therapy may be long-term, you may only be able to evaluate based on whether or not the client began the process.

Additionally, you should evaluate the client's level of self-care. Does the client have the knowledge to maintain sexual health? Is the client aware of resources to obtain further information or to manage the present or future problems?

KEY PRINCIPLES

- The biological, psychological, social, and cultural influences one experiences throughout life have a significant impact on human sexuality.
- Physiological, psychosocial, and developmental factors affect sexuality.
- Self-assessment of your attitudes, preferences, and prejudices should precede assessment of the client's sexuality.
- Sexuality is a major part of many life processes.
- Sexual needs vary in health and illness for clients across the life span.
- The PLISSIT model (permission, limited information, specific suggestion, and intensive therapy) is an appropriate model to use for nursing intervention.

BIBLIOGRAPHY

Alexander, L.L., Treiman, K., & Clark, P. (1996). A national survey of nurse practitioner: Chlamydia knowledge and treatment practices of female patients. Comment. *Nurse Practitioner, 21*(10), 8.

American Heart Association. (1995). Sex and heart disease. Dallas: Author.

*American Psychiatric Association (1994). *Diagnostic and Statistical Manual of Mental Disorders* (4th ed.). (DSM-IV). Washington, DC: Author.

*Annon, J.S. (1976). The PLISSIT model: A proposed conceptual scheme for the behavioral treatment of sexual problems. *Journal of Sex Education and Therapy, 2*(1), 211–15.

*Bancroft, J. (1991) *Human sexuality and its problems* (2nd ed.). New York: Churchill Livingstone.

Carpenito, L.J. (1997). *Nursing diagnosis: Application to clinical practice* (7th ed.) Philadelphia: J.B. Lippincott Co.

Eliason, M.J. (1996). *Institutional barriers to health care for lesbian, gay, & bisexual persons.* Pub. No. 14-6762. New York: NLN Press.

Fogel, C. (1998). Women and sexuality. In E. Yangkin & M. Davis (Eds.). *Women's health* (pp 105-123). Stamford, CT: Appleton & Lange.

Gorman, L.J., Sultan, D.F., & Raines, M.L. (1996). *Davis's manual of psychosocial nursing for general patient care.* Philadelphia: F.A. Davis.

*James, T., Harding, I., & Corbett, K. (1994). Biased care? *Nursing Times, 90*(51):28–31.

Jones, R.E. (Ed.). (1997). *Human reproductive biology.* San Diego: Academic Press.

Luckmann, J. (Ed.). (1997). *Saunders manual of nursing care.* Philadelphia: W.B. Saunders Co.

*Masters, W., & Johnson, V. (1966). *Human sexual response.* Boston: Little, Brown.

*Matocha, L.K., & Waterhouse, J.K. (1993). Current nursing practice related to sexuality. *Research in Nursing & Health, 16*(5), 371–378.

National Alliance of Breast Cancer Organizations (NABCO). (1998). *Facts about breast cancer in the USA.* New York: Author.

Sharts-Hopko, N.C. (1997). STDs in women: What you need to know. *American Journal of Nursing, 97*(4) 46–54.

*Shively, M.G., & DeCecco, J. (1977). Components of sexual identity. *Journal of Homosexuality, 3,* 41–48.

Spector, R.E. (1996). *Cultural diversity in health & illness* (4th ed.). Stamford, CT: Appleton & Lange.

Tierney, L.M., McPhee, S.J., & Papadakis, M.A. (Eds.). (1997). *Current medical diagnosis and treatment.* Stamford, CT: Appleton & Lange.

Taylor, C. (1998). A grain of salt: Some new annotations to "lessons of the new genetics." *Networker,* March/April, 42–43.

*World Health Organization. (1975). *Education & treatment in human sexuality: The training of health professionals.* Report of a WHO Meeting, Technical Report Series No. 572. Geneva: Author.

Zimbler, E.R. (1997). *Psychiatric nursing: Promoting mental health.* Stamford, CT: Appleton & Lange.

*Asterisk indicates a classic or definitive work on this subject.

UNIT 14

Coping–Stress-Tolerance Pattern

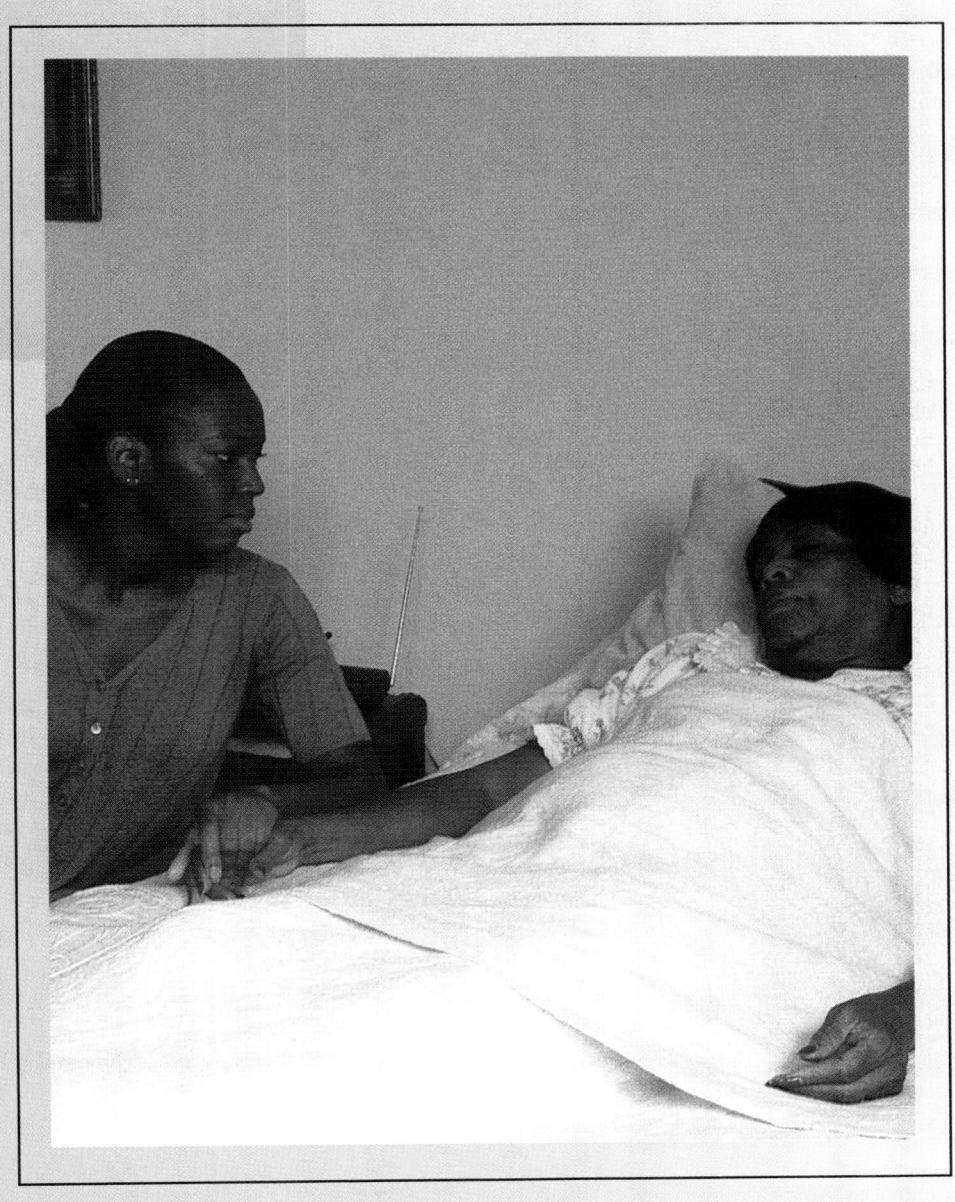

Coping–Stress Tolerance

Carolyn Chambers Clark and V. Doreen Wagner

Key Terms

adaptation
coping
crisis
defense mechanism
developmental crisis
eustress
hardiness

homeostasis
psychoneuroimmunology
resilience
situational crisis
stress
stressor

LEARNING OBJECTIVES

After studying this chapter, you should be able to:

1. Describe physiological and psychological concepts of stress.

2. Identify two challenges to coping skills and a variety of commonly used methods of coping.

3. Describe at least three factors affecting coping skills, including physiological, developmental, and psychological factors.

4. Discuss the assessment of a client's stress tolerance and coping skills.

5. Write a stress-related nursing diagnosis for a client and distinguish between related diagnoses.

6. Plan for goal-directed interventions to reduce stress.

7. Evaluate a client's progress toward stress tolerance and coping.

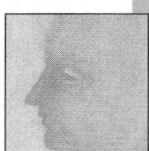

Billy Osceola is a 55-year-old, diabetic, Native American man recovering from a left below-knee amputation performed 10 days ago. During your first home health nursing visit, you see a liquor bottle open on the table. He raises his voice angrily when you try to talk to him about following a diabetic menu plan. Alcohol is on his breath. When you question him about it, he grunts and angrily asks you to leave, shouting that he doesn't need any nurse coming to see him. He refuses to let you near him. You go, telling him you'll be back to see him the next morning.

The next day, Mr. Osceola is polite and sober but basically noncommunicative. You are concerned when you see him put a stained, damp rag on his stump over the remains of a surgical dressing. When you ask him about it, he says his leg hurts and he's trying to fix it with an herbal potion he got from the shaman. He refuses to talk further about his leg and says there is no need to come see him.

Mr. Osceola is stressed. He is having difficulty accepting his current situation. His behavior has the potential to interfere with wound healing and prevent him from taking positive action to manage his health. You consider a stress-related nursing diagnosis (see accompanying chart) for this client.

STRESS-RELATED NURSING DIAGNOSES

Ineffective Individual Coping: Inability to form a valid appraisal of the stressors, inadequate choices of practiced responses, and/or inability to use available resources.

Ineffective Denial: The state of a conscious or unconscious attempt to disavow the knowledge or meaning of an event to reduce anxiety/fear to the detriment of health.

From North American Nursing Diagnosis Association. (1999). NANDA nursing diagnoses: Definitions and classification 1999–2000. Philadelphia: Author.

CONCEPTS OF STRESS

Stress is a physiological response produced by the normal wear and tear of bodily processes and external and internal demands. Examples of normal wear and tear are stress on bones and muscles from exercise, demands on circulation to meet metabolic needs, and the energy required to digest food. Selye (1956) described stress as a nonspecific physiological response—that is, the nature of the response is the same regardless of the demand. Selye was the first to recognize the role of the adrenal cortex and pituitary gland in the stress response. He also coined the term **stressor** as the description of a stress-causing agent. Examples of stressors include extreme hot or cold, an argument, a virus, an exam, cigarette smoke, a death, or any of the countless demands of the environment. To the extent that stress is an etiological factor in disease, illness can be thought of as an imbalance that occurs when the body fails to adapt to complex physical and emotional stressors in the internal and external environment.

Imbalance can result from many different stressors. Anxiety or lack of rest, or any other lack or challenge, can affect homeostasis and create an imbalance. **Homeostasis** is the tendency of biological systems to maintain relatively constant conditions in the internal environment while continuously interacting with and adjusting to changes originating within or outside the system. Thus, it describes a healthy, more or less stable, physiological state in which there is no undue imbalance. Think of homeostasis as a fluctuating condition or dynamic state in which there is no continuing imbalance between a cell's or a person's internal and external environments. Stress results from attempts to balance internal and external environmental demands.

One way the human body seeks to maintain homeostasis is through physiological responses. For example, sympathetic nervous system activity increases heart rate, cardiac output, respiratory rate, muscle tension, mental alertness, and glucose levels. The pituitary gland stimulates the adrenal cortex and thyroid gland. The thyroid gland manipulates metabolism. And the kidneys and adrenal glands maintain a balance of fluid and electrolytes.

Physiological Stress Response

Clearly, the physiological stress response is a complex neuroendocrine phenomenon (Fig. 52–1). Selye (1956) described this phenomenon as three physiological stages of the stress response and called them the *general adaptation syndrome*. The three stages are the alarm reaction stage, resistance stage, and exhaustion stage. In the alarm reaction stage, the sympathetic nervous system initiates the fight-or-flight response and activates defense mechanisms. Adrenaline surges, the heart speeds, and the body prepares for fighting or running away. This fight-or-flight response is sustained by the hypothalamic-pituitary-adrenal axis, which releases cortisone, norepinephrine, and epinephrine into the blood.

In the resistance stage, the body attempts to adapt to the stressor. The parasympathetic nervous system modulates the body's response by opposing the actions of the sympathetic nervous system. Resulting from the resistance stage, the person either recovers or becomes exhausted, thus entering the exhaustion stage. The body cannot function defensively against the stressor and physiological regulation decreases. If the stress continues in this stage of exhaustion, death can result.

Although the general adaptation response is helpful in understanding the physiological response to acute stress, situations of chronic stress are too complex to be explained by a single model. Stress is an elusive concept because it can be chronic or acute, physical or psychological, mild or severe. Also, what is stressful for one person may not be stressful for another. And what is stressful at one point in time may not be at another point.

Interaction of Physiological and Psychosocial Stressors

A stressor that affects any aspect of your being affects your whole self. Research clearly shows that psychological stress can lead to increased susceptibility to disease by suppressing the immune response. The higher the level of reported stress, the greater the probability of that suppressed immune response. Negative moods, such as anxiety and depression, are

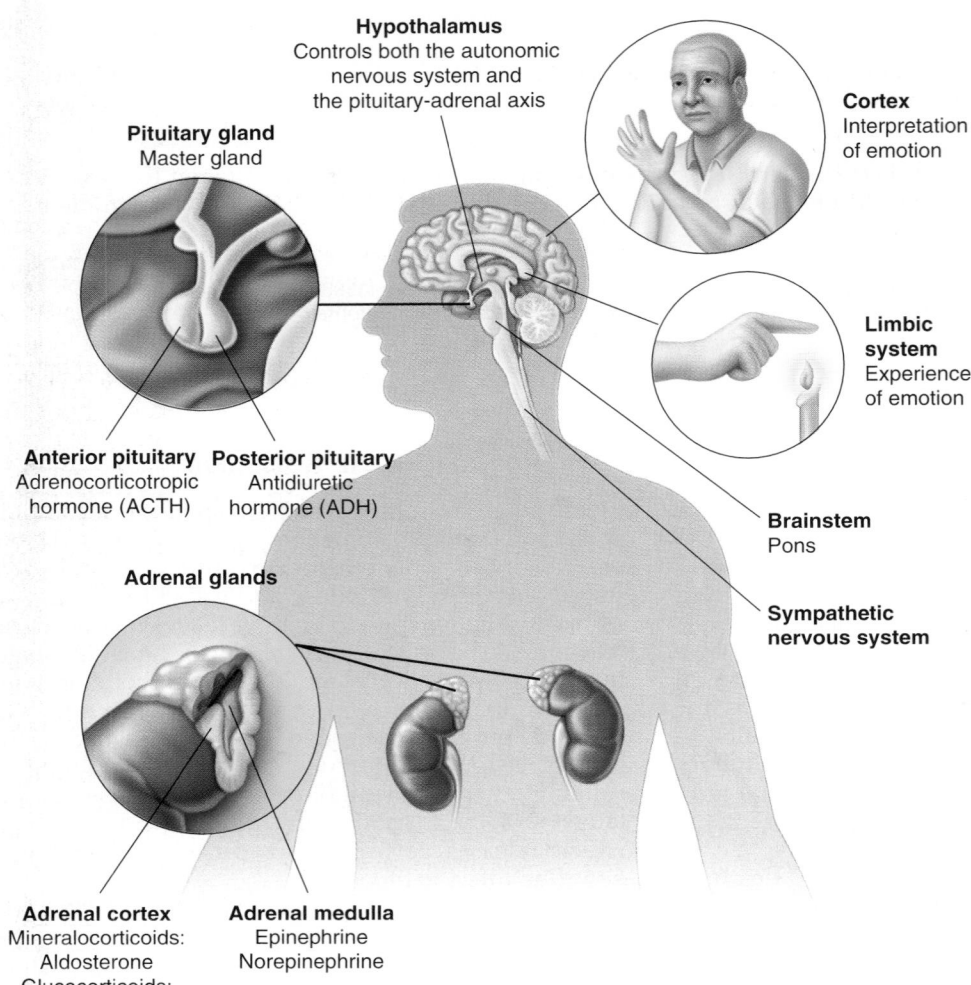

Hypothalamus
Controls both the autonomic
nervous system and
the pituitary-adrenal axis

Pituitary gland
Master gland

Cortex
Interpretation
of emotion

Anterior pituitary
Adrenocorticotropic
hormone (ACTH)

Posterior pituitary
Antidiuretic
hormone (ADH)

**Limbic
system**
Experience
of emotion

Brainstem
Pons

Adrenal glands

**Sympathetic
nervous system**

Adrenal cortex
Mineralocorticoids:
Aldosterone
Glucocorticoids:
Cortisol

Adrenal medulla
Epinephrine
Norepinephrine

Figure 52–1. The physiological
stress response is a complex neuroendocrine phenomenon.

associated with reduced immune function and are considered to be distress. Mild stress, such as regular exercise, can enhance immune function and is called eustress. **Eustress** refers to stress that results in positive outcomes.

Stress and Illness

Stress can cause some diseases and exacerbate others. For example, stress contributes to hypertension by increasing peripheral vascular resistance and the heart's workload. Prolonged stress from major burn injuries or critical illness can cause stress ulcers. And stress worsens such disorders as ulcerative colitis and rheumatoid arthritis.

Likewise, illness can cause stress. An ill person may not eat, and nutritional imbalances may introduce additional stress. When illness occurs, there is an attempt at both the physiological and psychological levels to strike a balance and achieve homeostasis. The ill person attempts to adapt to physical changes. Depending on the actions taken, wellness or additional illness can result.

Although much is still unknown about the relationship of stress to disease, researchers agree that stress affects the immune response. Over the past decade, investigators have been generating new, exciting findings about the many links between the nervous system and the immune system. Stress has become an important psychological variable in the field of psychoneuroimmunology. **Psychoneuroimmunology** is the study of the interface between the brain and immunology. Evidence of the effects of stress on immune competence provides compelling support for the link between the brain and immune system.

CONCEPTS OF COPING

Another way humans strive to achieve balance or homeostasis is through psychosocial coping. **Coping** is any effort directed toward management of dangerous, threatening, or challenging situations. It includes cognitive, affective, and behavioral responses that are situation specific and should be analyzed within the context of interpersonal transactions (Lazarus & Folkman, 1984). Coping is believed to be a major component in the relationship between the experience of stress and health. Coping is a similar concept to adaptation. **Adaptation** is a process through which individuals accommodate changes in the internal or external environment to preserve functioning and pursue goals.

People learn to cope or adapt to stressors by using methods that were successful in the past. For example, if a client learned in the past that he could escape from an unpleasant situation and return to homeostasis by going to bed, sleeping occurs in response to stress.

Challenges to Coping Skills

Both anxiety- and crisis-provoking situations challenge a person's coping skills. In both experiences, finding coping skills inadequate, the individual intensifies coping efforts and may develop new skills.

Anxiety

Anxiety is a vague, uneasy feeling, the source of which is often nonspecific or unknown to the individual. The feeling of discomfort ranges from mild apprehension to panic. The hospitalized client may experience anxiety from pain, fear of death, and actual or imagined losses, such as disfigurement or the inability to return to a previous lifestyle.

People experience anxiety when they expect one thing to happen and something different occurs. For example, if a client expected to have a biopsy and was then told that he needs more-radical surgery, anxiety can narrow the perceptual field and interfere with successful coping. People who are unable to perform or think they will be unable to perform to their expecta-

tions experience a form of anxiety called performance anxiety. See Chapter 47 for more information on anxiety.

When you discover that he did not have breakfast, Mr. Osceola agrees to let you prepare lunch for him. A proud man, he refuses to use the crutches that lie at his bedside. When he gets out of bed, he gets around in an old wheelchair a neighbor loaned him. While preparing lunch, how would you assess Mr. Osceola further for anxiety and the methods he uses to cope?

Crisis

A **crisis** is an upset in a balanced or stable state for which the usual methods of adaptation and coping are not sufficient. Crises usually occur secondary to unusual or threatening situations that demand a decrease in stressors or a reallocation of energy. A person in crisis is faced with overwhelming adaptive tasks. As anxiety rises, the person's ability to perceive what is happening declines steadily. Internal disorganization and feelings of helplessness occur. Feelings of grief and shame can also be associated with a crisis.

There are two major types of crises: developmental and situational. A **developmental crisis** occurs when a person is unable to complete the tasks needed for a particular developmental level. A developmental crisis can occur at any stage of life and may result from a wide range of stressors (Table 52–1). A **situational crisis** is a physically or psychologically hazardous situation that is not easily antici-

TABLE 52–1
Developmental Crises

Developmental Level	Approximate Age	Stressors That Could Precipitate a Crisis
Infancy	Birth to about 2 years	• Lack of unconditional love. • Lack of basic needs being met. • Lack of ability to make beginning environmental manipulations.
Childhood	About 2 to 6 years	• Inability to influence others with verbal communication. • Inability to delay satisfaction. • Inability to increase motor control. • Refusal of others to grant autonomy.
Juvenile	6 to 9 years	• Entry into school. • Inability to learn appropriate roles. • Inability to produce assignments. • Difficulty with pal relationship. • Inability to compete, compromise, or cooperate. • Blocks to increasing motor, social, and/or physiological growth.
Preadolescence	9 to 12 years	• Confusion about physiological (sex) changes.
Adolescence	12 to 21+ years	• Blocks to evaluation of strengths and limitations.
Adulthood	21+ to death	• Inability to produce children. • Parenthood, especially firstborn. • Blocks to communication with other age groups. • Inability to achieve personal concept of success. • Inability to adapt to success.
Old age	Varies	• Extreme physical, social, or economic restrictions. • Blocks to reassessing life experiences. • Inability to face death. • Social or sensory deprivation.

pated and for which a person is inadequately prepared. Even events that many people consider positive, such as graduation, a promotion, or the holidays can precipitate a crisis.

A crisis of either type has the following characteristics:

- Disturbs homeostasis
- Involves loss
- Does not respond to usual adaptive activities
- Is perceived as overwhelming or life-threatening
- Is self-limiting
- Demands a relatively immediate response
- Produces openness to change
- Brings unresolved problems to the foreground
- Is associated with increased affect and decreased communication abilities
- Follows a definite sequence: shock, scattered attempt at problem-solving, failure, tension further increased, disorganization, resolution (precrisis level of functioning, depression and withdrawal, or growth)
- Requires intervention to reach equilibrium

Because of its emergency qualities, a crisis usually lasts no more than 24 or perhaps 48 hours. In crisis, the person's mind, body, and spirit attempt to return to a balanced state of homeostasis. Being confronted by a crisis event or events requires new responses to adapt to the situation. These new responses may be internal competencies, such as new ways to think through a problem, or they may be external social skills, such as phoning a suicide prevention center. Either the problem is solved or the person adapts to the lack of a solution. In either case, a new state of balance is reached. Because of the temporary state of disorganization, the person in crisis is likely to remember old problems related to the present event.

Methods of Coping

However, not all stressors produce a crisis. People respond to stress in many ways, all intended to alleviate the stress and increase their level of comfort. Stress that is primarily psychological or interpersonal can be dealt with by thought or mental mechanisms. Most of these mechanisms are used to varying degrees by all people at some time in their lives. In fact, people tend to use whatever coping devices are familiar to them, whether those devices are ultimately helpful or not. Difficulties, including crisis, may occur if a person has only a few coping strategies and these are not useful in a situation. Any coping mechanism, when used to an extreme, can distort reality and foster problematic relationships.

Common coping behaviors include the following:

- Listening to music or other rhythm forms
- Talking it out with another person
- Sleeping
- Engaging in leisure activities, such as vacationing
- Using emotional releases, such as crying, swearing, fighting, singing, laughing, or whistling
- Being touched or stroked or having sex

Keep in mind that some people are aware of what they do to protect themselves and maintain homeostasis. Others react so automatically that they are not always aware of what they do to reduce stress.

Besides coping strategies, people also respond to stress by using defense mechanisms (Table 52–2). **Defense mechanisms** are mental processes used, without planning or even full awareness, to protect or defend one's (psychological) self from stress and maintain psychological homeostasis. Most defense mechanisms are automatic. Although using defense mechanisms does not imply imbalance or mental illness, if the pat-

TABLE 52–2
Defense Mechanisms

Mechanism	Description
Compensation	Excelling in one area to overcome a real or imagined deficit
Conversion	Converting feelings into a physical disability or symptom
Denial	Avoiding emotional conflicts by refusing to acknowledge anything that might cause intolerable emotional pain
Depersonalization	Losing a sense of identity; having feelings of being someone else
Displacement	Shifting feelings from a less socially acceptable or more threatening object or person to a more acceptable or less threatening one
Identification	Modeling oneself after an admired person
Intellectualization	Denying feelings by answering with detailed impersonal statements
Projection	Attributing unacceptable thoughts or feelings to others
Rationalization	Using an excuse to justify behavior while disguising an unconscious motive
Reaction formation	Acting directly opposite to one's wishes, feelings, or desires
Regression	Behaving in ways that were appropriate at earlier developmental periods
Repression	Placing traumatic situations out of awareness so they cannot be consciously remembered
Sublimation	Redirecting an unacceptable tendency to a more acceptable one
Suppression	Deciding consciously not to act
Transference	Acting toward a stranger as if he or she were a significant other

tern of behavior is sufficiently dominant so as to limit function, defense mechanisms are harmful.

FACTORS AFFECTING STRESS TOLERANCE

While every person has a unique response to stress, some people have more reserve or capacity to resist challenges to self-integrity. This is partly because how a person tolerates and copes with stress is influenced by genetics, lifestyle, culture, developmental stage, physiological characteristics, and psychological traits. In the Cross-Cultural Care chart, we see one man's unique experience with stress in which he displays both effective and ineffective coping.

To help people cope with stressors you need to understand the characteristics of people who are successful in managing stress. Three factors you should con-

sider are perception of the stressful event, resilience, and hardiness.

Perception of a Stressful Event

Stressors are neither positive nor negative but are only stressful if perceived on some level as stressful. Consequently, the stimuli needed to produce stress are individualized. Because the perception of what is stressful, as well as the response to the situation, is highly individualized and fluid, one person may miss a bus to work and start to worry about being fired. Another person may miss the same bus, pull out a novel, and read until the next bus appears. Likewise, a person can be in a state of balance at one moment and imbalance the next. It all depends on the demands of the internal and external environment.

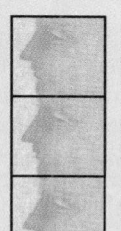

CROSS-CULTURAL CHART
CARING FOR A NATIVE AMERICAN CLIENT

Billy Osceola, the client presented in this chapter, is a Native American of the Seminole tribe. He has always lived on the Big Cypress reservation in Florida. Mr. Osceola runs a smoke shop for the reservation. A number of values and beliefs that Mr. Osceola exhibits tend to be common in Native Americans of the Seminole tribe. Although every client is unique, many members of the Seminole tribe tend to hold the following values and beliefs:

- The shaman relies on a number of medicinal plants and herbs, including St. John's wort, willow, and ginseng. Herbal potions are often used in conjunction with lengthy chants.
- Eating should coincide with hunger rather than being set at three meals a day.
- Family is very important, with extended family the norm.
- Use of silence indicates respect for the other person.
- Eye contact is avoided because it is a sign of disrespect.
- Sacred myths and legends provide spiritual guidance. Religion and healing practices are blended together.
- Illness is caused by disequilibrium with nature. Everything that happens is the result of something else.

Julianna, Mr. Osceola's night nurse, is aware of many of these Seminole values. Let's see how she demonstrates cultural sensitivity with Mr. Osceola:

Julianna: Well, good evening! Was your day better today?

Mr. Osceola: [Nods his head affirmatively]

Julianna: [Observing his downcast eyes and his hand rubbing his left leg slightly above the dressing] Is your leg giving you some trouble tonight?

Mr. Osceola: It hurts still in my foot and calf. I think that is why it is so hard to believe that it is gone. I knew my drinking would get me one day.

Julianna: You are experiencing normal feelings. Our bodies talk to us, don't they? Did you know they call those pains in a missing part phantom pain?

Mr. Osceola: Phantom pain . . . hmmm. I wonder what my shaman would say about phantom pain. He may have some herbs I can take.

Julianna: He may have something for the pain. However, he is not here tonight and I can tell that you are very uncomfortable. May I bring you some of the hospital medicine for tonight?

Mr. Osceola: [Nods his head affirmatively]

Critical Thinking Questions

- What might have happened if Julianna hadn't recognized the importance of respecting Mr. Osceola's beliefs about his shaman and the use of herbs?
- What behaviors did Mr. Osceola exhibit that meet the valued characteristics of the Seminole Native American?
- Why might Mr. Osceola appreciate the theory of phantom pain?

References

Leininger, M. (1991). *Culture care diversity and universality: A theory of nursing.* New York: National League for Nursing Press.
Website URL: *www.seminoletribe.com* Hollywood, Florida, ©1997.

Resilience

The concept of resilience helps to explain individual differences in response to stressors. Haase (1997) defined **resilience** as the process of identifying or developing resources and strengths to flexibly manage stressors to gain a positive outcome, a sense of confidence, mastery, and self-esteem. She and her research team interviewed adolescents with cancer and other chronic illnesses through two cross-sectional studies of courage and resilience. Factors identified as important to resilience included the following:

- Individual protective factors, such as courageous coping, which includes optimistic and confrontative strategies, hope, and spiritual perspective
- Family protective factors, including family adaptation and cohesion
- Social protective factors, including health resources and social connectedness with peers and others with the same or a similar condition

Hardiness

The concept of psychological hardiness is another attempt to explain why some people are less prone to stress than others. Psychological **hardiness,** or the ability to survive stress, is composed of three ingredients:

- Commitment to self, work, family, and important values
- A sense of personal control over one's life
- The ability to see change in one's life as a challenge to master

Levels of basal pituitary-adrenal hormones and beta-endorphins, the body's natural tranquilizers, correlate closely with self-esteem, hardiness, and affective stability (Zorrilla, DeRubeis, & Redei, 1995). Individual and family hardiness are resources that help a person to resist stress (Fig. 52–2).

Mr. Osceola is flushed. He picks at his lunch and rubs the damp rag with herbal potion around and around on his stump. He chants

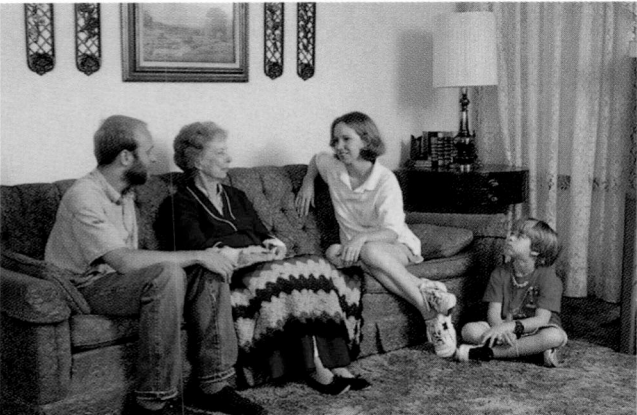

Figure 52–2. Individual and family hardiness are resources that help a person to resist stress.

repeatedly under his breath. You ask to see the herbal cloth so you can visualize the stump dressing better. Mr. Osceola holds it out, but won't let you hold the cloth. You can see drainage on the old dressing. An odor seems to be coming from the wound too. You ask to test his blood for "sugar" and finally touch his hand. Mr. Osceola's skin is burning hot. Have you noticed the signs of hardiness in Mr. Osceola?

ASSESSMENT

Assessment of a client under stress will include obtaining subjective and objective data. A general assessment of the client's coping abilities and stress tolerance can be incorporated in the health history and physical examination. From those assessment findings, you will then focus your assessment activities.

General Assessment of Stress Tolerance and Coping

Health History

Gathering health history information to determine stress tolerance and coping is done by interview. To have a successful interview, you must respect the client, provide privacy, and ensure confidentiality. Throughout the interview, you will begin to build a therapeutic relationship with the client and begin to understand the source of stress. During the interview, ask questions designed to assess the client's stress tolerance and coping, such as those in Box 52-1.

Physical Examination

This portion of the client assessment provides objective data. (For a full discussion of physical examination techniques, review Chapter 10.) Physical signs of

---

BOX 52–1

SAMPLE INTERVIEW QUESTIONS TO ASSESS STRESS TOLERANCE AND COPING

- What has been the most stressful event that has happened to you during this hospitalization/holiday season?
- How do you feel when you are stressed?
- Have you experienced any recent changes in your life (in the last year) related to your health, family, lifestyle habits, daily activities, work, or finances? Have you had any losses?
- How would you rate these life changes on a scale of 1 to 10 (from least stressful to most stressful)?
- How have you coped with similar stressors before? What do you do to make yourself feel less stressed?
- Have you received treatment for any stress-related problems in the past?

stress would be observed during this examination. Cardiovascular signs of the stress response are an increased heart rate, increased blood pressure, and palpitations. Also, the client may complain of headaches, muscle tension, and gastrointestinal disturbances. The client also may complain of disturbed sleep, unusual fatigue, restlessness, and poor cognitive function. However, these physical signs alone cannot justify a conclusion that the client has a stress response.

Focused Assessment for Ineffective Individual Coping

Assess the client's stressors carefully, because you cannot judge the effectiveness of the client's coping strategies if you incorrectly identify the problem or stressor. First, find out how the client views the situation. Further assessment of the client's perception of the stress will help the client make proper choices among coping behaviors. Also, determine what external and internal environmental demands are being placed on the client. Does the client use too little or too much energy in attempting to adapt? Talk with the client's significant others to determine their perception of the stressful event. Does the situation seem threatening or overwhelming to the client? These data are essential to effectively assess and then analyze the client's situation. After this assessment, if you believe that the client demonstrates inadequate coping behaviors and problem-solving abilities, you would make a nursing diagnosis of *Ineffective individual coping*.

Defining Characteristics

Characteristics for the diagnosis of *Ineffective individual coping* are observable data in three categories. First, ineffective coping can be defined as a change in the person's usual pattern of behaving. This change may be in the usual communication pattern, the ability to meet role expectations, or the use of social supports. Second, ineffective coping can be observed as signs and symptoms of distress such as tension, fatigue, sleep disturbance, poor concentration, ineffective problem-solving, or inability to meet basic needs. Third, ineffective coping is seen in the form of self-destructive behavior such as substance abuse, risk-taking behavior, or other coping mechanisms that hinder resolution of the problem.

Related Factors

Coping with stress is related to the need to manage thinking patterns, alleviate the physical manifestations of stress, and develop coping strategies. First, the ability to cope with stressors depends on the person's cognitive appraisal of the situation. Cognitive appraisal means the worth or value assigned by thoughts and feelings—in other words, how you think about something. Second, the discomfort of stress results from signs and symptoms of the physiological stress response. Energy is directed at managing the somatic signs of tension and is not available for effective cop-

ing responses. Last, successful coping depends on the repertoire of coping skills.

Focused Assessment for Ineffective Denial

At certain stages of coping with and adapting to a stressful event, denial is a useful and healthy defense mechanism that permits the client to retain hope. Assess the degree of denial and its effectiveness as a coping strategy by asking yourself questions such as the following. Has the client delayed seeking care to the detriment of his health? Does the client refuse treatment even after saying that he understands its benefits? Does the client's nonverbal behavior show fear even though he says he has no fear? Has the client been abusing alcohol or other substances? If you find many positive responses to these questions, the client has probably used denial inappropriately with untoward health effects. If that is the case, then you would make a nursing diagnosis of *Ineffective denial*.

Defining Characteristics

Defining characteristics of ineffective denial are the evidence that the person is denying that a problem exists, the manifestations of the problem, or the effects of the problem. Additionally, there must be evidence of negative effects from the denial. Denial can result in a client delaying to seek health care or refusing health care. It can also result in noncompliance with a potentially helpful therapeutic regimen.

Related Factors

Factors related to the nursing diagnosis *Ineffective denial* may be anxiety, fear of death, loss of autonomy, and defense against a perceived threat. Nursing interventions are aimed at reducing anxiety, helping the person develop the perception of control, and reducing the perception of threat.

You are unable to test Mr. Osceola's blood glucose level. He says that he did not have any insulin in the house anyway. He wants you to leave because, "You are trying to do things I don't need." You tell him you'll leave, but you have to replace the dressing on his leg first. "Fine, hurry up and do it so you will leave me be!" You recognize that Mr. Osceola is denying the need for your help out of fear of the consequences of the infection. How can you reduce his fear and establish trust?

DIAGNOSIS

After reviewing all assessment data, such as reports of a recent loss of a loved one, heart palpitations, and inability to sleep, you must cluster the data to distinguish the relevant data from irrelevant data. The determination of patterns and recognition of cues or defining characteristics will assist you in making an appropriate diagnosis, as shown in the data clustering chart.

Use the diagnosis *Ineffective individual coping* when the client's diagnostic cues include observable anxiety,

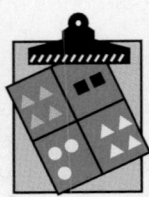

CLUSTERING DATA TO MAKE A NURSING DIAGNOSIS
STRESS-RELATED PROBLEMS

Data Cluster	Diagnosis
26-year-old female is admitted to emergency department with foot laceration resulting from accidental injury. History reveals complaints of poor appetite, poor concentration, neck and back pain, and insomnia. Works 32 hours per week and attends college full time. Single mother of two children.	*Ineffective individual coping* related to situational crisis
Mr. E., age 70, was diagnosed with prostate cancer 2 weeks after the death of his wife 1 year ago. No children, but cousin lives nearby. Refused cancer therapy because, "I don't have any prostate problems." Client's cousin brought him to doctor's office when he complained of not urinating for 2 days.	*Ineffective denial* related to fear of death and personal loss
33-year-old female seeking care in the emergency department. Pacing, wringing hands, and crying. Sweating profusely. Blood pressure and pulse elevated with respirations at 32 and shallow. Says that husband left 2 weeks ago, she recently lost her job, and, "I'm afraid I'm going crazy."	*Anxiety* related to stress of lifestyle change

his behavior and language are disorganized and difficult to understand, and he is experiencing a life event that tends to produce crisis. However, when the client delays seeking health care to the point of harm, refuses treatment after hearing the benefits of care, and shows signs of physiological imbalance, consider using the nursing diagnosis *Ineffective denial.* The differentiating factor between the two diagnoses is the inappropriate use of denial as a coping behavior.

PLANNING

Together, you and your client will need to develop realistic, measurable goals and outcomes designed to help the client better tolerate stressful events by using effective coping skills. Planning for a client who is experiencing stress would include the following overall goals:

- The client is able to identify potential stressors.
- The client demonstrates, both verbally and behaviorally, decreased stress.
- The client develops effective methods of coping with stress.

Expected Outcomes for the Client With Ineffective Individual Coping

The client whose coping and problem-solving abilities interfere with his life will need assistance with setting realistic outcomes. Basic expected outcomes for the client with ineffective individual coping include those listed as follows:

- The client will demonstrate effective coping behaviors as evidenced by identifying the stressor, identifying usual coping behaviors, discussing coping alternatives, and choosing and using a coping strategy in an actual situation.
- The client will effectively solve an identified problem, as evidenced by identifying the problem, discussing the steps of the problem-solving process, applying the problem-solving process to the problem in discussion, and implementing the problem-solving process.
- The client will return to a previous level of functioning, as evidenced by the client maintaining an adequate balance of rest and sleep, achieving an appropriate level of social interaction and daily activities, and developing problem-solving techniques to decrease the effects of stress.

Expected Outcomes for the Client With Ineffective Denial

Denial can be a useful coping mechanism to defend oneself from a stressful event. Rather than setting a goal of eliminating denial, you will need to help the client increase stress tolerance and use of healthy coping skills. Expected outcomes for a client with ineffective denial may include the following:

- The client will demonstrate a low to moderate anxiety level, as evidenced by reduced signs and symptoms secondary to relaxation techniques.
- The client will use the facts of his health status to achieve his full health potential, as evidenced by the client receiving the facts of his illness in a supported manner and using that information in a way that allows compliance with the health care regimen.

Mr. Osceola will not look at his leg while you rapidly change the dressing. You note that the amputation incision is coming open in the center and producing large amounts of foul, purulent drainage from the opening. The skin is red and edematous around the incision. You place a new dressing on the leg and ask Mr. Osceola if he knows that his leg is infected. Can you write an expected outcome that would indicate Mr. Osceola is making progress toward acceptance of the seriousness of his condition?

INTERVENTION

Effective nursing actions are based on an understanding of the concepts of stress and coping behaviors. Interventions either increase coping skills, reduce the physical signs and symptoms of stress, or manage stressors to prevent stress.

Interventions to Increase Coping Skills

The interventions to increase coping skills require establishing a therapeutic relationship and mutual goal-setting with the client. Together the nurse and client analyze the problem (the situation and coping behaviors), define the problem, define goals, and work through and modify coping so it brings a sense of well-being (Heim, 1995). You can help the client effectively cope by using social supports, protecting a vulnerable self, and learning new information. Recent research suggests that increasing a client's coping skills can have a direct relationship with his health status, as described in the State of Nursing Science chart.

Enhancing Social Supports

Positive support, given with unconditional positive regard, provided by a client's social circle is important for effective coping. Encourage and enlist the involvement of family and significant others to help the client tolerate the stressful event. Teach or role model effective support.

If the client has little or no social support, contact appropriate support groups, clergy, or social services to aid the client with further coping strategies. You as the nurse can also enhance social support by listening and using therapeutic communication, teaching techniques, and using supportive behaviors. You can also provide support to the client by ensuring his access to telephones, by encouraging expansion of his social and personal contacts, and by helping significant others gain access to special visitations during critical care or prolonged hospitalizations.

Protecting a Vulnerable Self

Because defense mechanisms may initially allow the client to protect or defend the self to reduce stress or anxiety, you should avoid breaking through the client's defenses unless you first teach him an alternative way to cope. You can use cognitive techniques to reframe the stressor in more acceptable terms, help the client identify strengths, or introduce information about the stressor in small, manageable amounts. When the client feels safe and his anxiety is controlled, you may be able to successfully help the client recognize the negative effects of defensive behavior.

A**ction** A**lert!**
Avoid confronting denial unless you have evidence that the client can cope with the loss of this defense mechanism.

Gaining Control Through Knowledge

A common source of anxiety and stress is the inability to control a situation that often accompanies a serious illness. Knowledge is power. While it may not change the situation, it can increase the sense of control. Fear of the unknown is a major contributor to stress. Provide information to help the client and family feel a sense of control. However, you must assess the client's readiness to receive information.

Interventions to Reduce the Physiological Stress Response

Relaxation is an intervention that nurses use to reduce stress when working with ill or healthy clients. Further interventions to consider include using suggestion, teaching coping thoughts, using guided imagery, teaching inner dialogue approaches, and practicing meditation.

Inducing the Relaxation Response

Relaxation therapy has been shown in research to reduce anxiety and stress in psychiatric clients and may be useful in reducing the length of hospital stay in surgical patients, as discussed in the Cost of Care chart. Clients sometimes are encouraged to develop their own relaxation and stress-reduction audiotapes. Progressive relaxation techniques include helping the client relax by focusing on breathing or other body sensations. These measures have been shown to reduce stress and enhance client coping (McCain, Zeller, Cella, Urbanski, & Novak, 1996).

Using Guided Imagery

The autonomic nervous system connects the mind with every cell in the body. Thus, a thought held in the mind can affect hormonal balance, blood flow, and metabolism. To a certain extent, an image can actually contribute to health or illness. Relaxation of the body facili-

THE STATE OF NURSING SCIENCE

STRESS AND COPING IN PATIENTS WITH CHRONIC ILLNESS

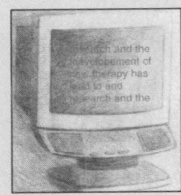

WHAT ARE THE ISSUES?

A chronic illness such as arthritis affects most aspects of a person's life, including self-care ability and relationships with others. To offer effective education and support for people with such chronic illnesses, you need to understand the subjective experience of the client, especially in the area of stress and coping.

WHAT RESEARCH HAS BEEN CONDUCTED?

Past research has identified some of the many stressors experienced by people with arthritis. These include pain, changes in mobility and self-care, and changes in relationships with others. People cope with such stressors in a variety of ways. Mahat (1997) surveyed 53 adults with rheumatoid arthritis to see what they identified as stressors and what they did to cope with them. Mahat also asked people to rate the effectiveness of the coping strategies they used.

To conduct this research, Mahat developed a checklist of 10 common stressors based on past reports in the literature. The coping scale used was previously developed based on Lazarus and Folkman's theory of stress. This theory identifies two major types of coping strategies: problem-focused and emotion-focused. Problem-focused strategies would be those used when the threat of the stressor could be changed. Emotion-focused strategies would be those used when the stressor could not be changed.

Downe-Wamboldt and Melanson (1998) conducted home-based interviews with 64 adults with rheumatoid arthritis and used path analysis to examine relationships among variables that might explain differences in the level of psychological well-being among the people studied. These variables included severity of impairment from the disease, social status, perceived stressors, coping strategies, and psychological well-being. One advantage of path analysis is that it considers the effect of many variables at one time. This is especially helpful when researchers are trying to understand something as complex as human adaptation to stress.

WHAT HAS THE RESEARCH CONCLUDED?

The most frequent stressors identified in Mahat's survey included pain, mobility changes, and difficulty in self-care. These are consistent with past research and what is known about the major features of rheumatoid arthritis. The most frequent coping strategies that subjects reported using were those categorized as "optimistic." Examples of "optimistic" strategies include using positive thinking or maintaining a positive outlook. These strategies are considered examples of emotion-focused coping. The second most frequent type of coping strategy

used was a confrontive strategy, such as problem-solving. These two types of coping strategies—optimistic and confrontive—were also rated the most effective for this sample of people with rheumatoid arthritis.

Mahat also found that the longer a person lived with rheumatoid arthritis, the more negatively family relationships were affected and the more likely evasive coping strategies were used. This study rated the two types of coping strategies noted above—optimistic and confrontive—as most effective for coping with the impact of the disease on family relationships.

Mahat concluded that, in addition to helping people develop effective coping strategies, nurses need to prioritize effective pain management as a goal for their patients with rheumatoid arthritis. The clients studied indicated that pain was their number-one stressor.

Downe-Wamboldt and Melanson found that the variables they studied helped them understand almost half of the difference in psychological well-being in the people with rheumatoid arthritis interviewed for their study. For example, people who perceived their illness as a challenge had increased psychological well-being, while those who perceived their illness as harmful had decreased psychological well-being. As in the study by Mahat, optimistic coping strategies were the ones used most frequently by people with rheumatoid arthritis.

Downe-Wamboldt and Melanson also examined the effect of severity of impairment on the other variables. They found that even when people had severe impairment from arthritis, they could still have higher scores in well-being if they reported perceiving their disease as a challenge rather than as harmful. Thus, current objective measures of the severity of symptoms of chronic disease do not always give us insight into how the person lives with the disease. For this, we need to ask people about their perceptions and respond to them as individuals.

WHAT IS THE FUTURE OF RESEARCH IN THIS AREA?

Now that research has identified sources of stress for people with arthritis, we need to study the outcomes of various types of coping strategies. It is also important to identify ways to help people develop effective coping strategies that will enable them to adapt to the changes that result from chronic disease. Researchers also need to develop better measurement tools for stress and coping.

REFERENCES

Downe-Wamboldt, B.L., & Melanson, P.M. (1998). A causal model of coping and well-being in elderly people with arthritis. *Journal of Advanced Nursing, 27*(6), 1109–1116.

Mahat, G. (1997). Perceived stressors and coping strategies among individuals with rheumatoid arthritis. *Journal of Advanced Nursing, 25*(6), 1144–1150.

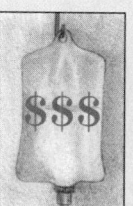
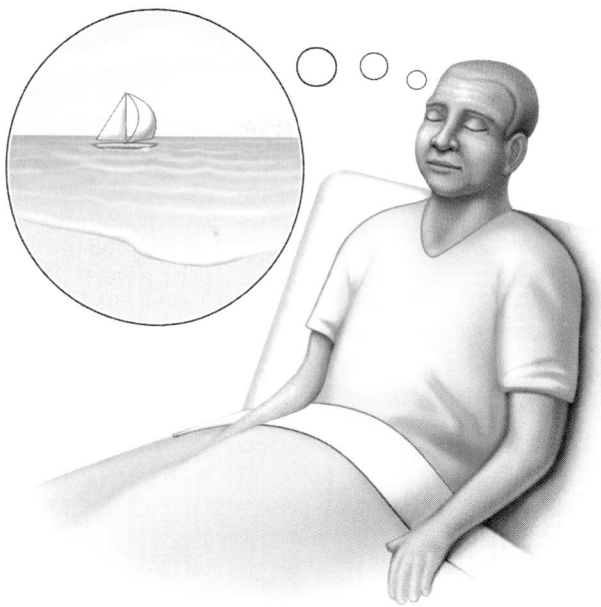

Figure 52–3. Relaxation facilitates the creation of positive internal images, which in turn signal the muscles to relax further and promote better health.

tates the creation of positive internal images, which in turn signal the muscles to relax and promote better health (Fig. 52–3). Imagery is also a tool for distraction when a person is under stress, in pain, or fearful.

Teaching specific stress-reduction methods can provide clients with strategies to offset ineffective individual coping and ineffective denial. By developing a repertoire of alternative skills, some of which are described in the Considering the Alternatives chart, a client can begin to have a realistic expectation of being able to cope.

Practicing Adaptive Thinking

Cognitive therapy refers to methods of treatment that help a person change attitudes, perceptions, and patterns of thinking from irrational to realistic thoughts about the self and situations. Here are two techniques.

SELF-SUGGESTION

To use suggestion for stress reduction, start by obtaining data on sources of the client's stress. Then agree on an individualized stress-reduction suggestion. Help the client to a relaxed state. Then repeat or ask the client to repeat the stress-reduction suggestion.

Once the stressful situation has been identified, you and the client decide which portion of the situation to focus on and how the suggestions can be worded most effectively for that client. For example, in a situation in which a client becomes highly stressed talking with a physician, the client may be taught to use the statement: "I can stay calm when talking with my doctor."

COPING THOUGHTS

Another stress reduction method that can be used for self-care purposes is teaching stress coping thoughts (Davis, McKay, & Eschelman, 1995). This approach is based on cognitive psychology theory, which holds that thoughts rule feelings. The way the future or present is imagined intensifies or decreases the feelings experienced. For example, being late for an assignment can result in stress for you or it may result in a calm, problem-focused response. Positively interpreting lateness will likely lead to feelings of calmness. Negatively interpreting the event can bring knots to the stomach and an increased heart rate and rapid respirations.

When working to reverse negative thoughts, coping statements can be used to reduce stress at various points in the stressful situation. For example, when anticipating the situation, you could say (or teach the client to say), "I'm going to be all right. I won't let this upset me." As the situation begins, you could say, "I'll take this step by step. I'm handling this right now."

CONSIDERING THE ALTERNATIVES
RELAXATION THERAPIES

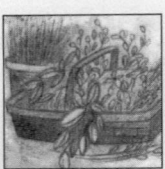

Stressful conditions have been shown in countless experiments in both animals and humans to have potentially harmful effects on immune function and resistance to disease (Brown, 1998). What makes the difference between whether or not a stressor harms the mind or body?—Our reactions. In this chart we will therefore examine how to enhance the ability—in both our clients and ourselves—to take charge of reactions to stressors so that we respond in a way that is more consistent with good health.

Relaxation comes in many forms, and people *do* many things to relax. This is healthy. Yet a very important form of relaxation involves *doing* very little, or even "nothing." This is difficult for many people. There are many forms or techniques one can practice to achieve relaxation, and there is ample evidence for the beneficial effects of relaxation on health. One master of *taijiquan (tai chi chuan)* and *qigong (chi kung)* calls relaxation "the fine art of doing nothing and achieving everything" (Ha & Olsen, 1996).

Researcher, author, and Harvard professor Herbert Benson, M.D., has studied and written extensively about stress and its effects. He coined the phrase "the relaxation response" to describe a potential physiological response, or ability, that we all have, which is essentially the opposite of the fight-or-flight response. The relaxation response can protect us against the harmful effects of stress because it can lower the heart rate (and in some cases blood pressure), lower the respiratory rate, and benefit homeostasis in general (Benson, 1993). In part, these changes occur because relaxation is related to increased parasympathetic activity, with a concomitant decrease in sympathetic nervous activity. In recent years the emerging field of psycho-neuro-immunology has lent credence to the existence of the relaxation response by documenting the mind-body effects of stress, our reactions to it, and the moderating effects of various interventions.

According to Benson, the relaxation response can be elicited in many ways. Dr. Benson developed a simple technique, drawn from a number of meditative disciplines. It combines a comfortable posture, relaxing the muscles of the body, and slow, natural breathing, with focus on a word or phrase that has personal "resonance." He recommends daily practice of 10 to 20 minutes.

To some, meditation sounds like an esoteric practice associated with religions of the Far East, such as Hinduism or Buddhism. In fact, meditative practice has been a part of most religions, including Judaism and Christianity. To many people, prayer, or religious contemplation, is a form of meditation. But meditation can be practiced without particular religious affiliation, as in the relaxation response and the practice of "mindfulness." According to Ha and Olsen (1996, p. 15), mindfulness is "a special attention to the moment that involves body, mind and spirit." Mindfulness is related to Buddhist meditation. While producing relaxation, its aim is "to nurture an inner balance of mind that allows you to face *all* life situations with greater stability, clarity, understanding, and even wisdom, and to act or respond effectively and with dignity out of that clarity and understanding" (Kabat-Zinn, 1993, p. 261). Jon Kabat-Zinn, Ph.D., has led groups in the practice of mindfulness and has found positive benefits for thousands of people as a complement to their medical care.

Qigong (chi kung) is a meditative practice in the Chinese tradition of the martial and healing arts. Literally meaning *energy* or *breath practice, qigong* focuses on developing and allowing the free circulation of *qi,* or internal energy. The various styles of *qigong* use breath, movement, postures, and mental focus to achieve this free circulation. Research has begun to support the use of *qigong* as a general practice, and adjunctively in the treatment of many medical conditions. For example, in hypertensive patients, *qigong* has been found effective in reducing the incidence of stroke and related mortality. Increases in hormone levels and bone density and improvements in a variety of blood chemistry parameters have been found with the practice of *qigong.* In China, where mainstream medicine tends to view *qigong* as beneficial, the practice is often taught to patients and advocated for a number of diseases, including cancer (Sancier, 1996). It has been estimated that up to 80 million Chinese practice some form of *qigong* daily (Mayer, 1996–1997).

(continued)

And when the situation ends, you could say, "I got through this and I did well. I'm able to handle this situation."

Once coping thoughts have been formulated, ask the client to write them on index cards and place them on the bedside table, tape them to the bathroom mirror, or place them in any spot routinely seen. Have the client read the coping thought cards frequently.

Action Alert!
Ward off stress burnout by designing some coping thought cards for yourself. Refer to them up to 20 times a day for greatest effectiveness.

CONSIDERING THE ALTERNATIVES
RELAXATION THERAPIES (continued)

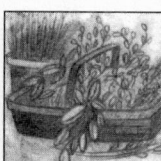 Biofeedback is a technique of teaching physiological self-control using instruments that measure bodily processes such as skin temperature, heart rate, muscle electrical activity, galvanic skin response, and sometimes brainwaves. The trainee is made aware of these measurements visually on a computer screen, or via audible tones, and learns to control these processes using techniques in many ways similar to those described above. Breathing, progressive muscle relaxation, a sense of "mindfulness," and an alert yet passive "letting go" attitude are all elements of biofeedback. The patient is taught the techniques and encouraged to practice them regularly on his or her own. With the instruments allowing the person to perceive "inside-the-skin" events, the techniques allow for voluntary control of autonomic, normally automatic and unconscious processes (Green & Green, 1977). One of the common techniques taught in biofeedback is hand-warming, which after a single session in one experiment resulted in increased cardiac output and decreased systemic vascular resistance in a group of clients with cardiac disorders (Moser, Dracup, Woo, & Stevenson, 1997). Biofeedback has been widely used in pain programs, by physical therapists, with clients who have respiratory conditions, and by many psychotherapists. Unlike many of the other techniques discussed in this chart, biofeedback training is often reimbursable by insurance carriers.

All of the practices that we have been discussing have a number of commonalities and similar aims. People may use other methods, such as yoga, *taijiquan,* quiet contemplation of nature or music, guided imagery, or simply whatever works for them to achieve relaxation. In fact, in one study, a variety of interventions were shown to be equally effective in reducing the symptoms of job stress, such as anxiety, depression, fatigue, and confusion (Field, Quintino, Henteleff, Wells-Kiefe, & Delvecchio-Feinberg, 1997). In the words of one meditation teacher, "I often compare the mind in meditation to a jar of muddy water: The more I leave the water without interfering or stirring it, the more the particles of dirt will sink to the bottom, letting the natural clarity of the water shine through" (Rinpoche, 1993, p. 2). What is

evident is that—however one achieves it—achieving quiet and relaxation has positive effects on many levels: mind, body, and spirit.

Resources

Publications that can expand and keep your knowledge of complementary and alternative medicine current:

Goleman, D., & Gurin, J. (1993). *Mind body medicine: How to use your mind for better health.* New York: Consumer Reports Books.
Green, E., & Green, A. (1997). *Beyond biofeedback.* Fort Wayne, IN: Knoll.
Ha, F., & Olsen, E. (1996). *Yiquan and the nature of energy: The fine art of doing nothing and achieving everything.* Berkeley, CA: Summerhouse.
Schafer, W. (1992). *Stress management for wellness* (2nd ed.). Orlando, FL: Harcourt Brace Jovanovich.

References

Benson, H. (1993). The relaxation response. In D. Goleman & J. Gurin (Eds.), *Mind body medicine: How to use your mind for better health* (pp 233–257). New York: Consumer Reports Books.
Brown, W.A. (1998). The placebo effect. *Scientific American, 278*(1), 90–95.
Field, T., Quintino, O., Henteleff, T., Wells-Kiefe, L., & Delvecchio-Feinberg, G. (1997). Job stress reduction therapies. *Alternative Therapies in Health and Medicine, 3*(4), 54–56.
Green, E., & Green, A. (1977). *Beyond biofeedback.* Fort Wayne, IN: Knoll.
Ha, F., & Olsen, E. (1996). *Yiquan and the nature of energy: The fine art of doing nothing and achieving everything.* Berkeley, CA: Summerhouse.
Kabat-Zinn, J. (1993). Mindfulness meditation: Health benefits of an ancient Buddhist practice. In D. Goleman & J. Gurin (Eds.), *Mind body medicine: How to use your mind for better health* (pp 259–275). New York: Consumer Reports Books.
Mayer, M. (1996–1997). Qigong and behavioral medicine: An integrated approach to chronic pain. *Qi—The Journal of Traditional Eastern Health and Fitness,* (Winter 1996–1997), 20–31.
Moser, D.K., Dracup, K., Woo, M.A., & Stevenson, L.W. (1997). Voluntary control of vascular tone by using skin-temperature biofeedback-relaxation in patients with advanced heart failure. *Alternative Therapies in Health and Medicine, 3*(1), 51–59.
Rinpoche, S. (1993). *The Tibetan book of living and dying.* New York: HarperCollins.
Sancier, K.M. (1996). Medical applications of Qigong. *Alternative Therapies in Health and Medicine, 2*(1), 40–46.
Schafer, W. (1992). *Stress management for wellness* (2nd ed.). Orlando, FL: Harcourt Brace Jovanovich.

Increasing Receptivity

INNER DIALOGUE

Inner dialogue may be of help to clients who are unable to verbalize their thoughts and feelings directly. People who use self-blame or guilt may find help through inner dialogue, too. It is a structured way of providing positive direction without focusing on self-destructive feelings. Clients who want to solve a work-related problem can turn to their inner "work" advisers.

Inner dialogue is based on the idea that everyone has an intuitive wisdom. Before using the inner adviser, clients must prepare. Have the client ask the following:

• If I had an inner adviser, what would he, she, or it look like?

- What characteristics would my inner adviser have that would be helpful to me?
- What is the best way to communicate with my inner adviser?
- What are my usual body symptoms that could be giving me messages about imbalances in my body or mind?
- In what ways have I been stressing myself lately?

The answers to these questions provide valuable clues to help the client create a dialogue with the self to become receptive to one's own intuitive wisdom.

Action **A**lert!
Use mutual goal-setting to explore interventions that are consistent with the client's values and beliefs.

MEDITATION

Meditation is an effective way to calm the body and mind. Meditation may be associated with religious practices or just a way of freeing the mind and focusing on positive messages. The practice of meditation is used to find a sense of oneness with the self, other people, the universe, or a god. The therapeutic benefits of meditation include relaxation, stress relief, decreased oxygen consumption, decreased heart rate and blood pressure, and improved immune system function.

Interventions to Manage Stress

Interventions to manage stress include preventing crises, intervening in crises, and teaching hardiness skills.

Preventing Crises

Preventing a crisis is always preferable to intervening in a crisis that already exists. To help prevent a crisis, make sure that all of the client's basic needs are met before you leave the unit or the client's home, or before the client leaves the clinic. Ask the client about his daily needs. Communicate clearly to staff regarding additional unmet needs prior to leaving for the day. Before discharge, make referrals to home health nurses after consulting with client about any anticipated unmet needs.

Anticipate situations that could precipitate a crisis. Tell the client you are available to talk. For example, before surgery, offer to talk with your client about his thoughts, feelings, and expected changes in his body or life. Prepare the client for expected changes. Refer the client to a discussion group or support group for pertinent life changes. The client may benefit from a new parent group, a pre-retirement group, a new ostomy group, or a group for newly diagnosed diabetics.

Intervening in Crises

If your client is already in crisis, realize that he is already overloaded with decisions, thoughts, and feelings. Use the following interventions to help him navigate the crisis successfully:

- Use a calm, slow tone of voice, attentive body posture, and eye contact. As needed, orient the client to who you are and where he is.
- Use short phrases to reduce sensory input.
- Avoid talking about the future. Instead, stay with what the client is experiencing at the moment.
- Point out any movement toward dealing with the crisis: "You're sounding calmer now."
- As the client's anxiety level declines (his speech slows, for example, or his pacing stops), begin to focus on problem-solving. Use such phrases as, "If I hear you right, the problem is that . . . ."
- Identify the client strengths as you observe them. Underline their importance in helping the client get through this crisis.

Once the problem is identified, locate resources to help with the crisis. For example, a possible resource might be a clinical specialist in psychiatric or mental health nursing. Another resource might be a friend who could bridge the gap between a hospital stay and going home by providing companionship for the discharged client. For a suicidal person, make sure he has the number of a 24-hour crisis line and agrees to call that number, you, or another health care professional at specific set times until the crisis passes. Tell a hospitalized suicidal client that you must share this information with other staff involved in the client's care, so they can help keep him safe.

Action **A**lert!
Suicidal and homicidal thoughts, feelings, or actions must be recorded in nursing notes and reported verbally to the nurse in charge and other caregivers.

Teaching Hardiness Skills

Hardiness is the ability to survive stress. Exercise is a good antidote to stress but may be short-term. Jogging or lifting weights after an argument can help that evening, but the next morning stress levels can rise if the stress-provoking situation still exists. Hardiness skills are long-term inoculations against stressors. Three techniques are especially helpful: focusing, reconstructing stressful situations, and compensating through self-improvement.

FOCUSING

Ask the client to focus on recognizing bodily signals that stress is interfering with comfort. To help the client focus, ask "Where do you carry stress in your body?" or "Where is the stress located in your body?" Ask the client to make a list of things that are bothering him today. After he completes the list, ask, "What is keeping you from feeling terrific today?" Develop affirmations such as, "This day is getting better and better," or provide other comfort measures in collaboration with the client to enhance his comfort.

RECONSTRUCTING

The client can enhance hardiness by reconstructing stressful situations in a way that puts the experience in perspective. Help the client reconstruct a stressful situation by asking the client to think about a recent episode of distress. Then have him write down three things that could have happened to make it turn out better. Finally, ask the client to write down three ways it could have gotten worse. This exercise increases the client's ability to put the situation in perspective, a useful procedure for reducing stress.

COMPENSATING

Compensating through self-improvement will lower a client's stress level. Compensation works most effectively with stressors that cannot be avoided, such as illness, impending divorce, unexpected death, or the loss of a loved one. The feeling of loss of control that results from this kind of event can be balanced by taking on a new challenge, such as learning to sew, teaching someone a skill, or helping someone else. These efforts can reassure the client that he can still cope with life.

EVALUATION

Maintaining the effectiveness of a client's coping abilities is an ongoing process that includes client input. Evaluation of the expected outcomes will let you know if your interventions and nursing care were effective. If stressors were not identified, stress was not reduced, and new coping behaviors were not effective, then the overall goals were not met. Reassess and adjust the care plan to meet the client's needs.

KEY PRINCIPLES

- Stress can be physiological, psychosocial, cultural, developmental, or situational. Stress, stressors, and adaptation interact in a highly individualized way to give a total mind, body, and spirit effect. What is stressful for one person may not be stressful for another.
- Homeostasis is a healthy, relatively balanced state that is maintained by physiological balancers, coping behaviors, defense mechanisms, resilience, and hardiness. You will support all attempts to cope, teaching new growth-promoting coping skills.
- Psychoneuroimmunology refers to the interface between the brain and immunology. The evidence for the effects of stress on immune competence is compelling.
- Coping is situation specific and a major component in the relationship between stress and health.
- Anxiety is a common reaction to stress in both clients and nurses. At higher levels, anxiety may precipitate a crisis.
- Illness can be thought of as an imbalance that occurs when the body cannot adapt to complex physical and emotional stressors in the environment.
- Crises are either developmental or situational and upset the balanced or stable state. Balance is restored either through solving the problem or adapting to the lack of a solution.
- Resilience is the process of identifying or developing resources and strengths to flexibly manage stressors to gain a positive outcome, a sense of confidence, mastery, and self-esteem.
- Hardiness explains why some people do not experience high levels of stress. Hardiness is composed of control, commitment, and challenge.

BIBLIOGRAPHY

Ashenberg, M.D., Maier, N.P., Lambert, S.A., & McAiley, L.G. (1996). Easing the wait: development of a pager program for families. *Pediatric Nursing, 22*(2), 103–107, 112–113.
Chalmers, K., Thomson, K., & Degner, L.F. (1996). Information, support, and communication needs of women with a family history of breast cancer. *Cancer Nursing, 19*(3), 204–213.
Chlan, L.L. (1995). Psychophysiolgic responses of mechanically ventilated patients to music: A pilot study. *American Journal of Critical Care, 4*(3), 233–238.
Clark, C.C. (1995). Exploring guided imagery. *The Nursing Spectrum, 5*(10), 9.
Clark, C.C. (1995). Stress management. *The Nursing Spectrum, 5*(2), 12–14.
Clark, C.C. (1996a). Stress management. In C.C. Clark (Ed.), *Wellness practitioner: Concepts, research, and strategies* (pp 68–95). New York: Springer Publishing Company.
Davis, M., McKay, M., & Eschelman, E.R. (1995). *The relaxation and stress reduction workbook.* Richmond, CA: New Harbinger Publications.
Ell, K. (1996). Social networks, social support and coping with serious illness: The family connection. *Social Science & Medicine, 42*(2), 173–183.
Galloway, S.C., & Graydon, J.E. (1996). Uncertainty, symptom distress, and information needs after surgery for cancer of the colon. *Cancer Nursing, 19*(2), 112–117.
Haase, J.E. (1997). Hopeful teenagers with cancer: Living courage. *Reflections, 23*(1), 20.
Hagerty, B.M., Williams, R.A., Coyne, J.C., & Early, M.R. (1996). Sense of belonging and indicators of social and psychological functioning. *Archives of Psychiatric Nursing, 10*(4), 235–244.
Heim, E. (1995). Coping-based intervention strategies. *Patient Education & Counseling, 26*(1), 145–151.
Houldin, A.D., & Wasserbauer, N. (1996). Psychosocial needs of older cancer patients: A pilot study abstract. *MEDSURG Nursing, 54*(4), 253–256.
Huang, C. (1995). Hardiness and stress: A critical review. *Maternal-Child Nursing Journal, 23*(3), 82–89.
Janelli, L.M., Kanask, G.W., Jones, H.M., & Kennedy, M.C. (1995). Exploring music intervention with restrained patients. *Nursing Forum, 30*(4), 12–18.
Janelli, L.M., Kanask, G.W., Jones, H.M., & Kennedy, M.C. (1996). What do cancer patients identify as supportive and unsupportive behaviour of nurses? A pilot study. *European Journal of Cancer Care, 5*(2), 103–110.
Lachman, V.D. (1996). Stress and self-care revisited: A literature review. *Holistic Nursing Practice, 19*(2), 1–12.
*Lazarus, R.S., & Folkman, S. (1984). *Stress, appraisal and coping.* New York: Springer Publishing Company.

*Asterisk indicates a classic or definitive work on this subject.

McCain, N.L., Zeller, J.M., Cella, D.F., Urbanski, P.A., & Novak, R.M. (1996). The influence of stress management training in HIV disease. *Nursing Research, 45*(4), 246–253.

McCarty, E.F. (1996). Caring for a parent with Alzheimer's disease: Process of daughter caregiver stress. *Journal of Advanced Nursing, 23*(4), 792–803.

Melanson, P.M., & Downe-Wamboldt, B. (1995). The stress of life with rheumatoid arthritis as perceived by older adults. *Activities, Adaptation & Aging, 19*(4), 33–47.

Miles, J.S., Carlson, J., & Funk, S.G. (1996). Sources of support reported by mothers and fathers of infants hospitalized in a neonatal intensive care unit. *Neonatal Network—Journal of Neonatal Nursing, 15*(3), 45–52.

*Norbeck, J.S. (1982). The Norbeck Social Support Questionnaire. *Write to:* Dean, School of Nursing, University of California, San Francisco, 521 Parnassus Avenue, San Francisco, CA 94103–0604.

Oakland, S., & Ostell, A. (1996). Measuring coping: A review and critique. *Human Relations, 49*(2), 133–155.

Seckel, M.M., & Birney, M.H. (1996). Social support, stress, and age in women undergoing breast biopsies. *Clinical Nurse Specialist, 10*(3), 137–143.

*Selye, H. (1956). *The stress of life.* New York: McGraw-Hill.

Tarkka, M., & Paunonen, M. (1996). Social support provided by nurses to recent mothers on a maternity ward. *Journal of Advanced Nursing, 23*(6), 1202–1206.

Tomlinson, P.S., Kirschbaum, M., Harbaugh, B., & Anderson, K.H. (1996). The influence of illness severity and family resources on maternal uncertainty during critical pediatric hospitalization. *American Journal of Critical Care, 5*(2), 140–146.

Ulmer, D. (1996). Prevention. Stress management for the cardiovascular patient: A look at current treatment and trends. *Progress in Cardiovascular Nursing, 11*(1), 21–29.

Zorrilla, E.P., DeRubeis, R.J., & Redei, E. (1995). High self-esteem, hardiness and affective stability are associated with high basal pituitary-adrenal hormone levels. *Psychoneuroendocrinology, 20*(6), 591–601.

53

Family Coping

Joanne H. Frey

Key Terms

binuclear family	intergenerational family
closed system	lesbian or gay family
communal family	nuclear family
extended family	open system
family	role conflict
family-centered nursing	role stress
family household	single-parent family
family systems theory	system
heterosexual cohabiting family	

LEARNING OBJECTIVES

After studying this chapter, you should be able to:

1. **Describe the concepts of family, family function, and family relationships.**
2. **Discuss the factors affecting family coping.**
3. **Assess the family, especially noting major stressors that may interfere with healthy coping, place the client at risk, or both.**
4. **Diagnose family problems that respond to nursing care.**
5. **Plan for goal-directed interventions to prevent or correct family problems identified by nursing diagnoses.**
6. **Evaluate outcomes that describe progress toward or resolution of family problems.**

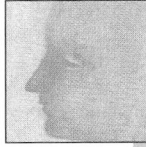

Mrs. Nora Harrington, age 35, was admitted to a hospital for evaluation of acute low back pain. She was overweight, looked older than her stated age, and appeared tense and pale. During her stay, Nora was visited by a Catholic priest and her oldest child, Alice, age 16. Her other children, Bobby, age 15; Flo, age 12; and Greg, age 11, did not visit her. Her husband, Mike Harrington, age 38, did not visit her because he had a "fear of hospitals."

Nora spent much of her time on the telephone giving Alice instructions about child care and household chores. Nora was discharged with no confirmed diagnosis. Alice drove her home.

When the home health nurse visited, Nora was lying on the sofa amid a clutter of plates, glasses, magazines, and tissues. She told the nurse that she was feeling better but could not perform her back exercises. Mr. Harrington came home during the visit, looking unkempt and emaciated, with yellow skin. Temporarily unemployed, he had shopped for groceries and beer. Nora visibly tensed on his arrival.

He poured a glass of beer and sat down, although he did not engage the nurse with eye contact or conversation. Nora stopped talking and looked at him. Mike half-jokingly stated he wouldn't burden them with his presence when he knew he wasn't wanted and abruptly left the room. Nora's eyes filled with tears.

In the kitchen, Alice was putting away groceries in an otherwise empty refrigerator. The nurse asked Alice if she had the day off from school, and the girl replied that she was the only help for her mother. She hoped to go to college when she graduated since she had a scholarship to the State University. She did not know if she could go, since there was a lot of extra work while her mother was ill.

The nurse was about to leave when Nora informed her that the family had a social worker at the neighborhood center. The nurse diagnoses *Ineffective family coping: Disabling.*

FAMILY COPING NURSING DIAGNOSES

Family Coping: Potential for Growth: Effective managing of adaptive tasks by family member involved with the client's health challenge, who now is exhibiting desire and readiness for enhanced health and growth in regard to self and in relation to the client.

Ineffective Family Coping: Compromised: A usually supportive primary person (family member or close friend) is providing insufficient, ineffective, or compromised support, comfort, assistance, or encouragement that may be needed by the client to manage or master adaptive tasks related to his/her health challenge.

Ineffective Family Coping: Disabling: Behavior of significant person (family member or other primary person) that disables his/her capacities and the client's capacities to effectively address tasks essential to either person's adaptation to the health challenge.

Altered Parenting: Inability of the primary caretaker to create an environment that promotes the optimum growth and development of the child.

Altered Family Processes: A change in family relationships and/or functioning.

Altered Family Processes: Alcoholism: The state in which the psychosocial, spiritual, and physiological functions of the family unit are chronically disorganized, leading to conflict, denial of problems, resistance to change, ineffective problem-solving, and a series of self-perpetuating crises.

Parental Role Conflict: The state in which a parent experiences role confusion and conflict in response to crisis.

From North American Nursing Diagnosis Association. (1999). NANDA nursing diagnoses: Definitions and classification 1999–2000. Philadelphia: Author.

CONCEPTS OF FAMILY

A **family** is two or more people united by a common goal to create a physical, cultural, spiritual, and nurturing bond that will promote the physical, mental, spiritual, and social development of each of its members, while maintaining cohesiveness as a unit. This unit, identifying itself as a family, can be forged by blood (genetics), law (marriage/adoption), or spirit.

The family is the basic social unit of society and has needs as a unit. You will have opportunities to assess families for threats to healthy family coping when either an individual or the family interacts with the health care delivery system.

Family Structure and Function

Family-centered nursing is health care that focuses on the health of the family as a unit, as well as the maintenance and improvement in the health and growth of each person in that unit. The recipient of care is the family itself. It is based on the family's response to actual or potential health problems or life processes that can be treated by nursing care. It involves intervening to help the family manage the impact of stressors on the family.

Family Structures

NUCLEAR FAMILY. The **nuclear family** is composed of husband, wife, and offspring living in a common household with one or both partners gainfully employed. In 1998, the U.S. Census Bureau reported almost 71 million family households and 31 million nonfamily households (69% and 31%) in the United States. A **family household** contains the householder and at least one other person related to the householder by birth, marriage, or adoption. The three types of family households are a married couple, a female householder with no spouse present, and a male householder with no spouse present. Overall, families had an average of 3.18 members, with Hispanic families at 3.92 members, African-American families at 3.42 members, and white families at 3.02 members (Casper & Bryson, 1998a; Clemen-Stone, McGuire, & Eigsti, 1998). In general, ethnic minority families will gain prominence in numbers in the years ahead.

The Harrington family is a nuclear family. Do they demonstrate the strengths generally associated with nuclear families?

INTERGENERATIONAL FAMILY. An **intergenerational family** includes more than one generation of a family living together in one residence or within a small geographical area. This type of family exists because of cultural values, the family's financial status, safety concerns, or because elderly parents or other disabled family members cannot care for themselves physically, financially, or emotionally. Multiple generations often enrich family life (Fig. 53–1).

EXTENDED FAMILY. The **extended family** unit includes the nuclear family as well as other relatives such as aunts, uncles, cousins, and grandparents who are committed to maintaining family ties. They may live in close proximity or in geographically different places. The defining characteristic is identification as a family unit and maintaining an inter-relatedness that is mutually supportive, such as caring for the elderly by younger members and caring for the young by older family members.

In 1998, almost 4 million children under age 18 (6%) lived in households headed by their grandparents in every socioeconomic and ethnic group. Overall, 27% of these families live in poverty; two-thirds live with only their grandmother. In contrast, 19% of children living in homes maintained by their parents are in poverty (Casper & Bryson, 1998a).

SINGLE-PARENT FAMILY. **Single-parent families** are households in which the children live with one parent, usually because of divorce, out-of-wedlock births, or the death of a spouse. This type of family usually is headed by a woman, often a teenager. Currently, at least half of children live in a single parent home for part of their life. In 1998, 27.3% of the U.S. households were composed of single parents living with their own children under age 18. There were 2.1 million father-child and 9.8 million mother-child family households. In the mother-child family households, 42.2% of mothers had never married.

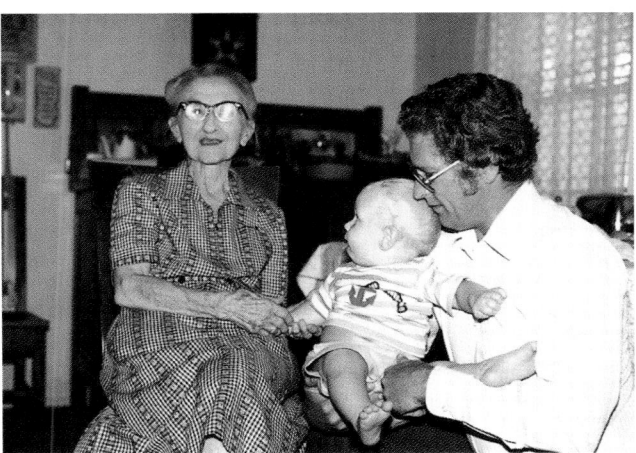

Figure 53–1. Multiple generations enrich family life.

About 42% of single-parent families, headed by women, live below the poverty line. Without a partner, it can be even harder to manage as a family unit since more energy may be required to meet basic needs. When parents feel powerless to protect and provide for their families, it can result in them experiencing low self-esteem, frustration, resignation, or fatalism. Without proper support and healthy coping skills, the parent may escape the resulting pain with alcohol, drugs, abusiveness, abandonment, or suicide (Casper & Bryson, 1998b; Pollack, 1997).

If Nora Harrington decided she could no longer tolerate her husband's alcoholism, what problems might she have as a result of becoming a single parent?

A*ction* A*lert!*
Identify the single-parent family for the purpose of understanding strengths and weaknesses. The single-parent family may be a functional, healthy family unit.

NONTRADITIONAL FAMILIES

There are many nontraditional family structures. A **binuclear family** exists where children are part of two nuclear families with coparenting and joint custody. A **heterosexual cohabiting family** is an unmarried couple living together with or without children. A **communal family** is a household of more than one monogamous couple with children, each of which shares resources and socializes the children as a group activity. A **lesbian or gay family** includes either a female or male couple living together with or without children. Recognition of various types of families and their strengths and weaknesses underlies family assessment (Clemen-Stone, McGuire, & Eigsti, 1998).

A*ction* A*lert!*
Be aware that your own family is not the only type of family structure or the only "correct" one. Prejudices or biases will prevent you from delivering effective family nursing care.

Family Functions

The family's organization and functioning are based on the mixture of societal and cultural behaviors and rituals. Families function to satisfy both the needs of individuals within the family and the family as a social unit. The primary functions include the affective function, socialization and social placement function, reproductive function, economic function, and health care function.

Affective needs are met by providing psychosocial protection and support of the family members. Families confer feelings of acceptance and value on their members through love, intimacy, nurturing, acceptance, caring, sharing, and support (Fig. 53–2). The socialization and social placement function includes socialization of children by helping them become productive members of their society, as well as the conferring of status on family members. Reproductive functions are to maintain family continuity over the

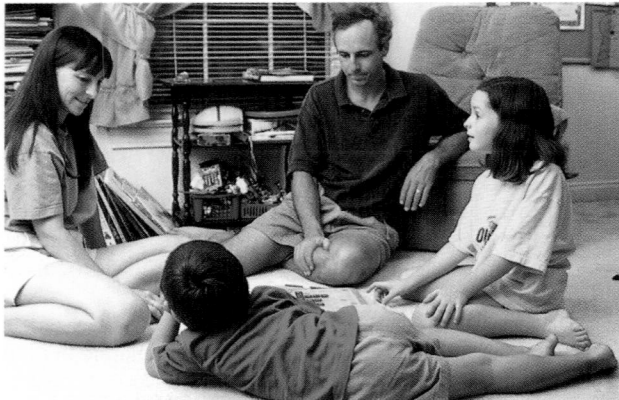

Figure 53–2. Families confer feelings of acceptance and value on their members by the development of love, intimacy, nurturing, acceptance, caring, sharing, and support.

generations as well as for societal survival. Providing for the economic needs of the family includes having sufficient resources and allocating these resources to provide for food, clothes, shelter, recreation, education, and quality of life. The health care function is to provide for nutrition, mental health, immunizations, and physical well-being (Friedman, 1998).

Role Stress and Conflict

In families, roles are structured for the division of labor and the distribution of power (Fig. 53–3). Power may be formally assigned by designating one person the head of the household. A woman may assign her husband the role of repairman by openly stating that she does not have the skill to do home repairs. Power can be used inappropriately in a manner that is destructive to others or mutually shared among family members to get both common and individual needs met.

Family functions can be compromised by role stress and role conflict. **Role stress** is an emotion that occurs when a person has difficulty meeting the demands of a role. It can occur when competing demands interfere, when the family structure is rigid, or when role expectations are unrealistic. **Role conflict** is incompatible expectations for behavior within a role, between two or more roles, or when a role is incongruent with a person's beliefs and values. Role conflict can be manifested as inter-role conflict, in which competing roles are in conflict. Intersender role conflict occurs when two people have different expectations of how the role will be performed. Personal role conflict is an inner conflict between values held internally that is the opposite of an external value the role demands.

What role stressors and conflicts can you imagine are present in the Harrington family?

Theoretical Approaches to Family

The application of nursing theories offers a conceptual approach to family assessment.

Family Systems Theory

The study of the family can be approached as the study of a system (family) with subsystems (individual members) interacting with each other. A **system** is a set of integrated, interacting parts that function as a whole, with structure and patterns of function that accomplish the work of the whole. It has boundaries that filter and regulate what passes through its boundaries as it tries to maintain balance or equilibrium. An **open system** exchanges matter, energy, and information with other systems and with the environment. A **closed system** is a set of integrated, interacting parts that function as a whole and do not interact with other systems or the environment.

The family is a set consisting of individual members who interact to create the family unit and who structure relationships for the division of labor and for meeting the needs of the family. The healthy family is an open system with complex interactions both within the family and in the external world. It controls its boundaries through its values, beliefs, attitudes, and rules. It is self-regulating and can adjust the family unit as the needs of its members change so that harmony and balance exist. When the open family system loses its balance, outside help can assist in its stabilization. The closed family system excludes others, functions in isolation, and is the pathological model.

When you assess the family as a system, you observe whether the system is working, whether the subsystems are functioning, and whether the system is open, available for input, or closed, having limited outside support or input.

Interactional Theory

Interactional theory emphasizes the internal dynamics of family life or how the individual members interact with one another and with the family as a whole. Interactionalists view the family as being relatively closed to outside systems and emphasize analysis of the internal aspects of family dynamics. The interactionalist would describe the family by describing roles, the decision-making process, communication, conflict, and reaction to stress. Rigidity, suppression, or lack of spontaneity, especially in a family member

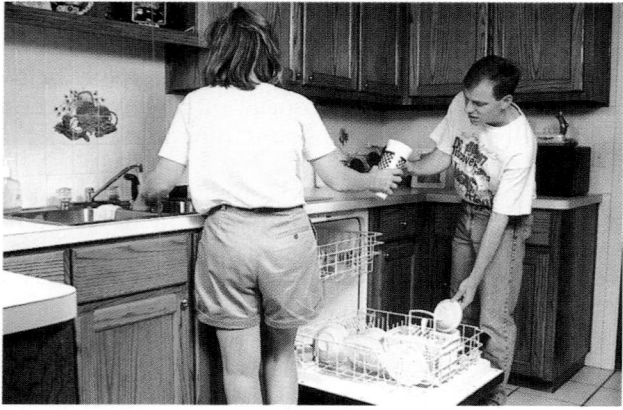

Figure 53–3. Family roles are structured for the division of labor and the distribution of power.

who is not interacting with any degree of balance, throws the family into disequilibrium.

Developmental Theories

Assessing a family from a developmental perspective is to look at family development throughout its generational life cycle. Knowing individual and family developmental tasks, you can determine the family unit's health by assessing the family's successful mas-

tery of appropriate tasks while also observing whether individual family members' actions are appropriate to their developmental level (Table 53–1).

FACTORS AFFECTING FAMILY COPING

General Factors

Many factors affect the family's ability to cope, including the family members' culture, religious values, so-

TABLE 53–1

Family Developmental Tasks by Developmental Stage and Age

Family Stage	Age of Children	Family Tasks
The family during pregnancy	Fetal development	• Maintaining health of fetus. • Allocating resources. • Dividing labor. • Transition of identity into parenthood. • Socialization of family members. • Maintaining order. • Maintaining motivation and morale.
The family with a neonate	Newborn	• Maintaining control over the childbirth events. • Communicating effectively with each other and significant others. • Maintaining a satisfying relation with each other and significant others. • Resolving the birthing experience. • Meeting physical and emotional needs of the neonate. • Assigning roles. • Incorporating the neonate into the family. • Reallocating resources.
The family with an infant	Oldest child 6 weeks to 1 year	• Promoting physical and emotional development. • Adapting lifestyle to the changing infant. • Incorporating new family structure into society. • Maintaining interpersonal relationship. • Establishing goals, priorities, and values.
The family with a toddler or preschooler	2 to 5 years	• Initiating and maintaining a home. • Maintaining physical growth and well-being (air, food, safety).
The family with a school-aged child	6 to 12 years	• Meeting the physical needs of the family. • Expanding family communications and activities. • Maintaining marital satisfactions. • Socialization and education of the children. • Developing the potential of all individual family members. • Communicating effectively with all family members.
The family with an adolescent	13 to 19 years	• Allowing for and providing for individual differences and needs. • Working out a system of financial and family responsibility. • Maintaining open communication among family members. • Widening the horizons of adolescents and their parents. • Maintaining family ethical and moral standards.
The family during the child's transition to adulthood	20 to 44 years	• Continuance of physical care. • Redefining need-response pattern. • Supporting maturation of the child. • Allocating resources. • Maintaining family relationships. • Establishing priorities and maintaining goals. • Evaluating and maintaining socioeconomic security for the future. • Evaluating and maintaining family accomplishments. • Changing and maintaining family relationships.
The family in senescence	45 to 75 years	• Maintaining socioeconomic security to death. • Reviewing family accomplishments. • Changing and maintaining family relationships. • Children are planning for or assuming care of parents.

cial values, communication patterns, support for each other, and communities. The accompanying Cross-Cultural Care chart illustrates the importance of culture for the Harrington family. When families are unable to educate their members, particularly the young, their coping ability is affected. In families with abnormal patterns of communication, for example, there may be an unspoken agreement not to share feelings or information about certain family problems that affect their coping abilities. When they are unable to protect the family from physical and mental harm, their ability to cope is affected.

Stressors

Family coping is the family unit's method of managing the stressors of family life. Family stress is defined as the family's response to any outside force—or stressor—that affects the family. The response to stressors creates a situation in which normal family processes, employed to attain goals and maintain status quo, are out of balance or in disequilibrium. Adaptation is the ability of the family to achieve this balance or equilibrium. Coping is the means the family uses to adapt to stress.

As a family progresses through the developmental stages, from forming a marriage to launching the youngest child into the adult world, each transition brings joys and stressors. The family makes adjustments, learns new coping strategies, and uses transitional crises as a means of family growth. Positive predictors of successful transition from one stage to the next include successful completion of the last developmental stage, a history of effective family support for family members in transition, willingness to redefine family roles and responsibilities, and a history of successes, individually and as a family.

Families are exposed to multiple situational stressors. Any relationship can be a stressor, and when an additional component is added, such as divorce or an out-of-wedlock birth, it can cause a loss of equilibrium for the members of a family. Other stressors include work and family conflicts, financial and job-related stress, and the struggle to care for elderly parents.

A*ction* A*lert!*
Stressors can be a threat or a challenge. The difference depends on how the family perceives them.

Effective Coping

Healthy families have resources for managing stress. Stress that is perceived as an opportunity is a positive experience for the family. Through good problem-solving skills, the family develops its coping skills. When one family member becomes ill and other family members must care for her, the family grows as

---

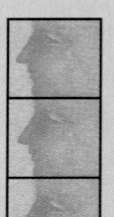

CROSS-CULTURAL CARE
CARING FOR AN IRISH-AMERICAN CATHOLIC CLIENT

If you ask Mike Harrington about his family, he will tell you he is Irish and proud of it. He remembers his grandmother telling stories about his family building this country by working on the railroads. However, he has no ties to an Irish community or to any family in Ireland. He does attribute his drinking to being Irish.

Although each client is unique, many Irish-Americans tend to share certain characteristics:

- Feel family loyalty and provide support to extended family.
- Many are Catholic, may also be Protestants.
- Outgoing, friendly manner, may exhibit stoicism.
- Characterized as drinkers, lovers, fighters, poets, and are known for their depressions.
- Proud of doing hard work and hard play.
- Catholics may avoid birth control and abortion.
- May desire visits from a priest and the Sacrament of the Sick if dying.
- Prefer that a dying newborn be baptized, even by a nurse, to aid the infant's entrance to heaven.

The nurse has the following conversation with Mike.

Nurse: Your drinking is causing problems in your family.

Mike: My wife just doesn't understand. The men in my family have always enjoyed their beer. We work hard and play hard. I always provide for my family.

Nurse: I know you love your family and want the best for them. Your daughter has a good mind and wants to go to college.

Mike: Yes, that girl is smart, alright. I am proud of her.

Nurse: She can't do it with all of the responsibility she has at home. Can you think of any ways you could help her?

Critical Thinking Questions

- The nurse is appealing to Mike's strength to make changes in the family. Do you think it will have an impact on Mike?
- As you read about the Harringtons, have you identified any other strengths?
- How would you approach this family to improve their ability to function as a family unit?

outlined in the State of Nursing Science chart. The family can feel good about the way they handled the stressor and can enhance their collective self-esteem. Effective management of stressors is a family strength.

Examples of strategies used by families who have effective coping skills include the following:

- Discussing problems and concerns among family members
- Demonstrating human emotional responses, such as crying and laughing
- Confronting stressors realistically
- Seeking professional guidance if necessary

Healthy families can reappraise and reorder priorities in work and private life based on family values. They work off stress and anger by doing meaningful tasks and using stress-reducing mechanisms such as prayer and meditation, yoga, deep-breathing exercises, relaxation tapes, imagery, or biofeedback.

Ineffective and Dysfunctional Coping

Unhealthy families lack resources for managing stress. Stress perceived by the family as a danger or a threat that could overwhelm their coping skills is negative stress. It can be caused by the number of stressors, the critical importance of the stressor, or the overwhelming threat of the stressor. Ineffective coping is the use of maladaptive defense mechanisms, poor communication, poor problem identification, and poor decision-making by one or more family members. Ineffective coping skills, such as the use of drugs, blur the reality of the situation until problems become overwhelming. Failure to satisfactorily resolve a stressor contributes to lowered self-esteem and increases the use of maladaptive coping skills in future stressful situations.

Dysfunctional families either cannot meet the needs of the family or function in a way that is harmful to its members. The family is usually in pain and functions at the expense of the individuals in the family. Physical or psychological abuse is a dysfunctional family problem.

ASSESSMENT

General Assessment of Families

Applying the philosophy of family-centered nursing, individual problems are also family problems. Your assessment identifies the coping abilities of both individual and family.

Your first visit to the family is definitive in establishing a trusting relationship. You need to be honest, nonthreatening, cordial, and caring with them to begin to form a family team. You interview families for a purpose. You will need to develop a systematized method for family assessment that includes the information you need but does not subject the family to unnecessary intrusion. You will need to be able to distinguish "healthy" family behavior from dysfunctional behavior.

Action Alert!
To prepare for a family home visit, first reflect on your values. What are your thoughts about the family? Do you possess any biases or prejudices that would prevent you from giving good nursing care?

The assessment begins with verifying the information on the referral sheet and obtaining family data. You will want to determine the family members, including their age, gender, developmental stage, and roles. You can obtain additional cues regarding the family's state of health. One of your challenges will be to determine whether or not the family works well together. When asking about the family, you obtain information through what they say and through observations of body gestures, vocal tones, facial expressions, and word selection. Your family assessment will determine whether the family is healthy or dysfunctional.

A healthy family will show genuine interest in learning to help the client. Their relationships are caring with a sense of togetherness and with a willingness to help in managing a problem.

Dysfunctional families have ineffective communications and living patterns, marginal health practices, strained or poor coping skills, and ineffective child rearing practices. Indicators of ineffective family coping include family members who deny or trivialize problems, detach themselves, or refuse to offer any help. When there is tension, the family may sit apart and not make eye contact. They may uneasily watch each other's movements and give very cautious responses to avoid or prompt conflict.

Action Alert!
Pay attention to your instincts. Tension and hostility can be felt. Think about situations you have experienced. When there was tension in the air, could you almost feel it?

You will make observations of the family's adaptive ability, communication patterns, ability to function as a system, physical needs, ability to protect their members, health promotion activities, and community support (Table 53–2).

Review this list of questions. What data would you gather for the Harringtons? How would you gather this data?

Focused Assessment for Family Coping: Potential for Growth

Family coping: Potential for growth is a wellness nursing diagnosis that allows you to be a family advocate, a teacher, an observer, and a tender of the sick. Families whose members are effectively managing adaptation to the health challenges of its members are given this diagnosis. It reflects families who demonstrate readiness for enhanced health and growth in regard to themselves and the client.

This diagnosis is also appropriate for a client who is ill. For example, when a client who has had his leg amputated states that he would like to change his

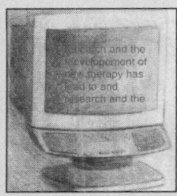

THE STATE OF NURSING SCIENCE

FAMILY AND CAREGIVER INVOLVEMENT IN INSTITUTIONAL SETTINGS

What Are the Issues?

When a person is admitted to a hospital or nursing home, the focus of assessment and care is usually on the individual client. Consideration of the needs and potential contributions of family and other caregivers is often neglected. However, interactions with these people can be times to gather important information about the client as an individual. These interactions can also help to educate family caregivers about how to care for clients, especially those who will return to the home for recovery or continued care. Understanding what family members and other caregivers need from nurses during hospitalization is a first step in developing effective ways to help.

What Research Has Been Conducted?

Laitinen and Isola (1996) used a qualitative approach to find out ways to encourage the participation of family members and other caregivers in the care of clients. (Qualitative approaches are useful when the research base is limited. The results of this type of study can be used to develop instruments for measuring important concepts in future quantitative studies.) The researchers categorized the responses from 369 subjects who were identified as family or other caregivers for clients in three different settings: a university hospital, a geriatric unit, and a nursing home.

Data were collected at three separate times over 3 years. The researchers found that people valued communication with nurses and looked to them for direction on how to help their loved ones. Effective communication was characterized by empathy, warmth, and trust. Barriers to participation included lack of communication, as well as negative attitudes on the part of nurses. Poor health of the family member and lack of willingness were also seen as barriers to participation.

Friedemann et al. (1997) focused exclusively on the needs of family members of clients admitted to nursing homes. They analyzed information from surveys received from 143 directors of nursing and from telephone interviews of 177 family members. The directors of nursing reported on the availability of activities in which family members might participate in their facility. The types of activities included team member functions, visitor/entertainer functions, and learner/client advocate functions (p. 529). The most frequently encouraged activities were "staff calling family for advice with resident problems, personal invitations to family activities, permission to call unit day or night, [and] meetings to plan care" (p. 531). Nursing homes that ranked higher in promoting family involvement were more likely to encourage such activities as "family group to help solve nursing home problems, instruction in client care for families, classes to learn about chronic illness, etc., support groups for families, advisory board open to family members, educational materials for families to borrow, [and] education about nursing home program" (p. 530).

(continued)

---

dressing because he wants to see if he can do it correctly, or if he will need help from his family when he goes home, this client is indicating the potential for growth.

Defining Characteristics

The family with potential for growth is recognized by health promoting behaviors. They may ask questions about health care, ask about resources for knowledge, or ask for assistance in other ways. You may recognize this family through discussions of the impact of a current crisis on individual family members' own values, priorities, goals, or relationships. They will recognize the impact and attempt to manage it.

Related Factors

When the family's needs are sufficiently gratified and adaptive tasks effectively addressed to enable goals of

self-actualization to surface, the family has the potential for growth. This "wellness" diagnosis is used when families indicate that they wish to retake control of a situation or when they show a willingness to be taught ways of seeking a higher level of wellness. The types of behaviors that are observed in healthy families indicate that the families and the family members have successfully achieved their appropriate developmental tasks. The family also has adequate support systems to achieve further personal and family growth. Healthy families effectively manage to adapt to health challenges of their family members.

Focused Assessment for Ineffective Family Coping: Compromised

The diagnosis of *Ineffective family coping: Compromised* indicates that a major crisis has occurred to alter the

THE STATE OF NURSING SCIENCE
FAMILY AND CAREGIVER INVOLVEMENT IN INSTITUTIONAL SETTINGS (continued)

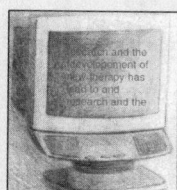

Information from the interviews with family members indicated that communication and lack of education and encouragement were the biggest problems related to family interaction. Characteristics of staff perceived as most family oriented included "being helpful, cooperation in problem solving, [and] mutual liking" (p. 534). Family members indicated that they valued nursing homes where activities to "maintain connectedness" (p. 535) were encouraged. These would include efforts by the staff to help the client stay a part of the family whenever possible.

What Has the Research Concluded?

Laitinen and Isola (1996) recommended that nurses include contact with family and other caregivers early in the client's admission as a way to sort out the potential contribution that family can make and what to expect from the nursing staff. Early in the admission is a good time to identify possible barriers to care such as poor health of the family member.

Friedemann et al. (1997) concluded that activities encouraging family involvement were, at least in part, meeting the needs of families for such involvement. When this was not true, families became concerned about the safety of their loved ones (p. 536).

What Is the Future of Research in This Area?

The pressure to shorten the length of stay for clients in hospital settings means that some client recovery will occur in other settings. Family members who are able may be called upon to provide direct care under the supervision of health care providers. As they assume this responsibility, it will be important for nurses to develop effective ways to help them function in this role. Certainly, hospitalization is the time to start such support. Future research must be conducted on the best ways to encourage and support family participation in care. Such encouragement includes both the communication between nurses and family members and institutional policies and procedures that promote family involvement.

Studies are needed on ways to improve the communication between nurses and family members so that family members feel valued and respected. Nurses need to learn more about how families perceive their role in caring for clients. With the common goal of meeting the needs of clients, nurses and family members can join together to make it happen.

References

Friedemann, M., Montgomery, R.J., Maiberger, B., & Smith, A.A. (1997). Family involvement in the nursing home: Family-oriented practices and staff-family relationships. *Research in Nursing & Health, 20,* 527–537.

Laitinen, P., & Isola, A. (1996). Promoting participation of informal caregivers in the hospital care of the elderly patient: Informal caregivers' perceptions. *Journal of Advanced Nursing, 23,* 942–947.

family's ability to function or support individuals within the family in a helpful manner. It can occur in reasonably functional families who have never had a major crisis or in a dysfunctional family whose support systems are under pressure, and who are unable to meet a health challenge.

Defining Characteristics

Defining characteristics for *Ineffective family coping: Compromised* include both objective and subjective elements. The family may or may not recognize that their coping is compromised. However, this family usually is trying to meet the needs of its members, but feels their efforts are not adequate. On the other hand, a significant person may be overly protective of the client, investing all of her energy into being sure that the client's needs are met. Other family members may be neglected.

The cues to compromised coping come from the client or significant other. For example:

- The client expresses or confirms a concern or complaint about a significant other's response to her health problem.
- A significant person describes or confirms an inadequate understanding or knowledge base, which interferes with effective assistive or supportive behaviors.
- A significant person describes preoccupation with personal reactions (such as fear, anticipatory grief, guilt, anxiety) to the client's illness, disability, or other situational or developmental crises.

This diagnosis should be considered when risk factors exist or when the client or another individual complains about the caretaker's inadequate abil-

TABLE 53–2
Family Assessment Criteria

Criteria	Assessment Questions
Physical needs	• Is the family shelter adequate? • Does the family shelter provide the basic essentials that will allow proper food consumption, such as a workable refrigerator and stove? • Is there an adequate water supply and is the water that flows from the faucet safe to drink? • Is the home warm and cool enough? • How is the home heated? • Is there money for gas, electricity, propane, or wood? • Is there a working toilet and a bathtub or shower where adequate hygiene measures can be carried out? • Is there enough money for soap? • Are there beds where each family member can be assured of a good night's sleep? • Can the family shelter offer room for activity, such as a television, a room where children can play, and toys? • Is there something pretty in the home or anything that makes the environment more homey and comfortable? • Is there adequate food in the refrigerator or cupboard? • If the family qualifies for food stamps or extra food, like a bag of wheat or flour, can someone prepare an adequate meal? • Are there proper cooking and eating utensils? • Are bathroom facilities easily accessible for the recovering client? • How many stairs must the client climb to get into the home? • Is the home clean, well-ventilated, and well kept, or is it dirty, unkempt, and lacking such essentials as a flushing toilet or hot water?
Protection	• If the family is fearful, what is the source of the fear? Is it outside, as in a dangerous neighborhood? Or is it inside, as in an abusive parent or mate? • What options are available for the fearful? • Is there a social worker in the picture? Collaborative work is sometimes essential when dealing with families that have multiple problems. • Are adults allowed to smoke where there are children? • Are safety belts and child seats used appropriately? • Are dangerous chemicals, medications, and matches safely stored out of reach of children?
Health promotion	• Do family members smoke, drink to excess, or use illegal drugs? • Do family members exercise, wear safety belts when driving, and wear helmets when bike riding? • Do family members eat well-balanced meals (ask for a sample daily menu), see a dentist, and get proper amounts of sleep? • When someone is ill, does the family have all the integrity and resources, physically, mentally, emotionally, and economically, to intelligently handle the stressors inherent in sickness and the individual autonomy to meet their own needs?
Communication	• Do family members feel understood by each other? • What is their communication network like? Can you observe basic communication errors? • Do all family members feel safe and important enough to share their feelings and opinions? Have they had a lot of practice? Do they do it well or superficially?

ity. Caretakers may be consumed with their own needs and unable to care for the client.

Related Factors

Related factors for *Ineffective family coping: Compromised* include the following:

• Temporary preoccupation by a significant person who is trying to manage emotional conflicts and personal suffering and is unable to perceive or act effectively in regard to the client's needs.

• Temporary family disorganization and role changes.

• Prolonged disease or disability progression that exhausts the supportive capacity of significant people.

• Other situational or developmental crises or situations the significant person may be facing.

• Inadequate or incorrect information or understanding by a primary person.

• Little support provided by the client, in turn, for the primary person.

TABLE 53–2
Family Assessment Criteria *Continued*

Criteria	Assessment Questions
	• How well does the family listen? How well do they receive the messages sent?
	• Are messages sent in an intimidating, manipulative way or are they "I think . . ." or "I feel . . ." statements?
	• Do family members assume they understand, or is there valuable feedback?
	• Does the family share, or do they have secrets? Is not sharing a power move or a destructive habit—a way to avoid conflict?
	• How does the family react to transmitted messages? Do they respect the feelings of the sender? Do they react inappropriately emotionally? Do they ask questions to get more information?
	• Do they value messages and apply them appropriately?
Family as a system	• Does the family interact with the community?
	• Does the family accept public assistance if it is needed?
	• Are the subsystems of the family (each family member) able to reach his or her own potential, or are they stifled in a closed system?
	• If there is a disrupting force, what mechanisms do they have to reach equilibrium?
Community support	• Is the community air quality within acceptable limits for pollution? Is the water safe to drink? Is there adequate garbage collection? Are police visible?
	• Is there transportation available, or are there stores close by to get essentials?
	• What does this community offer in shared values and ethnicity of your client? Are there places to worship, hospitals, and other support systems that help in a crisis?
	• How is the fire station and ambulance service? How far away are they?
	• Is there a newspaper to support the community's communication system?
	• Are there cultural offerings in which the entire family can participate and enjoy?
	• Are there parks and playgrounds?
	• Are there organized sports and places children can go to after school, such as a YMCA, a Boy's Club, or the Girl Scouts? Is there a good school system, with an active parent-teacher association?
	• Can students walk safely or ride a short distance to school? Is public transportation available?
	• What services are available for the old and infirm?
	• Does the community offer intellectual stimulation with theater, plays, and museums? Is it a friendly town where children can run and play? Is it safe?
	• Will this community support your client and the family?
Adaptive abilities	• Who is identified as the client?
	• Do all family members have their physical, mental, emotional, socioeconomic, and spiritual needs met within the context of the family?
	• Is a stressor seen by the family as an opportunity to grow or does it throw a family's functional ability into disequilibrium?
	• Can a family help itself when out of balance?
	• Can family members accept help when their needs overwhelm their resources?
	• Are family members flexible in adapting or adopting roles?
	• Does the family communicate effectively?
	• How does the client like being cared for at home?

Focused Assessment for Ineffective Family Coping: Disabling

Ineffective family coping: disabling is a diagnosis that indicates that the destructive behavior of family members has disrupted the family's ability to function. Family members often have significant physical, cognitive, or psychological problems. Examples include family members with psychiatric disorders, illegal drug use, rebellion against authority, abusive relationships, or geographical or social isolation.

Defining Characteristics

When a crisis has disabled the family's coping abilities, the signs of lack of family function are more dramatic. The client may not be getting her needs met. The person in the caregiving role may behave with intolerance, aggression, or hostility toward the client, providing care in a harsh manner. On the other hand, the client may be neglected.

The primary caregiver may either become overly involved with the client's care, neglecting other family members and especially the self, or the family may deny the seriousness of the illness or that the client needs extensive care and continue with their lives as though nothing has changed, thus failing to provide adequate care.

Relationships within the family may suffer. Family members other than the client may develop illnesses or complain of symptoms. They may make decisions that are detrimental to the family's economic or social well-being.

The disabled function may be manifested in the client. A client who is overly demanding or dependent and who disregards the needs of the family can be a sign of disabled family functioning.

Related Factors

Related factors for *Ineffective family coping: Disabling* include the following:

- Unresolved family issues
- Ineffective family communication
- Differing coping styles in family members
- Relationship problems among family members

Focused Assessment for Altered Parenting

Altered parenting occurs when parents either have inadequate parenting skills or experience crises that have interfered with their adjustment to parenting.

Defining Characteristics

Defining characteristics for *Altered parenting* include those for the infant or child and those for the parent. Characteristics that apply to the infant or child include the following:

- Poor cognitive development and academic performance
- Frequent illness or accidents
- Evidence of physical and psychological trauma or abuse
- Lack of attachment, running away
- Failure to thrive
- Behavioral disorders
- Poor social competence
- Lack of separation anxiety

Characteristics that apply to the parent include the following:

- Inappropriate child care arrangements
- Rejection or hostility to the child, overly punitive, inconsistent behavior management
- Statements of inability to meet the child's needs
- Inflexibility to meet the needs of the child or situation
- Poor or inappropriate caretaking skills, inconsistent care
- Child neglect, abuse, or abandonment
- Inadequate child health maintenance, including unsafe home environment

- Verbalization of inability to control child or role, inadequacy, frustration
- Negative statements about the child
- Inappropriate visual, tactile, or auditory stimulation
- Insecure or lack of attachment to infant, little cuddling
- Deficient or poor mother-child or parent-child interaction

Related Factors

A great number of factors may be related to *Altered parenting*. Parents who are physically, mentally, or cognitively impaired or from dysfunctional and abusive families themselves may have difficulty bonding with their infants. Parents may be unable to nurture their children if they have never been nurtured. Interruptions in family life, especially through separation, divorce, or death, can cause poor care or neglect of children. Parents may have unrealistic expectations (perfectionism) of themselves, their infant, or their partner and attempt to control their environment.

In general, factors related to *Altered parenting* are contained in five main categories:

- *Social,* which includes such factors as lack of access to resources, social isolation, job problems, marital conflict, lack of social support, poor coping and problem-solving skills, and problems with being or acting as a parent
- *Knowledge,* which includes such factors as inadequate knowledge of child health and parenting skills, unrealistic expectations, and inability to recognize an infant's cues
- *Physiological,* which includes physical illness
- *Infant or child,* which includes premature birth, illness, prolonged separation from parent, difficult temperament or "wrong" gender, unwanted pregnancy, and physical or developmental abnormality
- *Psychological,* which includes a history of substance abuse, disability, depression, difficult labor and delivery, adolescent parent, and poor prenatal care

DIAGNOSIS

You will need to group all the data collected about a family into clusters to arrive at appropriate nursing diagnoses, as outlined in the accompanying data clustering chart. Indeed, when working with a family, you may need to use a wide variety of nursing diagnoses. The key to determining accurate nursing diagnoses is in obtaining all relevant information, verifying it, and then clustering it appropriately.

Mrs. Harrington's nurse obtained additional information from the social worker at the community center. She found that Mr. Harrington's abuse of alcohol has caused major problems for the family. He is a daily drinker. He recently lost his job because he was drinking at work. He was the major breadwinner of the family, so the family is in a financial crisis. The nurse selects the nursing di-

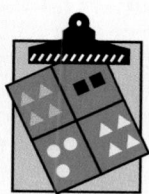

CLUSTERING DATA TO MAKE A NURSING DIAGNOSIS
FAMILY COPING PROBLEMS

Data Clusters	Nursing Diagnosis
Martha has three children, ages 3, 5, and 9. The 3-year-old has been diagnosed with cystic fibrosis. Martha has been a devoted mother, enjoying creating fun activities for the children and being a Girl Scout leader. Currently she is focusing her attention on the youngest child. The 9-year-old is expected to feed and dress the 5-year-old.	*Altered parenting* related to overwhelming care needs of child with cystic fibrosis.
Mitch Reeves is a 55-year-old man who has had quadruple coronary artery bypass grafting and has residual heart failure. He is on extended medical leave. His wife is planning to build a new, larger house and expects him to be able to negotiate with the builders. She has previously been a realistic and thoughtful homemaker.	*Ineffective family coping: Disabling,* related to wife's denial of possible long-term effects from open heart surgery
Rebecca, age 75, has been living with her mother, age 95, and providing financial and emotional support. The relationship has been mutually satisfying and beneficial to both Rebecca and her mother. Her mother had been healthy and active until she recently fractured her ankle. Rebecca tells the nurse that she does not know how to manage her mother's care. Rebecca's diabetes is out of control and she is learning to give herself insulin.	*Ineffective family coping: Compromised,* related to recent injury confounding the care situation
Mary Elizabeth has a 7-year-old child diagnosed with attention deficit hyperactivity disorder. She has just been accepted in a community college semiconductor technology program. She needs the training to obtain a better job because she is recently divorced.	*Risk for altered parenting* related to multiple stressors
John is 35 years old. His wife has recently died from cancer. He has two children, ages 6 and 10. John has been working long hours in an effort to manage his grief. He often comes home after his own mother has put the children to bed. On weekends he spends time on household chores. The 6-year-old has started wetting the bed again, and the 10-year-old is acting out in school. John says he can't deal with any problems, that his mother will have to handle it.	*Altered family processes* related to situational crisis of wife's death
Linda has a 4-year-old child. She is a single mother and works at a minimum-wage job. She attends college. She is currently in the hospital with a ruptured appendix. She tells the nurse that she is unable to be an adequate mother to her child.	*Parental role conflict* related to crisis precipitated by acute illness

agnosis *Altered family processes: Alcoholism.* There was also great concern voiced by the social worker for Bobby, the 15-year-old, who was expelled from school and has been arrested for being drunk in public and shoplifting. Alice, the daughter, is frequently absent from school to take care of the family. With this additional information from the social worker, some of this dysfunctional family's major problems are coming to light. What would be your plan of care for this family?

PLANNING

Expected Outcomes for the Family With Family Coping: Potential for Growth

Interventions are dependent on the goals identified and the nursing tasks needed to reach the desired outcome. They may require that each family member adapt to the reality of the family's new situation. Examples of outcomes are that the family realistically appraise the changes that the health situation will mean for them. The family will understand the meaning of the health situation, share thoughts and feelings about it, plan together, and take effective action to manage it and the necessary changes in family function.

Expected Outcomes for the Family With Ineffective Family Coping: Compromised

Always plan with the family, not for the family. Reinforce their efforts. Help the family anticipate what they may need and help them identify their strengths and resources. Assess the family's communication ability and coping skills. Goals may be that the family will realistically appraise their situation, identify their strengths and weakness, verbalize their fears, and identify and prioritize the needs of each family member. They will work cooperatively and agree on compromises to meet the most important needs of each family member.

Expected Outcomes for the Family With Ineffective Family Coping: Disabling

If the family meets the criteria for a "disabling" diagnosis, they are not functioning well at all. There are desired goals that the family must attempt to reach. First, with your assistance, the family must look honestly at the communication skills, problem-solving techniques, and decision-making skills that resulted in this disabling condition. Outcomes include the expectation that individuals in the family will identify their own developmental and situational needs and discuss with the family appropriate means to achieve them. The family will have a realistic understanding of the expectations of the client and be more appropriate in their care for her.

The Harrington family could be described using the diagnosis *Ineffective family coping: Disabling*. Or, in managing Mike's alcoholism, the more specific diagnosis of *Ineffective family coping: Alcoholism* could be used.

Expected Outcomes for the Family With Altered Parenting

The following are examples of goals for *Altered parenting* with a parent/child role conflict involved:

- The parents will gain an understanding of their nurturing role during a specific illness.

- The parents will prioritize the importance of meaningful and truthful communication of their feelings and expectations regarding the situation.
- The parents will be able to discuss the balance needed between business and personal responsibilities while being a support to each other and to other family members.
- The parents will be able to identify what they need for support both internally and externally to function as a family.

INTERVENTION

Interventions to Establish a Nurse-Family Relationship

Nursing interventions used to establish a nurse-family relationship include establishing trust, listening actively, overcoming family resistance, and reinforcing family strengths. To successfully intervene with families, you need to develop a working relationship with all family members based on trust. A full explanation of your role and the services you offer should be given at the level of the family's understanding. Establishing trust in a closed family system is a slow process. You will need to use active listening to understand the problem from the family's perspective.

Active listening involves hearing what the family is saying and using your communication skills to help family members express and explore thoughts and feelings but not pressing for information if a person is reluctant to talk. The initial meeting with a family is used to establish you as an informed resource who will honor the family's confidences and respect the family's members. You can begin by offering non-threatening general information regarding parenting, developmental stages, relationships, or caregiving as appropriate to the family's needs. You will use your communication skills, such as reflection, to make sure you understand what each family member is expressing. You will need to reinforce the family's strengths and help them overcome resistance to change.

When behavior patterns are well established, resistance to outside help and to change is a normal reaction. Resistance can be overcome by having the family assume control through the process of mutual goal-setting. You must know how to sensitively approach the family. Your level of understanding of their power structure and their cultural influences could garner support or promote family resistance. Give a description of your nursing interventions and what will likely happen if the interventions are successful, or what will continue to happen if they fail. Provide support and praise for the family strengths as developmental or situational stressors are managed. Reinforcing family strengths will help the family grow and change (Fig. 53–4).

Interventions to Help Solve Family Problems

Nursing interventions to help families with problem-solving are defining the problem, acknowledging feel-

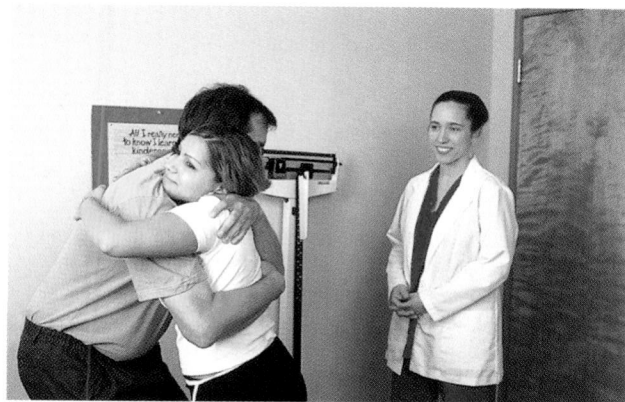

Figure 53–4. Reinforcing family strengths will help the family grow and change.

ings, exploring coping skills, limiting the scope of the problem, and exploring solutions. With your help, family members should start to define the problems or stressors and how they affect their ability to function. You can help the family identify areas of family coping that keep them vulnerable and discuss ways to strengthen their defenses. You can help them by listening actively and attempting to identify the underlying feelings that may be keeping the family from working out a solution.

The family may want to start by discussing how they interacted before the current situation arose (family illness, birth of a baby) to see if they understand the negative interactions they have been using with each other. When a family is faced with a problem that is long-term or extensive, seeing the problem in its entirety can be overwhelming. Stay in the "now," and keep the family in reality. Offer information related to a specific problem. By the time the family has worked together to identify their problems and has defined the source of the problems, many ideas for solutions have probably been offered. Plans to implement these proposed solutions should be made. You should support any strengths the family may have identified.

Interventions to Change Family Behaviors

Interventions to change family behaviors include role-modeling effective behaviors, providing education, and identifying destructive behaviors. You must always remember your role-modeling status and demonstrate skills and distribute information in a professional manner. Be careful not to show negative reactions to clients' behaviors.

A key to providing effective education for clients is identifying their readiness to learn. Information provided when the family is stressed or not focused may not be remembered or may be rejected. The topics are based on the identified family problems and the family's need for knowledge to understand their problems, to identify solutions, and to implement needed changes to accomplish their goals.

Role-modeling is an effective method of teaching caregiving skills. This is true for parents of infants and young children (Fig. 53–5) and families caring for members who are sick. Hopefully, you have developed a trusting relationship with the family so they allow you to function as a role model. You can begin demonstrating parenting skills, or specific nursing skills needed to meet the ill family member's needs. When this occurs, you will be able to gain better insight into the family's stressors.

Helping family members identify destructive behavior is an advanced nursing skill but is essential to help the family with destructive behaviors. The alcoholic family is a good example of a family with destructive behavior. Begin by asking the family to recall all past concrete events that caused them worry, concern, or grief that was related to the alcoholic member of the family. A "family session" could discuss the personal growth and goals of each family member that has been affected by the alcoholic member. Allow them time to vent their feelings and respect the perspective of each family member. Then the family may be gently eased into identifying the specific destructive behaviors and other maladaptive coping skills that may have been utilized by the family to deny reality. By making a list of all problems that have affected their dysfunctional alcoholic family, they would have a resource to use in the "recall exercise" if they should begin to regress into denial. You must identify those members in denial, those who are resistant, and those who are hostile to change. If they are not identified, their sabotage behavior could ruin all the good that has been accomplished. They may feel very loyal to the alcoholic member or may also be alcoholic. Whatever the cause, they need extra time to ask questions and get further information. Changing destructive behavior requires long-term work with the family.

EVALUATION

Evaluation is the last stage of the nursing process and is an ongoing process. After your family assessment is completed, your nursing diagnoses require certain goals and interventions, as shown in the accompanying Nursing Care Planning chart. The family is evalu-

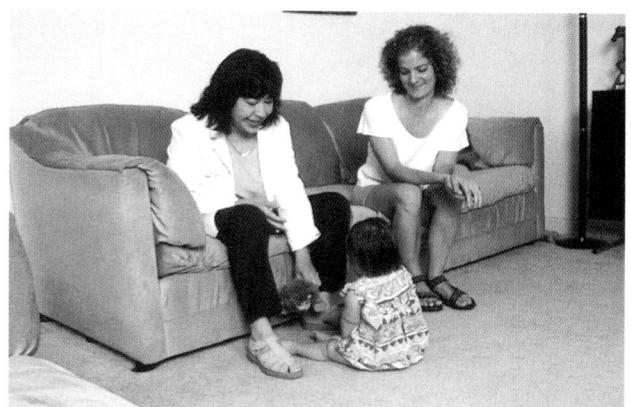

Figure 53–5. Role-modeling is an effective method of teaching caregiving skills.

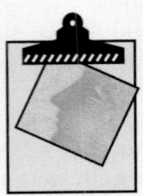

NURSING CARE PLANNING
A FAMILY WITH AN ALCOHOLIC MEMBER

Consultation With Social Worker

The social worker reports that she has been working with the Harrington family for several years. Mike is frequently out of work. She believes their problems are escalating. Nora would like Mike to go into an alcohol rehabilitation program. The social worker has made the arrangements. She asks the nurse to participate in an intervention to get Mike to enter the program.

Nursing Assessment Mike's long history of alcoholism makes it doubtful he will be successful in remaining sober, even if he completes the rehabilitation program. However, his drinking is placing the family at risk. Will participate in confronting Mike about his drinking and help him enter the program.

NURSING CARE PLAN

Nursing Diagnosis	Outcome Criteria	Interventions	Evaluation
Ineffective family coping: Alcoholism	Family identifies the manifestations of alcoholism and agrees that alcoholism is a problem for their family.	Interview and educate family and any significant others regarding the alcoholism.	The family cites examples of alcoholic behaviors described by the nurse.
	All family members state readiness to intervene.	Have each member list, in concrete terms, behaviors shown by the alcoholic member that concerned them. *Motivation to intervene is to be helpful and loving, not judgmental or punishing.*	Each family member shares and rehearses the problems caused by Mike's alcoholism.
	Alcoholic family member will be confronted about drinking by a united family.	Arrange convenient date and private place. Make sure unsuspecting alcoholic member will be present.	Nora and her children agree to confront Mike on Monday.
	Family will agree on treatment modality.	Arrange admission for inpatient detoxification for intervention date; family commits to consequence for noncompliance (i.e., move out of house).	Nora and her children agree to move to a new apartment without Mike if he does not comply.

Continued

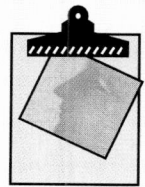

NURSING CARE PLANNING

A FAMILY WITH AN ALCOHOLIC MEMBER *(continued)*

NURSING CARE PLAN *(continued)*

Nursing Diagnosis	Outcome Criteria	Interventions	Evaluation
	The family will follow basic rules of an intervention.	Review basic rules: no name calling, no backing out or minimizing problems. A professional intervener, or an appointed family member, in charge, should explain to the suspected alcoholic *that all are here because of their love and concern;* then ask him to please not talk until everyone has spoken. Add that he will then have time to speak at the end. Each member, in turn, should read his list, using an "I feel . . ." or "It made me feel . . ." type statement.	The family, social worker, and nurse gather at the home and ask Mike to join them. Bobby refuses to participate. He says his father will never stop drinking. Each family member tells Mike how his drinking is affecting them.
		There should be no accusing, no name-calling, or judgmental attitudes. Be honest. His belief that he drinks moderately and has been fooling everyone is challenged.	The social worker assumes the role of arbitrator. She has to remind Nora several times to refrain from judgment. Mike tries to deny how much he drinks.
		Have alcoholic sign an agreement—this is very important—so that the alcoholic does not later renege, minimizing or denying the problem.	Mike agrees to enter the rehabilitation program.
		The family will support each other. Have clothes packed; transport immediately to the detoxification unit.	The nurse and social worker drive him there. Mike signs himself in.

Italicized interventions indicate culturally specific care.

Critical Thinking Questions

1. How do you think Mike will respond to this family intervention?
2. What kind of support will the family need if Mike does not agree to seek help?
3. Do you see signs that this family has personal resources to support them in the decision to move to a new location if Mike does not seek help?

ated after each nursing intervention. Assuming that the goals are realistic and comprehensive, a noticeable improvement should result.

Factors that have an impact on the evaluation stage of the nursing process are the compliance of the client and family, the quality control of the care given, the consistency of the support systems, and a realistic time frame for reaching the goals. When the goals are not met, you need to re-evaluate every step of the nursing process. Was the assessment comprehensive, validated, and clustered correctly? Was the diagnosis appropriate and complete? Were the goals realistic and attainable for the client as well as the family? Were there enough sustained support systems? Did everyone do his job? Did the interventions achieve what you and the family expected and wanted? If the family has been involved in the process, they will be willing to reassess and continue. Point out the family successes and identify the areas where more work is needed. Families will respond, especially when they can see that their efforts have been recognized and appreciated.

KEY PRINCIPLES

- The family as a client is the essence of family-centered nursing care.
- Family nursing care is based on the family response to actual or potential health problems.
- Family roles are structured for the division of labor and the distribution of power.
- Family function can be compromised by role stress and role conflict.
- The healthy family is an open system with complex interactions both within the family and within the external world.
- The interactionist would describe the family by describing roles, the decision-making process, communication, conflict, and reaction to stress.
- Knowing individual and family developmental tasks, nurses can determine the family unit's health by assessing the family's successful mastery of appropriate tasks while also observing whether individual family members' actions are appropriate to their developmental level.
- Stressors can be a threat or a challenge. It depends on how the family perceives them.
- Healthy families have resources for managing stress.
- Ineffective coping can be caused by the number of stressors and the critical importance of or the overwhelming threat of the particular stressor.
- A healthy family is one whose members are genuinely interested in what the nurse has to say and are willing to help the client.
- Indicators of ineffective family coping are family members who deny or trivialize problems, detach themselves, or refuse to offer any help.

- The *Family coping: Potential for growth* diagnosis is a wellness nursing diagnosis that is observed in families whose members are effectively managing adaptation to a health challenge of one of its members.
- The key to determining accurate nursing diagnoses is obtaining all relevant information, verifying it, and then clustering it appropriately.
- You will need to establish a nurse-client relationship based on trust.
- Interventions to establish a nurse-family relationship are establishing trust, listening actively, overcoming resistance, and reinforcing family strengths.
- Interventions for problem-solving are defining the problem, acknowledging feelings, exploring coping skills, limiting the scope, and exploring solutions to problems.
- Interventions to change behaviors are role-modeling effective behaviors, providing education, and identifying destructive behaviors.

BIBLIOGRAPHY

Appiah, K.A., & Gates, H.L. (eds). (1997). *Dictionary of global culture*. New York: Knopf.

Beauchesne, M., Kelly, B., & Gauthier, M.A. (1997). The genogram: A health assessment tool. *Nurse Educator, 22*(3), 9.

Casper, L.M., & Bryson, K. (1998a). Current Population Reports: Population Characteristics. U.S. Economics and Statistics Bureau: Department of Commerce. Available from: http://www.census.gov/population/www.socdemo/hh-fam.html. 12/18/98

Casper, L.M., & Bryson, K. (1998b). Co-resident Grandparents and Their Grandchildren: Grandparent Maintained Families. U.S. Census Bureau. Available from: http://www.census.gov/population/www/documentation/twps0026/twps0026.html 12/20/98

Clark, C. C. (1997). Posttraumatic stress disorder: How to support healing. *American Journal of Nursing, 97*(8), 27–32.

Clemen-Stone, S., McGuire, S.L., & Eigsti, D.G. (1998). *Comprehensive community health nursing: Family, aggregate, & community practice*. St. Louis: Mosby.

Cravener, P.A. (1997). Promoting active learning in large lecture classes. *Nurse Educator, 22*(3), 23.

Fink, S. (1995). The influence of family resources and family demands on the strains and well-being of caregiving families. *Nursing Research, 44*(3), 139–146.

Friedman, M.M. (1998). *Family nursing: Theory, research, and practice*. Stamford, CT: Appleton & Lange.

Gordon, M. (1997). *Manual of nursing diagnosis 1997–1998*. St Louis: Mosby.

Hatton, D.C. (1997). Managing health problems among homeless women with children in a transitional shelter. *Image: Journal of Nursing Scholarship, 29*(1), 33–37.

Holaday, B. (1997). What causes stress in mothers of chronically ill children? *Reflections, 97*(1), 24.

Katz, J.R. (1997). Back to basics: Providing effective patient teaching. *American Journal of Nursing, 97*(5), 33–36.

Lockhart, J.S., & Resick, L.K. (1997). Teaching cultural competence. *Nurse Educator, 22*(3), 27.

Lynch, S. (1997). Elder abuse: What to look for, how to intervene. *American Journal of Nursing, 97*(1), 27.

McInerney, C. (1998). Is someone hurting you? *On Call, 1*(3), 25.

North American Nursing Diagnosis Association. (1999). *NANDA nursing diagnosis: Definitions & classification 1999–2000.* Philadelphia: Author.

Orem, D.E. (1995). *Nursing: Concepts of practice* (5th ed.). St. Louis: Mosby-Year Book.

Pollock, R. (1997). *Family U.S.A.* A National Health Consumer Advocacy Group.

Quigley, L.A., & Marlatt, G.A. (1996). Drinking among young adults: Prevalence, patterns, and consequences. *Alcohol, Health and Research World, 20*(3), 185–191.

Shea, C.A., Mahoney, M., & Lacey, J.M. (1997). Breaking through the barriers to domestic violence intervention. *American Journal of Nursing, 97*(6), 26–33.

Thompson, S.K. (1997). Community health strategies. *Nurse Educator, 22*(4), 11–14.

Windle, M. (1996). Effects of parental drinking on adolescents. *Alcohol Health & Research World, 20*(3), 181–184.

Zucker, R., Ellis, D., Bingham, C.R., & Fitzgerald, H. (1996). The development of alcoholic subtypes: Risk variation among alcoholic families during the early childhood years. *Alcohol Health & Research World, 20*(1), 46–54.

The Caregiver Role

Laura Roddy Redic

Key Terms

caregiver
caregiver burden
caregiver burnout
caregiver stress
caring

coping patterns
family dynamics
objective caregiver burden
subjective caregiver burden

LEARNING OBJECTIVES

After studying this chapter, you should be able to:

1. Describe the concepts of caregiving and *Caregiver role strain*.
2. Discuss a variety of factors affecting an individual's ability to provide care.
3. Describe the assessment of caregivers, including clients experiencing or at risk for role strain.
4. Differentiate among the variety of diagnoses that may be appropriate for caregiving clients.
5. Plan for goal-directed nursing interventions directed at preventing or reducing *Caregiver role strain*.
6. Evaluate the outcomes of nursing care provided to clients experiencing *Caregiver role strain*.

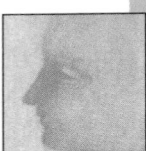

Mrs. LaVerne Roddy, age 76, was married to Laurence for 60 years. After his death 2 years ago, LaVerne felt overwhelmed by her transition to widowhood. She lost weight, had difficulty sleeping, and became uncharacteristically forgetful, anxious, and angry. She stopped attending church regularly, doing her beloved yard work, socializing with family and friends, and going to the senior center.

At first, her family attributed this change of behavior to her grief over the loss of her husband. As time passed, they became increasingly concerned about her and had her evaluated by the nurse practitioner who was her primary care provider. After an extensive work-up, the nurse practitioner informed the family that Mrs. Roddy had primary degenerative dementia of the Alzheimer's type.

The nurse gave the family a referral for a home evaluation. The home health nurse performed a functional assessment of Mrs. Roddy and established a plan of care. Sadly, the client failed to respond to the nursing interventions and progressively declined from independence to total dependence. The family refused to place her in a skilled nursing facility because of their close and loving relationship with Mrs. Roddy, as well as their cultural and spiritual beliefs. They were at *Risk for caregiver role strain* (see Caregiver Nursing Diagnoses chart).

CAREGIVER NURSING DIAGNOSES

Caregiver Role Strain: A caregiver's felt or exhibited difficulty in performing the family caregiver role.

Risk for Caregiver Role Strain: A caregiver is vulnerable for felt difficulty in performing the family caregiver role.

From North American Nursing Diagnosis Association. (1999). NANDA Nursing diagnoses: Definitions and classification 1999–2000. Philadelphia: Author.

CONCEPTS OF CAREGIVING

Although caregivers can be both professional and nonprofessional, the focus of this chapter is on non-professional caregivers who have family or personal ties to clients who receive care. Given this scope, a **caregiver** is defined as one who provides care to a dependent or partially dependent family member or friend.

The family caregiver role is not new. Before health care facilities existed, families routinely cared for their ill members themselves or hired help if they were financially able. Changes in health care delivery in recent years (such as shorter hospital stays and increased technological advances) have led to the increased use of family caregivers and home care. There are more than 25 million family caregivers in the United States who provide two-thirds of all the home care. These caregivers provide $300 billion dollars of free service every year to their family members who require care in the home (Agenet, 1999; NFCA, 1998).

Characteristics of Caregivers

The Family Caregiver Alliance (FCA, 1999), the National Family Caregivers Association (NFCA, 1998), the National Alliance for Caregiving, and the American Association of Retired Persons (NAC & AARP, 1997) all report similar demographic findings about caregivers (see Box 54–1). The typical caregiver is a married, middle-aged, female family member who lives with the person receiving care. The typical caregiver has multiple responsibilities, including full or part-time work, child care, and household chores. Nearly half of caregivers are caring for a spouse, about a quarter care for a parent, about 1 in 5 care for a child, and about 1 in 10 care for another person, such as a sibling, friend, or neighbor (Fig. 54–1). These caregivers are commonly frustrated, and they have an increased risk of depression. Their greatest needs are for emotional support and respite care.

In many cases, caregivers enter their roles with ambivalent feelings. Love for family members and the satisfaction derived from helping coexist with feelings of resentment about their loss of privacy and frustration at believing they have no control over what happens. The caregiving responsibility is not always assumed by

---

BOX 54–1

DEMOGRAPHIC PROFILE OF FAMILY CAREGIVERS

Although estimates vary depending on the definitions of caregivers and the types of surveys used, the following statistics should give you a good idea of today's typical caregivers.

- 72 to 81% are female.
- 66 to 79% are married.
- 70% are between ages 40 and 60.
- More than half who are under age 65 work.
- 42% reduced their work hours and 18% quit their jobs to give care.
- 77% have multiple responsibilities (including full- or part-time employment, child care, and household chores).
- 69 to 78% live with the care receiver.
- 48 to 54% care for a spouse.
- 21 to 24% care for a parent.
- 17 to 19% care for a child.
- 9% care for a sibling, friend, or other.
- 34% receive no help from family or friends.
- Median household income is $20,000–$35,000.
- The most pressing caregiver needs are emotional support (87%) and respite care (76%).
- 49 to 58% show clinically significant depressive symptoms.
- 69% consider frustration their most frequent emotion.

Data from National Alliance for Caregiving & American Association of Retired Persons. (NAC & AARP, 1997). Family caregiving in the U.S.: Findings from a national study final report. Available from: http://caregiving.org/content/repsprods.asp 3/10/97.

---

choice but because of a blend of responsibility, desire, and family or sociocultural expectations.

Caregivers may experience a greater burden when they also hold a job. Immeasurable financial losses occur when they are forced to reduce work hours or quit working so they can care for a family member (see the Cost of Care chart).

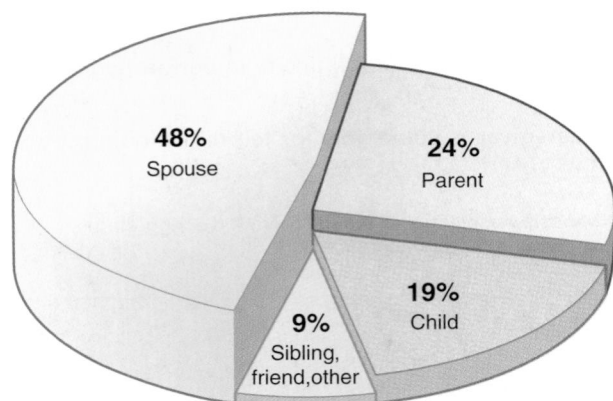

Figure 54–1. For whom do caregivers care? (Data from National Family Caregivers Association Member Survey 1997: A profile of caregivers. Available at: http://www.nfcacares.org/survey.html.)

Caring

Caring is a universal behavior observed in human beings and influenced by society, culture, values, and gender. When we care, we consider another's point of view, their objective needs, and what they expect of us. Our attention, our mental engrossment, is on the cared-for, not ourselves. Caring "for" includes those actions and behaviors that are associated with "doing for" the receiver of care. Caring "about" involves positive and unconditional regard for the recipient of care.

Many caregivers feel inadequate when they are able to care "for" but unable to care "about" the receiver of care. An example is the caregiver and the care receiver who have a history of incompatibility. They may find it difficult to care "about" each other. The stress from such a relationship can lead to *Caregiver role strain*.

> A*ction* A*lert!*
> During your initial and ongoing assessments, be alert to clues about how family caregivers feel about the caring role.

Caregiver Role Strain

Caregivers are at increased risk for role strain when they have trouble performing the caregiver role (NANDA, 1999). This strain is associated with the burden and responsibilities involved in the care of dependent family members. It can result from the developmental level of the caregiver (too young to provide the care), the living environment (inadequate space), situational stressors (financial problems), or a need for extensive care (family member has Alzheimer's disease).

Strain can also occur when there are unresolved conflicts between the caregiver and care recipient or when there is resentment, anger, and guilt about taking on the role of caregiver. For example, the wife of an elderly brain-impaired care recipient may resent being in the caregiver role because of an earlier history of abuse from her husband. The burden of this arrange-

ment may be especially trying and energy-depleting for her.

Caregiver role strain can also occur when a caregiver neglects her own health and lets existing conditions worsen. In a recent survey, the loss of leisure time, feelings of isolation, and changes in family dynamics were reported to be the most burdensome aspects of caregiving (NFCA, 1997).

Caregiver role strain may be minimized when the recipient and the caregiver predetermine how and by whom the care will be provided. The caregiver agrees to accept the role and makes preparations.

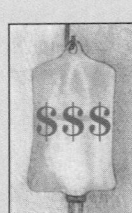

THE COST OF CARE
THE ECONOMIC IMPACT OF CAREGIVING IN AMERICA

There are 25 million family caregivers in the United States. These caregivers provide at least two-thirds of all home care. Only 10 to 20% of family caregivers use formal services through public or private agencies. The National Family Caregivers Association (NFCA) estimates that these home care services are valued at $300 billion annually.

Caregivers, Inc. (1997) studied the impact of caregiving on the workforce in America. The findings revealed that variables affecting caregivers were time lost from work, decreased productivity, and lost opportunities (such as career advancement missed because of caregiving obligations). Because of concerns regarding their caregiving obligations, 20% of workers reduce their work hours, 27% work less effectively, 58% work more slowly, and 1 in 7 quit work to become a full-time caregiver. Others use unpaid time off from work to cope. Some must continue to work to pay for the care of their loved ones.

The study noted that employers lose more than $3,100 yearly on each employee who has caregiving responsibilities. Factors related to caregiving that lead to the employer's financial losses include absenteeism, problems of job retention, lost productivity, employee stress, problems of employee well-being, and an aging workforce.

References

AgeNet. (1999). *Family caregivers: Who are they?* Available from: http://www.agenet.com/Who_Are_They.html 3/18/99.

Caregivers, Inc. (1997). *Caregivers and the workplace: What you should know as an employer.* Caregivers, Inc. Available from: http://www.caregivr.com/carelinks.html 3/18/99.

National Family Caregivers Association. (NFCA, 1998). *Fact sheet: Selected caregiver statistics.* Kensington, MD: Author.

$\mathcal{A}ction\ \mathcal{A}lert!$
You must be knowledgeable and alert to the cues that indicate family *Caregiver role strain*.

Caregiver Burden

Caregiver burden refers to the unrelenting physical, psychological, social, or financial problems that occur when a caregiver provides for the health needs of an impaired family member or friend (Jones, 1996). **Subjective caregiver burden** refers to the caregiver's personal appraisal of a caregiving situation and the extent to which the person perceives it to be a burden. **Objective caregiver burden** refers to the observable, tangible costs to the caregiver in behaviors required or disruptions experienced (Jones, 1996). Both subjective and objective burdens place the caregiver at risk for increased stress.

Caregiver Stress

Stress is a stimulus that a person perceives as challenging or harmful. **Caregiver stress** refers to the caregiver's reaction to physical, emotional, sociocultural, financial, and environmental stressors brought on by the caregiving experience. Caregivers who are under stress suffer physical and emotional disabilities that interfere with their caregiver capabilities. Because of this, you should educate caregivers about the dangers of stress and offer them self-help strategies to eliminate it or reduce its effects.

$\mathcal{A}ction\ \mathcal{A}lert!$
Offer caregivers self-help strategies to reduce the detrimental effects of caregiver stress.

Caregiver Burnout

Caregiver burnout is a depletion of physical and mental energy caused by providing care for a chronically ill person over a long period of time. The more complicated the treatment program or needs of the receiver, the greater the risk for caregiver burnout. Caregiver behaviors that suggest burnout include ongoing and constant fatigue, decreasing interest in work and work production, withdrawal from social contacts, increasing fear of death, increasing use of stimulants and alcohol, sleep disturbances, change in eating patterns, and feelings of helplessness and depression.

Family caregivers who experience burnout are generally involved in unrelenting daily care of family members as opposed to several hours per day for a few days a week. They may feel unable to divorce themselves from the caregiving situation because of family, cultural, personal, or financial obligations.

It is important for you to intervene before burnout occurs in family caregivers. Helping caregivers recognize unrealistic expectations of themselves and the need for respite care are essential nursing interventions.

$\mathcal{A}ction\ \mathcal{A}lert!$
Be aware of the emotional upheavals experienced by caregivers and be prepared to support them in their problem-solving and decision-making activities.

FACTORS AFFECTING CAREGIVING
Social Factors
Social Support System

When caregivers have an inadequate social support system, they are more likely to experience *Caregiver role strain*. The caregiver's social support system may include relatives, friends, and others who will help in caring for the dependent family member. Support can include financial, emotional, or daily caregiving assistance. The accompanying chart describes one caregiver's view of support and what it can mean.

Caregiver stressors can originate from intrafamily, interfamily, or extrafamily sources. One common intrafamily stressor is a lack of time for oneself. Research has shown that many caregivers have no leisure time and receive inconsistent or no help from family or friends. Another intrafamily stressor is lack of appreciation for one's efforts. Caregiver surveys indicate that many caregivers feel taken for granted and unappreciated (NFCA, 1998; FCA, 1997).

An example of an interfamily stressor is when a caregiver has feelings of unrelenting stress from caring for a dependent family member. An example of an extrafamily stressor is when a caregiver quits work to care for a family member and then experiences a financial hardship.

Caregivers who cannot get beyond the burdens, responsibilities, isolation, and stressors of caregiving will begin to perceive caregiving as a solitary journey. The length and intensity of this journey is alleviated when each family member takes a proactive role in the care of the recipient.

Family Dynamics

Family dynamics are the forces at work within the family that result in particular coping behaviors. Family dynamics can suffer when interactions and relationships stop working to efficiently accomplish the family's functions and tasks. The stress created by caring for a dependent family member causes new roles to emerge. The extent and complexity of the caregiving process can exhaust family coping behaviors and place the family at risk. Examples of cues that the family is at risk for *Caregiver role strain* include the resurfacing of childhood issues with siblings, tension between spouses when one takes on additional family responsibilities, and resentment from children when parents have less time and energy for them.

It is important for you to help families recognize when they are at risk for *Caregiver role strain*. Encourage and support family members when they have reached the limit of their capabilities or resources for caregiving. Help them by discussing available short-term care

"IT HELPS—AND HURTS—TO REMEMBER WHO THEY WERE"

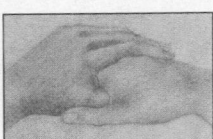 Not long after my wife of 42 years retired from her job at the district court, she began to show what I thought were signs of depression. We were leaving our 10-room house, now emptied of seven children, for a smaller, cozier place, and she was having difficulty packing. She was more quiet and forgetful, just seemed to be losing her zip. She'd also had a car accident. Nothing serious—just a momentary lapse of attention. She also misplaced things. I found a bank book in her raincoat pocket, a plastic bag with several of her rings in the pocket of a jacket she seldom wore. Seven years later, I'm still trying to find her engagement ring.

Before her annual physical, I tipped off the internist about her symptoms. He referred us to a neurologist, who ordered an extensive series of tests: thyroid cocktail, x-rays, EEG, EKG, MRI, and an extensive psychoneurological examination. Ruling out any physiological problem left only one possibility: Alzheimer's.

I immediately joined the Alzheimer's Association, got a medical ID bracelet for my wife, contacted social service agencies, and talked with my colleagues at the Visiting Nurses Association. They told me to start looking at rest homes immediately, which I did. Before long, I applied at a facility that offered both day care and full-time care. Good advice; there's a long waiting list now.

One day my wife slipped out of the house and then couldn't find her way back. Because of her work at the courthouse, the police knew her and brought her home. That's when I had alarms installed on the doors. Over a period of months, she lost all ambition—no longer cooked, so we went out to eat. I was still working full-time as a pharmacist, and she would call me repeatedly at work wanting to know where I was and when I was coming home.

I hired a companion for her who claimed to have cared for a grandmother with Alzheimer's; she didn't work out for us, however. Then I hired a neighbor who had worked in a day care facility for Alzheimer's patients. That worked until the neighbor said my wife needed to be in day care full-time. A good solution temporarily. She adjusted very well to the structured routine and simple exercises.

The rages began at home. She would throw things and strike out at me, although at 4'11" tall, she wasn't much of a threat to my 6', 200-pound frame. And she would be up, prowling the house in the middle of the night. When the final stages of incontinence began, my macho "I can take care of anything" attitude crumbled. I knew she needed more care than I could provide.

Six years after the diagnosis, she became a resident at the same place where she had been in day care. It was an easy transition. A year later, her speech is now very limited. Every day, I say, "I love you. Do you love me?"

She says, "Yep."

Yesterday I told her, "I've got good news."

She said, "What is it?"

"You're a grandmother for the fifteenth time." She smiled but didn't reply so I don't know how much she understood.

Since her diagnosis, our lives have been pretty much like the book *The 36-Hour Day*. The disease varies from person to person. The wife of a friend of mine deteriorated rapidly, yet others in the facility with my wife have been there 5 or 6 years. The experts say Alzheimer's patients don't suffer physical pain, but every family suffers. Depression and guilt are common. What makes the biggest difference for the caregiver is support—or lack of it—by family and friends. We're blessed with wonderful kids—six daughters and a son. For our fortieth wedding anniversary, before disaster struck, they sent us to Europe for 2 weeks. The ones who live nearby visit her often. They pay to have my house cleaned and keep my freezer stocked with food. They call often. They've told me: "You did more than you should. You needed help sooner." I feel guilty when I go to my monthly support group meetings and hear stories of family members so much worse off.

People find it hard to visit Alzheimer's patients—even family members. As soon as my wife went into the rest home, I called her three closest friends. Not one has gone to see her.

She gets wonderful care. The place is mostly staffed with RNs. But regardless of how good the care is, you need to be there every day to keep an eye on the little things. Massachusetts has a good system for monitoring all convalescent homes. When I asked the Department of Public Health for the report on my wife's facility, they sent an eight-page review. Out of a possible score of 80, the place rated 79.

Outside each resident's room, there's a brief biography of that person. You find people from all walks of life: a Federal district court judge, a nun who taught French, a nun who ran a convalescent home, an attorney, the owner of a bus company, a PhD educator, a hospital chaplain, and a former football player. It helps—and hurts—to remember who they were.

I know three other fellows with wives in a similar situation. Once a week, we go out for an inexpensive meal, share a bottle of wine, and talk about other things. As with me, their wives were "the brains of the organization." Now we're having to learn to do all the things they did for us. When I owned a business, my wife did all the book-keeping, all the buying, plus shopping for and raising seven kids, then worked 20 years at the county courthouse. She was amazing.

I have a lot of faith in God. I pray a lot, but I cry a lot, too. Work helps. I still put in 26 hours a week at a pharmacy. I garden, and I love to read. Sure, I'm losing my hair, and I have dentures and orthotics, but I work out on my Alpine Climber 3 days a week. Not bad for a man of 71.

options, such as respite care, private nurses, and adult day health. As appropriate, also discuss long-term care options such as skilled nursing facilities.

Action Alert!
Assess families involved in caregiving for how well they are coping.

Cultural/Religious Factors

Cultural expectations may also place caregivers at risk for *Caregiver role strain.* Conflicts may exist between what is expected from one's culture and what can actually be accomplished (Jones, 1995). In some cultures, women are expected to care for dependent relatives. Such cultural practices may have been conceived during an era when women were expected to remain at home and were not part of the workforce. Today, such expectations may not be feasible. When working women try to assume all expected roles, *Caregiver role strain* may occur.

Picot (1995b) studied the physiological aspects of caregiving on African-American female caregivers. She determined that African-American caregivers perceived greater levels of reward, mediated by the comfort of religion and prayer, than Caucasians. Further findings revealed that caregivers with a higher level of education (whether African-American or Caucasian) reported fewer rewards than those with less education.

Mackinnon, Gien, and Durst (1996) interviewed 10 first-generation Chinese elderly care recipients and found four major areas of concern: loneliness and isolation, reduced resources in which to reciprocate the care-receiving relationship, an expressed need for meaningful relationships and roles within the family, and the desire for greater independence.

Studies such as the preceding indicate that you must be culturally sensitive when developing nursing interventions to prevent *Caregiver role strain* and care recipient stress.

Socioeconomic Factors

The financial cost associated with caregiving can cause many families to experience financial difficulties. Financial setbacks are especially prevalent in families whose members have to leave the workforce in order to care for a dependent family member. These families are placed at risk for *Caregiver role strain* due to financial instability.

The Family Caregiver Alliance (FCA, 1997) reported that 40% of caregivers incur additional financial expenses for care-related products, services, and activities. Twenty-six percent of caregivers spent up to 10% of their monthly income on caregiving. Thirty-one percent incurred bills for travel, 24% for special diets for the care recipient, and 25% for telephone and utility charges.

The costs of caregiving in terms of lost productivity from caregivers who are employed full-time is estimated at about $11.4 billion per year. When part-time and long-distance caregivers are included, this figure rises to about $29 billion each year (FCA, 1997).

Psychological Factors

Meeting the needs of dependent family members is emotionally taxing for caregivers. Although most caregivers experience some type of psychological distress while they perform caregiver duties, their coping patterns and the quality and quantity of support provided by their social network can minimize their stress. The more serious and demanding the care is, the greater the likelihood the caregiver will experience psychological problems.

Studies have shown that nearly half of all caregivers become clinically depressed. The Family Caregiver Alliance (FCA, 1997) reported that caregivers use prescription drugs to alleviate their depression, anxiety, and insomnia more than twice as often as noncaregivers. About 80% of caregivers reported that they experienced emotional strain as a result of caregiving.

Coping Patterns

Coping patterns are the specific protective behaviors used by an individual or a family to respond to stressful situations. When caregivers and families are under stress, both cognitive and noncognitive processes direct their coping behavior. If their usual coping patterns are ineffective because of a crisis, the family becomes vulnerable to damaging stress.

Psychoneuroimmunology and Health

Micozzi (1996) reports that higher cognitive centers and limbic emotional centers are capable of regulating virtually all aspects of the immune system and, therefore, have a profound effect on health and illness. Thoughts, feelings, emotions, and perceptions can alter immunity. Each thought and feeling has a chemical consequence in the brain. As little as 5 minutes in a stressful situation was observed to cause a rise in cortisol levels in research animals. You need to be knowledgeable concerning the relationship between the psychoneuroimmune pathways, stress, and health in order to prevent or alleviate the consequences of long-term caregiving.

Action Alert!
Assess the stress levels of elderly caregivers because the aging immune system is already compromised. Additional stressors could result in accelerated debilitation in the aging caregiver.

Locus of Control

Locus of control also affects the caregiving role. An internal locus of control is the belief that you can control the circumstances in your life. An external locus of control is the belief that other people, destiny, or luck controls your circumstances. For example, a caregiver with an external locus of control may be burdened by the belief that "bad luck" placed him in the position of caregiver. This thought process places him at high risk for depression.

On the other hand, a caregiver with an internal locus of control is more likely to take responsibility for his decision to serve as caregiver. Taking responsibility for one's actions helps to alleviate the stress associated with caregiving. Take time to assess caregivers' beliefs about the causes for their circumstances.

ASSESSMENT

General Assessment of the Caregiver

In most settings, caregivers are not considered clients, so their specific needs may go unmet. To prevent *Caregiver role strain*, however, you need to assess the needs of both caregiver and the ill family member as well as the community resources available to them.

To determine the needs of a caregiver, you will need to assess her perceptions of the caregiving process. This includes her understanding of her responsibilities as a caregiver, her expectations (and her family's expectations) of the caregiving duties, her relationship with the care receiver, and her other responsibilities, such as work and child care.

Several caregiver assessment tools are available to help you collect these data. Some assess the caregiver's physical and mental health, and others assess family dynamics, perceptions of caregiving, the adequacy of social support systems, and cultural expectations. One measurement tool that assesses positive and negative feelings of caregivers is the Picot Caregiver Rewards Scale (Fig. 54–2). The purpose of this tool is to measure the level of positive rewards in the caregiver's relationship with the care recipient. The higher the level of rewards, the lower the level of caregiver costs and depression.

Focused Assessment for Caregiver Role Strain

Defining Characteristics

Defining characteristics for the diagnosis *Caregiver role strain* include the following:

- Apprehension about the care receiver's future health and the caregiver's ability to provide care
- Apprehension about the possible need to institutionalize the care receiver
- Apprehension about the care receiver's care when caregiver becomes ill or dies
- Difficulty performing required activities
- Inability to complete caregiving tasks
- Preoccupation with the care routine
- Altered caregiving activities
- Altered caregiver health status

Additional objective cues that may indicate *Caregiver role strain* are the following:

- The caregiver is not as attentive to personal appearance.

- The caregiver pays attention to details in caregiving but not to other activities (poor concentration at work, school, other activities).
- The caregiver has difficulty making positive statements about self since taking on caregiver role.
- The caregiver is inappropriately cheerful or in denial of the seriousness of the situation.

*A*ction *A*lert!
The caregiver who contracts stress-related or opportunistic illnesses (such as herpes zoster, hypertension, gastric distress, infections, or colds) may be experiencing *Caregiver role strain*.

Related Factors

Factors that contribute to the caregiver's effectiveness in performing the unrelenting or complex care requirements of the care receiver may be classified as pathophysiological, psychosocial, developmental, and situational (Table 54–1).

Focused Assessment for Related Nursing Diagnoses

When caregiving families cannot manage internal or external stressors caused by inadequate resources, there is the potential for abusive or neglectful care of family members. This behavior is particularly observed in the care of the elderly and young children and situations wherein domestic abuse may escalate between couples who had unstable relationships before the caregiving began. In such situations, the diagnosis *Ineffective family coping* may apply.

Caregiving families are at risk for the diagnosis *Altered family processes* whenever they experience a stressor that disrupts their usual state of functioning. Role changes from illness and disruption of family routines can have a great impact on the family functioning. Further, socioeconomic losses and other detrimental factors can lead to *Caregiver role strain*, role burden, and role stress.

The caregiver role, which crosses all developmental levels, is very taxing for parents. In many cases, parents are members of the "sandwich generation": They have both children and elderly parents who require their attention or care. Because of the need to play dual roles—caregiver and parent—they may be at risk for *Parental role conflict*.

When the negative stressors are so great that a person cannot see an alternative solution to the problem, he is at risk for the diagnosis *Hopelessness*. He is unable to make decisions and has little energy to dispense on activities. His appearance may change from well-kept to poorly groomed. It is difficult for him to maintain interest or eye contact. *Hopelessness* can be seen in both the caregiver and the care recipient. It is possible for a client in this state to become suicidal.

A person is in a state of *Social isolation* when the desire to be involved with others goes unmet because of physiological, situational, or maturational problems.

ID# _____

Now I'd like to talk to you about some of the ways people feel about caring for another person. Please tell me how you feel now about caring for your [ELDER]. Choose only one answer for each statement from the following: A great deal [4], Quite a lot [3], Somewhat [2], A little [1], or Not at all [0].

	Great deal	Quite a lot	Some-what	A little	Not at all
1. I feel God will bless me.	4	3	2	1	0
2. I feel better about myself.	4	3	2	1	0
3. I feel I have become a stronger, tolerant, and/or patient person around persons with sickness or handicaps.	4	3	2	1	0
4. I feel having others say that taking care of my relative is the right thing to do is important.	4	3	2	1	0
5. I feel that my relative will remember me in his/her will for my care.	4	3	2	1	0
6. I feel someone will take care of me when I need it.	4	3	2	1	0
7. I feel nurses, doctors, and social workers work harder to care for my [ELDER] too.	4	3	2	1	0
8. I feel that placing my [ELDER] in a nursing home will be avoided.	4	3	2	1	0
9. I feel that doctors, nurses and social workers do not know everything about my [ELDER]'s chances for getting better.	4	3	2	1	0
10. I feel receiving a smile, touch, or eye contact from my [ELDER] is important.	4	3	2	1	0
11. I feel I have a closer relationship with my [ELDER].	4	3	2	1	0
12. I feel I have an opportunity to repay my [ELDER] for a past debt.	4	3	2	1	0
13. I feel receiving a "thank you" from my [ELDER] is important.	4	3	2	1	0
14. I feel I have become a better person by learning new information.	4	3	2	1	0
15. I feel I have become a better person by learning new ways to care for the elderly.	4	3	2	1	0
16. I feel that I have made many new friends.	4	3	2	1	0
17. I feel more important.	4	3	2	1	0
18. I feel I have the freedom to make decisions that matter.	4	3	2	1	0
19. I feel I do not need to hold a job.	4	3	2	1	0
20. I feel that receiving praise and admiration for my efforts from doctors, nurses and social workers is important.	4	3	2	1	0
21. I feel I can now plan my own schedule each day.	4	3	2	1	0
22. I feel happier now than I did before I started caring for my [ELDER].	4	3	2	1	0
23. I feel that caring for my [ELDER] has made our family grow and work closer together.	4	3	2	1	0
24. I feel my family members now look up to me because of my efforts under difficult circumstances.	4	3	2	1	0

[IF CARE RECEIVER LIVES WITH RESPONDENT:]

25. I feel having my relative live with me means added money coming into the house.	4	3	2	1	0

Figure 54–2. The Picot Caregiver Reward Scale. (Copyright 1995 by Sandra J. Fulton Picot.)

TABLE 54–1
Factors Affecting Caregiver Effectiveness

Category	Examples of Influential Factors
Developmental	• Caregiver developmentally not ready for caregiver role, as when a young adult must care for a middle-aged parent. • Developmental delay of the receiver or caregiver. • Family's stage of development conflicts with caregiving requirements, as when a newly married couple must care for a sick sibling rather than preparing for child rearing.
Psychosocial	• Psychosocial or cognitive problems in the receiver of care. • Marginal coping patterns in caregiver. • History of poor relationship between caregiver and care receiver. • Caregiver is spouse. • Care receiver exhibits bizarre behavior. • Relationship of caregiver to receiver (spouse, sibling, parent, child, friend, other relative, acquaintance). • Family coping patterns. • Spiritual, religious, or cultural beliefs. • Financial risk borne by caregiver.
Situational	• Abuse or violence in the family. • Situational stressors such as loss, disaster, crisis, poverty, or major life events such as birth, hospitalization, leaving home, returning home, marriage, divorce, employment, retirement, or death. • Poor family dynamics before caregiving began. • Duration of caregiving required. • Inadequate physical environment for providing care (housing, transportation, community services, equipment). • Family or caregiver isolation. • Lack of respite and recreation for caregiver. • Inexperience with caregiving. • Caregiver's competing role commitments. • Complexity and amount of caregiving tasks required.
Physiological	• Severity of the recipient's illness. • Addiction or codependency. • Premature birth or congenital defect. • Discharge from health care facility with significant home care needs. • Impaired caregiver health. • Unpredictable course of illness or unstable caregiver health.

Caregivers are at risk for this condition because of the restrictions placed on them by caregiving. The more intensive the caregiving needed, the more likely the person will be socially isolated. This condition can also occur in both the caregiver and the care recipient.

DIAGNOSIS

The diagnosis of *Caregiver role strain* is used when family caregivers feel or exhibit difficulty in performing their family caregiver roles. The diagnosis *Risk for caregiver role strain* is used when family caregivers are vulnerable for felt difficulty in performing their family caregiver roles (NANDA, 1999). It represents the burden of caregiving on the physical and emotional health of family caregivers and the effects on their families and the social systems of caregivers and care receivers.

PLANNING

Because of changes in the health care system and the movement to managed care, nursing care managers are required to conduct collaborative multidisciplinary conferences in which caregivers participate. The focus of the planning session is to provide quality, safe, and cost-effective care to the homebound client and to customize the plan of care to meet the specific needs of the client and caregiver.

After a thorough assessment of the client, caregivers, and resources, a care plan is established with expected care outcomes. The outcomes may include sharing frustrations, identifying support systems, identifying ways to improve daily life, conveying empathy, establishing support plans, and being able to listen to the caregiver without giving advice (Carpenito, 1997).

The plan of care that the family is given upon discharge from an acute care setting is evaluated in the home setting and revised as needed to meet the needs of the family.

Mrs. Roddy developed a urinary tract infection and needed to be hospitalized. While there, she developed acute respiratory failure and required mechanical ventilation. Attempts to wean her from the ventilator failed, and the family faced the decision of whether to bring her home or admit her to a long-term care facility. What factors did the family need to consider in deciding whether to care for Mrs. Roddy at home?

INTERVENTION

Interventions to Reduce Caregiver Role Strain

Providing Empathy

Assessment data may reveal that the caregivers need to ventilate or to be told that they are doing a good job. Performing the tasks of a caregiver is a lonely, isolating experience that can prompt feelings that no one understands the difficulties and demands of the job. When visiting a caregiver, allow time to share feelings. Convey admiration for positive behaviors that you observe, such as devotion, love, a little job well done, or the client's sense of satisfaction and involvement in family life. Listen to the caregiver's feelings, communicate understanding, and promote a sense of competency not just once but as often as is needed to achieve

positive results. Encourage the family and support them in their decision-making.

Help the caregiver appreciate the task she has undertaken by giving information about the difficulties of the caregiving responsibilities. Educate the caregiver about self-care activities that can be used to alleviate *Caregiver role strain* (see teaching strategies in Box 54–2).

Promoting Realistic Appraisal

Caregivers may have unrealistic goals and objectives for the caregiving situation. You can help a caregiver assess the reality of the length of time care will be needed, how much recovery is possible, how much cooperation or self-help can be expected from the recipient of care, and what elements of care are essential. The caregiver may be in denial or just uninformed about the demands of the situation.

Many caregivers do not have insight into the role responsibilities involved in the day-to-day care of a dependent care receiver. Asking them to describe a typical day or their involvement in social or leisure activi-

---

BOX 54–2

TEACHING STRATEGIES FOR REDUCING CAREGIVER ROLE STRAIN

Establish Partnerships in Your Family Member's Care

- Establish good relationships with health care providers. They can make sure your family member receives good health care, and they can provide information about the person's medical condition, what to expect in the future, and available community resources.
- Contact a professional with whom you feel comfortable talking about the frustrations of providing care. Clergy, social workers, psychologists, and psychiatric nurses are trained to provide counseling on caregiving issues.
- Join a caregiver support group. This is another good place to share your frustrations and obtain help in managing your stress, locating resources, reducing feelings of isolation, and obtaining support.
- If you have an employee assistance program at work, use it to obtain help with feelings about your caregiver role and to learn about community resources that can help to alleviate your stress.
- Involve your family from the beginning by sharing your concerns with them and dividing up, when possible, the caregiving responsibilities.
- Take time to consider how you might take better care of yourself.

Take Care of Yourself

- Set realistic goals. Trying to balance caregiving with time for yourself, work, and other obligations is difficult. Determine your priorities and turn to others for help with your caregiving responsibilities.
- Carve time out for yourself, even an hour a day. Do something you enjoy, such as reading a book or going to lunch with a friend. Do not give up your favorite pastimes or withdraw from your friends.
- Accept your feelings. Recognize that you may be grieving. Talk about your feelings with a family member, close friend, or counselor.
- Recognize signs of stress. Are you feeling irritable, helpless, hopeless? Do minor things upset you or make you cry? Are you having trouble sleeping, gaining or losing weight, or feeling exhausted all the time? Are you getting ill more often than you used to? Use a support group, get counseling, and use respite care.
- Get some exercise each day. Take a walk, take stairs instead of an elevator, walk when you are on the phone, put energy into housework, mow the lawn, and so on.
- Recognize your limits. Maybe you will not be able to provide care until the care recipient dies. Learn to "let go" from the start and share your caregiver burdens with other family members or professional caregivers.

From National Alliance for Caregiving. (NAC, 1998). Caregiving tips. Available at: http://caregiving.org/content/tips.asp 3/17/99.

ties helps them to understand that the responsibilities are tremendous and in some cases overwhelming. Help the caregiver be realistic about the personal effects of maintaining the present schedule and responsibilities. The caregiver should make plans for maintaining physical health, emotional status, and relationships with family and friends. You can help the caregiver develop a plan for scheduling needed respite time. The caregiver needs to have "me" time to unwind from the pressures of the caregiving role and maintain good health.

Using Resources

Much of *Caregiver role strain* may stem from a lack of knowledge about available resources or unwillingness to accept assistance. Many caregivers try to take care of their loved one alone or with a few family members. They are unaware of the resources available to them in the community or how to request help from others. Provide information about volunteer resources, health insurance benefits, and Medicare or Medicaid benefits. Volunteers can be used to sit with the recipient of care while the caregiver goes to the grocery store, has lunch with friends, or otherwise takes a break from the caregiving role.

Some caregivers decline help because they associate asking for help with "begging" or not being able to manage their own affairs. Statements such as "I never depend on anyone to help me" or "We aren't destitute" demand investigation. Make sure that the caregiver understands the relationship between over-extending herself as a caregiver and the high probability that she will suffer the ill effects of excessive stress. Encourage her to take care of herself so she can continue to effectively take care of her loved one.

If you can, talk to family members separately from the caregiver. Interesting facts may surface during this discussion. For example, other family members may not be aware that the primary caregiver is at risk for caregiver role stain. Sometimes, when family members become aware of the difficulties the primary caregiver is experiencing, they are willing to provide help with caregiving. For family members who cannot provide direct care, providing emotional support to the primary care provider with visits or phone calls may help to reduce *Caregiver role strain*.

Providing Direct Assistance

You may need to develop interventions to help the caregiver obtain information and instrumental support. First, assess the type of services the caregiver is providing. Typically, the caregiver provides personal care and treatments, prepares meals, cleans house, does yard work, makes appointments, takes the person to medical appointments, and manages finances. Help the caregiver identify both professional and volunteer (family, friends, neighbors, church) resources. It may help the caregiver if you give her permission to

ask for help from family and friends by discussing how most people feel good when they provide a "little help."

When a care recipient can no longer remain in the home, you will need to help identify options available for placement such as nursing home placement. Discuss the advantages and disadvantages of each option but allow control in decision-making to remain with the caregiver. Support her decisions to help minimize the guilt feelings she may experience when the care recipient needs to be placed in a facility.

Interventions to Prevent Caregiver Role Strain

Engaging Assistance From Family and Friends

When possible and with the permission of the caregiver, engage other family members in the appraisal of the caregiver's situation. Allow each member the opportunity to share their frustration and concerns about the changes in family function created by the need for caregiving. Stress that in many situations there are no problems to be solved, only pain to be shared. You are in a good position to help other family members recognize the needs of both caregiver and care recipient. You can help them identify the kinds of support they can give. Emphasize the importance of emotional support—that is, regular phone calls, cards, letters, and visits. Discuss the need to give the caregiver "permission" to enjoy herself (respite care, vacations, day trips).

For caregivers who have access to the Internet, you can encourage its use as a support system. It can give them easy access to resources that meet their needs, such as information about their family member's health problems. It can provide them with Internet caregiver support groups. And it can serve as a diversionary intervention for caregivers unable to leave the home at regular intervals.

One such Internet site is the Caregiver Survival Resources. It is available at on the World Wide Web at http://www.caregiver911.com. Caregivers can consult with "Dr. Caregiver," correspond via e-mail with other caregivers, and learn about workshops, books, tapes, and other resources that may prevent them from experiencing *Caregiver role strain*.

Encouraging Social Support and Advocacy

Encourage caregivers to use a social support system to help manage their emotional needs. Support groups, in particular, can help caregivers appraise the reality of their situations and provide information about methods of care and resources. You can link caregivers with social support resources.

Many caregiver advocacy groups are recruiting members who will speak out and demand an improvement in the quality and quantity of caregiving services at the local, state, and federal levels. The opportunity to join with other caregivers and advocates for caregivers can be a satisfying social outlet for some caregivers.

Mrs. Roddy's family attended a discharge planning conference in which the discharge team discussed Mrs. Roddy's deteriorating condition and the health care options available for the family. Because Mrs. Roddy had expressed a desire to remain in her home and had not wanted to go to a nursing home, the family decided to try home care. After the family caregivers were instructed in the care of a ventilator-dependent client and declared competent caregivers, Mrs. Roddy was discharged home with a tracheostomy, gastrostomy tube feedings, Foley catheter, heparin lock, and therapeutic bed. A home health nurse collaborated with the family and the home health team. What interventions on the part of the home health nurse might help to prevent *Caregiver role strain?*

EVALUATION

In collaboration with caregivers, evaluate progress toward preventing or reducing *Caregiver role strain.* Based on that information, revise nursing diagnoses, outcomes, and plans of care. As part of your evaluation, assess the effectiveness of your interventions. Did you successfully reduce the caregiver's apprehension about her ability to provide care? Did the caregiver receive the type of help she needed to take care of herself?

Caregiver role strain can have a strong detrimental influence on caregivers and their families. Successful nursing care can prevent caregiver burnout and the physical and emotional disorders associated with it. Your care can make a tremendous difference in the lives of caregiving families.

KEY PRINCIPLES

- Caregivers are at risk for role strain from the burden, responsibilities, and stress associated with caregiving.
- Caregivers are not clients of the health care system; as such, their specific needs may go unmet.
- Nurses need to be alert to the unmet needs of caregivers as well as care recipients.
- The diagnosis *Caregiver role strain* is used when family caregivers feel or exhibit difficulty in performing their family caregiver roles.
- The diagnosis *Risk for caregiver role strain* is used when family caregivers are vulnerable for felt difficulty in performing their family caregiver roles.
- The Picot Caregiver Reward Scale is used to determine caregivers' positive feelings and perceived rewards in their caregiving experiences.
- Nursing interventions are based first on establishing a trusting relationship with the caregiver.
- Nurses interventions include helping the caregiver identify when she needs to examine other options, such as respite care, nursing home placement, or hospice care.

- Evaluation is a systematic ongoing process where you and the caregiver evaluate progress toward preventing or reducing *Caregiver role strain.*

BIBLIOGRAPHY

Acton, G.J., & Miller, E.W. (1996). Affiliated-individuation in caregivers of adults with dementia. *Issues in Mental Health Nursing, 17*(3), 245–260.

AgeNet. (1999). *Family caregivers: Who are they?* Available from: http://www.agenet.com/Who_Are_They.html 3/18/99.

Bock, D.J. (1995). A case manager's practical tips for family caregivers. *Journal of Case Management, 4*(4), 128–131.

Boland, D.L., & Sims, S.L. (1996). Family care giving at home as a solitary journey. *Image: Journal of Nursing Scholarship, 28*(1), 55–58.

Caregivers, Inc. (1997). *Caregivers and the workplace: What you should know as an employer.* Caregivers, Inc. Available from: http://www.caregivr.com/carelinks.html 3/18/99.

Carpenito, L. (1997). *Nursing diagnosis: Applications to clinical practice* (7th ed.). Philadelphia: Lippincott Williams & Wilkins.

Cox, C.B. (1996). Discharge planning for dementia patients: Factors influencing caregiver decisions and satisfaction. *Health and Social Work, 21*(2), 97–104.

Doenges, M., Moorhouse, M., & Burley, J. (1995). *Application of nursing process and nursing diagnosis: An interactive text for diagnostic reasoning* (2nd ed.). Philadelphia: F.A. Davis.

England, M. (1996). Sense of relatedness and interpersonal network of adult offspring caregivers: Linkages with crisis, emotional arousal, and perceived health. *Archives of Psychiatric Nursing, 10*(2), 85–95.

Family Caregiver Alliance. (FCA, 1999). *Caregivers at risk.* Available from: http://www.caregiver.org/stat_risk.html 3/15/99.

Family Caregiver Alliance. (FCA, 1998). *Fact sheet: Selected caregiver statistics.* Available from: http://www.caregiver.org/factsheets.medica_source/caregiver_statsC.html 3/17/99.

Family Caregiver Alliance. (FCA, 1997). *California resource center survey.* San Francisco: Author.

Fink, S.V. (1995). The influence of family resources and family demands on the strains and well-being of caregiving families. *Nursing Research, 44*(3), 139–146.

Hawkins, B. (1996). Daughters and caregiving: Taking care of our own. *Journal of the American Association of Occupational Health Nursing, 44*(9), 433–437.

Hibbard, J., Neufeld, A., & Harrison, M.J. (1996). Gender differences in the support networks of caregivers. *Journal of Gerontological Nursing, 22*(9), 15–23.

Holden, K. (1999). Caregiver and stress. *Self-Help & Psychology Magazine.* Available from: http://www.shpm.com/cgi-bin/library/searchindex 3/16/99.

Holicky, R. (1996). Caring for the caregivers: The hidden victims of illness and disability. *Rehabilitation Nursing, 21*(5), 247–252.

Jones, P.S. (1995). Paying respect: Care of elderly parents by Chinese and Filipino American women. *Health Care for Women International, 16*(5), 385–398.

Jones, S.L. (1996). The association between objective and subjective caregiver burden. *Archives of Psychiatric Nursing, 10*(2), 77–84.

Mackinnon, M.E., Gien, L., & Durst, D. (1996). Chinese elders speak out: Implications for practice. *Clinical Nursing Research, 5*(3), 326–342.

McKibbon, J., Genereux, L., & Seguin-Roberge, G. (1996). Who cares for the caregivers? *Canadian Nurse, 92*(3), 38–41.

Micozzi, M. (1996). Fundamentals of complimentary and alternative medicine. New York: Churchill Livingstone.

National Alliance for Caregiving. (NAC, 1998a). *Caregiving tips.* Available from: http://caregiving.org/content/tips.asp 3/17/99.

National Alliance for Caregiving. (NAC, 1998b). *The caregiving boom: Baby boomer women giving care.* Bethesda, MD: Author.

National Alliance for Caregiving & American Association of Retired Persons. (NAC & AARP, 1997). *Family caregiving in the U.S.: Findings from a national study final report.* Available from: http://caregiving.org/content/repsprods.asp 3/10/97.

National Family Caregivers Association. (NFCA, 1998). *Caregiver survey report.* Kensington, MD: Author.

National Family Caregivers Association. (NFCA, 1996). *The resourceful caregiver: Helping family caregivers help themselves.* St. Louis: Mosby Year Book Inc.

North American Nursing Diagnosis Association. (NANDA, 1999). *Nursing diagnoses: Definitions and classification 1999–2000.* Philadelphia: Author.

Picot, S. (1995a). Choice and social exchange theory and the rewards of African American caregivers. *Journal of the National Black Nurses' Association, 7*(2), 29–40.

Picot, S.J. (1995b). Rewards, costs, and coping of African American caregivers. *Nursing Research, 44*(3), 147–152.

Thobaben, M. (1999). Anticipatory guidance for family caregivers. *Home Health Care Management & Practice,* in press.

Wagner, D.L. (1998). *Comparative analysis of caregiver data for caregivers to the elderly (1997).* Bethesda, MD: National Alliance for Caregiving.

Weeks, S., & O'Connor, P.C. (1996). Taking on the family caregiver role: Nurses' sensitivity to the needs of prospective family caregivers. *Rehabilitation Nursing Research, 5*(1), 16–22.

Value-Belief Pattern

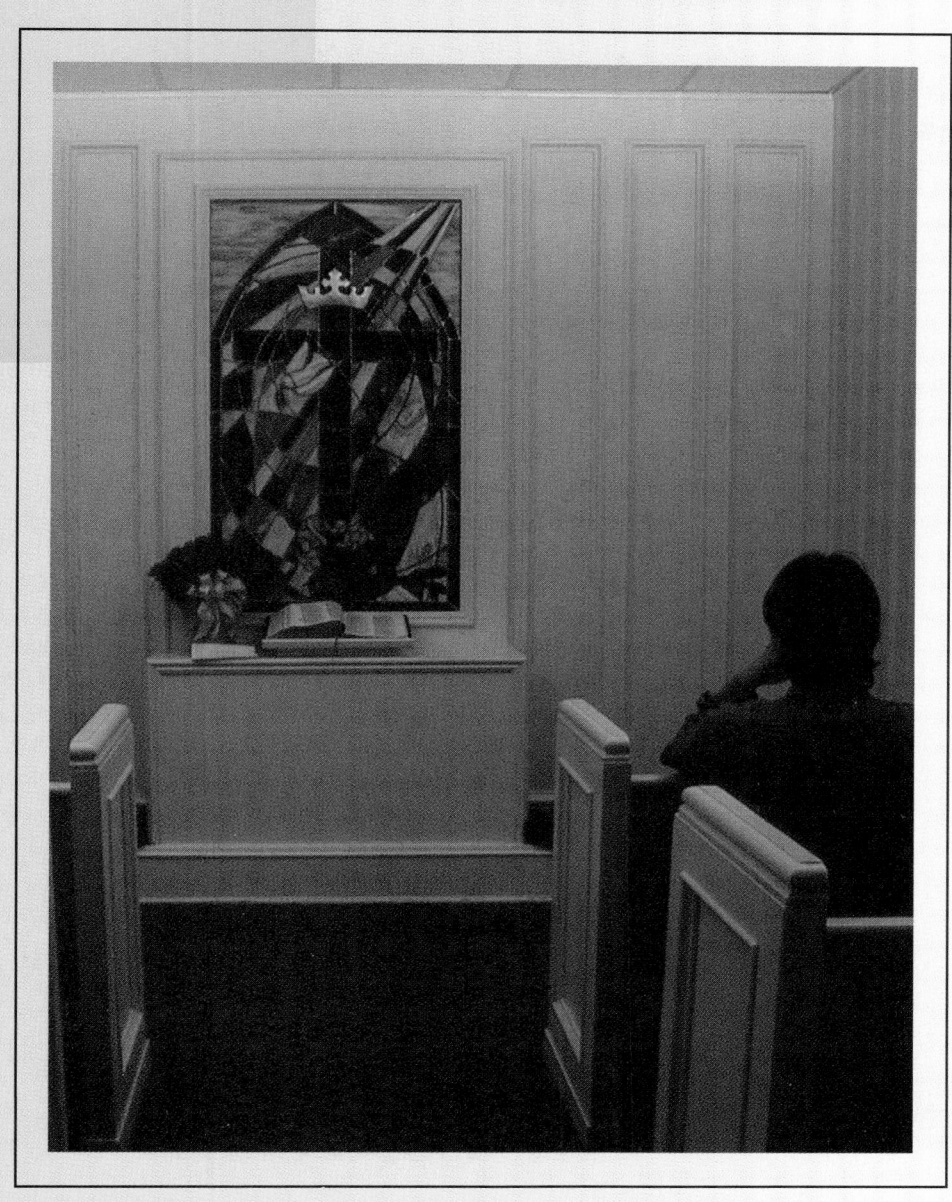

Spirituality

Virginia Nehring and Martha Meraviglia

Key Terms

agnostic
atheist
faith
hope
monotheism

polytheism
religion
spiritual distress
spiritual well-being
spirituality

LEARNING OBJECTIVES

After studying this chapter, you should be able to:

1. Relate the concepts of spirituality, religion, and faith with the concept of providing spiritual care in nursing.
2. Discuss the factors affecting a client's spiritual needs.
3. Assess a client for spiritual well-being.
4. Make a nursing diagnosis for a client in spiritual distress.
5. Plan care for a client experiencing spiritual distress.
6. Discuss nursing interventions for enhancing spiritual well-being.
7. Evaluate interventions for relieving spiritual distress.

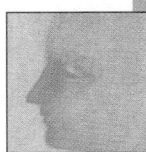

Mr. Groves is a 56-year-old master electrician who has just returned home from the hospital after a radical prostatectomy for invasive carcinoma 4 days ago. His suprapubic wound has a 3-cm opening that requires daily wound care. You make plans to assist Mr. Groves in managing his wound care and supporting his recovery from surgery. You discover that Mr. Groves has spiritual needs in addition to his obvious physical and psychological needs. You consider the diagnosis of *Spiritual distress* (see the chart, Spirituality Nursing Diagnoses).

SPIRITUALITY
NURSING DIAGNOSES

Spiritual Distress: Disruption in the life principle that pervades a person's entire being and that integrates and transcends one's biological and psychological nature.

Risk for Spiritual Distress: At risk for an altered sense of harmonious connectedness with all of life and the universe in which dimensions that transcend and empower the self may be disrupted.

Potential for Enhanced Spiritual Well-Being: Spiritual well-being is the process of an individual's developing/unfolding of mystery through harmonious interconnectedness that springs from inner strengths.

From North American Nursing Diagnosis Association. (1999). NANDA nursing diagnoses: Definitions and classification 1999–2000. Philadelphia: Author.

CONCEPTS OF SPIRITUALITY
Spirituality

Spirituality is a process and sacred journey, the essence or life principle of a person, a belief that relates a person to the world, and a way of giving meaning to existence. It is any personal transcendence beyond the present context of reality, a personal quest to find meaning and purpose in life, and a relationship or sense of connection with Mystery, Higher Power, God, or Universe (Burkhardt, 1989) Table 55–1 lists characteristics of spirituality.

Spirit is the essence of a person, which connects to all living things. Spirituality is the core of the human that interprets and unifies the whole person. Spirituality shapes and gives meaning to life and to what one can be.

Spirituality is seen in everything one is, one knows, and one does. Spirituality involves not only being but knowing and doing. Spirituality encompasses a person's sense of meaning and purpose in life in addition to religious beliefs or behaviors, such as prayer (Fig. 55–1). However, this idea transcends any structured religion.

Stallwood and Stoll (1975) created a model in which the person is viewed in a holistic fashion, with the spiritual dimension as the central and integrative dimension. They believe spirituality is the means by which a person stays in relationship with the self, other people, the environment, and God or a higher power.

TABLE 55–1
Characteristics of Spirituality

Characteristic	Elements
General	• Connectedness to all things • Unity or wholeness permeating all of life and manifested through becoming and connecting; cannot occur in isolation
Being (important relationships and sense of connection with oneself)	• Going inward • Being in touch with self • Sense of communion with others, God, and the world • Being open to new things • Feeling of inner synchrony and harmony
Knowing (what and how one knows)	• Evolving understanding of the processes and events of life • Receptive openness to life • Active seeking and discovering • Trusting in one's own experiences
Doing (what one does and how one acts)	• Connection with something bigger than the self • Activities such as prayer, going to church, meditation, rituals • Being with others, assisting friends, raising children, caring for parents • With the earth, gardening, recycling, composting

Information from Burkhardt, M.A. (1994). Becoming and connecting: Elements of spirituality for women. Holistic Nursing Practice, 8(4), 12–21.

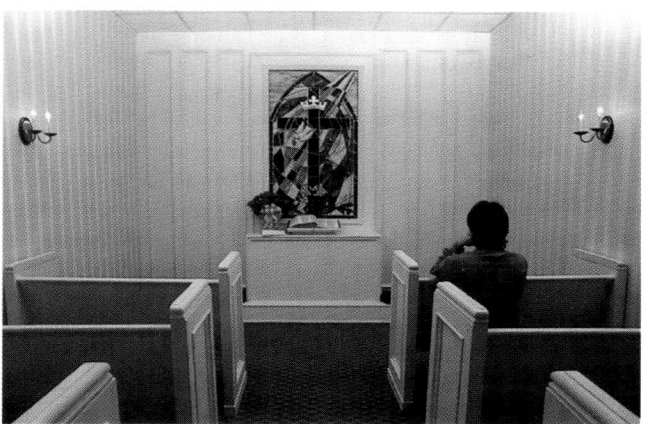

Figure 55–1. Spirituality encompasses a person's sense of meaning and purpose in life, in addition to religious beliefs or behaviors, such as prayer.

Religion

Religion is a belief system, including dogma, rituals, and traditions (Legere, 1984). Religion can also mean a social institution in which people participate together, rather than an individual searching alone for meaning in life. Typically, religion includes the personal commitment to and serving of God or a transcendent power with worshipful devotion and conduct in accordance with divine commands, especially as found in sacred writings or declared by authoritative teachers. Religion can therefore be viewed as a service to God, organized within a specified set of beliefs and practices.

Spiritual and religious expressions are not necessarily synonymous. A person can be spiritual without being religious and religious without being spiritual. Spirituality has to do with experience; religion has to do with the conceptualization of that experience. Spirituality focuses on what happens in the heart, whereas religion tries to capture and explain that experience.

Many religions of the world, such as Islam, are based on a belief in a singular God. **Monotheism** is the belief in the existence of one God who created and rules the universe. Other faiths, such as many Native American beliefs, perceive many spirits in the world. **Polytheism** is the belief in more than one god. Still others, such as Hindu, see many gods coexisting, but all as manifestations of the one Absolute God.

An **atheist** is a person who believes there is no God or higher power. Such a person denies the possible existence of God. Atheists may find meaning for life through relationships, work, or secular humanism, which is a set of beliefs about the world without the notion of God. However, some people do not believe in a God and feel no need to find an alternative set of principles.

An **agnostic** is a person who is undecided about the existence of God or a higher power. Because God is not provable, agnostics believe silence on the issue is the only wise position. Some agnostics argue that the only meaning in life is the meaning individuals invest in life. There is no ultimate meaning. All such decisions are a matter of choice and faith.

Faith

Faith is belief in or commitment to something or someone that helps a person realize purpose. By definition, faith is belief without proof. Each person chooses what to believe. Faith is universal, a part of living, a part of acting, and a part of self-understanding (Fowler & Keen, 1985).

Faith is always in relationship to others, to the environment, and to the ultimate conditions of existence. Faith is the awareness, the intuition, and the conviction of relatedness to something or someone more than the mundane or everyday world. Although faith is always an inner knowing, it always includes a social or interpersonal dimension.

Faith relates the boundaries and depths of experience to a source, center, and standard of values in life. It involves the total self. The content—or images, values, beliefs, symbols, and rituals—of a person's faith is of central importance in informing behavior and shaping personality.

Hoshiko's Model

Hoshiko's (1991) model illustrates the relationships each person possesses (Fig. 55–2). The person is related to other people, to an ultimate reality or God, to the environment, and to time. The arrow from past to present to future indicates the dynamic nature of the world view as time passes, as well as a person's present relationship to both the past and the future. Forgiveness does not change what has happened, but does change the person's relationship to the past—and some would say to the present and future as well. The circular arrow to the self demonstrates reflection and change as a person grows and redefines the self.

Fowler's Stages

Fowler (1974) analyzed the development of faith over the life span. Each developmental stage has its own particular wholeness, grace, and integrity:

STAGE 0. UNDIFFERENTIATED. In an infant, faith is acceptance of love and trust in the caregiver. If the infant is not loved consistently, doubt, anxiety, dread, and terror result.

STAGE I. INTUITIVE-PROJECTIVE. With awareness of the religious practices of the family, the child imitates religious behaviors with little distinction of fact from fantasy. Stories, gestures, and symbols are absorbed as

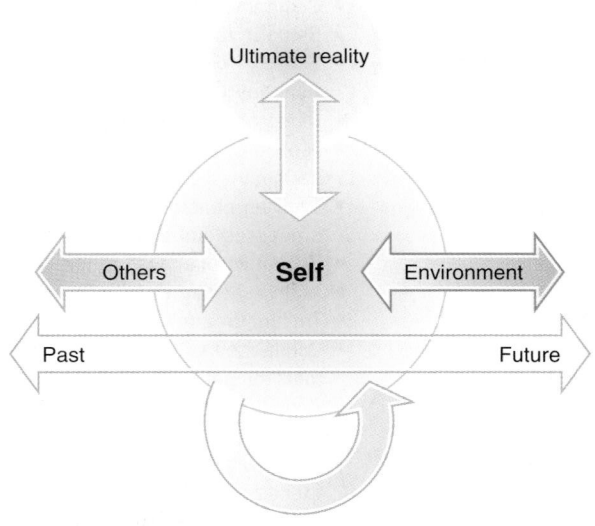

Figure 55–2. Hoshiko's model of the person as a spiritual being. The circular arrow to the self demonstrates reflection and change as a person grows and redefines the self. (Redrawn from Hoshiko, B. [1991]. Worldview as a model of spirituality. In Shelly, J.A. Teaching spiritual care [2nd ed., pp. 19–31]. Madison, Nurses Christian Fellowship.)

long-lasting images. Feeling and knowing are fused in the young child. Thinking about a deity is in pre-anthropomorphic imagery and is highly personal. For example, God is everywhere, like the wind.

STAGE II. MYTHIC-LITERAL. The child begins to differentiate between fact and fantasy, primarily through questioning a trusted adult. When the child hears inconsistent beliefs, the child chooses which to believe, based on affection for the person presenting it. Stories help dramatize beliefs. Anthropomorphic imagery is used to describe deity—God is like a father, for example.

STAGE III. SYNTHETIC-CONVENTIONAL. The adolescent recognizes that different settings have their own rules and that beliefs and symbols can have more than one meaning. The adolescent uses personal judgment to choose and evaluate the reliability of adults and hence their version of truth. Constructs about spirituality are broadened. For example, the adolescent recognizes both deity and the self as spirit.

STAGE IV. INDIVIDUATING-REFLECTIVE. For those whose faith continues to develop, the young adult finds that appealing to authority, trying to achieve consensus with others, or compartmentalization through believing one thing in one setting and another thing in another setting all fail. Institutional religion is seen as conventional, and other belief systems may be examined. The person takes responsibility and may choose to become committed to a particular faith.

STAGE V. POLAR-DIALECTICAL OR PARADOXICAL-CONSOLIDATE. The adult with extensive spiritual experiences sees the paradoxical—affirms the beliefs, symbols, and rituals of a particular faith while recognizing that these are but symbols, a way of approaching the deity. The adult can acknowledge and respect the beliefs, symbols, and rituals and traditions of other faith groups.

STAGE VI. UNIVERSALIZING. This stage, reached by very few, represents a love for and communion with God that is not self-conscious and is fully integrated into a life of service and practical concern for all peoples regardless of faith traditions. Mother Theresa might be seen as an example of such a person.

Spirituality and Health

The human-environment connection is a mutual process in which persons exist in open participation with the universe and become more than, and different from, the sum of their parts. This concept of a person expands the definition of health. Holistic health is affected by our spirituality and is created through harmony with the universe.

Spiritual experiences can enhance feelings of compassion, peace of mind, and harmony with the environment (Dossey & Guzetta, 1995). These feelings represent a balance between inner and outer aspects of human experience. Beliefs about spirituality, life after death, and purpose in life are important aspects of high-level wellness. For example, Kaczorowski (1989) found that anxiety is lower in highly spiritual persons

confronting life-threatening illness. Additionally, people who are spiritually well report less depression, less loneliness, and an overall feeling of well-being despite the presence of illness (Reed, 1987).

Germere (1996) found that psychiatric clients described four spiritual needs: a means to understand death, a way to cope with suffering, a source of moral values, and a connection with transcendent love. The clients identified seven activities useful in meeting spiritual needs. These were praying or meditating, participating in church or organized religion, reading inspirational literature, attending self-help groups, interacting with children, listening to inspirational music, and being in nature. The predominant theme of the participants was how uncommon it was to discuss spirituality, although they felt it was very beneficial because they could learn from each other, could express difficult emotions in a supportive atmosphere, and could gain motivation to work on this area of life.

It is the spirit that synthesizes the total personality and provides some sense of energizing direction and order to live by, and the sense of selflessness and a willingness to do more for others than for yourself. **Spiritual well-being** is a process of being and becoming that surrounds the totality of a person's inner resources, the wholeness of spirit and unifying dimension, a process of transcendence, and the perception of life as having meaning (Burkhardt, 1989). Spiritual well-being includes

- A concern for others and self
- A sense of meaning and enjoyment in life
- A commitment to purposes greater than the self
- A sense of relatedness
- A means for moving through debilitating guilt, anger, or anxiety
- Life-affirming relationships or harmonious interconnectedness with deity, self, community, and environment

Spiritual well-being is closely related to hope. **Hope** is an interpersonal process created through trust and nurtured by a trusting relationship with others, including God. Hope is belief, expectancy, or trust that things will be better. Hope is believed to be necessary for persons to survive illness or difficult times.

Spiritual health refers to the state of wholeness of a spiritual dimension. It includes

- A sense of personal fulfillment
- A sense of peace with the self and the world
- A sense of fulfillment in life and interaction with self and others
- The ability to discover and articulate basic purpose in life
- The ability to experience love, joy, peace, and fulfillment
- An ability to live in wholeness consistent with the values of community and self

Spiritual distress is a disruption that pervades the entire being and that integrates and transcends biological and social nature (Burkhardt, 1989) resulting in distress of the human spirit. Spiritual distress is a factor crucial to healing and health care.

Spirituality in Nursing

Nursing recognizes the spiritual aspect of human nature as an integral component of a person's sense of wellness. Spiritual well-being is one approach to attain and maintain holistic health. Nursing theorists recognize the importance of spirituality.

Travelbee (1971) underscored the significance of spiritual values by emphasizing the importance of finding meaning in illness, thus suggesting that spirituality is essential to human health. She described inherent contradictions in people as creatures who have to confront and endure conflict but who have the innate ability to transcend the material aspects of their nature.

Paterson and Zderad (1988) elaborated on the inherent contradictions that are part of being human. By emphasizing the conflict between the spiritual and material dimensions of the self, this theory supports the dimension of assisting clients to confront spiritual dilemmas.

Watson (1985) incorporated the abstract spiritual concepts of soul, spirit, and transcendence to explain the nature of a person and the goals of nursing. Spirituality is a developmental phenomenon growing and changing through life experiences. Maintaining faith, hope, and altruistic values aids this developmental change process.

Roy (1988) states that one assumption about the healing process was the premise that human nature is rooted in relatedness to the absolute truth of the creator. Although not stated in Roy's original theory, implicit in her work is that healing involves a relationship with a deity.

Newman (1986) characterized spiritual growth as movement toward a state of absolute consciousness in which the spatial-temporal self is transcended. In this state the person is aware of a unity that includes but is greater than the self, and there is an experience of unconditional love. As development of the physical self becomes more restricted with aging, former methods of coping no longer work. Transcendence offers an alternative to the spiritual impasse that the elderly or severely ill may experience: an awareness that extends beyond the physical self. Spirituality is integral to the health process at all ages but particularly in later life.

Most nurses claim to give holistic care, but several studies confirm that nurses commonly avoid addressing spirituality. Fewer than 15% of nurses include spirituality in the care of clients (Piles, 1990). In a study by Boutell and Bozett (1990), most nurses said that they assessed clients' spiritual needs. Fears, sources of strength, and feelings of hope were the most frequently assessed. Nurses over age 50 were more likely than younger nurses to assess the spiritual realm. Perhaps as nurses grow closer to their own death, and experience the deaths of loved ones, they become more sensitive to the spiritual needs of clients in their care.

Overview of Major Religions

Health care will include clients who practice a diversity of religions. If the client states a faith, you should know resources for obtaining more information about that faith, especially the most common faiths (Table 55–2). All religions fulfill the purpose of describing and explaining spiritual experiences. You need to be aware of the particular beliefs and practices of each religion to assess and care for the spiritual needs of clients.

Hinduism

Hinduism is a complex belief system from India dating back 3,000 years. Within this religion the individual is seen as being on a spiritual journey to discover the self or consciousness. The self is considered to be absolute truth. The true nature of the self is connected with the supreme consciousness of the cosmos known as Brahma. Brahma, then, is the source of all existence, literally the godhead of creation. Hindus worship many gods, such as Vishnu and Shiva, which are believed to be the embodiment of the godhead.

A key concept within Hinduism is Maya. Maya refers to the world that appears to us, the material objects around us. It represents an illusion of time and space. For Hindus, Maya impedes an awareness of the self by keeping one's focus on the things of the world.

Rebirth is another belief central to Hinduism. When anyone dies, he is reborn as another creature based on deeds in a previous existence. When a person performs perfect deeds, attains perfection, knowledge,

TABLE 55–2

The Ten Largest Religions in the United States (Self-Identification, 1990)

Religion	Estimated Adult Population	Estimated Percentage of Adult Population
Christianity	151,225,000	86.2%
Nonreligious	13,116,000	7.5%
Judaism	3,137,000	1.8%
Agnostic	1,186,000	0.7%
Islam	527,000	*0.5%
Unitarian Universalist	502,000	0.3%
Buddhism	401,000	*0.4%
Hinduism	227,000	*0.2%
Native American Religion	47,000	—
Scientologist	45,000	—

*Islam, Buddhist, and Hindu figures adjusted upward to account for possible undercount.

From Adherents.com. Available at: http://www.adherents.com/rel_USA.html#religions. Accessed November 4, 1999.

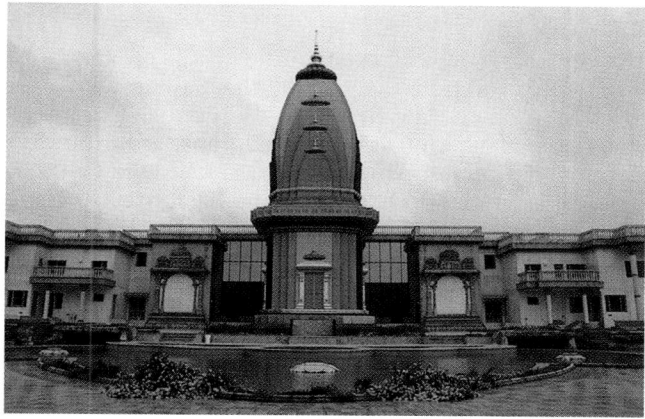

Figure 55–3. In Hinduism, believers gather in Hindu temples to chant prayers or scripture.

or is extremely ascetic, he will earn salvation from the process of rebirth.

Hinduism has many religious practices for the spiritual journey of finding the self. Yoga is one such practice that helps people integrate mind, body, and spirit so that they can encounter the self and attain perfect knowledge. Within yoga there are steps for achieving integration, such as physical posturing, breathing control, concentration, meditation, and enlightenment.

The rituals of worship facilitate the spiritual journey. Worship is primarily done individually by meditating to encounter the self. Believers also gather in temples to chant prayers or scripture (Fig. 55–3).

Hinduism is not just a religion but represents both a lifestyle and social structure for its followers. Because of this, the beliefs have implications for spiritual care. The law of karma is an example of Hinduism's influence on the lifestyle by the understanding of personal health and well-being. Karma is the belief that for every action there is a corresponding reaction. For Hindus, karma is central to health and all thoughts and actions have effects on the body and mind. Personal harmony is maintained by following this law of nature. Physical illness is explained by previous actions, even actions in another life (Martin, 1989).

Buddhism

Buddhism originated with the teachings of Buddha Gautama in approximately 550 BC in India. Gautama followed the early beliefs of Hinduism to find enlightenment through yoga practices. After a long period of spiritual growth, he began to teach the people about his experiences and his transformation to Buddha. Central to Buddhism are the Four Noble Truths, which include

- Life is suffering
- Suffering is a result of one's desires for pleasure, power, and existence
- To stop suffering, one must stop desiring
- The way to stop desiring, and thus suffering, is to follow the Eightfold Path. It includes right views,

right intention, right speech, right action, right livelihood, right effort, right awareness, and right concentration

Through this process, one experiences a state of release known as nirvana. To Buddha, there was no encounter with the self or godhead as in Hinduism. When he died, Buddha is believed to have entered a final state of nirvana.

Over the years there have arisen several traditions of Buddhism. The Theravada tradition emphasizes the composite nature of all things and the absence of gods to help. This tradition has spread throughout Southeast Asia. The Mahayana tradition stresses an expanded understanding of the universe with celestial beings and a godhead. This tradition is the predominate type of Buddhism throughout East Asia, including China, Korea, and Japan. The Tantrayana sect of Buddhism is the major type in Tibet and Mongolia. This tradition describes a visualized god and uses tantric rituals to experience nirvana, such as sacred gestures and sounds (Britannica Online, 1998).

Because of the various sects of Buddhism with differing beliefs, they cannot be assessed as a group when providing spiritual care. You need to assess the specific beliefs the Buddhist holds and then consider those beliefs and practices when caring for the client's spiritual needs.

Buddhists use yoga meditation as a religious practice. The concept of balance is important to Buddhists. They stress the middle path in life, emphasizing self-control and discipline. The Chinese believe that yin, the shady side of the mountain, and yang, the sunny side, demonstrate this idea of balance. Along with this understanding of life is the notion of the dynamic flow of the energy in the universe. There is also a feeling of unity with all of the people and things in the world. Buddhists want to be aware of the unity but remain nonattached (Martin, 1989).

Taoism

Taoism dates back over 2,500 years in China to a man known as Lao Tzu. This man professed unique ideas that developed into a religion. Taoism encourages a positive attitude toward life that includes an accepting outlook and yielding character.

Taoism has three meanings for Tao. First, Tao means ultimate reality, which is beyond human comprehension. Second, Tao means the way of the universe as the power in and behind everything in nature. Finally, Tao is the way of human life. Taoism focuses on the way of life when one encounters the power and energy in the universe.

Taoists believe in three gods, including the originator Lao Tzu. They also use metaphysical practices such as magic to tap into the power of the universe. The religion has shamans and high priests to carry out the rituals for encountering the energy in the universe.

The idea of ch'i is central to Taoist beliefs and practices. Ch'i is the vital energy or life force in the universe and within each person. Much focus is placed on increasing ch'i and removing the blocks to its flow. Practices such as the use of herbal medicines, acupuncture, and meditation are advocated for increasing the amount and flow of ch'i through the mind and body.

Taoist beliefs have implications for you in terms of health and spiritual care. In Taoism, health represents the harmony in the universe. The concept of ch'i is foundational to the Chinese system of medicine with alternative forms of medical treatment. Being sensitive to the contrast between Western and Chinese medicine will enable you to provide health and spiritual care for clients who embrace these beliefs.

Judaism

As with most major religions, Judaism represents a religion and a way of life that influence the community of believers through conduct and culture. Judaism began well over 4,000 years ago when God, the creator of the universe, called Abraham into a covenant relationship. The covenant extends to all of Abraham's descendants, making them a kingdom of priests and a holy nation.

The fundamental teachings of Judaism are grouped around the concept of monotheism. Central to the religion is the belief that people are at the core of God's creation. Judaism also believes that people are basically good because they are made in God's image. God is seen as just, merciful, and compassionate. The Jewish people are called to be like God and to worship God through their lives. The Torah (sacred writings of the Law) and the Talmud (Oral Law) are viewed as divine revelations on the rules for living and the experiences of others with God.

There are several Jewish sects, which adopt differing religious practices that you need to be aware of in providing spiritual care. Orthodox Jews comply with the traditional beliefs and practices of Judaism. They strictly follow the Torah and Talmud, which include practices of daily worship, dietary regulations (no pork, and foods be prepared in a kosher, proper manner), traditional prayers in Hebrew, study of the Torah, special clothing and head covering, and observance of the Sabbath. Conservative Jews follow the traditional practices of Orthodox Judaism with some modifications. They adhere to most of the dietary regulations and the Sabbath. Conservative Judaism provided a middle ground to the liberal Reform Judaism that abandoned the traditional practices for modernization. Reformed Jews believe in the one true God and practice the ethical principles of Judaism but have removed the lifestyle restrictions of Orthodox Judaism.

In caring for a Jewish client, you will need to determine the specific beliefs and practices embraced by the person. Providing privacy for daily prayers is very important for many Jewish clients, as is the need to keep the Sabbath by refraining from physical and recreational activities. Knowledge of the client's dietary restrictions and the need for kosher food items is imperative in providing for health and spiritual care.

Christianity

The central figure in Christianity is Jesus of Nazareth. Jesus is considered the Christ, the Savior who was foretold and expected by the Jewish people. Christianity is one of the largest world religions, with the predominant groups being the Roman Catholic Church, the Protestant churches, and the Eastern Orthodox Church.

Christianity's primary beliefs include

- Focus on Jesus Christ as the son of God
- Trinitarian God (Father, Son, and Holy Spirit)
- Redemption of people from sin through the death and resurrection of Jesus
- Holy Spirit of God given to all believers
- Revelation of God's word in Bible
- Final judgment by God at the end of one's life

Each group within Christianity has unique beliefs and practices. The Roman Catholic Church relies on scripture and tradition for its beliefs and practices. Members must attend church services regularly and participate in the sacraments of the faith, which include baptism, confirmation, communion, confession, and extreme unction. The Eastern Orthodox Church is similar to the Roman Catholic Church except leadership is with the patriarchs instead of the pope, priests can marry instead of remaining celibate, and members do not say Rosary prayers.

The Protestant churches have many denominations with a variety of differing beliefs. Primarily, Protestant churches rely on the Bible instead of tradition as the basis for beliefs and practices. Another unique belief of Protestant Christians is the forgiveness of all believers' sins through faith in Jesus Christ, with good deeds not contributing to salvation.

You need to identify the specific beliefs and practices of Christian clients in order to provide appropriate spiritual care. Based on a detailed assessment, you can determine the spiritual needs of the client and establish effective interventions to meet those needs. With Christian clients, you should be sensitive to their need for quiet prayer time. Roman Catholics and Eastern Orthodox Christians may desire a priest to administer communion, extreme unction, or anointing for healing. They may want pictures of saints or angels in the room for spiritual and emotional comfort. Protestants may want to talk about life and illness openly in regard to their relationship with Jesus.

Islam

The religion of Islam began with Muhammad during the 600s in Arabia. He began to have visions and revelations while meditating in the caves around Mecca in which the angel Gabriel delivered messages from God, known as Allah, about God's greatness and human beings' sinful nature. Allah is viewed as the only God, one who created the universe and sustains its inhabitants. Muhammad is considered the last prophet of God in a long line of prophets, which include Abraham, Isaiah, and Jesus.

The revelations from Allah were written down and form the sacred book of the Qur'an for the Muslims. Most of the book includes the Islamic laws concerning the spiritual life of daily prayers, fasting, pilgrimage to Mecca, giving, and attaining salvation; and social laws on inheritance, crime, personal conduct, and marriage. The Qur'an includes stories from the Hebrew Bible about Adam and Eve, Abraham, and Joseph.

Muhammad and his successors conquered vast territories and imposed the religious and governmental laws of Islam on the people. The religion spread very rapidly into the Middle East, India, Europe, and Africa. There are currently two main sects of Islam, which include the traditionalist Sunni (the largest group) and the Shi'ite. The predominate difference between the sects is that the Sunni have combined regional customs with the Qur'an Law. There are four subgroups of Sunni in the Islam community (Britannica Online, 1998).

Islamic religious practices include the Five Pillars of Islam, which the believer is to practice faithfully. The Five Pillars include

- Recite the creed, "There is no God but Allah, and Muhammad is the messenger of Allah."
- Observe the five prayer times each day.
- Give at least 2.5% of one's income to help the poor.
- Fast during the day in the month of Ramadan.
- Go once during one's lifetime on a pilgrimage to Mecca.

The Law or Shari'ah describes the way of life for Muslims, including beliefs and practices.

The Islamic religion has special implications for you in caring for a Muslim client. You must be aware of the spiritual need for daily prayer time at sunrise, noon, midafternoon, sunset, and bedtime. Muslims must wash before each prayer time even if they are sick. They are forbidden to eat pork and drink alcohol. Muslim women are required to cover all of their body and maintain modesty in all situations.

Native American Religion

The Native American people known as American Indians were separated by over 500 languages but shared similar religious beliefs. The people worshiped many gods and the objects that surrounded them, such as the sun and moon. They worshiped a sacred power represented in mythological beings. Many Native Americans believed in good and evil forces, which were manifested through spirits.

Most tribes had a shaman or medicine man on whom they relied for spiritual knowledge. The shaman performed special rituals to ensure tribal survival and prosperity. The Native American people worshipped the land and held tribal grave sites as sacred. The Native American Church is the most widespread religious group today among Native Americans. This religion is also known as Peyotism for its use of the hallucinogenic substance, peyote. The beliefs of the religion combine ideas from Christianity and primitive Indian beliefs, such as the belief in one God, known as the Great Spirit, and belief in the Peyote Spirit, which is similar to Jesus. Peyote is eaten to enhance communication with God and to receive spiritual power (Britannica Online, 1998).

An understanding of the general spiritual beliefs of Native Americans will help you care for their spiritual needs. You need to assess each client's personal beliefs to provide care unique to that person. Always maintaining an unbiased attitude to unique spiritual beliefs will allow you to care for clients.

FACTORS AFFECTING SPIRITUALITY

The spiritual needs of the clients you will care for vary greatly depending on their spiritual beliefs, stage of faith, degree of illness, and adaptation to illness. The predominant spiritual needs of people are a search for meaning, a sense of hope, forgiveness, love, connectedness, and a sense of purpose. Many factors can affect spiritual needs. The four types of factors included here are developmental, cultural, psychosocial, and physiological.

Developmental Factors

Children

Meeting the spiritual needs of children usually is concerned with teaching children and helping them apply religious principles in their daily lives. Children do not have a spiritual crisis in the same sense as adults. The defining characteristics of *Spiritual distress* do not fit children. Children sometimes feel a sense of confusion about God when prayers do not seem to be answered. For example, the child may pray for a parent with cancer to get well, but the parent may die anyway. However, children who are victims of abuse or other impossibly difficult family situations and who appear to be hurting at their inner core could be described as being in spiritual distress. You can do much to help meet the spiritual needs of these and all children (Fig. 55–4).

Adolescents and Young Adults

Adolescence is a time of questioning the meaning of life and the religious teachings that may have been a part of childhood. Some degree of spiritual distress is a normal part of adolescence. The adolescent needs someone who will listen without judging or offering advice while the questions of faith are explored. Spiritual distress is closely related to depression and suicide, both of which have a high incidence in adolescence.

Young adults often separate themselves from family, culture, and religion when they leave home for college or after getting a job. When the young adult is a long way from home, it is easy to stop the religious

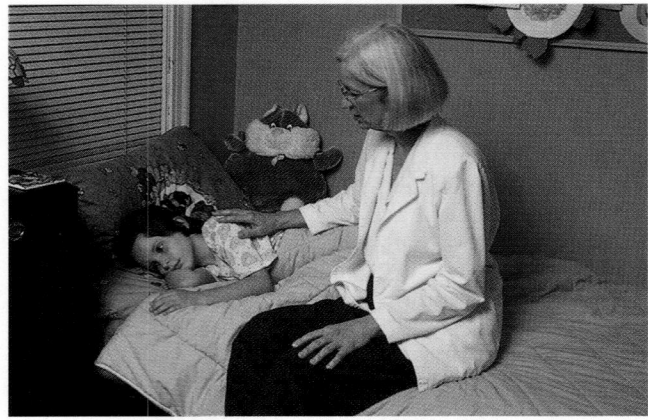

Figure 55–4. Nurses can have an important role in meeting the spiritual needs of children who are sick or suffering from spiritual distress.

practices that have been a part of childhood. When a crisis occurs, they are not in touch with a source of spiritual strength. Young adulthood is a time of seeking to be in touch with the spiritual self and exploring alternative forms of spiritual guidance such as astrology, eastern religions, and New Age methods.

Middle Adults

The American dream has led many people to pursue financial success, an appealing appearance, and social recognition as the path to a full and satisfying life. However, Kasser and Ryan (1996) have confirmed the common wisdom that extrinsic signs of success are not necessarily associated with happiness. Close interpersonal relationships may actually be more important. Middle-aged adults often re-evaluate life priorities and develop other aspects of the self. During midlife, success-driven adults may shift their values to friends and family.

Spirituality becomes more important as middle-aged adults discover discontent with their lives. The uneasiness or dissatisfaction with life can be a significant impetus for exploring spiritual beliefs. For many middle-aged adults, this time in life is for connecting with the values and beliefs from their childhood. For others the transition of middle age is a time for expanding and refining spiritual ideas. The opportunity to explore spirituality can provide adults with a foundation for healthier living as old age approaches.

Older Adults

Religion tends to become increasingly important as the person ages. In fact, religion is the key to life satisfaction for many older adults. A sense of the encompassing love of God is a basic emotional security and firm spiritual foundation for the elderly at the end of life.

Older adults have an enhanced reasoning ability to transcend the immediate and derive meaning from conflict (Reed, 1991). The elderly are more than problem-solvers; they are problem transformers. The elderly are often more concerned with why than what

or how to. There is transcendence of preoccupation with the physical self and increased awareness of the spiritual self. As an individual grows older, there is less emotional investment in externals and more attention to the inner self and perception and organization of life and its events.

It is important for the elderly person to be respected as a spiritual being because of the spiritual perception of the self. The elderly become concerned about the meaning of the past. The way an older adult remembers the past, lives in the present, and anticipates the future often reflects spiritual views. The elderly seem to need

- A sense of worth despite physical decline
- A sense of trust in self and trust in an ultimate other
- A sense of forgiveness toward self and others

TABLE 55–3

Characteristics of Spiritual Well-Being in the Older Adult: Relationships and Time

Characteristic	Elements
Relationships	
An ultimate other	• Believes in a supreme being. • Trusts in God. • Communicates with God through prayer. • Participates in religious practices.
The nature of others	• Accepts or tolerates differences with others. • Expresses mutual love and concern. • Expresses mutual forgiveness. • Accepts and gives help. • Appreciates nature.
Self	• Accepts self and situations in life. • Values inner self. • Values self determination. • Has a positive attitude. • Expresses life satisfaction.
Time	
Past	• Recognizes parental and other influences. • Expresses sociocultural ties with past situations and outcomes. • Describes ties with a formal belief system. • Describes past religious practices and rituals. • Expresses growth and change over time.
Present	• Lives up to potential. • Expresses congruency between values and practice. • Open to growth and change. • Participates in communal prayers or rituals. • Finds meaning and purpose in life.
Future	• Sets goals. • Hopes in ultimate integration. • Hopes in afterlife. • Searches for meaning and purpose in life.

Hungelmann, J., Kenkel-Rossi, E., Klassen, L., & Stollenwerk, R. (1985). Spiritual well-being in older adults: Harmonious interconnectedness. Journal of Religion and Health, 24(2), 147–153.

- An affirmation of meaning in the life the person has lived
- A transcendence of losses to enable the person to live more fully in the present
- Love and care for the self as well as others

Table 55–3 lists characteristics of spiritual well-being in the older adult.

Research has confirmed that involvement of older adults in organized religion is positively correlated with health status and functional capacity (Ainlay & Smith, 1984). Seriousness of illness or number of diagnosed health problems correlate positively with extent of spiritual involvement. In other research, spirituality was found to be a basic social process of older adults in general, regardless of health status (Hungelmann, Kenkel-Rossi, Klassen, & Stollenwerk, 1985).

In older adults, feelings such as happiness, usefulness, and life satisfaction are positively correlated with religious participation and other forms of spirituality.

Further, spirituality is the predominant coping strategy used by the elderly to enhance well-being (Koenig, George, & Siegler, 1988). Spiritual or religious beliefs help to transcend the negative stereotypes of aging and maintain or gain a sense of meaning and autonomy in society. However, spiritual expression tends to change in later life. Organized religious practices diminish and more personal forms of religious or spiritual expression increase.

Cultural Factors

The broader culture and subculture to which a client belongs can influence spiritual needs, as discussed in the accompanying Cross-Cultural Care chart. The beliefs and religious practices of the group will determine what type of spirituality is most appropriate. As pointed out in the overview of world religions, all religious beliefs and practices are bound to the culture and guide the group's lifestyle.

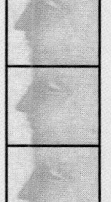

CROSS-CULTURAL CHART
CARING FOR A MEXICAN-AMERICAN CLIENT

Jesse Groves, the client whose story we've been following throughout the chapter, is of Mexican descent. His family immigrated to Arizona in the early 1900s and settled near Tucson. Although each person is unique, Mexican-Americans have a tendency to value the following:

- Traditional values of family roles, including men heading the family and women taking care of the family.
- Working hard, even under difficult situations, to support the family.
- Providing direct help to family and extended family members.
- Following the rules.
- Stoicism, not complaining about discomfort.
- Putting the needs of other family members before their own.
- Denying the severity of health related issues.

Let's watch how Sam, the nurse caring for Mr. Groves, demonstrates sensitivity to Mr. Groves' cultural values:

Sam: Hello, Mr. Groves. How are you today?

Mr. Groves: I'm much better. My wound seems to be healing well.

Sam: [Assesses the wound before cleaning it] Have you had much discomfort since I last did wound care?

Mr. Groves: Oh no! The wound doesn't hurt at all. I don't have any discomfort.

Sam: How are you feeling about your cancer?

Mr. Groves: I'm doing so much better now. You've really helped me. I can see I have a future, that this cancer is not going to get me.

Sam: That's good, Mr. Groves. Can you tell me a little about your thoughts of God during the last few days?

Mr. Groves: Well, I did what you suggested and called the church down the road. The secretary took my name and number and later that day the minister called. He sounds real nice and is coming by tomorrow to visit me.

Sam: That's good. What do you think you'll talk about?

Mr. Groves: I'm going to run some of my ideas by him to see what he thinks about God causing diseases like cancer.

Sam: I'm glad that you've thought about what you want to discuss with him. Will your wife be here when he comes?

Mr. Groves: I don't know. Why?

Sam: I think it might be a good idea to talk with the minister alone so you can share your feelings and ideas more openly instead of holding back in consideration of your wife and her beliefs.

Mr. Groves: That sounds good to me too.

Critical Thinking Questions

- What might have happened if Sam hadn't considered the Mexican-American cultural value of stoicism when discussing discomfort with Mr. Groves?
- Why did Sam ask what Mr. Groves was going to talk to the minister about during their visit?
- What do you think was the reason Sam suggested Mrs. Groves not be present when Mr. Groves talks with the minister?

CONSIDERING THE ALTERNATIVES
AYURVEDA

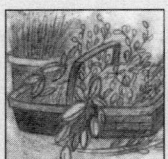

Ayurveda, which means the science or lore of life, is the predominant medical system of ancient India and has survived to the present day. Many Ayurvedic concepts and earliest works probably predate both Greek and Chinese medicine; they share some roots and concepts with the Hippocratic tradition. The earliest mention of Ayurveda was in the ancient Hindu scriptures known as the Vedas, which are perhaps 5,000 years old. The most important Ayurvedic texts, the *Charaka Samhita,* and the surgical text *Sushruta Samhita,* have been variously dated as 8th or 10th century B.C. or the first millennium A.D. (Svoboda & Lade, 1995; Trawick, 1992). Although originating in the Hindu tradition, Ayurveda is not now generally associated with a particular religion.

Like Greek and Chinese medicine, Ayurveda is a humoral medicine, meaning that part of the theory attempts to relate the aspects of the outer world to the world within our bodies. The five humors or elements of Ayurveda are earth, water, air, fire, and ether. The last, ether, "is both the source of all matter and the space in which it exists. . . . Our physical bodies are also made up of these Five Great Elements . . . everything that exists in the vast external universe, the macrocosm, also appears in the internal cosmos of the human body, the microcosm, in altered form" (Svoboda & Lade, 1995). Although the specific humors or elements differ in the different systems (for example, in traditional Chinese medicine the five elements are earth, metal, water, wood, and fire), they always represent ways of categorizing and describing mental and physical function and applying therapy.

Ayurvedic medicine was already practiced at the time of the Buddha and experienced a long period of fruitful development through the first millennium A.D. There were Ayurvedic hospitals, a number of branches of specialized practice, including surgery, and universities where students could study. A number of Ayurvedic texts were written during this period. Muslim invasion of India in the 10th century and British rule in the 18th and 19th centuries nearly caused Ayurvedic practice to disappear. However, in the last century, along with a resurgence of Indian nationalism, Ayurveda has come back into practice. Like traditional medicine in China, it has redeveloped both as an alternative to modern medicine and sometimes as a complement to it.

Ayurveda posits a need for balance and harmony to maintain optimum health. *Prana* is considered the life force, somewhat akin to *qi* in Chinese medicine, a force that empowers function and activity in the body and can be cultivated through various practices. When the *prana* is abundant and flowing, it concentrates in the chakras, or energy centers.

One of the most important theories of Ayurveda is that of the three *doshas.* The *doshas* are described as three psychosomatic types, *Vata, Pitta,* and *Kapha.* Each person is felt to be a combination of the three types, with one type predominating. For example, a *Vata* person has a narrow body frame, rarely sweats, and prefers warm temperatures. A *Pitta* person has a medium build, sweats profusely, and prefers a cool climate. A *Kapha* person is broad framed, sweats moderately, and likes the change from season to season. Health is a state of "balance between the elements of the mind and body that correspond to *Vata, Pitta,* and *Kapha*" (Badmaev & Majeed, 1996).

The philosophical views of the culture toward a higher power, sin, salvation, health, and the future affect how clients will respond to changes in health. For example, a client from India, raised a dedicated Hindu, would express a fatalistic belief in the future and his lack of control over future events. A Jewish client from America might appear more optimistic about his future because he believes he can cry out for God's mercy.

The leadership pattern of the subculture may affect clients' spiritual needs as well. People tend to follow the advice of leaders. You need to be aware of the potential influence of leadership patterns when assessing clients' spiritual needs.

Psychosocial Factors

Various psychological and social factors can influence spiritual needs. Socially, a support system and social roles can influence spiritual responses to illness. Psychologically, a personality type, outlook on life, coping style, and meaning ascribed to life affects spirituality. Keep in mind that clients may adhere to many different ways of thinking about personalities and how they relate to health, as discussed in the Considering the Alternatives chart.

A client's general outlook on life stems from his personality. Both of these psychological factors influence the client's coping ability in times of distress or illness. Coping styles that might interfere with effective management of a crisis include denial, minimizing, self-blame, and regression. You need to be aware of these psychological factors in assessing clients' spirituality.

How a client views and adapts to an illness can be directly influenced by a previous experience with illness. For example, if a client was seriously injured in

AYURVEDA (continued)

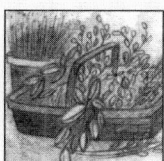

Ayurveda does have a spiritual component, stressing a need for each person to have a healthy spiritual understanding, relation to God or the divine, and thus an awareness of one's place in what we perceive as objective reality. This understanding allows a connection and flow with universal energies, which helps to maintain health. Medication is often the tool used to achieve this.

Ayurveda stresses the importance of living a natural lifestyle and consuming a healthy diet. Sickness may first be treated by diet alone; if that is insufficient, medicines may be tried. Foods, like medicines, will be recommended according to what will help the client achieve balance. Thus, what is helpful to one person may lead to imbalance in another. This is usually determined by which *dosha* is prominent, and by making recommendations according to the different tastes and their effects on the *doshas*.

Most of the research on Ayurvedic medicine has been focused on herbal medicine. Studies have been carried out on combinations of herbs and on single herbs. For example, a formula known as Padma 28 was shown to improve memory and general well-being in a group of 21 elderly clients (Panjwani, Priestley, & Lewis, 1987). Many individual herbs have been shown to possess antidiabetic properties. For example, the herb *Gymnema sylvestre* has shown positive effects in both type I and type II diabetes. In the former it appeared to enhance the function of insulin and allowed decreased insulin dosages. In the latter it allowed reduction and in some cases discontinuance of oral hypoglycemic agents (Mur-

ray, 1998). A number of other herbs have also shown promise in treating diabetes (Majeed & Prakash, 1998). These and other studies indicate a wealth of possible health applications from Ayurvedic remedies, as well as potential wisdom to be gained from the holistic perspective of Ayurvedic teachings.

Resources

Publications that can expand and keep your knowledge of complementary and alternative medicine current:

Chopra, D. (1991). *Creating health.* Boston: Houghton Mifflin.
Leslie, C., & Young, A. (Eds.). (1992). *Paths to Asian medical knowledge.* University of California Press, 2120 Berkeley Way, Berkeley, CA 94720.
Svoboda, R., & Lade, A. (1995). *Tao and Dharma, Chinese medicine and Ayurveda.* Lotus Press, P.O. Box 325, Twin Lakes, WI 53181.

References

Badmaev, B., & Majeed, M. (1996, February). The dosha theory of Ayurvedic medicine. *Health Supplement Retailer.* 22–34.
Majeed, M., & Prakash, L. (1998, April). Anti-diabetic herbs. *Health Supplement Retailer,* 35.
Murray, M. (1998). Diabetes mellitus. *Natural Medicine Journal, 1*(3), 4–18.
Panjwani, H.K., Priestely, J., & Lewis, A.E. (1987). Clinical evaluation of Padma 28 in treatment of senility and other geriatric circulatory disorders: A pilot study. *Alternative Medicine, 2*(1), 11–17.
Svoboda, R., & Lade, A. (1995). *Tao and dharma: Chinese medicine and Ayurveda.* Twin Lakes, WI: Lotus Press.
Trawick, M. (1992). Death and nurturance in Indian systems of healing. In C. Leslie & A. Young (Eds.), *Paths to Asian medical knowledge.* Berkeley: University of California Press.

---

an automobile accident and experienced spiritual growth during that time, the thought of a critical illness might not pose such a threat to his sense of spiritual well-being.

Physiological Factors

Many illnesses are perceived as a threat to a sense of well-being, which can initiate a spiritual conflict. Diseases that are life-threatening or chronic are especially capable of stimulating such a crisis. For example, when a person is initially diagnosed with cancer, doubts and fears may arise about the future. The meaning and purpose of the disease may also be questioned.

Pain can present a challenge to spiritual beliefs. The presence of extensive or uncontrollable pain has long been understood to initiate spiritual as well as mental pain. For example, a client who experiences an automobile accident with serious physical injury may call into question beliefs in a God who caused such

discomfort. Pain can prevent a client's usual involvement in religious activities as well.

When Mr. Groves returns home from the hospital after his surgery, you are assigned to conduct an admission assessment. What types of questions will you ask to assess Mr. Grove's spirituality? Do you expect his diagnosis of prostate cancer will affect his sense of spiritual well-being? Are Mr. Groves' religious practices important in his recovery from surgery?

ASSESSMENT

Because nursing involves the whole person, you are responsible for supporting the power of the spirit as a tool for client healing. Clients who despair or feel hopeless are more likely to die, or die sooner, even when there is little physiological disease to justify the death. Those who are joyful are more likely to live even in the face of overwhelming physiological illness. We begin the nursing process portion of this chapter with assessment of spiritual needs.

General Assessment of Spirituality

Data about the client's spiritual condition are most frequently obtained through observation and from discussion with the client. The major factors that influence spiritual assessment are time constraints and client acuity. Nurses are sometimes so busy with the hectic pace of health care that they do not take the time to care for the spiritual needs of clients (Fig. 55–5).

During your assessment of Mr. Groves, you discover that he used to attend a nondenominational Christian church but stopped 12 years ago when he got a divorce. He and his present wife do not practice "all that church stuff." He says his wife is an agnostic. What can you ask Mr. Groves to find out more about his spiritual beliefs? Do you think Mrs. Groves' disbelief has influenced Mr. Groves' spiritual beliefs?

Health History

The nursing history in most settings asks if the client has a religious preference. To gain more than this limited information you need to ask additional questions about belief or unbelief.

Specific objective data can be sought, such as asking openly about current religious practices, whether the client would like to visit the chapel or have a cleric, rabbi, or other religious leader visit. These are acceptable, nonthreatening questions. The client may be asked about the appropriate care for a religious item to prevent its loss and yet have it readily available to the client. Sometime just asking, "How can I help you?" is sufficient.

You can encourage the client to express thoughts and feelings. You can listen to stories the client tells to help determine the role of spirituality in his life and health. The accompanying A Patient's View chart offers one such example of an individual client's story. From stories like these, you can determine how clients perceive their lives and their relationships with themselves, others, and the rest of creation.

In summary, then, you must use client cues to formulate open-ended, nonjudgmental questions and statements that facilitate the creation of a trusting nurse-client relationship in which spiritual needs—such as those of purpose, love, belonging, and self-worth—can be examined and interventions planned.

After talking more with Mr. Groves, you learn that he has begun to pray after learning about his cancer. Mr. Groves also tells you that he has been thinking about going to church when he can drive again. What can you say to encourage Mr. Groves in pursuing the fulfillment of his spiritual needs? Would you offer to provide him spiritual care?

Assessment Tools

Care for spiritual needs is increasingly being seen as central to nursing and to healing. The spiritual nature of a person cannot be directly observed or measured. Yet, in the company of someone profoundly depressed, the void created by lack of spirit has an infectious, dampening effect on your spirit. Likewise, the high-spirited, ebullient individual who bubbles over with life and enthusiasm is easily recognized (Carson, 1993). If you are to give holistic care to a spiritual being, knowing how to assess the need for such care is crucial.

Spiritual assessment is difficult because spirituality is elusive. Because of the pluralism of ideologies, philosophies, and creeds, discrepancies may occur between your beliefs and those of the client. Your own beliefs may interfere with identifying subtle cues to the client's spiritual needs. The confusion between religion and spirituality also can complicate assessment.

To appraise a client's spiritual needs, ask questions such as the following:

- Is God important to you right now? Has God been important in the past?
- Are your religious practices meaningful for you now? In the past?
- Have you found your prayers to be helpful now? In the past?
- Has your current illness affected your spiritual experiences?

The format of these questions provides you with an efficient and effective means for assessing the client's current spiritual needs. In this way you are prepared to address a client's specific needs.

The most widely known assessment tool in nursing consists of a series of questions addressing personal beliefs (Stoll, 1979). The tool is a challenging instrument requiring extensive time and thought to complete. It provides you with significant information about the client's spirituality to plan for spiritual nursing care. Box 55-1 gives guidelines for spiritual assessment.

As you finish providing wound care, Mr. Groves begins to tell you his concerns about dying from cancer. What can you say in response to his fears of dying? How will your own spiritual beliefs about life and death affect your care of Mr. Groves? What are the defining characteristics Mr. Groves is exhibiting? What nursing diagnosis do you think is most appropriate?

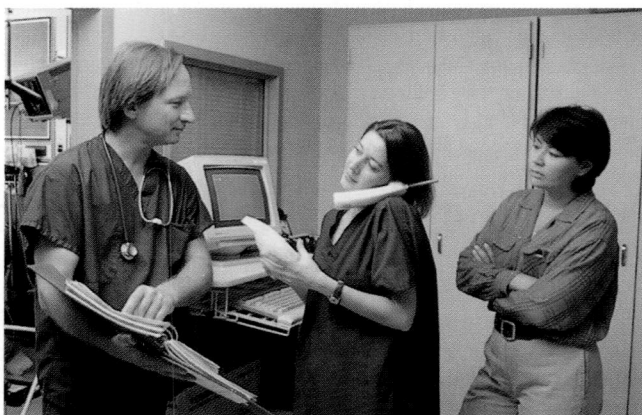

Figure 55–5. Nurses are sometimes so busy with the hectic pace of health care that they do not take the time to care for the spiritual needs of clients.

A PATIENT'S VIEW
"I WALK BY FAITH, NOT JUST BY WHAT I SEE"

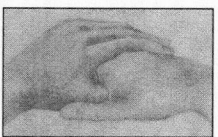 In 1956, people had begun to think of polio as history. I was 4 years old and had been given two out of three doses of the Salk vaccine, so no one thought I could have polio. But they were wrong. I don't remember much about the early months in the hospital but my parents said it was touch and go for a while. I do remember the rehabilitation, however. My mother had me doing intensive exercises with sandbags, mostly to strengthen my right leg.

Those exercises paid off. I recovered full use of my legs and was able to play sports, so we thought it was just a "mild" case. I was an active, happy kid, successful in school, went to college, married right after graduation, and went East with my wife to enter seminary.

After growing up in a small town in California's gold country, life in a major urban center was a totally new experience. At first we didn't pay a lot of attention to the city's problems—poverty, drugs, crime—assuming that we would move on after I finished seminary. Twenty-four years and four sons later, we're still here, committed to our church and to the importance of renewing this city and other cities across the country.

Over the years we've seen a tremendous flight from the city, but we've also seen that "you can run but you can't hide." Decay follows those who flee. We've seen how crucial it is for people to make a serious commitment to live, work, and shop in the city, not abandon it. Our sons don't regret being raised here. They've faced urban crime and feel prepared to deal with city life. Serving this church in this city gives you a sense that what you're involved with really matters, that you can make a difference, a sense that this is what God has called you to do. That sense of mission—that commitment—and my faith in God and Christ have helped me cope during the past 3 years since history came back to haunt me.

During a general examination in late 1994, the doctor said my blood pressure was too high and told me to lose weight, so I started working out. That's when the unexplained falling started. When I fell and broke my finger the following spring, I thought I had slipped on the steps but then realized that my legs felt weak, especially the right leg. The doctor did some manual strength tests and referred me to a neurologist. More tests followed. By July 1995 the diagnosis of post-polio syndrome came as no surprise. The strength was (and is) deteriorating in both legs, but it's more acute in the left leg because of all those years favoring the right leg.

Unlike many people with post-polio syndrome, I'm not in pain. But the weakness in my legs and the crushing fatigue (the most common symptom) have imposed limits I feel I'm too young to accept at age 46. My running days are over, so tennis is gone. I have trouble going down steps or even a slope because my quadriceps are shot. Last winter, I decided it was time to wear a brace on my right knee. Now that summer is here and I sometimes wear shorts, I've begun to experience what it means to be visibly imperfect. People treat you differently. They don't know what to do or say. I realize how easily we categorize someone as handicapped—not quite a person—how wrong it is to define a person in terms of an affliction, and how important it is to recognize there's lots more to a person than meets the eye.

The fatigue is more than physical. It's also brain fatigue that renders you incapable of doing anything. It has affected the quality and quantity of my work. And I have a terrible time sleeping (also a common problem), so I'm working with a sleep disorders clinic. To conserve my flagging energy, I'm talking with the other two pastors in the church about reducing my workload. I'm a private person by nature, someone who prefers to work alone, so it's more than a little painful to hand things over to someone else. This experience has brought me into a new and deeper level of understanding of how much I need other people and their God-given talents and abilities. It's made me ask: What will it take to pastor this church? The obvious answer: a team approach. That's good news.

One of the biggest challenges of this condition is the uncertainty, the unpredictability of the problem. No one knows whether the deterioration will continue, perhaps to paralysis, or whether it will abate at some point. The progression is different in every person affected. Thinking too far ahead discourages me, so I just try to focus on today. I pray to sustain that focus. And I count my blessings.

My wife and family give me enormous support and a fair amount of laughter. My parents offer tremendous encouragement. They exemplify grace under pressure, especially my mom, who's lived with lupus since 1964. She's a model of what it means to live the life you have with grace and trust in God even when your body doesn't work right and you're in pain. My father has cared for her and encouraged her. I've learned so much from their lives. My mom has taught me to press on, to do what you can do and not be undone by what you can't do. I haven't totally mastered that; I bounce around a lot. My mom is also a great woman of prayer and I've learned from that too. A lot of people pray for me on a regular basis and I'm convinced that it helps.

My congregation is very much aware of what's going on with me. They know I suffer, and they seem to hear me differently as a result. There's a stronger link between us. Just like all the parts of our body need each other, community develops where there's weakness and suffering. When I was depending on my intellect, en-

(continued)

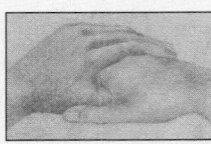

A PATIENT'S VIEW
"I WALK BY FAITH, NOT JUST BY WHAT I SEE" (continued)

ergy, skills and abilities, being totally self-reliant, I hadn't seemed to need God all that much. I believe God is often hidden to the proud and strong but makes Himself known to the humble and weak.

This experience has brought me into a deeper relationship with God and you can't put a price on that. My relationship with Christ means accepting both the good and the bad. I may not understand how this disease fits in but it doesn't make me question the relationship. I see a parallel in my relationship with my teenage sons. We may not always understand each other and they may not like what I tell them to do but we all know that I love them like nothing else.

I feel blessed that I can get around, that I'm not crippled. This is just one thing in my life. It's real—and the most pressing thing I have to face—but it's just one thing. I'm laboring not to let this condition define me. This affliction has caused me to stop and think about what I'm doing with my life—what's most important. I'm starting to get a clearer picture. But meanwhile, I walk by faith, not just by what I see. That's the heart of Christian life.

Focused Assessment for Spiritual Distress

Defining Characteristics

Spiritual distress incorporates the five spiritual needs of forgiveness, love, hope, trust, and meaning and purpose in life. Defining characteristics for *Spiritual distress* are observed as a natural part of a therapeutic relationship. The client expresses this distress both verbally and behaviorally. Sometimes it is even a direct expression of loss of faith, anger at God, or questioning the meaning of life/death.

Often the subject is more likely to arise when the client cannot sleep, is crying, or has other obvious signs of distress. Misdirected anger or hostility may occur out of spiritual distress.

BOX 55–1
GUIDELINES FOR SPIRITUAL ASSESSMENT

To Determine Client's Beliefs, Values, and Concept of God or Divine Being

- Is religion or God significant to you? If yes, can you describe how?
- Is prayer helpful to you? What happens when you pray?
- Does a God or deity function in your personal life? If yes, can you describe how?
- How would you describe your God or what you worship?

To Determine Client's Sources of Hope and Strength

- Who is the most important person to you?
- To whom do you turn when you need help? Are they available?
- In what ways do they help?
- What is your source of strength and hope?
- What helps you the most when you feel afraid to need special hope?

To Determine Client's Religious Practices

- Do you feel your faith (or your religion) is helpful to you? If yes, would you tell me how?
- Are there any religious practices that are important to you?
- Has being sick made any difference in your practice of praying?
- Has being sick made any difference in your religious practices?
- What religious books or symbols are helpful to you?

To Determine Client's Perceived Relation Between Spiritual Beliefs and Health

- What has bothered you most about being sick (or what is happening to you)?
- What do you think caused this to happen to you?
- Has being sick (or what has happened to you) made any difference in your feelings about God or the practice of your faith?
- Is there anything that is especially frightening or meaningful to you?

Stoll, R. (1979). Guidelines for spiritual assessment. American Journal of Nursing, 79(9), 1574–1577.

Related Factors

Factors related to *Spiritual distress* include the following:

- Challenged belief and value system (e.g., due to moral/ethical implications of therapy or to intense suffering)
- Separation from religious/cultural ties

Clients who are experiencing a crisis are susceptible to spiritual distress. Some treatment factors can cause spiritual distress. Depending on the client's religious faith, abortion, blood transfusions, amputation, or even being in isolation can create spiritual conflict.

Antecedents to spiritual distress include loneliness, fear of the unknown, guilt or expressions of regret, anger toward God or a higher power, loss of hope, and a change in relationships, values, and beliefs. Any client verbalizing such feelings is at high risk for spiritual distress. The risk factors for spiritual distress also include anxiety, blocks to self-love, inability to forgive, stress, substance abuse, and disasters.

Focused Assessment for Related Nursing Diagnoses

Spiritual may not be the most obvious presenting need. However, many nursing diagnoses can have an element of spiritual distress.

Ineffective Individual Coping

A nursing diagnosis frequently confused with spiritual needs is *Ineffective individual coping*, which is the impairment of adaptive behaviors and problem-solving abilities in meeting life's demands and roles. The defining characteristics of *Ineffective individual coping* demonstrate that the client is not dealing with life events appropriately. If the client exhibits increased anxiety, unhappiness, pessimism, nonperformance of activities of daily living, or drug abuse, then the client's primary diagnosis should be *Ineffective individual coping*.

Hopelessness

Occasionally you may use the diagnosis of *Hopelessness* when *Spiritual distress* is more appropriate for the client's needs. Hopelessness is a state in which the person sees limited or no alternatives or personal choices available and is unable to mobilize energy. The characteristics are behavioral including passivity, slow response, decreased affect, and despondency. Spiritual distress, with a loss of belief in God or a higher power, may be a related factor for feelings of hopelessness. By conducting a thorough assessment of the spiritual domain, you can distinguish between spiritual distress and hopelessness.

Dysfunctional Grieving

To differentiate between *Dysfunctional grieving* and *Spiritual distress*, you need to conduct a complete assessment of the psychological and spiritual dimensions. Dysfunctional grieving is a process of maladaptive and excessive emotional responses after experiencing a significant loss. It can lead to spiritual distress with questions revolving around the meaning of life and death. The characteristics of dysfunctional grieving are separate from those of spiritual distress. These behaviors include alterations in lifestyle, such as eating, sleeping, activity, physical symptoms of fear and anxiety, and distorted emotional reactions, such as anger, denial, and low self-esteem.

DIAGNOSIS

Spiritual needs can be confused with psychological or social needs, thus leading to the wrong diagnosis and plan of care. You need to differentiate spiritual distress from related nursing diagnoses, such as *Fear, Dysfunctional grieving, Hopelessness, Ineffective individual coping,* and *Anxiety.* By focusing on the defining characteristics, you can determine which diagnosis is most appropriate for the client's needs. For the spiritual nursing diagnoses, the major issues are one's relationship to God or a higher power, beliefs and values, and the search for meaning and purpose in life.

In finalizing a diagnosis, keep in mind that you may tend to feel comfortable with cues that support your diagnosis and overlook or deny those that do not (Lunney, 1990). Self-knowledge is crucial when trying to understand a client, interact appropriately, and cluster data to arrive at appropriate diagnoses, as suggested by the Data Clustering chart. Therefore, you must be aware of and open to your own spiritual biases and beliefs. In addition to promoting positive spirituality, you must possess positive spirituality.

During your next visit, you talk with Mr. Groves about your nursing diagnosis of *Spiritual distress* and your tentative plans for spiritual care. Mr. Groves is very pleased you will be helping him with his spiritual needs, but Mrs. Groves expresses her disagreement with the plans. What will you say to the couple, because their needs are quite different?

PLANNING

Establish expected outcomes for clients who have spiritual distress in conjunction with the client. Given the complex nature of the spiritual domain, a specific target date for achieving outcomes may not be realistic.

The overall expected outcome for the client with spiritual distress is that the client will develop an inner spiritual peace and a sense of spiritual well-being. Additional expected outcomes are based on individual needs. If the client has discussed anger toward God, then an appropriate outcome would be that the client expresses anger and related feelings with an impartial person.

An expected outcome for a client who expresses questions about the meaning of life or suffering would be that the client will experience a greater sense of meaning, purpose, and hope in living with an illness.

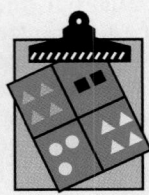

CLUSTERING DATA TO MAKE A NURSING DIAGNOSIS
SPIRITUAL PROBLEMS

Data Cluster	Diagnosis
Young African-American woman who recently lost her infant expresses disbelief in God, confusion about her former beliefs, and guilt about the child's death.	*Spiritual distress* related to loss of child, sense of guilt, and conflict about beliefs
A Native American man is talking about suicide after losing his wife and son in an automobile accident. He has been treated for bipolar disease for 10 years, has resumed drinking since their deaths, and is angry at God for taking them.	*Ineffective individual coping* related to loss of loved one, psychiatric disorder, and drinking problem
An elderly immigrant from Vietnam is diagnosed with ovarian cancer that has metastasized. She understands her condition and expresses a readiness for death.	*Potential for enhanced spiritual well-being* related to terminal cancer
A recently retired man suffers a massive stroke with complete left hemiparesis. He talks about his lack of spiritual beliefs, sense of things being unreal, feelings of anger, and denial about lost health.	*Dysfunctional grieving* related to multiple losses, including employment, career, health, and physical independence
A 13-year-old girl is being evaluated for sexual abuse by her stepfather. She talks about her anger at God, recent nightmares, and meaning of her life.	*Spiritual distress* related to sexual abuse and confusion with meaning in life

For a client expressing inner conflict about beliefs, an outcome would be that the client will have a clearer understanding of personal beliefs and values. When a person has talked about a conflict in his relations with God or a higher power, then an appropriate outcome would be that the client will establish meaningful relations with his deity, himself, and others.

There are four goals for you in helping a client confront spiritual distress. First, you may help the client create, maintain, or renew relationships. As people review their lives, they may experience guilt as they consider unfulfilled expectations for themselves or acts of omission or commission toward themselves or others. To relieve this spiritual pain, there must be a sense of forgiveness. Persons of all belief systems should be assisted in resolving human differences and renewing relationships whenever these are recognized as sources of spiritual pain.

Second, all humans have a need for love expressed through relationships and seen in words and acts of kindness. This positive regard or love must be unconditional even for those who are unpleasant or apparently unresponsive to the family's or your efforts.

Third, you can help the client search for meaning. However helpful you wish to be, though, in the final analysis the person himself must create personal meaning. You can engage in supportive actions, such as accompaniment and listening, even when the final outcome is the client's submission to suffering and death.

Last, there is always the need for hope, which suggests the possibility of future good. Hope can be as simple as freedom from pain or the ability to perform certain tasks. Even a dying person can hope for a reunion with deceased loved ones, union with God, or at least a superior alternative to the current painful situation. Those who do not believe in an afterlife may believe in the transfer of physical energy, being remembered by others, or leaving a legacy to their children or community. You can help the client see hope in each remaining moment and the chance to make a positive difference while such moments continue.

You provide spiritual care for Mr. Groves on each subsequent home visit. What spiritual interventions are most appropriate for Mr. Groves? What spiritual interventions are available for Mrs. Groves?

INTERVENTION
Interventions to Relieve Spiritual Distress

Thinking about meaning should not be perceived as a problem. Spiritual distress can be an opportunity for growth and change. Spiritual distress is not pathological but is part of experiencing the meaning and fullness of life. Recognizing that all persons face crises at times throughout life allows you to care for clients who are struggling to both understand and shape the meaning of life. Initial interventions can be implemented even by a beginning nurse.

Communicating About Spiritual Needs

Communicating about spiritual needs requires sensitivity, concern, empathy, a willingness to listen, and a nonjudgmental attitude. It also requires communication that is direct, specific, and clear. For example, if a client asks if he is going to die, you can refocus the question onto the client's fear of dying. On the other hand, listening to the client can be healing in and of itself. A client experiencing spiritual distress does not require answers but needs someone who will listen and hear with empathy. Listening with unconditional, positive regard is the single most therapeutic action you can take.

If listening to clients debating the meaning of life makes you anxious, you will need to examine your own beliefs so that you are comfortable in them and capable of listening without feeling anxious or defensive. It is important to acknowledge the client's true feelings, even when they are negative. Any person with an illness may suddenly be faced with doubts and fears concerning being dependent or dying. Common responses include grief over loss, unbearable anxiety, or anger at God. Dwelling on such feelings may cause considerable spiritual distress. You can help a great deal simply by acknowledging how terrible such feeling and fears can be. Be sure to stress that grappling with strong feelings, such as anger, fear, or despair, is normal when facing severe illness or hospitalization. Finally, continue to comfort with your physical presence, demonstrating availability and caring.

Using Yourself Therapeutically

It is very easy for you to avoid using yourself therapeutically. You can do this by giving pain or sleep medication, making it clear that you are too busy to talk, ignoring nonverbal cues, or refusing to hear the true message of what a client is saying. Even prayer can be misused if rote recitations are used to respond to hard questions or as a means of closing the discussion rather than dealing with feelings or issues.

It is also easy for your own feelings to interfere with your ability to listen. Feelings of isolation, fear, guilt, anger, grief, or being overwhelmed may require you to temporarily leave the situation until you can address your personal feelings. You cannot expect to always be able to listen to deep emotions. Time out is acceptable so that you will be able to continue giving quality care at a later time.

Using yourself therapeutically requires connection with each client. This connection includes such caring behaviors as taking time, touching, listening, being present and available, giving "good" nursing care, extra attention, and being understanding and accepting. Perhaps most important is that clients perceive these caring behaviors even in the midst of routine nursing activities.

Lack of spiritual care is often attributed to time constraints. However, one study found that spiritual care typically was not time-consuming, nor did it require extensive knowledge of different religions and philosophies. Brief comments about a supreme being's care, an encouraging word or touch, and visits of 5 to 10 minutes were all remembered by clients as significant spiritual care even years after the event (Conco, 1995). Spiritual care was associated with a caregiver with whom the recipient sensed a relationship. Therapeutic use of the self will help give meaning, purpose, hope, and connectedness to clients.

Accompanying the Client

Taylor and Ferszt (1990) use the concept of *accompaniment*. You can view being with clients as accompanying them on their journey. Thus, you have a vital role even when unable to alter what is happening to the client physically. Taylor and Ferszt change the traditional definition of nursing care from "doing" to "being."

Donley (1991) believes accompaniment is an important aspect of the caregiver's role. Being with the client requires you to enter into the reality of suffering to develop a sense of communion with the sufferer. You offer quiet sharing of your presence and help the person bear the burden of suffering. Accompaniment involves both your presence and comforting the client.

Promoting a Therapeutic Environment

Minor alterations in the hospital environment can bring the client tremendous spiritual comfort. Encourage family or friends to bring in inspirational art, such as paintings or prints. For example, paintings or photographs depicting a spiritual leader can be a source of comfort. Personal religious objects such as prayer beads, statues, and incense also may relieve spiritual distress, as do may sacred texts such as the Bible, Qur'an, a book of prayers, or sacred poetry. Music can be used therapeutically. In addition to suggesting religious television or radio programs, encourage family and friends to bring the client CDs or tapes of chants, hymns, or other inspirational music.

The internal environment may also be manipulated. For example, you can teach the client to use meditation, relaxation, and guided imagery. Meditation is an act of surrender, of letting go of usual preoccupations. Besides having positive psychological and physiological effects, it is a means by which the client can sense and experience directly or know intuitively what the conscious mind may deny or avoid. Many hospitals have relaxation or guided imagery audio or videotapes, with images such as a flickering fire or waves on a beach.

Providing Access to Spiritual Advisors

It is your responsibility to make sure that the client receives care by being supportive and helpful. It is not always your responsibility to personally give care. If you feel unable to be supportive, you may call another nurse who is more comfortable with spiritual issues or you may ask the client if he would like to speak with a member of the pastoral care staff or another spiritual advisor (Fig. 55–6).

When illness requires a client to engage in behaviors usually avoided, it is often helpful to have a spiritual leader discuss the spiritual restrictions in relation to therapeutic requirements. For example, a client can be excused from a spiritual fast if food is needed for healing. Having a spiritual leader discuss the exemption after you explain the purpose of the therapy is often helpful.

Even for those who do not consider themselves religious, when a clergy member or chaplain appears, the client's imagination and memories of their spiritual tradition and heritage may be triggered. A therapeutic interaction may result. In many hospitals in the United States, a visit by a Christian minister is routine. Be aware that such a visit may not be welcomed by clients of a different faith. Ask such clients if they would like you to contact their own spiritual advisor. In any case, it is always acceptable to simply ask if a visit with a cleric would be helpful or if the client would like to visit the hospital chapel.

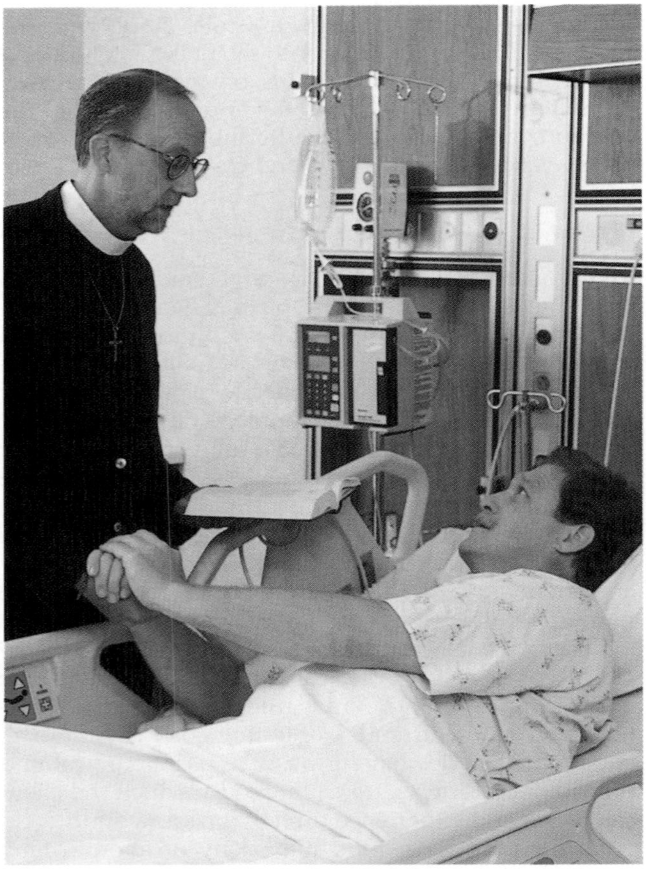

The chapel itself can be very helpful. Quiet time alone in a pew can sometimes help a client pray with a better sense that God is listening. Religious symbols are often therapeutic. Clients imaging God, a Higher Power, or the reality of love surrounding them will often feel better even when nothing else can be done. The feeling of being alone is reduced in such a setting.

Any request by a client for a spiritual counselor should be honored. Especially in emergency cases, clergy must be called. Most religious leaders know how to support the client without interfering in medical interventions, even in such acute care settings as the operating room or emergency department.

Helping the Client Maintain Relationships

Illness commonly causes isolation. The loss of ongoing contact with family, friends, and worshipers at church or other spiritual centers is often acutely felt. Being cut off from others is a form of suffering. Clients who identify themselves in relation to their faith community may be particularly vulnerable to a sense of spiritual isolation. You can help relieve the client's spiritual distress by recommending that family members contact the client's spiritual community and arrange for visits, phone calls, or gifts of cards or flowers as appropriate.

Supporting the Client's Faith Practices

Research has demonstrated that many clients use prayer as an effective coping strategy for dealing with health crises. Other helpful faith practices that were frequently cited included placing one's faith and trust in God and obtaining strength from God (Koenig, George, & Siegler, 1988).

There are varying levels of commitment to religion. Some people follow the rituals of their religion very closely; others accept the beliefs but feel that certain rituals are outdated. A discussion of religious practices with the client will help you provide appropriate care.

Religious leaders of most faiths wear specific clothing and are often addressed by a specific title to indicate their religious position. To demonstrate your respect and support for the client's faith, determine the proper title for religious leaders of that faith and call the leader by that title.

Rituals and religious practices can sustain the client. Rituals bring a sense of unity, providing identification with the past and hope for the future. Healing rituals are a part of the practice of most forms of religion. Many clerics are willing to have a healing service in the hospital, either at the bedside or in the chapel, with both client and family present. You may help the client engage in a ritual or celebrate a holy day by contacting the spiritual advisor, discussing the ritual with

Figure 55–6. If you feel unable to meet the spiritual needs of clients, you can ask the client if he would like to speak with a member of the pastoral care staff or another spiritual adviser.

other members of the health care team, and planning the day's activities around the planned ritual.

Other religious interventions may be planned according to the client's religious preferences. Many books are available that give the implications of typical nursing interventions for persons of various faiths. For example, in relation to cleanliness, Jewish men wash their hands before daily prayers and before and after meals. To support the practice, you may offer to supply a warm, wet washcloth before and after prayers and meals.

Prayer has been called the raising of the mind and heart to God. For many clients, it is a source of strength as well as a cry for understanding, for the power to endure, and for the wisdom to grow. Praying for help and healing is an action accepted in almost all cultures, although the objective of such prayers may differ. You can offer to say a prayer personally, to be present while the client prays, or to request that a minister, priest, or rabbi be present to share in the prayer. Many clients have favorite texts from sacred writings that they recite as a prayer when words otherwise fail. When clients are very ill or weak, or have impaired vision, you may offer to read their favorite prayers aloud for them.

Helping the Client Explore Meaning

While giving routine care, you can also help clients explore their thoughts about the meaning of illness, suffering, or life. Simple questions can help the client focus on meaning, as can the therapeutic techniques of reminiscence, visualization, life-review processes, and contemplation of literature.

Both you and the client may recognize the importance of illness in growth. Through pain, the person is alerted to be quiet, to allow the process to ferment, and to be inspired by the quiet. In aloneness, the person discovers the need for the presence and touch of another. Because most humans are ambivalent and somewhat unsure about the meaning of life, the client may need a supportive listener to encourage exploration of the meaning of this experience. It is often not the experience itself but its meaning that is important. Your reflective listening can allow your clients to explore their beliefs and feelings.

An intervention you can use to help clients find meaning is the use of *reminiscence.* Through reminiscence the client can examine his life experiences to discover new meanings or reconnect to forgotten moments that represent significant meaning. Finding meaning through reminiscence helps the client maintain ego integrity.

Another method for exploring meaning is to encourage the client to engage in a *life review.* Although the immediate results can be an autobiography to be given to family members or stories of childhood events to be given to children or grandchildren, the most important outcome is the client's own increased understanding of his life. Such an understanding may help the client accept current circumstances, regardless of the expected long-term outcome.

You can also help clients explore meaning through literature, including myth, metaphor, biographies, poetry, and song lyrics. When clients come to the end of one stage in life and the beginning of a new one, as occurs with traumatic injury or debilitating illness, they may experience tremendous anxiety, pain, and turmoil. Myths deal with the thresholds of such passages (Campbell, Moyers, & Flowers, 1988) and function to bring the person into harmony with destiny. You can offer to read such literature aloud or to leave books at the bedside for the client to read.

Stories that use subtle metaphors allow a truth to be shared without the glare of reality. Using metaphor in search of truth, meaning, and significance allows clients to confront issues of self-identify gently and helps them to see the universality of their suffering. Biographies are less subtle but equally revealing and inspiring. Some clients find poetry and songs a source of understanding when they reveal the insights of others whose sufferings were similar to their own.

To be able to transcend the present situation and perceive higher meaning and purpose in the situation may require that you share personal past situations of suffering and ways that you discovered meaning and purpose. Examining meaning and purpose in life through inward reflection is advocated for you to be able to help clients articulate their inward struggles.

After 6 weeks, Mr. Groves' suprapubic wound has healed and he will be discharged from home care. He tells you that he will need radiation therapy for the treatment of metastatic cancer. He appears quite distressed about the change in his condition and voices doubts about God's care of him. What plans can you make for Mr. Groves' spiritual needs after his discharge from your care?

Interventions to Enhance Spiritual Well-Being

Encouraging Hope

Hope is the means by which a person maintains integrity while being in the midst of illness and disease. Hope helps a client cope. Hope has been found predictive of favorable outcomes. A person without hope is in critical condition. Because hope is necessary for life, you must confirm that there is always hope.

Especially for an older person, you may have to help the client confront the possibility of death and yet have hope. Elements of this concept are presented in the State of Nursing Science chart. One approach is to encourage the client to be aware of nature's cycle. Suggest that the client take the time to watch the changes in the sky, the rising and setting of the sun, the falling of leaves, and the beginning of new growth. Watching the daily and seasonal changes can help put into perspective the cycle of life and death, dying and rebirth, year after year. Humankind is part of the cycle of life and death, too.

You can teach the client *reality surveillance.* By reconstructing past events and reasoning about them, the client searches for clues that hope is feasible. The

THE STATE OF NURSING SCIENCE
HOPE IN OLDER ADULTS

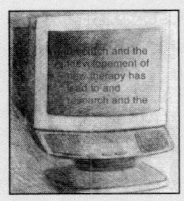

WHAT ARE THE ISSUES?

A holistic approach to working with people includes the spiritual dimension. This concept of spiritual dimension means more than just a person's religion. It includes how a person views relationships with oneself, other people, and God (Dyson, Cobb, & Forman, 1997, p. 1183). A part of one's spirituality is hope. Life-threatening illnesses and the aging process itself can challenge a person's sense of hopefulness. To provide holistic care, you need to understand what hope looks like in older adults before you can help people maintain hope in difficult circumstances.

WHAT RESEARCH HAS BEEN CONDUCTED?

Several researchers have explored hope in older adults. They all used self-report measures to estimate levels of hope under various health conditions. Farran, Wiken, and Fidler (1995) compared several measures of hope, social support, and health between a sample of community-dwelling older adults and those admitted to a geropsychiatric unit. Fehring, Miller, and Shaw (1997) studied the relationships among spiritual well-being, religiosity, hope, and depression in older adults with cancer. Fowler (1997) selected a brief tool on hope and one on health promotion to use with a sample of adults with Parkinson's disease. Most of her subjects were over age 65.

WHAT HAS THE RESEARCH CONCLUDED?

Farran, Wiken, and Fidler (1995) found that older adults admitted to a geropsychiatric unit had much lower levels of hope, social support, mental and physical health, and function in activities of daily living, and higher levels of stressful life events than did community-dwelling older adults. A second part of this study looked at how the level of hope changed at discharge from the unit. The researchers found that, upon discharge from the unit, the older adults in their study had an increase in hope that approached the levels of the community-dwelling older adults. The researchers hypothesized that interactions with staff contributed to the increase in hope.

The older adults with cancer in the study by Fehring, Miller, and Shaw (1997) had a positive relationship between hope and intrinsic religiosity. The researchers found that intrinsic religiosity related to such things as having meaning and purpose in one's life. Both hope and religiosity appeared to serve as coping measures for people with cancer. The researchers encouraged nurses to assess levels of hope in their clients and to look for ways to encourage them to draw on sources of hope.

The adults with Parkinson's disease studied by Fowler (1997) reported high levels of hope as well as health-promoting behaviors. The results on the subscale of spiritual growth in the instrument that measured health-promoting lifestyles were positively related to levels of hope. This supported previous research. Fowler suggested that nurses look for ways to help people maintain hope, such as encouraging social support through participation in religious activities, if they are identified as meaningful to the person (1997, p. 115).

WHAT IS THE FUTURE OF RESEARCH IN THIS AREA?

With reliable measures of hope, researchers can examine what nursing interventions might influence levels of hope. Interventions may need to be individualized based on the health condition of the older adult. In addition to helping people maintain hope, nurses need to see how hopefulness might affect a person's overall sense of well-being (Fowler, 1997, p. 116).

REFERENCES

Dyson, J., Cobb, M., & Forman, D. (1997). The meaning of spirituality: A literature review. *Journal of Advanced Nursing, 26,* 1183–1188.

Farran, C.J., Wiken, C.S., & Fidler, R. (1995). A study of hope in geriatric patients. *Journal of Nursing Science, 1*(1–2), 16–26.

Fehring, R.J., Miller, J.F., & Shaw, C. (1997). Spiritual well-being, religiosity, hope, depression, and other mood states in elderly people coping with cancer. *Oncology Nursing Forum, 24*(4), 663–671.

Fowler, S.B. (1997). Hope and a health-promoting lifestyle in persons with Parkinson's disease. *Journal of Neuroscience Nursing, 29*(2), 111–116.

client may need help in devising and revising goals, such as small steps in physical progress or defining tasks to be done or relationships that need renewal. Small goals can be set to help make each day more positive. For example, humanity's unlimited potential for becoming provides a continuous reason to hope. The client can hope to be the best person possible today. Or the person can look forward to a specific event, such as a wedding or family reunion. If there is reason to believe the client may not be able physically to participate in the event, the client can personally dictate an audiotape or write a letter to those who will be present to express love and good wishes. You can encourage expression using symbolic imagery in art, music, poetry, or stories.

Hope refers to the belief that whatever the outcome of a specific illness, everything will be all right. Such hope can be fostered when you share stories about people who have overcome great difficulties or personal events of overcoming troubles. Self-disclosure can help clients feel that they know the caregiver much better. Consequently, clients can feel that they can transcend the present situation to a hoped-for better future.

Many books are available that may give hope and joy to clients, even those who are dying. Such books are often very uplifting and optimistic because they demonstrate continued growth and development, love, and enjoyment of life until the end. Regardless of the specific illness or disease, there are probably books written by people suffering the same problem, which helps confirm that the client is not alone in suffering. Such books may also give hints as to coping mechanisms that proved helpful to another.

Helping the Client Interpret Crises as Spiritual Growth

Physical illness can be a crisis that forces clients to seek meaning in the chaos they are feeling. It may prompt clients to try to resolve interpersonal problems, their relationship with God, or feelings of failure from not having achieved certain life goals. Your first duty in such situations is to help clients achieve clarity about the problem.

Smucker (1996) described three stages of spirituality from her study of people experiencing some type of crisis. The first stage is "breaking the web of life." It happens when an event occurs unexpectedly. Feelings during this stage range from anxiety to fearfulness. The client may express concern as he tries to make sense of the circumstances. With the passage of time and with personal effort, the second stage begins.

Smucker calls the second stage "rebuilding the web of life." During this stage of spiritual crisis, people focus on the return of stability to their life. They became aware of the changes that have occurred in their life and choose to find meaning in these events. Many people feel their faith deepen and become more real during this time.

The third stage is known as "wondering." In this stage, people describe awe at the mysteries of life as they realize that they have not found answers. Rather than being frustrated at the limits of human knowing, however, they conclude that the ways of God are unfathomable. Believing in a higher being helps them to live even without rational answers.

Mr. Groves has undergone 4 weeks of radiation therapy to his pelvis. It causes diarrhea and a skin breakdown near his anus. You are reinstated to provide wound care and pain management.

How does spiritual distress and suffering affect the management of pain? Why would you want to differentiate between spiritual, emotional, and physical pain and suffering?

Helping the Client Deal With Suffering

You can help clients interpret the causes of suffering and determine what the appropriate responses might be (Donley, 1991). Pain is a physical response to injury and is easy to alleviate by comfort measures and medical treatment, such as drugs or surgery. It is much harder to reduce suffering, which is the client's personal interpretation of the pain.

To effectively intervene with a suffering client, you need to understand the meaning of suffering. Different religions emphasize different meanings for suffering, but it is most commonly perceived as punishment, mystery, or redemption. Punishment is often the first thought. Many clients ask, "What did I do to deserve this?" Most of us realize that some lifestyle behaviors can lead directly to illness, and many people believe that strong faith can lead to healing. Therefore, clients may blame themselves for their bad habits or not having sufficient faith to achieve healing. Assess for self-blame from the client or the client's family, and reassure them that the true causes of most illnesses are unknown.

Some religions place suffering in the realm of mystery. According to these traditions, the meaning of illness is not really understandable. The question is not, "Why me?" but, "Why not me?" Other ancient traditions suggest that suffering is instructive, that a person will learn by suffering, and that suffering will bring about a reordering of personal values that leads to redemption. Many recent theorists propose that some illnesses may be chosen by the soul for an important spiritual purpose, such as to advance the sufferer's spiritual development.

You can help your clients identify and explore their own interpretation of suffering. By being present with clients you can allow them to verbalize their concerns about the meaning of their suffering. Listening and clarifying the interpretations of suffering can help clients deal with the suffering. Also, you can encourage clients to find some positive aspects to their suffering. As they discuss their suffering with you and their family and friends, clients will feel some release from the extreme burden of the suffering.

EVALUATION

To evaluate the plan of care, you must always ask the client if the outcomes have been achieved, as suggested in the Nursing Care Planning chart. Spiritual health and a sense of spiritual well-being constitute a process that spans an entire lifetime. It is only appropriate for you to evaluate the expected outcomes for evidence of individual improvement.

When the client has been successful in confronting spiritual distress, it can be expected that the person will continue in his relationship with his God and engage in spiritual practices not detrimental to his health. Rather than express negative feelings of fear, guilt, or anxiety, they will express harmony and wholeness. Lastly, they may verbalize hope, trust, inner peace, and satisfaction with their spiritual condition. Their life will have meaning and purpose.

If your interventions are successful, the client will show signs of spiritual health. Carson (1989) created a

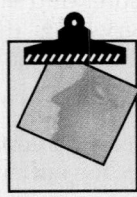

NURSING CARE PLANNING
A CLIENT WITH SPIRITUAL DISTRESS

Initial Data

Mr. Groves is a 56-year-old master electrician who has just returned home from the hospital after a radical prostatectomy for invasive carcinoma 4 days ago. His suprapubic wound has a 3-cm opening that requires daily wound care.

Nursing Assessment

As the nurse, you make plans to assist Mr. Groves in managing his wound care and supporting his recovery from surgery. You discover that Mr. Groves has spiritual needs in addition to the obvious physical and psychological needs. During your assessment you also find out that he used to attend a non-denominational Christian church but stopped 12 years ago when he got a divorce. He and his present wife do not practice "all that church stuff." He says his wife is an agnostic. After talking more with Mr. Groves, he tells you he has begun to pray again since learning about his cancer. Mr. Groves also tells you he has been thinking about going to church when he can drive again. As you finish providing wound care, Mr. Groves begins to tell you about his concerns about dying from the cancer.

NURSING CARE PLAN

Nursing Diagnosis	Expected Outcomes	Interventions	Evaluation (After 2 Weeks)
Spiritual distress related to conflict about spiritual beliefs, diagnosis of prostate cancer, and concern about relationship with God.	Client will experience a greater sense of meaning and hope in living with cancer.	Listen to client's concerns and feelings. Provide time to be with client. *Ask about previous beliefs and spiritual experiences.*	Client discusses his sense of meaning in life with cancer. Client shares about his previous beliefs.
	Client will have a sense of belonging.	*Encourage client to contact church of interest to have home visit with clergy. Encourage visits from spiritual counselor.*	Client calls a nearby church and minister comes to visit him.
	Client will have a clearer understanding of personal beliefs.	*Allow client to verbalize previous beliefs.* Provide opportunity for client to explore new spiritual beliefs.	Client talks about previous and potential spiritual beliefs and experiences.
	Client will establish meaningful relationship with himself, God, and others.	Encourage client to take responsibility for own life. *Encourage client to pray.*	Client begins to accept life with cancer. Client reports great satisfaction from his prayers.
		Encourage client to contact spiritual family members and friends during recovery.	Client contacts former friend with strong spiritual beliefs.

Italicized interventions indicate culturally sensitive care.

Critical Thinking Questions
1. Do you expect Mr. Groves' diagnosis of prostate cancer will affect his sense of spiritual well-being?
2. Do you think Mrs. Groves' disbelief has influenced Mr. Groves' spiritual beliefs and practices?
3. What can you say to encourage Mr. Groves in pursuing the fulfillment of his spiritual needs?
4. How will your own spiritual beliefs about life and death affect your care of Mr. Groves?

list of characteristics indicative of spiritual well-being, including the following:

- Sense of inner peace
- Compassion for others
- Reverence for life
- Gratitude
- Appreciation of both unity and diversity
- Humor
- Wisdom
- Generosity
- Ability to transcend the self
- Capacity for unconditional love

Hungelmann, Kenkel-Rossi, Klassen, and Stollenwerk (1985), in their analysis of spiritual well-being in older adults, found that well-being requires a relationship with self, others, the environment, and an ultimate other or God. The person looks simultaneously to the past, lives in the present, and hopes for the future.

Conco (1995) interviewed clients to discover how spiritual care was perceived. The clients said that being ill made them receptive to spiritual care. Anyone who spent brief moments with clients and gave spiritual care was remembered months and years later as a spiritual caregiver. The clients described these caregivers as full of love, accepting, and spiritually focused. The participants said that spiritual care was important to their coping with illness and to their recovery. Some felt it brought them through the experience.

Mrs. Groves calls to tell you Mr. Groves has been admitted to the hospital for management of his pain. She expresses her fears of his dying. How can you provide emotional support while being sensitive to Mrs. Groves' spiritual beliefs? Will this cause you any distress?

KEY PRINCIPLES

- Spirituality is a process and sacred journey, the experience of the radical truth of things, and a belief that relates a person to the world and gives meaning to existence.
- Religion is a belief system, including dogma, rituals, and traditions. It is also a social institution in which people participate to search for meaning in life.
- Faith is belief in or commitment to something or someone that helps a person realize purpose and meaning in life.
- Spiritual health enables and motivates us to search for meaning and purpose in life, to seek the supernatural or some meaning, which transcends us.
- Nursing care of a client's spiritual needs should always be based on respect for the person and his personal beliefs.
- Barriers to spiritual nursing care include lack of preparation, objective empathy, lack of time, confusion of spiritual needs with psychosocial needs,

materialism, empiricism, and lack of personal spiritual beliefs.
- The major religions of North America include Christianity, Judaism, Hinduism, Buddhism, Taoism, Islam, and Native American religions.
- Developmental, cultural, psychosocial, and physiological factors affect individual spiritual needs.
- Based on a thorough assessment, you can plan spiritual care for clients with the nursing diagnoses *Spiritual distress, Risk for spiritual distress,* and *Potential for enhanced spiritual well-being.*
- *Spiritual distress* is a state in which a person experiences a disruption in the life principle that pervades the entire being and that integrates and transcends one's biological and psychological nature.
- Interventions to relieve spiritual distress include establishing a therapeutic relationship, promoting an environment for sharing, providing access to spiritual advisors, helping the client maintain relationships, supporting the client's faith practices, and helping the client explore meaning.
- Interventions to enhance spiritual well-being are encouraging hope, helping the client interpret crisis as spiritual growth, and helping the client deal with suffering.
- Evaluation of the nursing process is based on an appraisal of the expected outcomes specified for and with the client.

BIBLIOGRAPHY

*Ainlay, S.C., & Smith, R. (1984). Aging and religious participation. *Gerontology, 39*(3), 357–363.

Barnum, B.S. (1996). *Spirituality in nursing.* New York: Springer.

Boutell, K., & Bozett, F. (1990). Nurses' assessment of patients' spirituality: Continuing education implications. *Journal of Continuing Education in Nursing, 21*(4), 172–176.

Britannica Online. (1998). *Britannica encyclopedia.* Chicago: Britannica Publishing.

*Burkhardt, M. (1989). Spirituality: An analysis of the concept. *Holistic Nursing Practice, 3*(3), 69–77.

*Burkhardt, M.A. (1994). Becoming and connecting: Elements of spirituality for women. *Holistic Nursing Practice, 8*(4), 12–21.

Campbell, J., Moyers, B., & Flowers, B.S. (Eds.). (1988). *The power of myth.* New York: Doubleday.

Carson, V. (1993). Spirituality: Generic or Christian. *Journal of Christian Nursing, 3,* 24–27.

*Carson, V.B. (1989). *Spiritual dimensions of nursing practice.* Philadelphia: W.B. Saunders.

Conco, D. (1995). Christian patients' views of spiritual care. *Western Journal of Nursing Research, 17*(3), 266–276.

Donley, R. (1991). Spiritual dimensions of health care: Nursing's mission. *Nursing and Health Care, 12*(4), 178–183.

Dossey, B.M., & Guzetta, C.E. (1995). *Holistic nursing* (2nd ed.). Gaithersburg, MD: Aspen.

*Ellison, C., & Paloutzion, R. (1982). Spiritual well-being: Conceptualization measurement. *Journal of Psychology and Theology, 11,* 330–340.

Encyclopedia Britannica. (1998). *1998 Britannica book of the year.* Chicago: Britannica Publishing.

Fehring, R.J. (1986). Validating diagnostic labels: Standardized methodology. In M.E. Hurley (Ed.), *Classification of nursing diag-*

*Asterisk indicates a classic or definitive work on this subject.

noses: Proceedings of the sixth conference (pp 183–190). St. Louis: Mosby.

*Fowler, J.W. (1974). Toward a developmental perspective on faith. *Religion Education, 69*(2), 207–219.

*Fowler, J., & Keen, S. (1985). *Life maps: Conversations on the journey of faith.* Waco, TX: Word Books.

Germere, V. (1996). Psychiatric patients' experience of spirituality in a group setting. *Image: Journal of Nursing Scholarship, 28*(3), 279.

Hensley, L. (1994). Spiritual distress: A validation study. In R.M. Carroll-Johnson & M. Paquette (Eds.), *Nursing diagnoses: Proceedings of the tenth conference.* Philadelphia: J.B. Lippincott.

Highfield, M.F., & Cason, C. (1983). Spiritual needs of patients: Are they recognized? *Cancer Nursing, 6*(3), 187–192.

Hoshiko, B. (1991). Worldview as a model of spirituality. In J.A. Shelly (Ed.), *Teaching spiritual care* (2nd ed.) (pp 19–31). Madison, WI: Nurses Christian Fellowship.

*Hungelmann, J., Kenkel-Rossi, E., Klassen, L., & Stollenwerk, R. (1985). Spiritual well-being in older adults: Harmonious interconnectedness. *Journal of Religion and Health, 24*(2), 147–153.

Kaczorowski, J.M. (1989). Spiritual wellbeing and anxiety in adults diagnosed with cancer. *Hospice Journal, 5*(3–4), 105–116.

Kasser, T., & Ryan, R.M. (1996). Further examining the American dream: Differential correlates of intrinsic and extrinsic goals. *Personality & Social Psychology Bulletin, 22*(3), 280–287.

Koenig, H.G., George, L.K., & Siegler, I.C. (1988). The use of religion and other emotion-regulating coping strategies among older adults. *The Gerontologist, 28*(3), 303–310.

*Legere, T.E. (1984). A spirituality for today. *Studies in Formative Spirituality, 5*(3), 375–383.

Lunney, M. (1990). Accuracy of nursing diagnosis: Concept development. *Nursing Diagnosis, 1*, 12–17.

*Martin, J.P. (1989). Eastern spirituality and health care. In V. Carson (Ed.), *Spiritual dimensions of nursing practice* (pp 113–131). Philadelphia: W.B. Saunders.

*Moberg, D.O. (1984). Subjective measures of spiritual well-being. *Review of Religious Research, 25*(4), 351–361.

Newman, M.A. (1986). *Health as expanding consciousness.* St. Louis: Mosby.

North American Nursing Diagnosis Association. (1999). *NANDA nursing diagnoses: Definitions and classification 1999–2000.* Philadelphia: Author.

Paterson, J.G., & Zderad, L.T. (1988). *Humanistic nursing.* New York: National League for Nursing.

Piles, C.L. (1990). Providing spiritual care. *Nurse Educator, 15*(1), 36–41.

*Reed, P.G. (1987). Spirituality and well-being in terminally ill hospitalized adults. *Research in Nursing & Health, 10*, 335–344.

Reed, P.G. (1991). Spirituality and mental health in older adults: Extant knowledge for nursing. *Family and Community Health, 14*(2), 14–25.

Roy, C. (1988). An explication of the philosophical assumptions of the Roy Adaptation Model. *Nursing Science Quarterly, 1*(1), 26–34.

Smucker, C. (1996). A phenomenological description of the experience of spiritual distress. *Nursing Diagnosis, 7*(2), 81–89.

*Stallwood, J., & Stoll, R. (1975). Spiritual dimension of nursing practice. In I.L. Beland & J.Q. Passos (Eds.), *Clinical nursing* (3rd ed.) (pp 1086–1098). New York: Macmillan.

*Stoll, R.I. (1979). Guidelines for spiritual assessment. *American Journal of Nursing, 79*(9), 1574–1577.

Taylor, P., & Ferszt, G. (1990). Spiritual healing. *Holistic Nursing Practice, 4*(4), 32–38.

Travelbee, J. (1971). *Interpersonal aspects of nursing* (2nd ed.). Philadelphia: F.A. Davis.

Watson, J. (1985). *Human science and human care* (p 46). Norwalk, CT: Appleton-Century Crofts.

Special Client Populations

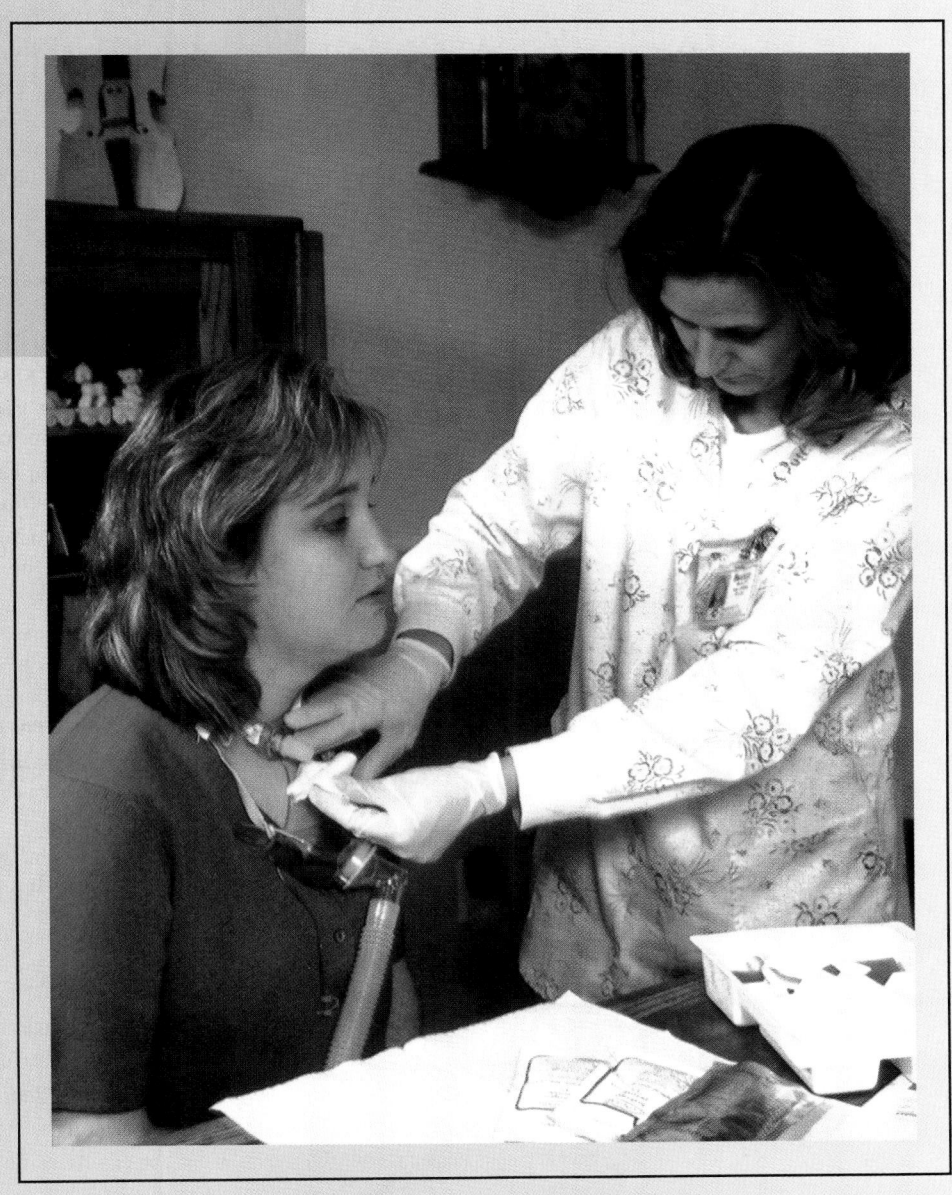

The Client With Functional Limitations

Kristen L. Easton and Margaret L. Bell

Key Terms

activities of daily living
chronic illness
chronicity
community reintegration
functional limitations

handicap
impairment
instrumental activities of daily
    living
rehabilitation

LEARNING OBJECTIVES

After studying this chapter, you should be able to:

1. Discuss several concepts related to rehabilitation.
2. Distinguish among the following terms: functional limitations, disability, impairment, and handicap.
3. State three major goals of rehabilitation.
4. Identify some common conditions that require rehabilitative services.
5. Contrast the roles of the members of the interdisciplinary team.
6. Compare a variety of care settings in which rehabilitation may be practiced.
7. Discuss the current costs and funding sources for those with disabilities.
8. Describe factors affecting ability and disability, including the client's environment, lifestyle, and culture.
9. Cite two assessment tools that could be used for a person with a functional limitation.
10. List three major nursing diagnoses for a person with a spinal cord injury.
11. Implement nursing interventions to provide quality care for people with physical limitations.
12. State several ways to evaluate whether or not rehabilitation outcomes have been met.

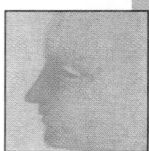

Eighteen-year-old Robert Baldwin sustained a complete C5-6 spinal cord injury as a result of hitting his head on the bottom of a shallow swimming pool. After stabilization in the acute care hospital, Robert spent about 2 months in a freestanding rehabilitation institute, learning to make the many adjustments required by the changes in his functional abilities resulting from tetraplegia. Once an active high school student, Robert now uses an electric wheelchair. He has fair to good shoulder movement and biceps activity, along with minimal wrist extension, but otherwise no active movement from just below the

(continued)

shoulders down. Robert requires 6 to 8 hours of attendant care daily for assistance with activities of daily living. He lives with his family, who help care for him. *Self-care deficit* and *Impaired physical mobility* are primary nursing diagnoses. Robert also struggles with feelings of powerlessness related to his inability to control many aspects of his life. He said to one of his friends, "I don't feel like I have control over anything in my life anymore." Robert has experienced a number of losses and is working through the grieving process. One of Robert's greatest challenges is reintegration into the school environment. This will require changes to be made in the external environment. The public school Robert attends has assigned a caregiver to help him during the school day. The school also put air conditioning in the parts of the building where Robert spends much of his day. This was necessary to accommodate his heat intolerance (common in spinal cord injury) during the summer months. A special door with an automatic opener was installed for Robert to enter the building. Once some of these adaptations were made, Robert adjusted quite well to his return. The social support from family, friends, teachers, and the community played a significant role in his ability to adapt to his limitations.

CONCEPTS OF FUNCTIONAL LIMITATION

Disabilities are present in about 1 in 5 Americans, with 10% of Americans having a serious disability. (Disabilities Affect One-Fifth of All Americans. Census Brief, U.S. Department of Commerce Bureau of the Census [1997]. www.census.gov/prod/3/97pubs/.) Disabilities can be a result of injury, chronic illness, congenital defect, or mental conditions. Adjustment to long-term health alterations is affected by many different factors such as socioeconomic status, environment, culture, educational level, lifestyle, resource availability, and a host of other factors.

Rehabilitation is defined as "the process of adaptation, or recovery, through which an individual suffering from a disabling condition, whether temporary or irreversible, participates to regain, or attempt to regain, maximum function, independence, and restoration" (Easton, 1999). According to this broad definition, clients may require rehabilitation for short-term problems, such as a broken arm or hip, or for a long-term problem, such as multiple sclerosis or another chronic, progressive disease. The goals are for the person to achieve maximal functional status and a satisfactory quality of life. An interdisciplinary team is a group of people working together with the client to achieve mutually established goals for rehabilitation.

Although people with physical challenges may have difficulty performing some tasks, they are still able to do many other tasks, or use adaptive equipment to complete tasks. Thus, use of the term *functional limitation* for such people suggests that it is not the person who is disabled, but just that a limitation in function exists (Fig. 56–1). **Functional limitation** refers to difficulties people may experience in performing activities of daily living (ADLs) or instrumental activities of daily living (IADLs). **Activities of daily living** can be defined as the basic activities usually performed in the course of a normal day in a person's life, such as eating, toileting, dressing, bathing, or brushing the teeth. **Instrumental activities of daily living** are food preparation, housekeeping, laundry, transporta-

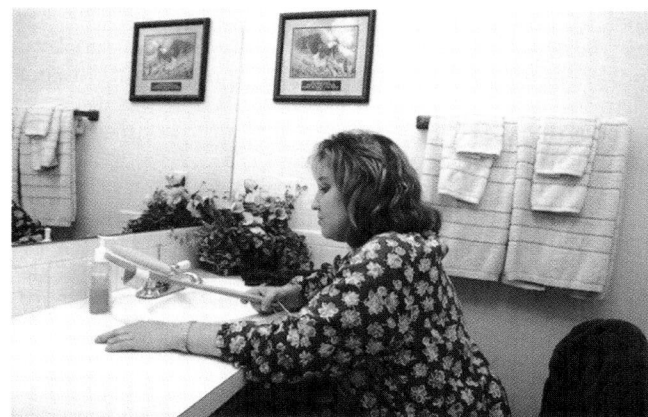

Figure 56–1. While people with physical challenges may have difficulty performing some tasks, they are still able to do many other tasks, sometimes with the use of adaptive equipment. Like this wheelchair-bound woman, these people are not "unable" or "disabled"; they have a functional limitation.

tion, using the telephone, shopping, and handling finances. *Functional limitations* is an appropriate term to describe the difficulties that people with physical challenges face in performing activities of daily living. The term *disability,* or *disabled,* is not preferred because it suggests that a person is not able, or the person is unable.

Impairment is a term used when discussing limitations resulting from any one of a variety of conditions, whether related to disease, trauma, or birth defect. An impairment relates to the physical or physiological cause of the limitation. For example, a person with a visual impairment may just need to wear glasses, or may be legally blind. The word *impairment* is similar to functional limitations.

Handicap suggests an interaction between the client with a disability and the environment. A **handicap** is a disadvantage experienced by a person as a result of impairment that limits the person's "normal" function. Health care professionals realize that this term carries negative overtones. Handicapped is a judgment that society places upon people when they view them as having a significant limitation. A handicap occurs at the societal level.

One important task for you to undertake is to ascertain the meaning of the limitation to the individual client. Some people who have lived with and adjusted to severe physical limitations for many years do not consider themselves disabled. Others may refer to themselves as crippled by comparatively minimal functional deficits. So while definitions are useful for your general and scientific knowledge, they do not replace the need for competent assessment in every area of the client's life to determine an individualized plan for quality care.

Many clients require rehabilitation due to functional limitations resulting from stable or progressive chronic illnesses. According to the Commission on Chronic Illness, **chronic illness** is defined as "all impairments or deviations from normal that have one or more of the following characteristics: are permanent, leave residual disability, are caused by a nonreversible pathological condition, require special training of the client for rehabilitation, or may be expected to require a long period of supervision, observation, or care" (Strauss, 1975).

Clients experiencing long-term health alterations require nursing care within a framework of chronicity. The word **chronicity** is a broad term that encompasses chronic illnesses as well as disease or congenital defects that permanently alter a person's previous health status (Lubkin, 1998; Easton, 1997).

Common Disabilities

There are several major areas in which common disabilities or functional limitations are seen. These include musculoskeletal impairments, neurological impairments, sensory/perceptual deficits, cognitive disorders, and chronic illnesses.

Musculoskeletal and neurological impairments occur across the life span. Childhood musculoskeletal impairments are often congenitally acquired, such as cerebral palsy. In the adolescent and young adult, spinal cord or brain injuries may be the cause. In the older adult, the impairment often results from arthritis or hip fractures. Stroke, Parkinson's disease, and multiple sclerosis are additional examples of common neurological impairments.

Interdisciplinary Team

Many different professionals make up the interdisciplinary team that helps those with disabilities down the road to recovery or adaptation. These include doctors, nurses, physical and occupational therapists, social workers, psychologists, and nutritionists. There are also auxiliary personnel who contribute to the team approach on an individualized care plan basis, although they may not be part of the usual team. These would include the pastoral care provider, recreational therapist, vocational counselor, audiologist, prosthetist, orthotist, and other specialists. The roles of

major team members are discussed in the following section.

Nurses who specialize in caring for people with disabilities or functional limitations are called *rehabilitation nurses*. "Rehabilitation nursing is a dynamic, creative specialty which promotes the positive adaptation of individuals with disabilities, through a holistic, nurturing environment, by combining your clinical skills, advanced knowledge, and resourcefulness with the perseverance, motivation, and strengths of the client to achieve maximal independence and an acceptable quality of life" (Easton, 1999). You should employ basic rehabilitative care in your daily practice.

Rehabilitation nurses share the following roles: teacher, caregiver, advocate, counselor, consultant, and researcher. Depending on your educational level and experience, these roles take on different degrees of emphasis. For example, an advanced practice nurse (APN) in rehabilitation may engage much more in the roles of teacher and consultant than direct caregiver, whereas a nurse with a doctorate may focus more on research.

Nurses who care for those with functional limitations become experts in several areas of assessment and care. These include physical and psychosocial assessment, bowel and bladder management, skin care, nutrition, behavior, teaching, and family participation. Education of clients and families is a key nursing skill when preparing people to re-enter the community after experiencing a long-term health alteration.

The Association of Rehabilitation Nurses (ARN) is the specialty organization in this field of interest. The ARN was founded in 1974, recognizing rehabilitation nursing as a specialty. Certification in rehabilitation is attained by successfully passing an examination that tests knowledge in the area of rehabilitation. Registered nurses with 2 years of current experience in rehabilitation and who meet other stated requirements can sit for the examination. The credential CRRN indicates Certified Rehabilitation Registered Nurse.

Physiatrists control the medical management of rehabilitation clients. They help evaluate overall functional progress, prescribe medications and treatments, and give medical direction and guidance to the team.

The *physical therapist* (PT) is a licensed professional who assists clients with activities involving the lower extremities. Assessing range of motion, mobility, strength, balance, and gait, as well as working with the person on ambulation activities are all within the physical therapist's role. PTs have expertise and training in muscle anatomy and physiology and can be a valuable resource for you. PTs deal with movement and may also help fit clients for adaptive devices, supervise whirlpool treatment for pressure ulcers or wounds, and perform dressing changes after whirlpool treatment. Pain management is another area in which PTs may function through the use of hot or cold packs, transcutaneous electrical nerve stimulation (TENS) units, and other modalities. Physical therapy assistants (PTAs) have less training and work under the direction of the PT to carry out the treatment plan.

The *occupational therapist* (OT) helps restore or maintain function, particularly in the upper extremities and areas that promote community re-entry and role adaptation. OTs assess the person's self-care skills such as bathing and dressing, and other ADLs. Working with clients on vocational and home management skills (such as cooking, doing laundry, shopping) is the job of the OT. Certified occupational therapy assistants (COTAs) also help provide care. COTAs have less training and education than OTs and work under their supervision to ensure quality client care.

The *speech therapist,* or speech-language pathologist, assesses swallowing, respiration, phonation and language ability. Speech therapists help clients improve communication, using a variety of treatment modalities, including auditory, verbal, visual, and motor processing (Fig. 56–2). The speech-language pathologist works with those having difficulty with verbal expression or cognitive problems. Common treatments include exercises of muscles used in speech and swallowing, thermal stimulation, and memory cues. Stroke clients with dysphagia or aphasia often require the services of a speech therapist to help them regain the use of oral-facial muscles needed for speaking and swallowing.

The *nutritionist* or dietitian plays an important role on the team for clients who may be receiving tube feedings, or those with nutritional deficits. Causes of *Altered nutrition: less than body requirements* may include dysphagia, aspiration, or malnutrition. Nutritionists can provide information on the contents of various nutritional supplements. They also educate about dietary modifications or restrictions, whether in a group setting or on a one-to-one basis.

The *social worker* focuses on assessment and evaluation of the client's social situation. *Case managers* may also function in this capacity, but may have a background in another discipline such as nursing. A comprehensive psychosocial history is taken. Insurance companies are contacted to arrange for medical coverage, arrange placement to another facility if needed, and order equipment for home use. Social workers engage in a large amount of client and family counseling, assisting people to utilize appropriate coping mechanisms, while keeping tabs on the pulse of family dynamics and the overall socioeconomic status of the family. Case managers and social workers also provide a valuable link to community resources and can recommend the most appropriate facilities placement. They answer questions related to insurance policies, reimbursement protocol, and documentation for other team members. Discharge planning and follow-up are additional skills.

Psychologists provide client and family counseling. Psychologists differ from psychiatrists (who may also be part of the interdisciplinary team) in that they are not medical doctors. The focus of the psychologist is on behavior modification and family adaptation. Such treatment is supportive and evaluative, helping the client and family utilize appropriate coping mechanisms during crisis situations. Psychologists may also assist the team itself directly by providing insight into group dynamics and the processes through which the team is working.

The *recreational therapist* plans a variety of activities to incorporate a therapeutic use of leisure time. Activities such as painting, making decorations for a party, horticulture, pet therapy, or music therapy are common. Entertainment and socialization are also key elements of a comprehensive recreational therapy program. Recreational therapists may help plan and implement community re-entry trips or outings. They arrange for special activities such as birthday parties, holidays, or group events like Wheelchair Olympics. Although not all facilities are able to afford the services of a qualified recreational therapist, the notion of this type of therapy should be included in every rehabilitation program and long-term care facility.

The client's *spiritual leader,* whether a priest, rabbi, minister, deacon, or lay person, is someone whom the client respects as a religious advisor. Many facilities have chaplains, deacons, or other spiritual guides available to sit with people or offer prayer. Some facilities offer religious services. Clients with long-term health alterations often use prayer as a coping mechanism and look to faith in God or another spiritual being for a source of comfort (Easton et al., 1995). The client's spiritual leader can help those experiencing symptoms of spiritual distress.

The *prosthetist* and *orthotist* are team members whose services are not required by every client. The prosthetist works with those needing a prosthesis, such as those with lower limb amputation who will be fitted with a prosthesis to promote ambulation (Fig. 56–3). The orthotist helps fit braces and orthoses, adaptive equipment to assist with normal movement and prevent secondary complications or corrective braces.

Settings of Care

Long-term care encompasses a variety of services that may be community or facility based. The most appro-

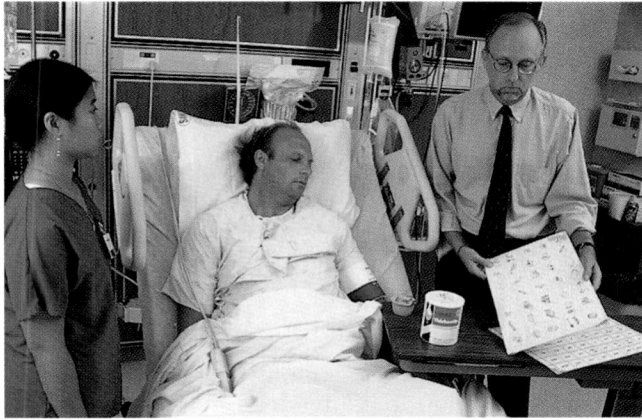

Figure 56–2. Speech therapists help clients improve communication, using a variety of treatment modalities, including auditory, verbal, visual, and motor processing.

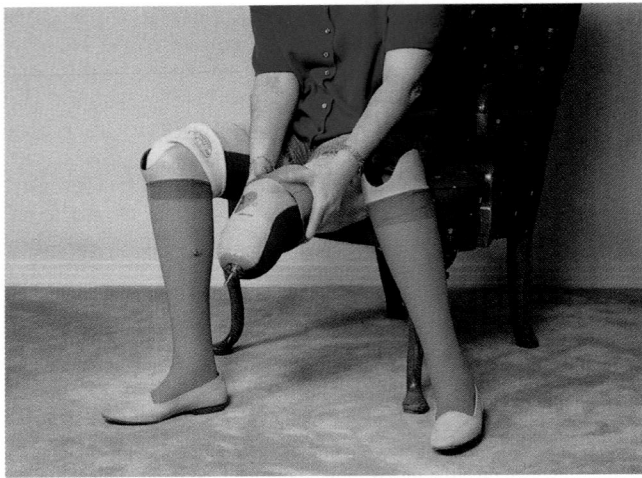

Figure 56–3. Prosthetists work with people needing prostheses, like this woman who has undergone a lower-limb amputation. Her lower-leg prosthesis promotes ambulation and offers a near-normal cosmetic appearance.

priate care setting for each person is determined by several factors, including the degree of functional impairment, personal preference, current living arrangements, financial resources, cost of services, and available family or informal caregiver support. Older adults should be encouraged to maintain independence as long as possible, but should long-term care become necessary, you should be aware of the types of services available.

Community-Based Services

Home delivered meals or Meals on Wheels is a service available for people unable to prepare adequate meals for themselves. These programs provide at least one nutritionally balanced meal daily, usually at noon. For the elderly person who can manage a simpler meal for breakfast and dinner, this service can help maintain independence while providing balanced nutrition. Some elderly people eat part of the meal at noon and save the rest for the evening meal.

Chore services offer help with home maintenance and include yard work, heavy housecleaning, minor house repairs, and errands and may be a key factor for some elderly people in being able to maintain independent living. Chore services are most often provided by family and friends. However, limited funding may be available for these services through a home health agency.

Homemaker services provide assistance with personal care, administration of medications, light housekeeping, shopping, and meal preparation. As with chore services, limited funding may be available.

Home health care programs provide more comprehensive services to people requiring medical care that can be managed at home. These services include physical, occupational, and speech therapy; skilled nursing care; and nursing assistant services to assist with personal care. Home health care is

warranted when a person is considered homebound.

Respite care is a temporary service enabling informal caregivers to take a break from their caregiving responsibilities. Caregiver time-off can be arranged for a few hours or a week or longer. Respite care is provided at home by homemaker and home health care services, or provided outside the home at a nursing home or hospital. Respite care reduces subjective caregiver burden, enhances caregiver well-being, and delays or decreases the likelihood of nursing home placement (Kosloski & Montgomery, 1995). Flexibility, choice, and consumer control are important features of effective respite programs because each family situation is different (Feinberg & Kelly, 1995).

Adult day care centers offer care in a protective setting away from the elder's home during daytime hours. This care includes health maintenance, restorative measures, and recreational activities. When 24-hour supervision or assistance is required and family caregivers have other day-time obligations, enrollment in an adult day care center makes it possible for the elder to continue living in a familiar environment with family and friends. These programs serve older adults who need supervision due to illness, disability, or the effects of aging. Elders may attend full or part-time. Adult day care is cost-effective and allows older adults to interact with others under professional supervision.

Facility-Based Services

Assisted living facilities combine shelter with other support services, such as meals, housekeeping, laundry, shopping, and some personal care. These facilities include adult foster care, board and care homes, group homes, residential care units managed by nursing homes, and assisted living units in retirement communities.

Long-term care facilities, or *nursing homes,* provide interdisciplinary care to people who do not require hospitalization but whose needs for care exceed available informal and formal community resources. Typical long-term care facilities provide several levels of care. Skilled nursing care provides rehabilitative and subacute care services, including measures such as intravenous fluids, medications, wound care, enteral feeding, and therapy. Intermediate care units offer custodial care. Nursing home placement may be emotionally difficult for both the client and the family member. Having an opportunity to evaluate available facilities helps alleviate the guilt and fear that may be associated with this decision. Questions to ask when evaluating a nursing home are presented in Box 56–1.

Americans With Disabilities Act

The Americans with Disabilities Act is a significant piece of legislation that advocates for those with disabilities. According to this law, employers must provide "reasonable accommodation" for workers with functional limitations or disabilities. An employee cannot be discriminated against nor fired on the basis of physical limitations. The employer must make reasonable efforts to accommodate the special needs of employees. For example, buildings must be accessible. If this means that a ramp needs to be installed for a worker in a wheelchair, then this must be done. If the sinks in the bathrooms must be raised so a wheelchair could go under them, then this is generally reasonable. If an employee cannot climb stairs due to a disability or injury, then an elevator may need to be installed. Businesses built since the enactment of the Americans with Disabilities Act are much more likely to be accessible to those with functional limitations.

BOX 56–1

QUESTIONS TO ASK WHEN EVALUATING A NURSING HOME

Ownership, Licenses, and Certification

- Who owns and manages the facility?
- Is it a for-profit or not-for-profit facility?
- What levels of care are provided?
- Does the facility have a current state license?
- Does the administrator have a current state license?
- Is the facility currently accredited by the Joint Commission on Accreditation of Healthcare Organizations?
- Is the facility Medicaid/Medicare certified?

Location

- Will the location enable family and friends to visit easily?
- Will the location enable continued use of a personal physician?
- Is there a hospital nearby?
- Is the facility located in a safe neighborhood?

Safety

- Is there evidence of accident prevention measures such as hand rails in the hallways, grab bars in the bathrooms, sturdy chairs, nonskid floors, and ample lighting?
- Is the facility currently in compliance with state and federal fire safety codes?
- What infection control measures are enforced?

Living Environment

- Are private bedrooms available?
- If residents share bedrooms, how are roommates assigned and what is the policy for resident conflict?
- Is storage space for clothing and personal belongings adequate?
- Does each bedroom have a bathroom with a shower and accommodation for a wheelchair?
- Are hallways large enough for two wheelchairs to pass easily?

Meals

- Does the staff include an onsite registered dietitian?
- Is attention given to special dietary needs and preferences?

- Is there an attractive, inviting dining room for ambulatory residents?
- Is socialization encouraged at meal time?
- Is the food adequate, tasty, and attractively served?

Nursing Service

- Is there commitment to individualized care and maintaining resident dignity?
- Is there positive support for restorative and rehabilitative care?
- Are staff well groomed, courteous, and respectful?
- What is the composition and educational preparation of the staff?
- What is the staff-to-resident ratio on day, evening, and night shifts?

Medical and Other Special Services

- Who are the staff physicians? Are they board certified in geriatric medicine?
- Is a physician readily available for emergencies?
- Are physical, occupational, speech, and respiratory therapies available?
- Are there provisions for eye, dental, and foot care?
- Does the staff include a social worker?
- Are beautician and barber services available?

Social, Educational, Recreational, and Religious Activities

- Are visiting hours flexible?
- Are there inside and outside common areas for visiting and walking?
- Is there a planned orientation for new admissions?
- Are there family programs such as support groups and educational programs?
- What recreational opportunities are provided?
- What provisions are made to meet religious needs?

Cost

- What is the daily basic rate?
- What services are included in the daily basic rate?
- What additional costs will there be?
- Are billing procedures and payment policies clearly explained?

FACTORS AFFECTING FUNCTIONAL LIMITATIONS

A wide range of factors influence a person's ability to cope with physical limitations and adjust to long-term health alterations. These may include lifestyle, environment, stage of growth and development, culture or ethnicity, religious influences, socioeconomic status, psychosocial factors, and physiological factors.

Lifestyle Factors

The onset of a health problem resulting in functional limitations often requires lifestyle changes. The person may have to learn a new job, modify the methods/means of transportation, or establish new communication systems. Adjustments may even be as basic as maintaining life functions. Lifestyle changes include adaptations in activities of daily living.

Environmental Factors

Environmental factors that can affect ability and disability are many. These may include the person's living situation, the workplace, or time spent in leisure activities. If a living situation is unsafe, either in a physical sense (if it adds to fall risk) or in a psychological sense (causes additional stress from abuse or neglect), the risk of disability may be increased. Workplaces can pose additional health threats, although employers are required to reveal potentially hazardous materials in the work environment to employees. Employers are to provide adequate protective equipment and education to minimize injury. Some individuals engage in high-risk behaviors with regard to leisure activities.

Lack of community resources also affects people with functional limitations. There may be many architectural barriers to overcome. Going out to dinner may require major time in planning and preparation. The person has to consider not only transportation issues but also accessibility to bathroom facilities, dining facilities, walkways, parking lots, and the like. You should know the resources available for people with physical limitations in their community to encourage community reintegration. **Community reintegration** is the return and acceptance of a disabled person as a participating member of the community.

Developmental Factors

A person's stage of growth and development certainly can influence the ability to adapt to change. The age at the onset of a functional limitation affects the person's knowledge and personal resources for coping with a change in functional capacity.

In the case study at the beginning of this chapter, the teenager with a spinal cord injury has major adjustments to make. Not only does he have to cope with the usual stresses of teenage life and high school, but after his injury there are many additional factors to deal with. Once an active teen, he is now paralyzed. What issues associated with Robert's developmental stage might the multidisciplinary team need to address? Consider issues related to sexuality and future goals for a career, marriage, and children. How might Robert's level of maturity influence his ability to deal with these life changes?

Cultural/Religious Factors

Culture and ethnicity may also influence ability and disability. Some ethnic groups are more likely to have a higher incidence of certain chronic illnesses. Additionally, cultural norms may influence how people seek treatment for illnesses. Also, some cultures do not believe in nursing home use (Clavon, 1986), preferring to care for their relatives at home, so a greater amount of client and family education may be needed. Intergenerational care may cause you to explore a variety of teaching options in dealing with a vast age range of caregivers.

Those in ethnic minority groups have more functional limitations, increased medical problems, poorer health, and more work-related disabilities (Damron-Rodriguez, Wallace, & Kington, 1994). They often rely more on informal health services such as folk cures and often have impaired access to professional health care. Elderly minority men have disproportionately higher rates of disease and death as a result of influenza, pneumonia, and chronic respiratory conditions such as bronchitis and emphysema (Tripp-Reimer, Johnson, & Rios, 1995).

Cultural norms, as well as religious beliefs, also influence a person's ability to adapt to disability and the support systems needed for maximal outcomes. You need to develop cultural sensitivity when dealing with people from ethnic or religious groups different from your own.

Psychosocial Factors

Many psychosocial factors influence long-term outcomes after a physical limitation is apparent. The client's previous coping patterns, their ability to adapt to change, and the amount of social support they have can positively or negatively affect their situation.

Socioeconomic status may affect the person's ability to pay for needed health care. Transportation and access to care often present barriers for people with physical limitations.

Some clients may feel that the health care system will not benefit them. They may not believe that the treatment prescribed will help. Certain cultural norms encourage the use of folk medicine and remedies prior to going to the physician. If a client does not believe that rehabilitation or other care is going to make a difference, he is less likely to participate. Likewise, if clients feel that they have little or no control over their situation, or that their actions make little difference, they are less likely to be ready to learn ways to help themselves.

Self-image and self-esteem are often affected by long-term physical problems. People may need to adjust to an altered body image.

How might Robert's self-image, self-esteem, and body image be affected by his tetraplegia?

Those with disfiguring burns, colostomies, or paralysis, or anyone who must use adaptive equipment may feel stigmatized. This is the negative way that society may view people who are different from the norm. Fighting such stigmas is hard enough for those with adequate coping mechanisms and family support, but for those without many resources, it can be devastating.

Physiological Factors

Many people have multiple co-existing illnesses or problems in addition to a physical limitation. For example, a person may have had an amputation of the lower leg because of diabetes and poor circulation. These chronic problems are generally progressive and can negatively influence a person's ability to adapt to a functional limitation. Likewise, if a person is legally blind from glaucoma, this factor may make it difficult to perform activities of daily living.

Physiological changes that occur as a normal part of the aging process contribute to the number of persons experiencing deficits in the ability to care for themselves. Also, people with physical limitations are living much longer than in past years. New problems are being discovered as a result of those who are aging with a disability that occurred decades ago. The probability of having multiple chronic conditions such as arthritis, hypertension, heart disease, hearing impairments, or orthopedic problems increases with advancing age. More than 80% of elderly people report at least one chronic problem (Eliopoulos, 1997; Zarle, 1989).

As the number of elderly in the population increases, so does the percentage of clients needing assistance with daily activities. As life expectancy increases, so does the number of elderly living with disabilities. The elderly (also the fastest growing age group in the United States) and the disabled include people from all racial, cultural, religious, and socioeconomic backgrounds, making the need to address the problems of aging and disability of primary and universal concern for the future in health care.

ASSESSMENT

General Assessment of Functional Limitations

When working with people with functional limitations, you need to have excellent assessment skills. While the entire interdisciplinary team aids in holistically assessing the client, you are primarily responsible for documentation in several key areas. One of these is the person's overall health and functional assessment.

Action **A**lert!
As a Registered Nurse, you have primary responsibility for documentation of a client's overall health status and functional assessment.

Health History

A thorough history is essential to assessment of the person with functional limitations. Ask direct questions about the onset of symptoms. Ask how long the person has had the particular limitations. Be sure to use the facility's form that documents how much help the person needs at home with ADLs. Ask specific questions about pain and how it is managed.

Assessing functional status is actually a team job. Functional status refers to a person's ability to perform self-care activities and other tasks that are necessary for independent living. A systematic approach to assessment of functional status enables objective appraisal to determine the kind of support needed and responses to such support.

A standardized tool is useful for objective comparison of the client's progress from admission to discharge, as well as for setting goals throughout the rehabilitation stay. Such instruments help "determine physical functional status, document the need for interventions and services, devise a treatment plan, and assess and monitor progress" (Kelly-Hayes, 1996, p. 146).

Many tools or scales are used to assess functional status; some of the more commonly used instruments include the Functional Independence Measure (FIM) scale, the Instrumental Activities of Daily Living Scale (Box 56–2), the Katz Index of Activities of Daily Living, the PULSES Profile, and the Barthel Index (Granger, Albrecht, & Hamilton, 1979).

The FIM scale is one of the most reliable and valid tools for measuring functional status. It measures disability in categories of both cognitive and motor functions. The team member rates the individual from being dependent (1) to complete independence (7) in several different categories. Scores can be totaled in several ways and compared. Many facilities have each team member complete specific sections. Team members may also keep more detailed FIM scores through separate documentation related specifically to their discipline. Having a quantitative measure is helpful for insurance coverage and can show progress in a numerical way, allowing for goals and outcome predictions.

The Katz Index of Activities of Daily Living (Box 56–3) is designed to evaluate six functions: bathing, dressing, toileting, transferring, continence, and feeding. Performance is rated as independent or dependent. This tool is easy to use and offers a quick assessment of the basic tasks needed for self-care.

BOX 56–2

INSTRUMENTAL ACTIVITIES OF DAILY LIVING SCALE

Action	Score
A. Ability to use telephone	
1. Operates telephone on own initiative: looks up and dials numbers, etc.	1
2. Dials a few well-known numbers	1
3. Answers telephone but does not dial.	1
4. Does not use telephone at all.	0
B. Shopping	
1. Takes care of all shopping needs independently.	1
2. Shops independently for small purchases.	0
3. Needs to be accompanied on any shopping trip.	0
4. Completely unable to shop.	0
C. Food preparation	
1. Plans, prepares, and serves adequate meals independently.	1
2. Prepares adequate meals if supplied with ingredients.	0
3. Heats and serves prepared meals, or prepares meals but does not maintain adequate diet.	0
4. Needs to have meals prepared and served.	0
D. Housekeeping	
1. Maintains home alone or with occasional assistance (e.g., "heavy work–domestic work").	1
2. Performs light daily tasks such dishwashing, bed-making.	1
3. Performs light daily tasks but cannot maintain acceptable level of cleanliness.	1
4. Needs help with all home maintenance tasks.	1
5. Does not participate in any housekeeping tasks.	0
E. Laundry	
1. Does personal laundry completely.	1
2. Launders small items: rinses socks, stockings, etc.	1
3. All laundry must be done by others.	0
F. Mode of transportation	
1. Travels independently on public transportation or drives own car.	1
2. Arranges own travel via taxi but does not otherwise use public transportation.	1
3. Travels on public transportation when assisted or accompanied by another.	1
4. Travel limited to taxi or automobile with assistance of another.	0
5. Does not travel at all.	0
G. Responsibility for own medications	
1. Is responsible for taking medications in correct dosage at correct time.	1
2. Takes responsibility if medication is prepared in advance in separate dosages.	0
3. Is not capable of dispensing own medication.	0
H. Ability to handle finances	
1. Manages financial matters independently (budgets, writes checks, pays rent, bills, goes to bank), collects and keeps track of income.	1
2. Manages day-to-day purchases but needs help with banking, major purchases, etc.	1
3. Incapable of handling money.	0

Physical Examination

Physical examination is essential to a good assessment. The examination should be thorough, and there may be a need to focus on neuromuscular function. A cranial nerve assessment should be done if neurological deficits are suspected. Standard assessments should include orientation, cognition and memory checks, grip strength, pupils, facial symmetry, and speech. Any abnormalities should be noted and conveyed to other team members. Assess the reflexes, motor function, and the strength of the muscles.

Action Alert!
Note any neurological abnormalities and convey them to other rehabilitation team members, particularly the physician.

You should also assess respiratory function, cardiac function, general nutritional status, condition of the skin, and elimination.

Diagnostic Tests

The purpose of diagnostic tests with regard to function is to establish a baseline. Then comparisons can be made to evaluate outcomes and progress. Practicality should be emphasized. That is, though measurements may be made with the help of tests and tools, the person's abilities to perform ADLs is more important.

The underlying cause of the limitation is of primary concern. Any diagnostic tests ordered by the physician will help determine cause of functional decline. These could include computed tomography (CT) scans or magnetic resonance imaging (MRI) for diagnosis of stroke, head injury, multiple sclerosis, or spinal cord injury. Many neurological disorders that affect function cannot be determined by any single diagnostic test. Laboratory results may or may not be helpful in diagnosis of some conditions.

You will look at the medical diagnosis to gain a perspective on what outcomes are reasonable for the

---

BOX 56–3

KATZ INDEX OF ACTIVITIES OF DAILY LIVING

The Index of Independence in Activities of Daily Living is based on an evaluation of the functional independence or dependence of patients in bathing, dressing, toileting, transferring, continence, and feeding. Specific definitions of functional independence and dependence appear below the index.

A—Independent in feeding, continence, transferring, toileting, dressing, and bathing.
B—Independent in all but one of these functions.
C—Independent in all but bathing and one additional function.
D—Independent in all but bathing, dressing, and one additional function.
E—Independent in all but bathing, dressing, toileting, and one additional function.
F—Independent in all but bathing, dressing, toileting, transferring, and one additional function.
G—Dependent in all six functions.
Other—Dependent in at least two functions, but not classifiable as C, D, E, or F.

Independence

Independence means without supervision, direction, or active personal assistance, except as specifically noted below. This is based on actual status and not on ability. A patient who refuses to perform a function is considered as not performing the function, even though she is deemed able.

BATHING (SPONGE, SHOWER, OR TUB)

Independent: assistance only in bathing a single part (such as the back or a disabled extremity) or bathes self completely)
Dependent: assistance in bathing more than one part of body; assistance in getting in or out of tub or does not bathe self

DRESSING

Independent: gets clothes from closets and drawers; puts on clothes, outer garments, braces; manages fasteners; act of tying shoes is excluded
Dependent: does not dress self or remains partly undressed

TOILETING

Independent: gets to toilet; gets on and off toilet; arranges clothes; cleans organs of excretion; (may manage own bedpan used at night only and may or may not be using mechanical supports)
Dependent: uses bed pan or commode or receives assistance in getting to and using toilet

TRANSFERRING

Independent: moves in and out of bed independently and moves in and out of chair independently (may or may not be using mechanical supports)
Dependent: assistance in moving in or out of bed and/or chair; does not perform one or more transfers

CONTINENCE

Independent: Urination and defecation entirely self-controlled
Dependent: partial or total incontinence in urination or defecation; partial or total control by enemas, catheters, or regulated use of urinals and/or bedpans

FEEDING

Independent: gets food from plate or its equivalent into mouth; (precutting of meat and preparation of food, as buttering bread are excluded from evaluation)
Dependent: assistance in act of feeding (see above); does not eat at all or needs parenteral feeding

From Katz, S., Ford, A.B., Moskowitz, R.W., Jackson, B.A., Jafe, M.W., & Cleveland, M.A. (1963). Studies of illness in the aged. The Index of ADL: A standardized measure of biological and psychosocial function. Journal of the American Medical Association, 185(12), 914–919.

person. However, the reason behind the functional limitation may be obvious if due to injury, such as with spinal cord injury. Other tests or tools such as those discussed previously may help "diagnose" functional limitations.

DIAGNOSIS

Many NANDA nursing diagnoses are frequently used in the care of those with functional limitations. A few of the more common diagnoses are discussed here.

The initial response to loss of function is feelings of helplessness and powerlessness. The client undergoing rehabilitation may express feelings of powerlessness through anger or apathy. The nursing diagnosis *Powerlessness* may therefore be appropriate for a client with a newly diagnosed functional limitation.

Self-care deficit is applicable to people experiencing impaired ability to perform any one of the basic self-care activities such as feeding, bathing/hygiene, and toileting. Dressing and grooming are additional activities that those with *Self-care deficit* may have difficulty with. Be sure to specify which ADLs are affected when using this diagnosis.

The diagnosis *Impaired physical mobility* focuses care on improving the person's mobility. Movement is fundamental to performing ADLs, so it is essential that interventions address maximizing rehabilitation potential as well as minimizing further loss of physical movement.

Activity intolerance is a relevant diagnosis to supplement *Self-care deficit* when reduced strength and endurance are major factors influencing the ability to perform ADLs. People with stroke, chronic airflow limitation, cardiovascular disease, arthritis, end-stage renal disease, lupus, and multiple sclerosis often experience activity intolerance. Activity intolerance may also be related to bedrest deconditioning. While there is a gradual decline in strength and endurance with advanced age, particularly after the age of 75, this problem is compounded by pathology.

When a person has impairments in sensory or perceptual areas that interfere with the ability for independent living, the nursing diagnosis *Sensory/perceptual alterations* may apply. Be sure to identify the specific alteration when using this diagnosis—whether visual, auditory, kinesthetic, gustatory, tactile, or olfactory. For example, people with glaucoma may have visual alterations, and people with hemiplegia as a result of a stroke might have tactile impairments.

Risk for injury is an important nursing diagnosis in managing care for clients with functional limitations, because risk for injury increases as functional ability declines. Falls are a common problem among older adults with reduced functional capacity and a major factor contributing to dependence. Fear of falling or loss of confidence also contributes to dependence because of self-imposed, unwarranted avoidance of activities. Specific preventive strategies are needed to reduce the risk of injury due to falls as well as measures to restore self-confidence.

What defining characteristics of *Impaired physical mobility* does Robert evidence? What cues suggest that he might have *Self-care deficit*? What type or types of *Self-care deficit* does he appear to have? What did Robert say to suggest that *Powerlessness* might be an appropriate diagnosis for him?

PLANNING

Goals in rehabilitation are aimed at maximizing function and preventing complications. Rehabilitation goals are the desired outcomes for each rehabilitation client. Goals are mutually established between team members and the client. They should be measurable, time-limited, and realistic. Goals are essential to the rehabilitation process and are long-term and short-term in nature. Individual team members will assist the client in establishing such objectives, and the entire team will also set goals that are worked on together, such as those in Box 56–4.

In the inpatient setting, other team members are present during the daytime hours, but nurses are present on all shifts, therefore you must be aware of the goals of all other team members to ensure continuity of care when therapists are not present. Weekly interdisciplinary team meetings allow you to stay current with the goals of other team members. Planning is done by each individual team member and discipline, but also as a group as it relates to discharge goals and dates.

When planning nursing care, you should keep in mind the goals of rehabilitation. Interventions should be directed at helping the person perform self-care, becoming or remaining independent, preventing complications, and promoting self-esteem. You should assist people to do everything they can for themselves, thus

---

BOX 56–4

GENERAL CLIENT GOALS OF THE INTERDISCIPLINARY REHABILITATION TEAM

- Fostering self-care, self-sufficiency.
- Encouraging maximal independence level.
- Maintaining function.
- Preventing complications.
- Restoring optimal function.
- Promoting maximal potential of function.
- Emphasizing abilities.
- Adaptation/adjustment.
- Promoting acceptable quality of life.
- Maintaining dignity.
- Re-education.
- Community reintegration, community re-entry.
- Promoting optimal wellness.

From Easton, K.L. (1999). *Gerontological rehabilitation nursing.* Philadelphia: W.B. Saunders.

promoting independence and autonomy. These activities will then promote quality of life and general feelings of well-being.

Typical outcomes for which to plan include improvement in mobility and functional status, as measured by a tool such as the FIM. You would also expect to see increased ability to perform self-care, increased independence, and increased self-esteem. Planning for home discharge is always a goal. You may need to arrange for caregivers. However, independence at home is not always possible, so alternate arrangements should be considered.

INTERVENTION

Interventions to Prevent Disability

The effectiveness of nursing interventions for clients with long-term problems has been well documented (Neal, 1995; Shiell, Kenny, & Farnworth, 1993). Nursing care plans that emphasize support and education help clients and family members cope with and adjust to the complications of long-term health problems. Nurses have been shown to make a positive impact related to outcomes for those with chronic illness and disabilities when rehabilitative interventions are employed. Thus, the importance of your practicing rehabilitative techniques within the interdisciplinary team cannot be overemphasized.

There are many physical problems that may cause or contribute to disability and necessitate rehabilitative services to maximize function. Additional factors, as previously discussed, contribute to disability and ability. Broad interventions that can be applied to a variety of situations are presented here, providing specific examples of implementation.

Addressing Factors That Contribute to Functional Limitations

Many factors influence the ability to cope with functional limitations. Instruct clients and families about how they can modify or change some of the factors. Examples of things they may change to improve the client's physical health include a diet low in cholesterol, increasing exercise, smoking cessation, maintaining an ideal weight, limiting alcohol consumption, and managing stress.

Several of these factors are related to psychosocial adjustment as well. Learning community resources is important to adjustment. Transportation may be a key issue if the person is in a wheelchair or cannot drive. Social support, including family, friends, and religious support, can help buffer the effects of stress. Other suggestions appear under the section Factors Affecting Function Limitations.

Teaching Clients and Families About Safety

There are several key areas for teaching in relation to safety. For people with paralysis or decreased sensory perception, the risk of injury is high.

Robert had no feeling from his level of injury down. Thus, Robert and his family would need to be instructed to avoid extremes in temperature to avoid burns. What specific measures might you teach Robert and his family to help him avoid sunburn and other burns? Robert would also be in danger of not feeling injuries, such as bumps or bruises caused by adaptive equipment. What would you need to teach Robert about the use of a wheelchair to help him avoid injury?

Stroke survivors also have a high risk for injury. Similar to the person with spinal cord injury, stroke survivors may not have feeling, or have decreased sensation on, one side of the body. *Neglect,* or a form of ignoring one's body part, is a relatively common phenomenon. Sometimes this is due to visual deficits. Other times the person does not recognize an arm or leg as being part of his body. Care must be taken to instruct clients and families to support hemiplegic arms and legs to promote safety.

Many people with functional impairments, even those with tetraplegia, may be able to drive. For people with spinal cord injury, hand controls may be used. Usually cognition is not a factor, so physical abilities would be developed. However, cognition is a factor for those with stroke and head injury. People with these types of problems may not realize that driving a vehicle would be unsafe. The team must carefully evaluate each individual to be sure that driving would be safe for them.

A commonly cited reason for seeking nursing home placement or protected living is fear of falls. Fractures from falls lead to decreased mobility, reduced independence, and major changes in lifestyle.

Psychological responses in the aftermath of a fall, even without serious injury, can cause the older person to make adjustments in lifestyle and living arrangements. Recognizing that serious injury could have occurred, the person responds emotionally to the fall and fears falling again. Anxiety results in loss of confidence. People may become overly cautious and restrict their activities, which results in social withdrawal or isolation. Feelings of vulnerability and fragility carry over into other dimensions of the person's life.

Concerns about death, becoming a burden to family or friends, or requiring institutionalization often weigh heavily on the person's mind. You can help clients and families decrease the risk for falls by identifying fall risk factors that may be present in the person's environment or related to health status.

Modifications may need to be made in the home environment. For example, throw rugs should be removed, and stairways clearly marked. Handrails may need to be installed. Non-skid shoes should be worn at all times, and the person should be encouraged to call for assistance or supervision at home if needed.

Interventions to Promote Self-Care

In working with clients and families in long-term care, or those with chronic health alterations, a large pro-

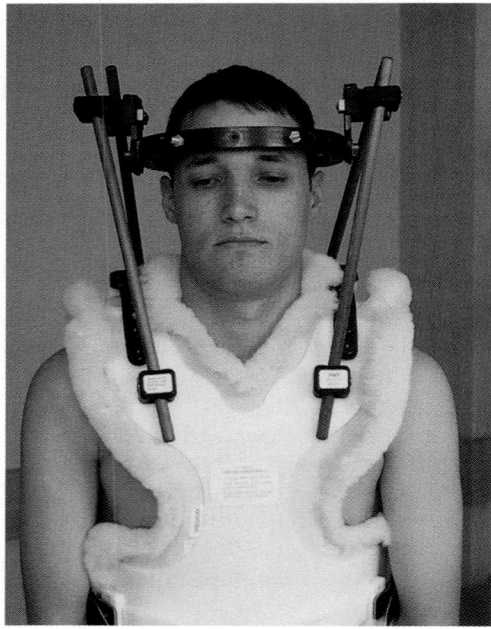

portion of your time will be spent in client/family teaching. Every member of the team assists with client education in each respective discipline, but you are in a unique position to reinforce the teaching of other disciplines. In inpatient facilities, nurses are the only team members present around the clock, so knowledge of what other therapists are working on with clients is important. Good communication among team members will be essential for optimum client outcomes.

All team members focus on assisting the person to perform self-care. This involves helping people find ways to adapt and adjust to changes in functional status and abilities. Adapting to the use of splints, braces, adaptive devices, and devices like halo traction are all part of the rehabilitation process (Fig. 56–4). In this section, a few of the more common tasks to promote self-care are discussed.

Assisting With Dressing and Grooming

The occupational therapist (OT) is the team member who works with the person learning to perform ADLs. This includes dressing and grooming. When an OT is not available, this task falls to you or the nursing assistant. Several techniques may be helpful to you in assisting people with dressing and hygiene.

People with one-sided weakness or paralysis should be reminded that when donning a shirt or dress, the weaker extremity goes in first. That is, the person uses the stronger arm to put the weaker arm into the sleeve. Likewise, the weaker leg is put into the trousers first, then the stronger.

Figure 56–4. Adapting to the use of splints, braces, adaptive devices, and devices like halo traction are all part of the rehabilitation process.

For some people, especially those with balance problems, dressing in bed may be easier than dressing in a chair. The OT will teach the client additional techniques, such as propping one leg on the knee of the other to put on or take off socks and avoid bending over, or using adaptive equipment such as reachers and grabbers to facilitate dressing. Likewise, to make grooming easier, long-handled sponges and one-handed showerheads may help with bathing. Having the toothpaste held on a suction cup base to keep it from moving, or having a Velcro handle for those with little grip strength are other common adaptations. You should teach the use of all such tools when they promote self-care.

You should remember that all ADLs will take considerably longer when a person is attempting to complete them independently after experiencing a disability. Extra time and patience are essential. Family members need to be encouraged to allow clients to do everything they can for themselves, even though it may be frustrating. Doing things for them encourages dependence on a caregiver and does not promote autonomy.

Action **A**lert!
Encourage clients to do what they can for themselves.

Assisting With Medication Management

One of the most important areas for nursing teaching is that of medications. Almost all people with long-term health problems or disabilities take medications. Many clients will be able to learn their medication schedule, but some, particularly those with cognitive deficits, may require the assistance of a caregiver. Two of the most useful tools for teaching medication management are the medication schedule and medication box. You should write out a schedule of the person's daily medications in large and simple print. The information should include the name of the medication, the dosage (whether number of pills or milligrams or both), the action (in simple terms), and side-effects or important information about the medication.

A medication box can assist the person in organizing daily medications. There are four compartments in most boxes, and seven separate containers, each of which can be removed for the person to take with him for the day. Thus, if a person cannot set up his own medications, the caregiver can set them up for a week at a time. Boxes can be modified for each individual if different time intervals are needed.

When teaching a client or family member to set up a medication box, the first step is to learn the medication schedule and use it as a guide. People will soon learn to recognize each pill by its color, shape, and size. Using this information as auditory and visual cues assists with learning. For example, you might say, "This is Lasix, your water pill, the small white one." When placing medications from the package or bottle into the box for set-up, the bottle should be checked at least before and after opening. You check each medication with the client and family and engage in teaching about the medication while the box is being set up. Additionally, having a routine, such as scheduling medications to be taken at meal time, helps reduce errors or forgetfulness.

Keeping a journal of blood glucose levels when the person takes daily insulin may be needed. Setting out pills and the needed supplies, as well as breakfast, may help an older person with minor memory problems to recall all that needs to be done. Giving step-by-step instructions may also be needed.

Reducing Unilateral Neglect

The client with unilateral neglect may have minor neglect or be experiencing a more severe form, in which a body part, most often a paralyzed arm, is not recognized as his own. Unilateral neglect may occur with several conditions, particularly after stroke or brain injury. People with this problem may need help with ADLs, self-feeding, and positioning. People with unilateral neglect need frequent cues to pay attention to the affected side. This means the person will be at high risk for injury. Proper positioning of the affected limb is essential. A flaccid arm should be placed in a sling, or supported by a lapboard or arm trough. It should never be allowed to dangle or pull on the shoulder joint, as this can cause subluxation, a painful dislocation at the socket.

A*ction* A*lert!*
When a client experiences unilateral neglect, proper positioning of the affected limb is essential.

The environment should be set up to maximize performance and success. A general rule to follow when working with people experiencing unilateral neglect is to work especially with the affected extremity during therapy and all interactions, and to place items on the unaffected side to avoid isolation when a caregiver is not present. If items such as the water pitcher or call light are placed on the affected side, the person may not see them or may not be able to get to them, thus contributing to a sense of isolation and helplessness. It should be remembered at all times that self-care is the key to rehabilitation, and all interventions should promote this concept. Sensory stimulation using multiple modalities should also be used during teaching, as each person has unique learning needs and capabilities.

Referring to Community Resources

One of the most important, yet simplest, ways for you to assist those with functional limitations is to be knowledgeable about community resources. Since people with functional limitations are largely influenced by the external environment, be aware of architectural barriers as well as accessible buildings within the community. Knowledge about available support groups and where they meet or key contact people for specific concerns is also needed. Providing lists of groups, mentors, transportation for those in wheelchairs, meal arrangements, or senior centers can help with community re-entry and reduce social isolation. You can also use the social worker and chaplain, as well as the local church or synagogue, as resources within the community.

EVALUATION

The evaluation phase of the nursing process with regard to people with functional limitations or disabilities is generally outcome focused. The most objective way to measure progress in functional status is by using scales or tools such as the FIM scale discussed earlier. Such tools provide quantifiable data with which to compare initial function to outcomes after therapy has been completed. Additionally, statistics such as these can provide valuable information about the client's progress toward recovery and help justify costs to insurance companies and other payers. Using a nationally recognized scale, different facilities can also compare their outcomes with those of similar institutions, allowing for some type of quality control measurements.

Other types of evaluation are less formal and results are more difficult to quantify. Changes in life satisfaction, perceived quality of life, and coping and adaptation skills are more difficult to measure. Although valid and reliable tools exist to measure such abstract constructs, most facilities lack the time and trained staff to routinely conduct the necessary studies for adequate outcome measures of these more intangible benefits of rehabilitation. You and other health care professionals may rely more on observations and clients' statements about their life having improved as a result of interventions to gauge success in meeting emotional, spiritual, and psychosocial needs.

KEY PRINCIPLES

- Rehabilitation should begin the first day a person is diagnosed.
- Chronic illness and disability affect every area of a person's life.
- Motivation is important to attaining maximum independence.
- Rehabilitation assists people to achieve the maximal level of independence possible.
- Emphasizing a person's strengths is a key to preventing powerlessness.
- Nursing should focus on working with what clients have left, not what they have lost.
- Activity is important in the prevention of the hazards of immobility.
- Care of people with functional limitations must be holistic in nature to be effective.

BIBLIOGRAPHY

*Clavon, A. (1986). The black elderly. *Journal of Gerontological Nursing, 12*(5), 6–12.

Damron-Rodriguez, J., Wallace, S., & Kington, R. (1994). Service utilization and minority elderly: Appropriateness, accessibility and acceptability. *Gerontology & Geriatrics Education, 15*(1), 45–62.

*Dittmar, S. (1989). *Rehabilitation nursing: Process and application.* St. Louis: Mosby.

Easton, K.L. (1997). Advanced practice nursing for individuals with chronic illness and disability. In K.M. Johnson (Ed.). *Advanced practice nursing in rehabilitation* (pp. 117–113). Glenview, IL: Association of Rehabilitation Nurses.

Easton, K.L. (1999). *Gerontological rehabilitation nursing.* Philadelphia: W.B. Saunders.

Easton, K., Rawl, S., Zemen, D., Kwiatkowski, S., & Burczyk, B. (1995). The effects of nursing follow-up on the coping strategies used by rehabilitation patients after discharge. *Rehabilitation Nursing Research, 4*(4), 119–127.

Eliopoulos, C. (1997). *Gerontological nursing.* Philadelphia: Lippincott.

Feinberg, L.F., & Kelly, K.A. (1995). A well-deserved break: Respite programs offered by California's statewide system of caregiver resource center. *The Gerontologist, 35,* 701–705.

*Fitzsimmons, B., & Bunting, L.K. (1993). Parkinson's disease: Quality of life issues. *Nursing Clinics of North America, 28*(4), 807–818.

Granger, C.V., Albrecht, G.L., & Hamilton, B.B. (1979). Outcome of comprehensive medical rehabilitation: Measurement by PULSES Profile and the Barthel Index. *Archives of Physical Medicine and Rehabilitation, 60,* 145–154.

Halper, J., & Costello, K.M. (1997). *Multiple sclerosis: Current therapies, future hope.* Baltimore: Paper presented at the meeting of the Association of Rehabilitation Nurses.

*Johnson, F., Foxall, M.J., Kelleher, E., Kentopp, E., Mannlein, E.A., & Cook, E. (1988). Comparison of mental health and life satisfaction of five elderly ethnic groups. *Western Journal of Nursing Research, 10*(5), 613–628.

Kelly-Hayes, M. (1996). Functional evaluation. In S. Hoeman (Ed.). *Rehabilitation nursing: Process and application* (pp. 144–155). St. Louis: Mosby.

Kosloski, K., & Montgomery, R.J.V. (1995). The impact of respite use on nursing home placement. *The Gerontologist, 35*(1), 67–74.

Levy, R.N., Levy, C.M., Snyder, J., & Digiovanni, J. (1995). Outcome and long-term results following total hip replacement in elderly patients. *Clinical Orthopaedics and Related Research, 316,* 25–30.

Lubkin, I.M. (1998). Chronic Illness: Impact and interventions. 4th ed. *The Jones and Bartlett Series in Nursing.* Boston: Jones and Bartlett.

*Namey, M., & Schwetz, K. (1993). What's new in multiple sclerosis management? Paper presented at the 1993 Association of Rehabilitation Nurses Annual Conference, Denver, Colorado.

Neal, L.J. (1995). The rehabilitation nursing team in the home health care setting. *Rehabilitation Nursing, 20*(1), 32–39.

Rawl, S., Easton, K.L., Zemen, D., Kwiatkowski, S., & Burczyk, B. (1998). The effectiveness of a nurse-managed follow-up program for rehabilitation patients after discharge. *Rehabilitation Nursing, 23*(4):204–209.

Rosebrough, A. (1997). Chronic neurological disorders: Multiple sclerosis, Parkinson's disease, myasthenia gravis, and Guillain-Barré Syndrome. In P.A. Chin, D. Finocchiaro, and A. Rosebrough (Eds.). *Rehabilitation nursing practice* (pp. 443–473). New York: McGraw-Hill.

Rush, S. (1996). Rehabilitation following ORIF of the hip. *Topics in Geriatric Rehabilitation, 12*(1), 38–45.

*Shiell, A., Kenny, P., & Farnworth, M.S. (1993). The role of the clinical nurse coordinator in the provision of cost-effective orthopaedic services for elderly people. *Journal of Advanced Nursing, 18,* 1424–1428.

*Sprinzeles, L.L. (1993). The effects of neurological impairment and rehabilitation on patients with Parkinson's Disease (PD) and their families. Paper presented at the 1993 Association of Rehabilitation Nurses Annual Conference, Denver, Colorado.

*Storck, I.F., & Thompson-Hoffman, S. (1991). Demographic characteristics of the disabled population. In S. Thompson-Hoffman & I.F. Storck (Eds.). *Disability in the United States: A portrait from national data* (pp. 1–12). New York: Springer.

Strauss, A.L. (1975). *Chronic illness and the quality of life.* St. Louis: C.V. Mosby Co.

Thomas, R.L. (1996). Management of hip fracture in the geriatric patient: A team approach in the institutional setting. *Topics in Geriatric Rehabilitation, 12*(1), 59–69.

Tripp-Reimer, T., Johnson, R. & Rios, H. (1995). Cultural dimensions in gerontological nursing. In M. Stanley & P. Beare (Eds.) *Gerontological nursing.* Philadelphia: F.A. Davis.

Weekly, N.J. (1995). Parkinsonism: An overview. *Geriatric Nursing, 16*(4), 169–172.

*Zarle, N.S. (1989). Continuity of care: balancing care of elders between health care settings. *Nursing Clinics of North America, 24*(3), 697–705.

---

*Asterisk indicates a classic or definitive work on this subject.

The Surgical Client

V. Doreen Wagner

Key Terms

ambulatory surgery
anesthesia
anesthesiologist
certified registered nurse
  anesthetist
circulating nurse
general anesthesia
intraoperative phase
local anesthesia
malignant hyperthermia

perioperative
perioperative nursing
postanesthesia care unit
postoperative phase
preoperative phase
regional anesthesia
registered nurse first assistant
scrub nurse

LEARNING OBJECTIVES

After studying this chapter, you should be able to:

1. **Describe the surgical experience using the perioperative phases as a framework.**

2. **Identify factors that may affect the surgical outcome of a perioperative client.**

3. **Conduct a preoperative nursing history and physical assessment to identify client strengths and factors that increase risks for perioperative complications.**

4. **Describe the nursing role in the psychological and educational preparation of the surgical client.**

5. **Differentiate between general, regional, and local anesthesia.**

6. **Discuss the role of the perioperative nurse when managing the intraoperative care of the surgical client.**

7. **Identify priority intraoperative nursing diagnoses.**

8. **Design an intraoperative nursing care plan.**

9. **List factors that may affect a postoperative client in the immediate recovery period.**

10. **Explain the nursing management of potential complications the client faces postoperatively.**

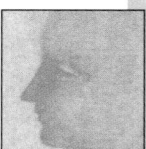

Berris Warren, an alert, oriented 61-year-old Afro-Caribbean man, has prostate cancer. His cancer was diagnosed by his primary physician in Jamaica 1 month ago, after an episode of not being able to urinate. He admitted having urinary difficulty for about 9 months. His daughter, a pediatric nurse practitioner, assisted him in getting a second opinion from a urologist in Atlanta, Georgia, where she and her family live. The cancer was confirmed and Mr. Warren was scheduled for a prostatectomy in 2 weeks. His surgical experience has begun.

CONCEPTS OF THE SURGICAL EXPERIENCE

Surgery is an invasive medical procedure performed on all parts of the human body to diagnose or treat illnesses, correct deformities and defects, repair injuries, and cure certain diseases. Clients who require surgery enter the health care setting in a wide variety of situations. A client may enter the facility feeling relatively healthy while awaiting planned elective surgery, or may be in much distress when facing emergency surgery for a traumatic injury. Surgical clients may be any age and at any point on the health-illness continuum.

Nurses assume important and active roles in caring for the client before, during, and after surgery. Collaborative and independent nursing care prevents complications and promotes optimal outcomes for the surgical client. The nursing process is used during each phase of the client's surgical experience to promote the recovery of health, prevent further injury or illness, and facilitate coping. Most importantly, however, nurses provide a familiar human touch and voice during a client's surgical journey.

Settings

In the past, the client was admitted to the hospital the day before a scheduled surgery for completion of preoperative assessments and laboratory testing. Surgery was usually performed in a hospital operating room (OR) and involved several days of recovery in the hospital. For some procedures, this is still the case. However, with the increased cost containment measures and technological advances, the majority of surgical clients are admitted on the day of surgery or are not admitted to a hospital at all.

An increasing number and type of surgical procedures are being performed as ambulatory procedures in emergency rooms, doctor's offices, free-standing surgery clinics, mobile surgical units, and outpatient surgical units in hospitals. **Ambulatory surgery** is same-day or outpatient surgery that can be performed with general or local anesthesia, usually takes less than 2 hours, and requires less than a 3-hour stay in a recovery area.

Ambulatory surgery has steadily increased over the last decade. Fewer laboratory tests, fewer preoperative and postoperative medications, smaller, less invasive incisions, less psychological stress, reduced cost, and less susceptibility to nosocomial infections are some of the reasons clients and physicians alike prefer ambulatory surgery. In some cases, ambulatory surgery has been mandated by third-party payers—private insurance companies, government insurers (Medicare and Medicaid), and health management organizations.

Classification of Surgical Procedures

Surgical procedures are classified according to the client's admission status, urgency, degree of risk, and purpose (Table 57–1). Classifications may overlap or be found in all classes. An elective procedure may be ambulatory and diagnostic, or the same procedure may be performed for different reasons on a hospitalized client.

Surgical procedures may also combine several classifications (such as a client who has sustained multiple traumatic injuries in an automobile accident and may require major, reconstructive, and emergency surgery). It is important to remember that regardless of the defined degree of risk, any surgical procedure imposes physical and psychological stress and seldom is considered minor by the client. The classification system indicates the type of nursing care a client might require.

Perioperative Phases

All clients progress through the surgical experience in three phases. The word **perioperative** is used to describe the preoperative, intraoperative, and postoperative phases of the surgical experience. **Perioperative nursing** is a specialized area of practice that describes the provision of care for the surgical client throughout the continuum of care. The concept of perioperative nursing stresses the importance of providing continuity of care for the surgical client using the nursing process. Historically, the term *operating room nursing* was used to describe the surgical care of clients. However, with the advent of technology, multiple surgical settings and managed care, the surgical care of the client is no longer based just in the operating room.

In many facilities, the perioperative nurse assesses a client's health status preoperatively, identifies specific client needs, teaches and counsels, attends to the client's needs intraoperatively in the OR, and then follows the client's entire recovery postoperatively. However, in other institutions, different nurses care for the surgical client during each phase of the surgical experience. Provision of safe, consistent, and effective nursing care during each phase of surgery is a major responsibility.

Preoperative Phase

The **preoperative phase** begins when the decision for surgical intervention is made. The range of nursing activities includes, but is not limited to, preoperative assessment of the client's physical, psychological, and social states, the planning of nursing care that is required to prepare the client for surgery, and the implementation and evaluation of nursing interventions. This phase ends when the client is safely transported into the OR for the surgical procedure.

Intraoperative Phase

The **intraoperative phase** begins with the client's entry into the OR and ends when the client is transferred to the recovery room or other areas where immediate post-surgical attention is given. During this phase, focus is on the continuing assessment and diagnosis of

TABLE 57–1
Classification of Surgical Procedures

Type	Description	Examples
Admission Status		
Ambulatory (outpatient)	Client enters setting, has surgical procedure, and is discharged on the same day	• Breast biopsy.
		• Cataract extraction.
		• Hemorrhoidectomy.
		• Scar revision.
Same day admit	Client enters hospital and undergoes surgery on the same day and remains for convalescence	• Carotid endarterectomy.
		• Cholecystectomy.
		• Mastectomy.
		• Vaginal hysterectomy.
Inpatient	Client is admitted to hospital, undergoes surgery, and remains in hospital for convalescence	• Amputation.
		• Heart transplant.
		• Laryngectomy.
		• Resection of aortic aneurysm.
Urgency		
Elective	Delay of surgery has no ill effects; surgery is performed on basis of client's preference	• Breast reconstruction.
		• Hernia repair.
		• Joint bunionectomy.
		• Tonsillectomy.
Urgent	Necessary for client's health and may prevent further damage; usually done within 24–48 hours	• Amputation.
		• Colon resection for obstruction.
		• Coronary artery bypass.
Emergency	Performed as soon as possible to save client's life or to preserve a body part or organ	• Control of hemorrhage.
		• Repair perforated ulcer.
		• Tracheostomy.
Degree of Risk		
Major (elective, urgent, or emergent)	To improve or maintain health, to restore function, or to preserve life. Includes opening the abdomen, thorax, or cranium	• Exploratory laparotomy.
		• Nephrectomy.
		• Traumatic injury repair.
Minor (usually elective)	Restores function or corrects deformities, such as lesions	• Arthroscopy.
		• Cataract extraction.
		• Dilatation and curettage.
		• Removal of warts.
		• Tooth extraction.
Purpose		
Diagnostic	Surgical exploration to assist in making a diagnosis (may involve biopsy)	• Breast biopsy.
		• Bronchoscopy.
		• Exploratory laparotomy.
		• Skin biopsy.
Ablative	Removal or excision of diseased body part or organ	• Amputation.
		• Appendectomy.
		• Colon resection.
		• Thyroidectomy.
Palliative	Reduces intensity of disease or illness symptoms but is not intended to be curative	• Arthroscopy.
		• Colostomy.
		• Debulking of malignant tumor.
		• Nerve root resection.
Constructive	Restores function in congenital anomalies	• Cleft palate repair.
		• Closure of atrial-septal heart defect.
Reconstructive	Restores function or appearance to traumatized tissue	• Breast reconstruction.
		• Internal fixation of fracture.
		• Scar revision.
		• Skin graft.
Transplant	Replaces malfunctioning organs	• Cornea.
		• Heart.
		• Joints.
		• Kidney.

the client's physiological and psychological responses and the implementation and evaluation of interventions to promote safety and privacy as well as prevent wound infection and promote healing.

Safe and effective intraoperative care requires a team effort (Fig. 57–1). Each member of the surgical team brings unique skills that must be coordinated to achieve desired client outcomes. Team members are categorized as sterile or nonsterile in relation to the sterile surgical field.

Sterile team members are those who scrub their hands and arms, don sterile attire, use sterile instruments and supplies, and work in the sterile surgical field. Members of the sterile surgical team include the surgeon; physician assistants and registered nurse first assistants; and the scrub person, who may be a registered nurse, a licensed vocational or practical nurse, or a surgical technician.

The **registered nurse first assistant** (RNFA) is an expanded nursing role, requiring additional education, in which the perioperative nurse works as a first assistant during the surgical procedure. The RNFA is a perioperative role that is gaining legislative acceptance as a way to serve the public's health care needs in a cost-effective manner. The RNFA replaces an assisting surgeon and therefore is more cost-effective when viewed by insurance reimbursement guidelines. The RNFA may perform the following functions during the surgical procedure: handling tissue and organs with instruments, providing exposure of surgical site, suturing tissue, and providing hemostasis. These functions are independent of the scrub nurse role, as the RNFA does not concur-

rently function as the scrub person. The RNFA may also be involved in preoperative and postoperative care of the client.

The **scrub nurse** is a registered nurse with special qualifications that include knowledge of aseptic technique, instruments and equipment, anatomy and physiology, and surgical procedures and, most importantly, promotion of client safety. This knowledge helps the scrub nurse anticipate needs of the surgical team and thus reduces the duration of anesthesia time for the client. The scrub nurse sets up and maintains the sterile field; hands supplies and instruments to the surgeon and assistants; keeps an accurate count of instruments, sponges, and sharps; monitors aseptic technique; and uses the nursing process to ensure client safety. The scrub nurse role is seen as an integral part of perioperative nursing practice. When the scrub role is performed by someone other than the nurse, that person is in a delegated technical role and under the supervision of a perioperative nurse. These technically trained unlicensed assistive personnel are called operating room technicians or surgical technicians.

Members of the nonsterile surgical team have responsibilities outside the sterile field and do not wear sterile attire. The nonsterile team members include, but are not limited to, the anesthesiologist, the nurse anesthetist, and the circulating nurse. The **circulating nurse,** or circulator, must be a registered nurse who assists the client to meet individual needs during all three phases of the surgical experience. The circulating nurse coordinates the care of the client, is the client's advocate, and manages activities outside the sterile

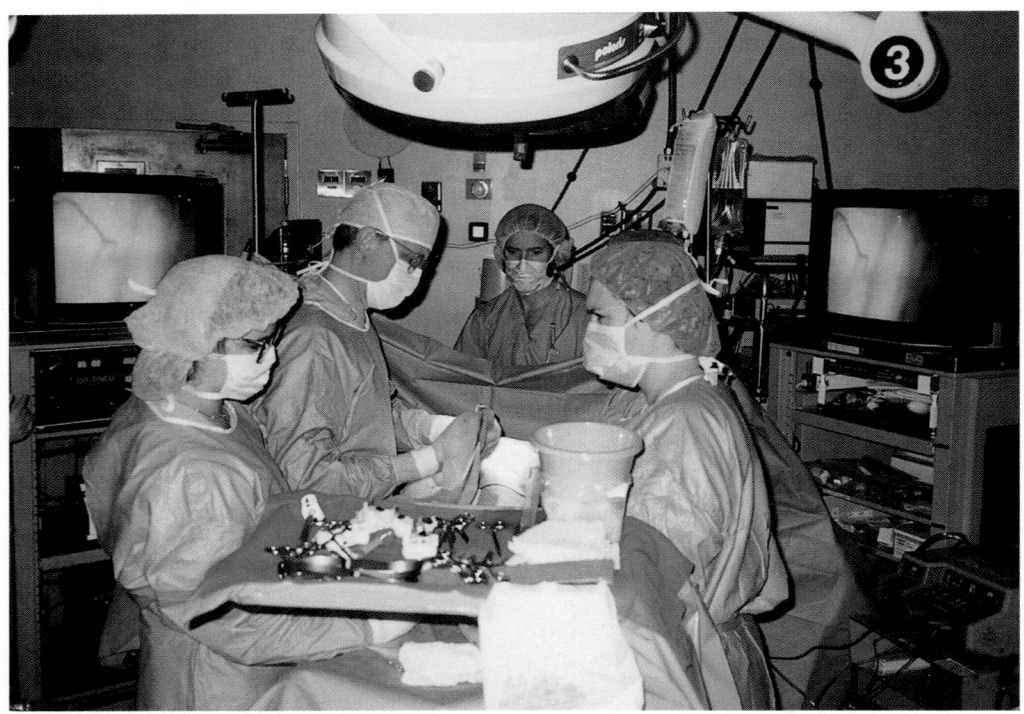

Figure 57–1. Safe, effective intraoperative care requires a team effort.

field. The nursing process is the framework used to meet client needs and achieve overall desired outcomes. The circulating nurse does the following:

- Provides emotional support to the client prior to induction of anesthesia
- Performs preoperative and ongoing client assessment
- Directs and assists with proper positioning of the client
- Performs the surgical skin preparation
- Creates and maintains a safe environment
- Implements and enforces policies and procedures to ensure client safety
- Administers medications and solutions to the sterile field
- Manages catheters, tubes, drains, and specimens
- Protects the client's privacy and dignity
- Documents client assessment data and care needs with outcomes
- Communicates relevant information to other team members and to the client's family

Other people that make up the nonsterile surgical team are radiology and laboratory technicians, perfusionists, perioperative educators, pathologists, nurse's aides, and personnel from materials management, environmental services, and central services. All participate in ensuring a safe surgical experience for the client. However, it is the perioperative nurse who coordinates the contributions of each surgical team member.

Postoperative Phase

The **postoperative phase** can be divided into two segments of care: the immediate and the ongoing postoperative periods. The immediate postoperative period includes an evaluative assessment by the perioperative nurse and admittance to the postanesthesia care unit. The **postanesthesia care unit** (PACU), previously known as the recovery room or postanesthesia room, is an area where clients remain until they regain consciousness from the effects of anesthesia. Most clients who receive general anesthesia, major regional anesthesia, or monitored local anesthesia care are transferred to a PACU. The perioperative nurse in some cases may actually provide care for the client in the PACU; however, it is more common for the perioperative nurse to give a transfer of care report to a postanesthesia nurse. The PACU nurse is skilled in the care of clients immediately after surgery and has in-depth knowledge of anesthetics, pain management, and surgical procedures.

Nursing care in the PACU involves immediate assessment of changes in the physical and psychological status of the client, along with appropriate planning and implementation of care, such as frequent monitoring of airway patency, vital signs, and neurological status; providing intravenous fluids and blood; accurately assessing output from all drains; and providing a thorough transfer report of the client's status to the

nurse receiving the client on the unit and to the client's family and friends.

After transfer to the surgical unit or ambulatory recovery area, the client is in the ongoing phase of postoperative care. This period includes all care given during the course of surgical convalescence to the time of discharge, and continues with assisted care or self-care at home.

Discharge planning, which includes teaching and referral, is also part of the ongoing care throughout the client's surgical experience. The client and family are prepared to assume any care that may be needed after discharge. If needed, community resources are used. A community or home health nurse is a valuable resource for the client with treatment needs after discharge.

Anesthesia

Anesthesia is the partial or complete loss of sensation with or without a loss of consciousness that results from administration of an anesthetic agent. Anesthetics are given by an **anesthesiologist,** a medical physician who specializes in anesthesiology, or by specifically trained physician assistants. Another anesthesia provider, the **certified registered nurse anesthetist** (CRNA) is an advanced practice registered nurse who has been specifically educated in the administration of anesthetic agents.

The role of the perioperative nurse in anesthesia management begins with the preoperative assessment and ends when the client recovers from the effects of anesthesia. An understanding of the following concepts enhances the perioperative nurse's ability to collaborate with anesthesia providers: anesthesia risk classifications, choice of anesthetic agents, client positioning principles, induction and intubation techniques, levels of general anesthesia, malignant hyperthermia, and client monitoring parameters during local and regional anesthesia procedures. These concepts are discussed further throughout this chapter. As the client's advocate, perioperative nurses also maintain a quiet environment once the client has entered the operating room and provide emotional support to help reduce client anxiety.

The anesthesiologist considers multiple factors when selecting anesthetic techniques and agents. Prior to surgery, the anesthesiologist evaluates the physical condition and age of the client, the presence of co-existing diseases, the type, site, and duration of the operation, the client's preference, and the surgeon's preference. The American Society of Anesthesiology (ASA) has developed a classification system to identify risk factors based on the client's health status (Table 57–2). As part of the preoperative evaluation, the anesthesiologist places the client in a class according to physical status. For example, a traumatically injured client with severe head and neck injuries who was evaluated by the neurosurgeon prior to surgery would be given a classification of P5. This identifies a client who is not expected to

TABLE 57–2
ASA Physical Status Classification System

P1	A normal healthy patient
P2	A patient with mild systemic disease
P3	A patient with severe systemic disease
P4	A patient with severe systemic disease that is a constant threat to life
P5	A moribund patient who is not expected to survive without the operation
P6	A declared brain-dead patient whose organs are being removed for donor purposes

American Society of Anesthesiologists. Available at: http://www.asahq.org/ProfInfo/PhysicalStatus.html. Accessed May 10, 1999.

survive 24 hours and is an extreme risk for anesthesia.

Preoperative medications may be ordered by the anesthesiologist or surgeon to reduce preoperative anxiety, minimize secretions in the respiratory tract, decrease acidity and production of gastric secretions, relieve pain, and decrease metabolism so that less anesthetic agent is necessary. Medications are selected on the basis of the preoperative assessment findings and demands of the intended surgical procedure.

Anesthesia is used to produce a loss of sensation with or without the loss of consciousness, and also provides analgesia, reflex loss, and muscle relaxation during a surgical procedure. Therefore, the goal of anesthesia is the elimination of pain and awareness at a level safe for the client. One of three types of anesthesia is used during surgical procedures: general anesthesia, regional anesthesia, or local anesthesia.

General Anesthesia

General anesthesia is produced by inhalation or by injection of anesthetic drugs in the bloodstream, or a combination of both, and causes the client to lose all sensation and consciousness. The client also experiences amnesia of surgical events. General anesthesia is accomplished in four phases. The phases are preinduction, induction, maintenance, and reversal.

The *preinduction phase* begins as soon as the client is brought into the actual operating room. Monitoring devices are applied to the client with a brief explanation of each device. Methods for intraoperative monitoring include the following:

- Electrocardiogram (ECG) continuously displayed
- Arterial blood pressure and heart rate determined and evaluated every 5 minutes or more
- Pulse oximetry
- Body temperature readings
- Respirometer and inspiratory pressure readings
- End-tidal CO_2 analysis

Based on the cardiovascular and pulmonary status of the client, the surgical procedure, and the chance of significant physiological changes, additional invasive monitors or special monitoring equipment may be used as deemed necessary.

The *induction phase* begins with the introduction of anesthetic agents and ends with endotracheal intubation and stabilization of the client. Induction involves putting the client safely to sleep. A patent airway and adequate ventilation must be ensured at all times.

The *maintenance phase* starts when stabilization is accomplished. During this period, the client is positioned for the procedure, the skin is prepared, and the surgery is performed. The anesthesiologist or CRNA maintains the proper depth of anesthesia while constantly monitoring physiological parameters such as vital signs and oxygen and carbon dioxide levels.

The final phase of anesthesia is the *reversal phase.* As the anesthetic agents are withdrawn or the effects are reversed pharmacologically, the client begins to awaken. The endotracheal tube is removed once the client is able to re-establish voluntary breathing. It is critical to ensure airway patency in this period, because extubation may cause bronchospasm or laryngospasm. Other potential problems during this phase include vomiting with risk for aspiration, slow spontaneous respirations, and uncontrolled reflex movements or shivering.

General anesthesia has both advantages and disadvantages. One advantage is that it can be used for clients of any age and for any surgical procedure, while leaving the client unaware of the physical trauma. Additionally, rapid excretion of the anesthetic agent and prompt reversal of its effects are considered advantageous.

Disadvantages of general anesthesia include risks associated with circulatory and respiratory depression. Clients with serious respiratory or circulatory diseases, such as emphysema or congestive heart failure, are at a high risk for complications during and after surgery.

Regional Anesthesia

When general anesthesia is contraindicated or not a desirable choice, regional anesthesia may be used. **Regional anesthesia** is a type of anesthesia in which medication is instilled into or around the nerves to block the transmission of nerve impulses in a particular area or region. Regional anesthesia produces analgesia, relaxation, and reduced reflexes. There are several techniques for regional anesthesia and the choice depends on the type and length of surgery, the preferences of the anesthesiologist and surgeon, and, if possible, the preference of the client. Regional anesthesia techniques require the skill of an anesthesiologist and may be used for complex procedures.

When receiving regional anesthesia, the client is awake during the procedure but does not perceive pain. Regional anesthesia is often supplemented with sedatives and narcotics to achieve one or more of the following: to decrease anxiety, to decrease awareness of the surroundings, to provide additional analgesia, and to improve cooperation. A screen is usually used to restrict the client's view of the surgical area and to protect the sterile field. Regional anesthesia may be classified further as follows.

NERVE BLOCK ANESTHESIA

Nerve block anesthesia involves injection of the anesthetic agent into and around a nerve group or nerve trunk to produce a lack of sensation over a specific body area. Major blocks involve multiple nerves like the brachial plexus or an axillary nerve block that would anesthetize the arm. Minor blocks involve a single nerve (a facial nerve, for example).

BIER BLOCK ANESTHESIA

Intravenous block anesthesia, otherwise known as Bier block anesthesia, is used most often for procedures involving the arm, wrist, and hand. An occlusion tourniquet is put on the extremity to prevent absorption of the injected intravenous drug beyond the involved extremity.

SPINAL ANESTHESIA

Spinal anesthesia is also known as a subarachnoid block. Surgeries of the lower abdomen, perineum, and lower extremities are likely candidates for this type of regional anesthesia. It requires a lumbar puncture through one of the interspaces between lumbar disk 2 (L2) and the sacrum (S1), such as at the L3-L4 interspace (Fig. 57–2A). Cerebrospinal fluid (CSF) dripping from the needle cannula confirms correct placement prior to injection of the anesthetic. With spi-

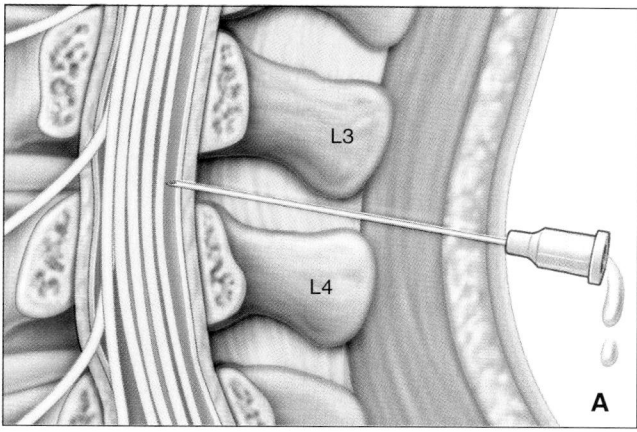

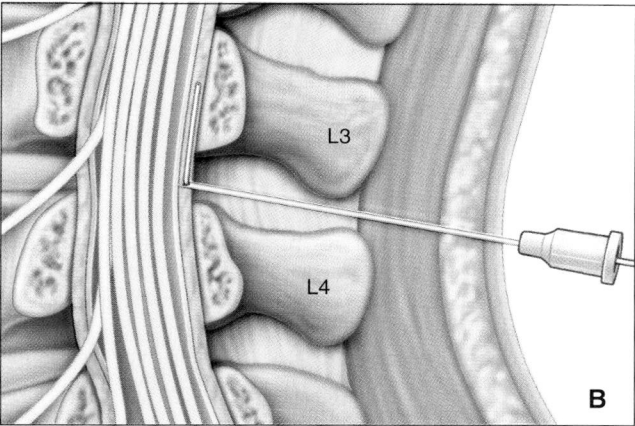

Figure 57–2. Placement of needle for spinal anesthesia *(A)* and catheter for epidural anesthesia *(B)*.

nal anesthesia, continued leakage of CSF from the needle insertion site may cause decreased CSF pressure and result in postoperative headaches. Bedrest with restrictions on elevating the head of the bed, maintaining hydration, and applying pressure to the infusion site combat this common side effect.

EPIDURAL ANESTHESIA

Epidural anesthesia occurs when local anesthetic agents are injected into the epidural space, which is located outside the dura mater of the spinal cord. This type of anesthesia is used frequently for surgeries involving the abdomen and lower extremities. Advantages of epidural anesthesia are reduced risk of headaches or hypotensive reactions. However, precise skill is required to introduce the catheter into the epidural space (Fig. 57–2B).

Local Anesthesia

Local anesthesia is any agent that induces a temporary loss of feeling due to the inhibition of nerve endings in a specific part of the body. Topical application and local (or extravascular) infiltration are the usual routes of local anesthesia techniques.

Topical surface anesthesia is applied to the mucous membranes or skin to block nerve impulses at that site. Minor wounds involving the skin or mucosa may be topically anesthetized using a cocaine solution (4 to 10% solution), lidocaine, or benzocaine prior to the operation.

Local nerve infiltration is achieved by the injection of an agent such as lidocaine or tetracaine around a local nerve to depress nerve sensation over a limited area of the body. This technique is used during minor surgical procedures such as skin and muscle biopsies, removal of superficial cysts, and suturing of small wounds.

The surgeon is frequently the one to administer local anesthesia and the client usually receives narcotic or selective supplemental medications. In many cases, anesthesia personnel are called on; these situations are referred to as monitored anesthesia care. The primary purpose of monitored anesthesia care is to provide support to the surgeon and to ensure client safety and comfort.

The Association of Operating Room Nurses (AORN) has guidelines that are applicable to situations in which the perioperative nurse cares for the client receiving local anesthesia with or without conscious sedation in the absence of anesthesia professionals (AORN, 1999). The perioperative nurse is then responsible for monitoring the client and for the administration of supplemental medications to sedate the client during the procedure. Many facilities require advanced cardiac life support certification of the nurses who monitor clients receiving local anesthesia.

Informed Consent

Prior to surgery, the surgeon is required to ask the client to sign a legal document stating the client's informed consent to have the operative procedure performed. Informed consent implies that the client has agreed to allow something to happen, such as surgery, based on a full disclosure of facts needed to make an intelligent decision. This document serves to legally protect the client, nurse, physician, and health care facility. Surgical informed consent includes the following information:

- Need for the procedure in relation to the diagnosis
- Description and purpose of the proposed procedure
- Possible benefits and potential risks
- Likelihood of a successful outcome
- Alternative treatments or procedures available
- Anticipated risks should the procedure not be performed
- Physician's advice as to what is needed
- Right to refuse treatment or withdraw consent

It is the legal responsibility of the surgeon who performs the procedure to obtain the client's informed consent. The signing of an official consent form primarily provides evidence that the consent process occurred and that the client is aware of the concept of informed consent. The signature of a member of the health care staff provides witness to the signature of the client. Therefore, the nurse's signature only confirms the signing of the consent form.

Facilitating the informed consent process is an important role, as you may be the last health care professional the client sees before having surgery. When validating informed consent status, ask the client if he understands the procedures for which consent has been given. If a client denies understanding, or you suspect he does not understand, notify the physician. Do not attempt to answer the client's questions regarding risks, benefits, or alternative treatment of the scheduled surgery. It is the surgeon's legal duty to discuss these matters with the client in the process of obtaining informed consent. In case law, it is considered detrimental to the client if another health care provider attempts to answer informed consent questions and is considered an intrusion into the physician-client relationship (Pryor, 1997).

Action Alert!

Notify the surgeon immediately if a client is unsure about the nature of the surgical procedure he is about to undergo. Act as a client advocate and do not allow the surgery to proceed if the client may not have been informed adequately.

Other times that consent is not informed are when the client is confused, unconscious, mentally incompetent, known to have chronic alcohol or drug abuse, or under the influence of sedatives. All consent forms must be signed before any preoperative sedation or narcotic medications are given (Pape, 1997). As the client advocate, you are responsible for recognizing and confirming that the client's decision is an informed one.

Clients must personally sign the consent form if they are of legal age (varies among states), under legal age but have a valid marriage certificate, designated as an emancipated minor (certain states), and not presently under legal guardianship. If the client is a minor or legally considered to be incompetent and not included in the aforementioned categories, a parent or legal guardian signs the consent form. If an adult is incapable of giving informed consent, consent must be obtained from the next of kin. The order of kin relationship for an adult is usually spouse, adult child, parent, and sibling.

In a life-threatening emergency, when consent cannot be obtained from the client or a family member, then the law generally agrees that consent is assumed. This is referred to as *implied consent*. In emergency situations, every effort is made to obtain consent from a family member or guardian. Telephone consent may be obtained and must be witnessed by two persons who hear the family member's oral consent.

After the consent form is completed in ink, verify that the correct date, time, and signatures are on the form and place it in the client's record. The record then accompanies the client to the operating room.

FACTORS AFFECTING SURGICAL OUTCOME

To determine the level of surgical risk, screening the client for factors affecting surgical outcome may help prevent perioperative complications. Lifestyle habits, cultural and religious practices, developmental stage, socioeconomic status, and physiological factors are all considered when determining a client's surgical outcome.

Lifestyle Factors

A nursing history gathered about the client's lifestyle provides valuable information regarding surgical risk and postoperative convalescence. Nurse researchers at Johns Hopkins University have increased understanding of women's recovery and rehabilitation after coronary artery bypass graft (CABG) surgery and have found meaningful interventions related to lifestyle changes postoperatively to prevent further disease (Allen, 1997). The areas assessed related to lifestyle are nutritional status; use of alcohol, tobacco, and recreational drugs; activities of daily living; and occupation. Lifestyle factors are critical to predicting recovery.

Nutrition

Normal tissue repair and resistance to infection depend on adequate nutrition. Surgery increases the body's need for nutrients. Both malnutrition and obesity increase surgical risk. Nutritional deficiencies of protein and vitamins A, C, and B complex are particularly significant because each of these substances is essential for wound healing. A malnourished client is prone to fluid and electrolyte imbalances, reduced energy stores, improper wound healing, and infection after surgery. Both the obese and the underweight client are at risk for intraoperatively acquired pressure ulcers at pressure points due to positioning required for surgery. Elective surgeries may be postponed until the client loses or gains weight and other nutritional deficiencies are corrected.

The obese client also has other possible complications to consider. Obese clients usually have reduced ventilatory and cardiac function, and positions required for surgery may limit ventilation further. Inhalation anesthesia is absorbed and stored by adipose tissue and then released postoperatively. Therefore, the obese client requires more anesthetic during surgery and recovers more slowly from its effects. Fatty tissue is also more difficult to suture and has less resistance to infection, which may lead to the postoperative complications of delayed wound healing, wound infection, and dehiscence of the wound.

Specifically ask clients about their vitamin, herbal, or supplement intake. Some popular nutritional supplements that may have a detrimental effect on surgical clients include, but are not limited to, garlic, vitamin E, and eicosapentaenoic acid (fish oil).

Garlic is used by clients to reduce cholesterol levels as well as treat infections and other ailments. Research has shown that garlic decreases platelet aggregation, increases clotting times, and decreases plasma viscosity. Garlic therefore has a potential to increase surgical bleeding. These bleeding effects will be magnified if clients also take antiplatelet medications such as aspirin or nonsteroidal anti-inflammatory drugs. Clients should stop taking garlic at least 1 week before surgery takes place (Petry, 1997).

Taking vitamin E is potentially hazardous to surgical clients because studies show that vitamin E reduces platelet adhesion. Studies also show that oral ingestion of vitamin E slows wound healing, particularly collagen synthesis. Clients undergoing abdominal wall surgery or tendon repairs are at special risk (Petry, 1997).

Similar to garlic and vitamin E, fish oil or eicosapentaenoic acid lowers a person's risk for developing cardiovascular disease by decreasing platelet aggregation and adhesion (Petry, 1997). While these effects are beneficial in the prevention of thrombotic cardiovascular events, the resultant increased bleeding time is detrimental during surgery.

Activity and Exercise

The quantity and quality of a client's rest and sleep habits as well as his or her exercise program are important considerations in facilitating recovery. Rest and sleep are essential to physical and mental restoration and recovery from the stress of surgery. A client with a well-established exercise program usually has improved body systems function, which decreases the risks of surgery. Information gained during a preoperative nursing history allows for individualizing interventions to promote rest, sleep, and exercise.

Substance Abuse

Although it may be difficult, ask the client about possible drug use, abuse, and addiction. The categories of agents most likely to be abused include tobacco, alcohol, opioids, marijuana, and cocaine. Encourage the client to answer truthfully and ask the interview questions in a matter-of-fact manner. When clients are informed of the potential interactions of these drugs and anesthetic medications, most clients will respond truthfully about their drug use. Clients whose alcohol intake is habitual and in large amounts require larger doses of anesthesia and postoperative analgesics. Clients who smoke are at higher risk for respiratory complications after surgery. The potential for postoperative complications is increased for clients who use, abuse, or are addicted to recreational drugs, alcohol, or tobacco.

Cultural and Religious Factors

Cultural influences on the surgical experience also affect the client's responses and perceptions to a surgical experience, as suggested in the Cross-Cultural Care chart. Nurses frequently care for clients whose cultural beliefs are different from their own. In the area of client education, ignorance of cultural differences can pose serious problems; without such cultural knowledge, you will alienate the very clients you want to teach and possibly run the risk of the teaching-learning process being ignored. Awareness of cultural backgrounds may require nursing interventions to meet needs in such areas as language spoken, foods eaten, family interactions and participation, personal space, and health beliefs and practices.

Knowledge of the meaning of religion for the client can help identify a possible source of support. Support the client's spiritual needs through acceptance, participation in prayer, or referral to clergy or chaplain. Faith in a higher being provides support and helps to reduce fears.

Developmental Factors

Infants and the elderly are greater surgical risks than children and young to middle-aged adults. The neonate has a lower total blood volume, which makes a small blood loss a serious situation because of the risk of dehydration. The infant also has difficulty maintaining a stable body temperature during surgery because the shivering reflex is not well developed, making potential hypothermia more likely.

With an increasingly older population undergoing surgical procedures, assessment of physiological changes is critical to providing safe holistic care to the elderly client. Geriatric clients are at additional risk from surgery because of impaired circulation from limited cardiac function and arteriosclerotic disease. Careful assessment and special attention to risk factors that threaten impending ventilatory, renal, metabolic, infectious, or thromboembolitic complications are im-

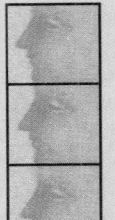

CROSS-CULTURAL CARE
CARING FOR AN AFRO-CARIBBEAN CLIENT

Berris Warren, the client we've been reading about in this chapter, is from Jamaica and of African descent. He was born in a small village outside of Kingston, Jamaica. His family has been on the island since the 17th century. They were some of the first slaves brought from Africa by the Spanish. Growing sugar cane and bananas has been a part of his life as long as he can remember. Although each client is unique, many Afro-Caribbeans hold the following values:

- Religion and spirituality
- Music
- Humor
- Extended family (especially in rural communities)
- A collective or communal view of society
- Community responsibility for children
- Playing down achievements to avoid standing out
- Enjoying life and finding immediate gratification
- Respecting others by looking away and covering one's mouth when laughing.

As you read below, take note how Mr. Warren's nurse, Darryl, demonstrates sensitivity to Mr. Warren's cultural values:

Darryl: Good morning, Mr. Warren. I am Darryl, your nurse for today. Good morning, Miss.

Mr. Warren: Whey yuh a seh! (Glances around at Darryl, roommate, and daughter and smiles). It is mi dawta.

Daughter: Good morning.

Darryl: I see you have a tape player. Have you and Mr. Arnold (roommate) been playing music all night?

Mr. Warren: Dat is mi bredda. Ha! (Looks away and covers his mouth.) We dance the night away. (Roommate laughs with Mr. Warren.)

Darryl: How did that make your incision feel, Mr. Warren?

Mr. Warren: Lawd have mercy! All better—mi a-go today! Mi girl hep me.

Daughter: We will be going home today. Father needs further instruction on his catheter and leg bag. I'm a nurse and can help him at home—it seems he will let me. He's recuperating at my house.

Darryl: Well, let's check your belly and catheter, Mr. Warren, so you can get home!

Critical Thinking Questions

- Did Mr. Warren exhibit any of the valued cultural tendencies listed earlier?
- Why did the nurse readily include the roommate in the conversation instead of remaining client focused?
- Do you think Mr. Warren values his daughter's assistance?
- Because of some language barriers, what educational strategies may work best for discharge teaching?

perative for the prevention of postoperative complications of the geriatric client (Lusis, 1996). Physiological changes related to aging decrease the older client's ability to respond to surgical stressors, alter the response to medications given perioperatively, and prolong or alter the healing process (Table 57–3). Energy reserves are usually limited, and hydration and nutritional status may be poor. The single most critical aspect that affects perioperative care is the decreased homeostatic capacity in the elderly client (Ruzicka, 1997).

Socioeconomic Factors

Economic factors influence both the immediate surgical intervention and the follow-up care. Make appropriate referrals to social workers early in the preoperative phase so that discharge planning can be initiated. Most surgical procedures require a delay in the client returning to work or may necessitate a change in the way a client supports self and family. Assess the client's occupational history to anticipate the effects surgery may have on recovery and eventual work perfor-

mance. Knowledge of a client's usual work and concerns regarding returning to work prepare you for making necessary referrals and individualizing teaching plans.

Physiological Factors

The client's medical history serves as a framework of care to be provided by the nurse, the anesthesia provider, and the surgeon. Illnesses, medications, and previous surgery are discussed as physiological factors that may affect surgical outcome.

Illnesses

Pre-existing illnesses can influence the client's ability to tolerate anesthesia and surgery and to reach a full recovery (Table 57–4). A review of the medical history will alert you to past hospitalizations and client outcomes. Pathologic changes associated with past and present illnesses increase surgical risk as well as the potential for postoperative complications. Clients planning for ambulatory surgery should also be

TABLE 57–3
How Physiological Changes of Aging Increase Surgical Risk

Body System	Changes	Risk
Pulmonary	• Reduced range of movement in diaphragm.	• Reduced vital capacity. • Diminished cough reflex.
	• Lung tissue stiffened. • Air spaces enlarged.	• Decreased oxygenation of blood.
Cardiovascular	• Degenerative changes in heart. • Rigidity of arterial walls. • Reduced innervation of heart. • Arterial walls thickened.	• Reduced cardiac reserve. • Predisposes to hemorrhage and rise in blood pressure. • Predisposes to thrombus formation.
Renal	• Reduced bladder capacity.	• Postoperative urine retention due to larger amount of urine that stays in bladder after voiding.
	• Reduced blood flow to kidneys.	• Increases danger of shock when blood loss occurs.
Neurological	• Decreased reaction time. • Sensory losses. • Increased pain tolerance.	• Confusion following anesthesia. • Less able to respond to early warning signs of postoperative complications.
Metabolic	• Lower basal metabolic rate. • Reduced number of red blood cells. • Change in total amounts of potassium and water volume.	• Reduces total oxygen consumption. • Reduces ability to carry oxygen to tissues. • Predisposes to fluid and electrolyte imbalances.
Integumentary	• Decreased vascularity and turgor of skin.	• Predisposes to pressure ulcers.
Gastrointestinal	• Decreased motility of gastrointestinal tract.	• Predisposes to constipation. • Raises the risk of paralytic ileus.

TABLE 57–4
Medical Conditions That Increase Surgical Risk

Medical Condition	Associated Risk
Respiratory disorders, such as asthma, bronchitis, and emphysema	• Hypoventilation and spasms of bronchus or larynx. • Respiratory depression from general anesthesia. • Reduced ability to compensate for acid-base imbalances.
Cardiovascular disorders, such as congestive heart failure or recent myocardial infarction	• Increased demands on myocardium (from stress of surgery) to maintain cardiac output. • Increased risk of myocardial infarction. • Increases risk of hemorrhage, shock, hypotension, thrombophlebitis, stroke, and fluid volume overload.
Diabetes mellitus	• Increased susceptibility to infection. • Delayed wound healing from altered glucose metabolism and circulatory impairment. • Increased risk for fluctuating blood glucose levels, possibly leading to life-threatening hypoglycemia or ketoacidosis.
Renal and liver disease	• Altered metabolism and elimination of drugs administered during surgery. • Poor tolerance for general anesthesia. • Increased risk for fluid, electrolyte, and acid-base imbalances. • Predisposed to hemorrhage and delayed wound healing.
Malnutrition	• Increased risk of organ failure and shock because client's metabolic reserves may not be sufficient to allow the body to respond to the physical stress of surgery. • Poor wound healing and infection from increased metabolic demands from surgery.
Obesity	• Delayed wound healing. • Infection and wound dehiscence. • Pneumonia and atelectasis. • Thrombophlebitis. • Arrhythmias and heart failure.
Alcoholism	• Probable malnourishment and possible delirium tremens (withdrawal symptoms). • Increased risk of infection and physical injury. • Possible need for increased dose of general anesthesia. • Liver damage may predispose to hemorrhage.
Nicotine abuse	• Respiratory complications, such as atelectasis, pneumonia, and bronchitis, from increased secretions and decreased ability to expectorate.

assessed for major medical problems that may raise their risk for complications. If the client is at increased risk, surgery as an outpatient may not be a consideration.

Although the presence of an acute infection usually results in the cancellation of elective surgery, clients with active chronic infections such as acquired immunodeficiency syndrome and tuberculosis may still have surgery. When preparing the client for surgery, remember that standard universal precautions need to be taken with every client.

Medications

Review of the client's current medication regimen is essential. It is important to recognize polypharmacy or the concurrent use of multiple medications. It occurs in all age groups but is more common with the elderly. Studies have shown that clients age 65 and over use an average of two to six prescribed medications and one to three over-the-counter (OTC) medications on a regular basis (Larson & Martin, 1999). The use of multiple medications predisposes clients to adverse drug reactions and interactions with other medications in the perioperative setting. Medication interactions are more likely to occur in the elderly than in the younger client because older adults tend to take more medications.

A number of pharmacological categories are used routinely during the client's surgical experience. These include anesthesia agents, antimicrobials, anticoagulants, hemostatic agents, oxytocics, steroids, diagnostic imaging dyes, diuretics, central nervous system agents, and emergency protocol medications. It has been reported that a seriously ill client may receive as many as 20 medications in a perioperative setting at one time (Larson & Martin, 1999). Large numbers of medications increase the chance of interactions.

It is also common for clients to use herbal remedies as alternative or complementary medicines. Ask clients about their use of herbal remedies, either as dietary supplements (several herbal supplements were discussed previously under nutritional factors) or as medicines. Unless specifically asked, some clients may not consider their natural remedies as medicines. Even though herbs are natural products, they act like medications and may interact or potentiate other medications or interfere with surgical procedures (Table 57–5).

Some medications may be canceled when a client goes to surgery. However, it is important to know the purposes and actions of drugs, as specific medications may be given to clients with diseases such as diabetes. The anesthesiologist in collaboration with the client's physician and surgeon will determine whether these medications should be taken the day of surgery as well as whether they should be taken postoperatively (Table 57–6).

Remember to assess for allergies to drugs that may be given during any phase of the surgical experience. Ask the client to tell you what exactly happened when they took a drug reported as an allergent. It is also important to inquire about nondrug allergies, including allergies to foods, chemicals, pollen, antiseptics used to prepare the skin for surgery, and latex rubber products. The client with a history of allergic responsiveness has a greater potential for demonstrating hypersensitivity reactions to anesthesia agents. Many facilities require that the client receive an allergy identification band to be worn before going to surgery. Flag the front of the client's chart to alert all health care providers to the client's allergy status.

Previous Surgery

A past experience with surgery can influence the physical and psychological responses to the planned surgery and can alert the nurse to special needs and possible risk factors. Complications such as anaphylaxis due to allergic reaction during previous surgery signals the need for preventive measures for the upcoming procedure. Complications such as thrombophlebitis or pneumonia after a prior surgery provide data needed to support preoperative teaching and careful postoperative monitoring. Reports of severe anxiety before previous surgery may indicate the need for additional emotional support and teaching.

TABLE 57–5

Preoperative Considerations for Commonly Used Herbs

Herb	Common Uses	Preoperative Considerations
Feverfew	• Migraine prevention.	• Has anticoagulation factors. • Preoperative assessment should include clotting studies. • Discontinue before surgery.
Ginger	• Motion sickness. • Cough. • Menstrual cramps. • Intestinal gas.	• Risk of prolonged clotting times. • Preoperative assessment should include clotting studies. • Discontinue before surgery.
St. John's wort	• Antidepressant. • Antiviral properties. • Anti-inflammatory action.	• Should not be used with other psychoactive drugs, monoamine oxidase inhibitors, or serotonin reuptake inhibitors. • Discontinue before surgery because of possible drug interactions.
Valerian root	• Sedative or tranquilizer effect. • Sleep aid.	• Should not be used with other sedatives or anxiolytics. • May increase effects of central nervous system depressants.

TABLE 57–6

Medications That May Influence the Intraoperative Course

Medication Type	Intraoperative Effects
Anticoagulants	• Alter normal clotting factors and thereby increase risk of hemorrhage.
Antihypertensives	• Interact with anesthetics to cause bradycardia, hypotension, and impaired circulation.
Antiarrhythmics	• Can reduce cardiac contractility and impair conduction during anesthesia.
Anticonvulsants	• Certain anticonvulsants (phenytoin and phenobarbital, for example) can alter metabolism of anesthetic agents after long-term use.
Corticosteroids	• With prolonged use, cause atrophy of adrenal glands, which decreases body's ability to withstand stress.
Insulin	• Diabetic client's need for insulin preoperatively is reduced because of fasting (NPO) status.
Diuretics	• Potentiate electrolyte and fluid imbalances.
Antidepressants	• Increase the hypotensive effects of anesthesia.
Antibiotics	• Potentiate the action of anesthetic drugs.

Psychological Factors

Client perceptions of the upcoming surgery, individual coping patterns, perceived body image, and sexuality issues all affect the surgical client psychologically. Understanding more about the client's psychological factors may influence the surgical outcome beneficially.

Perceptions of the Surgical Procedure

A well-informed client knows what to expect and in general accepts and copes more effectively with surgery and recovery. Misconceptions about the surgical outcome or the actual perioperative process can cause undue stress and fear. Because people respond on the basis of their perceptions, it is important to find out exactly how the surgery is perceived. Identify the client's perceptions of the procedure to better plan for teaching and emotional preparation measures.

A client's perceptions of and reactions to the surgical experience are also influenced by sociocultural factors, including family health beliefs and practices, economic factors, and cultural background. Assessing the social situation of the client and family is particularly important if you are incorporating the family as part of the client's plan of care during the perioperative period. If a client who requires surgery has been brought up in a family that believes surgery is the last option in treating an illness, he or she may refuse to have surgery or may be convinced that death will result. The resulting anxiety and physical condition make this particular client even more susceptible to surgical risk.

Reactions to teaching, physical care, and pain are also influenced by family values.

Coping Patterns and Support Systems

Surgery is a significant and stressful event in the life of the client and family. The client is concerned about the surgery and whether it will improve health. Hospitalization and the convalescent period may be lengthy and costly. Clients often feel they have very little control over their situation. Determine the client's coping patterns, support systems, and sociocultural needs to better understand the impact surgery has on a client's and family's emotional health.

Determine whether family members can provide support. The effect of others on the client's level of anxiety needs to be determined. Encourage significant others to be part of the surgical experience if they are able to provide support before and after surgery.

Body Image

Surgery can leave permanent disfigurement or alteration in body function. Concern over mutilation or loss of a body part compounds a client's fears. Removal of certain body parts may affect the client's feelings about appearing feminine, masculine, or even as a whole person. Determination of the client's perceptions regarding alterations of his or her body from surgery is an important assessment consideration.

Sexuality

The physical and psychological aspect of a client's sexuality is often affected by surgery. Excision of a breast, a colostomy, or removal of the prostate gland may affect a client's sexuality. Even minor surgeries such as a hernia repair or a cervical biopsy force clients to temporarily refrain from sexual intercourse. Encourage clients to express sexuality concerns. The client facing even temporary sexual dysfunction requires support. Include the client's sexual partner in discussions about sexuality to provide the couple a shared understanding on how to cope with sexual function limitations.

PREOPERATIVE PHASE

After the client decides to have surgery, preoperative preparation begins. Assessment is the first step in the preoperative preparation of the client. Analysis of assessment data allows for determination of risk factors, prevention measures needed, particular nursing intervention, and a probable surgical outcome.

Mr. Warren, accompanied by his wife and daughter, is at the hospital completing his diagnostic testing and preoperative teaching. This is his first surgery and hospitalization. He received only minimal preoperative education from the urologist. Mr. Warren is asking the perioperative nurse many questions about the upcoming surgical events. Based on this information, what nursing diagnosis might the nurse want to consider to assist Mr. Warren and his family to cope with the rapidly approaching surgery?

PREOPERATIVE NURSING DIAGNOSES

Anxiety: A vague uneasy feeling of discomfort or dread accompanied by an autonomic response; the source is often nonspecific or unknown to the individual; a feeling of apprehension caused by anticipation of danger. It is an altering signal that warns of impending danger and enables the individual to take measures to deal with threat.

Anticipatory Grieving: Intellectual and emotional responses and behaviors by which individuals, families, and communities work through the process of modifying self-concept based on the perception of potential loss.

Risk for Latex Allergy Response: At risk for an allergic response to natural latex rubber products.

Knowledge Deficit: Absence or deficiency of cognitive information related to a specific topic.

From North American Nursing Diagnosis Association. (1999). NANDA nursing diagnoses: Definitions and classification 1999–2000. Philadelphia: Author.

ASSESSMENT

The importance of preoperative assessment cannot be overemphasized. It is an interdisciplinary activity, and responsibility for the assessment extends to all members of the health care team. The analysis of the preoperative assessment information is used to prepare the client physically and mentally for surgery and to communicate pertinent information to other surgical team members. Preoperative data are also used throughout the intraoperative and postoperative phases.

General Assessment of the Preoperative Client

Approach assessment of the preoperative client in a holistic manner, by gathering information about the physiological, psychological, spiritual, and social needs of the client and family or significant others. From these baseline data, identify surgical risk factors, physical and psychological support needs, and teaching needs, and determine the priority of nursing care. Assessment of the preoperative client is done by taking a nursing history and health history, performing a physical examination, and analyzing laboratory data. This initial patient database demonstrates the holistic assessment approach needed to determine care priority of the surgical client.

Health History

NURSING HISTORY
When taking a history, you are screening the preoperative client for risks that may cause complications during the perioperative period. The nursing history is an assessment of risk factors and strengths in the client's physical and psychosocial status. Other sources of information are the client's family or significant others. Data that are significant to the surgical experience

include the health history, lifestyle, coping patterns and support systems, and client perceptions of self and of the surgical procedure.

The nursing history interview often is a time when cues from verbal and nonverbal communication may be used to identify fears and concerns related to the client's perception of the surgery, and to plan interventions to provide information and emotional support necessary for successful recovery from surgery. Therapeutic communication skills are essential in establishing a trusting nurse-client relationship necessary to identify and resolve fears. The reduction of fear is of major importance in preoperative preparation, because emotional stress added to the physical stress of surgery increases surgical risk.

SURGICAL HEALTH HISTORY
A health history is taken by the surgeon to determine pathological conditions and to provide a basis for planning surgical care. The collection of data about the client before surgery is probably completed in the surgeon's office. If a client has chronic medical problems (cardiac, pulmonary, renal), a medical physician, possibly a specialist, may also be consulted to provide *medical clearance* for the client prior to surgery. This clearance usually involves further diagnostic testing to determine the level of surgical risk related to his chronic status. The term *medical clearance* implies that the client is rated as a low surgical risk.

Physical Examination

Clients should be in optimal physical condition before surgery. A thorough examination of all body systems should be performed to assess the client's status (Table 57–7). Collect physiological data preoperatively to obtain baseline data for comparison during the intraoperative and postoperative phases of care and to identify potential problems that may require preventive nursing interventions before, during, and after surgery.

TABLE 57–7
Preoperative Physical Assessment

System	Assessment	Purpose
General survey	Height	Determination of nutritional status
	Weight	Baseline data for preoperative and postoperative phases
	Vital signs	Indication of underlying imbalances or infection
	General	Reflects energy levels and physical and emotional status
Integumentary	Skin turgor	Evidence of hydration
	Bony prominences	Indication of potential for injury or pressure ulcers
	Mucous membranes	Indication of hydration and oxygenation
Respiratory	Breathing rate, depth, and rhythm; adventitious sounds; diameter and shape of thorax	Abnormalities may indicate a pre-existing condition that could raise the risk of respiratory trouble during surgery or of atelectasis or pneumonia after surgery
Cardiovascular	Peripheral pulses and apical pulse, rate, rhythm, character	Baseline data for intraoperative and postoperative phases of care
	Presence of edema or other abnormal finding	Abnormal findings indicate possible complications, such as thrombophlebitis, emboli, or arrhythmias
Neurological	Level of consciousness and level of motor and sensory function	Provides baseline data for postoperative assessments and identifies limitations to activity
Abdomen	Size, shape, bowel sounds, and last bowel movement	Provides baseline data for postoperative assessments

Diagnostic Tests

Clients may undergo preoperative preparation several days prior to surgery or immediately before surgery if the procedure is done on an emergency basis. Usually, preadmission testing is done in the hospital, the physician's office, or an outpatient laboratory. Many facilities have written protocols for preoperative tests. The surgeon orders preoperative radiological and other laboratory tests (Box 57–1).

Abnormalities may warrant treatment before the client has surgery. Check the physician's orders carefully and see that they are carried out to ensure that the results are obtained before surgery. In many institutions, the nurse screens the test results for abnormalities and informs the surgeon and anesthesiologist as appropriate. The window of time for laboratory and diagnostic testing acceptability is the 4 months before surgery if all results were normal (Patton, 1999).

With the testing completed, the client anticipating a scheduled surgery usually enters the hospital the day surgery is performed. The traditional preoperative routine, with the client entering the hospital the day before surgery, is not usually done now unless the client has special therapy or testing needs. Regardless of the method of entry into the setting, you must be able to properly prepare the client for surgery.

Focused Assessment for Anxiety

Anxiety is present in most surgical clients to a certain degree. It is a state in which a person experiences generalized feelings of unease and apprehension that are triggered by an actual or perceived threat. Anxiety in-

BOX 57–1
COMMONLY ORDERED PREOPERATIVE TESTS

Blood studies
  Red blood cell count
  Hematocrit
  Hemoglobin
  White blood cell count with differential
Prothrombin or partial thromboplastin time
Type and crossmatch
Creatinine
Blood urea nitrogen
Electrolytes
Human chorionic gonadotropin (pregnancy test)
Fasting glucose level
Urinalysis
Chest x-ray
Electrocardiogram

terferes with the client's ability to concentrate, recall information, and process new information. Assessment that focuses on identification of the nursing diagnosis *Anxiety* as soon as the client consents to surgery provides an opportunity to work with the client and family members in developing a plan of care that addresses anxiety management.

Responses to stressors or anxiety can be adaptive or maladaptive. Adaptive behaviors are purposeful.

The client adapts to a stressful situation by preparing to face it or by removing the threat. Maladaptive behaviors result from the inability to adapt to a stressful situation. Stress responses are cumulative and an increasing number of stressors can eventually drain adaptive energy. The newly admitted surgical client who has been confronted with many stressors before admission is more likely to react with a high level of anxiety as new stressors are encountered. Identify anxiety in a client by looking for the objective signs and listening for the subjective cues of anxiety. Encourage the client to be open in expression and communication of thoughts and feelings. Ask clients about past hospital experiences that frightened them or that cause them to have concern about their current surgery. Some of these concerns are quite valid. In a study on preoperative anxiety in women, one woman talked about her lungs collapsing during surgery as a child and about how frightened she was about the required use of a ventilator to assist her breathing during her upcoming surgery (Wiens, 1998). Chapter 47 discusses this nursing diagnosis fully.

Focused Assessment for Anticipatory Grieving

Anticipatory grieving is the expectation by the client that he or she will experience a disruption in familiar patterns concerning other people, possessions, job, status, home, and parts and processes of the body after surgery. Anticipatory grieving is the grief response seen in a client anticipating a personal loss. Chapter 50 provides more information about loss.

Focus the preoperative assessment to determine the sequence of subjective states in which there is the expectation of, or actual, loss of life, bodily function, or activity. Discussing with the client the type of loss expected, feelings about control of the situation, and his or her usual patterns of coping with loss leads to individualizing the plan of care for the client.

Clients consenting to surgery for removal of a body part (internal or external) often grieve before surgery because of this anticipated loss. As an example, it is common for a woman to grieve before mastectomy for the expected loss of her breast. For many, the loss of a breast signifies the loss of femininity.

Focused Assessment for Risk for Latex Allergy Response

Focused assessment of risk factors will help you identify clients who need the nursing diagnosis *Risk for latex allergy response*. An accurate assessment of the client's past experience is imperative to identify those at risk for a systemic reaction, such as stories of complicated anesthesia events, hives from blowing up a balloon, or severe swelling of the labia with a urinary catheterization.

When latex glove use was dramatically increased in the late 1980s with the advent of Universal Precautions (now called Standard Precautions), latex allergies response became much more common. Basically, every health care worker wears gloves. Most gloves are powdered to facilitate donning. The powder adsorbs protein allergens from latex gloves and deposits them on skin and into surgical wounds; it also aerosolizes the protein allergens. Aerosolized latex allergens are carried in ventilation systems and cause further need for prevention measures.

Latex allergy is classified into three categories: irritant reaction, type IV allergic reaction, and type I allergic reaction. The most commonly recognized is actually a nonallergic irritant reaction. Type IV allergic reactions to latex are a cell-mediated response to the chemical irritants found in latex products. The true latex allergy is a type I allergic reaction and occurs shortly after exposure to the proteins in latex rubber. Type I reaction is an IgE-mediated systemic reaction and occurs when latex proteins are touched, inhaled, or ingested.

Factors influencing the diagnosis *Risk for latex allergy response* are the person's susceptibility and the route, duration, and frequency of latex exposure (Kleinbeck et al., 1998). Risk factors for latex allergy response include the following:

- History of anaphylactic reaction of unknown etiology during a medical or surgical procedure
- Multiple surgical procedures (especially from infancy)
- Food allergies (specifically kiwi, bananas, avocados, chestnuts)
- A job with daily exposure to latex (medical, nursing, food handlers, tire manufacturers)
- Conditions needing continual or intermittent catheterization
- History of reactions to latex (balloons, condoms, gloves)
- Allergy to poinsettia plant
- History of allergies and asthma

Focused Assessment for Knowledge Deficit

The nursing diagnosis *Knowledge deficit* means the client or family is demonstrating an inability to learn and comprehend information about the surgical experience or inability to perform skills as needed to improve the client's level of wellness. Knowledge deficit of perioperative activities related to a lack of exposure is a common nursing diagnosis during the preoperative phase of care and may continue throughout the client's surgical experience in some form.

Identify the client's learning needs and you can individualize the plan of care through the determination of related factors. At times, *Knowledge deficit* may be related to psychosociological barriers, such as denial of a health situation, the impending surgery, or both. Many times knowledge deficits occur because it is the client's first surgical experience (Fig. 57–3). The client may have received inaccurate information or be unable to understand information concerning the surgi-

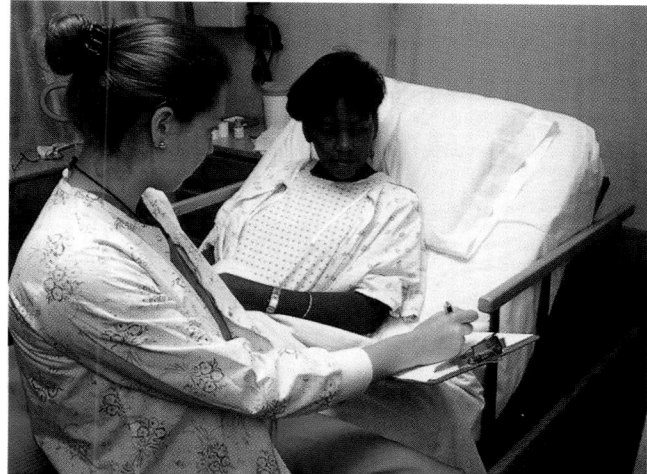

Figure 57–3. Many times, knowledge deficits occur when the client is undergoing her first surgical experience.

cal experience related to the mode of presentation (such as when you talk faster than the client can follow). When the client denies the illness or injury, he may have a lack of desire to learn about the surgical experience. Anxiety also has a strong effect on a client's ability to learn and is a common denominator for knowledge deficit in the surgical client.

DIAGNOSIS

Cluster data as suggested in the data clustering chart on the preoperative assessment of the surgical client to

identify nursing diagnoses and related factors for the client and family. Diagnosis gives direction for specific care interventions provided during the surgical experience. Preoperative nursing care includes the physical and psychological care given before a surgical procedure to promote comfort and prevent complications during or following surgery. To effectively manage the course of a surgical client, preventive care is essential. The nature and type of surgery, as well as the client's health status, affect the choice of nursing diagnoses.

In the preoperative phase, the client may experience emotional distress that can affect his or her surgical experience in numerous ways. Risk factors may be present without the client presenting signs and symptoms. Many preoperative nursing diagnoses reflect assessment of potential risk and are made to provide interventions to also meet client needs during the intraoperative and postoperative phases. Nursing care throughout the perioperative period must be consistent and documented, as the preoperative nursing diagnoses are the basis for consistent holistic care from admission through recovery. Preventive care is essential to manage the surgical client effectively. The nature and type of surgery, as well as the client's health status, suggest defining characteristics for many diagnoses.

PLANNING

The planning process includes setting priorities, establishing client goals or expected outcomes, and selecting nursing interventions for care of the surgical client. The focus of perioperative nursing is to minimize the

---

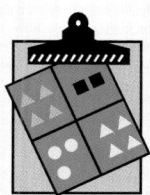

CLUSTERING DATA TO MAKE A NURSING DIAGNOSIS
PERIOPERATIVE PROBLEMS

Data Cluster	**Diagnosis**
A 26-year-old registered nurse in outpatient clinic for cervical cone biopsy discussing preoperative data with the admitting nurse. Recent rash on her hands, swelling of eyelids at end of each day at work, and allergic to bananas.	*Risk for latex allergy response* related to history of recent sensitivity to latex items and history of allergies
A 71-year-old librarian diagnosed with breast cancer weighs 88 pounds and is 5'3" in height. Scheduled for mastectomy this morning.	*Risk for perioperative positioning injury* related to emaciated state
A 2-day-old infant for heart defect repair that requires only 40 minutes to repair.	*Risk for altered body temperature* related to extreme of age and lack of organ development
Client says, "I can't go home! I'm so sick and need extra help." Refuses to get out of bed and complete morning care. Abdominal incision healing without complications.	*Delayed surgical recovery* related to perception of needing more time to recover in the hospital setting

client's risks before and during surgery to maximize the potential for positive outcomes during postoperative recovery. However, the overall goal of the preoperative phase is that the client is psychologically and physically prepared for surgery. Specific expected outcome criteria to evaluate achievement of these goals and the effectiveness of nursing interventions follow.

Expected Outcomes for the Client With Anxiety

The overall expected outcome for the preoperative client experiencing *Anxiety* is that the client will demonstrate, both verbally and behaviorally, a decrease in anxiety. The client may verbalize the experience of anxiety, describe past coping methods that were successful, exhibit a reduction in physical symptoms of anxiety, interact with others in a focused manner, or choose a decisive course of action from a list of alternatives.

Since *Anxiety* may be present throughout the entire perioperative period, the expected outcomes that the client attains may be new methods of coping with stress and controlling anxiety. Some examples of outcome criteria include identifying sources of anxiety, describing symptoms of increasing anxiety, verbalizing long-term coping strategies (exercise, meditation, relaxation techniques), and discussing methods to enlarge or make use of an existing support system.

Expected Outcomes for the Client With Anticipatory Grieving

The outcome expected for *Anticipatory grieving* is that the client will adjust or adapt to the expected loss and reinvest energy and activities in living a productive and meaningful life. This would be a progressive movement through stages of grief toward resolution and adaptation to the diagnoses, treatment regimen, and possible surgical outcome.

Expected Outcomes for the Client With Risk for Latex Allergy Response

The outcome for a client with the nursing diagnosis *Risk for latex allergy response* is that the client will not experience a latex allergy response. This outcome includes all classifications of latex allergy: irritant reaction, type IV reaction, and type I reaction.

Expected Outcomes for the Client With Knowledge Deficit

The expected outcome for the diagnosis *Knowledge deficit* is that the client verbalizes adequate knowledge and understanding of expected preoperative procedures and care, intraoperative routines, and procedures to be performed postoperatively to prevent complications. Teaching is continued and reinforced throughout the

entire surgical experience. Refer to Chapter 16 for further information on teaching the client.

For the surgical client, outcomes for the preoperative phase include communication of a lack of knowledge and desire to know, setting of realistic learning goals, and expression of new knowledge and decreased anxiety related to fear of unknowns, misconceptions, or misinformation.

Outcomes for the intraoperative phase include description of the surgical procedure and its purpose in general terms, identification of routine monitoring to be done intraoperatively, and verbalization of events and sensations expected in the OR.

Outcomes for the postoperative phase include accurate demonstration of desired postoperative skills (use of incentive spirometer and turning-coughing-deep breathing [TCDB] exercises), verbalization of expectations and understanding of usual postoperative pain control and alternative comfort measures (patient-controlled analgesia [PCA] pump usage and splinting incision), discussion of signs and symptoms of wound infection, and verbalization of lifestyle modifications needed to follow prescribed postoperative regimen.

INTERVENTION

The perioperative nurse performs nursing interventions according to the priorities established for the nursing diagnoses. The focus of preoperative intervention is to assist the client with both psychological and physical preparation for surgery and postoperative recovery. Many of these interventions are continued throughout the client's surgical experience.

Interventions to Reduce Anxiety

Because most clients experience some form of *Anxiety* when confronted with surgery, help the client identify the source of his or her anxiety and suggest strategies for managing the anxiety. Interventions should focus on providing information about the impending surgery, clarifying misinformation the client may have, teaching the client relaxation techniques, helping the client explore the source of anxiety, and communicating the client's psychosocial status to the other health care team members. Include interventions that provide support to the client, particularly during the immediate preoperative period. Gentle physical contact, a quiet and unhurried environment, soothing words, and provision of amenities, such as a warm blanket and head phones for listening to music, help the client deal with his anxiety.

Anxiety level will influence how you prepare the client preoperatively. The purpose of preoperative teaching is to help decrease client anxiety that might result from a lack of information about the surgery. Because of short hospital stays, discharge teaching must be initiated during the preoperative period. Be aware of the effects of anxiety on learning and allow time for repetition, reinforcement, and verification of the client's understanding.

Preoperative information helpful to most clients relates to preoperative tests and activities, events related to the surgery itself, and what will happen in the postoperative phase of surgery. Clients are less anxious and participate more readily if they know the reasons for perioperative activities. Allowing clients to participate in decision making concerning their care when that is a realistic option helps the client maintain some control over the perioperative events.

Teach clients activities that help to decrease anxiety and to gain a sense of control. The most common approaches include relaxation exercises, music therapy, and guided imagery. Use therapeutic communication skills and techniques to establish a supportive and trusting nurse-client relationship and to facilitate psychological safety and security. Listen carefully, give the client time to talk, and watch for clues of disabling anxiety. Provide an empathetic, private environment for the client to cry and express anger. The client may also be provided preferred music or a familiar personal object to soothe anxiety.

Interventions to Promote Functional Grieving

When a client is confronted with surgery and a perceived loss, grieving on a functional level is necessary, as well as physically and emotionally healthy. Conversely, dysfunctional grieving has a negative impact on the well-being of the client. Dysfunctional grief can lead to physical and psychological imbalance.

Identify *Anticipatory grieving* and help the client move along the grief continuum to a point where he or she is able to deal with the stressors of surgery. Assist the client in identifying with the grief and understanding that grieving is common. Discuss the stages of grieving with the client and provide encouragement to set goals in response to the expected loss. This enhances the client's understanding of the normalcy of grief and his or her ability to cope.

If defining characteristics of *Anticipatory grieving* are present, document and communicate the findings to the appropriate members of the health care team such as psychologists, pastoral services, and social workers. Encourage the client to seek help from these resources. Listen and show empathy if the client exhibits behaviors such as crying, anger, or sorrow. This shows concern, understanding, and support for the client. If not contraindicated because of the client's cultural practices, establish body contact with the client by touching the hand or shoulder and explain that feelings of loss are normal.

Interventions to Prevent Latex Allergy Response

To provide a latex-safe environment for susceptible clients, all surgical clients should be screened for the *Risk for latex allergy response* before admission. Identifica-

tion of clients at risk is the initial step in providing prevention.

When a client with a suspected or known latex allergy is scheduled for surgery, all potential risk areas (latex use) are avoided and the client is admitted directly to the OR as the first case of the day if possible. Many facilities have converted isolation rooms into latex-safe environments for care of the perioperative client with latex allergy. Ensure that everyone on the health care team is aware that a client is, or may be, latex allergic. Place a medical alert band or allergy band around the client's wrist and clearly flag the chart about the latex reaction status. Remove all natural rubber latex products from a known or suspected latex-allergic client's care area. Use latex-free pharmaceutical measures to prepare the client's medications. Have a crash cart standing by stocked with latex-free equipment, supplies, and drugs for treating anaphylaxis. As ordered, give prophylactic treatment with glucocorticoid steroids and antihistamines to latex-allergic clients preoperatively. Box 57–2 lists interventions for the care of perioperative clients with a risk for latex allergy response.

The risk for the health care worker becoming sensitized to latex ranges from 8 to 17% (Kim et al., 1998). You need to know about the risks of latex to protect clients, latex-sensitive colleagues, and yourself. Wash,

---

BOX 57–2

RESPONDING TO A CLIENT'S RISK FOR LATEX ALLERGY

Latex-Alert Client (High Risk for Allergic Response)

- No required premedications.
- No special pharmaceutical protocols required.
- Use nonlatex gloves.
- Use latex-safe supplies.
- Keep a latex-safe supply cart available in client's area.

Latex-Allergy Client (Suspected or Known Allergic Response)

- Administer prophylactic treatment with steroids and antihistamines preoperatively.
- Prepare a latex-safe environment, include latex-safe supply cart and crash cart.
- Apply cloth barrier to client's arm under a blood pressure cuff.
- Use medications from glass ampules.
- Do not puncture rubber stoppers with needles.
- Wear synthetic gloves.
- Use latex-free syringes.
- Use latex-safe (polyvinyl chloride) IV tubing.
- Do not use latex preparation on IV bags.

rinse, and dry hands thoroughly after removing gloves or between glove changes. Never wear oil-based lotions with latex gloves. Oil breaks down latex, damages the glove as a barrier, and releases additional allergens. Non-oil-based products are compatible with latex.

Interventions to Increase Client Knowledge

Assess the client's level of understanding and willingness to learn to determine the level of *Knowledge deficit* before implementing preoperative teaching. Minimally, knowledge concerning surgical routines, nothing-by-mouth (NPO) requirements, TCBD exercises, wound site splinting, postoperative pain management, postoperative leg exercise, and discharge instructions should be identified. Go over written material with the client. Validate comprehension of the information by asking questions and requesting return demonstrations. Remember that anxiety can interfere with comprehension.

Teaching postoperative activities is done in the preoperative phase and is the nurse's responsibility. Clients and families need to know about the surgical events and sensations, how to manage pain, and how to perform the physical activities necessary to decrease postoperative complications and facilitate recovery. The teaching-learning process should be individualized to meet both specific and common needs of surgical clients.

The timing of teaching is a significant consideration; teaching that is done too far in advance of surgery or when the client is highly anxious will be less effective. Many facilities provide preoperative teaching sessions prior to admission so that the client is prepared for surgery. Whether done before or after admission, a preoperative teaching checklist gives nurses organized and comprehensive guidelines for instruction. Check at your clinical facility to see an example of teaching items found on a preoperative checklist.

Teaching the Client About Surgical Events and Sensations

Clients and their families need to know when surgery is scheduled, approximate length of surgery, time spent in the recovery room, and what will be done before, during, and after surgery. An explanation of surgical events includes a description of the various members of the perioperative health care team. Preparatory information helps clients and their families anticipate the steps of a procedure and form a realistic mental picture of the surgical experience. When events occur as predicted, the client is better able to cope.

Clients also need to know about sensations typically experienced before, during, and after surgery. Informing the client about sensations in the OR will reduce anxiety before the client is anesthetized. Sensations will differ depending on the type of surgery, but teaching should include descriptions of the following:

- Feelings experienced from preoperative medications, such as drowsiness and a dry mouth

- Sights and sensations like bright lights and cold temperatures that are commonplace in the OR
- Information about the numerous monitoring devices that will be placed on the client before being anesthetized, such as a blood pressure cuff, pulse oximeter, and ECG pads
- Sensations that normally occur after surgery and anesthesia, such as a sore throat from an endotracheal tube, blurred vision from ophthalmic ointment, incisional pain, and tightness of the dressings

Teaching the Client About Pain Management

Pain is an expected and normal part of the surgical experience and an area of great concern for the client and family. Inform the client that pain medicine will be available to assist with pain management postoperatively. Encourage the client to use the pain medication as often as needed to achieve an optimal activity level postoperatively. Surgical clients may avoid taking pain medications for fear of becoming addicted. The client should be informed that most drug dosages and the required intervals between them are not sufficient to cause dependence.

Pain medications allow the client to manage pain and raise his ability to carry out activities and exercises necessary to recovery. Explore with the client effective coping mechanisms used to manage pain such as medications, position changes, back rubs, wound splinting, relaxation, biofeedback, and warm moist or dry heat applied to the painful site. Introduce the client to the technique of rating pain on a scale of 0 (no pain) to 10 (worst possible pain) to allow the nurse and client better communication and evaluation of pain management.

If intramuscular or oral analgesics will be used, the client needs to know the schedule for these drugs. Pain medications usually are ordered on an as-needed (p.r.n.) basis, with a time restriction between doses (such as every 3 to 4 hours). Pain medications are usually given parenterally for the first few days and as long as a client is NPO; with food intake and decreasing pain levels, oral pain medications are then administered.

Patient-controlled analgesia (PCA) is commonly used and provides the client with control over pain. The PCA medications may be either intravenous or via epidural catheter. Instruct the client on how to operate the PCA pump and the importance of self-administering medication as soon as pain becomes noticeable and prior to any activity. If the client or nurse waits until the postoperative pain is at an excruciating level, an analgesic will not provide relief. The time intervals between doses and the amount of medication that can be used within a given period are programmed into the device. You are responsible for assessing the effectiveness of the pain relief. Alternate methods of pain control are also encouraged for use with the PCA for better relief of pain after surgery (Fig. 57–4). Chapter 42 discusses pain in detail.

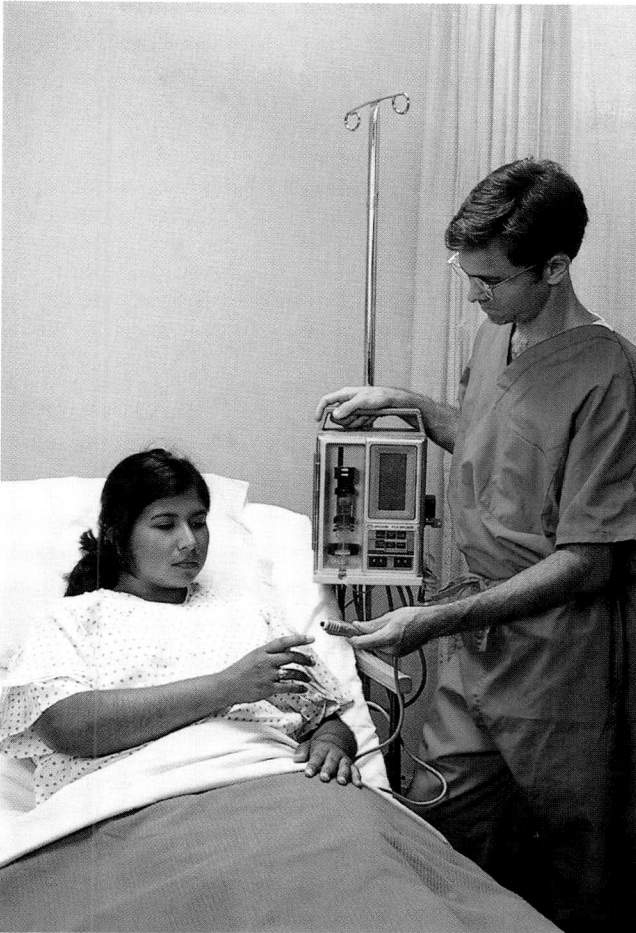

Figure 57–4. Teach the client how to operate the PCA pump, stressing the importance of self-administering pain medication as soon as pain becomes noticeable.

Teaching the Client About Postoperative Physical Exercises

Given a rationale for postoperative activities and procedures, the client is better prepared to participate in his own care. Every preoperative teaching program should include explanations and demonstrations of postoperative exercises designed to prevent postoperative complications. The most common causes of postoperative complications are pulmonary and cardiovascular alterations, including atelectasis, pneumonia, thrombophlebitis, and emboli.

Pulmonary complications are the leading cause of postoperative morbidity and mortality. The two most common postoperative pulmonary complications after abdominal or cardiothoracic surgery are nosocomial pneumonia and atelectasis. Brooks-Brunn (1997) identified risk factors having a significant association with postoperative pulmonary complications. It was significant to have two or more of these risk factors:

- Age 60 or over
- Impaired preoperative cognitive function
- History of smoking in previous 8 weeks
- History of cancer

- Incision above or both above and below the umbilicus
- Body mass index of 27 or greater (healthy index is 18 to 25)

Physical activities to decrease the potential for complications are taught in the preoperative phase. The client should be able to verbalize and demonstrate the activities prior to surgery. TCDB and leg exercises are described subsequently.

TURNING EXERCISES
Turning in bed improves venous return and respiratory function and increases gastrointestinal peristalsis. Incisional pain makes moving and turning in bed difficult and this activity should be practiced before surgery. The client should turn from side to side every 2 hours.

COUGHING
Coughing facilitates removal of retained mucus from the respiratory airways and usually is taught in conjunction with the deep-breathing exercise. A deep cough is more beneficial than merely clearing the throat. The client must anticipate incisional discomfort and understand the importance of coughing. Splinting an incision minimizes pain during coughing exercises (Fig. 57–5). Advise the client to perform exercises during the period when pain medication has reached its peak effectiveness.

DEEP BREATHING
While under general anesthesia, the cough reflex is suppressed, mucus accumulates in the tracheobronchial passages, and the lungs do not fully ventilate. After the surgical procedure, respirations are often less effective because of the anesthesia, pain medications, and pain from the incision. As a result, alveoli do not inflate and may collapse and secretions are retained, increasing the potential for atelectasis and pneumonia.

Diaphragmatic breathing improves lung expansion and oxygen delivery without using excess energy. The client learns to use the diaphragm during deep-

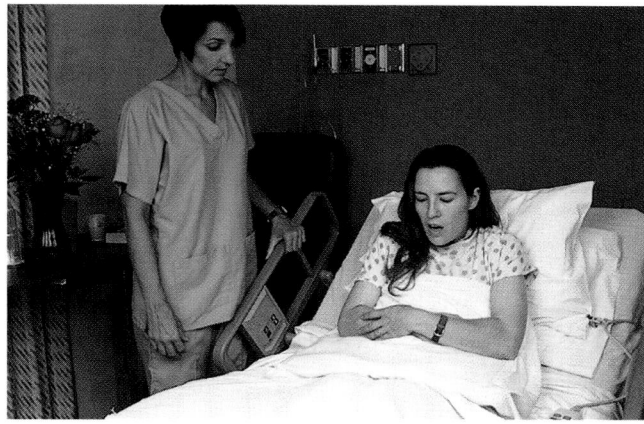

Figure 57–5. Preoperatively, teach the client to splint her incision to minimize pain during coughing.

breathing exercises and eventually the client's lung volume improves.

To facilitate deep-breathing, the physician often orders an incentive spirometer for the client's use. Incentive spirometry encourages forced inspiration and helps reinflate collapsed alveoli and remove secretions. The therapy is effective in preventing postoperative atelectasis. Chapter 39 discusses respiratory function in depth.

LEG EXERCISES

During surgery, venous blood return from the legs slows; some surgical positions also may decrease venous return. Postoperative bedrest potentiates this decreased venous blood return, and venous stasis occurs. With circulatory stasis of the legs, thrombophlebitis and resultant emboli are potential complications. Leg exercises increase venous return through flexion and contraction of the quadriceps and gastrocnemius muscles.

Leg exercises should be encouraged 10 to 12 times every 1 to 2 hours. These exercises should be done with you assisting the client for the first 24 to 48 hours after surgery and as necessary thereafter, depending on risk factors and the client's status. Crossed legs, pillows behind the knees, and elevation of the bed's knee gatch must be avoided. Leg exercises must be individualized to client needs, physical condition, physician preference, and hospital protocol.

Some surgeons routinely order elastic stockings or mechanical sequential compression devices to stimulate and enhance the actions to the veins when leg muscles contract. These aids are useless if the legs are not exercised and may actually impair circulation if the legs remain inactive or the stockings or devices are inappropriately sized or applied.

Teaching the Client About Preoperative Physical Preparation

The physical preparation of the preoperative client depends on the client's health status, type of surgical procedure, and physician's orders. You, as the nurse, are responsible for the preparation and safety of the client on the day of surgery in the areas of nutrition and fluid balance, skin preparation, elimination, and rest and sleep. Independent as well as interdependent nursing interventions will be needed to prepare the client physically for surgery.

MAINTAINING NUTRITION AND FLUID BALANCE

Clients need to be well nourished and hydrated prior to surgery to counteract the fluid and electrolyte loss intraoperatively and to promote healing postoperatively. Preoperative assessment data provide the information for individualizing interventions regarding the need for preoperative supplemental nutrition, fluids, or electrolytes. If the client's laboratory results show a hemoglobin level of less than 10 g/dL and hematocrit less than 30%, blood may be ordered by the physician to be given preoperatively to maintain volume and increase oxygenation of tissues during surgery.

The diet ordered for the preoperative client will depend on the type of procedure and the choice of anesthesia. Clients having general anesthesia or major regional anesthesia are placed NPO up to 8 hours before the surgery. Approximately 6 hours of fasting leaves the client's gastrointestinal tract relatively empty of food content, so the risks for vomiting or aspirating emesis during surgery are minimized greatly by the NPO status. The risk for aspiration of gastric fluids still remains. You should explain the rationale for being NPO, remove all food and fluids from the bedside, and place a sign above the bed to notify others of the restriction. The client who is at home the night before surgery must also understand the importance of not taking food or fluids and be willing to follow these restrictions. Notify the surgeon and the anesthesiologist if the client eats or drinks during this fasting period.

It is common practice to give antacids (to raise gastric fluid pH) or histamine blockers (to decrease gastric acid production) to high-risk clients, such as those with obesity, pregnancy, traumatic injury, intestinal obstruction, hiatal hernia, or active gastrointestinal bleeding, on the morning of surgery. This is a measure to prevent damage to tracheobronchial mucosa if aspiration occurs. There are other situations in which the client will be allowed to take oral medications, either preoperative or maintenance, with sips of water while on NPO status preoperatively.

PREPARING THE SKIN

An alteration in skin integrity, such as a surgical incision, provides a potential site for infection. Surgical site infections are the second most common type of nosocomial infection and account for close to one third of all hospital-acquired infections. Surgical site infection is a risk for all perioperative clients and is considered during each phase of the surgical experience.

Without proper skin preparation, the risk for the development of a postoperative skin infection increases. Bathing the evening before surgery with an antimicrobial or bacteriostatic soap, with particular attention to the proposed surgical site, is believed to reduce the incidence of postoperative wound infections. If the surgery involves the head, neck, or upper chest area, the client may be required to shampoo the hair.

The incisional site is usually shaved prior to surgery since hair is a reservoir for bacteria. Wet or dry razor shaves, hair clippers, or depilatory creams may be used to remove hair. Shaving the skin was once done the night before surgery, but is now most often done immediately before the procedure in the surgical holding area. This change in practice is based on findings that the increased time for growth of bacteria raises potential for infection. Each agency or facility should have policies and protocols regarding the timing, method, and people responsible for the preoperative skin preparation of surgical clients. Preoperative nursing actions taken to reduce the potential for infection include proper client preparation to reduce the amount of pathogenic organisms.

PREPARING THE BOWEL AND BLADDER

Use assessment data to establish the preoperative baseline related to the client's elimination pattern and determine the need for an order for further bowel elimination. If the client has not had a bowel movement for several days or has had barium diagnostic testing, an enema helps prevent postoperative constipation. Bowel surgery, such as a colon resection, often necessitates a preoperative bowel evacuation to empty the bowel of feces, as an empty bowel prevents contamination of the surgical area during surgery. Manipulation of the bowel during abdominal surgery results in absence of peristalsis for up to 24 hours and sometimes longer. Enemas and cathartics cleanse the gastrointestinal tract to prevent incontinence and contamination during surgery.

The bladder is usually not prepared until immediately prior to surgery. Instruct the client to void just before transferring to the holding room. If the client has to void after receiving preoperative sedative medications, a bedpan or urinal is provided to prevent injury from falls. An empty bladder minimizes incontinence during surgery. Indwelling urinary catheters increase the risk for urinary tract infections and are not routinely inserted for all surgical procedures. However, a catheter may be placed for clients undergoing intestinal, gastrointestinal, obstetrical, and gynecological surgery. It is important for the bladder to remain empty and decreased in size during these procedures to avoid injury to the bladder when the surgeon is working in the pelvic region. Indwelling catheters, if ordered, are usually inserted in the OR immediately after the client has been anesthetized.

PROMOTING REST AND SLEEP

Rest and sleep are important for reducing stress before surgery and are essential for normal healing and recovery after surgery. Promote rest and sleep in the preoperative phase by assisting the client in meeting psychological needs, by providing a quiet environment, and by keeping to the client's usual bedtime routine as much as possible. Frequently the physician orders a sedative-hypnotic or antianxiety agent to be taken the night before surgery. An advantage to ambulatory or same-day surgery is that the client is able to sleep at home the night before surgery and will probably sleep better in the familiar environment.

ENSURING PHYSICAL READINESS

The day of surgery preparation varies greatly depending on whether the client is admitted to a facility or presents as an ambulatory surgical client. If the client is previously admitted to the hospital, you provide the physical readiness of the client for surgery. If ambulatory status, the client or family member will share in the preoperative preparation activities. Immediately before surgery, you are responsible for the final preparation of the client, as well as determining that all orders have been carried out and that the medical record is complete and ready to accompany the client to the OR.

A preoperative checklist outlines the responsibilities on the day of surgery, and these activities must be completed before the client is transferred to surgery (Box 57–3). This list helps to ensure that no preoperative detail has been omitted that may affect the client's intraoperative and recovery periods. It is especially important to determine that all preoperative orders

---

BOX 57–3

EXAMPLES OF ITEMS ON A PREOPERATIVE CHECKLIST

Day Before Surgery

(Check the items that are completed and document why if not complete)

☐ Consent forms: Admission, general, surgical, anesthesia, blood
☐ Allergies: Medications, foods, environmental, latex
☐ History and physical on chart or dictated
☐ Admission database in chart
☐ Pre-anesthesia evaluation completed
☐ Old chart obtained
☐ Lab work completed and results in chart
☐ Blood ordered: type & screen, type & crossmatch, no. of units, autologous, directed donor
☐ ECG results in chart
☐ X-ray results in chart or films with chart
☐ Surgeon notification if abnormal lab work
☐ Advance directives
☐ Addressograph plate on chart

Day of Surgery

(Check the items that are completed and document why if not complete)

☐ NPO since: _____
☐ Voided/catheter emptied
☐ Shave/skin prep (nail polish, makeup, and hairpins removed)
☐ Antiembolism stockings/sequential compression device
☐ Dentures, hearing devices, contacts/glasses, prosthesis, jewelry
☐ Preoperative teaching completed and documented
☐ IV started and infusing
☐ Preoperative medications administered and documented

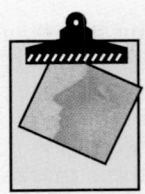

NURSING CARE PLANNING
A PREOPERATIVE CLIENT

Preoperative Data

Mr. Warren is scheduled for surgery in 5 days. He is in the preadmissions office of the hospital's admitting area. The preoperative nurse is gathering assessment data and assisting Mr. Warren with preoperative preparation. He has many questions about the intraoperative and postoperative events of his surgical experience. Mr. Warren states that his doctor told him the reasons for the surgery and the outcome probabilities. He knows what the doctor is going to do and why but is unsure of the rest of the process. Mr. Warren's daughter acts as translator periodically because of his heavy Jamaican patois.

Physician's Orders

Admit morning of scheduled surgery
Surgical procedure: nerve sparing radical retropubic prostatectomy
Admitting diagnosis: prostate cancer
Routine preoperative labs: CBC with differential, chest x-ray, ECG, prothrombin and partial thromboplastin time, type and crossmatch with 4 units specify available, creatinine, blood urea nitrogen, electrolytes
Attach last week's ultrasonography report, biopsy results, urology studies, and office labs
NPO
Finger stick glucose testing at 7:30 AM
Pentobarbital 100 mg IM on call to OR
Start IV 1000 mL D$_5$ Lactated Ringer's at 100 mL/hr
To OR with thigh-high anti-embolism stockings and sequential compression stockings

Nursing Assessment

61-year-old Jamaican man diagnosed with prostate cancer. Awake, alert, and oriented ×3 and to situation. History of arthritis and recently diagnosed with diabetes. Says he takes no medications for diabetes. Takes occasional aspirin for arthritis pain—"Only when it flares up." No complaints of arthritis pain at present. Reports last aspirin dose 2 weeks ago. Takes no vitamins or dietary supplements. However, does take some herbals: sarsparilla tea for arthritis and corn silk tea for bladder problems. Denies ingestion of herbs over last 2 weeks. Anesthesia informed of herbal usage. Temperature 98.4°F, pulse 84, respirations 20, BP 138/88 sitting. Skin intact, warm, and dry with pink, moist oral mucosa. Lungs clear bilaterally. Heart sounds regular in rate and rhythm. Abdomen soft, nondistended, with normoactive bowel sounds auscultated. No complaints of pain, only comments about slow flow of urine, difficulty in starting stream, and occasional burning with urination. Reports recent notice of vague heavy feeling in his back. Asking multiple questions about perioperative course of events. Wife and daughter in attendance. Daughter translates some of her father's phrases for clarity. Scheduled for prostatectomy in 5 days. This is client's first surgical experience.

Continued

and procedures have been completed and documentation is complete before any preoperative medications are given to the client. Verify the presence of a signed informed consent for surgery, laboratory data, history and physical examination report, baseline vital signs, and completed nurse's notes.

Prosthetic devices of any type may be damaged or lost during surgery. Therefore, the client must remove all removable prosthetics, including partial and complete dentures and artificial eyes and limbs. If the client has a brace, check with the surgeon to determine whether the brace should remain on the client during surgery.

In some agencies, nurses inventory all removable client devices and secure the items. It is common for family members to keep the items, or you may secure the devices at the client's bedside or in the facility's safe. Refer to institutional policies regarding securing the client's personal items.

Removing dentures can be embarrassing for the client; therefore, if dentures are to be removed prior to surgery, privacy should be offered. Document and inform surgical team members of the client's feelings about removal and of denture location. Dentures are placed into a container labeled with client's name for safekeeping after removal. In some instances, dentures

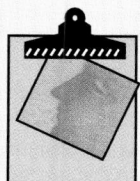

NURSING CARE PLANNING
A PREOPERATIVE CLIENT *(continued)*

NURSING CARE PLAN

Nursing Diagnosis	Expected Outcomes	Interventions	Evaluation
Knowledge deficit related to perioperative care events related to lack of exposure secondary to first surgical experience	Will describe four events that occur in holding area and OR.	Provide teaching booklets "Prostate Surgery and You" and "The Surgical Experience" *Encourage daughter to read booklets.*	Handed booklets to daughter and asked for verbalization about the areas and the events. Discuss perioperative course of events.
		Explain events that will occur in holding area (e.g., shave prep, monitoring vital signs) and in OR (e.g., cold, OR bed, anesthesia)	Listened intently and looked at daughter frequently. Held wife's hand. Asked questions during and at end of the explanation.
	Will describe routine postoperative nursing care events.	Explain and demonstrate common activities that occur postoperatively in the PACU and on the surgical unit (monitoring, catheter care, activity, diet, pain control, sequential compression stockings)	Client asked questions regarding catheter and compression stockings. Stated he understood.
	Will demonstrate postoperative exercises, splinting, and use of patient-controlled analgesia (PCA) pump.	Demonstrate turning-coughing-deep breathing (TCDB) exercises, splinting incision, and PCA pump usage	Daughter emphasized the PCA usage to her father. Client return-demonstrated all activities properly.

Italicized interventions indicate culturally specific care.

Critical Thinking Questions

1. Why do you think Mr. Warren handed the booklets about his surgery and surgical experience to his daughter? How would you determine the usefulness of the booklets to Mr. Warren?
2. Mr. Warren is from Jamaica and plans to recuperate at his daughter's home in Atlanta after discharge from the hospital. What other teaching may be needed related to home care?
3. Prostatectomy can sometimes cause impotence. How would you approach discussion about postoperative sexual activities and coping with possible sexual dysfunction?

are left in place until after the first stages of anesthesia. Having well-fitted dentures in place can provide a better seal for ventilation prior to intubation in the OR.

Anything in or around the eye may irritate or injure the eye during surgery; therefore contact lenses, false eyelashes, and eye make-up must be removed. Glasses and hearing aids are also removed; for the severely hearing impaired, this should not be done until immediately after induction of anesthesia. Allowing the client to be able to see and hear with the use of these aids facilitates communication and raises the client's sense of control in the preoperative setting.

EVALUATION

Evaluate preoperative outcomes before the client goes to surgery, as suggested in the accompanying Nursing Care Planning chart. Evaluation of several outcomes continues into the postoperative period. Frequently, there is limited time for evaluation, as the client's surgery may be emergent, or tests are barely completed by the time the client is sent to surgery. The plan of care for a preoperative client is effective and the outcomes are met if the client is physically and emotionally prepared for surgery.

INTRAOPERATIVE PHASE

The intraoperative phase of the client's surgical experience begins when the client enters the OR and ends when he is transferred to a recovery area. The perioperative nurse is the client's advocate during surgery. Knowledge of the client gained through assessment provides information necessary to provide care specifically for that client. You, the perioperative nurse, compensate for the client's inability to provide self-care by devising a nursing care plan to protect the client during surgery.

The holding area is busy with numerous clients and health care personnel talking and doing various activities of preparation. Mr.

Warren has spoken with the surgeon and has been thoroughly assessed by anesthesia personnel and the circulator. His lower abdominal incision site has been shaved. Intravenous fluids are infusing and the CRNA just gave another medication through the line. Mr. Warren is very drowsy but is holding his wife's hand very tightly. His daughter is rubbing his forehead. The circulating nurse arrives at his side and announces it is time to go for his procedure. His family kiss him and he is taken to the OR suite prepared for him by the CRNA and the circulator.

During his assessment, the circulator determines that *Risk for perioperative positioning injury* is an important nursing diagnosis for Mr. Warren. Why might that be an appropriate diagnosis, given Mr. Warren's health history? What other nursing diagnoses might be appropriate?

INTRAOPERATIVE NURSING DIAGNOSES

Risk for Infection: The state in which an individual is at increased risk for being invaded by pathogenic organisms.

Risk for Perioperative Positioning Injury: A state in which the client is at risk for injury as a result of the environmental conditions found in the perioperative setting.

Risk for Injury: A state in which an individual is at risk of injury as a result of environmental conditions interacting with the individual's adaptive and defensive resources.

Risk for Altered Body Temperature: The state in which an individual is at risk for failure to maintain body temperature within normal range.

From North American Nursing Diagnosis Association. (1999). NANDA nursing diagnoses: Definitions and classification 1999–2000. Philadelphia: Author.

ASSESSMENT

The focus of nursing care during this phase is to ensure client privacy and safety. Maintaining a safe environment includes protecting the client from injury, infection, and complications arising from anesthesia and the surgery itself.

The holding area, a unit usually connected to the OR suites, is where the surgical team further prepares the client for surgery. The circulator is usually the first member of the surgical team encountered by the client. Assessment activities and certain interventions are conducted in the holding area before the client is taken to the OR suite.

General Assessment of the Intraoperative Client

Assessment data are obtained from a combination of chart review, client and family interviews, observations, and physical and psychosocial assessments. The intraoperative assessment of the client begins with verification and analysis of preoperative data to determine priority of care. A nursing history and brief

physical examination are usually completed immediately prior to the surgery.

Health History

While the client is in the holding area, establish baseline assessment data for intraoperative and postoperative care. The assessment data provided by the client and data from the nursing units (outpatient and inpatient) are important. The preoperative assessment information, preoperative checklist, type of surgery scheduled, and immediate client needs influence the intraoperative plan of care. You may also carry out immediate preoperative care, possibly including skin preparation, starting intravenous fluids, and giving medications.

Chart assessment and identification of the surgical client requirements vary with each facility, client condition, and specific surgical procedures. This assessment activity is a final validation of medical record contents and identification of the client and surgical site. The following is usually included in this validation process:

- Identification of the client
- Identification of the surgical site

- History and physical examination report
- Operative consent form
- Preoperative medications
- Last intake of food and fluids
- Urinalysis
- Pregnancy status
- Complete blood count and electrolyte values
- Chest x-ray and electrocardiogram
- Values or beliefs that may require intraoperative care adjustments
- Communication impairments
- Location of valuables and prostheses
- Location of family and significant others

Physical Examination

Physical assessment data important to intraoperative nursing care include vital signs, height, weight, age, allergic reactions, condition of skin, skeletal and muscle impairments, perceptual difficulties, level of consciousness, and any source of pain. Baseline vital signs are important data when anesthetics and other drugs are administered. The surgical team is guided by height and weight of the client regarding dosages of anesthetic drugs and even for the width and length of the operating table. Age can indicate special needs for clients, such as warming units/lights for neonates or special padding for the frail skin of elderly clients. Allergic reactions can be avoided with measures as simple as a change in the solution to prepare the skin or as extensive as providing a latex-safe environment for latex-allergic clients. The condition and cleanliness of the skin determine the amount and type of intraoperative skin preparation and will alert the surgical team to the potential for infection or skin integrity breakdown. Knowledge of skeletal and muscle impairments helps prevent positional injuries. Vision or hearing impairments may lead you to adapt communication techniques to meet individual client needs. Increased safety measures may be necessary when a client presents with an altered mental status or decreased level of consciousness. Identify and communicate sources of pain to others in the surgical team to prevent unnecessary discomfort for the client.

Once the client has been properly identified and thoroughly assessed, discuss the next step in his care with some details and basic information about the operating room itself. Fear of the unknown, fear of losing control, and misconceptions can increase the client's anxiety. Perceptions about surgery can still be influenced quite significantly at this point.

Transport the client from the holding area into the operating room prepared specifically for that client's surgical procedure. The client is usually still awake and will see several people in complete surgical attire, which includes masks, protective eyewear, gowns, and sterile gloves. There are rows of shiny, silver instruments on tables and the room is cold. Provide emotional and physical support to the client by providing reassurance, further explanations, warm blankets, and a caring touch on the hand or shoulder. De-

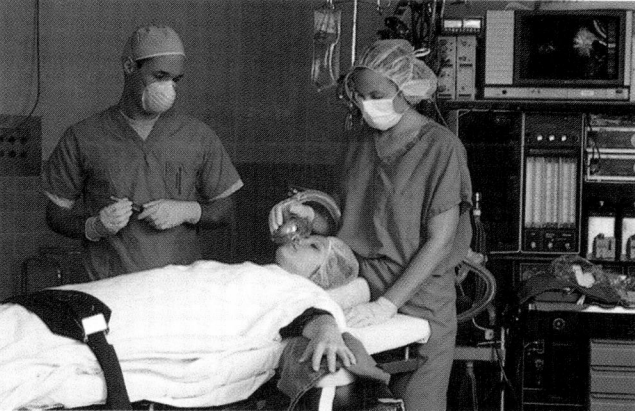

Figure 57–6. During induction of anesthesia, stand by the client and provide reassurance.

pending on the type of procedure, assist the client to the operating bed and place a safety strap across the client's thighs. The surgical procedure will begin after induction of anesthesia and positioning of the client takes place. As the circulating nurse, assist the anesthesia provider with the induction of anesthesia and intubation. Stand by the client and reassure him while at the bedside (Fig. 57–6). Fear of never awakening and fear of the unknown are uppermost in the client's mind at this time. Your presence will reduce anxiety and provide emotional support during induction. Remain as the client's advocate throughout this intraoperative stage of care through continued assessment and intervention of the client's physical and emotional status.

Mr. Warren is transported to the OR via stretcher. He is assisted to the OR bed. What steps should the nurse take to ensure client safety and warmth?

Focused Assessment for Risk for Infection

The skin, which is the body's first line of defense, is violated by a surgical incision. Although the incision is aseptically created and controlled, the risk for wound infection is increased by the presence of a portal of entry for pathogenic microorganisms. Other factors that may indicate a higher chance for postoperative infection, such as those listed subsequently, should also be assessed.

Definition

The intraoperative nursing diagnosis *Risk for infection* is defined as the accentuated risk of invasion of a surgical wound by pathogenic organisms from either exogenous or endogenous sources. Exogenous infection is acquired from organisms outside the client's body. Endogenous infections come from the large number of microorganisms found in and on the client's body.

Risk Factors

Besides the skin incision, other risk factors that can influence a client's risk for wound infection include malnutrition, obesity, extremes of age, inadequate tissue perfusion (large blood loss), history of exposure to infectious diseases and inadequate secondary defenses (immunosuppression, reduced hemoglobin concentration, leukopenia), substance abuse, wound classification (contaminated or infected), and a break in surgical aseptic technique.

Focused Assessment for Risk for Perioperative Positioning Injury

Positioning of the client for surgery is one of the most important aspects of perioperative nursing. Surgical positioning is securing the client's body into a place that allows for optimal exposure of surgical site and the least compromise in both physiological functions and mechanical stresses. The client is vulnerable to positioning injury, particularly when the procedure is performed under general anesthesia. Physiological, musculoskeletal, and integumentary systems can be severely compromised at a time when the client is unable to alert you to a problem.

Assessment relative to positioning includes gathering data about the scheduled procedure, age, height, weight, activity level, muscle tone, nutritional status, skin condition, and cardiopulmonary status. Assess skin status of clients of all ages with particular attention to the very young and the very old. Assess medical history, pre-existing mobility, and range of motion. Principles of client positioning are grounded in knowledge of anatomy and physiology, range of motion (ROM), vulnerable points and positions, and nursing assessment.

Definition

When the client is at risk for injury as a result of the environmental conditions found in the perioperative setting, the nursing diagnosis of *Risk for perioperative positioning injury* is made. During surgery and owing to surgical positioning, the accentuated risk of impaired gas exchange, neuromuscular impingement, vascular compromise, or tissue injury is possible for all clients.

Risk Factors

The degree of risk for positioning injury depends on whether the client receives general or regional anesthesia, on the type and length of procedure, on the required position, and on the client's overall condition at the time of surgery. Anesthetic agents and muscle relaxants depress the pain and pressure receptors and cause loss of tone and muscle relaxation. The normal defense mechanisms cannot guard against joint damage and muscle stretch and strain. When an anesthetized client is positioned with exaggerated range of motion, injury may occur. Evidence of hyperextension injury can range from mild postoperative discomfort to dislocation.

During surgery, clients are immobile and cannot reposition themselves to relieve discomfort from prolonged pressure. The period of immobility is even longer than the length of the surgical procedure, given that prolonged pressure may begin with sedation, include the time the client is in the preoperative area, during surgery, and in the immediate recovery period. Therefore, surgery is one of the few times when a client who is not normally at risk for pressure ulcers is at high risk. Anesthetic agents also disrupt normal vasodilation and constriction, decreasing the perfusion to bony prominences.

Figure 57–7 illustrates some common perioperative positions and the padding provided to relieve pressure in each position. Extreme positions such as Trendelenburg, in which the head and upper body are lower than the feet, affect circulation and oxygen–carbon dioxide exchange. Positions can also decrease compliance of the lung and the ability of the thoracic cage to expand, with hypoventilation resulting.

Because anesthetics commonly cause dilation of peripheral vessels, venous blood tends to pool in areas that are dependent. During some procedures, extremities may be in a dependent position for an extended amount of time, causing significant pooling to occur.

Administration of anesthetics also results in nervous system depression. As a client advocate, you must be aware that when nervous system depression takes place, the body's compensatory actions are no longer functioning. Failure to recognize and relieve pressure to peripheral nerves may result in minor sensory motor loss to permanent paralysis.

Other *Risk for perioperative positioning injury* factors include chronic diseases, vascular surgery (blood perfusion may already be compromised by the client's disease process), existing or previous trauma or injury, paralysis and muscle weakness or motor deficits, impaired immune function, and an altered metabolic or nutritional state.

Focused Assessment for Risk for Injury

Besides perioperative positioning injury, the possibility of injury to the client during the intraoperative phase of the surgical experience may be related to retained foreign objects or electrical or burn hazards. The OR is one of the most technically driven areas in a health care facility and contains sophisticated and potentially hazardous equipment. Safe practices in the use of supplies, instrumentation, and electronic devices will prevent needless injuries.

Extraneous objects such as sponges, sharps (needles, blades), and instruments left inadvertently in the client during surgery can result in postoperative pain, infection, obstruction, extended hospital stay or readmittance, additional surgery and cost, and delayed surgical recovery. One way to reduce the potential for retained foreign objects is surgical counts.

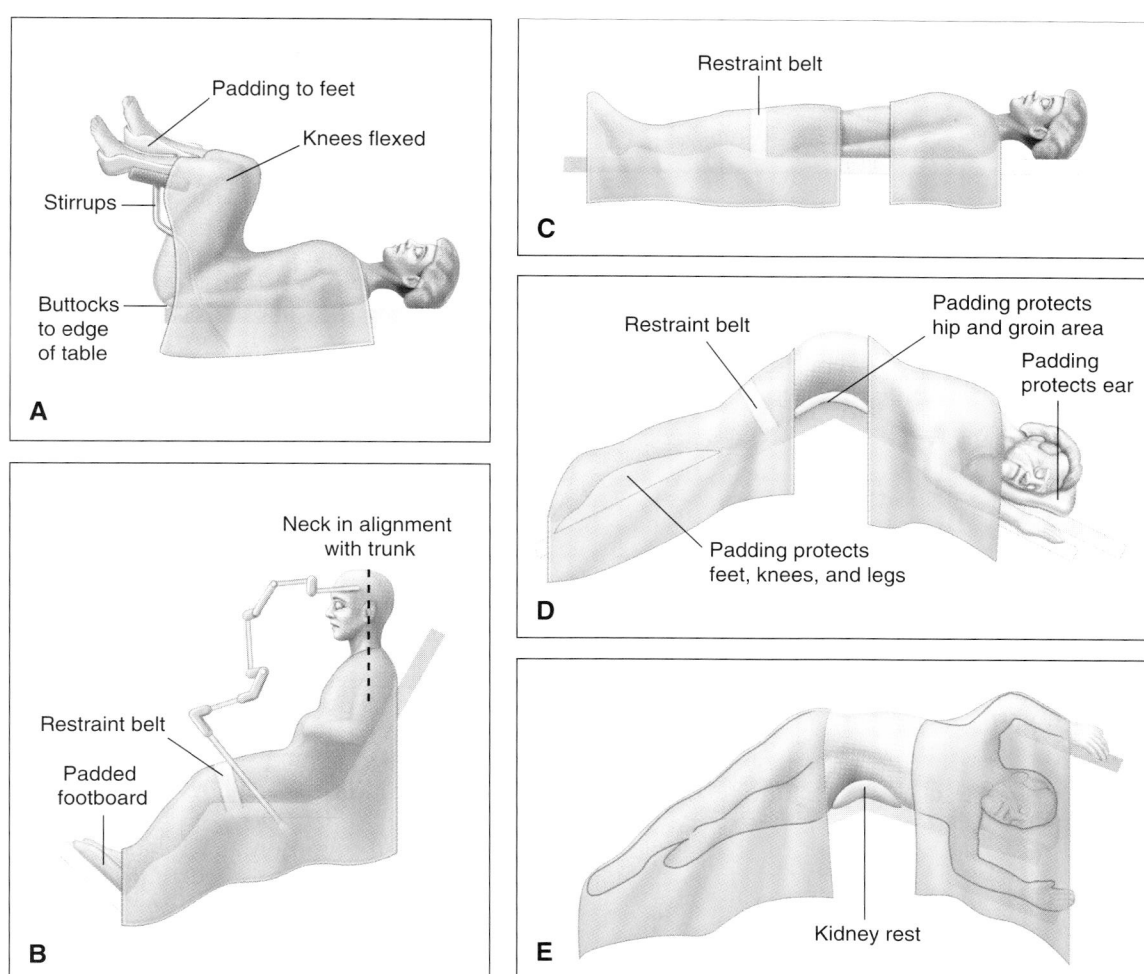

Figure 57–7. Common perioperative positions and the padding provided to relieve pressure in each position. *A,* Lithotomy position, used for vaginal and perineal procedures. *B,* Sitting position, used for neurological procedures. *C,* Supine position (the most common position). Potential pressure points are the occiput, scapula, olecranon, thoracic vertebrae, sacrum, coccyx, and calcaneus. *D,* Jack-knife position, used for gluteal and anorectal surgeries. *E,* Lateral kidney position, used for procedures requiring a retroperitoneal approach.

Recommended Practices for Perioperative Nursing: Counts—Sponge, Sharp, and Instrument (AORN, 1999) advises that sponges, sharps, and instruments be counted for all surgical procedures, that counts be documented, and that counting be enforced through institution policy and procedure. The need for bypassing surgical counts exists only in extreme emergency situations and should be documented as such.

Electrocautery as a means of controlling bleeding is practiced routinely in most of the surgical cases today. Radiofrequency electrical current is passed through the body for the purpose of cutting tissue or coagulating bleeding tissues by a hand-held *active electrode* (commonly called Bovie or cautery). The amount of power and the type of current (cut, coagulate, combination), are regulated by controls on the electrocautery unit and the active electrode. A grounding pad, or *dispersive pad,* is provided to complete the electrical circuit through the body and back to the generator or the electrosurgical unit. Injuries can occur at the dispersive site, at the active

electrode, or elsewhere, such as ECG electrode sites or a body part touching metal.

Lasers provide another method for hemostasis during surgery. Lasers deliver high-beam energy directly onto tissues. The water in cells evaporates so quickly that the cell actually explodes and vaporizes. This thermal effect cuts, cauterizes, and sterilizes tissue. Laser use during surgery is the responsibility of the entire surgical team. Lasers can cause thermal reactions that can lead to fire, skin burns, and optical damage by either direct or scattered radiation. Specific laser safety precautions must be followed to prevent injury.

Definition

The diagnosis *Risk for injury* is defined as a state in which a person is at risk of injury as a result of environmental conditions interacting with the client's adaptive and defensive resources. The use of sponges, sharps, instruments, and electrical devices, inherent to the OR environment, constitutes environmental risk.

Risk Factors

Risk factors related to retained foreign objects include the following:

- The complexity of the procedure
- Depth of the surgical wound and the body cavities or organs opened
- An emergency procedure that precludes counts
- Intraoperative hemorrhage that requires immediate use of multiple uncounted sponges
- Change of nursing staff during the procedure

Risk factors related to electrical or burn hazards on the electrosurgical unit include the following:

- Excessive body hair, scar tissue, or damaged tissue
- Presence of internal metal prosthetic device at the dispersive site
- Obesity (fat does not conduct electricity as well as muscle tissue)
- Use of ECG lead pads and rectal temperature probes
- Exposed metal touching client's skin (includes heavy metal jewelry at pierced sites)
- Defective grounding pad or inappropriate pad placement

Risk factors related to electrical or burn hazards on the laser unit include the following:

- Movement during laser operation
- Use of reflective instruments (refracts the laser beam)
- Inadequate eye protection for the client (surgical team's eyes can be injured as well)
- Use of dry sponges at laser site of operation
- Use of non–laser safe endotracheal tube during respiratory or digestive tract surgery
- Use of flammable skin preparation agents
- Use of flammable draping materials

Focused Assessment for Risk for Altered Body Temperature

All intraoperative clients are at risk for alteration in body temperature regulation. Hypothermia is the most common alteration and is described as a core body temperature below 95°F (35°C). Hyperthermia is when an individual's body temperature is elevated above 99°F and is not as commonly seen in the intraoperative setting.

Anesthetic agents interfere with the body's temperature-regulating mechanism and metabolic rate, causing hypothermia. Exposure to a cool or cold environment, medications causing vasodilation, inadequate clothing, evaporation from skin in cool environment, decreased metabolic rate, inability or decreased ability to shiver, and inactivity are all intrinsic to the OR. Research indicates that 90% of surgical clients experience some degree of hypothermia (Huber & Slade, 1999). Intraoperatively induced hypothermia causes postoperative complications that lengthen time spent in the PACU and potentially lengthen hospital stays. Complications include postoperative vasoconstriction and shivering, with increased postoperative pain, impaired wound healing, increased clotting time resulting in postoperative bleeding, decreased drug metabolism and clearance, and increased cardiac output.

Signs that indicate hypothermia include reduction in body temperature below the normal range, pallor, cool skin, cyanotic nail beds, piloerection (goosebumps), slow capillary refill, tachycardia, and hypertension. Assess the client for malnutrition, extremes of age, chronic illness, or trauma, as these conditions further increase the risk for hypothermia.

Anesthetic agents may also trigger a hyperthermic response known as malignant hyperthermia. **Malignant hyperthermia** (MH) is a rare, autosomal dominant inherited syndrome that is life-threatening. It is triggered by anesthetic inhalation agents and neuromuscular blocking medications used to induce general anesthesia. It is characterized by a rapid rise in temperature, with temperatures rising as high as 110°F (Dunn, 1997).

The syndrome or crisis may develop during induction of anesthesia, 12 hours after receiving anesthesia, and may recur up to 48 hours after treatment (Vermette, 1998).

A delay in recognition and treatment can result in sudden death of the surgical client from cardiac arrest, brain damage, body system failure, or disseminated intravascular coagulation (Dunn, 1997).

Definition

Altered body temperature is the state in which a person is at risk for failure to maintain body temperature within the normal range. All surgical clients are at risk for hypothermia during the intraoperative phase of care. It is uncommon to see hyperthermia as a complication intraoperatively, but when it occurs it can be a serious problem for the client.

Risk Factors

High-risk clients include those with altered metabolic rate, illness or trauma, medications causing vasoconstriction or vasodilation, inappropriate clothing for environmental temperature, inactivity, extremes of weight, extremes of age, dehydration, and sedation, and those with family history of malignant hyperthermia and endocrine disorders. Cold solutions such as intravenous fluids, skin preparation solutions, and wound irrigation solutions add to the risk for hypothermia. Hyperthermia may occur from overuse of heating blankets and heating lamps or from malignant hyperthermia. Clients at risk for MH usually have large, bulky muscles and muscular defects as seen in inguinal hernias and ptosis. MH is most often seen in children and men.

*A*ction *A*lert!

If a client develops malignant hyperthermia, bring the MH cart right away. Immediately assist with termination of anesthesia and surgery. Assist the anesthesia provider by preparing drugs from the MH cart. Dantrolene sodium is the primary drug given during the crisis. Prepare to begin active cooling. Use iced saline to lavage any open body cavities, and cool the body further with cooling blankets and ice packs at the groin, neck, axillae, and head.

DIAGNOSIS

Nursing diagnoses from the preoperative phase are reviewed after the intraoperative assessment and modified to individualize the care plan for the client in the operating room. Additional diagnoses are added to provide direction for the intraoperative and postoperative care of the client. Client problems common during the intraoperative period are potential nursing diagnoses, and prevention of these problems is essential. These possible diagnoses are related to the incision, OR environment, effects of anesthesia, and the provision of client comfort, safety, and support during the intraoperative period.

PLANNING

The overall focus of intraoperative planning is the safety of the client. During the planning of care, the environment, equipment, and supply needs are prioritized according to the availability of assessment data. Procedural basics for the surgical team's care of the client can be anticipated based on the client's age, scheduled procedure, and surgeon's preferences of instrumentation and supplies. Once the client is assessed, an individualized plan of care is made.

Expected Outcomes for the Client With Risk for Infection

The expected outcome for the diagnosis *Risk for infection* is that the client remains free from surgical site infection. Surgical asepsis will be maintained during the client's surgical procedure. The client's temperature will remain below 100°F with other vital signs and laboratory values remaining within normal limits. The incision site will be free of erythema, induration, undue tenderness, and purulent drainage. The edges of the incision maintain approximation, and dehiscence of the wound will not occur.

Expected Outcomes for the Client With Risk for Perioperative Positioning Injury

The outcome for *Risk for perioperative positioning injury* is for the client to remain free from injury related to positioning during surgery. This includes the following outcome criteria:

- Effective breathing patterns with no restrictions to ventilation

- Adequate cardiac output with no significant episodes of hypertension or hypotension
- Surgical positioning that facilitates adequate gas exchange and maintains adequate ventilation/perfusion ratio
- Skin integrity maintained to avoid physical breakdown
- No evidence of neurological musculoskeletal or vascular compromise, including numbness, tingling, weakness, or pain of positioned limbs not present preoperatively
- No alteration in tissue perfusion, such as reddened, ulcerated, edematous, or excoriated skin areas

Expected Outcomes for the Client With Risk for Injury

The outcome for the client with the diagnosis *Risk for injury* is for the client to remain free from injury related to retained foreign objects or electrical or burn hazards. The client will not have any retained sponges, instruments, or sharps following wound closure—unless such placement was deliberate and recorded. The client will be free from injury related to the use of electrical equipment as evidenced by absence of skin lesions, burns, neuromuscular damage, and signs of electrical shock.

Expected Outcomes for the Client With Risk for Altered Body Temperature

The expected outcome for the client with *Risk for altered body temperature* is that the client will maintain core body temperature ranging from 97.3°F to 98.8°F during perioperative care. The client also shows no complications associated with hypothermia, such as soft tissue injury, dehydration, or hypovolemic shock when rewarmed. Any genetic disposition for malignant hyperthermia is known and there will be no diaphoresis, shivering, or tachycardia. Adequate oxygen will also be delivered to tissues.

INTERVENTION

The *Standards and Recommended Practices for Perioperative Nursing* (AORN, 1999) describe standards of perioperative care and provide specific guidelines for perioperative nurses to ensure positive outcomes for surgical clients. Among these guidelines, recommendations for instrument and supply sterilization, use of aseptic technique principles to create a sterile field, prevention of physical injury, and adequate skin preparation of the surgical client are provided. Follow these standards, recommended practices, and specific hospital policies during perioperative nursing intervention. Interventions for the aforementioned nursing diagnoses will be based on the AORN *Standards and Recommended Practices.*

Interventions to Prevent Infection

Decrease risk for wound infection by using sterile technique and following recommended practices and your facility's policies. Interventions that reduce the client's potential for developing surgical site infections include maintaining a sterile field and monitoring and controlling the client's environment. Initiate corrective measures when a break in technique occurs, as contamination of the sterile field may lead to wound contamination and subsequent infection.

Classify the surgical wound according to the degree of contamination of the wound and surrounding tissue (Table 57–8). Classification helps to assess the risk of wound infection from an endogenous source and determine the need for antibiotic therapy.

Administer antibiotics as ordered because intraoperative administration of antibiotics can reduce the incidence of wound infection and lessen its severity. The presence of pathogenic microorganisms is verified by processing intraoperative aerobic and anaerobic cultures for laboratory analysis.

Timeliness and preparedness of the surgical team can decrease operative time, thus reducing the amount of time a client has an open surgical wound. Also, it is important to ensure that all surgical team members wear appropriate operating room attire, as the human body is a major source of microbial contamination. Maintain an operating room temperature of 68° to 75°F (20° to 23.9°C) and a relative humidity at 50% ± 10%, unless contraindicated, because cooler air temperatures and lower humidity inhibit microbial growth.

The surgical skin preparation is intended to prevent introduction of exogenous microbes into the incision site and should incorporate aseptic technique. Intraoperative routines for skin preparation should also comply with institutional protocol. The AORN *Recommended Practices for Skin Preparation* of clients may be used to base a generic plan of care for operative site preparation before the incision is made (AORN, 1999). An ideal skin preparation agent should be easy to apply, dry quickly, and deliver broad-spectrum antimicrobial protection throughout the duration of the surgery. The choice of antimicrobial agent and skin preparation technique may vary from institution to institution.

Assess and document the condition of the client's skin before beginning the skin preparation. Allergies, especially to chemicals, should be documented. Maintain the client's privacy by exposing only the area to be prepared. Don sterile gloves. The area of the "prep" should be wide enough to include the surgical site and a substantial area surrounding it. The center of the sterile field is the surgical incision site. Start the preparation at the incision site, moving outward in continually expanding circles away from the surgical site and not returning to the original site with the prep sponge. Time, area, solutions used, and skin condition are charted. After preparation of the skin, sterile members of the surgical team drape the area intended for incision. Only the site to be incised is left exposed.

The perioperative nursing documentation provides necessary data for further intervention to prevent postoperative infection. It is important to communicate to other health care members through verbalization and documentation. Document nursing assessments, interventions, and outcomes during the operative procedure. Documentation includes the operative procedure, type of anesthesia, surgical times, wound classification, antibiotics given, presence of packing, drains, indwelling catheters and other invasive devices, implants and tissue or organ transplants, type of dressing applied, estimated blood loss, and evaluation of each expected outcome. Most facilities have forms that ensure that the appropriate documentation of nursing process is carried out.

Interventions to Prevent Perioperative Positioning Injury

Positioning the client for surgery is a shared responsibility. The surgeon, perioperative nurse, and anesthesia provider all communicate to determine positioning needs. Positioning usually follows induction of general anesthesia and when an alternative anesthetic technique (such as regional or local) is used, then the anesthesia provider indicates the time for positioning of the client to protect the integrity of the airway. Positioning should provide physiological alignment for all points, while at the same time providing protection from the sequelae of pressure, abrasion, prolonged stretching or compression of nerves, and other injuries. When positioning the client for surgery, pay particular attention to the following goals:

- Provide for adequate thoracic excursion
- Provide for correct body alignment

TABLE 57–8
Surgical Wound Classifications

Type of Wound	Definition
Clean	• No break in aseptic technique. • Gastrointestinal, genitourinary, or respiratory tract not entered. • No inflammation present.
Clean-contaminated	• Minor break in aseptic technique. • Gastrointestinal, genitourinary, or respiratory tract entered without spillage.
Contaminated	• Major break in aseptic technique. • Gross spillage from gastrointestinal tract or infected biliary or genitourinary tracts.
Dirty-infected	• Acute inflammation present. • Traumatic wound with devitalized tissue or foreign body. • Fecal contamination with delayed treatment. • Established infection before surgery.

- Prevent pressure on bony prominences, skin, and eyes
- Prevent occlusion of arteries and veins
- Avoid stretching and compression of nerve tissue
- Avoid unnecessary exposure of the client's body
- Allow for previously assessed aches, pains, or deformities

Provide adequate padding, positional devices, and support for the client during positioning for surgery. Possible pressure areas and bony prominences are given special attention and may be given extra padding to prevent complications. There are numerous positions in which the client may be placed. The supine position is the most common position used. The lithotomy position is used for pelvic and perineal surgeries. The prone position provides access for back surgeries (laminectomy). Other positions include Trendelenburg, lateral, kidney, jack-knife, and sitting.

Attachments and padding are used to keep extremities within the client's anatomic range of motion. The position of extremities and positioning devices should be rechecked during longer procedures to ensure no displacement has occurred. Monitor and document the circulation to all four extremities. During long surgical procedures, intervene with changes in the client's position at least every 2 hours to increase circulation and relieve pressure at pressure areas to prevent circulatory compromise and intraoperatively acquired pressure ulcers.

Action Alert!
Protect all bony prominences and pressure areas carefully. You have a key role in recognizing and preventing intraoperatively acquired pressure ulcers. Pressure ulcers that develop in the OR typically develop 1 to 3 days postoperatively. The damage from intraoperative pressure originates deep within the tissues at the bone and not on the skin surface like other pressure ulcers.

Interventions to Prevent Injury

Perform sponge, sharp, and instrument counts according to institutional protocol. Perform counts at change of shift or during any personnel relief. Only x-ray detectable sponges are used in the wound. Items deliberately left in the body are documented, such as nasal packing. When an incorrect count occurs, inform the surgeon and recount. Enlist all surgical team members to assist in locating the missing item. Common policy is that if a count remains incorrect after search, an incident report is filed, and an x-ray is taken. If the x-ray reveals the retained object, appropriate measures are taken to retrieve it, and surgery is completed. Document counts taken, any corrective action, and results of subsequent counts.

During the preparation for the client's procedure, check all electrical equipment and alarms for proper working order. Assess the client's skin integrity before and after electrosurgical unit use, especially at posi-

tional pressure points and under the dispersive pad. If the client is repositioned at all during the procedure, reconfirm the integrity of the dispersive pad placement. Position the client free from contact with metal surfaces.

Following surgery, remove the dispersive pad slowly to prevent denuding of the skin. Check the client for incidental burns with particular attention given to ECG electrode sites.

The perioperative nurse ensures that only qualified personnel operate the laser, provides a safe and properly functioning laser unit, monitors the use of protective devices, and protects the client and surgical team from laser injury. Cover the eyes of the client with appropriate cover and follow all precautions for the use of lasers.

Interventions to Prevent Altered Body Temperature

The most common body temperature alteration seen in the OR is hypothermia. The cool OR environment, the client's inactivity and lack of clothing, extensive and invasive surgical procedures, and decreased metabolic rate from drugs all lower the client's body temperature. There are several intraoperative interventions to preserve or even increase the client's temperature. Place warm coverings on the client's body, extremities, and head. A warming blanket (hyperthermia unit) may be placed on the OR bed, if not contraindicated by the need for x-rays during the procedure. Use warm saline irrigation to decrease the amount of body core temperature loss. Heat lamps may also be used to provide additional warmth. Continuous temperature monitoring is important. If large volumes of intravenous fluids are given, provide a fluid warmer unit.

EVALUATION

Upon closure of the wound and placement of a sterile dressing, perform a postoperative evaluation of the client as outlined in the accompanying Nursing Care Planning chart. Document specific evaluative findings on the intraoperative record. Evaluation data will continue to be gathered postoperatively because some complications (e.g., wound infection) may occur days after the procedure. Intraoperative care of the client focuses on risk management and prevention of injury related to anesthesia, positioning and equipment, environment, and the actual surgical procedure itself. The intraoperative nurse's notes are documentation of client care in the OR.

The plan of care for an intraoperative client is effective and outcomes are met if the client is physically safe and complications are prevented. However, responsibility to the client does not end for the perioperative nurse in the OR with the application of a sterile dressing. Perioperative nursing care continues during the postoperative phase.

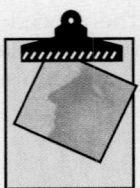

NURSING CARE PLANNING
AN INTRAOPERATIVE CLIENT

Intraoperative Data

Mr. Warren is transported via stretcher to his OR suite. He notices how cool it is and comments on all the equipment and masked people he sees. The circulator reminds him that his room was specially prepared for him and that she will be with him from start to finish. They reach OR #14 and go through the double doors. The nurse and anesthesia personnel help Mr. Warren move safely over to the OR bed. A safety strap is applied and warm blankets are placed over him. He states that he puts himself in God's hands and holds the circulator's hand tightly. Mr. Warren breathes deeply from the oxygen mask that is placed over his mouth and nose.

Physician's Orders

Insert 22 Fr. Foley cath to drainage
Use prostatectomy procedure card for routine orders and particulars for this surgeon

Nursing Assessment

Mr. Warren, a 61-year-old Afro-Caribbean man, was admitted this AM for nerve-sparing radical retropubic prostatectomy with admitting diagnosis of prostate cancer. Prostate ultrasound, biopsy, and urology reports in chart. Other lab results within normal limits. 4 units O-negative blood available. Height: 5'10" Weight: 220. History of arthritis and recently diagnosed with diabetes. Glucose test reading: 148 at 7:30 AM. Reports on no medications with occasional aspirin usage. Last aspirin usage 2 weeks ago. Ambulatory with full range of motion to extremities. Finger joints slightly enlarged with minimal decrease in range of motion. No complaints of joint pain, just stiffness reported. States recent "heavy feeling" in his lower back. NPO since last night. IV infusing left forearm. Voided "best I could" prior to leaving preop admitting area. TED hose and sequential stockings on client, who states "keeping me warm." Skin intact, dry and slightly cool to touch. Provided warm blankets and OR cap for head. Peripheral pulses palpable and equal. Wife and daughter at side of stretcher before transfer to OR. To OR #14 via stretcher.

NURSING CARE PLAN

Nursing Diagnosis	Expected Outcomes	Interventions	Evaluation
Risk for perioperative positioning injury related to history of arthritis and diabetes	Will remain free from injury related to positioning during surgery.	Assess mobility and range of motion (ROM), skin integrity, and neurovascular status before positioning.	Decreased joint movement in hands and feet. Shoulder and hip ROM full, but client complains of feeling stiff—arthritis. Reports recent lower back discomfort. Diabetic. Skin integrity intact.

Continued

POSTOPERATIVE PHASE

The immediate postoperative phase of nursing care begins as soon as the surgical procedure is concluded. The postoperative course involves both the immediate postoperative period and the ongoing postoperative convalescence. For an ambulatory client, the immediate postoperative period lasts only 1 to 2 hours and convalescence will occur at home. For a hospitalized client, the immediate postoperative period may last several hours, with convalescence taking 1 or more days in the hospital setting, depending on the extent of surgery and the client's response. Further recovery will then take place at home or perhaps in a long-term care facility.

ASSESSMENT

Assessment of postoperative clients includes the critical variables that affect recovery and convalescence. Knowledge of preoperative condition, anesthesia type, length of operation, amount of blood loss, and the organ system involved in the surgery will help direct the plan of care for the postoperative client. You must be skilled at recognizing change in the client's status, as

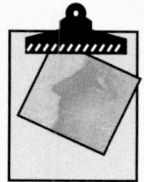

NURSING CARE PLANNING
AN INTRAOPERATIVE CLIENT *(continued)*

NURSING CARE PLAN

Nursing Diagnosis	Expected Outcomes	Interventions	Evaluation
		Reassess mobility and ROM, skin integrity, and neurovascular status 24 hours postoperatively.	Client expressed no complaints of pain, numbness, or change in ROM. Able to raise arms above head. No pressure point signs of breakdown. Will reassess in 48 hours.
	Skin integrity maintained with no physical breakdown.	Use special high-risk positioning aids for extra support and padding during care.	Placed gel pads at occiput and sacrum, foam protectors to heels and elbows, and pillow under knees. No signs of redness or excoriation noted post procedure. Will re-evaluate in 72 hours.
	No evidence of neurological, musculoskeletal, or vascular compromise.	Compare preop assessment data to postop assessment data 24 hours after surgery.	Peripheral pulses remained intact and same during perioperative course. No numbness, tingling, or pain reported. No signs of skin breakdown. Will re-evaluate in 48 hours.

Critical Thinking Questions

1. Why do you think the antiembolism stockings and the sequential compression device are in place during the surgical procedure? Does the length of the procedure make a difference to the client's circulation? Why or why not?
2. The nurse took extra precautions with the client when positioning. Why would you consider Mr. Warren to be at risk for positioning injury?
3. Once the client is in final position, the perioperative nurse should do an overall check to ensure that positioning will not cause injury. Describe at least four factors that the perioperative nurse should assess.

any variation from normal may be the onset of complications. Therefore, assessment is key in prevention of postoperative complications.

General Assessment of the Immediate Postoperative Client

While applying humidified oxygen and various monitoring devices (such as a cardiac monitor, pulse oximeter, or blood pressure cuff), perform a rapid initial assessment of the client's airway, breathing, and circulatory adequacy immediately upon receiving the client in the PACU. The anesthesia provider

gives a report to the PACU nurse about the client's surgical status. The American Society of PeriAnesthesia Nurses (ASPAN, 1995) recommends that a comprehensive report from anesthesia providers include the following:

- Relevant preoperative status (vital signs, laboratory values, allergies)
- Anesthesia technique used during the procedure
- Type of surgical procedure performed
- Anesthetic agents used
- Length of time anesthesia was administered
- Time that reversal agents were given
- Estimated blood loss and replacement fluids given

The circulating nurse corroborates previously reported data about the preoperative status of the client and includes information about the presence of tubes, drains and catheters, wound status, any surgical complications, and the types of communication with the client's family members. During this report, the client is continuously monitored.

After reviewing events occurring in the OR, assess the client's status on a continual basis and initiate interventions immediately as needed. The PACU nursing care plans are designed to do the following:

- Determine the client's physiological status at the time of admission to the PACU
- Re-evaluate the client so that physiological trends become apparent
- Establish the client's baseline parameters
- Assess the ongoing status of the surgical site
- Assess recovery from anesthesia
- Compare current client status with discharge criteria

The goal of postanesthesia care is to identify actual and potential client problems that may occur as a result of anesthetic administration and surgery and to intervene appropriately. ASPAN (1995) has defined *Standards of Postanesthesia Nursing Practice* to guide the PACU nurse in the care of adult, pediatric, and geriatric clients. Care of the immediate postanesthesia client usually occurs over a 1- to 3-hour period. Assisting the client to a safe physiological level of function after anesthesia is the main objective, with basic care prioritized in relation to the client's airway, breathing, and circulation. Common postoperative problems in the immediate recovery stage include airway compromise, respiratory insufficiency, cardiac compromise, neurological compromise, hypothermia, pain, and nausea and vomiting.

Action Alert!
Laryngospasm is a respiratory emergency caused by reflex contractions of the pharyngeal muscles, which cause spasms of the vocal cords and prevent the client from a positive-pressure inspiration. Signs and symptoms include dyspnea, hypoxia, hypoventilation, absence of breath sounds, and hypercarbia. Laryngospasm requires immediate response and intervention. Hyperextend the client's head and begin positive-pressure ventilation. Medications that are used in the treatment of laryngospasm include lidocaine, steroids, and atropine. Endotracheal intubation is required if the laryngospasm persists or if hypoxia cannot be corrected.

The client may be discharged from the PACU to an inpatient unit, intensive care unit, ambulatory care unit, or home. The choice of the site will be based on client acuity, access to follow-up care, and the potential for postoperative complications. Clients are ready for discharge from the PACU when they have demonstrated recovery from the effects of anesthesia; have a patent airway, stable vital signs, and minimal wound or other drainage; have returned to preoperative level of consciousness; have adequate urinary output; and

have no unresolved acute problems. Following evaluation and documentation of the client's condition, the client is discharged according to written protocols and discharge criteria. Many times, a numeric scoring system is used to reflect the client's readiness for discharge.

Ongoing General Assessment of the Postoperative Client

Mr. Warren is transferred by nurses from the stretcher to his bed in a semi-private room. He spent 2 hours in the PACU prior to transfer. He remains drowsy but responds appropriately to questions and simple commands. Mr. Warren hums, sings, and dozes. Vital signs remain stable. His abdominal dressing is dry and intact, with a Jackson-Pratt drain on the right side collecting bright red bloody drainage. He has a Foley catheter in traction and patent with pink to red urine draining. No clots in the tubing are noted. IV fluids are infusing, and PCA is in use. The client is not complaining of pain upon transfer. What immediate postoperative teaching about PCA would be appropriate for Mr. Warren? What nursing diagnoses might be appropriate for Mr. Warren in the immediate postoperative phase?

The client is received in the unit room and safely transferred to a bed by the PACU nurse and the unit nurse. Report is given about the client's surgical and PACU course with a review of the PACU record and clarification of physician orders. The unit nurse completes a set of immediate vital signs for comparison to postanesthesia findings before the PACU nurse leaves the room. Minor vital sign changes normally occur after transporting a client.

Your first assessment of the client's general condition includes respiratory and cardiovascular status, level of consciousness, condition of dressings and drains, intravenous fluid status, skin integrity, and comfort level. Institutional protocol for assessment routines should be followed. Common time frames for continuing postoperative assessment activities are every 15 minutes the first hour, every 30 minutes for 2 hours, every hour for 4 hours, and then every 4 hours as needed. Assessments may be more frequent depending on the client's condition. The initial findings are used as a baseline for identifying any postoperative changes.

After you complete the first assessment of the client and determine stability, allow the family to visit. Explain the purpose of the frequent postoperative procedures. Inform the family of the client's condition and that the client may fall in and out of sleep (common after general anesthesia) for most of the day. The family is also instructed and enlisted to maintain safety for the client, such as keeping the side rails up, the call bell in reach, and the bed in its lowest position.

A number of potential complications may occur during the postoperative phase on the surgical unit. These have been described in the preoperative and intraoperative sections of this chapter. Nursing management activities are also based on an awareness of po-

POSTOPERATIVE NURSING DIAGNOSES

Ineffective Airway Clearance: Inability to clear secretions or obstructions from the respiratory tract to maintain a clear airway.

Altered Tissue Perfusion: A decrease in oxygen resulting in failure to nourish the tissues at the capillary level.

Pain: An unpleasant sensory and emotional experience arising from actual or potential tissue damage or described in terms of such damage (International Association for the Study of Pain); sudden or slow onset of any intensity from mild to severe with an anticipated or predictable end and a duration of less than 6 months.

Altered Urinary Elimination: The state in which an individual experiences a disturbance in urine elimination.

Nausea: An unpleasant, wave-like sensation in the back of the throat or epigastrium or throughout the abdomen that may or may not lead to vomiting.

Risk for Constipation: At risk for a decrease in a person's normal frequency of defecation accompanied by difficult or incomplete passage of stool and/or passage of excessively hard, dry stool.

Body Image Disturbance: Confusion in the mental picture of one's physical self.

Delayed Surgical Recovery: An extension of the number of postoperative days required for individuals to initiate and perform on their own behalf activities that maintain life, health, and well-being.

From North American Nursing Diagnosis Association. (1999). NANDA nursing diagnoses: Definitions and classification 1999–2000. Philadelphia: Author.

tential complications of surgery in general, as well as complications specific to the client's surgical procedure itself.

Focused Assessment for Ineffective Airway Clearance

Assess the patency of the airway, respiratory rate, patterns of respiratory work, and breath sounds to identify potential alterations in respiratory function. Results should be compared to the client's preoperative status.

Assess the intensity of breath sounds and for the presence of adventitious breath sounds. Monitor for the client's use of accessory muscles. Note the amount and quality of secretions, as these will indicate the presence of respiratory infection and hydration of the mucociliary blanket. Chapter 39 gives a more detailed discussion on respiratory conditions.

The postoperative client is at particular risk for *Ineffective airway clearance.* A common cause of ineffective airway clearance is airway obstruction due to relaxation of the tongue on the posterior pharyngeal wall. Residual effects of anesthesia drugs and muscle relaxants affect muscle control over the tongue and jaw and may decrease cough and gag reflexes.

Postoperative immobility or even the expected decreased mobility can cause clients to take shallow breaths. Many postoperative clients, especially those who have had major abdominal or thoracic surgery, have a tendency to take shallow breaths and to avoid coughing because of the pain it causes. The postoperative development of atelectasis and pneumonia is directly related to hypoventilation, constant recumbent position, ineffective coughing, and smoking. Without medical and nursing intervention, atelectasis can progress to pneumonia when microorganisms grow in the stagnant mucus and an infection develops. Other related factors include airway spasm; presence of artificial airway; excessive secretions; coexisting respiratory disease; tracheobronchial irritation (endotracheal intubation and anesthetic agents); obesity; flow of blood, vomitus, or secretions into airway; and alteration in level of consciousness caused by continued sedation.

Focused Assessment for Altered Tissue Perfusion

General assessment activities of tissue perfusion include monitoring of the client's blood pressure, heart rate, pulses, and skin temperature and color. Results should be compared with preoperative baseline status of the surgical client. Review the chart for information regarding the surgical procedure performed, and equipment used for positioning during the surgery, as these factors are involved in the postoperative client's risk for altered tissue perfusion. Assess the client for postoperative dehydration due to inadequate fluid replacement, intraoperative blood loss and postoperative bleeding, vomiting, or wound drainage. Fluid volume deficit leads to decreases in cardiac output and tissue perfusion.

Blood clots may form in the leg veins as a result of inactivity, pressure, and body position, all of which lead to stasis and decreased tissue perfusion. Because it may lead to pulmonary embolism, deep vein thrombosis is a potentially life-threatening complication. Deep vein thrombosis is seen more commonly in the older client, the obese client, and the immobilized client.

Fainting or syncope in the postoperative client may indicate decreased cardiac output, fluid deficits, or defects in cerebral tissue perfusion. Syncope develops when the postoperative client sits up rapidly or during the first ambulation attempts.

Perfusion may be compromised by the interruption of arterial or venous flow. Cerebral perfusion may be altered by intracranial pressure changes caused by space-taking lesions, edema, decreased systemic blood pressure, hypoxia, and direct interruption of cerebral flow by a thrombus or embolus. Clients with previous history of atherosclerosis, malnutrition, obesity, and cigarette smoking are commonly seen with perfusion problems. Inadequate exchange problems that occur with hypothermia, hypoventilation, and immobility can alter tissue perfusion. Anesthesia agents and other medications are related to perfusion compromise because of vasodilation and vasoconstriction properties. Hypovolemia due to hemorrhage or dehydration can cause life-threatening perfusion alterations. Renal or gastrointestinal perfusion problems in clients may be related to abdominal aortic aneurysms or occlusion conditions of the ureters and bowels.

Focused Assessment for Pain

Postoperative pain is caused by injured nerve fibers in incised or traumatized tissue. Assessment of pain is ongoing throughout the postoperative phase and often begins as the client returns to consciousness in the PACU. A surgical client's pain increases as the effects of anesthesia wear off.

According to the Agency for Health Care Policy and Research's pain management guideline (AHCPR, 1992), an individualized pain management plan should be established for every postoperative client. The plan is guided by assessment of the client's pain.

The most important information in pain assessment is the client's report. Although observation of a client's behavioral symptoms provides objective information, it cannot be considered conclusive evidence to the identification of pain. Assess and reassess pain frequently during the postoperative period. Determine the frequency of assessment based on complaints of pain, severity, and operation performed. Increase frequency of assessment if pain is poorly controlled or if interventions are changed.

Observe for indications of pain such as restlessness or grimacing. Question the client about the characteristics and degree of pain. Note the onset, site, duration, intensity, associated aggravating and alleviating factors, and the client's description of the pain. Ask the client to rate his pain using a pain scale. Pain assessment begins in PACU and continues during postoperative convalescence. Chapter 42 has further information regarding pain.

The incision may be only one source of pain. Surgical manipulation, presence of irritating drainage tubes, tight dressings or casts, and the muscular strains from positioning on the OR table are all factors that may make the client express high levels of pain. Severity of pain may be related to the type of surgical procedure performed. Severity of pain is also associated with the type of anesthetic agent used. Clients who received regional anesthesia may not experience pain in the PACU, but will do so later.

Precipitating factors of pain include motion affecting the incision area, such as when the client turns, coughs, and deep breathes. Fear of and the expectation of pain seem to intensify one's response to pain, as do cultural ways of expressing and coping with pain. Clients who had chronic pain prior to surgery may or may not have a higher tolerance for pain.

Factors associated with aggravating the client's pain threshold are fatigue, position changes, environmental stressors, and inadequate pain relief measures. If the client is in pain, simple activities or procedures that normally do not cause pain will be intolerable to the client.

Focused Assessment for Altered Urinary Elimination

Assess intake and output including all potential sources of intake and output. Observe color, clarity, and odor of urine. Assess for signs of dehydration. Assess the bladder by palpating the lower abdomen to ascertain distention, especially for clients who have received spinal or epidural anesthesia or undergone urinary tract instrumentation (Fig. 57–8).

Urinary elimination can be altered by anesthesia, manipulation of pelvic structures during surgery, inactivity and a recumbent position, and altered food and fluid intake during the perioperative period. Urinary retention and urinary tract infections are common postoperative complications.

Alteration in urinary function can result postoperatively from the recent changes in intake and output of fluids, urinary tract infection, anatomic obstruction, overdistention of the bladder, sensory motor impairment, changes in blood volume, and changes in secretion of antidiuretic hormone (ADH). Common factors that increase ADH secretion and reduce urine output include emotional stress, surgery, pain, hemorrhage, anesthesia agents, and opioids used for pain relief.

Operative trauma, anesthesia, and analgesics cause decreased nerve stimulation to the bladder and the external urinary sphincter. Bedrest may also interfere

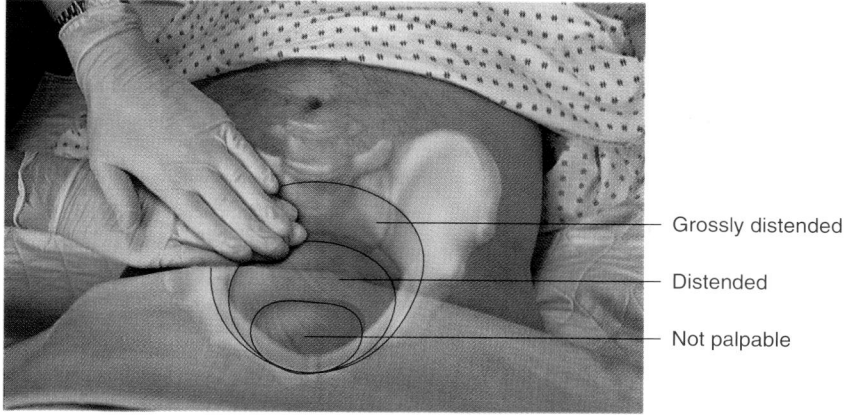

Grossly distended

Distended

Not palpable

Figure 57–8. Assess the bladder by palpating the lower abdomen for distention.

with normal bladder tone by causing decreased nerve stimulation and inadequate output.

Focused Assessment for Nausea

Nausea is an unpleasant sensation, reportedly wave-like, in the back of the throat, epigastrium, or throughout the abdomen that may or may not lead to vomiting. Nausea is a postoperative problem that affects a large number of clients. It may begin in the PACU and continue for several days postoperatively.

Assess the client carefully to differentiate between nausea that is narcotic-induced and nausea caused by improper gastric emptying. Assess the abdomen visually for distention. Assess the client's ability to tolerate diet and determine whether the client is vomiting. Look for possible complications from vomiting, which include fluid and electrolyte imbalances, increased pain, or aspiration.

Post-surgical nausea can be caused by multiple factors. Anesthesia agents and opiate narcotics can stimulate chemoreceptors in the inner ear and the vomiting center in the brain. Many anesthetics are retained in fat cells, so the obese client may be more prone to nausea and vomiting. Clients with a history of motion sickness are likely candidates for post-surgical nausea and vomiting. If a client reports nausea after a previous surgery, he will more than likely be nauseated after this surgery.

Manipulation of the intestines during abdominal surgery decreases bowel activity postoperatively. Inactivity postoperatively maintains a sluggish bowel. If bowel peristalsis does not occur, gastric juices, liquids, and any food taken are unable to leave the stomach through the bowel, so they are regurgitated or vomited. Fluid volume deficit and electrolyte imbalances may also cause nausea and vomiting.

Focused Assessment for Risk for Constipation

Frequently bowel elimination is altered after abdominal or pelvic surgery and sometimes after other surgical procedures as well. Return to normal gastrointesti-

nal function may be delayed by general anesthesia, narcotic analgesia, decreased mobility, or altered fluid and food intake during the perioperative period. The *Risk for constipation* is commonly present in the postoperative client.

The essential assessment for gastrointestinal function postoperatively is the auscultation of the abdomen to determine the presence, frequency, and characteristics of the client's bowel sounds. Bowel sounds are diminished or frequently absent in the immediate postoperative period when peristalsis is decreased.

Motility of the large intestine may be reduced for 3 to 5 days, although small intestine motility resumes within 24 hours. Swallowed air and gastrointestinal secretions may accumulate in the colon, producing flatulence and gas pains. A distended abdomen with absent or high-pitched bowel sounds may indicate paralytic ileus, which is an absence of peristalsis with resultant intestinal obstruction.

Action **A**lert!
Assess bowel sounds carefully. The intestinal obstruction and abdominal distention of paralytic ileus is painful and the client faces possible surgical intervention to release the obstruction. Paralytic ileus is first treated nonsurgically by bowel decompression, which is the insertion of a nasogastric tube with intermittent to constant suction.

Risk Factors

Risk factors for developing constipation postoperatively include the following:

- Recent abdominal or pelvic surgery
- Recent environmental changes
- Decreased physical activity
- Emotional stress
- Insufficient fluid intake
- Decreased fiber intake
- Change in usual foods or eating patterns
- Decreased gastrointestinal motility
- Medications, such as sedatives, nonsteroidal anti-inflammatory drugs, antacids, or opiates
- Post-surgical obstruction, such as paralytic ileus
- Electrolyte imbalances

Focused Assessment for Body Image Disturbance

Assessment of the client's and family's perception of the surgery and its altering effects is important. Be alert for signs of postoperative anxiety and depression. These responses may develop in any client as part of the grief response to a loss of a body part or organ or as a disturbance in body image. Clients may show a revulsion toward their appearance such as refusing to look at an incision.

If surgery led to an impairment of a body function, the client's role within the family can change significantly. The fear of not being able to return to a functional role in the family may cause the client to even avoid participating in the plan of care for discharge to home. The family plays a crucial role in the efforts to improve the client's self-concept.

Focused Assessment for Delayed Surgical Recovery

When clients extend the number of postoperative days usually required to self-perform the activities that maintain life, health, and well-being, the nursing diagnosis of *Delayed surgical recovery* is made. Failure of the client to become actively involved in recovery adds to the risk of delayed healing and the increased incidence of complications. Clients are usually apprehensive about postoperative recovery and the possible complications that can occur. The more complicated the surgical procedure, the more anxious the client is about assuming self-care activities. Sometimes this apprehension may interfere with surgical recovery. However, postoperative complications and knowledge deficits are usually the cause of *Delayed surgical recovery.*

Evaluate the client's general condition, chronic disease processes, and laboratory test results. The incidence of wound sepsis is higher in clients who are older, immunosuppressed, or malnourished or have had a lengthy surgical procedure (longer than 3 hours) or a prolonged hospital stay. Monitor vital signs because elevated temperatures can occur any time postoperatively and may mean different things. Transient low-grade fever is considered normal. If inflamed tissue was excised during the operation, you should expect a constant elevated temperature for 3 to 5 days postoperatively. Gradually the temperature will return to normal. A temperature that is intermittently high, called a spiking temperature, may mean something more serious. Determining the source of the fever is crucial. Spiking temperatures during the first 2 days postoperatively are usually pulmonary in origin. Auscultate lung sounds for adventitious noise or decreased sounds and encourage coughing and deep-breathing exercises. From the fourth to seventh day, suspect wound complications if temperatures are spiking. Thrombophlebitis can cause a fever from the sixth to the 10th day.

Ongoing assessment of the client's surgical site also identifies early signs and symptoms of wound infection. Evidence of a wound infection usually is not apparent before the third to fifth postoperative day. The local manifestations are redness, swelling, increasing pain, or tenderness at the site. Systemic signs are fever and leukocytosis.

Assessment of the surgical wound requires knowledge of the type of wound, the specific surgical procedure, and basic knowledge of wound healing principles. Assess for wound pain. When incisional pain is accompanied by an increased or purulent flow of drainage, it usually indicates delayed healing or presence of infection. Incisional pain is usually most severe for the first 3 days and then it should progressively diminish. Assess the amount, color, odor, and consistency of wound drainage from the wound, on the dressings, and in drainage reservoirs.

Use the database completed preoperatively to assess the client's needs related to learning abilities and support resources. The client may be sent home with continued need for special supplies, equipment, assistance with activities of daily living, special medications, or dressing changes. Assess for the particular needs and determine the teaching and referrals needed for continued care.

Defining Characteristics

The diagnostic cues of *Delayed surgical recovery* are evidence of interrupted healing, continued spiking of fever, loss of appetite with or without nausea, requiring moderate to full assistance to complete self-care, reports of pain at high levels, and postponement of returning to employment or work activities.

Related Factors

The stress of inadequate nutrition, impaired circulation, and metabolic alterations raises the risk for delayed healing during the postoperative period. The physical stresses to the wound during coughing, vomiting, distention, and general movement of body parts are also key factors specific to delayed recovery. The general related factors of *Delayed surgical recovery* are lack of knowledge, depression, malnutrition, and postoperative complications, such as paralytic ileus, pneumonia, thrombophlebitis, and wound infection.

DIAGNOSIS

Determine the status of identified preoperative and intraoperative problems and cluster new assessment data to identify additional postoperative diagnoses. The focus of postoperative nursing care is again prevention of complications. Previously diagnosed problems such as *Knowledge deficit* and *Risk for infection* usually continue as postoperative nursing diagnoses.

PLANNING

Care of the postoperative client is planned to maximize the potential for positive recovery outcomes.

Specific outcome criteria used for evaluation of goal achievement and effectiveness of the intervention are discussed here.

Expected Outcomes for the Client With Ineffective Airway Clearance

The overall expected outcome for *Ineffective airway clearance* is for the client's airway to remain patent. The client will show no signs of pulmonary compromise and adventitious breath sounds are absent upon auscultation (Fig. 57–9). Oxygen level is in the normal range, arterial blood gas levels remain at baseline, and ventilation is adequate.

The client will experience no alterations in respiratory function as evidenced by the following criteria:

- Alert, oriented, and displays no agitation or somnolence
- Shows no signs of aspiration
- Respiratory rate stays within ±5 of baseline rate
- Auscultation reveals no adventitious breath sounds
- Coughs effectively and expectorates normal sputum

Expected Outcome for the Client With Altered Tissue Perfusion

The expected outcome for the client with *Altered tissue perfusion* is to return tissue perfusion and cellular oxygenation to or maintain them within normal parameters as evidenced by the following:

- All pulses palpable
- Extremities warm with normal color
- No complaints of pain or tingling to limbs
- Vital signs normal for client
- Bowel sounds present
- 1,500 to 3,000 mL output daily or equivalent to intake

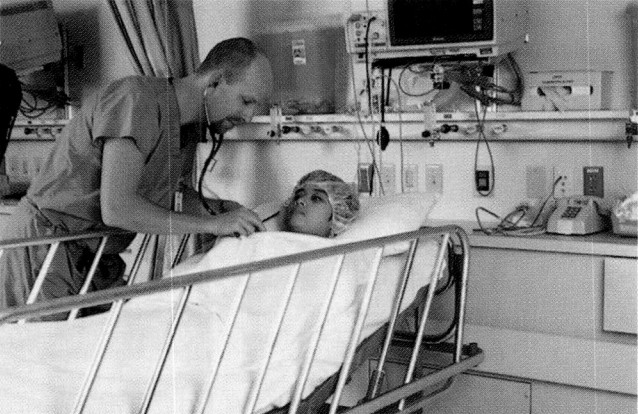

Figure 57–9. Expected outcomes for the postoperative client with ineffective airway clearance include the absence of adventitious breath sounds on auscultation.

- Alert with recent memory normal
- Hemoglobin 15.5 ± 1.1 g/dL in men and 13.7 ± 1.0 g/dL in women
- Partial thromboplastin time 25 to 39 seconds
- Arterial blood gases within normal limits

Expected Outcomes for the Client With Pain

The overall expected outcome for *Pain* is that the client will verbalize that pain is relieved or adequately controlled. Specific criteria include that the location and nature of the pain are described; factors that worsen or relieve the pain experience are identified; and the client describes and carries out appropriate interventions for pain relief.

Expected Outcomes for the Client With Altered Urinary Elimination

The client with *Altered urinary elimination* will have the expected outcome that his bladder will not be palpable after voiding. The following criteria will also be met: voiding occurs in 150- to 400-mL amounts; absence of dribbling or dysuria is reported; post-void residual is less than or equal to 100 mL; and difficulties with urinating are reported promptly.

Expected Outcomes for the Client With Nausea

The overall expected outcome for the client with *Nausea* is that the client reports that the nausea is relieved. Further outcome criteria to be met may include the ability to take fluids and food, identification of the factors that worsen or alleviate nausea, and vomiting does not occur.

Expected Outcomes for the Client With Risk for Constipation

The expected outcome for the client at *Risk for constipation* is that the client's bowel schedule returns to normal patterns. Further goals to be met include the client evacuating soft, formed stool without undue straining, drinking 2,000 to 3,000 mL of fluid daily, and describing normal bowel function and how fluids, diet, and exercise affect function.

Expected Outcomes for the Client With Body Image Disturbance

The overall expected outcome is that the client will use adaptive behaviors in response to alterations in psychosocial function. Specific goals may include the client expressing comfort with his own body image, verbalizing ways to cope with the alteration, demonstrating ways to enhance relaxation and stress reduction, and discussing feelings, and coping effectiveness as a family unit.

Expected Outcomes for the Client With Delayed Surgical Recovery

The overall expected outcome for the client with *Delayed surgical recovery* is that the client will return to a functional state of health within limits posed by surgery. The client will participate in the recovery process by actively participating in planning for discharge, performing activities related to postoperative care, and progressively demonstrating self-care activities.

INTERVENTION

Dramatic and life-threatening changes can occur in the early postoperative phase. Prevention of complications is inherent in postoperative care, while prompt recognition and immediate intervention are imperative in the continued well-being and recovery of the client. Interventions for selected postoperative nursing diagnoses are discussed subsequently.

Interventions to Maintain the Airway

Determine the cause of the compromised airway and initiate corrective action. Perform endotracheal suctioning when secretions are present. Endotracheal suctioning should be done only when the real need for it exists, as it may traumatize the airway. Note stridor, a change in skin color, and any change in mental alertness.

> **A**ction **A**lert!
> Determine the cause of the ineffective airway and correct the problem immediately. The first step is recognition; the second is an open airway. The client's tongue may be relaxed because of anesthesia, narcotics, and muscle relaxants. Or it may become edematous because of an allergic reaction or surgical manipulation. Blood or secretions may be compromising the airway as well.

If the client is nauseated or still stuporous, place the client on one side so that secretions or vomit can flow out of the mouth. If level of consciousness and conditions allow, position the client with his head slightly elevated. This position promotes chest expansion and better ventilation. Administer oxygen as needed and as warranted. Some clients, such as compromised trauma clients, may remain on the mechanical ventilator postoperatively. Mechanically ventilated clients will require critical care by specially educated nurses.

Monitor vital signs, as changes from baseline may indicate increased respiratory and cardiac work related to increased airway resistance, hypoxemia, or the presence of respiratory infection. Monitor arterial oxygen tension (PaO_2) and hemoglobin saturation via pulse oximetry. Hypoxemia or decreased saturation may be related to decreasing ventilation from accumulated secretions in the airways. Improvements in these values could be related to effective coughing or suctioning. Stimulate the client and ask him to take deep breaths.

Turning, coughing, and deep breathing exercises help the client prevent alveolar collapse and move secretions to large airway passages for easier expectoration. Splinting the incision with a pillow or rolled blanket provides support to the incision and facilitates a deeper cough with expectoration of secretions. Adequate and frequent pain medications should be given because incisional pain often is the greatest deterrent to client participation in ambulation and TCDB exercises. Provide emotional support during these exercises by maintaining contact through touch and communication.

Instruct the client to use the incentive spirometer for maximum inspiration. Encourage early ambulation to increase chest wall expansion and stimulate respiratory rate and circulation. Educate the client about the essential need to maintain hydration, parenteral or oral, to keep secretions thin and loose. Provide oral hygiene frequently for the client to maintain integrity of mucous membranes.

Interventions to Promote Tissue Perfusion

Promotion of tissue perfusion is accomplished with simple interventions for the most part. Monitor the client's blood pressure, heart rate, pulses, and skin temperature and color. Compare findings with the preoperative baseline status of the surgical client. Facilitate venous return from the lower extremities by helping the client with leg exercises and ambulation.

Some surgeons prescribe elastic antithromboembolitic stockings or sequential compression devices to stimulate venous return in the legs. Sequential compression devices used with antiembolic stockings are especially effective in reducing deep vein thrombosis in general surgical high-risk clients.

> **A**ction **A**lert!
> Assess for complaints of swelling, inflammation, aching, or pain in the calf with walking or with dorsiflexion of the foot (Homans' sign). These complaints are symptoms of thrombophlebitis.

Promote cerebral perfusion and prevention of syncope by making changes slowly in the client's position. Progression to ambulation can be achieved by first raising the head of the client's bed, assisting the client to a sitting position on the bedside with legs dangling, and then assisting the client to a standing position by the bed. If the client voices no complaints and no change in vital signs occurs, start ambulation. If faintness occurs, help the client to a sitting position and then with lying down. Many times the physician will order that the client stand at the bedside the evening of surgery with ambulation beginning the first postoperative day. Progressive increases in levels of activity promote tissue perfusion and the client will usually feel less faint with each activity (Fig. 57–10).

Interventions to Reduce or Alleviate Pain

Pain is expected after surgery. Nevertheless, the client should receive substantial relief from and control of

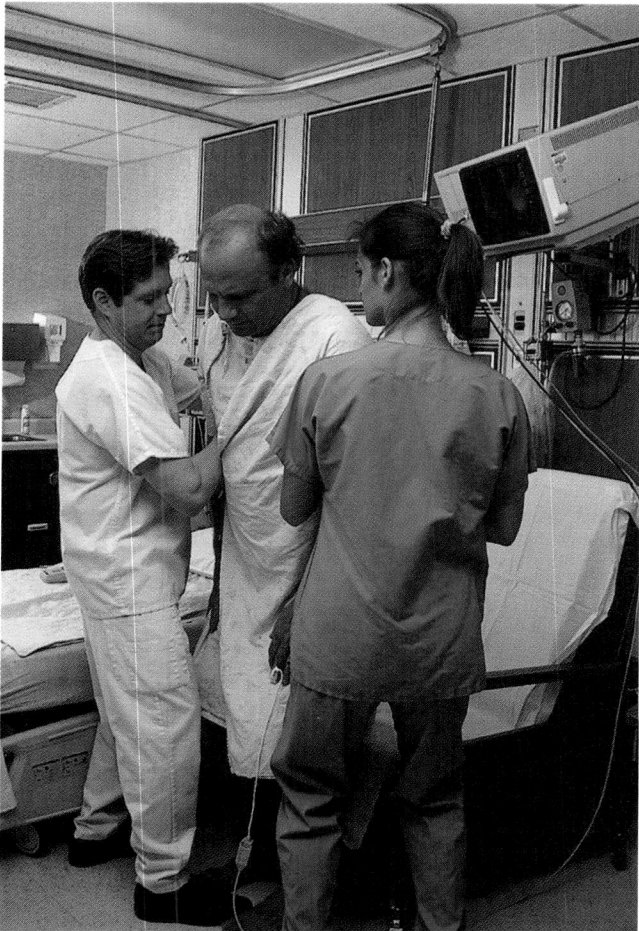

Figure 57–10. Progressive increases in levels of postoperative activity promote tissue perfusion.

this pain. Managing acute postoperative pain is an important nursing intervention before, during, and after surgery. Excellent pain control techniques not only can lead to improved client outcomes but also can reduce the cost of care, as shown in the accompanying chart. Successful pain management involves the cooperative effort of the client, physician, and nurse and begins with preoperative education.

Interventions for pain include pharmacological and behavioral actions. The most rapid relief from pain is provided through intravenous narcotics, while more sustained relief may be through the use of epidurals, PCA, or regional anesthesia techniques. Many clients achieve adequate pain relief through intramuscular or oral administration of analgesic medications. Documentation of the medication's effectiveness is important.

Various nonpharmacological approaches to pain management are used alone or in conjunction with drug therapy to control acute postoperative pain. Relaxation, distraction, massage, acupuncture, and therapeutic touch are several approaches of pain management. Transcutaneous electrical nerve stimulation (TENS) has also been successful in decreasing postoperative pain for many clients.

Interventions to Promote Urinary Elimination

The urine of the postoperative client should be examined for both quantity and quality, with the urine color, amount, consistency, and odor noted. Indwelling urinary catheters should be assessed for patency, with urine output at least 0.5 mL/kg per hour. Urine output is one of the most valuable clinical indicators of renal perfusion. A drop in renal arterial pressure and flow produces renal arterial vasoconstriction and results in decreased glomerular filtration and decreased urine output. Normal urine flow is 50 mL/hour.

If no voiding occurs within 6 to 8 hours after surgery, the lower abdomen should be inspected and the bladder palpated and percussed for distention.

Low urine output (800 to 1,500 mL) in the first 24 hours postoperatively may be expected, regardless of fluid intake, because of the physiological stress of surgery, preoperative fluid restriction, and loss of fluids during surgery. The inability to urinate, with urinary

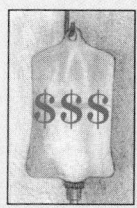

THE COST OF CARE
PAIN MANAGEMENT

Recent studies have shown that improved pain control techniques not only can lead to improved client outcomes but also can reduce the cost of care. Advances in surgical techniques and pain management have led to an increased number of outpatient surgeries and it is estimated that in the near future, over 85% of all surgical procedures will be on an outpatient basis.

A study was made of the effect of using intraoperative local anesthetics versus general anesthesia on postoperative pain and length of stay for inguinal hernia repairs. It was found that the use of one of the local anesthetics investigated (bupivacaine) reduced the required dosage of narcotics intraoperatively and also led to a very significant reduction in postoperative narcotics, from an average equivalent of 10.64 mg of morphine sulfate to 0.05 mg.

There was also a concurrent reduction in postoperative nausea from 47% for the general anesthesia case to 0% for the cases using bupivacaine and a respective reduction in average length of stay from 171 to 61 minutes. Thus, not only did the clients experience an improved outcome through the reduction of pain, but the combination of the replacement of expensive narcotics with inexpensive local anesthetics, the elimination of general anesthesia, and the greatly reduced length of stay reduced costs through decreased use of labor and supplies.

Reference

Roberge, C.W., & McEwen, M. (1998). The effects of local anesthetics on postoperative pain. *AORN Journal, 68*(6), 1003–1012.

retention, may occur postoperatively as a result of the recumbent position, effects of anesthesia and narcotics, inactivity, nervous tension, or surgical manipulation in the pelvic region. Incisional pain may alter perceptions and interfere with the client's awareness of the less intense sensation arising as the bladder fills with urine.

Oliguria, the diminished output of urine related to intake, is associated with acute renal failure and is a less common complication, although a more serious problem if it occurs after surgery. It may result from renal ischemia caused by inadequate renal perfusion or altered cardiovascular function.

Nursing interventions promoting the return of normal urinary elimination include the following:

- Monitor intake and output balance.
- Assist with the assumption of a normal position to void (sitting for women and standing for men).
- Provide reassurance regarding ability to void and use the techniques to assist in voiding (such as running water or pouring warm water over the perineum).
- Maintain ordered rate of intravenous fluids.
- Encourage oral fluids, when ordered.
- Provide privacy when the client is using a bedpan, commode, or bathroom.
- Assess for bladder distention if the client has not urinated within 6 hours after surgery or if client voids in amounts less than 100 mL.
- Insert a straight or indwelling catheter as ordered.

Interventions to Reduce or Alleviate Nausea

Determine the onset, duration, and frequency of nausea symptoms. Is it associated with anesthesia agents or narcotic pain medications? Administer appropriate medications. If the client is actively vomiting, choose a route other than by mouth for drug administration.

Ask the client what he usually does when he is nauseated. Provide a cool cloth for the neck or forehead. Place an emesis basin and call bell within reach, turn off lights, and allow the client to rest quietly. Attempt to rid the room of strong odors or food smells.

Auscultate for gurgling and rumbling sounds in all four quadrants to indicate return of peristalsis. Ask clients whether or not they have passed flatus, as both bowel sounds and active flatus indicate active peristalsis.

If the client is unable to take fluids by mouth or is actively vomiting, monitor hydration status and intravenous infusions carefully. Keep an accurate intake and output record. Monitor laboratory findings such as electrolytes and hematocrit for signs of fluid volume deficit. Electrolyte imbalances can also be the cause of nausea with vomiting.

Interventions to Prevent Constipation

Preventing constipation is preferable to treating it. Assess for the return of peristalsis by auscultating bowel sounds every 4 hours when the client is awake. When the abdomen is distended, it will feel taut or tight to palpation. Ask the client about his ability to pass flatus or stool. Encourage and assist with early ambulation if it is not contraindicated. Unless there is a medical condition to restrict fluids (such as renal failure), facilitate daily fluid intake of 2,500 to 3,000 mL by offering fluids of the client's choice and placing a ready supply at bedside. Encourage the intake of high-fiber foods unless contraindicated by diet restrictions. Maintain privacy at all times when clients use the bathroom, bedpan, or commode. Assist the client with a more normal position for defecation on a bedpan by raising the head of the bed if not contraindicated. Discourage the use of irritant or stimulant type laxatives because they irritate the entire bowel. Administer glycerin suppositories or mineral oil enemas as ordered for constipation.

Interventions to Promote Realistic Body Image

To facilitate coping and to promote a realistic body image, provide the client with privacy and accept each client as an individual. Identify through verbal and nonverbal cues who may be at risk for inability to cope with an alteration in his or her body and offer opportunities for clients and families to verbalize their feelings about the change. Encourage the client to be part of decision-making throughout the postoperative experience and provide honest information to the client and family about all aspects of care. Collaborate with other members of the health care team and provide referrals to meet psychosocial needs as necessary.

Interventions to Promote Surgical Recovery

You have an important role in the recovery of the postoperative client. You are usually the first to recognize postoperative problems. Frequent assessment enables you to detect postoperative complications, initiate treatment or referrals, and promote surgical recovery.

The most significant general nursing measure to prevent postoperative complications is early ambulation. It has been nearly 50 years since it was first advocated and the value of early ambulation is still just as significant. The exercise associated with walking increases muscle tone, improves gastrointestinal and urinary tract function, stimulates circulation, and maintains normal respiratory function.

Nursing care of surgical wounds is directed at preventing and monitoring for wound complications, including the following:

- Maintain aseptic technique in dressing changes and care of drains and tubes.
- Use medical asepsis (hand-washing protocols).
- Maintain nutritional status; encourage diet selection high in carbohydrates, proteins, calories, and vitamins.
- Maintain hydration.

Assess the wound for approximation of wound edges, color of the wound and surrounding area, drains or tubes, condition of sutures or staples, and signs of dehiscence or evisceration.

A*ction* A*lert!*
Cover the wound and call the surgeon immediately if the client's wound shows dehiscence and evisceration.

As the client enters the discharge period of postoperative care to recuperate outside the hospital setting, provide individualized information and support to aid the client in meeting self-care needs (Fig. 57–11). Postoperatively, the client will be able to perform many self-care activities and will be encouraged to do those activities and more. Raise the client's confidence and involvement in the recovery process by encouraging participation in care planning preoperatively for the client's eventual discharge from the hospital. All teaching activities should be accompanied by written information and guidelines for the client to refer to while at home.

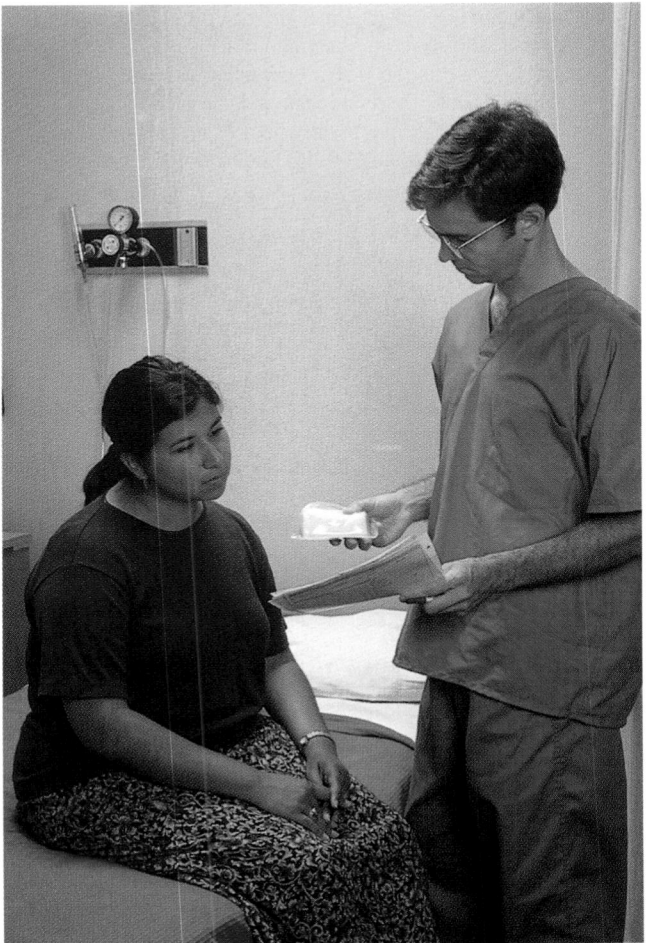

Figure 57–11. In preparation for discharge, provide individualized information and support for the postoperative client.

This is important when a large amount of detailed information is presented, such as a complicated open wound dressing change.

Because the hospital stay is often very brief, you must make an organized, coordinated effort to educate the client and family members. Specifics and teaching needs may vary, but the most common needs include the following:

- Care of wound site and any dressings
- Signs and symptoms of a wound infection and when to call the physician
- Symptoms to be reported that may occur in other parts of the body
- Medications and why, when, and how to take them
- Activities allowed and restricted (such as driving, sexual intercourse, returning to work) and when various activities may be resumed
- When and where to return for follow-up care (provide phone number if needed)
- Specific questions and concerns on individual basis

The client must be accompanied by a responsible adult at discharge. Written and verbal instructions and immediate supplies are given to the client. A follow-up evaluation of the client's status may be made by telephone several days later, and any specific concerns are addressed at that time.

If the client has delayed surgical recovery, he or she may need to be transferred to a long-term or extended care facility or have home health nursing visits. Collaboration and further education of the client and the family will be needed prior to the client's leaving the hospital. Assessment of and planning for special needs and supplies should be reflected in the transfer or discharge documentation. Continued care and evaluation of recovery will continue until the client returns to his or her optimal level of health.

EVALUATION

Evaluate the postoperative client thoroughly, as shown in the accompanying Nursing Care Planning chart. Keep in mind, however, that postoperative evaluation of outcomes is not always readily apparent. The client's stay is usually short and access to the client for outcome evaluation is sometimes difficult. Approach evaluation of care collaboratively, as nursing care provided intraoperatively related to a preoperative diagnosis may not have progressed to the evaluation stage until the client is preparing for postoperative discharge.

In the evaluation of *Risk for infection* or *Delayed surgical recovery,* you may need to call the client at home and ask specific questions, or perhaps you will evaluate the client's outcomes in collaboration with the surgeon's office after the client's first postoperative office visit. Documentation of postoperative evaluation of outcomes is placed in the client's chart.

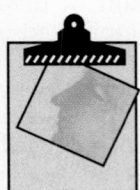

NURSING CARE PLANNING
A POSTOPERATIVE CLIENT

Postoperative Data

Mr. Warren arrived on the GU unit at 2:30 PM on the day of his surgery. The transfer from PACU went smoothly and the client was stable. At 4:00 AM, Mr. Warren was having dry heaves and complaining of the worst "sickness in my belly and brain" that he has ever experienced. The nurse works with the client to determine the cause of the nausea.

Physician's Orders

Vital signs q30 minutes ×4, q1h ×4, q2h ×2, then q4h
NPO until awake, then clear liquid diet as tolerated
Nothing per rectum
Maintain Foley traction, do not manipulate catheter. Strict intake and output.
No irrigation of Foley—if low output or clots, call physician STAT
D_5 ½ NS 1000 mL at 125 mL/hr alternate with D_5 LR at 125 mL/hr
Drain Jackson-Pratt drain q4h and record
CBC and platelet count, electrolytes, blood urea nitrogen, and creatinine on 3rd postop day
Kefzol 1 g q8h for 5 days
PCA orders and pain control per anesthesia department
Phenergan 50 mg IM q4h prn nausea
Antiembolism stockings with sequential compression device—until ambulating in halls

Nursing Assessment

Client complaining of severe nausea and presenting with dry heaves. Emesis basin at bedside. Placed cool cloth on forehead. Skin cool, clammy, and ashen in color. BP 108/70, pulse 88, respirations 26, and axillary temperature 97.2°F. Bowel sounds hypoactive ×4 quadrants with abdomen softly distended. Lower abdominal dressing bulky, dry, and intact. Jackson-Pratt drain to right of dressing with sanguineous drainage. Foley catheter traction intact and draining pink urine with occasional small bloody clots. IV fluids infusing left forearm without redness, edema, or pain. PCA intact with client using button q30 minutes to q1 hour. Reports lower abdominal incision pain at 4 on scale of 0–10. Sequential hose over TED hose in progress. Daughter at bedside.

NURSING CARE PLAN

Nursing Diagnosis	Expected Outcomes	Interventions	Evaluation (First Day Postoperative)
Nausea related to ineffective gastric emptying, narcotic medications, or both	Identifies factors that worsen or alleviate nausea.	Ask client to identify what makes the nausea worse and what makes it better.	Client says "Lawd have mercy—it bad" while lying very still. States never had motion sickness problems in past. PCA morphine in progress. *Daughter applying cool cloth to forehead.*
		Administer antiemetic medications.	Phenergan 50 mg IM given with marked decrease in nausea. Able to sit on side of bed and do TCDB exercises 40 minutes after administration of antiemetic.

Continued

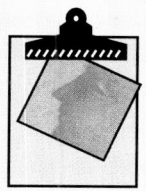

NURSING CARE PLANNING
A POSTOPERATIVE CLIENT *(continued)*

NURSING CARE PLAN

Nursing Diagnosis	Expected Outcomes	Interventions	Evaluation (First Day Postoperative)
		Consult physician for a change in pain medication.	Called physician and requested change to Dilaudid for client. Received orders to change IV medication in PCA pump to Dilaudid (noted to cause less nausea) for pain relief. Change PCA pump to Dilaudid at 8 AM.
	Has active bowel sounds upon auscultation.	Auscultate bowel sounds carefully in all four quadrants as frequently as needed, then q4h.	Faint hypoactive bowel sounds auscultated in all four quadrants. Denies passing flatus.
	Has no vomiting.	Provide cool cloth for neck, forehead, or both. Place emesis basin and call bell within reach.	Client has not vomited, just had dry heaves. Comfort measures were welcomed.
		If vomiting, monitor hydration status and continue IV infusions.	Not vomiting, but while nauseated, continued IV infusions and monitored hydration status. *Daughter said she would help keep track of any intake and output.*
	Able to take fluids and food.	Offer only cool clear liquids and progress as client tolerates.	First day postop orders for clear liquids only. Took sips on 7–3 shift and progressed to 600 mL intake on 3–11 shift.
	Reports the nausea is relieved.	Assess complaint of nausea for onset, duration, and frequency as needed.	Complained of severe nausea at 4:00 AM and moderate nausea at 9:00 AM. After giving antiemetic ×2 and changing PCA medication at 8:00 AM, client reported relief of nausea.

Italicized interventions indicate culturally specific care.

Critical Thinking Questions

1. What do you think may be causing Mr. Warren's nausea? What other nursing measures besides those mentioned above may help the client with his nausea?
2. If Mr. Warren began vomiting, it would affect his hydration status. How do you assess for hydration status? Would dehydration cause additional problems because of his particular type of surgery?
3. The dry heaves Mr. Warren is experiencing can cause abdominal incision pain because of the abdominal muscle use during retching. How could you assist the client with supporting the abdominal incision during this type of situation?

KEY PRINCIPLES

- Clients confronted with impending surgery face both psychological and physiological stressors.
- The anticipation of surgery may cause anxiety for many clients, who associate surgery with pain, possible disfigurement, loss of independence, and even death.
- Previous illnesses, chronic diseases, and past surgeries influence the ability of the client to tolerate surgery.
- The geriatric client is at higher surgical risk because of declining physiological status.
- The time before, during, and after surgery is called the perioperative period; it is divided into preoperative, intraoperative, and postoperative phases.
- Preoperative assessment data gathered about the surgical client provide an important baseline with which to compare intraoperative and postoperative assessment data.
- Nursing diagnoses of the surgical client may have implications for nursing care during one or all phases of perioperative care.
- Primary responsibility for informed consent rests with the surgeon. However, verification of informed status is an advocacy responsibility of the nurse.
- Structured and timely preoperative teaching positively influences the recovery of surgical clients.
- A major focus of perioperative nursing care during the intraoperative phase is maintenance of client safety through advocacy and prevention of complications.
- Immediate postoperative nursing care in the PACU focuses on prevention of complications from anesthesia and surgery.
- Ongoing postoperative care of the surgical client is planned to facilitate recovery from surgery and to teach the client how to cope with alterations.
- Evaluation of all perioperative care is at times difficult because the client may be discharged from your care before the outcome is ready for evaluation.

BIBLIOGRAPHY

*Agency for Health Care Policy and Research. (1992). *Clinical Practice Guideline. Acute pain management: Operative or medical procedures and trauma.* Rockville, MD: U.S. Dept. of Health and Human Services.

Allen, J. (1997). Lifestyle impacts recovery. *Reflections, 23*(1), 18.

Alleyne, M. (1996). *Africa: Roots of Jamaican culture.* Chicago: Research Associates School Times Publications.

American Nurses Association (1996). *Latex allergy: Protect yourself—protect your patients* (brochure): Author.

American Society of PeriAnesthesia Nurses. (1995). *ASPAN: Standards for post-anesthesia nursing practice.* Virginia: Author.

Association of Operating Room Nurses. (1999). *AORN standards and recommended practices for perioperative nursing.* Colorado: Author.

Brooks-Brunn, J.A. (1997). Surgery: Protecting the lungs. *Reflections, 23*(1), 16.

Brumfield, V.C., Kee, C.C., & Johnson, J.Y. (1996). Preoperative client teaching in ambulatory surgery settings. *AORN Journal, 64*(6), 941–952.

Butts, J.D., & Wolford, E.T. (1997). Timing of perioperative antibiotic administration. *AORN Journal, 65*(1), 109–112, 114–115.

Campese, C. (1996). Development and implementation of a pain management program. *AORN Journal, 64*(6), 931–940.

Crenshaw, J. (1999). Research for practice: New guidelines for preoperative fasting. *American Journal of Nursing, 99*(4), 49.

Dunn, D. (1997). Malignant hyperthermia. *AORN Journal, 65*(4), 728–762.

Gruendemann, B.J., & Fernsebner, B. (1995). *Comprehensive perioperative nursing: Principles. Volume 1.* Sudbury, MA: Jones and Bartlett.

Huber, P., & Slade, A. (1999). Intraoperative hypothermia length of stay in the postanesthesia care unit. *Surgical Services Management, 5*(1), 46–50.

Hutchinsson, B., Baird, M.G., & Wagner, S. (1998). Electrosurgical safety. *AORN Journal, 68*(5), 830–844.

Killen, A.R., Kleinbeck, S.V., Golar, K., Takahashi Schuchardt, J., and Uebele, J. (1997). The prevalence of perioperative nurse clinical judgements. *AORN Journal, 65*(1), 101–108.

Kim, K., Graves, P., Safadi, G., Alhadeff, G., & Metcalfe, J. (1998). Implementation recommendations for making health care facilities latex safe. *AORN Journal, 67*(3), 615–632.

Kleinbeck, S., English, N., Sherley, M., & Howes, R. (1998). A criterion-referenced measure of latex allergy knowledge. *AORN Journal, 68*(3), 384–392.

Larson, P., & Martin, J. (1999). Polypharmacy and elderly patients. *AORN Journal, 69*(3), 619–628.

Lusis, S. (1996). The challenges of nursing elderly surgical patients. *AORN Journal, 64*(6), 954–962.

McDougal, W.S. (1996). *Prostate disease: The most comprehensive, up-to-date information available to help you understand your condition, make the right treatment choices, and cope effectively.* New York: Times Books.

Meeker, M.H., & Rothrock, J.C. (Eds.). (1995). *Alexander's care of the client in surgery* (10th ed.). St. Louis: Mosby-Year Book.

Morse, J.M., Bottorff, J.L., & Hutchinson, S. (1995). The paradox of comfort. *Nursing Research, 44*(1), 14–19.

North American Nursing Diagnosis Association (1999). *NANDA nursing diagnoses: Definitions & classification 1999–2000.* Philadelphia: Author.

Pape, T. (1997). Legal and ethical considerations of informed consent. *AORN Journal, 65*(6), 1122–1127.

Patton, C. (1999). Preoperative nursing assessment of the adult patient. *Seminars in Perioperative Nursing, 8*(1), 42–47.

Petry, J. (1997). Nutritional supplements and surgical patients. *AORN Journal, 65*(6), 1117–1121.

*Porter, J., & Jick, H. (1980). Addiction rare in patients treated with narcotics. *New England Journal of Medicine, 302*, 123.

Pryor, F. (1997). Key concepts in informed consent for perioperative nurses. *AORN Journal, 65*(6), 1105–1110.

Rothrock, J.C. (1996). *Perioperative nursing care planning* (2nd ed.). St. Louis: Mosby-Year Book.

Ruzicka, S. (1997). The impact of normal aging processes and chronic illness on perioperative care of the elderly. *Seminars in Perioperative Nursing, 6*(1), 3–13.

Stein, R.H. (1995). The perioperative nurse's role in anesthesia management. *AORN Journal,62*(5), 794–798, 801, 803–804.

Vermette, E. (1998). Malignant hyperthermia. *American Journal of Nursing, 98*(4), 45.

Wiens, A. (1998). Preoperative anxiety in women. *AORN Journal, 68*(1), 74–88.

Whitley, G.G., & Tousman, S.A. (1996). A multivariate approach for validation of anxiety and fear. *Nursing Diagnosis, 7*(3), 116–124.

*Asterisk indicates a classic or definitive work on this subject.

58

The Emergency Client

Betty Samford

Key Terms

acuity rating
acute area
against medical advice
emergency
hemodynamic monitoring
interfacility transfer

intrafacility transfer
nonacute area
nonurgent
semi-urgent
triage
urgent

LEARNING OBJECTIVES

After studying this chapter, you should be able to:

1. Describe the concept of emergency care.
2. Discuss the concept of triage and the roles of the triage nurse.
3. Identify factors affecting the outcome of emergency care, including lifestyle, culture, and socioeconomics.
4. Describe the assessment of the emergency department client.
5. Write nursing diagnoses for a client who has an emergent respiratory problem, cardiac problem, or a risk of violence directed at self or others.
6. Plan for specific goal-oriented nursing intervention in emergent respiratory problems, cardiac problems, or violence directed at self or others.
7. Describe fundamental emergency nursing care to the client with a change in respiratory, cardiac, or psychosocial status.
8. Evaluate the outcomes of goal-oriented nursing care for the emergency client.

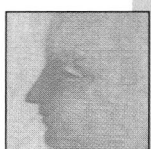

Barry, a homeless middle-aged man, was found unconscious on the street in 17°F weather. An emergency medical services crew transported him to the emergency department, as they would for any homeless person in need of acute medical care. As Barry began to regain consciousness in the ambulance, he tried to fight with the paramedics and was subsequently restrained to prevent harm to himself and others. This is his first admission to the emergency department.

Barry is typical of the homeless culture. He has a high school education with a year of technical training as an automobile mechanic. He was laid off from his job 4 years ago and has since been separated from his wife, child, and home. He has a 10-year history of diagnosed clinical depression but has not taken his antidepressive medication for 3 years. He has been without a home for 2 years.

The behavioral characteristics of depression, hopelessness, and despair are an outcome of Barry's lifestyle and inability to provide for himself on a long-term basis. The violent behavior stems from his anger and chronic use of alcohol. Barry was startled as the paramedics tried to help him; he has been physically assaulted on the streets many times. Barry's diagnosis of *Risk for violence* is one of the three most common acute nursing diagnoses that require immediate, often life-saving, intervention.

EMERGENCY NURSING DIAGNOSES

Decreased Cardiac Output: A state in which the blood pumped by the heart is inadequate to meet the metabolic demands of the body.

Impaired Gas Exchange: Excess or deficit in oxygenation and/or carbon dioxide elimination at the alveolar-capillary membrane.

Risk for Violence: Directed at Others: Behaviors in which an individual demonstrates that he/she can be physically, emotionally, and/or sexually harmful to others.

Risk for Violence: Self-Directed: Behaviors in which an individual demonstrates that he/she can be physically, emotionally, and/or sexually harmful to self.

From North American Diagnosis Association. (1999). NANDA nursing diagnoses: Definitions and classification 1999–2000. Philadelphia: Author.

CONCEPTS OF EMERGENCY CARE

An **emergency** is a serious health situation that arises suddenly and either threatens life or would result in serious complications without prompt treatment. Emergencies can be medical, surgical, traumatic, or psychiatric events. Medical emergencies are acute physiological events that are treated primarily with medicine. Surgical emergencies are events for which surgery is required to protect the client's life. Traumatic emergencies are injuries commonly caused by blunt or penetrating impact to the body from motor vehicle collisions, knives, or guns. Psychiatric events are acute mental health problems that precipitate a crisis.

Types of Facilities

A hospital emergency department's primary function is to treat clients who are experiencing emergencies (also called emergent problems), as described previously, although emergency department staff also treat clients for nonemergent problems. Freestanding urgent-care facilities are usually neighborhood clinics where clients receive care for problems that do not require immediate or advanced treatments. These facilities reduce the strain on community resources designed for true emergencies, and they commonly reduce the overall cost of health care. Most communities are actively engaged in attempts to reduce health care costs, as described in the accompanying Cost of Care chart.

An emergency department may be classified as a trauma center according to the types of medical resources available on a 24-hour basis. As examples, level I and II trauma centers have a full trauma surgical team readily available around the clock. Level III and IV hospital emergency departments may have a full surgical team available, but the members may neither specialize in trauma nor be in the hospital 24 hours a day. Although not all emergency departments meet the criteria for a major trauma center, they do provide life-saving care until the client can be transferred to a facility more appropriately equipped and staffed.

Treatment Areas

Usually, emergency department treatment areas are physically and conceptually divided into acute areas and nonacute areas, although the terminology may vary among facilities. The **acute area** is the physical space where clients with life-threatening health problems are treated. These problems might include multiple trauma, cardiac problems, respiratory distress, or psychiatric emergencies. The **nonacute area** is used for clients who present with all other types of health problems. These may include urgent, semi-urgent, or nonurgent problems. An **urgent** problem is one for which the client requires prompt care, although a wait of 20 to 60 minutes will not affect the outcome of treatment. One example is a fracture of an extremity in a child. A **semi-urgent** problem is one for which the client requires timely treatment within 4 to 6 hours. An example of a semi-urgent problem includes a small laceration that requires sutures. A **nonurgent** problem is one for which the amount of time a person delays treatment is not a critical issue. An example is a client who needs a refill of a prescription medication.

The staff in an emergency department must continually strive to meet the needs of nonacute clients while providing prompt, life-saving treatment for emergencies. The needs of both the acute and non-acute client can be met by the nurse who stays organized and wisely uses available resources (Box 58–1). Some general goals of an emergency department are to

- Resuscitate and stabilize clients with acute problems.
- Reduce suffering for all clients.
- Provide holistic, including emotional, support to families.
- Educate clients before discharge.

Triage

A sick or injured client who comes to an emergency department expects to receive safe and organized care

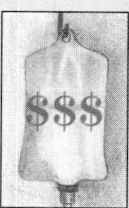

THE COST OF CARE

USING VOLUNTEERS TO HELP STAFF AN EMERGENCY DEPARTMENT

By pursuing a path of resourcefulness, a rural emergency department successfully solved a financial problem. After building its new emergency department, the 142-bed rural hospital in Sterling, Illinois, found that it needed an additional staff member to act as client advocate and assist clients in public relations-type activities.

However, the hospital could not afford to hire another person because of the cost of building the new department. Instead, officials recruited volunteers—54 of them—to act as liaisons with clients. They helped to keep clients' families informed, controlled traffic in the emergency department, helped with transportation, obtained blankets for clients, and spent time with children as they waited.

At the close of the program's first year, hospital officials took a survey of the emergency department staff, the liaison staff, and the registration staff to evaluate the program. On a scale of 1 to 5 (with a 5 being the best), emergency department staff gave the program a score of 4.18, liaisons gave it a score of 4.00, and registration staff gave it a score of 5.00. Using these results, officials pronounced the program a success.

Overall, the hospital saved $17,064 in staff salaries for the year. Plus, the emergency department had the added benefit of satisfied clients, emergency department staff, and registration staff.

Reference

Wolford, S. (1995). Emergency department patient liaison volunteers: A cost containment and visitor satisfaction strategy. *Journal of Emergency Nursing, 21,* 17–21.

ority rating based on the severity of the illness or injury, the client then proceeds with registration or is taken into the treatment area for immediate care (Fig. 58–1). For example, a 46-year-old man with a minor arm laceration would receive a nonacute rating and proceed to the registration counter, while a 68-year-old woman with substernal chest pain radiating to her left arm would be taken directly to the acute treatment area.

Roles of the Triage Nurse

The triage assignment requires a registered nurse who can function under pressure as a nurse-clinician, educator, and manager. In the role of clinician, the triage nurse uses physical assessment techniques, effective communication, and decision-making skills to initiate treatment for nursing diagnoses, and to monitor for changes in status. As an educator, the nurse gives information about managing the present illness and adopting pertinent health practices. A visit to the emergency department may be the first contact with the health care system for some clients, and the only opportunity for health education. The third role of the triage nurse is to assist in the management of client flow in the department.

Some of the most challenging responsibilities of the triage nurse are to communicate effectively with clients and families to increase their understanding of waiting times, to inform families about the condition of sick or injured loved ones, and to explain priorities that may require clients to be seen by a physician outside the chronological order of their arrival. One individual may be seen by the physician before another individual. The triage nurse and all staff working in the emergency department must know how to organize priorities, manage fearful or angry clients, and be effective in education and public relations.

FACTORS AFFECTING THE OUTCOME OF EMERGENCY CARE
Lifestyle Factors

A client's lifestyle may ultimately influence the outcome of care. Lifestyle factors important to the emergency department are those that will prevent the current problem from recurring, ensure that the client will receive follow-up care, and keep the client safe. Teaching in the emergency department includes the use of motorcycle helmets and automobile seat belts, prevention of cardiovascular disease, and accidental poisons.

Socioeconomic Factors

Socioeconomic factors prompt some clients to seek routine care in an emergency department. Although these clients receive the same quality treatment as the acute client, the outcomes may differ because of the client's inability to pay for medications or follow-up

in a timely manner. **Triage** is the decision-making process used to determine client treatment priorities based on the severity of injury and priority for treatment. A French term, it means "to sort into three groups." Historically, the military used this concept to sort the near-fatally wounded from the walking wounded. The most severely injured soldiers were left to die, the moderately injured received hospital treatment, and the least severely injured were treated and returned to the battlefield.

This concept partially describes the function of the triage nurse in a modern emergency department. Within minutes of entering an emergency department, each client is briefly assessed based on the chief complaint. Depending on the client's **acuity rating,** a pri-

---

BOX 58-1

TIPS FOR ORGANIZING NURSING INTERVENTIONS

- Maintain an awareness of ongoing activities, such as client acuity ratings, the times still needed for ongoing procedures, and the needs of clients who will require teaching.
- Perform the least time-consuming tasks first. For example, when possible administer oral medications before intravenous medications, because the latter requires more time.
- Consolidate your activities and interventions to make the most of every client contact. For example, assess a client's vital signs when assessing for pain relief. Or teach a client about the signs and symptoms of infection while applying a wound dressing.
- Be flexible.
- If necessary, care for a demanding client first, rather than waste time in a power struggle.

- Use technology effectively by "piggy-backing" appropriate intravenous medications on an infusion pump instead of standing at the bedside to give medications.
- Use resources effectively; for example, have the client read printed handouts before you provide verbal discharge instructions.
- Delegate tasks appropriately and maintain communication with team members.
- Store commonly used supplies in a convenient location and keep extra supplies readily available. Take steps to anticipate the need for additional supplies.
- Ask your charge nurse for help if you feel overwhelmed; remember that even the most experienced nurses feel stress.

---

care. Most emergency departments have a social worker on hand to assist clients who have social and financial needs.

Cultural Factors

Cultural factors may influence the outcomes of emergency care. Especially in the culture of poverty and homelessness, the emergency department is a source of care in the absence of other avenues for receiving care. Consequently, emergency department staff may

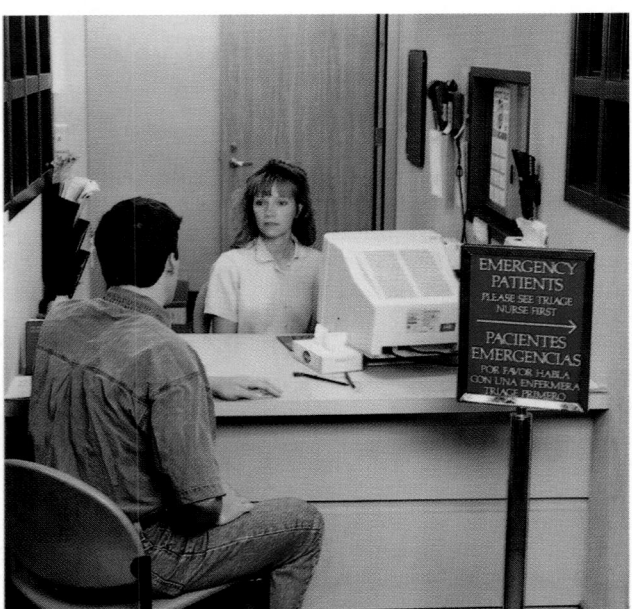

Figure 58-1. Registration in the emergency department.

need to address other medical needs along with the chief complaint if the outcomes are to be positive, as described in the Cross-Cultural Care chart. Additionally, outcomes are affected by the delay in seeking care because of lack of access or lack of financial resources, and often resulting in a higher likelihood of urgent or semi-urgent problems.

The client's religious practices also may influence outcomes. For example, the client may believe that illness is a punishment. Or the client may oppose receiving blood or blood products. Although you may believe that these practices will adversely influence the client's outcome, you must honor the diverse cultural practices of clients who come to the emergency department.

ASSESSMENT

The triage nurse performs a general survey, takes a brief history, and performs a limited physical assessment, focusing on the client's chief complaint or stated reason for seeking medical care. The objectives of the triage assessment are to collect baseline data and establish priorities for the client's care.

General Assessment of the Client Presenting for Emergency Care

When a client approaches the triage area, the nurse visually surveys the client's ability to breathe, level of consciousness, motor functions, and skin color. The survey also includes observation of the client's hygiene, appropriateness of dress, posture, and facial expressions. The mood of the client and family may be important.

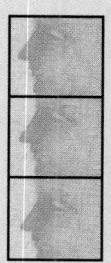

CROSS-CULTURAL CARE
CARING FOR A HOMELESS MAN

Barry is a homeless man who was brought to the emergency department by emergency medical personnel. He is separated from his wife and child and has been homeless for 2 years. He has a history of clinical depression. However, Barry has not taken his antidepressant medication for at least 3 years.

Homelessness is a national health concern that affects men, women, and children of all ages. Although all clients are unique, homeless people tend to share certain cultural health characteristics, such as the following:

- Difficulty meeting daily basic needs, such as finding food, toileting, and securing a safe place to sleep.
- A focus on the present moment, not the future.
- The need to live an invisible life to avoid street dangers.
- Health problems that usually relate to environmental conditions, such as upper respiratory infections, malnutrition, and hypothermia.
- The need to seek primary health care from local emergency departments because of the 24-hour availability of treatment without the need to pay for it.
- Decreased self-esteem, depression, powerlessness, hopelessness, and an apathetic attitude caused by the loss of a functional role in society.
- High stress levels, which can lead to anger, irritability, and feelings of despair.
- Positive response to nonjudgmental, nonthreatening health care environments.
- Benefits gained from a referral to a social service agency that addresses the person holistically.

The staff in an emergency department setting have frequent contact with homeless people. See how Susan, an emergency department nurse, talks with Barry in a manner that meets his cultural needs:

Susan: Barry, you are in the emergency department now. The paramedics brought you here when they found you lying in the street. We're going to make sure that you didn't suffer any damage in this cold weather. Okay?

Barry: Okay, but don't tie me up with those ropes any more.

Susan: Barry, they're not ropes. They're padded restraints, and they were put on you because you fought with the paramedics as they were trying to help you. Do you understand?

Barry: Yeah, I get it. But I'm okay. I just feel asleep in the street because I had nowhere else to go. The shelter is full tonight. I'm okay.

Susan: Yes, you seem okay. But it's important to us that you weren't injured by the cold weather. The only way we can find out is to run some blood tests and monitor your heart for a little while. Is that okay?

Barry: Yes, but I'm leaving here anytime I want to. I don't have to stay here.

Susan: [As Barry is attached to the cardiac monitor, pulse oximeter, and automatic blood pressure machine, an emergency technician prepares to start an intravenous line and draw blood.] We know you don't have to stay here. We're going to give you some warm fluids. Later, when we know you're okay, we'll order you some food and get you in touch with the social worker. Will you stay here and stay calm so we can help you?

Barry: Yeah. It would be nice to have some hot food from someone who cares.

Critical Thinking Questions

- Is the emergency department an appropriate setting to make sure that a homeless client has a proper meal, referral to a social worker, and temporary shelter?
- Considering that homeless people tend to feel powerless, anxious, and hopeless, how did Susan help or hinder Barry in coping with these problems?
- In your opinion, how did Susan manage Barry's potential for anger?

Reference

Davis, R.E. (1996). Tapping into the culture of homelessness. *Journal of Professional Nursing, 12,* 176–183.

Action Alert!
Make a quick survey of the client's ability to breathe and level of consciousness when the client first approaches triage.

Health History

The keys to obtaining a concise but careful health history at triage are to listen to the subjective data and ask specific questions to focus the client's chief complaint.

Closed-ended or open-ended questions may be asked to help the client describe the reason for seeking care. Note the client's psychological affect while obtaining the health history.

Quickly establishing rapport with clients of diverse cultural, ethnic, and personal traits can be challenging. Dialects, slang, street talk, and foreign languages complicate your efforts to obtain a history. Additionally, the fear associated with a serious illness or injury can produce defensive, angry behaviors.

Physical Examination

The primary goals in the physical examination are to assess the immediate threat from the chief complaint and to set priorities for care. Vital signs are essential baseline information to assess physiological integrity. If you have doubts as to which vital signs to assess, err on the side of completeness.

A complete set of vital signs in a client age 12 or older includes blood pressure, pulse, respiratory rate, and temperature. In clients under age 12, the weight (recorded in kilograms) is usually substituted for the blood pressure. However, blood pressure is taken on all clients with a history of a head injury or multiple trauma. All clients under age 16 should be weighed.

Diagnostic Tests

A wide variety of tests can be done in the emergency department to aid rapid diagnosis. The following diagnostic studies are most commonly ordered.

PULSE OXIMETRY. Any client with a high risk for low plasma oxygenation is monitored with pulse oximetry. An oxygen saturation (SaO_2) below 90% warrants immediate attention. Pediatric clients with a respiratory illness should have a pulse oximetry reading done to detect a low SaO_2.

PEAK EXPIRATORY FLOW RATE. This test uses a peak expiratory flow meter to provide a baseline measure of airflow obstruction (Fig. 58–2). Administer it before and after giving bronchodilators to a client with reactive airway disease, such as an asthma attack.

COMPLETE BLOOD COUNT. This test assesses for infection and internal bleeding in clients with acute problems and clients who may need surgery, particularly those with bleeding or abdominal pain.

ELECTROLYTE LEVELS. This test is ordered for clients with acute problems and those with a history of vomiting and diarrhea. It helps reveal the causes of problems such as cardiac dysrhythmia, altered mental status, or syncope.

SERUM GLUCOSE LEVEL. Ordered for clients with an altered level of consciousness, this test screens for uncontrolled glucose levels. It also may be ordered for any client who seems inebriated or who has symptomatic diabetes mellitus.

BLOOD UREA NITROGEN (BUN) AND SERUM CREATININE LEVELS. These tests assess kidney function. While BUN may also be altered by dehydration, serum creatinine is specific to kidney function.

LIPASE AND AMYLASE LEVELS. A physician may order this test for a client with abdominal pain, especially if the client has a history of pancreatitis or alcohol abuse.

CARDIAC ENZYMES. Because damaged cardiac tissue produces enzymes, this test is ordered for clients who have chest pain. The test may include levels of troponin T, troponin I, and serum myoglobin.

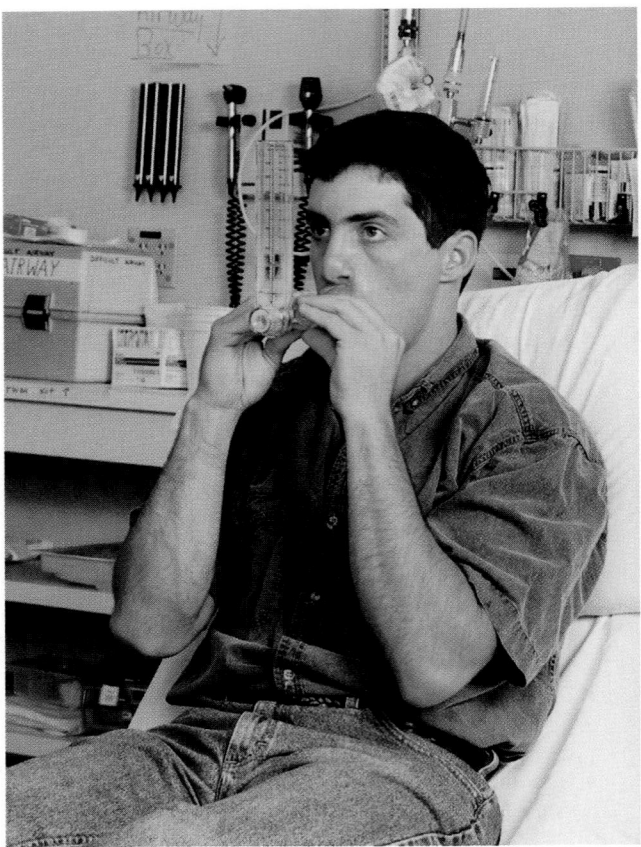

Figure 58–2. Determining a client's peak expiratory flow rate with a peak expiratory flow meter is a common diagnostic test used in the emergency department.

COAGULATION STUDIES. These tests, ordered to monitor anticoagulation therapy, may include a prothrombin time for a client taking warfarin (Coumadin) or a partial prothrombin time as a baseline for a client that may receive heparin.

ARTERIAL BLOOD GAS LEVELS. This test provides a more detailed and more accurate view of the client's respiratory function than pulse oximetry.

TOXICOLOGY SCREEN. Depending on the client's signs and symptoms, a physician may order a serum ethanol level or serum or urine tests for barbiturates, benzodiazepines, amphetamines, opiates, cannabis, acetaminophen, and salicylates. A toxicology screen is commonly ordered for a client who may have overdosed on drugs or for an older adult with a sudden change in mental status.

RADIOLOGICAL STUDIES. Extremity films, chest x-rays, and abdominal films are common x-rays obtained from the emergency department. The x-ray department is usually adjacent to the emergency department and used to obtain other diagnostic studies.

Focused Assessment for Impaired Gas Exchange

Impaired gas exchange can result in hypoxemia, a medical emergency that arises when the client has a plasma oxygen saturation (PO_2) of less than 90% (Consensus Conference, 1996). A hypoxemic state can lead to respiratory arrest, cardiac arrest, or both.

Naturally, if a client is in obvious respiratory distress, your assessment should begin with the airway. A person can die within a few minutes if his airway is totally occluded. Consequently, in life-threatening respiratory distress, you will collect subjective and objective data at the same time that you begin rendering immediate respiratory care.

Objective data include overall appearance, posture, level of consciousness, and skin color. The client in respiratory distress will sit upright or lean forward, appear anxious, and have visible, exaggerated movements of the chest wall. Other signs include use of accessory muscles, a prolonged expiratory phase, rapid respiratory rate, and shallow breathing. In severe hypoxia, the client's skin will feel cold and clammy, and the client may lose consciousness. Breath sounds in a client with severe respiratory distress may be decreased or absent.

Gather subjective data in a brief and direct manner to save time and to minimize the client's oxygen needs (Box 58–2). When the client can converse without respiratory distress, ask the following questions to obtain a more complete subjective database.

- How long have you had a breathing problem? Do you normally have shortness of breath?
- Do you have a cough? If so, is it productive? What color is the sputum?
- Do you hurt anywhere? (If so, use the PQRST mnemonic for further assessment; see Chapter 37.)

BOX 58–2

GATHERING DATA FROM A CLIENT WITH RESPIRATORY DISTRESS

The following is a list of direct, closed-ended questions you may use to obtain data from a client in respiratory distress:

- *Can you speak?* A client with a complete airway obstruction will not be able to speak.
- *Do you have a history of a respiratory problem?* The most basic treatment for any respiratory problem is to give oxygen. However, the amount and route differ according to the client's respiratory history.
- *Are you on oxygen at home?* A client on home oxygen may have a chronic respiratory disease and an inability to tolerate high-flow oxygen.
- *Do you take any medication for this respiratory problem?* As needed, obtain or make a list of the client's respiratory and other medications.

- Do you smoke? If so, how many packs per day for how many years?
- Have you had a recent change in living or environmental conditions?

Defining Characteristics

Defining characteristics for *Impaired gas exchange* may include the following:

- Dyspnea, nasal flaring, or abnormal rate, rhythm, or depth of breathing
- Abnormal arterial blood gases
- Hypoxia
- Pale, dusky skin (possible cyanosis in neonates)
- Restlessness, somnolence, irritability, confusion, sweating, visual disturbances, or headache upon awakening
- Tachycardia

Related Factors

A low PO_2 can be the result of any medical condition that alters the ventilation-perfusion relationship in the lungs or the function of the alveolar-capillary membrane. People with head trauma, crushing chest injuries, chronic obstructive pulmonary disease, complete cervical fracture, asthma, burns with smoke inhalation, or high blood alcohol levels are at risk for hypoxemia.

A*ction* A*lert!*
The absence of adventitious breath sounds does not rule out respiratory distress. Consider all respiratory parameters.

Focused Assessment for Decreased Cardiac Output

The definition of decreased cardiac output is a volume of blood less than 5.6 liters pumped from the left ventricle per minute. Standard objective measures can be used to assess the adequacy of the client's cardiac output. Any condition that impairs cardiac output warrants immediate assessment because the client's survival is at risk.

When assessing a client who may have decreased cardiac output, ask the following key questions:

- Do you have heart problems? If yes, what is the medical diagnosis?
- Do you have swelling in your ankles or feet? If yes, for how long?
- Have you had recent dizziness or fainting?

Inspect the client's general appearance. Observe for cyanotic, clammy, pale skin. The client may have an altered level of consciousness and may appear anxious and tired. Observe the nail beds, lips, and toenails for decreased blood flow (cyanosis, decreased capillary refill, coldness). Look for signs of dehydration, such as reduced skin turgor and dry mucous membranes.

Defining Characteristics

Defining characteristics for *Decreased cardiac output* may include the following:

- Dysrhythmias, tachycardia, chest pain, abnormal cardiac enzymes
- Dyspnea, orthopnea, use of accessory muscles of respiration
- Fatigue, restlessness, altered mental state
- Jugular vein distention
- Oliguria, edema, weight gain
- Crackles, wheezing, coughing
- Reduced peripheral pulses and cold, clammy skin
- Variations in blood pressure readings.

Related Factors

Consider the diagnosis of *Decreased cardiac output* for clients with myocardial infarction, cardiac dysrhythmias, poisoning, spinal shock, hemorrhage, and heart failure. In coronary artery disease, it may be the result of left ventricular damage or dysrhythmia. In a poisoning, it may be related to the cardiotonic properties of the substance. In spinal shock, it may be the result of loss of sympathetic tone. In heart failure, it results from the failure of the heart as a pump.

Focused Assessment for Risk for Violence

Violence includes harm to the self, other clients, visitors, family members, and staff. Emergency department nurses should be alert to the signs that a client is at risk for violence. Especially in the emergency department, violence is not terribly unusual. In a Philadelphia hospital, 67% of surveyed emergency department nurses reported at least one assault during their professional careers, and 36% reported having been assaulted during the previous year (Burgess, Burgess, & Douglas, 1994). These statistics seem staggering, but they show the need for recognizing and managing potential violence.

A*ction* A*lert!*
If a client threatens violence, perform a focused assessment for the underlying cause.

To ensure a safe environment, recognize the potential for violence before it occurs. Before gathering subjective data, assess each client's general appearance. How is the client dressed? Is he disheveled or neat? Does he appear agitated or have trouble maintaining eye contact? Does he seem to understand what is being said? Does he seem to be under the influence of drugs? Does he smell of alcohol? Does he have pockets or a bag that could contain a weapon?

If you determine that your client has the potential for violence, approach him in a calm and self-assured manner. Simply ask, "How can I help you?" in a quiet and low-toned voice. When obtaining subjective data, use periods of silence to prevent the client from becoming overwhelmed. Also ask injury-specific questions. The following may serve as a guideline:

- Do you have any drugs or weapons with you?
- Did you drink or take any substances that could harm you?
- Do you physically hurt anywhere?
- Have you ever tried to harm yourself or someone before now?
- Are you hearing voices or seeing anything unusual?
- Tell me more about what happened.

A*ction* A*lert!*
Make sure a violent client has no access to hospital supplies or personal items that could be used as a weapon.

Before proceeding with a physical examination, you must be convinced that the client's risk for aggression is under control. When you begin the physical examination, explain why, where, and how you are going to touch the client. Start with basic vital signs. And be sure to assess objective data that could explain behavioral changes, such as the client's blood glucose level.

Defining Characteristics

Defining characteristics for *Risk for violence* to self or others may include the following:

- Cognitive impairment
- Conflicts in interpersonal relationships, sexual orientation, or gender identity
- History of antisocial behavior
- History of childhood abuse
- History of drug or alcohol abuse
- History of witnessing family violence
- History of violence or threats of violence
- Poor social supports
- Suicidal behavior
- Symptoms of psychosis, such as hallucinations, delusions, and loose association
- Unemployment or recent loss of job

Related Factors

Violence in the emergency department occurs for many reasons. A client involved in domestic violence who seeks medical care and solace may be followed to the emergency department by the abuser. An older adult may come to the emergency department agitated and shouting obscenities secondary to a hypoxic state. A suicidal client may have a hidden weapon and attempt self-harm when you leave the room. The client may feel anger from a previous emergency department visit. He may be under the influence of alcohol or other drugs, such as phencyclidine (PCP). He may have an existing psychiatric history, such as paranoid schizophrenia, or he may suffer from an acute organic psychosis.

A*ction* A*lert!*
Never leave a suicidal client alone. Find a sitter if you must leave the room.

In the acute area, you provide initial nursing care to Barry by beginning with a brief explanation of where he is and why he was brought to the emergency department. You assess his lung and heart sounds and take his vital signs. After helping him undress and put on a hospital gown, you take a basic health history. Barry is attached to the cardiac monitor, pulse oximeter, and automatic blood pressure machine. An intravenous saline lock is started and blood is drawn at the same time for a complete blood count, electrolyte test, and toxicology screen. Why and how would you assess his risk for violence?

Focused Assessment for Related Nursing Diagnoses

Related nursing diagnoses can be identified for both the family and the client. An experience in an emergency department elicits many feelings, and emotions are often labile. You may consider the following nursing diagnoses: *Spiritual distress, Anxiety, Powerlessness,* and *Hopelessness.* In A Caregiver's View, the wife of a severely injured client describes her experience.

Spiritual Distress

Clients and family members will react differently to a crisis based on their past experiences, spiritual belief system, life values, and personal attachment to the actual loss. Clients and family members may ask to talk with the hospital chaplain or their personal spiritual counselor. You can assist clients in spiritual distress by assessing the need for spiritual resources and care, contacting the spiritual counselor, and continuing to monitor the client's and family's need for spiritual counseling.

Anxiety

Anxiety is one of the most common responses to the need for emergency care. It can be a functional emotion at low levels. At higher levels, however, it can lead to physical and cognitive dysfunction. Anxiety can be manifested by behavioral expressions ranging from crying to verbal threats. Recognize the stressors involved for a lay person in a noisy, closed-in, fast-paced emergency setting. Assess for signs of anxiety, such as restlessness or nervousness, by asking, "How may I help you?"

Action Alert!
The question, "How may I help you?" is comforting to a client in emotional distress.

Powerlessness

Powerlessness can have a physiological cause, such as an inability to communicate after a stroke, or a situational cause, such as a lack of knowledge about the problem that needs emergency care. Refusal of medication and procedures can be a response to a feeling of powerlessness. Avoid power struggles with the client and assess for the underlying cause. Listen, and then problem-solve together.

Hopelessness

Clients who feel hopeless see no positive solutions to a problem (Carpenito, 1995). In an emergency setting, this is sometimes a reality. The loss of an infant or child, the sudden death of a loved one, or the frequent exacerbation of a chronic illness can lead to overwhelming feelings of hopelessness and despair. Assess for feelings of despair and ideas of suicide. A comforting touch and kind words are sometimes all it takes to show caring. Consult clergy, social workers, or counselors as resources.

Barry shows signs of anxiety while he is in the emergency department by displaying an occasional outburst of angry feelings and blaming others. His voice trembles as he speaks, and he seems to be on the edge of crying. Barry repeatedly states that he wants to know everything you're doing to him. At times, he loudly announces, "I can leave this place anytime I want to." Barry is displaying signs of both anxiety and powerlessness. How would you respond?

DIAGNOSIS

The nature of emergency nursing presents obstacles to the formal use of nursing diagnoses. These include clients with multisystem complaints in an environment that addresses a chief complaint, rapid turnover of clients, and the lack of a formal written care plan. Although the written record does not always reflect the process, it is advantageous and quite feasible to use nursing diagnoses. However, the clustering of data, as shown in the accompanying chart, continues to guide the setting of priorities and selection of interventions.

PLANNING

The emergency department has plans for groups or categories of clients in the form of protocols for management. Additionally, the nursing staff plans for nursing needs that are common to all emergency department clients. Long-term and short-term goals have a specific meaning in the emergency department.

For example, in hypoxemia, the immediate goal is to ensure an oxygen saturation above 95%. An intermediate outcome is that the client maintains respiratory function while the etiology of the hypoxemia is determined. The long-term expected outcome is identification and treatment of the etiology.

Barry might have developed hypoxemia if he had vomited and aspirated while still on the street. The short-term outcome for Barry is to have an oxygen saturation above 95% immediately after arriving at the emergency department. The intermediate outcome is that high saturation levels are maintained while diagnostic tests and physical examinations are performed. The long-term expected outcome is that Barry suffers no permanent cerebral or tissue damage from hypoxia.

The immediate goal for a client with a decreased cardiac output is the stabilization of vital signs at a

A CAREGIVER'S VIEW

I HAD NO IDEA HOW THIS ACCIDENT WAS GOING TO CHANGE OUR LIVES

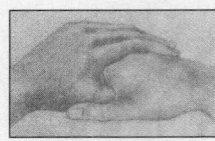

I was at work when the phone call came. My husband Mike had been rushed to the hospital, unconscious. While evaluating the roof of an apartment building, he had fallen through a skylight onto a concrete floor 25 feet below.

The next few hours are a blur. As soon as I got to the hospital, someone gave me Mike's wedding ring. I put it on my hand and kept it there. A hospital volunteer stayed with me for the first couple of hours. I was in shock. I didn't cry, didn't talk much, just prayed a lot. As family members came in, the volunteer explained to them what had happened and that Mike was in a coma.

Then a nurse took me into the emergency room to see Mike. He was almost unrecognizable. His whole head and face were swollen and discolored, his right ear was crumpled and black. He looked like a big plum. His right arm was in a cast because he had fallen on his right side and broken his wrist. He had tubes everywhere. The doctors told me he had a 50-50 chance of living through the night and that they were going to do a CT scan to check for paralysis. That's when I fell apart. I hadn't even thought about the possibility of paralysis. Mike was only 29 years old. I was 22. I had no idea how this accident was going to change our lives; I just wanted him to live.

After he survived the first 24 hours, the ICU nurses told me that the next 3 days would be critical. I stayed at the hospital but I couldn't sleep until those 3 days were up. He lay in a coma for 21 days, cared for by an amazing, wonderful team of ICU nurses. Most of them

took time to explain the how and why of every procedure. I needed that reassurance, needed to trust that he was getting the best possible care. They talked to Mike, not knowing whether he could hear or understand, and they talked with me, asked how I was doing.

Mike spent 99 days in the hospital, and I visited him every day. I stayed with him every night until he was out of the coma—an incredibly difficult time. Our parents were taking turns looking after the children, and it was hard for them to understand just what was going on, especially our daughter, who was just 18 months old.

When Mike came out of the coma, he had episodes of violence, punching at people, trying to run away. He even tried to break out of the restraints, so they assigned one-on-one nurses, most of them male, to be with him so I could get away for a little rest. These nurses were great companions to both of us, very understanding and supportive.

The rehabilitation team was wonderful too. They never gave up on him. They encouraged him, praised his progress—and that helped keep me going. When Mike was in rehab, I took our 6-year-old son and our daughter to see him for the first time. My son seemed relieved to see Mike. I think until then he had believed his dad was dead.

Looking back on that experience, I realize how much I came to depend on the nurses for information and support, and how much I appreciated their patience, honesty, and basic human kindness. Most of them were so gentle with him when they bathed him and shaved his face. And they spent time with me too, asked how I

(continued)

level that produces adequate tissue perfusion. This goal is achieved by giving such medications as vasoconstrictors (to increase blood pressure) and inotropic agents (to strengthen the heart). The long-term expected outcome is identification and treatment of the cause.

Examples of these outcomes in Barry show an immediate increase in cardiac output as evidenced by stable vital signs and an increase in his SaO_2 level; an intermediate outcome is that his cardiac output is maintained while the diagnostic tests are reviewed and appropriate resources consulted. The long-term outcome is that his lack of cardiac output causes no permanent organ damage.

The short-term expected outcome for a client at risk for violence is immediate physical and emotional safety. The intermediate outcome is to maintain calm and nonviolent behaviors while diagnostic tests, physical assessment, and appropriate resources are

consulted. The long-term outcome is that the etiology of the behavior is determined and treated appropriately.

With Barry, the short-term outcome is that he and those around him experience no physical harm. The intermediate outcome is that he remains calm after the physical restraints are removed, his laboratory values are determined, and he begins to verbalize his reasons for the violent behavior. The long-term outcome is that he remains nonviolent and receives a social service follow-up for his self-abusive and violent behavior.

INTERVENTION

Interventions for the Acute Area

The acute treatment area demands constant vigilance to detect rapid changes in a client's status. Electronic monitoring of heart rate and rhythm, blood pressure readings, and pulse oximetry are standard procedure.

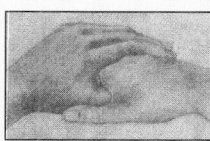

was doing, asked about the children, and talked with me about our life before this happened. One nurse brought in books and articles to help me understand what was happening with Mike. Others told me about patients with similar injuries and how they and their families had coped.

There were a few nurses—just a few—who could have done a better job. Some of them just seemed to give up on Mike and told me I might never get him back. That outright negativity was unacceptable. Once they found out how young I was, they didn't give me credit for being able to handle the situation. One night a nurse came in and told me to go home, didn't introduce herself or anything, but kept repeating: "You need to go home and get some rest." I couldn't explain why I couldn't go home, why I needed to be there, and so we got into an argument. That was awful.

It's been almost a year since the accident and Mike is doing well. He looks the same as ever and is walking and talking fine. He's come a long way. After he came out of the coma, he didn't know me; he thought I was one of the nurses. Telling him over and over about our life together has helped rebuild his memory, especially about the children. He remembered our son and mine from a previous relationship. But he didn't remember that the daughter we have together is his own. He's very sweet, but he didn't remember me, and he's not the person I remember. We've gone from being mother/child to sister/brother, but it's like starting over in the marriage. With therapy and counseling, he's slowly be-

ginning to remember things. Sometimes he surprises me by remembering something on his own, and it's like getting a present.

I see progress here and there all the time. He behaves much more like an adult now. For a while he couldn't even watch scary movies. But the first seizure after he got home set him back a lot. He's on medication to control the seizures, and that makes him tired. His EEGs are good but he does have scar tissue on the brain. There were four fractures and damage to the frontal and side lobes. However, we both hope that eventually he'll be able to work again. Memory is the main concern. Sometimes you can talk with him and 10 minutes later he won't remember the conversation. And he goes off the subject sometimes or makes immature comments. Working on two different things at once is a struggle for him too.

This has been a big wake-up call for me. It made me realize that life is short and you never know what someone else is going through. Things like this happen to people every day. Worker's compensation has been a blessing in taking care of expenses, but this has been a huge financial setback. Family and friends have helped a lot but we're basically living on my salary. I'm a secretary, not a big wage earner. The hardest part is being responsible for everything—house, finances, children—and not having any time for myself. It's lonely, and that's the biggest change. Whenever I feel like I'm about to "lose it," I talk with Mike's therapist or with my family or friends, and that helps. My faith in God has truly seen me through all of this. I'm doing better, but I wonder about the future and how long I can do all this by myself.

Emergency department nurses must constantly watch for rapid declines or gradual changes that demonstrate a trend of deterioration.

Emergency nurses commonly recognize warning signs and symptoms and initiate treatments before a full arrest occurs. Other interventions may include improving gas exchange, increasing cardiac output, and reducing the risk for violence.

Initiating Cardiopulmonary Resuscitation

Your role requires quick thinking and fast acting in an emergent situation. The most crucial nursing intervention is initiating life-saving techniques. This could be as simple as opening an airway for an infant who is not breathing or as intense as giving cardiopulmonary resuscitation (CPR) with a full arrest procedure to an adult. Remember, a fully trained staff and physician are readily available to assist in emergent situations (Procedure 58–1).

In a health care setting, CPR is initiated by the person who finds the victim. The rescuer determines that the client is unresponsive, calls a code, and begins CPR. The CPR team usually includes a respiratory therapist, an intensive care nurse, an experienced general duty nurse, and a physician. Someone to draw blood for the laboratory and a technician with a portable x-ray machine may also respond to the code. Each person involved with the CPR procedure has a specific task assigned in advance. The tasks include the following:

- Inserting an endotracheal tube and ventilating the client with a bag-valve mask
- Performing chest compressions
- Starting an intravenous line
- Setting up intravenous solutions
- Preparing and administering medications
- Attaching a heart monitor and pulse oximeter
- Recording the procedure for legal documentation
- Caring for the family

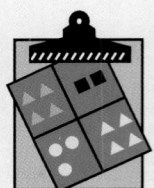

CLUSTERING DATA TO MAKE A NURSING DIAGNOSIS
EMERGENT PROBLEMS

Data Cluster	Diagnosis
A 67-year-old client has a history of chronic respiratory disease, upright posture, and labored breathing. Respirations are 26; SaO_2 is 82% on room air. There are decreased lung sounds in all fields.	*Impaired gas exchange* related to hypoxia
A middle-aged male presents to the emergency department complaining of chest pain for the past 4 hours. The pain is of sudden onset and radiates to the left arm. Blood pressure is 92/62, pulse 102 and irregular, respirations 22, temperature 99.2°F orally; SaO_2 is 89% room air. Peripheral pulses are faint, and skin is clammy and pale.	*Decreased cardiac output* related to myocardial infarction
A 26-year-old client ingested 30 tricyclic antidepressant pills 2 hours ago in a suicide attempt and is now unconscious. Blood pressure is 84/68, pulse 132 and irregular, respirations 12 and shallow, temperature 100.2°F rectally. SaO_2 is 94% on 100% oxygen.	*Decreased cardiac output* related to tricyclic cardiac toxicity
A client is brought to the emergency department after being arrested for fighting in a tavern. He acts inebriated and has alcohol on the breath and clothes. Blood pressure is 168/102, pulse 96, respirations 28, temperature 97.7°F tympanic. The client is screaming obscenities and trying to get out of four-point restraints.	*Risk for violence: directed at others,* related to substance abuse

- Making contact with a physician, laboratory, x-ray technician, and electrocardiogram operator

Improving Gas Exchange

The client in an emergency department may need interventions to restore and monitor his respiratory function. Interventions to treat hypoxemia are aimed at oxygenation of tissues. The team works together to establish the client's airway, breathing, and circulation; administer supplemental oxygen; deliver intravenous fluids, blood products, and medications; monitor vital signs, cardiac function, and oxygen level; perform diagnostic tests; and assist with endotracheal intubation and mechanical ventilation.

PROVIDING SUPPLEMENTAL OXYGEN
According to the American Heart Association, any client in respiratory distress with the potential for decreased PO_2 should receive supplemental oxygen (Cummins, 1997). The amount and delivery device will vary depending on the client's underlying medical condition and clinical symptoms.

*A*ction *A*lert!
Always assess for a history of chronic obstructive pulmonary disease before administering supplemental oxygen. Giving too much oxygen or giving it too quickly could actually depress this client's respiratory drive.

MINIMIZING OXYGEN DEMANDS
Besides giving oxygen to keep the client's oxygen saturation above 90%, you will need to minimize the client's oxygen demand to help maintain his physiological state. Simple ways to reduce oxygen demand are to place the client in a comfortable position, encourage the client not to talk, and allow the client to stay in one place. For example, place the urinal and all personal items within reach. Anticipating the client's needs and concerns reduces the need for the client to attempt communication.

Another intervention to minimize oxygen demand is to administer intravenous sedatives and analgesics. The medications work by decreasing sympathetic nervous system activity and reducing the total energy expenditure and work of breathing. You must monitor

Cardiopulmonary Resuscitation

TIME TO
ALLOW
▼
Novice:
4 minutes
Expert:
4 minutes

If you discover that a client has stopped breathing, that his heart has stopped beating, or both, you will need to "call a code" and start cardiopulmonary resuscitation (CPR). Done correctly, this procedure helps keep oxygenated blood flowing to the client's brain and other tissues until help arrives.

Delegation Guidelines

The nursing assistant may be the first caregiver to discover a client with cardiopulmonary arrest. Most institutions therefore require assistive personnel to be competent in CPR or basic life support. The trained nursing assistant may initiate CPR and call for help. Upon the arrival of help, the nursing assistant will be relieved of resuscitative duties and employed to gather and assemble the necessary emergency equipment or summon other expertise as needed. In an institutional setting, the roles of personnel in such emergencies are often delineated in advance of an actual event.

Equipment Needed

- Bag-valve mask, if available

1 Assess the person for unresponsiveness.

To see if the person is responsive, tap his shoulder or gently shake him while loudly speaking his name.

2 If the person fails to respond, call for help by activating the emergency response system according to your facility's policy.

In most facilities, you will ask the switchboard operator to announce a certain code along with the client's location. If you are in the community, you will most likely call 911 or a local emergency response system.

3 Make sure the person has an open airway.

a. Position the client on his back on a hard, flat surface, if possible. Place his arms at his sides.

This position maximizes the effectiveness of CPR. If you must roll the person over, use a log-roll maneuver, in which the person's entire body rolls as a unit. This process minimizes the risk of twisting his spine.

b. Open the airway using the head tilt–chin lift maneuver or the jaw thrust maneuver.

An unconscious person faces a high risk that his tongue and soft tissues of the pharynx will obstruct his airway. If the person may have a neck injury, use the jaw thrust maneuver rather than the head tilt–chin lift.

c. Remove visible food or vomitus from the person's mouth.

If the person has liquid in his mouth, cover your index and middle fingers with a cloth and sweep his mouth. If the person has solid material in his mouth, use your index finger to remove it.

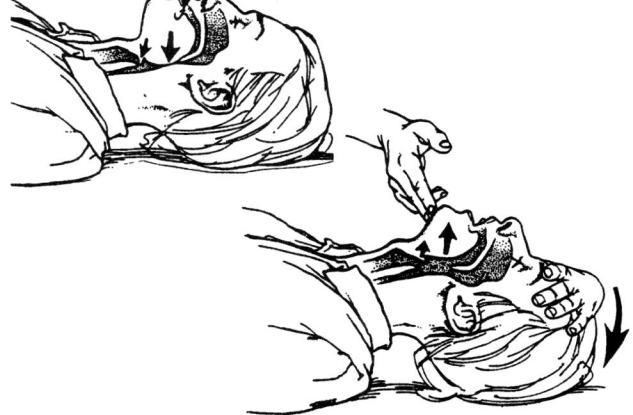

Opening the airway using the head tilt–chin lift maneuver. (From Emergency Cardiac Care Committee and Subcommittees [1992]. AHA guidelines for cardiopulmonary resuscitation and emergency cardiac care. JAMA, 268, 2193. Copyright 1992, American Medical Association.)

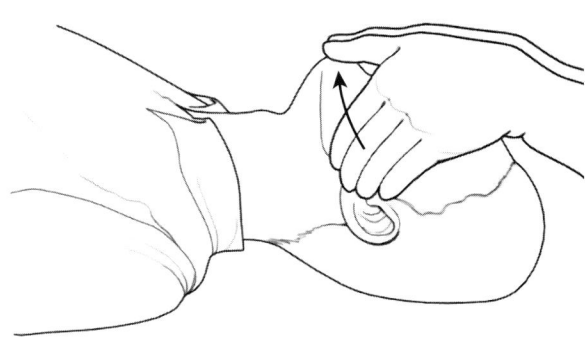

Opening the airway using the jaw thrust maneuver.

Continued

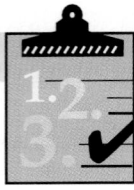
Cardiopulmonary Resuscitation

4 Determine whether the person is breathing.

This process should take about 3 to 5 seconds. Remember to keep the person's airway open while you assess his breathing.

a. Look to see whether the person's chest rises and falls.

If you notice that the person is trying to breathe but cannot, make sure that you have successfully opened his airway. Remember that reflex gasping, which occurs early in cardiac arrest, is not adequate to oxygenate the person's blood.

b. Position your ear over the person's mouth and nose. Listen for exhaled air and see if you can feel air escaping onto your face.

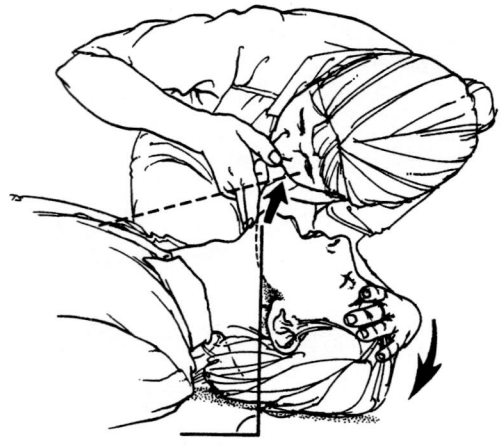

Listening and feeling for exhalation. (From Emergency Cardiac Care Committee and Subcommittees [1992]. AHA guidelines for cardiopulmonary resuscitation and emergency cardiac care. JAMA, 268, 2193. Copyright 1992, American Medical Association.)

If you determine that the person is breathing and he has not sustained a traumatic injury, log-roll him onto his side (the recovery position) and continue to watch him closely until either he revives or additional help arrives.

5 If the victim is not breathing, begin administering breaths.

If possible, use a bag-valve mask or another type of barrier device to administer breaths. If this is not possible, perform mouth-to-mouth, mouth-to-nose, or mouth-to-stoma breathing. Exhaled air contains enough oxygen to support brain and tissue function. Throughout rescue breathing, remember to keep the person's airway open.

a. To administer effective mouth-to-mouth breaths, you will need to keep air from escaping through

the person's nose. To do so, use the thumb and index finger of the hand resting on the person's forehead to gently pinch his nose closed.

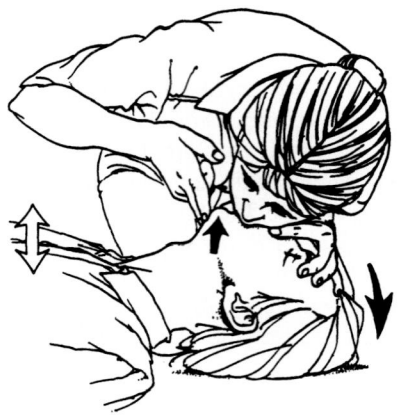

Performing mouth-to-mouth breathing. (From Textbook of Basic Life Support for Healthcare Providers, 1994. Copyright American Heart Association.)

b. Likewise, to administer effective mouth-to-nose breaths, you will need to keep air from escaping through the person's mouth. To do so, use the hand resting below the person's chin to hold his mouth closed.

c. Take a deep breath and place your lips around the victim's mouth or nose.

Make sure that your lips have created an airtight seal. If you are using a bag-valve mask, hold the edges of the mask against the person's face to make an airtight seal.

d. Give two slow breaths. Inhale between breaths if you are not using a bag-valve mask.

Each breath should last 1½ to 2 seconds, long enough to fill the person's lungs. You should see the person's chest rise with each breath. Avoid administering breaths too quickly or forcefully because excessive pressure can cause air to enter the person's stomach rather than his lungs.

e. After delivering each breath, turn your head so your ear is positioned over the person's mouth and nose. Listen and feel for exhaled air.

If you do not hear or feel the exhalation, reposition the person, make sure his airway is open (by repositioning his head and removing foreign matter as needed), and try again. If you are administering mouth-to-nose breaths, you may need to open the person's mouth to allow exhalation.

6 Check for a pulse at the person's carotid artery

This process should take about 5 to 10 seconds.

a. Locate the carotid artery in the groove between the trachea and the large muscles along the sides of the neck. Place two or three fingers in this groove.

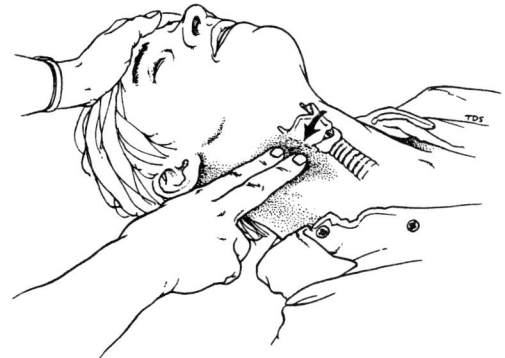

Feeling for the carotid pulse. (From Emergency Cardiac Care Committee and Subcommittees [1992]. AHA guidelines for cardiopulmonary resuscitation and emergency cardiac care. JAMA, 268, 2193. Copyright 1992, American Medical Association.)

Keep the person's head in its tilted position to maintain an open airway during this process.

b. If you feel a pulse but the person is not breathing, resume rescue breathing at 10 to 12 breaths per minute (one every 5 to 6 seconds).

Remember that the person may have a slow pulse, a weak or thready pulse, or an irregular pulse. Palpate carefully before deciding that the person has no pulse.

c. If you feel no pulse and the person is not breathing, begin chest compressions.

7 Assume the proper position for chest compressions.

To maximize the effectiveness of chest compressions, make sure the person's head is not elevated above his feet, and make sure he is lying on a hard surface.

a. Place the heel of one hand on the bottom half of the person's sternum, just above the xiphoid process.

To reduce the risk of fracturing the person's ribs, position the long axis of the heel of your hand on the long axis of the person's sternum.

b. Place your other hand on top of the first, so your hands are parallel.

c. Raise your fingers off of the person's chest, so only the heels of your hands rest on his sternum.

If you prefer, you can twine your fingers together to help keep them off the person's chest wall.

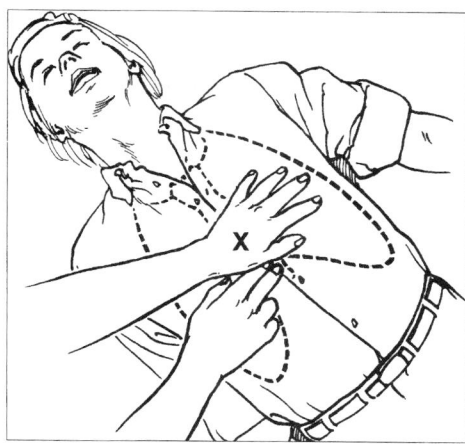

Finding the correct position for external chest compressions. (From Textbook of Basic Life Support for Healthcare Providers, 1994. Copyright American Heart Association.)

d. Lock your elbows and keep your arms straight. Position your shoulders directly over the person's sternum, so you form a straight line from your shoulders through your arms to your hands on the person's sternum.

Compressing the chest straight down is most effective. In this position, you can use your body weight to help compress the chest. Also, compressing straight down helps keep the person from rolling.

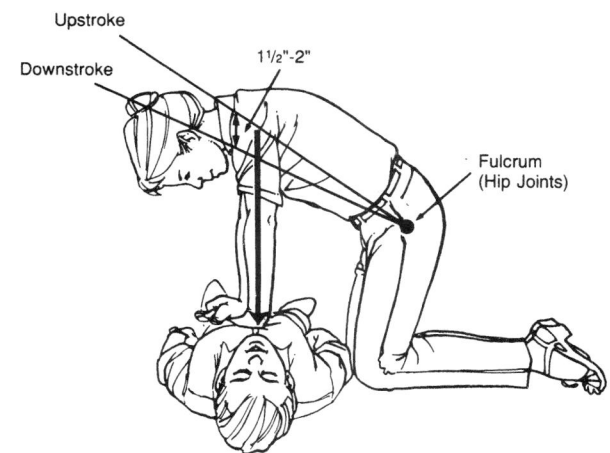

Performing chest compressions. (From Textbook of Basic Life Support for Healthcare Providers, 1994. Copyright American Heart Association.)

8 Administer chest compressions.

a. With each compression, apply enough force to depress the person's chest by about 1½ to 2 inches.

Continued

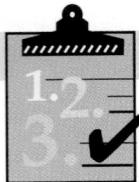

Cardiopulmonary Resuscitation

For a very small person, you may not need this degree of compression. For a large person, you may need more force to create a palpable carotid or femoral pulse. Ideally, a colleague will monitor the person's femoral pulse to make sure that your compressions are forceful enough to produce a pulse.

b. Between compressions, release the pressure fully and allow the person's chest to return to its normal position.

This allows blood to flow to the person's heart and chest.

c. Deliver 15 compressions at a rate of 80 to 100 compressions per minute.

The use of 80 to 100 compressions per minute makes it more likely that you will maintain compression for 50% of the cycle, which will maximize arterial pressure. Properly performed, chest compressions can produce systolic arterial blood pressure peaks of 60 to 80 mm Hg.

d. While giving compressions, count "one and, two and, three and, four and, five and, six and, seven and, eight and, nine and, ten and, eleven and, twelve and, thirteen and, fourteen and, fifteen."

9 Begin the standard cycle of chest compressions and rescue breaths.

a. After 15 compressions, open the person's airway and give two slow rescue breaths.

b. Find the proper hand position and give 15 more compressions at a rate of 80 to 100 per minute.

c. After four complete cycles of 15 compressions and two breaths, reassess the client.

If you detect no carotid pulse, continue with chest compressions and rescue breaths until help arrives. If you detect a pulse, check to see if the person is breath-

ing. If not, administer rescue breaths at a rate of 10 to 12 per minute and monitor the person's pulse closely.

10 If a colleague arrives to help you before the full emergency team is ready, coordinate your rescue efforts.

a. After giving 15 chest compressions, open the person's airway and begin rescue breathing. At this point, your colleague can take over the chest compressions

b. When you complete the two rescue breaths, your colleague can begin chest compressions counting out loud, "one and, two and, three and, four and, five."

The first compression will produce exhalation. Deliver chest compressions at a rate of 80 to 100 per minute. Because of the time needed to administer breaths, the person will actually receive about 60 compressions per minute. To help maintain the proper hand position, the person delivering chest compressions should not take her hands away from the person's chest.

c. As the person's chest is rising after receiving the fifth compression, give one breath.

d. At the end of each minute, reassess for a pulse and spontaneous breathing.

In a hospital, a heart monitor can be used to track the person's heart beat. However, continue to monitor the femoral artery pulse to track the effectiveness of compressions.

e. When the emergency team arrives, interrupt CPR just long enough for the person to receive an endotracheal tube, which allows for a well-controlled airway. Connect the bag-valve mask to 100% oxygen at a high flow rate.

Based on CPR guidelines in American Heart Association (1997): Basic Life Support for Healthcare Providers. Dallas: Author.

the client's respiratory and cardiac status carefully to ensure proper gas exchange. Inform the family that the client needs to reduce oxygen needs by remaining quiet. While giving physical care, help to maintain a low anxiety level by explaining where the client is and what is being done. Use a comforting touch. Even sedated clients may respond in a positive way to a gentle voice and touch.

MONITORING

Once the client's respiratory status and vital signs are stabilized, the primary nursing interventions are aimed at reassessment and monitoring using a holistic nursing approach. Continual monitoring of the client's physiological state includes frequent assessment of respirations, blood pressure, cardiac rhythm, heart rate, and mental status.

ENDOTRACHEAL INTUBATION

Endotracheal intubation is indicated to establish and maintain an airway in clients with acute respiratory failure or respiratory arrest. The procedure is usually performed by a physician. Your role in endotracheal intubation is to make the equipment available and to initiate breathing with an Ambu bag. Intravenous sedatives and paralyzing agents may be given to the conscious client to allow rapid intubation.

The client is placed on a mechanical ventilator by the respiratory therapist. Continuously monitor the client's condition, especially his cardiac and respiratory status. Escort the client's family or significant others from the room before the procedure begins. Place them in a quiet area and keep them informed about the client's condition.

A*ction* A*lert!*
Offer emotional support to the family of an intubated client.

Increasing Cardiac Output

The basic goals for a client with *Decreased cardiac output* are to promote a cardiac output adequate to meet systemic metabolic needs and to treat the cause of the decreased output. Usually, interventions include continuous monitoring, supplemental oxygen, monitoring urinary output, giving medications, and hemodynamic monitoring.

CONTINUOUS MONITORING

The client will need continuous monitoring for early detection of hypoxia, hypotension, tachycardia, cardiac arrhythmias, pulmonary edema, and shock. Monitoring includes drawing blood for a complete blood count, electrolytes, cardiac enzymes, and clotting studies. Monitoring is initiated with a pulse oximeter unit, cardiac monitor (Fig. 58–3), automatic blood pressure cuff, and indwelling urinary catheter. Chest x-rays, a 12-lead electrocardiogram, and arterial blood gas measurements are taken.

ADMINISTERING OXYGEN

Oxygen is administered for clients with decreased cardiac output to increase the oxygen level in vital organs. The risk of hypoxemia in clients experiencing a decrease in cardiac output makes the administration of oxygen a top priority.

MONITORING URINARY OUTPUT

Low perfusion causes a decrease in urinary output. This is because the renal system responds to decreased cardiac output by vasoconstriction in the nephrons. You will need to titrate the delivery of intravenous fluids to maintain a urine output of at least 30 mL per hour to avoid renal failure. An indwelling urinary catheter is inserted to monitor urinary output.

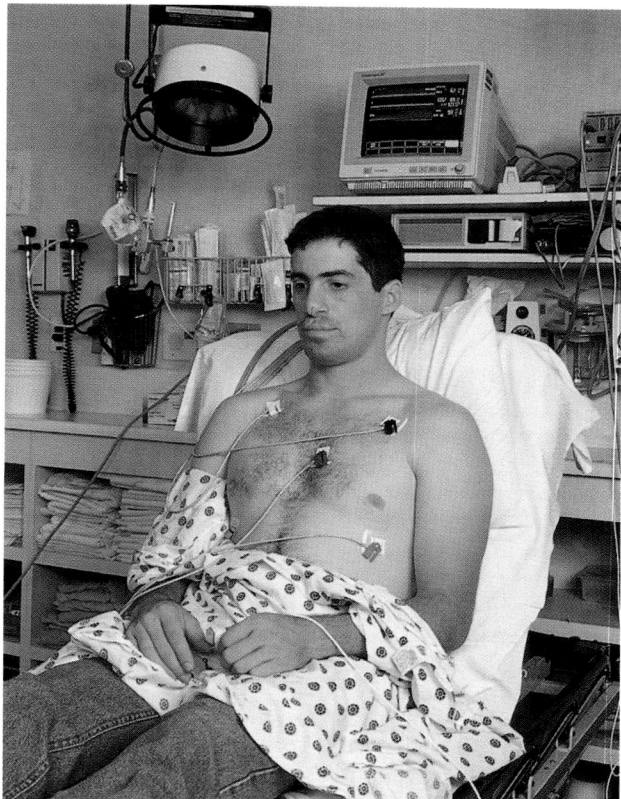

Figure 58–3. Continuous cardiac monitoring is initiated for a client experiencing decreased cardiac output.

ADMINISTERING MEDICATION

The goals in drug therapy are to increase the strength of contraction, maintain the heart rate and rhythm, and maintain blood pressure. Vasoactive drugs are used to increase cardiac output in hemodynamically unstable clients. You must have a sound knowledge of each drug's mechanism of action, indications, dosage, side effects, and appropriate administration techniques.

A*ction* A*lert!*
Administration of oxygen and vasoconstricting medications are two primary actions in working with clients with decreased cardiac output.

HEMODYNAMIC MONITORING

Hemodynamic monitoring involves using invasive procedures and sophisticated equipment to monitor the client's cardiac output, arterial pressure, and central venous pressures. Basic nursing responsibilities in hemodynamic monitoring are to prepare the client for the procedure, assist the physician with inserting either a central venous or arterial catheter, provide continuous assessment and monitoring of the client and equipment until the person is transferred from the emergency department, and provide nursing interventions based on the client's hemodynamic changes.

Reducing the Risk for Violence

The first priority with clients at risk for violent behavior is to ensure safety for the client, visitors, and staff. The secondary goal is to determine the cause of the behavior. The three safety interventions are verbal control, physical restraint, and chemical restraint. A fourth option is a combination of chemical and physical restraint.

VERBAL CONTROL

The initial approach to the client should be calm verbal intervention to immediately defuse the situation. Box 58–3 contains a list of general guidelines for approaching a verbally abusive person. Remember that some clients are out of touch with reality or under the influence of substances.

Maier (1996) discusses a talk-down procedure called *overdosing* to de-escalate a potentially violent client. Overdosing saturates the client with agreement. Do not argue. Establish verbal contact with the client using soft but assertive statements. Be aware of your own body posture, facial expressions, and attitude. Use the client's first name. Try to verbally give the client a positive sense, such as telling the person you are here to help. Avoid making the situation worse by eliminating any reason for the client to argue.

Maier (1996) states that this process of agreement gives the client an opportunity to make a choice. Each choice the client has to ponder decreases the energy expended in anger or hostility. Even if you have to agree to disagree with the client, it still allows the client more self-control and a sense of power over the situation. Look for cues that the person is de-escalating.

BOX 58–3

GUIDELINES FOR APPROACHING A VERBALLY ABUSIVE CLIENT

- Approach the client in a calm manner.
- Acknowledge the client's feelings.
- Let the client do most of the talking.
- Limit the number of other people around the client.
- Stay at least 2 feet away from the client.
- Stand to the side of the client, not directly in front.
- Stand near the door.
- Maintain eye contact, but do not stare.

Adapted from Sanchez-Gallegos, D., & Viens, D.C. (1995). When the client is armed or dangerous: Management of violent and difficult clients in primary care. Nurse Practitioner, 20(6), 26–32.

The client's body will appear more relaxed, and his arms will fall to his sides. At this time, discuss viable options for a solution. The process may only take a few minutes. It gives the angry person a chance to establish contact with one specific person, to ventilate anger without interruption, and to calm down enough to gain self-control. Keep in mind that clients who are under the influence of substances may not respond to this procedure (Maier, 1996).

PHYSICAL RESTRAINT

Physically restraining a client who is out of control is a potential hazard for you and the staff. Only properly trained persons should attempt to restrain a physically abusive client. Most emergency departments have security guards trained to handle crisis situations, and many staff members are trained in how to physically restrain an aggressive person.

Once the client is secure in restraints, it is a nursing function to make sure the client remains safe. Each emergency department has guidelines regarding the frequency of vital sign measurement, neurovascular checks, and time out for toileting (if appropriate). If the client has had a chemical restraint while in a physical restraint, you must be doubly careful to safeguard his respiratory, circulatory, and psychological status. Aspiration of vomitus, permanent nerve damage, and emotional pain and suffering are potential problems for a client who is improperly restrained. It is legally important for the staff to strictly follow the hospital's policies and procedures when caring for a physically restrained client.

CHEMICAL RESTRAINT

Chemical restraint refers to the administration of medication as a means of controlling behavior. This decision is made after all attempts to verbally calm the client have failed. Chemically restraining a client who is actively inflicting harm to self or others is one of the most appropriate and safest methods of controlling dangerous behavior. The medication is always ordered by the physician. Basic nursing guidelines to be observed when caring for a chemically restrained client appear in Box 58–4.

> **A**ction **A**lert!
> A physically or chemically restrained client must be reassessed frequently, according to the hospital's policies and procedures.

You are gentle yet deliberate in giving care to Barry. The primary nursing interventions needed—after Barry's vital signs, respiratory status, and cardiac status became stable—consist of giving warm intravenous fluids, ordering him a full meal, and monitoring his physiological status. You give priority to Barry's potential for violent behavior. He is not physically or chemically restrained because he displays no signs of harming himself or others. You realize the occasional outbursts are Barry's method of gaining control over his personal situation. Talk to him in a gentle voice, and reassure him that you are there to help him. Although Barry may leave the emergency department at any time, he has stayed in the

GUIDELINES FOR THE CARE OF A CHEMICALLY RESTRAINED CLIENT

- Remember that an abusive or violent client already feels powerless. However, this does not alter the need for restraints if the client is uncontrollable.
- Chemical restraints are ordered by an emergency physician and administered by an emergency nurse.
- Usually, the client is physically restrained to allow administration of the medication and to ensure safety for the client and staff.
- The client's respiratory, neurovascular, and mental status must be assessed routinely according to the emergency department's policy regarding restraints.
- Certain safety measures should be in place for any sedated client. For example, physical restraints may be placed on the client, and side rails should be raised at all times. Ideally, a family member should stay at the bedside to help calm the client if he awakens suddenly. Check the client's vital signs frequently.
- A psychological or psychiatric referral should be made for any emergency department client who requires restraint.

warm environment. What would you do if he said he wanted to leave?

Interventions for Discharge

Discharge from the emergency department considers the client's and family's ongoing needs and safety, whether the discharge is to home, to another facility, to another area of the hospital, or to the morgue and funeral home. It is legally imperative that you ensure the client's well-being and safety by following nursing standards for discharge.

Discharging Against Medical Advice

A client who leaves the emergency department (or any hospital department) against the advice of a physician and without proper written discharge instructions has been discharged **against medical advice** (AMA). A client may leave the emergency department for many reasons. He may grow tired of waiting for a nonacute treatment room. A physician may deny a desired treatment, as when a person with drug-seeking behaviors walks out when denied narcotics. When possible, you should have a client who leaves AMA sign a legal form stating that the hospital is not responsible for the client's welfare after he leaves. Document that the cli-

ent left AMA and was willing (or unwilling) to sign the appropriate form. Note the condition of the person upon leaving.

Discharging Home

All clients discharged from the emergency department must be able to care for themselves without difficulty or must be accompanied by a competent caregiver. Procedures for client discharge stress the importance of ethical and legal responsibilities for the client's safety. Upon discharge, the client should be in an improved physical and psychosocial condition compared to when he entered the emergency department.

The process of discharging a person home begins with obtaining subjective and objective evaluation data. Ask the client if he is feeling well enough to go home, who will provide home care, and how the client is getting home. Reassess the chief complaint, take vital signs, and document pain relief. The physician orders the discharge and gives specific instructions for home care. Give appropriate instructions to the client and caregiver in written and verbal form, explaining the medical diagnosis, home care needed, name of a follow-up physician, and information about prescription medicines. The record should reflect that the client received and understood the written instruction and has a responsible person driving him home.

Action Alert!
A client discharged home must be able to perform self-care or must have a competent caregiver.

Discharging Interfacility

In 1985, the Consolidated Omnibus Budget Reconciliation Act (COBRA) was passed. It is a Federal law stating that the transfer of clients from one health facility to another must be done using certain guidelines to ensure client safety and well-being. The COBRA law governs **interfacility transfer,** which is the transfer of an emergency department client from one health care facility to another.

In general, this law mandates that certain clients be assessed before being transferred, and that a physician accepts the client at the receiving hospital. This law also states that client hospital records must accompany the client and that qualified persons will care for the client during the transport process. Essentially, COBRA prohibits client "dumping" and imposes a financial penalty on facilities that violate the guidelines.

Action Alert!
Transfer clients only with an accepting physician, written informed client consent, and assured safety measures during transport.

A client may be transferred to a skilled nursing facility, long-term care, or mental health institution that may or may not require the same legal documents as a hospital-to-hospital transfer. The primary nursing responsibility in any client transfer is to make sure the client is physiologically and psychologically safe. For example, a client would not be transferred to a mental health facility with an unstable blood pressure and pulse from acute alcohol intoxication. Likewise, interfacility transfer would not take place if the client refused to go to the receiving facility.

The physician is responsible to write the transfer order and, in a collaborative effort, you and the physician will perform specific interventions to make sure that the client is ready for the transfer. As in any discharge, you will reassess the client, complete the proper forms, and call a report to the receiving facility.

Discharging Intrafacility

Intrafacility transfer is when a client is transferred within the same general facility as the emergency department. The client still needs to be discharged from the emergency department and admitted to the appropriate area in the same facility. You will need to keep the client in the emergency department until a physician examines the person and writes orders for admission. Perform a reassessment of the client and report to the receiving nurse caring for the client.

If the client is admitted to a specialty intensive care unit, then you probably will escort the client to the unit with portable monitoring devices in place in case an emergency arises en route. If the client needs surgery, you will prepare the person by witnessing the operative permit, performing diagnostic tests or giving medication ordered by the surgeon, and calling a report to the nurse who will care for the client after surgery.

Discharging to a Funeral Home

Death is an inevitable part of an emergency setting. When a client dies, one of your priorities is to meet the needs of the family or significant other. See Chapter 50 for a discussion of death, loss, and grief.

Clients who die in the emergency department are transported to the hospital morgue or remain in the emergency department until a funeral home representative receives the body. It is your responsibility to care for the body. If the client died as a result of violence or for an unknown reason, the medical examiner and police must be notified. Care for the body in a manner that preserves evidence; for example, any clothing removed from the client is handled while wearing gloves, bagged a specific way, and given to the law enforcement officer.

You may assist the family by calling the funeral home of their choice. Ask if the family would like you to call a priest, chaplain, or spiritual counselor of their choice. Accompany the family to view the body so you can provide emotional support and to preserve any legal evidence. Give any jewelry removed from the client (if not needed as evidence) to the family, and document the transaction on the client's record. According to protocol, you or the physician may approach the family about organ donation.

*A*ction *A*lert!
The family is high priority when a client dies in the emergency department. Offer support and call the spiritual counselor of their choice.

EVALUATION

Since most clients are in the emergency department only for a few hours, short-term evaluation is most applicable to this population. Ask yourself the following questions by way of evaluation:

- Was the client triaged in a timely manner after entering the emergency department?
- Was the problem treated in a timely manner?
- Was the client discharged in better condition than when admitted?
- Was the client satisfied with the care received?
- Is the client free of preventable complications?
- Was the initial assessment complete and appropriate to the client's condition?
- Was the client included in setting realistic goals?
- Were the family's needs met?
- Was the family fully used to support the client?
- Was care provided according to facility policies?
- Were discharge instructions fully explained and understood?
- Were appropriate precautions taken for a safe discharge?

Any client who needs long-term evaluation will be admitted to the hospital, transferred to a more appropriate facility, or given a referral for community follow-up. Any physically and emotionally stable client may go home with a community follow-up. Long-term evaluation includes social service follow-up, specialty physician referral, immunization clinic referral, or physical therapy treatments.

In Barry's case, evaluation took place in the acute area until he was warmed by fluids and hot meal, displayed calm behavior, and showed no physiological instability. After that, he was placed in the nonacute area and monitored until plans were made for a community follow-up. The social worker secured a place for him to sleep that evening and made sure he had community referrals for food, shelter, and further health care.

The Nursing Care Planning chart summarizes the application of the nursing process to Barry.

KEY PRINCIPLES

- The concept of emergency care includes treating acute, life-threatening conditions as well as nonacute (urgent, semi-urgent, and nonurgent) conditions.
- Triage is a nursing activity that involves separating and prioritizing clients to ensure that clients in life-threatening situations receive prompt treatment.
- The roles of the emergency nurse include clinician, educator, manager, and client advocate.

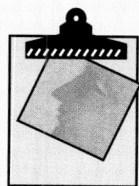

NURSING CARE PLAN
A CLIENT AT RISK FOR VIOLENCE

Admission Data

Barry is admitted to the emergency department with a risk for violence to himself and others. As he became responsive, he fought with paramedics, who placed him in four-point restraints to protect himself and others from harm. The restraints are removed in the emergency department. Barry has calmed, but he states "I'm not going to stay here."

Emergency Standing Orders

Cardiac monitoring and pulse oximetry
Complete VS with rectal temperature
Oxygen per nasal cannula @ 3 L/min

IV saline lock and blood drawn to hold for physician's orders

Physician's Orders

CBC and electrolytes
ECG
Chest x-ray

Full diet
Restrain as needed

Nursing Assessment

Barry is calm at the moment. He does not appear to have a realistic understanding of his situation. Needs social service referral.

NURSING CARE PLAN

Nursing Diagnosis	Expected Outcomes	Interventions	Evaluation
Risk for violence	Client demonstrates calm behavior and self control	Establish trusting relationship with client. *Approach client in calm and reassuring manner.* Keep ED room quiet. Use restraints as ordered.	Client remains calm and cooperative.
	Client acknowledges feelings and behaviors regarding potential violence	Encourage verbalizations regarding feelings. Encourage calm behavior.	Client verbalizes feelings and remains calm.
	Client agrees to follow up with the social worker	Arrange consult with social worker.	Social worker forms discharge plan

Italicized interventions indicate culturally specific care.

Critical Thinking Questions
1. What assessment data would predict the probability that Barry will follow up with a social worker?
2. In your opinion, what would be the optimal living arrangement to protect Barry from himself?
3. From Barry's point of view, what objection might he have to the living arrangement you envisioned?

- The three highest priorities in caring for an emergency department client are to ensure adequate oxygenation, circulation, and safety.
- Hypoxemia is the result of any pathophysiological process that reduces arterial oxygen saturation.
- A decrease in cardiac output is the result of any pathophysiological process that impairs the amount of blood ejected from the left ventricle.

- Violence in the emergency department can result from situational, developmental, or organic crisis, and may involve the client, visitors, or staff.
- Nursing interventions in the emergency department are instituted to treat life-threatening symptoms, determine the cause, and provide holistic support until the client is discharged from the emergency department.

BIBLIOGRAPHY

Badger, J.M. (1995). Reaching out to the suicidal patient. *American Journal of Nursing, 95*(3).

*Burgess, A.W., Burgess, A.G., & Douglas J.E. (1994). Examining violence in the workplace. *Journal of Psychosocial Nursing, 32*(7), 11–18.

Carpenito, L.J. (1995). *Nursing diagnosis: Application to clinical practice* Philadelphia: J.B. Lippincott Company.

Consensus Conference (1996). Tissue hypoxia: How to detect, how to correct, how to prevent. *American Journal of Respiratory and Critical Care Medicine, 154,* 1573–1578.

Cummins, R. (Ed). (1997). Advanced cardiac life support. *American Heart Association.*

Davis, R.E. (1996). Tapping into the culture of homelessness. *Journal of Professional Nursing, 12,* 176–183.

Driscoll, A., Shanahan, A., Crommy, L., & Gleeson, A. (1995). The effect of patient position on the reproducibility of cardiac output measurements. *Heart & Lung, 24*(1), 38–44.

Erstad, B.L., Grier, D.G., Scott, M.E., Esser, M.J., & Joshi, P. (1996). Recognition and treatment of ethanol abuse in trauma patients. *Heart & Lung, 25*(4), 330–336.

Furukawa, M.M. (1996). Meeting the needs of the dying patient's family. *Critical Care Nurse, 16*(1), 51–57.

Guilliatt-Herbert, A. & Mahaffey, T. (1995). Nurse-physician collaboration: A win-win survival strategy. *American Journal of Nursing (Suppl. September),* 34–37.

Hill, B., & Geraci, S.A. (1998). A diagnostic approach to chest pain based on history and ancillary evaluation. *The Nurse Practitioner, 23*(4), 20–45.

Keep, N.B., & Gilbert, C.P. (1995). How safe is your ED? *American Journal of Nursing, 95*(9), 45–51.

Kitt, S., Selfridge-Thomas, J., Proehl, J.A., & Kaiser, J. (1995). *Emergency nursing: A physiologic and clinical perspective.* Philadelphia: W.B. Saunders.

Maier, G.J. (1996). Managing threatening behavior: The role of talk down and talk up. *Journal of Psychosocial Nursing, 34*(6), 25–30.

Pakieser, R.A., Lenaghan, P.A., & Muelleman, R.L. (1998). Battered women: Where they go for help? *Journal of Emergency Nursing, 24,* 16–19.

Puntillo, K.A., & Neighbor, M.L. (1997). Two methods of assessing pain intensity in English-speaking and Spanish-speaking emergency department patients. *Journal of Emergency Nursing, 23,* 597–601.

Radwin, L.E. (1995). Knowing the patient: A process model for individualized intervention. *Nursing Research, 44,* 364–370.

Sanchez-Gallegos, D., & Viens, D.C. (1995). When the client is armed or dangerous: Management of violent and difficult clients in primary care. *Nurse Practitioner, 20*(6), 26–32.

Volsko, T.A., Chatburn, R.L., & Kallstrom, T.J. (1996). Evaluation of a commercial standard for checking pulse oximeter performance. *Respiratory Care, 41*(2), 100–104.

Wolford, S. (1995). Emergency department patient liaison volunteers: A cost containment and visitor satisfaction strategy. *Journal of Emergency Nursing, 21,* 17–21.

Zerwic, J.J. (1998). Symptoms of acute myocardial infarction: Expectations of a community sample. *Heart & Lung, 27*(2), 75–81.

*Asterisk indicates a definitive or classic work on this subject.

The Community as a Client

Phyllis Russo Wells

Key Terms

community
community forum
community health nursing
epidemiology
focus group
key informant
Omaha system

opinion survey
parish nurse
participant observation
public health nursing
vulnerable population
windshield survey

LEARNING OBJECTIVES

After studying this chapter, you should be able to:

1. Describe basic concepts of community health nursing as it applies to the community as the client.
2. Discuss factors that affect community health.
3. Describe several methods and types of data used in assessing communities.
4. Identify two approaches to nursing diagnosis for groups, populations, or communities.
5. Describe methods used in planning care for a community.
6. Identify goal-directed interventions that promote health and prevent disease in a community.
7. Identify methods of evaluation used to measure outcomes of community health interventions.

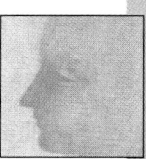

ABC Day School is a day care center for children ages 18 months through 11 years. It provides care from 7:00 AM to 6:00 PM, Monday through Friday. These past 2 weeks, many of the children and several of the staff have had diarrhea. A community health nurse from the county health department has been called to assess the situation, identify the cause or causes, and advise on methods of prevention.

COMMUNITY HEALTH NURSING DIAGNOSES

Knowledge Deficit (Specify): Absence or deficiency of cognitive information related to specific topic.

Health-Seeking Behaviors (Specify): A state in which an individual in stable health is actively seeking ways to alter personal health habits and/or the environment to move toward a higher level of health.

From North American Nursing Diagnosis Association. (1999). NANDA nursing diagnoses: Definitions and classification 1999–2000. Philadelphia: Author.

CONCEPTS OF COMMUNITY AS CLIENT

To understand the concept of the community as a client, one needs to define community and community health nursing. A **community** is a geographic location, or an aggregate or population of individuals who have one or more personal or environmental characteristics in common (Hunt & Zurek, 1997). In other words, a community is defined by location, people, and social systems. As a location, a community is defined by its boundaries, such a city, county, or nation, or by political boundaries, such as a precinct or ward. A community can also be defined as a group of people or a population with a common interest, culture, religion, or race, such as people working together to make a playground safe for children, a Native American group, or a Jewish community. Communities can vary in size, from a small group to the global community around the world.

Community health nursing is the field of nursing that promotes and preserves the health of these populations by (1) understanding and applying concepts of public health and community, (2) working with community organizations to assist in community development, (3) providing generalist care to selected individuals, families, and groups, and (4) providing health promotion, health maintenance, health education, and coordination of care.

It is a synthesis of nursing theory and public health theory aimed at preserving and promoting the health of communities. When nursing practice is focused on a group or community, the group or community is the client. Nursing care directed to individuals or families contributes to the health of the total population, but the goal in community health nursing is to have an impact on the group or community as a whole. Other definitions of community health nursing are based on where health care activities take place, such as in a client's home or at a neighborhood location such as a school, rather than locations considered to be health agencies, such as public and private health facilities (American Nurses Credentialing Center, 1998).

In the literature, the term *community health nursing* may be used interchangeably with *public health nursing*. **Public health nursing** is more strictly defined as the practice of promoting and protecting the health of populations through nursing activities to improve the quality of life (including its physical, mental, and social aspects), to prevent disease, and to control communicable disease consistent with available knowledge and resources.

Community health nursing draws heavily on the concept of primary health care. Both involve community participation in decision-making, focus on health promotion and disease prevention, are accessible to all, and include what is called an "intersectoral" approach to planning and implementing programs (World Health Organization & United Nations International Children's Emergency Fund, 1978; Barnes et al., 1995; Stanhope & Lancaster, 1996).

Settings and Agencies for Community Health Nursing

Settings and agencies where health care delivery takes place have changed remarkably over the last several years. These changes have been attributed to increasing health care costs, the changing face of the population, and the varieties of illnesses that health care providers confront. Health care is now being provided in many nontraditional settings.

Community health nurses are being employed in businesses, industrial settings, schools, prisons, day care centers, churches, residential centers, and mental health centers. They provide hospice care at home and in acute care settings. They also provide care in long-term-care facilities, day clinics, ambulatory settings, and shelters for battered women and homeless people. Community health nurses travel in vans, providing care to those who are not able to come to the health care facilities. Nurses also provide care through 24-hour telephone advisory services, as shown in the Cost of Care Chart. And finally, community health nurses continue to provide care in county and state public health departments.

Roles of Nurses in Community Health Nursing

In most nursing specialties, nurses have many roles, including caregiver, educator, manager, researcher, consultant, role model, leader, and client advocate. Community health nurses continue to perform in

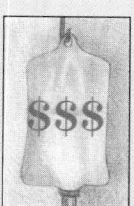

THE COST OF CARE
PEDIATRIC HOTLINE VERSUS EMERGENCY ROOM ADMISSION

A children's hospital in Toronto, Canada, was faced with the problem of identifying a cost-effective way to "provide parents with reassurance and treatment guidelines that allowed them to care for their children at home." When various hospital services received calls from parents with questions about their children's health, it was typically easier and safer to suggest a visit to the emergency department because these health care providers usually did not have the "time and expertise required to provide adequate assessment and advice to parents." This placed an additional strain on the already overburdened and expensive emergency department.

To solve this problem, a 24-hour telephone advisory service called the Medical Information Center (MIC) was developed and staffed by experienced registered nurses with expertise in pediatrics and critical care. Specific protocols for assessment, diagnosis, intervention,

and documentation were created so that parents could be referred to the advisory service rather than the emergency department. When a language barrier or other factor made it difficult for the nurses to obtain information, parents were directed to their family doctor or the emergency department.

The MIC has resulted in extensive savings in health care costs. In 1991, the cost per call to the MIC was approximately $7.00, compared to the cost of a walk-in clinic at $50.00 per visit and an emergency department at $100.00 per visit. These figures do not include the cost of tests performed during emergency department admissions. Based on 1991 figures, the MIC saved the Ontario health care system $2,393,632.

Reference

Wilkins, V.C. (1993). Pediatric hotline: Meeting community needs while conserving health care dollars. *Journal of Nursing Administration, 23*(3), 26–28.

---

these roles. However, the settings and agencies of practice differ from typical acute care settings. These differences in settings influence the roles of the community health nurse.

Home health nurses provide direct care to clients and families. They teach clients and families the "how-tos" and "whys" of self-care. There has been an increase in home health visiting because the cost for home visits is lower than for institutional care; fewer family member caregivers are available to mobile families; many clients are homebound but not ill enough to be hospitalized; and more elderly clients are in need of home care because of our increased life expectancy. Home health nurses care for the chronically ill, the terminally ill, and those who need "high-tech" care, such as ventilators.

School nurses provide immunizations, health screenings (vision, hearing, and so on), counseling, administration of medications, basic care (first aid) for minor complaints, and education in environmental health and school safety. They also take part in case finding and case management, as well as health promotion and preventive health care campaigns.

Occupational health nurses promote the health and safety of workers through worksite programs. They provide direct care and treatment for job-related illnesses or injuries. They coordinate health education programs for smoking cessation, healthy diets, exercise, and weight control. They participate in employee assistance programs for substance abuse and coping with personal problems. They act as employee advocates for job safety and keep records of occupational health histories.

Discharge planning nurses help clients in the process of moving from one health care setting to another.

These nurses must know about the resources available to clients so they can coordinate the delivery of those resources (Box 59–1).

Case management nurses coordinate access and utilization of health services. They are responsible for the client's care from entry into the health care system through discharge.

Nurse epidemiologists are detectives of illness and disease. **Epidemiology** is the study of the cause and distribution of disease, disability, and death among groups of people. The nurse epidemiologist uses the *epidemiological triangle* in solving health care mysteries (Fig. 59–1). The triangle represents the relationship among agent, host, and environment necessary for disease to occur. Elimination of any one of these may eliminate the occurrence of disease.

The nurse epidemiologist uses many sources of information to look for trends in health issues. These include reports of vital statistics, morbidity and mortality reports, demographic statistics, and biostatistics. Trends can be seen over time, in a specific geographic area, and affecting a population. This information is helpful in making changes for healthful outcomes.

The nurse epidemiologist may conduct case studies, field investigations, and field surveys and may assist in surveillance or monitoring activities. Through these projects, information is reported to local health authorities and passed on to district, state, provincial, and national officials.

Challenges of Community Health Nursing

Promotion of healthful living is an important component of community health nursing. Health promotion

BOX 59–1

ACTIVITIES OF DISCHARGE PLANNING NURSES, CASE MANAGEMENT NURSES, AND NURSE EPIDEMIOLOGISTS IN THE COMMUNITY

Discharge Planning Nurses

- High-risk or referral screening.
- Assessment for anticipated needs post-discharge.
- Assessment of resources: What is available, accessible, and affordable for client.
- Interdisciplinary, family, client, and provider conferencing.
- Goal setting.
- Referral and coordination of resources and providers.
- Education of client and caregivers.
- Monitoring of outcomes.
- Documentation of process and outcomes in client records.

Case Management Nurses

- Casefinding.
- Screening.
- Assessment.
- Identification of problems.
- Prioritizing problems and planning.

- Advocation of client's interest.
- Arrangement for service delivery.
- Monitoring of clients during service.
- Reassessment.
- Evaluation and documentation.

Nurse Epidemiologists

- Case studies, in which the nurse assesses a client's environment, including family, community, and health history.
- Field investigations, in which the nurse gathers information regarding variables surrounding a problem or disease, then looks for causal relationships.
- Field surveys, in which the nurse acts as a part of a team to determine the frequency of a problem or disease at a specified time or the amount of the problem or disease in an entire population group.
- Surveillance, in which the nurse monitors the incidence and prevalence of communicable diseases through accurate recordkeeping and data collection.

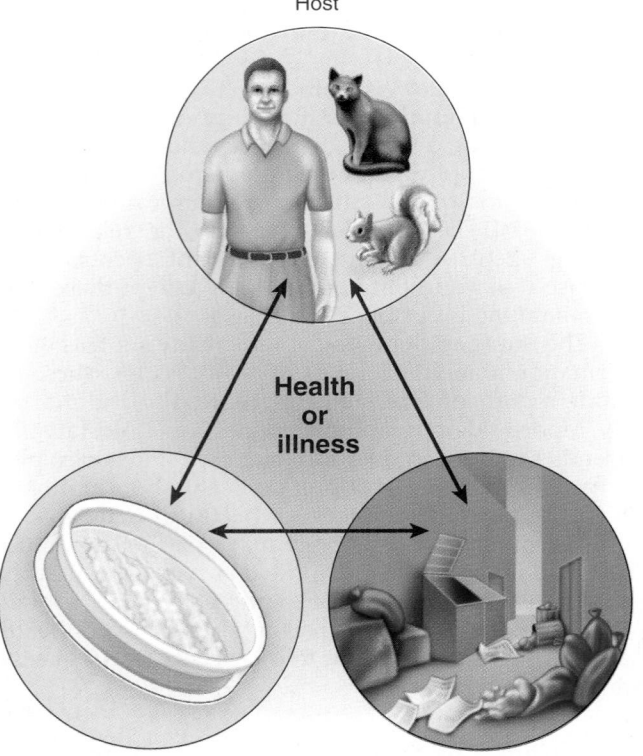

Host

Health
or
illness

Agent

Environment

Figure 59–1. In an epidemiological triangle, the *agent* is an animate or inanimate factor whose presence or absence may lead to disease, disability, and death. It is most often viral, bacterial, fungal, or protozoal. The *host* is a living species—human or animal—susceptible to disease, disability, or death. The *environment* includes all external conditions and influences affecting the living species, which in turn can affect transmission of the disease.

activities sustain or improve the health and well-being of individuals, families, and communities. Activities include education, demonstration, and encouragement of healthful practices. These activities can be affected by public policy, environmental characteristics, and the ability of the community to take action.

Influencing Public Policy

Public policy is one way to make changes to promote health. Public policy is a planned course of action taken to address selected issues or problems. The policy-making process assesses the problem, plans programs, finds resources for programs, implements programs, and evaluates programs. Public health policy allocates and distributes resources to meet the health needs of a population (Clark, 1996).

A nurse may participate in policy-making in several ways. These include calling or writing to a political representative, testifying at a public hearing, serving on committees, or educating clients about proposed changes in laws that affect health care.

Promoting a Supportive Environment

A supportive environment is essential to changing health care. Steps to build the supportive environment include distributing information to inform as well as to recruit. Nurses can help establish a supportive environment by contacting key persons in the community, especially those persons who have relationships with the groups targeted for change. Having a solid rapport with these persons helps build a base of support. Most important, maintaining open communication and supplying current and accurate information regarding developments are essential to successful change.

Encouraging Community Participation and Action

Community action is an integral component when making changes to promote health. The community must acknowledge the changes to be made and become a part of those changes. These programs are successful when people living in the community participate. Community members who are knowledgeable and motivated take part in assessing, planning, implementing, and evaluating health programs.

A*ction* A*lert!*
If community members fail to see value or worth in a change, the community will not work as efficiently toward the end goals.

Community partnerships are a means of participation and involvement in a community to make health care changes. Models of community participation include community activation (Wickizer et al., 1993), participatory action research (Rains & Ray, 1995), and community partnership primary care (Courtney et al., 1996). In these models of participation, communities join in a partnership, alliance, or contract with health care facilities, churches, schools, universities, workplaces, or governmental institutes. Communities or

groups are given opportunities to express opinions, clarify needs, assist in developing health care programs, and empower themselves to continue with community self-care (Kulig & Wilde, 1996). Community participation "increases access to health care; provides for greater efficiency, effectiveness, and coordination of services; and leads to equity and self-reliance" (Sawyer, 1995, p. 21).

However, there are obstacles or limitations to community participation and involvement. These are related to "power, resources, and control" (Sawyer, 1995, p. 18). There may be inequalities of these factors in a given group that will affect the group's ability to agree on or reach specific goals. These partnership models will be discussed later under Interventions.

Collaborating With Other Disciplines and Sectors

When devising plans and interventions to improve the health of a community, the focus cannot remain on physical health alone. Other aspects of life affecting health must also be considered. Interdisciplinary collaboration is needed among health care providers (nurses, physicians, physical therapists, occupational therapists, nutritionists, and so on). Intersectoral collaboration is needed as well.

This type of collaboration involves other sectors of the community that affect health. People who are influential in areas affecting the environment, industry, housing, sanitation, politics, education, and social services of the community are examples of those whose collaboration can be most important to creating change in the community. The various sectors must have mutually agreed upon goals to have successful outcomes.

Using Appropriate Technology

Technological determinants of health have had positive and negative outcomes. Increases in complex and expensive forms of technology have had a tremendous impact on health and health care. Infants born after only 23 weeks (rather than the full 40 weeks) of gestation are surviving thanks to high-tech procedures and newly developed medications. However, the hospital stay for these premature infants may extend from 3 to 5 months after birth, at a cost of up to $500,000. Other outcomes of technology include improved quality and prolonged life of the chronically ill, disabled, and elderly. Faster and more accurate diagnoses means a better chance of survival when facing serious, life-threatening illnesses.

The Internet information highway and ever-improving computer technology connects community health nurses and clients with resources easily and quickly. The latest medical techniques and data are available at one's fingertips. Telehealth is the use of technologies to support the education of community members and health professionals as well as offering clinical applications. Telemedicine is the use of electronic communication to provide clinical care. It

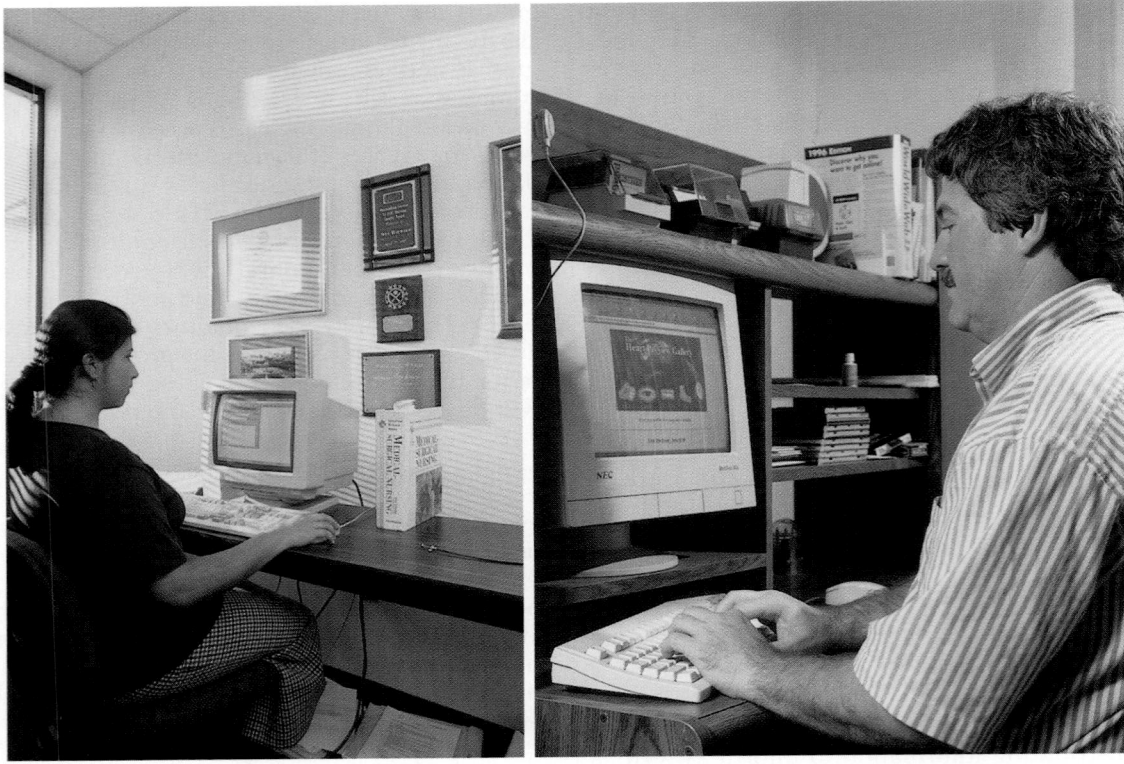

Figure 59–2. Through on-line computer links, clients can connect with community health practitioners in physicians' offices and home health agencies.

ranges from using the telephone or fax to share information (such as a written description or a photo of a wound) to interactive video conferencing.

Advances in technology are allowing more agencies to provide client care at home. Examples include on-line computer links that connect clients in their homes with community health practitioners in physicians' offices and home health agencies (Fig. 59–2), remote-controlled drug delivery devices, and point of care diagnostics, such as x-ray films transmitted in real time over a modem. There is an ongoing process of experimentation, evaluation, and implementation of telemedicine applications in many urban and rural areas. However, reimbursement for such services is currently the exception rather than the rule. The communication infrastructure that supports them is not universally available, and the efficacy of methods has not been fully demonstrated (National Rural Health Association, 1998; Thobaben, 1998b).

Adopting a Holistic Approach

Care of a community must be holistic. In providing that care, the nurse must be able to see the bigger picture. Health care cannot be separated from other facets of life. Factors such as housing, sanitation, employment, and education affect health and therefore must be included in efforts to promote health. Health promotion is a societal goal as well as an individual goal. The fact that health affects so many facets of life directs commu-nity health care providers to recognize health promotion as a philosophy or way of life. It should be a continuous and ongoing application and goal.

Promoting Accessibility

Accessibility to health care refers to the availability of health services and the equality of delivery to all. In the United States, there are many barriers to access. These include lack of health insurance, lack of finances, lack of transportation to the location of services, language barriers, care unavailable at hours convenient to clients, long waits in clinics, housing in areas where health care services are not readily available, a rising cost of services, limited knowledge of existing services, and negative attitudes and beliefs about delivery of services (Barker et al., 1994; Northam, 1996).

There are several **vulnerable populations** who have increased difficulty in obtaining health care. These are subgroups of a larger population that have an increased risk of health problems because of exposure or other health or nonhealth problems. These include the poor, the homeless, cultural minorities, and those who live in rural communities. Also affected are groups of people stigmatized for their personal situations, their particular illnesses, or both (Hunt & Zurek, 1997). These include the mentally ill, persons infected with the human immunodeficiency virus (HIV), and persons with acquired immunodeficiency syndrome (AIDS).

Populations Commonly Served by Community Health Nurses

With the changes now taking place in the delivery of health care, an increased amount of health care once provided in acute care settings is now being provided in varied community settings. These types of care include chemotherapy, dialysis, physical therapy, occupational therapy, and postoperative rehabilitation. However, several populations historically have been and continue to be served by community health nurses.

Community health nurses "provide education, case management and primary care to individuals and families who are members of vulnerable populations and high risk groups" (American Public Health Association, Public Health Nursing Section, 1996). These vulnerable groups are affected by decreased finances and access to care, leading to poorer health outcomes. They include the poor, the homeless, the elderly, pregnant adolescents, the uninsured, mothers and infants, and children of all ages. Other groups or aggregates with more specific health concerns served by community health nurses are listed below.

Poor Clients

The inability to pay for health care services is a major barrier to access. The poor suffer from a "higher rate of chronic illness, higher infant morbidity and mortality rates, shorter life expectancy, [and] more complex health problems" (Stanhope & Lancaster, 1996, p. 653). The populations or aggregates most affected by inadequate finances include women, children, the elderly, the homeless, and those living in rural communities. Although the poor have had Medicaid insurance available since 1966, only about half of people living below the poverty level qualify for Medicaid. Even for those who do qualify, several factors have decreased coverage.

- Health care costs increased by inflation have not been matched by Medicaid.
- Many providers have stopped accepting Medicaid because insufficient benefits are paid (PEW Health Professions Commission, 1991).
- Deductibles and copayments continue to increase (Barker et al., 1994).

Homeless Clients

An increasing number of homeless people can be found in both urban and rural areas. The rise in homelessness over the past 15 to 20 years results from a growing shortage of affordable rental housing and a simultaneous increase in poverty (Fig. 59–3). Poor people are frequently unable to pay for housing, food, child care, and health care. They are forced to accept impossible choices between food, shelter, and other basic needs. Housing, which absorbs a high proportion of income, sometimes must be dropped.

Being poor means being a paycheck or an illness away from living on the streets. Estimates of the num-

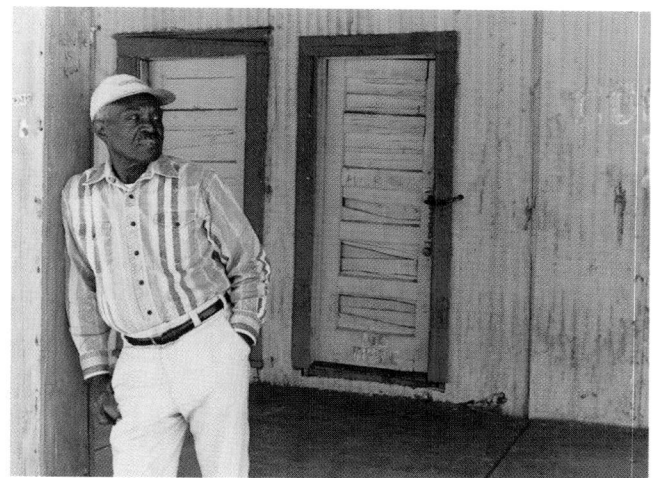

Figure 59–3. The homeless are among the groups served by community health nurses.

ber of homeless people in the United States are as high as three million and increasing. Families are now the fastest growing group in the homeless population, especially women and children. Health problems among the homeless include tuberculosis, skin infestations, respiratory infections, chronic physical disorders (such as asthma, anemia, and malnutrition) and mental disorders (anxiety and depression). Homeless people are more vulnerable to accidental injury and assault and are unable to get adequate rest, exercise, and nutrition. Homeless children may go without immunizations, may be developmentally delayed, and may show signs of behavioral problems. Homeless women use more illegal drugs, alcohol, and cigarettes (Link et al., 1994; National Coalition for the Homeless, 1998; Thobaben, 1998a; Wagner, Menke, & Ciccone, 1995).

Migrant Workers

In the United States, there are approximately 4.2 million migrant farm workers and their families. Migrant workers face health problems similar to those of the homeless. Even if they can find health services, the transient nature of their work makes it difficult to provide continuity of care. They work in one of the most hazardous occupations. They are exposed to occupational dangers, such as falls and machinery accidents. They have a high incidence of respiratory illnesses, including hypersensitivity pneumonitis, or "farmer's lung." Their exposure to pesticides and chemicals increases their risk of contracting a variety of malignant and nonmalignant chronic diseases. Many migrant workers are uninsured, unaware of existing health care services, or unable to use services because of a lack of bicultural or bilingual health care providers. They also may lack transportation to these services and may fear deportation if they are "illegally" in the United States (Clemen-Stone, McGuire, & Eigsti, 1998; Stanhope & Lancaster, 1996).

Minority Clients

African-Americans, American Hispanics, Appalachian-Americans, Asian-Americans, and Native Americans are among the cultural and ethnic minorities that have difficulty accessing health care. Reasons may vary for these groups but quite often include language barriers and communication patterns, a lower level of education, use of folk health practitioners instead of scientific medicine, limited job opportunities (which, in turn, decreases personal finances and opportunities for health care insurance), and cultural beliefs and values regarding health and illness (Clark, 1996).

Rural Clients

Accessing health care for people in rural communities is difficult for several reasons. Access is limited because of poverty, the need to travel long distances, lack of transportation, long waiting times, and lack of available health care providers and facilities (Clark, 1996). According to a report of The PEW Health Professions Commission, "metropolitan areas have five times the rate of hospital-based physicians and almost twice the rate of office-based physicians as nonmetropolitan counties." Also, "of the 545 hospitals closed in the United States between 1981 and 1988, about one-third were rural community hospitals" (Shugars, O'Neil, & Bader, 1991, p. 26).

Stigmatized Populations

Certain other aggregates of people have difficulty accessing health care because of "prejudice, discrimination, and lack of status or power" (Hunt & Zurek, 1997, p. 83). They may have illnesses that are feared and misunderstood, such as HIV infection, AIDS, and severe mental illness. Other groups have personal life situations that may be looked down upon. These groups of people include pregnant adolescents, substance abusers, and emotionally or physically abused people in addition to the poor, homeless, migrant, and minority clients mentioned previously (Clark, 1996; Stanhope & Lancaster, 1996).

Pregnant Adolescents

One million teenage girls in America get pregnant every year. Most of these pregnancies are unplanned, and most of these girls will remain single parents (Cockey, 1997). The medical complications related to teen pregnancies include low birth weight, preterm labor and delivery, poor maternal weight gain, pregnancy-induced hypertension, anemia, and sexually transmitted diseases. Lack of prenatal care accounts for these poor outcomes. Other factors associated with poor pregnancy outcomes—such as poverty, lack of education, and poor family support—add to the complications caused by inadequate prenatal care (Carter et al., 1994; Stanhope & Lancaster, 1996; Cockey, 1997).

Mothers, Infants, and Children

Women and children are cared for by community health nurses throughout their life span. However, women of childbearing age, infants, and school-aged children are groups targeted by community health nurses. Diagnoses commonly seen in women of childbearing age are in areas related to reproductive health, including preconception counseling, family planning, and prenatal care. Community health nurses care for, or refer for assistance, women with diagnoses related to sexually transmitted diseases; chronic diseases, such as heart disease, arthritis, and osteoporosis; depression; breast, cervical, and uterine cancers; domestic violence; occupational work hazards; problems of weight control; and menopause.

Community health nurses can influence the health of future generations by caring for infants and children. Diagnoses for infants and children stem from problems related to preterm and low-birth-weight infants, congenital anomalies, HIV infection and AIDS, accidental injuries, developmental and chronic conditions, attention deficit hyperactivity disorder, child abuse, fetal alcohol syndrome, poor nutrition, lack of immunizations, and environmental hazards. Other diagnoses may be related to language barriers, homelessness, drug addiction, violence, and lack of primary health care (Hawkins, Hayes, & Corliss, 1994; Bekemeier, 1995).

Elderly Clients

Many older adults lack preventive and health maintenance services because of decreased finances, lack of transportation and mobility, and inadequate knowledge about prevention.

Clients With HIV and AIDS

Persons infected with HIV and those with AIDS are more susceptible to further health and socioeconomic risks and discrimination. They have an increased risk of developing cancer (such as Kaposi's sarcoma) and other opportunistic diseases because of their weakened immune systems. Many of these people are left poor, homeless, and without family support. Community health nurses continue to care for a portion of this population in shelters (U.S. Department of Health and Human Services, Public Health Service. CDC Division of HIV/AIDS, 1998).

Clients With Tuberculosis

Despite advances in controlling tuberculosis in the population at large, it has resurfaced in several population groups. People at increased risk of contracting tuberculosis include those infected with HIV, those who have AIDS, the homeless, immigrants, refugees, substance abusers, and prisoners (Kitazawa, 1995; Mayo, White, Oates, & Franklin, 1996). Tuberculosis is a community health concern, especially because of the rise of multi-drug resistant strains.

Clients With Chronic Health Problems

Several groups of people have more specific health concerns that put them at increased risk for additional health problems. People with chronic health problems, such as diabetes, hypertension, heart and lung disease, and mental illness, can benefit from the care of community health nurses. Community health nurses educate, counsel, and case-manage those with chronic health problems.

Not only are individuals and families affected by these diseases, but population groups and society in general are also affected by the results of chronic health problems as seen in mortality and morbidity, years of life lost, and financial costs (Clark, 1996).

FACTORS AFFECTING COMMUNITY HEALTH

Health and the health care of individuals, families, and communities are influenced by social, cultural, economic, political, and environmental factors (Fig. 59–4). These factors affect how health is defined, who is healthy, who is at increased risk for certain health problems, what health care costs will be, how health care is paid for, who has access to health care, and who makes the laws affecting health care.

Social and Cultural Factors

Socioeconomic and cultural factors that influence health and health care include lifestyle practices, such as smoking, use of alcohol, use of illegal substances, exercise habits, and eating habits. Stresses from occu-

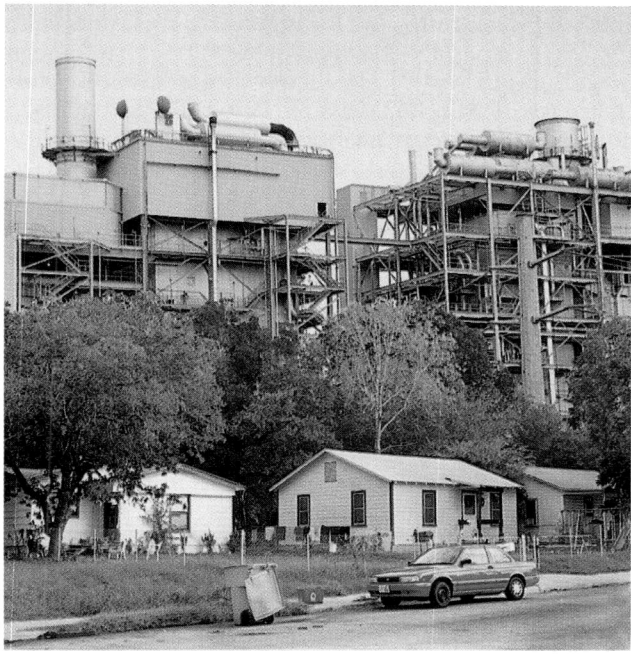

Figure 59–4. Many factors affect the health of individuals, families, and communities. In this community, families live with the possible health risks associated with proximity to a chemical plant.

pation, family life, and peer pressure affect health. Beliefs and values, as well as level of education and knowledge, affect health and health practices. Where people live can also affect their health status. Generally, urban areas have increased violence and crime, whereas rural areas have less access to health care facilities and personnel (Wagner, Menke, & Ciccone, 1995; Northam, 1996).

Economic Factors

Economic influences on health and health care come from private, public, and governmental sectors. After World War II, the United States was affected by price inflation for all goods and services, including health care (Stanhope & Lancaster, 1996). Health care inflation continued into the 1980s. However, with the introduction of diagnosis-related groups (commonly known as DRGs) in 1983, health care spending began to decline. DRGs based insurance reimbursement on a fixed price per case and served as the catalyst for the cost-containment movement still evident today.

The annual cost of health care has grown "from less than $143 per person in 1960 to $2,808 per person in 1991" (U.S. Department of Commerce, cited in Clark, 1996). The continuing increase in the cost of health care results from several factors, including the use of new and expensive technology, the increased cost of insurance premiums, and the need for continued care of many chronically ill, disabled, and elderly people.

The people with financial power in a community have the ability to affect where money might be used in improving health. They will be influential in decisions to clean the environment, build new health care facilities, or promote healthful living projects.

The litigious atmosphere in some areas of practice affects cost of health care by increasing insurance premiums for both providers and consumers of health care. The fear of legal action from alleged malpractice commonly leads health care providers to order more procedures or tests than they otherwise might, just to eliminate all possibilities of medical neglect.

Changes in the ways health care is financed have greatly affected access to health care. For those who can afford to either pay directly or obtain adequate health insurance, access is typically easy. However, many working poor are uninsured, underinsured, or unable to qualify for Medicaid. Personal economic factors that influence health include the employment status of persons and populations. The unemployed typically do not have health insurance. Many small businesses do not offer health insurance to their employees. Consequently, even working people are experiencing decreasing health care benefits as a result of cost-containing measures (reduced company contributions, limited coverages, or increased deductibles).

Political Factors

Political influences affect the areas in which federal, state, and local governments carry out health care functions: providing direct health care services, financing health care, collecting and disseminating health care information, and setting health care policy. Providing direct care includes programs for immunization; providing health care to Native Americans, veterans, and members of the military (Champus); and running specialized clinics (as for tuberculosis).

The government finances research; direct care through Medicare, Medicaid, and Social Security programs; and special programs, such as the special supplementary food program for women, infants, and children. Collection and dissemination of health information by the government includes gathering vital statistics, compiling morbidity and mortality data, taking census reports, and undertaking numerous other topics of surveillance and reporting. The purpose of government policy setting is to prevent problems, solve problems, or both. An example of policy setting was the passage of amendments to the Social Security Act in 1965 that established Medicare and Medicaid (public health care insurance programs for the elderly, poor, and disabled). In the ongoing process to decrease the federal government's budget deficit, governmental programs—including those affecting health care—are under scrutiny for elimination or redesign.

Environmental Factors

The environment of a community influences health. Clean, well-built housing and adequate energy and water supplies as well as sanitation services are important to health. Safety services, such as fire, police, and emergency medical services are essential. Well-maintained roads and transportation services, and adequate communication media (radio, TV, newspapers, postal service); accessible educational, religious, and recreational facilities; and restaurants, grocery stores, and general shopping facilities all affect a community's health. Additional services such as Meals-on-Wheels, school nutrition programs, Big Brother/Big Sister programs, crisis intervention programs, and day care programs add to the improved health and well-being of a community. Lacking the essential services can put a community at risk for poor health outcomes.

ASSESSMENT

A community or group health assessment is the initial step in the problem-solving process to promote health or prevent illness in a population. Assessment identifies elements that contribute to or detract from the health of the group. Several factors affect the type and scope of assessment to be done. These are seen in Box 59–2.

Assessments vary in the types of data or information collected and the avenues by which it is collected. When assessing communities, the nurse needs to collect data that reflect what the community thinks it needs as well as what the health care provider might think is important.

BOX 59–2

FACTORS AFFECTING THE TYPE AND SCOPE OF COMMUNITY ASSESSMENT

- Purpose of assessment.
- Size of community or group.
- Location of community or group.
- Available time to complete the assessment.
- Personnel and expertise of personnel directing the assessment.
- Political environment (if applicable) within community or group.
- Cost/benefit relationship of results.

Assessment Data

When assessing the community or group as the client, a broader scheme or framework of assessment must be used. Types of data to be collected include environmental, cultural, socioeconomic, political, and demographic data as well as health data (Fig. 59–5).

Environmental data may include location, climate, physical geography, housing, sanitation, water supply, toxic hazards, public utilities, transportation, industrial versus residential areas, public services (such as police and fire departments and emergency services), health care facilities and services available, schools, libraries, grocery stores, and other types of stores.

Cultural data may include types of ethnic groups and religious groups (including their beliefs and value systems), language barriers, alternative health care practices and use of alternative healers, and dietary customs. Identifying existing priorities and motivations is an important step in assessing a community.

Socioeconomic and political data may include income status, educational level, educational resources, employment status, employment availability, unemployment rates, governmental structure, formal and informal community leaders (including distribution and use of power), community history, community harmony and violence, media and communication avenues, community stressors, leisure and recreational activities available, and political processes.

Demographic data may include information collected through the census, such as race, age, numbers of persons living in specific locations, population growth, and family statistics. Other sources of information include birth and death certificates, crime reports, morbidity and mortality reports, and secondary data from previously collected information.

Methods of Data Collection

Methods of collecting data include windshield surveys, participant observations, focus groups, inter-

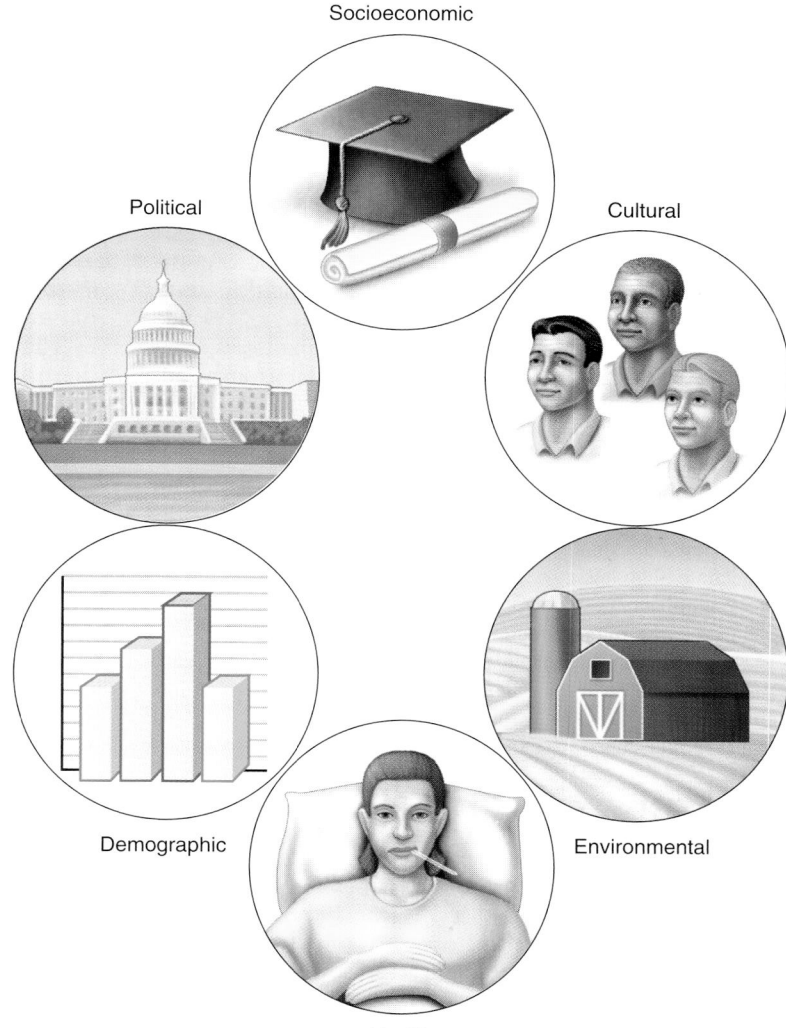

Figure 59–5. Types of data to collect when assessing a community or group.

viewing key informants, community forums, opinion surveys, and secondary data analysis. Also, research data and statistics from previous studies on similar health problems can be highly beneficial in assessing, diagnosing, planning, and evaluating.

A **windshield survey** is a method of data collection in which the researcher drives through a neighborhood to conduct a general assessment of that neighborhood through observation. It is a quick way to get an objective view of the neighborhood environment and the observable facets of community living conditions.

Participant observation is a method of community assessment that examines formal and informal social systems at work. The researcher (nurse, social worker, or other) shares in the life activities of the group while observing and collecting data. The data collector takes part in the life of the community and observes how health and health care may be affected by identified conditions.

A **focus group** is a method of data collection in which six to 12 people from a group or aggregate are brought together for discussion, guided when neces-

sary by a skilled, nonjudgmental leader. The leader listens carefully and guides the group only when necessary. Through the use of focus groups, the participants' opinions, beliefs, and experiences can be recorded and analyzed to be used in making health care decisions. Focus groups can stimulate research questions, develop recruitment strategies, validate data from other sources, and evaluate outcomes of interventions (Stevens, 1996).

A **key informant** is a community leader, professional, politician, or business person who possesses knowledge of the needs of the community and who can act as a useful source of data and a supporter of new programs. These persons may have access to important information and may also be influential in persuading certain sectors to make health care changes.

An **opinion survey** is a method of data collection performed through telephone interviews, mailed questionnaires, door-to-door interviews, or at clinic sites. These are more expensive forms of data collection, and they also limit the type of persons who will respond. Some people have no telephone, some people cannot read (and therefore cannot answer a questionnaire), and some people simply prefer not to take part in a survey (Taylor & Haley, 1996).

A **community forum** is an open meeting where members of a community or group may come to share opinions and concerns about a particular issue. Information gathered here may be different from that gathered by other means because these meetings are open to the general public.

Finally, the nurse may access secondary data gathered on previous occasions. This may include data from records of schools, health departments, police and fire departments, or volunteer organizations such as the American Cancer Society, Planned Parenthood, or a community domestic violence hotline.

Returning to the day care center story introduced earlier, the community health nurse has been completing the assessment of occupants and environment to identify the causes of and risk factors for infectious diarrhea. The nurse used participant observation to collect data about the day care center. This entailed spending several hours observing the children and staff. Assessment data that appeared in the nurse's report are summarized in Box 59–3.

By researching the topic of infectious diseases in day care settings, the nurse identified several factors that could put this population at increased risk for infectious diarrhea. And she noted resources and constraints that could influence the situation.

DIAGNOSIS

Physicians used the term *community diagnosis* as early as the 1950s in applying the medical diagnosis of disease to groups of people (McGavran, 1956). Formulating a diagnosis for a community is somewhat different from formulating a diagnosis for an individual. Difficulties in defining a community diagnosis may result from the following:

- Differences in the definition of health among populations.
- Variations in defining community.
- Related etiologies (social, economic, political, and environmental) that health care providers may not be able to address.
- The entity or unit of care being assessed (one person as a member of the community versus the community as a whole).
- Variations in importance among primary, secondary, and tertiary prevention (Neufeld & Harrison, 1995).

There are a number of different approaches to formulating a diagnosis in community health nursing. The diagnosis can be an actual or potential problem affecting the specified group or population with specific etiology and effects. Neufeld and Harrison (1995; 1996) describe this type of nursing diagnosis as a *deficit diagnosis.*

In continuing with the focus of community health nursing to promote health, Neufeld and Harrison (1995; 1996) also recommend the use of a *wellness diagnosis.* A wellness diagnosis describes positive healthful responses, listing related factors that sustain the healthful response. This type of diagnosis directs nurses toward actions that support the promotion and maintenance of health.

Therefore, the components of a community nursing diagnosis include (1) the name of the community or group with a statement of the problem (actual or potential) or the healthful response, (2) related factors identified for that problem or healthful response, and (3) signs and symptoms that characterize the problem or the positive, healthful actions for promoting or maintaining health.

The purpose of making a diagnosis is not only to identify the problem or healthful actions. A diagnosis also gives direction for planning interventions, encouraging positive actions, and evaluating outcomes. Two approaches commonly used in making nursing diagnoses are proposed by the North American Nursing Diagnosis Association (NANDA) and the Omaha System.

NANDA Diagnoses

NANDA diagnoses have traditionally focused on the individual or family. Unfortunately, most NANDA classifications do not include diagnostic statements for population groups, nor do they fit health promotion or wellness situations. However, you can use a *Knowledge deficit* or *Health-seeking behavior* diagnosis for a group.

After examining the information gathered through the assessment of the day care center and reviewing research studies pertaining to infectious diarrhea, the community health nurse decided on the following NANDA nursing diagnoses for these day care groups:

> *Knowledge deficit* related to age of population as evidenced by lack of awareness and ability to practice proper hygiene
> *Knowledge deficit* related to inadequate training in personal and environmental hygiene as evidenced by day care staff not washing hands after changing infants' diapers.

Omaha System

In the 1970s, a system of diagnoses was developed with the intention of being broad enough to identify external health factors as well as physical factors. Called the **Omaha system,** it was a nursing diagnosis system developed by the Visiting Nurses Association of Omaha, Nebraska. It allows flexibility in defining diagnoses or problems for groups as well as individuals, and it can also be used in many alternative health care settings (Martin & Scheet, 1992).

The three components of the Omaha system are the problem classification scheme, the intervention scheme, and the problem rating scale for outcomes. The problem classification scheme contains four domains, each with several client health problems or conditions. It also includes descriptive signs and symptoms. The intervention scheme focuses on four categories of nursing actions or activities. These actions are directed by such target areas as caretaking

BOX 59–3

PLANNING CARE FOR A POPULATION WITH AN OUTBREAK OF INFECTIOUS DIARRHEA

Notification of Outbreak

ABC Day School is a day care center for children ages 18 months through 11 years. It provides care from 7:00 AM to 6:00 PM Monday through Friday. During the past 2 weeks, many of the children and several of the staff have had diarrhea. A community health nurse from the county health department has been called to assess the situation, identify the cause or causes of the outbreak, and advise on methods of prevention.

Nursing Assessment of Population Group

The children are divided by ABC Day Care into the following general age groups:

18 months	20 children
2 years	21 children
3 years	21 children
3.5 years	23 children
4 years	24 children
5–11 years	34 children

Although the total number of children at this time is 143, not all children are necessarily at day care every day. Also, the children ages 5 to 11 are present only before and after their regular school hours: 7:00 to 8:30 AM and 3:00 to 6:00 PM. Generally, the children come from upper middle class families. Most live with both parents, although a few are from single-parent homes. Most children are here for care while parents are working.

Each class has a certain amount of structured learning to it, depending on the age group. Activities vary and may include playtime (indoors and outdoors), arts and crafts, naptime, and lunchtime. Each age group has its own room (with bathroom included) and playground, where the majority of their time is spent. There is a common lunchroom. All rooms are carpeted except for the lunchroom and the room reserved for 18-month-old children. A total of 20 teachers and other personnel have contact with the children. A total of 20 children and three staff members had complaints of diarrhea. No particular age group was affected more than another.

Identified Risks

Identified risk factors related to the children:

- Forty-one children under 3 years old (the age group at highest risk for infectious diarrhea).
- Lack of knowledge and practice of proper hygiene (not bowel-trained).
- Immature and inexperienced immune system.

Identified risk factors related to the caregivers:

- Inadequate training in personal and environmental hygiene.

- Breaks in sanitary routines because of frequent, spontaneous, and urgent demands from children.
- Cross-coverage of different child age groups can facilitate transfer of organisms from one group to another.
- Inadequate screening for chronic infectious diseases.

Identified risk factors related to the environment and economics:

- Close physical interactions between children and between children and caregivers.
- Less-than-optimal hygiene from use of bowel-training chairs that promote environmental contamination; poorly designed placement of sinks, diaper-changing area, and food handling areas; and common use of moist art supplies and communal water play.
- Economic pressure to decrease staff/child ratio to limit the cost of child care.
- Work pressures on parents to bring ill children to day care facility.

Resources and Constraints

Resources or beneficial aspects:

- Management at the day-care center is eager to make it a healthier, safer place for the children.
- Staff is willing to attend inservices to increase their knowledge of preventive measures against infectious diseases.
- Children are divided into groups by age and usually have the same two teachers (leaving them less open to cross-infections from other groups).

Constraints or Deterrents:

- Enteric pathogens can be spread directly by person-to-person transmission or indirectly by the hands of staff, fomites, environmental contamination, or contaminated food.
- The criteria of an outbreak of diarrheal illness have not been established.
- Many parents send their children to day care not knowing that the diarrhea their child has is infectious.

NANDA Nursing Diagnoses

- *Knowledge deficit* related to age of population as evidenced by lack of awareness and ability to practice proper hygiene.
- *Knowledge deficit* related to inadequate training in personal and environmental hygiene as evidenced by day care staff not washing hands after changing infants' diapers.

Continued

BOX 59-3

PLANNING CARE FOR A POPULATION WITH AN OUTBREAK OF INFECTIOUS DIARRHEA (continued)

Omaha Nursing Diagnoses

Domain	Problem	Signs and Symptoms
Environmental	Sanitation: precautions against infection or disease	Infectious agent
Psychosocial	Caretaking: providing care for dependent child	Difficulty providing preventive health care
Physiological	Bowel function: ability to evacuate waste	Abnormal frequency/consistency of stool (20 persons with diarrhea in 2 weeks)
Health-related behaviors	Personal hygiene: individual practice conducive to health and cleanliness	Inadequate hand-washing by children and day care personnel

Interventions

- Conduct weekly inservice for 4 weeks to educate day care personnel in the principles of general hygiene to reduce the development and spread of infection. Inservice will include information on the mode of transmission of infectious agents, the importance and techniques of proper hand-washing (a video tape is available for viewing), disposal or cleaning of materials and surfaces contaminated with body secretions, food handling and meal service, and diaper changing and toileting.
- Wash, on a regular basis, toys and other objects that children handle or put in their mouths.
- Assign same cots and linens to same children during naptime. These also should be washed on a regular basis.
- Separate any child who becomes ill from the other children until the ill child can be sent home.
- Develop an information letter for parents regarding infectious diarrhea and how to prevent it from spreading.
- Establish criteria for exclusion of ill children by defining what constitutes diarrhea.
- Establish policies for readmission of previously ill children.
- Establish policies for administration of medication to children who have been diagnosed.
- Monitor compliance of preventive hygiene practices taught.
- Monitor outbreaks of infectious diarrhea and other infectious diseases.

These plans will be put into action over a period of 4 weeks. The daily interventions will continue for the next 3 months with a monthly monitoring.

Evaluation

Four months after inception of the program (1 month to establish interventions and 3 months to use interventions) an outcomes evaluation was completed. The goal of fewer than 3.85 episodes per month of infectious diarrhea was met, with only two episodes in the first month, two episodes in the second month, and three episodes in the third month. The outcomes of knowledge, behavior, and health status all improved.

	Before Interventions	After Interventions
Knowledge	2—Minimal	4—Adequate
Behavior	3—Inconsistently appropriate	5—Consistently appropriate
Health Status	2—Severe signs and symptoms	4—Minimal signs and symptoms

For an explanation of numerical scores, see Table 59–1.

The ABC Day School will continue with the interventions suggested as well as offer an annual review of this prevention program for its staff.

Critical Thinking Question

What would you do if the episodes of infectious diarrhea exceeded 3.85 per month?

TABLE 59–1
The Omaha Problem Rating Scale for Outcomes

Concept	1	2	3	4	5
Knowledge The ability of the client to remember and interpret information	No knowledge	Minimal knowledge	Basic knowledge	Adequate knowledge	Superior knowledge
Behavior The observable responses, actions, or activities of the client fitting the occasion or purpose	Never appropriate	Rarely appropriate	Inconsistently appropriate	Usually appropriate	Consistently appropriate
Status The condition of the client in relation to objective and subjective defining characteristics	Extreme signs and symptoms	Severe signs and symptoms	Moderate signs and symptoms	Minimal signs and symptoms	No signs and symptoms

From Martin, K.S., & Scheet, N.J. (1992). The Omaha System: Applications for community health nursing. Philadelphia: W.B. Saunders Co.

and parenting skills, communication, education, and nutrition. The problem rating scale for outcomes (Table 59–1) is an evaluation tool using a Likert-type scale (evaluating a specific outcome on a 1 to 5 scale with 1 equaling a poor outcome and 5 equaling an excellent outcome) to measure outcomes for specific diagnoses or health problems related to client knowledge, behavior, and health status (Martin & Scheet, 1992). The problem rating scale can be used to evaluate the client before, during, and after completion of an intervention. With this type of diagnosis system, the nurse is able to describe wellness as well as deficit diagnoses.

Four problems were identified for this day care group using the Omaha system's problem classification scheme (see Box 59–3). These problems were all inter-related, involving sanitation, caretaking, bowel function, and personal hygiene. The intervention scheme and problem rating scale for outcomes will be discussed in the sections that follow.

PLANNING

General Principles for Working With Groups

When identifying goals and planning interventions for groups, the community health nurse needs to have certain knowledge, skills, and attitudes. These include the following:

- The ability to identify existing community networks.
- An understanding of subcultures.
- Assessing whether goals, interests, and motivation of the community are the same as those of the health care providers.
- Understanding how to build community consensus and cohesiveness.

- Recognizing that external factors or determinants have an impact on a group's health.
- Acknowledging the need for ongoing assessment during planning and implementation.

When working with groups, you must recognize, value, and respect the group's capabilities, strengths, intelligence, uniqueness, and goals. Working successfully with community groups requires measures to ensure community participation. Through community participation comes community development and community empowerment. The concept of community participation grew from historic roots in democratic theory and government. In the 1960s and 1970s, it was recognized with such names as grass-roots mobilization; consumer, social, or citizen participation; and neighborhood activism.

In community development, health care providers and community groups work together to define problems, identify resources, and use existing community leaders and organizations to carry out interventions toward health goals. Empowering a community entails teaching skills, supplying information, and providing access to community resources so the community has the tools and opportunities to make change through educated and informed decisions (Altman, 1995; Barnes et al., 1995; May, Mendelson, & Ferketich, 1995; Stanhope & Lancaster, 1996). Empowering a community increases a "sense of community connectedness, commitment, and coherence" (Altman, 1995, p. 232). An empowered community is able to improve the quality of life for its members.

Using Research to Identify Goals and Plan Interventions for Population Groups

In planning health care interventions for population groups, the community health nurse will certainly use the information gathered during the assessment process. However, an important source of information that can be very useful when identifying goals and planning interventions for population groups is research previously done on other groups with the same or similar diseases or health problems. Previous research studies may provide baseline standards to measure against, identify risks for certain populations, reveal rates of specific diseases or health problems, and provide suggestions for outcomes. Past studies may also provide information essential in preventing and controlling the disease or health problem as well as methods of monitoring the effectiveness of the interventions used.

The community health nurse, keeping in mind the information from the assessment of this day care center community, continued to review what was available in research to help plan for interventions and goals. In one study, diarrhea attack rates were significantly higher for children from birth through age 1 year (76%) and those ages 13 to 24 months (23%), with 1.24 episodes of diarrhea per child per year (Pickering, Bartlett, & Woodward, 1986). Another study found the incidence of diarrhea among children under age 3 to be 17 times greater than that among older children, with 1.02 episodes of diarrhea per child per year (Bartlett et al., 1985).

The nurse used these rates as a basis to set a goal of a decreased incidence of diarrheal episodes for the day care center. She multiplied the figure 41 (children in the high-risk age group) by 1.13 (the average result of the studies mentioned above), and divided by 12 (months) to arrive at a potential incidence rate for the ABC Day School of 3.85 episodes of diarrhea per month. But there were 23 cases of diarrhea reported in 2 weeks, according to the nurse's assessment data. This is 7.6 more cases than the potential incidence rate.

The objective or goal for ABC Day School was stated as follows: The children of ABC Day School will have a rate of infectious diarrhea of less than 3.85 episodes per month 3 months after interventions are incorporated.

INTERVENTION

Interventions are actions or activities implemented to reach goals or objectives or to solve a problem. Interventions used to promote, improve, or maintain health for communities include community participation, development, and empowerment; community outreach programs; health promotion and education activities; and activities that promote social change.

Interventions Within Community Groups

Community Activation

Community activation emphasizes the involvement and coordination of major community institutions (such as schools, universities, and local health departments) to mobilize community leadership and resources for health promotion and to improve public awareness of health issues. It includes organized efforts to increase community awareness and agreement about health problems, increase coordinated planning of prevention and environmental change programs,

increase allocation of resources between organizations, and increase citizen involvement in these processes (Wickizer et al., 1993).

For example: The local health department collaborated with the town's church ministry board to coordinate a program to identify and refer people with hypertension for treatment. Nursing students from the university were recruited to help with this project by assisting with advertising the program, taking blood pressures, and taking part in presentations on preventing hypertension. The goal was accomplished through awareness, screening, and education programs.

Participatory Action Research

Participatory action research is a research model that relies on local community knowledge. It empowers group members to develop their leadership potential. It is a combination of community involvement, research, and action that supports local ability and judgment in solving community problems. It is a flexible and collaborative effort between the researcher and the community (Rains & Ray, 1995).

For example: Community members from a rural town joined a research team (which included a nurse) to identify health problems in their community. The community members were involved in the entire process, including compiling research questions, constructing and distributing survey tools, analyzing findings, and taking action on the results. After identifying several health problems in their community, one specific problem was identified as the most "winning" healthful change issue. This was to reduce the number of smokers and the amount of smoking in their town. This town voted in policy changes and initiated strategies of primary prevention related to decreasing smoking (Rains & Ray, 1995).

Community Partnership Primary Care

Community partnership primary care emphasizes community development and community empowerment. In this model of community participation, health professionals and the community work together to identify strengths, problems, and needs in the community. They then develop strategies to improve the health of the community. Health professionals work toward empowering people toward self-care to improve health, supporting communities to take action on their own behalf to promote health and prevent or reduce problems (Courtney et al., 1996).

For example: In an urban Hispanic community, a nurse practitioner met with a group of neighborhood women who were attending a Bible study group at a local church. The nurse used an empowerment education approach with the women's group to help them develop their own self-care strengths.

Parish and Neighborhood Nursing

Parish nursing and neighborhood nursing are forms of community outreach. This type of care is useful in primary prevention and health promotion.

*A*ction *A*lert!
Parish and neighborhood nurses are in key positions in the community to improve accessibility to care.

A **parish nurse** is a registered nurse who is employed by (or volunteers at) a religious or health care organization for the purpose of providing nursing care to members of a church congregation. The nurse operates through churches to promote wellness through holistic care. This revival of church-based health care occurred in 1983 with the development of parish nursing by Lutheran chaplain Granger Westberg (Westberg, 1990).

Parish nurses address not only the physical but also the emotional and spiritual needs of congregational community members. Parish nurses do not provide home health care services or perform invasive nursing procedures. They do provide education, advocacy, counseling, and screening. They also train and coordinate volunteers, make referrals to community resources, and develop and facilitate support groups (Miskelly, 1995; Dunkle, 1996; Schank, Weis, & Matheus, 1996).

Churches are effective sites for health promotion and disease prevention programs because of the greater accessibility for the congregations. Parish nurses collaborate with community and public health agencies to increase health care access to members of their congregations. Parish nursing may be financed through a church or health care institution, or the parish nurse may volunteer time, but it is still coordinated by the church or institution.

Neighborhood nursing is an outgrowth of the idea of district nursing that seeks to promote healthy communities by collaborating with people where they live, work, and go to school. Today it is also referred to as block nursing. Neighborhood-oriented nursing can provide broad-based case management and care coordination. Neighborhood nurses can detect problems early on, before they become crises. They can work in partnership with social agencies and health professionals (Zerwekh, 1993). Some examples of community-focused activities by neighborhood nurses include participation in health fairs, developing and presenting health education programs, initiating volunteer programs, presenting talks on health topics to community groups, and participating in developing and testing a town disaster plan (Reinhard et al., 1996). Neighborhood nurses can invite key community members to identify community needs, resources, and strategies. However, the biggest single factor limiting the growth and success of neighborhood nursing is how it can be financed. Some projects have been financed by county grants and donations (Reinhard et al., 1996). Others have trouble obtaining financing.

Interventions to Promote Health

Health promotion interventions are used to increase the health and well-being of individuals, families, and communities. Health promotion activities may include

Teaching for WELLNESS

HAND-WASHING INSTRUCTIONS FOR A DAY CARE CENTER

Purpose: To prevent transmission of infectious agents.

Rationale: Proper hand-washing can help prevent the spread of pathogens. Specific teaching can reinforce video and verbal instructions from nurse.

Expected Outcome: Staff at the day care center will continue to use proper hand-washing technique and the incidence of infectious disease will decline.

Client Instructions

- Stand well away from the sink so your hands and clothes do not touch the sink surface.
- Using warm water, wet your hands and wrists thoroughly, holding them angled downward in the sink so water will run toward your fingertips.
- Place soap (preferably antibacterial) on your hands and rub vigorously for 15 to 30 seconds, massaging all skin areas, joints, fingernails, and areas between fingers. If you are wearing rings, slide them up and down while rubbing your fingers to work the soap under them. If you are using bar soap, hold the bar in your hands throughout the lathering process.
- Rinse your hand and wrists thoroughly.
- Use a clean, dry paper towel to dry from your fingers to your wrists and arms. Discard the towel.
- Use another clean, dry paper towel to turn off the faucet. Discard the towel.
- The entire hand-washing process should take 2 to 4 minutes.

using health appraisals, encouraging healthy lifestyle behaviors, providing healthy environments, developing effective coping skills, and educating to promote healthful decision-making (Clark, 1996). On a broader scale, health promotion activities often require changes involving health policy, economic conditions, legislation, or funding. The goals for these changes may take longer to be accomplished.

Health promotion and illness prevention are the primary goals of community health nursing. They are considered the primary level of prevention in nursing to maintain health. As seen in the day care example in this chapter, proper hand-washing is the best way to prevent the spread of disease. The Teaching for Wellness chart outlines proper hand-washing technique.

Health promotion encourages actions to achieve optimal health. Examples include educating people about the hazards of smoking and encouraging them to stop smoking. Illness prevention measures provide a means to prevent or block a disease process. Examples include receiving immunizations against infectious diseases and brushing your teeth to prevent tooth decay.

Secondary and tertiary levels of prevention have traditionally been considered levels of prevention seen in hospitals and long-term-care facilities. More and more, however, these types of care are being seen in community health settings as well. The secondary level of prevention entails identifying an illness or disease process and eliminating or reducing it. Examples include blood pressure screening and mammograms. Once a disease process is identified, treatment can begin to eliminate or reduce the problem. The tertiary level of prevention also includes rehabilitative care. People with some form of permanent disability or terminal illness will strive to maintain their optimal health in this level of care. Examples include helping an amputee learn to walk with a prosthetic leg or recommending a support group for a woman who has undergone a mastectomy.

These three levels of health promotion and illness prevention can be applied to groups as well as individuals. Immunizations, health screening, and education and support groups are all examples of community health interventions that can be used to promote health and prevent illness in groups.

Interventions to Educate the Community

Health education interventions come in many forms. Communities can be educated through health fairs, the media, entertainment venues, and programs in the workplace, schools, school-based or school-linked clinics, and community clinics. The ultimate goal of health education is to develop the ability and create an environment that enables communities to promote health and prevent and manage disease (Steckler et al., 1995).

Dillion and Sternas define a health fair as "a voluntary, community-based, cost-effective event used to detect health problems, identify risk factors, and provide educational information and supportive resources to promote healthy lifestyles of its participants" (1997, p. 2). Health fairs are offered by a variety of sponsors. Often a health care organization will collaborate with a community organization, such as a school, church, or radio or television station, to present health information and exhibits. They usually are open to the public. Besides the uses listed above, it is hoped that attendees will gain an awareness of health and health problems and an interest in adopting behaviors that improve health and reduce illness and injuries (Dillion & Sternas, 1997).

Use of the media is a powerful tool to communicate health information to the public. Electronic (radio, television, and Internet) and print (newspapers and magazines) media influence decisions, opinions, and behaviors. The media can provide information to the public about health education programs, screenings

and other events, and research results. Many newspapers have "lifestyle" sections that include information about health and health care. The news media are considered credible sources of information and often have extensive coverage about an issue that can effectively influence public perceptions and attitudes (Steckler et al., 1995).

A public information campaign is an intervention useful in creating awareness about a variety of problems, such as drinking and driving, the use of illegal drugs, cancer, AIDS, violence, and crime prevention. These campaigns make use of television, radio, posters, pamphlets, videotapes, booklets, and comic books. Information is also relayed through billboards, print ads, and displays in commercial and public places.

Enter-education (also called edutainment) is an intervention that combines education with entertainment. It is used to make positive changes in behaviors and attitudes. Audiences are educated via popular television programs and films on such topics as drinking and driving, AIDS, and using mammograms to screen for breast cancer. Audiences often relate strongly to their favorite television characters or talk-show host. They may imitate their behaviors or follow their advice (Steckler et al., 1995).

Interventions to Promote Social Change

When working to educate groups of people, "the most effective community health education strategy is one that raises the level of awareness and concerns for groups at risk of ill health and enables them to devise their own strategies to reduce risk" (Steckler et al., 1995, p. 313). The health care provider must take into account the local values, norms, beliefs, and behavior patterns when attempting to change health attitudes and behavior. Also, the provider must acknowledge that health and health promotion activities are affected by many external determinants and require the collaborative involvement of other disciplines and sectors in providing interventions (Neufeld & Harrison, 1995).

Several intervention strategies are useful in making smooth, well-ordered changes. For one, you can use social structures to support healthful changes. These include churches, informal social networks, voluntary associations, and neighborhoods. For another, you can use linking agents. These are "individuals who act as gatekeepers in reaching community members and organizations" (Steckler et al., 1995, p. 313). These people help enlist community members in participating in healthful changes. They provide social support and help increase access for certain vulnerable groups.

Community coalitions, such as Healthy Cities, focus on "mobilizing local resources and political, professional, and community members to improve the health of the community" (Stanhope & Lancaster, 1996, p. 334). Together these coalitions can work to increase access to care, develop healthy public policy, and strengthen community action toward healthful goals (Stanhope & Lancaster, 1996).

Nurses who work with communities and population groups may identify the need for change in social, political, economic, or health care systems. Interventions to change these systems as well as the physical environment often require policy change. These policy changes take time, personnel, energy, and finances. You must carefully assess the situation, work effectively with the community system, and recognize the many variables (such as resistant community officials or scarce funds) that could affect the change process and outcomes. Change is more readily accepted when information is disseminated in ways compatible with the community's norms, values, and customs. Finally, once again, by developing and strengthening community participation and action, health care providers will promote a community's ability and opportunity to take appropriate action to protect and improve the health of its members (Stanhope & Lancaster, 1996).

The community health nurse and staff of the day care center met to discuss ways to decrease the spread of infectious diarrhea. This meeting promoted cooperation with the staff, allowed the nurse to assess what the staff knew about the subject, and resulted in a list of interventions agreed on by all present (see Box 59–3). These interventions were appropriate to address the NANDA diagnoses and the Omaha system.

The director of the day care center was concerned about what costs might be incurred for these interventions. These included purchasing or renting a video to show hand-washing technique; printing a letter to parents regarding infectious diarrhea; obtaining additional supplies for cleaning hands, toys, linens, and so on; and compensating the health education instructor for inservice classes.

EVALUATION

Evaluation is the process of determining whether the goals or objectives of a program have been met. To evaluate the outcomes of health interventions, goals or objectives must first be identified. These goals are identified by assessing the community or group and identifying diagnoses and related factors.

Evaluation of interventions or programs can be accomplished while in progress. This is called *formative evaluation.* Evaluation completed at the end of interventions or programs is called *summative evaluation.* There are four general types of results or goals that may be evaluated: outcomes, outputs, impact, and efficiency. *Outcomes* refers to the quality and the consequences of the program. (Were the end goals or objectives accomplished?) *Outputs* refers to quantity. (How many people were served?) *Impact* refers to the effect on the total community or group and what changes might occur in the future. (How did the intervention affect the community, and could it continue to affect future members of the community?) *Efficiency* refers to how effectively resources were employed. (What did the goals cost in money, time, and personnel?)

Methods of Evaluation

Several methods—including case study, observation, and survey—are useful in evaluating programs and interventions, but no one method addresses all four of the results. A *case study* evaluates a program through observation of program activity, review of reports prepared during the program, and conversations with program personnel. Data collected can be both objective and subjective.

Observational methods are another means to evaluate programs. In *participatory observation,* the observer actually takes part in the program. In *nonparticipatory observation,* the observer remains outside of the program, observing only at specified times. *Surveys* are an evaluation tool that can be used to describe and analyze the results of a program. These can be completed through questionnaires or by personal interviews. *Pretest–intervention–post-test* is an evaluation method used to identify whether changes in knowledge, behavior, or attitudes have taken place after an intervention is applied or a program completed. A *cost-benefit analysis* and a *cost-effectiveness analysis* are two methods of evaluating the economic costs and benefits of a program. These are formal analytic techniques for comparing the positive and negative effects of a program (Anderson & McFarlane, 1995). It is important to know and understand how each of these methods can help you evaluate a community health intervention program while planning the program, before it begins.

Health Goals and Objectives

Health goals may involve a variety of areas, including community and environmental changes, policy level changes, individual behavior changes, and group health improvements. The American Nurses' Association defined outcome criteria (results or goals) as a "focus on the end results of nursing care; a measurable change in the state of health of a community, family, or individual; the end product of a professional process; a change in the environment or in the attitude of the client toward health care" (1986, p.18).

Thompson (1992, p. S70) described health improvement goals as the following:

- Reducing inequities in health.
- Adding life to years (increasing level of wellness and coping, especially among the elderly and the disabled).
- Adding health to life (reducing illness, disease, and disability).
- Adding years to life (reducing premature death).

Measuring the outcomes of community health has not been an easy task. Stanhope and Lancaster noted that "community health nursing has been involved primarily in evaluating program outcomes to justify program expenditures rather than in evaluating client outcomes" (1996, p. 427). Measuring outcomes in community health may be difficult because of the empha-

CONSIDERING THE ALTERNATIVES
ALTERNATIVE OR COMPLEMENTARY?

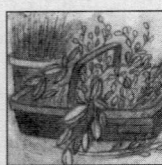 "The structural reasons that medical pluralism is a prominent feature of health care throughout the world are that biomedicine, like Ayurveda and every other therapeutic system, fails to help many patients. Every system generates discontent with its limitations and a search for alternative therapies. Similarly, moral conflicts dispose people to different interpretations of illnesses. Ayurveda, biomedicine, and other traditions provide different rhetorics for responsibility and different meanings for suffering" (Leslie, 1992, p. 205).

Placed throughout this textbook has been a series of charts like this one describing the most common ideas and practices in the field of complementary and alternative medicine. Some of these ideas and practices are ancient, some modern. Their distance from the mainstream is varied and changing. How much a particular treatment or therapy is viewed as an alternative to mainstream biomedicine, and how much it is viewed as complementary to mainstream practice, varies with one's viewpoint. This too is changing. Some argue that the application of specific complementary and alternative medical practices apart from their philosophy of origin and their place within a coherent system reduces healing to a cookbook of remedies and techniques with diminished value. But—differences of opinion, practice, and philosophy notwithstanding—those in the healing professions have similar goals: relieving suffering and promoting health.

Some people are very critical of complementary and alternative medicine and of the beliefs and research that underlie them. Sometimes the virulence of the attacks on complementary and alternative medicine betrays the beliefs, biases, and fears of the attackers. Historically, changes in science and medicine have been difficult and have created tensions and controversies among everyone involved. During such times of change, ideology often substitutes for open-mindedness, and a spirit of condemnation replaces one of healthy skepticism (Dossey, 1998; Achterberg, 1998; Leskowitz, 1998).

Were we to turn our focus away from complementary and alternative medicine for a moment and turn the spotlight back onto mainstream medical practices, we would find that "only about 20 percent of modern medical remedies in common use have been scientifically proved to be effective." Thus, the accusation that complementary and alternative medicine works only by

the placebo effect can also be applied to much of mainstream medicine. Interestingly, many complementary and alternative therapies even attempt to foster the placebo effect, which has been repeatedly shown to be quite powerful (Brown, 1998).

Spirituality is an area often overlooked in traditional Western medicine. Ayurvedic and Chinese medicine, on the other hand, do not draw strong distinctions among body, mind, and spirit. Interestingly, a person's sense of connectedness with others and a sense of spirit—however one defines it—has been found to be important for health. For example, many people pray as part of their religious practice and beliefs, without giving much thought to its efficacy. Now researchers are examining whether prayer may have positive effects on health, whether for those praying, those prayed for, or both (Dossey, 1993). Although the research is controversial scientifically, there is a growing body of provocative evidence that prayer yields positive effects. Some say that these positive effects may relate in some cases to the placebo effect or to self-healing abilities. Nevertheless, some research seems to demonstrate positive effects of prayer even for people who did not know they were being prayed for (Byrd, 1988). Whatever forthcoming research demonstrates, these initial findings remind us of the inter-relationship (and possible unity) of body, mind, and spirit. This inter-relationship is important for us to understand, both for ourselves in our personal lives, and for our clients, so that we may do a better job of caring for the whole person.

There have probably always been controversies in medicine. In the minds of some, the germ theory of disease, pioneered by Pasteur and Koch in the late 1800s, put to rest an idea espoused by traditional Chinese medicine and even by Hippocrates that illness results from lack of harmony between an individual and the environment. It seemed that diseases were caused by specific organisms, and therefore could be cured by a specific medicine. Yet despite the advances that resulted from the advent of the germ theory, many diseases do not fit this model. As René Dubos wrote, "In reality, the search for *the* cause may be a hopeless pursuit because most disease states are the indirect outcome of a constellation of circumstances rather than the direct result of single determinant factors." Claude Bernard, a pioneering physiologist, believed that health depends on a continual interplay between a person's internal and external environments. In 1959, Dubos wrote that the ancient doctrines of harmony—abstract though they

CONSIDERING THE ALTERNATIVES

ALTERNATIVE OR COMPLEMENTARY? (continued)

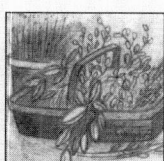 seemed compared with the cause-and-effect germ theory—were re-entering scientific discussion (Dubos, 1959). And in a recent article, Spiegel, Stroud, and Fyfe (1998) point out that while the cause-and-effect thinking underlying the germ theory of disease has worked powerfully for Western medicine in acute, curable diseases, it does not work well in the context of chronic, progressive diseases. This leaves patients, and those providing treatment, unsatisfied. Moreover, it has led people to search for alternatives.

In our time, people want safe and effective ways to treat disease and maintain health. This desire drives the increased use of complementary and alternative medicine today. And this desire may be leading to an important shift in thinking: An increasing portion of the practices described in the "Considering the Alternatives" charts placed throughout this book are now being viewed as complementary rather than alternative. Information is an important factor in this shift. In fact, the exchange of information is growing to become an essential part of the relationship between health care providers and clients. Clients who are better informed and more able to participate in decisions about their own health experience better outcomes (Galland, 1997). At the time of this writing, 53 medical schools in the United States have either elective courses or informal discussion groups and lectures on complementary and alternative medicine (Moore, 1998). Computer technology has enabled clients to inform themselves about their illnesses, and they are often the ones to inform their physicians of some developments. Nurses and physicians themselves are reaching out for more information and more tools to help consumers. Learning is often a two-way process.

The integration of complementary and alternative medicine into certain areas continues. For example, many hospitals now employ massage therapists. Pain management programs often include biofeedback and sometimes acupuncture, along with other therapies. In China, many patients with cancer use modern biomedicine as well as herbal medicine and *qigong*. In Japan, many hospitalized patients take herbal as well as pharmaceutical medicines. In Europe, many physicians prescribe herbal medicines, and large numbers of patients take herbs. One Oklahoma physician has estimated that utilization of herbs in an HMO for which he works could save between $500,000 and $750,000 yearly in drug costs (Kinchelow, 1997). If cost savings such as

these can be demonstrated consistently, they will no doubt further the use of complementary and alternative medicine.

We have seen how important it is for health care providers to be aware of the therapies and remedies, including vitamins and minerals, their clients use. However, clients will more likely share this information if they sense that it will be received open-mindedly by the provider.

Resources

Publications that can expand and keep your knowledge of complementary and alternative medicine current:

The American Holistic Nurses' Association, P.O. Box 2130, Flagstaff, AZ 86003-2130; 800-278-AHNA; e-mail: AHNA-flag@flaglink.com; Internet: http://www.ahna.org *Publishers of the* Journal of Holistic Nursing, *as well as a newsletter; also, developers of a certificate program in holistic nursing.*

Dossey, L. (1993). *Healing words: The power of prayer and the practice of medicine.* New York: HarperCollins.

Dubos, R. (1959). *Mirage of health: Utopias, progress, and biological change.* New York: Harper and Row.

Integrative medicine: Integrating conventional and alternative medicine. Quarterly journal. Elsevier Science, Inc. 655 Avenue of the Americas, New York, NY 10010-5107. (888) 437-4636.

References

Achterberg, J. (1998). Between lightning and thunder: The pause before the shifting paradigm. *Alternative Therapies in Health and Medicine, 4*(3), 62–66.

Brown, W.A. (1998). The placebo effect. *Scientific American, 278*(1), 90–95.

Byrd, R.C. (1988). Positive therapeutic effects of intercessory prayer in a coronary care unit population. *Southern Medical Journal, 81*(7), 826–829.

Dossey, L. (1993). *Healing words: The power of prayer and the practice of medicine.* New York: HarperCollins.

Dossey, L. (1998). The right man syndrome: Skepticism and alternative medicine. *Alternative Therapies in Health and Medicine, 4*(3), 12–9, 108–114.

Dubos, R. (1959). *Mirage of health: Utopias, progress, and biological change.* New York: Harper and Row.

Galland, L. (1997). *The four pillars of healing.* New York: Random House.

Kinchelow, L. (1997). Herbal medicines can reduce costs in HMO. *HerbalGram, #41,* 49.

Leskowitz, E. (1998). Un-debunking therapeutic touch. *Alternative Therapies in Health and Medicine, 4*(4), 101–102.

Leslie, C. (1992). *Paths to Asian medical knowledge.* Los Angeles: University of California Press.

Moore, N.G. (1998). A review of alternative medicine courses taught at US medical schools. *Alternative Therapies in Health and Medicine, 4*(3), 90–101.

Spiegel, D., Stroud, P., & Fyfe, A. (1998). Complementary medicine. *Western Journal of Medicine, 168,* 241–247.

sis on health promotion and disease prevention (Zlot-nick, 1992). Also, outcomes are influenced by uncontrollable factors, such as the environment. Deal concluded that "the absence of definitive outcome data associated with many community-based nursing interventions weakens statements about the effectiveness of these efforts" (1994, p. 318).

In 1991, however, two works were published that set forth national standards and objectives for health by the year 2000. The American Public Health Association (APHA) published *Healthy Communities 2000: Model Standards for Community Attainment of the Year 2000 National Health Objectives.* Local communities may apply the model standards in planning to meet local needs, to establish community-specific measurable health objectives, to encourage communication and coordination of community efforts, and to help communities justify needed programs and budgets to legislative bodies (American Public Health Association, 1991; Stanhope & Lancaster, 1996).

The U.S. Department of Health and Human Services, Public Health Service, also published *Healthy People 2000: National Health Promotion and Disease Prevention Objectives.* This work includes educational and community-based programs that address lifestyles and environmental or regulatory measures to protect large population groups. These two publications can be used as guides for communities to identify objectives for healthful changes. The next segment of this program, Healthy People 2010, will address such issues as changing demographics, advances in preventive therapies, and new technologies (Stanhope & Lancaster, 1996; U.S. Department of Health and Human Services, Public Health Service, 1991; U.S. Department of Health and Human Services, Public Health Service, 1998).

With more and more health care being provided in community settings, researchers need to evaluate and validate healthful outcomes. Steckler and colleagues stated, "To scientifically assess the effects of community-level interventions, studies need to involve multiple communities in both experimental and control conditions . . . this can be extremely expensive and difficult to do" (1995, p. 315). More research is needed to identify effective evaluation methods for interventions when the community is the client.

Four months after the inception of the day care center's program (1 month to establish interventions and 3 months to use interventions), an outcomes evaluation was completed to evaluate whether the goal of fewer than 3.85 episodes per month of infectious diarrhea was met. The information needed was obtained through monthly monitoring. The goal was met with only two episodes in the first month, two episodes in the second month, and three episodes in the third month. Using the Omaha system's problem rating scale for outcomes of knowledge, behavior, and health status, improvements were seen in all three areas (see Box 59–3). The ABC Day School will continue with the interventions suggested as well as offer an annual review of this prevention program for its staff.

KEY PRINCIPLES

- A community is a group of people, or a population, who have one or more personal or environmental characteristics in common.
- Community health nursing is a combination of nursing and public health science designed to promote health and prevent illness in population groups.
- Community health care takes place in many non-traditional settings, including businesses, schools, and shelters. It is brought to communities through mobile health care vans.
- A community health nurse's roles include caregiver, educator, counselor, referral source, role model, advocate, case finder, case manager, coordinator, liaison, discharge planner, leader, change agent, researcher, and epidemiologist.
- A community health nurse must have the knowledge, skills, and attitude to bring people together in a coalition to be effective in promoting health and preventing illness in the community.
- Providing community health care presents challenges in developing public policy, promoting access to health care, using appropriate technology, collaborating with many disciplines, and encouraging community participation.
- Community health nurses provide primary care, education, and case management to individuals and families who belong to vulnerable populations and high-risk groups.
- A population's health is influenced by cultural, social, economic, political, and environmental factors.
- Methods of collecting data for a community assessment include windshield surveys, participant observations, focus groups, key informants, community forums, opinion surveys, and secondary data analysis.
- A community nursing diagnosis includes the name of the group, the specific problem (actual or potential), and the related factors. It may also include signs and symptoms of the problem.
- NANDA diagnoses and Omaha system diagnoses are two approaches used by community health nurses in identifying problems in population groups.
- In solving health care problems, research provides baseline standards to measure against; identify risks for certain populations; reveal rates of specific diseases or health problems; and provide suggestions for outcomes.
- Interventions employed to promote, improve, or maintain community health include community participation, development, and empowerment; community outreach programs; health promotion and health education activities; and activities that promote social change.
- Community participation is a key concept of community health care and is concerned with the vari-

ous ways members of a group are involved in health care planning.

- Evaluation is the process of determining whether a program's goals or objectives have been met. Formative evaluation is done while the program is in progress. Summative evaluation is done at the completion of the program.

BIBLIOGRAPHY

Altman, D.G. (1995). Strategies for community health intervention: Promises, paradoxes, pitfalls. *Psychosomatic Medicine, 57*(3), 226–233.

American Nurses Credentialing Center. (1998). *Community Health Nurse.* Available from http://www.nursingworld.org/ancc/generalist/gb2.html. 11/2/98

*American Nurses' Association. (1986). *Standards of community health nursing practice.* Kansas City, MO: Author.

*American Public Health Association. (1991). *Healthy Communities 2000: Model standards for community attainment of the year 2000 national health objectives* (3rd ed.). Washington, DC: Author.

Anderson, E.T., & McFarlane, J.M. (1995). *Community-as-partner: Theory and practice in nursing.* Philadelphia: J.B. Lippincott Co.

*Barker, J.B., Bayne, T., Higgs, Z.R., Jenkin, S.A., Murphy, D., & Synoground, G. (1994). Community analysis: A collaborative community practice project. *Public Health Nursing, 11*(2), 113–118.

Barnes, D., Eribes, C., Juarbe, T., Nelson, M., Proctor, S., Sawyer, L., Shaul, M., & Meleis, A.I. (1995). Primary health care and primary care: A confusion of philosophies. *Nursing Outlook, 43*(1), 7–16.

*Bartlett, A.V., Moore, M., Gary, G.W., Starko, K.M., Erben, J.J., & Meredith, B.A. (1985). Diarrheal illness among infants and toddlers in day care centers. *The Journal of Pediatrics, 107*(4), 495–502.

Bekemeier, B. (1995). Public health nurses and the prevention of and intervention in family violence. *Public Health Nursing, 12*(4), 222–227.

*Carter, D.M., Felice, M.E., Rosoff, J., Zabin, L.S., Beilenson, P.L., & Dannenberg, A.L. (1994). When children have children: The teen pregnancy predicament. *American Journal of Preventive Medicine, 10*(2), 108–113.

Clark, M.J. (1996). *Nursing in the Community* (2nd ed.). Stamford, CT: Appleton & Lange.

Clemen-Stone, S., McGuire, S.L., Eigsti, D.G. (1998). *Comprehensive community health nursing: Family, aggregate, & community practice* (5th ed.). St. Louis: Mosby.

Cockey, C.D. (1997). Preventing teen pregnancy. *AWHONN - Lifelines, 1*(3), 32–40.

Courtney, R., Ballard, E., Fauver, S., Gariota, M., & Holland, L. (1996). The partnership model: Working with individuals, families, and communities toward a new vision of health. *Public Health Nursing, 13*(3), 177–186.

*Deal, L. (1994). The effectiveness of community health nursing interventions: A literature review. *Public Health Nursing, 11*(5), 315–323.

Dillion, D.L., & Sternas, K. (1997). Designing a successful health fair to promote individual, family, and community health. *Journal of Community Health Nursing, 14*(1), 1–14.

Dunkle, R.M. (1996). Parish nurses help patients—body and soul. *RN,* May 1996, 55–57.

Hawkins, J.W., Hayes, E.R., & Corliss, C.P. (1994). School nursing in America, 1902–1994: A return to public health nursing. *Public Health Nursing, 11*(6), 416–425.

Hunt, R., & Zurek, E.L. (1997). *Introduction to community based nursing.* Philadelphia: Lippincott-Raven.

Kitazawa, S. (1995). Tuberculosis health education in homeless shelters. *Public Health Nursing, 12*(6), 409–416.

Kulig, J.C., & Wilde, I. (1996). Collaboration between communities and universities: Completion of a community needs assessment. *Public Health Nursing, 13*(2), 112–119.

*Link, B.G., Susser, E., Stueve, A., Phelan, J., Moore, R.E., & Struening, E. (1994). Lifetime and five-year prevalence of homelessness in the United States. *American Journal of Public Health, 84*(12), 1907–1912.

*Martin, K.S., & Scheet, N.J. (1992). *The OMAHA System: Applications for community health nursing.* Philadelphia: W.B. Saunders Co.

May, K.M., Mendelson, C., & Ferketich, S. (1995). Community empowerment in rural health care. *Public Health Nursing, 12*(1), 25–30.

Mayo, K., White, S., Oates, S.K., & Franklin, F. (1996). Community collaboration: Prevention and control of tuberculosis in a homeless shelter. *Public Health Nursing, 13*(2), 120–127.

McGavran, E.G. (1956). Scientific diagnoses and treatment of a community as a patient: *Journal of the American Medical Association, 163*(8), 773–777.

Miskelly, S. (1995). A parish nursing model: Applying the community health nursing process in a church community. *Journal of Community Health Nursing, 2*(1), 1–14.

National Coalition for the Homeless. (1998). NCH Fact Sheet #1: Why Are People Homeless? Available from: http://www.2.ari.net/home/nch/causes.html. 11/8/98

National Rural Health Association. (1998). *The role of telemedicine in rural health care.* Available from: http://www.nrharural.org/pagefile/issuepapers/ipager7.html. 11/8/98

Neufeld, A., & Harrison, M.J. (1995). Integrating nursing diagnoses for population groups within community health nursing practice. *Nursing Diagnosis, 6*(1), 37–41.

Neufeld, A., & Harrison, M.J. (1996). Educational issues in preparing community health nurses to use nursing diagnosis with population groups. *Nurse Education Today, 16*(3), 221–226.

North American Nursing Diagnoses (NANDA). (1999). *NANDA Nursing Diagnoses: Definitions and Classifications 1999–2000.* Philadelphia: Author.

Northam, S. (1996). Access to health promotion, and disease prevention among impoverished individuals. *Public Health Nursing, 13*(5), 353–364.

*Pickering, L.K., Bartlett, A.V., & Woodward, W.E. (1986). Acute infectious diarrhea among children in day care: Epidemiology and control. *Reviews of Infectious Diseases, 8*(4), 539–547.

Rains, J.W., & Ray, D.W. (1995). Participatory action research for community health promotion. *Public Health Nursing, 12*(4), 256–261.

Reinhard, S.C., Christopher, M.A., Mason, D., McConnell, K., Rusca, P., & Toughill, E. (1996). Promoting healthy communities through neighborhood nursing. *Nursing Outlook, 44*(5), 223–228.

Sawyer, L.M. (1995). Community participation: Lip service? *Nursing Outlook, 43*(1), 17–22.

Schank, M.J., Weis, D., & Matheus, R. (1996). Parish nursing: Ministry of healing. *Geriatric Nursing, 17*(1), 11–13.

*Shugars, D.A., O'Neil, E.H., & Bader, J.D. for the PEW Health Professions Commission. (1991). *Healthy America: Practitioners for 2005, an agenda for action for U.S. health professional schools.* Durham: The PEW Health Professions Commission.

Stanhope, M., & Lancaster, J. (1996). *Community health nursing: Process and practice for promoting health* (4th ed.). St. Louis: Mosby-Year Book.

Steckler, A., Allegrante, J.P., Altman, D., Brown, R., Burdine, J.N., Goodman, R.M., & Jorgensen, C. (1995). Health education intervention strategies: Recommendations for future research. *Health Education Quarterly, 22*(3), 307–328.

Stevens, P.E. (1996). Focus groups: Collecting aggregate-level data to understand community health phenomena. *Public Health Nursing, 13*(3), 170–176.

Thobaben, M. (1998a). Medical-surgical nursing in multiple settings. In F. Monahan & M. Neighbors (Eds.), *Medical-surgical nursing: Foundations for clinical practice* (2nd ed., pp. 17–30) Philadelphia: W.B. Saunders Co.

Thobaben, M. (1998b). Health care technology issues in home care. *Home Care Provider, 3*(5), 244–245.

*Asterisk indicates a classic or definitive work on this subject.

*Thompson, J.C. (1992). Program evaluation within a health promotion framework. *Canadian Journal of Public Health, 83*(Supplement 1), S67–S71.

U.S. Bureau of the Census. *Resident population of the United States: Estimates by age and sex.* Available from: http://www.census.gov/population/ estimates/nation/intfile2-1.txt. 9/7/98

U.S. Department of Health and Human Services, Public Health Service. CDC Division of HIV/AIDS. (1998). *Living With HIV/AIDS.* Available from http://www.cdc.gov/nchstp/hiv_aids/dhap.htm. 11/8/98.

*U.S. Department of Health and Human Services, Public Health Service. (1991). *Healthy People 2000: National health promotion and disease prevention objectives.* Washington: US Department of Health and Human Services, Public Health Service.

Wagner, J.D., Menke, E.M., & Ciccone, J.K. (1995). What is known about the health of homeless rural families? *Public Health Nursing, 12*(6), 400–408.

*Westberg, G.E. (1990). *The parish nurse: providing a minister of health for your congregation.* Minneapolis: Augsburg Fortress.

*Wickizer, T.M., VonKorff, M., Cheadle, A., Maeser, J., Wagner, E.H., Pearson, D., Beery, W., & Psaty, B.M. (1993). Activating communities for health promotion: A process evaluation method. *American Journal of Public Health, 83*(4), 561–567.

*Wilkins, V.C. (1993). Pediatric hotline. Meeting community needs while conserving health care dollars. *Journal of Nursing Administration, 23*(3), 26–28.

*World Health Organization (WHO) & United Nations International Children's Emergency Fund (UNICEF). (1978). Primary health care: Report of the International Conference on Primary Health Care. Geneva: World Health Organization.

*Zerwekh, J.V. (1993). Commentary: Going to the people - public health nursing today and tomorrow. *American Journal of Public Health, 83*(12), 1676–1678.

*Zlotnick, C. (1992). A public health quality assurance system. *Public Health Nursing, 9*(2), 133–137.

60

The Homebound Client

Deborah K. Zastocki

LEARNING OBJECTIVES

After studying this chapter, you should be able to:

1. Describe concepts important to home care nursing, including accreditation, reimbursement, and scope of services.
2. Describe factors affecting the outcomes of home care.
3. Write effective nursing diagnoses that are consistent with reimbursement guidelines for the homebound client.
4. Describe expected outcomes for homebound clients.
5. Describe types of nursing interventions employed to achieve typical expected outcomes for homebound clients.
6. Document evaluation data that promote the expected outcomes of home health care.

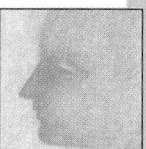

Cynthia Mullen, a Slavic/German-American, is a 35-year-old female with a history of type I diabetes mellitus controlled by insulin. Cynthia has been monitoring her blood glucose levels and administering her own injections of insulin in the morning and before her evening meal. Cynthia's spouse has been very supportive but is seldom available because his job as a truck driver requires him to make long trips away from home. Recently, Cynthia developed an ulcer on her right foot that required hospitalization for surgical débridement. The stress of surgery and the wound on her foot resulted in fluctuating blood glucose levels that were difficult to control.

The home care nurse plans to help Mrs. Mullen manage the effects of her illness and support her recovery. Because the home environment may be a factor in Mrs. Mullen's ability to control her diabetes and care for her wound, the nurse makes the diagnosis of *Impaired home maintenance management.*

THE HOMEBOUND CLIENT **NURSING DIAGNOSIS**	**Impaired Home Maintenance Management:** Inability to independently maintain a safe, growth-promoting immediate environment. From North American Nursing Diagnosis Association. (1999). NANDA nursing diagnoses: Definitions and classification 1999–2000. Philadelphia: Author.

CONCEPTS OF HOME CARE NURSING

Home care nursing represents one of the most exciting practice areas for the future of nursing. Acute care continues to consolidate and refocus, causing decreases in length of stay and hospitalizations. As a result more clients will require home care. In addition, the aging population and advances in technology represent increasing needs and options for delivering care in the home. Home care nursing practice will continue to require increasingly technical skills as well as creativity and flexibility in planning care needs for a diverse client base.

Home care nursing requires a broad array of skills. You will need to maintain sensitivity to culture, race, gender, sexual orientation, social class, and economic factors (Meleis, 1995). You will need knowledge of the normal life span. Additionally, you will need skill in the delivery of technologically complex care that was once provided only in a hospital. Your skill will need to extend to assessing the effects of the home environment on the client's health and promoting a healing home environment. Clearly, the trend in home care nursing is one of growing diversity and scope.

Terminology of Home Care Nursing

The evolution of home-based nursing practice has been in the form of district nursing, public health nursing, community health nursing, and home care nursing or home health nursing. The distinctions among these types of nursing practice tend to blur. However, there are some differentiating characteristics.

Chapter 59 has defined community health nursing; home care nursing is one aspect of community health nursing. **Home care nursing** is a comprehensive, holistic field of nursing focused on the client and family (or support system) and delivered in the client's home. It requires skills in health assessment, health maintenance, health promotion, restoration, rehabilitation, and terminal care. As family-centered care, it requires understanding of the family system. Because it often focuses on health promotion and prevention, many professionals prefer to call it *home health care* rather than simply home care.

Home care refers to any of a variety of services provided to clients and families in their places of residence for the purpose of treating illness, restoring health, rehabilitating, promoting health, and palliating. In this chapter, home care nursing refers to the broad scope of nursing practiced within home care

services. The roles of nurses in public health, community health, or home health may overlap with the roles described for home health care nursing. A home care provider is a person or organization (often called an agency) that delivers home care.

Regulation of Home Care Nursing

Home care is affected by the political and social forces that act on health care. Accreditation is important to protect the safety of the public using home care services, and it impacts the nature and quality of the services offered. Additionally, the reimbursement policies of third-party payors affects the nature of services provided.

Accreditation of Home Care Agencies

Although accreditation is a means of promoting quality by voluntarily meeting national standards, it is almost mandatory because it is typically a requirement for receiving third-party reimbursement. Home care agencies have been subject to accreditation by three boards:

- The Joint Commission on Accreditation of Health-Care Organizations
- The Community Health Accreditation Program
- The National Home Caring Council

Reimbursement Issues in Home Care Nursing

As home care developed in the last quarter of the 20th century, home care nurses felt the challenge of meeting the client's and family's needs within tightly controlled reimbursement criteria.

MEDICARE AND MEDICAID

As a leading provider of services in home care, Medicare and Medicaid tend to set the standards for the industry. Medicare and Medicaid regulations have specific criteria for home care reimbursement and have created a clear shift to a medical model of practice. The focus is one of disease treatment. For a client to receive reimbursable home care services, the regulations require the following:

- The person be under a physician's care
- The physician confirm the need for home care and write orders that outline the plan of treatment, including frequency and duration of services
- The person be homebound

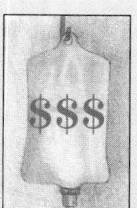

THE COST OF CARE
MEDICARE HMOs

In 1983, Medicare health maintenance organizations (HMO) were introduced as a cost-saving measure for the Medicare program. The fee-for-service system was thought to be fragmented, focused on acute care, likely to duplicate services and, therefore, ill-prepared to control costs while meeting the health and social needs of an aging population.

Now, however, there is concern about whether the current capitated systems are truly cost-effective and can offer integrated care models adequate to address the needs of the elderly, particularly those with the greatest needs, such as the frail elderly.

Seeking answers to these sorts of questions, Experton (1997) examined the differences in health care usage and cost among a group of frail elderly clients under the three primary payor/provider systems: Medicare fee-for-service, Medicare HMO, and dual Medicare-Medicaid enrollment.

Experton's analyses revealed no differences in total expenditures for fee-for-service enrollees and HMO enrollees. Expenditures for Medicare-Medicaid beneficiaries were about 50% higher than for enrollees in either of the other two reimbursement systems. HMO enroll-ees were more likely to have two or more hospitalizations and received fewer home health services than Medicare fee-for-service enrollees.

Discussion

To evaluate this research, consider the following questions. Are there differences in the populations using these three methods of reimbursement? Could the lower use of home health services account for the increased hospital admissions for HMO enrollees? Is the population studied representative of all Medicare clients? If the overall cost of fee-for-service and HMO enrollees is the same, does it matter whether costs are incurred in hospital or home settings? Why might dual Medicare-Medicaid beneficiaries incur greater overall costs? What other research would be helpful to conduct on this subject?

Reference

Experton, B., et al. (1997). The impact of payor/provider type on health care use and expenditures among the frail elderly. *American Journal of Public Health, 87*(2), 210–216.

- The person require skilled care (as specifically defined by Medicare)

The referring physician is required to plan, review, and certify that care is necessary.

These requirements threatened the rich heritage of the nursing model of health promotion and disease prevention in rendering these services unreimbursable. Thus, home care nurses were faced with the need to respond holistically to client and family needs while practicing under a system in which reimbursement required a multidisciplinary approach.

Support services (such as assistance with shopping and cleaning for the homebound) were not endorsed. The home care nurse faced the crisis of attempting to find or create other support services to enable the client to remain at home.

In addition to ensuring quality and safety, the home care nurse evaluates the most cost-effective approach to providing care. Reimbursement issues and financial constraints of the family may require alternative sources for equipment and supplies. This part of the home health nurse's responsibility requires you to be aware of various religious, charitable, and voluntary organizations that often provide free or lower-cost equipment or that make loans of equipment for those in the population served. The local church or branch of the American Cancer Society, for example, can be a valuable resource for both equipment and support.

Scope of Home Care Services

Home care services are characterized by diversity. The trend has been described as an extension of institutional medical care into the home. As a home care nurse, you will work to create a caring environment despite the presence of high-technology equipment and services.

The Family as Client

The family, which includes both traditional family members and significant others, represents the infrastructure upon which the client's plan of care can be based. Applying the concepts from systems theory, the impact of the family is readily apparent. The family serves as the client's caregiver, connection with the community and outside agencies, and emotional support, as advocate, provider of resources, and so on. Consequently, to plan care properly, your initial assessment requires a focus on both the client and the family.

Action Alert!
Perform an environmental and family system assessment in the initial stages of planning care to determine the need for consultations with additional professionals.

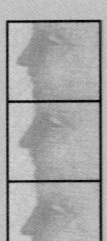

CROSS-CULTURAL CARE
CARING FOR A SLAVIC/GERMAN-AMERICAN CLIENT

Mrs. Mullen, whose story we are following in this chapter, is of Slavic/German descent. Her husband is of German descent. Leininger (1991) has identified certain values that tend to be important to people of this background:

- Being clean and neat.
- Being orderly and well-organized.
- Being stoic, not complaining, and not asking for help.
- Adhering to routines and rules.

The home environment and lifestyle of a controlled and orderly life is important to both Mr. and Mrs. Mullen. Equally important is a high degree of self-reliance and stoicism. Mr. Mullen relies on Mrs. Mullen to maintain the household.

In preparation for hospital discharge, the home care coordinator met with Mr. and Mrs. Mullen to prepare for continuing care in their home. The home care coordinator then communicated with Judy Page, the home care nurse responsible for Mrs. Mullen's care. In addition to ensuring that the necessary supplies and equipment would be available for the first home visit, the home care nurse initiated the therapeutic relationship with a telephone call to the Mullen home on the day of discharge.

The following conversation occurred between the home care coordinator and Mrs. Mullen during the first home visit.

Judy: I am here to work with you to be sure you get the care you will need.

Mrs. Mullen: I don't think I will need any help. I have been taking care of myself for a long time.

Judy: Tell me what has happened to you.

Mrs. Mullen: I have this little sore on my foot. It won't heal. I guess it's because I have diabetes.

Critical Thinking Questions

- If you were Judy, what would you say next?
- Do you think that Mrs. Mullen's behavior is a result of her culture, or do you think it has another meaning?
- How can you help Mrs. Mullen to improve the chances that her wound will heal?

Reference

Leininger, M. (1991). *Culture care diversity and universality: A theory of nursing.* New York: National League for Nursing Press.

Types of Services

Required services can range from medically oriented services to self-care assistance and wellness services. Medically oriented care is based on a physician's order and involves such high-technology services and equipment as nutrition support, intravenous therapy, renal dialysis, respiratory support, and rehabilitation (Fig. 60–1). Clients typically have been discharged from an acute care setting or have long-term disabilities. Although self-care assistance from homemakers, home health aides, and companions may prevent institutional care, reimbursment by third-party payors requires documentation for possible coverage.

Additionally, wellness—or health promotion—services that focus on the health-oriented consumer are not reimbursed by third-party payors. Services include health education (such as teaching about nutrition and stress management), self-improvement, diagnostic screening (such as monitoring of blood pressure and blood cholesterol level), illness prevention (such as assistance with smoking cessation), and promotion of fitness.

Although many of the traditionally reimbursed services require a skilled nursing level and homebound status, the impact of health maintenance organizations (HMOs) and telemedicine is slowly expanding the scope of reimbursed services. For example, many HMO contracts allow a home visit for the postpartum mother and infant. Perinatal home care is expanding as well, enabling many pregnant women—even those with high-risk pregnancies—to be managed at home. These clients would traditionally have been hospitalized for such high-risk conditions as preterm labor, pregnancy-induced hypertension, or hyperemesis. By means of high-technology monitoring equipment, the client can use a telephone modem to transmit uterine contractions. Through a minipump, the client can receive regularly scheduled as well as preprogrammed boluses of medication.

Telemedicine and the focus on disease management for chronically ill clients with diabetes, cardiac disorders, and lung diseases permit remote monitoring of vital signs and heart and lung function. These services link nurses and other professionals to various sites and can include videoconferencing for client education. Populations that benefit most from this technology include the elderly, postnatal clients, postsurgical clients, and clients with chronic conditions.

In the course of a day, the home care nurse may see a wide variety of clients with varying needs, including the following:

- A new mother and infant for their first postpartum and infant care visit
- A child who requires long-term mechanical ventilation in a family learning to plan for long-term care needs

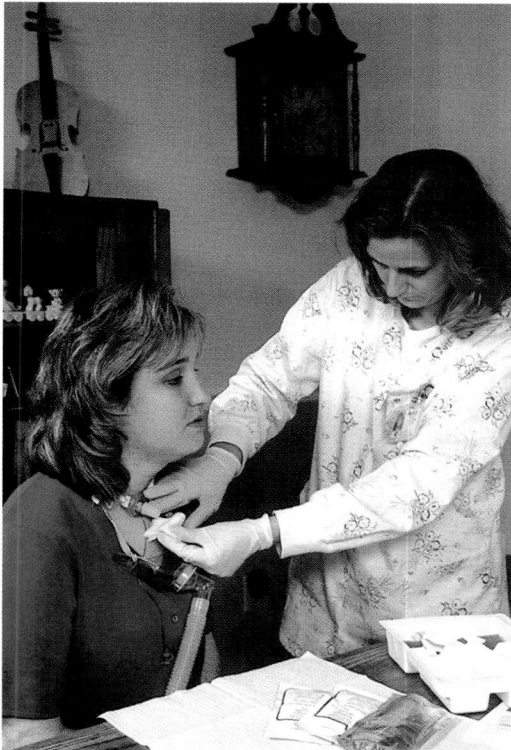

Figure 60–1. Clients requiring high-technology care can now receive that care at home.

- An adolescent adjusting to a new diagnosis of type I diabetes mellitus who requires a plan that includes family support for meal planning
- A person with a mental health disorder who requires medication adjustment
- A person recovering from surgery who requires assistance with wound management
- A person recovering from a cerebrovascular accident who requires rehabilitation to perform activities of daily living
- A person with arthritis who needs to learn to use assistive devices to achieve independence in the home
- A terminally ill person who needs care to promote quality of life and pain control while at home.

Of those using home care, clients over age 65 represent the largest and fastest growing group in the United States. The higher ratio of chronic illness and disability among elderly people and the limited availability of family caregivers are just two reasons behind the growing use of home health services by the elderly.

Another important group in need of home care is people with acquired immune deficiency syndrome (AIDS), a disease that has had a dramatic impact on the health care system in the United States. Naturally, as the number of people with AIDS increases, the demand for treating them in the home will also increase.

Home Care Nursing Practice

As home health care evolves, so too does home care nursing. Working as a generalist, the home care nurse cares for clients from birth to death and throughout the health-illness continuum. To perform this role, you must use knowledge and skills needed to provide acute care, chronic illness care, palliation, mental health promotion, rehabilitation, and care needed to address age-specific problems in the community.

Home care nursing also allows clinical specialization in such areas as gerontology, maternal-child care, diabetes, hospice, and parenteral infusion therapy. These options require a strong knowledge base and a holistic approach to promote successful acute care while preventing the development of a "minihospital" environment in the home. You assume the roles of the technically skilled provider of care, educator, advocate, collaborator, leader, and case manager. Box 60–1 lists key skills essential to home care nursing.

A Model for Home Care Nursing Practice

Home care nursing practice results from several theoretical models, such as general systems, self-care, and adaptation theories. Systems theory is used to assist the family to function effectively as a system. Self-care theory is used to develop the means to assist the client toward independence. Adaptation theory is used to help the client make changes to produce optimum function in the face of disabling health problems. The Albrecht Nursing Model for Home Health Care (Fig. 60–2) incorporates these theories into a framework for home nursing practice.

This model assumes that clients and their families participate actively, capably, and responsibly in their care. It also addresses the complex and changing relationships inherent in home care. In short, it uses the interaction of structural elements and process elements to predict the outcomes of care (Albrecht, 1990).

Structural elements include the client, family, agency, nurse, and health team. They may be affected by such factors as client acuity, costs, and demand.

Process elements include the focus and intensity of care, coordination of care by the nurse, and intervention. Outcomes (the responses to care) include satisfaction, quality of care, cost-effectiveness, health status, and self-care capability (Albrecht, 1990). This professional nursing model clearly advances home care nursing practice and research.

Goals of Home Care Nursing

Home care nursing takes place within a multidisciplinary delivery system, in which the nurse (a case manager) manages care delivered in the client's home. The home care nurse strives to do the following:

- Restore the client's health by helping the client resume an appropriate level of functioning
- Maintain the client's health by preserving the client's functional abilities and independence

BOX 60–1

KEY SKILLS FOR HOME CARE NURSING

Communication and Family System Dynamics

- Assessing interactions among client and family members.
- Identifying best methods to communicate and teach the client for mutual goal setting.
- Establishing realistic goals with client and family.

Wound Care

- Assessing wound healing.
- Providing wound care, including sterile dressings, débridement, and irrigation.
- Teaching clients and families about wound care.

Intravenous Therapy

- Assessing and managing fluid balance.
- Inserting catheter and drawing blood for studies.
- Administering medications, blood products, and parenteral nutrition.

Elimination

- Using enterostomal therapy skills.
- Teaching clients and families about special appliances and skin care products.
- Inserting urinary catheter.

- Teaching clients and families about catheter insertion techniques and proper maintenance.

Rehabilitation

- Assessing the need for assistive equipment, range-of-motion exercises, and ambulation.
- Instructing clients and families in the use of equipment, exercises, and ambulation.

Pediatric/Maternal-Child Health

- Assessing prenatal and postpartum clients.
- Using fetal monitoring techniques.
- Assessing normal growth and development.
- Evaluating family system dynamics.

Cardiac

- Assessing cardiovascular status.
- Instructing clients and families in pulse-taking.

Oncology

- Administering intravenous therapy and chemotherapeutic agents.
- Assisting clients and families with trying to cope with grief, loss, and bereavement.

- Promote the client's health by minimizing the effects of illness
- Improve the client's health by helping the client achieve a higher level of functioning than previously existed (Stewart, 1979).

Case Management

To accomplish these goals, the nurse must marshal the appropriate resources (both personnel and equipment) and employ them together in a coordinated plan.

Case management requires the ability to do the following:

- Function independently, make decisions, solve problems, and manage emergencies in the home
- Coordinate, collaborate with, consult with, and direct other health care providers, contracted providers of equipment or services, and community resources, and to decide when to contact the physician
- Develop a plan of care to help the client and family achieve clearly defined, measurable, client-centered outcomes by an estimated date based on negotiation among the client, family, and nurse

- Think in terms of family interaction and dynamics
- Implement appropriate protocols for all procedures and equipment
- Communicate verbally, through interviewing, teaching, and providing feedback, and in writing, through documentation of skilled care provided by nurses and others and the client's response to care
- Function cost-effectively through a sound understanding of the economics of health care and the legislation and regulations imposed on it (Rovinski & Zastocki, 1989).

Nurse-Client Relationship

The nature of the nurse-client relationship is modified somewhat by the home environment. Always remember that you are a guest in your clients' homes. As such, you need to respect the customs and lifeways of the family, such as by calling the client by a preferred name (formal or informal), addressing the decision-maker even if that person is not the client, or even removing your shoes at the door if that is the family custom. Portraying a nonjudgmental attitude toward appearances, sounds, and smells in the home promotes the beginning of a therapeutic relationship.

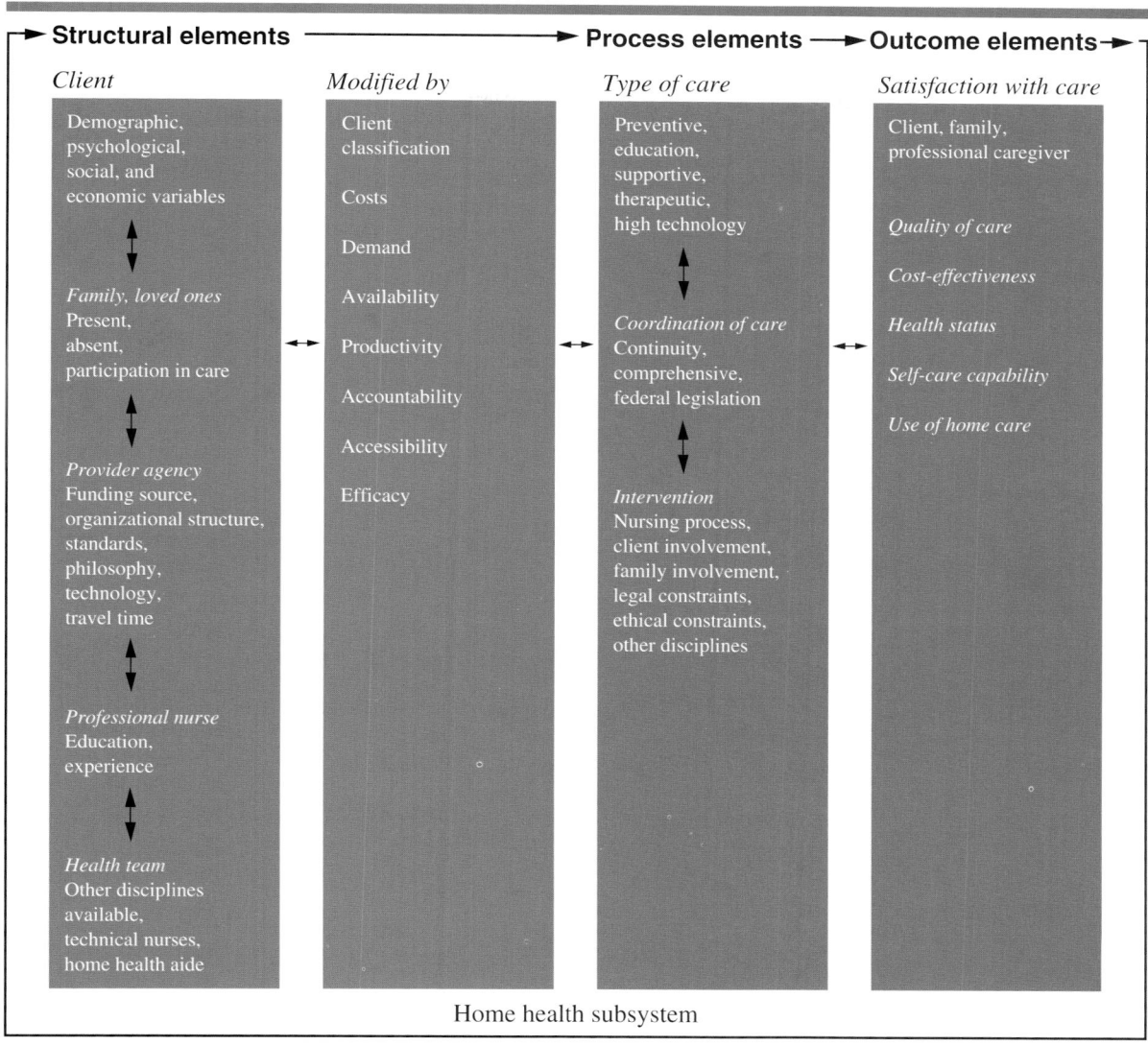

Structural elements ──────────────────────→		Process elements ──→	Outcome elements ──→
Client	*Modified by*	*Type of care*	*Satisfaction with care*
Demographic, psychological, social, and economic variables	Client classification	Preventive, education, supportive, therapeutic, high technology	Client, family, professional caregiver
	Costs		
	Demand		*Quality of care*
Family, loved ones Present, absent, participation in care	Availability	*Coordination of care* Continuity, comprehensive, federal legislation	*Cost-effectiveness*
	Productivity		*Health status*
	Accountability		*Self-care capability*
	Accessibility		*Use of home care*
Provider agency Funding source, organizational structure, standards, philosophy, technology, travel time	Efficacy	*Intervention* Nursing process, client involvement, family involvement, legal constraints, ethical constraints, other disciplines	
Professional nurse Education, experience			
Health team Other disciplines available, technical nurses, home health aide			

Home health subsystem

Figure 60–2. The Albrecht Nursing Model for Home Health Care. (From Mary Nies Albrecht, Ph.D., RN [1990]. The Albrecht nursing model for home health care: Implications for research, practice, and education. Public Health Nursing, 7[2], 118–126. Reprinted by permission of Blackwell Scientific Publications, Inc.)

At the same time, you have entered the home to offer professional services. Respecting the client's home environment does not preclude you from asking to have the volume lowered on a television or radio or requesting some quiet, undisturbed time.

Try to maintain as much of the client's usual routine as possible. Minimizing perceived barriers to the treatment plan will promote compliance.

Protecting Personal Safety

Safety—yours as well as your clients'—is a primary concern in home care nursing. Escorts are usually provided for travel in high-risk environments. Traveling to these locations requires constant awareness of your surroundings. Your agency should have your exact schedule and location of all visits. Wearing jewelry and carrying a purse or money is not recommended.

Ask that unfriendly pets be secured during the visit. Avoid placing personal clothing, such as your coat, in an area where home infestation can occur.

FACTORS AFFECTING THE OUTCOME OF HOME CARE

Lifestyle factors, environmental factors, developmental factors, cultural and religious factors, socioeconomic factors, psychological factors, and physiologic factors have the potential to affect the client's outcomes.

Lifestyle Factors

Understanding the client's beliefs about health as well as lifestyle behaviors is pivotal in defining realistic goals and appropriate intervention strategies. If the client does not perceive susceptibility to or the seriousness of damaging lifestyle behaviors, simply saying, "doing this is good for you" will not be effective. You must design strategies that realistically address perceived susceptibility and seriousness, promote the perceived benefits of action, and minimize the perceived barriers.

Environmental Factors

Health is affected by the client's environment as well. Living in a physical environment that promotes health is critical to both short-term and long-term health goals. You will work with the client and family to maintain an environment that enhances rather than damages health.

Unlike the controlled environment of a hospital or other institution, the home environment represents both potentially healing and damaging elements. From a systems theory and self-care perspective, you will want to maximize the elements that promote safety and healing, such as cleanliness, electricity, running water, refrigeration, and temperature control.

Developmental Factors

Clients of all ages require home care services. Various disease processes can have a temporary or long-term developmental impact. In illness, children may regress to previous developmental stages. Developmental factors are particularly important in terms of learning theory. Teaching sessions for children should be short and allow for child participation. Adolescents have the beginning of abstract thinking and, at times, may project a rather cavalier attitude toward your teaching content.

Adults typically learn best when they see a need and an immediate use for what is to be learned. Learner motivation is stimulated by focusing on perceived "need to know," as compared with "nice to know," information. Elderly clients experience varying degrees of change in cerebral function, reduced auditory and visual activity, and reduced tactile sensitivity and motor dexterity.

Cultural/Religious Factors

Cultural competence skills include cross-cultural communication, cultural assessment, cultural interpretation, and intervention. Communicating with the client in the home requires careful attention to conversational style and pacing, personal space, eye contact, touch, and time orientation (Lipson, 1997).

Care planning incorporates each client's sense of modesty, personal hygiene, special clothing or amulets, food beliefs, and rituals. Include family relationships, expectations of family members, visitor expectations, illness beliefs, and health practices in how you will carry out your plan.

Socioeconomic Factors

Sensitivity to socioeconomic factors is essential in effective care planning. The client may be unfamiliar with neighborhood or community resources. Support systems for transportation to shop for supplies, lifting heavy equipment, or giving expert advice may be lacking.

In addition to seeking social service and community support when appropriate, helping the client to use that support cost-effectively is equally important. Assess the cost/benefit ratio for the client and family when choosing equipment and supplies. For example, a long-term client may benefit from an expensive piece of equipment, which provides longer service and higher reliability. A client with short-term needs may not require the same caliber of equipment.

A*ction* A*lert!*
Be familiar with the criteria for third-party reimbursement for home care. Your skill in documentation of needs may affect the client's eligibility for reimbursement.

Psychological Factors

Each client has different life experiences, values, needs, goals, and beliefs. Combined with the client's developmental level, life perspective defines the psychological factors to consider in planning care. Additionally, illness may overtax a client and family that usually functions well psychologically.

As the home care nurse, you must be aware of the client's or family's ongoing capacity to manage the illness and treatment plan. Changes in role functioning are particularly disruptive to family routines. For a client with mental illness, the family may be reluctant to reach out for help. You should be prepared to help the family identify when to seek outside help.

Physiological Factors

The nature and severity of the disease process may influence the client's outcomes on both a short-term and long-term basis. Additionally, complicating chemical imbalances and impaired homeostasis may result from medication administration and other treatment modalities. Ongoing communication with the physician is necessary for adjustments in the medical regimen.

ASSESSMENT

Assessment of the homebound client and family includes biopsychosocial and environmental status as well as functional abilities to help predict the client's needs. On your first visit to a client's home, you will be assessing health needs that have already been identified through a referral or the client's request for services. The assessment data that you collect will help you develop a plan to meet health needs of the client and family. Data are collected through a systematic health history interview and a physical examination. The focus for the assessment may be narrowed by any available medical history and diagnostic tests.

*A*ction *A*lert!
As you collect information, record it in organized patterns for easy identification of nursing diagnoses. Develop a framework for assessment based on nursing problems so you can automatically identify nursing problems.

General Assessment of the Homebound Client

You will organize assessment findings into strengths and limitations or deficits. Intervention strategies designed to incorporate strengths will increase the probability of positive outcomes. Care is planned to compensate for limitations or deficits. Positive findings are strengths that can be capitalized on during the intervention phase. These strengths can serve to facilitate the resolution of the client's problem.

Negative findings are limitations, deficits, or weaknesses. If the client and family are coping with these negative findings, no action is warranted. If coping is ineffective, these limitations form the basis for the nursing diagnostic statement and are critical for establishing eligibility for service. Table 60–1 summarizes the assessment guidelines for home care nursing.

Health History

The health history in the homebound client expands beyond the illness or disease process to include how the client and family will meet the current health challenge in the home environment. Components of the health history include psychosocial assessment, functional assessment, affective (emotional) assessment, and environmental assessment.

Recall the case of Mrs. Mullen, introduced at the beginning of the chapter. The nursing assessment for Mrs. Mullen on the first home visit was as follows:

> Client experiencing fluctuating blood glucose levels after recent surgical débridement of an ulcer on her right foot. She has been given crutches to prevent weight-bearing on the right foot. Pedal pulses on both feet are present and equally strong. Blood glucose 225. Wound size is 2 cm located beneath right great toe/plantar area. Wound site reveals viable moist pink tissue with no redness or swelling in the skin surrounding the wound. Concerned about ability to manage wound care and using crutches in the home.

What additional data would you collect to plan Mrs. Mullen's care?

PSYCHOSOCIAL ASSESSMENT
Begin the history with the client's perception of the reason for your visit and the identified problem. Allow the client and designated caregiver to describe the

TABLE 60–1
Assessment Guidelines for Home Care Nursing

The parameters for completing the learner assessment are summarized for quick reference:
Biopsychosocial
  Age, sex, developmental level.
  Medical diagnoses, nursing diagnoses.
  Ethnicity, race, culture, religion, language.
  Socioeconomic status, living arrangements.
  Support systems, marital relationship, roles of family members.
  Relationship with health care provider.
Environmental
  Occupation, job-related issues.
  Home and community resources.
Functional abilities and limitations
  Psychomotor areas.
  Sensory status.
  Mobility, dexterity.
  Comfort: psychological, physical, and energy level.
Cognitive areas
  Ability to learn, identified *best* way to learn.
  Educational background, reading ability, functional illiteracy.
  Knowledge of disease and therapeutic plan.
Affective (emotional) areas
  Patient's and family's reactions and adjustment to patient's illness.
  Health beliefs and values.
  Compliance issues.
  Readiness and motivation for learning, prior learning experiences.
  Patient's self-image, personality.

From Zastocki, D.K., & Rovinski, C.A. (2000). Home care: Patient and family instructions (2nd ed.). Philadelphia: W.B. Saunders Co.

events that have created a need for services. The client and family may have concerns that are different from the problem that justified the visit from the third-party payor's perspective. Also, listening and validating the story may be therapeutic.

As you actively listen to the client's and family's perception of their needs, psychosocial assessment data may become evident. For example, a family member may say, "We asked the doctor for a referral to a home health agency because Mother lives alone, we live 60 miles away, and we can't come here every day to be with her." This need for social support for the parent is a different perspective than the medical need for managing wound care. To make the family feel understood, you will need to postpone the focus on the physical need and spend time discussing the problem from the family's perspective.

*A*ction *A*lert!
Keep your assessment organized by developing the art of gently guiding the client and family through the systematic assessment while actively listening to their perceptions of the problem.

ASSESSMENT OF FUNCTIONAL ABILITIES

Functional abilities and limitations are at least partially revealed during the history and physical examination. Hearing, vision, mobility, memory, and other functional problems that become apparent can affect the outcome of the nursing care plan. For example, blindness in a person newly diagnosed with type 1 diabetes mellitus modifies the person's needs. Functional abilities and limitation of family caregivers may also be important.

After completing the physical examination, you can return to functional problems and perform a more detailed examination. For example, vision can be tested by asking the client to read samples of written instructions in several type sizes. To determine the personal safety of a client who uses a walker, you will need to know if the person can get to the telephone, the toilet, the refrigerator, and possibly to activate an emergency response system. Actually observing the client using the walker will provide additional information about the client's mobility.

Functional assessment includes a focus on activities of daily living, such as when and how well the client can bathe, toilet, dress, eat, sleep, move about, cook, clean, and communicate with caregivers. You will document functional abilities by noting whether the client is completely independent; requires assistance from devices, equipment, or another person; or is totally dependent (see Chapters 37 and 56).

ASSESSMENT OF THE ENVIRONMENT

Environmental assessment identifies the client's capacity to establish and maintain a safe home environment that supports the success of treatment goals. Assessment tools are available to help you evaluate the safety of a client's home environment. The characteristics of an unsafe home environment are found below under the diagnosis of *Impaired home maintenance management*.

Physical Examination

Because most home health visits are for an identified medical need, your physical examination will most likely start with the identified problem and proceed to areas that may be tangentially related to the reason for the visit, based on the results of your nursing history. The physical examination may need to be thorough, or it may be modified by the client's description of need.

Because you will be in the client's home without the immediate presence of other colleagues, your physical assessment skills must be highly proficient. Based on the general needs of clients seen frequently at home, assessment skills in the following systems are essential:

- Heart, pressures, and pulses
- Thorax and lungs
- Musculoskeletal structures
- Peripheral vascular system
- Nervous system

- Mental status
- Skin
- Specific findings for infants, children, and elderly people

Focused Assessment for Impaired Home Maintenance Management

The home health client who is elderly, has functional disabilities, and lives alone on a fixed income is at risk for being unable to independently maintain a safe, health-promoting immediate environment. You should assess the client's ability to maintain the home.

Defining Characteristics

Cues can be identified in subjective statements by the client and family members and objective observations of the household to determine home maintenance needs. Subjective statements include indirect expressions of difficulty in maintaining the home in a comfortable fashion, reports of outstanding debts or financial crisis, or direct requests for assistance with home maintenance. You will need well-developed communication skills to reduce barriers to the discussion of personal problems and to gain insight into specific areas where assistance is needed.

Objective observations of the household include the presence of offensive odors and the accumulation of dirt, food, dirty laundry, or unhygienic wastes. A room temperature that is too high or low for the season represents a clear safety risk, as does the presence of rodents or insects. Lack of cooking or health care equipment, even with the most well-intentioned family support system, will also require immediate attention. An important observation involves the health status of household members and includes assessment of the coping skills and physical abilities of the family caregiver. Areas of concern include anxiety, depression, exhaustion, and repeated hygienic disorders, infestations, or infections.

The diagnosis of *Impaired home maintenance management* is made when the client or family needs assistance to do the following:

- Modify the home for disability by installing rails in stairways or hallways, mounting grab bars in bathrooms, constructing ramps, raising the toilet seat, or widening a doorway.
- Clean the house or yard or both for the purpose of eliminating health hazards.
- Rid the premises of rodents, roaches, or other vermin that are producing a health hazard.
- Maintain an interior temperature for warmth in the winter and coolness in the summer.
- Eliminate hazards from the home, such as carbon monoxide from faulty furnaces, fire hazards, broken rails on stairs, exposed lead-based paint, faulty open space heaters, and faulty wiring.
- Learn sanitation methods.

- Acquire safety features like smoke alarms, carbon monoxide alarms, or an emergency response system.
- Acquire indoor plumbing and a water supply.
- Pay the utility bills.
- Insulate the home.

The specific definition of the need for assistance may vary depending on the philosophy of the nurse, the employing agency, and the community. Agencies that provide public assistance and volunteer agencies have specific definitions of need that control the distribution of limited resources.

Related Factors

The related or etiological factor is commonly the physical inability to maintain the home environment. The physiological implications of impaired cognitive or emotional functioning, substance abuse, chronic debilitating disease, and client/family disease or injury can result in limited home management capabilities. Measures to restore or improve health are part of the solution to the problem. The client may have additional personal factors that impede home maintenance. Lack of knowledge, lack of motivation, and lack of role modeling are areas for nursing intervention.

Mrs. Mullen demonstrates understanding of sick-day rules and is able to adjust to changes in her insulin regimen. Your interview reveals that Mrs. Mullen's ulcer resulted from not wearing proper footwear. What may this information tell you concerning education needs?

DIAGNOSIS

Use data collected during the assessment phase to support the assignment of nursing diagnoses that communicate the client's and family's needs. Because the basic goal of care in the home is to maximize the client's independence and maintain safety, *Impaired home maintenance management* is one of the nursing diagnoses used most often in home care nursing. Diagnoses may also reflect the philosophy of the family as the focus of nursing care. Other frequently used nursing diagnoses apply to clients and families of all ages and at all levels of wellness.

Because Mrs. Mullen is normal weight, she will need to decrease her usual 2,000-kilocalorie American Diabetic Association (ADA) diet to 1,500 calories because of her decreased activity. The home environment appears safe, as Mrs. Mullen demonstrates safe crutch-walking and adequate support for food shopping and supplies. Her anxiety seems to be alleviated as a result of discussing her concerns about wound care and managing at home. What nursing diagnoses are suggested by these data?

Physical Needs

Nursing diagnoses for physical needs are closely associated with the medical need for the home health visit.

The following are example diagnoses for physical needs:

- *Impaired skin integrity* related to infected wound healing by third intention
- *Ineffective airway clearance* related to ineffective cough secondary to a tracheostomy
- *Chronic pain* related to terminal, progressive cancer of prostate
- *Altered health maintenance* related to new treatment regimen of insulin to control diabetes

Other physical diagnoses may be present that are not directly reimbursable. You will need to provide third-party payors with data that support the cost-effectiveness of treating these diagnoses. As an example, consider the following diagnosis: *Altered nutrition: less than body requirements, related to 30-pound weight loss secondary to cancer of the prostate.*

If you can document that by treating this diagnosis the client will be more likely to attain adequate self-care, the diagnosis could become reimbursable. For example, the client who manages parenteral therapy for pain may become more active and independent as a result of improved nutrition, thus reducing the need for pain medication.

Psychosocial Needs

Psychosocial nursing diagnoses are made to identify problems that result directly from the medical need for home care or that interfere with the client's ability to manage needed care. Cost-effective results can be achieved. The following are examples:

- *Ineffective family coping (disabling or compromised) related to lack of respite from care of a chronically ill family member.* Treatment for this diagnosis could reduce the need for services by enabling family members to continue as caregivers.
- *Ineffective individual coping related to failure of multiple attempts to properly adhere to the prescribed ADA diet.* Treatment for this diagnosis could reduce complications and the need for emergency care for a newly diagnosed client with diabetes.

Nursing diagnoses that reflect a client's affective needs can sometimes be directly connected to the medical problem that justified the home visit. An example is *Anxiety related to a complex medical regimen.*

Functional Needs

To be reimbursable, nursing diagnoses that reflect a client's functional status must be directly treatable by a prescription for the underlying medical problem. Examples of reimbursable diagnoses include the following:

- *Activity intolerance related to chronic oxygen deficit.* (Part of the treatment is oxygen therapy.)
- *Risk for injury related to lack of experience using a walker.* (Treatment includes teaching the client to use a walker.)

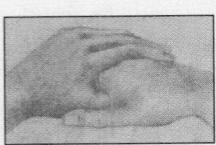
Depending on each client's circumstances, and in the absence of a definitive medical treatment, some diagnoses may not be reimbursable. Examples include the following:

- *Self-care deficit related to chronic confusion*
- *Risk for infection related to a compromised immune system*

Providing interventions for nursing diagnoses related to improving the environment can prevent illness and should lower health care costs. For example, resolving the diagnosis of *Impaired home maintenance management related to lack of financial resources to maintain a warm home* could reduce the likelihood of hospitalization for pneumonia.

PLANNING

Planning logically flows from the critical thinking process involved in defining the nursing diagnoses. For a client recovering from an acute condition, the goal is to return to the previous level of functioning. For a client with a long-term condition, the goal is to maintain the maximum level of functioning.

Expected Outcomes for the Client Recovering From an Acute Illness

The overall expected outcome for recovery from an acute illness is that the client resume the previous level of functioning and health status. The client recovering from total hip replacement surgery, for example, will require planning to coordinate assistive devices and home adaptive equipment, such as a raised toilet seat. In addition, the plan focuses on rehabilitation in conjunction with physical therapy.

Outcomes for clients recovering from acute illnesses may include the following:

- Demonstrates wound care technique
- Demonstrates safe mobility
- States that he or she will follow medication plan

A client plan for postsurgical recovery is typically short-term. A pregnant client may require a plan that covers both prenatal and postpartum care.

The physician's order includes washing the wound with saline, changing the dressing daily, and packing the wound with wet-to-wet saline dressings. Mrs. Mullen's plan will be daily visits the 1st week and three visits the 2nd week. How will you begin teaching to prepare Mrs. Mullen for increased self-care? What types of instruction will you give Mrs. Mullen about when to call you or her doctor about her blood glucose levels or the appearance of her wound?

Expected Outcomes for the Client With a Long-Term Condition

The goal for a client with a long-term condition is to maintain maximum functioning. For example, the plan may focus on pain relief and comfort measures if the client has a terminal illness that requires palliation.

Additional support requires careful planning for coordination of providers: pharmacy services for intravenous therapy, a dietitian for nutritional assessment for clients throughout the life span, from infants through geriatrics.

Typical outcomes for clients with long-term conditions include the following:

- Experiences an alleviation of pain and related symptoms
- Maintains optimal functional abilities appropriate to the disease stage
- Adapts to lifestyle changes as a result of the disease
- Achieves optimal biopsychosocial/sensory motor rehabilitation within the limits imposed by the disease

INTERVENTION

Using the Albrecht model, nursing interventions can be examined based on the expected outcomes for home health nursing. Intervention is discussed for the outcomes of client and family satisfaction, self-care, and quality of care.

Interventions to Enhance Client and Family Satisfaction

Active client and family participation in the planning process, and the incorporation of setting mutual goals,

promotes trust and satisfaction. Compliance will be increased through client and family involvement in goal setting.

Setting Mutual Goals

During home care, you will work with the client and family to establish realistic short-term and long-term goals that meet the client's health needs. However, satisfaction increases when care is provided within the values and expectations of the family setting.

In this process, give the client and family a large measure of control. Their wishes and abilities should drive the planning of care. Members of the multidisciplinary team are guests in the home and are obligated to respect the family's structure, environment, and culture. Asking the client and family what they expect as a result of the care plan forms the basis for a trusting professional relationship.

Writing a Contract

Mutual goal setting and compliance are increased by the use of a contract—an agreement between two or more parties that something will or will not be done. You can formalize the nursing care plan as a contract with the client or family by writing into the plan the activities that you will perform and those that the client or family will perform. The family then signs the care plan with you.

The care plan or contract also states outcomes in measurable behaviors so that both parties have the same expectation for outcome achievement. As an example of the necessary specificity, a partial list of measurable criteria for a client with the diagnosis *Risk for infection related to long-term use of a urinary catheter* would be written as follows:

- Client or family identifies signs and symptoms of urinary tract infection within two visits.
- Client or family demonstrates appropriate daily catheter care; that is, daily soap and water cleansing, within two visits.

Teaching "Survival Skills"

Establishing goals in a realistic and reimbursable manner requires a focus on "survival skills" (Stern, 1991). These are essential aspects of care needed to help the client and family manage the therapeutic regimen safely and within defined parameters. The survival skill philosophy is useful, for example, in planning to meet learning needs. It helps you avoid giving the client and family too much information—an action that may be overwhelming to the client.

Focusing teaching about safety and the steps needed to maintain and improve health is more likely to meet the client's and family's needs as well as to be reimbursed. This approach supports professional standards if the essential elements of teaching are correctly chosen.

One element essential to the client's safety and sense of well-being is knowing when to call for help.

The client and family alone in the home, without nursing or medical knowledge, will derive a sense of security from knowing whom and when to call for help. As appropriate, give the client and family a list of signs and symptoms that suggest a need for professional intervention.

Interventions to Increase Self-Care Capacity

Promoting a maximal level of independence requires focused interventions to build on the client's and family's strengths while designing approaches to minimize deficits.

Providing Client Teaching

Teaching is inherent in providing care in the home because the goal is to make the client independent in self-care. You and other team members are only in the home for part of a day or week; therefore, the client must learn to manage without professional assistance.

Teaching is focused on behavior change that you consider essential to health maintenance in the home. Areas to consider for teaching opportunities include self-care skills necessary for maintenance of a new treatment regimen, understanding body system changes that result from a disease process, managing a therapeutic diet, effective use of medications, and activity planning.

Your teaching plan must be coordinated with all disciplines that provide care. Clients become confused when they receive seemingly contradictory information or when information provided by the physician, nurse, physical therapist, and other health team members varies too widely.

Teaching in the home setting has some advantages over the hospital or clinic setting. For example, it allows you to demonstrate and the client and family to practice new skills with the equipment and supplies that will actually be used in the setting where they will be used. This realism offers an advantage over the more theoretical teaching that can be done in an acute care setting. Additionally, the client feels more relaxed and in control at home and may feel more ready to take charge of the procedure.

On the other hand, some home teaching situations demand a creative approach. For example, to promote compliance with a complex medication regimen, you may need to design a system to help the client organize medications and remember to take them. A clean, empty egg carton can be labeled for various medications and the times they should be taken. Or a medication reminder can be obtained from the drug store. The client would have to agree to fill each slot in the morning with the appropriate medications and would have to be able to understand that the medication should be taken on time, so that all slots are empty by bedtime.

Another idea is to label a monthly calendar to prompt the client to adhere to a schedule. It is important to adapt the treatment regimen, to whatever extent possible, to the client's and family's daily routine.

Insisting that the client adhere to the arbitrary medication times used in an acute care setting can adversely affect compliance.

Use of written material that can be left in the home reinforces information and promotes compliance. Written material should contain easy-to-follow directions, preferably written at no higher than the eighth-grade reading level for most clients. The use of illustrations, when possible, is helpful for any client, especially for the client who is illiterate or who reads poorly. It may be helpful to print instructions with enough white space to hand-write individualized instructions. Elderly clients may need large-print versions of instruction sheets.

Counseling the Client

Counseling is an interactive helping process based on a therapeutic relationship established through mutual trust and respect. Like teaching, counseling includes providing information and helping to change behaviors. However, counseling implies that the relationship is part of the therapeutic process, that the client enters into the relationship to achieve a desired change, and therefore that the client is an active participant.

Because successful home nursing often requires that the family be viewed as the client, a therapeutic relationship should be established with the entire family.

Successful counseling requires that you understand the client's beliefs and values to help work toward behavioral changes that are consistent with the client's self system. Beliefs and values are most often derived from the larger social and cultural context. The health beliefs and values held by the family and client can seem problematic when they differ from the beliefs and values held by the new practitioner.

A*ction* A*lert!*
Focus on the client and family as people first, and on their different beliefs and values as secondary, to remove barriers to the therapeutic relationship.

Interventions to Ensure Quality Care

Quality care is a subjective concept; that is, it means different things to different people. For this reason, client satisfaction is commonly used as an indicator of quality. Other indicators of quality include care that is efficient, well coordinated, safe, and effective in solving the client's problem.

In a client's home, quality of care is achieved when the following occurs:

- Therapeutic nursing actions are based on the established plan of care and are consistent with and supportive of the medically prescribed treatment regimen.
- The nurse maintains competence in performing therapeutic nursing activities.
- The methods of the therapeutic nursing actions are appropriate to the home setting.

To provide quality home care, nursing actions must be based on a specific body of knowledge. Therapeutic nursing activities include clinical technical skills, teaching, counseling, and coordination of care. Direct-care skill requirements vary greatly with the client's environment, the technology required, and the capabilities of the client and family.

The home setting is an autonomous practice setting, typically lacking in direct supervision. You must be prepared to perform psychomotor skills by established guidelines, to make decisions, and to modify procedures in unique home environments. You may work in a homeless shelter, a house without running water, or an expansive three-story house where the kitchen is far from the bedroom.

Thus, application of clinical skills in the home setting requires a shift in perspective from that of the acute care approach. For example, in the home, you are concerned with providing infection control in the client's usual microbial environment.

Coordinating Care

Coordination is essential to quality because it helps maintain continuity of care between service agencies and among providers of care. Coordination provides a link between acute care and home care. In an increasingly high-technology environment, the multitude of providers, services, and equipment can easily result in duplicated or omitted care.

In addition to coordinating the actions of team members, you also are responsible for supervising nonlicensed staff, such as home health aides. The home health aide needs clearly defined assignments with expected outcomes. You will evaluate the client's and family's reports about services provided by the aide, and you may observe those services directly from time to time.

An established plan of care facilitates planning for the most appropriate team member to provide services while also ensuring that the client receives the needed care. Your primary role may be to establish the plan and delegate care to the team member best qualified to provide it.

Between home visits, telephone contact will help to monitor the client's status and maintain interaction with other members of the care team. As case manager, you will monitor and evaluate each component of the care plan to ensure that all actions complement each other. You also will function as an advocate to ensure that the client's and family's rights and confidentiality are protected.

Making Referrals

When care needed in the home exceeds your scope of practice, your expertise, or the services of the home health agency, a referral for additional services is essential. As a home health nurse, you need to be able to recognize health problems that are beyond the scope of nursing practice and that should be referred to a physician. This does not mean that you need to be able to diagnose medical problems.

You also make a referral when a nutritionist, physical therapist, respiratory therapist, or occupational therapist has more skill in managing a particular problem. Although home health agencies often provide an array of services, the referral may need to be between agencies.

Referrals are most successful when you have a relationship with the agency or person to whom you refer the client. You can better match services with the client's needs when you are familiar with the services provided and with the expertise of an agency or person. Keep a file of local agencies with information about their services. A computerized contact management program or a database can allow easy access to agency information to make the best match of client to services.

Providing for Safety

Understanding the elements of the home environment is essential in planning appropriately for the client's safety, particularly on discharge from the acute setting to the home. The client may have impaired mobility from a variety of conditions, including cardiopulmonary, neurological, and musculoskeletal problems. The need to climb stairs to enter or leave the home, use the bathroom, or function in the kitchen may pose significant challenges. Other safety hazards may exist in the home environment as well. You can be helpful with suggestions for modifying routine, changing work habits to conserve energy, or ways for working safely.

To keep Mrs. Mullen's right foot elevated and maximize safety, how would you help her organize her activities and personal space?

Modifying the Care Plan

Home care nursing makes maximum use of the client's strengths and resources to ensure safe and effective care. It is care in the *client's home,* the place where people expect to be themselves and live by their own schedule. Therefore, it cannot be provided by a standardized formula for time, place, methods, or equipment. Rather, the nurse works to bring all the elements of the situation together and modifies the care plan accordingly.

For example, developing a routine that maximizes the client's support system can promote safety. For some clients, bathing activities are best scheduled when someone is available in the home to provide assistance if needed. Age-specific environmental concerns vary from the small child who is exploring a new environment to the elderly with diminished hearing or vision and impaired mobility.

Interventions to Assist With Home Maintenance Management

Although nurses typically do not provide direct assistance with home maintenance, helping the client find assistance can be an important intervention in the overall maintenance of the client's health. Plans for treating the illness or condition are developed in the context of the home environment. Therefore, obtaining needed services and coordinating care is an integral nursing role.

Rather than giving direct assistance, you will intervene to help the client and family evaluate their home for health hazards and physical safety problems. You should be familiar with potential safety hazards associated with health problems and functional disabilities. Familiarity with the home safety checklist in Chapter 28 will help you promote a safe home environment.

In most cases, the client or family is responsible for modifying the home environment. If they cannot do so, however, you may need to provide assistance in obtaining a needed service. Because home modifications exceed the expertise of most nurses, you should make yourself familiar with community resources for homemaker services, repair services, laundry, and pest control. Information or assistance may be obtained through a referral to the local health department, public utility safety engineers, or community programs for safe housing. Examples of services that may be enlisted include the following:

- Hands on Housing
- Caritas
- Habitat for Humanity
- Housekeeping services
- Volunteer programs

EVALUATION

Your evaluation should demonstrate that the elements of the nursing process are present. It should be evident that the client's needs were comprehensively and appropriately assessed, that a plan was developed with the client and family, that the client received needed care, and that the care resulted in the expected outcomes (or evidence that explains why the outcomes were not achieved.) Process evaluation relies heavily on documentation.

Documentation records data that suggest the client's and family's progress or lack of progress toward established outcomes. Therefore, it is part of the evaluation of the effectiveness of the plan of care. In documenting home care nursing, always state facts rather than opinions. Make note of skilled nursing interventions (activities within the scope and practice of the registered professional nurse), including the following:

- Assessment
- Observation
- Evaluation of signs and symptoms
- Planning of individualized goal-directed care
- Teaching self-care to promote independence
- Using clinical skills in the application of treatments and the provision of direct care

Documentation is the primary method by which you demonstrate legal and professional accountability.

Upon discharge from home care, Mrs. Mullen's wound reveals consistent buildup of granulation tissue that requires only a transparent dressing. The diabetes plan reflects a return to increasing activity and a dietary adjustment back to a 2,000-kilocalorie ADA diet and insulin on a split mixed dosages of:

AM 15 units NPH and 4 units regular
PM 6 units NPH and 2 units regular
No coverage

For a 2-week period Mrs. Mullen will call her physician every Tuesday with the results of her blood glucose monitoring. She will alternate performing blood glucose monitoring at breakfast and dinner one day and lunch and bedtime the following day. She will demonstrate an understanding of when to call the physician for insulin or wound-care issues. In addition, she will verbalize the proper foot care needed to prevent injuries in the future.

Although discharge planning begins during the assessment and planning phases, preparation for discharge from home care receives increasing emphasis as outcomes near achievement. Planning for discharge from home care is just as important as planning for discharge from acute care. Legal and ethical issues involving abandonment are relevant in both environments. The relationship formed between you, the client, and family members requires skillful preparation before termination, whether the client is leaving acute care or home care services.

Documentation of evaluation data is used to determine the need for continuation of services.

In your documentation, describe the exact nature or circumstances of the client's condition, keeping in mind the financial ramifications of the terms that you use. For example, if you describe the client as "up ad lib," the client's homebound status may be forfeited. However, if you document that the client can walk about 20 feet before developing extreme shortness of breath, you will have demonstrated why the person has trouble leaving the home.

Documentation should reveal the answers to the following questions:

- Why does the client need the skills of a professional nurse for health care?
- What clinical findings demonstrate that the client's condition is not stable?
- Why is the client unable to manage self-care needs?
- Why is the documented plan of care reasonable and essential in light of the applicable medical diagnoses?

KEY PRINCIPLES

- Home care services include nursing care, social work, physical therapy, respiratory therapy, speech therapy, occupational therapy, registered dietitian counseling, laboratory services, and home health aide services.
- People of all ages and varying socioeconomic backgrounds may need a variety of home care services.

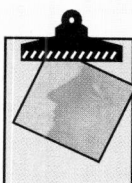

NURSING CARE PLANNING
A HOMEBOUND DIABETIC CLIENT WITH A FOOT WOUND

Assessment Data

During the first home visit for Mrs. Mullen, the home nurse immediately began the assessment. A partial listing of the admission assessment data included the following:

- 35-year-old well-developed white female.
- Right foot wound located on the dorsum measuring 2.5 cm × 3.5 cm.
- Wound exhibits no signs of infection.
- Right foot and toes warm to touch.
- Blood glucose monitoring results range from 180 to 240.
- Urine, free of ketones.
- T 98.8 degrees F, BP 130/74, P 74, R 18.
- Height and weight: 5 ft. 7 in., 135 lb.
- States no numbness or pain in right foot wound.
- States, "I can't get my housework done when I'm on these crutches. I need to get this foot healed up. Look at this house. It's a mess!"
- Dirty dishes and pans all over kitchen counter, on table, and in sink; laundry piled up on and near washing machine in kitchen; house generally unkempt and dusty.

Physician's Orders   Wound care
Monitor diabetes

NURSING CARE PLAN

Nursing Diagnosis	Expected Outcomes	Interventions	Evaluation
Impaired home maintenance management related to effects of chronic debilitating disease, foot ulcer	Wound healing: Foot and toes warm to touch; States no numbness or pain; Wound pink with absence of redness, swelling, tenderness, odor, or purulent drainage; Wound healing continues without signs of infection	Teach signs and symptoms of wound infection; Teach importance of maintaining dressing dry and intact and wound free from contamination; Perform wound care; Teach wound care techniques; Assess stages of wound healing; *Encourage client to take responsibility for care; give praise for independence*	Wound 2.5 cm × 3.5 cm; Granulation present over all surfaces; No drainage; *Mrs. Mullen is pleased to demonstrate how well she can change the dressing and describe the wound. Technique is impeccable.*
	Able to bear weight bilaterally without crutches	Teach when to begin weight bearing	Client able to bear weight bilaterally without crutches
	States increased satisfaction with own ability to maintain home	Arrange for temporary assistance with housework (until able to bear weight bilaterally)	States, "Its so good to be up and around again. See, no more dirty dishes!"

Italicized interventions indicate culturally specific care.

Critical Thinking Questions

1. What is the significance of the presence of granulation tissue in the wound?
2. What reaction would you expect to the suggestion that Mrs. Mullen could benefit from someone to help her with housework? How would you respond?
3. How would you alter the plan of care if, at the time of your evaluation, Mrs. Mullen's wound were red and tender?

- The home care nurse assumes the roles of technically skilled direct care provider, educator, advocate, collaborator, leader, and case manager.
- The Albrecht nursing model for home health care assumes that clients and their families are active and responsible participants in their care.
- The goals of home care nursing are to restore health and help the client return to an appropriate level of functioning, maintain health and preserve functional abilities and independence, promote health and minimize effects of illness, and improve health and help the client achieve a higher level of functioning.
- The professional nurse, as the case manager, collaborates and coordinates care with other members of the multidisciplinary health care team.
- Factors affecting the outcome of home care include lifestyle, environmental, developmental, cultural, religious, socioeconomic, psychological, and physiological factors.
- Assessment includes psychosocial, physical, functional, and environmental factors.
- The most frequently encountered nursing diagnosis in home care nursing is *Impaired home maintenance management.*
- Planning home care requires focusing on what can be realistically achieved in the family system.
- Expected outcomes for clients recovering from acute illness may be very different from clients with long-term needs.
- Home care nursing interventions are designed to plan for client and family satisfaction, ensure cost-effective care, ensure quality of care, increase self-care capability, enhance health status, ensure effective use of home care services, and assist with home maintenance management.
- During evaluation, the measurement and documentation of outcomes must be discussed with the client and family.
- Home care implies a philosophy of promoting independence in a qualitative and cost-effective manner.

BIBLIOGRAPHY

Adams, C.E. et al. (1997). Home health nurse patient care and coordination time: Health maintenance organization versus fee-for-service. *Journal of Nursing Administration, 27*(3), 21–27.

*Albrecht, M.N. (1990). The Albrecht nursing model for home health care: Implications for research, practice, and education. *Public Health Nursing, 7*(2), 118–126.

*Albrecht, M.N., & Perry, K.M. (1992). Home health care. *Clinical Nursing Research, 1*(3), 305–311.

*American Nurses' Association. (1986). *Standards of home health nursing practice*. Kansas City, MO: Author.

*American Nurses' Association. (1996). *Standards of community health nursing practice*, Washington, D.C.: Author.

*Arno, P.S. et al. (1994). The economic impact of high-technology home care. *Hastings Center Report, 24*(5), S15–S19.

*Arras, J.D., & Dubler, N.N. (1994). Bringing the hospital home: Ethical and social implications of high-tech home care. *Hastings Center Report, 24*(5), S19–S28.

Bowles, K.H., & Naylor, M.D. (1996). Nursing intervention classification systems. *Image: Journal of Nursing Scholarship, 28*(4), 303–308.

Brent, N.J. (1997). Home healthcare fraud: Implications for the home healthcare agency and nurse. *Home Healthcare Nurse, 15*(1), 38–40.

Bryan, Y.E. et al. (1997). Preparing to change from acute to community-based care. *Journal of Nursing Administration, 27*(5), 35–44.

Burns, L.R. et al. (1996). Impact of integrated community nursing services on hospital utilization and costs in a Medicare risk plan. *Inquiry, 33*(1), 30–41.

Byrd, M.E. (1997). A typology of the potential outcomes of maternal-child home visits: A literature analysis. *Public Health Nursing, 14*(1), 3–11.

Campinha-Bacote, J. et al. (1996). The challenge of cultural diversity for nurse educators. *Journal of Continuing Education in Nursing, 27*(2), 59–64.

Capone, L.J. (1998). Home care: A family affair. *Home Healthcare Nurse, 15*(1), 49–51.

Churness, V.H. et al. (1991). Home health patient classification system. *Home Healthcare Nurse, 9*(2), 14–22.

Clemen-Stone, S. et al. (1995). Comprehensive community health nursing. St. Louis: Mosby-Year Book.

Department of Health and Human Services. (1996). Health care financing administration: Medical home health agency manual. *Transmittal*, April.

Experton, B. et al. (1997). The impact of payor/provider type on healthcare use and expenditures among the frail elderly. *American Journal of Public Health, 87*(2), 210–216.

Gagnon, A.J. et al. (1997). A randomized trial of a program of early postpartum discharge with nurse visitation. *American Journal of Obstetrics and Gynecology, 176*(1), 205–211.

Grobe, S.J. (1996). The nursing intervention lexicon and taxonomy: Implications for representing nursing care data in automated patient records. *Holistic Nursing Practice, 11*(1), 48–63.

*Harris, M.D. (1994). Handbook of Home Health Care Administration. Gaithersberg, MD: Aspen Publishers, Inc.

Harris, M.D. (1996). Medical home health agency manual revisions. *Home Healthcare Nurse, 14*(9), 696–697.

Harris, M.D., & Dugan, M. (1996). Evaluating the quality of home care services using patient outcome data. *Home Healthcare Nurse, 14*(6), 463–468.

Hays, B.J. et al. (1997). Measuring the need for nursing care in older adults living at home. *Public Health Nursing, 14*(1), 37–41.

Hilgendorf, P.M. (1996). Profile of the successful home health nurse case manager. *Nursing Management, 27*(10), 32Q–R, 32U–V.

Hoeman, S. (1996). Intraethnic diversity. *Home Healthcare Nurse, 14*(7), 568.

Joint Commission on Accreditation of Health-Care Organizations (1999). *Comprehensive accreditation manual for home care*. Oakbrook Terrace, IL: Author.

Jones, E. (1997). Telemedicine fosters home care. *Health Measures, 2*(1), 20–25, 37.

Lang, N.M. (Ed.). (1995). Nursing data systems: An emerging framework. In *Data System Advances for Clinical Nursing Practice*. Washington, DC: American Nurses Publishing.

Leeka, A.B. (1995). Ethical delivery of specialized care beyond hospital walls. *Caring*, September, 18–22.

Lipson, J. (1996). Self-care nursing in multicultural context. Thousand Oaks, CA: Sage.

Lipson, J. et al. (1997). Culture and nursing care: A pocket guide. San Francisco: USC San Francisco Nursing Press.

*Livengood, W.S. et al. (1983). The impact of DRGs on home health care. *Home Healthcare Nurse, 1*(1), 29–31, 34.

Love, M., & Khanna, R. (1996). Home healthcare, managed care, and capitation. *Healthcare Information Management, 10*(2), 57–60.

Meleis, A. et al. (1995). Diversity, marginalization, and culturally competent health care: Issues in knowledge development. Washington, D.C.: American Academy of Nursing.

---

*Asterisk indicates a classic or definitive work on this subject.

Meyer, H. (1997). Home care goes corporate. *Hospitals and Health Networks, 71*(9), 20–26.

Morrall, K. (1996). Home care: Possibilities, profits, and problems. *Hospital and Health Networks, 70*(6), 81.

*Rovinski, C.A., & Zastocki, D.K. (1989). *Home care: A technical manual for the professional nurse.* Philadelphia: W.B. Saunders Co.

*Saba, V.K. et al. (1991). A nursing intervention taxonomy for home health care. *Nursing and Health Care, 12*(6), 296–299.

Saint Pierre, M., & Dittbrenner, H. (1995). HCFA's home health initiative: The first comprehensive reassessment of the medicare home health benefit. *Caring,* March, 22–27.

*Schmele, J.A. (1989). Standards: The state of the art. In C.G. Meisenheimer (Ed.). *Quality assurance for home health care* (pp 56–64). Rockville, MD: Aspen.

Snow, C. (1997). Here comes PPS. *Modern Healthcare, 27*(8), 40–45.

*Speigel, A.D. (1983). *Home health care: Home birthing to hospice care.* Baltimore: National Health Publishing.

*Stanhope, M.K. (1989). Home care past perspectives and implications for the present and future. In C.G. Meisenheimer (Ed.). *Quality assurance for home health care* (pp 3–12). Rockville, MD: Aspen.

*Stern, T.E. (1991). An early discharge program: An entrepreneurial nursing practice becomes a hospital affiliated agency. *Journal of Perinatal and Neonatal Nursing, 59*(1), 1–8.

*Stewart, J.E. (1979). *Home health care.* St. Louis: C.V. Mosby.

*Swanson, C., & Rodarte, M. (1994). Hospital-based home care: Delivering success. *Medical Surgical Nursing, 3*(5), 403–405.

Turner, B.K. (Ed.). (1995). *Multifaith information manual* (3rd ed.). Toronto: Multifaith Counsel on Spiritual and Religious Care.

Wilson, R., & Fulmer, T. (1997). Introduction of wireless, pen-based computing among visiting nurses in the inner city: A qualitative study. *Journal of Community Health Nursing, 14*(1), 23–37.

Winter, A., & Winter, R. (1993). Consumer's guide to free medical information. Englewood Cliffs, NJ: Prentice Hall.

Zablocki, E. (1997). Adapting to the evolution of risk sharing. *Home Healthcare Today, 3*(2), 14–21.

*Zastocki, D.K., & Rovinski, C.A. (2000). *Home care: Patient and family instructions* (2nd ed.). Philadelphia: W.B. Saunders Co.

Zink, M.R., & Greaves, P. (1996). Home care accreditation with the community health accreditation program: Part II: The process. *Home Healthcare Nurse, 14*(9), 684–688.

Appendices

APPENDIX 1

Recommended Dietary Allowances,* Revised 1989

Designed for the maintenance of good nutrition of practically all healthy people in the United States

Category	Age (Years) or Condition	Weight† (kg)	Weight† (lb)	Height† (cm)	Height† (in)	Protein (g)	Fat-Soluble Vitamins Vitamin A (µg RE)‡	Vitamin D (µg)§	Vitamin E (mg α-TE)¶	Vitamin K (µg)	Water-Soluble Vitamins Vitamin C (mg)	Thiamin (mg)	Riboflavin (mg)	Niacin (mg NE)**	Vitamin B₆ (mg)	Folate (µg)	Vitamin B₁₂ (µg)	Minerals Calcium (mg)	Phosphorus (mg)	Magnesium (mg)	Iron (mg)	Zinc (mg)	Iodine (µg)	Selenium (µg)
Infants	0.0–0.5	6	13	60	24	13	375	7.5	3	5	30	0.3	0.4	5	0.3	25	0.3	400	300	40	6	5	40	10
	0.5–1.0	9	20	71	28	14	375	10	4	10	35	0.4	0.5	6	0.6	35	0.5	600	500	60	10	5	50	15
Children	1–3	13	29	90	35	16	400	10	6	15	40	0.7	0.8	9	1.0	50	0.7	800	800	80	10	10	70	20
	4–6	20	44	112	44	24	500	10	7	20	45	0.9	1.1	12	1.1	75	1.0	800	800	120	10	10	90	20
	7–10	28	62	132	52	28	700	10	7	30	45	1.0	1.2	13	1.4	100	1.4	800	800	170	10	10	120	30
Males	11–14	45	99	157	62	45	1,000	10	10	45	50	1.3	1.5	17	1.7	150	2.0	1,200	1,200	270	12	15	150	40
	15–18	66	145	176	69	59	1,000	10	10	65	60	1.5	1.8	20	2.0	200	2.0	1,200	1,200	400	12	15	150	50
	19–24	72	160	177	70	58	1,000	10	10	70	60	1.5	1.7	19	2.0	200	2.0	1,200	1,200	350	10	15	150	70
	25–50	79	174	176	70	63	1,000	5	10	80	60	1.5	1.7	19	2.0	200	2.0	800	800	350	10	15	150	70
	51+	77	170	173	68	63	1,000	5	10	80	60	1.2	1.4	15	2.0	200	2.0	800	800	350	10	15	150	70
Females	11–14	46	101	157	62	46	800	10	8	45	50	1.1	1.3	15	1.4	150	2.0	1,200	1,200	280	15	12	150	45
	15–18	55	120	163	64	44	800	10	8	55	60	1.1	1.3	15	1.5	180	2.0	1,200	1,200	300	15	12	150	50
	19–24	58	128	164	65	46	800	10	8	60	60	1.1	1.3	15	1.6	180	2.0	1,200	1,200	280	15	12	150	55
	25–50	63	138	163	64	50	800	5	8	65	60	1.1	1.3	15	1.6	180	2.0	800	800	280	15	12	150	55
	51+	65	143	160	63	50	800	5	8	65	60	1.0	1.2	13	1.6	180	2.0	800	800	280	10	12	150	55
Pregnant						60	800	10	10	65	70	1.5	1.6	17	2.2	400	2.2	1,200	1,200	320	30	15	175	65
Lactating	1st 6 months					65	1,300	10	12	65	95	1.6	1.8	20	2.1	280	2.6	1,200	1,200	355	15	19	200	75
	2nd 6 months					62	1,200	10	11	65	90	1.6	1.7	20	2.1	260	2.6	1,200	1,200	340	15	16	200	75

*The allowances, expressed as average daily intakes over time, are intended to provide for individual variations among most normal persons as they live in the United States under usual environmental stresses. Diets should be based on a variety of common foods in order to provide other nutrients for which human requirements have been less well defined.

†Weights and heights of Reference Adults are actual medians for the U.S. population of the designated age, as reported by NHANES II. The use of these figures does not imply that the height-to-weight ratios are ideal.

‡Retinol equivalents. 1 retinol equivalent = 1 µg retinol or 6 µg β-carotene.

§As cholecalciferol. 10 µg cholecalciferol = 400 IU of vitamin D.

¶Tocopherol equivalents. 1 mg d-α tocopherol = 1 α-TE.

**1 NE (niacin equivalent) is equal to 1 mg of niacin or 60 mg of dietary tryptophan.

Reprinted with permission from Recommended Dietary Allowances: 10th edition. Copyright 1989 by the National Academy of Sciences. Courtesy of the National Academy Press, Washington, DC.

Recommended Nutrient Intake for Canadians, 1990

Summary of Examples of Recommended Nutrients Based on Energy Expressed as Daily Rates

Age	Sex	Energy (kcal)	Thiamin (mg)	Riboflavin (mg)	Niacin (NE)*	n-3 PUFA† (g)	n-6 PUFA (g)
Months							
0–4	Both	600	0.3	0.3	4	0.5	3
5–12	Both	900	0.4	0.5	7	0.5	3
Years							
1	Both	1100	0.5	0.6	8	0.6	4
2–3	Both	1300	0.6	0.7	9	0.7	4
4–6	Both	1800	0.7	0.9	13	1.0	6
7–9	M	2200	0.9	1.1	16	1.2	7
	F	1900	0.8	1.0	14	1.0	6
10–12	M	2500	1.0	1.3	18	1.4	8
	F	2200	0.9	1.1	16	1.2	7
13–15	M	2800	1.1	1.4	20	1.5	9
	F	2200	0.9	1.1	16	1.2	7
16–18	M	3200	1.3	1.6	23	1.8	11
	F	2100	0.8	1.1	15	1.2	7
19–24	M	3000	1.2	1.5	22	1.6	10
	F	2100	0.8	1.1	15	1.2	7
25–49	M	2700	1.1	1.4	19	1.5	9
	F	1900	0.8‡	1.0‡	14‡	1.1‡	7‡
50–74	M	2300	0.9	1.2	16	1.3	8
	F	1800	0.8‡	1.0‡	14‡	1.1‡	7‡
75+	M	2000	0.8	1.0	14	1.1	7
	F§	1700	0.8‡	1.0‡	14‡	1.1‡	7‡
Pregnancy (additional)							
1st Trimester		100	0.1	0.1	1	0.05	0.3
2nd Trimester		300	0.1	0.3	2	0.16	0.9
3rd Trimester		300	0.1	0.3	2	0.16	0.9
Lactation (additional)		450	0.2	0.4	3	0.25	1.5

Recommended Nutrient Intake for Canadians, 1990 *Continued*

Summary Examples of Recommended Nutrient Intake Based on Age and Body Weight Expressed as Daily Rates

Age	Sex	Weight (kg)	Protein (g)	Vita-min A (RE)¶	Vita-min D (μg)	Vita-min E (mg)	Vita-min C (mg)	Folate (μg)	Vita-min B₁₂ (μg)	Cal-cium (mg)	Phos-phorus (mg)	Magne-sium (mg)	Iron (mg)	Iodine (μg)	Zinc (mg)
Months															
0–4	Both	6.0	12**	400	10	3	20	25	0.3	250††	150	20	0.3‡‡	30	2‡‡
5–12	Both	9.0	12	400	10	3	20	40	0.4	400	200	32	7	40	3
Years															
1	Both	11	13	400	10	3	20	40	0.5	500	300	40	6	55	4
2–3	Both	14	16	400	5	4	20	50	0.6	550	350	50	6	65	4
4–6	Both	18	19	500	5	5	25	70	0.8	600	400	65	8	85	5
7–9	M	25	26	700	2.5	7	25	90	1.0	700	500	100	8	110	7
	F	25	26	700	2.5	6	25	90	1.0	700	500	100	8	95	7
10–12	M	34	34	800	2.5	8	25	120	1.0	900	700	130	8	125	9
	F	36	36	800	2.5	7	25	130	1.0	1100	800	135	8	110	9
13–15	M	50	49	900	2.5	9	30§§	175	1.0	1100	900	185	10	160	12
	F	48	46	800	2.5	7	30§§	170	1.0	1000	850	180	13	160	9
16–18	M	62	58	1000	2.5	10	40§§	220	1.0	900	1000	230	10	160	12
	F	53	47	800	2.5	7	30§§	190	1.0	700	850	200	12	160	9
19–24	M	71	61	1000	2.5	10	40§§	220	1.0	800	1000	240	9	160	12
	F	58	50	800	2.5	7	30§§	180	1.0	700	850	200	13	160	9
25–49	M	74	64	1000	2.5	9	40§§	230	1.0	800	1000	250	9	160	12
	F	59	51	800	2.5	6	30§§	185	1.0	700	850	200	13	160	9
50–74	M	73	63	1000	5	7	40§§	230	1.0	800	1000	250	9	160	12
	F	63	54	800	5	6	30§§	195	1.0	800	850	210	8	160	9
75+	M	69	59	1000	5	6	40§§	215	1.0	800	1000	230	9	160	12
	F	64	55	800	5	5	30§§	200	1.0	800	850	210	8	160	9
Pregnancy (additional)															
1st trimester			5	0	2.5	2	0	200	0.2	500	200	15	0	25	6
2nd trimester			15	0	2.5	2	10	200	0.2	500	200	45	5	25	6
3rd trimester			24	0	2.5	2	10	200	0.2	500	200	45	10	25	6
Lactation (additional)			22	400	2.5	3	25	100	0.2	500	200	65	0	50	6

*Niacin equivalents.
†PUFA, polyunsaturated fatty acids.
‡Level below which intake should not fall.
§Assumes moderate (more than average) physical activity.
¶Retinol equivalents.
**Protein is assumed to be from breast milk and must be adjusted for infant formula.
††Infant formula with high phosphorus should contain 375 mg calcium.
‡‡Breast milk is assumed to be the source of the mineral.
§§Smokers should increase vitamin C by 50%.
Reprinted with permission of Health Canada, Health Protection Branch.

DIETARY REFERENCE INTAKES

In 1997 and 1998, the National Academy of Sciences issued the first and second of a series of reports on Dietary Reference Intakes (DRIs), which update and expand the Recommended Dietary Allowances (RDAs) set by the Academy since 1941. The reports recommend intake levels for U.S. and Canadian individuals and population groups and, for the first time, set maximum-level guidelines to reduce the risk of adverse health effects from overconsumption of a nutrient. Additional reports on antioxidants, macronutrients, trace elements, electrolytes and water, and other food components will follow.

Unlike the RDAs, which established the minimal amounts of nutrients needed to be protective against possible nutrient deficiency, the new values are designed to reflect the latest understanding about nutrient requirements based on optimizing health in individuals and groups. The new recommendations include four categories of reference intakes:

- *Recommended Dietary Allowance:* The intake that meets the nutrient need of almost all of the healthy individuals in a specific age and gender group. The RDA should be used in guiding individuals to achieve adequate nutrient intake aimed at decreasing the risk of chronic disease. It is based on estimating an average requirement plus an increase to account for the variation within a particular group. The amount of scientific evidence available allowed the committee to calculate RDAs for phosphorus and magnesium.
- *Adequate Intake:* When sufficient scientific evidence is not available to estimate an average requirement, Adequate Intakes (AIs) have been set. Individuals should use the AIs as a goal for intake where no RDA exists. The AI is derived through experimental or observational data that show a mean intake that appears to sustain a desired indicator of health, such as calcium retention in bone for most members of a population group. For example, AIs have been set for infants through 1 year of age using the average observed nutrient intake of populations of breast-fed infants as the standard. The committee set AIs for calcium, vitamin D, and fluoride.
- *Estimated Average Requirement (EAR):* The intake that meets the estimated nutrient need of half the individuals in a specific group. This figure is to be used as the basis for developing the RDA and is to be used by nutrition policy-makers in the evaluation of the adequacy of nutrient intakes of the group and for planning how much the group should consume.
- *Tolerable Upper Intake Level:* The maximum intake by an individual that is unlikely to pose risks of adverse health effects in almost all healthy individuals in a specified group. This figure is not intended to be a recommended level of intake, and

Criteria and Dietary Reference Intake Values for Calcium by Life-Stage Group

Life-Stage Group*	Criterion	AI (mg/day)
0–6 months	Human milk content	210
6–12 months	Human milk + solid food	270
1–3 years	Extrapolation of maximal calcium retention from 4 through 8 years	500
4–8 years	Maximal calcium retention	800
9–13 years	Maximal calcium retention	1,300
14–18 years	Maximal calcium retention	1,300
19–30 years	Maximal calcium retention	1,000
31–50 years	Calcium balance	1,000
51–70 years	Maximal calcium retention	1,200
>70 years	Extrapolation of maximal calcium retention from 51 through 70 years	1,200
Pregnancy		
<19 years	Bone mineral mass	1,300
19–50 years	Bone mineral mass	1,000
Lactation		
<19 years	Bone mineral mass	1,300
19–50 years	Bone mineral mass	1,000

*All groups except Pregnancy and Lactation include males and females.

there is no established benefit for individuals to consume nutrients at levels above the RDA or AI. For most nutrients, this figure refers to total intakes from food, fortified food, and nutrient supplements.

Criteria and Dietary Reference Intake Values for Phosphorus by Life-Stage Group

Life-Stage Group*	Criterion	EAR (mg/day)	RDA (mg/day)	AI (mg/day)
0–6 months	Human milk content	—	—	100
6–12 months	Human milk + solid food	—	—	275
1–3 years	Factorial approach	380	460	—
4–8 years	Factorial approach	405	500	—
9–13 years	Factorial approach	1,055	1,250	—
14–18 years	Factorial approach	1,055	1,250	—
19–30 years	Serum P(e,i)	580	700	—
31–50 years	Serum P(i)	580	700	—
51–70 years	Extrapolation of serum P(i) from 19 through 50 years	580	700	—
>70 years	Extrapolation of serum P(i) from 19 through 50 years	580	700	—
Pregnancy				
<19 years	Factorial approach	1,055	1,250	—
19–50 years	Serum P(i)	580	700	—
Lactation				
<19 years	Factorial approach	1,055	1,250	—
19–50 years	Serum P(i)	580	700	—

*All groups except Pregnancy and Lactation include males and females.
P(e,i), inorganic phosphate concentration.

Criteria and Dietary Reference Intake Values for Magnesium by Life-Stage Group

Life-Stage Group	Criterion	EAR (mg/day) Male/Female	RDA (mg/day) Male/Female	AI (mg/day) Male/Female
0–6 months	Human milk content	—/—	—/—	30/30
6–12 months	Human milk + solid food	—/—	—/—	75/75
1–3 years	Extrapolation of balance from older children	65/65	80/80	—
4–8 years	Extrapolation of balance from older children	110/110	130/130	
9–13 years	Balance studies	200/200	240/240	
14–18 years	Balance studies	340/300	410/360	
19–30 years	Balance studies	330/255	400/310	
31–50 years	Balance studies	350/265	420/320	
51–70 years	Balance studies	350/265	420/320	
>70 years	Intracellular studies; decreases in absorption	350/265	420/320	
Pregnancy				
<19 years	Gain in lean mass	—/335	—/400	
19–30 years	Gain in lean mass	—/290	—/350	
31–50 years	Gain in lean mass	—/300	—/360	
Lactation				
<19 years	Balance studies	—/300	—/360	
19–30 years	Balance studies	—/255	—/310	
31–50 years	Balance studies	—/265	—/320	

Criteria and Dietary Reference Intake Values for Vitamin D by Life-Stage Group

Life-Stage Group*	Criterion	AI (μg/day)†‡
0–6 months	Serum 25(OH)D	5
6–12 months	Serum 25(OH)D	5
1–3 years	Serum 25(OH)D	5
4–8 years	Serum 25(OH)D	5
9–13 years	Serum 25(OH)D	5
14–18 years	Serum 25(OH)D	5
19–30 years	Serum 25(OH)D	5
31–50 years	Serum 25(OH)D	5
51–70 years	Serum 25(OH)D	10
>70 years	Serum 25(OH)D	15
Pregnancy		
<19 years	Serum 25(OH)D	5
19–50 years	Serum 25(OH)D	
Lactation		
<19 years	Serum 25(OH)D	5
19–50 years	Serum 25(OH)D	

*All groups except Pregnancy and Lactation include males and females.
†As cholecalciferol: 1 μg cholecalciferol = 40 IU vitamin D.
‡In the absence of adequate exposure to sunlight.

Criteria and Dietary Reference Intake Values for Fluoride by Life-Stage Group

Life-Stage Group	Criterion	AI (mg/day) Male/Female
0–6 months	Human milk content	0.01/0.01
6–12 months	Caries prevention	0.5/0.5
1–3 years	Caries prevention	0.7/0.7
4–8 years	Caries prevention	1.1/1.1
9–13 years	Caries prevention	2.0/2.0
14–18 years	Caries prevention	3.2/2.9
19–30 years	Caries prevention	3.8/3.1
31–50 years	Caries prevention	3.8/3.1
51–70 years	Caries prevention	3.8/3.1
>70 years	Caries prevention	3.8/3.1
Pregnancy		
<19 years	Caries prevention	—/2.9
19–50 years	Caries prevention	—/3.1
Lactation		
<19 years	Caries prevention	—/2.9
19–50 years	Caries prevention	—/3.1

Tolerable Upper Intake Levels (UL), by Life-Stage Group

Life-Stage Group	Calcium (g/day)	Phosphorus (g/day)	Magnesium* (mg/day)	Vitamin D (μg/day)†	Fluoride (mg/day)
0–6 months	ND‡	ND	ND	25	0.7
6–12 months	ND	ND	ND	25	0.9
1–3 years	2.5	3	65	50	1.3
4–8 years	2.5	3	110	50	2.2
9–18 years	2.5	4	350	50	10
19–70 years	2.5	4	350	50	10
>70 years	2.5	3	350	50	10
Pregnancy					
<19 years	2.5	3.5	350	50	10
19–50 years	2.5	3.5	350	50	10
Lactation					
<19 years	2.5	4	350	50	10
19–50 years	2.5	4	350	50	10

*The UL for magnesium represents intake from a pharmacological agent only and does not include intake from food and water.
†As cholecalciferol: 1 g cholecalciferol = 40 IU vitamin D.
‡ND: Not determinable due to lack of data on adverse effects in this age group and concern with regard to lack of ability to handle excess amounts. Source of intake should be from food only to prevent high levels of intake.

Recommended Levels for Individual Intake, B Vitamins and Choline

Life-Stage Group	Thiamin (mg/d)	Riboflavin (mg/d)	Niacin (mg/d)*	Vitamin B_6 (mg/d)	Folate (μg/d)†	Vitamin B_{12} (μg/d)	Pantothenic Acid (mg/d)	Biotin (μg/d)	Choline‡ (mg/d)
Infants									
0–5 months	0.2	0.3	2	0.1	65	0.4	1.7	5	125
6–11 months	0.3	0.4	3	0.3	80	0.5	1.8	6	150
Children									
1–3 years	**0.5**	**0.5**	**6**	**0.5**	**150**	**0.9**	2	8	200
4–8 years	**0.6**	**0.6**	**8**	**0.6**	**200**	**1.2**	3	12	250
Males	**0.9**	**0.9**	**12**	**1.0**	**300**	**1.8**	4	20	375
9–13 years									
14–18 years	**1.2**	**1.3**	**16**	**1.3**	**400**	**2.4**	5	25	550
19–30 years	**1.2**	**1.3**	**16**	**1.3**	**400**	**2.4**	5	30	550
31–50 years	**1.2**	**1.3**	**16**	**1.3**	**400**	**2.4**	5	30	550
51–70 years	**1.2**	**1.3**	**16**	**1.7**	**400**	**2.4**§	5	30	550
>70 years	**1.2**	**1.3**	**16**	**1.7**	**400**	**2.4**§	5	30	550
Females									
9–13 years	**0.9**	**0.9**	**12**	**1.0**	**300**	**1.8**	4	20	375
14–18 years	**1.0**	**1.0**	**14**	**1.2**	**400**¶	**2.4**	5	25	400
19–30 years	**1.1**	**1.1**	**14**	**1.3**	**400**¶	**2.4**	5	30	425
31–50 years	**1.1**	**1.1**	**14**	**1.3**	**400**¶	**2.4**	5	30	425
51–70 years	**1.1**	**1.1**	**14**	**1.5**	**400**¶	**2.4**§	5	30	425
>70 years	**1.1**	**1.1**	**14**	**1.5**	**400**	**2.4**§	5	30	425
Pregnancy (all ages)	**1.4**	**1.4**	**18**	**1.9**	**600****	**2.6**	6	30	450
Lactation (all ages)	**1.5**	**1.6**	**17**	**2.0**	**500**	**2.8**	7	35	550

NOTE: This table presents Recommended Dietary Allowances (RDAs) in bold type and Adequate Intakes (AIs) in ordinary type. RDAs and AIs may both be used as goals for individual intake. RDAs are set to meet the needs of almost all (97–98%) individuals in a group. For healthy breastfed infants, the AI is the mean intake. The AI for other life-stage groups is believed to cover their needs, but lack of data or uncertainty in the data prevents clear specification of this coverage.

*As niacin equivalents: 1 mg of niacin = 60 mg of tryptophan.

†As dietary folate equivalents (DFE). 1 DFE = 1 μg food folate = 0.6 μg of folic acid (from fortified food or supplement) consumed with food = 0.5 μg of synthetic (supplemental) folic acid taken on an empty stomach.

‡Although AIs have been set for choline, there are few data to assess whether a dietary supply of choline is needed at all stages of the life cycle, and it may be that the choline requirement can be met by endogenous synthesis at some of these stages.

§Since 10 to 30% of older people may malabsorb food-bound B_{12}, it is advisable for those older than 50 years to meet their RDA mainly by taking foods fortified with B_{12} or a B_{12}-containing supplement.

¶In view of evidence linking low folate intake with neural tube defects in the fetus, it is recommended that all women capable of becoming pregnant consume 400 μg of synthetic folic acid from fortified foods and/or supplements in addition to intake of food folate from a varied diet.

**It is assumed that women will continue taking 400 μg of folic acid until their pregnancy is confirmed and they enter prenatal care, which ordinarily occurs after the end of the periconceptual period—the critical time for formation of the neural tube.

Adapted courtesy of the National Academy of Sciences–Institute of Medicine.

MetLife Height and Weight Tables

Men*					Women*				
Height		Small Frame	Medium Frame	Large Frame	Height		Small Frame	Medium Frame	Large Frame
Feet	Inches				Feet	Inches			
5	2	128–134	131–141	138–150	4	10	102–111	109–121	118–131
5	3	130–136	133–143	140–153	4	11	103–113	111–123	120–134
5	4	132–138	135–145	142–156	5	0	104–115	113–126	122–137
5	5	134–140	137–148	144–160	5	1	106–118	115–129	125–140
5	6	136–142	139–151	146–164	5	2	108–121	118–132	128–143
5	7	138–145	142–154	149–168	5	3	111–124	121–135	131–147
5	8	140–148	145–157	152–172	5	4	114–127	124–138	134–151
5	9	142–151	148–160	155–176	5	5	117–130	127–141	137–155
5	10	144–154	151–163	158–180	5	6	120–133	130–144	140–159
5	11	146–157	154–166	161–184	5	7	123–136	133–147	143–163
6	0	149–160	157–170	164–188	5	8	126–139	136–150	148–167
6	1	152–164	160–174	168–192	5	9	129–142	139–153	149–170
6	2	155–168	164–178	172–197	5	10	132–145	142–156	152–173
6	3	158–172	167–182	176–202	5	11	135–148	145–159	155–176
6	4	162–176	171–187	181–207	6	0	138–151	148–162	158–179

To Approximate Your Frame Size

Bend forearm upward at a 90° angle. Keep fingers straight and turn the inside of your wrist toward your body. Place thumb and index finger of other hand on the two prominent bones on either side of the elbow. Measure space between your fingers on a ruler. (A physician would use a caliper.) Compare with tables below listing elbow measurements for *medium-framed* men and women. Measurements lower than those listed indicate small frame. Higher measurements indicate large frame.

Elbow Measurements for Medium Frame

Height in 1" Heels Men	Elbow Breadth	Height in 1" Heels Women	Elbow Breadth
5′2″–5′3″	2½″–2⅞″	4′10″–4′11″	2¼″–2½″
5′4″–5′7″	2⅝″–2⅞″	5′0″–5′3″	2¼″–2½″
5′8″–5′11″	2¾″–3″	5′4″–5′7″	2⅜″–2⅝″
6′0″–6′3″	2¾″–3⅛″	5′8″–5′11″	2⅜″–2⅝″
6′4″	2⅞″–3¼″	6′0″	2½″–2¾″

*Source of basic data: 1979 Build Study, Society of Actuaries and Association of Life Insurance Medical Directors of America, 1980. Copyright 1980 by the Society of Actuaries, Schaumburg, IL. Reprinted with permission.

Physical Growth From Birth to 18 Years

Age	Percentile, Boys								Percentile, Girls						
	5th	*10th*	*25th*	*50th*	*75th*	*90th*	*95th*		*5th*	*10th*	*25th*	*50th*	*75th*	*90th*	*95th*
At birth	**46.4**	**47.5**	**49.0**	**50.5**	**51.8**	**53.5**	**54.4**	**Length (cm)**	**45.4**	**46.5**	**48.2**	**49.9**	**51.0**	**52.0**	**52.9**
	18¼	18¾	19¼	20	20½	21	21½	Length (in.)	17¾	18¼	19	19¾	20	20½	20¾
	2.54	**2.78**	**3.00**	**3.27**	**3.64**	**3.82**	**4.15**	**Weight (kg)**	**2.36**	**2.58**	**2.93**	**3.23**	**3.52**	**3.64**	**3.81**
	5½	6¼	6½	7¼	8	8½	9¼	Weight (lb)	5¼	5¾	6½	7	7¾	8	8½
	32.6	**33.0**	**33.9**	**34.8**	**35.6**	**36.6**	**37.2**	**Head circumference (cm)**	**32.1**	**32.9**	**33.5**	**34.3**	**34.8**	**35.5**	**35.9**
	12¾	13	13¼	13¾	14	14½	14¾	Head circumference (in.)	12¾	13	13¼	13½	13¾	14	14¼
3 months	**56.7**	**57.7**	**59.4**	**61.1**	**63.0**	**64.5**	**65.4**	**Length (cm)**	**55.4**	**56.2**	**57.8**	**59.5**	**61.2**	**62.7**	**63.4**
	22¼	22¾	23½	**24**	24¾	25½	25¾	Length (in.)	21¾	22¼	22¾	23½	24	24¾	25
	4.43	**4.78**	**5.32**	**5.98**	**6.56**	**7.14**	**7.37**	**Weight (kg)**	**4.18**	**4.47**	**4.88**	**5.40**	**5.90**	**6.39**	**6.74**
	9¾	10½	11¾	13¼	14½	15¾	16¼	Weight (lb)	9¼	9¾	10¾	12	13	14	14¾
	38.4	**38.9**	**39.7**	**40.6**	**41.7**	**42.5**	**43.1**	**Head circumference (cm)**	**37.3**	**37.8**	**38.7**	**39.5**	**40.4**	**41.2**	**41.7**
	15	15¼	15¾	16	16½	16¾	17	Head circumference (in.)	14¾	15	15¼	15½	16	16¼	16½
6 months	**63.4**	**64.4**	**66.1**	**67.8**	**69.7**	**71.3**	**72.3**	**Length (cm)**	**61.8**	**62.6**	**64.2**	**65.9**	**67.8**	**69.4**	**70.2**
	25	25¼	26	26¾	27½	28	28½	Length (in.)	24¼	24¾	25¼	26	26¾	27¼	27¾
	6.20	**6.61**	**7.20**	**7.85**	**8.49**	**9.10**	**9.46**	**Weight (kg)**	**5.79**	**6.12**	**6.60**	**7.21**	**7.83**	**8.38**	**8.73**
	13¾	14½	15¾	17¼	18¾	20	20¾	Weight (lb)	12¾	13½	14½	16	17¼	18½	19¼
	41.5	**42.0**	**42.8**	**43.8**	**44.7**	**45.6**	**46.2**	**Head circumference (cm)**	**40.3**	**40.9**	**41.6**	**42.4**	**43.3**	**44.1**	**44.6**
	16¼	16½	16¾	17¼	17½	18	18¼	Head circumference (in.)	15¾	16	16½	16¾	17	17¼	17½
12 months	**71.7**	**72.8**	**74.3**	**76.1**	**77.7**	**79.8**	**81.2**	**Length (cm)**	**69.8**	**70.8**	**72.4**	**74.3**	**76.3**	**78.0**	**79.1**
	28¼	28¾	29¼	30	30½	31½	32	Length (in.)	27½	27¾	28½	29¼	30	30¾	31¼
	8.43	**8.84**	**9.49**	**10.15**	**10.91**	**11.54**	**11.99**	**Weight (kg)**	**7.84**	**8.19**	**8.81**	**9.53**	**10.23**	**10.87**	**11.24**
	18½	19½	21	22½	24	25½	26½	Weight (lb)	17¼	18	19½	21	22½	24	24¾
	44.8	**45.3**	**46.1**	**47.0**	**47.9**	**48.8**	**49.3**	**Head circumference (cm)**	**43.5**	**44.1**	**44.8**	**45.6**	**46.4**	**47.2**	**47.6**
	17¾	17¾	18¼	18½	18¾	19¼	19½	Head circumference (in.)	17¼	17¼	17¾	18	18¼	18½	18¾
18 months	**77.5**	**78.7**	**80.5**	**82.4**	**84.3**	**86.6**	**88.1**	**Length (cm)**	**76.0**	**77.2**	**78.8**	**80.9**	**83.0**	**85.0**	**86.1**
	30½	31	31¾	32½	33¼	34	34¾	Length (in.)	30	30½	31	31¾	32¾	33½	34
	9.59	**9.92**	**10.67**	**11.47**	**12.31**	**13.05**	**13.44**	**Weight (kg)**	**8.92**	**9.30**	**10.04**	**10.82**	**11.55**	**12.30**	**12.76**
	21¼	21¾	23½	25¼	27¼	28¾	29½	Weight (lb)	19¾	20½	22¼	23¾	25½	27	28¼
	46.3	**46.7**	**47.4**	**48.4**	**49.3**	**50.1**	**50.6**	**Head circumference (cm)**	**45.0**	**45.6**	**46.3**	**47.1**	**47.9**	**48.6**	**49.1**
	18¼	18½	18¾	19	19½	19¾	20	Head circumference (in.)	17¾	18	18¼	18½	18¾	19¼	19¼

Table continued on following page

Physical Growth From Birth to 18 Years *Continued*

	Percentile, Boys								Percentile, Girls						
Age	***5th***	***10th***	***25th***	***50th***	***75th***	***90th***	***95th***		***5th***	***10th***	***25th***	***50th***	***75th***	***90th***	***95th***
24 months	**82.3**	**83.5**	**85.6**	**87.6**	**89.9**	**92.2**	**93.8**	**Length (cm)**	**81.3**	**82.5**	**84.2**	**86.5**	**88.7**	**90.8**	**92.0**
	32½	32¾	33¾	34½	35½	36¼	37	Length (in.)	32	32½	33¼	34	35	35¾	36¼
	10.54	**10.85**	**11.65**	**12.59**	**13.44**	**14.29**	**14.70**	**Weight (kg)**	**9.87**	**10.26**	**11.10**	**11.90**	**12.74**	**13.57**	**14.08**
	23¼	24	25¾	27¾	29¾	31½	32½	Weight (lb)	21¾	22½	24½	26¼	28	30	31
	47.3	**47.7**	**48.3**	**49.2**	**50.2**	**51.0**	**51.4**	**Head circumference (cm)**	**46.1**	**46.5**	**47.3**	**48.1**	**48.8**	**49.6**	**50.1**
	18½	18¾	19	19¼	19¾	20	20¼	Head circumference (in.)	18¼	18¼	18½	19	19¼	19½	19¾
36 months	**91.2**	**92.4**	**94.2**	**96.5**	**98.9**	**101.4**	**103.1**	**Length (cm)**	**90.0**	**91.0**	**93.1**	**95.6**	**98.1**	**100.0**	**101.5**
	36	36½	37	38	39	40	40½	Length (in.)	35½	35¾	36¾	37¾	38½	39¼	40
	12.26	**12.69**	**13.58**	**14.69**	**15.59**	**16.66**	**17.28**	**Weight (kg)**	**11.60**	**12.07**	**12.99**	**13.93**	**15.03**	**15.97**	**16.54**
	27	28	30	32½	34¼	36¾	38	Weight (lb)	25½	26½	28¾	30¾	33¼	35¼	36½
	48.6	**49**	**49.7**	**50.5**	**51.5**	**52.3**	**52.8**	**Head circumference (cm)**	**47.6**	**47.9**	**48.5**	**49.3**	**50.0**	**50.8**	**51.4**
	19¼	19¼	19½	20	20¼	20¼	20¾	Head circumference (in.)	18¾	18¾	19	19½	19¾	20	20¼
4 years	**95.8**	**97.3**	**100.0**	**102.9**	**105.7**	**108.2**	**109.9**	**Stature (cm)**	**95.0**	**96.4**	**98.8**	**101.6**	**104.3**	**106.6**	**108.3**
	37¾	38¼	39¼	40½	41½	42½	43¼	Stature (in.)	37½	38	39	40	41	42	42¾
	13.64	**14.24**	**15.39**	**16.69**	**17.99**	**19.32**	**20.27**	**Weight (kg)**	**13.11**	**13.84**	**14.80**	**15.96**	**17.56**	**18.93**	**19.91**
	30	31½	34	36¾	39¾	42½	44¾	Weight (lb)	29	30½	32¾	35¼	38¾	41¾	44
5 years	**102.0**	**103.7**	**106.5**	**109.9**	**112.8**	**115.4**	**117.0**	**Stature (cm)**	**101.1**	**102.7**	**105.4**	**108.4**	**111.4**	**113.8**	**115.6**
	40¼	40¾	42	43¼	44½	45½	46	Stature (in.)	39¾	40½	41½	42¾	43¾	44¾	45½
	15.27	**15.96**	**17.22**	**18.67**	**20.14**	**21.70**	**23.09**	**Weight (kg)**	**14.55**	**15.26**	**16.29**	**17.66**	**19.39**	**21.23**	**22.62**
	33¾	35¼	38	41¼	44½	47¾	51	Weight (lb)	32	33¾	36	39	42¾	46¾	49¾
6 years	**107.7**	**109.6**	**112.5**	**116.1**	**119.2**	**121.9**	**123.5**	**Stature (cm)**	**106.6**	**108.4**	**111.3**	**114.6**	**118.1**	**120.8**	**122.7**
	42½	43¼	44¼	45¾	47	48	48½	Stature (in.)	42	42¾	43¾	45	46½	47½	48¼
	16.93	**17.72**	**19.07**	**20.69**	**22.40**	**24.31**	**26.34**	**Weight (kg)**	**16.05**	**16.72**	**17.86**	**19.52**	**21.44**	**23.89**	**25.75**
	37¼	39	42	45½	49½	53½	58	Weight (lb)	35½	36¾	39¼	43	47¼	52¾	56¾
8 years	**118.1**	**120.2**	**123.2**	**127.0**	**130.5**	**133.6**	**135.7**	**Stature (cm)**	**116.9**	**118.7**	**122.2**	**126.4**	**130.6**	**134.2**	**136.2**
	46½	47¼	48½	50	51½	52½	53½	Stature (in.)	46	46¾	48	49¾	51½	52¾	53½
	20.40	**21.39**	**23.09**	**25.30**	**27.91**	**31.06**	**34.51**	**Weight (kg)**	**19.62**	**20.45**	**22.26**	**24.84**	**27.88**	**32.04**	**34.71**
	45	47¼	51	55¾	61½	68½	76	Weight (lb)	43¼	45	49	54¾	61½	70¾	76½

10 years														
Stature (cm)	149.5	147.2	142.9	138.3	133.6	129.5	127.5	148.1	145.5	141.6	137.5	133.4	130.1	127.7
Stature (in.)	58¾	58	56¼	54½	52½	51	50¼	58¼	57¼	55¾	54¼	52½	51¼	50¼
Weight (kg)	47.17	43.70	37.53	32.55	28.71	25.76	24.36	45.27	40.80	35.61	31.44	28.07	25.52	24.33
Weight (lb)	104	96¼	82¾	71¾	63¼	56¾	53¾	99¾	90	78½	69¼	62	56¼	53¾
12 years														
Stature (cm)	162.7	160.0	155.8	151.5	147.0	142.3	139.8	162.3	159.4	154.6	149.7	144.4	140.3	137.6
Stature (in.)	64	63	61¼	59¾	57¾	56	55	64	62¾	60¾	59	56¾	55¼	54¼
Weight (kg)	60.81	55.99	48.07	41.53	36.52	32.53	30.52	58.09	52.73	45.77	39.78	35.09	31.46	29.85
Weight (lb)	134	123½	106	91½	80½	71¾	67¼	128	116¼	101	87¾	77¼	69¼	65¾
14 years														
Stature (cm)	171.3	168.7	164.6	160.4	155.9	151.5	148.7	176.7	173.8	168.5	163.1	156.9	151.8	148.8
Stature (in.)	67½	66½	64¾	63¼	61½	59¾	58½	69½	68½	66¼	64¼	61¾	59¾	58½
Weight (kg)	73.08	66.04	57.09	50.28	44.54	40.11	37.76	72.13	65.57	58.31	50.77	45.21	40.64	38.22
Weight (lb)	161	145½	125¾	110¾	98¼	88½	83¼	159	144½	128½	112	99¾	89½	84¼
16 years														
Stature (cm)	173.3	171.1	166.9	162.4	157.8	154.1	151.6	185.4	182.4	178.1	173.5	168.7	163.9	161.1
Stature (in.)	68¼	67¼	65¾	64	62¼	60¾	59¾	73	71¾	70	68¼	66½	64½	63¾
Weight (kg)	80.99	71.68	62.29	55.89	50.09	45.78	43.41	85.62	77.97	70.26	62.10	56.16	51.16	47.74
Weight (lb)	178½	158	137¼	123¼	110½	101	95¾	188¾	172	155	137	123¾	112¾	105¼
18 years														
Stature (cm)	173.6	171.0	167.6	163.7	159.6	156.0	153.6	187.6	185.3	181.2	176.8	172.3	168.7	165.7
Stature (in.)	68¼	67¼	66	64½	62¾	61½	60½	73¾	73	71¼	69½	67¾	66½	65¼
Weight (kg)	82.47	72.25	62.78	56.62	51.39	47.47	45.26	95.76	88.41	76.04	68.88	62.61	57.89	53.97
Weight (lb)	181¾	159¼	138½	124¾	113¼	104¾	99¾	211	195	167¾	151¾	138	127¾	119

From National Center for Health Statistics, Health Resources Administration, DHEW, Hyattsville, MD. Data from Fels Research Institute, Yellow Springs, Ohio; smoothed by least squares-cubic-spline technique. Conversion of metric data to inches and pounds by Ross Laboratories.

Glossary

abrasion a superficial injury caused by rubbing or scraping of the skin against another surface (Chap. 32)

abstract a short summary that contains brief information about the purpose of the study, the number of subjects, the methodology used to select subjects, the type of study being conducted, and the major results from the study (Chap. 18)

access a complex construct representing the personal use of health care services and the structures or processes that facilitate or impede that use (Chap. 5)

accommodation a process of change, or modifying old ways of thinking to fit new situations (Chap. 19)

accountability the obligation to provide an accounting or rationale for personal actions or the actions of others (Chap. 17)

accreditation a process that monitors an educational program's ability to meet predetermined standards for student outcomes (Chap. 2)

acting-out behaviors inappropriate or unexpected client behaviors that communicate a message about the client's true or subconscious feelings and concerns (Chap. 15)

action stage the stage of change in which the person changes risky behaviors and the context of the behavior (environment, experience) and makes significant efforts to reach goals (Chap. 25)

active listening participation in a conversation with a client in which the nurse attends to what the client says and has a part in helping the client clarify, elaborate, and give additional pertinent information (Chap. 8)

active processing a systematic series of mental actions to analyze and interpret information about a client (Chap. 8)

active transport an active process by which molecules move from an area of lower concentration to an area of higher concentration through an expenditure of energy (Chap. 31)

activities of daily living (ADLs) the basic activities usually performed in the course of a normal day in a person's life, such as eating, toileting, dressing, bathing, or brushing the teeth (Chap. 56)

acuity rating a priority rating based on the severity of the illness or injury (Chap. 58)

acute area the physical space in an emergency department where clients with life-threatening problems are treated (Chap. 58)

acute pain short-term, self-limited pain with a probable duration of less than 6 months; expected to resolve when the tissue heals (Chap. 42)

adaptation the change that occurs as a result of assimilation and accommodation, also called coping behavior (Chap. 19); a process through which individuals accommodate changes in the internal or external environment to preserve functioning and pursue goals (Chap. 52)

adjuvant analgesic any medication that may increase analgesic efficacy, thus allowing for a smaller opioid dosage (Chap. 42)

admit note the opening nurse's note acknowledging the arrival of a new client (Chap. 14)

adolescence the period of transition between childhood and adulthood that includes rapid growth and dramatic change, both physically and psychologically (Chap. 21)

advance directive a written document that provides direction for health care when a person is unable to make his or her own treatment choices (Chap. 2)

adverse effect serious medication ef-fect that may or may not be expected and is potentially dangerous to the client (Chap. 26)

affect the observable expression of feelings or emotions (Chap. 45)

affective learning domain the learning domain that relates to ethics or principles that guide moral behavior and to reasoning that determines right behavior (Chap. 16)

afterload the final determinant of stroke volume, defined as the pressure against which the left ventricle pumps (aortic systolic pressure); higher aortic pressure forces the heart to work harder, and less blood is ejected from the ventricles with each contraction (Chap. 40)

against medical advice term used to indicate that a client has left the emergency department against the advice of the physician and without proper written discharge instructions (Chap. 58)

ageism a stereotype, prejudice, or discrimination against people, especially older adults, based on their age (Chap. 23)

agnosia the failure to recognize or identify objects despite an intact sensory ability (Chap. 45)

agnostic a person who is undecided about the existence of God or a higher power (Chap. 55)

agonist analgesic an opioid that stimulates activity at an opioid receptor site to produce analgesia (Chap. 42)

alopecia loss of hair and baldness (Chap. 36)

ambulatory care center facility that provides health services on an outpatient basis to those who visit a hospital or other health care facility and depart after treatment on the same day (Chap. 5)

ambulatory surgery same-day or outpatient surgery that can be performed with general or local anesthesia, usually takes less than 2 hours, and requires less than a 3-hour stay in a recovery area (Chap. 57)

amino acids compounds composed of carbon, hydrogen, oxygen, and an amino group and classified as essential or nonessential depending on whether the body can manufacture them from other sources (Chap. 29)

analgesia reduction of the perception or experience of pain (Chap. 42)

anaphylaxis a severe allergic reaction that requires immediate intervention to prevent possible death (Chap. 26)

androgyny an anthropological term meaning that a person may display both male and female characteristics and may relate to both a male and a female gender identity and role (Chap. 51)

anesthesia partial or complete loss of sensation, with or without loss of consciousness, as a result of being given an anesthetic agent (Chap. 57)

anesthesiologist a medical physician who specializes in anesthesiology and provides anesthesia for surgical clients (Chap. 57)

anion a negatively charged ion, such as chloride, bicarbonate, phosphate, sulfate, or proteinate (Chap. 31)

anorexia lack of appetite (Chap. 30)

anorexia nervosa a syndrome characterized by self-induced weight loss driven by a morbid fear of becoming fat (Chap. 21)

antagonist a drug, such as naloxone, that blocks activity at μ and κ receptors by displacing opioid analgesics currently attached to them (Chap. 42)

antagonistic effect an effect that occurs when one drug reduces or negates the effect of another, which may be accidental or purposeful (Chap. 26)

anthropometric measurements measurements of physical characteristics of the body (such as height and weight), as well as the amount of muscle or fat tissue in the body (Chap. 29)

antibiotic a drug that kills bacteria (Chap. 27)

antibody a circulating protein that recognizes and destroys foreign invaders or immunoglobulins (Chap. 27)

anticipatory grief intellectual and emotional responses and behaviors by which individuals, families, and communities attempt to work through the process of modifying self-concept based on the perception of potential loss (Chap. 50)

antidiuretic hormone substance produced by the hypothalamus and secreted by the posterior pituitary gland that causes the kidneys to retain water (Chap. 40)

antimicrobial the ability to limit the spread of microorganisms (Chap. 27)

anuria the absence of urine (Chap. 35)

anxiety a diffuse, highly uncomfortable, sometimes vague sense of apprehension or dread accompanied by one or more physical sensations (Chap. 47)

anxiety disorder the production of anxiety that indicates a relentless, ineffective mechanism designed to compel a person to lessen the supposed danger that is triggering the anxiety response (Chap. 47)

anxiolytics an antianxiety medication used primarily to treat anxiety disorders (Chap. 47)

aphasia a language disorder resulting from brain damage or disease to speech centers in the brain resulting in a variety of difficulties in formulating, expressing, and understanding language (Chap. 44)

apical pulse the heart rate counted at the apex of the heart on the anterior chest (Chap. 9)

APIE charting a method of charting that evolved from the problem-oriented type of medical record and that is designed to allow documentation using the nursing process; the acronym stands for *a*ssessment, *p*roblem identification, *i*nterventions, and *e*valuation (Chap. 14)

apraxia the inability to carry out motor activities despite the functional ability to perform them (Chap. 45)

arousal erotic excitement that precedes sexual response and occurs in the presence of physically and emotionally pleasurable stimuli (Chap. 51)

articulation the process of molding sounds into enunciated words and phrases (Chap. 44)

aspiration the inspiration of foreign material into the airway (Chaps. 28 and 30)

assault an attempt or threat to touch another person unjustly (Chap. 2)

assessment the process of gathering data about the client's health status to identify the concerns and needs that can be treated or managed by nursing care (Chap. 8)

assimilation the process of learning from new experiences (Chap. 19)

atheist a person who believes there is no God or higher power (Chap. 55)

atherosclerosis pathological condition in which fat and plaque are deposited on the intimal surface of arteries (Chap. 40)

atrophy a decrease in the size of a normally developed tissue or organ as a result of inactivity or diminished function (Chap. 38)

attachment development of strong ties of affection of an infant with a significant other (mother, father, sibling, caretaker) (Chap. 19)

attending behaviors nursing behavior that show that you are paying attention to and listening to what the client is saying (Chap. 15)

attention the ability to focus on an object or activity (Chap. 45)

attention-deficit/hyperactivity disorder a neuropsychological disorder associated with disturbances in attention, impulsivity, and hyperactivity (Chap. 20)

atypical analgesic a drug not primarily indicated for managing pain but used to treat specific types of pain, such as an anticonvulsant to treat neuropathic pain (Chap. 42)

auditory the sensation of hearing (Chap. 43)

auscultation the process of listening to sounds generated within the body (Chap. 10)

auscultatory gap absence of a second Korotkoff sound, a common finding in hypertension (Chap. 9)

authority the ability or legitimate power to make decisions, implement strategies, and elicit work (Chap. 17)

autonomy the right to make our own choices, that is, to self-determine (Chap. 3)

awareness the state of being awake and alert enough to react to stimuli, also known as consciousness (Chap. 45)

bacterium a single-celled organism that can reproduce outside of cells (Chap. 27)

bacteriuria the presence of bacteria in the urine (Chap. 35)

baroreceptors specialized cells located in the aorta and carotid arteries that detect pressure changes in the vascular system (Chap. 40)

basal metabolic rate the amount of energy needed to maintain essential basic body functions expressed as calories per hour per square meter of body surface (Chap. 9)

battery the actual willful touching of another person that may or may not cause harm (Chap. 2)

bedrest a prescribed or self-imposed restriction to bed for therapeutic reasons (Chap. 38)

beneficence the promotion of good by the performance of actions that benefit others (Chap. 3)

bereave "to rob" or make desolate, traditionally defined as "being deprived through death," such as a widow who is deprived by the death of her husband (Chap. 50)

binuclear family two nuclear families with joint children, coparenting, and joint custody (Chap. 53)

biographical data information that identifies and describes a person, such as name, address, age, gender, religious affiliation, race, or occupation (Chap. 8)

biotransformation the process of inactivating and breaking down a drug, also called drug metabolism (Chap. 26)

bisexual sexual orientation in which one may be sexually attracted to members of either gender (Chap. 51)

blanchable erythema a reddened area that turns white or pale temporarily when pressure is applied (Chap. 32)

body image a person's perception of his or her body; the physical dimension of self-concept or how a person perceives and evaluates appearance and function of self (Chap. 46)

body language nonverbal communication behaviors that are accomplished by the movement of the body or body parts, by the presentation of ourselves to the world, and by the use of our personal space (Chap. 15)

bonding a process of forming an attachment between parent and newborn (Chap. 19)

bowel incontinence inability to voluntarily control the passage of feces and gas (Chap. 34)

bradycardia a pulse rate of less than 60 beats per minute in an adult (Chap. 9)

bradypnea a respiratory rate below 12 breaths per minute for an adult (Chap. 9)

breakthrough pain intermittent episodes of pain that occur despite continued use of an analgesic (Chap. 42)

Broca's area the center of motor speech control, located in the frontal lobe of the brain and responsible for controlling muscles of the mouth, tongue, and larynx, which produce speech (Chap. 44)

bronchospasm spasm of the smooth muscles of the bronchi and/or the bronchioles that results in decreased airway diameter (Chap. 39)

bruxism a parasomnia characterized by violent, repetitive grinding of the teeth that occurs during the lighter stages of sleep or during partial arousals (Chap. 41)

bulimia nervosa a disorder characterized by binge eating coupled with

purging via emetics, laxatives, or self-induced vomiting (Chap. 21)

burns injury caused by excessive exposure to heat, electricity, chemicals, gases, radioactivity, or thermal agents (Chap. 28)

calorie a measure of the energy content of food, also called a kilocalorie (Chap. 29)

carbohydrate a simple or complex compound composed of carbon, oxygen, and hydrogen (Chap. 29)

cardiac output the amount of blood pumped by the ventricles of the heart per minute (Chap. 40)

cardinal signs and symptoms data of greatest significance in diagnosing a particular illness, disease, or health problem (Chap. 8)

care plan conference the action of a group conferring or consulting together to plan care for the client (Chap. 12)

caregiver one who provides care to a dependent or partially dependent family member or friend (Chap. 54)

caregiver burden unrelenting physical, psychological, social, or financial problems that occur when a caregiver provides for the health needs of an impaired family member or friend (Chap. 54)

caregiver burnout depletion of physical and mental energy caused by providing care for a chronically ill person over a long period of time (Chap. 54)

caregiver stress the caregiver's reaction to physical, emotional, sociocultural, financial, and environmental stressors brought on by the caregiving experience (Chap. 54)

caries a destructive process causing decalcification of the tooth enamel and leading to continued destruction of the enamel and dentin with resulting cavitation of the tooth (Chap. 36)

caring a universal behavior observed in human beings and influenced by society, culture, values, and gender (Chap. 54)

case management a care delivery system that focuses on the management of client care across an episode of illness (Chap. 13)

catabolism production of glucose from the breakdown of muscle and lean body mass in a process known as glyconeogenesis (Chap. 30)

cathartic a medication, stronger than a laxative, used to induce emptying of the bowel (Chap. 34)

cation a positively charged ion, such as sodium, potassium, calcium, magnesium, or hydrogen (Chap. 31)

cephalocaudal a normal pattern of

neuromuscular growth and development, which starts at the head and moves toward the feet (Chap. 19)

certification a voluntary process by which a nurse can be granted recognition for meeting certain criteria established by a nongovernment association (Chap. 2)

certified registered nurse anesthetist an advanced practice registered nurse who has been specifically educated in the administration of anesthetic agents and provides anesthesia for clients under an anesthesiologist's supervision (Chap. 57)

cerumen waxy secretion of the glands of the external acoustic meatus; commonly known as ear wax (Chap. 36)

charting by exception a method of charting that provides documentation in progress notes only if data are significant or abnormal (Chap. 14)

chemical name the name that precisely describes the chemical and molecular structure of a medication (Chap. 26)

chemoreceptors specialized cells, such as taste buds and olfactory cells, that are adapted for excitation or stimulation by various chemicals (Chap. 43)

chest percussion using cupped hands to rhythmically clap on the chest wall over various segments of the lungs to mobilize secretions (Chap. 39)

chest physiotherapy an approach to mobilizing and draining secretions from gravity-dependent areas of the lung that uses a combination of postural drainage, chest percussion, and vibration (Chap. 39)

chief complaint the problem that caused the client to seek health services, call the doctor, or request a visit with a nurse, in the client's own words (Chap. 8)

choking an internal obstruction of the airway by food or a foreign body (Chap. 28)

chronic illness all impairments or deviations from normal that have one or more of the following characteristics: are permanent, leave residual disability, are caused by a nonreversible pathological condition, require special training of the client for rehabilitation, or may be expected to require a long period of supervision, observation, or care (Chap. 56)

chronic pain long-term, constant, or recurring pain without an anticipated or predictable end and a duration of more than 6 months (Chap. 42)

chronicity a broad term that encompasses chronic illnesses as well as disease or congenital defects that permanently alter a person's previous health status (Chap. 56)

circadian rhythm a biorhythmic pattern that is regularly repeated at 24-hour intervals (Chap. 41)

circulating nurse a registered nurse (also called a circulator) who helps clients meet individual needs during all three phases of the surgical experience, coordinates the client's care, acts as the client's advocate, and manages activities outside the sterile field (Chap. 57)

civil law regulates disputes between individuals or between individuals and groups (Chap. 2)

claudication cramp-like pains in the calves caused by poor circulation of the blood to the leg muscles (Chap. 40)

client advocate a nursing role in which the nurse assists clients in expressing their rights whenever necessary (Chap. 1)

clinical judgment a conclusion or an opinion that a problem or situation requires nursing care; determines the cause of the problem, distinguishes between similar problems, or discriminates between two or more courses of action (Chaps. 7 and 11)

clinical pathway a standardized multidisciplinary care plan that projects the expected course of the client's treatment and progress over the hospital stay (Chap. 12)

closed question question that calls for a specific response from the client (Chap. 8)

closed system a set of integrated, interacting parts that function as a whole and do not interact with other systems or the environment (Chap. 53)

code status a term used to identify the specific orders for a client regarding whether to begin resuscitative actions, and the extent of those actions, at the time of a cardiac or respiratory arrest (Chap. 50)

cognition the process of knowing and interacting with the world, also known as thought (Chap. 45)

cognitive development a progression of mental abilities from illogical thinking to logical thinking, from simple to complex problem-solving, and from understanding concrete ideas to understanding abstract ideas (Chap. 19)

cognitive learning domain the learning domain that encompasses knowledge, comprehension, and critical thinking skills (Chap. 16)

collaboration the act of two or more health care professionals performing work cooperatively to achieve a common goal (Chap. 12)

collaborative problem a clinical problem that cannot be solved by the nurse alone (or by the nursing staff), but requires treatments or medications that the nurse is not able to do or not licensed to order (Chap. 11)

colloid a macromolecule, such as a protein, that is too large to pass through a cell membrane and that does not readily dissolve into a solution (Chap. 31)

colloid osmotic pressure osmotic pressure exerted by large molecules, such as protein (Chap. 31)

colostomy a surgical procedure involving the creation of an opening between the colon and the abdominal wall (Chap. 34)

common law standards and rules applicable to our interactions with one another that are recognized, affirmed, and enforced through judicial decisions (Chap. 2)

communal family a household of more than one monogamous couple with children, each of which shares resources and socializes the children as a group activity (Chap. 53)

communication a complex process in which information is exchanged between two or more individuals, called senders and receivers (Chap. 44)

community a geographic location, or an aggregate or population of individuals who have one or more personal or environmental characteristics in common (Chap. 59)

community approach a nursing approach for vulnerable populations that emphasizes the provision of resources for disease prevention, treatment, and rehabilitation, with a consequent decrease in exposure to risk factors for health-related problems (Chap. 48)

community forum an open meeting where members of a community or group may come to share opinions and concerns about a particular issue (Chap. 59)

community health nursing nursing that promotes and preserves the health of populations by (1) understanding and applying concepts of public health and community, (2) working with community organizations to assist in community development, (3) providing generalist care to selected individuals, families, and groups, and (4) providing health promotion, health maintenance, health education, and coordination of care (Chap. 59)

community reintegration the return and acceptance of a disabled person as a participating member of the community (Chap. 56)

computerized care plan a standardized care plan or a care plan created from a computer program (Chap. 12)

conceptual framework a group of related concepts that support a particular viewpoint or focus (Chap. 6)

conceptual model a graphic explanation of theoretical relationships (Chap. 6)

concrete operations stage of cognitive development at which children begin to project the self into other people's situations and realize that their own way of thinking is not the only way (Chap. 20)

concurrent audit an evaluation method to inspect the nursing staff's compliance with predetermined standards and criteria while the nurses are providing care (Chap. 13)

confidentiality the client's right to privacy in the health care delivery system; as a nurse, you have an ethical obligation to maintain client confidentiality (Chap. 2)

confusion the state in which the individual experiences or is at risk of experiencing a disturbance in cognition, altered memory, and orientation of an undetermined origin or onset (Chap. 45)

consciousness the state of being awake and alert enough to react to stimuli, also known as awareness (Chap. 45)

conservation a child's ability to understand that changing the shape of a substance does not change its quality (Chap. 20)

constipation a condition in which feces are abnormally hard and dry and evacuation is abnormally infrequent (Chap. 34)

constitutional delay of puberty an absence of early signs of puberty, such as Tanner stage II breasts by age 13 for girls or Tanner stage II genitalia by age 14 for boys (Chap. 21)

consultation the act of two or more health care professionals deliberating for the purpose of making decisions (Chap. 12)

contemplation stage the stage of change in which the individual intends to change within the next 6 months (Chap. 25)

context the condition under which a communication occurs (Chap. 15)

continuing education informal courses that assist professional nurses in developing and maintaining clinical expertise and knowledge that promotes the quality of nursing care (Chap. 1)

continuous quality improvement a systematic approach to control and to improve quality from both professionals' and clients' perspectives (Chap. 13)

contract an agreement between two or more individuals creating certain rights and obligations in exchange for goods or services (Chap. 2)

contracture an abnormal shortening of muscle fibers or their associated connective tissue that results in resistance to stretching and eventually in permanent fixation (Chap. 38)

controlled substance a drug that affects the mind or behavior, may be habit-forming, and has a high potential for abuse, including narcotics, barbiturates, and illegal drugs (Chap. 26)

coping patterns specific protective behaviors used by an individual or family to respond to stressful situations (Chap. 54)

coping the ability to deal with dangerous, threatening, or challenging situations (Chap. 52)

cough a sudden audible, forceful expulsion of air from the lungs, usually an involuntary, reflexive action in response to an irritant (Chap. 39)

counseling a method of communication that actively involves the client in the recognition of personal risk factors and management of necessary behavior changes (Chap. 25)

credentialing methods by which the nursing profession attempts to ensure and maintain the competency of its practitioners (Chap. 2)

criminal law defines specific behaviors determined to be inappropriate in the orderly functioning of society (Chap. 2)

crisis an upset in a balanced or stable state for which the usual methods of adaptation and coping are not sufficient (Chap. 52)

critical periods periods of time when a person has an increased vulnerability to physical, chemical, psychological, or environmental influences (Chap. 19)

critical thinking purposeful, self-regulatory judgment that gives reasoned and reflective consideration to evidence, contexts, conceptualizations, methods, and criteria (Chap. 7)

cue an indicator of the presence or existence of a problem or condition that represents a client's underlying health status (Chaps. 8 and 11)

cultural competence having enough knowledge of cultural groups that are different from your own to be able to interact with a member of a group in a manner that makes the person feel respected and understood (Chap. 4)

culture a patterned behavioral response developed over time as a consequence of imprinting the mind through social and religious structures and intellectual and artistic manifestations (Chap. 4)

cyanosis a blue color to the skin that results from the concentration of deoxygenated hemoglobin close to the surface of the skin (Chap. 39)

data pieces of subjective or objective information about the client or the signs and symptoms of disease (Chap. 8); information that a researcher is interested in collecting (Chap. 18)

data collection the process by which the researcher acquires subjects and collects the information necessary to answer the research question (Chap. 18)

database all of the information that has been collected about the client and recorded in the health record as a baseline for the initial plan of care (Chap. 8)

débridement the removal of dirt, foreign matter, and dead or devitalized tissue from a wound (Chap. 32)

decentering accommodation a child's ability to adapt thought processes to perceive more than one reason for a person's actions (Chap. 20)

decision-making choosing between two or more options as a means to achieve a desired result (Chap. 7)

decoder (receiver) the person to whom a message is aimed (Chap. 15)

deep vein thrombosis the condition caused when a blood clot (thrombus) develops in the lumen of a deep leg vein, such as the tibial, popliteal, femoral, or iliac vein (Chap. 38)

defamation either a false communication or a careless disregard for the truth that results in damage to someone's reputation (Chap. 2)

defendant the person against whom a lawsuit is filed (Chap. 2)

defense mechanism method used to protect oneself from stress and maintain psychological homeostasis (Chap. 52)

defining characteristic descriptor of a client's behavior that determines whether a nursing diagnosis is present and whether a particular diagnosis is appropriate or accurate (Chap. 11)

deglutition the reflex passage of food, fluids, or both from the mouth to the stomach, also known as swallowing (Chap. 30)

dehiscence partial or total separation of the edges of a wound (Chap. 32)

delegation assigning responsibility for certain tasks to other people, thereby allowing the manager to concentrate on organizational goals and productivity (Chap. 17)

delirium a disturbance in consciousness and a change in cognition that develops over a short period of time (Chap. 45)

delusions false personal beliefs (Chap. 45)

dementia multiple cognitive deficits that include impairment of memory and judgment resulting in a progressive decline in intellectual functioning, synonymous with chronic confusion (Chap. 45)

demographic data factual information that can be counted to describe populations of clients (Chap. 8)

dentures a complement of teeth, either natural or artificial; ordinarily used to designate an artificial replacement for the natural teeth (Chap. 36)

deontology a theory that is not concerned with the consequences of an act but rather with the obligation or duty to perform the act (Chap. 3)

dependent variable the variable hypothesized to change with treatment and thus to have been caused by an independent variable (Chap. 18)

development a progression of behavioral changes that involve the acquisition of appropriate cognitive, linguistic, and psychosocial skills (Chap. 19)

developmental crisis occurs when a person is unable to complete the tasks of a developmental level (Chap. 52)

developmental milestones the predictable patterns of normal development according to age (Chap. 19)

developmental task an important activity that arises at a certain period in life (Chap. 19)

diagnosis-related group a system of classification or grouping of patients according to medical diagnosis for purposes of paying hospitalization costs (Chap. 5)

diagnostic label a concise term or phrase that represents a pattern of related signs and symptoms, otherwise known as a nursing diagnosis (Chap. 11)

diagnostic reasoning the process of clustering assessment data into meaningful sets and generating hypotheses about the client's human responses (Chaps. 7 and 11)

diaphragmatic (abdominal) breathing breathing in which the majority of ventilatory work is accomplished by the diaphragm and abdominal muscles; deliberate use of the diaphragm and abdominal muscles to control breathing (Chap. 39)

diarrhea rapid movement of fecal matter through the intestine, resulting in poor adsorption of water, nutrients, and electrolytes and producing abnormally frequent evacuation of watery stools (Chap. 34)

diastole relaxation of the ventricles of the heart (Chap. 40)

diastolic blood pressure the constant pressure in the arteries during myocardial relaxation (Chap. 9)

differential cell count breaks down the number of white cells into their different types (Chap. 27)

differential diagnosis the process of deciding among several possible diagnoses to most accurately describe the client's problem (Chap. 11)

differentiated development a normal pattern of development, which becomes increasingly differentiated over time, starting with a generalized response and progressing to a skilled specific response (Chap. 19)

diffusion a passive process by which molecules move through a cell membrane from an area of higher concentration to an area of lower concentration without the expenditure of energy (Chap. 31)

direct care intervention a treatment performed through interaction with the client (Chap. 12)

disaccharide a molecule that forms when two monosaccharides condense and join together to form a double sugar (Chap. 29)

discharge note a nursing note that reflects the circumstances around the release of a client from a facility (Chap. 14)

discharge planning preparation for moving a client from one level of care to another within or outside of the current health care agency (Chap. 12)

disease a specific disorder characterized by a recognizable set of signs and symptoms, attributable to heredity, infection, diet, or environment (Chap. 24)

disenfranchised grief grief that lacks social acknowledgment, validation, and support for the bereaved (Chap. 50)

disuse to stop using organs or body parts, to restrict activities, or to be immobile (Chap. 38)

diuresis increased secretion of urine (Chap. 35)

diversity differences in modes or patterns of care between cultures, including specific patterns of care within cultural groups (Chap. 4)

documentation the recording of information relevant to data collection, planning, implementation, and client response to care given (Chap. 14)

durable power of attorney for health care document that designates a person to make decisions about the client's medical treatment in the event that the client becomes unable to do so, also called a proxy directive (Chap. 3)

dysarthria impaired articulation (Chap. 44)

dysfunctional grief extended, unsuccessful use of intellectual and emotional responses by which individuals, families, and communities attempt to work through the process of modifying self-concept based on the perception of potential loss (Chap. 50)

dysphagia difficulty in swallowing (Chaps. 30 and 44)

dysphonia difficulty in producing vocal sounds (Chap. 44)

dyspnea the subjective sensation of difficulty in breathing (Chap. 39)

dysrhythmia abnormalities of heart rate or rhythm (Chap. 40)

dyssomnia any sleep disturbance that involves the amount, quality, or timing of sleep, such as insomnia or hypersomnia (Chap. 41)

dysuria difficult or painful urination (Chap. 35)

edema abnormal accumulation of fluid in the interstitial spaces of tissues; commonly known as swelling (Chap. 40)

egocentrism the tendency to spend so much time thinking about and focusing on your own thoughts and changes in your own body that you come to believe that others are focused on them as well (Chap. 21)

electrolyte a substance that, when placed in water or another solvent, separates into electrically charged particles (ions) (Chap. 31)

emergency a serious health situation that arises suddenly and either threatens life or would result in serious complications without prompt treatment (Chap. 58)

emic dimension a person's or social group's subjective perception and

experiences related to health (Chap. 25)

empathy accurate perception of the client's feelings (Chap. 15)

encoder (sender) the person who initiates a transaction to exchange information, convey thoughts and feelings, or engage another (Chap. 15)

endorphin an internally secreted opioid-like substance released by a signal from the cerebral cortex that attaches to opioid receptors and blocks transmission of the pain signal (Chap. 42)

endotracheal tube a catheter passed through the nose or mouth into the trachea for the purpose of establishing an airway (Chap. 39)

enteral nutrition provision of nutrition through a tube in the gastrointestinal tract (Chap. 30)

enuresis recurrent involuntary urination that occurs during sleep (Chap. 35)

epidemiology study of the cause and distribution of disease, disability, and death among groups of people (Chap. 59)

epidural analgesia method of analgesia in which a catheter is placed between the spinal vertebrae and the dura mater to allow the diffusion of an analgesic drug across the dura mater into the cerebrospinal fluid (Chap. 42)

epithelialization movement of epithelial cells to the wound bed (Chap. 32)

equianalgesia a dosage that provides the same amount of pain relief independent of the drug or route (Chap. 42)

eschar thick, leathery, necrotic devitalized tissue (Chap. 32)

ethics a branch of philosophy that attempts to determine what constitutes good, bad, right, and wrong in human behavior (Chap. 3)

ethnic describing a group of people of the same race or national origin within a larger cultural system who are distinctive based on traditions of religion, language, or appearance (Chap. 4)

ethnicity reflections of the characteristics a group may share in some combination (Chap. 4)

ethnocentricism the belief that one's own ethnic beliefs, customs, and attitudes are correct and thus superior ones (Chap. 4)

etic dimension the objective interpretation of health by a scientifically trained practitioner (Chap. 25)

etiology the cause of a disease (Chap. 24)

eupnea a normal rate of breathing (Chap. 9)

eustress stress that results in positive outcomes (Chap. 52)

evaluation a systematic and ongoing process of examining whether expected outcomes have been achieved and whether nursing care has been effective (Chap. 13)

evisceration protrusion of internal organs through an incision (Chap. 32)

exclusive provider organization a type of group health care practice in which enrollees are restricted to the list of preferred providers of health care called "exclusive providers" (Chap. 5)

excoriation an injury to the epidermis caused by abrasion, scratching, a burn, or chemicals, such as sweat, wound drainage, feces, or urine coming in contact with skin (Chap. 38)

experimental research a study in which the researcher manipulates a treatment or intervention, randomly assigns subjects to either a control or an experimental group, and has control over the research situation (Chap. 18)

extended family family unit that includes the nuclear family and other relatives, such as aunts, uncles, cousins, and grandparents, who are committed to maintaining family ties (Chap. 53)

exteroceptors sensory receptors located in the skin and mucous membranes that are stimulated by touch, light pressure, pain, temperature, odor, sound, and light (Chap. 43)

exudate fluid and cells that have escaped from blood vessels during the inflammatory response and are left in surrounding tissues (Chap. 32)

faith belief in or commitment to something or someone that helps a person realize purpose without proof of its existence (Chap. 55)

false imprisonment involves the restraining, with or without force, of another person against his or her wishes (Chap. 2)

familial short stature a height below the third percentile on the growth chart (Chap. 21)

family two or more people united by a common goal to create a physical, cultural, spiritual, and nurturing bond that will promote the physical, mental, spiritual, and social development of each of its members, while maintaining cohesiveness as a unit (Chap. 53)

family-centered nursing health care that focuses on the health of the family as a unit, as well as the maintenance and improvement in the health and growth of each person in that unit (Chap. 53)

family dynamics the forces at work within the family that result in particular coping behaviors (Chap. 54)

family household a unit that includes the householder and at least one other person related to the householder by birth, marriage, or adoption (Chap. 53)

family systems theory the study of the family approached as the study of a system (family) with subsystems (individual members) interacting with each other (Chap. 53)

fecal impaction a collection of putty-like or hardened feces in the rectum or sigmoid colon that prevents the passage of normal stool and becomes more and more hardened as the colon continues to absorb water from it (Chap. 34)

feces body waste discharged from the intestine, also called stool, excreta, or excrement (Chap. 34)

feedback the process by which effectiveness of communication is determined (Chap. 15)

fetal alcohol syndrome a distinct cluster of physical and mental impairments caused by prenatal exposure to alcohol (Chap. 22)

fever a regulated rise in temperature that is mediated by a rise in temperature set-point (Chap. 33)

fiber the structure of which plants are composed, including cellulose, hemicellulose, pectins, gums, and mucilages (Chap. 29)

fidelity honoring agreements and keeping promises (Chap. 3)

filtration the passage of water and certain smaller particles through a semipermeable membrane assisted by hydrostatic or capillary pressure (Chap. 31)

first pass effect partial metabolism of opioid analgesics by the liver before they reach the systemic circulation, thereby resulting in a decrease in opioid availability (dosage) (Chap. 42)

fistula an abnormal passage between two internal organs or between internal organs and the external skin surface (Chap. 32)

flaccid the state of being weak, soft, and flabby, lacking normal muscle tone, or having no ability to contract (Chap. 37)

flatulence the presence of abnormal amounts of gas in the gastrointestinal tract, causing abdominal distention and discomfort (Chap. 34)

flatus gases normally found in the gastrointestinal tract and passed through the anus (Chap. 34)

flow sheet a form used to document data that can be more easily followed in graphic or tabular form (Chap. 14)

focus charting a method of charting that addresses client problems or needs and includes a column that summarizes the focus of the entry (Chap. 14)

focus group method of data collection in which 6 to 12 people from a group or aggregate are brought together for discussion, guided when necessary by a skilled, nonjudgmental leader (Chap. 59)

footdrop a contracture deformity in which the muscles of the anterior foot are lengthened and the muscles of plantar flexion along with the Achilles tendon are shortened, resulting in plantar flexion of the foot (Chap. 38)

formal operations the ability to reason abstractly (Chap. 21)

fraud the false representation of some fact with the intention that it will be acted upon by another person (Chap. 2)

friction injury injury in which the epidermal layer of skin is rubbed off, possibly from a restraint, a dressing, or a tube (Chaps. 32 and 38)

functional health patterns the positive and negative behaviors a person uses to interact with the environment and maintain health (Chap. 8)

functional limitations difficulties that people with physical challenges face in performing activities of daily living (Chap. 56)

gate control theory hypothesis of an alteration in the transmission of the ascending pain signal by a spinal gating mechanism located in the dorsal horn; the pain signal may be inhibited or facilitated by multiple variables (Chap. 42)

gender a person's sex, either male or female (Chap. 51)

gender identity the internal belief or sense that one is male or female (Chap. 51)

gender role the outward appearance, behaviors, attitudes, and feelings deemed culturally appropriate for males and females (Chap. 51)

general anesthesia loss of all sensation, consciousness, and memory of the surgical event as a result of inhaling an anesthetic drug, having it injected into the bloodstream, or both (Chap. 57)

generic name the name (also called a nonproprietary name) assigned to a drug by the United States Adopted Names Council when the drug is first manufactured (Chap. 26)

gingivitis inflammation of the gums, usually manifested by the primary symptom of bleeding of the gums (Chap. 36)

glycogen the form in which carbohydrates are stored in the muscle tissue of humans and animals (Chap. 29)

Gram's stain a specific microscopic test used to obtain rapid results on a culture sent to the laboratory (Chap. 27)

grief emotional, physical, cognitive, and behavioral responses to bereavement, separation, or loss (Chap. 50)

grief attack unexpected, involuntary resurgence of acute grief-related emotions and behaviors triggered by routine events, sometimes accompanied by uncontrollable crying or emotional display (Chap. 50)

grief work efforts (necessary to complete the normal grieving and mourning process) by a grieving person to acknowledge the physical and psychological pain of bereavement and to integrate the loss into the future (Chap. 50)

growth the physiological development of a living being and the quantitative (measurable) change seen in the body (Chap. 19)

guaiac test test used to check for occult blood, usually performed by a nurse after obtaining a fecal or urine sample (Chap. 34)

gustatory the sensation of taste (Chap. 43)

gynecomastia a benign increase in breast tissue associated with puberty (Chap. 21)

hallucinations sensory reactions in the absence of real stimuli (Chap. 45)

handicap a disadvantage experienced by a person as a result of impairment that limits the person's "normal" function (Chap. 56)

hardiness the ability to survive stress based on three ingredients: commitment to self, work, family, and important values; a sense of personal control over one's life; and the ability to see change in one's life as a challenge to master (Chap. 52)

health goals outline broadly what needs to be done to achieve health for individuals, families, and communities (Chap. 24)

health-illness continuum a range that extends from high-level wellness (an optimal state of mental and physical well-being), to a neutral state in which the person cannot be considered either healthy or ill, to illness and premature death (Chap. 24)

health maintenance organization a type of group health care practice that provides basic and supplemental health maintenance and treatment services to voluntary enrollees who prepay a fixed periodic fee set without regard to the amount or kind of services received (Chap. 5)

health perception the knowledge and experience of one's state of wellness and well-being (Chap. 24)

health promotion the advancement of health through the encouragement of activities that enhance the wellness of individuals, families, and communities (Chap. 24)

health status the third domain of the Vulnerable Populations Conceptual Model; it includes age- and gender-specific morbidity and mortality (Chap. 48)

health within illness an event that can expand human potential by providing an opportunity for personal growth and well-being despite having an illness (Chap. 24)

heat exhaustion a rise in body temperature that is usually related to inadequate fluid and electrolyte replacement during physical activity (Chap. 33)

heat stroke an elevation of body temperature that is usually above 40.6°C (105°F) with altered central nervous system function (Chap. 33)

hematoma an accumulation of bloody fluid beneath tissue (Chap. 32)

hematuria the presence of blood in the urine (Chap. 35)

hemiparesis a numbness or other abnormal or impaired sensation experienced on only one side of the body and that limits activities of daily living (Chap. 37)

hemiplegia paralysis of one side of the body (Chap. 37)

hemodynamic monitoring the use of invasive procedures and sophisticated equipment to monitor a client's cardiac output, arterial pressure, and central venous pressure (Chap. 58)

hemoptysis coughing and spitting up blood as a result of bleeding from any part of the lower respiratory tract (Chap. 39)

hemorrhage bleeding from a wound bed or site (Chap. 32)

heterosexual sexual orientation in which one is sexually attracted to members of the opposite gender (Chap. 51)

heterosexual cohabiting family an unmarried couple living together with or without children (Chap. 53)

home care services provided to clients and families in their place of residence for the purpose of treating illness, restoring health, rehabilitating, promoting health, and palliating (Chap. 60)

home care nursing comprehensive, holistic nursing focused on the client and family (or support system) and delivered in the client's home (Chap. 60)

homeostasis a healthy, more or less stable, physiologic state in which there is no undue imbalance (Chap. 52)

homophobia a fear of becoming homosexual through contact with lesbians and gay men or even having close or intimate feelings toward someone of the same sex (both of which are myths) (Chap. 51)

homosexual sexual orientation in which one is sexually attracted to members of the same gender (Chap. 51)

hope an interpersonal process created through trust and nurtured by a trusting relationship with others, including God (Chap. 55)

hospice a cluster of special services that address the special needs of dying persons and their families (Chaps. 5 and 50)

human capital a dimension of the Resource Availability domain of the Vulnerable Populations Conceptual Model; it includes income, jobs, education, and housing (Chap. 48)

human response patterns descriptions of people in relation to their environment (Chap. 8)

humanistic care understanding and knowing a client in as natural or human a way as possible while helping or guiding the client to achieve certain goals, make improvements, reduce discomforts, or face disability or death (Chap. 4)

hydrostatic pressure pressure exerted by the fluid within a compartment that results from the weight of the fluid (Chap. 31)

hypercapnia high carbon dioxide level in the blood, usually resulting from failure of the lungs to remove carbon dioxide (Chap. 39)

hypersensitivity reaction a mild allergic reaction to a drug (Chap. 26)

hypersomnia a dyssomnia characterized by excessive sleepiness (Chap. 41)

hypertension a condition in which blood pressure is constantly elevated and compensatory mechanisms continue to produce hormones that increase blood volume and vessel constriction (Chap. 9)

hyperthermia an elevation in body temperature related to an imbalance between heat gain and heat loss (Chap. 33)

hypertonic having an osmotic pressure greater than that of the solution to which it is being compared (Chap. 31)

hyperventilation increase in the rate and depth of breathing, clinically defined as $PaCO_2$ less than 35 mm Hg; also known as hyperpnea (Chap. 39)

hypnotic a drug that acts on the central nervous system to shorten sleep onset, reduce night-time wakefulness, or decrease anxiety when insomnia is associated with increased anxiety (Chap. 41)

hypomotility decreased peristalsis from lack of stimulation of the gastrocolic reflex and from the food bolus activating the parasympathetic nervous system (Chap. 38)

hypostatic pneumonia inflammation of the lungs caused by stasis of secretions, which become a medium for bacteria growth (Chap. 38)

hypotension a condition in which lowered blood pressure results from lowered circulating blood volume, commonly caused by blood loss, shock, or dehydration (Chap. 9)

hypothermia a state in which body temperature is reduced below normal (Chap. 33)

hypothesis a tentative prediction of the relationship between two or more variables being studied (Chap. 18)

hypotonic having an osmotic pressure lower than that of the solution to which it is being compared (Chap. 31)

hypoventilation decrease in the rate and depth of breathing, clinically defined as $PaCO_2$ greater than 45 mm Hg (Chap. 39)

hypoxemia deficient oxygenation of the blood (Chap. 39)

hypoxia deficient oxygenation of body tissues (Chap. 39)

idiosyncratic response an unexplained and unpredictable response to a medication (Chap. 26)

ileostomy a surgical procedure involving the creation of an opening between the ileum and the abdominal wall (Chap. 34)

illness a personal experience of feeling unhealthy and involves changes in a person's state of well-being and social function (Chap. 24)

immobility the inability to move the whole body or a body part (Chap. 38)

immunization medication administered to activate an immune response before exposure to the disease agent (Chap. 27)

immunosuppression use of medications to suppress the body's immune system (Chap. 27)

impairment limitations resulting from any one of a variety of conditions, whether related to disease, trauma, or birth defect (Chap. 56)

inactivity defined as not performing or being of use; usually defines the individual who is not active but sedentary or inert (Chap. 38)

incentive spirometer a device that provides a visual goal for and measurement of inspiration, thus encouraging the client to execute and sustain maximal inspiration (Chap. 39)

independent variable the variable that may change during a study, but the change is expected to remain constant or to cause change in another variable (Chap. 18)

indirect care intervention a treatment performed away from the client but on behalf of a client or group of clients (Chap. 12)

individualized care plan a plan written specifically for each client who enters a health care facility and developed from the admission history, physical and functional assessments, and problems anticipated from the physician's treatment plan (Chap. 12)

infant a child between the ages of 1 month and the end of 12 months (Chap. 19)

infection clinical syndrome caused by the invasion and multiplication of pathogens (Chap. 27)

inference the process of attaching meaning to data or reaching a conclusion about data; based on a premise that supports or helps support a conclusion (Chap. 8)

inflammatory response a localized reaction to injury that is activated when there is tissue damage (Chap. 27)

informed consent the legal right of a client to receive adequate and accurate information about his or her medical condition and treatment (Chap. 2), or of a potential research participant to receive sufficient information about a research project to enable him or her to consent voluntarily to participate or decline to participate (Chap. 18)

injury trauma or damage to some part of the body (Chap. 28)

inotropic agent a medication that increases the contractility of the heart muscle, thereby increasing cardiac output (Chap. 40)

insomnia a dyssomnia characterized by difficulty initiating or maintaining sleep (Chap. 41)

inspection the systematic visual examination of the client (Chap. 10)

institutional review board a committee whose duties include making sure that proposed research meets the federal requirements for ethical research (Chap. 18)

instrumental activities of daily living food preparation, housekeeping, laundry, transportation, using the telephone, shopping, and handling finances (Chap. 56)

instruments the tools a researcher uses to conduct a study (Chap. 18)

interface pressure pressure created in tissues that are compressed between the bones and a support surface by the weight of the body (Chap. 38)

interfacility transfer the transfer of an emergency department client from one health care facility to another (Chap. 58)

intergenerational family more than one generation of a family living together in one residence or within a small geographical area (Chap. 53)

interoceptors sensory receptors located in the viscera and blood vessels that provide visceral information regarding pain, cramping, and fullness (Chap. 43)

interval or progress note a nursing note that is entered at various times during a shift that reflects any aspect of change in client condition, or anything affecting the client such as tests, stat or prn medications, and procedures (Chap. 14)

interview a planned series of questions designed to elicit information for a particular purpose (Chap. 8)

intradermal route injection into the dermis layer of the skin (abbreviated ID) (Chap. 26)

intrafacility transfer the transfer of a client within the same general facility as the emergency department (Chap. 58)

intramuscular route injection into muscle tissue (abbreviated IM) (Chap. 26)

intraoperative phase surgical phase that starts with the client's entry into the operating room and ends when the client is transferred to the recovery room or other area to receive immediate post-surgical attention (Chap. 57)

intrathecal analgesia method of analgesia in which a catheter is placed in the subarachnoid space between the dura mater and the spinal cord to allow immediate drug diffusion into the cerebrospinal fluid (Chap. 42)

intravenous route injection into a vein (abbreviated IV) (Chap. 26)

intrusive memory vivid, realistic, commonly disturbing memory of events surrounding a death that return to the bereaved unexpectedly and unintentionally, overriding existing conscious thinking (Chap. 50)

intuition an ability to understand the whole without having systematically examined the parts (Chap. 8)

invasion of privacy occurs when the client's private affairs are unreasonably intruded upon by the nurse (Chap. 2)

ischemia decreased supply of oxygenated blood to tissues (Chap. 40)

isolation identification of a client who has an infection and implementation of precautions to prevent the spread of that infection (Chap. 27)

isometric exercise a form of active exercise that increases muscle tension by applying pressure against stable resistance, where there is no joint movement and the length of the muscle remains unchanged, but the tone and strength are maintained or increased (Chap. 37)

isotonic having an osmotic pressure equal to that of the solution to which it is being compared (Chap. 31)

isotonic exercise a form of active exercise in which the muscle contracts and moves with little change in resistance (Chap. 37)

judgment the ability to make rational decisions (Chap. 45)

justice moral rightness, fairness, or equity (Chap. 3)

Kegel exercises exercises performed to strengthen the pelvic and vaginal muscles to help control stress incontinence in women (Chap. 35)

key informant a community leader, professional, politician, or business person who has knowledge of the needs of the community who can act as a useful source of data and a supporter of new programs (Chap. 59)

kinesthetic the sensation of position (Chap. 43)

Korotkoff's sounds five distinct sounds heard while measuring blood pressure (Chap. 9)

kyphosis an abnormal condition of the vertebral column characterized by increased convexity in the thoracic spine when viewed from the side (Chap. 37)

laceration a wound caused by penetration of a sharp object, resulting in an open wound with jagged edges (Chap. 32)

language a set of words having meanings that are comprehensible within a group (Chap. 15)

latchkey children children in elementary school who spend some part of their time before or after school without the supervision of an adult (Chap. 20)

law a body of rules of action or conduct prescribed by a "controlling authority," which is the government (Chap. 2)

laxative a medication, less potent than a cathartic, used to induce emptying of the bowel (Chap. 34)

leadership showing others the way, directing others in a course of action, going before others, or going with and inspiring others (Chap. 17)

leading question a question that suggests a possible appropriate response (Chap. 8)

learned helplessness a perception that further efforts would be useless based on the failure of previous efforts (Chap. 49)

learning the acquisition of knowledge, behavior, or skill through experience, practice, study, or instruction (Chap. 16)

learning contract an agreement in which each party (nurse and client) agrees to contribute certain things; the nurse provides information and the client agrees to use that information (Chap. 16)

learning disability a lifelong disorder that affects the manner in which people with normal or above-average intelligence select, retain, and express information (Chap. 20)

learning objective a statement that describes the intended results of learning rather than the process of instruction (Chap. 16)

lesbian or gay family female or male couples living together with or without children (Chap. 53)

lesion a wound, injury, or pathological change in the body (Chap. 10)

liability the legal obligation or responsibility to provide care to a client that meets the accepted standards of care (Chap. 2)

libido the conscious or unconscious sex drive; desire for pleasure or satisfaction (Chap. 51)

license grants the owner formal permission from a constituted authority to practice a particular profession (Chap. 2)

lifestyle a behavior or group of behaviors, chosen by the person, that may have either a positive or a negative influence on health (Chap. 25)

living will document that provides written instructions about when life-sustaining treatment should be terminated (Chap. 3)

loading dose an initial medication dose that exceeds the maintenance or therapeutic dose (Chap. 26)

local anesthesia a temporary loss of feeling in an area of the body caused by the inhibition of nerve endings after being given a certain type of anesthetic drugs, usually by topical application or local (or extravascular) infiltration (Chap. 57)

longevity statistics report of the life expectancy of the population and groups within the population, a well-established measure of community health (Chap. 24)

loss the removal, change, or reduction in value of something valued or held dear, and the feelings that result (Chap. 50)

maceration a softening of the epidermis caused by prolonged contact with moisture, such as a wet sheet or diaper (Chap. 38)

maintenance stage the stage of change that takes place during the 6 months after the person changes the high-risk behavior (Chap. 25)

malaise a feeling of indisposition (Chap. 33)

malignant hyperthermia a rare, life-threatening, autosomal dominant inherited syndrome that rapidly causes a very high temperature after anesthetic inhalation agents and neuromuscular blocking medications used to induce general anesthesia are given (Chap. 57)

malnutrition a disorder characterized by insufficient or excessive nourishment of body tissue caused by improper diet or impaired absorption or metabolism of nutrients (Chap. 30)

malpractice acts of negligence by a professional person as compared to the actions of another professional person in similar circumstances (Chap. 2)

managed care a system that combines the functions of health insurance and the actual delivery of care in which costs and utilization of services are controlled (Chap. 5)

management implementation of strategies that promote effective and efficient use of resources (human, technological, supplies, and time) to achieve organizational goals (Chap. 17)

Medicaid a welfare program providing partial health care services for indigent people; is supported jointly by federal and state governments (Chap. 5)

medical asepsis practices to reduce the numbers of pathogenic microorganisms in a person's environment (Chap. 27)

Medicare a federally funded national health insurance program in the United States for people over 65 years of age (Chap. 5)

memory the retention or storage of information learned about the world (Chap. 45)

menarche the time of the first menstrual period (Chap. 21)

menopause the second stage in the female climacteric, during which hormone production is reduced, the ovaries stop producing eggs, and menstruation ceases (Chap. 22)

message the content a sender wishes another person (the receiver) to receive in the process of communication (Chap. 15)

metabolic acidosis a pathological condition caused by an increase in noncarbonic acids, a decrease in bicarbonate in the extracellular fluid, or both (Chap. 31)

metabolic alkalosis a pathological condition caused by an increase in bicarbonate, a decrease in acid in the extracellular fluid, or both (Chap. 31)

metabolism the process by which energy from nutrients is used by the cells or stored for later use (Chap. 29)

metaparadigm the incorporation of the most abstract or broad knowledge elements of a discipline; consists of more than one paradigm (Chap. 6)

micturition the process of emptying the bladder (Chap. 35)

middle adulthood the period of time between ages 35 and 64 (Chap. 22)

midlife crisis a stressful life period during middle adulthood, precipitated by the review and re-evaluation of one's past, including goals, priorities, and life accomplishment, during which the person experiences inner turmoil, self-doubt, and major restructuring of personality (Chap. 22)

milliequivalent one-thousandth of a chemical equivalent; the measurement used to express the chemical activity or combining power of an ion (Chap. 31)

milliosmole the amount of dissolved particles needed to produce a unit of force (Chap. 31)

minerals inorganic elements present in small amounts in virtually all body fluids and tissues (Chap. 29)

minimum data set the least information allowable to be collected on every client entering an institution or being admitted to a particular service within the institution (Chap. 8)

mixed agonist-antagonist analgesic— analgesic that attaches to both the κ and μ opioid receptor sites, simultaneously providing analgesia at the κ site and blocking activity at the μ site if given after the client receives a morphine-like drug (Chap. 42)

model a symbolic and physical visualization of some aspect of reality (Chap. 6)

modulation an internal or external restraining of the nociceptive process that inhibits transmission of the pain signal at any place along the transmission pathway (Chap. 42)

monosaccharide a six-carbon sugar (a subunit of carbohydrates), such as glucose, fructose, or galactose (Chap. 29)

monotheism belief in the existence of one God who created and rules the universe (Chap. 55)

morals standards of conduct that represent the ideal in human behavior to which society expects its members to adhere (Chap. 3)

mourning social and cultural acts used by a bereaved person to express thoughts and feelings of sorrow (Chap. 50)

multicultural society a society composed of more than one culture or subculture (Chap. 4)

multiple sleep latency test a direct, objective measure of sleepiness used to evaluate excessive somnolence and daytime sleepiness (Chap. 41)

narcolepsy striking hypersomnia characterized by abnormal sleep tendencies and pathological rapid eye movement sleep, manifested as excessive daytime sleepiness, disturbed night-time sleep, cataplexy, sleep paralysis, and hypnagogic hallucinations (Chap. 41)

narrative charting a method of charting that provides information in the form of statements that describe events surrounding client care (Chap. 14)

necrosis localized death of tissues caused by disease, oxygen deficit, or injury (Chap. 40)

negligence occurs when harm or injury is caused by an act of either omission or commission by a lay person (Chap. 2)

neologism the creation of words that are meaningless to the listener, a common language problem of the aphasic client (Chap. 44)

neuropathic pain transmission of a pain signal from the site of injury to the higher brain centers via a nervous system that has been damaged in some way (Chap. 42)

newborn a child who was born within the previous 28 days (Chap. 19)

nightmare a vivid or frightening dream that occurs during rapid eye movement sleep, awakens the person from sleep, and can be easily recalled (Chap. 41)

nociception transmission of a pain signal from a site of tissue damage to areas of the brain where perception occurs (Chap. 42)

nociceptive pain pain transmitted from a site of injury to the higher brain centers via an intact nervous system (Chap. 42)

nociceptor primary afferent fiber that initiates the pain experience when stimulated by tissue damage (Chap. 42)

nocturia the term used for nighttime urination (Chap. 35)

nocturnal emission a discharge of semen during sleep (Chap. 21)

nonacute area area of the emergency department used for clients with non-life-threatening conditions; subclassified as urgent, semi-urgent, or non-urgent (Chap. 58)

nonelectrolyte substance that does not ionize and thus does not carry an electrical charge, such as glucose (Chap. 31)

nonexperimental research a type of study in which the researcher collects data without the introduction of a treatment or intervention (Chap. 18)

nonmaleficence requires the practitioner to do no harm (Chap. 3)

nonopioid analgesic a drug that provides analgesia at the peripheral level by a mechanism other than the opioid receptor sites (Chap. 42)

nonprescription medication a drug that can be purchased without a prescription to enhance personal health or treat common health problems, also known as an over-the-counter medication (Chap. 26)

non–rapid eye movement sleep a sleep state in which a quiet brain functions in an active body (Chap. 41)

nonurgent a problem for which the amount of time a person delays treatment is not a critical issue (Chap. 58)

nonverbal communication a set of behaviors that conveys messages either without words or by supplementing verbal communication (Chap. 15)

nosocomial infection an infection that is acquired from a reservoir in the hospital (Chap. 27)

nuclear family husband, wife, and offspring living in a common household with one or both partners gainfully employed (Chap. 53)

nurse manager a nurse responsible for managing the operation and expenses of a health care organization that employs nurses as the means to produce health (Chap. 17)

nurse-initiated intervention an intervention within the scope of nursing practice and prescribed by the nurse independent of the physician (Chap. 12)

nursing an accountable discipline guided by science, theory, a code of ethics, and the art of care and comfort to treat human responses to health and illness (Chap. 1)

nursing care plan a guide for client care that identifies client problems in need of nursing care (specified by nursing diagnoses), predicts outcomes that are sensitive to nursing care, and lists interventions that will result in the expected outcomes (Chap. 12)

nursing diagnosis a clinical judgment about individual, family, or community responses to actual or potential health problems or life processes (Chap. 11)

nursing history a narrative of the client's past health and health practices that focuses on information needed to plan nursing care while a medical history focuses on illness and the treatment of disease (Chap. 8)

nursing intervention any treatment, based on clinical judgment and knowledge, that a nurse performs to enhance client outcomes (Chap. 12)

nursing process a clinical decision-making framework that includes critical thinking, diagnostic reasoning, and clinical judgment; composed of five interwoven phases: assessment, diagnosis, planning, intervention, and evaluation (Chap. 7)

nutrient a biochemical substance used by the body for growth, maintenance, and repair (Chap. 29)

nutrition the science of food and nutrients, and the processes by which an organism takes them in and uses them for energy to grow, maintain

function, and renew itself (Chap. 29)

nutritional status the condition of the body resulting from its use of the essential nutrients available to it (Chap. 29)

obesity body weight or body fat percentage that exceeds a chosen reference point (Chap. 21)

object permanence the awareness that unseen objects do not disappear, evidenced by the infant searching for an object that has been moved out of sight (Chap. 19)

objective caregiver burden the observable, tangible costs to the caregiver in behaviors required or disruptions experienced (Chap. 54)

objective data characteristics about the client that you can observe directly (Chap. 8)

obstructive sleep apnea a sleep disorder manifested by periodic cessation of airflow at the nose and mouth during inspiration and that arouses the person from sleep (Chap. 41)

occult blood an amount of blood too small to be seen without a microscope (Chap. 34)

official name the name assigned by the Food and Drug Administration (often the same as the generic name) after a drug is approved (Chap. 26)

older adult any person over age 65 (Chap. 23)

olfactory the sensation of smell (Chap. 43)

oliguria a diminished, scanty amount of urine (Chap. 35)

Omaha system a nursing diagnosis system developed by the Visiting Nurses Association of Omaha, Nebraska (Chap. 59)

open system system that exchanges matter, energy, and information with other systems and with the environment (Chap. 53)

open-ended question a question that allows the client freedom in the manner of response (Chap. 8)

operational definition the meaning of a concept precisely as it is being used in a study, defined in a manner that specifies how concepts will be measured (Chap. 18)

ophthalmoscope an instrument used to visualize the retina, including the optic disk, macula, and retinal blood vessels through the pupil (Chap. 10)

opinion survey a method of data collection performed through telephone interviews, mailed questionnaires, door-to-door interviews, or at clinic sites (Chap. 59)

opioid analgesic any morphine-like drug that attaches to the opioid receptors and produces analgesia by

blocking substance P, a powerful neurotransmitter of the pain signal (Chap. 42)

opioid naive no or minimal previous exposure to opioid analgesics (Chap. 42)

opioid receptor portion of a nerve cell to which an opioid or opioid-like substance can bind (Chap. 42)

orgasm sexual tension evidenced by muscular spasm and engorgement of blood vessels reaching maximum intensity; a highly pleasurable and totally involuntary response (Chap. 51)

orientation awareness of person, place, and time (Chap. 45)

orientation phase a brief exchange to establish the purpose, the procedure, and the nurse's role as a phase of the interview process (Chap. 8)

orthostatic hypotension a drop in systolic blood pressure of 20 mm Hg or more and a drop in diastolic blood pressure of 10 mm Hg or more for 1 or 2 minutes after a client stands up; a temporary condition of low blood pressure caused by the failure of compensatory mechanisms to regulate pressure as the person moves from a lying to a sitting or standing position (Chap. 38)

osmolality the number of milliosmoles per kilogram of water (Chap. 31)

osmolarity the number of milliosmoles per liter of solution (Chap. 31)

osmosis the movement of water through a semipermeable membrane from an area of lower concentration of particles to an area of higher concentration of particles (Chap. 31)

osteoporosis a condition in which there is a decreased mass per unit volume of normally mineralized bone, primarily from a loss of calcium, that makes bones brittle and porous (Chap. 38)

ostomy a surgical procedure that creates an opening through the abdomen into the intestine to allow fecal matter to exit the intestine from a site other than the anus (Chap. 34)

otoscope a hand-held instrument used to examine the external ear, the eardrum, and, through the eardrum, the ossicles of the middle ear (Chap. 10)

ototoxic a damaging effect on cranial nerve VIII or the organs of hearing and balance (Chap. 43)

pain an unpleasant sensory and emotional experience associated with actual and potential tissue damage; described in terms of such damage (Chap. 42)

pain behavior anything a person says or does that implies the presence of pain (Chap. 42)

palpation a form of touch or feeling with the hand used to obtain information about temperature, moisture, texture, consistency, size, shape, position, and movement (Chap. 10)

paradigm set of philosophical assumptions from which a scientist studies natural phenomena (Chap. 6)

paralanguage the nonverbal components of spoken language, which give speech its rhythm and humanness and include stress, accent, pitch, pause, intonation, rate, volume, and quality (Chap. 15)

paralytic ileus a temporary stoppage of peristalsis caused by direct handling of the bowel during surgery (Chap. 34)

paraparesis a numbness or other abnormal or impaired sensation in the legs and trunk (Chap. 37)

paraphasia a word substitution problem of the aphasic client who speaks fluently (Chap. 44)

paraplegia paralysis characterized by motor or sensory loss in the legs and trunk (Chap. 37)

parasomnia abnormal movements and behaviors that occur during sleep, such as somnambulism, sleep terrors, sleep enuresis, nightmares, and bruxism (Chap. 41)

parenteral nutrition provision of total nutrition through a central or peripheral intravenous catheter (Chap. 30)

parenteral route a route for medication administration that is outside the gastrointestinal tract (Chap. 26)

parish nurse a registered nurse who is employed by (or volunteers at) a religious or health care organization for the purpose of providing nursing care to members of a church congregation (Chap. 59)

participant observation a method of community assessment that examines formal and informal social systems at work, in which the researcher shares in the life activities of the group while observing and collecting data (Chap. 59)

pathogen a disease-producing microorganism (Chap. 27)

pathological anxiety a disproportionate anxiety response to a given stimulus by virtue of its intensity or duration (Chap. 47)

patient-controlled analgesia a drug delivery approach that employs an external infusion pump to deliver an opioid dose on a "client demand" basis (Chap. 42)

peer review the evaluation of the performance of one staff member by another staff member to judge the quality of care provided (Chap. 13)

perceived barriers perceived negative aspects of a health action or perceived impediments to undertaking the recommended behaviors (Chap. 25)

perceived benefits perceptions and beliefs about the effectiveness of the recommended actions in preventing the health threat (Chap. 25)

perceived severity perceived seriousness of contracting an illness or leaving it untreated (Chap. 25)

perceived susceptibility subjective perception of the risk of contracting a health condition (Chap. 25)

perception conscious mental recognition or registration of a sensory stimulus, as, for example when a person smells a sweet fragrance and gets the mental image of a cherry (Chap. 43)

perceptual learning domain the ability to perceive (see, hear, understand, and respond) written words, spoken words, pictures, or symbols (Chap. 16)

percussion the use of short, sharp strikes to the body surface to produce palpable vibrations and characteristic sounds (Chap. 10)

performance appraisal a systematic and standardized evaluation of an employee's work contribution, quality of work, and potential for advancement, made by the employee's supervisor (Chap. 13)

perineum the pelvic floor and associated structures of the pelvic outlet, bounded anteriorly by the symphysis pubis, laterally by the ischial tuberosities, and posteriorly by the coccyx (Chap. 36)

perioperative the term used to describe the preoperative, intraoperative, and postoperative phases of the surgical experience (Chap. 57)

perioperative nursing a specialized area of practice that describes the provision of care for the surgical client throughout the continuum of care (Chap. 57)

peristalsis rhythmic smooth muscle contractions of the intestinal wall that propel the intestinal contents forward toward the anus (Chap. 34)

personal identity the organizing principle of the personality that accounts for the unity, continuity, consistency, and uniqueness of an individual (Chap. 46)

personal space a private zone or "bubble" around our body that we believe is an extension of ourselves and belongs to us (Chap. 15)

pharmacokinetics the activity of a drug from the time it enters the body until it leaves (Chap. 26)

phonation the production of sound by the vibration of the vocal cords (Chap. 44)

physical dependence an involuntary physiological phenomenon that occurs after repeated exposure to an opioid analgesic that causes withdrawal symptoms if the opioid is abruptly withdrawn or an opioid antagonist is administered (Chap. 42)

physician-initiated intervention an intervention within the scope of nursing practice but that requires a physician's order for the nurse to implement (Chap. 12)

PIE charting like APIE charting, a method of charting that evolved from the problem-oriented type of medical record and that is designed to allow documentation using the nursing process; the acronym stands for *p*roblem identification, *i*nterventions, and *e*valuation (Chap. 14)

plaintiff the party bringing a lawsuit that alleges certain facts and outcomes (Chap. 2)

plaque a soft, thin film of food debris, mucin, and dead epithelial cells that is deposited on the teeth and provides a medium for the growth of bacteria (Chap. 36)

point of maximum impulse the point where the heart comes the closest to the chest wall at the apex of the heart (Chap. 10)

poisoning an adverse condition or physical state resulting from the administration of a toxic substance (Chap. 28)

policy a set of rules and regulations that govern nursing practice and nursing care (Chap. 13)

polypharmacy the use of more drugs than indicated (Chap. 23)

polysaccharide a group of monosaccharides joined together in a chain that can be converted back to monosaccharides through a process called acid hydrolysis (Chap. 29)

polysomnography the continuous measurement and recording of physiological activity during sleep using electroencephalogram, electro-oculogram, electrocardiogram, and electromyogram tracings to monitor brain activity, eye movements, heart rate and rhythm, and muscle movements (Chap. 41)

polytheism belief in more than one god (Chap. 55)

polyuria a large amount of urine usually associated with diabetes mellitus or diabetes insipidus (Chap. 35)

population health the consideration of health problems encountered as a result of being a part of a group, and the focus on interventions for a population rather than for an individual (Chap. 24)

positive listening understanding the auditory messages sent by a sender (Chap. 15)

postanesthesia care unit an area where clients remain until they regain consciousness from the effects of anesthesia, previously known as the recovery room or postanesthesia room (Chap. 57)

postoperative phase period following an operation, which can be divided into two segments of care: the immediate postoperative period includes an evaluative assessment by the perioperative nurse and admittance to the postanesthesia care unit; the ongoing postoperative period includes all care given during the course of surgical convalescence to the time of discharge, continuing with assisted care or self-care at home (Chap. 57)

postural drainage a technique in which the client assumes one or more positions that will facilitate the drainage of secretions from the bronchial airways (Chap. 39)

PQRST model a model for the assessment of pain: P stands for provoking incident; Q stands for quality; R stands for region, radiation, or relieving factors; S stands for severity; and T stands for timing (Chap. 37)

precontemplation stage the first stage in the change process, in which a person does not intend to change a high-risk behavior in the foreseeable future (the next 6 months), primarily because he is unaware of the long-term consequences of the behavior (Chap. 25)

precordium the area on the anterior chest overlying the heart and great vessels (Chap. 10)

preferred provider organization an organization of physicians, hospitals, and pharmacists whose members discount their health care services to subscriber patients; may be organized by a group of physicians, an outside entrepreneur, an insurance company, or a company with a self-insurance plan (Chap. 5)

preload the amount of blood in the left ventricle immediately before contraction; the main force that stretches cardiac muscle fibers (Chap. 40)

preoperative phase phase that begins with the decision for surgical intervention and ends when the client is safely transported into the operating room for a surgical procedure (Chap. 57)

preparation stage the third stage in the change process, in which a person intends to take action in the very near future, usually within the next month (Chap. 25)

presbycusis a sensorineural hearing loss of high-frequency tones that occurs in the elderly and may lead to a loss of all hearing frequencies (Chap. 43)

presbyopia loss of near vision in older people that results from reduced elasticity in the lens and weakened ciliary muscles (Chap. 43)

preschooler a child in the developmental stage between 3 and 5 years of age (Chap. 20)

prescription an order for a medication that contains the client's name, medication name, dose, route, frequency, amount of the medication to be dispensed, number of refills allowed (if any), and the physician's signature (Chap. 26)

pressure ulcer any lesion caused by unrelieved pressure that leads to damage of underlying tissues (Chaps. 32 and 38)

preventive health care the recognition of the risk of disease and actions taken to reduce that risk (Chap. 24)

primary health care all care necessary to people's lives and health, including health education, nutrition, sanitation, maternal and child health care, immunizations, prevention, and control of endemic disease (Chap. 24)

primary prevention actions that are considered true prevention because they precede disease or dysfunction and are applied to clients considered physically and emotionally healthy to protect them from health problems (Chap. 24)

private law controls the relationships between private individuals and/or private organizations (Chap. 2)

problem-oriented medical records a form of documentation originally designed to organize information according to identified client problems, with all members of the health team documenting information sequentially (Chap. 14)

problem-solving defining a problem, selecting information pertinent to its conclusion (recognizing stated and unstated assumptions), formulating alternative solutions, drawing a conclusion, and judging the validity of the conclusion (Chap. 7)

procedural law establishes the manner of proceeding used to enforce a specific legal right or obtain redress (Chap. 2)

procedure a detailed description of a specific method of performing nursing care (Chap. 13)

professional misconduct a violation of the nurse practice act that can result in disciplinary action against a nurse (Chap. 2)

professionalism behavior that upholds the status, methods, character, and standards of a given profession (Chap. 1)

proprioception sensation pertaining to stimuli originating from within the body regarding spatial position and muscular activity or to the sensory receptors that they activate (Chap. 37)

proprioceptors sensory receptors located chiefly in the muscle, tendons, and inner ear that convey a sense of position movement and muscle coordination (Chap. 43)

prospective payment system a payment system in which the amount to be paid for a specific service is predetermined (Chap. 5)

protein a compound containing polymers of amino acids linked together in a chain to form polypeptide bonds (Chap. 29)

protocol a detailed set of guidelines for nursing care for a client with a specific condition (Chap. 13)

proximodistal a normal pattern of skill development, which moves from the midline of the body outward (Chap. 19)

pseudodementia depression that is misinterpreted as dementia (Chap. 45)

psychological dependence (addiction) a chronic disorder demonstrated by overwhelming involvement with obtaining and using a drug for its mind-altering effects (Chap. 42)

psychomotor learning domain the learning domain concerned with physical and motor skills (Chap. 16)

psychoneuroimmunology the study of the interface between the brain and immunology (Chap. 52)

psychosocial development development that involves subjective feelings and interpersonal relationships (Chap. 19)

puberty the sequence of physiological

events that cause the reproductive organs to mature, making conception and childbirth possible (Chap. 21)

public health nursing the practice of promoting and protecting the health of populations through nursing activities to improve the quality of life (including its physical, mental, and social aspects), to prevent disease, and to control communicable disease consistent with available knowledge and resources (Chaps. 59 and 60).

public law regulates the relationship of individuals to government agencies and may be administrative, constitutional, or statutory (Chap. 2)

pulmonary embolus condition that results when a piece of a deep vein thrombus breaks free, floats in the blood stream to the pulmonary circulation, and lodges in a pulmonary blood vessel (Chap. 38)

pulse deficit the condition of the apical pulse rate exceeding the radial pulse rate (Chap. 9)

pulse oximeter a device for measuring the oxygen saturation of functional hemoglobin in the blood (Chap. 39)

pulse pressure the difference between systolic and diastolic blood pressure readings (Chap. 9)

pursed-lip breathing a technique of mouth breathing that creates slight resistance to exhalation by contracting the lips to reduce the size of the opening, thus maintaining an even reduction of intrathoracic pressure during exhalation (Chap. 39)

pyrogen any agent that causes or stimulates a fever (Chap. 33)

quadriparesis a numbness or other abnormal or impaired sensation in all four limbs and the trunk (Chap. 37)

quadriplegia an abnormal condition characterized by paralysis of the arms, legs, and trunk below the level of an associated injury to the spinal cord (Chap. 37)

qualifier a word such as *impaired, altered, decreased, ineffective, acute,* or *chronic* that gives greater specificity to a nursing diagnosis (Chap. 11)

qualitative research a type of study that uses ideas analyzed as words (Chap. 18)

quality assurance a process of evaluating the outcome of care measured against predetermined standards and implementing methods of improvement (Chap. 13)

quantitative research a type of study that uses variables analyzed as numbers (Chap. 18)

quasiexperimental research a type of study in which the researcher manipulates a treatment or intervention but is unable to randomize subjects into groups or lacks a control group (Chap. 18)

range-of-motion exercises any body action (active or passive) involving the muscles, joints, and natural directional movements, such as abduction, extension, flexion, pronation, and rotation (Chap. 37)

rapid eye movement sleep a sleep state in which a highly active brain functions in an immobilized body (Chap. 41)

reactive hyperemia reddening of the skin caused by blood rushing back into ischemic tissues (Chap. 32)

recommended dietary allowance the level of a nutrient that is adequate to meet the needs of almost all healthy people, as determined by the Food and Nutrition Board of the National Research Council (Chap. 29)

referral a process designed to provide the client with access to health care and supportive services that are not available from the sending institution (Chap. 25)

referred pain pain experienced at a distant site from the injured tissue (Chap. 42)

reflex incontinence unexpected voiding without awareness of the need to void, specific to the client with a spinal cord injury (Chap. 35)

regional anesthesia a type of anesthesia that produces analgesia, relaxation, and reduced reflexes after medication is instilled into or around the nerves to block the transmission of nerve impulses (Chap. 57)

registered nurse first assistant an expanded nursing role that requires additional education in which the perioperative nurse works as a first assistant during the surgical procedure (Chap. 57)

registration a process by which an applicant provides specific information to the state agency administering the nursing registration process (Chap. 2)

rehabilitation the process of adaptation, or recovery, through which an individual suffering from a disabling condition, whether temporary or irreversible, participates to regain, or attempt to regain, maximum function, independence, and restoration (Chap. 56)

related factors factors that appear to be related to a nursing diagnosis and help define how the problem should be managed (Chap. 11)

relative risk the second domain of the Vulnerable Populations Conceptual Model; considered to be the ratio of the risk of poor health among populations who do not receive resources and are exposed to risk factors compared with those populations who do receive resources and are not exposed to these risk factors (Chap. 48)

religion a belief system that includes dogma, rituals, and traditions, and also a social institution in which people participate together rather than alone (Chap. 55)

relocation stress syndrome a set of physiological or psychosocial disturbances (or both) caused by transferring a person from one environment to another (Chap. 49)

renal calculi stones formed in the kidney when the excretion rate of calcium or other minerals is high, as when osteoclastic activity releases calcium from the bones during immobility (Chap. 38)

rescue dose administration of as-needed doses of an immediate-release analgesic in response to breakthrough pain and in addition to the scheduled analgesic dosage (Chap. 42)

research design a researcher's strategy for testing a hypothesis (Chap. 18)

research problem an observation, situation, occurrence, or even a hunch that an investigator chooses to research (Chap. 18)

resilience the process of identifying or developing resources and strengths to flexibly manage stressors to gain a positive outcome, a sense of confidence, mastery, and self-esteem (Chap. 52)

resonance the forced vibration of a structure that is related to a source of sound and results in changes in the quality of the sound (Chap. 44)

resource availability the first domain of the Vulnerable Populations Conceptual Model; it includes the availability of socioeconomic and environmental resources (Chap. 48)

respiration the exchange of oxygen and carbon dioxide between the atmosphere and the cells of the body; a series of metabolic activities by which living cells break down carbohydrates, amino acids, and fats to produce energy in the form of ATP (adenosine triphosphate) (Chap. 39)

responsibility being held answerable for personal actions or the actions of others as defined by the organizational structure and the level of assigned authority (Chap. 17)

rest a state of being physically and mentally relaxed while awake and alert (Chap. 41)

resting energy expenditure the basal metabolic rate plus the energy needed for minimal activity (Chap. 30)

restless legs syndrome an intrinsic sleep disorder characterized by intense, abnormal, lower extremity sensations and irresistible leg movements that delay sleep onset (Chap. 41)

restraint a device (usually a wristlet, anklet, or other type of strap) intended for medical purposes that limits movement to the extent necessary for treatment, examination, or protection of the client (Chap. 28)

reticular activating system portion of the midbrain and thalamus that keeps the brain aroused and controls the sleep-wake cycle, level of consciousness, the ability to direct attention to specific tasks, and the perception of sensory input that might alter behavior (Chap. 43)

retirement the permanent withdrawal from one's job (Chap. 23)

retrospective audit an evaluation method to inspect the medical record for documentation of compliance with the standards (Chap. 13)

risk factors internal or external environmental factors that increase the vulnerability of a person, family, or community to an unhealthful event (Chap. 11)

risk-for nursing diagnosis describes human responses that *may* develop in a vulnerable person, family, or community (Chap. 11)

risk management a process of identifying, evaluating, and reducing or financing the cost of predictable losses, including loss from litigation (Chap. 17)

role a homogeneous set of behaviors, attitudes, beliefs, principles, and values that are normatively defined and expected of a person in a given social position or status in a group (Chap. 49)

role conflict incompatible expectations for behavior within a role, between two or more roles, or when a role is incongruent with a person's beliefs and values (Chaps. 49 and 53)

role distance the condition in which the client carries out role behaviors that differ from those expected in the client's current cultural or societal situation (Chap. 49)

role failure the absence of role behaviors or ineffective role behaviors re-

sulting in a lack of success in a role (Chap. 49)

role performance the roles a person assumes or is given, including the actions, thoughts, and feelings associated with those roles. Roles are defined in terms of relationship to others (Chap. 46)

role strain the condition in which a person feels unable to accomplish the tasks required of a role or of multiple roles (Chap. 49)

role stress emotion that occurs when a person has difficulty meeting the demands of a role (Chap. 53)

role transition the state in which a person has started to take on the behaviors of a role but has not fully developed the expected behaviors (Chap. 49)

sampling the process of selecting subjects from the population being studied (Chap. 18)

sandwich generation middle-aged adults caught between the needs of adjacent generations, caring for ill or frail parents while handling the competing demands of children and employment (Chap. 22)

school-aged child a child in the developmental stage between 6 and 11 years of age (Chap. 20)

scoliosis a structural lateral curvature of the spine (Chap. 21)

scrub nurse a registered nurse with special qualifications that include knowledge of aseptic technique, instruments, and equipment; anatomy and physiology; surgical procedures; and most importantly, promotion of client safety (Chap. 57)

searching in the context of the grief reaction, conscious and unconscious efforts by the bereaved to negate the reality of the loss through finding the deceased alive and well (Chap. 50)

secondary prevention actions that focus on the early diagnosis and prompt treatment of people with health problems or illnesses and who are at risk for developing complications or worsening conditions (Chap. 24)

sedative a drug that exerts a soothing, tranquilizing effect on the central nervous system, resulting in a shortened sleep onset and the alleviation of anxiety (Chap. 41)

selective attention the act of consciously choosing when and to whom a person will give attention to a loss and allow thoughts and feelings to enter the conscious mind (Chap. 50)

self-concept a relatively enduring set of attitudes and beliefs about both

the physical self and the psychological self (Chap. 46)

self-efficacy the conviction that one can successfully execute a behavior required to produce the outcomes (Chap. 25)

self-esteem the degree to which a person has a positive evaluation of self based on her perceptions of how she is viewed by others as well as on her view of herself (Chap. 46)

semi-urgent a problem for which the client requires timely treatment within 4 to 6 hours (Chap. 58)

sensation the reception of stimulation through receptors of the nervous system (Chap. 43)

sense of presence nonthreatening, comforting perception by the bereaved of the presence of the deceased through one or more of the senses or in dreams, fortuitous events, or conversations (Chap. 50)

sensory channel the means by which a message is sent; the three primary sensory channels are visual, auditory, and kinesthetic (Chap. 15)

sensory deprivation inadequate reception or perception of environmental stimuli (Chap. 43)

sensory overload excessive environmental stimuli or when the stimulus is beyond the person's ability to absorb or comprehend (Chap. 43)

sensory stimulation the activation and exhilaration of the senses (Chap. 19)

septicemia infection in the bloodstream (Chap. 27)

set-point the temperature that thermoregulatory mechanisms attempt to maintain (Chap. 33)

sexual desire a wish participate in sexual intimacy that is activated by thoughts, fantasies, emotions, and psychological wants and needs (Chap. 51)

sexual dysfunction a change or disruption in sexual health or function that the affected person views as unrewarding or inadequate (Chap. 51)

sexual identity a perception of self as male or female (Chap. 51)

sexual orientation description of a person's sexual attraction and feelings of erotic potential toward a partner or toward members of either gender (heterosexual, homosexual, or bisexual) (Chap. 51)

sexual patterns a person's chosen expressions of sexuality (Chap. 51)

sexual response cycle phases of response in relation to sexual stimuli (Chap. 51)

sexuality the state or quality of being sexual, including the collective characteristics that distinguish male and female (Chap. 51)

shearing force (shear) a mechanical force that acts on a skin area in a direction parallel to the body's surface (Chaps. 32 and 38)

sibling rivalry the competition of brothers and sisters for the attention, approval, and affection of the parents (Chap. 20)

side effect an unintended or unplanned effect of a medication that typically is not dangerous (Chap. 26)

signs characteristics of disease or dysfunction that can be observed directly as objective data (Chap. 8)

single-parent family a household where children live with one parent (Chap. 53)

situational crisis a hazardous situation that is not easily anticipated and for which a person is inadequately prepared (Chap. 52)

sleep a reversible behavioral state in which perceptions of and responses to environmental stimuli are decreased and the body is relatively quiet (Chap. 41)

sleep deprivation a state resulting when an individual does not get enough sleep

sleep enuresis bedwetting during sleep (Chap. 41)

sleep terrors a parasomnia (also known as night terrors) that occurs during slow-wave sleep and is characterized by arousal, agitation, and signs of sympathetic nervous system activity, such as dilated pupils, increased sweating, tachypnea, and tachycardia (Chap. 41)

slow-wave sleep also called deep sleep and characterized by high-voltage electroencephalographic activity and a high arousal threshold, which can make it difficult to arouse the sleeper (Chap. 41)

SOAP charting a method of charting used to record progress notes with problem-oriented medical records; includes *s*ubjective data, *o*bjective data, *a*ssessment, and *p*lan (Chap. 14)

social integration a dimension of the Resource Availability domain of the Vulnerable Populations Conceptual Model; it refers to having a harmonious relationship with society in which the person participates as a full member of the society (Chap. 48)

social status a dimension of the Resource Availability domain of the Vulnerable Populations Conceptual Model; it refers to the position of an individual in relation to others in the society; reflected in power to control the political process and the distribution of resources (Chap. 48)

social support the subjective feeling of belonging, or being accepted, loved, esteemed, valued, and needed for oneself, not for what one can do for others (Chap. 25)

somatic pain well-localized pain, usually from bone or spinal metastases or from injury to cutaneous or deep tissues (Chap. 42)

somesthetic pertains to sensations and sensory structures of the body (Chap. 43)

somnambulism a slow-wave sleep parasomnia associated with stereotypical "sleepwalking" behaviors (Chap. 41)

source-oriented medical records a type of medical record with separate divisions according to health discipline (e.g., medicine, nursing, laboratory, respiratory care) (Chap. 14)

spastic describes muscle contractions caused by reflex activity rather than by central nervous system control (Chap. 37)

spiritual distress a disruption that pervades a person's being and that integrates and transcends one's biological and social nature, resulting in distress of the human spirit (Chap. 55)

spiritual well-being a process of being and becoming that surrounds the totality of a person's inner resources, the wholeness of spirit and unifying dimension, a process of transcendence, and the perception of life as having meaning (Chap. 55)

spirituality a process and sacred journey, an essence or life principle of a person, the experience of the radical truth of things, and a belief that relates a person to the world and gives meaning to existence (Chap. 55)

sputum mucus secreted from the lungs, bronchi, and trachea; may include epithelial cells, bacteria, and debris (Chap. 39)

standard precautions a set of actions, including hand-washing and the use of barrier precautions, designed to reduce transmission of infectious organisms (Chap. 27)

standardized care plan a care plan developed commercially or by an individual health care facility (Chap. 12)

standards of care authoritative statements that describe a competent level of clinical nursing practice demonstrated through assessment, diagnosis, outcome identification, planning, implementation, and evaluation (Chap. 13)

standards of client care the essential elements of nursing care prescribed for specific client populations (Chap. 13)

standards of practice the aspects of nursing care that nursing staff should assess, plan, implement, and evaluate during daily and ongoing care for specific client populations (Chap. 13)

standards of professional performance authoritative statements that describe a competent level of behavior in the professional role, including activities related to quality of care, performance appraisal, education, collegiality, ethics, collaboration, research, and resource utilization (Chap. 13)

starch the form in which plants store glucose (Chap. 29)

statutory law law enacted by the state or federal legislative branch of government (Chap. 2)

steatorrhea gray stool mixed with observable fat and mucus and caused by malabsorption of fat (Chap. 34)

stereotyping the assumption that an attribute present in some members of a group is present in all members of a group (Chap. 4)

stoma a surgically created opening between the abdominal wall and intestine through which fecal material passes (Chap. 34)

strangulation constriction of the airway from an external cause (Chap. 28)

stress a physiological response produced by the normal wear and tear of bodily processes and external and internal demands (Chap. 52)

stress incontinence the reported or observed dribbling of urine with increased abdominal pressure (Chap. 35)

stressor a cause of stress, such as extreme hot or cold, an argument, a virus, an examination, cigarette smoke, a death, or any of the countless demands of the environment (Chap. 52)

stroke volume amount of blood ejected from the heart with each contraction (Chap. 40)

subcutaneous route injection of medication into subcutaneous tissue, which lies directly underneath the dermis of the skin (abbreviated SC or SQ) (Chap. 26)

subjective caregiver burden a caregiver's personal appraisal of a caregiving situation and the extent to which the person perceives it to be a burden (Chap. 54)

subjective data information that is provided by the client and cannot be directly observed (Chap. 8)

substantive law the part of law that actually stipulates one's rights and duties, in contrast to procedural law, which guides enforcement of one's rights (Chap. 2)

suffering an unpleasant emotional response to pain (Chap. 42)

suffocation lack of oxygen caused either by airway obstruction or by oxygen starvation from insufficient atmospheric oxygen (Chap. 28)

sundowning the nocturnal exacerbation of disruptive behaviors and agitation associated with clients who have dementia (Chap. 41)

symbolic play pretend or imaginative play that enables the preschooler to recreate experiences and to try out roles (Chap. 20)

symptoms subjective information that is indicative of disease as perceived by the client (Chap. 8)

synergistic effect the result of one drug enhancing or increasing the effect of another drug, which may be accidental or purposeful (Chap. 26)

synovium the inner layer of the articular capsule surrounding a freely movable joint that is loosely attached to the external fibrous capsule and secretes a thick fluid to lubricate the joint and absorb shock (Chap. 37)

system a set of integrated, interacting parts that function as a whole, with structure and patterns of function that accomplish the work of the whole (Chap. 53)

systole contraction of the ventricles of the heart (Chap. 40)

systolic blood pressure the maximum force of blood in the arteries during myocardial contraction (Chap. 9)

tachycardia heart rate above 100 beats per minute (Chap. 40)

tachypnea a respiratory rate above 20 breaths per minute for an adult (Chap. 9)

tactile the sensation of touch (Chap. 43)

target organ the type of body tissue affected by a medication (Chap. 26)

tartar a yellowish film of calcium phosphate, carbonate, food particles, and other organic matter deposited on the teeth by saliva (Chap. 36)

taxonomy a system of identification, naming, and classification of phenomena (Chap. 11)

teaching a set of planned activities performed to influence knowledge, behavior, or skill (Chap. 16)

teaching plan an organized, individualized, written presentation of what the client must learn and how the instructions and information needed will be provided (Chap. 16)

teleology a set of theories that postulate that the outcomes or conse-

quences of an action determine its value (Chap. 3)

teratogen an agent or influence that causes physical defects in the developing fetus (Chap. 19)

teratogenic potential the possibility that a medication will harm a developing fetus (Chap. 26)

termination the last phase of an interview or a nurse-client relationship; marked by ensuring that the expectations are met and that client satisfaction is present (Chap. 8)

termination stage the stage of change in which the person is no longer tempted to engage in old behavior (Chap. 25)

tertiary prevention actions taken when a defect or disability is permanent and irreversible. It involves minimizing the effects of the disease or disability by interventions directed at preventing complications and deterioration (Chap. 24)

thanatology the discipline of study and research that deals with death and death-related topics (Chap. 50)

theoretical framework a logical but abstract structure that suggests the relationship among the variables in a research study (Chap. 18)

theory a group of propositions used to describe, explain, or predict a phenomenon (Chap. 6)

therapeutic effect the intended effect or action of a medication (Chap. 26)

therapeutic rapport a special bond that exists between a nurse and a client who have established a sense of trust and a mutual understanding of what will occur in their relationship (Chap. 15)

therapeutic relationship a helping relationship in which nurses are helpers and clients are those seeking help; personal, client-focused, and aimed at realizing mutually determined goals (Chap. 15)

thermogenesis the generation of heat from the chemical reactions that take place in cellular activity (Chap. 9)

thermolysis the processes through which heat is dispersed from the body through radiation, conduction, convection, and evaporation (Chap. 9)

third spacing the movement of fluid into an area that makes it physiologically unavailable, such as the peritoneal space (ascites), the pericardial space (pericardial effusion), the pleural space (pleural effusion), or the vesicles produced by a burn wound (Chap. 31)

toddler a child between ages 1 and 3 (Chap. 19)

tolerance an involuntary physiological

phenomenon that occurs after repeated exposure to an opioid analgesic in which pain relief decreases despite a stable or escalating opioid dosage (Chap. 42)

topical route method of administering a medication directly to a body site, such as the skin, eyes, ears, nose, throat, vagina, or rectum (Chap. 26)

tort a civil wrong committed by one person against another person or his or her property; can be intentional or unintentional (Chap. 2)

total incontinence inability to control urination, usually in immobile cognitively impaired persons, in which undergarments or bed are almost continually wet (Chap. 35)

toxic effect an effect that results from an accumulation of a medication in the body (Chap. 26)

trade name the name given by a manufacturer to a medication it produces, also known as a trade name (Chap. 26)

transcultural nursing culturally competent nursing care focused on differences and similarities among cultures with respect to caring, health, and illness based on the client's cultural values, beliefs, and practices (Chap. 4)

transfer note a nursing note that reflects the movement of a client from one location to another either within the agency or to another agency (Chap. 14)

trauma a physical injury or wound caused by a forceful, disruptive, or violent action (Chap. 28)

triage a decision-making process used to determine client treatment priorities based on the severity of injury and priority for treatment (Chap. 58)

triglyceride three fatty acids and a glycol unit that constitute the chief form of fat in the diet and the main form of fat transport in the blood (Chap. 29)

trochanter roll the roll of a sheet placed under a client's hip to prevent external rotation of the trochanter (hip joint) in the supine position (Chap. 38)

turgor a reflection of the skin's elasticity, measured as the time it takes for the skin to return to normal after being pinched lightly between the thumb and forefinger (Chap. 10)

unconditional positive regard respect for the client that is not dependent on the client's behavior (Chap. 15)

universality a common mode or value of caring or a prevailing pattern of care across cultures (Chap. 4)

urge incontinence the reported or observed sudden desire to urinate and immediate seeking of toileting facilities (Chap. 35)

urgent a problem for which the client requires prompt care, although a wait of 20 to 60 minutes will not affect the outcome of treatment (Chap. 58)

urinalysis a physical, chemical, and microscopic examination of the urine (Chap. 35)

urinary frequency urination that occurs at shorter-than-usual intervals without an increase in daily urine output (Chap. 35)

urinary incontinence involuntary passage of urine (Chap. 35)

urinary retention the inability to pass all or part of the urine that has accumulated in the bladder (Chap. 35)

urinary urgency a sudden, forceful urge to urinate (Chap. 35)

urination the term commonly used for the act of micturition (Chap. 35)

validation substantiating or confirming the accuracy of the information against another source or by another method (Chap. 8)

values ideals, beliefs, and patterns of behavior that are prized and chosen by a person, group, or society (Chap. 3)

values clarification a process that allows us to identify our personal values and develop self-awareness (Chap. 3)

variance any deviation from a clinical pathway (Chap. 13)

vascular resistance the resistance of blood vessels to distention (Chap. 9)

ventilation the process of exchanging air between the ambient air and the lungs; *pulmonary ventilation* refers to the total exchange of air, whereas *alveolar ventilation* refers to the effective ventilation of the alveoli (Chap. 39)

veracity adherence to the truth, thus requiring consistent, continual truth-telling (Chap. 3)

verbal communication the use of words to convey messages (Chap. 15)

vibration a technique of chest physiotherapy whereby the chest wall is set in motion by oscillating movements of the hands or a vibrator for the purpose of mobilizing secretions (Chap. 39)

virtue a practice of conforming life and conduct to moral and ethical principles (Chap. 3)

virtue theory an ethical theory that focuses on the characteristics that are intrinsic to the person performing the action (Chap. 3)

virus a microorganism much smaller than a bacterium that can only replicate inside the cell of a host, such as a human (Chap. 27)

visceral pain poorly localized pain that results from nociceptor activation by stretching, distention, or contraction of smooth muscle walls; ischemia of the visceral wall; irritation or inflammation; or torsion or traction on mesenteric attachment organs (Chap. 42)

viscosity the relative ability of a fluid to flow (Chap. 40)

visual the sensation of sight (Chap. 43)

vitamin an organic substance found in food that serves as a coenzyme in enzymatic reactions (Chap. 29)

void a term synonymous with micturition and urination that is used most often in clinical settings (Chap. 35)

vulnerable population a subgroup of a larger population that has an increased risk of health problems because of exposure or other health or nonhealth problems (Chap. 59)

well-being a subjective perception of a good and satisfactory existence in which the individual has a positive experience of personal abilities, harmony, and vitality (Chap. 24)

wellness a state of optimal health or optimal physical and social functioning (Chap. 24)

wellness nursing diagnosis a nursing diagnosis that describes human responses to levels of wellness in a person, family, or community that have the potential for growth or enhancement to a higher state of well-being (Chap. 11)

Wernicke's area the portion of the brain that helps control the content of speech and affects auditory and visual comprehension (Chap. 44)

windshield survey a method of data collection in which the researcher drives through a neighborhood to conduct a general assessment of that neighborhood through observation (Chap. 59)

working phase a phase of the interview process in which the client and the nurse work together to review the client's health history and establish potential and actual problems that will be addressed as part of the care plan (Chap. 8)

wound a disruption of the normal anatomical structure and function that results from pathological processes that arise internally or externally to the involved organ(s) (Chap. 32)

wrist drop a contracture of the wrist in the flexed position (Chap. 38)

young adulthood the period of time between ages 20 and 35 (Chap. 22)

INDEX

Note: Page numbers in *italics* refer to illustrations. Page numbers followed by the letter b refer to boxed material; those followed by t refer to tables.

Psychosocial factors *(Continued)*
  in grief response, 1363
  in home care nursing, assessment of, 1605, 1605t
  in hygiene, 935–936
  in pain management, 1181
  in sexuality, 1391, *1393*
  in spirituality, 1472–1473
  in stress, interaction with physiological stressors, 1413–1414
  in urinary elimination, 891
Psychosocial needs assessment, for homebound clients, 1607
Psychosocial status, documentation of, 289
Psychosocial well-being, altered, nursing care plan for, in older
    adults, 473
Puberty, definition of, 426
  delayed, constitutional, 428–429
    pathological, 429
  onset of, 1387
  stages of, *427*
Pubic hair, female, inspection of, 215
  male, inspection of, 217
Public health nursing. See also *Community health nursing.*
  definition of, 1574
Public law, 27
Public policy, influence of community health nurses in, 1577
Pulmonary. See also *Lung(s).*
Pulmonary disorders. See *Respiratory problem(s).*
Pulmonary edema, from extracellular fluid excess, 752
Pulmonary embolism, related to deep vein thrombosis, 1016
  signs and symptoms of, 1016
Pulmonary function tests, 1054, 1055t
Pulmonic valve, heart sounds related to, 198, *200*
Pulp, dental, 928
Pulse(s), apical, assessment of, 199
    measurement of, 157–158, *158*
  apical-radial, measurement of, 158
  assessment of, for neurovascular status, 985t
  characteristics of, 154–155
  deficit of, 158
  definition of, 150
  factors affecting, 154t
  measurement of, 155–158
  palpation of, factors affecting, 158, 158t
  patterns of, 154t
  peripheral, assessment of, 205–206
    measurement of, 155–156, *155*
  quality of, 158
  radial, measurement of, 156–157
  rate of, average range for, by age group, 146t
    characteristics of, 154–155, 154t
    documenting, 147, *147*
  rhythm of, characteristics of, 155
  strength of, 155
Pulse oximetry, in emergency care, 1556
  in respiratory disease, 1055–1056, *1056*
Pulse pressure, definition of, 160
PULSES Profile, of activities of daily living, 1495
Pulsus alternans, definition of, 154t
Pulsus paradoxus, definition of, 154t, 155
  detection of, during blood pressure measurement, 163
Pupil(s), accommodation of, 181
  response of, to light, 181
Pure Food and Drug Act of 1906, 525
Pursed-lip breathing, 1070–1072
Purulent exudate, 787
Pustule(s), characteristics of, *785*
Pyrogen(s), definition of, 831
  endogenous vs. exogenous, 831

Qi, in Chinese medicine, 70b
  in Taoism, 1467–1468
Qigong (chi kung), 1424
Quadriparesis, definition of, 977
Quadriplegia, definition of, 977

Quality, of nursing care, standards for evaluation of, 267–277
  of voice, as paralanguage element, 314
Quality assurance, documentation's role in, 275
  for home care, interventions for ensuring, 1610–1611
  in evaluation of compliance with standards, 275
  management of, 350–352
    goals and objectives for, 350–351
    mission statement for, 350, 350b
    policies and procedures for, 351–352, *351*
  retrospective and concurrent audits in, 275, 276
Quality improvement, based on nursing research, 379
  continuous, in evaluation of compliance with standards, 276
  goals for, 93
  initiatives for, incident or adverse occurrence reports in, 38, 94
    risk management programs in, 38, 94
Questions, types of, in interviews, 134

Radial pulse(s), measurement of, 156–157
Radiation, as heat loss mechanism, *829*
  for sterilization, 614t
Radiation injury, epidemiology of, 651
Radiation therapy, wound healing affected by, 800
Radiography, for musculoskeletal problems, 985
  in emergency care, 1556
  in impaired skin integrity, 794
  of bowel, 857–858
  of chest, in respiratory disease, 1054
Random sampling, for research studies, 374–375
Range of motion, assessment of, 979, 980t–984t
  exercises for improving, active, 1022
    active vs. passive, 993
    against resistance, 1022
    home care considerations in, 995
    passive, machine for performing, 1022, *1022*
    procedure for, 994–995
Rapport, therapeutic, 308
  with clients, 133–134
Rapport talk, as communication method of women, 316
Rate of speech, as paralanguage element, 314
Raynaud's disease, 1111
Reabsorption, of body fluids, 734
Readiness to learn, 333
Reading, helping children with, 421
Reality, helping clients maintain, 324
  presenting, in therapeutic communication, 324
Reality surveillance, for encouraging hope, 1481–1482
Reasoned action, theory of, as model of behavioral change, 500
Reasoning, confidence in, in critical thinking, 118
  diagnostic, clinical judgment in, 227
    critical thinking process in, 114, 227
    process of, 226–231
    steps in, 227–231, 228b–229b
  in assessment, 131–132
  inferential, in assessment, 131–132, 131b
Recall, total, in critical thinking, 115
Recognition, in cultural competence, 61
Recognition phase, of grief response, 1365–1366
Recommended dietary allowance. See also *Dietary reference intakes.*
  above-average levels in, 692
  definition of, 692, 1620
  for promoting nutrition, 695
  for vitamins and minerals, 1617t
Recommended nutrient intake, for Canadians, 1618t–1619t
Reconstructing, as hardiness improvement method, 1427
Recreational therapist, 1491
Rectal tube, for flatulence, 876–877
Rectocele, inspection for, 216
Rectum, assessment of, 214–215, *215*
  digital examination of, for fecal impaction, 861
  instillation of medication in, 589, 594–595
  temperature measurement via, 150, 152
Rectus femoris, as site for intramuscular injections, 572, *572*